INSTRUCTOR RESOURCES FOR NURSING EXCELLENCE

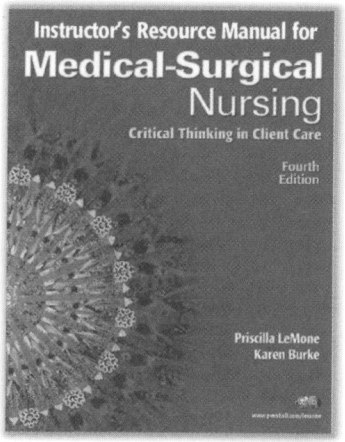

Instructor's Resource Manual for
Medical-Surgical
Nursing
Critical Thinking in Client Care
Fourth Edition

Priscilla LeMone
Karen Burke

Instructor's Resource Manual
ISBN: 0-13-198572-8
This manual helps faculty plan and manage the medical-surgical nursing course. It includes a brand new "Strategies for Success" module which discusses Learning Theories, Planning for Instruction, How to Use Effective Pedagogies, Assessing Learning, and more!
Presented in an easy-to-use tabular format, the manual includes

- detailed lecture notes organized by learning objectives
- Suggestions for Classroom Activities
- Suggestions for Clinical Activities
- Test Item File with comprehensive rationales

Instructor's Resource DVD-ROM
ISBN: 0-13-198569-8
This DVD-ROM includes all the textbook resources that instructors need to teach medical-surgical nursing courses.

- Comprehensive **PowerPoint** presentations that integrate lecture slides, images, animations or videos, and other resources into a single file
- **Classroom Response System** questions set in PowerPoint slides (Ask your Prentice Hall representative for more information about hardware to enhance your presentation)
- Complete **Image Gallery** in PowerPoint
- **TestGen** Test Item Files with questions in all NCLEX-RN® formats, including questions mapped to the chapter learning objectives and the clinical competencies
- Link to the **Prentice Hall Instructor's Resource Center** for additional resources
  Alternate CD-ROM versions are available to faculty who cannot use the DVD-ROM version. ISBN: 0-13-235058-0

Online Course Management Systems

For Students	**For Instructors**
Exam Review Questions	Test Item Files
Case Studies	PowerPoint Presentations
Media Gallery Resources	Discussion Board
MediaLinks	Class Announcements
Email Communication	

For a Preview, go to:

 http://cms.prenhall.com/webct/ index.html

 http//cms.prenhall.com/ blackboard/index.html

Student Assessment...Real Nursing Skills...Remediation...The path to student success and nursing excellence!

An easy-to-use adaptive online tool that allows instructors and students to measure performance and adapt course content without investing additional time or resources! Nursing instructors today need to

measure student competence and understanding of nursing concepts as they progress through the curriculum. *MyNursingLab* saves instructors time by providing quality feedback and ongoing individualized assessments for students, and an easy to use method to organize and adapt course materials including assignable homework. *MyNursingLab* is a user-friendly site giving students the opportunity to test themselves on key concepts and skills. Students can track their own progress through the course and use their customized study plan activities to remediate and help them achieve success in the classroom, in clinicals, and ultimately on the NCLEX-RN®.
To take a tour and see the power of *MyNursingLab*, go to **www.prenhall.com/nursing**.

Ask your Prentice Hall Representative about package options for your curriculum.

HOW YOUR BOOK IS ORGANIZED

BUILD YOUR CLINICAL COMPETENCE TO ACHIEVE NURSING EXCELLENCE

1. BUILD UPON YOUR FOUNDATIONAL KNOWLEDGE

Building upon your experience from anatomy, physiology, and fundamentals courses, each body system unit begins with an assessment chapter. Reviewing this chapter gives you the foundation for the nursing care chapters that follow.

ANATOMY AND PHYSIOLOGY REVIEW ▶

The Anatomy and Physiology Review for each body system reviews structures and functions essential for understanding the assessment, pathophysiology, and nursing care that come later.

424   UNIT 4 / Responses to Altered Integumentary Structure and Function

Figure 15–1 ■ Anatomy of the skin.

cells, nerve fibers, and lymphatic vessels. Most of the hair follicles, sebaceous glands, and sweat glands are located in the dermis. The dermis consists of a papillary and a reticular layer. The papillary layer contains ridges that indent the overlying epidermis. It also contains capillaries and receptors for pain and touch. The deeper, reticular layer contains blood vessels, sweat and sebaceous glands, deep pressure receptors, and dense bundles of collagen fibers. The regions between these bundles form lines of cleavage in the skin. Surgical incisions parallel to these lines of cleavage heal more easily and with less scarring than incisions or traumatic wounds across cleavage lines.

Superficial Fascia

A layer of subcutaneous tissue called the superficial fascia lies under the dermis. It consists primarily of adipose (fat) tissue and helps the skin adhere to underlying structures.

Glands of the Skin

The skin contains sebaceous (oil) glands, sudoriferous (sweat) glands, and ceruminous glands. Each of these glands has a different function.

Sebaceous glands are found all over the body except on the palms and soles. These glands secrete an oily substance called **sebum**, which usually is ducted into a hair follicle. Sebum softens and lubricates the skin and hair and also decreases water loss from the skin in low humidity. Sebum also protects the body from infection by killing bacteria. The secretion of sebum is stimulated by hormones, especially androgens. If a sebaceous gland becomes blocked, a pimple or whitehead appears on the surface of the skin; as the material oxidizes and dries, it forms a blackhead. Acne vulgaris is an inflammation of the sebaceous glands.

There are two types of sweat glands: eccrine and apocrine. Eccrine sweat glands are more numerous on the forehead, palms, and soles. The gland itself is located in the dermis; the duct to the skin rises through the epidermis to open in a pore at the surface. Sweat, the secretion of the eccrine glands, is composed mostly of water but also contains sodium, antibodies, small amounts of metabolic wastes, lactic acid, and vitamin C. The production of sweat is regulated by the sympathetic nervous system and serves to maintain normal body temperature. Sweating also occurs in response to emotions.

Most apocrine sweat glands are located in the axillary, anal, and genital areas. The secretions from apocrine glands are similar to those of sweat glands, but they also contain fatty acids and proteins. Apocrine glands are a remnant of sexual scent glands. Ceruminous glands are modified apocrine sweat glands. Located in the skin of the external ear canal, they secrete yellow-brown waxy cerumen. This substance provides a sticky trap for foreign materials.

◀ GENETIC CONSIDERATIONS

This box lists specific genetic issues for each body system that help you incorporate relevant questions when you take a client health history.

GENETIC CONSIDERATIONS
Neurologic Disorders

- In all types of spinocerebellar ataxia, there is degeneration of the spinal cord and cerebellum, resulting in loss of muscular coordination and spasticity.
- One recently confirmed risk factor for Parkinson disease is a positive family history of the disease. This neurodegenerative disease affects more than half a million people, manifested by tremor, muscular stiffness, and difficulty with balance and walking.
- Although multiple sclerosis (MS) is not directly inherited, genetic factors may influence a predisposition to MS within families as well as the severity and course of the disease
- Narcolepsy, a sleep disorder, does have a familial connection.
- Huntington disease is an inherited degenerative disorder that leads to dementia. It currently affects approximately 30,000 Americans, with an additional 150,000 at risk for inheriting the disease from their parents.
- Fredreich's ataxia is a rare inherited disease that causes a progressive loss of voluntary muscle coordination and enlargement of the heart.
- Essential tremor, as a primary disorder, affects as many as 3 to 4 million people. In more than half of cases, essential tremor is inherited as an autosomal dominant trait, meaning that children of an individual with the disease have a 50% chance of also developing the disorder.
- Epilepsy is one of the most common neurological diseases, characterized by abnormal cell firing in the brain that causes recurring seizures. Recent evidence suggests that there may be a genetic predisposition in up to 70% of cases.
- Charcot-Marie-Tooth syndrome is the most common inherited peripheral neuropathy in the world, characterized by a slowly progressive degeneration of the muscles of the foot, lower leg, hand, and forearm.
- Alzheimer's disease (AD) is a leading cause of death in adults, increasing in incidence with age and more common in women. AD tends to run in families, with mutations in 4 genes believed to be responsible for the disease.
- Amyotrophic lateral sclerosis (ALS) is a neurologic disease that causes progressive degeneration of motor neurons in the brain and spinal cord, resulting in paralysis and death. Chromosome abnormalities have been linked to familial ALS.
- Although Tay-Sachs disease is most often considered a disease of children, there is a chronic adult form that causes neuron dysfunction and psychosis.

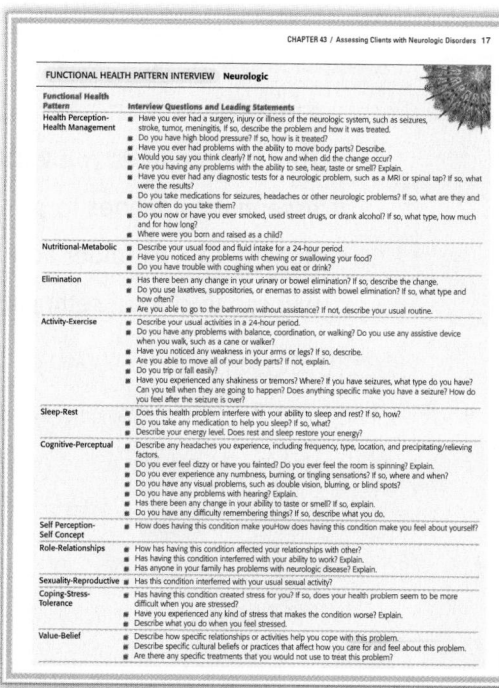

◀ DIAGNOSTIC TESTS

This table summarizes key diagnostic tests used for disorders of each body system and the related nursing care.

▲ ASSESSMENTS WITH ABNORMAL FINDINGS

Organized in a new, two-column format, the assessment section provides easy-to-follow steps that include normal findings, as well as abnormal findings that might be present.

▲ FUNCTIONAL HEALTH PATTERN INTERVIEW

This table provides you with sample assessment questions related to functional health patterns so you can plan your interviews during a client health history and physical assessment.

2. HONE YOUR CLINICAL SKILLS

Use the special application boxes to help prepare for clinical experiences.

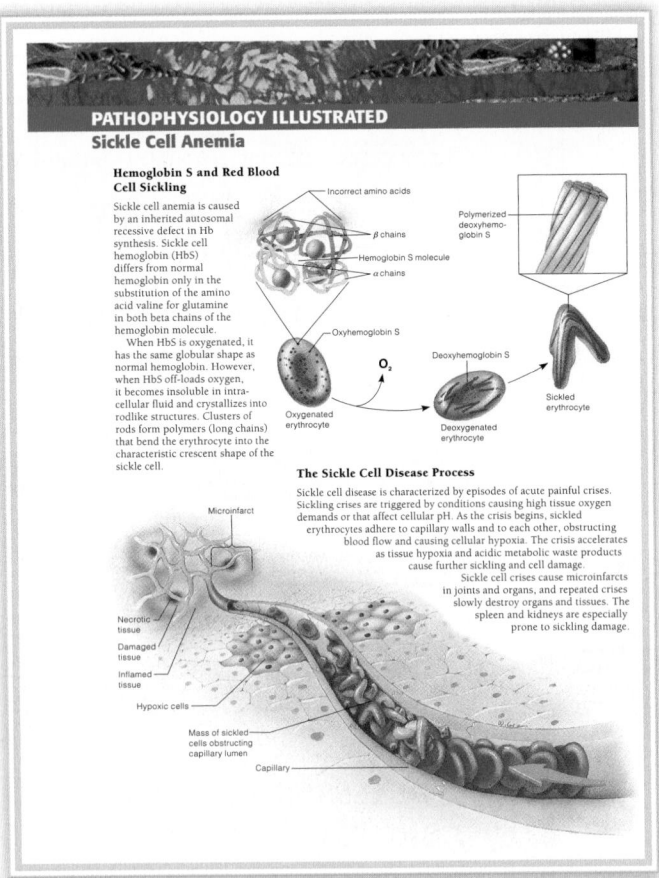

PATHOPHYSIOLOGY ILLUSTRATED

Sickle Cell Anemia

Hemoglobin S and Red Blood Cell Sickling

Sickle cell anemia is caused by an inherited autosomal recessive defect in Hb synthesis. Sickle cell hemoglobin (HbS) differs from normal hemoglobin only in the substitution of the amino acid valine for glutamine in both beta chains of the hemoglobin molecule.

When HbS is oxygenated, it has the same globular shape as normal hemoglobin. However, when HbS off-loads oxygen, it becomes insoluble in intracellular fluid and crystallizes into rodlike structures. Clusters of rods form polymers (long chains) that bend the erythrocyte into the characteristic crescent shape of the sickle cell.

Incorrect amino acids

β chains

Hemoglobin S molecule

α chains

Polymerized deoxyhemo-globin S

Oxyhemoglobin S

O₂

Deoxyhemoglobin S

Sickled erythrocyte

Oxygenated erythrocyte

Deoxygenated erythrocyte

The Sickle Cell Disease Process

Sickle cell disease is characterized by episodes of acute painful crises. Sickling crises are triggered by conditions causing high tissue oxygen demands or that affect cellular pH. As the crisis begins, sickled erythrocytes adhere to capillary walls and to each other, obstructing blood flow and causing cellular hypoxia. The crisis accelerates as tissue hypoxia and acidic metabolic waste products cause further sickling and cell damage.

Sickle cell crises cause microinfarcts in joints and organs, and repeated crises slowly destroy organs and tissues. The spleen and kidneys are especially prone to sickling damage.

Microinfarct

Necrotic tissue

Damaged tissue

Inflamed tissue

Hypoxic cells

Mass of sickled cells obstructing capillary lumen

Capillary

NURSING CARE OF THE OLDER ADULT
Fluid Volume Deficit

Fluid volume deficit, or dehydration, is a common reason for hospitalization of people over age 65 who live either in the community or in a long-term care setting. Older adults have a significant number of risk factors for fluid volume deficit (see the preceding section of this chapter). In addition, the older adult has fewer intracellular reserves, contributing to rapid development of dehydration. Without intervention, mortality from dehydration can exceed 50% in the older adult population (Suhayda & Walton, 2002).

Manifestations of fluid volume deficit may be more difficult to recognize in the older adult. A change in mental status, memory, or attention may be an early sign. Skin turgor is less reliable as an indicator of dehydration, although assessing turgor over the sternum or on the inner aspect of the thigh may be more effective. Dry oral mucous membranes and tongue furrows also are indicative of dehydration. Orthostatic vital signs may not demonstrate typical changes in the dehydrated older adult.

▲ NURSING CARE OF THE OLDER ADULT

This box prepares you with essential guidelines to provide nursing care for older adults you will see in clinical settings.

▲ PATHOPHYSIOLOGY ILLUSTRATED

The 3-D art brings the concepts to life—visual illustrations of disease processes help you better understand pathophysiology and its impact on the body.

▲ NURSING RESEARCH BOXES

These evidence-based practice boxes focus on research into specific topics and relate it to current nursing care. Critical thinking questions show you how research can be applied to nursing care.

▲ MEDICATION ADMINISTRATION BOXES

This box prepares you to administer the most common drugs you will encounter in treating disorders within the chapter, as well as related nursing responsibilities and client-family teaching.

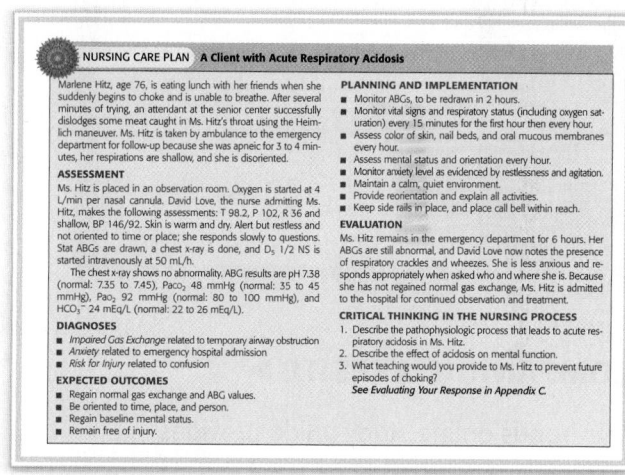

▲ NURSING CARE PLANS

Learn how to construct nursing care plans by studying the case study model presented in your book, including assessment, diagnoses, expected outcomes, planning and implementation, and evaluation. Critical thinking questions give you more opportunity to apply what you learn.

3. PREPARE FOR NCLEX-RN® SUCCESS

Take advantage of multiple opportunities to prepare yourself for the NCLEX-RN®. We offer unique sets of test questions at the end-of-chapter, on the student Prentice Hall Nursing MediaLink DVD-ROM, on your textbook Companion Website, and in the Study Guide.

TEST YOURSELF NCLEX-RN® REVIEW ▶

At the end of each chapter, test your application and analysis of the chapter concepts within NCLEX®-style review questions. Answers and comprehensive rationales appear in Appendix C.

TEST YOURSELF NCLEX-RN® REVIEW

1. The key difference between emergencies and disasters is that:
   1. emergencies are controlled.
   2. disasters result from man-made errors.
   3. emergencies can typically be handled by available emergency services.
   4. disasters typically involve the local emergency services and no other agencies.
2. Which of the following is NOT true regarding nurses' responsibilities in disaster preparedness?
   1. Nurses have a responsibility to the public to be knowledgeable about disaster preparedness and response.
   2. Nurses must have a personal and family plan as a part of their disaster preparedness and response plan.
   3. Nurses will be the leaders in the incident command structure set up at the site of the disaster.
   4. Nurses who are prepared for disasters will be better able to help themselves, their families, and their communities in a

5. Which of the equipment
   1. PPE pr
   2. Eye, fac PPE pr
   3. PPE sh and/or
   4. Healthc strict ha
6. Which of th
   1. Decont downw
   2. Decont the disa
   3. Decont hospital
   4. Decont

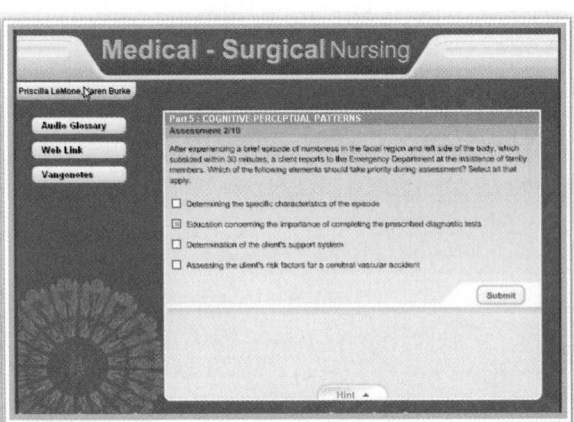

◀ PRENTICE HALL NURSING MEDIALINK DVD-ROM

Packaged with your textbook, the Student DVD-ROM provides you with additional practice NCLEX®-style tests and feedback with rationales for right and wrong answers. Each question is coded to the step in the Nursing Process, Cognitive Level, and the Category of Client Need according to the NCLEX-RN® Test Plan.

A CD-ROM version of this student resource can be purchased online at www.MyPearsonStore.com using ISBN: 0-13-235057-2

COMPANION WEBSITE ▶

This bonus online study guide provides even more NCLEX-RN® review questions with instant feedback, and rationales for all answers help you learn the material and prepare you for course exams.

www.prenhall.com/lemone

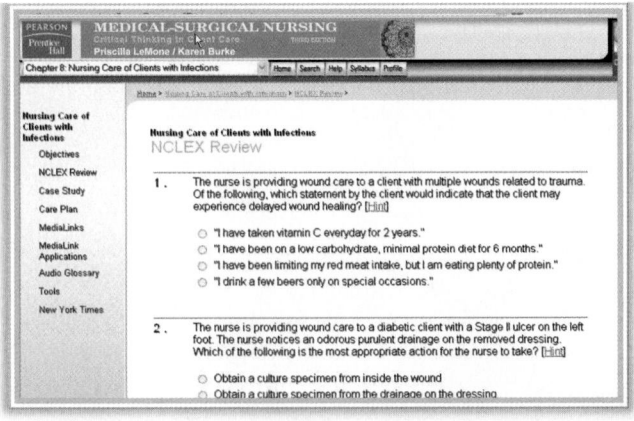

STUDENT STUDY GUIDE

ISBN: 0-13-198570-1

Using your Study Guide, you can test yourself with NCLEX-RN® review questions in each chapter.

4. BUILD YOUR CLINICAL COMPETENCE

Finally, to achieve nursing excellence, you need to synthesize and apply the concepts you learned from all the chapters in a body system unit. At the end of each unit in your textbook, Building Clinical Competence gives you the opportunity to pull the unit material together by practicing skills needed to care for multiple patients simultaneously. This activity has three parts:

FUNCTIONAL HEALTH PATTERN ACTIVITY ▶

Through this activity you will learn more about how disorders discussed in the unit affect clients' functional health status. The Functional Health Pattern is further defined, priority nursing diagnosis are identified, and critical thinking questions allow you to apply your learning.

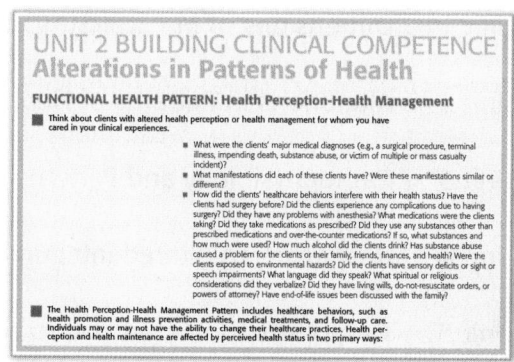

CLINICAL SCENARIO ▶

Each clinical scenario presents you with multiple clients. The critical thinking questions ask you to set priorities while managing multiple clients, preparing you for NCLEX® questions that test prioritization and safe nursing care. To be successful, you need to apply not only knowledge from across the unit but also principles related to setting priorities and maintaining patient safety.

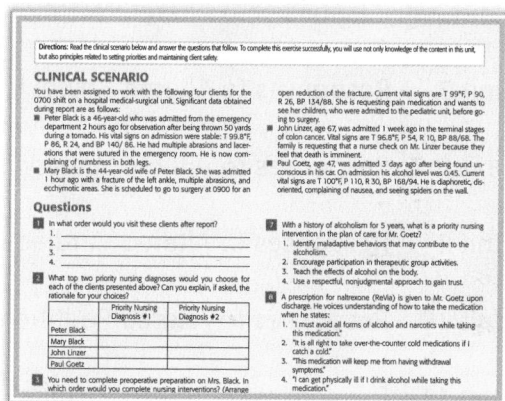

CASE STUDY WITH CONCEPT MAP ▶

Read the Case Study and review the Concept Map that diagrams the priority diagnosis. Go to the student DVD-ROM and use the concept mapping software to practice organizing and representing a priority nursing diagnosis in a concept map that you build on your own.

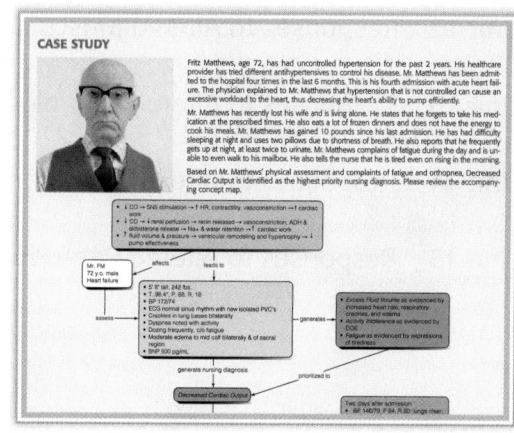

On the Next Page, *you will find a list of all the* **Building Clinical Competence** *activities and where to find them in your textbook.*

BUILDING CLINICAL COMPETENCE

Use the Building Clinical Competence features to review for unit exams in your course.

BUILD YOUR CLINICAL COMPETENCE TO ACHIEVE NURSING EXCELLENCE

Medical-Surgical
Nursing
Critical Thinking
in Client Care

FOURTH EDITION

Priscilla LeMone, RN, DSN, FAAN
Associate Professor Emeritus
Sinclair School of Nursing
University of Missouri–Columbia
Columbia, Missouri

Karen Burke, RN, MS
Education Consultant
Oregon State Board of Nursing
Portland, Oregon

PEARSON

Prentice
Hall

Upper Saddle River, New Jersey 07458

Library of Congress Cataloging-in-Publication Data

Medical-surgical nursing : critical thinking in client care / [edited by] Priscilla LeMone, Karen Burke.—4th ed.

p. ; cm.

Includes bibliographical references and index.

ISBN-13: 978-0-13-171308-6 (alk. paper)

ISBN-10: 0-13-171308-6 (alk. paper)

1. Nursing. 2. Surgical nursing. 3. Critical thinking. I. LeMone, Priscilla. II. Burke, Karen M.

[DNLM: 1. Nursing Process. 2. Nursing Care. 3. Patient Care Planning. 4. Perioperative Nursing. WY 100 M4892 2008]

RT41.M493 2008

617′.0231—dc22   2006101508

Publisher: Julie Levin Alexander

Publisher's Assistant: Regina Bruno

Editor-in-Chief: Maura Connor

Acquisitions Editor: Pamela Fuller

Editorial Assistant: Melisa Baez

Development Editor: Kim Wyatt

Managing Editor, Development: Marilyn Meserve

Managing Production Editor: Patrick Walsh

Production Liaison: Cathy O'Connell

Production Editor: Lynn Steines, Carlisle Publishers Services

Manufacturing Manager: Ilene Sanford

Design Director and Cover Designer: Mary Siener

Photographer: Patrick Watson

Director of Marketing: Karen Allman

Senior Marketing Manager: Francisco Del Castillo

Marketing Coordinator: Michael Sirinides

Associate Editor: Michael Giacobbe

Media Development Editor: John J. Jordan

New Media Project Manager: Tina Rudowski

Composition: Carlisle Publishing Services, Inc.

Printer/Binder: RR Donnelley Willard

Cover Printer: Phoenix Color

Cover photo: Kaleidoscope: Caribbean Blues, Paula Nadelstern, artist; Karen Bell, photographer

Notice: Care has been taken to confirm the accuracy of information presented in this book. The authors, editors, and the publisher, however, cannot accept any responsibility for errors or omissions or for consequences from application of the information in this book and make no warranty, express or implied, with respect to its contents. The authors and publisher have exerted every effort to ensure that drug selections and dosages set forth in this text are in accord with current recommendations and practice at time of publication. However, in view of ongoing research, changes in government regulations, and the constant flow of information relating to drug therapy and drug reactions, the reader is urged to check the package inserts of all drugs for any change in indications of dosage and for added warnings and precautions. This is particularly important when the recommended agent is a new and/or infrequently employed drug.

Pearson Education Ltd.

Pearson Education Singapore, Pte. Ltd.

Pearson Education Canada, Ltd.

Pearson Education—Japan

Pearson Education Australia PTY, Limited

Pearson Education North Asia Ltd.

Pearson Educación de Mexico, S.A. de C.V.

Pearson Education Malaysia, Pte. Ltd.

Pearson Education, Upper Saddle River, New Jersey

10 9 8 7 6 5 4 3 2 1

ISBN-13: 978-0-13-171308-6

ISBN-10: 0-13-171308-6

Dedication

I dedicate this book to Oz, who fills my days with sunshine.

Priscilla LeMone

I dedicate this book to Louise, mentor and friend; the woman who sets the standard for always striving to make a difference for the future of nursing.

Karen Burke

ABOUT THE AUTHORS

PRISCILLA LEMONE, RN, DSN, FAAN

Priscilla LeMone spent most of her career as a nurse educator, teaching medical-surgical nursing and pathophysiology at all levels from diploma to doctoral students. She has a diploma in nursing from Deaconess College of Nursing (St. Louis, Missouri), baccalaureate and master's degrees from Southeast Missouri State University, and a doctorate in nursing from the University of Alabama–Birmingham. She is retired as an Associate Professor Emeritus, Sinclair School of Nursing, University of Missouri–Columbia, but continues to keep up to date in nursing as an author of nursing textbooks.

Dr. LeMone had numerous awards for scholarship and teaching during her more than 30 years as a nurse educator. She is most honored for receiving the Kemper Fellowship for Teaching Excellence from the University of Missouri–Columbia, the Unique Contribution Award from the North American Nursing Diagnosis Association, and for being selected as a Fellow in the American Academy of Nursing.

She believes that her education gave her solid and everlasting roots in nursing. Her work with students has given her the wings that allow her love of nursing and teaching to continue through the years.

Recently married after 8 years of widowhood, Dr. LeMone lives in Ohio. When she has time, she enjoys traveling, gardening, and reading fiction.

KAREN M. BURKE, RN, MS

Karen Burke has practiced nursing in direct care and as a nurse educator and administrator. She is currently the Education Consultant for the Oregon State Board of Nursing. In this role, she serves as a consultant to new and existing nursing education programs in the state.

Ms. Burke entered nursing with a diploma from Emanuel Hospital School of Nursing in Portland, Oregon, later completing baccalaureate studies at Oregon Health & Science University (OHSU), and a master's degree at the University of Portland. She retired as the Director of Health Occupations at Clatsop Community College in Astoria, Oregon. Ms. Burke currently is a member of the steering committee for the Oregon Consortium for Nursing Education, and is actively involved in the Education Committee of the Oregon Nursing Leadership Council. She is coauthor of another text, *Medical-Surgical Nursing Care* (2nd edition) with Priscilla LeMone, Elaine Mohn-Brown, and Linda Eby.

Ms. Burke strongly values the nursing profession and the importance of providing a strong education in the art and science of nursing for all students preparing to enter the profession. Her diverse experience has prepared her to relate to nursing students at all levels and in diverse programs.

Ms. Burke divides her time between a house in the country with her husband Steve and spoiled cat, and a small condo in the city. She and Steve love to garden, travel, and spend time with their extended family. Ms. Burke enjoys a passion for quilting, accumulating and gradually completing multiple UFOs (unfinished objects).

CONTRIBUTORS

We extend a deep, sincere thanks to our contributors, who gave their time, effort, and expertise so willingly to the development and writing of chapters and resources that help foster our goal of achieving nursing excellence through building your clinical competence.

TEXTBOOK CONTRIBUTORS

Jane Bostick, PhD, RN
Assistant Professor of Clinical Nursing
University of Missouri–Columbia
Columbia, Missouri
Chapter 6: Nursing Care of Clients with Problems of Substance Abuse

Nancy R. Bowers, MSN, RN, CNS
Associate Professor
University of Cincinnati–Raymond Walters College
Cincinnati, Ohio
Chapter 8: Genetic Implications of Adult Health Nursing

Cheryl DeGraw, MSN, RN, CRNP, CNE
Nursing Instructor
Florence–Darlington Technical College
Florence, South Carolina
End-of-Unit features

Mei R. Fu, PhD, RN, MS, MA, APRN-BC, BS, BA
Assistant Professor, Course Coordinator
New York University
New York, New York
Chapter 14: Nursing Care of Clients with Cancer

Joanne C. Langan, PhD, RN
Chair, Division of Mental Health, Family, Community, and Systems Nursing
Assistant Professor
Saint Louis University, School of Nursing
St. Louis, Missouri
Chapter 7: Nursing Care of Clients Experiencing Disasters

Elaine Mohn-Brown, EdD, RN
Nursing Professor
Chemeketa Community College
Salem, Oregon
Chapter 17: Nursing Care of Clients with Burns

Helen Sandkuhl, MSN, CEN, TNS, FAEN
Director of Nursing, Emergency Services
Saint Louis University Hospital
St. Louis, Missouri
Chapter 11: Nursing Care of Clients Experiencing Trauma and Shock

Marjorie Whitman, MSN, RN, AOCNS
Nurse Clinician
University of Missouri Hospital
Columbia, Missouri
Chapter 4: Nursing Care of Clients Having Surgery
Chapter 9: Nursing Care of Clients Experiencing Pain
Chapter 12: Nursing Care of Clients with Infections
Chapter 13: Nursing Care of Clients with Altered Immunity
Chapter 19: Nursing Care of Clients with Endocrine Disorders
Chapter 20: Nursing Care of Clients with Diabetes Mellitus

STUDENT AND INSTRUCTIONAL RESOURCE CONTRIBUTORS

Katrina Allen, MSN, RN, CCRN
Nursing Instructor
Faulkner State Community College
Bay Minette, Alabama
Companion Website

Christina Baumer, PhD, RN, CNOR, CHES
Division Chair, Continuing Education
Program Director, Surgical Technology
Lancaster General College of Nursing and Health Sciences
Lancaster, Pennsylvania
Study Guide

Sharon F. Beasley, MSN, RN
Nursing Instructor
Technical College of the Lowcountry
Beaufort, South Carolina
Companion Website
Student DVD-ROM

Michelle Buchman, RN, BSN, BC
Educational Support Services LLC
St. John's Marian Center
Chesterfield, Missouri
Study Guide

Donna L. Bumpus, MSN
Assistant Professor
Lamar University
Beaumont, Texas
Instructor's Resource Manual

Joy Burnard, MSN, RN, CDE
Adjunct Faculty
Point Loma Nazarene University
Bakersfield, California
Companion Website

Barbara M. Carranti, MS, RN, CNS
Instructor, Department of Nursing
Le Moyne College
Syracuse, New York
Companion Website

Kim Cooper, MSN, RN
Nursing Department Chair, Assistant Professor
Ivy Tech Community College of Indiana
Terre Haute, Indiana
Student DVD-ROM

Nina R. Cuttler, MSN, APRN, BC
Nursing Instructor
Central Carolina Technical College
Sumter, South Carolina
Student DVD-ROM

Vera Dauffenbach, EdD, MSN, RN
Associate Professor, Director of the Graduate Program
Bellin College of Nursing
Green Bay, Wisconsin
Companion Website

Katherine H. Dimmock, EdD, MSN, RN, JD
Nursing Dean and Professor
Columbia College of Nursing
Milwaukee, Wisconsin
Companion Website
Student DVD-ROM

Susan A. Erlewine, MSN, RN, CHPN
Assistant Professor
Hocking College School of Nursing
Nelsonville, Ohio
Companion Website

Pamela Fowler, MSN, BSN
Assistant Professor of Nursing
Rogers State University
Claremore, Oklahoma
Instructor's Resource Manual

Polly C. Haigler, PhD, RN, BC
Clinical Associate Professor
University of South Carolina
Columbia, South Carolina
Student DVD-ROM

Amy Herrington, MSN, RN, CEN
Critical Care Staff Development Specialist
University of Kentucky Healthcare
Lexington, Kentucky
Companion Website

Ann Isaacs, MS, APRN, BC
Professor of Nursing
Luzerne County Community College
Nanticoke, Pennsylvania
Companion Website
Student DVD-ROM

Tricia Jenkins, RN, MBA, PhD
Assistant Professor
Florida Atlantic University
Boca Raton, Florida
Instructor's Resource CD-ROM

Cathleen E. Kunkler, MSN, RN, ONC
Instructor, Nurse Education
Corning Community College
Corning, New York
Companion Website

Mary Ann Siciliano McLaughlin, MSN, RN
Nurse Educator
Hospital of the University of Pennsylvania
Philadelphia, Pennsylvania
Companion Website

Linda Oakley-Clancy, MSN, RN
Assistant Professor
Manatee Community College
Bradenton, Florida
Companion Website

Tami J. Rogers, DVM, MSN, BSN
Professor of Nursing
Valencia Community College
Orlando, Florida
Companion Website
Student DVD-ROM

Christine M. Thomas, MSN, DNSc, RN
Assistant Professor
West Chester University
West Chester, Pennsylvania
Companion Website
Student DVD-ROM

Loretta Wack, MSN, RN
Associate Professor
Blue Ridge Community College
Weyers Cave, Virginia
Companion Website

Julie Will, MSN, RN
Associate Professor
Ivy Tech Community College
Terre Haute, Indiana
Companion Website

Kathleen Wilson, MSN, RN
Nursing Professor
Houston Community College
Houston, Texas
Companion Website
Student DVD-ROM

Charlotte Wisnewski, PhD, RN, BC, CDE
Assistant Professor
University of Texas Medical Branch
Galveston, Texas
Student DVD-ROM

Nancy H. Wright, RN, BS, CNOR
Professor of Nursing
Virginia College
Birmingham, Alabama
Instructor's Resource Manual

Annette Zampelli, MSN, CRNP
Nursing Professor
Pennsylvania State Hershey Medical
Center and School of Nursing
Hershey, Pennsylvania
Companion Website
Instructor's Resource Manual

Dawn Zwick, MSN, RN, CNP
Lecturer, Graduate Program
Kent State University
Kent, Ohio
Student DVD-ROM

THANK YOU

Our heartfelt thanks go out to our colleagues from schools of nursing across the country who have given their time generously during the past two years to help us create this exciting new edition of our book. These individuals helped us plan and shape this textbook and resources by reviewing chapters, art, designs, and more. **Medical-Surgical Nursing: Critical Thinking in Client Care,** fourth edition, has reaped the benefit of your collective experience as nurses and teachers, and we have made many improvements due to your efforts, insights, suggestions, objections, encouragement, and inspiration. Among those who gave us their encouragement and comments are the following:

ACADEMIC REVIEWERS

Theresa Adelman, MSN, RN, CEN, TNS,
Methodist College of Nursing

Sheila Alexander, PhD, RN,
University of Pittsburgh

Catherine A. Andrews, PhD, RN,
Edgewood College

Vivian E. Austin, RN, MSN,
Macon State College

Michael Beach, MSN, APRN,
University of Pittsburgh

Deborah Becker, MSN, CRNP, BC,
University of Pennsylvania

Margaret Bellak, MN,
Indiana University of Pennsylvania

Carol Bence, MS, RN,
Indiana Wesleyan University

Alice Blazeck, RN, DNSC,
University of Pittsburgh

Donna Bowles, EdD, MSN, RN,
Indiana University Southeast

Judith E. Breitenbach, MS, RN,
Towson University

Debra J. Brown, PhD, RN, FNP, ANP, BC,
University of North Carolina–Chapel Hill

Michelle Buchman, RN, BSN, BC,
St. John's Marian Center

Donna L. Bumpus, MSN, RN,
Lamar University

Susan E. Caulkins, MSN, APRN, BC,
Central Carolina Technical College

Cynthia L. Dakin, PhD, RN,
Northeastern University

Barbara Ann D'Anna, DSL, MSN, RN, CNOR,
Anne Arundel Community College

Maggie Davis, MSN, RN,
Central Florida Community College

Rosalinda DeLuna, RN, CCRN,
Indiana University Northwest

Linda Denison, APRN, BC,
University of Wisconsin

Wanda Dooley, MSN, APRN, BC, FNP,
Northern Virginia Community College

Phyllis Dubendorf, MSN, RN, CRNP,
University of Pennsylvania

Elizabeth Farren Corbin, PhD, FNP, RN,
Baylor University

Marianne Fasano, Med, MSN, RN, CRNI, CWOCN, PCCN,
Pasco–Hernando Community College

Patricia Fowler, MSN, RNC, CNS,
University of Texas–El Paso

Kathleen W. Free, MSN, RNC, ARNP,
Indiana University Southeast

Arlinda Garner, MS, RN,
College of the Mainland

Janet Goeldner, MSN, RN, AOCN,
University of Cincinnati–Raymond Walters College

Sung Hi Gwak, MSN, CCRN, RN, BC,
Borough of Manhattan Community College

Becky Haglund, MN, RN,
Santa Ana College

Polly Haigler, PhD, RN, BC,
University of South Carolina

Barbara A. Hannah, EdD, MS, CPAN, BS,
University of Oklahoma

Anne Helm, MSN, RN,
Owens Community College

Carolyn Insley, MS, MN, RN, BSN,
Fort Hays State University

Vanessa Johnson, PhD, MS, BSN,
University of Oklahoma

Catherine B. Kaesburg, MSN, RN, CNS,
Illinois State University

Sarah Keeling, MN, RN, BSN,
Georgia Perimeter College

Bonnie Kirkpatrick, MS, RN, CNS,
Ohio State University

Andrea Knesek, MSN, BC,
Macomb Community College

Cheryl Lantz, MS, RN, BSN,
Dickinson State University

Rhonda Lawes, RN, MS,
University of Oklahoma

Catherine Lazo-Miller, MS, RN,
Indiana University Northwest

Jennifer Leisegang, MSN, RN, ARNP,
Whatcom Community College

Christine Linert, MSN, RN, OCN,
Collin County Community College

Kit Mallow, MSN, RN,
Gogebic Community College

Hyacinth Martin, MSED, MA, RN,
Borough of Manhattan Community College

Jill M. Mayo, MSN, RN,
Mississippi College

Ellen McAvoy, MA, RN,
Hillsborough Community College

Arlene McGrory, DNSc, RN,
University of Massachusetts–Lowell

Gail Meagher, MSN, RN,
Odessa College

Ann Merrill, MS, MA, BSN,
University of Oklahoma

Brenda Michel, EdD, MS, RN,
Lincoln Land Community College

Sue Miller, MSN, RNC, CNS,
Catawba Valley Community College

Jo Mizzi, MBA, RN,
Highline Community College; Bellevue Community College; Overlake Hospital and Medical Center

Elise Muller-Lindgren, RN, MN, CHPN,
Highline Community College

Judy Ogans, MS, RN,
University of Oklahoma

Gina Oliver, PhD, RN,
University of Missouri–Columbia

Wendi Palermo, MSN, RN,
McNeese State University

Karen Peel, MN, CCRN,
University of South Carolina

Rebecca A. Phillips, PhD, RN,
University of Oklahoma

Bill Powell, PhD, RN, FNP,
University of North Carolina–Chapel Hill

Tara McMillan Queen, RN, AA, BSN, MN, ANP-C, GNP,
Mercy School of Nursing

Colleen Quinn, MSN, RN,
Broward Community College

Anita K. Reed, MSN, RN,
St. Elizabeth School of Nursing

Tami J. Rogers, BSN, MSN, DVM,
Valencia Community College

Pamela Johnson Rowsey, PhD, RN,
University of North Carolina–Chapel Hill

Megan Sary, MSN, RN,
Merritt College

Jeannie Short, MSN, RN,
Indiana Wesleyan University

Annette S. Stacy, MSN, RN, AOCN,
Arkansas State University

Judith Stauder, MSN, RN,
Stark State College of Technology

Cecilia Tolson, MSN, CNOR, RN,
Owens Community College

Shirley E. Van Zandt, MSN, MPH, CRNP,
Johns Hopkins University

Benita Walton-Moss, DNS, APRN, BC,
Johns Hopkins University

Antoinette Willsea, MSN, RN,
Piedmont College

Kathleen M. Woodruff, MS, CRNP,
Johns Hopkins University

Annette Zampelli, MSN, CRNP,
Penn State Hershey Medical Center

CLINICAL REVIEWERS

Randall Beaton, PhD, EMT,
University of Washington

Pamela Bilyeu, RN, BSN, CNOR, CURN, ONC,
Saint Vincent Healthcare

William P. Carrick, MSN, BSN,
McLean Hospital; Cab Health and Recovery

Cynthia Christensen, MSN, CVN, ARNP-BC,
Ben Collins D.O.

Cathy Cormier, MN, RN,
Southeastern Louisiana State University

Caroline Kuhlman, MSN, APRN-BC, ACON,
Massachusetts General Hospital

Debra J. Lenhart, MSN, RN,
Oklahoma University

Connie Miller, MSN, FNP-C, CDE, BC-ADM,
Cheyenne Crossroads Clinic

Bonnie Pedraza, MSN, RN, CCRN,
University of Wisconsin–Milwaukee

Joanne Farley Serembus, EdD, RN, CCRN,
Roxborough Memorial Hospital

Colleen Marie Totero, MSN, RN, ANCC, APNP, CCRN,
University of Wisconsin

Denise York, MEd, MS, CNS, RNC,
Columbus State Community College

STUDENT REVIEWERS

Julie Bauder,
Johns Hopkins University School of Nursing

Lorna Benoit,
Essex Community College

Lori Bunalski,
The College of New Jersey

Marla Greco,
Pennsylvania State University

Jessica Kramer,
The College of New Jersey

Kristina Smith,
University of Maryland

Emily Watson,
The College of New Jersey

Melissa Whitty,
The College of New Jersey

This is a wonderful time to become a nurse! We have all heard about the nursing shortage, especially as it relates to the aging of the population. In fact, the need for new nurses is projected to be at or greater than one million by 2010. While this problem will have to be faced as a society as a whole, it means that your knowledge and skills will be in great demand to meet healthcare needs well into the future. We wrote this book to help you build those skills.

Nursing students are expected to build on knowledge of basic sciences, social sciences, and the fundamentals of nursing to synthesize and critically analyze new skills necessary to ensure clinical competence. We revised and updated the fourth edition of *Medical-Surgical Nursing: Critical Thinking in Client Care* to provide you with the knowledge and skills you need to care for adult clients to promote health, facilitate recovery from illness and injury, and provide support when coping with disability or loss.

Throughout the text, we make every effort to communicate that both nurses and adult clients may be male or female; and that clients require holistic, individualized care regardless of their age or racial, cultural, or socioeconomic background.

OUR GOAL—HELPING YOU ACHIEVE CLINICAL COMPETENCE BY BUILDING ON YOUR SKILLS

Our focus in writing this book is to provide you with knowledge that provides a base for clinical judgment and that can be applied to provide safe, individualized, and competent clinical nursing care. Our easily understood, straightforward style will help you integrate concepts in pathophysiology, pharmacology, and interdisciplinary healthcare interventions into prioritized nursing care. We developed multiple learning strategies to help you succeed—audio, illustrations, teaching tips, and video and animation media. We include boxes, tables, special features and illustrations, as well as synthesis and critical thinking exercises, so you can build your skills for class, for clinical, for NCLEX®, and for practice.

We believe that students learn best within a nursing model of care with consistent organization and understandable text. Starting with the first edition, we have held fast to our vision that this textbook:

- Maintains a strong focus on nursing care as the essential element in learning and doing nursing, regardless of the age of the client or the setting for care.
- Provides a proper balance of physiology, pathophysiology, pharmacology, and interdisciplinary care on which to base safe, competent, and individualized nursing care.
- Emphasizes the nurse's role as an essential member of the interdisciplinary healthcare team.
- Uses functional health patterns and the nursing process as the structure for providing nursing care in today's world by prioritizing nursing diagnoses and interventions specific to altered responses to illness.

- Fosters critical thinking and decision-making skills as the basis for nursing excellence in clinical practice.
- Continues to believe that the person receiving care has not only a personal experience with health and illness, but is also an active participant in maintaining and/or regaining health. Within this philosophy, we regard that person as a client, rather than a patient, in this textbook. The client may be an individual, a family, or a community.

ORGANIZATION

The book is organized into 52 chapters in six major parts, organized by functional health patterns. Each part opens with a concept map illustrating the relationship of each functional health pattern to possible nursing diagnoses. The parts are then divided into units based on alterations in human structure and function. Each unit with a focus on altered health states opens with an assessment chapter. On the accompanying DVD-ROM, students find a comprehensive review of anatomy and physiology complete with animations, three-dimensional structures, and exercises. This draws upon the student's prerequisite knowledge, and serves to reinforce basic principles of anatomy and physiology as applied to physical assessment.

Following the assessment chapter in each unit, the nursing care chapters provide information about major conditions and diseases. Each of these nursing care chapters follows a consistent format, including three key components:

PATHOPHYSIOLOGY The discussion of each *major* illness or condition begins with incidence and prevalence with an overview of pathophysiology, followed by manifestations and complications. *Focus on Cultural Diversity* boxes demonstrate how race, age, and gender affect differences in incidence, prevalence, and mortality. *Pathophysiology Illustrated* art brings physiologic processes to life.

INTERDISCIPLINARY CARE Interdisciplinary care considers treatment of the illness or condition by the healthcare team. The section includes information about specific tests necessary for diagnosis, medications, surgery and treatments, fluid management, dietary management, and complementary and alternative therapies.

NURSING CARE Because illness prevention is critical in health care today, this section begins with health promotion information. We discuss nursing care within a context of priority nursing diagnoses and interventions, with rationales provided for each intervention. Boxes that present information essential to client care are *Nursing Care, Meeting Individualized Needs, Practice Alerts, Medication Administration, Nursing Research,* and *NANDA, NIC, and NOC Linkages.* Last, for each major disorder or condition, we provide a narrative *Nursing Care Plan* that begins with a brief case study, followed by the steps of the nursing process. Critical thinking questions specific to the care plan conclude with a section called *Evaluate Your Response* that provides additional guidance for critical thinking. Suggested guidelines are found in Appendix C.

CHAPTER REVIEW This end-of-chapter section concludes with ten multiple-choice review questions to reinforce comprehension of the chapter content. (The correct answers with rationales are found in Appendix C.) The *EXPLORE MediaLink* feature encourages students to use the DVD-ROM and the Companion Website to apply what they have learned from the textbook through critical thinking and interactive exercises.

What's New in the Fourth Edition

We carefully reviewed the third edition of this book to ensure current content and the necessary knowledge to educate the next generation of nurses. New features of the fourth edition include:

- We divided the chapter objectives into Learning Outcomes and Clinical Competencies. Learning Outcomes show you the knowledge you'll gain, while Clinical Competencies demonstrate how you will apply that knowledge.
- We changed the heading "Collaborative Care" to "Interdisciplinary Care" to better illustrate the role of each member of the healthcare team in providing safe, research-based, client-centered care.
- We added a list of key terms to the beginning of each chapter, and these terms are then printed in bold type and defined at the first occurrence within text. You can learn the correct pronunciation of all terms on the Audio Glossary, found on the textbook's Companion Website.
- We added new chapters and content to make the book absolutely current and clinically relevant.
  - Chapter 7: Nursing Care of Clients Experiencing Disasters
  - Chapter 8: Genetic Implications of Adult Health Nursing
  - Chapter 38: Nursing Care of Clients with Ventilation Disorders
  - Chapter 39: Nursing Care of Clients with Gas Exchange Disorders
- We redesigned the assessment chapters that begin each body system unit to provide students with a more structured, easy-to-use overview for assessment of that body system. The new format includes:
  - A list of needed equipment at the beginning of each chapter.
  - Increased review of normal anatomy and physiology of the system being assessed.
- The assessment section of the chapter is divided as follows:
  - *Diagnostic Tests* This section includes diagnostic test tables and a narrative summary. The tables include the name of the test, the purpose and description of the test, and related nursing care.
  - *Genetic Considerations* This section reminds you of the relevant genetic-based information to gather during the health history.
  - *Health Assessment Interview* This interview not only summarizes and prioritizes the questions to ask, but also provides an interview guide based on functional health patterns.
  - The *Physical Assessment* section is in a new, easy-to-read two-column format that demonstrates how to perform the assessment, with normal and abnormal findings.
- We added a box titled *Fast Facts* to highlight and summarize important data about the prevalence and incidence of selected disorders and other featured content.
- An end-of-unit review for each of the 15 units, called *Building Clinical Competence,* synthesizes what you've learned in the unit and applies the knowledge to specific cases. The feature includes:
  - A functional health pattern expansion that includes further discussion and critical thinking questions;
  - A clinical scenario involving a priority issue reflection piece that synthesizes underlying concepts and includes a variety of questions that allow students to apply different skills; and
  - A case study with concept map that further synthesizes material using the nursing process.

SPECIAL FEATURES

MEDICATION ADMINISTRATION

NANDA, NIC, AND NOC

NURSING CARE OF THE OLDER ADULT

NURSING CARE PLAN

NURSING RESEARCH: EVIDENCE-BASED PRACTICE

SAMPLE DOCUMENTATION

CONTENTS

PART V COGNITIVE AND PERCEPTUAL PATTERNS 1500

PART I

Medical-Surgical Nursing Practice

Functional Health Patterns with Related Nursing Diagnoses

HEALTH PERCEPTION-HEALTH MANAGEMENT

- Perceived health status
- Perceived health management
- Healthcare behaviors: health promotion and illness prevention activities, medical treatments, follow-up care

VALUE-BELIEF

- Values, goals, or beliefs (including spirituality) that guide choices or decisions
- Perceived conflicts in values, beliefs, or expectations that are health related

COPING-STRESS-TOLERANCE

- Capacity to resist challenges to self-integrity
- Methods of handling stress
- Support systems
- Perceived ability to control and manage situations

NUTRITIONAL-METABOLIC

- Daily consumption of food and fluids
- Favorite foods
- Use of dietary supplements
- Skin lesions and ability to heal
- Condition of the integument
- Weight, height, temperature

PART I
MEDICAL-SURGICAL NURSING PRACTICE NANDA NURSING DIAGNOSES

- Latex Allergy Response
- Caregiver Role Strain
- Chronic Sorrow
- Compromised Family Coping
- Death Anxiety
- Anxiety
- Decisional Conflict
- Disturbed Body Image
- Fatigue
- Fear
- Deficient Fluid Volume
- Excess Fluid Volume
- Ineffective Health Maintenance
- Health-Seeking Behaviors
- Risk for Infection
- Deficient Knowledge
- Nausea
- Acute Pain
- Chronic Pain
- Risk for Injury
- Powerlessness
- Disturbed Personal Identity
- Ineffective Protection
- Delayed Surgical Recovery
- Self-Care Deficit
- Low Self-Esteem
- Disturbed Sleep Pattern
- Ineffective Therapeutic Regimen Management
- Disturbed Thought Processes
- Risk for Violence

SEXUALITY-REPRODUCTIVE

- Satisfaction with sexuality or sexual relationships
- Reproductive pattern
- Female menstrual and perimenopausal history

ELIMINATION

- Patterns of bowel and urinary excretion
- Perceived regularity or irregularity of elimination
- Use of laxatives or routines
- Changes in time, modes, quality or quantity of excretions
- Use of devices for control

ROLE-RELATIONSHIPS

- Perception of major roles, relationships, and responsibilities in current life situation
- Satisfaction with or disturbances in roles and relationships

ACTIVITY-EXERCISE

- Patterns of personally relevant exercise, activity, leisure, and recreation
- ADLs that require energy expenditure
- Factors that interfere with the desired pattern (e.g., illness or injury)

SELF-PERCEPTION–SELF-CONCEPT

- Attitudes about self
- Perceived abilities, worth, self-image, emotions
- Body posture and movement, eye contact, voice and speech patterns

SLEEP-REST

- Patterns of sleep and rest-/relaxation in a 24-h period
- Perceptions of quality and quantity of sleep and rest
- Use of sleep aids and routines

COGNITIVE-PERCEPTUAL

- Adequacy of vision, hearing, taste, touch, smell
- Pain perception and management
- Language, judgment, memory, decisions

Adapted from *Nursing Diagnosis: Process and Application*, 3rd ed., by M. Gordon, pp. 80–96. Copyright © 1994, with permission from Elsevier Science.

Dimensions of Medical-Surgical Nursing

CHAPTER 1 Medical-Surgical Nursing

LEARNING OUTCOMES

- Describe the core competencies for healthcare professionals: patient-centered care, interdisciplinary teams, evidence-based practice, quality improvement, and informatics.

- Apply the attitudes, mental habits, and skills necessary for critical thinking when using the nursing process in client care.

- Explain the importance of nursing codes and standards as guidelines for clinical nursing practice.

- Explain the activities and characteristics of the nurse as caregiver, educator, advocate, leader and manager, and researcher.

CLINICAL COMPETENCIES

- Demonstrate critical thinking when using the nursing process to provide knowledgeable, safe client care.

- Provide clinical care within a framework that integrates, as appropriate, the medical-surgical nursing roles of caregiver, educator, advocate, leader/manager, and researcher.

MEDIALINK

Resources for this chapter can be found on the Prentice Hall Nursing MediaLink DVD-ROM accompanying this textbook, and on the Companion Website at http://www.prenhall.com/lemone

Medical-surgical nursing is the health promotion, health care, and illness care of adults based on knowledge derived from the arts and sciences and shaped by knowledge (the science) of nursing. The adult client—the person with whom and for whom nursing care is designed and implemented—ranges in age from the late teens to the early 100s. Medical-surgical nursing focuses on the adult client's response to actual or potential alterations in health. The wide range of ages and the variety of healthcare needs specific to individual clients make medical-surgical nursing an ever-changing and challenging area of nursing practice.

In this textbook, discussions of the human responses are structured within the framework of functional health patterns, and nursing care is presented within the context of nursing diagnoses. The term **client** is used throughout the text, based on a philosophy that individuals are active participants in health and illness as well as consumers of healthcare services.

Regardless of the type of healthcare service or setting, medical-surgical nurses must use knowledge and skills to be competent and safe when providing client care. Nursing care is structured by the activities planned and carried out through critical thinking within the nursing process, is based on ethics and standards established by nursing organizations, and is focused on returning the client to a state of functional health. This chapter provides a broad overview of the clinical practice of medical-surgical nursing, including core competencies, framework and guidelines for care delivery, and the roles of the nurse in medical-surgical care.

CORE COMPETENCIES FOR SAFE AND EFFECTIVE HEALTH CARE

The healthcare system in North America faces numerous challenges, including an increasingly older client population, changing consumer desires and expectations, rapidly expanding information and technologies, and a focus on improving quality and safety of care. After examining a number of studies about these challenges, the Institute of Medicine (IOM) (2001) found that although misuse of services and injuries resulting from errors are becoming more common, the safety and quality problems exist largely because of problems within the system and not because of highly dedicated healthcare professionals.

To meet the challenges, the National Academy of Sciences (2003) proposed a set of five **core competencies** that all healthcare professionals should possess, regardless of their discipline, to meet the needs of the 21st-century healthcare system. The competencies are based on using communication, knowledge, technical skills, critical thinking, and values in clinical practice. The core competencies with a description of related activities are outlined in Table 1–1.

TABLE 1–1 Core Competencies for Healthcare Professionals

COMPETENCY	DESCRIPTION OF ACTIVITIES
Provide client-centered care	■ Identify, respect, and care about client's differences, values, preferences, and needs. ■ Relieve pain and suffering. ■ Coordinate care. ■ Listen to, communicate with, and educate clients. ■ Advocate disease prevention, wellness, and promotion of healthy lifestyles.
Work in interdisciplinary teams	■ Cooperate, collaborate, communicate, and integrate care in teams to ensure that care is continuous and reliable.
Use evidence-based practice	■ Integrate best research findings with clinical expertise and client values for optimum care. ■ Participate in learning and research activities to the extent possible.
Apply quality improvement	■ Identify errors and hazards in care. ■ Understand and implement basic safety principles. ■ Understand and measure quality of care in terms of structure, process, and outcomes in relation to patient and community needs. ■ Design and test interventions to change processes and systems of care, with the objective of improving quality.
Use informatics	■ Communicate, manage knowledge, decrease error, and support decision making (critical thinking) using information technology.

Source: Data from National Academy of Sciences. (2003). *Executive summary: Health professions education: A bridge to quality* (pp. 1–15). Retrieved from www.nap.edu

FRAMEWORK FOR PRACTICE: CRITICAL THINKING IN THE NURSING PROCESS

The **nursing process** is the series of critical thinking activities nurses use as they provide care to clients. These activities define a nursing model of care, differentiating nursing from other helping professions. The nursing process can be used in any setting. The purpose of care may be to promote wellness, maintain health, restore health, or facilitate coping with disability or death. Regardless of the purpose of care, the planned process of nursing allows for the inclusion of specific, individualized, and holistic activities.

Critical Thinking

Critical thinking is, most basically, thinking about one's own thinking. It is self-directed thinking that is focused on what to believe or do in a specific situation. It involves attitudes and skills. Critical thinking occurs when the nurse uses scientific knowledge and the nursing process to consider a client care situation and then make judgments and decisions about what to do in that situation. As you practice critical thinking, you must consider:

- The purpose of the thinking (e.g., is it to collect more data or is it to report the data to someone else?)
- Your level of acquired knowledge
- Prejudices that may influence thinking (e.g., believing that all people in poverty are dirty or that the aged are incapable of learning how to care for themselves, or letting emotions affect decision making)
- Information that is needed from other sources such as faculty members, a skilled clinical nurse, a textbook or journal article, or the policies of the healthcare agency
- The ability to identify other possible options, evaluate the alternatives, and reach a conclusion
- Personal values and beliefs.

Critical thinking takes practice so that it becomes an integral component of the nurse's attitudes and skills. Critical thinking exercises are included throughout this book to provide that practice.

Attitudes and Mental Habits Necessary for Critical Thinking

Thinking critically involves more than just cognitive (knowledge) skills. It is strongly influenced by one's attitudes and mental habits. To think critically, you must focus your attention on your attitudes and how they affect your thinking. These attitudes and mental habits include the following:

- Being able to think independently so that you make clinical decisions based on sound thinking and judgment. This means, for example, that you are not influenced by negative comments from other healthcare providers about a client.
- Being willing to listen to and be fair in your evaluation of others' ideas and beliefs. This involves listening carefully to other ideas and thoughts, and making a decision based on what you learn instead of how you feel.
- Having empathy by being able to put yourself in the place of another to better understand that other person. For example, if you put yourself in the place of the person with severe pain, you are better able to understand why he or she is so upset when pain medications are late.
- Being fair minded and considering all viewpoints before making a decision through a sense of justice and being humble. This means you consider the viewpoints of others that may be different from yours before reaching a conclusion. You also realize that you are constantly learning from others. You are not afraid to say, "I don't know the answer to that question, but I will find out and let you know."
- Being disciplined so that you do not stop at easy answers, but continue to consider alternatives.
- Being creative and self-confident. Nurses often need to consider different ways of providing care and constantly look for better, more cost-effective methods. Confidence in one's decisions is gained through critical thinking.

Critical Thinking Skills

The major critical thinking skills are divergent thinking, reasoning, clarifying, and reflection. A description of each follows.

Divergent thinking is having the ability to weigh the importance of information. This means that when you collect data from a client, you can sort out the data that are relevant for the care of your client from the data that are not relevant and then explore alternatives to draw a conclusion. Abnormal data are usually considered relevant; normal data are helpful but may not change the care you provide.

Reasoning is having the ability to discriminate between facts and guesses. By using known facts, problems are solved and decisions are made in a systematic, logical way. For example, when you take a pulse you must know the facts of normal pulse rate for a person of this age, types of medications the client is taking that may alter the pulse rate, and the emotional and physical state of the client. Based on these facts, you are able to decide if the pulse rate is normal or abnormal.

Clarifying involves noting similarities and differences to sift out unnecessary information to help focus on the present situation. For example, when caring for a client with chronic pain, you must know the definition of chronic pain and the similarities and differences between acute pain and chronic pain.

Reflection occurs when you take time to think about something, comparing different situations with similar solutions. It cannot take place in an emergency situation. As you reflect on your experiences in nursing, many of those experiences may in turn become alternatives when caring for a different client.

Critical thinking is an expected ability of all nurses. Using critical thinking to provide care that is structured by the nursing process allows the nurse to provide safe, effective, holistic, and individualized care. See Table 1–2 for nursing process steps and corresponding critical thinking applications.

The Nursing Process

The nursing process benefits nurses who provide care, clients who receive care, and settings where care is provided. As nurses gain increasing autonomy in their practice, the use of the nursing process helps them identify their independent practice domain. The nursing process also provides a common reference system and a common terminology to serve as a base for improving clinical practice through research. In addition, the nursing process can serve as a framework for the evaluation of quality care.

TABLE 1–2 Using Critical Thinking in the Nursing Process

NURSING PROCESS STEP	CRITICAL THINKING SKILLS	QUESTIONS TO CHECK YOUR THINKING
Assessment	Making reliable observations Distinguishing relevant from irrelevant data Distinguishing important from unimportant data Validating data Organizing data Categorizing data according to a framework Recognizing assumptions	What assumptions am I making about the patient? Is my data correct and accurate? How reliable are my sources? What data is important? Relevant? What biases do I have that might cause me to miss important information? Am I listening carefully to get the patient's and family's perspective? Do I have all the facts? What other data might I need?
Diagnosis	Finding patterns and relationships among cues Identifying gaps in the data Making inferences Suspending judgment when lacking data Making interdisciplinary connections Stating the problem Examining assumptions Comparing patterns with norms Identifying factors contributing to the problem	Do I know what is within normal limits for the data? Do I have enough data to make a valid inference? What biases might I have that could affect how I see the patient's problems? Do I have enough data to make a nursing diagnosis or should I make a "possible" diagnosis? What other problems might this data suggest other than the one that seems most obvious to me?
Planning	Forming valid generalizations Transferring knowledge from one situation to another Developing evaluative criteria Hypothesizing Making interdisciplinary connections Prioritizing client problems Generalizing principles from other sciences	Do I need help to plan interventions, or am I qualified to do it? Did I remember to give high priority to the problems the patient and family identified as important? What are the most important problems we need to solve? What interventions worked in similar situations? Is this situation similar enough to merit using them with this patient? Are there other plans that might be more agreeable to the patient, and therefore more likely to work? Why do I expect these interventions to be effective? Based on what knowledge?
Implementation	Applying knowledge to perform interventions Using interventions to test hypotheses	Has the patient's condition changed since the plan was made? Have I overlooked any new developments? What is the patient's initial response to the intervention? Are there any safety issues I have overlooked?
Evaluation	Deciding whether hypotheses are correct Making criterion-based evaluations	What are the patient responses after the interventions? Have I overlooked anything? Does the data indicate that goals were met? Does the patient feel the goals were met? Does the patient trust me enough to give honest answers? Am I sure the problem is really resolved? What might we have done that would have been more effective? What nursing care is still needed, if any?

Source: Used with permission from *Nursing Process and Critical Thinking* (4th ed.) by J. M. Wilkinson, 2005. Reprinted by permission of Pearson Education, Inc. Upper Saddle River, NJ.

The nursing process also benefits the client receiving care and the agency or institution providing that care. The client receives planned, individualized interventions; participates in all steps of the process; and is assured continuity of care through the written care plan. The nursing process benefits the healthcare institution through better resource utilization, increased client satisfaction, and improved documentation of care.

The five steps or phases in the nursing process are assessment, diagnosis, planning, implementation, and evaluation. These steps are interrelated and interdependent. The steps are most often used cyclically, as illustrated in Figure 1–1 ■. The steps have been legitimized by the American Nurses Association (ANA) Standards of Practice, state nursing practice acts, and licensing examinations that are structured on a nursing model of care based on the nursing process.

This textbook assumes that the student already has a basic understanding of the nursing process and is now ready to expand and apply that knowledge to adult clients with medical-surgical health problems. The following discussion is intended to serve only as a review; for more information, consult books specifically focused on the use of the nursing process, and read the case studies in the nursing care chapters throughout this textbook.

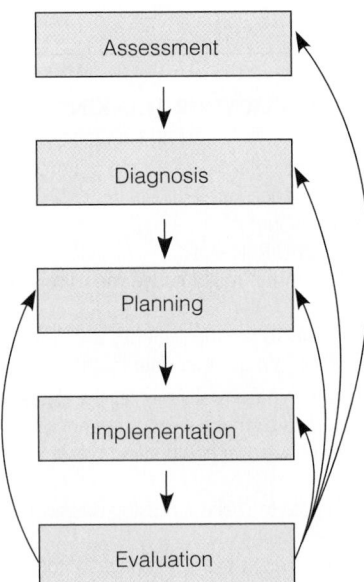

Figure 1–1 ■ Steps of the nursing process. Notice that the steps are interrelated and interdependent. For example, evaluation of the client might reveal the need for further assessment, additional nursing diagnoses, and/or a revision of the plan of care.

In addition to nursing care plans that are based on a client care situation and describe each step of the process, charts are included throughout the text that illustrate the relationship of nursing diagnoses (NANDA), nursing interventions (NIC), and nursing outcomes (NOC). Categorized as the NNN Alliance, the links between and among NANDA, NIC, and NOC represent the collaborative relationship between the North American Nursing Diagnosis Association (NANDA) and the Center for Nursing Classification and Clinical Effectiveness (Nursing Interventions Classification [NIC] and Nursing Outcomes Classification [NOC]) at the University of Iowa. "The goal of this alliance is to advance the development, testing, and refinement of nursing language" (Dochterman & Bulechek, 2004, p. 7).

Assessment

Assessment is usually listed as the first step of the nursing process, but in actuality it is a critical element in each of the steps. It begins with the client's first encounter with the healthcare system and continues as long as the client requires care. During assessment, data (pieces of information) about health status are collected, validated, organized, clustered into patterns, and communicated either verbally or in written form. Assessment serves as the basis for deriving accurate nursing diagnoses, for planning and implementing both initial and ongoing individualized care, and for evaluating care.

The data that the nurse collects must be holistic; that is, the nurse must carefully consider all dimensions of an individual. The data collected are both objective and subjective. Information that the nurse perceives by the senses is *objective data*; it is seen, heard, touched, or smelled, and can be verified by another person (e.g., blood pressure, temperature, pulse, or the presence of infected drainage). Information that is perceived only by the person experiencing it (e.g., pain, dizziness, or anxiety) is *subjective data*.

Nurses assess clients in two ways: through an initial assessment and through focused assessments. The initial assessment of the client, conducted through a nursing history and physical assessment, is necessary to accumulate comprehensive data about health responses, identify specific factors that contribute to these responses in an individual, and facilitate mutually established goals and outcomes of care.

Focused assessments are ongoing and continuous, occurring whenever the nurse interacts with the client. They enable the nurse to evaluate nursing actions and make decisions about whether to continue or change interventions to meet outcomes. They also provide structure for documenting nursing care. In addition, focused assessments enable the nurse to identify responses to a disease process or treatment modality not present during the initial assessment, or to monitor the status of an actual or potential problem previously identified (Alfaro, 2005).

To make accurate and holistic assessments, nurses must have and use a wide variety of knowledge and skills. The ability to assess the physical status of the client is essential, as is the ability to use effective communication techniques. Nurses must be knowledgeable in pathophysiology and pharmacology and be able to identify abnormal laboratory and diagnostic test data. Finally, nurses must have a solid foundation of nursing knowledge and skill that will enable them to interpret assessment data and to use that interpretation as the basis for individualized care.

Diagnosis

The ANA defines nursing as "the diagnosis and treatment of human responses to actual or potential health problems" (1980, p. 9). The nurse labels each response with a nursing diagnosis, defined by the North American Nursing Diagnosis Association (NANDA, 2003) as a clinical judgment about individual, family, or community responses to actual or potential health problems/life processes. Nursing diagnoses provide the basis for selection of nursing interventions to achieve outcomes for which the nurse is accountable. Nurses develop and implement a plan of care for actual responses; they also plan interventions to support health concerns and prevent illness concerns for potential human responses.

The nurse analyzes data collected during the assessment step to support appropriate nursing diagnoses. During analysis, the nurse clusters data into categories of information that can be used to identify actual or potential alterations in health. Data can be organized within a variety of frameworks and methods for identifying patterns of human behavior (Wilkinson, 2005). Methods commonly used are basic human needs (Maslow, 1970), body systems, human response patterns, and functional health patterns (Gordon, 1982). The broad organizational structure used to categorize information in this book is based on functional health patterns, outlined in Box 1–1.

Making a diagnosis is a complex process that always involves uncertainty. Therefore, the nurse uses diagnostic reasoning to choose nursing diagnoses that best define the individual client's health problems. Diagnostic reasoning is a form of clinical judgment used to make decisions about which label (or diagnosis) best describes the patterns of data. Elements of the clinical judgment process include data gathering and validation, data categorization, intuition, and prior clinical experience.

BOX 1–1 Functional Health Patterns

1. *Health perception–health management pattern.* Describes client's perceived pattern of health and well-being and how health is managed.
2. *Nutritional-metabolic pattern.* Describes pattern of food and fluid consumption relative to metabolic need and pattern indicators of local nutrient supply.
3. *Elimination pattern.* Describes pattern of excretory function (bowel, bladder, and skin).
4. *Activity-exercise pattern.* Describes pattern of exercise, activity, leisure, and recreation.
5. *Cognitive-perceptual pattern.* Describes sensory-perceptual and cognitive patterns.
6. *Sleep-rest pattern.* Describes patterns of sleep, rest, and relaxation.

7. *Self-perception–self-concept pattern.* Describes self-concept pattern and perceptions of self (e.g., body comfort, body image, feeling state).
8. *Role-relationship pattern.* Describes patterns of role engagements and relationships.
9. *Sexuality-reproductive pattern.* Describes client's patterns of satisfaction and dissatisfaction with sexuality; describes reproductive patterns.
10. *Coping–stress tolerance pattern.* Describes general coping pattern and effectiveness of the pattern in terms of stress tolerance.
11. *Value-belief pattern.* Describes patterns of values, beliefs (including spiritual), or goals that guide choices or decisions.

Source: Adapted from *Nursing Diagnosis: Process and Application* (3rd ed.) by M. Gordon, 1994, St. Louis: Mosby-Year Book. Used with permission.

Although there is no universal list of diagnoses used in nursing, the work of NANDA is widely accepted. The diagnoses are classified by a taxonomy; that is, they are grouped into classes and subclasses based on patterns and relationships. Work on both the nursing diagnoses and the taxonomy is ongoing. The NANDA system was accepted in 1988 by the ANA as the official system of diagnosis for the United States. Nursing diagnoses within the NANDA taxonomy are used in this book.

A diagnosis is written in two parts joined by the phrase "related to." The first part of the statement is the particular human response that has been identified from the analysis of data. It identifies what needs to change in a specific client as a result of nursing interventions, and it also identifies the client outcomes that measure the change. The part of the statement that follows the "related to" phrase identifies the physical, psychosocial, cultural, spiritual, and/or environmental factors (etiologies) that cause or contribute to the occurrence of the response.

Many nurses write nursing diagnoses using a method known as PES (Gordon, 1994). Diagnoses written with this method have three components:

1. The problem (P), which is the NANDA label
2. The etiology (E) of the problem, which names the related factors and is indicated by the phrase "related to"
3. The signs and symptoms (S), which are the defining characteristics and are indicated by the phrase "as manifested by."

Examples of nursing diagnoses written with the PES method are as follows:
- *Anxiety* related to hospitalization as manifested by statements of nervousness and by crying
- *Bowel Incontinence* related to loss of sphincter control as manifested by involuntary passage of stool
- *Fatigue* related to the side effects of chemotherapy as manifested by the inability to carry out normal daily routines and statements of overwhelming exhaustion.

Planning

During the planning step, the nurse develops a list of nursing interventions (actions) and client outcomes to promote healthy responses and to prevent, reverse, or decrease unhealthy responses. *Outcomes*, which are mutually established by the client and nurse, identify what the client will be able to do as a result of the nursing interventions. Both outcomes and nursing interventions are documented in a written plan of care that directs nursing activities and documentation and provides a tool for evaluation (Alfaro, 2005). The plan of care may be documented in a variety of formats.

Nurses plan interventions for two types of client problems: those that require nursing management, stated as nursing diagnoses; and those that require collaborative management, which may be referred to as collaborative or clinical problems. Nursing diagnoses provide the basis for selecting nurse-initiated interventions to achieve outcomes for which the nurse is accountable. Collaborative problems are most often based on medical diagnoses (such as hemorrhage) that nurses monitor to detect onset or changes in status.

Outcome criteria for nursing diagnoses are client centered, time specific, and measurable. They are classified into three domains: cognitive (knowing), affective (feeling), and psychomotor (doing). The nurse considers all three domains to ensure holistic care.

Outcome criteria for collaborative problems are nursing goals, usually written as statements that begin with "to detect and report early signs and symptoms of potential complications of . . ." and "to implement preventive and corrective nursing interventions ordered by . . ." (Alfaro, 2005). In many instances, these goals are not written as part of the plan of care. Preventive and corrective nursing interventions for collaborative problems may be ordered by the physician or by institutional policy, procedures, protocols, or standards.

The nursing interventions planned must be specific and individualized. If, for example, the nurse identifies that a client is at risk for fluid volume deficit, it is not enough for the nurse to simply encourage the client to drink increased amounts of fluid. The nurse and the client together must identify those liquids the client prefers, the times that will be best for drinking them, and the amount of fluid (in ounces or milliliters); this information must be documented as a nursing order on the written care plan. Only then does care truly become a part of the plan of care.

Implementation

The implementation step is the action or "doing" phase of the nursing process, during which the nurse carries out planned interventions. Ongoing assessment of the client before, during, and after the intervention is an essential component of implementation. Although the plan may be appropriate, many variables can modify or negate any planned intervention, making a change in the plan necessary. For example, the nurse would not be able to force fluids if the client were nauseated or vomiting.

When implementing the planned interventions, the nurse follows several important principles:

- Set daily priorities, based on initial assessments and on the client's condition as reported during the change of shift report and/or documented in the client's chart. Ensure that critical assessments (such as status of invasive lines, fluids infusing, or changes in health status during the preceding shift) take first priority.
- Be aware of the interrelated nature of nursing interventions. For example, while giving a bath the nurse can also assess physical and psychologic status, use therapeutic communication, teach the client, do range-of-motion exercises, and provide skin care.
- Determine the most appropriate interventions for each client, based on health status and illness treatment. Examples of appropriate interventions include:
  - Directly performing the activity for the client.
  - Assisting the client to perform the activity.
  - Supervising the client/family while they are performing the activity.
  - Teaching the client/family about health care.
  - Monitoring the client at risk for potential complications or problems.
- Use available resources to provide interventions that are realistic for the situation and practical in terms of equipment available, financial status of the client, and resources available (including staff, agency, family, and community resources).

Documenting interventions is the final component of implementation, and it is a legal requirement. Many different methods are used to document care. Narrative source-oriented and problem-oriented charting methods are used, as are focused charting, charting by exception, and computer-assisted documentation.

Evaluation

The evaluation step allows the nurse to determine whether the plan was effective and either to continue the plan, to revise the plan, or to terminate the plan. The outcome criteria that were established during the planning step provide the basis for evaluation. Although evaluation is listed as the last part of the nursing process, it takes place continuously throughout client care.

To evaluate a plan, the nurse collects data from the client and the client's chart. The nurse then compares the status of the client with the written outcomes. If the outcomes have been accomplished, the nurse may either continue or terminate the plan. If the outcomes have not been accomplished, the nurse must modify the nursing diagnoses, outcomes, or plan.

The Nursing Process in Clinical Practice

With experience, the nurse does not consciously stop and consider each step. Rather, using the process as a framework, care is based on the client's specific, individualized needs. For example, when caring for a client who is hemorrhaging, the nurse uses all five steps simultaneously to meet critical, life-threatening needs. In contrast, when considering long-term needs for a client with a chronic illness or disability, the nurse makes in-depth assessments, mutually determines goals with the client, and provides documentation through a written plan of care that can be developed and revised as necessary by all nurses providing care. As a nurse becomes an expert practitioner, the nursing process becomes so much a part of the nurse that he or she may not even consciously consider it while providing care; the practice is the process (Benner, 1984).

GUIDELINES FOR NURSING PRACTICE

Nursing practice is structured by codes of ethics and standards that guide nursing practice and protect the public. Individual nursing practice is held to these standards in a court of law. The guidelines are especially important because nurses encounter legal and ethical problems almost daily.

Codes for Nurses

An established **code of ethics** is one criterion that defines a profession. **Ethics** are principles of conduct. Ethical behavior is concerned with moral duty, values, obligations, and the distinction between right and wrong. Codes of ethics for nurses provide a frame of reference for "professionally valued and ideal nursing behaviors that are congruent with the principles expressed in the Code for Nurses" (Ketefian, 1987, p. 13).

The large number of ethical issues facing nurses in clinical practice makes the established codes for nurses critical to moral and ethical decision making. The codes also help to define the roles of nurses. The codes of ethics presented here were developed by and for members of the International Council of Nurses (ICN) and the ANA.

The ICN Code

The ICN Code of Ethics for Nurses (2006) helps guide nurses in setting priorities, making judgments, and taking action when they face ethical dilemmas in clinical practice. The ICN code specifies what nurses are accountable for in terms of people, practice, society, coworkers, and the profession. The philosophical base for the ICN code is that nurses are responsible for promoting health, preventing illness, and alleviating suffering.

BOX 1–2 **The American Nurses Association Code of Ethics for Nurses**

- The nurse, in all professional relationships, practices with compassion and respect for the inherent dignity, worth, and uniqueness of every individual, unrestricted by considerations of social or economic status, personal attributes, or the nature of health problems.
- The nurse's primary commitment is to the patient, whether an individual, family, group, or community.
- The nurse promotes, advocates for, and strives to protect the health, safety, and rights of the patient.
- The nurse is responsible and accountable for individual nursing practice and determines the appropriate delegation of tasks consistent with the nurse's obligation to provide optimum patient care.
- The nurse owes the same duties to self as to others, including the responsibility to preserve integrity and safety, to maintain competence, and to continue personal and professional growth.

- The nurse participates in establishing, maintaining, and improving health care environments and conditions of employment conducive to the provision of quality health care and consistent with the values of the profession through individual and collective action.
- The nurse participates in the advancement of the profession through contributions in practice, education, administration, and knowledge development.
- The nurse collaborates with other health professionals and the public in promoting community, national, and international efforts to meet health needs.
- The profession of nursing, as represented by associations and their members, is responsible for articulating nursing values, for maintaining the integrity of the profession and its practice, and for shaping social policy.

Source: Reprinted with permission from American Nurses Association, *Code of Ethics for Nurses with Interpretive Statements,* © 2001, American Nurses Publishing. American Nurses Foundation/American Nurses Association, Washington, DC.

The ANA Code

The ANA Code of Ethics for Nurses (2001) states principles of ethical concern, guiding the behavior of nurses and also defining nursing for the general public (Box 1–2).

Standards of Nursing Practice

A **standard** is a statement or criterion that can be used by a profession and by the general public to measure quality of practice. Established standards of nursing practice make each individual nurse accountable for practice. This means that each nurse providing care has the responsibility or obligation to account for his or her own behaviors within that role. Professional nursing organizations develop and implement standards of practice to identify clearly the nurse's responsibilities to society.

The ANA standards of nursing practice (2004b) are outlined in Box 1–3. These standards allow objective evaluation of nursing licensure and certification, institutional accreditation, quality assurance, and public policy.

BOX 1–3 **ANA Standards of Practice**

STANDARDS OF PRACTICE

- *Assessment:* The nurse collects comprehensive data pertinent to the patient's health or the situation.
- *Diagnosis:* The nurse analyzes the assessment data to determine the diagnosis or issues.
- *Outcome identification:* The nurse identifies expected outcomes for a plan individualized to the patient or the situation.
- *Planning:* The nurse develops a plan that prescribes strategies and alternatives to attain expected outcomes.
- *Implementation:* The nurse implements the identified plan, coordinates care delivery, employs strategies to promote health and a safe environment. The advanced practice registered nurse also provides consultation and uses prescriptive authority and treatment.
- *Evaluation:* The nurse evaluates progress toward attainment of outcomes.

STANDARDS OF PROFESSIONAL PRACTICE

- *Quality of practice:* The nurse systematically enhances the quality and effectiveness of nursing practice.
- *Practice evaluation:* The nurse evaluates one's own practice in relation to professional practice standards and guidelines, relevant statutes, rules, and regulations.
- *Education:* The nurse attains knowledge and competency that reflect current nursing practice.
- *Collegiality:* The nurse interacts with and contributes to the professional development of peers and colleagues.
- *Collaboration:* The nurse collaborates with patient, family, and others in the conduct of nursing practice.
- *Ethics:* The nurse integrates ethical provisions in all areas of practice.
- *Research:* The nurse integrates research findings into practice.
- *Resource utilization:* The nurse considers factors related to safety, effectiveness, cost, and impact on practice in the planning and delivery of nursing services.
- *Leadership:* The nurse provides leadership in the profession and the professional practice setting.

Source: Adapted from *ANA Standards of Practice and Professional Performance* (2003). American Nurses Association, Washington, DC. Used with permission.

LEGAL AND ETHICAL DILEMMAS IN NURSING

A **dilemma** is a choice between two unpleasant, ethically troubling alternatives. Nurses who provide medical-surgical nursing care face dilemmas almost daily—so many, in fact, that a complete discussion of them is impossible here. However, many commonly experienced dilemmas involve confidentiality, client rights, and issues of dying and death. The nurse must use ethical and legal guidelines to make decisions about moral actions when providing care in these and in many other situations.

Nurses respect the right to confidentiality of client information found in the client's record or secured during interviews. (In most instances, state nursing practice acts legally require nurses to uphold this right.) Rights of the client as an individual, however, can result in dilemmas for the nurse in the clinical setting. For example, the right to privacy and confidentiality creates a dilemma when it conflicts with the nurse's right to information that may affect personal safety. This may happen when the nurse does not know a client's HIV status. The law in most states mandates that HIV test results can be given to another person only if the client provides written consent for the release of that information. Many healthcare providers believe that this law violates their own right to personal safety and are actively working to change the law.

The right to refuse treatment (including surgery, medication, medical therapy, and nourishment) is another client right that raises nursing dilemmas. The situation, the alternatives, and the potential harm from refusal must be carefully explained. By law, the client must establish an advance directive on admission to a healthcare agency stating the client's choice about preserving or prolonging life. An **advance directive**, or living will, is a document in which a client formally states preferences for health care in the event that he or she later becomes mentally incapacitated. The client also names a person who has durable power of attorney to serve as a substitute decision maker to implement the client's stated preferences. This document becomes a part of the client's hospital record and is honored even if the client becomes incompetent during the period of treatment. The dilemma arises when the client's preferences conflict with the law. For example, the client may indicate that there is to be no food or fluids given during end-of-life care. However, several states assert that artificial feeding is not a procedure that may be rejected under living will statutes. The nurse is faced with the dilemma of carrying out the client's wishes or following the law.

The issues surrounding dying and death have become increasingly pressing as advances in technology extend the lives of people with chronic debilitating illness and major trauma. These changes have altered concepts of living and dying, resulting in ethical conflicts regarding quality of life and death with dignity versus technologic methods of preserving life in any form.

Even if the client is competent and requests that no heroic measures be used to maintain life, many questions arise in nursing care. What constitutes a heroic measure? Should nursing interventions to provide comfort include administering narcotics at a level known to depress respirations? Should a feeding tube be placed in the client who is terminally ill? These and other questions are being debated not only within the healthcare system but also in the courts.

ROLES OF THE NURSE IN MEDICAL-SURGICAL NURSING PRACTICE

Health care today is a vast and complex system. It reflects changes in society, changes in the populations requiring nursing care, and a philosophical shift toward health promotion rather than illness care. The roles of the medical-surgical nurse have broadened and expanded in response to these changes. Medical-surgical nurses are not only caregivers but also educators, advocates, leaders and managers, and researchers. The nurse assumes these various roles to promote and maintain health, to prevent illness, and to facilitate coping with disability or death for the adult client (a person requiring healthcare services) in any setting.

The Nurse as Caregiver

Nurses have always been caregivers. However, the activities carried out within the caregiver role have changed tremendously in the 21st century. From 1900 to the 1960s, the nurse was almost always female and was regarded primarily as the person who gave personal care and carried out physicians' orders. This dependent role has changed as a result of the increased education of nurses, research in and the development of nursing knowledge, and the recognition that nurses are autonomous and informed professionals.

The caregiver role for the nurse today is both independent and collaborative. Nurses independently make assessments and plan and implement client care based on nursing knowledge and skills. Nurses also collaborate with other members of the healthcare team to implement and evaluate care (Figure 1–2 ■).

As a caregiver, the nurse is a practitioner of nursing both as a science and as an art. Using critical thinking in the nursing

Figure 1–2 ■ The healthcare team discusses the individualized plan of care and outcomes.

Source: Cindy Charles/PhotoEdit Inc.

BOX 1–4 Culturally Sensitive Nursing

The primary focus of nursing care is the client as the client relates to the environment and experiences events or situations related to health or illness. These experiences are given shape and personal meaning by culture—the socially inherited characteristics of a human group. These characteristics include the beliefs, practices, habits, likes, dislikes, customs, and rituals people learn from their families and pass on to their children. Cultural background is an essential component of a person's ethnic identity. A person's ethnic identity includes belonging to a social group within a culture and a social system and sharing a common religion, language, ancestry, and physical characteristics.

The healthcare system encompasses clients who are culturally diverse. This diversity includes differences in country of origin, health beliefs, sexual orientation, race, socioeconomic level, and age. Despite increasing diversity, nursing has been slow to address the need for culturally sensitive care. Many different factors account for this inattention, including ethnocentrism (people's belief that their own cultural group's beliefs and values are the only acceptable ones) and prejudice. The healthcare system is itself a culture, primarily, of white middle-class people, and it often serves as a barrier to culturally sensitive care.

The 1992 American Academy of Nursing Expert Panel on Culturally Competent Nursing Care identified several reasons why it has become increasingly important that nurses plan culturally sensitive care:

- The demographic and ethnic composition of the population of the world in general, and the United States in particular, has changed markedly, and there is a lack of ethnic representation in healthcare professionals in the healthcare system. Information on and knowledge about values, beliefs, experiences, and healthcare needs of various populations is limited.
- There is a growing awareness and acceptance of diversity and an increased willingness to maintain and support ethnic and cultural heritage.

- People of color and immigrants are facing increasing unemployment, decreasing opportunity, and limited access to health care. These conditions may contribute to the establishment of new minorities, such as the homeless.
- The international focus on providing health care for all people (within the context of inequity, barriers, and lack of access) may have raised the consciousness of healthcare professionals to some of the inequities inherent in healthcare systems in both developing countries and developed countries.
- Nurses comprise the largest force in the delivery of health care and therefore have the potential to contribute to the changing inequities in and inaccessibility to health care.
- Consumers are becoming increasingly aware of what is competent and sensitive health care.

This same panel of experts proposed general principles for nurses for becoming sensitive to cultural diversity and providing culturally sensitive care. For example:

- Nurses must learn to appreciate intergroup and intragroup cultural diversity and commonalties in racial/ethnic minority populations.
- Nurses must understand how social structure factors shape health behaviors and practices among members of racial/ethnic minorities.
- Nurses must confront their own ethnocentrism and racism.
- Nurses must begin rehearsing, practicing, and evaluating services provided to cross-cultural populations.

People of every culture have the right to have their cultural values known, respected, and addressed appropriately in nursing and other healthcare services (Leininger, 1991). To provide nursing care that is culturally sensitive, nurses must develop a sensitivity to personal fundamental values about health and illness; must accept the existence of differing values; and must be respectful of, interested in, and understanding of other cultures without being judgmental.

---

process as the framework for care, the nurse provides interventions to meet not only the physical needs but also the psychosocial, cultural, spiritual, and environmental needs of clients and families. See Box 1–4 for a discussion of culturally sensitive nursing care. Considering all aspects of the client ensures a holistic approach to nursing. Holistic nursing care is based on a philosophical view that interacting wholes are greater than the sum of their parts. A holistic approach also emphasizes the uniqueness of the individual.

In providing comprehensive, individualized care, the nurse uses critical thinking skills to analyze and synthesize knowledge from the arts, the sciences, and nursing research and theory. The science (knowledge base) of nursing is translated into the art of nursing through caring. Caring is the means by which the nurse is connected with and concerned for the client (Benner & Wrubel, 1989). Thus, the nurse as caregiver is knowledgeable, skilled, empathic, and caring.

The Nurse as Educator

The nurse's role as educator is becoming increasingly important for several reasons. Healthcare providers and consumers as well as local, state, and federal governments are placing greater

emphasis on health promotion and illness prevention; hospital stays are becoming shorter; and the number of people with chronic illnesses in our society is increasing. Early discharge of clients from the hospital setting to home care means that family caregivers must learn how to perform complex skills. All of these factors make the educator role essential to maintaining the health and well-being of clients.

The framework for the role of educator is the teaching–learning process. Within this framework, the nurse assesses learning needs, plans and implements teaching methods to meet those needs, and evaluates the effectiveness of the teaching. To be an effective educator, the nurse must have effective interpersonal skills and be familiar with adult learning principles (Figure 1–3 ■).

A major component of the educator role today is discharge planning. Discharge planning, which begins on admission to a healthcare setting, is a systematic method of preparing the client and family for exit from the healthcare agency and for maintaining continuity of care after the client leaves the setting. Discharge planning also involves making referrals, identifying community and personal resources, and arranging for necessary equipment and supplies for home care.

Figure 1–3 ■ The nurse's role as educator is an essential component of care. As part of the discharge planning process, the nurse is responsible for teaching for self-care at home.

Source: Barros & Barros/Getty Images, Inc.—Image Bank.

The Nurse as Advocate

The client entering the healthcare system may be unprepared to make independent decisions. However, today's healthcare consumer is better educated about options for care, and may have very definite opinions. The nurse as client advocate actively promotes the client's rights to autonomy and free choice. The nurse as advocate speaks for the patient, mediates between the patient and other persons, and/or protects the patient's right to self-determination (Ellis & Hartley, 2004). The goals of the nurse as advocate are to:

- Assess the need for advocacy.
- Communicate with other healthcare team members.
- Provide client and family teaching.
- Assist and support client decision making.
- Serve as a change agent in the healthcare system.
- Participate in health policy formulation.

The nurse must practice advocacy based on the belief that clients have the right to choose treatment options, based on information about the results of accepting or rejecting the treatment, without coercion. The nurse must also accept and respect the decision of the client, even though it may differ from the decision the nurse would make.

The Nurse as Leader and Manager

All nurses are leaders and managers. They practice leadership and they manage time, people, resources, and the environment in which they provide care. Nurses carry out these roles by directing, delegating, and coordinating nursing activities. Nurses must be knowledgeable about how and when to delegate, as well as the legal requirements of delegation. Nurses also evaluate the quality of care provided.

Models of Care Delivery

Nurses are leaders and managers of client care within a variety of models of care delivery. Examples are primary nursing, team nursing, and case management. The nursing shortage made the combination of primary and team nursing more economically feasible.

PRIMARY NURSING Primary nursing allows the nurse to provide individualized direct care to a small number of clients during their entire inpatient stay. This model was developed to reduce the fragmentation of care experienced by the client and to facilitate family-centered continuity of care. In primary nursing, the nurse provides care; communicates with clients, families, and other healthcare providers; and carries out discharge planning.

TEAM NURSING Team nursing is practiced by teams of variously educated healthcare providers. For example, a team may consist of a registered nurse, a licensed practical nurse, and two unlicensed assistive personnel (UAPs). The registered nurse is the team leader. The team leader is responsible for making assignments and has overall responsibility for patient care by team members. All team members work together, each performing the activities for which he or she is best prepared.

CASE MANAGEMENT Case management focuses on management of a caseload (group) of clients and the members of the healthcare team caring for those clients. The purpose of case management is to maximize positive outcomes and contain costs. The nurse who is case manager is usually a clinical specialist, and the caseload consists of clients with similar healthcare needs. As case manager, the nurse makes appropriate referrals to other healthcare providers and manages the quality of care provided, including accuracy, timeliness, and cost. The case manager also is in contact with clients after discharge, ensuring continuity of care and health maintenance.

Delegation

Delegation is carried out when the nurse assigns appropriate and effective work activities to other members of the healthcare team. When the nurse delegates nursing care activities to another person, that person is authorized to act in the place of the nurse, although the nurse retains the accountability for the activities performed. Delegation skills are becoming increasingly important in health care as agencies restructure and implement cost containment measures. More categories of healthcare workers with often minimal nursing education and experience are being hired to assist the registered nurse as *nurse extenders,* or *UAPs.* Guidelines for delegation (Ellis & Hartley, 1998) include the following:

- Know the level of competence of each member of the healthcare team, the complexity of the task to be assigned, and the amount of time available to supervise the tasks.
- Know the level of nursing judgment and evaluation required for the task.
- Consider the potential harm and difficulty of performing the task.
- Know the state's nurse practice act and any practice limitations that may exist.
- Know the job descriptions for each category of worker.
- Assign the right job to the right person. Tasks that are routine and standard are the best to assign to others.
- Give clear and complete directions for assignments. Ask questions to be sure directions have been understood.
- Give the team member the authority to complete the task.
- Monitor the outcomes of the care provided and give constructive evaluation if necessary.

Evaluating Outcomes of Nursing Care

CRITICAL PATHWAYS A **critical pathway** (also called a clinical path or pathway) is a healthcare plan designed to provide care with a multidisciplinary, managed action focus. Such pathways are generally developed for specific diagnoses—usually high-volume, high-risk, and high-cost case types—with the collaboration of members of the healthcare team. This client care management tool describes how resources will be used to achieve predetermined outcomes. It also establishes the sequence of multidisciplinary interventions, including education, discharge planning, consultations, medication administration, diagnostics, therapeutics, and treatments.

The goals of critical pathways are to:
- Achieve realistic, expected client and family outcomes.
- Promote professional and collaborative practice and care.
- Ensure continuity of care.
- Guarantee appropriate use of resources.
- Reduce costs and length of stay.
- Provide the framework for continuous improvement.

Critical pathways are often used in conjunction with case management models and/or quality improvement efforts. The overall goal is to design pathways that facilitate a reproducible standard of care for specific client populations and improve the quality and proficiency of that care.

The agency determines the process for developing a critical pathway. Information imperative to the development of any critical pathway includes literature reviews, chart reviews, expert opinion, and insurance reimbursements for the designated case type. A typical approach is to first identify high-cost, high-volume, and high-risk case types for the agency. Next, a multidisciplinary team, which includes physicians, develops a consensus around the management of the case type and a critical pathway. The pathway is then piloted with a designated group of clients, and revisions are based on the number and types of variances. The goal is to develop a pathway that best meets the needs of clients in the particular practice setting.

When clients do not achieve expected outcomes, variances (deviations from the established plan) from the critical pathways are recorded and studied by the multidisciplinary team. In many agencies, critical pathways are designed so that interventions and variances can be easily documented. Most documentation systems require a check off when interventions are performed or variances occur.

In many agencies, critical pathways are replacing traditional nursing care plans. The advantages of critical pathways are that they are outcome driven and provide a timeline to achieve specified goals. Additionally, critical pathways provide opportunities for healthcare workers to collaborate and establish dynamic plans of care that consider all of the clients' needs. Although initially developed for acute hospitalizations, critical pathways are now developed to manage clients in home health, outpatient, and long-term settings.

QUALITY ASSURANCE As a leader and manager, the nurse is responsible for the quality of client care through a process called **quality assurance**. This process consists of the quality control activities that evaluate, monitor, or regulate the standard of services provided to the consumer. Clients are assured of quality care through professional and technical licensure of individual care providers; accreditation of hospitals (e.g., by the Joint Commission on Accreditation of Healthcare Organizations [JCAHO]); licensure of hospitals, pharmacies, and nursing homes; and certification in specialty areas.

Quality assurance methods also are used to evaluate client care. They commonly evaluate actual care against an established set of standards of care. Nurses and other healthcare providers make this evaluation by reviewing documentation, by conducting client surveys and nurse interviews, and/or by direct observation of nurse or client performance. The data are then used to identify differences between actual practice and established standards and to develop a plan of action to resolve any differences. The actions are then assessed through internal peer review or by an external medical review organization, called a utilization and quality control peer review organization (PRO), to determine whether they were effective in improving practice. These reviews have resulted in such healthcare changes as an increase in outpatient surgeries with a resultant decrease in the number of inpatient surgeries.

The Nurse as Researcher

Nurses have always identified problems in client care. Although they have developed interventions to meet specific needs, the activities often have not been conducted within a scientific framework or communicated to other nurses through nursing literature. To develop the science of nursing, nursing knowledge must be established through clinical research and then published, so that the findings can be used by all nurses to provide evidence-based client care.

To be relevant, nursing research must have a goal to improve the care that nurses provide clients. This means that all nurses must consider the researcher role to be integral to nursing practice. Summaries of relevant nursing research are included in almost all of the nursing care chapters of this textbook. After the summary and discussion of each study, a critical thinking section specifically related to the findings of the study encourages the student to apply the findings to the clinical setting.

EXPLORE MEDIALINK

Prentice Hall Nursing MediaLink DVD-ROM
Audio Glossary
NCLEX-RN® Review

COMPANION WEBSITE www.prenhall.com/lemone
Audio Glossary
NCLEX-RN® Review
Care Plan Activity: Nursing Process
Case Studies
Advance Directive
Critical Thinking in the Nursing Process
MediaLink Applications
Medication and Healthcare Needs Assist Programs
Nursing Code of Ethics
Links to Resources

CHAPTER HIGHLIGHTS

■ Recommended core competencies for all healthcare professionals include providing client-centered care, working in interdisciplinary teams, using evidence-based practice, applying quality improvement, and using informatics.

■ The nursing process is the cyclical series of critical thinking activities used by nurses to provide client care to promote wellness, maintain health, restore health, or facilitate coping with disability or death. The five steps of the nursing process are assessment, diagnosis, planning, implementation, and evaluation.

■ The clinical practice of nursing is guided by codes for nurses and standards of practice.

■ Nurses function as caregivers, educators, advocates, leaders and managers, and researchers to promote and maintain health, to prevent illness, and to facilitate coping with disability or death for the adult client.

TEST YOURSELF NCLEX-RN® REVIEW

1 The National Academy of Sciences has proposed a set of core competencies for healthcare professionals. What is the primary purpose of these competencies?
1. to make all healthcare professionals equal
2. to improve safety and quality of care
3. to reduce the number of medical lawsuits
4. to maintain public faith in physicians

2 What does the nurse use in the practice setting to make clinical judgments and decisions?
1. nursing process
2. standards of care
3. nursing ethics
4. critical thinking

3 Which of the following statements is true of outcomes developed during the planning phase of the nursing process?
1. Outcomes are mutually established by the client and the nurse.
2. Outcomes are mutually established by the nurse and the physician.
3. Outcomes are mandated by institutional policies and standards.
4. Outcomes are written by clients and family members.

4 The steps of the nursing process are used when providing care to clients. From the list below, select the order in which the steps are most often used.
1. outcomes
2. assessment
3. evaluation
4. implementation
5. planning

5 When nurses discuss the "science of nursing," what does this phrase mean?
1. clinical competency
2. holistic care
3. knowledge base
4. practice component

6 What role does the nurse demonstrate when developing and providing health information?
1. advocate
2. caregiver
3. researcher
4. educator

7 What goal is a component of the nurse's role as advocate?
1. assisting and supporting client decision making
2. conducting research about the effects of exercise
3. delegating responsibilities for client care to others
4. performing range-of-motion exercises

8 A nurse assigns appropriate work activities to other members of her team. What role is being illustrated?
1. advocate
2. leader/manager
3. researcher
4. caregiver

9 A method of establishing a standard of care and evaluating outcomes of that standard involves:
1. writing a dress code policy for a healthcare agency.
2. creating a critical pathway for a specific type of client.
3. establishing quality assurance regulations.
4. implementing a new procedure to change dressings.

10 A nurse delegates vital sign assessment to a UAP. Who is accountable for the assessment findings?
1. the UAP
2. the client
3. the nurse
4. the physician

See Test Yourself answers in Appendix C.

BIBLIOGRAPHY

Alfaro, R. (2005). *Applying nursing process: A tool for critical thinking* (6th ed.). Philadelphia: Lippincott.

American Nurses Association. (1980). *A social policy statement.* Kansas City, MO: Author.

_____. (2001). *Code of ethics for nurses.* Washington, DC: Author.

_____. (2003). *Nursing's social policy statement* (2nd ed.). Washington, DC: Author.

_____. (2004a). *Managed care: Challenges & opportunities for nursing.* Retrieved from http://nursingworld.org/readroom/fsmgdcar.htm

_____. (2004b). *Nursing: Scope and standards of practice.* Washington, DC: Author.

_____. (2005). *ANA's health care agenda 2005.* Washington, DC: Author.

Benner, P. (1984). *From novice to expert: Excellence and power in clinical nursing practice.* Redwood City, CA: Addison-Wesley Nursing.

Benner, P., & Wrubel, J. (1989). *The primacy of caring: Stress and coping in clinical nursing practice.* Redwood City, CA: Addison-Wesley Nursing.

Chitty, K. (2004). *Addressing diversity.* Retrieved from http://www.aoa.dhhs.gov/prof/adddiv/adddiv.asp

_____. (2005). *Professional nursing: Concepts & challenges* (4th ed.). Philadelphia: Saunders.

Dochterman, J. M., & Bulechek, G. M. (2004). *Nursing interventions classification (NIC)* (4th ed.). St. Louis, MO: Mosby.

Ellis, J., & Hartley, C. (1998). *Nursing in today's world: Challenges, issues, and trends* (6th ed.). Philadelphia: Lippincott.

_____. (2004). *Managing and coordinating nursing care* (4th ed.). Philadelphia: Lippincott.

Federal Interagency Forum on Aging-Related Statistics. (2004). *Older Americans 2004: Key indicators of well-being.* Washington, DC: U.S. Government Printing Office.

Gordon, M. (1982). *Nursing diagnosis: Process and application.* New York: McGraw-Hill.

_____. (1994). *Nursing diagnosis: Process and application* (3rd ed.). St. Louis, MO: Mosby.

Greggs-McQuilkin, D. (2003). The specialty of medical-surgical nursing: The solid rock, not the stepping stone. *MEDSURG Nursing, 12*(1), 5, 26.

Institute of Medicine Committee on Good Quality of Health Care in America. (2001). *Crossing the quality chasm: A new health system for the 21st century.* Washington, DC: National Academy Press.

International Council of Nurses (2006). *The ICN Code of ethics for nurses.* Geneva: Author.

Ketefian, S. (1987). Moral behavior in nursing. *Advances in Nursing Science, 9*(1), 10–19.

Klenner, S. (2000). Mapping out a clinical pathway. *RN, 63*(6), 33–36.

Leininger, M. (1991). Transcultural care principles, human rights, and ethical considerations. *Journal of Transcultural Nursing, 3*(1), 21–23.

Maslow, A. (1970). *Motivation and personality.* New York: Harper & Row.

NANDA International. (2003). Nursing diagnoses: Definitions & classification. Philadelphia: Author.

National Academy of Sciences. (2003). *Executive summary: Health professions education: A bridge to quality* (pp. 1–18). Retrieved from http://www.nap.edu

Radwin, L. (1990). Research on diagnostic reasoning in nursing. *Nursing Diagnosis, 1*(2), 70–77.

Spector, R. (2004). *Cultural diversity in health and illness* (6th ed.). Upper Saddle River, NJ: Prentice Hall.

Spotlight on medical-surgical nursing. (2003). *NURSING, 33*(4), 88–R2.

Wilkinson, J. M. (2005). *Nursing process and critical thinking.* (4th ed.) Upper Saddle River, NJ: Pearson Education, Inc.

World Health Organization. (1974). *Constitution of the World Health Organization: Chronicle of the World Health Organization.* Geneva: Author.

CHAPTER 2 Health and Illness in the Adult Client

LEARNING OUTCOMES

- Define health, incorporating the health–illness continuum and the concept of high-level wellness.

- Explain factors affecting functional health status.

- Discuss the nurse's role in health promotion.

- Describe characteristics of health, disease, and illness.

- Describe illness behaviors and needs of the client with acute illness and chronic illness.

- Describe the primary, secondary, and tertiary levels of illness prevention.

- Compare and contrast the physical status, risks for alterations in health, assessment guidelines, and healthy behaviors of the young adult, middle adult, and older adult.

- Explain the definitions, functions, and developmental stages and tasks of the family.

CLINICAL COMPETENCIES

- Include knowledge of developmental levels and of activities to promote, restore, and maintain health when planning and implementing care for adult clients.

- Include family members in teaching to promote and maintain health of the adult client.

MEDIALINK

Resources for this chapter can be found on the Prentice Hall Nursing MediaLink DVD-ROM accompanying this textbook, and on the Companion Website at http://www.prenhall.com/lemone

The human responses that nurses must consider when planning and implementing care result from changes in the structure and/or function of all body systems, as well as the interrelated effects of those changes on the psychosocial, cultural, spiritual, economic, and personal life of the client.

The World Health Organization (WHO) defines **health** as "a state of complete physical, mental, and social well-being, and not merely the absence of disease or infirmity" (WHO, 1974, p. 1). However, this definition does not take into account the various levels of health a person may experience, or that a person may be clinically described as ill yet still define oneself as well. These additional factors, which greatly influence nursing care, include the health–illness continuum and high-level wellness.

THE HEALTH–ILLNESS CONTINUUM AND HIGH-LEVEL WELLNESS

The **health–illness continuum** represents health as a dynamic process, with high-level **wellness** at one extreme of the continuum and death at the opposite extreme (Figure 2–1 ■). Individuals place themselves at different locations on the continuum at specific points in time.

Dunn (1959) expanded the concept of a continuum of health and illness in his description of high-level wellness. Dunn conceptualized wellness as an active process influenced by the environment. He differentiated good health from wellness:

> Good health can exist as a relatively passive state of freedom from illness in which the individual is at peace with his environment. . . . Wellness is an integrated method of functioning, which is oriented toward maximizing the potential of which the individual is capable, within the environment where he is functioning. (1959, p. 4)

A variety of factors influence wellness, including self-concept, environment, culture, and spiritual values. Providing care based on a framework of wellness facilitates active involvement by both the nurse and the client in promoting, maintaining, or restoring health. It also supports the philosophy of **holistic health care**, in which all aspects of a person (physical, psychosocial, cultural, spiritual, and intellectual) are considered as essential components of individualized care.

Factors Affecting Health

Many different factors affect a person's health or level of wellness. These factors often interact to promote health or to become risk factors for alterations in health. The factors affecting health are described next.

Genetic Makeup

Each person's genetic makeup influences health status throughout life. Genetic makeup affects personality, temperament, body structure, intellectual potential, and susceptibility to the development of hereditary alterations in health. Examples of chronic illnesses that are associated with genetic makeup include sickle cell disease, hemophilia, diabetes mellitus, and cancer.

Cognitive Abilities and Educational Level

Although cognitive abilities are determined prior to adulthood, the level of cognitive development affects whether people view themselves as healthy or ill; cognitive levels also may affect health practices. Injuries to and illnesses affecting the brain may alter cognitive abilities. Educational level affects the ability to understand and follow guidelines for health. For example, if an individual is functionally illiterate, written information about healthy behaviors and health resources is worthless.

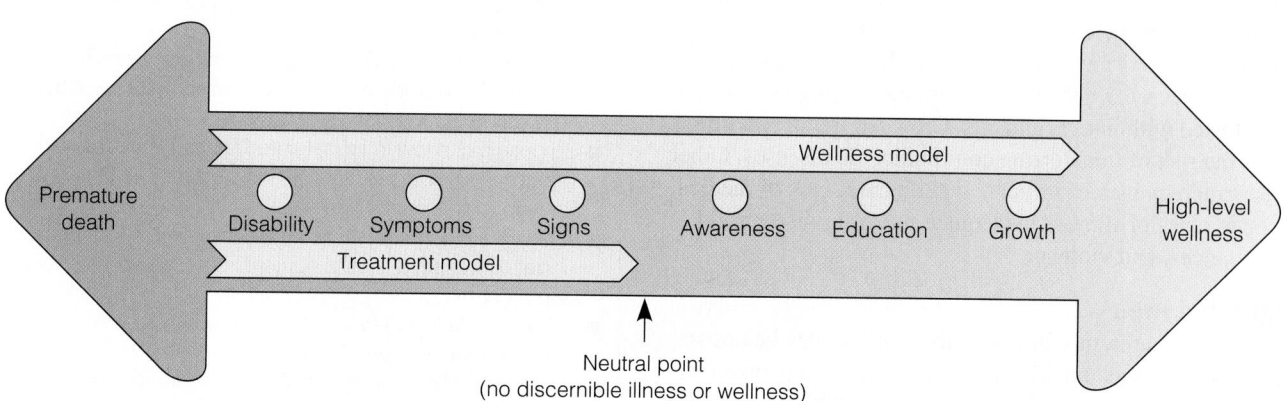

Figure 2–1 ■ The health–illness continuum.

Source: From *Wellness Workbook* by J. W. Travis and R. S. Ryan, 1998, Berkeley, CA: Ten Speed Press. Used with permission.

Race, Ethnicity, and Cultural Background

Certain diseases occur at a higher rate of incidence in some races and ethnic groups than in others. For example, in the United States, hypertension is more common in African Americans, tuberculosis and diabetes mellitus are among the leading causes of illness in Native Americans, and eye disorders are more prevalent in Chinese Americans. The ethnic and cultural background of an individual also influences health values and behaviors, lifestyle, and illness behaviors. Every culture defines health and illness in a way that is unique; in addition, each culture has its own health beliefs and illness treatment practices.

Age, Gender, and Developmental Level

Age, gender, and developmental level are factors in health and illness. Cardiovascular disorders are uncommon in young adults, but the incidence increases after the age of 40. Myocardial infarctions are more common in men than women until women are postmenopausal. Some diseases occur only in one gender or the other (e.g., prostate cancer in men and cervical cancer in women). The older adult often has increased incidence of chronic illness and increased potential for serious illness or death from infectious illnesses such as influenza and pneumonia.

Lifestyle and Environment

The components of a person's lifestyle that affect health status include patterns of eating, use of chemical substances (alcohol, nicotine, caffeine, legal and illegal drugs), exercise and rest patterns, and coping methods. Examples of altered responses are the relationship of obesity to hypertension, cigarette smoking to chronic obstructive pulmonary disease, a sedentary lifestyle to heart disease, and a high-stress career to alcoholism. The environment has a major influence on health. Occupational exposure to toxic substances (such as asbestos and coal dust) increases the risk of pulmonary disorders. Air, water, and food pollution increase the risk of respiratory disorders, infectious diseases, and cancer. Environmental temperature variations can result in hypothermia or hyperthermia, especially in the older adult.

Socioeconomic Background

Both lifestyle and environmental influences are affected by one's income level. The culture of poverty, which crosses all racial and ethnic boundaries, negatively influences health status. Living at or below the poverty level often results in crowded, unsanitary living conditions or homelessness. Housing often is overcrowded, lacks adequate heating or cooling, and is infested with insects and rats. Crowded living conditions increase the risk of transferring communicable diseases. Other problems include lack of infant and child care, lack of medical care for injuries or illness, inadequate nutrition, use of addictive substances, and violence.

Geographic Area

The geographic area in which one lives influences health status. Such illnesses as malaria are more common in tropical areas of North America, whereas multiple sclerosis occurs with greater frequency in the northern United States and Canada. Other geographic influences are seen in the number of skin cancers in people living in sunny, hot areas and sinus infections in people living in areas of high humidity.

Health Promotion and Maintenance

For many years, the emphasis in nursing was on care of the acutely ill client in the hospital setting. With changes in society and in health care, this emphasis is shifting toward preventive, community-based care. Although the focus of this textbook is not community health nursing, the importance of teaching health-promoting behaviors is an essential component of medical-surgical nursing.

Healthy Living

Practices that are known to promote health and wellness include the following:

- Eat three balanced meals a day, following the guidelines developed jointly by the U.S. Department of Agriculture (USDA) and the U.S. Department of Health and Human Services (DHHS) (Box 2–1). It is also helpful to follow a general guideline of what to eat each day, such as with the Food Guide Pyramid illustrated in Figure 2–2 ■. The food pyramid was revised in 2005, with recommendations for a greater emphasis on monounsaturated and polysaturated fats, the inclusion of whole-grain foods with each meal, and increased intake of fish and vegetables. The goal of the revision is to reduce obesity and cardiovascular disease. A web site is available to individualize the plan by helping consumers choose foods and amounts. After entering their age, gender, and activity level, consumers get their own plan at an appropriate calorie level, and can print out a miniposter and worksheet to track progress.
- Exercise moderately and regularly.
- Sleep 7 to 8 hours each day.
- Limit alcohol consumption to a moderate amount, and favor red wine.
- Eliminate smoking.

BOX 2–1 Dietary Guidelines for Health

- Eat a variety of foods to get the energy, proteins, vitamins, minerals, and fiber needed for good health.
- Balance intake of food with physical activity. Maintain or improve body weight to reduce the risks of high blood pressure, heart disease, stroke, certain cancers, and type 2 diabetes mellitus.
- Choose a diet with plenty of grain products, vegetables, and fruits, which provide needed fiber and complex carbohydrates and can help lower intake of fat.
- Choose a diet low in fat, saturated fat, and cholesterol to reduce the risk of heart attack and certain types of cancer, and to help maintain a healthy weight.
- Choose a diet moderate in sugars. Increased sugar intake can increase weight, decrease nutrient intake, and contribute to tooth decay.
- Choose a diet moderate in salt and sodium to help reduce the risk of high blood pressure.
- Drink alcoholic beverages, if at all, in moderation. Alcohol provides non-nutrient calories, may be addicting, and causes many health problems.

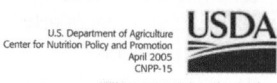

Figure 2–2 ■ The revised Food Guide Pyramid is designed to be used as a method of helping Americans make healthy food choices and be active every day.

From *U.S. Department of Agriculture and U.S. Department of Health and Human Services. (2005).* http://www.mypyramid.gov/downloads/miniposter.pdf

- Keep sun exposure to a minimum.
- Maintain recommended immunizations (Table 2–1).

The nurse promotes health by teaching the activities that maintain wellness, by providing information about the characteristics and consequences of diseases when risk factors have been identified, and by supplying specific information about decreasing risk factors (Pender, Parsons, & Murdaugh, 2006).

The nurse also promotes health by following healthy practices and serving as a role model.

National Health Promotion

The DHHS (2000) published national health objectives for the year 2010. Goals and leading health indicators are described in Box 2–2.

TABLE 2–1 Recommended Immunizations for Adults

VACCINE	INDICATIONS	DO NOT GIVE TO
Measles-mumps-rubella	Anyone born after 1956 and never infected, or those likely to be exposed, such as those entering college or the military.	Pregnant women, immunocompromised people, or anyone with a history of anaphylactic reaction to egg protein or neomycin.
Tetanus and diphtheria toxoids	Anyone who has never been vaccinated should have the primary series, followed by booster every 10 years.	None identified.
Hepatitis B	Anyone likely to have repeated exposure (such as healthcare providers or sex partners of a known carrier) or who have had exposure (such as a needle-stick injury to a healthcare worker).	People with a history of anaphylactic reaction to common baker's yeast.
Influenza A	Anyone at high risk for complications, healthcare providers, and those wanting immunity.	Those with a high fever, or a history of anaphylactic reaction to egg protein.
Pneumococcal pneumonia	Anyone at high risk for pneumococcal disease, those over 65 years of age.	Pregnant women.
Varicella	Anyone never infected, especially healthcare providers and child care workers.	Pregnant women, immunocompromised people, those who have received an immune globulin or a blood transfusion within 5 months, or those with a history of anaphylactic reactions to neomycin or gelatin.

BOX 2–2 Goals and Leading Health Indicators: *Healthy People 2010*

Healthy People 2010 has two major goals: to increase the quality and years of healthy life and to eliminate health disparities.

The major goals are divided into 28 focus areas, with each area having a specific goal. For example, for cancer, the goal is to reduce the number of new cancer cases as well as the illness, disability, and death caused by cancer.

The leading indicators used to measure the expected goals are as follows:

- Physical activity
- Overweight and obesity
- Tobacco use
- Substance abuse
- Responsible sexual behavior
- Mental health
- Injury and violence
- Environmental quality
- Immunization
- Access to health care

Source: Data from *Healthy People 2010* by U.S. Department of Health and Human Services, 2000, Washington, DC.

Disease and Illness

Disease and *illness* are terms that are often used interchangeably, but in fact they have different meanings. In general, nursing is concerned with illness, whereas medicine is concerned with disease.

Disease

Disease (literally meaning "without ease") is a medical term describing alterations in structure and function of the body or mind. Diseases may have mechanical, biologic, or normative causes. Mechanical causes of disease result in damage to the structure of the body and are the result of trauma or extremes of temperature. Biologic causes of disease affect body function and are the result of genetic defects, the effects of aging, infestation and infection, alterations in the immune system, and alterations in normal organ secretions. Normative causes are psychologic but involve a mind–body interaction, so that physical manifestations occur in response to the psychologic disturbance.

The cause of many diseases is still unknown. The following are generally accepted as common causes of disease:

- Genetic defects
- Developmental defects resulting from exposure to viruses, chemicals, or drugs that affect the developing fetus
- Biologic agents or toxins (including viruses, bacteria, rickettsia, fungi, protozoa, and helminths)
- Physical agents such as temperature extremes, radiation, and electricity
- Chemical agents such as alcohol, drugs, strong acids or bases, and heavy metals
- Generalized response of tissues to injury or irritation
- Alterations in the production of antibodies, resulting in allergies or hypersensitivities
- Faulty metabolic processes (e.g., a production of hormones or enzymes above or below normal)
- Continued, unabated stress.

Diseases may be classified as acute or chronic, communicable, congenital, degenerative, functional, malignant, psychosomatic, idiopathic, or iatrogenic. These classifications are defined in Table 2–2. In all types of disease, alterations in structure or function cause signs and symptoms (**manifestations**) that prompt a person to seek treatment from a physician or traditional healer. Although both subjective symptoms and objective signs commonly appear with disease, objective signs often predominate. Examples of objective signs include bleeding, vomiting, diarrhea, limitation of movement, swelling, visual disturbances, and changes in elimination. However, pain (a subjective symptom) is often the primary reason that prompts a person to seek health care.

Illness

Illness is the response a person has to a disease. This response is highly individualized, because the person responds not only to his or her own perceptions of the disease but also to the perceptions of others. Illness integrates pathophysiologic alterations; psychologic effects of those alterations; effects on roles,

---

TABLE 2–2 Disease Classifications and Definitions

CLASSIFICATION	DEFINITION
Acute	A disease that has a rapid onset, lasts a relatively short time, and is self-limiting
Chronic	A disease that has one or more of these characteristics: (1) is permanent, (2) leaves permanent disability, (3) causes nonreversible pathophysiology, (4) requires special training of the client for rehabilitation, (5) requires a long period of care
Communicable	A disease that can spread from one person to another
Congenital	A disease or disorder that exists at or before birth
Degenerative	A disease that results from deterioration or impairment of organs or tissues
Functional	A disease that affects function or performance but does not have manifestations of organic illness
Malignant	A disease that tends to become worse and cause death
Psychosomatic	A psychologic disease that is manifested by physiologic symptoms
Idiopathic	A disease that has an unknown cause
Iatrogenic	A disease that is caused by medical therapy

relationships, and values; and cultural and spiritual beliefs. A person may have a disease and not categorize himself or herself as ill, or may validate feelings of illness through the comments of others ("You don't look as though you feel well today").

ACUTE ILLNESS An **acute illness** occurs rapidly, lasts for a relatively short time, and is self-limiting. The condition responds to self-treatment or to medical-surgical intervention. Clients with uncomplicated acute illnesses usually have full recovery and return to normal preillness functioning.

Illness behaviors are the way people cope with the alterations in health and function caused by a disease. Illness behaviors are highly individualized and are influenced by age, gender, family values, economic status, culture, educational level, and mental status. A sequence of illness behaviors (Suchman, 1972) follows:

1. *Experiencing symptoms.* In the first stage of an acute illness, a person experiences one or more manifestations that serve as cues for an awareness that a change in normal health is occurring. The most significant manifestation is pain. Examples of other symptoms that signal an illness are bleeding, swelling, fever, or difficulty with breathing. If the manifestations are mild or are familiar (such as symptoms of the common cold or influenza), the person usually uses over-the-counter medications or a traditional remedy for self-treatment. If the symptoms are relieved, no further action is taken; however, if the symptoms are severe or become worse, the person moves to the next stage.

2. *Assuming the sick role.* In the second stage of the sequence, the person assumes the sick role. This role assumption signals acceptance of the symptoms as proof that an illness is present. The person usually validates this belief with others and seeks support for the need to have professional treatment or to stay at home from school or work. Self-preoccupation is characteristic of this stage, and the person focuses on alterations in function resulting from the illness. If the illness is resolved, the person validates a return to health with others and resumes normal activities; however, if manifestations remain or increase in severity and others agree that no improvement has occurred, the person moves to the next stage by seeking medical care.

3. *Seeking medical care.* In our society, a physician or other healthcare provider most often provides validation of illness. People who believe themselves to be ill (and who are encouraged by others to contact a healthcare provider) make the medical contact for diagnosis, prognosis, and treatment of the illness. If the medical diagnosis is of an illness, the person moves to the next stage. If the medical diagnosis does not support illness, the client may return to normal functioning or may seek validation from a different healthcare provider.

4. *Assuming a dependent role.* The stage of assuming a dependent role begins when a person accepts the diagnosis and planned treatment of the illness. As the severity of the illness increases, so does the dependent role. It is during this stage that the person may enter the hospital for treatment and care. The responses of the person to care depend on many different variables: the severity of the illness, the degree of anxiety or fear about the outcome, the loss of roles, the support systems available, individualized reactions to stress, and previous experiences with illness care.

5. *Achieving recovery and rehabilitation.* The final stage of an acute illness is recovery and rehabilitation. Institutional health care focuses on the acute care needs of the ill client, with recovery beginning in the hospital and completed at home. This focus makes client education and continuity of care a major goal for nursing. It has also contributed to the shift in settings for nursing care, with increasing numbers of nurses providing care in community settings and the home. The person now gives up the dependent role and resumes normal roles and responsibilities. As a result of education during treatment and care, the person may be at a higher level of wellness after recovery is complete. There is no set timetable for recovery from an illness. The degree of severity of the illness and the method of treatment both affect the length of time required, as does the person's compliance with treatment plans and motivation to return to normal health.

CHRONIC ILLNESS **Chronic illness** is a term that encompasses many different lifelong pathologic and psychologic alterations in health. It is the leading health problem in the world today, and the number of people with chronic illnesses is estimated to triple by the year 2040. Current trends affecting an increased incidence of chronic illnesses include diseases of aging, diseases of lifestyle and behavior, and environmental factors.

Most descriptions of chronic illness are based on the definition by the National Commission on Chronic Illness, which states that a chronic illness is any impairment or deviation from normal functioning that has one or more of the following characteristics:

- It is permanent.
- It leaves permanent disability.
- It is caused by nonreversible pathologic alterations.
- It requires special training of the client for rehabilitation.
- It may require a long period of care.

Chronic illness is also characterized by impaired function in more than one body system; responses to this impaired function may occur in sensory perception, self-care abilities, mobility, cognition, and social skills. The demands on the individual and family as a result of these responses are often lifelong (Miller, 2000).

The intensity of a chronic illness and its related manifestations range from mild to severe, and the illness is usually characterized by periods of remission and exacerbation. During periods of **remission**, the person does not experience symptoms, even though the disease is still clinically present. During periods of **exacerbation**, the symptoms reappear. These periods of change in symptoms do not appear in all chronic diseases.

Each person with a chronic illness has a unique set of responses and needs. The response of the person to the illness is influenced by the following factors:

- The point in the life cycle at which the onset of the illness occurs
- The type and degree of limitations imposed by the illness
- The visibility of impairment or disfigurement
- The pathophysiology causing the illness
- The relationship between the impairment and functioning in social roles
- Pain and fear.

These factors are highly complex. They are interrelated within each person, resulting in individualized illness behaviors and needs. Because there are so many different chronic diseases and because the experience of each person with the illness is a composite of individualized responses, it is difficult to generalize about needs. However, almost all people with a chronic illness will need to:

- Live as normally as possible, despite the symptoms and treatment that make the person with a chronic illness feel alienated, lonely, and different from others without the illness.
- Learn to adapt activities of daily living and self-care activities.
- Grieve the loss of physical function and structure, income, status, roles, and dignity.
- Comply with a medical treatment plan.
- Maintain a positive self-concept and a sense of hope.
- Maintain a feeling of being in control.
- Confront the inevitability of death. (Miller, 2000)

Some people with chronic illness successfully meet health-related needs, whereas others do not. Research indicates that adaptation is influenced by variables such as anger, depression, denial, self-concept, locus of control, hardiness, and disability. Nursing interventions for the person with a chronic illness focus on education to promote independent functioning, reduce health-care costs, and improve well-being and quality of life.

ILLNESS PREVENTION Activities to prevent illness include any measures that limit the progression of an illness at any point of its course. Three levels of illness prevention have been defined (Leavell & Clark, 1965). Each level of prevention occurs at a distinct point in the development of a disease process and requires specific nursing interventions (Edelman & Mandle, 2006). The levels are as follows:

1. *Primary level of prevention.* This level includes generalized health promotion activities as well as specific actions that prevent or delay the occurrence of a disease. Following are examples of primary prevention activities:
   - Protecting oneself against environmental risks, such as air and water pollution
   - Eating nutritious foods
   - Protecting oneself against industrial hazards
   - Obeying seat belt and helmet laws
   - Obtaining sex counseling and practicing safer sex
   - Obtaining immunizations
   - Undergoing genetic screenings
   - Eliminating the use of alcohol and cigarettes.
2. *Secondary level of prevention.* This level involves activities that emphasize early diagnosis and treatment of an illness that is already present, to stop the pathologic process and enable the person to return to his or her former state of health as soon as possible. Following are examples of secondary prevention activities:
   - Having screenings for diseases such as hypertension, diabetes mellitus, and glaucoma
   - Obtaining physical examinations and diagnostic tests for cancer
   - Performing self-examination for breast and/or testicular cancer

- Obtaining tuberculosis skin tests
- Obtaining specific treatment for illness (e.g., the treatment of streptococcal infections of the throat will prevent secondary infections involving the heart and/or kidneys).

3. *Tertiary level of prevention.* This level focuses on stopping the disease process and returning the affected individual to a useful place in society within the constraints of any disability. The activities primarily revolve around rehabilitation. Following are examples of tertiary prevention measures:
   - Obtaining medical or surgical treatment for an illness
   - Enrolling in specific rehabilitation programs for cardiovascular problems, head injuries, and strokes
   - Joining work training programs following illness or injury
   - Educating the public to employ rehabilitated people to the fullest possible extent.

MEETING HEALTH NEEDS OF ADULTS

The adult years commonly are divided into three stages: the young adult (ages 18 to 40), the middle adult (ages 40 to 65), and the older adult (over age 65). Although developmental markers are not as clearly delineated in the adult as in the infant or child, specific changes do occur with aging in intellectual, psychosocial, and spiritual development, as well as in physical structures and functions.

The developmental theories specific to the adult, with related stages and tasks, are listed in Table 2–3. Applying a variety of developmental theories is important to the holistic care of the adult client as nurses perform assessments, implement care, and provide teaching.

The Young Adult

From ages 18 to 25, the healthy young adult is at the peak of physical development. All body systems are functioning at maximum efficiency. Then, during the 30s, some normal physiologic changes begin to occur. A comparison of physical status for young adults during their 20s and 30s is shown in Table 2–4.

Risks for Alterations in Health

The young adult is at risk for alterations in health from accidents, sexually transmitted infections, substance abuse, and physical or psychosocial stressors. These risk factors may be interrelated.

INJURIES Unintentional injuries are the leading cause of injury and death in people between ages 15 and 24 (Centers for Disease Control and Prevention, [CDC], 2003). Most injuries and fatalities occur as the result of motor vehicle crashes; but injuries and death also result from assaults (homicide), drowning, fire, guns, occupational accidents, and exposure to environmental hazards. Accidental injury or death is often associated with the use of alcohol or other chemical substances, or with psychologic stress. Intentional self-harm (suicide) is the third leading cause of death in young adults of both genders.

SEXUALLY TRANSMITTED INFECTIONS Sexually transmitted infections include genital herpes, chlamydia, gonorrhea, syphilis, and HIV/AIDS. The young adult who is sexually active with a variety of partners and who does not use condoms is at greatest risk for development of these diseases. Nursing care of clients with sexually transmitted infections is discussed in Chapter 52 ∞.

TABLE 2–3 Theories of Adult Development

	THEORIST	AGE	TASK
Psychosocial Development	Erikson	18–25	Identity versus role confusion ■ Establishing an intimate relationship with another person ■ Committing oneself to work and to relationships
		25–65	Generativity versus stagnation ■ Accepting one's own life as creative and productive ■ Having concern for others
		65–death	Integrity versus despair ■ Accepting worth of one's own life ■ Accepting inevitability of death
Spiritual Development	Fowler	After 18	■ Having a high degree of self-consciousness ■ Constructing one's own spiritual system
		After 30	■ Being aware of truth from a variety of viewpoints
	Westerhoff	Young adult	Searching faith ■ Acquiring a cognitive and an affective faith through questioning one's own faith
		Middle–older adult	Owned faith ■ Putting faith into action and standing up for beliefs
Moral Development	Kohlberg	Adult	Postconventional level Social contract/legalistic orientation ■ Defining morality in terms of personal principles ■ Adhering to laws that protect the welfare and rights of others Universal-ethical principles ■ Internalizing universal moral principles ■ Respecting others; believing that relationships are based on mutual trust
Developmental Tasks	Havighurst	18–35	■ Selecting and learning to live with a mate ■ Starting a family and rearing children ■ Managing a home ■ Starting an occupation ■ Taking on civic responsibility ■ Finding a congenial social group
		35–60	■ Achieving civic and social responsibility ■ Establishing and maintaining an economic standard of living ■ Assisting teenage children in becoming responsible and happy adults ■ Developing leisure-time activities ■ Relating to one's spouse as a person ■ Accepting and adjusting to the physiologic changes of middle age ■ Adjusting to aging parents
		60 and over	■ Meeting civic and social obligations ■ Establishing an affiliation with one's own age group ■ Establishing satisfactory physical living arrangements ■ Adjusting to decreasing physical strength, health, retirement, reduced income, death of spouse

Source: Data from *Childhood and Society* (2nd ed.) by E. Erickson, 1963. New York: Norton; *Stages of Faith: The Psychology of Human Development and the Quest for Meaning* by J. W. Fowler, 1981, New York: Harper & Row; *Human Development and Education* (3rd ed.) by R. J. Havighurst, 1972, New York: Longman; *The Meaning and Measurement of Moral Development* by L. Kohlberg, 1979, New York: Clark University; *and Will Our Children Have Faith?* by J. Westerhoff, 1976, New York: Seabury Press.

SUBSTANCE ABUSE Substance abuse is a major cause for concern in the young adult population. Although alcohol abuse occurs at all ages, it is greater in the 20s than during any other decade of the life span. Alcohol contributes to motor vehicle crashes and physical violence, and it is damaging to the developing fetus in pregnant women. It can also cause liver disease and nutritional deficits.

Other substances that are commonly abused include nicotine, marijuana, amphetamines, cocaine, and crack. Smoking increases the risk of respiratory and cardiovascular diseases.

Cocaine and crack can cause death from cardiovascular effects (increased heart rate and ventricular dysrhythmias), and can lead to addiction and health problems in the baby born to an addicted mother. Nursing care of clients with problems of substance abuse is discussed in Chapter 6 ∞.

PHYSICAL AND PSYCHOSOCIAL STRESSORS Physical stressors that increase the risk of illness include environmental pollutants and work-related risks (e.g., electrical hazards, mechanical injuries, or exposure to toxins or infectious agents). Other physical stressors include exposure to the sun,

TABLE 2–4 Physical Status and Changes in the Young Adult Years

ASSESSMENT	STATUS DURING THE 20S	STATUS DURING THE 30S
Skin	Smooth, even temperature	Wrinkles begin to appear
Hair	Slightly oily, shiny Balding may begin	Graying may begin Balding may begin
Vision	Snellen 20/20	Some loss of visual acuity and accommodation
Musculoskeletal	Strong, coordinated	Some loss of strength and muscle mass
Cardiovascular	Maximum cardiac output 60–90 beats/min Mean BP: 120/80	Slight decline in cardiac output 60–90 beats/min Mean BP: 120/80
Respiratory	Rate: 12–20 Full vital capacity	Rate: 12–20 Decline in vital capacity

ingestion of chemical substances (e.g., caffeine, alcohol, nicotine), and pregnancy.

Many different and individualized psychosocial stressors may affect the young adult. Choices must be made about education, occupation, relationships, independence, and lifestyle. The young adult without adequate education or job skills may face unemployment, poverty, homelessness, and limited access to health care. Divorces in the United States are increasing. Three of every five marriages end in divorce, and this number is even higher among young adults (Edelman & Mandle, 2006). Divorce often results in loneliness, feelings of failure, financial difficulties, domestic violence, and child abuse. The inability of the young adult to cope with these stressors may result in suicide, which ranks next to accidents as a major cause of death in this age group. Although difficult to prove, it is believed that some accidental deaths, especially when associated with substance abuse, are actually suicides.

Assessment Guidelines

The following guidelines are useful in assessing the achievement of significant developmental tasks in the young adult. Does the young adult:

- Feel independent from parents?
- Have a realistic self-concept?
- Like oneself and the direction in which life is going?
- Interact well with family?
- Cope with the stresses of constant change and growth?
- Have well-established bonds with significant others, such as marriage partners or close friends?
- Have a meaningful social life?
- Have a career or occupation?
- Demonstrate emotional, social, and economic responsibility for own life?
- Have a set of values that guide behavior?
- Have a healthy lifestyle?

Physical assessment of the young adult includes height and weight, blood pressure, and vision. During the health history, the nurse should ask specific questions about substance use, sexual activity and concerns, exercise, eating habits, menstrual history and patterns, coping mechanisms, any familial chronic illnesses, and family changes.

Promoting Healthy Behaviors in the Young Adult

The nurse promotes health in the young adult by teaching the behaviors listed in Box 2–3. Health information for the young adult is primarily provided in community settings. Examples are as follows:

- Health-related courses and seminars at colleges and universities include information on the use of sports and exercise facilities, alcohol and drug abuse, smoking cessation, mental health, and sexual health.
- Workplace programs include blood pressure monitoring, exercise, smoking cessation, cafeteria nutrition guidelines, and stress reduction activities.
- Community programs include media information, health fairs, support groups, and information about risk factors for disease and injury.

The Middle Adult

The middle adult, ages 40 to 65, has physical status and function similar to that of the young adult. However, many changes take place between ages 40 and 65. Table 2–5 lists the physical changes that normally occur in the middle years.

Risks for Alterations in Health

The middle adult is at risk for alterations in health from obesity, cardiovascular disease, cancer, substance abuse, and physical and psychosocial stressors. These factors may be interrelated.

OBESITY The middle adult often has a problem maintaining a healthy weight. Weight gain in middle adulthood is usually the result of continuing to consume the same number of calories while decreasing physical activity and experiencing a decrease in basal metabolic rate. Obesity affects all of the major organ systems of the body, increasing the risk of atherosclerosis, hypertension, elevated cholesterol and triglyceride levels, and diabetes. Obesity is also associated with heart disease, osteoarthritis, and gallbladder disease.

CARDIOVASCULAR DISEASE The major risk factors, especially for coronary artery disease, include age, male gender, physical inactivity, cigarette smoking, hypertension, elevated blood cholesterol levels, and diabetes. Other contributing factors include obesity, stress, and lack of exercise. The middle

BOX 2–3 Healthy Behaviors in the Young Adult

- Choose foods from all food groups, and eat a variety of foods.
- Choose a diet low in fat (30% or less of total calories), saturated fat (less than 10% of calories), and cholesterol (less than 300 mg daily).
- Choose a diet that each day includes at least three servings of vegetables, two servings of fruits, and six servings of grains.
- Use sugar, salt, and sodium in moderation.
- For females, increase to or maintain 18 mg of iron daily in the diet, and 400 mg of folic acid per day through diet or supplements.
- Make exercise a regular part of life, carrying out activities that increase the heart rate to a set target, and maintain that rate for 30–60 minutes three or four times a week.
- Include exercise as part of any weight reduction program.

- Have regular physical examinations, including assessment for cancer of the thyroid, ovaries, lymph nodes, and skin (every 3 years).
- Have a vision examination every 2–4 years.
- Have an annual dental checkup.
- For females between ages 20 and 39 have a clinical breast examination by a healthcare professional every 3 years.
- For females, have Pap tests as recommended by a physician: annually until three or more consecutive normal results, and then at physician's discretion.
- For males, have testicular and prostate examinations every 5 years.
- Conduct breast self-examination or testicular self-examination monthly.
- Maintain immunizations.

---

adult is at risk for peripheral vascular, cerebrovascular, and cardiovascular disease.

CANCER Cancer is the third leading cause of death in adults between ages 25 and 64 in the United States, with one-third of cases occurring between ages 35 and 64. Cancers of the breast, colon, lung, and reproductive system are common in the middle years. The middle adult is at risk for cancer as a result of increased length of exposure to environmental carcinogens, as well as alcohol and nicotine use. Nursing care of the client with cancer is discussed in Chapter 14 ∞.

SUBSTANCE ABUSE Although the middle adult may abuse a variety of substances, the most commonly abused are alcohol, nicotine, and prescription drugs. Excess alcohol use in the middle adult contributes to an increased risk of liver cancer, cirrhosis, pancreatitis, hyperlipidemia, and anemia. Alcoholism also increases the risk of accidental injury or death and disrupts careers and relationships. Cigarette smoking increases the risk of cancer of the larynx, lung, mouth, pharynx, bladder, pancreas, esophagus, and kidney; of chronic obstructive pulmonary disorders; and of cardiovascular disorders.

PHYSICAL AND PSYCHOSOCIAL STRESSORS The middle adult years are ones of change and transition, frequently resulting in stress. Both men and women must adapt to changes in physical appearance and function and accept their own mortality. Children may leave home or choose to remain at home longer than they are welcome. Parents are aging, with illness probable and death inevitable. The middle adult thus becomes part of what has been called "the sandwich generation," caught between the need to care for both children and aging parents. Both men and women may make career changes, and approaching retirement becomes a reality. Divorce in the middle years is a major emotional, social, and financial stressor.

TABLE 2–5 Physical Changes in the Middle Adult Years

ASSESSMENT	CHANGES
Skin	■ Decreased turgor, moisture, and subcutaneous fat result in wrinkles. ■ Fat is deposited in the abdominal and hip areas.
Hair	■ Loss of melanin in hair shaft causes graying. ■ Hairline recedes in males.
Sensory	■ Visual acuity for near vision decreases (presbyopia) during the 40s. ■ Auditory acuity for high-frequency sounds decreases (presbycusis); more common in men. ■ Sense of taste diminishes.
Musculoskeletal	■ Skeletal muscle mass decreases by about age 60. ■ Thinning of intervertebral discs results in loss of height (about 2.5 cm [1 inch]). ■ Postmenopausal women may have loss of calcium and develop osteoporosis.
Cardiovascular	■ Blood vessels lose elasticity. ■ Systolic blood pressure may increase.
Respiratory	■ Loss of vital capacity (about 1 L from age 20 to 60) occurs.
Gastrointestinal	■ Large intestine gradually loses muscle tone; constipation may result. ■ Gastric secretions are decreased.
Genitourinary	■ Hormonal changes occur: menopause, women (↓ estrogen); andropause, men (↓ testosterone).
Endocrine	■ Gradual decrease in glucose tolerance occurs.

BOX 2–4 Healthy Behaviors in the Middle Adult

- Choose foods from all food groups, and eat a variety of foods.
- Choose a diet low in fat (30% or less of total calories), saturated fat (less than 10% of calories), and cholesterol (less than 300 mg daily). Adjust daily calorie intake to maintain healthy weight.
- Choose a diet that each day includes at least three servings of vegetables, two servings of fruits, and six servings of grains.
- Use sugar, salt, and sodium in moderation.
- Increase calcium intake (in perimenopausal women) to 1,200 mg daily.
- Consume high-fiber foods.
- Make exercise a part of life, carrying out regular exercise that is moderately strenuous, is consistent, and avoids overexertion; exercise for 30 minutes at least 4 to 5 times a week.
- Include exercise as part of any weight reduction program.
- Have an annual vision examination.
- Have an annual dental checkup.

- Have a physical examination annually, including assessment for cancer of the thyroid, testes, prostate, mouth, ovaries, skin, lymph nodes, and for cholesterol and blood glucose levels.
- For females, have a mammogram every year from age 40 on. Have a clinical breast examination annually.
- For females, have a Pap test as recommended for the young adult (see Box 2–3).
- Have an annual stool blood test; or a digital rectal examination (DRE) and a flexible sigmoidoscopy every 5 years; or a colonoscopy and DRE every 10 years or a double-contrast barium enema and a DRE every 5–10 years.
- For males, have testicular and prostate examinations annually, including a DRE, after age 50.
- Conduct breast self-examination or testicular self-examination every month. (The perimenopausal woman should set a specific date each month for the exam, as menstrual periods may be irregular or absent.)

Assessment Guidelines

The following guidelines are useful in assessing the achievement of significant developmental tasks in the middle adult. Does the middle adult:

- Accept the aging body?
- Feel comfortable with and respect him- or herself?
- Enjoy some new freedom to be independent?
- Accept changes in family roles?
- Enjoy success and satisfaction from work and/or family roles?
- Interact well and share companionable activities with a partner?
- Expand or renew previous interests?
- Pursue charitable and altruistic activities?
- Consider plans for retirement?
- Have a meaningful philosophy of life?
- Follow preventive healthcare practices?

Physical assessment of the middle adult includes all body systems, including blood pressure, vision, and hearing. Monitoring for risks and onset of cancer symptoms is essential. During the health history, the nurse should ask specific questions about food intake and exercise habits, substance abuse, sexual concerns, changes in the reproductive system, coping mechanisms, and family history of chronic illnesses.

Promoting Healthy Behaviors in the Middle Adult

The nurse promotes health in the middle adult by teaching the behaviors listed in Box 2–4. Information about health for the middle adult may be provided in a variety of community settings, including outpatient clinics, occupational health clinics, and private practice. Examples are as follows:

- Specific programs emphasize accepting responsibility for one's own health. This type of teaching can be in a seminar or on a one-to-one basis, and includes information specific to a group of individuals with an identified need, such as smokers, women who have just entered the workforce, or men nearing retirement.
- The community and industries provide information about safety hazards in the home and workplace, as well as during leisure activities.

- Literature about community resources is available for health promotion, including programs offered at alcohol/drug abuse treatment centers, clinics and health centers, counseling services, crisis intervention centers, spouse abuse programs, and health education and promotion agencies (e.g., American Red Cross, American Cancer Society, American Heart Association, YWCA, YMCA).

The Older Adult

The older adult period begins at age 65, but it can be further divided into three periods: the young-old (ages 65 to 74), the middle-old (ages 75 to 84), and the old-old (age 85 and over). With increasing age, a number of normal physiologic changes occur, as listed in Table 2–6.

The older adult population is increasing more rapidly than any other age group. In the last century, the number of adults in the United States living to age 65 or older increased from 4% in 1900 to 12.3% in 2003. There will be 71 million older adults by the year 2030, more than twice the number in 2000. The average life expectancy in the United States is 72 years for men and 79 years for women (Administration on Aging, 2003; American Association of Retired Persons, 2004).

FAST FACTS
Diversity in Older Adults

- Currently, minority older adults comprise over 16.1% of all older Americans.
- By 2030, the minority older adult population is projected to increase by 217%, compared with 81% for the older adult white population.
- Minority elders will increase as follows: African Americans = 128%, Asians = 301%, Hispanic Americans = 322%, American Indians and Alaska Natives = 193%.

Source: Data from Administration on Aging. (2004). *Addressing diversity.* Retrieved from www.aoa.dhhs.gov/prof/addiv/addiv_pf.asp

TABLE 2–6 Physical Changes in the Older Adult Years

ASSESSMENT	CHANGES
Skin	■ Decreased turgor and sebaceous gland activity result in dry, wrinkled skin. Melanocytes cluster, causing "age spots" or "liver spots."
Hair and nails	■ Scalp, axillary, and pubic hair thins; nose and ear hair thickens. Women may develop facial hair. ■ Nails grow more slowly; may become thick and brittle.
Sensory	■ Visual field narrows, and depth perception is distorted. ■ Pupils are smaller, reducing night vision. ■ Lenses yellow and become opaque, resulting in distortion of green, blue, and violet tones and increased sensitivity to glare. ■ Production of tears decreases. ■ Sense of smell decreases. ■ Age-related hearing loss progresses, involving middle- and low-frequency sounds. ■ Threshold for pain and touch increases. ■ Alterations in proprioception (sense of physical position) may occur.
Musculoskeletal	■ Loss of overall mass, strength, and movement of muscles occurs; tremors may occur. ■ Loss of bone structure and deterioration of cartilage in joints results in increased risk of fractures and in limitation of range of motion.
Cardiovascular	■ Systolic blood pressure rises. ■ Cardiac output decreases. ■ Peripheral resistance increases, and capillary walls thicken.
Respiratory	■ Continued loss of vital capacity occurs as the lungs become less elastic and more rigid. ■ Anteroposterior chest diameter increases; kyphosis. ■ Although blood carbon dioxide levels remain relatively constant, blood oxygen levels decrease by 10–15%.
Gastrointestinal	■ Production of saliva decreases, and decreased number of taste buds decrease accurate receptors for salt and sweet. ■ Gag reflex is decreased, and stomach motility and emptying are reduced. ■ Both large and small intestines have some atrophy, with decreased peristalsis. ■ The liver decreases in weight and storage capacity; gallstones increase; pancreatic enzymes decrease.

Genitourinary	■ Kidneys lose mass, and the glomerular filtration rate is reduced (by nearly 50% from young adulthood to old age).
	■ Bladder capacity decreases, and the micturition reflex is delayed. Urinary retention is more common.
	■ Women may have stress incontinence; men may have an enlarged prostate gland.
	■ Reproductive changes in men occur:
	  —Testosterone decreases.
	  —Sperm count decreases.
	  —Testes become smaller.
	  —Length of time to achieve an erection increases; erection is less full.
	■ Reproductive changes in women occur:
	  —Estrogen levels decrease.
	  —Breast tissue decreases.
	  —Vagina, uterus, ovaries, and urethra atrophy.
	  —Vaginal lubrication decreases.
	  —Vaginal secretions become alkaline.

Endocrine	■ Pituitary gland loses weight and vascularity. ■ Thyroid gland becomes more fibrous, and plasma T_3 decreases. ■ Pancreas releases insulin more slowly; increased blood glucose levels are common. ■ Adrenal glands produce less cortisol.

The increase in numbers of older adults has important implications for nursing. Clients needing health care in all settings will be older, requiring nursing interventions and teaching specifically designed to meet needs that differ from those of young and middle adults. Although gerontologic nursing (care of the older adult) is a nursing specialty area, it is also an integral component of medical-surgical nursing (Figure 2–3 ■).

Risks for Alterations in Health

The older adult is at risk for alterations in health from a variety of causes. Most older adults have one chronic health problem, while many have multiple illnesses. The most frequently occurring conditions in the older adult are hypertension, arthritis, heart diseases, cancer, sinusitis, and diabetes. The leading causes of death are heart disease, cancer, and stroke. Like the middle adult, the older adult is at risk for alterations in health from obesity and a sedentary lifestyle. Other risk factors specific to this age group include accidental injuries, pharmacologic effects, and physical and psychosocial stress.

INJURIES Injuries in the older adult cause many different problems: illness, financial burdens, hospitalization, self-care

Figure 2–3 ■ The older adult population is increasing more rapidly than any other age group, making gerontologic nursing an integral component of medical-surgical nursing practice.

deficits, loss of independence, and even death. The risk of injury is increased by normal physiologic changes that accompany aging, pathophysiologic alterations in health, environmental hazards, and lack of support systems. The three major causes of injury in the older adult are falls, fires, and motor vehicle crashes. Of these, falls with resultant hip fractures are the most significant in terms of long-term disability and death.

PHARMACOLOGIC EFFECTS A number of risk factors predispose the older adult to experiencing drug toxicity. Age-related changes in tissue and organ structure and function alter the absorption of both oral and parenteral medications. Low nutritional levels and decreased liver function may alter drug metabolism. The aging kidney may not excrete drugs at the normal clearance rate. Self-administration of both prescribed and over-the-counter medications presents risks for error resulting from confusion, forgetfulness, or misreading the directions. The older adult may take several drugs at once, and it is difficult to know how drugs interact with each other (Weitzel, 2001). In addition, the older adult living on a fixed income may have to make a choice between buying medications or food, resulting in undermedication and treatment of an illness.

PHYSICAL AND PSYCHOSOCIAL STRESSORS The older adult is exposed to the same environmental hazards as the young and middle adult, but the accumulation of years of exposure may now appear. For example, exposure to the sun in earlier years may be manifested by skin cancer, and the long-term effects of exposure to noise pollution can result in impaired hearing. The older adult (especially the older male) is at increased risk for respiratory disorders as a result of years of smoking, or from such pollutants as coal or asbestos dust. Living conditions and economic constraints may prevent the older adult from having necessary heating and cooling, contributing to thermal-related illnesses and even death. Elder abuse and neglect further increase the risk of injury or illness.

Psychosocial stressors for the older adult include the illness or death of a spouse, decreased or limited income, retirement, isolation from friends and family because of lack of transportation or distance, return to the home of a child, or relocation to a long-term healthcare facility. A further stressor may be role loss or reversal—for example, when the wife becomes the caretaker of her chronically ill husband.

Assessment Guidelines

The following guidelines are useful in assessing the achievement of significant developmental tasks in the older adult. Does the older adult:

- Adjust to the physiologic changes related to aging?
- Manage retirement years in a satisfying manner?
- Have satisfactory living arrangements and income to meet changing needs?
- Participate in social and leisure activities?
- Have a social network of friends and support persons?
- View life as worthwhile?
- Have high self-esteem?
- Have the abilities to care for self or to secure appropriate help?
- Gain support from a value system or spiritual philosophy?
- Adapt lifestyle to diminishing energy and ability?
- Accept and adjust to the death of significant others?

Physical assessment of the older adult includes a careful examination of all body systems. During the health history, the nurse should ask specific questions about usual dietary patterns; elimination; exercise and rest; use of alcohol, nicotine, over-the-counter medications, and prescription drugs; sexual concerns; financial concerns; and support systems.

Promoting Healthy Behaviors in the Older Adult

The nurse promotes health in the older adult by teaching the behaviors listed in Box 2–5. Older adults get the same benefits from health teaching as young adults and middle adults; they should never be viewed as being "too old" for healthy living practices. However, nurses should structure teaching activities to meet age-related physiologic changes, such as using charts and literature with large print. Health education for the older adult is provided in hospitals, long-term care facilities, retirement centers, outpatient clinics, senior citizen centers, and other community settings. Examples are as follows:

- Educational seminars teach about accident prevention in the home, in automobiles, and when taking public transportation.
- Health screenings and information from health fairs can specifically aid the older adult.
- Community programs provide immunization for influenza and pneumonia.
- Literature is available about financial assistance for health care, crisis hot lines, community services and resources (as described earlier for the middle adult), transportation, and nutrition (such as the Meals-on-Wheels program).

THE FAMILY OF THE ADULT CLIENT

Although some clients are totally alone in the world, most have one or more people who are significant in their lives. These significant others may be related or bonded to the client by birth, adoption, marriage, or friendship. Although not always meeting

BOX 2–5 Healthy Behaviors in the Older Adult

■ Eat a variety of nutrient-dense foods and beverages within and among the basic food groups while choosing foods that limit the intake of saturated and trans fats, cholesterol, added sugars, salt, and alcohol.

■ Choose a diet low in fat (30% or less of total calories), saturated fat (less than 10% of calories), and cholesterol (less than 300 mg daily). Choose foods high in fiber, low in sodium, and high in potassium.

■ People with dark skin and those with little sunlight exposure should consume extra vitamin D from fortified foods or supplements.

■ Individuals with hypertension and African Americans should consume no more than 1,500 mg of sodium each day.

■ If weight loss is needed, aim for a slow, steady loss by decreasing caloric intake while maintaining an adequate nutrient intake and increasing physical activity.

■ Increase calcium intake to 1,200 mg daily.

■ Make exercise a part of life, carrying out regular exercise that is moderately strenuous, is consistent, and avoids overexertion; exercise for 30 to 60 minutes every day, if possible.

■ Have an annual vision examination, including a test for glaucoma. (*Medicare covers a test for glaucoma every 12 months for people at high risk.*)

■ Practice good oral hygiene with teeth brushing and flossing and have a dental checkup one to two times a year.

■ Have a physical examination annually, including blood studies for glucose and cholesterol. (*Medicare covers a one-time physical examination if conducted within the first 6 months of having Medicare Part B. Tests for diabetes are covered, with number of times per year depending on number of risk factors. Medicare covers costs for cholesterol, lipids, and triglyceride levels every 5 years.*)

■ For women, have a bone density examination. (*Bone density examinations are covered by Medicare every 24 months [or more if medically necessary] for those at risk for osteoporosis.*)

■ For women, have a mammogram every year. Perform a breast self-examination every month and have a breast examination

annually. (*Medicare covers mammograms once every 12 months for all women age 40 and older.*)

■ For women, have an annual pelvic examination and Pap test as recommended by their healthcare provider. Women who have had a total hysterectomy (with removal of the uterus and cervix) may choose to stop having Pap tests unless the surgery was done to treat cervical precancer or cancer. Women who are at high risk for hereditary nonpolyposis colon cancer should be offered a screening for endometrial cancer with endometrial biopsy beginning at age 35. (*Medicare covers a pelvic examination and Pap test every 24 months for all women and once every 12 months for those at high risk.*)

■ For men, a prostate-specific antigen (PSA) blood test and a digital rectal examination (DRE) should be offered annually. Men at high risk (African-American men and those who have a family history of father or brothers diagnosed with prostate cancer at an early age) should begin testing at age 45. (*Medicare covers a DRE and PSA test once every 12 months for all men over age 50.*)

■ Have one of the following to screen for colon cancer: yearly fecal occult blood test (FOBT) or fecal immunochemical test (FIT); flexible sigmoidoscopy every 5 years; yearly FOBT or FIT plus flexible sigmoidoscopy every 5 years; double-contrast barium enema every 5 years; or colonoscopy every 10 years. Individuals who have an increased risk of colon cancer because of colon cancer, a personal history of chronic inflammatory bowel disease, a family history of colon cancer, or who have had adenomatous polyps should have screening more often. (*Medicare pays for one or more of these depending on the test prescribed and the level of risk.*)

■ Use sunscreen and avoid sunburn.

■ Obtain an annual influenza immunization and have the pneumonia vaccine at age 65. (*Medicare pays for an annual influenza shot once a year in the fall or winter and covers the cost of the pneumococcal shot, which most people only need once.*)

Note: Medicare pays costs of examinations only for people who are enrolled in the program.

---

traditional definitions, people (or even pets) significant to the client are the client's family. The nurse includes the family as an integral component of care in all healthcare settings.

Definitions and Functions of the Family

What is a **family**? The definitions of a family are changing as society changes. According to one definition, a family is a unit of people related by marriage, birth, or adoption (Duvall, 1977). A more comprehensive definition is that a family is composed of two or more people who are emotionally involved with each other and live in close geographical proximity. In a global society, it may not be possible for family members to live in close proximity, but they do remain emotionally involved.

Although every family is unique, all families have certain structural and functional features in common. Family structure (family roles and relationships) and family function (interactions among family members and with the community) provide the following:

■ *Interdependence.* The behaviors and level of development of individual family members constantly influence and are influenced by the behaviors and level of development of all other members of the family.

■ *Maintaining boundaries.* The family creates boundaries that guide its members, providing a distinct and unique family culture. This culture, in turn, provides values.

■ *Adapting to change.* The family changes as new members are added, current members leave, and the development of each member progresses.

■ *Performing family tasks.* Essential tasks maintain the stability and continuity of the family. These tasks include physical maintenance of the home and the people in the home, the production and socialization of family members, and the maintenance of the psychologic well-being of members.

Family Developmental Stages and Tasks

The family, like the individual, has developmental stages and tasks. Each stage brings change, requiring adaptation; each new stage also brings family-related risk factors for alterations in health. The nurse must consider the needs of the client both at a specific developmental stage and within a family with specific developmental tasks. Family developmental stages and developmental tasks are described next; related risk factors and health problems for each stage are listed in Table 2–7.

Couple

Two people, living together with or without being married, are in a period of establishing themselves as a couple. The developmental tasks of the couple include adjusting to living together as a couple, establishing a mutually satisfying relationship, relating to kin, and deciding whether to have children (in those of child-bearing age).

Family with Infants and Preschoolers

The family with infants or preschoolers must adjust to having and supporting the needs of more than two members. Other developmental tasks of the family at this stage are developing an attachment between parents and children, adjusting to the economic costs of having more members, coping with energy depletion and lack of privacy, and carrying out activities that enhance growth and development of the children.

TABLE 2–7 Family-Related Risk Factors for Alterations in Health

STAGE	RISK FACTORS	HEALTH PROBLEMS
Couple, or Family with Infants and Preschoolers	■ Lack of knowledge about family planning, contraception, sexual and marital roles ■ Inadequate prenatal care ■ Altered nutrition: inadequate nutrition, overweight, underweight ■ Smoking, alcohol/drug abuse ■ First pregnancy before age 16 or after age 35 ■ Low socioeconomic status ■ Lack of knowledge about child health and safety ■ Rubella, syphilis, gonorrhea, AIDS	Premature pregnancy Low-birth-weight infant Birth defects Injury to infant or child Accidents
Family with School-Age Children	■ Unsafe home environment ■ Working parents with inappropriate or inadequate resources for child care ■ Low socioeconomic status ■ Child abuse or neglect ■ Multiple, closely spaced children ■ Repeated infections, accidents, and hospitalizations ■ Unrecognized and unattended health problems ■ Poor or inappropriate nutrition ■ Toxic substances in the home	Behavior problems Speech and vision problems Learning disabilities Communicable diseases Physical abuse Cancer Developmental delay Obesity, underweight
Family with Adolescents and Young Adults	■ Family values of aggressiveness and competition ■ Lifestyle and behavior leading to chronic illness (substance abuse, inadequate diet) ■ Lack of problem-solving skills ■ Conflicts between parent and children	Violent death and injury Alcohol/drug abuse Unwanted pregnancy Suicide Sexually transmitted infections Domestic abuse
Family with Middle Adults	■ High-cholesterol diet ■ Overweight ■ Hypertension ■ Smoking, alcohol abuse ■ Physical inactivity ■ Personality patterns related to stress ■ Exposure to environment: sunlight, radiation, asbestos, water or air pollution ■ Depression	Cardiovascular disease (coronary artery disease and cerebral vascular disease) Cancer Accidents Suicide Mental illness
Family with Older Adults	■ Age ■ Depression ■ Drug interactions ■ Chronic illness ■ Death of spouse ■ Reduced income ■ Poor nutrition ■ Lack of exercise ■ Past environment and lifestyle	Impaired vision and hearing Hypertension Acute illness Chronic illness Infectious diseases (influenza, pneumonia) Injuries from burns and falls Depression Alcohol abuse

Family with School-Age Children

The family with school-age children has the developmental tasks of adjusting to the expanded world of children in school and encouraging educational achievement. A further task is promoting joint decision making between children and parents.

Family with Adolescents and Young Adults

The developmental tasks of the family with adolescents and young adults focus on transition. While providing a supportive home base and maintaining open communications, parents must balance freedom with responsibility and release adult children as they seek independence.

Family with Middle Adults

The family with middle adults (in which the parents are middle aged and children are no longer at home) has the developmental tasks of maintaining ties with older and younger generations and planning for retirement. If the family consists of just the middle-aged couple, they have the developmental task of reestablishing the relationship and (if necessary) acquiring the role of grandparents.

Family with Older Adults

The older adult family has the developmental tasks of adjusting to retirement, adjusting to aging, and coping with the loss of a spouse. If a spouse dies, further tasks include adjusting to living alone or closing the family home.

The Family of the Client with a Chronic Illness

The client with a chronic illness may be hospitalized for diagnosis and treatment of acute exacerbations, but the care of the client is primarily provided at home. Chronic illness in a family member is a major stressor that may cause changes in family structure and function, as well as changes in performing family developmental tasks.

Many different factors affect family responses to chronic illness; family responses in turn affect the client's response to and perception of the illness. Factors influencing response to chronic illness include personal, social, and economic resources; the nature and course of the disease; and demands of the illness as perceived by family members.

Support for the family is essential. The following information should be considered when performing any family assessment and developing a client's plan of care:

- Cohesiveness and communication patterns within the family
- Family interactions that support self-care
- Number of friends and relatives available
- Family values and beliefs about health and illness
- Cultural and spiritual beliefs
- Developmental level of the client and family.

It is important to remember that standardized teaching plans may not be effective. Rather, clients with chronic illnesses and their families should be given the freedom to choose appropriate literature, self-help or support groups, and interactions with others who have the same illness.

EXPLORE MEDIALINK

Prentice Hall Nursing MediaLink DVD-ROM
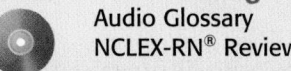
    Audio Glossary
    NCLEX-RN® Review

COMPANION WEBSITE www.prenhall.com/lemone

    Audio Glossary
    NCLEX-RN® Review
    Care Plan Activity: Family-Centered Care in Chronic Illness
    Case Studies
       Care Across the Lifespan
       Developing Teaching Programs
    MediaLink Applications
    Links to Resources

CHAPTER HIGHLIGHTS

- Health, an ever-changing state, is affected by genetic makeup; cognitive abilities and educational level; race, ethnicity, and cultural background; age, gender, and developmental level; lifestyle and environment; socioeconomic background; and geographic area.
- The emphasis of nursing has shifted from acute illness care in the hospital setting to preventive community-based care. An essential component of medical-surgical nursing is teaching health-promoting behaviors to promote and maintain functional health status.
- Illnesses may be acute or chronic, with behaviors of illness individualized within a fairly predictable sequence of experiencing symptoms, assuming the sick role, seeking medical help, assuming a dependent role, and achieving recovery and rehabilitation.

- Young adults are at risk for alterations in health from injuries, sexually transmitted infections, substance abuse, workplace exposure to pollutants, sun exposure, and psychologic stressors.
- Middle adults are at risk for alterations in health from obesity, cardiovascular disease, cancer, substance abuse, and the stresses of change and transition.
- Older adults are at risk for alterations in health from chronic illnesses (including hypertension, heart disease, cancer, and stroke), injuries, drug toxicities, and changes in income and marital status.
- The family is an integral component in planning and implementing nursing care for the adult client.

TEST YOURSELF NCLEX-RN® REVIEW

1 Which definition best describes wellness?
   1. a complete absence of disease
   2. depends on number of chronic illnesses
   3. never having to take medications
   4. actively practicing healthy behaviors

2 Many different factors affect the health of an individual. Which of the following are included? (Select all that apply.)
   1. genetic makeup
   2. cognitive abilities
   3. height
   4. age
   5. race

3 Which of the following diseases has a genetic basis?
   1. tuberculosis
   2. sickle cell disease
   3. appendicitis
   4. indigestion

4 Primary levels of prevention are general health promotion actions that prevent or delay the occurrence of a disease. Which of the following is a primary preventive activity?
   1. practicing safer sex
   2. having a screening for hypertension
   3. doing a self-breast examination
   4. having surgery

5 You call your instructor to say you have the "flu" and will not be in class. What level of illness behavior are you demonstrating?
   1. experiencing symptoms
   2. assuming the sick role
   3. seeking medical care
   4. assuming a dependent role

6 Your nephew was born with a heart defect. How would this disorder be classified?
   1. an acute illness
   2. a malignant illness
   3. an iatrogenic illness
   4. a congenital illness

7 Of the following descriptors, which is specific to a chronic illness?
   1. occurs rapidly
   2. lasts for a lifetime
   3. self-limiting
   4. lasts for a short time

8 Mr. Jones, age 50, is 30 pounds overweight, smokes, and rarely exercises. As a middle adult, these factors increase his risk for disorders of which body system?
   1. cardiovascular
   2. renal
   3. gastrointestinal
   4. nervous

9 You have been asked to present a health-related program at the local senior center. What would be an appropriate topic?
   1. the hazards of substance abuse
   2. accident prevention in the home
   3. family roles and tasks
   4. treating acute illness

10 Which of the following developmental tasks are a part of the life of a family with older adults if a spouse dies? (Select all that apply.)
   1. coping with lack of privacy
   2. planning for retirement
   3. adjusting to aging
   4. coping with loss
   5. relating to kin

See Test Yourself answers in Appendix C.

BIBLIOGRAPHY

Administration on Aging, U.S. Department of Health and Human Services. (2003). *Statistics: A profile of older Americans, 2003.* Retrieved from http://www.aoa.dhhs.gov/prof/Statistics/profile/2003/3_pf.asp

Administration on Aging. (2004). *Addressing diversity.* Retrieved from www.aoa.dhhs.gov/prof/adddiv/adddiv_pf.asp

American Association of Retired Persons. (2004). *Profile of older Americans, 2004.* Washington, DC: Resource Services Group.

American Cancer Society. (2004). *ACS cancer detection guidelines.* Retrieved from http://www.cancer.org/docroot/PE_2_3X_ACS_Cancer_Detectopm_Guidelines_36. . .

Centers for Disease Control and Prevention. (2003). *Preliminary data for 2003.* Washington, DC: U.S. Department of Health and Human Services.

D'Cruz, P. (2003). Family-focused interventions in health and illness. *Journal of Health Management, 5*(1), 37–56.

Dunn, H. (1959). High-level wellness for man and society. *American Journal of Public Health, 49,* 786–972.

Duvall, E. (1977). *Marriage and family development.* Philadelphia: Lippincott.

Edelman, C., & Mandle, C. (2006). *Health promotion throughout the lifespan* (6th ed.). St. Louis, MO: Mosby.

Eliopolous, C. (2004). *Gerontological nursing* (6th ed.). Philadelphia: Lippincott.

Erikson, E. (1963). *Childhood and society* (2nd ed.). New York: Norton.

Federal Citizen Information Center. (2004). *The food guide pyramid.* Retrieved from http://www.pueblo.gsa.gov/cic_text/food/food-pyramid/main.htm

Fowler, J. (1981). *Stages of faith: The psychology of human development and the quest for meaning.* New York: Harper & Row.

Freidman, M., Bowden, V., & Jones, E. (2003). *Family nursing: Research, theory and practice.* Upper Saddle River, NJ: Prentice Hall.

Havighurst, R. (1972). *Human development and education* (3rd ed.). New York: Longman.

Heitman, L. (2004). Social support and cardiovascular health in families. *Journal of Cardiovascular Nursing, 19*(1), 86–91.

Kohlberg, L. (1979). *The meaning and measurement of moral development.* New York: Clark University.

Leavell, H., & Clark, A. (1965). *Preventive medicine for doctors in the community.* New York: McGraw-Hill.

Lubkin, I., & Larsen, P. (2006). *Chronic illness: Impact and interventions* (6th ed.). Boston: Jones & Bartlett.

Miller, C. (2003). Safe medication practices: Nursing assessment of medications in older adults. *Geriatric Nursing, 24*(5), 314–315, 317.

_____. (2004). *Nursing for wellness in older adults: Theory and practice* (4th ed.). Philadelphia: Lippincott.

Miller, J. (2000). *Coping with chronic illness: Overcoming powerlessness* (3rd ed.). Philadelphia: F. A. Davis.

National Vital Statistics Reports. (2005, March 7). Table 1. Deaths, percentage of total deaths, and death rates for the 10 leading causes of death in selected age groups, by race and sex, United States, 2002. *National Vital Statistics Report, 53*(17), 13–14.

Pender, N., Parsons, M., & Murdaugh, C. (2006). *Health promotion in nursing practice* (5th ed.). Upper Saddle River, NJ: Prentice Hall.

Senior Site. (2004). *Learning to cope with chronic illness.* Retrieved from http://seniors-site.com/coping/chronic.html

Strauss, A., et al. (1984). *Chronic illness and the quality of life.* St. Louis, MO: Mosby.

Suchman, E. (1972). Stages of illness and medical care. In E. Jaco (Ed.), *Patients, physicians and illness.* New York: Free Press.

U.S. Department of Health and Human Services. (2000). *Healthy people 2010.* Washington, DC: Author.

Weitzel, E. A. (2001). Risk for poisoning: Drug toxicity. In M. Maas, K. Buckwalter, M. Hardy, T. Tripp-Reimer, M. Titler, & J. Specht (Eds.), *Nursing care of older adults: Diagnoses, outcomes, & interventions* (pp. 34–46). St. Louis, MO: Mosby.

Westerhoff, J. (1976). *Will our children have faith?* New York: Seabury Press.

World Health Organization. (1974). *Constitution of the World Health Organization: Chronicle of the World Health Organization.* Geneva: Author.

CHAPTER 3 Community-Based and Home Care of the Adult Client

LEARNING OUTCOMES

- Differentiate community-based care from community health care.
- Discuss selected factors affecting health in the community.
- Describe services and settings for healthcare consumers receiving community-based and home care.
- Describe the components of the home healthcare system, including agencies, clients, referrals, physicians, reimbursement, legal considerations, and nursing care.
- Compare and contrast the roles of the nurse providing home care with the roles of the nurse in medical-surgical nursing discussed in Chapter 1.
- Explain the purpose of rehabilitation in health care.

CLINICAL COMPETENCIES

- Provide client care in community-based settings and the home.
- Apply the nursing process to care of the client in the home.

MEDIALINK

Resources for this chapter can be found on the Prentice Hall Nursing MediaLink DVD-ROM accompanying this textbook, and on the Companion Website at http://www.prenhall.com/lemone

Health care is provided by medical-surgical nurses in a variety of settings. There are approximately 6,000 hospitals, 17,000 residential and long-term care providers, and more than 20,000 home care providers in the United States. Currently, only clients requiring complex surgery, who are acutely ill or seriously injured, or who are having babies are hospitalized and then only for a minimum period of time. As a result, most healthcare services are provided in settings outside the hospital. Those settings include clinics, schools, prisons, day care centers for children and seniors, offices, and homes. The discussion in this chapter focuses on selected community services and settings and home care.

People requiring healthcare services may access and use the system through a variety of providers and settings, including hospital-based outpatient care, community-based offices and clinics, and home care. In the healthcare system of the 21st century, hospitals are primarily acute care providers with services focused on high-technology care for severely ill or injured people or for people having major surgery. Even those clients rarely remain in the hospital for long. They are moved as rapidly as possible to less acute care settings within the hospital and then to community-based and home care. Health care has become a managed care, community-based system. Although many nurses are still employed in hospitals, they are increasingly providing nursing care outside of the acute care, in-hospital setting.

COMMUNITY-BASED NURSING CARE

A community may be a small neighborhood in a major urban city or a large area of rural residents. Communities are formed by the characteristics of people, area, social interaction, and common ties. Each community, however, is unique. People who live in a community may share a culture, history, or heritage. Although a community is where people live, have homes, raise families, and carry on daily activities, its members often cross community boundaries to work or to seek health care. Nurses who provide care within a community must know the composition and characteristics of the clients with whom they will work.

In contrast to community health nursing, which focuses on the health of the community, **community-based care** centers on individual and family healthcare needs. The nurse practicing community-based care provides direct services to individuals to manage acute or chronic health problems and to promote self-care. The care is provided in the local community, is culturally competent, and is family centered. The philosophy of community-based nursing directs nursing care for clients wherever they are, including where they live, work, play, worship, and go to school.

Nurses provide community-based care in many different ways and locations, ranging from leading support groups in a hospital (for individuals and family members diagnosed with such illnesses as cancer or diabetes) to managing a freestanding clinic to providing care at the client's home. Box 3–1 illustrates the varied settings within the community in which a nurse may provide care.

Factors Affecting Health in the Community

Many factors can affect the health of individuals in a community. These factors include social support systems, the community healthcare structure, environmental factors, and economic resources.

BOX 3–1 **Community-Based Nursing Care Settings**

- Hospitals
    - Outpatient (ambulatory) surgery
    - Outpatient diagnostics and treatments
    - Cardiac rehabilitation
    - Support groups
    - Education groups
- County health departments
- Senior centers
- Long-term care
- Parish nursing
- Adult day care centers
- Homeless shelters
- Mobile vans
- Mental health centers
- Schools
- Crisis intervention centers
- Ambulatory surgery centers
- Alcohol/drug rehabilitation
- Healthcare provider offices
- Healthcare clinics
- Free clinics
- Urgent care centers
- Rural health centers
- Home care
- Hospice care
- Industry
- Jails and prisons

Social Support Systems

A person's social support system consists of the people who lend assistance to meet financial, personal, physical, or emotional needs. In most instances, family, friends, and neighbors provide the best social support within the community. To understand the community social structure, the nurse needs to know what support is available for health care for the client and family, including neighbors, friends, their church, organizations, self-help groups, and professional providers. The nurse also must know and respect the cultural and ethnic background of the community.

Community Healthcare Structure

The healthcare structure of a community has a direct effect on the health of the people living and working within it. The size of the community often determines the type of services provided as well as the access to the services. For example, urban residents have various means of transportation to a variety of community healthcare providers, whereas rural residents must often travel long distances for any type of care. The financial base of the community is also important, often determining state and county funding of services.

Nurses who provide community-based care must know about public health services, the number and kind of health screenings offered, the location and specialty of healthcare professionals within the community, and the availability and accessibility of services and supplies. Other factors to consider include facilities (e.g., day care and long-term care), housing, and the number and kind of support agencies providing assistance (e.g., housing, shelter, and food).

Environmental Factors

The environment within which a person lives and works may have both helpful and harmful effects on health. Air and water quality differs across communities. Air pollution may occur across a large area or may be limited to the home. Within the home, pollution may occur from such sources as molds, pesticides, and fumes from new carpet. The water source also varies, with water supplies coming from rivers, lakes, reservoirs, or wells. Regardless of the source, chemical runoff or bacteria may contaminate water. It is critical to determine whether clients have a safe supply of running water.

Household and community safety and health resource accessibility are also important. Nurses must consider lighting; street, sidewalk, and road upkeep and conditions; effects of ice and snow; condition of stairs and floors; and usefulness and availability of bathroom facilities. Physical barriers to accessing community resources include lack of transportation, distance to services, and location of services.

Economic Resources

Economic resources encompass the financial and insurance coverages that provide the means to have health care within the community. As private medical insurance becomes more and more expensive, fewer citizens have it; and many U.S. citizens have no insurance at all. Most unskilled jobs do not provide healthcare benefits, resulting in a substantial percentage of what might be labeled "the working poor," those who have no

financial assistance for illness care or healthcare screenings from an employer. Older adults with fixed or limited incomes often find their monthly income consumed by medicines and medical supplies.

Medicare and Medicaid are health assistance programs created by 1965 Social Security amendments. Medicare is a federal health insurance plan designed to help with the acute care needs of people with disabilities and those over 65 years of age. This plan covers some services provided in hospitals, long-term facilities, and the home; however, many necessary healthcare components are not covered fully or at all, including adaptive equipment for safety, such as shower seats or raised toilet seats. Since January, 2006, those who receive Medicare, regardless of income, health status, or prescription drug usage have had access to prescription drug coverage. Coverage for care at home continues only as long as skilled providers are needed, and the person is not considered homebound even if he or she needs a wheelchair and assistance from others to leave the home. Medicaid is a state-run health insurance program for people with limited incomes. Each state has different benefits and criteria for coverage.

COMMUNITY-BASED HEALTHCARE SERVICES

Community-based healthcare services can take many forms. Selected examples are discussed in the following sections.

Community Centers and Clinics

Community centers and clinics may be directed by physicians, advanced practice nurses in collaboration with physicians, or advanced practice nurses working independently (depending on state regulations). These healthcare settings may be located within a hospital, be part of a hospital but located in another area, or be independent of a hospital base. Healthcare centers and clinics provide a wide range of services and often meet the health needs of clients who are unable to access care elsewhere. This group includes the homeless, the poor, those with substance abuse problems, those with sexually transmitted infections, and the victims of violent or abusive behavior.

Day Care Programs

Day care programs, such as senior centers, are usually located where people gather for social, nutritional, and recreational purposes. They may provide care for older adults with physical disabilities or mild Alzheimer's disease while family caregivers are at work. These programs vary among communities. Meals may be provided at low cost.

Parish Nursing

Parish nursing is a nontraditional, community-based way of providing health promotion and health restoration nursing interventions to specific groups of people. It meets the needs of people who are often underserved by the traditional healthcare system.

A nurse who practices parish nursing works with the pastor and staff of a faith community to promote health and healing through counseling, referrals, teaching, and assessment of healthcare needs. A parish nurse may be employed by a hospital and contracted by a church, be employed directly by a church, or work as a volunteer with the congregation of a church. The parish nurse helps bridge gaps between members of the church and the healthcare system.

Meals-on-Wheels

Many communities have a food service, usually called Meals-on-Wheels, for older people who do not have assistance in the home for food preparation. A hot, nutritionally balanced meal is delivered once a day, usually at noon. Volunteers often deliver the meals, providing not only nutrition but also a friendly, caring visit each day.

HOME CARE

Home care is not easily defined. It is not simply illness care at home, nor is it the act of setting up a hospital room in someone's house. The National Association for Home Care (NAHC) (2000) defines **home care** as services for people who are recovering, disabled, or chronically ill and who are in need of treatment or support to function effectively in the home environment. The U.S. Department of Health and Human Services places home care along a continuum of health care. Home care is provided in the client's place of residence for the purpose of promoting, maintaining, or restoring health or of maximizing the level of independence while minimizing the effects of disability and illness, including terminal illness.

Home care encompasses both health and social services provided to the person who is chronically ill, disabled, or recovering in his or her own home. Home care is usually provided when a person needs help that cannot be provided by a family member or friend. Among clients who benefit from home care services are those who:

- Cannot live independently at home because of age, illness, or disability.
- Have chronic, debilitating illnesses such as congestive heart failure, heart disease, kidney disease, respiratory diseases, diabetes mellitus, or muscle-nerve disorders.
- Are terminally ill and want to die with comfort and dignity at home.
- Do not need inpatient hospital or nursing home care but require additional assistance.
- Need short-term help at home for postoperative care.

The services provided in the home may include professional nursing care, care provided by home care aides, physical therapy, speech therapy, occupational therapy, medical social worker services, and nutritional services. Clients receiving home care services are usually under the care of a physician, with the focus of care being treatment or rehabilitation. Registered nurses or licensed practical nurses provide nursing care based on physician orders. These nurses give direct care, supervise other care providers, coordinate client care with the physician, advocate for the client and family, and teach family members and friends how to care for the client to assist the nurse as well as when professional services are no longer necessary.

Home care is both professional and technical. Professional home care is provided by people who are practice driven, licensed, certified, and/or have special qualifications. Nurses, therapists, social workers, and home aides are considered professional providers. Durable medical equipment companies (businesses that deliver medical equipment to homes) are technical providers. Technical home care providers are business and product driven. Customer satisfaction, field service, reimbursement, and profits are their primary concerns.

Brief History of Home Care

Many milestones marked the growth and development of home care in the United States. The passage of Medicare in 1965, Medicaid in 1970, the addition of hospice benefits in 1973, and the introduction of diagnosis-related groups (DRGs) in 1983 dramatically affected home care. Medicare legislation entitled the nation's elderly to home care services, primarily skilled nursing and other curative or restorative therapies. This same benefit was extended to certain younger Americans with disabilities in 1973.

The introduction of DRGs to help control healthcare costs greatly increased home care. DRGs are categories for reimbursement of inpatient services. The DRG system pays the same predetermined amount of money for the care of different persons with the same medical diagnosis. Many changes in the healthcare system have been attributed to the introduction of DRGs, including earlier discharge from hospitals and the increased need for home care services.

Hospice and Respite Care

Hospice care is a special component of home care, designed to provide medical, nursing, social, psychologic, and spiritual care for clients who are terminally ill and their families. Hospice care relies on a philosophy of relieving pain and suffering and allowing the client to die with dignity in a comfortable environment. Licensed nurses, medical social workers, physicians, occupational and physical therapists, and volunteers provide care. Hospice care is discussed in Chapter 5 ∞.

Respite care provides short-term or intermittent home care, often using volunteers. These services exist primarily to give the family member or friend who is the primary caregiver some time away from care. Respite care does much to relieve the burden of full-time caregiving.

The Home Care System

Nurses who practice home care do so within a system that includes home healthcare agencies, clients, referral sources, physicians, reimbursement sources, and legal considerations. The system is interactive and, like any other, functions best when its members communicate, cooperate, and collaborate with one another.

Types of Home Health Agencies

Home care agencies are either public or private organizations engaged in providing skilled nursing and other therapeutic services in the client's home. The several different types of home care agencies differ only in the way their programs are organized and

---

MEETING INDIVIDUALIZED NEEDS **The Client Being Discharged from Acute Care to Home Care**

QUESTIONS FOR CONSIDERATION

- Does the client need follow-up therapy, treatments, or additional education?
- What equipment, supplies, or information about community resources is necessary?
- What teaching materials can be sent home? Are they written at an acceptable reading level? Do they come in other languages?
- What cognitive abilities do the client and the caregiver seem to have? Are there any sensory deprivations that impede learning?

- Who will be the principal caregiver in the home? Is there one? Are all caregivers comfortable in doing what needs to be done? If not, what support do they need to become comfortable?
- Was the caregiver present during and included in instruction? How have the client and caregiver responded to health teaching thus far? Have they comprehended what has been taught? Was their stress level such that they could not listen?
- Has a devastating diagnosis and/or prognosis just been determined?
- Is high-technology intervention necessary?

---

administered. All home care agencies are similar in that they must meet uniform standards for licensing, certification, and accreditation. Home care agencies include the following:

- *Official or public agencies.* State or local governments operate these agencies, which are financed primarily by tax funds. Most official agencies offer home care, health education, and disease prevention programs in the community.
- *Voluntary or private not-for-profit agencies.* Donations, endowments, charities such as the United Way, and third-party (insurance company) reimbursement support these agencies. They are governed by a volunteer board of directors, which usually represents the community they serve.
- *Private, proprietary agencies.* Most of these agencies are for-profit organizations governed by either individual owners or national corporations. Although some participate in third-party reimbursement, others rely on clients paying their own bills (often called out-of-pocket expenses).
- *Institution-based agencies.* These agencies operate under a parent organization, such as a hospital. The home care agency is governed by the sponsoring organization and the mission of both is similar. Often, the majority of home care referrals come from the parent organization.

Home care agency personnel typically include administrators, managers, care providers (these may be experienced in social work, medical-surgical care, mental health care, or infusion services), and business office staff. Depending on the agency and geographic location, professional providers may include registered nurses, practical nurses, nurse practitioners, enterostomal therapists, physical therapists, occupational therapists, speech therapists, respiratory therapists, social workers, a chaplain or pastoral minister, dietitians, and home care aides. It is not unusual for clients to require the services of several professionals simultaneously. No matter how many providers are in the home, the responsibility for case coordination (also called case management) remains with the registered nurse.

Clients

The client in home care is the person receiving care and the person's family. The recognition that the family is also a client acknowledges the powerful influence that families exert on health. A client's family is not limited to persons related by birth, adoption, or marriage. In the home, family members may include lovers, friends, colleagues, other significant people, and even animals that hold the potential of greatly affecting the healthcare environment.

Age and functional disability are the primary predictors of need for home care services. Information from a national survey conducted by the Agency for Health Care Policy and Research found that about half of all home care clients are over the age of 65 and that the number of home care services that clients need seems to increase with age.

The old adage that discharge plans begin at admission makes more sense today than ever before. With shortened lengths of hospital stay, it is imperative for nurses to evaluate all clients for their ability to manage at home. Nurses preparing to send clients home must consider many of the questions outlined in the Meeting Individualized Needs box on this page.

Referrals

A **referral source** is a person recommending home care services and supplying the agency with details about the client's needs. The source may be a physician, nurse, social worker, therapist, or discharge planner. Families sometimes generate their own referrals, either by approaching one of the sources already mentioned or by calling a home care agency directly to make an inquiry. When the family seeks a referral and the agency believes that the client qualifies for services, usually the agency contacts the client's physician and requests a referral on the client's behalf.

The nurse may make a referral to either a home care agency, a hospice, or a community resource if the client seems to need formal follow-up beyond the present clinical setting. Hospital discharge planners, social workers, organizations for older adults, and local nonprofit agencies usually have a good command of the services and support groups available in their communities.

The nurse must talk to clients and their caregivers about concerns related to home management. It is not unusual for one family member to think that no additional help is necessary and for another to feel differently.

The nurse can facilitate an informal family meeting in which everyone shares concerns and can make inquiries about the family's insurance coverage for home care. Suggesting services that families cannot afford only adds to the problem. For clients with limited means, the nurse can consult with staff in the institution who are most knowledgeable about funding. In every instance, it is important that the nurse avoid making assumptions: Well-educated and financially secure clients can be just as overwhelmed by illness as clients who are poor and less learned. Everyone is a referral candidate.

If the family believes that no help is necessary and the nurse believes otherwise, then the nurse may ask the family to consider an evaluation visit, explaining how the situation may look different once the client is home. If family members continue to refuse, the nurse can let them know that the door is never closed and give them contacts in the community that they can access independently should their needs change.

Physicians

Home care cannot begin without a physician's order, nor can it proceed without a physician-approved treatment plan. This is a legal and reimbursement requirement. Only after a referral is made and an initial set of physician orders is obtained can a nursing assessment visit be scheduled to identify the client's needs. If the input of another provider, such as a physical therapist, is necessary to complete the initial assessment, then the nurse arranges for this visit.

At the nursing assessment visit, the nurse begins to formulate the plan of care. Box 3–2 lists Medicare's required data for the nursing plan of care. Once formulated, the nurse sends the plan of care back to the physician for review and approval. The physician's signature on the plan of care authorizes the home care agency's providers to continue with services and also serves as a contract indicating agreement to participate in the care of the client on an ongoing basis. The plan is reviewed as necessary, but at least once every 60 days.

Reimbursement for Services

A reimbursement source pays for home care services. Medicare is home care's largest single reimbursement source, although other sources exist (Medicaid, other public funding, private insurance, and public donation). The reimbursement source evaluates each treatment plan to determine if the goals and plans set forth by the professional providers match the needs assessed. Only interventions identified on the treatment plan are covered. Periodically the reimbursement source may ask for the home care provider's notes to substantiate what is being done in the home. This is one reason why accurate documentation is critical.

Medicare does not reimburse visits made to support general health maintenance, health promotion, or clients' emotional or socioeconomic needs. Both client and nurse must meet specific criteria to secure Medicare reimbursement. The client must meet all of the following criteria:

- The physician must decide that the client needs care at home and make a plan for home care.
- The client must need at least one of the following: intermittent (not full-time) skilled nursing care, physical therapy, speech language pathology services, or occupational therapy.
- The client must be homebound. This means leaving the home is a major effort. When leaving the home, it must be infrequent, for a short time, to get medical care, or to attend religious services.
- The home care agency must be Medicare approved.

Medicare will reimburse only when the skilled provider performs at least one of the following tasks:

- Teaching about a new or acute situation
- Assessing an acute process or a change in the client's condition
- Performing a skilled procedure or a hands-on service requiring the professional skill, knowledge, ability, and judgment of a licensed nurse (Figure 3–1 ■).

The reimbursement guidelines present problems because they are not sensitive to the full scope of nursing practice. Many of the client and family needs that nurses encounter during home visits are complex and time consuming, reflecting both intense psychosocial and economic concerns. This situation presents a profound dilemma. How are nurses to reconcile spending time on issues for which their agency will receive no payment? How are they to meet agency home visit productiv-

---

BOX 3–2 Medicare's Required Data for the Plan of Care

1. All pertinent diagnoses
2. A notation of the beneficiary's mental status
3. Types of services, supplies, and equipment ordered
4. Frequency of visits to be made
5. Client's prognosis
6. Client's rehabilitation potential
7. Client's functional limitations
8. Activities permitted
9. Client's nutritional requirements
10. Client's medications and treatments
11. Safety measures to protect against injuries
12. Discharge plans
13. Any other items the home health agency or physician wishes to include

Source: Data from Medicare Health Insurance Manual-11, Section 204.2.

Figure 3–1 ■ The home health nurse provides client and caregiver education. This nurse is teaching the client and family how to apply dressings.

ity standards when each home they enter requires more and more from them? How are they to document activities and interventions that are not considered "skilled"? There are no easy answers to these questions.

Legal Considerations

The legal considerations in home care center around issues of privacy and confidentiality, the client's access to health information, the client's freedom from unreasonable restraint, witnessing of documents, informed consent, and matters of negligence and/or malpractice. Numerous sources suggest that nurses can best avoid lawsuits by familiarizing themselves with the standards of practice, providing care that is consistent with both the standards and their agency's policies, and documenting all care fully and accurately according to agency guidelines.

Home care nurses are responsible for adhering to the same codes and standards that guide all other nurses. These codes and standards guide nursing practice and protect the public. In addition to these guidelines, other codes and statements give specific guidance on issues that affect care in the home.

The American Nurses Association (ANA) Standards for Home Health Nursing Practice are used in conjunction with the ANA Standards of Community Health Nursing as a basis for the practice of nursing in the home. The standards address the nursing process, interdisciplinary collaboration, quality assurance, professional development, and research. The standards speak to two levels of practitioners (the generalist, who is prepared on the baccalaureate level, and the specialist, who is prepared on the graduate level) and outline what achievements are expected of the professional nurse in the home.

Another source of guidance regarding home care is the NAHC Bill of Rights. Its use is a federal requirement for all home care agencies. Although they are permitted to make additions to the NAHC's original Bill of Rights, home care agencies are required by law to address the concepts in the NAHC Bill of Rights with all home care clients on the initial visit. The Bill of Rights is shown in Box 3–3.

BOX 3–3 Example of a Home Health Agency's Bill of Rights

The agency acknowledges the client's rights and encourages the client and family to participate in their plan of care through informed decision making. In accordance with this belief, each client/family member will receive, prior to admission, the following bill of rights and responsibilities.

1. The client and the client's property will be treated with respect by the program's staff.
2. The client will receive care without regard to race, color, creed, age, sex, religion, national origin, or mental or physical handicap.
3. The client has the right to be free from mental and physical abuse.
4. The client's medical record and related information is maintained in a confidential manner by the program.
5. The client will receive a written statement of the program's objectives, scope of services, and grievance process prior to admission.
6. The client, family, or guardian has the right to file a complaint regarding the services provided by the program without fear of disruption of service, coercion, or discrimination.
7. The client will be advised of the following in advance of service:
   a. Description of services and proposed visit frequency
   b. Overview of the anticipated plan of care and its likely outcome
   c. Options that may be available.
8. The client/family is encouraged to participate in the plan of care. The client will receive the necessary information concerning the client's condition and will be encouraged to participate in changes that may arise in care.
9. The program shall provide for the right of the client to refuse any portion of planned treatment to the extent permitted by law without relinquishing other portions of the treatment plan, except where medical contraindications exist. The client will be informed of the expected consequences of such action.
10. The client has a right to continuity of care:

a. Services provided within a reasonable time frame
b. A program that is capable of providing the level of care required by the client
c. Timely referral to alternative services, as needed
d. Information regarding impending discharge, continuing care requirements, and other services, as needed.
11. The client will be informed of the extent to which payment will be expected for items or services to be furnished to clients by Medicare, Medicaid, and any other program that is funded partially or fully with federal funds. Upon admission, the client will be informed orally and in writing of any charges for items and services that the program expects will not be covered upon admission. The client will be informed of any change in this amount as soon as possible, but no later than within 25 days after the program is made aware of the change.
12. Upon request, the client may obtain:
   a. An itemized bill
   b. The program's policy for uncompensated care
   c. The program's policy for disclosure of the medical record
   d. Identity of healthcare providers with which the program has contractual agreements, insofar as the client's care is concerned
   e. The name of the responsible person supervising the client's care and how to contact this person during regular business hours.
13. The client has the right to obtain medical equipment and other health-related items from the company of the client's choice and assumes financial responsibility for such. The program's staff will assist in obtaining supplies and physician approvals as needed.
14. The client/family is responsible for:
   a. Giving the program accurate, necessary information
   b. Being available and cooperative during scheduled visits
   c. Assisting, as much as possible, in the plan of care
   d. Alerting the staff to any problems as soon as possible.

The Nursing Process in Home Care

The nursing process used in home care is no different from that practiced in any other setting. The unique challenges of home care present themselves chiefly in the implementation step. Generally, the differences lie in assessing how the home's unique environment affects the need or problem and using outcome criteria and mutual participation to plan goals and interventions.

Assessment

In home care, nursing assessment and data collection center chiefly around the first home visit. This is not to say that nurses do not collect information on an ongoing basis, but because most agencies require the submission of a plan of care within 48 hours of the initial evaluation, the first visit carries tremendous weight. Under ideal circumstances, a preliminary review of background information initiates the assessment process; the reality in home care, however, is that few clients are referred with copies of either their medical records or their discharge summaries. If the client has received home care services in the past, records may be available, but often all the nurse has prior to initiating care is the referral form describing the present problem, some notations about past medical history, and a projection of the skilled interventions needed. Therefore, it falls to the nurse to try to obtain as complete a clinical picture as possible when meeting the client.

Assessment begins when the nurse calls the client to arrange a visit. This initial telephone call can yield much information to the nurse who pays close attention. For example:

- How alert, oriented, and stressed does the client (and/or family) seem to be?
- Does the client know the reason for the home care referral?
- How open to intervention do the client and family seem to be?
- Have they encountered any difficulties since discharge from the prior setting?
- Do they need any supplies on the first visit?

During the visit, much of the assessment process centers around collecting the information requested on the tools and forms contained in the agency's admission packet. These packets usually include a physical and psychosocial database; a medication sheet; forms for pain assessment, spiritual assessment, and financial assessment; and a family roster. It is extremely important that the data collected be as complete and accurate as possible and reflect subjective, objective, current, and historical information. Through interviewing, direct observation, and physical assessment, the nurse can achieve the goal of the initial visit, namely, to gain as clear and accurate a clinical picture of the client as possible.

Diagnosis

After completing the initial assessment, the nurse identifies the real and/or potential client problems that emerge from the data. Nursing diagnoses describing the client's health problems and needs, based on data collection, must be part of the home care record both to organize care and to justify reimbursement.

In almost all home care situations, *Deficient Knowledge* is an appropriate nursing diagnosis. Nursing interventions for this diagnosis specific to a client with Alzheimer's disease and the client's family can be found in the Meeting Individualized Needs box on the following page.

Planning

Planning in home care includes setting priorities, establishing goals, and deciding on intervention strategies designed to meet the needs of the client. The greatest level of success is achieved when clients feel an ownership of the suggested plan. For this reason, planned interventions and outcome criteria should be client centered, realistic, achievable, and mutually accepted. The nurse works with the client to:

- Identify significant issues and needs.
- Set mutually agreed-on goals (outcome criteria).
- Make and initiate acceptable plans to meet the goals.

Outcome criteria should be verbally stated to clients and documented clearly and concisely, in timed, measurable, and observable terms. These measures help clients and care providers to better focus their work together and evaluate the effectiveness of care. In addition, outcome criteria provide the reimbursement source a measurable standard from which to judge the appropriateness of the plan of care.

Implementation

The home care nurse implements most of the planned interventions, although some may be carried out by another agency provider, a paraprofessional introduced into the setting by the nurse case manager, or the client.

Nurses and clients reach an agreement about the implementation of care through a process called **contracting**, the negotiation of a cooperative working agreement between the nurse and client that is continuously renegotiated. Contracting is a concept used often in, but not exclusively by, many home and community health settings. Contracting can occur both formally and informally. It involves exploring a need, establishing goals, evaluating resources, developing a plan, assigning responsibilities, agreeing on a time frame, evaluating, and deciding to continue or terminate the plan. Contracting requires the nurse to relinquish control as the expert and consider the client as an equal partner in the process.

Contracting is not appropriate with all clients. It is certainly inadvisable if the nurse–client relationship is to be no more than two visits or if the client has limited cognitive abilities. However, contracting is useful for clients who demonstrate a willingness to be active participants in their health care. It is empowering, can save time, and keeps the nursing care goals directed and focused.

Evaluation

Evaluation in home care is both formative and summative. Formative evaluation is the systematic ongoing comparison of the plan of care with the goals actually being achieved from visit to visit. In summative evaluation, the nurse reviews the total plan of care and the client's progress toward goals to determine the client's eligibility for discontinuation of services.

Reimbursement guidelines may be helpful in driving the evaluation process. Because reimbursement sources require that all skilled services be justified, many home care agencies have designed their clinical notes to include areas for evalua-

MEETING INDIVIDUALIZED NEEDS **Family Home Care for the Older Adult with a Dementing Disorder**

NURSING DIAGNOSIS
Deficient Knowledge related to lack of information about Alzheimer's disease process and care

OUTCOME CRITERIA
Short term: Adequate knowledge, as evidenced by family's stating of disease progression and treatment (expected within 1 week)
Long term: Adequate knowledge, as evidenced by family's following of the recommended interventions throughout illness course (within 1 month) or by discharge from home health

INTERVENTIONS
■ Alert the family to both environmental hazards and client habits that could threaten safety. (first visit)
■ Provide the family with specific recommendations for keeping the client safe, for example, serving foods warm, not hot; allowing the client to eat with fingers; cutting food in small pieces; wearing an ID bracelet; discouraging daytime sleep. (first visit)
■ Discuss the disease course (degenerative), the prognosis (incurable), typical issues of concern (promoting adequate nutrition, activity, rest, safety, and independence); supporting cognitive function; communication, socialization, and family caregiving; the supportive care available; and the ultimate need for long-term placement with disease progression. (first visit)
■ Discuss local resources, including adult day care, support groups, and Alzheimer's Disease Association. Give family a list of these resources. (first visit)

■ Include all family members or significant persons in teaching and planning care. (each visit)
■ Prepare the family for typical types of Alzheimer's disease behaviors: forgetfulness, disorientation, agitation, screaming, crying, physical or verbal abuse, accusations of infidelity. (subsequent visits)
■ Teach the family specific interventions for dealing with these behaviors: calm, unhurried manner, music, stroking, rocking, structuring the environment, distracting the client. (subsequent visits)
■ Stress the importance of both exercise and recreation in terms of quality of life and decreasing nighttime restlessness. (subsequent visits)
■ Reinforce the client's continued needs for socialization and intimacy. (subsequent visits)
■ Suggest specific interventions for meeting socialization needs: limiting visitors to one or two at a time, pet therapy, use of the phone. (subsequent visits)
■ Suggest useful interventions that are described in the literature and/or that are utilized in more formal Alzheimer's disease settings and may also be helpful in the home. (subsequent visits)
■ Keep the environment safe for the client.
■ Use reality orientation with client several times a day, and post clocks, calendars, and telephone numbers within easy sight of the client.
■ Give client simple directions, using simple sentences and a quiet, monotone voice so as not to excite the client.
■ Allow the use of the telephone, because calls will help orient the client.

tion of the client's response to the visit's interventions and documentation of a plan of care for the next scheduled visit.

Roles of the Home Care Nurse

The role expectations of the home care nurse are similar to those of the professional nurse in any setting. On behalf of clients in the home, the nurse serves as an advocate, a provider of direct care, an educator, and a coordinator of services (see Chapter 1 ∞).

Advocate

As client advocate, the nurse explores, informs, supports, and affirms the choices of clients. Advocacy begins on the first visit, when the nurse discusses advance directives, living wills, and durable power of attorney for health care. The home care agency's Bill of Rights also needs to be discussed. During the course of care, clients may need help negotiating the complex medical system (especially in regard to medical insurance), accessing community resources, recognizing and coping with required changes in lifestyle, and making informed decisions. When the family's desires differ from the client's, advocacy can be a challenge. If a conflict arises, the nurse must remain the client's primary advocate.

In the home, there are no colleagues present to consult, to assist, or to rely on for support. The home is a practice setting

where nurses learn to trust their theoretical and intuitive knowledge and to be totally accountable.

Provider of Direct Care

Home care nurses usually are not involved in providing personal care for clients (bathing, changing linens, and so on). Family members often provide routine personal care, or the nurse may arrange for a home care aide. If a personal care need arises during the course of the skilled visit (e.g., if a client has an incontinent episode), the nurse typically either bathes and changes the client or assists the caregiver to do so before moving on to the skilled activities planned for the visit.

As a provider of direct care, the nurse uses the nursing process to assess, diagnose, plan care, intervene, and evaluate client needs. During the course of this process, home care nurses frequently are involved in performing specific procedures and treatments such as physical assessments, care of intravenous lines, ostomy care, wound care, and pain management.

Personal health habits, living conditions, resources, and support systems may leave much to be desired. It is not unusual for home care nurses to face unchanged dressings, under-treated infections, off-and-on self-medication, poor nutrition, filthy conditions, and unreliable caregivers. No matter how vigilant nurses may be, practice settings like these work against their best efforts. If the conditions cannot be changed,

Figure 3–2 ■ Home visits offer opportunities to work on health promotion. This nurse takes a client's blood pressure while visiting for an unrelated condition.

Source: Don Mason/Corbis Bettman.

the nurse may withdraw from the situation or continue to practice within the environment and report substandard care by caregivers.

Educator

Most of the home care nurse's time is spent teaching. Many nurses believe that their role as teacher is the crux of their nursing practice and that nurses in the home are always teaching (Figure 3–2 ■). For this reason, it is important that home care nurses develop expertise in the theory and principles of client education.

The greatest educational challenge may be motivating the client. Discovering what it takes to make the client want to learn and focusing the client on what is most important can tax the ingenuity of even the most dedicated nurse. Despite the work involved, nurses are rewarded by the knowledge that through their efforts, clients have learned to manage independently. Because the nurse's role as educator is becoming increasingly important, guidelines for community-based care are included in the discussion of each major disorder addressed in this textbook.

When preparing clients for discharge to home, the nurse focuses on safety and survival first. Even if health education is to continue with home care, a day or two may elapse before the nurse arrives, and clients must be able to manage by themselves until then. The nurse must not discharge clients without giving them the correct information and supplies to get them through the first few days at home. Additionally, clients should not be discharged without phone numbers and complete written information about their medications and the manifestations of complications they should report to their doctor or the nurse who discharged them. Finally, all clients should be able to at least minimally manage any necessary treatments. Management includes not only performing procedures safely but also knowing how to obtain necessary supplies in the community.

Clients need help understanding their situations, making healthcare decisions, and changing health behaviors. It is unrealistic, however, to believe that clients can be taught everything

they need to know during today's shortened hospital stays. The nurse should therefore recommend a home care referral for anyone in need of follow-up teaching. Prioritized teaching is essential: Even under the best of circumstances, clients generally forget about one-third of what is said to them, and their recall of specific instructions and advice is less than 50%. Comprehensive information related to client and family teaching is included in most of the following chapters in this textbook. This can be used as a guide in planning teaching.

Coordinator of Services

As coordinator of services, the home care nurse is the main contact with the client's physician and all other providers involved in the treatment plan. It is the responsibility of the registered nurse case coordinator (or clinical case manager) to report client changes, discuss responses, and develop and secure treatment plan revisions on an ongoing basis. This is accomplished both formally, through scheduled case and team conferences, and informally (often over the phone) with concerned providers. Documentation of all coordination activities is legally required.

Special Considerations in Home Care Nursing

Nursing practice in the home is a unique experience that differs in many ways from nursing practice in a hospital setting. The word *home* generates strong feelings of ownership, control, security, family history, independence, comfort, protection, and conflict. The family perceives a sharing of self when they consistently allow entry to a stranger. Because clients and nurses most often meet during periods of vulnerability and crisis, and because socializing is such an integral part of the home visit process, nurse providers are often perceived as friends or extended family members, blurring the boundaries of practice.

Nurses are invited into homes. Nurses are guests and cannot assume entry, as they do in formal clinical settings. The environment belongs to the client, who retains control. Every nursing action must communicate respect for these boundaries. To negotiate both repeated entry and a share of power in the client's domain, the nurse must establish trust and rapport quickly. This is often difficult, because most home care nurses are with each client for only 1 hour a few times a week.

During the course of establishing rapport and getting to know each other as people, the nurse–client relationship often becomes something more. Nurses and clients end up giving to each other and learning from each other. By connecting as human beings, they touch each other's spirits in profound ways (Carson, 1989). In home health, it is not unusual for nurses to realize suddenly not only that they do things to create a healing environment but also that their very presence has become the healing environment.

Over time, as the nurse becomes a familiar presence and the family's behavior relaxes, the nurse can gain a clearer and more complete picture of family relationships, dynamics, lifestyle choices, and coping patterns. Multigenerational behavior patterns are more obvious, and working around them can become quite a feat.

Today, more older adults are living alone. Some may have current or potential caregivers nearby, whereas others, for any of various reasons, have no one. These people often require considerable nursing support to remain strong, independent, and resourceful. Caring for "families of one" can take a toll on even the strongest home care nurse. Some nurses have reported calling between visits, keeping in touch after discharge, and driving by on days off because they have such difficulty "letting go" of their concerns about these clients.

Caregiver burden is not easily hidden in the home. In more than 22 million American households, people are taking care of relatives and friends with disabilities (Administration on Aging, 2003b). Many of these caregivers are themselves older adults. Healthcare planners visualize the home as a place where all kinds of medical services can occur but may give little thought to how people manage. Few ever ask whether families can cope with the level of care they are expected to assume. Caregiving has only recently been acknowledged as a complex activity, requiring adjustment in family living patterns, relationships, and finances. For some families, the crisis of caregiving is short lived, but for others it lasts for years. As a result, caregivers are at great risk for both physical and emotional illness. Because the success of home care depends heavily on the supports in place, addressing the needs of the support network is imperative.

Nursing Interventions to Ensure Competent Home Care

Despite differences in the setting, nursing care for clients in their homes is a highly rewarding clinical practice. The following discussion provides practical information for competent care with successful outcomes.

Establish Trust and Rapport

To establish trust and rapport in the client's home, nurses must try to find common ground and to let go of ethnocentric ("My culture's way is the best way") views. Nurses must be sure everything they say and do communicates an understanding that they are guests—offering suggestions in a way that acknowledges the client's right to say no, sensing and honoring "where people are in their situation," maintaining a respectful distance, and noticing and honoring family customs ("I see that no one wears shoes in your house; I'll take mine off, too."). Nurses should try to negotiate their schedules around the family's needs; nursing should enhance family coping, not complicate it. Above all, nurses should validate clients' illness experiences, remembering that everyone needs someone who is willing to listen and say, "I hear what you are saying, and I think I have a sense of how you feel."

Proceed Slowly

The nurse must enter the home with an awareness that the first contact is important. On the first nursing visit, the nurse can suggest to clients that they have someone else present "to help them listen." To avoid overwhelming clients with too much information, the nurse stresses the essential information and repeats it on subsequent visits. When making suggestions, the nurse offers clients the pluses and minuses of each alternative. Informed decisions are difficult to make if people are too overwhelmed to think of their options. The nurse speaks slowly, directly, and within the client's range of vision (the client may have to lip-read) and refrains from shouting at clients who have hearing impairments. The nurse must allow time for families to process new information.

Set Goals and Boundaries

The nurse explores clients' expectations of home care. In particular, the nurse explains the primary goal (to achieve self-care), defines nurse and client roles within this framework, and discusses limitations. The nurse may make statements such as "No, a home care nurse is not the same as a private duty nurse" and "Home care nurses do not routinely do that, but today I will make an exception." It is important for the nurse to stress mutual accountability, choice, and negotiation as part of the process.

Assess the Home Environment

The nurse surveys the overall home environment, using common sense, intuition, and imagination. Among the variables to note are sights, sounds, smells, dress, tone of voice, body language, and the use of touch; visiting patterns among family members; significant relationships; what is sacred and what is not; the appearance of the house, yard, sidewalk, and neighborhood; and the effect of illness on the family. The nurse asks questions and listens carefully to stories and offhand remarks.

Set Priorities

It is important that nurses be flexible and realize they cannot tackle everything. Although it is necessary to enter the home with a plan in mind, nurses must be prepared to modify the plan according to conditions they encounter once inside. Safety, issues that are of concern to clients, and those problems that can most easily be solved should be addressed first. Alternatively, the nurse can focus on safety first, then short-term and long-term goals. If the priorities that are set are primarily the nurse's and not the client's, then they may not be met.

Promote Learning

Instead of just teaching the client, the nurse tries actively to promote the client's ability to learn by, for example, identifying what is most important to the client and teaching that. Survival takes first priority; the nurse teaches the information people need to ensure their safety until the next visit. The nurse prioritizes material on a needs-to-know, wants-to-know, ought-to-know basis, assessing and responding to learner readiness.

Timing is important; people who are not ready to listen cannot be taught. In addition, the nurse must allow a sufficient amount of time to teach, ask clients how and when they learn best, use appropriate methods and materials when possible, and capitalize on clients' frustrations and desires to regain control of self-care. When possible, the nurse teaches while providing care.

The nurse can empower clients to learn by talking them through learning tasks, encouraging them to listen to their own bodies and to ask questions, and urging them to write thoughts and questions about their care and have them ready for the next visit or doctor's appointment.

Limit Distractions

Homes are full of events or circumstances that may divert attention from the job at hand. Such distractions as children, animals, noise, clutter, and mannerisms that are controlling, manipulative, or aggressive can try even the most experienced nurse. However, environmental and behavioral distractions can yield useful information about people, their relationships, and their values. For example, a dirty house could indicate a lack of interest in housekeeping, outright neglect and abuse, depression, or increased disability.

Distractions should be limited as much as possible. For example, the nurse might ask a client, "May I please turn off your television while we visit?" or "I would like to schedule my next visit for a time when the children are in school. Is that all right with you?" The nurse must be truthful about allergies, fear of a client's pet, or difficulty hearing in a particular room, but should not debate the priority of the visit over the distraction (such as a favorite television show). The nurse may not change the client's views and may also risk losing the client's trust and rapport. If all efforts at limiting distractions fail, the nurse should leave the home and return on another day: "I can see this is not going to work for us today. I will need to leave."

If any distraction originates with the nurse, such as fear of harm, reaction to the client's lifestyle, preoccupation with role, or a feeling of being overwhelmed by the situation in the home, the nurse should seek out a colleague to discuss the problem. Often, another perspective helps when dealing with the issue.

Put Safety First

Safety assessment in the home is a nursing responsibility and a legal requirement. Nurses cannot close their eyes to an unsafe environment. Upon entering the home and on a continuing basis, it is imperative that the nurse alert the family to unsafe and hazardous conditions, suggest remedies, and document in the clinical record the family's response to the nurse's suggestions. See Box 3–4 for a sample home safety assessment list. In particular, nurses must remain alert to:

- How clients handle stairs
- How clients manage their own care if they are alone

- The presence of a smoke detector in the home
- The presence of bathroom safety equipment
- Electrical hazards
- Slippery throw rugs, clutter, or a furniture arrangement that may cause a fall
- A supply of expired medications
- Inappropriate clothing or shoes
- Cooking habits that may precipitate a fire
- An inadequate food supply
- Poorly functioning utilities
- Chipping paint
- Signs of abusive behavior

Nurses cannot go into homes and change the family's living space and lifestyle, but they can register their concern and react appropriately if the situation suggests that an injury is about to occur or if they suspect abuse or neglect. In the home and community setting, ignoring an unsafe environment is considered nursing negligence.

The disposal of toxic medications and sharp objects (such as needles used for injections) is also a safety issue in the home, especially if young children are present. Once again, it is imperative that the nurse address this with the client, demonstrate safe disposal, and provide the necessary equipment to accomplish that end. Documentation should address what information the nurse has covered, the family's response to the teaching, and assessment of the family's ongoing practice of safety precautions.

Nurses must focus on safety and survival first, for themselves as well as their clients, in all that they do. When traveling in the community, the nurse takes such precautions as keeping car doors locked, having a cellular phone, keeping supplies out of sight, and staying inside the car in potentially dangerous situations. Colleagues, families, and community members can offer useful guidelines for maintaining safety and self-protection.

Make Do

Nurses must learn to be resourceful and cost conscious with equipment, supplies, and services in the home. When needing to make do or improvise, they should do so in a low-key manner to avoid causing the family additional anxiety. The nurse must make

---

BOX 3–4 Home Safety Assessment Checklist

General Household Safety
1. Do stairwells and halls have good lighting?
2. Do staircases have handrails on both sides?
3. Are rugs securely tacked down?
4. Is the telephone readily accessible? Is the dial easy to read?
5. Are electrical cords in good condition and out of the way?
6. Is furniture sturdy?
7. Is the temperature of the home comfortable?
8. Are protective screens in front of fireplaces or heating devices?
9. Are smoke detectors and carbon monoxide detectors present and working?

Bathroom
1. Are grab bars present in the tub and/or shower? Around the toilet?

2. Are toilet seats high enough?
3. Are nonskid materials (rugs, mats) on the floor, tub/shower?
4. Are medications stored safely? Out of the reach of children?
5. Is the water temperature safe?
6. Are electrical outlets and appliances a safe distance from the tub?

Kitchen
1. Are floors slippery? Are nonskid rugs used?
2. Is the stove in good working order?
3. Is the refrigerator in good working order? Clean?
4. Are electrical outlets overloaded with appliance cords?
5. Are sharp objects kept in a special container or safe area?
6. Is food storage adequate? Clean?
7. Are cleaning materials stored safely?

every effort to convey the message that the situation is under control; after leaving the home, the nurse can react as necessary.

Control Infection

Infection control in the home centers around protecting clients, caregivers, and the community from the spread of disease. Within the home, nurses may encounter clients with infectious or communicable diseases, clients who are immunocompromised, and/or clients having multiple access devices, drainage tubes, or draining wounds. The home presents a challenging environment in which to practice infection control for several reasons: Families typically are set in their own ways of doing things; caregivers often lack any formal education on the subject; the setting itself may not be conducive; and the facilities for even the most basic of aseptic practices (hand washing) may be lacking. Without a doubt, the single most important nursing intervention in controlling infection is health teaching. Clients and caregivers need to know the importance of effective hand washing, the effective use of gloves, proper disposal of wastes and soiled dressings, proper handling of linens, and the practice of standard precautions. Unfortunately, the imparting of important information does not always bring about a change in behavior. Trying to change a family's values frequently demands a great deal of ingenuity from the nurse.

REHABILITATION

Rehabilitation is the process of learning to live to one's maximum potential with a chronic impairment and its resultant functional disability. Rehabilitation nursing is based on a philosophy that each person has a unique set of strengths and abilities that can enable that person to live with dignity, self-worth, and independence. Nursing care to promote rehabilitation primarily focuses on clients with chronic illnesses or impairments. Rehabilitation most often begins in the acute phase of an illness or injury.

The terms *impairment, disability,* and *handicap* are often used as synonyms, but they have different meanings. An **impairment** is a disturbance in structure or function resulting from physiologic or psychologic abnormalities. A **disability** is the degree of observable and measurable impairment. A **handicap** is the total adjustment to disability that limits functioning at a normal level (Stanhope & Lancaster, 2006). For example, following a motorcycle accident, a client had damage to her left leg that resulted in an impairment in the ability to flex her knee. This resulted in a 50% disability of that leg and caused a handicap, because the client was a school bus driver and could no longer operate the bus safely.

Rehabilitation promotes reintegration into the client's family and community through a team approach. Many different aspects of the client's life are included in the plan of care, including physical function, mental health, interpersonal relationships, social interactions, family support, and vocational status. This comprehensive consideration of the client requires the expertise of a team of healthcare providers, who usually meet weekly to discuss the achievement of client goals.

Assessment of the client and family includes functional health level and self-care abilities, educational needs, psychosocial needs, and the home environment. It is critical to determine the priorities of needs from the client and family perspective before establishing any plan of care. The nurse assesses the client's level of physical function, goals, concerns, stage of loss, home environment, and available resources.

Interventions to facilitate rehabilitation are revised to meet client and family needs as the client progresses toward reintegration. In general, interventions are planned and implemented to prevent complications, assist in achieving a realistic level of independence, educate the client and family about home care, and make referrals to community agencies (for nursing care, special equipment or supplies, support groups, counseling, physical therapy, occupational therapy, respiratory therapy, vocational guidance, house cleaning, meals).

EXPLORE MediaLink

Prentice Hall Nursing MediaLink DVD-ROM
 Audio Glossary
 NCLEX-RN® Review

COMPANION WEBSITE www.prenhall.com/lemone
 Audio Glossary
 NCLEX-RN® Review
 Care Plan Activity: Home Health Assessment
 Case Study: Safety in the Home
 MediaLink Application: Home Nursing Care Strategies
 Links to Resources

CHAPTER HIGHLIGHTS

■ In contrast to community health, which focuses on the health of a population, community-based care focuses on individual and family healthcare needs. Services are provided in many different settings and by various programs, including community centers and clinics, day care programs, parish nursing, and Meals-on-Wheels.

- Factors affecting health in the community include social support systems, community healthcare structures, the environment, and economic resources.
- Home care is defined as services for people who are recovering, disabled, or chronically ill and who are in need of treatment or support to function effectively in the home environment.
- Two special components of home care are hospice care and respite care.
- The home care system includes agencies, clients, referral sources, physicians, reimbursement sources, and legal considerations.

- The roles of the home care nurse include advocate, provider of direct care, educator, and coordinator of services.
- Nursing interventions to ensure competent care include those used to establish trust and rapport, proceed slowly, set goals and boundaries, assess the home environment, set priorities, promote learning, limit distractions, put safety first, and control infection.
- Rehabilitation is the process of learning to live to one's maximum potential with a chronic health impairment and its resultant disability.

TEST YOURSELF NCLEX-RN® REVIEW

1 What is the focus of community-based nursing care?
1. the function of the community
2. the health of the community
3. individual and family health
4. older adult needs and services

2 One way in which urban and rural residents may differ is:
1. access to healthcare services.
2. age and gender of residents.
3. family tasks and values.
4. ability to follow directions.

3 What is the name given to nursing care provided by a faith community to promote health and healing?
1. respite care
2. parish nursing
3. block nursing
4. day care

4 Which of the following services helps relieve the stress of full-time caregiving?
1. parish nursing
2. block nursing
3. day care
4. respite care

5 Home health care provides care to clients with a wide variety of healthcare needs. Which of the following clients would benefit from home care? (Select all that apply.)
1. Mrs. Jones, age 78, has broken her hip and cannot live independently at home.
2. Miss Ace, age 18, has had surgery for an infected appendix.
3. Mr. Strip, age 52, has a terminal illness and wants to die at home.
4. Miss Taylor, age 35, living alone, has had major abdominal surgery.
5. Mr. Wines, age 80, has some weakness from arthritis.

6 While making the first home health visit, the nurse discusses advance directives, living wills, and durable power of attorney for health care. These topics are part of which nursing role?
1. provider of direct care
2. coordinator of services
3. educator
4. advocate

7 Which of the following home health agency personnel is responsible for care coordination?
1. physician
2. social worker
3. home health aide
4. registered nurse

8 What agency is the largest single reimbursement source for home care?
1. Medicare
2. Medicaid
3. private insurance
4. self-pay

9 Nurses practicing in the home provide teaching for a variety of topics. Which of the following teaching areas is essential to maintaining infection control?
1. fire and smoke detectors
2. hand washing
3. uncluttered floors and stairs
4. medications

10 What element of home care is a requirement of reimbursement?
1. family member approval
2. completion of agency forms
3. physician's order
4. treatment plan

See Test Yourself answers in Appendix C.

BIBLIOGRAPHY

Administration on Aging, U.S. Department of Health and Human Services. (2003a). *Hospice care*. Retrieved from http://www.aoa.dhhs.gov
_____. (2003b). *National family caregiver support program*. Retrieved from http://www.aoa.dhhs.gov
American Nurses Association. (1998). *Scope and standards of parish nursing practice*. Washington, DC: Author.
_____. (1999). *Scope and standards of home health nursing practice*. Washington, DC: Author.
Bryant, R. (2002). Evidence-based health care in home care. *Caring, 21*(6), 6–8.
Carson, V. (1989). *Spiritual dimensions of nursing practice*. Philadelphia: Saunders.
Cho, S. (2005). Older people's willingness to use home care nursing services. *Journal of Advanced Nursing, 51*(2), 166–173.
Clemen-Stone, S., McGuire, S., & Eigsti, D. (2002) *Comprehensive community health nursing: Family,*

aggregate and community practice (6th ed.). St. Louis, MO: Mosby.
Collier, E., & Harrington, C. (2005). Discharge planning, nursing home placement, and the Internet. *Nursing Outlook, 53*(2), 95–102.
Health Care Financing Administration. (2003). *Managed care in Medicare and Medicaid. Fact sheet*. Washington, DC: U.S. Department of Health and Human Services.
Hoare, K. (2004). Care home placement: Can admission direct from acute hospital be justified? *Nursing Older People, 16*(6), 14–17.
Medicare. (2004). Long-term care. Retrieved from http://www.medicare.gov/LongTermCare/Static/TypesOverview.asp
National Association for Home Care. (2000). *How to choose a home care provider. What are my rights as a patient?* Retrieved from http://www.nahc.org

Naylor, M., Stephens, C., & Bixby, M. (2005). Cognitively impaired older adults: From hospital to home. *American Journal of Nursing, 105*(2), 52–62.
North American Nursing Diagnosis Association. (2005). *Nursing diagnoses: Definitions and classification 2005–2006*. Philadelphia: Author.
Stanhope, M., & Lancaster, J. (2006). *Foundations of nursing in the community* (2nd ed.). St. Louis, MO: Mosby.
U.S. Department of Health and Human Services. (2004). *Medicare and home health care* (Pub. No. CMS-10969). Baltimore, MD: Centers for Medicare & Medicaid Services.
_____. (2005). *Medicare & you 2005*. Washington, DC: Author.
Wilkinson, J. (2005). *Prentice Hall nursing diagnosis handbook with NIC interventions and NOC outcomes*. Upper Saddle River, NJ: Prentice Hall.

UNIT 1 BUILDING CLINICAL COMPETENCE
Dimensions of Medical-Surgical Nursing

FUNCTIONAL HEALTH PATTERN: Health Perception-Health Management

■ Think about clients with altered health perception or health management for whom you have cared in your clinical experiences.

> ■ What were the clients' major medical diagnoses (e.g., hypertension, diabetes mellitus, cancer, chronic obstructive pulmonary disease, stroke, or alcoholism)?
> ■ What manifestations did each of these clients have? Were these manifestations similar or different?
> ■ How did the clients' healthcare behaviors interfere with their health status? Did they have yearly physical examinations and routine eye examinations? Did they obtain recommended immunizations? Did they use preventive measures, such as conducting breast or testicular self-examinations, applying sunscreen, following dietary recommendations, decreasing alcohol intake, stopping smoking, beginning to exercise regularly, practicing safer sex, using stress reduction activities? Did they achieve developmental tasks appropriate for their age? Did they interact well with family and friends?

■ The Health Perception-Health Management Pattern includes healthcare behaviors, such as health promotion and illness prevention activities, medical treatments, and follow-up care. Individuals are at different locations on the illness–wellness continuum at specific points in time. Health perception and health maintenance are affected by factors that influence the individual's health status or level of wellness in two primary ways:

> ■ Factors affecting health that may be altered to prevent disease processes are diet (e.g., osteoporosis), substance abuse (e.g., alcoholism), smoking (e.g., chronic obstructive pulmonary disease, lung cancer), socioeconomic status (e.g., communicable disease, violence or abuse), or occupational exposure (e.g., pulmonary disease due to asbestos, tuberculosis).
> ■ Factors affecting health that cannot be altered and may result in disease processes are genetics (e.g., sickle cell disease, hemophilia), age (e.g., type 2 diabetes mellitus, myocardial infarction), or race (e.g., hypertension).

■ A client's perceived pattern of health and well-being affects how health is managed. Improper health management affects the body's ability to maintain homeostasis, leading to manifestations such as:

> ■ Vomiting (caused by a variety of factors, including ingestion of chemicals, toxic materials, or infectious materials; chronic liver or kidney disease, and allergic responses to medications)
> ■ Bleeding (as from trauma or decreased platelets or deficient clotting factors ► resulting in the delay of activation or inability to activate the clotting pathway ► causing loss or leakage of blood)
> ■ Pain (resulting from many physical factors, including trauma, edema, and changes in pH or inflammatory changes ► which may cause tissue damage that stimulates pain receptors ► which transmit pain impulses to the brain).

■ Priority nursing diagnoses within the Health Perception-Health Management functional health pattern that may be appropriate for clients include:

> ■ *Health-Seeking Behaviors* as evidenced by making dietary changes as prescribed, decreasing alcohol intake, stopping smoking, and joining a health club to participate in an exercise program
> ■ *Deficient Knowledge: Healthy Behaviors* as evidenced by lack of interest in learning about health care, inability to understand healthcare teaching (developmental level), and misinterpretation of healthcare teaching completed
> ■ *Ineffective Health Maintenance* as evidenced by smoking, drinking alcohol or other substance abuse, sedentary lifestyle, and not seeking routine health care
> ■ *Risk for Injury* related to poor hygiene habits, self-treatment of illnesses, not taking prescribed medications, and participating in risk-taking behaviors.

■ Two nursing diagnoses from other functional health patterns often are of high priority for the client with deficits in Health Perception-Health Management:

> ■ *Self-Care Deficit* (Activity/Exercise)
> ■ *Situational Low Self-Esteem* (Self-Perception/Self-Concept)

CLINICAL SCENARIO

You have been assigned to work with the following home healthcare clients on the day shift. Significant data obtained during report are as follows:

- Mrs. Cora Clark is a 76-year-old woman with a prolapsed uterus. She uses a pessary to keep her uterus in place but the pessary fell out last night. You will need to replace it today because her uterus is prolapsing without it in place.
- Tom Smith is a 19-year-old man who is at home due to osteomyelitis in the left leg from a previous leg fracture obtained in a motorcycle–motor vehicle crash. You need to change his left leg dressing and administer IV vancomycin (Vancocin), which is to be given every 12 hours.

- Marguerite Garcia is an 86-year-old Hispanic woman who has hypertension, type 2 diabetes mellitus, and congestive heart failure. She is to have her blood pressure taken and a glucometer check done for her blood sugar level. You will need to make sure she is taking her prescribed medications and set up her medications for the week.
- Sebastian Huian is a 56-year-old Asian man who had a stroke that left him with left-sided weakness and some speech difficulties. He speaks little English. He is being discharged from the rehabilitation unit this morning. You will be doing an intake at the first home health visit to determine what his needs will be and how much assistance he will need from home health.

Questions

1 In what order would you visit these clients after report?
1. _____
2. _____
3. _____
4. _____

2 What top two priority nursing diagnoses would you choose for each of the clients presented above? Can you explain, if asked, the rationale for your choices?

	Priority Nursing Diagnosis #1	Priority Nursing Diagnosis #2
Cora Clark		
Tom Smith		
Marguerite Garcia		
Sebastian Huian		

3 The priority nursing diagnosis for Mrs. Clark is:
1. *Risk for Infection*
2. *Self-Care Deficit*
3. *Anxiety*
4. *Disturbed Body Image*

4 Mrs. Garcia understands the preventive teaching done by the nurse when she states:
1. "I will take my antihypertensive medication on a daily basis."
2. "I will walk on the days the weather is warm and dry."
3. "I will keep my doctor's appointments as scheduled."
4. "I will check my blood sugar every other day."

5 The nurse explains a diet of low-sodium foods to Mrs. Garcia. She understands this diet when she picks which meal plan?
1. Spanish rice with canned tomatoes, peppers, and onions
2. tacos with ground beef, lettuce, tomatoes, and salsa
3. burritos with beans, meat, and cheese
4. fajitas with lean beef, peppers, tomatoes, onions

6 What role is the nurse demonstrating when performing the home health intake evaluation on Mr. Huian?
1. educator
2. caregiver
3. advocate
4. manager

7 The tertiary level of prevention focuses on stopping the disease process and returning the affected client to a useful place in society. Which is an example of a tertiary level of prevention for Mr. Huian?
1. eating a nutritious diet to promote healing and gain more strength

2. having screenings for other disease processes, such as hypertension
3. enrolling in a work training program for individuals with extremity weakness
4. eliminating the use of tobacco and alcohol

8 Nursing interventions to ensure competent home care for Mr. Huian include: (Select all that apply.)
1. establish trust and rapport
2. have his 14-year-old son translate for him
3. assess the home environment for safety
4. discuss having family members feed him due to his left arm weakness
5. set goals for home health care and rehabilitation

9 Changing Tom Smith's dressing and administering the IV antibiotics demonstrates which part of the nursing process?
1. assessment
2. planning
3. implementation
4. evaluation

10 Tom Smith's family will be involved in planning and implementing his nursing care. What is the most important information to consider when assessing the family and developing a plan of care for him?
1. family interactions that are cohesive, communicative, and support self-care
2. family member roles and developmental stages and tasks
3. number of friends or relatives who will be available to assist
4. family's ability to adapt to change and ability to perform tasks

11 A client with a terminal illness has advanced directives stating no procedures or feedings for end-of-life care. On rounds, you find a nurse giving the client a tube feeding. What interventions should you carry out first?
1. Notify the supervisor and the physician about the nurse feeding the client.
2. Notify the family to change the advance directive.
3. Talk to the nurse about the client's advance directives and discuss why the nurse is feeding the client.
4. Ignore that you saw the nurse feeding the client and continue with your client care.

12 The nursing process is a reference system for improving clinical practice and evaluating quality of nursing care. Benefits for the client receiving nursing care are that the client: (Select all that apply.)
1. receives planned, individualized interventions.
2. is ensured continuity of care.
3. does not need to participate in the process.
4. has increased satisfaction in care.
5. is ensured quality of care.

CASE STUDY

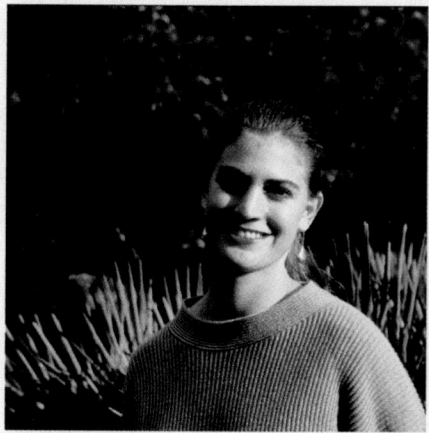

Betty Jo Moore is a 20-year-old woman who is admitted to the women's health unit for treatment of lower abdominal pain, chills, and foul-smelling vaginal discharge. During the admission assessment she states that she is unmarried and has been sexually active for the past three years with multiple sexual partners. Vital signs are T 100.4°F, P 92, R 22, BP 118/76. Lab studies drawn in the emergency department indicate a WBC count of 25,000 mm³, an erythrocyte sedimentation rate of 22 mm/h, and a positive C-reactive protein. She is to begin antibiotic therapy and needs education about safer sex practices.

Ms. Moore is diagnosed with pelvic inflammatory disease. The pathophysiology of pelvic inflammatory disease is as follows: pathogenic microorganisms enter the vagina during intercourse or other sexual activity and alter the cervical mucosa, allowing the microorganisms to travel to the uterus, the fallopian tubes, and the ovaries. Multiplication of the microorganisms results in infection and possibly abscess formation. Manifestations of pelvic inflammatory disease include fever, chills, purulent vaginal discharge, vaginal bleeding, severe lower abdominal pain, pain on movement of the cervix, and dysuria. Complications that can occur from pelvic inflammatory disease are pelvic abscess, infertility, ectopic pregnancy, chronic pelvic pain, pelvic adhesions, and dyspareunia. Based on Ms. Moore's medical diagnosis and treatment plan, *Deficient Knowledge: Safer Sex* is identified as the priority nursing diagnosis at this time.

BJM
20 y.o. female
PID

← affects —

- Pathogenic organisms enter the vagina through sexual activity
- Changes occur in the cervical mucosa, decreasing protection
- Microorganisms travel to the uterus, fallopian tubes, and ovaries
- Microorganisms multiply and invade mucous membranes, causing infection and abscesses

leads to ↓

— assess →

- States she has had unprotected sexual activity with multiple partners
- T 100.4 F,
- Lower abdominal pain (8 on a scale of 1 to 10) on abdominal palpation
- Thick, odorous, green vaginal discharge

— generates →

- Acute Pain related to inflammation as evidenced by statements of pain on abdominal palpation
- Ineffective Health Maintenance related to unprotected sexual activity with multiple partners as evidenced by pelvic infection
- Risk for Injury related to pelvic infection

generate nursing diagnosis ↓

prioritized to →

Deficient Knowledge: Safer Sex

expected outcomes ↓

- Normal oral temperature
- Lab values within normal limits
- Takes total prescribed antibiotic dose
- Verbalize understanding of STIs
- Verbalize need for male partner to wear condom during sexual intercourse

— evaluate →

- Temperature within normal range
- Lab values within normal ranges
- Completes entire dose of prescribed medications
- Verbalizes understanding of cause, effects, and treatment of STIs
- Demonstrates correct application of male condom

Interdisciplinary Interventions
- Monitor lab values on return to clinic

Independent Interventions
- Instruct to call clinic if oral temperature is over 100° F
- Explain rationale for taking all of prescribed antibiotic even when manifestations are gone
- Teach cause, manifestations, complications, and treatment for PID caused by a sexually transmitted organism
- Provide information about safer sex, including how to apply a male condom

UNIT 2

Alterations in Patterns of Health

CHAPTER 4

Nursing Care of Clients Having Surgery

LEARNING OUTCOMES

- Discuss the differences and similarities between outpatient and inpatient surgery.
- Describe the various classifications of surgical procedures.
- Identify diagnostic tests used in the perioperative period.
- Describe nursing implications for medications prescribed for the surgical client.

- Provide appropriate nursing care for the client in the preoperative, intraoperative, and postoperative phases of surgery.
- Identify variations in perioperative care for the older adult.
- Describe principles of pain management specific to acute postoperative pain control.
- Use the nursing process as a framework for providing individualized care for the client undergoing surgery.

CLINICAL COMPETENCIES

- Assess the physiologic health status of clients for surgery to determine their ability to tolerate surgery and risks for complications.
- Assess the psychosocial health status of the client and family.
- Transfer the client safely within the operating room and throughout the postoperative stay.
- Participate in client and family teaching prior to anesthesia and prior to discharge from the facility.
- Create and maintain a sterile field in the operating room and use universal precautions to prevent infections.

- Provide equipment and supplies based on client need.
- Perform sponge, sharps, and instrument counts before discharging the client from the operating room.
- Physiologically monitor the client during surgery. As part of the interdisciplinary team, promote safe practice and client rehabilitation.
- Monitor and control the environment to prevent accidents or injury to the client and the healthcare team. Respect the client's rights, including privacy, at all times (AORN, 2005b).

Surgery is an invasive medical procedure performed to diagnose or treat illness, injury, or deformity. Although surgery is a medical treatment, the nurse assumes an active role in caring for the client before, during, and after surgery. Interdisciplinary care and independent nursing care together prevent complications and promote the surgical client's optimal recovery. **Interdisciplinary care** refers to healthcare services provided by professionals in addition to physicians and surgeons including nurses, pharmacists, social workers, medical technologists, dietitians, chaplains, physical therapists, and occupational therapists. The interdisciplinary team addresses client issues beyond a strictly medical focus. **Independent nursing care** is care provided by nurses within the scope of their practice without the direction or supervision of a physician. Dependent nursing care refers to interventions by nurses that must have a physician order for the action to be legal.

Perioperative nursing is a specialized area of practice. It incorporates the three phases of the surgical experience: preoperative, intraoperative, and postoperative. The **preoperative phase** begins when the decision for surgery is made and ends when the client is transferred to the operating room. The **intraoperative phase** begins with the client's entry into the operating room and ends with admittance to the postanesthe-

sia care unit (PACU), or recovery room. The **postoperative phase** begins with the client's admittance to the PACU and ends with the client's complete recovery from the surgical intervention.

Surgical procedures can be classified according to purpose, risk factor, and urgency (Table 4–1). Based on this information, nursing care can be individualized to best meet client needs.

Although the perioperative nurse works in collaboration with other healthcare professionals to identify and meet the client's needs, the perioperative nurse has the primary responsibility and accountability for nursing care of the client undergoing surgery.

SETTINGS FOR SURGERY

Surgical patients may be inpatients or outpatients. The complexity of the surgery and recovery and the expected disposition of the client following the surgery are the major differences. Sometimes outpatients (i.e., clients intending to be discharged home immediately following surgery) are admitted to the hospital. Cataract removal with or without lens implants, hernia repairs, tubal ligations, vasectomies, dilation

TABLE 4–1 Classification of Surgical Procedures

	CLASSIFICATION	FUNCTION	EXAMPLES
Purpose	Diagnostic	Determine or confirm a diagnosis	Breast biopsy, bronchoscopy
	Ablative	Remove diseased tissue, organ, or extremity	Appendectomy, amputation
	Constructive	Build tissue/organs that are absent (congenital anomalies)	Repair of cleft palate
	Reconstructive	Rebuild tissue/organ that has been damaged	Skin graft after a burn, total joint replacement
	Palliative	Alleviate symptoms of a disease (not curative)	Bowel resection in client with terminal cancer
	Transplant	Replace organs/tissue to restore function	Heart, lung, liver, kidney transplant
Risk Factor	Minor	Minimal physical assault with minimal risk	Removal of skin lesions, dilation and curettage (D&C), cataract extraction
	Major	Extensive physical assault and/or serious risk	Transplant, total joint replacement, cholecystectomy, colostomy, nephrectomy
Urgency	Elective	Suggested, though no foreseen ill effects if postponed	Cosmetic surgery, cataract surgery, bunionectomy
	Urgent	Necessary to be performed within 1 to 2 days	Heart bypass surgery, amputation resulting from gangrene, fractured hip
	Emergency	Performed immediately	Obstetric emergencies, bowel obstruction, ruptured aneurysm, life-threatening trauma

and curettage (D&C), hemorrhoidectomies, and biopsies are commonly performed outpatient surgeries.

Inpatient and outpatient surgeries are performed in the same operating suites in most hospitals. There are also **freestanding outpatient surgical facilities**, which are not physically connected to a hospital. Surgeons may practice in both hospital and freestanding surgical facilities. Some outpatient surgeries are performed in surgeons' offices rather than surgical centers. The number of outpatient surgeries has grown rapidly in the past decade as part of the effort to contain the high costs of surgery. Moreover, increasingly complex surgeries on clients with complicated medical problems are now commonly performed on an outpatient basis. This increase in number of procedures and acuity level of the clients has presented a challenge to the perioperative nurse, the client, and the family.

Outpatient surgery potentially offers several advantages:
- Decreased cost to the client, hospital, and insuring agency
- Reduced risk of hospital-acquired infection
- Less interruption in the client's and family's routine
- Possible reduction in time lost from work and/or other responsibilities
- Less physiologic stress to the client and family.

Outpatient surgery also presents some disadvantages:
- Less time for the nurse to establish rapport with client and family
- Less time for the nurse to assess, evaluate, and teach the client and family
- Lack of opportunity for the nurse to assess for the risk of postoperative complications that may occur after discharge
- Less time for adequate pain control before discharge.

Many similarities exist between nursing care of the inpatient and outpatient surgical clients. Physical care is provided in much the same manner in the preoperative, intraoperative, and postoperative phases of surgery. The major differences lie in the degree of teaching and emotional support that must be provided for outpatient surgical clients and their families. In addition to the physiologic insult of surgery, the outpatient surgical client must cope with the additional stress of needing to learn a great deal of information in a short span of time. The nurse teaches the client and family in both the preoperative and postoperative periods to enable the client to perform self-care following discharge. More extensive teaching and emotional support is mandated as clients requiring more complex surgical procedures and experiencing more complicated health problems undergo outpatient surgery.

PRACTICE ALERT

Clients having outpatient surgery should wear or bring clothing that will be easy to put on after surgery and accommodate any dressings or appliances. Furthermore, despite being NPO, clients must bring any medications including herbal preparations they regularly use (especially those prescribed by other providers), such as steroids, antibiotics, anticoagulants, antivirals, diuretics, oral contraceptives, hypotensives, cardiotonics, hypoglycemics, asthma medications, seizure medications, and analgesics. Clients should consult with the surgeon and anesthesiologist before taking these medications.

Following outpatient surgery, the client is discharged after meeting the institution's criteria:
- Vital signs are stable.
- Client is able to stand and begin to walk without dizziness or nausea.
- Pain is controlled or alleviated.
- Client is able to urinate.
- Client is oriented.
- Client and/or significant other demonstrates understanding of postoperative instructions.

LEGAL REQUIREMENTS

It is the responsibility of the surgeon who performs the procedure to obtain the client's consent for care. The surgeon should discuss the procedure with the client and family in language they can understand. **Informed consent** is disclosure of risks associated with the intended procedure or operation to the client, and includes a legal document required for certain diagnostic procedures or therapeutic measures, including surgery. The language of the document varies according to statutory and common law of each state. This legal document protects the client, nurse, physician, and healthcare facility. Informed consent includes the following information:
- Need for the procedure in relation to the diagnoses
- Description and purpose of the proposed procedure
- Possible benefits and potential risks
- Likelihood of a successful outcome
- Alternative treatments or procedures available
- Anticipated risks should the procedure not be performed
- Physician's advice as to what is needed
- Right to refuse treatment or withdraw consent.

Ideally, the nurse should be present when the preceding information is provided. Later, the nurse can discuss the information with the client and family, if necessary. If the client has questions or concerns that were not discussed or made clear, or if the nurse questions the client's understanding, the surgeon is responsible for supplying further information. If these situations arise, the nurse should contact the surgeon before having the client sign a consent for operation and special procedures. Following a thorough discussion of the consent for operation or special procedures, the nurse witnesses the client's voluntary signature on the form (Figure 4–1 ■). The nurse also signs the form, indicating that the correct person is signing the form and that the client was alert and aware of what was being signed.

Perioperative Risk Factors

Prior to planning and implementing care for the surgical client, the nurse must first assess the client's needs and the factors that may increase the risks associated with surgery. The type of surgical procedure directs the assessment and interventions planned by the nurse. However, a complete assessment is also necessary to identify *risk factors* and to determine the client's overall health status. Table 4–2 lists common risk factors for the client undergoing surgery, and the related nursing interventions and implications. For example, when a client is admitted for

M.R. # _____

Saint Francis Medical Center

Informed Consent to Operation, Administration of Anesthetics, and to the Rendering of Other Medical Services

1. I do hereby authorize and direct _____ M.D./D.O./D.D.S., my physician, and/or such associates or assistants of his choice, to perform the following operation or procedure:

_____

_____

upon _____ (patient's name). I understand that the above named physician and his associates or assistants are employed by me and will be occupied solely with performing such operation or procedure.

2. The nature of the operation or procedure has been explained to me and no warranty or guarantee has been made as to result or cure. I have been advised that additional surgical and/or medical procedures or treatment may be deemed necessary during the course of the operation or procedure consented hereto, and I fully consent to such additional procedures and treatment which, in the opinion of my physician, are deemed necessary or desirable for the well-being of the patient. The possible risks and complications of the operation or procedure have been explained to me. The physician has explained to me the above medical terminology and I satisfactorily understand the type of operation/procedure.

3. I hereby authorize and direct the above named physician and/or his associates or assistants or those working under his direction to provide for _____ (patient's name) such additional services as he or they may deem reasonable and necessary, including, but not limited to, the administration and maintenance of anesthesia, blood or blood derivatives, and the performance of services involving pathology and radiology and I hereby consent thereto. The possible risks and complications of blood transfusions and the administration of anesthetics have also been explained to me.

4. I understand also that the persons in attendance at such operation or procedure for the purpose of administering anesthesia, and the radiologists in attendance at such operation or procedure for the purpose of performing radiological (X-ray) service are not the agents, servants, or employees of St. Francis Medical Center nor of any physician, but are independent healthcare providers who are employed by me in the same way that my surgeon and physician are employed by me.

5. I hereby authorize the Medical Center pathologist or personnel to use their discretion in the disposal of any severed tissue or member.

6. I hereby grant permission for St. Francis Medical Center to obtain clinical photographs for educational purposes or for my patient record as deemed necessary by my physician.

7. The **exception to this consent:** (If none, write "none".) _____ _____ and I assume full responsibility for these exceptions.

_____   _____
PATIENT'S SIGNATURE   **DATE**

If the patient is a minor or incompetent or is unable to sign, the following must be completed:

I hereby certify that I am the (relationship) _____ of the above named patient

who is unable to sign because _____ ,

and I am fully authorized to give the consent herein granted.

_____   _____
SIGNATURE   DATE

_____   _____
WITNESSED BY/date   **WITNESSED BY/date**

If signed in the physician's office, the following MUST be completed by the Medical Center.

_____   _____
REVIEWED BY (patient name) **/date**   **WITNESSED BY /date**

Figure 4–1 ■ Informed consent form.

TABLE 4–2 Nursing Implications for Surgical Risk Factors

FACTOR	ASSOCIATED RISK	NURSING IMPLICATIONS
Advanced age	Older adults have age-related changes that affect physiologic, cognitive, and psychosocial responses to the stress of surgery; decreased tolerance of general anesthesia and postoperative medications; and delayed wound healing.	Selected nursing interventions are summarized in Table 4–6.
Obesity	The obese client is at increased risk for delayed wound healing, wound dehiscence, infection, pneumonia, atelectasis, thrombophlebitis, arrhythmias, and heart failure.	Promote weight reduction if time permits. Monitor closely for wound, pulmonary, and cardiovascular complications postoperatively. Encourage coughing, turning, and diaphragmatic breathing exercises and early ambulation.
Malnutrition	Reserves may not be sufficient to allow the body to respond satisfactorily to the physical assault of surgery; organ failure and shock may result. Increased metabolic demands may result in poor wound healing and infection.	With the physician and dietitian, promote weight gain by providing a well-balanced diet high in calories, protein, and vitamin C. Administer total parenteral nutrition intravenously, nutritional supplements, and tube feedings as prescribed. Daily weights and calorie counts also may be ordered.
Dehydration/ electrolyte imbalance	Depending on the degree of dehydration and/or type of electrolyte imbalance, cardiac dysrhythmia or heart failure may occur. Liver and renal failure may also result.	Administer intravenous fluids as ordered. Monitor I&O. Monitor client for evidence of electrolyte imbalance (see Chapter 10 ∞).
Cardiovascular disorders	Presence of cardiovascular disease increases the risk of hemorrhage and shock, hypotension, thrombophlebitis, pulmonary embolism, stroke (especially in the older client), and fluid volume overload.	Diligently monitor vital signs, especially pulse rate, regularity, and rhythm, and general condition of the client. Closely monitor fluid intake (oral and parenteral) to prevent circulatory overload. Assess skin color. Assess for chest pain, lung congestion, and peripheral edema. Observe for signs of hypoxia, and administer oxygen as ordered. Early postoperative ambulation and leg exercises reduce the risk of vascular problems, such as thrombophlebitis and pulmonary embolism.
Respiratory disorders	Respiratory complications such as bronchitis, atelectasis, and pneumonia are some of the most common and serious postoperative complications. Respiratory depression from general anesthesia and acid–base imbalance may also occur. Clients with pulmonary disease are more at risk for developing these complications.	Closely monitor respirations, pulse, and breath sounds. Also assess for hypoxia, dyspnea, lung congestion, and chest pain. Encourage coughing, turning, and diaphragmatic breathing exercises and early postoperative ambulation. Encourage the client to quit smoking or at least to reduce the number of cigarettes smoked.
Diabetes mellitus	Diabetes causes an increased risk for fluctuating blood glucose levels, which can lead to life-threatening hypoglycemia or ketoacidosis. Diabetes also increases the risk for cardiovascular disease, delayed wound healing, and wound infection.	Monitor the client closely for signs and symptoms of hypoglycemia and hyperglycemia. Monitor blood glucose levels every 4 hours or as ordered. Administer insulin as prescribed. Encourage intake of food at the designated meal and snack times.
Renal and liver dysfunction	The client with renal or liver dysfunction may poorly tolerate general anesthesia, have fluid/electrolyte and acid–base imbalances, decreased metabolism and excretion of drugs, increased risk for hemorrhage, and delayed wound healing.	Monitor for fluid volume overload, intake and output (I&O), and response to medication. Evaluate closely for drug side effects and evidence of acidosis or alkalosis.
Alcoholism	The client may be malnourished and experience delirium tremens (acute withdrawal symptoms). More general anesthesia may be required. Hemorrhage and delayed wound healing can result from liver damage and poor nutritional status.	Monitor closely for signs of delirium tremens. Encourage well-balanced diet. Monitor for wound complications. Administer supplemental nutrients parenterally as ordered.

(continued)

TABLE 4–2 Nursing Implications for Surgical Risk Factors (continued)

FACTOR	ASSOCIATED RISK	NURSING IMPLICATIONS
Nicotine use	Cigarette smokers are at increased risk for respiratory complications such as pneumonia, atelectasis, and bronchitis because of increased mucous secretions and a decreased ability to expel them.	Ideally, the client should quit smoking. Be supportive of the client, and monitor closely for respiratory difficulties. Coughing, turning, and diaphragmatic breathing exercises with early ambulation are very important. Increase daily fluid intake to 2500–3000 mL (unless contraindicated) to help liquefy respiratory secretions to aid expectoration. A nicotine patch may help the client tolerate withdrawal during the postoperative period.
Adolescence	Diversity in age, and physical, cognitive, and psychologic maturation makes preparation for surgery vary in content and inclusion of significant others. Increased need for control, privacy, and peer interaction poses special challenges in the acute care setting.	Adapt assessment and interventions to the development level of individual clients, involving them in preparation and care to the extent possible. Allow for regressive and independent behavior including rejection of adult support.
Medications	Anesthesia interaction with some medications can cause respiratory difficulties, hypotension, and circulatory collapse. Other medications can produce side effects that may increase surgical risk.	Inform the anesthesiologist of all prescribed or over-the-counter medications.
Anticoagulants (including aspirin)	May cause intraoperative and postoperative hemorrhage.	Monitor for bleeding. Assess PT/PTT values.
Diuretics (particularly thiazides)	May lead to fluid and electrolyte imbalances, producing altered cardiovascular response and respiratory depression.	Monitor I&O and electrolytes. Assess cardiovascular and respiratory status.
Antihypertensives (particularly phenothiazines)	Increase the hypotensive effects of anesthesia.	Closely monitor blood pressure.
Antidepressants (particularly monoamine oxidase inhibitors)	Increase the hypotensive effects of anesthesia.	Closely monitor blood pressure.
Antibiotics (particularly the "mycin" group)	May cause apnea and respiratory paralysis.	Monitor respirations.
Herbal supplements	Some may prolong the effects of anesthesia. Others may increase the risks of bleeding or raise blood pressure.	Inquire about the use of herbs or other dietary supplements. These should be discontinued at least 2 weeks before surgery.
Temperature variations	Deviations from normothermia, either hypothermia or hyperthermia, may cause infection, cardiac morbidity, myocardial ischemia, surgical bleeding, skin damage, or client discomfort.	Monitor core temperatures and prevent chilling or overheating. Remove wet drapes and test the temperature of fluids used.

surgery on the right knee, it should be of concern to the nurse if this client has diabetes, smokes 1.5 packs of cigarettes per day, has numbness in the right foot, and takes insulin. This information should be incorporated into a care plan, using appropriate nursing diagnoses and interventions to meet all of the client's needs and assist the client toward full postoperative recovery.

Risks are associated with all surgical interventions. For example, transporting the client to and from the operating suite requires assessment of the needs of the client for supplemental oxygen, intravenous therapy, cardiac monitoring, and safety issues pertaining to the means of transport. Many clients enter the operating suite highly anxious and may benefit from medication to help them relax prior to administration of anesthesia. This can

be discussed with the anesthetist. Chemicals, electrical equipment, and environmental hazards in the surgical area have the potential for harm and must be monitored and maintained carefully.

Unfortunately, there is a risk of performing the wrong surgery on the wrong client: wrong site, wrong procedure, wrong person (Gibbs, 2005). In 2004, the Joint Commission on Accreditation of Healthcare Organizations (JCAHO) issued a universal protocol mandating preoperatively (1) verifying the procedure, (2) physically marking and initialing the site, and (3) taking a "time out" before starting any procedure. The goal of the time out is to ensure the right procedure will be performed on the right client on the correct site with the necessary and correct healthcare providers in attendance. A time out is an intentional stoppage of the preparation for the operation, in the operating suite, before the patient is anesthetized. All participants are introduced and encouraged to ask any questions or express any concerns before the surgery is commenced. This strategy was adopted from the airline industry, where accidents can lead to fatal outcomes.

Another potential error is retained foreign bodies such as instruments, needles, or sponges. The incidence of this problem increased after airport security was enhanced in 2001 and surgical instruments were discovered in former clients when they were boarding airplanes. To prevent accidental retention the American College of Surgeons recommends consistent application and adherence to standardized procedures for counting of objects used in the surgery, methodical wound exploration before closing the site, using x-ray detectable materials in the wound, maintenance of optimal OR environments to allow focused surgical performance, employing technological methods to ensure no unintended item remains, and suspension of these measures as needed in life-threatening situations (Gibbs, 2005). Like wrong site injury, foreign body retainment seems to be linked to poor communication among perioperative care providers and faulty processes of care in the operating room.

A complete history of medications the client has been taking regularly is vital information. Over-the-counter medicines and herbal preparations as well as prescription medications may interact with drugs given during surgery, putting a client at increased risk (Bailey & Dresser, 2004). As part of the preoperative planning and teaching, early consideration of complementary and alternative medicine is important. This information should be obtained in a matter of fact and nonjudgmental manner, because a judgmental attitude could cause the client to withhold information.

Anticoagulant medications should be discontinued by the client prior to surgery to prevent excessive blood loss during surgery. These include aspirin and nonsteroidal anti-inflammatory drugs. If laboratory tests of bleeding time, PT, PTT, and INR are elevated, the surgery may be cancelled. Guidelines for discontinuing use vary according to the particular medication; it is generally recommended that aspirin or products containing aspirin be discontinued 5 days or longer before surgery. Similarly, herbs or nutritional supplements that impair clotting should be discontinued 2 weeks prior to surgery (Norred & Brinker, 2001; Saper, 2005). The most common self-prescribed medicines that may inhibit coagulation are vitamin E, garlic, ginkgo, ginseng, fish oil, and chamomile (Norred & Brinker, 2001). Many plants contain coumarins with the potential to interact with warfarin and inhibit coagulation. Others inhibit platelet aggregation or prevent the conversion of fibrinogen to fibrin. All of these create a risk for bleeding.

Clients taking warfarin for the risk of blood clots due to atrial fibrillation will be counseled about the appropriate time to withdraw warfarin. If surgery is urgent due to trauma or sudden onset of morbidity, the impact of anticoagulants needs to be evaluated with PT, PTT, and INR before the operation and appropriate support for clotting administered.

In addition to clotting impairment, excessive consumption of herbal medicines or dietary supplements can produce levels of chemicals that interact with conventional medications, exacerbating or impairing the intended effect. Anesthesia drugs often decrease hepatic blood flow and interfere with metabolism and elimination of medications (Bailey & Dresser, 2004; Bressler, 2005). This increases the risk of adverse drug–herbal supplement interactions during surgery. Cardiovascular instability, impaired glucose control, increased metabolism of perioperative medication, and unpredictable response to anesthesia are categories of adverse reactions of perioperative herbal use (Saper, 2005; Wren et al., 2002).

In the perioperative period, hypothermia and hyperthermia are risks. Typically, surgical suites are maintained quite cold. Lowering environmental temperature is common in surgical suites, but research shows that normothermia (core body temperature in the range of 36.0 to 37.5°C [Porth, 2005]) in the client provides less risk to the client for infection, cardiac morbidity, myocardial ischemia, surgical bleeding, and client discomfort. Methods to minimize the risk of hypothermia include:

- Apply warm blankets on arrival in the surgical area and after sterile drapes are removed.
- Limit the amount of skin exposed during positioning and skin preparation.
- Limit the time of skin exposure between prepping and draping.
- Prevent surgical drapes from becoming wet.
- Adjust the room temperature for normothermia.
- Monitor client's temperature to avoid overheating.
- Use heat-maintenance devices such as warming units, stockings, caps, and leggings.
- Warm irrigation or infusion solutions as needed.
- Humidify the airway.

The anesthetized client loses heat intraoperatively and is unable to restore temperature through the normal mechanisms of shivering or muscle contractions. Hyperthermia should also be avoided. Heating of fluids or use of heating units necessitates accurate measurement of the temperature and assessment of the client's skin integrity. Body temperature is best evaluated through core temperature monitoring, which includes esophageal or tympanic assessment (AORN Recommended Practices Committee, 2000).

Interpreting and responding to identified risk factors require nursing judgment. It is important to bring information to the attention of the surgeons and anesthesiologists prior to surgery, so necessary modifications can be made for the patient.

PRACTICE ALERT
Remind diabetic clients that the stress of surgery increases rather than decreases blood sugar. Coordinate insulin injection and/or hypoglycemic medication with the client, surgeon, and anesthesiologist.

Interdisciplinary Care

The client undergoing surgery receives care from a number of healthcare providers. Surgeons, nurses, scrub persons, anesthetists, phlebotomists, x-ray technicians, registration clerks, and transporters are often involved in securing the safety and health of clients. Case managers, social workers, and spiritual care providers are available based on client need and desire. This interdisciplinary approach focuses on placing the client in the best possible health status before, during, and after surgery.

Diagnosis

Diagnostic tests performed prior to surgery provide baseline data or reveal problems that may place the client at additional risk during and after surgery. Because of the trend toward shortened hospital stays, many diagnostic studies and procedures are performed in a preadmission clinic within a week prior to elective surgery.

Complete blood counts, electrolyte studies, coagulation studies, and urinalysis are the most commonly performed preoperative laboratory tests. Table 4–3 discusses the significance and nursing implications of abnormal findings for these common tests. Additional diagnostic tests may be performed as the history and physical findings indicate. For example, if the

client has a low hemoglobin and hematocrit, and significant blood loss during surgery is anticipated, then the surgeon may order a type and crossmatch of the client's blood for a possible transfusion.

In addition to laboratory tests, older clients or those with risk factors related to heart and lung function typically have a chest x-ray. This radiologic procedure provides baseline information about the size, shape, and condition of the heart and lungs. Pulmonary complications such as lung disease, tuberculosis, calcification, infiltration, or pneumonia may require that surgery be postponed to allow the client to undergo further evaluation or treatment. If findings are abnormal and the surgery cannot be postponed, information from the chest x-ray study can be used to determine the safest form of anesthesia.

Another commonly performed preoperative diagnostic procedure is the electrocardiogram (ECG). This test is ordered routinely on clients undergoing general anesthesia when they are over 40 years of age or have cardiovascular disease. The ECG

TABLE 4–3 Laboratory Tests for Perioperative Assessment

TEST	SIGNIFICANCE OF INCREASED VALUES	SIGNIFICANCE OF DECREASED VALUES	NURSING IMPLICATIONS
Hemoglobin (Hgb) and hematocrit (Hct)	Dehydration, excessive fluid plasma loss, polycythemia vera	Fluid overload, excessive blood loss, anemia	Monitor oxygenation, (I&O), and vital signs; assess for bleeding.
Glucose and Hemoglobin-A	Impaired glucose metabolism, stress, or infection	Inadequate glucose intake in relation to insulin	If decreased, monitor for signs and symptoms of hypoglycemia. Notify surgeon if <70 mg/dL or >180 mg/dL.
White blood cell (WBC) count	Infectious/inflammatory processes, leukemia	Immune deficiencies	Monitor for signs of inflammation; monitor drainage, temperature, and pulse. Use strict universal precautions.
Platelet count	Malignancies, polycythemia vera	Clotting deficiency disorders, chemotherapy	If decreased, assess for bleeding at incision sites and drainage tubes, and assess for hematomas.
Carbon dioxide (CO_2)	Emphysema, chronic bronchitis, asthma, pneumonia, respiratory acidosis, vomiting, nasogastric suctioning	Metabolic acidosis, hyperventilation	Monitor respiratory status and arterial blood gases (ABGs).
Electrolytes Potassium (K^+)	Kidney dysfunction, dehydration, suctioning	Side effects of diuretics, vomiting, NG suctioning	Monitor K^+ level, cardiac and neurologic function, and preoperative diuretic therapy.
Sodium (Na^+)	Kidney dysfunction, normal saline-containing intravenous fluids	Side effects of diuretics, vomiting, NG suctioning	Monitor Na^+ level and I&O; assess for peripheral edema and effects of perioperative diuretic therapy.
Chloride (Cl^-)	Kidney dysfunction, dehydration, alkalosis	Side effects of diuretics, vomiting, NG suctioning	Monitor Cl^- level and I&O; assess for peripheral edema and perioperative diuretic therapy.
Prothrombin time (protime, or PT) and partial thromboplastin time (PTT)	Defect in mechanism for blood clotting, anticoagulant therapy (aspirin, heparin, warfarin), side effect of other drugs affecting clotting time	Hypercoagulability of the blood may lead to thrombus formation in the veins	If clotting time is elevated, monitor PT/PTT values. Assess for bleeding at incision site and drainage tubes and for hematomas. If clotting time is decreased, monitor for thrombus formation (pulmonary emboli, thrombophlebitis), and evaluate PT and PTT values.
Urinalysis	Varied	Varied	Used to detect abnormal substances (e.g., protein, glucose, red blood cells, or bacteria) in the urine. Notify surgeon if abnormalities are detected.

provides data for evaluation about either new or preexisting cardiac conditions. The client's surgery may be cancelled or postponed if a life-threatening cardiac condition is discovered.

In addition to the chest x-ray study and ECG, other diagnostic tests may be performed preoperatively to gather further assessment data. For example, for clients who have chronic obstructive pulmonary disease, pulmonary function studies often are performed to determine the extent of respiratory dysfunction. This information guides the anesthesiologist before and during surgery in choosing the type of anesthetic to be used, and it guides the surgeon and nursing staff in the recovery phase.

Creatine clearance (the calculated amount of creatinine in a 24-hour urine collection) is the best indicator of renal function (Pagana & Pagana, 2002). As clients age, muscle mass decreases and serum creatinine may be falsely low because of decreased muscle turnover. A low serum creatinine is an indicator of good renal function, so the creatinine value must be confirmed in the urine. Older adults are especially susceptible to renal insufficiency, which puts them at risk for volume overload in the perioperative period and accumulation of metabolic by-products and medications dependent on renal clearance (Loran et al., 2005).

Medications

The client having surgery receives medications before, during, and after surgery to achieve specific therapeutic outcomes. Traditionally, all medication orders are cancelled when the client goes to surgery and must be rewritten by the physician when the client returns to the postsurgical care unit.

The surgical client usually is given preoperative medications 45 to 70 minutes before the scheduled surgery. Any delay in administration should be reported promptly to the surgical department. Preoperative medications may also be given in the surgical holding room to produce the desired effects.

An increasingly common strategy to prevent intense or lingering pain is the use of *preemptive analgesia*. Preemptive analgesia prevents sensitization of the central and peripheral nervous system by painful stimuli by blocking the pain pathways with local, regional, or epidural analgesia prior to incision. Sensitization to pain prolongs the painful experience; blocking the sensitization throughout the perioperative period results in decreased pain in the postoperative period, shortened hospital stay, quicker return to self-care, and decreased residual pain (Gottschalk & Smith, 2001).

A combination of preoperative drugs may be ordered to achieve the desired outcomes with minimal side effects. Such outcomes include sedation, reducing anxiety, inducing amnesia to minimize unpleasant surgical memories, increasing comfort during preoperative procedures, reducing gastric acidity and volume, increasing gastric emptying, decreasing nausea and vomiting, and reducing the incidence of aspiration by drying oral and respiratory secretions.

Antibiotic prophylaxis is effective in the prevention of postoperative complications in many surgeries (Andersen et al., 2005; Bedouch et al., 2004; Bratzler et al., 2005; Silber et al., 2005). Table 4–4 outlines commonly prescribed preoperative medications.

Decisions about which of the client's routine medications to administer prior to surgery when the client is NPO require careful analysis. The best guideline is to confer with the surgeon and anesthetist about specific medications. The reason for caution has to do with potential interactions between anesthesia and medications and the effect on the client if drugs such as steroids, antiseizure medications, and tranquilizers are discontinued abruptly. Generally, insulin is withheld when the client is NPO, but depending on the anticipated length of the surgery, the dosage may be adjusted for the previous evening as well as the morning of surgery. Under anesthesia the signs and symptoms of hypoglycemia (insulin reaction) are absent, so withholding insulin the morning of surgery when the client is NPO is advisable. Plasma glucose is monitored intermittently during surgery with the goal of maintaining normal blood sugar level (see Table 4–2). Clients who ordinarily manage their diabetes mellitus with oral medications often experience hyperglycemia perioperatively. It has been common to manage hyperglycemia with sliding scale insulin. Evidence-based practice supports subcutaneous basal insulin administration for hyperglycemic clients to maintain glycemia below 180 mg/dL throughout the perioperative period. This practice is associated with better healing, fewer infections, and shorter hospital stays (Odom-Forren, 2006).

Assessment of medications the client uses is vital prior to anesthesia. In addition to medications prescribed by a physician, assessment should include over-the-counter preparations (including aspirin and illegal drugs) and herbal medications (see Table 4–2).

INTRAOPERATIVE MEDICATIONS **Anesthesia** is used to produce unconsciousness, analgesia, reflex loss, and muscle relaxation during a surgical procedure. General anesthesia produces these effects, whereas regional anesthesia results in analgesia, reflex loss, and muscle relaxation but does not cause the client to lose consciousness. An anesthesiologist (physician) or certified registered nurse anesthetist (CRNA) administers anesthetics during the intraoperative phase of surgery.

General Anesthesia **General anesthesia** is most commonly administered by inhalation and, to a lesser extent, by the intravenous route. It produces central nervous system depression. As a result, the client loses consciousness and does not perceive pain, skeletal muscles relax, and reflexes diminish.

Advantages to general anesthesia include rapid excretion of the anesthetic agent and prompt reversal of its effects when desired. Additionally, general anesthesia can be used with all age groups and any type of surgical procedure. It produces amnesia.

Disadvantages of general anesthesia include risks associated with circulatory, respiratory, hepatic, and renal side effects. Clients with serious respiratory or circulatory diseases, such as emphysema or congestive heart failure, are at greater risk for complications. Clients with renal or hepatic disease cannot metabolize and eliminate anesthetics safely.

General anesthesia is provided with inhalation agents or total intravenous anesthesia (TIVA). Clients with a history of malignant hyperthermia (MH) avoid inhalation agents because they

TABLE 4–4 Preoperative Medications

GENERIC	TRADE	DOSE AND ROUTE	ACTION BY CATEGORY	NURSING IMPLICATIONS
Antibiotics	Cefazolin	1–2 g IV ½–2 hr. preop	Prevents surgical site infections in orthopedic and general surgeries and associated with lower risk of mortality in elderly clients	Clients with Beta-Lactam allergies receive Vancomycin (1 g) or Clindamycin (600–900 mg)
Benzodiazepines				
Midazolam	Versed	3–5 mg IM	Decreases anxiety and produces sedation to some extent	Monitor for respiratory depression, hypotension, drowsiness, and lack of coordination.
Diazepam	Valium	2–10 mg PO	Induces amnesia	
Lorazepam	Ativan	1–4 mg IM or IV	May induce substantial amnesia	
Opioid Analgesics				
Morphine	Morphine	5–15 mg IM	Decreases anxiety, provides analgesia	Monitor for respiratory depression and safety if ambulating.
Fentanyl	Sublimaze	25–50 mcg IV, IM	Rapid onset, short duration	Less nausea and vomiting than morphine sulfate.
Oxycodone	Roxicodone	5–10 mg PO	Immediate release only available in 5 mg tabs	Mild to moderate pain; client cannot be NPO.
Hydrocodone	Vicodin	5–10 mg PO	Includes acetaminophen	Mild to moderate pain; client cannot be NPO.
Tramadol	Ultram	50–100 mg PO	Antidepressant effects with acetaminophen	Moderate to severe pain; antiemetics may be needed.
Codeine	Tylenol with Codeine	7.5, 15, or 30 mg		Very constipating, mild to moderate pain.
Nonopioid Analgesics Antacids				
Sodium citrate	Bicitra	15–30 mL PO	Increases the pH and reduces volume of gastric fluid; used in clients with GERD and/or trauma	No significant factors in this setting.
H₂ Receptor Antagonists				
Cimetidine	Tagamet	300 mg IV, IM, or PO	Reduces gastric acid volume and concentration	Monitor for confusion and dizziness in older adults.
Famotidine	Pepcid	20 mg IV		
Ranitidine	Zantac	50 mg IV, IM, or PO		
Gastric Acid Pump Inhibitors				
Lansoprazole	Prevacid	15–60 mg PO	Suppresses gastric acid secretion	Monitor for dizziness and headache, rash, or thirst.
Omeprazole	Prilosec	20–40 mg PO		
Antiemetics				
Metoclopramide	Reglan	10 mg IV	Enhances gastric emptying	Monitor for sedation and extrapyramidal reaction (involuntary movement, muscle tone changes, and abnormal posture).
Droperidol	Inapsine	10–15 mg PO 0.625–2.5 mg IM	Tranquilizer	
Anticholinergics				
Atropine sulfate	Atropine sulfate	0.4–0.6 mg IM or IV	Reduces oral and respiratory secretions to decrease risk of aspiration; decreases vomiting and laryngospasm	Monitor for confusion, restlessness, and tachycardia. Prepare client to expect a dry mouth.
Glycopyrrolate	Robinul	0.1–0.3 IM mg or IV		
Scopolamine	Scopolamine	0.4–0.6 mg IM or IV		

can trigger MH (Box 4–1). With the increase in ambulatory and minimally invasive surgeries, anesthetics are used that enable shorter recovery phases. *Fast-tracking* involves a rapid recovery phase, often bypassing the PACU (Hassan & Fahy, 2005).

The phases of general anesthesia are divided into three distinct categories: induction, maintenance, and emergence. During the induction phase, the client receives the anesthetic agent intravenously or by inhalation. During this phase, airway patency

BOX 4–1 Malignant Hyperthermia (MH)

Malignant hyperthermia (MH) is a rare but serious reaction to volatile inhalational anesthetic gases and succinylcholine, a depolarizing neuromuscular blocker. The client manifests the following signs and symptoms: unexplained rise in end-tidal carbon dioxide that does not respond to ventilation, hyperthermia, tachypnea, tachycardia, and sustained skeletal muscle contraction (Carter-Templeton, 2005). If unchecked the condition will progress to hyperkalemia, myoglobinuria, disseminated intravascular coagulation, congestive heart failure, bowel ischemia, and compartment syndrome in the limbs. Dantrolene sodium is the drug that inhibits the muscular pathology and prevents death.

Because the condition is inherited, susceptibility testing is available but the testing is expensive and the most accurate test involves an invasive procedure. The "gold standard" involves biopsy of thigh skeletal muscle tissue to determine sensitivity to caffeine and halothane (CHCT) (Litman & Rosenberg, 2005). Genetic testing is not as sensitive and reliable as CHCT but will be improved with the discovery of more causative mutations. Clients with muscle myopathies such as muscular dystrophy sometimes experience early

signs of MH and respond well to dantrolene. Because the symptoms of MH may manifest with other pathologies, it is important for clients to know if they have a genetic susceptibility to MH which could affect all members of the family (Brandom, 2005).

MH can develop during an operation or when the client returns to the PACU. If the early symptoms of MH (e.g., escalating temperature, increased carbon dioxide production) are suspected, immediately administer 100% oxygen with a non-rebreather mask, stay with the patient, ensure good IV access, and summon the anesthesia provider. The anesthesia provider will order 2.5 mg/kg of dantrolene which can be given IV push. The dantrolene can be repeated up to 10 mg/kg until the signs and symptoms of MH diminish. Measures to decrease core body temperature should be started at once and continued until core temperature is 36.0°C. A urinary catheter should be placed to monitor urine output and blood drawn for testing. Blood gases should be drawn to measure pH; sodium bicarbonate is given to correct metabolic acidosis. Insulin may be ordered to decrease serum potassium. Expect this client to be transferred to the ICU for continued monitoring and doses of dantrolene every 4–6 hours.

is achieved and maintained with either endotracheal intubation or newer devices including the laryngeal mask airway (LMA) esophageal-tracheal Combitube, or lighted stylet or wand (Hassan & Fahy, 2005). These alternative methods of airway maintenance do not require direct visualization of the vocal cords for placement and allow ventilation. Intubation is difficult with some clients and these devices are an option to avoid creation of a surgical airway with a cricothyroidotomy or tracheostomy.

The next phase of general anesthesia is maintenance. During this period, the client is positioned, the skin is prepared, and surgery is performed. The anesthesiologist maintains the proper depth of anesthesia while constantly monitoring physiologic parameters such as heart rate, blood pressure, respiratory rate, temperature, and oxygen and carbon dioxide levels. The final phase of anesthesia is the client's emergence from this altered physiologic state. As the anesthetic agents are withdrawn or the effects reversed pharmacologically, the client begins to awaken. The endotracheal tube or laryngeal mask is removed (extubated) once the client is able to reestablish voluntary breathing. It is critical to ensure airway patency during this period, because extubation may cause bronchospasm or laryngospasm.

Regional Anesthesia **Regional anesthesia** is a type of local anesthesia in which medication instilled around the nerves blocks transmission of nerve impulses in a particular area. Regional anesthesia produces analgesia, relaxation, and reduced reflexes. The client is awake and conscious during the surgical procedure but does not perceive pain. Regional anesthesia may be classified in several ways:

- Local nerve infiltration is achieved by injecting lidocaine or tetracaine around a local nerve to depress nerve sensation over a limited area of the body. This technique may be used when a skin or muscle biopsy is obtained or when a small wound is sutured.

- Nerve blocks are accomplished by injecting an anesthetic agent at the nerve trunk to produce a lack of sensation over a specific area, such as an extremity.
- Epidural blocks are local anesthetic agents injected into the epidural space, outside the dura mater of the spinal cord. This type of intraspinal anesthesia provides safe and effective pain relief for surgeries for clients of all ages with less risk of adverse effects than general anesthesia. It is indicated for surgeries of the arms and shoulders, thorax, abdomen, pelvis, and lower extremities (Schwartz, 2006). The epidural catheter is often left in place for pain relief in the postoperative period; it is also used for chronic pain management.

Spinal anesthesia is administered similarly to epidural except the anesthetic medication is infused in a single injection. Spinal anesthesia is effective for approximately 90 minutes. Surgeries of the lower abdomen, perineum, and lower extremities are likely to use this type of regional anesthesia. Leakage of cerebrospinal fluid (CSF) into the epidural space causes reduced CSF pressure and postoperative headaches. Treatment may include hydration, caffeine, analgesics, or administration of an epidural blood patch (Schwartz, 2006). Hypotension is common with epidural and spinal anesthesia. Monitor BP and, if critical hypotension occurs, alert the anesthesia provider and expect to increase intravenous fluids and administer vasoactive medications.

Conscious Sedation An increasing number of surgical and diagnostic procedures are being performed using **conscious sedation**. This type of anesthesia provides analgesia, amnesia, and moderate sedation. The pharmacologic effects are produced by administering a combination of intravenous medications with opioids (such as morphine sulfate, meperidine hydrochloride [Demerol], and fentanyl [Sublimaze]) or sedatives (such as diazepam [Valium] and midazolam [Versed]). During conscious sedation the client is able to independently maintain an open airway. This allows the client to respond to verbal and physical stimulation. Physician supervision is always required and a registered nurse must be prepared to initiate rescue if sedation becomes too deep. Institutions base their credentialing requirements on professional organization guidelines, regulatory agency requirements, and state law (O'Donnell et al., 2003).

Assessment prior to conscious sedation includes evaluating the appropriateness of the client based on physical status. Clients with compromised circulation or airway, a history of sleep apnea or snoring, a history of problems with anesthesia or analgesia, or medications that would potentially interact with conscious analgesia medications may need an anesthesiologist to manage the effects of anesthesia. Clients need to be appropriately fasting, and baseline vital signs must be taken prior to giving a sedative. A consent form must be signed by the client, and a patent IV line must be in place. Equipment to rescue the client should be available if sedation becomes too deep. Monitor oxygen saturation, pulse, breathing, and level of consciousness throughout the procedure.

Common adverse side effects include venous thrombosis, phlebitis, local irritation, confusion, drowsiness, hypotension, and apnea. Reversal agents (naloxone hydrochloride [Narcan] and flumazenil [Romazicon]) are used as needed to enhance the safety of conscious sedation.

POSTOPERATIVE MEDICATIONS Management of acute postoperative pain by medication improves with greater understanding of pain physiology and the development of better methods to deliver adequate pain medication. For more information on pain management, see the nursing care section later in this chapter on managing acute postoperative pain and also see Chapter 9 ∞.

Established, persistent, severe pain is more difficult to treat than pain that is at its onset. Therefore, postoperative analgesics should be administered at regular intervals around the clock (ATC) to maintain a therapeutic blood level. Administering analgesics as needed (prn) lowers this therapeutic level; delays in medication administration further increase pain intensity. Therefore, prn administration of analgesics is not recommended in the first 36 to 48 hours postoperatively. Patients using patient-controlled analgesia (PCA) or patient-controlled epidural analgesia (PCEA) in the postoperative period need to be taught the importance of using the allowed dosages regularly to prevent increasing pain levels.

In the immediate postoperative period, older adult clients benefit from the same protocol for morphine titration as do younger clients. Intravenous morphine may be initiated at a slightly reduced dose and then titrated to the same protocol for younger patients. Morphine-related adverse effects such as nausea, vomiting, respiratory depression, urinary retention, pruritus, and allergy or sedation are similar among varying age groups. However, older adult clients require fewer opioids than younger clients in the later postoperative period. PCEA may be more effective for older adult clients and is associated with earlier improved mental status and bowel activity (Loran et al., 2005).

> **PRACTICE ALERT**
> Nurses are responsible for assessing clients' pain level and administering pain medication. Work collaboratively with surgeons to schedule postoperative analgesics rather than rely on prn administration orders.

Nonsteroidal anti-inflammatory drugs (NSAIDs) treat mild to moderate postoperative pain. This category of drugs should be given soon after surgery (orally, parenterally, or rectally) along with opioids unless contraindicated. Although NSAIDs may not be sufficient to control pain completely, they allow lower doses of opioid analgesics and, therefore, fewer side effects. NSAIDs can be given safely to older clients, but observe closely for side effects, particularly gastric and renal toxicity.

Opioid analgesics, such as morphine, are considered the foundation for managing moderate to severe postoperative pain. Opioid dosage requirements vary greatly from one client to another, so the dosage must be individually tailored. Later in the postoperative recovery period, opioid analgesics (oral or intramuscular) may be given prn. In this way, pain relief can be maintained, while the potential for drug side effects is decreased.

Contrary to the belief of many healthcare providers (including nurses), physical dependence and tolerance to opioid analgesics is uncommon in short-term postoperative use. Additionally, opioid analgesics, when used to treat acute pain, rarely lead to psychologic dependence and addiction. According to the World Health Organization ladder, acute pain is appropriately treated with opioids, tapering to acetaminophen as healing progresses. Chronic pain, in contrast, increases from acetaminophen to opioids as tolerance develops or the condition worsens. The opioid-naïve client will tolerate and achieve analgesia with a lower dose of opioid than the client who is opioid-tolerant and uses opioids for chronic pain (Ersek et al., 2004).

Older clients tend to be more sensitive to the analgesic effects of opioids, experiencing a higher peak effect with a longer duration of pain control. Nursing Research: Evidence-Based Practice on the following page provides additional information.

> **PRACTICE ALERT**
> Oral analgesia requires a significantly greater dose than parenteral for most analgesics. Teach clients who are being discharged and their caregivers the relative strength of oral analgesics. (Caution them to not rely on trade names to gauge effectiveness. Two Tylenol with codeine (30 mg) is *equianalgesia* to 10 mg parenteral morphine; however, oral Demerol 100 mg does not provide equianalgesia with 10 mg parenteral morphine. (See Chapter 9 ∞ for details about equianalgesia.)

Surgical Environment

MEMBERS OF THE SURGICAL TEAM Because of the complexity of the intraoperative environment, members of the surgical team must function as a coordinated unit. The surgeon, surgical assistant(s), anesthesiologist or CRNA, circulating nurse, and

NURSING RESEARCH | **Evidence-Based Practice: Assisting Older Adults to Communicate Postoperative Pain**

Nurses rely heavily on clients' assessments of the pain they are experiencing. Pain is a subjective experience—a symptom rather than a sign. Rating of pain intensity by the client is the gold standard for knowing when to provide an intervention to decrease pain, and it is considered more accurate than nurses' evaluations of behavioral manifestations of pain. Older clients who believe that healthcare providers know best how to manage their pain are at risk for inadequately treated pain.

McDonald and colleagues (2005) used a program for coaching older adults about postoperative pain communication and management. In this study older adults preparing for single-knee replacement surgery attended a preoperative joint replacement class where they learned about recovering from the surgery and pain management. Forty subjects greater than age 65 were randomly assigned either to the regular class, which included pain management information, or an intervention class, which included both information on pain management and skills to effectively communicate about pain.

The subjects in the communication skills class were taught to enhance pain communication with several strategies consistent with communication accommodation theory (CAT). CAT holds that people adjust their communication based on their own needs and the perceived behavior of others. Skills to enhance communication include evaluating whether the other person (the nurse) has understood the message being given about pain and is willing to include the client as a team member in controlling the pain. Language to describe pain intensity, location, and sensation is modeled. Clients must report their pain because they are the experts about their own pain experience.

The groups were post-tested on postoperative days 1 and 2 and on days 1 and 7 after discharge, using the Brief Pain Inventory Short Form (BPI-SF). This instrument consists of 15 questions that measure pain severity, extent of interference with activities, and pain relief in response to treatment. The group that received the communication skill information had significantly less pain interference with activity and greater pain relief with treatments on postoperative day 1 than the comparison group. On postopera-

tive day 2, pain interference was similar for both groups and pain relief with treatment was greater for the comparison group. Pain severity scores were similar for both groups on postoperative days 1 and 2. There was no significant difference between the two groups in the postdischarge measures of any pain dimension.

IMPLICATIONS FOR NURSING

Findings from this study highlight the importance of coaching older adults to report their pain experience candidly, particularly in the immediate postoperative period. Establishing trust within the nurse–client relationship is critical to relieving pain. Coaching older clients to describe their pain location, intensity, and sensation gives them permission to communicate in a manner with which they may feel uncomfortable at first. Coaching is necessary to dispel myths about professional expertise and to allow clients control and independence so that they are willing to ask for pain medications. Exploring with older clients their perception of pain, as well as the significance it has for recovery from illness, are necessary elements in providing adequate pain relief and restoring health.

CRITICAL THINKING IN CLIENT CARE

1. What physiologic changes make pain management more difficult for an 80-year-old client following surgery than for a 30-year-old?
2. Your older client says: "I deserved this pain, so I don't want to take anything to make it better." What would be your response and why?
3. A man of Native American descent, age 76, replies that "something doesn't feel right" when asked to rate his pain on a scale of 0 to 10. His pulse is increased and he is protective of his abdominal incision. What could you ask or do to accurately assess his pain?
4. If your grandfather were having surgery tomorrow, what would you like him to be taught about pain management?
5. An independent, 85-year-old woman has a PCA pump for analgesia following major surgery. She continuously presses the pump button, but continues to complain of severe pain. What do you do now?

scrub person or operating room technician (Figure 4–2 ■) constitute the surgical team. Each member provides specialized skills and is essential to the successful outcome of the surgery. Risks to members of the surgical team from bloodborne pathogens or injury are minimized when the surgical team is well organized and prepared.

The surgeon is the physician performing the procedure. As head of the surgical team, the surgeon is responsible for all medical actions and judgments.

The surgical assistant works closely with the surgeon in performing the operation. The number of assistants varies according to the complexity of the procedure. The assistant may be another physician, a nurse, a physician assistant, or other trained personnel. The assistant performs such duties as exposing the operative site, retracting nearby tissue, sponging and/or

suctioning the wound, ligating bleeding vessels, and suturing or helping suture the surgical wound.

The anesthesiologist or certified registered nurse anesthetist relieves the surgeon of the responsibility for the client's general well-being, thus allowing the surgeon to focus on the technical aspects of the procedure. The anesthesiologist or CRNA evaluates the client preoperatively, administers the anesthesia and other required medications, transfuses blood or other blood products, infuses intravenous fluids, continuously monitors the client's physiologic status, alerts the surgeon to developing problems and treats them as they arise, and supervises the client's recovery in the PACU.

The **circulating nurse** is a highly experienced registered nurse who coordinates and manages a wide range of activities before, during, and after the surgical procedure. For example,

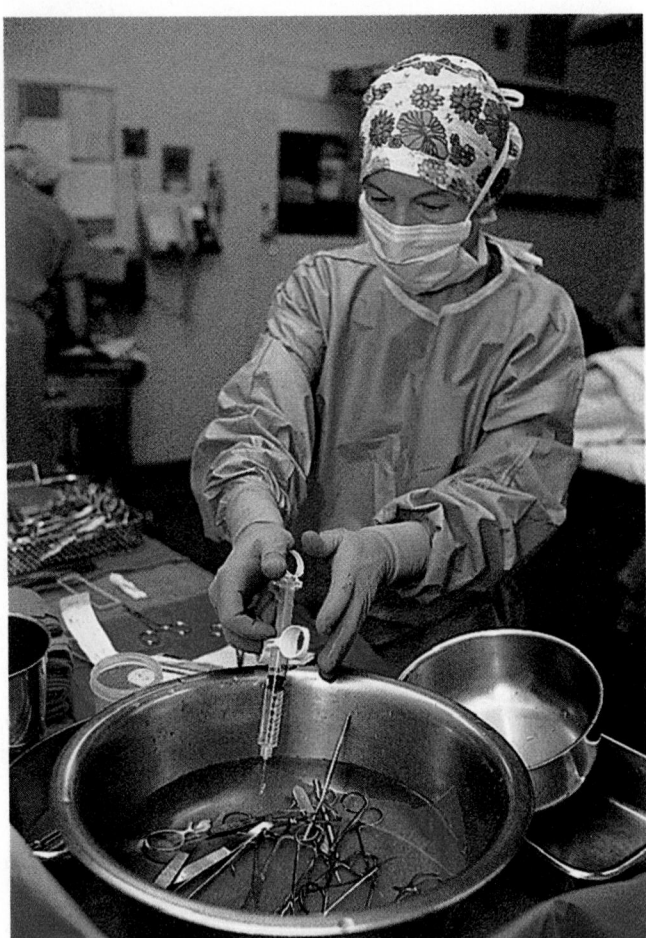

Figure 4–2 ■ A scrub nurse in the operating room.

the circulating nurse oversees the physical aspects of the operating room itself, including the equipment. The circulating nurse also assists with transferring and positioning the client, prepares the client's skin, ensures that no break in aseptic technique occurs, and counts all sponges and instruments. The circulating nurse assists all other team members, including the anesthesiologist or CRNA. Thorough documentation in the surgical area is essential, and the circulating nurse is responsible for documenting intraoperative nursing activities, medications, blood administration, placement of drains and catheters, and length of the procedure. The circulating nurse also formulates a care plan based on physiologic and psychosocial assessments of the client. Finally, the circulating nurse is at all times an advocate for the safety and well-being of the client.

The role of the **scrub person** primarily involves technical skills, manual dexterity, and in-depth knowledge of the anatomic and mechanical aspects of a particular surgery. The scrub person handles sutures, instruments, and other equipment immediately adjacent to the sterile field. The role of the scrub person may be assumed by a registered nurse or an operating room technician (ORT), depending on hospital policy and the complexity of the surgery. Registered nurses are responsible for patient outcomes including the performance of the role of scrub person. AORN believes that registered nurses should maintain an active presence in

the role of scrub person to ensure appropriate delegation and supervision of scrub duties and to maintain an integral link between scrub and circulating responsibilities (AORN, 2005a).

The role of nurses in surgery continues to evolve to improve client care. Although not participating in the surgical procedure, PACU nurses are part of the surgical team. In recent years, nurses have begun to specialize within the already specialized field of perioperative nursing. Specialty surgical teams are developing in response to the demands of increasingly complex technical surgeries. For example, a designated open heart surgical team may be responsible for all open heart cases and ordinarily not be involved with other procedures. The use of specialty surgical teams allows nurses to become highly skilled in a particular range of procedures.

SURGICAL ATTIRE Strict dress codes are necessary in the surgical department to provide infection control within the operating room suites, reduce cross-contamination between the surgery department and other hospital units or departments, and promote both personnel and client health and safety. Based on research and recommendations by hospital infection control authorities, guidelines for attire differ among surgical facilities. Following institutional guidelines, all personnel in the surgical department must be in proper surgical attire. The design and composition of the surgical attire minimize bacterial shedding, thus reducing wound contamination. The area in the surgical department is divided into *unrestricted, semirestricted,* and *restricted* zones. The unrestricted zones permit access by those in hospital uniforms or street clothes. These areas may also allow limited access for communicating with operating room personnel.

The semirestricted zones require scrub attire, including a scrub suit, shoe covers, and a cap or hood (Figure 4–3 ■). Hallways, work areas, and storage areas are considered semirestricted. New guidelines exist for attire in the semirestricted and restricted areas of the OR. Previously, each person had to disrobe and don hospital-laundered scrubs. Today, home-laundered scrubs are accepted by many institutions. There is controversy about this, but the infection control decision to allow home laundry was based on data comparing hospital and home-laundered apparel. These items are covered with sterile gowns in the restricted areas only if the person is "scrubbed in" for the surgery. Only fabrics that are woven or disposable and will not harbor bacteria are allowed and all items of apparel must be covered by appropriate fabric. Anything that can be covered with a scrub jacket is acceptable under these guidelines and no fabric other than the approved scrub uniform fabric can be exposed to the environment. AORN guidelines (AORN Recommended Practices Committee, 2005) suggest that home-laundered scrubs be brought to the OR in a clean covering and donned at the facility, not worn into the hospital from home. Institutions vary in their interpretation of these guidelines.

Artificial nails are discouraged in surgery and anywhere the nurse will have direct contact with high-risk clients. These nails are associated with glove tears and even after careful hand washing can harbor potential pathogens (Church, 2003).

Restricted zones are within operating rooms. Personnel wear masks, sterile gowns, and gloves in addition to appropriate scrub attire if they are participating at the operating table.

Figure 4–3 ■ Surgical attire. *A,* Scrub attire includes scrub suit, shoe covers, and cap or hood to cover hair. *B,* Sterile attire includes scrub suit, shoe covers, and cap or hood, plus gown, gloves, and mask.

The outer sterile covering is changed between procedures or when it becomes soiled or wet.

THE SURGICAL SCRUB The surgical scrub is performed to render hands and arms as clean as possible in preparation for a procedure. All personnel who participate directly in the procedure must perform a surgical scrub with a brush and antimicrobial soap. Skin cannot be rendered sterile, but it can be considered "surgically clean" following the scrub. The purposes of the surgical scrub are to:

- Remove dirt, skin oils, and transient microorganisms from hands and forearms.
- Increase client safety by reducing microorganisms on surgical personnel.
- Leave an antimicrobial residue on the skin to inhibit growth of microbes for several hours.

Following the 5- to 10-minute surgical scrub, hands and arms are dried with sterile towels.

Client Preparation

Although much preparation has taken place prior to the client's transfer to the surgical department, additional activities such as shaving and positioning may be performed. The skin preparation, which usually includes cleansing the area with a prescribed antimicrobial agent, already may have been performed either by the client or by nursing personnel before the transfer to the surgical department. Additional skin cleansing is performed in the surgical department to further decrease microorganisms on the skin and thereby reduce the possibility of wound infection.

The surgeon also may order the skin shaved in and around the proposed incision area (Figure 4–4 ■). Shaving may be completed preoperatively, but more often it is performed in the surgical department. The extent of shaving varies. Generally, the area shaved is wider than the planned incision because of the possibility of unexpected extension of the incision. Disposable, sterile supplies are used, in accordance with aseptic techniques. However, the benefit of shaving the incisional site has become controversial. Physical trauma to the shaved area can weaken the client's defense against organisms, thus increasing the chance of wound infection. An altered body image also may result from the physiologic trauma of a surgical shave, particularly if the shave involves the head or groin area. Hospital policy and surgeon preference should be followed.

Preparing the client for surgery also includes **positioning** the client on the operating table. Table 4–5 shows frequently used positions and describes corresponding surgical procedures and possible adverse effects. Positioning exposes the operative site and provides access for anesthesia administration. Proper positioning is imperative to prevent injury to the client. Pressure, rubbing, and/or shearing forces can cause injury to the tissue over bony prominences. If positioning causes normal joint range of motion to be exceeded, injury to muscles and joints can occur. Improper positioning also can lead to sensory and motor dysfunction, resulting in nerve damage. Pressure on peripheral blood vessels can decrease venous return to the heart and negatively affect the client's blood pressure. Additionally, oxygenation of the blood can be decreased if the client is not properly positioned to promote lung expansion.

Because the anesthetized client cannot respond to discomfort, it is the surgical team's responsibility to position the client not only for the best surgical advantage but also for client safety and comfort. The circulating nurse refers to hospital policy, the surgeon's preference, and the client's history to ensure optimal positioning, and continuously assesses the client.

INTRAOPERATIVE AWARENESS Prior to induction of anesthesia, the circulating nurse establishes rapport with the client to assess the client's psychologic status. This assessment is continued throughout the surgical procedure. After anesthetic medications have been given, the client may appear oblivious to the surroundings; however, anesthesiologists are concerned about patient awareness with recall of intraoperative events (Hassan & Fahy, 2005). Monitors of depth of anesthesia are based on the knowledge that general anesthesia induction is usually accompanied by increased high-frequency electroencephalogram (EEG) activity, which results in increasing sedation and eventual loss of consciousness. The bispectral index monitor (BIS) and the entropy module are types of monitors used to measure the depth of anesthesia and prevent awareness. These devices are based on EEG activity to indicate level of consciousness and depth of anesthesia (White et al., 2006). Intraoperative awareness is the client's subconscious awareness of what is being said and done during surgery. White et al. (2006) compared the aforementioned monitors and reported that no patient had intraoperative recall at 24-hour follow-up interview. Although most clients do not consciously remember what happened or what was said, psychologic trauma can result. Because loss of consciousness is gradual, conversations during surgery should be professional.

Figure 4–4 ■ Areas to be shaved. *A*, Head surgery. *B*, Abdominal surgery. *C*, Thoracoabdominal surgery. *D*, Gynecologic surgery. *E*, Genitourinary surgery. *F*, Forearm, elbow, or hand surgery. *G*, Hip surgery. *H*, Lower leg or foot surgery.

PRACTICE ALERT
Do not say anything while the client is unconscious that would be inappropriate if the client were awake. Maintain a respectful, professional demeanor throughout the operative period.

SPECIAL CONSIDERATIONS FOR THE OLDER ADULT
Because of cardiovascular and tissue changes that result from aging, surgeries longer than 2 hours place the older adult at increased risk for complications. The older adult is more prone to hypotension, hypothermia, and hypoxemia resulting from anesthesia and the cool temperature in the operating room.

Positioning may also cause complications in the older adult. Intraoperative positioning of arthritic joints can cause postoperative joint pain unrelated to the operative site. Also, the longer the surgery, the greater the chance of decubitus ulcer (pressure sore) formation. The older client is at increased risk for developing pressure sores because of decreased subcutaneous fat tissue and reduced peripheral circulation.

TABLE 4–5 Common Surgical Positions

POSITION AND USE	POSSIBLE ADVERSE EFFECTS AND NURSING INTERVENTIONS
(a) The *dorsal recumbent* (or *supine*) *position* is used for many abdominal surgeries (e.g., colostomy and herniorrhaphy) as well as for some thoracic surgeries (e.g., open heart surgery) and some surgeries on the extremities. 	This position may cause excessive pressure on posterior bony prominences, such as the back of the head, scapulae, sacrum, and heels. Pad these areas with soft materials. To avoid compression of blood vessels and sluggish circulation, ensure that the knees are not flexed. Use trochanter rolls or other padding to avoid internal or external rotation of the hips and shoulders.
(b) The *semisitting position* is used for surgeries on the thyroid and neck areas. 	This position can lead to postural hypotension and venous pooling in the legs. It may promote skin breakdown on the buttocks. Sciatic nerve injury is possible. Assess for hypotension. Ensure that knees are not sharply flexed. Use soft padding to prevent nerve compression.
(c) The *prone position* is used for spinal fusions and removal of hemorrhoids. 	This position causes pressure on the face, knees, thighs, anterior ankles, and toes. Pad bony prominences, and support the feet under the ankles. To promote optimum respiratory function, raise the client's chest and abdomen, and support with padding. Corneal abrasion could occur if the eyes are not closed or are insufficiently padded.
(d) The *lateral chest position* is used for some thoracic surgeries, as well as hip replacements. 	This may cause excessive pressure on the bony prominences on the side on which the client is positioned. Ensure adequate padding and support, especially of the downside arm. The weight of the upper leg may cause peroneal nerve injury on the downside leg. Both legs must therefore be padded.
(e) The *lithotomy position* is used for gynecologic, perineal, or rectal surgeries. 	This position causes an 18% decrease (from a standing position) in vital capacity of the lungs. Monitor respirations, and assess for hypoxia and dyspnea. The lithotomy position can lead to joint damage, peroneal nerve damage, and damage to peripheral blood vessels. To avoid injury, ensure adequate padding, and manipulate both legs into the stirrups simultaneously.
(f) The *jackknife position* is used for proctologic surgeries, such as removal of hemorrhoids, and for some spinal surgeries. 	This position causes a 12% decrease (from a standing position) in vital capacity of the lungs. Monitor respirations, and assess for hypoxia and dyspnea. In this position, the greatest pressure is felt at the bends in the table. Therefore, the client is supported with pads at the groin and knees, as well as at the ankles. Padding of the chest and knees helps prevent skin breakdown. Padding and proper positioning help prevent pressure on the ear, the neck, and the nerves of the upper arm.

Finally, the older adult often has some degree of hearing and/or visual impairment. These impairments coupled with a strange environment can make the operating room a frightening, disorienting place. By effectively communicating with the client, the nurse can provide support and reassurance to minimize these factors. To decrease confusion and assist in communication, hearing aids and glasses should be used when appropriate and possible.

Nutrition

Wound healing after surgery depends on adequate nutritional intake. During the immediate postoperative phase, dietary intake is withheld until evidence of peristalsis is found and the client can tolerate liquids without nausea and vomiting. While intravenous fluids maintain hydration and electrolyte balance, they do not provide nutrition. Some clients believe that intravenous fluids are the same as intravenous "feeding," but this is a myth. Unless balanced nutrition through gastrointestinal intake can be reestablished within 3 to 4 days, parenteral hyperalimentation is critical for homeostasis and wound healing.

- Protein, calories, and vitamins are needed for wound healing and recovery from surgery.
- Low-fat, high-fiber diets are important for chronic cardiovascular fitness, but are contraindicated in the wound healing phase following surgery.
- Failure to use the gastrointestinal tract for more than 4 or 5 days allows the intestinal mucosa to atrophy, putting the client at risk for infection.

Fluid administered through peripheral veins must be isotonic or only moderately hypertonic to prevent sclerosing the small peripheral veins. Solutions of 10% dextrose are tolerable peripherally for a short time but do not provide adequate calories for healing and maintenance. To provide adequate nutrition, central vein access must be established and solutions must be prepared with protein, carbohydrates, lipids, vitamins, and minerals. This is important for clients who have extended recovery periods without eating after surgery.

Parenteral nutrition has serious risks. Central vein access may cause infection and sepsis. Normal stimulation to the intestinal tract is lost when the parenteral approach is used alone. Using the gut is better than using the vein because it (1) prevents intestinal atrophy, which results in a very thin bowel wall poorly suited to absorb nutrients; (2) prevents bacteria and inert particles from translocating across the bowel lining into the bloodstream; (3) introduces fats and other large particles into the lymphatic circulation and stimulates the immune system; and (4) is safer and far less expensive than parenteral nutritional support (Heimburger & Weinsier, 1997; Lindgren & Ames, 2005). Education and counseling to support adequate nutritional intake should be ongoing throughout the preoperative and postoperative period.

NURSING CARE

The following section will discuss nursing care in each of the three phases of surgery. A case study at the end of the section follows one client through the postoperative experience, bringing this information together. Perioperative nursing diagnoses are provided in Box 4–2 to assist in identifying the

---

BOX 4–2 Examples of Perioperative Nursing Diagnoses

PREOPERATIVE	INTRAOPERATIVE	POSTOPERATIVE
■ Knowledge, Deficient	■ Knowledge, Deficient	■ Knowledge, Deficient
■ Anxiety	■ Anxiety	■ Pain
■ Fear	■ Fear	■ Breathing Pattern, Ineffective
■ Decisional Conflict	■ Airway Clearance, Ineffective	■ Airway Clearance, Ineffective
■ Coping, Ineffective	■ Aspiration, Risk for	■ Skin Integrity, Impaired
■ Sexuality Patterns, Ineffective	■ Cardiac Output, Decreased	■ Nutrition Imbalanced: Less than Body Requirements
■ Sleep Pattern, Disturbed	■ Hypothermia	■ Sexuality Patterns, Ineffective
■ Thought Processes, Disturbed	■ Infection, Risk for	■ Sleep Pattern, Disturbed
■ Family Processes, Interrupted	■ Thought Processes, Disturbed	■ Fatigue
■ Spiritual Distress	■ Gas Exchange, Impaired	■ Urinary Retention
	■ Urinary Elimination, Impaired	■ Urinary Elimination, Impaired
	■ Fluid Volume, Deficient	■ Adjustment, Impaired
	■ Fluid Volume, Excess	■ Body Image, Disturbed
	■ Communication: Verbal, Impaired	■ Mobility: Physical, Impaired
		■ Activity Intolerance, Risk for
		■ Injury, Risk for
		■ Health Maintenance, Ineffective
		■ Diversional Activity, Deficient
		■ Social Isolation
		■ Spiritual Distress

needs of the surgical client. This is not an exhaustive list, but it can serve as a guide in identifying possible nursing diagnoses.

Preoperative Nursing Care

The client's response to planned surgery varies greatly. When planning and implementing nursing care, consider individual psychologic and physical differences, the type of surgery, and the circumstances surrounding the need for surgery. A thorough nursing assessment is needed to determine the most appropriate care for each client undergoing surgery.

Before planning and implementing care for the surgical client, gather assessment information by taking a nursing history and performing a physical examination. Use this information to establish baseline data, identify physical needs, determine teaching needs and psychologic support for the client and family, and prioritize nursing care. The type of surgical procedure directs the assessment and intervention planned by the nurse.

PRACTICE ALERT
Be sure to assess information about use of over-the-counter medications including herbal supplements. These drugs can interact with medications administered in the perioperative period.

Surgery is a significant and stressful event. Regardless of the nature of the surgery (whether major or minor), the client and family will be anxious. Some clients and their families seek care from a spiritual provider during this time. The degree of anxiety they will feel is not necessarily proportional to the magnitude of the surgical procedure. For example, a client scheduled to have a biopsy to rule out cancer, which is considered minor surgery, may be more anxious than a client undergoing gallbladder removal, which is considered major surgery.

The nurse's ability to listen actively to both verbal and nonverbal messages is imperative to establishing a trusting relationship with the client and family. Therapeutic communication can help the client and family identify fears and concerns. The nurse can then plan nursing interventions and supportive care to reduce the client's anxiety level and assist the client to cope successfully with the stressors encountered during the perioperative period.

Preoperative Client and Family Teaching

Client teaching is an essential nursing responsibility in the preoperative period. Client education and emotional support have a positive effect on the client's physical and psychologic well-being, both before and after surgery. In an analysis of 102 studies, surgical clients receiving client education and/or supportive interventions had less pain and anxiety, experienced fewer complications, were discharged sooner, were more satisfied with their care, and returned to normal activities sooner than clients who did not receive this type of care. These positive outcomes may be attributed in part to the sense of control the client gains through the nurse's teaching.

Client teaching should begin as soon as the client learns of the upcoming surgery. Teaching may begin as early as in the physician's office or at the time of preadmission testing. Although education continues during postoperative care, most teaching is done before surgery, because pain and the effects of anesthesia can greatly diminish the client's ability to learn.

The amount of information desired varies from client to client. Therefore, assess the client's need for and readiness to accept information. The teaching will be directed in part by the particular surgical procedure that is being performed and by the type of anesthesia. The information in Box 4–3 is relevant to most clients undergoing major surgery.

In addition to teaching the client and family about measures that will decrease the risk of complications, provide other preoperative information to prepare the client and family for surgery. This information should include the following:

- Diagnostic tests—reasons and preparations
- Arrival time if surgery is scheduled in early morning
- Preparations for surgery after midnight prior to a morning surgery, skin preparation, indwelling catheter or bladder elimination, start of intravenous infusion, preoperative medication, handling of valuables (rings, watch, money)
- Sedative/hypnotic medication to be taken the night before surgery to promote rest and sleep
- Counseling on whether to take significant medications the morning of surgery
- Informed consent
- Expected timetable for surgery and the recovery room
- Method to inform family of progress throughout surgery
- Transfer to the surgery department
- Location of the surgical waiting room
- Transfer to recovery room
- Anticipated postoperative routine and devices or equipment (drains, tubes, equipment for IV infusions, oxygen or humidifying mask, dressings, splints, casts)
- Plans for postoperative pain control

PRACTICE ALERT
Researchers report that many clients experience unnecessarily long preoperative fasts.

The American Society of Anesthesiologists provides guidelines for preoperative fasting in healthy clients undergoing elective procedures; they are available online. Withdrawal from caffeine in beverages such as coffee or colas may cause headaches and irritability. Dehydration, hypovolemia, and hypoglycemia are other recognized side effects. Thirst, worry, and hunger are reported by clients to be related to fasting. Fasting does not ensure that the stomach will be empty or that the gastric contents will be less acidic.

Preoperative Client Preparation

A preoperative surgical checklist serves as an outline for finalizing preparation of the client for surgery in most institutions. Complete the checklist before the client is transported to surgery. Nursing responsibilities the day of surgery are as follows:

- Assist with bathing, grooming, and changing into operating room gown.
- Ensure that the client takes nothing by mouth (NPO). Provide additional teaching, and reinforce prior teaching.

BOX 4–3 **Preoperative Client Teaching**

Diaphragmatic Breathing Exercise

Diaphragmatic (abdominal) breathing exercises are taught to the client who is at risk for developing pulmonary complications, such as atelectasis or pneumonia. Risk factors for pulmonary complications include general anesthesia, abdominal or thoracic surgery, history of smoking, chronic lung disease, obesity, and advanced age.

In diaphragmatic breathing, the client inspires deeply while allowing the abdomen to expand outward. On expiration, the abdomen contracts inward as air from the lungs is expelled.

1. Explain to the client that the diaphragm is a muscle that makes up the floor of the abdominal cavity and assists in breathing. The purpose of diaphragmatic breathing is to promote lung expansion and ventilation and enhance blood oxygenation.
2. Position the client in a high or semi-Fowler's position (see figure below).
3. Ask the client to place the hands lightly on the abdomen.
4. Instruct the client to breathe in deeply through the nose, allowing the chest and abdomen to expand.
5. Have the client hold the breath for a count of 5.
6. Tell the client to exhale completely through pursed (puckered) lips, allowing the chest and abdomen to deflate.
7. Have the client repeat the exercise five times consecutively.

Encourage the client to perform diaphragmatic breathing exercises every 1 to 2 waking hours, depending on the client's needs and institutional protocol.

Coughing Exercise

Coughing exercises are also taught to the client who is at risk for developing pulmonary complications. The purpose of coughing is to loosen, mobilize, and remove pulmonary secretions. Splinting the incision decreases the physical and psychologic discomfort associated with coughing.

1. Assist the client in following steps 1 through 4 for diaphragmatic breathing.
2. Ask the client to splint the incision with interlocked hand or pillow (see figure below).
3. Tell the client to take three deep breaths and then cough forcefully.
4. Have the client repeat the exercise five times consecutively every 2 hours while awake, taking short rest periods between coughs, if necessary.

Diaphragmatic breathing exercise.

Splinting abdomen while coughing.

- Remove nail polish, lipstick, and makeup to facilitate circulatory assessment during and after surgery.
- Ensure that identification, blood, and allergy bands are correct, legible, and secure.
- Remove hair pins and jewelry; a wedding ring may be worn if it is removed from the finger, covered with gauze, replaced, and then taped to the finger.
- Complete skin or bowel preparation as ordered.
- Insert an indwelling catheter, intravenous line, or nasogastric tube as ordered.
- Remove dentures, artificial eye, and contact lenses, and store them in a safe place.

- Leave a hearing aid in place if the client cannot hear without it, and notify the operating room nurse.
- Verify that the informed consent has been signed prior to administering preoperative medications.
- Weigh the client and record height and weight in the chart (for dosage of anesthesia).
- Verify that all ordered diagnostic test reports are in the chart.
- Have the client empty the bladder immediately before the preoperative medication is administered (unless an indwelling catheter is in place).
- Administer preoperative medication as scheduled (refer to "Medications" earlier in the chapter and Table 4–4).

BOX 4–3 **Preoperative Client Teaching (continued)**

Leg, Ankle, and Foot Exercises

Leg exercises are taught to the client who is at risk for developing thrombophlebitis (inflammation of a vein, which is associated with the formation of blood clots). Risk factors for developing thrombophlebitis include decreased mobility preoperatively and/or postoperatively; a history of difficulties with peripheral circulation; and cardiovascular, pelvic, or lower extremity surgeries.

The purpose of leg exercises is to promote venous blood return from the extremities. As the leg muscles contract and relax, blood is pumped back to the heart, promoting cardiac output and reducing venous stasis. These exercises also maintain muscle tone and range of motion, which facilitate early ambulation.

Teach the client to perform the following exercises while lying in bed:

1. Muscle pumping exercise: Contract and relax calf and thigh muscles at least 10 times consecutively.
2. Leg exercises:
   a. Bend the knee and raise it toward the chest (see figure below).
   b. Straighten out leg and hold for a few seconds before lowering the leg back to the bed.
   c. Repeat exercise five times consecutively prior to alternating to the other foot.
3. Ankle and foot exercises:
   a. Rotate both ankles by making complete circles, first to the right and then to the left (see figure below).
   b. Repeat five times and then relax.
   c. With feet together, point toes toward the head and then to the foot of the bed (see figure below).
   d. Repeat this pumping action 10 times, and then relax.

Encourage the client to perform leg, ankle, and foot exercises every 1 to 2 hours while awake, depending on the client's needs and ambulatory status, the physician's preference, and institutional protocol.

Turning in Bed

The client who is at risk for circulatory, respiratory, or gastrointestinal dysfunction following surgery is taught to turn in bed. Although this may be a simple task prior to surgery, after surgery (particularly after abdominal surgery) the client may find it a difficult procedure. To make the procedure more comfortable, the client may need to splint the incision by using the hand placed on a small pillow or blanket. Additionally, the client should be taught that analgesics can be given to ease postoperative discomfort involved with turning. Encourage the client to turn every 2 hours while awake.

1. Tell the client to grasp the side rail toward the direction to be turned, to rest the opposite foot on the mattress, and to bend the knee.
2. Instruct the client to roll over in one smooth motion by pulling on the side rail while pushing off with the bent knee.
3. Pillows may need to be positioned behind the client's back to help the client maintain a side-lying position. The older client may also need padding over pressure points between the knees and ankles to decrease the chance of decubitus ulcer formation from pressure.

1 Flexed **2** Straight out **3** Then down

Leg exercises.

Ankle and foot exercises.

- Ensure the safety of the client once the medication has been given by placing the client on bed rest with raised side rails and by placing the call light within reach.
- Obtain and record vital signs.
- Provide ongoing supportive care to the client and the client's family.
- Document all preoperative care in the appropriate location, such as the preoperative surgical checklist, the medication record, and the narrative preoperative nursing notes.
- Verify with the surgical personnel the client's identity, and verify that all client information is documented appropriately.
- Help the surgical personnel transfer the client from the bed to the stretcher.

- Prepare the client's room for postoperative care, including making the surgical bed and ensuring that the anticipated supplies and equipment are in the room.

Intraoperative Nursing Care

The intraoperative phase of surgery begins when the client enters the operating room and ends when the client is transferred to the postanesthesia care unit. Nursing care in this phase focuses on keeping the client and the environment safe and providing physiologic monitoring and psychologic support. Circulating nurses and scrub nurses, according to specific role definitions, support and care for the client and assist the surgeons.

PRACTICE ALERT
Objects on the sterile drape are considered sterile. Remain a minimum of 12 inches away from draped tables and sterile fields to avoid contamination if you are not attired in sterile gown and gloves.

Postoperative Nursing Care

Immediate Postoperative Care

Immediate postoperative care begins when the client has been transferred from the operating room to the PACU. The PACU nurse is part of the surgical team and monitors the client's vital signs and surgical site to determine the response to the surgical procedure and to detect significant changes. Assessing mental status and level of consciousness is another ongoing nursing responsibility, and the client may require repeated orientation to time, place, and person. Emotional support also is essential, because the client is in a vulnerable and dependent position. Assessing and evaluating hydration status by monitoring intake and output is crucial to detecting cardiovascular or renal complications. In addition, the PACU nurse assesses the client's pain level. Careful administration of analgesics provides comfort without compounding the potential side effects from the anesthesia.

Care When the Client Is Stable

When awake and after being stabilized, the client is transferred to his or her room. The PACU nurse communicates information about the client's condition and postoperative orders to the floor nurse prior to the client's arrival. This prepares the floor nurse for additional problems or needed equipment.

Immediate and continuing assessment is essential to detect and/or prevent complications. In documenting assessment findings, the nurse completes a flow record of the individual client's situation. Baseline data are obtained and compared with preoperative data. A postoperative head-to-toe assessment includes but may not be limited to the following:

- General appearance
- Vital signs
- Level of consciousness
- Emotional status
- Quantity of respirations
- Skin color and temperature
- Discomfort/pain
- Nausea/vomiting
- Type of intravenous fluids and flow rate
- Dressing site
- Drainage on the dressing and/or bed linen
- Urinary output (catheter or ability to urinate)
- Ability to move all extremities.

The hospital policy or physician's orders dictate the frequency of follow-up assessments. After major surgery, the nurse generally assesses the client every 15 minutes during the first hour and, if the client is stable, every 30 minutes for the next 2 hours, and then every hour during the subsequent 4 hours. Assessments are then carried out every 4 hours, subject to change according to the client's condition and protocol for the particular surgical procedure. It is critically important to inform the surgeon immediately if the assessment reveals any signs of impending shock or other life-threatening changes.

After carrying out the initial assessment and ensuring the client's safety by lowering the bed, raising the side rails, and placing the call light within reach, the nurse notes the physician's postoperative orders. These orders guide the nurse in the care of the postoperative client. For example, the orders specify activity level, diet, medications for pain and nausea, antibiotics, continuation of preoperative medications, frequency of vital sign assessments, administration of intravenous fluids, and laboratory tests such as hemoglobin and potassium level. In most institutions, orders written prior to surgery must be re-ordered following surgery because the client's condition is presumed to have changed.

Nursing Care of Common Postoperative Complications

Several factors place the client at risk for postoperative complications. Nursing care before, during, and after surgery is aimed at preventing and/or minimizing the effects of these complications.

Preoperative care and teaching to decrease postoperative complications have been discussed. The following section addresses postoperative cardiovascular, respiratory, and wound complications, and problems associated with elimination.

Cardiovascular Complications

Common postoperative cardiovascular complications include shock, hemorrhage, deep venous thrombosis, and pulmonary embolism.

SHOCK Shock is a life-threatening postoperative complication. It results from an insufficient blood flow to vital organs, an inability to use oxygen and nutrients, or the inability to rid tissues of waste material. Hypovolemic shock, the most common type in the postoperative client, results from a decrease in circulating fluid volume. Decreased fluid volume develops with blood or plasma loss or, less commonly, from severe prolonged vomiting or diarrhea. Symptoms vary according to the severity of the shock; the greater the loss of fluid volume, the more severe the symptoms. Chapter 11 ∞ provides a detailed discussion of nursing care of the client with various types of shock.

HEMORRHAGE Hemorrhage is an excessive loss of blood. A concealed hemorrhage occurs internally from a blood vessel that is no longer sutured or cauterized or from a drainage tube that has eroded a blood vessel. An obvious hemorrhage occurs externally from a dislodged or ill-formed clot at the wound. Hemorrhage also may result from abnormalities in the blood's ability to clot; these abnormalities may result from a pathologic condition, or they may be a side effect of medications.

Hemorrhage from a venous source oozes out quickly and is dark red, whereas an arterial hemorrhage is characterized by bright red spurts of blood pulsating with each heartbeat.

Whether the hemorrhage is from a venous or an arterial source, hypovolemic shock will occur if sufficient blood is lost from the circulation.

Common assessment with hemorrhage depends on the amount and rate of blood loss. Restlessness and anxiety are observed in the early stage of hemorrhage. Frank bleeding will be present if the hemorrhage is external. The client will have symptoms characteristic of shock.

Care of the client who is hemorrhaging centers around stopping the bleeding and replenishing the circulating blood volume. Nursing care includes providing care for shock and one or more of the following:

- Applying one or more sterile gauze pads and a snug pressure dressing to the area
- Applying pressure with gloved hands (may be necessary for severe external bleeding)
- Preparing client and family for emergency surgery (in severe situations when bleeding cannot be stopped).

DEEP VENOUS THROMBOSIS Deep venous thrombosis (DVT) is the formation of a thrombus (blood clot) in association with inflammation in deep veins. This complication most often occurs in the lower extremities of the postoperative client. It may result from the combination of several factors, including trauma during surgery, pressure applied under the knees, and sluggish blood flow during and after surgery. Clients particularly at risk for developing DVT include those who are over age 40 and who:

- Have undergone orthopedic surgery to lower extremities; urologic, gynecologic, or obstetric surgeries; or neurosurgery.
- Have varicose veins.
- Have a history of thrombophlebitis or pulmonary emboli.
- Are obese.
- Have an infection.
- Have a malignancy.

Common assessment findings reveal pain or cramping in the involved calf or thigh. Redness and edema of the entire extremity may occur along with a slightly elevated temperature. The client may have a positive Homans' sign (pain in the calf on dorsiflexion of the affected foot).

Nursing care of the client with DVT focuses on preventing a portion of the clot from dislodging and becoming an embolus (traveling blood clot) circulating to the heart, brain, or lungs; preventing other clots from forming; and supporting the client's own physiologic mechanism for dissolving clots. Nursing care includes the following measures:

- Administer anticoagulants and analgesics as prescribed. (NSAIDs are not usually given along with anticoagulants, because doing so increases the anticoagulant effects.)
- Monitor laboratory values for clotting times.
- Maintain bed rest and keep affected extremity at or above heart level.
- Apply thigh-high antiemboli stockings or devices to stimulate venous return.
- Ensure that the affected area is not rubbed or massaged.
- Apply heat as prescribed.
- Record bilateral calf or thigh circumferences every shift.

- Teach and support the client and family.
- Assess color and temperature of involved extremity every shift.

PULMONARY EMBOLISM A pulmonary embolism is a dislodged blood clot or other substance that lodges in a pulmonary artery. For the postoperative client with DVT, the threat that a portion of the thrombus may dislodge from the vein wall and travel to the lung, heart, or brain is a constant concern. Early detection of this potentially life-threatening complication depends on the nurse's astute, continuing assessment of the postoperative client.

Common assessment findings of the client experiencing a pulmonary embolism include mild to moderate dyspnea, chest pain, diaphoresis, anxiety, restlessness, rapid respirations and pulse, dysrhythmias, cough, and cyanosis. The severity of the symptoms is determined by the degree of pulmonary vascular blockage. Sudden death can occur if a major pulmonary artery becomes completely blocked.

Stabilizing respiratory and cardiovascular functioning while preventing the formation of additional emboli is of utmost importance in the care of the client with a pulmonary embolism. Nursing care includes the following measures:

- Immediately notify the physician and nursing supervisor.
- Frequently assess and record general condition and vital signs.
- Maintain the client on bed rest, and keep the head of the bed elevated.
- Provide oxygen as ordered and monitor pulse oximetry.
- Administer prescribed intravenous fluids to maintain fluid balance while preventing fluid overload.
- Administer prescribed anticoagulants.
- Maintain comfort by administering analgesics and sedatives (use caution to prevent respiratory depression).
- Provide supportive measures for the client and family.

Refer to Chapter 39 ∞ for a detailed discussion of pulmonary embolism.

Respiratory Complications

Common postoperative respiratory complications include pneumonia and atelectasis.

PNEUMONIA Pneumonia is an inflammation of lung tissue. Inflammation is caused either by a microbial infection or by a foreign substance in the lung, which leads to an infection. Numerous factors may be involved in the development of pneumonia, including aspiration infection, retained pulmonary secretions, failure to cough deeply, and impaired cough reflex and decreased mobility.

Common assessment findings of the postoperative client with pneumonia are as follows:

- High fever
- Rapid pulse and respirations
- Chills (may be present initially)
- Productive cough (may be present depending on the type of pneumonia)
- Dyspnea
- Chest pain
- Crackles and wheezes.

Treating the pulmonary infection, supporting the client's respiratory efforts, promoting lung expansion, and preventing the organisms' spread are the goals in the care of the client with pneumonia. Nursing care includes the following measures:

- Obtain sputum specimens for culture and sensitivity testing.
- Position client with the head of the bed elevated.
- Encourage the client to turn, cough, and perform deep-breathing exercises at least every 2 hours.
- Assist with incentive spirometry, intermittent positive pressure breathing (IPPB), and/or nebulizer treatments as ordered.
- Ambulate client as condition permits and as prescribed.
- Administer oxygen as ordered.
- Assess vital signs, breath sounds, and general condition.
- Maintain hydration to help liquefy pulmonary secretions.
- Administer antibiotics, expectorants, antipyretics, and analgesics as ordered.
- Provide or assist with frequent oral hygiene.
- Prevent the spread of microorganisms by teaching proper disposal of tissues, covering mouth when coughing, and good hand washing technique.
- Provide supportive measures for the client and family. Chapter 39 ∞ provides a detailed discussion of pneumonia.

ATELECTASIS Atelectasis is an incomplete expansion or collapse of lung tissue resulting in inadequate ventilation and retention of pulmonary secretions. Common assessment findings include dyspnea, diminished breath sounds over the affected area, anxiety, restlessness, crackles, and cyanosis.

Promoting lung expansion and systemic oxygenation of tissues is a goal in the care of the client with atelectasis. Nursing care includes these tasks:

- Position the client with the head of bed elevated.
- Administer oxygen as prescribed.
- Encourage coughing, turning, and deep breathing every 2 hours.
- Ambulate the client as condition permits and as prescribed.
- Assist with incentive spirometry or other pulmonary exercises, such as inflating a balloon, as ordered.
- Administer analgesics as prescribed.
- Promote hydration.
- Provide supportive measures to the client and family.

Wound Complications

Discussion of the complications associated with surgical wounds follows an overview of wound healing, wound drainage, and nursing care of wounds.

Wounds heal by either *primary, secondary,* or *tertiary intention* (Figure 4–5 ■). Healing by primary intention takes place when the wound is uncomplicated and clean and has sustained little tissue loss. The edges of the incision are well approximated (have come together well) with sutures, staples, or superglue for drain holes or superficial wounds (Zide, 2005). This type of surgical incision heals quickly, and very little scarring is expected.

Secondary intention refers to the healing that occurs when the wound is large, gaping, and irregular. Tissue loss prevents wound edges from approximating; therefore, granulation fills in the wound. This type of wound takes longer to heal, is more prone to infection, and develops more scar tissue.

Primary intention

Clean incision   Early suture   "Hairline" scar

Secondary intention

Gaping wound with blood clot   Granulation tissue fills in wound   Large scar

Tertiary intention

Contaminated wound   Granulation tissue   Closure with wide scar

Figure 4–5 ■ Wound healing by primary, secondary, and tertiary intention.

Stages of Wound Healing

- *Stage I: from surgery through day 2.* Inflammatory process occurs to prepare the surrounding tissue for healing. Blood vessels constrict, and clotting occurs. Vasodilation follows, bringing more blood, white blood cells, and fibroplastin to the wound site. Epithelial cells begin to form and reestablish blood flow in the wound tissue. A mild temperature elevation is normal.
- *Stage II: day 3 through day 14 following surgery.* Fewer white blood cells are present. Collagen tissue forms in the wound tissue. Granulation tissue, red with a rich blood supply, is established.
- *Stage III: day 15 to week 6 following surgery.* Collagen fibers continue to strengthen the wound. As the blood supply decreases, the scar tissue appears pink and somewhat raised.
- *Stage IV: several months to a year following surgery.* As the wound tissue constricts, the scar becomes flat, smaller, and white.

If enough time passes before a wound is sutured, healing by tertiary intention occurs. Infection is more likely to take place. Because the wound edges are not approximated, tissue is regenerated by the granulation process. Closure of the wound results in a wide scar.

From the time the surgical incision is made until the wound is completely healed, all wounds progress through four stages of healing. However, healing time varies according to many factors, such as age, nutritional status, general health, and the type and location of the wound. Figure 4–5 provides a summary of the stages of wound healing.

Wound drainage (exudate) results from the inflammatory process in the first two stages of wound healing. The drainage is from the rich blood supply that surrounds the wound tissue and is composed of escaped fluid and cells. The drainage is described as serous, sanguineous, or purulent.

- Serous drainage contains mostly the clear serous portion of the blood. The drainage appears clear or slightly yellow and is thin in consistency.
- Sanguineous drainage contains a combination of serum and red blood cells and has a thick, reddish appearance. This is the most common type of drainage from a noncomplicated surgical wound.
- Purulent drainage is composed of white blood cells, tissue debris, and bacteria. Purulent drainage is the result of infection and tends to be of a thicker consistency, with various colors specific to the type of organism. It also may have an unpleasant odor.

Box 4–4 describes and illustrates various types of wound drainage devices. These devices decrease pressure in the wound area by removing excess fluid, which promotes healing and decreases complications.

Nursing care of the postoperative client with a surgical wound focuses on preventing and monitoring for wound complications. The nurse assumes a leading role in supporting the wound healing process, providing emotional support to the client and teaching wound care to the client.

Common assessment findings of an infected wound include pain; purulent, odorous discharge and redness; warmth; tenderness; and edema around the edges of the incision. Additionally, the client may have a fever, chills, and increased respiratory and pulse rates. Nursing care includes the following measures:
- Maintain medical asepsis (e.g., by using good hand washing technique).
- Follow Centers for Disease Control and Prevention guidelines for wound care.

BOX 4–4 Wound Drainage Devices

A Penrose drain, used for passive wound drainage, promotes healing from the inside to the outside (see figure A below). The use of the drain decreases the chance of abscess formation. The safety pin in the Penrose drain prevents the exposed end from slipping down into the wound. Wound care focuses on cleaning around the drain with a prescribed solution, such as sterile normal saline, and replacing the precut gauze dressing as necessary to keep the surrounding skin dry and encourage further drainage. An absorbent dressing is placed over the drain and gauze (not shown).

Wound suction devices promote drainage of fluid from the incision site, decreasing pressure on healing tissues and reducing abscess formation. Shown are the Jackson-Pratt and Hemovac wound suction devices (see figures B and C below).

The frequency with which the nurse empties the device depends on the time elapsed since surgery, type of surgery, amount of drainage, and hospital policy. For example, immediately after surgery the nurse may empty the device every 15 to 60 minutes. With time, as drainage decreases, the device is emptied every 2 to 4 hours (per hospital policy). Amount, color, consistency, and odor of drainage are documented.

Usually, the drain is removed on the second to fourth day after surgery. Removal causes minor client discomfort. The drain site is cleaned, superglue may be applied to the hole, and a sterile dressing is applied.

Wound drainage devices. *A*, Penrose passive wound drainage device. *B*, Jackson-Pratt wound suction device. *C*, Hemovac wound suction device.

- Observe aseptic technique during dressing changes and handling of tubes and drains.
- Assess vital signs, especially temperature.
- Evaluate the characteristics of wound discharge (color, odor, and amount).
- Assess the condition of the incision (approximation of the edges, sutures, staples, or drains).
- Clean, irrigate, and pack the wound in the prescribed manner. Sterile normal saline is often prescribed; povidone-iodine (Betadine) is no longer recommended for wound care.
- Maintain the client's hydration and nutritional status.
- Culture the wound prior to beginning antibiotic therapy.
- Administer antibiotics and antipyretics as prescribed.
- Provide supportive measures to client and family.

Dehiscence is a separation in the layers of the incisional wound (Figure 4–6A ■). Treatment depends on the extent of wound disruption. If the dehiscence is extensive, the incision must be resutured in surgery. **Evisceration** is the protrusion of body organs from a wound dehiscence (Figure 4–6B). These serious complications may result from delayed wound healing or may occur immediately following surgery. They also may occur after forceful straining (coughing, sneezing, or vomiting). When dehiscence occurs, immediately cover the wound with a sterile dressing moistened with normal saline. Emergency surgery is performed to repair these conditions.

Either the nurse, physician, physician assistant (PA), or nurse practitioner (NP) removes sutures or staples after the wound has healed sufficiently (usually 5 to 10 days after surgery). Removal is performed using medical aseptic technique. Additional support may be provided to the incision by applying strips of tape (or Steri-Strips) as directed by institutional policy or by the physician.

Although widely used, wound vacuums are not used to accelerate healing when normal healing is expected. When complications occur in surgically created wounds or a wound occurs traumatically, accelerated granulation stimulated by a wound vacuum may be beneficial. The wound vacuum, along with appropriate antimicrobial therapy and surgery, speeds healing (Antony & Terrazas, 2004).

Complications Associated with Elimination

Common postoperative complications associated with elimination include urinary retention and altered bowel elimination. The inability to urinate with urinary retention may occur postoperatively as a result of the recumbent position, effects of anesthesia and narcotics, inactivity, altered fluid balance, nervous tension, or surgical manipulation in the pelvic area. Nursing care centers on promoting normal urinary elimination and includes the following measures:

- Assess for bladder distention if the client has not voided within 7 to 8 hours after surgery or if the client is urinating small amounts frequently.
- Assess the amount of urine in the bladder with a portable ultrasound scanner. This noninvasive procedure provides information to prevent unnecessary catheterization and decreases the potential for urinary tract infections and urethral trauma from repeated catheterizations.
- Monitor intake and output.
- Maintain intravenous infusion if fluids are prescribed.
- Increase daily oral fluid intake to 2500 to 3000 mL if the client's condition permits.
- Insert a straight or indwelling catheter if ordered.
- Promote normal urinary elimination by:
  a. Assisting and providing privacy when the client uses a bedpan.
  b. Helping the client use the bedside commode or walk to the bathroom.
  c. Assisting male clients to stand to void.
  d. Pouring a measured amount of warm water over the perineal area. (If urination occurs, subtract the amount of water from the total amount for an accurate output measurement.)

Bowel elimination frequently is altered after abdominal or pelvic surgery and sometimes after other surgeries. Return to normal gastrointestinal function may be delayed by general anesthesia, narcotic analgesia, decreased mobility, or altered fluid and food intake during the perioperative period.

Nursing care centers on the return of normal bowel function and includes the following measures:

- Assess for the return of normal peristalsis:
  a. Auscultate bowel sounds every 4 hours while the client is awake.
  b. Assess the abdomen for distention. (A distended abdomen with absent or high-pitched bowel sounds may indicate paralytic ileus.)
  c. Determine whether the client is passing flatus.
  d. Monitor for passage of stool, including amount and consistency.

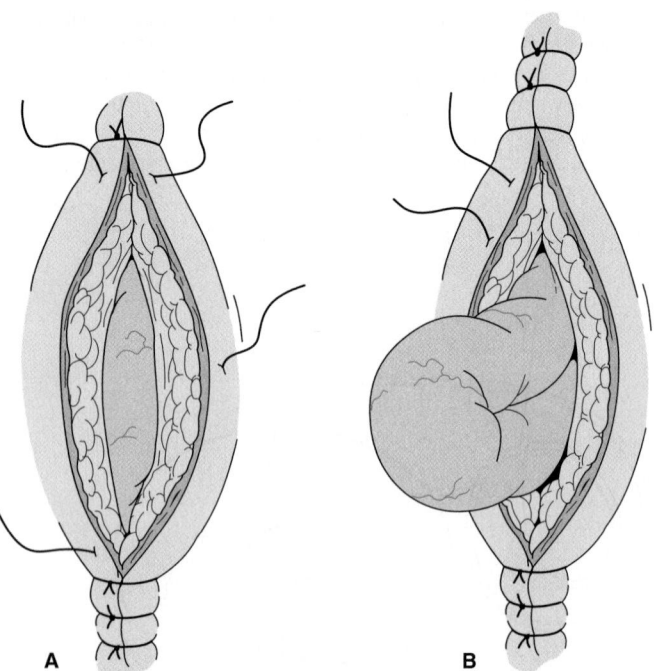

Figure 4–6 ■ Wound complications. *A*, Dehiscence is a disruption in the incision resulting in a separation of the layers of the wound. *B*, Evisceration is a protrusion of a body organ through a surgical incision.

- Encourage early ambulation within prescribed limits.
- Facilitate a daily fluid intake of 2500 to 3000 mL (unless contraindicated).
- Provide privacy when the client is using the bedpan, bedside commode, or bathroom.

If no bowel movement has occurred within 3 to 4 days after surgery, a suppository or an enema may be ordered.

Special Considerations for Older Adults

Physiologic, cognitive, and psychosocial changes associated with the aging process place the older adult at increased risk for postoperative complications. These age-related changes with selected nursing interventions are summarized in Table 4–6. With an ever-increasing population of older adults, particularly the very old, the nurse must be aware of these normal changes and modify nursing care accordingly in an effort to provide safe, supportive care.

Managing Acute Postoperative Pain

Pain is expected after surgery. It is neither realistic nor practical to eliminate postoperative pain completely. Nevertheless, the client should receive substantial relief from and control of this discomfort. Controlling postoperative pain not only promotes comfort but also facilitates coughing, turning, deep-breathing exercises, earlier ambulation, and decreased length of hospitalization, resulting in fewer postoperative complications, and therefore reducing healthcare costs. Despite the apparent benefits and methods of effective pain control and improved understanding of pain physiology, many postoperative clients do not receive adequate pain relief or control (MacLellan, 2004; Schechter, 2004).

Managing acute postoperative pain is an important nursing role before, during, and after surgery. Successful pain management involves the cooperative efforts of the client, physician, and nurse. The American Society of Anesthesiologists suggests six specific guidelines for perioperative pain management. These include education and training for healthcare providers, monitoring of patient outcomes, 24-hour availability of anesthesiologists providing perioperative pain management, and use of a dedicated acute pain service. Preoperatively, the client should learn how much pain to anticipate and what methods are available to control pain. After discussing options with the client, healthcare providers must respect the client's personal preferences.

Postoperative medications were discussed earlier in the chapter. Various nonpharmacologic approaches to pain management are used alone or in combination to control acute postoperative pain. Relaxation, music, distraction, and imagery techniques can decrease mild pain and anxiety. Massage and the

TABLE 4–6 Nursing Interventions for Older Surgical Clients

SYSTEM	AGE-RELATED CHANGES	NURSING INTERVENTIONS
General appearance	Change in height, weight, and fat distribution	Assess physical parameters. Provide for warmth. Turn frequently.
Integument	Diminished integrity secondary to loss of subcutaneous fat and decreased oil production, elasticity, and hydration	Provide careful preoperative preparation to avoid trauma. Use other means to assess oxygenation and hydration, such as evaluation of mucous membranes, laboratory studies, and urine output.
Sensory-perceptual	Decline in vision and hearing ability; dryness of mouth	Compensate for sensory deficits: speak low, not loud; minimize noise in environment; provide adequate room light; stay within client's field of vision when speaking; encourage client to wear hearing aid to the operating room. Provide comfort measures when NPO.
Respiratory	Decreased efficiency of cough reflex and decreased aeration of lung fields	Teach and encourage coughing and diaphragmatic breathing exercises. Assess baseline parameters. Constantly monitor lung sounds and respiratory status.
Cardiovascular	Less efficient, decreased adaptation to stress	Monitor for hypotension and shock. Assess for thrombus formation, cardiac dysrhythmias, peripheral pulses, and edema.
Gastrointestinal	Decline in gastric motility	Encourage intake of adequate fluids, nutritious meals, soft diet. Assist with feeding; monitor bowel function.
Genitourinary	Decreased efficiency of kidney; loss of bladder control	Monitor I&O and electrolyte levels. Assess for drug side effects. Assist with voiding as needed.
Musculoskeletal	Stiffness of joints; decrease in strength; brittleness of bones	Carefully position on OR table. Move carefully and gently. Prevent pressure sores.
Cognitive-psychosocial	Decreased reaction time; stable intellectual ability; proneness to delirium and altered mental status while in hospital	Provide ample time for making decisions. Implement safety measures. Talk to client as adult, not as child. Orient frequently.

Source: Adapted from "Perioperative Nursing Care for the Elderly Surgical Patient" by C. Dellasea and C. Burgunder, 1991, *Today's O.R. Nurse, 13*(6), 12–17.

application of heat or cold can also relieve postoperative pain (McRee et al., 2003). Transcutaneous electrical nerve stimulation (TENS) has been used successfully to decrease postoperative incisional pain. Other approaches include acupuncture, acupressure, and therapeutic touch. Additional information on pain management techniques is found in Chapter 9 .

Opioid dosage requirements vary greatly from one client to another and by the route they are taken. Remember that oral doses of analgesics are not equal to parenteral doses. Oral doses need to be higher to provide **equianalgesia**. (See Table 9–4 regarding equianalgesics.)

The client's input and participation in assessing pain and pain relief is essential to a successful pain control regime. For example, the client can rate the pain on a scale of 0 to 10 (where 0 signifies no pain and 10 signifies unbearable pain). Assess and document pain at scheduled intervals to determine the degree of pain control, to observe for drug side effects, and to assess the need for changes in the dosage and/or frequency of medication administration. When a range of dosage is ordered, carefully titrate opioid dosages based on individual assessments of need and response to therapy.

Using NANDA, NIC, and NOC

Chart 4–1 shows links between NANDA nursing diagnoses, NIC, and NOC when caring for the postoperative client.

Community-Based Care

Because the postoperative phase does not end until the client has recovered completely from the surgical intervention, the nurse plays a vital role as the client nears discharge. As the client prepares to recuperate at home, provide information and support to help the client successfully meet self-care demands. All aspects of teaching should be accompanied by written guidelines, directions, and information. This is particularly helpful when a large amount of unfamiliar, detailed information is presented. Because the hospital stay is often brief, make an organized, coordinated effort to educate the client and family. Teaching needs vary, but the most common needs include:

- How to perform wound care. Teaching is more effective if the nurse first demonstrates and explains the procedure for the client and family or other caregiver. The client and family should then participate in the care. To evaluate the effectiveness of the teaching, ask the client or caregiver to demonstrate the procedure in return. Ideally, teaching is carried out over several days, evaluated, and periodically reinforced.

NANDA, NIC, AND NOC LINKAGES
CHART 4–1 The Postoperative Client

NANDA

Acute Pain

↓

NIC

Medication Administration (IM)

Medication Administration (IV)

Patient-Controlled Analgesia (PCA)

Pain Management

Postanesthesia Care

↓

NOC

Pain Level

Pain Control

Symptom Control

Data from *NANDA's Nursing Diagnoses: Definitions & classification 2005–2006* by NANDA International (2003), Philadelphia; *Nursing Interventions Classification (NIC)* (4th ed.) by J. M. Dochlerman & G. M. Bulechek (2004), St. Louis, MO: Mosby; and *Nursing Outcomes Classification (NOC)* (3rd ed.) by S. Moorhead, M. Johnson, and M. Maas (2004), St. Louis, MO: Mosby.

- Signs and symptoms of a wound infection. The client should be able to determine what is normal and what should be reported to the physician.
- Method and the frequency of taking one's temperature.
- Limitations or restrictions that may be imposed on such activities as lifting, driving, bathing, sexual activity, and other physical activities.
- Control of pain. If analgesics are prescribed, instruct the client in the dosage, frequency, purpose, common side effects, and other side effects to report to the physician. Reinforce the use of relaxation, distraction, imagery, or other pain control techniques that the client has found useful in controlling postoperative pain.

NURSING CARE PLAN   A Client Having Surgery

Martha Overbeck is a 74-year-old widow of German descent who lives alone in a senior citizens' housing complex. She is active there, as well as in the Lutheran Church. She has been in good health and is independent, but she has become progressively less active as a result of arthritic pain and stiffness. Mrs. Overbeck has degenerative joint changes that have particularly affected her right hip. On the recommendation of her physician and following a dis-

cussion with her friends, Mrs. Overbeck has been admitted to the hospital for an elective right total hip replacement. Her surgery has been scheduled for 8:00 A.M. the following day.

Mrs. Eva Jackson, a close friend and neighbor, accompanies Mrs. Overbeck to the hospital. Mrs. Overbeck explains that her friend will help in her home and assist her with the wound care and prescribed exercises.

NURSING CARE PLAN A Client Having Surgery (continued)

ASSESSMENT

Gloria Nobis, RN, is assigned to Mrs. Overbeck's care on return to her room. Ms. Nobis performs a complete head-to-toe assessment and determines that Mrs. Overbeck is drowsy but oriented. Her skin is pale and slightly cool. Mrs. Overbeck states she is cold and requests additional covers. Ms. Nobis places a warmed cotton blanket next to Mrs. Overbeck's body, adds another blanket to her covers, and adjusts the room's thermostat to increase the room temperature. Mrs. Overbeck states that she is in no pain and would like to sleep. She has even, unlabored respirations and stable vital signs as compared to preoperative readings.

Mrs. Overbeck is NPO. An intravenous solution of dextrose and water is infusing at 100 mL/h per infusion pump. No redness or edema is noted at the infusion site. Ms. Nobis notes that the antibiotic ciprofloxacin hydrochloride (Cipro) is to be administered by mouth when the client is able to tolerate fluids. Mrs. Overbeck has a large gauze dressing over her right upper lateral thigh and hip with no indications of drainage from the wound. Tubing protrudes from the distal end of the dressing and is attached to a passive suctioning device (Hemovac). Ms. Nobis empties 50 mL of dark red drainage from the suctioning device and records the amount and characteristics on a flow record. Mrs. Overbeck has a Foley catheter in place with 250 mL of clear, light amber urine in the dependent gravity drainage bag.

When assessing Mrs. Overbeck's lower extremities, Ms. Nobis finds her feet slightly cool and pale with rapid capillary refill time bilaterally. Dorsalis pedis and posterior tibial pulses are strong and equal bilaterally. Ms. Nobis notes slight pitting edema in the right foot and ankle as compared with the left extremity. She also notes sensation and ability to move both feet and toes, without numbness or tingling (paresthesia).

Ms. Nobis records the above findings on a postoperative flowsheet. After ensuring that Mrs. Overbeck is safely positioned and can reach her call light, Ms. Nobis gives Mrs. Overbeck's friend, Mrs. Jackson, a progress report. They then go into Mrs. Overbeck's room.

DIAGNOSES

Ms. Nobis makes the following postoperative nursing diagnoses for Mrs. Overbeck.

- *Risk for Infection* of right hip wound related to disruption of normal skin integrity by the surgical incision
- *Risk for Injury* related to potential dislocation of right hip prosthesis secondary to total hip replacement
- *Pain* related to right hip incision and positioning of arthritic joints during surgery

EXPECTED OUTCOMES

The expected outcomes established in the plan of care specify that Mrs. Overbeck will:

- Regain skin integrity of the right hip incision without experiencing signs or symptoms of infection.
- Demonstrate (along with Mrs. Jackson) proper aseptic technique while performing the dressing change.
- Verbalize signs and symptoms of infection to be reported to her physician.
- Describe measures to be taken to prevent dislocation of right hip prosthesis.

- Report control of pain at incision and in arthritic joints.
- Remain afebrile.

PLANNING AND IMPLEMENTATION

Ms. Nobis develops a care plan that includes the following interventions to assist Mrs. Overbeck during her postoperative recovery.

- Use aseptic technique while changing dressing.
- Monitor temperature and pulse every 4 hours to assess for elevation.
- Assess wound every 8 hours for purulent drainage and odor. Assess edges of wound for approximation, edema, redness, or inflammation in excess of expected inflammatory response.
- Teach Mrs. Overbeck and Mrs. Jackson how to use aseptic technique while assessing the wound and performing the dressing change.
- Teach Mrs. Overbeck and Mrs. Jackson the signs and symptoms of infection and when to report findings to the physician.
- Review and discuss with Mrs. Overbeck the written materials on total hip replacement.
- Convey empathetic understanding of Mrs. Overbeck's incisional and arthritic joint pain.
- Medicate Mrs. Overbeck every 4 hours (or as ordered) to maintain a therapeutic analgesic blood level.

EVALUATION

Throughout Mrs. Overbeck's hospitalization, Ms. Nobis works with Mrs. Overbeck and Mrs. Jackson to ensure that Mrs. Overbeck can care for herself after discharge from the hospital. Five days after her surgery, Mrs. Overbeck is discharged with a well-approximated incision with no indications of an infection. Prior to discharge, Ms. Nobis is confident that with Mrs. Jackson's help, Mrs. Overbeck can properly assess the incision. With minimal help, Mrs. Overbeck is able to replace the dressing using aseptic technique. She can cite the signs and symptoms of an infection, take her own oral temperature, and describe preventive measures to decrease the chances of dislocating her prosthetic hip. Because of her reduced mobility the past 5 days, Mrs. Overbeck says she can tell the arthritis in her "old bones" is "acting up." She reports less pain in her right hip than before the surgery. Mrs. Overbeck tells Ms. Nobis she will be back the following winter to have her left hip replaced.

CRITICAL THINKING IN THE NURSING PROCESS

1. Describe risk factors for Mrs. Overbeck's safety; what changes in her home environment would you suggest to promote safety until she recovers more fully?
2. Why is Mrs. Overbeck placed on the antibiotic Cipro although she has no indications of an infection? What teaching would you do?
3. Mrs. Overbeck's clotting time is slightly elevated as a result of an ordered anticoagulant. Why would this medication be ordered? Consider the client's age and the area of surgery.
4. Mrs. Overbeck is 30 pounds above her ideal weight and has osteoarthritis. Develop a care plan for the nursing diagnosis *Ineffective Health Maintenance* related to intake in excess of metabolic requirements.

See Evaluating Your Response in Appendix C.

EXPLORE MediaLink

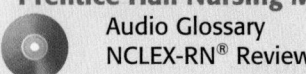

Prentice Hall Nursing MediaLink DVD-ROM
Audio Glossary
NCLEX-RN® Review

Animation/Video
Epidural Placement

COMPANION WEBSITE www.prenhall.com/lemone
Audio Glossary
NCLEX-RN® Review
Care Plan Activity: Providing Postoperative Care
Case Study: The Circulating Nurse
MediaLink Applications
Anesthesia and Outpatient Surgery
Consent Forms
Joint Replacement Patient Education Program
Links to Resources

CHAPTER HIGHLIGHTS

- Surgeries take place in traditional and nontraditional settings with increasing use of minimally invasive procedures that expedite discharge, facilitate healing, and increase client satisfaction.

- Surgery is an invasive procedure and legal guidelines must be followed to protect the client and the healthcare providers. The surgical team includes surgeons, anesthetists, nurses, and technicians; all are responsible for the safety of the client and the progression of the surgery.

- The focus on safety during surgery continues to increase with attention directed to preventing wrong site, wrong patient surgeries. Procedures are established to verify that the right patient will have the correct surgery. A team approach to safety works best; each member of the team must feel accountable for the results of the surgery and entitled to share observations and concerns as the procedure progresses.

- Inpatient clients have relatively short stays, which are best achieved by early ambulation, pain control, and proper nutrition. Providing information for self-care is challenging with the shortened stays and rate of admissions and discharges. From the time of entry to the surgical setting, the client's discharge must be planned and prepared.

- Client teaching prior to and following surgery empowers clients to achieve successful recovery, discharge, and rehabilitation. Most of

the care clients receive during healing is either provided by self or a caregiver outside the healthcare environment. Clients and their families need to know appropriate assessments and interventions to monitor the healing process.

- Pain management is offered prior to, during, and after surgery with methods designed to give the best therapeutic response. While acute pain occurs related to the surgery, many clients also experience chronic pain that affects their response to pain management therapies.

- Behaviors characteristic of older adult clients and ethnically diverse populations increase the need for individualized care. Assessment of physical and emotional status can be more difficult when clients have hearing or visual impairments or when individuals speak and understand a foreign language. Surgery can be frightening to clients and their families and they need reassurance and interventions to decrease pain, relieve anxiety, and promote healing.

- Operating room and postanesthesia care nursing are professional specialties that require unique orientation and education. These professionals make careful assessments of the risks each client faces and make plans to ensure safe, successful surgical outcomes. Special attention is focused on early recognition and treatment of postoperative complications associated with cardiopulmonary function, respiratory function, wound healing, elimination, and pain.

TEST YOURSELF NCLEX-RN® REVIEW

1 The nurse's primary responsibility related to informed consent is:
1. defining the risks and benefits of the surgery.
2. witnessing the client's signature on the consent form.
3. explaining the right to refuse treatment or withdraw consent.
4. advising the client and family about what is needed for the diagnosis.

2 Obtaining a preoperative blood pressure measurement serves the following purpose:
1. Fulfills a legal requirement.
2. Informs anesthesiologist so proper level of anesthesia can be given.
3. Prevents atelectasis.
4. Provides a baseline to compare postoperative blood pressure levels.

3 Nonsteroidal anti-inflammatory drugs are given in the postoperative period to:
1. stimulate appetite.
2. increase amnesia.
3. potentiate analgesia.
4. improve renal function.

4 Discharge planning for a client following general surgery will include dietary management guidelines. Specifically, the client will eat a diet:
1. low in cholesterol, high in fat.
2. high in protein, moderate in calories.
3. low in fat, high in fiber.
4. diet that is regular, but without dairy products.

5 In the immediate postoperative period for knee surgery, assessment distal to the site includes:
1. urinary Ph.
2. rebound tenderness.
3. Chvostek's sign.
4. neurovascular assessment.

6 In the postoperative period, medications the client is prescribed prior to surgery must be:
1. continued after surgery.
2. decreased by half for 36 hours.
3. ordered anew prior to administration.
4. withheld until evidence of anesthesia is absent.

7 The client with diabetes mellitus who is NPO prior to surgery:
1. has no risk for hyperglycemia.
2. should receive sliding-scale insulin prescriptions.
3. will benefit from hypoglycemia during anesthesia.
4. will fail to manifest signs of hypoglycemia under anesthesia.

8 Acute pain management medications in the immediate postoperative period generally
1. progress from NSAIDs to opioids.
2. progress from oral to parenteral routes.
3. should be scheduled rather than prn to promote control.
4. induce a strong sedative effect to decrease the risk of nausea.

9 Lengthy operative procedures can put the older client at risk for:
1. memory loss due to blood loss.
2. hearing loss due to extended anesthesia.
3. weight loss due to lack of nutritional intake.
4. pressure sores and joint pain from operative positioning.

10 Hypothermia in the perioperative period
1. decreases cardiac ischemia.
2. reduces the risk for wound infection.
3. increases client comfort and analgesia.
4. requires interventions to prevent and relieve.

See Test Yourself answers in Appendix C.

BIBLIOGRAPHY

American Society for Pain Management Nursing and the American Pain Society. (2004). Consensus statement: The use of "as needed" range orders for opioid analgesics in the management of acute pain. Retrieved January 9, 2005, from http://www.ampainsoc.org/advocacy/range.htm

American Society of Anesthesiologists. (2004). Practice guidelines for acute pain management in the perioperative setting. An updated report by the American Society of Anesthesiologists Task Force on Acute Pain Management. *Anesthesiology, 100,* 1573–1581.

Andersen, B. R., Kallehave, F. L., & Andersen, H. K. (2005). Antibiotics versus placebo for prevention of postoperative infection after appendicectomy (Review). *The Cochrane Database of Systematic Reviews, 4.*

Antony, S., & Terrazas, S. (2004). A retrospective study: Clinical experience using vacuum-assisted closure in the treatment of wounds. *Journal of the National Medical Association, 96*(8), 1073–1077.

AORN. (2005a). AORN position statement on the role of the scrub person. AORN official statements. Retrieved January 21, 2006, from http://www.aorn.org/about/positions/default.htm

AORN. (2005b). Competency statements, 21–35. Standards, recommended practices, and guidelines. Denver, CO: AORN, Inc.

AORN Recommended Practices Committee. (2005). Recommended practices for surgical attire. *AORN Journal, 81,* 413–420.

AORN Recommended Practices Committee. (2000). Recommended practices for safety through identification of potential hazards in the perioperative environment. *AORN Journal, 72,* 690–692, 695, 697–698.

Arndt, K. (1999). Inadvertent hypothermia in the OR. *AORN Journal, 70,* 204–214.

Asher, M. E. (2004). Surgical considerations in the elderly. *Journal of Perianesthesia Nursing, 19*(6), 406–414.

Bailey, D. G., & Dresser, G. K. (2004). Natural products and adverse drug reactions. *Canadian Journal of Medicine, 170*(4), 1531–1532.

Banks, R. R., & Danks, B. (2004). Laryngeal mask airway: Review of indications and use. *Journal of Emergency Nursing, 30*(1), 30–35.

Bedouch, P., Labarere, J., Chirpaz, E., Allenet, B., Lepape, A., Fourny, M., et al. (2004). Compliance with guidelines on antibiotic prophylaxis in total hip replacement surgery: Results of a retrospective study of 416 patients in a teaching hospital. *Infection Control & Hospital Epidemiology, 25*(4), 302–307.

Bhattacharyya, T., Yeon, H., & Harris, M. B. (2005). The medical-legal aspects of informed consent in orthopaedic surgery. *The Journal of Bone and Joint Surgery, 87A*(11), 2395–2400.

Brandom, B. W. (2005). The genetics of malignant hyperthermia. *Anesthesiology Clinics of North America, 23,* 615–619.

Bratzler D. W., & Houck, P. M. (2005). Surgical Infection Prevention Guideline Writers Workgroup. Antimicrobial prophylaxis for surgery: An advisory statement from the National Surgical Infection Prevention Project. *American Journal of Surgery, 189*(4), 395–404.

Bressler, R. (2005). Herb-drug interactions: Interactions between Kava and prescription medications. *Geriatrics, 60*(9), 24–25.

Brown, B., Riippa, M., & Shaneberger, K. (2001). Promoting patient safety through preoperative patient verification. *AORN Journal, 74*(5), 690–698.

Busen, N. H. (2001). Perioperative preparation of the adolescent surgical patient. *AORN Journal, 73,* 337–363.

Carless, P., Moxey, A., O'Connell, D., & Henry, D. (2004). Autologous transfusion techniques: A systematic review of their efficacy. *Transfusion Medicine, 14*(2), 123–144.

Carter-Templeton, H. (2005). Malignant hyperthermia. *Nursing, 35*(6), 88.

Church, N. (2003). Ban on artificial nails recommended for anyone having direct patient contact. *Oregon Nurse, 68*(1), 5.

Cohen, M. J., & Schecter, W. P. (2005). Perioperative pain control: A strategy for management. *Surgical Clinics of North America, 85,* 1243–1257.

Crensha, J. T., & Winslow, E. H. (2002). Preoperative fasting: Old habits die hard. *American Journal of Nursing, 102*(5), 36–45.

Danter, J. H. (2003). Put a realistic spin on geriatric assessment. *Nursing, 33*(12), 52–55.

Dunn, D. (2004). Preventing perioperative complications in an older adult. *Nursing 2004, 34*(11), 36–42.

Ersek, M., Cherrier, M. M., Overman, S. S., & Irving, G. A. (2004). The cognitive effects of opioids. *Pain Management Nursing, 5*(2), 75–93.

Evans, C. (2004). Improving assessment of pain in older people. *Emergency Nurse, 12*(5), 18–21.

Gibbs, V. C. (2005). Patient safety practices in the operating room: Correct-site surgery and nothing left behind. *Surgical Clinics of North America, 85,* 1207–1319.

Gottschalk, A., & Smith, D. S. (2001). New concepts in acute pain therapy: Preemptive analgesia. *American Family Physician, 63*(10), 1979–1984.

Graham, I. D., Fergusson, D., Dokainish, H., Biggs, J., McAuley, L., & Laupacis A. (1999). Autologous versus allogeneic transfusion: Patients' perceptions and experiences. *Canadian Medical Association Journal, 160*(7), 989–995.

Hartrick, C. T. (2004). Multimodal postoperative pain management. *American Journal of Health-System Pharmacology, 61*(S1), S4–S10.

Hassan, Z., & Fahy, B. G. (2005). Anesthetic choices in surgery. *Surgical Clinics of North America, 85,* 1075–1089.

Heimberger, D. C., & Weinsier, R. L. (1997). *Handbook of clinical nutrition* (3rd ed.). St. Louis, MO: Mosby.

Ireland, D. (1997). Legal issues in ambulatory surgery. *Nursing Clinics of North America, 32*(2), 469–476.

Joint Commission. (2004). *Comprehensive accreditation manual for hospitals: the official handbook.* Oak Brook Terrace, IL: Joint Commission Resources, Inc.

Lindgren, V. A., & Ames, N. (2005). Caring for patients on mechanical ventilation: What research indicates is best practice. *American Journal of Nursing, 105*(5), 50–60.

Litman, R. S., & Rosenberg, H. (2005). Malignant hyperthermia: Update on susceptibility testing. *Journal of the American Medical Association, 293*(23), 2918–2924.

Loran, D. B., Hyde, B. R., & Zwischenberger, J. B. (2005). Perioperative management of special populations: The geriatric patient. *Surgical Clinics of North America, 85,* 1259–1266.

MacLellan, K. (2004). Postoperative pain: Strategy for improving patient experiences. *Journal of Advanced Nursing, 46*(2), 179–193.

McDonald, D. D., Thomas, G. J., Livingston, K. E., & Severson, J. S. (2005). Assisting older adults to communicate their postoperative pain. *Clinical Nursing Research, 14*(2), 109–126.

McRee, L. D., Noble, S., & Pasvogel, A. (2003). Using massage and music therapy to improve postoperative outcomes. *AORN, 78*(3), 433–447.

Monarch, S., & Wren, K. (2004). Geriatric anesthesia implications. *Journal of Perianesthetia Nursing, 19*(6), 379–384.

Norred, C. L., & Brinker, F. (2001). Potential coagulation effects of preoperative complementary and alternative medicines. *Alternative Therapies in Health & Medicine, 7*(6), 58–67.

Odom-Forren, J. (2006). Preventing surgical site infections. *Nursing, 36*(6), 58–63.

O'Donnell, J. M., Bragg, K., & Sell, S. (2003). Procedural sedation: Safely navigating the twilight zone. *Nursing, 33*(4), 36–44.

Olson, D. M., Cheek, D. J., & Morgenlander, J. C. (2004). The impact of bispectral index monitoring on rates of propofol administration. *AACN Clinical Issues, 15*(1), 63–73.

Pagana, K. D., & Pagana, T. J. (2002). *Mosby's manual of diagnostic and laboratory tests* (2nd ed.). St. Louis, MO: Mosby.

Phillips, N. (2004). *Berry & Kohn's operating room technique* (10th ed.). St. Louis, MO: Mosby.

Porth, C. (2005). *Pathophysiology: Concepts of altered health states* (7th ed.). Philadelphia: Lippincott.

Reitman, C. A., Watters, W. C. III, & Sassard, W. R. (2004). The Cell Saver in adult lumbar fusion surgery: A cost–benefit outcomes study. *Spine, 29*(14), 1580–1583.

Saper, R. B. (2005). *Overview of herbal medicine.* UpToDate online. Retrieved January 9, 2006, from http://www.uptodate.com

Saufl, N. M. (2004). Preparing the older adult for surgery and anesthesia. *Journal of Perianesthesia Nursing, 19*(6), 372–378.

Schechter, L. N. (2004). Clinical advances in the management of postoperative pain: Introduction. *American Journal of Health-System Pharmacy, 61,* S1, S3–S4.

Schwartz, A. J. (2006). Learning the essentials of epidural anesthesia. *Nursing, 36*(1), 44–50.

Silber, J. H., Rosenbaum, P. R., Trudeau, M. E., Chen, W., Zhang, X., Lorch, S. A., et al. (2005). Preoperative antibiotics and mortality in the elderly. *Annals of Surgery, 242*(1), 107–114.

Stringer, B., Infante-Revard, C., & Hanley, J. (2001). Quantifying and reducing the risk of bloodborne pathogen exposure. *AORN Journal, 73,* 1135–1146.

Tappen, R. M., Muzic, J., & Kennedy, P. (2001). Preoperative assessment and discharge planning for older adults undergoing ambulatory surgery. *AORN Journal, 73,* 464–474.

Walton, J. (2001). Helping high-risk surgical patients beat the odds. *Nursing 2001, 31*(3), 54–59.

White, P. F., Tang, J., Romero, G. F., Wender, R. H., Naruse, R., Sloninsky, A., et al. (2006). A comparison of state and response entropy versus bispectral index values during the perioperative period. *Anesthesia & Analgesia, 102,* 160–167.

Whitman, M. (2000). The starving patient. *Clinical Journal of Oncology Nursing, 4*(3), 121–125.

Wren, K. R., Kimbrall, S., & Norred, C. L. (2002). Use of complementary and alternative medications by surgical patients. *Journal of Perianesthesia Nursing, 17*(3), 170–177.

Zide, B. M. (2005). Seven more tips for the operating room. *Plastic & Reconstructive Surgery, 115*(3), 973–975.

CHAPTER 5

Nursing Care of Clients Experiencing Loss, Grief, and Death

LEARNING OUTCOMES

- Differentiate loss, grief, and mourning.
- Compare and contrast theories of loss and grief.
- Explain factors affecting responses to loss.
- Discuss legal and ethical issues in end-of-life care.
- Describe the philosophy and activities of hospice.

CLINICAL COMPETENCIES

- Identify physiological changes in the dying client.
- Provide nursing interventions to promote a comfortable death.
- Provide individualized care for clients and families experiencing loss, grief, or death.

MEDIALINK

Resources for this chapter can be found on the Prentice Hall Nursing MediaLink DVD-ROM accompanying this textbook, and on the Companion Website at
http://www.prenhall.com/lemone

anticipatory grieving, *86*
bereavement, *92*
chronic sorrow, *97*
death, *85*
death anxiety, *97*
do-not-resuscitate order, *91*

durable power of attorney, *90*
end-of-life nursing care, *89*
euthanasia, *91*
grief, *85*
grieving, *85*
healthcare surrogate, *90*

hospice, *91*
living will, *90*
loss, *85*
mourning, *85*
palliative care, *92*

Loss may be defined as an actual or potential situation in which a valued object, person, body part, or emotion that was formerly present is lost or changed and can no longer be seen, felt, heard, known, or experienced. A loss may be temporary or permanent, complete or partial, objectively verifiable or perceived, physical or symbolic. Only the person who experiences the loss can determine the meaning of the loss. Although the order of importance varies with the person, people most commonly fear the losses listed in Box 5–1.

Loss always results in change. The stress associated with the loss may be the precipitating factor leading to physiologic or psychologic change in the person or family. The effective or ineffective resolution of feelings surrounding the loss determines the person's ability to deal with the resulting changes.

Grief is the emotional response to loss and its accompanying changes. Grief as a response to loss is an inevitable dimension of the human experience. The loss of a job, a role (e.g., the loss of the role of spouse, as occurs in divorce), a goal, body integrity, a loved one, or the impending loss of one's own life may trigger grief. Loss is also integral to death. Although death is the ultimate loss, losses that occur in any phase of the life cycle may produce grief responses as intensely painful as those observed in the death experience.

Grieving may be thought of as the internal process the person uses to work through the response to loss. **Mourning** describes the actions or expressions of the bereaved, including the symbols, clothing, and ceremonies that make up the outward manifestations of grief. Both grieving and mourning are healthy responses to loss because they ultimately lead the person to invest energy in new relationships and to develop positive self-regard.

Death is defined in many ways. One commonly used definition of death is an irreversible cessation of circulatory and respiratory functions or irreversible cessation of all functions of the entire brain, including the brainstem. With the current life support systems available, the most often used criterion for determining death is whole-brain death (permanent irreversible cessation of the functioning of all areas of the brain). The criteria for whole-brain death are listed in Chapter 11 ∞.

Although death is an inevitable part of life, it is often an immensely difficult loss for the person who is dying and for his or her loved ones. Death may be accidental (such as from trauma) or come at the end of a long and painful struggle with a terminal illness such as cancer or AIDS. It may also be intentional, if a person commits suicide.

THEORIES OF LOSS AND GRIEF

Medical-surgical nurses often care for clients exhibiting responses typical of various stages of the grieving process. Highly individual in quality and duration, the grief process may range from discomforting to debilitating, and it may last a day or a lifetime, depending on what the loss means to the person experiencing it. Although each person experiences loss in a different manner, knowledge of some of the major theories of loss and grief can give the nurse a framework for holistic care of the client and family anticipating or experiencing a loss. Table 5–1 summarizes the theories discussed next.

Freud: Psychoanalytic Theory

Freud (1917/1957) wrote about grief and mourning as reactions to loss. Freud described the process of mourning as one in which the person gradually withdraws attachment from the lost object or person. He observed that with normal grieving, this withdrawal of attachment is followed by a readiness to make new attachments. In comparing melancholia (prolonged gloominess, depression) with the "normal" emotions of grief and its expression in mourning, Freud observed that the "work of mourning" is a nonpathologic condition that reaches a state of completion after a period of inner labor.

Bowlby: Protest, Despair, and Detachment

Bowlby (1973, 1980) believed that the grieving process initiated by a loss or separation from a loved object or person successfully ends when the grieving person experiences feelings of emancipation from the lost object or person. He divided the grieving process into three phases and identified behaviors characteristic of each phase.

- *Protest.* The protest phase is marked by a lack of acceptance of the loss. All energy is directed toward protesting the loss. The person experiences feelings of anger toward self and others, and feelings of ambivalence toward the lost object or person. Crying and angry behaviors characterize this phase.

BOX 5–1 **Types of Losses**

- Death
- Health
- Body part
- Social status
- Lifestyle
- Marital relationship (i.e., through divorce)
- Reproductive function
- Sexual function

TABLE 5–1 Summary of Theories of Loss

THEORIST	DYNAMICS
Freud	Grief and mourning are reactions to loss. Grieving is the inner labor of mourning a loss. Inability to grieve a loss results in depression.
Bowlby	The successful grieving process initiated by a loss or separation during childhood ends with feelings of emancipation from the lost person or object.
Engel	After the person perceives and evaluates the loss, the person adapts to it. Shock and disbelief, developing awareness, and restitution occur during the first year following the loss; in the months following, the person puts the lost relationship into perspective.
Lindemann	A sequence of responses is experienced following a catastrophic event; concepts of anticipatory grieving and morbid grief reactions are defined.
Caplan	Periods of psychologic crisis are precipitated by hazardous circumstances; successful resolution of grief involves feelings of hope and engaging in activities of ordinary living.
Kübler-Ross	Five stages define the response to loss: denial, anger, bargaining, depression, and acceptance. Stages are not necessarily sequential.

- *Despair.* The person's behavior becomes disorganized. Despair mounts as efforts to deny the loss compete with acceptance of permanent loss. Crying and sadness, coupled with a desire for the lost object or person to return, result in disorganized thoughts as the client recognizes the reality of the loss.
- *Detachment.* As the person realizes the permanence of the loss and gradually relinquishes attachment to the lost object, a reinvestment of energy occurs. Both the positive and negative aspects of the relationship are remembered. Expressions of hopefulness and readiness to move forward are characteristic of this phase.

Engel: Acute Grief, Restitution, and Long-Term Grief

Engel (1964) related the grief process to other methods of coping with stress: After the person perceives and evaluates the loss (the stressful event), the person adapts to it. Engel's recognition of the impact of cognitive factors on the grieving process was an important contribution to our understanding of grieving.

Engel described three main stages in the grief process: an acute stage, a restitution stage, and a long-term stage. The acute stage is initiated by shock and disbelief and is manifested by denial, which may help the person to cope with the overwhelming pain. As the shock and disbelief begin to fade, the loss becomes a reality, and pain, anguish, anger, guilt, and blame surface.

Culturally patterned behaviors, such as maintaining a stoic pose in public or weeping openly, characterize this phase.

The acute stage is followed by a stage of restitution, in which the mourning is institutionalized. Friends and family gather to support the grieving person through rituals dictated by the culture. The mourner continues to feel a painful void and is preoccupied with thoughts of the loss. The mourner may join a support group or seek other social support for coping with the loss. This stage lasts about 1 year, after which the mourner begins to come to terms with the loss and interests in people and activities are renewed.

Lindemann: Categories of Symptoms

Lindemann (1944) interviewed people who had lost a loved one during the course of medical treatment, disaster victims, and relatives of members of the armed forces who had died. Lindemann's research led him to describe normal grief, anticipatory grieving, and morbid grief reactions. He placed symptoms characteristic of normal grief into categories of somatic (physical symptoms without an organic cause) distress, preoccupation with the image of the deceased, feelings of guilt, hostile reactions, and loss of patterns of conduct.

Anticipatory grieving was defined as a cluster of predictable responses to an anticipated loss. These responses include the range of feelings experienced by the person or family preoccupied with an anticipated loss. The term *morbid grief reaction* described delayed and dysfunctional reactions to loss; a variety of debilitating health problems were seen in people who displayed excessive or delayed responses to loss.

Caplan: Stress and Loss

Caplan's (1990) theory of stress and its relationship to loss is useful in understanding the grief process. He expanded the focus of the grief process to include not only bereavement but also other episodes of stress that people experience, such as the stress that can result from surgery or childbirth. Caplan described three factors that influence the person's ability to deal with a loss:

- The psychic pain of the broken bond and the agony of coming to terms with the loss
- Living without the assets and guidance of the lost person or resource
- The reduced cognitive and problem-solving effectiveness associated with the distressing emotional arousal.

He believed these factors might cause distress for a year or more following the loss.

Caplan described the process of building new attachments to replace those that have been lost. This process involves two elements: a feeling of hope and the assumption of regular activity as a form of participating in ordinary living.

Kübler-Ross: Stages of Coping with Loss

Kübler-Ross's (1969, 1978) research on death and dying provided a framework for gaining insight about the stages of coping with an impending or actual loss. According to Kübler-Ross, not all people dealing with a loss go through these stages, and those who do may not experience the stages in the sequence described. In identifying the stages of death and dying, Kübler-Ross (1978) repeatedly stressed the danger of prematurely labeling a "stage" and emphasized that her goal was to describe her observations of how people come to terms with situations of loss.

Some or all of the following reactions may occur during the grieving process and may reappear as the person experiences the loss:

- *Denial.* A person may react with shock and disbelief after receiving word of an actual or potential loss. After receiving a terminal diagnosis, notification of a death, or other serious loss, people may make such statements as "This can't be happening to me" or "This can't be true."
- *Anger.* In the anger stage, the person resists the loss. The anger is often directed toward family and healthcare providers.
- *Bargaining.* The bargaining stage serves as an attempt to postpone the reality of the loss. The person makes a secret bargain with God, expressing a willingness to do anything to postpone the loss or change the prognosis.
- *Depression.* The person enters a stage of depression as the full impact of the actual or perceived loss is realized. The person prepares for the impending loss by working through the struggle of separation. While grieving over "what cannot be," the person may either talk freely about the loss or withdraw from others.
- *Acceptance.* The person begins to come to terms with the loss and resumes activities with an air of hopefulness for the future. Some dying people reach a stage of acceptance in which they may appear to be almost devoid of emotion. The struggle is past, and the emotional pain is gone.

FACTORS AFFECTING RESPONSES TO LOSS

A variety of factors affect a person's responses to loss. These include age, social support, families, cultural and spiritual practices, and rituals of mourning.

Age

The understanding of and reaction to loss is influenced by the age of the person experiencing the loss. In general, as people experience life transitions, their ability to understand and accept the losses associated with the transitions increases. From the age of 3 years, the development of the concept of death as a loss proceeds rapidly. Table 5–2 outlines the development of the concept of death throughout the life span.

Social Support

Grieving is painful and lonely. One's social support system is important because of its potentially positive influence on the successful resolution of grief. Some losses may lead to social isolation, placing clients at high risk for dysfunctional grief reactions. For example, loved ones of people who die from AIDS often report feeling excluded by the deceased person's family and by healthcare providers. Characteristic factors that can interfere with successful grieving include the following:

- Perceived inability to share the loss
- Lack of social recognition of the loss

TABLE 5–2 Development of the Concept of Death

AGE	BELIEFS/ATTITUDES ABOUT DEATH
3	Fears separation; lacks comprehension of permanent separation.
3 to 5	Believes death is like sleeping and is reversible. Expresses curiosity about what happens to the body.
6 to 10	Understands finality of death. Views own death as avoidable. Associates death with violence. Believes wishes can be responsible for death.
11 to 12	Reflects views of death expressed by parents. Expresses interest in afterlife as an understanding of mortality develops. Recognizes death as irreversible and inevitable.
13 to 21	Usually has a religious and philosophic view of death but seldom thinks about it. Views own death as distant or a challenge, acting out defiance through reckless behavior. Previously held developmental awareness of death may still be present.
22 to 45	Does not think about death unless confronted with it. Emotionally distances self from death. Attitude toward death influenced by religious and cultural beliefs.
46 to 65	Experiences the death of parents or friends. Accepts own mortality. Experiences waves of death anxiety. Puts life in order to prepare for death and decrease anxiety.
66 and older	Fears lingering, incapacitating illness. Views death as inevitable but from a philosophical view point: that is, as freedom from pain and illness or as a spiritual reunion with deceased friends and loved ones.

- Ambivalent relationships prior to the loss
- Traumatic circumstances of the loss.

A move, a divorce, or even the death of a pet can cause a person to feel extremely isolated, yet the person experiencing these types of loss does not ordinarily receive the same social support offered to the person mourning the death of a loved one. A woman having an abortion or giving up a child for adoption seldom receives the same social support as the mother of a child who died at birth. It is therefore especially important for the nurse *not* to place a value on the client's loss when assessing the need for support.

The painful nature of grief can cause the client to withdraw from a previously established social support system, thereby increasing the feelings of loneliness caused by the loss. A recently widowed woman, for example, may refuse invitations involving married couples with whom she had socialized while her husband was alive. The client's needs for social interaction, however, remain similar to those established before the loss.

Families

A well-functioning family usually rallies after the initial shock and disbelief and provides support for each other during all phases of the grieving process. After a loss, the functional family is able to shift roles, levels of responsibility, and ways of communicating.

The family may have negative as well as positive effects. For example, the dying client may request that someone the family perceives as an outsider be near, and the family may respond with anger to the perceived "intrusion." Similarly, certain family members may express hurt feelings or anger if the client is unresponsive to other family members. Well-meaning family members also may try to shield the client from the pain of grieving. It is rare for the family and the client to experience anger, denial, and acceptance in unison. While one member is in denial, another may be angry because "not enough is being done."

Cultural and Spiritual Practices

The influence of culture and ethnic identity on communication, family values, and beliefs about and practices related to illness and death are important considerations when providing nursing care. As described by Spector (2004), there are countless ethnocultural and religious differences in the way people observe dying, death, and mourning. For example, regional differences in the way death is expressed in the United States include "passed away," "died peacefully," "departed this life," "went home to be with God," and "passed from this life." Objects such as masks, statues, and photos are also used to express death and death rituals. Examples of cultural rites related to death (Spector, 2004) include:

- *China:* Initial burial is in a coffin; after 7 years, the body is exhumed and cremated, and the urn is reburied in a tomb.
- *Iraq:* Iraqis follow Muslim rites, with the body generally cared for, washed, and wrapped in a white cloth. The body generally remains at home.
- *Israel:* Relatives remain with the dying person and the body is never left alone. The eyes must be closed at death. The body is buried in the ground within 24 hours except on the Sabbath (Saturday).
- *Mexico:* Family members stay with the dying person around the clock and their grief may be expressive.

Clients who are dying often ask questions of themselves and others as to what their life has meant, why this illness has affected them, and what will happen to them when they die. They may feel abandoned by God, or worry that their behavior caused the illness resulting in death. These questions and concerns lead to spiritual distress, which if unresolved may lead to hopelessness, anxiety, and depression. When spiritual distress is resolved, clients can die more peacefully.

Spirituality is at the core of human existence, integrating and transcending the physical, emotional, intellectual, and social dimensions (Reed, 1996). The principles, values, personal philosophy, and meaning of life by which the client has pursued goals and self-actualization may be called into question when

the client responds to an actual or perceived loss. Because of a fear of intruding on the personal spiritual beliefs and practices of the client, the nurse often feels at a loss in implementing interventions that would be helpful to the client responding to a loss. The following questions (using the mnemonic FICA) may be used to assess a client's spiritual or religious practices (Lynn, Schuster, & Kabcenell, 2000).

- *Faith.* What is your faith or belief? Do you consider yourself a spiritual or a religious person? Does religious faith or spirituality play an important part in your life? What do you believe gives your life meaning?
- *Influence.* How does your religious faith or spirituality influence your thoughts about health? How does it affect the way that you take care of yourself?
- *Community.* Do you consider yourself part of a spiritual or religious community or congregation? How is that community or congregation a source of support for you?
- *Address.* Do you have any special religious or spiritual issues or concerns that you would like me to address with you? Is there someone else you would like to speak to about these matters?

It is often difficult for clients with an incurable illness to maintain hope and a sense that their lives have had meaning. To meet spiritual needs, nurses can help clients accept the uncertainty that comes with their illness and future death, and respect the spiritual beliefs and practices of clients and their families. Clients who are religious need opportunities for prayer, devotions, and religious rituals. Other resources for spirituality include meditation, guided imagery, music, and art. Privacy and space for these activities should be provided without question.

Rituals of Mourning

Through participation in religious ceremonies such as baptism, confirmation, and bat or bar mitzvah, people joyously celebrate progression to a new stage of life and loss of a former way of being. The funeral ceremony serves many of the same purposes in meeting the needs of the bereaved as people gather to share loss. Through the ceremony, people symbolically express triumph over death and deny the fear of death. Culture is the primary factor that dictates the rituals of mourning. See Focus on Cultural Diversity on the following page for examples of terminal illness care in selected cultures.

Nurses' Response to Clients' Loss

Nurses care for clients and families at various stages of the grief process and may feel that crisis situations are not the time for self-reflection. However, because the nurse's conscious or unconscious reactions to the client's responses to the loss will influence the outcome of any interventions, nurses need to take time to analyze their own feelings and values related to loss and the expression of grief. The nurse can promote self-awareness by reflecting on the following questions:

- What are my personal feelings about how grief should be expressed?
- Am I making judgments about the meaning of this loss to the client?
- Are unresolved losses in my own life preventing me from relating therapeutically to the client?

FOCUS ON CULTURAL DIVERSITY   Cultural Aspects of Terminal Illness Care

Culture/Ethnicity	Nursing Interventions
American Indian	Some tribes prefer not to openly discuss terminal prognosis and DNR decisions, because negative thoughts may make inevitable loss occur sooner. Suggest a family meeting to discuss care and end-of-life issues. If the family feels comfortable, all members of the family and close friends may remain 24 hours a day (eating, joking, singing). Mourning is done in private, away from the dying person. After death, the family may hug, touch, sing, and stay close to the deceased.
Black/African American	Suggest that the family have a family meeting or talk with a minister or family elder. Client may decide to have older family member disclose a poor prognosis. Care for the dying family member is often done at home until death is imminent.
Chinese American	Ensure the head of the family is present when terminal illness is discussed. The client may not want to discuss approaching death. Special amulets or cloths may be brought from home. Family members may prefer to bathe the body after death.
Iranian	Information about a terminal illness should be presented by a trusted member of the healthcare team to the family, and never to the client when he or she is alone. Most Iranians believe in tagdir (will of God) in life and death as a predestined journey. When death occurs, notify the head of the family first. DNR decisions are often made by the family. The family may want to bathe the body.
Mexican American	Based on the belief that worry may make health worse, the family may want to protect the client from seriousness of illness. The information is often handled by an older daughter or son. Extended family members are obligated to pay respects to the sick and dying, although pregnant women do not care for dying persons or attend funerals. May prefer the client die at home. Prayers, amulets, and rosary beads are used, and the priest should be notified. Death is seen as an important spiritual event. The family may bathe the body and spend time with the body.
Vietnamese	Consult head of family before telling client about a terminal illness. Entire family will make DNR decision, often with assistance from a priest or monk. Clients often prefer to die at home. Family should have extra time with the body, and may cry loudly and uncontrollably. Spiritual/religious rites are often conducted in the room.

Source: Adapted from *Culture & Nursing Care: A Pocket Guide* by J. G. Lipson, S. L. Dibble, & P. A. Minarik (Eds.), 1996, San Francisco: UCSF Nursing Press; *Cultural Diversity in Health & Illness,* 6e, R. E. Spector. 2004, Upper Saddle River, N.J.: Prentice Hall Health.

The following resources may be useful in helping nurses provide care to dying clients:

- DyingWell
- National Hospice and Palliative Care Organization
- International Association for Hospice and Palliative Care
- National Foundation for Treatment of Pain.

END-OF-LIFE CARE

End-of-life (the final weeks of life when death is imminent) **nursing care** that ensures a peaceful death was mandated by the International Council of Nurses (1997) and further supported by the AACN (1999). Following are selected competencies necessary for nurses to provide high-quality end-of-life care as defined by the AACN (1999):

- Promote the provision of comfort care to the dying as an active, desirable, and important skill, and an integral component of nursing care (Figure 5–1 ■).
- Communicate effectively and compassionately with the patient, family, and healthcare team members about end-of-life issues.
- Recognize one's own attitudes, feelings, values, and expectations about death and the individual, cultural, and spiritual diversity existing in those beliefs and customs.

MediaLink End-of-Life Resources

Figure 5–1 ■ The nurse helps the client visualize the hospital room as a safe, comfortable place to die by surrounding the client with familiar pictures and objects.

NURSING RESEARCH   **Evidence-Based Practice: End-of-Life Care**

End-of-life care is emerging as a major concern in the United States. Although many people die in the hospital, little research has been done about deaths in the critical care unit (CCU). Clients are not admitted to the CCU to die, but approximately 20% of critical care clients do not live to be discharged from the hospital. Most deaths in the CCU occur in undesirable situations, for example, when clients do not respond to the advanced technology and decide to forgo further treatment, or are comatose or receiving mechanical ventilation. In most instances, clients dying in the CCU are isolated from family members. The purpose of this study (Kirchhoff et al., 2000) was to address the largely unstudied area of CCU nursing care by conducting focus groups of CCU nurses.

IMPLICATIONS FOR NURSING

Regardless of the setting for end-of-life care, nurses need to ensure that clients are as free from pain as possible, and that the comfort and dignity of the client are maintained. In addition, family members should be given time to begin to accept the dying process. This may be facilitated by having the family member provide physical care and lie in bed with the client, and by providing time and space for family rituals and saying good-bye. Nurses also need to show the family that they care and are involved. However, nurses face the dilemmas of sometimes having a less optimistic outlook than physicians, of approving or not approving the use of extraordinary measures to preserve life, and of not wanting to share feelings following a death or sharing too much.

CRITICAL THINKING IN CLIENT CARE

1. What environmental differences are present between a regular hospital unit and a critical care unit that might make quality end-of-life care more difficult for nurses?
2. The family of a client in the CCU says to you, "Uncle Al is going to die, isn't he?" What would you need to know before responding? How would you respond?
3. A CCU client who previously had been improving suddenly dies. The staff are saddened, and several are in tears. A more experienced nurses says, "Oh, you just have to go on. There's nothing else to do." Do you agree? Why or why not?

Source: Data from Kirchhoff, K., Spuhler, V., Walker, L., Hutton, A., Cole, B., & Clemmer, T. (2000). Intensive care nurses' experiences with end-of-life care. *American Journal of Critical Care, 9*(1), 35–42.

- Demonstrate respect for the patient's views and wishes during end-of-life care.
- Use scientifically based standardized tools to assess symptoms (e.g., pain, dyspnea, constipation, anxiety, fatigue, nausea/vomiting, and altered cognition) experienced by patients at the end of life.
- Use data from symptom assessment to plan and intervene in symptom management using state-of-the-art traditional and complementary approaches.
- Assist the patient, family, colleagues, and one's self to cope with suffering, grief, loss, and bereavement in end-of-life care.

Nursing Considerations for End-of-Life Care

Nurses care for the dying client in critical care units, emergency rooms, hospital units, long-term care facilities, and the home. (See Nursing Research: Evidence-Based Practice above for research about intensive care nurses' experiences with end-of-life care.) Regardless of the setting, the client's wishes about death should be respected. The Dying Person's Bill of Rights states that each person has "the right to be cared for by caring, sensitive, knowledgeable people who will attempt to understand my needs and will be able to gain some satisfaction in helping me face my death" (Barbus, 1975).

Legal and Ethical Issues

Issues such as those involved in advance directives and living wills, euthanasia, and quality of life are especially important to nurses in upholding the specific care requests of their clients.

ADVANCE DIRECTIVES Advance directives are legal documents that allow a person to plan for health care and/or financial affairs in the event of incapacity. They include living wills, healthcare surrogates, and durable power of attorney.

FAST FACTS
Types of Advance Directives
- **Living will:** A document that provides written directions about life-prolonging procedures to provide instructions when a person can no longer communicate in a life-threatening situation.
- **Healthcare surrogate:** An individual selected to make medical decisions when a person is no longer able to make them for himself or herself.
- **Durable power of attorney:** A document that can delegate the authority to make health, financial, and/or legal decisions on a person's behalf. It must be in writing and must state that the designated person is authorized to make healthcare decisions.

A living will is a legal document that formally expresses a person's wishes regarding life-sustaining treatment in the event of terminal illness or permanent unconsciousness. It is not a type of durable power of attorney and usually does not designate a substitute decision maker. It is the responsibility of the nurse as client advocate to request and record the client's preference for care and include it in the plan of care. The nurse's documentation helps communicate these preferences to the other members of the healthcare team.

All facilities that receive Medicare and Medicaid funds are required to provide all clients with written information and counseling about advance directives and the institution's policies governing them. The specific terms of this requirement are found in the Patient Self-Determination Act (PSDA). A copy of the signed advance directive must be kept in the client's medical record, but clients do not have to sign it in order to be treated. Nurses are the ones in close contact with clients, so they are often left with unresolved feelings about the moral, ethical, and legal aspects of their actions. Although advance directives do not ease the pain of seeing clients die, they do help nurses provide clients with the care that the clients have chosen.

DO-NOT-RESUSCITATE ORDERS A **do-not-resuscitate** (DNR, or "no-code") **order** is written by the physician for the client who has a terminal illness or is near death. This order is usually based on the wishes of the client and family that no cardiopulmonary resuscitation be performed for respiratory or cardiac arrest. A comfort-measures-only order indicates that no further life-sustaining interventions are necessary and that the goal of care is a comfortable, dignified death. Agency protocols should be established that define "comfort care" for consistency in nursing care. Confusing or conflicting DNR orders create dilemmas, because nurses are involved in resuscitation and either begin CPR or ensure that unwanted attempts do not occur. The American Nurses Association (ANA) has made specific recommendations related to a DNR order (Box 5–2). The ANA further recommends that guidelines and policies be developed to help resolve conflicts between clients and their families, between clients and healthcare professionals, and among healthcare professionals.

BOX 5–2 The ANA Position on Nursing Care and Do-Not-Resuscitate Decisions

- The choices and values of the competent patient should always be given highest priority, even when these wishes conflict with those of healthcare providers and families.
- In the case of the incompetent or never competent patient, any existing advance directives or the decisions of surrogate decision makers acting in the patient's best interest should be determinative.
- The DNR decision should always be a subject of explicit discussion among the patient, the family, any designated surrogate decision maker acting in the patient's best interest, and the healthcare team. The decision should include consideration of the efficacy and desirability of CPR, a balancing of benefits and burdens to patients, and therapeutic goals.
- DNR orders must be clearly documented, reviewed, and updated periodically to reflect changes in the patient's condition.
- Nurses have a responsibility to educate patients and their families about various forms of advance directives such as living wills and durable power of attorney.
- If it is the nurse's personal belief that his or her moral integrity is compromised by professional responsibility to carry out a particular DNR order, the nurse should transfer the responsibility for the patient's care to another nurse.

Source: From *Task Force on the Nurse's Role in End of Life Decisions* by ANA Board of Directors, 1992.

EUTHANASIA **Euthanasia** (from the Greek for painless, easy, gentle, or good death) is now commonly used to signify a killing prompted by some humanitarian motive. There are many arguments for and against euthanasia, and nurses have often found themselves at the center of the debate. As a result, nurses have pushed for the development of appropriate guidelines and procedures for DNR orders. When no such orders exist, the nurse faces a dilemma. Certainly, there are situations in which the nurse's role is clear. For example, it is considered malpractice to participate in "slow codes" (in which the nurse does not hurry to alert the emergency team when a terminally ill client who does not have a DNR order stops breathing).

The natural death laws seek to preserve the notion of voluntary versus involuntary euthanasia. In voluntary euthanasia, the competent adult client and a physician, nurse, or adult friend or relative make the decision to terminate life. Involuntary euthanasia ("mercy killing") is performed without the client's consent. Because care settings offer many complex and technologic interventions, it is not likely that the ethical aspects of euthanasia will soon be resolved. However, advance directives do give clients a much more active role in decisions about their own care.

Settings and Services for End-of-Life Care

Settings and services for end-of-life care range from the critical care unit in a hospital to the client's own home. Two methods of providing end-of-life care—hospice and palliative care—are described in this section.

Hospice

Hospice is a philosophy of care rather than a program of care. It is "comprehensive and coordinated care for clients with limited life expectancy, provided both at home and in institutional settings" (Fine, 2004, p. 1) that reaffirms the right of every client and family to fully participate in the final stages of life. Provided by hospice agency nurses and other members of a healthcare team (including social workers, ministers, home health aides, and volunteers), it is based on a philosophy of death with comfort and dignity, encompassing biomedical, psychosocial, and spiritual aspects of the dying experience. Although most hospice care is provided in the home, it may also be provided in hospitals, long-term care facilities, or other community-based settings.

The American hospice movement was originally led by volunteers (many of whom were nurses) who wanted to make life better for those who were dying. These devoted volunteers promoted the dignity of patients during their death and decreased their institutionalization. In 1986, Congress passed the Medicare Hospice Benefit and also gave states the option of including hospice services in their Medicaid programs.

There are approximately 2,500 hospice agencies in the United States, with most services and care reimbursed by a Medicare hospice benefit (National Association for Home Care & Hospice, 2004). Services are reimbursed by Medicare for an initial 90-day period, followed by a subsequent 90-day period, and an unlimited number of 60-day periods as long as the patient continues to meet eligibility requirements. The average length of service is 47 days (CDC, 2006). Hospice services usually begin when the patient has 6 months or less to live and ends with the family 1 year after the death of the patient. This continuation of care for the family is called bereavement care (**bereavement** is the time of mourning experienced after a loss).

To be eligible for hospice benefits from Medicare or Medicaid, the client must have a serious, progressive illness with a limited life expectancy. In most cases, a family (or other) caregiver must be continuously in the home with the client. The client must have Medicare, waive traditional Medicare benefits for the terminal illness, have physician certification of a terminal illness, and care must be provided by a Medicare-certified hospice agency or program.

Palliative Care

Palliative care is an area of care that has evolved out of the hospice experience, but exists outside of hospice programs, is not restricted to the end of life, and is used earlier in the disease experience. Palliative care, which can be used in all types of healthcare settings, is focused on the relief of physical, mental, and spiritual distress for individuals who have an incurable illness. The goal of palliative care is to prevent and relieve suffering by early assessment and treatment of pain and other physical, psychosocial, and spiritual needs to improve the client's quality of life.

Although palliative care may be provided by a single person, it usually involves the combined efforts of an interdisciplinary team, including physicians, nurses, social workers, chaplains, home health aides, and volunteers. Care is provided in the client's home (or long-term care facility, senior living facility, or hospital). The expected outcomes of care are directed by interventions to manage current manifestations of the illness and to prevent new manifestations from occurring.

Physiologic Changes in the Dying Client

Death is a highly individualized process, and may occur rapidly or slowly. Physiologic changes are a part of the dying process. These changes result in any or all of the manifestations listed in the box below as death nears. Although each person responds differently, certain manifestations are common in the dying process, regardless of the trauma or disease process that is causing death. The discussion that follows includes treatments and related nursing care.

Pain

A common problem for clients at the end of life, pain is what people often say they fear the most. Pain, a subjective experience, is influenced by the client's emotions, previous experiences with pain, and family and culture. Unfortunately, pain is often undertreated at the end of life (Tierney et al., 2004), because physicians and nurses fear they will cause addiction or cause harm from the high dose of opioids necessary to control pain at the end of life. However, nearly all pain at the end of life can be managed without causing addiction or hastening death through respiratory depression. It is of utmost importance to keep the client comfortable through general comfort measures (Box 5–3) and by administering ordered medications for pain, neuropathic pain (which is rarely relieved by opioids), seizures, and/or anxiety. The pathophysiology, treatment, and nursing care of clients experiencing pain are fully described in Chapter 9 ∞.

PRACTICE ALERT

There is no maximum allowable dose at end of life for opioids such as morphine sulfate; the dose should be increased to whatever is necessary to relieve pain. Meperidine (Demerol) is not useful for chronic pain because it has a short half-life and a toxic metabolite that can cause irritability and seizures (Tierney et al., 2004).

Dyspnea

Respiratory changes, including dyspnea, are normal as death nears. Dyspnea is a subjective experience, and the client often reports having a feeling of suffocation, shortness of breath, or tightness in the chest. Up to 50% of dying clients have severe dyspnea, especially those with lung tumors (primary or metastatic), restrictive lung disease, or pleural effusion (Tierney et al., 2004). Regardless of the terminal illness or fatal injury, the final cause of death is a lack of oxygen to the brain.

MANIFESTATIONS of Impending Death

- Difficulty talking or swallowing
- Nausea, flatus, abdominal distention
- Urinary and/or bowel incontinence, constipation
- Decreased sensation, taste, and smell
- Weak, slow, and/or irregular pulse
- Decreasing blood pressure
- Decreased, irregular, or Cheyne-Stokes respirations
- Changes in level of consciousness
- Restlessness, agitation
- Coolness, mottling, and cyanosis of the extremities.

BOX 5–3 Providing Comfort for the Client Nearing Death

- Maintain clean skin and bed linens.
- Use a draw sheet to turn the client as often as possible so the client is comfortable.
- Position the client to promote comfort and protect bony areas with padding. Reposition the client and raise the head of the bed if fluids accumulate in the upper airways and back of the throat.
- Use bed pads or insert a Foley catheter (if ordered) for urinary incontinence.
- Use gentle massage to improve circulation and shift edema.
- Provide small, frequent sips of fluids, ice chips, or Popsicles.
- Provide oral care, using a soft moist brush or glycerin swab.
- Clean secretions from the eyes and nose.
- Administer ordered pain medications as needed to maintain comfort.
- Administer oxygen as prescribed to relieve dyspnea.

As death nears, respirations often become fast or slow, shallow and labored. The client may have apnea or Cheyne-Stokes respirations (regular periods of deep, rapid breathing followed by no breaths for 5 to 30 seconds). Fluid may accumulate in the lungs causing rales and rhonchi, especially in clients who are well hydrated and are having difficulty swallowing or coughing. These sounds are not painful for the client, but they may be treated with oxygen, opioids (to improve respirations and decrease anxiety), and medications to decrease secretions (atropine, scopolamine, hyoscyamine, or glycopyrrolate). Note that oxygen and suctioning are only temporary measures, and (especially with suctioning) may even be traumatic for the client. Nursing care to improve respirations includes keeping the head of the bed elevated. Keeping the room cool and providing a breeze from a fan often makes the client more comfortable.

PRACTICE ALERT

Morphine is the medication of choice for palliative treatment of dyspnea. Nebulized morphine may be used, and is often more effective than that given by other routes, but it increases the risk of bronchospasm. Nebulized morphine is contraindicated in clients with chronic obstructive pulmonary disease because of the risk of respiratory depression and increasing hypercapnia.

Anorexia, Nausea, and Dehydration

Although anorexia and a decrease in food and fluid intake are normal in the dying client, the family often views this as "giving up." Anorexia may be a protective mechanism; the breakdown of body fats results in ketosis, which leads to a sense of well-being and helps decrease pain. Parenteral or enteral feedings do not improve symptoms or prolong life and may actually cause discomfort. As weakness and difficulty swallowing progress, the gag reflex is decreased and clients are at increased risk for aspiration if oral foods or fluids are given.

Nausea, with or without vomiting, is a common problem in dying clients. Nausea and vomiting may be caused by reduced gastric emptying, constipation, bowel obstruction, a side effect of morphine, uremia, or hypercalcemia. If the client is conscious and complains of nausea, antiemetics such as prochlorperazine (Compazine) or odansetron (Zofran) should be administered.

Dehydration is less of a problem than overhydration. Forcing fluids or initiating intravenous fluids for hydration may in turn increase fluid in the lungs, peripheral edema, ascites, and vomiting. Dehydration in the client nearing death primarily causes discomfort from dry mouth and thirst. The client should be given small sips of water, or an atomizer can be used to spray the inside of the mouth. Oral care should be given at least every 2 hours, and more often if the client is breathing through his or her mouth. Glycerin swabs may be used to keep the lips less dry.

Altered Levels of Consciousness

Neurologic dysfunction results from any or all of the following: decreased cerebral perfusion, hypoxemia, metabolic acidosis, sepsis, an accumulation of toxins from liver and renal failure, the effects of medications, and disease-related factors. These changes may result in a decreased level of consciousness or ag-

itated delirium. Clients with terminal delirium may be confused, restless, or agitated. Moaning, groaning, and grimacing often accompany the agitation and may be misinterpreted as pain. Level of consciousness often decreases to the point where the client cannot be aroused. Although decreased consciousness and agitation are both normal states at the end of life, they are very distressing to the client's family.

If possible, confusion or agitation is treated based on its cause; for example, by relieving pain or dyspnea. Other medications include low doses of neuroleptics, tranquilizers, or antianxiety medications. A client near death often has altered cerebral function, so the nurse must stand near the bedside and speak clearly. Hearing is thought to be the last sense a dying client loses, so the nurse should never whisper or engage in conversation with the family as if the client were not there. Nursing care for the comatose client includes:
- Using artificial tears if the client does not blink
- Keeping lights at a low level
- Keeping skin clean and dry
- Covering only with a light blanket
- Using adult incontinence pads or pants for incontinence
- Turning every 2 hours and maintaining joint positions.

Hypotension

As death nears, the cardiac output decreases, as does intravascular blood volume. As a result, blood pressure gradually decreases and the pulse is often rapid and irregular. The extremities are cooler, and cyanosis is present in nail beds, skin, and lips. The skin on the legs and in dependent areas may become mottled in color. Renal perfusion decreases and the kidneys cease to function. Urinary output is scanty. The client will have tachycardia, hypotension, cool extremities, and cyanosis with skin mottling.

Support for the Client and Family

As the client's condition deteriorates, the nurse's knowledge of the client and family guides the care provided. It may be necessary to provide opportunities for clients to express personal preferences about where they want to die and about funeral and burial arrangements. If the family feels that this is morbid, the nurse explains that it helps clients to keep a sense of control as they approach death.

The client needs the opportunity to say good-bye to others. The nurse encourages and supports the client and family as they terminate relationships as a necessary part of the grief process. The nurse acknowledges that termination is painful and, if the client or family desires, stays with them during this time. Family members are often afraid to be present at the moment of death, yet dying alone is the greatest fear expressed by clients.

Death

The manifestations listed on page 94 are seen after death occurs, and are the basis for pronouncing death. They appear gradually and not in any special order. Pronouncement of death is legally required by a physician or other healthcare provider to confirm death. The time of death, with any related data, is documented in the client's chart.

> ### MANIFESTATIONS of Death
>
> - Absence of respirations, pulse, and heartbeat
> - Fixed and dilated pupils; eyes may stay open
> - Release of stool and urine
> - Waxen color (pallor) as blood settles to dependent areas
> - Body temperature drops
> - Lack of reflexes
> - Flat encephalogram

The nurse may also fear being present at the moment of the client's death. In fact, Kübler-Ross (1969) noted that the nurse's fear of death frequently interferes with the ability to provide support for the dying client and family. Thoughts such as "Please, God, don't let him die on my shift" are common, and they express the nurse's emotional turmoil in dealing with the task. Nurses who have worked through their own feelings about death and dying are more at ease in assisting the dying client toward a peaceful death.

After the death, the family is encouraged to acknowledge the pain of loss. The nurse's presence and support as the bereaved express their sorrow, anger, or guilt can help them resolve their grief. It is important for the bereaved not to suppress the pain of grieving with drugs. By accepting variations in the expression of grief, the nurse supports the family's grief reactions and helps prevent dysfunctional grieving. Dysfunctional grieving is an extended and unsuccessful resolution of grief.

Resolution of grief begins with acceptance of the loss. The nurse can encourage this acceptance by maintaining open, honest dialogue and by providing the family with the opportunity to view, touch, hold, and kiss the person's body. As family members realize the finality of the death, they are often comforted by the presence of the nurse who cared for the client during the final days.

Postmortem Care

The nurse documents the time of death (required for the death certificate and all official records), notifies the physician, and assists the family (if needed) in choice of a funeral home. If the client dies at home, death must be pronounced before the body is removed. In some states and in some situations, nurses can pronounce death; for specifics, consult state practice acts, laws, and agency policy. All jewelry is removed and given to the family unless they ask that it be left on. The body is kept in place until the family is ready and gives permission. If an autopsy is required or requested, the body must be left undisturbed (e.g., do not remove any tubes) for transportation to the medical examiner.

Documentation of the death is completed by sending a completed death certificate to the funeral home (for a death in the home), or by completing the required paperwork and sending the body to the morgue or funeral home (for a death in the hospital or long-term care setting).

Nurses' Grief

The nurse who has developed a close relationship with the client who has died may experience strong feelings of grief. Sharing grief with the family after the death of a loved one helps both the

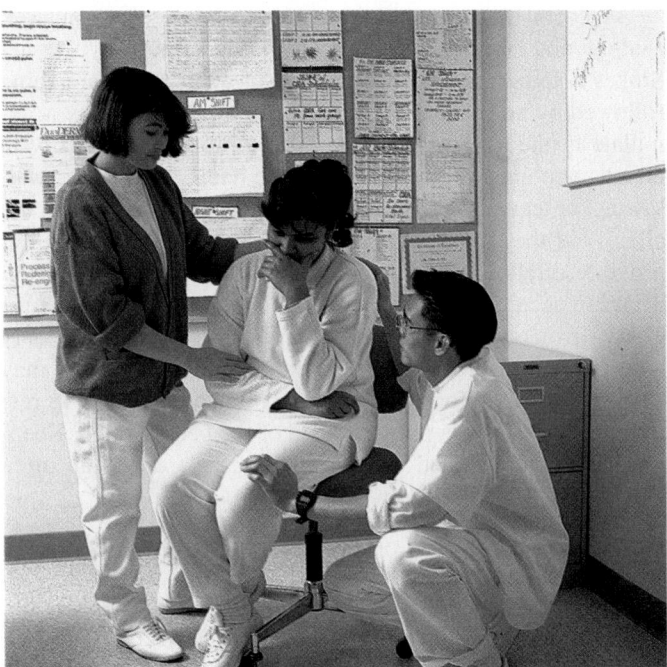

Figure 5–2 ■ Nurses who work with dying clients need support from their colleagues to work through their often overwhelming feelings of grief.

nurse and family to cope with their feelings about the loss. Taking time to grieve after the death of a client provides a release that can help prevent "blunting" of feelings, a problem often experienced by nurses who care for clients who are terminally ill.

> **PRACTICE ALERT**
> Crying with families, at one time considered unprofessional, is now recognized as simply an expression of empathy and caring.

Nurses working with clients who are critically or terminally ill should be aware that witnessing a client's death and the family's grief may reactivate feelings about some unresolved grief in their own lives. In these cases, nurses may need to reflect on their responses to their own losses. Also, nurses who work with dying clients need support from peers and other professionals to work through the often overwhelming feelings that result from dealing with death, grief, and loss (Figure 5–2 ■).

Interdisciplinary Care

Interventions for loss and grief may be planned and implemented by any or all members of the healthcare team. Nurses and social workers provide interventions to help clients or families adapt to a loss. They also make referrals to mental health professionals (grief counselors, social services), support groups, chaplains, or legal or financial assistance agencies.

Grieving clients frequently enter the healthcare system with significant somatic symptoms. In some cases, the symptoms of grief and loss are overlooked until the client reaches a crisis state requiring psychiatric medical intervention. Collaborative care by the physician and the nurse early in the normal grieving process can help the client achieve an early and effective resolution of grief and avoid physical or psychiatric health problems.

Nursing Care

Nurses practicing in all types of settings care for clients who are in various stages of the grieving process. Grief is highly individual. The grief process may range from uncomfortable to debilitating, and it may last for a day or a lifetime, depending on what the loss means to the person experiencing it.

Health Promotion

In planning and implementing nursing care for the client experiencing a loss, the nurse considers the individual responses, which may vary greatly. In an era of short acute care stays for clients, nurses may feel that an elaborate grief assessment is impossible or, at the least, impractical. But research and clinical experience suggest that clients who delay the grieving process after a loss are prone to have health problems that may last a lifetime. See Nursing Care of the Older Adult below for an end-of-life checklist for older adults.

Assessment

Knowledge of the expected physical reactions to loss provides the nurse with a basis for identifying reactions that require further assessment. To assess the extent of somatic distress, the nurse observes for changes in sensory processes and asks questions about the client's sleeping and eating patterns, activities of daily living, general health status, and pain.

Physical Assessment

Clients may experience one or more predictable somatic symptoms as they become aware of a loss. Gastrointestinal symptoms occur frequently and may include indigestion, nausea or vomiting, anorexia, weight gain or loss, constipation, or diarrhea. The shock and disbelief that accompany a loss may cause shortness of breath, a choking sensation, hyperventilation, or loss of strength. Some clients also report insomnia, preoccupation with sleep, fatigue, and decreased or increased activity level.

Crying and sadness are observed during normal grief states. Crying may make the client feel exhausted and interfere with carrying out activities of daily living. However, a person who is unable to cry may have difficulty completing the mourning process. If the client does not express feelings of grief, somatic symptoms may increase.

It is imperative that the client's concerns about pain be assessed, especially if the client has cancer or another painful illness. Knowledge of pain theories and pain assessment can help the nurse assess the need for pain medication (see Chapter 9 ∞). During the last stages of dying, the client usually becomes very weak, and sensations and reflexes decrease; these changes call for careful assessment of the client's physical needs.

Reactions to loss are not always obvious. For example, in clients who experience an illness following a serious loss, assessment may reveal somatic complaints related to the grief state as well as the illness. When a person who has been healthy begins to develop patterns of increased illness, the nurse should be aware that this may signal dysfunctional grieving. This is especially common in the loss and grieving associated with a change in body image. In addition to making a physical assessment, assess the client's perception of the alteration in body image. The loss of a body part, weight gain or loss, and scars from surgery or trauma can be difficult for the client to accept. Some clients may grieve hair loss that accompanies chemotherapy used in cancer treatment.

NURSING CARE OF THE OLDER ADULT   End-of-Life Checklist

- Take time a day or so before appointments with your healthcare provider to think about the questions you need answered and concerns you want to discuss. It is often a good idea to keep a pad of paper and a pen handy so you can write down things as they come to you.
- Do not hesitate to have your doctor explain your diagnosis again if you didn't understand the explanation the first time or if you missed some key points. The same goes for details about using medications and possible side effects.
- You may wish to have a friend or family member go with you to medical appointments.
- When you visit the doctor, take an up-to-date list of all the medications (prescribed and over-the-counter) you are currently taking.
- If you have physical pain, tell your healthcare provider. You will probably be asked to rate your pain on a scale of 1 (no pain) to 10 (severe pain). Your rating helps determine what pain relief measures are appropriate.

- It is a good idea to ask your healthcare provider about hospice services well before you are likely to need them.
- Your family and close friends should be aware of your treatment preferences (such as the existence of a DNR order). You might consider documenting your wishes in a living will.
- Think about asking and appointing someone you trust to make your healthcare decisions, in case the moment comes when you can no longer make them yourself.
- If you are feeling depressed or anxious or need emotional support, consider talking to a pastor, chaplain, rabbi, or other trusted person in your faith community. If necessary, ask your healthcare provider to recommend someone to help you sort out your feelings.
- Avoid withdrawing from social activities. Keep communicating with your family, friends, and the people who help care for you. If you are open with them you are more likely to get the care you need.

Source: Data from the United States Senate Special Committee on Aging. (2000). *End-of-Life Care Checklist for Seniors.* Retrieved from www.advancedseniorsolutions.com/end_of_life_care%20v2.htm

Spiritual Assessment

Because spiritual beliefs and practices greatly influence people's reaction to loss, it is important to explore them with the client when assessing a loss. The spiritually healthy client has inner resources that help work through the grief process. Faith, prayer, trust in God or a superior being, perception of a purpose in life, or belief in immortality are examples of the inner resources that may sustain the client during an actual or perceived loss.

Assessing the client's spiritual life and its significance to the client and family helps identify spiritual support systems. Some nurses are uncomfortable with assessing the client's spiritual needs; the following questions may be helpful:

- What are the spiritual aspects of the client's philosophy about life? Death?
- Are the values and beliefs about life and death congruent with those of people who are important to the client?
- Which spiritual resources and rituals have significance for the client?

Belief systems that are incompatible with those of family members can be an additional source of stress for clients dealing with a loss. The anger and resentment often observed among families faced with decisions concerning dying members may be avoided if the nurse assesses the potential effect of differing beliefs.

Clients coping with a loss often perceive that it is a punishment from God for their wrongdoing or for their failure to remain faithful to their religious practices. Therefore, it is important to assess the level of guilt the client or family expresses. Assessing the client's comments regarding feelings of responsibility for the loss helps determine whether these feelings are an expected phase of grieving or indicate dysfunctional grieving.

Clients who had not considered themselves religious before the actual or perceived loss often turn to religion to seek comfort or to cope with feelings of despair, helplessness, hopelessness, or guilt. They may utter anguished statements such as "Why, God?" or "Please help me, God." The nurse continues to assess the client's verbalization of such feelings to determine the best interventions to help the client cope with the loss.

Psychosocial Assessment

When working through the grief process, clients can be overwhelmed by the fears associated with the loss and the changes it will produce. The client responding to an actual or perceived loss commonly expresses anxiety (fear of the unknown). An extreme level of anxiety can threaten the client's well-being. Assessment includes helping clients openly acknowledge their fears. Some clients may fear the feelings they experience while proceeding through the grief process more than the loss itself. The most common fear expressed by clients facing a loss is that of losing self-control.

Focusing on the meaning of the loss to the client is more important than attempting to place the client in a sequence or phase of grief. The degree of caring and sensitivity shown when asking questions about the meaning of the loss influences the amount of information the client will be willing to reveal. Asking questions such as "Why do you feel this way?" or "What does this loss mean to you?" is less helpful than making a statement such as "This must be difficult for you." The latter more effectively conveys a genuine interest in hearing how the client feels about the loss.

Awareness of the altered sensorium observed during the stage of shock and disbelief provides parameters for assessment. The nurse may note in the client feelings of numbness, unreality, emotional distance, intense preoccupation with the lost object, helplessness, loneliness, and disorganization. As awareness of the loss begins to develop, preoccupation with the lost person or object may increase, and self-accusation and ambivalence toward the lost person or object may follow.

Nursing Diagnoses and Interventions

A variety of nursing diagnoses may be appropriate for the client experiencing loss and grief, as well as for the client who is nearing death. Nurses practicing medical-surgical nursing will most often provide interventions for *Anticipatory Grieving, Chronic Sorrow,* and *Death Anxiety.*

Anticipatory Grieving

Anticipatory grieving is a combination of intellectual and emotional responses and behaviors by which people adjust their self-concept in the face of a potential loss. Anticipatory grieving may be a response to one's own future death; to potential loss of body parts or functions; to potential loss of a significant person, animal, or possession; or to potential loss of a social role. Nursing interventions are designed to assist with grief resolution.

- Assess for factors causing or contributing to the grief. Ask about support systems, how many losses have occurred, relationship with the lost person, significance of the body part, and previous experiences with loss and grief. *Grief and mourning occur when a person experiences any type of loss.*
- Use open-ended questions to encourage the person to share concerns and the possible effect on the family. *Grief resolution cannot occur until the client acknowledges the loss.*
- Promote a trusting nurse–client relationship: Allow enough time for communications; speak clearly, simply, and concisely; listen; be honest in responses to questions; do not give unrealistic hope; offer support; and demonstrate respect for the person's age, culture, religion, race, and values. *An effective nurse–client relationship begins with acceptance of the client's feelings, attitudes, and values related to the loss. If the client is ready to talk, listening and being present are the most appropriate interventions.*
- Ask about strengths and weaknesses in coping with the anticipated loss. *Current responses are influenced by past experiences with loss, illness, and death. Socioeconomic and cultural background, as well as cultural and spiritual beliefs and values, affect a person's ability to adapt to loss.*
- Teach the client and family the stages of grief. *This helps them to be aware of their emotions in each stage and reassures them that their reactions are normal.*
- Provide time for decision making. *In periods of stress, people may need extra time to make informed decisions.*
- Provide information about appropriate resources, including support from family, friends, and support groups, community resources, and legal/financial aids. *Support from others decreases feelings of loneliness and isolation and facilitates grief work.*

Chronic Sorrow

Chronic sorrow is a cyclical, recurring, and potentially progressive pattern of pervasive sadness experienced in response to continual loss, throughout the trajectory of an illness or disability. It is triggered by situations that bring to mind the person's losses, disappointments, or fears. It may be experienced by a client, parent or caregiver, or person with chronic illness or disability.

- Explain the difference between chronic sorrow and chronic grieving. *Grieving is time limited and ends in adaptation to the loss. Chronic sorrow may vary in intensity, but it persists as long as the person with the disability or chronic sorrow condition lives.*
- Encourage verbalization of feelings about the loss, and about the personal relevance of the changes to hopes for the future. *Expressing feelings is normal and necessary to decrease the emotional pain.*
- Help identify triggers that intensify the sorrow, such as birthdays, anniversaries, and holidays. *When triggers have been identified, role-playing may make the events less painful.*
- Refer to appropriate community support groups. *Participating in support groups with others experiencing grief is helpful in coping with loss.*
- Encourage use of personal, family, significant other, and spiritual support systems *to facilitate coping with loss.*

Death Anxiety

Death anxiety is worry or fear related to death or dying. It may be present in clients who have an acute life-threatening illness, who have a terminal illness, who have experienced the death of a family member or friend, or who have experienced multiple deaths in the same family.

- Explore the client's knowledge of the situation. For example, ask, "What has your doctor told you about your condition?" *This informs you of the client's knowledge base about the condition and about his or her ability to make informed decisions.*
- Ask the client to identify specific fears about death. *This provides data about any unrealistic expectations or misperceptions.*
- Determine the client's perceptions of strengths and weaknesses in coping with death. *Identifying past strengths can help the client cope with loss, illness, and death.*
- Ask the client to identify needed help. *This determines whether available resources are adequate.*
- Encourage independence and control in decisions about treatment and care. *This promotes self-esteem, decreases feelings of powerlessness, and allows the client to retain dignity in dying.*
- Facilitate access to culturally appropriate spiritual rituals and practices. *This provides spiritual comfort.*
- Explain advance directives and assist with them if necessary. *Advance directives help ensure that the client's wishes for end-of-life care are carried out.*
- Encourage life review and reminiscence. *Life review is self-affirming.*
- Encourage activities such as listening to music, aromatherapy, massage, or relaxation exercises. *These activities decrease anxiety.*
- Suggest keeping a journal or leaving a written legacy. *A written document provides continuing support to others after death.*

Using NANDA, NIC, and NOC

Chart 5–1 shows linkages between NANDA, NIC, and NOC when caring for the client experiencing loss, grief, and death.

Community-Based Care

In addition to teaching clients and families to carry out the physical skills that are necessary to the client's care, nurses also provide information on identifying signs of deterioration and additional sources of support. General guidelines for teaching clients and families about grief include those suggested in the Meeting Individualized Needs box on page 98. In addition, suggest the following resources:

- Hospice
- Home health agencies
- Support groups
- Public health departments
- Church, synagogue, or mosque
- Pastoral counseling centers
- Mental health agencies.

MediaLink Grief Resources

NANDA, NIC, AND NOC LINKAGES
CHART 5–1 **The Client Experiencing Death Anxiety**

NANDA

Death Anxiety

↓

NIC

Dying Care

Spiritual Support

Coping Enhancement

Anxiety Reduction

Emotional Support

Hope Instillation

↓

NOC

Acceptance: Health Status

Anxiety Control

Depression Level

Dignified Dying

Fear Control

Hope

Data from *NANDA's Nursing Diagnoses: Definitions & classification 2005–2006* by NANDA International (2003), Philadelphia; *Nursing Interventions Classification (NIC)* (4th ed.) by J. M. Dochterman & G. M. Bulecheck (2004), St. Louis, MO: Mosby; and *Nursing Outcomes Classification (NOC)* (3rd ed.) by S. Moorhead, M. Johnson, and M. Maas (2004), St. Louis, MO: Mosby.

MEETING INDIVIDUALIZED NEEDS Teaching for Clients Experiencing a Loss

- Encourage both children and adults to discuss expected or impending loss and to express feelings.
- Teach problem-solving skills: Define what the possible changes and problems are related to the predicted loss, develop potential strategies for dealing with problems, list pros and cons of each strategy, and decide which strategies might be most useful to try first to solve potential problems associated with loss.
- Teach individuals and families how to support a person who is dealing with an impending loss.

- Explain what to expect with a loss: sadness, fear, rejection, anger, guilt, loneliness.
- Teach signs of grief resolution:
  - No longer living in the past, becoming future oriented
  - Breaking ties with the lost object or person (Acute stage often shows signs of resolving in 6 to 12 months.)
  - The possibility of having painful "waves" of grief years after the loss, especially on the anniversary of the loss and in response to "triggers" such as pictures, events, songs, or memories.

NURSING CARE PLAN A Client Experiencing Loss and Grief

Pearl Rogers is a 79-year-old African-American woman who is admitted to the Methodist Home Nursing Center. Mrs. Rogers lived with her husband of 58 years until his death 9 months ago. She had one son who died in an auto accident 2 years ago, and she has one daughter who lives nearby. After her husband's death, Mrs. Rogers lived with her daughter until her admission to the nursing center. Mrs. Rogers has become increasingly agitated and helpless, complaining constantly of pain. Her daughter states that Mrs. Rogers is chronically constipated, has difficulty sleeping, and has stopped engaging in all social activities, including weekly church services. She cries frequently. Extensive medical testing prior to her admission to the nursing center revealed Mrs. Rogers has arthritis but no other pathologic disorder.

ASSESSMENT

On admission to the nursing center, Mrs. Rogers says, "I'm a sick woman, and no one will listen to me! I can't walk, I'm so weak. My head hurts, and I'm always sick at my stomach. I haven't had a bowel movement in a week, and I never sleep more than 3 hours a night." Physical assessment findings include swollen knees and ankles, with limited mobility of the lower extremities.

DIAGNOSES

- *Dysfunctional Grieving* related to stress of husband's death
- *Disturbed Sleep Pattern* related to grieving
- *Constipation* related to inactivity

EXPECTED OUTCOMES

- Engage in normal grief work: Work through grief process, discuss reality of losses, use nondestructive coping mechanisms, and discuss positive and negative aspects of the loss.
- Experience adequate and restful sleep: Fall asleep 20 to 30 minutes after retiring and awaken feeling rested after 7 to 8 hours of sleep.
- Have a bowel movement with soft formed stools at least every other day.

PLANNING AND IMPLEMENTATION

- Promote trust: Show empathy and caring, demonstrate respect for her culture and values, offer support and reassurance, be honest, engage in active listening.

- Assist in labeling her feelings: anger, fear, loneliness, guilt, isolation.
- Explore previous losses and the ways in which the client has coped.
- Encourage review of her relationship with her dead husband.
- Reinforce expressions of behaviors associated with normal grieving.
- Encourage participation in usual spiritual practices.
- Encourage participation in a grief group that meets at the facility.
- Consult with the physical and recreational therapist to help the nursing staff provide afternoon activities.
- Provide measures that assist in bowel evacuation: Encourage exercise as tolerated, including walks and rocking in a rocking chair. Offer foods that stimulate bowel movements. Offer privacy: Close the door, ensuring that the emergency call bell is within reach, and do not interrupt.
- Administer a mild laxative and/or stool softener, if necessary, but discontinue as soon as possible.

EVALUATION

After 4 weeks at the nursing center, Mrs. Rogers states, "I don't feel any better, but I know I have to accept my situation." Although Mrs. Rogers states that she doesn't feel better, she is walking the length of the hall, sleeping better, and having regular bowel movements. Mrs. Rogers is also less withdrawn and has openly discussed her feelings related to her husband's death, including her anger at the loss of her son and her husband less than 2 years apart. She has attended the grief group once and has attended chapel services on Sunday for the past 2 weeks. Her daughter visits her each Saturday and takes her in a wheelchair to the shopping mall.

CRITICAL THINKING IN THE NURSING PROCESS

1. What common physical manifestations of grief did Mrs. Rogers experience?
2. How might Mrs. Rogers's daughter be more involved in developing and implementing her mother's plan of care?
3. Suppose Mrs. Rogers says that she does not want any help, that she just wants to be left alone to die. How would you respond?
See Evaluating Your Response in Appendix C.

EXPLORE MediaLink

Prentice Hall Nursing MediaLink DVD-ROM
Audio Glossary
NCLEX-RN® Review

COMPANION WEBSITE www.prenhall.com/lemone
Audio Glossary
NCLEX-RN® Review
Care Plan Activity: Anticipatory Grieving
Case Study: Do-Not-Resuscitate
MediaLink Applications
DNR Regulations
Explore Your Feelings about Death
Grieving Process
Hospice: Purpose and Benefits
Links to Resources

CHAPTER HIGHLIGHTS

- Grief is the emotional response to a loss, experienced by a person as grieving. Bereavement, a form of depression accompanied by anxiety, is a common response to loss of a loved one by death. Death, although inevitable, is an immensely difficult loss.

- There are many different theories of how people respond to loss and grief. These theories are useful when providing nursing care to clients and their families.

- A person's response to loss is influenced by age, social support, family members, cultural and spiritual beliefs, and rituals of mourning. Nurses need to assess the way in which they respond to loss to better care for clients.

- Legal and ethical issues involved in end-of-life care include advance directives (living wills, healthcare surrogate, and durable power of attorney), do-not-resuscitate orders, and euthanasia.

- Hospice, a model of care for clients and their families when faced with limited life expectancy, supports a dignified and peaceful death. Palliative care is focused on the relief of physical, mental, and spiritual distress for people with an incurable illness.

- To provide knowledgeable and compassionate care at the end of life, nurses must recognize physiologic changes as the client nears death, support the client and family, provide postmortem care, and resolve their own grief.

- Nursing care of clients experiencing an actual or potential loss includes accurate physical, spiritual, and psychosocial assessment; and interventions for the human responses of anticipatory grieving, chronic sorrow, and/or death anxiety.

TEST YOURSELF NCLEX-RN® REVIEW

1 Which of the following statements best describes loss?
1. It is determined by one's cultural values.
2. It is largely dependent on support of family and friends.
3. It can be determined only by the person who experiences it.
4. It is the same as grief and mourning.

2 Kübler-Ross believed that one usually first responds to a situation of loss with:
1. anger.
2. bargaining.
3. depression.
4. denial.

3 What is an important factor in the successful resolution of grief?
1. social isolation
2. support systems
3. triggers of grief
4. loss acknowledgment

4 What is the primary factor that dictates the rituals of mourning?
1. culture
2. age
3. gender
4. religion

5 What document expresses a person's wishes for life-sustaining treatment in the event of terminal illness or permanent unconsciousness?
1. durable power of attorney
2. living will
3. no-code order
4. healthcare surrogate

6 Which of the following statements is true of hospice?
1. Hospice is a special place of care.
2. Hospice care is a lifelong type of care.
3. Hospice is a model of care rather than a place of care.
4. Hospice is designed for clients with serious chronic illness.

7 A client nearing death requests that no medication be given that would cause a loss of consciousness, including pain medication. What would a nurse do to provide the best end-of-life care in this situation?
1. Give the medication; comfort is the highest priority.
2. Give half the ordered dose to provide compassionate care.
3. Discuss this with family members and follow their wishes.
4. Respect the client's wishes and withhold pain medications.

8 Which of the senses is believed to be the last one lost as a person nears death?
1. hearing
2. vision
3. touch
4. smell

9 Which of the following statements best describes the treatment of pain at the end of life?
1. As client nears death, no pain is perceived and no medications are necessary.
2. It is important to withhold pain medications if the client has respiratory changes.
3. There is no maximum allowable dose for opioids during end-of-life care.
4. Nurses should not administer opioids to the dying client.

10 A woman, recently widowed, tells the nurse, "I just can't even get out of bed in the mornings anymore." What response would be most helpful in resolving her grief?
1. "I don't know why you feel that way."
2. "This must be a difficult time for you."
3. "Why do you think you feel this way?
4. "After you get up, you will feel better."

See Test Yourself answers in Appendix C.

BIBLIOGRAPHY

American Association of Colleges of Nursing. (1999). *Peaceful death: Recommended competencies and curricular guidelines for end-of-life nursing care.* Washington, DC: Author.

_____. (2004). *Position statement: Moral distress.* Available from info@aacn.org

American Association of Retired Persons. (2003). *End of life: Talking about your final wishes.* Retrieved from http://www.aarp.org/life/endoflife/Articles/a2003-12-02-endoflife-finalwishes.html

American Geriatrics Society. (2002). *Position statement: The care of dying patients.* Retrieved from http://americangeriatrics.org/products/positionpapers/careofd.html

American Nurses Association. (1992a). *Position statement on nursing and the Patient Self-Determination Act.* Kansas City: Author.

_____. (1992b). *Report from the task force on the nurse's role in end of life decisions.* Kansas City: Author.

_____. (2003). *Position statements: Pain management and control of distressing symptoms in dying patients.* Retrieved from http://www.nursingworld.org/readroom/position/ethics/etpain.htm

Barbus, A. J. (1975). The Dying Person's Bill of Rights. *American Journal of Nursing, 75*(1), 99.

Bialk, J. (2004). Ethical guidelines for assisting patients with end-of-life decision making. *MEDSURG Nursing, 13*(2), 87–90.

Bowlby, J. (1973). *Attachment and loss: Separation, anxiety, and anger* (Vol. 2). New York: Basic Books.

_____. (1980). *Attachment and loss: Loss, sadness, and depression* (Vol. 3). New York: Basic Books.

Caplan, G. (1990). Loss, stress, and mental health. *Community Mental Health Journal, 26*(1), 27–48.

Centers for Disease Control & Prevention: *Hospice care.* (2006) Retrieved from http://www.cdc.gov/nchs/fastats/hospicecare.htm

Collins, F. (2004). An evaluation of palliative care services in the community. *Nursing Times, 100*(33), 34–37.

Dochterman, J., & Bulechek, G. (2004). *Nursing interventions classification (NIC)* (4th ed.). St. Louis, MO: Mosby.

Dunne, K. (2004). Grief and its manifestations. *Nursing Standard, 18*(45), 45–53.

Engel, G. (1964). Grief and grieving. *American Journal of Nursing, 64*, 93.

Ferrell, B., & Coyle, N. (2002). An overview of palliative nursing care. *American Journal of Nursing, 102*(5), 26–31.

Fine, P. (2004). *What is hospice?* Medscape from WebMD. Retrieved from http://www.medscape.com/viewarticle/4187401

Florida Department of Elder Affairs and the Florida Partnership for End-of-life Care. (2004). *Making choices: Beginning to plan for end-of-life care.* Retrieved from http://elderaffairs.state.fl.us

Freud, S. (1917/1957). Mourning and melancholia. In J. Strachey & A. Tyson (Eds.), *The complete psychological works of Sigmund Freud* (Vol. 14). London: Hogarth Press.

Given, B., Wyatt, G., Given, C., Sherwood, P., Gift, A., DeVoss, D., et al. (2004). Burden and depressions among caregivers of patients with cancer at the end of life. *Oncology Nursing Forum, 31*(6), 1105–1117.

Hennemann, E., & Karras, G. (2004). Determining brain death in adults: A guideline for use in critical care. *Critical Care Nurse, 24*, 50–56. Retrieved from http://ccn.aacnjournals.org/cgi/contents/full/24/5/50

Hospice Foundation of America. (2005). *The dying process: A guide for caregivers.* Washington, DC: Hospice Foundation of America.

International Council of Nurses. (1997). *Basic principles of nursing care.* Washington, DC: American Nurses Publishing.

Kirchhoff, K., Spuhler, V., Walker, L., Hutton, A, Cole, B., & Clemmer, T. (2000). Intensive care nurses' experiences with end-of-life care. *American Journal of Critical Care, 9*(1), 35–42.

Kruse, B. (2004). The meaning of letting go: The lived experience for caregivers of persons at end of life. *Journal of Hospice and Palliative Nursing, 6*(4), 215–222.

Kübler-Ross, E. (1969). *On death and dying.* New York: Macmillan.

_____. (1978). *To live until we say goodbye.* Englewood Cliffs, NJ: Prentice Hall.

_____. (1997). *On death and dying: What the dying have to teach doctors, nurses, clergy, and their own families.* New York: Simon & Schuster.

Lewis, I., & McBride, M. (2004). Anticipatory grief and chronicity: Elders and families in racial/ethnic minority groups. *Geriatric Nursing, 25*(1), 44–47.

Lindemann, E. (1944). Symptomatology and management of acute grief. *American Journal of Psychiatry, 32*, 141.

Living wills and health care proxies. (2004). *Harvard Women's Health Watch, 11*(5), 6–7.

Lynn, J., Schuster, J., & Kabcenell, A. (2000). *Sourcebook: Improving care for the end of life.* Oxfordshire, England: Oxford University Press.

Mazanec, P., & Tyler, M. (2003). Cultural considerations in end-of-life care: How ethnicity, age, and spirituality affect decisions when death is imminent. *American Journal of Nursing, 103*(3), 50–58.

Merck Manual of Geriatrics. (2005). *Chapter 13: Care of the Dying Patient.* Retrieved from http://www.merck.com/mrkshared/mmg/sec1/ch13.jsp

Moorhead, S., Johnson, M., & Maas, M. (2003). *Nursing outcomes classification (NOC)* (3rd ed.). St. Louis, MO: Mosby.

National Association for Home Care & Hospice. (2004). *Hospice facts & statistics.* Washington, DC: Author.

Poor, B., & Poirrier, G. (2001). *End of life nursing care.* Boston: Jones & Bartlett.

Pomeranz, J., & Brustman, M. (2005). When's the time right to enter hospice care? *Nursing, 55*(8), 43.

Rancour, P. (2002). Catapulting through life stages: When younger adults are diagnosed with life-threatening illnesses. *Journal of Psychosocial Nursing and Mental Health Services, 40*(2), 32–37, 52–53.

Reed, P. G. (1996). Transcendence: Formulating nursing perspectives. *Nursing Science Quarterly, 9*(1), 2–4.

Spector, R. (2004). *Cultural diversity in health and illness* (6th ed.). Upper Saddle River NJ: Prentice Hall.

Teasdale, K. (2004). Care of the bereaved when postmortems are required. *Nursing Times, 100*(36), 32–33.

Tierney, L. M., McPhee, S. J., & Papadakis, M. A. (2004). *Current medical diagnosis & treatment* (43rd ed.). New York: McGraw Hill.

Tuttas, C. (2002). The facts of end-of-life care. *Journal of Nursing Care Quality, 16*(2), 10–16.

Wiese, K. (2003). Grief, loss and bereavement. *Prairie Rose, 72*(4), 20–27.

Wilkinson, J. (2005). *Prentice Hall nursing diagnosis handbook with NIC interventions and NOC outcomes* (8th ed.). Upper Saddle River, NJ: Prentice Hall.

Yetman, L. (2004). Helping patients make their wishes known. *Home Healthcare Nurse, 22*(8), 576.

CHAPTER 6 Nursing Care of Clients with Problems of Substance Abuse

LEARNING OUTCOMES

- Explain risk factors associated with substance abuse.
- Recognize the signs and symptoms of potential substance abuse in coworkers.
- Describe common characteristics of substance abusers.
- Classify major addictive substances.
- Explain the effects of addictive substances on physiologic, cognitive, psychologic, and social well-being.

- Support interdisciplinary care for the client with substance abuse problems, including diagnostic tests, emergency care for overdose, and treatment of withdrawal.
- Develop a framework for providing individualized nursing care for clients experiencing problems with substance abuse using the nursing process.

CLINICAL COMPETENCIES

- Assess functional health status of clients with substance abuse.
- Monitor, document, and report physical manifestations of substance abuse.
- Assess for signs of withdrawal and monitor for life-threatening conditions.
- Use evidence-based research to plan and implement nursing care for clients experiencing withdrawal symptoms.
- Derive priority nursing diagnoses from assessment data.

- Formulate appropriate goals and implement individualized nursing interventions for clients with problems of substance abuse.
- Provide skilled nursing care during detoxification period.
- Collaborate with other disciplines when caring for clients with substance abuse problems.
- Educate client about stress management, coping skills, nutrition, relapse prevention, and healthy lifestyle choices.
- Revise plan of care as needed to promote, maintain, or restore functional health status to clients with substance abuse problems.

MEDIALINK

Resources for this chapter can be found on the Prentice Hall Nursing MediaLink DVD-ROM accompanying this textbook, and on the Companion Website at http://www.prenhall.com/lemone

Substance abuse refers to the use of any chemical in a fashion inconsistent with medical or culturally defined social norms despite physical, psychologic, or social adverse effects. Anxiety and depressive disorders frequently occur with substance abuse, and more than 90% of people who commit suicide have a depressive or substance abuse disorder (National Institute of Mental Health, 2004). According to the *Results from the 2004 National Survey on Drug Use and Health: National Findings* (Substance Abuse and Mental Health Services Administration [SAMHSA], 2005), 9.4% of the American population ages 12 or older (22.5 million Americans) reported problems with substance dependence or abuse in 2004.

The *Diagnostic and Statistical Manual of Mental Disorders,* fourth edition, text revision (DSM-IV-TR) (American Psychiatric Association, 2000) includes a classification scheme for distinguishing between substance abuse and substance dependence. **Substance dependence** refers to a severe condition occurring when the use of the chemical substance is no longer under an individual's control for at least 3 months. Continued use of the substance usually persists despite adverse effects on the person's physical condition, psychologic health, and interpersonal relationships. The DSM-IV-TR criteria deal with the behavioral as-

pects and the maladaptive patterns of substance use, emphasizing the physical symptoms of **tolerance** and **withdrawal**. Tolerance is a cumulative state in which a particular dose of the chemical elicits a smaller response than before. With increased tolerance, the individual needs higher and higher doses to obtain the desired effect. When a person is physically addicted to the drug and stops taking it, **withdrawal symptoms** can occur within hours. Withdrawal is an uncomfortable state lasting several days, manifested by tremors, diaphoresis, anxiety, high blood pressure, tachycardia, and possibly convulsions. An overview of the DSM-IV-TR diagnostic criteria for substance abuse and substance dependence is shown in Box 6–1.

The human tendency to seek pleasure and avoid stress and pain is partially responsible for substance abuse. Although far from definite, evidence implicates the endogenous opioid system in the development and maintenance of addictive behaviors. Currently available data suggest that ethanol increases opioid neurotransmission and that this activation is part of the mechanism responsible for its reinforcing effect (Oswald & Wand, 2004). Although most studies have focused on the role of dopamine D(1) and D(2) receptors in sustaining the addictive danger of drugs, recent stud-

BOX 6–1 Substance Abuse versus Substance Dependence

SUBSTANCE ABUSE	SUBSTANCE DEPENDENCE
Maladaptive pattern of substance use leading to clinically significant impairment or distress, manifested by **one or more** of the following within a 12-month period: 1. Failure to fulfill major role obligations at work, school, and home. 2. Involvement in physically hazardous situations while impaired (driving while intoxicated, operating a machine, exacerbation of physical symptoms such as ulcers). 3. Recurrent legal or interpersonal problems. 4. Continued use despite recurrent social and interpersonal problems.	Maladaptive pattern of substance use leading to clinically significant impairment or distress, manifested by **three or more** of the following within a 12-month period: 1. Presence of tolerance to the drug. 2. Presence of withdrawal symptoms. 3. Substance is taken in larger amounts or for longer periods than is intended. 4. Unsuccessful or persistent desire to cut down or control substance use. 5. More time spent in getting, taking, and recovering from the substance. May withdraw from family or friends and spend more time using substance in private. 6. Decline in or absence of important social, occupational, or recreational activities. 7. Continued use of substance despite knowledge of adverse effects.

Source: Adapted from *Diagnostic and Statistical Manual of Mental Disorders* (4th ed., text rev.) (DSM-IV-TR) by American Psychiatric Association, 2000, Washington, DC: Author.

ies have also shown that the dopamine D(3) receptor is involved in drug-seeking behavior (Heidbreder et al., 2004). The reinforcing properties of drugs can create a pleasurable experience and reduce the intensity of unpleasant experiences.

The craving one has for a particular substance may also be heightened by a phenomenon known as the "kindling" effect. **Kindling** refers to long-term changes in brain neurotransmission that occur after repeated detoxifications (Bayard et al., 2004). Recurrent detoxifications increase neuron sensitivity and are thought to intensify obsessive thoughts or cravings for a substance. Eventually the brain responds spontaneously in a dysfunctional manner even when the substance is no longer being used (Stuart & Laraia, 2005). This phenomenon may explain why subsequent episodes of withdrawal from a substance tend to worsen progressively.

Although there is no greater prevalence of psychiatric illness in substance abusers than in the general population, co-occurring disorders are often present. The term **co-occurring disorders** refers to the coexistence of substance abuse or dependence and a psychiatric disorder in one individual. **Dual diagnosis** and **dual disorder** are older terms that were previously used to describe

individuals with co-occurring disorders. One disorder can be an indication of another, such as the relationship between alcoholism and depression. Alcohol dependence and major depression commonly occur together and research suggests that both illnesses pose a significant risk for the development of the other disorder within 1 year's time (Gilman & Abraham, 2001). A depressed person may use self-medication in the form of alcohol to treat the depression, or the alcoholic person may become depressed. One study, describing the prevalence and characteristics of co-occurring serious mental illness (SMI) and substance abuse or dependence, found that most common co-occurring disorders in adult mental health clients were (1) alcohol and/or cannabis abuse with psychoses and heroin and/or (2) alcohol abuse or dependence with depression (Virgo et al., 2001). Compared with other SMI clients, those who were dually diagnosed were younger, more often male, in less stable accommodations, more likely to be unemployed, and more likely to have more than one psychiatric diagnosis and personality disorder. They also tended to have more crises and pose greater risk to themselves and others (Virgo et al., 2001). Box 6–2 lists terminology associated with substance abuse.

BOX 6–2 Terminology Associated with Substance Abuse

TERM	DEFINITION	TERM	DEFINITION
Abstinence	Voluntarily going without drugs or alcohol	Korsakoff's psychosis	Secondary dementia caused by thiamine (B_1) deficiency that may be associated with chronic alcoholism; characterized by progressive cognitive deterioration, confabulation, peripheral neuropathy, and myopathy
Addiction	A disease process characterized by the continued use of a specific chemical substance despite physical, psychologic, or social harm (used interchangeably with substance dependence)		
		Physical dependence	A state in which withdrawal syndrome will occur if drug use is discontinued
Codependence	A cluster of maladaptive behaviors exhibited by significant others of a substance-abusing individual that serves to enable and protect the abuse at the expense of living a full and satisfying life	Polysubstance abuse	The simultaneous use of many substances
		Psychologic dependence	An intensive subjective need for a particular psychoactive drug
Co-occurring disorders	Concurrent diagnosis of a substance use disorder and a psychiatric disorder. One disorder can precede and cause the other, such as the relationship between alcoholism and depression	Substance abuse	Continued use of a chemical substance in a fashion inconsistent with medical or social norms, for at least 1 month, despite related problems
Cross-tolerance	Tolerance to one drug confers tolerance to another	Substance dependence	A severe condition occurring when the use of the chemical substance is no longer under control, for at least 3 months; continued use persists despite adverse effects (used interchangeably with addiction)
Delirium tremens	A medical emergency usually occurring 3 to 5 days following alcohol withdrawal and lasting 2 to 3 days. Characterized by paranoia, disorientation, delusions, visual hallucinations, elevated vital signs, vomiting, diarrhea, and diaphoresis		
		Tolerance	State in which a particular dose elicits a smaller response than it formerly did. With increased tolerance the individual needs higher and higher doses to obtain the desired response
Detoxification	The process of helping an addicted individual safely through withdrawal		
Dual diagnosis	The coexistence of substance abuse/ dependence and a psychiatric disorder in one individual (used interchangeably with dual disorder and co-occurring disorders)	Wernicke's encephalopathy	Caused by thiamine (B_1) deficiency, characterized by nystagmus, ptosis, ataxia, confusion, coma, and possible death. Thiamine deficiency is common in chronic alcoholism
Kindling	Brain sensitization to events such as stress, trauma, or the effects of substance use	Withdrawal syndrome	Constellation of signs and symptoms that occurs in physically dependent individuals when they discontinue drug use

RISK FACTORS

Various risk factors help explain why one person becomes addicted while another does not. Genetic, biologic, psychologic, and sociocultural factors shed light on how a person may abuse or become dependent on a substance.

- *Genetic factors* include an apparent hereditary factor, especially with alcohol use and dependence. Most of the related genetic research has focused on alcoholism. Evidence supports the D(2) dopamine receptor gene (DRD2 A1 allele) as a genetic marker in adolescent males with increased risk for developing substance use problems (Conner et al., 2005). The discovery in 1990 that the DRD2 A1 allele gene appeared to be associated with alcoholism has led to a growing body of genetic research into substance abuse disorders (Stuart & Laraia, 2005). Women drink less alcohol and have fewer alcohol-related problems than men. In addition, women are less likely to have characteristics associated with heavy drinking including aggressiveness, drinking to reduce distress, and antisocial tendencies (Nolen-Hoeksema, 2004). See the Genetics Consideration box on this page.
- *Biologic factors* were first identified by Jellinek in his *Disease Model of Alcoholism*. He hypothesized that addiction to alcohol may have a biochemical basis and identified specific phases of the disease (Jellinek, 1946). Expanding on Jellinek's early work, researchers have implicated low levels of dopamine and serotonin in the development of alcohol dependence (Czermak et al., 2004; Guardia et al., 2000; Nellissery et al., 2003). Dopamine and dopamine receptor sites are intricately involved in the complex workings between the nervous system and abusive substances. Any drug's ability to

have an impact on the biochemical mechanism of the brain must be able to do so at a receptor site or at a number of receptor sites (Figure 6–1 ■). Most abused substances either mimic or block the brain's most important neurotransmitters at their respective receptor sites. For example, heroin and other opiates mimic natural opiate-like neurotransmitters such as endorphin, enkephalin, and dynorphin. In contrast, cocaine and other stimulants block the reuptake of dopamine, serotonin, and norepinephrine (Stuart & Laraia, 2005).

- *Psychologic factors* attempt to explain substance abuse through a combination of psychoanalytic, behavioral, and family system theories. Psychoanalytic theorists view substance abuse as a fixation at the oral stage of development, whereas behavioral theorists see addiction as a learned, maladaptive behavior. Family system theory focuses on the pattern of family relationships throughout several generations. No addictive personality type has been identified; however, several common factors seem to exist among alcoholics and drug users. Another type of alcoholism may be more environmentally influenced and is linked with onset after the age of 25, inability to stop after one drink, and a passive-dependent personality (Stuart & Laraia, 2005). Many substance abusers have experienced sexual or physical abuse in their childhood and as a result have low self-esteem and difficulty expressing emotions. A link also exists between substance abuse and psychiatric disorders such as depression, anxiety, and antisocial and dependent personalities. The habit of using a substance becomes a form of self-medication

GENETIC CONSIDERATIONS
Alcoholic Fathers and Their Sons

Genetic research has determined that children of alcoholics (COAs) are at higher risk for developing substance use problems (Conner et al., 2005). This is primarily true with male relatives. One type of alcoholism seen mostly in the sons of alcoholic fathers is associated with an early onset, inability to abstain, and an antisocial personality (Stuart & Laraia, 2005). Results of one study revealed that adolescent boys of alcoholics with the D(2) dopamine receptor gene (DRD2 A1 allele) tried and got intoxicated on alcohol more often than boys without this genetic marker. In addition, they tried more, and used more substances overall. Boys with the allele developed a more serious tobacco habit and experienced a marijuana high at an earlier age than boys without the allele (Conner et al., 2005).

CRITICAL THINKING IN CLIENT CARE

1. Why is it important to ask your clients if they have a family history of substance abuse?

2. What questions should you ask when assessing for increased risk of substance abuse?

3. Does having a positive family history of substance abuse indicate that a person will develop a substance abuse problem? Why or why not?

Agonistic effects

Drug induces increase in synthesis of neurotransmitter

Drug increases release of transmitter

Drug activates receptors that normally respond to neurotransmitter

Drug

Receptor site

Antagonistic effects

Drug interferes with release of neurotransmitter

Drug acts as a false transmitter, occupying receptor sites normally sensitive to neurotransmitter

Drug causes leakage of neurotransmitter from synaptic vesicles

Synaptic vesicle

Drug

Receptor site

Figure 6–1 ■ Action of abusive substances at brain receptor sites.

FOCUS ON CULTURAL DIVERSITY   Substance Use and Ethnicity

Ethnic identity plays a unique role in drug use behavior. Patterns of substance use are influenced by cultural norms and practices, in addition to other environmental and biologic factors. Adolescents in particular are influenced by ethnic and cultural practices. Positive ethnic identity (i.e., strong ethnic affiliation, attachment, and pride) may "protect" adolescents against drug use and help them form resistant behaviors to substance abuse (Marsiglia et al., 2004). A higher number of black and Hispanic children are exposed to alcohol problems in the home than white children (Ramisetty-Mikler & Caetano, 2004). Adolescent use of tobacco, alcohol, and illicit drugs was reportedly different in racial and ethnic groups. On average, Native American high school seniors revealed the highest levels of tobacco, alcohol, and illicit drug use, while Latin American, African American, and Asian Americans showed less drug use (Wallace et al., 2002). Another study reported that Asian American college students had a lower rate of alcohol dependence than Caucasian college students (Luczak et al., 2004). The highest rates of past-year methamphetamine use were found among Native Hawaiians or other Pacific Islanders (2.2%), American Indians or Alaska Natives (1.7%), and persons reporting two or more races (1.9%) (SAMHSA, 2005) (Figure 6–2 ■). Past-year methamphetamine use among whites (0.7%) and Hispanics (0.5%) was higher than among blacks (0.1%) or Asians (0.2%) (Office of Applied Studies [OAS], 2005a). Substance abuse and type 2 diabetes are serious health problems among Native Americans (Leonardson et al., 2005).

Critical Thinking in Client Care

1. You are a school nurse with a large population of Native Americans, Latin Americans, and African Americans in the commu-

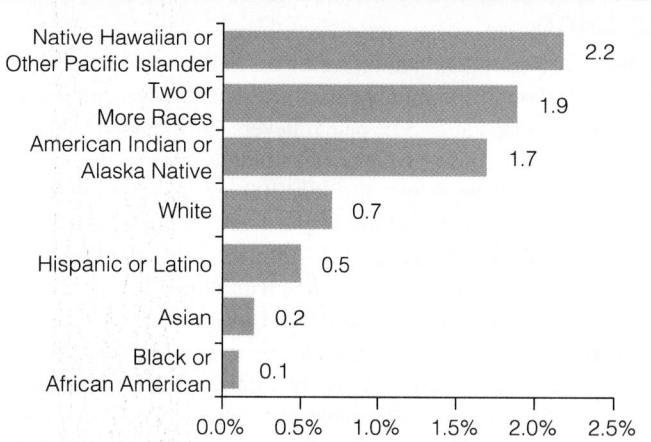

Source: SAMHSA, 2002, 2003, and 2004 NSDUH.

Figure 6–2 ■ Methamphetamine use by race/ethnicity: 2002, 2003, and 2004.

nity. An increasing problem with alcohol use and binge drinking among the high school students has become evident. The school superintendent has asked you for ideas to address this problem. How would you respond?

2. You are caring for a 23-year-old Asian American female brought to the emergency room by her boyfriend who tells you they were at a college party where she had alcohol for the first time. She is weak, her face is flushed, and she is vomiting violently. What would you do?

---

to cope with day-to-day problems, and over time develops into an addiction.

- *Sociocultural factors* often influence individuals' decisions as to when, what, and how they use substances. Ethnic differences in the way alcohol is metabolized may explain why some individuals choose not to drink. It is hypothesized that the Asian population has a deficiency of aldehyde dehydrogenase (ADH), the chemical in the brain that breaks down alcohol acetaldehyde (Cook et al., 2005). A buildup of acetaldehyde in the brain causes toxic symptoms characterized by vomiting, flushing, and tachycardia. Compared to other ethnic groups, Asian Americans report the lowest prevalence of family history of alcoholism (Ebberhart et al., 2003). Caucasians, Hispanics, and African Americans, on the other hand, have sufficient aldehyde dehydrogenase for metabolizing alcohol, and report higher alcoholism rates (Bersamin et al., 2005). Religious background may also correlate with the likelihood that a person will abuse alcohol. Among major religions, people of Jewish faith have the lowest rate of alcoholism while Roman Catholics have the highest rate. See the Focus on Cultural Diversity box above.

Many factors place a person at risk for substance use, abuse, and dependence. No single cause can explain why one individual develops a pattern of drug use and another person does not. Thorough assessment of these factors is necessary to understand the whole person and plan appropriate interventions.

CHARACTERISTICS OF ABUSERS

As mentioned, no addictive personality type exists; however, many abusers have several characteristics in common. Addictive behavior associated with alcoholism and other substances is characterized by compulsive preoccupation with obtaining the substance, loss of control over consumption, and development of tolerance and dependence as well as impaired social and occupational functioning (Weiss & Porrino, 2002). There is a tendency for drug users to indulge in impulsive, risk-taking behaviors. Abusers often have a low tolerance for frustration and pain. Often, drug users are rebellious against social norms and engage in various antisocial and risky behaviors such as stealing, promiscuity, driving while intoxicated, and violence against others. There is also a tendency toward anxiety, anger, and low self-esteem in substance abusers. Many people have a desire for social acceptance and initiate drug use to "fit in" with a peer group. Others may suffer from social anxiety and need drugs or alcohol to feel less inhibited while interacting with others.

ADDICTIVE SUBSTANCES AND THEIR EFFECTS

Caffeine

Caffeine is a stimulant that increases the heart rate and acts as a diuretic. Although commonly consumed daily in soft drinks, coffee, tea, chocolate, and some pain relievers, an excessive amount of caffeine can cause negative physiologic effects, especially cardiac-related risks. Approximately 300 mg per day is safe for most people, but over 600 mg is considered excessive and not recommended (Kneisl et al., 2004). Individuals with a history of cardiac disease are advised to cut down or eliminate caffeine intake altogether. Caffeine, if consumed in large quantities, can also cause higher total cholesterol levels and insomnia.

Many people in today's society recognize the adverse effects of too much caffeine in the system and voluntarily cut down on caffeine by drinking decaffeinated beverages. A caffeine-addicted person who abruptly withdraws from caffeine will most likely experience headaches and irritability. A rising number of adolescents are developing caffeine dependence by consuming sizable quantities of soft drinks and coffee. In a study investigating caffeine dependence in teenagers, researchers found that 15 out of 36 subjects reported tolerance to caffeine, described withdrawal symptoms after cessation of caffeine intake, reported unsuccessful attempts to control use, and endorsed use despite knowledge of physical or psychologic problems associated with caffeine (Bernstein et al., 2002). These results are significant due to the vast number of teens who consume caffeinated beverages.

Nicotine

Nicotine is found in tobacco and enters the system via the lungs (cigarettes and cigars) and oral mucous membranes (chewing tobacco as well as smoking). In low doses, nicotine stimulates nicotinic receptors in the brain to release norepinephrine and epinephrine, causing vasoconstriction. As a result, the heart rate accelerates and the force of ventricular contractions increases. Gastrointestinal (GI) effects include an increase in gastric acid secretion, tone and motility of GI smooth muscle, and promotion of vomiting. Nicotine acts on the central nervous system (CNS) as a stimulant, binding to acetylcholine receptors in the brain and causing the release of dopamine and norepinephrine. Quitting smoking is thought to be difficult because of dopamine release, which, in turn, reinforces the addictive craving for more. Smoking cessation can pose a problem for hospitalized clients. See the Nursing Research: Evidence-Based Practice for Smoking Cessation in Hospitalized Patients box below.

Initially, nicotine increases respiration, mental alertness, and cognitive ability, but eventually it depresses these responses (Kneisl et al., 2004). Moderate doses of nicotine can cause tremors. With high doses, such as acute poisoning from insecticides, convulsions and death can occur.

Tolerance can develop to nausea and dizziness, but not to the cardiovascular effects. Nicotine dependence results from chronic use with withdrawal seen as craving, nervousness, restlessness, irritability, impatience, increased hostility, insomnia, impaired concentration, increased appetite, and weight gain. Gradual reduction in nicotine use seems to prolong suffering. Chronic health problems from smoking have been well established in the form of cancer, heart disease, emphysema, hypertension, and death (Kneisl et al., 2004).

Since the 1990s, smoking rates among adult women have steadily increased. Smoking is now the number one cause of preventable death and disease among women. According to a

---

NURSING RESEARCH | **Evidence-Based Practice for Smoking Cessation in Hospitalized Patients**

Despite the well-publicized deleterious health effects posed by cigarette smoking and the legally restricted access to cigarettes, smoking remains a persistent problem. Smoking has been banned in stores, malls, hospitals, office buildings, and even a number of restaurants. Admission to the hospital provides an excellent opportunity for nurses to assist patients to quit smoking. Patients in hospitals may find it easier to quit in an environment where smoking is restricted or prohibited. In addition, individuals may be more open to cessation efforts when faced with the risks associated with surgery. In a review of the literature, researchers found that high-intensity behavioral interventions that include at least 1 month of follow-up contact were effective in helping hospitalized patients quit smoking (Rigotti et al., 2005). Healthcare professionals, especially nurses, can be very instrumental in smoking cessation efforts.

Another literature review provided evidence that nursing interventions for smoking cessation have potential benefits (Rice & Stead, 2005). Nicotine replacement therapy (NRT) also increases quit rates with or without additional counseling (Rice & Stead, 2005; Silagy et al., 2005). NRT aims to reduce withdrawal from tobacco products by replacing nicotine in the blood. All forms of NRT, available as chewing gum, skin patches, nose spray, inhalers, and tablets increase the likelihood that a person will succeed in quitting smoking (Silagy et al., 2005). Effective nursing strategies include asking patients about their tobacco use, counseling those who want to quit, reinforcing cessation efforts, and early follow-up with those who quit smoking. This evidence points to the important role nurses play in encouraging their clients to quit smoking and the need for nurses to incorporate smoking cessation interventions as part of their standard practice.

CRITICAL THINKING IN CLIENT CARE

1. You are caring for a 55-year-old man recently hospitalized for acute angina who asks you what is the best way to stop smoking. What would you do?
2. Why do you think nurses and other healthcare professionals should (or should not) quit smoking?
3. You are caring for a 12-year-old girl who tells you she has smoked cigarettes occasionally and believes it makes her more popular with her older friends. She admits that she knows that smoking is supposed to be bad for you but doesn't see the harm in smoking a few cigarettes every day. How would you respond?

recent report by the surgeon general, far more women are dying of lung cancer than of breast cancer, and around 165,000 women died prematurely from smoking-related diseases such as cancer, stroke and heart disease (U.S. Department of Health and Human Services, 2005). Women are also confronted with unique health concerns from smoking during pregnancy. Secondhand effects from smoking have been demonstrated, especially to fetuses during pregnancy. Smoking during pregnancy leads to increased risks for infants such as low birth weight, spontaneous abortions, perinatal mortality, and sudden infant death.

Cannabis

Cannabis sativa is the source of marijuana. The greatest psychoactive substances are in the flowering tops of the cannabis plant. Marijuana (also know as grass, weed, pot, dope, joint, and reefer) and hashish are the most common derivatives. The psychoactive component of marijuana is an oily chemical known as delta-9-tetrahydrocannabinol (THC). THC activates specific cannabinoid receptors in the brain. Evidence suggests that marijuana may act like opioids and cocaine in producing a pleasurable sensation, probably by causing release of endogenous opioids and then dopamine (Kneisl et al., 2004). Marijuana use can trigger psychosis in schizophrenic clients and, according to recent research, cannabis use may be a risk factor in developing future psychotic symptoms (Ferdinand et al., 2005).

Physiologic effects of cannabis are dose related and can cause an increase in heart rate and bronchodilation in short-term use. Chronic long-term use can lead to airway constriction, bronchitis, sinusitis, asthma, and increased risk for respiratory cancer (Watson et al., 2000). The reproductive system is also affected by marijuana; it causes decreased spermatogenesis and testosterone levels in males and suppresses follicle-stimulating, luteinizing, and prolactin hormones in females, making breast-feeding for new mothers impossible. Birth defects may also be associated with cannabis use. Marijuana crosses the placental barrier and is spread to fetal tissues. When a pregnant woman smokes marijuana, she increases the risk of abnormalities in the fetus such as CNS disturbances, low birth weight, decreased length, smaller head circumference, and fetal death (Kneisl et al., 2004). Subjective effects of marijuana include euphoria, sedation, and hallucinations. In addition, chronic use of marijuana can result in amotivational behaviors such as apathy, dullness, poor grooming, reduced interest in achievement, and disinterest. At extremely high doses, tolerance and physical dependence result.

Alcohol

Alcohol is the most commonly used and abused substance in the United States. Alcohol and other CNS depressants act on other neurotransmitters in the brain such as gamma-aminobutyric acid (GABA). GABA is the most prevalent inhibitory neurotransmitter in the brain and has a major role in decreasing neuronal excitability. Alcohol creates an additive effect with GABA, further inhibiting arousal and depressing the autonomic nervous system. This may explain why cross-tolerance effects occur when alcohol and other CNS depressants are used in combination (Varcarolis, 2002). When taken together, alcohol and other CNS depressants such as benzodiazepines and barbiturates can lead to respiratory depression and death.

Two-thirds of the nation's adult population consumes alcohol regularly. An estimated 14 million Americans (approximately 1 in every 13 adults) abuse alcohol or are alcoholic (National Institute on Alcohol Abuse and Alcoholism, 2004).

Although the legal drinking age in all 50 states is 21, many underage people obtain and use alcohol. Of the 14 million adults who abused alcohol in 2003, 95% started drinking alcohol before age 21 (SAMHSA, 2004). During 2004, an estimated 142,701 alcohol-related emergency department (ED) visits were made by patients ages 12 to 20 (OAS, 2006). Table 6–1 lists the top 10 drugs most frequently found in combination with alcohol in ED visits of patients ages 12 to 20.

MediaLink Case Study: Alcohol Withdrawal

TABLE 6–1 Top 10 Combination Drugs Found in Alcohol-Related ED Visits

RANK	DRUG	VISITS	PERCENT OF VISITS
	Total alcohol with other drugs	*45,282*	*100%*
1	Marijuana	22,244	49%
2	Cocaine	10,066	22%
3	Stimulants (amphetamine/methamphetamine)	3,805	8%
4	Alprazolam	3,057	7%
5	Drug unknown	1,835	3%
6	Ibuprofen	1,585	3%
7	Acetaminophen	1,524	3%
8	Methylenedioxymeth-amphetamine (MDMA)	1,502	3%
9	Acetaminophen-hydrocodone	1,436	3%
10	Heroin	1,323	3%

Source: Office of Applied Studies, SAMHSA, Drug Abuse Warning Network, 2004.

Alcohol is absorbed in the mouth, stomach, and digestive tract. The liver metabolizes approximately 95% of the ingested alcohol and the rest is excreted via the skin, kidney, and lungs. Generally, an individual can break down approximately 1 ounce of whiskey every 90 minutes. Factors such as body mass, food intake, and liver function can affect the rate of alcohol absorption.

When used in moderation, certain types of alcohol can have positive physiologic effects by decreasing coronary artery disease and protecting against stroke. However, when consumed in excess, alcohol can severely diminish one's ability to function and will ultimately lead to life-threatening conditions. Chronic use of alcohol can cause severe neurologic and psychiatric disorders. Severe damage to the liver occurs with chronic alcohol abuse, and can progress from fatty liver to other liver diseases such as hepatitis or cirrhosis. Chronic alcoholism is the major cause of fatal cirrhosis. Alcohol causes damaging effects to many other systems including myocardial disease, erosive gastritis, acute and chronic pancreatitis, sexual dysfunction, and an increased risk of breast cancer.

Malnutrition is another serious complication of chronic alcoholism; thiamine (B_1) deficiency in particular can result in neurologic impairments. Thiamine depletion is thought to cause the Wernicke-Korsakoff syndrome observed in chronic alcoholics (Stuart & Laraia, 2005). Severe cognitive impairment is a principal feature of **Wernicke's encephalopathy** and **Korsakoff's psychosis**. Although Wernicke's and Korsakoff's are sometimes considered to be two distinctive disorders, they are actually different phases of the same disease, commonly called Wernicke-Korsakoff syndrome. Wernicke's encephalopathy indicates the "acute" stage of the illness, and Korsakoff's psychosis indicates the "chronic" stage.

Although alcohol is a CNS depressant, it actually disrupts sleep, thus altering the sleep cycle, decreasing the quality of sleep, intensifying obstructive sleep apnea, and reducing total sleeping time. Heavy drinkers have a higher mortality rate and many fatalities occur from alcohol-related accidents. Blood alcohol levels (BALs) are highly predictive of CNS effects. Eu-

phoria, reduced inhibitions, impaired judgment, and increased confidence are seen at 0.05% (Kneisl et al., 2004). The legal level of intoxication in many states is 0.10%, although there is a trend toward lowering the level to 0.08% in other states. Toxic levels in excess of 0.5% can cause coma, respiratory depression, peripheral collapse, and death (Kneisl et al., 2004). Chronic consumption of alcohol produces tolerance and creates cross-tolerance to general anesthetics, barbiturates, benzodiazepines, and other CNS depressants. If alcohol is withdrawn abruptly, the brain becomes overly excited because receptors previously inhibited are no longer inhibited (Bayard et al., 2004). This hyperexcitability manifests clinically as anxiety, tachycardia, hypertension, diaphoresis, nausea, vomiting, tremors, sleeplessness, and irritability. Severe manifestations of alcohol withdrawal include seizures, convulsions, and **delirium tremens (DT)**. Episodes of delirium tremens have a mortality rate of 1% to 5% (Kasser et al., 2004).

CNS Depressants

Central nervous system depressants including barbiturates, benzodiazepines, paraldehyde, meprobamate, and chloral hydrate are also subject to abuse. Cross-dependence exists among all CNS depressants and cross-tolerance can develop to alcohol and general anesthetics. Chronic users of barbiturates require progressively higher doses to achieve subjective effects as tolerance develops, but they develop little tolerance to respiratory depression. The depressant effects related to barbiturates are dose dependent and range from mild sedation to sleep to coma to death. With larger doses over time and a combination of alcohol and barbiturates, the risk of death increases greatly. The risk of accidental overdose and death resulting from barbiturates has resulted in decreased use, yet barbiturates are still clinically useful for seizure disorders and alcohol withdrawal. Benzodiazepines have replaced barbiturates as the drugs of choice for anxiety-related disorders. Benzodiazepines alone are safer than barbiturates, because an overdose of oral benzodiazepines rarely results in death. However, CNS depressants when taken together (for example, alcohol and benzodiazepines) can result in death.

Psychostimulants

Psychostimulants such as cocaine and amphetamines have a high potential for abuse. Euphoria is the main subjective effect associated with cocaine and amphetamines, leading to addiction. **Cocaine** powder has been "snorted" (inhaled through the nostrils) for thousands of years, but a more dangerous method used nowadays is called freebasing. Cocaine base (freebased cocaine, or "crack") is heat stable and is usually "cooked" in a baking soda solution and smoked (freebasing). Cocaine hydrochloride (HCl) is diluted or cut before sale and the pure form ("rocks") is administered intranasally (snorted) or injected intravenously. "Skin popping" is a subcutaneous method many substance abusers are using to administer drugs, perhaps leading to the formation of abscesses under the skin. Mild overdose of cocaine produces agitation, dizziness, tremor, and blurred vision. Severe overdose produces anxiety, hyperpyrexia, convulsions, ventricular dysrhythmias, severe hypertension, and hemorrhagic stroke with possible angina or myocardial infarction (MI).

The use of cocaine during pregnancy is especially problematic, because the drug crosses the placenta and enters the fetal bloodstream. Spontaneous abortion, premature delivery, retardation of intrauterine growth, congenital abnormalities, and fetal addiction can result. Long-term intranasal use of cocaine can cause atrophy of the nasal mucosa, necrosis and perforation of the nasal septum, and lung damage. The growing practice of crack cocaine injection requires serious attention, because this new drug use behavior is associated with increased rates of high-risk behaviors. Recent research indicates that injection drug users (IDUs) exhibited significantly higher rates of risky health behaviors. High-risk sexual behaviors were especially prevalent among female crack cocaine injectors. Higher self-reported rates of adverse health outcomes, such as sexually transmitted infections (STIs), hepatitis C, and abscesses among crack injectors, were found, although no differences in rates of HIV infection were self-reported (Buchanan et al., 2006).

Amphetamine use is on the rise and poses a severe health risk to society due to its devastating physical and neurologic consequences, including amphetamine-induced mental disorders. Methamphetamine is illegally manufactured, distributed, and abused and is currently the most widespread amphetamine used in the United States (OAS, 2005a). Methamphetamine is a powerful stimulant drug commonly referred to as *speed, crystal, crank, go,* and, most recently, *ice,* a smokable form of methamphetamine. The manufacture of methamphetamine is a relatively simple process and can be carried out by individuals without special knowledge or expertise in chemistry. Methamphetamine is often taken in combination with other drugs such as cocaine and marijuana and, like heroin and cocaine, can be inhaled, injected, ingested, or smoked.

In 2004, an estimated 1.4 million persons ages 12 or older (0.6% of the population) had used methamphetamine in the past year, and 600,000 persons (0.2% of the population) had used methamphetamine in the past month (OAS, 2005a). The highest rate of methamphetamine use in the past year was found among young adults between the ages of 18 and 25 (1.6%). Methamphetamine use among males (0.7%) was slightly higher than for females (0.5%) (Figure 6–3 ■).

It appears that methamphetamine is an "equal opportunity" drug for addiction without regard to gender, age, race, or sexual preferences. With regard to race or ethnicity, the highest percentage rates of methamphetamine use were found among Native Hawaiians or other Pacific Islanders (2.2%), people reporting two or more races (1.9%), and American Indians or Alaska Natives (1.7%) (OAS, 2005a). The lowest rates of methamphetamine use were among whites (0.7%), Hispanics (0.5%), Asians (0.2%), and African Americans (0.1%).

Methamphetamine use has been linked with HIV infection and high rates of STIs in homosexual, heterosexual, and bisexual men and women all over the United States (AIDS Alert, 2005; Brown et al., 2005; Semple et al., 2004; Shoptaw et al., 2005). Heterosexual men and women displayed severe to moderate depressive symptoms due to perceived stigma associated with methamphetamine use, emphasizing the importance of identifying and treating depression in this population (Semple et al., 2005). An interesting finding from the 2004 *National Survey*

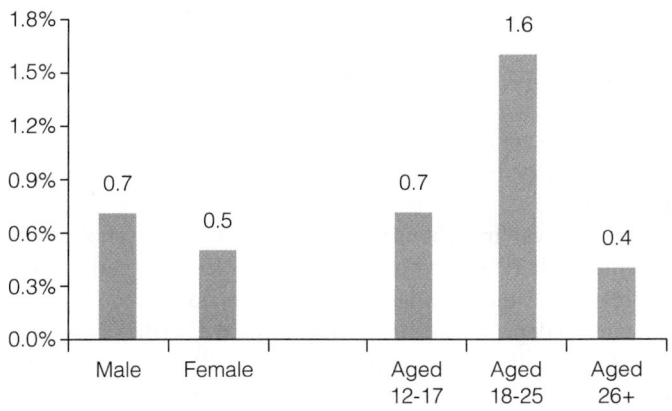

Source: SAMHSA, 2002, 2003, and 2004 NSDUH.

Figure 6–3 ■ Methamphetamine use by gender and age: 2002, 2003, and 2004.

on Drug Use and Health (NSDUH) was that the western half of the United States reported the highest levels of methamphetamine use from 2002 through 2004 (OAS, 2005a). Twelve states including Nevada (2.2%), Wyoming, and Montana (1.5% each) ranked highest for past-year methamphetamine use. Connecticut (less than 0.1%), New York, and North Carolina (0.12% each) were among the states with the lowest rates (Figure 6–4 ■).

Amphetamines cause arousal and an elevation of mood with a sense of increased strength, mental capacity, self-confidence, and a decreased need for food and sleep. Methamphetamine users in treatment have reported physical symptoms associated with the use of methamphetamine including weight loss, tachycardia, tachypnea, hyperthermia, insomnia, and muscular tremors (OAS, 2005a). The behavioral and psychiatric symptoms reported most often include violent behavior, repetitive activity, memory loss, paranoia, delusions of reference, auditory hallucinations, and confusion or fright. A psychotic state with hallucinations and paranoia are common with long-term

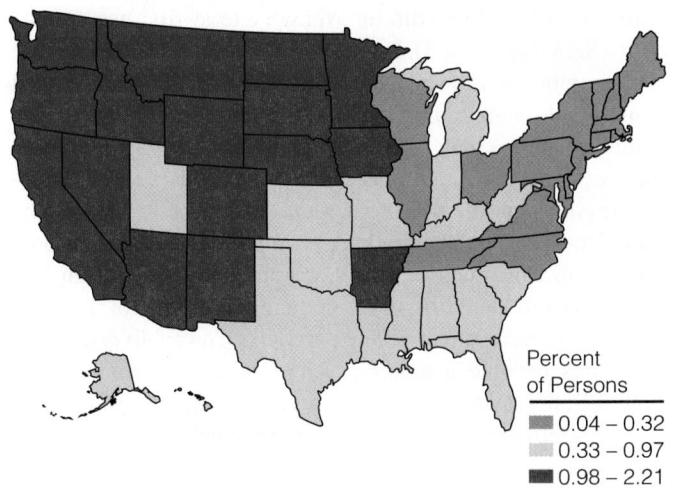

Percent of Persons
- 0.04 – 0.32
- 0.33 – 0.97
- 0.98 – 2.21

Source: SAMHSA, 2002, 2003, and 2004 NSDUH.

Figure 6–4 ■ Methamphetamine use by state: 2002, 2003, and 2004.

use, requiring treatment similar to other psychotic disorders. The cardiovascular effects of amphetamines are comparable to those of cocaine, including vasoconstriction, tachycardia, hypertension, angina, and dysrhythmias. Tolerance to mood elevation, appetite suppression, and cardiovascular effects develops with amphetamines; however, dependence is more psychologic than physical.

Withdrawal from amphetamines produces dysphoria and craving with fatigue, prolonged sleep, excessive eating, and depression. Although a large number of people cope with amphetamine dependence worldwide, limited evidence exists for effective treatment (Srisurapanont et al., 2005). In a systematic review of treatment measures for amphetamine dependence and abuse, antidepressants provided little benefit concerning amphetamine use. Both biologic and psychosocial treatments should be further investigated (Srisurapanont et al., 2005). Brief cognitive behavioral therapy (CBT) was reported to improve methamphetamine users' attempts to resist the urge to use methamphetamine in stressful interpersonal situations (Yen et al., 2004). A culturally tailored CBT program was more effective than standard CBT in reducing methamphetamine use and high-risk sexual behaviors (Shoptaw et al., 2005).

Opiates

Opiates such as morphine, meperidine, codeine, hydrocodone, and oxycodone are narcotic analgesics. Examples of some common brand names include Vicodin, Percocet, OxyContin, and Darvon. Narcotic analgesics are a type of pain reliever derived from natural or synthetic opiates. A small percentage of individuals are originally exposed to opiates in the context of prescription pain management; however, most people use opiates under social or illicit circumstances. The urban poor constitute the majority of abusers, although opiates are used and abused by people at all socioeconomic levels. The problem of abuse of and addiction to prescribed narcotics has resurfaced as a major issue for the United States in the early 2000s and has worsened during the past few years (Compton & Volkow, 2006). In 2004, the number of new nonmedical users of Oxy-Contin was 615,000, with an average age at first use of 24.5 years (SAMHSA, 2005). Figure 6–5 ■ shows a steady increase in the number of initiates from 1995, when OxyContin was first available, through 2003. This increase in opiate abuse seems to reflect, in part, changes in medication prescribing practices, changes in drug formulations, and fairly easy access via the Internet. Although the use of narcotic analgesics for acute pain management looks benign, long-term use has been associated with significant rates of abuse or addiction. OxyContin is a controlled-released form of oxycodone prescribed for the management of moderate to severe pain. OxyContin diversion and abuse has become a major problem in certain areas of the United States, particularly rural areas and Appalachia (Hays, 2004). A retrospective review of 534 medical records revealed that 27% of patients admitted and discharged from an addiction detoxification unit were dependent on prescription opiate medications (Miller & Greenfeld, 2004). The most frequently mentioned medication was Vicodin (hydrocodone) followed by OxyContin (oxycodone). According to data collected by the

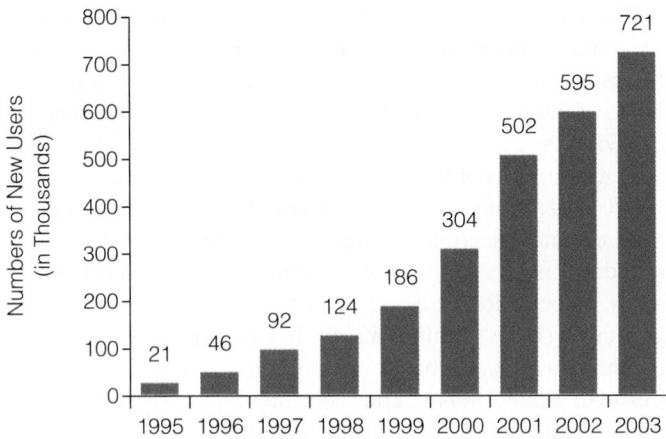

Source: SAMHSA, 2002, 2003, and 2004 NSDUH.

Figure 6–5 ■ Annual numbers of new nonmedical users of OxyContin, 1995–2003.

Drug Abuse Warning Network (DAWN), drug abuse–related emergency department visits involving narcotic analgesics increased 153% in the nation (from 42,857 visits in 1995 to 108,320 ED visits in 2002) (SAMHSA, 2004). The greatest increases during this period occurred for oxycodone (512%), methadone (176%), hydrocodone (159%), and morphine (116%). Illicit or nonmedical use of OxyContin has been widely cited in recent media reports; however, nonmedical use was found in only 0.4% of the population in 2001 and rarely led to the abuse of other drugs (Sees et al., 2005).

Heroin has been abused for many centuries and is usually administered intravenously. It induces a "rush" or "kick" that lasts less than a minute, followed by a sense of euphoria lasting several hours. Tolerance develops to the euphoria, respiratory depression, and nausea but not to constipation and miosis. Physical dependence occurs with long-term use of opiates. Initial withdrawal symptoms such as drug craving, lacrimation, rhinorrhea, yawning, and diaphoresis usually take 10 days to run their course, with the second phase of opiate withdrawal lasting for months with insomnia, irritability, fatigue, and potential GI hyperactivity and premature ejaculation as problems. Methadone is a synthetic opiate used to treat chronic pain and addiction to other opiates. Methadone does not hinder one's ability to function productively as other narcotics do and is a viable support for withdrawal (Stuart & Laraia, 2005).

Hallucinogens

Hallucinogens are also called psychedelics and include phencyclidine (PCP), 3,4-methylenediosy-methamphetamine (MDMA), D-lysergic acid diethylamide (LSD), mescaline, dimethyltryptamine (DMT), and psilocin. Psychedelics bring on the same types of thoughts, perceptions, and feelings that occur in dreams. PCP (also called angel dust and peace pill) was developed in the 1950s as an anesthetic similar to ketamine, but due to its severe side effects, its development for human use was discontinued. PCP is known for inducing violent behavior and for inducing negative physical reactions such as seizures, coma, and death (OAS,

2005c). The most common route of administration is smoking to-bacco, marijuana, or herbal cigarettes laced with PCP powder or the liquid form of PCP.

MDMA, commonly known as Ecstasy, was very popular in the 1980s as a recreational "club drug" associated with dance clubs or "raves" and has reappeared in recent years as a date or rape drug. According to 2003 NSDUH data, approximately 2.1 million persons ages 12 or older (0.9%) used Ecstasy during the past year; however, its use has declined from 3.2 million users in 2002 (SAMHSA, 2005). The rate of past-year Ecstasy use was significantly greater among 18- to 25-year-olds (3.7%) than among 12- to 17-year-olds (1.3%) or persons ages 26 or older (0.3%) (SAMHSA, 2005). Parties where other drugs such as marijuana or alcohol are present may lead to easier access or availability of Ecstasy, thereby increasing the chances for first-time Ecstasy use. One study suggests that cannabis use is a powerful risk factor for subsequent first onset of Ecstasy use (Zimmerman et al., 2005). Another study reported approximately 20% of youths ages 16 to 23 admitted to using one or more of the following drugs: methamphetamine, Ecstasy, LSD, ketamine, GHB (gamma-hydroxybutyrate), and flunitrazepam (Rohypnol) (Wu et al., 2006). Females were more likely than males to report using multiple club drugs. Staying in school and getting married were associated with decreased odds of club drug use. On the other hand, use of club drugs was increased by criminal behaviors and recent alcohol abuse or dependence.

LSD was first used to simulate psychosis. It affects sero-tonin receptors at multiple sites in the brain and spinal cord. LSD is usually taken orally but can be injected or smoked, as in tobacco- or marijuana-laced cigarettes. The individual's re-sponse to a "trip," the experience of being high on LSD, cannot be predicted and psychologic effects and "flashbacks" are com-mon. Serotonin imbalance is thought to affect impulse control and may be responsible for uninhibited sexual responses in women who have been given the drug without their knowledge. Other hallucinogens are similar to LSD but with different po-tency and course of action. Because physical dependence to hallucinogens does not appear to occur, withdrawal symptoms are not present.

Inhalants

Inhalants are categorized into three types: anesthetics, volatile nitrites, and organic solvents. Nitrous oxide (laughing gas) and ether are the most abused anesthetics. Amyl nitrite, butyl nitrite, and isobutyl nitrite are volatile nitrites used especially by homo-sexual males to induce venodilation and anal sphincter relax-ation. Amyl nitrite is manufactured for medical use, but butyl and isobutyl nitrites are sold for recreational use. Other names for butyl and isobutyl nitrites are *climax, rush,* and *locker room.* Street names for amyl nitrite are *poppers* or *snappers* (Box 6–3). Brain damage or sudden death can occur the first, tenth, or hun-dredth time an individual uses an inhalant, resulting in "sudden sniffing death." This danger makes the use of inhalants more hazardous than some other substances.

Another danger is the wide assortment of organic solvents that are available to and inhaled by young children. Organic solvents are ingested by three different methods: bagging, huff-

ing, or sniffing. *Bagging* involves pouring the solvent in a plas-tic bag and inhaling the vapor. *Huffing* refers to pouring the sol-vent on a rag and inhaling. *Sniffing* refers to inhaling the solvent directly from the container. Common organic solvents are toluene, gasoline, lighter fluid, paint thinner, nail polish re-mover, benzene, acetone, chloroform, and model airplane glue. The effects from inhaling organic solvents are similar to those of alcohol, with prolonged use leading to multiple toxicities and an increased risk for abusing other substances. Children who used inhalants before the age of 14 were twice as likely to initiate opiate use compared to those who had never tried opi-ates (Storr et al., 2005). There are no antidotes for these in-halants; therefore, management of overdose is supportive.

INTERDISCIPLINARY CARE

Effective treatment of substance abuse and dependence results from the efforts of an interdisciplinary team specializing in the treatment of psychiatric and substance abuse disorders. Thera-pies may include detoxification, aversion therapy to maintain ab-stinence, group and/or individual psychotherapy, psychotropic medications, cognitive-behavioral strategies, family counseling, and self-help groups. Clients suffering from substance abuse can

---

BOX 6–3 Common Street Names for Abused Substances

SUBSTANCE	STREET NAME
Alcohol	Booze, brew, spirits, juice, hootch
Amphetamines	Bennies, crystal, crystal meth, crank, dexies, diet pills, dolls, eye-openers, ice, lid poppers, pep pills, purple hearts, speed, uppers
Barbiturates	Barbs, beans, black beauties, blue angels, candy, downers, goof balls, ludes, nebbies, reds, sleepers, tranks, yellow jackets, yellows
Benzodiazepines	Bennies, blues, rainbows, reds, sopors, yellows
Cocaine	Bernice, bernies, big C, blow, Charlie, coke, dust, girl, heaven, jay, lady, nose candy, nose powder, snow, sugar, white lady Crack: Conan, freebase, rock, toke, white cloud, white tornado
Hallucinogens	Acid, big D, blotter, blue heaven, cap D, deeda, flash, L, mellow yellows, microdots, paper acid, sugar, ticket, yello, Ecstasy
Heroin, morphine	H, horse, harry, boy, M, Miss Emma, scag, "shit," smack, stuff, white junk, white stuff
Marijuana	Acapulco gold, Aunt Mary, broccoli, dope, grass, grunt, hay, hemp, herb, J, joint, joy stick, killer weed, Mary Jane, pot, ragweed, reefer, smoke, weed, "shit"
Opiates	Meperidine (Demerol), hydrocodone (Vicodin), Percocet, oxycodone (OxyContin), and Darvon

be treated in either inpatient or outpatient settings. A substance overdose is a life-threatening condition that requires emergency hospitalization to stabilize the client medically before implementing any of the interventions mentioned. Several diagnostic tests can provide valuable information about the client's physical condition and set the course for treatment.

Diagnostic Tests

The body fluids most often tested for drug content are blood and urine, although saliva, perspiration, and even hair can be tested. The simplest method of detecting blood alcohol content is by using a Breathalyzer. More invasive procedures such as serum drug levels are useful in the emergency department and other hospital settings to treat drug overdoses or complications. A urine drug screen (UDS) and/or BAL are the main biologic measures for assessment purposes. Urine drug screening (UDS) is noninvasive and the preferred method for detecting substances in the body. Companies often require a UDS of prospective employees before hiring them. In addition, professional and college athletes are now required to submit to random drug testing. Results of UDS are also used within the court system to determine drug use in relation to criminal activity. The length of time that drugs can be found in blood and urine varies according to dosage and metabolic properties of the drug. All traces of the drug may disappear within 24 hours or may still be detectable 30 days later. The psychoactive substance found in marijuana, THC, is stored in fatty tissues (especially the brain and reproductive system) and can be detected in the body for up to 6 weeks (Kneisl et al., 2004).

Knowledge of the BAL is helpful in ascertaining the level of intoxication, the level of tolerance, and whether the person accurately reported recent drinking. At 0.10% (after 5 to 6 drinks in 1 to 2 hours), voluntary motor action becomes clumsy and reaction time is impaired. The degree of impairment varies with gender, weight, and food ingestion. Small women who drink alcohol on an empty stomach will experience intoxication more rapidly than large males who have eaten a full meal. At 0.20% (after 10 to 12 drinks in 2 to 4 hours), function of the motor area in the brain is depressed, causing staggering and ataxia (Kneisl et al., 2004). A level above 0.10% without associated behavioral symptoms indicates the presence of tolerance. A BAL greater than 0.10% (or 0.08% in some states) is considered legal intoxication. High tolerance is a sign of physical dependence. Assessing for withdrawal symptoms is important when the BAL is high. Medications given for treatment of withdrawal from alcohol are usually not started until the BAL is below a set norm (usually below 0.10%) unless withdrawal symptoms become severe. BAL may be repeated several times, several hours apart, to determine the body's metabolism of alcohol and when it is safe to give the client medication to minimize the withdrawal symptoms.

Emergency Care for Overdose

The care of a client who has overdosed on any substance is a serious medical emergency. Respiratory depression may require mechanical ventilation. The client may become severely sedated and difficult to arouse. Every effort must be made to keep the client awake; however, stupor and coma may often result. A seizure is another serious complication that requires emergency treatment. If the overdose was intentional, the client must be constantly monitored for further signs of suicidal ideation. Never leave an actively suicidal client alone. Signs of overdose and withdrawal from major substances are summarized in Table 6–2 along with recommended treatments.

Treatment of Withdrawal

All CNS depressants, including alcohol, benzodiazepines, and barbiturates, have a potentially dangerous progression of withdrawal. Alcohol and the entire class of CNS depressants share the same withdrawal syndrome. Early signs of withdrawal appear within a few hours following cessation of the drug, peak after 24 to 48 hours, and then rapidly disappear unless the withdrawal progresses to delirium tremens. Severe withdrawal or delirium tremens is a medical emergency that usually occurs 2 to 5 days following alcohol withdrawal and persists for 2 to 3 days. The symptoms of severe withdrawal include disorientation, paranoid delusions, visual hallucinations, and marked withdrawal symptoms. Seizures may also occur, requiring the use of emergency equipment. Treatment of severe withdrawal during detoxification is mostly symptomatic through acetaminophen, vitamins, and medications to minimize discomfort.

In managing alcohol withdrawal, the goal is to minimize adverse outcomes, such as patient discomfort, seizures, delirium and mortality, and to avoid the adverse effects of withdrawal medications, such as excess sedation (Kasser et al., 2004). Close monitoring is essential to ensure protection of the patient. Critical care monitoring may be indicated to manage alcohol withdrawal delirium, particularly when very high doses of benzodiazepines are needed, or when there are significant concurrent medical conditions. Medications such as benzodiazepines are effectively used to minimize the discomfort associated with alcohol withdrawal and prevent serious adverse effects, in particular seizures (Ntais et al., 2005). A symptom-triggered approach to the administration of benzodiazepines during alcohol withdrawal results in less total medication use and requires a shorter duration of treatment (Bayard et al., 2004). The Clinical Institute Withdrawal Assessment for Alcohol (CIWA-Ar) is currently recommended to manage the symptoms of acute alcohol withdrawal (McKay et al., 2004). In a symptom-triggered regimen, medication is given only when the CIWA-Ar score is higher than 8 points (Bayard et al., 2004).

Two unique medications used to treat alcoholism are disulfiram (Antabuse) and naltrexone (ReVia, Depade). Disulfiram is a form of aversion therapy that prevents the breakdown of alcohol, causing physical illness (intense vomiting) if taken while drinking alcohol. All forms of alcohol, including over-the-counter cough and cold preparations, must be avoided. Naltrexone can help reduce the craving for alcohol by blocking the pathways to the brain that trigger a feeling of pleasure when alcohol and other narcotics are used. Because naltrexone blocks opiate receptors, clients should avoid taking any narcotics, such as codeine, morphine, or heroin, while on naltrexone. Clients should also discontinue all narcotics 7 to 10 days before starting on naltrexone. It is also recommended that clients wear a medical alert bracelet stating they are on naltrexone, in case

TABLE 6–2 Signs and Treatment of Overdose and Withdrawal

	OVERDOSE		WITHDRAWAL	
DRUG	**SIGNS**	**TREATMENT**	**SIGNS**	**TREATMENT**
CNS Depressants Alcohol Barbiturates Benzodiazepines	Cardiovascular or respiratory depression or arrest (mostly with barbiturates) Coma Shock Convulsions Death	*If awake:* Keep awake Induce vomiting Activated charcoal to absorb drug VS q 15 minutes *Coma:* Clear airway, intubate IV fluids Gastric lavage Seizure precautions Possible hemo or peritoneal dialysis Frequent VS Assess for shock and cardiac arrest	Nausea and vomiting Tachycardia Diaphoresis Anxiety or agitation Tremors Marked insomnia Grand mal seizures Delirium (after 5–15 years of heavy use)	Carefully titrated detoxification with similar drug NOTE: Abrupt withdrawal can lead to death.
Stimulants Cocaine-crack Amphetamines	Respiratory distress Ataxia Hyperpyrexia Convulsions Coma Stroke Myocardial infarction (MI) Death	Antipsychotics Management for: 1. Hyperpyrexia 2. Convulsions 3. Respiratory distress 4. Cardiovascular shock 5. Acidify urine (ammonium Cl for amphetamine)	Fatigue Depression Agitation Apathy Anxiety Sleepiness Disorientation Lethargy Craving	Antidepressants (desipramine) Dopamine agonist Bromocriptine
Opiates Heroin Meperidine Morphine Methadone	Pupil dilation due to anoxia Respiratory depression-arrest Coma Shock Convulsions Death	Narcotic antagonist (Narcan) quickly reverses CNS depression	Yawning, insomnia Irritability Rhinorrhea Panic Diaphoresis Cramps Nausea and vomiting Muscle aches Chills and fever Lacrimation Diarrhea	Methadone tapering Clonidine-naltrexone detoxification Buprenorphine substitution
Hallucinogens Lysergic acid diethylamide (LSD)	Psychosis Brain damage Death	Low stimuli with minimal light, sound, activity Have one person "talk down client," reassure Speak slowly and clearly Diazepam or chloral hydrate for anxiety	No pattern of withdrawal	
Phencyclidine piperidine (PCP)	Possible hypertensive crisis Respiratory arrest Hyperthermia Seizures	Acidify urine to help excrete drug (cranberry juice, ascorbic acid); in acute stage: ammonium chloride Minimal stimulis Do NOT attempt to talk down, speak slowly in low voice Diazepam or Haldol		
Inhalants Volatile Solvents such as butane, paint thinner, airplane glue, or nail polish remover	Intoxication: 1. Excitation 2. Drowsiness 3. Disinhibition 4. Staggering 5. Lightheadedness 6. Agitation Side effects: 1. Damage to nervous system 2. Death	Support affected systems	No pattern of withdrawal	
Nitrites	Enhance sexual pleasure	Neurologic symptoms may respond to vitamin B_{12} and folate		
Anesthetics such as nitrous oxide	Giggling, laughter Euphoria	Chronic users may experience polyneuropathy and myelopathy		

of emergency medical treatment. While on disulfiram or naltrexone, psychosocial treatments such as Alcoholics Anonymous meetings, individual counseling, or group therapy are important, because the desire to "take a break" from treatment can overcome the client's motivation to continue taking the medication.

Withdrawal symptoms from opiates and stimulants can be very unpleasant but are generally not life threatening. The client experiencing an acute phase of cocaine withdrawal may become suicidal. Common drugs used in the treatment of substance abuse and withdrawal are presented in Table 6–3.

NURSING CARE

Nurses may interact with clients experiencing substance abuse or substance dependence in a variety of settings. The most common setting, of course, is an alcohol and drug abuse (ADA) treatment program where clients are hospitalized for 20 to 30 days for detoxification and inpatient therapy. These clients may be voluntarily admitted but most are court-ordered to undergo treatment after charges of driving under the influence (DUI) or driving while intoxicated (DWI). Clients with substance abuse or dependence have impaired senses and risk-taking behaviors that lead to injuries from falls and accidents requiring medical attention. Therefore, hospital emergency departments as well as medical and surgical units are places where nurses will frequently encounter these clients. Occupational nurses and community health nurses will also interact with substance-abusing clients in employee assistance programs and community health departments. Urgent care, pain clinics, and ambulatory care centers are other settings in which clients with substance abuse disorders will frequently appear for minor health problems associated with chronic disorders related to substance abuse or dependence.

Health Promotion

Nursing care of the client with substance abuse or dependence is challenging and requires a nonjudgmental atmosphere promoting trust and respect. Health promotion efforts are aimed at preventing drug use among children and adolescents and reducing the risks among adults. Adolescence is the most common phase for the first experience with drugs (Stuart & Laraia, 2005), therefore teenagers are a vulnerable population, often succumbing to peer pressure. Healthy lifestyles, parental support, stress management, good nutrition, and information about ways to steer clear of peer pressure are important topics for the nurse to provide in school programs.

Nurses should provide adults with information on healthy coping mechanisms, relaxation, and stress reduction techniques to decrease the risks of substance abuse. Nurses have a responsibility to educate their clients about the physiologic effects of substances on the body as well as ways to manage stress and anxiety. Nurses must encourage and support periods of abstinence while assisting clients to make major changes in lifestyles, habits, relationships, and coping methods. See Meeting Individualized Needs on page 115 for a discussion of older clients with substance abuse problems.

Assessment

A comprehensive approach to the assessment of substance use is essential to ensure adequate and appropriate intervention. Three important areas to assess are a history of the client's past substance use, medical and psychiatric history, and the presence of psychosocial concerns. Ask questions in a nonthreatening, matter-of-fact manner, phrased as to not imply wrongdoing (Henderson-Martin, 2000). For instance, a nonthreatening question such as "How much alcohol do you

TABLE 6–3 Drugs Used in the Treatment of Substance Withdrawal/Abuse

DRUG	DOSE	PURPOSE
Benzodiazepines		
1. Chlordiazepoxide (Librium)	15–100 mg	Diminishes anxiety and has anticonvulsant qualities to
2. Diazepam (Valium)	4–40 mg	provide safe withdrawal. May be ordered q4h or prn to
3. Oxazepam (Serax)	30–120 mg	manage adverse effects from withdrawal, then dose is
4. Lorazepam (Ativan)	2–6 mg	tapered to zero.
Vitamins		
1. Thiamine (vitamin B$_1$)	100 mg/day	Prevents Wernicke's encephalopathy
2. Folic acid	1 mg/day	Corrects vitamin deficiency caused by heavy long-term alcohol abuse
3. Multivitamins	1 tab/cap daily	
Anticonvulsants		
1. Phenobarbital	30–320 mg	For seizure control and sedation
2. Magnesium sulfate	1 g q6h	Reduces postwithdrawal seizures
Abstinence medications		
1. Disulfiram (Antabuse)	250 mg/day	Prevents breakdown of alcohol
2. Naltrexone (ReVia)	50 mg/day	Diminishes cravings for alcohol and opioids
3. Acamprosate (Campral)	666 mg BID	Decreases alcohol craving
4. Methadone	40 mg/day	Blocks craving for heroin
Antidepressants		
1. Fluoxetine (Prozac)	20–80 mg/day	Enhances and stabilizes mood and diminishes anxiety
2. Sertraline (Zoloft)	50–200 mg/day	

MEETING INDIVIDUALIZED NEEDS Substance Abuse in the Older Adult

Substance abuse in older adults is likely to increase over subsequent decades as baby boomers reach retirement age. The number of older adults in need of substance abuse treatment is estimated to increase from 1.7 million in 2001 to 4.4 million in 2020 (Gfroerer et al., 2003). People of any age can have substance abuse problems, but the consequences in older adults can be more critical. Falls and accidents can rob older adults of their independence, and substance abuse increases the risk of falls by affecting alertness, judgment, coordination, and reaction time. In addition, older adults (especially older women) are more likely than younger people to use prescription or over-the-counter medicines, which can be harmful when mixed with alcohol and/or illicit drugs (Lantz, 2005; Simoni-Wastila & Strickler, 2004). Alcohol and drug abuse can also make certain medical problems hard to diagnose, for example, by dulling a pain sensation that might warn of a heart attack.

Although substance abuse and dependence are not as common in older adults as in younger ones, it is less likely to be recognized. Unfortunately, a substance abuse problem in an older adult can be difficult to detect because many of the symptoms of abuse (e.g., insomnia, depression, loss of memory, anxiety, musculoskeletal pain) may be confused with conditions commonly seen in older clients (Lantz, 2005). Healthcare professionals frequently attribute these symptoms to the aging process and fail to address the misuse and abuse of substances in the elderly. Often, the *symptoms* of substance abuse are treated rather than confronting the abuse itself. Older adults are also at greater risk for numerous physical problems and premature death because alcohol negatively interacts with the natural aging process to increase risks for injuries, hypertension, cardiac dysrhythmias, cancers, gastrointestinal problems, cognitive deficits, bone loss, and emotional challenges, most notably depression (Stevenson, 2005). Because depression and alcohol abuse are the most frequently found disorders in completed suicides, nurses should routinely screen older adults for both substance abuse and mental disorders.

CRITICAL THINKING IN CLIENT CARE

1. You are caring for an 85-year-old man who tells you that since his wife died 6 months ago, he only feels like drinking to dull the pain of her loss. How would you respond?
2. Why do you think nurses and other healthcare professionals often fail to recognize and address substance abuse problems in the older adult?
3. You are caring for an older adult who denies that alcohol has become a serious problem, even though this is the third hospitalization for this client in 6 months due to accidents, falls, and blackouts. What would you do?

BOX 6–4 Examples of Open-Ended Questions for Assessment

- On average, how many days per week do you drink alcohol or use drugs?
- On a typical day when you use drugs or alcohol, how many hits or drinks do you have?
- What is the greatest number of drinks you have had at any one time during the past month?
- What drug(s) did you take before coming to the hospital or clinic?
- How long have you been using the substances?
- How often and how much do you usually use?
- What kinds of problems has substance use caused for you, your family, friends, finances, and health?

---

drink?" is preferable to the judgmental question, "You don't drink too much alcohol, do you?" Open-ended questions that elicit more than a simple yes or no answer help to determine the direction of future counseling. Examples of open-ended questions are provided in Box 6–4. Use therapeutic communication techniques to establish trust prior to the assessment process.

History of Past Substance Use

A thorough history of the client's past substance use is important to ascertain the possibility of tolerance, physical dependence, or withdrawal syndrome. The following questions are helpful in eliciting a pattern of substance use behavior:

- How many substances has the client used simultaneously (**polysubstance abuse** or simultaneous use of many substances) in the past?
- How often, how much, and when did the client first use the substance(s)?
- Is there a history of blackouts, delirium, or seizures?
- Is there a history of withdrawal syndrome, overdoses, and complications from previous substance use?
- Has the client ever been treated in an alcohol or drug abuse clinic?
- Has the client ever been arrested for driving under the influence or charged with any criminal offense while using drugs or alcohol?
- Is there a family history of drug or alcohol use?

Medical and Psychiatric History

The client's medical history is another important area for assessment and should include the existence of any concomitant physical or mental condition (e.g., HIV, hepatitis, cirrhosis, esophageal varices, pancreatitis, gastritis, Wernicke-Korsakoff syndrome, depression, schizophrenia, anxiety, or personality disorder). Ask about prescribed and over-the-counter medications as well as any allergies or sensitivity to drugs. A brief overview of the client's current mental status is also significant.

- Is there a history of abuse (physical or sexual) or family violence?
- Has the client ever tried to commit suicide?
- Is the client currently having suicidal or homicidal ideation?

Psychosocial Issues

Information about the client's level of stress and other psychosocial concerns can help in the assessment of substance use problems.

- Has the client's substance use affected his or her ability to hold a job?
- Has the client's substance use affected relationships with spouse, family, friends, or coworkers?
- How does the client usually cope with stress?
- Does the client have a support system that helps in time of need?
- How does the client spend his or her leisure time?

Screening Tools

Several screening tools such as the Michigan Alcohol Screening Test (MAST) (Pokorny et al., 1972) and the Brief Drug Abuse Screening Test (B-DAST) (Skinner, 1982), may help the nurse determine the degree of severity of substance abuse or dependence (Figure 6–6 ■). These screening tools provide a nonjudgmental, brief, and easy method to ascertain patterns of substance abuse behaviors.

- *Michigan Alcohol Screening Test (MAST) Brief Version* is a 10-question, dichotomous, self-administered questionnaire that takes 10 to 15 minutes to complete. An answer of yes to 3 or more questions indicates a potentially dangerous pattern of alcohol abuse.
- *The CAGE questionnaire* (Ewing, 1984), is more useful when the client may not recognize he or she has an alcohol problem or is uncomfortable acknowledging it. This questionnaire is designed to be a self-report of drinking behavior or may be administered by a professional. One affirmative response indicates the need for further discussion and follow-up. Two or more yes answers signify a problem with alcohol that may require treatment.
  - Have you ever felt you should *Cut* down on your drinking?
  - Have people *Annoyed* you by criticizing your drinking?
  - Have you ever felt bad or *Guilty* about your drinking?
  - Have you ever had a drink first thing in the morning (an "*Eye-opener*") to steady your nerves or to get rid of a hangover?

Brief MAST Scoring Yes to 3 or more indicates alcoholism

1. Do you feel you are a normal drinker?
2. Do friends or relatives think you are a normal drinker?
3. Have you ever attended a meeting of Alcoholics Anonymous?
4. Have you ever gotten in trouble at work because of drinking?
5. Have you ever lost friends or girlfriends/boyfriends because of drinking?
6. Have you ever neglected your obligations, your family, or your work for 2 or more days in a row because of your drinking?
7. Have you ever had delirium tremens (DTs), severe shaking, or heard voices or seen things that were not there after heavy drinking?
8. Have you ever gone to anyone for help about your drinking?
9. Have you ever been in a hospital because of your drinking?
10. Have you ever been arrested for drunken driving or other drunken behavior?

B-DAST The following questions concern information about your involvement with drugs *not including alcoholic beverages* during the past 12 months.

In the statements, "drug abuse" refers to (1) the use of prescribed or OTC drugs in excess of the directions and (2) any nonmedical use of drugs. The various classes of drugs may include cannabis, solvents, antianxiety drugs, sedative-hypnotics, cocaine, stimulants, hallucinogens, and narcotics. Remember *do not include alcoholic beverages*.

Have you used drugs other than those required for medical purposes?	Yes ___	No ___
Do you abuse more than one drug at a time?	Yes ___	No ___
Are you always able to stop using drugs when you want to?	Yes ___	No ___
Have you had "blackouts" or "flashbacks" as a result of drug use?	Yes ___	No ___
Do you ever feel bad about your drug abuse?	Yes ___	No ___
Does your spouse (or parents) ever complain about your involvement with drugs?	Yes ___	No ___
Have you neglected your family because of your use of drugs?	Yes ___	No ___
Have you engaged in illegal activities in order to obtain drugs?	Yes ___	No ___
Have you ever experienced withdrawal symptoms (felt sick) when you stopped taking drugs?	Yes ___	No ___
Have you had medical problems as a result of your drug use (e.g., memory loss, hepatitis, convulsions, bleeding, etc.)?	Yes ___	No ___

Scoring: one positive response warrants further evaluation

Figure 6–6 ■ Screening tools for alcohol and drug abuse.

Source: Adapted from "The Brief MAST: A Shortened Version of the Michigan Alcohol Screening Test" by A. D. Porkorny, B. A. Miller, and H. B. Kaplan, 1972, *American Journal of Psychiatry,* 129, pp. 342–345. Copyright 1972 by the American Psychiatric Association; and *Brief Drug Abuse Screening Test* (B-DAST) (p. 363) by H. A. Skinner, 1982, Langford Lance, England: Elsevier Science LTd. Copyright 1982. Both reprinted by permission.

- *Brief Drug Abuse Screening Test (B-DAST)* is a yes/no self-administered questionnaire that is useful in identifying people who are possibly addicted to drugs other than alcohol. A positive response to one or more questions suggests significant drug abuse problems and warrants further evaluation. Because self-report tools are not always answered truthfully, all clients who screen positive for drug addiction should be evaluated according to other diagnostic criteria.

Withdrawal Assessment Tools

Nurses working in medical-surgical units, psychiatric units, and special substance abuse units routinely care for patients experiencing acute alcohol or opiate withdrawal. Several assessment tools are available to determine the severity of withdrawal symptoms and indicate the need for pharmacologic treatment to manage withdrawal symptoms. Examples of withdrawal assessment tools are the revised *Clinical Institute Withdrawal Assessment of Alcohol–Revised (CIWA-Ar)* (Sullivan et al., 1989) and the *Clinical Opiate Withdrawal Scale (COWS)* (Wesson & Ling, 2003).

- The *Clinical Institute Withdrawal Assessment of Alcohol–Revised (CIWA-Ar)* (Sullivan et al., 1989) (Figure 6–7 ■) is used widely in clinical and research settings for initial assessment and ongoing monitoring of alcohol withdrawal signs and symptoms. The CIWA-Ar scale is a validated 10-item assessment tool that can be used to monitor and medicate patients going through alcohol withdrawal. The CIWA-Ar assesses for several alcohol withdrawal symptoms (e.g., high blood pressure, rapid pulse and respirations, tremors, insomnia, irritability, sweating, and convulsions) and results in a score that is used to direct the administration of benzodiazepines or other drugs to relieve associated symptoms of withdrawal and prevent seizures. A score of 8 points or fewer corresponds to mild withdrawal symptoms. Scores of 9 to 15 points indicate moderate withdrawal, whereas a score of 15 or greater denotes severe withdrawal and an increased risk of delirium tremens and seizures.
- *Clinical Opiate Withdrawal Scale (COWS)* (Wesson & Ling, 2003) rates 11 common signs or symptoms of opiate withdrawal. The summed total score of the 11 items can be used to assess the intensity of opiate withdrawal and determine the extent of a patient's physical dependence on opioids. A score of less than 12 on the COWS indicates mild or no opiate withdrawal symptoms, whereas a score of 13 or more indicates moderate to severe withdrawal symptoms.

Nursing Diagnoses and Interventions

The primary nursing diagnoses and interventions for clients with substance abuse problems are listed below. Implications for nursing care in acute and home care settings are combined in this discussion. See the Nursing Care Plan on page 119 for more on the client experiencing withdrawal from alcohol.

Risk for Injury and Risk for Violence

- Assess client's level of disorientation to determine specific risks to safety. *Knowledge of the client's level of cognitive functioning is essential to the development of an appropriate plan of care.*

- Obtain a drug history as well as urine and blood samples for laboratory analysis of substance content. *Subjective history is often not accurate and knowledge regarding substance use is important for accurate assessment.*
- Place client in a quiet, private room to decrease excessive stimuli, but do not leave client alone if excessive hyperactivity or suicidal ideation is present. *Excessive stimuli increase client's agitation.*
- Frequently orient client to reality and the environment, ensuring that potentially harmful objects are stored outside the client's access. *Client may harm self or others if disoriented and confused.*
- Monitor vital signs every 15 minutes until stable and assess for signs of intoxication or withdrawal. *The most reliable information about withdrawal symptoms are vital signs; they provide information about the need for medication during detoxification.*

Ineffective Denial

- Be genuine, honest, and respectful of the client. Keep all promises and convey an attitude of acceptance of the client. *The development of a nonjudgmental, therapeutic nurse–client relationship is essential to gain the client's trust.*
- Identify maladaptive behaviors or situations that have occurred in client's life and discuss how the use of substances may have been a contributing factor. *The first step in combating denial is for the client to recognize the relationship between substance use and personal problems.*
- Do not accept the use of defense mechanisms such as rationalization or projection as the client attempts to blame others or make excuses for his or her behavior. Use confrontation with caring to avoid placing the client on the defensive. *Confrontation interferes with the client's ability to use denial.*
- Encourage client participation in therapeutic group activities such as co-occurring disorder or Alcoholics Anonymous (AA) meetings with other people who are experiencing or have experienced similar problems. *Peer feedback is often more accepted than feedback from authority figures.*

Ineffective Coping

- Establish a trusting relationship. *Trust is essential to the nurse–client relationship.*
- Set limits on manipulative behavior and maintain consistency in responses. *Client is unable to set own limits and must begin to accept responsibility without being manipulative.*
- Encourage client to verbalize feelings, fears, or anxieties. Use attentive listening and validate client's feelings with observations or statements that acknowledge feelings. *Verbalization of feelings helps client to develop insight into behaviors and long-standing problems.*
- Explore methods of dealing with stressful situations other than resorting to substance use. Provide encouragement for changing to a healthier lifestyle. Teach healthy coping mechanisms (e.g., physical exercise, progressive muscle relaxation, deep breathing exercises, meditation, and imagery). *Client needs knowledge about how to adapt to stress without resorting to drug use.*

Clinical Institute Withdrawal Assessment of Alcohol Scale, Revised (CIWA-Ar)

Patient:_____ Date: _____ Time: _____ (24 hour clock, midnight = 00:00)

Pulse or heart rate, taken for one minute:_____ Blood pressure:_____

NAUSEA AND VOMITING -- Ask "Do you feel sick to your stomach? Have you vomited?" Observation.
0 no nausea and no vomiting
1 mild nausea with no vomiting
2
3
4 intermittent nausea with dry heaves
5
6
7 constant nausea, frequent dry heaves and vomiting

TREMOR -- Arms extended and fingers spread apart. Observation.
0 no tremor
1 not visible, but can be felt fingertip to fingertip
2
3
4 moderate, with patient's arms extended
5
6
7 severe, even with arms not extended

PAROXYSMAL SWEATS -- Observation.
0 no sweat visible
1 barely perceptible sweating, palms moist
2
3
4 beads of sweat obvious on forehead
5
6
7 drenching sweats

ANXIETY -- Ask "Do you feel nervous?" Observation.
0 no anxiety, at ease
1 mild anxious
2
3
4 moderately anxious, or guarded, so anxiety is inferred
5
6
7 equivalent to acute panic states as seen in severe delirium or acute schizophrenic reactions

AGITATION -- Observation.
0 normal activity
1 somewhat more than normal activity
2
3
4 moderately fidgety and restless
5
6
7 paces back and forth during most of the interview, or constantly thrashes about

TACTILE DISTURBANCES -- Ask "Have you any itching, pins and needles sensations, any burning, any numbness, or do you feel bugs crawling on or under your skin?" Observation.
0 none
1 very mild itching, pins and needles, burning or numbness
2 mild itching, pins and needles, burning or numbness
3 moderate itching, pins and needles, burning or numbness
4 moderately severe hallucinations
5 severe hallucinations
6 extremely severe hallucinations
7 continuous hallucinations

AUDITORY DISTURBANCES -- Ask "Are you more aware of sounds around you? Are they harsh? Do they frighten you? Are you hearing anything that is disturbing to you? Are you hearing things you know are not there?" Observation.
0 not present
1 very mild harshness or ability to frighten
2 mild harshness or ability to frighten
3 moderate harshness or ability to frighten
4 moderately severe hallucinations
5 severe hallucinations
6 extremely severe hallucinations
7 continuous hallucinations

VISUAL DISTURBANCES -- Ask "Does the light appear to be too bright? Is its color different? Does it hurt your eyes? Are you seeing anything that is disturbing to you? Are you seeing things you know are not there?" Observation.
0 not present
1 very mild sensitivity
2 mild sensitivity
3 moderate sensitivity
4 moderately severe hallucinations
5 severe hallucinations
6 extremely severe hallucinations
7 continuous hallucinations

HEADACHE, FULLNESS IN HEAD -- Ask "Does your head feel different? Does it feel like there is a band around your head?" Do not rate for dizziness or lightheadedness. Otherwise, rate severity.
0 not present
1 very mild
2 mild
3 moderate
4 moderately severe
5 severe
6 very severe
7 extremely severe

ORIENTATION AND CLOUDING OF SENSORIUM -- Ask "What day is this? Where are you? Who am I?"
0 oriented and can do serial additions
1 cannot do serial additions or is uncertain about date
2 disoriented for date by no more than 2 calendar days
3 disoriented for date by more than 2 calendar days
4 disoriented for place/or person

Total **CIWA-Ar** Score _____
Rater's Initials _____
Maximum Possible Score 67

The CIWA-Ar is not copyrighted and may be reproduced freely. This assessment for monitoring withdrawal symptoms requires approximately 5 minutes to administer. The maximum score is 67 (see instrument). Patients scoring less than 10 do not usually need additional medication for withdrawal.

Figure 6–7 ■ Assessment tool for alcohol withdrawal.

Source: From "The Revised Clinical Institute Withdrawal Assessment for Alcohol scale (CIWA-Ar)" by J. T. Sullivan, K. Sykora, J. Schneiderman, C. A. Naranjo, & E. M. Sellers, 1989, *British Journal of Addictions,* 84, 1353–1357. Reprinted by permission.

NURSING CARE PLAN   A Client Experiencing Withdrawal from Alcohol

George Russell, age 58, fell at home and broke his arm. His wife took him to the ER and an open reduction internal fixation (ORIF) of his right wrist was performed under general anesthetic in the operating room. He was admitted to the postoperative unit for observation following surgery because he required large amounts of anesthesia during the procedure.

Mr. Russell has a ruddy complexion and looks older than his stated age. He discloses that he was laid off from his factory job 2 years ago and has been working odd jobs until last week when he was hired by a local assembly plant. His father was a recovering alcoholic and his 30-year-old son has been treated for alcohol abuse in the past. Mr. Russell states that he knows alcoholism runs in the family, but he feels that he has his drinking under control. However, he cannot remember the events that led up to his fall and how he might have broken his arm.

ASSESSMENT

During the nursing assessment, Mr. Russell is hesitant to provide information and refuses to make eye contact. Prior to his operation, a BAL was drawn because the ER nurse detected alcohol on his breath. His BAL was 0.40% which is five times the legal limit for intoxication in many states. His vital signs are within the upper limits of normal, but he is confused and disoriented with slurred speech and a slight tremor of the hands. He is 6 feet tall and weighs 140 pounds. His total albumin is 2.9 mg and he has elevated liver enzymes. His wife states that he rarely eats the meals she prepares because he is usually drinking and has no appetite for food.

DIAGNOSES

- *Ineffective Individual Coping* related to possible hereditary factor and personal vulnerability
- *Risk for Injury* related to aggressive behavior, unsteady gait, and impaired motor responses
- *Ineffective Denial* related to inability to recognize maladaptive behaviors caused by substance use
- *Imbalanced Nutrition: Less than Body Requirements* related to anorexia manifested by decreased weight and low serum protein levels

EXPECTED OUTCOMES

- Client will express his true feelings associated with using alcohol as a method of coping with stressful situations.
- Client will identify three adaptive coping mechanisms he can use as alternatives to alcohol in response to stress.
- Client will verbalize the negative effects of alcohol and agree to seek professional help with his drinking.

- Client will be free of injury as evidenced by steady gait and absence of subsequent falls.
- Client will gain 1 lb (0.45 kg) per week without evidence of increased fluid retention. Serum albumin levels will return to normal range.

PLANNING AND IMPLEMENTATION

- Establish trusting relationship with client and spend time with him discussing his feelings, fears, and anxieties.
- Consult with a physician regarding a schedule for medications during detoxification and observe for signs of withdrawal syndrome.
- Explain the effects of alcohol abuse on the body and emphasize that prognosis is closely associated with abstinence.
- Teach a relaxation technique that the client feels is useful.
- Provide community resource information about self-help groups and, if client is receptive, a list of meeting times and phone numbers.
- Consult with a dietitian to determine number of calories needed to provide adequate nutrition and realistic weight gain. Document intake, output, and calorie count.
- Consult with physician to begin vitamin B_1 (thiamine) and dietary supplements.

EVALUATION

Mr. Russell was discharged from the postoperative unit without complications. He successfully underwent detoxification and contacted the Employee Assistance Program at his new place of employment. He was on medical leave while his arm completely healed and now attends Alcoholics Anonymous meetings 5 days a week. He reports that he enjoys taking long walks with his wife in the warm weather and that his appetite has returned. He has gained 10 pounds in the past 6 weeks and feels physically better than he has in many years.

CRITICAL THINKING IN THE NURSING PROCESS

1. Explain why it would be important to include questions about Mr. Russell's medication history and his use of other medications during the initial nursing assessment.
2. Mr. Russell asks you to explain the risks of taking disulfiram (Antabuse). What should you tell him?
3. Develop a care plan for Mr. Russell for the nursing diagnosis of *Imbalanced Nutrition: Less than Body Requirements*. Why is this necessary?

See Evaluating Your Response in Appendix C.

Imbalanced Nutrition: Less than Body Requirements

- Administer vitamins and dietary supplements as ordered by physician. *Vitamin B_1 is necessary to prevent complications from chronic alcoholism such as Wernicke's syndrome.*
- Monitor lab work (e.g., total albumin, complete blood count, urinalysis, electrolytes, and liver enzymes) and report significant changes to physician. *Objective laboratory tests provide necessary information to determine the extent of malnourishment.*

- Collaborate with dietitian to determine number of calories needed to provide adequate nutrition and realistic weight gain. Document intake, output, and calorie count. Weigh daily if condition warrants. *Weight loss or gain is important assessment information so that an appropriate plan of care can be developed.*
- Teach the importance of adequate nutrition by explaining the Food Guide Pyramid (see Chapter 2) and relating the physical effects of malnutrition on body systems. *Client may have inadequate knowledge of proper nutritional habits.*

Chronic Low or Situational Low Self-Esteem

- Spend time with client and convey an attitude of acceptance. Encourage client to accept responsibility for own behaviors and feelings. *An attitude of acceptance enhances self-worth.*
- Encourage client to focus on strengths and accomplishments rather than weaknesses and failures. *Minimize attention to negative ruminations.*
- Encourage participation in therapeutic group activities. Offer recognition and positive feedback for actual achievements. *Success and recognition increase self-esteem.*
- Teach assertiveness techniques and effective communication techniques such as the use of "I feel" rather than "You make me feel" statements. *Previous patterns of communication may have been aggressive and accusatory, causing barriers to interpersonal relationships.*

Deficient Knowledge

- Assess client's level of knowledge and readiness to learn the effects of drugs and alcohol on the body. *Baseline assessment is required to develop appropriate teaching material.*
- Develop teaching plan that includes measurable objectives. Include significant others, if possible. *Lifestyle changes often affect all family members.*
- Begin with simple concepts and progress to more complex issues. Use interactive teaching strategies and written materials appropriate to the client's educational level. Include information on physiologic effects of substances, the propensity for physical and psychologic dependence, and the risks to a fetus if the client is pregnant. *Active participation and handouts enhance retention of important concepts.*

Disturbed Sensory Perceptions

- Observe for withdrawal symptoms. Monitor vital signs. Provide adequate nutrition and hydration. Place on seizure precautions. *These actions provide supportive physical care during detoxification.*
- Assess level of orientation frequently. Orient and reassure client of safety in presence of hallucinations, delusions, or illusions. *Client may be frightened.*
- Explain all interventions before approaching client. Avoid loud noises and talk softly to client. Decrease external stimuli by dimming lights. *Excessive stimuli increase agitation.*
- Administer prn medications according to detoxification schedule. *Benzodiazepines help to minimize the discomfort of withdrawal symptoms.*

Disturbed Thought Processes

- Give positive reinforcement when thinking and behavior are appropriate or when client recognizes that delusions are not based in reality. *Drugs and alcohol can interfere with client's perception of reality.*
- Use simple, step-by-step instructions and face-to-face interaction when communicating with client. *Client may be confused or disoriented.*
- Express reasonable doubt if client relays suspicious or paranoid beliefs. Reinforce accurate perception of people or situations. *It is important to communicate that you do not share that false belief as reality.*
- Do not argue with delusions or hallucinations. Convey acceptance that the client believes a situation to be true, but that the nurse does not see or hear what is not there. *Arguing with the client or denying the belief serves no useful purpose, because delusions are not eliminated.*
- Talk to client about real events and real people. Respond to feelings and reassure client that he or she is safe from harm. *Discussions that focus on the delusions may aggravate the condition. Verbalization of feelings in a nonthreatening environment may help the client develop insight.*

Using NANDA, NIC, and NOC

Charts 6–1, 6–2, and 6–3 show links between NANDA, NIC, and NOC when caring for the client with a substance abuse problem.

Community-Based Care

The community provides many options for treating substance abuse including a mixture of individual, group, and family therapy. Medical detoxification can occur in hospitals, psychiatric units, special substance abuse units, methadone clinics, or outpatient settings. Less restrictive environments include residential rehabilitation programs, halfway houses, and partial hospitalization programs. These programs provide structured environments for the recovering substance abuser while maintaining a viable presence in the community. In addition, clients

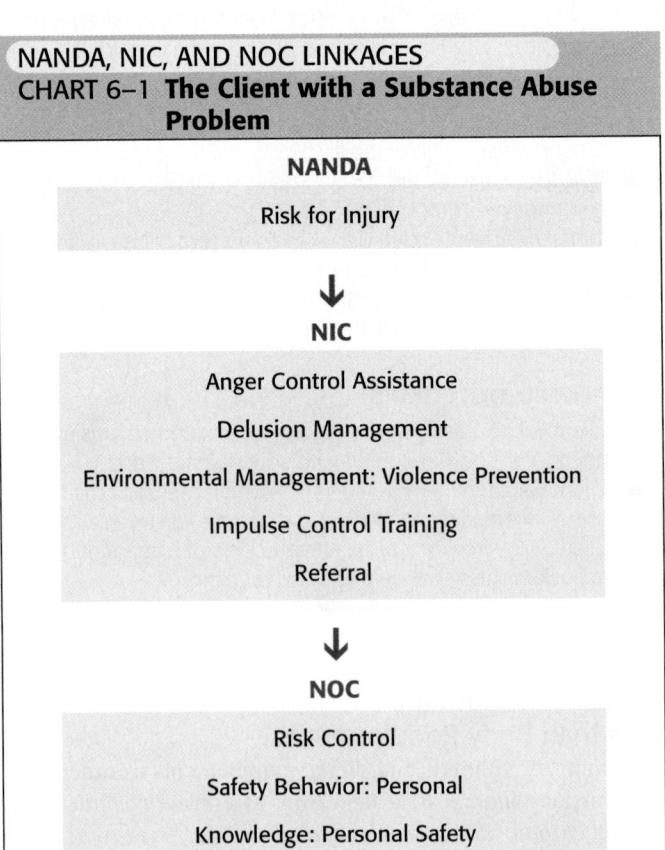

NANDA, NIC, AND NOC LINKAGES
CHART 6–1 The Client with a Substance Abuse Problem

NANDA

Risk for Injury

↓

NIC

Anger Control Assistance

Delusion Management

Environmental Management: Violence Prevention

Impulse Control Training

Referral

↓

NOC

Risk Control

Safety Behavior: Personal

Knowledge: Personal Safety

Data from *NANDA's Nursing Diagnoses: Definitions & classification 2005–2006* by NANDA International (2003), Philadelphia; *Nursing Interventions Classification (NIC)* (4th ed.) by J. M. Dochterman & G. M. Bulechek (2004), St. Louis, MO: Mosby; and *Nursing Outcomes Classification (NOC)* (3rd ed.) by S. Moorhead, M. Johnson, and M. Maas (2004), St. Louis, MO: Mosby.

can obtain vocational counseling, become involved in self-help groups such as Alcoholics Anonymous or Narcotics Anonymous, and receive drug and health education.

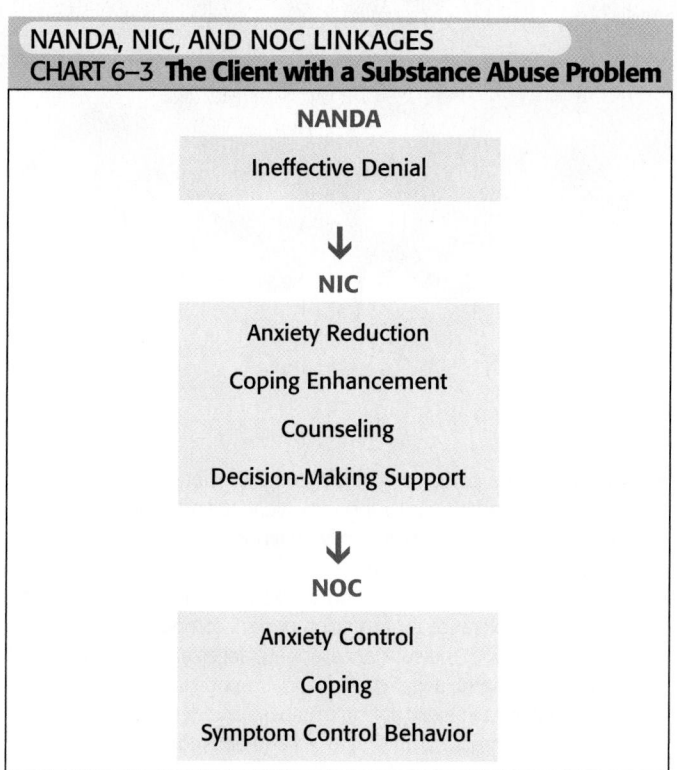

NANDA, NIC, AND NOC LINKAGES
CHART 6–2 The Client with a Substance Abuse Problem

NANDA

Imbalanced Nutrition: Less than Body Requirements

↓

NIC

Nutritional Counseling

Nutritional Monitoring

Weight Gain Assistance

↓

NOC

Nutritional Status

Data from *NANDA's Nursing Diagnoses: Definitions & classification 2005–2006* by NANDA International (2003), Philadelphia; *Nursing Interventions Classification (NIC)* (4th ed.) by J. M. Dochterman & G. M. Bulechek (2004), St. Louis, MO: Mosby; and *Nursing Outcomes Classification (NOC)* (3rd ed.) by S. Moorhead, M. Johnson, and M. Maas (2004), St. Louis, MO: Mosby.

NANDA, NIC, AND NOC LINKAGES
CHART 6–3 The Client with a Substance Abuse Problem

NANDA

Ineffective Denial

↓

NIC

Anxiety Reduction

Coping Enhancement

Counseling

Decision-Making Support

↓

NOC

Anxiety Control

Coping

Symptom Control Behavior

Data from *NANDA's Nursing Diagnoses: Definitions & classification 2005–2006* by NANDA International (2003), Philadelphia; *Nursing Interventions Classification (NIC)* (4th ed.) by J. M. Dochterman & G. M. Bulechek (2004), St. Louis, MO: Mosby; and *Nursing Outcomes Classification (NOC)* (3rd ed.) by S. Moorhead, M. Johnson, and M. Maas (2004), St. Louis, MO: Mosby.

Teaching the client and family includes:
- The negative effects of substance abuse including physical and psychologic complications of substance abuse
- The signs of relapse and the importance of after-care programs and self-help groups to prevent relapse
- Information about specific medications that help to reduce the craving for alcohol (naltrexone [ReVia]) and maintain abstinence (disulfiram [Antabuse]), including the potential side effects, possible drug interactions, and any special precautions to be taken (e.g., avoiding over-the-counter medications such as cough syrup that may have alcohol content)
- Ways to manage stress including techniques such as progressive muscle relaxation, abdominal breathing techniques, imagery, meditation, and effective coping skills.

In addition, suggest the following resources:
- Alcoholics Anonymous, Narcotics Anonymous, and other self-help groups
- Employee assistance programs
- Individual, group, and/or family counseling
- Community rehabilitation programs
- National Alliance for the Mentally Ill.

PRACTICE ALERT

Clients are at highest risk for relapse within the first few months after stopping the abused substance. An acronym that can assist the client in recognizing behaviors that lead to relapse is **HALT: h**ungry, **a**ngry, **l**onely, and **t**ired. Nurses should emphasize the importance of a balanced diet, adequate sleep, healthy recreation activities, and a caring support system to prevent relapse.

IMPAIRED NURSES

Healthcare providers are as susceptible as anyone else to developing substance abuse. By the very nature of their roles, dentists, pharmacists, physicians, and nurses are in frequent contact with drugs and are at high risk for substance abuse problems. One study exploring family history of alcohol and drug use in healthcare professionals found that nurses reported a higher prevalence of alcoholism in their families than dentists and physicians (Kenna & Wood, 2005). However, no significant differences were found in healthcare professionals' drinking levels. As a rule, nurses experience many pressures in the workplace and have easy access to drugs. Trinkoff and colleagues (2000) found that nurses reported higher substance use if they had easy access to prescription drugs, increased role strain, and close social connections with substance abusers. Two factors, stronger religious practices and treatment for depressive symptoms, were associated with reduced substance abuse. Substance abuse and dependence can lead to impaired professional practice; therefore, nurses must act responsibly when coworkers display signs of substance abuse. Healthcare professionals have a higher risk for opiate abuse than other professionals due to the high accessibility of opiates in their line of work (Trinkoff et al., 2000). If colleagues are showing signs of a substance abuse problem, information about impaired nurse programs is available through state boards of nursing to help individual nurses. Warning signs of impaired nurses in the workplace are listed in Table 6–4.

TABLE 6–4 Warning Signs of Impaired Nurses in the Workplace

AT-RISK SITUATIONS	OBSERVABLE WARNING SIGNS
Easy access to prescription drugs	Inaccurate narcotic counts or frequent missing drugs Clients complain of ineffective pain control, deny receiving pain meds Excessive "wasting" of drugs Volunteering to give medications to clients Frequent trips to the bathroom
Role strain	Frequent tardiness or absenteeism, especially before and after scheduled days off Haphazard, shoddy charting Client care judgment errors Unorganized, erratic behavior; unkempt appearance
Depression	Irritability, unable to focus or concentrate Abrupt mood swings Isolating self, taking long breaks Apathetic, depressed, lethargic Unexplained absences from assigned unit
Signs of alcohol or drug use	Smell of alcohol on breath Excessive use of perfumes, mouthwash, or mints Slurred speech, flushed face, reddened eyes, unsteady gait Wearing long sleeves in hot weather to cover up arms
Signs of withdrawal	Tremors, restlessness, sweating Watery eyes, runny nose, stomachaches

EXPLORE MediaLink

Prentice Hall Nursing MediaLink DVD-ROM
Audio Glossary
NCLEX-RN® Review

Animation
Cocaine

COMPANION WEBSITE www.prenhall.com/lemone
Audio Glossary
NCLEX-RN® Review
Care Plan Activities
  Alcohol Withdrawal
  Tobacco Cessation
Case Study: Alcohol Withdrawal
MediaLink Applications
Links to Resources

CHAPTER HIGHLIGHTS

■ Substance abuse is the unsanctioned use of any chemical despite adverse effects on the individual's physical, psychological, interpersonal, or social health.

■ Substance dependence occurs when control over the chemical substance is lost and the individual must use increasing amounts to produce the desired effect (tolerance) and must use the substance to avoid or relieve uncomfortable symptoms (withdrawal).

■ Combinations of genetic, biologic, psychological, and sociocultural factors contribute to substance abuse or dependence. Addictive behavior has been linked to biochemical changes in dopamine and serotonin brain levels as well as heredity, ethnic differences, and peer pressure. Thorough assessment of individual risk factors is necessary to plan and deliver appropriate nursing interventions.

■ Adolescents are particularly influenced by society and peers to use substances; predominantly tobacco, alcohol, and illicit drugs. A positive ethnic identity and family environment act as "protective" deterrents for substance use.

■ Substance abusers have common characteristics including risk-taking behavior, low tolerance for frustration or pain, compulsive preoccupation with the substance, anxiety, anger, and low self-esteem. Stress management, anger control, social support, and counseling are helpful strategies to avoid substance abuse and dependence.

■ Alcohol is the most commonly used and abused substance; however, polysubstance abuse is frequent in many individuals. Substances such as marijuana, cocaine, and methamphetamine are often used in conjunction with alcohol. Prescription anti-anxiety agents have been abused in the past; and there is a growing trend in prescription narcotic analgesic abuse.

- Nursing care of clients experiencing substance abuse problems includes health promotion efforts to prevent substance abuse: comprehensive physical, spiritual, and psychosocial assessment; and interventions for the human responses of ineffective coping and denial, imbalanced nutrition, low self-esteem, disturbed thought processes, disturbed sensory perception, and risk for injury or violence.

- Nurses are susceptible to substance abuse due to pressures in the workplace and easy access to drugs. Nurses need to assess their response to stress and seek early treatment for depressive symptoms to avoid impaired professional practice.

TEST YOURSELF NCLEX-RN® REVIEW

1 What is the minimum level of alcohol in the blood for an individual to be considered intoxicated?
1. 0.05%
2. 0.08%
3. 0.50%
4. 1.00%

2 Which of the following questions is *most* appropriate when interviewing the client who is suspected of alcohol abuse problems?
1. "Typically, how many days per week do you drink alcoholic beverages?"
2. "Have you been drinking lately?"
3. "You don't drink much alcohol, do you?"
4. "Has your drinking caused a lot of problems between you and your spouse?"

3 What is the rationale behind ordering thiamine (vitamin B$_1$) for a person with a history of chronic alcoholism?
1. to prevent acute pancreatitis
2. to prevent cirrhosis of the liver
3. to prevent hepatic encephalopathy
4. to prevent Wernicke's encephalopathy

4 Which of the following substances present the highest medical danger during withdrawal?
1. CNS stimulants and amphetamines
2. opiates and marijuana
3. alcohol and CNS depressants
4. amphetamines and hallucinogens

5 What is the rationale for prescribing disulfiram (Anatabuse) for a person who suffers from alcohol abuse?
1. to decrease the discomfort of withdrawal symptoms
2. to decrease the pleasant, reinforcing effects of alcohol
3. to prevent the breakdown of alcohol, thereby inhibiting impulsive drinking
4. to block the signs and symptoms of alcohol withdrawal

6 Which is NOT a warning sign of substance abuse in the nurse?
1. impaired motor coordination, slurred speech, bloodshot eyes
2. unkempt appearance; disorganized, erratic behavior
3. clients consistently report effective pain control
4. frequent absenteeism or tardiness, unexplained absences from the unit

7 Which of the following statements is FALSE?
1. Smoking is the leading known cause of preventable death and disease among women.
2. The smoking rates for women have steadily declined since the 1950s.
3. Women who smoke during pregnancy have a higher risk for spontaneous abortions.
4. Women who smoke have an increased risk for stroke and heart disease.

8 Which statement by the client illustrates an understanding of your teaching regarding naltrexone (ReVia)?
1. "I should read labels of over-the-counter cold medicines to make sure they don't have alcohol."
2. "I should stop taking all pain medications before starting on naltrexone."
3. "I should go to my Narcotics Anonymous meetings for 1 month, then I can stop going."
4. "I should wear a medical alert bracelet that states I'm taking naltrexone."

9 Which of the following is a realistic goal for a client with substance abuse?
1. The client will identify ways to deal with stressful situations instead of resorting to substance use.
2. The client will refrain from using substances until craving for the substance has been eliminated.
3. The client will focus on negative aspects of past behaviors and interpersonal relationships.
4. The client will be able to use alcohol or drugs in moderation.

10 An appropriate nursing diagnosis for a client with substance abuse problems is:
1. *Imbalanced Nutrition: Greater than Body Requirements* related to food intake in excess of energy expenditure
2. *Excess Fluid Volume* related to increased intake of vitamins and dietary supplements
3. *Ineffective Denial* related to inability to recognize maladaptive behaviors related to substance use
4. *Disturbed Thought Processes* related to infectious process and pain

See Test Yourself answers in Appendix C.

BIBLIOGRAPHY

AIDS Alert. (2005). Studies show link between meth use and HIV infections: Resurgence of STDs tied to drug's use. *AIDS Alert, 20*(9), 97, 99–101.

American Psychiatric Association (2000). *Diagnostic and statistical manual of mental disorders* (4th ed., text revision). Washington, DC: Autuor.

Bayard, M., McIntyre, J., Hill, K., & Woodside J. (2004). Alcohol withdrawal syndrome. *American Family Physician, 69*(6), 1443–1450.

Bernstein, G. A., Carroll, M. E., Thuras, P. D., Cosgrove, K. P., & Roth, M. E. (2002). Caffeine dependence in teenagers. *Drug and Alcohol Dependence, 55*(1), 1–6.

Bersamin, M., Paschall, M. F., & Flewelling, R. L. (2005). Ethnic differences in relationships between risk factors and adolescent binge drinking: a national study. *Prevention Science, 6*(2), 127–137.

Brown, A. H., Domier, C. P., & Rawson, R. A. (2005). Stimulants, sex, and gender. *Sexual Addiction & Compulsivity, 12*(2–3), 169–180.

Buchanan, D., Tooze, J. A., Shaw, S., Kinzly, M., Heimer, R., & Singer, M. (2006). Demographic, HIV risk behavior, and health status characteristics of "crack" cocaine injectors compared to other injection drug users in three New England cities. *Drug and Alcohol Dependence, 81*(3), 221–229.

Compton, W. M., & Volkow, N. D. (2006). Major increases in opioid analgesic abuse in the United States: Concerns and strategies. *Drug and Alcohol Dependence, 81*(2), 103–107.

Conner, B. T., Noble, E. P., Berman, S. M., Ozkaragoz, T., Ritchie, T., Antolin, T., et al. (2005). DRD2 genotypes and substance use in adolescent children of alcoholics. *Drug and Alcohol Dependence, 79*(3), 379–387.

Cook, T. A., Luczak, S. E., Shea, S. H., Ehlers, C. L., Carr, L. G., & Wall, T. L. (2005). Associations of ALDH2 and ADH1B genotypes with response to alcohol in Asian Americans. *Journal of Studies on Alcohol, 66*(2), 196–204.

Czermak, C., Lehofer, M., Wagner, E. M., Prietl, B., Lemonis, L., Rohrhofer, A., et al. (2004). Reduced dopamine D_4 receptor mRNA expression in lymphocytes of long-term abstinent alcohol and heroin addicts. *Addiction, 99*(2), 251–257.

Dochterman, J. M., & Bulechek, G. M. (Eds.). (2004). *Nursing interventions classification (NIC)* (4th ed.). St. Louis, MO: Mosby.

Ebberhart, N. C., Luczak, S. E., Avenecy, N., & Wall, T. L. (2003). Family history of alcohol dependence in Asian Americans. *Journal of Psychoactive Drugs, 35*(3), 375–377.

Ewing, J. A. (1984). Detecting alcoholism: The CAGE questionnaire. *Journal of the American Medical Association, 252*(14), 1905–1907.

Ferdinand, R. F., Sondeijker, F., van der Ende, J., Selten, J., Huizink, A., & Verhulst, F. C. (2005). Cannabis use predicts future psychotic symptoms, and vice versa. *Addiction, 100*(5), 612–618.

Gfroerer, J., Penne, M., Pemberton, M., & Folsom, R. (2003). Substance abuse treatment need among older adults in 2020: The impact of the aging baby-boom cohort. *Drug and Alcohol Dependence, 69*(2), 127–135.

Gilman, S. E., & Abraham, H. D. (2001). A longitudinal study of the order of onset of alcohol dependence and major depression. *Drug & Alcohol Dependence, 63*(3), 277–286.

Guardia, J., Catafau, A. M., Battle, F., Martin, J. C., Segura, L., Gonzalvo, B., et al. (2000). Striatal dopaminergic D_2 receptor density measured by [123I] iodobenzamide SPECT in the prediction of treatment outcome of alcohol-dependent patients. *American Journal of Psychiatry, 157*, 127–129.

Hays, L. R. (2004). A profile of OxyContin addiction. *Journal of Addictive Diseases, 23*(4), 1–9.

Heidbreder, C. A., Andreoli, M., Marcon, C., Thanos, P. K., Ashby, C. R., & Gardner, E. L. (2004). Role of dopamine D3 receptors in the addictive properties of ethanol. *Drugs of Today, 40*(4), 355–365.

Henderson-Martin, B. (2000). No more surprises: Screening patients for alcohol abuse. *American Journal of Nursing, 100*(9), 26–32.

Jellinek, E. (1946). *Phases in the drinking history of alcoholics.* New Haven, CT: Hillhouse Press.

Kasser, C., Geller, A., Howell, E., & Wartenberg, A. (2004). *Detoxification: Principles and protocols.* Chevy Chase, MD: American Society of Addiction Medicine.

Kenna, G. A., & Wood, M. D. (2005). Family history of alcohol and drug use in healthcare professionals. *Journal of Substance Use, 10*(4), 225–238.

Kneisl, C. R., Wilson, H. S., & Trigoboff, E. (2004). *Contemporary psychiatric–mental health nursing.* Upper Saddle River, NJ: Pearson-Prentice Hall.

Lantz, S. M. (2005). Prescription drug and alcohol abuse in an older woman. *Clinical Geriatrics, 12*(1), 39–43.

Leonardson, G. R., Kemper, E., Ness, F. K., Koplin, B. A., Daniels, M. C., & Leonardson, G. A. (2005). Validity and reliability of the audit and CAGE-AID in Northern Plains American Indians. *Psychological Reports, 97*(1), 161–166.

Luczak, S. E., Wall, T. L., Cook, T. A., Shea, S. H., & Carr, L. G. (2004). ALDH2 status and conduct disorder mediate the relationship between ethnicity and alcohol dependence in Chinese, Korean, and White American college students. *Journal of Abnormal Psychology, 113*(2), 271–278.

Marsiglia, F. F., Kulis, S., Hecht, M. L., & Sills, S. (2004). Ethnicity and ethnic identity as predictors of drug norms and drug use among preadolescents in the U.S. Southwest. *Substance Use & Misuse, 39*(7), 1061–1094.

McKay, A., Koranda, A., & Axen, D. (2004). Using a symptom-triggered approach to manage patients in acute alcohol withdrawal. *Med-Surg Nursing, 13*(1), 15–21.

Miller, N. S., & Greenfeld, A. (2004). Patient characteristics and risk factors for development of dependence on hydrocodone and oxycodone. *American Journal of Therapeutics, 11*(1), 26–32.

Moorhead, S., Johnson, M., & Maas, M. (Eds.). (2004). *Nursing outcomes classification (NOC): Iowa outcomes project* (3rd ed.). St. Louis, MO: Mosby.

National Institute of Mental Health. (2004). *The numbers count: Mental disorders in America* (NIH Publication No. 01–4584). Bethesda, MD: Author. Retrieved February 9,

2005, from http://www.nimh.nih.gov/publicat/numbers.cfm

National Institute on Alcohol Abuse and Alcoholism. (2004). *Alcoholism: Getting the facts* (NIH Publication No. 96-4153). Bethesda, MD: Author. Retrieved February, 9, 2005, from http://www.niaaa.nih.gov/publications/booklet.htm

Nellissery, M., Feinn, R. S., Covault, J., Gelernter, J., Anton, R. F., Pettinati, H., et al. (2003). Alleles of a functional serotonin transporter promoter polymorphism are associated with major depression in alcoholics. *Alcoholism: Clinical and Experimental Research, 27*(9), 1402–1408.

Nolen-Hoeksema, S. (2004). Gender differences in risk factors and consequences for alcohol use and problems. *Clinical Psychology Review, 24*(8), 981–1010.

Ntais, C., Pakos, E., Kyzas, P., & Ioannidis, J. P. (2005). Benzodiazepines for alcohol withdrawal. *The Cochrane Database of Systematic Reviews,* Issue 4, The Cochrane Collaboration. New York: John Wiley & Sons.

North American Nursing Diagnosis Association. (2003). *Nursing diagnoses: Definitions & classification 2003–2004.* Philadelphia: Author.

Office of Applied Studies. (2004). Narcotic analgesics, 2002 update. *The Drug Abuse Warning Network (DAWN) Report,* September, 2004. Rockville, MD: Substance Abuse Mental Health Services Administration.

_____. (2005a). Methamphetamine use, abuse, and dependence: 2002, 2003 & 2004. *The NSUDH Report,* September 16, 2005. Rockville, MD: Substance Abuse and Mental Health Services Administration.

_____. (2005b). Substance use among past year Ecstasy users. *The NSUDH Report,* April 29, 2005. Rockville, MD: Substance Abuse and Mental Health Services Administration.

_____. (2005c). Trends in admissions for PCP: 1993–2003. *The NSUDH Report,* October 28, 2005. Rockville, MD: Substance Abuse and Mental Health Services Administration.

_____. (2006). Emergency department visits involving underage drinking. *The Drug Abuse Warning Network (DAWN) Report,* Issue 1. Rockville, MD: Substance Abuse Mental Health Services Administration.

Oswald, L. M., & Wand, G. S. (2004). Opioids and alcoholism. *Physiology & Behavior, 81*(2), 339–358.

Pokorny, A. D., Miller, B. A., & Kaplan, H. B. (1972). The brief MAST: A shortened version of the Michigan Alcohol Screening Test. *American Journal of Psychiatry, 129,* 342–345.

Ramisetty-Mikler, S., & Caetano, R. (2004). Ethnic differences in the estimates of children exposed to alcohol problems and alcohol dependence in the United States. *Journal of Studies on Alcohol, 65*(5), 593–599.

Reneman, L., Booij, J., de Bruin, K., Reitsma, J. B., de Wolff, F. A., Gunning, W. B., et al. (2001). Effects of dose, sex, and long-term abstention from use on toxic effects of MDMA (Ecstasy) on brain serotonin neurons. *Lancet, 358*(9296), 1864–1869.

Rice, V. H., & Stead, L. F. (2005). Nursing interventions for smoking cessation. *The Cochrane Database of Systematic Reviews,* Issue 4, The Cochrane Collaboration. New York: John Wiley & Sons.

Rigotti, N. A., Munafo, M. R., Murphy, M. F. G., & Stead, L. F. (2005). Interventions for smoking cessation in hospitalized patients. *The Cochrane Database of Systematic Reviews,* Issue 4, The Cochrane Collaboration. New York: John Wiley & Sons.

Sees, K. L., Di Marino, M. E., Ruediger, N. K., Sweeney, C. T., & Shiffman, S. (2005). Non-medical use of OxyContin tablets in the United States. *Journal of Pain & Palliative Care Pharmacotherapy, 19*(2), 13–23.

Semple, S. J., Grant, I., & Patterson, T. L. (2004). Female methamphetamine users: Social characteristics and sexual risk behavior. *Women & Health, 40*(3), 35–50.

Semple, S. J., Patterson, T. L., & Rant, I. (2005). Methamphetamine use and depressive symptoms among heterosexual men and women. *Journal of Substance Use, 10*(1), 31–47.

Shoptaw, S., Reback, C. J., Peck, J. A., Yang, X., Rotheram-Fuller, E., Larkins, S., et al. (2005). Behavioral treatment approaches for methamphetamine dependence and HIV-related sexual risk behaviors among urban gay and bisexual men. *Drug and Alcohol Dependence, 78*(2), 125–134.

Silagy, C., Lancaster, T., Stead, M., & Fowler, G. (2005). Nicotine replacement therapy for smoking cessation. *The Cochrane Database of Systematic Reviews,* Issue 4, The Cochrane Collaboration. New York: John Wiley & Sons.

Simoni-Wastila, L., & Strickler, G. (2004). Risk factors associated with problem use of prescription drugs. *American Journal of Public Health, 94*(2), 266–268.

Siqueira, L., Diab, M., Bodian, C., & Rolnitzky, L. (2001). The relationship of stress and coping methods to adolescent use. *Substance Abuse, 22*(3), 157–166.

Skinner, H. A. (1982). *Drug Abuse Screening Test (DAST)* (p. 363). Langford Lance, England: Elsevier Science Ltd.

Srisurapanont, M., Jarusuraisin, N., & Kittirattanapalboon, P. (2005). Treatment for amphetamine dependence and abuse. *The Cochrane Database of Systematic Reviews,* Issue 4, The Cochrane Collaboration. New York: John Wiley and Sons.

Stevenson, J. S. (2005). Alcohol use, misuse, abuse, and dependence in later adulthood. *Annual Review of Nursing Research, 23,* 245–280.

Storr, C. L., Westergaard, R., & Anthony, J. C. (2005). Early onset inhalant use and risk for opiate initiation by young adulthood. *Drug and Alcohol Dependence, 78*(3), 253–261.

Stuart, G. W., & Laraia, M. T. (2005). *Stuart & Sundeen's principles and practice of psychiatric nursing* (8th ed.). St. Louis, MO: Mosby.

Substance Abuse and Mental Health Services Administration. (2003). *Results from the 2002 National Survey on Drug Use and Health: National findings* (Office of Applied Studies, NSUDH Series H-22, DHHS Publication No. SMA 03-3836). Rockville, MD: Author.

_____. (2004). *Results from the 2003 National Survey on Drug Use and Health: National findings* (Office of Applied Studies, NSDUH Series H-25, DHHS Publication No. SMA 04-3964). Rockville, MD: Author.

_____. (2005). *Results from the 2004 National Survey on Drug Use and Health: National findings* (Office of Applied Studies, NSDUH Series H-28, DHHS Publication No. SMA 05-4062). Rockville, MD: Author.

Sullivan, J. T., Sykora, K., Schneiderman, J., Naranjo, C. A., & Sellers, E. M. (1989). Assessment of alcohol withdrawal: The revised Clinical Institute Withdrawal Assessment for Alcohol scale (CIWA-Ar). *British Journal of Addictions, 84,* 1353–1357.

Trinkoff, A. M., Zhou, Q., Storr, C. L., & Soeken, K. L. (2000). Workplace access, negative proscriptions, job strain, and substance use in registered nurses. *Nursing Research, 49*(2), 83–90.

U.S. Department of Health and Human Services. (2005). *At a glance: Women and smoking: A report of the surgeon general–2001.* Rockville, MD: Centers for Disease Control and Prevention, National Center for Chronic Disease Prevention and Health Promotion, Office on Smoking and Health. Retrieved February 9, 2005, from http://www.cdc.gov/tobacco/sgr/sgr_forwomen/ataglance.htm

Varcarolis, E. (2002). *Foundations of psychiatric mental health nursing: A clinical approach* (4th ed.). Philadelphia: W.B. Saunders.

Virgo, N., Bennett, G., Higgins, D., Bennett, L., & Thomas, P. (2001). The prevalence and characteristics of co-occurring serious mental illness (SMI) and substance abuse or dependence in the patients of Adult Mental Health and Addictions Services in eastern Dorset. *Journal of Mental Health, 10*(2), 175–188.

Wallace, J. M., Bachman, J. G., O'Malley, P. M., Johnston, L. D., Schulenberg, J. E., & Cooper, S. M. (2002). Tobacco, alcohol, and illicit drug use: Racial and ethnic differences among U.S. high school seniors. *Public Health Reports, 117*(Suppl 1), S67–S75.

Watson, S. J., Benson, J. A. & Joy, J. E. (2000). Marijuana and medicine: Assessing the science base: A summary of the 1999 Institute of Medicine Report. *Archives of General Psychiatry, 57*(4), 547–552.

Weiss, F., & Porrino, L. J. (2002). Behavioral neurobiology of alcohol addiction: Recent advances and challenges. *Journal of Neuroscience, 22*(9), 3332–3337.

Wesson, D. R., & Ling, W. (2003). The clinical opiate withdrawal scale (COWS). *Journal of Psychoactive Drugs, 35*(2), 253–259.

Wu, L. T., Schlenger, W. E., & Gavin, D. M. (2006). Concurrent use of methamphetamine, MDMA, LSD, ketamine, GHB, and flunitrazepam among American youths. *Drug and Alcohol Dependence, 84*(1), 102–113.

Yen, C., Wu, H., Yen, J., & Ko, C. (2004). Effects of brief cognitive-behavioral interventions on confidence to resist the urges to use heroin and methamphetamine in relapse-related situations. *Journal of Nervous and Mental Disease, 192*(11), 788–791.

Zimmerman, P., Wittchen, H., Waszak, F., Nocon, A., Hofler, M., & Lieb, R. (2005). Pathways into Ecstasy use: The role of prior cannabis use and Ecstasy availability. *Drug and Alcohol Dependence, 79*(3), 331–341.

CHAPTER 7 Nursing Care of Clients Experiencing Disasters

LEARNING OUTCOMES

- Distinguish the difference between an emergency and a disaster.
- Describe the types of injuries or symptoms that are associated with biologic, chemical, or radiologic terrorism.
- Evaluate nursing interventions for the treatment of injuries related to biologic, chemical, or radiologic terrorism.
- Explain the rationale for reverse triage in disasters versus conventional triage in emergencies.

- Discuss situations requiring the need for client isolation or client decontamination.
- Discuss the role of the nurse in disaster planning, response, and mitigation.
- Identify ways that nurses are able to provide care to clients with special considerations.

CLINICAL COMPETENCIES

- Assess health status of clients who have experienced a disaster and monitor, document, and triage to the appropriate level of care.
- Use evidence-based research to plan and implement nursing care for clients with injuries suffered as a result of a disaster.
- Using assessment skills, determine priority nursing diagnoses, implement, and evaluate individualized nursing interventions for clients who are victims of disasters.
- Provide skilled nursing care to treat disaster-related injuries.
- Integrate interdisciplinary care of clients with an understanding of local, state, and federal systems of disaster response.

- Evaluate and revise plan of care and interventions based on client's condition, environmental factors, and resources to promote, maintain, or restore functional health status to clients who have sustained injuries due to a disaster.
- Provide education to promote prevention of disaster-related injuries.

MEDIALINK

Resources for this chapter can be found on the Prentice Hall Nursing MediaLink DVD-ROM accompanying this textbook, and on the Companion Website at http://www.prenhall.com/lemone

All nurses will be expected to care for victims of disasters whether they work in acute care settings, ambulatory sites, long-term care facilities, or at home in their communities. There is no way to know where or when disasters may strike. Because of this, nurses must be prepared to assist clients, families, friends, healthcare workers, first responders, and communities in their recovery from disastrous events. There are a number of basic competencies that nurses should be cognizant of related to disaster preparedness.

CORE EMERGENCY AND DISASTER PREPAREDNESS COMPETENCIES FOR NURSES

The International Nursing Coalition for Mass Casualty Education (INCMCE) was founded to ensure a competent nurse workforce to respond to mass casualty incidents (MCIs) by facilitating the development of policies related to mass casualty events as they influence the public health infrastructure and impact on nursing practice, education, research, and regulation.

In August 2003, the INCMCE published *Educational Competencies for Registered Nurses Responding to Mass Casualty Incidents*. The purpose of this publication is to provide registered nurses with the awareness of critical competencies necessary to respond effectively to mass casualty events (Box 7–1). Nurses are expected to have sufficient knowledge to recognize the potential for a disaster event, when such an event has occurred, and what nurses can do to protect themselves, family members, and community members from harm or from potential exacerbation of conditions. Nurses must be aware of their role in disaster planning, response, and mitigation. Equally important, nurses must be aware of professional limitations and be able to respond to MCIs appropriately within the scope of nursing practice. It is strongly recommended that these core competencies be introduced in basic nursing curricula and be offered as continuing education for those who have completed their basic education.

DEFINITIONS
Types of Disasters

Disasters may be natural or man-made. Noji (1997) defines disasters as "events that require extraordinary efforts beyond those needed to respond to everyday emergencies." **Natural disasters**

BOX 7–1 Educational Competencies for Registered Nurses Responding to Mass Casualty Incidents

Core Competencies
1. Critical thinking
2. Assessment
3. Technical skills
4. Communication

Core Knowledge Areas
1. Health promotion, risk reduction, and disease prevention
2. Healthcare systems and policy
3. Illness and disease management
4. Information and healthcare technologies
5. Ethics
6. Human diversity

Professional Role Development
1. A description of nursing roles in MCIs
2. Identification of the most appropriate or most likely healthcare role for oneself during an MCI

Source: INCMCE (2003).

---

are caused by acts of nature or emerging diseases. They may be predictable through advanced meteorologic technologies or unexpected. One of the greatest natural disasters in recorded history ravaged the province of Banda Aceh, Indonesia, which was less than 150 kilometers from the epicenter of a 9.15 earthquake that triggered a tsunami and killed more than 200,000 people in December 2004. Hurricane Katrina hit landfall on August 29, 2005, along the Central Gulf Coast. The hurricane caused vast devastation as its storm surge breached the levee system that protected New Orleans from Lake Ponchartrain and the Mississippi River. Most of the New Orleans area was flooded, and heavy damage was also inflicted on the coasts of Mississippi and Alabama. Katrina is considered the most destructive and costliest natural disaster in the history of the United States (U.S. Department of Homeland Security, 2005). **Man-made disasters** are either accidental or intentional. They include complex emergencies, technologic disasters, material shortages, and other disasters not caused by natural hazards (Noji, 1997). Examples of man-made or human-generated disasters include war; chemical, biologic, radiologic, and nuclear terrorism; transportation accidents; group violence; food or water contamination; deforestation; and building collapses. Contamination of large amounts of vegetables at a grocery store is an example of a deliberate or *intentional* man-made disaster. A campfire that has been left unattended such that the embers are carried by high winds to the dry trees and brush nearby creating a massive forest fire is an example of a man-made *accidental* disaster.

An **emergency** is distinguished from a disaster in that an emergency encompasses an unforeseen combination of circumstances calling for immediate action for a range of victims from one to many. For example, a motor vehicle accident may call for emergency assistance for a small number of individuals whose injuries are minor to very severe or fatal. Emergencies are generally accommodated within the emergency management system. Disasters seldom involve a single victim. Instead, disasters are complex emergencies that significantly overwhelm available hospitals, emergency medical services, facilities, and resources. Disasters are typically labeled as **multiple casualty incidents** with more than 2 but fewer than 100 persons injured or **mass casualty incidents** in which 100 or more casualties are involved (Beachley, 2000). An example of a mass casualty incident is that of an entire community affected by the release of a hazardous material such as a chemical as a result of a train derailment. With human fatalities of approximately 200,000 and 1300 in Banda Aceh and the Gulf Coast, respectively, the tsunami in Indonesia and Hurricane Katrina are prime examples of mass casualty incidents (American Red Cross, 2006). In summary, the key difference between an emergency and a disaster is that an emergency can be handled by the usual emergency management systems already in place, while a disaster overwhelms general emergency systems and requires additional resources.

Hazardous materials pose a potential risk to life, health, or property if they are released because of their chemical, biologic, or physical nature. The hazard exists during any stage of use, from the production and storage of these substances to their transportation, use, or disposal. Hazardous materials accidents range from the unintentional release of household hazardous materials to chemical spills on highways to groundwater contamination by naturally occurring methane gas (Langan, 2005a).

Terrorism

Another classification of man-made, intentional disaster is terrorism. **Terrorism** is defined by the U.S. Department of Defense as the "calculated use of violence or the threat of violence to inculcate fear; intended to coerce or to intimidate governments or societies in the pursuit of goals that are generally political, religious or ideological" (Payne, 2003). One of the goals of terrorism is to cause psychologic effects that reach a much wider audience than the immediate victims or object of an attack. High-profile acts draw attention to the terrorists and their cause. It is thought that terrorists seek to obtain leverage, influence, and power through the publicity generated by their violence (Hoffman, 2003).

The weapons terrorists use are often described as conventional and nonconventional. **Conventional weapons** include bombs and guns. Car and truck bombs have become powerful weapons in suicide attacks such as the Oklahoma City bombing of the Alfred P. Murrah Federal Building on April 19, 1995. Terrorists use explosive bombs such as letter and parcel bombs as well as incendiary bombs such as Molotov cocktails. Other types of conventional terrorist weapons include handguns, rifles, semi-automatic weapons, hand grenades, rocket-propelled devices, and even surface-to-air, shoulder-fired missiles that can bring down helicopters, fighter aircraft, and civilian airliners (United Nations Office for Drug Control and Crime Prevention, 2002).

Nonconventional terrorist weapons include those in the chemical, biologic, and nuclear categories. Chemical terrorism attacks may manifest as the release of a toxin into highly populated areas, bodies of water, and unventilated areas. Another type of chemical terrorism is a specific attack on a particular product, especially a food product. This is accomplished by introducing a toxic chemical substance directly into the product. The anthrax attacks against U.S. public officials after 9/11 illustrate how these small amounts of "white powder" can encourage mass panic and hysteria in the public (Simonsen & Spindlove, 2004). (See Box 7–2.)

Another name for biologic terrorism is **bioterrorism**. Biologic terrorism is the "use of etiological agents (disease) to cause harm or kill a population, food, and/or livestock. Biological terrorism includes the use of organisms such as bacteria, viruses, and rickettsia and the use of products of organisms—toxins" (Maniscalco & Christen, 2002, p. 144). The main purpose of biologic weapon use is mass devastation. Unfortunately, it is not uncommon for the results of a biologic attack not to be known for several hours or days after the attack because aerosolized biologic particles are odorless, colorless, and tasteless. Unless the terrorists announce the biologic attack, it may remain unknown until clients begin to present at emergency departments or physicians' offices a few days or weeks after the release of the agent. Detection is difficult because of the numerous different healthcare facilities available for client treatment. Surveillance is essential to detect such an event. **Surveillance** is "collecting and analyzing data to establish a baseline and determine a point at which there is a change or trend in the health of the population" (Rebmann, 2005, p. 204). The goal of the surveillance system is to determine the status of the public's health and detect any sudden change in that status. Fortunately, biologic weapons are not as common, accessible, or available as chemical weapons.

Healthcare providers must be alert to the recognition, reporting, and treatment of high-priority biologic agents. A disaster preparedness plan should be established in every healthcare facility that outlines the protocol and procedures to be taken with a suspected bioterrorism attack. Hospital staff will alert the infection control nurse when subtle changes or trends in symptoms among clients are seen. The public health department is also given these data. When an unusual disease pattern presents itself, laboratories perform tests on cultures that would normally be discarded as contaminants. Laboratory personnel report unusual clusters of laboratory results. Special laboratories have been established to perform a battery of tests on suspicious specimens of rarely seen bacteria, toxins, viruses, or increased numbers of a particular strain or specimen. The Centers for Disease Control and Prevention (CDC) have created detailed "Fact Sheets" about bioterrorism agents and diseases for healthcare providers.

MEDIALINK Bioterrorism Resources

BOX 7–2 Biologic Threat Infections

Following the terrorist attacks on September 11, 2001, and the development of anthrax cases in the United States, concern has arisen about the possible use of biologic weapons. The most likely pathogens to be used for this purpose include anthrax, smallpox, botulism, pneumonic plague, and viral hemorrhagic fevers.

Anthrax is an acute bacterial infection caused by *Bacillus anthracis*, a gram-positive, spore-producing organism that occurs in inhaled, cutaneous, and gastrointestinal forms. The spores are impervious to temperature and sunlight, and remain viable for years.

Inhalation anthrax carries the highest mortality rate because spores of 1 to 5 microns are easily inhaled and deposited in the alveoli. The client initially exhibits influenza-like symptoms such as fever, nonproductive cough, headache, and malaise that advances to respiratory distress, x-ray evidence of mediastinal widening, and hemodynamic collapse in 3–5 days. Death may occur shortly thereafter. Untreated clients die in 2 to 3 days. The characteristic lesion of cutaneous anthrax progresses from an itching papule to a painless, serosanguineous-filled vesicle that forms a black necrotic center. Clients who ingest the anthrax bacillus develop nausea, vomiting, severe abdominal pain, and bloody diarrhea. Diagnosis is confirmed by a positive blood culture, polymerase chain reaction, and serology. On confirmation of anthrax exposure, prophylaxis is initiated with oral ciprofloxacin (Cipro) or doxycycline (Doxycin) for 60 days; people with confirmed systemic anthrax cases must receive anti-infectives intravenously (CDC, 2006).

Healthcare workers risk exposure to anthrax through direct contact with a contaminated surface, contact with exposed persons' contaminated clothes, or direct unprotected contact with the open lesions of cutaneous anthrax. Guidelines for decontamination of extensively exposed persons include removal of clothing and storage in a sealed plastic bag, and showering with soap and water. If gross contamination with the agent occurs and soap and water decontamination is ineffective, use a bleach solution (1:10 dilution of household bleach/final hypochlorite concentration 0.5%) and rinse after 10 to 15 minutes (Heymann, 2004).

In 1980, the World Health Organization certified that *smallpox* was eradicated. Routine smallpox vaccination was discontinued in 1972, leaving people under the age of 30 at risk for this disease if it reappears or is used as a weapon. Smallpox spreads by direct contact or by inhalation of respiratory droplets. Symptoms include a high fever, headache, and malaise, followed by a vesicular/pustular rash appearing simultaneously on the face and extremities. Once the lesions break open and spread large amounts of the virus into the mouth and throat, people are highly contagious and should be placed in negative-pressure rooms. Anyone exposed to the client should be vaccinated and monitored closely. Vaccination up to 4 days of exposure provides almost complete protection.

Healthcare providers should be alert to illness patterns that could indicate an unusual infectious disease outbreak. Indicators of a biologic agent release include increased disease incidence among people in the same geographic area (e.g., people who attended the same event); the disease pattern is inconsistent with client age, such as chickenpox among adults; and a client presents with symptoms of a rare disease. The presence of one or more of these indicators should be reported to public health authorities to determine the infectious disease source and to prevent further exposure (World Health Organization, 2006).

PRACTICE ALERT

Healthcare providers should become suspicious when increased numbers of clients present to the emergency department with flu-like symptoms and retailers notice an increase in purchases of over-the-counter flu and diarrhea medications.

Nuclear/Radiologic Terrorism

The **nuclear** category of nonconventional terrorist weapons encompasses the use of a nuclear device to cause mass murder and devastation. This category of terrorism includes the use or threat of the use of fissionable radioactive materials in an attack. An explosion at a nuclear power plant is an example of this type of terrorism. Using conventional weapons against one of the many nuclear reactors in the world could cause an explosion that would cause extensive and possibly irreversible environmental damage. Damage to the reactors could cause radioactive matter to be released into the atmosphere, potentially endangering large population centers (U.S. Department of State, 2006).

The **radiologic dispersion bomb** is probably the most accessible nuclear device to be used by terrorists. Another name for this device is **dirty bomb** because it consists of a conventional explosive and radioactive waste by-products from nuclear reactors. The dirty bomb discharges deadly radioactive particles into the environment. It is cheaper to make than a nuclear bomb and radioactive waste material is relatively easy to obtain.

Radioactive waste is found throughout the world and is typically not as well guarded as nuclear weapons (Harris, 2005).

TYPES OF DISASTERS AND COMMON INJURIES

Hurricane and Tsunami-Related Injuries

A **hurricane** is a type of tropical cyclone. It is a low-pressure system that generally forms in the tropics. Hurricanes can wreak havoc on coastlines as well as several hundred miles inland. Hurricanes and tropical storms can also spawn tornadoes, create storm surges along the coast, and cause extensive damage from heavy rainfall. Floods are deadly and destructive. Excessive rain can trigger landslides or mudslides, especially in mountainous regions. Flooding on rivers and streams may persist for several days or more after the storm (Federal Emergency Management Agency, 2005).

Common physical effects include asphyxia due to drowning; wounds; bone, joint, and muscle injuries; aggravation of chronic illnesses; stress-related symptoms; upper respiratory infections; gastrointestinal illnesses; clean-up injuries; animal, snake, and insect bites; skin irritations and infections; obstetrical complications; and waterborne and insect-borne diseases from contaminated water supplies and insect breeding grounds (Clark, 2003a; Smith & Maurer, 2000). See Table 7–1 for injury-specific nursing interventions.

TABLE 7–1 Types of Disasters and Common Injuries

TYPE OF DISASTER	COMMON INJURIES	NURSING IMPLICATIONS
Hurricane-Related Injuries	Drowning; clean-up injuries; aggravation of chronic illnesses; stress-related symptoms; upper respiratory infections; gastrointestinal illnesses; animal, snake, and insect bites; obstetrical complications; contaminated water supplies and insect-breeding grounds; heat-related illnesses; lack of sanitation and safe housing	Asphyxia can occur along with wounds; bone, joint, and muscle injuries; and infections. Also possible are skin irritations and infections; waterborne and insect-borne diseases; dehydration; starvation or malnutrition, and diseases and injuries.
Tsunami-Related Injuries	"Tsunami lung," a severe infection caused by swallowing muddy, bacteria-laden water	Requires aggressive respiratory and ventilator management, blood transfusions, antibiotics, and other medical support.
Thunderstorm-Related Injuries	Resistance of body tissues to electrical current *Least resistance:* nerves, blood, mucous membranes, muscle *Intermediate resistance:* dry skin *Most resistance:* tendon, fat, bone	Potential for tissue destruction with longer duration of contact with high-voltage current; if energy current is dissipated at the skin surface, significant surface burns result, especially in calloused areas.
Tornado-Related Injuries	Flying debris; injuries similar to hurricane-related injuries	Injuries and fatalities can occur.
Earthquake-Related Injuries	High incidence of mortality and morbidity; explosions	May result in stress-related symptoms; wounds; bone, joint, and muscle injuries; clean-up injuries; gastrointestinal and respiratory problems; aggravation of chronic illnesses; obstetrical complications; burns.
Snowstorm-Related Injuries	Overexertion and exhaustion	Myocardial infarction can occur.
Disaster-Related Eye Injuries	"Specks" of dust or debris; cuts, punctures, or stuck objects; blows to the eye	Administer eyewash or flushing versus rubbing; stabilize eye with rigid shield. Apply cold compress, no pressure; client should visit healthcare professional to rule out serious injury or internal eye damage.
Blast Injuries	Auditory	Tympanic membrane rupture, ossicular disruption, and cochlear damage occur; damage from foreign body can occur.
	Eye, orbit, face	Perforated globe, air embolisms, fractures are common; damage from foreign body can occur.
	Respiratory	May result in blast lung, hemothorax, pneumothorax, pulmonary contusion and hemorrhage, atrioventricular fistulas (source of air embolism), airway epithelial damage, aspiration pneumonitis, sepsis.
	Digestive	May result in bowel perforation, hemorrhage, ruptured liver or spleen, sepsis, mesenteric ischemia from air embolism.
	Circulatory	Cardiac contusion, myocardial infarction from air embolism, shock, vasovagal hypotension, peripheral vascular injury, and air embolism-induced injury can occur.
	Central nervous system injury	Concussion, closed and open brain injury, stroke, spinal cord injury, air embolism-induced injury can occur.
	Renal injury	May result in renal contusion, laceration, acute renal failure due to rhabdomyolysis, hypotension, and hypovolemia.
	Extremity injury	Traumatic amputation, fractures, crush injuries, compartment syndrome, burns, cuts, lacerations, acute arterial occlusion, air embolism-induced injury can occur.
Blunt Trauma	Head and torso blunt trauma, penetrating trauma	Fractured limbs and spinal injury can occur.
Pressure Trauma	Lungs	Tearing of the alveoli cause swelling, fluid accumulation, possible pulmonary emboli, eventual hypoxia.
	Ear and bowel injury: ear pain, hearing loss	Keep auditory canal clean, make the client comfortable.

(continued)

TABLE 7–1 Types of Disasters and Common Injuries (continued)

TYPE OF DISASTER	COMMON INJURIES	NURSING IMPLICATIONS
Radiological Dispersion Bomb (Dirty Bomb) Blast	Radiation sickness	Get rid of contaminated clothes, shower, and evacuate the area within a day of a small or medium blast. Those close to the blast could suffer radiation sickness and require hospital care.
Nuclear Detonation	Thermal burns	May involve only the epidermis and upper layers of dermis with short duration of heat exposure.
Bright Light Flash of Nuclear Detonation	Eye burn injuries	May blind the client momentarily, effects will disappear with time, can impair a client's ability to perform self-care and other ADLs.
Radiation Exposure Injury	Bone marrow and blood cell damage	A reduction in the blood's oxygen-carrying capacity results in nausea, fatigue, and a general feeling of malaise. Reduced platelet production causes clotting disorders and possibly hemorrhage. When the body's white blood cells are destroyed, it is important to reduce the client's exposure to infection. Infection at the time of reduced WBC production can be severe and even fatal.
	Bowel	Cells that reproduce the bowel lining are damaged, resulting in nausea, loss of appetite, vomiting, diarrhea, fluid loss, and malaise in the acute stage; later, dehydration, malnutrition, bowel hemorrhage, and perforation may occur; if radiation exposure is not exacerbated by other injury or pathology, clients will generally survive.
	Integument	Erythema or generalized reddening of the skin occurs when skin cells are damaged, with the appearance of a sunburn; more serious burns may occur with persistent exposure or extremely high radiation doses.
	Nervous and cardiovascular systems	With acute radiation exposure, blood vessel and nerve cells are damaged and the client is incapacitated and experiences cardiovascular collapse, confusion, and even an "on fire" sensation throughout the body; symptoms this severe generally do not permit survival.
Chemical Burns	Range from minor to life-threatening injuries	Remove clothing from injury site as well as any jewelry; flush chemical from skin with thorough decontamination; cover wounds loosely with a dry, sterile, or clean cloth.

Source: Adapted from *Centers for Disease Control and Prevention* (2003a), Cooper (1995), DeLorenzo & Porter (2000), and Harris (2005).

As a result of Hurricane Katrina, many people lost their homes, family members, friends, and the environment that supported their daily routines. Many basic physical needs in the aftermath of the hurricane could not be met, which put survivors at risk of dehydration, starvation or malnutrition, heat-related illnesses, and diseases and injuries related to lack of sanitation and safe housing (Myers-Walls, 2005). The CDC offers a number of specific strategies to promote health and safety after a hurricane.

A **tsunami**, a seismic sea wave, is a series of ocean waves characterized by having a long period and wavelength and the ability to travel at speeds greater than 500 miles per hour. As the tsunami encounters shallow water, its height increases drastically, resulting in a sudden increase in sea level, thereby flooding low-lying coastal areas (Pacific Tsunami Museum, 2001). Injuries are similar to those seen with hurricanes.

Thunderstorm-Related Injuries

Risk of a lightning strike is possible during a thunderstorm. The short duration of a lightning strike results in a very short flow of current internally, despite the high voltage of lightning. Additionally, the almost immediate flashover of current around the body usually results in very little, if any, skin breakdown or burning of tissues (Cooper, 1995). Note, however, that the longer the duration of contact with high-voltage current, the greater the potential for tissue destruction.

High electrolyte and water content in the body conduct the greatest electrical current. Hence, the greatest conductors of electrical current in the body are the nerves, muscle, and blood vessels. High resistors to electric current are bone, tendon, and fat, due to their tendency to heat up and coagulate instead of transmitting current. Much of the energy current may be dissipated at the skin surface. This results in significant surface burns, especially in calloused areas (Cooper, 1995). Care providers should realize that a person who has been struck by lightning does not carry an electrical charge that can shock other people.

Tornado-Related Injuries

Flying debris causes most fatalities and injuries in tornadoes. Additionally, the following physical effects may be seen: bone, muscle, and joint injuries; fractures; aggravation of chronic illnesses, obstetrical complications, stress-related symptoms; upper respiratory infections and those associated with fiberglass; clean-up wounds; and gastrointestinal illnesses (Smith & Maurer, 2000).

Earthquake-Related Injuries

Earthquakes have a high incidence of mortality and morbidity. The most common health effects experienced by victims of earthquakes include stress-related symptoms; wounds; bone, joint, and muscle injuries; burns from explosions; clean-up injuries; gastrointestinal and respiratory problems; aggravation of chronic illnesses; obstetrical complications; and death (Smith & Maurer, 2000).

Snowstorm-Related Injuries

Overexertion and exhaustion are major problems during the snow shoveling that is done following a snowstorm. The exertion required to shovel heavy snow in the extreme cold may cause a myocardial infarction.

Disaster-Related Eye Injuries

Clients should be cautioned not to rub the eye that has "specks" of dust or debris in it. They should instead use an eyewash, flushing the eye with copious amounts of water. However, if there are cuts, punctures, or objects stuck in the eye, clients should not wash the eye or try to remove an object stuck in the eye. The eye should be stabilized with a rigid shield without pressure. The bottom half of a paper cup can be used as a shield. When there are complaints of blows to the eye, cold compresses should be applied without pressure. A plastic bag full of crushed ice can be taped to the forehead to rest gently on the injured eye. All of these clients should see a physician to rule out serious injury or internal eye damage (National Institute for Occupational Safety and Health, 2001).

Blast Injuries

Blast injuries are the result of explosive munitions, often involving car or package bombs. Care for persons injured by blast injuries typically focuses on abdominal and lung injuries, penetrating wounds, traumatic amputations, and burns (Scott et al., 2005).

Radiologic Dispersion Bomb (Dirty Bomb) Blast

The dirty bomb consists of a conventional explosive such as trinitrotoluene (TNT) packed with radioactive waste by-products from nuclear reactors. When detonated, the dirty bomb will discharge deadly radioactive particles into the environment. When the dirty bomb explodes, the radioactive material spreads in the wind like a dust cloud. In this way, it reaches far wider areas than the initial explosion (Harris, 2005).

As Harris (2005) explains, the long-term destructive force of the dirty bomb would be caused by the ionizing radiation from the radioactive material. In a person's body, an ion's electrical charge may lead to unnatural chemical reactions inside the cells. The charge can break DNA chains. Cells with broken DNA strands either die or the DNA develops a mutation. Diseases develop as the result of widespread cell death. If the DNA mutates, a cell may become cancerous. The cancer may spread and the cells may malfunction. This series of events may result in a wide variety of symptoms collectively referred to as **radiation sickness**. While this condition can be deadly, it is survivable with bone marrow transplantation (Harris, 2005).

People are exposed to ionizing radiation frequently, but in small doses, with little if any ill effects. Some of the sources of this everyday exposure are outer space, the stars, sun, natural radioactive isotopes, and x-ray machines. The risk of cancer and radiation sickness would be increased by exposure to a dirty bomb and the subsequent rise in radiation levels above normal. The fatal effects of the dirty bomb may not be apparent in the short term after exposure, but could kill people years later (Harris, 2005).

Thermal Burns

A thermal burn is the most common mechanism resulting in injury and death associated with nuclear detonation. A tremendous amount of thermal energy is created by a nuclear reaction. This energy travels unimpeded through the air. The energy is absorbed by the contact surface. It may create burns or ignite combustibles. The burns may involve only the epidermis and upper layers of dermis because of the short duration of heat exposure.

Thermal burn injuries can be severe and are treated as any other burn. Radiation suppresses the immune system, so special care must be taken to reduce the potential infection often associated with full-thickness burns (DeLorenzo & Porter, 2000). More information on burn care can be found in Chapter 17 ∞ .

Radiation Exposure Injury

Radiation exposure results in injury from ionizing radiation altering some cell structures. Cells are damaged from the changes in DNA in bone marrow, blood, bowel, skin, and nervous and cardiovascular systems (DeLorenzo & Porter, 2000).

The major activities performed for clients who have suffered a nuclear casualty are triage, evacuation or sheltering, search and rescue, radioactive monitoring, decontamination, and direct client care. The client will be assessed for injuries such as burns or blunt trauma. Pressure injuries such as lung injury, difficult breathing, or minor stroke-like symptoms (air emboli) must be assessed quickly. There may be some early complaints of radiation exposure such as nausea or fatigue. The signs and symptoms of serious radiation exposure may not occur for several hours and do not suggest imminent death. Since radiation has a cumulative danger, shorter exposure times are less damaging.

The victim should be evacuated from the exposure area, along with the healthcare provider and first responders (DeLorenzo & Porter, 2000). Wind shifts are monitored continuously to minimize exposure. Triage is done to classify the clients into categories of immediate, delayed, and minimal. Comfort measures, such as psychologic support and empathy, are given to clients.

Flash blindness to the eyes caused by a detonation blast lasts only a few minutes during daylight and up to 30 minutes at night. Reassure clients that their eyesight will return and have someone remain with them until their sight is restored (DeLorenzo & Porter, 2000).

INTERDISCIPLINARY CARE

DISASTER PLANNING, RESPONSE, AND MITIGATION

In the United States, disaster preparedness has been a priority issue for government and military agencies. These efforts have been expanded to public and private healthcare sectors. Healthcare professionals are among the essential personnel in addressing disaster preparations and in dealing with the consequences of a disaster. Nurses comprise the largest group of healthcare professionals, and will play key roles in disaster relief whether they work in hospitals, residential facilities, ambulatory care, schools, or simply at home in their communities. The general public looks to nurses for information and trusts that what nurses advise is true and accurate. Nurses have a responsibility to be educated and to assimilate the new skills and demands necessary to assist clients, families, and communities in preparing for and responding to disastrous situations effectively.

Numerous disaster agencies are involved in disaster planning, response, and mitigation depending on the severity of the disaster and the resultant necessary response:

- A *Level I disaster* is dealt with effectively by local emergency response personnel and organizations.
- A *Level II disaster* requires mutual aid from surrounding communities and regional efforts.
- A *Level III disaster* overwhelms local and regional assets and statewide or federal assistance is required (Goolsby, Kulkarni, & Mothershead, 2006).

Agencies that may become involved include the Federal Emergency Management Agency (FEMA), the U.S. Army Corps of Engineers, the U.S. Department of Health and Human Services (DHHS), the American Red Cross (an international disaster relief agency), United Nations Headquarters of the Disaster Relief Organization, Pan American Health Organization (PAHO), International Reserve Committee, and local volunteer organizations such as the Boy Scouts of America, Goodwill Industries, and Volunteers of America. National agencies have state and local offices that respond to disasters. However, the most immediate response is from the local groups and organizations. Individual states may request aid from neighboring states or the federal government if the disaster exceeds local and state resources. The local disaster response organizations include fire departments, police departments, public health departments, public works, emergency services, and the local branch of the American Red Cross.

Local disaster response plans include action plans for various types of disaster situations, designation of the overall incident commander, and identification of community resources. The local emergency management agency is also represented in the state management planning efforts.

Hospitals and other healthcare agencies develop their own disaster plans. However, it is very important that each agency understands its role within the larger community disaster plan. When disasters occur, competing healthcare systems must put the competition aside and work collaboratively in the response effort to ensure favorable outcomes following the impact of the disaster.

STAGES AND PHASES OF A DISASTER

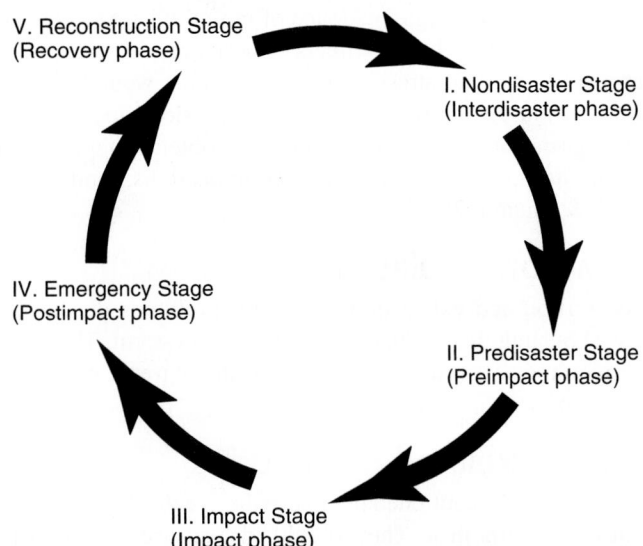

- V. Reconstruction Stage (Recovery phase)
- I. Nondisaster Stage (Interdisaster phase)
- II. Predisaster Stage (Preimpact phase)
- III. Impact Stage (Impact phase)
- IV. Emergency Stage (Postimpact phase)

Figure 7–1 ■ The stages of a disaster are cyclical. After a disaster, the planning cycle begins again, with evaluation of the current disaster plan and community response, debriefing with all disaster response agencies and personnel, and modifying disaster plans based on lessons learned.

Source: Illustration by Christina Langan Dalton.

The five stages of disaster preparedness are the *nondisaster* or *interdisaster* stage, the *predisaster* stage, the *impact* stage, the *emergency* stage, and the *reconstruction* or *rehabilitation* stage (Noji, 1997) (See Figure 7–1 ■). The nondisaster stage is the time for planning and preparation as the threat of a disaster is still in the future. It is a time for prevention, preparedness, and mitigation activities. The predisaster stage occurs when there is knowledge about an impending disaster that has not yet occurred. Activities during this stage include warning, preimpact mobilization, and evacuation if appropriate. The impact stage is a time when the disaster event has occurred and the community experiences the immediate effects. The emergency stage involves the immediate response to the effects of the disaster. The community relies on local assistance or aid because outside sources of aid have not yet arrived. In the reconstruction or recovery stage, restoration, reconstitution, and mitigation take place. This stage involves rebuilding and returning to some semblance of "normalcy" but also includes mitigation activities or planning to prevent subsequent disasters or to minimize the effects of future disasters (Langan, 2005b).

The key to effective disaster management is predisaster planning and preparation. Clark (2003a) states that the two purposes of disaster planning are to "reduce the community's vulnerability to the disaster and to prevent it, if possible, and to ensure that resources are available for effective response in the event of a disaster" (p. 634). A comprehensive emergency management plan addresses four major areas: mitigation, preparedness, response, and recovery.

Mitigation is the action taken to prevent or reduce the harmful effects of a disaster on human health or property. It involves future-oriented activities to prevent subsequent disasters or to minimize their effects. Mitigation may take the form of reinforcing highway overpasses and levees, sandbagging, developing communication strategies as backup systems to what is currently in place, and educating professionals and the public regarding preparation and response to disasters. A key nursing activity related to mitigation is the active participation in learning about the major aspects of disasters to remain current in their knowledge base and be able to teach the general public. Another mitigation activity is the anticipation of needed resources and policies to assist nurses and other professionals in implementing an effective disaster response.

Preparedness is having a comprehensive disaster plan in place that coordinates efforts among many people, agencies, and levels of government. The plan will be based on familiarity with possible disaster agents based on previous experiences, as well as experiences of others from various regions and countries. It is imperative that all persons and agencies who may be involved in the disaster response be involved in the planning. In this way, information is shared and representatives from each agency explain and offer their respective resources and expertise and note deficiencies in the plan. Planning committees will exist on all levels—federal, regional, state, local, and individual agency. Nurses participate in this facet of disaster planning by having a nurse representative on the planning committee at least at the agency level.

Response to disasters happens in the emergency stage, after the disaster event has occurred. The community has been rapidly assessed for damage, and the types and extent of injuries suffered as well as the immediate needs of the community have been determined. Hospital disaster planners must plan for the possibility that the next disaster may involve the hospital. The hospital's response may include the evacuation of clients as well as relocating and operating from an independent facility. **Surge capacity** is the healthcare system's ability to rapidly expand beyond normal services to meet the increased demand for qualified personnel, medical care, and public health in the event of a large-scale disaster. The Agency for Healthcare Research and Quality (2005) has published a report discussing the use of former "shuttered" hospitals to expand surge capacity during mass casualty events. Hospitals must be constantly aware of the number of beds available, which clients may be discharged, staffing, equipment, other resources, and their overall ability to manage casualties quickly.

The local community provides assistance or aid initially, because outside sources of aid have not yet arrived. Assistance from outside of the affected area arrives later and search and rescue operations commence as well as first aid, emergency medical assistance, establishment or restoration of communication and transportation, assessment of infectious diseases and mental health problems, and evacuation of residents, if necessary. Nurses should follow the disaster plan of their agencies, communities, and the local emergency management agency. This includes having a disaster plan for the nurse's immediate family. In this way, the nurse will feel secure in the fact that the immediate family is situated safely and the nurse can respond to the staging area to await instructions. Nurses use their expertise in infectious disease control and in assessing physical as well as psychosocial needs. In a disaster, mental health issues are extremely significant for victims, families, friends, first respon-

ders, and all healthcare workers. Nurses will ensure that clients receive follow-up care for both physical wounds and mental health concerns. Advanced practice nurses may take on significantly greater responsibilities especially if they are competent and prepared in emergency and trauma care. Protocols and standards of care are in place to guide the practice of all nurses. It is imperative that nurses determine the boundaries of their practice in times of emergencies when mass numbers of victims must be treated without the luxury of an on-site physician.

The **recovery** aspect of disaster response is also called **reconstruction**. During this stage, restoration, reconstitution, and mitigation take place. Restoration includes rebuilding, replacing lost or damaged property, returning to school and work, and continuing life without those who were killed in the disaster. Reconstitution occurs when the life of the community returns to a new "normal." The final stage of recovery is mitigation, which is also an activity in the preparation and planning aspects of the nondisaster stage. This illustrates the cyclical nature of planning and disaster response. The work is never complete. Future-oriented activities take place to prevent subsequent disasters or to minimize their effects. Some of these activities may include increased security and surveillance measures. Nurses may suggest ideas for responding to the victims of disasters more effectively and efficiently. For example, nurses may communicate the need for carts stocked with specific items that will assist them in treating clients faster. They may also suggest a more efficient method of tracking clients as they enter the healthcare system and move from area to area based on the clients' acuity and condition. Nurses will participate in mock disasters, read updated protocols, and practice their skills repeatedly to maintain competence. Mock disasters or disaster drills can take the form of tabletop exercises/discussions or simulated drills with "mock" victims. Mock disaster drills allow the participants to become familiar with the plan, and the areas that need strengthening in the plan will become evident (Langan, 2005b).

CASUALTY MANAGEMENT

During a disaster, nurses may be expected to perform triage. Nurses perform triage every day in every emergency department. **Triage** means sorting. A very basic triage system is to categorize or label victims needing the most support and emergency care as "red." Those less critical but still in need of transport to emergency centers for care are classified as "yellow." Victims who have minor injuries and do not warrant transport to an emergency center are categorized as "green." Victims who are least likely to survive or are already deceased are color coded as "black." (See Table 7–2.) These are the triage levels given to clients under normal circumstances or when there are only a few victims. However, when there is a mass casualty event with greater than 100 victims, **reverse triage** may be instituted. Reverse triage works on the principle of the greatest good for the greatest number. For example, if there were a collision between a train full of railroad cars filled with toxic chemicals and a full tour bus in a highly populated area, this disaster would likely be called a mass casualty event. In this case, those persons who were the most ambulatory and least injured would be transported or instructed to

TABLE 7–2 Simple Triage and Rapid Transport (START) System

Red (Immediate)	Critically injured, with problems that will require immediate intervention to correct. (Clients with a respiratory rate above 30 are tagged "red." If their respirations are below 30, assess their circulatory status. If capillary refill takes more than 2 seconds, tag them "red." If it is below 2 seconds, assess mental status.)
Yellow (Delayed)	Injured, and will require some medical attention, but they will not die if care is delayed while you care for other clients; not ambulatory and will require a stretcher for transportation. (Clients who can follow simple commands such as hand grips are tagged as "yellow." Clients who cannot follow simple commands are tagged "red.")
Green (Ambulatory)	Not critically injured, and can walk and care for themselves. (Have them walk to a safe place, but do not lose track of them; every client triaged at an incident is tracked to the best of the responder's ability.)
Black (Expectant)	Deceased, or have such catastrophic injuries that they are not expected to survive to be transported. (If the client is not breathing, open the airway manually. If they remain apneic, tag them "black"; if they begin breathing, they are tagged "red.")

Source: Adapted from Streger (n.d.). *Prehospital Triage.* Retrieved from http://www.emsmagazine.com/articles/emsarts/triage.html

move quickly to the warm zone, away from the immediate accident site to get decontaminated and processed first. (See Box 7–3.) Those with minor injuries would be decontaminated next. Those with more severe to most severe injuries would be treated in that order. In this way, the most victims with the greatest chance of survival could be saved most efficiently with limited resources. Many emergency personnel will share the difficulty of making these decisions at disaster sites when the first inclination might be to rescue the most severely injured.

Triage is a continuous process in which priorities are reassigned as needed treatments, time, and the condition of the victims change. This process must balance human lives with the realities of the situation, such as supplies and personnel. (See Box 7–4.) The triage role requires a person who is able to rapidly assess clients' conditions under stressful, often adverse conditions and assign a category. Those assigned to triage are expected to function independently, yet as part of a coordinated team effort (James et al., 2005). It has been suggested that emergency personnel should triage/categorize the victims so that physicians and nurses can be best utilized in the treatment area, performing client care. Advanced practice personnel will continue to triage and perform more complete assessments.

BOX 7–4 Key Triage Points to Remember

1. Use a triage system that is easy to learn, easy to implement in stressful conditions, and does not require advanced diagnostic skills yet allows for basic client interventions.
2. Use the Incident Management System on every incident and wear personnel identification vests.
3. Get accurate preliminary and final client counts and relay this information to the incident commander.
4. Use some type of visual color-coded identification system to indicate client priority.
5. Do not fall into the trap of using your time providing one-to-one client care.
6. Retriage clients frequently, at the incident, on arrival at the treatment area, and periodically thereafter.
7. Make certain the walking-wounded are gathered and treated.
8. Preplan for potential incidents that may occur.
9. Be aware that emergency responders may be potential targets.
10. Practice, practice, practice.

Source: Adapted from Streger (n.d.). *Prehospital Triage.* Retrieved from http://www.emsmagazine.com/articles/emsarts/triage.html

BOX 7–3 Hot, Warm, and Cold Zones

The site of the disaster where a weapon was released or where the contamination occurred is called the **hot zone**. It is considered contaminated and only those persons in the appropriate **personal protective equipment** (PPE) may enter this zone. PPE is equipment used for the protection of personnel including gloves, masks, goggles, gowns, and biologic disposal bags (Maniscalco & Christen, 2002). Typically, fire, police, and military personnel will collect evidence and begin their investigation in this zone. The **warm zone** is adjacent to the hot zone. Another name for this area is the *control zone*. This area is where decontamination of victims or triage and emergency treatment take place. The level of PPE required is based on the dynamic risk assessment of the threat and agent involved. The **cold zone** is considered to be the safe zone. It is adjacent to the warm zone and is the area where a more in-depth triage of victims would occur. Survivors may find shelter in this area, and the command and control vehicles would be found here as well as the emergency transport vehicles.

Isolation and Personal Protective Equipment

Persons suspected of having smallpox or some other highly contagious disease will need to be isolated from other clients, visitors, or healthcare personnel. For example, persons with pulmonary tuberculosis and a severe illness requiring hospitalization should be placed in a private room with negative-pressure ventilation. Clients are taught to cover their nose and mouth when coughing or sneezing. Persons entering the room (including nurses and other healthcare personnel) should wear personal respiratory protective devices capable of filtering submicron particles. Decontamination of the air may be achieved through ventilation and supplemented by ultraviolet light (Heymann, 2004).

Gas masks are used in a broad range of military, industrial, and emergency situations to protect the user from hazardous dust, gas, or other aerosols. Biologic contaminants that are spread through aerosolized droplets create a threat to those not wearing PPE. A gas mask may be considered a high-performance respirator and is usually equipped with both eye protection and air supply protection or treatment. A hood, helmet, or headgear is generally worn to protect the skin, eyes, airways, and respiratory systems. Protective clothing is made to guard against mild irritants and even serious lethal materials. Some protective suits are disposable, intended for one use only. Others are durable, multilayered fabrics that are completely impermeable and are reusable. The Occupational Safety and Health Administration (OSHA) has issued guidelines to inform healthcare workers and first responders about the correct level of PPE for various situations. The Chemical, Biological, Radiological, and Nuclear (CBRN) Personal Protection Equipment Selection Matrix for Emergency Responders and other information specific to PPE can be located online at the OSHA website.

In addition to the isolation of clients, special air handling systems are used in the isolation rooms to prevent the spread of the contaminated droplets into the general hospital air vents. Many hospitals also have the capability to shut off airflow in contaminated areas to prevent the spread of contaminants to other "clean" areas of the hospital. The heating, ventilation, air conditioning, and refrigeration (HVAC) systems are closely monitored and can be shut down in designated areas to avoid air intake from the outside as well, especially in cases of outdoor environmental contamination.

Recording Victim Data

The CDC has created a Mass Trauma Data Instrument (Figure 7–2 ■) to record data about victims of disasters. The categories on the data sheet include demographics, circumstances of the injury, injury conditions, and disposition and details of the conditions. The completion of this form will be initiated by the triage nurse and completed by the nurse who implements the treatment or transfers the client to another unit/department.

Crowd Control

When a disaster occurs, many people converge on the site. Those who come are the curious and those who truly mean to assist in the rescue and recovery of victims. However, this crowd of people needs to be controlled by authorities in charge of the site and rescue and recovery. Similarly, crowds may arrive at the hospital or healthcare delivery sites when injured or even when they just think they may be injured or contaminated in some way. The job of crowd control is not under the auspices of nurses or other healthcare personnel. The agency's security personnel and/or the local police force must control these crowds. If control is not maintained, chaos ensues and those in greatest need of medical assistance may be unable to reach healthcare providers in order to avoid further declines in their health status. In fact, nurses, physicians, and other healthcare workers should not enter an area that has not been secured. To put one's safety at risk jeopardizes the potential treatment of many. Additionally, social services personnel or psychiatric service providers should be available to assist the "worried well" cope with the trauma they have experienced or witnessed or simply heard about through the news media.

Psychosocial Needs

The importance of mental health services for victims, the public, first responders, and healthcare workers cannot be overstated. Both those persons directly affected by the disaster as well as those indirectly affected will seek medical care and advice. Many who seek medical attention are simply anxious about the threat of injury. At times, reassurance is all that is necessary. However, with large numbers of people seeking health care, the system is quickly overwhelmed. Mental health experts may quickly assess individual needs, offer immediate advice, and refer for follow-up care if deemed appropriate.

People react to disasters in a variety of ways, both physically and behaviorally. Their reactions depend on the severity of the threat and their proximity to the area of direct impact. The closer the person is to the area of impact and the longer the exposure, the greater the likelihood of a more severe reaction to the event. Table 7–3 summarizes the normal initial responses aimed at survival (Ganong, 1999; Murray & Zentner, 2001; Selye, 1965, 1980).

TABLE 7–3 Responses to Stress: General Adaptation Syndrome (Gas) and Levels of Anxiety

GAS STAGE	PHYSICAL RESPONSE	BEHAVIORS RELATED TO ANXIETY
Alarm Stage	Pupils dilate; blurred vision. Hearing sharper or diminished.	Misinterpret stimuli. Confusion. Poor concentration. Selective inattention. Need for assistance.
Severe Anxiety or Panic	Stronger, faster heart rate and respirations. Palpitations, arrhythmias, elevated blood pressure.	Feeling of impending doom. Terror. Fearful. Agitation. Irritability. Demanding. Impulsive. Paresthesias.
	Muscle tone increased. Headaches.	Muscle tension. Excitable, restless movements. Tremors. Rigidity. Weakness.
	Basal metabolism rate increased. Body temperature elevated. Perspiration. Altered glucose, protein, and lipid metabolism. Increased startle response.	Insomnia. Urgency of speech and movement. Fatigue. Dehydration. Weight loss. Appetite changes. Smooth muscle of gastrointestinal and urinary tracts less motile, interfering with digestion and elimination of wastes.
	Hypoglycemia from glycogenolysis due to high energy demands.	Blood glucose increase. Appetite changes. Dehydration. Fatigue. Poor concentration.
	Increased blood clotting and suppressed immune response if Stage persists.	Blood stasis; thrombus formation. Resistance to infection and disease reduced.

Abstractor _____   Case#_____

Mass Trauma Data Instrument

Demographics

Facility: _____   **Date:** ___ / ___ / ___   **Time:**_____ (24 hour)

Last Name: _____   **DOB:** ___ / ___ / ___   **Age:** _____ Yrs Months

First Name: _____   **Sex:** M   F   No Data

Medical Record #: _____   **Other:**_____

Circumstances of Injury

Reason for Visit: _____

How did the injury happen? _____

What was s/he doing? _____

Where did the injury occur? _____

Was the injury caused by the event?   ☐ Direct Effect   ☐ Indirect Effect   ☐ Not Event Caused   ☐ No Data

How Patient Arrived: ☐ Ambulance   ☐ Public Transportation   ☐ Private Vehicle

           ☐ Walked / Carried   ☐ Other: _____   ☐ No Data

Summary Information

Injury Condition(s): (Check all that apply)

☐ Amputation   ☐ Poisoning: _____
☐ Brain Injury (concussion)   ☐ Smoke Inhalation
☐ Burn: ____% ___Degree   ☐ Sprain / Strain / Dislocation
☐ Crush   ☐ Superficial (scrape/bruise)
☐ Cut / Open Wound
☐ Drowning / Submersion
☐ Foreign Body
☐ Fracture   ☐ Other: _____
☐ Overexertion   ☐ No Data

Other Condition(s): (Check all that apply)

☐ Abdominal Pain / N / V / Diarrhea
☐ Altered Mental Status / Coma
☐ Breathing Problem
☐ Chest Pain   ☐ Psychological Problem
☐ Eye / Vision Problem   ☐ Rash
☐ Fever
☐ Hearing Problem
☐ Neurologic Problem   ☐ Other: _____
☐ Pregnancy   ☐ No Data

Disposition: ☐ Hospitalized   ☐ Discharged Home   ☐ Transported to Other Medical Facility   ☐ Left / AMA

              ☐ Died   ☐ Other: _____   ☐ No Data

Details of Conditions

Condition #1: _____   **Body Part(s):**_____

Condition #2: _____   **Body Part(s):**_____

Condition #3: _____   **Body Part(s):**_____

Condition #4: _____   **Body Part(s):**_____

Figure 7–2 ■ The CDC's Mass Trauma Data Instrument.

Retrieved from http://www.bt.cdc.gov/masstrauma/word/rapidassessmentform.doc

Most people exhibit great coping mechanisms and resilience in the aftermath of a disaster. However, mechanisms should be developed for identifying and referring those who need psychologic counseling. After the September 2001 terrorist attacks on the World Trade Center and the Pentagon, it was reported that 71% of the persons surveyed felt depressed, 49% had difficulty concentrating, and 33% had trouble sleeping at night. Most (92%) felt sad when watching news coverage of the event, yet 63% stated a compulsion to continue to watch the news (Pew Research Center for the People and the Press, 2001). Reactions to terrorist events and disasters in general are influenced by developmental level and maturity, prior experiences with disasters, and cultural background (McLaughlin et al., 2005).

NURSING CARE

The Role of the Nurse in Disaster Relief

Because nurses have an obligation to keep current in new and emerging trends in health care and threats to society, learning about the prevention and mitigation of disasters is essential. Nurses must be aware of the roles they play in all aspects of disaster preparedness and response (Box 7–5.) It is imperative that nurses first know how to take care of themselves in order to assist others. By educating oneself and being proactive in regular drills and practice of skills, nurses take an active role in helping others to save lives and fulfill an important obligation to society.

Applying basic first aid skills can be very helpful in immediate disaster relief efforts until emergency help can be obtained. The American Red Cross invites nurse volunteers and will provide the necessary training. Many nurses have taken advantage of online disaster certificate programs, and efforts are being made to integrate disaster preparedness content into nursing courses.

BOX 7–5 Roles of Nurses in Disasters

1. Prepare selves, families, friends, and communities for disasters in conjunction with the local disaster preparedness plan.
2. Continue educating self on various types of disasters and appropriate response.
3. Provide emergency services with consideration of victims' abilities, deficits, culture, language, or special needs.
4. Assist in the mobilization of healthcare personnel, food, water, shelter, medication, clothing, and other assistive devices.
5. Collaborate with agencies in authority including local, state, and federal representatives to deploy resources based on the greatest good for the greatest number.
6. Consider needs of victims including shelter both temporary and permanent, as well as psychologic, economic, legal, and spiritual factors.
7. Become involved with local, state, and national disaster planning agencies to schedule regular meetings to continually review and modify disaster plans.

In many different practice settings, nurses serve on disaster preparedness and response planning committees. Nurses are receiving in-service education on biologic, chemical, and radiologic threats to client health as well as surveillance and reporting of suspicious activities. Although nursing professionals may not be asked to don decontamination gear to decontaminate victims, nurses should be aware of decontamination basics so that they will remain safe from exposure and be able to direct others when threatened with contamination. Some nurses choose to be actively involved with disaster medical assistance teams as part of the National Disaster Medical System.

In a true mass casualty event, it is impossible to have physicians present at every station where they are needed. Nurses may have to assume expanded roles in making decisions for the most appropriate treatment of casualties. Discussions should take place among physicians, nurses, and policy makers regarding the necessity of the nurses' expanded roles in crisis situations. As noted earlier in the chapter, these agency policies must be documented in the agency-wide plan. Additionally, all healthcare personnel must receive any specialized training required to be safe and competent practitioners of the expanded duties. This training must be practiced and updated and those participating in the training must be tracked and notified of additional requirements as necessary. See the Nursing Research box on page 138.

Implications for Nurses Working with Victims of Disasters

The role of the nurse in a disaster depends greatly on a number of variables including the nature of the disaster, the number of victims and severity of injuries, the location of the disaster as well as the location of the nurse, the availability of supplies, rescue and command personnel, and other necessary resources. The nurse must be able to perform under stressful conditions but will not be expected to endanger self, other nurses, or other rescuers.

If it is safe to do so, the nurse begins by triaging and assessing the victims for the best care and best use of available resources. Very quick, direct treatment may be given, or the nurse may be involved in extended periods of time with a mobile surgical unit. Local authorities such as the police, fire, and emergency medical services will guide the nurse in securing the area and determining the safe zone for the nurse and others to work. The National Disaster Medical System is the agency responsible for coordinating disaster relief with local fire, police, and emergency medical services to provide overall disaster assistance. Victim assistance may be offered in the field in mobile shelters, in local clinics, in hospitals, or in makeshift buildings.

Nurses take on a variety of roles based on their expertise and the needs of the victims. Nurses will be expected to follow the emergency preparedness plans outlined in their communities and in their agencies of employment. When a disaster occurs, it is not a time for individual creativity. However, individual nurses should be the leaders in their communities in discussing emergency preparedness and contingency plans.

NURSING RESEARCH   Evidence-Based Practice: Disaster Education

The nursing profession has recognized the need to develop resources to teach practicing and future nurses to improve their response to victims of radiologic, biologic, and chemical terrorism. However, nursing students may have different perceptions about working with disaster victims. The purpose of a descriptive study (Young & Persell, 2004) was to identify student nurses' major concerns and learning needs in working with victims of terrorism. Ninety-five junior and senior baccalaureate nursing students participated in the study by completing an anonymous questionnaire regarding their concerns about terrorism and how their lives had changed following September 11, 2001. The students' main concern was for the safety of themselves and their families. The students indicated they would not be willing to care for victims if there was a lack of protection for all types of terrorist agents for themselves and their families. The students did not demonstrate an accurate understanding of the pathogenic nature of many terrorist agents even though the nursing faculty members had provided self-education articles for the students. The students' concerns for specific infectious agents appeared to be based on unnecessary fear or inappropriate confidence.

IMPLICATIONS FOR NURSING

If nurses do not believe that a terrorist event is a real threat in their communities, they may not be motivated to become more pre-

pared for terrorist events. The nation's emergency healthcare planners and trauma nurses will have a major challenge preparing more nurses for disasters, especially mass casualty events. During a terrorist attack, the general public will seek information about the event from all healthcare providers. The public will also expect nurses to deliver safe and competent care to the victims of terrorism. Disaster care information should be a part of the curriculum in all basic nursing education schools. Continuing education and elective courses should continue to be planned. Basic disaster preparedness competencies should be required for all new graduate nurses so that they have a solid foundation on which to build.

CRITICAL THINKING IN CLIENT CARE

1. Make a list of all the barriers that nursing students and practicing nurses might express as reasons they do not need or value disaster/terrorism education and preparation.
2. Discuss the rationale for including basic disaster preparedness content in all basic nursing education programs.
3. Consider the results of this study. What could have been done differently to assist the nursing students in learning facts and the pathogenic nature of the terrorist agents presented in the articles?

Source: Adapted from "Biological, Chemical, and Nuclear Terrorism Readiness: Major Concerns and Preparedness of Future Nurses" by C. F. Young & D. Persell, 2004, *Disaster Management & Response, 2*(4), pp. 109–114.

Clients who have experienced disasters will present with a variety of individualized needs. Nursing diagnoses that may apply include:

- *Anxiety*
- *Communication, Verbal, Impaired*
- *Coping, Ineffective*
- *Fear*
- *Post-Trauma Syndrome, Risk for*
- *Powerlessness*
- *Injury, Risk for*
- *Trauma, Risk for*

Special Considerations

Older Adults

It is not appropriate to generalize needs to all older adults. Many are quite independent and active into their 90s. However, some older persons lack the physical stamina to recover quickly from disastrous events. The nurse must assess the individual's ability to cope with and recover from unexpected events, socioeconomic factors, support systems, potential healthcare needs, and resources. See the accompanying Nursing Care Plan.

Teaching about disaster preparedness is important in all communities. Older adults need to determine the appropriateness of "sheltering in place" should there be an environmental event outside of their homes, or of being evacuated if they are unable to care for themselves for extended periods of time. This becomes a very real issue when roads become impassable or usual modes of transportation and communication are disrupted.

A current list of medications, doses, and times of administration should be kept in an easily accessible, secure place. The names and phone numbers of significant persons, relatives, those with power of attorney, healthcare providers, or any others to be notified in case of emergency should also be kept in an easily accessible place. Additionally, the following materials should be considered essential in keeping with the person should evacuation to a shelter be necessary: eyeglasses and eyeglass prescriptions, style and serial numbers of medical devices such as pacemakers, healthcare policies and numbers, identification, list of allergies, blood type, checkbook, credit cards, insurance agent's name and number, driver's license, 72-hour supply of medications, dentures, list of special dietary needs, sturdy shoes, warm clothing, blankets, incontinence briefs, prostheses, hearing aids, hearing aid batteries, extra wheelchair batteries, oxygen, and other assistive devices (American Red Cross, n.d.).

Immunocompromised Clients

Clients who are immunocompromised pose special problems to the healthcare community especially if these persons are unable to access health care quickly in a disaster situation. A compromised immune system may be due to treatments such as chemotherapy or immunosuppressants or from an underlying disease such as HIV. The immunocompromised population would be at greater risk for complications and death than the general population should a bioterrorist attack occur. For example, a potential complication following smallpox vaccination is generalized vaccinia. It is believed to result from a

NURSING CARE PLAN   A Client with Injuries to Hands, Foot, and Suffering from Trauma of Natural Disaster

Mr. Ed Jones, a 75-year-old widower, is retired from his job as a cabinetmaker. He continues to work with wood as a hobby in the basement of his home located on the banks of the Deep River. He sells small toys at craft fairs and flea markets in nearby communities. His daughter lives approximately 20 minutes away and checks in on him at least every weekend. Mr. Jones is independent and sees his primary care physician occasionally for monitoring of his blood pressure, which is controlled with antihypertensive medications. Following a week of heavy rainstorms, flash flooding occurred in the area and Mr. Jones's basement sustained much water damage and ruined most of his stored wood, wooden toy products, and the woodworking machinery. Mr. Jones waded through the waist-deep water to get to the rescue boat rather than wait for the boat to get to him. He is subsequently admitted to the medical/surgical unit due to concerns from the EMTs who triaged him at the fire station 5 miles inland from Mr. Jones's neighborhood.

ASSESSMENT

Lisa Smith, RN, obtains a nursing assessment. Mr. Jones states that he has been on antihypertensive medications for "a few years" but only takes his medication "once in awhile" since it has been some time since his last office visit and he wants his remaining pills "to last" until he can get back to the doctor. He has had numerous cuts to his hands from his woodworking and has had a big ulcer on his right foot "for a few weeks" caused by a tool that fell on his foot. He did not seek medical care because he believed it would get better on its own. "It looks worse than it is. It really doesn't even hurt."

When asked about his home he stated, "Everything is gone. My wife is gone, my wood, my tools . . . it's all over."

Physical assessment findings include T 100.7°F PO, P 96, R 20, and BP 178/100. Skin cool and dry with multiple lesions on both hands and a Stage II ulcer on his right dorsal foot with yellow-green exudate. Pain rated at a 2 on a 10 scale with 10 being the worst pain there could be. Lungs are clear, heart rate regular. No edema noted. Abdominal assessment is normal. Neurologically intact. Weight is normal for height and frame. A culture is ordered and taken of the yellow-green exudate of the right foot.

Preliminary blood work results show WBCs at 15,000/mm³. A peripheral IV is initiated with continuous fluids and IV antibiotics are ordered every 6 hours. An antihypertensive medication is ordered on a regular schedule plus a prn antihypertensive for systolic >180 and diastolic >90.

DIAGNOSES

- *Impaired Skin Integrity* of the right foot and hands related to lesions (cuts) on the hands and Stage II ulcer with exudates on the right foot
- *Powerlessness* related to perceived loss of control over life situation
- *Ineffective Thermoregulation* related to trauma
- *Acute Pain* related to expression of pain secondary to skin lesions

EXPECTED OUTCOMES

- Regain skin integrity—ulcer on right foot and lesions on hands will heal.
- Identify aspects of his life still under his control.
- Maintain body temperature at normothermic levels.
- Express feeling of comfort and relief from pain.

PLANNING AND IMPLEMENTATION

- Inspect skin every shift; describe and document skin condition; report changes.
- Perform prescribed treatment regimen for skin condition. Clean lesions on hands and right foot every 8 hours and assess healing.
- Arrange psychosocial consult(s).
- Guide the client through a life review. Encourage reflection on past achievements.
- Help the client identify the aspects of his life that are still under his control.
- Allow the client the right to express feelings.
- Monitor client's body temperature every 4 hours, more often if indicated.
- Monitor and record client's heart rate and rhythm, blood pressure, and respiratory rate every 4 hours.
- Administer analgesics, antipyretics, and medications as indicated. Monitor and record their effectiveness.
- Maintain hydration; monitor intake and output.
- Assess client's signs and symptoms of pain and administer pain medication as prescribed. Monitor and record the medication's effectiveness and adverse effects.

EVALUATION

Mr. Jones was hospitalized for 3 days, receiving intravenous antibiotic therapy, analgesics, an antidepressant, monitoring of his cardiac response to a new antihypertensive medication, wound care, and sessions with the social services representative and his daughter. His hand lesions are healed, the foot ulcer has developed new granulation tissue with no signs of infection, he is afebrile, and his blood pressure is maintained within normal limits. He will be discharged to his daughter's home until his home can be assessed for the extent of the water damage and feasibility of repair. He has agreed to visit a therapist to work through his feelings of grief and loss. He has expressed an interest in attending monthly support group meetings with his neighbors who also experienced losses in this disaster.

CRITICAL THINKING IN THE NURSING PROCESS

1. What action did Mr. Jones take that probably exacerbated his skin lesions?
2. What other testing might you anticipate related to Mr. Jones's delayed healing?
3. What were the contributing factors to Mr. Jones's fever?
4. What life situations contributed to Mr. Jones's attitude about life?

See Evaluating Your Response in Appendix C.

vaccinia viremia with skin manifestations. In noncompromised persons, generalized vaccinia consists of vesicles or pustules appearing on normal skin distant from the vaccination site. The rash is generally self-limited and usually requires only supportive therapy. However, immunocompromised clients may have a toxic course and require vaccinia immune globulin (VIG), available only from the CDC (Cono et al., 2003).

An additional issue the nurse should discuss with this population is their preparation for disaster events related to infection control. Clients should carry treatment calendars with them at all times so that any healthcare provider can determine where they are in their treatment program and disease process. Clients should plan a backup location to visit for chemotherapy if their usual office is inaccessible. Nurses should also assess their clients' knowledge level regarding the avoidance of raw seafood or possibly contaminated water. Bottled water should be ready so the client can avoid drinking water of questionable purity. Bone marrow transplant clients are instructed not to eat fresh fruits and vegetables due to the risk of contamination and subsequent infection. It is safest for this population of clients to consume processed or canned foods if they can be heated to the proper temperatures.

Clients with Sensory, Speech, or Literacy Deficits

Persons who have sensory deficits, speech or language impairments, or who are illiterate must be assessed for the most effective means of communicating steps to be taken in the case of a disaster. One cannot generalize that all people with hearing impairments or speech impairments will choose a particular means of communication. This may be an individual preference. A multitude of communication means are available through technological support systems as well as written and visual cue boards. Public service announcements may inform the general public about impending natural disasters and about proper steps to be taken to be safely rescued or sheltered. Nurses are in the position of alerting community leaders about special needs of members of their communities. Public service personnel, including fire, police, and emergency services, should be alerted to extenuating circumstances and needs of specific individuals in the community. The collaborative planning efforts of the individual, family members, caregivers, and emergency service personnel will help alleviate any undue pain and suffering caused by the lack of understanding of emergency messages and directives.

Clients with Mobility and Sensory Deficits

The U.S. Department of Health and Human Services (2005) has estimated that 13% of the U.S. population experiences some form of activity limitation due to a chronic condition. Many persons require the use of assistive technology devices (ATDs) to accommodate mobility and other impairments. Careful planning must be in place in order to provide necessary support during and after a disaster. Arrangements must be made in advance to provide adequate numbers of volunteers or staff to assist

when this group must be relocated or regrouped in a safe room or shelter. These individuals or their caregivers must provide input to service personnel to determine what kind of support services would be necessary in an emergency or disaster. Emergency personnel or rescue teams may need to learn a few basic phrases in American Sign Language. Something as simple as carrying a notepad and pencil or directions in large print may be just what is necessary to share information with people who have hearing impairments or visual impairments, respectively.

Non-English-Speaking Clients

The literacy of non-English-speaking clients should be assessed in both their own language and in English. One cannot assume that individuals are literate in their own language. It is ideal to obtain the assistance of an interpreter, preferably an interpreter with whom the client is familiar, to assist in translating information for the client. Communication aids can be prepared in advance of disasters to be used during emergencies. The communication aids or disaster preparedness and response procedures should be practiced on a regular basis prior to an emergency. The use of visual aids is very helpful. Do not use children as interpreters if adults are available. The stress of interpretation can be overwhelming to the children and place an unnecessary burden on them.

Spiritual Considerations

Religion tends to be a source of comfort for those who are experiencing the threat of loss of life, property, or way of living. Churches, synagogues, and clergy become active in supporting their congregations in times of disaster. Religious leaders should be actively involved in community planning for disaster preparedness especially if certain religious considerations should be strictly followed. For example, in some religions, the human body and all of its parts are considered sacred. To be sensitive to this religious belief, all tissues and blood would be collected at the site of a disaster by those trained to collect such material versus washing this matter away from the scene. In general, rescue personnel would need to be informed of specific religious obligations or rights to be able to be sensitive to the individual's religious beliefs and practices.

Summary

Nurses are invaluable in disaster relief efforts whether they are answering questions from their neighbors regarding the water supply in their communities or assisting in complex care using their advanced practice knowledge in a hospital.

Nurses have a responsibility to the public to maintain competence in nursing practice and to be cognizant of evolving threats to the public's health. Nurses must learn about anticipated and unexpected disasters as well as their vital roles in emergency preparedness and response. Nurses will play a role in disaster response whether they work in acute care settings, long-term care, ambulatory care or in the community, and at home.

EXPLORE MediaLink

Prentice Hall Nursing MediaLink DVD-ROM
Audio Glossary
NCLEX-RN® Review

COMPANION WEBSITE www.prenhall.com/lemone
Audio Glossary
NCLEX-RN® Review
Care Plan Activity: Clients Experiencing Disasters
Case Study: Disaster Scenario
MediaLink Applications
Links to Resources

CHAPTER HIGHLIGHTS

- Disasters require extraordinary efforts beyond those needed to respond to everyday emergencies.
- Nurses have an obligation to keep current in new and emerging trends in health care and threats to society.
- Learning about the prevention and mitigation of bioterrorism and disasters in general is essential.
- Reverse triage is used in mass casualty events instead of traditional triage in order to do the greatest good for the greatest number.

- Nurses will be actively engaged in assessing the physical as well as the mental needs of victims, their families, first responders, and other healthcare personnel.
- Nurses need to have their own family disaster plans in place to be able to assist others in times of disasters.
- Nurses are actively involved in disaster mitigation, planning, and response efforts by learning and practicing their communities' and agencies' disaster preparedness systems.

TEST YOURSELF NCLEX-RN® REVIEW

1 The key difference between emergencies and disasters is that:
1. emergencies are controlled.
2. disasters result from man-made errors.
3. emergencies can typically be handled by available emergency services.
4. disasters typically involve the local emergency services and no other agencies.

2 Which of the following is NOT true regarding nurses' responsibilities in disaster preparedness?
1. Nurses have a responsibility to the public to be knowledgeable about disaster preparedness and response.
2. Nurses must have a personal and family plan as a part of their disaster preparedness and response plan.
3. Nurses will be the leaders in the incident command structure set up at the site of the disaster.
4. Nurses who are prepared for disasters will be better able to help themselves, their families, and their communities in a disaster situation.

3 The purpose of reverse triage is to:
1. save scarce resources for future use.
2. test first responders on their triage classification categories.
3. save those persons who are in the most critical condition.
4. do the greatest good for the greatest number with limited resources.

4 It is important to assess clients' literacy in their primary language because:
1. they are most comfortable speaking in their primary language.
2. they are most comfortable reading in their primary language.
3. they may not be able to read and comprehend in their primary language.
4. they may be too shy to communicate in English if it is not their primary language.

5 Which of the following is true about personal protective equipment (PPE)?
1. PPE protects by creating a barrier against hazards.
2. Eye, face, head, foot, and hand protection are addressed in PPE programs.
3. PPE should reduce the likelihood of occupational injury and/or illness.
4. Healthcare workers do not need to wear PPE if they follow strict hand washing protocol and universal precautions.

6 Which of the following is NOT true about decontamination?
1. Decontamination corridors should be set up in an area downwind from the hospital entrance.
2. Decontamination begins in the hot zone, closest to the site of the disaster.
3. Decontamination must take place before the client enters the hospital.
4. Decontaminating a person should be done by sweeping strokes away from you and the client.

7 Another name for a radiological dispersion bomb is:
1. a dirty bomb.
2. an ionization radiation bomb.
3. a nonfiltered bomb.
4. a radio-controlled remote bomb.

8 One of the results of DNA mutation inside cells exposed to ionizing radiation that can be deadly, but is survivable with bone marrow transplantation, is a description of:
1. ionizing sickness.
2. radiation sickness.
3. TNT sickness.
4. compromised immune sickness.

9 Nurses should assess the special needs of older adults as part of the emergency preparedness plan because:
1. all older adults will need some kind of special support.
2. some older adults will take the lead in evacuation efforts in nursing homes.
3. not all older adults need the same level of support in emergencies and disasters.
4. some older adults will be unable to evacuate even with multiple support agencies.

10 Nurses may need the assistance of a mental health worker following a disaster because:
1. all nurses need the help of a mental health worker at one point or another in their nursing careers.
2. nurses are often suffering from loss during a disaster while caring for survivors.
3. the nurse may feel as overwhelmed and traumatized as the population for whom she or he is caring.
4. b and c.

See Test Yourself answers in Appendix C.

BIBLIOGRAPHY

Agency for Healthcare Research and Quality. (2005, September). *Use of former ("shuttered") hospitals to expand surge capacity.* Retrieved January 16, 2006, from http://www.ahrq.gov/research/shuttered/

American Red Cross. (2006). *American Red Cross and IOM open new homes in Indonesia.* Retrieved October 20, 2006 from http://www.redcross.org/article/0,1072, 0_332_5110,00.html

American Red Cross. (2001). *Disaster preparedness for seniors by seniors.* Retrieved May 15, 2005, from http://www.redcross.org/services/disaster/beprepared/ seniors.html

American Red Cross. (n.d.). *Your evacuation plan.* Retrieved January 16, 2006, from http://www.redcross.org/services/ disaster/0,1082,0_6_,00.html

Beachley, M. (2000). Nursing in a disaster. In C. M. Smith & F. A. Maurer (Eds.), *Community health nursing* (pp. 424–445). Philadelphia: W. B. Saunders.

Centers for Disease Control and Prevention. (2003a, March 17). *Explosions and blast injuries: A primer for clinicians.* Retrieved May 14, 2005, from http://www.bt.cdc.gov/ masstrauma/explosions.asp

Centers for Disease Control and Prevention. (2003b, June 2). *Mass trauma data instrument.* Retrieved May 14, 2005, from http://www.bt.cdc.gov/masstrauma/word/ rapidassessmentform.doc

Centers for Disease Control and Prevention. (2006, February 22). *Fact sheet: Anthrax information for health care providers.* Retrieved July 31, 2006, from http://www.bt.cdc.gov/ agent/anthrax/anthrax-hcp-factsheet.asp#cutaneous

Centers for Disease Control and Prevention. (n.d.). Key facts about hurricane recovery: Protect your health and safety after a hurricane. Retrieved January 16, 2006, from http://www.bt.cdc.gov/disasters/hurricanes/recovery.asp

Clark, M. J. (2003a). Care of clients in disaster settings. In M. J. Clark, *Community health nursing: Caring for populations* (4th ed., pp. 623–653). Upper Saddle River, NJ: Pearson/Prentice Hall.

Clark, M. J. (2003b). Information on selected communicable diseases. In M. J. Clark, *Community health nursing: Caring for populations* (4th ed., pp. 781–782). Upper Saddle River, NJ: Pearson/Prentice Hall.

Cono, J., Casey, C. G., & Bell, D. M. (2003). Smallpox vaccination and adverse reactions. *MMWR, 52*(RR04), 1–28.

Cooper, M. A. (1995, September). *Emergent care of lightning and electrical injuries.* Retrieved May 14, 2005, from http://www.uic.edu/abs/lightninginjury/treatment.html

County of Henrico (n.d.). *Community disaster preparedness manual.* Retrieved April 27, 2005, from http://www.co. henrico.va.us/fire/cpm_man.pdf

DeLorenzo, R. A., & Porter, R. S. (2000). *Weapons of mass destruction: Emergency care.* Upper Saddle River, NJ: Prentice Hall Health.

Federal Emergency Management Agency. (2005). *Are you ready? Hurricanes.* Retrieved January 31, 2006, from http://www.fema.gov/areyouready/hurricanes.shtm

Ganong, W. (1999). *Review of medical physiology* (19th ed.). Stamford, CT: Appleton and Lange.

Ganor, B. (n.d.). *Biological terrorism.* Retrieved May 14, 2005, from http://www.ict.org.il/inter_ter/noncon.htm#biological

Goolsby, C., Kulkarni, R., & Mothershead, J. L. (2006). *Disaster planning.* Retrieved August 1, 2006, from http://www. emedicine.com/emerg/topic718.htm

Harris, T. (2005). *How dirty bombs work.* Retrieved April 23, 2005, from http://www.howstuffworks.com/ dirty-bomb1.htm

Heymann, D. L. (2004). *Control of communicable diseases manual* (18th ed., pp. 20–25, 568–569). Washington, DC: American Public Health Association.

Hoffman, B. (2003). Terrorism. *In Microsoft Encarta Online Encyclopedia 2003.* Retrieved February 22, 2003, from http://encarta.msn.com/encnet/frefpages/RefArtTextOnly. asp?refid=761564344&print=3

International Nursing Coalition for Mass Casualty Education. (2003, August). *Educational competencies for registered nurses related to mass casualty incidents.* Retrieved May 1, 2005, from http://www.aacn.nche.edu/Education/pdf/ INCMCECompetencies.pdf

James, D. C., Langan, J. C., Sandkuhl, H., & Benbenishty, J. (2005). Preparing staff and inactive registered nurses to manage casualties. In J. C. Langan & D. C. James (Eds.), *Preparing nurses for disaster management* (pp. 95–123). Upper Saddle River, NJ: Pearson/Prentice Hall.

Langan, J. C. (2005a). Disasters: A basic overview. In J. C. Langan & D. C. James (Eds.), *Preparing nurses for disaster management* (pp. 1–16). Upper Saddle River, NJ: Pearson/Prentice Hall.

Langan, J. C. (2005b). Planning for disasters. In J. C. Langan & D. C. James (Eds.), *Preparing nurses for disaster management* (pp. 17–33). Upper Saddle River, NJ: Pearson/Prentice Hall.

Maniscalco, P. M., & Christen, H. T. (2002). *Understanding terrorism and managing the consequences.* Upper Saddle River, NJ: Pearson/Prentice Hall.

McLaughlin, D. E., Murray, R. B., & Benbenishty, J. (2005). Promoting mental health: Predisaster and postdisaster. In J. C. Langan & D. C. James (Eds.), *Preparing nurses for disaster management* (pp. 55–77). Upper Saddle River, NJ: Pearson/Prentice Hall.

Murray, R. B., & Zentner, J. (2001). *Health promotion strategies through the life span* (7th ed.). Upper Saddle River, NJ: Pearson/Prentice Hall.

Myers-Walls, J. A. (2005). Children as victims of Hurricane Katrina. Retrieved February 12, 2006, from http:// www.ces.purdue.edu/cfs/topics/HD/ChildrenVictims HurrKatrina.pdf

National Institute for Occupational Safety and Health. (2001, September). *Eye safety for emergency response and disaster recovery.* Retrieved May 11, 2005, from http://www.cdc.gov/niosh/eyesafe.html

National Institute of Mental Health. (2002). *Mental health and mass violence: Evidence-based early psychological interventions for victims/survivors of mass violence. A workshop to reach consensus on best practices* (NIH Publication No. 02-5138). Washington, DC: U.S. Government Printing Office.

Noji, E. K. (1997). The nature of disaster: General characteristics and public health effects. In E. K. Noji (Ed.), *The public health consequences of disasters* (pp. 3–20). New York: Oxford University Press.

North Carolina Department of Health and Human Services. (n. d.). *After the storm: Injury prevention.* Retrieved May 14, 2005, from http://www.dhhs.state.nc.us/docs/ hurricanepreventinjury.htm

Occupational Safety and Health Administration. (2004, August 30). *CBRN personal protective equipment selection matrix for emergency responders.* Retrieved May 14, 2005, from http://www.osha.gov/SLTC/emergency preparedness/ cbrnmatriz/index.html

Pacific Tsunami Museum. (2001). *Tsunami glossary.* Retrieved February 12, 2006, from http://www.tsunami.org/ definitions.htm

Payne, C. (2003, September). Definition of terrorism. *World Conflict Quarterly.* Retrieved April 23, 2005, from http://www.globalterrorism101.com/UTDefinition.html

Pew Research Center for the People and the Press. (2001). *American psyche reeling from terror attacks.* Retrieved August 24, 2005, from http://people-press.org/reports/ display.php3?ReportID=3

Pryor, T. (2005). Remembering the tsunami: Story of hope. *Reflections on Nursing Leadership,* 4th Quarter, pp. 26–27.

Rebmann, T. (2005). The role of the infection control nurse in disaster preparedness. In J. C. Langan & D. C. James (Eds.), *Preparing nurses for disaster management* (pp. 199–218). Upper Saddle River, NJ: Pearson/Prentice Hall.

Scott, S. G., Vanderploeg, R. D., Belanger, H. G., & Scholten, J. D. (January, 2005). Blast injuries: Evaluating and treating the postacute sequelace. *Federal Practitioner, 67–75.*

Selye, H. (1965). Stress syndrome. *American Journal of Nursing, 65*(3), 97–99.

Selye, H. (1980). The stress concept today. In I. C. Kutash and L. B. Schlesinger (Eds.), *Handbook on stress and anxiety* (pp. 127–144). New York: Jossey Bass.

Simonsen, C. E., & Spindlove, J. R. (2004). *Terrorism today.* Upper Saddle River, NJ: Pearson/Prentice Hall.

Smith, C. M., & Maurer, F. A. (2000). *Community health nursing: Theory and practice* (2nd ed.). Philadelphia: W. B. Saunders.

Sparks Ralph, S., & Taylor, C. M. (2005). *Nursing diagnosis: Reference manual* (6th ed.). Philadelphia: Lippincott Williams & Wilkins.

Stevens, J., & Slone, L. (2005). *Tsunami and mental health: What can we expect?* Retrieved January 16, 2006, from http://www.ncptsd.va.gov/facts/disasters/fs_tsunami_ Mental_Health.html

United Nations Office for Drug Control and Crime Prevention. (2002). *Conventional terrorist weapons.* Retrieved April 23, 2005, from http://www.undcp.org/odccp/terrorism_ weapons_conventional.html

U.S. Department of Health and Human Services. (2005). *Health United States, 2005.* Washington, DC: Author.

U. S. Department of Homeland Security. (2005). *Emergencies & disasters.* Retrieved August 14, 2006, from http://www.dhs.gov/interwlb/assetlibrary/Katrina.htm

U.S. Department of State. (2006). *Fact sheet: Guidance for responding to radiological and nuclear incidents.* Washington, DC. Retrieved July 31, 2006, from http://travel.state.gov/travel/tips/health/health_1184.html

World Health Organization. (2006). *Smallpox.* Retrieved August 1, 2006, from http://www.who.int/mediacentre/ factsheets/smallpox/en/index.html

Young, C. F., & Persell, D. (2004). Biological, chemical, and nuclear terrorism readiness: Major concerns and preparedness of future nurses. *Disaster Management & Response, 2*(4), 109–114.

UNIT 2 BUILDING CLINICAL COMPETENCE
Alterations in Patterns of Health

FUNCTIONAL HEALTH PATTERN: Health Perception-Health Management

■ Think about clients with altered health perception or health management for whom you have cared in your clinical experiences.

- What were the clients' major medical diagnoses (e.g., a surgical procedure, terminal illness, impending death, substance abuse, or victim of multiple or mass casualty incident)?
- What manifestations did each of these clients have? Were these manifestations similar or different?
- How did the clients' healthcare behaviors interfere with their health status? Have the clients had surgery before? Did the clients experience any complications due to having surgery? Did they have any problems with anesthesia? What medications were the clients taking? Did they take medications as prescribed? Did they use any substances other than prescribed medications and over-the-counter medications? If so, what substances and how much were used? How much alcohol did the clients drink? Has substance abuse caused a problem for the clients or their family, friends, finances, and health? Were the clients exposed to environmental hazards? Did the clients have sensory deficits or sight or speech impairments? What language did they speak? What spiritual or religious considerations did they verbalize? Did they have living wills, do-not-resuscitate orders, or powers of attorney? Have end-of-life issues been discussed with the family?

■ The Health Perception-Health Management Pattern includes healthcare behaviors, such as health promotion and illness prevention activities, medical treatments, and follow-up care. Individuals may or may not have the ability to change their healthcare practices. Health perception and health maintenance are affected by perceived health status in two primary ways:

- Factors that interfere with health care are lack of understanding of basic health practices (e.g., altered cognition, altered coping), inability to take responsibility for meeting health needs (e.g., alcoholism, substance abuse), or lack of communication skills (e.g., non-English-speaking, illiterate).
- Factors that interfere with the desire to seek a higher level of wellness are inability to change declining health status (e.g., cancer, kidney failure, impending death), need for treatment (e.g., surgery), catastrophic events (e.g., motor vehicle crash injuries, weather-related event injuries, thermal or chemical burns).

■ A client's perceived pattern of health and well-being affects how health is managed. Unexpected events can alter the client's health status, leading to manifestations such as:

- Anxiety (uneasy feeling of the unknown ► resulting in sympathetic nervous system responses)
- Grief (physical and emotional responses ► due to loss or impending loss ► resulting in withdrawal of attachment)
- Death (irreversible condition ► resulting from cessation of circulatory and respiratory functions or irreversible cessation of all functions of the brain).

■ Priority nursing diagnoses within the Health Perception and Health Management Pattern that may be appropriate for clients include:

- *Impaired Skin Integrity* as evidenced by surgical incisions, injuries due to accidents or falls, physical immobility, and skin changes in older adults
- *Risk for Injury* related to misuse of drugs and alcohol, environmental hazards, intraoperative complications, and inadequate postoperative care
- *Ineffective Therapeutic Regimen Management* as evidenced by economic difficulties, lack of knowledge of health care, and mistrust of healthcare personnel
- *Powerlessness* as evidenced by expressed inability to carry out treatment regimen, loss of control due to chronic or debilitating conditions, and dependency on others.

■ Two nursing diagnoses from other functional health patterns often are of high priority for the client with deficits in Health Perception-Health Management:

- *Impaired Verbal Communication* (Cognitive-Perceptual)
- *Ineffective Individual Coping* (Coping-Stress-Tolerance)

CLINICAL SCENARIO

You have been assigned to work with the following four clients for the 0700 shift on a hospital medical-surgical unit. Significant data obtained during report are as follows:

- Peter Black is a 46-year-old who was admitted from the emergency department 2 hours ago for observation after being thrown 50 yards during a tornado. His vital signs on admission were stable: T 99.8°F, P 86, R 24, and BP 140/ 86. He had multiple abrasions and lacerations that were sutured in the emergency room. He is now complaining of numbness in both legs.
- Mary Black is the 44-year-old wife of Peter Black. She was admitted 1 hour ago with a fracture of the left ankle, multiple abrasions, and ecchymotic areas. She is scheduled to go to surgery at 0900 for an open reduction of the fracture. Current vital signs are T 99°F, P 90, R 26, BP 134/88. She is requesting pain medication and wants to see her children, who were admitted to the pediatric unit, before going to surgery.
- John Linzer, age 67, was admitted 1 week ago in the terminal stages of colon cancer. Vital signs are T 96.8°F, P 54, R 10, BP 88/68. The family is requesting that a nurse check on Mr. Linzer because they feel that death is imminent.
- Paul Goetz, age 47, was admitted 3 days ago after being found unconscious in his car. On admission his alcohol level was 0.45. Current vital signs are T 100°F, P 110, R 30, BP 168/94. He is diaphoretic, disoriented, complaining of nausea, and seeing spiders on the wall.

Questions

1 In what order would you visit these clients after report?

1. _____
2. _____
3. _____
4. _____

2 What top two priority nursing diagnoses would you choose for each of the clients presented above? Can you explain, if asked, the rationale for your choices?

	Priority Nursing Diagnosis #1	Priority Nursing Diagnosis #2
Peter Black		
Mary Black		
John Linzer		
Paul Goetz		

3 You need to complete preoperative preparation on Mrs. Black. In which order would you complete nursing interventions? (Arrange your choices in order from first to last.)

1. Remove nail polish.
2. Have client void.
3. Get operative permit signed.
4. Administer preoperative medication as ordered.
5. Document all preoperative care.

4 Mrs. Black understands the postoperative teaching done by the nurse when she states:

1. "I will need to stay still in the bed to prevent pain."
2. "I will need to cough frequently to remove fluids from my lungs."
3. "Since I will have a PCA machine for pain medication, I will not have to ask for pain medication."
4. "I will be able to eat and drink as soon as I return from surgery."

5 The nurse explains to Mrs. Black that a diet of protein, increased calories, and vitamins are necessary for healing wounds after surgery. Mrs. Black understands this diet when she picks which meal plan?

1. hamburger, french fries, and a cola beverage
2. tossed salad, chocolate pudding, and iced tea
3. fried chicken, broccoli and cheese, and lemonade
4. salmon patty, baked potato, and milk

6 After assessing Mr. Black, which nursing intervention should the nurse perform first?

1. Call the physician to report the numbness in his legs.
2. Have Mr. Black perform active exercises to prevent thrombosis in his legs.
3. Ambulate Mr. Black in the hall to promote circulation to his legs.
4. Medicate Mr. Black for pain so he can move his legs better.

7 With a history of alcoholism for 5 years, what is a priority nursing intervention in the plan of care for Mr. Goetz?

1. Identify maladaptive behaviors that may contribute to the alcoholism.
2. Encourage participation in therapeutic group activities.
3. Teach the effects of alcohol on the body.
4. Use a respectful, nonjudgmental approach to gain trust.

8 A prescription for naltrexone (ReVia) is given to Mr. Goetz upon discharge. He voices understanding of how to take the medication when he states:

1. "I must avoid all forms of alcohol and narcotics while taking this medication."
2. "It is all right to take over-the-counter cold medications if I catch a cold."
3. "This medication will keep me from having withdrawal symptoms."
4. "I can get physically ill if I drink alcohol while taking this medication."

9 When Mr. Goetz was admitted to the emergency department, which laboratory studies would you expect to have been drawn? (Select all that apply.)

1. UDS
2. electrolytes
3. ALK
4. complete blood cell count
5. AST
6. BAL

10 To prepare the family for Mr. Linzer's death, the nurse institutes the following interventions:

1. Teach the stages of coping with the loss of their family member.
2. Explain the physical symptoms they may see as death approaches.
3. Discuss funeral and burial arrangements with the family.
4. Refer family to appropriate support groups to assist in dealing with death.

11 When preparing for the role the nurse will play in disaster relief, the nurse must first:

1. be able to apply basic first aid skills.
2. be aware of decontamination procedures.
3. serve on disaster preparedness committees.
4. know how to take care of himself or herself.

12 Older adult clients are at increased risk for complications from surgery. Which complications does the nurse need to be prepared to treat, if they occur?

1. hypotension, hypothermia, and hypoxemia
2. hypertension, hyperthermia, and aspiration
3. tachycardia, hypertension, and tachypnea
4. bradycardia, hypotension, and bradypnea

CASE STUDY

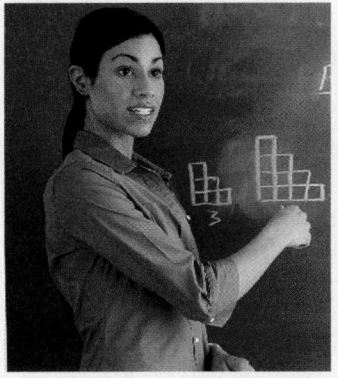

Mrs. Maria Rodriguez is admitted to the emergency department with open left fractures of the tibia and fibula, left upper quadrant pain, and reddened areas across the left shoulder, neck, and chest. According to the paramedics, she was involved in a multiple-car crash on an icy highway. On initial assessment she is found to be a non-English-speaking Hispanic, 28 years of age, is 5' 2" in height, and weighs 120 pounds. Her vital signs are T 100°F, P 100, R 28 and shallow, BP 150/86. She indicates her pain scale level as 9 out of 10, even after being medicated with morphine in the ambulance.

After chest, abdominal, and leg x-rays, Mrs. Rodriguez is diagnosed with crushing injury and comminuted fractures of the left tibia and fibula, a hematoma on her spleen, and bruising across the shoulder, neck, and chest due to the seat belt. With the use of a translator, the physician explains that she will have to have surgery to repair her fractures. Mrs. Rodriguez begins crying and wringing her hands after speaking with the physician.

Blood is drawn for the following laboratory studies: complete blood count (CBC) with differential, electrolytes, prothrombin time (PT), partial thromboplastin time (PTT), and blood gases. A urine specimen is sent to the laboratory for a urinalysis. Preoperative preparation is completed. The nurse tries to calm the client and answer any questions she has regarding the surgery and what will happen in the postoperative period. The nurse attempts to contact family members and a priest to see the client before she goes to surgery. At the ordered time, the nurse administers prescribed preoperative medication and Mrs. Rodriguez is sent to the operating room.

Due to difficulty understanding the English language, pain, and the need for surgery, Mrs. Rodriguez is very anxious. The nursing diagnosis of *Anxiety* is appropriate for guiding preoperative nursing care. Anxiety is an uneasy feeling of not knowing what is going to happen. The pathophysiology of anxiety is anticipation of danger or a threat to health status that leads to a "fight-or-flight" response from the sympathetic nervous system. Manifestations of anxiety are restlessness, tachycardia, rapid breathing, facial flushing, increased perspiration, weakness, tremors, and impaired attention and concentration. Complications of anxiety are nausea, vomiting, diarrhea, loss of appetite, insomnia, immobility, and powerlessness that can lead to panic or phobias.

Based on Mrs. Rodriguez's medical diagnosis and treatment plan, *Anxiety* is identified as the priority nursing diagnosis at this time.

Pathophysiology
- Anxiety may occur in response to a situational stressor.
- In severe anxiety, the person experiences a sense of doom and terror.

affects → **Mrs. R**
28 y.o. female
Trauma/fractures

leads to ↓

assess →
- Open fractures of left lower fibula and tibia
- Severe pain in leg and abdomen
- Crying, wringing hands, agitated
- P 90, R 32
- Family not present
- Only speaks Spanish

generates →
- Acute Pain related to fractures and abdominal injury
- Risk for Infection related to injury to left lower leg
- Impaired Tissue Integrity related to open fractures of left lower leg

generate nursing diagnosis ↓   *prioritized to* →

Anxiety

expected outcomes ↓

- Crying lessens and agitation decreases
- Pulse and respirations decrease
- Verbalize anxiety about going to surgery
- Priest will visit prior to surgery
- Family will be at bedside following surgery

evaluate →
- Crying and agitation decreased
- Pulse and respiratory rates decreased
- Verbalizes fear of loss of job and caring for children after surgery
- Family contacted and on their way to the hospital

Interdisciplinary Interventions
- Request interpreter to explain what is happening and what will be done
- Request visit by priest prior to surgery
- Request assistance from social service in locating family

Independent Interventions
- Approach with a calm, reassuring manner and use a soft voice and touch as appropriate
- Use therapeutic communications to encourage verbalization of fears
- Use interpreter to explain all preoperative and postoperative care
- Assist in taking slow, deep breaths

UNIT
3

Pathophysiology and Patterns of Health

CHAPTER 8 Genetic Implications of Adult Health Nursing

LEARNING OUTCOMES

- Discuss the role of genetic concepts in health promotion and health maintenance.

- Apply knowledge of the principles of genetic transmission and risk factors for genetic disorders.

- Describe the significance of delivering genetic education and counseling follow-up in a professional manner.

- Identify the implications of genetic advances on the role of nurses with particular attention to spiritual, cultural, ethical, legal, and social issues.

- Identify the significance of recent advances in human genetics and the impact on healthcare delivery.

CLINICAL COMPETENCIES

- Integrate genetic physical assessment and the use of a pedigree family history into delivery of nursing care.

- Identify clients or families with actual or potential genetic conditions and initiate referrals to a genetics professional.

- Prepare clients and their families for a genetic evaluation and facilitate the genetic counseling process.

- Integrate basic genetic concepts into client and family education and the reinforcement of information provided to clients by genetic professionals.

The genetic knowledge obtained from the Human Genome Project (Box 8–1) has changed not only the way disease treatment is approached but, more importantly, how nurses look at health promotion and health maintenance. DNA is at the center of the state of our health (Figure 8–1 ■). We now know that good health is associated with genes functioning properly and if genes are not functioning properly, disease or an increased risk for disease can result. This includes not only the traditional genetic disorders, but also common complex diseases such as heart disease, stroke, diabetes, and several kinds of cancer. The knowledge gained from **human genome** research has and will have a profound impact on the prevention, diagnosis, and treatment of genetic disorders and complex diseases.

INTEGRATING GENETICS INTO NURSING PRACTICE

Genetic knowledge will continue to revolutionize how persons perceive themselves as well as their health status and their health potential. Therefore, nurses must integrate new genetic knowledge into their nursing practice. This expectation has been defined in the ANA/ISONG *Statement on the Scope and Standards of Genetics Clinical Nursing Practice* (Box 8–2). In addition, a national interdisciplinary group known as the National Coalition for Health Professional Education in Genetics (NCHPEG) has developed competencies to encourage health-

BOX 8–1 **Human Genome Project**

In 1986, the U.S. Department of Energy (USDOE) announced the Human Genome initiative, and in 1990 the USDOE joined with the National Institutes of Health (NIH) to develop the Human Genome Project (HGP). The ultimate goal was to sequence the human genome and to identify all human genes. The completion of a high-quality reference sequence was announced in April 2003. Information obtained through the sequencing of the human genome has had a tremendous impact on finding the genes associated with human disease. Future research will now be directed toward understanding the complex functions of cellular regulation, human variation, and the interplay of genes and environment and how all the cell organelles, genes, and proteins work together in life's functions (USDOE Genome Programs, 2003).

Trillions of cells

Each cell:
- 46 human chromosomes
- 2 meters of DNA
- 3 billion DNA subunits (the bases: A, T, C, G)
- 25,000 genes code for proteins that perform all life functions

DNA the molecule of life

Cell

Chromosomes

Protein

Gene

DNA

Figure 8–1 ■ Each cell nucleus throughout the body contains the genes, DNA, and chromosomes that make up the majority of an individual's genome. The remaining portion of the human genome is in the mitochondria.

MEDIALINK   Human Genome Project Animation

MediaLink   National Coalition for Health Professional Education in Genetics (NCHPEG) Core Competencies

BOX 8-2 ANA/ISONG Standards of Genetics Clinical Nursing Practice Statement

ANA/ISONG *Statement on the Scope and Standards of Genetics Clinical Nursing Practice:*

All licensed registered nurses, regardless of their practice setting, have a role in the delivery of genetics services and the management of genetic information. Nurses require genetic knowledge to identify, refer, support, and care for persons affected by, or at risk for manifesting or transmitting, genetic conditions. As the public becomes more aware of the genetic contribution to health and disease, nurses in all areas of practice will be increasingly asked to address basic genetics-related questions, service needs, or both.

Source: Used with permission from American Nurses Association and International Society of Nurses in Genetics. Copyright 1998, p. 2. Washington, DC: American Nurses Publishing.

BOX 8-3 Using the People-First Approach

The nurse must incorporate a "people-first" philosophy and use genetic terminology that is sensitive to the maintenance of an individual's positive self-image. This can be accomplished by using "unaltered" or "wild-type" gene instead of "normal" gene and "altered" gene; "altered, disease-producing gene" or "gene alteration," instead of the term "mutated" or "abnormal" gene when communicating genetic concerns to clients, other healthcare providers, or the public.

wild type = normal = expected = unaltered
versus
mutated = abnormal = defective = unexpected = altered

care providers to integrate genetic knowledge, skills, and attitudes while delivering care to clients.

Nurses must have basic genetic knowledge to care for the needs of clients and their families with known or suspected genetic disease. Basic level nursing practice that meets the standard of genetic nursing includes:

- Identifying simple risk factors by completing a genetics focused family history and also drawing a three-generation pedigree
- Incorporating a genetics focus into physical assessments
- Applying concepts of health promotion and health maintenance to assist the client and family to make informed decisions and lifestyle choices
- Collaborating with the client to perform interventions that include advocacy, supporting the client's decisions, teaching, making referrals, clarifying information, and providing information about available resources and services
- Partnering with the community to educate the public and supporting legislation that protects genetic information and those with genetic conditions from discrimination
- Completing an evaluation of the delivery of care for the client
- Applying knowledge of the ethical, legal, and social implications of genetic information.

Through the application of fundamental genetic concepts, nurses can significantly improve the nursing care provided to clients.

GENETIC BASICS

A basic knowledge of the cell, DNA, cell division, chromosomes, and genes is essential to deliver the genetic standard of care to the adult client (Box 8-3).

The cell is the basic unit of life and it is the working unit of all living systems. Life starts as a single cell, but the developed human body is made up of trillions of cells. These cells share common features such as a nucleus that contains 46 chromosomes, and organelles such as mitochondria. There are many different types of "specialized" cells that function differently depending on their location. For example, pancreatic cells have a very different function than that of nerve cells.

All human cells, except mature red blood cells, contain a complete set of deoxyribonucleic acid (DNA) molecules. DNA molecules consist of long sequences of nucleotides or bases represented by the letters A, G, T, and C. The order of these bases gives the exact instructions for the functioning of that particular cell. Writing the correct order of the bases using the above abbreviations represents the sequence of the bases in DNA. All of the DNA in a human cell is referred to as the human genome, or the complete set of inheritance for an individual. The human genome includes the DNA in the cell nucleus as well as the DNA found in the mitochondria, which will be discussed later in this section. Each person's genome is unique. Identical (monozygotic) twins are the exception because they develop from only one fertilized ovum and share identical DNA (Guttmacher & Collins, 2002).

The cell nucleus contains about 6 feet of DNA that is tightly wound and packaged into 23 pairs of chromosomes making a complete set of 46 **chromosomes**. The structure and number of chromosomes can be shown by a karyotype, or picture, of an individual's chromosomes (Figure 8-2 ■) There are two copies of each chromosome. One copy, or half of the complete set of these 46 chromosomes, is inherited from the mother and the other copy, or the other half of the 46 chromosomes, is inherited from the father. For example, an individual will have two of chromosome 1, one inherited from her mother and one inherited from her father. These two copies or pairs of inherited chromosomes are called **homologous chromosomes**. Chromosomes are numbered according to size, with chromosome 1 being the largest and chromosome 22 being the smallest. The first 22 pairs of chromosomes, known as **autosomes**, are alike in males and females. The 23rd pair, the **sex chromosomes**, determines an individual's gender. A female has two copies of the X chromosomes (one copy inherited from each parent) and a male has one X chromosome (inherited from his mother) and a Y chromosome (inherited from his father).

Cell Division

Mitosis and meiosis are the two types of cell division in human cells. **Mitosis** is the process of making new cells and it takes place in the **somatic**, or tissue, **cells** of the body. Cell division through mitosis heals wounds and replaces cells lost daily on skin surfaces and in the lining of gastrointestinal and respiratory

Figure 8–2 ■ A karyotype is a picture of an individual's chromosomes. It shows the chromosomal structure and number of the 22 pairs of autosomes and the sex chromosomes.

tracts. In addition, mitosis is responsible for development. The mitotic activity of the zygote and its daughter cells is the foundation for a human's growth and development. The zygote undergoes mitosis to form a multicellular embryo, then fetus, then infant. Cell division through mitosis results in two cells called *daughter cells* that are genetically identical to the original cell, or *mother cell*, and each other.

Meiosis is also known as the reduction division of the cell. Meiosis occurs only in the sex cells of the testes and ovaries and results in the formation of the sperm and oocyte (gametes). Meiosis is very similar to mitosis in that it is a form of cell division; however, through a series of complex mechanisms, the amount of genetic material is reduced in half (23 chromosomes). This is very important because when the two sex cells combine during fertilization, the total number of chromosomes (46) is present in the offspring's cells. The purposes of meiosis is to produce gametes, to reduce the number of chromosomes by half, and also to make new combinations of genetic material from crossing over and independent assortment processes, which allows diversity in the human population.

Chromosomal Alterations

Alterations in chromosomes often occur during cell division (meiosis or mitosis) and are classified as either alterations in the number of chromosomes or structural alterations. They involve either part of or the whole chromosome. The clinical consequences of number and structural changes in the chromosomes in an individual vary depending on the amount and type of DNA affected by the alterations.

Alterations in Chromosome Number

An increase or decrease in chromosomal numbers can occur during meiosis or mitosis (Box 8–4). Alterations occur often during meiosis because meiosis is a highly specific and complex process and each new daughter cell must contain exactly one chromosome from each homologous pair of chromosomes. During meiosis, the paired chromosomes may fail to separate, resulting in daughter cells with either two copies or no copies of that chromosome. This

---

BOX 8–4 Variations in Chromosomal Number

Aneuploidy—the condition when extra or missing chromosomes exist; if there is an addition or deletion of chromosome number and the individual lives, physical abnormalities and/or mental retardation is common.
Monosomy—the loss of a single chromosome from a pair; i.e., Turner syndrome (45,XO)
Trisomy—the gain of a single chromosome, making a total of three copies of a certain chromosome; i.e., trisomy 21 or Down syndrome
Euploidy—the presence of the normal number of 46 chromosomes
Polyploidy—the condition when more than two pairs of all the chromosomes are present

---

is known as **nondisjunction**. This creates an egg or sperm cell with either two copies or no copies of a particular chromosome. When these egg or sperm cells are fertilized by a normal gamete that contains 23 copies of all of the chromosomes, a zygote that is monosomic (one member of the chromosome pair is missing) or trisomic (having three chromosomes instead of the usual two) results. These circumstances produce such conditions as Turner syndrome (**monosomy**) or **trisomy 21** (Down syndrome).

Alterations in Chromosome Structure

Alterations in chromosome structure include inversions, deletions and duplications, and translocations. In a chromosomal inversion a segment of a chromosome is reversed, changing the DNA sequence for that portion of the chromosome. It occurs when a chromosome breaks in two places and the piece between the breaks turns upside down and reattaches within the same chromosome. The clinical consequences of an inversion depend on how much chromosomal material is involved, where the inversion occurs, and what type of inversion is present.

A chromosomal alteration that includes a missing (deletion) or additional (duplication) whole chromosome or segment of a chromosome is an unbalanced rearrangement. An unbalanced rearrangement can result in missing genes, confusing directions from the genes, or too much gene product, which often results in a condition that is not compatible with life or altered physical and/or mental development. An example is *cri du chat* syndrome (mental retardation, crying that sounds like a cat mewing, and low-set ears), which results from a large deletion on chromosome 5.

Translocation (chromosomal reshuffling) occurs when a segment of a chromosome transfers or moves and attaches itself to another chromosome. An example is the reciprocal translocation that is found in 95% of clients with chronic myelogenous leukemia (CML). The contributing translocation occurs between chromosomes 9 and 22 and is known as the Philadelphia chromosome (Ph 1). Unlike the translocation responsible for Down syndrome, which occurs in the germ cells, the translocation responsible for CML occurs in somatic cells and therefore is not inheritable (National Cancer Institute, 2005; Nussbaum et al., 2001).

Genes

The nurse must also have knowledge of genes—what they are, the role genes play in homeostasis, as well as the consequences of gene alterations. How these gene alterations are inherited is also important for nursing interventions and teaching the client who is at risk for or who has a known gene (DNA-based) condition. Knowledge of the function and inheritance of genes is implicit in health promotion as well as health maintenance of the client and his or her family.

A **gene** is a small portion (segment) of the nucleotide (base) sequence of a chromosome DNA molecule that can be identified as having a particular function or characteristic. These segments of DNA within each gene have specific directions for the functioning of the gene. This specific sequence of nucleotides (the genes and the variations therein) is referred to as the individual's **genotype**. Each chromosome contains numerous genes arranged in a linear order. Researchers currently believe there are about 20,000 to 25,000 genes in the human genome. The number of genes present on each chromosome varies. Chromosome 1 is the largest chromosome and has the largest number of genes with 2,968. The Y chromosome has the smallest number of genes with 231 (Human Genome Project [HGP], 2004a).

All genes come in pairs because chromosomes come in pairs. The only exception to all genes being paired are the genes on the sex chromosomes (X and Y) present in males. All genes have a specific location on a specific chromosome. This is known as the **genetic locus**. For example, one of the many genes located on chromosome 19 is a gene for eye color. There may be slight variations or different forms of a gene, for instance, green versus blue eye color, and these different forms or versions of genes are called **alleles**. When an individual has two identical forms (alleles) of a gene they are said to be **homozygous** (homo = same). If an individual has two different forms (alleles) of the gene, they are said to be **heterozygous** (hetero = different). Genes can be described as *altered* or *mutated,* when a change has taken place, or

expressed, when the gene has an impact on the outward appearance of an individual and/or the functioning of cells. The observable, outward expression of an individual's entire physical, biochemical, and physiologic makeup, as determined by their genotype (alleles) and environmental factors, is referred to as **phenotype**. Phenotype may be expressed or observed as curly or straight hair or the presentation of signs and symptoms of a disease.

Function and Distribution of Genes

Although the function of more than 50% of the genes in the human genome is unknown, we do know that about 2% of the genes give directions to parts of the cell for how to make proteins, what type of proteins to make, and how much of a protein to make (HGP, 2004a). These protein-directing genes are very important to life and functioning as a human being because proteins are very specialized and perform a variety of functions within the cell. These functions include transmitting messages between cells, fighting infection, directing genes to turn "on" or "off," forming structures, as well as sensing light, taste, and smell (Jegalian, 2000). Some gene activities change from moment to moment in response to tens of thousands of intra- and extracellular environmental signals (USDOE Genome Programs, 2003). An example of this is the feedback mechanism that stimulates a cell to produce insulin after eating a candy bar. After eating, a gene on chromosome 11 directs pancreatic cells to produce, modify, and secrete insulin. Although the gene for producing insulin is present in all nucleated cells of the body, it is only functional in insulin-secreting pancreatic cells (Guttmacher & Collins, 2002).

Mitochondrial Genes

Chromosomes in the cell nucleus are not the only site where genes reside. Several dozen that are involved in energy metabolism are located in the cell mitochondria (the "powerhouse" of the cell). **Mitochondria** are concerned with energy production and metabolism. Some cells contain more mitochondria than others, but each mitochondrion contains its own copies of DNA identified as mitochondrial DNA (mtDNA). Because ova have many mitochondria and sperm do not (most mitochondria are located in the tail of the sperm that detaches after fertilization), mtDNA is primarily inherited from the mother. Therefore, mitochondrial genes and any diseases due to DNA alterations on those genes are transmitted through the mother in a matrilineal pattern. This pattern of inheritance is very different from the pattern of inheritance of genes found in the nucleus of the cell (Guttmacher & Collins, 2002). Thus, an affected female will pass the mtDNA mutation to all of her children; however, an affected male will not pass the mtDNA mutation to any of his children (Nussbaum et al., 2001). Signs and symptoms of conditions as a result of mitochondrial gene alterations are primarily involved in high-energy tissues and organs such as skeletal muscles, liver, kidney, brain and nerve cells, ears, eyes, endocrine system, and heart muscle. Symptoms develop over years as unhealthy or dying cells are not replaced. Hypertrophic cardiomyopathy, heart block, seizures, and deafness are also associated with mtDNA gene alterations (Nussbaum et al., 2001).

Gene Alterations and Disease

A protein will malfunction and in many cases cause disease if any kind of alteration (mutation or change) is present in the order of the DNA sequence within a gene. These gene alterations can be inherited from one or both parents or they can be acquired. *Mutations* inherited from a parent (hereditary mutations) are also known as *germline mutations* because the mutation exists in the reproductive sperm or ova of the parent. Consequently, the DNA in every cell of that offspring will have the gene alteration and also can be inherited from generation to generation.

The second kind of gene alteration is an *acquired mutation* or *somatic mutation*. These alterations occur in the DNA of cells of the individual throughout their life. They can result from errors during cell division (mitosis) or from environmental influences such as radiation or toxins (National Institutes of Health [NIH], 1995).

Today, we know that gene alterations are responsible for approximately 6000 hereditary diseases. However, different gene alterations within a particular gene can result in a wide variety of signs and symptoms. For example, the *CFTR* gene for cystic fibrosis is a very large gene located on chromosome 7. More than 800 different mutations of this gene have been reported to cause cystic fibrosis (Wine et al., 2001). The area of the *CFTR* gene that controls mucous production can have more than 300 different gene alterations resulting in a variety of symptoms ranging from mild, to severe, or no symptoms at all (NIH, 1995). Gene alterations, not the genes themselves, cause genetic diseases and conditions.

Other situations where gene alterations cause illness and disease are through gene interaction with the environment. These genes and conditions are referred to as multifactorial (Jegalian, 2000). Alterations in regulatory genes may also occur. Regulatory genes play a part in maintaining homeostasis or normal functioning. A regulatory gene mutation might lead to the loss of expression of a gene, to unexpected expression in a tissue in which it is usually silent, or a change in the time when a gene is usually expressed. An example of a regulatory gene mutation associated with disease includes the insulin gene region that increases the risk of type 1 diabetes (Guttmacher & Collins, 2002).

Gene Alterations That Decrease Risk of Disease

Although it is common to associate gene mutations with disease, it is important to remember that gene mutations can also be helpful and decrease the risk of disease. Gene alterations and genetic variations may also have a protective role in the expression of diseases. A common example is the protective value of the gene alteration that causes sickle cell disease. Those individuals with this gene alteration have protection against malaria. Another, less common example of a "protective" gene alteration is the one on the receptor gene named *CCR5*. This mutation consists of a deletion within the DNA sequence. Persons who are homozygous for the *CCR5* mutation (have two copies of the altered gene) are almost completely resistant to infection with HIV type I, and those who are heterozygous for the deletion (have one copy of the altered gene) progress much slower from the stage of HIV infection to AIDS

(Guttmacher & Collins, 2002). As genomic research continues, more and more of these types of beneficial gene alterations will be identified.

Single Nucleotide Polymorphisms

Single nucleotide polymorphisms, or SNPs ("snips"), are one-letter (base pair) variations in the DNA sequence that occur in greater than 1% of the population. In all people, 99.9% of the DNA is identical; SNPs are responsible for differences among individuals. **Polymorphisms** are DNA sequences that have many forms but give the genetic "directions" for the same thing. Most of these differences have no effect on the individual. Some cause subtle differences in numerous characteristics in appearance such as widow's peak, tongue rolling, and attached ear lobes. Other SNPs, however, affect an individual's risk for certain diseases and have a major impact on how the individual responds to environmental factors such as toxins, microbes, and medications. Scientists are mapping these areas of SNPs in order to move to the next step of identifying the multiple genes that are associated with diseases that are not caused by single-gene alterations, but the complex diseases caused by multiple genes such as cancer, cardiovascular disease, some forms of mental illness, and diabetes (HGP, 2004c; Jegalian, 2000).

PRINCIPLES OF INHERITANCE

Knowledge of inheritance allows the nurse to not only offer and reinforce genetic information to clients and their families but also to assist them in managing their care and in making reproductive decisions. The basic underlying principles of inheritance that nurses can apply to inheritance risk assessment and teaching include (1) all genes are paired, (2) only one gene of each pair is transmitted (passed on) to an offspring, and (3) one copy of each gene in the offspring comes from the mother and the other copy comes from the father. Understanding the Mendelian patterns of inheritance is made easier by relating these principles.

Mendelian Pattern of Inheritance

Conditions that are caused by a mutation or alteration of a single gene are known as *monogenic* or *single-gene disorders*. There are more than 6000 known single-gene disorders occurring in about 1 per 200 births (HGP, 2003). The most common gene alterations that result in genetic disorders are categorized into Mendelian inheritance patterns, because they are predictably passed on from generation to generation following Mendel's laws of inheritance. These single-gene mutations follow an autosomal dominant, autosomal recessive, **X-linked recessive**, or **X-linked dominant** inheritance pattern. The first three of these patterns are the most common. Modes of transmission or inheritance for thousands of conditions resulting from monogenic alterations have been identified (Online Mendelian Inheritance in Man, 2003).

Recessive vs. Dominant Disorders

The distinction between recessive and dominant phenotypes or disease presence (expression) is in the amount of gene product (usually proteins) from the unaltered (**wild-type** or normal) gene. When the individual is heterozygous (has one unaltered

Figure 8–3 ■ This Punnett square shows potential gene combinations (genotypes) and resulting phenotypes of children from parent genotypes with an autosomal dominant altered gene. Phenotypes are expressed (affected) when a male *or* female has one copy of the gene alteration.

BOX 8–5 Autosomal Dominant Mendelian Inheritance Characteristics

(Examples: neurofibromatosis, breast and ovarian cancer, autosomal dominant polycystic kidney disease, Marfan syndrome, Huntington disease, familial hypercholesterolemia)

When the nurse gathers a family history, the nurse should assess for any of the following characteristics of autosomal dominant inheritance:

1. Both males and females are affected.
2. Males and females are usually affected in equal numbers.
3. An affected child will have an affected parent and/or all generations will have an affected individual (appearing as a vertical pattern of affected individuals on the family pedigree).
4. Unaffected children of an affected parent will have unaffected offspring.
5. A significant proportion of isolated cases are due to a new mutation.

---

gene and one altered gene), the altered gene as well as the disease is classified as recessive if half of the product produced from the unaltered gene is enough to maintain homeostasis and perform the expected function. Therefore, two altered genes must be present to cause a diseased state. If the altered gene causes disease even though the unaltered gene is producing the gene product, then the altered gene as well as the disease is classified as dominant (Nussbaum et al., 2001).

Autosomal Dominant

Autosomal dominant (AD) conditions are the result of an altered gene on any of the 22 autosomes or non–sex chromosomes (Figure 8–3 ■). More than half of the known Mendelian conditions are autosomal dominant. In AD conditions, disease occurs in spite of the fact that there exists one unaltered or normal gene. Also, homozygous dominant conditions are generally much more severe than heterozygous dominant conditions and are often lethal. Because homozygous dominant conditions are usually lethal and would result from *both parents being affected*, the nurse should consider an individual exhibiting an autosomal dominant condition as heterozygous. See Box 8–5 for characteristics of an AD pattern of inheritance.

Autosomal Recessive

A gene or genetic condition is considered recessive when two copies of altered genes are needed to express the condition. Autosomal recessive (AR) conditions are the result of an altered gene on any of the 22 autosomes or non–sex chromosomes (Figure 8–4 ■). An individual with a recessive condition has inherited one altered gene from his mother and one from his father. In most cases, neither of the parents is affected and, therefore,

each of the parents must have a single gene alteration on one chromosome of a pair and the normal, wild-type or unaltered form of the gene on the other chromosome. These parents would be known as **carriers** of the condition and they do not usually exhibit any signs and symptoms of the condition. Because the gene alteration occurs on a non–sex chromosome, both males and females have an equal chance of inheriting the altered gene from their parent. Generally, conditions that are autosomal recessive are more severe and have an earlier onset than conditions with other patterns of inheritance. Most inborn errors in metabolism or metabolic conditions are autosomal recessive. Many are enzyme defects and the functioning of the unaltered gene is sufficient to

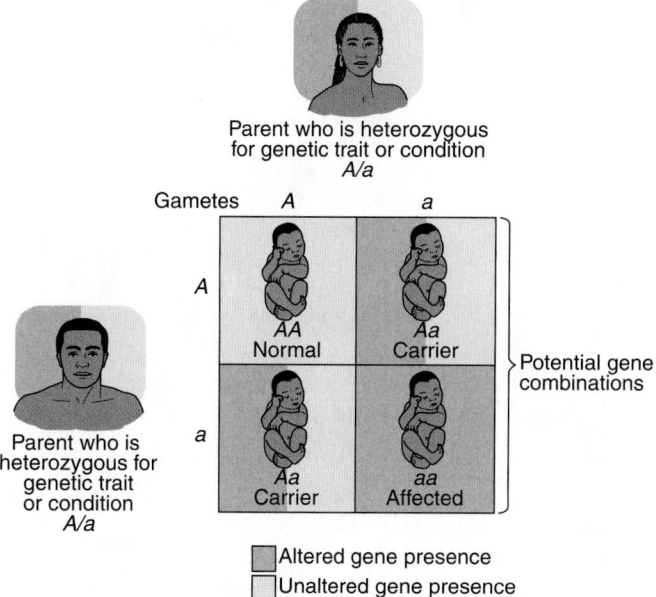

Figure 8–4 ■ This Punnett square shows potential gene combinations (genotypes) and resulting phenotypes of children from parent genotypes with an autosomal recessive altered gene. Phenotypes are expressed (affected) when a male *or* female has two copies of the gene alteration.

provide normal functioning in the person who is heterozygous or the carrier of one copy of the altered gene (Lashley, 2005). See Box 8–6 for characteristics of an AR pattern of inheritance.

X-Linked Recessive

X-linked conditions are the result of an altered gene on the X chromosome. Unlike the autosomes, the sex chromosome, X,

---

BOX 8–6 Autosomal Recessive Mendelian Inheritance Characteristics

(*Examples: hemochromatosis type 1, cystic fibrosis, phenylketonuria, sickle cell anemia*)

When the nurse gathers a family history, the nurse should assess for any of the following characteristics of autosomal recessive inheritance:

1. Both males and females are affected.
2. Males and females are usually affected in equal numbers.
3. An affected child will have an unaffected parent but may have affected siblings (appearing as a horizontal pattern of affected individuals on the family pedigree).
4. The condition may appear to skip a generation.
5. The parents of the affected child may be consanguineous (close blood relatives).
6. The family may be descendants of a certain ethnic group that is known to have a more frequent occurrence of a certain genetic condition.

---

is unevenly distributed to males and females. The female has two X chromosomes and the male has only one. Thus, the family history and pattern of inheritance has a characteristic distribution pattern among the males and females in the family (Figure 8–5 ■). Because the male has only one copy of any gene on the X chromosome, it becomes the only copy available to give direction for those particular functions of these genes regardless of whether it is considered dominant or recessive in the female. Thus, if any of these genes are altered, an unaltered counterpart is not present to "override" the altered functioning gene.

The consequences of the altered gene on an X chromosome will be expressed in all males. Females, on the other hand, will have two copies and the unaltered gene generally compensates for the altered gene, making the female a carrier. The male receives his X chromosome from his mother and his Y chromosome from his father. The female offspring receives an X chromosome from each of her parents. Thus, all affected males will pass on the altered X chromosome to all of his daughters who will be carriers of the altered gene. A male can never transmit an altered gene on the X chromosome to his sons because the male will transmit only the Y chromosome to his sons. Because of these transmission patterns, the most commonly occurring transmission of an X-linked condition is through a female who is a carrier of an altered gene. See Box 8–7 for characteristics of an X-linked recessive pattern of inheritance.

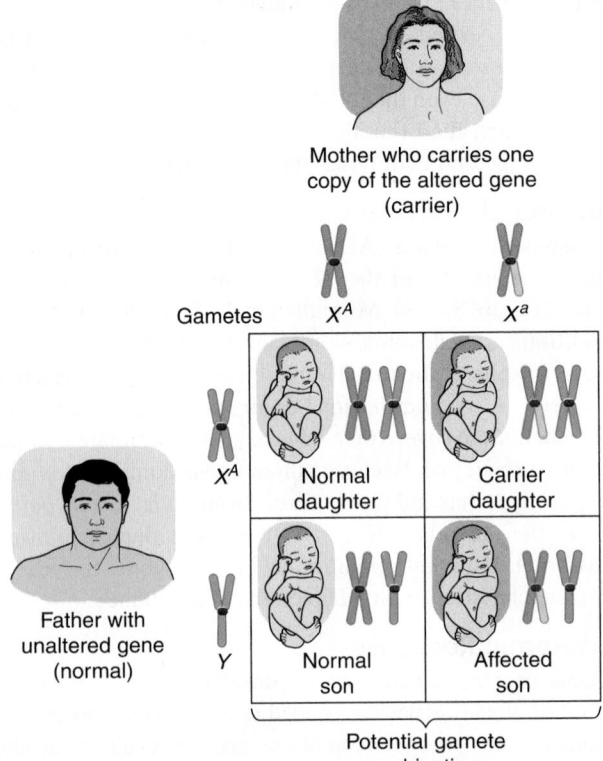

Figure 8–5 ■ These Punnett squares show potential gene combinations (genotypes) and resulting phenotypes of children from different parent genotypes with an X-linked recessive altered gene. Phenotypes are expressed (affected) in a male with only one copy of the gene alteration and in a female with two copies of the altered gene.

BOX 8–7 X-Linked Recessive Mendelian Inheritance Characteristics

(Examples: hemophilia A; Duchenne muscular dystrophy)

When the nurse gathers a family history, the nurse should assess for any of the following characteristics of X-linked recessive inheritance:

1. More males will be affected than females; rarely seen in females.
2. An affected male will have all carrier daughters.
3. There is no male-to-male inheritance.
4. Affected males are related by carrier females.
5. Females may report varying milder symptoms of the condition.
6. A new sporadic case could be due to a new mutation.

X-Linked Dominant

X-linked dominant conditions also exist but these conditions are very rare. If a male is affected, the condition is severe and often lethal. A family history of multiple male miscarriages may be a sign of an X-linked dominant condition.

Variability in Classic Mendelian Patterns of Inheritance

Along with understanding the classic Mendelian inheritance patterns, several other concepts are also important for families to understand when the nurse is assisting clients with or at risk for inheriting a genetic disorder. These include the following exceptions or variations to the traditional Mendelian patterns of inheritance.

Penetrance

Penetrance is the probability that a gene will be expressed phenotypically. It is an "all or none" concept in that, either the gene will be expressed (even if mildly expressed) or it will not be expressed at all. Penetrance can be measured in the following way. In a certain group of individuals with the same genotype, what percentage of them will exhibit at least some signs and/or symptoms of the condition? If the number is less than 100%, then that condition is said to show reduced penetrance. For example, the gene alterations that cause achondroplasia exhibit 100% penetrance and all individuals with one copy of the gene alteration will exhibit signs and symptoms of the disease (Nussbaum et al., 2001).

New Mutation

When there is no previous history of a condition including even subtle signs and symptoms of the disease in any other immediate or distant family member, the disease may be caused by a spontaneous new mutation. This case is usually called *de novo* mutation. New mutations of a gene are most frequently seen in autosomal dominant conditions because one copy of an altered gene is all that is necessary to elicit a state of altered health. Autosomal dominant diseases known to have high mutation rates include neurofibromatosis, achondroplasia (dwarfism), and Marfan syndrome. New mutations are also possible in autosomal recessive diseases although rarely expressed because two altered genes are necessary for signs and symptoms to appear.

Finally, new mutations are often seen in X-linked recessive disorders, such as hemophilia A, since the male with just one altered gene will demonstrate the disease.

Anticipation

Anticipation is said to occur when successive generations of a family exhibit more severe signs and symptoms of certain diseases and the disease often has an earlier onset. An example is myotonic dystrophy type 1, an autosomal dominant condition characterized by a range of signs and symptoms including myotonia, muscle weakness, cataracts, and cardiac dysrhythmias. The congenital form is severe, causing mental retardation and may be life threatening. Most children with this congenital form of myotonic dystrophy have a mildly affected mother who may not even be aware she has the disease (Nussbaum et al., 2001). The severity of the condition as well as the age of onset is determined by the number of trinucleotide repeats. Trinucleotide repeats are short DNA sequences such as the CTG base sequence of the gene *DMPK* that are repeated to greater than 2000 times, which results in alterations in the protein products produced by the gene and varying signs and symptoms.

Variable Expressivity

Expressivity is used to describe the severity of the **gene expression** of the phenotype. When people with the same genetic makeup (genotype) exhibit signs and/or symptoms with varying degrees of severity the phenotype is described as *variable expression* (Nussbaum et al., 2001).

Variable expression is common in the autosomal dominant condition, neurofibromatosis. Although neurofibromatosis has 100% penetrance, variable expressivity can occur within family members with each family member exhibiting a variety of signs and/or symptoms.

Multifactorial (Polygenic or Complex) Disorders

Many birth defects such as cleft lip and palate, as well as many adult-onset conditions such as cancer, mental illnesses, asthma, diabetes, obesity, heart disease, and Alzheimer's disease, have a multifactorial cause. **Multifactorial conditions** occur as a result of several gene (polygenic) variations, lifestyle, and environmental influences that work together. The polygenic concept is illustrated with the multiple genes involved in an individual's susceptibility for breast cancer. These genes have been identified on chromosomes 6, 11, 13, 14, 15, 17, and 22. Exactly which genes interrelate and how many environmental influences are enough to cause the presentation of many of the common complex diseases or conditions is not known. However, it is believed that by 2010, the major contributing genes for many common complex conditions will be identified (HGP, 2004a).

Multifactorial conditions accumulate in families but these conditions do not follow the characteristic Mendelian pattern of inheritance seen with single-gene conditions. Inheritable recurrence risks vary in multifactorial conditions. With information gathered from a family history, basic occurrence risks can be assessed for an individual. For instance, premature death in a first-degree relative, two affected first-degree relatives, and two second-degree maternal or paternal relatives with at least one individual having premature onset of the disease are all considered high inheritance risks. Moderate risks include an individual having a first-degree relative with late or unknown disease onset or two second-degree relatives from the same lineage with late or unknown disease onset. An individual having no affected relatives or a negative family history, only one affected second-degree relative from one or both sides of the pedigree is considered average or general population risk (Scheuner et al., 1997).

Recurrence risks refer to whether or not a condition will occur again in subsequent pregnancies. Because a Mendelian pattern is not present, statistical percentages can be used to represent the chance that parents have a condition that will occur in another child. The risk of recurrence is higher when more than one family member is affected. The recurrence risk after the first affected child is 4.0%, whereas the recurrence risk after a second affected child increases to 10%. It is also known that the recurrence risk increases with an increase in severity of the defect.

INTERDISCIPLINARY CARE

Many health professionals work together in screening, diagnosis, identification, and treatment of genetic disorders. The goals of collaborative care are early diagnosis through testing and assessment, and development of an effective treatment plan, combined with psychosocial support to enhance coping and referral to a genetic specialist when needed.

Genetic Testing

Genetic testing may be used for a client's clinical management, for making personal decisions, or for assisting in reproductive choices. A genetic test is very different from other types of clinical tests. Genetic tests involve the analysis of DNA, RNA, chromosomes, and serum levels of specific enzymes or metabolites. Enzymes and metabolites are part of the protein products that genes produce. DNA, RNA, and/or chromosomes are very unique for each individual and the results have personal, social, financial, and legal implications. Some genetic tests are diagnostic, while others are predictive or inform the individual of an increased risk of acquiring a disease or condition. A "positive" genetic test may indicate that the asymptomatic individual will develop a genetic condition, but a prediction of the onset or severity of the condition cannot be made.

Complications also arise in client understanding because a negative test result cannot guarantee the disease or condition might not develop in the future, often because environmental influences cannot be measured or controlled. Also, the genetic test may have only been able to detect the most common gene mutations and not all of the disease-producing gene alterations are known or available for inclusion in clinical testing. Clients may learn they will develop a genetic condition such as Huntington disease, for which there is no treatment. Clients may find out through genetic testing that they are a carrier and they have unknowingly passed the altered disease-producing gene on to their children.

Finally, the implications of genetic test results are far reaching. While confidentiality and autonomy for the client always

are foremost for the nurse, the implications to the client's children, grandchildren, siblings, and other extended family members who share a percentage of the same genes can be life altering. This information may be very confusing and very different from how they have perceived health care in the past and how they perceived the implications of a simple "blood test."

TYPES OF GENETIC TESTS The nurse should understand that genetic tests can be classified into two categories: screening and diagnostic. A positive screening genetic test result notifies the client of an increased risk or probability but must always be confirmed by diagnostic testing. Screening genetic tests are most commonly completed in prenatal, newborn, and carrier circumstances. In contrast, a diagnostic test can definitively validate or eliminate a genetic disorder in the symptomatic client and then direct clinical management. Box 8–8 lists some of the positive and negative aspects of genetic testing.

Several categories of genetic tests included as subcategories of screening and diagnostic genetic tests follow:
- *Newborn screening* is carried out on large sections of the newborn population and provides a means to identify children who have an increased risk for developing a genetic disease such as phenylketonuria, sickle cell disease, or maple syrup urine disease.
- *Carrier testing* is completed on asymptomatic individuals who may be carriers of one copy of a gene alteration that can be transmitted to future children in an autosomal recessive or X-linked pattern of inheritance. This may be part of a couple's premarriage or preconception planning if they belong to a particular ethnic group with known incidence to genetic disorders such as sickle cell anemia and Tay-Sachs disease. It may be necessary to determine the exact gene mutation

---

BOX 8–8 Positive and Negative Outcomes Related to Genetic Testing

Benefits of Genetic Testing

Provide for:
- Early screening and preventive measures
- Future planning and life preparation
- Lifestyle adaptations
- Decreased confusion and anxiety
- Psychologic stress relief
- Reproductive choices
- Informed extended family members
- Early medical and/or surgical intervention
- Cost of medical follow-up reduced (if negative result)

Possible Negative Outcomes of Genetic Testing
- Survivor guilt
- Loss of identity
- No treatment may exist
- Employability and insurability affected
- Confusion about accessing health care and resources
- Risk for invasion of confidentiality and privacy
- Social stigmatization

Source: Data from Secretary's Advisory Committee on Genetic Testing (SACGT), National Institutes of Health, 2000.

from an affected family member prior to carrier testing. This is often completed through lineage analysis.

- *Preimplantation genetic diagnosis (PGD)* involves the detection of disease-causing gene alterations in human embryos just after *in vitro* fertilization and before implantation in the uterus, thus providing an opportunity for preselection of unaffected embryos for implantation. This type of genetic testing is most often used by parents who are both carriers of a single-gene recessive disorder and who wish to implant into the uterus only the embryo(s) without the disease-causing gene alteration. PGD is usually not covered by insurance, is very costly, and is available at only a small number of centers and for only a small number of disorders (GeneTests, 2004). More recently it has also been used to determine tissue type for donation of tissue such as bone marrow to a sibling or parent (Javitt et al., 2004).

- *Predictive genetic testing* is usually made available to the asymptomatic individual and includes both predispositional and presymptomatic testing. A positive predispositional testing result will indicate there is an increased risk that the individual might eventually develop the disease. Common examples include breast cancer and hereditary nonpolyposis colorectal cancer. A presymptomatic test is performed when development of the disease is certain if the gene alteration is present. These tests are medically indicated when the seriousness and mortality of the disease can be reduced with knowledge of the gene alteration. An example of this would be hereditary hemochromatosis or familial hypercholesterolemia. Life planning and lifestyle choices can be influenced by predictive testing.

- Other uses of genetic testing include organ transplantation tissue typing and pharmacogenetic testing, which involves predicting or studying the client's response to particular medications (Javitt et al., 2004). For example, pharmacogenetic testing has shown that individuals who have Alzheimer's disease and carry two copies of a particular altered gene do not respond well to a drug frequently used in the treatment of Alzheimer's disease. However, if the individual only has one copy of the altered gene, the drug is effective in slowing the progression of the disease (Secretary's Advisory Committee on Genetic Testing, 2000a).

DIAGNOSING CHROMOSOMAL ALTERATIONS Microscopic examination of chromosomes through a karyotype can reveal chromosomal alterations such as chromosomal additions, deletions, gross breaks, and rearrangements or rejoinings (translocations) (USDOE Genome Programs, 2003). Among other things, these chromosomal alterations are responsible for many forms of cancer and, more importantly, particular tumor types. Chromosomal diagnostic examination can be accomplished with a simple blood sample and skin or buccal cell sampling. A karyotype is completed in a cytogenetics laboratory. Chromosomes can be identified by their size and unique light and dark banding patterns. The pairs of autosomal chromosomes are arranged from 1 to 22 according to each chromosome's size, unique banding patterns, and centromere position. The sex chromosomes complete the picture, with the X chromosome(s) first, then the Y chromosome (if present). The karyotype shows all of the chromosome pairs lined up and positioned on a piece of paper allowing for visual chromosomal analysis. (See Figure 8–2 earlier in this chapter.) The final report contains numerical data that includes the total number of chromosomes present. If there is an additional or deleted chromosome, it is identified with a plus (+) or minus (−) symbol. For example, the male individual with 47, XY, +18 has 47 chromosomes (instead of the expected number of 46) that include an additional chromosome 18.

DIAGNOSING GENE ALTERATIONS With the rapidly expanding advances in technology and the identification of genes in the human genome, the availability of genetic, DNA (gene)-based tests has grown tremendously. Currently, more than 900 genetic tests are available with more becoming available each day (US-DOE Genome Programs, 2003). **DNA-based tests** involve new, sophisticated technology that permits the examination of the DNA itself. Genetic testing that is DNA based can be obtained from blood, bone marrow, amniotic fluid, fibroblast cells of the skin, or buccal cells from the mouth. Genetic testing includes different types of DNA-based tests. The appropriate genetic tests may be testing for a specific mutation. This would be used if a family member was known to have a genetic condition and could therefore be tested for that particular gene alteration. Another way to examine DNA is by running a panel of mutations. This is done when there are a specific number of identified genes that the majority of individuals with a genetic condition have, for instance, a panel of the three mutations on the *BRCA1* gene that are common in the Ashkenazi Jewish population. A third type of DNA-based test is a complete gene sequence (GeneTests, 2004).

QUALITY AND ACCURACY OF GENETIC TESTS Genetic nurses have expressed concerns that genetic tests are becoming available too quickly with no regulation of the companies that are offering genetic tests. The quality, accuracy, and reliability of genetic test results are not measured against any common standard. Individuals often make hard and irrevocable life-altering decisions after receiving test results so accuracy and reliability are essential. Also, in most cases, minimal or no education is provided for the individual undergoing testing, nor is there any quality counseling or follow-up after the results are given to the individual. Genetic tests are often offered by laboratories before the tests have been proven safe, effective, and practical. Because the majority of genetic conditions are rare, there is often only one laboratory offering the genetic test that is needed. Recently, concerns have been voiced about "direct to consumer" genetic testing. Genetic tests are being offered at "walk-in" locations and also via the Internet. Individuals can receive results of genetic tests in private without a physician's order and fear of discrimination, but also without education or knowledge of the implications of the test results.

Concerns also exist related to test validity, test sensitivity and specificity, the quality of the laboratory performing the test, and the competence of the client's healthcare provider to interpret the test results. **Test sensitivity** refers to how specifically the test identifies (positive test result) individuals who are affected and/or who have the disease phenotype. A test with a high degree of sensitivity has very few false negatives and many true positives. **Test specificity** refers to how specifically the test does not identify (negative test result) individuals who are unaffected or do not have the disease phenotype. A test with a high degree of specificity has very few false positives (SACGT, 2000). The laboratory selected for the genetic test should have a CLIA88 (Clinical Laboratories Improvement Amendments of 1988) certification (Javitt et al., 2004).

 NURSING CARE

The Role of the Nurse in Genetic Testing

With knowledge of available genetic tests and the many implications related to genetic testing, the nurse can assist clients as they weigh choices regarding genetic testing. As consumers of multimedia, clients often have unreliable sources for information related to genetic testing. They may form many misconceptions about the types of genetic tests available and what information these different types of genetic tests are able and not able to provide. When managing genetic information about genetic testing, the nurse must include education for the individual and the family. Communication with the client about genetic testing should include an assessment of the positive and negative outcomes of the test. Are there existing treatments for the condition being tested? Psychologic issues should also be emphasized. Who will be affected by the test results? Will the test results be shared with extended family members?

The nurse is responsible for alerting clients of their right to make an informed decision prior to any genetic testing with consideration of the special circumstances arising from the family, culture, and community life. All genetic testing should be voluntary and it is the nurse's responsibility to ensure that the consent process includes discussion of the risks and benefits of the test, including any physical harm as well as potential psychologic and societal injury by stigmatization, discrimination, and emotional stress (Beskow et al., 2001; International Society of Nurses in Genetics, 2000).

Above all, nurses have a responsibility to fully educate clients about the multiple issues related to genetic testing. Clients should engage in genetic testing with full knowledge, confidentiality, and autonomously. Informed consent may be given verbally, although some laboratories require written consent. Prior to the testing, the client should have an idea of the probability for a positive or negative result if one can be determined by the client's or family history (GeneTests, 2004). To deliver the expected standard of care, it is imperative that the nurse include these issues when developing an educational plan for the client anticipating the use of genetic testing and as part of the informed consent process.

Ensuring Confidentiality and Privacy for Genetic Testing

Although confidentiality and privacy are integral parts of delivery of care for all nurses, this issue is of even more concern as it relates to genetic information. Results of genetic tests can be far reaching and can affect employment and insurance options. Will the results affect the client's ability to obtain and/or maintain insurance coverage? Can an employer refuse to hire or promote an individual because of genetic testing results? Can genetic information be released to the courts, military, schools, or adoption agencies? Would a client with a known gene alteration for Huntington disease be offered a college scholarship to the best law school? There is debate over whether genetic privacy is different from medical privacy. The nurse should inform clients of their rights and responsibility to know who will have access to the genetic test results. Those providing the genetic tests must provide the client with assurance that the results will be handled confidentially, and that there will be no access to the genetic information by a third party without written permission of the individual being tested.

Results of genetic tests should only be communicated directly to the individual who gave the consent. No outside governmental, employment, or insurance organizations should ever have access to genetic test results without the written permission of clients. Clients should confirm how they will receive the test results. Clients should ask who will have access to the test results and what will happen to the DNA sample after the test is completed. In the majority of cases, results of genetic tests should not be shared with extended family members without written permission. Healthcare providers are legally liable to maintain that confidence. Exceptions to the individual's privacy may be made only when the individual refuses to inform extended family members when a very high probability of irreversible harm exists for the extended family member and informing the family member can prevent the harm (National Human Genome Research Institute, 2005). Every effort should be made to educate the individual about the benefits of informing extended family members if applicable. Genetic testing should ideally be accompanied by pretest and post-test counseling by genetic specialists or by another knowledgeable healthcare provider.

Psychosocial Issues

Although family and individual anxiety may be decreased with a negative test result, potential problems do exist and the nurse must be prepared to address them. Concerns about carrier status may interfere with development of intimacy and interpersonal relationships. Nonpaternity may be revealed through genetic testing. For example, the parents of a child born with an autosomal recessive condition will be considered carriers of the altered gene the majority of the time. To counsel the parents about future pregnancies, the parents would be tested to confirm their genotype, and nonpaternity may become an issue. A positive test result may lead to feelings of unworthiness, confusion, anger, depression, and self-image disturbance. Survivor guilt may affect adults with negative results if their siblings are positive. The individual carrying a gene alteration for a late-onset disease may have an increased tendency for risky behaviors and may choose not to be a positive member of society. Relatives of an individual affected with a genetic disorder may be very frightened when they realize what their own future might be (SACGT, 2000a). The individual who has inherited an altered disease-producing gene may foster deep resentment toward the parent who carries the altered gene. Parents and older generations may feel tremendous guilt for passing the altered gene to their children and grandchildren (Wertz et al., 1994).

Economic Issues

The nurse should consider the cost of genetic tests, which can range from hundreds to thousands of dollars, depending on the size of the gene being tested. Most insurance companies do not cover genetic tests but if there is insurance coverage, the individual must weigh the cost of allowing the insurance company to have access to the genetic information (HGP, 2005).

Genetic tests differ from routine medical tests in many ways. The risks and benefits of genetic testing are numerous and complicated. Nurses have an obligation to maintain their knowledge regarding genetic testing to advocate for the client as well as maintain ethical standards of care. Above all, nurses must be able to recognize the limits of their expertise and how to refer a client to genetic specialists and additional resources.

Assessment

Health Promotion and Health Maintenance

Health promotion and health maintenance of the client are viewed as the foundations of all nursing care. However, most individuals do not know their complete genetic makeup. Some know they carry an altered gene that causes a specific disease, but the majority of individuals do not know with certainty what their future health status will be. With no sure knowledge of genetic makeup or whether a certain alteration in health status will occur (heart disease, for example), healthy lifestyles are not always a priority. Imagine, then, if people knew their statistical risks for developing or inheriting disease by having complete access to the types of genes in their cells? Health promotion and health maintenance teaching and nursing interventions would be based on specific genes. The nurse could provide important, life-saving nutritional information to their clients based on their specific risks, and clients then might be more inclined to maintain a proper diet, give up their sedentary lifestyle, increase exercise, and decrease fast-food intake. Personal lifestyle choices would become more personal and monitoring health might take on a new meaning.

With knowledge of genetic conditions, the nurse can ensure health teaching and early detection of complications from genetic conditions with emphasis on primary and secondary care interventions. For example:

- A woman with a strong family history and/or mutations in the *BRCA1* and *BRCA2* tumor suppressor genes should begin monthly self breast exams, and have screening clinical breast exams and mammographies at an earlier age than the general population.
- A man with a strong family history and/or mutations in the *BRCA1* and *BRCA2* tumor suppressor genes should report

any mass, tenderness, or swelling in the breast tissue and maintain early screening for prostate cancer.
- Aggressive colonoscopy screening every 1 to 2 years beginning at age 25 is important for the individual with a positive family history and/or mutations in the *MLH1/MSH2* gene, which increases the risk for hereditary nonpolyposis colorectal cancer.

Clients receiving early intervention and health promotion-focused care can live longer and with a much better quality of life that those who do not. The nurse must be able to identify both community-based and genetic-based resources that are available to assist the client in strategies to support both health promotion and health maintenance activities.

By simply integrating into practice the genetic aspects of assessment, observation, and history gathering, the nurse can improve the standard of care delivered and have a very positive impact on the client. The nurse does not need to be a genetic expert, but with heightened awareness, appropriate inquiries and referrals to genetic specialists can be completed.

Client Intake and History

Nurses can improve the standard of nursing care and have a positive impact on clients by integrating genetic concepts into their existing practice of inspection, observation, and history gathering. Nurses do not need to be genetic experts, but they should be able to recognize genetic features of physical assessment, basic patterns of inheritance, and predisposition to development of disease. As nurses integrate genetic concepts into their delivery of care, appropriate inquiries and referrals to genetic specialists can be completed.

Although family history has long been a part of nursing assessment, the relative importance of this assessment piece has recently increased as our knowledge of the interaction of genes and the environment has expanded. In phenotypically "healthy" individuals, an accurate and complete family history can identify a single-gene (Mendelian) disorder or a mitochondrial, multifactorial, or chromosomal inheritance pattern as well as guide the prevention, diagnosis, and treatment of common complex diseases such as cardiovascular disease and cancer. A family history illustrates the interaction of genes and the environment for an individual and consequently provides a basis for individualized disease prevention (Guttmacher et al., 2004). Although an individual's inheritance risks from his or her genotype are nonmodifiable, knowledge of an individual's increased risk for chronic disease can influence lifestyle choices, clinical management, and sometimes risk reduction and prevention of the disease. Knowledge of a family history can also guide diagnostic workups and clinical treatment (Guttmacher et al., 2004).

Pedigrees

A nurse should know how to take a family history, record the history in a pedigree, and think "genetically." A pedigree is a pictorial representation or diagram of the medical history of a family. Multiple symbols are utilized to present this picture (Figure 8–6 ■) and the finished pedigree presents a family's medical data and biologic relationship information at a glance

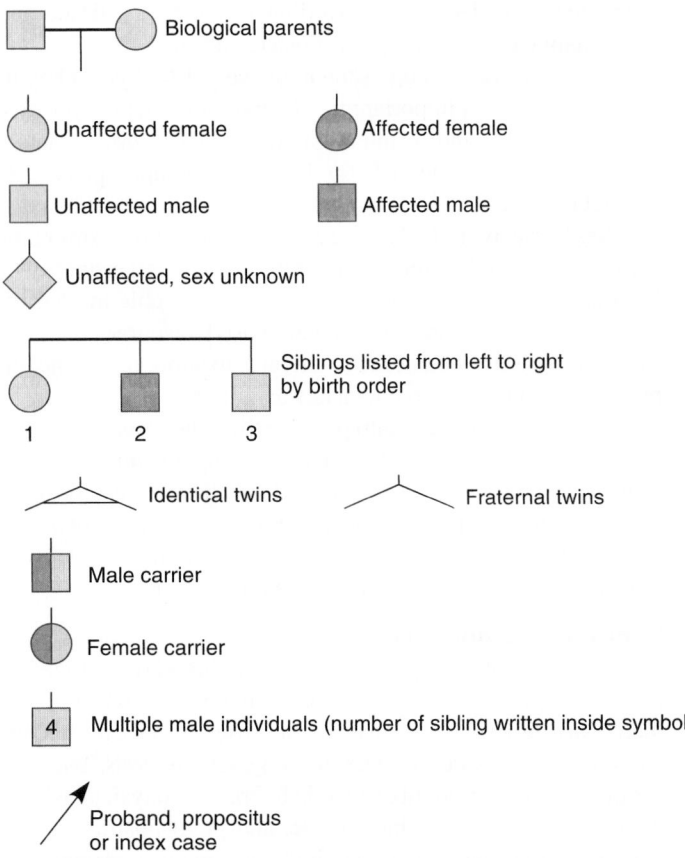

Figure 8–6 ■ Selected standardized symbols for use in drawing a pedigree.

(Figure 8–7 ■). A pedigree provides the nurse, genetic counselor, or geneticist with a clear, visual representation of relationships of affected individuals to the immediate and extended family. It can identify other individuals in the family who might benefit from a genetic consultation. It also can identify a single-gene alteration pattern of inheritance or a cluster of multifactorial conditions, and a referral and/or reproductive risk teaching for the individual and family can result. A family's learning can be enhanced by the visual teaching contribution a pedigree can provide and also clarify any inheritance misunderstandings or misconceptions. Box 8–9 lists steps for creating a family pedigree. If completed correctly and completely, a pedigree allows all healthcare professionals working with the client or family to quickly see what history and background information has been collected (Box 8–10).

It is important to gather a three-generation family pedigree even if the nurse believes this is a first occasion of the condition within a family (Figure 8-7). A condition without any identifiable inheritance pattern on the pedigree may be due to a new mutation or variable expressivity. Throughout the process of gathering family history assessment data, the nurse must remember family confidentiality at all times: All information related to a pedigree is confidential information. The history may reveal sensitive details that include infertility problems, elective termination of pregnancies, or nonpaternity. This information may not even be known by a current partner or immediate and extended family members. Other sensitive issues include pregnancies conceived by technology, a history of suicides, drug or alcohol abuse, and same-sex relationships. Box 8–11 lists ethical implications of genetic information.

Challenges inherent in recalling the family history include the client's inability to remember any conditions that may have been surgically repaired and then forgotten, or reporting conditions that may have been attributed incorrectly to other causes. Also, the family history may contain information previously unknown to extended family members. Reproductive decisions may have been made that were against the family's religious or cultural beliefs. Both immediate and extended family members may be unaware of these "family skeletons" and the client may be very reluctant to reveal this information (Bennett, 1999; Bowers, 2002).

Genetic Physical Assessment

An assessment of newborns and children with a genetics focus of minor and major anomalies is essential. A minor anomaly or malformation is an unusual or morphologic feature that in itself is of no serious medical or cosmetic concern to the individual or family. A major anomaly is a serious structural defect at birth that may interfere with normal functioning of body systems and may lead to a lifelong disability or even an early death (Aase, 1992).

Some children grow into adults whose physical features may or may not have been recognized as potential links to genetic conditions. Anomalies that exist after a person is beyond expected developmental and cognitive milestones may go unnoticed, but they may still be important. The nurse can pick up cues to genetic problems by inspecting the client and other family members. If practical, nurses should ask to look at family photographs and examine them for common dysmorphic features and family traits. Subjective assessment data can also be valuable. A client's complaints of fatigue and joint pain may indicate the onset of hereditary hemochromatosis. A physical assessment that includes a genetics focus is important for nurses when caring for any age client. An undiagnosed genetic condition may also have implications for reproductive decisions the client makes. However, genetic assessments and genetic referrals are important throughout the life span.

Nursing Diagnosis and Interventions

Nurses are responsible for comprehensively delivering the correct standard of care to clients, but at the same time being aware of the limitations of their own knowledge and expertise. In addition to the continuous integration of genetic aspects into nurses' assessments of family history and physical assessment, nurses are also responsible for carrying out interventions that include initiating referrals to genetic specialists and delivering care to the individual or family in any of the following ways. Nursing diagnoses to consider include:

- *Anticipatory Grieving*
- *Anxiety*
- *Disturbed Body Image*
- *Ineffective Coping*
- *Decisional Conflict*

A

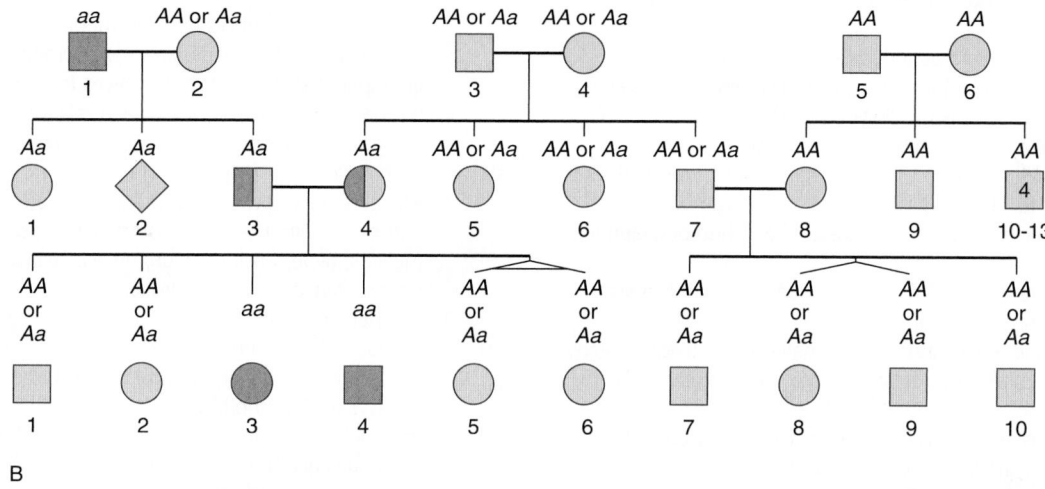

B

(A) A representative pedigree for a single character or genetic condition through three generations.
(B) The most probable genotypes of each individual in the pedigree for an autosomal recessive condition, represented by AA, Aa, or aa.

Figure 8–7 ■ Sample three-generation pedigree.

Source: Redrawn from Klug, W. S., & Cummings, M. R. (2003). *Concepts of genetics* (7th ed., p. 63). Upper Saddle River, NJ: Prentice Hall.

- *Interrupted Family Processes*
- *Ineffective Health Maintenance*
- *Deficient Knowledge*
- *Powerlessness*
- *Spiritual Distress*

Genetic Referrals and Counseling

After gathering assessment data that incorporates genetic concepts, the nurse is able to initiate a referral to genetic specialists if there are indicators for a genetic referral (Box 8–12). The nurse should provide the client with information about the advantages of a referral to genetic specialists, and the disadvantages of not following through with the referral. The nurse should inform the client that a genetic referral can provide information and answer many questions they may have concerning genetic health. Questions regarding the conditions, inheritance, availability of treatment, as well as economic, insurance, and future implications can be addressed.

Clients who are concerned about genetic disease may benefit from a genetic consultation whether or not genetic testing is available for that condition. Many people seek information and coping strategies as much as they do test results. Referral of a client with a suspected genetic problem to a geneticist, genetic clinical nurse specialist, or genetic clinic is an expected nursing responsibility in the same way as referrals to a dietitian or a social worker. When in doubt, the nurse should contact the advanced practice genetic clinical nurse, genetic counselor, or geneticist to discuss concerns.

CLIENT PREPARATION FOR GENETIC REFERRALS AND GENETIC COUNSELING Not knowing what to expect from a genetic referral is common, and the fear of the unknown may cause anxiety for the client. To facilitate the referral to a genetic specialist, the nurse should educate the client so that he or she knows what to expect during as well as after a genetic evaluation.

BOX 8–9 Steps in Drawing a Pedigree

I. How to:
1. Work in pencil.
   a. Family historians often remember additional relatives and details only after questioning is almost completed.
II. Organization:
1. Begin recording data in the middle of the sheet of paper.
   a. Allow enough room for both the maternal and paternal sides of the family.
2. Use only standard pedigree symbols.
   a. For example, males are represented by squares and females by a circle.
3. The male individual in a couple is placed on the left of the relationship line and the paternal side of the family also goes on the left-hand side of the paper.
III. Determining Family Relationships:
1. The nurse should determine the relationships within the family by asking questions such as:
   ■ Do you have a partner or are you married?
   ■ How many biologic brothers and sisters do you have?
   ■ How many children do you have?
   ■ Do all the children have the same biologic father?
   ■ Do all the children share the same mother and father?
2. Referral to "the baby's father or mother" can be helpful until a relationship or marriage is established between the parents.
3. Referral to a "union" if marriage does not exist can also help communication.
4. Determine if each individual is married, has children, signs and symptoms, etc., before continuing on to the next individual.
5. Always ask if there is any chance the mother could be related to the father or if any other parents in the family are blood relatives.
   ■ To determine consanguinity.
IV. Who Should or Should Not Be Included:
1. To ensure accuracy, the pedigree should include the parents, offspring, siblings, aunts, uncles, grandparents, and first cousins of the individual seeking counseling.
2. Detailed information about the spouses of the proband's family can be omitted unless there is a history of some kind of disorder or condition.
3. Eliminating persons or any information that does not contribute any valuable information can help keep the pedigree small and more manageable.
V. Recording the Family History:
1. Determine the approximate size of the family.

2. Record the family's ethnic background at the top of the page.
3. The initial drawing should begin with the proband, or the person who is affected with the genetic condition.
   a. Usually the reason someone is seeking a genetic referral.
4. The proband is marked with an arrow on the pedigree.
5. Draw and mark the symbols for the brothers and sister of the proband. Draw the relationship line, the line of descent, marriage or union line, and symbols for parents of the proband.
   a. Repeat this step for any children of the proband or children of the proband's brothers and sisters.
6. Children resulting from a mating (siblings) should be recorded in descending order of their birth with oldest sibling on the left.
7. Continue with symbols for all immediate relatives drawn previously and then draw and mark symbols for paternal grandparents and indicated relatives followed by the same for the maternal grandparents and relatives.
8. A legend key should contain all of the correct symbols for each indicated disease.
9. Record the age of onset of common and complex diseases and/or conditions such as coronary heart disease; diabetes mellitus; hypertension; colon, breast, ovarian, or endometrial cancer; and stroke.
10. The pedigree should include at least three generations.
    a. Generations are symbolized by Roman numerals along the left-hand side of the paper with the first generation marker, I, at the top.
    b. Each person in the generation should follow an imaginary horizontal line from left to right.
11. The names of each individual (maiden names in case of married women) and their dates of birth should be included along with half-siblings, pregnancy losses, still births, previous marriages, and adopted children.
VI. Other:
1. Consanguinity may be suspected if the historian repeatedly gives the same last name on both sides of the family.
   a. Consanguinity can be confirmed by asking if any relatives in the family have ever had a child together.
VII. Completing the Pedigree:
1. When completed, the pedigree should be dated and signed with the name, credentials, and position of the person drawing it.

Source: Data from Bennett, R. L. (1999). *The practical guide to the genetic family history.* New York: Wiley-Liss.

Usually before the first genetic evaluation visit, the client will be contacted to provide a detailed medical and family history and to make an appointment for genetic consultation. The client should be prepared to give as exact a family history as possible so that a detailed three-generation pedigree can be constructed. The client should be informed that a genetic consultation usually lasts several hours. During the appointment, a genetic clinical nurse, genetic counselor, and/or a physician will perform an initial interview with the client. A geneticist will examine the client in order to establish an accurate diagnosis. Tests may be ordered. These may include chromosome (cytogenetic) analysis, DNA-based testing, x-rays, biopsy, biochemical tests, and linkage studies (Lashley, 2005). After the exam and the completion of any applicable testing, the

BOX 8–10 Specific Facts and Health Information to Include in a Pedigree

- Age/birth date or year of birth
- Age of death (year, if known)
- Cause of death
- Age at diagnosis
- Full siblings versus half or step-siblings
- Pregnancy with gestational age (LMP) or estimated date of delivery (EDD)
- Infertility versus no children by choice
- Pregnancy complications with gestational ages noted (e.g., 6 wks, 32 wks)
- Miscarriage (SAB)

- Stillbirth (SB)
- Pregnancy termination (TOP)
- Relevant health information (e.g., height and weight)
- Affected/unaffected status—define shading of symbols in a legend key
- Ethnic background
- Consanguinity
- Date pedigree taken or updated
- Name of person who took pedigree and credentials
- Key or legend

geneticist and/or genetic counselor will discuss the findings with the client and make recommendations. The discussion will include the natural history of the condition, the inheritance patterns, the current preventive or treatment options, and the risks to the client and/or family. The visit will also include opportunities for questions and answers as well as the assessment and evaluation of the client's understanding. It is typical for the information retention of a client facing a new genetic diagnosis to be very low. This makes it imperative for the nurse to take advantage of opportunities to reinforce genetic concepts at a later time when the client is ready.

As the visit concludes, the client can expect appropriate referrals to be made, discussion of available services or research studies, and possible scheduling of a follow-up visit. A summary of the information is usually sent to the client and the client's healthcare provider will receive a report if requested by the client.

Genetic healthcare providers present the client with information to promote informed decisions. They are also sensitive to the importance of protecting the individual's autonomy. A challenge during any visit to a genetic specialist is providing nondirective counseling. Clients should be permitted to make decisions that are not influenced by any biases or values from the nurse, counselor, or geneticist. Many clients are accustomed to practitioners and nurses providing direction and guidance in their decision making, and clients may be very uncomfortable with the nondirectional approach of the nurse. They may believe that the nurse or healthcare provider is withholding very bad news. The nurse should discuss the positives and negatives of each decision and present as many options as possible through the use of therapeutic listening and communication skills (Cunniff, 2001).

Client Teaching

The nurse must be aware of available genetic resources and participate in the education of genetic disorders as well as health promotion and prevention. Informing clients of what to expect from a genetic referral as well as clarifying and/or reinforcing information obtained during a genetic referral or from genetic test results is also important.

The cultural and religious beliefs and values of the client must be assessed by the nurse prior to teaching. Are the gene alterations viewed as uncontrollable and believed to be occurring secondary to cultural belief such as a stranger looking at the client? Or, are the gene alterations considered a "punishment"? A client's readiness to learn can be influenced by cultural or religious beliefs and values. Obtaining educational materials in the native language of the client will also help facilitate the teaching-learning experience.

The nurse must be aware of common inheritance misconceptions such as a client's belief that with a 25% recurrence risk, after one child is affected, the next three children will be unaffected or with a 50% recurrence risk, every other child will be affected. The recurrence risk *for each pregnancy* should be continually stressed by the nurse. Clients often believe that a family member has inherited the genetic condition because they look or "take after" a relative with a genetic condition. When new gene alterations or mutations are discussed, clients will often exhibit surprise because no one else in the family has the condition so they perceive that the trait or condition cannot possibly be inherited (Bennett, 1999). Helping clients to understand these genetic concepts is fundamental to delivering the standard of genetic nursing care.

Psychosocial Care

To meet the client's psychosocial needs, the nurse should identify the client's expectations and needs as well as the client's cultural, spiritual, value, and belief system. From where does the client receive strength? Denial of the genetic diagnosis is common and nurses must be aware of the client's state of acceptance. Individuals often will not believe that a chronic genetic condition exists. Nurses must also provide care to help alleviate any anxiety and/or guilt in the client. Anxiety of the unknown is common when awaiting diagnosis or test results, but individuals also experience anxiety from not understanding the future implications of a confirmed genetic disease. Guilt may be associated with knowledge of the existence of a genetic condition in a family. The nurse must support clients as they contemplate telling extended family members, friends, and neighbors about a confirmed diagnosis. Clients often do not want to tell extended family members until they are ready. The nurse should encourage open discussions and the expression of fears and concerns. Guilt and shame are very common as a client deals with the loss of the expectation and dream of a healthy, productive life.

BOX 8–11 Ethical Implications of Genetic Information

The nurse must consider the enormity of the ethical issues facing all families who have knowledge of their genetic makeup. The ethical issues a nurse may have to discuss with the client are numerous. A few of the issues are listed below.

Access to Information

- Who should have access to personal genetic information, and how will it be used?
- Do insurers, employers, courts, law enforcement, schools, universities, adoption agencies, and the military have a right to access this information?

Self-Perception

- How does personal genetic information affect an individual's perception of self?
- How does personal genetic information affect society's perceptions of that individual?
- How does personal genetic information affect an individual's cultural identity?
- How is self-identity and self-worth affected by a confirmed genetic risk or condition?

Family Roles and Relationships

- Should an individual be tested for an autosomal dominant condition if the siblings and/or parents are opposed to knowing if they, themselves, have the altered gene?
- Should potential mates have genetic information?
- Should two people with increased genetic risk be prohibited from having children?
- Should a child be tested?
- Should the father be told if genetic testing and/or genetic counseling reveals nonpaternity?
- Should adoption records contain a complete genetic history of the biologic parents?
- Is there an obligation to tell other family members if an altered gene that demands a change in lifestyle (nutrition, exercise, smoking, etc.) is diagnosed?
- Is there an obligation to tell other family members if an altered gene that causes early debilitation and/or death is diagnosed?

Informed Consent

- Are all individuals receiving true informed consent and do they understand all of the consequences of agreeing to even a simple blood test in the doctor's office that may reveal a diagnosis or increased risk for a genetic condition?

Health and Life Insurance

- Should insurance companies have access to genetic test results?
- Should medical insurance costs be higher for persons with a known gene disease-producing alteration?
- Should medical insurance costs be higher for persons with a known increased risk for disease because of any gene alteration?
- Should medical insurance costs be higher for persons with known increased risk for disease because of any gene alteration if they make unhealthy lifestyle choices and do nothing to lower their risk?
- Should the individual be covered by medical insurance at all?
- Should individuals pay higher costs if they have children?
- Should individuals be required to have a large life insurance policy to financially protect their families?

Financial

- Should the child be eligible for government grants or any scholarship money?
- Should society be expected to financially support children through government programs or private insurance?
- What is the motivation to save money for the future?

Employment

- Should an employer have access to an individual's genetic profile?
- Should a young adult be hired even though she/he will burden the company with multiple sick days, higher insurance financial support, etc.?
- Should the individual receive promotional opportunities and increased job responsibilities if the employer knows there will be a great deal of lost work days?
- Will the individual's productivity be affected by the genetic condition?

Reinforce to clients that genetic alterations are caused by changes within a gene and not by superstitions related to sin or other cultural beliefs. However, it is important to remember that everyone has superstitions or beliefs and the nurse must remain nonjudgmental. As mothers, fathers, siblings, and extended family members provide continuous care for the client with a genetic condition, depression can result. Depression also can occur in the individual with the chronic condition. The nurse must maintain awareness of the possibility of depression and be proactive in obtaining support for the client or family.

The nurse also is responsible for assessing the client's coping mechanisms as well as available family, spiritual, cultural, and community support systems. Genetic conditions can cause a permanent strain on family dynamics and relationships. The nurse may need to help the client reaffirm his or her self-worth and value (Lashley, 2005). If seen in an academic setting, clients may feel they are part of a "production line" even though they are present for a very private problem (Cunniff, 2001). Nurses must be sensitive to these perceptions, provide open communication, and encourage discussion of feelings. Growth and development and meeting adult developmental milestones can be altered by actual or potential genetic disorders. Especially unique is the potential or actual inheritance of a late-onset condition such as Huntington disease. The client with this altered gene may not meet any of the developmental tasks in moving through adulthood. Should the client get married, attend college, save money, or worry about future? The nurse must identify the impact of genetic knowledge on activities of daily living but also movement through developmental milestones. Both client and family strengths need to be identified.

BOX 8–12 Adult Indicators for a Referral to a Genetic Specialist

Adult History Assessment Data Concerns

- Several closely related individuals affected with the same or related conditions:
  - Breast and ovarian cancer
  - Colon and endometrial cancer
  - Diabetes
  - Hypertension
  - Coronary heart disease
  - Thyroid cancer
  - Colon polyps
- A common disorder with earlier age of onset than typical (increase concern if it occurs in more than one family member):
  - Breast cancer: < 45–50 years of age or premenopausal
  - Colon cancer: < 45–50 years of age
  - Prostate cancer: < 45–60 years of age
  - Vision loss: < 55 years of age
  - Hearing loss: < 50–60 years of age
  - Dementia: < 60 years of age
  - Heart disease: < 40–60 years of age
  - Stroke: < 60 years of age
- A sudden or unexpected death in someone who "seemed" healthy

- Renal disease
- Asthma
- Suicides

An Individual with:

- Two or more conditions
- A medical condition and dysmorphic features
- Developmental delay with dysmorphic features and/or physical birth anomalies
- Learning disabilities
- Behavioral problems
- Unexplained:
  - Movement disorders
  - Seizures
  - Hypotonia
  - Ataxia
  - Infertility
- Disproportionate tall or short stature
- Proportionate short stature with dysmorphic features
- Atypical sexual development
- Premature ovarian failure

Source: American Medical Association. (2004). *Family medical history in disease prevention*. Retrieved March 12, 2005, from http://www.ama-assn.org/go/familyhistory

---

The nurse can refer the client to a support group. However it is important to have permission from the client if the nurse is providing a support group with the client's name and contact information.

Another key role for the nurse is to help clients with the often difficult task of communicating genetic information such as inheritance patterns to extended family members. Cultural values of autonomy and privacy are impacted when a client must consider whether to communicate genetic information to extended family members who may also carry the altered gene. The history of a genetic alteration that may or may not cause disease can be extensive within a family, affecting multiple family members. Family members often have difficulty understanding that some genetic conditions have variable expressivity. Members of the extended family often are shocked and feel a profound sense of guilt that they are the one who has carried the gene alteration that caused their loved one to have a genetic condition.

Careful self-assessment of feelings is essential for the nurse. The nurse must continually advocate for clients and support their decisions even if the decisions contradict the nurse's own ideals and morals. Coping with genetic revelations and making genetic-related treatment decisions are difficult activities for everyone. The nurse must remember that clients will need resources and support, and also help in gathering information about reproductive options.

Evaluation

Expected outcomes of delivering nursing care with a genetic focus include:

- The client will make informed and voluntary decisions related to genetic health issues.
- The client will accurately identify:
  - Basic genetic concepts and simple inheritance risk probabilities
  - What to expect from a genetic referral.
  - The influence of genetic factors in health promotion and health maintenance.
  - Differences between medical and genetic tests.
  - Social, legal and ethical issues related to genetic testing.

VISIONS FOR THE FUTURE

Nurses are often the primary caregivers to whom clients turn for information, guidance, and clarification of ideas. This nursing role is essential not only in providing direct nursing care but as a member of the community. As more information about the genetic revolution becomes available to consumers—in areas such as pharmacogenomics, gene transfer, ethics, genetic engineering, and stem cell research—the role of nurses remains not only vital but grows enormously. Nurses should remain educated, informed, knowledgeable, and ready to discuss trends and changes with clients and their families.

MEDIALINK Case Study: Genetic Resources

EXPLORE MediaLink

Prentice Hall Nursing MediaLink DVD-ROM
Audio Glossary
NCLEX-RN® Review

Animation
Human Genome Project

COMPANION WEBSITE www.prenhall.com/lemone
Audio Glossary
NCLEX-RN® Review
Care Plan Activity: Genetic Implications of Adult Health
    Nursing Care
Case Study: Genetic Implications
MediaLink Application: Create and Analyze a Family Pedigree
Links to Resources

CHAPTER HIGHLIGHTS

■ Nurses are responsible for basic genetic knowledge and delivering the expected standard of genetic nursing care.

■ When cell division does not occur as expected, chromosomal alterations on the autosomes or sex chromosomes can result.

■ Chromosomal alterations can be seen in a human karyotype.

■ Protein-directing genes are very important to life and functioning as a human being because proteins are very specialized and perform a variety of functions within the cell.

■ Different forms of genes are alleles.

■ An individual may be identified as heterozygous or homozygous for a single gene.

■ Some gene alterations cause disease and some are protective from disease.

■ Mitochondrial gene alterations are inherited from the mother and are primarily involved in high-energy organs such as skeletal muscles, brain, and heart muscle.

■ Multifactorial inheritance does not follow Mendelian inheritance patterns.

■ Genetic healthcare providers present the individual and their family with information to promote informed decisions.

■ Many types of genetic tests are available and they differ from routine medical tests.

■ All genetic tests have special considerations related to social, financial, ethical, and legal implications.

■ Basic genetic nursing care involves family risk assessment through a detailed family history, drawing a three-generation pedigree, and integrating genetic concepts into a physical assessment.

■ Basic genetic nursing involves initiating a referral to a genetic specialist.

■ Knowledge of the principles of inheritance allows the nurse to not only offer and reinforce genetic information to clients and their families but also to assist them in managing their care and in making reproductive decisions.

■ Genetic concepts can be applied to health promotion and health maintenance.

■ The nurse must be aware of the social, ethical, cultural, and spiritual issues related to the delivery of genetic nursing care.

TEST YOURSELF NCLEX-RN® REVIEW

1 The client is discussing the inheritance of an autosomal dominant trait. The client has the condition and the client's wife does not. They have one child without the condition. The nurse would be correct in explaining to the client that he is most likely which genotype?
1. FF
2. Ff
3. ff
4. X_fY

2 The male client diagnosed with Fabry disease is admitted to the unit. Which statement made by the client would indicate to the nurse that the client understands Mendelian inheritance concepts? "I have the disease because . . ." (Select all that apply.)
1. my mother had Fabry and my father did not."
2. my father's mother had Fabry disease."
3. my grandmother's brother had Fabry disease."
4. my father has Fabry disease."

3 The nurse is providing information regarding genetic testing to a couple who believe they are carriers of an autosomal recessive gene alteration. Which statement by the nurse is appropriate?
1. "If both of you are carriers, all of your sons will be affected and all of your daughters will be carriers."
2. "Chromosomal studies will reveal if you are actually a carrier."
3. "Newborn screening will reveal if your child is affected."
4. "During the genetic evaluation, you will be asked to provide at least a three-generation family history."

4 The nurse knows that which assessment data obtained during a family history may suggest a genetic condition or inherited susceptibility to a common disease? (Select all that apply.)
1. breast cancer at age 33
2. a sibling who died unexpectedly while playing basketball at age 66
3. colon polyps in four third-degree relatives
4. a brother's unexplained infertility

5 When analyzing a family pedigree, the nurse notes the pedigree demonstrates that successive generations contain affected individuals, both males and females are affected, and there is no father-to-offspring inheritance. What is the most likely pattern of inheritance?
1. autosomal dominant
2. autosomal recessive
3. x-linked recessive
4. multifactorial
5. mitochondrial

6 When the nurse is developing a teaching plan, which statement is a correct rationale regarding the health promotion and health maintenance benefits from an assessment of family history? (Select all that apply.)
1. Clinical treatment options can be more focused.
2. Prophylactic treatments can be started early.
3. Specific diet, exercise regimen, and genotype can be determined.
4. Single-gene alteration can be diagnosed.

7 The nurse is recording a family pedigree. Which would be correct to include in drawing the pedigree?
1. Detailed information is important for all persons recorded on the pedigree.
2. The maternal side of the family should be placed on the left of the page.
3. The proband is marked with an arrow and a "P."
4. Two generations should be recorded and labeled with Roman numerals.

8 The nurse would consider which assessment finding(s) as minor anomalies? (Select all that apply.)
1. café au lait spots
2. ear pits
3. atrial septal defect (ASD)
4. hypertelorism

9 Which are appropriate concepts for the nurse to include when developing a teaching plan for the client prior to genetic testing? (Select all that apply.)
1. Predispositional genetic tests are medically indicated when the seriousness and mortality of the disease can be reduced with knowledge of the gene alteration.
2. To meet quality assurance, laboratories should hold a CLIA88 certification.
3. A mutation panel contains the most common gene alterations but it may not include all of the disease-causing mutations.
4. Family members affected by genetic test results have a legal right to the test results.

10 The client asks the nurse if a genetic referral is necessary. Which information would be appropriate for the nurse to provide? Most likely genetic specialists will: (Select all that apply.)
1. provide direction for important decision making.
2. complete chromosomal studies.
3. ask to see photographs of relatives.
4. provide information about the natural history of the condition.

See Test Yourself answers in Appendix C.

BIBLIOGRAPHY

Aase, J. (1992). Dysmorphic diagnosis for the pediatric practitioner. *Pediatric Clinics of North America, 39*, 135–156.

American Nurses Association and International Society of Nurses in Genetics, Inc. (1998). *Statement on the scope and standards of genetics clinical nursing practice.* Washington, DC: American Nurses Publishing.

American Society of Human Genetics. (1998). ASHG statement: Professional disclosure of familial genetic information. *American Journal of Human Genetics, 62*, 474–483.

American Society of Human Genetics & American College of Medical Genetics. (1995). Points to consider: Ethical, legal, and psychosocial implications of genetic testing in children and adolescents. *American Journal of Human Genetics, 57*, 1233–1241.

Bennett, R. L. (1999). *The practical guide to the genetic family history.* New York: Wiley-Liss.

Bennett, R. L., Steinhaus, K. A., Uhrich, S. B., O'Sullivan, C. K., Resta, R. G., Lochner-Doyle, D., et al. (1995). Recommendations for standardizing human pedigree nomenclature. *American Journal of Human Genetics, 56*, 745–752.

Beskow, L., Burke, W., Merz, J., Barr, P., Terry, S., Penchaszadeh, V., et al. (2001). Informed consent for population based research involving genetics. *Journal of the American Medical Association, 286*, 2315–2321.

Bird, T. D. (2004, August 9). Myotonic dystrophy type I. In *GeneReviews at GeneTests: Medical Genetics Information Resource* [Online database]. Copyright, University of Washington, Seattle. 1997–2005. Retrieved April 10, 2005, from http://www.genetests.org

Bowers, N. R. (2002). Meeting the standard of genetic nursing care. *JSPN: The Journal for Specialists in Pediatric Nursing, 7*, 123–126.

Burke, W. (2004). Genetic testing in primary care. *Annual Review Genomics: Human Genetics, 5*, 1–14.

Chinnery, P. F. (2005, April 12). Leber hereditary optic neuropathy. In *GeneReviews at GeneTests: Medical Genetics Information Resource* [Online database].

Copyright, University of Washington, Seattle. 1997–2005. Retrieved April 17, 2005, from http://www.genetests.org

Cohen, B. H., & Gold, D. R. (2001). Mitochondrial cytopathy in adults: What we know so far. *Cleveland Clinic Journal of Medicine, 68*, 625–642.

Collins, F. S. (2000). Shattuck lecture—medical and societal consequences of the human genome project. *New England Journal of Medicine, 341*(1), 28–37.

Collins, F. S., Green, E. D., Guttmacher, A. E., & Guyer, M. S. (2003). A vision for the future of genomic research [Electronic version]. *Nature, 422*, 835–847.

Cunniff, C. (2001, October). *Culture and genetic health care.* Paper presented at the meeting of the International Society of Nurses in Genetics 14th Annual Educational Conference, San Diego, CA.

Cutler, C. (2003). Glucose-6-phosphate dehydrogenase deficiency. *Medline Plus.* Retrieved April 28, 2005, from http://www.nlm.nih.gov/medlineplus/ency/article/000528.htm

Dietz, H. C. (2003, September 22). Marfan syndrome. In *GeneReviews at GeneTests: Medical Genetics Information Resource* [Online database]. Copyright, University of Washington, Seattle. 1997–2005. Retrieved April 4, 2005, from http://www.genetests.org

GeneCare Medical Genetics Center. (2002). *FISH* [Brochure]. Chapel Hill, NC: Author.

Gene reviews. In *GeneTests: Medical Genetics Information Resource* [Online database]. Copyright, University of Washington, Seattle. 1993–2005. Retrieved April 2005 from http://www.genetests.org

GeneTests. (2004). *About genetic services.* Retrieved April 22, 2005, from http://www.genetests.org

Genetics Home Reference: Your Guide to Understanding Genetic Conditions [Online reference]. Available at http://ghr.nlm.nih.gov/

Greendale, K., & Pyeritz, R. E. (2001). Empowering primary care health professionals in medical genetics: How soon? How fast? How far? *American Journal of Medical Genetics, 106*, 223–232.

Guttmacher, A. E., & Collins, F. (2002). Genomic medicine: A primer. *New England Journal of Medicine, 347*, 1512–1527.

Guttmacher, A. E., Collins, F. S., & Carmona, R. H. (2004). The family history—more important than ever. *New England Journal of Medicine, 351* (22), 2333–2336.

Guttmacher, A. E., Jenkins, J., & Uhlman, W. R. (2001). Genomic medicine: Who will practice it? A call to open arms. *American Journal of Medical Genetics, 106*, 216–222.

Guttmacher, A. E., & McDonald, J. (2004, March 16). Hereditary hemorrhagic telangiectasia (HHT). In *GeneReviews at GeneTests: Medical Genetics Information Resource* [Online database]. Copyright, University of Washington, Seattle. 1997–2005. Retrieved April 9, 2005, from http://www.genetests.org

Human Genome Project. (2002). *The Human Genome Project partners with minority community leaders for genomics education.* Retrieved April 27, 2005, from http://www.ornl.gov/sci/techresources/Human_Genome/publicat/jmmbbag.pdf

Human Genome Project. (2003). *Genetic disease information—pronto!* Retrieved April 27, 2005, from http://www.ornl.gov/techresources/Human_Genome/medicine/assist.shtml

Human Genome Project. (2004a). *From genome to the proteome.* Retrieved April 27, 2005, from http://www.ornl.gov/sci/techresources/Human_Genome/project/info.shtml

Human Genome Project. (2004b). *Gene testing.* Retrieved April 27, 2005, from http://www.ornl.gov/sci/techresources/Human_Genome/medicine/genetest.shtml

Human Genome Project. (2004c). *SNP fact sheet.* Retrieved April 27, 2005, from http://www.ornl.gov/techresources/Human_Genome/faq/snps.shtml

International Society of Nurses in Genetics. (2000). *Position statement: Informed decision-making consent: The role of the nurse.* Retrieved April 27, 2005, from http://www.isong.org/about/position_statements/index.html

Javitt, G., Stanley, E., & Hudson, K. (2004). Direct-to-consumer genetic tests, government oversight, and the first amendment: What the government can (and can't) do to protect the public's health. *Oklahoma Law Review, 57,* 251–302. Retrieved April 9, 2005, from http://www.law.ou.edu/lawrevs/olr/

Jegalian, K. (2000). *Genetics the future of medicine* (NIH Publication No. 00-4873). Washington, DC: National Human Genome Research Institute, National Institutes of Health.

Jones, K. L. (1997). *Smith's recognizable patterns of human malformations* (5th ed.). Philadelphia: Saunders.

Klug, W. S., & Cummings, M. R. (2003). *Concepts of genetics* (7th ed.). Upper Saddle River, NJ: Pearson/Prentice Hall.

Lashley, F. R. (2005). *Clinical genetics in nursing practice* (3rd ed.). New York: Springer.

Loyd, J. E., & Phillips, J. A. (2004, Novermber 2). BMPR2 related primary pulmonary hypertension. In *GeneReviews at GeneTests: Medical Genetics Information Resource* [Online database]. Copyright, University of Washington, Seattle. 1997–2005. Retrived April 17, 2005, from http://www.genetests.org

National Cancer Institute. (2005). *Chronic myelogenous leukemia: Treatment.* Retrieved April 27, 2005, from http://www.cancer.gov/cancertopics/pdq/treatment/CML/HealthProfessional

National Coalition for Health Professional Education in Genetics. (2000, updated 2005). *Core competencies in genetics essential for all health-care professionals.* Retrieved April 29, 2005, from http://www.nchpeg.org

National Human Genome Research Institute. (2004). *Researchers discover use of novel mechanism preserves Y chromosome genes.* Retrieved April 27, 2005, from http://www.genome.gov/11007628

National Human Genome Research Institute, National Institutes of Health. (1997). In N. Holtzman & M. Watson (Eds.), *Promoting safe and effective genetic testing in the United States.* Retrieved April 9, 2005, from http://www.genome.gov/10002393

National Institutes of Health. (1987). *Consensus development conference statement: Neurofibromatosis.* (Volume 6, Number 12).

National Institutes of Health & National Cancer Institute. (1995). *Understanding gene testing* (NIH Publication No. 96-3905). Washington, DC: U.S. Department of Health and Human Services, National Institutes of Health.

Nussbaum, R. L., McInnes, R. R., Willard, H. F., & Boerkoel, C. F. (2001). *Thompson & Thompson genetics in medicine* (6th ed.). Philadelphia: Saunders.

Online Mendelian Inheritance in Man. (2003). McKusick-Nathans Institute for Genetics Medicine, Johns Hopkins University (Baltimore, MD) and National Center for Biotechnology Information Library of Medicine (Bethesda, MD). Retrieved from http://www.ncbi.nlm.nih.gov/omim/

Pyeritz, R. E., & Gasner, C. (1994). *The Marfan syndrome* (4th ed.). New York: National Marfan Foundation.

Scanlon, C., & Fibison, W. (1995). *Managing genetic information: Implications for nursing practice.* Washington, DC: American Nurses Publishing.

Scheuner, M. T., Wang, S. J., Raffel, L. J., Larabell, S. K., & Rotter, J. I. (1997). Family history: A comprehensive genetic risk assessment method for the chronic conditions of adulthood. *American Journal of Medical Genetics, 71,* 315–324.

Secretary's Advisory Committee on Genetic Testing, National Institutes of Health. (2000). *Enhancing the oversight of genetic tests: Recommendations of the SACGT.* Retrieved April 22, 2005, from http://www4.od.nih.gov/oba/sacgt/GTDocuments.html

U.S. Department of Energy Biological and Environmental Research Source. (2003). *Gene gateway—Exploring genes and genetic disorders.* Retrieved April 27, 2005, from http://www.ornl.gov/TechResources/Human_Genome/posters/chromosome/

U.S. Department of Energy Genome Programs. (2003). *Genomics and its impact on science and society: The human genome project and beyond.* Retrieved April 28, 2005, from http://www.ornl.gov/hgmis/publicat/primer/

Wenstrup, R. J. (2001, July). *The Ehlers-Danlos syndromes.* Paper presented at the 2nd Biennial Genetics Update Workshop, Cincinnati, OH.

Wertz, D., Famos, J., & Reilly, P. (1994). Genetic testing for children and adolescents: Who decides? *Journal of American Medical Association, 272,* 875–881.

Wine, J., Kuo, E., Hurlock, G., & Moss, R. (2001). Comprehensive mutation screening in cystic fibrosis center. *Pediatrics, 107,* 280–286.

CHAPTER 9 Nursing Care of Clients Experiencing Pain

LEARNING OUTCOMES

- Describe the neurophysiology of pain.

- Compare and contrast definitions and characteristics of acute, chronic, breakthrough, central, phantom, and psychogenic pain.

- Discuss factors affecting individualized responses to pain.

- Clarify myths and misconceptions about pain.

- Discuss interdisciplinary care for the client in pain, including medications, surgery, transcutaneous electrical nerve stimulation, and complementary therapies.

- Use the nursing process as a framework for providing individualized nursing care for clients experiencing pain.

CLINICAL COMPETENCIES

- Assess client's pain intensity; quality; location; pattern; intensifiers; nullifiers; side effects of analgesics; effect on physical, psychologic, and social function, mood, and support for managing pain.

- Determine client's desire and preference for pain management.

- Intervene with client-approved pharmacologic and nonpharmacologic methodologies. Administer medications knowledgeably and safely.

- Utilize equianalgesia tables for transitioning among opioid analgesics. Match continuous pain with around-the-clock, long-acting dosing and intermittent pain with short-acting medications.

- Provide client and family teaching about effective pain control.

- Evaluate effectiveness of interventions to relieve pain; retreat or adjust doses of medication and interventions as necessary.

- Revise plan of care according to client's response to interventions and need for control.

MEDIALINK

Resources for this chapter can be found on the Prentice Hall Nursing MediaLink DVD-ROM accompanying this textbook, and on the Companion Website at http://www.prenhall.com/lemone

Pain is a subjective response to both physical and psychologic stressors. All people experience pain at some point during their lives. Although pain usually is experienced as uncomfortable and unwelcome, it also serves a protective role, warning of potentially health-threatening conditions. For this reason, pain is increasingly referred to as the *fifth vital sign*, with recommendations to assess pain with each vital sign assessment. The Joint Commission on Accreditation of Healthcare Organizations (JCAHO) (2001) has established pain standards that identify the relief of pain as a client right and requires healthcare facilities to implement specific procedures for, and provider education on, pain assessment and management.

Each individual pain event is a distinct and personal experience influenced by physiologic, psychologic, cognitive, sociocultural, and spiritual factors. Pain is the symptom most associated with describing oneself as ill, and it is the most common reason for seeking health care. The International Association for the Study of Pain defines pain as an unpleasant sensory and emotional experience associated with actual or potential tissue damage, or described in terms of such damage. Although there are many definitions and descriptors of pain, the one most relevant is that pain is "whatever the person experiencing it says it is, and existing whenever the person says it does" (McCaffery, 1979, p. 11). This definition acknowledges the client as the only person who can accurately define and describe his or her own pain and serves as the basis for nursing assessment and care of clients in pain. It also supports the values and beliefs about pain necessary for holistic nursing care, including the following:

- Only the person affected can experience pain; that is, pain has a personal meaning.
- If the client says he or she has pain, the client is in pain. All pain is real.
- Pain has physical, emotional, cognitive, sociocultural, and spiritual dimensions.
- Pain affects the whole body, usually negatively.
- Pain may serve as both a response to and a warning of actual or potential trauma.

NEUROPHYSIOLOGY AND THEORIES OF PAIN

Neurophysiology

The peripheral nervous system is composed of two types of neurons: sensory and motor. Pain is perceived through the sensory neurons and responded to through the motor neurons. Connections or synapses occur within the spinal cord and again within the central nervous system (CNS), where cognitive analysis of the painful stimulus leads to a response. A highly intense pain may prompt an immediate reflex response that precedes awareness of the pain.

Nerve receptors for pain are called **nociceptors** (Figure 9–1 ■). They are located at the ends of small afferent neurons and are woven throughout all tissues of the body except the brain. Nociceptors are especially numerous in the skin and muscles. Pain occurs when biologic, mechanical, thermal, electrical, or chemical factors stimulate nociceptors (Table 9–1). The intensity and duration of the stimuli determine the sensation. Long-lasting, intense stimulation produces greater pain than brief, mild stimulation.

Nociceptors are stimulated either by persistent mechanical, chemical, or thermal stimuli to the cell or by the local release of biochemicals secondary to cell injury. *Bradykinin,* a polypeptide element of the kinin protein system (McCance & Huether, 2002), appears to be the most abundant and potent pain-producing chemical; other biochemical sources of pain include prostaglandins, histamine, hydrogen ions, and potassium ions. These biochemicals are thought to bind to nociceptors in response to noxious stimuli, causing the nociceptors to initiate pain impulses.

TABLE 9–1 Pain Stimuli

CAUSATIVE FACTOR	EXAMPLE
Microorganisms (e.g., bacteria, viruses)	Meningitis
Inflammation	Sore throat
Impaired blood flow	Angina
Invasive tumor	Colon cancer
Radiation	Therapy for cancer
Heat	Sunburn
Obstruction	Kidney stone
Spasm	Colon cramping
Compression	Carpal tunnel syndrome
Decreased movement	Pain after cast removal
Stretching or straining	Sprained ankle
Fractures	Fractured hip
Swelling	Arthritis
Deposits of foreign tissue	Endometriosis
Chemicals	Skin rash
Electricity	Electrical burn
Conflict, difficulty in life	Psychogenic pain

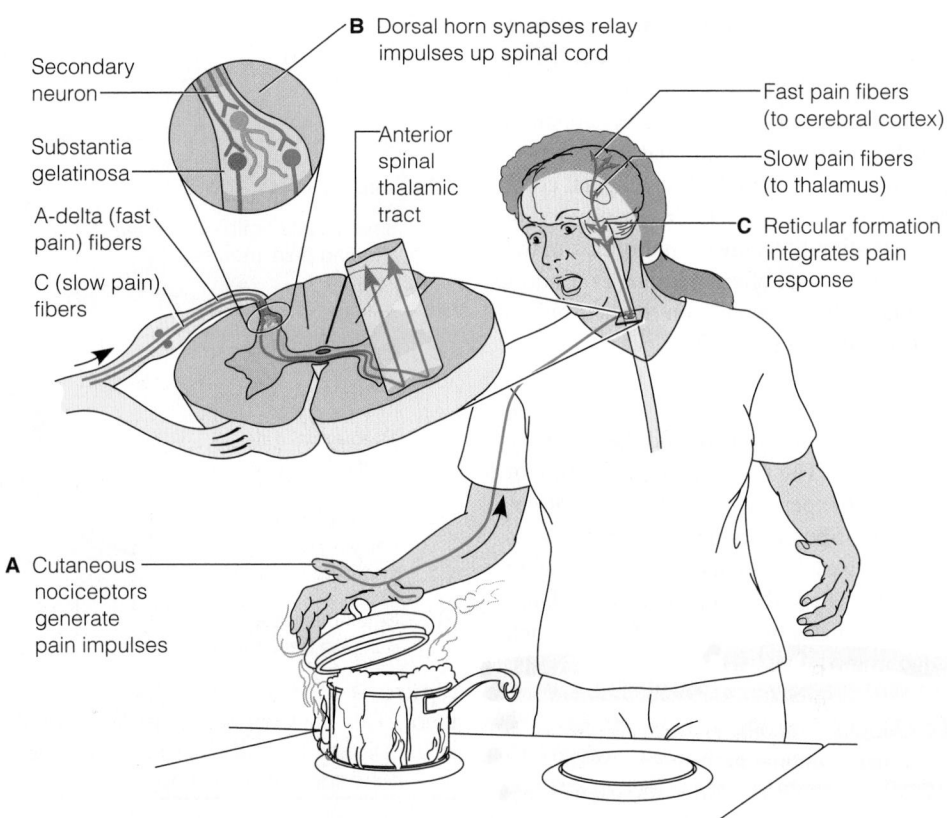

Figure 9–1 ■ *A*, Cutaneous nociceptors generate pain impulses that travel via A-delta and C fibers to the spinal cord's dorsal horn. *B*, Secondary neurons in dorsal horn pass impulses across spinal cord to anterior spinothalamic tract. *C*, Slow pain impulses ascend to the thalamus, while fast pain impulses ascend to the cerebral cortex. The reticular formation in the brainstem integrates the emotional, cognitive, and autonomic responses to pain.

Pain Pathway

The neural pathway of pain is illustrated in Figure 9–1 and is summarized as follows:

1. Pain is perceived by the nociceptors in the periphery of the body, for example, in the skin or viscera. Cutaneous pain is transmitted through small afferent A-delta and even smaller C nerve fibers to the spinal cord. A-delta fibers are myelinated and transmit impulses rapidly. They produce sharp, well-defined pain sensations, such as those that result from cuts, electric shocks, or the impact of a blow. A-delta fibers are associated with acute pain. C fibers are not myelinated and thus transmit pain impulses more slowly. The pain from deep body structures (such as muscles and viscera) is primarily transmitted by C fibers, producing diffuse burning or aching sensations. C fibers are associated with chronic pain. Both A-delta and C fibers are involved in most injuries. For example, if a person bangs the elbow, A-delta fibers transmit this pain stimulus within 0.1 second. The person feels this pain as a sharp, localized, smarting sensation. One or more seconds after the blow, the person experiences a duller, aching, diffuse sensation of pain impulses carried by the C fibers.
2. Secondary neurons transmit the impulses from the afferent neurons through the dorsal horn of the spinal cord, where they synapse in the substantia gelatinosa. The impulses then cross over to the anterior and lateral spinothalamic tracts.
3. The impulses ascend the anterior and lateral spinothalamic tracts and pass through the medulla and midbrain to the thalamus.
4. In the thalamus and cerebral cortex, the pain impulses are perceived, described, localized, and interpreted, and a response is formulated. A noxious impulse becomes pain when the sensation reaches conscious levels and is perceived and evaluated by the person experiencing the sensation.

Some pain impulses ascend along the paleospinothalamic tract in the medial section of the spinal cord. These impulses enter the reticular formation and the limbic systems, which integrate emotional and cognitive responses to pain. Interconnections in the autonomic nervous system may also cause an autonomic response to the pain. In addition, deep nociceptors often converge on the same spinal neuron, resulting in pain that is experienced in a part of the body other than its origin.

Inhibitory Mechanisms

Efferent fibers run from the reticular formation and midbrain to the substantia gelatinosa in the dorsal horns of the spinal cord. Along these fibers, pain may be inhibited or modulated. The analgesia system is a group of midbrain neurons that transmits impulses to the pons and medulla, which in turn stimulate a pain inhibitory center in the dorsal horns of the spinal cord. The exact nature of this inhibitory mechanism is unknown.

The most clearly defined chemical inhibitory mechanism is fueled by *endorphins* (endogenous morphines), naturally occurring opioid peptides present in neurons in the brain, spinal cord, and gastrointestinal tract. Endorphins in the brain are released in response to afferent noxious stimuli, whereas endorphins in the spinal cord are released in response to efferent impulses. Endorphins work by binding with opiate receptors on the neurons to inhibit pain impulse transmission (Figure 9–2 ■).

Pain Theories

Several theories explain the response to pain and the diversity of human experiences with pain. The meaning or perception of pain can be modified by past experiences, motivation, attention, personality, and culture. Specificity and pattern theories describe nerve impulses of varying intensity terminating in pain centers in the forebrain. These theories provide explanations of the neurophysiologic basis of pain. In 1965, Melzack and Wall postulated gate-control theory (Porth, 2005). A gating mechanism exists at the spinal cord level where nerve transmission may be blocked by competing impulses. This explains the ability for even low-intensity stimulation such as light brushing of the skin to successfully block the experience of pain. Pain perception results from the interaction of two systems: the substantia gelatinosa in the dorsal horns of the spinal cord (Figure 9–3 ■), which regulates impulses entering or leaving the spinal cord, and an inhibitory system within the brain stem.

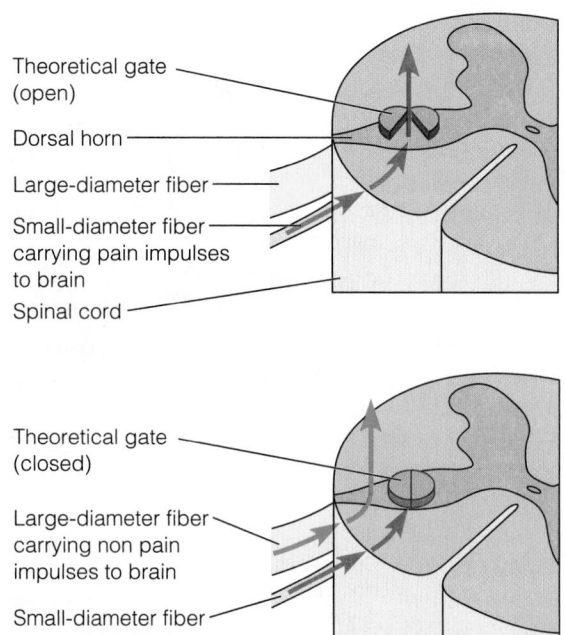

Figure 9–3 ■ The spinal cord component of the gate-control theory. Pain transmission by small-diameter fibers is blocked when large-diameter fibers carrying touch impulses dominate, closing the gate in the substantia gelatinosa.

Small-diameter A-delta and C fibers in the spinal cord carry fast and slow pain impulses. In addition, large-diameter A-beta fibers carry impulses for tactile stimulation from the skin. In the substantia gelatinosa, these impulses encounter a "gate" thought to be opened and closed by the domination of either the large-diameter touch fibers or the small-diameter pain fibers. If impulses along the small-diameter pain fibers outnumber impulses along the large-diameter touch fibers, the gate is open, and pain impulses travel unimpeded to the brain. If impulses from the touch fibers predominate, they will close the gate, and the pain impulses will be "turned away" at the gate. This explains why light stimulation such as massaging a stubbed toe can reduce the intensity and duration of the pain.

The second system described by gate-control theory, the inhibitory system, is thought to be located in the brain stem. It is believed that cells in the midbrain, activated by a variety of stimuli such as opiates, psychologic factors, or even simply the presence of pain itself, signal receptors in the medulla. These receptors in turn stimulate nerve fibers in the spinal cord to block the transmission of impulses from pain fibers.

Ongoing research demonstrates that the control and modulation of pain is much more complex than the description supplied by gate-control theory, which served as a basis for further research about pain-modulating systems. Tactile information is now known to be transmitted by both large- and small-diameter fibers, and interactions between sensory neurons is known to occur at multiple levels of the CNS. Melzack subsequently developed the neuromatrix theory of pain to integrate cultural and genetic factors with basic neurophysiologic function (Porth, 2005).

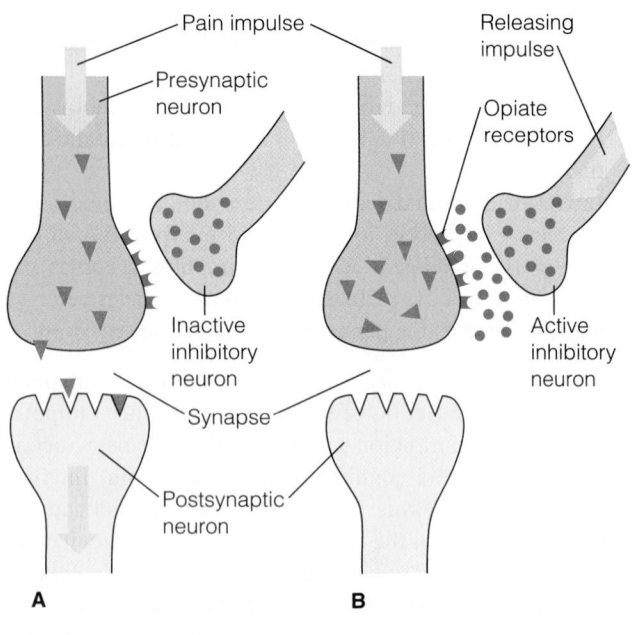

▲ = Neurotransmitters   ● = Endorphins

Figure 9–2 ■ *A*, Pain impulse causes presynaptic neuron to release burst of neurotransmitters across synapse. These bind to postsynaptic neuron and propagate impulse. *B*, Inhibitory neuron releases endorphins, which bind to presynaptic opiate receptors. Neurotransmitter release is inhibited, and pain impulse is interrupted.

One pain theory that is quite significant in clinical terms describes the effect of sensitizing the central and peripheral nervous system to painful stimuli. According to this theory, painful signals create a cascade of changes in the nervous system, which in turn increase the responsiveness of the peripheral and central neurons. These changes, in turn, increase the response to future signals and amplify pain (Dahl & Møiniche, 2004). Studies of infants undergoing painful procedures show that those who received analgesia experienced reduced sensitivity to future painful events, while those who did not receive analgesia experienced greater sensitivity (Taddio & Katz, 2005). Sensitization occurs from nociceptive barrage as well as inflammation that follows the injury or incision. In adults this theory indicates the value of preventing sensitization as well as treating perceived pain with multi-modal pain therapy. Local and regional anesthesia used in combination with central anesthesia prior to incision to diminish sensitization of these pathways results in significantly reduced consumption of intravenous morphine by patient-controlled analgesia in the 5 days following surgery (Hartrick, 2004).

TYPES AND CHARACTERISTICS OF PAIN
Acute Pain

Acute pain has a sudden onset, is usually temporary, and is localized. Pain that lasts for less than 6 months and has an identified cause is classified as acute pain. The onset is usually sudden, most often resulting from tissue injury from trauma, surgery, or inflammation. The pain is usually sharp and localized, although it may radiate. The three major types of acute pain are as follows:

- *Somatic pain* arises from nerve receptors originating in the skin or close to the surface of the body. Somatic pain may be either sharp and well localized, or dull and diffuse. It is often accompanied by nausea and vomiting.

- *Visceral pain* arises from body organs. Visceral pain is dull and poorly localized because of the low number of nociceptors. The viscera are sensitive to stretching, inflammation, and ischemia but relatively insensitive to cutting and temperature extremes. Visceral pain is associated with nausea and vomiting, hypotension, and restlessness. It often radiates or is referred. It may be described as cramping, intermittent pain, or colicky pain.

- *Referred pain* is pain that is perceived in an area distant from the site of the stimuli. It commonly occurs with visceral pain as visceral fibers synapse at the level of the spinal cord, close to fibers innervating other subcutaneous tissue areas of the body (Figure 9–4 ■). Pain in a spinal nerve may be felt over the skin in any body area innervated by sensory neurons that share that same spinal nerve route. Body areas defined by spinal nerve routes are called *dermatomes* (see Chapter 43 ∞).

Acute pain warns of actual or potential injury to tissues. As a stressor, it initiates the fight-or-flight autonomic stress response. Characteristic physical responses include tachycardia, rapid and shallow respirations, increased blood pressure, dilated pupils,

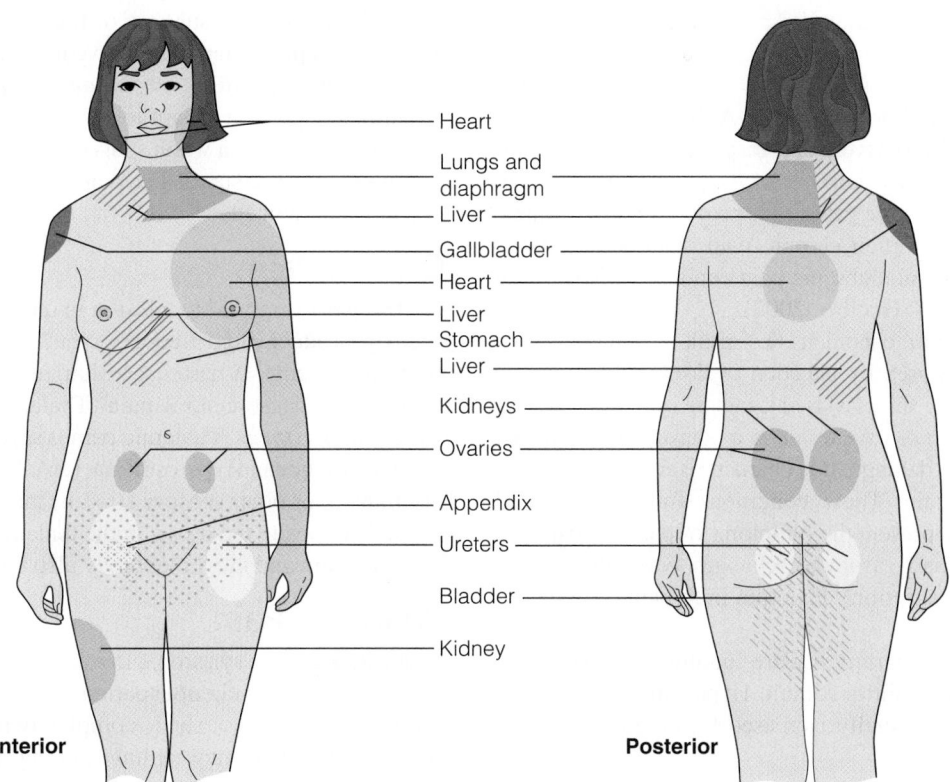

Heart
Lungs and diaphragm
Liver
Gallbladder
Heart
Liver
Stomach
Liver
Kidneys
Ovaries
Appendix
Ureters
Bladder
Kidney

Anterior

Posterior

Figure 9–4 ■ Referred pain is the result of the convergence of sensory nerves from certain areas of the body before they enter the brain for interpretation. For example, a toothache may be felt in the ear, pain from inflammation of the diaphragm may be felt in the shoulder, and pain from ischemia of the heart muscle (angina) may be felt in the left arm.

sweating, and pallor. The person experiencing the pain responds to this threat with anxiety and fear. This psychologic response may further increase the physical responses to acute pain.

Chronic Pain

Chronic pain is prolonged pain, usually lasting longer than 6 months. It is not always associated with an identifiable cause. The heart rate and blood pressure may fall within normal ranges due to physiologic adaptation, but hormonal stress responses to pain persist. Chronic pain lowers the pain threshold as a result of the depletion of serotonin and endorphin levels in the neurons; this leads to depression and irritability (Schaffer & Yucha, 2004). Unlike acute pain, chronic pain has a much more complex and poorly understood purpose.

Chronic pain can be subdivided into four categories:

- *Recurrent acute pain* is characterized by relatively well-defined episodes of pain interspersed with pain-free episodes. Examples of recurrent acute pain include migraine headaches and sickle cell crises.
- *Ongoing time-limited pain* is identified by a defined time period. Some examples are cancer pain, which ends with control of the disease or death, and burn pain, which ends with rehabilitation or death.
- *Chronic nonmalignant pain* is non–life-threatening pain that nevertheless persists beyond the expected time for healing. Chronic lower back pain falls into this category.
- *Chronic intractable nonmalignant pain syndrome* is similar to simple chronic nonmalignant pain but is characterized by the person's inability to cope well with the pain and sometimes by physical, social, and/or psychologic disability resulting from the pain.

The client with chronic pain often is depressed, withdrawn, immobile, irritable, and/or controlling. Although chronic pain may range from mild to severe and may be continuous or intermittent, the unrelenting presence of the pain often results in the pain itself becoming the pathologic process requiring intervention. The most common chronic pain condition is lower back pain. Other common chronic pain conditions include the following (McCance & Huether, 2002):

- *Neuralgias* are painful conditions that result from damage to a peripheral nerve caused by infection or disease. Postherpetic neuralgia (following shingles) is an example.
- *Complex regional pain syndrome* is a neuropathic pain that results from nerve damage. It is characterized by continuous severe, burning pain. These conditions follow peripheral nerve damage and present the symptoms of pain, vasospasm, muscle wasting, and vasomotor changes (vasodilation followed by vasoconstriction). Phantom limb pain is an example (Porth, 2005).
- *Hyperesthesias or hyperalgesias* are conditions of oversensitivity to tactile and painful stimuli. Hyperesthesias result in diffuse pain that is usually increased by fatigue and emotional lability.
- *Myofascial pain syndrome* is a common condition marked by injury to or disease of muscle and fascial tissue. Pain results from muscle spasm, stiffness, and collection of lactic acid in the muscle. Fibromyalgia is an example.

- Cancer often produces chronic pain, usually due to factors associated with the advancing disease. These factors include a growing tumor that presses on nerves or other structures, stretching of viscera, obstruction of ducts, or metastasis to bones. The malignant tumor also may mechanically stimulate pain or the production of biochemicals that cause pain. Pain also may be associated with treatments such as chemotherapy and radiation therapy.
- Chronic postoperative pain is rare but may occur following incisions in the chest wall, radical mastectomy, radical neck dissection, and surgical amputation.
- Clients with chronic pain may also suffer from breakthrough pain, incident pain, end-of-dose pain, and acute pain. Breakthrough and incident pain, discussed next, are associated with coughing or activity but may be spontaneous without an identifiable cause. End-of-dose pain refers to an increasing awareness of pain prior to the next scheduled dose of controlled-release analgesia.

Breakthrough Pain

Breakthrough pain is pain that exceeds baseline treated or untreated pain (Svendsen et al., 2005). It is often described as a sudden flare that exceeds the analgesic effect of long-acting pain medications; it is sometimes associated with end of dose of an **analgesic**. Whether the pain is **malignant** or nonmalignant in origin, treated or untreated, breakthrough pain is temporary and often debilitating. An increase in the baseline dose of analgesic to prevent breakthrough or administration of doses timed in relation to patterns of breakthrough may be needed.

Incident pain is a subtype of breakthrough pain. It is predictable pain precipitated by an event or activity such as coughing, changing position, or being touched. Clients at rest sometimes report their pain to the prescriber as very tolerable only to cry out in pain when subsequently attempting to change positions in bed or stand. The pain is experienced when an activity is commenced.

Central Pain

Central pain is related to a lesion in the brain that may spontaneously produce high-frequency bursts of impulses that are perceived as pain. A vascular lesion, tumor, trauma, or inflammation may cause central pain. Thalamic pain is one of the most common types. Thalamic pain is severe, spontaneous, and often continuous. Hyperesthesia (an abnormal sensitivity to touch, pain, or other sensory stimuli) may occur on the side of the body opposite the lesion in the thalamus. The perception of body position and movement may also be lost.

Phantom Pain

Phantom pain is a syndrome that occurs following amputation of a body part. The client experiences pain in the missing body part even though he or she is completely mentally aware that it is gone. This pain may include itching, tingling, or pressure sensations, or it may be more severe, including burning or stabbing sensations. In some cases, the client may describe a sensation that an amputated limb is twisted or cramped. It is thought that this type of pain may be due to stimulation of the severed nerves at the site of the amputation. Treatment is complex and often unsuccessful.

Psychogenic Pain

Psychogenic pain is experienced in the absence of any diagnosed physiologic cause or event. Typically psychogenic pain involves a long history of severe pain. It is thought that the client's emotional needs prompt the pain sensations. Psychogenic pain is real, and may in turn lead to physiologic changes, such as muscle tension, which may produce further pain. This condition may result from interpersonal conflicts, a need for support from others, or a desire to avoid a stressful or traumatic situation. Depression is often present.

FACTORS AFFECTING RESPONSES TO PAIN

Physical response to pain involves specific and often predictable neurologic changes. In fact, everyone has the same pain *threshold* and perceives pain stimuli at the same stimulus intensity. For example, heat is perceived as painful at 44° to 46° C, the range at which it begins to damage tissue. What varies is the person's *tolerance,* which is based on perception of and reaction to pain. The individualized response to pain is shaped by multiple and interacting factors, including age, sociocultural influences, emotional status, past experiences with pain, the source and meaning of the pain, and the client's knowledge base.

When one describes a person as highly sensitive to pain, one is referring to the person's **pain tolerance**, which is the amount of pain a person can endure before outwardly responding to it. The ability to tolerate pain may be decreased by repeated episodes of pain, fatigue, anger, anxiety, and sleep deprivation. Medications, alcohol, hypnosis, warmth, distraction, and spiritual practices may increase pain tolerance.

Age

Age influences a person's perception and expression of pain. Dangerous misconceptions exist regarding the management of pain in older adults. The foremost misconception is that normal aging decreases neurophysiologic sensitivity to pain. There is no evidence that **nociception** is altered by age. Studies of elderly nursing home residents found daily, persistent pain among them,

with 40% of those who reported pain on the first assessment still in pain 60 to 180 days later (Teno et al., 2002). There is evidence of decreased glomerular filtration and decreased activity of the cytochrome P450 system responsible for the activation and metabolism of many opioids (Yarbro et al., 2005). Individual opioids have differing patterns of metabolism, and doses need to be adjusted to accommodate the decline in glomerular filtration rate and specific metabolisms. This response is different from concluding that older adult patients do not perceive pain and therefore have no need for pain medications.

The second and equally damaging belief is one held by nurses. This is the belief that opioids cause excessive respiratory depression in older adults and that pain and discomfort are unavoidable aspects of aging (Closs, 1996). While peripheral vascular disease or diabetes may lead to neuropathy and interfere with normal nerve impulse transmission, neuropathy can manifest as hyperesthesias as well as hypoesthesias. Both of these manifestations cause discomfort. Individuals in this age group may fail to acknowledge pain, believing that pain is inevitable or fearing dependency if they alarm their loved ones (Sheehan & Schirm, 2003).

Often believing that pain is a part of growing older, the client may ignore pain or self-medicate with over-the-counter medications. As a result of these behaviors, the older adult is at increased risk of injury or serious illness. Table 9–2 lists some age-related changes and their effects on pain. Despite the changes, older adults need and tolerate the same dosing formula for intravenous morphine as younger patients without greater adverse effects or sedation (Loran et al., 2005).

Older adult clients may hesitate to ask for pain medicine because they fear narcotic **addiction** and loss of independence. They may not understand the burden of untreated pain and the benefits of regular analgesia (Brown, 2004). Furthermore, assessment of pain in older adults may be difficult when the client is cognitively impaired and has difficulty communicating descriptions of pain. Nurse researchers have found, however, that even some adults with cognitive impairments were able to describe current, usual, or worse pain when a standardized pain scale was used. The MDS pain assessment scale is reportedly easier to administer to older clients than the visual analog scale (Fries et al., 2001).

Delirium in the acutely ill patient and dementia, which occurs in approximately 50% of adults over age 85, are barriers

TABLE 9–2 Nursing Care of the Older Adult: Age-Related Changes and Their Effects on Pain

FACTORS RELATED TO AGING	EFFECTS	OUTCOMES
Decreased blood flow	Ischemia, decreases in brain function	Client forgets to take medication
Changes in neurotransmitters related to sleep and mood	Decreased sleep resulting in vulnerability to pain	Greater risk of chronic pain, fatigue, increased withdrawal
Reduced levels of norepinephrine	Lowered transmission of pain	Less likely to notice an injury
Changes in sensory interpretation	Lowered pain sensation	Client may not take appropriate protective action
Decreased peripheral nerve conduction	Lowered response to pain	Not seeking appropriate care
Slowed reaction time	Slower avoidance response	Client receives more serious injury
Reduced movement	Increased risk for muscle wasting	May cause immobility

to assessing pain. Recommended methods for pain assessment include (1) behavioral observations for which no tool has been validated, (2) documenting baseline behavior and activity patterns and monitoring changes that might indicate further pain assessment, and (3) conducting an empiric analgesia trial. The analgesia trial is made in relation to potentially painful procedures or in the presence of known pathology, or when pain is suspected. Acetaminophen 500 mg is administered three to four times daily. A decrease in pain-related behaviors or resumption of usual patterns of activity could suggest that pain is being controlled and that the client may need around-the-clock analgesic administration (Herr, 2002).

Sociocultural Influences

Ethnopharmacology, a developing science, focuses on the effects of ethnicity (the combination of genetics and culture) on drug absorption, metabolism, distribution, and excretion (Munoz & Hilgenberg, 2005). It is important to consider cultural influences in order to effectively assess and treat clients in pain.

Each person's response to pain is strongly influenced by the family, community, and culture. Sociocultural influences affect the way in which a person tolerates pain, interprets the meaning of pain, and reacts verbally and nonverbally to the pain. For example, if the client's family believes that males should not cry and must tolerate pain stoically, the male client often will appear withdrawn and refuse pain medication. If a family encourages open and intense emotional expression, the client may cry freely and appear comfortable requesting pain medication.

Cultural standards also teach an individual how much pain to tolerate, what types of pain to report, to whom to report the pain, and what kind of treatment to seek. For example, clients of northern European ancestry may value "being a good patient," which may cause them to avoid "complaining" about their pain, whereas clients of Jewish ancestry may value seeking information about their pain, which may cause them to discuss their pain often and in detail. Note, however, that behaviors vary greatly within a culture and from generation to generation. The nurse should approach each client as an individual, observing the client carefully, taking the time to ask questions, and avoiding assumptions.

The nurse also has a set of sociocultural values and beliefs about pain. If these values and beliefs differ from those of the client, the assessment and management of pain may be based on the values of the nurse rather than on the needs of the client. The nurse must be familiar with ethnic and cultural diversity in pain expression and management and respect cultural differences. It is particularly important to remember that pain behaviors are not an objective indicator of the amount of pain present for any individual client. Finally, most experts agree that cultural differences in the expression of, response to, and interpretation of the meaning of pain need further research.

Emotional Status

Emotional status influences the pain perception. The sensation of pain may be blocked by intense concentration (during sports activities, for example) or may be increased by anxiety or fear.

Pain often is increased when it occurs in conjunction with other illnesses or physical discomforts such as nausea or vomiting. The presence or absence of support people or caregivers that genuinely care about pain management also may alter emotional status and the perception of pain.

Anxiety may increase the perception of pain, and pain may in turn cause anxiety. In addition, the muscle tension common with anxiety can create its own source of pain. This association explains why nonpharmacologic interventions such as relaxation or guided imagery are helpful in relieving or decreasing pain.

Fatigue, lack of sleep, and depression also are related to pain experiences. Pain interferes with a person's ability to fall asleep and stay asleep and thus induces fatigue. In turn, fatigue can lower pain tolerance. Depression is clearly linked to pain: Serotonin, a neurotransmitter, is involved in the modulation of pain in the CNS. In clinically depressed people, serotonin is decreased, leading to an increase in pain sensations. The reverse is also true: In the presence of pain, depression is common.

Past Experiences with Pain

Previous experiences with pain are likely to influence the person's response to a current pain episode. If supportive adults responded to childhood experiences with pain appropriately, the adult usually will have a healthy attitude to pain. If, however, the person's pain was responded to with exaggerated emotions or neglectful indifference, that person's future responses to pain may be exaggerated or denied.

The responses of healthcare providers to the person in pain can influence the person's response during the next pain episode. If providers respond to pain with effective strategies and a caring attitude, the client will remain more comfortable during any subsequent pain episode, and anxiety will be avoided. If, however, the pain is not adequately relieved, or if the client feels that empathetic care was not given, anxiety about the next pain episode sets up the client for a more complex and therefore more painful event.

Source and Meaning

The meaning associated with the pain influences the experience of pain. For example, the pain of labor to deliver a baby is experienced differently from the pain following removal of a major organ for cancer. Because pain is the major signal for health problems, it is strongly linked to all associated meanings of health problems, such as disability, loss of role, and death. For this reason, it is important to explain to clients the etiology and prognosis for the pain assessed.

If the client perceives the pain as deserved (e.g., "just punishment for sins"), the client may actually feel relief that the "punishment" has commenced. If the client believes that the pain will relieve him or her from an unrewarding job, dangerous military service, or even stressful social obligations, there may similarly be a feeling of relief. In contrast, pain that is perceived as meaningless—for example, chronic low back pain or the unrelieved pain of arthritis—can cause anxiety and depression.

Knowledge

A lack of understanding of the source, outcome, and meaning of the pain can contribute negatively to the pain experience. The nurse needs to assess the client's readiness to learn, use methods of teaching that are effective for the client and family, and evaluate learning carefully. Teaching must include the process of the pain, its predictable course (if possible), and the proposed plan of care. In addition, encourage clients to communicate preferences for pain relief. Learning how to let significant others know of the presence of pain and how to use their help can also promote effective pain management.

MYTHS AND MISCONCEPTIONS ABOUT PAIN

Myths and misconceptions about pain and its management are common in both healthcare providers and clients. Some of the most common of these myths are included here:

- *Pain is a result, not a cause.* According to the traditional view of pain, pain is only a symptom of a condition. However, it is now recognized that unrelieved or poorly relieved pain itself sets up further responses, such as immobility, anger, and anxiety; pain may also delay healing and rehabilitation.
- *Chronic pain is really a masked form of depression.* Serotonin plays a chemical role in pain transmission and is also the major modulator of depression. Therefore, pain and depression are chemically related, not mutually exclusive. It is common to find them coexisting.
- *Narcotic medication is too risky to be used to treat chronic pain.* This common misconception often deprives clients of the most effective source of pain relief. It is true that other methods should be tried first; if, however, they prove ineffective, narcotics should be considered as an appropriate alternative.
- *It is best to wait until a client has pain before giving medication.* It is now widely accepted that anticipating pain has a noticeable effect on the amount of pain a client experiences. Offering pain relief before a pain event is well on its way can lessen the pain.
- *Many clients lie about the existence or severity of their pain.* Very few clients lie about their pain.
- *Postoperative pain is best treated with intramuscular injections.* The most commonly used postoperative pain relief for many years was meperidine (Demerol) given intramuscularly. However, meperidine has many adverse effects, such as irritating tissues and producing the CNS stimulant normeperidine. In addition, meperidine is short acting. Most contemporary experts do not recommend its use to manage postoperative pain (Cohen & Schecter, 2005).
- *Pain relief interferes with diagnosis.* There is a prevailing attitude in the emergency department (ED) that pain relief can interfere with diagnosis. Research about treating pain with analgesics in the ED consistently shows no impact on physical assessment findings or diagnosis (Pasero, 2003). Despite a prevailing attitude that pain management is an essential part of quality medical care, pain management in the ED is difficult because of the short-term associations with clients, increased vigilance against drug abuse, and the myth that diagnosis is impaired by pain relief.

INTERDISCIPLINARY CARE

Effective pain relief results from collaboration among healthcare providers. Pain clinics are centers staffed by a team of healthcare professionals who use a multidisciplinary approach to managing chronic pain. Therapies may include traditional pharmacologic agents as well as herbs, vitamins, and other dietary supplements; nutritional counseling; psychotherapy; biofeedback; hypnosis; acupuncture; massage; and other treatments. Hospices for dying clients also provide a multifaceted approach to pain management. Chapter 5 provides information about pain management during end-of-life care.

Medications

Medication is the most common approach to pain management. A variety of drugs with many kinds of delivery systems are available. These drugs include nonnarcotic analgesics, nonsteroidal anti-inflammatory drugs (NSAIDs), narcotics, synthetic narcotics, antidepressants, and local anesthetic agents. In addition to administering the prescribed medications, the nurse may act independently in choosing the dosage and timing. The nurse is also responsible for assessing the side effects of the medications, evaluating the medication's effectiveness, and providing client teaching. The nurse's roles in pain relief are those of client advocate and direct caregiver.

The World Health Organization (WHO) "ladder of analgesia" effectively guides the use of medications (WHO, 1986/1990) (Figure 9–5 ■). NSAIDs and narcotic pain medications are used progressively until pain is relieved, reflecting

Figure 9–5 ■ The WHO analgesic ladder illustrates the process for selection of analgesic medications for pain management.

From *Cancer Pain Relief and Palliative Care* by World Health Organization, 1990 (Technical Report Series, no. 804) Geneva: WHO. Reprinted by permission.

the interactive nature of these two types of analgesics. Box 9–1 describes terms associated with pain medication.

NONNARCOTIC ANALGESICS Nonnarcotic analgesics such as acetaminophen (Tylenol) produce analgesia and reduce fever. The exaction mechanism of action is unknown. They are used to treat mild to moderate pain. A newer class of centrally acting nonopioid analgesics is used for moderate to moderately severe pain. Included in this class is the widely used tramadol (Ultram). Its analgesic effect is comparable to that of codeine, yet is less powerful than that of morphine. Serious side effects are rare, but do include seizures (Lehne, 2004).

NSAIDS NSAIDs act on peripheral nerve endings and minimize pain by interfering with prostaglandin synthesis. Examples include aspirin and ibuprofen. The NSAIDs have anti-inflammatory, analgesic, and antipyretic actions. NSAIDs are the treatment of choice for mild to moderate pain and continue to be effective when combined with narcotics for moderate to severe pain. Examples of NSAIDs and factors to consider when selecting an NSAID are provided in Table 9–3. The cyclooxygenase-2 (COX-2) selective NSAIDs are newer formulations; although less harmful to gastric mucosa, their usage has been questioned because of cardiac-associated adverse reactions and some have been taken off the market. Nursing implications for NSAIDs are found in the Medication Administration box on the next page.

NARCOTICS (OPIOIDS) Narcotics, or opioids, are derivatives of the opium plant. These drugs (and their synthetic forms) are

TABLE 9–3 Factors to Consider When Selecting an NSAID

CHEMICAL CLASS	HALF LIFE (HOURS)	ONSET OF ACTION (HOURS)	USUAL DOSING INTERVAL (TIMES PER DAY)	USUAL DAILY DOSE (MG)
Salicylates				
Acetylated				
Aspirin	0.25	0.25–0.50	4–6	325–1000
Aspirin, buffered				
Aspirin, enteric coated				
Aspirin, sustained release				
Nonacetylated				
Choline salicylate (Arthropan)		1–2	2–4	1200
Choline magnesium trisalicylate				
(Trilisate)	2–19	2	2–4	1200
Diflunisal (Dolobid)	8–12	2–3	2–3	250–500
Salsalate (Disalcid)	2–19	—	2–3	325–3000
Magnesium salicylate		—	3–4	Various
Sodium salicylate			4–6	Various
Propionic Acids				
Fenoprofen (Nalfon)	2–3	—	3–4	300–600
Flurbiprofen (Ansaid)	5.7	—	2–3	100
Ibuprofen (Motrin, others)	2	0.5	3–4	300–800
Ketoprofen (Orudis)	1.6–4	—	3–4	25–75
Ketoprofen SR (Oruvail)		—	1	200
Naproxen (Naprosyn)	13	1	2	250–500
Naproxen sodium (Anaprox)	13–15	1–2	2	250–500
Oxaprozin (Daypro)	21–25	1–2	1–2	600
Acetic Acids				
Diclofenac sodium (Voltaren)	1.2–2	0.5	3	50
Etodolac (Lodine)	6–7	0.5	3	200–400
Indomethacin (Indocin)	4–6	0.5	2–4	25–50
Indomethacin SR (Indocin SR)	—	2–4		150
Ketoralac (Toradol)	4–6	0.5–1	4–6	10–30
Sulindac (Clinoril, others)	8	—	2	150–200
Tolmetin (Tolectin)	5	—	3	400
Fenamates (Anthranilic Acids)				
Meclofenamate (Meclomen)	2–3	—	3–4	50
Mefenamic acid (Ponstel)	2	—	4	250
Oxicams				
Piroxicam (Feldene)	24	2–4	1–2	10–20
Nonacidic (Naphthylkanone)				
Nabumetone (Relafen)	22	—	1–2	500–1000
Pyrazolones				
Phenylbutazone (Butazolidin)	40–60	0.5–1	3–4	100–600

BOX 9–1 Terms Associated with Pain Medication

- *Addiction:* The compulsive use of a substance despite negative consequences, such as health threats or legal problems.
- *Drug abuse:* The use of any chemical substance for other than a medical purpose.
- *Physical drug dependence:* A biologic need for a substance. If the substance is not supplied, physical withdrawal symptoms occur.
- *Psychologic drug dependence:* A psychologic need for a substance. If the substance is not supplied, psychologic withdrawal symptoms occur.

- *Drug tolerance:* The process by which the body requires a progressively greater amount of a drug to achieve the same results.
- *Equianalgesic:* Having the same pain-killing effect when administered to the same individual. Drug dosages are equianalgesic if they have the same effect as morphine sulfate 10 mg administered intramuscularly.
- *Pseudoaddiction:* Behavior involving drug seeking; a result of receiving inadequate pain relief.

---

the pharmacologic treatment of choice for moderate to severe pain. Examples are morphine, codeine, and fentanyl (Duragesic, Actiq). Narcotic analgesics produce analgesia by binding to opioid receptors both within and outside the CNS. A summary of narcotic drugs, their usual dosages, peak effect, and nursing implications is provided in Table 9–4.

A common myth among healthcare professionals is that using narcotics for pain treatment poses a real threat of addiction. Actually, when the medications are used as recommended, there is little to no risk of addiction. Rather, if pain is not adequately treated, the client may seek more and more narcotic relief, thus increasing the risk of an adversarial relationship with the provider and a weakening of the trust relationship between client and provider (Trame, 2002) (Box 9–2). Nursing implications for narcotics are found in the Medication Administration box on page 182.

ANTIDEPRESSANTS Antidepressants within the tricyclic and related chemical groups act on the production and retention of serotonin in the CNS, thus inhibiting pain sensation. They also promote normal sleeping patterns, further alleviating the suffering of the client in pain. They are useful with neuropathic pain.

ANTICONVULSANTS Similar to antidepressants, some seizure medications such as gabapentin (Neurontin) and carbamazepine (Tegretol) are useful with neuropathic pain, including shingles (herpes zoster), migraine headaches, and diabetic neuropathic pain. These drugs reduce pain and sleep disruption. Drugs that are primarily used to treat epilepsy (seizures) have been used to treat nerve pain conditions and migraine headache for several decades. Many anticonvulsant drugs have been shown in clinical studies to be effective.

LOCAL ANESTHETICS Drugs such as benzocaine and xylocaine are part of a large group of substances that block the initiation and transmission of nerve impulses in a local area, thus blocking pain as well. They are sometimes used to enable a client to begin moving and using a painful area to diminish long-term pain.

Local anesthetics can be delivered by a variety of methods. Delivery can be made directly to the sheath of a nerve through a peripheral nerve catheter. During surgery, a soaker-type catheter can be inserted along a surgical incision to deliver local relief; this method may decrease the need for opioids and allow the client to resume activity sooner (D'Arcy, 2005).

MEDICATION ADMINISTRATION   Nonsteroidal Anti-Inflammatory Drugs

Examples of NSAIDs are:
aspirin (acetylsalicylic acid)
fenoprofen calcium (Nalfon)
ibuprofen (Motrin)
rofecoxib (Vioxx)
diflunisal (Dolobid)
ketorolac tromethamine (Toradol)
naproxen (Naprosyn)
indomethacin (Indocin)

The NSAIDs have anti-inflammatory, analgesic, and antipyretic effects. It is believed that they inhibit the enzyme cyclooxygenase, thereby decreasing synthesis of prostaglandins. These drugs provide analgesic effects by reducing inflammation and by perhaps blocking the generation of noxious impulses.

Nursing Responsibilities
- Do not administer aspirin with other NSAIDs.

- Assess and document if the client is taking a hypoglycemic agent or insulin; the NSAIDs may increase the hypoglycemic effect.
- Administer with meals, milk, or a full glass of water to decrease gastric irritation.
- Assess clients who are also taking anticoagulants for bleeding; the NSAIDs increase this risk.

Health Education for the Client and Family
- Drugs may cause gastrointestinal bleeding (report nausea, vomiting of blood, dark stools), visual disturbances (report blurred or diminished vision), hearing problems, dizziness, skin rash, and renal problems (report weight gain or edema).
- Take medications with meals to decrease gastric irritation.
- Avoid drinking alcohol or taking any over-the-counter drug unless approved by the healthcare provider.
- The desired effects may not appear for 3–5 days, and the full effects may not appear for 2–4 weeks.
- Maintain regular healthcare appointments.

TABLE 9–4 Equianalgesic Drug Chart

ANALGESIC	DOSAGE (MG)	PEAK (MIN)	DURATION (H)	NURSING CONSIDERATIONS
Morphine sulfate	10 IM 30–60 PO	30–60 IM 60–120 PO	4–5 IM 4–5 PO	PO dose is 3–6 times the IM dose. A lower dose may be appropriate for older clients with chronic pain. Contraindicated in clients with acute bronchial asthma or upper airway obstruction.
Butorphanol tartrate (Stadol)	2 IM N/A PO	30–60 IM	3–4 IM	May cause withdrawal in clients physically dependent on narcotics. May cause hallucinations. Increases cardiac workload. Contraindicated in clients with myocardial infarction.
Codeine	130 IM 200 PO	30–60 IM 60–120 PO	4 IM 4 PO	PO dose is about 1.5 times the IM dose. Often given synergistically with aspirin or acetaminophen for best effect. More toxic in high doses than morphine. Causes more nausea and vomiting than morphine and is constipating.
Hydromorphone HCl (Dilaudid)	1.5 IM 7.5 PO	15–30 IM 30 PO	4 IM 4 PO	PO dose is 5 times IM dose. Shorter acting than morphine. May cause loss of appetite. Contraindicated in clients with increased intracranial pressure or status asthmaticus.
Levorphanol tartrate (Levo-Dromoran)	2 IM 4 PO	60 IM 90–120 PO	4–5 IM 4–5 PO	Longer acting than morphine when given in repeated, regular doses. Accumulates, so analgesic effect may increase. SC recommended over IM route. Warn client drug has bitter taste. Contraindicated in clients with respiratory depression, asthma, alcoholism, or increased intracranial pressure.
Meperidine HCl (Demerol)	75 IM 300 PO	30–50 IM 60–90 PO	2–4 IM 2–4 PO	Metabolized to normeperidine, a toxic CNS stimulant that may cause CNS hyperexcitability. Normeperidine's effects increased, not reversed, by naloxone. Use with caution in clients with renal disease. PO dose of 300 not recommended.
Methadone HCl (Dolophine)	10 IM 20 PO	60–120 IM 90–120 PO	4–6 IM 4–6 PO	Initial PO dose is twice IM dose. Accumulates, so analgesic effect may increase. Warn client drug has bitter taste. Also used for heroin detoxification and temporary maintenance. Oral liquid form is legally required in maintenance programs.
Nalbuphine HCl (Nubain)	10 IM N/A PO	30–60 IM	3–6 IM	Longer acting and less likely to cause hypotension than morphine. Respiratory depression does not increase with increased dosages as compared to morphine. Similar to butorphanol, but does not increase cardiac workload.
Oxycodone HCl	N/A IM 30 PO	60 PO	3–6 PO	Available as a single-entity product in tablet or liquid form. Also available in 5-mg dose in drugs such as Percodan and Percocet. Has faster onset and higher peak effect than most PO narcotics.
Oxymorphone HCl (Numorphan)	1–1.5 IM N/A PO	30–60 IM	3–6 IM	Also available as rectal suppository (10 mg equianalgesic), but more effective if given IM.
Pentazocine HCl	60 IM 180 PO	30–60 IM 30–90 PO	3–4 IM 3–4 PO	PO dose is 3 times IM dose. May produce withdrawal in clients physically dependent on narcotics. May cause confusion, hallucinations, anxiety. Contraindicated in clients with head injury or increased intracranial pressure. Use with caution in clients with cardiac problems.
Propoxyphene HCl (Darvon)	N/A IM 500 PO	120 PO	4–6 PO	Available only in oral form in United States. Never give as much as 500 mg PO. PO dose of 65–130 mg recommended. Used for mild to moderate pain. May cause false decreases in urinary steroid excretion tests. Report suspected propoxyphene abuse; propoxyphene in excessive doses ranks second to barbiturates as a cause of drug-related deaths.

Note: Morphine sulfate 10 mg IM is the analgesic dose to which all other IM and PO doses in this table are considered equianalgesic.

BOX 9–2 Pain Management and Drug Abuse History

Clients addicted to pain relievers often experience inadequate dosing of medications for pain. When providers suspect or learn of drug abuse, they tend to order lower doses than they would for a person of similar size and injury. Despite significant data showing very little addiction as the result of treating pain with adequate analgesia, prescribers still undertreat pain in clients with addictions. Addiction is a neurophysiologic disease; when clients with addiction have injuries they usually need greater doses of pain medication because of the tolerance they have developed from repeated exposure to opioids. Even clients without an addiction may exhibit behaviors suggesting addiction when pain is undertreated (Trame, 2002).

Cook et al. (2004) report an experiment to evaluate provider attitudes about prescribing analgesics for those in acute pain with a history of drug abuse. They sent questionnaires to 745 physicians in one county and received 120 responses. Sixty-six of the responders received the case of a seriously burned client with no mention of addiction; 54 responders received the case of an acutely burned client with heroin addiction. The physicians were provided the same selection of analgesics and dosages for both clients in the case studies. The physicians' prescribing practices were significantly different for the two clients; the client with heroin addiction was prescribed significantly more nonopioid analgesics than the nonaddicted client.

Furthermore, there was no significant difference in the dosages prescribed for the two clients despite the risk for greater tolerance to opiates by the heroin-addicted client. The authors suggest that prescribers may be uninformed about the pathophysiology of addiction and increased need for analgesia in addiction. They also observe that analgesics may be rationed to addicted persons in an effort to wean them from their addiction. During the acute stress of injury or infection, however, withholding pain medication is an added stressor. The client will benefit from detoxification and recovery management after the acute phase is over. Nurses attempting to advocate for the comfort needs of an addicted client may encounter increased resistance without good explanations. This creates an ethical as well as a professional dilemma.

Providing analgesics for a client with chronic pain who has a history of addiction or ongoing addiction may be even more challenging. Clients may be fearful that their pain will be undertreated or that addiction will return or increase if the pain is treated with opioids (Compton & Athanasos, 2003). It is important to clearly communicate all needed information about medications and accessibility to providers. Dose escalation may be monitored with careful assessment and random urine screens. Treatment for addiction should be included in the care plan to minimize the risk of addiction or relapse.

BISPHOSPHONATES AND RADIOPHARMACEUTICALS These medications target malignant tumors growing in bone. Referred to as *osseous metastases*, these expanding, painful tumors impair function. Bisphosphonates stabilize bone, slowing or preventing the development of tumors, and have a pain-relieving benefit which exceeds that of steroids and NSAIDs. Pamidronate is effective with breast cancer metastases and multiple myeloma; a newer generation bisphosphonate, zoledronic acid, is useful with bony metastases secondary to lung, prostate, renal cell, and other solid tumors (Cahill, 2005).

Radiopharmaceuticals are unsealed substances produced in a nuclear reactor that emit a beta particle or an electron. The radioactivity is particularly damaging to malignant cells and is a safe and effective treatment for bony metastases. The most commonly used is samarium-153 (Quadramet). A flare reaction may follow administration; it is a temporary increase in bony pain prior to the therapeutic response. More serious side effects include myelosuppression from radiation of adjacent bone marrow and disseminated intravascular coagulation (DIC) (Silberstein et al., 2001). These treatments may be given intravenously or orally. Care of clients treated with radiopharmaceuticals must follow radiation precautions, disposing of all body fluids quickly and thoroughly.

DURATION OF ACTION Each of the pharmacologic agents has a unique absorption and duration of action. The nurse caring for the client in pain must understand that no drug will have a totally predictable course of action, because each person absorbs, metabolizes, and excretes medications at different dosage levels. The only way to obtain reliable data about the effectiveness of the medication for the individual client is to assess how that client responds. Therefore, the best choice is to individualize the dosing schedule.

The two major descriptors of dosing schedules are around-the-clock (ATC) or as necessary (PRN), meaning *pro re nata*, Latin for "as circumstances may require.") ATC administration is appropriate if the client experiences pain constantly and predictably during a 24-hour period. In contrast, prn administration is appropriate for pain that is not predictable or constant. Note that prn medication should be administered as soon as the pain begins or prior to onset, when increased pain is anticipated, such as when an activity is planned. PRN dosing is also appropriate when the expected direction of ATC doses falls short. Dosing with short-acting opioids for this type of pain should be administered as needed in addition to the ATC dose for chronic, persistent pain (Ferrell, 2000).

Giving analgesics before the pain occurs or increases gives the client confidence in the certainty of pain relief and thereby avoids some of the untoward effects of pain. The benefits of a preventive approach can be summarized as follows:

- The client may spend less time in pain.
- Frequent analgesic administration may allow for smaller doses and less analgesic administration.
- Smaller doses will in turn mean fewer side effects.
- The client's fear and anxiety about the return of pain will decrease.
- The client will probably be more physically active and avoid the difficulties caused by immobility.

The side effects of a drug can become difficult to manage if the dosage is too high, and clients may suffer unnecessary pain because of reluctance to endure side effects. The best formula for adequate dosage is a balance between effective pain relief

MEDICATION ADMINISTRATION   Narcotic Analgesics

Examples of narcotic analgesics are:

buprenorphine HCl (Buprenex)
codeine
hydromorphone HCl (Dilaudid)
meperidine HCl (Demerol)
morphine sulfate
nalbuphine HCl (Nubain)
oxycodone
oxymorphone HCl (Numorphan)
pentazocine (Talwin)
propoxyphene napsylate (Darvocet-N)

Narcotic analgesics are used to treat severe pain. The drugs in this category include opium morphine, codeine, opium derivatives, and synthetic substances. Morphine and codeine are pure chemical substances isolated from opium. These drugs decrease the awareness of the sensation of pain by binding to opiate receptors in the brain and spinal cord. It is also believed that they diminish the transmission of pain impulses by altering cell membrane permeability to sodium and by affecting the release of neurotransmitters for efferent nerves sensitive to noxious stimuli. Narcotic analgesics affect the central nervous system, causing analgesia, euphoria, drowsiness, mental clouding, and lethargy. They also have various other effects: Depending on the drug used, the narcotics depress respirations, stimulate the vomiting center, depress the cough reflex, induce peripheral vasodilatation (resulting in hypotension), constrict the pupil, and decrease intestinal peristalsis. The narcotics are addictive, causing psychologic and physical dependence.

NURSING RESPONSIBILITIES

- Narcotics are regulated by federal law; the nurse must record the date, time, client name, type and amount of the drug used, and sign the entry in a narcotic inventory sheet. If the drug must be wasted after it is signed out, the act must be witnessed and the narcotic sheet signed by the nurse and the witness. Computerized narcotic documentation methods are also available.
- Keep a narcotic antagonist, such as naloxone, immediately available to treat respiratory depression.
- Assess allergies or adverse effects from narcotics previously experienced by the client.

- Meperidine (Demerol) is associated with CNS toxicity and thus involves significant patient risk. For any client who is receiving more than one dose, monitor for nervousness, restlessness, tremors, twitching, shakiness, myoclonic jerks, diaphoresis, changes in level of awareness, agitation, disorientation, confusion, delirium, hallucinations, violent shivering, and/or seizures. This toxicity can occur with any route of administration or any dosing regimen. This risk is increased with oral administration and in clients with decreased renal function (including normal changes with aging). Report these manifestations to the physician.
- Assess for any respiratory disease, such as asthma, that might increase the risk of respiratory depression.
- Assess the characteristics of the pain and the effectiveness of drugs that have been previously used to treat the pain.
- Take and record baseline vital signs before administering the drug.
- Administer the drugs, following established guidelines.
- Monitor vital signs, level of consciousness, papillary response, nausea, bowel function, urinary function, and effectiveness of pain management.
- Teach noninvasive methods of pain management for use in conjunction with narcotic analgesics.
- Provide for client safety.

HEALTH EDUCATION FOR THE CLIENT AND FAMILY

- The use of narcotics to treat severe pain is unlikely to cause addiction.
- Do not drink alcohol.
- Do not take over-the-counter medications unless approved by the healthcare provider.
- Increase intake of fluids and fiber in the diet to prevent constipation.
- The drugs often cause dizziness, drowsiness, and impaired thinking; use caution when driving or making decisions.
- Report decreasing effectiveness or the appearance of side effects to the physician.

---

and minimal side effects. Within prescribed limits, the nurse can choose the correct dose according to the client's response. It is also the role of the nurse to inform the physician if the prescribed dosage does not meet the client's needs.

ROUTES OF ADMINISTRATION The route of administration significantly affects how much of the medication is needed to relieve pain. For example, oral doses of some narcotics must be up to five times greater than parenteral doses to achieve the same degree of pain relief. Different narcotics have different recommended dosages. Consulting an equianalgesic dosage chart helps ensure that dosages of different narcotics administered by different routes will have the same analgesic effect when administered to the same client. Dosage for transitioning from intravenous or oral analgesia to transdermal application is determined by using equianalgesic data. These charts are based on a comparison of an analgesic to 10 mg

(IM) of morphine. Table 9–4 is an example of an equianalgesic chart.

Oral The simplest route for both client and nurse is the oral (PO) route. Special nursing care is still required, because some medications must be given with food, some are irritating to the gastrointestinal system, and some clients have trouble swallowing pills. Liquid and timed-release forms are available for special applications.

Rectal The rectal route is helpful for clients who are unable to swallow. Several of the opioid narcotics are available in this form. The rectal route is effective and simple, but the client and family may not accept it. To be effective, any rectal medication must be placed above the rectal sphincter.

Transdermal The **transdermal**, or "patch," form of medication is increasingly being used because it is simple, painless,

Figure 9–6 ■ The transdermal patch administers medication in predictable doses.

Figure 9–7 ■ PCA units allow the client to self-manage severe pain. The units may be portable or mounted on intravenous poles.
Courtesy of Baxter Healthcare Corporation.

and delivers a continuous level of medication (Figure 9–6 ■). Transdermal medications are easy to store and apply. Reapplication every 72 hours enhances compliance. Additional short-acting medication is often needed for breakthrough pain. Overdosage can occur as well with this route. It is important to start with a low dose and **titrate** (which means to increase or decrease dose in small increments) to the effective level. It is lipid soluble and may be stored in fat cells longer than expected. Monitor level of sedation and respiratory effort.

To apply a medication transdermally, the nurse or client must clip any hair from the area, clean the site (which should be on the upper torso) with clear water, dry the cleansed area, apply the patch immediately upon opening the package, and ensure that the contact is complete, especially around the edges. The effectiveness of a patch lasts about 72 hours, and the next patch should be applied on a different site. When first applying a transdermal medication, expect 12 to 24 hours until therapeutic level is absorbed; similarly, when discontinuing expect a gradual decline in level because of medication reservoir in the skin. When the client has fever or inflammation of the skin, expect increased rate of absorption. Exercise and use of electric blankets or heating pads also may accelerate absorption.

Intramuscular Once the most popular route for pain medication administration, the intramuscular (IM) route is being reconsidered. Its disadvantages include uneven absorption from the muscle, discomfort on administration, and time consumed to prepare and administer the medication.

Intravenous The intravenous (IV) route provides the most rapid onset, usually ranging from 1 to 15 minutes. Medication can be given by drip, bolus, or patient-controlled analgesia (PCA), a pump with a control mechanism that affords the client self-management of pain (Figure 9–7 ■). The advantages of PCA are dose precision, timeliness, and convenience. The patient does not have to wait for a nurse to assess the need for pain medication, then procure and deliver the analgesia (Strassels et al., 2005). Respiratory depression and sedation are minimized when plasma levels of opioids are steady (Lehne, 2004). PCA, especially with basal dosing (continuous infusion of a very

small dose), facilitates frequent small dosing. Several drugs are available for this route. The disadvantages are the nursing care needed for any intravenous line, the potential for infection, and the cost of disposable supplies. The PCA method of administration requires careful client teaching and monitoring.

Subcutaneous The subcutaneous (SC) route is accepted, but it is less commonly used than other methods. Its advantages and disadvantages are similar to those of the intramuscular route.

Epidural The epidural route is invasive and requires more extensive nursing care but may provide better analgesia and postoperative recovery than intravenous delivery. When a combination of local anesthetics and opioids is infused by the epidural route, patients experience better pain relief, earlier bowel recovery, earlier mobility, and decreased length of hospital stay than with the intravenous route (Mann et al., 2003). See page 184 for nursing implications for clients receiving epidural analgesia.

Nerve Blocks In a nerve block, anesthetics, sometimes in combination with steroidal anti-inflammatory drugs, are injected by a physician or nurse anesthetist into or near a nerve, usually in an area between the nociceptor and the dorsal root. The procedure may be performed to determine the precise location of the source of the pain: Pain relief indicates that the injection site is the site of the source of the pain.

Temporary (local) nerve blocks may give the client enough relief to (1) develop a more hopeful attitude that pain relief is possible, (2) allow local procedures to be performed without causing discomfort, or (3) exercise and move the affected part. Nerve blocks may also be performed to predict the results of neurosurgery. For long-term pain relief, a permanent neurolytic agent is used. Neurolytic blocks usually are reserved for terminally ill clients because of the risks of weakness, paralysis, and bowel and bladder dysfunction.

Surgery

As a pain relief measure, surgery usually is performed only after all other methods have failed. Clients need thorough knowledge of the implications of the use of surgery for pain relief. For

NURSING CARE OF THE CLIENT   Receiving Intraspinal Analgesia

Intraspinal analgesia is used to manage chronic and intractable cancer and severe postoperative pain. The intraspinal route may be either intrathecal (into the subarachnoid space) or epidural (into the epidural space). With the infusion of a narcotic into these spaces, there is a direct effect on the opiate receptors in the dorsal horn of the spinal cord; the narcotics are also absorbed systemically and affect the brain. This method provides complete pain relief but has some potentially dangerous side effects.

PROCEDURE
The physician places a catheter into the epidural space. Tubing is attached to an infusion pump, and the prescribed medication is administered. A portable or implantable pump may be used for narcotic administration that lasts more than a few days.

NURSING CARE
- Monitor vital signs every 15 minutes for the first 2–3 hours and every hour for the first 24 hours; the client is at risk for respiratory depression, which may not manifest itself for several hours.
- Ensure that naloxone, a narcotic antagonist, is immediately available to reverse respiratory depression.
- Monitor the effectiveness of the pain management.
- Monitor intake and output. Intraspinal narcotics may block the micturition reflex, causing urinary retention and necessitating the insertion of a Foley catheter.
- Use sterile technique to care for the catheter.

Placement of the catheter in the epidural space.

---

example, motor function loss is an unwelcome side effect of some surgeries. Surgical procedures used to relieve pain are shown in Figure 9–8 ■ and include the following:

CORDOTOMY A *cordotomy* is an incision into the anterolateral tracts of the spinal cord to interrupt the transmission of pain. Because it is difficult to isolate the nerves responsible for upper body pain, this surgery is most often performed for pain in the abdominal region and legs, including severe pain from terminal cancer. A percutaneous cordotomy produces lesions of the anterolateral surface of the spinal cord by means of a radio-frequency current.

NEURECTOMY A *neurectomy* is the removal of a nerve. It is sometimes used for pain relief. A peripheral neurectomy is the severing of a nerve at any point distal to the spinal cord.

SYMPATHECTOMY The sympathetic nerves play an important role in producing and transmitting the sensation of pain. A

sympathectomy involves destruction by injection or incision of the ganglia of sympathetic nerves, usually in the lumbar region or the cervicodorsal region at the base of the neck.

RHIZOTOMY A *rhizotomy* is surgical severing of the dorsal spinal roots. It is most often performed to relieve the pain of cancer of the head, neck, or lungs. A rhizotomy may be performed not only by surgically cutting the nerve fibers but also by injecting a chemical such as alcohol or phenol into the subarachnoid space or by using a radio-frequency current to selectively destroy pain fibers.

Transcutaneous Electrical Nerve Stimulation
A transcutaneous electrical nerve stimulation (TENS) unit consists of a low-voltage transmitter connected by wires to electrodes placed by the client as directed by the physical therapist (Figure 9–9 ■). The client experiences a gentle tapping or vi-

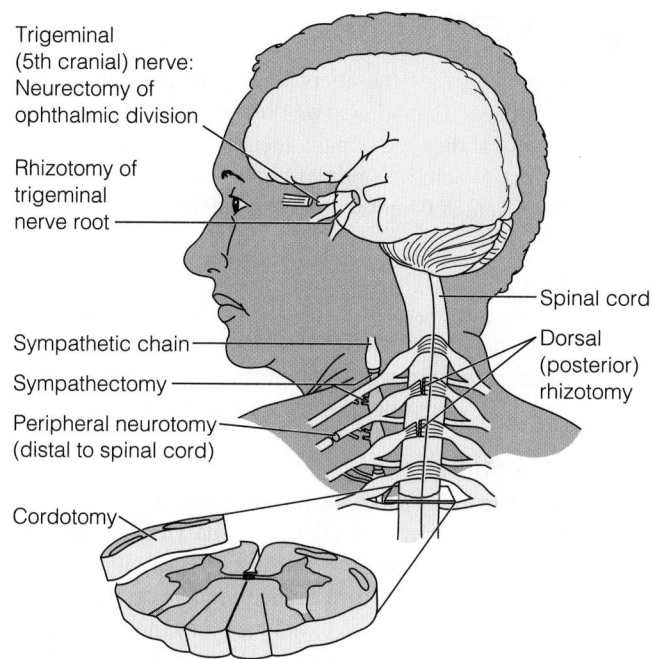

Trigeminal
(5th cranial) nerve:
Neurectomy of
ophthalmic division

Rhizotomy of
trigeminal
nerve root

Sympathetic chain

Sympathectomy

Peripheral neurotomy
(distal to spinal cord)

Cordotomy

Spinal cord

Dorsal
(posterior)
rhizotomy

Figure 9–8 ■ Surgical procedures are used to treat severe pain that does not respond to other types of management. They include cordotomy, neurectomy, sympathectomy, and rhizotomy.

brating sensation over the electrodes. The client can adjust the voltage to achieve maximum pain relief.

The gate-control theory clarifies how TENS works. It is believed that TENS electrodes stimulate the large-diameter A-beta touch fibers to close the gate in the substantia gelatinosa. It is also theorized that TENS stimulates endorphin release by inhibitory neurons.

A TENS unit is most commonly used to relieve chronic benign pain and acute postoperative pain. In either case, thorough

Figure 9–9 ■ The TENS unit is believed to assist in pain management through the gate-control theory. Electrodes that deliver low-voltage electrical stimuli are placed directly on the client over painful areas.

Source: Rehabilicare, Inc./Complex Technologies.

client teaching is essential, including an explanation of manufacturer's directions, instructions on where to place the electrodes, and the importance of placing the electrodes on clean, unbroken skin. The client should assess the skin daily for signs of irritation.

TENS offers several advantages: avoidance of drug side effects, client control, and good interaction with other therapies. Disadvantages are its cost and the need for expert training for initiation.

Complementary Therapies

ACUPUNCTURE Acupuncture is an ancient Chinese system involving the stimulation of certain specific points on the body to enhance the flow of vital energy (chi) along pathways called meridians. Acupuncture points can be stimulated by the insertion and withdrawing of needles, the application of heat, massage, laser, electrical stimulation, or a combination of these methods. Only care providers with special training can use this method. Acupuncture is becoming a more widely accepted therapy, especially for the treatment of pain.

BIOFEEDBACK Biofeedback is an electronic method of measuring physiologic responses, such as brain waves, muscle contraction, and skin temperature, and then "feeding" this information back to the client. Most biofeedback units consist of electrodes placed on the client's skin and an amplification unit that transforms data into visual cues, such as colored lights. The client thus learns to recognize stress-related responses and to replace them with relaxation responses. Eventually, the client learns to repeat independently those actions that produce the desired brain wave effect.

Relaxation helps the client avoid the anxiety that often accompanies and complicates pain. Additionally, biofeedback gives the client a measure of control over the response to pain.

HYPNOTISM Hypnosis is a trance state in which the mind becomes extremely suggestible. To achieve hypnosis, the client sits or lies down in a dimly lit, quiet room. The therapist suggests that the client relax and fix attention on an object. The therapist then repeats in a calm, soothing voice simple phrases, such as instructions to relax and listen to the therapist's voice. The client gradually becomes more and more relaxed and falls into a trance in which the client is no longer aware of the physical environment and hears only the therapist's voice. During this state, the therapist may make suggestions to encourage pain relief. It is possible to achieve complete anesthesia or to modify pain in a variety of ways through hypnotism. For the technique to work, however, the client must be fully relaxed and must want to be hypnotized.

Advantages include client control and lack of side effects. Disadvantages include the need for a skilled practitioner. However, some clients can learn to hypnotize themselves to achieve pain relief.

RELAXATION Relaxation involves learning activities that deeply relax the body and mind. Relaxation distracts the client, lessens the effects of stress from pain, increases pain tolerance, increases the effectiveness of other pain relief measures, and increases perception of pain control. In addition, by teaching the client relaxation techniques, the nurse acknowledges the client's pain and provides reassurance that the client will receive help in managing the pain (Schaffer & Yucha, 2004). Examples of relaxation activities include:

- *Diaphragmatic breathing* can relax muscles, improve oxygen levels, and provide a feeling of release from tension. The use of diaphragmatic breathing is more effective when the client either lies down or sits comfortably, remains in a quiet environment, and keeps the eyelids closed. Inhaling and exhaling slowly and regularly are also helpful. The technique for diaphragmatic breathing is described and illustrated in Chapter 4 ∞ .

- *Progressive muscle relaxation* may be used alone or in conjunction with deep breathing to help manage pain. The client should be taught to tighten one group of muscles (such as those of the face), hold the tension for a few seconds, and then relax the muscle group completely. The client should repeat these actions for all parts of the body. This method is also more effective when the client lies or sits comfortably, is in a quiet environment, and keeps the eyelids closed. Tapes are available to help the client with this relaxation process.

- *Guided imagery*, also called creative visualization, is the use of the imaginative power of the mind to create a scene or sensory experience that relaxes the muscles and moves the attention of the mind away from the pain experience. To use guided imagery, the client must be able to concentrate, use the imagination, and follow directions. The nurse can facilitate this technique by asking the client for some descriptions of what the client finds most relaxing. The nurse then speaks to the client in a calm, soothing voice about those places or situations. The client usually must close the eyes to reduce visual stimulation so that the mind can picture the situation in as much detail as possible. Tapes are available to assist the client with guided imagery.

- *Meditation* is a process whereby the client empties the mind of all sensory data and, typically, concentrates on a single object, word, or idea. This activity produces a deeply relaxed state in which oxygen consumption decreases, muscles relax, and endorphins are produced. At its deepest level, the meditative state may resemble a trance. A variety of exercises can induce the meditative state, and all are relatively easy to learn. Many books and tapes are available commercially.

DISTRACTION Distraction involves the redirection of the client's attention away from the pain and onto something that the client finds more pleasant. Examples of distracting activities are practicing focused breathing, listening to music, or doing some form of rhythmic activity to music. For example, the client using recorded music for distraction may sing along with the song, tap out the rhythm with the fingers or foot, clap to the music, conduct the music, or add harmony. Full participation in the music is key to pain relief.

Participating in an activity that promotes laughter, such as reading a joke book or viewing a comedy, has been found to be highly effective in pain relief. Laughing for 20 minutes or more is known to produce an increase in endorphins that may continue pain relief even after the client stops laughing.

CUTANEOUS STIMULATION It is believed that stimulation of the skin is effective in relieving pain because it prompts closure of the gate in the substantia gelatinosa. Cutaneous stimulation may be accomplished by massage, vibration, application of heat and cold, and therapeutic touch.

NURSING CARE

Nursing care of the client with pain presents perhaps more of a challenge than almost any other type of illness or injury. Regardless of the type of pain, the goal of nursing care is to assist the client to achieve optimal control of the pain. See the Nursing Care Plan: A Client with Chronic Pain on page 191.

Assessment

A comprehensive approach to pain assessment is essential to ensure adequate and appropriate interventions. The four assessment areas are client perceptions, physiologic responses, behavioral responses, and the client's attempts to self-manage the pain.

Client Perceptions

The most reliable indicator of the presence and degree of pain is the client's own statement about the pain. The McGill Pain Questionnaire is a useful tool in assessing the client's subjective experience of the pain. It asks the client to locate the pain, to describe the quality of the pain, to indicate how the pain changes with time, and to rate the intensity of the pain (Figure 9–10 ■). Several tools are available to assess specific pain qualities (Brunton, 2004; Jensen, 2006).

The client's perception of the pain can also be assessed by using the PQRST technique (Jimenez, 1998):

- P = What precipitated (triggered, stimulated) the pain? Has anything relieved the pain? What is the pattern of the pain?
- Q = What are the quality and quantity of the pain? Is it sharp, stabbing, aching, burning, stinging, deep, crushing, viselike, gnawing?
- R = What is the region (location) of the pain? Does the pain radiate to other areas of the body?
- S = What is the severity of the pain?
- T = What is the timing of the pain? When does it begin, how long does it last, and how is it related to other events in the client's life?

The most common method to assess the severity of pain is a pain rating scale. Several scales are illustrated in Figure 9–11 ■. For clients who do not understand English or numerals, a scale using colors (e.g., light blue for no pain through bright red for worst possible pain) or pictures may be helpful. The following nursing interventions will help the nurse use a pain rating scale to achieve optimal results:

- To ensure consistent communication, explain the specific pain rating scale being used. If a word descriptor scale is used, verify that the client can read the language being used. If a numerical scale is used, be sure the client can count to 10. If the client is not able to report pain because of communication difficulties, intubation, emotional disturbances, or cognitive impairments, follow these guidelines (Pasero & McCaffery, 2000):
  - Be sure the client is unable to report pain. Researchers have found that even nursing home residents with cognitive impairments can validly self-report pain (Horgas & Elliott, 2004).
  - Consider pathologic conditions and procedures that might cause pain and treat the client for pain.

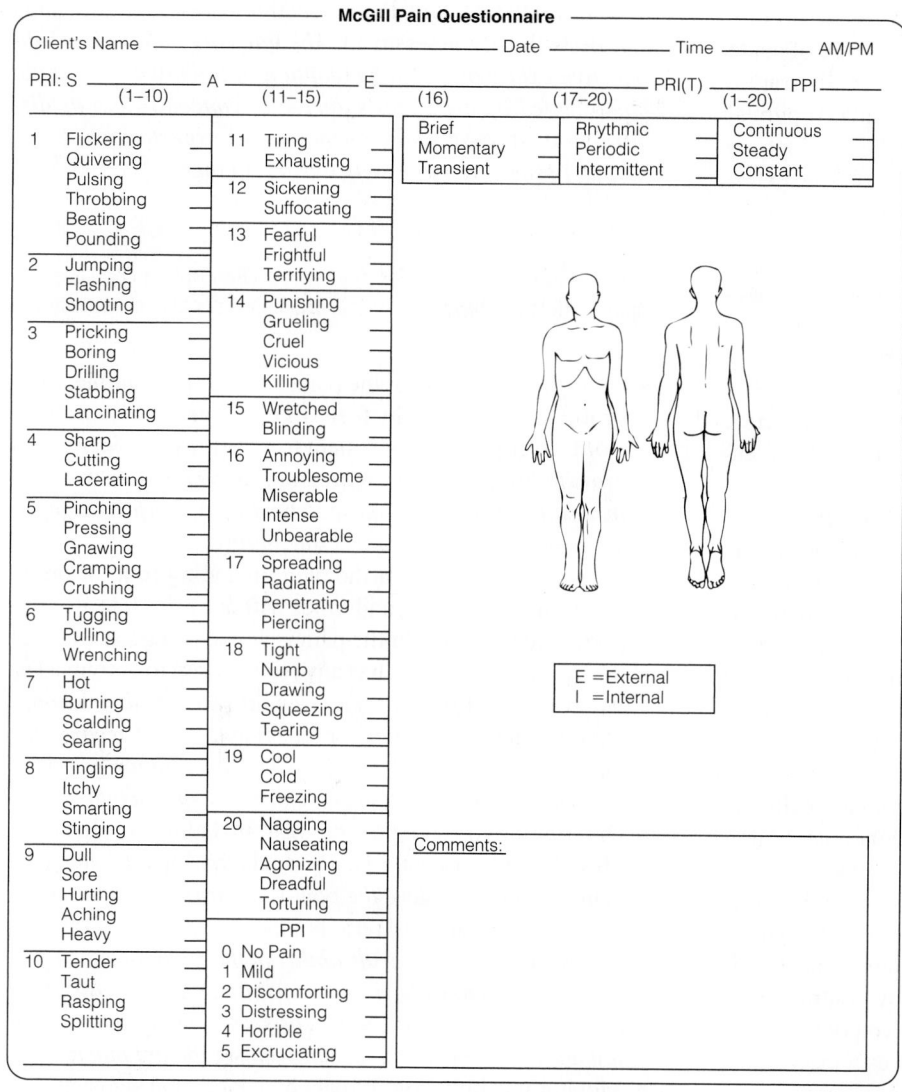

Figure 9–10 ■ The McGill Pain Questionnaire.

From *Pain Measurement and Assessment* by R. Melzack, 1983, New York: Raven. Reprinted by permission.

Figure 9–11 ■ Examples of commonly used pain scales.

- Look for indicators of pain, such as grimacing, restlessness, stillness, verbal or nonverbal vocalizations, and holding on to an object tightly (Horgas & Elliott, 2004).
- Ask a family member or caretaker if they suspect the client is having pain to serve as a proxy pain rating.
- Discuss the definition of the word *pain* to ensure that the client and the provider are communicating on the same level. It is often helpful to use the client's own words when describing the pain.
- Explain that the report of pain is important for promoting recovery, not just for achieving temporary comfort.
- Ask the client to establish a comfort-function goal. This is a level of pain that does not interfere with or prevent the performance of essential activities of recovery or living. Often, pain assessment is made while a client is sedentary. In this state the client may experience less pain than when active and falsely estimate tolerable pain ratings. Provide guidelines for setting goals. Researchers found that pain ratings higher than 3 (scale of 0–10) interfered significantly with patients' activities, and scores of 6 and 7 decrease quality of their life (Slaughter et al., 2002).

Physiologic Responses

Predictable physiologic changes occur in the presence of acute pain. These may include muscle tension; tachycardia; rapid, shallow respirations; increased blood pressure; dilated pupils; sweating; and pallor. Over time, however, the body adapts to the pain stimulus, and these physiologic changes may be extinguished in clients with chronic pain.

Behavioral Responses

Some behaviors are so typical of people in pain that the behaviors are referred to as *pain behaviors*. They include bracing or guarding the painful part, taking medication, crying, moaning, grimacing, withdrawing from activity and socialization, becoming immobile, talking about pain, holding the painful area, breathing with increased effort, exhibiting a sad facial expression, and being restless.

Behavioral responses to pain may or may not coincide with the client's report of pain and are not very reliable cues to the pain experience. For example, one client may rate pain at an 8 on a 1–10 scale while laughing or walking down the hall; another may deny pain completely while tachycardic, hypertensive, and grimacing. Discrepancies between the client's report of pain and behavioral responses may be the result of cultural factors, coping skills, fear, denial, or the utilization of relaxation or distraction techniques.

Clients may deny pain for a variety of reasons, including fear of injections, fear of drug/narcotic addiction, misinterpretation of terms (the client may not think that aching, soreness, or discomfort qualify as pain), or the misconception that healthcare providers know when clients experience pain. Some clients may deny pain as part of an attempt to deny that there is something wrong with them. Other clients, by contrast, may think that "as-needed" medications will be given only if their pain rating is high. Clients may also use pain as a mechanism to gain attention from family and healthcare providers.

Self-Management of Pain

The client's attempts to manage pain are useful additions to the assessment database. This information is individualized and client specific, including many factors such as culture, age, and client knowledge. Get detailed descriptions of actions the client or significant others took, when and how these measures were applied, and how well they worked.

Nursing Diagnoses and Interventions

The primary nursing diagnoses for clients in pain are acute pain and chronic pain. The interventions for these diagnoses are combined in this discussion.

Acute Pain or Chronic Pain

- Assess the characteristics of the pain by asking the client to:
  - Point to the pain location or mark the pain location on a figure drawing. *Pain location provides information about the etiology of the pain and the type of pain being experienced.*
  - Rate the intensity of the pain by using a pain scale (1 to 10, with 10 being the worst pain ever experienced), a visual analog scale (a scale on which pain is marked on a continuum from no pain to severe pain), or with word descriptors

(such as the McGill Pain Questionnaire). Use the same scale with each assessment. *The intensity of pain is a subjective experience. The perception of the intensity of pain is affected by the client's degree of concentration or distraction, state of consciousness, and expectations. Some body tissues are more sensitive than others.*

PRACTICE ALERT
Do not assume that the older client or the client with a cognitive impairment is not having pain or is unable to identify its intensity.

- Describe the quality of the pain, saying, for example, "Describe what your pain feels like." If necessary, provide word descriptors for the client to select. *Descriptive terms provide insight into the nature and perception of the pain. In addition, the location and type of pain (for example, acute versus chronic) affect the quality.*
- Describe the pattern of the pain, including time of onset, duration, persistence, and times without pain. It is also important to ask whether the pain is worse at regular times of the day and whether it has any relationship to activity. *The pattern of pain provides clues about cause and location.*
- Describe any precipitating or relieving factors. *Precipitating factors include sleep deficits, anxiety, temperature extremes, excessive noise, anxiety, fear, depression, and activity.*
- Describe the meaning of the pain, including its effects on lifestyle, self-concept, roles, and relationships. *Clients with acute pain may believe the pain is a normal response to injury or that it signals serious illness and death. Pain is a stressor that may affect the ability of the client to cope effectively. The client with chronic pain often has concerns about addiction to pain medication, costs, social interactions, sexual activities, and relationships with significant others.*
- Monitor manifestations of pain by taking vital signs; assessing skin temperature and moisture; observing pupils; observing facial expressions, position in bed, guarding of body parts; and noting restlessness. *Autonomic responses to pain may result in increased blood pressure, tachycardia, rapid respirations, perspiration, and dilated pupils. Other responses to pain include grimacing, clenching the hands, muscle rigidity, guarding, restlessness, and nausea. The client with chronic pain may have an unexpressive, tired facial appearance.*

PRACTICE ALERT
Consider pain the fifth vital sign and assess clients for pain every time you check temperature, pulse, respirations, and blood pressure.

- Communicate belief in the client's pain by verbally acknowledging the presence of the pain, listening carefully to the description of pain, and acting to help the client manage the pain. *Because pain is a personal, subjective experience, the nurse must convey belief in the client's pain. By conveying belief in the client's pain, the nurse reduces anxiety and thereby lessens pain.* See the Nursing Research box on the following page.
- Provide optimal pain relief with prescribed analgesics, determining the preferred route of administration. Provide

NURSING RESEARCH   Evidence-Based Practice for the Client Experiencing Pain

Pain that is not adequately managed is the focus of regulatory agencies, professional healthcare organizations, and consumer groups. Despite well-defined guidelines for pain management, there is a gap between guideline standards of care and implementation of care. Observational studies of pain management are valuable because they are time sensitive. Relying on nurses' self-report of pain management introduces bias and loses currency. In the study by Manias et al. (2005) nurses were observed in 2-hour periods of high environmental, patient, and nursing activity. Examination of the collected observations by independent analysts revealed six categories of response to patients' pain. The pain was (1) responded to effectively; (2) prioritized as less important than completing medication administration, vital sign assessment, taking telephone calls, or dressing changes; (3) ignored because cues were missed; (4) treated as part of the medication administration regimen and given or withheld according to schedule; (5) prevented through comfort measures, medicating before pain was present or was going to occur as with dressing changes, teaching the importance of early communication about pain; and (6) was only addressed reactively, after the painful experience.

Because pain management is mandatory with regulatory agencies such as JCAHO, attention to patients' self-reported pain scores is increasing. It is valuable to have the informative detail this study provides. Communication among nurses, physicians, and clients is key to pain relief. Knowledge of pharmacology and the nonpharmacology of pain relief needs to be taught and reviewed regularly.

Environmental distractions and interruptions are associated with less attention to pain management. Few conditions have higher priority for the client than pain relief, but the study revealed that nurses accept pain as a normal component of the postoperative surgery experience. Administrators need to be aware that competing responsibilities impact nurses' ability to provide effective pain management. Those responsibilities include documentation, admitting new patients, and completing discharge teaching and arrangements. Pain management is an important component of professional nursing; nurses should be supported in their efforts to address pain with compassion and efficiency.

CRITICAL THINKING IN CLIENT CARE

1. Reflect on your own experiences with pain. Will those experiences facilitate or hinder your assessments and interventions for clients in pain?
2. You are caring for a young man who has multiple injuries from a motorcycle accident. He tells you his pain is so bad that "he just wants to die." How would you respond?
3. You are caring for an 80-year-old man with diabetes who has had his left foot amputated for gangrene. He is restless and moaning. Another nurse tells you to only give one-half of the ordered dose of narcotics because "he is old and there is a danger of respiratory depression." What would you do?
4. Why do you think nurses tend to underestimate and undermedicate pain?

---

pain-relieving measures for severe pain on a regular around-the-clock basis or by self-administration (such as with a PCA pump). *The client is part of the decision-making process and can exert some control over the situation by choosing the administration route. Analgesics are usually most effective when they are administered before pain occurs or becomes severe. Around-the-clock administration has been proven to provide better pain management for both acute and chronic pain. Do not crush or break or allow patients to chew controlled-release oral preparations; a dose meant to be slowly absorbed that is absorbed rapidly may lead to a toxic overdose and death. Capsules containing pellets for controlled-release medications can be opened and sprinkled over soft foods; the pellets should not be crushed, chewed, or dissolved (Vallerand, 2003).*

■ Evaluate and monitor the effects of analgesics and other pain-relieving measures and teach family members or significant others to be alert for adverse reactions to pain medications. Sedation, constipation, nausea, and dizziness are common side effects. *Excessive sedation can progress to significant respiratory depression (Pasero & McCaffery, 2002). Check oxygen saturation q2 at the beginning of opioid therapy and after increasing dosage (Pasero & McCaffery, 2002). Prevent falls that may result from sedation or dizziness. If the client has symptoms of excessive opioid dosage, antidotes are available. Narcan (naloxone) is used for morphine overdose. Use caution to titrate Narcan slowly. Never*

push an entire dose all at once. Administer only enough Narcan to eliminate adverse effects such as respiratory depression or excessive sedation. If excessive Narcan is administered, the client may experience acute withdrawal and will have no pain relief. It may take considerable time to reestablish a therapeutic comfort level.

■ Determine the level of sedation the client with tolerate. *For clients with chronic pain or cancer pain who need high doses of opioids, sedation may interfere with quality of life and neither the client nor the family want the client so sedated.* Several classes of drugs are being used to counteract sedation. They are usually given in the morning so they will not interfere with sleep throughout the night. Amphetamines, especially methylphenidate (Ritalin), are the most commonly used; modafinil (Provigil) has been used for several years, and donepezil (Aricept), which is used for the symptoms of Alzheimer's disease, reduces sedation and fatigue (Bourdeanu et al., 2005).

■ Teach the client and family nonpharmacologic methods of pain management, such as relaxation, distraction, and cutaneous stimulation. *These techniques are especially useful when used in conjunction with pain medications and may also be useful in managing chronic pain.*

■ Provide comfort measures, such as changing positions, back massage, oral care, skin care, and changing bed linens. *Basic comfort measures for personal cleanliness, skin care, and mobility promote physical and psychosocial well-being, lessening the perception of pain.*

■ Provide client and family teaching, and make referrals if necessary to assist with coping, financial resources, and home care. *The client (and family) with pain requires information about medications, noninvasive techniques for pain management, and sources of assistance with home-based care. The client with acute pain requires information about the expected course of pain resolution.*

Using NANDA, NIC, and NOC

Linkages between NANDA, NIC, and NOC when caring for the client in pain are illustrated in Chart 9–1.

Community-Based Care

Teaching of the client and family includes:

■ Specific drugs to be taken, including the frequency, potential side effects, possible drug interactions, and any special precautions to be taken (such as taking with food or avoiding alcohol)
■ How to take or administer the drugs (Box 9–3)
■ The importance of taking pain medications before the pain becomes severe
■ An explanation that the risk of addiction to pain medications is very small when they are used for pain relief and management
■ The importance of scheduling periods of rest and sleep.
   In addition, suggest the following resources:
■ Pain clinics
■ Community support groups
   ■ American Cancer Society
   ■ American Pain Society.

NANDA, NIC, and NOC Linkages
CHART 9–1 **The Client with Chronic Pain**

NANDA

Chronic Pain

↓

NIC

Medication Administration

Pain Management

Meditation Facilitation

Cutaneous Stimulation

↓

NOC

Comfort Level

Pain Control

Pain: Disruptive Effects

Depression Level

Data from *NANDA's Nursing Diagnoses: Definitions & Classification 2005–2006* by NANDA International (2005), Philadelphia; *Nursing Interventions Classification (NIC)* (4th ed.) by J. M. Dochterman & G. M. Bulechek (2004), St. Louis, MO: Mosby; and *Nursing Outcomes Classification (NOC)* (3rd ed.) by S. Moorhead, M. Johnson, and M. Maas (2004), St. Louis, MO: Mosby.

BOX 9–3 **Providing Long-Term Analgesia at Home**

ROUTE	DRUG	NURSING IMPLICATIONS
Oral	Oxycodone (OxyContin)	Available in a timed-release formulation for 12-hour dosing and as fast-acting formulations (OxyIR, OxyFAST) for breakthrough pain.
Oral	Morphine (Kadian)	Formulated of timed-release particles in a capsule. If client can't swallow the capsule, may be sprinkled over food or given by nasogastric or gastric tube.
Transdermal	Fentanyl (Duragesic)	Absorbed slowly through the skin; allows 72-hour dose schedule. Up to 14 hours to achieve therapeutic level; when discontinued therapeutic effect will decay slowly.
Transdermal	Lidocaine (Lidoderm)	Effective for 12 hours for various neuropathic pains. Monitor clients also taking Class 1 antiarrhythmic drugs for increased effects.
Transmucosal	Fentanyl citrate (Actiq)	A lozenge formulation used to treat breakthrough cancer pain in opioid-tolerant clients.

NURSING CARE PLAN A Client with Chronic Pain

Susan Akers, age 37, is currently being seen at an outpatient clinic for chronic nonmalignant pain. She works at a local paper factory. She has a 3-year history of neck and shoulder pain that usually is accompanied by headaches. She believes the pain is related to lifting objects at work, but it is now precipitated by activities of daily living. Susan is absent from work approximately three times a month and states that the absences are due to her pain and headaches. She has been seeking care in the local emergency department on the average of twice monthly for injections for pain. She does not regularly use medications but does take Darvocet-N 100 and Valium as needed (usually two to three times a day). Ms. Akers is divorced and has two children. She states that she has several friends in the area, but her parents and siblings live in another part of the United States.

ASSESSMENT

During the nursing history, Susan rates her pain during an acute episode as a 7 on a 1 to 10 scale. She states that lifting objects and moving her hands and arms above shoulder level precipitate sharp pain. The pain never really goes away, but it does decrease with upper extremity rest. She says that when she lifts a lot at work, she has difficulty sleeping that night. She takes two Darvocet-N 100 tablets every 4 hours when the pain is severe, but does not get complete relief.

DIAGNOSIS

■ *Chronic Pain* related to muscle inflammation

EXPECTED OUTCOMES

■ Return for follow-up visits with a journal of activities and pain experiences.
■ After 3 to 5 days on regularly scheduled doses of pain medication, report a decrease in the level of pain from 7 to 3 or 4 on a 1 to 10 scale.
■ Decrease number of absences from work.
■ Modify activities at work and at home, especially when pain is intense.

PLANNING AND IMPLEMENTATION

■ Encourage discussion of pain, and acknowledge belief in Susan's report of pain.
■ Consult with a physician for a nonnarcotic analgesic with a minimum of side effects, and instruct in maintaining regular dosing schedules.
■ For episodes of acute pain, take narcotic analgesics as soon as the pain begins and every 4 hours; while continuing the dosage of nonnarcotic analgesic.
■ Teach one relaxation technique that is personally useful.
■ Explore distraction techniques such as listening to music, watching comedies, or reading.
■ Provide clinic phone number and instruct to call if pain is unrelieved with narcotic and nonnarcotic analgesics.

EVALUATION

Susan returns for scheduled follow-up visits with a completed journal of her activities and associated pain. She reports that taking oral narcotic analgesics has relieved her pain and that within 3 weeks nonnarcotic analgesics brought her pain under control. She also reports that her supervisor has reassigned her to a position that requires no lifting. She now rates her pain at 2 or 3 on a 1 to 10 scale. She has missed only 1 day of work in the last 3 months and reports that her children and friends have helped with her household tasks when she has requested they do so.

CRITICAL THINKING IN THE NURSING PROCESS

1. Describe three factors that support the statement "Pain is a personal experience."
2. Susan asks you how often she should take her pain medications. You tell her to (a) take them on a regular basis or (b) wait until she experiences pain. Which action would you choose, and why?
3. Develop a care plan for Susan for the nursing diagnosis of *Risk for Constipation*. Why is this necessary?
See Evaluating Your Response in Appendix C.

EXPLORE MediaLink

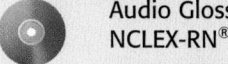

Prentice Hall Nursing MediaLink DVD-ROM
Audio Glossary
NCLEX-RN® Review

Animation/Video
Epidural Placement
Morphine
Naproxen
Reflex Arc

COMPANION WEBSITE www.prenhall.com/lemone
Audio Glossary
NCLEX-RN® Review
Care Plan Activity: The Client in Pain
Case Study: Assessing the Client in Pain
MediaLink Applications
Links to Resources

CHAPTER HIGHLIGHTS

- Pain is perceived in the central nervous system. Opioids and other analgesics block the perception of pain; NSAIDs and most nonpharmacologic interventions block or decrease the transmission of pain from the periphery to the CNS. Measures to block the sensitization of pain-transmitting fibers are being used prior to painful procedures and incision in surgery.

- There are many types of pain, and treatment varies according to the type and combination of types. Acute pain usually decreases as healing progresses; chronic pain has acute exacerbations and compounds acute pain. Breakthrough pain is recognized as an increase in pain intensity that occurs when the peak and duration of medications are reached. Incident pain occurs in relation to a change or increase in activity. Central pain results from CNS lesions. Phantom pain occurs after amputations, seeming to originate in the missing limb. Psychogenic pain has no identifiable physiologic origin.

- Ethnicity (genetics and culture) and gender impact pain perception and behavior. Behavioral assessment of pain intensity is less accurate than a client's report of pain intensity.

- Myths and misconceptions exist about pain and its management; the client's perceived cause of pain and the best self-care method to relieve pain provide pertinent assessment information.

- Clients also respond to pain on the basis of their emotional state, past experiences with pain, and the meaning of the painful experience. Clients with malignant diagnoses may have significantly different interpretations of pain than clients with benign disease.

- Older adult clients perceive pain as intensely as younger adults. They need the same amount of opioids in the immediate postoperative period but may have difficulty metabolizing or eliminating medications.

- Assertively assess pain in older clients. Older clients may hesitate to report pain for fear of losing independence or being considered a bother. Cognitive impairment following CVA, dementia, or delirium makes self-report of pain less reliable. Behavioral scales for assessing pain are useful when clients cannot give self-reports.

- Addiction is a neurophysiologic disease. Clients with addiction to opioids may need greater doses of opioids to control pain because of the tolerance they may have developed through usage.

- Emergency department physicians and nurses are constrained in the prescription of opioids by the risk of overmedicating clients who are drug seeking and by the myth that pain management interferes with diagnosis.

- Pain management includes assessment, intervention, and evaluation. It is important to verify that interventions have been effective. If not, interventions must be identified that bring pain down to a level of intensity with which the client feels satisfied.

TEST YOURSELF NCLEX-RN® REVIEW

1. Your neighbor has had lower back pain for 9 months. How would this pain be categorized?
   1. acute pain
   2. chronic pain
   3. referred pain
   4. somatic pain

2. Which of the following statements is a pain myth?
   1. It is best to wait until a client has pain before giving medication.
   2. Anxiety can cause pain; pain can cause anxiety.
   3. Meperidine (Demerol) is no longer recommended for postoperative pain.
   4. The rationale for use of a TENS unit is supported by the gate-control theory.

3. You are taking a health history for a client who has taken a NSAID for several years. What would be an appropriate question to ask?
   1. "Do you understand what this drug could do to you?"
   2. "Have you ever vomited blood or had very dark stools?"
   3. "Do you know that you may become addicted to this drug?"
   4. "Have you noticed any problems with your breathing?"

4. You are replacing a transdermal pain medication. Where on the body would you place it?
   1. On one side of the buttocks
   2. Below the navel, midline on the abdomen
   3. On the anterior thigh
   4. On the upper torso

5. Which of the following statements would be most useful in determining the *quality* of a client's pain?
   1. "Tell me where you hurt."
   2. "Rate your pain on a scale of 0 to 10."
   3. "Describe what your pain feels like."
   4. "Tell me how this pain affects your sleep."

6. The client has orders for intravenous patient-controlled analgesia (PCA). The following principles are true EXCEPT:
   1. basal doses are continuous.
   2. overdose cannot occur.
   3. a 10-minute lockout each hour allows six bolus doses.
   4. unused bolus doses cannot accumulate.

7. The most common side effects of opioid analgesics are:
   1. anuria, diplopia, and cough.
   2. constipation, nausea, and sedation.
   3. pruritus, constipation, and hallucinations.
   4. dysphagia, fever, and gastritis.

8. The preferred route of opioid administration for chronic pain is:
   1. transdermal.
   2. oral.
   3. intravenous.
   4. rectal.

9. The equivalent dose of an oral drug compared to the intravenous preparation of the same drug is:
   1. equal dosage.
   2. twice the intravenous dose.
   3. varies according to the drug but usually greater.
   4. one-half the intravenous dose.

10. Clients treated for chronic pain may need additional pain management strategies for:
    1. breakthrough pain.
    2. acute pain.
    3. end-of-dose pain.
    4. all of the above.

See Test Yourself answers in Appendix C.

BIBLIOGRAPHY

American Pain Society. (2006). *Pain: The fifth vital sign.* Retrieved from http://ampainsoc.org

Arnstein, P. (2006). Placebo: No relief for Ms. Mahoney's pain. *American Journal of Nursing, 106*(2), 54–57.

Bourdeanu, L., Loseth, D. B., & Funk, M. (2005). Management of opioid-induced sedation in patients with cancer. *Clinical Journal of Oncology Nursing, 9*(6), 705–711.

Brown, D. (2004). A literature review exploring how healthcare professionals contribute to the assessment and control of postoperative pain in older people. *International Journal of Older People Nursing, 13*(6b), 74–90.

Brunton, S. (2004). Approach to assessment and diagnosis of chronic pain. *Journal of Family Practice, 53*(10 Supplement), S3–S10.

Cahill, B. A. (2005). Management of cancer pain. In C. H. Yarbro, M. H. Frogge, & M. Goodman (Eds.), *Cancer nursing*, (6th ed., pp 662–697). Boston: Jones & Bartlett.

Carpenito, L. (2000). *Nursing diagnosis: Application to clinical practice* (8th ed.). Philadelphia: Lippincott.

Closs, S. J. (1996). Pain and elderly patients: a survey of nurse's knowledge and experiences. *Journal of Advanced Nursing, 23*(2), 237–242.

Cohen, M. J., & Schecter, W. P. (2005). Perioperative pain control: A strategy for management. *Surgical Clinics of North America, 85*, 1243–1257.

Compton, P., & Athanasos, P. (2003). Chronic pain, substance abuse and addiction. *Nursing Clinics of North America, 38,* 525–537.

Cook, L., Sefcik, E., & Stetina, P. (2004). Pain management in the addicted population: A case study comparison of prescriptive practice. *Journal of Addictions Nursing, 15,* 11–14.

Dahl, J. B., & Møiniche, S. (2004). Pre-emptive analgesia. *British Medical Bulletin, 71,* 13–27.

Dalton, J. A., & Coyne, P. (2003). Cognitive-behavioral therapy: Tailored to the individual. *Nursing Clinics of North America, 38,* 465–476.

D'Arcy, Y. (2005). Conquering pain: Have you tried these new techniques? *American Journal of Nursing, 35*(3), 36–42.

Evans, C. (2004). Improving assessment of pain in older people. *Emergency Nurse, 12*(5), 18–21.

Ferrell, B. (2000). *A nurse's guide to breakthrough cancer pain.* Pyros Education Group. Chatham, N.J.: Medimedia USA.

Fries, B. E., Simon, S. E., Morris, J. N., Flodstrom, C., & Bookstein, F. L. (2001). Pain in U.S. nursing homes: Validating a pain scale for the minimum data set. *Gerontologist, 41*(2): 173–179.

International Association for the Study of Pain. (1994). Definitions. Retrieved from http://www.iasp-pain.org/terms-p.html#Pain

Gottschalk, A., & Smith, D. S. (2001). New concepts in acute pain therapy: Preemptive analgesia. *American Family Physician, 63*(10), 1979–1984.

Grace, P. (2006). Ethical issues: The clinical use of placebos. *American Journal of Nursing, 106*(2), 58–61.

Hartrick, C. T. (2004). Multimodal postoperative pain management. *American Journal of Health-System Pharmacology, 61*(S1), S4–S10.

Haugh, R. (2005). Hospitals and clinicians confront a new imperative: Pain management. *Hospitals & Health Networks, 79*(4), 51–52, 54, 56.

Herr, K. (2002). Pain assessment in cognitively impaired old adults: New strategies and careful observation help pinpoint unspoken pain. *American Journal of Nursing, 102*(12), 65–67.

Horgas, A. L., & Elliott, A. F. (2004). Pain assessment and management in persons with dementia. *Nursing Clinics of North America, 39,* 593–606.

Jensen, M. P. (2006). Using pain quality assessment measures for selecting analgesic agents. *Clinical Journal of Pain, 22*(1), Supplement, 59–513.

Jimenez, S. L. M. (1998). Pain and comfort assessment: The key to effective pain management. *The Journal of Perinatal Education, 7*(1), 35–38.

Joint Commission on Accreditation of Healthcare Organizations. (2001). *Joint Commission on Accreditation of Healthcare Organizations pain standards for 2004.* Available from http://www.jcaho.org

Kodiath, M. (1997). Chronic pain: Contrasting two cultures. *Clinical Excellence for Nurse Practitioners, 1*(1), 59–61.

Lehne, R. A. (2004). *Pharmacology for nursing care* (5th ed.). St. Louis, MO: W. B. Saunders.

Loran, D. B., Hyde, B. R., & Zwischenberger, J. B. (2005). Perioperative management of special populations: The geriatric patient. *Surgical Clinics of North America, 85,* 1259–1266.

Manias, E., Bucknall, T., & Botti, M. (2005). Nurses strategies for managing pain in the postoperative setting. *Pain Management Nursing, 6*(1), 18–29.

Mann, C., Pouzeratte, Y., & Eledjam, J. J. (2003). Postoperative patient-controlled analgesia in the elderly: Risks and benefits of epidural versus intravenous administration. *Drugs & Aging, 20*(5), 337–345.

McCaffery, M. (1979). *Nursing management of the patient with pain.* Philadelphia: Lippincott.

McCaffery, M., & Arnstein, P. (2006). Pain control: The debate over placebos in pain management. *American Journal of Nursing, 106*(2), 62–65.

McCaffery, M., & Pasero, C. (1999). *Pain: Clinical manual* (2nd ed.). St. Louis, MO: Mosby.

McCance, K., & Huether, S. (2002). *Pathophysiology: The biologic basis for disease in adults and children.* (4th ed.). St. Louis, MO: Mosby.

Melzack, R. (1975). The McGill Pain Questionnaire: Major properties and scoring methods. *Pain, 1,* 277.

Merboth, M. K., & Barnason, S. (2000). Managing pain: The fifth vital sign. *Nursing Clinics of North America, 35*(2), 375–383.

Munoz, C., & Hilgenberg, C. (2005). Ethnopharmacology: Understanding how ethnicity can affect drug response is essential to providing culturally competent care. *American Journal of Nursing, 105*(8), 40–48.

O'Donnell, J. M., Bragg, K., & Sell, S. (2003). Procedural sedation: Safely navigating the twilight zone. *Nursing, 33*(4), 36–44.

Palos, G. R., Mendoza, T. R., Cantor, S. B., Aday, L. A., & Cleeland, C. S. (2004). Perceptions of analgesic use and side effects: What the public values in pain management. *Journal of Pain and Symptom Management, 28*(5), 460–473.

Pasero, C. (2003). Pain in the emergency department. Withholding pain medication is not justified. *American Journal of Nursing, 103*(7), 73–74.

Pasero, C., & McCaffery, M. (2000). Pain control: When patients can't report pain. *American Journal of Nursing, 100*(9), 22–23.

Pasero, C., & McCaffery, M. (2002). Pain control: Monitoring sedation: It's the key to preventing opioid-induced respiratory depression. *American Journal of Nursing, 102*(2), 67, 69.

Pasero, C., & McCaffery, M. (2004). Pain control. Comfort-function goals: A way to establish accountability for pain relief. *American Journal of Nursing, 104*(9), 77–78, 81.

Portenoy, R. K., Ugarte, C., Fuller, I., & Haas, G. (2004). Population-based survey of pain in the United States: Differences among white, African American, and Hispanic subjects. *Journal of Pain, 5*(6), 317–328.

Porth, C. (2005). *Pathophysiology: Concepts of altered health states* (7th ed.). Philadelphia: Lippincott.

Schaffer, S. D., & Yucha, C. B. (2004). Relaxation & pain management. *American Journal of Nursing, 104*(8), 75–76, 78–79, 81–82.

Sheehan, D. K., & Schirm, V. (2003). End-of-life care of older adults. *American Journal of Nursing, 103*(11), 48–59.

Silberstein, E. B., Saenger, E. L., & Saenger, S. R. (2001). Painful osteoblastic metastases: The role of nuclear medicine. *Oncology, 15*(2), 157–163.

Slaughter, A., Pasero, C., & Manworren, R. (2002). Unacceptable pain levels. *American Journal of Nursing, 102*(5), 75–77.

Strassels, S. A., McNicol, E., & Suleman, R. (2005). Postoperative pain management: A practical review, part 1. *American Journal of Health-System Pharmacy, 62*(18), 1904–1916.

Svendsen, K. B., Andersen, S., Arnason, S., Arnér, S., Breivik, H., Heiskanen, T., et al. (2005). Breakthrough pain in malignant and non-malignant diseases: A review of prevalence, characteristics and mechanisms. *European Journal of Pain, 9,* 195–206.

Taddio, A., & Katz, J. (2005). The effects of early pain experience in neonates on pain responses in infancy and childhood. *Pediatric Drugs, 7*(4), 245–257.

Tariman, J. D. (2005). Multiple myeloma. In C. H. Yarbro, M. H. Frogge, & M. Goodman (Eds.), *Cancer nursing* (6th ed., pp. 1461–1489). Boston: Jones & Bartlett.

Teno, J., Bird, C., & Mor, V. (2002). *The prevalence and treatment of pain in U.S. nursing homes.* Providence, RI: Center for Gerontology and Health Care Research, Brown University.

Trame, C. (2002). Pharmacology consult: Just what are we treating—addiction or pain? *Clinical Nurse Specialist, 16*(1), 295–297.

U.S. Department of Health and Human Services. (1992). *Acute pain management: Operative or medical procedures and trauma* (AHCPR Publication No. 92-0032). Rockville, MD: Agency for Health Care Policy and Research, Public Health Service.

Vallerand, A. H. (2003). The use of long-acting opioids in chronic pain management. *Nursing Clinics of North America, 38,* 435–445.

Watt-Watson, J., Garfinkel, P., Gallop, R., Stevens, B., & Streiner, D. (2000). The impact of nurses' empathic responses on patients' pain management in acute care. *Nursing Research, 49*(4), 191–200.

Wilsey, B., Fishman, S., Rose, J. S., & Papazian, J. (2003). Pain management in the ED. *American Journal of Emergency Medicine, 22*(1), 51–57.

Wilson, B. A., Shannon, M. T., & Stang, C. L. (2006). *Nursing drug guide 2006.* Upper Saddle River, NJ: Prentice Hall.

World Health Organization. (1986/1990). *Cancer pain relief.* Geneva: Author.

Yarbro, C., Frogge, M. H., & Goodman, M. (Eds.) (2005). *Cancer nursing: Principles & practice* (6th ed.). Boston: Jones & Bartlett.

CHAPTER 10

Nursing Care of Clients with Altered Fluid, Electrolyte, and Acid–Base Balance

LEARNING OUTCOMES

- Describe the functions and regulatory mechanisms that maintain water and electrolyte balance in the body.

- Compare and contrast the causes, effects, and care of the client with fluid volume or electrolyte imbalance.

- Explain the pathophysiology and manifestations of imbalances of sodium, potassium, calcium, magnesium, and phosphorus.

- Describe the causes and effects of acid–base imbalances.

CLINICAL COMPETENCIES

- Assess and monitor fluid, electrolyte, and acid–base balance for assigned clients.

- Administer fluids and medications knowledgeably and safely.

- Determine priority nursing diagnoses, based on assessment data, to select and implement individualized nursing interventions.

- Provide client and family teaching about diet and medications used to restore, promote, and maintain fluid, electrolyte, and acid–base balance.

- Integrate interdisciplinary care into care of clients with altered fluid, electrolyte, and acid–base balance.

MEDIALINK

Resources for this chapter can be found on the Prentice Hall Nursing MediaLink DVD-ROM accompanying this textbook, and on the Companion Website at
http://www.prenhall.com/lemone

acidosis, *238*	**bases,** *238*	**Kussmaul's**
acids, *238*	**buffers,** *238*	**respirations,** *244*
active transport, *200*	**dehydration,** *203*	**orthopnea,** *209*
alkalis, *238*	**diffusion,** *199*	**osmosis,** *198*
alkalosis, *238*	**dyspnea,** *209*	**Paco$_2$,** *239*
anasarca, *209*	**edema,** *209*	**Pao$_2$,** *239*
anion gap, *243*	**electrolytes,** *196*	**polyuria,** *209*
arterial blood gases (ABGs), *213*	**filtration,** *200*	**serum bicarbonate,** *239*
ascites, *209*	**fluid volume deficit (FVD),** *203*	**stridor,** *231*
atrial natriuretic peptide	**fluid volume excess,** *209*	**tetany,** *229*
(ANP), *202*	**glomerular filtration rate,** *214*	**third spacing,** *203*
base excess (BE), *239*	**homeostasis,** *195*	**volatile acids,** *238*

Changes in the normal distribution and composition of body fluids often occur in response to illness and trauma. These changes affect fluid balance of the intracellular and extracellular compartments of the body, the concentration of electrolytes within fluid compartments, and the body's hydrogen ion concentration (pH). Normal physiologic processes depend on a relatively stable state in the internal environment of the body. The fluid volume, electrolyte composition, and pH of both intracellular and extracellular spaces must remain constant within a relatively narrow range to maintain health and life.

Homeostasis is the body's tendency to maintain a state of physiologic balance in the presence of constantly changing conditions. Homeostasis is necessary if the body is to function optimally at a cellular level and as a total organism. Homeostasis depends on multiple factors in both the external and internal environments, such as available oxygen in the air and nutrients in food, as well as normal body temperature, respiration, and digestive processes. The normal volume, composition, distribution, and pH of body fluids reflect a state of homeostasis.

Changes in the normal volume of fluids, their composition, distribution, and relative acidity or alkalinity have the potential to disrupt most functional health patterns. Imbalances of fluids, electrolytes, and pH affect the ability to maintain activities of daily living (the Activity-Exercise Pattern), think clearly (the Cognitive-Perceptual Pattern), and engage in self-care (the Health Perception-Health Management Pattern). Conversely, alterations in a number of health patterns affect the ability to maintain homeostasis. Alterations in the Nutritional-Metabolic Pattern affect the ability to consume adequate food and fluids. Disruptions of the Elimination Pattern may lead to retention or loss of excess amounts of fluids and electrolytes. Disrupted heart or respiratory function, which falls within the Activity-Exercise Pattern, has the potential to affect fluid, electrolyte, and acid–base balance.

The goal in managing fluid, electrolyte, and acid–base imbalances is to reestablish and maintain a normal balance. Nursing care includes identifying and assessing clients who are likely to develop imbalances, monitoring clients for early manifestations, and implementing collaborative and nursing interventions to prevent or correct imbalances. Effective nursing interventions require an understanding of the multiple processes that maintain fluid, electrolyte, and acid–base balance and an understanding of the causes and treatment of imbalances that occur.

Mechanisms that maintain normal fluid and electrolyte balance are discussed first, followed by sections on fluid imbalances and electrolyte imbalances. Discussion of normal acid–base balance precedes discussion of acid–base imbalances. Case studies related to selected fluid, electrolyte, and acid–base disorders are found throughout the chapter.

OVERVIEW OF NORMAL FLUID AND ELECTROLYTE BALANCE

Fluid and electrolyte balance in the body involves regulatory mechanisms that maintain the composition, distribution, and movement of fluids and electrolytes. This section provides an overview of fluid and electrolyte balance in the body. It is followed by discussion of fluid volume and electrolyte balance disorders.

Body Fluid Composition

Body fluid is composed of water and various dissolved substances (solutes).

Water

Water is the primary component of body fluids. It functions in several ways to maintain normal cellular function. Water:

- Provides a medium for the transport and exchange of nutrients and other substances such as oxygen, carbon dioxide, and metabolic wastes to and from cells.
- Provides a medium for metabolic reactions within cells.
- Assists in regulating body temperature through the evaporation of perspiration.
- Provides form for body structure and acts as a shock absorber.
- Provides insulation.
- Acts as a lubricant.

Total body water constitutes about 60% of the total body weight, but this amount varies with age, gender, and the amount of body fat. Total body water decreases with aging; in people over age 65, body water may decrease to 45% to 50% of total body weight. Fat cells contain comparatively little water: In the

TABLE 10–1 Balanced Fluid Gain and Loss for an Adult

	SOURCE	AMOUNT (mL)
Gain	Fluids taken orally	1200
	Water in food	1000
	Water as by-product of food metabolism	300
		↓
	Total	2500
		↑
Loss	Urine	1500
	Feces	200
	Perspiration	300
	Respiration	500

person who is obese, the proportion of water to total body weight is less than in the person of average weight; in a person who is very thin, the proportion of water to total body weight is greater than in the person of average weight. Adult females have a greater ratio of fat to lean tissue mass than adult males; therefore, they have a lower percentage of body water content.

To maintain normal fluid balance, body water intake and output should be approximately equal. The average fluid intake and output usually is about 2500 mL over a 24-hour period. Food and fluids consumed provide the majority of water gain; carbohydrate metabolism and other metabolic processes produce an additional small amount.

Urine production and excretion account for most water loss. The average daily urine output is 1500 mL in adults. At least 400 mL of highly concentrated urine per day is required to excrete metabolic wastes produced by the body. *Insensible* water loss (which normally cannot be measured) occurs through the skin, lungs, and feces. These losses, while normally small, can increase significantly during exercise, when environmental temperatures are high, and during illness that increases the respiratory rate, perspiration, or gastrointestinal (GI) losses (particularly diarrhea). Table 10–1 shows the sources of fluid gain and loss.

Electrolytes

Body fluids contain both water molecules and chemical compounds. These chemical compounds can either remain intact in solution or separate (dissociate) into discrete particles. **Electrolytes** are substances that dissociate in solution to form charged particles called ions. *Cations* are positively charged electrolytes; *anions* are negatively charged electrolytes. For example, sodium chloride (NaCl) in solution dissociates into a sodium ion, a cation carrying a positive charge (Na^+); and a chloride ion, an anion carrying a negative charge (Cl^-). Electrolytes may be *univalent,* with only one unit of electrical charge, such as sodium (Na^+) and chloride (Cl^-); or they may be *divalent,* carrying two units of electrical charge, such as magnesium (Mg^{2+}) and phosphate (HPO_4^{2-}).

Electrolytes have many functions. They:
- Assist in regulating water balance.
- Help regulate and maintain acid–base balance.
- Contribute to enzyme reactions.
- Are essential for neuromuscular activity.

The concentration of electrolytes in body fluids generally is measured in milliequivalents per liter of water (mEq/L). A *milliequivalent* is a measure of the chemical combining power of the ion. For example, 100 mEq of sodium (Na^+) can combine with 100 mEq of chloride (Cl^-) to form sodium chloride (NaCl). Sodium, potassium, and chloride usually are measured in milliequivalents. In some cases, the amount of an electrolyte in body fluid may be measured by weight in milligrams per 100 mL (1 deciliter [dL]) of water (mg/dL). Calcium, magnesium, and phosphorus often are measured by weight in milligrams per deciliter. Other laboratories use the International System of Measurements, or SI units.

Body Fluid Distribution

Body fluid is classified by its location inside or outside of cells. *Intracellular fluid* (ICF) is found within cells. It accounts for approximately 40% of total body weight (Figure 10–1 ■). ICF is essential for normal cell function, providing a medium for metabolic processes. *Extracellular fluid* (ECF) is located outside of cells. It accounts for approximately 20% of the total body weight. ECF is classified by location:
- Interstitial fluid is located in the spaces between most of the cells of the body. It accounts for approximately 15% of total body weight.
- Intravascular fluid, called *plasma*, is contained within the arteries, veins, and capillaries. It accounts for approximately 5% of total body weight.

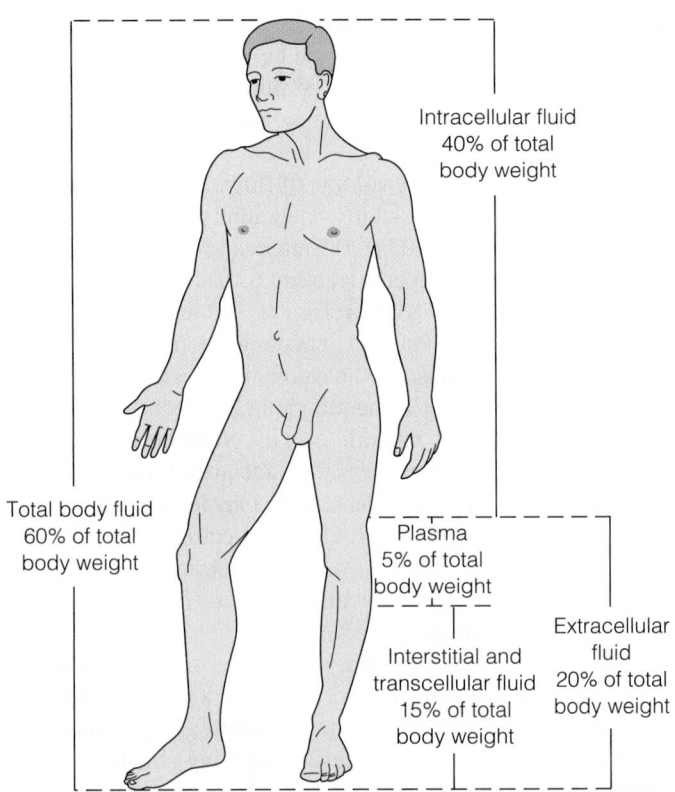

Intracellular fluid 40% of total body weight

Total body fluid 60% of total body weight

Plasma 5% of total body weight

Interstitial and transcellular fluid 15% of total body weight

Extracellular fluid 20% of total body weight

Figure 10–1 ■ The major fluid compartments of the body.

- Transcellular fluid includes urine; digestive secretions; perspiration; and cerebrospinal, pleural, synovial, intraocular, gonadal, and pericardial fluids.

A trace amount of water is found in bone, cartilage, and other dense connective tissues; this water is not exchangeable with other body fluids.

ECF is the transport medium that carries oxygen and nutrients to and waste products from the cells. For example, plasma transports oxygen from the lungs and glucose from the digestive system to the tissues. These solutes diffuse through the capillary wall into the interstitial space, and from there across the cell membrane into the cells. Waste products of metabolism (e.g., carbon dioxide and hydrogen ion) diffuse from the intracellular space into the interstitial space, and from there into plasma via the capillary walls. Plasma then transports these waste products to the lungs and kidneys for elimination.

Although the overall concentration of solutes in ICF and ECF is nearly identical, the concentration of specific electrolytes differs significantly between these compartments, as shown in Figure 10–2 ■. ICF contains high concentrations of potassium (K^+), magnesium (Mg^{2+}), and phosphate (PO_4^{2-}), as well as other solutes such as glucose and oxygen. Sodium (Na^+), chloride (Cl^-), and bicarbonate (HCO_3^-) are the principal extracellular electrolytes. The high sodium concentration in ECF is essential to regulating body fluid volume. The concentration of potassium in ECF is low. There is a minimal difference in electrolyte concentration between plasma and interstitial fluid. Normal values for electrolytes in plasma are shown in Table 10–2.

The body fluid compartments are separated by several types of membranes:

- Cell membranes separate interstitial fluid from intracellular fluid.
- Capillary membranes separate plasma from interstitial fluid.
- Epithelial membranes separate transcellular fluid from interstitial fluid and plasma. These membranes include the mucosa of the stomach, intestines, and gallbladder; the pleural, peritoneal, and synovial membranes; and the tubules of the kidney.

A cell membrane consists of layers of lipid and protein molecules. The layering of these molecules controls the passage of fluid and solutes between the cell and interstitial fluid. The cell membrane is selectively permeable; that is, it allows the passage of water, oxygen, carbon dioxide, and small water-soluble molecules, but bars proteins and other intracellular colloids.

The capillary membrane separating the plasma from the interstitial space is made of squamous epithelial cells. Pores in the membrane allow solute molecules (such as glucose and sodium), dissolved gases, and water to cross the membrane. Minute amounts of albumin and other proteins can also pass through the pores of a capillary membrane, but normally plasma proteins stay in the intravascular compartment.

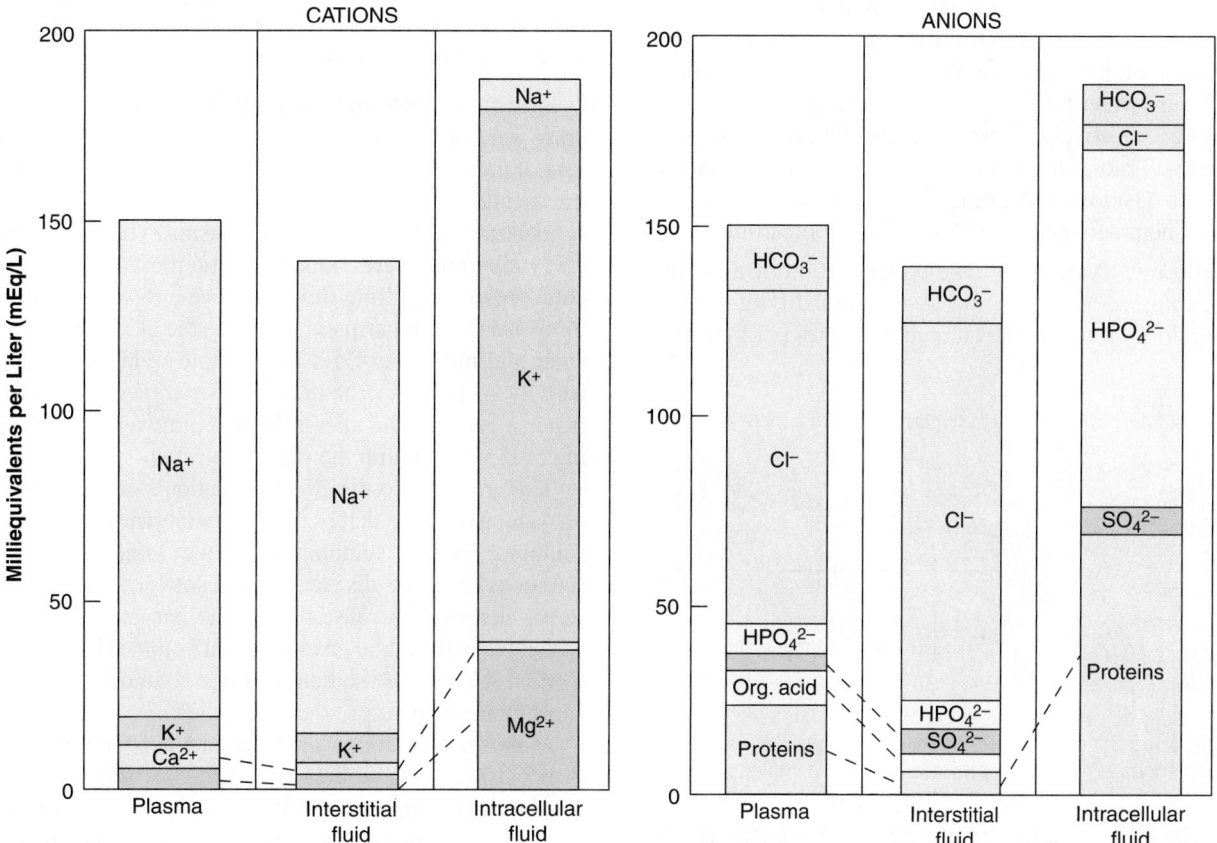

Figure 10–2 ■ Electrolyte composition (cations and anions) of body fluid compartments.

TABLE 10–2 Normal Values for Electrolytes and Serum Osmolality

SERUM COMPONENT	VALUES	
	CONVENTIONAL	SI
Electrolytes		
Sodium (Na^+)	135–145 mEq/L	135–145 mmol/L
Chloride (Cl^-)	98–106 mEq/L	98–106 mmol/L
Bicarbonate (HCO_3^-)	22–26 mEq/L	22–26 mmol/L
Calcium (Ca^{2+}) (total)	8.5–10 mg/dL	2.1–2.6 mmol/L
Potassium (K^+)	3.5–5.0 mEq/L	3.5–5.0 mmol/L
Phosphate/inorganic phosphorus (PO_4^{-2})	1.7–2.6 mEq/L (2.5–4.5 mg/dL)	0.8–1.5 mmol/L
Magnesium (Mg^{2+})	1.6–2.6 mg/dL (1.3–2.1 mEq/L)	0.8–1.3 mmol/L
Serum osmolality	275–295 mOsm/kg	275–295 mmol/kg

Body Fluid Movement

Four chemical and physiologic processes control the movement of fluid, electrolytes, and other molecules across membranes between the intracellular and interstitial space and the interstitial space and plasma. These processes are osmosis, diffusion, filtration, and active transport.

OSMOSIS The process by which water moves across a selectively permeable membrane from an area of lower solute concentration to an area of higher solute concentration is **osmosis** (Figure 10–3 ■). A *selectively permeable membrane* allows water molecules to cross but is relatively impermeable to dissolved substances (*solutes*). Osmosis continues until the solute concentration on both sides of the membrane is equal. For example, if pure water and a sodium chloride solution are separated by a selectively permeable membrane, then water molecules will move across the membrane to the sodium chloride solution. Osmosis is the primary process that controls body fluid movement between the ICF and ECF compartments.

Osmolarity and Osmolality The concentration of a solution may be expressed as the osmolarity or osmolality of the solution. *Osmolarity* refers to the amount of solutes per liter of solution (by volume); it is reported in milliosmoles per liter (mOsm/L) in a solution. *Osmolality* refers to the number of solutes per kilogram of water (by weight); it is reported in milliosmoles per kilogram (mOsm/kg). Because osmotic activity in the body is regulated by the number of active particles (solutes) per kilogram of water, osmolality is used to describe the concentration of body fluids. The normal osmolality of both ICF and ECF ranges between 275 and 295 mOsm/kg. The osmolality of the ECF depends chiefly on sodium concentration. Serum osmolality may be estimated by doubling the serum sodium concentration (approximately 142 mEq/L). Glucose and urea contribute to the osmolality of ECF, although to a lesser extent than sodium.

Osmotic Pressure and Tonicity The power of a solution to draw water across a membrane is known as the *osmotic pressure* of the solution. The composition of interstitial fluid and intravascular plasma is essentially the same except for a higher concentration of proteins in the plasma. These proteins (especially albumin) exert colloid osmotic pressure (also called oncotic pressure), pulling fluid from the interstitial space into the intravascular compartment. Because the osmolality of intravascular and interstitial fluid is essentially identical, the osmotic activity of plasma proteins is important in maintaining fluid balance between the interstitial and intravascular spaces, helping hold water within the vascular system.

Tonicity refers to the effect a solution's osmotic pressure has on water movement across the cell membrane of cells within that solution. *Isotonic* solutions have the same concentration of solutes as plasma. Cells placed in an isotonic solution will neither shrink nor swell because there is no net gain or loss of water within the cell, and no change in cell volume (Figure 10–4A ■). Normal saline (0.9% sodium chloride solution) is an example of an isotonic solution.

Hypertonic solutions have a greater concentration of solutes than plasma. In their presence, water is drawn out of a cell, causing it to shrink (Figure 10–4B). A 3% sodium chloride solution is hypertonic. *Hypotonic* solutions (such as 0.45% sodium chloride) have a lower solute concentration than plasma (Figure 10–4C). When red blood cells are placed in a

Higher solute concentration   Lower solute concentration

H_2O

H_2O

H_2O

Dissolved substances

Selectively permeable membrane

Water molecules

Figure 10–3 ■ Osmosis. Water molecules move through a selectively permeable membrane from an area of low solute concentration to an area of high solute concentration.

A Isotonic solution

B Hypertonic solution

C Hypotonic solution

Figure 10–4 ■ The effect of tonicity on red blood cells. *A,* In an isotonic solution, RBCs neither gain nor lose water, retaining their normal biconcave shape. *B,* In a hypertonic solution, cells lose water and shrink in size. *C,* In a hypotonic solution, cells absorb water and may burst (hemolysis).

hypotonic solution, water moves into the cells, causing them to swell and rupture (*hemolyze*).

The concepts of osmotic draw and tonicity are important in understanding the pathophysiologic changes that occur with fluid and electrolyte imbalances, as well as treatment measures. For example, an increased sodium concentration of extracellular fluid pulls water from the ICF compartment into the ECF compartment, causing cells to shrink. In this case, administer-

ing a hypotonic intravenous solution to reduce the sodium concentration and osmolality of ECF will facilitate water movement back into the cells.

DIFFUSION The process by which solute molecules move from an area of high solute concentration to an area of low solute concentration to become evenly distributed is **diffusion** (Figure 10–5 ■). The two types of diffusion are simple and facilitated diffusion. *Simple diffusion* occurs by the random

Higher solute concentration   Lower solute concentration

Dissolved
substance

Semipermeable
membrane

Figure 10–5 ■ Diffusion. Solute molecules move through a semipermeable membrane from an area of high solute concentration to an area of low solute concentration.

movement of particles through a solution. Water, carbon dioxide, oxygen, and solutes move between plasma and the interstitial space by simple diffusion through the capillary membrane. Water and solutes move into the cell by passing through protein channels or by dissolving in the lipid cell membrane. *Facilitated diffusion*, also called carrier-mediated diffusion, allows large water-soluble molecules, such as glucose and amino acids, to diffuse across cell membranes. Proteins embedded in the cell membrane function as *carriers*, helping large molecules cross the membrane.

The rate of diffusion is influenced by a number of factors, such as the concentration of solute and the availability of carrier proteins in the cell membrane. The effect of both simple and facilitated diffusion is to establish equal concentrations of the molecules on both sides of a membrane.

FILTRATION The process by which water and dissolved substances (solutes) move from an area of high hydrostatic pressure to an area of low hydrostatic pressure is **filtration**. This usually occurs across capillary membranes. *Hydrostatic pressure* is created by the pumping action of the heart and gravity against the capillary wall. Filtration occurs in the glomerulus of the kidneys, as well as at the arterial end of capillaries.

A balance of hydrostatic (filtration) pressure and osmotic pressure regulates the movement of water between the intravascular and interstitial spaces in the capillary beds of the body. Hydrostatic pressure within the arterial end of the capillary pushes water into the interstitial space. Hydrostatic pressure within the interstitial space opposes this movement to some degree. At the venous end of the capillary, the osmotic force of plasma proteins draws fluid back into the capillary (Figure 10–6 ■).

ACTIVE TRANSPORT **Active transport** allows molecules to move across cell membranes and epithelial membranes against a concentration gradient. This movement requires energy (adenosine triphosphate, or ATP) and a carrier mechanism to maintain a higher concentration of a substance on one side of the membrane than on the other. The sodium-potassium pump is an important example of active transport (Figure 10–7 ■). High concentrations of potassium in intracellular fluids and of sodium in extracellular fluids are maintained because cells actively transport potassium from interstitial fluid (where the concentration of potassium is about 5 mEq/L) into intracellular fluid (where the potassium concentration is about 150 mEq/L).

Body Fluid Regulation

Homeostasis requires several regulatory mechanisms and processes to maintain the balance between fluid intake and excretion. These include thirst, the kidneys, the renin–angiotensin–aldosterone mechanism, antidiuretic hormone, and atrial natriuretic peptide. These mechanisms affect the volume, distribution, and composition of body fluids.

Thirst

Thirst is the primary regulator of water intake. Thirst plays an important role in maintaining fluid balance and preventing dehydration. The thirst center, located in the brain, is stimulated when the blood volume drops because of water losses or when serum osmolality (solute concentration) increases (Figure 10–8 ■).

The thirst mechanism is highly effective in regulating extracellular sodium levels. Increased sodium in ECF increases

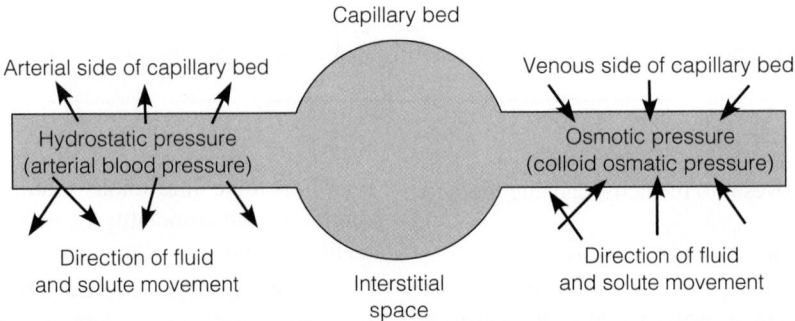

Capillary bed

Arterial side of capillary bed

Venous side of capillary bed

Hydrostatic pressure
(arterial blood pressure)

Osmotic pressure
(colloid osmatic pressure)

Direction of fluid
and solute movement

Direction of fluid
and solute movement

Interstitial
space

Figure 10–6 ■ Fluid balance between the intravascular and interstitial spaces is maintained in the capillary beds by a balance of filtration at the arterial end and osmotic draw at the venous end.

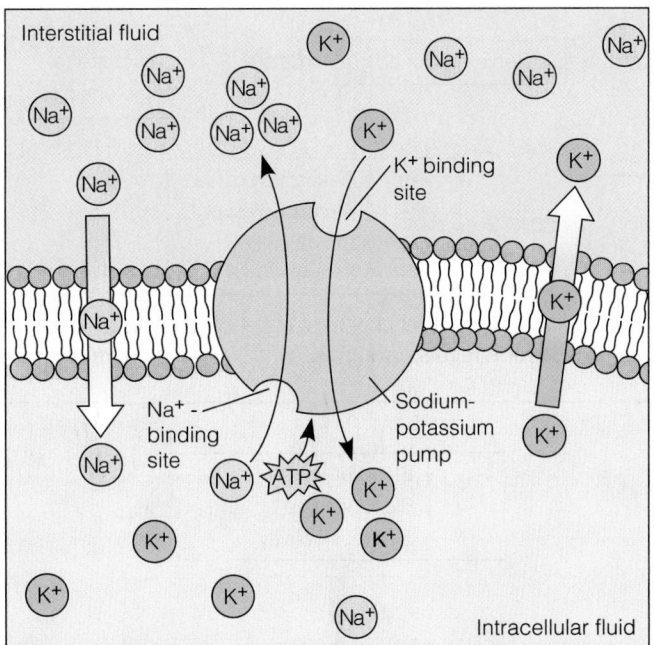

Figure 10–7 ■ The sodium-potassium pump. Sodium and potassium ions are moved across the cell membranes against their concentration gradients. This active transport process is fueled by energy from ATP.

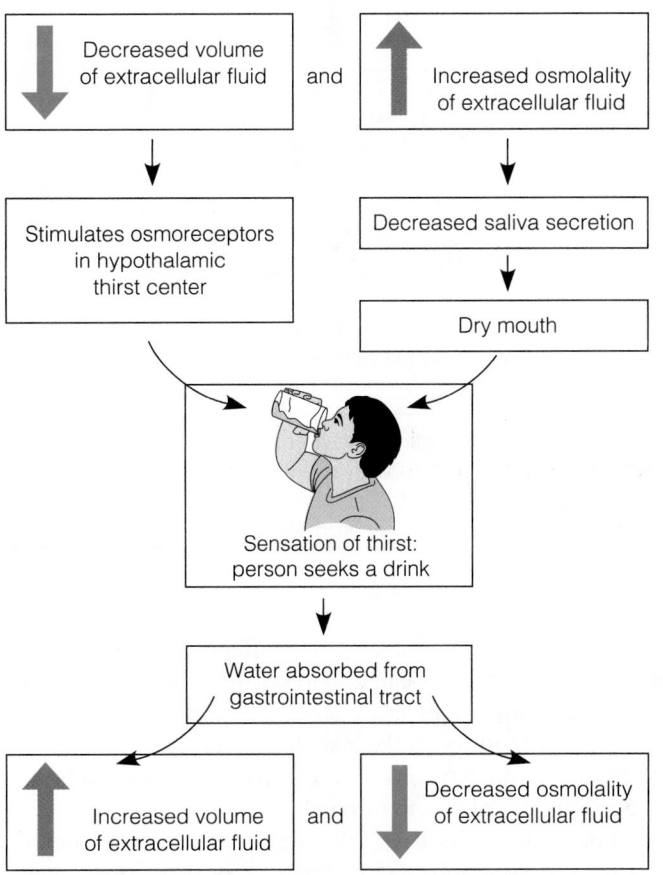

Figure 10–8 ■ Factors stimulating water intake through the thirst mechanism.

serum osmolality, stimulating the thirst center. Fluid intake in turn reduces the sodium concentration of ECF and lowers serum osmolality. Conversely, a drop in serum sodium and low serum osmolality inhibit the thirst center.

PRACTICE ALERT
The thirst mechanism declines with aging, making older adults more vulnerable to dehydration and hyperosmolality (high serum osmolality). Clients with an altered level of consciousness or who are unable to respond to thirst also are at risk.

Kidneys
The kidneys are primarily responsible for regulating fluid volume and electrolyte balance in the body. They regulate the volume and osmolality of body fluids by controlling the excretion of water and electrolytes. In adults, about 170 L of plasma are filtered through the glomeruli every day. By selectively reabsorbing water and electrolytes, the kidneys maintain the volume and osmolality of body fluids. About 99% of the glomerular filtrate is reabsorbed, and only about 1500 mL of urine is produced over a 24-hour period.

Renin–Angiotensin–Aldosterone System
The renin–angiotensin–aldosterone system works to maintain intravascular fluid balance and blood pressure. A decrease in blood flow or blood pressure to the kidneys stimulates specialized receptors in the juxtaglomerular cells of the nephrons to produce *renin*, an enzyme. Renin converts angiotensinogen (a plasma protein) in the circulating blood into angiotensin I. Angiotensin I travels through the bloodstream to the lungs, where it is converted to angiotensin II by angiotensin-converting enzyme (ACE). Angiotensin II is a potent vasoconstrictor; it raises the blood pressure. It also stimulates the thirst mechanism to promote fluid intake and acts directly on the kidneys, causing them to retain sodium and water. Angiotensin II stimulates the adrenal cortex to release aldosterone. Aldosterone promotes sodium and water retention in the distal nephron of the kidney, restoring blood volume (Figure 10–9 ■).

Antidiuretic Hormone
Antidiuretic hormone (ADH), released by the posterior pituitary gland, regulates water excretion from the kidneys. Osmoreceptors in the hypothalamus respond to increases in serum osmolality and decreases in blood volume, stimulating ADH production and release. ADH acts on the distal tubules of the kidney, making them more permeable to water and thus increasing water reabsorption. With increased water reabsorption, urine output falls, blood volume is restored, and serum osmolality drops as the water dilutes body fluids (Figure 10–10 ■).

In addition to decreased blood volume and increased serum osmolality, increased amounts of ADH are released in response to stress, pain, surgery and anesthesia, some medications such as morphine and barbiturates, and mechanical ventilation. Its release is inhibited by ethanol, medications such as phenytoin, as well as increased circulating blood volume and decreased serum osmolality (Suhayda & Walton, 2002).

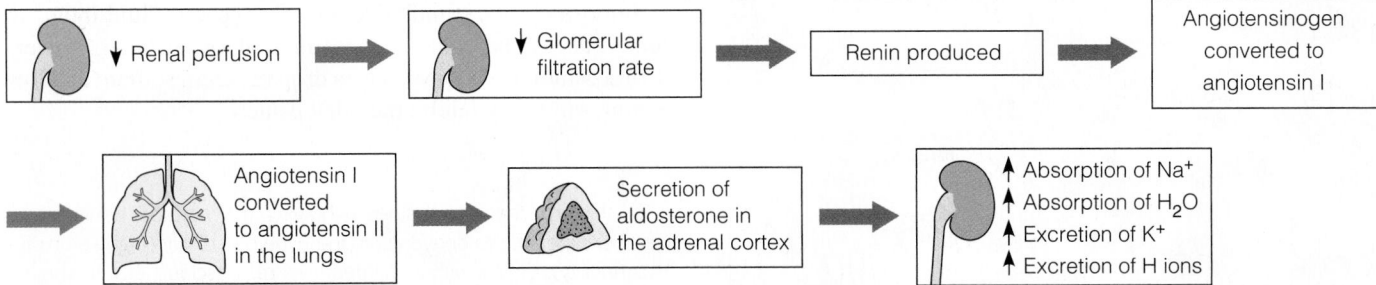

Figure 10–9 ■ The renin–angiotensin–aldosterone system. Decreased blood volume and renal perfusion set off a chain of reactions, leading to release of aldosterone from the adrenal cortex. Increased levels of aldosterone regulate serum K^+ and Na^+, blood pressure, and water balance through effects on the kidney tubules.

Two disorders of ADH production illustrate the effect of ADH on water balance and urine output. First, diabetes insipidus is a condition characterized by deficient ADH production. The lack of ADH causes the distal tubules and collecting ducts of the kidney to be impermeable to water, so little water is reabsorbed into the bloodstream. As a result, copious, very dilute urine is excreted. Water loss leads to increased concentration of the plasma, or increased serum osmolality. ADH is not released in response to the serum hyperosmolality, but the thirst mechanism is stimulated and the client drinks additional fluids, maintaining high urine output. In the other condition, the syndrome of inappropriate ADH secretion (SIADH), excess ADH is released. Increased water reabsorption causes increased fluid volume and scant, concentrated urine output. These diseases of the pituitary gland are discussed in Chapter 19 ∞.

Atrial Natriuretic Peptide

Atrial natriuretic peptide (ANP) is a hormone released by atrial muscle cells in response to distention from fluid overload. ANP affects several body systems, including the cardiovascular, renal, neural, gastrointestinal, and endocrine systems, but it primarily affects the renin–angiotensin–aldosterone system. ANP opposes this system by inhibiting renin secretion and blocking the secretion and sodium-retaining effects of aldosterone. As a result, ANP promotes sodium wasting and diuresis (increased urine output) and causes vasodilation.

CHANGES IN THE OLDER ADULT

A number of changes commonly occurring with aging affect homeostasis. In older adults, the percentage of total body water is lower than in younger or middle age adults. Lean muscle mass is lower in older adults, and the percentage of body fat is higher; as a result water accounts for about 50% of the total body weight (TBW) of an older man and about 45% TBW of an older woman. Sodium and water regulation become less efficient with aging. Renal blood flow and glomerular filtration decline with aging; consequently, the kidneys are less able to effectively concentrate the urine and conserve sodium and water. The perception of thirst decreases, interfering with the thirst mechanism. Consequently, the older adult may become dehydrated without being aware of the need to increase fluid intake. Aging affects temperature regulation as well.

Figure 10–10 ■ Antidiuretic hormone (ADH) release and effect. Increased serum osmolality or a fall in blood volume stimulates the release of ADH from the posterior pituitary. ADH increases the permeability of distal tubules, promoting water reabsorption.

Functional changes of aging also affect fluid balance:
- Fear of incontinence can lead to self-limiting of fluid intake.
- Physical disabilities associated with age-related illnesses, such as arthritis or stroke, may limit access to fluids.
- Cognitive impairments can interfere with recognition of thirst and the ability to respond to it.

Older adults who have self-care deficits, or who are confused, depressed, tube fed, on bed rest, or taking medications (such as sedatives, tranquilizers, diuretics, and laxatives) are at greatest risk for fluid volume imbalance. Older adults without air conditioning are at risk during extremely hot weather.

FLUID AND ELECTROLYTE IMBALANCES

FLUID IMBALANCE
The Client with Fluid Volume Deficit

Fluid volume deficit (FVD) is a decrease in intravascular, interstitial, and/or intracellular fluid in the body. Fluid volume deficits may be due to excessive fluid losses, insufficient fluid intake, or failure of regulatory mechanisms and fluid shifts within the body. FVD is a relatively common problem that may exist alone or in combination with other electrolyte or acid–base imbalances. The term **dehydration** refers to loss of water alone, even though it often is used interchangeably with fluid volume deficit.

FAST FACTS

- Water loss of as little as 1–2% impairs cognition and physical performance
- Loss of 7% of body water can lead to circulatory collapse
- Dehydration is one of the ten most common hospital admitting diagnoses for older adults (Suhayda & Walton, 2002)

Pathophysiology

The most common cause of fluid volume deficit is excessive loss of gastrointestinal fluids from vomiting, diarrhea, gastrointestinal suctioning, intestinal fistulas, and intestinal drainage. Other causes of fluid losses include:

- Excessive renal losses of water and sodium from diuretic therapy, renal disorders, or endocrine disorders
- Water and sodium losses during sweating from excessive exercise or increased environmental temperature
- Hemorrhage
- Chronic abuse of laxatives and/or enemas.

Inadequate fluid intake may result from lack of access to fluids, inability to request or to swallow fluids, oral trauma, or altered thirst mechanisms. Older adults are at particular risk for fluid volume deficit (see Nursing Care of the Older Adult box on this page).

Fluid volume deficit can develop slowly or rapidly, depending on the type of fluid loss. Loss of extracellular fluid volume can lead to *hypovolemia,* decreased circulating blood volume. Electrolytes often are lost along with fluid, resulting in an *isotonic fluid volume deficit.* When both water and electrolytes are lost, the serum sodium level remains normal, although levels of other electrolytes such as potassium may fall. Fluid is drawn into the vascular compartment from the interstitial spaces as the body attempts to maintain tissue perfusion. This eventually depletes fluid in the intracellular compartment as well.

Hypovolemia stimulates regulatory mechanisms to maintain circulation. The sympathetic nervous system is stimulated, as is the thirst mechanism. ADH and aldosterone are released, prompting sodium and water retention by the kidneys. Severe fluid loss can lead to cardiovascular collapse.

Two other types of fluid volume deficit, hypovolemic fluid volume deficit and hypertonic fluid volume deficit, are discussed as effects of sodium imbalance in that section of this chapter.

NURSING CARE OF THE OLDER ADULT
Fluid Volume Deficit

Fluid volume deficit, or dehydration, is a common reason for hospitalization of people over age 65 who live either in the community or in a long-term care setting. Older adults have a significant number of risk factors for fluid volume deficit (see the preceding section of this chapter). In addition, the older adult has fewer intracellular reserves, contributing to rapid development of dehydration. Without intervention, mortality from dehydration can exceed 50% in the older adult population (Suhayda & Walton, 2002).

Manifestations of fluid volume deficit may be more difficult to recognize in the older adult. A change in mental status, memory, or attention may be an early sign. Skin turgor is less reliable as an indicator of dehydration, although assessing turgor over the sternum or on the inner aspect of the thigh may be more effective. Dry oral mucous membranes and tongue furrows also are indicative of dehydration. Orthostatic vital signs may not demonstrate typical changes in the dehydrated older adult.

THIRD SPACING **Third spacing** is a shift of fluid from the vascular space into an area where it is not available to support normal physiologic processes. The trapped fluid represents a volume loss and is unavailable for normal physiologic processes. Fluid may be sequestered in the abdomen or bowel, or in such other actual or potential body spaces as the pleural or peritoneal space. Fluid may also become trapped within soft tissues following trauma or burns.

In many cases, fluid is sequestered in interstitial tissues and thus unavailable to support cardiovascular function. Surgery triggers adaptive stress responses and the release of stress hormones (ACTH, cortisol, and catecholamines). These hormones increase blood glucose levels to provide increased fuel for metabolic processes and lead to vasoconstriction that redistributes blood to vital organs (the heart and brain). Renal blood flow falls, stimulating the renin–angiotensin–aldosterone system. This promotes sodium and water retention to maintain intravascular volume. The blood vessel and tissue damage caused by surgery stimulate the release of inflammatory mediators such as histamine and prostaglandins. These substances lead to local vasodilation and increased capillary permeability, allowing fluid to accumulate in interstitial tissues.

Assessing the extent of FVD resulting from third spacing is difficult. It may not be reflected by changes in weight or intake-and-output records, and it may not become apparent until after organ malfunction occurs (Metheny, 2000).

Manifestations

With a rapid fluid loss (such as hemorrhage or uncontrolled vomiting), manifestations of hypovolemia develop rapidly. When the loss of fluid occurs more gradually, the client's fluid volume may be very low before symptoms develop. The *Multisystem Effects of Fluid Volume Deficit* are illustrated on the following page.

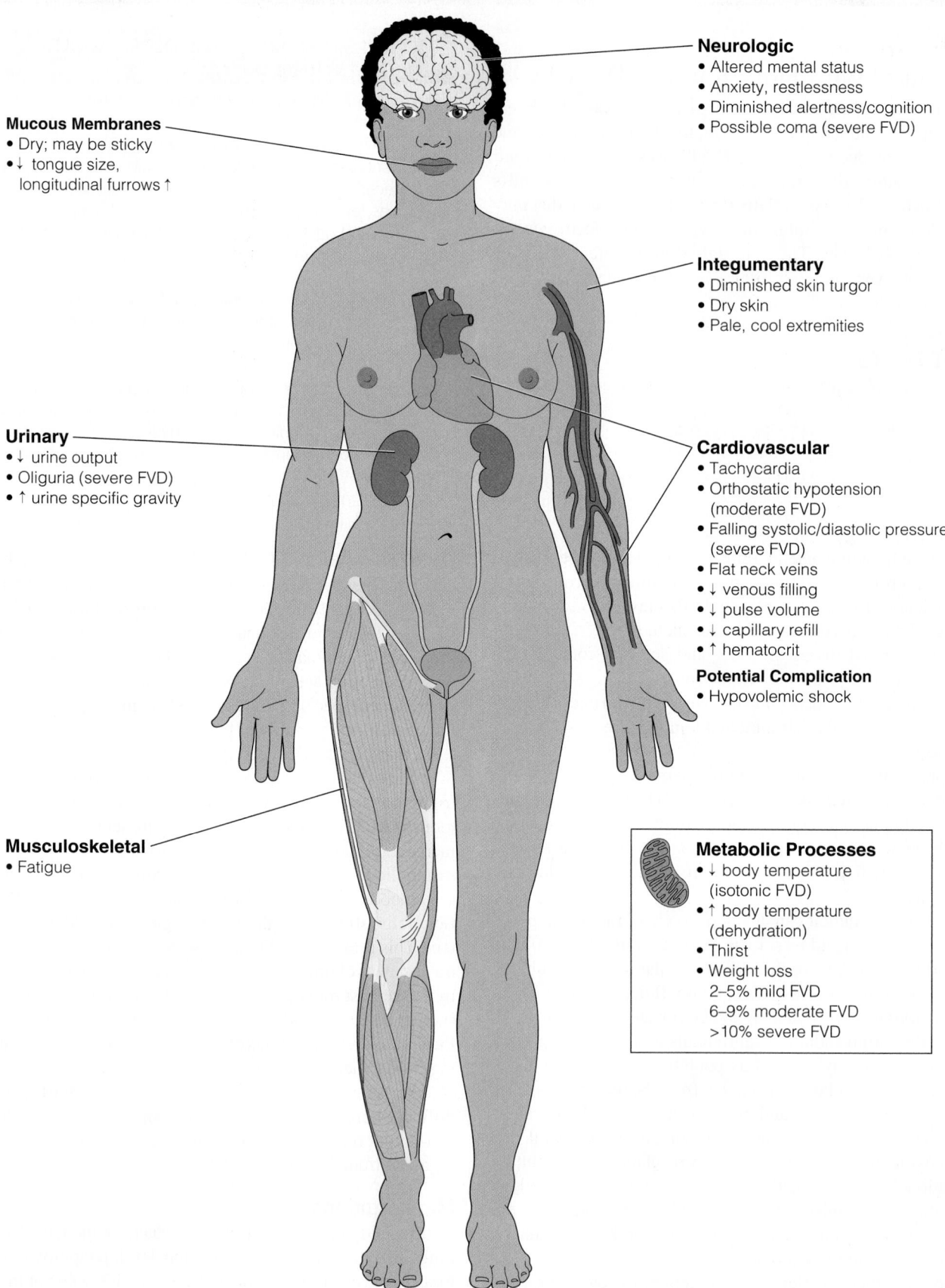

Neurologic
- Altered mental status
- Anxiety, restlessness
- Diminished alertness/cognition
- Possible coma (severe FVD)

Mucous Membranes
- Dry; may be sticky
- ↓ tongue size, longitudinal furrows ↑

Integumentary
- Diminished skin turgor
- Dry skin
- Pale, cool extremities

Urinary
- ↓ urine output
- Oliguria (severe FVD)
- ↑ urine specific gravity

Cardiovascular
- Tachycardia
- Orthostatic hypotension (moderate FVD)
- Falling systolic/diastolic pressure (severe FVD)
- Flat neck veins
- ↓ venous filling
- ↓ pulse volume
- ↓ capillary refill
- ↑ hematocrit

Potential Complication
- Hypovolemic shock

Musculoskeletal
- Fatigue

Metabolic Processes
- ↓ body temperature (isotonic FVD)
- ↑ body temperature (dehydration)
- Thirst
- Weight loss
  2–5% mild FVD
  6–9% moderate FVD
  >10% severe FVD

Rapid weight loss is a good indicator of fluid volume deficit. Each liter of body fluid weighs about 1 kg (2.2 lb). The severity of the fluid volume deficit can be estimated by the percentage of rapid weight loss: a loss of 2% to 5% of total body weight represents a mild FVD; 6% to 9%, moderate FVD; and 10% or greater, severe FVD.

Loss of interstitial fluid causes skin turgor to diminish. When pinched, the skin of a client with FVD remains elevated. Loss of skin elasticity with aging makes this assessment finding less accurate in older adults. Tongue turgor is not generally affected by age; therefore, assessing the size, dryness, and longitudinal furrows of the tongue may be a more accurate indicator of FVD.

Postural or orthostatic hypotension is a sign of hypovolemia. A drop of more than 15 mmHg in systolic blood pressure when changing from a lying to standing position often indicates loss of intravascular volume. Venous pressure falls as well, causing flat neck veins, even when the client is recumbent. Loss of intravascular fluid causes the hematocrit to increase.

Compensatory mechanisms to conserve water and sodium and maintain circulation account for many of the manifestations of fluid volume deficit, such as tachycardia; pale, cool skin (vasoconstriction); and decreased urine output. The specific gravity of urine increases as water is reabsorbed in the tubules. Table 10–3 compares assessment findings for fluid deficit and fluid excess.

INTERDISCIPLINARY CARE

The primary goals of care related to fluid volume deficit are to prevent deficits in clients at risk and to correct deficits and their underlying causes. Depending on the acuity of the imbalance, treatment may include replacement of fluids and electrolytes by the intravenous, oral, or enteral route. When possible, the oral or enteral route is preferred for administering fluids. In acute situations, however, intravenous fluid administration is necessary.

TABLE 10–3 Comparison of Assessment Findings in Clients with Fluid Imbalance

ASSESSMENT	FLUID DEFICIT	FLUID EXCESS
Blood pressure	Decreased systolic Postural hypotension	Increased
Heart rate	Increased	Increased
Pulse amplitude	Decreased	Increased
Respirations	Normal	Moist crackles Wheezes
Jugular vein	Flat	Distended
Edema	Rare	Dependent
Skin turgor	Loose, poor turgor	Taut
Output	Low, concentrated	May be low or normal
Urine specific gravity	High	Low
Weight	Loss	Gain

Diagnosis

Laboratory and diagnostic tests may be ordered when fluid volume deficit is suspected. Such tests measure:

- *Serum electrolytes.* In an isotonic fluid deficit, sodium levels are within normal limits; when the loss is water only, sodium levels are high. Decreases in potassium are common.
- *Serum osmolality.* Measurement of serum osmolality helps to differentiate isotonic fluid loss from water loss. With water loss, osmolality is high; it may be within normal limits with an isotonic fluid loss.
- *Hemoglobin and hematocrit.* The hematocrit often is elevated due to loss of intravascular volume and hemoconcentration.
- *Urine specific gravity and osmolality.* As the kidneys conserve water, both the specific gravity and osmolality of urine increase.
- *Central venous pressure (CVP).* The CVP measures the mean pressure in the superior vena cava or right atrium, providing an accurate assessment of fluid volume status. The technique for measuring CVP is outlined in Box 10–1.

Fluid Management

Oral rehydration is the safest and most effective treatment for fluid volume deficit in alert clients who are able to take oral fluids. Adults require a minimum of 1500 mL of fluid per day or approximately 30 mL per kg of body weight (ideal body weight is used to calculate fluid requirements for obese clients) for maintenance. Fluids are replaced gradually, particularly in older adults, to prevent rapid rehydration of the cells. In general, fluid deficits are replaced at a rate of approximately 30% to 50% of the deficit per 24 hours.

For mild fluid deficits in which the loss of electrolytes has been minimal (e.g., moderate exercise in warm weather), water alone may be used for fluid replacement. When the fluid deficit is more severe and when electrolytes have also been lost (e.g., FVD due to vomiting and/or diarrhea, strenuous exercise for longer than an hour or two), a carbohydrate/electrolyte solution such as a sports drink, ginger ale, or a rehydrating solution (e.g., Pedialyte or Rehydralyte) is more appropriate. These solutions provide sodium, potassium, chloride, and calories to help meet metabolic needs.

INTRAVENOUS THERAPY When the fluid deficit is severe or the client is unable to ingest fluids, the intravenous route is used to administer replacement fluids. Table 10–4 describes the types, tonicity, and uses of commonly administered intravenous fluids. Isotonic electrolyte solutions (0.9% NaCl or Ringer's solution) are used to expand plasma volume in hypotensive clients or to replace abnormal losses, which are usually isotonic in nature. Normal saline (0.9% NaCl) tends to remain in the vascular compartment, increasing blood volume. When administered rapidly, however, this solution can precipitate acid–base imbalances, so balanced electrolyte solutions such as lactated Ringer's solution are preferred to expand plasma volume.

Five percent dextrose in water (D_5W) or 0.45% NaCl (one-half normal saline or 1/2 NS) are given to provide water to treat total body water deficits. D_5W is isotonic (similar in tonicity to the plasma) when administered and thus does not provoke hemolysis

BOX 10–1 Measuring Central Venous Pressure with a Manometer

CVP is a hemodynamic monitoring method for evaluating fluid volume status. It measures mean right atrial pressure by means of a catheter. The CVP catheter is inserted by a physician, most often at the client's bedside, into the antecubital, internal jugular, or subclavian vein. Either a hemodynamic monitoring system (see Chapter 32 ∞) or a manual system may be used to measure the CVP. Nursing responsibilities in measuring CVP are as follows:

1. Explain to the client and family what is being done.
2. Prior to the first measurement, take baseline vital signs, and measure the level of the right atrium on the client's thorax. This is usually at the fourth intercostal space on the lateral chest wall, midway between the anterior and posterior chest. This site, called the *phlebostatic axis,* is marked and used as the reference point for all measurements.
3. If possible, place the bed in the same position for each reading, usually with the client supine and the head of the bed flat. Elevating the head of the bed to as much as 60 degrees usually does not affect the accuracy of the CVP reading in clients who are hemodynamically stable (Urden et al., 2006).
4. Use a carpenter's level to check the level of the measuring device to make sure the transducer or the 0 on the manometer is level with the phlebostatic axis (see figure).
5. Remove any air bubbles in the line.
6. If using a manometer, turn the stopcock so that fluid flows into the manometer, filling it a few centimeters above the expected reading. Then turn the stopcock to open the line between the manometer and the client. The fluid level will fall and then reach a point at which it fluctuates with the client's respirations. This point is recorded as the CVP.

7. After the measurement is taken, turn the stopcock so that the fluid can again flow from the fluid source to the client.

Normal Values

When CVP is measured by a manometer, normal values range from 2 to 8 cm water. With a hemodynamic monitoring system, the normal CVP range is 2 to 5 mmHg. A low CVP indicates inadequate venous return from fluid deficit and hypovolemia or due to peripheral vasodilation. A high CVP indicates fluid overload, cardiac problems that decrease cardiac contractility, or pulmonary disorders that increase pulmonary vascular resistance.

of red blood cells. The dextrose is metabolized to carbon dioxide and water, leaving free water available for tissue needs. Hypotonic saline solution (0.45% NaCl with or without added electrolytes) or 5% dextrose in 0.45% sodium chloride (D₅ 1/2 NS) are used as maintenance solutions. These solutions provide additional electrolytes such as potassium, a buffer (lactate or acetate) as needed, and water. When dextrose is added, they also provide a minimal number of calories.

FLUID CHALLENGE A fluid challenge, the rapid administration of a designated amount of intravenous fluid, may be performed to evaluate fluid volume when urine output is low and cardiac or renal function is questionable. A fluid challenge helps prevent fluid volume overload resulting from intravenous fluid therapy when cardiac or renal function is compromised. Nursing responsibilities for a fluid challenge are as follows:

1. Obtain and document baseline vital signs, breath sounds, urine output, and mental status.
2. Administer (by IV infusion) an initial fluid volume of 200 to 300 mL over 5 to 10 minutes.
3. Reevaluate baseline data at the end of the 5- or 10-minute infusion period.
4. Administer additional fluid until a specified volume is infused or the desired hemodynamic parameters are achieved.

NURSING CARE

Nurses are responsible for identifying clients at risk for fluid volume deficit, initiating and carrying out measures to prevent and treat fluid volume deficit, and monitoring the effects of therapy.

Health Promotion

Health promotion activities focus on teaching clients to prevent fluid volume deficit. Discuss the importance of maintaining adequate fluid intake, particularly when exercising and during hot weather. Advise clients to use commercial sports drinks to replace both water and electrolytes when exercising during warm weather. Instruct clients to maintain fluid intake when ill, particularly during periods of fever or when diarrhea is a problem.

Discuss the increased risk for fluid volume deficit with older adults (see page 203) and provide information about prevention. Teach older adults (and their caretakers) that thirst decreases with aging and urge them to maintain a regular fluid intake of about 1500 mL per day, regardless of perception of thirst.

Carefully monitor clients at risk for abnormal fluid losses through routes such as vomiting, diarrhea, nasogastric suction, increased urine output, fever, or wounds. Monitor fluid intake in clients with decreased level of consciousness, disorientation, nausea and anorexia, and physical limitations.

TABLE 10–4 Commonly Administered Intravenous Fluids

	FLUID AND TONICITY	USES
Dextrose in Water Solutions	5% dextrose in water (D$_5$W) Isotonic	Replaces water losses Provides free water necessary for cellular rehydration Lowers serum sodium in hypernatremia
	10% dextrose in water (D$_{10}$W) Hypertonic	Provides free water Provides nutrition (supplies 340 kcal/L)
	20% dextrose in water (D$_{20}$W) Hypertonic	Supplies 680 kcal/L May cause diuresis
	50% dextrose in water (D$_{50}$W) Hypertonic	Supplies 1700 kcal/L Used to correct hypoglycemia
Saline Solutions	0.45% sodium chloride Hypotonic	Provides free water to replace hypotonic fluid losses Maintains levels of plasma sodium and chloride
	0.9% sodium chloride Isotonic	Expands intravascular volume Replaces water lost from extracellular fluid Used with blood transfusions Replaces large sodium losses (as from burns)
	3% sodium chloride Hypertonic	Corrects serious sodium depletion
Combined Dextrose and Saline Solution	5% dextrose and 0.45% sodium chloride Isotonic	Provides free water Provides sodium chloride Maintenance fluid of choice if there are no electrolyte imbalances
Multiple Electrolyte Solutions	Ringer's solution Isotonic (electrolyte concentrations of sodium, potassium, chloride, and calcium are similar to plasma levels)	Expands the intracellular fluid Replaces extracellular fluid losses
	Lactated Ringer's solution Isotonic (similar in composition of electrolytes to plasma but does not contain magnesium)	Replaces fluid losses from burns and the lower gastrointestinal tract Fluid of choice for acute blood loss

Assessment

Collect assessment data through the health history interview and physical examination.

- *Health history:* Risk factors such as medications, acute or chronic renal or endocrine disease; precipitating factors such as hot weather, extensive exercise, lack of access to fluids, recent illness (especially if accompanied by fever, vomiting, and/or diarrhea); onset and duration of symptoms.
- *Physical assessment:* Weight; vital signs including orthostatic blood pressure and pulse; peripheral pulses and capillary refill; jugular neck vein distention; skin color, temperature, turgor; level of consciousness and mentation; urine output. See Box 10–2 for physical assessment changes in the older adult.

BOX 10–2 Assessing Older Adults: Fluid Volume Deficit

With aging, the elasticity of skin decreases. As a result, turgor diminishes, even in the well-hydrated older adult. This makes skin turgor less reliable when assessing for fluid volume deficit. In addition, some older adults experience postural hypotension, even when well hydrated. Allow the older adult to stand quietly for a full minute before rechecking blood pressure and pulse when measuring orthostatic vital signs.

- *Diagnostic tests:* Serum osmolality and electrolytes, hemoglobin and hematocrit (expect values to fall with rehydration), urine specific gravity and osmolality, central venous pressure readings.

Nursing Diagnoses and Interventions

The focus for nursing diagnoses and interventions for the client with fluid volume deficit is on managing the effects of the deficit and preventing complications.

Deficient Fluid Volume

Clients with a fluid volume deficit due to abnormal losses, inadequate intake, or impaired fluid regulation require close monitoring as well as immediate and ongoing fluid replacement.

- Assess intake and output accurately, monitoring fluid balance. In acute situations, hourly intake and output may be indicated. *Urine output should be 30 to 60 mL per hour (unless renal failure is present). Urine output of less than 30 mL per hour indicates inadequate renal perfusion and an increased risk for acute renal failure and inadequate tissue perfusion.*

PRACTICE ALERT
Report a urine output of less than 30 mL per hour to the primary healthcare provider.

NURSING RESEARCH Evidence-Based Practice for Clients with Imbalanced Fluid Volume

Nurses caring for clients with a fluid volume imbalance frequently monitor both 24-hour intake and output records and daily weights. These measurements require caregiver time, and may be providing redundant data. Nurse managers on three nursing units compared the results of continuous 48-hour intake and output records with daily weights for a total of 73 selected clients on their units. Their findings suggest that even when compliance with recording accurate intake and output is optimal, it is an unreliable measure of actual fluid balance (Wise et al., 2000).

IMPLICATIONS FOR NURSING

A significant shortage of licensed nurses is predicted for the early part of the 21st century. Tight nursing resources will require efficient nursing practice to maintain quality care. This study suggests that for the majority of clients (the exceptions being clients with kidney disease or who are on a fluid restriction), measuring accurate daily weights is a better indicator of fluid balance than intake and output records.

CRITICAL THINKING IN CLIENT CARE

1. What factors can you identify that would affect the accuracy of intake and output records?
2. What measures can you and your institution take to ensure accurate daily weight measurements?
3. Compare intake and output records and daily weights for your assigned clients. Is the balance between intake and output accurately reflected by day-to-day weight changes? If not, what factors can you identify that might account for this discrepancy?

Source: Adapted from "Evaluating the Reliability and Utility of Cumulative Intake and Output" by L. C. Wise et al., 2000, *Journal of Nursing Care Quality, 14*(3), pp. 37–42.

- Assess vital signs, CVP, and peripheral pulse volume at least every 4 hours. *Hypotension, tachycardia, low CVP, and weak, easily obliterated peripheral pulses indicate hypovolemia.*
- Weigh daily under standard conditions (time of day, clothing, and scale). *In most instances (except third spacing), changes in weight accurately reflect fluid balance.* See the Nursing Research box on this page.
- Administer and monitor the intake of oral fluids as prescribed. Identify beverage preferences and provide these on a schedule. *Oral fluid replacement is preferred when the client is able to drink and retain fluids.*
- Administer intravenous fluids as prescribed using an electronic infusion pump. Monitor for indicators of fluid overload if rapid fluid replacement is ordered: dyspnea, tachypnea, tachycardia, increased CVP, jugular vein distention, and edema. *Rapid fluid replacement may lead to hypervolemia, resulting in pulmonary edema and cardiac failure, particularly in clients with compromised cardiac and renal function.*
- Monitor laboratory values: electrolytes, serum osmolality, blood urea nitrogen (BUN), and hematocrit. *Rehydration may lead to changes in serum electrolytes, osmolality, BUN, and hematocrit. In some cases, electrolyte replacement may be necessary during rehydration.*

Ineffective Tissue Perfusion

A fluid volume deficit can lead to decreased perfusion of renal, cerebral, and peripheral tissues. Inadequate renal perfusion can lead to acute renal failure. Decreased cerebral perfusion leads to changes in mental status and cognitive function, causing restlessness, anxiety, agitation, excitability, confusion, vertigo, fainting, and weakness.

- Monitor for changes in level of consciousness and mental status. *Restlessness, anxiety, confusion, and agitation may indicate inadequate cerebral blood flow and circulatory collapse.*
- Monitor serum creatinine, BUN, and cardiac enzymes, reporting elevated levels to the physician. *Elevated levels may indicate impaired renal function or cardiac perfusion related to circulatory failure.*

- Turn at least every 2 hours. Provide good skin care and monitor for evidence of skin or tissue breakdown. *Impaired circulation to peripheral tissues increases the risk of skin breakdown. Turn frequently to relieve pressure over bony prominences. Keep skin clean, dry, and moisturized to help maintain integrity.*

Risk for Injury

The client with fluid volume deficit is at risk for injury because of dizziness and loss of balance resulting from decreased cerebral perfusion secondary to hypovolemia.

- Institute safety precautions, including keeping the bed in a low position, using side rails as needed, and slowly raising the client from supine to sitting or sitting to standing position. *Using safety precautions and allowing time for the blood pressure to adjust to position changes reduce the risk of injury.*
- Teach client and family members how to reduce orthostatic hypotension:
  a. Move from one position to another in stages; for example, raise the head of the bed before sitting up, and sit for a few minutes before standing.
  b. Avoid prolonged standing.
  c. Rest in a recliner rather than in bed during the day.
  d. Use assistive devices to pick up objects from the floor rather than stooping.

Teaching measures to reduce orthostatic hypotension reduces the client's risk for injury. Prolonged bed rest increases skeletal muscle weakness and decreases venous tone, contributing to postural hypotension. Prolonged standing allows blood to pool in the legs, reducing venous return and cardiac output.

Using NANDA, NIC, and NOC

Chart 10–1 shows linkages between NANDA nursing diagnoses, nursing interventions classification (NIC), and nursing outcomes classification (NOC) for the client with fluid volume deficit.

Community-Based Care

Depending on the severity of the fluid volume deficit, the client may be managed in the home or residential facility, or may be

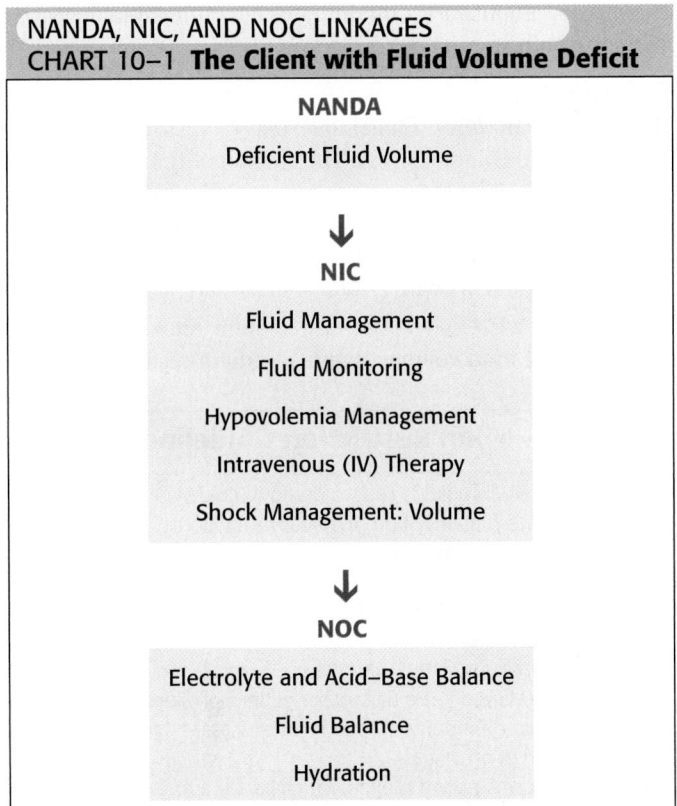

NANDA, NIC, AND NOC LINKAGES
CHART 10–1 The Client with Fluid Volume Deficit

NANDA

Deficient Fluid Volume

↓

NIC

Fluid Management

Fluid Monitoring

Hypovolemia Management

Intravenous (IV) Therapy

Shock Management: Volume

↓

NOC

Electrolyte and Acid–Base Balance

Fluid Balance

Hydration

Data from *NANDA's Nursing Diagnoses: Definitions & classification 2005–2006* by NANDA International (2003), Philadelphia; *Nursing Interventions Classification (NIC)* (4th ed.) by J. M. Dochterman & G. M. Bulechek (2004), St. Louis, MO: Mosby; and *Nursing Outcomes Classification (NOC)* (3rd ed.) by S. Moorhead, M. Johnson, and M. Maas (2004), St. Louis, MO: Mosby.

admitted to an acute care facility. Assess the client's understanding of the cause of the deficit and the fluids necessary for providing replacement. Address the following topics when preparing the client and family for home care:

- The importance of maintaining adequate fluid intake (at least 1500 mL per day; more if extra fluid is being lost through perspiration, fever, or diarrhea)
- Manifestations of fluid imbalance, and how to monitor fluid balance
- How to prevent fluid deficit:
  - Avoid exercising during extreme heat.
  - Increase fluid intake during hot weather.
  - If vomiting, take small frequent amounts of ice chips or clear liquids, such as weak tea, flat cola, or ginger ale.
  - Reduce intake of coffee, tea, and alcohol, which increase urine output and can cause fluid loss.
- Replacement of fluids lost through diarrhea with fruit juices or bouillon, rather than large amounts of tap water
- Alternate sources of fluid (such as gelatin, frozen juices, or ice cream) for effective replacement of lost fluids.

THE CLIENT WITH FLUID VOLUME EXCESS

Fluid volume excess results when both water and sodium are retained in the body. Fluid volume excess may be caused by fluid overload (excess water and sodium intake) or by impairment of the mechanisms that maintain homeostasis. The excess fluid can lead to excess intravascular fluid (hypervolemia) and excess interstitial fluid (**edema**).

Pathophysiology

Fluid volume excess usually results from conditions that cause retention of both sodium and water. These conditions include heart failure, cirrhosis of the liver, renal failure, adrenal gland disorders, corticosteroid administration, and stress conditions causing the release of ADH and aldosterone. Other causes include an excessive intake of sodium-containing foods, drugs that cause sodium retention, and the administration of excess amounts of sodium-containing intravenous fluids (such as 0.9% NaCl or Ringer's solution). This *iatrogenic* (induced by the effects of treatment) cause of fluid volume excess primarily affects clients with impaired regulatory mechanisms.

In fluid volume excess, both water and sodium are gained in about the same proportions as normally exists in extracellular fluid. The total body sodium content is increased, which in turn causes an increase in total body water. Because the increase in sodium and water is isotonic, the serum sodium and osmolality remain normal, and the excess fluid remains in the extracellular space.

Stress responses activated before, during, and immediately after surgery commonly lead to increased ADH and aldosterone levels, leading to sodium and water retention. In the immediate postoperative period, however, this additional fluid tends to be sequestered in interstitial tissues and unavailable to support cardiovascular and renal function (see earlier "Third Spacing" section in this chapter). This sequestered fluid is reabsorbed into the circulation within about 48 to 72 hours after surgery. Although it is then normally eliminated through a process of diuresis, clients with heart or kidney failure are at risk for developing fluid overload.

Manifestations and Complications

Excess extracellular fluid leads to hypervolemia and circulatory overload. Excess fluid in the interstitial space causes peripheral or generalized edema. The following manifestations of fluid volume excess relate to both the excess fluid and its effects on circulation:

- The increase in total body water causes weight gain (more than 5% of body weight) over a short period.
- Circulatory overload causes manifestations such as:
  - A full, bounding pulse
  - Distended neck and peripheral veins
  - Increased central venous pressure (>11–12 cm of water)
  - Cough, **dyspnea** (labored or difficult breathing), **orthopnea** (difficulty breathing when supine)
  - Moist crackles (rales) in the lungs; pulmonary edema (excess fluid in pulmonary interstitial spaces and alveoli) if severe
  - Increased urine output (**polyuria**)
  - **Ascites** (excess fluid in the peritoneal cavity)
  - Peripheral edema, or if severe, **anasarca** (severe, generalized edema).
- Dilution of plasma by excess fluid causes a decreased hematocrit and BUN.
- Possible cerebral edema (excess water in brain tissues) can lead to altered mental status and anxiety.

Heart failure is not only a potential cause of fluid volume excess, but it is also a potential complication of the condition if the heart is unable to increase its workload to handle the excess blood volume. Severe fluid overload and heart failure can lead to pulmonary edema, a medical emergency. See Chapter 32 ∞ for more information about heart failure and pulmonary edema.

INTERDISCIPLINARY CARE

Managing fluid volume excess focuses on prevention in clients at risk, treating its manifestations, and correcting the underlying cause. Management includes limiting sodium and water intake and administering diuretics.

Diagnosis

The following laboratory tests may be ordered.
- *Serum electrolytes* and *serum osmolality* are measured. Serum sodium and osmolality usually remain within normal limits.
- *Serum hematocrit* and *hemoglobin* often are decreased due to plasma dilution from excess extracellular fluid.

Additional tests of *renal* and *liver function* (such as serum creatinine, BUN, and liver enzymes) may be ordered to help determine the cause of fluid volume excess if it is unclear.

Medications

Diuretics are commonly used to treat fluid volume excess. They inhibit sodium and water reabsorption, increasing urine output. The three major classes of diuretics, each of which acts on a different part of the kidney tubule, are as follows:
- Loop diuretics act in the ascending loop of Henle.
- Thiazide-type diuretics act on the distal convoluted tubule.
- Potassium-sparing diuretics affect the distal nephron.

The nursing implications for diuretics are outlined in the Medication Administration box below.

Treatments

FLUID MANAGEMENT Fluid intake may be restricted in clients who have fluid volume excess. The amount of fluid allowed per day is prescribed by the primary care provider. All fluid intake must be calculated, including meals and that used to administer medications orally or intravenously. Box 10–3 provides guidelines for clients with a fluid restriction.

DIETARY MANAGEMENT Because sodium retention is a primary cause of fluid volume excess, a sodium-restricted diet of-

---

BOX 10–3 **Fluid Restriction Guidelines**

- Subtract requisite fluids (e.g., ordered IV fluids, fluid used to dilute IV medications) from total daily allowance.
- Divide remaining fluid allowance:
  - Day shift: 50% of total
  - Evening shift: 25% to 33% of total
  - Night shift: Remainder
- Explain the fluid restriction to the client and family members.
- Identify preferred fluids and intake pattern of client.
- Place allowed amounts of fluid in small glasses (gives perception of a full glass).
- Offer ice chips (when melted, ice chips are approximately half the frozen volume).
- Provide frequent mouth care.
- Provide sugarless chewing gum (if allowed) to reduce thirst sensation.

MEDICATION ADMINISTRATION   **Diuretics for Fluid Volume Excess**

Diuretics increase urinary excretion of water and sodium. They are categorized into three major groups: loop diuretics, thiazide and thiazide-like diuretics, and potassium-sparing diuretics. Diuretics are used to enhance renal function and to treat vascular fluid overload and edema. Common side effects include orthostatic hypotension, dehydration, electrolyte imbalance, and possible hyperglycemia. Diuretics should be used with caution in the older adult. Examples of each major type follow.

LOOP DIURETICS

Furosemide (Lasix)	**Ethacrynic Acid (Edecrin)**
Bumetanide (Bumex)	**Torsemide (Demadex)**

Loop diuretics inhibit sodium and chloride reabsorption in the ascending loop of Henle (see Chapter 27 ∞ for the anatomy of the kidneys). As a result, loop diuretics promote the excretion of sodium, chloride, potassium, and water.

THIAZIDE AND THIAZIDE-LIKE DIURETICS

Bendroflumethiazide (Naturetin)
Chlorothiazide (Diuril)
Hydrochlorothiazide (HydroDIURIL, Oretic)
Metolazone (Zaroxolyn)
Polythiazide (Renese)
Chlorthalidone (Hygroton)
Trichlormethiazide (Naqua)
Indapamide (Lozol)

Thiazide and thiazide-like diuretics promote the excretion of sodium, chloride, potassium, and water by decreasing absorption in the distal tubule.

POTASSIUM-SPARING DIURETICS

Spironolactone (Aldactone)
Amiloride HCl (Midamor)
Triamterene (Dyrenium)

Potassium-sparing diuretics promote excretion of sodium and water by inhibiting sodium-potassium exchange in the distal tubule.

Health Education for the Client and Family

- The drug will increase the amount and frequency of urination.
- The drugs must be taken even when you feel well.
- Take the drugs in the morning and afternoon to avoid having to get up at night to urinate.
- Change position slowly to avoid dizziness.
- Report the following to your primary healthcare provider: dizziness; trouble breathing; or swelling of face, hands, or feet.
- Weigh yourself every day, and report sudden gains or losses.
- Avoid using the salt shaker when eating.
- If the drug increases potassium loss, eat foods high in potassium, such as orange juice and bananas.
- Do not use salt substitute if you are taking a potassium-sparing diuretic.

ten is prescribed. Americans typically consume more than 4 or 5 g of sodium every day; recommended sodium intake is 500 to 2400 mg per day. The primary dietary sources of sodium are the salt shaker, processed foods, and foods themselves (Box 10–4).

A mild sodium restriction can be achieved by instructing the client and primary food preparer in the household to reduce the amount of salt in recipes by half, avoid using the salt shaker during meals, and avoid foods that contain high levels of sodium (either naturally or because of processing). In moderate and severely sodium-restricted diets, salt is avoided altogether, as are all foods containing significant amounts of sodium.

NURSING CARE

Nursing care focuses on preventing fluid volume excess in clients at risk and on managing problems resulting from its effects. See the Nursing Care Plan: A Client with Fluid Volume Excess on the following page.

Health Promotion

Health promotion related to fluid volume excess focuses on teaching preventive measures to clients who are at risk (e.g., clients who have heart or kidney failure). Discuss the relation-ship between sodium intake and water retention. Provide guidelines for a low-sodium diet, and teach clients to carefully read food labels to identify "hidden" sodium, particularly in processed foods. Instruct clients at risk to weigh themselves on a regular basis, using the same scale, and to notify their primary care provider if they gain more than 5 lb in a week or less.

Carefully monitor clients receiving intravenous fluids for signs of hypervolemia. Reduce the flow rate and promptly report manifestations of fluid overload to the physician.

Assessment

Collect assessment data through the health history interview and physical examination.

- *Health history:* Risk factors such as medications, heart failure, acute or chronic renal or endocrine disease; precipitating factors such as a recent illness, change in diet, or change in medications. Recent weight gain; complaints of persistent cough, shortness of breath, swelling of feet and ankles, or difficulty sleeping when lying down.
- *Physical assessment:* Weight; vital signs; peripheral pulses and capillary refill; jugular neck vein distention; edema; lung sounds (crackles or wheezes), dyspnea, cough, and sputum; urine output; mental status.
- *Diagnostic tests:* Monitor serum electrolytes and osmolality, hemoglobin and hematocrit, urine specific gravity.

Nursing Diagnoses and Interventions

Nursing diagnoses and interventions for the client with fluid volume excess focus on the multisystem effects of the fluid overload.

Excess Fluid Volume

Nursing care for the client with excess fluid volume includes collaborative interventions such as administering diuretics and maintaining a fluid restriction, as well as monitoring the status and effects of the excess fluid volume. This is particularly critical in older clients because of the age-related decline in cardiac and renal compensatory responses.

- Assess vital signs, heart sounds, CVP, and volume of peripheral arteries. *Hypervolemia can cause hypertension, bounding peripheral pulses, a third heart sound (S_3) due to the volume of blood flow through the heart, and high CVP readings.*
- Assess for the presence and extent of edema, particularly in the lower extremities, the back, sacral, and periorbital areas. *Initially, edema affects the dependent portions of the body—the lower extremities of ambulatory clients and the sacrum in bedridden clients. Periorbital edema indicates more generalized edema.*

> **PRACTICE ALERT**
> Assess urine output hourly. Maintain accurate intake and output records. Note urine output of less than 30 mL per hour or a positive fluid balance on 24-hour total intake and output calculations. Heart failure and inadequate renal perfusion may result in decreased urine output and fluid retention.

- Obtain daily weights at the same time of day, using approximately the same clothing and a balanced scale. *Daily weights are one of the most important gauges of fluid balance. Acute*

BOX 10–4 Foods High in Sodium

High in Added Sodium

Processed Meat and Fish
- Bacon
- Luncheon meat and other cold cuts
- Sausage
- Smoked fish

Selected Dairy Products
- Buttermilk
- Cheeses
- Cottage cheese
- Ice cream

Processed Grains
- Graham crackers
- Most dry cereals

Most Canned Goods
- Meats
- Soups
- Vegetables

Snack Foods
- Salted popcorn
- Potato chips/pretzels
- Nuts
- Gelatin desserts

Condiments and Food Additives
- Barbecue sauce
- Catsup
- Chili sauce
- Meat tenderizers
- Worcestershire sauce
- Saccharin
- Pickles
- Soy sauce
- Salted margarine
- Salad dressings

Naturally High in Sodium
- Brains
- Kidney
- Clams
- Crab
- Lobster
- Oysters
- Shrimp
- Dried fruit
- Spinach
- Carrots

NURSING CARE PLAN   A Client with Fluid Volume Excess

Dorothy Rainwater is a 45-year-old Native American woman hospitalized with acute renal failure that developed as a result of acute glomerulonephritis. She is expected to recover, but she has very little urine output. Ms. Rainwater is a single mother of two teenage sons. Until her illness, she was active in caring for her family, her career as a high school principal, and community activities.

ASSESSMENT

Mike Penning, Ms. Rainwater's nurse, notes that she is in the oliguric phase of acute renal failure, and that her urine output for the previous 24 hours is 250 mL; this low output has been constant for the past 8 days. She gained 1 lb (0.45 kg) in the past 24 hours. Laboratory test results from that morning are sodium, 155 mEq/L (normal 135 to 145 mEq/L); potassium, 5.3 mEq/L (normal 3.5 to 5.0 mEq/L); calcium, 7.6 mg/dL (normal 8.0 to 10.5 mg/dL), and urine specific gravity 1.008 (normal 1.010 to 1.030). Ms. Rainwater's serum creatinine and blood urea nitrogen (BUN) are high; however, her ABGs are within normal limits.

In his assessment of Ms. Rainwater, Mike notes the following:
- BP 160/92; P 102, with obvious neck vein distention; R 28, with crackles and wheezes; head of bed elevated 30 degrees; T 98.6°F
- Periorbital and sacral edema present; 3+ pitting bilateral pedal edema; skin cool, pale, and shiny
- Alert, oriented; responds appropriately to questions
- Client states she is thirsty, slightly nauseated, and extremely tired.

Ms. Rainwater is receiving intravenous furosemide and is on a 24-hour fluid restriction of 500 mL plus the previous day's urine output to manage her fluid volume excess.

DIAGNOSES

- *Excess Fluid Volume* related to acute renal failure
- *Risk for Impaired Skin Integrity* related to fluid retention and edema
- *Risk for Impaired Gas Exchange* related to pulmonary congestion
- *Activity Intolerance* related to fluid volume excess, fatigue, and weakness

EXPECTED OUTCOMES

- Regain fluid balance, as evidenced by weight loss, decreasing edema, and normal vital signs.

- Experience decreased dyspnea.
- Maintain intact skin and mucous membranes.
- Increase activity levels as prescribed.

PLANNING AND IMPLEMENTATION

- Weigh at 0600 and 1800 daily.
- Assess vital signs and breath sounds every 4 hours.
- Measure intake and output every 4 hours.
- Obtain urine specific gravity every 8 hours.
- Restrict fluids as follows: 350 mL from 0700 to 1500; 300 mL from 1500 to 2300; 100 mL from 2300 to 0700. Prefers water or apple juice.
- Turn every 2 hours, following schedule posted at the head of bed. Inspect and provide skin care as needed; avoid vigorous massage of pressure areas.
- Provide oral care every 2 to 4 hours (can brush her own teeth, caution not to swallow water); use moistened applicators as desired.
- Elevate head of bed to 30 to 40 degrees; prefers to use own pillows.
- Assist to recliner chair at bedside for 20 minutes two or three times a day. Monitor ability to tolerate activity without increasing dyspnea or fatigue.

EVALUATION

At the end of the shift, Mike evaluates the effectiveness of the plan of care and continues all diagnoses and interventions. Ms. Rainwater gained no weight, and her urinary output during his shift is 170 mL. Her urine specific gravity remains at 1.008. Her vital signs are unchanged, but her crackles and wheezes have decreased slightly. Her skin and mucous membranes are intact. Ms. Rainwater tolerated the bedside chair without dyspnea or fatigue.

CRITICAL THINKING IN THE NURSING PROCESS

1. What is the pathophysiologic basis for Ms. Rainwater's increased respiratory rate, blood pressure, and pulse?
2. Explain how elevating the head of the bed 30 degrees facilitates respirations.
3. Suppose Ms. Rainwater says, "I would really like to have all my fluids at once instead of spreading them out." How would you reply, and why?
4. Outline a plan for teaching Ms. Rainwater about diuretics.
See Evaluating Your Response in Appendix C.

---

weight gain or loss represents fluid gain or loss. Weight gain of 2 kg is equivalent to 2 L of fluid gain.
- Administer oral fluids cautiously, adhering to any prescribed fluid restriction. Discuss the restriction with the client and significant others, including the total volume allowed, the rationale, and the importance of reporting all fluid taken. *All sources of fluid intake, including ice chips, are recorded to avoid excess fluid intake.*
- Provide oral hygiene at least every 2 hours. *Oral hygiene contributes to client comfort and keeps mucous membranes intact; it also helps relieve thirst if fluids are restricted.*
- Teach client and significant others about the sodium-restricted diet, and emphasize the importance of checking

before bringing foods to the client. *Excess sodium promotes water retention; a sodium-restricted diet is ordered to reduce water gain.*
- Administer prescribed diuretics as ordered, monitoring the client's response to therapy. *Loop or high-ceiling diuretics such as furosemide can lead to rapid fluid loss and signs of hypovolemia and electrolyte imbalance.*
- Promptly report significant changes in serum electrolytes or osmolality or abnormal results of tests done to determine contributing factors to the fluid volume excess. *Gradual correction of serum electrolytes and osmolality is expected, however, aggressive diuretic therapy can lead to overcorrection.*

Risk for Impaired Skin Integrity

Tissue edema decreases oxygen and nutrient delivery to the skin and subcutaneous tissues, increasing the risk of injury.

- Frequently assess skin, particularly in pressure areas and over bony prominences. *Skin breakdown can progress rapidly when circulation is impaired.*
- Reposition the client at least every 2 hours. Provide skin care with each position change. *Frequent position changes minimize tissue pressure and promote blood flow to tissues.*
- Provide an egg-crate mattress or alternating pressure mattress, foot cradle, heel protectors, and other devices to reduce pressure on tissues. *These devices, which distribute pressure away from bony prominences, reduce the risk of skin breakdown.*

Risk for Impaired Gas Exchange

With fluid volume excess, gas exchange may be impaired by edema of pulmonary interstitial tissues. Acute pulmonary edema is a serious and potentially life-threatening complication of pulmonary congestion.

- Auscultate lungs for presence or worsening of crackles and wheezes; auscultate heart for extra heart sounds. *Crackles and wheezes indicate pulmonary congestion and edema. A gallop rhythm (S_3) may indicate diastolic overloading of the ventricles secondary to fluid volume excess.*
- Place in Fowler's position if dyspnea or orthopnea is present. *Fowler's position improves lung expansion by decreasing the pressure of abdominal contents on the diaphragm.*
- Monitor oxygen saturation levels and **arterial blood gases (ABGs)** for evidence of impaired gas exchange ($SaO_2 < 92\%$ to 95%; $PaO_2 < 80$ mmHg). Administer oxygen as indicated. *Edema of interstitial lung tissues can interfere with gas exchange and delivery to body tissues. Supplemental oxygen promotes gas exchange across the alveolar-capillary membrane, improving tissue oxygenation.*

Community-Based Care

Teaching for home care focuses on managing the underlying cause of fluid volume excess and preventing future episodes of excess fluid volume. Address the following topics when preparing the client and family for home care:

- Signs and symptoms of excess fluid and when to contact the care provider
- Prescribed medications: when and how to take, intended and adverse effects, what to report to care provider
- Recommended or prescribed diet; ways to reduce sodium intake; how to read food labels for salt and sodium content; use of salt substitutes, if allowed (Box 10–5)
- If restricted, the amount and type of fluids to take each day; how to balance intake over 24 hours
- Monitoring weight; changes reported to care provider
- Ways to decrease dependent edema:
    a. Change position frequently.
    b. Avoid restrictive clothing.
    c. Avoid crossing the legs when sitting.
    d. Wear support stockings or hose.
    e. Elevate feet and legs when sitting.

BOX 10–5 Client Teaching

Low-Sodium Diet

- Reducing sodium intake will help the body excrete excess sodium and water.
- The body needs less than one-tenth of a teaspoon of salt per day.
- Approximately one-third of sodium intake comes from salt added to foods during cooking and at the table; one-fourth to one-third comes from processed foods; and the rest comes from food and water naturally high in sodium.
- Sodium compounds are used in foods as preservatives, leavening agents, and flavor enhancers.
- Many nonprescription drugs (such as analgesics, cough medicine, laxatives, and antacids) as well as toothpastes and mouthwashes contain high amounts of sodium.
- Low-sodium salt substitutes are not really sodium free and may contain half as much sodium as regular salt.
- Use salt substitutes sparingly; larger amounts often taste bitter instead of salty.
- The preference for salt will eventually diminish.
- Salt, monosodium glutamate, baking soda, and baking powder contain substantial amounts of sodium.
- Read labels.
- In place of salt or salt substitutes, use herbs, spices, lemon juice, vinegar, and wine as flavoring when cooking.

- How to protect edematous skin from injury:
    a. Do not walk barefoot.
    b. Buy good-fitting shoes; shop in the afternoon when feet are more likely to be swollen.
- Using additional pillows or a recliner to sleep, to relieve orthopnea.

SODIUM IMBALANCE

Sodium is the most plentiful electrolyte in ECF, with normal serum sodium levels ranging from 135 to 145 mEq/L. Sodium is the primary regulator of the volume, osmolality, and distribution of ECF. It also is important to maintain neuromuscular activity. Because of the close interrelationship between sodium and water balance, disorders of fluid volume and sodium balance often occur together. Sodium imbalances affect the osmolality of ECF and water distribution between the fluid compartments. When sodium levels are low (hyponatremia), water is drawn into the cells of the body, causing them to swell. In contrast, high levels of sodium in ECF (hypernatremia) draw water out of body cells, causing them to shrink.

Overview of Normal Sodium Balance

Most of the body's sodium comes from dietary intake. Although a sodium intake of 500 mg per day is usually sufficient to meet the body's needs, the average intake of sodium by adults in the United States is about 6 to 15 g per day (Porth, 2005). Other sources of sodium include prescription drugs and certain self-prescribed remedies. Sodium is primarily excreted by the kidneys. A small amount is excreted through the skin and the gastrointestinal tract.

The kidney is the primary regulator of sodium balance in the body. The kidney excretes or conserves sodium in response to changes in vascular volume. A fall in blood volume prompts several mechanisms that lead to sodium and water retention:

- The renin–angiotensin–aldosterone system (see Figure 10–9) is stimulated. Angiotensin II prompts the renal tubules to reabsorb sodium. It also causes vasoconstriction, slowing blood flow through the kidney and reducing glomerular filtration. This further reduces the amount of sodium excreted. Angiotensin II promotes the release of aldosterone from the adrenal cortex. In the presence of aldosterone, more sodium is reabsorbed in the cortical collecting tubules of the kidney, and more potassium is eliminated in the urine.
- ADH is released from the posterior pituitary (see Figure 10–10). ADH promotes sodium and water reabsorption in the distal tubules of the kidney, reducing urine output and expanding blood volume.

In contrast, when blood volume expands, sodium and water elimination by the kidneys increases.

- The **glomerular filtration rate** (the rate at which plasma is filtered through the glomeruli of the kidney) increases, allowing more water and sodium to be filtered and excreted.
- ANP is released by cells in the atria of the heart. ANP increases sodium excretion by the kidneys.
- ADH release from the pituitary gland is inhibited. In the absence of ADH, the distal tubule is relatively impermeable to water and sodium, allowing more to be excreted in the urine. Table 10–5 summarizes the causes and effects of sodium imbalances.

The Client with Hyponatremia

Hyponatremia is a serum sodium level of less than 135 mEq/L. Hyponatremia usually results from a loss of sodium from the body, but it may also be caused by water gains that dilute ECF.

Pathophysiology

Excess sodium loss can occur through the kidneys, gastrointestinal tract, or skin. Diuretic medications, kidney diseases, or adrenal insufficiency with impaired aldosterone and cortisol production can lead to excessive sodium excretion in urine. Vomiting, diarrhea, and gastrointestinal suction are common causes of excess sodium loss through the GI tract. Sodium may also be lost when gastrointestinal tubes are irrigated with water instead of saline, or when repeated tap water enemas are administered (Porth, 2005). Excessive sweating or loss of skin surface (as with an extensive burn) can also cause excessive sodium loss.

Water gains that can lead to hyponatremia may occur with:

- Systemic diseases such as heart failure, renal failure, or cirrhosis of the liver
- Syndrome of inappropriate secretion of antidiuretic hormone (SIADH), in which water excretion is impaired
- Excessive administration of hypotonic intravenous fluids.

Hyponatremia causes a drop in serum osmolality. Water shifts from ECF into the intracellular space, causing cells to swell and reducing the osmolality of intracellular fluid. Many of the manifestations of hyponatremia can be attributed to cellular edema and hypo-osmolality.

Manifestations

The manifestations of hyponatremia depend on the rapidity of onset, the severity, and the cause of the imbalance. If the condition develops slowly, manifestations are usually not experienced until the serum sodium levels reach 125 mEq/L. In addition, the manifestations of hyponatremia vary, depending on extracellular fluid volume. Early manifestations of hyponatremia include muscle cramps, weakness, and fatigue from its effects on muscle cells. Gastrointestinal function is affected, causing anorexia, nausea and vomiting, abdominal cramping, and diarrhea.

As sodium levels continue to decrease, the brain and nervous system are affected by cellular edema. Neurologic mani-

TABLE 10–5 Causes and Manifestations of Sodium Imbalances

IMBALANCE	POSSIBLE CAUSES	MANIFESTATIONS
Hyponatremia Serum sodium < 135 mEq/L Critical value < 120 mEq/L *Other Lab Values* Serum osmolality < 280 mOsm/kg Critical value < 250 mOsm/kg	■ Excess sodium loss through kidneys, GI tract, or skin ■ Water gains related to renal disease, heart failure, or cirrhosis of the liver ■ SIADH ■ Excessive hypotonic IV fluids	■ Anorexia, nausea, vomiting, abdominal cramping, and diarrhea ■ Headache ■ Altered mental status ■ Muscle cramps, weakness, and tremors ■ Seizures and coma
Hypernatremia Serum sodium > 145 mEq/L Critical value > 160 mEq/L *Other Lab Values* Serum osmolality > 295 mOsm/kg Critical value > 325 mOsm/kg	■ Altered thirst ■ Inability to respond to thirst sensation or obtain water ■ Profuse sweating ■ Diarrhea ■ Diabetes insipidus ■ Oral electrolyte solutions or hyperosmolar tube-feeding formulas ■ Excess IV fluids such as normal saline, 3% or 5% sodium chloride, or sodium bicarbonate	■ Thirst ■ Increased temperature ■ Dry, sticky mucous membranes ■ Restlessness ■ Weakness ■ Altered mental status ■ Decreasing level of consciousness ■ Muscle twitching ■ Seizures

festations progress rapidly when the serum sodium level falls below 120 mEq/L and include headache, depression, dulled sensorium, personality changes, irritability, lethargy, hyperreflexia, muscle twitching, and tremors. If serum sodium falls to very low levels, convulsions and coma are likely to occur.

When hyponatremia is associated with decreased ECF volume, the manifestations are those of hypovolemia (*hypotonic dehydration*). In hyponatremia associated with fluid volume excess, manifestations include those of hypervolemia.

INTERDISCIPLINARY CARE

Interdisciplinary management of hyponatremia focuses on restoring normal blood volume and serum sodium levels.

Diagnosis
The following laboratory tests may be ordered.
- *Serum sodium* and *osmolality* are decreased in hyponatremia (serum sodium < 135 mEq/L; serum osmolality < 275 mOsm/kg).
- A *24-hour urine specimen* is obtained to evaluate sodium excretion. In conditions associated with normal or increased extracellular volume (such as SIADH), urinary sodium is increased; in conditions resulting from losses of isotonic fluids (e.g., sweating, diarrhea, vomiting, and third-space fluid accumulation), by contrast, urinary sodium is decreased.

Medications
When both sodium and water have been lost (hyponatremia with hypovolemia), sodium-containing fluids are given to replace both water and sodium. These fluids may be given by mouth, nasogastric tube, or intravenously. Isotonic Ringer's solution or isotonic saline (0.9% NaCl) solution may be administered. Cautious administration of intravenous 3% or 5% NaCl solution may be necessary in clients who have very low plasma sodium levels (110 to 115 mEq/L).

Loop diuretics are administered to clients who have hyponatremia with normal or excess ECF volume. Loop diuretics promote an isotonic diuresis and fluid volume loss without hyponatremia (see page 210). Thiazide diuretics are avoided because they cause a relatively greater sodium loss in relation to water loss.

In addition, drugs to treat the underlying cause of hyponatremia may be administered.

Fluid and Dietary Management
If hyponatremia is mild, increasing the intake of foods high in sodium may restore normal sodium balance (see Box 10–4). Fluids often are restricted to help reduce ECF volume and correct hyponatremia (see Box 10–3).

NURSING CARE

Nursing care of the client with hyponatremia focuses on identifying clients at risk and managing problems resulting from the systemic effects of the disorder.

Health Promotion
People at risk for mild hyponatremia include those who participate in activities that increase fluid loss through excessive per-spiration (diaphoresis) and then replace those losses by drinking large amounts of water. This includes athletes, people who do heavy labor in high environmental temperatures, and older adults living in non–air-conditioned settings during hot weather. Teach the following to clients who are at risk:
- Manifestations of mild hyponatremia, including nausea, abdominal cramps, and muscle weakness
- The importance of drinking liquids containing sodium and other electrolytes at frequent intervals when perspiring heavily, when environmental temperatures are high, and/or if watery diarrhea persists for several days.

Assessment
Assessment data related to hyponatremia include the following:
- *Health history:* Current manifestations, including nausea and vomiting, abdominal discomfort, muscle weakness, headache, other symptoms; duration of symptoms and any precipitating factors such as heavy perspiration, vomiting, or diarrhea; chronic diseases such as heart or renal failure, cirrhosis of the liver, or endocrine disorders; current medications.
- *Physical assessment:* Mental status and level of consciousness; vital signs including orthostatic vitals and peripheral pulses; presence of edema or weight gain.
- *Diagnostic tests:* Serum sodium and osmolality; serum potassium.

Nursing Diagnoses and Interventions
Risk for Imbalanced Fluid Volume
Because of its role in maintaining fluid balance, sodium imbalances often are accompanied by water imbalances. In addition, treatment of hyponatremia can affect the client's fluid balance.
- Monitor intake and output, weigh daily, and calculate 24-hour fluid balance. *Fluid excess or deficit may occur with hyponatremia.*

> ### PRACTICE ALERT
> Carefully monitor clients receiving sodium-containing intravenous solutions for signs of hypervolemia (increased blood pressure and CVP, tachypnea, tachycardia, gallop rhythm [S_3 and/or S_4 heart sounds], shortness of breath, crackles). Hypertonic saline solutions can lead to hypervolemia, particularly in clients with cardiovascular or renal disease.

- Use an intravenous flow control device to administer hypertonic saline (3% and 5% NaCl) solutions; carefully monitor flow rate and response. *Hypertonic solutions can increase the risk of pulmonary and cerebral edema due to water retention. Careful monitoring is vital to prevent these complications and possible permanent damage.*
- If fluids are restricted, explain the reason for the restriction, the amount of fluid allowed, and how to calculate fluid intake. *Teaching increases the client's sense of control and compliance.*

For additional nursing interventions that may apply to the client with hyponatremia, review the discussions of fluid volume deficit and fluid volume excess.

Risk for Ineffective Cerebral Tissue Perfusion

The client with severe hyponatremia experiences fluid shifts that cause an increase in intracellular fluid volume. This can cause brain cells to swell, increasing pressure within the cranial vault.

- Monitor serum electrolytes and serum osmolality. Report abnormal results to the care provider. *As serum sodium levels fall, the manifestations and neurologic effects of hyponatremia become increasingly severe.*
- Assess for neurologic changes, such as lethargy, altered level of consciousness, confusion, and convulsions. Monitor mental status and orientation. Compare baseline data with continuing assessments. *Serum sodium levels of 115 to 120 mEq/L can cause headache, lethargy, and decreased responsiveness; sodium levels less than 110 to 115 mEq/L may cause seizures and coma.*
- Assess muscle strength and tone, and deep tendon reflexes. *Increasing muscle weakness and decreased deep tendon reflexes are manifestations of increasing hyponatremia.*

> **PRACTICE ALERT**
> Maintain a quiet environment, and institute seizure precautions in clients with severe hyponatremia. Severe hyponatremia can lead to seizures. A quiet environment reduces neurologic stimulation. Safety precautions, such as ensuring that side rails are up and having an airway readily available, reduce risk of injury from seizure.

Community-Based Care

Teaching for home care focuses on the underlying cause of the sodium deficit and often on prevention. Teach clients who have experienced hyponatremia and those who are at risk for developing hyponatremia about the following:

- Manifestations of mild and more severe hyponatremia to report to the primary care provider
- The importance of regular serum electrolyte monitoring if taking a potent diuretic or on a low-sodium diet
- Types of foods and fluids to replace sodium orally if dietary sodium is not restricted.

The Client with Hypernatremia

Hypernatremia is a serum sodium level greater than 145 mEq/L. It may develop when sodium is gained in excess of water, or when water is lost in excess of sodium. Either fluid volume deficit or fluid volume excess often accompany hypernatremia.

Pathophysiology

Two regulatory mechanisms protect the body from hypernatremia: (1) Excess sodium in ECF stimulates the release of ADH so more water is retained by the kidneys; and (2) the thirst mechanism is stimulated to increase the intake of water (Metheny, 2000). These two factors increase extracellular water, diluting the excess sodium and restoring normal levels. Because of the effectiveness of these mechanisms, hypernatremia almost never occurs in clients who have an intact thirst mechanism and access to water.

Water deprivation is a cause of hypernatremia in clients who are unable to respond to thirst due to altered mental status or physical disability. Excess water loss may occur with watery diarrhea or increased insensible losses (due to fever, hyperventilation, excessive perspiration, or massive burns). Unless water is adequately replaced, clients with diabetes insipidus (see Chapter 19 ∞) also may develop hypernatremia. Excess sodium intake can result from ingestion of excess salt or hypertonic intravenous solutions. Clients who experience near-drowning in seawater are at risk for hypernatremia, as are clients with heatstroke.

Manifestations

Hypernatremia (also known as *hypertonic dehydration*) causes hyperosmolality of ECF. As a result, water is drawn out of cells, leading to cellular dehydration. The most serious effects of cellular dehydration are seen in the brain. As brain cells contract, neurologic manifestations develop. The brain itself shrinks, causing mechanical traction on cerebral vessels. These vessels may tear and bleed. Although the brain rapidly adapts to hyperosmolality to minimize the water loss, acute hypernatremia can cause widespread cerebral vascular bleeding (Metheny, 2000).

Thirst is the first manifestation of hypernatremia. If thirst is not relieved, the primary manifestations relate to altered neurologic function (see Table 10–5). Initial lethargy, weakness, and irritability can progress to seizures, coma, and death in severe hypernatremia. Both the severity of the sodium excess and the rapidity of its onset affect the manifestations of hypernatremia.

INTERDISCIPLINARY CARE

Treatment of hypernatremia depends on its cause. Hypernatremia is corrected slowly (over a 48-hour period) to avoid development of cerebral edema secondary to a shift of water into the brain cells.

Diagnosis

The following laboratory and diagnostic tests may be ordered:

- *Serum sodium levels* are greater than 145 mEq/L in hypernatremia.
- *Serum osmolality* is greater than 295 mOsm/kg in hypernatremia.
- The *water deprivation test* may be conducted to identify diabetes insipidus. Water and all other fluids are withheld for a specified period of time. During this time, urine specimens are obtained for osmolality and specific gravity. No change in these values supports the diagnosis of diabetes insipidus.

Medications

The principal treatment for hypernatremia is oral or intravenous water replacement. Hypotonic intravenous fluids such as 0.45% NaCl solution or 5% dextrose in water (which is isotonic when administered, but provides pure water when the glucose is metabolized) may be administered to correct the water deficit. Diuretics may also be given to increase sodium excretion.

NURSING CARE

The primary focus of nursing care related to hypernatremia is prevention. Measures to prevent hypernatremia include identifying risk factors, teaching clients and caregivers, monitoring laboratory test results, and working with the interdisciplinary team to reduce the potential for hypernatremia.

Health Promotion

Clients at risk for hypernatremia, as well as their care providers, need teaching to prevent this electrolyte disorder. Instruct caregivers of debilitated clients who are unable to perceive thirst or unable to respond to it to offer fluids at regular intervals. If the client is unable to maintain adequate fluid intake, contact the primary care provider about an alternate route for fluid intake (e.g., a feeding tube). Teach care providers the importance of providing adequate water for clients receiving tube feedings (many of which are hypertonic).

Assessment

Assessment data related to hypernatremia include the following:
- *Health history:* Duration of symptoms and any precipitating factors such as water deprivation, increased water loss due to heavy perspiration, temperature or rapid breathing, diarrhea, excess salt intake, or diabetes insipidus; current medications; perception of thirst.
- *Physical assessment:* Vital signs including temperature; mucous membranes; altered mental status or level of consciousness; manifestations of fluid volume excess or fluid volume deficit.
- *Diagnostic tests:* Monitor serum sodium and osmolality, serum potassium.

Nursing Diagnoses and Interventions
Risk for Injury

Mental status and brain function may be affected by hypernatremia itself or by rapid correction of the condition that leads to cerebral edema. In either case, closely monitor the client and take precautions to reduce risk of injury.

- Monitor and maintain fluid replacement to within the prescribed limits. Monitor serum sodium levels and osmolality; report rapid changes to the care provider. *Rapid water replacement or rapid changes in serum sodium or osmolality can cause fluid shifts within the brain, increasing the risk of bleeding or cerebral edema.*
- Monitor neurologic function, including mental status, level of consciousness, and other manifestations such as headache, nausea, vomiting, elevated blood pressure, and decreased pulse rate. *Both hypernatremia and rapid correction of hypernatremia affect the brain and brain function. Careful monitoring is vital to detect changes in mental status that may indicate cerebral bleeding or edema.*
- Institute safety precautions as necessary: Keep the bed in its lowest position, side rails up and padded, and an airway at bedside. *Clients with sodium disorders are at risk for injury due to seizure activity and changes in mental status.*

- Keep clocks, calendars, and familiar objects at bedside. Orient to time, place, and circumstances as needed. Allow significant others to remain with the client as much as possible. *An unfamiliar environment and altered thought processes can further increase the client's risk for injury. Significant others provide a sense of security and reduce the client's anxiety.*

Community-Based Care

When preparing the client who has experienced hypernatremia for home care, discuss the following topics:
- The importance of responding to thirst and consuming adequate fluids (If the client is dependent on a caregiver, stress the importance of regularly offering fluids to the caregiver.)
- If prescribed, guidelines for following a low-sodium diet (see Box 10–5)
- Use and effects (intended and unintended) of any prescribed diuretic or other medication
- The importance of following a schedule for regular monitoring of serum electrolyte levels and reporting manifestations of imbalance to care provider.

POTASSIUM IMBALANCE

Potassium, the primary intracellular cation, plays a vital role in cell metabolism, and cardiac and neuromuscular function. The normal serum (ECF) potassium level is 3.5 to 5.0 mEq/L.

Overview of Normal Potassium Balance

Most potassium in the body is found within the cells (ICF), which have a concentration of 140 to 150 mEq/L. This significant difference in the potassium concentrations of ICF and ECF helps maintain the resting membrane potential of nerve and muscle cells; either a deficit or an excess of potassium can adversely affect neuromuscular and cardiac function. The higher intracellular potassium concentration is maintained by the sodium-potassium pump.

To maintain its balance, potassium must be replaced daily. Normally, potassium is supplied in food. Virtually all foods contain potassium, although some foods and fluids are richer sources of this element than others (Box 10–6).

The kidneys eliminate potassium very efficiently; even when potassium intake is stopped, the kidneys continue to excrete it. Because the kidneys do not conserve potassium well, significant amounts may be lost through this route. However, because the kidneys are the principal organs involved in the elimination of potassium, renal failure can lead to potentially serious elevations of serum potassium.

Aldosterone helps regulate potassium elimination by the kidneys. An increased potassium concentration in ECF stimulates aldosterone production by the adrenal gland. The kidneys respond to aldosterone by increasing potassium excretion. Changes in aldosterone secretion can profoundly affect the serum potassium level.

Normally only small amounts of potassium are lost in the feces, but substantial amounts may be lost from the gastrointestinal

BOX 10–6 Foods High in Potassium

Fruits
- Apricots
- Avocados
- Bananas
- Cantaloupe
- Dates
- Oranges
- Raisins

Vegetables and Vegetable Juices
- Carrots
- Cauliflower
- Mushrooms
- Peas
- Potatoes
- Spinach
- Tomatoes
- V-8 Juice

Meats and Fish
- Beef
- Chicken
- Kidney
- Liver
- Lobster
- Pork loin
- Tuna
- Turkey
- Salmon

Milk Products
- Buttermilk
- Chocolate milk
- Evaporated milk
- Low-fat yogurt
- Milk

brane potential of cells. Resting membrane potential, in turn, is necessary for transmitting nerve impulses. Potassium imbalances affect transmission and conduction of nerve impulses, maintenance of normal cardiac rhythms, and contraction of skeletal and smooth muscle (McCance & Huether, 2006).

As the primary intracellular cation, potassium plays a major role in regulating the osmolality of ICF, and it is involved in metabolic processes. Potassium is necessary for the storage of glycogen in skeletal muscle cells. Table 10–6 summarizes potassium imbalances, their causes, and manifestations.

The Client with Hypokalemia

Hypokalemia is an abnormally low serum potassium (less than 3.5 mEq/L). It usually results from excess potassium loss, although hospitalized clients may be at risk for hypokalemia because of inadequate potassium intake.

Pathophysiology

Excess potassium may be lost through the kidneys or the gastrointestinal tract. These losses deplete total potassium stores in the body.

- Excess potassium loss through the kidneys often is secondary to drugs such as potassium-wasting diuretics, corticosteroids, amphotericin B, and large doses of some antibiotics. Hyperaldosteronism, a condition in which the adrenal glands secrete excess aldosterone, also causes excess elimination of potassium through the kidneys. Glucosuria and osmotic diuresis (e.g., associated with diabetes mellitus) also cause potassium wasting through the kidneys (Metheny, 2000).

tract with diarrhea or through drainage from an ileostomy (a permanent opening into the small bowel).

Potassium constantly shifts into and out of the cells. This movement between ICF and ECF can significantly affect the serum potassium level. For example, potassium shifts into or out of the cells in response to changes in hydrogen ion concentration (pH, discussed later in this chapter) as the body strives to maintain a stable acid–base balance.

The significant difference between intracellular and extracellular potassium concentrations is vital to the resting mem-

TABLE 10–6 Causes and Manifestations of Potassium Imbalances

IMBALANCE	CAUSES	MANIFESTATIONS
Hypokalemia Serum potassium < 3.5 mEq/L Critical value < 2.5 mEq/L	■ Excess GI losses: vomiting, diarrhea, ileostomy drainage ■ Renal losses: diuretics, hyperaldosteronism ■ Inadequate intake ■ Shift into cells: alkalosis, rapid tissue repair	Cardiovascular ■ Dysrhythmias ■ ECG changes Gastrointestinal ■ Nausea and vomiting ■ Anorexia ■ Decreased bowel sounds ■ Ileus Musculoskeletal ■ Muscle weakness ■ Leg cramps
Hyperkalemia Serum potassium > 5.0 mEq/L Critical value > 6.5 mEq/L	■ Renal failure ■ Potassium-sparing diuretics ■ Adrenal insufficiency ■ Excess potassium intake (e.g., excess potassium replacement) ■ Aged blood ■ Shift out of cells: cell and tissue damage, acidosis	Cardiovascular ■ Tall, peaked T waves, widened QRS ■ Dysrhythmias ■ Cardiac arrest Gastrointestinal ■ Nausea and vomiting ■ Abdominal cramping ■ Diarrhea Neuromuscular ■ Muscle weakness ■ Paresthesias ■ Flaccid paralysis

- Gastrointestinal losses of potassium result from severe vomiting, gastric suction, or loss of intestinal fluids through diarrhea or ileostomy drainage.

Potassium intake may be inadequate in clients who are unable or unwilling to eat for prolonged periods. Hospitalized clients are at risk, especially those on extended parenteral fluid therapy with solutions that do not contain potassium. Clients with anorexia nervosa or alcoholism may develop hypokalemia due to both inadequate intake and loss of potassium through vomiting, diarrhea, or laxative or diuretic use.

A *relative* loss of potassium occurs when potassium shifts from ECF into the cells. This usually is due to loss of hydrogen ion and alkalosis, although it also may occur during periods of rapid tissue repair (e.g., following a burn or trauma), in the presence of excess insulin (insulin promotes potassium entry into skeletal muscle and liver cells), during acute stress, or because of hypothermia. In these instances, the total body stores of potassium remain adequate.

Manifestations

Hypokalemia affects the transmission of nerve impulses, interfering with the contractility of smooth, skeletal, and cardiac muscle, as well as the regulation and transmission of cardiac impulses.

- Characteristic electrocardiogram (ECG) changes of hypokalemia include flattened or inverted T waves, the development of U waves, and a depressed ST segment (Figure 10–11 ■). The most serious cardiac effect is an increased risk of atrial and ventricular *dysrhythmias* (abnormal rhythms). Hypokalemia increases the risk for digitalis toxicity in clients receiving this drug used to treat heart failure (see Chapter 32 ∞).
- Hypokalemia affects both the resting membrane potential and intracellular enzymes in skeletal and smooth muscle cells. This causes skeletal muscle weakness and slowed peristalsis of the gastrointestinal tract. Muscles of the lower extremities are affected first, then the trunk and upper extremities. This effect of hypokalemia is magnified when serum calcium levels are above normal.
- Carbohydrate metabolism is affected by hypokalemia. Insulin secretion is suppressed, as is the synthesis of glycogen in skeletal muscle and the liver.

Hypokalemia also can affect kidney function, particularly the ability to concentrate urine. Severe hypokalemia can lead to *rhabdomyolysis*, a condition in which muscle fibers disintegrate, releasing myoglobin to be excreted in the urine.

Manifestations of hypokalemia are more pronounced when potassium losses occur acutely. When hypokalemia develops gradually, potassium shifts out of the cells, helping maintain the ratio of intracellular to extracellular potassium. As a result, the neuromuscular manifestations of hypokalemia are less severe. The *Multisystem Effects of Hypokalemia* are summarized on the following page.

INTERDISCIPLINARY CARE

The management of hypokalemia focuses on prevention and treatment of a deficiency.

(a) Normal ECG

(b) ECG in hypokalemia

(c) ECG in hyperkalemia

Figure 10–11 ■ The effects of changes in potassium levels on the electrocardiogram (ECG). *A,* Normal ECG; *B,* ECG in hypokalemia; *C,* ECG in hyperkalemia.

Diagnosis

The following laboratory and diagnostic tests may be ordered:
- *Serum potassium* (K^+) is used to monitor potassium levels in clients who are at risk for or who are being treated for hypokalemia. A serum K^+ of 3.0 to 3.5 mEq/L is considered

MULTISYSTEM EFFECTS **of Hypokalemia**

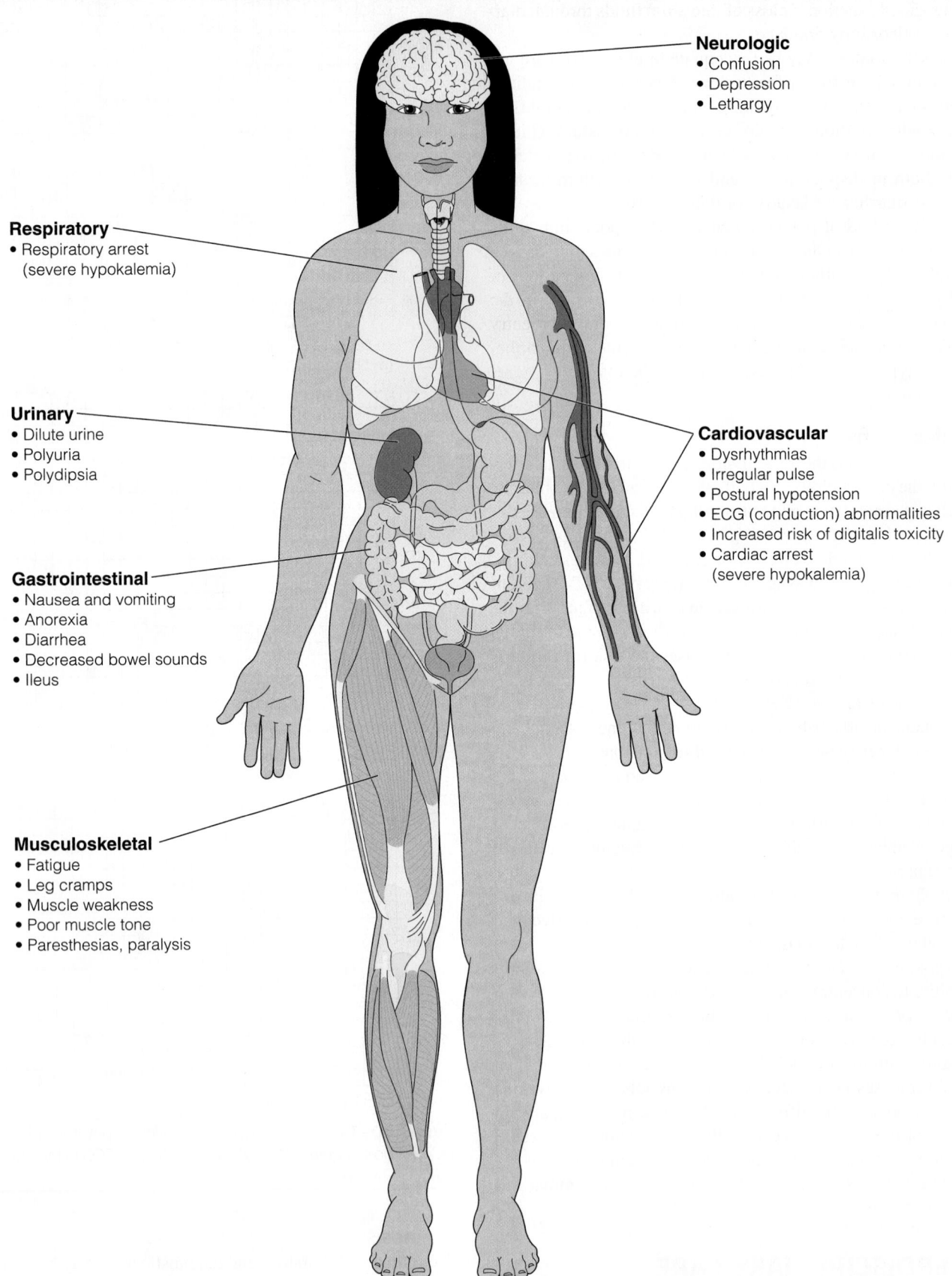

Neurologic
- Confusion
- Depression
- Lethargy

Respiratory
- Respiratory arrest
  (severe hypokalemia)

Urinary
- Dilute urine
- Polyuria
- Polydipsia

Gastrointestinal
- Nausea and vomiting
- Anorexia
- Diarrhea
- Decreased bowel sounds
- Ileus

Musculoskeletal
- Fatigue
- Leg cramps
- Muscle weakness
- Poor muscle tone
- Paresthesias, paralysis

Cardiovascular
- Dysrhythmias
- Irregular pulse
- Postural hypotension
- ECG (conduction) abnormalities
- Increased risk of digitalis toxicity
- Cardiac arrest
  (severe hypokalemia)

mild hypokalemia. Moderate hypokalemia is defined as a serum K^+ of 2.5 to 3.0 mEq/L, and severe hypokalemia as a serum K^+ of less than 2.5 mEq/L (Metheny, 2000).

- *Arterial blood gases (ABGs)* are measured to determine acid–base status. An increased pH (alkalosis) often is associated with hypokalemia. (See Table 10–10 later in this chapter for normal ABG values.)
- *Renal function studies*, such as *serum creatinine* and *blood urea nitrogen (BUN)*, may be ordered to evaluate for potential causes or effects of hypokalemia.
- *ECG recordings* are obtained to evaluate the effects of hypokalemia on the cardiac conduction system.

Medications

Oral and/or parenteral potassium supplements are given to prevent and, as needed, treat hypokalemia. To prevent hypokalemia in the client taking nothing by mouth, 40 mEq of potassium chloride per day is added to intravenous fluids. The dose used to treat hypokalemia includes the daily maintenance requirement, replacement of ongoing losses (e.g., gastric suction), and additional potassium to correct the existing deficit. Several days of therapy may be required. Commonly prescribed potassium supplements, their actions, and nursing implications are described in the Medication Administration box below.

Nutrition

A diet high in potassium-rich foods is recommended for clients at risk for developing hypokalemia or to supplement drug therapy (see Box 10–6).

NURSING CARE

See the following page for a Nursing Care Plan: A Client with Hypokalemia.

Health Promotion

When providing general health education, discuss using balanced electrolyte solutions (e.g., Pedialyte or sports drinks) to replace abnormal fluid losses (excess perspiration, vomiting, or severe diarrhea). Discuss the necessity of preventing hypokalemia with clients at risk. Provide diet teaching and refer clients with anorexia nervosa for counseling. Stress the potassium-losing effects of taking diuretics and using laxatives to enhance weight loss. Discuss the potassium-wasting effects of most diuretics with clients taking these drugs, and encourage a diet rich in high-potassium foods, as well as regular monitoring of serum potassium levels.

Assessment

Assessment data related to hypokalemia include the following:

- *Health history:* Current manifestations, including anorexia, nausea and vomiting, abdominal discomfort, muscle weakness or cramping, other symptoms; duration of symptoms and any precipitating factors such as diuretic use, prolonged vomiting or diarrhea; chronic diseases such as diabetes, hyperaldosteronism, or Cushing's syndrome; current medications.
- *Physical assessment:* Mental status; vital signs including orthostatic vitals, apical and peripheral pulses; bowel sounds, abdominal distention; muscle strength and tone.
- *Diagnostic tests:* Serum electrolytes, K^+, Na^+, and Ca^{2+} in particular, arterial pH and other ABG results, renal function tests (creatinine and BUN), ECG changes.

Nursing Diagnoses and Interventions

The effects of hypokalemia on cardiac impulse transmission and cardiac and skeletal muscle function are the highest priority nursing care focus.

MEDICATION ADMINISTRATION Hypokalemia

POTASSIUM SOURCES
Potassium acetate (Tri-K)
Potassium bicarbonate (K + Care ET)
Potassium citrate (K-Lyte)
Potassium chloride (K-Lease, Micro-K 10, Apo-K)
Potassium gluconate (Kaon Elixir, Royonate)

Potassium is rapidly absorbed from the gastrointestinal tract; potassium chloride is the agent of choice, because low chloride often accompanies low potassium. Potassium is used to prevent and/or treat hypokalemia (e.g., with parenteral nutrition and potassium-wasting diuretics, and prophylactically after major surgery).

Nursing Responsibilities
- When giving oral forms of potassium:
  a. Dilute or dissolve effervescent, soluble, or liquid potassium in fruit or vegetable juice or cold water.
  b. Chill to increase palatability.
  c. Give with food to minimize GI effects.
- When giving parenteral forms of potassium:
  a. Administer slowly.
  b. Do *not* administer undiluted.

  c. Assess injection site frequently for signs of pain and inflammation.
  d. Use an infusion control device.
- Assess for abdominal pain, distention, gastrointestinal bleeding; if present, do not administer medication. Notify healthcare provider.
- Monitor fluid intake and output.
- Assess for manifestations of hyperkalemia: weakness, feeling of heaviness in legs, mental confusion, hypotension, cardiac dysrhythmias, changes in ECG, increased serum potassium levels.

Health Education for the Client and Family
- Do not take potassium supplements if you are also taking a potassium-sparing diuretic.
- When parenteral potassium is discontinued, eat potassium-rich foods.
- Do not chew enteric-coated tablets or allow them to dissolve in the mouth; this may affect the potency and action of the medications.
- Take potassium supplements with meals.
- Do not use salt substitutes when taking potassium (most salt substitutes are potassium based).

NURSING CARE PLAN A Client with Hypokalemia

Rose Ortiz is a 72-year-old widow who lives alone, although close to her daughter's home. Ms. Ortiz has mild heart failure and is being treated with digoxin (Lanoxin) 0.125 mg, furosemide (Lasix) 40 mg PO daily, and a mildly restricted sodium diet (2 g daily). For the last several weeks, Ms. Ortiz has complained that she feels weak and sometimes faint, light-headed, and dizzy. Serum electrolyte tests ordered by her physician reveal a potassium level of 2.4 mEq/L. Potassium chloride solution (Kaochlor 10%, 20 mEq/15 mL) PO twice daily is prescribed, and Ms. Ortiz is referred to Nancy Walters, RN, for follow-up care.

ASSESSMENT

Ms. Ortiz's health history reveals that she has rigidly adhered to her sodium-restricted diet and has been compliant in taking her prescribed medications, with the exception of occasionally taking an additional "water pill" when her ankles swell. She takes a laxative every evening to ensure a daily bowel movement. She states that she is reluctant to take the potassium chloride the doctor has ordered because her neighbor complains that his potassium supplement upsets his stomach. Physical assessment findings included T 98.4, P 70, R 20, and BP 138/84. Muscle strength in her upper extremities is normal and equal; lower extremity strength is weak but equal. Sensation is normal.

DIAGNOSES

- *Risk for Injury* related to muscle weakness
- *Risk for Ineffective Health Maintenance* related to lack of knowledge about how diuretic therapy and laxative use affect potassium levels

EXPECTED OUTCOMES

- Maintain potassium level within normal limits (3.5 to 5.0 mEq/L).
- Regain normal muscle strength.
- Remain free of injury.
- Verbalize understanding of the effects of diuretic therapy and laxatives on potassium levels.

- Identify measures to avoid gastrointestinal irritation when taking oral potassium.
- Identify potassium-rich foods.

PLANNING AND IMPLEMENTATION

- Explain need to use caution when ambulating, particularly when climbing or descending stairs.
- Discuss side effects of furosemide, and explain how taking additional tablets may have contributed to hypokalemia.
- Discuss alternative measures to prevent constipation without using laxatives on a regular basis (e.g., high-fiber diet, adequate fluid intake).
- Explain purpose of the prescribed potassium and its role in reversing muscle weakness.
- Teach to take potassium supplement after breakfast and supper, diluted in 4 oz of juice or water, and to sip it slowly over a 5- to 10-minute period. Advise to call if gastric irritation occurs.
- Discuss dietary sources of potassium; provide a list of potassium-rich foods.

EVALUATION

On a follow-up visit 1 week later, Ms. Ortiz states that her muscle weakness, dizziness, and other symptoms have resolved. She is taking the prescribed drugs as directed and is using laxatives only two or three times a week. Ms. Ortiz reports that she has increased her intake of potassium-rich foods and fluids and of high-fiber foods. Her potassium level is within normal limits.

CRITICAL THINKING IN THE NURSING PROCESS

1. What is the pathophysiologic basis for Ms. Ortiz's muscle weakness and dizziness?
2. How might the chronic overuse of laxatives contribute to hypokalemia?
3. Describe the interaction of digitalis, diuretics, and potassium.
4. Develop a plan of care for Ms. Ortiz for the nursing diagnosis of *Perceived Constipation.*
   See Evaluating Your Response in Appendix C.

Decreased Cardiac Output

Hypokalemia affects the strength of cardiac contractions and can lead to dysrhythmias that further impair cardiac output. Hypokalemia also alters the response to cardiac drugs, such as digitalis and the antidysrhythmics.

- Monitor serum potassium levels, particularly in clients at risk for hypokalemia (those with excess losses due to drug therapy, gastrointestinal losses, or who are unable to consume a normal diet). Report abnormal levels to the care provider. *Potassium must be replaced daily, because the body is unable to conserve it. Either lack of intake or abnormal losses of potassium in the urine or gastric fluids can lead to hypokalemia.*
- Monitor vital signs, including orthostatic vitals and peripheral pulses. *As cardiac output falls, the pulse becomes weak and thready. Orthostatic hypotension may be noted with decreased cardiac output.*

PRACTICE ALERT

Place clients with severe hypokalemia on a cardiac monitor. Closely monitor cardiac rhythm and observe for characteristic ECG changes of hypokalemia (ST segment depression, flattened T waves, and U waves). Report rhythm changes and treat as indicated. Severe hypokalemia can cause life-threatening dysrhythmias.

- Monitor clients taking digitalis for toxicity. Monitor response to antidysrhythmic drugs. *Hypokalemia potentiates digitalis effects and increases resistance to certain antidysrhythmics.*
- Dilute intravenous potassium and administer using an electronic infusion device. In general, potassium is given no faster than 10 to 20 mEq/h. Closely monitor intravenous flow rate and response to potassium replacement. *Rapid potassium administration is dangerous and can lead to hyperkalemia and cardiac arrest.*

Activity Intolerance

Muscle cramping and weakness are common early manifestations of hypokalemia. The lower extremities are usually affected initially. This muscle weakness can cause the client to fatigue easily, particularly with activity.

■ Monitor skeletal muscle strength and tone, which are affected by moderate hypokalemia. *Increasing weakness, paresthesias, or paralysis of muscles or progression of affected muscles to include the upper extremities or trunk can indicate a further drop in serum potassium levels.*

■ Monitor respiratory rate, depth, and effort; heart rate and rhythm; and blood pressure at rest and following activity. *Tachypnea, dyspnea, tachycardia, and/or a change in blood pressure may indicate decreasing ability to tolerate activities. Report changes to the care provider.*

■ Assist with self-care activities as needed. *Increasing muscle weakness can lead to fatigue and affect the ability to meet self-care needs.*

Risk for Imbalanced Fluid Volume

■ Maintain accurate intake and output records. *Gastrointestinal fluid losses can lead to significant potassium losses.*

■ Monitor bowel sounds and abdominal distention. *Hypokalemia affects smooth muscle function and can lead to slowed peristalsis and paralytic ileus.*

Acute Pain

Discomfort is common when intravenous potassium chloride at a concentration of more than 40 mEq/L is given into a peripheral vein.

■ When possible, administer intravenous KCl through a central line. *The rapid blood flow through central veins dilutes the KCl solution, decreasing discomfort.*

■ Spread the total daily dose of KCl over 24 hours to minimize the concentration of intravenous solutions. *High concentrations of KCl are irritating to vein walls, particularly if inflammation is present.*

■ Discuss with the physician using a small amount of lidocaine prior to or with the infusion. *Both a lidocaine bolus given at the infusion site and a small amount of lidocaine in the intravenous infusion have been shown to at least partially relieve discomfort associated with concentrated potassium solutions* (Metheny, 2000).

Using NANDA, NIC, and NOC

Chart 10–2 shows links between NANDA nursing diagnoses, NIC, and NOC for a client with a potassium imbalance.

Community-Based Care

The focus in preparing the client with or at risk for hypokalemia is prevention. Discharge planning focuses on teaching self-care practices. Include the following topics when preparing the client and family for home care.

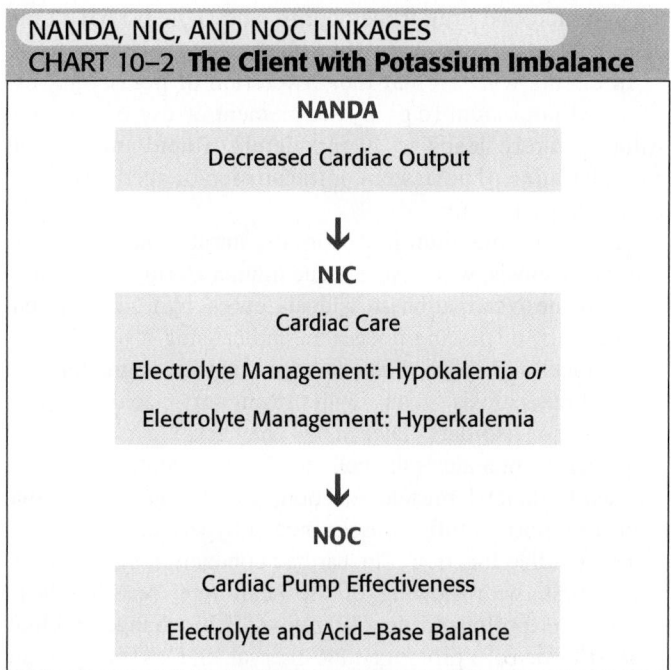

NANDA, NIC, AND NOC LINKAGES
CHART 10–2 The Client with Potassium Imbalance

NANDA

Decreased Cardiac Output

↓

NIC

Cardiac Care

Electrolyte Management: Hypokalemia *or*

Electrolyte Management: Hyperkalemia

↓

NOC

Cardiac Pump Effectiveness

Electrolyte and Acid–Base Balance

Data from *NANDA's Nursing Diagnoses: Definitions & classification 2005–2006* by NANDA International (2003), Philadelphia; *Nursing Interventions Classification (NIC)* (4th ed.) by J. M. Dochterman & G. M. Bulechek (2004), St. Louis, MO: Mosby; and *Nursing Outcomes Classification (NOC)* (3rd ed.) by S. Moorhead, M. Johnson, and M. Maas (2004), St. Louis, MO: Mosby.

■ Recommended diet, including a list of potassium-rich foods

■ Prescribed medications and potassium supplements, their use, and desired and unintended effects

■ Using salt substitutes (if recommended) to increase potassium intake; avoiding substitutes if taking a potassium supplement or potassium-sparing diuretic

■ Manifestations of potassium imbalance (hypokalemia or hyperkalemia) to report to healthcare provider

■ Recommendations for monitoring serum potassium levels

■ If taking digitalis, manifestations of digitalis toxicity to report to healthcare provider

■ Managing gastrointestinal disorders that cause potassium loss (vomiting, diarrhea, ileostomy drainage) to prevent hypokalemia.

The Client with Hyperkalemia

Hyperkalemia is an abnormally high serum potassium (greater than 5 mEq/L). Hyperkalemia can result from inadequate excretion of potassium, excessively high intake of potassium, or a shift of potassium from the intracellular to the extracellular space. *Pseudohyperkalemia* (an erroneously high serum potassium reading) can occur if the blood sample hemolyzes, releasing potassium from blood cells, before it is analyzed. Hyperkalemia affects neuromuscular and cardiac function.

Pathophysiology

Impaired renal excretion of potassium is a primary cause of hyperkalemia. Untreated renal failure, adrenal insufficiency (e.g., Addison's disease or inadequate aldosterone production), and medications (such as potassium-sparing diuretics, the antimicrobial drug trimethoprim, and some NSAIDs) impair potassium excretion by the kidneys.

In clients with normal renal excretion of potassium, excess oral potassium (e.g., by supplement or use of salt substitutes) rarely leads to hyperkalemia. Rapid intravenous administration of potassium or transfusion of aged blood can lead to hyperkalemia.

A shift of potassium ions from the intracellular space can occur in acidosis, with severe tissue trauma, during chemotherapy, and due to starvation. In acidosis, excess hydrogen ions enter the cells, displacing potassium and causing it to shift into the extracellular space. The extent of this shift is greater with metabolic acidosis than with respiratory acidosis (see "Acid–Base Disorders" later in this chapter).

Hyperkalemia alters the cell membrane potential, affecting the heart, skeletal muscle function, and the gastrointestinal tract. The most harmful consequence of hyperkalemia is its effect on cardiac function. The cardiac conduction system is affected first, with slowing of the heart rate, possible heart blocks, and prolonged depolarization. ECG changes include peaked T waves, a prolonged PR interval, and widening of the QRS complex (see Figure 10–11). Ventricular dysrhythmias develop, and cardiac arrest may occur. Severe hyperkalemia decreases the strength of myocardial contractions.

Skeletal muscles become weak, and paralysis may occur with very high serum potassium levels. Hyperkalemia causes smooth muscle hyperactivity, leading to gastrointestinal disturbances.

The seriousness of hyperkalemia is based on the serum potassium (K^+) level and ECG changes.

- *Mild hyperkalemia:* serum K^+ between 5 and 6.5 mEq/L; ECG changes limited to peaked T wave
- *Moderate hyperkalemia:* serum K^+ between 6.5 and 8 mEq/L; ECG changes limited to peaked T wave
- *Severe hyperkalemia:* serum K^+ greater than 8 mEq/L; ECG shows absent P waves and widened QRS pattern.

Manifestations

The manifestations of hyperkalemia result from its effects on the heart, skeletal, and smooth muscles. Early manifestations include diarrhea, colic (abdominal cramping), anxiety, paresthesias, irritability, and muscle tremors and twitching. As serum potassium levels increase, muscle weakness develops, progressing to flaccid paralysis. The lower extremities are affected first, progressing to the trunk and upper extremities. The heart rate may be slow (bradycardia) and irregular. The ECG shows T-wave changes and, at high serum potassium levels, widening of the QRS complex and absence of P waves.

INTERDISCIPLINARY CARE

The management of hyperkalemia focuses on returning the serum potassium level to normal by treating the underlying cause and avoiding additional potassium intake. The choice of therapy for existing hyperkalemia is based on the severity of the hyperkalemia.

Diagnosis

The following laboratory and diagnostic tests may be ordered:

- *Serum electrolytes* show a serum potassium level greater than 5.0 mEq/L. Low calcium and sodium levels may increase the effects of hyperkalemia; therefore, these electrolytes are usually measured as well.
- *ABGs* are measured to determine if acidosis is present.
- An *ECG* is obtained and *continuous ECG monitoring* is instituted to evaluate the effects of hyperkalemia on cardiac conduction and rhythm.

Medications

Medications are administered to lower the serum potassium and to stabilize the conduction system of the heart. For moderate to severe hyperkalemia, calcium gluconate is given intravenously to counter the effects of hyperkalemia on the cardiac conduction system. While the effect of calcium gluconate lasts only for 1 hour, it allows time to initiate measures to lower serum potassium levels. To rapidly lower these levels, regular insulin and 50 g of glucose are administered. Insulin and glucose promote potassium uptake by the cells, shifting potassium out of ECF. In some cases, a β_2-agonist such as albuterol may be given by nebulizer to temporarily push potassium into the cells. Sodium bicarbonate may be given to treat acidosis. As the pH returns toward normal, hydrogen ions are released from the cells and potassium returns into the cells.

To remove potassium from the body, sodium polystyrene sulfonate (Kayexalate), a resin that binds potassium in the gastrointestinal tract, may be administered orally or rectally. If renal function is normal, diuretics such as furosemide are given to promote potassium excretion. Commonly prescribed drugs, their actions, and nursing implications are listed in the Medication Administration box on the following page.

Dialysis

When renal function is severely limited, either peritoneal dialysis or hemodialysis may be implemented to remove excess potassium. These measures are invasive and typically used only when other measures are ineffective. See Chapter 29 ∞ for more information about dialysis.

 NURSING CARE

Nursing care focuses related to hyperkalemia include identifying clients at risk, preventing hyperkalemia, and addressing problems resulting from the systemic effects of hyperkalemia. A Nursing Care Plan: A Client with Hyperkalemia is found on page 226.

Health Promotion

Clients at the greatest risk for developing hyperkalemia include those taking potassium supplements (prescribed or over-the-counter), using potassium-sparing diuretics or salt substitutes, and experiencing renal failure. Athletes participating in competition sports such as body building and using anabolic steroids, muscle-building compounds, or "energy drinks" also may be at risk for hyperkalemia.

MEDICATION ADMINISTRATION Hyperkalemia

DIURETICS

Potassium-wasting diuretics, such as furosemide (Lasix), may be used to enhance renal excretion of potassium.

Nursing Responsibilities
- Monitor serum electrolytes.
- Monitor and record weight at regular intervals under standard conditions (same time of day, balanced scale, same clothing).
- Monitor intake and output.

INSULIN, HYPERTONIC DEXTROSE, AND SODIUM BICARBONATE

Insulin, hypertonic dextrose (10% to 50%), and sodium bicarbonate are used in the emergency treatment of moderate to severe hyperkalemia. Insulin promotes the movement of potassium into the cell, and glucose prevents hypoglycemia. The onset of action of insulin and hypertonic dextrose occurs within 30 minutes and is effective for approximately 4 to 6 hours.

Sodium bicarbonate elevates the serum pH; potassium is moved into the cell in exchange for hydrogen ion. Sodium bicarbonate is particularly useful in the client with metabolic acidosis. Onset of effects occurs within 15 to 30 minutes and is effective for approximately 2 hours.

Nursing Responsibilities
- Administer intravenous insulin and dextrose over prescribed interval of time using an infusion pump.
- Administer sodium bicarbonate as prescribed. It may be administered as an intravenous bolus or added to a dextrose-in-water solution and given by infusion.
- In clients receiving sodium bicarbonate, monitor for sodium overload, particularly in clients with hypernatremia, heart failure, and renal failure.

- Monitor the ECG pattern closely.
- Monitor serum electrolytes (K^+, Na^+, Ca^{2+}, Mg^{2+}) frequently during treatment.

CALCIUM GLUCONATE AND CALCIUM CHLORIDE

Intravenous calcium gluconate or calcium chloride is used as a temporary emergency measure to counteract the toxic effects of potassium on myocardial conduction and function.

Nursing Responsibilities
- Closely monitor the ECG of the client receiving intravenous calcium, particularly for bradycardia.
- Calcium should be used cautiously in clients receiving digitalis, because calcium increases the cardiotonic effects of digitalis and may precipitate digitalis toxicity, leading to dysrhythmias.

SODIUM POLYSTYRENE SULFONATE (KAYEXALATE) AND SORBITOL

Sodium polystyrene sulfonate (Kayexalate) is used to treat moderate or severe hyperkalemia. Categorized as a cation exchange resin, Kayexalate exchanges sodium or calcium for potassium in the large intestine. Sorbitol is given with Kayexalate to promote bowel elimination. Kayexalate and sorbitol may be administered orally, through a nasogastric tube, or rectally as a retention enema. The usual dosage is 20 g three or four times a day with 20 mL of 70% sorbitol solution.

Nursing Responsibilities
- Because Kayexalate contains sodium, monitor clients with heart failure and edema closely for water retention.
- Monitor serum electrolytes (K^+, Na^+, Ca^{2+}, Mg^{2+}) frequently during therapy.
- Restrict sodium intake in clients who are unable to tolerate increased sodium load (e.g., those with CHF or hypertension).

Teach all clients to carefully read food and dietary supplement labels. Discuss the importance of taking prescribed potassium supplements as ordered, and not increasing the dose unless prescribed by the care provider. Advise clients taking a potassium supplement or potassium-sparing diuretic to avoid salt substitutes, which usually contain potassium. Discuss the importance of maintaining an adequate fluid intake (unless a fluid restriction has been prescribed) to maintain renal function to eliminate potassium from the body.

Assessment

Assessment data related to hyperkalemia include the following:
- *Health history:* Current manifestations, including numbness and tingling, nausea and vomiting, abdominal cramping, muscle weakness, palpitations; duration of symptoms and any precipitating factors such as use of salt substitutes, potassium supplements, or reduced urine output; chronic diseases such as renal failure or endocrine disorders; current medications.
- *Physical assessment:* Apical and peripheral pulses; bowel sounds; muscle strength in upper and lower extremities; ECG pattern.
- *Diagnostic tests:* Serum electrolytes, potassium, sodium, and calcium in particular; ABGs; digitalis levels; ECG.

Nursing Diagnoses and Interventions

The effects of excess potassium on the electrical conduction and contractility of the heart are the highest priority for nursing care, particularly when the serum potassium level is 6.5 mEq/L or higher.

Risk for Decreased Cardiac Output

Hyperkalemia affects depolarization of the atria and ventricles of the heart. Severe hyperkalemia can cause dysrhythmias with ventricular fibrillation and cardiac arrest. The cardiac effects of hyperkalemia are more pronounced when the serum potassium level rises rapidly. Low serum sodium and calcium levels, high serum magnesium levels, and acidosis contribute to the adverse effects of hyperkalemia on the heart muscle.

PRACTICE ALERT

Monitor the ECG pattern for development of peaked, narrow T waves, prolongation of the PR interval, depression of the ST segment, widened QRS interval, and loss of the P wave. Notify the physician of changes. Progressive ECG changes from a peaked T wave to loss of the P wave and widening of the QRS complex indicate an increasing risk of dysrhythmias and cardiac arrest.

NURSING CARE PLAN A Client with Hyperkalemia

Montigue Longacre, a 51-year-old African-American male, has end-stage renal failure. He arrives at the emergency clinic complaining of shortness of breath on exertion and extreme weakness.

ASSESSMENT

Mr. Longacre tells the nurse, Janet Allen, RN, that he normally receives dialysis three times a week. He missed his last treatment, however, to attend his father's funeral. During the last several days, he has eaten a number of fresh oranges he received as a gift. Physical assessment findings include T 99.2, P 100, R 28, BP 168/96, 2+ pretibial edema, and a 6-lb (3.6-kg) weight gain since his last hemodialysis treatment 4 days ago. Laboratory and diagnostic tests show the following abnormal results.

- K^+ 6.5 mEq/L (normal 3.5 to 5 mEq/L)
- BUN 118 mg/dL (normal 7 to 18 mg/dL)
- Creatinine 14 mg/dL (normal 0.7 to 1.3 mg/dL)
- HCO_3^- 17 mEq/L (normal 22 to 26 mEq/L)
- Peaked T wave noted on ECG.

Mr. Longacre is placed on continuous ECG monitoring, and the physician prescribes hemodialysis. As an interim measure to lower the serum potassium, the physician prescribes $D_{50}W$ (25 g of dextrose), one ampule, to be administered intravenously with 10 units of regular insulin over 30 minutes.

DIAGNOSES

- *Activity Intolerance* related to skeletal muscle weakness
- *Risk for Decreased Cardiac Output* related to hyperkalemia
- *Risk for Ineffective Health Maintenance* related to inadequate knowledge of recommended diet
- *Excess Fluid Volume* related to renal failure

EXPECTED OUTCOMES

- Gradually resume usual physical activities.
- Maintain serum potassium level within normal range.

- Verbalize causes of hyperkalemia, the importance of hemodialysis treatments as scheduled, and the role of diet in preventing hyperkalemia.

PLANNING AND IMPLEMENTATION

- Monitor intake and output.
- Monitor serum potassium and ECG closely during treatment.
- Teach causes of hyperkalemia and the relationship between hemodialysis and hyperkalemia.
- Discuss the importance of avoiding foods high in potassium to prevent or control hyperkalemia.

EVALUATION

Following emergency treatment and hemodialysis, Mr. Longacre's ECG and serum potassium level have returned to normal. His muscle strength has returned to near normal, and he verbalizes an understanding of his prescribed hemodialysis regimen. Janet Allen provides verbal and written information about hyperkalemia, the importance of complying with the hemodialysis regimen, and the importance of limiting intake of dietary sources of potassium in renal failure. She also furnishes a list of foods high in potassium and cautions against using potassium-containing salt substitutes and nonprescription drugs.

CRITICAL THINKING IN THE NURSING PROCESS

1. What information given by Mr. Longacre indicated that he might be experiencing hyperkalemia?
2. Why was continuous ECG monitoring instituted as an emergency measure?
3. What additional emergency measures might have been instituted if Mr. Longacre's serum potassium level had been 8.5 mEq/L and his ECG had showed changes in impulse conduction?
4. Develop a care plan for Mr. Longacre for the nursing diagnosis of *Anxiety*.

See Evaluating Your Response in Appendix C.

- Closely monitor the response to intravenous calcium gluconate, particularly in clients taking digitalis. *Calcium increases the risk of digitalis toxicity.*

Risk for Activity Intolerance

Both hypokalemia (low serum potassium levels) and hyperkalemia (high serum potassium levels) affect neuromuscular activity and the function of cardiac, smooth, and skeletal muscles. Hyperkalemia can cause muscle weakness and even paralysis.

- Monitor skeletal muscle strength and tone. *Increasing weakness, muscle paralysis, or progression of affected muscles to affect the upper extremities or trunk can indicate increasing serum potassium levels.*
- Monitor respiratory rate and depth. Regularly assess lung sounds. *Muscle weakness due to hyperkalemia can impair ventilation. In addition, medications such as sodium bicarbonate or sodium polystyrene sulfonate can cause fluid retention and pulmonary edema in clients with preexisting cardiovascular disease.*

- Assist with self-care activities as needed. *Increasing muscle weakness can lead to fatigue and affect the ability to meet self-care needs.*

Risk for Imbalanced Fluid Volume

Renal failure is a major cause of hyperkalemia. Clients with renal failure also are at risk for fluid retention and other electrolyte imbalances.

- Closely monitor serum potassium, BUN, and serum creatinine. Notify the physician if serum potassium level is greater than 5 mEq/L, or if serum creatinine and BUN levels are increasing. *Serum creatinine and BUN are the primary indicators of renal function. Levels of these substances rise rapidly in acute renal failure, more slowly in chronic renal failure (see Chapter 29 ∞).*
- Maintain accurate intake and output records. Report an imbalance of 24-hour totals and/or urine output less than 30 mL/hour. *Oliguria (scant urine) or anuria (no urine output) may indicate renal failure and an increased risk for hyperkalemia and fluid volume excess.*

- Monitor clients receiving sodium bicarbonate for fluid volume excess. *Increased sodium from injection of a hypertonic sodium bicarbonate solution can cause a shift of water into the extracellular space.*
- Monitor clients receiving cation exchange resins and sorbitol for fluid volume excess. *The resin exchanges potassium for sodium or calcium in the bowel. Excessive sodium and water retention may occur.*

Community-Based Care

Preventing future episodes of hyperkalemia is the focus when preparing the client for home care. Include the family, a significant other, or a caregiver when teaching the following topics:

- Recommended diet and any restrictions including salt substitutes and foods high in potassium
- Medications to be avoided, including over-the-counter and fitness supplements
- Follow-up appointments for lab work and evaluation.

CALCIUM IMBALANCE

Calcium is one of the most abundant ions in the body. The normal adult total serum calcium concentration is 8.5 to 10.0 mg/dL.

Overview of Normal Calcium Balance

Calcium is obtained from dietary sources, although only about 20% of the calcium ingested is absorbed into the blood. The remainder is excreted in feces. Extracellular calcium is excreted by the kidneys. Approximately 99% of the total calcium in the body is bound to phosphorus to form the minerals in bones and teeth. The remaining 1% is in extracellular fluid. About half of this extracellular calcium is ionized (free); it is this ionized calcium that is physiologically active. The remaining extracellular calcium is bound to protein or other ions.

Ionized calcium is essential to a number of processes:

- Stabilizing cell membranes
- Regulating muscle contraction and relaxation
- Maintaining cardiac function
- Blood clotting.

Serum calcium levels are regulated by the interaction of three hormones: parathyroid hormone (PTH), calcitonin, and calcitriol (a metabolite of vitamin D). When serum calcium levels fall, the parathyroid glands secrete PTH, which mobilizes skeletal calcium stores, increases calcium absorption in the intestines, and promotes calcium reabsorption by the kidneys (Figure 10–12 ■). Calcitriol facilitates this process by stimulating calcium release from the bones, absorption in the intestines, and reabsorption by the kidneys. Calcitonin is secreted by the thyroid gland in response to high serum calcium levels. Its effect on serum calcium levels is the opposite of PTH: It inhibits the movement of calcium out of bone, reduces intestinal absorption of calcium, and promotes calcium excretion by the kidneys.

Serum calcium levels are also affected by acid–base balance. When hydrogen ion concentration falls and the pH rises (alkalosis), more calcium is bound to protein. While the total

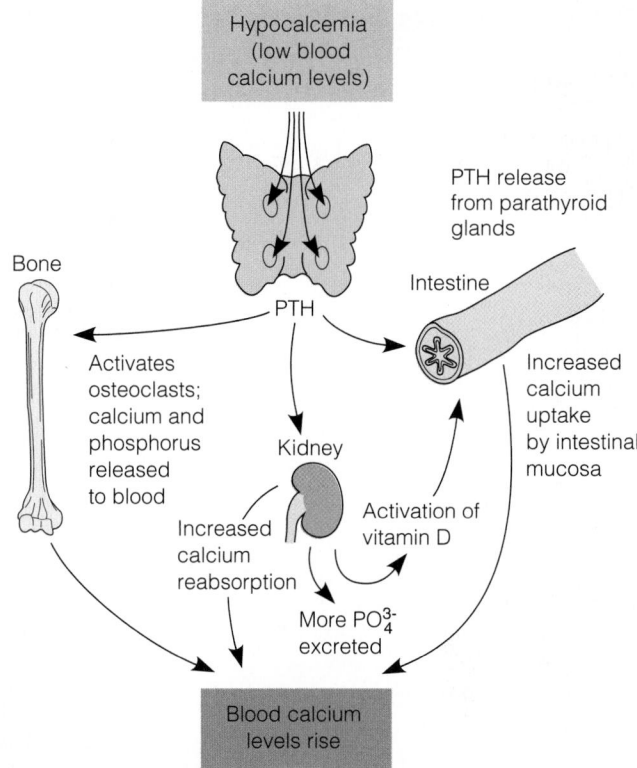

Figure 10–12 ■ Low calcium levels (hypocalcemia) trigger the release of parathyroid hormone (PTH), increasing calcium ion levels through stimulation of bones, kidneys, and intestines.

serum calcium remains unchanged, less calcium is available in the ionized, active form. Conversely, when hydrogen ion concentration increases and the pH falls (acidosis), calcium is released from protein, making more ionized calcium available.

Finally, the total amount of calcium in blood plasma fluctuates with plasma protein levels, particularly the albumin level. As the albumin level falls, the total amount of plasma calcium declines. Table 10–7 summarizes the causes and manifestations of calcium imbalances.

The Client with Hypocalcemia

Hypocalcemia is a total serum calcium level of less than 8.5 mg/dL. Hypocalcemia can result from decreased total body calcium stores or low levels of extracellular calcium with normal amounts of calcium stored in bone. The systemic effects of hypocalcemia are caused by decreased levels of ionized calcium in extracellular fluid.

Risk Factors

Certain populations of people are at greater risk for hypocalcemia: people who have had a parathyroidectomy (removal of the parathyroid glands), older adults (especially women), people with lactose intolerance, and those with alcoholism. Older adults often consume less milk and milk products (good sources of calcium) and may have less exposure to the sun (a source of vitamin D). Older adults also may be less active, promoting calcium loss from bones. They are more likely to be

TABLE 10-7 Causes and Manifestations of Calcium Imbalances

IMBALANCE	CAUSES	MANIFESTATIONS
Hypocalcemia Serum calcium < 8.5 mg/dL or 4.3 mEq/L Critical value < 6.0 mg/dL	■ Parathyroidectomy or neck surgery ■ Acute pancreatitis ■ Inadequate dietary intake ■ Lack of sun exposure ■ Lack of weight-bearing exercise ■ Drugs: loop diuretics, calcitonin ■ Hypomagnesemia, alcohol abuse ■ Acute renal failure 　with hyperphosphatemia	Neuromuscular ■ Tetany 　■ Paresthesias 　■ Muscle spasms 　■ Positive Chvostek's sign 　■ Positive Trousseau's sign 　■ Laryngospasm 　■ Seizures ■ Anxiety, confusion, psychoses Cardiovascular ■ Decreased cardiac output ■ Hypotension ■ Dysrhythmias Gastrointestinal ■ Abdominal cramping ■ Diarrhea
Hypercalcemia Serum calcium >10 mg/dL or 5.3 mEq/L Critical value >13.0 mg/dL	■ Hyperparathyroidism ■ Some cancers ■ Prolonged immobilization ■ Paget's disease ■ Excess milk or antacid intake ■ Chronic renal failure 　with associated 　hyperparathyroidism	Neuromuscular ■ Muscle weakness, fatigue ■ Decreased deep tendon reflexes Behavioral ■ Personality changes ■ Altered mental status ■ Decreasing level of consciousness Gastrointestinal ■ Abdominal pain ■ Constipation ■ Anorexia, nausea, vomiting Cardiovascular ■ Dysrhythmias ■ Hypertension Renal ■ Polyuria, thirst

taking drugs that interfere with calcium absorption or promote calcium excretion (e.g., furosemide). Older women are at particular risk after menopause because of reduced estrogen levels. Intolerance to lactose (found in milk and milk products) causes diarrhea and often limits the intake of milk and milk products, leading to possible calcium deficiency. Ethanol, or drinking alcohol, has a direct effect on calcium balance, reduces its intestinal absorption, and interferes with other processes involved in regulating serum calcium levels.

Pathophysiology

Common causes of hypocalcemia are hypoparathyroidism (see Chapter 19 ∞) resulting from surgery (parathyroidectomy, thyroidectomy, radical neck dissection) and acute pancreatitis. In the client who has undergone surgery, symptoms of hypocalcemia usually occur within the first 24 to 48 hours, but may be delayed.

PRACTICE ALERT
Carefully monitor clients who have undergone neck surgery for manifestations of hypocalcemia. Check serum calcium levels, and report changes to the care provider.

Additional causes of hypocalcemia include other electrolyte imbalances (such as hypomagnesemia or hyperphosphatemia), alkalosis, malabsorption disorders that interfere with calcium absorption in the bowel, and inadequate vitamin D (due to lack of sun exposure or malabsorption). Hyperphosphatemia often occurs in acute renal failure, with reciprocal hypocalcemia. Massive transfusion of banked blood also can lead to hypocalcemia. Citrate is added to blood to prevent clotting and as a preservative. When blood is administered faster than the liver can metabolize the citrate, it can bind with calcium, temporarily removing ionized calcium from circulation. Many drugs increase the risk for hypocalcemia, including loop diuretics (such as furosemide), anticonvulsants (such as phenytoin and phenobarbital), phosphates (including phosphate enemas), and drugs that lower serum magnesium levels (such as cisplatin and gentamicin) (Metheny, 2000).

Extracellular calcium acts to stabilize neuromuscular cell membranes. This effect is reduced in hypocalcemia, increasing neuromuscular irritability. The threshold of excitation of sensory nerve fibers is lowered as well, leading to paresthesias (altered sensation). The nervous system becomes more excitable, and muscle spasms develop. In the heart, this change in cell membranes can lead to dysrhythmias such as ventricular tachycardia and cardiac arrest. Hypocalcemia decreases the contractility of cardiac muscle fibers, leading to decreased cardiac output.

Manifestations and Complications

The most serious manifestations of hypocalcemia are **tetany** (tonic muscular spasms) and convulsions. Numbness and tingling around the mouth (circumoral) and in the hands and feet develop. Muscle spasms of the face and extremities occur, and deep tendon reflexes become hyperactive. Chvostek's sign, contraction of the facial muscles produced by tapping the facial nerve in front of the ear (Figure 10–13A ■), and Trousseau's sign, carpal spasm induced by inflating a blood pressure cuff on the upper arm to above systolic blood pressure for 2 to 5 minutes (Figure 10–13B), indicate increased neuromuscular excitability in clients without obvious symptoms.

A

B

Figure 10–13 ■ *A,* Positive Chvostek's sign. *B,* Positive Trousseau's sign.

Tetany can cause bronchial muscle spasms, simulating an asthma attack, and visceral muscle spasms, producing acute abdominal pain. Cardiovascular manifestations include hypotension, possible bradycardia (slow heart rate), and ventricular dysrhythmias.

Serious complications of hypocalcemia include airway obstruction and possible respiratory arrest from laryngospasm, ventricular dysrhythmias and cardiac arrest, heart failure, and convulsions.

INTERDISCIPLINARY CARE

Management of hypocalcemia is directed toward restoring normal calcium balance and correcting the underlying cause.

Diagnosis

The following laboratory and diagnostic tests may be ordered when hypocalcemia is known or suspected. Measurements include:

- *Total serum calcium,* the amount of ionized (active) calcium available, usually is estimated. In critically ill clients, however, *ionized calcium* may be directly measured using ion-selective electrodes. Direct measurement of ionized calcium requires special handling of the blood specimen, including placing the specimen on ice and analyzing it immediately.
- *Serum albumin,* because the albumin level affects serum calcium results. When the albumin level is low (hypoalbuminemia), the amount of ionized calcium may remain normal even though the total calcium level is low.
- *Serum magnesium,* because hypocalcemia is often associated with hypomagnesemia (serum magnesium < 1.6 mg/dL). In this case, normal magnesium levels must be restored to correct the hypocalcemia.
- *Serum phosphate;* hyperphosphatemia (serum phosphate > 4.5 mg/dL) can lead to hypocalcemia because of the inverse relationship between phosphorus and calcium (as phosphate levels rise, calcium levels fall).
- *Parathyroid hormone (PTH),* to identify the possible diagnoses of hyperparathyroidism.
- An *ECG,* to evaluate the effects of hypocalcemia on the heart, such as a prolonged ST segment.

Medications

Hypocalcemia is treated with oral or intravenous calcium. The client with severe hypocalcemia is treated with intravenous calcium to prevent life-threatening problems such as airway obstruction. The most common intravenous calcium preparations include calcium chloride and calcium gluconate. Although calcium chloride contains more elemental calcium than calcium gluconate, it also is more irritating to the veins and may cause venous sclerosis (hardening of the vein walls) if given into a peripheral vein. Intravenous calcium preparations can cause necrosis and sloughing of tissue if they extravasate into subcutaneous tissue. Rapid drug administration can lead to bradycardia and possible cardiac arrest due to overcorrection of hypocalcemia with resulting hypercalcemia. See the Medication Administration box on the next page for further information about calcium administration.

MEDICATION ADMINISTRATION   Calcium Salts

CALCIUM SALTS
Calcium carbonate (BioCal, Calsam, Caltrate, OsCal, Tums, others)
Calcium chloride
Calcium citrate (Citrical)
Calcium glubionate
Calcium gluceptate
Calcium gluconate (Calcinate)
Calcium lactate

Calcium salts are given to increase calcium levels when there is a deficit (a total body deficit or inadequate levels of extracellular calcium). Calcium is necessary to maintain bone structure and for multiple physiologic processes including neuromuscular and cardiac function as well as blood coagulation. In the presence of vitamin D, calcium is well absorbed from the gastrointestinal tract. Severe hypocalcemia is treated with intravenous calcium preparations.

Nursing Responsibilities
Oral calcium salts:
- Administer 1 to 1.5 hours after meals and at bedtime.
- Give calcium tablets with a full glass of water.

Intravenous calcium salts:
- Assess IV site for patency. Do not administer calcium if there is a risk of leakage into the tissues.
- May be given by slow IV push (dilute with sterile normal saline for injection prior to administering) or added to compatible parenteral fluids such as NS, lactated Ringer's solution, or D_5W.
- Administer into the largest available vein; use a central line if available.
- Do not administer with bicarbonate or phosphate.
- Continuously monitor ECG when administering IV calcium to clients taking digitalis due to increased risk of digitalis toxicity.
- Frequently monitor serum calcium levels and response to therapy.

Health Education for the Client and Family
- Take calcium tablets with a full glass of water 1 to 2 hours after meals. Do not take with food or milk. If possible, do not take within 1 to 2 hours of other medications.
- Maintain adequate vitamin D intake through diet or exposure to the sun to promote calcium absorption.
- Calcium carbonate can cause constipation. Eat a high-fiber diet and maintain a generous fluid intake to prevent constipation.

Oral calcium preparations (calcium carbonate, calcium gluconate, or calcium lactate) are used to treat chronic, asymptomatic hypocalcemia. Calcium supplements may be combined with vitamin D, or vitamin D may be given alone to increase gastrointestinal absorption of calcium.

Nutrition
A diet high in calcium-rich foods may be recommended for clients with chronic hypocalcemia or with low total body stores of calcium. Box 10–7 lists foods that are high in calcium.

NURSING CARE

Health Promotion
Because of the large stores of calcium in bones, most healthy adults have a very low risk of developing hypocalcemia. A deficit of total body calcium is often associated with aging, however, increasing the risk of osteoporosis, fractures, and disability. Women have a higher risk for developing osteoporosis than men due to lower bone density and hormonal influences.

BOX 10–7 Foods High in Calcium

■ Cottage cheese	■ Canned sardines and salmon
■ Cheese	■ Rhubarb
■ Milk	■ Broccoli
■ Cream	■ Collard greens
■ Yogurt	■ Soy flour
■ Ice cream	■ Spinach
■ Molasses	■ Tofu

Teach women of all ages the importance of maintaining adequate calcium intake through diet and, as needed, calcium supplements. Stress the relationship between weight-bearing exercise and bone density, and encourage women to engage in a regular aerobic and weight-training exercise regime. Discuss hormone replacement therapy and its potential benefits during and after menopause. See Chapter 42 ∞ for more information about osteoporosis.

Assessment
Assessment data related to hypocalcemia include the following:
- *Health history:* Current manifestations, including numbness and tingling around mouth and of hands and feet, abdominal pain, shortness of breath; acute or chronic diseases such as pancreatitis, liver or kidney disease; current medications.
- *Physical assessment:* Muscle spasms; deep tendon reflexes; Chvostek's sign and Trousseau's sign; respiratory rate and depth; vital signs and apical pulse; heart rate and rhythm; presence of convulsions.
- *Diagnostic tests:* Serum electrolytes (calcium, magnesium, phosphate, and potassium in particular), serum albumin, thyroid and parathyroid hormone levels; ECG.

Nursing Diagnoses and Interventions
The effect of hypocalcemia on neuromuscular irritability, with the risk for muscle spasm and convulsions, is the highest priority for nursing care of the client.

Risk for Injury
The client with hypocalcemia is at risk for injury from possible laryngospasm, cardiac dysrhythmias, or convulsions. In addition, too rapid administration of intravenous calcium or ex-

travasation of the medication into subcutaneous tissues can lead to injury.

- Frequently monitor airway and respiratory status. Report changes such as respiratory **stridor** (a high-pitched, harsh inspiratory sound indicative of upper airway obstruction) or increased respiratory rate or effort to the physician. *These changes may indicate laryngeal spasm due to tetany.*

PRACTICE ALERT
Laryngeal spasm is a respiratory emergency, requiring immediate intervention to maintain ventilation and gas exchange.

- Monitor cardiovascular status including heart rate and rhythm, blood pressure, and peripheral pulses. *Hypocalcemia decreases myocardial contractility, causing reduced cardiac output and hypotension. It also can cause bradycardia or ventricular dysrhythmias. Cardiac arrest may occur in severe hypocalcemia.*
- Continuously monitor ECG in clients receiving intravenous calcium preparations, especially if the client also is taking digitalis. *Rapid administration of calcium salts can lead to hypercalcemia and cardiac dysrhythmias. Calcium administration increases the risk of digitalis toxicity and resultant dysrhythmias.*
- Provide a quiet environment. Institute seizure precautions such as raising the side rails and keeping an airway at bedside. *A quiet environment reduces central nervous system stimuli and the risk of convulsions in the client with tetany.*

Community-Based Care

In preparing the client with hypocalcemia for discharge and home care, consider the circumstances leading to low serum calcium levels. Discuss risk factors for hypocalcemia specific to the client, and provide information about managing these risk factors to avoid future episodes of hypocalcemia. Teach about prescribed medications, including calcium supplements. Provide a list of foods high in calcium, as well as sources of vitamin D if recommended. Discuss symptoms to report to the care provider, and stress the importance of follow-up care as scheduled.

The Client with Hypercalcemia

Hypercalcemia is a serum calcium value greater than 10.0 mg/dL. Excess ionized calcium in ECF can have serious widespread effects.

Pathophysiology

Hypercalcemia usually results from increased resorption of calcium from the bones. The two most common causes of bone resorption are hyperparathyroidism and malignancies. In hyperparathyroidism, excess PTH is produced. This causes calcium to be released from bones, as well as increased calcium absorption in the intestines and retention of calcium by the kidneys. Hypercalcemia is a common complication of malignancies. It may develop as a result of bone destruction by the tumor or due to hormone-like substances produced by the tumor itself. Prolonged immobility and lack of weight bearing

also cause increased resorption of bone with calcium release into extracellular fluids. Self-limiting hypercalcemia also may follow successful kidney transplant. Levels of parathyroid hormone may be altered in chronic renal failure, leading to increased serum calcium levels.

Increased intestinal absorption of calcium also can lead to hypercalcemia. This may result from excess vitamin D, overuse of calcium-containing antacids, or excessive milk ingestion. Renal failure and some drugs such as thiazide diuretics and lithium can interfere with elimination of calcium by the kidneys, causing high serum calcium levels.

The effects of hypercalcemia largely depend on the degree of serum calcium elevation and the length of time over which it develops. In general, higher serum calcium levels are associated with more serious effects. Calcium has a stabilizing effect on the neuromuscular junction; hypercalcemia decreases neuromuscular excitability, leading to muscle weakness and depressed deep tendon reflexes. Gastrointestinal motility is reduced as well. In the heart, calcium exerts an effect similar to digitalis (see Chapter 32 ∞), strengthening contractions and reducing the heart rate. Hypercalcemia affects the conduction system of the heart, leading to bradycardia and heart blocks. The ability of the kidneys to concentrate urine is impaired by hypercalcemia, causing excess sodium and water loss and increased thirst.

Extremely high serum calcium levels affect mental status. This is thought to be due to increased calcium in cerebrospinal fluid. Behavioral effects range from personality changes to confusion, impaired memory, and acute psychoses.

Manifestations and Complications

Manifestations of hypercalcemia relate to its effects on neuromuscular activity, the central nervous system, the cardiovascular system, and the kidneys. Decreased neuromuscular excitability causes muscle weakness and fatigue, as well as gastrointestinal manifestations such as anorexia, nausea, vomiting, and constipation. Central nervous system (CNS) effects may include confusion, lethargy, behavior or personality changes, and coma. Cardiovascular effects include dysrhythmias, ECG changes, and possible hypertension. Hypercalcemia causes polyuria and, as a result, increased thirst.

Complications of hypercalcemia can affect several different organ systems. Peptic ulcer disease may develop due to increased gastric acid secretion. Pancreatitis can occur as a result of calcium deposits in pancreatic ducts. Excess calcium can precipitate out of urine to form kidney stones. Hypercalcemic crisis, an acute increase in the serum calcium level, can lead to cardiac arrest.

INTERDISCIPLINARY CARE

The management of hypercalcemia focuses on correcting the underlying cause and reducing the serum calcium level. Treatment is particularly important in clients who have one or more of the following: serum calcium levels greater than 12 mg/dL, overt symptoms of hypercalcemia, compromised renal function, and inability to maintain an adequate fluid intake.

Diagnosis

The laboratory and diagnostic tests that may be ordered and the resultant findings are as follows:

- *Serum electrolytes* show a total serum calcium greater than 10.0 mg/dL.
- *Serum PTH levels* are measured to identify or rule out hyperparathyroidism as the cause of hypercalcemia.
- *ECG* changes in hypercalcemia include a shortened QT interval, shortened and depressed ST segment, and widened T wave. Bradycardia or heart block may be identified on the ECG.
- *Bone density scans* may be done to monitor bone resorption and the effects of treatment measures on mineralization of bone.

Medications

Measures to promote calcium elimination by the kidneys and reduce calcium resorption from bone are used to treat hypercalcemia. In acute hypercalcemia, intravenous fluids are given (see "Fluid Management" section that follows) with a loop diuretic such as furosemide to promote elimination of excess calcium. Calcitonin, which promotes the uptake of calcium into bones, also may be used to rapidly lower serum calcium levels.

A number of drugs that inhibit bone resorption are available. The bisphosphonates (pamidronate and etidronate) are commonly used to treat hypercalcemia associated with malignancies. These drugs also are used to prevent and treat osteoporosis. Nursing implications for calcitonin and bisphosphonate drugs are presented in the Medication Administration boxes in Chapter 42 ∞. When a bisphosphonate drug is ineffective to correct hypercalcemia, mithramycin, a chemotherapeutic agent, may be used.

Rapid reversal of hypercalcemia in emergency situations may be accomplished by intravenous administration of sodium phosphate or potassium phosphate. Calcium binds to phosphate, thus decreasing serum calcium levels. Paradoxically, complications of this therapy can include fatal hypocalcemia resulting from binding of the ionized calcium and soft tissue calcifications.

Other drug therapies include the use of intravenous plicamycin (Mithracin) to inhibit bone resorption. Glucocorticoids (cortisone), which compete with vitamin D, and a low-calcium diet may be prescribed to decrease gastrointestinal absorption of calcium, inhibit bone resorption, and to increase urinary calcium excretion. Also, calcitonin may be prescribed to decrease skeletal mobilization of calcium and phosphorus and to increase renal output of calcium and phosphorus. See Chapter 19 ∞ for more information about and nursing implications of glucocorticoid therapy.

Fluid Management

Intravenous fluids, usually isotonic saline, are administered to clients with severe hypercalcemia to restore vascular volume and promote renal excretion of calcium. Isotonic saline is used because sodium excretion is accompanied by calcium excretion. Careful assessment of cardiovascular and renal function is done prior to fluid therapy; the client is carefully monitored for evidence of fluid overload during treatment.

NURSING CARE

Health Promotion

Identify and monitor clients at risk for hypercalcemia. Promote mobility in clients when possible. Assist hospitalized clients to ambulate as soon as possible. In the home setting, discuss the benefits of regular weight-bearing activity with clients, families, and caregivers. Encourage a generous fluid intake of up to 3 to 4 quarts per day. Encourage clients at risk to limit their intake of milk and milk products, as well as calcium-containing antacids and supplements. In addition, clients with prolonged immobility or hypercalcemia are encouraged to consume fluids that increase the acidity of urine (which inhibits calcium stone formation), such as cranberry or prune juice.

Assessment

Assessment data related to hypercalcemia include the following:

- *Health history:* Current manifestations, including weakness or fatigue, abdominal discomfort, nausea or vomiting, increased urination and thirst; changes in memory or thinking; duration of symptoms and any risk factors such as excess intake of milk or calcium products, prolonged immobility, malignancy, renal failure, or endocrine disorders; current medications.
- *Physical assessment:* Mental status and level of consciousness; vital signs including apical pulse; bowel sounds; muscle strength of upper and lower extremities; deep tendon reflexes.
- *Diagnostic tests:* Serum electrolytes, urinary calcium, ECG, and cardiac rhythm monitoring.

> **PRACTICE ALERT**
> Remember, calcium has a stabilizing or sedative effect on neuromuscular transmission. Therefore:
>
> Hypocalcemia → Increased neuromuscular excitability, muscle twitching, spasms, and possible tetany
> Hypercalcemia → Decreased neuromuscular excitability, muscle weakness, and fatigue

Nursing Diagnoses and Interventions

Risk for Injury

Clients with hypercalcemia are at risk for injury due to changes in mental status, the effects of hypercalcemia on muscle strength, and loss of calcium from bones.

- Institute safety precautions if confusion or other changes in mental status are noted. *Changes in mental status may impair judgment and the client's ability to maintain own safety.*

> **PRACTICE ALERT**
> Monitor cardiac rate and rhythm, treating and/or reporting dysrhythmias as indicated. Prepare for possible cardiac arrest; keep emergency resuscitation equipment readily available. Hypercalcemia can cause bradycardia, various heart blocks, and cardiac arrest. Immediate treatment may be necessary to preserve life.

- Observe for manifestations of digitalis toxicity, including vision changes, anorexia, and changes in heart rate and rhythm. Monitor serum digitalis levels. *Hypercalcemia increases the risk of digitalis toxicity.*
- Promote fluid intake (oral and/or intravenous) to keep the client well hydrated and maintain dilute urine. Encourage fluids such as prune or cranberry juice to help maintain acidic urine. *Acidic, dilute urine reduces the risk of calcium salts precipitating out to form kidney stones.*
- If excess bone resorption has occurred, use caution when turning, positioning, transferring, or ambulating. *Bones that have lost excess calcium may fracture with minimal stress or trauma (pathologic fractures).*

Risk for Excess Fluid Volume

Large amounts of isotonic intravenous fluid often are administered to help correct acute hypercalcemia, leading to a risk for hypervolemia. Clients with preexisting cardiac or renal disease are at particular risk.

- Closely monitor intake and output. *A loop diuretic such as furosemide may be necessary if urinary output does not keep up with fluid administration.*
- Frequently assess vital signs, respiratory status, and heart sounds. *Increasing pulse rate, dyspnea, adventitious lung sounds, and an S_3 on auscultation of the heart may indicate excess fluid volume and potential heart failure.*
- Place in semi-Fowler's to Fowler's position. *Elevating the head of the bed improves lung expansion and reduces the work of breathing.*
- Administer diuretics as ordered, monitoring response. *Loop diuretics may be ordered to help eliminate excess fluid and calcium.*

Community-Based Care

Discuss the following topics when preparing the client for discharge:

- Avoid excess intake of calcium-rich foods and antacids.
- Use prescribed drugs to prevent excess calcium resorption. Discuss their dose, use, and desired and possible adverse effects.
- Increase fluid intake to 3 to 4 quarts per day; increase the intake of acid ash foods (meats, fish, poultry, eggs, cranberries, plums, prunes); increase dietary fiber and fluid intake to prevent constipation.
- Maintain weight-bearing physical activity to prevent hypercalcemia.
- Report early manifestations of hypercalcemia to care provider.
- Follow recommended schedule for monitoring serum electrolyte levels.

MAGNESIUM IMBALANCE

Only about 1% of the magnesium in the body is in extracellular fluid; the rest is found within the cells and in bone. The normal serum concentration of magnesium ranges from 1.6 to 2.6 mg/dL (1.3 to 2.1 mEq/L).

Overview of Normal Magnesium Balance

Magnesium is obtained through the diet (it is plentiful in green vegetables, grains, nuts, meats, and seafood) and excreted by the kidneys. Magnesium is vital to many intracellular processes, including enzyme reactions and synthesis of proteins and nucleic acids. Magnesium exerts a sedative effect on the neuromuscular junction, decreasing acetylcholine release. It is an essential ion for neuromuscular transmission and cardiovascular function. The physiologic effects of magnesium are affected by both potassium and calcium levels. Approximately 65% of extracellular magnesium is ionized; the remainder is bound to protein. Table 10–8 summarizes common causes and manifestations of magnesium imbalances.

The Client with Hypomagnesemia

Hypomagnesemia is a magnesium level of less than 1.6 mg/dL. It is a common problem, particularly in critically ill clients. Hypomagnesemia may be caused by deficient magnesium intake, excessive losses, or a shift between the intracellular and extracellular compartments.

Risk Factors

Loss of gastrointestinal fluids, particularly from diarrhea, an ileostomy, or intestinal fistula is a major risk factor for hypomagnesemia. Disruption of nutrient absorption in the small intestine also increases the risk. Chronic alcoholism is the most common cause of deficient magnesium levels in the United States (Metheny, 2000). Multiple factors associated with alcoholism contribute to hypomagnesemia: deficient nutrient intake, increased gastrointestinal losses, impaired absorption, and increased renal excretion. Other risk factors for hypomagnesemia include:

- Protein-calorie malnutrition or starvation
- Endocrine disorders including diabetic ketoacidosis
- Drugs such as loop or thiazide diuretics, aminoglycoside antibiotics, amphotericin B, and cyclosporine
- Rapid administration of citrated blood (banked blood)
- Kidney disease.

Pathophysiology

Magnesium deficiency usually occurs along with low serum potassium and calcium levels. The effects of hypomagnesemia relate not only to the magnesium deficiency but also to hypokalemia and hypocalcemia.

Hypomagnesemia causes increased neuromuscular excitability, with muscle weakness and tremors. The accompanying hypocalcemia contributes to this effect. In the central nervous system, this increased neural excitability can lead to seizures and changes in mental status.

Deficient intracellular magnesium in the myocardium increases the risk of cardiac dysrhythmias and sudden death. Hypokalemia increases this risk. Hypomagnesemia also increases the risk of digitalis toxicity. Chronic hypomagnesemia may contribute to hypertension, probably due to increased vasoconstriction.

TABLE 10-8 **Causes and Manifestations of Magnesium Imbalances**

IMBALANCE	CAUSES	MANIFESTATIONS
Hypomagnesemia Serum magnesium < 1.6 mg/dL Critical value < 1 mg/dL	■ Chronic alcoholism ■ GI losses: intestinal suction, diarrhea, ileostomy ■ Impaired absorption ■ Inadequate replacement ■ Increased excretion: drugs, renal disease, osmotic diuresis	Neuromuscular ■ Muscle weakness, tremors ■ Tetany, seizures Gastrointestinal ■ Dysphagia ■ Anorexia, nausea, vomiting, diarrhea Cardiovascular ■ Tachycardia ■ Dysrhythmias ■ Hypertension CNS ■ Mood and personality changes ■ Paresthesias
Hypermagnesemia Serum magnesium > 2.6 mg/dL or 2.1 mEq/L Critical value > 4.7 mg/dL	■ Renal insufficiency or failure ■ Excess intake of antacids, laxatives ■ Excess magnesium administration	Neuromuscular ■ Muscle weakness ■ Depressed deep tendon reflexes Gastrointestinal ■ Nausea and vomiting Cardiovascular ■ Hypotension ■ Bradycardia ■ Cardiac arrest CNS ■ Respiratory depression ■ Coma

Manifestations and Complications

Neuromuscular manifestations of hypomagnesemia include tremors, hyperreactive reflexes, positive Chvostek's and Trousseau's signs (see Figure 10–13), tetany, paresthesias, and seizures. CNS effects include confusion, mood changes (apathy, depression, agitation), hallucinations, and possible psychoses.

An increased heart rate and ventricular dysrhythmias are common, especially when hypokalemia is present or the client is taking digitalis. Cardiac arrest and sudden death may occur. Gastrointestinal manifestations include nausea, vomiting, anorexia, diarrhea, and abdominal distention.

INTERDISCIPLINARY CARE

Hypomagnesemia is diagnosed by measuring serum electrolyte levels. The ECG shows a prolonged PR interval, widened QRS complex, and depression of the ST segment with T-wave inversion.

Treatment is directed toward prevention and identification of an existing deficiency. Magnesium is added to intravenous total parenteral nutrition solutions to prevent hypomagnesemia.

In clients able to eat, a mild deficiency may be corrected by increasing the intake of foods rich in magnesium (Box 10–8), or with oral magnesium supplements. Oral magnesium supplements may cause diarrhea, however, limiting their use.

Clients with manifestations of hypomagnesemia are treated with parenteral magnesium sulfate. Treatment is continued for several days to restore intracellular magnesium levels. Magnesium may be given intravenously or by deep intramuscular in-

---

BOX 10–8 **Foods High in Magnesium**

- Green, leafy vegetables
- Seafood
- Meat
- Wheat bran
- Milk
- Legumes
- Bananas

- Oranges
- Grapefruit
- Chocolate
- Molasses
- Coconut
- Refined sugar

---

jection. Renal function is evaluated prior to administration, and serum magnesium levels are monitored during treatment. The intravenous route is used for severe magnesium deficiency or if neurologic changes or cardiac dysrhythmias are present. See the Medication Administration box on the next page for the nursing implications of parenteral magnesium sulfate.

NURSING CARE

Health Promotion

Discuss the importance of maintaining adequate magnesium intake through a well-balanced diet, particularly with clients at risk (people with alcoholism, malabsorption, or bowel surgery). Many hospitalized clients are at risk for hypomagnesemia due to protein-calorie malnutrition and other disorders. Monitor serum magnesium levels, reporting changes to the healthcare provider.

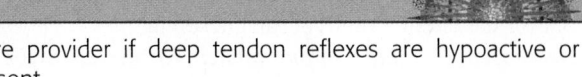

MEDICATION ADMINISTRATION   **Magnesium Sulfate**

Magnesium sulfate is used to prevent or treat hypomagnesemia. It also is used as an anticonvulsant in severe eclampsia or preeclampsia. It may be given intravenously or by intramuscular injection.

Nursing Responsibilities
■ Assess serum magnesium levels and renal function tests (BUN and serum creatinine) prior to administering. Notify the care provider if magnesium levels are above normal limits or renal function is impaired.
■ Frequently monitor neurologic status and deep tendon reflexes during therapy. Withhold magnesium and notify the

care provider if deep tendon reflexes are hypoactive or absent.
■ Monitor intake and output.
■ Administer IM doses deep into the ventral or dorsal gluteal sites.
■ Intravenous magnesium sulfate may be given by direct IV push or by continuous infusion.

Health Education for the Client and Family
Explain purpose and duration of treatment. Discuss reason for frequent neurologic and reflex assessments.

Assessment

In addition to asking questions related to risk factors for hypomagnesemia, use the guidelines for assessing clients with hypokalemia and hypocalcemia for subjective and objective assessment data. Monitor diagnostic studies such as serum electrolytes, serum albumin levels, and the ECG.

Nursing Diagnoses and Interventions

Nursing care for clients with hypomagnesemia focuses on careful monitoring of manifestations and responses to treatment, promoting safety, client and family teaching, and administering prescribed medications.

Risk for Injury

■ Monitor serum electrolytes, including magnesium, potassium, and calcium. *Magnesium deficiency often is accompanied by deficiencies of potassium and calcium.*
■ Monitor gastrointestinal function, including bowel sounds and abdominal distention. *Hypomagnesemia reduces gastrointestinal motility.*
■ Initiate cardiac monitoring, reporting and treating (as indicated) ECG changes and dysrhythmias. In clients receiving digitalis, monitor for digitalis toxicity. *Low magnesium levels can precipitate ventricular dysrhythmias, including lethal dysrhythmias such as ventricular fibrillation.*
■ Assess deep tendon reflexes frequently during intravenous magnesium infusions and prior to each intramuscular dose. *Depressed tendon reflexes indicate a high serum magnesium level.*
■ Maintain a quiet, darkened environment. Institute seizure precautions. *Increased neuromuscular and CNS irritability can lead to seizures. A quiet, dark environment reduces stimuli.*

Community-Based Care

Prior to discharge, instruct the client to increase dietary intake of foods high in magnesium and provide information about magnesium supplements. In addition, if alcohol abuse has precipitated a magnesium deficit, discuss alcohol treatment options, including inpatient treatment and support groups such as Alcoholics Anonymous, Al-Anon, and/or Al-a-Teen.

The Client with Hypermagnesemia

Hypermagnesemia is a serum magnesium level greater than 2.6 mg/dL. It is much less common than hypomagnesemia. Hypermagnesemia can develop in renal failure, particularly if magnesium is administered parenterally or orally (e.g., magnesium-containing antacids or laxatives). Older adults are at risk for hypermagnesemia as renal function declines with aging and they are more likely to use over-the-counter laxatives and other preparations that contain magnesium.

Pathophysiology and Manifestations

Elevated serum magnesium levels interfere with neuromuscular transmission and depress the central nervous system. Hypermagnesemia also affects the cardiovascular system, potentially causing hypotension, flushing, sweating, and bradydysrhythmias.

Predictable manifestations occur with increasing serum magnesium levels. With lower levels, nausea and vomiting, hypotension, facial flushing, sweating, and a feeling of warmth occur. As levels increase, signs of CNS depression appear (weakness, lethargy, drowsiness, weak or absent deep tendon reflexes). Marked elevations cause respiratory depression, coma, and compromised cardiac function (ECG changes, bradycardia, heart block, and cardiac arrest).

INTERDISCIPLINARY CARE

The management of hypermagnesemia focuses on identifying and treating the underlying cause. All medications or compounds containing magnesium (such as antacids, intravenous solutions, or enemas) are withheld. In the client with renal failure, hemodialysis or peritoneal dialysis is instituted to remove the excess magnesium.

Calcium gluconate is administered intravenously to reverse the neuromuscular and cardiac effects of hypermagnesemia. The client may require mechanical ventilation to support respiratory function, and a pacemaker to maintain adequate cardiac output.

NURSING CARE

Nursing care includes instituting measures to prevent and identify hypermagnesemia in clients at risk, monitoring for critical effects of hypermagnesemia, and providing measures to ensure the client's safety. Consider the following nursing diagnoses for the client with hypermagnesemia:

- *Decreased Cardiac Output* related to altered myocardial conduction
- *Risk for Ineffective Breathing Pattern* related to respiratory depression
- *Risk for Injury* related to muscle weakness and altered level of consciousness
- *Risk for Ineffective Health Maintenance* related to lack of knowledge about use of magnesium-containing supplements, antacids, laxatives, and enemas.

Community-Based Care

Discharge teaching and planning focus on instructions to avoid magnesium-containing medications, including antacids, mineral supplements, cathartics, and enemas (Box 10–9).

PHOSPHATE IMBALANCE

Although most phosphate (85%) is found in bones, it is the primary intracellular anion. About 14% is in intracellular fluid, and the remainder (1%) is in extracellular fluid. The normal serum phosphate (or phosphorus) level in adults is 2.5 to 4.5 mg/dL. Phosphorus levels vary with age, gender, and diet.

Overview of Normal Phosphate Balance

Phosphate is essential to intracellular processes such as the production of ATP, the fuel that supports muscle contraction, nerve cell transmission, and electrolyte transport. Phosphate is vital for red blood cell function and oxygen delivery to tissues; nervous system and muscle function; and the metabolism of fats, carbohydrates, and protein. It also assists in maintaining acid–base balance.

Phosphorus is ingested in the diet, absorbed in the jejunum, and primarily excreted by the kidneys. When phosphate intake is low, the kidneys conserve phosphorus, excreting less. An inverse relationship exists between phosphate and calcium levels: When one increases, the other decreases. Regulatory mechanisms for calcium levels (parathyroid hormone, calcitonin, and vitamin D) also influence phosphate levels. The causes and manifestations of phosphate imbalances are summarized in Table 10–9.

The Client with Hypophosphatemia

Hypophosphatemia is a serum phosphorus of less than 2.5 mg/dL. Low serum phosphate levels may indicate a total body deficit of phosphate or a shift of phosphate into the intracellular space, the most common cause of hypophosphatemia. Decreased gastrointestinal absorption of phosphate or increased renal excretion of phosphate also can cause low phosphate levels. Hypophosphatemia often is *iatrogenic,* that is, related to treatment. Selected causes of hypophosphatemia include the following:

- *Refeeding syndrome* can develop when malnourished clients are started on enteral or total parenteral nutrition. Glucose in the formula or solution stimulates insulin release, which promotes the entry of glucose and phosphate into the cells, depleting extracellular phosphate levels.
- Medications frequently contribute to hypophosphatemia, including intravenous glucose solutions, antacids (aluminum- or magnesium-based antacids bind with phosphate), anabolic steroids, and diuretics.

BOX 10–9 Medications Containing Magnesium

Antacids	Laxatives
■ Gelusil	■ Milk of Magnesia
■ Maalox No.1	■ Magnesium oxide
■ Maalox Plus	■ Haley's M-O
■ Riopan	■ Magnesium citrate
■ Milk of Magnesia	■ Epsom salts
■ Mylanta	
■ Di-Gel	
■ Gaviscon	

TABLE 10–9 Causes and Manifestations of Phosphate Imbalances

IMBALANCE	CAUSES	MANIFESTATIONS
Hypophosphatemia Serum phosphorus < 2.5 mg/dL Critical value < 1 mg/dL	■ Shift of phosphorus into cells ■ IV glucose administration ■ Total parenteral nutrition without phosphorus ■ Aluminum- or magnesium-based antacids ■ Diuretic therapy ■ Alcoholism	■ Paresthesias ■ Muscle weakness ■ Muscle pain and tenderness ■ Confusion, decreasing LOC ■ Seizures ■ Bone pain, osteomalacia ■ Anorexia, dysphagia ■ Decreased bowel sounds ■ Possible acute respiratory failure
Hyperphosphatemia Serum phosphate > 4.5 mg/dL Critical value > 90 mg/dL	■ Renal failure ■ Chemotherapy ■ Muscle tissue trauma ■ Sepsis ■ Severe hypothermia ■ Heat stroke	■ Circumoral and peripheral paresthesias ■ Muscle spasms ■ Tetany ■ Soft tissue calcification

- Alcoholism affects both the intake and absorption of phosphate.
- Hyperventilation and respiratory alkalosis cause phosphate to shift out of extracellular fluids into the intracellular space.
- Other causes include diabetic ketoacidosis with excess phosphate loss in the urine, stress responses, and extensive burns.

Pathophysiology and Manifestations

Most effects of hypophosphatemia result from depletion of ATP and impaired oxygen delivery to the cells due to a deficiency of the red blood cell enzyme 2,3-DPG. Severe hypophosphatemia affects virtually every major organ system:

- *Central nervous system:* Reduced oxygen and ATP synthesis in the brain causes neurologic manifestations such as irritability, apprehension, weakness, paresthesias, lack of coordination, confusion, seizures, and coma.
- *Hematologic:* Oxygen delivery to the cells is reduced. Hemolytic anemia (excessive RBC destruction) may develop due to lack of ATP in red blood cells.
- *Musculoskeletal:* Decreased ATP causes muscle weakness and release of creatinine phosphokinase (CPK, a muscle enzyme); acute rhabdomyolysis (muscle cell breakdown) can develop. Muscle cell destruction, in turn, can lead to acute renal failure as myoglobin, a muscle cell protein, exerts a toxic effect on the kidney tubule.
- *Respiratory:* Chest muscle weakness can interfere with effective ventilation, leading to respiratory failure.
- *Cardiovascular:* Hypophosphatemia decreases myocardial contractility; decreased oxygenation of the heart muscle can cause chest pain and dysrhythmias.
- *Gastrointestinal:* Anorexia can occur, as well as dysphagia (difficulty swallowing), nausea and vomiting, decreased bowel sounds, and possible ileus due to reduced gastrointestinal motility.

INTERDISCIPLINARY CARE

Treatment for hypophosphatemia is directed at prevention, treating the underlying cause of the disorder, and replacing phosphate. An improved diet and oral phosphate supplement (such as Neutra-Phos or Neutra-Phos K capsules) may restore normal phosphate levels in clients with a mild to moderate deficiency. Intravenous phosphate (sodium phosphate or potassium phosphate) is given when serum phosphate levels are less than 1 mg/dL. Oral phosphate supplements are then continued for up to 1 week to restore intracellular phosphate levels (Metheny, 2000).

NURSING CARE

Nurses can be instrumental in identifying clients at risk for phosphate deficiency and preventing it from developing. Nurses should closely monitor serum electrolyte values in clients at risk, including those who are malnourished, receiving intravenous glucose solutions or total parenteral nutrition, or being treated with diuretic therapy or antacids that bind with phosphate. Nursing diagnoses that may be appropriate for the client with hypophosphatemia include:

- *Impaired Physical Mobility* related to muscle weakness and poor coordination
- *Ineffective Breathing Pattern* related to weakened muscles of respiration
- *Decreased Cardiac Output* related to reduced myocardial contractility
- *Risk for Injury* related to muscle weakness and altered mental status.

Community-Based Care

In preparing for discharge, teach the client and family about the causes and manifestations of hypophosphatemia. Discuss the importance of avoiding phosphorus-binding antacids, unless prescribed. Stress a well-balanced diet to maintain an adequate intake of phosphate.

The Client with Hyperphosphatemia

Hyperphosphatemia is a serum phosphate level greater than 4.5 mg/dL. As with other electrolyte imbalances, it may be the result of impaired phosphate excretion, excess intake, or a shift of phosphate from the intracellular space into extracellular fluids.

- Acute or chronic renal failure is the primary cause of impaired phosphate excretion.
- Rapid administration of phosphate-containing solutions can increase serum phosphate levels. This can include phosphate enemas. In addition, excess vitamin D increases phosphate absorption and can lead to hyperphosphatemia in clients with impaired renal function.
- A shift of phosphate from the intracellular to extracellular space can occur during chemotherapy, due to sepsis or hypothermia, or because of extensive trauma or heat stroke.
- Because phosphate levels are affected by serum calcium concentrations, disruption of the mechanisms that regulate calcium levels (e.g., hypoparathyroidism, hyperthyroidism, or vitamin D intoxication) can lead to hyperphosphatemia.

Pathophysiology and Manifestations

Excessive serum phosphate levels cause few specific symptoms. The effects of high serum phosphate levels on nerves and muscles (muscle cramps and pain, paresthesias, tingling around the mouth, muscle spasms, tetany) are more the result of hypocalcemia that develops secondary to an elevated serum phosphorus level. The phosphate in the serum combines with ionized calcium, and the ionized serum calcium level falls.

Calcification of soft tissues can occur with high phosphate levels. Phosphates bind with calcium to precipitate in soft tissues such as the kidneys and other organs. Soft tissue calcification can impair the function of affected organs.

INTERDISCIPLINARY CARE

Treatment of the underlying disorder often corrects hyperphosphatemia. When this is not feasible, phosphate-containing drugs are eliminated and intake of phosphate-rich foods such as organ meats and milk and milk products is restricted. Agents that bind with phosphate in the gastrointestinal tract (such as calcium-containing antacids) may be prescribed. If renal function is adequate, intravenous normal saline may be given to promote renal excretion of phosphate. Dialysis may be necessary to reduce phosphate levels in clients with renal failure.

NURSING CARE

When providing nursing care for the client with hyperphosphatemia, monitor the client for laboratory data revealing an excess of phosphorus and a deficit of calcium, as well as the signs of hypocalcemia.

Community-Based Care

Discuss the risk of hyperphosphatemia related to using phosphate preparations as laxatives or enemas, particularly with clients who have other risk factors for the disorder. When preparing the client for discharge, teach about the use of phosphate-binding preparations as ordered and dietary phosphate restrictions.

ACID–BASE DISORDERS

Homeostasis and optimal cellular function require maintenance of the hydrogen ion (H^+) concentration of body fluids within a relatively narrow range. Hydrogen ions determine the relative acidity of body fluids. **Acids** release hydrogen ions in solution; **bases** (or **alkalis**) accept hydrogen ions in solution. The hydrogen ion concentration of a solution is measured as its pH. The relationship between hydrogen ion concentration and pH is inverse; that is, as hydrogen ion concentration increases, the pH falls, and the solution becomes more acidic. As hydrogen ion concentration falls, the pH rises, and the solution becomes more alkaline or basic. The pH of body fluids is slightly basic, with the normal pH ranging from 7.35 to 7.45 (a pH of 7 is neutral).

REGULATION OF ACID–BASE BALANCE

A number of mechanisms work together to maintain the pH of the body within this normal range. Metabolic processes in the body continuously produce acids, which fall into two categories: volatile acids and nonvolatile acids. **Volatile acids** can be eliminated from the body as a gas. Carbonic acid (H_2CO_3) is the only volatile acid produced in the body. It dissociates (separates) into carbon dioxide (CO_2) and water (H_2O); the carbon dioxide is then eliminated from the body through the lungs. All other acids produced in the body are *nonvolatile acids* that must be metabolized or excreted from the body in fluid. Lactic acid, hydrochloric acid, phosphoric acid, and sulfuric acid are examples of nonvolatile acids. Most acids and bases in the body are weak; that is, they neither release nor accept a significant amount of hydrogen ion.

Three systems work together in the body to maintain the pH despite continuous acid production: buffers, the respiratory system, and the renal system.

Buffer Systems

Buffers are substances that prevent major changes in pH by removing or releasing hydrogen ions. When excess acid is present in body fluid, buffers bind with hydrogen ions to minimize the change in pH. If body fluids become too basic or alkaline, buffers release hydrogen ions, restoring the pH. Although buffers act within a fraction of a second, their capacity to maintain pH is limited. The major buffer systems of the body are the bicarbonate-carbonic acid buffer system, phosphate buffer system, and protein buffers.

The bicarbonate-carbonic acid buffer system can be illustrated by the following equation:

$$CO_2 + H_2O \leftrightarrow H_2CO_3 \leftrightarrow H^+ + HCO_3^-$$

Bicarbonate (HCO_3^-) is a weak base; when an acid is added to the system, the hydrogen ion in the acid combines with bicarbonate, and the pH changes only slightly. Carbonic acid (H_2CO_3) is a weak acid produced when carbon dioxide dissolves in water. If a base is added to the system, it combines with carbonic acid, and the pH remains within the normal range. Although the amounts of bicarbonate and carbonic acid in the body vary to a certain extent, as long as a ratio of 20 parts bicarbonate (HCO_3^-) to 1 part carbonic acid (H_2CO_3) is maintained, the pH remains within the 7.35 to 7.45 range (Figure 10–14 ■).

The normal serum bicarbonate level is 24 mEq/L, and that of carbonic acid is 1.2 mEq/L. Thus, the ratio of bicarbonate to carbonic acid is 20:1. It is this ratio that maintains the pH within the normal range. Adding a strong acid to extracellular fluid depletes bicarbonate, changing the 20:1 ratio and causing the pH to drop below 7.35. This is known as **acidosis**. Addition of a strong base depletes carbonic acid as it combines with the base. The 20:1 ratio again is disrupted and the pH rises above 7.45, a condition known as **alkalosis**.

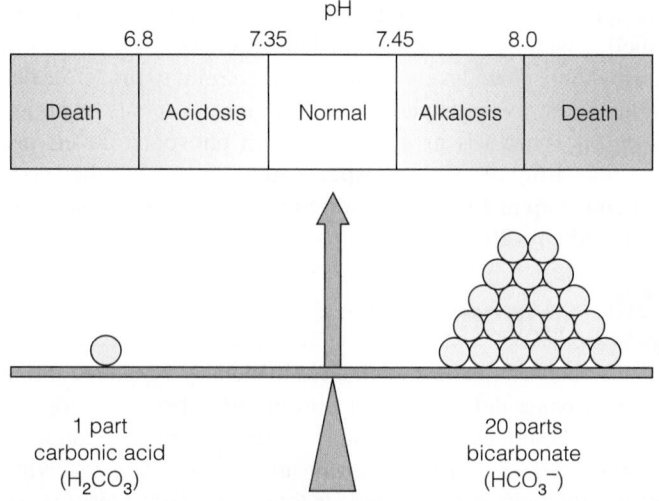

Figure 10–14 ■ The normal ratio of bicarbonate to carbonic acid is 20:1. As long as this ratio is maintained, the pH remains within the normal range of 7.35 to 7.45.

hydrogen ion. Excess hydrogen ions also enter the cells, displacing potassium from the intracellular space to maintain the balance of cations and anions within the cells. The effect of both processes is to increase serum potassium levels. Also in acidosis, calcium is released from its bonds with plasma proteins, increasing the amount of ionized (free) calcium in the blood. Magnesium levels may fall in acidosis.

Manifestations

Metabolic acidosis affects the function of many body systems. Its general manifestations include weakness and fatigue, headache, and general malaise. Gastrointestinal function is affected, causing anorexia, nausea, vomiting, and abdominal pain. The level of consciousness declines, leading to stupor and coma. Cardiac dysrhythmias develop, and cardiac arrest may occur. The skin is often warm and flushed. Skeletal problems may develop in chronic acidosis, as calcium and phosphate are released from the bones. Manifestations of compensatory mechanisms are seen. The respirations are deep and rapid, known as **Kussmaul's respirations**. The client may complain of shortness of breath or dyspnea. See the Manifestations box below.

INTERDISCIPLINARY CARE

Management of metabolic acidosis focuses on treating the underlying cause of the disorder and correcting the acid–base imbalance.

Diagnosis

The following laboratory and diagnostic tests may be ordered.
- *ABGs* generally show a pH of less than 7.35 and a bicarbonate level of less than 22 mEq/L. A compensatory decrease in $PaCO_2$ to less than 35 mmHg is usually present.
- *Serum electrolytes* demonstrate elevated serum potassium levels and possible low magnesium levels. The total calcium may remain unchanged, although more physiologically active ionized calcium is available. Sodium, chloride, and bicarbonate levels are used to calculate the anion gap.
- The *ECG* may show changes that reflect both the acidosis (particularly when severe) and the accompanying hyperkalemia.
- Other diagnostic studies such as the blood glucose and renal function studies may be ordered to identify the underlying cause of metabolic acidosis.

MANIFESTATIONS of Metabolic Acidosis

- Anorexia
- Nausea and vomiting
- Abdominal pain
- Weakness
- Fatigue
- General malaise
- Decreasing levels of consciousness
- Dysrhythmias
- Bradycardia
- Warm, flushed skin
- Hyperventilation (Kussmaul's respirations)

Medications

An alkalinizing solution such as bicarbonate may be given if the pH is less than 7.2 to reduce the effects of the acidosis on cardiac function. Sodium bicarbonate is the most commonly used alkalinizing solution; others include lactate, citrate, and acetate solutions (which are metabolized to bicarbonate). Alkalinizing solutions are given intravenously for severe acute metabolic acidosis. In chronic metabolic acidosis, the oral route is used.

The client treated with bicarbonate must be carefully monitored. Rapid correction of the acidosis may lead to metabolic alkalosis and hypokalemia. Hypernatremia and hyperosmolality may develop as well, leading to water retention and fluid overload.

PRACTICE ALERT

As metabolic acidosis is corrected, potassium shifts back into the intracellular space. This can lead to hypokalemia and cardiac dysrhythmias. Carefully monitor serum potassium levels during treatment.

Treatment for diabetic ketoacidosis includes intravenous insulin and fluid replacement (see Chapter 20 for the treatment of diabetic ketoacidosis). Alcoholic ketoacidosis is treated with saline solutions and glucose. Treatment for lactic acidosis from decreased tissue perfusion (e.g., shock or cardiac arrest) focuses on correcting the underlying problem and improving tissue perfusion. Clients with chronic renal failure and mild or moderate metabolic acidosis may or may not require treatment, depending on the pH and bicarbonate levels. When metabolic acidosis is due to diarrhea, treatment includes correcting the underlying cause and providing fluid and electrolyte replacement.

NURSING CARE

Nurses frequently provide care for clients with metabolic acidosis, although the focus of care often is the disorder underlying the acidosis (e.g., diabetes mellitus, renal failure) rather than the acidosis itself. For this reason, it is vital for the nurse to be aware of the effects of the acidosis and its implications for nursing care.

Health Promotion

To promote health in clients at risk for metabolic acidosis, discuss management of their underlying disease process (e.g., type 1 diabetes or renal failure) to prevent complications such as diabetic ketoacidosis and metabolic acidosis. Because early manifestations of metabolic acidosis (e.g., fatigue, general malaise, anorexia, nausea, abdominal pain) resemble those of common viral disorders such as "the flu," stress the importance of promptly seeking treatment if these symptoms develop.

Assessment

Assessment data related to metabolic acidosis include the following:
- *Health history:* Current manifestations, including anorexia, nausea, vomiting, abdominal discomfort, fatigue, lethargy,

TABLE 10–12 Compensation for Simple Acid–Base Imbalances

PRIMARY DISORDER	CAUSE	COMPENSATION	EFFECT ON ABGS
Metabolic acidosis	Excess nonvolatile acids; bicarbonate deficiency	Rate and depth of respirations increase, eliminating additional CO_2	$\downarrow$pH $\downarrow$$HCO_3^-$ $\downarrow$ $Paco_2$
Metabolic alkalosis	Bicarbonate excess	Rate and depth of respirations decrease, retaining CO_2	$\uparrow$ pH $\uparrow$ HCO_3^- $\uparrow$ $Paco_2$
Respiratory acidosis	Retained CO_2 and excess carbonic acid	Kidneys conserve bicarbonate to restore carbonic acid:bicarbonate ratio of 1:20	$\downarrow$ pH $\uparrow$ $Paco_2$ $\uparrow$ HCO_3^-
Respiratory alkalosis	Loss of CO_2 and deficient carbonic acid	Kidneys excrete bicarbonate and conserve H^+ to restore carbonic acid:bicarbonate ratio	$\uparrow$ pH $\downarrow$ $Paco_2$ $\downarrow$ HCO_3^-

drogen ions are produced, forming lactic acid. Both oxygen and glucose are necessary for normal cell metabolism. When intracellular glucose is inadequate due to starvation or a lack of insulin to move it into cells, the body breaks down fatty tissue to meet its metabolic needs. In this process, fatty acids are released, which are converted to ketones; ketoacidosis develops. Aspirin (acetylsalicylic acid) breaks down into salicylic acid in the body. Substances such as aspirin, methanol (wood alcohol), and ethylene (contained in antifreeze and solvents) cause a toxic increase in body acids by either breaking down into acid products (salicylic acid) or stimulating metabolic acid production (Porth, 2005). Renal failure impairs the body's ability to excrete excess hydrogen ions and form bicarbonate.

Excess metabolic acids increase the hydrogen ion concentration of body fluids. The excess acid is buffered by bicarbonate, leading to what is known as a high **anion gap** acidosis (Box 10–11).

The pancreas secretes bicarbonate-rich fluid into the small intestine. Intestinal suction, severe diarrhea, ileostomy drainage, or fistulas can lead to excess losses of bicarbonate. Hyperchloremic acidosis can develop when excess chloride solutions (such as NaCl or ammonium chloride) are infused, causing a rise in chloride concentrations. It also may be related to renal disease or administration of carbonic anhydrate inhibitor diuretics. The anion gap remains normal in metabolic acidosis due to bicarbonate loss or excess chloride.

Acidosis depresses cell membrane excitability, affecting neuromuscular function. It also increases the amount of free calcium in ECF by interfering with protein binding. Severe acidosis (pH of 7.0 or less) depresses myocardial contractility, leading to a fall in cardiac output. If kidney function is normal, acid excretion and ammonia production increase to eliminate excess hydrogen ions.

Acid–base imbalances also affect electrolyte balance. In acidosis, potassium is retained as the kidney excretes excess

BOX 10–11 Unraveling the Anion Gap

Calculation of the anion gap can help identify the underlying mechanism in metabolic acidosis if it is unclear.

The number of cations (positively charged ions) and anions (negatively charged ions) in ECF normally is equal (refer to Figure 10–2). Not all of these ions, however, are measured in laboratory testing (e.g., organic acids and proteins). The anion gap is calculated by subtracting the sum of two measured anions, chloride and bicarbonate, from the concentration of the major cation, sodium (see figure). The normal anion gap is 8 to 12 mEq/L.

Excess acids in ECF are buffered by bicarbonate, reducing serum bicarbonate levels and the total measured concentration of anions. This increases the anion gap (B in figure). When bicarbonate is lost from the body or chloride levels increase, however, the anion gap remains within normal limits (C in figure). This occurs because an increase or decrease in one of these negatively charged ions causes a corresponding change in the other to maintain balance (e.g., $\downarrow HCO_3^- \leftrightarrow \uparrow Cl^-$), and there is no change in the amount of unmeasured anions.

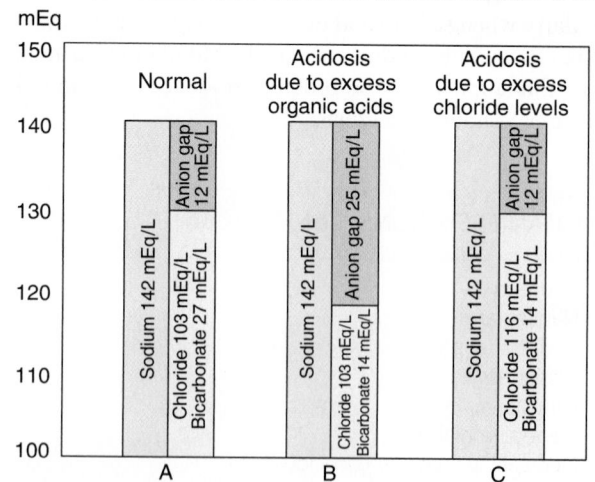

Illustration of the anion gap in metabolic acidosis. *A*, Normal anion gap. *B*, High anion gap caused by excess acids. *C*, Normal anion gap with hyperchloremia.

Intracellular and plasma proteins also serve as buffers. Plasma proteins contribute to buffering of extracellular fluids. Proteins in intracellular fluid provide extensive buffering for organic acids produced by cellular metabolism. In red blood cells, hemoglobin acts as a buffer for hydrogen ion when carbonic acid dissociates. Inorganic phosphates also serve as extracellular buffers, although their roles are not as important as the bicarbonate-carbonic acid buffer system. Phosphates are, however, important intracellular buffers, helping to maintain a stable pH within the cells.

Respiratory System

The respiratory system (and the respiratory center of the brain) regulates carbonic acid in the body by eliminating or retaining carbon dioxide. Carbon dioxide is a potential acid; when combined with water, it forms carbonic acid (see previous equation), a volatile acid. Acute increases in either carbon dioxide or hydrogen ions in the blood stimulate the respiratory center in the brain. As a result, both the rate and depth of respiration increase. The increased rate and depth of lung ventilation eliminate carbon dioxide from the body, and carbonic acid levels fall, bringing the pH to a more normal range. Although this compensation for increased hydrogen ion concentration occurs within minutes, it becomes less effective over time. Clients with chronic lung disease may have consistently high carbon dioxide levels in their blood.

Alkalosis, by contrast, depresses the respiratory center. Both the rate and depth of respiration decrease, and carbon dioxide is retained. The retained carbon dioxide then combines with water to restore carbonic acid levels and bring the pH back within the normal range.

Renal System

The renal system is responsible for the long-term regulation of acid–base balance in the body. Excess nonvolatile acids produced during metabolism normally are eliminated by the kidneys. The kidneys also regulate bicarbonate levels in extracellular fluid by regenerating bicarbonate ions as well as reabsorbing them in the renal tubules. Although the kidneys respond more slowly to changes in pH (over hours to days), they can generate bicarbonate and selectively excrete or retain hydrogen ions as needed. In acidosis, when excess hydrogen ion is present and the pH falls, the kidneys excrete hydrogen ions and retain bicarbonate. In alkalosis, the kidneys retain hydrogen ions and excrete bicarbonate to restore acid–base balance.

Assessment of Acid–Base Balance

Acid–base balance is evaluated primarily by measuring arterial blood gases.

PRACTICE ALERT

Arteries are high-pressure vessels in contrast to veins. Obtaining an arterial blood sample requires specialized training. It may be done by a registered nurse, respiratory therapist, or laboratory technician who has been trained in drawing ABGs. Apply firm pressure to the puncture site for 2 to 5 minutes after the needle is withdrawn to prevent bleeding into the surrounding tissues.

Arterial blood is used because it reflects acid–base balance throughout the entire body better than venous blood. Arterial blood also provides information about the effectiveness of the lungs in oxygenating blood. The elements measured are pH, the $Paco_2$, the Pao_2, and bicarbonate level.

PRACTICE ALERT

You will see the abbreviations $Paco_2$ and Pao_2 used interchangeably with Pco_2 and Po_2. The P stands for partial pressure: the pressure exerted by the gas dissolved in the blood. The a indicates that the sample is arterial blood. Because these measurements rarely are done on venous blood, the a often is deleted from the abbreviation.

The **$Paco_2$** measures the pressure exerted by dissolved carbon dioxide in the blood. The $Paco_2$ reflects the respiratory component of acid–base regulation and balance. The $Paco_2$ is regulated by the lungs. The normal value is 35 to 45 mmHg. A $Paco_2$ of less than 35 mmHg is known as *hypocapnia;* a $Paco_2$ greater than 45 mmHg is *hypercapnia.*

The **Pao_2** is a measure of the pressure exerted by oxygen that is dissolved in the plasma. Only about 3% of oxygen in the blood is transported in solution; most is combined with hemoglobin. However, it is the dissolved oxygen that is available to the cells for metabolism. As dissolved oxygen diffuses out of plasma into the tissues, more is released from hemoglobin. The normal value for Pao_2 is 80 to 100 mmHg. A Pao_2 of less than 80 mmHg is indicative of *hypoxemia.* The Pao_2 is valuable for evaluating respiratory function, but is not used as a primary measurement in determining acid–base status.

The **serum bicarbonate** (HCO_3^-) reflects the renal regulation of acid–base balance. It is often called the metabolic component of arterial blood gases. The normal HCO_3^- value is 22 to 26 mEq/L.

The **base excess (BE)** is a calculated value also known as *buffer base capacity.* The base excess measures substances that can accept or combine with hydrogen ion. It reflects the degree of acid–base imbalance by indicating the status of the body's total buffering capacity. It represents the amount of acid or base that must be added to a blood sample to achieve a pH of 7.4. This is essentially a measure of increased or decreased bicarbonate. The normal value for base excess for arterial blood is -3.0 to $+3.0$. Normal ABG values are summarized in Table 10–10.

ABGs are analyzed to identify acid–base disorders and their probable cause, to determine the extent of the imbalance, and to monitor treatment. When analyzing ABG results, it is important to use a systematic approach. First evaluate each individual measurement, then look at the interrelationships to determine the client's acid–base status (Box 10–10).

ACID–BASE IMBALANCE

Acid–base imbalances fall into two major categories: acidosis and alkalosis. Acidosis occurs when the hydrogen ion concentration increases above normal (pH below 7.35). Alkalosis

TABLE 10-10 Normal Arterial Blood Gas Values

VALUE	NORMAL RANGE	SIGNIFICANCE
pH	7.35 to 7.45	Reflects hydrogen ion (H^+) concentration ■ < 7.35 = acidosis ■ > 7.45 = alkalosis
$Paco_2$	35 to 45 mmHg	Partial pressure of carbon dioxide (CO_2) in arterial blood ■ < 35 mmHg = hypocapnia ■ > 45 mmHg = hypercapnia
Pao_2	80 to 100 mmHg	Partial pressure of oxygen (O_2) in arterial blood ■ < 80 mmHg = hypoxemia
HCO_3^-	22 to 26 mEq/L	Bicarbonate concentration in plasma
BE	−3 to +3	Base excess; a measure of buffering capacity

occurs when the hydrogen ion concentration falls below normal (pH above 7.45).

Acid–base imbalances are further classified as *metabolic* or *respiratory* disorders. In metabolic disorders, the primary change is in the concentration of bicarbonate. In metabolic acidosis, the amount of bicarbonate is decreased in relation to the amount of acid in the body (Figure 10–15A ■). It can develop as a result of abnormal bicarbonate losses or because of excess nonvolatile acids in the body. The pH falls below 7.35 and the bicarbonate concentration is less than 22 mEq/L. Metabolic alkalosis, by contrast, occurs when there is an excess of bicarbonate in relation to the amount of hydrogen ion (Figure 10–15B). The pH is above 7.45 and the bicarbonate concentration is greater than 26 mEq/L.

In respiratory disorders, the primary change is in the concentration of carbonic acid. *Respiratory acidosis* occurs when carbon dioxide is retained, increasing the amount of carbonic acid in the body (Figure 10–16A ■). As a result, the pH falls to less than 7.35, and the $Paco_2$ is greater than 45 mmHg. When too much carbon dioxide is "blown off," carbonic acid levels fall and *respiratory alkalosis* develops (Figure 10–16B). The pH rises to above 7.45 and the $Paco_2$ is less than 35 mmHg.

Acid–base disorders are further defined as *primary* (simple) and *mixed*. Primary disorders usually are due to one cause. For example, respiratory failure often causes respiratory acidosis due to retained carbon dioxide; renal failure usually causes metabolic acidosis due to retained hydrogen ion and impaired

---

BOX 10-10 Interpreting Arterial Blood Gases

1. Look at the pH.
   - ■ pH < 7.35 = acidosis
   - ■ pH > 7.45 = alkalosis
2. Look at the $Paco_2$.
   - ■ $Paco_2$ < 35 mmHg = hypocapnia; more carbon dioxide is being exhaled than normal
   - ■ $Paco_2$ > 45 mmHg = hypercapnia; carbon dioxide is being retained
3. Evaluate the pH–$Paco_2$ relationship for a possible respiratory problem.
   - ■ If the pH is < 7.35 (acidosis) and the $Paco_2$ is > 45 mmHg (hypercapnia), retained carbon dioxide is causing increased H^+ concentration and *respiratory acidosis*.
   - ■ If the pH is > 7.45 (alkalosis) and the $Paco_2$ is < 35 mmHg (hypocapnia), low carbon dioxide levels and decreased H^+ concentration are causing *respiratory alkalosis*.
4. Look at the bicarbonate.
   - ■ If the HCO_3^- is < 22 mEq/L, bicarbonate levels are lower than normal.
   - ■ If the HCO_3^- is > 26 mEq/L, bicarbonate levels are higher than normal.
5. Evaluate the pH, HCO_3^-, and BE for a possible metabolic problem.
   - ■ If the pH is < 7.35 (acidosis), the HCO_3^- is < 22 mEq/L, and the BE is < −3 mEq/L, then low bicarbonate levels

and high H^+ concentrations are causing *metabolic acidosis*.
   - ■ If the pH is > 7.45 (alkalosis), the HCO_3^- is > 26 mEq/L, and the BE is > +3 mEq/L, then high bicarbonate levels are causing *metabolic alkalosis*.
6. Look for compensation.
   - ■ *Renal compensation:*
      - ■ In respiratory acidosis (pH < 7.35, $Paco_2$ > 45 mmHg), the kidneys retain HCO_3^- to buffer the excess acid, so the HCO_3^- is > 26 mEq/L.
      - ■ In respiratory alkalosis (pH > 7.45, $Paco_2$ < 35 mmHg), the kidneys excrete HO_3^- to minimize the alkalosis, so the HCO_3^- is < 22 mEq/L.
   - ■ *Respiratory compensation*
      - ■ In metabolic acidosis (pH < 7.35, HCO_3^- < 22 mEq/L), the rate and depth of respirations increase, increasing carbon dioxide elimination, so the $PaCo_2$ is < 35 mmHg.
      - ■ In metabolic alkalosis (pH > 7.45, HCO_3^- > 26 mEq/L), respirations slow, carbon dioxide is retained, so the $Paco_2$ is > 45 mmHg.
7. Evaluate oxygenation.
   - ■ Pao_2 < 80 mmHg = hypoxemia; possible hypoventilation
   - ■ Pao_2 > 100 mmHg = hyperventilation

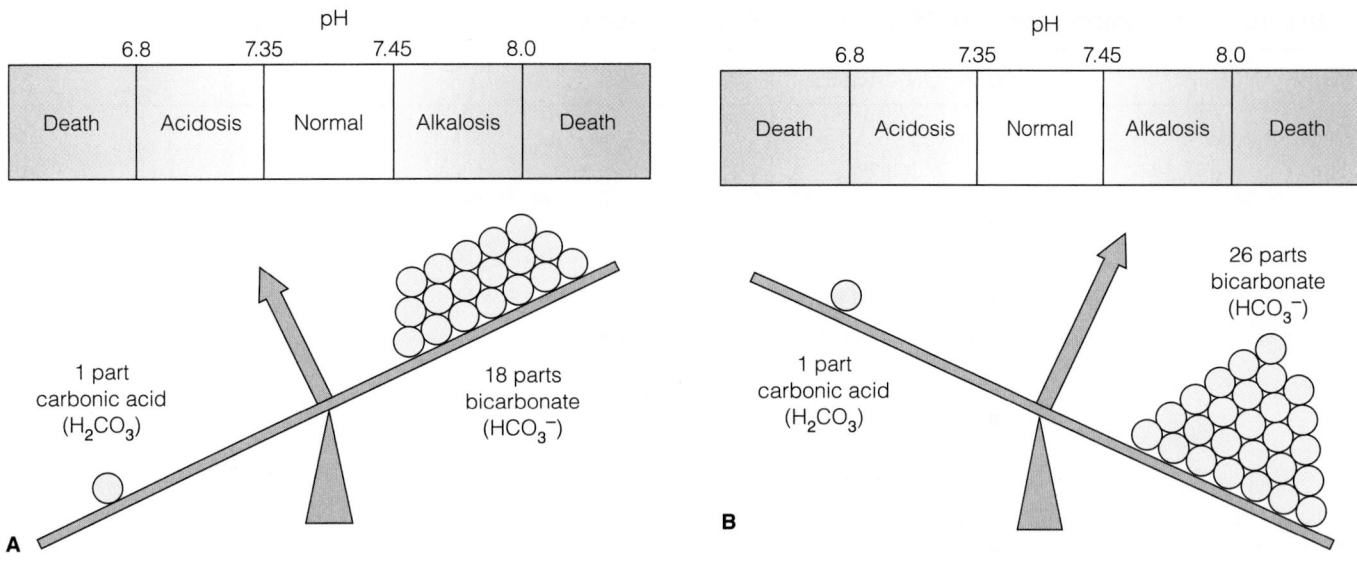

Figure 10–15 ■ Metabolic acid–base imbalances. *A,* Metabolic acidosis. *B,* Metabolic alkalosis.

bicarbonate production. Table 10–11 summarizes primary acid–base imbalances with common causes of each. Mixed disorders occur from combinations of respiratory and metabolic disturbances. For example, a client in cardiac arrest develops a mixed respiratory and metabolic acidosis due to lack of ventilation (and retained CO_2) and hypoxia of body tissues that leads to anaerobic metabolism and acid by-products (excess nonvolatile acids).

FAST FACTS

- Simple acid–base imbalances are more commonly seen than mixed imbalances. Common causes of simple acid–base imbalances include:
  - Diabetic ketoacidosis (metabolic acidosis)
  - Chronic obstructive lung disease (respiratory acidosis)
  - Anxiety-related (psychogenic) hyperventilation (respiratory alkalosis)
- Critically ill clients are at higher risk for mixed acid–base imbalances.

Compensation

With primary acid–base disorders, compensatory changes in the other part of the regulatory system occur to restore a normal pH and homeostasis. In metabolic acid–base disorders, the change in pH affects the rate and depth of respirations. This, in turn, affects carbon dioxide elimination and the Pa_{CO_2}, helping restore the carbonic acid to bicarbonate ratio. The kidneys compensate for simple respiratory imbalances. The change in pH affects both bicarbonate conservation and hydrogen ion elimination (Table 10–12).

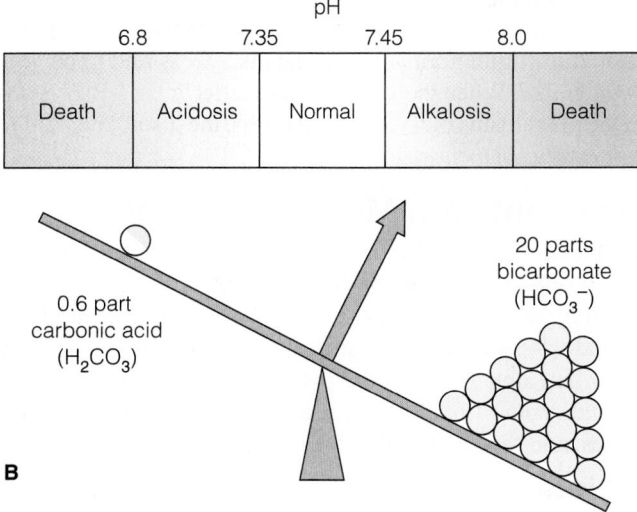

Figure 10–16 ■ Respiratory acid–base imbalances. *A,* Respiratory acidosis. *B,* Respiratory alkalosis.

TABLE 10–11 Common Causes of Primary Acid–Base Imbalances

IMBALANCE	COMMON CAUSES

Metabolic acidosis
pH < 7.35
HCO₃⁻ < 22 mEq/L
Critical values
pH < 7.20
HCO₃⁻ < 10 mEq/L
	↑ Acid production
	  ■ Lactic acidosis
	  ■ Ketoacidosis related to diabetes, starvation, or alcoholism
	  ■ Salicylate toxicity
	↓ Acid excretion
	  ■ Renal failure
	↑ Bicarbonate loss
	  ■ Diarrhea, ileostomy drainage, intestinal fistula
	  ■ Biliary or pancreatic fistulas
	↑ Chloride
	  ■ Sodium chloride IV solutions
	  ■ Renal tubular acidosis
	  ■ Carbonic anhydrase inhibitors

Metabolic alkalosis
pH > 7.45
HCO₃⁻ > 26 mEq/L
Critical values
pH > 7.60
HCO₃⁻ > 40 mEq/L
	↑ Acid loss or excretion
	  ■ Vomiting, gastric suction
	  ■ Hypokalemia
	↑ Bicarbonate
	  ■ Alkali ingestion (bicarbonate of soda)
	  ■ Excess bicarbonate administration

Respiratory acidosis
pH < 7.35
Pa$_{CO_2}$ >45 mm Hg
Critical values
pH < 7.2
Pa$_{CO_2}$ > 77 mmHg
	Acute respiratory acidosis
	  ■ Acute respiratory conditions (pulmonary edema, pneumonia, acute asthma)
	  ■ Opiate overdose
	  ■ Foreign body aspiration
	  ■ Chest trauma
	Chronic respiratory acidosis
	  ■ Chronic respiratory conditions (COPD, cystic fibrosis)
	  ■ Multiple sclerosis, other neuromuscular diseases
	  ■ Stroke

Respiratory alkalosis
pH > 7.45
Pa$_{CO_2}$ < 35 mm Hg
Critical values
pH > 7.60
Pa$_{CO_2}$ < 20 mmHg
	■ Anxiety-induced hyperventilation (e.g., anxiety)
	  ■ Fever
	  ■ Early salicylate intoxication
	  ■ Hyperventilation with mechanical ventilator

Compensatory changes in respirations occur within minutes of a change in pH. These changes, however, become less effective over time. The renal response takes longer to restore the pH, but is a more effective long-term mechanism. If the pH is restored to within normal limits, the disorder is said to be *fully compensated*. When these changes are reflected in ABG values but the pH remains outside normal limits, the disorder is said to be *partially compensated*.

The Client with Metabolic Acidosis

Metabolic acidosis (bicarbonate deficit) is characterized by a low pH (<7.35) and a low bicarbonate (<22 mEq/L). It may be caused by excess acid in the body or loss of bicarbonate from the body. When metabolic acidosis develops, the respiratory system attempts to return the pH to normal by increasing the rate and depth of respirations. Carbon dioxide elimination increases, and the Pa$_{CO_2}$ falls (<35 mmHg).

Risk Factors

Metabolic acidosis rarely is a primary disorder; it usually develops during the course of another disease:

- *Acute lactic acidosis* usually results from tissue hypoxia due to shock or cardiac arrest.
- Clients with type 1 diabetes mellitus are at risk for developing *diabetic ketoacidosis*. (See Chapter 20 ∞ for more information about diabetes and its complications.)
- *Acute* or *chronic renal failure* impairs the excretion of metabolic acids.
- Diarrhea, intestinal suction, or abdominal fistulas increase the risk for excess *bicarbonate loss*.

Other common causes of metabolic acidosis are listed in Table 10–11.

Pathophysiology

Three basic mechanisms that can cause metabolic acidosis are:
- Accumulation of metabolic acids
- Excess loss of bicarbonate
- An increase in chloride levels.

An accumulation of metabolic acids can result from excess acid production or impaired elimination of metabolic acids by the kidney. Lactic acidosis develops due to tissue hypoxia and a shift to anaerobic metabolism by the cells. Lactate and hy-

other symptoms; duration of symptoms and any precipitating factors such as diarrhea, ingestion of a toxin such as aspirin, methanol, or ethylene; chronic diseases such as diabetes or renal failure, cirrhosis of the liver, or endocrine disorders; current medications.
- *Physical assessment:* Mental status and level of consciousness; vital signs including respiratory rate and depth; apical and peripheral pulses; skin color and temperature; abdominal contour and distention; bowel sounds; urine output.
- *Diagnostic tests:* ABGs, serum electrolytes, tests for underlying disorders.

Nursing Diagnoses and Interventions

Nursing management of clients with metabolic acidosis often focuses on the primary disorder (e.g., diabetic ketoacidosis or renal failure); however, the acidosis itself has effects that must be attended to when providing care.

Decreased Cardiac Output

Metabolic acidosis affects cardiac output by decreasing myocardial contractility, slowing the heart rate, and increasing the risk for dysrhythmias. The accompanying hyperkalemia increases the risk for decreased cardiac output as well (see earlier discussion about hyperkalemia).
- Monitor vital signs, including peripheral pulses and capillary refill. *Hypotension, diminished pulse strength, and slowed capillary refill may indicate decreased cardiac output and impaired tissue perfusion. Poor tissue perfusion can increase the risk for lactic acidosis.*
- Monitor the ECG pattern for dysrhythmias and changes characteristic of hyperkalemia. Notify the physician of changes. *Progressive ECG changes such as widening of the QRS complex indicate an increasing risk of dysrhythmias and cardiac arrest. Dysrhythmias further decrease cardiac output, possibly intensifying the degree of acidosis.*
- Monitor laboratory values, including ABGs, serum electrolytes, and renal function studies (serum creatinine and BUN). *Frequent monitoring of laboratory values allows evaluation of the effectiveness of treatment as well as early identification of potential problems.*

Risk for Excess Fluid Volume

Administering bicarbonate to correct acidosis increases the risk for hypernatremia, hyperosmolality, and fluid volume excess.
- Monitor and maintain fluid replacement as ordered. Monitor serum sodium levels and osmolality. *Bicarbonate administration can cause hypernatremia and hyperosmolality, leading to water retention.*
- Monitor heart and lung sounds, CVP, and respiratory status. *Increasing dyspnea, adventitious lung sounds, a third heart sound (S_3) due to the volume of blood flow through the heart, and high CVP readings are indicative of hypervolemia and should be reported to the care provider.*
- Assess for edema, particularly in the back, sacral, and periorbital areas. *Initially, edema affects dependent tissues—the back and sacrum in clients who are bedridden. Periorbital edema indicates more generalized edema.*

- Assess urine output hourly. Maintain accurate intake and output records. Note urine output less than 30 mL/hour or a positive fluid balance on 24-hour total intake and output calculations. *Heart failure and inadequate renal perfusion may lead to decreased urine output.*
- Obtain daily weights using consistent conditions. *Daily weights are an accurate indicator of fluid balance.*
- Administer prescribed diuretics as ordered, monitoring the client's response to therapy. *Loop or high-ceiling diuretics such as furosemide can lead to further electrolyte imbalances, especially hypokalemia. This is a significant risk like that seen during correction of metabolic acidosis.*

Risk for Injury

Mental status and brain function are affected by acidosis, increasing the risk for injury.
- Monitor neurologic function, including mental status, level of consciousness, and muscle strength. *As the pH falls, mental functioning declines, leading to confusion, stupor, and a decreasing level of consciousness.*
- Institute safety precautions as necessary: Keep the bed in its lowest position, side rails raised. *These measures help protect the client from injury resulting from confusion or disorientation.*
- Keep clocks, calendars, and familiar objects at bedside. Orient to time, place, and circumstances as needed. Allow significant others to remain with the client as much as possible. *An unfamiliar environment and altered thought processes can further increase the risk for injury. Significant others provide a sense of security and reduce anxiety.*

Nursing care also includes measures to treat the underlying disorder, such as diabetic ketoacidosis. Refer to the chapters on diabetes (Chapter 20 ∞) and renal failure (Chapter 29 ∞) for specific interventions.

Community-Based Care

Discharge planning and teaching focus on the underlying cause of the imbalance. The client who has developed ketoacidosis as a result of diabetes mellitus, starvation, or alcoholism needs interventions and teaching to prevent future episodes of acidosis. Diet, medication management, and alcohol dependency treatment are vital teaching areas. When metabolic acidosis is related to renal failure, the client should be referred for management of the renal failure itself. Clients who have experienced diarrhea or excess ileostomy drainage leading to bicarbonate loss need information about appropriate diarrhea treatment strategies and when to call their primary care provider.

The Client with Metabolic Alkalosis

Metabolic alkalosis (bicarbonate excess) is characterized by a high pH (>7.45) and a high bicarbonate (>26 mEq/L). It may be caused by loss of acid or excess bicarbonate in the body. When metabolic alkalosis develops, the respiratory system attempts to return the pH to normal by slowing the respiratory rate. Carbon dioxide is retained, and the Pa_{CO_2} increases (>45 mmHg).

Risk Factors

As is the case with other acid–base imbalances, metabolic alkalosis rarely occurs as a primary disorder. Risk factors include hospitalization, hypokalemia, and treatment with alkalinizing solutions (e.g., bicarbonate).

Pathophysiology

Hydrogen ions may be lost via gastric secretions, through the kidneys, or because of a shift of H^+ into the cells. Metabolic alkalosis due to loss of hydrogen ions usually occurs because of vomiting or gastric suction. Gastric secretions are highly acidic (pH 1 to 3). When these are lost through vomiting or gastric suction, the alkalinity of body fluids increases. This increased alkalinity results both from the loss of acid and selective retention of bicarbonate by the kidneys as chloride is depleted. (Chloride is the major anion in ECF; when it is lost, bicarbonate is retained as a replacement anion.)

Increased renal excretion of hydrogen ions can be prompted by hypokalemia as the kidneys try to conserve potassium, excreting hydrogen ion instead. Hypokalemia contributes to metabolic alkalosis in another way as well. When potassium shifts out of cells to maintain extracellular potassium levels, hydrogen ions shift into the cells to maintain the balance between cations and anions within the cell.

Excess bicarbonate usually occurs as a result of ingesting antacids that contain bicarbonate (such as soda bicarbonate or Alka-Seltzer) or overzealous administration of bicarbonate to treat metabolic acidosis. Common causes of metabolic alkalosis are summarized in Table 10–11.

In alkalosis, more calcium combines with serum proteins, reducing the amount of ionized (physiologically active) calcium in the blood. This accounts for many of the common manifestations of metabolic alkalosis. Alkalosis also affects potassium balance: Hypokalemia not only can cause metabolic alkalosis (see above), but it also can result from metabolic alkalosis. Hydrogen ions shift out of the intracellular space to help restore the pH, prompting more potassium to enter the cells and depleting ECF potassium. The high pH depresses the respiratory system as the body retains carbon dioxide to restore the carbonic acid to bicarbonate ratio.

Manifestations and Complications

Manifestations of metabolic alkalosis (see the box below) occur as a result of decreased calcium ionization and are similar to those of hypocalcemia, including numbness and tingling around

MANIFESTATIONS of Metabolic Alkalosis

- Confusion
- Decreasing level of consciousness
- Hyperreflexia
- Tetany
- Dysrhythmias
- Hypotension
- Seizures
- Respiratory failure

the mouth, fingers, and toes; dizziness; Trousseau's sign; and muscle spasm. As the respiratory system compensates for metabolic alkalosis, respirations are depressed and respiratory failure with hypoxemia and respiratory acidosis may develop.

INTERDISCIPLINARY CARE

Interdisciplinary management of metabolic alkalosis focuses on diagnosing and correcting the underlying cause.

Diagnosis

The following laboratory and diagnostic tests may be ordered.

- *ABGs* show a pH greater than 7.45 and bicarbonate level greater than 26 mEq/L. With compensatory hypoventilation, carbon dioxide is retained, and the $Paco_2$ is greater than 45 mmHg.
- *Serum electrolytes* often demonstrate decreased serum potassium (<3.5 mEq/L) and decreased chloride (<95 mEq/L) levels. The serum bicarbonate level is high. Although the total serum calcium may be normal, the ionized fraction of calcium is low.
- *Urine pH* may be low (pH 1 to 3) if metabolic acidosis is caused by hypokalemia. The kidneys selectively retain potassium and excrete hydrogen ion to restore ECF potassium levels. Urinary chloride levels may be normal or greater than 250 mEq/24 hours.
- The *ECG pattern* shows changes similar to those seen with hypokalemia. These changes may be due to hypokalemia or to the alkalosis.

Medications

Treatment of metabolic alkalosis includes restoring normal fluid volume and administering potassium chloride and sodium chloride solution. The potassium restores serum and intracellular potassium levels, allowing the kidneys to more effectively conserve hydrogen ions. Chloride promotes renal excretion of bicarbonate. Sodium chloride solutions restore fluid volume deficits that can contribute to metabolic alkalosis. In severe alkalosis, an acidifying solution such as dilute hydrochloric acid or ammonium chloride may be administered. In addition, drugs may be used to treat the underlying cause of the alkalosis.

NURSING CARE

Health Promotion

Health promotion activities focus on teaching clients the risks of using sodium bicarbonate as an antacid to relieve heartburn or gastric distress. Stress the availability of other effective antacid preparations and the need to seek medical evaluation for persistent gastric symptoms.

In the hospital setting, carefully monitor laboratory values for clients at risk for developing metabolic alkalosis, particularly clients undergoing continuous gastric suction.

Assessment

Focused assessment data related to metabolic alkalosis include the following:

- *Health history:* Current manifestations, such as numbness and tingling, muscle spasms, dizziness, other symptoms; duration of symptoms and any precipitating factors such as bicarbonate ingestion, vomiting, diuretic therapy, or endocrine disorders; current medications.
- *Physical assessment:* Vital signs including apical pulse and rate and depth of respirations; muscle strength; deep tendon reflexes.
- *Diagnostic tests:* ABGs, serum electrolytes.

Nursing Diagnoses and Interventions

As with metabolic acidosis, nursing care of the client with metabolic alkalosis often focuses on intervening for client responses to the primary problem, rather than the alkalosis itself. However, the risk for impaired gas exchange is a priority problem, especially with severe metabolic alkalosis.

Risk for Impaired Gas Exchange

Respiratory compensation for metabolic alkalosis depresses the respiratory rate and reduces the depth of breathing to promote carbon dioxide retention. As a result, the client is at risk for impaired gas exchange, especially in the presence of underlying lung disease.

- Monitor respiratory rate, depth, and effort. Monitor oxygen saturation continuously, reporting an oxygen saturation level of less than 95% (or as ordered). *The depressed respiratory drive associated with metabolic alkalosis can lead to hypoxemia and impaired oxygenation of tissues. Oxygen saturation levels of less than 90% indicate significant oxygenation problems.*
- Assess skin color; note and report cyanosis around the mouth. *Central cyanosis, seen around the mouth and oral mucous membranes, indicates significant hypoxia.*
- Monitor mental status and level of consciousness (LOC). Report decreasing LOC or behavior changes such as restlessness, agitation, or confusion. *Changes in mental status or behavior may be early signs of hypoxia.*
- Place in semi-Fowler's or Fowler's position as tolerated. *Elevating the head of the bed facilitates alveolar ventilation and gas exchange.*
- Schedule nursing care activities to allow rest periods. *The client who is hypoxemic has limited energy reserves, necessitating frequent rest and limited activities.*
- Administer oxygen as ordered or necessary to maintain oxygen saturation levels. *Supplemental oxygen can help maintain blood and tissue oxygenation despite depressed respirations.*

Deficient Fluid Volume

Clients with metabolic alkalosis often have an accompanying fluid volume deficit.

PRACTICE ALERT
Assess intake and output accurately, monitoring fluid balance. In acute situations, hourly intake and output may be indicated. Urine output of less than 30 mL/hour indicates inadequate tissue perfusion, inadequate renal perfusion, and an increased risk for acute renal failure.

- Assess vital signs, CVP, and peripheral pulse volume at least every 4 hours. *Hypotension, tachycardia, low CVP, and weak, easily obliterated peripheral pulses indicate hypovolemia.*
- Weigh daily under standard conditions (time of day, clothing, and scale). *Rapid weight changes accurately reflect fluid balance.*
- Administer intravenous fluids as prescribed using an electronic infusion pump. Monitor for indicators of fluid overload if rapid fluid replacement is ordered: dyspnea, tachypnea, tachycardia, increased CVP, jugular vein distension, and edema. *Rapid fluid replacement may lead to hypervolemia, resulting in pulmonary edema and cardiac failure, particularly in clients with compromised cardiac and renal function.*
- Monitor serum electrolytes, osmolality, and ABG values. *Rehydration and administration of potassium chloride will affect both acid–base and fluid and electrolyte balance. Careful monitoring is important to identify changes.*

Community-Based Care

When preparing the client with metabolic alkalosis for discharge, consider the cause of the alkalosis and any underlying factors. For example, provide teaching about the following:

- Using appropriate antacids for heartburn and gastric distress
- Using potassium supplements as ordered or eating high-potassium foods to avoid hypokalemia if taking a potassium-wasting diuretic or if aldosterone production is impaired
- Contacting the primary care provider if uncontrolled or extended vomiting develops.

The Client with Respiratory Acidosis

Respiratory acidosis is caused by an excess of dissolved carbon dioxide, or carbonic acid. It is characterized by a pH less than 7.35 and a $PaCO_2$ greater than 45 mmHg. Respiratory acidosis may be either acute or chronic. In chronic respiratory acidosis, the bicarbonate is higher than 26 mEq/L as the kidneys compensate by retaining bicarbonate.

Risk Factors

Acute or chronic lung disease (e.g., pneumonia or chronic obstructive pulmonary disease [COPD]) is the primary risk factor for respiratory acidosis. Other conditions that depress or interfere with ventilation, such as excess narcotic analgesics, airway obstruction, or neuromuscular disease, also are risk factors for respiratory acidosis. Selected causes of respiratory acidosis are listed in Table 10–11.

Pathophysiology

Both acute and chronic respiratory acidosis result from carbon dioxide retention caused by alveolar hypoventilation. Hypoxemia (low oxygen in the arterial blood) frequently accompanies respiratory acidosis.

ACUTE RESPIRATORY ACIDOSIS Acute respiratory acidosis occurs due to a sudden failure of ventilation. Chest trauma, aspiration of a foreign body, acute pneumonia, and overdoses of narcotic or sedative medications can lead to this condition. Because acute respiratory acidosis occurs with the sudden onset of hypoventilation—for example, with cardiac arrest—the

Paco$_2$ rises rapidly and the pH falls markedly. A pH of 7 or lower can occur within minutes (Metheny, 2000). The serum bicarbonate level initially is unchanged because the compensatory response of the kidneys occurs over hours to days.

Hypercapnia (increased carbon dioxide levels) affects neurologic function and the cardiovascular system. Carbon dioxide rapidly crosses the blood–brain barrier. Cerebral blood vessels dilate and, if the condition continues, intracranial pressure increases and *papilledema* (swelling and inflammation of the optic nerve where it enters the retina) develops (Porth, 2005). Peripheral vasodilation also occurs, and the pulse rate increases to maintain cardiac output.

CHRONIC RESPIRATORY ACIDOSIS Chronic respiratory acidosis is associated with chronic respiratory or neuromuscular conditions such as COPD, asthma, cystic fibrosis, or multiple sclerosis. These conditions affect alveolar ventilation because of airway obstruction, structural changes in the lung, or limited chest wall expansion. Most clients with chronic respiratory acidosis have COPD with chronic bronchitis and emphysema. (See Chapter 39 ∞ for more information about COPD.) In chronic respiratory acidosis, the Paco$_2$ increases over time and remains elevated. The kidneys retain bicarbonate, increasing bicarbonate levels, and the pH often remains close to the normal range.

The acute effects of hypercapnia may not develop because carbon dioxide levels rise gradually, allowing compensatory changes to occur. When carbon dioxide levels are chronically elevated, the respiratory center becomes less sensitive to the gas as a stimulant of the respiratory drive. The Pao$_2$ provides the primary stimulus for respirations. Clients with chronic respiratory acidosis are at risk for developing *carbon dioxide narcosis,* with manifestations of acute respiratory acidosis, if the respiratory center is suppressed by administering excess supplemental oxygen.

PRACTICE ALERT
Carefully monitor neurologic and respiratory status in clients with chronic respiratory acidosis who are receiving oxygen therapy. Immediately report a decreasing LOC or depressed respirations.

Manifestations

The manifestations of acute and chronic respiratory acidosis differ. In acute respiratory acidosis, the rapid rise in Paco$_2$ levels causes manifestations of hypercapnia. Cerebral vasodilation causes manifestations such as headache, blurred vision, irritability, and mental cloudiness. If the condition continues, the level of consciousness progressively decreases. Rapid and dramatic changes in ABGs can lead to unconsciousness and ventricular fibrillation, a potentially lethal cardiac dysrhythmia. The skin of the client with acute respiratory acidosis may be warm and flushed, and the pulse rate is elevated.

The manifestations of chronic respiratory acidosis include weakness and a dull headache. Sleep disturbances, daytime sleepiness, impaired memory, and personality changes also may be manifestations of chronic respiratory acidosis (see the box on this page).

MANIFESTATIONS of Respiratory Acidosis

Acute Respiratory Acidosis
- Headache
- Warm, flushed skin
- Blurred vision
- Irritability, altered mental status
- Decreasing level of consciousness
- Cardiac arrest

Chronic Respiratory Acidosis
- Weakness
- Dull headache
- Sleep disturbances with daytime sleepiness
- Impaired memory
- Personality changes

INTERDISCIPLINARY CARE

Clients with acute respiratory failure usually require treatment in the emergency department or intensive care unit. The focus is on restoring adequate ventilation and gas exchange. Hypoxemia often accompanies acute respiratory acidosis, so oxygen is administered as well. Supplemental oxygen is administered with caution to clients with chronic respiratory acidosis.

Diagnosis

The following laboratory and diagnostic tests may be ordered.
- *ABGs* show a pH of less than 7.35 and a Paco$_2$ of more than 45 mmHg. In acute respiratory acidosis, the bicarbonate level is initially within normal range but increases to greater than 26 mEq/L if the condition persists. In chronic respiratory acidosis, both the Paco$_2$ and the HCO$_3^-$ may be significantly elevated.
- *Serum electrolytes* may show hypochloremia (chloride level < 98 mEq/L) in chronic respiratory acidosis.
- *Pulmonary function tests* may be done to determine if chronic lung disease is the cause of the respiratory acidosis. These studies would not be done during the acute period, however.

Additional diagnostic tests may be done to identify the underlying cause of the respiratory acidosis. *Chest x-ray* and *sputum studies* (cytology and culture) may be ordered to identify an acute or chronic lung disorder. If drug overdose is suspected, *serum levels* of the drug may be obtained.

Medications

Bronchodilator drugs may be administered to open the airways and antibiotics prescribed to treat respiratory infections. If excess narcotics or anesthetic has caused acute respiratory acidosis, drugs to reverse their effects (such as naloxone) may be given.

Respiratory Support

Treatment of respiratory acidosis, either acute or chronic, focuses on improving alveolar ventilation and gas exchange. Clients with severe respiratory acidosis and hypoxemia may require intubation and mechanical ventilation (see Chapter 39 ∞ for more information about these procedures). The $Paco_2$ level is lowered slowly to avoid complications such as cardiac dysrhythmias and decreased cerebral perfusion. In clients with chronic respiratory acidosis, oxygen is administered cautiously to avoid carbon dioxide narcosis.

Pulmonary hygiene measures, such as breathing treatments or percussion and drainage, may be instituted. Adequate hydration is important to promote removal of respiratory secretions.

NURSING CARE

See the Nursing Care Plan: A Client with Acute Respiratory Acidosis below.

Health Promotion

Health promotion activities related to respiratory acidosis focus on identifying, monitoring, and teaching clients at risk. Carefully monitor clients receiving anesthesia, narcotic analgesics, or sedatives for signs of respiratory depression. Monitor the response of clients with a history of chronic lung disease to oxygen therapy. Teach clients who have an identified risk for respiratory acidosis (such as people using narcotic analgesia for cancer pain and people with chronic lung disease) and their

families about early manifestations of respiratory depression and acidosis, and instruct them to immediately contact their care provider if manifestations develop.

Assessment

Assessment data related to respiratory acidosis include the following:
- *Health history:* Current manifestations, including headache, irritability or lethargy, difficulty thinking, blurred vision, and other symptoms; duration of symptoms and any precipitating factors such as drug use or respiratory infection; chronic diseases such as cystic fibrosis or COPD; current medications.
- *Physical assessment:* Mental status and level of consciousness; vital signs; skin color and temperature; rate and depth of respirations, pulmonary excursion, lung sounds; examination of optic fundus for possible papilledema.
- *Diagnostic tests:* ABGs, serum electrolytes; white blood cell count (indicator of infection), sputum culture results, serum drug and toxicology results.

Nursing Diagnoses and Interventions

Restoring effective alveolar ventilation and gas exchange is the priority of interdisciplinary and nursing care for clients with respiratory acidosis.

NURSING CARE PLAN A Client with Acute Respiratory Acidosis

Marlene Hitz, age 76, is eating lunch with her friends when she suddenly begins to choke and is unable to breathe. After several minutes of trying, an attendant at the senior center successfully dislodges some meat caught in Ms. Hitz's throat using the Heimlich maneuver. Ms. Hitz is taken by ambulance to the emergency department for follow-up because she was apneic for 3 to 4 minutes, her respirations are shallow, and she is disoriented.

ASSESSMENT

Ms. Hitz is placed in an observation room. Oxygen is started at 4 L/min per nasal cannula. David Love, the nurse admitting Ms. Hitz, makes the following assessments: T 98.2, P 102, R 36 and shallow, BP 146/92. Skin is warm and dry. Alert but restless and not oriented to time or place; she responds slowly to questions. Stat ABGs are drawn, a chest x-ray is done, and D_5 1/2 NS is started intravenously at 50 mL/h.

The chest x-ray shows no abnormality. ABG results are pH 7.38 (normal: 7.35 to 7.45), $Paco_2$ 48 mmHg (normal: 35 to 45 mmHg), Pao_2 92 mmHg (normal: 80 to 100 mmHg), and HCO_3^- 24 mEq/L (normal: 22 to 26 mEq/L).

DIAGNOSES

- *Impaired Gas Exchange* related to temporary airway obstruction
- *Anxiety* related to emergency hospital admission
- *Risk for Injury* related to confusion

EXPECTED OUTCOMES

- Regain normal gas exchange and ABG values.
- Be oriented to time, place, and person.
- Regain baseline mental status.
- Remain free of injury.

PLANNING AND IMPLEMENTATION

- Monitor ABGs, to be redrawn in 2 hours.
- Monitor vital signs and respiratory status (including oxygen saturation) every 15 minutes for the first hour then every hour.
- Assess color of skin, nail beds, and oral mucous membranes every hour.
- Assess mental status and orientation every hour.
- Monitor anxiety level as evidenced by restlessness and agitation.
- Maintain a calm, quiet environment.
- Provide reorientation and explain all activities.
- Keep side rails in place, and place call bell within reach.

EVALUATION

Ms. Hitz remains in the emergency department for 6 hours. Her ABGs are still abnormal, and David Love now notes the presence of respiratory crackles and wheezes. She is less anxious and responds appropriately when asked who and where she is. Because she has not regained normal gas exchange, Ms. Hitz is admitted to the hospital for continued observation and treatment.

CRITICAL THINKING IN THE NURSING PROCESS

1. Describe the pathophysiologic process that leads to acute respiratory acidosis in Ms. Hitz.
2. Describe the effect of acidosis on mental function.
3. What teaching would you provide to Ms. Hitz to prevent future episodes of choking?
See Evaluating Your Response in Appendix C.

Impaired Gas Exchange

- Frequently assess respiratory status, including rate, depth, effort, and oxygen saturation levels. *Decreasing respiratory rate and effort along with decreasing oxygen saturation levels may signal worsening respiratory failure and respiratory acidosis.*

> **PRACTICE ALERT**
> Frequently assess level of consciousness. A decline in LOC may indicate increasing hypercapnia and the need for increasing ventilatory support (such as intubation and mechanical ventilation).

- Promptly evaluate and report ABG results to the physician and respiratory therapist. *Rapid changes in carbon dioxide or oxygen levels may necessitate modification of the treatment plan to prevent complications of overcorrection of respiratory acidosis.*
- Place in semi-Fowler's to Fowler's position as tolerated. *Elevating the head of the bed promotes lung expansion and gas exchange.*
- Administer oxygen as ordered. Carefully monitor response. Reduce the oxygen flow rate or percentage and immediately report increasing somnolence. *Supplemental oxygen can suppress the respiratory drive in clients with chronic respiratory acidosis.*

Ineffective Airway Clearance

- Frequently auscultate breath sounds (whether on or off a mechanical ventilator). *Increasing adventitious sounds or decreasing breath sounds (faint or absent) may indicate worsening airway clearance due to obstruction or fatigue.*
- Encourage the client with chronic respiratory acidosis to use pursed-lip breathing. *Pursed-lip breathing helps maintain open airways throughout exhalation, promoting carbon dioxide elimination.*
- Frequently reposition and encourage ambulation as tolerated. *Repositioning, sitting at the bedside, and ambulation promote airway clearance and lung expansion.*
- Encourage fluid intake of up to 3000 mL per day as tolerated or allowed. *Fluids help liquefy secretions and hydrate respiratory mucous membranes, promoting airway clearance.*
- Administer medications such as inhaled bronchodilators as ordered. *Inhaled bronchodilators help relieve bronchial spasm, dilating airways.*
- Provide percussion, vibration, and postural drainage as ordered. *Pulmonary hygiene measures such as these help loosen respiratory secretions so they can be coughed out of airways.*

Using NANDA, NIC, and NOC

Chart 10–3 shows links between NANDA nursing diagnoses, NIC, and NOC when caring for a client with respiratory acidosis.

Community-Based Care

Planning and teaching for home care focuses on the problem that caused the client to develop respiratory acidosis. The client who developed acute respiratory acidosis as a result of acute pneumonia or chest trauma may only require teaching to prevent future problems. If acute respiratory acidosis occurred secondarily

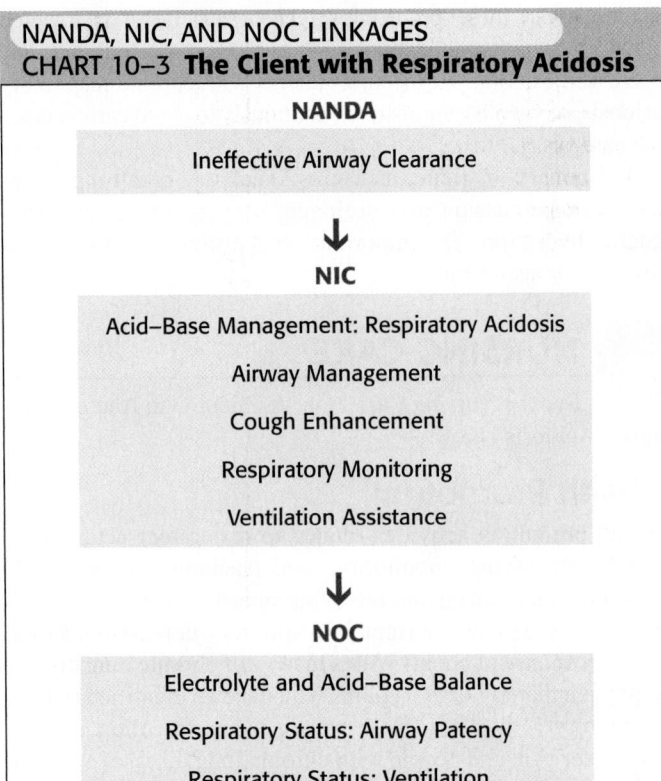

NANDA, NIC, AND NOC LINKAGES
CHART 10–3 The Client with Respiratory Acidosis

Data from *NANDA's Nursing Diagnoses: Definitions & classification 2005–2006* by NANDA International (2003), Philadelphia; *Nursing Interventions Classification (NIC)* (4th ed.) by J. M. Dochterman & G. M. Bulechek (2004), St. Louis, MO: Mosby; and *Nursing Outcomes Classification (NOC)* (3rd ed.) by S. Moorhead, M. Johnson, and M. Maas (2004), St. Louis, MO: Mosby.

to a narcotic overdose, determine if the drug was prescribed for pain or if it was an illicit street drug. Provide teaching to the client who requires narcotic medication on a continuing basis. Refer the client using illicit drugs to a substance abuse counselor, treatment center, or Narcotics Anonymous as appropriate.

For clients with chronic lung disease, discuss ways to avoid future episodes of acute respiratory failure. Encourage the client to be immunized against pneumococcal pneumonia and influenza. Discuss ways to avoid acute respiratory infections and measures to take when respiratory status is further compromised.

The Client with Respiratory Alkalosis

Respiratory alkalosis is characterized by a pH greater than 7.45 and a $PaCO_2$ of less than 35 mmHg. It is always caused by hyperventilation leading to a carbon dioxide deficit.

Risk Factors

Anxiety with hyperventilation is the most common cause of respiratory alkalosis; therefore, anxiety disorders increase the risk for this acid–base imbalance. In the client who is critically ill, mechanical ventilation is a risk factor for respiratory alkalosis.

Pathophysiology

In acute respiratory alkalosis, the pH rises rapidly as the $PaCO_2$ falls. Because the kidneys are unable to rapidly adapt to the change in pH, the bicarbonate level remains within normal limits. Anxiety-based hyperventilation is the most common cause of acute respiratory alkalosis. Other physiologic causes of hyperventilation include high fever, hypoxia, gram-negative bacteremia, and thyrotoxicosis. Early salicylate intoxication (aspirin overdose), encephalitis, and high progesterone levels in pregnancy directly stimulate the respiratory center, potentially leading to hyperventilation and respiratory alkalosis. Hyperventilation also can occur during anesthesia or mechanical ventilation if the rate and tidal volume (depth) of ventilations is excessive.

If hyperventilation continues, the kidneys compensate by eliminating bicarbonate to restore the bicarbonate to carbonic acid ratio. The bicarbonate level is lower than normal in chronic respiratory alkalosis, and the pH may be close to the normal range.

Alkalosis increases binding of extracellular calcium to albumin, reducing ionized calcium levels. As a result, neuromuscular excitability increases and manifestations similar to hypocalcemia develop. Low carbon dioxide levels in the blood cause vasoconstriction of cerebral vessels, increasing the neurologic manifestations of the disorder.

Manifestations

The manifestations of respiratory alkalosis include light-headedness, a feeling of panic and difficulty concentrating, circumoral and distal extremity paresthesias, tremors, and positive Chvostek's and Trousseau's signs. The client also may experience tinnitus, a sensation of chest tightness, and palpitations (cardiac dysrhythmias). Seizures and loss of consciousness may occur. (See the Manifestations box on this page.)

INTERDISCIPLINARY CARE

Management of respiratory alkalosis focuses on correcting the imbalance and treating the underlying cause.

Diagnosis

ABGs generally show a pH greater than 7.45 and a $PaCO_2$ of less than 35 mmHg. In chronic hyperventilation, there is a compensatory decrease in serum bicarbonate to less than 22 mEq/L and the pH may be near normal.

Medications

A sedative or antianxiety agent may be necessary to relieve anxiety and restore a normal breathing pattern. Additional drugs to correct underlying problems other than anxiety-induced hyperventilation may be ordered.

Respiratory Therapy

The usual treatment for anxiety-related respiratory alkalosis involves instructing the client to breathe more slowly and having the client breathe into a paper bag or rebreather mask. This allows rebreathing of exhaled carbon dioxide, increasing $PaCO_2$ levels and reducing the pH. If excessive ventilation by a mechanical ventilator is the cause of respiratory alkalosis, ventilator settings are adjusted to reduce the respiratory rate and tidal volume as indicated. When hypoxia is the underlying cause of hyperventilation, oxygen is administered.

MANIFESTATIONS **of Respiratory Alkalosis**

- Dizziness
- Numbness and tingling around mouth, hands, and feet
- Palpitations
- Dyspnea
- Chest tightness
- Anxiety/panic
- Tremors
- Tetany
- Seizures, loss of consciousness

NURSING CARE

Health Promotion

Identify clients at risk in the hospital (e.g., clients on mechanical ventilation or who have a fever or infection), and monitor assessment data and ABGs to identify early manifestations of hyperventilation and respiratory alkalosis.

Assessment, Diagnoses, and Interventions

Ineffective Breathing Pattern

The usual cause of hyperventilation and respiratory alkalosis is psychologic, although physiologic disorders also can lead to hyperventilation. It is important to not only address the hyperventilation, but also to identify the underlying cause.

- Assess respiratory rate, depth, and ease. Monitor vital signs (including temperature) and skin color. *Assessment data can help identify the underlying cause, such as a fever or hypoxia.*
- Obtain subjective assessment data such as circumstances leading up to the current situation, current health and recent illnesses or medication use, and current manifestations. *Subjective data provide cues to the cause and circumstances of the hyperventilation response.*
- Reassure the client that he or she is not experiencing a heart attack and that symptoms will resolve when breathing returns to normal. *Manifestations of hyperventilation and respiratory alkalosis such as dyspnea, chest tightness or pain, and palpitations can mimic those of a heart attack.*
- Instruct the client to maintain eye contact and breathe with you to slow the respiratory rate. *These measures help to make the client aware of respirations and provide a sense of support and control* (Ackley & Ladwig, 2006).
- Have the client breathe into a paper bag. *This allows the client to rebreathe exhaled carbon dioxide, increasing the $PaCO_2$ and decreasing the pH.*
- Protect the client from injury. *If hyperventilation continues to the point at which the client loses consciousness, respirations will return to normal, as will acid–base balance.*
- If the client has experienced repeated episodes of hyperventilation or has a chronic anxiety disorder, refer for counseling. *Counseling can help the client develop alternative strategies for dealing with anxiety.*

Community-Based Care

Planning and teaching for home care is directed toward the underlying cause of hyperventilation. If anxiety precipitated the episode, discuss anxiety management strategies with the client. Refer the client and family to a counselor if appropriate. Teach the client to identify a hyperventilation reaction, and how to breathe into a paper bag to manage it at home.

EXPLORE MEDIALINK

Prentice Hall Nursing MediaLink DVD-ROM

Audio Glossary
NCLEX-RN® Review

Animations
Acid–Base Balance
Fluid Balance
Furosemide
Membrane Transport

COMPANION WEBSITE www.prenhall.com/lemone
Audio Glossary
NCLEX-RN® Review
Care Plan Activities
   Fluid Volume Deficit
   Hypocalcemia
Case Studies
   Third Spacing
   Hypernatremia
MediaLink Applications
   Metabolic Acidosis and Type 1 Diabetes
   Alterations in Electrolytes, Medications, Fluid Volumes
Links to Resources

CHAPTER HIGHLIGHTS

- The volume and composition of body fluid is normally maintained by a balance of fluid and electrolyte intake; elimination of water, electrolytes, and acids by the kidneys; and hormonal influences. Change in any of these factors can lead to a fluid, electrolyte, or acid–base imbalance that adversely impacts health.
- Fluid, electrolyte, and acid–base imbalances can affect all body systems, especially the cardiovascular system, the central nervous system, and the transmission of nerve impulses. Conversely, primary disorders of the respiratory, renal, cardiovascular, endocrine, or other body systems can lead to an imbalance of fluids, electrolytes, or acid–base status.
- Fluid and sodium imbalances commonly are related; both affect serum osmolality.
- Potassium imbalances are commonly seen in clients with acute or chronic illnesses. Both hypokalemia and hyperkalemia affect cardiac conduction and function. Carefully monitor cardiac rhythm and status in clients with very low or very high potassium levels.
- Calcium imbalances primarily affect neuromuscular transmission: Hypocalcemia increases neuromuscular irritability; hypercalcemia

- depresses neuromuscular transmission. Magnesium imbalances have a similar effect.
- Acid–base imbalances may be caused by either metabolic or respiratory problems. Simple acid–base imbalances (respiratory or metabolic acidosis or alkalosis) are more commonly seen than mixed imbalances.
- Buffers, lungs, and kidneys work together to maintain acid–base balance in the body. Buffers respond to changes almost immediately; the lungs respond within minutes; the kidneys, however, require hours to days to restore normal acid–base balance.
- The lungs compensate for metabolic acid–base imbalances by excreting or retaining carbon dioxide. This is accomplished by increasing or decreasing the rate and depth of respirations.
- The kidneys compensate for respiratory acid–base imbalances by producing and retaining or excreting bicarbonate, and by retaining or excreting hydrogen ions.
- Careful monitoring of respiratory and cardiovascular status, mental status, neuromuscular function, and laboratory values is an important nursing responsibility for all clients with fluid, electrolyte, or acid–base imbalances.

TEST YOURSELF NCLEX-RN® REVIEW

1 A client is admitted to the emergency department with hypovolemia. Which intravenous solution would the nurse anticipate administering?
   1. Ringer's solution
   2. 10% dextrose in water
   3. 3% sodium chloride
   4. 0.45% sodium chloride

2 When assessing a client with fluid volume deficit, the nurse would expect to find:
   1. increased pulse rate and blood pressure.
   2. dyspnea and respiratory crackles.
   3. headache and muscle cramps.
   4. orthostatic hypotension and flat neck veins.

3 The nurse caring for a client with acute hypernatremia includes which of the following in the plan of care? (Select all that apply.)
1. Conduct frequent neurologic checks.
2. Restrict fluids to 1500 mL per day.
3. Orient to time, place, and person frequently.
4. Maintain intravenous access.
e. Limit length of visits.

4 Laboratory results for a client show a serum potassium level of 2.2 mEq/L. Which of the following nursing actions is of highest priority for this client?
1. Keep the client on bed rest.
2. Initiate cardiac monitoring.
3. Start oxygen at 2 L/min.
4. Initiate seizure precautions.

5 The nurse evaluates teaching about calcium supplement therapy as effective when the client states that she will take her calcium tablets:
1. all at one time in the morning.
2. with meals.
3. as needed for tremulousness.
4. with a full glass of water.

6 A client who is known to be an alcoholic presents with confusion, hallucinations, and a positive Chvostek's sign. Which medication(s) should the nurse anticipate administering?
1. magnesium sulfate
2. calcium chloride
3. insulin and glucose
4. sodium bicarbonate

7 Arterial blood gas results for a client show pH 7.21, PaO_2 98 mmHg, $Paco_2$ 32 mmHg, and HCO_3^- 17 mEq/L. The nurse correctly interprets these values as indicative of which of the following acid–base imbalances?
1. metabolic acidosis
2. metabolic alkalosis
3. respiratory acidosis
4. respiratory alkalosis

8 A client is admitted with a suspected heroin overdose and a respiratory rate of 5 to 6 per minute. Which of the following assessment data would the nurse anticipate? (Select all that apply.)
1. pH 7.29
2. alert and oriented
3. $Paco_2$ 54 mmHg
4. HCO_3^- 32 mEq/L
e. skin warm and flushed

9 The nurse caring for a client undergoing several days of gastric decompression recognizes that the client is at risk for which of the following acid–base imbalances?
1. metabolic acidosis
2. metabolic alkalosis
3. respiratory acidosis
4. respiratory alkalosis

10 A client undergoing mechanical ventilation following a severe chest wall injury and flail chest complains of chest tightness, anxiety, and feeling as though she cannot get enough air. She is afraid she is having a heart attack. The nurse should first
1. administer prescribed analgesic.
2. contact respiratory therapy to evaluate ventilator settings.
3. obtain arterial blood gases.
4. notify the physician.

See Test Yourself answers in Appendix C.

BIBLIOGRAPHY

Ackley, B. J., & Ladwig, G. B. (2006). *Nursing diagnosis hand book: A guide to planning care* (7th ed.). St. Louis: Mosby.

Astle, S. M. (2005). Restoring electrolyte balance. *RN, 68*(5), 34–40.

Beers, M. H., & Berkow, R. (Eds.). (2004). *The Merck manual of diagnosis and therapy* (17th ed.). Merck & Co., Inc. Internet edition provided by Medical Services, USMEDSA, USHH.

Bennett, J. A., Tomas, V., & Riegel, B. (2004). Unrecognized chronic dehydration in older adults: Examining prevalence rate and risk factors. *Journal of Gerontological Nursing, 30*(11), 22–28, 52–53.

Burger, C. M. (2004a). Emergency. Hyperkalemia: Averting crisis with early recognition and intervention. *American Journal of Nursing, 104*(11), 61–65.

Burger, C. M. (2004b). Emergency. Hyperkalemia: When serum K⁺ is not okay. *American Journal of Nursing, 104*(10), 66–70.

Call-Schmidt, T. (2001). Interpreting lab results: A primer. *MEDSURG Nursing, 10*(4), 179–184.

Carmichael, K. A., & Alper, B. S. (2004). State consult. Hypercalcemia. *Clinical Advisor, 7*(12), 67–69.

Copstead, L. C., & Banasik, J. L. (2005). *Pathophysiology* (3rd ed.). St. Louis, MO: Elsevier/Saunders.

Danner, K. (2000). Acid/base balance: Making sense of pH. *CIN PLUS* (On-line serial), *3*(1), 3.

Dochterman, J., & Bulechek, G. (2004). *Nursing interventions classification (NIC)* (4th ed.). St. Louis, MO: Mosby.

Edwards, S. (2001). Regulation of water, sodium and potassium: Implications for practice. *Nursing Standard, 15*(22), 36–44.

Edwards, S. L. (2005). Maintaining calcium balance: Physiology and implications. *Nursing Times, 101*(19), 58–61.

Elgart, H. N. (2004). Assessment of fluids and electrolytes. *AACN Clinical Issues: Advanced Practice in Acute and Critical Care, 15*(4), 607–621.

Hayes, D. D. (2004). Calcium in the balance. *Nursing Made Incredibly Easy!, 2*(2), 46–53.

Holman, C., Roberts, S., & Nicol, M. (2005). Promoting adequate hydration in older people. *Nursing Older People, 17*(4), 31–32.

Hughes, E. (2004). Principles of post-operative patient care. *Nursing Standard, 19*, 43–51, 53.

Johnson, A. L., & Criddle, L. M. (2004). Pass the salt: Indications for and implications of using hypertonic saline. *Critical Care Nurse, 24*(5), 36–38, 40–44, 46+.

Kasper, D. L., Braunwald, E., Fauci, A. S., Hauser, S. L., Longo, D. L., & Jameson, J. L. (Eds.). (2005). *Harrison's principles of internal medicine* (16th ed.). New York: McGraw-Hill.

Krueger, D., & Tasota, F. J. (2003). Eye on diagnostics. Keeping an eye on calcium levels. *Nursing, 33*(6), 68, 70.

Larson, K. (2003). Home health care. Fluid balance in the elderly: Assessment and intervention—Important role in community health and home care nursing. *Geriatric Nursing, 24*(5), 306–309.

Lehne, R. A. (2004). *Pharmacology for nursing care* (5th ed.). Philadelphia: W. B. Saunders.

McCance, K. L., & Huether, S. E. (2006). *Pathophysiology: The biologic basis for disease in adults and children* (5th ed.). St. Louis, MO: Mosby.

Metheny, N. M. (2000). *Fluid and electrolyte balance: Nursing considerations* (4th ed.). Philadelphia: Lippincott.

Mitchell, D. (2004). Consult stat. Here's an easy way to make sense of IV fluid therapy. *RN, 67*(10), 65–67, 39.

Moorhead, S., Johnson, M., & Maas, M. (2004). *Nursing outcomes classification (NOC)* (3rd ed.). St. Louis, MO: Mosby.

NANDA International. (2005). *Nursing diagnoses: Definitions and classification 2005–2006.* Philadelphia: Author.

Oh, H., Suh, Y., Hwang, S., & Seo, W. (2005). Effects of nasogastric tube feeding on serum sodium, potassium and glucose levels. *Journal of Nursing Scholarship, 37*(2), 141–147.

O'Keeffe, S. (2005). Clinician's guide to interpreting arterial blood gases (ABG's). *Clinical Times, 2*(3), 3.

Porth, C. M. (2005). *Pathophysiology: Concepts of altered health states* (7th ed.). Philadelphia: Lippincott.

Pruitt, W. C., & Jacobs, M. (2004). Interpreting arterial blood gases: Easy as ABC. *Nursing, 34*(8), 50–53.

Simpson, H. (2004). Respiratory nursing. Interpretation of arterial blood gases: A clinical guide for nurses. *British Journal of Nursing, 13*(9), 522–528.

Stanner, S. (2005). Preventing undernutrition and dehydration in older people. *Nursing & Residential Care, 7*(1), 17–19.

Suhayda, R., & Walton, J. C. (2002). Preventing and managing dehydration. *MEDSURG Nursing, 11*(6), 267–278.

Sweeney, J. (2005a). Clinical queries. What causes hyponatremia? *Nursing, 35*(6), 18.

Sweeney, J. (2005b). Clinical queries. What causes sudden hypokalemia? *Nursing, 35*(4), 12.

Tierney, L. M., McPhee, S. J., & Papadakis, M. A. (2005). *Current medical diagnosis and treatment* (44th ed.). New York: Lange Medical Books/McGraw-Hill.

Urden, L. D., Stacy, K. M., & Lough, M. E. (2006). *Thelan's critical care nursing: Diagnosis and management* (5th ed.). St. Louis, MO: Mosby.

van Wissen, K., & Breton, C. (2004). Perioperative influences on fluid distribution. *MEDSURG Nursing, 13*(5), 304–311.

Whitney, E. N., & Rolfes, S. R. (2002). *Understanding nutrition* (9th ed.). Belmont, CA: Wadsworth.

Wilkinson, J. M. (2005). *Nursing diagnosis handbook with NIC interventions and NOC outcomes* (8th ed.). Upper Saddle River, NJ: Prentice Hall Health.

Wise, L. C., Mersch, J., Racioppi, J., Crosier, J., & Thompson, C. (2000). Evaluating the reliability and utility of cumulative intake and output. *Journal of Nursing Care Quality, 14*(3), 37–42.

Woodrow, P. (2003). Assessing fluid balance in older people: Fluid replacement. *Nursing Older People, 14*(10), 29–30.

Woodrow, P. (2004). Continuing professional development. Arterial blood gas analysis. *Nursing Standard, 18*(21), 45–52, 54–55.

Yucha, C. (2004). Renal regulation of acid–base balance. *Nephrology Nursing Journal, 31*(2), 201–208.

Zembrzuski, C. (2004). Try this: Best practices in nursing care to older adults. Nutrition and hydration. *MEDSURG Nursing, 13*(1), 60–61.

CHAPTER 11 Nursing Care of Clients Experiencing Trauma and Shock

LEARNING OUTCOMES

- Describe the components and types of trauma.

- Discuss causes, effects, and initial management of trauma.

- Describe steps of the primary survey to diagnose and manage life-threatening injuries.

- Discuss diagnostic tests used in assessing clients experiencing trauma and shock.

- Describe collaborative interventions for clients experiencing trauma and shock, including medications, blood transfusion, and intravenous fluids.

- Explain organ donation and forensic implications of traumatic injury or death.

- Discuss the risk factors, etiologies, and pathophysiologies of hypovolemic shock, cardiogenic shock, obstructive shock, and distributive shock.

- Use the nursing process as a framework for providing individualized care to clients experiencing trauma and shock.

- Describe the role of the nurse in trauma prevention education and evaluate a plan of care to restore the functional health status of trauma clients.

- Understand and comply with guidelines related to the Uniform Anatomical Gift Act.

CLINICAL COMPETENCIES

- Obtain initial data about the trauma client to include history taking, assessment, review of past medical history, and communication with prehospital and other healthcare providers and family members.

- Evaluate client response to medical and surgical interventions for clients sustaining multiple trauma and shock.

- Communicate significant data and changes in the condition of a client who has sustained trauma.

- Formulate nursing diagnoses based on manifestations recognized during the nursing assessment.

- Develop a plan of care for the trauma client based on scientific knowledge and client diversity.

- Advocate for clients' rights as indicated by documents that address end-of-life issues.

THE CLIENT EXPERIENCING TRAUMA

Trauma is defined as injury to human tissues and organs resulting from the transfer of energy from the environment. In the past the term *trauma* has been associated with the word *accident*. *Accident* means that the injury occurred without intent, a result of random chance. We now know that a considerable number of injuries are preventable and not of random chance. Intentional and nonintentional trauma encompass a variety of injuries resulting from motor vehicle crashes, pedestrian injuries, gunshot wounds, falls, violence toward others, or self-inflicted violence. The injuries, disabilities, and deaths resulting from these acts constitute a major health-care challenge.

FAST FACTS
- Trauma kills more people between the ages of 1 and 44 than any other disease or illness.
- 62 percent of all deaths from ages 15 to 24 are due to trauma. (NIGMS, 2006)

Trauma usually occurs suddenly, leaving the client and family with little time to prepare for its consequences. Nurses provide a vital link in both the physical and psychosocial care for the injured client and family. In caring for the client who has experienced trauma, nurses must consider not only the initial physical injury, but also its long-term consequences, including rehabilitation. Trauma may alter the client's previous way of life, potentially affecting independence, mobility, cognitive thinking, and appearance.

Components of Trauma

Trauma results from an abnormal exchange of energy between a host and a mechanism in a predisposing environment. The *host* is the person or group at risk of injury. Multiple factors influence the host's potential for injury: age, sex, race, economic status, preexisting illnesses, and use of substances such as street drugs and alcohol.

The *mechanism* is the source of the energy transmitted to the host. The energy exchanged can be mechanical, gravitational, thermal, electrical, physical, or chemical. Table 11–1 lists the most common mechanisms for each type of energy. Mechanical energy is the most common type of energy transferred to a

TABLE 11–1 Common Mechanisms of Injury by Energy Source

ENERGY SOURCE	COMMON MECHANISMS OF INJURY
Mechanical	Motor vehicles Firearms Machines
Gravitational	Falls
Thermal	Heating appliances Fire Freezing temperatures
Electrical	Wires, sockets, and other electrical objects Lightning
Physical	Fists, feet, and other body parts (as in physical assault) Sharp objects, such as knives Ultraviolet radiation Ionizing radiation Water (drowning) Other submersion agents (e.g., grain) Explosions
Chemical	Drugs Poisons Industrial chemicals

host in trauma. The most common mechanical source of injury in all adult age groups is the motor vehicle.

Guns are another common mechanical source of injury. Trauma from gunshot wounds has steadily increased during the past 20 years and remains a major reason for emergency department and trauma center admissions, especially in large cities.

When describing a traumatic injury, *intention* is included as a component. Most gunshot and stab wounds are examples of intentional injuries. It is important to remember, however, that some gunshot wounds are unintentional, such as those that occur when children play with their parents' guns. Other common unintentional injuries result from motor vehicle crashes, falls, drowning, and fires. Although hunting accidents are rare in comparison to the number of people participating in the sport, hunting-related deaths and injuries have decreased with the implementation of mandatory "hunting safety" courses in some states.

The final component of trauma is the *environment*. For example, a road that has become slippery after a snowstorm is a physical environment that may contribute to an injury. Occupation is an important environmental factor to consider. Those in certain occupations face a high risk of trauma; examples include police officers, firefighters, professional athletes, race car drivers, and taxi cab drivers. One's social environment also influences risk for injury; see the Meeting Individualized Needs box below for one example, domestic violence.

Types of Trauma

Minor trauma causes injury to a single part or system of the body and is usually treated in a physician's office or in the hospital emergency department. A fracture of the clavicle, a small second-degree burn, and a laceration requiring sutures are examples of minor trauma. Major or **multiple trauma** involves serious single-system injury (such as the traumatic amputation of a leg) or multiple-system injuries. Multiple trauma is most often the result of a motor vehicle crash.

Trauma is further classified as either blunt or penetrating. **Blunt trauma** occurs when there is no communication between the damaged tissues and the outside environment. It is caused by various forces including *deceleration* (a decrease in the speed of a moving object), *acceleration* (an increase in the speed of a moving object), *shearing* (forces occurring across a plane, with structures slipping across each other), *compression*, and *crushing*. Blunt forces often cause multiple injuries that can affect the head, spinal cord, bones, thorax, and abdomen. Blunt trauma is frequently caused by motor vehicle crashes, falls, assaults, and sports activities.

Penetrating trauma occurs when a foreign object enters the body, causing damage to body structures. Structures commonly affected include the brain, lungs, heart, liver, spleen, the intestines, and the vascular system. Examples of penetrating trauma are gunshot or stab wounds and impalement.

Other types of trauma include inhalation injuries from gases, smoke, or steam; burn or freezing injuries; and blast injuries from explosions. Blast injuries result from the temperature and velocity of air movement and the force of projectiles from the explosion. Blast injuries are more severe in water than in air because blast waves travel farther and faster in water. Trauma from blast injuries includes pulmonary edema and hemorrhage, damage to abdominal organs, burns, penetrating injuries, and ruptured tympanic membranes.

Outcome studies show a correlation between survival rates of multiple trauma victims and rapid response times by prehospital providers coupled with appropriate decision making with regard to transporting the victim to a facility capable of treating their injuries (Han et al., 2003). As a result, a system was devised to assist prehospital providers to make the appropriate decisions. Trauma clients are classified as class 1, 2, or 3 based on factors including mechanism of injury, vehicle speed, height of falls, and location of penetrating injuries. Class 3 trauma is the least severe. An example would be a same-level fall without loss of consciousness or significant injury. Class 1 trauma involves life-threatening injuries likely to require medical specialists or immediate surgical intervention. While any hospital emergency department should be capable of caring for class 3 trauma clients, clients meeting class 1 or 2 criteria should be transported to a designated trauma center when possible. Facilities designated as trauma centers have medical specialists and surgical coverage available or on call 24 hours a day.

MEETING INDIVIDUALIZED NEEDS   Assessing Elder Abuse and Intimate Partner Violence (IPV)

IPV

Most IPV incidents are not reported, thus it is believed that the available data greatly underestimate the true magnitude of the problem. It is estimated that more than 5.3 million women are beaten by male partners every year, resulting in 1300 deaths annually. IPV is the single largest cause of injury to women in the United States. Among men, 3.2 million IPV episodes occur annually, accounting for approximately 800,000 men raped or physically assaulted by an intimate partner.

IPV is a widespread problem that occurs regardless of age, sex, race, socioeconomic status, or education. IPV is also referred to as partner abuse or spousal abuse (CDC, 2003). In 2001, intimate partner violence made up 20% of violent crime against women. The same year, intimate partners committed 3% of all violent crimes against men.

VIOLENCE AND THE ELDERLY

Elder abuse is defined as anything that endangers the life of an elderly person. This can range from physical or emotional assault to intimidation, neglect, or financial exploitation. Willful deprivation of food or medical care is also included. The National Elder Abuse Incidence study found that approximately 551,000 persons aged 60 or older were abused or neglected in a 1-year period. Persons 80 years of age and older experienced abuse and neglect at two to three times their proportion in the older population. The perpetrator is a family member in 90% of the cases.

The general approach to diagnosis in abuse situations is challenging and many times hidden. As with spousal, elder, or child abuse, the task of identification is complex. The following are clues to identify violence-related injuries:

■ Injuries that do not correlate with the history
■ Injuries that suggest a defensive posture
■ Injuries during pregnancy
■ Pattern injuries
■ Pattern burns
■ Sexual abuse/rape
■ Unusual or unexplained fractures
■ Signs of confinement
■ Unusual interaction between client and caregiver
■ Lack of medical attention; immunizations not up to date; poor dental health
■ Unexplained dehydration or malnutrition

Source: From Bureau of Justice Statistics Crime Data, *Intimate Partner Violence, 1993–2001*, February 2003; Retrieved March 30, 2006, from http://www.aoa.gov/eldfam/Elder_Rights/Elder_Abuse/Elder_Abuse_pf.asp

Effects of Traumatic Injury

Death is a common result of serious traumatic injury, and may be immediate, early, or late. Immediate death happens at the scene from such injuries as a torn thoracic aorta or decapitation. Early death occurs within several hours of the injury from, for example, shock or delay in recognizing injuries. Late death generally occurs 1 or more days after the injury and results from multiple organ failure, sepsis, and coagulopathies.

Because of the serious consequences of trauma, it is important to rapidly identify the client's injuries and institute appropriate interventions quickly. Following are common results of trauma and interventions necessary for good outcomes.

Airway Obstruction

Assessment of the airway is the highest priority in the trauma client. Other distracting injuries may take the inexperienced practitioner away from the airway, but if the airway is not patent and the client is unable to deliver oxygen to vital organs, all other interventions are futile.

Assessment includes determining airway patency. If the client is unresponsive, manual opening of the airway using a jaw-thrust or chin-lift maneuver is necessary. Once the airway is opened, the practitioner must identify any potential obstruction from the tongue, loose teeth, foreign bodies, bleeding, secretions, vomitus, or edema. If the client is responsive and can vocalize, that is a good indication that the airway is clear.

Any time the nurse performs an intervention it is important to reassess the effectiveness of the intervention. For example, if the nurse suctions the airway to remove vomitus, he or she would reassess the airway after suctioning to determine if that intervention was successful or if the airway needs to be suctioned a second time.

All trauma clients should receive high-flow oxygen until stabilized. Assessment of breathing effectiveness is paramount. Assessment should include whether the client has spontaneous breathing, good rise and fall of the chest, determination of skin color, general rate and depth of respirations, use of abdominal or accessory muscles, position of the trachea, observation of chest wall integrity and presence of jugular vein distention, bilateral breath sounds, and the presence of any surface trauma.

In addition to suctioning, other available airway adjuncts include oral or nasal pharyngeal airways, oxygen delivery devices, laryngeal mask airways, Combitubes, and endotracheal intubation (Figure 11–1 ■). Intubation is the preferred method of airway management if the client is unable to maintain oxygenation or an open airway.

Trauma clients may exhibit several aspects of airway management that are unique and require special preparation and precautions, as discussed below.

CLOSED HEAD INJURY Changes in hemodynamics, oxygenation, and ventilation should be minimized in order to maintain adequate cerebral perfusion pressure. Laryngoscopy causes a marked increase in intracranial pressure (ICP).

The goal is to maintain a $PaCO_2$ of 30 to 35 mmHg. Lidocaine administered 3 to 5 minutes prior to intubation can blunt an increase in ICP that is secondary to laryngeal stimulation. In

Figure 11–1 ■ Placement of an oral endotracheal tube (ETT) for intubation. When the ETT is in place, air or oxygen can be blown into the external opening of the tube and enter the trachea.

a normotensive client, beta-blockers are given 2 to 3 minutes prior to intubation to attenuate the sympathetic response. Effective induction agents such as Etomidate or thiopental have not been shown to increase ICP.

MAXILLOFACIAL TRAUMA Significant distortion of normal anatomy occurs in facial trauma, and respiratory compromise is not uncommon. Even in clients who present with mild respiratory compromise, rapid deterioration from edema or hemorrhage can occur. A surgical airway may be the only alternative.

DIRECT AIRWAY TRAUMA Penetrating trauma to the neck is associated with a high degree of morbidity and mortality. Airway involvement includes dyspnea, cyanosis, subcutaneous emphysema, hoarseness, or air bubbling from the wound. Orotracheal intubation with rapid sequence intubation is the technique of choice. The key is early identification of the need for intubation before the client has no airway at all. Tracheobronchial injury occurs in approximately 10% to 20% of clients with penetrating neck injuries.

CERVICAL SPINE INJURY Securing an airway in the presence of a presumed C-spine injury is recommended. Approximately 3% to 6% of major trauma victims have clinically significant C-spine injuries. Oral intubation with manual in-line axial head and neck stabilization is a safe method. The probability of C-spine injury is decreased if the following criteria are met:

- Absence of midline cervical spine tenderness
- Normal alertness
- Absence of intoxication
- Absence of a painful distracting injury
- No focal neurologic defects.

BURNS Burn clients with airway compromise require aggressive management. Upper airway edema associated with inhalation or enclosed-space fires can progress during the postburn phase. Securing an airway sooner rather than later is the goal. See Chapter 17 ∞ for nursing care of the client with burns.

Tension Pneumothorax

A **pneumothorax** results when air enters the potential space between the parietal and visceral pleura. The thorax is completely filled by the lungs. Surface tension between the pleural surfaces holds the lungs to the chest wall. Air present in the pleural space will eventually collapse the lungs. A **tension pneumothorax** is a special type of pneumothorax that is life threatening and requires immediate intervention. On inspiration, air enters the pleural space, does not escape on expiration, and increases the intrapleural pressure. This pressure collapses the injured lung and shifts the mediastinal contents, compressing the heart, great vessels, trachea, and eventually the uninjured lung. In turn, this causes the following signs and symptoms:

- Severe respiratory distress
- Hypotension
- Jugular vein distention
- Tracheal deviation toward the uninjured side
- Cyanosis.

Figure 11–2 ■ A needle thoracostomy may be used in the emergency treatment of a tension pneumothorax. *A*, A large gauge needle is introduced, and air and fluid are aspirated. *B*, Alternatively, a chest tube may be inserted and connected to a chest drainage system.

The immediate short-term lifesaving intervention is a needle thoracostomy, in which a large-bore needle is inserted into the second intercostal space at the midclavicular line. See Figure 11–2 ■.

Hemorrhage

When the client has suffered an injury that causes external hemorrhage, such as severing of an artery, the bleeding must be controlled immediately. This may be done by applying direct pressure over the wound and applying pressure over arterial pressure points (Figure 11–3 ■).

Internal hemorrhage may result from either blunt or penetrating traumatic injury. Discovering the cause and location of the injury, as well as the extent of related blood loss, are the most important concerns. Several potential spaces in the body can accommodate large amounts of blood that may accumulate (called *third spacing*) following injury. For example, bleeding into the pleural space may occur with chest trauma, and bleeding into the abdominal cavity may occur with abdominal trauma. A pelvic fracture may cause massive hemorrhaging into the retroperitoneal region. Once the source of internal hemorrhage has been recognized, interventions are initiated, including operative control of bleeding and continual assessment of the client. Hemorrhage may result in hypovolemic shock (discussed later in the chapter).

Integumentary Effects

Injuries to the integument generally are not as serious as other injuries, with the exception of burns (see Chapter 17 ∞). The primary organ involved in integumentary trauma is the skin;

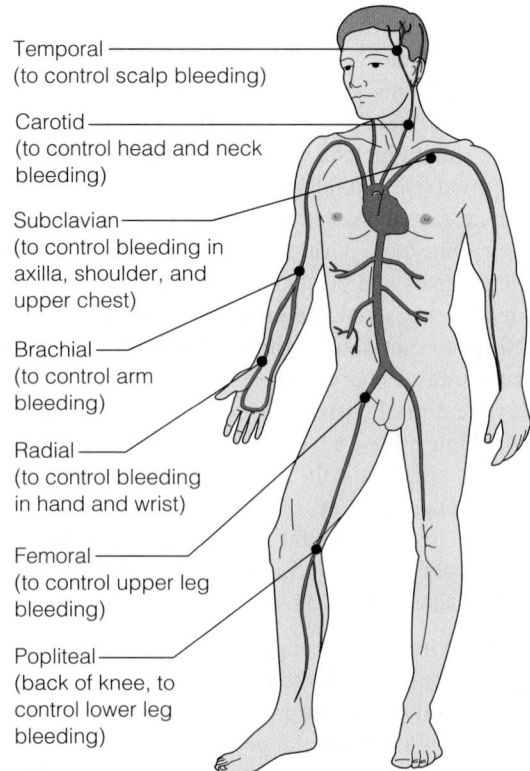

Temporal
(to control scalp bleeding)

Carotid
(to control head and neck bleeding)

Subclavian
(to control bleeding in axilla, shoulder, and upper chest)

Brachial
(to control arm bleeding)

Radial
(to control bleeding in hand and wrist)

Femoral
(to control upper leg bleeding)

Popliteal
(back of knee, to control lower leg bleeding)

Figure 11–3 ■ The major pressure points used for the control of bleeding.

however, underlying structures may also be injured. Injuries may result from either blunt or penetrating sources. It is important to evaluate all injuries to the integument, because they may indicate a more serious injury such as an open fracture. Additionally, large wounds may contribute to significant blood loss.

Five specific injuries to the integument are contusions, abrasions, puncture wounds, lacerations, and full-thickness avulsion injuries (Figure 11–4 ■). **Contusions**, or superficial tissue injuries, result from blunt trauma that causes the breakage of small blood vessels and bleeding into the surrounding tissue. **Abrasions**, or partial-thickness denudations of an area of integument, generally result from falls or scrapes. **Puncture wounds** occur when a sharp or blunt object penetrates the integument. **Lacerations** are open wounds that result from sharp cutting or tearing. Injuries to the integument are at risk for contamination from dirt, debris, or foreign objects. Infection may cause further physical stress to the client with multiple injuries. **Full-thickness avulsion injuries** are injuries that result in loss of all of the layers of the skin, causing fat and muscle to be exposed. The size of the wound impacts both the length of time necessary for healing to take place as well as the risk for infection. These types of injuries are treated by suturing the wound together, reattaching avulsed skin, or by skingrafting.

Abdominal Effects

The abdomen contains both solid organs (liver, spleen, and pancreas) and hollow organs (stomach and intestines). Direct trauma to the abdomen can lacerate and compress the solid organs and cause burst injuries to the hollow organs. Blood vessels may be torn and organs may be displaced from their blood supply, producing life-threatening hemorrhage. Damage to the mesenteric vessels supplying the bowel can result in bowel ischemia and infarction. Injury to the stomach, pancreas, and small bowel may allow digestive enzymes to leak into the abdominal cavity. Rupture of the large bowel results in escape of feces, which causes peritonitis. Blunt or penetrating trauma to the abdomen may also cause rupture of the diaphragm with herniation of the abdominal organs into the thoracic cavity. The immediate threat following abdominal trauma is hemorrhage; the later threat is peritonitis.

Musculoskeletal Effects

Musculoskeletal injuries may occur alone or with multiple injuries as the result of blunt or penetrating trauma. Musculoskeletal injuries usually are not considered a high priority in the care of the client with multiple injuries. Exceptions are the life- or limb-threatening musculoskeletal injury, such as a dislocated hip, pulseless extremity, or significant blood loss such as from a femur or pelvic fracture. Musculoskeletal injuries may provide clues to the presence of other serious injuries; for example, a fractured clavicle may indicate an associated thoracic injury. Care of the client who has suffered a musculoskeletal injury is discussed in Chapter 41 ∞ .

Neurologic Effects

Head injuries are a common type of injury sustained as the result of trauma. Injuries to the spinal cord resulting in loss of neurologic function are devastating outcomes of trauma, but they are much less common than head injuries. Most head and spinal cord injuries result from blunt trauma and are sustained in motor vehicle crashes. Falls, sports injuries, and assault are other sources of neurologic injury. Care of the client with a neurologic injury is discussed in Chapters 44, 45, and 46 ∞ .

Multiple Organ Dysfunction Syndrome

Multiple organ dysfunction syndrome (MODS) is a common complication of severe injury and a frequent cause of death in intensive care units. MODS is a progressive impairment of two or more organ systems. This is the result of an uncontrolled inflammatory response to severe injury or illness.

Clients at risk for MODS are those with a disturbance in homeostasis resulting from one or a combination of the following conditions:

- Infection
- Injury
- Inflammation
- Ischemia
- Immune response
- Intoxication of substances
- Iatrogenic factors.

The primary organ systems involved in MODS are the respiratory, renal, hepatic, hematologic, cardiovascular, gastrointestinal, and neurologic systems. Supportive therapy depends on the identification of correctable causes. It may be one or a combination of several therapies. Surgical intervention, antibiotic administration, corticosteroid administration, and correction coagulopathies are some of the therapies used for this condition. MODS following injuries produce more than half of the late mortality following trauma.

Figure 11–4 ■ Traumatic injuries to the skin include *A*, contusion; *B*, abrasion; *C*, puncture wound; *D*, laceration.

Effects on the Family

Trauma usually occurs suddenly and with little warning. It may result in death or cause injury serious enough to alter both the client's and the family's lives. The suddenness and seriousness of the event are precipitating factors in the development of a psychologic crisis. During the past decade, some emergency departments have instituted care plans that allow families to be present during resuscitation. This type of care is not without controversy, but it should be considered when appropriate.

INTERDISCIPLINARY CARE

Interdisciplinary care of the trauma client depends on a team approach. Providing trauma care with a team focus helps each team member know his or her role. Prompt delegation of tasks and responsibilities improves the client's chances for survival and decreases the morbidity that may result from traumatic injuries.

Prehospital Care

The major functions of prehospital care include injury identification, critical interventions, and rapid transport.

INJURY IDENTIFICATION Emergency care of the client experiencing trauma is based on rapid assessment to identify injuries and begin appropriate interventions. Injuries that indicate the need for trauma center care include:

- Penetrating injuries to the abdomen, pelvis, chest, neck, or head
- Spinal cord injuries with deficit
- Crushing injuries to the abdomen, chest, or head
- Major burns
- Injuries leading to airway compromise or obstruction.

Many methods help healthcare providers determine the seriousness of the client's injuries and the potential for survival. Scoring systems such as the Champion Revised Trauma Scoring System can be helpful (Table 11–2). A rapid but comprehensive trauma assessment, completed on the scene, includes:

- *Airway and breathing assessments* to determine if the airway is patent, maintainable, or nonmaintainable, and if ventilations are impeded, such as by rib fractures or a collapsed lung
- *Circulation assessment* to palpate peripheral and central pulses; to assess capillary refill, skin color, and temperature; and to identify any external sources of bleeding
- *Level of consciousness* and *pupillary function assessment*
- Assessment for any obvious injuries.

The Glasgow Coma Scale is another scoring system that is used to quantify the level of consciousness following traumatic brain injury. See Chapter 43 ∞.

CRITICAL INTERVENTIONS As life-threatening problems are identified during the primary assessment, appropriate on-the-scene interventions must be performed immediately. These include providing life support, immobilizing the cervical spine, managing the airway, and treating hemorrhage and shock.

Immobilization of the client's cervical spine is a primary intervention. The client is placed on a spine board, and a cervical collar and a head immobilizer are applied (Figure 11–5 ■). The

TABLE 11–2 Champion Revised Trauma Scoring System

TEST	SCORE	CODED VALUE
Glasgow Coma Scale*	13 to 15	4
	9 to 12	3
	6 to 8	2
	4 to 5	1
	3	0
Systolic blood pressure	>89	4
	76 to 89	3
	50 to 75	2
	1 to 49	1
	0	0
Respiratory rate	10 to 29	4
	>29	3
	6 to 9	2
	1 to 5	1
	0	0
	Total score:	_____

The highest possible total score is 12. The lowest possible score is 0. The higher the total score, the greater the chance of survival.

*See Chapter 43 for instructions for using the Glasgow Coma Scale.
Source: From "A Revision of the Trauma Score" by H. Champion et al., 1989, Journal of Trauma, 29(5), 624. Used with permission.

cervical spine may also be immobilized by logrolling the client onto a board, placing towel rolls or a head immobilizer along the sides of the client's head, and securing the client to the board. If the client was wearing a helmet at the time of injury, the helmet should remain on until the client arrives at the hospital, unless the client's airway is at risk. If necessary, healthcare personnel at the scene will remove the helmet by

Figure 11–5 ■ Immobilization of the cervical spine at the scene of the accident is essential to prevent further injury to the spinal cord. The combined use of a hard cervical collar, head blocks, and tape best restricts flexion, extension, rotation, and lateral bending of the neck.

Source: Spencer Grant/Photo Researchers, Inc.

manipulating it over the client's nose and ears while holding the client's head and neck immobile; safe removal requires at least two people. Improper removal risks injury or additional injury to the spinal cord.

If the client's airway is patent, oxygen is administered. Ventilations may be assisted with a bag-valve-mask resuscitator until airway management is achieved. Active external bleeding is controlled by direct pressure. Measures to reverse shock (discussed later in the chapter) are initiated.

RAPID TRANSPORT Clients who have multiple injuries must be transported as soon as possible to a regional trauma center. The most common modes of rapid transport are ground ambulance and air ambulance, which includes helicopters specially staffed and equipped to care for trauma victims. Figure 11–6 ■ shows a flight nurse assessing a client. Stable clients within access of a ground ambulance are best transported by ground. Unstable clients and those injured in the wilderness or other areas in which ground access is difficult may best be transported by air. When these transport systems are unavailable, the client is transported by any possible means. Morbidity and mortality rates are reduced when the client is transported to a facility that can manage their injuries within an hour of the injury. In trauma, this time is referred to as the "Golden Hour."

Emergency Department Care

DIAGNOSIS The diagnostic tests ordered once the client reaches the hospital depend on the type of injury the client has sustained. Tests that may be ordered for victims of trauma include the following:

- *Blood type and crossmatch* involves typing the client's blood for ABO antigens and Rh factor, screening the blood for antibodies, and crossmatching the client's serum and donor red blood cells.
- *Blood alcohol level* measures the amount of alcohol in a client's blood. Studies have found that between 20% and 50% of people who are injured may be intoxicated. Alcohol alters the client's level of consciousness and response to pain (NHTSA, 2006).
- *Urine drug screen* may also be ordered. Like alcohol, such drugs as cocaine alter the client's level of consciousness and overall response to the primary survey.
- *Pregnancy test* for any woman of childbearing age rules out the potential for pregnancy and fetal injury.
- The primary goal of the *focused assessment by sonography in trauma (FAST)* exam is to evaluate the presence of blood in body cavities where it is not supposed to be. Primary focus is on the peritoneum. It is also helpful in identification of blood in the pleura and pericardium.
- *Diagnostic peritoneal lavage* determines the presence of blood in the peritoneal cavity, which may indicate abdominal injury. This test is generally done in the emergency department. A local anesthetic (such as lidocaine) is injected subcutaneously, and a small incision is made in the lower abdomen. A catheter is placed into the peritoneal cavity, and any free blood is aspirated. If 10 mL of blood is found, the client is taken to the operating room for exploratory surgery. If no free blood is aspirated, 1 L of a warm isotonic solution (Ringer's solution or normal saline) is rapidly infused into the peritoneal cavity and then allowed to drain by gravity. If the solution returns pink and is found to have a red blood cell count of 100,000 mm^3, a white blood cell count of >500, or bile, food, or feces, the test is considered positive and the client is taken to the operating room for exploratory surgery. This procedure has been used less since the inception of the FAST exam.
- *Computerized tomography (CT) scans* can discover injuries to the brain, skull, spine, spinal cord, chest, and abdomen.
- *Magnetic resonance imaging (MRI) scans* can discover injuries to the brain and spinal cord.

Figure 11–6 ■ Flight nurses provide initial assessment, stabilization, and support for clients with trauma.

MEDICATIONS Medications used to treat the client who has experienced trauma depend on the type and severity of the injuries, as well as the degree of traumatic shock that is present. The following general categories of medications may be used. (Fluid administration and the drugs listed are covered later in the chapter in discussion of the collaborative care of the client in shock.)

- Blood components and crystalloids are administered intravenously in the initial treatment of traumatic shock to replace intravascular volume.
- Inotropic drugs (drugs that increase myocardial contractility) are given to increase cardiac output and improve tissue perfusion. These drugs, administered only after fluid volume restoration, include dopamine (Dopastat, Intropin), dobutamine (Dobutrex), and isoproterenol (Isuprel).
- Vasopressors may be administered in conjunction with fluid replacement to treat neurogenic, septic, or anaphylactic shock. Examples of vasopressors include dopamine, epinephrine, norepinephrine, and phenylephrine.
- Opioids, administered by bolus or continuous infusion, are used to treat pain as soon as possible. However, the effects of the pain medications may alter client responses to injury and mask potential injuries. If pain medications are administered, they must be carefully regulated, and the client must be closely monitored.
- If the client has penetrating and open wounds, tetanus immunization status must be determined. If the client is unable to remember when the last tetanus immunization was given or is unable to answer, tetanus prophylaxis is given.

BLOOD TRANSFUSIONS Blood and blood components are initially produced in the body and then donated for use by another person through a **transfusion** (an infusion of blood or blood components). A client may be given whole blood, packed red blood cells (RBCs), platelets, plasma, albumin, clotting factors, prothrombin, or cryoprecipitate (Table 11–3). Blood and blood components increase the amount of hemoglobin available to carry oxygen to the cells, improve hemoglobin and hematocrit levels during active bleeding, increase intravascular volume, and replace deficient substances such as platelets and clotting factors.

Each person has one of four blood types: A, B, AB, or O. The blood group antigens A and B, present on RBC membranes, form the basis for the ABO blood categorization. The presence or absence of these inherited antigens determines one's blood type. People with blood type A have A antigens, those with type B have B antigens, those with type AB have both antigens, and those with neither antigen have blood type O (called a universal donor).

FAST FACTS
- Type AB blood is the "universal recipient."
- Type O blood is the "universal donor."

ABO antibodies develop in the serum of people whose RBCs lack the corresponding antigen; these antibodies are called anti-A and anti-B. The person with blood type B has A antibodies, the person with type A has B antibodies, the person with type O has both types of antibodies, and the person with blood type AB has no antibodies (called a universal recipient).

A third antigen on the RBC membrane is D. People who are Rh positive have the D antigen, whereas people who are Rh negative do not. These antigens and antibodies may cause ABO and Rh incompatibilities.

A transfusion of incompatible blood causes hemolysis (breakdown) of the RBCs and agglutination of erythrocytes. (*Agglutination* is the clumping of cells that results from their interaction with specific antibodies.) The ABO blood group names and compatibilities are listed in Table 11–4.

Before RBCs or whole blood can be administered, a series of procedures determine donor and recipient ABO types and Rh groups. These procedures, called a *type and crossmatch*, are performed by mixing the donor cells with the recipient's serum and watching for agglutination. If none occurs, the blood is considered compatible.

Despite meticulous procedures for matching blood types and antigens, blood transfusion reactions may still occur. The most common is a *febrile reaction*. Antibodies within the client receiving the blood are directed against the donor's white blood cells, causing fever and chills. Febrile reactions typically begin during the first 15 minutes of the transfusion. Using leukocyte-poor blood avoids future febrile reactions.

Hypersensitivity reactions result when antibodies in the client's blood react against proteins, such as immunoglobulin A, in the donor blood. Hypersensitivity reactions may appear during or after the transfusion. The manifestations of hypersensitivity reaction include *urticaria* (the appearance of reddened wheals of various sizes on the skin) and itching.

Hemolytic reactions, the most dangerous transfusion reactions, usually result from an ABO incompatibility. Clumping RBCs block capillaries, decreasing blood flow to vital organs. In addition, macrophages engulf the clumped RBCs, releasing free hemoglobin into the circulating blood; the hemoglobin is then filtered by the kidneys and may block the renal tubules, causing renal failure. Hemolytic reactions usually begin after infusion of 100 to 200 mL of the incompatible blood. Manifestations of a hemolytic reaction include flushing of the face, a burning sensation along the vein, headache, urticaria, chills, fever, lumbar pain, abdominal pain, chest pain, nausea and vomiting, tachycardia, hypotension, and dyspnea. If any of these manifestations appear, the blood transfusion must be immediately discontinued.

Other risks to clients receiving blood include circulatory overload, electrolyte imbalances, and infectious diseases such as hepatitis or cytomegalovirus.

Clients who have experienced trauma of any severity have had substantial blood loss and are usually in hypovolemic shock. Blood replacement is the treatment of choice to restore oxygen-carrying capacity. Clients in severe shock with active bleeding are given universal, type O red blood cells immediately. Clients with less severe injuries or bleeding may be stabilized with other types of fluids until type-specific or crossmatched blood is available.

Some emergency departments and trauma centers use autotransfusion to provide blood for transfusions for the client with multiple injuries and/or severe shock. Autotransfusion is a method of blood administration in which special equipment collects and returns the client's own blood. The chest cavity is the typical source of blood to be autotransfused.

TABLE 11–3 Volume Resuscitation Therapies

COMPONENT	INDICATIONS	ADVANTAGES	DISADVANTAGES
Ringer's lactate	Restoration of circulating volume Replacement of electrolyte deficits	Good availability Safe to use Low cost Aids in buffering acidosis	Rapid movement from the intravascular to the extravascular space, leading to three or more times requirement for replacement
Normal saline	Restoration of circulating volume Vehicle compatible with administration of blood	Good availability Low cost Safe to use	Hyperchloremic acidosis associated with prolonged use of sodium solutions
Whole blood	Replaces blood volume and oxygen-carrying capacity in hemorrhage and shock	Contains RBCs, plasma proteins, clotting factors, and plasma	Contains few platelets or granulocytes; deficient in clotting factors V and VII Greatest risks are for incompatibility or circulatory overload
Packed RBCs	Restoration of intravascular volume Replacement of oxygen-carrying capacity	One unit of RBCs should increase the hemoglobin of a 70-kg adult by approximately 1 g/dL in the absence of volume overload or continuing blood loss	Red cells require compatibility testing Risk of transmitting bloodborne pathogens Should be warmed to prevent hypothermia
Platelets	Significant thrombocytopenia (platelet count less than 20,000–50,000/mm^3) Continued hemorrhage	Compatibility testing is not required Typical platelet transfusion should raise the platelets of a 70-kg adult approximately 30,000–50,000/UL	Postexposure prophylaxis with anti-Rh immune globulin should be considered following Rh$^+$ platelet transfusion to an Rh$^-$ woman
Albumin	Expends blood volume in shock and trauma	Good availability	Is not a substitute for whole blood Hypersensitivity reactions can occur
Fresh frozen plasma (FFP)	Documented coagulopathy Restoration of clotting factors Supplies plasma proteins	Crossmatching and Rh compatibility not required	Must be thawed in a 37°C water bath for approximately 30 minutes Should be ABO compatible
Cryoprecipitate	Coagulopathy with low fibrinogen Restoration of fibrinogen	Rh type not important	Risk of transmitting bloodborne pathogens Contains hemagglutinins If large volume of ABO incompatible cryoprecipitate are administered, intravascular hemolysis can occur

Nursing considerations for blood transfusion therapy are described in the Medication Administration box on the following page.

Emergency Surgery

Immediate surgical intervention is indicated when the client remains in shock despite resuscitation and there is no obvious external sign of blood loss. Abdominal and chest x-ray, ultrasound studies, diagnostic peritoneal lavage, or CT scan may be performed to help identify the potential source of the blood loss. It is important for the emergency or trauma nurse to speak with the family as soon as possible and keep them informed about what is happening to their family member. Unfortunately, the need for emergency surgery may not allow time for family members or significant others to see their loved one before transfer to the operating room.

Organ Donation

The Uniform Anatomical Gift Act (1968, 1987) requires that people be informed about their options for organ donation.

TABLE 11–4 Blood Group Types and Compatibilities

BLOOD GROUP	RBC AGGLUTINOGENS	SERUM AGGLUTINOGENS	COMPATIBLE DONOR BLOOD GROUPS	INCOMPATIBLE DONOR BLOOD GROUPS
A	A	Anti-B	A, O	B, AB
B	B	Anti-A	B, O	A, AB
AB	A, B	None	A, B, AB, O	None
O	None	Anti-A, anti-B	O	A, B, AB

Note: Group O is often called the universal donor, and group AB is called the universal recipient.

MEDICATION ADMINISTRATION   Blood Transfusion

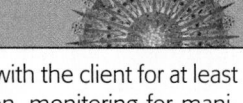

The risk for and seriousness of blood transfusion reactions require that extreme caution be taken when blood is administered. Most fatal transfusion reactions are the result of human error. Although general guidelines are provided here, each institution has specific policies and procedures that must be followed. Prior to beginning the transfusion, the nurse must determine that typed and crossmatched blood is available and collect the needed equipment: a Y-tubing blood administration set with a filter, a large-bore intravenous catheter (usually 18 or 19 gauge), and normal saline solution. Only normal saline is used with a blood transfusion. Dextrose causes clumping of RBCs, and distilled water causes hemolysis.

Nursing Responsibilities
- Obtain client consent.
- Assess for any previous reactions to blood.
- Explain the procedure to the client, and answer any questions.
- Prepare the intravenous equipment. Shut off one side of the Y tubing, and attach the other side to the saline solution. Flush the tubing and filter with the saline.
- If venous access is not already in place, insert the intravenous needle (following body substance precautions), and begin administering the saline.
- Using institutional procedure, obtain the blood from the blood bank or laboratory. Administer the blood immediately; if this is not possible, return it to the blood bank or laboratory.
- Check and document that the donor and recipient blood have been tested and are compatible. This usually involves two nurses, each verifying that:
  a. An order for blood has been written.
  b. Type and crossmatch have been done.
  c. The name of the client and the name on the blood bag are identical.
  d. The number assigned to the unit of blood is identical to the one on the requisition for the blood.
  e. Blood type and Rh factor are compatible.
  f. The blood has not exceeded its expiration date.
  g. The unit of blood is intact and has no bubbles or discoloration.
- Identify the client by reading the armband and, if conscious, asking the client to tell you his or her name. Check the armband against the unit of blood.
- Gently invert the blood bag several times to mix the plasma and RBCs.
- Take and record vital signs as a baseline.
- Attach the open side of the Y tubing to the blood unit, and begin the transfusion at a slow rate of about 2 mL/min. (Some trauma clients may have blood infused at a rapid rate. If blood is infused rapidly, it may need to be warmed prior to adminis-

tration to prevent hypothermia.) Stay with the client for at least the first 15 minutes of the transfusion, monitoring for manifestations of a reaction and taking the client's vital signs.
- Continue to monitor the client during the transfusion, assessing for manifestations of hypersensitivity or hemolytic reactions and taking and recording vital signs as directed by institutional policy.
- After the first 15 minutes, the rate of infusion is increased. If there is no danger of fluid volume overload, most clients can tolerate an infusion of a unit of blood (ranging from 250 to 500 mL, depending on the blood component administered) in 2 hours. The unit of blood must be administered within 3 to 4 hours; after this time, it has warmed and begins to deteriorate.
- Take the following actions if manifestations of a reaction occur:
  a. Stop the infusion of blood immediately, and notify the physician. Continue to infuse the saline.
  b. Take vital signs and assess manifestations.
  c. Compare the blood slip with the unit of blood to ensure that an identification error was not made.
  d. Save the blood bag and any remaining blood for return to the laboratory for further tests to determine the cause of the reaction.
  e. Follow institutional policy for collecting urine and venous blood samples.
  f. Continue to monitor the client and provide prescribed interventions to treat hypersensitivity or hemolytic manifestations.

Health Education for the Client and Family
- The possible risks of blood transfusions include transmission of infectious diseases and acquired immune deficiency syndrome (AIDS). However, because of careful handling and storage of blood, bacterial contamination is rare. Although hepatitis may be transmitted by contaminated blood, new tests for hepatitis antibodies in donor blood are reducing this risk. Many people are afraid of contracting AIDS from blood; however, donor screening and HIV-antibody testing of donor blood has virtually eliminated the transmission of HIV by blood transfusion. A new risk that has been identified is the transmission of West Nile Virus through blood transfusions. Screening for this risk is asking potential donors about the presence of symptoms indicative of West Nile Virus.
- During the transfusion, immediately report any warm feelings, chills, itching, feelings of weakness or fainting, or difficulty breathing.
- Report any signs of a delayed transfusion reaction: chills, fever, cough, difficulty breathing, hives, itching, or changes in circulation, and seek medical care immediately.

Under this act, consent for organ donation may be given not only by the donor but also by a spouse, adult children, parents, adult siblings, guardian, or any adult authorized to do so. The act also encourages people to carry donor cards.

The increased success of organ transplant has made it a more common and valuable method of prolonging and improving life; however, many people are still waiting for organs, and

many people who may be suitable organ donors die each year from trauma. Organs and tissues that may be transplanted include bones, eyes, liver, lungs, skin, muscles and tendons, pancreas, intestines, kidneys, heart, and heart valves.

The organ donation process begins with identification of the potential organ donor. Most people are potential organ donors. Exceptions include those who:

- Currently abuse intravenous drugs
- Have preexisting untreated infections, such as septicemia
- Have any malignancy other than a primary brain tumor
- Have active tuberculosis.

In the past HIV-positive clients were excluded as donors. Recent legislative changes now allow HIV-positive clients to donate to HIV-positive recipients.

The family needs to be made aware of the client's prognosis and presented with the option of donating the client's organs. Both the family's and the client's feelings about organ donation must be explored. Even if the client carries an organ donation card, many institutions will not remove any organs without a signature from a family member or other authorized person. The nurse must always respect the family's concerns and feelings during this process. Some members of certain cultural groups may have religious constraints or issues of mistrust that may interfere with the donation process.

Box 11–1 lists **brain death criteria**. Once brain death has been confirmed, the family must also understand the diagnosis and be allowed time to accept the client's death.

When caring for an adult client who is an organ donor, the nurse carries out the following:

- Maintain systolic blood pressure of 90 mmHg to keep the client's organs perfused until removal.
- Maintain urine output at >30 mL/h. This is usually accomplished by administering fluids and/or inotropic agents such as dopamine.
- Maintain oxygen saturation at 90% or greater.

Forensic Considerations

Injuries often happen under circumstances that require legal investigation. Many injuries, particularly penetrating trauma, may involve criminal activity. Therefore, the nurse must recognize the need to identify, store, and properly transfer potential evidence for medicolegal investigations.

Each item of clothing removed from the client must be placed in a breathable container, such as a paper bag, and documented appropriately. Bullets or knives should be labeled, with their source specified, and given to the proper authorities. Holes found in clothing should not be disturbed. When it is necessary to cut off clothing, these areas should be avoided and never cut through if at all possible.

BOX 11–1 Brain Death Criteria

Clinical Signs
- Irreversible condition
- Apnea with a $PaCO_2$ greater than 60 mmHg
- No response to deep stimuli
- No spontaneous movement (some spinal cord reflexes may be present)
- No gag or corneal reflex
- No oculocephalic or oculovestibular reflex
- Absence of toxic or metabolic disorders

Confirmatory Tests
- Cerebral blood flow study
- Electroencephalogram

The client's hands may yield important evidence, such as powder burns or residue on the skin or tissue or hair samples beneath the fingernails. In the case of death, it is recommended that paper bags be placed over the client's hands if the presence of evidence is suspected; otherwise, the evidence should be collected from nail clippings.

Identify all wounds and document these findings with pictures, diagrams, or written descriptions. Once the evidence has been collected, identified, and properly stored, ensure that it is given to the appropriate authorities. A chain of custody needs to be maintained throughout the entire process. All evidence must be identified and labeled, and documentation procedures must chronicle where and in whose possession the evidence has been. For the chain of custody to remain intact, the evidence must remain in the continuous possession of identified people and be marked and sealed in tamper-proof containers.

NURSING CARE

Nursing care of the client who has been injured begins with a primary assessment and the initiation of collaborative interventions for any life-threatening injuries. Nursing care is directed toward the client's specific responses to trauma.

Health Promotion

Prevention efforts can reduce the incidence and severity of trauma. Areas of health promotion and trauma prevention interventions for individuals and communities include the following:

- *Motor vehicle safety:* seat belts, air bags, helmets, driving under the influence of alcohol or drugs, reckless driving, visual or cognitive deficits in the older adult, cell phone use, driver fatigue
- *Home safety:* snow and ice removal, electrical wiring, falls, burns, drowning
- *Farm safety:* operating heavy equipment, safe storage of chemicals such as fertilizers
- *Work safety:* operating work equipment, wearing safety equipment, removal of jewelry
- *Relationships:* domestic violence, child abuse, elder abuse, or neglect
- *Communities:* gun control, gangs, condition of streets, neighborhood safety.

(In providing information about trauma prevention to members of the community, the nurse serves as a healthcare educator, political activist, and safety advocate.)

Assessment

See Interdisciplinary Care for assessment of the client experiencing trauma.

Nursing Diagnoses and Interventions

The trauma client has many complex and interrelated actual or potential alterations in health. The nursing care in this section focuses on client and family problems with respirations, infection, immobility, spirituality, and stress. Nursing interventions for decreased cardiac output and altered perfusion are discussed in the section of the chapter on nursing care of the client in shock. See the accompanying Nursing Care Plan on page 266.

MediaLink Case Study: A Client Experiencing Trauma

NURSING CARE PLAN   A Client with Multiple Injuries

Jane Souza is a 25-year-old married woman with two children who provides day care for preschool children in her home. As she is driving the interstate at 65 miles per hour, a car crosses the median and strikes her vehicle head-on. Jane, who is not wearing a seat belt, is thrown forward against the steering wheel. The front of her car is pushed up against her by the car that struck her, entrapping her lower extremities.

After extensive efforts to extricate her from the car, Jane is transported to the local trauma center. She is still conscious, is receiving high-flow oxygen by mask, and has one intravenous line in place. Her vital signs are a palpable systolic blood pressure of 80, a pulse rate of 120, and a respiratory rate of 36. On arrival, she states that she is having difficulty breathing.

ASSESSMENT

- *Airway:* Maintainable with high-flow oxygen in place.
- *Breathing:* Respiratory rate of 36, multiple bruising and abrasions on right side of her chest, decreased breath sounds on the right side.
- *Circulation:* No palpable radial pulses; palpable brachial pulses. Monitor shows sinus tachycardia. No active external bleeding noted. Skin color pale, cool to the touch, and diaphoretic.
- *Neurologic:* Moved her fingers when asked; complains of difficulty breathing; denies that she is hurt. Pupils 4 mm, equal, and react to light. Has a broken right arm and an open fracture of the left ankle; because of these injuries, extremity movement is limited.

Because of Jane's respiratory distress, she is intubated and ventilated with 100% oxygen. Another intravenous line is inserted and O-negative blood administered.

DIAGNOSES

- *Ineffective Breathing Pattern* related to multiple bruises and abrasions on the right side of the chest, and respiratory difficulty

- *Deficient Fluid Volume* related to acute internal blood loss (presumed because no active bleeding can be found)
- *Risk for Injury* related to trauma resuscitation

EXPECTED OUTCOMES

- Maintain adequate oxygenation.
- Maintain adequate circulating blood volume.

PLANNING AND IMPLEMENTATION

- Monitor airway and assist in any needed airway management.
- Explain all procedures.
- Monitor the effects of fluid and blood administration, including any changes in blood pressure and pulse.
- Prepare for transfer to the operating room for emergency surgery.
- Keep family informed about her condition.

EVALUATION

Jane is transferred to the operating room, where it is determined that she has a ruptured spleen and a serious pelvic fracture. Jane's treatment continues in the operating room.

CRITICAL THINKING IN THE NURSING PROCESS

1. Is the nursing diagnosis *Deficient Fluid Volume* appropriate for Jane Souza? Why or why not?
2. The assessment of a client who has experienced trauma is, in order: A = airway, B = breathing, and C = circulation. What is the rationale for this sequence?
3. Following surgery, Jane is moved to the surgical intensive care unit. She is very anxious and restless. What assessments would you make to identify the cause of her restlessness?
4. Infection is a common complication for the trauma client. Describe five risks for infection that are present from the time of injury to the time of hospital discharge.

See Evaluating Your Response in Appendix C.

Ineffective Airway Clearance

The client with multiple injuries is at great risk for developing airway obstruction and apnea. Facial injuries, loose teeth, blood, and vomitus increase the risk for aspiration and obstruction. Neurologic injuries and cerebral edema alter the client's respiratory drive and ability to keep the airway clear.

- Assess if airway is patent, maintainable, or nonmaintainable. Assess for manifestations of airway obstruction: stridor, tachypnea, bradypnea, cough, cyanosis, dyspnea, decreased or absent breath sounds, changes in oxygen levels, and changes in level of consciousness. *Assessing the airway and initiating interventions are the first steps in managing the client with multiple injuries.*
- Monitor oxygen saturation by applying a pulse oximeter. Adjust oxygen flow to maintain oxygen saturation from 94% to 100%. *Changes in oxygen saturation as measured by the pulse oximeter indicate the effectiveness of the client's airway. Pulse oximetry in clients who have been exposed to carbon monoxide (i.e., house fires) is unreliable since it cannot differentiate carboxyhemoglobin from oxyhemoglobin.*

- Monitor level of consciousness. *An early sign of an ineffective airway is change in the client's behavior. If the client becomes restless, anxious, combative, or unresponsive, the effectiveness of the airway needs to be immediately evaluated and appropriate interventions initiated.*

Risk for Infection

Traumatic injuries are considered dirty wounds. Projectiles enter the body through dirty surfaces and clothing, carrying dirt and debris into the wound. Open fractures provide a portal for the entry of bacteria and dirt. Even with surgical intervention, the wounds often remain contaminated.

- Use careful hand washing practices. *Hand washing remains the single most important factor in preventing the spread of infection.*
- Use strict standard precautions and aseptic technique when caring for wounds. *Standard precautions are essential to protect the client and the nurse from infection.* In addition:
  - Monitor wounds for odor, redness, heat, swelling, and copious or purulent drainage.

- Monitor hidden wounds, such as those under casts, by asking the client whether the pain has increased and observing for increased drainage and heat over the area of the wound.
- Ensure that cross-contamination between wounds does not occur. Collect drainage in ostomy bags if it is copious. *The skin is the first line of defense against infection. Wounds provide a portal of entry for organisms. Risk factors for wound infection include contamination, inadequate wound care, and the condition of the wound at the time of closure. Aseptic techniques used in applying and changing dressings reduce the entry of organisms.*
- Take and record vital signs, including temperature, every 2 to 4 hours. *Vital signs, particularly an elevated body temperature, indicate the presence of an infection.*
- Provide adequate fluids and nutrition. *Adequate fluids, calories, and protein are essential to wound healing.*
- Assess for manifestations of gas gangrene: fever, pain, and swelling in traumatized tissues; drainage with a foul odor. *Gas gangrene is usually caused by the organism* Clostridium perfringens. *This bacterium is found in the soil and can be introduced into the body during a traumatic injury. The organism grows in the tissues, causing necrosis; hydrogen and carbon dioxide are released, with resultant swelling of tissues. If the infection continues, tissues are progressively destroyed, and sepsis and death may result.*
- Assess status of tetanus immunization and administer tetanus toxoid or human toxin-antitoxin as prescribed. *Tetanus is caused by an exotoxin produced by* Clostridium tetani, *usually introduced through an open wound. The organism is commonly found in the soil.*
- Use strict aseptic technique when inserting catheters, suctioning, administering parenteral medications, or performing any other invasive procedure. *Using aseptic technique during invasive procedures reduces the risk of entry of organisms.*

Impaired Physical Mobility

The client with trauma injuries is often unable to change positions independently and is at risk for complications of the integumentary, cardiovascular, gastrointestinal, respiratory, musculoskeletal, and renal systems. Clients at greatest risk are those who have had multiple injuries, spinal cord injuries, peripheral nerve injuries, and traumatic amputations. Collaborate with the physical therapist and occupational therapist (if available) to determine the most effective types and schedule of exercises and assistive devices.

- If active bleeding or edema is not present, provide active or passive exercises to affected and unaffected extremities at least once every 8 hours. *Exercise improves muscle tone, maintains joint mobility, improves circulation, and prevents contractures.*
- Help the client turn, cough, and deep breathe and use the incentive spirometer at least every 2 hours. *Changing positions, coughing, deep breathing, and incentive spirometry reduce the risk of integumentary and respiratory complications.*
- If the client is unable to be moved and positioned, consider a specialty bed, such as the kinetic continuous rotation bed

(Figure 11–7 ■). *The kinetic continuous rotation bed allows continuous turning of the client; the motion decreases pulmonary complications, venous stasis, postural hypotension, urinary stasis, muscle wasting, and bone demineralization.*

- Monitor the lower extremities each day for manifestations of deep venous thrombosis: heat, swelling, and pain. Measure and record the circumference of the thigh and calf each day. If antiemboli stockings or intermittent compression stockings are used, remove them for 1 hour during each shift and assess the skin. *Venous stasis results when surrounding muscles are unable to contract and help move the blood through the veins. Thrombus (clot) formation in deep veins is a major risk for pulmonary embolism.*

Spiritual Distress

Trauma generally strikes without warning and carries potentially devastating consequences, including severe alterations in the lives of the victim and family, and death. The traumatic death of a loved one may be the most difficult event a family may ever experience. The decision to cease life support systems or to donate organs challenges the family's belief systems and psychologic stability. Nursing care of the family (or client) experiencing spiritual distress includes the following:

- Give the family information about the option to donate the client's organs. *The decision to donate organs needs to be based on information about the client's condition, prognosis, and criteria by which brain death is determined. It is*

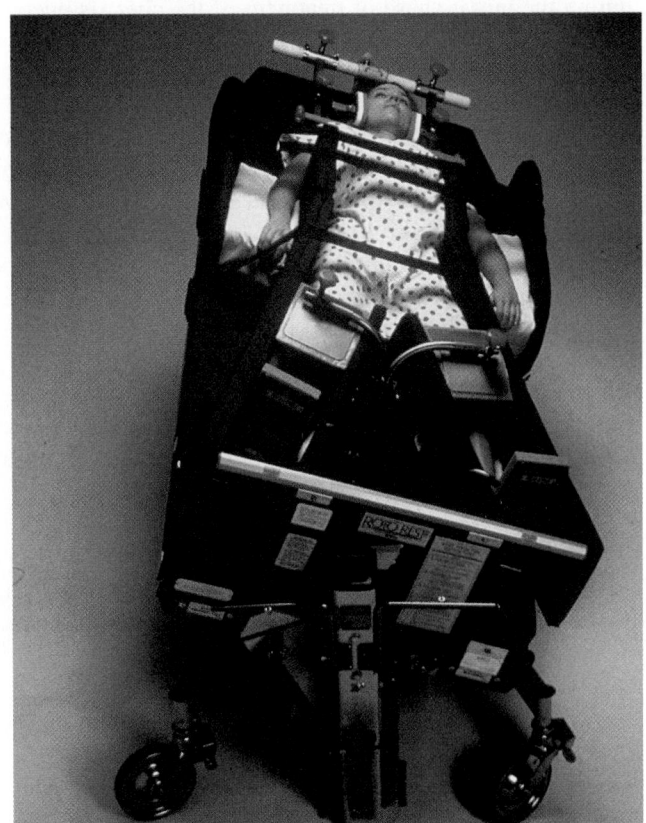

Figure 11–7 ■ A kinetic continuous rotation bed provides a means of turning the client with multiple injuries to decrease the hazards of immobility.

Courtesy of Kinetic Concepts, Inc.

important to convey to family members that organ donation is only an option and that they should not feel they are obligated to consent or are doing something wrong if they do not consent.

- Encourage the family to ask questions and express their feelings about the traumatic event and/or organ donation. *Allowing families to express their feelings may help prevent long-term consequences such as guilt.*
- Refer the family for follow-up care. Long-term follow-up is important for the family facing the sudden death of a loved one. *Grieving is not an overnight process, and providing the family with resources that may be used in the future may help prevent future crises and dysfunction.* (For more information, see Chapter 5 ∞.)

Post-Trauma Syndrome

Post-trauma syndrome is an intense, sustained emotional response to a disastrous event. It is characterized by emotions that range from anger to fear and by flashbacks or psychic numbing. In the initial stage, the client may be calm or may express feelings of anger, disbelief, terror, and shock. In the long-term phase, which begins anywhere from a few days to several months after the event, the client often experiences flashbacks and nightmares of the traumatic event. The client may call on ineffective coping mechanisms, such as alcohol or drugs, and withdraw from relationships.

- Assess emotional responses while providing physical care. Observe for crying, sleep problems, suspiciousness, and fear during the initial phase of treatment. If the client is unconscious, encourage family members and friends to express their feelings. *These assessments provide valuable information about the client's ability to cope with the trauma.*
- Be available if the client wishes to talk about the trauma, and encourage expression of feelings. *The client may initially deny negative feelings; this denial is a coping mechanism in the initial phase of recovery.*
- Teach relaxation techniques, such as deep breathing, progressive muscle relaxation, or imagery (see Chapter 9 ∞). *These techniques are often useful in coping when thoughts of the trauma recur.*
- Refer the client and family members for counseling, psychotherapy, or support groups as appropriate. *Continued therapy may be necessary in assisting the client and family to resolve the acute and long-term effects of trauma.*

Using NANDA, NIC, and NOC

Chart 11–1 shows links between NANDA nursing diagnoses, NIC, and NOC when caring for the client with multiple injuries.

Community-Based Care

Address the following topics to prepare the client and family for home care:

- The type of home environment to which the client will be returning, including any changes that will be required to let the client function in that environment
- Medications, dressings, wound care, equipment, and supplies
- Special diet, if needed
- Rehabilitation plan and its effect on the client's family

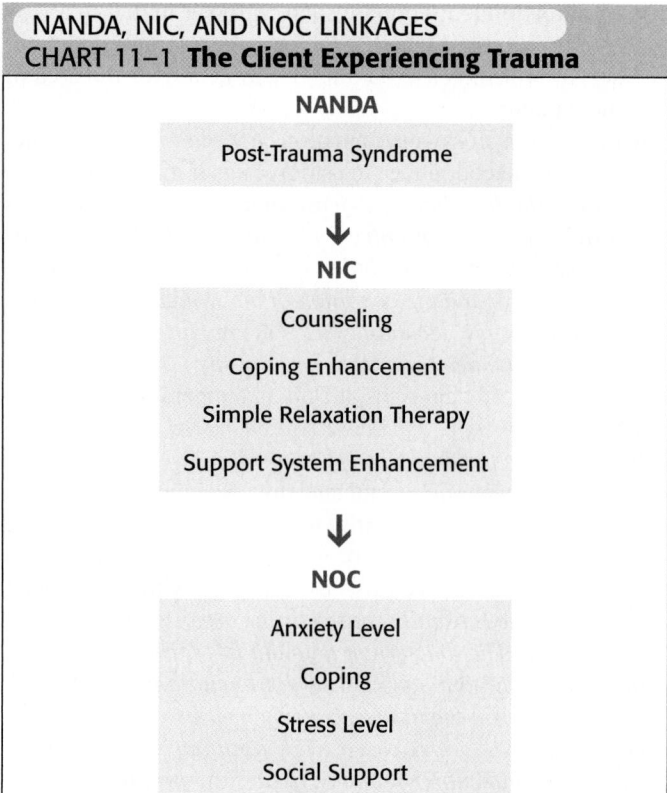

NANDA, NIC, AND NOC LINKAGES
CHART 11–1 **The Client Experiencing Trauma**

NANDA

Post-Trauma Syndrome

↓

NIC

Counseling

Coping Enhancement

Simple Relaxation Therapy

Support System Enhancement

↓

NOC

Anxiety Level

Coping

Stress Level

Social Support

Data from *NANDA's Nursing Diagnoses: Definitions & Classification 2005–2006* by NANDA International (2005), Philadelphia; *Nursing Interventions Classification (NIC)* (4th ed.) by J. M. Dochterman & G. M. Bulechek (2004), St. Louis, MO: Mosby; and *Nursing Outcomes Classification (NOC)* (3rd ed.) by S. Moorhead, M. Johnson, and M. Maas (2004), St. Louis, MO: Mosby.

- Follow-up appointments with the physician or at the trauma clinic
- Emotional changes that the client may undergo as a result of the trauma
- Helpful resources:
  - Home health care
  - Community support groups
  - National Institute of Neurological Disorders and Stroke.

THE CLIENT EXPERIENCING SHOCK

Shock is a clinical syndrome characterized by a systemic imbalance between oxygen supply and demand. This imbalance results in a state of inadequate blood flow to body organs and tissues, causing life-threatening cellular dysfunction.

Overview of Cellular Homeostasis and Hemodynamics

To maintain cellular metabolism, cells of all body organs and tissues require a regular and consistent supply of oxygen and the removal of metabolic wastes. This homeostatic regulation is maintained primarily by the cardiovascular system and depends on four physiologic components:

1. A cardiac output sufficient to meet bodily requirements
2. An uncompromised vascular system, in which the vessels have a diameter sufficient to allow unimpeded blood flow

and have good tone (the ability to constrict or dilate to maintain normal pressure)

3. A volume of blood sufficient to fill the circulatory system, and a blood pressure adequate to maintain blood flow

4. Tissues that are able to extract and use the oxygen delivered through the capillaries.

In a healthy person, these components function as a system to maintain tissue perfusion. During shock, however, one or more of these components are disrupted. An understanding of basic hemodynamics is necessary to understand the pathophysiology of shock:

- **Stroke volume (SV)** is the amount of blood pumped into the aorta with each contraction of the left ventricle.
- **Cardiac output (CO)** is the amount of blood pumped per minute into the aorta by the left ventricle. CO is determined by multiplying the stroke volume (SV) by the heart rate (HR): CO = SV × HR.

PRACTICE ALERT
Cardiac output (CO) = stroke volume (SV) × heart rate (HR).

- **Mean arterial pressure (MAP)** is the product of cardiac output and systemic vascular resistance (SVR): MAP = CO × SVR. When CO, SVR, or total blood volume rises, MAP and tissue perfusion increase. Conversely, when CO, SVR, or total blood volume falls, MAP and tissue perfusion decrease.
- The sympathetic nervous system maintains the smooth muscle surrounding the arteries and arterioles in a state of partial contraction called *sympathetic tone*. Increased sympathetic stimulation increases vasoconstriction and SVR; decreased sympathetic stimulation allows vasodilatation, which decreases SVR.

Pathophysiology

When one or more cardiovascular components do not function properly, the body's hemodynamic properties are altered. Consequently, tissue perfusion may be inadequate to sustain normal cellular metabolism. The result is the clinical syndrome known as shock. The manifestations of shock result from the body's attempts to maintain vital organs (heart and brain) and to preserve life following a drop in cellular perfusion. However, if the injury or condition triggering shock is severe enough or of long enough duration, then cellular hypoxia and cellular death occur.

Shock is triggered by a sustained drop in mean arterial pressure. This drop can occur after a decrease in cardiac output, a decrease in the circulating blood volume, or an increase in the size of the vascular bed due to peripheral vasodilatation. If intervention is timely and effective, the physiologic events that characterize shock may be stopped; if not, shock may lead to death. See Table 11–5 for classifications of shock.

Stage I: Early, Reversible, and Compensatory Shock
The initial stage of shock begins when baroreceptors in the aortic arch and the carotid sinus detect a sustained drop in MAP of less than 10 mmHg from normal levels. The circulating blood volume may decrease (usually to less than 500 mL), but not enough to cause serious effects.

The body reacts to the decrease in arterial pressure as it would to any physical stressor. The cerebral integration center initiates the body's response systems, causing the sympathetic nervous system to increase the heart rate and the force of cardiac contraction, thus increasing cardiac output. Sympathetic stimulation also causes peripheral vasoconstriction, resulting in increased systemic vascular resistance and a rise in arterial pressure. The net result is that the perfusion of cells, tissues, and organs is maintained.

Symptoms are almost imperceptible during the early stage of shock. The pulse rate may be slightly elevated. If the injury is minor or of short duration, arterial pressure is usually maintained, and no further symptoms occur.

Compensatory shock begins after the MAP falls 10 to 15 mmHg below normal levels. The circulating blood volume is reduced by 25% to 35% (1000 mL or more), but compensatory mechanisms are able to maintain blood pressure and tissue perfusion to vital organs, thereby preventing cell damage.

- Stimulation of the sympathetic nervous system results in the release of epinephrine from the adrenal medulla and the release of norepinephrine from the adrenal medulla and the sympathetic fibers. Both hormones rapidly stimulate the alpha- and

TABLE 11–5 Classification of Hemorrhagic Shock and Client Presentation

	COMPENSATED/ CLASS I	MILD/CLASS II	MODERATE/CLASS III	SEVERE/CLASS IV
Blood loss	Up to 750 mL	750–1500 mL	1500–2000 mL	>2000 mL
Percent of blood volume loss	Up to 15%	15–30%	30–40%	>40%
Heart rate	<100	>100	>120	>140
Blood pressure	Normal or increased	Normal	Decreased	Markedly decreased
Pulse pressure	Normal or increased	Decreased	Decreased	Decreased
Capillary refill	Normal	Mild increase	Usually delayed	Delayed
Respiratory rate	Normal	Mild increase	Moderate tachypnea	Markedly tachypnea
Urine output (mL/h)	>30 mL	20–30 mL	5–15 mL	Anuria
Mental status	Normal–slightly anxious	Mildly anxious–agitated	Anxious–confused	Lethargic–obtunded

beta-adrenergic fibers. Stimulated alpha-adrenergic fibers cause vasoconstriction in the blood vessels supplying the skin and most of the abdominal viscera. Perfusion of these areas decreases. Stimulated beta-adrenergic fibers cause vasodilatation in vessels supplying the heart and skeletal muscles (beta₁ response), and increase the heart rate and force of cardiac contraction (beta₂ response). Further, blood vessels in the respiratory system dilate, and the respiratory rate increases (beta₂ response). Thus, stimulation of the sympathetic nervous system results in increased cardiac output and oxygenation of these tissues.

- The renin–angiotensin response occurs as the blood flow to the kidneys decreases. Renin released from the kidneys converts a plasma protein to angiotensin II, which causes vasoconstriction and stimulates the adrenal cortex to release aldosterone. Aldosterone causes the kidneys to reabsorb water and sodium and to lose potassium. The absorption of water maintains circulating blood volume while increased vasoconstriction increases SVR, maintaining central vascular volume and raising blood pressure.

- The hypothalamus releases adrenocorticotropic hormone, causing the adrenal glands to secrete aldosterone. Aldosterone promotes the reabsorption of water and sodium by the kidneys, preserving blood volume and pressure.

- The posterior pituitary gland releases antidiuretic hormone, which increases renal reabsorption of water to increase intravascular volume. The combined effects of hormones released by the hypothalamus and posterior pituitary glands work to conserve central vascular volume.

- As MAP falls in the compensatory stage of shock, decreased capillary hydrostatic pressure causes a fluid shift from the interstitial space into the capillaries. The net gain of fluid raises the blood volume.

Working together, these compensatory mechanisms can maintain MAP for only a short period of time. During this period, the perfusion and oxygenation of the heart and brain are adequate. If effective treatment is provided, the process is arrested, and no permanent damage occurs. However, unless the underlying cause of shock is reversed, these compensatory mechanisms soon become harmful, and shock perpetuates shock.

Stage II: Intermediate or Progressive Shock

The progressive stage of shock occurs after a sustained decrease in MAP of 20 mmHg or more below normal levels and a fluid loss of 35% to 50% (1800 to 2500 mL of fluid). Although the compensatory mechanisms in the previous state remain activated, they are no longer able to maintain MAP at a level sufficient to ensure perfusion of vital organs.

The vasoconstriction response that first helped sustain MAP eventually limits blood flow to the point that cells become oxygen deficient. To remain alive, the affected cells switch from aerobic to anaerobic metabolism. The lactic acid formed as a by-product of anaerobic metabolism contributes to an acidotic state at the cellular level. As a result, adenosine triphosphate, the source of cellular energy, is produced inefficiently. Lacking energy, the sodium-potassium pump fails. Potassium moves out of the cell, while sodium and water move inward. As this

process continues, the cell swells, cell membrane integrity is lost, and cell organelles are damaged. Lysosomes within the cell spill out their digestive enzymes, which disintegrate any remaining organelles. Some enzymes spread to adjacent cells, where they erode and rupture cell membranes.

The acid by-products of anaerobic metabolism dilate the precapillary arterioles and constrict the postcapillary venules. This causes increased hydrostatic pressure within the capillary, and fluid shifts back into the interstitial space. The capillaries also become increasingly permeable, allowing serum proteins to shift from the vascular space into the interstitium. The buildup of plasma proteins increases the osmotic pressure in the interstitium, further accelerating the fluid shift out of the capillaries.

Throughout this period, the heart rate and vasoconstriction increase; however, perfusion of the skin, skeletal muscles, kidneys, and gastrointestinal organs is greatly diminished. Cells in the heart and brain become hypoxic while other body cells and tissues become ischemic and anoxic. A generalized state of acidosis and hyperkalemia ensues (see Chapter 10 ∞). Unless this stage of shock is treated rapidly, the client's chances of survival are poor.

Stage III: Refractory or Irreversible Shock

If shock progresses to the irreversible stage, tissue anoxia becomes so generalized and cellular death so widespread that no treatment can reverse the damage. Even if MAP is temporarily restored, too much cellular damage has occurred to maintain life. Death of cells is followed by death of tissues, which results in death of organs. Death of vital organs contributes to subsequent death of the body.

Effects of Shock on Body Systems

Whatever its causes, shock produces predictable effects on the body's organ systems. (See *Multisystem Effects of Shock* on the following page.)

CARDIOVASCULAR SYSTEM The perfusion and oxygenation of the heart are adequate in the early stages of shock. As shock progresses, myocardial cells become hypoxic, and myocardial muscle function diminishes. Initially, the blood pressure may be normal or even slightly elevated (as a result of compensatory mechanisms) and the heart rate only slightly increased. Sympathetic stimulation increases the heart rate (a sinus tachycardia of 120 beats per minute is common) in an effort to increase cardiac output. As a result of vasoconstriction and decreased blood volume, the palpated pulse is rapid, weak, and thready; as shock progresses, peripheral pulses are usually nonpalpable.

Tachycardia reduces the time available for left ventricular filling and coronary artery perfusion, further reducing cardiac output. With progressive shock, altered acid–base balance, hypoxia, and hyperkalemia damage the heart's electrical systems and contractility. Consequently, cardiac dysrhythmias may develop. Decreased blood volume with decreased venous return also decreases cardiac output, and blood pressure falls.

The blood pressure changes produced by shock are characterized by a progressive decrease in both systolic and diastolic pressures and a narrowing pulse pressure. Auscultation of

MULTISYSTEM EFFECTS of Shock

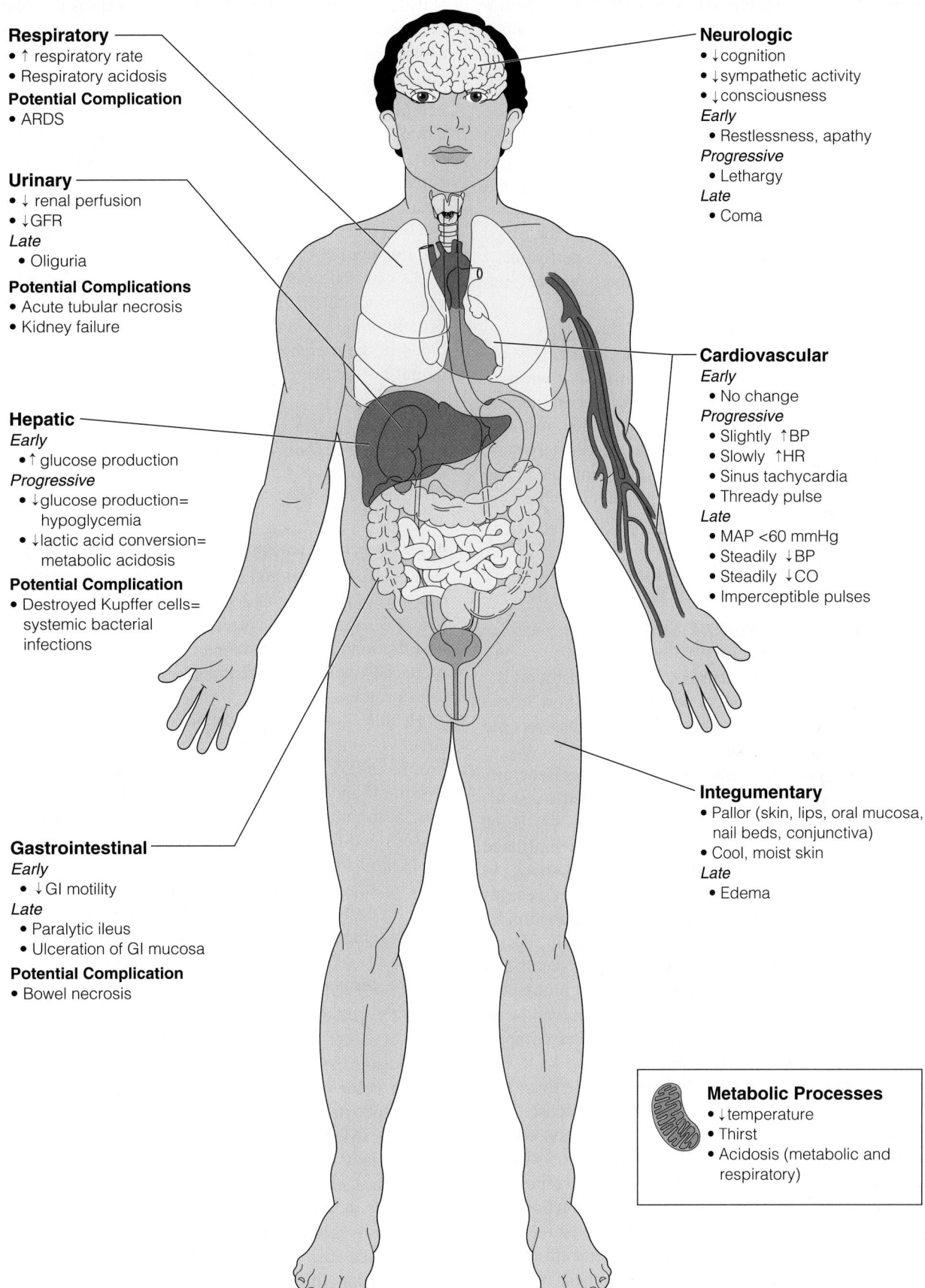

Respiratory
- ↑ respiratory rate
- Respiratory acidosis

Potential Complication
- ARDS

Urinary
- ↓ renal perfusion
- ↓GFR

Late
- Oliguria

Potential Complications
- Acute tubular necrosis
- Kidney failure

Hepatic

Early
- ↑ glucose production

Progressive
- ↓glucose production= hypoglycemia
- ↓lactic acid conversion= metabolic acidosis

Potential Complication
- Destroyed Kupffer cells= systemic bacterial infections

Gastrointestinal

Early
- ↓ GI motility

Late
- Paralytic ileus
- Ulceration of GI mucosa

Potential Complication
- Bowel necrosis

Neurologic
- ↓cognition
- ↓sympathetic activity
- ↓consciousness

Early
- Restlessness, apathy

Progressive
- Lethargy

Late
- Coma

Cardiovascular

Early
- No change

Progressive
- Slightly ↑BP
- Slowly ↑HR
- Sinus tachycardia
- Thready pulse

Late
- MAP <60 mmHg
- Steadily ↓BP
- Steadily ↓CO
- Imperceptible pulses

Integumentary
- Pallor (skin, lips, oral mucosa, nail beds, conjunctiva)
- Cool, moist skin

Late
- Edema

Metabolic Processes
- ↓temperature
- Thirst
- Acidosis (metabolic and respiratory)

blood pressure is often difficult or impossible and is an inaccurate reflection of blood pressure status. For this reason, hemodynamic monitoring is usually instituted to follow the client's cardiovascular status accurately.

RESPIRATORY SYSTEM During shock, oxygen delivery to cells may be impaired by a drop in circulating blood volume or, in the case of blood loss, by an insufficient number of red blood cells that carry oxygen. Although the respiratory rate increases because of compensatory mechanisms that promote oxygenation, the number of alveoli that are perfused decreases, and gas exchange is impaired. As a result, oxygen levels in the blood decrease, and carbon dioxide levels increase. As perfusion of the lungs diminishes, carbon dioxide is retained, and respiratory acidosis occurs.

A complication of decreased perfusion of the lungs is acute respiratory distress syndrome (ARDS), or "shock lung." The exact mechanism that produces ARDS is unknown, but some contributing factors have been identified. The pulmonary capillaries become increasingly permeable to proteins and water, resulting in noncardiogenic pulmonary edema. Production of surfactant (which controls surface tension within alveoli) is impaired, and the alveoli collapse or fill with fluid. This potentially lethal form of respiratory failure may result from any condition that causes hypoperfusion of the lungs, but it is more common in shock caused by hemorrhage, severe allergic responses, trauma, and infection. (ARDS is discussed further in Chapter 39 ∞.)

GASTROINTESTINAL AND HEPATIC SYSTEMS The gastrointestinal organs normally receive 25% of the cardiac output through the splanchnic circulation. Shock constricts the splanchnic arterioles and redirects arterial blood flow to the heart and brain. Consequently, gastrointestinal organs become ischemic and may be irreversibly damaged.

Gastric mucosa tends to ulcerate when it becomes ischemic. Lesions of the gastric and duodenal mucosa (called *stress ulcers*) can develop within hours of severe trauma, sepsis, or burns (Porth, 2005). Gastrointestinal ulcers may hemorrhage within 2 to 10 days following the original cause of shock. In addition, the permeability of damaged mucosa increases, allowing enteric bacteria or their toxins to enter the abdominal cavity and then progress to the circulation, resulting in sepsis.

Gastric and intestinal motility is impaired during shock, and paralytic ileus may result. If the episode of shock is prolonged, necrosis of the bowel may occur. In many cases, alterations in the structure and function of the gastrointestinal tract impair absorption of nutrients, such as protein and glucose.

Shock also alters the metabolic functions of the liver. Initially, *gluconeogenesis* (the process of forming glucose from noncarbohydrate sources) and *glycogenolysis* (the breakdown of glycogen into glucose) increase. This process allows blood glucose levels to increase as the body attempts to respond to the stressor; however, as shock progresses, liver functions are impaired, and hypoglycemia develops. Metabolism of fats and protein is impaired, and the liver can no longer effectively remove lactic acid, contributing to the development of metabolic acidosis.

The destruction of the liver's reticuloendothelial Kupffer cells (phagocytes that destroy bacteria) causes a further problem. Bacteria may proliferate within the circulatory system, causing overwhelming bacterial infection and toxicity.

NEUROLOGIC SYSTEM The primary effects of shock on the neurologic system involve changes in mental status and orientation. Cerebral hypoxia produces altered levels of consciousness, beginning with apathy and lethargy and progressing to coma. A common early symptom of cerebral hypoxia is restlessness. Continued ischemia of brain cells eventually causes swelling, resulting in cerebral edema, neurotransmitter failure, and irreversible brain cell damage.

As cerebral ischemia worsens, the sympathetic activity and vasomotor centers are depressed. This leads to a loss of sympathetic tone, causing systemic vasodilatation and pooling of blood in the periphery. As a result, venous return and cardiac output further decrease.

> **PRACTICE ALERT**
> An early sign of shock is a change in the level of consciousness. Late signs of shock include mental status changes, hypotension, and marked tachycardia.

RENAL SYSTEM Blood that normally perfuses the kidneys is shunted to the heart and brain during the progressive stage of shock, resulting in renal hypoperfusion. The drop in renal perfusion is reflected in a corresponding decrease in the glomerular filtration rate. Urine output is reduced, and the urine that is produced is highly concentrated. Oliguria of <20 mL/h indicates progressive shock.

Healthy kidneys can tolerate a drop in perfusion for only about 20 minutes; thereafter, acute tubular necrosis develops (Porth, 2005). As tubular necrosis occurs, epithelial cells slough off and block the tubules, disrupting nephron function. The accumulating loss of functional nephrons eventually causes renal failure. Without normal renal function, metabolic waste products are retained in the plasma.

If treatment restores renal perfusion, the kidneys can regenerate the lost epithelial cells in the tubules, and renal function usually returns to normal. However, in a client who is older or chronically ill or in sustained shock, loss of renal function may become permanent.

EFFECTS ON SKIN, TEMPERATURE, AND THIRST In most types of shock, blood vessels supplying the skin are vasoconstricted, and the sweat glands are activated. As a result, changes in skin color occur. The skin of Caucasian clients becomes pale. In people with darker skin (such as those of African, Hispanic, or Mediterranean descent), shock-related skin color changes may be assessed as paleness of the lips, oral mucous membranes, nail beds, and conjunctiva. The skin is usually cool and moist and, in the later stages of shock, often edematous.

The body temperature decreases as shock progresses, the result of a decrease in overall body metabolism. Some people in shock become thirsty, probably a response to decreased blood volume and increased serum osmolality (Porth, 2005).

Types of Shock

Shock is identified according to its underlying cause. All types of shock progress through the same stages and exert similar effects on body systems. Any differences are noted in the following discussion.

Hypovolemic Shock

Hypovolemic shock is caused by a decrease in intravascular volume of 15% or more (Porth, 2005). In hypovolemic shock, the venous blood returning to the heart decreases, and ventricular filling drops. As a result, stroke volume, cardiac output, and blood pressure decrease. Hypovolemic shock is the most common type of shock, and it often occurs simultaneously with other types.

The decrease in circulating blood volume that triggers hypovolemic shock may result from:

- Loss of blood volume from hemorrhage (from surgery, trauma, gastrointestinal bleeding, blood coagulation disorders, ruptured esophageal varices)
- Loss of intravascular fluid from the skin due to injuries such as burns (see Chapter 17 ∞)
- Loss of blood volume from severe dehydration
- Loss of body fluid from the gastrointestinal system due to persistent and severe vomiting or diarrhea, or continuous nasogastric suctioning
- Renal losses of fluid due to the use of diuretics or to endocrine disorders such as diabetes insipidus
- Conditions causing fluid shifts from the intravascular compartment to the interstitial space
- Third spacing due to such disorders as liver diseases with ascites, pleural effusion, or intestinal obstruction

Hypovolemic shock affects all body systems. Its effects vary depending on the client's age, general state of health, extent of injury or severity of illness, length of time before treatment is provided, and the rate of volume loss.

The manifestations of hypovolemic shock result directly from the decrease in circulating blood volume and the initiation of compensatory mechanisms (Figure 11–8 ■). The loss of circulating blood volume reduces cardiac output by decreasing venous return to the heart. As a result, blood pressure drops. The carotid and cardiac baroreceptors sense the decrease in blood pressure and communicate it to the vasomotor centers in the brainstem. The vasomotor centers then induce the sympathetic compensatory responses. If the fluid loss is less than 500 mL, activation of the sympathetic response is generally adequate to restore cardiac output and blood pressure to near normal, although the heart rate may remain elevated.

With a sustained loss of blood volume (1000 mL or more), the shock stage progresses. Heart rate and vasoconstriction increase, and blood flow to the skin, skeletal muscles, kidneys, and abdominal organs decreases. Several renal mechanisms and a decline in capillary pressure help conserve blood volume. Eventually, the amount of blood flowing to cells is too low to oxygenate them and sustain production of cellular energy. Anaerobic metabolism begins, producing an acidotic environment for cells. As a result, cells lose their physical integrity. If

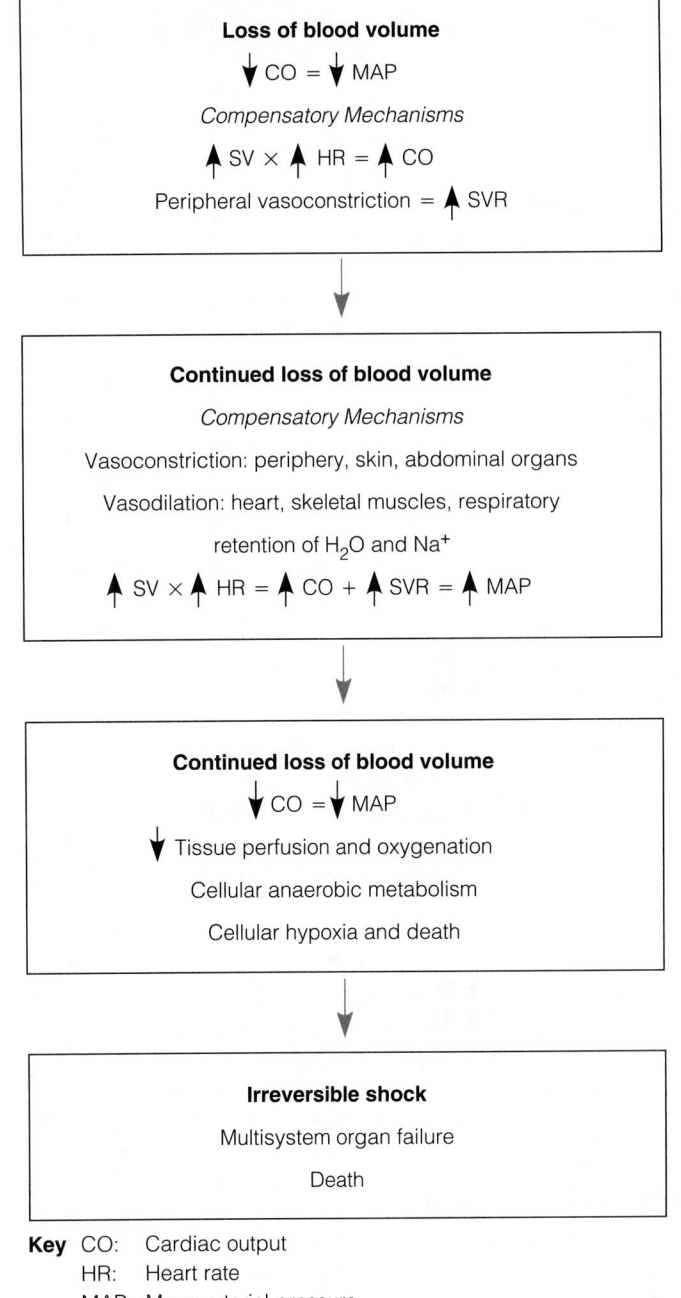

Figure 11–8 ■ The stages of hypovolemic shock.

untreated, shock causes multiple organ failure, and death results. Manifestations of various stages of hypovolemic shock are listed in the box on the following page.

OLDER ADULTS EXPERIENCING HYPOVOLEMIA With aging comes a relative decrease in sympathetic activity in relation to the cardiovascular system. Cardiac compliance also decreases with age. Atherosclerosis affects many vital organs' sensitivity to even the slightest reduction in blood flow. Many elderly people experience secondary volume depletion due to chronic diuretic

MANIFESTATIONS of Hypovolemic Shock

INITIAL STAGE
- Blood pressure: normal to slightly decreased
- Pulse: slightly increased from baseline
- Respirations: normal (baseline)
- Skin: cool, pale (in periphery), moist
- Mental status: alert and oriented
- Urine output: slight decrease
- Other: thirst, decreased capillary refill time

COMPENSATORY AND PROGRESSIVE STAGES
- Blood pressure: hypotension
- Pulse: rapid, thready
- Respirations: increased
- Skin: cool, pale (includes trunk); poor turgor with fluid loss, edematous with fluid shift
- Mental status: restless, anxious, confused, or agitated
- Urine output: oliguria (less than 30 mL/h)
- Other: marked thirst, acidosis, hyperkalemia, decreased capillary refill time, decreased or absent peripheral pulses

IRREVERSIBLE STAGE
- Blood pressure: severe hypotension (often, systolic pressure is below 80 mmHg)
- Pulse: very rapid, weak
- Respirations: rapid, shallow; crackles and wheezes
- Skin: cool, pale, mottled with cyanosis
- Mental status: disoriented, lethargic, comatose
- Urine output: anuria
- Other: loss of reflexes, decreased or absent peripheral pulses

use or malnutrition. Also, clients prescribed beta-blockers may not present with tachycardia as an early indicator of shock. This important sign can be masked due to beta-adrenergic blockade. These clients will require early invasive monitoring in order to avoid excessive or inadequate volume restoration. This should be considered early in the treatment phase.

Cardiogenic Shock

Cardiogenic shock occurs when the heart's pumping ability is compromised to the point that it cannot maintain cardiac output and adequate tissue perfusion. Cardiac disorders are discussed in Chapters 30 and 32 ∞; this section focuses only on the effects of shock caused by these disorders.

The loss of the pumping action of the heart may be caused by the following conditions:
- Myocardial infarction
- Cardiac tamponade
- Restrictive pericarditis
- Cardiac arrest
- Dysrhythmias, such as fibrillation or ventricular tachycardia
- Pathologic changes in the valves
- Cardiomyopathies from hypertension, alcohol, bacterial or viral infections, or ischemia
- Complications of cardiac surgery
- Electrolyte imbalances (especially changes in normal potassium and calcium levels)

- Drugs affecting cardiac muscle contractility
- Head injuries causing damage to the cardioregulatory center.

Myocardial infarction is the most common cause of cardiogenic shock. Clients admitted to the hospital for treatment of myocardial infarction or cardiac surgery are at risk for cardiogenic shock. The severity and progression of shock are related to the amount of myocardial damage.

Whatever the cardiogenic cause, the decrease in cardiac output causes a decrease in MAP. Heart rate may increase in response to compensatory mechanisms. However, tachycardia increases myocardial oxygen consumption and decreases coronary perfusion. The myocardium becomes progressively depleted of oxygen, causing further myocardial ischemia and necrosis. The typical sequence of shock is essentially unchanged in cardiogenic shock.

Cyanosis, however, is more common in cardiogenic shock, because stagnating blood increases extraction of oxygen from the hemoglobin at the capillary beds. As a result, the skin, lips, and nail beds may appear cyanotic. As cardiac failure and cardiogenic shock progress, left ventricular end-diastolic pressure increases. The increase is transmitted to the pulmonary capillary bed, and pulmonary edema may occur. Retention of blood in the right side of the heart increases right atrial pressure, which leads to jugular venous distention as a result of backflow through the vena cava. Manifestations of cardiogenic shock are listed in the box below.

Obstructive Shock

Obstructive shock is caused by an obstruction in the heart or great vessels that either impedes venous return or prevents effective cardiac pumping action. The causes of obstructive shock are impaired diastolic filling (e.g., pericardial tamponade or pneumothorax), increased right ventricular afterload (e.g., pulmonary emboli), and increased left ventricular afterload (e.g., aortic stenosis, abdominal distention). The manifestations are the result of decreased cardiac output and blood pressure, with reduced tissue perfusion and cellular metabolism.

Distributive Shock

Distributive shock (also called **vasogenic shock**) includes several types of shock that result from widespread vasodilatation and decreased peripheral resistance. Because the blood volume does not change, relative hypovolemia results.

MANIFESTATIONS of Cardiogenic Shock

- Blood pressure: hypotension
- Pulse: rapid, thready; distention of veins of hands and neck
- Respirations: increased, labored; crackles and wheezes; pulmonary edema
- Skin: pale, cyanotic, cold, moist
- Mental status: restless, anxious, lethargic progressing to comatose
- Urine output: oliguria to anuria
- Other: dependent edema; elevated central venous pressure (CVP); elevated pulmonary capillary wedge pressure; arrhythmias

MediaLink   Case Study: Identifying Types of Shock

Septic Shock

Septic shock, the leading cause of death for clients in intensive care units, is one part of a progressive syndrome called *systemic inflammatory response syndrome* (SIRS). This condition is most often the result of gram-negative bacterial infections (i.e., *Pseudomonas, E. coli, Klebsiella*), but may also follow gram-positive infections from *Staphylococcus* and *Streptococcus* bacteria. Gram-negative sepsis has greatly increased in the past 10 years, with a 60% mortality rate despite treatment. The pathophysiology of septic shock is complex and not completely understood.

Clients at risk for developing infections leading to septic shock include those who are hospitalized, have debilitating chronic illnesses, or have poor nutritional status. The risk is heightened after invasive procedures or surgery. Other clients at risk of septic shock include older adults and those who are immunocompromised. Portals of entry for infection that may lead to septic shock are as follows:

- *Urinary system:* catheterizations, suprapubic tubes, cystoscopy
- *Respiratory system:* suctioning, aspiration, tracheostomy, endotracheal tubes, respiratory therapy, mechanical ventilators
- *Gastrointestinal system:* peptic ulcers, ruptured appendix, peritonitis
- *Integumentary system:* surgical wounds, intravenous catheters, intra-arterial catheters, invasive monitoring, decubitus ulcers, burns, trauma
- *Female reproductive system:* elective surgical abortion, ascending infections from transmission of bacteria during the intrapartal and postpartal periods, tampon use, sexually transmitted infections.

Septic shock begins with *septicemia* (the presence of pathogens and their toxins in the blood). As pathogens are destroyed, their ruptured cell membranes allow endotoxins to leak into the plasma. The endotoxins disrupt the vascular system, coagulation mechanism, and immune system and trigger an immune and inflammatory response (see Chapter 12 ∞ for more information). For this reason, the initial effects of septic shock differ from those of hypovolemic and cardiogenic shock; cardiac output is high and systemic vascular resistance is low.

Endotoxins directly damage the endothelial lining of small blood vessels first; the small blood vessels of the kidneys and lungs are most susceptible. Cellular damage stimulates the release of vasoactive proteins and activates coagulation factor XII. The vasoactive proteins stimulate peripheral vasodilatation and increase capillary permeability; the activation of coagulation factors results in the production of multiple intravascular blood clots.

As a result of the increased capillary permeability and vasodilatation, fluid shifts from the intravascular space to the interstitial space. Hypovolemia results as fluid volume is lost from the circulating blood. Hypovolemia and intravascular coagulation alter oxygenation and cellular metabolism, leading to anaerobic metabolism, lactic acidosis, and cellular death.

Septic shock has an early phase and a late phase. In early septic shock (sometimes called the *warm phase*), vasodilatation results in weakness and warm, flushed skin, and the sep-ticemia often causes high fever and chills. In late septic shock (sometimes called the *cold phase*), hypovolemia and activity of the compensatory mechanisms result in typical shock manifestations, including cold, moist skin; oliguria; and changes in mental status. Death may result from respiratory failure, cardiac failure, or renal failure. Manifestations of septic shock are listed in the box below.

Toxic shock syndrome is an especially virulent form of septic shock, occurring most frequently in menstruating women who use tampons. It is thought that bacterial toxins diffuse from the site of infection in the vagina into the circulation. The toxins then trigger a widespread inflammatory response and septic shock. The manifestations of toxic shock syndrome include extreme hypotension, hyperpyrexia, headache, myalgia, confusion, skin rash, vomiting, and diarrhea (Porth, 2005).

Disseminated intravascular coagulation (DIC), a generalized response to injury, is a potential risk in septic shock. This condition is characterized by simultaneous bleeding and clotting throughout the vasculature. Sepsis injures blood cells, causing platelet aggregation and decreased blood flow. As a result, blood clots form throughout the microcirculation. The clotting slows circulation further while stimulating excess fibrinolysis. As the body's stores of clotting factors are depleted, generalized bleeding begins. DIC is further discussed in Chapter 34 ∞.

Neurogenic Shock

Neurogenic shock is the result of an imbalance between parasympathetic and sympathetic stimulation of vascular smooth muscle. If parasympathetic overstimulation or sympathetic understimulation persists, sustained vasodilatation occurs, and blood pools in the venous and capillary beds.

Neurogenic shock causes dramatic reduction in systemic vascular resistance as the size of the vascular compartment increases. As systemic vascular resistance decreases, pressure in the blood vessels becomes too low to drive nutrients across capillary membranes, and cellular metabolism is impaired.

MANIFESTATIONS of Septic Shock

EARLY (WARM) SEPTIC SHOCK
- Blood pressure: normal to hypotension
- Pulse: increased, thready
- Respirations: rapid and deep
- Skin: warm, flushed
- Mental status: alert, oriented, anxious
- Urine output: normal
- Other: increased body temperature; chills; weakness; nausea, vomiting, diarrhea; decreased CVP

LATE (COLD) SEPTIC SHOCK
- Blood pressure: hypotension
- Pulse: tachycardia, arrhythmias
- Respirations: rapid, shallow, dyspneic
- Skin: cool, pale, edematous
- Mental status: lethargic to comatose
- Urine output: oliguria to anuria
- Other: normal to decreased body temperature; decreased CVP

The following conditions can cause neurogenic shock by increasing parasympathetic stimulation or inhibiting sympathetic stimulation of the smooth muscle of blood vessels:

- Head injury
- Trauma to the spinal cord (spinal shock, a form of neurogenic shock, is described in Chapter 45 ∞)
- Insulin reactions (which cause hypoglycemia, decreasing glucose to the medulla)
- Central nervous system depressant drugs (such as sedatives, barbiturates, or narcotics)
- Anesthesia (spinal and general)
- Severe pain
- Prolonged exposure to heat.

Bradycardia occurs early, but tachycardia begins as compensatory mechanisms are initiated. Central venous pressure drops as veins dilate, venous return to the heart decreases, stroke volume decreases, and MAP falls. In early stages, the extremities are warm and pink (from the pooling of blood), but as shock progresses, the skin becomes pale and cool. Manifestations of neurogenic shock are listed in the box below.

Anaphylactic Shock

Anaphylactic shock is the result of a widespread hypersensitivity reaction (called *anaphylaxis*). The pathophysiology in this type of shock includes vasodilatation, pooling of blood in the periphery, and hypovolemia with altered cellular metabolism. These physiologic alterations occur when a sensitized person has contact with an *allergen* (a foreign substance to which an individual is hypersensitive). Many different allergens can cause anaphylactic shock, including medications, blood administration, latex, foods, snake venom, and insect stings.

Anaphylactic shock does not occur with the first exposure to an allergen. With the first exposure to a foreign substance (the *antigen*), the body produces specific immunoglobulin E (IgE) antibodies against this antigen. The person is thus sensitized to that specific antigen. With subsequent exposure, the antigen reacts with the already formed IgE antibodies, disrupting cellular integrity. In addition, large amounts of histamine and other vasoactive amines are released and distributed through the circulatory system. These substances cause increased capillary permeability and massive vasodilatation, resulting in profound hypotension and eventual vascular collapse.

Histamine also causes constriction of smooth muscles in the bladder, uterus, intestines, and bronchioles. Respiratory distress, bronchospasm, laryngospasm, and severe abdominal cramping result. Serotonin (a neurotransmitter with vasoconstrictive properties) is released, further affecting respiratory status by increasing capillary permeability in the lungs. As a result, plasma leaks into the alveoli, gas exchange is impaired, and pulmonary edema may occur.

Anaphylactic shock begins and progresses rapidly. Manifestations may begin within 20 minutes of contact with an antigen. Unless appropriate intervention is provided, death can occur within a matter of minutes. Because anaphylaxis is rapid and potentially lethal, people with known allergies should carry some form of warning (such as a Medic-Alert bracelet) informing others of their susceptibility. Healthcare providers should be extremely careful to assess and document allergies or previous drug reactions. Manifestations of anaphylactic shock are listed in the box below.

INTERDISCIPLINARY CARE

Medical care for the client in shock focuses on treating the underlying cause, increasing arterial oxygenation, and improving tissue perfusion. Depending on the cause and type of shock, interventions include emergency care measures, oxygen therapy, fluid replacement, and medications. Emergency care is often the first course of collaborative action taken to arrest shock, as discussed earlier in this chapter.

Diagnosis

The following diagnostic tests can help identify the type of shock and assess the client's physical status. Measurements include:

- *Blood hemoglobin* and *hematocrit*. Changes in hemoglobin and hematocrit concentrations usually occur in hypovolemic shock. These changes reflect the underlying etiology. In hypovolemic shock resulting from hemorrhage, the hemoglobin and hematocrit concentrations are lower than normal. In hypovolemic shock resulting from intravascular fluid loss, by contrast, the hemoglobin and hematocrit concentrations are higher than normal.
- *Arterial blood gases (ABGs)*, to determine oxygen and carbon dioxide levels and pH. The effects of shock and of the body's compensatory mechanisms cause a decrease in pH (indicating acidosis), a decrease in the partial pressure of

---

MANIFESTATIONS **of Neurogenic Shock**

- Blood pressure: hypotension
- Pulse: slow and bounding
- Respirations: vary
- Skin: warm, dry
- Mental status: anxious, restless, lethargic progressing to comatose
- Urine output: oliguria to anuria
- Other: lowered body temperature

MANIFESTATIONS **of Anaphylactic Shock**

- Blood pressure: hypotension
- Pulse: increased, dysrhythmias
- Respirations: dyspnea, stridor, wheezes, laryngospasm, bronchospasm, pulmonary edema
- Skin: warm, edematous (lips, eyelids, tongue, hands, feet, genitals)
- Mental status: restless, anxious, lethargic to comatose
- Urine output: oliguria to anuria
- Other: paresthesias; pruritus; abdominal cramps, vomiting, diarrhea

oxygen (PaO_2) and in total oxygen saturation, and an increase in the partial pressure of carbon dioxide ($PaCO_2$).

■ *Serum electrolytes,* to monitor the severity and progression of shock. As shock progresses, glucose levels decrease, sodium levels decrease, and potassium levels increase.

■ *Blood urea nitrogen (BUN), serum creatinine levels, urine specific gravity,* and *osmolality,* to check renal function. As perfusion of the kidneys is decreased and renal function is reduced, the BUN and creatinine levels increase as does urine specific gravity and osmolality.

■ *Blood cultures,* to identify the causative organism in septic shock.

■ *White blood cell (WBC) count* and *differential,* in the client with septic or anaphylactic shock. The total WBC count is increased in septic shock. Elevated neutrophils indicate acute infection, increased monocytes indicate a bacterial infection, and increased eosinophils indicate an allergic response.

■ *Serum cardiac enzymes,* which are elevated in cardiogenic shock: lactate dehydrogenase (LDH), creatine phosphokinase (CPK), and serum glutamic-oxaloacetic transaminase (SGOT).

■ *Central venous catheter,* to aid in the differential diagnosis of shock and to provide information about the preload of the heart. A pulmonary artery catheter may be inserted to monitor cardiac dynamics, fluid balance, and the effects of vasoactive medications.

Other diagnostic tests may be ordered to determine the extent of injury or damage or to locate the site of internal hemorrhage. These tests might include x-ray studies, CT scans, MRI, endoscopic examinations, and echocardiograms. Newer diagnostic methods for hypoperfusion include gastric tonometry and sublingual $PaCO_2$. Gastric tonometry measures the partial pressure of carbon dioxide in the gastric lumen. The measurement of sublingual carbon dioxide correlates well with decreased MAP (Sole et al., 2001).

Medications

When fluid replacement alone is not sufficient to reverse shock, vasoactive drugs (drugs causing vasoconstriction or vasodilatation) and inotropic drugs (drugs improving cardiac contractility) may be administered. When used to treat shock, these drugs increase venous return through vasoconstriction of peripheral vessels; they also improve the pumping ability of the heart by facilitating myocardial contractility and by dilating coronary arteries to increase perfusion of the myocardium.

Drugs used to treat shock are discussed in the Medication Administration box on page 278. Other drugs that may be administered to the client in shock include:

■ Diuretics to increase urine output after fluid replacement has been initiated
■ Sodium bicarbonate to treat acidosis
■ Calcium to replace calcium lost as a result of blood transfusions
■ Antiarrhythmic agents to stabilize heart rhythm
■ Broad-spectrum antibiotics to suppress organisms responsible for septic shock

■ A cardiotonic glycoside (such as digitalis) to treat cardiac failure
■ Corticosteroids to treat anaphylactic shock
■ Morphine to dilate veins and decrease anxiety.

Oxygen Therapy

Establishing and maintaining a patent airway and ensuring adequate oxygenation are critical interventions in reversing shock. All clients in shock (even those with adequate respirations) should receive oxygen therapy (usually by mask or nasal cannula) to maintain the PaO_2 at greater than 80 mmHg during the first 4 to 6 hours of care. If the client's unassisted respiration cannot maintain PaO_2 at this level, ventilatory assistance may be necessary. Care of the client requiring ventilatory assistance is discussed in Chapter 38 ∞.

Fluid Replacement

The most effective treatment for the client in hypovolemic shock is the administration of intravenous fluids or blood. Fluids also treat septic and neurogenic shock. However, the client with cardiogenic shock may require either fluid replacement or restriction, depending on pulmonary artery pressure.

Various fluids may be administered alone or in combination as part of fluid replacement therapy in treating shock. Whole blood or blood products increase the oxygen-carrying capacity of the blood and thus increase oxygenation of cells. Fluid replacements, such as crystalloid and colloid solutions, increase circulating blood volume and tissue perfusion. Fluid replacements are administered in massive amounts through two large-bore peripheral lines or through a central line.

CRYSTALLOID SOLUTIONS Crystalloid solutions contain dextrose or electrolytes dissolved in water; they are either isotonic or hypotonic. Isotonic solutions include normal saline (0.9%), lactated Ringer's solution, and Ringer's solution. Hypotonic solutions include one-half normal saline (0.45%) and 5% dextrose in water (D_5W).

All crystalloid solutions increase fluid volume in both the intravascular and the interstitial space. Of the total amount infused, only about 25% remains in the intravascular system; the remaining 75% moves into the interstitial space. Consequently, fluid volume is only minimally expanded and the potential for peripheral edema is increased when crystalloid solutions are used. However, Ringer's lactate (an electrolyte solution) and 0.9% saline are the fluids of choice in treating hypovolemic shock, especially in the emergency phase of care while blood is being typed and crossmatched. Large amounts of these solutions may be infused rapidly, increasing blood volume and tissue perfusion.

COLLOID SOLUTIONS Colloid solutions contain substances (colloids) that should not diffuse through capillary walls. Hence, colloids tend to remain in the vascular system and increase the osmotic pressure of the serum, causing fluid to move into the vascular compartment from the interstitial space. As a result, plasma volume expands. Colloid solutions used to treat shock include 5% albumin, 25% albumin, hetastarch, plasma protein fraction, and dextran.

MEDICATION ADMINISTRATION   The Client in Shock

ADRENERGICS (SYMPATHOMIMETICS)
Vasoconstrictors
   Norepinephrine (Levophed)
   Metaraminol (Aramine)
Inotropes
   Dopamine (Inotropin)*
   Dobutamine (Dobutrex)
   Isoproterenol (Isuprel)

Adrenergic drugs (also called sympathomimetics) mimic the fight-or-flight response of the sympathetic nervous system, selectively stimulating alpha-adrenergic and beta-adrenergic receptors. Many of these drugs have both vasopressor (vasoconstricting) effects and positive inotropic effects (Table 11–6). Stimulation of alpha-adrenergic receptors results in vasoconstriction and increased systemic blood pressure. Stimulation of beta-adrenergic receptors increases the force and rate of myocardial contraction.

The physiologic effect of these drugs includes improved perfusion and oxygenation of the heart, with increased stroke volume and heart rate, and increased cardiac output. Increased cardiac output in turn increases tissue perfusion and oxygenation. The major disadvantage is that increases in stroke volume and heart rate also increase the oxygen requirements of the myocardium. These drugs may be used in the early stages of shock, especially in types of shock characterized by vasodilation.

Nursing Responsibilities
- Carefully monitor responses in the older adult, who may be especially sensitive to sympathomimetics and require lower doses.
- When administering these drugs by the subcutaneous route, carefully aspirate the injection site to avoid injecting the drug directly into a blood vessel.
- Use the intravenous route only with continuous infusion pumps. Carefully adjust the dose to accommodate the client's cardiovascular status (as ordered by the physician or by written protocol).
- Document lung sounds, vital signs, and hemodynamic parameters before starting the medication, and then according to institutional policy (usually every 5 to 15 minutes).

TABLE 11–6 Adrenergic Drugs Used to Treat Shock

ACTION	DRUG	RECEPTOR
Vasoconstrictors	Norepinephrine (Levophed)	A
	Metaraminol (Aramine)	A
Inotropes	Dopamine (Inotropin)*	A, B^1
	Dobutamine (Dobutrex)	B^1
	Isoproterenol (Isuprel)	B^1, B^2

Receptors are dose dependent.

- Record and monitor urine output. Report output of less than 30 mL/h.
- Be aware that the sympathomimetics are incompatible with sodium bicarbonate or alkaline solutions.
- When administering drugs that cause vasoconstriction, such as norepinephrine (Levophed) and metaraminol (Aramine), monitor the intravenous insertion site for infiltration. If infiltration does occur, stop the infusion and notify the physician immediately. (Infiltration may cause ischemia and necrosis of tissue.)

Health Education for the Client and Family
- Because these drugs mimic a physiologic reaction to stress, they may cause feelings of anxiety.
- Close monitoring to adjust the dose will be carried out by qualified nurses using written protocols.
- Report heart palpitations or chest pain immediately.

VASODILATORS
Nitroglycerin (Tridil)
Nitroprusside (Nipride)

Drugs that cause vasodilation act directly on smooth muscle, affecting both arterioles and veins. Peripheral resistance, cardiac output, and pulmonary wedge pressure are all reduced as a result of the vasodilation. These effects decrease the oxygen need of the heart and decrease pulmonary congestion. Vasodilators are used primarily in the treatment of cardiogenic shock and may be combined with a sympathomimetic (e.g., dopamine).

Nursing Responsibilities
- Protect these drugs from light by wrapping the intravenous bag in the package that is provided.
- Mix with D$_5$W only.
- Infuse with an infusion pump, and use within 4 hours of reconstitution.
- Do not add other medications to the solution.
- Assess mental status, blood pressure, and pulse prior to initiating medication. Thereafter, assess blood pressure and pulse according to institutional policy (usually every 5 minutes initially, then every 15 minutes until stable, and then every hour).
- Monitor for confusion, dizziness, tachycardia, arrhythmias, hypotension, and adventitious breath sounds. Report these immediately if they occur, and slow infusion to a keep-open rate.
- Monitor for signs of thiocyanate poisoning (nausea, disorientation, muscle spasms, decreased or absent reflexes) if infusion lasts longer than 72 hours.
- Keep client in bed with side rails up.

Health Education for the Client and Family
- It is important to stay in bed and change positions slowly to avoid dizziness.
- The blood pressure and pulse are taken frequently to adjust the dose of medication.
- Headache is a common side effect.

Colloid products reduce platelet adhesiveness and have been associated with reductions in blood coagulation. Consequently, the client's prothrombin time (PT), International Normalized Ratio (INR), platelet count, and activated partial thromboplastin time (APTT) should be monitored when these solutions are administered. Normal values are as follows:

PT	10–15 seconds
INR	1–1.2 seconds
Platelets	150,000–400,000
APTT	<35 seconds

MEDICATION ADMINISTRATION Colloid Solutions

COLLOID SOLUTIONS (PLASMA EXPANDERS)
Albumin 5% (Albuminar-5, Buminate 5%)
Albumin 25% (Albuminar-25, Buminate 25%)
Dextran 40 (Gentran 40)
Dextran 70 (Gentran 70, Macrodex)
Dextran 75 (Gentran 75)
Hetastarch (Hespan [HES])
Plasma protein fraction (Plasmanate, Plasma-Plex, Plasmatein, Protenate)

These solutions are blood volume expanders and are used to treat hypovolemic shock due to surgery, hemorrhage, burns, or other trauma. Albumin and plasma protein fraction are prepared from healthy blood donors. Dextran and hetastarch are synthetically prepared large molecules. The solutions promote circulatory volume and tissue perfusion by rapidly expanding plasma volume. Dextran solutions are infrequently used.

Nursing Responsibilities
- Before infusion begins, establish baseline of vital signs, lung sounds, heart sounds, and (if possible) CVP and pulmonary artery wedge pressure.
- Start administration of ordered intravenous fluids, using a large-gauge (18- or 19-gauge) infusion needle.
- Take and record vital signs as required by institutional policy (usually every 15 to 60 minutes) and client status.
- Take and record intake and output every 1 to 2 hours.
- Monitor for manifestations of congestive heart failure or pulmonary edema (dyspnea, cyanosis, cough, crackles, wheezes).

If these manifestations appear, stop the fluids and notify the physician immediately.
- Monitor for bleeding from new sites; an increase in blood pressure may cause bleeding in severed vessels that did not bleed with decreased blood pressure.
- Monitor for manifestations of dehydration (dry lips; scant, dark-colored urine; loss of skin turgor). Increased intravenous fluids are usually ordered if the client becomes dehydrated.
- Monitor for manifestations of circulatory overload (jugular vein distention, increase in CVP, increase in pulmonary artery wedge pressure). If these manifestations occur, slow rate of infusion and notify physician.
- Monitor prothrombin time, partial thromboplastin time, and platelet counts.
- If administering dextran or plasma protein fraction, have epinephrine and antihistamines readily available for any manifestations of a hypersensitivity reaction (fever, chills, rash, headache, wheezing, flushing).
- Maintain client on bed rest with side rails elevated.

Health Education for the Client and Family
- The solutions are given to replace lost serum protein, which helps maintain the volume of blood.
- The vital signs are taken frequently to ensure the safety of the client.

See the Medication Administration box above for further information about colloid solutions and associated nursing responsibilities and client teaching.

BLOOD AND BLOOD PRODUCTS If hypovolemic shock is due to hemorrhage, the infusion of blood and blood products may be indicated. The goal of blood administration is to keep the hematocrit at 30% to 35% and the hemoglobin level between 12.5 and 14.5 g/100 mL. Available blood and blood products include fresh whole blood, stored whole blood, packed RBCs, platelet concentrate, fresh-frozen plasma, and cryoprecipitate. Often, packed RBCs are given to provide hemoglobin concentration and are supplemented with crystalloids to maintain an adequate circulatory volume. (See discussion of blood administration earlier in the chapter.)

NURSING CARE

Nursing assessments and interventions to prevent shock are an essential part of the nursing care of every client. The primary nursing interventions to prevent shock are assessment and monitoring.

Health Promotion and Assessment

Nursing assessments are critical in preventing shock. Identifying clients at risk and making focused assessments are essential. Although shock may occur at any age, physiologic changes with aging make the older adult a high-risk population. (See the Nursing Care of the Older Adult box on page 280.)

- *Hypovolemic shock:* Clients who have undergone surgery, have sustained multiple traumatic injuries, or have been seriously burned are most likely to develop hypovolemic shock. Monitoring fluid status is essential in preventing shock and includes daily assessments of weight, fluid intake by all routes, measurable fluid loss (e.g., urine, vomitus, wound drainage, gastric drainage, and chest tube drainage), and fluid loss that must be estimated, such as fluid lost via profuse perspiration and wound drainage. Assessments for the critically ill client are ongoing and include fluid balance, hemodynamic values, and vital signs.
- *Cardiogenic shock:* Clients with left anterior wall myocardial infarctions are at risk for developing cardiogenic shock. Nursing care to prevent the development of cardiogenic shock focuses on maintaining or improving myocardial oxygen supply by providing immediate pain relief, maintaining rest, and administering supplemental oxygen.
- *Neurogenic shock:* The risk of neurogenic shock is increased in clients who have spinal cord injuries and those who have received spinal anesthesia. Preventive nursing care includes maintaining immobility of clients with spinal cord trauma and elevating the head of the bed 15 to 20 degrees following spinal anesthesia. Elevations of more than 20 degrees, however, can potentiate headaches following spinal anesthesia and should be avoided.
- *Anaphylactic shock:* Prevent anaphylactic shock by collecting information about allergies and drug reactions during the

---

NURSING CARE OF THE OLDER ADULT **Variations In Assessment Findings—Shock**

- Cardiac changes may include a thickened left ventricular wall, decreased elasticity of the myocardium, and more rigid valves. These changes result in a decreased stroke volume and cardiac output, thus decreasing responses to shock in general and increasing the risk of cardiogenic shock.
- Decreased arterial wall elasticity and vasomotor tone reduce the older adult's ability to respond to a decrease in oxygenation.

- Decreased elasticity and turgor of the skin make assessments of skin turgor more difficult.
- Previous medication and blood administration increase the risk of anaphylactic shock.
- Decreased immune system response increases the risk of septic shock.

---

health history. Note these allergies clearly on all documents and place a special armband on the client. Careful and frequent assessments during blood administration may prevent serious reactions to blood or blood products.

- *Septic shock:* Clients who are hospitalized, are debilitated, are chronically ill, or have undergone invasive procedures or tube insertions are at high risk for septic shock. Nursing care to prevent septic shock includes careful and consistent hand washing, the use of aseptic techniques for procedures (e.g., catheterizations, suctioning, changing dressings, starting and maintaining intravenous fluids or medications), and monitoring for local and systemic manifestations (e.g., WBC and differential counts) of infection.

Nursing Diagnoses and Interventions

Nursing care for the client in shock focuses on assessing and monitoring overall tissue perfusion and on meeting psychosocial needs of the client and the family. This section discusses nursing diagnoses that are appropriate for the client with hypovolemic shock. See accompanying Nursing Care Plan on the following page.

Decreased Cardiac Output

Decreased cardiac output is the primary problem for the client in shock. Although much of the care related to this diagnosis is collaborative, many independent nursing interventions are critical to the care of the client in shock.

NURSING RESEARCH **Evidence-Based Practice for Care of ICU Clients Sustaining Multiple Trauma**

Ventilator-associated pneumonia (VAP) is an important client safety issue in critically injured clients. The purpose of this study (Dodek, 2005) was to develop an evidence-based guideline for prevention of ventilator-assisted pneumonia.

Data extraction consisted of gathering physical, positional, and pharmacologic interventions that may influence the development of VAP. The authors searched for pertinent randomized trials and case reviews that involved clients on mechanical ventilation. The study was isolated to include only adults, and only studies published before April 1, 2003, were considered.

Physical strategies included:
- Route of endotracheal intubations
- Systematic search for maxillary sinusitis
- Frequency of ventilator circuit changes
- Airway humidification
- Endotracheal suctioning system
- Sublette secretion drainage
- Chest physiology
- Timing of tracheotomy.
  Positional strategies included:
- Kinetic bed therapy
- Semirecumbent positioning
- Prone positioning.
  Pharmacologic strategies included:
- Stress ulcer prophylaxis
- Prophylactic antibiotics, including selective decontamination of the digestive track.

IMPLICATIONS FOR NURSING
The following section identifies pertinent findings to support the conclusion that effectively implemented guidelines may decrease the morbidity, mortality, and costs of VAP in mechanically ventilated clients.

Based on direct evidence the following recommendations are encouraged:
- Orotracheal intubation is the route of choice when intubation is necessary.
- Recommend that new circuits for each client be instituted and changed if the circuits become soiled.
- Weekly changes of heat and moisture exchangers on equipment providing mechanical ventilation.
- Recommend the use of closed endotracheal suction systems that are changed for each new client and as clinically indicated.
- Recommend that clinicians consider the use of subglottic secretion drainage.
- Recommend that clinicians consider the use of kinetic beds.
- Recommend the use of semirecumbent positioning, with a goal of 45 degrees, in clients without contraindications.
  The pharmacologic strategies that were studied were unfounded and not recommended for the VAP guideline.

CRITICAL THINKING IN CLIENT CARE
1. Considering the information from this study, how would you communicate the recommendations to the medical staff for the client with mechanical ventilation?
2. What is the rationale behind the above recommendations?

NURSING CARE PLAN A Client with Septic Shock

Huang Mei Lan is a 43-year-old unmarried female who lives alone in a major West Coast city. Ms. Huang came to America 15 years ago from China and now speaks English well. Her family still lives in China. She worked in a neighborhood sewing shop until 3 years ago, when she was diagnosed with breast cancer. Her treatment included mastectomy of the affected breast and follow-up chemotherapy.

Last month, Ms. Huang experienced a recurrence of cancer in the lymph glands of the affected side. Surgery to remove the glands was performed and chemotherapy started. Ms. Huang has a central line, a urinary catheter, and a surgical incision. She is underweight, weak, and depressed. Although she has multiple physical problems, she never complains or asks for any kind of medication.

ASSESSMENT

Ms. Huang's primary nurse, Robert O'Brien, enters her room early in the morning to make an initial assessment. He finds Ms. Huang huddled in the middle of the bed, shivering violently. Her vital signs are T 104°F, P 110, R 30, and BP 106/66. Her skin is hot, dry, and flushed with poor turgor. She is alert and oriented, but is restless and appears anxious. Ms. Huang states she is nauseated and suddenly begins vomiting and is incontinent of liquid stool. Laboratory data indicate leukocytosis, respiratory alkalosis, and reduced platelet count. Blood cultures, as well as cultures of Ms. Huang's sputum, urine, and wound drainage, are conducted. She is diagnosed as having septic shock.

Hetastarch is ordered per intravenous line, and intravenous broad-spectrum antibiotics are begun until the organism and its portal of entry can be determined. Despite treatment, Ms. Huang's condition worsens. Her blood pressure continues to drop, her skin becomes cool and cyanotic, and she begins to have periods of disorientation. She is transferred to the critical care unit. As she is being prepared for the transfer, she begins to cry and asks, "Am I going to die?"

DIAGNOSES

- *Deficient Fluid Volume* related to vomiting, diarrhea, high fever, and shift of intravascular volume to interstitial spaces
- *Ineffective Breathing Pattern* related to rapid respirations and progression of septic shock
- *Ineffective Tissue Perfusion* related to progression of septic shock with decreased cardiac output, hypotension, and massive vasodilatation

- *Anxiety* related to feelings that illness is worsening and is potentially life threatening, and the transfer to the critical care unit

EXPECTED OUTCOMES

- Maintain adequate circulating blood volume.
- Regain and maintain blood gas parameters within normal limits.
- Regain and maintain stable hemodynamic levels.
- Verbalize increased ability to cope with stressors.

PLANNING AND IMPLEMENTATION

- Monitor neurologic status, including mental status and level of consciousness.
- Monitor cardiovascular status, including arterial blood pressure; rate, rhythm, and quality of pulses; central venous pressure; pulmonary artery pressure; and cardiac output.
- Monitor color and character of skin.
- Monitor results of ABGS, blood counts, clotting times, and platelet counts.
- Monitor respiratory status, including respiratory rate, rhythm, and breath sounds.
- Monitor body temperature every 2 hours.
- Monitor urinary output hourly, reporting any output of <30 mL/h.
- Explain procedures and provide comfort measures (oral care, skin care, turning, positioning).

EVALUATION

Despite intensive nursing and medical care, Ms. Huang's condition remains critical. The interventions are continued.

CRITICAL THINKING IN THE NURSING PROCESS

1. Vasopressors may be used in the treatment of septic shock. Explain the rationale for their use.
2. While monitoring Ms. Huang's ABGS, the nurse notes that her PaO_2 is <60 mmHg and her $PaCO_2$ is >50. What do these findings indicate, and why have they occurred?
3. Ms. Huang has been given large amounts of colloids intravenously. Hemodynamic monitoring indicates a higher than normal CVP and pulmonary artery pressure. What do these findings indicate? What physical assessments would you make to confirm the changes?

See Evaluating Your Response in Appendix C.

- Assess and monitor cardiovascular function via the following:
  - Blood pressure
  - Heart rate and rhythm
  - Pulse oximetry
  - Peripheral pulses
  - Hemodynamic monitoring of arterial pressures, pulmonary artery pressures, and central venous pressures (CVPs).

  A baseline assessment is necessary to establish the stage of shock. If palpable peripheral pulses and audible (to auscultation) blood pressure are lost, inserting central arterial, venous, and pulmonary artery catheters is essential to establish progression of shock accurately and to evaluate the client's response to therapy.

- Measure and record intake and output (total output and urinary output) hourly. *A decrease in circulating blood volume with hypotension and the effect of the compensatory mechanisms associated with shock can cause renal failure. Urinary output of <30 mL/h in an acutely ill adult indicates reduced renal blood flow.*
- Monitor bowel sounds, abdominal distention, and abdominal pain. *Decreased splanchnic blood flow reduces bowel motility and peristalsis; paralytic ileus may result.*
- Monitor for sudden sharp chest pain, dyspnea, cyanosis, anxiety, and restlessness. *Hemoconcentration and increased platelet aggregation may result in pulmonary emboli.*
- Maintain bed rest and provide (to the extent possible) a calm, quiet environment. Place in a supine position with the legs

elevated to about 20 degrees, trunk flat, and head and shoulders elevated higher than the chest (about 10 degrees) (Figure 11–9 ■). *Limiting activity and ensuring rest decreases the workload of the heart. The supine position with legs elevated increases venous return; however, this position should not be used for clients in cardiogenic shock. The Trendelenburg position is no longer recommended, because it causes the abdominal organs to press against the diaphragm (limiting respirations), decreases filling of the coronary arteries, and initiates aortic and carotid sinus reflexes.*

Ineffective Tissue Perfusion

As shock progresses, diminished tissue perfusion causes ischemia and hypoxia of major organ systems. As shock worsens, blood flow and oxygenation of the lungs, heart, and brain are also impaired. Hypoxia and ischemia result from decreased tissue perfusion in the kidneys, brain, heart, lungs, gastrointestinal tract, and the periphery.

■ Monitor skin color, temperature, turgor, and moisture. *Decreased tissue perfusion is evidenced by the skin becoming pale, cool, and moist; as hemoglobin concentrations decrease, cyanosis occurs.*
■ Monitor cardiopulmonary function by assessing/monitoring the following:
  ■ Blood pressure (by auscultation or by hemodynamic monitoring)
  ■ Rate and depth of respirations
  ■ Lung sounds
  ■ Pulse oximetry
  ■ Peripheral pulses (brachial, radial, dorsalis pedis, and posterior tibial); include presence, equality, rate, rhythm, and quality (If unable to palpate pulses, use a device such as a Doppler ultrasound flowmeter to assess peripheral arterial blood flow.)
  ■ Jugular vein distention
  ■ CVP measurements.
  Baseline vital signs are necessary to determine trends in subsequent findings. As shock progresses, the blood pressure decreases, and the pulse becomes rapid, weak, and thready. As perfusion of the lungs decreases, crackles, wheezes, and dyspnea are commonly assessed. Capillary refill is prolonged, and peripheral pulses are weak or nonpalpable. Neck veins that cannot be seen when the client is in the supine position indicate decreased intravascular volume. CVP is an accurate means of determining fluid status in the client in shock;

the findings will be low (5 to 15 cm of water is normal) in hypovolemic shock because of the decreased blood volume. (See Chapter 10 ∞ for a discussion of CVP.)

■ Monitor body temperature. *An elevated body temperature increases metabolic demands, depleting reserves of bodily energy. It also increases myocardial oxygen demand and may place the client with previous cardiac problems at even greater risk for hypoperfusion.*
■ Monitor urinary output per Foley catheter hourly, using a urometer. *Urine output is a reliable indicator of renal perfusion.*
■ Assess mental status and level of consciousness. *The appropriateness of the client's behavior and responses reflects the adequacy of cerebral circulation. Restlessness and anxiety are common early in shock; in later stages, the client may become lethargic and progress to a comatose state. Altered levels of consciousness are the result of both cerebral hypoxia and the effects of acidosis on brain cells.*

Anxiety

Many clients in hypovolemic shock have experienced some form of major trauma and may have life-threatening, multiple injuries. Following on-the-scene treatment, the client is usually admitted to the healthcare setting through the emergency department. Surgery may be required to treat injuries, followed by care in a critical care unit. Throughout this sequence of crisis events, treatment is invasive, and contact with family is minimal. Client and family responses to these situations of uncertainty, instability, and change include anxiety, fear, and powerlessness. These responses are affected by age, developmental level, cultural and ethnic group, experience with illness and the healthcare system, and support systems.

■ Assess the cause(s) of the anxiety, and manipulate the environment to provide periods of rest. *Reducing stimuli that cause anxiety is calming and facilitates rest, which is necessary in the client at risk for bleeding.*
■ Administer prescribed pain medications on a regular basis. *Pain precipitates and/or aggravates anxiety.*
■ Provide interventions to increase comfort and reduce restlessness:
  ■ Maintain a clean environment.
  ■ Provide skin and oral care.
  ■ Monitor the effectiveness of ventilation or oxygen therapy.
  ■ Eliminate all nonessential activities.
  ■ Remain with the client during procedures.
  ■ Speak slowly and calmly, using short sentences.
  ■ Use touch to provide support.
  Unfamiliar sounds, sights, and odors can increase anxiety. Damp skin or a dry mouth increases discomfort. Inadequate gas exchange with a decrease in oxygen or an increase in carbon dioxide in the blood may cause the client to experience a "feeling of doom." Activity increases the body's need for oxygen. Listening and touch provide support in an environment in which the client often feels alone and abandoned. Severe anxiety interferes with the ability to understand others and to respond appropriately.
■ Provide support for the client and family:
  ■ Provide time, space, and privacy for family members.

Figure 11–9 ■ The client in shock should be positioned with the lower extremities elevated approximately 20 degrees (knees straight), trunk horizontal, and the head elevated about 10 degrees.

- Allow family members access to the client when feasible.
- Encourage the expression of feelings and concerns. Provide anticipatory guidance to prepare for recovery or death and to support realistic hope.
- Acknowledge the beliefs, values, and expectations of the client and family.

Allowing the family access to the client reduces anxiety and gives both the client and the family some feeling of control. If prognosis is poor, access and involvement allow the family to begin the grieving process. If recovery is expected, contact provides the client and family with a feeling of hope. Supporting the client and family facilitates concrete problem solving, promotes acceptance of the illness and its implications, and helps them begin to establish ways of managing the illness experience.

- Provide information about the current setting to both the client and family; give the family information about available resources (such as pastoral care, social services, temporary housing, meals). *Knowing what to expect and how to control the environment to meet basic needs reduces anxiety.*

Using NANDA, NIC, and NOC

Chart 11–2 shows links between NANDA nursing diagnoses, NIC, and NOC when caring for the client who is experiencing shock.

Community-Based Care

Home care for the client who has experienced shock is highly individualized, depending on the cause and the illness or injury that caused shock. Therefore, topics for consideration are not included in this section.

NANDA, NIC, AND NOC LINKAGES
CHART 11–2 The Client in Shock

NANDA

Ineffective Tissue Perfusion: Cerebral

NIC

Acid-Base Monitoring

Cerebral Perfusion Monitoring

Fluid/Electrolyte Management

Hypovolemia Management

Shock Management

NOC

Tissue Perfusion: Cerebral

Circulation Status

Vital Signs

Neurologic Status

Data from *NANDA's Nursing Diagnoses: Definitions & Classification 2005–2006* by NANDA International (2005), Philadelphia; *Nursing Interventions Classification (NIC)* (4th ed.) by J. M. Dochterman & G. M. Bulechek (2004), St. Louis, MO: Mosby; and *Nursing Outcomes Classification (NOC)* (3rd ed.) by S. Moorhead, M. Johnson, and M. Maas (2004), St. Louis, MO: Mosby.

EXPLORE MEDIALINK

Prentice Hall Nursing MediaLink DVD-ROM
Audio Glossary
NCLEX-RN® Review

Animation/Video
Administering Blood
Hypovolemic Shock
Trauma Injuries

COMPANION WEBSITE www.prenhall.com/lemone
Audio Glossary
NCLEX-RN® Review
Care Plan Activity: Clients Experiencing Trauma and Shock
Case Studies
A Client Experiencing Trauma
Identifying Types of Shock
MediaLink Applications
Injury Prevention
Organ Donation
Shock
Links to Resources

CHAPTER HIGHLIGHTS

- Traumatic injuries affect human tissues and organs resulting from a transfer of energy from the environment. Energy sources can be mechanical, gravitational, thermal, electrical, physical, or chemical.
- Trauma can be categorized as minor trauma, which causes minimal damage to underlying tissues, or major trauma, which can involve a serious single system injury or multiple trauma. Trauma is further categorized into blunt and penetrating trauma. Blunt trauma is caused by various forces such as deceleration, acceleration, shearing, compression, or crushing. Penetrating trauma occurs when a foreign object enters the body.
- Airway assessment is the highest priority in the trauma patient and supersedes all other interventions.
- During the primary survey the nurse identifies all life-threatening injuries and performs appropriate interventions. In the secondary survey, the nurse identifies all injuries in order to prioritize care.
- Shock is a clinical condition in which there is an imbalance between oxygen supply and demand. This imbalance results in inadequate blood flow to organs and tissues causing life-threatening cellular dysfunction.
- An early sign of shock is a change in the level of consciousness with restlessness being a common symptom of cerebral hypoxia.
- There are three stages of shock: compensatory (stage I) which is an early and reversible stage; progressive (stage II) which is

- when fluid loss is 35–50% and affected cells switch from aerobic to anerobic metabolism in order to remain alive; and the final stage is irreversible (stage III) in which tissue anoxia and cellular death become so widespread that no treatment can reverse the damage.
- Hypovolemic shock is the most common type of shock and is caused by a decrease in the circulating blood volume by 15% or greater. Treatment consists of stopping the bleeding, getting oxygen to the cellular level, and restoring blood volume. This is accomplished by providing high-flow oxygen to the patient, surgical intervention, and transfusion of blood products.
- Cardiogenic shock is caused when the pumping ability of the heart is compromised to the point that the heart cannot maintain adequate cardiac output and tissue perfusion.
- Septic shock is a part of a progressive syndrome called systemic inflammatory response syndrome (SIRS), a condition most often caused by gram–negative infections.
- Anaphylactic shock results in vasodilatation, pooling of blood in the periphery and hypovolemia which leads to altered cellular metabolism. This condition is the result of a fulminating hypersensitivity reaction to a foreign substance.

TEST YOURSELF NCLEX-RN® REVIEW

1 What is the most common mechanical source of injury in adults of all ages?
1. gunshot wounds
2. fire
3. drowning
4. motor vehicles

2 Severe facial injuries, such as those resulting from going through a windshield, increase the risk for all of the following. Which would you assess first?
1. airway obstruction
2. hemorrhage
3. contusions
4. fractures

3 Which on-the-scene intervention would be a priority?
1. Determine cause of injury.
2. Assess airway patency.
3. Assess peripheral capillary refill.
4. Palpate for internal hemorrhage.

4 You are monitoring blood administration to a trauma victim in shock. Which of the following assessments indicate a dangerous transfusion reaction?
1. red raised areas (wheals) on the skin that itch
2. an increase in body temperature by 3°
3. decreasing blood pressure and dyspnea
4. increasing blood pressure and pulse

5 What type of shock causes widespread vasodilatation and decreased peripheral resistance?
1. cardiogenic shock
2. septic shock
3. hypovolemic shock
4. obstructive shock

6 What is the best method to manage uncontrolled bleeding?
1. apply direct pressure
2. clamp a visible vessel
3. apply a tourniquet
4. elevate the injured part

7 Trauma is defined as:
1. injury to human tissues from the transfer of energy.
2. result of random chance.
3. accidental injury.
4. an intentional injury.

8 Which of the following is not a risk from a blood transfusion?
1. AIDS
2. West Nile Virus
3. transfusion reaction
4. weight gain

9 Distributive shock is caused by:
1. blood loss.
2. widespread vasodilatation.
3. ineffective cardiac pumping action.
4. hypersensitivity reaction.

10 Shock is defined as:
1. a systemic imbalance between oxygen supply and demand.
2. sufficient cardiac output.
3. hemorrhage.
4. abnormal blood pressure.

See Test Yourself answers in Appendix C.

BIBLIOGRAPHY

Adewale, A. (2004). Evaluation and management of blunt and penetrating thoracic trauma. *Trauma Reports, 5*(2). Atlanta, GA: Thomson/American Health Consultants.

American College of Emergency Physicians. (2003). *Fact sheet: Domestic violence*. Dallas, TX: Author.

American Red Cross Northern Ohio Blood Services Region. (2005). *What's your blood type?* Cleveland, OH: Author.

Aminzadeh, F., & Edwards, N. (2003). Exploring senior's views on the use of assistive devices in fall prevention. *Public Health Nursing, 15*(4), 297–304.

Andrew, L. B. (2004). *Depression & suicide*. Retrieved May 17, 2005, from http://www.emedicine.com/emer/topic129.htm

Baker, W. E., & Wassermann, J. (2004). Unsuspected vascular trauma: Blunt arterial injuries. *Emergency Medicine Clinics of North America, 22*(4), 1081–1098.

Bickley, L. S., & Szilagy, P. G. (2004). *Bates' guide to physical examination and history taking* (8th ed.). Philadelphia: Lippincott Williams & Wilkins.

Chang, E. (2006). *Pathophysiology applied to nursing* (1st ed.). St. Louis, MO: Mosby-Yearbook.

Christian, C. (2003). Recognition of child abuse in the pediatric patient. *Trauma Reports, 1*(3). Atlanta, GA: Thomson/American Health Consultants.

Cohen, S. (2003). *Trauma nursing secrets*. Philadelphia: Hanley & Belfus. *Common reactions to trauma*. Retrieved May 17, 2005, from http://www.ncptsd.va.gov/facts/disasters/fs_foa_handout.html

Corpron, C. (2004, January/February). Delayed or missed diagnoses: Avoiding these pitfalls in the trauma patient. *Trauma Reports, 5*(1). Atlanta, GA: Thomson/American Health Consultants.

Crain, E. F., & Gershel, J. C. (2003). *Clinical manual of emergency pediatrics* (4th ed.). New York: McGraw-Hill.

Dodek, P. (2005). Improving patient safety in critical care: Big challenge, exciting opportunity. *Canadian Journal of Anesthesia, 52*(5), 459–462.

Emergency Nurses Association. (2003). *CATN II. A conceptual approach to injury and illness* (2nd ed.). Dubuque, IA: Kendall/Hunt.

_____. (2004). *Emergency nursing pediatric course* (3rd ed.). Des Plaines, IL: Author.

_____. (2006). *Emergency nurse core course* (5th ed.). Des Plaines, IL: Author.

EMSC Grant Panel. (2004). Clinical policy: Evidence-based approach to pharmacological agents used in pediatric sedation and analgesia in the emergency department. *Journal of Emergency Nursing, 30*(5), 447–461.

Gestring, M., Johnson, J., & Stafford, P. (2001). Current concepts in the diagnosis and early management of abdominal trauma. *Trauma Reports, 2*(2). Atlanta, GA: Thomson/American Health Consultants.

Han, Y. Y., Carcillo, J. A., Dragotta, M. A., Bills, D. M., Watson, R. S., Westerman, M. E., et al. (2003). Early reversal of pediatric-neonatal shock by community physicians is associated with improved outcomes. *Pediatrics, 221*(4), 79–89.

Hemorrhagic shock. Retrieved May 17, 2005, from http://www.emedicine.com/emerg/topic531.htm

Hohenhaus, S. M. (2004). An informal discussion of emergency nurses clinical practice: What's new and what works. *Journal of Emergency Nursing, 30*(5), 475–477.

Huether, S. (2004). *Understanding pathophysiology* (3rd ed.). St. Louis, MO: Mosby-Yearbook.

Introduction to the FAST exam. Retrieved May 17, 2005 from http://www.cpr.orgtw/ettc/fast_exam.htm

Kaide, C., & Hollingsworth, J. (2003, March/April). Current strategies for airway management in the trauma patient. *Trauma Reports, 4*(2). Atlanta, GA: Thomson/American Health Consultants.

Karch, A. (2004). *Nursing drug guide*. Philadelphia: Lippincott Williams & Wilkins.

Kelley, D. (2004). *Transfusion medicine update: Update on plasma and cryoprecipitate transfusion*. Retrieved from http://www.itxm.org/tmu2004-1.htm

Kovacs, G. L., Law, J. A., Ross, J., Tallon, J., MacQuarrie, K., Petrie, D., et al. (2004). Acute airway management in the emergency department by non-anesthesiologists. *Canadian Journal of Anesthesia, 51*(2), 174–180.

Lovett, P. (2004). *Types of shock*. Retrieved May 17, 2005, from http://cc.manscache.com/cache.aspx?g+2798586333573&lang+en-us&mkt=en-us&for

Malineni, K. C., & McCullough, P. A. (2004). *Sudden cardiac death*. Retrieved March 7, 2005, from http://www.emedicine.com/med/topic276.htm

Mandavia, D. P., & Joseph, A. (2004). Bedside echocardiography in chest trauma. *Emergency Medicine Clinics of North America, 22*(3), 601–619.

McKenna, B. G., Smith, N. A., Poole, S. J., & Coverdale, J. H. (2003). Horizontal violence; Experiences of registered nurses in their first year of practice. *Journal of Advanced Nursing, 42*(1), 90–96.

Mokhlesi, B., & Corbridge, T. (2003). Toxicology in the critically ill patient. *Clinics in Chest Medicine, 24*(4), 689–711.

National Highway Traffic Safety Administration. (2004). *National standardized child passenger safety training program curriculum*. Washington, DC: Author.

_____. (2004). Retrived October 2, 2006 from http://www.nhtsa.gov

National Institute of General Medical Sciences (NIGMS), National Institutes of Health. (2006). Fact sheet: Trauma, shock, burn and injury: Fact and Figures. Retrieved October 2, 2006, from http://publications.nigms.nih.gov/factsheets/trauma_burn_facts.html

National Institute on Alcohol Abuse and Alcoholism. (2003). *Underage drinking: A major public health challenge*. Retrieved May 16, 2005, from http://www.niaa.nih.gov/publications/aa59.htm

National Institute on Drug Abuse. (2004). *InfoFacts: High school and youth trends*. Retrieved May 16, 2005, from http://drugabuse.gov/Infofax/HSYouthtrends.html

Newgard, C. D., Lewis, R. J., & Kraus, J. F. (2005). Steering wheel deformity and serious thoracic or abdominal injury among drivers and passengers involved in motor vehicle crashes. *Annals of Emergency Medicine, 45*(1), 43–50.

Porth, C. (2005). *Pathophysiology: Concepts of altered health states* (7th ed.). Philadelphia: Lippincott.

Reid, C. L., Perrey, C., Pravica, V., et al. (2003). Genetic variation in pro-inflammatory and anti-inflammatory cytokine production in multiple organ dysfunction syndrome. *Critical Care Medicine, 30*, 2216.

Rossoll, L. W. (2004). Invasive hemodynamic monitoring. In J. A. Proehl (Ed.), *Emergency nursing procedures* (3rd ed., pp. 413–431). Philadelphia: Saunders.

Rozycki, G. S. (2004). What's new in trauma and critical care. *Journal of American College of Surgeons, 198*(5), 798–805.

Sawyer, M. A., & Sawyer, E. M. (2004). *Blunt chest trauma*. Retrieved May 17, 2005, from http://www.emedicine.com/med/topic3658.htm

Schultz, J. M., & Trunkey, D. D. (2004). Blunt cardiac injury. *Critical Care Clinics, 20*(1), 57–70.

Sibai, B. (2004). Diagnosis, controversies, and management of the syndrome of hemolysis, elevated liver enzymes, and low platelet count. *Obstetrics and Gynecology, 103*(5), 981–991.

Sole, M. L., Byers, J. F., Ludy, J. E., Zhang, Y., Banta, C. M., & Brummel, K. (2003). A multisite survey of suctioning techniques and airway management practices. *American Journal of Critical Care, 12*(3), 220–230.

Sole, M. L., Lamborn, M. L., & Hartshorn, J. C. (Eds.). (2001). *Introduction to critical care nursing* (3rd ed.). Philadelphia: Saunders.

Teague, H., Swencki, S., & Tang, D. (2005, March/April). The burned patient: assessment, diagnosis, and management in the ED. *Trauma Reports, 6*(2). Atlanta, GA: Thomson/American Health Consultants.

Verklan, M. T., & Walden, M. (2004). *Core curriculum for neonatal intensive care nursing* (3rd ed.). St. Louis, MO: Elsevier Saunders.

Vinas, F. C., & Philitis, J. (2004). *Penetrating head trauma*. Retrieved May 17, 2005, from http://www.emedicine.com/med/topic2888.htm

Voils, C. M., Kim, K. S., & Wittbrodt, E. T. (2004). Recent trends in the management of ventilator-associated pneumonia. *Journal of Pharmacy Practice, 18*(1), 53–62.

Walls, R. M. (Ed.). (2004). *Manual of emergency airway management*. Philadelphia: Lippincott Williams & Wilkins.

Wanek, S., & Mayberry, J. C. (2004). Blunt thoracic trauma: Flail chest, pulmonary contusion, and blast injury. *Critical Care Clinics, 20*(1), 71–81.

Wilson, B., Shannon, M., & Stang, C. (2005). *Nursing drug guide 2001*. Upper Saddle River, NJ: Prentice Hall.

CHAPTER 12 Nursing Care of Clients with Infections

LEARNING OUTCOMES

- Discuss the components and functions of the immune system and the immune response.

- Compare antibody-mediated and cell-mediated immune responses.

- Describe the pathophysiology of wound healing, inflammation, and infection.

- Identify factors responsible for nosocomial infections.

- Use the nursing process as a framework to provide individualized care to clients with inflammation and infection.

CLINICAL COMPETENCIES

- Apply universal precautions, particularly hand washing, to prevent the spread of infection within the client, to other clients in the facility, and to members of the interdisciplinary team and visitors.

- Assess for signs and symptoms of inflammation or infection.

- Determine priority nursing diagnosis, based on assessment data, to select and implement individualized nursing interventions for clients with infections.

- Integrate interdisciplinary care into care of clients with infection.

- Promote therapeutic levels of anti-inflammatory and anti-infective medication through prompt administration and client and family teaching.

- Be alert for hypersensitivities to anti-infectives prior to administering and during administration.

- Provide teaching for clients with inflammation or an infection and their families.

- Revise plan of care as needed to provide effective care to promote, maintain, or restore functional health patterns to clients with infections.

MEDIALINK

Resources for this chapter can be found on the Prentice Hall Nursing MediaLink DVD-ROM accompanying this textbook, and on the Companion Website at http://www.prenhall.com/lemone

The human body is continually threatened by foreign substances, infectious agents, and abnormal cells. The immune system is the body's major defense mechanism against infectious organisms and abnormal or damaged cells. Recent years have seen the emergence of resistant microorganisms such as methicillin-resistant *Staphylococcus aureus* and altered strains of familiar diseases, such as multiple-drug-resistant tuberculosis. New diseases have also emerged, such as Lyme disease, *Clostridium difficile,* and human immunodeficiency virus (HIV).

A thorough knowledge of the immune system increases understanding of the local and systemic inflammatory response, resistance to infectious disease, and the importance of immunization. This foundation can help the nurse teach clients and families to follow recommended treatment regimens, to promote and maintain health, and to prevent disease. In addition, the nurse can prescribe appropriate rehabilitative measures, such as increased rest and attention to optimal nutrition.

OVERVIEW OF THE IMMUNE SYSTEM

The immune system is a complex and intricate network of specialized cells, tissues, and organs. Cells of the immune system seek out and destroy damaged cells and foreign tissue, yet recognize and preserve host cells (Porth, 2005). The immune system performs the following functions:

- Defends and protects the body from infection by bacteria, viruses, fungi, and parasites.
- Removes and destroys damaged or dead cells.
- Identifies and destroys malignant cells, thereby preventing their further development into tumors.

The immune system is activated by minor injuries, such as small lacerations or bruises, or by major injuries, such as burns, surgeries, and systemic diseases (e.g., pneumonia). The response of the immune system may be nonspecific or specific. Nonspecific responses prevent or limit the entry of invaders into the body, thereby limiting the extent of tissue damage and reducing the workload of the immune system. Inflammation is a nonspecific response activated by both minor and major injuries. When the inflammatory process is unable to destroy invading organisms or toxins, a more specific response, called the immune response, is activated.

Immune System Components

The immune system consists of molecules, cells, and organs that produce the immune response (Table 12–1). These components may be involved in the nonspecific inflammatory response, the specific immunologic response, or both.

Leukocytes

Leukocytes, or white blood cells (WBCs), are the primary cells involved in both nonspecific and specific immune system responses. Like all blood cells, leukocytes derive from stem cells, the hemocytoblasts, in the bone marrow (Figure 12–1 ■). Unlike red blood cells (RBCs), which are confined to the circulation, leukocytes use the circulation to transport themselves to the site of an inflammatory or immune response. As the mobile units of the immune system, leukocytes detect, attack, and destroy anything that is recognized as "foreign." They are able to move through tissue spaces, locating damaged tissue and infection by responding to chemicals released by other leukocytes and damaged tissue.

The normal number of circulating leukocytes is 4,500 to 10,000 cells per cubic millimeter (mm^3) of blood. Many more leukocytes are marginated; that is, they adhere to vascular epithelial cells along the vessel walls, in other tissue spaces, or in the lymph system. In the presence of an attack such as an infection, additional WBCs are released from the bone marrow, leading to **leukocytosis,** a WBC count of greater than $10,000/mm^3$. As WBCs move out of the bone marrow into the blood, the bone marrow increases its production of additional leukocytes. A decrease in the number of circulating leukocytes, known as **leukopenia,** occurs when bone marrow activity is suppressed or when leukocyte destruction increases.

Leukocytes are divided into three major groups: granulocytes, monocytes, and lymphocytes. The granulocytes and monocytes derive from the myeloid stem cells of the bone marrow and are instrumental in the inflammatory response. Lymphocytes derive from the lymphoid stem cells of the bone marrow and are the primary cells involved in the specific immune response. In laboratory tests, the WBC count indicates the total number of circulating leukocytes. The WBC differential identifies the portion of the total represented by each type of leukocyte.

TABLE 12–1 Cells and Tissues of the Immune System

COMPONENT	LOCATION	FUNCTION
Leukocytes		
Granulocytes		
Neutrophils	Circulation	Phagocytosis and chemotaxis
Eosinophils	Circulation, respiratory tract, and gastro-intestinal tract	Phagocytosis
		Protection against parasites
		Involved in allergic response
Basophils	Circulation	Release of chemotactic substances
Monocytes and macrophages	Circulation (monocytes) and body tissue, such as skin (histocytes), liver (Kupffer cells), alveoli, spleen, tonsils, lymph nodes, bone marrow, brain	Trapping and phagocytizing of foreign substances and cellular debris
		Secretion of interleukin-1 to stimulate lymphocyte growth
Lymphocytes		
T cells (mature in thymus gland)	Circulation, lymph system, tissues	Activation of T and B cells
		Control of viral infections and destruction of cancer cells
		Involved in hypersensitivity reactions and graft tissue rejection
B cells (mature in bone marrow)	Circulation, spleen	Production of antibodies (immunoglobulins) to specific antigens
NK (natural killer) cells	Circulation	Cytotoxic; killing of tumor cells, fungi, viral-infected cells, and foreign tissue
Lymphoid Tissues		
Primary or central lymphoid structures	Bone marrow and thymus gland	Production of immune cells; sites for cell maturation
Secondary or peripheral lymphoid structures	Lymph nodes, spleen, tonsils, intestinal lymphoid tissue, lymphoid tissue in other organs	Sites for activation of immune cells by antigens

GRANULOCYTES Granulocytes constitute 60% to 80% of the total number of normal blood leukocytes. Their cytoplasm has a granular appearance, and their nuclei are distinctively multi-lobular (see Figure 12–1). Granulocytes have a short life span, measured in hours to days, compared to the life span of mono-cytes, which is measured in months to years. Granulocytes play a key role in protecting the body from harmful microorganisms during acute inflammation and infection. There are three types of granulocytes: neutrophils, eosinophils, and basophils.

Neutrophils, also called polymorphonuclear leukocytes (PMNs or polys), are the most plentiful of the granulocytes, constituting 55% to 70% of the total number of circulating leukocytes. Neutrophils are *phagocytic* cells, responsible for engulfing and destroying foreign agents, particularly bacteria and small particles. Neutrophils are the first phagocytic cells to arrive at the site of invasion, drawn by chemicals released by damaged tissue and invading organisms.

Neutrophils are produced in the bone marrow and released into the circulation when they mature. Segmented neutrophils (or segs) are mature forms, and usually account for about 55% of total leukocytes. *Bands* are immature neutrophils and usually comprise 5% of leukocytes. As neutrophils mature, their nucleus changes from round to kidney bean shaped (banded) and then the nucleus separates into small, attached segments, thus the designations "banded" versus "segmented" neutrophils. It takes about 10 days for a neutrophil to mature and be released into the circulation. Once released, neutrophils have a circulating half-life of 6 to 10 hours. They cannot replicate and must be replaced constantly to maintain adequate numbers in the circulation. They do not return to the bone marrow.

Eosinophils account for 1% to 4% of the total number of circulating leukocytes. They mature in the bone marrow in 3 to 6 days before being released into the circulation. Eosinophils have a circulating half-life of 30 minutes and a tissue half-life of 12 days. They too are phagocytic cells, but are less efficient at this process than neutrophils. Eosinophils are found in large numbers in the respiratory and gastrointestinal tracts, where they are thought to be responsible for protecting the body from parasitic worms, including tapeworms, flukes, pinworms, and hookworms. Eosinophils surround the parasite and release toxic enzymes from their cytoplasmic granules. The parasite, although too large to be phagocytized, is destroyed. Eosinophils are also involved in a hypersensitivity response, inactivating some of the inflammatory chemicals released during the inflammatory response.

Basophils constitute about 0.5% to 1% of the circulating leukocytes. These cells are not phagocytic. Granules within basophils contain proteins and chemicals such as heparin, histamine, bradykinin, serotonin, and a slow-reacting substance of anaphylaxis (leukotrienes). These substances are released into the bloodstream during an acute hypersensitivity reaction or stress response.

MONOCYTES, MACROPHAGES, AND DENDRITIC CELLS These cells are the mediators of immunity. They recognize foreign matter (from molecules to cells) and initiate immune responses. *Monocytes* are the largest of the leukocytes and constitute 2% to 3% of circulating leukocytes. After their release from the bone marrow,

Figure 12–1 ■ The development and differentiation of leukocytes from hemocytoblasts.

monocytes circulate in the serum for 1 to 2 days. They then migrate to various tissues throughout the body, attaching themselves to the tissues, where they remain for months or even years until they are activated. Monocytes mature into **macrophages** after settling into the tissues. Once they have migrated and matured, macrophages are differentiated by the tissues in which they reside. *Histiocytes* are tissue macrophages in loose connective tissue, *Kupffer cells* are found in the liver, *alveolar macrophages* in the lungs, and *microglia* in the brain. Tissue macrophages are also found in the spleen, tonsils, lymph nodes, and bone marrow. Dendritic cells are star-shaped cells that originate in both the myeloid and the lymphoid cell lines. Langerhans cells are specialized dendritic cells in the skin. Monocytes, macrophages, and dendritic cells are antigen-presenting cells (APCs), which activate immune responses in both B and T lymphocytes.

Monocytes, macrophages, and dendritic cells are actively phagocytic, with the capacity to phagocytize large foreign particles and cell debris. Once they are in the tissue, macrophages can multiply to encapsulate and trap foreign matter that cannot be phagocytized. Dendritic cells have long processes that can capture antigens and migrate to lymphoid tissue. They serve as sentinels for antigens in most organs including heart, lungs, liver, kidney, and gastrointestinal tract (Goldsby et al., 2003). Like neutrophils, macrophages are drawn to an inflamed area by chemicals released from damaged tissue, a process known

as chemotaxis. Monocytes and macrophages activate the immune response against chronic infections such as tuberculosis, viral infections, and certain intracellular parasitic infections; dendritic cells activate T cells against cancer, assist B lymphocytes to produce antibodies, and downregulate the immune system (DeMeyer & Buchsel, 2005).

LYMPHOCYTES Small and nondescript cells, the **lymphocytes** account for 20% to 40% of circulating leukocytes. Lymphocytes are the principal effector and regulator cells of specific immune responses to protect the body from microorganisms, foreign tissue, and cell mutations or alterations. Through a process known as immune surveillance, lymphocytes monitor the body for cancerous cells and eliminate or destroy them.

Like other leukocytes, lymphocytes derive from the stem cells in the bone marrow (Figure 12–2 ■). Lymphocytes have "homing" patterns: They constantly circulate, then return to concentrate in lymphoid tissues (the lymph nodes, spleen, thymus, tonsils, Peyer's patches in the submucosa of the distal ileum, and the appendix). On contact with an antigen, B lymphocytes are activated and mature into either plasma cells, which secrete antibodies, or memory cells. On contact with APCs, T lymphocytes mature into active T_{helper} cells, cytotoxic T cells, or memory T cells. Memory cells stay inactive, sometimes for years, but activate immediately with subsequent

Figure 12–2 ■ The development and differentiation of lymphocytes from the lymphoid stem cell (lymphoblasts).

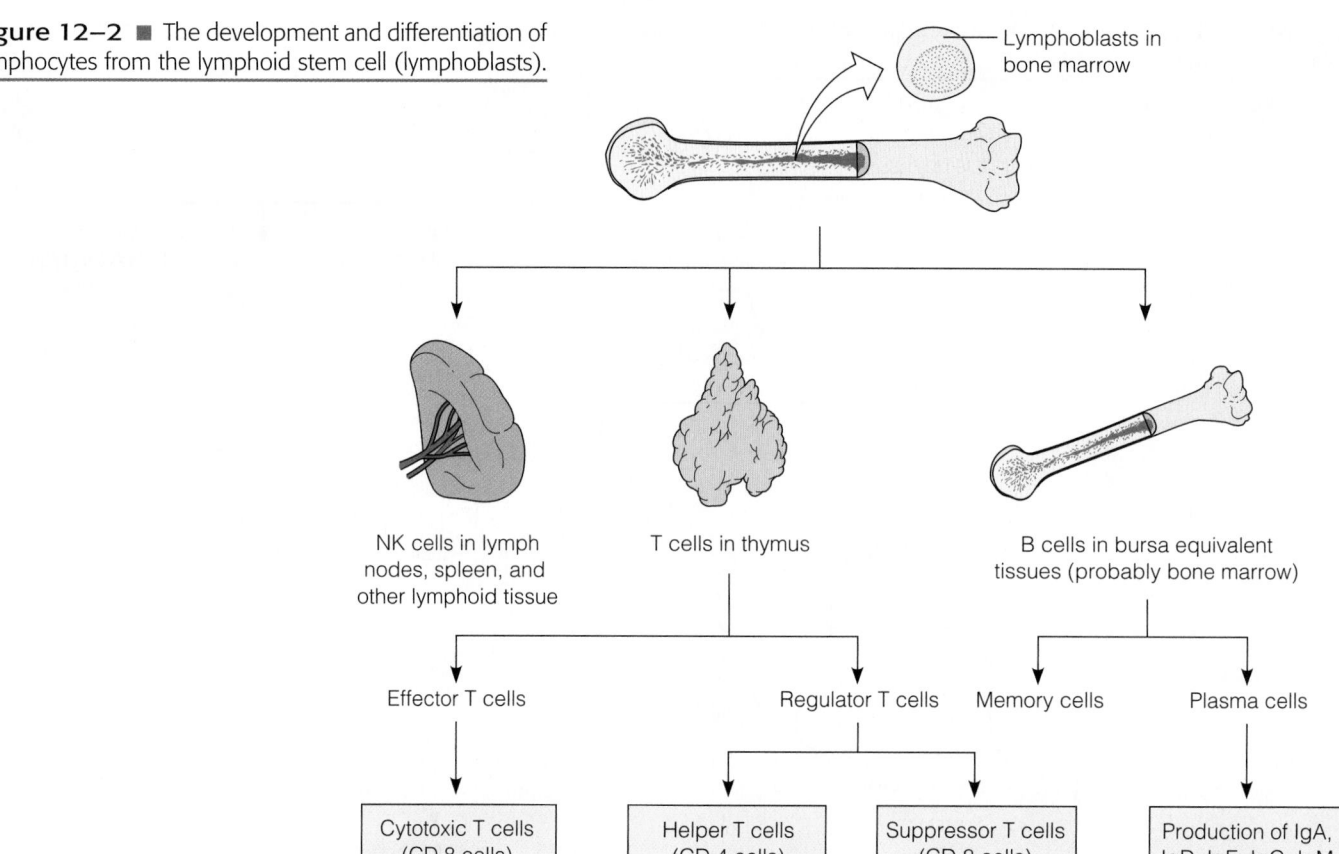

exposure to the same antigen. They then proliferate rapidly, producing an intense immune response. Memory cells are responsible for providing acquired immunity.

Lymphocyte types are difficult to distinguish by appearance. They have distinct differences in how and where they mature, and in life cycle, surface characteristics, and function.

The three types of lymphocytes are **T lymphocytes (T cells)**, **B lymphocytes (B cells)**, and **natural killer cells (NK cells** or **null cells)**. None of these cells acts independently. Their functions are closely interrelated.

T cells mature in the thymus gland, whereas B cells complete their maturation in the bone marrow. T cells and B cells are integral to the specific immune response and are discussed further in that section of this chapter.

NK cells are large, granular cells found in the spleen, lymph nodes, bone marrow, and blood. They constitute 15% of circulating lymphocytes. NK cells provide immune surveillance and resistance to infection, and they play an important role in the destruction of early malignant cells. Like B cells and T cells, NK cells are cytotoxic, but unlike T cells do not require connection with an APC to become activated and kill cancer cells, virus-infected cells, and cells infected with microbes (Porth, 2005). Fortunately, NK cells are inhibited when contact is made with normal host cells.

ANTIGENS Substances that are recognized as foreign or "nonself" are called **antigens**; they provoke a specific immune response when introduced into the body. Typically, antigens are large protein molecules, although polysaccharides, polypeptides, and nucleic acids may also be antigenic. Many antigens are proteins found on the cell membrane or cell wall of microorganisms or tissues such as transplanted tissue or organs, incompatible blood cells, vaccines, pollen, egg white, and insect or snake venom.

Complete antigens, known as immunogens, have two characteristics:

■ *Immunogenicity* is the ability to stimulate a specific immune response.
■ *Specific reactivity* is the stimulation of specific immune system components.

The portion of an antigen that incites a specific immune response is called its antigenic determinant site (*epitope*). Complete antigens typically are large molecules with multiple antigenic sites; examples include proteins and certain polysaccharides. Small molecules (e.g., chemical toxins, drugs, and dust) that cannot evoke an antigenic response alone may link to proteins to function as complete antigens. These proteins to which they link are known as haptens.

When an antigen is encountered in the body, generation of an effective immune response involves two major groups of cells: lymphocytes and APCs. Dendritic cells are APCs; two specific types of dendritic cells develop from pluripotent stem cells in the bone marrow. DC1s arise from monocytes, myeloid-type immune cells, and DC2s derive from lymphocyte precursors (DeMeyer & Buchsel, 2005). DC1s activate T cells against cancer cells. DC2s assist B lymphocytes to produce antibodies and to downregulate the immune system (Kimball, 2005). Downregulation is very important to avoid autoimmune diseases.

Antigen-presenting cells are recognized by a specific receptor on a lymphocyte, and an immune response is generated by the lymphocytes. Two separate but overlapping immune responses may occur, depending on the antigen itself and the type of immune cell activated by contact with the antigen. The B cell or humoral branch of the immune system mainly eliminates extracellular antigens such as bacteria, bacterial toxins, and free viruses through the production of **antibodies**, molecules that bind with the antigen and inactivate it. There are five classes of antibodies: IgG, IgA, IgM, IgD, and IgE. These proteins make up the **antibody-mediated (humoral) immune response**. Intracellular pathogens, such as viral-infected cells, cancer cells, and foreign tissue, activate T lymphocytes, which are the primary agents of the **cell-mediated (cellular) immune response**. In this immune response, the lymphocytes themselves, in the form of helper T cells, cytotoxic T cells, and NK cells, inactivate the antigen, either directly or indirectly.

Lymphoid System

The *lymphoid system* consists of the lymph nodes, spleen, thymus, tonsils, lymphoid tissue scattered in connective tissues and mucosa, and the bone marrow. The thymus and bone marrow, in which T cells and B cells mature, are considered central lymphoid organs. The spleen, lymph nodes, tonsils, and other peripheral lymphoid tissue are peripheral lymphoid organs (Figure 12–3 ■). This system exists to recover proteins such as albumin for the vascular system and to protect the bloodstream from invading organisms. Cells of the immune system such as neutrophils, macrophages, and dendritic cells carry antigens from interstitial space to lymph nodes for immune surveillance in the lymphatic circulation. Unlike the vascular tree, which has tight epithelial junctions, lymphatic epithelium is replete with open junctions that promote lymphocyte access and effectively protect the bloodstream from antigen entry.

Lymph nodes, the most numerous elements of the lymphoid system, are small, round, or bean-shaped encapsulated bodies that vary in size from 1 mm to 2 cm. Distributed throughout the body, lymph nodes generally occur in groups at the junction of the lymphatic vessels. They can be found in the neck, axillae, abdomen, and groin.

Lymph nodes have two functions: (1) to filter foreign products or antigens from the lymph and (2) to house and support proliferation of lymphocytes and macrophages. Lymph, a clear, protein-containing fluid transported within lymph vessels, enters the node through afferent lymphatic vessels. Inside the node, the lymph flows through sinuses in the cortex of the lymph node where T and B lymphocytes and macrophages are abundant, then through sinuses of the medulla of the lymph node, which contains macrophages and plasma cells. The presence of a foreign antigen stimulates lymphocytes and macrophages to proliferate in the lymph nodes. Macrophages destroy the antigen by phagocytosis. Immune cells and lymph then leave the lymph node through efferent vessels. An abundant blood supply to the node also facilitates lymphocyte movement.

The *spleen* is the largest lymphoid organ in the body and the only lymphoid organ that can filter blood. The spleen is located in the upper left quadrant of the abdomen. The spleen has two kinds of tissue, white pulp and red pulp. White pulp is lymphoid tissue that serves as a site for lymphocyte proliferation and immune surveillance. B cells predominate in the white pulp. Blood filtration occurs in the red pulp. In blood-filled venous sinuses, phagocytic cells dispose of damaged or aged RBCs and platelets. Other debris and foreign matter, such as bacteria, viruses, and toxins, are also removed from the blood. The spleen also stores blood and the breakdown products of RBCs for future use. The spleen is not essential for life. If it is removed because of disease or trauma, the liver and the bone marrow assume its functions.

The *thymus gland* is located in the superior anterior mediastinal cavity beneath the sternum. It reaches its maximum size at puberty, then begins to atrophy slowly. By adulthood, it is difficult to differentiate from surrounding adipose tissue even though it remains active. In the elderly, the vast majority of thymus tissue has been replaced by adipose and fibrous connective tissue. During fetal life and childhood, the thymus serves as a site for the maturation and differentiation of thymic lymphoid cells, the T cells. Thymosin, an immunoregulatory hormone of the thymus, stimulates lymphopoiesis, the formation of lymphocytes or lymphoid tissue.

Bone marrow is soft organic tissue found in the hollow cavity of the long bones, particularly the femur and humerus, as well as the flat bones of the pelvis, ribs, and sternum. Bone marrow produces and stores hematopoietic stem cells, from which all cellular components of the blood are derived (see Figure 12–1).

Lymphoid tissues are also located at key sites of potential invasion by microorganisms: the submucosa of the genitourinary, respiratory, and gastrointestinal tracts and the skin. Plasma cells in these lymphoid tissues defend the body against bacterial

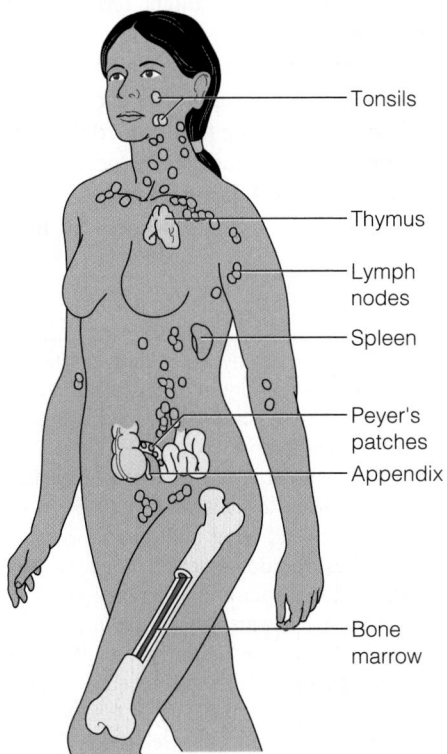

Tonsils

Thymus

Lymph nodes

Spleen

Peyer's patches

Appendix

Bone marrow

Figure 12–3 ■ The lymphoid system: the central organs of the thymus and bone marrow, and the peripheral organs, including the spleen, tonsils, lymph nodes, and Peyer's patches.

invasion at areas exposed to the external environment. In general, these tissues are known as *mucosa-associated lymphoid tissue* (MALT). Diffuse collections of lymphocytes, plasma cells, and phagocytes are scattered throughout the respiratory tract, concentrating at bifurcations of the bronchi and bronchioles. Peyer's patches, or gut-associated lymphoid tissue (GALT), comprises the largest collection of immune cells in the body (Bourlioux et al., 2003). Ingestion and absorption of solid foodstuffs and liquids continually expose the lining of the gut to resident microflora and infectious pathogens. Unlike peripheral lymph nodes, which respond to pathogens with acute inflammatory responses, GALT processes common intestinal antigens without producing acute inflammation. Collections of immune cells make up the GALT. Intraepithelial lymphocytes fill the spaces between mucosal epithelial cells. Beneath the basement membrane of gut epithelium lie abundant T cells and mature plasma cells, which are sources of IgA. Peyer's patches hold dense collections of lymphocytes in lymphoid nodules. As naïve B and T cells migrate through Peyer's patches, they are sensitized to specific antigens. In mesenteric lymph nodes these sensitized cells proliferate and circulate throughout the vascular tree where they produce secretory IgA. Secretory IgA coats mucosal cells and prevents attachment of intraluminal bacteria in the intestine, upper respiratory tract, the bronchi, mammary ducts, and salivary glands. Thus the GALT collection of immune cells effectively protects mucosa throughout the body that is exposed to resident and foreign pathogens.

Tonsils and adenoids protect the body from inhaled or ingested foreign agents. Skin-associated lymphoid tissue contains lymphocytes and dendritic cells such as Langerhans cells in the epidermis, which transport antigens to regional lymph nodes for destruction and development of specific immunity to the antigen.

Nonspecific Inflammatory Response

Barrier protection is the body's first line of defense against infection. The skin is the primary barrier. When intact, it prevents invasion by external organisms. When the skin is damaged or lost (e.g., as a result of injury, surgery, or burns), infection is much more likely. The membranes lining inner surfaces of the body are protected by a barrier of mucus, which traps microorganisms and other foreign substances. These can then be removed by other protective mechanisms, such as ciliary movement or the washing action of tears or urine. In addition, many body fluids contain bactericidal substances that provide barrier protection. These include acid in gastric fluid, zinc in prostatic fluid, and lysozyme in tears, nasal secretions, saliva, and sweat (Porth, 2005; Rink & Gabriel, 2000).

When these first-line defenses are breached, resulting tissue damage or foreign material entering the body induces a nonspecific immune response known as inflammation. **Inflammation** is an adaptive response to injury that brings fluid, dissolved substances, and blood cells into the interstitial tissues where the invasion or damage has occurred. The response is called *nonspecific* because the same events occur regardless of cause of the inflammatory process. Through the inflammatory reaction, the invader is neutralized and eliminated, destroyed tissue removed, and the process of healing and repair initiated.

The inflammatory response has three stages: (1) a vascular response characterized by vasodilation and increased permeability of blood vessels, (2) a cellular response and phagocytosis, and (3) healing (tissue repair).

Vascular Response

After tissue cells are damaged, local blood vessels briefly constrict. Vasodilation follows almost immediately as inflammatory mediators such as histamine and kinins are released from damaged tissue (Box 12–1). Increased blood flow causes vasocongestion at the injury site with resultant redness and heat. The congestion also increases local hydrostatic pressure. This, along with increased vessel permeability that results from chemical mediators, moves fluid out of the capillaries and into the interstitial spaces of the tissue. The escaping fluid, called fluid exudate, contains large amounts of protein and causes local edema. Fluid exudate has three functions: (1) It provides protection to the injured tissue by bringing certain nutrients needed for tissue healing;

BOX 12–1 **Inflammatory Mediators**

Many of the manifestations of inflammation are produced by *inflammatory mediators,* which are chemicals released as a result of immunologic processes or tissue injury or damage. These inflammatory mediators are broadly classified as follows:

- Vasoactive substances produce smooth muscle constriction, postcapillary vasodilation, and increased capillary permeability.
- Chemotactic factors attract leukocytes to the damaged tissue.
- Plasma enzymes activate the clotting cascade, plasminogen system, and complement system.
- Miscellaneous cell products (e.g., oxygen metabolites and lysosomal enzymes) damage surrounding tissue.

Many of the outward manifestations of inflammation result from vasoactive substances such as *histamine, serotonin,* and *leukotrienes* (formerly known as slow-reacting substance of anaphylaxis, or SRS-A). Stored in mast cells, basophils, and platelets, histamine is released when an injury occurs or with stimulation by the immune system. An important component of the early inflammatory response, histamine causes vasodilation and vascular permeability in the affected area. His-

tamine is also a key factor in many hypersensitivity reactions. Serotonin is released from platelets and produces effects similar to those of histamine. The leukotrienes play a significant vasoactive role in the later stages of the inflammatory response.

Prostaglandins are chemotactic substances that draw leukocytes to the inflamed tissue. In addition, they play a vasoactive role and are pain and fever inducers. Aspirin and other nonsteroidal anti-inflammatory drugs (NSAIDs) as well as the glucocorticoids inhibit prostaglandin synthesis, thereby reducing fever, pain, and inflammation.

Plasma factors such as Hageman factor activate the clotting cascade, plasminogen system (involved in the lysis of clots), and complement system. With activation of the clotting cascade, bacteria and other foreign substances are trapped in the area of tissue damage. Fibrin, which has vasoactive by-products, is also released. (See Chapter 34 for a full description of the clotting process.) The complement system serves a chemotactic role and facilitates the phagocytic process.

Major chemical mediators of inflammation are summarized in Table 12–7 on page 304.

(2) it dilutes bacterial toxins; and (3) it transports cells needed for phagocytosis. Mild tissue damage such as a blister produces a *serous* exudate of primarily plasma fluid and a few proteins. With moderate to severe tissue damage, fluid exudate is *sanguineous* or *hemorrhagic,* containing large amounts of RBCs. A mixture of RBCs and serum is referred to as *serosanguineous* exudate. *Fibrinous* exudate forms a thick, sticky meshwork of fibrinogen, in effect "walling off" inflamed tissues and preventing the spread of infection (Porth, 2005). In more severe or acute inflammation, the fluid contains fibrin, RBCs, and dead and live bacteria. This type of exudate, called *purulent* exudate, has an odor and color characteristic of the bacteria present.

The vascular response localizes invading bacteria and keeps them from spreading. Increased capillary permeability enhances the release of clotting factors such as fibrinogen, which converts to fibrin threads, entrapping the bacteria and walling them off from contact with the rest of the body.

Cellular Response

The cellular stage of the inflammatory process begins within less than an hour after the injury. This stage is marked by the margination and emigration of leukocytes into the damaged tissue, chemotaxis, and phagocytosis (Porth, 2005).

As serous fluid escapes the capillaries, the viscosity of blood in the area increases and its flow becomes more sluggish. Leukocytes marginate, moving to the edges of the blood vessels, and begin to adhere to the capillary endothelium. This process is known as *pavementing*. After margination and pavementing, leukocytes emigrate from the blood vessel into the tissue spaces (Figure 12–4 ■). Within hours, millions of leukocytes emigrate into the area of inflammation (Price & Wilson, 2003).

Once leukocytes have emigrated, they are drawn to the damaged or inflamed tissues by chemotactic signals. Infectious agents, damaged tissues, and activated plasma substances such as complement fractions provide chemotaxic signals that attract an army of neutrophils, monocytes, and macrophages to the injury site.

The number of neutrophils around the site increases to about 15,000 to 25,000/mm³, and they begin their role in phagocytosis within a few hours. Monocytes become transient macrophages to augment the activity of the fixed macrophages and dendritic cells; together they engulf dead cells, damaged tissue, nonfunctioning neutrophils, and invading bacteria.

Phagocytosis

Phagocytosis is a process by which a foreign agent or target cell is engulfed, destroyed, and digested. Neutrophils, macrophages, and dendritic cells, known as *phagocytes,* are the primary cells involved in phagocytosis. Once attracted to the inflammatory site, phagocytes select and engulf foreign material.

The following factors or processes help phagocytes differentiate foreign tissue from normal cells:

- *Smooth surface.* Normal tissue has a smooth surface that is resistant to phagocytosis, whereas the rough surface of a foreign agent or target cell promotes phagocytosis.
- *Surface charge.* Healthy body cells present an electronegative surface charge that repels phagocytes. Cellular debris and foreign agents, by contrast, have an electropositive charge that attracts them.

A Leukocytes in circulation

B Margination and pavementing

C Emigration

Figure 12–4 ■ The process of leukocyte emigration at the site of inflammation. *A,* Normal blood flow with free movement of formed elements. *B,* As blood flow slows, leukocytes move toward the periphery of stream and begin to cling to capillary endothelium, a process known as margination and pavementing. *C,* Leukocytes emigrate from the vessel into inflamed tissues.

- *Opsonization.* This immune system process coats the surface of bacteria or target cells with a substance (an opsonin) as in the complement system (Box 12–2). Opsonization enables the phagocyte to bind tightly with the foreign tissue, facilitating phagocytosis (Figure 12–5A ■).

Phagocytes engulf the foreign agent or target cell by projecting pseudopodia ("false feet") in all directions around it (Figure 12–5B). This produces a chamber called a *phagosome* containing the antigen, which is ingested into the cytoplasm (Figure 12–5C). Once the phagosome has been engulfed, lysosomes fuse with the phagosome, killing any live organism and releasing digestive enzymes, which destroy the antigen (Figure 12–5D).

Phagocytes—in particular, neutrophils and macrophages—contain bactericidal agents that kill most of the bacteria they ingest before the bacteria can multiply and destroy the phagocyte itself. The phagocyte kills bacteria in a number of ways; for

BOX 12–2 The Complement System

The *complement system* consists of approximately 20 complex plasma proteins that are activated by a tissue injury or antigen–antibody reaction. The complement system is involved in both nonspecific and specific immune responses. Its activation results in the production of effector molecules that are involved in the processes of inflammation, phagocytosis, and cell lysis or destruction (Goldsby et al., 2003; Porth, 2005). Specifically, complement activation leads to the following:

■ *Mediation of the inflammatory response.* When the complement system is activated, chemical mediators such as histamine are released from mast cells and basophils, leading to smooth muscle contraction, increased vascular permeability and edema, and the attraction of leukocytes.

■ *Opsonization (or coating) of antigen–antibody complexes to facilitate phagocytosis.*

■ *Alteration of the cell membrane or viral capsule.* When the cell surface is altered, lysis results. Bacteria and viruses are destroyed; certain normal cells, such as RBCs, platelets, and lymphocytes, that are damaged or old may also be destroyed through this process.

The complement system has three "arms," or pathways, of protein and enzyme reactions. The *classic pathway* is activated by antibody-containing immunoglobulins and other substances such as DNA and C-reactive protein. The *alternate and lectin pathways* do not use antibodies, are activated by tissue injury, polysaccharides, or enzymes, and are part of the nonspecific immune system (Porth, 2005). When either pathway is activated, the result is mediation of the inflammatory process, attraction of phagocytes, facilitation of phagocytosis, and lysis of microbes.

---

example, it alters the intracellular pH and produces bactericidal agents. Oxidizing agents, such as superoxide, hydrogen peroxide, and hydroxyl ions, are bactericidal. Two lysosomal substances that kill bacteria are lysozyme and phagocytin.

Some antigens, such as the tubercle bacterium, have coats or secrete substances that are resistant to lysosomal and bactericidal agents. To destroy such antigens, lysosomes release digestive enzymes into the phagosome. The lysosomes of neutrophils and macrophages contain an abundance of proteolytic (protein-destroying) enzymes that digest bacteria and other foreign protein components. The macrophage's lysosomes also contain lipases (fat-splitting enzymes) capable of digesting the thick lipid

Figure 12–5 ■ The process of phagocytosis. *A,* Opsonization coats the surface of the bacterium with IgG (an antibody) and complement. *B,* The bacterium is bound to and engulfed by the phagocyte. *C,* The phagosome is ingested into the cytoplasm of the phagocyte. *D,* Lysosomes fuse with the phagosome, releasing digestive enzymes and destroying the antigen.

membranes of such bacteria as *Mycobacterium tuberculosis* and *Mycobacterium leprae.*

Once neutrophils have ingested toxic substances to their capacity, they in turn are killed. Neutrophils have the capacity to phagocytize 5 to 20 bacteria before they become inactive. Macrophages then digest the dead neutrophils. Monocytes or macrophages are capable of phagocytizing up to 100 bacteria. Because of their size, they can ingest larger particles than neutrophils can ingest, such as whole RBCs, necrotic tissue, cell fragments, malarial parasites, and dead neutrophils. Dendritic cells are also phagocytic and secrete Il-12, which is an important cytokine in the maturation of T$_{helper}$ cells (Kimball, 2005). Macrophages have the ability to extrude (release) the toxic substances and lysosomal enzymes within their phagosomes. As a result, they can continue to function for months and even years.

Healing

Inflammation is the first phase of the healing process. During the inflammatory process, particulate matter, bacteria, damaged cells, and inflammatory exudate are removed by phagocytosis. This process, called *debridement*, prepares the wound for healing. Adequate nutrition is essential for inflammation and healing to proceed. Protein, glucose, and oxygen are needed by leukocytes for chemotaxis, phagocytosis, and intercellular killings. Persons with diabetes are at risk for poor healing of wounds. Probable causes for this risk may be small vessel disease, which impairs microcirculation and increased affinity for oxygen common to glycosylated hemoglobin. Oxygen circulation is impaired as well as release of oxygen to the cells (McCance & Huether, 2002).

The second phase of the healing process, known as *reconstruction*, may overlap the inflammatory phase. The ideal result of the healing process is *resolution*, the restoration of the original structure and function of the damaged tissue. Simple resolution occurs when there is no destruction of the normal tissue and the body is able to neutralize and remove the offending agent through the inflammatory process.

Resolution may also occur when the damaged tissue is capable of regeneration. The ability to regenerate, or replace lost *parenchyma* (functional tissue) with new, functional cells varies by tissue and cell type.

- *Labile cells* continue to regenerate throughout life. These cells are found in tissues where there is a daily turnover of cells—namely, bone marrow and the epithelial cells of the skin, mucous membranes, cervix, gastrointestinal tract, and genitourinary tract.
- *Stable cells* normally stop replicating when growth ceases, but are capable of regeneration when stimulated by an injury. Osteocytes (which are found in bone) and parenchymal cells of the kidneys, liver, and pancreas are stable cells.
- *Permanent* or *fixed cells* are unable to regenerate. When these cells are destroyed, they are replaced by fibrous scar tissue. Nerve cells, skeletal muscle cells, and cardiac muscle cells are fixed cells (Porth, 2005). Researchers are searching for signaling molecules that will stimulate repair of permanent cells, allowing regeneration. Paralysis from spinal cord injury is often the stimulus for this research focus. When regeneration and complete resolution are not possible, healing occurs by replacement of the destroyed tissue with collagen scar tissue. This process is known as *repair*. Although tissue that has undergone repair lacks the physiologic function of the destroyed tissue, the scar fills the lesion and provides tensile tissue strength. The healing process is discussed further in Chapter 4 ∞.

Specific Immune Response

The introduction of antigens into the body causes a more specific reaction than the nonspecific inflammatory response. On the first exposure to an antigen, a change occurs in the host, resulting in a specific and rapid response following subsequent exposures. This specific response is known as the *immune response.*

The immune response to an antigen has the following distinctive properties:

- The immune response typically is directed against materials recognized as foreign (i.e., from outside the body) and is not usually directed against the self (i.e., cells or structures produced by the body). This property is known as *self-recognition*.
- The immune response is *specific*. It is initiated by and directed against particular antigens (such as a specific virus, bacterium, or transplanted tissue).

- Unlike a localized inflammatory response, the immune response is systemic. Immunity is generalized; it is not restricted to the initial site of infection or entry of foreign tissue.
- The immune response has memory. Repeated exposures to an antigen produce a more rapid response.

A client whose immune system is able to identify antigens and effectively destroy or remove them is said to be **immuno-competent**. Health problems may occur when the immune response is altered (see Chapter 13 ∞ for further discussion).

Antibody-Mediated Immune Response

The antibody-mediated (humoral) immune response is produced by B lymphocytes (B cells). B cells are constantly replaced through cell division and proliferation in the bone marrow. It is believed that B cells mature in the bone marrow and then migrate to the spleen to await activation. They normally constitute 10% to 15% of circulating lymphocytes.

B cells are activated by contact with an antigen and by T cells (discussed in the next section). Each B cell has receptor sites for a specific antigen or antigens. When the antigen is encountered, the activated B cell proliferates and differentiates into antibody-producing plasma cells and memory cells (Figure 12–6 ■). Plasma cells are short lived, lasting only about 1 day. While alive, however, they can produce thousands of antibody molecules per second. Memory cells retain antibody-producing information, allowing a rapid response if the antigen is again encountered.

An antibody is an **immunoglobulin (Ig)** molecule with the ability to bind to and inactivate a specific antigen. Immunoglobulins comprise the gamma globulin portion of the blood proteins. The immune system produces numerous antibodies, each active against a specific antigen. As mentioned earlier, antibodies fall into five classes of immunoglobulins: IgG, IgA, IgM, IgD, and IgE. Each has a slightly different structure and function. Their roles are summarized in Table 12–2.

TABLE 12–2 Immunoglobulin Characteristics and Functions

CLASS	PERCENTAGE OF TOTAL	CHARACTERISTICS AND FUNCTION
IgG	75%	Most abundant Ig; also known as gamma globulin; found in blood, lymph, and intestines Active against bacteria, bacterial toxins, and viruses Activates complement The only Ig to cross the placenta, providing immune protection to neonate
IgA	10% to 15%	Found in saliva, tears, and bronchial, gastrointestinal, prostatic, and vaginal secretions, as well as blood and lymph Provides local protection on exposed mucous membrane surfaces and potent antiviral activity by preventing binding of the virus to cells of the respiratory and gastrointestinal tracts Levels decrease during stress
IgM	5% to 10%	Found in blood and lymph First antibody produced with primary immune response High concentrations early in infection, decreases within about a week Mediates cytotoxic response and activates complement
IgD	<1%	Found in blood, lymph, and surfaces of B cells Exact function unknown; may be receptor-binding antigens to B-cell surface
IgE	<0.1%	Found on mast cells and basophils Involved in release of chemical mediators responsible for immediate hypersensitivity (allergic and anaphylactic) response

Figure 12–6 ■ Antibody-mediated (humoral) immunity. On initial exposure to the antigen, B cells with appropriate receptor sites are activated to become plasma cells and produce antibodies or memory cells. This is known as the primary response. With subsequent exposures, memory cells respond rapidly with antibody production. This is known as the secondary response.

Antibodies are Y-shaped molecules with two light and two heavy polypeptide chains (Figure 12–7 ■). The top portion of the Y, called the *Fab* or *antigen-binding fragment,* is chemically variable and specific to the antigen. The lower portion, the F_c, or *crystallized fragment,* is constant for its class of immunoglobulin and directs the biologic activity of the immunoglobulin (the manner in which it functions). For example, the lower portion of immunoglobulin molecules produced against hepatitis A and hepatitis B are the same (IgG), but the upper portion is different and specific to the virus.

The antibodies produced by B cells (see Figure 12–7) link with the antigen (Figure 12–8 ■) and inactivate it through one of the following processes:

■ Promoting phagocytosis of the antigen by neutrophils
■ Precipitation: combining with soluble antigens to form an insoluble complex or precipitate

■ Neutralization: combining with a toxin to neutralize its effects; the antigen–antibody complex is then destroyed by the process of phagocytosis
■ Lysis of the antigen cell membrane caused by combination with antibodies and complement proteins
■ Agglutination (clumping) of antigens to form a noninvasive aggregate
■ Opsonization: coating of the antigen with antibodies and complement, making them more susceptible to phagocytosis.

The complete antibody-mediated response occurs in two phases. With initial exposure to an antigen, the primary response develops. B cells are activated to proliferate and begin producing antibodies. There is a latency period of 3 to 6 days before antibodies become detectable in the blood. Levels then continue to rise, peaking at 10 to 14 days after the initial exposure. With many illnesses (e.g., chickenpox), this peak correlates with recovery.

Figure 12–7 ■ An antibody molecule. The Fab section is unique, providing an antigen-specific binding site. The F$_c$ section is common to each class of immunoglobulin (IgG, IgA, IgM, IgD, IgE).

Subsequent exposure to the same antigen elicits a secondary response. Memory cells (see Figure 12–6) formed during the primary response stimulate the production of plasma cells, and an almost immediate rise in antibody levels occurs (Figure 12–9 ■). This rapid secondary response is the basis of acquired immunity and is instrumental in preventing disease. It is also the mechanism through which vaccines provide protection from disease.

Cell-Mediated Immune Response

Many antigens cannot stimulate the antibody-mediated response or are "hidden" from it because they live inside the body's cells (viruses and mycobacteria are examples of such antigens). The immune response providing protection against these antigens is the cell-mediated immune response, also called *cellular immunity*. T lymphocytes (T cells) initiate this type of immune response.

Approximately 70% to 80% of circulating lymphocytes are T cells. T cells migrate to the thymus during fetal and early life,

Figure 12–8 ■ Antigen–antibody binding. The unique Fab site on the antibody binds with specific receptor sites on the antigen. As shown, more than one kind of antibody may be produced to an antigen.

Figure 12–9 ■ Antibody production in the primary and secondary responses of the antibody-mediated immune response. Note the more rapid and effective production following subsequent exposure.

establishing the lifetime pool of cells. T cells have a life span measured in years, maintaining their numbers through proliferation, primarily in the lymph nodes.

T cells are much more complex than B cells. There are two major classes of T cells, *effector cells* and *regulator cells*. The main effector T cell is the *cytotoxic cell*, also called the *killer T cell*. Regulator T cells are further classified into two groups: *helper T cells* and *suppressor T cells*.

T cells are antigen specific; that is, each subset is activated by a particular antigen. The antigens that activate T cells must be presented on another cell surface, such as pieces of virus presented on the surface of an infected cell, or the histocompatibility locus antigen on a cell of transplanted tissue. When activated, T cells divide and proliferate, forming antigen-specific *clones* (Figure 12–10 ■). A clone is an exact copy of another cell.

Cytotoxic T cells bind with cell surface antigens on virus-infected or foreign cells. Killer T cells destroy the identified cell by combining with it and then either destroying its cell membrane or releasing cytotoxic substances into the cell. They are vital in the control of viral and bacterial infections.

Regulator T cells play a key role in controlling the immune response. The majority of regulator T cells are helper T cells. They stimulate the proliferation of other T cells, amplify the cytotoxic activity of killer T cells, and activate B cells to proliferate and differentiate. They interact directly with B cells to promote their multiplication and conversion into plasma cells capable of producing antibodies. The other regulatory T-cell group, suppressor T cells, provides negative feedback, making the immune response a self-limiting process.

On activation, both effector and regulator T cells synthesize and release lymphokines, a type of soluble protein. Lymphokines are a subgroup of nonspecific defense mechanisms known as **cytokines** (Box 12–3). Lymphokines secreted by cytotoxic and helper T cells are important in amplifying the immune response and the nonspecific inflammatory response. They stimulate the following:

■ B cells to become plasma cells and produce antibodies
■ Macrophages to become activated macrophages (the most aggressive phagocyte)
■ Proliferation of killer T cells.

Figure 12–10 ■ Cellular immune response. *A,* An infected cell, abnormal cell, or phagocyte presents antigen on its surface that binds with a receptor site on a killer T cell or a helper T cell. The killer T cell is activated to proliferate into memory cells or mature cytotoxic cells. *B,* The helper T cell is activated to augment the cytotoxic response and stimulate the antibody-mediated immune response.

Suppressor T cells release lymphokines, which inhibit the activity of other T cells and B cells.

Although T cells can be activated only by specific antigens, much of the resulting effect is nonspecific—in other words, an enhanced inflammatory response. Like the antibody-mediated response, the cell-mediated response has memory. Subsequent exposures to an antigen result in a more rapid and effective inflammatory response and more effective phagocytosis by macrophages. This memory provides the basis for skin testing. A client previously exposed to tuberculosis, for example, develops a more pronounced inflammatory response when minute amounts are injected under the skin.

The Client with Natural or Acquired Immunity

Immunity refers to the protection of the body from disease. Immunity to disease may be either natural or acquired, active or passive.

Immunity develops from the activation of the body's immune response. Depending on the antigen, antibody-mediated or cell-mediated responses are activated. The immune response typically involves components of both. In the immunocompetent client, these responses inactivate and remove the antigen, allowing recovery to occur or preventing the development of disease. Clients with suppressed or impaired immune function

are more susceptible to disease and require protection from exposure to environmental elements. Isolation techniques are employed to prevent the spread of disease and to protect immune-suppressed clients.

Pathophysiology

The processes of antibody-mediated and cell-mediated immunity result in the development of **acquired immunity** or **active immunity**. Active immunity occurs when the body produces antibodies or develops immune lymphocytes against specific antigens. Memory cells, which can produce an immediate immune response on reexposure to the antigen, provide long-term immunity.

Active immunity can be naturally acquired, resulting from contact with the disease-producing antigen and subsequent development of the disease. Naturally acquired immunity is common for diseases such as chickenpox and hepatitis A, making the risk of developing the disease a second time very low.

For many diseases, the potential consequences of a single disease episode on the individual and society make prevention desirable, especially for highly contagious diseases capable of causing epidemics. In these instances, immunization or vaccination is used to provide artificially acquired immunity. The purpose of vaccination is to establish adequate levels of antibody and/or memory cells to provide effective immunity (Goldsby et al., 2003). Vaccination introduces the

BOX 12–3 **Cytokines**

Cytokines are hormone-like polypeptides produced primarily by cells of the immune system. Cytokines are also produced in small quantities in many different tissues throughout the body. Cytokines act as messengers of the immune system, facilitating communication between the cells to adjust or vary the inflammatory reaction or to initiate immune cell proliferation and differentiation. Cytokines are an essential component of an adequate immune response. The major cytokines and their functions are summarized in Table 12–3.

Interferons are a class of cytokine with broad antiviral and anticancer effects. A number of different forms of interferon exist, broadly grouped as alpha, beta, and gamma interferons. Interferon is synthesized by cells infected with a virus and secreted into extracellular fluid. It then binds to specific receptors on uninfected neighboring cells, protecting them from infection. The spread of the virus is thus inhibited, and recovery from infection enhanced. It appears that interferons also moderate the activity of NK cells and may be involved in preventing the spread of abnormal malignant cells.

---

disease-producing antigen into the body in a manner that will stimulate the immune system to form antibodies and memory cells but will not produce disease. Vaccines may be made of killed organisms or of live organisms that have been attenuated or modified to reduce their disease-producing capability. Typhoid is an example of a killed organism vaccine; measles-mumps-rubella (MMR) vaccine, by contrast, is made from attenuated organisms. Many newer vaccines use subunits of the antigen; these are portions of the organism that have antigenic properties but are unable to produce disease.

Passive immunity provides temporary protection against disease-producing antigens. Passive immunity is provided by antibodies produced by other people or animals. These acquired antibodies are used up; they either combine with the antigen or are naturally degraded by the body, and their protection is grad-

ually lost. Naturally acquired passive immunity is provided by the transfer of maternal antibodies via the placenta and breast milk to the infant. Rabies human immune globulin and hepatitis B immune globulin (HBIG) are examples of immunizations used to provide artificially acquired passive immunity. The types of active and passive immunity are summarized in Table 12–4.

INTERDISCIPLINARY CARE

Collaborative care focuses primarily on assessing the client's immune status and ensuring acquired immunity to prevent disease.

Diagnosis

A number of diagnostic tests can be performed to assess the client's immune status.

TABLE 12–3 **Major Cytokines and Their Functions**

CYTOKINE	WHERE PRODUCED	PRIMARY FUNCTIONS
Interleukin-1 (IL-1)	Monocytes and macrophages; other cells	Activates T and B cells Induces fever and tissue catabolism Enhances NK activity Attracts neutrophils, macrophages, and lymphocytes Stimulates endothelial cell growth, collagen, and collagenases
Interleukin-2 (IL-2)	Helper T cells	Stimulates T and B cell proliferation Activates killer T and NK cells
Interleukin-3 (IL-3)	T cells	Stimulates growth and differentiation of bone marrow stem cells
Interleukin-4 (IL-4)	Activated helper T cells	Stimulates proliferation of T and B cells Increases IgE secretion by B cells
Interleukin-5 (IL-5)	T cells and activated mast cells	Promotes differentiation of B cells and eosinophils Stimulates production of IgA
Gamma interferon	T and NK cells	Stimulates phagocytosis by neutrophils and macrocytes Activates NK cells Augments B cell proliferation, enhancing both cellular and humoral immune responses
Alpha and beta interferons	Virus-infected cells; macrophages	Activate macrophages and endothelial cells Augment NK cell activity Act at gene level to protect neighboring cells from invasion by intracellular parasites, such as viruses, rickettsia, malaria
Tumor necrosis factor (TNF)	Activated macrophages, T cells, and NK cells	Major chemical mediator of inflammatory response Stimulates T-cell activation, antibody production, and accumulation of leukocytes at inflammatory site Directly cytotoxic to some tumor cells Induces fever

TABLE 12–4 Types of Acquired Immunity

TYPE OF IMMUNITY		HOW DEVELOPED	EXAMPLES
Active Immunity	Natural	Acquired by infection with an antigen, resulting in the production of antibodies	Chickenpox, hepatitis A
	Artificial	Acquired by immunization with an antigen, such as attenuated live virus vaccine	MMR, polio, DPT, hepatitis B vaccines
Passive Immunity	Natural	Acquired by transfer of maternal antibodies to the fetus or neonate via the placenta or breast milk	Neonate initially protected against MMR if mother immune
	Artificial	Acquired by administration of antibodies or antitoxins in immune globulin	Gamma globulin injection following hepatitis A exposure

■ *Serum protein* measures the total protein in the blood including albumin and globulins. Normal levels for the adult are 6 to 8 g/dL; albumin is approximately 60% (3.2 to 4.5 g/dL) of the total serum protein, and globulins are normally 2.3 to 3.4 g/dL. Total protein levels, albumin, and globulin are decreased in malnutrition and liver disease. Decreased globulin levels are noted with immunologic deficiencies.

■ *Protein electrophoresis* analyzes protein content especially for albumin and gamma globulin and is used to assess immune function. Gamma globulins subjected to further electrophoresis separate into immunoglobulins: IgA, IgD, IgE, IgG, and IgM (see Table 12–2). Analysis of specific levels of each provides clues about the immune status of the client. IgG levels are increased during acute infection. Decreased levels of IgG, IgA, and IgM are found in malignancies.

■ *Antibody testing* is ordered to determine if a client has developed antibodies in response to an infection or immunization. Antibodies for hepatitis, HIV, rubella, toxoplasmosis, and *Treponema pallidum* (the organism causing syphilis) can be identified. An elevated titer level for hepatitis and rubella indicates immunity. For the other disorders and hepatitis, it may also be used to determine if the client has the disease.

■ *Skin testing* can assess cell-mediated immunity. A known antigen such as streptokinase, tuberculin purified protein derivative, or candida is injected intradermally. The site is then observed for induration and erythema, which typically peaks at 24 to 48 hours. An induration of at least 10 mm in diameter is a positive reaction indicating previous exposure and sensitization to the antigen. (See Chapter 13 ∞ for further information on skin testing for hypersensitivity reactions.) No reaction, or **anergy**, indicates depressed cell-mediated immunity.

Immunizations

Vaccines are suspensions of whole or fractionated bacteria or viruses that have been treated to make them nonpathogenic. Vaccines are given to induce an immune response and subsequent immunity. Although vaccine development has been a major factor in improving public health, no vaccine is completely effective or entirely safe. Table 12–5 outlines the vaccines recommended for the adult client to maintain optimal health and immune status.

Adults born before 1956 are generally considered to be immune to measles, mumps, and rubella by prior infection. For persons born after 1956 whose immunologic status is unclear or who are at significant risk of exposure to these diseases (e.g., persons entering healthcare careers), reimmunization is recommended (Centers for Disease Control and Prevention [CDC], 2002c).

Tetanus and diphtheria toxoids are combined in a single immunization. The pediatric form of the vaccine is known as DT; the adult form is Td. The vaccine stimulates active immunity by inducing the production of antibodies and antitoxins. After an initial series of three immunizations, an intramuscular (IM) booster injection of 0.5 mL is recommended every 10 years to maintain protection. Older clients, particularly those who never entered the workforce (e.g., older female adults), may have never received the initial series of DT vaccine.

Hepatitis B (HB) vaccine is given as a series of three immunizations to promote active immunity to hepatitis B. This vaccine is recommended for everyone at high risk for exposure through blood or other body fluids. It is mandated by the Occupational Health and Safety Administration (OSHA) for all healthcare workers at risk. Other high-risk populations include intravenous drug users, sexual partners of infected individuals, clients on hemodialysis, prison guards, and athletic coaches.

Influenza vaccine is recommended for persons at high risk for serious sequelae of influenza, including older adults, persons with lung disease or other chronic illness, and immunosuppressed individuals. The antigenic strain included in influenza vaccine varies each year according to the predicted predominant strains affecting the population. Yearly reimmunization is therefore required.

Pneumococcal vaccine is generally recommended for the same populations as influenza vaccine. A single dose of this vaccine confers lifetime immunity, although repeating immunization every 6 years may be considered for high-risk clients. Pneumococcal vaccine for all senior citizens is a U.S. public health and Medicare goal. The purpose of immunization is to prevent respiratory infections and hospitalizations (CMS, 2003; Quinley & Shih, 2004; Shorr, 2005).

In addition to routine immunizations, people traveling outside the United States and Canada should receive vaccines against diseases that are endemic in certain regions of the world.

Other immunologic substances may be administered as indicated. Immune globulins provide passive immunity as protection against a known or potential exposure to an antigen. Standard immune globulin is given to household contacts of clients with hepatitis A and persons traveling to areas in which

TABLE 12–5 Recommended Immunizations for Adults

VACCINE	TYPE	DOSE	INDICATIONS	PRECAUTIONS AND NURSING IMPLICATIONS
Measles-mumps-rubella (MMR)	Live virus	0.5 mL SC	All adults born after 1956, particularly those who are at risk for infection, such as college students and military recruits. Measles and mumps vaccination particularly recommended for males without history of previous infection; rubella vaccination recommended for all seronegative females.	As a live virus vaccine, should not be administered to pregnant women or immunocompromised clients. Do not administer to clients with a history of anaphylactic reaction to egg protein or neomycin.
Tetanus and diphtheria toxoids (Td)	Inactivated toxins	0.5 mL IM	Initial series of 3 injections (2 doses, 4 to 6 weeks apart; third dose 6 to 12 months after dose 2) if never immunized; booster every 10 years; following a major or contaminated wound if more than 5 years since last booster.	Do not give in first trimester of pregnancy or to clients with a history of anaphylactic reaction to horse serum; administer deep IM in deltoid of dominant arm.
Hepatitis B (HB)	Inactive viral antigen	1.0 mL IM	Series of 3 doses: initial and at 1 and 6 months. Recommended for anyone at risk for exposure and for postexposure prophylaxis.	Use with caution in pregnant or lactating females, older clients, and clients with active infection; have epinephrine 1:1000 available on unit in case of anaphylaxis and laryngospasm.
Influenza	Inactivated virus or viral components	0.5 mL IM	Yearly for all clients over age 65 and those at risk for complications, including debilitated clients and clients with chronic disease.	Do not administer to acutely ill clients or clients with history of anaphylactic reaction to egg protein.
Pneumococcal	Bacterial polysaccharides	0.5 mL IM or SC	One dose for clients over age 65 and those at risk for pneumococcal pneumonia, including clients with chronic lung disease or other chronic diseases.	Do not administer to pregnant women.

it is endemic. HBIG contains higher titers of antibody to hepatitis B virus and is used for persons exposed by blood or sexual contact. Following confirmed or suspected contact with a pathogen, selected vaccines may be administered to stimulate an immediate immune response (Table 12–6).

For most vaccines, a sensitivity test should be performed prior to administration to detect sensitivity to substances such as horse serum or eggs. The substance is injected intradermally; if after 20 minutes there is no evidence of a reaction, the selected vaccine can be administered.

Moderate to severe local reactions may occur following administration of an immunization. Common reactions include redness, swelling, tenderness, and muscle ache. Administering the vaccine in the dominant arm of the client helps minimize local reactions, because use and movement of the arm facilitates absorption of the solution. Applying heat to the site is also beneficial. Occasionally local ulcerations occur; when they do, warm, wet pack, or sterile wet-to-dry dressings may be prescribed.

NURSING CARE

Maintaining a population that is fully immunized against common, potentially epidemic, and devastating diseases is a major public health task for nursing. Nurses not only rec-ommend and administer vaccines to individual clients and their families, but also plan and implement preventive care for whole communities.

Although this process may appear to be straightforward, multiple issues affect society's ability to immunize the entire population. For some people, for example, religious beliefs may preclude the use of immunizations to prevent disease. Also, people who are not citizens and the medically indigent population have difficulty accessing immunization services. Lack of immunization not only puts the individual at increased risk for infectious disease, but also increases the cost of medical services and the possibility of exposing immunocompromised people to disease.

Health Promotion

In the public health setting, the nurse looks at the immunization needs and illness risk for an entire community. Communities include not only cities and localities but also groups of people, such as college populations and employees in a workplace. Public education needs may be met through presentations to groups of people, feature articles in newspapers and other local publications, advertising, radio presentations and public service announcements, and one-to-one discussion and teaching.

TABLE 12–6 Preparations for Postexposure Prophylaxis

DISEASE	PREPARATION AND DOSE	INDICATIONS
Hepatitis A	Human immune globulin (IG), 0.02 mL/kg IM	Contacts in day care centers, households, custodial institutions; patrons of eating establishments known to have been exposed by infected food worker
Hepatitis B	Hepatitis B immune globulin (HBIG), 0.06 mL/kg IM	Possible percutaneous or sexual contact with blood or body fluids of an infected individual; usually given concurrently with hepatitis B vaccine
Varicella	Varicella-zoster immune globulin (VZIG), 12.5 units/kg; minimum dose 125 units, maximum 625 units	Susceptible adults exposed to varicella virus (e.g., chickenpox or shingles)
Tetanus	Tetanus immune globulin (TIG), 500 to 3000 units IM (part infiltrated around wound)	Clients with major or contaminated wounds who have no history of tetanus immunization or an unclear one that is not up to date; Td usually given as well
Rabies	Human rabies immune globulin (HRIG), 20 IU/kg, half IM, half infiltrated around wound	Persons with a significant exposure to a rabid or potentially rabid animal; followed with 5-dose course of rabies vaccine
Measles	Human immune globulin (IG), 0.25 mL/kg IM	Susceptible close contacts, especially people who are immunosuppressed; postpone immunization with measles vaccine until 3 months after IG
Rubella	Human immune globulin (IG), 0.55 mL/kg IM	Pregnant women exposed in first trimester when termination of pregnancy is not an option; does not ensure protection of fetus

Source: Table adapted from Harrison's Principles of Internal Medicine (14th ed.) by A. S. Fauci et al. (Eds.), 1998, New York: McGraw-Hill.

Assessment

Collect the following data through the health history and physical examination. Further focused assessments are described with nursing interventions in the next section.

- *Health history:* age, medication use (corticosteroids and antibiotics) and blood transfusion, nutrition, allergies, infection, immunizations, autoimmune disorders, chronic diseases such as diabetes mellitus, cancer
- *Physical assessment:* skin lesions or rashes, breath sounds, respiratory rate.

Nursing Diagnoses and Interventions

Nursing care focuses on preventing injury from the immunization and educating the client. See the accompanying Nursing Care Plan on the following page.

Health-Seeking Behaviors: Immunization

For individual clients and their families, nurses promote immunocompetence by assessing immune status, recommending appropriate immunizations, and administering vaccines as ordered or indicated. Once a person reaches adulthood, routine immunizations often become a neglected part of health care.

- Determine knowledge level, understanding, attitudes, and religious beliefs about immunization. *This provides a basis for further education and determines if religious beliefs may contraindicate immunization.*
- Discuss the value and reasons for recommended immunizations. *Understanding promotes adherence.*
- Reinforce positive health-seeking behaviors. *This will help promote future health maintenance activities.*

- Using recommended immunization schedules, develop a plan to attain optimal immunization status. *Adherence with recommended schedules for immunization is important in preventing disease and disability.*
- Do not administer MMR or influenza vaccine if allergic to eggs, or tetanus antitoxin if sensitive to horse serum. *Vaccines prepared from chicken or duck embryos are contraindicated in clients who are allergic to eggs. Tetanus antitoxin is prepared from horse serum. Both will cause a severe allergic reaction.*
- Withhold administration of active immunologic products in the presence of an upper respiratory infection or other infection. *Active immunizations can cause a greater inflammatory reaction in the presence of infections.*
- Do not administer oral polio vaccine, MMR, or any live virus vaccine to immunosuppressed clients or to clients who are in close household contact with an immunosuppressed person. *Live virus vaccines can cause disease in the immunosuppressed client. The virus may be transmitted from close household contacts during the initial postvaccination period.*
- Do not administer live attenuated virus vaccines and passive immunizations such as gamma globulin simultaneously. *Passive antibodies interfere with the response of the live attenuated virus.*
- Prior to administering prescribed vaccine, check the expiration date and manufacturer's instructions. *Outdated vaccines cannot provide adequate immunization protection. Certain injection sites have better absorption than others.*
- Keep epinephrine 1:1000 readily available for subcutaneous injection when administering immunizations. *Epinephrine causes vasoconstriction and reduces laryngospasm; in acute anaphylaxis, it can be lifesaving.*

NURSING CARE PLAN A Client with Acquired Immunity

Terry Adams is a 48-year-old executive who is planning a trip to central Africa. In preparation, he contacts his local healthcare provider to obtain the necessary immunizations. Jane Wong, the registered nurse in the clinic, obtains a nursing history of Mr. Adams.

ASSESSMENT

Mr. Adams's history reveals that he has always been very healthy and active, apart from a mild case of asthma. As an adult, he has had little problem with his asthma "except for those rare occasions on which I am dumb enough to smoke more than one cigarette!" He is divorced and is not currently in a continuing relationship. He has two grown daughters with whom his relationship is good. Since contracting hepatitis A several years ago, he drinks alcohol only rarely, and never more than one or two drinks at any one time. He confesses to little organized exercise but plays golf two or three times a week and states that he is such a hyperactive workaholic that he rarely sits for any length of time. Mr. Adams has not seen a physician since recovering from the hepatitis and is unsure when he last received any immunizations. He does not know if he had all recommended childhood immunizations, but recalls getting both Salk and Sabin polio vaccines when they became available. His physical examination reveals an alert and healthy individual with no abnormalities noted. His vital signs are as follows: T 97.4°F, P 64, R 14, and BP 142/82.

The physician orders the following immunizations for Mr. Adams:

- Measles-mumps-rubella (MMR)
- Combined tetanus and diphtheria toxoids (Td)
- Yellow fever vaccine
- Typhoid vaccine
- Meningococcal meningitis vaccine

DIAGNOSES

- *Health-Seeking Behaviors: Immunization* related to impending international travel
- *Ineffective Health Maintenance* related to apparent lapse in immunization status
- *Risk for Injury* related to adverse response to immunization

EXPECTED OUTCOMES

- Obtain necessary immunizations.
- Verbalize a schedule for maintaining up-to-date immunization status.
- Experience no significant adverse effects from immunization.

PLANNING AND IMPLEMENTATION

- Administer MMR, Td, and meningococcal meningitis vaccines prior to discharge from clinic.
- Observe closely for 30 minutes following immunization for potential adverse responses.
- Schedule return visit in 1 week for typhoid vaccine.
- Provide referral to a registered vaccination center for yellow fever vaccine and documentation of vaccination.
- Provide instructions for comfort measures to relieve local and systemic adverse effects of vaccines. Provide written instructions on manifestations that should be reported to the physician.
- Document immunizations on a permanent record at the clinic and for the client.

EVALUATION

Terry Adams completes his prescribed immunizations without major adverse effects, although he does complain of fever, malaise, and general achiness for several days following the typhoid vaccination. His trip to Africa is successful, and he returns to the United States without contracting any infectious diseases.

CRITICAL THINKING IN THE NURSING PROCESS

1. Explain why it is important for adults to continue receiving immunizations throughout their life span.
2. If a client says to you, "I don't believe in immunizations. I hear they are dangerous," how would you respond?
3. When should a client contact the primary caregiver after receiving an immunization?
   See Evaluating Your Responses in Appendix C.

PRACTICE ALERT

Observe the client for 20 to 30 minutes following inoculation to monitor for possible adverse reactions.

Community-Based Care

Educating individual clients, families, and the public about the maintenance of immune status is a significant nursing responsibility. For individual clients and their families, instructions focus on the following areas:

- Appropriate immunizations and recommended schedules for initial vaccination and boosters
- How and where to obtain immunizations
- The need to observe the client for up to 30 minutes following a vaccination for possible adverse reactions
- Possible side effects and adverse effects of the immunization administered

- Self-care measures for side effects and postvaccination discomfort
- Responses to immunization that should be reported immediately to the primary care provider
- Maintenance of a permanent immunization record
- Beneficial resources:
  - County or public health departments
  - Centers for Disease Control and Prevention National Immunization Program
  - National Institute of Allergy and Infectious Diseases

NORMAL IMMUNE RESPONSES
The Client with Tissue Inflammation

As noted, inflammation is a nonspecific response to injury that serves to destroy, dilute, or contain the injurious agent or damaged tissue. Inflammation may be either acute or chronic.

Acute inflammation is a short-term reaction of the body to all types of tissue damage. It is immediate and aimed at protecting the body and preventing further invasion or injury. Acute inflammation usually lasts less than 1 to 2 weeks. Once the injurious agent is removed, the inflammation subsides. Healing with tissue repair or scar formation occurs, and the body functions in normal or near-normal capacity.

Chronic inflammation is slower in onset and may not have an acute phase. Its clinical manifestations occur over months or years. It involves cell proliferation and is debilitating, with long-term adverse effects. There is increased cellular exudate, necrosis, fibrosis, and sometimes tissue scarring, resulting in severe tissue damage.

Pathophysiology of Tissue Inflammation

The tissue damage that evokes an inflammatory response may be caused by specific or nonspecific agents. These agents may be *exogenous,* from outside the body, or *endogenous,* from within the body. Causes of inflammation include the following:

- Mechanical injuries, such as cuts or surgical incisions
- Physical damage, such as burns
- Chemical injury from toxins or poisons
- Microorganisms, such as bacteria, viruses, or fungi
- Extremes of heat or cold
- Immunologic responses, such as hypersensitivity reactions
- Ischemic damage or trauma, such as a stroke or myocardial infarction.

Acute Inflammation

Regardless of the cause, location, or extent of the injury, the acute inflammatory response follows the previously outlined sequence of vascular response, cellular and phagocytic response, and healing.

Many of the manifestations of inflammation are produced by inflammatory mediators such as histamine and prostaglandins released when tissue is damaged (see Table 12–7 and Box 12–1 on inflammatory mediators).

The cardinal signs of inflammation include the following:

- Erythema (redness)
- Local heat caused by the increased blood flow to the injured area (hyperemia)
- Swelling due to accumulated fluid at the site
- Pain from tissue swelling and chemical irritation of nerve endings
- Loss of function caused by the swelling and pain.

The degree of functional loss depends on the location and extent of the injury. With increased tissue damage, more fluid exudate is formed, resulting in more swelling, pain, and functional impairment. Pain may be immediate or delayed. Prostaglandins intensify and prolong the pain. Kinins cause irritation to the nerve endings and contribute to the pain sensation.

Dead neutrophils, necrotic tissue, and, if the tissue is infected, digested bacteria accumulate as a result of inflammation and phagocytosis, forming *pus.* Pus usually forms and remains until after the infection subsides. Pus may push itself to the surface of the body or become internalized. In the latter case, pus is gradually autolyzed (self-digested) by enzymes over a period of days. The end product is then absorbed by the body. On occasion, pus may remain after the infection is resolved. Pockets of pus, called abscesses, may need to be artificially drained with a procedure called *incision and drainage (I&D).* Ectopic calcifications are another possible result of residual collections of pus.

Systemic responses to inflammation include an increase in the size of lymph nodes due to the proliferation of macrophages within the nodes in response to microorganisms in the lymph. Enlarged lymph nodes are usually noted in the groin, axillae, and neck (Figure 12–11 ■). Fever, often precipitated by inflammatory mediators or bacterial toxins, inhibits the growth of many microorganisms and increases tissue repair functions. Loss of appetite and fatigue may occur in the effort to conserve energy during the inflammatory process. Leukocytosis occurs with increased WBC production to support inflammation and phagocytosis.

Local and systemic manifestations of inflammation are summarized in the box below.

MANIFESTATIONS of Inflammation

Local Manifestations
- Erythema
- Warmth
- Pain
- Edema
- Functional impairment

Systemic Manifestations
- T > 100.4°F (38°C) or <96.8°F (36°C)
- P > 90/min
- R > 20/min (tachypnea)
- WBC > 12,000/mm^3 or >10% bands

TABLE 12–7 Major Chemical Mediators of Inflammation

FACTOR	SOURCE	EFFECT
Histamine	Mast cells, basophils, and platelets	Vasodilation and increased capillary permeability, producing tissue redness, warmth, and edema
Kinins (bradykinin and others)	Plasma protein factors	Histamine-like effects; chemotaxis and pain inducers
Prostaglandins	Metabolism of arachidonic acid from cell membranes	Histamine-like effects; chemotaxis, pain, and fever inducers
Leukotrienes	Arachidonic acid metabolism	Smooth muscle constriction (especially bronchoconstriction), increased vascular permeability, chemotaxis

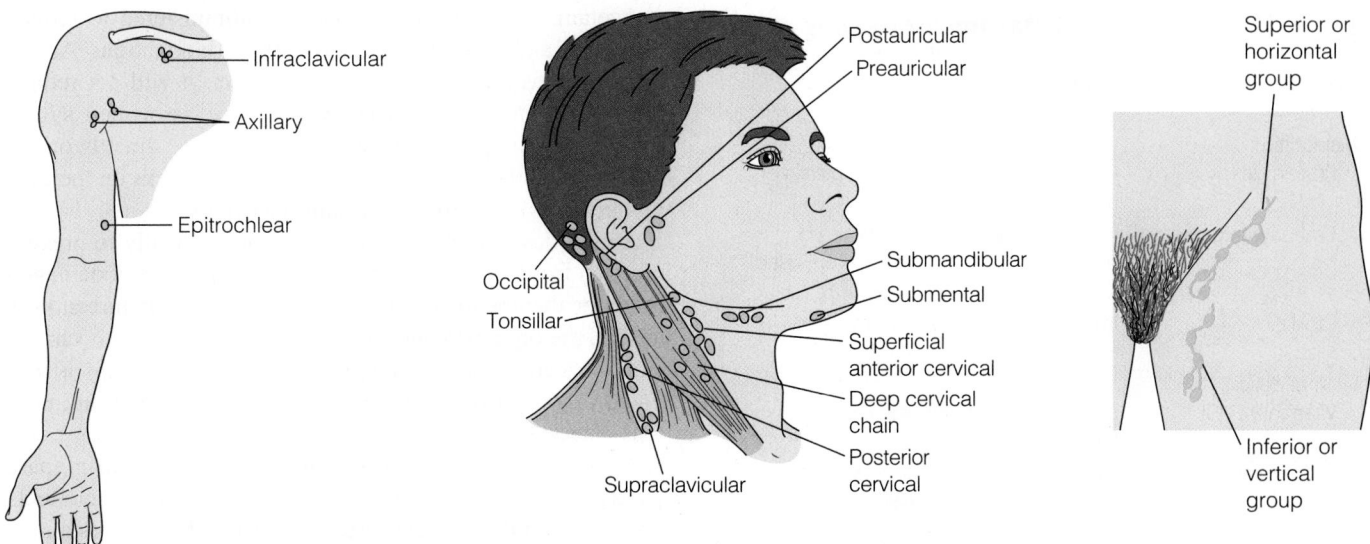

Figure 12–11 ■ Lymph nodes that may be assessed by palpation.

Chronic Inflammation

Whereas acute inflammation is a self-limiting process lasting less than 2 weeks, chronic inflammation tends to be self-perpetuating, lasting weeks to months or years. Chronic inflammation may develop when the acute inflammatory process has been ineffective in removing the offending agent. For example, mycobacteria have cell walls with high lipid and wax content, making them resistant to phagocytosis. Chronic inflammation and granuloma formation is common with *Mycobacterium tuberculosis* infection. Persistent irritation by chemicals, particulate matter, or physical irritants such as talc, asbestos, or silica may also result in chronic inflammation.

The chronic inflammatory process is characterized by a dense infiltration of the site by lymphocytes and macrophages. The macrophages mass or coalesce to form a multinucleated giant cell surrounded by lymphocytes, in a lesion called a *granuloma*. The granuloma is effective in walling off the offending agent, isolating it from the rest of the body; however, the infectious agent or offending irritant may not be destroyed and can survive within the granuloma for a long period of time. The granuloma formed in tuberculosis is called a tubercle. *M. tuberculosis* can survive for many years within the tubercle, emerging when the client's immune system is no longer able to contain it.

Osteoarthritis is another condition hallmarked by chronic inflammation. Inflammation in the joint capsule makes movement of the joint very painful. The capsule is enlarged with inflammatory exudates, which cause stretching of the capsule for movement to occur. This is not an infectious process; it is a disease process that stimulates the inflammatory processes.

Complications

Inflammation and wound healing are highly metabolic processes that may be affected by a number of factors. Without adequate nutrition, blood supply, and oxygenation, tissues cannot effectively complete the process. Impaired inflammatory and immune processes can interfere with phagocytosis and preparation of the wound for healing. Infection prolongs the inflammatory process and delays healing.

Chronic diseases may also impair healing. Diabetes mellitus is a prominent example. With high blood glucose levels associated with poorly controlled diabetes, chemotaxic and phagocytic function are decreased. Collagen formation and tensile strength of the wound are also impaired. Small blood vessel disease is common in people with diabetes, a factor that further impairs the healing process.

Drug therapy, particularly corticosteroid medications, may suppress the immune and inflammatory responses, delaying healing (Porth, 2005). Other external factors, such as exposure to ionizing radiation and wound cleansing agents, can also affect healing. Table 12–8 summarizes major factors that affect the inflammatory process and wound healing.

INTERDISCIPLINARY CARE

Management of the client with inflamed tissue focuses on promoting healing. Care is generally supportive, allowing the client's own physiologic processes to remove foreign matter and damaged cells. Wound care may be minimal, involving only simple cleaning, or extensive, involving irrigations and debridement. The client is encouraged to rest, to increase fluid intake, and to eat a well-balanced, nutritious diet. Anti-inflammatory medications are administered only when the inflammatory process has become problematic. With orthopedic cases, anti-inflammatory medications are avoided because they may retard bone formation and healing (Dahners & Mullis, 2004). Antibiotics may also be prescribed to help eliminate infectious causes of inflammation.

Diagnosis

The following diagnostic tests may be ordered to identify the source and extent of inflammation. An important part of the

TABLE 12–8 Factors That May Impair Healing

FACTOR	EFFECT
Malnutrition	
Protein deficit	Prolongs inflammation and impairs healing process
Carbohydrate and kilocalorie deficit	Impairs metabolic processes and promotes catabolism; proteins are used for energy rather than for healing
Fat deficit	Impairs cell membrane synthesis in tissue repair
Vitamin deficits	
Vitamin A	Limits epithelialization and capillary formation
B-Complex	Inhibits enzymatic reactions that contribute to wound healing
Vitamin C	Impairs collagen synthesis
Tissue hypoxia	Associated with an increased risk of infection and impaired healing, because oxygen is required to support cell function and collagen synthesis
Impaired blood supply	Inadequate delivery of oxygen and nutrients to healing tissues and removal of waste products
Impaired inflammatory and immune processes	Decreased phagocytosis and wound debridement; increased risk of infection; delayed healing

assessment of the client with an inflammation is monitoring the results of these tests.

- *WBC with differential* provides information about the type and extent of inflammatory response. The differential count (the percentage of the total WBC made up by each type of leukocyte) provides further clues about inflammatory processes (Table 12–9).
- *Erythrocyte sedimentation rate* (*ESR* or *sed rate*) is a nonspecific test to detect inflammation. The rate at which RBCs fall to the bottom of a vertical tube is an indicator of inflammation. An increased ESR may indicate acute or chronic inflammation, tuberculosis, autoimmune disorders, some malignancies, and nephritis. Decreased ESR is found in congestive heart failure, sickle cell anemia, and polycythemia vera.
- *C-reactive protein (CRP) test* is used to detect CRP. This abnormal glycoprotein is produced by the liver and is excreted into the bloodstream during the acute phase of an inflammatory process. The expected result of this test is negative for CRP. A positive result indicates an acute or chronic inflammatory process. It may also indicate the client's response to therapy, because it decreases when inflammation subsides.

In addition to the above diagnostic tests, cultures of the blood and other body fluids may be ordered to determine if infection is the cause of inflammation.

Medications

Medications may be prescribed for the client with an inflammatory response to help alleviate distressing symptoms or destroy infectious agents.

Acetaminophen (Tylenol) may be administered to reduce the fever and pain associated with inflammation. Acetaminophen has no anti-inflammatory effect; it will not reduce the inflammatory process but will relieve associated symptoms. Acetaminophen decreases fever by acting directly on the hypothalamus heat-regulating center. It also works on the central nervous system to relieve pain sensations.

Antibiotics may be used either prophylactically to prevent infection from interfering with the healing process of damaged tissue, or therapeutically to treat the infection. If infection is present, the organism and its response or sensitivity to various antibiotics are used to guide therapy. Antibiotic therapy is presented in greater depth in the section of this chapter on infectious diseases.

Although inflammation is a beneficial process to prepare acutely injured tissue for healing, it can have damaging effects as well. When these effects are a concern or the manifestations of inflammation are deleterious to the client, anti-inflammatory medications may be prescribed. Anti-inflammatory medications fall into three broad groups: salicylates, such as aspirin; other nonsteroidal anti-inflammatory drugs (NSAIDs); and corticosteroids.

Aspirin (also called acetylsalicylic acid, or ASA) is an NSAID that has antipyretic, analgesic, and antiplatelet effects. Its beneficial effects are largely dose related. Low doses (as little as 81 mg/day) inhibit platelet aggregation and normal blood clotting. Higher doses (650 to 1000 mg 4 to 5 times per day) are required to accomplish its anti-inflammatory effects. However, 650 mg of aspirin is an effective analgesic and antipyretic dosage. To relieve pain, aspirin acts primarily on peripheral sensory nerves by inhibiting the synthesis of prostaglandins and kinins, which are chemical stimuli of sensory nerves. As an antipyretic, aspirin acts both centrally and peripherally. It inhibits the formation of pyrogenic substances that raise the hypothalamic thermostat. It also dilates peripheral blood vessels and promotes diaphoresis, increasing the dissipation of heat (Wilson, 2006).

In therapeutic doses, aspirin mediates the inflammatory process by inhibiting the synthesis of prostaglandins and acting on the mobility and activation of leukocytes. Inflammation is reduced, along with the swelling, redness, and impaired function that accompanies it.

The other NSAIDs have activity similar to that of aspirin. They inhibit prostaglandin synthesis, reducing the inflammatory and pain response. NSAIDs fall into the following classifications:

- *Salicylates,* which include aspirin and related compounds
- *Acetic acids,* including indomethacin (Indocin), ketorolac (Toradol), sulindac (Clinoril), and tolmetin (Tolectin)
- *Propionic acids,* including ibuprofen (Motrin and numerous nonprescription preparations), fenoprofen (Nalfon), and naproxen (Naprosyn)
- *Fenamates,* including meclofenamate (Meclomen)
- *Pyrazoles,* including phenylbutazone (Butazolidin)
- *Oxicams,* including piroxicam (Feldene).

Each group has a slightly different mode of action for prostaglandin inhibition. Clients may have varying degrees of relief with different NSAIDs; sometimes, several different

TABLE 12–9 The White Blood Cell Count and Differential

CELL TYPE AND NORMAL VALUE	INCREASED	DECREASED
Total WBCs: 4000 to 10,000 per mm³	*Leukocytosis:* Infection or inflammation, leukemia, trauma or stress, tissue necrosis	*Leukopenia:* Bone marrow depression, overwhelming infection, viral infections, immunosuppression, autoimmune disease, dietary deficiency
Neutrophils (segs, PMNs, or polys): 55% to 70%	*Neutrophilia:* Acute infection or stress response, myelocytic leukemia, inflammatory or metabolic disorders	*Neutropenia:* Bone marrow depression, overwhelming bacterial infection, viral infection, Addison's disease
Eosinophils (eos): 1% to 4%	*Eosinophilia:* Parasitic infections, hyper-sensitivity reactions, autoimmune disorders	*Eosinopenia:* Cushing's syndrome, autoimmune disorders, stress, certain drugs
Basophils (basos): 0.5% to 1%	*Basophilia:* Hypersensitivity responses, chronic myelogenous leukemia, chickenpox or smallpox, splenectomy, hypothyroidism	*Basopenia:* Acute stress or hypersensitivity reactions, hyperthyroidism
Monocytes (monos): 2% to 8%	*Monocytosis:* Chronic inflammatory disorders, tuberculosis, viral infections, leukemia, Hodgkin's disease, multiple myeloma	*Monocytopenia:* Bone marrow depression, corticosteroid therapy
Lymphocytes (lymphs): 20% to 40%	*Lymphocytosis:* Chronic bacterial infection, viral infections, lymphocytic leukemia	*Lymphocytopenia:* Bone marrow depression, immunodeficiency, leukemia, Cushing's syndrome, Hodgkin's disease, renal failure

Source: Data from Corbett, J. V. (2004). Laboratory tests and diagnostic procedures with nursing diagnoses (6th ed.), Upper Saddle River, NJ: Prentice Hall and *Diagnostic and Laboratory Test Reference* (3rd ed.) by K. D. Pagana and T. J. Pagana, 1997, St. Louis, MO: Mosby-Year Book.

agents must be tried before the most effective is identified. Side effects also differ to a certain extent; however, all have a potential cross-sensitivity with aspirin, all irritate the gastrointestinal tract, and all cause some degree of sodium and water retention. They also are more costly than aspirin, but they have a longer duration of action; therefore, fewer daily doses are required to achieve the desired effect. Indomethacin and phenylbutazone are the most toxic of the NSAIDs. Their use is limited to short-term therapy. (See Chapter 9 ∞ for further information on NSAIDs.)

For acute hypersensitivity reactions, such as reactions to poison oak, or for inflammation that cannot be managed by aspirin or NSAID therapy, corticosteroid therapy may be prescribed. The glucocorticoids are hormones produced by the adrenal cortex that have widespread effects on body metabolism and the immune response. Glucocorticoids inhibit inflammation and may be lifesaving in acute fulminating or chronic progressive inflammation. They do not cure disease; they are palliative to manage the inflammatory process.

When glucocorticoids are prescribed to manage inflammation, the following principles are used to guide therapy:
- The smallest possible effective dose is used.
- If a local-acting preparation such as a topical agent or intra-articular injection will be effective, it is prescribed.
- To minimize suppression of adrenal gland activity, an alternate-day dose schedule is used when possible.
- High-dose corticosteroid therapy is rarely stopped abruptly, but tapered, allowing the client's adrenal glands to resume normal function.

The incidence of potentially harmful side effects increases with higher doses and prolonged therapy.

The nursing implications of caring for a client receiving corticosteroid medications are discussed in Chapter 26 ∞.

Nutrition

Healing depends on cell replication, protein synthesis, and the function of specific organs—the liver, heart, and lungs in particular. Weight loss and protein depletion are risk factors for poor healing and wound complications. Even a few days of severely impaired nutritional intake can noticeably affect healing.

The client with an inflammatory process or healing wound requires a well-balanced diet of sufficient kilocalories to meet the metabolic needs of the body (see Table 12–8). Inflammation often produces *catabolism,* a state in which body tissues are broken down. Healing, by contrast, is a process of *anabolism,* or building up. Without sufficient kilocalories and nutrients, catabolism may predominate, impairing healing.

Carbohydrates are important to meet energy demands, as well as to support leukocyte function. However, hyperglycemia experienced in diabetes may impair healing. In diabetes, the glucose molecules bind the oxygen more tightly to the hemoglobin molecule and prevent adequate release of oxygen to the tissues for healing. In diabetes this is at least the partial explanation for impaired healing (McCance & Huether, 2002). Adequate protein is necessary for tissue healing and the production of antibodies and WBCs. Lack of adequate protein increases the risk of infection. Complete protein sources, those that provide the essential amino acids, are preferred. Dietary fats are used in the synthesis of cell membranes.

Vitamins A, B-complex, C, and K are also important to the healing process. Vitamin A is necessary for capillary formation and epithelialization. B-complex vitamins promote wound healing, and vitamin C is necessary for collagen synthesis. Vitamin K provides a vital component for the synthesis of clotting factors in the liver.

Although it has been established that minerals contribute to the inflammatory and healing processes, less is known about required amounts. Zinc appears to be important for tissue growth, skin integrity, cell-mediated immunity, and other general immune mechanisms (Arnold & Barbul, 2006). However, the use of zinc supplements in smokers is cautioned against and sources in whole foods are recommended over supplements. (See Chapter 21 ∞ for a detailed discussion on nutrition.)

NURSING CARE

Acute inflammation may be self-limiting or extensive and require hospitalization. Nursing care includes teaching clients with acute and chronic inflammatory conditions self-management at home.

Health Promotion

Health promotion activities to prevent inflammation focus on reducing the risk for accidents and exposure to harmful agents that can result in subsequent injury. It is important to educate the public about potential hazards in both the work and home environments. In addition, safety education guidelines such as not drinking and driving, wearing a protective helmet when riding a bicycle, and using a safety belt in the car are important areas for discussion. Because most injuries occur at home, it is also important to discuss ways to make the home safer.

Assessment

The following data are collected through the health history and physical examination. Further focused assessments are described with nursing interventions in the next section.

- *Health history:* risk factors, nutrition, medication use (anti-inflammatory and corticosteroids), location, duration, and type (redness, heat, pain, swelling, and impaired function) of symptoms
- *Physical assessment:* movement of injured area, circulation, wounds, lymph nodes.

Nursing Diagnoses and Interventions

The nursing care needs of the client with an inflammatory process are related to the manifestations of inflammation (pain in particular) and altered tissue integrity. Priority nursing diagnoses include *Pain, Impaired Tissue Integrity,* and *Risk for Infection.*

Pain

Along with redness, warmth, swelling, and impaired function, pain is one of the cardinal manifestations of inflammation. Depending on the cause, affected area, and degree of inflammation, pain may be acute and immobilizing or chronic and demoralizing. It is important to remember that pain is a subjective experience and that client responses to pain vary. (Refer to Chapter 9 ∞ for more information about pain and pain management.)

- Assess pain using a scale of 0 to 10, with 0 being no pain and 10 being the worst pain; note the character and location of the pain. *Because pain is subjective, the client provides the most accurate information regarding his or her pain experience.*
- Use physical and nonverbal cues to further assess the level of pain. *This intervention is especially important if the client is nonverbal or tends to underreport pain.*

- Administer anti-inflammatory medications as prescribed. *These medications help reduce the pain resulting from acute inflammation.*
- Administer analgesic medications as prescribed. *Although most analgesics do little to reduce inflammation, they provide additional pain relief by reducing the perception of pain.* Chest infections such as pneumonia may compromise breathing. Do not hesitate to administer opioids to ease the pain of breathing. In addition to applying oxygen at appropriate levels (low for those with chronic obstructive pulmonary disease to preserve the oxygen drive to breathe), relieving pain helps increase the depth and slow the rate of respirations. Because opioids can depress respirations, it is important to monitor oxygen saturation and encourage the patient to take deep breaths to keep oxygen saturation adequate.
- Monitor effectiveness of interventions. *Results may call for modifications in the regimen.*
- Provide comfort measures, such as back rubs, position changes, or relaxation techniques. *These measures reduce muscle tension, relieve areas of pressure, and provide distraction.*
- Encourage activities such as reading, watching television, and taking part in social interactions. *Such activities provide distraction from the pain experience.*
- Encourage rest. *Strenuous activity or exercising an inflamed body part may increase discomfort and tissue damage.*
- Provide cold or heat as pain-relief measures, as ordered. *For an acute injury, cold reduces swelling and relieves pain; after the initial stage, heat increases blood flow to the affected tissue and relieves pain and swelling by promoting absorption of edema. Either heat or cold may be contraindicated with some inflammatory processes; for example, if the appendix is acutely inflamed, applying heat to the abdomen may prompt the appendix to rupture, increasing the risk of peritonitis. If unsure, check with the client's primary care provider.*

> **PRACTICE ALERT**
> Use heat or cold application cautiously in older clients who have fragile skin and are at risk for tissue injury.

- Elevate the inflamed area if possible. *Elevation promotes venous return and reduces swelling.*
- Teach about the appropriate use and expected effects of anti-inflammatory medications. *If the client's pain continues after the initial doses of anti-inflammatory medication, he or she may become discouraged and stop taking the medication before it becomes fully effective.*

Impaired Tissue Integrity

The inflammatory response can either precipitate or result from an impairment in the integrity of skin, support, or other tissues. Whatever the cause of the tissue alteration, it is vital that the nurse consider this alteration in delivering care.

- Assess general health and nutritional status. *Poor general health or chronic diseases such as diabetes mellitus or renal failure interfere with the healing processes and increase the risk of infection.*

- Assess circulation to the affected area. *Adequate tissue perfusion and oxygenation are necessary for healing.*
- Monitor the skin and surrounding tissue for increased signs of inflammation. *Inflammation can spread to adjacent tissues leading to conditions such as cellulitis.*
- Provide protection and support for inflamed tissue. *This reduces discomfort and decreases the risk of further tissue damage.*
- Clean inflamed tissue gently; if possible, use water, normal saline, or nontoxic wound cleansers such as Comfeel (Coloplast Corporation) only. *Soap and harsh cleansers such as povidone-iodine (Betadine) and hydrogen peroxide can cause further drying and tissue damage. Granulation tissue in a healing wound is fragile and easily damaged.* (See Chapter 4 ∞ for further discussion of wound care.)
- Keep the inflamed area dry, and expose it to air as much as possible. *This promotes healing and helps prevent infection.*
- Balance rest with the tolerable degree of mobility. *Rest decreases metabolic demands and allows for cell regeneration while mobility helps to promote oxygenation and perfusion of the tissues.*
- Provide supplemental oxygen as ordered. *Supplemental oxygen improves tissue oxygenation and reduces hypoxia.*
- Provide a well-balanced diet with adequate kilocalories to meet the body's metabolic and healing needs. If the client is allowed nothing by mouth (NPO), suggest parenteral or enteral nutrition. For the client who is unable to consume an adequate diet, consult with a dietitian for between-meal supplements and/or multivitamin supplements. *Careful attention to diet and nutrient intake is important to provide the nutrients necessary for immune function and healing and to prevent catabolism.*

Risk for Infection

The inflammatory response often indicates that body defense mechanisms have been set in motion to protect against invading microorganisms. Wounds, whether traumatic or surgical in nature, are typically contaminated, as attested to by subsequent wound infections. The client with a healing wound is at particular risk for infection.

- Assess the wound for specific signs of infection, including purulent drainage, odor, and poor healing. *The normal inflammatory response can indicate infection and, on occasion, mask its presence.*
- Evaluate complete blood counts for adequate WBC response. *Leucocytosis may indicate infection or healthy response to injury and protection from infection. Immune-impaired clients may not respond with increased WBCs; signs of inflammation may be diminished in those individuals.*
- Monitor temperature, pulse, and respirations at least every 4 hours. *In response to the inflammatory process the temperature rises, usually in the range of 99°F (37.2°C) to 100.9°F (38.2°C). A temperature of 101.0°F (38.3°C) or above indicates infection. Fever is usually accompanied by increased heart and respiratory rates.*
- Culture purulent or odorous wound drainage. *Wound culture is used to determine the infectious organism and to direct antibiotic therapy.*

- Apply dry or moist heat to the affected area for no longer than 20 minutes several times a day. *Heat increases the circulation of blood to and from the inflamed tissue. Time is limited to prevent burns.*
- Provide fluid intake of 2500 mL/day. *Adequate hydration promotes blood flow and nutrient supply to the tissues and also dilutes and removes waste products from the body.*
- Ensure adequate nutrition. *Adequate nutrition enhances the function and production of T cells and B cells, which are important in the immune response.*
- Use good hand washing techniques. *Hand washing removes transient microorganisms and is the best mechanism to prevent the spread of infection to a susceptible person.*
- Wear sterile gloves when providing wound care. *Using sterile gloves helps prevent further contamination of the wound and the spread of infection to other clients.*

Community-Based Care

Client and family teaching enhances understanding of the inflammatory process, its cause, and its management. Teaching is also important to prevent further compromise that could result in infection.

Instructions, verbal and written, should include the following:
- Increase fluid intake to 2500 mL (approximately 2.5 quarts) per day.
- Eat a well-balanced diet high in vitamins and minerals and with adequate protein and kilocalories for healing.
- Use good hand washing techniques, particularly when caring for wounds or inflamed tissue and after using the bathroom.
- Elevate the inflamed area to reduce swelling and pain.
- Apply heat or cold for no longer than 20 minutes at a time to reduce the risk of tissue damage from burns or frostbite.
- Take all medications as prescribed, notifying the physician if adverse effects or hypersensitivity responses are noted. (See Nursing Research: Evidence-Based Practice on page 310).
- Rest acutely inflamed tissue; do not engage in strenuous activity until the inflammation has subsided.

The Client with an Infection

Microorganisms—including bacteria, viruses, fungi, and parasites—often invade the human body and proliferate if undetected and controlled or eliminated by inflammatory and immune responses. In most cases, contact between humans and microorganisms is incidental and may even be beneficial to both organisms. Resident bacteria of the skin, mucous membranes, and gastrointestinal tract are an important part of the body's defense system. However, many microorganisms are virulent; that is, they have the ability to cause disease. **Pathogens** are virulent organisms rarely found in the absence of disease. Some microorganisms, known as opportunistic pathogens, rarely, if ever, cause harm to persons with intact immune systems, but are capable of producing infectious disease in the immunocompromised host (Porth, 2005).

Infectious disease has been pervasive throughout history. Modern medicine, antibiotic therapy, immunizations, and other public health measures to protect food and water supplies have

NURSING RESEARCH   Evidence-Based Practice for Antibiotics and Infection

Nurses discharging clients from outpatient and acute care settings frequently teach clients to take a complete prescribed dose of oral antibiotics to manage acute infectious illness. Ingesting less than complete doses exposes clients to the risk of resistant infections and less than therapeutic outcomes. There are many potential restraining forces to the completion of antibiotic dosing: cost of purchase; difficulty swallowing the pills; multiple, frequent doses; and the potential for adverse, unpleasant side effects.

Because adherence is so important and nurses are client educators, Aronson (2005) studied in depth the experience of 11 clients who had just completed a short-term antibiotic regimen to treat a variety of acute infectious illnesses with various antibiotic regimens. The 11 subjects represent diverse gender and cultural backgrounds. They participated in 30-minute interviews within 2 weeks of completing their antibiotic regimen. The interviews were audiotaped and evaluated for themes. This qualitative study is the first part of a research program to evaluate an intervention to promote adherence to taking antibiotics for a short-term period. The clients' descriptions, views, and experiences are the unique aspect of this research on adherence to antibiotic self-administration. Most studies of adherence have been conducted from the prescribers' rather than the clients' perspective.

Aronson analyzed the client descriptions of their experience taking their prescribed antibiotics by organizing the responses into categories of consistent themes; a second colleague experienced in qualitative research independently analyzed the data and the results were compared until the categories were agreed on. The central theme that emerged was successful antibiotic self-administration. The clients integrated the dosing into their daily schedules and adapted to any unplanned circumstances. The primary categories involved in self-administration were

(1) medication-taking behaviors, (2) factors influencing adherence, and (3) attitudes and beliefs about the medication and the value of completing the prescribed dose. Subcategories were identified for each of these main categories.

Clients described methods for remembering to take the medication, methods of dealing with anticipated or experienced side effects, and factors that build trust in their relationship with the prescriber. The severity of the symptoms that led to antibiotic prescription made them more likely to report intention to adhere to the dosing regimen.

IMPLICATIONS FOR NURSING

Nurses teach clients about short-term antibiotic self-administration in outpatient and inpatient settings. The findings from this study can be used to guide educational interactions. Based on the findings in this study, encourage client involvement in the decision to take short-term antibiotic medications to strengthen the relationship with the prescriber. Ask clients to identify the method they will use to remind themselves of each dose; inquire about their knowledge of and plans to manage side effects from the medication.

CRITICAL THINKING IN CLIENT CARE

1. Identify methods that clients can use to remind themselves of dosing schedules.
2. An 86-year-old woman is being discharged to her home following a respiratory infection. Identify the information she will need about short-term antibiotic medication when she is discharged.
3. Discuss potential side effects of short-term antibiotics on the gastrointestinal tract.
4. Discuss the interrelationship between malnutrition and immune system function.

Data from Aronson, B. (2005). Medication management behaviors of adherent short-term antibiotic users. *Clinical Excellence for Nurse Practitioners, 9*(1), 23–30.

significantly reduced the prevalence of infectious diseases in many parts of the world. In spite of these advances, many infections, including malaria, typhoid, and tuberculosis, remain prevalent in developing nations. Sexually transmitted infections rage through modern cities and industrialized populations. New varieties and strains of pathogens, such as HIV, evolve to cause disease.

To a certain extent, modern medicine has contributed to the development of infectious diseases caused by antibiotic-resistant strains of microorganisms. Tuberculosis is on the rise in the United States, partially because organisms have become resistant to standard therapies. Clients receive immunosuppressive therapy following organ or tissue transplant or in the treatment of neoplasms, making them more susceptible to infection. Metal and plastic prosthetic devices are implanted, providing potential sites for colonization by disease-producing organisms (Fauci et al., 1998). It has also become apparent that many diseases long considered unrelated to microorganisms may actually be infectious; for example, colonization of the gastric mucosa with *Hel-*

icobacter pylori is the predominant cause of peptic ulcer disease, and oncogenic viruses have the ability to transform normal cells into malignant cells.

Pathophysiology

Infection occurs when an organism is able to colonize and multiply within a host. The host can be any organism capable of supporting the nutritional and physical growth requirements of the microorganism—for example, humans. When the host experiences injury, pathologic changes, inflammation, or organ dysfunction in response to an infection or from intoxication by cellular poisons produced by a pathogen, the host is said to have an infectious disease.

For a microorganism to cause infection, it must have disease-causing potential (virulence), be transmitted from its reservoir, and gain entry into a susceptible host. This is known as the chain of infection (Figure 12–12 ■).

PATHOGENS Pathogens capable of infecting and causing disease in a susceptible host include bacteria, viruses, mycoplasma, rick-

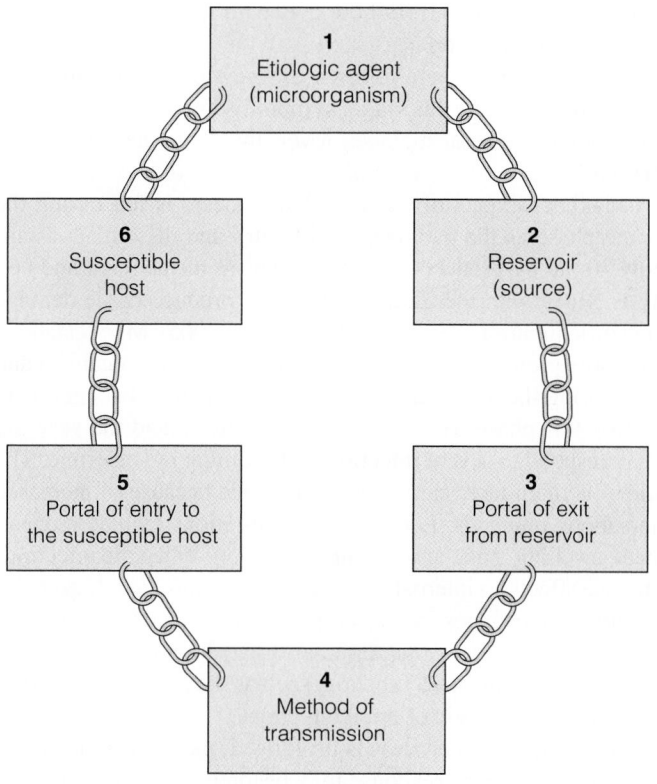

Figure 12–12 ■ The chain of infection.

ettsia, chlamydia, fungi, and parasites such as protozoa, helminths (worms), and arthropods (Box 12–4). Each organism causes a different specific reaction in the host.

A number of different mechanisms have evolved in pathogens to facilitate their transmission and increase their ability to invade the host and cause disease. Factors influencing the transmission of an organism include its resistance to drying and to variations in environmental temperature. For example, spore-forming organisms are extremely resistant to drying.

Many microorganisms are capable of producing toxins or enzymes to facilitate their invasion of the host, increase their resistance to host defenses, and increase their ability to cause disease. Adhesion factors produced by or incorporated into the cell wall or membrane of the pathogen improve its ability to attach and colonize the host. Pathogens may also produce enzymes to enhance their spread to local tissues, chemicals to block specific immune processes or deplete neutrophils and macrophages, or extracellular capsules to discourage phagocytosis.

Pathogens are often capable of producing toxins that alter or destroy the normal function of host cells and promote colonization, proliferation, and invasion by the pathogen. Toxins often increase the disease-producing capability of the pathogen and, in some cases, are totally responsible for it; for example, cholera, tetanus, and botulism result from bacterial toxins, not from the direct effects of the infection. **Exotoxins** are soluble proteins secreted into surrounding tissue by the microorganism.

BOX 12–4 **Pathogenic Organisms**

Bacteria

Bacteria are single-celled organisms capable of autonomous reproduction. Relatively small and simple organisms, they contain a single chromosome. A flexible cell membrane and rigid cell wall surrounds their cytoplasm, giving them a distinctive shape; some also have an extracellular capsule for additional protection. Bacteria have different characteristics and growth requirements: *aerobes* require oxygen for survival, whereas *anaerobes* cannot survive in the presence of oxygen; *gram-positive* bacteria stain purple when subjected to crystal violet stain, whereas *gram-negative* bacteria do not stain with crystal violet but turn red when subjected to safranin stain; the colonies formed by replicating bacteria differ from one another.

Viruses

Viruses are obligate intracellular parasites that are incapable of reproducing outside of a living cell. Viruses consist of a protein coat around a core of either DNA or RNA. Some viruses are shed continuously from infected cell surfaces; others, after inserting their genetic material into that of the infected cell, remain latent until they are stimulated to replicate. Viruses may or may not cause lysis and death of the host cell during replication. Oncogenic viruses are able to transform normal cells into malignant cells.

Mycoplasma

Although similar to bacteria, mycoplasma are smaller and have no cell wall, making them resistant to antibiotics that inhibit cell wall synthesis (e.g., penicillins).

Rickettsia and Chlamydia

As obligate intracellular parasites with a rigid cell wall, rickettsia and *Chlamydia* have some features of both bacteria and viruses. Rather than depending on the host cell for reproduction, they use vitamins, nutrients, or products of metabolism (e.g., ATP) from the host. *Chlamydia* are transmitted by direct contact, whereas many rickettsiae infect the cells of arthropods (e.g., fleas, ticks, and lice) and are transmitted from these vectors to humans.

Fungi

Fungi are prevalent throughout the world, but few are capable of causing disease in humans. Most fungal infections are self-limited, affecting the skin and subcutaneous tissue. Some fungi, such as *Pneumocystis carinii*, can cause life-threatening opportunistic infections in the immunocompromised host.

Parasites

The term *parasite* is typically applied to members of the animal kingdom that infect and cause disease in other animals. Protozoa, helminths, and arthropods are considered parasites. Protozoa are single-celled organisms transmitted via direct or indirect contact or an arthropod vector. Helminths are wormlike parasites: roundworms, tapeworms, and flukes are examples. They gain entry into humans primarily through ingestion of fertilized eggs or penetration of larvae through the skin or mucous membranes. Arthropod parasites, such as scabies (mites), lice, and fleas, typically infest external body surfaces, causing localized tissue damage and inflammation. Transmission is by direct contact with the arthropod or its eggs.

Source: Data summarized from *Pathophysiology: Concepts of Altered Health States* (7th ed.) by C. M. Porth, 2005, Philadelphia: Lippincott Williams & Wilkins.

Exotoxins are highly poisonous, causing cell death or dysfunction. **Endotoxins** are found in the cell wall of gram-negative bacteria and are released only when the cell is disrupted. Endotoxins have less specific effects than exotoxins, but they act as activators of many human regulatory systems, producing fever, inflammation, and potentially clotting, bleeding, or hypotension when released in large quantities.

RESERVOIR AND TRANSMISSION The reservoir or source, where the pathogen lives and multiplies, may be either endogenous or exogenous. Organisms that reside on skin or mucosal surfaces of the host are endogenous. Exogenous sources can include other humans, animals, soil, water, intravenous fluid, or equipment. Infectious diseases are usually transmitted from human sources, that is, persons who have clinical disease or carriers with subclinical infection. Carriers harbor the pathogen without showing evidence of clinical disease. Pathogens exit human hosts via respiratory secretions, body fluids from the gastrointestinal and genitourinary tracts, skin or mucous membrane lesions, the placenta, and blood.

Organisms may be transmitted from the source to the susceptible host by direct or indirect contact, droplet or airborne transmission, or a vector. Direct contact includes person-to-person spread or contact with infected body fluids, as well as transmission from contaminated food or water. Indirect contact occurs when the infectious agent is contracted by use of inanimate objects, such as dirty eating utensils. Sneezing, talking, and coughing allow transmission by droplet contact when the host is within 2 to 3 feet of the source. Smaller respiratory particles that stay suspended in air and are carried via air currents allow airborne transmission. Vectors are insects and animals such as flies, mosquitoes, or rodents that act as intermediate hosts between the source and host. Microorganisms usually first colonize the portal of entry: nonintact skin, wounds, mucous membranes, and the respiratory, gastrointestinal, or genitourinary tracts.

HOST FACTORS The susceptible host is the final link in the chain of infection. Exposure to pathogens does not automatically cause infection or infectious disease. The outcome of contact with a pathogenic microorganism is determined by the balance of microbial virulence and host resistance. Factors that can enable the host to resist infection include the following:
- Physical barriers, such as the skin and mucous membranes
- The hostile environment created by acid stomach secretions, urine, and vaginal secretions
- Antimicrobial factors in saliva, tears, and prostatic fluid
- Respiratory defenses, including humidification, filtration, the mucociliary escalator, cough reflex, and alveolar macrophages
- Specific and nonspecific immune responses to pathogenic invasion.

Stages of the Infectious Process
When infectious disease develops in the host, it typically follows a predictable course with stages based on the progression and intensity of manifestations.

The initial stage is the incubation period, during which the pathogen begins active replication but does not yet cause symptoms. Depending on the organism and host factors, the incubation period may last from hours, as with salmonella, to years, as with HIV infection.

The prodromal stage follows, during which symptoms first begin to appear. At this stage, symptoms are often nonspecific and include general malaise, fever, myalgias, headache, and fatigue.

Maximal impact of the infectious process is felt during the acute phase as the pathogen proliferates and disseminates rapidly. Toxic by-products of microorganism metabolism and cell lysis, along with the immune response, produce tissue damage and inflammation during this stage (Porth, 2005). Manifestations are more pronounced and specific to the infecting organism and site during the acute stage. Fever and chills may be significant during this phase. However, alcoholic clients and the very old may respond to severe infection by becoming hypothermic. The client is often tachycardic and tachypneic because of increased metabolic demands. Localized manifestations include redness, heat, swelling, pain, and impaired function. When the infectious disease affects an internal organ, manifestations are related to inflammatory changes in that organ and surrounding tissue. The client may experience tenderness to palpation over the site or show signs of impaired function, such as the hematuria and proteinuria characteristic of renal infections.

If the infectious process is prolonged, manifestations of the continuing immune response may become apparent. Catabolic and anorexic effects of the infection can lead to loss of body fat and muscle wasting. Immune complexes may be deposited at sites other than the primary infection, resulting in an inflammatory process. Glomerulonephritis (e.g., following strep throat) and vasculitis are possible results. Another possible consequence of prolonged infection and immune response is the triggering of an autoimmune disease process (discussed in Chapter 13 ∞), such as rheumatic cardiomyopathy or celiac disease. Type 1 diabetes mellitus is thought to be the result of such a response (Porth, 2005).

As the infection is contained and the pathogen eliminated, the convalescent stage of the disease occurs. During this stage, affected tissues are repaired and manifestations resolve. Resolution of the infection is total elimination of the pathogen from the body without residual manifestations. If a balance between organism and host factors occurs with neither predominating, chronic disease may develop or the organism may be driven into a protected site, such as an abscess. A carrier state develops when host defenses eliminate the infectious disease but the organism continues to multiply on mucosal sites (Fauci et al., 1998).

Complications
Multiple and varied complications are associated with infectious diseases. They are typically specific to the infecting organism and the body system affected.

Acute invasion of the blood by certain microorganisms or their toxins can result in septicemia and septic shock. Whereas bacteremia, the presence of bacteria in the blood, may not have serious effects, septicemia refers to systemic disease associated with their presence or toxins. Septic shock indicates a state of hypotension and impaired organ perfusion resulting from sepsis. Unless treated aggressively, septic shock leads to diffuse cell and tissue injury, and potentially to organ failure. See Chapter 11 ∞ for an in-depth discussion of septic shock, other shock syndromes, and their management.

Nosocomial Infections

Nosocomial infections are acquired in a healthcare setting, such as a hospital or nursing home. Also called healthcare-associated infections (HAIs), nosocomial infections account for an estimated 2 million infections, 90,000 deaths, and $4.5 billion in excess healthcare costs annually. HAIs add hospital days, reduce admissions by occupying available beds, and add to the cost of health care (Stone et al., 2005).

FAST FACTS

- Nosocomial infections typically manifest after 48 hours of hospitalization. Infections that manifest within 48 hours of hospitalization are attributed to community sources.
- Urinary tract infection is the most common type of HAI, leading to the most frequent cause of gram-negative septicemia in hospitalized patients.
- Pneumonia is the second most common hospital-acquired infection and has a mortality rate of 20% to 50%. It is associated with mechanical ventilators, tracheostomies, and endotracheal intubation (Porth, 2005).
- Bacteremia is associated with intravascular and urinary catheters. Because of the risk of infection, insertion of central lines as well as urinary catheters is conducted as a sterile procedure with careful attention to preventing contamination.
- *Clostridium difficile*–associated diarrhea is a frequently acquired nosocomial infection. It is an antibiotic-associated diarrhea and the risk of acquiring it increases with length of hospital stay, especially in an intensive care unit (ICU).

Clients entering hospitals are often the least able to mount immune defenses to infection. Immunologic responses may be compromised and normal defenses impaired in clients with, for example, cancer or chronic diseases, pressure ulcers, or organ transplants (Tierney et al., 2006). Nosocomial infections also occur when antibiotic therapy has altered natural defenses and impaired resistance to harmful microorganisms. Endogenous organisms outside their normal habitats (such as in *Escherichia coli* in the urinary tract) become a threat to the client. Other pharmacologic and therapeutic procedures such as chemotherapy, the use of corticosteroids, or radiation therapy also contribute to nosocomial infections. Gram-negative enteric bacteria and gram-positive *Staphylococcus aureus* are the most common bacteria responsible.

Invasive procedures and altered immune defenses are the main factors contributing to infection. Urinary catheterization is the number one cause; cardiac catheterization, peripheral and central intravenous lines, respiratory care procedures, and surgical procedures are also closely linked to nosocomial infection. Consequently, the urinary tract, surgical wounds, the respiratory tract, and invasive catheter sites on the skin are most often affected by hospital-acquired infection. Hospital-acquired pneumonia is the second most common nosocomial infection, accounting for 15% to 20% of these serious infections. Usually associated with ICU

residency and mechanical ventilation, Sopina and Sobria (2005) found hospital-acquired pneumonia in non-ICU clients with severe underlying disease and a hospital stay greater than 5 days. Organisms causing the infection are often resistant to many drugs, not responding to antibiotics usually effective in treating infections acquired outside the hospital.

PRACTICE ALERT

Since October 2002, alcohol-based hand rub has been recommended by the CDC as the preferred method for hand hygiene (CDC, 2002a). Antiseptic soaps and detergents are the next most effective agents and nonantiseptic soaps are the least effective. A soap and water wash is recommended for visibly soiled hands. Wearing gloves does not eliminate the need for hand washing.

Prevention is the most important control measure for nosocomial infections. The pathogens causing these infections are transmitted primarily by contact with hospital personnel and contaminated inanimate objects (Posani, 2004). *Effective hand washing is the single most important measure in infection control.* Although infections may also be transmitted by the airborne route, contaminated equipment, or from the environment, these are less significant causes. Invasive procedures and equipment should be used only when absolutely necessary; for example, it is not appropriate to insert an indwelling catheter when the only indication is incontinence. Peripheral intravenous equipment and sites must be kept clean and changed regularly: intravenous bags and bottles every 24 hours, tubing every 24 to 96 hours, and sites every 2 to 3 days according to agency policy (CDC, 2002b; Evans-Smith, 2005).

Antibiotic-Resistant Microorganisms

Antibiotic-resistant microorganisms are increasing at an alarming rate primarily due to prolonged or inappropriate use of antibiotic therapy. Although antibiotic therapy is expected to eradicate all targeted microorganisms, sometimes a few bacteria survive, leading to bacteria that reproduce with antibiotic resistance already encoded into their genetic makeup (Lehne, 2004). Other bacteria produce enzymes that inactivate drugs, change drug binding sites, or alter their cell membrane to prevent drug absorption.

Some of the current resistant strains include:

- Methicillin-resistant *S. aureus* (MRSA)
- Multidrug-resistant tuberculosis (MDR-TB)
- Penicillin-resistant *Streptococcus pneumoniae* (PRSP)
- Vancomycin-resistant *Enterococci* (VRE)
- Vancomycin intermediate or resistant *S. aureus* (VISA or VRSA)
- Extended-spectrum beta-lactamase (ESBL) (Kjonegaard & Myers, 2005).

MRSA exists not only in hospitals but also is becoming more prevalent in the community setting where young people such as children in day care or amateur and professional athletes share equipment. MRSA colonizes in the nares and skin. Healthcare personnel often transmit *S. aureus* unknowingly on their hands for it is transmitted primarily by direct physical contact, not through respiratory droplets (Kjonegaard & Myers, 2005). Most

S. aureus strains resist treatment by methicillin and other similar drugs, the treatment of choice for *S. aureus* infections. Vancomycin has been the only uniformly effective drug for hospital-acquired MRSA; however, community-acquired MRSA is sensitive to antibiotics such as tetracycline, doxycycline, clindamycin, and sulfamethoxazole-trimethoprim. The community-acquired MRSA is also resistant to cephalexin, dicloxacillin, erythromycin, and quinolones. Soft-tissue infections with MRSA may manifest as abscesses, furuncles, or cellulitis and may be mistaken for a spider bite.

In 1997, a new form of *S. aureus* emerged with resistance to vancomycin, known as vancomycin intermediate or resistant *S. aureus*. Today VISA or VRSA has been identified; both VISA and VRSA are resistant to methicillin. Clients with MRSA, VISA, or VRSA are isolated in a private room using contact precautions.

Enterococci are part of the normal flora of the gastrointestinal and female genital tracts. Frequent use of vancomycin caused *Enterococci* to develop resistance, leading to vancomycin-resistant *Enterococci*. Direct transmission occurs on the hands of healthcare personnel or contact with contaminated equipment. Stringent infection control measures are instituted; care is provided using contact precautions and clients are placed either alone or with other VRE-infected clients.

Streptococcus pneumoniae, the most common cause of community-acquired pneumonia, has developed into its resistant form, penicillin-resistant *S. pneumoniae*. Unlike MRSA and VRE, PRSP is transmitted by droplets from the respiratory tract and requires transmission-based droplet precautions.

Clostridium difficile is an organism that has developed very resistant and highly morbid strains associated with frequent use of broad-spectrum antibiotics in hospitals. A common cause of nosocomial diarrhea, it is usually treated with metronidazole or vancomycin (Rao & Bradley, 2003). An even more virulent strain has been identified that is resistant to both metronidazole and vancomycin (Warny et al., 2005).

Extended-spectrum beta-lactamase–producing microorganisms are resistant to third-generation cephalosporins and include gram-negative *Klebsiella* and *E.coli*. These organisms colonize indwelling urinary catheters or gastrostomies and also mechanical ventilators. They spread by direct and indirect contact.

Universal precautions, most importantly hand washing, and modest use of antibiotics are critical actions for stopping the spread of these diseases. Equipment such as stethoscopes, blood pressure cuffs, and thermometers should be restricted to use by each patient identified with one of these diseases. Personal protective gear used and disposed of appropriately are important safeguards.

Biological Threat Infections

Following the terrorist attacks on September 11, 2001, and the development of anthrax cases in the United States, concern has arisen about the possible use of biological weapons. The most likely pathogens to be used for this purpose include anthrax, smallpox, botulism, pneumonic plague, and viral hemorrhagic fevers. (See Chapter 7 ∞ for more on biological terrorism.)

Infectious Process in Older Adults

Older adults, particularly those over the age of 75 years, are at greater risk of acquiring an infection than younger people. Although the incidence of septicemia in the United States is increasing in all age groups, the greatest increase is among people over the age of 65 years (Baine, Yu, & Summe, 2001). Physiologic changes of aging that put the elderly at increased risk for infection include the following:

- *Cardiovascular changes:* decreased cardiac output, loss of capillaries, and decreased tissue perfusion delaying inflammatory response and healing
- *Respiratory system changes:* decreased mucociliary escalator, decreased elastic recoil, and a diminished cough reflex leading to decreased clearance of respiratory secretions
- *Genitourinary changes:* loss of muscle tone, reduced bladder contractility, altered bladder reflexes, and prostatic hypertrophy in men leading to reduced bladder capacity and incomplete emptying
- *Gastrointestinal system changes:* impaired swallow reflex, decreased gastric acidity, and delayed gastric emptying thus increasing the risk of aspiration
- *Skin and subcutaneous tissue changes:* thinning of skin, decreased cushioning, and decreased sensation leading to increased risk of injury and ulceration
- *Immune changes:* decreased phagocytosis, reduced inflammatory response, slowed or impaired healing processes leading to reduced immunity.

In addition to the previous physiologic changes, other factors that may contribute to the older adult's increased risk for infectious disease are as follows:

- Decreased activity level related to musculoskeletal, neurologic, or balance problems
- Poor nutrition and an increased risk of dehydration
- Chronic diseases, such as diabetes mellitus, cardiac disease, and renal disease
- Chronic medication use
- Lack of recent immunizations against preventable infectious diseases
- Altered mentation and dementias
- Hospitalization or residence in a long-term care facility
- Presence of invasive devices, such as indwelling urinary catheters and gastric tubes.

In addition, the thymus gland atrophies and by age 50 to 60 years thymic hormone levels are undetectable. Although the exact relationship of these events to T-cell function is unclear, some T-cell populations decrease or decline in function as the person ages. The ability of T cells to proliferate following activation also declines with advancing age; in addition, a portion of T cells cannot be activated in the elderly (Porth, 2005). With these changes, cell-mediated immune function declines. The client has reduced resistance to antigens such as *M. tuberculosis,* influenza and varicella-zoster viruses, malignant cells, and tissue grafts.

Immunoglobulin levels remain relatively stable, but primary and secondary antibody responses decline with aging. This diminished antibody production has clinical implications in that immunizations (single-dose and booster) may not produce the expected protective immune response.

The older adult is not only at increased risk for infection, but also may not exhibit the classic manifestations of inflammation and infection. Older adults are likely to take NSAIDs and corticosteroids that interfere with inflammation and healing. The cardinal signs of inflammation—redness, heat, and swelling—tend to be diminished or absent in older adults. The classic signs of infection—fever and chills—may be absent altogether because of age-related changes in the immune system, loss of central temperature control mechanisms, decreased muscle mass, and loss of shivering ability. The older adult may have only subtle signs of sepsis, including changes in mental status, disorientation, and tachypnea (Porth, 2005). Infectious diseases commonly seen in the elderly client are outlined below.

INTERDISCIPLINARY CARE

The goals of care for the client with an infection are to identify the organ system affected by the infection, to identify the causative agent, and to achieve a cure by the least toxic, least expensive, and most effective means. Fortunately, most infectious diseases are self-limiting and will resolve with little or no medical care. However, medical treatment can be lifesaving in an overwhelming infection or immunocompromised host.

The body part or organ system affected by the infection is often obvious from the client's history and presenting signs and symptoms. Identifying the system allows the range of possible infecting organisms to be narrowed to those known to affect that system. The manner of presentation provides further cues as to the diagnosis. For example, pneumococcal pneumonia typically presents with an acute onset of chills, fever, and cough in a previously healthy adult, whereas the client with viral pneumonia relates a gradual onset of symptoms, with systemic manifestations such as muscle aches and headache often predominant. A history of recent activities also provides clues. Family members who all vomit and have diarrhea within 12 hours after a picnic probably do not have the flu.

NURSING CARE OF THE OLDER ADULT | Infections

Because immune function declines with aging, older adults are more susceptible to infections. In fact, infections are among the top 10 causes for hospitalization and 1 of the 5 leading causes of death among people over 65 years of age.

Age-related changes may obscure the presentation of infection in older adults. Rather than an elevated temperature to signal an infection, confusion and subtle changes in behavior such as restlessness may be observed. The WBC count may be slightly elevated.

In addition to monitoring for changes in the client's mental status or behavior, the nurse should collect data on the amount of fluids consumed, urinary output, activity levels, complaints of fatigue, and respiratory status. A thorough assessment is necessary to facilitate an early diagnosis and prompt treatment that will improve outcomes for the older adult. Delay in treating infection may prolong the client's immobility and reduce the ability to perform activities of daily living.

Urinary Tract Infections
Urinary tract infection (UTI) is not only the most common infection but also the leading cause of bacteremia and sepsis in older adults. Factors that contribute to UTI include poor hygiene, incomplete bladder emptying, inadequate fluid intake, and long-term indwelling catheters. In addition, chronic conditions and medications may contribute to retention, which can result in urinary tract infection.

Respiratory Tract Infections
The leading causes of pneumonia in older adults include *S. pneumoniae, Haemophilus influenzae, Klebsiella pneumoniae, S. aureus,* and pneumococci. As a result of physiologic changes, the older adult with pneumonia may not present with cough or sputum production. Influenza A and B are prevalent in the aged; however, strain A accounts for greater illness severity and death (Eliopoulos, 2005). Both pneumonia and influenza cause high mortality rates in the older person.

Frail older adults, especially those with chronic respiratory conditions such as emphysema, are at risk for developing pneumonia as a complication of influenza. To prevent this complication, all persons over 65 should receive an annual immunization for influenza. In addition, pneumonia caused by pneumococcus bacteria can be deadly for older adults. Therefore, it is recommended that individuals over 65 also receive the pneumococcal immunization.

Tuberculosis has a relatively high incidence in older adults, especially those living in long-term care facilities. It often occurs as reactivation or secondary tuberculosis when the immune system can no longer contain the bacteria.

Other Infections
Older adults have the highest incidence of gangrene of the appendix and gallbladder. Diverticulitis increases due to chronic constipation and changes in the intestinal wall. Postoperative wound infections and decubitus ulcers are also most prevalent in older adults.

Nosocomial Infections
Nosocomial infections are more common in older adults. Nursing interventions should focus on prevention strategies such as (1) avoiding prolonged bed rest unless the medical condition contraindicates mobilization, (2) encouraging clients to take deep breaths, (3) providing adequate fluids, and (4) providing regular toileting schedules with good hygiene. The nurse must steadfastly adhere to principles of infection control.

Home Care
To prevent infection, the older adult should be taught to:
- Eat a well-balanced diet.
- Drink adequate fluids.
- Get adequate rest.
- Obtain an annual influenza immunization.
- Use good hand washing techniques.

Older adults and families should be taught to seek medical attention if they:
- Develop a fever or other signs and symptoms of infection.
- Exhibit changes in mental status and/or behavior.
- Experience fatigue or changes in activity levels.

Once the infecting agent has been identified, either positively or by probability, therapy can be specifically tailored to the client's needs. Viral infections often resolve without treatment other than supportive care, such as providing rest and fluids. Skin infections may respond to a topical agent, avoiding the potential adverse effects of one administered systemically.

Diagnosis

To assess the client's response to infection, identify the infecting organism, and monitor the progress of therapy, the following diagnostic tests may be ordered:

- *WBC count* provides clues about the infecting organism and the body's immune response to it (see Table 12–9).
- *WBC differential* is also ordered (see Table 12–9). Neutrophilia, increased numbers of circulating neutrophils (or PMNs), is a common response with infection as the bone marrow responds to an increased need for phagocytes. Along with neutrophilia, a shift to the left is common in acute infection. This means that there are more immature neutrophils in circulation than normal (Figure 12–13 ■), indicating an appropriate bone marrow response.
- *Procalcitonin (CTpr)* is a precursor of the hormone calcitonin. Procalcitonin increases dramatically during infection and sepsis and is accepted as both a marker of sepsis and a harmful mediator in lower respiratory tract and systemic infections (Christ-Crain et al., 2004; Müller & Becker, 2001).
- *Cultures of the wound, blood, or other infected body fluids* are used to identify probable microorganisms by their characteristics, such as shape, growth patterns, and Gram-staining qualities. After the organism is cultured, it is subjected to various antibiotics known to be effective against its particular strain to determine which antibiotic is likely to be most effective. This is known as sensitivity testing. Generally 24 to 48 hours are required to grow the organ-

ism, potentially delaying the institution of therapy. Because antibiotics (and possibly oxygen therapy) can alter the ability to culture an organism, specimens should be obtained before instituting therapy.

- *Serologic testing* provides an indirect means of identifying infecting agents by detecting antibodies to the suspected organism. When the antibody titer against a specific organism rises during the acute phase of an infectious disease and begins to fall during convalescence, the diagnosis is supported. Although it is not as accurate as culture, serology is particularly useful for organisms that cannot easily be cultured, such as hepatitis B or HIV (Porth, 2005).
- *Direct antigen detection methods* are in the process of being developed. These tests use monoclonal antibodies, which are purified antibody forms, to detect antigens in specimens from the diseased host (Porth, 2005). See Box 12–5. These tests offer rapid and accurate identification of the offending microorganism.
- *Antibiotic peak and trough levels* monitor therapeutic blood levels of the prescribed medication(s). The therapeutic range, that is, the minimum and maximum blood levels at which the drug is effective, is known for a given drug. By measuring blood levels at the predicted peak (1 to 2 hours after oral administration, 1 hour after intramuscular administration, and 30 minutes after intravenous administration) and trough (lowest level, usually a few minutes before the next scheduled dose), healthcare personnel can determine that the client is maintaining a level within the therapeutic range at all times, ensuring maximal effect from the drug. It is also possible to determine whether the drug is reaching a toxic or harmful level during therapy, increasing the likelihood of adverse effects.
- *Radiologic examination of the chest, abdomen, or urinary system* may be ordered to detect organ abnormalities indicating an inflammatory response or tissue damage.

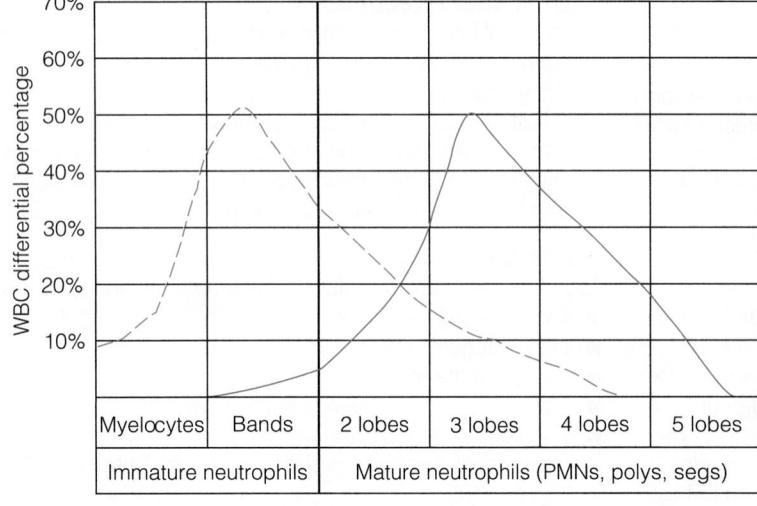

Type of WBC	Normal differential	Shift to left
Myelocytes	0%	Present
Band neutrophils (bands)	3% to 5%	Increased
Segmented neutrophils (segs, polys, PMNs)	50% to 65%	May be stable, increased, or decreased

Figure 12–13 ■ Neutrophils by stage of maturity and normal distribution in the blood.

BOX 12–5 Monoclonal Antibodies

Antigens typically have numerous antigenic determinant sites, each capable of stimulating a different subset of B cells. Each clone secretes a slightly different antibody from the others. The immunoglobulin produced as a result is therefore *polyclonal,* with multiple different antibodies. In 1975, researchers devised a technique for making a single clone of "immortal" B cells that could be maintained indefinitely in a laboratory and would produce a single antibody to a specific antigen (see figure below). This pure antibody, known as a *monoclonal* antibody, offers the following advantages:

- It can target specific antigens.
- It has a single, constant binding affinity for the antigen.
- It can be diluted to a specific titer or concentration, because it is not mixed with other antibodies.
- It can be purified to avoid adverse responses (McCance & Huether, 2002).

In addition to their use in providing passive protection from disease, multiple other uses are being identified for monoclonal antibodies, including the diagnosis and treatment of cancer, immunosuppression to prevent rejection of transplanted tissue or organs, immune response analysis, imaging techniques for diagnostic uses, and the early detection of viral infections (Lehne, 2004; McCance & Huether, 2002).

Source: Figure adapted from *The World of the Cell* by W. Becker & D. Deane, 1986, Redwood City, CA: Benjamin Cummings; *Textbook of Diagnostic Microbiology* by C. R. Mahon & G. Manuselis Jr., 1995, Philadelphia: W.B. Saunders. Reprinted by permission.

- *Lumbar puncture* is performed to obtain cerebrospinal fluid (CSF) for examination and culture if a central nervous system (CNS) infection, such as meningitis or encephalitis, is suspected.
- *Ultrasonic examination* is a noninvasive diagnostic test to evaluate organ function such as an echocardiogram or renal ultrasonography.

Medications

Once the infecting organism and affected body system have been identified, specific therapy to cure the infectious disease can be instituted. The number of antimicrobial agents available makes choosing the appropriate one seem overwhelming. The perfect anti-infective agent would destroy pathogens while preserving host cells, would be effective against many different organisms while not promoting the development of resistance, would distribute to necessary tissues, and would remain in the body for relatively long periods.

Because no currently available antimicrobial meets all the above criteria, physicians look for the agent that will be effective, has little toxicity, can be administered with relative convenience, and is cost effective. Characteristics of both the host and the infecting organism are considered in making the selection. The following host factors are considered in choosing an antimicrobial agent:

- *History of hypersensitivity.* Previous hypersensitivity responses to an antimicrobial contraindicate the use of that agent or one of its class.
- *Age and childbearing status of the client.* Sulfonamides and tetracyclines as well as some less common agents are contraindicated for pregnant women due to their possible effects on the fetus. Some drugs may cross into breast milk.
- *Renal function.* Because most antimicrobials are excreted through the kidneys, renal function is important. Impaired renal function may contraindicate a specific drug, such as an aminoglycoside, because of its nephrotoxicity, or it may call for a reduced dosage.
- *Hepatic function.* Because hepatic function may alter the metabolism of a particular antimicrobial, the risk of toxicity increases. Again, certain drugs are avoided with impaired hepatic function; others may dictate a reduced dosage.
- *Site of the infection.* The infection site is critical in choosing both the antimicrobial to be used and the route by which it is administered. Antimicrobials can be applied topically or administered by oral, intramuscular, intravenous, interperitoneal, intrathecal, or intramedullary routes. Oral and intravenous routes are most commonly used.
- *Other host factors.* Chronic diseases or other medications in the treatment regimen are also considered.

Antimicrobial preparations are broadly classified as bacteriostatic or bactericidal. **Bacteriostatic agents** inhibit the growth of the microorganism, leaving its destruction to the host's immune system. These agents are generally not indicated for the immunocompromised host. Tetracyclines, erythromycin, and chloramphenicol are bacteriostatic preparations. **Bactericidal agents** are capable of killing the organism without immune system intervention. These include the penicillins, cephalosporins, and aminoglycoside antibiotics.

The activity of antimicrobial agents on bacteria, fungi, and viruses falls under five basic mechanisms:

- Impairing cell wall synthesis, leading to lysis and cell destruction
- Inhibiting protein synthesis, causing impaired microbial function
- Altering cell membrane permeability, causing intracellular contents to leak
- Inhibiting the synthesis of nucleic acids
- Inhibiting cell metabolism and growth.

Obviously, agents that work on the cell wall will not be effective against organisms that have no cell wall, such as mycoplasma and viruses. The antimicrobial's spectrum of activity is also considered in making a selection. Therapy is often initiated with a broad-spectrum antimicrobial until the specific organism is identified.

Finally, many microorganisms have the ability to develop resistance to an anti-infective agent; that is, the pathogen continues to live and grow in the presence of the anti-infective. Resistance develops as a result of a chance mutation by the pathogen, al-

lowing a subpopulation of cells to survive. The chance of an organism's becoming resistant to an agent is partially related to the dose delivered. Resistance is less likely to occur when a lethal dose is administered; therefore, it is vital that clients understand the need to take all doses of the prescribed drug as ordered.

Antimicrobial medications are generally classified as antibacterial or antibiotic, antiviral, antifungal, and antiparasitic.

ANTIBIOTICS Medications used to treat bacterial infections are generally known as antibiotics. Their development and use began before World War II and has proliferated rapidly since. Most antibiotics are biologic substances, that is, substances produced by other microorganisms. Antibiotics fall into classes of drugs with related chemical structure and activity. Some are effective against only gram-positive bacteria, and others are effective against only gram-negative organisms. Newer broad-spectrum antibiotics have activity against a wide variety of bacteria, including both gram-positive and gram-negative forms. No antibiotic is totally safe. Hypersensitivity responses occur, and some drugs are toxic to organ systems, exhibiting hepatotoxicity, nephrotoxicity, ototoxicity, or bone marrow suppression. Therefore, always check for allergies before administering the first dose. The antibiotics presented in the Medication Administration box are organized according to their antibacterial action.

ANTIVIRALS Antiviral therapy is a relatively new phenomenon. Most antibiotics have little effect on viruses, because the virus has no cell wall and no cytoplasm, produces no enzymes, and sequesters itself in a host cell to reproduce. Antiviral agents must be very selective in differentiating normal cellular activity from viral activity. In addition, the immune function of the host is a vital component in fighting viral infections; antiviral therapy may be relatively ineffective in the severely immunocompromised host. Making a timely diagnosis to allow institution of antiviral therapy can be an additional problem, because viruses are less easily identified using laboratory techniques. Antiviral agents in common use are summarized in the Medication Administration box on page 322. Antiretroviral agents used in the management of HIV and AIDS are presented in Chapter 13 ∞.

ANTIFUNGALS Antifungal agents are available in both topical and systemic forms. They act by interfering with the cytoplasmic membrane of the fungus. Topical agents include preparations for cutaneous use to treat candidiasis, tineas, and ringworm. Vaginal preparations to treat vulvovaginal candidiasis are also available, as are several nonprescription topical and vaginal antifungal agents.

Amphotericin B (Fungizone) is a systemic antifungal agent for parenteral administration. It is used to treat severe, life-threatening fungal infections including histoplasmosis, blastomycosis, and candidiasis. Another systemic antifungal in current use is flucytosine (Ancobon). Unlike amphotericin B, flucytosine can be administered orally. It is used to treat severe candidiasis infections such as candida septicemia, endocarditis, pulmonary or urinary tract infections, and *Cryptococcus* meningitis.

Fluconazole (Diflucan) has the broadest use as an antifungal agent. It can be administered either orally or parenterally and is

MEDICATION ADMINISTRATION Antibiotic Therapy

I. Cell Wall Synthesis Inhibitors

PENICILLINS

Penicillin G	Dicloxacillin (Dynapen)
Penicillin V	Methicillin (Staphcillin)
Amoxicillin (Amoxil)	Mezlocillin (Mezlin)
Amoxicillin and potassium	Nafcillin (Unipen)
clavulanate (Augmentin)	Oxacillin (Prostaphlin)
Ampicillin (Polycillin)	Piperacillin (Pipracil)
Carbenicillin (Geopen, Geocillin)	Ticarcillin (Ticar)

Penicillins are bactericidal and interfere with cell wall synthesis and the enzymes involved in cell division and synthesis. They are more effective on gram-positive than gram-negative organisms. Resistance is now more common among *Streptococci* and *Staphylococci.* They are considered to be safe, effective, and of low toxicity.

Nursing Responsibilities

- Monitor for hypersensitivity responses such as local erythema and itching at the site of injection, skin rashes, urticaria (hives), itching, fever, chills, and anaphylaxis.
- Observe clients receiving parenteral penicillin for at least 30 minutes.
- Discontinue the drug immediately if any hypersensitivity response occurs. Be prepared to administer antihistamines or corticosteroids for a mild reaction. Anaphylaxis is treated with epinephrine subcutaneously or intravenously and airway support.
- Do not administer penicillin to anyone with a history of a severe allergic reaction to any form of the drug; a cross-reactivity may occur in clients allergic to cephalosporin or carbapenem antibiotics.
- Assess for superinfection (vaginitis, stomatitis, or diarrhea) due to elimination of resident bacteria.
- Monitor for therapeutic response.

Health Education for the Client and Family

- Notify the physician if you see white patches on the oral mucosa or if vaginitis develops. An antifungal drug may be prescribed and the antibiotic continued.
- Consuming yogurt or buttermilk may prevent superinfection. Do not take these products within 1 hour of taking the drug.

CEPHALOSPORINS

1st Generation	2nd Generation
Cephalexin (Keflex)	Cefotetan (Cefotan)
Cefazolin (Ancef)	Cefaclor (Ceclor)
	Cefmetazole (Zefazone)

3rd Generation	4th Generation
Cefoperazone (Cefobid)	Cefepime (Maxapime)
Ceftazidime (Fortaz)	
Ceftriaxone (Rocephin)	

Cephalosporins are structurally similar to the penicillins and also inhibit cell wall synthesis. They are divided into four groups, or generations. First-generation cephalosporins act primarily against gram-positive organisms. Second- and third-generation drugs are more effective against gram-negative organisms than against gram-positive ones. Fourth-generation cephalosporins act effectively against both gram-positive and gram-negative organisms.

Nursing Responsibilities

- Monitor for previous hypersensitivity response to cephalosporins or penicillins.
- Assess intravenous site for phlebitis; intramuscular site may cause local pain.
- Monitor laboratory results for adverse response, such as leukopenia and thrombocytopenia, nephrotoxicity (elevated BUN and serum creatinine), or hepatotoxicity (elevated bilirubin, LDH, ALT, AST, and alkaline phosphatase).
- Assess for signs of superinfections.

Health Education for the Client and Family

- Take the medication on an empty stomach, 1 hour before or 2 hours after meals.
- Avoid alcohol while using cefmetazole, cefoperazone, or cefotetan because alcohol intolerance can develop with these antibiotics. These same drugs intensify bleeding tendencies.
- Space doses of the medication relatively evenly throughout the day and evening hours.
- Increase consumption of buttermilk or yogurt to prevent intestinal superinfection.

CARBAPENEMS

This newer class of antibiotics includes only three drugs and all must be given parenterally. Imipenem has the broadest antimicrobial spectrum of any drug (Lehne, 2004). This makes it especially useful against mixed organism infections. Imipenem, meropenem, and ertapenem cross the meninges and achieve therapeutic doses in CSF; they are effective against MRSA. These antibiotics cause bacterial cell wall lysis and subsequent death of the bacteria. Side effects include nausea and vomiting, diarrhea, hypersensitivity reactions, occasional superinfections with bacteria or fungi, and, rarely, seizures.

Nursing Responsibilities

Ertapenem should not be mixed with dextrose or other drugs containing dextrose. IV infusions should be slow and given over at least 30 minutes. The dosage of all three drugs should be reduced if there is evidence of renal impairment.

- Check for history of hypersensitivity to cephalosporins and penicillins and monitor for signs of reactions.
- Assess for signs of superinfection.
- Monitor laboratory indicators of renal function.

Health Education for the Client and Family

- Instruct client to report any signs or symptoms of allergy such as skin rash, itching, or hives.

VANCOMYCIN

This antibiotic inhibits cell wall synthesis and is used for serious infections. It is only effective against gram-positive bacteria, especially *S. aureus* and *Staphylococcus epidermidis* including the strains resistant to methicillin. *C. difficile* is also susceptible to this antibiotic, but infection with *C. difficile* is often treated first with metronidazole to delay emergence of resistance to vancomycin.

Nursing Responsibilities

- Infuse slowly over 60 minutes or more to avoid "red man" syndrome. The syndrome is characterized by erythematous rash, flushing, tachycardia, and hypotension. Clients may become dizzy and agitated. The occurrence is usually associated with a first dose of vancomycin and is seen within 4 to 6 minutes of the start of a dose or after completion.
- Ototoxicity is a more serious adverse effect of vancomycin because hearing loss may be irreversible. Clients may report a

(continued)

sensation of fullness in their ears; this is evidence that ototoxicity is developing.

OXAZOLIDINONES

Linezolid is the first antibiotic in a new class of antibiotics called oxazolidinones. This antibiotic is significant because it is effective against organisms that are resistant to both vancomycin and methicillin. Because of its usefulness against those organisms, these drugs should be reserved for infections caused by VRE and MRSA (Lehne, 2004).

Nursing Responsibilities

This drug is generally well tolerated. Common side effects include nausea, diarrhea, and headache. It can cause reversible myelo-suppression if used for longer than 2 weeks. It is a weak inhibitor of monoamine oxidase, creating risk for hypertension. It also prevents serotonin uptake so it increases the risk of serotonin syndrome when taken with selective serotonin reuptake inhibitors.

Health Education for the Client and Family

It can be taken with or without food. Avoid taking ephedrine, pseudoephedrine, methylphenidate, or cocaine with this drug. Hypertension may develop. Large amounts of foods containing tyramine should be avoided because the combination could cause headaches. Tyramine is generally found in foods that have been preserved or aged. Using leftovers with soy sauce or salami that have been refrigerated more than 24 to 48 hours may cause headaches.

B-LACTAMASE INHIBITORS

Clavulanic acid sulbactam

Combination agents

Unasyn

Timentin

Zosyn

Augmentin

II. Bacterial Protein Synthesis Inhibitors

TETRACYCLINES

Tetracycline HCl   **Minocycline HCl (Minocin)**

Doxycycline (Vibramycin) **Oxytetracycline (Terramycin)**

Tetracyclines are active against many gram-positive and gram-negative bacteria, such as *Mycoplasma, Rickettsia*, and *Chlamydia*. They are bacteriostatic, interfering with microbial protein synthesis. Tetracycline binds readily with metal and solid elements in the bowel, limiting its absorption when administered with food; the other preparations are highly soluble in lipids and can be administered with food.

Nursing Responsibilities

- Schedule doses 1 hour before or 2 hours after meals. Do not give with milk or milk products or antacids.
- Monitor for signs of superinfection.
- If the client is taking an anticoagulant, monitor prothrombin time and for signs of bleeding.

Health Education for the Client and Family

- Avoid excessive sun exposure to reduce the risk of photosensitivity reactions.

MACROLIDES

Erythromycin (E-Mycin)   **Clarithromycin**

Azithromycin (Zithromax)   **Erythromycin salts (Ilosone, E.E.S., Erythrocin)**

Macrolides are bacteriostatic and act effectively against gram-positive and gram-negative organisms. Erythromycin is used to treat streptococcal pharyngitis in clients who are allergic to penicillin. Azithromycin is ordered more frequently because the client takes the drug for 5 days, increasing client adherence.

Nursing Responsibilities

- Administer erythromycin on an empty stomach or immediately before meals.
- Give the drug with a full glass of water. Do not administer with acidic fruit juice.

Health Education for the Client and Family

- Gastric distress is a common side effect with erythromycin.

AMINOGLYCOSIDES

Amikacin (Amikin)   **Gentamicin (Garamycin)**

Kanamycin (Kantrex)   **Netilmicin (Netromycin)**

Streptomycin   **Tobramycin (Nebcin)**

Aminoglycosides are bactericidal, interfering with protein synthesis in the pathogen. They are especially effective against gram-negative organisms. To provide a broader spectrum of activity, they are often combined with other antibiotics, especially penicillins. Aminoglycosides can be administered in multiple or single daily doses. They are ototoxic and nephrotoxic; the risk is highest for older adults, clients with preexisting renal disease, and persons receiving other ototoxic or nephrotoxic drugs.

Nursing Responsibilities

- Assess renal function before and during aminoglycoside therapy. Monitor intake and output, daily weight, BUN, and serum creatinine.
- Assess for adverse effects on hearing such as loss of perception of high tones, tinnitus, and vertigo.
- Notify the physician if the client is receiving other nephrotoxic or ototoxic drugs such as furosemide (Lasix) and ethacrynic acid (Edecrin).
- Administer intravenous preparations separately from other drugs; flush tubing before and after administration.

Health Education for the Client and Family

- Monitor for a sudden weight gain that may indicate adverse effects on the kidney and report it to the physician.

III. Bacterial Nucleic Acid Inhibitors

FLUOROQUINOLONES

Ciprofloxacin (Cipro)   **Gatifloxacin (Tequin)**

Levofloxacin (Levaquin)

Fluoroquinolones are bactericidal and especially active against gram-negative and some gram-positive organisms. They are used to manage infections of the respiratory, gastrointestinal, and genitourinary tracts.

Nursing Responsibilities

- Increase fluid intake to 2000 to 3000 mL/day unless contraindicated to prevent crystalluria.
- Monitor laboratory results for hepatotoxicity (elevated ALT, AST).

Health Education for the Client and Family

- Drink six to eight glasses of water per day.
- Avoid exposure to sunlight while taking these drugs.

MEDICATION ADMINISTRATION Antibiotic Therapy (continued)

SULFONAMIDES AND TRIMETHOPRIM
Sulfamethizole (Thiosulfil Forte)
Sulfamethoxazole (Gantanol; in combination with trimethoprim, TMP-SMZ, Bactrim, Septra)
Sulfisoxazole (Gantrisin)

Sulfonamides are bacteriostatic. Trimethoprim is an antibiotic effective against most gram-positive and many gram-negative organisms. It is often combined with sulfamethoxazole to manage urinary tract infections, *P. carinii* pneumonia, and otitis media. Skin rashes and pruritus are the most common hypersensitivity reactions. Severe reactions include exfoliative dermatitis and Stevens-Johnson syndrome.

Nursing Responsibilities
- Assess for history of hypersensitivity to sulfonamides and related medications, such as thiazide diuretics and hypoglycemic preparations.
- Monitor intake and output. Maintain a fluid intake of at least 1500 mL/day.
- Assess for evidence of bleeding, easy bruising, or systemic infection, and monitor blood count for possible bone marrow depression.

Health Education for the Client and Family
- Take medication on an empty stomach with a full glass of water. Maintain a fluid intake of at least 2 quarts per day.
- Protect the skin from excessive sun exposure with clothing and sunscreens to reduce the risk of photosensitivity.

METRONIDAZOLE (FLAGYL)
Metronidazole is effective against anaerobic gram-negative bacteria and protozoan infections caused by amebiasis, giardiasis, and trichomoniasis. It is commonly used to prevent and treat infections following intestinal surgery, and is the drug of first choice with *C. difficile*.

Nursing Responsibilities
- Monitor for CNS effects of dizziness, headache, ataxia, confusion, depression, and peripheral neuropathy.
- Administer with food to minimize gastric distress and metallic taste. Infuse intravenous metronidazole over 60 minutes.
- Discontinue the medication and notify the physician if neurologic reactions occur.
- Increase fluid intake to 2500 mL/day to minimize the risk of nephrotoxicity.

Health Education for the Client and Family
- This medication may turn urine reddish brown; caution client that this is expected and not harmful.
- Discontinue the drug and notify the physician if hypersensitivity reaction or adverse effects occur, such as changes in mentation or coordination, painful or frequent urination, painful or difficult intercourse, impotence.
- Do not drink alcohol while taking this medication; an Antabuse-type reaction (flushing, sweating, headache, vomiting, and abdominal cramps) may occur.
- Maintain a fluid intake of 2.5 to 3 quarts per day.
- When the drug is prescribed for *Trichomonas* infections, treatment of both partners is necessary.
- While taking metronidazole, use condoms to prevent cross-contamination during intercourse.

---

used to treat candidiasis infections as well as *Cryptococcus* meningitis. It is generally better tolerated than other systemic antifungal medications.

ANTIPARASITICS Drugs used to treat parasitic infections are as varied as the organisms that cause them. Generally, agents classified as antiparasitic are both expensive and likely to be toxic. Quinine was one of the first antiparasitic drugs developed in the treatment of malaria. Quinine is highly toxic, but newer forms such as chloroquine (Aralen, Chlorocon) and hydroxychloroquine (Plaquenil) are widely used as antimalarial drugs. Metronidazole (e.g., Flagyl) is used to treat infections of protozoan parasites (see the Medication Administration box above).

Isolation Techniques

Controlling the spread of infectious diseases in the hospital or long-term care setting is particularly important to preventing nosocomial infection. Hand washing remains the single most important factor in preventing the transmission of infections. Not all infectious diseases spread readily, necessitating special techniques or procedures. However, diseases such as chickenpox (varicella) and pulmonary tuberculosis are highly contagious and are spread by the airborne route, requiring special precautions to protect other hospitalized clients. Two newer airborne threats are SARS and avian flu. These are addressed in Chapter 37 ∞.

In determining the need for isolation precautions, healthcare personnel consider the usual reservoir or source of the microorganism, the mode of transmission, and susceptibility of hospital staff and other clients. For example, clients with *P. carinii* pneumonia do not require isolation, because immunocompetent persons are not susceptible to this infection.

The CDC has published guidelines for isolation precautions to be used in healthcare facilities (Glover, 2000). These guidelines include both *standard precautions* and *category-specific isolation precautions*.

Standard Precautions

Standard Precautions, published by the Hospital Infection Control Practices Advisory Committee of the Centers for Disease Control in 1996, provides guidelines for the handling of blood and other body fluids. These guidelines are used with all clients, regardless of whether they have a known infectious disease. The guidelines were developed in light of the realization that many clients with an infectious disease such as HIV or hepatitis B have no apparent symptoms, but can transmit the disease to others. Standard precautions are used by all healthcare workers who have direct contact with clients or with their body fluids or have indirect contact, such as by emptying trash, changing linens, or cleaning the room.

MEDICATION ADMINISTRATION — Antiviral Agents

AMANTADINE (SYMMETREL)
Amantadine is used to prevent and treat influenza A. It has been shown to be 55% to 80% or more effective in preventing the disease. When administered within 24 to 72 hours after the onset of symptoms, it reduces common manifestations of influenza. It is generally well tolerated; minimal CNS side effects, such as dizziness, anxiety, insomnia, and difficulty concentrating, may occur.

ACYCLOVIR (ZOVIRAX) AND GANCICLOVIR (CYTOVENE)
Acyclovir and ganciclovir are related compounds used primarily in the treatment of herpes viruses. Acyclovir is prescribed mainly in the treatment of genital herpes simplex infections. Although it does not kill the virus, acyclovir is effective in reducing the severity, duration, and frequency of recurrence of symptoms. Ganciclovir is indicated primarily in the treatment of cytomegalovirus infection. Although acyclovir is generally well tolerated with little toxicity, ganciclovir may profoundly suppress bone marrow function, and its use is therefore limited.

ZIDOVUDINE (AZT, RETROVIR)
Zidovudine inhibits replication of HIV, although it does not kill it. Zidovudine's use is limited to clients with symptomatic HIV infection or CD4 cell counts of less than 200/mm^3. Zidovudine may be administered either orally or parenterally. Many clients are unable to tolerate recommended doses because of the drug's adverse effects, including nausea, anorexia, malaise, severe anemia, and granulocytopenia. Zidovudine is usually administered in combination with other antiretroviral medications.

VIDARABINE (VIRA-A)
Vidarabine inhibits viral DNA synthesis and is effective against many herpesvirus infections. Its primary use is in treatment of herpes simplex encephalitis.

INTERFERONS
Interferons are naturally produced cytokines whose use as antiviral agents is being explored. When administered intranasally, interferons have been shown to be effective in preventing rhinovirus upper respiratory infections. Other uses being explored include treatment of human papillomavirus (genital warts) and preventing or reducing Kaposi's sarcoma in clients with AIDS. They are also used in combination biotherapy regimens for malignant melanoma.

Standard precautions apply to the following:

- Blood
- All body fluids, secretions, and excretions, regardless of whether they contain visible blood
- Nonintact skin
- Mucous membranes.

Barrier protection is used to prevent exposing skin and mucous membrane surfaces to blood and body fluids. Barrier protection involves using gloves for touching or handling body fluids, and adding other protection such as gowns, masks, and goggles if splashing or spraying is likely. Needles and other sharp objects are not recapped or bent, but disposed of in puncture-proof containers to prevent inadvertent percutaneous (needle-stick) exposure. Standard precautions are presented in Appendix A.

Transmission-Based Precautions
In addition to hand washing and standard precautions, the nature and spread of some infectious diseases require that special techniques be used to protect uninfected clients and workers. The CDC identifies three types of transmission-based precautions: airborne, droplet, and contact precautions. Transmission-based precautions may be combined for diseases that have multiple routes of transmission. Indications for the use of transmission-based isolation precautions and the specific measures to be taken are outlined in Table 12–10.

NURSING CARE

Nursing management related to infectious disease has two foci: (1) *prevention* and (2) *health promotion and maintenance*. Prevention focuses on assessing the client's risk for infection based on underlying conditions, immune response, and prophylactic measures such as immunizations.

Health Promotion
Preventing infection requires education of not only healthcare personnel but also the general public. Part of an education program includes understanding the importance of immunizations, the guidelines for using antibiotics to prevent drug-resistant microorganisms, and the ways to prevent the spread of infection. Check immunization records for all family members and encourage them to keep immunizations up to date. Increase public awareness regarding appropriate antibiotic use. Guidelines for preventing the spread of infection to others include the following:

- Avoid crowds and contact with susceptible persons, especially those who are immunosuppressed (e.g., persons who have HIV infection, who are undergoing therapy for cancer, or who have had an organ transplant).
- Use disposable tissues to contain respiratory secretions when coughing or sneezing.
- Use appropriate food-handling precautions for diseases spread via the fecal–oral route, such as hepatitis A.
- Avoid contact with or sharing of body fluids. For example, do not share needles or razors; use a condom during sexual activity, or abstain; have each person clean their own blood spills or wounds if possible.

Assessment
The following data are collected through the health history and physical examination. Further focused assessments are described with nursing interventions in the next section.

TABLE 12–10 Transmission-Based Precautions

CATEGORY	INFECTIOUS DISEASES	PURPOSE	PRECAUTIONS
Airborne precautions	Pulmonary tuberculosis, chickenpox (with contact precautions), measles, respiratory infections (pneumonia)	Reduce risk of airborne transmission of infectious agents. Airborne transmission occurs by dissemination of either airborne droplet nuclei or dust particles containing the infectious agent.	Private room with hand washing and toilet facilities, and special ventilation that does not allow air to circulate to general hospital ventilation; mask or special filter respirator for everyone entering room.
Droplet precautions	Meningitis, pertussis	Reduce risk of droplet transmission of infectious agents. Droplet transmission involves contact of conjunctivae of the eyes or mucous membranes of the nose or mouth with large-particle droplets generated during coughing, sneezing, talking, or procedures such as suctioning.	Private room with hand washing and toilet facilities; mask, eye protection, and/or face shields worn by everyone entering room.
Contact precautions	Acute diarrhea, chickenpox (with airborne precautions), respiratory syncytial virus (RSV); skin, wound, or urinary tract infection with multidrug-resistant organisms; S. aureus infections	Reduce risk of transmission by direct or indirect contact. Direct contact transmission involves skin-to-skin contact and physical transfer of organisms. It may occur between clients or during direct care activities such as bathing or turning clients. Indirect contact involves contact with a contaminated object.	Private room with hand washing and toilet facilities; gowns and protective apparel to provide barrier protection; disposable supplies or decontamination of all articles leaving room.

- *Health history:* age, medication use (antipyretics and anti-infectives), nutrition, exposure to infectious persons, immunizations, invasive procedures and therapies, chronic diseases such as diabetes mellitus, cancer
- *Physical assessment:* vital signs, body system(s) where infection is suspected, lymph node enlargement, and tenderness.

Nursing Diagnoses and Interventions

Clients with an infection may be managed in the hospital or at home. During the acute phase, nursing care includes administering prescribed antibiotics, implementing and maintaining aseptic technique and infection control measures, and encouraging a balance of rest and activity, good nutritional intake, and other general health measures to support immunologic function and healing. The key nursing diagnoses are *Risk for Infection, Anxiety, Hyperthermia,* and *Pain.*

Risk for Infection

The spread of infection is a risk in any facility that houses many people. It is a particular risk in hospitals, where many clients have at least some degree of immunosuppression and many drug-resistant strains of pathogens are prevalent. It is vital that nurses use good hand washing techniques at all times, employ standard precautions with all clients, and use category-specific isolation techniques as indicated to prevent infectious spread to other clients, themselves, and their families.

- Admit clients with known or suspected infections to a private room. *This is important to minimize the risk to other clients.*
- Wash hands on entering and leaving the client's room, using a 10- to 15-second vigorous scrub with soap or antibacterial scrub solution. *A 10- to 15-second scrub removes transient microorganisms from the skin and helps prevent transmission of infection to or from the client.*
- Use standard precautions and personal protective devices to reduce the risk of transmission. *Gloves, gowns, and masks are to be worn whenever there is a risk of skin or mucous membrane contamination by direct contact with infectious material, airborne spread of organisms, or droplet nuclei.*
- Explain the reasons for and importance of isolation procedures during hospitalization. *Clients with isolation precautions may feel neglected, dirty, or shunned. Explanation of reasons and procedures can enhance the client's and family's understanding and acceptance.*
- Place a mask on the client and/or cover all infectious lesions or wounds completely when transporting the client to other parts of the facility for diagnostic or treatment procedures. *These measures help minimize air contamination and the risk to visitors and personnel.*
- Collect a culture and sensitivity (C&S) specimen as ordered or indicated by purulent drainage, pyuria, or other manifestations of infection. *C&S is performed to determine the presence and type of infectious organisms as well as antibiotics most likely to be effective in eradicating it.*

PRACTICE ALERT
Collect the specimen before the first dose of antibiotics is administered to ensure adequate organisms for culture.

- Administer prescribed anti-infective agents. *Anti-infectives are used to destroy the invading microorganism.*
- Inform all personnel having contact with the client of the diagnosis. *This is particularly important for a client with a disease requiring category-specific isolation so that personnel can take appropriate precautions.*
- Ensure that visitors don appropriate protective wear before they enter the client's room. *Protective wear reduces their risk of infection.*
- Use appropriate measures for disposing of contaminated tissues, dressings, or other material and for removing soiled linens and equipment from the client's room. *Check hospital policy or published guidelines for category-specific isolation.*
- Teach the importance of complying with prescribed treatment for the entire course of the regimen. *Because anti-infective agents kill only a portion of the pathogen population with each dose, completion of the entire course of therapy is necessary to reduce the risk of relapse and of creating drug-resistant organisms.*

Anxiety

The client with an infectious disease may experience anxiety related to his or her manifestations, treatment measures, the prognosis, and expected outcome of the disease. The diagnosis of an infection can be traumatic, causing feelings of uneasiness, isolation, guilt (e.g., in regard to sexually transmitted infections), apprehension, or depression.

- Assess level of anxiety. *The level of anxiety influences the client's response to and interpretation of the situation and degree of threat it poses.*
- Discuss the infection, treatments, prognosis, and outcomes. *Discussions help to allay fears and misconceptions.*
- Support and enhance the client's coping strategies. *A person uses intrapersonal and interpersonal mechanisms to reduce or relieve anxiety.*
- Include significant others in the plan of care. *Inclusion of the client and family members provides assurance and confidence, and promotes understanding of the unknown.*
- Explain isolation procedures, and answer any concerns. *Isolation may be necessary to prevent the spread of infection but can cause great anxiety for the client and family members.*
- Provide referrals as needed for continuing care, for example, to home health agencies or for dressing changes or periodic assessment. *Referrals are often necessary to provide ongoing interventions and maintain continuity of care.*

Hyperthermia

Hyperthermia is an expected consequence of the infectious disease process. Fever may produce mild, short-term effects or, when prolonged, may cause serious life-threatening effects.

- Monitor temperature especially during episodes of chills; note heart rate and rhythm. *Chills indicate a rising temperature. Hyperthermia can cause dysrhythmias.*

PRACTICE ALERT
Monitor temperature between 5 P.M. and 7 P.M. because the body's daily temperature cycle peaks at this point.

- Administer prescribed antipyretic as indicated for elevated temperature. *Although antipyretics lower the temperature and enhance comfort for the client, this benefit must be weighed against the possible beneficial effect of an elevated temperature in the immune response. Fever increases the motility and activity of WBCs, stimulates the production of interferon, and activates T cells. In addition, temperatures above the normal range inhibit the growth of many microorganisms (Porth, 2005).*
- Promote body cooling through lowering the room temperature. *Rapid cooling stimulates the hypothalamus to increase the body's temperature; this increases both shivering and metabolic rate.*

PRACTICE ALERT
Use ice packs, cool/tepid baths, or hypothermia blanket with caution to prevent unnecessary shivering.

- Monitor fluid loss; encourage increased fluid and electrolyte intake either orally or intravenously. *Hyperthermia causes fluid loss from evaporation and may result in dehydration and electrolyte imbalance.*
- If diaphoretic, bathe and provide dry clothing and bedding. *These measures increase client comfort and decrease further water evaporation.*
- Promote rest periods. *Rest increases energy reserve that is depleted by an increased metabolic, heart, and respiratory rate.*

Pain, Acute

Pain often accompanies infections as part of the inflammatory process or secondary to delayed healing. *Increasing pain in a wound may signal infection, especially if accompanied by erythema or purulence. Keep the wound clean and dry and administer prescribed antibiotics to promote healing and decrease pain.*

Using NANDA, NIC, and NOC

Chart 12–1 shows links between NANDA, NIC, and NOC when caring for the client with an infection.

Community-Based Care

Client and family teaching is directed toward helping the client recover from the infection or disease, preventing its spread to others, and preventing life-threatening complications. Instructions should include the following points:

- Use good hand washing techniques, particularly after touching infected wounds or lesions, coughing, sneezing, blowing the nose, or using the bathroom. Wash hands thoroughly before eating or performing any procedures such as dressing changes. Wash hands with soap and water before and after preparing food or eating and before and after using the toilet or handling diapers. Do not share eating utensils.
- Take all prescribed antibiotics as ordered even after symptoms have subsided. Take the prescription at intervals around the clock as directed.
- Never allow anyone else to use your medications and never use anyone else's prescription even if they appear to be the same.

NANDA, NIC AND NOC LINKAGES
CHART 12–1 **The Client with an Infection**

NANDA

Delayed Surgical Recovery

NIC

Infection Control

Medication Administration

Vital Signs Monitoring

Wound Care

NOC

Infection Severity

Wound Healing: Primary Intention

Post Procedure Recovery Status

Data from *NANDA's Nursing Diagnoses: Definitions & Classification 2005–2006* by NANDA International (2003), Philadelphia; *Nursing Interventions Classification (NIC)* (4th ed.) by J. M. Dochterman & G. M. Bulechek (2004), St. Louis, MO: Mosby; and *Nursing Outcomes Classification (NOC)* (3rd ed.) by S. Moorhead, M. Johnson, and M. Maas (2004), St. Louis, MO: Mosby.

- If instructed to stop taking a medication, destroy any that remains by flushing in toilet or garbage disposal
    Notify your healthcare provider if:
  - Symptoms do not improve within 24 to 48 hours after antibiotic therapy is instituted, or they worsen.
  - Signs of antibiotic allergy (itching, rash, difficulty breathing or swallowing, swelling of the face or tongue) occur. Discontinue medication and contact prescriber.
  - Adverse responses, such as gastrointestinal distress, interfere with completion of the prescription.
  - Signs of superinfection (vaginitis, oral candidiasis, or diarrhea) occur.
  - Manifestations of infection recur after completing prescribed antibiotic.
- Report redness, swelling, or drainage around wounds or persistent high fever.
- Increase fluid intake to at least 2500 mL (2.5 quarts) per day.
- Report any signs of opportunistic infections: loose, watery, and foul-smelling diarrhea; vaginal discharge or itching; fuzzy growth or white plaques in mouth or on tongue; blood in urine, chills, fever, or unusual cough.
- In addition, suggest the following resources:
  - County or public health department
  - Centers for Disease Control and Prevention

EXPLORE MediaLink

Prentice Hall Nursing MediaLink DVD-ROM
Audio Glossary
NCLEX-RN® Review

Animations/Video
Inflammatory Response
Penicillin
White Blood Cells

COMPANION WEBSITE www.prenhall.com/lemone
Audio Glossary
NCLEX-RN® Review
Care Plan Activity: Postoperative Infection
Case Study: The Client with an Infection
MediaLink Applications
   Antibiotic-Resistant Organisms
   Hopsital-Acquired Infections
Links to Resources

CHAPTER HIGHLIGHTS

- The human body has a remarkable capacity to survive in an environment of deadly microorganisms and pathogens that can weaken and kill the body. Both natural barriers and the immune system prevent the invasion and replication of pathogens. The lymphatic system provides conduits for pathogens, isolating them from the bloodstream where they would grow rapidly.

- The adaptability and specificity of immune responses is possible because immune cells are genetically encoded to capture pathogens, move them to lymph nodes, and develop specific immune reactions. However, if the immune system's self-recognition fails, highly damaging autoimmune diseases can develop.

- A revolutionary increase in knowledge and understanding of the immune system has enabled progress in clinical medicine. Through scientific research concerning T and B lymphocytes, cytokines, antibodies, and other elements of the immune system, treatments are evolving for cancer, AIDs, organ transplantation, autoimmune diseases, infectious disease, and vaccines.
- Inflammation is a protective mechanism designed to prevent pathogens from entering the bloodstream and populating functional tissues such as heart, liver, and kidney. Pain acts as a signal that tissue has been damaged and stimulates protective responses such as cleansing wounds and limiting function while healing progresses. Restoration occurs as the inflammatory process isolates the injury and repairs damaged tissue.
- Localized infections may damage tissue and create pain, but systemic infections are life-threatening if they progress to septic shock. Unfortunately, hospitals are hazardous environments populated with collections of pathogens. Hospital-borne infections are often introduced into the body by medical procedures.
- Hygiene, protection from harm, and nutrition support the immune defenses. Antimicrobial medications limit the spread of pathogens, but can lose their effectiveness when microbes mutate and develop resistance.

TEST YOURSELF NCLEX-RN® REVIEW

1 When a client receives gamma globulin following exposure to hepatitis A, the nurse expects the client to develop:
  1. natural passive immunity. *wrong intact*
  2. natural active immunity.
  3. acquired passive immunity.
  4. acquired active immunity.

2 When performing a physical assessment of a client, the nurse should expect which of these findings related to a systemic infection?
  1. erythema
  2. enlarged lymph nodes
  3. pain
  4. decreased heart rate

3 Which one of the following medications is known to inhibit prostaglandin synthesis?
  1. acetaminophen (Tylenol)
  2. prednisone
  3. penicillin
  4. aspirin

4 The client with an acute infection shows a shift to the left on the WBC differential count. The nurse recognizes a shift to the left because of which laboratory finding?
  1. increased band neutrophils
  2. increased eosinophils
  3. decreased leukocytes
  4. decreased monocytes

5 A client is admitted with methicillin-resistant *Staphylococcus aureus* in a draining sacral wound. The client should be placed in which type of isolation precautions?
  1. droplet precautions
  2. contact precautions
  3. airborne precautions
  4. protective precautions

6 The T cells of the immune system adapt to kill:
  1. intracellular organisms.
  2. interstitial microbes.
  3. extracellular viruses.
  4. protozoans.

7 Thrombocytosis is best explained as:
  1. increased platelets.
  2. decreased clotting time.
  3. decreased platelets.
  4. average number of platelets.

8 The nursing diagnosis *Risk for Infection* pertains to:
  1. the infected patient only.
  2. healthcare workers in the facility.
  3. patients hospitalized at the same time.
  4. the infected patient, healthcare workers, and other patients.

9 When administering antibiotics, the primary nursing role is monitoring for:
  1. compliance.
  2. therapeutic levels.
  3. oxygen desaturation.
  4. hypersensitivities and teaching.

10 Standard isolation techniques are employed for all hospitalized patients. These include:
  1. hand washing, use of masks, and recapping needles.
  2. use of masks and gowns, and spraying of disinfectant regularly.
  3. use of gloves, gowns, and goggles with contaminated body fluids.
  4. use of alcohol-based hand rub for visibly dirty or blood contaminated hands.

See Test Yourself answers in Appendix C.

BIBLIOGRAPHY

Andreoli, T., Bennett, J., Carpenter, C., Griggs, R. C., & Lose, J. (Eds.). (2004). *Cecil essentials of medicine* (6th ed.). Philadelphia: W. B. Saunders.

Arnold, M., & Barbul, A. (2006). Nutrition and wound healing. *Plastic and Reconstructive Surgery, 117*(7 Suppl), 42S–58S.

Aronson, B. (2005). Medication management behaviors of adherent short-term antibiotic users. Clinical Excellence for Nurse Practitioners, 9(1), 23–30.

Baine, W. B., Yu, W., & Summe, J. P. (2001). The epidemiology of hospitalization of elderly Americans for septicemia or bacteremia in 1991–1998. Application of Medicare claims data. *Annals of Epidemiology, 11*(2), 118–126.

Bourlioux, P., Koletzko, B., Guarner, F., & Braesco, V. (2003). The intestine and its microflora are partners for the protection of the host: Report on the Danone Symposium "The Intelligent Intestine," held in Paris, June 14, 2002. *American Journal of Clinical Nutrition, 78*(4), 675–683.

Centers for Disease Control and Prevention. (2000). *Preventing emerging infectious diseases. A strategy for the 21st century.* Retrieved from http://www.cdc.gov/mmwr/preview/mmwrhtml/00054779.htm

_____. (2001, October). Update: Investigation of anthrax associated with intentional exposure and interim public health guidelines. *MMWR, 50*(41), 889–897.

_____. (2002a). Guidelines for hand hygiene in health-care settings. *MMWR Recommendations and Reports, 51*(RR 16), 1–44.

_____.(2002b). *Guidelines for the prevention of intravascular catheter-related infections.* Retrieved from http://www.cdc.gov/mmwr/preview/mmwrhtml/mm5132a9.htm

_____. (2002c). *Recommended adult immunization schedule, United States, 2002–2003.* Retrieved from http://www.cdc.gov/mmwr/preview/mmwrhtml/mm5140a5.htm

_____. (2003). Prevention and control of influenza: Recommendations of the Advisory Committee on Immunizations Practices (ACIP). *MMWR Morbidity and Mortality Weekly Report, 52* (RR08), 1–36.

_____. (2004). National Nosocomial Infections Surveillance (NNIS) System Report, data summary from January 1992 through June 2004, issued October 2004, *American Journal of Infection Control, 32*, 470–485.

Christ-Crain, M., Jaccard-Stolz, D., Bingisser, R., Gencay, M. M., Huber, P. R., Tamm, M., et al. (2004). Effect of procalcitonin-guided treatment on antibiotic use and outcome in lower respiratory tract infections: Cluster-randomised, single-blinded intervention trial. *Lancet, 363*(9409), 600–607.

CMS. (2003). Retrieved from http://www.aha.org/aha/key_issues/patient_safety/contents/Pneumonia_project.pdf

Coleman, E. A. (2001). Anthrax. *American Journal of Nursing, 101*(12), 48–52.

Dahners L. E., & Mullis, B. H. (2004). Effects of nonsteroidal anti-inflammatory drugs on bone formation and soft-tissue healing. *Journal of the American Academy of Orthopaedic Surgeons, 12*(3), 139–143.

DeMeyer, E. S., & Buchsel, P. C. (2005). A dendritic cell primer for oncology nurses. *Clinical Journal of Oncology Nursing, 9*(4), 460–464.

Dochterman, J., & Bulechek, G. (2004). *Nursing interventions classification (NIC)* (4th ed.). St. Louis, MO: Mosby.

Eliopoulos, C. (2005). *Gerontological nursing* (6th ed.). Philadelphia: Lippincott Williams & Wilkins.

Evans-Smith, P. (Ed.). (2005). *Taylor's clinical nursing skills: A nursing process approach.* Philadelphia: Lippincott Williams & Wilkins.

Fauci, A. et al. (1998). *Harrison's principles of internal medicine* (14th ed.). New York: McGraw-Hill.

George, E. L. (2005). Does a high WBC count signal infection? *Nursing2005, 35*(1), 20–21.

Glover, T. L. (2000). How drug-resistant microorganisms affect nursing. *Othopaedic Nursing, 19*(2), 19–26.

Goldsby, R. A., Kindt, T. J., Osborne, B. A., & Kuby, J. (2003). *Immunology* (5th ed.). New York: W. H. Freeman.

Gordin, F. M., Schultz, M. E., Huber, R. A., & Gill, J. A. (2005). Reduction in nosocomial transmission of drug-resistant bacteria after introduction of an alcohol-based handrub. *Infection Control and Hospital Epidemiology, 26*(7), 650–653.

Hazzard, W., Blass, J. R., Halter, J. B., Ouslander, J. G., & Tinetti, M. E. (Eds.). (2003). *Principles of geriatric medicine and gerontology* (5th ed.). New York: McGraw-Hill.

Johnson, M., Maas, M., & Moorhead, S. (2000). *Iowa outcomes project: Nursing outcomes classification (NOC)* (2nd ed.). St. Louis, MO: Mosby.

Kasper, D. L., et al. (2005). *Harrison's principles of internal medicine* (16th ed.). New York: McGraw-Hill.

Kimball, J. (2005). *Kimball's biology pages.* Retrieved from http://biology-pages.info

Kjonegaard, R., & Myers III, F. E. (2005). Arresting drug-resistant organisms. *Nursing 2005, 35*(6), 48–50.

Lehne, R. A. (2004). *Pharmacology for nursing care* (4th ed.). St. Louis, MO: Saunders/Elsevier.

Lutz, C., & Przytulski, K. (2001). *Nutrition and diet therapy* (3rd ed.). Philadelphia: F. A. Davis.

McCance, K., & Huether, S. (2002). *Pathophysiology: The biologic basis for disease in adults and children* (4th ed.). St. Louis, MO: Mosby.

McCloskey, J., & Bulechek, G. (2000). *Iowa intervention project: Nursing interventions classification (NIC)* (3rd ed.). St. Louis, MO: Mosby.

McKibben, L., Horan, T. C., Tokars, J. I., Fowler, G., Cardo, D. M., Pearson, M. I., et al. (2005). Guidance on public reporting of healthcare-associated infections: Recommendations of the Healthcare Infection Control Practices Advisory Committee: A special report. *Infection Control and Hospital Epidemiology, 26*(6), 580–587.

Moorhead, S., Johnson, M., & Maas, M. (2003). *Nursing outcomes classification (NOC)* (3rd ed.). St. Louis, MO: Mosby.

Müller, B., & Becker, K. L. (2001). Procalcitonin: How a hormone became a marker and mediator of sepsis. *Swiss Medical Weekly, 131*, 595–602.

Pagana, K. D., & Pagana, T. J. (2002). *Mosby's manual of diagnostic and laboratory tests* (2nd ed.). St. Louis, MO: Mosby.

Porth, C. (2005). *Pathophysiology: Concepts of altered health states* (6th ed.). Philadelphia: Lippincott Williams & Wilkins.

Posani, T. (2004). *Clostridium difficile:* Causes and interventions. *Critical Care Nursing Clinics of North America, 16*(4), 547–551.

Price, S., & Wilson, L. (2003). *Pathophysiology: Clinical concepts of disease processes* (6th ed.). St. Louis, MO: Mosby.

Rao, A. S., & Bradley, S. F. (2003). *Clostridium difficile* in older adults and residents of long-term care facilities. *Annals of Long-Term Care, 11*(5), 42–47.

Quinley, J. C., & Shih, A. (2004). Improving physician coverage of pneumococcal vaccine: A randomized trial of a telephone intervention. *Journal of Community Health, 29*(2), 103–115.

Rink, L., & Gabriel, P. (2000). Zinc and the immune system. *Proceedings of the Nutrition Society, 59*(4), 541–552.

Sandhu, S. K., & Mossad, S. B. (2001). Influenza in the older adult. *Geriatrics, 56*(1), 43–44, 47–48, 51.

Shorr, A. F. (2005). Preventing pneumonia: The role for pneumococcal and influenza vaccines. *Clinics in Chest Medicine, 26*(1), 123–134.

Silverblatt, F. J., Tibert, C., Mikolich, D., Blazek-D'Arezzo, J., Alves, J., Tack, M., et al. (2000). Preventing the spread of vancomycin-resistant enterococci in a long-term care facility. *Journal of the American Geriatrics Society, 48*(10), 1211–1214.

Sopena, N., & Sabria, M. (2005). Multicenter study of hospital-acquired pneumonia in non-ICU patients. *Chest, 127*(1), 213–219.

Stone, P. W., Hedblom, E. C., Murphy, D. M., & Miller, S. B. (2005). The economic impact of infection control: Making the business case for increased infection control resources. *American Journal of Infection Control, 33*(9), 542–547.

Thames, D., & Meiner, S. E. (2006). Infection. In S. E. Meiner & A. G. Lueckenotte (Eds.), *Gerontologic nursing* (3rd ed., pp. 328–343). St. Louis, MO: Mosby Elsevier.

Tierney, L., McPhee, S., & Papadakis, M. (Eds.). (2006). *Current medical diagnosis & treatment* (44th ed.). Stamford, CT: Appleton & Lange.

Todd, B. (2006). Emerging infections: Preventing bloodstream infection. *American Journal of Nursing, 106*(1), 29–30.

Turkoski, B. B. (2005a). Fighting infection: An ongoing challenge. Part I. *Orthopaedic Nursing, 24*(1), 40–46.

Turkoski, B. B. (2005b). Fighting infection: An ongoing challenge, Part 2—Antibacterials. *Orthopaedic Nursing, 24*(3), 210–221.

Walker, B. W. (2004). Assessing gastrointestinal infections. *Nursing 2004, 34*(5), 48–52.

Warny, M., Pepin, J., Fang, A., Killgore, G., Thompson, A., Brazier, J., et al. (2005). Toxic production by an emerging strain of *Clostridium difficile* associated with outbreaks of severe disease in North America and Europe. *Lancet, 366*, 1079–1083.

Weber, D. J., Sickbert-Bennett, E., Gergen, M. F., & Rutala, W. A. (2003). Efficacy of selected hand hygiene agents used to remove *Bacillus atrophaeus* (a surrogate of *Bacillus anthracis*) from contaminated hands. *Journal of the American Medical Association, 289*(10), 1274–1277.

Wilkinson, J. (2005). *Prentice Hall nursing diagnosis handbook with NIC interventions and NOC outcomes* (8th ed.). Upper Saddle River, NJ: Prentice Hall Health.

Wilson, B. A., Shannon, M. T., & Stang, C. L. (2006). *Nursing drug guide 2006.* Upper Saddle River, NJ: Prentice Hall.

CHAPTER 13 Nursing Care of Clients with Altered Immunity

LEARNING OUTCOMES

- Review normal anatomy and physiology of the immune system.
- Describe the four types of hypersensitivity reactions.
- Discuss the pathophysiology of autoimmune disorders and tissue transplant rejection.
- Discuss the characteristics of immunodeficiencies.
- Identify laboratory and diagnostic tests used to diagnose and monitor immune response.

- Describe pharmacologic and other collaborative therapies used in treating clients with altered immunity.
- Correlate the pathophysiologic alterations with the manifestations of HIV/AIDS infection.
- Use the nursing process as a framework to provide individualized care to clients with altered immune responses.

CLINICAL COMPETENCIES

- Assess functional health status of clients with altered immunity and monitor, document, and report abnormal manifestations.
- Use evidence-based practice to plan and implement nursing care for clients with AIDS.
- Assess for hypersensitivities and anticipate treatment if signs and symptoms develop.
- Provide client teaching about hypersensitivities, avoidance of sensitizing agents, and prophylactic treatment.
- Determine priority nursing diagnoses, based on assessment data, to select and implement individualized nursing interventions and teaching for clients with altered immunity.
- Protect clients who are immune suppressed.

- Recognize manifestations of developing anaphylaxis.
- Recognize manifestations of infection and minimize nosocomial exposure.
- Utilize universal precautions to protect self and clients from HIV exposure.
- Recognize the burden and benefit of HAART for the client with HIV infection.
- Integrate interdisciplinary care into care of the client with altered immunity.
- Revise plan of care as needed to provide effective interventions to promote, maintain, or restore functional health status to clients with altered immunity.

MEDIALINK

Resources for this chapter can be found on the Prentice Hall Nursing MediaLink DVD-ROM accompanying this textbook, and on the Companion Website at http://www.prenhall.com/lemone

Recent years have seen the emergence of new diseases affecting the immune system. These diseases include human immunodeficiency virus (HIV) infection and altered strains of familiar diseases such as multiple-drug-resistant tuberculosis. At the same time, our understanding of the components of the immune system and specific immune responses is increasing. It is therefore vital that today's nurses understand the foundations of the immune system and the immune response.

OVERVIEW OF THE IMMUNE SYSTEM

The immune system functions to protect the body from invasion by foreign antigens, to identify and destroy potentially harmful cells, and to remove cellular debris. These functions are accomplished by the lymphoid organs and specifically designed lymphocytes through the processes of antibody-mediated immune response and cell-mediated immune response.

The effectiveness of the immune system depends on its ability to differentiate normal host tissue from abnormal or foreign tissue. Body cells, tissues, and fluids have unique antigenic properties recognized by the immune system as "self." External agents, such as microorganisms, cells and tissues from other humans or animals, and some inorganic substances, have antigenic properties recognized by the immune system as "non-self."

Each body cell displays specific cell surface characteristics, or markers, that are unique to each person. These are known as human leukocyte antigens (HLAs). A person's HLA characteristics are coded within a large cluster of genes known as the major histocompatibility complex (MHC) located on chromosome 6. Recall that chromosomes are paired; each person inherits one member of the pair from each parent. A chromosome pair contains multiple genes, each carrying instructions for production of one polypeptide chain. The number of genes in the MHC results in a multitude of HLA combinations. As a result, the possibility of two people having the same HLA type is extremely remote. Identical twins may be the exception, and some siblings have very similar HLA patterns. In tissue grafting and organ transplants, matching the HLA type as closely as possible tends to decrease rejection.

Immunocompetent clients have an immune system that identifies antigens and effectively destroys or removes them. When the immune system functions improperly, the result may be an overreaction or deficiency, resulting in health problems. Overreaction of the immune system leads to hypersensitivity disorders, such as allergies. When the immune system loses the ability to recognize self, autoimmune disorders may ensue (Table 13–1). Immunodeficiency diseases or malignancies can develop when the immune system is incompetent or unable to respond effectively, as is the case with acquired immunodeficiency disorder. These alterations in immunity are discussed later in this chapter.

As discussed previously in Chapter 12 ∞, the *antibody-mediated immune response* is accomplished by B lymphocytes (B cells) that are further divided into memory cells and plasma cells. They are activated by contact with an antigen and by T cells. B cells produce antibodies, also known as immunoglobulins (see Table 12–2), and serve to inactivate an invading antigen. One immunoglobulin in particular, IgM, forms natural antibodies, such as those for ABO blood group antigens, and is an important component of the immune system complexes seen in autoimmune disorders. Memory cells "remember" an antigen, and, when exposed to it a second time, immediately initiate the immune response. This action provides the foundation of acquired immunity.

In contrast, *cell-mediated immunity* acts at the cellular level by attacking antigens directly and by activating B cells. T lymphocytes comprise the cell-mediated immune response and are subdivided into effector cells and regulator cells. The cytotoxic cell or killer T cell is the primary effector cell. Regulator T cells are divided into two subsets known as helper T cells and suppressor T cells.

Proteins on the surface of the T cell help define its function and also provide a marker that can be used to identify the cell class. These proteins are known as the cluster of differentiation antigen or *CD antigen.* The two primary CD proteins are CD4 and CD8. Both cytotoxic and suppressor T cells carry the CD8 antigen. Helper T cells have the CD4 antigen and are often called CD4 cells. CD4 cells are the most numerous of the T lymphocytes, making up 70% of the circulating population.

Helper T cells initiate the immune response, whereas suppressor T cells limit it. Helper T cells accomplish their role by promoting growth of additional T cells, by stimulating proliferation of B cells, and by activating killer T cells. It is believed that suppressor T cells are important in preventing autoimmune disorders. Proper immune system function depends on the correct balance between helper and suppressor T cells.

In addition to destroying viruses and bacteria, cytotoxic T lymphocytes also attack malignant cells. They also are responsible for the rejection of transplanted organs and grafted tissues.

TABLE 13–1 Selected Autoimmune Disorders

More organ specific	Hashimoto's thyroiditis	A chronic progressive inflammatory disease of the thyroid with lymphocyte infiltration and gradual destruction of the gland. See Chapter 19.
	Primary myxedema	Thyroid deficiency resulting from destruction of the thyroid gland due to an autoimmune process, often Hashimoto's thyroiditis. See Chapter 19.
	Thyrotoxicosis	Hyperthyroidism resulting from thyroid-stimulating immunoglobulins that stimulate activity of the gland. See Chapter 19.
	Pernicious anemia	Anemia resulting from absence of intrinsic factor associated with loss of parietal cells; most clients have antibodies to parietal cells. See Chapter 34.
	Addison's disease	Atrophy and hypofunction of the adrenal cortex, probably autoimmune in origin. See Chapter 19.
	Myasthenia gravis	A disease characterized by episodic muscle weakness caused by antibodies to the acetylcholine receptor of the neuromuscular junction. See Chapter 46.
	Insulin-dependent diabetes mellitus	Impaired insulin secretion, often the result of islet cell destruction by antibodies directed at the cell surface or cytoplasm. See Chapter 20.
	Goodpasture's syndrome	A type II hypersensitivity disorder with pulmonary hemorrhage and progressive glomerulonephritis characterized by circulating antiglomerular basement membrane antibodies. See Chapter 29.
	Multiple sclerosis	A probable autoimmune process resulting in disseminated patches of demyelination in the brain and spinal cord and varied neurologic manifestations. See Chapter 46.
	Idiopathic thrombocytopenic purpura	A chronic disorder characterized by petechiae, purpura, mucosal bleeding, and antibodies against platelets. See Chapter 34.
	Primary biliary cirrhosis	Inflammation and fibrosis of the bile ducts, probably of autoimmune origin. See Chapter 24.
	Active chronic hepatitis	A serious liver disease often resulting in hepatic failure and/or cirrhosis; may be autoimmune with infiltration by T cells and plasma cells. See Chapter 24.
Less organ specific	Ulcerative colitis	A chronic inflammatory disease of colon mucosa, possibly of autoimmune origin. See Chapter 26.
	Sjögren's syndrome	A systemic inflammatory disorder characterized by dryness of the mouth, eye, and other mucous membranes with lymphocyte infiltration of affected tissues. See Chapter 42.
	Rheumatoid arthritis	A chronic syndrome with inflammation of peripheral joints and generalized manifestations, characterized by infiltration of synovium by lymphocytes and plasma cells. See Chapter 42.
	Scleroderma	Diffuse fibrosis, degenerative changes, and vascular abnormalities of skin, joint structures, and internal organs; probably of autoimmune origin. See Chapter 42.
Non–organ specific	Systemic lupus erythematosus	An inflammatory connective tissue disorder characterized by the presence of antinuclear antibodies. See Chapter 42.

CHANGES IN IMMUNE FUNCTION IN THE OLDER ADULT

Immune function declines with aging, although many of the mechanisms leading to this decline are not clear. External factors, such as nutritional status and the effects of chemical exposure, ultraviolet radiation, and environmental pollution, affect the older adult's immune status. Internal factors affect it as well, including genetics, the function of the neurologic and endocrine systems, chronic and prior illnesses, and individual anatomic and physiologic variations. These myriad influences make it difficult to determine the effect of aging on the immune system. In some older individuals, the immune system is as effective as that of younger persons.

Whereas the antibody response to foreign antigens is diminished, autoantibodies (antibodies that react to the client's own tissues) are more common in older persons. The presence of autoantibodies suggests impaired regulation of the immune system, but it is not associated with an increased incidence of autoimmune disorders (Murasko & Gardner, 2003). The hypersensitivity response is also reduced or delayed.

ASSESSMENT OF ALTERED IMMUNE SYSTEM FUNCTION

Unlike body systems that are composed of a few closely related organs, the immune system is diverse and scattered. Optimal immune function depends on intact skin and mucous membrane barriers, adequate blood cell production and differentiation, a functional system of lymphatics and the spleen, and the ability to differentiate foreign tissue and pathogens from normal body tissue and flora. Because of this diversity of organs and function, assessment of the immune system is often integrated throughout the history and physical examination.

Health History

Prior to interviewing the client, review the biographic data, including age, sex, race, and ethnic background. This information can provide valuable clues about possible immunologic disorders. For example, many autoimmune disorders are more prevalent in women than in men. Family history is also important because there is a genetic component in the etiology of many disorders affecting the immune system.

Many interview questions related to the immune system and disorders that affect it are of a sensitive nature. Be sure to provide for privacy prior to the interview. If family members are present, request that they leave as well. Establish a trusting relationship with the client prior to asking the most sensitive questions (e.g., those related to the use of illicit drugs or sexual activity). Epidemiological data show that social and racial groups have peculiar risks for HIV infection; cultural sensitivity is necessary for effective communication.

Physical Assessment

The techniques of inspection and palpation are especially important in assessing a client's immune system.

- Assess the general appearance. Note whether the client's stated and apparent age coincide. Evident fatigue or weakness may indicate acute or chronic illness or immunodeficiency. Assess height, weight, and body type for apparent weight loss or wasting. Observe ease of movement and note any evident stiffness or difficulty moving. Check vital signs. *An elevated temperature may indicate an infection or inflammatory response.*
- Inspect the mucous membranes of the nose and mouth for color and condition. *Pale, boggy (edematous) nasal mucosa is often associated with chronic allergies. Note petechiae, white patches, or lacy white plaques in the oral mucosa; they may indicate hemolysis or immunodeficiency.*
- Assess skin color, temperature, and moisture. *Pale or jaundiced skin may indicate a hemolytic reaction. Pallor may also indicate bone marrow suppression with accompanying immunodeficiency. Inspect the skin for evidence of rashes or lesions, such as petechiae, numerous bruises, purple or blue patches or lesions indicative of Kaposi's sarcoma, and wounds that are infected, inflamed, or unhealed. Note the location and distribution of any rashes or lesions.*
- Inspect and palpate the cervical lymph nodes for evidence of lymphadenopathy (swelling) or tenderness. *Palpate the nodes of the axillae and groin as well* (see Figure 12–11).
- Assess the musculoskeletal system by inspecting and palpating the joints for redness, swelling, tenderness, or deformity. *Such changes may indicate an autoimmune disorder such as rheumatoid arthritis or systemic lupus erythematosus. Check joint range of motion as well, including that of the spine.*

ALTERED IMMUNE RESPONSES

Considering the complexity of the immune system, it is not surprising that abnormal or harmful responses occur. Altered immune system responses include those characterized by hyperresponsiveness of the immune system and those characterized by an impaired immune response. Allergies, autoimmune disorders, and reactions to organ or tissue transplants are all examples of hyperresponsive immune function. AIDS and other immunodeficiency disorders result from impairment of the immune system.

THE CLIENT WITH A HYPERSENSITIVITY REACTION

Hypersensitivity is an altered immune response to an antigen that results in harm to the client. When the antigen is environmental or exogenous, it is called an **allergy**, and the antigen is referred to as an *allergen*. The tissue response to a hypersensitivity reaction may be simply irritating or bothersome, causing a runny nose or itchy eyes, or it may be life threatening, leading to blood cell hemolysis or laryngospasm.

Hypersensitivity reactions are primarily classified by the type of immune response that occurs on contact with the allergen. They may also be classified as immediate or delayed hypersensitivity responses. Anaphylaxis and transfusion reactions are examples of immediate hypersensitivity reactions; contact dermatitis is a typical delayed response. Allergies are sometimes referred to by the affected organ system (e.g., allergic rhinitis) or the allergen involved, as in hay fever. Classification by immunologic response is the preferred means of studying allergies. Although more than one type of reaction may occur simultaneously, it is practical and insightful to study and treat allergy by classified types (King et al., 2005).

Pathophysiology

In a hypersensitivity reaction, an antigen–antibody or antigen–lymphocyte interaction causes a response that is damaging to body tissues. Antigen–antibody responses characterize types I, II, and III, also known as immediate hypersensitivity responses. Type IV hypersensitivity is an antigen–lymphocyte reaction, resulting in a delayed hypersensitivity response.

Type I IgE-Mediated Hypersensitivity

Common hypersensitivity reactions, such as allergic asthma, allergic rhinitis (hay fever), allergic conjunctivitis, hives, and anaphylactic shock, are typical of type I or IgE-mediated hypersensitivity. This type of hypersensitivity response is triggered when an allergen interacts with IgE bound to mast cells and basophils. The antigen–antibody complex prompts release of histamine and other chemical mediators, complement, acetylcholine, kinins, and chemotactic factors (Figure 13–1 ■).

When a potent allergen such as bee or wasp venom or a drug is injected, resulting in widespread antibody–antigen reaction and response to these chemical mediators, a systemic response such as anaphylaxis, urticaria, or angioedema results.

Sensitization stage

Antigen (allergen) invades body.

Plasma cells produce large amounts of class IgE antibodies against allergen.

IgE antibodies attach to mast cells in body tissues.

Subsequent (secondary) responses

More of same allergen invades body.

Allergen combines with IgE attached to mast cells, which triggers release of histamine (and other chemicals) from mast cell granules.

Histamine causes blood vessels to dilate and become leaky, which promotes edema; stimulates release of large amounts of mucus; and causes smooth muscles to contract (if respiratory system is site of allergen entry, asthma may ensue).

Mast cell with fixed IgE antibodies

IgE

Granules containing histamine

Antigen

Mast cell granules release contents after antigen binds with IgE anitbodies

Histamine and other chemical mediators

Outpouring of fluid from capillaries

Release of mucus

Constriction of small respiratory passages (bronchioles)

Figure 13–1 ■ Type I IgE-mediated hypersensitivity response.

Anaphylaxis is an acute systemic type I response that occurs in highly sensitive persons following injection of a specific antigen. Substances known to trigger anaphylaxis are summarized in Box 13–1. Anaphylaxis rarely follows oral ingestion, although this is possible. Food allergies are the cause of 150 deaths per year in the United States (Tierney et al., 2005). The reaction begins within minutes of exposure to the allergen and may be almost instantaneous. The release of histamine and other mediators causes vasodilation and increased capillary permeability, smooth muscle contraction, and bronchial constriction. These chemical mediators cause the client to experience the typical manifestations of ana-

phylaxis. Initially, a sense of foreboding or uneasiness, lightheadedness, and itching palms and scalp may be noted. Hives may develop, along with angioedema (localized tissue swelling) of the eyelids, lips, tongue, hands, feet, and genitals. Swelling can also affect the uvula and larynx, impairing breathing. This is further complicated by bronchial constriction. The client exhibits air hunger, stridor and wheezing, and a barking cough. These respiratory effects can be lethal if the reaction is severe and intervention is not immediately available. Vasodilation and fluid loss from the vascular system can lead to impaired tissue perfusion and hypotension, a condition known as *anaphylactic shock*.

Antigen attaches to foreign cell or tissue.

Plasma cells produce IgG or IgM antibodies, which bind to antigens.

Binding of antigens with antibodies stimulates complement activation.

Complement activation results in destruction of the target cell by lysis, phagocytosis, or activation of killer T cells.

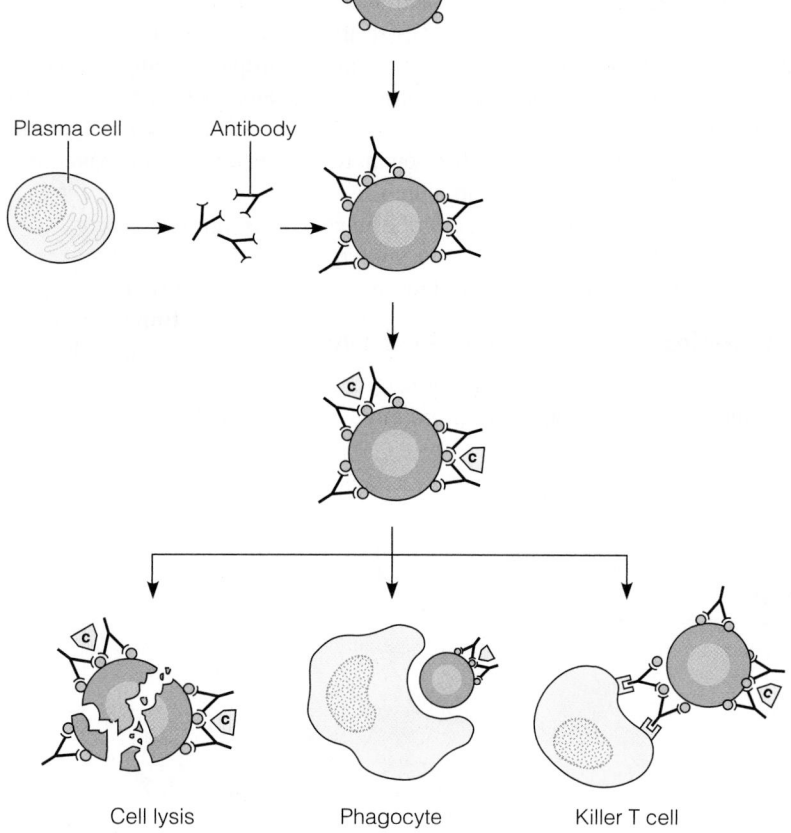

Antigen

Plasma cell   Antibody

Figure 13–2 ■ Type II cytotoxic hypersensitivity response.

Cell lysis   Phagocyte   Killer T cell

BOX 13–1 Substances Known to Trigger Anaphylaxis in Sensitized Persons

Hormones
- Insulin
- Vasopressin
- Parathormone

Enzymes
- Trypsin
- Chymotrypsin
- Penicillinase

Pollens
- Ragweed
- Grass
- Trees

Foods
- Eggs
- Seafoods
- Nuts
- Grains
- Beans
- Cottonseed oil
- Chocolate

Vitamins
- Thiamine
- Folic acid

Insect Venom
- Yellow jacket
- Hornet
- Paper wasp
- Honey bee

Occupational Agents
- Rubber products
- Industrial chemicals (ethylenes)

Antibiotics
- Penicillins
- Cephalosporins
- Amphotericin B
- Nitrofurantoin

Local Anesthetics
- Procaine
- Lidocaine

Medical Diagnostic Agents
- Sodium dehydrocholate
- Sulfobromophthalein

Antiserum
Antilymphocyte gamma globulin

Fortunately, localized responses are more common manifestations of type I hypersensitivity. These are typically atopic responses; that is, they have a strong genetic predisposition. Atopic reactions are the result of localized, rather than systemic, IgE-mediated responses to an allergen. They are prompted by contact of the allergen with cell-bound IgE in the bronchial tree, nasal mucosa, and conjunctival tissues. Chemical mediators are released locally, producing symptoms such as asthma, allergic rhinitis (hay fever), conjunctivitis, or atopic dermatitis. Allergens commonly associated with atopic reactions of this type include pollens, fungal spores, house dust mites, animal dander, and feathers (Porth, 2005). Food allergens can also cause localized responses such as diarrhea or vomiting. If the gastrointestinal mucosa is altered by a local allergic response, then the allergen may be absorbed, leading to a systemic reaction. Urticaria (hives) is the most common systemic response to food allergies.

Type II Cytotoxic Hypersensitivity

A hemolytic transfusion reaction to blood of an incompatible type is characteristic of a type II or cytotoxic hypersensitivity reaction. IgG or IgM type antibodies are formed to a cell-bound antigen such as the ABO or Rh antigen. When these antibodies bind with the antigen, the complement cascade is activated, resulting in destruction of the target cell (Figure 13–2 ■). Hemolytic disease of the newborn is caused by this type of reaction.

Type II reactions may be stimulated by an exogenous antigen, such as foreign tissue or cells, or a drug reaction, in which the drug forms an antigenic complex on the surface of a blood cell, stimulating the production of antibodies. The affected cell is then destroyed in the resulting antigen–antibody reaction; for example, hemolytic anemia is sometimes associated with the administration of drugs such as penicillins, cephalosporins, and streptomycin. Withdrawal of the drug stops the reaction and cell destruction (Goldsby et al., 2003).

Endogenous antigens can also stimulate a type II reaction, resulting in an autoimmune disorder such as Goodpasture's syndrome, in which antigens are formed to specific tissues in the lungs and kidneys. Hashimoto's thyroiditis and autoimmune hemolytic anemia are additional examples of autoimmune type II reactions.

Type III Immune Complex–Mediated Hypersensitivity

Type III hypersensitivity reactions result from the formation of IgG or IgM antibody–antigen immune complexes in the circula-tion. When these complexes are deposited in vessel walls and ex-travascular tissues, complement is activated and chemical media-tors of inflammation such as histamine are released. Chemotactic factors attract neutrophils to the site of inflammation. When neu-trophils attempt to phagocytize the immune complexes, lysosomal enzymes are released, increasing tissue damage (Figure 13–3 ■).

Either systemic or local responses may be seen with type III reactions. For example, serum sickness is a systemic response, so named because it was first identified after administration of foreign serum (e.g., horse antitetanus toxin). Although foreign serums are no longer administered, serum sickness still occurs in response to some drugs, such as penicillin and sulfon-amides. Immune complexes are deposited in walls of small blood vessels, the kidneys, and joints. Manifestations of serum sickness include fever, urticaria or rash, arthralgias, myalgias, and lymphadenopathy.

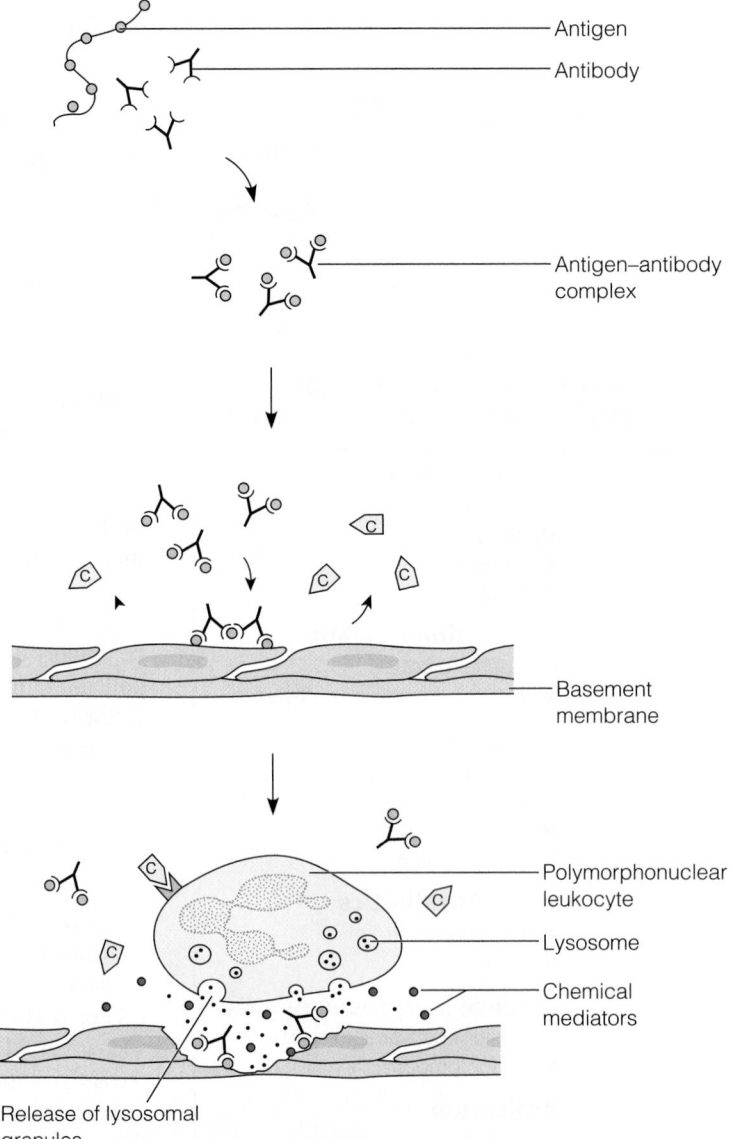

Antigens invade body and bind to antibodies in circulation. Antigen–antibody complexes are formed.

Antigen

Antibody

Antigen–antibody complex

Antigen–antibody complexes are deposited in the basement membrane of vessel walls and other body tissues, activating complement.

Basement membrane

Complement activation leads to release of inflammatory chemical mediators. Infiltration of polymorphonuclear leukocytes (PMNs) is followed by release of lysozymes. Tissue damage may be extensive.

Polymorphonuclear leukocyte

Lysosome

Chemical mediators

Release of lysosomal granules

Figure 13–3 ■ Type III immune complex–mediated hypersensitivity response.

Localized responses may occur at a number of different sites. As immune complexes accumulate in the glomerular basement membrane of the kidneys—for example, following a streptococcal infection or with systemic lupus erythematosus—glomerulonephritis develops. When an antigen such as dust from moldy hay is inhaled, an acute alveolar inflammatory response can occur. This condition can develop in agricultural workers.

Type IV Delayed Hypersensitivity

Type IV reactions differ from other hypersensitivity responses in two ways. First, these reactions are cell mediated rather than antibody mediated, involving T cells of the immune system. Second, type IV reactions are delayed rather than immediate, developing 24 to 48 hours after exposure to the antigen. Type IV hypersensitivity responses result from an exaggerated interaction between an antigen and normal cell-mediated mechanisms. This exaggerated interaction results in the release of soluble inflammatory and immune mediators (from the lysozymes within the macrophages) and recruitment of killer T cells, causing local tissue destruction (Figure 13–4 ■).

Contact dermatitis is a classic example of a type IV reaction. Intense redness, itching, and thickening affect the skin in the area exposed to the antigen. Fragile vesicles are often present as well. Many antigens can provoke this response; poison ivy is a prime perpetrator. In the healthcare setting, an allergic response to latex can also produce contact dermatitis. An estimated 8% to 13% of healthcare workers are allergic to latex (National Institute of Occupational Safety and Health [NIOSH], 2005). Other examples of cell-mediated responses include a positive tuberculin test and graft rejection episodes.

Latex Allergy

Although protective against infection, the repetitive use of latex gloves creates a persistent exposure to latex for healthcare workers. When gloves are powdered with cornstarch to facilitate donning and removing gloves, the cornstarch particles aerosolize when the gloves are removed. The cornstarch includes latex particles. This creates a respiratory exposure as well as dermal exposure to latex. In addition, chemicals used in the manufacture of latex products may be irritating. Products such as balloons, condoms, and rubber bands are commonly made of latex.

Antigen-presenting cell encounters cytotoxic T cell.

Antigen-presenting cell

T cell

Interaction causes release of lympho-kines, which attract macrophages.

Lymphokines

Lysozymes

Macrophage

Macrophages release lysozymes, resulting in local tissue damage.

Figure 13–4 ■ Type IV delayed hypersensitivity response.

Sensitivity to latex develops without the user being aware until a rash appears on the hands. Type IV hypersensitivity (contact dermatitis) can progress to type I systemic allergic reactions without previous symptoms signaling an escalation. It is important to protect the client and the healthcare worker who is allergic to latex. Prevention is aided by employers who select products free of latex. Nonlatex gloves are recommended for use where there is no contact with infectious materials or blood. Workers should be screened periodically to detect symptoms of allergy and educated about latex sources. Hand washing after using latex products limits exposure (NIOSH, 2005).

INTERDISCIPLINARY CARE

The focus of care for clients with allergic responses is on the following:
- Minimize exposure to the allergen.
- Prevent a hypersensitivity response.
- Provide prompt, effective interventions for allergic responses when they occur.

Identifying allergens for the individual to reduce the likelihood of exposure is a key aspect of management. A complete history of the client's allergies is obtained, including medications, foods, animals, plants, and other materials. The type of hypersensitivity response is documented, as is its onset, manifestations, and usual treatment.

When a documented or suspected hypersensitivity reaction occurs, the allergen (e.g., intravenous medication or transfusion) is withdrawn immediately. With a type I hypersensitivity response, managing the client's airway takes highest priority, followed by maintaining cardiac output. Type II hypersensitivity responses may necessitate aggressive management of bleeding or renal failure. A type III (immune complex) reaction is treated by removing the offending antigen and interrupting the inflammatory response.

With a hypersensitivity response, supportive care is important to relieve discomfort. This often involves the administration of selected antihistamine or anti-inflammatory medications. Other therapies, such as plasmapheresis, may be prescribed in selected instances.

Diagnosis

To identify possible allergens or hypersensitivity reactions, the following laboratory tests may be ordered:
- *White blood cell (WBC) count with differential* can detect high levels of circulating eosinophils. Normally, eosinophils constitute a very small percentage (1% to 4%) of the total WBCs. Eosinophilia, however, is often present in clients with type I hypersensitivities.
- *Radioallergosorbent test (RAST)* measures the amount of IgE directed toward specific allergens. Test results are compared with control values and used to identify hypersensitivities. RAST poses no risk for an anaphylactic reaction. It is particularly useful in detecting allergies to some occupational chemicals and toxic allergens (Goldsby, 2003).
- *Blood type and crossmatch* are ordered prior to any anticipated transfusions. The client's ABO blood group and Rh status are determined. Two major antigens, designated A and B, may be present on RBCs. Clients with the A antigen are designated as blood type A; those with blood type B have the B antigen. When neither antigen is found on the RBCs, the person is identified as type O. A third major RBC antigen is the Rh antigen. Persons with this antigen are called Rh positive; those without are Rh negative. Because a blood transfusion is actually a transplant of living tissue, antigen matching is vital to prevent significant hypersensitivity reactions. Once blood type is determined, a sample of the client's blood is mixed with a sample of matching donor blood and observed for antigen–antibody reactions in the crossmatch portion of this test. Although this procedure greatly reduces the risk of a hemolytic transfusion reaction (type II hypersensitivity), it does not totally eliminate it.
- *Indirect Coombs' test* detects the presence of circulating antibodies (other than ABO antibodies) against RBCs. The client's serum is mixed with the donor's RBCs. If the client's serum contains antibodies to an RBC antigen, agglutination (clumping together) will occur. This is called a positive response. The normal value is negative, or no agglutination. This test is also part of the crossmatch of a blood "type and crossmatch."
- *Direct Coombs' test* detects antibodies on the client's RBCs that damage and destroy the cells. This is used following a suspected transfusion reaction to detect antibodies coating the transfused RBCs. It can also identify hemolytic anemia when the cause is unknown. In the direct Coombs' test, the client's RBCs are mixed with Coombs' serum, which contains antibodies to IgG and several complement components. Agglutination will occur if the client's RBCs are coated with antibodies, resulting in a positive test. As with the indirect Coombs' test, the normal test result is negative.
- *Immune complex assays* may be performed to detect the presence of circulating immune complexes in suspected type III hypersensitivity responses. The assays are particularly useful in diagnosing suspected autoimmune disorders. Nonspecific assays of IgG-, IgM-, and IgA-containing immune complexes, which do not detect specific antibodies, as well as specific antibody assays may be done. The normal result is a test negative for circulating immune complexes. A negative test does not, however, rule out an immune complex hypersensitivity response. In some cases, a negative result may indicate that the disease process has reached a later stage, in which complexes are no longer circulating but have initiated extensive tissue damage, such as glomerulonephritis (Kasper et al., 2005).
- *Complement assay* is also useful in detecting immune complex disorders. In these disorders, complement is, in effect, used up by the development of antigen–antibody complexes. Decreased levels are seen on examination. Both total complement level and amounts of individual components of the complement cascade can be determined.

Skin tests are also used to determine causes of hypersensitivity reactions. These tests are used to identify specific allergens to which a person may be sensitive. Allergens for testing are selected according to the client's history. Test solutions made from extracts of inhaled, ingested, or injected materials, such as pollens, mites, venoms, or some drugs, are used for the prick test and intradermal testing. Epicutaneous testing (prick testing) is generally done first to avoid a systemic reaction; it is followed by intradermal testing of allergens with a negative response to prick testing (Tierney et al., 2005). If the large-dose intradermal test were initially made, individuals highly allergic to a substance would be at increased risk for an anaphylactic reaction. Substances that cause a reaction to the prick test should not be tested intradermally.

- *Prick (epicutaneous or puncture) test:* A drop of diluted allergenic extract is placed on the skin, and the skin is then pricked or punctured through the drop. With a positive test, a localized pruritic wheal and erythema occur. The response is maximal at 15 to 20 minutes.
- *Intradermal:* A small amount (just enough to create a wheal) of allergen extract at a 1:500 or 1:1000 dilution is injected on the forearm or intrascapular area. If several allergens are being tested, injections are spaced 0.25 to 0.5 apart. As control measures, plain diluent (negative control) and histamine (positive control) are also injected. If there is no response to a particular allergen at 15 to 20 minutes, the test is negative. The appearance of a wheal and erythema, with a wheal diameter at least 5 mm greater than that produced by the control, indicates a positive response (Figure 13–5 ■).
- *Patch:* A 1-inch patch impregnated with the allergen (e.g., perfume, cosmetics, detergents, or clothing fibers) is applied to the skin for 48 hours. Absence of a response indicates a negative test result. Positive responses are graded from mild (erythema in the exposed area) to severe (erythema, papules, vesicles, or ulceration).
- *Food allergy testing* is performed when a food allergy is suspected but the source or implicated food item has not been clearly identified. Food allergy symptoms are typically demonstrated within hours of eating. Initially, the client is asked to keep a diary of foods consumed and allergic responses for a week. An elimination diet is then prescribed. The diet excludes most common food allergens and all suspected foods for 1 week. Any foods that may contain allergens in combination, such as breads, are also eliminated. If symptoms do not improve, a different variation of the elimi-

Figure 13–5 ■ Skin testing on the forearm showing induration and erythema typical of a positive response to an antigen.
Source: Southern Illinois University/Photo Researchers, Inc.

nation diet is prescribed. If symptoms are relieved, foods are reintroduced to the diet one at a time until symptoms recur, indicating allergy to that food.

Medications

When it is impossible to avoid the offending allergen and allergic manifestations are severe or disrupt the client's activities of daily living (ADLs), pharmacologic intervention is prescribed. *Immunotherapy,* also called hyposensitization or desensitization, consists of injecting an extract of the allergen(s) in gradually increasing doses. Immunotherapy is used primarily for allergic rhinitis or asthma related to inhaled allergens. It has also been shown to be effective in preventing anaphylactic responses to insect venom. With weekly or biweekly subcutaneous injections of the allergen, the client develops IgG antibodies to the allergen that appear to block effectively the allergic IgE-mediated response. Once a therapy plateau is reached, injections are continued indefinitely either monthly or bimonthly.

Antihistamines are the major class of drugs used in treating the symptoms of hypersensitivity responses, type I in particular. They are also useful to some extent in relieving manifestations (such as urticaria) of some type II and type III reactions.

Antihistamines block H_1-histamine receptors, acting as a competitive antagonist to histamine, but they do not affect the production or release of histamine. The prototype antihistamine is diphenhydramine (Benadryl). It and other antihistamines alleviate the systemic effects of histamine such as urticaria and angioedema. They are also useful in relieving allergic rhinitis, although they are not effective in all clients. Antihistamines are available in both prescription and nonprescription preparations. The preferred route of administration is oral, although diphenhydramine and others can be given parenterally, particularly when immediate action is needed, as in anaphylaxis. They also dry respiratory secretions through an anticholinergic effect. Their use is limited by their side effects, especially drowsiness and dry mouth. Antihistamines are not effective in relieving asthmatic responses to allergens and may actually worsen symptoms by their drying effect on respiratory secretions.

Antihistamines are often combined with a sympathomimetic agent such as pseudoephedrine to improve their decongestant activity and counteract their sedative effect. Antihistamines and decongestants are discussed further in Chapter 37 ∞.

The immediate treatment for anaphylaxis is parenteral epinephrine, an adrenergic agonist (sympathomimetic) drug that has both vasoconstricting and bronchodilating effects. These qualities, combined with its rapid action, make epinephrine ideal for treating an anaphylactic reaction. For mild reactions with wheezing, pruritus, urticaria, and angioedema, a subcutaneous injection of 0.3 to 0.5 mL of 1:1000 epinephrine is generally sufficient. For clients with an injected toxin such as a bee sting, an additional amount equivalent to one-half the above may be injected directly into the site of the sting and a tourniquet applied above it to prevent further systemic absorption. Intravenous epinephrine using a 1:100,000 concentration may be used in the client with a more severe anaphylactic reaction.

Clients who have experienced an anaphylactic reaction to insect venom or other potentially unavoidable allergens should carry a kit (commonly called a bee sting kit) for immediate treatment of future exposures. This kit typically includes a pre-filled syringe of epinephrine and an epinephrine nebulizer, allowing prompt self-treatment.

Cromolyn sodium (Intal, NasalCrom) is a drug used to treat allergic rhinitis and asthma. Cromolyn sodium acts by stabilizing the mast cell membrane, thus preventing chemical mediator release (Lehne, 2004). It is most effective when applied directly to involved tissue by inhaler or nasal spray. It has few side effects and a wide margin of safety, making it a good choice for clients in whom it is effective (Tierney et al., 2005).

Glucocorticoids (corticosteroids) are used in both systemic and topical forms for many types of hypersensitivity responses. Their anti-inflammatory effects, rather than their immunosuppressive effects, are of most benefit. A short course of corticosteroid therapy is often used for severe asthma, allergic contact dermatitis, and some immune-complex disorders (Tierney et al., 2005). Corticosteroids in topical forms or delivered by inhaler may be used for longer periods of time with few side effects; however, systemic absorption can occur.

Other Therapies

Other treatments used for hypersensitivity responses are generally dictated by the severity of the response and the organ system affected. Airway management takes highest priority for the client with an acute anaphylactic reaction. Insertion of an endotracheal tube or emergency tracheostomy may be required to maintain airway patency with severe laryngospasm. Because anaphylaxis places the person at risk for vasomotor collapse and significant hypotension, it is necessary to insert an intravenous line and initiate fluid resuscitation with an isotonic solution such as Ringer's lactate.

Plasmapheresis, removal of harmful components in the plasma, may be used to treat immune complex responses such as glomerulonephritis and Goodpasture's syndrome. Plasma and the glomerular-damaging antibody–antigen complexes are removed by passing the client's blood through a blood cell separator. The RBCs are then returned to the client along with an equal amount of albumin or human plasma. This procedure is usually done in a series rather than as a one-time treatment. It is not without risk, and informed consent is required. Potential complications of plasmapheresis include those associated with intravenous catheters, shifts in fluid balance, and alteration of blood clotting.

NURSING CARE

Nursing care related to hypersensitivity reactions is primarily directed toward prevention, early identification, and providing prompt, effective treatment.

Health Promotion

Health promotion activities include helping clients to identify possible allergens that prompt a hypersensitivity response and discussing possible strategies to avoid these allergens. Anyone with severe food allergies may need assistance from a dietitian to discuss necessary dietary changes and ways to continue

meeting nutrient needs. It is important that persons with hypersensitivities inform healthcare personnel of all allergens. People who experience anaphylactic reactions should wear a Medic-Alert bracelet or tag at all times to identify the substance(s) that provokes this response.

Assessment

Collect the following data through the health history and physical examination. Further focused assessments are described with nursing interventions in the next section.

■ *Health history:* risk factors, hypersensitivities (medications, household dust, bee stings, etc.), reaction (rash, hives, difficulty breathing), type of treatment for hypersensitivity reactions; allergy skin testing; asthma, hay fever, or dermatitis

■ *Physical assessment:* mucous membranes of nose and mouth, skin for lesions or rashes, eyes (tearing and redness), respiratory rate, and adventitious breath sounds.

Nursing Diagnoses and Interventions

Priority nursing diagnoses will vary according to the type of hypersensitivity reaction experienced by the client. Because nurses are most likely to become involved with a client experiencing a type I or type II response, this section focuses on diagnoses for these clients. Airway, breathing, and circulation (the ABCs) are of greatest importance for the client with an anaphylactic reaction. When a hemolytic reaction to an incompatible blood transfusion occurs, the client is at risk for injury.

Ineffective Airway Clearance

> **PRACTICE ALERT**
> Placing the client in Fowler's to high-Fowler's position allows optimal lung expansion and ease of breathing.

In anaphylactic reactions, the airway may be obstructed due to facial angioedema, bronchospasm, or laryngeal edema. Establishing and maintaining a patent airway is of highest priority.

■ Administer oxygen per nasal cannula at a rate of 2 to 4 L/min. Apply oxygen emergently and obtain a physician order for oxygen administration. *This increases the alveolar oxygen and its availability to cells of the body.*

■ Assess respiratory rate and pattern, level of consciousness and anxiety, nasal flaring, use of accessory muscles of respiration, chest wall movement, audible stridor; palpate for respiratory excursion; auscultate lung sounds and any adventitious sounds, such as wheezes. *Extreme anxiety or agitation, nasal flaring, stridor, and diminished lung sounds indicate air hunger and possible airway obstruction, necessitating immediate intervention.*

■ Insert a nasopharyngeal or oropharyngeal airway, and arrange for immediate intubation as indicated. *Ensuring an adequate airway is vital to preserve life.*

■ Administer subcutaneous epinephrine 1:1000, 0.3 to 0.5 mL, as prescribed. This may be repeated in 20 to 30 minutes if necessary. Administer parenteral diphenhydramine (deep intramuscular or intravenous) as prescribed. *Epinephrine is a potent vasoconstrictor and bronchodilator, counteracting the effects of histamine. Diphenhydramine is an antihista-mine that blocks histamine receptors and their effect. These medications can be effective in rapidly reversing manifesta-tions of anaphylaxis.*

- Provide calm reassurance. *Hypoxemia and air hunger are terrifying for the client. Anxiety can impair the client's abil-ity to cooperate with treatment and can increase the respira-tory rate, making breathing less effective.*

Decreased Cardiac Output

Peripheral vasodilation and increased capillary permeability from the release of histamine can significantly impair cardiac output. When it falls to the degree that tissue perfusion be-comes impaired and hypoxia results, a state of anaphylactic shock exists.

- Monitor vital signs frequently, noting fall in blood pressure, decreasing pulse pressure, tachycardia, and tachypnea. *These vital sign changes may indicate shock.*
- Assess skin color, temperature, capillary refill, edema, and other indicators of peripheral perfusion. *As cardiac output falls, peripheral vessels constrict and tissue perfusion is impaired.*
- Monitor level of consciousness. *A change in level of con-sciousness (lethargy, apprehension, or agitation) is often the first indicator of decreased cardiac output.*
- Insert one or more large-bore (18-gauge or larger) intravenous catheters. *It is important to insert intravenous catheters as soon as possible to provide sites for rapid fluid replacement.*
- Administer warmed intravenous solutions of lactated Ringer's or normal saline, as prescribed. *These isotonic so-lutions help maintain intravascular volume. Warmed solu-tions are used to prevent hypothermia from the rapid administration of large amounts of fluid at room temperature (about 70°F, or 21.1°C).*
- Insert an indwelling catheter, and monitor urinary output fre-quently. *As the cardiac output drops, the glomerular filtra-tion rate (GFR) falls. With an output of less than 30 mL/h, the client is at risk for acute renal failure from ischemia.*

PRACTICE ALERT
Aggressive fluid therapy may lead to hypervolemia and pulmonary edema; assess for shortness of breath and crackles in the lungs.

- Place a tourniquet above the site of an injected venom (such as a bee sting), and infiltrate the site with epinephrine as pre-scribed. *Use of a tourniquet and the vasoconstriction result-ing from epinephrine infiltration reduce further absorption of the allergen.*
- Once breathing is established, place the client flat with the legs elevated. *This position enhances perfusion of the central organs, such as the brain, heart, and kidneys.*

Risk for Injury

As noted, the potential for hypersensitivity responses is high in clients subjected to medical treatments. Because a blood trans-fusion is a transplant of living tissue, the risk for adverse im-munologic response and injury is particularly significant.

- Obtain and record a thorough history of previous blood trans-fusions and any reactions experienced, *no matter how mild.* Alert the physician if previous transfusion reactions have oc-curred. *The client who has received prior blood transfusions is at increased risk for a hypersensitivity reaction, because antibody production may have been stimulated by prior ex-posure to antigens.*

PRACTICE ALERT
Begin a blood transfusion within 30 minutes of its delivery from the blood bank to reduce bacterial contamination.

- Check for a signed informed consent to administer blood or blood products. *It is important to obtain informed consent for this invasive and risky procedure.*
- Using two licensed healthcare professionals, double-check patient identity, blood type, Rh factor, crossmatch, and expi-ration date for all blood and blood components received from the blood bank with the client's data. *This is an important safety measure to reduce the risk of a hemolytic transfusion reaction due to incompatible blood types.*
- Take and record vital signs within 15 minutes prior to initi-ating the blood infusion. Acetaminophen and diphenhy-dramine are prescribed and administered prior to beginning a blood transfusion to decrease inflammation and increase client comfort. The medications will not mask serious reac-tions. *This provides a baseline for evaluating any changes re-lated to the blood transfusion.*
- Infuse blood into a site separate from any other intravenous infusion. Use at least 20-gauge catheter for the infusion to promote flow. *This reduces the risk of damage to the blood cells due to incompatibility with other intravenous solutions or physical trauma. When blood is administered with dex-trose solutions (e.g., D_5W, D_5NS), blood cell hemolysis and aggregation occur; administration with lactated Ringer's can cause agglutination of cells. Administer with normal saline to prime intravenous tubing.*
- Administer 50 mL of blood during the first 15 minutes of the transfusion. *Reactions generally occur within the first 15 minutes.*
- During transfusion, monitor for complaints of back or chest pain, an increase in the temperature of more than 1.8°F, chills, tachycardia, tachypnea, wheezing, hypotension, hives, rashes, or cyanosis. *These signs may indicate an ad-verse reaction to the blood transfusion.*
- Stop the blood transfusion immediately if a reaction occurs, no matter how mild. Remove the blood bag and the tubing with blood in it. Flush new intravenous tubing with normal saline, keeping the intravenous line open. Notify the physi-cian and the blood bank.
- If a reaction is suspected, send the blood and administration set to the laboratory with a freshly drawn blood sample and urine specimen from the client. *These will be used to identify the cause of the reaction as well as its effect on the client.*
- If no adverse reaction occurs, administer the transfusion over 2 to 4 hours. *This time frame is important to limit the risk of bacterial growth.*

Community-Based Care

The vast majority of hypersensitivity responses are appropriately treated by the client or family members with little or no medical intervention. Teaching, therefore, is a vital component of care. If the client is at risk for anaphylaxis, involving the family in teaching is essential because the response may occur with such rapidity that the client will be unable to provide self-care.

Include the following points in teaching the client and family about managing hypersensitivities:

- When and how to use an anaphylaxis kit containing epinephrine and antihistamines in injectable, inhaler, and oral forms
- When to seek medical attention
- Use and adverse reactions of prescription and nonprescription antihistamines and decongestants
- Advantages of autologous blood transfusion if future surgery is scheduled
- Preventing an immune complex reaction such as glomerulonephritis
- Skin care to prevent contact dermatitis, including:
  - Expose affected areas to air and sun as much as possible.
  - Avoid direct contact with people who have an infection.
  - Wear cool, light, nonrestrictive clothing of natural fibers, such as cotton, to avoid irritating affected areas.
  - Avoid exposure to extremes of heat or cold.
  - Use bath oils or plain water instead of soaps and detergents.
  - Take tub baths in cool to lukewarm water rather than showers.
  - To decrease pruritus, maintain a cool environment and avoid exercising.
  - Trim fingernails to reduce the risk of skin damage.
- Helpful resources:
  - ALERT, Inc., Allergy to Latex Education and Resource Team
  - Food Allergy Network

THE CLIENT WITH AN AUTOIMMUNE DISORDER

Maintaining optimal health and preventing disease depend not only on the immune system's ability to recognize and destroy foreign tissues and other antigens, but also on the immune system's ability to recognize self. When this self-recognition is impaired and immune defenses are directed against normal host tissue, the result is an **autoimmune disorder**.

Autoimmune disorders can affect any tissue in the body. Some are tissue or organ specific, affecting particular tissue or a particular organ. Hashimoto's thyroiditis is an example of an organ-specific autoimmune disorder. Circulating antibodies are formed to certain thyroid components, resulting ultimately in destruction of the gland. In other disorders, autoantibodies are formed that are not tissue specific, but tend to accumulate and cause an inflammatory response in certain tissue, for example, the renal glomerulus or the hepatic small bile ductules. Autoimmune disorders may also be systemic, with neither antibodies nor the resulting inflammatory lesions confined to any one organ. Rheumatologic disorders, such as rheumatoid arthritis and systemic lupus erythematosus (SLE), are characteristic of systemic autoimmune disorders (Goldsby et al., 2003). A list of selected autoimmune disorders is included in Table 13–1.

Pathophysiology

The mechanism that causes the immune system to recognize host tissue as a foreign antigen is not clear. The following factors are under study as possible contributors to the development of autoimmune disorders:

- The release of previously "hidden" antigens into the circulation, such as DNA or other components of the cell nucleus, which elicits an immune response
- Chemical, physical, or biologic changes in host tissue that cause self-antigens to stimulate the production of autoantibodies
- The introduction of an antigen, such as a bacteria or virus, whose antigenic properties closely resemble those of host tissue, resulting in the production of antibodies that target not only the foreign antigen but also normal tissue. Heart damage in rheumatic fever and encephalitis following rabies vaccination are examples of the development of antibodies against normal tissue (Goldsby et al., 2003).
- A defect in normal cellular immune function that allows B cells to produce autoantibodies unchecked
- Initiation of the autoimmune response by very slow-growing mycobacteria.

Although the exact mechanism producing autoimmunity is unclear, several characteristics of autoimmune diseases are known. It is apparent that genetics plays a role because a higher incidence is seen in family members of people with autoimmune disorders. Autoimmune disorders are far more prevalent in females than in males. The disorders tend to overlap, so that the client with one autoimmune disorder may develop another or some manifestations of another. The onset of an autoimmune disorder is frequently associated with an abnormal stressor, either physical or psychologic. Autoimmune disorders are frequently progressive relapsing-remitting disorders characterized by periods of exacerbation and remission.

Specific autoimmune disorders are discussed in the sections of this textbook related to the affected organ systems or functional disruption.

INTERDISCIPLINARY CARE

For the most part, the diagnosis of an autoimmune disorder is based on the client's clinical manifestations. Serum assays are useful to identify autoantibodies. Other diagnostic tests are generally specific to the suspected disorder and to identifying the degree of tissue damage and destruction. Although the manifestations of these disorders can often be managed, a cure typically is not possible unless the affected target tissue is removed (e.g., colectomy for the client with ulcerative colitis).

Diagnosis

Serologic assays are used to identify and measure antibodies directed toward host tissue antigens or normal cellular components. Many detectable autoantibodies are not specific to a single autoimmune disorder and are used to establish the autoimmune process rather than the specific disorder. Although healthy people often have low levels of autoantibodies, levels are much higher in clients affected by an autoimmune disorder. The following serologic assays may be ordered:

- *Antinuclear antibody (ANA)* detects antibodies produced to DNA and other nuclear material. These antibodies can cause tissue damage characteristic of autoimmune disorders, such as SLE. The client's serum is combined with nuclear material and tagged antihuman antibody to detect ANA-antihuman antibody complexes. A negative, or normal, result is a titer <1:20. When complexes are detected at higher titer levels (>1:20), the test is positive for ANA. This test is not specific for SLE, because high levels of ANA may be present in rheumatoid arthritis (RA) and cirrhosis of the liver; nevertheless, 95% of clients with SLE have a positive ANA titer.
- *Lupus erythematosus (LE) cell test* is also used to detect SLE and monitor its treatment. Neutrophils that contain large masses of phagocytized DNA from the nuclei of PMNs are called LE cells. Like the ANA, the LE cell prep is nonspecific for SLE. A positive result may also be seen in RA or with medications such as isoniazid, penicillin, phenytoin, procainamide, streptomycin, or sulfonamide drugs.
- *Rheumatoid factor (RF)* is an immunoglobulin present in the serum of approximately 80% of clients with rheumatoid arthritis. Low titer levels (<1:20) may be present in the elderly. An RF titer 1:80 or higher indicates RA. A titer between 1:20 and 1:80 could indicate SLE, scleroderma, or liver cirrhosis (Pagana & Pagana, 2002).
- *Complement assay* may also be useful in identifying autoimmune disorders. In these disorders, complement may be consumed in the development of antigen–antibody complexes. Decreased levels are seen on examination. Both total complement level and amounts of individual components of the complement cascade can be determined.

Medications

Various approaches are used in the treatment of autoimmune disorders. Anti-inflammatory medications such as aspirin, nonsteroidal anti-inflammatory drugs (NSAIDs), and corticosteroids may be prescribed to reduce the inflammatory response and minimize tissue damage. (Refer to Chapter 9 ∞ for additional detail on these drugs.) When these agents are not effective or well tolerated by the client, slow-acting anti-inflammatory medications may be prescribed. Slow-acting or antirheumatic drugs include such medications as gold salts, hydroxychloroquine (Plaquenil), and penicillamine. Their use is further detailed in Chapter 42 ∞. Cytotoxic drugs may be used in combination with plasmapheresis in treating many autoimmune disorders. Cytotoxic drugs are discussed in further detail in the next section of this chapter. Disease modifying antirheumatic drugs (DMARDs) reduce signs and symptoms, reduce or prevent joint damage, and preserve the structure and function of the joints in patients with RA. These drugs may reduce health costs for clients with RA and allow them to remain active and productive. The most common DMARDs in current use are methotrexate (Rheumatrex), sulfasalazine (Azulfidine), hydroxychloroquine (Plaquenil), leflunomide (Arava), and cyclosporine (Sandimmune, Neoral).

Another class of antirheumatic drugs, referred to as *biologicals* or *biological response modifiers,* consists of laboratory-produced proteins that decrease the inflammatory process. These antibodies bind tumor necrosis factor alpha (TNF-α) and interleukin-1, both inflammatory elements. These medications include infliximab (Remicade) or adalimumab (Humira), etanercept (Enbrel), and anakinra (Kineret).

NURSING CARE

Nursing care measures for the client with an autoimmune disorder are individualized and tailored to needs dictated by manifestations of the disorder. Nurses often will be involved with the client in an outpatient setting such as an office or home, evaluating the client's response to therapy and self-care management.

Consider the following nursing diagnoses in planning care for the client with an autoimmune disorder:

- *Activity Intolerance* related to inflammatory effects of autoimmune disorder
- *Ineffective Coping* related to chronic disease process
- *Interrupted Family Processes* related to lack of understanding about autoimmune disorder and its effects
- *Ineffective Protection* related to disordered immune function
- *Risk for Ineffective Therapeutic Regimen Management* related to lack of understanding

Community-Based Care

Because many autoimmune disorders are chronic, teaching the client and family about the disorder and its management is a key nursing care component. The client may be taking drugs with multiple side effects or long-term effects, necessitating effective teaching. Clients with autoimmune disorders often do not appear to be ill, making it difficult for friends and families to understand their care needs. The chronicity of these disorders also puts the client at high risk for unproven remedies and quackery. Provide psychologic support, listening, and teaching. In addition, suggest resources such as local support groups and the American Autoimmune Related Diseases Association.

THE CLIENT WITH A TISSUE TRANSPLANT

Since the first kidney transplant was performed from one identical twin to the other in 1954, organ and tissue transplantation have become increasingly popular and viable treatment options. The transplantation of avascular tissues, such as skin, cornea, bone, and heart valves, is considered routine, with little need for tissue matching and **immunosuppression**. Transplants of organs (e.g., the kidney, heart, heart and lung, liver, and bone marrow) are increasingly common and are no longer considered experimental or extraordinary procedures. Common organ transplants are outlined in Table 13–2.

Transplant success is closely tied to obtaining an organ with tissue antigens as close to those of the recipient as possible. As noted earlier in this chapter, every body cell has cell surface antigens known as human leukocyte antigens that are unique to the individual. Although identical twins may have the same

TABLE 13–2 Organ Transplants

ORGAN	GRAFT TYPE	INDICATIONS FOR TRANSPLANT	SUCCESS RATE
Kidney	Allograft; may be isograft	End-stage renal disease	81–89% at 5 years
Heart	Allograft	End-stage cardiac disease refractory to medical management	72.5% at 5 years
Lung	Allograft	Pulmonary hypertension, cystic fibrosis, pulmonary fibrosis, chronic obstructive pulmonary disease	46% at 5 years
Liver	Allograft	Severe liver dysfunction due to chronic active hepatitis, primary biliary cirrhosis, sclerosing cholangitis	72–78% 5-year survival
Bone marrow	Autograft or allograft	Leukemia, aplastic anemia, congenital immunologic defects	30–70% cure
Skin	Autograft, allograft, or xenograft	Severe burns, plastic surgery	>95% at 5 years
Cornea	Allograft	Corneal ulceration and opacification	>95% at 5 years
Pancreas	Allograft	Pancreatic insufficiency, diabetes	80.3% pancreas
Islet cells	Allograft (multiple donor)	Type 1 diabetes mellitus	100% >2 years

Source: Data from *Current Medical Diagnosis and Treatment* (44th ed.) by L. M. Tierney, S. J. McPhee, and M. A. Papadakis, 2005, New York: Lange Medical Books/McGraw-Hill; US Transplant.org; Scientific registry of transplant recipients, accessed 10/23/05. http://www.ustransplant.org/

HLA type, the chance is reduced to 1 in 4 for siblings, and less than 1 in several thousand for unrelated individuals (Tierney et al., 2005). Matching the HLA type of the donor and recipient as closely as possible decreases the potential for rejection of the transplanted organ or tissue but does not eliminate it.

Pathophysiology

An **autograft**, a transplant of the client's own tissue, is the most successful type of tissue transplant. Skin grafts are the most common examples of autografts. Increasingly, autologous bone marrow transplants and blood transfusions are being used to reduce immunologic responses. When the donor and recipient are identical twins, the term **isograft** is used. Because of the high likelihood of an HLA match, the success of these grafts is good and rejection episodes are mild. Few people, however, have an identical twin to provide tissue for donation; and when the need is for an organ such as the heart, liver, or lungs, a living-donor transplantation is not possible. Most often, organ and tissue transplants are **allografts**, which are grafts between members of the same species but who have different genotypes and HLA. Allografts may come from living donors; examples are bone marrow, blood, and a kidney. Most often, however, organs for transplantation are obtained from a cadaver. Donors are typically people who meet the criteria for brain death; are less than 65 years old; and are free of systemic disease, malignancy, or infection, including HIV, hepatitis B, or hepatitis C. The organ is removed immediately before or after cardiac arrest and preserved until it is transplanted into the waiting recipient. Finally, **xenograft** is a transplant from an animal species to a human. These transplants are the least successful but may be used in selected instances, such as the use of pig skin as a temporary covering for a massive burn.

Tissue typing is used to determine **histocompatibility**, the ability of cells and tissues to survive transplantation without immunologic interference by the recipient. Tissue typing is performed in an attempt to match the donor and recipient as closely as possible for HLA type and blood type (ABO, Rh) and to identify preformed antibodies to the donor's HLA.

Both antibody-mediated and cell-mediated immune responses are involved in the complex process of transplant rejection. Host macrophages process donor antigen, presenting it to T and B lymphocytes. Activated lymphocytes (B and T cells) produce both antibody- and cell-mediated effects. Killer T cells bind with cells of the transplanted organ, resulting in cell lysis. Helper T cells stimulate the multiplication and differentiation of B cells, and antibodies are produced to graft endothelium. Complement activation or antibody-dependent cell-mediated cytotoxicity leads to transplant cell destruction. Rejection typically begins after the first 24 hours of the transplant, although it may present immediately. Rejection episodes are characterized as hyperacute, acute, or chronic, as summarized in Table 13–3.

Hyperacute tissue rejection occurs immediately to 2 to 3 days after the transplant of new tissue. Hyperacute rejection is due to preformed antibodies and sensitized T cells to antigens in the donor organ. Hyperacute rejection is most likely to occur in clients who have had a previous organ or tissue transplant, such as a blood transfusion. Hyperacute rejection may be evident even before the transplant procedure is completed. The grafted organ initially appears pink and healthy, but soon becomes soft and cyanotic as blood flow is impaired. Organ function deteriorates rapidly, and symptoms of organ failure develop.

Acute tissue rejection is the most common and treatable type of rejection episode. It occurs between 4 days and 3 months after the transplant. Acute rejection is mediated primarily by the cellular immune response, resulting in transplant cell destruction. The client experiencing acute rejection demonstrates manifestations of the inflammatory process, with fever, redness, swelling, and tenderness over the graft site. Signs of impaired function of the transplanted organ may be noted (e.g., elevated blood urea nitrogen [BUN] and creatinine, liver enzyme and bilirubin elevations, or elevated cardiac enzymes and signs of cardiac failure).

Chronic tissue rejection occurs from 4 months to years after transplant of new tissue. Chronic rejection is most likely the re-

TABLE 13–3 Transplant Rejection Episodes

TYPE	CAUSE	PRESENTATION	TREATMENT
Hyperacute	Preexisting antibodies to donor ABO or HLA antigens	Occurs within minutes to hours or days of the transplant Rapid deterioration of organ function	The transplant usually cannot be saved; prevent with crossmatch, and use antimetabolites or anti-inflammatory drugs before surgery.
Acute	Primarily a cell-mediated immune response to HLA antigens; antibody-mediated response may also contribute	Occurs within days to months after the transplant Signs of inflammation and impaired organ function	Increase immunosuppression using steroids, cyclosporine, monoclonal antibodies, or antilymphocyte globulins.
Chronic	Probably antibody-mediated response; may also involve inflammatory damage to vessel endothelium	Occurs 4 months to years after the transplant Gradual deterioration of organ function	None; loss of graft will occur, requiring retransplant.

sult of antibody-mediated immune responses. Antibodies and complement are deposited in transplant vessel walls, causing narrowing and decreased function of the organ due to ischemia. The gradual deterioration of transplanted organ function is seen with chronic tissue rejection.

Graft-versus-host disease (GVHD) is a frequent and potentially fatal complication of bone marrow transplant. When there is no close match between donor and recipient HLA, immunocompetent cells in the grafted tissue recognize host tissue as foreign and mount a cell-mediated immune response. If the host is immunocompromised, as is often the case when a bone marrow transplant is performed, host cells are unable to destroy the graft and instead become the targets of destruction. Of clients with very closely matched bone marrow, 30% to 60% nevertheless develop GVHD. Acute GVHD occurs within the first 100 days following a transplant and primarily affects the skin, liver, and gastrointestinal tract. The client develops a maculopapular pruritic rash beginning on the palms of the hands and soles of the feet. The rash may spread to involve the entire body and lead to desquamation. Gastrointestinal manifestations include abdominal pain, nausea, and bloody diarrhea. GVHD that lasts longer than 100 days is said to be chronic. If it is limited to the skin and liver, the prognosis is good. If multiple organs are involved, the prognosis is poor (Porth, 2005).

INTERDISCIPLINARY CARE

Pretransplant care and post-transplant care are directed toward reducing the risk that transplanted tissue will be rejected or result in GVHD. Diagnostic studies are directed first at identifying a suitable donor, then at monitoring the immune response to the transplant. Immunosuppressive therapy with medications is a vital part of post-transplant care. Indeed, the development of effective immunosuppressive drugs is responsible for the success of organ transplants using allografts.

Diagnosis

The following diagnostic tests may be ordered prior to organ or tissue transplantation:

- *Blood type and Rh factor* of both the donor and recipient are determined. Although there is some question about the benefit of histocompatibility testing prior to transplant of a cadaver organ, there is no question about the need for ABO blood group compatibility.
- *Crossmatching* of the client's serum against the donor's lymphocytes is performed to identify any preformed antibodies against antigens on donor tissues. If present, these antibodies would likely result in an immediate or hyperacute graft rejection with probable loss of the transplant.
- *HLA histocompatibility testing* identifies donors with an HLA type close to that of the recipient. It is used primarily to identify living donors for bone marrow and kidney transplant. Because of GVHD, histocompatibility tests to identify an identical or very close HLA match are particularly important in bone marrow transplant. HLA tests are performed using lymphocytes from a blood sample. The sample should not be obtained within 72 hours of a blood transfusion, because this will interfere with results.
- *Mixed lymphocyte culture (MLC) assay tests* also are used to determine histocompatibility between the donor and the recipient. This test identifies whether mononuclear cells of the recipient will react against the potential donor's leukocyte antigens. The disadvantage of this test is that results cannot be obtained until 7 to 10 days later (Chernecky & Berger, 2004). If the intended recipient is severely immunocompromised, the results may be falsely negative. Clients treated with chemotherapy within 2 weeks of specimen collection are potentially immunocompromised.
- *Ultrasonography* or *magnetic resonance imaging (MRI)* of the transplanted organ may be performed to evaluate its size, perfusion, and function.
- *Tissue biopsies* of the transplanted organ are performed routinely to assess for evidence of tissue rejection.

Medications

Prior to transplantation, several antibiotic and antiviral drugs may be prescribed, including the following:

- Trimethoprim-sulfamethoxazole (Septra, Bactrim), which decreases the incidence of gram-negative bacterial infections

- Acyclovir (Zovirax), which prevents the development of herpes simplex virus pneumonia in bone marrow transplant recipients
- Ganciclovir (Cytovene), which prevents the development of cytomegalovirus (CMV) pneumonia with bone marrow transplant recipients.

The mainstays of drug therapy for clients following a tissue or organ transplant are immunosuppressive agents. Varying regimens of these drugs are used, depending on the transplanted tissue and the medical center; however, a combination of corticosteroids and cyclosporine is common for maintenance therapy. Antilymphocyte therapy and the use of monoclonal antibodies are increasingly common in the immediate post-transplant period and for treating steroid-resistant rejection episodes.

Corticosteroids, primarily prednisone (Deltasone, others) and methylprednisolone (Solu-Medrol, others), were among the first medications used to prevent transplant rejection, and they remain important agents today. Although the exact anti-inflammatory and immunosuppressive activity of corticosteroids is unknown, they are known to suppress production of interleukin-1 and -2, decrease monocyte migration, and suppress proliferative and cytotoxic T-cell activity. Although they are very effective, large doses of corticosteroids used post-transplant are associated with significant adverse effects. Wound healing is impaired, and the metabolism of fats, proteins, and carbohydrates is altered. Blood glucose increases with steroid use, impairing glucose control. Fat distribution changes, producing a cushingoid appearance with moon facies, increased truncal fat, and "buffalo hump." Fluid retention and hypertension are potential problems, as are osteoporosis, gastrointestinal bleeding, and emotional disturbances.

Azathioprine (Imuran) has been in use as an immunosuppressant for more than 25 years and continues to be a component of many regimens. Azathioprine inhibits both cell-mediated and antibody-mediated immunity, although its activity is more specific for T cells than B cells. Because it is rapidly metabolized by the liver, azathioprine can be given to clients with impaired renal function but may not be effective in clients with impaired hepatic function. Bone marrow suppression is the most common adverse effect of this drug, necessitating frequent evaluation of the complete blood count (CBC). Hepatotoxicity, pancreatitis, and increased risk of neoplasm are also associated with azathioprine administration. Nursing responsibilities related to azathioprine are listed in the Medication Administration box on the following pages. Clients who cannot tolerate azathioprine may receive a newer immunosuppressant, mycophenolate mofetil (CellCept). Primarily, it is prescribed following renal and cardiac transplants. See Figure 13–6 ■.

Cyclosporine has contributed significantly to the success of organ transplantation since its introduction in the 1970s. Cyclosporine inhibits T-cell function and the normal cell-mediated immune response. The incidence of cyclosporine toxicity and side effects is related to blood levels, so blood levels are monitored closely. Cyclosporine is both nephrotoxic and hepatotoxic, especially at high doses. Observable toxic effects include hypertension and CNS symptoms such as

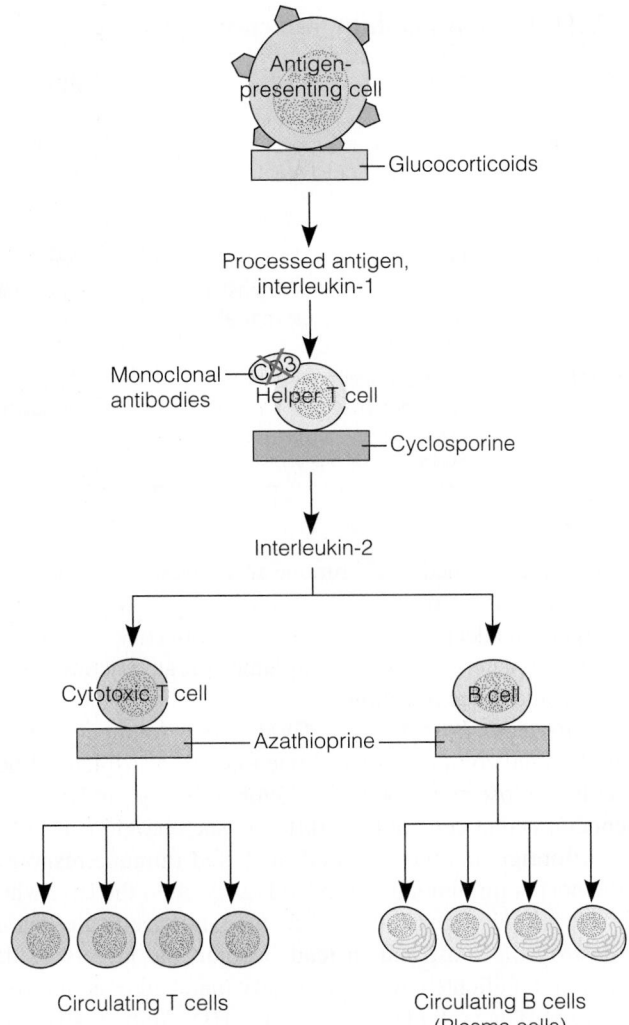

Figure 13–6 ■ Sites of action of immunosuppressive agents.

flushing or tingling of the extremities, confusion, visual disturbances, and seizures or coma.

Muromonab-CD3, also known as OKT3 or Orthoclone, is the first monoclonal antibody produced for therapeutic use in humans. As a monoclonal antibody, OKT3 is specific to T cells, blocking their generation and function. It binds with a surface antigen on T cells, inactivating and removing them from circulation. It also blocks killer T cells attached to the graft. Because of significant side effects, the use of OKT3 is limited primarily to treatment of steroid-resistant rejection. Two newer monoclonal antibodies, basiliximab (Simulect) and daclizumab (Zenapax), are a combination of mouse and human antibodies and cause fewer side effects.

Polyclonal antilymphocyte antibodies are also used as adjunctive immunosuppressant therapy. These are administered as antilymphocyte globulin (ALG) or antithymocyte globulin (ATG). These globulins contain antibodies against both T and B cells, as well as other mononuclear leukocytes. When administered, they deplete circulating lymphocytes, platelets, and granulocytes.

MEDICATION ADMINISTRATION Immunosuppressive Agents

T-CELL SUPPRESSORS
Cyclosporine (Sandimmune)
Tacrolimus (Prograf)
Sirolimus (Rapamune)
These drugs inhibit T-cell development and activation. They are given concurrently with a glucocorticoid and in combination with other immunosuppressants and inhibit immune system activity and organ rejection.

Nursing Responsibilities
- Monitor BUN and creatinine for evidence of nephrotoxicity.
- Teach the signs and symptoms of infection unique to immune-suppressed individuals. A temperature of 100.6°F is significant evidence of infection. A sore throat may be a manifestation. Other signs and symptoms of inflammation and infection may be absent.
- Teach clients good hygiene to avoid infection with special emphasis on hand washing and avoiding infected individuals.
- Monitor blood pressure and availability and use of antihypertensive medications.
- Teach to avoid grapefruit juice, which can raise cyclosporine levels by 50% to 200% and increase the risk of toxicity. Sirolimus should not be taken with grapefruit juice. Sirolimus increases cholesterol and triglycerides. Lipid-lowering drugs may be necessary to prevent hyperlipidemias.

CYTOTOXIC AGENTS
Azathioprine (Imuran)
Cyclophosphamide (Cytoxan)
Methotrexate (Rheumatrex, Trexall)
Mycophenolate (CellCept)
Certain drugs that are identified as cytotoxic or antineoplastic agents are effective as immunosuppressive agents. They act by decreasing the proliferation of cells within the immune system and are widely used to prevent rejection following a tissue or organ transplant. They are usually administered concurrently with corticosteroid therapy, allowing lower doses of both preparations and resulting in fewer side effects.

Nursing Responsibilities
- Monitor blood count, with particular attention to the WBC and platelet counts. Notify the physician if WBCs fall below 4000 or platelets below 75,000.
- Monitor renal and liver function studies, including creatinine, BUN, creatinine clearance, and liver enzymes. Report abnormal levels to the physician.
- Administer the drug as ordered. Administer oral preparations with food to minimize gastrointestinal effects. Antacids may be ordered.
- Have client increase fluids to maintain good hydration and urinary output, void frequently, and avoid taking in the evening, which promotes dwelling of the drug in the bladder overnight.
- Monitor intake and output.
- Monitor for signs of abnormal bleeding, bleeding gums, bruising, petechiae, joint pain, hematuria, and black or tarry stools.
- Use meticulous hand washing and other appropriate measures to protect the client from infection. Assess for signs of infection.

- Pulmonary fibrosis is a rare (<1%) potential adverse effect of cyclophosphamides. Therefore, monitor respiratory function using pulmonary function studies and monitor for clinical signs of dyspnea or cough.

Health Education for the Client and Family
- Avoid large crowds and situations where exposure to infection is probable.
- Report signs of infection, such as chills, fever, sore throat, fatigue, or malaise, to the physician.
- Use contraceptive measures to prevent pregnancy while on immunosuppressive therapy; these drugs are teratogenic.
- Avoid the use of aspirin or ibuprofen while taking these drugs. Report any signs of bleeding to the physician. Many over-the-counter products contain aspirin; check labels for aspirin.
- With cyclophosphamide, amenorrhea may occur. The menses will resume after the drug is discontinued.
- If taking cyclophosphamide, report difficulty breathing or cough to the physician.

MONOCLONAL ANTIBODY
- Muromonab-CD3 or OKT3 (Orthoclone); Basiliximab and Daclizumab
This monoclonal antibody against T cells is formed by immunizing a mouse with an antigen to produce a specific antibody. Lymphocytes producing the antibody, OKT3, are cloned, and the antibody is harvested. When injected into humans, OKT3 binds with a surface antigen on T cells, removing them from circulation and inactivating those bound to allograft cells. Due to the high incidence of adverse effects, the first two doses of OKT3 are administered by a physician and the client closely observed for 2 hours following each dose.

Nursing Responsibilities
- Be sure a chest x-ray has been performed within 24 hours preceding initiation of OKT3 therapy and that no congestion is present. The risk of anaphylaxis is greater in the client with fluid overload.
- Premedicate as ordered with hydrocortisone, acetaminophen, and diphenhydramine to reduce potential adverse effects.
- Position a crash cart or code cart with emergency medications in the client's room or in proximity to it.
- After each of the first two doses, monitor vital signs every 15 minutes for 2 hours, then every 30 minutes for 2 hours.
- After the first two doses, administer a 2.5- to 10-mg dose by intravenous push over 1 to 2 minutes.
- Observe closely for potential adverse effects, including chills and fever; tachycardia; headache and tremor; hypertension or hypotension; nausea, vomiting, and diarrhea; chest pain, dyspnea, and wheezing.
- OKT3 can also cause anaphylaxis; observe for evidence of urticaria, angioedema, laryngeal edema, wheezing, or other signs of anaphylactic reaction.
- Monitor CBC for evidence of leukopenia or pancytopenia.
- Assess for infection. Remember that typical signs of infection, including symptoms such as fever and inflammation, may be masked or reduced by immunosuppressive therapy.

(continued)

MEDICATION ADMINISTRATION Immunosuppressive Agents (continued)

Health Education for the Client and Family
- Teach about the drug and its purpose.
- Discuss potential adverse and side effects, and emphasize the need to report symptoms promptly.
- Inform the client that adverse effects are most likely to occur following the first two doses, necessitating close observation at that time. Reassure the client that this is standard protocol for this medication.

ANTILYMPHOCYTE GLOBULINS
Antithymocyte globulin or ATG (ATGAM)
Antilymphocyte globulin or ALG

These globulins containing antilymphocyte antibodies are produced by immunizing horses (the main source), rabbits, or sheep with human lymphocytes to stimulate production of antibodies (see figure at right). Serum from the animal is then recovered, and the active IgG fraction is isolated, purified, and administered parenterally to the client. It binds with peripheral lymphocytes and mononuclear cells, removing them from circulation.

ATG or ALG is used both to induce immunosuppression immediately following a transplant and to treat steroid-resistant rejection episodes. As with monoclonal antibody, multiple side effects are associated with ATG or ALG.

Nursing Responsibilities
- Perform a skin test for sensitivity to horse serum prior to initial dose. Report any positive reaction to the physician and hold administration until desensitization therapy has been completed.
- Premedicate as ordered with acetaminophen and diphenhydramine prior to each dose. Steroids may also be administered before the initial dose. Have epinephrine and hydrocortisone injections available at the bedside in case of anaphylactic reaction.
- Administer by intravenous infusion into a central line over 4 to 6 hours.
- Monitor vital signs hourly while medication is infusing.
- Assess for adverse effects, including chills and fever, erythema, and pruritus. Notify the physician; these may be treated symptomatically.
- Monitor CBC daily, notify the physician if WBC falls to less than $3000/mm^3$ or platelet count to less than $100,000/mm^3$. The medication may be stopped or reduced.
- Assess renal function studies to monitor for serum sickness. Report complaints of joint pain.
- Monitor for signs of infection, and report any signs promptly.

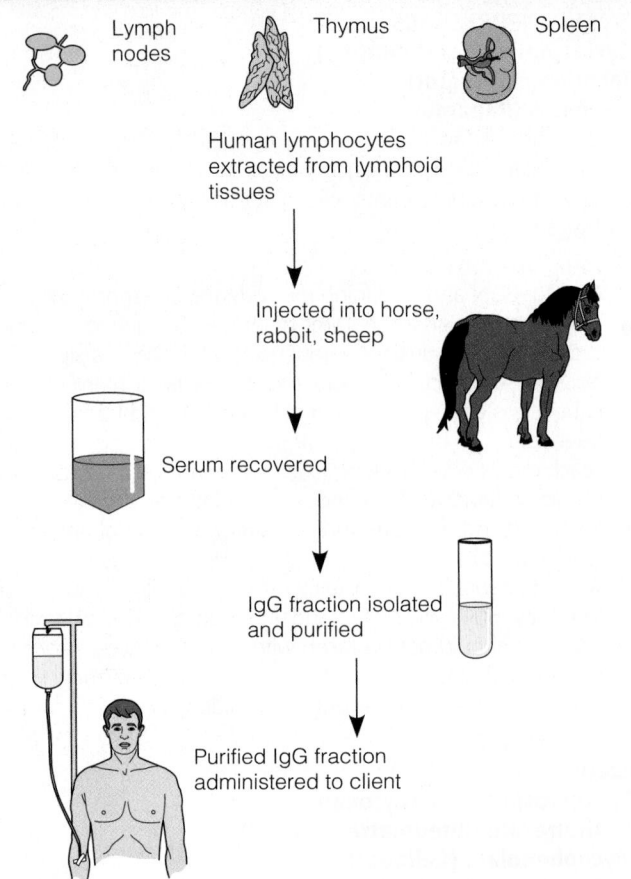

A horse is inoculated with washed human lymphocytes, stimulating the production of immunoglobulin with polyclonal antilymphocyte antibodies. These are then extracted from horse serum, purified, and administered intravenously to the client.

Health Education for the Client and Family
- Explain the need for special precautions and close monitoring while this drug is being administered.
- Instruct the client to report any adverse effects, including malaise or joint pain, promptly.
- Ask the client to report any evidence of easy bruising, bleeding gums, or black stools.
- Teach family members about the importance of not exposing the client to persons with infectious diseases.

NURSING CARE

The client who has an organ or tissue transplant has both immediate and long-term nursing care needs. Both the client and the family must be considered in providing nursing care.

Health Promotion

Part of the health promotion activities focus on preventing the need for a tissue transplant. It is important to increase public awareness regarding unhealthy lifestyle behaviors, such as excessive alcohol consumption and illegal drug use, and their relationship to organ failure. Clients with chronic diseases such as diabetes mellitus and hypertension must understand that inadequate management of these disorders could lead to end-stage renal disease. Other risk factors may simply relate to a person's heredity; understanding how heredity could affect future health might influence the client's lifestyle choices.

Assessment

Assessment data collected following a tissue transplant focus on identifying potential rejection episodes. Further focused assessments are described with nursing interventions in the next section.

Nursing Diagnoses and Interventions

Because of the continuing risk of transplant rejection and the need for immunosuppression, *Ineffective Protection* and *Risk for Impaired Tissue Integrity* are priority nursing care foci. The client's underlying disease process, the transplant, and the continuing need for immunosuppressive drug therapy also have emotional and psychologic consequences. Many nursing diagnoses, such as *Powerlessness* or *Ineffective Coping,* may be appropriate. The diagnosis *Anxiety* related to potential transplant rejection is considered in this section.

Ineffective Protection

Ineffective protection is a problem for the transplant client at all stages. Before the transplant occurs, failure of the affected organ may put the client at risk for infection and other multisystemic problems. Incisions and invasive perioperative procedures impair skin and mucous membrane protection from infectious organisms and other antigens. Immunosuppressive drugs given postoperatively to prevent graft rejection disarm the immune response to a certain extent, increasing the risk of infections and neoplastic growths.

PRACTICE ALERT
Use strict aseptic technique in changing dressings and caring for invasive catheters such as intravenous lines and indwelling urinary catheters to protect against external and resident host microorganisms.

- Wash hands on entering room and before providing direct care. *Hand washing removes transient organisms from the skin, reducing the risk of transmission to the client.*
- Assess frequently for signs and symptoms of infection. Monitor the temperature and vital signs every 4 hours. Assess for evidence of inflammation, abnormal wound drainage, changes in urine or other body secretions, complaints of pain, or behavior changes that may indicate infection. Culture abnormal wound drainage. *The client on immunosuppressive therapy is more susceptible to infection, and usual signs and symptoms may not be evident. Both the temperature and inflammatory response can be suppressed by therapy. Prompt identification and intervention for infection is important in the immunosuppressed client.*
- Monitor laboratory values, including CBC and tests of organ function; report changes to the physician. *An elevation in the WBC count with increased numbers of immature cells (bands) or a decline in function of the transplanted organ (e.g., a rising BUN and creatinine in the renal transplant client) may be early indications of infection or transplant failure.*
- Initiate reverse or protective isolation procedures as indicated by the client's immune status. *These procedures further protect the severely immunocompromised client from infection.*
- Instruct ill family members and visitors to avoid contact with the client. *A "minor" upper respiratory infection can be a significant illness in the immunocompromised host.*

- Help ensure adequate nutrient intake, offering supplementary feedings as indicated or maintaining parenteral nutrition if necessary. *Adequate nutrition is important for healing and immune system function.*
- Change intravenous bags and tubing at least every 24 hours, and change peripheral intravenous sites every 48 to 72 hours, unless contraindicated. Remove invasive catheters and lines as soon as they are no longer necessary. *Changing lines and sites is important to reduce bacterial contamination. Fewer invasive lines provide fewer sites for bacterial invasion of the body.*
- Emphasize the importance of washing hands thoroughly after using the bathroom and before eating. *This reduces the risk of infection with endogenous organisms.*
- Provide good mouth care. *Good mouth care reduces the population of oral microorganisms and helps maintain an intact mucous membrane lining.*
- Monitor for potential adverse effects of medications:
  - Thrombocytopenia and possible bleeding
  - Fluid retention with edema and possible hypertension
  - Loss of bone density, osteoporosis, and possible pathologic fractures
  - Renal or hepatic toxicity
  - Cardiac effects, particularly in the presence of fluid retention and hypervolemia.
  Medications used to maintain immunosuppression and preserve the allograft have many potential adverse effects that can alter normal protective and homeostatic mechanisms.

Risk for Impaired Tissue Integrity: Allograft

As noted, the risk for transplant rejection is highest in the initial postoperative period, but it is never completely eliminated for the client who has had an allograft. The client who has had a bone marrow transplant has the additional risk of developing GVHD, which can affect the integrity of skin, mucous membranes, and other organs.

- Administer immunosuppressive therapy as prescribed. *Suppression of the immune response is necessary to reduce the risk of graft destruction by normal immune responses and to preserve the graft's function.*
- Assess for evidence of graft rejection, including tenderness, erythema, and swelling over the site; sudden weight gain, edema, and hypertension; chills and fever; malaise; and an increased WBC count and sedimentation rate. Report any changes immediately. *Early identification of rejection allows adjustment of medication regimens and, possibly, preservation of the graft.*
- Monitor results of laboratory studies for function of the transplanted organ. *With a functional graft, results (e.g., renal or liver function studies) will improve; a functional decline may be an early indicator of rejection.*
- Assess for and report signs of GVHD immediately, including maculopapular rash, erythema of the skin and possible desquamation, hair loss, abdominal cramping and diarrhea, or jaundice with elevated bilirubin and liver enzymes (AST, ALT). *GVHD is a potentially lethal complication in the immunosuppressed client and necessitates immediate intervention.*

- Stress the importance of maintaining immunosuppressive therapy and reporting signs of graft rejection promptly to the physician. *Continued immunosuppression and prompt treatment of rejection are vital to preserving graft function.*

Anxiety

The client who undergoes an organ or tissue transplantation often faces the unwelcome choices of death from organ failure or receiving an organ that his or her body will likely attempt to reject. In most cases, the client understands that to receive this transplant, someone else must die and be willing to give up an organ. When the transplant comes from a living donor (bone marrow or kidney), the client may worry not only about himself or herself, but also about the condition of the donor. Fear of rejection and guilt may be even greater in this instance.

- Assess level of anxiety by noting such cues as expressions of apprehension, fear, or inadequacy; facial expression, tension, or shakiness; difficulty focusing; helplessness; poor eye contact; and restlessness. *Clients may have difficulty identifying or verbalizing feelings of fear and anxiety. Nonverbal cues are often useful in recognizing states of anxiety.*
- Provide opportunities to express feelings. Use opening statements such as "Facing an organ transplant must be very stressful." Listen attentively. *Encouragement and active listening allow the client to express feelings of anxiety or fear.*
- Arrange tasks to allow as much time with the client as possible. When leaving, tell the client when you will return. *Time spent with the client facilitates the development of trust.*
- Provide clear, concise directions. *Highly anxious clients have difficulty focusing and retaining information.*
- Encourage involvement in care but do not request unnecessary decisions. *The client needs to feel a sense of control but may become irritated if asked to make decisions unrelated to the situation.*
- Encourage family members to remain with the client as much as possible. *This can help reduce the client's anxiety.*
- Encourage the use of coping behaviors that have been effective for the client in the past. *Coping mechanisms and behaviors help lower anxiety to a more acceptable level.*

- Reduce or eliminate environmental stressors to the extent possible. *This gives the client a better sense of control.*
- Assist with stress reduction and relaxation techniques, such as guided imagery, meditation, and muscle relaxation. *These techniques help the client gain control over physical responses to anxiety.*
- Arrange for a counselor or mental health specialist to work with the client. *Counseling can help the client identify and deal with his or her feelings.*
- Assess the client's preference and desire for spiritual counseling prior to transplant. *Because there is a risk of death if the transplant fails, the client may want to discuss his or her concerns with a spiritual counselor.*

Community-Based Care

Teaching of the client and family regarding an organ or tissue transplant begins well before the transplant and continues throughout hospitalization and follow-up treatment.

Initial teaching focuses on the options, risks, and potential benefits of the transplant itself. Include the procedure by which the organ is selected and obtained, as well as the procedure by which it is transplanted into the client. If a living related donor is an option, discuss the risks and benefits for both the client and the donor. Outline the post-transplant treatment regimen, including any lifestyle changes that may be necessary.

Following the transplant, provide verbal and written instructions, including the following:

- Manifestations of transplant rejection and the importance of notifying the physician
- Immunosuppressive drug regimen and side effects
- Wound care
- Avoiding exposure to infectious diseases, particularly respiratory infections, and wearing a mask when going outside
- Meticulous personal hygiene, hand washing technique, and frequent mouth care
- Wearing a Medic-Alert bracelet or tag
- Follow-up visits to the physician or clinic
- Helpful resources:
  - American Council on Transplantation
  - Local and state support groups related to specific organ transplant, such as the National Kidney Foundation.

IMPAIRED IMMUNE RESPONSES

Disorders of impaired immune system responses may be either congenital or acquired. Often the function of either T or B cells is impaired, reducing the body's ability to defend against foreign antigens or abnormal host tissue.

No matter what the cause, clients with immunodeficiency disorders demonstrate an unusual susceptibility to infection. When the antibody-mediated response is primarily affected, the client is at particular risk for severe and chronic bacterial infections. These clients also do not develop long-lasting immunity to such diseases as chickenpox and are prone to recurrent cases. Clients with a defect of cell-mediated immunity tend to develop disseminated viral infections such

as herpes simplex and CMV. Candidiasis and other fungal infections are also common. Because T cells are involved with activating antibody-mediated immune responses as well, overwhelming bacterial infections may occur. Immunodeficiency in its most severe form occurs when both antibody-mediated and cell-mediated responses are impaired. Clients with combined immunodeficiency are susceptible to all varieties of infectious organisms, including those not normally considered to be pathogens.

Most immunodeficiency diseases are genetically determined and rare. They affect children more than adults. The noted exception is AIDS, an infectious disease caused by a virus.

THE CLIENT WITH HIV INFECTION

In 1981, five cases of *Pneumocystis carinii* pneumonia (PCP) and 26 cases of a rare cancer, Kaposi's sarcoma, were diagnosed in young, previously healthy homosexual males in Los Angeles and New York City. The term **acquired immunodeficiency syndrome (AIDS)** was ascribed to this new phenomenon to describe the immune system deficits associated with these opportunistic disorders. Prior to this time, both PCP and Kaposi's had been seen only in elderly, debilitated, or severely immunodeficient people. Other groups at risk for AIDS were soon identified: injection drug users, persons with hemophilia, recipients of blood transfusions, and immigrants from Haiti.

Research to identify the cause of this apparently new disease progressed feverishly, and in 1983, a common antibody was identified in clients with AIDS. The **human immunodeficiency virus (HIV)** was isolated in 1984. It then became apparent that AIDS was the final, fatal stage of HIV infection.

It began, like so many epidemics, with a few isolated cases, and has become a worldwide plague. (See the accompanying Focus on Cultural Diversity box.) AIDS invades our lives in ways we never imagined—testing our scientific knowledge, probing our private values, and eluding a vaccine or a cure. Progression of HIV-positive disease to AIDS has slowed because of the effectiveness of highly active antiretroviral therapy (HAART) (Centers for Disease Control and Prevention [CDC], 2006). This change in progression to AIDS makes monitoring of AIDS less useful as an indicator of infected cases. For that reason, the CDC developed new surveillance methods based on infection rates in high-risk populations.

Although the incidence of HIV has leveled and mortality due to AIDS has declined, the epidemic is far from over. In the United States it continues to disproportionately affect African Americans, males who have sex with males (MSM), and high-risk heterosexuals. High-risk heterosexuals are those who have sex with individuals known to be infected with HIV or with high risk for having HIV. Two separate elements are reported in the surveillance data: HIV infection rate and AIDS occurrence. HIV infection is dependent on exposure to the virus; conversion to AIDS is related to access and use of HAART. HIV new cases are highest among MSM and high-risk heterosexuals; AIDS occurrence continues among MSM, high-risk heterosexuals, and African Americans. (CDC, 2006).

Incidence and Prevalence

Through 2004, the CDC (2004) estimated that 1,039,000 to 1,185,000 persons in the United States were living with HIV/AIDS, with 24% to 27% undiagnosed and unaware of their HIV infection. By the end of December 2004, a cumulative total of 944,305 cases of AIDS had been reported. Deaths among people with AIDS had decreased from 50,610 in 1995 to 15,798 in 2004, more than likely the result of improved treatments rather than a decline in spread of the disease (CDC, 2006). A continued decline in deaths is dependent on access to quality care and treatment and continued development of treatments for those already heavily treated (Tierney et al., 2005).

The risk factors for HIV infection are behavioral. Among adults in the United States, 60% of reported cases are in men who have sex with other men, including homosexuals, bisexuals, and such groups as prison populations. Unprotected anal intercourse is the major route of transmission in this group. Injection drug use is the second leading risk factor, accounting for approximately 25% of cases. Sharing of needles and other drug paraphernalia is the primary route of transmission in this group. Heterosexual intercourse with an infected drug user and exchanging sex for drugs are major risk factors for women. Hemophiliacs who require large amounts of intravenous clotting factors and people infected through blood transfusion account for a small number of cases, approximately 2% (CDC, 2004).

The majority of women were infected through heterosexual contact (75%) with the remaining 25% through injection drug use. Among risk groups, the most rapid increases are noted in young gay and bisexual men, women, and inner-city injection drug users, especially African Americans and Hispanics (CDC, 2004). In the United States, the rate of male adult/adolescent HIV/AIDS cases (per 100,000 population) reported was 131.6 among African Americans, 60.2 among Hispanics, 20.8 among American Indians/Alaska Natives, 18.7 among Caucasians, and 13.9 among Asians/Pacific Islanders (CDC, 2004). The rapid increase of AIDS cases among women is of special concern; those numbers increased from 7% of cases in 1985 to 27% of newly reported cases in 2003 (CDC, 2004).

In addition, AIDS in the adult over age 50 accounts for approximately 10% of all reported cases in the United States (CDC, 2004). Declining immune system function in older adults significantly increases their risk for contracting HIV/AIDS, along with the belief that they cannot be affected by it. Just as younger persons with HIV/AIDS contract the diseases primarily through sexual intercourse, so does the elderly population. Because older adults are beyond childbearing years, they often fail

---

FOCUS ON CULTURAL DIVERSITY
HIV/AIDS

There are an estimated 36.2 million people infected with AIDS worldwide, with virtually every country in the world reporting cases of AIDS (Joint United Nations Programme on HIV/AIDS, 2000). The highest incidence is found in sub-Saharan Africa, South and Southeast Asia, the United States, western Europe, South America, and Canada. Approximately 70% of all people infected with HIV or who have AIDS live in sub-Saharan Africa, and another 16% live in South and Southeast Asia, largely in Thailand and India. The most common mode of transmission is heterosexual intercourse. The cofactors of general health status, the presence of genital ulcers, and the number of sexual partners correlate with incidence (Tierney et al., 2005).

Critical Thinking Questions

1. How accurate is informed consent for a clinical trial in Third World countries if investigators are dependent on translators? What factors could impact the validity of the consent?

2. Do you think it is ethical to do clinical trials in countries outside the origin of a product?

to use condoms when engaging in sexual activity. Manifestations may be overlooked by healthcare professionals, leading to a delayed diagnosis and increased severity of the disease.

HIV is a retrovirus transmitted by direct contact with infected blood and body fluids. Significant concentrations of the virus are present in blood, semen, vaginal and cervical secretions, and cerebrospinal fluid (CSF) of infected individuals. It is also found in breast milk and saliva. Sexual contact is the primary mode of transmission. HIV is also transmitted through contact with infected blood via needle sharing during injection drug use or by transfusion. Approximately 13% to 40% of infants born to HIV-positive mothers are infected perinatally. Breast-feeding is a route of transmission and should be avoided (Tierney et al., 2005).

Less than 0.04% of people voluntarily donating blood (a process that generally excludes people with high-risk behavior) are found to be HIV positive. HIV is not transmitted by casual contact, nor is there any evidence of its transmission by

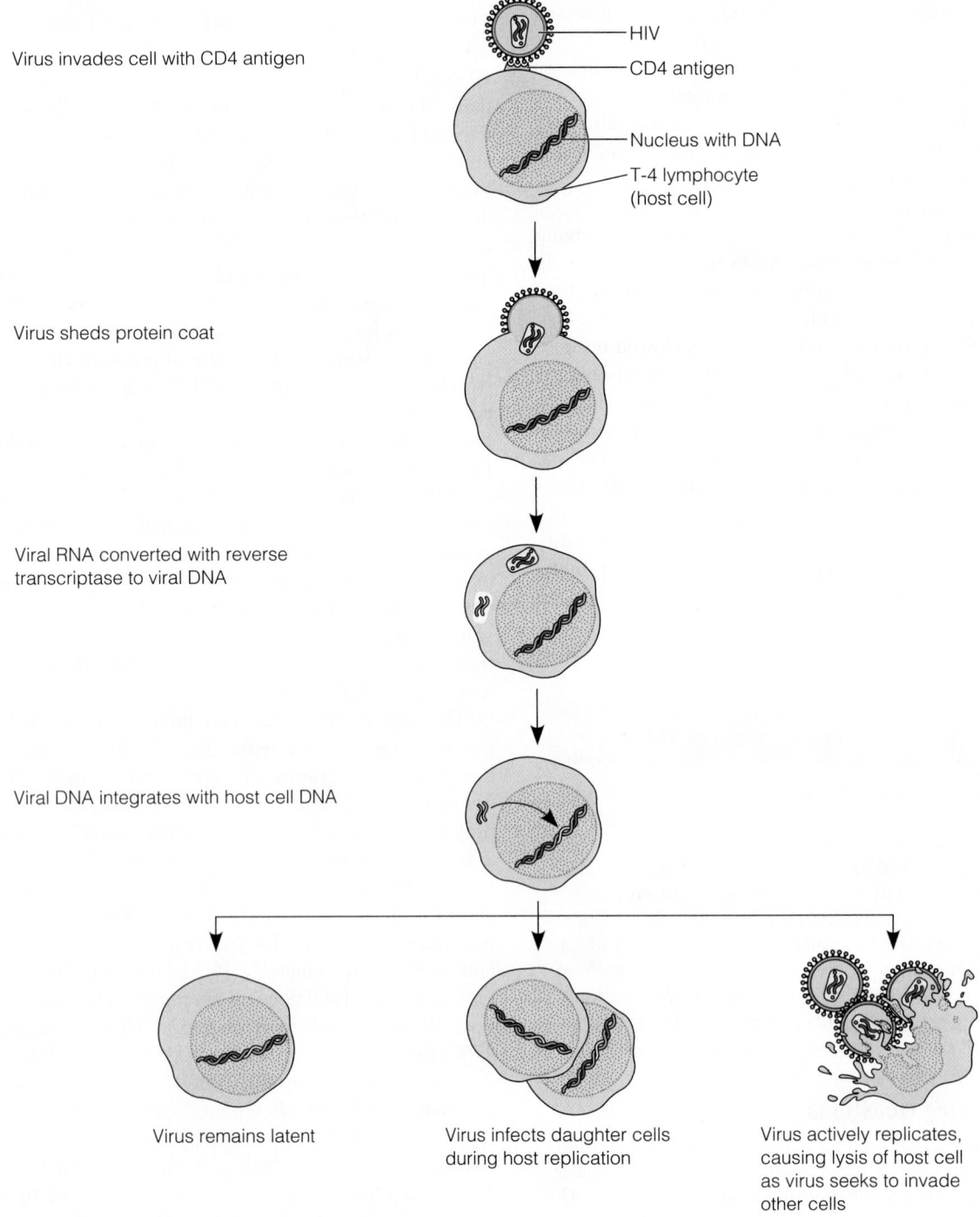

Virus invades cell with CD4 antigen

— HIV
— CD4 antigen
— Nucleus with DNA
— T-4 lymphocyte (host cell)

Virus sheds protein coat

Viral RNA converted with reverse transcriptase to viral DNA

Viral DNA integrates with host cell DNA

Virus remains latent

Virus infects daughter cells during host replication

Virus actively replicates, causing lysis of host cell as virus seeks to invade other cells

Figure 13–7 ■ How HIV infects and destroys CD4 cells.

vectors such as mosquitoes. Blood donation also poses no risk of contracting HIV to the donor, because only new sterile equipment is used. A small but real occupational risk exists for healthcare workers. Percutaneous exposure to infected blood or body fluids through a needle-stick injury or nonintact skin is the primary route of transmission. Documented evidence indicates that parenteral exposure poses a 0.3% risk of becoming HIV positive (Carrico, 2001; Tierney et al., 2005). Mucosal exposures, such as splashing in the eyes or mouth, pose a much smaller risk.

Pathophysiology and Manifestations

As mentioned, HIV is a retrovirus, meaning it carries its genetic information in RNA. On entry into the body, the virus infects cells that have the CD4 antigen. Once inside the cell, the virus sheds its protein coat and uses an enzyme called *reverse transcriptase* to convert the RNA to DNA (Figure 13–7 ■). This viral DNA is then integrated into host cell DNA and duplicated during normal processes of cell division. Within the cell, the virus may remain latent or become activated to produce new RNA and to form *virions*. The virus then buds from the cell surface, disrupting its cell membrane and leading to destruction of the host cell.

Although the virus may remain inactive in infected cells for years, antibodies are produced to its proteins, a process known as **seroconversion**. These antibodies are usually detectable 6 weeks to 6 months after the initial infection. Helper T or CD4 cells are the primary cells infected by HIV. It also infects macrophages and certain cells of the CNS. Helper T cells play a vital role in normal immune system function, recognizing foreign antigens and infected cells and activating antibody-producing B cells. They also direct cell-mediated immune activity and influence the phagocytic activity of monocytes and macrophages. The loss of these helper T cells leads to the immunodeficiencies seen with HIV in-

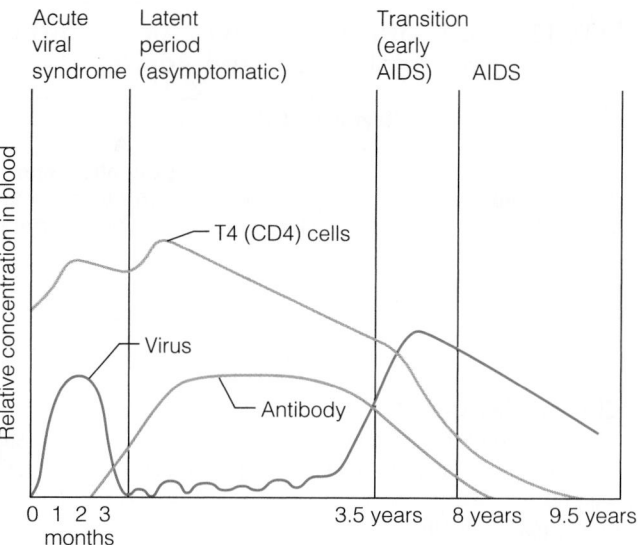

Figure 13–8 ■ The progression of HIV infection. Acute illness develops shortly after the virus is contracted, corresponding with a rapid rise in viral levels. Antibodies are formed and remain present throughout the course of infection. Late in the disease, viral activation results in a marked increase in virus while CD4 (T4) cells diminish as they are destroyed with viral replication. Antibody levels gradually decrease as immune function is impaired.

fection (Porth, 2005). Figure 13–8 ■ illustrates the typical course of HIV infection.

The clinical manifestations of HIV infection range from no symptoms to severe immunodeficiency with multiple opportunistic infections and cancers (see the Manifestations box below). It appears that the majority of clients develop an acute mononucleosis-type illness within days to weeks after contracting the virus. Typical manifestations include fever, sore throat,

---

MANIFESTATIONS **of HIV Infection and AIDS**

I. Acute Retroviral Syndrome (ARS) or Primary HIV Infection
   ■ Fever
   ■ Sore throat
   ■ Arthralgias and myalgias
   ■ Headache
   ■ Rash
   ■ Nausea, vomiting, and abdominal cramping
II. Asymptomatic Infection
   ■ None; converts to seropositive status
III. Persistent Generalized Lymphadenopathy
   ■ Enlargement of two or more extrainguinal sites for more than 3 months
IV. Other Acute Disease Symptoms
   ■ General malaise, fatigue
   ■ Low grade fever
   ■ Night sweats
   ■ Involuntary weight loss
   ■ Skin dryness, or rashes

V. Other Diseases and AIDS
   A. *AIDS Dementia Complex*
   B. *Secondary Infectious Diseases*
      ■ *Pneumocystis carinii* pneumonia
      ■ *Mycobacterium* tuberculosis
      ■ *Mycobacterium avium* complex
      ■ Candidiasis
      ■ Cryptosporidiosis
      ■ Cryptococcosis
      ■ Toxoplasmosis
      ■ Herpes simplex or herpes zoster
      ■ Cytomegalovirus
   C. *Secondary Cancers*
      ■ Kaposi's sarcoma
      ■ Non-Hodgkin's lymphoma
      ■ Cervical dysplasia and cervical cancer
   D. *Other Conditions*
      ■ Pelvic inflammatory disease
      ■ Human papillomavirus

BOX 13–2 Classification System for HIV Infection and Expanded AIDS Surveillance Case Definition for Adolescents and Adults

	Diagnostic Categories	Clinical Categories	
CD4 + T-cell Categories	**A** **Asymptomatic, Acute (Primary) HIV or Persistent Generalized Lymphadenopathy (PGL)**	**B** **Symptomatic, Not (A) or (C) Conditions**	**C** **AIDS-Indicator Conditions**
(1) ≥500/mm³	A1	B1	C1
(2) 200–499/mm³	A2	B2	C2
(3) <200/mm³	A3	B3	C3

As of January 1, 1993, people with AIDS-indicator conditions (clinical category C) and those in categories A3 or B3 were considered to have AIDS.

Clinical Category A

One or more of the following conditions in an adolescent or adult with documented HIV infection and without conditions in categories B and C:

- Asymptomatic HIV infection
- Persistent generalized lymphadenopathy
- Acute HIV infection with accompanying illness or history of acute HIV infection

Clinical Category B

Examples of conditions but are not limited to:

- Candidiasis, oral (thrush), or vulvovaginal (persistent, frequent, or poorly responsive to therapy)
- Cervical dysplasia/cervical carcinoma *in situ*
- Constitutional symptoms, such as fever (38.5°C) or diarrhea exceeding 1 month duration
- Hairy leukoplakia
- Herpes zoster involving at least two distinct episodes
- Pelvic inflammatory disease
- Peripheral neuropathy

Clinical Category C

- Candidiasis of bronchi, trachea, or lungs; esophagus
- Coccidioidomycosis
- Cryptococcosis
- Cryptosporidiosis with persistent diarrhea
- Cytomegalovirus infection (other than of liver, spleen, or lymph nodes)
- CMV retinitis
- HIV encephalopathy
- Herpes simplex: chronic ulcers or bronchitis, pneumonitis, or esophagitis
- *Mycobacterium avium* complex or disseminated
- *Mycobacterium tuberculosis*
- *Pneumocystis carinii* pneumonia
- Progressive multifocal leukoencephalopathy
- *Salmonella* septicemia
- Toxoplasmosis of the brain
- Kaposi's sarcoma
- Cervical cancer, invasive
- Lymphoma
- HIV wasting syndrome

Source: Adapted from "Revised Classification System for HIV Infection and Expanded Case Definition for AIDS Among Adolescents and Adults," 1993, *MMWR, CDC Recommendations and Reports, 41*(RR 17), pp. 1–19.

arthralgias and myalgias, headache, rash, and lymphadenopathy. Pathologic changes are also noted in the CNS of many infected individuals although the mechanism of neurologic dysfunction is unclear. The client may also experience nausea, vomiting, and abdominal cramping. The client often attributes this initial manifestation of HIV infection to a common viral illness such as influenza, upper respiratory infection, or stomach virus.

Following this acute illness, clients enter a long-lasting asymptomatic period. Although the virus is present and can be transmitted to others, the infected host has few or no symptoms. Clearly, the majority of HIV-infected persons are in this stage of the disease. The length of the asymptomatic period varies widely, but its mean length is estimated to be 8 to 10 years.

Some clients with few other symptoms develop persistent generalized lymphadenopathy. This is defined as enlargement of two or more lymph nodes outside the inguinal chain with no other illness or condition to account for the lymphadenopathy.

The move from asymptomatic disease or persistent lymphadenopathy to AIDS is often not clearly defined. The client may complain of general malaise, fever, fatigue, night sweats, and involuntary weight loss. Persistent skin dryness and rash

may be a problem. Diarrhea is common, as are oral lesions such as hairy leukoplakia, candidiasis, and gingival inflammation and ulceration. The development of advanced HIV typically occurs 10 to 11 years after initial infection; this varies according to the viral load, rate of disease progression, and the development of resistance to antiretroviral therapy (Kenny, 2004).

With the development of significant constitutional disease, neurologic manifestations, or opportunistic infections or cancers, the client has manifestations that are characteristic of AIDS and a very poor prognosis. HIV infection and AIDS may be classified by using the CDC's matrix classification system. Under this system, HIV disease is determined by the presence of clinical symptoms (clinical categories A, B, and C) and by T4 cell counts (categories 1, 2, and 3) (Box 13–2). When a client's T4 cell count falls to <200, he or she has late-stage AIDS, <50 is end stage AIDS (Coyne, Lyne, & Watson, 2002).

When clinical manifestations develop, the outcome varies. With antiretroviral therapy (ART), many clients are living longer after being diagnosed with AIDS. Today PCP is most commonly diagnosed in those who are undiagnosed or have a late diagnosis of HIV infection or who fail to take prophylactic antibiotics when their CD4 count is <200. ART is credited with decreasing the incidence of opportunistic infections and improving survival (CDC, 2004). The time of survival has increased from about 13 months at the start of the AIDS epidemic; however, survival after diagnosis of HIV-related lymphomas still averages less than 8 months.

AIDS Dementia Complex and Neurologic Effects

Neurologic manifestations of HIV are common, affecting 40% to 60% of clients with AIDS. Included among the manifestations are dementia, delirium, and seizures. They result from both the direct effects of the virus on the nervous system and opportunistic infections.

AIDS dementia complex is the most common cause of mental status changes for clients with HIV infection. This dementia results from a direct effect of the virus on the brain and affects cognitive, motor, and behavioral functioning. Fluctuating memory loss, confusion, difficulty concentrating, lethargy, and diminished motor speed are typical manifestations of AIDS dementia complex. Clients become apathetic, losing interest in work and social and recreational activities. As the complex progresses, the client develops severe dementia with motor disturbances such as ataxia, tremor, spasticity, incontinence, and paraplegia (Kasper et al., 2005; Porth, 2005).

Infections and lesions common with AIDS may also affect the CNS. Toxoplasmosis and non-Hodgkin's lymphoma are space-occupying lesions that may cause headache, altered mental status, and neurologic deficits. Cryptococcal meningitis and CMV infection also are common in people with AIDS. CNS complications have declined with the use of HAART therapy (Tierney et al., 2005).

Peripheral nervous system manifestations are also common in HIV-infected clients. Sensory neuropathies with manifestations of numbness, tingling, and pain in the lower extremities affect about 30% of clients with AIDS. A Guillain-Barré type of inflammatory demyelinating polyneuropathy can also occur, resulting in progressive weakness and paralysis.

Opportunistic Infections

Opportunistic infections are the most common manifestations of AIDS, often occurring simultaneously. The risk of opportunistic infections is predictable by the T4 or CD4 cell count. The normal CD4 cell count is greater than $1000/mm^3$. When the CD4 count falls to less than $500/mm^3$, manifestations of immunodeficiency are seen. With a count of less than $200/mm^3$, opportunistic infections and cancers are likely.

PNEUMOCYSTIS CARINII PNEUMONIA *Pneumocystis carinii* pneumonia is the most common opportunistic infection affecting clients with AIDS. Approximately 75% to 80% of clients develop PCP at some point in their disease (Tierney et al., 2005). It tends to be recurrent, and is the cause of death in about 20% of clients with AIDS. PCP is caused by a common environmental fungus that is not pathogenic in clients with intact immune systems.

Unlike many pneumonias, the manifestations of PCP are nonspecific and may progress insidiously. Clients often present with fever, cough, dyspnea, tachypnea, and tachycardia. Complaints of mild chest pain and sputum may also be present. Breath sounds may initially be normal. With severe disease, the client may present with cyanosis and significant respiratory distress.

TUBERCULOSIS An estimated 4% of clients with AIDS develop tuberculosis, contributing significantly to the rise in incidence of this disease in the United States. In some clients, active tuberculosis results from reactivation of a prior infection. In other clients, it is a new, primary disease facilitated by impaired immune function. Rapid progression, diffuse pulmonary infiltrates, and disseminated disease occur more commonly in clients with AIDS. Multiple-drug-resistant strains of tuberculosis present a significant problem (Tierney et al., 2005).

Clients with pulmonary tuberculosis present with a cough productive of purulent sputum, fever, fatigue, weight loss, and lymphadenopathy. Disseminated disease affects the bone marrow, bone, joints, liver, spleen, CSF, skin, kidneys, gastrointestinal tract, lymph nodes, brain, and other sites.

CANDIDIASIS *Candida albicans* infection is a common opportunistic infection in clients with AIDS. It is usually manifested as oral thrush or esophagitis. In women, vaginal candidiasis is frequent and often recurrent. Oral thrush presents as white, friable plaques on the buccal mucosa or tongue and, in the HIV-infected client, is often the first indication of progression to AIDS. Clients with esophagitis have difficulty swallowing and substernal pain or burning that increases with swallowing.

MYCOBACTERIUM AVIUM COMPLEX *Mycobacterium avium* complex (MAC) affects up to 25% of clients with AIDS, typically occurring late in the course of the disease when CD4 cell counts are less than $50/mm^3$. MAC is more common in women than men. MAC is caused by organisms commonly found in food, water, and soil. It is a major cause of "wasting syndrome" in persons with AIDS (Figure 13–9 ■). Manifestations of MAC include chills and fever, weakness, night sweats, abdominal pain and diarrhea, and weight loss. Nearly every organ can be infected, and most people with MAC develop disseminated disease.

OTHER INFECTIONS Herpes virus infections are common in clients with AIDS and may be severe. CMV can affect the retina, the gastrointestinal tract, or lungs. Disseminated herpes simplex or herpes zoster may occur, although severe mucocutaneous manifestations are more common.

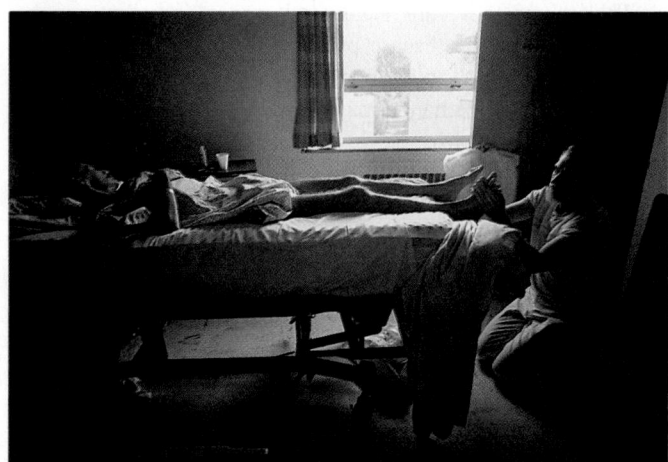

Figure 13–9 ■ Wasting syndrome in a client with AIDS.

Parasitic infections with *Toxoplasma gondii* and *Cryptococcus neoformans* commonly affect the CNS. Toxoplasmosis occurs as encephalitis or an intracerebral mass lesion. Changes in mental status, focal neurologic signs, and seizures may result. *Cryptococcus* infection may present as either meningitis or disseminated disease, primarily affecting the lungs. *Cryptosporidium,* a protozoon affecting the gastrointestinal tract, is an important cause of prolonged diarrhea in AIDS clients. Bacterial salmonella infections are also a relatively common cause of diarrhea.

Women with AIDS have a high incidence of pelvic inflammatory disease (PID). Although the pathogens appear to be the same as those in PID affecting non-HIV-infected women, the disease is more severe. Inpatient treatment with intravenous antibiotics is often necessary.

Secondary Cancers

As cell-mediated immune function declines, the risk of malignancy increases. The CDC classification of AIDS currently includes four cancers: Kaposi's sarcoma, non-Hodgkin's lymphoma, primary lymphoma of the brain, and invasive cervical carcinoma.

KAPOSI'S SARCOMA **Kaposi's sarcoma (KS)** is often the presenting symptom of AIDS. It remains the most common cancer associated with the disease. Kaposi's sarcoma is caused by a virus called the Kaposi sarcoma-associated herpesvirus, also known as human herpesvirus 8. Men who have sex with men not only have a risk of HIV infection, but are also more likely to be infected with the virus responsible for KS. Women who have sex with these men also have a risk of HIV and KS. The virus associated with KS appears to be mainly transmitted through sexual contact, although cases have also been reported in injection drug users. People whose immune system is suppressed because they have received an organ transplant have a 1 in 200 risk of developing KS (American Cancer Society, 2005).

A tumor of the endothelial cells lining small blood vessels, KS presents as vascular macules, papules, or violet lesions affecting the skin and viscera (Figure 13–10 ■). The face is a common site for skin lesions, especially the tip of the nose and pinnae of the ears. Common sites for visceral disease include the gastrointestinal tract, lungs, and lymphatic system.

The lesions of KS are usually painless initially, but may become painful as the disease progresses. Internally, the tumors may obstruct organ function or cause bleeding. When the lungs are involved, gas exchange may be severely impaired, resulting in pulmonary hemorrhage. This disease may progress slowly or rapidly. KS is an indicator of late-stage HIV disease, with an average survival time of 18 months after diagnosis.

LYMPHOMAS Lymphomas are malignancies of the lymphoid tissue, including lymphocytes, lymph nodes, and the lymphoid organs such as the spleen and bone marrow. In AIDS, two lymphomas are common, non-Hodgkin's lymphoma (including Burkitt's lymphoma) and primary lymphoma of the brain. Hodgkin's disease also occurs five times more frequently in clients with HIV infection than in those without. The CNS is the usual site for these lymphomas, although they may be found in the bone marrow, gastrointestinal tract, liver, skin, and mu-

Figure 13–10 ■ Kaposi's sarcoma lesions.
Source: Zeva Oelbaum/Peter Arnold, Inc.

cous membranes. They are aggressive tumors, growing and spreading rapidly. Headache and changes in mental status are common early symptoms of lymphomas affecting the CNS.

CERVICAL CANCER Of women with HIV infection, 40% have cervical dysplasia. Cervical cancer develops frequently and tends to be aggressive. Women with concurrent HIV infection and cervical cancer usually die of the cervical cancer, not AIDS. Because of this, it is recommended that women with HIV infection have Papanicolaou (Pap) smears every 6 months and aggressive treatment of cervical dysplasia with colposcopic examination and cone biopsy.

INTERDISCIPLINARY CARE

Although multiple research studies to identify a cure for HIV infection and AIDS are under way, no cure is currently available. This fact, plus the apparent universally fatal nature of the disease, make prevention a vital strategy in HIV care. New treatments are under investigation (Box 13–3).

The goals of care for the client with HIV disease are as follows:

- Early identification of the infection
- Promoting health-maintenance activities to prolong the asymptomatic period as long as possible
- Prevention of opportunistic infections
- Treatment of disease complications, such as cancers
- Providing emotional and psychosocial support.

Diagnosis

Diagnostic testing is used to screen and identify the infection, as well as to monitor the client's disease and immune status. The following diagnostic tests may be ordered. The likelihood that a positive screening test truly indicates the presence of HIV infection decreases as HIV prevalence in the tested population becomes lower. Therefore, false-positive HIV test results are more likely in settings where the tested population prevalence is lower than in settings where the tested population prevalence is higher. When a preliminary, positive rapid test is explained to clients, phrases like "a good chance of being infected" or "very likely infected" can be used to indicate the likelihood of

BOX 13-3 Investigational Immune-Based Treatment for HIV

HIV infection progressively alters the function of and destroys CD4 + lymphocytes. CD4 + cells are essential to the function of the immune system, including the body's ability to respond to infections. These cells initiate, direct, and regulate immune responses and may also directly attack infected cells. They also are a source of cytokines, the chemical messengers of the immune system. Destruction of CD4 + cells by HIV devastates the immune system, facilitating the development of fatal infections and neoplasms in the infected person. Immune-based treatments indirectly affect the HIV by improving the function of the immune system through actions that inhibit cytokines, replenish cytokines, or restore immune function. These treatments, used alone or in combination with antiretroviral drugs, are being investigated for use in the treatment of HIV.

Inhibiting Cytokines

Tumor necrosis factor alpha (TNF-α) is a cytokine secreted by activated monocytes and macrophages in response to infection, infestation, or tumor growth. It causes a proliferation of B cells and T cells. However, high levels of this cytokine may actually facilitate the development of disease by blocking the normal inflammatory response. It is believed that blocking the effect of TNF-α can suppress HIV production, although caution must be used.

Replenishing Cytokines

Some cytokines (interleukin-2, interleukin-12, and interferon alpha) may be helpful in treating HIV by stimulating the production of killer cells as well as increasing the function of lymphocytes. The interferons are part of the body's first line of defense against viruses. All of these agents have toxic side effects, requiring careful nursing assessment and care.

Restoring Immune System Function

HIV infection not only destroys CD4 + cells, but also eventually destroys the lymphoid organs, such as bone marrow and the thymus gland. Lymphocytes, including the CD4 + cells, are derived from stem cells in bone marrow and mature in the thymus. Two investigational treatments to restore the immune system are bone marrow transplant and thymus transplant. Bone marrow transplants have been used to correct other types of immune disorders (such as leukemia or lymphoma) but have yet to be effective in persons with HIV. A few thymus transplants have been done in HIV-infected persons, but have provided only temporary benefits.

HIV infection and qualified based on the HIV prevalence in the setting and the client's individual risk

Further testing is always required to confirm a reactive screening test result.

- *Enzyme-linked immunosorbent assay (ELISA)* is the most widely used screening test for HIV infection. The ELISA test was developed in 1985 to screen blood donors. ELISA tests for HIV antibodies; it does not detect the virus. Therefore, a client may have a negative ELISA test early in the course of infection, before detectable antibodies have developed. The test has a 99.5% or higher sensitivity when performed at least 13 weeks after infection. This means that more than 99.5% of tests performed on blood containing HIV antibodies will show a positive result. False positives can occur; therefore, an initial positive result is always tested repeatedly and confirmed using a different method of antibody detection, usually the Western blot.

  The FDA has licensed more than one rapid test; these are widely used because results can be given immediately. Immediate notification is critical because many clients tested for HIV do not return to learn the results; many cannot be located to give the test results and educate about safe behaviors whether they are positive or negative for HIV. Although confirmation of results is dependent on testing with a second source, ELISA or Western blot test, learning results immediately gives the client more information to make wise choices about his or her behaviors and self-care.

- *Western blot antibody testing* is more reliable but more time consuming and more expensive than ELISA. When combined with ELISA, however, a specificity of greater than 99.9% is achieved. Specificity is a measure of the probability that a negative test result indicates that no antibodies are present. In this test, the client's serum is mixed with HIV proteins to detect reaction. If antibodies to HIV are present, a detectable antigen–antibody response will occur.

- *HIV viral load tests* measure the amount of actively replicating HIV. Levels correlate with disease progression and response to antiretroviral medications. Levels greater than 5000 to 10,000 copies/mL indicate the need for treatment.

- *CBC* is performed to detect anemia, leukopenia, and thrombocytopenia, which are often present in HIV infection. Lymphopenia (or low levels of lymphocytes) is especially common in this disease.

- *CD4 cell count* is the most widely used test to monitor the progress of the disease and guide therapy. The CD4 cell count correlates very closely with the immunodeficiency disorders seen in AIDS. AIDS is now defined not only by the presence of opportunistic infections and other diseases indicative of immunodeficiency, but also by HIV-seropositive status and a CD4 count of less than 200/mm^3 or a percentage of CD4 lymphocytes of less than 14%. CD4 counts are recommended every 3 to 6 months for all people with HIV disease.

  In addition to these widely used tests, several other diagnostic tests may be performed:

- *Blood culture for HIV* provides the most specific diagnosis but is an expensive and cumbersome test that is not widely available in the United States.

- *Immune-complex-dissociated p24 assay* is a test for p24 (HIV) antigen in the blood. This antigen indicates active reproduction of HIV and tends to be positive prior to seroconversion and with advanced disease. It is most useful in monitoring disease progression and the antiviral activity of experimental medications (Pagana & Pagana, 2002; Tierney et al., 2005).

Other diagnostic tests are used primarily to detect secondary cancers and opportunistic infections in the client with HIV. Tests ordered are both general and specific to the client's manifestations and may include the following:

- *Tuberculin skin testing* to detect possible tuberculosis infection
- *MRI* of the brain to identify lymphomas
- *Specific cultures and serology examinations for opportunistic infections* such as PCP, toxoplasmosis, and others
- *Pap smears* every 6 months for early detection of cervical cancer in women with cervical dysplasia (Tierney et al., 2005).

Medications

Pharmacologic management of the client with HIV disease has four primary foci: (1) to suppress the infection itself, decreasing symptoms and prolonging life, (2) to provide prophylaxis of opportunistic infections, (3) to stimulate hematopoietic response, and (4) to treat opportunistic infections and malignancies. Effectiveness of treatment is monitored by viral load and CD4 cell counts; positive results are indicated by a reduction in viral load along with preserving the CD4 count above 350 mm^3. Treatment is recommended when the CD4 count falls below 200 mm^3. Clients with symptoms of severe disease are treated regardless of their CD4 level or viral load, so monitoring these individuals may reveal higher levels of CD4 or lower viral load. Initiating therapy in asymptomatic individuals with higher CD4 levels did not show protective effect and was thought to perhaps increase viral resistance. Today the drugs have been combined and dosing schedules simplified, which helps clients adhere to medication administration schedules. Currently, researchers are using clinical trials of asymptomatic clients receiving HAART to evaluate alternating drug regimens to prevent drug resistance by the viral organisms (Martinez-Picado et al., 2003).

Four classes of drugs used in antiretroviral treatment include nucleoside reverse transcriptase inhibitors (NRTIs), nonnucleoside reverse transcriptase inhibitors (NNRTIs), protease inhibitors (PIs), and entry inhibitors. HAART combines three or four antiretroviral drugs to reduce the incidence of drug resistance. Combination therapies increase the likelihood of decreasing viral load and symptoms but also burden clients with complicated and expensive medication schedules. Clients beginning the HAART protocol must understand the benefits, risks, costs, and effects on daily life. HAART does not eradicate HIV infection. HAART medications are expensive, the newer triple combinations such as Trizivir cost about $1030 for 60 doses, a 30-day supply. This costs approximately $13,400 per year, and does not include medications to prevent or treat opportunistic infections or cancer (Tierney et al., 2005). These medications are scheduled for specific times throughout the day; therefore, leading a normal life becomes a challenge. In addition, all HAART medications cause major adverse reactions leading to less than perfect adherence, as with most chronic diseases, but in this case, the outcome could be fatal.

Each client must be able to adhere to the treatment regimen. It may be preferable to delay initiating therapy until the client is able to agree to adhere so irregular dosing does not lead to viral resistance. Some providers gauge client ability to follow the HAART regimen by the client's success with prophylaxis for an opportunistic infection.

Several methods to promote and ensure adherence are being used and studied. Wroe and Thomas (2003) found it helpful to distinguish between intentional and unintentional nonadherence and treat them as separate entities. Clients' beliefs and internal logic were found to impact intentional nonadherence; preparing clients for the effects of HAART therapy by focusing on lessening clients' reasons for not taking medication is believed to reduce intentional nonadherence. Enriquez and McKinsey (2004) emphasize the role of nursing in preventing drug resistance by assessing patients' readiness to adhere to the treatment regimen and intervening to overcome identified barriers to adherence prior to initiating therapy.

Another approach to adherence is the use of electronic monitoring devices (EMD) (Bova et al., 2005). By placing a microprocessor in a medication cap, records are created of the time, date, and frequency of bottle opening. Although this method does not guarantee that the medication will be taken even if the cap is removed, the record created is a source for follow-up and discussion between the provider and the client. Whether the client is asked to keep a diary of taking the medication, using an EMD to keep a record, or relying on pill count, adherence to medication regimen is critically important.

Ingersoll and Heckman (2005) found the most effective provider–client relationship for fostering adherence is a balance of appropriate challenge and support. Providers who were never confrontational seem to be perceived by clients as giving permission to be less adherent. Although depression, substance use, and financial considerations undoubtedly influence adherence to HAART therapy, and need to be addressed, provider–client relationships seem to have the most influence on adherence behavior.

NUCLEOSIDE REVERSE TRANSCRIPTASE INHIBITORS The NRTIs (also called nucleoside analogs) inhibit the action of viral reverse transcriptase, a retroviral enzyme that catalyzes the substrates for conversion and copying of viral RNA to DNA sequences. This enzyme is necessary for viral integration into cellular DNA and replication. The nucleoside analogs act as a chemical decoy for building blocks of the formation of the DNA copy, preventing the RNA from being copied into DNA. Each drug substitutes for a particular nucleoside base at different points on the chain. See the accompanying Medication Administration guidelines below for this group of drugs.

Zidovudine (Retrovir, AZT) was the first antiretroviral agent approved for use with HIV infection. It remains in widespread use and has been shown to decrease symptoms and prolong the lives of clients with AIDS. Zidovudine is often given to clients with a CD4 cell count of less than 500 because of evidence that it slows the progression to severe disease (Tierney et al., 2005). Zidovudine may also be used prophylactically following a documented parenteral exposure to HIV. AZT is used in combination with ddI, ddC, or 3TC.

- Didanosine (ddI, Videx) also inhibits reverse transcriptase and viral replication. It is used in combination therapy with AZT.
- Stavudine (d4T, Zerit) is a retroviral inhibitor that has been shown to increase CD4 cell counts and decrease serum p24

MEDICATION ADMINISTRATION   Antiretroviral Nucleoside Analogs

ZIDOVUDINE (AZT, AZIDOTHYMIDINE)

Zidovudine is the first antiretroviral agent developed to treat HIV infection. It interferes with reverse transcriptase, thus inhibiting replication of the virus. The usual dose is 300 mg twice daily. It is administered orally. Dose-limiting side effects are anemia and neutropenia.

Nursing Responsibilities

- Assess for possible contraindications to therapy including allergic response or a CD4 count of greater than 350/mm^3.
- Administer by mouth, instructing the client to swallow capsules whole.
- Assess for adverse effects. Nausea and headache are common. They may be self-limiting, decreasing with time, or significant and continuing, necessitating a change of therapy. Nausea and neutropenia are treated with erythropoietin (epoetin alpha) and G-CSF (filgrastim).
- Assess CBC with differential and creatine phosphokinase. Notify the physician of significant changes.

Health Education for the Client and Family

- Zidovudine will not cure HIV infection but slows its progress and reduces significant symptoms.
- Take the drug at least 0.5 hour before or 1 hour after meals if tolerated.
- With this and all antiretroviral drugs, it is important to emphasize that the client is still infective and can pass the infection to others. Use safer sex practices and other measures to prevent transmission to partners. Do not donate blood or breast-feed.
- Notify the physician if signs of an infection or adverse response to zidovudine develop: sore throat, swollen lymph glands, fever; unusual fatigue or weakness; easy bruising, bleeding gums, or an injury that will not heal; persistent or intractable nausea; muscle pain or wasting.
- Continue all scheduled follow-up visits and laboratory studies to monitor for drug toxicity.
- Check with the physician before taking any prescription or over-the-counter drug.

DIDANOSINE (DDI, VIDEX)

As with zidovudine, didanosine does not kill HIV but inhibits its replication within the cells. Its activity is similar to that of zidovudine. Didanosine has been shown to increase CD4 cell counts and lower p24 antigen levels (Tierney et al., 2005). Didanosine is used alone for clients who are intolerant or resistant to zidovudine. It is also being used with zidovudine in combination therapy regimens. Didanosine does not cause the anemia associated with zidovudine, but it may cause neutropenia. Didanosine is also associated with an increased risk of pancreatitis, peripheral neuropathy, and dry mouth.

Nursing Responsibilities

- Assess for possible contraindications to didanosine therapy, including previous episodes of pancreatitis and impaired renal or liver function.
- Administer as directed. Tablets are to be chewed thoroughly or dissolved in 1 ounce of water at room temperature. The powder form is dissolved in water prior to administration, and diarrhea is attributable to the buffering agent used in this formula.
- Administer with caution to clients taking vincristine, rifampin, pentamidine, ethambutol, or metronidazole; the action of both drugs may be affected by concurrent administration. Intravenous pentamidine and trimethoprim-sulfamethoxazole taken concurrently may increase the risk of acute and fatal pancreatitis.
- Didanosine interferes with the absorption of ketoconazole and dapsone. Doses of these drugs should be scheduled at least 2 hours apart from didanosine doses.
- Evaluate for therapeutic response and possible adverse effects. Notify the physician if manifestations of peripheral neuropathy, diarrhea, depression, or other adverse effects develop.
- Stop the drug and notify the physician immediately if the client develops manifestations of pancreatitis or hepatic failure, including nausea and vomiting, severe abdominal pain, elevated bilirubin, or elevated serum enzymes (e.g., amylase, AST, ALT).

Health Education for the Client and Family

- Take the drug as directed. The prescribed two-tablet dose must always be taken to get the required amount of antacid to prevent the drug from being destroyed by stomach acid.
- Take on an empty stomach, at least 1 hour before or 2 hours after meals.
- Do not use alcohol while taking didanosine; alcohol may increase the risk of pancreatitis.
- Stop the drug and call the doctor immediately if nausea, vomiting, abdominal pain, or diarrhea develops. These may indicate pancreatitis.
- Call the doctor if extremity pain, weakness, numbness, or tingling occurs. These side effects usually disappear when didanosine is discontinued.
- Other side effects to report to the physician include unusual bleeding or bruising, fatigue, weakness, fever, or persistent sore throat.

ABACAVIR

Abacavir is a nucleoside analog with activity against some HIV strain resistant to other nucleoside drugs. It is prepared in combination with zidovudine and lamivudine (Trizivir), and one tablet is taken twice daily. This combination drug is composed exclusively of nucleoside analogs, lacking NNRTIs or PIs. As such it is less effective at decreasing viral load and allowing immune system enhancement, but the ease of administration makes it a useful drug for clients who cannot adhere to more complex regimens. The main toxicity is a hypersensitivity response in approximately 5% of clients manifested with flulike symptoms. Avoid repeated use in those individuals.

Nursing Responsibilities

- Assess for possible hypersensitivity reactions, anemia, and neutropenia.
- Evaluate for desired effect of increased CD4 counts and lower blood levels of p24 antigen.
- Notify the physician if the client develops evidence of pancreatitis, impaired hepatic function, or painful peripheral neuropathy.

Health Education for the Client and Family

- Take without regard to food or water.
- Check with the physician before taking any other prescription or over-the-counter medication.
- Report all signs and symptoms of hypersensitivity to this drug.
- Report to the physician signs of infection or changes in condition.

antigen levels. Current use is for clients who are intolerant of AZT.

- Lamivudine (3-TC, Epivir) is used for low CD4 cell counts or symptomatic disease as a first-line treatment in combination with AZT.
- Abacavir (Ziagen) is a potent inhibitor of reverse transcriptase; however, it may cause serious hypersensitivity reactions.
- Zidovudine plus lamivudine (Combivir) is a combination drug in use to decrease HIV zidovudine-resistant strains.

PROTEASE INHIBITORS Protease is a viral enzyme necessary for the formation of specific viral protein needs for viral assembly and maturation. PIs bond chemically with protease to block the function of the enzyme and result in the production of immature, noninfectious viral particles. When combined with other antiviral drugs, these chemicals increase the chance of eliminating the virus by interfering with different stages of its life cycle. However, viral resistance occurs rather quickly. PIs inhibit and induce metabolism of other drugs, so their use with other medications and the dose of those medications must be carefully planned. Some drugs will circulate longer because their metabolism is inhibited; others will be speedily metabolized and eliminated.

Protease inhibitors and nucleoside analogs are associated with serious metabolic derangements. These include elevated cholesterol and triglycerides, insulin resistance and diabetes mellitus, and changes in body fat composition, which are particularly distressing to the clients. These body fat changes are primarily abdominal obesity and skeletal wasting. This set of symptoms is referred to as lipodystrophy (Tierney et al., 2005). Elevated cholesterol should be treated with pravastatin or atorvastatin. Lovastatin and simvastatin react to PIs, so they need to be avoided. Reduction of dietary sources of cholesterol should be made.

- Saquinavir (Invirase) is used in combination with nucleoside analogs to treat progression of the disease.
- Ritonavir (Norvir) is used in combination with nucleoside analogs to treat progression of the disease.
- Indinavir (Crixivan) is used in combination with nucleoside analogs to treat progression of the disease.
- Nelfinavir (Viracept) is used in cases of failure of or intolerance to other protease inhibitors.
- Amprenavir (Agenerase) is the newest protease inhibitor.
- Lopinavir/Ritonavir (Kaletra) is the first combination of protease inhibitors active against some HIV strains resistant to other protease inhibitors.

NONNUCLEOSIDE REVERSE TRANSCRIPTASE INHIBITORS Nevirapine (Viramune), delavirdine (Rescriptor), and efavirenz (Sustiva) are NNRTIs that may be used in combination with nucleoside analogs and protease inhibitors. However, one limitation to NNRTIs is the high incidence of cross-resistance to NRTIs. Some studies have shown that nevirapine and efavirenz may significantly reduce serum levels of the protease inhibitors. Only one NNRTI should be used at the same time. Nevirapine has a reported risk for liver toxicity and Stevens-Johnson syndrome (Bartlett & Weber, 2005).

ENTRY INHIBITORS: ENFUVIRTIDE (FUZEON) This new class of drugs became available in 2003. These entry or fusion inhibitors prevent HIV from entering target cells by binding to the protein envelope that surrounds the virus. When bound to the drug, the virus cannot morph in order to fit and adhere to cell membranes (Covington, 2005). Adding this new class of drug to the regimen of heavily pretreated individuals improves CD4 counts and lowers viral loads (Tierney et al., 2005).

Other agents may also be administered in combination with antiretroviral therapy. Interferons, which are naturally occurring lymphokines, have been used alone and in combination. Alpha-interferon may be used to treat KS and in combination with zidovudine to slow disease progression. Gamma-interferon is also used. As more drugs become available, the burden to choose the best regimen increases for the healthcare provider. The most important limiting factor when choosing a regimen is client adherence. Second to that is selecting an effective combination of drugs without overlapping toxicities or toxicities so debilitating that adherence will be further impaired.

Some clients undergoing HAART are developing body composition changes and metabolic abnormalities associated with the therapy, especially the PIs. Increased fat deposition in the midsection, breasts, and neck with atrophy in the face, buttocks, and extremities describes the body composition changes; metabolic abnormalities include increased low-density lipoprotein cholesterol and triglycerides and insulin resistance. The combination of changes is consistent with metabolic syndrome, which increases the risk of cardiovascular disease and diabetes. These conditions are commonly treated with medications. Robinson (2005) has observed these serious changes in HIV-positive clients and hopes to prevent and treat the changes with diet and exercise without adding to the polypharmacy already experienced by those undergoing HAART.

A number of pharmacologic agents are used to prevent and treat opportunistic infections and malignancies in the client with HIV. These agents are outlined in Table 13–4.

Many clients at some point require an implanted venous access device, such as a Groshong catheter, to facilitate blood sampling, intravenous medication administration, transfusions, and parenteral nutrition. See Chapter 14 ∞ for nursing care of the client with an intravenous access device implant.

It is recommended that all HIV-infected clients receive pneumococcal, influenza, hepatitis B, and *Haemophilus influenzae b* vaccines. Persons with a positive PPD and negative chest x-ray are given prophylactic isoniazid. When the client's CD4 cell count falls to less than 200, prophylactic treatment for PCP is begun, usually with trimethoprim-sulfamethoxazole. Clients with a CD4 count of less than 100 are started on prophylactic treatment for MAC.

NURSING CARE

The client with HIV and AIDS has many care needs, including both physical and psychosocial support (see the Nursing Research box on page 360). Because there is as yet no cure or effective treatment for HIV disease, many of these needs fall within the realm of nursing to promote knowledge and understanding, self-care, comfort, and quality of life. As with many diseases that have an ultimately fatal outcome, the course of HIV infection may well be affected by the client's

TABLE 13–4 Pharmacologic Treatment of Common Opportunistic Infections and Malignancies in HIV Disease

CONDITION	TREATMENT	POTENTIAL ADVERSE EFFECTS
Infections		
Pneumocystis carinii pneumonia	Trimethoprim/sulfamethoxazole	Rash, neutropenia, anemia, thrombocytopenia, Stevens-Johnson syndrome
	Pentamidine	Hypotension, altered blood glucose levels, hypocalcemia, anemia and leukopenia, liver and renal toxicity, pancreatitis
Tuberculosis	Combination drug therapy using isoniazid, rifampin, ethambutol, pyrazinamide, or streptomycin	Multiple; see Chapter 38
Candidiasis Oral thrush	Clotrimazole troches Nystatin suspension	Few toxic responses noted for either medication
Esophagitis or recurrent vaginitis	Ketoconazole	Hepatitis, adrenal insufficiency
	Fluconazole	Hepatitis
	Amphotericin B	Bone marrow toxicity, acute renal or hepatic failure; nausea, vomiting; chills, fever, headache
Mycobacterium avium complex	Combination therapy using • Clarithromycin, plus	• Hepatitis, nausea, diarrhea
	• Clofazimine	• Diarrhea, nausea, vomiting; skin discoloration, pruritus, rash
	• Ethambutol	• Thrombocytopenia, hepatitis, optic neuritis
	• Rifampin	• Bone marrow depression, renal failure, hepatitis
	• Ciprofloxacin	• Nausea, rash
	• Amikacin	• Bone marrow depression, renal failure, ototoxicity, hepatitis
Cytomegalovirus	Ganciclovir	Bone marrow depression, fever
	Foscarnet	Renal failure, electrolyte imbalances, seizures
Herpes simplex or herpes zoster	Acyclovir	Nausea, vomiting, diarrhea; CNS effects; renal failure
Toxoplasmosis	Pyrimethamine, plus sulfadiazine or clindamycin and folinic acid	Bone marrow depression, rash; respiratory failure; nausea, vomiting, abdominal pain; hematuria
Malignancies		
Kaposi's sarcoma	Intralesional vinblastine	Inflammation and pain at injection site
Lymphoma	Combination chemotherapy	Nausea, vomiting; bone marrow toxicity; alopecia

social support systems, control, perceived self-efficacy in management, and coping mechanisms.

As the epidemic continues, nurses are providing care for increasing numbers of clients with HIV infection at various stages of disease. These clients are not only in special care settings, but also on general units, maternal–child units, hospice, and home settings. As clients with HIV disease live longer, nurses will increasingly encounter clients in whom HIV disease is a secondary diagnosis, with another primary diagnosis, for example, seizures, heart disease, diabetes mellitus, or an operative procedure.

Prevention

To date, no safe immunization to protect against HIV infection has been developed. Education, counseling, and behavior modification are the primary tools for AIDS prevention. The benefit of education and behavior modification is evident in the homosexual male population. The incidence of new HIV infections in this population has declined dramatically in high-prevalence cities. Nurses play a vital role in providing education about this epidemic and infection prevention for individuals and communities.

All sexually active individuals need to know how HIV is spread. Following are the only *totally* safe sex practices:

- No sex
- Long-term mutually monogamous sexual relations between two uninfected people
- Mutual masturbation without direct contact

Clients who do engage in sexual activity need to know and practice safer sex (Box 13–4). Reducing the number of sexual partners—for example, by entering into and remaining in a long-term mutually monogamous relationship with an uninfected partner—reduces the risk. Clients should not engage in unprotected sex, especially if the HIV status of the partner is unknown. Latex condoms have been shown to reduce the risk of transmitting HIV. Their effectiveness is improved when nonoxynol-9, a spermicide, is used for lubrication; however, it may cause genital ulcers which can facilitate HIV transmission. To be effective, condoms must be used with every sexual encounter involving vaginal, oral, or anal intercourse. They also need to be applied and removed properly. A female condom is also available for use.

Healthcare workers exposed to HIV infection or adults who experience a high-risk exposure to HIV may choose postexposure prophylaxis. Risk of exposure for healthcare workers may

MEDIALINK Case Study: HIV Prevention

NURSING RESEARCH Evidence-Based Practice and Nurses' Willingness to Care for People with AIDS

As reported by the Centers for Disease Control and Prevention, the number of deaths from AIDS has declined. This is believed to be the result of both the slowing of the epidemic and of improved treatment, which has lengthened the life span of people with AIDS. However, as treatment continues to improve survival, a key challenge will be the increasing number of people living with HIV and AIDS—and the additional resources needed for services, treatment, and care.

Several studies have found that some professional nurses and students are resistant to caring for clients with AIDS. One study by Sherman (1996) examined relationships among moral choices and nurses' willingness to care for clients with AIDS. The willingness to provide care for clients with this illness involves moral choices about one's own mortality (death anxiety), spirituality, and social support. In a survey of 220 registered nurses employed in eight hospitals in the New York Metropolitan area, Sherman found that willingness to care for AIDS patients was positively correlated with spirituality and perceived social support and negatively correlated with death anxiety. It is suggested that nurses' willingness to care for people with AIDS may be related not only to nurses' personal values and beliefs (expressed in spirituality) but also to their professional identity and role expectations.

Addressing nursing reluctance to treat clients with HIV infection, nursing educators Valois, Turgeon, Godin, Blondeau, and Cote (2001) researched the impact of persuasive messages on nursing students' beliefs and attitudes about caring for HIV-positive clients. Nursing education certainly increases knowledge and awareness of the science of HIV infection, but it may not modify attitudes or behaviors. According to the underlying theory of the research, individuals who receive evidence-based persuasive messages may develop favorable beliefs that will alter their willingness to perform a given behavior. Three main types of beliefs were considered in this study: behavioral belief (related to the expected consequences of adopting a behavior); normative belief (related to perceived social pressures by significant others resulting from adopting a behavior); and control belief (related to resources or barriers that seem to facilitate or hamper adoption of the behavior).

In three sessions, the student nurses in the experimental group were given positive persuasive messages about caring for HIV-infected clients. The persuasive messages were compelling and specific to caring for clients with HIV; case studies provided opportunities for the students to discuss the elements of the case within the framework of the persuasive messages. Students in the control group studied the science of caring for clients with HIV but did not receive the persuasive messages. When beliefs and attitudes about caring for HIV-positive clients were compared, the researchers found significantly greater willingness to provide care in the experimental group. Nursing students proved to be well prepared and motivated to receive this information.

IMPLICATIONS FOR NURSING

Standards of professional nursing clearly state that nurses will care for people with AIDS. To increase nurses' willingness to do so, students need to be better socialized into their roles and responsibilities. Providing information within an evidence-based framework, analyzing and defining effective nursing care in client cases, and utilizing the standards of professional nursing support the development of positive attitudes. Discussions within the classroom and clinical settings provide a safe means of bringing fears into the open and sharing experiences. Student groups can serve as support groups, improving communications, decreasing isolation and anxiety, and improving self-esteem and morale. Within the work setting, perceived support from colleagues and administrators as well as increased contact with people with AIDS are important factors in making caring a rewarding and positive experience.

CRITICAL THINKING IN CLIENT CARE

1. These studies were of student nurses and registered nurses. What differences do you think might have been found between the two groups today?
2. Carefully consider each of the following clients with AIDS and write a brief paragraph about how you would feel if you were assigned to care for them:
   a. A heterosexual female, age 25
   b. A homosexual male, age 35
   c. A newborn baby girl
   d. A 40-year-old single mother of three teenagers
   e. A 30-year-old homeless drug user
   f. A 17-year-old male with hemophilia, infected by blood transfusions

be through needle sticks or cuts with a sharp object, contact with mucous membrane or nonintact skin, semen, vaginal secretions, fluids contaminated with visible blood, and possibly CSF, synovial fluid, and pleural, peritoneal, pericardial, or amniotic fluids. CDC guidelines recommend treatment with HAART, which includes two NRTIs for lower risk exposures and the addition of a third drug for higher risk exposure. A 4-week course of treatment is recommended and should be started within 72 hours, preferably within 2 to 3 hours of exposure (Bartlett & Weber, 2005).

The most difficult group of high-risk people to reach and educate has been injection drug users. People in this group should never share needles, syringes, or other drug paraphernalia. Many cities have initiated needle-exchange programs, providing a sterile needle and syringe in exchange for a used one. A fresh solution of household bleach and water in a 1:10 ratio is effective to clean paraphernalia when sterile supplies are not available. It is important to also teach people in this population about safer sex practices, because most heterosexual HIV transmission occurs between injection drug users and their partners.

Screening of voluntary blood donors and donated blood supplies has reduced the risk of transmission by transfusion to 1 in 100,000. Because current blood-screening methods use antibody testing, receiving donated blood continues to carry a small risk. Clients in the *window period* between contraction of the virus and the development of detectable antibodies are able to transmit the virus to others, even though they do not yet test positive for HIV. This window period usually lasts from 6 weeks to 6 months; rarely, it lasts up to 1 year. When possible, encourage clients to use autologous transfusion, donating their own blood prior to an anticipated surgery. Seeking donations from family members is not encouraged for several reasons.

BOX 13–4 Guidelines for Safer Sex

- Practice mutual monogamy; if you are not in a mutually monogamous relationship, limit the number of sexual partners.
- Do not engage in unprotected sex, especially if HIV status of your partner is unknown. (Remember that a person may be infected and infective for up to 6 months before converting to seropositive status.)
- When entering into a new monogamous relationship, both partners should undergo HIV testing initially. If both are negative, practice abstinence or safer sex for 6 months, followed by retesting. If results still indicate that both partners are negative, sexual activity can probably be considered safe.
- Use latex condoms for oral, vaginal, or anal intercourse; avoid natural or animal skin condoms, which allow passage of HIV.
- For vaginal or anal sex, lubricate the condom with the spermicidal agent nonoxynol-9 for additional protection.
- Do not use an oil-based lubricant such as petroleum jelly, which can result in condom damage; water-based lubricants are acceptable.

- Women should carry and use a female condom.
- Remember that use of other means of birth control, such as oral contraceptives, provide no protection against HIV; barrier protection with a condom is necessary.
- Engage in safer sexual practices that are less damaging to sensitive tissues (e.g., mutual masturbation, avoiding anal or oral sex).
- Do not use drugs or alcohol.
- Do not share needles, razors, toothbrushes, sexual toys, or other items that may be contaminated with blood or body fluids.
- If HIV positive:
   a. Do not engage in unprotected sexual activity.
   b. Inform all current and former sexual partners of HIV status.
   c. Inform all healthcare personnel—primary care providers, physicians, and dentists in particular—of HIV status.
   d. Do not donate blood, plasma, blood products, sperm, organs, or tissue.
   e. If female, do not become pregnant.

Family members may have engaged in high-risk behaviors but lie about their risk because of embarrassment or fear of discovery. Furthermore, the family member may have a different blood type or have other contraindications to donating.

Encourage HIV-positive clients to abstain from donating blood, organs, or sperm. They should understand tactics to avoid exchange of body fluids by not sharing needles or other drug paraphernalia, not sharing razors, and not obtaining a tattoo. Stress the importance of informing all medical personnel providing direct care (especially anyone performing a dental, surgical, or obstetric procedure) about the diagnosis.

Healthcare workers can prevent most exposures to HIV by using standard precautions (refer to Appendix A and see Figure 13–11 ■). Testing to determine HIV status remains voluntary and relies on the use of antibody-screening methods. It is therefore impossible to identify every client who is HIV positive. With standard precautions, all clients are treated alike, eliminating the need to know the client's HIV status. All high-risk body fluids are treated as if they are infectious, and barrier precautions are used to prevent skin, mucous membrane, or percutaneous exposure to them. Counseling and testing are provided to healthcare workers with a documented needle-stick exposure. Some clinicians and facilities recommend prophylactic AZT therapy after needle-stick or splash exposure; however, it must be initiated immediately, and its effectiveness has yet to be established.

Assessment

Collect the following data through health history and physical examination. Further focused assessments are described with nursing interventions below.

- *Health history:* risk factors (transfusion, unprotected sex, needle exposure), infections (sexually transmitted infections, hepatitis, tuberculosis), medications, recreational drug use, foreign travel, pets
- *Physical assessment:* height, weight, nutrition, skin and mucous membranes, vision, lymph nodes, breath sounds,

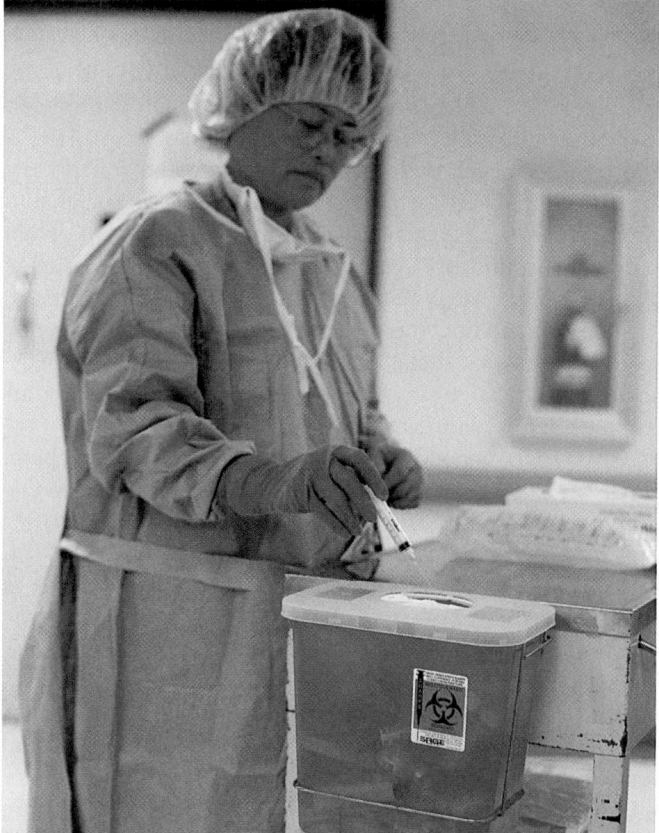

Figure 13–11 ■ This nurse is disposing of a needle and syringe in a special container, a necessary practice to avoid the transmission of HIV through needle sticks with contaminated needles.

abdominal tenderness, motor strength, coordination, cranial nerves, gait, deep tendon reflexes, genitourinary examination, mental status. Remember that symptoms must be interpreted and reported by the client. Like pain, the presence and severity of dyspnea are determined and reported by the client. We must believe what the client tells us. Assessment is the basis for differential diagnosis; fitting appropriate treatment to the correct etiology is critical. For example, delirium is an acute confusional state and, unlike dementia, is reversible. There are effective nursing interventions for these conditions (Coyne et al., 2002).

Nursing Diagnoses and Interventions

Nursing care needs for the client with HIV infection change over the course of the disease. Preventive healthcare measures, health maintenance activities, education, and support of coping mechanisms are important in the early stages of the disease. Counseling the client with a new diagnosis of HIV infection is vital. HIV infection and AIDS continue to carry a social stigma that may interfere with the client's usual support systems and coping mechanisms. As the disease progresses and the client experiences more physical symptoms, direct care needs become more important while the need for psychosocial support continues. Acute exacerbation of opportunistic infections may necessitate hospitalization, but typically the client is managed at home. See the accompanying Nursing Care Plan on page 363.

Ineffective Coping

On receiving the test results indicating HIV seropositive status, the person with HIV infection is faced with multiple issues rarely affecting other clients. First and foremost, HIV is a disease for which there is no known cure and which is, at this time, thought to be almost universally fatal. Social support systems, family relationships, and the ability to obtain and retain useful work and health insurance may be disrupted by the disease. The client may experience guilt about his or her lifestyle and how the disease was contracted. As the disease progresses, social isolation, fatigue, body image changes, medication side effects, and multiple other issues affect the client's abilities to cope.

- Assess social support network and usual methods of coping. *This will help both the nurse and the client identify people and mechanisms that can help the client cope more effectively with the disease.*
- If possible, assign a primary nurse, whether the setting is home health, hospice, or acute care. *This helps promote the development of a therapeutic and trusting relationship and provides for continuity of care.*
- Plan for consistent, uninterrupted time with the client. *Time and a consistent presence encourage the client to express feelings and work through issues related to HIV infection.*
- Interact at every opportunity outside of providing specific nursing care treatments. *This purposeful interaction communicates caring and acceptance without fear of HIV disease.*
- Support the client's social network. *Nontraditional families may offer more support than the traditional family. This in turn may necessitate a liberal interpretation of the term family if unit policy is immediate family only.*
- Promote interaction between the client, significant others, and family. *Hospitalization and manifestations of HIV disease may bring about isolation from others and decrease the client's ability to cope.*

- Encourage involvement in making care decisions. *This gives the client a greater sense of self-worth and control over the situation, increasing coping abilities.*
- Set and maintain limits on manipulative and other destructive behaviors. *The client who is unable to limit inappropriate behaviors needs the external control established by setting limits.*
- Assist to accept responsibility for actions without blaming others. *Effective coping cannot occur without accepting responsibility for one's actions.*
- Support positive coping behaviors, decisions, actions, and achievements. *As self-esteem is enhanced, coping improves* (Côté & Pepler, 2005).

Impaired Skin Integrity

Dryness, malnutrition, immobility from fatigue, and skin lesions on pressure sites contribute to impaired integrity of the skin for the client with HIV disease. Maintaining skin integrity is important because of the progressive and debilitating nature of the disease. It is also a consideration both as the first line of defense against infection in an immunosuppressed client and as a site for secondary manifestations such as KS and herpes.

- Monitor the skin frequently for lesions and areas of breakdown. *Early identification of impaired skin integrity allows prompt intervention.*
- Monitor lesions for signs of infection or impaired healing. *Infection or poor tissue perfusion not only impairs healing but may lead to further skin breakdown.*
- Turn at least every 2 hours, more frequently if necessary. *Turning decreases unrelieved pressure on bony prominences and improves circulation to the tissues.*
- Use pressure-relieving devices, such as pressure and egg-crate mattresses, or sheep skin pads for elbows and heels. *These devices provide prophylactic relief of pressure.*
- Keep skin clean and dry using mild, nondrying soaps or oils for cleansing. *Night sweats and diarrhea, if present, can cause breakdown and damage to the skin. Frequent cleansing with nondrying products discourages bacterial growth, thus reducing the risk of infection.*

PRACTICE ALERT
Applying protective creams to reddened areas in the rectal area protects skin from the caustic effects of diarrhea.

- Massage around but not over affected pressure sites to increase circulation to the surrounding tissue. *Massaging over the affected area can cause skin breakdown.*
- If blisters are noted, leave intact, and dress with a hydrocolloid (DuoDERM) dressing. *Blisters provide natural sterile coverings for damaged tissue, improving healing and preventing bacterial invasion.*
- Caution against scratching. If confused, trim fingernails and use mitts or soft restraints to prevent scratching. Check for circulation of hands and fingers frequently if mitts or restraints are used. *Scratching and skin damage allow bacteria to be introduced into lesions, increasing the risk of infection. Tight or restrictive restraints or mitts may compromise circulation.*

NURSING CARE PLAN   A Client with HIV Infection

Sara Lu is a 26-year-old elementary school teacher who lives with her parents and two younger sisters. Ms. Lu is very close to her parents and sisters; they share everything with each other. During the required physical for admission to graduate school, Ms. Lu tells her physician that lately she has felt fatigued. She also states that she has had a persistent sore throat, intermittent bouts of diarrhea, and mild shortness of breath for about a month. She takes no routine medications other than a daily multivitamin and an occasional acetaminophen tablet for a headache. She is active in a drama club in her community, and she jogs 3 miles three to four times a week. She is engaged to be married; her wedding date is 6 months away. Her fiancé is the only person with whom she has had sexual relations. Her sexual activity has been unprotected. Ms. Lu has a history of open heart surgery 7 years ago to correct a congenital valve defect. She has been physically healthy since that time, until about a month or two ago. The physician orders a mononucleosis test, ELISA, Western blot analysis, CD4 T-cell count, a p24 antigen test, and an erythrocyte sedimentation rate (ESR). She has been asked to return in 1 week for follow-up.

ASSESSMENT

On Ms. Lu's follow-up visit, Carole Kee, RN, obtains her nursing history. Ms. Lu continues to have flulike symptoms but has improved somewhat. She states that she just has not been as active as usual and is worried about her health. Her appetite has decreased because of soreness in her mouth, and she has noted some whitish patches on her tongue and cheeks.

A chest x-ray film reveals no abnormality. The results of her laboratory tests are as follows:

- ELISA: positive for antibodies against HIV
- Western blot analysis: positive for antibodies against HIV
- p24 antigen test: positive for circulating HIV antigens
- ESR: increased to 25 mm/h (normal for women is 15 to 20 mm/h; normal for men is 10 to 15 mm/h)
- CD4 T-cell count: 599/mm^3 (normal range is 600 to 1200 mm^3).

Ms. Lu's physical examination reveals that she has enlarged lymph nodes in her neck and white patches on her oral mucosa. Her skin is warm to the touch. Her vital signs are as follows: T 99.9°F (37.7°C), P 84, R 20, and BP 120/78.

Ms. Lu is told of the results of her laboratory tests and the medical diagnosis of HIV infection. Ms. Lu is obviously distressed and wants to know how this happened, its meaning, whether she has infected her loved ones, and whether she will get better.

DIAGNOSES

- *Imbalanced Nutrition: Less than Body Requirements* related to soreness in mouth
- *Risk for Deficient Fluid Volume* related to decreased fluid intake and diarrhea
- *Risk for Infection* related to altered immune protection
- *Anxiety* related to diagnosis and fear
- *Deficient Knowledge* about the HIV disease process

EXPECTED OUTCOMES

- Maintain adequate nutrition for optimal body and cellular function.

- Consume at least 2500 mL of fluid per day.
- Remain free of infections and their complications.
- Verbalize anxiety and use appropriate coping mechanisms.
- Verbalize and demonstrate knowledge of HIV disease.
- Verbalize measures to prevent HIV transmission to others, including safer sex practices.

PLANNING AND IMPLEMENTATION

- Monitor daily weight and intake and output.
- Monitor dietary habits and serum albumin levels.
- Teach Ms. Lu the importance of consuming a nutritionally balanced diet and maintaining adequate fluid intake.
- Suggest strategies for coping with anorexia and nausea.
- Provide dietary consultation referral.
- Encourage oral care before and after meals.
- Assess bowel sounds and monitor elimination pattern.
- Administer antiemetic and antimotility medications as ordered.
- Monitor for signs of dehydration, such as poor skin turgor, oliguria, and orthostatic hypotension.
- Increase fluid to 2500 mL daily.
- Use strict aseptic technique for all invasive procedures.
- Teach Ms. Lu to avoid exposure to infection and people with known illnesses.
- Administer antiretroviral medications and antibiotics as prescribed, and monitor response.
- Encourage maintenance of regular physical exercise.
- Provide opportunities for Ms. Lu to verbalize her feelings.
- Avoid false reassurances.
- Provide appropriate and adequate information about HIV/AIDS.
- Teach safer sex practices and other measures to prevent HIV transmission.
- Teach anxiety-controlling techniques, such as deep breathing and meditation.

EVALUATION

Ms. Lu is eager to learn about her illness and wants her family to come with her for further explanation. She states that she is sure her fiancé will be available as well. Ms. Lu is taking home antifungal medication, diet plans, and a schedule for increased exercise. She will return in 1 week for counseling and in 1 month for a follow-up physical.

CRITICAL THINKING IN THE NURSING PROCESS

1. How does age affect the body's response to fighting HIV? What other factors affect the risk of HIV infection and its progression?
2. Are the laboratory results for Ms. Lu a true indication that she is HIV positive? What additional tests might be ordered?
3. What is the most likely source of Ms. Lu's infection? What measures are used to reduce this risk, and how did she contract HIV? What is another possible source of Ms. Lu's HIV infection?
4. Ms. Lu says that her fiancé would like to have a child. How will you counsel her regarding pregnancy and childbearing?
See Evaluating Your Response in Appendix C.

- Avoid the use of heat or occlusive dressings. *Heat can further dry and damage the skin; occlusive dressings may impair circulation and lead to ulceration.*
- Prevent skin shearing by using a turnsheet and adequate personnel when repositioning. *Shearing causes tissue trauma that can lead to decubitus ulcers.*
- Encourage ambulation if possible; if the client is confined to bed, encourage active or passive range-of-motion exercises. *Activity increases circulation, decreases pressure and skin breakdown, and helps maintain muscle tone.*
- Monitor nutritional intake and albumin levels. *Maintenance of optimal nutrition decreases the risk of tissue breakdown and improves resistance to infection.*

Imbalanced Nutrition: Less than Body Requirements

Many factors associated with HIV disease, including manifestations of the disease itself, put the client at risk for altered nutrition and weight loss. Nausea and anorexia may be manifestations of the disease or the result of antiretroviral therapy. Chronic diarrhea is a common manifestation of constitutional HIV disease. Wasting syndrome is also common. It is manifested by involuntary weight loss of greater than 10% to 15% of baseline weight, severe diarrhea, fever, and chronic fatigue and weakness. The exact cause of wasting syndrome is unclear, but the diarrhea and fatigue contribute, as does the increased metabolic rate associated with fever. Oral and esophageal candidiasis and KS of the gastrointestinal tract may cause painful swallowing, making eating difficult and thereby contributing to anorexia. Poor nutritional status in the client with HIV can ultimately result in altered comfort, a change in body image, muscle wasting, increased risk of infection, and higher mortality and morbidity.

- Assess nutritional status, including weight; body mass; caloric intake; and laboratory studies, such as total protein and albumin levels, hemoglobin, and hematocrit. *These factors provide a baseline to determine the effectiveness of interventions.*
- Identify possible causes of altered nutrition. *Identification of causes provides direction for planned interventions.*
- Administer prescribed medications for candidiasis and other manifestations as ordered. *Eliminating this opportunistic infection improves comfort and facilitates food intake. Topical viscous anesthetic can help reduce pain and improve oral intake.*
- Administer antidiarrheal medications after stools and antiemetics prior to meals. Provide antipyretics as needed to control fever. *Reducing diarrhea will improve nutrient absorption; preprandial medication with an antiemetic reduces nausea and improves food intake. Reduction of fever lowers the body's metabolic demands.*

PRACTICE ALERT
High-fiber foods can increase intestinal motility and the incidence of diarrhea.

- Provide a diet high in protein and kilocalories. *A high-protein, high-kilocalorie diet provides the necessary nutrients to meet metabolic and tissue healing needs.*

- Offer soft foods and serve small portions. *Soft foods are easily digested. Small portions are more appealing to the anorectic or nauseated client.*
- Involve in meal planning and encourage significant others to bring favorite foods from home. *The client is more likely to consume adequate amounts of preferred foods. Allowing food choices enhances the client's sense of control.*
- Assist with eating as needed. *Fatigue and weakness can prevent the client from eating an adequate amount of food.*
- Provide supplementary vitamins and enteral feedings, such as Ensure. *This improves nutritional status and caloric intake.*
- Provide or assist with frequent oral hygiene. *Oral hygiene improves comfort and appetite, and reduces the risk of mucosal lesions.*
- Administer appetite stimulants, such as megestrol (Megace) and dronabinol (Marinol) as ordered. *Both drugs may increase appetite and promote weight gain.*

Ineffective Sexuality Patterns

The diagnosis of HIV infection can significantly alter the client's expressions of sexuality. Guilt over the diagnosis may interfere with libido. The client may be angry with a significant other or partner if that person was the probable source of infection. The client may fear spreading the disease to others via sexual relations. As the disease progresses, its manifestations can affect body image and self-esteem, impairing sexuality. Other symptoms, such as nausea, fatigue, and weakness, may also interfere with libido and sexual satisfaction.

- Examine your feelings about sexuality, your role in dealing with a client's sexuality, the client's lifestyle, and sexual preferences. *To deal effectively with the client's concerns, it is vital that the nurse be comfortable with his or her own feelings of sexuality and be able to accept the client's lifestyle. Referring the client to another nurse or counselor may be necessary.*
- Establish a trusting, therapeutic relationship through the use of time, active listening, caring, and self-disclosure. Maintain a nonthreatening, nonjudgmental attitude toward the client. *Sexuality is a private issue that will be uncomfortable or impossible for the nurse and client to discuss without a mutually trusting relationship.*
- Provide factual information about HIV infection and its effects. *This helps the client separate fears and myths from reality.*
- Discuss safer sex practices, including hugging, cuddling, nonsexual contact, the use of latex condoms and spermicidal lubricant, and mutual masturbation. *Alternative forms of sexual activity and expressing affection can allow the client and significant other to remain close throughout the course of the disease.*
- Encourage discussion of fears and concerns with significant other. *Open communication helps them to deal with issues related to sexuality.*
- For the client without a significant other, stress the need to continue to meet people and develop social relationships while practicing safer sex. *The risk of isolation is high in the client with HIV infection, and relationships with others help the client to cope with the disease.*

- Refer the client and significant other to local support groups for people and partners of people with HIV. *Support groups provide a social and support network of people facing the same issues.*

Using NANDA, NIC, and NOC

Chart 13–1 shows links between NANDA, NIC, and NOC when caring for the client with AIDS.

Community-Based Care

Teaching needs for both the client and significant other are extensive. The primary need is information about the disease, its spread, and its expected course. The client and family need current factual information to plan realistically and to combat myths, misperceptions, and prejudices. At the same time, it is important to include information about current research and progress in treating the disease to maintain a sense of hopefulness.

The following topics should be discussed with the client and family to prepare for home care:

- Guidelines for safer sex practices
- Nutrition, rest and exercise, stress reduction, lifestyle changes, and maintaining a positive outlook
- Infection prevention and transmission including hand washing and wearing gloves when handling client's secretions or excretions
- Importance of regular medical follow-up and monitoring of immune status
- Signs and symptoms of opportunistic infections and malignancies, as well as other symptoms that should be reported
- Medications and adverse effects
- Use and care of implanted venous access devices, total parenteral nutrition, intravenous pumps and continuous medication delivery systems, and intravenous or aerosolized medications
- Cessation of smoking, alcohol, and recreational or illicit drug use
- Home health services

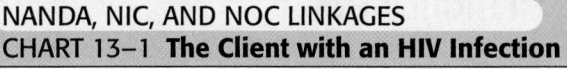

NANDA, NIC, AND NOC LINKAGES
CHART 13–1 The Client with an HIV Infection

NANDA

Fatigue

NIC

Energy Management

Nutrition Management

Support System Enhancement

NOC

Endurance

Nutritional Status: Energy

Stress Level

Data from *NANDA's Nursing Diagnoses: Definitions & Classification 2005–2006* by NANDA International (2003), Philadelphia; *Nursing Interventions Classification (NIC)* (4th ed.) by J. M. Dochterman & G. M. Bulechek (2004), St. Louis, MO: Mosby; and *Nursing Outcomes Classification (NOC)* (3rd ed.) by S. Moorhead, M. Johnson, and M. Maas (2004), St. Louis, MO: Mosby.

- Hospice and respite care services
- Community resources, such as support groups, social agencies, and counselors
- Helpful resources:
  - CDC National AIDS Hotline
  - Gay Men's Health Crisis Network
  - National Association of People with AIDS
  - National Organization for HIV over Fifty.

MEDIALINK AIDS/HIV Support and Resources

EXPLORE MEDIALINK

Prentice Hall Nursing MediaLink DVD-ROM
Audio Glossary
NCLEX-RN® Review
Crossword Puzzle: The Immune System

Animation/Video
Histamine
Immune System
Immune System in the Older Adult

COMPANION WEBSITE www.prenhall.com/lemone
Audio Glossary
NCLEX-RN® Review
Care Plan Activity: A Client with AIDS
Case Study: HIV Prevention
MediaLink Application: At Risk for HIV/AIDS
Links to Resources

CHAPTER HIGHLIGHTS

- The immune system is a complex combination of cellular and humoral components that protect against disease. Immunity develops when the body recognizes foreign proteins as "non-self" and develops nonspecific inflammatory responses and specific cellular responses to each foreign antigen.
- Clients suffer when the immune system is excessively or inadequately responsive, or when recognition of self fails and reactions escalate against self. The latter occurs in autoimmune diseases.
- With aging, there is a general decline in the sensitivity and regulation of the immune system, often resulting in autoimmune disease.
- Hypersensitivities are excessive responses to antigens that result in harm to the client. These range from benign to severely life threatening. Damage to host tissue is caused by chemicals of the immune response, destruction of cells, or creation of large antigen–antibody complexes that accumulate in the kidney glomerular capillaries.
- Allergic reactions are treated pharmacologically to prevent or moderate allergic responses. Another method of dampening allergic responses is by desensitization, a weekly process of introducing increasing amounts of known allergens subdermally.
- Clients must be taught that the safest practice is to avoid contact with all known allergens.
- Latex allergy is a problem for healthcare professionals. Repeated exposure to latex-containing equipment and gloves results in delayed hypersensitivity.

- Any type of allergic reaction has the potential to escalate to anaphylaxis. Respiratory arrest and cardiac failure are risks with full blown allergic reactions. Nurses must recognize early signs and symptoms and immediately signal for emergency care.
- Intentional immunosuppression is an essential step in preventing transplant rejection. The client receiving a transplanted organ will be treated with immune-suppressing drugs to prevent initial rejection, to maintain the transplant, and to halt any rejection process that may develop. Clients will take the immune-suppressing, antirejection drugs for their lifetime. The drugs prevent cytokine production that upregulates an immune reaction and targets the transplanted organ. Most immunosuppressing drugs are nephrotoxic; immunosuppression places clients at greater risk for infection and cancers.
- HIV/AIDS continues to spread and many clients are unaware they have the virus. AIDs is a profoundly immune-suppressed condition that results from viral destruction of cellular components of host immunity.
- A major change in the AIDS epidemic is the disease profile, which has benefited from HAART. HAART is a combination of drugs that limits viral replication and host susceptibility to opportunistic infections and cancer. Clients are living much longer with the disease without progression to AIDS. "Pill burden" refers to the number of pills the client must take daily to maintain immune function; side effects of the combination of drugs which make up HAART are appearing as clients live longer. In addition to increased susceptibility to infections and cancers, clients suffer from a dementia peculiar to AIDs.

TEST YOURSELF NCLEX-RN® REVIEW

1. Which one of the following conditions is caused by a type I IgE-mediated hypersensitivity reaction?
   1. autoimmune hemolytic anemia
   2. systemic lupus erythematosus
   3. graft rejection
   4. anaphylaxis

2. A client received a liver transplant 1 day ago. If the client were to develop an acute transplant rejection episode, when should the nurse expect to see the manifestations?
   1. approximately 4 days to 3 months later
   2. approximately 2 days later
   3. within the first 24 hours
   4. within the first 8 hours

3. The nurse notes a cough, shortness of breath, and tachypnea in a client with AIDS. Which opportunistic infection is probably causing these manifestations?
   1. *Toxoplasma gondii*
   2. cytomegalovirus
   3. *Pneumocystis carinii*
   4. *Cryptococcus neoformans*

4. Which of the following explanations should the nurse give to a client who has tested positive for HIV?
   1. "You have been diagnosed with AIDS."
   2. "At this point, AIDS is not active in your blood."
   3. "This means that you will not develop AIDS in the future."
   4. "Antibodies to the AIDS virus are present in the blood."

5. Clients taking zidovudine (Retrovir) should be monitored for which of the following adverse reactions?
   1. cardiotoxicity
   2. leukopenia
   3. nephrotoxicity
   4. polycythemia

6. The order of administering antigens in allergy testing is based on prevention of anaphylaxis. Which method should be used first?
   1. inhalation
   2. prick test
   3. intradermal injection
   4. subcutaneous injection

7. If a hypersensitivity response is suspected when blood products are infusing, the nurse should:
   1. discard the product immediately.
   2. replace all tubing and attach a new line with NS.
   3. backflush the line and run the NS attached at the Y tubing.
   4. remove the intravenous catheter and establish access distal to the site.

8. Protease inhibitors and nucleoside analogs share correlations to metabolic abnormalities including:
   1. lactose intolerance.
   2. diabetes mellitus.
   3. Hashimoto's thyroiditis.
   4. systemic lupus erythematosus.

9 The priority when initiating or changing HIV drug therapy regimens is:
1. cost of therapy.
2. access to dental care.
3. toxicities associated with each drug.
4. client willingness to adhere to the drug regimen.

10 Clients receiving kidney transplants will receive immunosuppressant therapy. The agent used to induce immunosuppression immediately following a transplant is often:
1. azathioprine.
2. corticosteroids.
3. muromonab-CD3.
4. antithymocyte globulin.

See Test Yourself answers in Appendix C.

BIBLIOGRAPHY

Ackley, B. J., & Ladwig, G. B. (2002). *Nursing diagnosis handbook* (5th ed.). St. Louis, MO: Mosby.

American Cancer Society. (2005). *Overviews: What is Kaposi's sarcoma?* Retrieved March 20, 2006, from http://www.nlm.nih.gov/medlineplus/kaposissarcoma.html

American Nurses Association. (1997). *Position statement: Needle exchange and HIV.* Washington, DC: Author.

Bartlett, J. G., & Weber, D. J. (2005). Management of adults exposed to HIV. UpToDate Online 13.2. Retrieved October 14, 2005, from http://222.utdol.com.

Binkley, H. M., Schroyer, T., & Catalfano, J. (2003). Latex allergies: A review of recognition, evaluation, management, prevention, education, and alternative product use. *Journal of Athletic Training, 38*(2), 133–140.

Bova, C. A., Fennie, K. P., Knafl, G. J., Dieckhaus, K. D., Wtrous, E., & Williams, A. B. (2005). Use of electronic monitoring devices to measure antiretroviral adherence: Practical considerations. *AIDS and Behavior, 9*(1), 103–110.

Carrico, R. M. (2001). What to do if you're exposed to a bloodborne pathogen. *Home Healthcare Nurse, 19*(6), 362–368.

Centers for Disease Control and Prevention. (1993). Revised classification system for HIV infection and expanded case definition for AIDS among adolescents and adults. *MMWR, Recommendations and Reports, 41*(RR-17), 1–19.

_____. (1996). Update: Provisional public health recommendations for chemoprophylaxis after occupational exposure to HIV. *MMWR, 45,* 468–472.

_____. (2004). Treating opportunistic infections among HIV-infected adults and adolescents. *MMWR Recommendations and Reports, 53*(RR-15), 1–113.

_____. (2006). *Statistics and surveillance.* Retrieved March 14, 2006, from http://www.cdc.gov/hiv/topics/surveillance/index.htm

Chernecky, C. C., & Berger, B. M. (2004). *Laboratory tests and diagnostic procedures* (4th ed.). Philadelphia: W. B. Saunders/Elsevier.

Côté J. K., & Pepler, C. (2005). Cognitive coping intervention for acutely ill HIV-positive men. *Journal of Clinical Nursing, 14*(3), 321–326.

Covington, L. W. (2005). Update on antiviral agents for HIV and AIDS. *Nursing Clinics of North America, 40*(1), 149–165.

Coyne, P. J., Lyne, M. E., & Watson, A. C. (2002). Symptom management in people with AIDS. *American Journal of Nursing, 102*(9), 48–57.

Dochterman, J., & Bulechek, G. (2004). *Nursing interventions classification (NIC)* (4th ed.). St. Louis, MO: Mosby.

Early HIV Infection Guideline Panel. (1994). *Evaluation and management of early HIV infection: Clinical practice guidelines* (AHCPR Publication No. 94-0572). Rockville, MD: AHCPR Public Health Service, USDHHS.

Enriquez, M., & McKinsey, D. (2004). Readiness for HIV treatment: Adherence is vital to managing disease and reducing resistance. *American Journal of Nursing, 104*(10), 81–84.

Goldsby, R. A., Kindt, T. J., Osborne, B. A., & Kuby, J. (2003). *Immunology.* (5th ed.). New York: W. H. Freeman.

Ingersoll, K. S., & Heckman, C. J. (2005). Patient-clinician relationships and treatment system effects on HIV medication adherence. *AIDS and Behavior, 9*(1), 89–101.

Johnson, M., Maas, M., & Moorhead, S. (2000). *Iowa outcomes project: Nursing outcomes classification (NOC)* (2nd ed.). Upper Saddle River, NJ: Prentice Hall Health.

Joint United Nations Programme on HIV/AIDS. (2000). *Men make a difference.* Press kit: World AIDS Day. HIV/AIDS in Africa. Retrieved from http://www.unaids.org/wac/2000/wad00/files/FS_Africa.htm

Kasper, D. L., Braunwald, E., Fauci, A., Hauser, S., Longo, D., & Jameson, J. L. (2005). *Harrison's principles of internal medicine* (16th ed.). New York: McGraw-Hill.

Katz, M. H., & Hollander, H. (2005). HIV infection. In L. M. Tierney, S. J. McPhee, & M. A. Papadakis (Eds.), *Current medical diagnosis and treatment* (Vol. 44). New York: Lange Medical Books/McGraw-Hill.

Kenny, P. E. (2004). The changing face of AIDS. *Nursing, 34*(8), 56–62.

King, H. C., Mabry, R. L., Mabry, C. S., Gordon, B. R., & Marple, B. F. (2005). *Allergy in ENT practice: The basic guide* (2nd ed.). New York: Thieme Medical Publisher.

Kirton, C. A., Ferri, R. S., & Eleftherakis, V. (1999). Primary care and case management of persons with HIV/AIDS. *Nursing Clinics of North America, 34*(1), 71–94.

Lehne, R. A. (2004). *Pharmacology for nursing care* (4th ed.). St. Louis: Saunders/Elsevier.

Lyon, D. E., & Munro, C. (2001). Disease severity and symptoms of depression in black Americans infected with HIV. *Applied Nursing Research, 14*(1), 3–10.

Martinez-Picado, J., Negredo, E., Ruiz, L., Shintani, A., Fumaz, C. R., Zala, C., et al. (2003). Alternation of antiretroviral drug regimens for HIV infection: A randomized, controlled trial. *Annals of Internal Medicine, 139*(2), 81–89.

McCloskey, J. C., & Bulechek, G. M. (2000). *Iowa interventions project: Nursing interventions classifications (NIC)* (3rd ed.). Upper Saddle River, NJ: Prentice Hall Health.

Moorhead, S., Johnson, M., & Maas, M. (2003). *Nursing outcomes classification (NOC)* (3rd ed.). St. Louis, MO: Mosby.

Muehlbauer, P., & White, R. (1998). Are you prepared for interleukin-2? *RN, 61*(2), 34, 36–38.

Murasko, D. M., & Gardner, E. M. (2003). Immunology of aging. In *Principles of geriatric medicine and gerontology* (5th ed.). New York: McGraw-Hill Professional.

National Center for HIV, STD, and TB Control. (2005). Divisions of HIV/AIDS prevention: Basic statistics. Retrieved October 23, 2005, from http://www.cdc.gov

National Institute of Allergy and Infectious Diseases. (2000). *HIV infection in women.* Bethesda, MD: National Institutes of Health.

National Institute of Occupational Safety and Health. (2005). Occupational latex allergy. Retrieved March 15, 2006, from http://www.cdc.gov/niosh/topics/latex

Novello, A. (1993, June). *Surgeon General's report to the American public on HIV infection and AIDS—extracts.* Rockville, MD: CDC National AIDS Clearinghouse.

Pagana, K. D., & Pagana, T. J. (2002). *Mosby's manual of diagnostic and laboratory tests* (2nd ed.). St. Louis, MO: Mosby.

Porth, C. (2005). *Pathophysiology: Concepts of altered health states* (6th ed.). Philadelphia: Lippincott.

Robinson, F. P. (2005). Body composition changes in patients with HIV. *American Journal of Nursing, 105*(13), 69–72.

Sherman, D. (1996). Nurses' willingness to care for AIDS patients and spirituality, social support, and death anxiety. *Image: Journal of Nursing Scholarship, 28*(3), 205–213.

Sowell, R. L., Moneyham, L., & Aranda-Naranjo, B. (1999). The care of women with AIDS. *Nursing Clinics of North America, 34*(1), 179–199.

Swenson, M. R. (2000). Autoimmunity and immunotherapy. *Journal of Intravenous Nursing, 23*(5S), S8–S13.

Szirony, T. A. (1999). Infection with HIV in the elderly population. *Journal of Gerontological Nursing, 25*(10), 25–31.

Thurlow, K. L. (2001). Latex allergies: Management and clinical responsibilities. *Home Healthcare Nurse, 19*(6), 369–376.

Tierney, L., McPhee, S., & Papadakis, M. (Eds.) (2005). *Current medical diagnosis & treatment* (44th ed.). New York: Lange Medical Books/McGraw-Hill.

Valdez, M. R. (2001). A metaphor for HIV-positive Mexican and Puerto Rican women. *Western Journal of Nursing Research, 23*(5), 517–535.

Valois, P., Turgeon, H., Godin, G., Blondeau, D., & Cote, F. (2001). Influence of a persuasive strategy on nursing students' beliefs and attitudes toward provisions of care to people living with HIV/AIDS. *Journal of Nursing Education, 40*(8), 354–358.

Wilkinson, J. (2005). *Prentice Hall nursing diagnosis handbook with NIC interventions and NOC outcomes* (8th ed.). Upper Saddle River, NJ: Prentice Hall Health.

Wroe, A. L., & Thomas, M. G. (2003). Intentional and unintentional nonadherence in patients prescribed HAART treatment regimens. *Psychology Health & Medicine, 8*(4), 453–463.

CHAPTER 14
Nursing Care of Clients with Cancer

LEARNING OUTCOMES

- Define cancer and differentiate benign from malignant neoplasms.
- Describe the theories of carcinogenesis.
- Explain and discuss known carcinogens and identify risk factors for cancer.
- Compare the mechanisms and characteristics of normal cells with those of malignant cells.
- Describe physical and psychologic effects of cancer.
- Describe and compare laboratory and diagnostic tests for cancer.

- Discuss the role of chemotherapy in cancer treatment and classify chemotherapeutic agents.
- Discuss the role of surgery, radiation therapy, and biotherapy in the treatment of cancer.
- Identify causes and discuss the nursing interventions for common oncologic emergencies.
- Design an appropriate care plan for clients with cancer and their families regarding cancer diagnosis, treatment, and coping strategies.

CLINICAL COMPETENCIES

- Assess functional health status of clients with cancer, and monitor, document, and report abnormal manifestations.
- Incorporate evidence-based research into the plan of nursing care for clients with cancer.
- Prioritize nursing diagnosis based on assessment data and implement appropriate nursing interventions for clients with cancer during cancer diagnosis, treatment, and rehabilitation.
- Administer chemotherapeutic medications and other medications for pain, nausea, and vomiting, mucositis, or anemia knowledgeably and safely.

- Use the nursing process as a framework for planning and providing individualized care and integrating interdisciplinary care for clients with cancer to meet their healthcare needs.
- Include cultural variation and diverse values in designing and implementing individualized plans of care for clients with cancer.
- Design and provide individualized client and family teaching to restore, promote, and maintain clients' functional status.
- Revise plan of care as needed to provide effective interventions for clients with cancer and their families.

MEDIALINK

Resources for this chapter can be found on
the Prentice Hall Nursing MediaLink DVD-ROM
accompanying this textbook, and
on the Companion Website at
http://www.prenhall.com/lemone

KEY TERMS

anaplasia, *374*
biotherapy, *396*
cachexia, *380*
cancer, *369*
carcinogenesis, *374*
carcinogens, *374*
cell cycle, *373*

chemotherapy, *389*
differentiation, *373*
dysplasia, *373*
hospice, *412*
hyperplasia, *373*
metaplasia, *373*
metastasis, *378*

neoplasms, *376*
oncogene, *374*
oncologic emergencies, *409*
oncology, *369*
radiation therapy, *395*
tumor marker, *383*
xerostomia, *408*

Cancer is a group of complex diseases with various manifestations depending on which body system is affected and the type of tumor cells involved. Cancer can affect people of any age, gender, ethnicity, or geographic region. Although the incidence and mortality rates of cancer have continued to decline since 1990, it remains one of the most feared diseases. The fear engendered by even the suggestion of a cancer diagnosis often evokes feelings of hopelessness and helplessness.

This chapter focuses on the general pathogenesis, pathophysiology, and etiology of cancer; identifies current diagnostic and treatment modalities; and discusses nursing care appropriate for clients with cancer. Discussions of cancers that affect specific body systems (e.g., leukemia, lung cancer) can be found in corresponding body system chapters in the text.

Cancer results when normal cells mutate into abnormal, deviant cells that then perpetuate within the body. Cancer can affect any body tissue. Nursing care of the client with cancer is holistic and comprehensive, focusing on cancer not as one disease, but as a constellation of many diseases. The nurse recognizes that cancer is a disruptive and life-threatening process that affects the whole person and that person's significant others. Nursing interventions are based on the understanding that cancer is a chronic disease that has acute episodes, that the client is often treated in the home, and that the client is usually treated with a combination of therapeutic modalities. Equally important, the nurse recognizes that caring for the client with cancer involves prevention, early detection, treatment, supportive care, long-term follow-up, and possibly end-of-life care (Oncology Nursing Society, 2006).

Oncology is the study of cancer. The term is derived from the Greek word *oncoma* ("bulk"). Oncologists specialize in caring for clients with cancer; they may be medical doctors, surgeons, radiologists, immunologists, or researchers. The oncology nurse is an important and significant member of the oncology team, who has received specialized training in cancer care and treatment. Oncology nurses have special skills in assisting the client and family with the psychosocial issues associated with cancer and terminal illness. Collaboration among healthcare professionals (e.g., surgeons, oncologists, nurses, social workers) ensures the most effective care and treatment for the client with cancer.

INCIDENCE AND MORTALITY

In the United States, about 1,399,790 new cancer cases are expected to be diagnosed in 2006 (American Cancer Society

[ACS], 2006a). One in every four deaths in the United States is caused by cancer and more than 1500 people die of cancer each day (ACS, 2006a). Mortality rates for different cancers vary. Lung cancer remains the leading cause of all cancer deaths in both men and women, accounting for approximately 29% of all cancer deaths (ACS, 2006a).

Due to advances in cancer prevention, early detection, and treatment, the 5-year survival rate for individuals with cancers continues to improve in the United States. However, minority ethnic groups such as African American and Asian American populations bear a disproportionate burden of cancer. African Americans have the highest mortality rate for all cancers and major cancers among all ethnic groups (ACS, 2006b). For example, although breast cancer occurs more commonly in Caucasian women than in African American women, the survival rate is 89% for Caucasian women compared to only 75% for African Americans; breast cancer death rates are 32% higher in African American women than in Caucasian women (ACS, 2006b). Similar disparities are seen in survival rates for colorectal, prostate, and endometrial cancers in these ethnic groups. Research has shown that lack of health insurance, lower incomes, unequal access to health care, knowledge deficit, and cultural beliefs and attitudes are influential factors contributing to cancer disparity among African Americans (Bach et al., 2002; Bradley et al., 2001; Li et al., 2002). For information about diversity and cancer risk and incidence see the Focus on Cultural Diversity box on the following page.

FAST FACTS
Cancer in the United States

- Breast cancer is the most frequently diagnosed cancer in women with an estimated incidence of 212,920 new cases in 2006.
- Prostate cancer is the most frequently occurring cancer in men with an estimated incidence of 234,460 new cases during 2006. The incidence rates of prostate cancer are significantly higher in African American men than in Caucasian men.
- Melanoma occurs mainly among Caucasian Americans; the incidence rates are more than 10 times higher among Caucasians than African Americans.
- The incidence of bladder cancer is about four times higher in men than in women, and almost two times higher in Caucasians than in African Americans.

Source: American Cancer Society. (2006a). *Cancer facts and figures—2006*. Atlanta: Author.

Risk Factors

Risk factors make an individual or a population vulnerable to a specific disease or other unhealthy outcome. Risk factors can be divided into those that are controllable and those that are not controllable. Knowledge and assessment of risk factors are especially important in counseling clients and families about measures to prevent cancer.

Heredity

It is estimated that 5% to 10% of cancers may have a hereditary component. The familial pattern of some breast and colon cancers has been well documented. Lung, ovarian, and prostate cancers have also shown some familial relationships. The Human Genome Project has identified new cancer-linked genes (Futreal et al., 2001). For most cancers, research has yet to distinguish true genetic transfer from environmental causes. So although further research is needed to identify cancers that are due to the inheritance of defective genes, familial predisposition to malignancies should be counted among risk factors so that people at risk can reduce behaviors that promote cancer. For example, a client with a family history of lung cancer should be counseled to avoid smoking, to avoid areas where smoking is allowed, and to avoid working in an occupation that may expose the client to inhaled carcinogens.

Age

Cancer is a disease associated with aging; 76% of cancer diagnoses occur after age 55 (ACS, 2006a). A number of factors are associated with this increased risk in older adults. One possible factor is that at least five cycles of genetic mutations seem necessary to cause permanent damage to the afflicted cells. In addition, long-term exposure to high doses of promotional agents is usually necessary to allow the cancer to take hold. In addition, the immune response alters with aging; its actions become more generalized and less specific (Blaylock, 1998). Another problem is that free radicals (molecules resulting from the body's metabolic and oxidative processes) tend to accumulate in the cells over time, causing damage and mutation.

Hormonal changes that occur with aging can be associated with cancer. Postmenopausal women receiving exogenous estrogen have an increased risk for breast and uterine cancers. Older men are at risk for prostate cancer, possibly due to breakdown of testosterone into carcinogenic forms. See the Nursing Care of the Older Adult box on the following page for a discussion about older adults and cancer.

Severe and/or cumulative losses also are implicated in promoting cancer. These losses, which are common to older adults, include the death of a spouse or friends, loss of position and status in society, and a decline in physical abilities (Rossi, 2004). These repeated stressors are related to changes in the immune system that may lead to the development of cancer.

Gender

Gender is a risk factor for certain types of cancer. Breast cancer is the most frequently diagnosed cancer in women; prostate cancer in men. The incidence of bladder cancer is about four times higher in men than in women (ACS, 2006a). Thyroid cancer occurs more commonly among females, whereas bladder cancer is seen more often among males (ACS, 2006a). See Chapters 50 ∞ and 51 ∞ for more information on gender-specific cancers.

Poverty

The poor are at higher risk for cancer than the population in general. Inadequate access to health care, especially preventive screening and counseling, may be a major factor. Although other factors that may be involved, such as diet and stress, usually come under the category of controllable risks, these risks are frequently uncontrollable in this population.

Stress

Continuous unmanaged stress that keeps hormones such as epinephrine and cortisol at high levels can result in systematic "fatigue" and impaired immunologic surveillance. When the body attempts to adapt to physiologic and psychologic stressors, it goes through a series of stages called the general adaptation syndrome (Rossi, 2004; Selye, 1984). First, the "alarm reaction" occurs, in which adrenal hormones increase, allowing the body to cope with the stressor. Eventually, the body reaches the "stage of resistance," in which the stress hormones are significantly reduced, indicating that adaptation has occurred. If the physiologic adaptation is supported by appropriate coping strategies, the stressor is considered managed and body systems return to prealarm functioning. However, if adaptation continues and the stress hormones remain elevated, the "stage of exhaustion" sets in. This stage will maintain life, but at great expense to body systems, resulting in general wear-and-tear and depression of the immune system (Rossi, 2004; Selye, 1984).

The role of personality in the causation of cancer is controversial. People with cancer-prone personalities are assumed to be people who have unhealthy coping behaviors for life stressors (Katz & Epstein, 2005). Cancer-prone people are identi-

NURSING CARE OF THE OLDER ADULT   Older Adults with Cancer

Nurses need to be aware of how cancer and cancer treatments affect older adults. Cancer is the second leading cause of death in people over age 65. The incidence of cancer increases with advancing age, probably as a result of the accumulated exposure to carcinogens and to age-related declines in the action of the immune system. The most commonly seen cancers in older women are colorectal, breast, lung, pancreatic, and ovarian. In older men, lung, colorectal, prostate, pancreatic, and gastric cancers occur most frequently.

The importance of screening and early detection of cancer does not diminish with age. Unfortunately, older adults may be less likely to undergo cancer screening or seek treatment for cancer due to fear, depression, cognitive impairments, poor access to health care, or financial constraints. Some older adults (and healthcare providers) mistake cancer symptoms for normal age-related changes. Believing that little can be done, they do not seek health care for their symptoms. Fear of the cancer diagnosis also keeps older adults from seeking appropriate health care. When they do seek treatment, chronic conditions frequently seen in older adults may make the diagnosis of cancer more difficult by masking or confounding the usual symptoms associated with cancer.

Older adults are at greater risk for side effects associated with cancer treatment because of age-related physiologic changes and chronic conditions associated with aging. This is particularly true for the side effects of chemotherapeutic agents. The incidence of toxic effects on the heart and central nervous system is increased. The side effects of chemotherapy can contribute to fatigue and cause problems related to immobility and functional decline. Alterations in the function of the immune system are also more frequent in older adults, which increases their risk for developing infection.

The problems associated with chemotherapy do not rule out its use, but the nurse must be aware of potential problems and monitor the client closely for the development of side effects. The nurse needs to consider the effect of aging on responses to the disease and its treatment.

Health Education for the Client and Family
- Discuss the warning signs of cancer.
- Stress the importance of seeking health care if any of the warning signs develop.
- Get an annual physical examination.
- For women, learn how to perform a monthly breast self-exam (BSE) and emphasize the importance of continuing BSE and regular mammography after menopause.
- Teach men the early signs of prostate cancer, and encourage them to have an annual digital rectal exam.

---

fied as those who tend to others' needs to the exclusion of their own and who rarely ask for help or support, even in personal crises. These people tend to be emotionally, and sometimes even physically, isolated and have a great deal of buried, unexpressed anger. It is thought that this kind of behavior pattern harms the immune system over time, promoting vulnerability to cancer. Depression is also considered a major risk factor, especially depression that is chronic or related to multiple or major losses. It is thought that depression and hopelessness tend to shut down the energizing chemicals in the body and depress immune responses (Kaye et al., 2000).

Diet
Some foods are considered genotoxic, such as the nitrosamines and nitrous indoles found in preserved meats and pickled, salted foods. Other foods, such as high-fat, low-fiber foods—the mainstay of many American diets—promote colon, breast, and sex hormone–dependent tumors. When fish and meat are excessively fried or broiled, potent carcinogenic compounds can form that may cause tumors in the mammary glands, colon, liver, pancreas, and bladder. Also, repeatedly using fat to fry foods at high temperatures produces high levels of polycyclic hydrocarbons, which increase cancer risk considerably. Although many people profess to have changed their dietary habits, one only has to observe the large number of people who still lunch on cheeseburgers and french fries (and who teach their children to do the same) to realize that much more educational and motivational work is needed in this area. Other food-related substances believed to increase cancer risk include sodium saccharine, red food dyes, and both regular and decaffeinated coffee.

Occupation
Occupational risk might be considered to be either controllable or uncontrollable. For many people, both education and ability limit their choice of occupation; during times of high unemployment, moreover, changing one's occupation because it poses risk factors may not be a viable option. Federal standards are designed to protect workers from hazardous substances, but many believe that these standards are not strict enough and that inspections are not frequent enough to prevent violations.

Specific risks vary according to the occupation. For example, outdoor workers such as farmers and construction workers are exposed to solar radiation; healthcare workers such as x-ray technicians and biomedical researchers are exposed to ionizing radiation and carcinogenic substances; and exposure to asbestos is a problem for people who work in old buildings with asbestos insulation in the walls. Table 14–1 correlates known carcinogens and occupations.

Infection
Because a number of viruses have been linked to some cancers, avoiding those specific infections will decrease risk. Although some infections may be unavoidable (Epstein-Barr, for example), others, such as genital herpes and papillomavirus-induced genital warts, can often be avoided by following safer sex practices (e.g., the use of condoms).

Tobacco Use
Lung cancer is considered highly preventable because of its relationship to smoking. The genotoxic carcinogenic substances in tobacco are considered weak; therefore, stopping smoking

TABLE 14–1 Chemical Carcinogens and Relationship to Occupation

CHEMICAL AGENT	ACTION	OCCUPATION AFFECTED
Polycyclic hydrocarbons (smoke, soot, tobacco, smoked foods) Benzopyrene	Genotoxic	Miners, coal/gas workers, chimney sweeps, migrant workers, workers in offices where smoking is allowed in closed areas
Arsenic	Genotoxic	Pesticide manufacturers, mining
Vinyl chloride polymers	Promotional	Plastics workers
		Artists
Methylaminobenzine	Genotoxic	Fabric workers
		Rubber and glue workers
Asbestos	Promotional	Construction workers, workers in old, run-down buildings with asbestos insulation, insulation makers
Wood and leather dust	Promotional	Woodworkers, carpenters, leather toolers
Chemotherapy drugs	Genotoxic	Drug manufacturers, pharmacists, nurses

can reverse the damage it causes. However, many other substances in tobacco are highly promotional, so that the larger the dose and longer the use, the higher the risk for developing cancer. Research has shown a significantly lower lung cancer death risk for former smokers compared to current smokers. Smokers who quit before middle age avoid more than 90% of the risk of lung cancer that can be attributed to tobacco (Peto et al., 2000).

Tobacco is also related to other forms of cancer. Smokers face an increased risk for oropharyngeal, esophageal, laryngeal, gastric, pancreatic, and bladder cancers. Pipe and cigar smokers are especially susceptible to oropharyngeal and laryngeal cancers. Oral and esophageal cancers are more common among those who chew tobacco or use snuff. Smokers who have a genetic decrease in alpha-$_1$-antitrypsin (an enzyme that protects lung tissue) that results in emphysema face an even higher cancer risk than smokers without this defect.

Additional research has documented the deleterious effects of secondhand tobacco smoke (Dietrich et al., 2002). Tobacco-specific nitrosamines were recovered in the urine of children living with smokers. It is now accepted that nonsmokers exposed to tobacco smoke over long periods of time, whether in the workplace or the home, have an increased risk for lung or bladder cancers.

Alcohol Use

Alcohol promotes cancer by enhancing the contact between carcinogens such as those in tobacco and the stem cells that line the oral cavity, larynx, and esophagus (Porth, 2005). People who both smoke and drink a considerable amount of alcohol daily have an increased risk for oral, esophageal, and laryngeal cancers.

Recreational Drug Use

Recreational drug use often promotes an unhealthy lifestyle that increases general cancer risk; for example, drug users often do not maintain adequate nutrition. Furthermore, recreational drugs are implicated as promoters because of their suppressive effect on the immune system. Although it has not been directly implicated in cancer development, marijuana has been demonstrated to cause chromosomal damage that may over time also result in cancer-causing DNA damage and ge-

netic mutations (Khalsa et al., 2002). Marijuana smoke is also much more injurious to lung tissue than tobacco smoke (Khalsa et al., 2002).

Obesity

Excessive body fat has been linked to an increased risk of hormone-dependent cancers. Because sex hormones are synthesized from fat, obese people often have excessive amounts of the hormones that feed hormone-dependent malignancies of the breast, bowel, ovary, endometrium, and prostate.

Sun Exposure

As the protective ozone layer thins, more of the sun's damaging ultraviolet radiation reaches the earth. As a consequence, the rate of skin cancers has increased. Sun-related skin cancers are now considered to be a problem for all people, regardless of skin color, but people of Northern European extraction with very fair skin, blue or green eyes, and light-colored hair are most vulnerable. Elderly people with decreased pigment are also more at risk, even those with darker skin.

Figure 14–1 ■ summarizes the interaction of factors that promote cancer.

PATHOPHYSIOLOGY

Cancer is a complex disease with hundreds of agents that can contribute to its pathogenesis. Advances in research have greatly increased the understanding of how cancer develops. It is now known that the development of cancer is a process in which normal cells are changed and acquire malignant properties. Before a discussion of the various theories of the causes of cancer, it is useful to review how normal cells divide and adapt to changing conditions.

Normal Cell Growth

Mature normal cells are uniform in size and have nuclei that are characteristic of the tissue to which the cells belong. Within the nucleus of normal cells, chromosomes containing deoxyribonucleic acid (DNA) molecules carry the genetic information that controls the synthesis of polypeptides (proteins). Genes are

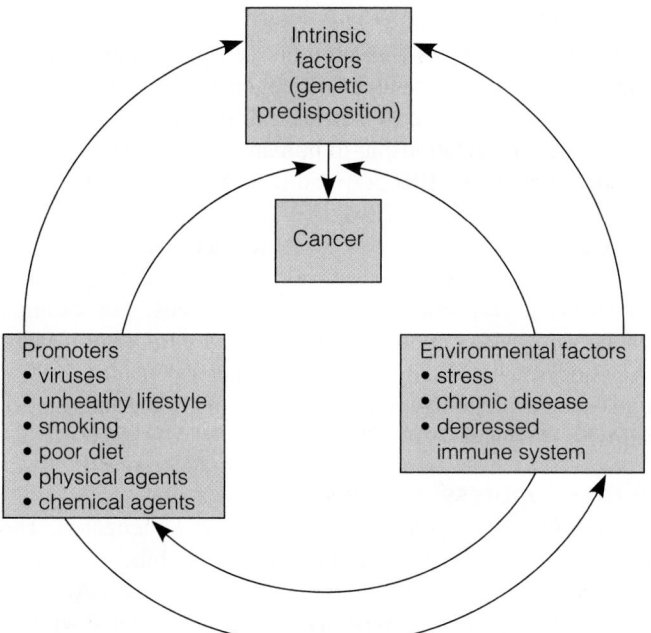

Figure 14–1 ■ Interaction of factors that promote cancer. Most people have immune systems that are competent enough to resist the establishment of cancer from an initiated cell. Cancer takes hold when a number of promotional factors occur together and over enough time to weaken immune resistance. Like factors are grouped together for ease of presentation but may occur in any combination.

subunits of chromosomes and consist of portions of DNA that specify the production of particular sets of proteins. Thus, genes control the development of specific traits. The genetic code in the DNA of every gene is translated into protein structures that determine the type, maturity, and function of a cell. Any change or disruption in a gene can result in an inaccurate "blueprint" that can produce an aberrant cell, which may then become cancerous. Box 14–1 lists some of the functions of DNA.

The Cell Cycle

Two coordinated events are responsible for cellular reproduction. Reproduction occurs as the result of replication of cellular DNA and mitosis, when the cell divides into two daughter cells with identical DNA.

The **cell cycle** consists of four phases. In the gap 1 or G_1 phase, the cell enlarges and synthesizes proteins to prepare for DNA replication. During this phase the cell prepares to replicate and enter into the synthesis phase. During the synthesis (S)

BOX 14–1 Functions of DNA

- Orders production of enzymes.
- Instructs cells to produce specific chemicals.
- Instructs cells to develop specific structures.
- Determines individual traits and characteristics.
- Controls other DNA by telling a cell to "switch on" and use some portion of the genetic information stored in it.

---

phase, DNA is replicated and the chromosomes in the cell are duplicated. During the next phase, gap 2 (G_2), the cell prepares itself for mitosis. Finally, with all preparation complete, the cell begins mitosis (M). This phase culminates in the division of the parent cell into two exact copies called daughter cells, each having identical genetic material. The cells then immediately enter G_1 where they begin the cell cycle again, or divert into a resting phase called G_0. The cell cycle is controlled by cyclins, which combine with and activate enzymes called cyclin-dependent kinases. Some cyclins cause a "braking" action and prevent the cycle from proceeding (Dunlop & Campbell, 2000). Checkpoints in the cell cycle ensure that it proceeds in the correct order.

A malfunction of any of these regulators of cell growth and division can result in the rapid proliferation of immature cells. In some cases, these cells are considered cancerous (malignant). Knowledge of cell cycle events is used in the development of chemotherapeutic drugs, which are designed to disrupt the cancer cells during different stages of their cell cycle. These drugs and their use are discussed later in the chapter.

Differentiation

Differentiation is a normal process occurring over many cell cycles that allows cells to specialize in certain tasks. For example, some epithelial cells lining the lungs develop into tall columnar cells with cilia. These columnar cells sweep potentially dangerous debris out of the lungs. When adverse conditions occur in body tissues during differentiation, protective adaptations can produce alterations in cells. Some of these alterations are helpful, but in other cases the cells mutate beyond usefulness and become liabilities (Porth, 2005). Following are potentially unproductive cellular alterations that occur during cell differentiation:

- **Hyperplasia** is an increase in the number or density of normal cells. Hyperplasia occurs in response to stress, increased metabolic demands, or elevated levels of hormones. Examples include the hyperplasia of myocardial cells in response to a prolonged increase in the body's demand for oxygen, and hyperplasia of uterine cells in response to rising levels of estrogen during pregnancy. Hyperplastic cells are under normal DNA control.

- **Metaplasia** is a change in the normal pattern of differentiation such that dividing cells differentiate into cell types not normally found in that location in the body. The metaplastic cell is normal for its particular type, but it is not in its normal location. Some metaplastic cells are less functional than the cells they replace. Metaplasia is a protective response to adverse conditions. Metaplastic cells are under normal DNA control and are reversible when the stressor or other disruptive condition ceases.

- **Dysplasia** represents a loss of DNA control over differentiation occurring in response to adverse conditions. Dysplastic cells show abnormal variation in size, shape, and appearance and a disturbance in their usual arrangement. Examples of dysplasia include changes in the cervix in response to continued irritation, such as from the human papillomavirus, or leukoplakia on oral mucous membranes in response to chronic irritation from smoking.

■ **Anaplasia** is the regression of a cell to an immature or undifferentiated cell type. Anaplastic cell division is no longer under DNA control. Anaplasia usually occurs when a damaging or transforming event takes place inside the dividing, still undifferentiated cell, leading to loss of useful function. Anaplasia may occur in response to overwhelmingly destructive conditions inside the cell or in surrounding tissue (Porth, 2005).

Although hyperplasia, metaplasia, and dysplasia often reverse after the irritating factor is eliminated, they can lead to malignancy under certain conditions. This is especially true of dysplasia, which represents a loss of DNA control. Anaplasia is not reversible, but the degree of anaplasia determines the potential risk for cancer.

ETIOLOGY

Intensive research efforts during the past several decades have led to an increased understanding of how cancer develops. The Human Genome Project, begun in 1990, has provided critical information about the development of cancer. Continuing research will provide information that will be key in the detection and prevention of cancer.

Cancer research has brought new options for cancer treatment and improved clients' overall survival rate. Almost daily, people hear of research studies indicating that certain foods, habits, or environmental factors may cause cancer. Although much of this is true and is inspiring a welcome preventive focus to health care, it is not true that one can determine the specific factors that cause cancer in any individual. Although taking responsibility for one's own health is a positive step, the emphasis on prevention may have a negative result if clients feel so guilty and blameworthy that they fail to seek out early and appropriate health care. Also, clients who feel that their bodies have failed them may become depressed, and such feelings can impair the functioning of an already stressed immune system.

Factors that cause cancer are both external (chemicals, radiation, and viruses) and internal (hormones, immune conditions, and inherited mutations). Causal factors may act together or in sequence to initiate or promote **carcinogenesis**. Ten or more years often pass between exposures or mutations and detectable cancer.

Theories of Carcinogenesis

Cellular Mutation

The theory of cellular mutation suggests that carcinogens cause mutations in cellular DNA. It is believed that the carcinogenic process has three stages: initiation, promotion, and progression. The initiation stage involves permanent damage in the cellular DNA as a result of exposure to a carcinogen (e.g., radiation, chemicals) that was not repaired or had a defective repair. Promotion may last for years and includes conditions, such as smoking or alcohol use, that act repeatedly on the already affected cells. In the progression stage further inherited changes acquired during the cell replication develop into a cancer.

Oncogenes

Oncogenes are genes that promote cell proliferation and are capable of triggering cancerous characteristics. Oncogenes can be classified according to their overall function. Several oncogenes and their relationship to human cancers have been identified. For example, BRCA-1 and BRCA-2 are associated with breast cancer (Surbone, 2001).

A decrease in the body's immune surveillance may allow the expression of oncogenes; this can occur during times of stress or in response to certain carcinogens. For example, clients with AIDS, who have a decreased number of T-helper lymphocytes, have a much higher than normal incidence of certain cancers, including non-Hodgkin's lymphoma and Kaposi's sarcoma (Donahue et al., 2000).

Tumor Suppressor Genes

Tumor suppressor genes normally suppress oncogenes. They can become inactive by deletion or mutation. Inherited cancers have been associated with tumor suppressor genes. An example is p53, a suppressor gene that has been associated with sarcoma and cancer of the breast and brain.

Central to these theories are two important concepts about the etiology of cancer. First, damaged DNA, whether inherited or from external sources, sets up the necessary initial step for cancer to occur. Second, impairment of the human immune system, from whatever cause, lessens its ability to destroy abnormal cells.

Known Carcinogens

A number of agents are known to cause cancer, or at least are strongly linked to certain kinds of cancers. These known carcinogens include viruses, drugs, hormones, and chemical and physical agents.

Carcinogens can be categorized in two groups: Genotoxic carcinogens directly alter DNA and cause mutations, and promoter substances cause other adverse biologic effects, such as cytotoxicity, hormonal imbalances, altered immunity, or chronic tissue damage. Promoter substances do not cause cancer in the absence of previous cell damage (initiation) and often require high-level and long-term contact with the altered cells (see Table 14–1).

Note also that although everyone comes into contact with a vast number of substances that are considered carcinogenic, not everyone develops cancer. Other factors, such as genetic predisposition, impairment of the immune response, and repeated exposure to the carcinogen, are necessary for a cancer to develop.

Viruses

Several viruses have been associated with the development of cancer. They damage cells and induce hyperplastic cell growth. Viral infection may play a role in cell mutation that can progress to malignant cells. Most people are able to suppress this progression (Spitalnick & diSant'Angnese, 2001). Box 14–2 identifies these viruses and the cancers with which they are associated.

In addition, viruses play a significant role in weakening immunologic defenses against neoplasms. For example, human

---

BOX 14–2 Cancers Associated with Different Viruses

Herpes Simplex Virus Types I and II (HSV-1 and HSV-2)
- Carcinoma of the lip
- Cervical carcinoma
- Kaposi's sarcoma

Human Cytomegalovirus (HCMV)
- Kaposi's sarcoma
- Prostate cancer

Epstein-Barr Virus (EBV)
- Burkitt's lymphoma

Human Herpesvirus-6 (HHV-6)
- Lymphoma

Hepatitis B Virus (HBV)
- Primary hepatocellular cancer

Papillomavirus
- Malignant melanoma
- Cervical, penile, and laryngeal cancers

Human T-Lymphotropic Viruses (HTLV)
- Adult T-cell leukemia and lymphoma
- T-cell variant of hairy-cell leukemia
- Kaposi's sarcoma

---

immunodeficiency virus (HIV), which infects T-helper lymphocytes and monocytes, impairs the person's protection against certain cancers such as lymphoma and Kaposi's sarcoma.

Other viruses have also been associated with human malignancies. Hepatitis B virus integrates its DNA with liver cell DNA and is believed to cause primary hepatocellular carcinoma. Papillomaviruses cause plantar, common, and flat warts, which are benign and usually regress spontaneously; however, they also cause genital warts and laryngeal papillomas, which are associated with malignant melanoma and cervical, penile, and laryngeal cancers. Retroviruses have been found to cause cancer in animals. Adult T-cell leukemia is the only human cancer known to be associated with a retrovirus (Hill, 2001).

Vaccines to prevent virus-induced cancers are being investigated. Preliminary results of the use of vaccines to treat malignancies, such as melanoma, have been encouraging (Berd, 2001).

Drugs and Hormones
Certain drugs can be either genotoxic or promotional. For example, chemotherapeutic drugs used to disrupt the cell cycle of malignant cells can be genotoxic for normal cells. They can also be promotional: By drastically reducing the number of leukocytes, they impair immune function. Examples of these chemotherapeutic drugs include busulfan, chlorambucil, and cyclophosphamide. Some recreational drugs also are implicated as carcinogens. These include the genotoxic betel nut chewed by many Pacific Islanders and the immunosuppressant promoters heroin and cocaine.

Hormones are also potential genotoxic carcinogens or promoters. Gonadotropic hormones often mediate cancers of the reproductive organs. Estrogen, both natural and synthetic, and diethylstilbestrol (DES) have been linked to cervical, endometrial, and breast cancers. Estrogen-containing contraceptive pills have been implicated in breast cancer, but they also have been shown to decrease the risk of ovarian cancer. Investigators have not reached a final conclusion about the cancer risk posed by contraceptives. Newer research suggests that alterations in the molecular structure of testosterone in older men may promote the development of prostate cancer. Also, glucocorticosteroids (cortisone) and anabolic steroids may act as promoters by altering the immune response or endocrine balance (Chapman & Goodman, 2000; Held-Warmkessel, 2000; Rubin et al., 2001).

Chemical Agents
Many chemicals have been demonstrated to be both genotoxic and promotional. Because many of these substances are encountered in the workplace, they constitute occupational hazards, which will be discussed more thoroughly. Examples of industrial and environmental carcinogens include polycyclic hydrocarbons, found in soot; benzopyrene, found in cigarette smoke; and arsenic, found in pesticides. These chemicals have some genotoxic action; some alter DNA replication. Other industrial and environmental chemicals are considered promotional agents. These include wood and leather dust, polymer esters (used in plastics and paints), carbon tetrachloride, asbestos, and phenol.

Natural substances in the body may also be carcinogenic or promotional. For example, end products of metabolism that are produced in excess amounts or are ineffectively eliminated, such as bile acids from a high-fat diet, may promote cancer.

Some foods contain carcinogens added during preparation or preservation. Examples include the sugar substitute sodium saccharine and nitrosamines and nitrous indoles, which are found in pickled, salted foods. In some cases, food contaminants produce carcinogenic chemicals. The *Aspergillus* fungi produce aflatoxin, a highly potent carcinogen. These organisms grow on improperly stored vegetable products, such as grains and peanuts.

Polycyclic aromatic hydrocarbons, nitrosamines, phenols, and other chemicals in tobacco act as either carcinogens or promoters of cancer (see Table 14–1).

Physical Agents
It has been well documented that excessive exposure to radiation causes increased rates of cancer by damaging the DNA in cells, by activating other oncogenetic factors, or by suppressing antitumor activity (protein inhibitors). Both solar radiation from ultraviolet rays and ionizing radiation from industrial or medical sources are carcinogenic. This fact has implications for workers exposed to these agents and for the population in general. Radon, a naturally formed radioactive gas found in the basements of many homes, is also a known carcinogen. People who have lived in areas where nuclear weapons have been tested or whose groundwater has been polluted by nuclear wastes are at risk for developing cancers. The effects of high-dose radiation exposure

and subsequent cancer development have been demonstrated in the survivors of the atomic bombs at Nagasaki and Hiroshima and in workers exposed to radiation during the cleanup of nuclear disasters such as Chernobyl.

Types of Neoplasms

A **neoplasm** is a mass of new tissue (a collection of cells) that grows independently of its surrounding structures and has no physiologic purpose. The term *neoplasm* is often used interchangeably with *tumor*, from the Latin word meaning "swelling." Neoplasms are said to be autonomous because of the following:

- They grow at a rate uncoordinated with the needs of the body.
- They share some of the properties of the parent cells but with altered size and shape.
- They do not benefit the host and in some cases are actively harmful.

Neoplasms are not completely autonomous, however, because they require a blood supply with nutrients and oxygen to sustain their growth. Neoplasms typically are classified as benign or malignant on the basis of their potential to damage the body and on their growth characteristics.

Benign Neoplasms

Benign neoplasms are localized growths. They form a solid mass, have well-defined borders, and frequently are encapsulated. Benign neoplasms tend to respond to the body's homeostatic controls. Thus, they often stop growing when they reach the boundaries of another tissue (a process called *contact inhibition*). They grow slowly and often remain stable in size. Because they are usually encapsulated, benign neoplasms often are easily removed and tend not to recur.

Although typically harmless, benign neoplasms nevertheless can be destructive if they crowd surrounding tissue and obstruct the function of organs. For example, a benign meningioma (from the meninges of the brain and spinal cord) can cause severely increased intracranial pressure (ICP), which progressively impairs the person's cerebral function. Unless the meningioma can be successfully removed, the steadily rising ICP will eventually lead to coma and death.

Malignant Neoplasms

In contrast to benign neoplasms, malignant neoplasms grow aggressively and do not respond to the body's homeostatic controls. Malignant neoplasms are not cohesive, and present with an irregular shape. Instead of slowly crowding other tissues aside, malignant neoplasms cut through surrounding tissues, causing bleeding, inflammation, and necrosis (tissue death) as they grow. This invasive quality of malignant neoplasms is reflected in the word origin of *cancer*, from the Greek *karkinos*, meaning "crab." Healthcare professionals are referring to a malignant neoplasm when they use the term *cancer*.

Malignant cells from the primary tumor may travel through the blood or lymph to invade other tissues and organs of the body and form a secondary tumor called a *metastasis*. This term also refers to the process by which such spreading of malignant neoplasms—perhaps their most destructive trait—occurs. Malignant neoplasms can recur after surgical removal

of the primary and secondary tumors and after other treatments. Table 14–2 compares benign and malignant neoplasms.

Malignant neoplasms vary in their degree of differentiation from the parent tissue. Highly differentiated cancer cells try to mimic the specialized function of the parent tissue, but undifferentiated cancers, consisting of immature cells, have almost no resemblance to the parent tissue and so perform no useful function. To make matters worse, undifferentiated cancers rob the body of its energy and nutrition as they grow. Undifferentiated anaplastic cells have little structural or functional relationship to the parent cells and are the basis of many malignant neoplasms. The degree of differentiation of anaplastic cells is a consideration in the classification and staging of neoplasms, discussed later in this chapter.

Characteristics of Malignant Cells

Malignant neoplasms may be identified by the following predictable cellular characteristics:

- *Loss of regulation of the rate of mitosis.* This results in rapid cell division and growth of the neoplasm.
- *Loss of specialization and differentiation.* Malignant cells do not perform typical cellular functions. Many produce hormones and enzymes similar to those of the parent tissue, but usually in excessive amounts, possibly revealing their presence.
- *Loss of contact inhibition.* Malignant cells do not respect other cellular boundaries. They easily invade and destroy other tissues.
- *Progressive acquisition of a cancerous phenotype.* Cellular mutation seems to be a sequential process involving successive generations of cells, each generation becoming more deviant than the previous one. Additionally, malignant cells seem to be "immortal"; that is, they do not stop growing and die, as do normal cells, which have a genetically determined life span.
- *Irreversibility.* The transformation into a malignant cell is irreversible. Rarely does a malignant neoplasm revert to a benign state.
- *Altered cell structure.* Cytologic examination of malignant cells reveals distinct differences in the cell nucleus and cyto-

TABLE 14–2 Comparison of Benign and Malignant Neoplasms

BENIGN	MALIGNANT
Local	Invasive
Cohesive	Noncohesive
Well-defined borders	Does not stop at tissue border
Pushes other tissues out of the way	Invades and destroys surrounding tissues
Slow growth	Rapid growth
Encapsulated	Metastasizes to distant sites
Easily removed	Not always easy to remove
Does not recur	Can recur

plasm as well as an overall cell shape that differs from that of normal cells of the particular tissue type.

- *Simplified metabolic activities.* The work of malignant cells is simpler than that of normal cells; they show an increased synthesis of substances needed for cell division, and they have no need to create proteins for the specialized functions of the tissues they invade.
- *Transplantability.* Malignant cells often break away from the primary tissue site and travel to other locations in the body, where they establish new growths.
- *Ability to promote their own survival.* Malignant cells may create ectopic sites to produce the hormones they need for their growth. By their very presence and their ability to initiate vascular permeability, malignant cells promote the development of nonneoplastic stroma, a connective tissue framework consisting of collagen and other components, which then supports the neoplasm. They may also create their own blood supply. Through a process called angiogenesis, tumor cells secrete a polypeptide angiogenic growth factor that stimulates blood vessels from surrounding normal tissue to grow into the tumor. Finally, malignant cells divert nutrition from the host to meet their own needs, by diffusion when the tumor is less than 1 mm and thereafter by means of the newly formed blood vessels. If unchecked, malignant cells eventually destroy their host.

The characteristics of malignant cells are summarized in Box 14–3.

Tumor Invasion and Metastasis

The ability of cancer cells to invade adjacent tissues and travel to distant organs is considered their most ominous characteristic. This quality makes treatment a considerable challenge (Hawkins, 2001).

BOX 14–3 **Characteristics of Malignant Cells**

- Loss of regulation of mitotic rate
- Loss of cell specialization
- Loss of contact inhibition
- Progressive acquisition of the cancerous phenotype and immortality
- Irreversibility of cancerous phenotype to greater aggressiveness
- Altered cell structure: differences in cell nucleus and cytoplasm
- Simplified metabolic activity
- Transplantability (metastasis)
- Ability to promote own survival

Invasion

Aggressive tumors possess several qualities that facilitate invasion (Figure 14–2 ■):

- *Ability to cause pressure atrophy.* The pressure of a growing tumor can cause atrophy and necrosis of adjacent tissues. The malignancy then moves into the vacated space.
- *Ability to disrupt the basement membrane of normal cells.* Many cancer cells can bind to elements of the basement membrane and secrete enzymes that degrade that physical barrier, thus facilitating their movement into normal tissues, lymph, and blood circulation.
- *Motility.* Because malignant cells are less tightly bound to each other than normal cells (reduced adhesiveness), they easily separate from the neoplasm and move into surrounding body fluids and tissues.

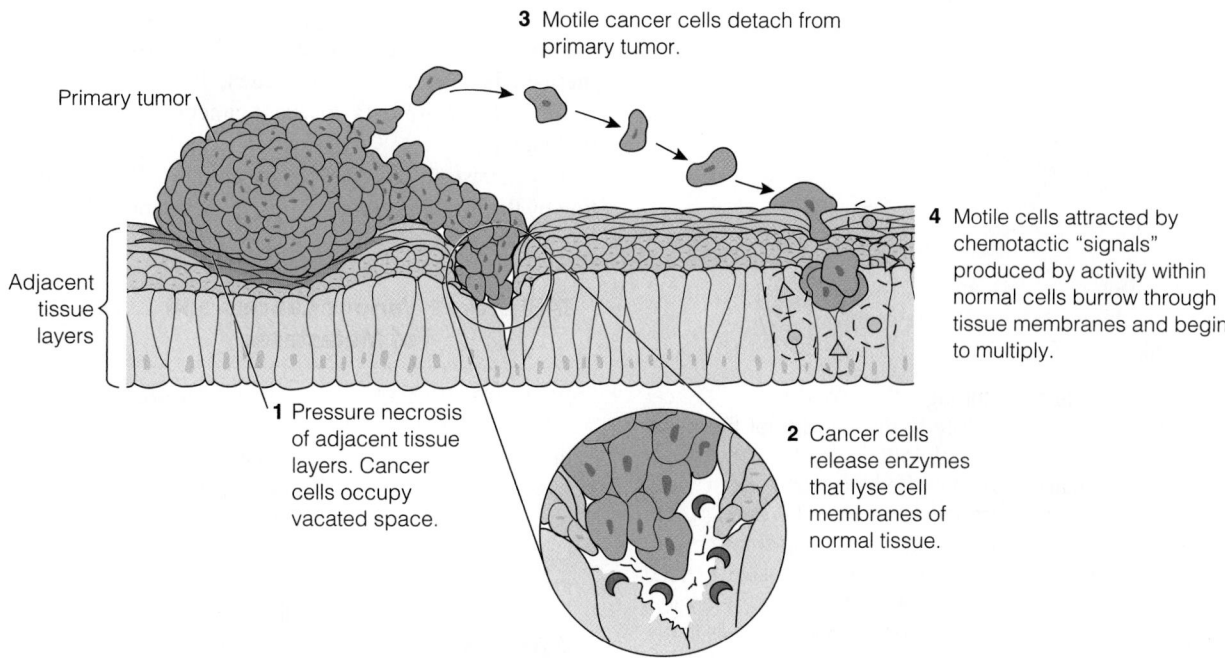

3 Motile cancer cells detach from primary tumor.

Primary tumor

4 Motile cells attracted by chemotactic "signals" produced by activity within normal cells burrow through tissue membranes and begin to multiply.

Adjacent tissue layers

1 Pressure necrosis of adjacent tissue layers. Cancer cells occupy vacated space.

2 Cancer cells release enzymes that lyse cell membranes of normal tissue.

Figure 14–2 ■ How cancer cells invade normal tissue.

- *Response to chemical signals from adjacent tissues.* Chemotaxis (the movement of cells in response to a chemical stimulus) calls the tumor cells into the normal tissues, possibly as a result of the degrading of the basement membranes of the normal cells. This breakdown of normal cellular membranes releases the chemical stimulus physiologically designed to draw normal phagocytic cells to clean up the debris. (See Chapter 12 ∞ on the inflammatory response for more information on chemotaxis.) Malignant cells are also known to respond chemotactically to the end product of cellular metabolism. Some cancer cells even produce a substance called autocrine motility factor, which calls other malignant cells to a normal tissue. The first invading cells produce this substance, which then actively draws other malignant cells from the primary tumor into the invaded normal tissue.

Metastasis

The factors that favor invasion also contribute to the process of metastasis. **Metastasis** can occur by means of one or more mechanisms including embolism in the blood or lymph or spread by way of body cavities.

A blood- or lymph-borne metastasis allows a new tumor to be established in a distant organ. Figure 14–3 ■ shows metastasis through the bloodstream. A tumor's ability to metastasize in this manner requires the following steps:

1. Intravasation of malignant cells through blood or lymphatic vessel walls and into the circulation

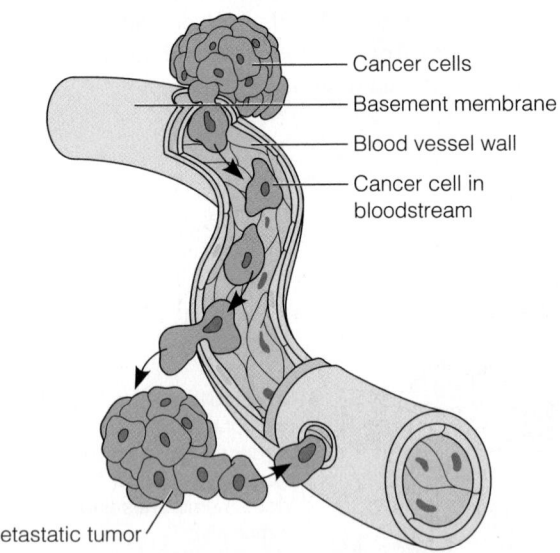

Metastatic tumor

Figure 14–3 ■ Metastasis through the bloodstream. Cancer cells secrete enzymes and a motility factor that disrupt the basement membrane in the blood vessel. In this way, the cancer cells gain access to the circulation. Once in the blood, only about 1 cell in 1000 escapes immune detection, but that can be enough. Undetected cells move out of the blood, again secreting enzymes and cutting through the vessel wall into new tissue. The tissue selected for establishing a new tumor may be downstream from the original tumor, or a chemical attraction may cause the malignant cells to target a specific site. Once in the new site, the malignant cells multiply and establish a metastatic tumor.

Cancer cells
Basement membrane
Blood vessel wall
Cancer cell in bloodstream

2. Survival of the malignant cells in the blood (To survive, the cells must escape the notice of the body's immune surveillance; only about 1 in 1000 cells does so.)
3. Extravasation from the circulation and implantation in a new tissue.

The tumor cells tend to clump together, forming an embolus, and continue growing until their size prevents further travel in the vessel or lymph channel. The growing neoplastic mass then uses its invasive abilities (secreting enzymes and motility factor) to move into the nearest organ.

About 60% of metastatic lesions tend to occur in a schema reflecting the pattern of blood or lymph circulation. However, it has been demonstrated that some malignant cells defy a bloodborne pattern and actually target specific organs to which they prefer to metastasize. For example, lung cancer frequently metastasizes to the adrenal glands, and breast cancer frequently metastasizes to bone.

Malignant cells that gain access to the lymph channels may travel to a preferred organ and then move into it the same way they emigrate through blood vessels. Alternatively, the malignant cells may become trapped in the lymph node and continue to grow. Eventually, the malignant cells replace the node's tissues. At this point, emboli from the cancerous node disseminate to other nodes, creating a cascade reaction. The malignant cascade causes widespread transfer of the tumor to uncharacteristic sites.

A malignant tumor may break through the walls of the organ in which it is primarily housed, shedding cells into the nearby body cavity. The cells then are free to establish new tumors in a distant area of that cavity. For example, malignant cells from a colon cancer may be seeded into the peritoneal cavity, establishing a new tumor in the mesenteric epithelium.

Metastatic lesions are differentiated from primary neoplasms by cell morphology: Metastatic cells do not resemble the tissue in which they reside. The most common sites of metastasis are the lymph nodes, liver, lungs, bones, and brain. Table 14–3 lists different cancers and common sites of metastasis.

For metastasis to occur, the cancerous cells must avoid detection by the immune system. Thus, impairment of the immune sys-

TABLE 14–3 Various Cancers and Sites of Metastases

PRIMARY TUMOR	COMMON METASTATIC SITES
Bronchogenic (lung)	Spinal cord, brain, liver, bone
Breast	Regional lymph nodes, vertebrae, brain, liver, lung, bone
Colon	Liver, lung, brain, ovary, bone
Prostate	Bladder, bone (especially vertebrae), liver
Malignant melanoma	Lung, liver, spleen, regional lymph nodes, brain

tem is a major factor in the establishment of metastatic lesions. Cells may escape detection in several different ways:

- Aggressive cancer cells may compile a large mass (greater than 1 cm) so rapidly that the immune system is unable to overcome the tumor before it takes hold in a new tissue.
- For tumor cells to be recognized as foreign by the immune system, they must display on their surface a special antigen called tumor-associated antigen (TAA). TAA marks tumor cells for destruction by the lymphocytes. Some oncogenic viruses depress the expression of TAA on infected cells. Also, some tumors in advanced stages of growth no longer display TAA. Thus, such tumor cells escape detection as they travel through the blood or lymph.
- If the person's immune response is weakened or altered, then a metastatic tumor may take hold with little opposition. Factors that may weaken or alter the immune response are listed in Box 14–4.

An estimated 50% to 60% of all cancers have already metastasized by the time the primary tumor is identified. This may account for the current 50% death rate and certainly supports the need for client education to facilitate early diagnosis. The time it takes for metastasis to occur is extremely variable and often difficult to predict. Some cancers, such as basal cell carcinomas, do not metastasize. The aggressiveness and location of the tumor, and the state of the person's immune system, determine whether and how rapidly metastasis takes place.

PHYSIOLOGIC AND PSYCHOLOGIC EFFECTS OF CANCER

Much of the nursing care for clients with cancer is related to the generalized effects of cancer on the body and the side effects of the treatments used to remove or destroy the cancer. Although pathophysiologic effects of the cancer vary with the type and location of the cancer, the following effects usually are observed.

Disruption of Function

Physiologic functioning can be upset by obstruction or pressure. For example, a large tumor in the bowel can stop intestinal motility, resulting in a bowel obstruction. Prostatic tumors can obstruct the bladder neck or urethra, resulting in urine retention. Intracranial pressure can be dangerously increased by a glioma.

Obstruction or pressure can cause anoxia and necrosis of surrounding tissues, which in turn cause a loss of function of the involved organ or tissue. For example, a kidney tumor may

---

BOX 14–4 **Factors That May Weaken or Alter the Immune Response**

- Accumulated stress
- Depression
- Increased age
- Pregnancy
- Chronic disease
- Chemotherapy treatment for the primary cancer

---

progress to renal failure. Pressure against the superior vena cava from an adjacent lung tumor or tumor-infiltrated lymph nodes can interrupt the blood flow to the heart.

In the liver, either a primary hepatocellular cancer or metastatic lesion can have several significant effects:

- In liver parenchymal tissue, it impairs the multiple life-sustaining functions of the liver, such as carbohydrate metabolism, synthesis of plasma proteins, detoxification, and immunologic functions. These functional impairments result in severe nutritional, hormonal, hematologic, and immunologic problems. (See Chapter 21 ∞ for a more complete discussion of liver functions and effects of disruption.)
- Because more than 1 L of blood per minute passes through the liver via the portal vein, obstruction to this flow by a tumor can cause portal hypertension. This results in backup of fluid and increased pressure in the splanchnic circulation. The end result is ascites (third-spaced fluid in the peritoneal cavity) and varices (friable, overdistended blood vessels) of the esophageal, gastric, mesenteric, and hemorrhoidal vessels.

Hematologic Alterations

Hematologic alterations can impair the normal function of blood cells. For example, in leukemia, a malignant proliferative disease of the hematopoietic (blood cell–producing) system, the immature leukocytes cannot perform the normal protective phagocytic functions and immunity is compromised. Additionally, the excessive numbers of immature leukocytes in the bone marrow diminish erythrocyte and thrombocyte (platelet) production, resulting in secondary anemia and clotting disorders (Scigliano et al., 2001).

Other examples of hematologic alteration include the following:

- Gastrointestinal tumors disrupt the absorption of vitamin B_{12} and iron.
- Growing tumors need purines and folate and have a unique ability to accumulate and store these substances. Thus, the tumor deprives the bone marrow of these substances, which are needed for erythropoiesis (red blood cell production).
- Renal cell carcinoma produces its own erythropoietin hormone, which causes an excessively large number of red blood cells to be produced and dumped into the bloodstream. The resulting polycythemia causes viscous blood, which impairs circulation, plugs small capillaries, and promotes thrombus formation.

Infection

If the tumor invades and connects two incompatible organs, such as the bowel and bladder, and thus creates a fistula, infection becomes a serious problem. As they destroy viable tissue and thus their source of nutrition, tumors may become necrotic and septicemia may result. Some tumors are less efficient in creating capillaries; as a consequence, the center of the tumor may become necrotic and infected. When a tumor grows near the surface of the body, it may erode through to the surface, thus breaking down the natural defenses of intact skin and mucous membranes and providing a site for the entry of microorganisms. Any malignant involvement of the organs or tissues of immunity—such as the liver, bone marrow, Peyer's patches in the small intestine, spleen, or lymph nodes—can seriously impair the immune response, allowing infections to develop in vulnerable tissues.

Hemorrhage

Tumor erosion through blood vessels can cause extensive bleeding, giving rise to severe anemia. Hemorrhage can be serious enough to cause life-threatening hypovolemic shock.

Anorexia-Cachexia Syndrome

A characteristic feature of cancer is the wasted appearance of its victims, called **cachexia**. In many cases, unexplained rapid weight loss is the first symptom that brings the client to a healthcare provider. This can be due to a variety of problems associated with cancer, such as pain, infection, depression, or the side effects of chemotherapy and radiation. Usually, however, the emaciation, malnutrition, and loss of energy are attributed to the anorexia-cachexia syndrome.

This syndrome is specific to cancer because of the effect of cancer cells on the host's metabolism. The neoplastic cells divert nutrition to their own use while causing changes that reduce the client's appetite. Early in the disease, glucose metabolism is altered, causing an increase in serum glucose levels. Through the process of negative feedback, *anorexia* (loss of appetite) results. In addition, the tumor secretes substances that decrease appetite by altering taste and smell and producing early satiety. Pain, infection, and depression also contribute to anorexia. Some types of cancers cause specific food aversions, such as to red meat, coffee, or chocolate.

Avaricious cancer cells support their growth through widespread catabolism of the body's tissue and muscle proteins. This catabolism, coupled with inadequate nutrient intake, results in the typical cachexia. Normally, a starvation state reduces the body's basal metabolic rate. However, in many people with cancer, the metabolic rate is increased, probably because of the hyperactive metabolic and reproductive activities of the malignant cells. One theory suggests that cytokinins the body produces in response to the tumor are responsible for both early satiety and cachexia. One specific cytokine, called tumor necrosis factor alpha or cachectin, is believed to enhance the increased metabolic consumption of nutrients. Cancers of the gastrointestinal system further promote anorexia-cachexia by decreasing absorption and use of nutrients; the side effects of some treatment modalities enhance this effect. Figure 14–4 ■ shows the characteristic appearance of a cachectic person.

Paraneoplastic Syndromes

Paraneoplastic syndromes are indirect effects of cancer. They may be early warning signs of cancer or indicate complications or return of a malignancy. The most frequently occurring paraneoplastic syndromes are endocrine, occurring when cancers set up ectopic sites of hormone production (Haapoja, 2000). Table 14–4 lists laboratory indicators of ectopic functioning. These ectopic sites produce excessive amounts of the hormone, which harm the host. Consider the following examples:

■ Breast, ovarian, and renal cancers may set up ectopic parathyroid hormone sites, causing severe hypercalcemia.

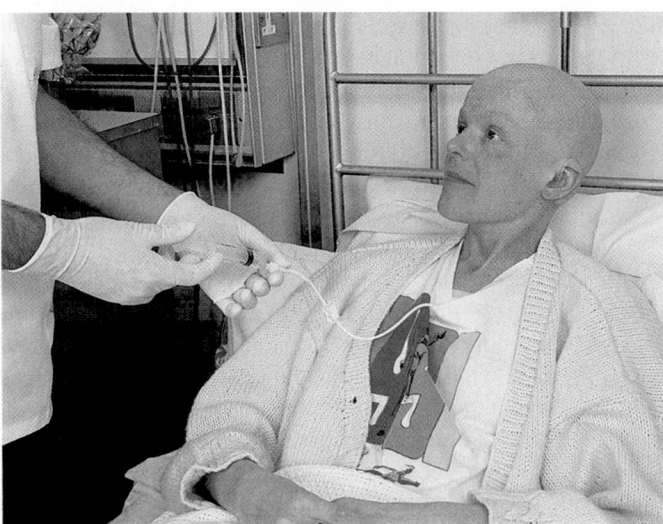

Figure 14–4 ■ Cachectic person. Cancer robs its host of nutrients and increases body catabolism of fat and muscle to meet its metabolic needs.
Source: Simon Fraser/SPL/Photo Researchers, Inc.

■ Oat cell and other lung cancers may produce ectopic secretions of insulin (causing hypoglycemia), parathyroid hormone (PTH), antidiuretic hormone (ADH, which causes excessive fluid retention, hypertension, and peripheral edema), and adrenocorticotropic hormone (ACTH). See Chapter 19 ∞ for the description of the multiple problems caused by excessive secretions of cortisone.

Other paraneoplastic syndromes include hematologic abnormalities such as anemia, thrombocytopenia, and coagulation abnormalities; nephrotic syndrome; cutaneous syndromes; and neurologic syndromes, such as distant tumors that produce increased ICP (Haapoja, 2000).

Pain

Pain is ranked as one of the most serious concerns of clients, families, and oncology healthcare professionals. Because pain

TABLE 14–4 Laboratory Indicators of Ectopic Functioning

HORMONE	SPECIFIC LABORATORY TEST
Antidiuretic hormone (ADH)	Serum and urine osmolality
Adrenocorticotropic hormone (ACTH)	Plasma ACTH ACTH suppression test ACTH stimulation test Urine catecholamines
Calcitonin	Serum calcitonin
Insulin	Serum glucose Glucose tolerance test
Parathyroid hormone (PTH)	Serum PTH Serum calcium
Thyroxine	Serum thyroid-stimulating hormone (TSH), T_3, T_4

management for people with cancer has a reputation for being ineffective, the anticipation of pain may engender fear in even the most stoic people. Most persons fear pain and suffering even more than possible death, although pain management strategies have improved tremendously. The findings from a 10-year study of more than 2000 patients in a palliative care program are encouraging. Following the World Health Organization guidelines for cancer pain relief, 88% of patients reported good to satisfactory pain relief (Zech et al., 1995). Research on pain with its devastating statistics has led to great improvement in pain management strategies.

Types of Cancer Pain

Cancer pain can be divided into two main categories, acute and chronic, with subgroupings. These classifications serve to indicate appropriate therapeutic approaches. Acute pain has a well-defined pattern of onset, exhibits common signs and symptoms, and is often identified with hyperactivity of the autonomic system. Chronic pain, which lasts more than 6 months, frequently lacks the objective manifestations of acute pain, primarily because the autonomic nervous system adapts to this chronic stress. Unfortunately, chronic pain often results in personality changes, alterations in functional abilities, and lifestyle disruptions that can seriously affect compliance with treatment and the quality of life.

Most cancer clients who cite acute pain as the primary symptom that led to the diagnosis tend to associate pain with the introduction to their disease. If these clients experience pain during the illness or after therapy, they often perceive the pain as introducing another cancer or as a recurrence of the original cancer. Other clients report experiencing pain as a component of cancer therapy. These clients often are able to endure the pain in anticipation of a successful outcome of treatment.

Chronic pain may be related to treatment or may indicate progression of the disease. Identifying the pain as treatment related rather than tumor related is extremely important because it has a definite effect on the client's psychologic outlook. For the client whose pain is due to the advancement of the disease, psychologic factors play an even more important role. Hopelessness and fear of impending death intensify physiologic pain and contribute to overall suffering (which goes well beyond just physical pain).

Three other categories used to classify clients with cancer pain are worth mentioning: clients with preexisting pain, those with a history of drug abuse, and dying clients with cancer-related pain. The first two groups may have altered perceptions of pain and may not have the anticipated response to pain medication. For the dying client, pain is strongly associated with both the client's and family's confrontation of issues of hopelessness and death. Confronting these issues can intensify the perception of pain (see Chapter 5 ∞).

Causes of Cancer Pain

Direct tumor involvement is the primary cause of the pain experienced by people with cancer. This includes metastatic bone disease, nerve compression, and involvement of visceral organs. The pain from tumor involvement is believed to be mechanical, resulting from stretching of tissues and compression.

Chemicals from ischemia or tumor metabolites and toxins that activate and sensitize nociceptors and mechanoreceptors are also responsible for tumor pain. See Chapter 9 ∞ for a more complete discussion of the mechanics of pain.

Side effects or toxic effects of cancer therapies (e.g., surgery, radiation, and chemotherapy) may also cause cancer pain. These are usually the result of traumatized tissue; one example of this is the oropharyngeal ulcerations that occur with some types of chemotherapy. However, these therapies may also be used to manage pain, such as radiation to decrease pain associated with bone metastasis.

Physical Stress

When the immune system discovers a neoplasm, it tries to destroy it using the resources of the body. The body mounts an all-out assault on the foreign invader, calling on many resources:

- Chemical mediators
- Hormones and enzymes
- Blood cells
- Antibodies
- Proteins
- Inflammatory and immune responses.

These protective responses also mobilize fluid, electrolytes, and nutritional systems. This massive effort requires tremendous energy. See Chapters 10 ∞ and 22 ∞ for specific information on these systems. If the neoplasm is small enough (i.e., microscopic), the immune system can destroy it, and a tumor will never manifest. A neoplasm of 1 cm is large enough to overwhelm most immune systems; however, the body will continue to try to fight it until it reaches the stage of exhaustion and is no longer capable (Selye, 1984). Thus, many clients with cancer present with fatigue, weight loss, anemia, dehydration, and altered blood chemistries (e.g., decreases in electrolytes).

Psychologic Stress

People confronted with the diagnosis of cancer exhibit a variety of psychologic and emotional responses. Some people see cancer as a death sentence and experience overwhelming grief, often giving up. Others may feel guilt, considering the cancer a punishment for past behaviors, such as smoking, unhealthy eating habits, or for delaying diagnosis or treatment. The person may experience anger, especially if the person believes that he or she had been practicing a healthful lifestyle; beneath that anger may reside feelings of powerlessness. Fear is common: fear of the outcome of the illness, fear of the effects of treatment, fear of pain, fear of death. Some people feel isolated because of the stigma of cancer and old beliefs of contagion. Body image concerns and sexual dysfunction may be present but often unexpressed, especially if the cancer is of the breast or sexual organs or causes visible body changes. Box 14–5 summarizes the physiologic and psychosocial effects of cancer.

INTERDISCIPLINARY CARE

Interdisciplinary care for the client with cancer begins with a variety of specialized laboratory and diagnostic tests.

BOX 14–5 Physiologic and Psychosocial Effects of Cancer

- Disruption of function (due to obstruction or pressure)
- Hematologic alterations
  a. Decreased leukocytes, erythrocytes, and thrombocytes
  b. Altered erythropoiesis
- Infections
  a. Fistula between noncompatible organs
  b. Necrosis of tumor center
  c. Malignant involvement of organs of immunity
- Hemorrhage (caused by erosion of neoplasm through blood vessels or surface of skin)
- Anorexia-cachexia syndrome
  a. Hyperglycemia
  b. Catabolism of tissue and muscle proteins
  c. Altered taste and smell
- Creation of ectopic sites of hormones
  a. PTH   c. ADH
  b. Insulin   d. ACTH
- Paraneoplastic syndromes
  a. Deep venous thrombosis
  b. Peripheral nerve problems
  c. Increased intracranial pressure
  d. Anorexia-cachexia syndrome
  e. Nephrotic syndrome
- Pain
  a. Acute and chronic
  b. Caused by direct tumor involvement or side effects of therapy
- Physical stress
  a. Increased general adaptation syndrome activity
  b. Increased immunologic activity
  c. Increased inflammatory response activity
  d. Nutritional, fluid, and electrolyte alterations
- Psychologic stress
  a. Grief   e. Fear
  b. Hopelessness   f. Isolation
  c. Guilt   g. Body image concerns
  d. Anger   h. Sexual dysfunction

Note: Manifestations depend on the type and location of the cancer.

Diagnosis

Several procedures are used to diagnose cancer. X-ray imaging, computed tomography (CT), ultrasonography, and magnetic resonance imaging (MRI) can locate abnormal tissues or tumors. However, only microscopic histologic examination of the tissue reveals the type of cell and its structural difference from the parent tissue. Tissue samples are acquired through biopsy, shedded cells (e.g., Papanicolaou smear), or collections of secretions (e.g., sputum). Lymph nodes are also biopsied to determine whether metastasis has begun. Simple screening procedures can be used to pick up substances secreted by the tumor, such as the prostatic-specific antigen (PSA) blood test now being used to identify early prostatic cancers. Increases in enzymes or hormones released by normal tissues when they are damaged can also contribute to the diagnosis. Increased alkaline phosphatase noted in bone metastases and osteosarcoma is one example of an enzyme increase associated with cancer. Recent research has identified tumor markers; they are used for early diagnosis, for tracking responses to therapy, and for devising immunologic treatments.

Some investigators studying chemical mediators of the immune system have noted that there seems to be communication between the chemical mediators and the emotional centers of the brain. A person who states "I feel I have cancer," should be listened to, and the complaint investigated thoroughly.

CLASSIFICATION To help standardize diagnosis and treatment protocols, an elaborate identification system has been developed. This consists of naming the tumor (classification) and describing its aggressiveness (grading) and spread within or beyond the tissue of origin (staging).

Tumors are classified and named by the tissue or cell of origin. Tumor nomenclature often incorporates the Latin stem identifying the tissue from which the tumor arises. For example, a carcinoma arises from epithelial tissue; adjectives are added to further specify the location. A glandular malignancy arising from epithelial tissue is classified as an adenocarcinoma. A tumor arising from supportive tissues is called a sarcoma; the specific type of tissue is added as a prefix. For example, a cancer of fibrous connective tissue is called fibrosarcoma, and a smooth muscle cancer is a leiomyosarcoma. A tumor from seminal or germ tissue is called a seminoma. Table 14–5 compares the nomenclature of benign and malignant neoplasms.

Other names for tumors incorporate the name of the discoverer of that particular cancer, such as Burkitt's lymphoma or Hodgkin's disease. Hematopoietic malignancies (also known as "liquid tumors") are usually named by the type of immature blood cell that predominates. An example is myelocytic leukemia, named for the immature form of the granulocyte that is predominant in this malignancy.

GRADING AND STAGING Grading evaluates the amount of differentiation (level of functional maturity) of the cell and estimates the rate of growth based on the mitotic rate. Cells that are the most differentiated—that is, most like the parent tissue and therefore the least malignant—are classified as grade 1 and are associated with a better prognosis. Grade 4 is reserved for the least differentiated and most aggressively malignant cells. Because of the differences inherent in tumor appearance and biologic behavior, grading criteria may vary with different locations and types of tumors.

Staging is used to classify solid tumors and refers to the relative size of the tumor and extent of the disease. The TNM classification system is an internationally recognized staging system: The T stands for the relative tumor size, depth of invasion, and surface spread; N indicates the presence and extent of lymph node involvement; and M denotes the presence or absence of distant metastases. Table 14–6 shows the basic outline of the TNM system; however, other systems are also used to differentiate types and locations of tumors (e.g., melanomas, cervical cancer, Hodgkin's disease).

CYTOLOGIC EXAMINATION For the malignant tissues to be identified by name, grade, and stage, they must first be subjected

TABLE 14–5 Nomenclature for Benign and Malignant Neoplasms

	TISSUE OF ORIGIN	BENIGN	MALIGNANT
Ectoderm/Endoderm	Epithelium	Papilloma	Carcinoma
	Gland	Adenoma	Adenocarcinoma
	Liver cells	Hepatocellular adenoma	Hepatocellular carcinoma
	Neuroglia	Glioma	Glioma
	Melanocytes	Melanoma	Malignant melanoma
	Basal cells		Basal cell carcinoma
	Germ cells	Tetroma	Seminoma
Mesoderm	Connective tissue		
	Adipose tissue	Lipoma	Liposarcoma
	Fibrous tissue	Fibroma	Fibrosarcoma
	Bone tissue	Osteoma	Osteosarcoma
	Cartilage	Chondroma	Chondrosarcoma
	Muscle		
	Smooth muscle	Leiomyoma	Leiomyosarcoma
	Striated muscle	Rhabdomyoma	Rhabdomyosarcoma
	Neural tissue		
	Nerve cells	Ganglioneuroma	Neuroblastoma
	Endothelial tissues		
	Blood vessels	Hemangioma	Angiosarcoma
			Kaposi's sarcoma
	Meninges	Meningioma	Malignant meningioma
Hematopoietic Tissues	Granulocytes	Granulocytosis	Leukemia
	Plasma cells		Multiple myeloma
	Lymphocytes		Lymphomas

TABLE 14–6 TNM Staging Classification System

	STAGE	MANIFESTATIONS
Tumor	T_0	No evidence of primary tumor.
	T_{IS}	Tumor *in situ.*
	T_1, T_2, T_3, T_4	Ascending degrees of tumor size and involvement.
Nodes	N_0	No abnormal regional nodes.
	N_{1a}, N_{2a}	Regional nodes—no metastasis.
	N_{1b}, N_{2b}, N_{3b}	Regional lymph nodes—metastasis suspected.
	N_x	Regional nodes cannot be assessed clinically.
Metastasis	M_0	No evidence of distant metastasis.
	M_1, M_2, M_3	Ascending degrees of metastatic involvement of the host including distant nodes.

to histologic and cytologic examination by light or electron microscope. Specimens are collected by three basic methods:

1. *Exfoliation from an epithelial surface.* Examples include scraping cells from the cervix (Pap smear) or bronchial washings.
2. *Aspiration of fluid from body cavities or blood.* Examples include white blood cells for evaluation of hematopoietic cancers, pleural fluid, and cerebrospinal fluid.

3. *Needle aspiration of solid tumors.* This could include the breast, lung, or prostate.

Cytologic examination is also carried out on specimens from biopsied tissues or tumors and on collected body secretions, such as sputum or urine.

After collection, specimens are spread on a glass slide, fixed, and stained if necessary. The morphologic features of the cells are examined, with special attention to the nucleus and cytoplasm. Other special pathologic procedures can be carried out on the specimen, but they must be ordered ahead of time if special preparations of the specimen are necessary.

Several special diagnostic cytologic procedures, such as cytogenetics, are proving useful in diagnosing and monitoring client response to treatment.

TUMOR MARKERS A **tumor marker** is a protein molecule detectable in serum or other body fluids. This marker is used as a biochemical indicator of the presence of a malignancy. Small amounts of tumor marker proteins are found in normal body tissues or benign tumors and are not specific for malignancy. However, high levels are suspicious and mandate follow-up diagnostic studies. Tumor marker tests are in the developmental and investigational phase and are most useful for monitoring the client's response to therapy and for detecting residual disease. However, one marker, PSA, has received a great deal of media attention as a detector of prostate cancer. As a result, many healthcare practitioners recommend screening for it in men over age 40, much as Pap smears and mammograms are recommended for women.

Tumor markers fall into two general categories: those derived from the tumor itself and those associated with host (immune) response to the tumor. Examples of tumor markers include the following:

- *Antigens.* These are present in fetal tissue but normally are suppressed after birth. Thus, their presence in large amounts may reflect an anaplastic process in tumor cells. Alpha-fetoprotein (AFP) and carcinoembryonic antigen (CEA) are oncofetal antigens.
- *Hormones.* Hormones are, of course, present in considerable amounts in human blood and tissues, but very high levels not related to other conditions may signify the presence of a hormone-secreting malignancy. Some common hormones seen as tumor markers include human chorionic gonadotropin (HCG), antidiuretic hormone (ADH), parathyroid hormone (PTH), calcitonin, and catecholamines.
- *Proteins.* These narrow down the type of tissue that may be malignant, although they can also be increased in hyperplastic disorders. Examples of tissue-specific proteins include serum immunoglobin and beta-2 microglobulin.
- *Enzymes.* Rapid, excessive growth of a tissue may cause some of the enzymes and isoenzymes normally present in that particular tissue to spill into the bloodstream. Elevated levels can point to either hyperplasia of the tissue or cancer. Prostatic acid phosphatase (PAP) and neuron-specific enolase (NSE) are examples. Table 14–7 compares selected tumor-derived markers with their presence in neoplasms and other conditions.

ONCOLOGIC IMAGING Because physical assessment usually cannot detect cancer until the tumor has reached a size that poses a major risk for metastasis, radiologic examination is extremely important in early diagnosis. This diagnostic process may involve routine x-ray imaging (usually for screening only), CT, MRI, ultrasonography, nuclear imaging, angiography, and positron emission tomography.

X-Ray Imaging Considered the least expensive and least invasive diagnostic procedure, film screen imaging (standard x-ray imaging) is the method of choice for screening such body areas as the breast (mammography), lung, and bone to identify changes in tissue density that may indicate malignancies. X-ray studies are limited in that they do not easily distinguish among calcifications, benign cystic growths, and true malignancies. However, as a screening tool, x-ray imaging can usually reassure the client if findings are negative or encourage follow-up studies if findings are suspicious. X-ray imaging is still the method of choice for lung cancer. Unfortunately, it does not usually reveal tumors until they have reached about 1 cm in size, which is late in their development.

Computed Tomography CT has vastly advanced the effectiveness of traditional x-ray methods. By applying computers and mathematics to diagnostic imaging, CT allows the visualization of cross sections of the anatomy. Because CT scans reveal subtle differences in tissue densities, they provide much greater accuracy in tumor diagnosis. This procedure, although more expensive than x-ray imaging, is useful in the screening for some cancers such as renal cell and most gastrointestinal tumors. CT scans are especially useful to evaluate possible lymph node involvement.

Magnetic Resonance Imaging Like CT, MRI involves computerized mathematical technology. The patient is placed within a strong magnetic field, pulsed radio waves are directed at the patient, and transmitted signals based on tissue characteristics are analyzed by a computer. Related diagnostic imaging procedures—positron emission tomography (PET) and single photon emission computed tomography (SPECT)—create visible images by measuring electrical impulses from different body structures. Although MRI is relatively expensive, it is the diagnostic tool of choice for both screening and follow-up of cranial and head and neck tumors.

Some clients become claustrophobic during the MRI procedure because they must be placed inside the diagnostic imaging machine, an experience that has been likened to being encased in a small tube. In addition, some machines make loud thumping sounds that can be frightening if the client is not informed beforehand that this is normal.

TABLE 14–7 Tumor-Derived Markers Associated with Specific Neoplasms

	TUMOR MARKER	ASSOCIATED NEOPLASM
Oncofetal Antigens	Carcinoembryonic antigen (CEA) Alpha-fetoprotein (AFP)	Adenocarcinomas of colon, lung, breast, ovary, stomach, pancreas Hepatocellular carcinoma, gonadal germ cell tumors (seminoma)
Hormones	Human chorionic gonadotropin (HCG) Calcitonin Catecholamines/metabolites	Gonadal germ cell tumors Medullary cancer of thyroid Pheochromocytoma
Isoenzymes	Prostatic acid phosphatase (PAP) Neuron-specific enolase (NSE)	Adenocarcinoma of prostate Small-cell lung carcinoma, neuroblastoma
Specific Proteins	Prostate-specific antigen (PSA) Immunoglobin CA 125 CA 19-9 CA 15-3	Adenocarcinoma of prostate Multiple myeloma Epithelial ovarian cancer Adenocarcinoma of pancreas, colon Breast cancer

Source: Adapted from "The Pathologic Evaluation of Neoplastic Disease" by J. D. Pfeifer and M. R. Wick, in *American Cancer Society Textbook of Clinical Oncology* (pp. 75–95) by A. I. Holleb, D. J. Fink, and G. P. Murphy, Eds., 1995, Atlanta: American Cancer Society.

Ultrasonography Ultrasonography is relatively safe and non-invasive. It measures sound waves as they bounce off various body structures, giving an image of normal anatomy as well as revealing abnormalities that indicate tumors. Ultrasonography has been adapted for diagnosing some specific tumors. For example, transrectal ultrasonography has provided excellent imaging of early prostate cancers and is used to guide needle biopsy. Ultrasound imaging is also more useful for detecting masses in the denser breast tissue of young women.

Nuclear Imaging Nuclear imaging involves the use of a special scintillation scanner in conjunction with the ingestion or injection of specific radioactive isotopes. This is an invasive but usually safe diagnostic method for identifying tumors in various body tissues. For the client with a newly diagnosed cancer, the procedure is often used to check for possible bone or other organ metastases. This evaluation helps the healthcare provider determine appropriate treatment.

The principle underlying the technology is that certain isotopes have an affinity for specific tissues; for example, radioactive iodine (I-131) has an affinity for the thyroid gland. Malignancies in these tissues sequester an abnormally large amount of the isotope, which then can be traced and measured by the scintillation scanner. This procedure is considered safe because the amount of isotope used is small enough not to damage normal cells.

The procedure is usually minimally distressing for clients. Drinking the isotope solution is not pleasant but is tolerable; some anxious clients may have difficulty lying still during the scan. Antianxiety medication may help. Some clients may experience nausea from drinking the isotope and require antiemetic drugs to complete the procedure. Client preparation may include allowing nothing by mouth or clear fluids only after midnight.

Angiography An expensive and invasive procedure, angiography is used infrequently for tumor diagnosis. Angiography is performed when the precise location of the tumor cannot be identified or there is a need to visualize the tumor's extent prior to surgery. The procedure involves injecting a radiopaque dye into a major blood vessel proximal to the organ or tissue to be examined. The movement of the dye through the vasculature of the organ or tissue is then traced by means of fluoroscopy or serial x-ray films. In some cases, small catheters are threaded through the vein under fluoroscopy to ensure the specific placement of the dye. Blockage to the flow of the dye indicates the tumor's location. Dye may also be used to identify blood vessels supplying a tumor, allowing the surgeon to know where to safely ligate vessels. Angiography requires preparation similar to that for minor surgery. This includes ensuring that the client takes in only fluids on the day of the examination, performing skin preparation at the insertion site, and administering sedative drugs prior to the procedure. Clients should be informed that injection of the dye used to enhance imaging may cause a hot, flushing sensation or nausea and vomiting. Although angiography is usually done on an outpatient basis, the client will be kept in a short-stay unit for several hours and monitored for such complications as bleeding at the catheter insertion site.

DIRECT VISUALIZATION Direct visualization procedures are invasive but do not require the use of radiography. Examples include the following:

- Sigmoidoscopy (viewing the sigmoid colon with a fiber-optic flexible sigmoidoscope)
- Cystoscopy (viewing the urethra and bladder)
- Endoscopy (viewing the upper gastrointestinal tract)
- Bronchoscopy (inspecting the tracheobronchial tree).

These methods allow the visual identification of the organs within the limits of the scope and usually permit biopsy of suspicious lesions or masses. Flexible fiber-optic scopes may be more useful, because they allow deeper penetration than do traditional scopes. These procedures all require some client preparation, cause moderate to considerable discomfort, and may require sedation or even anesthesia, as in the case of bronchoscopy. Some procedures, such as sigmoidoscopy and cystoscopy, may be performed in the physician's office and therefore cost less, making them more accessible screening procedures.

Client preparation includes a thorough bowel cleansing prior to the sigmoidoscopy and cystoscopy; the client may ingest only liquids the morning of the procedure. Because anesthesia may be required, clients undergoing bronchoscopy and endoscopy may be instructed to have nothing by mouth from midnight until the procedure. These procedures are discussed in greater detail in later chapters of this textbook. A more radical method of direct visualization for suspected malignancies is exploratory surgery with biopsy. The client undergoes the usual preoperative preparation (see Chapter 4) for the type of surgery anticipated. When the tumor is exposed, a sample of tissue (biopsy) is sent to the pathology laboratory for a "frozen-section" histologic examination. This can be done rapidly while the client remains on the operating table under anesthesia. If the initial report is negative, the benign mass is usually removed to prevent further symptoms. If the report is positive for cancer, the tumor and, often, adjacent lymph nodes are resected, along with any other suspicious tissue. The tumor, nodes, and any other specimens are sent to the pathology laboratory for more in-depth analysis. The client then receives the usual postoperative care.

LABORATORY TESTS Most laboratory tests of blood, urine, and other body fluids are used to rule out nutritional disorders and other noncancerous conditions that may be causing the client's symptoms. For example, a complete blood count (CBC) helps screen for such problems as anemia, infection, and impaired immunity. Blood chemistries can point out nutritional disturbances and electrolyte imbalances. However, in conjunction with other diagnostic studies, some laboratory tests can be quite useful either in screening for other pathologic conditions or for validating the cancer diagnosis (Kee, 2002). These tests include evaluating levels of enzymes such as alanine aminotransferase (ALT), aspartate aminotransferase (AST), and lactic dehydrogenase (LDH) for liver metastases. Special protein tumor markers such as PSA for prostate cancer and CEA for colon cancer are also used. Table 14–8 identifies some useful laboratory tests, their normal values, and their possible indications.

TABLE 14–8 Laboratory Tests Used for Cancer Diagnosis*

TEST	REFERENCE VALUE	ABNORMALITY INDICATED
Acid phosphatase (ACP)	0.0 to 0.8 unit/L	Elevated in prostate, breast, and bone cancer and in multiple myeloma
Adrenocorticotropic hormone (ACTH)	8 to 80 pg/mL	Decreased in adrenal cancer Elevated in pituitary cancer or with tumor that secretes ACTH (bronchiogenic cancer)
Alanine aminotransferase (ALT)	5 to 35 unit/mL (Frankel)	Moderate elevation in liver cancer
Albumin	3.5 to 5.0 g/dL	Decreased in malnutrition, metastatic liver cancer
Alkaline phosphatase (ALP)	20 to 90 unit/L	Elevated in cancer of liver, bone, breast, and prostate, in leukemia, and in multiple myeloma
Alpha-fetoprotein (AFP)	Male and nonpregnant female: <15 ng/mL	Elevated in germ cell tumors (e.g., seminoma), testicular cancer
Aspartate aminotransferase (AST)	5 to 40 unit/mL (Frankel)	Elevated in liver cancer
Bilirubin	Total: 0.1 to1.2 mg/dL Direct: 0.0 to 0.3 mg/dL	Elevated in liver and gallbladder cancer
Bleeding time	Ivy method: 3 to 7 minutes	Prolonged in leukemia and metastatic liver cancer
Blood urea nitrogen (BUN)	5 to 25 mg/dL	Decreased in malnutrition; increased in renal cancer
Calcitonin	Male: <40 pg/mL Female: <20 pg/mL	Elevated to >500 pg/mL in thyroid medullary cancer, breast cancer, and lung cancer
Calcium (Ca)	4.5 to 5.5 mEq/L 9.0 to 11.0 mg/dL	Elevated in bone cancer and ectopic parathyroid hormone production (paraplastic syndrome)
Carcinoembryonic antigen (CEA)	2.5 ng/mL in nonsmokers 5 ng/mL in smokers; >12 ng/mL neoplasms	Elevated with GI cancers, lung, breast, bladder, kidney, cervical, leukemias Used to evaluate effectiveness of cancer treatment
Chloride (Cl)	95 to 105 mEq/L	Decreased in vomiting, diarrhea, syndrome of inappropriate antidiuretic hormone (SIADH)
C-reactive protein	>1:2 titer is positive	Elevated in metastatic cancer and Burkitt's lymphoma
Creatinine	0.5 to 1.5 mg/dL	Decreased in malnutrition; elevated in most cancers
Dexamethasone suppression test	>50% reduction in plasma cortisol	Nonsuppression in adrenal cancer and ACTH-producing tumors, severe stress
Estradiol-serum	Female: 20 to 300 pg/mL Menopausal female: <20 pg/mL Male: 15 to 50 pg/mL	Elevated in estrogen-producing tumors and testicular tumors
Fibrinogen	200 to 400 mg/dL	Decreased in leukemia and as a side effect of chemotherapy
Gamma glutamyltransferase (GGT)	Male: 10 to 80 international unit/L Female: 5 to 25 international unit/L	Elevated in cancer of liver, pancreas, prostate, breast, kidney, lung, and brain
Fasting blood sugar	70 to 110 mg/dL	Decreased in malnutrition, cancer of stomach, liver, and lung
Haptoglobin	20 to 240 mg/dL	Elevated in Hodgkin's disease and cancer of lung, large intestine, stomach, breast, and liver
Hematocrit (Hct)	Male: 40% to 54% Female: 36% to 46%	Decreased in anemia, leukemia, Hodgkin's disease, lymphosarcoma, multiple myeloma, and malnutrition and as a side effect of chemotherapy
Hemoglobin (Hgb)	Male: 13.5 to 18 g/dL Female: 12 to 16 g/dL 1:3 ratio of Hgb:Hct	Decreased in anemia, many cancers, Hodgkin's disease, leukemia, and malnutrition and as a side effect of chemotherapy
Human chorionic gonadotropin (HCG)	Nonpregnant female <0.01 international unit/L	Elevated in choriocarcinoma
Insulin	5 to 25 microunit/mL	Elevated in insulinoma (islet cell tumor) and insulin-secreting cancers (e.g., lung cancer)
Lactic dehydrogenase (LDH)	100 to 190 international unit/L	Elevated in liver, brain, kidney, muscle cancers, acute leukemia, anemia

*All values refer to serum values unless otherwise indicated. Values are approximate; check the reference standards specified by your own agency's laboratory.

TABLE 14–8 Laboratory Tests Used for Cancer Diagnosis* (continued)

TEST	REFERENCE VALUE	ABNORMALITY INDICATED
Occult blood	Negative	Positive in gastric and colon cancers
Serum osmolality	280 to 300 mOsm/kg H_2O	Decreased in SIADH
Urine osmolality	50 to 1200 mOsm/kg H_2O	Increased in SIADH
Parathyroid hormone (PTH)	400 to 900 pg/mL	Increased in PTH-secreting tumors
Platelet (thrombocyte) count	150,000/mm^3 to 400,000/mm^3	Decreased in bone, gastric, and brain cancer, in leukemia, and as a side effect of chemotherapy
Potassium (K)	3.5 to 5.0 mEq/L	Decreased in vomiting and diarrhea and in malnutrition
Prostatic-specific antigen (PSA)	0 to 4 ng/mL	Elevated from 10 to 120+ in prostate cancer
Total protein	6.0 to 8.0 g/dL	Decreased in malnutrition, gastrointestinal cancer, Hodgkin's disease; elevated in vomiting, diarrhea, multiple myeloma
Red blood cells (RBCs)	Male: 4.6 to 6.0 million/mm^3 Female: 4.0 to 5.0 million/mm^3	Decreased in anemia, leukemia, infection, multiple myeloma
Sodium (Na)	135 to 145 mEq/L	Decreased in SIADH, vomiting; elevated in dehydration
Uric acid	Male: 3.5 to 8.0 mg/dL Female: 2.8 to 6.8 mg/dL	Increased in leukemia, metastatic cancer, multiple myeloma, Burkitt's lymphoma, after vigorous chemotherapy
White blood cells (WBC)		
Total leukocytes	4500/mm^3 to 10,000/mm^3	Elevated in acute infection, leukemias, tissue necrosis; decreased as a side effect of chemotherapy
Neutrophils	50% to 70%	Elevated in bacterial infection and Hodgkin's disease; decreased in leukemia and malnutrition and as a side effect of chemotherapy
Eosinophils	1% to 3%	Elevated in cancer of bone, ovary, testes, and brain
Basophils	0.4% to 1.0%	Elevated in leukemia and healing stage of infection
Monocytes	4% to 6%	Elevated in infection, monocytic leukemia and cancer; decreased in lymphocytic leukemia and as a side effect of chemotherapy
Lymphocytes	25% to 35%	Elevated in lymphocytic leukemia, Hodgkin's disease, multiple myeloma, viral infections, and chronic infections; decreased in malnutrition, cancer, and other leukemias and as a side effect of chemotherapy

PSYCHOLOGIC SUPPORT DURING DIAGNOSIS Preparing for and awaiting the results of diagnostic tests can create extreme anxiety. Many clients compare the experience to that of a prisoner awaiting trial and sentencing: After they know what the "sentence" is, then they can prepare for the future. In addition to coping with the possibility of a life-threatening disease, or at least a life-altering one, clients often also face the prospect of uncomfortable, even painful, diagnostic procedures. They have important decisions to make that depend on the outcome of those tests. Many unspoken questions may exist, including the following:

- Do I have cancer?
- If so, what kind, and how serious?
- Has it spread?
- Will I survive?
- What kind of treatment is needed?
- How will this affect my lifestyle?
- How will this affect family members and friends?

Denial or intellectualization serve some clients well, but others display signs of anxiety and stress as they attempt to cope. The nurse can provide valuable support during this very difficult stage by helping clients become actively involved in managing their life and disease. Talk with clients as soon as they enter the healthcare system, asking what they know already about what is going to happen and soliciting questions from them. Taking this approach and encouraging clients to share what knowledge and experience they have allows them to maintain control. From there, the nurse can provide the information needed.

It is essential that clients thoroughly understand the preparation required for their tests, especially if they will be preparing at home. They also need to be informed of any unusual effects that may occur as a result of the procedure, such as nausea from radioactive dye. If possible, a phone call the evening before to verify the client's understanding of the procedure and to answer questions can be helpful and supportive.

As clients begin to feel more comfortable with the nurse, they may express concerns, fears, and other emotions. The nurse should actively listen and be supportive, but avoid giving advice and false reassurance, providing appropriate information when needed. For clients who are not ready to discuss concerns or for those who appear angry, being nonjudgmental and providing nonverbal support may facilitate more open communication. An atmosphere of calmness, warmth, caring, and respect can ease the tension and often unspoken terror of this initial period.

Support of and communication with the client's significant others is extremely important. Often they try to be strong for the client but have many fears and emotional concerns that they do not feel comfortable expressing. The nurse needs to be available to the family while the client is undergoing diagnostic procedures. Allowing them to talk without the need to edit for the client's benefit can help them manage their own difficulties in coping with their loved one's potential cancer diagnosis.

Cancer Treatment

The goals of cancer treatment are aimed at cure, control, or palliation of symptoms. These goals may overlap. Cancer may be treated through surgery, chemotherapy, radiation therapy, biotherapy, photodynamic therapy, bone marrow and stem cell transplants, and complementary therapies. Once cancer is diagnosed, the initial focus is on surgical and medical treatment. The goals of treatment are:

- Eliminating the tumor or malignant cells
- Preventing metastasis
- Reducing cellular growth and the tumor burden
- Promoting functional abilities and providing pain relief to those whose disease has not responded to treatment.

SURGERY Surgery was once considered the only treatment for cancer before the mechanisms of cancer were understood. Today, surgery remains an important approach in cancer care. Surgical resection is used for diagnosis and staging of more than 90% of all cancers and for primary treatment of more than 60% of cancers. The goals of surgery have also expanded to include prophylaxis, diagnosis, treatment, reconstruction, and palliation.

Prophylactic surgery aims to remove tissues or organs that are likely to develop cancer. Advances in identification of genetic markers make prophylactic surgery an option for individuals with a strong family history and genetic predisposition for the development of cancer. For example, a woman with a strong history of breast cancer, positive findings of BRCA-1 or BRCA-2, and abnormal finding on mammography may consider prophylactic mastectomy as one of the selective options. Other examples of prophylactic operations include colectomy and oophorectomy. With limited research on the long-term physiologic and psychologic effects on individuals undergoing prophylactic surgery for cancer, it is vitally important for nurses and other healthcare professionals to discuss thoroughly with the client and family potential risks and postoperative outcomes of the prophylactic surgery prior to the surgery. Nurses should respect the client's decision whether or not to pursue the prophylactic surgery. For those clients who choose prophylactic surgery as a preventive measure for cancer, comprehensive preoperative teaching and counseling should be provided and long-term postoperative follow-up should be ensured to monitor the client's physiologic and psychologic adjustment to the prophylactic surgery.

Diagnostic surgery aims to ensure histologic diagnosis and staging of cancer through biopsy, endoscopy, laparoscopy, and open surgical exploration. Table 14–9 provides information about common surgical diagnostic procedures.

As a primary treatment for cancer, the goal of surgery is to remove the entire tumor and involved surrounding tissue and lymph nodes as much as possible and feasible. This sometimes necessitates mutilation of the body and the creation of new structures to assume function of the lost structures. For example, removal of the distal sigmoid colon and rectum requires a new means of bowel elimination, so the remaining healthy segment of the bowel is brought out through a created opening (stoma) in the abdominal wall, resulting in a permanent colostomy (see Chapter 26 ∞). In like manner, when the bladder is removed, the ureters are transplanted into a created pouch just under the abdominal wall. This serves as a continent ileostomy, a substitute reservoir for urine (see Chapter 28 ∞). Surgery can also destroy sensitive nerve plexuses, resulting in alteration or loss of normal functioning; for example, prostate surgery may result in incontinence and impotence. Surgical removal of involved regional lymph nodes can also lead to long-term lymphedema (swelling in the affected area) that greatly impacts cancer survivors' quality of life, for instance, lymphedema following surgery for breast cancer and melanoma (Armer et al., 2004; Fu, 2004, 2005).

Not all surgery results in such radical changes in functioning. The following surgeries can eliminate cancer successfully with less distressing results:

- Removing a nonessential portion of the organ or tissue containing the tumor, such as *in situ* small-bowel tumors
- Removing an organ whose function can be replaced chemically, such as the thyroid
- Resecting one of a pair of organs when the unaffected organ can take over the function of the missing one, such as a lung.

Although the removal of any major body part has physiologic and psychologic consequences, the alternative—terminal disease—is usually less desirable.

TABLE 14–9 Surgical Diagnostic Procedures

PROCEDURE	EXPLANATION
Fine-needle biopsy	Use of a very thin needle to aspirate a small amount of tissue from the tumors
Needle core biopsy	Use of a slightly larger needle than that used for a fine-needle biopsy to extract a small amount of tissue from tumors that cannot be aspirated by fine-needle aspiration
Incisional biopsy	Removal of part of a larger tumor by cutting through the skin
Excisional biopsy	Removal of an entire tumor through operation
Endoscopy	Use of a small viewing lens or video camera through natural body openings to view tumors such as cancer of the esophagus, stomach, or colon
Laparoscopy	Use of a small viewing lens or video camera through a small incision in the abdominal wall

If the tumor is in a nonresectable location or deeply invasive with metastases, surgery may be only a palliative measure to allow the involved organs to function as long as possible, to relieve pain and provide comfort, or to bypass an obstruction. Surgery may also be done to reduce the bulk of the tumor in advanced disease, both at primary and metastatic sites. Decreasing the tumor size enhances the ability to control the remaining disease through other modalities. Surgery is often used in conjunction with other treatments to effect a cure. For example, in cases when extensive removal of tissue is contraindicated (e.g., in surgical removal of a brain tumor), radiation may be used prior to surgery in an attempt to shrink the tumor before it is removed.

Surgical intervention may also be used for reconstruction and rehabilitation to achieve more desirable functional and cosmetic effect after curative or radical surgery. One example is the construction of transabdominal myocutaneous (TRAM) flaps in conjunction with or following modified radical mastectomy (see Chapter 51 ∞). For surgical interventions for cancers affecting specific body systems, refer to later chapters.

Surgical oncologists are working with researchers to identify premalignant disease earlier in high-risk populations and to conduct studies on ways to reverse oncogenic cell activity. Surgeons also work with molecular biologists using sophisticated techniques to develop monoclonal antibodies. Laser technology is being explored for use in different types of cancer surgery because it minimizes blood loss, reduces deformity, increases the accuracy of tissue resection, and enhances healing. Lasers are currently being used to treat radical prostatectomy in order to preserve urinary continence and sexual functioning. Another collaborative strategy under development is intraoperative radiation therapy, in which radiosensitive, nondiseased organs that may be damaged by radiation therapy are moved away from the radiation field and shielded. Radiation is then administered while the patient is on the operating table. This technique allows more penetrating radiation to be directed to the malignant tumor with less trauma to normal, vulnerable tissues or organs.

Nursing responsibilities focus on preparing the client physically and psychologically for the specific surgery, as well as teaching routine postoperative care in which the client is expected to participate. For example, the nurse teaches the client about respiratory care and the use of the incentive spirometer to improve postoperative ventilation, early ambulation to prevent circulatory problems, and how the client will receive fluids and nutrition (intravenously or orally, depending on the type of surgery). In addition, the nurse explains the specific surgical procedure and any anticipated alterations to the client's body, especially those that require major lifestyle adjustments, such as a colostomy. Before surgery, the nurse should give the client the opportunity to ask questions and to discuss concerns and fears. In some cases, the client may want to discuss alternative treatment options. In the latter case, the nurse should avoid trying to persuade the client to accept any one option; rather, the nurse should contact the oncologist and the surgeon and set up a conference for the client before surgery.

CHEMOTHERAPY **Chemotherapy** involves the use of cytotoxic medications to cure some cancers, such as leukemias, lymphomas, and some solid tumors; to decrease tumor size, adjunctive to surgery or radiation therapy; or to prevent or treat suspected metastases. Chemotherapy may also be used in conjunction with biotherapy. All chemotherapy has side effects or toxic effects. The type and severity depend on the drugs used.

Chemotherapy disrupts the cell cycle in various phases by interrupting cell metabolism and replication. It also works by interfering with the ability of the malignant cell to synthesize vital enzymes and chemicals. Phase-specific drugs work during only some phases of the cell cycle; non–phase-specific drugs work through the entire cell cycle. Figure 14–5 ■ lists some of the drugs useful in each phase of the cell cycle.

Most chemical treatment involves combinations of drugs in specific protocols given over varying periods of time. For example, one protocol for adult acute lymphocytic leukemia (ALL) uses the acronym DVPA: daunorubicin given on days 1 through 3; vincristine given on days 1, 8, 15, and 22; prednisone given on days 1 through 28, and asparaginase given on days 17 through 28. The treatment regimen is given in cycles with rest periods allowed, especially if toxic effects such as liver dysfunction or severe neutropenia occur. The treatment

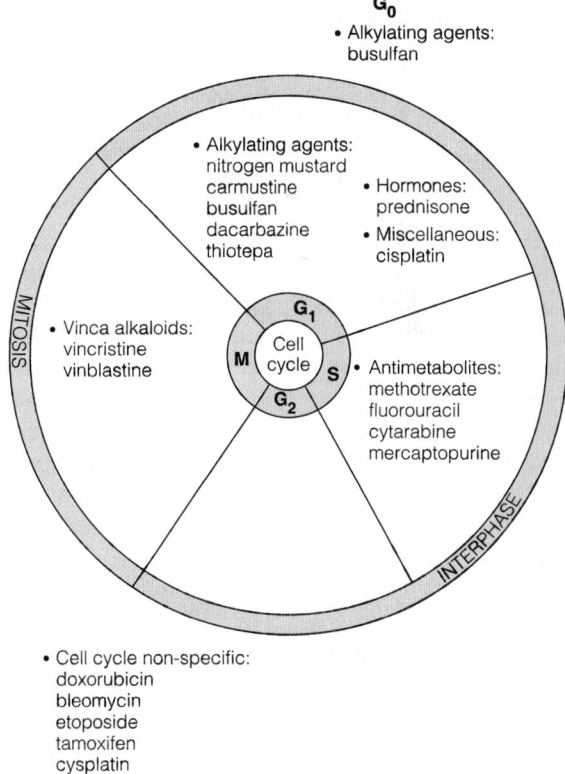

Figure 14–5 ■ Chemotherapeutic drugs useful in each phase of the cell cycle. Based on their chemical makeup and biologic activity, different drugs used for cancer treatment act in specific phases and subphases of the cell cycle. Some drugs, called non–phase-specific drugs, are generalized and act throughout the cycle. Chemotherapy often involves combinations of drugs designed to attack the cancer cells at many different times in the cycle and thus to enhance effectiveness.

is continued until the disease goes into remission. If the disease progresses, the particular protocol is abandoned and a new one may be tried.

Researchers have examined the possibility of basing chemotherapy administration on the body's circadian rhythms. Some drugs work better if they follow the normal cyclic fluctuations of body hormones during the night, whereas others are more effective when given during daytime hours. Chemotherapy administration that follows circadian rhythms appears to be more effective and causes fewer side effects with some types of cancer. A study of people with advanced colon cancer who were treated in this cyclic fashion (circadian rhythmic delivery, or CRD) demonstrated a 51% shrinkage in their tumors, compared with a shrinkage of only 28% in people who received chemotherapy in a steady dosage over 24 hours. In addition, the frequency and severity of side effects was decreased in the CRD group (Misset & Levi, 1995).

The cell-kill hypothesis explains why several courses of chemotherapy are necessary. A 1-cm tumor contains about 10^9 (10 billion) total cells, most of which are viable. During each cell cycle, the chemotherapy kills a fixed percentage of cells, always leaving some behind. With each reduction, the tumor burden of cells decreases until the number of viable, clonogenic cells (i.e., those that are able to clone daughter cells) becomes small enough to allow the body's immune system to finish the job. For this reason, oncologists usually give the maximum amount of chemotherapy tolerated by the client. High-dose chemotherapy remains controversial. A recent systematic review of 13 randomized controlled trials compared high-dose chemotherapy versus conventional chemotherapy for women with early poor prognosis breast cancer (Farquhar et al., 2006). Of the 2535 women randomized to receive high-dose chemotherapy and 2529 randomized to receive conventional chemotherapy, a statistically significant benefit was shown in event-free survival for women in the high-dose group at 3 and 4 years. Morbidity was more common and more severe in the high-dose group. However, there was no statistically significant difference between the groups with respect to the incidence of second cancers at 5 to 7 years' follow-up. Women in the high-dose group reported significantly worse quality-of-life scores immediately after treatment, but few statistically significant differences were found between the groups by 1 year.

Classes of Chemotherapy Drugs
Chemotherapeutic agents can be classified either by the effects of the agent on the cell or by the pharmacologic properties of the agent. According to the effects of the agent on the cell, chemotherapeutic agents can be divided into cell cycle–specific and cell cycle–nonspecific agents. Cell cycle-specific agents are effective at a specific phase (for example, S and M phases) in the cell cycle to prevent cell replication by damaging cellular DNA and blocking production of protein necessary for DNA and RNA synthesis. Cell cycle–nonspecific agents are effective throughout all the phases of the cell cycle, including the resting phase. Both cell cycle–specific and cell cycle–nonspecific agents are effective in rapidly dividing cells to prohibit the growth of fast-growing tumors.

The most common way of classifying chemotherapeutic agents is based on pharmacologic properties of the agent. The classifications include alkylating agents, antimetabolites, antitumor antibiotics, mitotic inhibitors, hormones and hormone antagonists, and miscellaneous agents.

Alkylating Agents. Alkylating agents are not phase specific and basically act on preformed nucleic acids by creating defects in tumor DNA. They cause crosslinking of DNA strands, which can permanently interfere with replication and transcription.

Alkylating agents work with both proliferating and nonproliferating cells (those in G_0 phase). Their toxicity relates to their ability to kill slowly cycling stem cells and manifests in delayed, prolonged, or permanent bone marrow failure. Toxicity can also cause a mutagenic effect on bone marrow stem cells, culminating in a treatment-resistant form of acute myelogenous leukemia. Because of the alkylating agents' effect on stem cells, they also cause irreversible infertility. Other common adverse effects include nephrotoxicity and hemorrhagic cystitis.

The several subclasses of alkylating agents include nitrogen mustard (mechlorethamine), nitrosoureas (carmustine), alkyl sulfonates (busulfan), triazines (dacarbazine), ethyleneimines (thiotepa), and cisplatin. Cisplatin is an alkylating agent containing platinum and chlorine atoms. It is most active in the G_1 subphase, but it is also not phase specific. Cisplatin binds to DNA and acts much like alkylating agents by forming intrastrand DNA crosslinks (gluing strands of DNA together so that they cannot separate). Its major toxic effect is reversible renal tubular necrosis. Cisplatin may be used alone or in combination with other chemotherapeutic drugs for testicular and ovarian cancers.

Antimetabolites. Antimetabolites, a group of somewhat diverse drugs, are phase specific, working best in the S phase and having little effect in G_0. They interfere with nucleic acid synthesis by either displacing normal metabolites at the regulatory site of a key enzyme or by substituting for a metabolite that is incorporated into DNA or RNA molecules.

Toxic effects usually do not occur until very high levels of the drug are administered. Toxicity is also more likely when the drugs accumulate in third-spaced fluid, such as pleural fluid (a characteristic that also makes them useful in treating malignant pleural effusions). Because the drug diffuses out slowly from the third-spaced fluid, exposure of the tissue to the drug is prolonged. Most toxic effects relate to rapidly proliferating cells, such as cells in the gastrointestinal tract, hair, and skin and white blood cells (WBCs). Signs and symptoms include the following:

- Nausea and vomiting
- Stomatitis
- Diarrhea
- Alopecia
- Leukopenia.

Some of the drugs can also cause liver and pulmonary toxicity.

The different types of antimetabolites include folic acid analogues (methotrexate), pyrimidine analogues (5-fluorouracil), cytosine arabinoside (ARA-C), and purine analogues (6-mercaptopurine).

Antitumor Antibiotics. Antitumor antibiotics are originally derived from natural sources that are generally too toxic to be used as antibacterial agents. They are not phase specific and act in several ways: They disrupt DNA replication and RNA transcription; create free radicals, which generate breaks in DNA and other forms of damage; and interfere with DNA repair. In addition, these drugs bind to cells and kill them, probably by damaging the cell membrane. Their main toxic effect is damage to the cardiac muscle. This limits the amount and duration of treatment. Examples of these antibiotics include actinomycin D, doxorubicin, bleomycin, mitomycin-C, and mithramycin.

Mitotic Inhibitors. Mitotic inhibitors are drugs that act to prevent cell division during the M phase. Mitotic inhibitors include the plant alkaloids and taxoids. Plant alkaloids consist of medications extracted from plant sources: Vinca alkaloids (e.g., vincristine and vinblastine) and etoposide (also called VP-16). The Vinca alkaloids are phase specific, acting during mitosis. They bind to a specific protein in tumor cells that promotes chromosome migration during mitosis and serves as a conduit for neurotransmitter transport along axons. The toxicity of these drugs is characterized by depression of deep tendon reflexes, paresthesias (pain and altered sensation), motor weakness, cranial nerve disruptions, and paralytic ileus. Etoposide acts in all phases of the cell cycle, causing breaks in DNA and metaphase arrest. Although etoposide may cause bone marrow suppression and nausea and vomiting, the most common toxic effect is hypotension resulting from too rapid intravenous administration.

The taxoids act during the G_2 phase to inhibit cell division. Paclitaxel is used for the treatment of Kaposi's sarcoma and metastatic breast and ovarian cancer. Taxotere is used for breast cancer. Toxicities associated with these drugs include alopecia, bone marrow depression, and severe hypersensitivity reactions (e.g., hypotension, dyspnea, and urticaria).

Hormones and Hormone Antagonists. The main hormones used in cancer therapy are the corticosteroids (e.g., prednisone), which are phase specific (G_1). These act by binding to specific intracellular receptors, repressing transcription of mRNA, and thereby altering cellular function and growth. Corticosteroids have multiple side effects such as impaired healing, hyperglycemia, hypertension, osteoporosis, and hirsutism.

Hormone antagonists work with hormone-binding tumors, usually those of the breast, prostate, and endometrium. They block the hormone's receptor site on the tumor and prevent it from receiving normal hormonal growth stimulation. These drugs do not cure, but do cause regression of the tumor in about 40% of breast and endometrial tumors and 80% of prostate tumors. Tamoxifen competes with estradiol receptors in breast tumors. Raloxifene blocks estrogen in the breast. Diethylstilbestrol competes with hormone receptors in endometrial and prostate tumors. Antiandrogen (flutamide) and luteinizing hormone–releasing hormone block testosterone synthesis in prostate cancers. The main side effects of these drugs are alterations of the secondary sexual characteristics.

Miscellaneous Agents. Several miscellaneous agents act at different phases in the cell cycle. L-Asparaginase and hydroxyurea are examples of miscellaneous agents.

Effects of Chemotherapeutic Drugs As described, the side effects and toxic effects of chemotherapy vary with the drug used and the length of treatment. Because most of these drugs act on fast-growing cells, the side effects are manifestations of damage to normal rapidly dividing somatic cells. The side effects of hormones express the action of the hormone used or suppression of the normal hormone, such as the masculinizing effects of male hormones administered for ovarian cancers.

Tissues usually affected by cytotoxic drugs include the following:

- Mucous membranes of the mouth, tongue, esophagus, stomach, intestine, and rectum. This may result in anorexia, loss of taste, aversion to food, erythema and painful ulcerations in any portion of the gastrointestinal tract, nausea, vomiting, and diarrhea.
- Hair cells, resulting in alopecia.
- Bone marrow depression affecting most blood cells (e.g., granulocytes, lymphocytes, thrombocytes, and erythrocytes). This results in an impaired ability to respond to infection, a diminished ability to clot blood, and severe anemia.
- Organs, such as heart, lungs, bladder, kidneys. This kind of damage is related to specific agents, such as cardiac toxicity with doxorubicin or pneumonitis with bleomycin.
- Reproductive organs, resulting in impaired reproductive ability or altered fetal development.

Table 14–10 gives the classifications of chemotherapeutic drugs, common examples, target malignancies, adverse effects and side effects, and nursing implications. Consult current pharmacology textbooks for additional drugs and for new combination therapies as they are developed.

Preparation and Administration Many states and individual hospitals require that personnel be trained and certified to administer chemotherapy. Pharmacists in large hospitals and independent home care agencies usually prepare chemotherapeutic drugs for parenteral administration under specific safety guidelines established by the federal government or the Oncology Nursing Society. In some agencies, nurses both prepare and administer these drugs. Because of the potential carcinogenic effects, it is usually recommended that the healthcare professional wear gloves, a mask, and gown while preparing and administering the drug and disposing of equipment. The nurse must use care when handling excretory products of clients undergoing chemotherapy and teach clients to dispose of their own body fluids safely. Oral medications pose a lesser risk of exposure, but a risk nonetheless, primarily through excretion in the urine.

Chemotherapeutic drugs can be administered orally, such as cyclophosphamide (Cytoxan) and chlorambucil (Leukeran). Other drugs, such as hormones or hormone-blocking agents, may also be given intramuscularly. However, many drugs require intravenous infusion or direct injection into intraperitoneal or intrapleural body cavities. Intravenous preparations can be given through large peripheral veins, but the risk of extravasation or irritation to the vein may preclude this method for

TABLE 14–10 Classifications of Chemotherapeutic Drugs

DRUG CLASSIFICATION	COMMON DRUGS	TARGET MALIGNANCIES	ADVERSE EFFECTS OR SIDE EFFECTS	NURSING IMPLICATIONS
Alkylating agents	Mechlorethamine (Mustargen)	Hodgkin's disease Lymphosarcoma Lung cancer Chronic leukemia	Nausea and vomiting Leukopenia Thrombocytopenia Hyperuricemia	Maintain good hydration. Alkalinize urine. Administer antiemetics prior to chemotherapy. Monitor WBC, uric acid. Assess for infection.
	Busulfan (Myleran)	Chronic myelogenous leukemia	Leukopenia Thrombocytopenia Renal failure Pulmonary fibrosis	Monitor WBCs, BUN. Maintain adequate fluid intake. Assess for infection. Assess lungs for fibrotic (coarse, loud) rales.
	Cyclophosphamide (Cytoxan)	Lymphomas Multiple myeloma Leukemias Adenocarcinoma of lung and breast	Hemorrhagic cystitis Renal failure Alopecia Stomatitis Liver dysfunction	Encourage daily fluid intake of 2 to 3 L during treatment. Monitor WBCs, BUN, liver enzymes. Teach ways to manage hair loss.
Antimetabolites	Methotrexate	Acute lymphoblastic leukemia Osteosarcoma Gestational trophoblastic carcinoma	Oral and gastrointestinal ulcerations Anorexia and nausea Leukopenia Thrombocytopenia Pancytopenia	Monitor CBC, WBC differential, BUN, uric acid, creatinine. Assess oral mucous membranes; treat ulcers prn. Assess for infection, bleeding.
	5-Fluorouracil (5-FU)	Colon carcinoma Rectal carcinoma Breast carcinoma Gastric carcinoma Pancreatic cancer	Stomatitis Alopecia Nausea and vomiting Gastritis Enteritis Diarrhea Anemia Leukopenia Thrombocytopenia	Monitor CBC with differential, BUN, uric acid. Administer antiemetics prn. Assess for bleeding; check stool occult blood. Evaluate hydration and nutrition status. Teach oral care for stomatitis. Assess for infection. Teach care for hair loss.
Antitumor antibiotics	Doxorubicin (Adriamycin)	Acute lymphoblastic leukemia (ALL) Acute myeloblastic leukemia Neuroblastoma Wilms' tumor Breast, ovarian, thyroid, lung cancer	Stomatitis Alopecia Nausea and vomiting Gastritis Enteritis Diarrhea Anemia Leukopenia Thrombocytopenia Cardiac toxicity	Monitor ECG; assess for arrhythmias, gallops, and congestive heart failure (CHF). Monitor CBC with differential, BUN, uric acid. Administer antiemetics prn. Assess for bleeding; check stool for occult blood. Evaluate hydration and nutrition status. Teach oral care for stomatitis. Assess for infection. Teach care for hair loss.

TABLE 14–10 **Classifications of Chemotherapeutic Drugs (continued)**

DRUG CLASSIFICATION	COMMON DRUGS	TARGET MALIGNANCIES	ADVERSE EFFECTS OR SIDE EFFECTS	NURSING IMPLICATIONS
	Bleomycin (Blenoxane)	Squamous cell carcinoma Lymphosarcoma Reticulum cell sarcoma Testicular carcinoma Hodgkin's disease	Mucocutaneous ulcerations Alopecia Nausea and vomiting Chills and fever Pneumonitis and pulmonary fibrosis	Check for fever 3 to 6 hours after administration. Have chest x-ray films taken every 2 to 3 weeks. Assess respiratory status, and check for coarse rales. Evaluate hydration and nutrition status. Teach oral care for stomatitis. Assess for infection. Teach care for hair loss.
Plant alkaloids	Vincristine (Oncovin)	Combination therapy for acute leukemia, Hodgkin's and non-Hodgkin's lymphomas, rhabdomyosarcoma, neuroblastoma, Wilms' tumor	Areflexia Muscle weakness Peripheral neuritis Constipation Paralytic ileus Mild bone marrow Depression	Assess neuromuscular function. Monitor CBC with differential. Evaluate gastrointestinal function. Manage constipation.
	Vinblastine (Velban)	Combination therapy for Hodgkin's disease, lymphocytic and histocytic lymphoma Kaposi's sarcoma, advanced testicular carcinoma, unresponsive breast cancer	Areflexia Alopecia Nausea and vomiting Bone marrow depression	Assess neuromuscular function. Monitor CBC with differential. Administer antiemetics prn. Teach ways to manage hair loss.
	Etoposide, also called VP-16 (VePesid)	Nonresponsive testicular tumors Small-cell lung cancer	Alopecia Hypotension with rapid infusion	Hydrate adequately before administration. Administer for 60 minutes. Monitor vital signs every 15 minutes during administration and every 2 to 4 hours thereafter. Teach ways to manage hair loss.
	Prednisone	Combination therapy for many tumors Leukemia Lymphoma	Fluid retention Hypertension Steroid diabetes Emotional lability Silent bleeding ulcers Increased risk for infection	Monitor vital signs. Administer diuretics prn. Check blood glucose regularly. Evaluate mental status. Administer oral medications with food. Administer hydrogen ion antagonist drugs (antacids) as ordered. Monitor WBC with differential. Check for signs of systemic infection.
	Diethylstilbestrol (DES)	Advanced breast and prostrate cancers	Fluid retention Feminization Uterine bleeding	Monitor vital signs. Administer diuretics prn as ordered. Explain reason for feminization to men, bleeding to women. Monitor for excessive bleeding.

(continued)

TABLE 14–10 Classifications of Chemotherapeutic Drugs (continued)

DRUG CLASSIFICATION	COMMON DRUGS	TARGET MALIGNANCIES	ADVERSE EFFECTS OR SIDE EFFECTS	NURSING IMPLICATIONS
Plant alkaloids *continued*	Tamoxifen (Nolvadex)	Breast cancer	Hot flashes Nausea and vomiting	Teach ways to manage hot flashes. Explain reason for hot flashes. Administer antiemetics as ordered.
Miscellaneous drugs	Cisplatin (CDDP) (Platinol)	Combination and single therapy for metastatic testicular and ovarian cancers, advanced bladder cancer, head and neck tumors, non–small-cell lung carcinoma, osteogenic sarcoma, neuroblastoma	Bone marrow depression: leukopenia and thrombocytopenia Renal tubular damage Deafness	Monitor WBC with differential and platelets, BUN, creatinine, uric acid. Watch for bleeding. Monitor for signs of infection. Evaluate hearing; check for tinnitus. Ensure that client is well hydrated before drug is administered. Encourage 2 to 3 L of fluid intake daily.

long-term therapy. Many clients now receive vascular access devices (VADs), especially if their treatment requires several cycles over weeks or months. VADs are also useful for adjunctive parenteral nutrition in the client who needs continuous intravenous infusions to manage pain or frequent blood drawing to monitor blood counts. Different types of VADs are available:

- Catheters that are inserted nonsurgically by threading them through a large peripheral vein into the vena cava. Called peripherally inserted central catheters (PICCs), they have multiple lumens that facilitate blood drawing. Placement is usually monitored by fluoroscopy.
- Catheters tunneled under the skin on the chest into a major vein, such as the subclavian vein. Hickman or Groshong catheters may be used.
- Surgically implanted ports, which are placed under the skin with a connected catheter inserted into a major vein. These are accessed by means of a special needle with a 90-degree angle inserted through the skin directly into the rubber dome of the port, which has a hard plastic back to prevent tissue damage. Figure 14–6 ■ shows examples of different catheters and vascular access ports.

Risk of infection, catheter obstruction, and extravasation are the main problems associated with VADs. Nurses therefore must teach clients and family members to observe for redness, swelling, pain, or exudate at the insertion site, which may indicate infection; to observe for swelling of the neck or skin near the VAD for extravasation and infiltration; and to flush catheters and provide site care (cleaning and dressing changes) on a regular basis. During each encounter with the client, the nurse always inspects the site; observes for infection, infiltration, and catheter occlusion; and provides site care when necessary.

Management of Clients Receiving Chemotherapy In addition to providing the above nursing interventions, nurses help identify and manage toxic effects or side effects of the drugs and provide psychosocial support. Careful assessment and monitoring of the client's signs and symptoms, including appropriate laboratory tests, alert the nurse to the onset of toxicity. Nausea and vomiting, diarrhea, inflammation and ulceration of oral mucous membranes, hair loss, skin changes, anorexia, and fatigue require specific medical and nursing actions. These actions are discussed later in this chapter under the appropriate nursing diagnoses. Indicators of organ toxicities, such as nephrotoxicity, neurotoxicity, or cardiac toxicity, must be reported immediately to the physician. Another aspect of managing clients undergoing chemotherapy is to teach them how to care for access sites and to dispose of used equipment and excretions safely. Nurses also teach clients to increase fluid intake to flush out the drugs; to get extra rest, which can both assist therapy and help the client avoid other illnesses; to identify major complications of their particular drug protocol; to know when to call the physician or emergency medical services; and, if their WBC count is low, to limit their exposure to other people, especially children or those with infections.

During chemotherapy, a number of psychologic issues that can cause moderate to severe emotional distress may arise. The need to plan activities around chemotherapy treatments and their side effects can impair the client's ability to work, manage a household or care for family members, function sexually, or participate in social and recreational activities. Weight loss and alopecia may prompt feelings of powerlessness and depression. The nurse can assist by carefully evaluating symptoms, providing specific interventions as indicated, and allowing clients

Figure 14-6 ■ Vascular access devices. *A,* Single- and double-lumen catheters. *B,* Triple-lumen and Groshong catheters.

Source: Photos A, B: Courtesy of Bard Access Systems, Salt Lake City, UT; Photo C, S/MS Deltec, Inc., St. Paul, MN; Photo D, Norfolk Medical, Skokie, IL.

opportunities to express their fears, concerns, and feelings. Clients should be encouraged to participate in their care and maintain control over their life as much as possible (McDaniel & Rhodes, 1998). Specific interventions will be discussed later in the chapter under the appropriate nursing diagnoses. Table 14–10 includes nursing implications for specific adverse effects of common chemotherapy drugs.

RADIATION THERAPY Still the treatment of choice for some tumors or by some oncologists, radiation may be used to kill the tumor, to reduce its size, to decrease pain, or to relieve obstruction. Lymph nodes and adjacent tissues are irradiated when beginning metastasis is suspected. **Radiation therapy** consists of delivering ionizing radiations of gamma and x-rays in one of two ways:

- *Teletherapy.* Also called external radiation, teletherapy involves delivery of radiation from a source at some distance from the client. A relatively uniform dosage is delivered to the tumor.
- *Brachytherapy.* In brachytherapy, the radioactive material is placed directly into or adjacent to the tumor, a technique that delivers a high dose to the tumor and a lower dose to the normal tissues. This allows delivery of high doses of radiation to the tumor while sparing adjacent tissue. Brachytherapy is also referred to as internal, interstitial, or intracavitary radiation.

For many common neoplasms, a combination of these two therapies is used.

Lethal injury to DNA is believed to be the primary mechanism by which radiation kills cells, especially cells in faster growing tumors and tissues. As a result, when given over time, radiation can destroy not only rapidly multiplying cancer cells but also rapidly dividing normal cells, such as those of the skin and mucous membranes. A malignant tumor is considered cured when there are no surviving tumor stem cells. The goal

of radiation therapy is to achieve maximum tumor control with a minimum of damage to normal tissue.

Implanted or ingested radiation can be dangerous for those living with, taking care of, or treating the client. Caregivers must use protection by, for example, shielding themselves from the source of radiation, limiting the time of exposure to the client, increasing the distance from the client, and using specific safety procedures for handling secretions. Box 14–6 identifies safety principles to be followed by those caring for clients undergoing internal radiation.

Tumors have differing sensitivities to radiation. Tumors that have the greatest number of rapidly proliferating cancer cells usually exhibit the best early response to radiation. The decision to use radiation rather than other modalities is based on balancing the probability of controlling the tumor against the probability of causing complications, such as tissue damage. The decision is usually made by risk–benefit analysis. Planning for radiation therapy includes assessing the disease site, tumor size, and histologic findings. Treatment schedules vary based on these factors (Neal & Hoskin, 1997). Box 14–7 lists the degree of radiosensitivity for selected cancers.

The client receiving external radiation may experience skin changes such as blanching, erythema, desquamation, sloughing, or hemorrhage. Ulcerations of mucous membranes may cause severe pain; in addition, oral secretions can decrease, making the client more vulnerable to infection and dental caries. Gastrointestinal effects include nausea and vomiting, diarrhea, or bleeding. Lungs may develop interstitial exudate, a condition called radiation pneumonia. Occasionally, external radiation therapy may cause fistulas or necrosis of adjacent tissues. Implanted radioactive materials can lead to similar problems; moreover, the excretory products of these clients are usually considered dangerous and need special disposal. See the Nursing Care box on page 397 for nursing implications for clients receiving radiation therapy.

BOX 14–6 Safety Principles for Radiation

These recommendations apply to caregivers working with clients receiving internal radiation (brachytherapy).

- Maintain the greatest possible distance from the source of radiation.
- Spend the minimum amount of time close to the radiation source.
- Shield yourself from the radiation with lead gloves and aprons when possible.
- If pregnant, avoid contact with radiation sources.
- If you work routinely near radiation, wear a monitoring device to measure whole-body exposure.
- Avoid direct exposure with radioisotope containers; for example, do not touch the container.
- Keep clients with implanted radioisotopes in a private room with private bath and as far away from other hospitalized persons as possible.
- Dispose of body fluids of clients with unsealed implanted radioisotopes with special care and in specially marked containers.
- Handle bed linen and clothing with care and according to agency protocol.
- Use long-handled forceps to place any dislodged implants into a lead container.
- Consult with the radiation therapy department for any questions or problems in caring for clients with radioactive implants.

BIOTHERAPY **Biotherapy** modifies the biologic processes that result in malignant cells, primarily through enhancing the person's own immune responses. The development of this therapy was based on the immune surveillance hypothesis. Although it has been established that a competent immune system is the body's most important defense against any disease, the role that various immune cells play in combating different types of ma-

BOX 14–7 Degree of Radiosensitivity for Selected Cancers

Very Radiosensitive
- Neuroblastoma
- Lymphomas
- Chronic leukemia

Moderately Radiosensitive
- Bronchogenic carcinoma
- Esophageal carcinoma
- Squamous cell carcinoma
- Prostate carcinoma
- Cervical carcinoma
- Testicular carcinoma

Nonradiosensitive
- Many adenocarcinomas
- Fibrosarcoma
- Osteogenic carcinoma

lignancies continues to be investigated. Currently, biotherapy is used for both hematologic malignancies, such as lymphoma and hairy-cell leukemia, and solid tumors, such as renal cancer and melanoma.

Tumor immunology has the following applications: detection screening in high-risk groups, differential diagnosis and classification of tumor cells, monitoring the course of the disease with early detection of recurrence, and active therapies to halt or limit the disease. The theory underlying tumor immunology is that most tumor cells have a structural appearance recognizable by the immune cells. Tumor-associated antigens exist on tumor cells but not on normal cells. TAAs elicit an immune response that, in a person with a competent immune system, destroys or inhibits tumor growth. Thus, TAAs can be isolated from serum and used for both diagnosis and various treatment modalities. The PSA is one such TAA currently in successful diagnostic use.

Tumor cells are often in a stage of arrested development (i.e., in the differentiation stage) for the cell type they represent; thus, they express antigens characteristic of that particular stage of development. The immaturity of the cells provides the physician with information about the relative aggressiveness of the cancer.

Another aspect of immunotherapy is the development of monoclonal antibodies that enhance the immune system's ability to fight the cancer. Monoclonal antibodies are developed by inoculating an animal with the tumor antigen and recovering the specific antibodies produced. The antibodies are then given to the person with that cancer to assist in the destruction of the tumor. Monoclonal antibodies are also re-created, or cloned, in the genetic laboratory by recombining DNA to produce the specific antibody. Techniques involving recombinant DNA have been used to combine these antibodies with toxins and drugs that are then delivered selectively to the tumor sites.

A number of cytokines (normal growth-regulating molecules) with antitumor activity have been synthesized. Alpha interferon (IFN-α), bacillus Calmette-Guérin (BCG, which has been used for many years as an inoculation against tuberculosis), and interleukin-2 (IL-2) have shown some therapeutic benefit in eliciting increased immune responses. Combination strategies have also helped stimulate the function of macrophages.

A most promising discovery has been the recently identified natural killer (NK) cells. These cells are like large granular lymphocytes, but have a cell surface phenotype different from that of T lymphocytes or macrophages. They have demonstrated a spontaneous cytotoxic effect on some types of cancer cells. They also provide a strong resistance to metastasis and secrete cytokines. When augmented by biologic response modifiers such as IL-2, they show increased tumor destructive activity (Battiato & Wheeler, 2000).

The use of hematopoietic growth factors (HGF) has been one of the most successful in biotherapy. HGF, such as granulocyte colony-stimulating factor and erythropoietin, offsets the suppression of granulocytes and erythrocytes that results from chemotherapy (Battiato & Wheeler, 2000).

Since the early 1990s, the combination of cytokines, particularly IFN-α and IL-2, with chemotherapy has been used in

NURSING CARE OF THE CLIENT Receiving Radiation Therapy

NURSING RESPONSIBILITIES FOR EITHER EXTERNAL OR INTERNAL RADIATION THERAPY

- Carefully assess and manage any complications, usually in collaboration with the radiation oncologist.
- Assist in documenting the results of the therapy; for example, clients receiving radiation for metastases to the spine will show improved neurologic functioning as tumor size diminishes.
- Provide emotional support, relief of physical and psychologic discomfort, and opportunities to talk about fears and concerns. For some clients, radiation therapy is a last chance for cure or even just for relief of physical discomfort.

EXTERNAL RADIATION

Prior to the start of treatments, the treatment area will be specifically located by the radiation oncologist and marked with colored semipermanent ink or tattoos. Treatment is usually given 5 days per week for 15 to 30 minutes per day over 2 to 7 weeks.

Nursing Responsibilities

- Monitor for adverse effects: skin changes, such as blanching, erythema, desquamation, sloughing, or hemorrhage; ulcerations of mucous membranes; nausea and vomiting, diarrhea, or gastrointestinal bleeding.
- Assess lungs for rales, which may indicate interstitial exudate. Observe for any dyspnea or changes in respiratory pattern.
- Identify and record any medications that the client will be taking during the radiation treatment.
- Monitor white blood cell counts and platelet counts for significant decreases.

Health Education for the Client and Family

- Wash the skin that is marked as the radiation site only with plain water, no soap; do not apply deodorant, lotions, medications, perfume, or talcum powder to the site during the treatment period. Take care not to wash off the treatment marks.
- Do not rub, scratch, or scrub treated skin areas. If necessary, use only an electric razor to shave the treated area.
- Apply neither heat nor cold (e.g., heating pad or ice pack) to the treatment site.
- Inspect the skin for damage or serious changes, and report these to the radiologist or physician.

- Wear loose, soft clothing over the treated area.
- Protect skin from sun exposure during treatment and for at least 1 year after radiation therapy is discontinued. Cover skin with protective clothing during treatment; once radiation is discontinued, use sun-blocking agents with a sun protection factor (SPF) of at least 15.
- External radiation poses no risk to other people for radiation exposure, even with intimate physical contact.
- Be sure to get plenty of rest and eat a balanced diet.

INTERNAL RADIATION

The radiation source, called an implant, is placed into the affected tissue or body cavity and is sealed in tubes, containers, wires, seeds, capsules, or needles. An implant may be temporary or permanent. Internal radiation may also be ingested or injected as a solution into the bloodstream or a body cavity or be introduced into the tumor through a catheter. The radioactive substance may transmit rays outside the body or be excreted in body fluids.

Nursing Responsibilities

- Place the client in a private room.
- Limit visits to 10 to 30 minutes, and have visitors sit at least 6 feet from the client.
- Monitor for side effects such as burning sensations, excessive perspiration, chills and fever, nausea and vomiting, or diarrhea.
- Assess for fistulas or necrosis of adjacent tissues.

Health Education for the Client and Family

- While a temporary implant is in place, stay in bed and rest quietly to avoid dislodging the implant.
- For outpatient treatments, avoid close contact with others until treatment has been discontinued.
- If the radiologist indicates the need for such measures, dispose of excretory materials in special containers or in a toilet not used by others.
- Carry out daily activities as able; get extra rest if feeling fatigued.
- Eat a balanced diet; frequent, small meals often are better tolerated.
- Contact the nurse or physician for any concerns or questions after discharge.

---

metastatic melanoma patients with promising results. Such a combination is referred to as either biochemotherapy or chemoimmunotherapy (Anderson et al., 1998; Cohen & Falkson, 1998; Legha et al., 1998). The rationale for biochemotherapy is based on the independent antitumor activity of both IFN-α and IL-2 against melanoma and their lack of cross-resistance with cytotoxic chemotherapy. Although the precise mechanism of antitumor effect of biochemotherapy regimens is less understood, two hypotheses have been proposed: (1) Chemotherapy enhances the antitumor effect of biologic agents and; (2) the biologic agents enhance the antitumor cytotoxic effect of chemotherapy (Anderson et al., 1998; Legha et al., 1998).

As promising as these biotherapies or biochemotherapies are, they are accompanied by serious side effects and toxicities

(Fu et al., 2002; Legha et al., 1998). IL-2 can cause acute alterations in renal, cardiac, liver, gastrointestinal, and mental functioning. IFN-α causes mental slowing, confusion, and lethargy and, when used in combination with 5-fluorouracil or IL-2, severe flulike symptoms—chills and fever of 103° to 106°F (39.4° to 41.1°C), nausea, vomiting, diarrhea, anorexia, severe fatigue, and stomatitis—may result. The toxic effects are probably exaggerations of the normal systemic effects that these substances cause when fighting infection. For example, IL-2 is known to raise body temperature substantially in an attempt to create a hostile environment for foreign invaders.

The Nursing Care box on the following page discusses nursing implications for clients receiving immunotherapy. For nursing care of specific problems, refer to the appropriate nursing diagnoses later in this chapter.

NURSING CARE OF THE CLIENT Receiving Immunotherapy

Immunotherapy can consist of various substances used alone, such as IL-2, or combination biotherapy, such as IFN-α with 5-fluorouracil. The nurse's role is to enhance the client's quality of life.

Nursing Responsibilities
- Monitor for side effects: IFN-α may cause mental slowing, confusion, and lethargy; combination therapy of 5-fluorouracil or IL-2 and IFN-α may cause severe flulike symptoms, with chills and fever of 103° to 106°F (39.4° to 41.1°C), nausea, vomiting, diarrhea, anorexia, severe fatigue, and stomatitis; erythropoietin may cause acute hypertension.
- Monitor enzymes and other appropriate biochemical indicators for acute alterations in renal, cardiac, liver, or gastrointestinal functioning, which can be side effects of IL-2.
- Evaluate response to therapy by conducting a thorough evaluation of clients' symptoms.
- Assess clients' coping behaviors and teach new strategies as needed.

- Manage fatigue and depression.
- Encourage self-care and participation in decision making.
- Provide close supervision for clients with altered mental functioning, either by caretakers or frequent nursing visits to the client's home.
- If client is unable to manage alone, teach medication administration and care of equipment to caregivers.

Health Education for the Client and Family
- Minimize symptoms by managing fever and flulike symptoms: increase fluid intake, take analgesic and antipyretic medications, and maintain bed rest until symptoms abate.
- Seek help for serious problems not managed by usual means, such as dehydration from diarrhea.
- Use correct techniques for providing subcutaneous injections.
- Identify how to work and care for ambulatory pumps when medication is administered through an intercatheter or vascular access device.

PHOTODYNAMIC THERAPY Photodynamic therapy is a method of treating certain kinds of superficial tumors. It is known by several different names: phototherapy, photoradiation, and photochemotherapy. Clients suffering from tumors growing on the surface of the bladder, peritoneal cavity, chest wall, pleura, bronchus, or head and neck are candidates for this treatment. The client is given an intravenous dose of a photosensitizing compound, Photofrin, which is selectively retained in higher concentrations in malignant tissue. This drug is activated by a laser treatment that is started 3 days after the drug injection and administered for 3 days. The drug interacts with oxygen molecules in the tissue to produce a cytotoxic oxygen molecule called singlet oxygen.

At the time of the first intravenous injection, clients are observed for adverse hypersensitivity reactions, such as nausea, chills, and hives. Systemic or long-term toxicities are rare. The main side effects are local skin reactions and temporary photosensitivity, transiently elevated liver enzymes, and inflammatory responses of the tissues being treated, such as peritoneal or pleural tissues. This treatment has been used successfully with early-stage lung cancer with response rates as high as 90% (Bruce, 2001).

The major nursing responsibilities associated with photodynamic therapy are to address the client and family's anxiety about undergoing a relatively new treatment procedure and to educate them in managing side effects. The drug remains in the subcutaneous tissues for 4 to 6 weeks after injection. Any direct or indirect exposure to the sun activates the drug, resulting in a chemical sunburn. Clients are taught to protect themselves from sunlight (even on cloudy days) by covering themselves from head to toe in opaque clothing, including a wide-brimmed hat, gloves, shoes and stockings, and sunglasses with 100% ultraviolet block. Long-term care of treated skin includes moisturizing lotions and protection from trauma or irritation.

BONE MARROW AND PERIPHERAL BLOOD STEM CELL TRANSPLANTATIONS Bone marrow transplantation (BMT) is an accepted treatment to stimulate a nonfunctioning marrow or to replace marrow. BMT is given as an intravenous infusion of bone marrow cells from donor to client. Most commonly used in leukemias, this therapy is being expanded to include treatment of other cancers including melanoma and testicular cancer. Chapter 34 ∞ provides an in-depth discussion of this procedure. Peripheral blood stem cell transplantation (PBSCT) is the process of removing circulating stem cells from the peripheral blood through apheresis and returning these cells to the patient after dose-intensive chemotherapy. PBSCT has fewer side effects, shorter hospitalization, and decreased cost compared to BMT.

COMPLEMENTARY THERAPIES Although advances in cancer treatment have increased 5-year survival rates, the uncertainty of cure of cancer and cancer reoccurrence often compels some clients to look for complementary therapies. It is estimated that approximately 30% to 50% of patients with cancer may have had the experience of using some kind of complementary therapy. Complementary therapies refer to therapies that clients choose as a complement to medical treatment. Common complementary therapies for cancer can be categorized into botanical agents, nutritional supplements, dietary regimens, mind–body modalities, energy healing, spiritual approaches, and miscellaneous therapies. Box 14–8 provides detailed information about complementary therapies.

To provide sensitive nursing care, nurses should be knowledgeable about common complementary therapies. Note that only half of the nation's state boards of nursing recognize selected complementary therapies as part of practice and approve safe delivery of those complementary therapies by registered nurses (Sparber, 2001). Nurses should use ethical principles of

BOX 14–8 Common Complementary Therapies for Cancer

TYPE	DESCRIPTION
Botanical agents	Herbs are believed to be the most "natural" and "safe" plants ingested with the hope for a cure of cancer. Commonly used botanical agents include echinacea, Essiac, ginseng, green tea, pau d'arco, and Hoxsey. The safety for many of these botanical agents has not been proven, especially as a complement to medical treatment.
Nutritional supplements	Chemical compounds include vitamins, minerals, enzymes, amino acids, and essential fatty acids, or proteins (such as shark cartilage). They are believed to have the ability to promote health and to help cure cancer. The safety of certain compounds such as vitamins has been established; however, in megadoses, many of the compounds can be toxic and have potential interactions with some therapeutic agents used for cancer such as chemotherapy.
Dietary regimens	The ingestion of only natural substances is believed to have the effect of purifying the body and slowing down the growth of cancer. Popular regimens include the grape diet, the carrot juice diet, and garlic, onions, and liver intake. However, the effectiveness of these dietary regimens remains to be established.
Mind–body modalities	The harmony of mind and body are believed to facilitate physiologic and psychologic healing. Such modalities include relaxation, meditation, or imagery. Recent research has shown that these modalities helped individuals with cancer adjust to the experience of cancer.
Energy healing	The human body is believed to be an energy field and cancer might be the result of a disturbed energy field. Energy therapies, such as therapeutic touch and healing touch, can affect the energy field of the human body and promote physiologic healing. Therapeutic touch uses the hands on or near the body with the intent to promote healing. Healing touch uses energy healing techniques to heal by restoring the harmony and balance of the body. Clinical practice and research on energy healing have shown positive findings of energy healing in a variety of patients.
Spiritual approaches	Faith in God or a higher power of the universe is believed to help cancer healing. Spiritual approaches include faith healing, prayer to God, prayer groups, and chain prayer. Research has shown that faith in God or a higher power also helped individuals with cancer to adjust to the experience of cancer.
Miscellaneous therapies	Aromatherapy has been used for clients with cancer to relieve nausea, vomiting, or retching and to decrease anxiety. However, aromatherapy might not be appropriate for clients who are highly sensitive to strong fragrance. Music, art, and humor therapies have also been used to help clients with cancer to reduce anxiety, to express feeling of loss, and to promote optimism.

autonomy, beneficence, nonmaleficence, and justice to guide their professional practice and care for clients who choose to use complementary therapies. It is also important for nurses to provide truthful, nonjudgmental responses to the questions or inquiries about complementary therapies from clients with cancer. Nurses should encourage clients to report the use of any complementary therapies to their oncologist to prevent potential interactions of the complementary therapies with their medical treatment.

Pain Management

Pain management is an important component of oncology care and is considered a crucial part of the collaborative treatment plan. It is estimated that 20% to 50% of clients with early-stage cancer and up to 95% of clients with advanced cancer experience pain that requires analgesia (Cady, 2001). There are three main categories of pain syndromes in clients with cancer, and the category influences the type of treatment:

- *Pain associated with direct tumor involvement.* The most common causes are metastases to bone, nerve compression or infiltration, and involvement of hollow visceral organs.
- *Pain associated with treatment.* This may include postsurgical incisional or wound pain; peripheral neuropathy, ulceration of

mucous membranes, and pain from herpes zoster outbreaks secondary to chemotherapy; and pain in nerve plexuses, muscles, and peripheral nerves from radiation therapy.

- *Pain from a cause not related to either the cancer or therapy,* such as diabetic neuropathy.

The goal of pain therapy is to provide relief that allows clients to function as they wish and, in the case of terminally ill clients, to die relatively free of pain. Drug therapy with opioid and nonopioid analgesics as well as adjuvant medications (those that enhance the effect of the analgesic) is the basis of most physician-guided pain management. Other therapies include injection of anesthetic drugs into spinal cord or specific nerve plexuses, surgical severing of nerves, radiation to reduce tumor size and pressure, and behavioral approaches. Pharmacologic pain management follows these steps:

1. Conduct careful initial and ongoing assessment of the pain.
2. Evaluate the client's functional goals.
3. Establish a plan with combinations of nonnarcotic drugs (such as aspirin or ibuprofen) with adjuvants (such as corticosteroids or antidepressants).
4. Evaluate the degree of pain relief.

MediaLink Case Study: Pain Management

5. Progress to stronger drugs as needed, from mild narcotics such as oxycodone (Percodan) or propoxyphene (Darvon) to strong narcotics such as morphine or hydromorphone (Dilaudid), and monitor side effects.

6. Continue to try combinations and escalate dosages until maximal pain relief balanced with client's need to function is achieved.

Medication usually is administered by the oral route as long as this route continues to be effective. Medication is given on a regular time schedule (e.g., every 4 hours) with additional medication prescribed to cover breakthrough pain. When the oral route alone becomes inadequate, the primary narcotic can be administered intramuscularly, subcutaneously, or rectally on an intermittent schedule or continuously by transdermal patches or intravenously by a continuous drip, usually controlled by an infusion pump. Some newer pumps are portable, deliver medication continuously, and allow clients to control their breakthrough pain with a limited number of boluses. When narcotic doses are increased gradually, there is no limit to the amount the client can receive, as long as adverse reactions can be managed. Clients have received up to 4800 mg daily (200 mg per hour) of morphine sulfate with up to six 200- to 400-mg breakthrough doses daily without major ill effects and with good pain control. The body develops tolerance to the sedative after a short period, and most clients are able to tolerate the level of medication needed to control the pain. Other side effects, such as constipation, nausea and vomiting, and itching, can be managed through the usual means and are discussed under the appropriate nursing diagnoses. If the client has persistent untoward side effects that do not respond to treatment, or if the client does not get adequate relief from the narcotic, different narcotics and combinations are tried. Morphine sulfate and transdermal fentanyl are the most commonly used drugs for relief of cancer pain (Ferrell & McCaffery, 1997).

Clients receiving high-dose narcotics should not have the medication abruptly stopped, because withdrawal symptoms will occur. If the drug needs to be stopped, it must be tapered gradually. For more information on pain management, and on alternative therapies in particular, see Chapter 9 ∞.

NURSING CARE

Nurses face a major challenge in educating clients about preventive measures and lifestyle changes to reduce the risk of cancer. At the same time, clients with cancer must be reassured that they are not responsible for having acquired cancer.

Once a cancer diagnosis is established, nurses help clients recover and support them during the rehabilitation phase. In cases of terminal cancer, nurses provide comfort and facilitate positive growth for the client and significant others.

Health Promotion

Early detection and treatment are considered the most important factors influencing the prognosis of those who have can-

cer. However, many people do not seek early diagnosis and treatment because of denial, fear and anxiety, stigma, or the absence of specific early signs such as pain or weight loss (which usually are late signs). For this reason, screening procedures such as mammograms, PSA, occult blood stool tests, and sigmoidoscopy may be lifesaving.

The American Cancer Society promotes early cancer detection through promotion of cancer awareness and guidelines for screening procedures. Although no longer in use by the ACS, the CAUTION model (Box 14–9) is helpful in promoting awareness of common symptoms that may indicate cancer. This model encourages people to seek medical attention when they discover signs and symptoms characteristic of cancer. For people without symptoms, the ACS recommends incorporating a cancer checkup into periodic health examinations. This general cancer checkup includes health counseling, teaching self-examination techniques when appropriate, and, depending on age and gender, examination for cancers of the thyroid, oral cavity, skin, lymph nodes, testes, and ovaries (ACS, 2006a).

If a person is at special risk due to heredity, environment, occupation, or lifestyle, special tests or more frequent examinations may be necessary. A routine cancer checkup should include counseling to improve health behaviors and physical examination with related tests of the breast, uterus, cervix, colon, rectum, testes, prostate, skin, thyroid, and lymph nodes. Box 14–10 lists the tests recommended for a cancer checkup. Nurses have a special role in public education and should encourage all with whom they come into contact to schedule cancer checkups. Nurses must be familiar with the ACS guidelines so that they can advise clients, their families, and significant others.

Assessment

Focused Interview

During this initial phase of the nursing process, collect the following significant data about the client:

- History of the client's disease, including the signs and symptoms that led the client to seek health care
- Other concurrent diseases, such as diabetes

BOX 14–9 American Cancer Society CAUTION Model: Seven Warning Signs of Cancer

Change in bowel or bladder habits
A sore that does not heal
Unusual bleeding or discharge
Thickening or lump in breast or elsewhere
Indigestion or difficulty swallowing
Obvious change in wart or mole
Nagging cough or hoarseness
　　　　If you have a warning signal, see your doctor!

Source: American Cancer Society.

BOX 14–10 American Cancer Society Guidelines for Cancer Screening

Breast Cancer
- Routine breast self-examination starting at age 20, prompt reporting of any change in breast tissue to healthcare provider
- Clinical breast examination every 3 years from ages 20 to 39 and yearly thereafter
- Annual screening mammography starting at age 40; women at increased risk may have more frequent mammography or other tests such as breast ultrasound exams

Colon and Rectum
Beginning at age 50, a combination of the following exams:
- Annual fecal occult blood test or fecal immunochemical test
- Flexible sigmoidoscopy every 5 years
- Colonoscopy every 10 years
- Double-contrast barium enema every 5 years

Cervix/Uterus
- Pelvic examination and Pap test every 2 years for sexually active girls and any woman over 18; less often for women with three consecutive negative results, more frequently if certain risk factors are present; women over age 70 who have had three or more consecutive normal Pap tests in previous 10 years may stop screening exams
- At age 35, women with risk for hereditary nonpolyposis colon cancer should be offered annual endometrial biopsy to screen for endometrial cancer

Prostate
Beginning at age 50; age 45 for African American men and those with a strong family history:
- Annual digital rectal exam
- PSA test

Source: American Cancer Society, 2006a.

BOX 14–11 Two Scales of Functional Status for Cancer Clients

Karnofsky Scale: Criteria of Performance Status (PS)
- 100 Normal; no complaints; no evidence of disease.
- 90 Able to carry on normal activity; minor signs or symptoms of disease.
- 80 Able to carry on normal activity with effort; some signs or symptoms of disease.
- 70 Cares for self; unable to carry on normal activity or to do active work.
- 60 Requires occasional assistance but is able to care for most of own needs.
- 50 Requires considerable assistance and frequent medical care.
- 40 Disabled; requires special care and assistance.
- 30 Severely disabled; hospitalization indicated, although death not imminent.
- 20 Very sick; hospitalization necessary; active supportive treatment necessary.
- 10 Moribund; fatal processes progressing rapidly.
- 0 Dead.

Eastern Cooperative Oncology Group Scale (ECOG)
- 0 Fully active, able to carry on all predisease activities without restriction. (Karnofsky 90 to 100)
- 1 Restricted in physically strenuous activity, but ambulatory and able to carry out work of a light or sedentary nature, for example, light housework or office work. (Karnofsky 70 to 80)
- 2 Ambulatory and capable of all self-care, but unable to carry out work activities. Up and about more than 50% of waking hours. (Karnofsky 50 to 60)
- 3 Capable of only limited self-care, confined to bed or chair 50% or more of waking hours. (Karnofsky 30 to 40)
- 4 Completely disabled, cannot carry out any self-care, totally confined to bed or chair. (Karnofsky 10 to 20)

Source: "Nitrogen Mustards in the Palliative Treatment of Carcinoma" by D. A. Karnofsky, L. Craver, & J. Burchenal, 1948. *Cancer 1*, pp. 634–656. Copyright © American Cancer Society. Reprinted by permission of Wiley-CISS, Inc. a subsidiary of John Wiley & Sons.

- Current physical or psychologic problems resulting from the cancer, such as pain or depression
- Understanding of the treatment plan
- Expectations of the treatment plan
- Functional limitations due to illness or treatment (Box 14–11)
- Effect of the disease on current lifestyle
- Reliable support systems or caretakers for the client
- Coping strategies and how well they are working.

INTERVIEW QUESTIONS The following are appropriate questions to ask the client during the initial interview and at subsequent assessments:
- "What brought you in to see the doctor?" Asking this question allows clients to tell their story in their own way, which may elicit more information than asking specific questions. The answer should elicit not only data about the signs and symptoms but also fears or concerns. If the cancer was discovered during a routine physical examination or checkup, the client may have some difficulty accepting the disease, especially if there were no symptoms. For clients who offer insufficient information in response to this open-ended ques-

tion, more specific questions may be necessary, such as "Did you have pain or any specific physical problems that caused you to seek health care?"
- "Do you have any other medical conditions or problems that are troubling you at this time?" It may be necessary to ask about specific diseases to help the client focus. For example, "Do you have high blood pressure?" or "Are you having any problems with your lungs?" Information gained from these questions can help you anticipate problems and formulate potential nursing diagnoses related to other diseases that may interact with the cancer.
- "What kinds of physical problems are you having at this time? Do you have pain? Are you nauseated? Have you lost a great deal of weight? Are you so tired you have difficulty carrying on your daily activities? Are you feeling blue or discouraged because of your illness?" For each positive response, ask follow-up questions to narrow down or define the

exact nature of the problem. Again, these data help identify what nursing diagnoses should be included in the care plan.

- "What options has your physician suggested for treating your cancer?" The answer will indicate clients' knowledge about their treatment and, possibly, their communication with the physician. Often, under the stress of a cancer diagnosis, clients do not hear or understand what the doctor is saying and are afraid to ask questions. Lack of knowledge indicates a need to collaborate with the physician to explain the information to the client so that the client can absorb and understand it. If the client has a good understanding of the treatment plan, discussing how he or she feels about it can be useful in exposing fears, concerns, and emotional responses.
- "What do you expect to happen as a result of this treatment?" The answer may reveal unrealistic expectations or lack of understanding of consequences of the treatment.
- "What effect is the disease and/or treatment having on your ability to carry on with your usual daily activities?" Additional questions may also be needed to pinpoint the types of limitations. The response to this question should provide information on the client's functional status such as those shown in Box 14–11. This information can also be used to identify the need to collaborate with professionals from other disciplines. For example, if the client is the sole financial support of the family and is unable to work, a social worker may be able to help with resources; if the client is extremely weak, referral to a physical therapist may help with energy conservation strategies and strengthening exercises.
- "Who is available to help you at home and run errands for you? Who can provide transportation for you to get to your appointments or treatments? Who can you rely on to be a good listener when you're sad or just to be a comfortable companion? Is there someone you would like to make healthcare decisions for you if there is a time when you are unable

to make them for yourself?" It often seems that the person with cancer is the one who takes care of everyone else; asking for help may be difficult for this person. This information can identify how much support and help the client has access to. The last question introduces the concept of advanced directives and durable power of attorney regarding health care (see Chapter 5 ∞).

- "How do you manage your stress or your feelings of discomfort? What helps you feel better? Do you think these measures work well for you?" The responses to these questions provide information about the client's coping strategies and may identify maladaptive strategies such as alcohol or drug use. Lack of appropriate coping methods can interfere with the client's response to treatment and decrease overall quality of life.

Other assessment questions may be useful at different stages of the client's illness. For example, if the client is not expected to survive the cancer, it is important to ask whether the client has made decisions about last wishes (e.g., for a funeral and burial), whether these have been discussed with significant others, and whether the client has made out a will.

Physical Assessment

As soon as the client is admitted to the healthcare service or agency, conduct a complete physical assessment to establish a baseline against which to evaluate later changes. It is especially important to document the nutritional status of the client using anthropomorphic measurements (i.e., frame size, height, weight, body fat, and muscle mass), and to evaluate laboratory results and note any specific signs and symptoms. Table 14–11 compares the manifestations of good nutrition with those of malnutrition.

It is also important to assess the client's hydration status, especially if the client is not taking oral food and fluids well or is having bouts of vomiting. Box 14–12 lists specific assessments for hydration status. Other recommended assessments are dis-

TABLE 14–11 Signs of Nutritional Status

SYSTEM	GOOD NUTRITION	POOR NUTRITION
General	Alert, energetic, good endurance, psychologically stable	Withdrawn, apathetic, easily fatigued, irritable
	Weight within range for height, age, body size	Over- or underweight
Integumentary	Skin glowing, good turgor, smooth, free of lesions	Skin dull, pasty, scaly-dry, bruises, multiple lesions
	Hair shiny, lustrous, minimal loss	Hair brittle, dull, falls out easily
Head, eyes, ears, nose, and throat	Eyes bright, clear, no fatigue circles	Eyes dull, conjunctiva pale, discoloration under eyes
	Oral mucous membranes pink-red and moist	Oral mucous membranes pale
	Gums pink, firm	Gums red, spongy, and bleed easily
	Tongue pink, moderately smooth, no swelling	Tongue bright to dark red, swollen
Abdomen	Abdomen flat, firm	Abdomen flaccid or distended (ascites)
Musculoskeletal	Firm, well-developed muscles	Flaccid muscles, wasted appearance
	Good posture	Stooped posture
	No skeletal changes	Skeletal malformations
Neurologic	Good attention span, good concentration, astute thought processes	Inattentive, easily distracted, impaired thought processes
	Good reflexes	Paresthesias, reflexes diminished or hyperactive

BOX 14–12 **Factors to Consider in Assessing Hydration Status**

- Intake and output
- Rapid weight changes
- Skin turgor and moisture
- Venous filling
- Vital sign changes
- Tongue furrows and moisture
- Eyeball softness
- Lung sounds
- Laboratory values

cussed under the specific nursing diagnoses that follow. They can also be found in other chapters that address specific body systems affected by the cancer.

Nursing Diagnoses and Interventions

Nursing goals focus on supporting the whole person and managing specific problems such as pain, poor nutrition, dehydration, fatigue, adverse emotional responses, altered individual and family coping, and the side effects of medical treatment. Nursing also focuses on improving the quality of life by promoting rehabilitation for survivors of cancer and helping those

who succumb to the disease maintain their dignity in the dying process. Because cancer affects the whole family, nursing care includes everyone involved with the client from the onset of diagnosis through the entire disease and treatment process and the ultimate outcome. Many diagnoses are pertinent to clients with cancer; this section addresses only the most common diagnoses. See the accompanying Nursing Care Plan. (Diagnoses specific to individual diseases can be found in their respective chapters.)

Anxiety

Early in the disease continuum, for example, during diagnosis and treatment, threats to or changes in health status, physical comfort, role functioning, or even socioeconomic status can cause anxiety. Later, anxiety may result from the anticipation of pain, disfigurement, or the threat of death. In particular, clients whose coping skills have been poor in the past (e.g., in managing anger) may find themselves at a loss to manage this current crisis. The client may manifest overt signs of anxiety: trembling, restlessness, irritability, hyperactivity, stimulation of the sympathetic nervous system (increased blood pressure, pulse, respiration, excessive perspiration, pallor), withdrawal, worried facial expressions, and poor eye contact. The client may report insomnia and feelings of tension and apprehension, or express concerns regarding perceived changes brought about by the disease and fear of future events.

NURSING CARE PLAN **A Client with Cancer**

James Casey, age 72, is of Northern European heritage. He has been receiving medical care for chronic obstructive pulmonary disease, chronic bronchitis, status postmyocardial infarction, and type I diabetes mellitus for over 15 years. He reports that he lost his wife from lung cancer 5 years ago and still "misses her terribly." He describes his bad habits as smoking two packs of cigarettes a day for 52 years (104 packs/year), one to two six-packs of beer a week, one "bourbon and water" a night, and "a lot of sugar-free junk food, like french fries." He assures the nurse that he quit smoking 2 years ago, when he could no longer walk a block without considerable shortness of breath, and just quit drinking alcohol a few weeks ago at his physician's insistence. About a year ago, he had a basal-cell carcinoma removed from his right ear. Six months ago, cancerous tumors were discovered in his bladder, and he underwent two 6-week chemotherapy courses of bladder instillations of BCG. His latest report indicates that the tumors have grown back and no further chemotherapy would be useful. The urologist had considered surgery but believed that Mr. Casey's other medical problems would compromise his chances of survival. Mr. Casey decides to let the disease run its course and to be managed at home through hospice care. Because he lives alone in a modest home, he asks his daughter, Mary, and her family to move in with him to provide care and support during his final months. The daughter accepts, saying she is glad to be able to spend this time with her father; she has been informed of the physical and emotional stress this will entail.

ASSESSMENT

Glynis Jackson, RN, the hospice nurse assigned as case manager for James Casey, completes a health history and physical exami-

nation during her first two visits in his home, 1 day apart. She gathers this information over 2 days to conserve his strength and allow more time for Mr. Casey and his daughter to talk about their concerns.

During the physical assessment, Glynis notes that Mr. Casey is pale with pink mucous membranes, thin with a wasted appearance and a strained, worried facial expression. He complains of severe back pain no longer adequately relieved by Percodan and Vicodin alternating every 2 to 4 hours. His blood pressure is 90/50, right arm in the reclining position with no significant orthostatic change; his apical pulse is 102, regular and strong; respiratory rate 24 and unlabored; breath sounds are clear but diminished in the bases; oral temperature is 96.8°F.

A tunnelled Groshong catheter as a VAD is present in the right anterior chest. There is no drainage, redness, or swelling at the site. The catheter was placed last week when the client was being evaluated at the anesthesiologist's office for pain management, but no medication is running via the VAD. Mary reports that his urinary output is adequate. Approximately 200 mL of yellow, cloudy, non-malodorous urine is present in the urinal at the bedside from his last voiding.

Mr. Casey states that he spends most of his time either in bed or sitting up in a chair in his room. He reports that he has no energy any more and is unable to walk to the bathroom unassisted, dress himself, or take care of his own personal hygiene. Glynis rates Mr. Casey's functional level at ECOG level 4: capable of only limited self-care, confined to bed or chair 50% or more of waking hours (Karnofsky 10 to 20). He tells the nurse that his daughter "is working day and night to help me and is looking awfully tired."

(continued)

NURSING CARE PLAN   A Client with Cancer (continued)

Mary reports that Mr. Casey is eating very poorly: He usually eats a small bowl of oatmeal with milk for breakfast and vegetable soup and crackers for lunch, but he tells her that he is too tired for dinner and wants only fruit juice. Mr. Casey tells the nurse that he has no appetite and eats just to please Mary. He does drink at least three to four glasses of water a day plus juice. His fingerstick blood sugars remain within normal range.

His current weight is 120 pounds at 67 inches tall, down from 180 pounds a year ago. He has lost about 30 pounds over the last 2 months.

Available laboratory values from his visit with the doctor show the following:

Total protein: 4.1 g/dL (normal range: 6.0 to 8.0 g/dL)
Albumin: 2.2 g/dL (normal range: 3.5 to 5.0 g/dL)
Hemoglobin: 10.2 g/dL (normal range: 13.5 to 18.0 g/dL)
Hematocrit: 30.5% (normal range: 40.0% to 54.0%)
BUN: 30 mg/dL (normal range: 5 to 25 mg/dL, slightly higher in older people)
Creatinine: 2.2 mg/dL (normal range: 0.5 to 1.5 mg/dL)

DIAGNOSES

- *Imbalanced Nutrition: Less than Body Requirements* related to anorexia and fatigue
- *Risk for Caregiver Role Strain* related to severity of her father's illness and lack of help from other family members
- *Chronic Pain* related to progression of disease process
- *Impaired Physical Mobility* related to pain, fatigue, and beginning neuromuscular impairment
- *Risk for Impaired Skin Integrity* related to impaired physical mobility and malnourished state

EXPECTED OUTCOMES

- Increase oral intake and show improvement in serum protein values.
- Daughter will be able to maintain supportive caretaking activities as long as Mr. Casey needs them.
- Minimal pain for the rest of his life.
- Able to continue his current activity level.
- Maintain intact skin.

PLANNING AND IMPLEMENTATION

- Ask about favorite foods, and ask Mary to offer a small portion of one of these foods each day.
- Encourage drinking up to four cans of liquid nutritional supplement with fiber a day, sipping them throughout the day.
- Talk with the physician about prescribing a medication to help stimulate the appetite.
- Plan to have a home health aide come to the home, give him a shower or bed bath daily, and assist his daughter with some of the household chores.
- Talk with Mary about having her adult son and daughter relieve her of the housework and stay with Mr. Casey so that she can get out of the house occasionally. Offer to talk with them if she is uncomfortable doing so.
- Request a volunteer to spend up to 4 hours a day, twice a week with Mr. Casey so that Mary can attend to outside activities and chores.
- Talk with the anesthesiologist, and work out a pain control program, using the VAD and a CADD-PCA infusion pump with a continuous morphine infusion.
- Call the infusion therapist to set up the equipment and supplies (including the medication) for the morphine infusion.
- Teach how to use the pump and about the side effects of the morphine infusion, including those that require a call to the nurse for assistance. Teach which untoward effects should be reported.
- Request a physical therapy consultation to evaluate current level of functioning and determine how to maintain current level.
- Instruct Mary to allow ample rest periods for James between activities.
- Order a hospital bed with electronic controls to be delivered to the house.
- Order a special foam pad for bed and chair and a bedside commode from the medical supply house.
- Instruct Mary and the home health aide to inspect skin daily, give good skin care with emollient lotion after bathing, and report any beginning lesions immediately to the nurse.

EVALUATION

James Casey did increase his oral intake a little, sometimes eating the special treats his daughter prepared and drinking one or two cans of liquid nutritional supplement a day. However, his weight did not increase; it stayed at about 120 pounds until his death 2 weeks later. His daughter was very grateful for the extra help from the home health aide and the volunteer, though she could not bring herself to ask her son and daughter for help and did not want the nurse to do so. She did become more rested and reported that "Dad and I had some wonderful 3:00 A.M. talks when he couldn't sleep."

Mr. Casey was started on 20 mg of morphine per hour with boluses of 10 mg 4 times a day, for breakthrough pain. This medication relieved his pain quite well; after 2 days he was alert enough most of the time to carry on a normal conversation and still walk to the bathroom with help up until 2 days before he died.

The hospital bed simplified Mr. Casey's care and made it much easier for him to rest comfortably and change position. His skin remained intact and in good condition.

Mary reported that Mr. Casey died peacefully in his sleep, about 2 weeks after care was started. She said spending the last weeks of his life together was a healing experience for both of them.

CRITICAL THINKING IN THE NURSING PROCESS

1. What other tests could be done to evaluate James Casey's nutritional status?
2. Mr. Casey had severe back pain. What were the possible pathophysiologic reasons for his pain?
3. One of the specified interventions was to consult the physician regarding medication to increase Mr. Casey's appetite. What medications might fulfill that function? What side effects might they have that would contraindicate these medications for him?
4. If Mr. Casey had developed signs and symptoms of sepsis, what manifestations would you expect to see? As the nurse making the home visits, what would be your nursing actions, and in what order of priority?

See Evaluating Your Response in Appendix C.

- Carefully assess the client's level of anxiety (moderate anxiety, severe anxiety, or panic) and the reality of the threats represented in the client's current situation. The level of anxiety and the reality of the perceived threat influence the type of intervention that is appropriate for the client. *A client in panic may need medical intervention with appropriate medications, whereas those with moderate or severe anxiety are often managed by the nurse through counseling and teaching new coping skills.*
- Establish a therapeutic relationship by conveying warmth and empathy and listening nonjudgmentally. *A client who feels safe in the relationship with the nurse more easily expresses feelings and thoughts. The client will be able to trust the nurse and perhaps be willing to try new behaviors as suggested. The amount of time this relationship may take to develop depends on the client's current emotional and mental state and the stage of the disease process.*
- Encourage the client to acknowledge and express feelings, no matter how inappropriate they may seem to the client. *Just by expressing their feelings, clients often can significantly diminish anxiety. Expressing feelings also allows the client to direct energy toward healing and thus has a positive therapeutic effect. Moreover, by acknowledging feelings, especially those the client considers unacceptable, the client can lay the groundwork for new coping behaviors.*
- Review the coping strategies the client has used in the past and build on past successful behaviors, introducing new strategies as appropriate. Explain why inappropriate strategies, such as repressing anger or turning to alcohol, are not helpful. *The client will be more willing to make changes that build on what has already worked in the past. The client will also be more willing to reject inappropriate strategies if he or she is given a persuasive reason why they have not had the desired effect in managing previous crises.*
- Identify resources in the community, such as crisis hotlines and support groups, that can help the client manage anxiety-producing situations. *The client may not have support systems available, or the client's significant others may be having their own difficulties in dealing with the cancer diagnosis. Programs such as "I Can Cope," sponsored by the American Cancer Society in most communities, provide education, counseling, and support in a group setting with other cancer clients.*
- Provide specific information for the client about the disease, its treatment, and what may be expected, especially for those clients with obvious misinformation. *Knowing what is to come gives the client a sense of control and enables the client to make decisions. Also, knowing that every effort will be made to keep the client as free of pain as possible can do a great deal to relieve anxiety.*
- Provide a safe, calm, and quiet environment for the client in panic. Remain with the client and administer antianxiety medications as ordered. *Staying with the client and displaying calmness and confidence can protect the client from injury and prevent further panic. If the panic does not subside with the nurse's presence and support, referral to the physician for medication management may be necessary.*
- Use crisis intervention theory to promote growth in the client and significant others, regardless of the outcome of the disease. *During a major crisis, people can, with assistance, transform the experience from one that causes defeat and despair to one that enhances personal and spiritual growth.* If you are not skilled in this area, a referral to an appropriate mental health professional may be helpful to the client and family.

Disturbed Body Image

Cancer and cancer treatments frequently result in major physiologic and psychologic body image changes. See the box on this page for manifestations of cancer. Loss of a body part (e.g., amputation, prostatectomy, or mastectomy), skin changes and hair loss from chemotherapy or radiation therapy, disfigurement of body part (e.g., lymphedema in the affected upper and lower extremities), or creation of unnatural openings on the body for elimination (e.g., colostomy or ileostomy) may have a major effect on the person's self-image. The gaunt, wasted appearance of the cachectic client or draining, malodorous lesions that result when cancer breaks through the skin are other significant etiologies of body image disturbance. This may also give rise to fear of rejection, which plays a major role in sexual dysfunction. In addition to all of the other afflictions the cancer brings about, the client may undergo major changes in appearance and function. The client may exhibit a visible physical alteration of some portion of the body, verbalize negative feelings about the body and/or fear of rejection by others, refuse to look at the affected site, and depersonalize the body change or lost part (e.g., by calling the colostomy "that thing").

- Discuss the meaning of the loss or change with the client. *Doing so helps the nurse discover the best approach for this particular client and involves the client more actively in interventions. A small, seemingly trivial loss may have a big impact, especially when viewed in light of the other changes that are occurring in the client's life. Likewise, a major loss may not be as important as the nurse might imagine. To ensure more appropriate and individualized care, evaluate each situation in terms of the reactions of the specific client.*
- Observe and evaluate interaction with significant others. *People who are important to the client may unintentionally reinforce negative feelings about body image; on the other hand, the client may perceive rejection where none exists.*

MANIFESTATIONS of Cancer

- Hair loss
- Depression
- Fever
- Bleeding gums
- Oropharyngeal ulcerations
- Stomatitis
- Anorexia
- Nausea and vomiting
- Diarrhea
- Emaciation
- General weakness
- Flaccid muscles
- Stooped posture
- Pallor
- Excessive bruising
- Radiation burns
- Visible tumor (abdomen)
- Odor of decay
- Hypotension

- Allow denial, but do not participate in the denial; for example, if a client does not want to look at the wound, the nurse may say, "I am going to change the dressing to your breast incision now." *During the initial stage of shock at the loss of a body part, denial is a protective mechanism and should not be challenged, nor should it be promoted. A matter-of-fact approach and an empathetic attitude will go far to facilitate the eventual acceptance of the change.*
- Assist the client and significant others to cope with the changes in appearance:
  a. Provide a supportive environment.
  b. Encourage the client and significant others to express feelings about the situation.
  c. Give matter-of-fact responses to questions and concerns.
  d. Identify new coping strategies to resolve feelings.
  e. Enlist family and friends in reaffirming the client's worth.
  A supportive, safe environment in which feelings are respected and new coping strategies can be tried promotes acceptance, as does reaffirming that the client's worth is not diminished by any physical changes.
- Teach the client or significant others to participate in the care of the afflicted body area. Provide support and validation of their efforts. *Active involvement in providing care, such as changing a dressing or emptying a colostomy bag, empowers the client and/or significant others. This intimate involvement also desensitizes feelings about disfigurement and promotes acceptance. Involving significant others reduces the risk of their rejecting the client and can promote closeness. Positive reinforcement from the nurse encourages them to continue these behaviors.*
- Teach strategies for minimizing physical changes, such as providing skin care during radiation therapy and dressing to enhance appearance and minimize change in the body part. *Early intervention can limit the negative side effects of treatment and actually promote recovery. Involving the client provides an additional way for the client to be in control of a difficult situation.*
- Teach ways to reduce the alopecia that results from chemotherapy and to enhance appearance until the hair grows back:
  a. Discuss the pattern and timing of hair loss. *This allows the client to cope with changes and incorporate them into daily activities.*
  b. Encourage wearing cheerful, brightly colored head coverings; assist in color coordinating them with usual clothing. *Attractive head coverings protect the bald head while allowing the client to feel stylish and well dressed.*
  c. Refer to a good wig shop before hair loss is experienced. *Hair color and texture can be matched to minimize obvious changes in appearance.*
  d. Refer to support programs such as "Look Good . . . Feel Better," which is sponsored by the American Cancer Society and the Cosmetic, Toilet, and Fragrance Association Foundation. *A support group can diminish feelings of isolation and provide practical tips for managing problems. For a list of community resources available to clients with cancer, refer to a local phone book.*
  e. Reassure that hair will grow back after chemotherapy is discontinued, but also inform that the color and texture of the new hair may be different. Hair loss has been identified as the most distressing symptom by many clients (Ferrell, 2000; Williams et al., 1999). *Interventions to reduce that loss can have a significant impact on body image concerns. Moreover, knowing what to expect may decrease anxiety and distress.*

Anticipatory Grieving

Anticipatory grieving is a response to loss that has not yet occurred. Overall, only 50% of people with cancer fully recover, and certain types of cancer have a much higher death rate; thus, the client with cancer is often confronted with facing death and making preparations for it. This can be a healthy response that allows the client and family to work through the dying process and achieve growth in the final stage of life. Perceived changes in body image and lifestyle also can prompt anticipatory grieving. The client or significant others may show sorrow, anger, depression, or withdrawal, expressing distress at the potential loss or verbalizing concern about unfinished life business. (See Chapter 5 ∞ for more on nursing care of the client who is grieving or dying.)

- Use the therapeutic communication skills of active listening, silence, and nonverbal support to provide an open environment for the client and significant others to discuss their feelings realistically and to express anger or other negative feelings appropriately. *This helps the client and family to get in touch with feelings and confront the possibility of the loss or death.*
- Answer questions about illness and prognosis honestly, but always encourage hope. *This allows for realistic appraisal of the situation and planning, and it also helps combat feelings of hopelessness and depression.*
- Encourage the dying client to make funeral and burial plans ahead of time and to be sure the will is in order. Make sure the necessary phone numbers can be easily located. *This gives a sense of control and relieves family members of these concerns at a time when the client is most in need of their support and when they themselves are extremely stressed.*
- Encourage the client to continue taking part in activities he or she enjoys, including maintaining employment as long as possible. *This gives a sense of continuity of life even in the face of severe losses.*

Risk for Infection

Malnutrition, impaired skin and mucous membrane integrity, tumor necrosis, and suppression of the white blood cells from chemotherapy or radiation may contribute to the risk for infection. Anorexia, as well as the disease itself, deprives the body of nutrients needed for healing, while impaired integrity of skin and mucous membranes (a result of chemotherapy and/or radiation therapy) compromise the first lines of defense against microbial invasion. Cells in the center of large or not very vascular tumors may die from malnutrition, eventually eroding through tissues to increase the risk of sepsis. Bone marrow depression resulting from the effects of certain types of cancers and from chemotherapy undermine the body's ability to respond to infection. The client may exhibit the classic signs of infection:

lassitude, fever, anorexia, pain in the affected area, and physical evidence of infection, such as a purulent, draining lesion or wound. If the bone marrow is compromised, the usual signs and symptoms of infection may be absent or reduced.

- Monitor vital signs. *Fever and sympathetic nervous system responses, such as increased pulse and respiration, are usual early signs of infection. However, severely immunosuppressed clients may be unable to mount a fever; therefore, the absence of fever cannot rule out infection.*
- Monitor WBC counts frequently, especially if the client is receiving chemotherapy known to cause bone marrow suppression. *This allows the nurse to notify the physician at the first sign of diminishing WBC counts so that corrective action can be taken.*
- Teach the client to avoid crowds, small children, and people with infections when WBC count is at nadir (lowest point during chemotherapy) and to practice scrupulous personal hygiene. *During periods of leukopenia, the client may lose immunity to his or her own natural flora. Careful attention to hygiene reduces the risk of infection. Crowds, which promote contact with a greater variety of infectious agents, and friends with minor infections can be very dangerous for the immunosuppressed. Small children should be avoided because they often have microbes to which most people are usually immune but which the client may not be able to resist.*
- Protect skin and mucous membranes from injury. Teach appropriate skin care measures, such as good hygiene, use of a moisturizing lotion to prevent dryness and cracking, frequent changes of position for the bed-bound, and immediate attention to skin breaks or lesions. *Ensuring intact skin strengthens the first line of defense against infection.*
- Encourage the client to consume a diet high in protein, minerals, and vitamins, especially vitamin C. *Improving nutrition decreases the risk of infection. Vitamin C has been shown to help prevent certain types of infection, such as colds.*

Risk for Injury

In addition to infection, cancer can pose a risk for injury from, for example, obstruction by a large tumor or one located in a limited body space (e.g., in the brain, bowel, or bronchial airways). If the cancer is one that creates ectopic sites of hormones, elevated levels of hormones that are not under the control of the pituitary gland can injure the client in a variety of ways. Signs of obstruction depend on the organ involved: Bowel obstruction presents with pain, distention, and cessation of bowel activities; obstruction in the brain gives signs of increased intracranial pressure or personality/behavioral change; bronchial obstruction manifests as respiratory distress, cyanosis, and altered arterial blood gases. Ectopic production of parathyroid hormone manifests as high serum calcium levels as well as signs of hypercalcemia; ectopic production of antidiuretic hormone causes fluid retention and manifests as hypertension and peripheral and pulmonary edema.

- Assess frequently for signs and symptoms indicating problems with organ obstruction. *Early detection of major problems allows the nurse to seek medical help before the problem evolves into a physiologic crisis.*

- Teach to differentiate minor problems from those of a serious nature. Encourage the client to consult with the nurse or physician if in doubt or to call 911 if the client becomes very ill. Box 14–13 provides guidelines to help clients identify serious problems. *Having guidelines for when to call the doctor provides an anxiety-reducing safety net for the client and family and promotes early detection of complications.*
- Monitor laboratory values that may indicate the presence of ectopic functioning and report abnormal findings to physicians immediately. (See Table 14–4 for laboratory indicators of ectopic functions.) *Early detection promotes early medical intervention and prevents serious consequences from the ectopic secretion.* Refer to Chapters 10, 19, and 20 ∞ for specific signs and symptoms of electrolyte imbalances and endocrine disorders.

Imbalanced Nutrition:
Less than Body Requirements

The anorexia-cachexia syndrome (described earlier in this chapter) is a common cause of malnutrition in cancer clients. Metabolism increases in response to increased cancer cell production while the cancer's parasitic activity reduces the nutrients available to the body. Loss of appetite, food aversion, nausea and vomiting, and painful oral lesions from chemotherapy or radiation may contribute to impaired nutrition. Tumors of the gastrointestinal tract that affect absorption also contribute to the problem. Manifestations include wasted appearance, considerable weight loss over a relatively short period of time, anthropometric measurements below 85% of standard for fat and muscle tissue, decreases in serum proteins, and negative responses to antigen testing.

BOX 14–13 When to Call for Help

Instruct the client or family member to call the nurse or physician if any of the following signs or symptoms occur:

- Oral temperature greater than 101.5°F (38.6°C)
- Severe headache; significant increase in pain at usual site, especially if the pain is not relieved by the medication regimen; or severe pain at a new site
- Difficulty breathing
- New bleeding from any site, such as rectal or vaginal bleeding
- Confusion, irritability, or restlessness
- Withdrawal, greatly decreased activity level, or frequent crying
- Verbalizations of deep sadness or a desire to end life
- Changes in body functioning, such as the inability to void or severe diarrhea or constipation
- Changes in eating patterns, such as refusal to eat, extreme hunger, or a significant increase in nausea and vomiting
- Appearance of edema in the extremities or significant increase in edema already present

Instruct the client or family member to call 911 if the client

- Is having much difficulty breathing or if the lips or face has a bluish tinge.
- Becomes unconscious or has a convulsion.
- Exhibits unmanageable behavior, such as being physically abusive, hurting self, or engaging in uncontrollable activity.

- Assess current eating patterns, including usual likes and dislikes, and identify factors that impair food intake. *This allows for a more individualized plan based on needs and preferences.*
- Evaluate degree of malnutrition:
  a. Check laboratory values for total serum protein, serum albumin and globins, total lymphocyte count, serum transferrin, hemoglobin, and hematocrit. *These values represent the laboratory values that are most likely to decrease with malnutrition.*
  b. Calculate nitrogen balance and creatinine-height index. Calculate skeletal muscle mass, and compare findings to normal ranges. *Urinary creatinine is an index of lean body mass and decreases in malnutrition. Lean muscle mass is catabolized for energy in clients with cancer.*
  c. Take anthropometric measurements and compare them to standards: height, weight, elbow breadth, arm circumference, triceps skinfold thickness, and arm muscle mass. *This estimates the degree of wasting; findings below 85% of standard are considered malnutrition.*
- Teach the principles of maintaining good nutrition by using the Food Guide Pyramid and adapting the diet to medical restrictions and current preferences. *This tailors the food plan to the client's needs and thereby promotes compliance.*
- Manage problems that interfere with eating:
  a. Encourage eating whatever is appealing and consider adding nutritional supplements such as Ensure Plus or Isocal to diet. *It is better to eat something even if it is not nutritionally balanced.*
  b. Eat small, frequent meals. *These are more easily digested and absorbed and usually better tolerated by the client with anorexia.*
  c. Encourage to try icy cold foods (such as ice cream) or those that are more highly seasoned if food has no taste. *Chemotherapy and radiation therapy may harm taste buds and prevent distinguishing the taste of foods. Strong seasonings and coldness make food more enjoyable to the client with diminished taste. However, spicy foods are not recommended for patients with stomatitis.*
  d. Encourage cold and bland semisoft and liquid foods with painful oropharyngeal ulcers; use a nonalcohol anesthetic mouthwash prior to eating. *These foods are less irritating to sensitive mucous membranes; deadening the pain can make chewing and swallowing easier.*
  e. Manage nausea and vomiting by administering antiemetic drugs (around-the-clock medication may be an effective preventive measure). Encourage client to eat small, frequent, low-fat meals with dry foods such as crackers and toast, to avoid liquids with meals, and to sit upright for an hour after meals. Remove emesis basins, and encourage oral hygiene before eating. *Dry, low-fat foods are more readily tolerated when nauseated. Removing vomiting cues, such as odor and supplies associated with vomiting, can reduce nausea.*
- Teach to supplement meals with nutritional supplements such as Ensure Plus or Isocal and to take multivitamin and mineral tablets with meals. Suggest increasing calories by adding ice cream or frozen yogurt to the liquid supplement or commercial protein-carbohydrate powders to milk or fruit juice. *Because the food intake is usually less than that needed to maintain or gain weight, these supplements can add calories in a manner often tolerated.*
- Teach to keep a food diary to document daily intake. *If the client can see how little is being consumed, he or she may eat more. A food diary also helps the nurse keep a calorie count and alert the physician if more drastic nutritional measures, such as a feeding tube or parenteral nutrition, need to be instituted.*
- Teach to administer parenteral nutrition via a central line or other VAD. Teach safety measures and care of the VAD, and explain how the pump delivering the solution works. Provide an emergency phone number for help with administration problems. (See Chapter 22 ∞ for safety guidelines for administering parenteral nutrition.) *The client with chronic or terminal cancer requiring parenteral nutrition is usually managed at home, so information on how to manage the entire process may be needed.*

Impaired Tissue Integrity

The most common impairment of tissue integrity occurs in the oral-pharyngeal-esophageal mucous membranes. It is secondary to the effects of some chemotherapeutic drugs and radiation treatment to the head and neck. The oral-pharyngeal-esophageal tissues are lined with cells with a high mitotic turnover rate and are therefore vulnerable to many chemotherapeutic drugs. Leukemias, bone marrow transplants, and herpes viral infections are other etiologic factors in the disruption of oral-pharyngeal-esophageal tissue. Manifestations of this problem may include the following:

- Small ulcers occur on the tongue and mucous membranes in the mouth and throat.
- Herpes simplex type 1 lesions or vesicles evolve into ulcerations.
- Fungal infections, such as thrush (due to *Candida* infections), are manifested by a white, yellow, or tan coating with dry, red, fissured tissue underneath.
- Red, swollen, friable gums bleed with minimal or no trauma.
- **Xerostomia** is excessive dryness of the mucous membranes (due to chemotherapy or radiation).

Manage such problems with the following interventions:

- Carefully assess and evaluate the type of tissue impairment present. Identify possible sources, such as chemotherapy or radiation therapy to head and neck. *This allows the nurse to implement corrective measures appropriate to the type of problem.*
- Implement and teach measures for preventing oropharyngeal infection:
  a. Observe for systemic signs of infection. Be suspicious of any fever that has no apparent cause. *This facilitates early identification of an infection before it spreads.*
  b. Encourage cleaning teeth gently and using a nonalcohol mouthwash several times a day. This can be done after waking up in the morning, after any oral intake, and before bedtime. Soak dentures nightly in hydrogen peroxide and floss gently with waxed floss after meals and

bedtime; this measure may be contraindicated for people with leukemia or thrombocytopenia. *Disrupted mucous membranes allow the normal oral bacterial flora into the systemic circulation, which can result in sepsis in the immunocompromised person. Reducing the oral flora by frequent hygiene decreases the risk of infection.*

   c. Culture any oral lesions, and report the problem to the physician. Herpes lesions may not follow a typical pattern in immunosuppressed clients. *Identifying the cause of the infection, whether viral, fungal, or bacterial, allows the physician to prescribe the appropriate treatment.*

■ Implement and teach measures for reducing trauma to delicate tissues:

   a. Counteract dry mouth (xerostomia) with lubricating and moisturizing agents, such as Gatorade, sugarless gum, and Blistex. *This protects mucous membranes from infection and trauma.*

   b. Avoid putting sharp instruments in the mouth. Use smooth plastic spoons and forks for eating, especially with a bleeding disorder. Dental work should be done by dental oncologists.

   c. Brush teeth with a very soft toothbrush and obtain a new toothbrush monthly. If gums are friable and bleeding, clean teeth with a soft cloth or toothpaste over finger. Chlorhexidine mouthwash (Peridex) may be used. *This protects gums from trauma and decreases risk of hemorrhage.*

■ Administer specific medications as ordered to control infection and/or pain:

   a. Acyclovir is often used to treat viral infections.

   b. Systemic antibiotics are used to treat bacterial infections.

   c. Nystatin or clotrimazole solution for "swish and swallow" or lozenges that dissolve slowly in the mouth are used for fungal infections.

   d. Use viscous Xylocaine or various combination mouthwashes before meals and as needed. These agents reduce pain and inflammation. See Box 14–14 for the ingredients of combination mouthwashes. *Knowing the contents of each mouthwash can prevent hypersensitivity reactions (e.g., to lidocaine) and assist in client teaching.*

Nursing Interventions for Oncologic Emergencies

In caring for clients with cancer, nurses may encounter a number of emergency situations in which their role may be pivotal to the client's survival. Most of these emergencies require astute observations, accurate judgments, and rapid action once the problem has been identified. A brief description of the more common **oncologic emergencies** with nursing interventions follows. In all cases, immediate notification of the physician or emergency team is the first step.

Pericardial Effusions and Neoplastic Cardiac Tamponade

Malignant pericardial effusion is an accumulation of excess fluid in the pericardial sac that compresses the heart, restricts heart movement, and results in a cardiac tamponade. The signs

---

BOX 14–14 Combination Mouthwashes for Oropharyngeal Pain Control

Kaiser Mouthwash
■ Nystatin
■ Hydrocortisone
■ Tetracycline

Stanford Mouthwash
■ Nystatin
■ Tetracycline
■ Lidocaine
■ Hydrocortisone

Xyloxylin Suspension
■ Benylin syrup
■ Lidocaine
■ Maalox suspension

Stomafate Suspension
■ Sucralfate
■ Sterile water
■ Benylin syrup
■ Maalox suspension

---

of cardiac tamponade are caused by compression of the heart, which leads to decreased cardiac output and impaired cardiac function. Signs include hypotension, tachycardia, tachypnea, dyspnea, cyanosis, increased central venous pressure, anxiety, restlessness, and impaired consciousness.

   Interventions include the following:

■ Start oxygen and alert respiratory therapy for other respiratory support as needed.
■ Insert an intravenous catheter if one is not already in place.
■ Monitor vital signs and initiate hemodynamic monitoring.
■ Prepare vasopressor drugs.
■ Bring emergency cart to bedside.
■ Set up for and assist physician with a pericardial tap (pericardiocentesis).
■ Reassure the client.

Superior Vena Cava Syndrome

The superior vena cava can be compressed by mediastinal tumors or adjacent thoracic tumors. The most common cause is small-cell or squamous-cell lung cancers. Occasionally the problem is caused by thrombus around a central venous catheter that then plugs up the vena cava, resulting in obstruction and backup of the blood flowing into the superior vena cava.

   Obstruction of the venous system causes increased venous pressure, venous stasis, and engorgement of veins that are drained by the superior vena cava. Signs and symptoms may develop slowly; facial, periorbital, and arm edema are early signs. As the problem progresses, respiratory distress, dyspnea, cyanosis, tachypnea, and altered consciousness and neurologic deficits may occur. Figure 14–7 ■ illustrates the superior venal cava syndrome.

   Emergency measures include the following:

■ Provide respiratory support with oxygen, and prepare for tracheostomy.
■ Monitor vital signs.
■ Administer corticosteroids (e.g., dexamethasone) to reduce edema.
■ If the disorder is due to a clot, administer antifibrinolytic or anticoagulant drugs.
■ Provide a safe environment, including seizure precautions.

After the emergency is managed, the client often receives radiation or chemotherapy to reduce the tumor size.

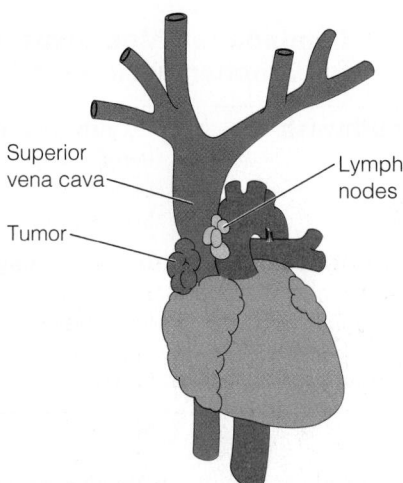

Figure 14–7 ■ The superior vena cava syndrome. The enlargement of a tumor adjacent to the superior vena cava (usually in the lung or mediastinum) compresses that major blood vessel, which leads into the right atrium of the heart. As a result, blood backs up into the venous system behind the obstruction, diminishing blood flow into the heart.

Sepsis and Septic Shock

Tumor necrosis, immune deficiency, antineoplastic therapy, malnutrition, and comorbid conditions can lead to the development of sepsis. Bacteria gain entrance to the blood, grow rapidly, and produce septicemia. Because malignant tumors are more likely to use anaerobic metabolic pathways, the bacteria of tumor sepsis are usually gram negative and damage the body through a combination of bacterial endotoxins and an uncontrolled immune reaction. Gram-negative sepsis progresses to systemic shock and eventually results in multisystem failure. Signs and symptoms appear in two phases. The first phase is characterized by vasodilation with vascular dehydration, high fever, peripheral edema, hypotension, tachycardia, tachypnea, hot flushed skin with creeping mottling beginning in the lower extremities, and anxiety or restlessness. Without treatment, the shock progresses to the second phase, which shows the more classic signs of shock: hypotension, rapid thready pulse, respiratory distress, cyanosis, subnormal temperature, cold clammy skin, decreased urinary output, and altered mentation. Identifying the problem while the client is still in the hyperdynamic state is crucial to the client's survival. See Chapter 11 ∞ for further discussion of septic shock.

Spinal Cord Compression

Spinal cord compression is most commonly associated with pressure from expanding tumors of the breast, lung, or prostate; lymphoma; or metastatic disease. Spinal cord compression constitutes an emergency because of the potential for irreversible paraplegia. Back pain is the initial symptom in 95% of the cases of spinal cord compression. This may progress to leg pain, numbness, paresthesias, and coldness. Later, bowel and bladder dysfunction occur and, finally, neurologic dysfunction progressing from weakness to paralysis.

Treatment often consists of radiation or surgical decompression, but early detection is essential. See Chapter 45 ∞ for further discussion of spinal cord compression.

Obstructive Uropathy

Clients with intra-abdominal, retroperitoneal, or pelvic malignancies, such as prostate, cervical, or bladder cancers, may experience obstruction of the bladder neck or the ureters. Bladder neck obstruction usually manifests as urinary retention, flank pain, hematuria, or persistent urinary tract infections, but ureteral obstruction is not often evident until the client is in renal failure. See Chapters 28 and 50 ∞ for further discussion of obstructive uropathy.

Hypercalcemia

Hypercalcemia in clients with cancer results from the excessive ectopic production of parathyroid hormone and is most commonly associated with cancers of the breast, lung, esophagus, thyroid, head, and neck and with multiple myeloma. Bone metastases may also cause hypercalcemia. When the rate of calcium mobilization from the bone exceeds the renal threshold for excretion, serum calcium levels can become dangerously elevated. Clients with hypercalcemia often present with nonspecific symptoms of fatigue, anorexia, nausea, polyuria, and constipation. Neurologic symptoms include muscle weakness, lethargy, apathy, and diminished reflexes. Without treatment, hypercalcemia progresses to alterations in mental status, psychotic behavior, cardiac arrhythmias, seizures, coma, and death (see Chapter 10 ∞).

Hyperuricemia

Hyperuricemia usually is a complication of rapid necrosis of tumor cells after vigorous chemotherapy for lymphomas and leukemias. Hyperuricemia may be related to increased uric acid production or to the tumor lysis syndrome associated with Burkitt's lymphoma. Uric acid crystals are deposited in the urinary tract, causing renal failure and uremia. Clients with hyperuricemia manifest with nausea, vomiting, lethargy, and oliguria.

Syndrome of Inappropriate Antidiuretic Hormone Secretion

Occurring in only about 2% of cancer clients, syndrome of inappropriate antidiuretic hormone secretion (SIADH) is related to an ectopic secretion of antidiuretic hormone that is usually associated with small-cell lung carcinoma, but also occasionally with prostate and adrenal cancers. The kidney secretes an excessive amount of sodium and conserves a disproportionate amount of free water, causing profound hyponatremia. Signs and symptoms include anorexia, nausea, muscle aches, and subtle neurologic symptoms that can progress to lethargy, confusion, seizures, and coma from cerebral edema.

Tumor Lysis Syndrome

Tumor lysis syndrome (TLS) is a life-threatening emergency for clients with cancer. TLS is characterized by a combination of two or more metabolic abnormalities, including hyperuricemia, hyperphosphatemia, hyperkalemia, and/or hypocalcemia (Cantril & Haylock, 2004; Holdsworth & Nguyen, 2003). The syndrome develops because of massive and rapid destruction or death of cancer cells caused by cytotoxic treatment such as chemotherapy, radiation, biologic therapy, hormonal therapy, and surgery (Habib & Saliba, 2002; Tanvetyanon & Choudhury, 2004). It can also occur spontaneously with sudden death of tumor cells (Jasek & Day, 1994). A high incidence of TLS occurs in patients with bulky, highly proliferating, and chemosensitive tumors such as high-grade lymphomas (Burkitt's lymphoma) and acute leukemia (ALL) (Beriwal et al., 2002; Habib & Saliba, 2002). Although the incidence of TLS in solid tumors is rare, cases of TLS following chemotherapy have been reported in patients with small-cell lung cancer, breast cancer, neuroblastoma, melanoma, and ovarian cancer (Habib & Saliba, 2002; Stoves et al., 2001).

The major cause of TLS is chemotherapy to tumors with a high proliferative rate, a relatively large tumor burden, and high sensitivity to cytotoxic agents, which leads to massive and rapid cell death. Usually, within a week of initiating chemotherapy, the body no longer can excrete the large amount of metabolic by-products from the cell death, resulting in the release of intracellular contents and metabolic by-products (such as potassium, phosphorus, and nucleic acid) into the bloodstream (Cairo & Bishop, 2004). As a result, a combination of metabolic derangements occurs, including hyperkalemia, hyperuricemia, and hyperphosphatemia with secondary hypocalcemia (Cairo & Bishop, 2004; Cantril & Haylock, 2004). These metabolic abnormalities put patients at risk for cardiac malfunction and renal failure.

Clinical manifestations of TLS include nausea, vomiting, lethargy, edema, fluid overload, congestive heart failure, cardiac dysrhythmias, seizures, muscle cramps, tetany, syncope, and possible sudden death (Cairo & Bishop, 2004; Cantril & Haylock, 2004). Diagnosis of TLS mainly depends on laboratory tests and clinical signs and symptoms. Prevention is crucial in management of TLS. Patients at risk for TLS include those with bulky chemosensitive cancer such as high-grade lymphomas and acute leukemia, elevated serum uric acid, potassium, phosphorus, and renal deficiency. Preventive and management measures include identifying patients at risk, administration of allopurinol to inhibit the conversion of nucleic acid to uric acid, hydration and diuretic therapy to promote urinary excretion of uric acid and phosphate, urine alkalinization to promote the urinary excretion of uric acid, administration of oral phosphate binder such as aluminium hydroxide to promote the excretion of phosphate through the bowel, administration of sodium polystyrene sulfonate (Kayexalate) to promote the excretion of potassium through the bowel, and initiation of hemodialysis to patients unresponsive to standard approaches to hyperkalemia, hyperuricemia, or hyperphosphatemia (Cairo & Bishop, 2004; Cantril & Haylock, 2004; Holdsworth & Nguyen, 2003).

Using NANDA, NIC, and NOC

Chart 14–1 shows links between NANDA, NIC, and NOC when caring for the client with cancer.

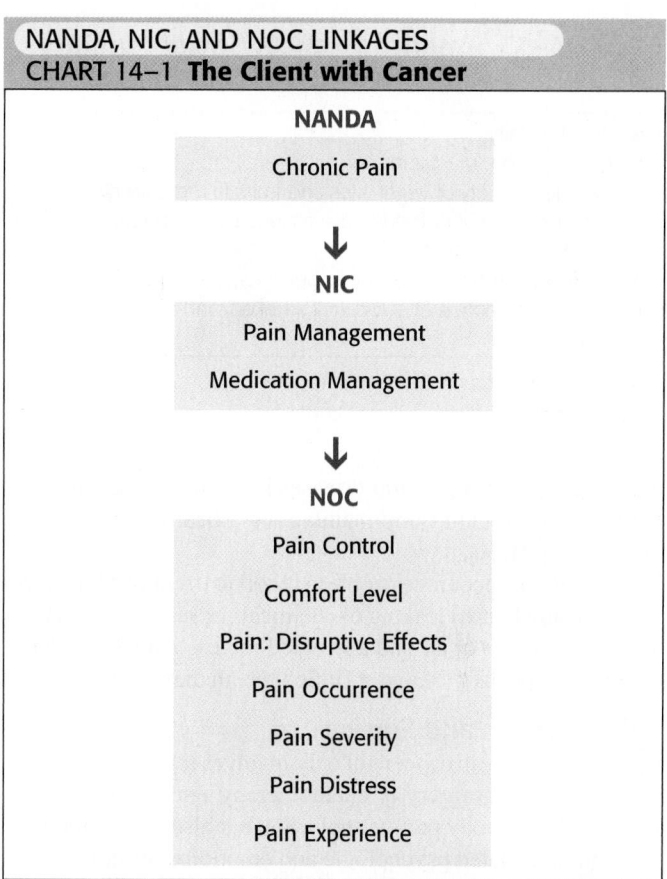

NANDA, NIC, AND NOC LINKAGES
CHART 14–1 The Client with Cancer

NANDA
Chronic Pain
↓
NIC
Pain Management
Medication Management
↓
NOC
Pain Control
Comfort Level
Pain: Disruptive Effects
Pain Occurrence
Pain Severity
Pain Distress
Pain Experience

Data from *NANDA's Nursing Diagnoses: Definitions & Classification 2005–2006* by NANDA International (2005), Philadelphia; *Nursing Interventions Classification (NIC)* (4th ed.) by J. M. Dochterman & G. M. Bulechek (2004), St. Louis, MO: Mosby; and *Nursing Outcomes Classification (NOC)* (3rd ed.) by S. Moorhead, M. Johnson, and M. Maas (2004), St. Louis, MO: Mosby.

Health Education for the Client and Family

Prevention

The ACS makes specific recommendations for cancer prevention in addition to the screening measures discussed earlier in this chapter. Based on these recommendations, nurses teach clients and families to decrease risk factors by:

- Avoiding tobacco and excessive alcohol use.
- Avoiding situations where secondhand smoke is abundant.
- Eating a low-fat, high-fiber diet.
- Consuming ample amounts of antioxidant foods, such as those containing beta carotene (a vitamin A precursor), vitamins E and C, and omega-3 oils.
- Avoiding foods with carcinogenic additives, dyes, or chemicals used in processing. Box 14–15 lists the ACS dietary guidelines.
- Taking certain medications and hormones, such as estrogen or tamoxifen, only under close medical supervision.
- Limiting exposure to radiation, including sun exposure.
- Using extreme caution if employed in an industry that uses carcinogenic chemicals or airborne particles (smoke). Seek new employment if at risk for related cancers.

BOX 14–15 **American Cancer Society Dietary Guidelines to Prevent Cancer**

- Avoid obesity.
- Cut down on total fat intake.
- Include a variety of vegetables and fruits in the daily diet.
- Eat more high-fiber foods, such as whole-grain cereals, vegetables, and fruits.
- Limit consumption of alcoholic beverages, if you drink at all.
- Limit consumption of salt-cured, smoked, and nitrate-cured foods.

Source: From the American Cancer Society, 2006.

- Protecting self from viral diseases known to cause cancer.
- Improving immunity by maintaining a healthy lifestyle and managing stress.

In addition, encourage people to report to the public health department any known leaking of chemicals or radioactive materials into the water or air and any noted increase in the incidence of cancer, especially of one specific type, in their communities.

Rehabilitation and Survival

Rehabilitation from cancer not only involves regaining strength, recovering from surgery or chemotherapy, and learning to live with an altered body part or appliance, but also entails recovering from associated psychologic and emotional turmoil.

Rehabilitation centers provide physical therapy, occupational therapy, speech therapy, job retraining, and an opportunity to recuperate before resuming full responsibilities. In addition, many clients go home to convalesce and receive in-home support in the form of nursing supervision, direct care, and teaching. Hygiene and home maintenance can be provided by a certified home health aide. Physical and occupational therapists provide muscle strengthening and mobility training (especially with prostheses), and home safety teaching.

Psychologic rehabilitation of cancer survivors addresses quality-of-life issues. Three "seasons of cancer survival" have been described (Mullan, 1985). The first starts with diagnosis but is dominated by treatment. The second stage is one of extended survival, which occurs when treatment ends and the watchful waiting period begins. This period is characterized by fear of recurrence. Permanent survival is said to begin when the survival period has gone on long enough that the risk of recurrence is small. In this period, the client has to deal with secondary problems related to health and social issues resulting from the cancer experience. Employment may be a problem, health insurance may be canceled, and life insurance may be difficult to get. Relationships may have suffered from the strain of the illness on significant others and the essential self-focusing required for recovery. However, both the client and significant others may have undergone a personal and spiritual growth that ushers in a new and enriching period of their lives.

New self-help groups are emerging in many communities to support others through their "seasons of survival." Many cancer survivors speak to groups about assisting other cancer survivors. Clients and families need to be informed about the many resources available through community agencies as well as the survivor support groups.

Community-Based Care

Before the client is discharged, teach both the client and significant others or caregivers to manage the client at home. Discuss problems that may result from the type of cancer and the treatment received, and provide information on how to manage these problems and when to call the physician.

- Teach wound care to the client with an open wound or draining lesion, and provide a referral to a home health nurse to monitor progress.
- Explain special diets clearly, or refer the client to a dietitian before discharge.
- Carefully review the physician's instructions with the client and family, making sure they understand medications to be taken, any other treatments, and when to see the doctor for follow-up care.
- Provide or order equipment and supplies needed for home care, especially any specialized bed or equipment to aid mobility and ensure safety in the home.
- For the client who will need complex care, such as parenteral nutrition, provide a referral to a home health nurse before discharge.

Because the hospital stay is often short, the client and family will benefit from follow-up phone calls at home for several days. People do not learn well under the stress of going home; give the client and family a number to call if they have concerns or questions.

Hospice Care

More and more cancer clients with terminal disease are electing to die at home. This decision has been made easier by the increased availability of **hospice** programs. When a client and family or significant others elect hospice care, they are usually precluding additional hospitalizations other than those required to manage reversible problems. Hospice clients also refuse resuscitation measures (CPR and other extraordinary measures).

Hospice care involves a multidisciplinary team and is designed to give the client comfort and to assist in a peaceful death with support to caretakers. The team usually consists of a nurse case manager, a physician, an anesthesiologist or pharmacist, an infusion therapist, a social worker, a physical therapist, a home health aide, and volunteers.

Many hospice services are connected with an inpatient respite care unit, where the client can receive 24-hour care for up to several weeks. This source provides the necessary care to the client if a family member becomes ill or needs to be relieved temporarily of the tremendous burden of caring for a dying loved one. Veterans Administration medical centers are very good models for these programs.

Studies of families that have participated in hospice services have found that family members were very positive about the experience (Teno et al., 2001). The aspects of hospice they most appreciated were the 24-hour accessibility and availability of the health team and the quality of communication from all team members. Family members emphasized that "the nurses listened, answered questions honestly, and prepared us for changes in the patient's condition." Team members were rated as very professional, but more relaxed and friendly than hospital staff; they talked with the family and displayed accepting, nonjudgmental attitudes. Team members were also seen as well informed, knowledgeable, and competent with excellent problem-solving skills. Chapter 5 ∞ provides more information on hospice care.

EXPLORE MediaLink

Prentice Hall Nursing MediaLink DVD-ROM
Audio Glossary
NCLEX-RN® Review

Animation/Video
Cancer
Cell Division
Mini-infusion Pumps

COMPANION WEBSITE www.prenhall.com/lemone
Audio Glossary
NCLEX-RN® Review
Care Plan Activity: Weight Loss and Chemotherapy
Case Studies
Cancer Therapies
Pain Management
MediaLink Applications
Cancer Research
Interpreting Lab Results
Links to Resources

CHAPTER HIGHLIGHTS

- One in every 4 deaths in the United States is caused by cancer and more than 1500 people die of cancer each day. Cancer can affect people of any age, gender, ethnicity, or geographic region.
- Cancer is the second leading cause of death in people over age 65. The incidence of cancer increases with advancing age. The most commonly seen cancers in older women are colorectal, breast, lung, pancreatic, and ovarian. In older men, lung, colorectal, prostate, pancreatic, and gastric cancers occur most frequently.
- Oncogenes are genes that promote cell proliferation and are capable of triggering cancerous characteristics. Several oncogenes, such as BRCA-1 and BRCA-2, are associated with breast cancer.
- Tumor suppressor genes, which normally suppress oncogenes, can become inactive by deletion or mutation. Inherited cancers have been associated with tumor suppressor genes, such as p53, a suppressor gene that has been associated with sarcoma and cancer of the breast and brain.
- The diagnosis and treatment of cancer is a pivotal life-changing event that prompts individuals to make immediate and ongoing adjustment to this life-threatening illness.
- Effective physical and psychosocial adjustment to cancer diagnosis and treatment has been shown to lead to successful completion of treatment, enhancement of cancer patients' ability to cope with disease, improvement of patients' quality of life, and ultimately, improvement of survival.

- The goals of cancer treatment are aimed at cure and control of cancer as well as management of cancer-related and treatment-related symptoms.
- Chemotherapy uses cytotoxic medications to cure or control cancer by interrupting cell metabolism and replication and by interfering with the ability of the malignant cell to synthesize vital enzymes and chemicals.
- Pain management is an important component of care for cancer patients. It is estimated that 20% to 50% of clients with early-stage cancer and up to 95% of clients with advanced cancer experience pain.
- Complementary therapies are therapies that clients choose as a complement to medical treatment. Common complementary therapies for cancer include botanical agents, nutritional supplements, dietary regimens, mind-body modalities, spiritual approaches, and miscellaneous therapies. To provide sensitive care, nurses should be knowledgeable about common complementary therapies.
- Tumor lysis syndrome (TLS), a combination of two or more metabolic abnormalities, is a life-threatening emergency for clients with cancer. Patients at risk for TLS include those with bulky chemosensitive cancer such as high-degrade lymphomas and acute leukemia, elevated serum uric acid, potassium, and phosphorus, and renal deficiency.

TEST YOURSELF NCLEX-RN® REVIEW

1 Mr. Lawrence has a history of colon cancer. Cells from the colon tumor have traveled to his liver. This process is called:
1. carcinogenesis.
2. dysplasia.
3. metastasis.
4. mutation.

2 A client diagnosed with lung cancer reports he is having difficulty sleeping and often feels tense. The most appropriate initial nursing intervention would be to:
1. encourage the client to express his feelings about the cancer diagnosis.
2. document the client's report of difficulty sleeping and tenseness in the chart.
3. obtain an order for medication for sleep from the physician.
4. offer an antianxiety drug such as Ativan (lorazepam).

3 Mr. Palacci is receiving external radiation for treatment of lung cancer. Client education for care of the skin in the marked area includes:
1. apply antibacterial ointment daily.
2. avoid contact with others.
3. avoid rubbing or scratching treated skin areas.
4. cleanse the skin with plain water.

4 Ms. Hernandez complains of nausea and vomiting following her daily chemotherapy treatment. The *most* appropriate nursing intervention would be to:
1. keep Ms. Hernandez NPO until her daily chemotherapy is completed.
2. provide antiemetic medication 30 to 40 minutes prior to each treatment.
3. provide clear liquids until the chemotherapy is completed.
4. schedule chemotherapy administration for bedtime.

5 Mrs. Smith experiences bone marrow depression as a result of chemotherapy. Which of the following would the nurse expect to find?
1. alopecia
2. nausea and vomiting
3. platelet count 50,000
4. temperature 102°F

6 Mr. Giosa, a 46-year-old businessman with a diagnosis of metastatic lung cancer, is going to have chemotherapy tomorrow. To help him better understand the role of chemotherapeutic agents in treating cancer, you have completed the teaching on chemotherapy with him. You determine that the teaching is effective, when Mr. Giosa states:
1. "Chemotherapy uses drugs that promote the normal growth of cells while killing the cancer cells."
2. "Chemotherapy only uses a single drug to treat cancer because drug resistance is rare."
3. "Chemotherapy includes drugs that not only attack cancer cells but also normal rapidly dividing cells."
4. "Chemotherapy is a preferred therapy because it has fewer adverse effects than radiation therapy."

7 During training for new radiation nurses, you have learned that the delivery of high-energy radiation (e.g., electrons, x-rays, photons) to kill cancer cells by using a machine to focus a beam of radiation on the body is called
1. external radiation therapy.
2. internal-beam radiation therapy.
3. brachytherapy.
4. biochemotherapy.

8 You are taking care of a client who just received the first cycle of chemotherapy for acute leukemia 2 days ago. As an oncology nurse, you are closely monitoring the client's laboratory tests of uric acid, potassium, phosphorus, and calcium based on the knowledge that the client is at risk for
1. spinal cord compression.
2. tumor lysis syndrome.
3. septic shock.
4. superior vena cava syndrome.

9 Replication of DNA to form two sets of chromosomes occurs in which phase of the cell cycle?
1. G_1
2. G_2
3. S
4. M

10 Oncogenes are genes
1. that promote cell growth when activated.
2. that block cell growth.
3. that stimulate a complex signaling process.
4. that are strictly regulated.

See Test Yourself answers in Appendix C.

BIBLIOGRAPHY

American Cancer Society. (2006a). *Cancer facts and figures—2006.* Atlanta: Author.

American Cancer Society. (2006b). *Cancer facts and figures for African Americans–2005–2006.* Atlanta: Author.

Anderson, C. M., Buzaid, A. C., Sussman, J. J., Lee, J. J., Ali-Osman, F., Braunschweiger, P. G., et al. (1998). Nitric oxide and neopterin levels and clinical response in stage III melanoma patients receiving concurrent biochemotherapy. *Melanoma Research, 8*(2), 149–155.

Armer, J., Fu, M. R., Wainstock, J. M., Zagar, E., & Jacobs, L. K. (2004). Lymphedema following breast cancer treatment, including sentinel lymph node biopsy. *Lymphology, 37,* 73–91.

Bach, P. B., Schrag, D., Brawley, O. W., Galaznik, A., Yakren, S., & Begg, C. B. (2002). Survival of blacks and whites after a cancer diagnosis. *JAMA, 287*(16), 2106–2113.

Battiato, L. A., & Wheeler, V. S. (2000). Biotherapy. In C. H. Yarbro, M. H. Frogge, M. Goodman, & S. L. Groenwald (Eds.), *Cancer nursing: Principles and practice* (5th ed., pp. 543–579). Boston: Jones & Bartlett.

Berd, D. (2001). Autologous, hapten-modified vaccine as a treatment for human cancers. *Vaccine, 19,* 2565–2570.

Bergh, J., Wiklund, T., Erikstein, B., Lidbrink, E., Lindman, H., Malmström, P., et al. (2000). Tailored fluorouracil, epirubicin, and cyclophosphamide compared with marrow-supported high-dose chemotherapy as adjuvant treatment for high-risk breast cancer: A randomised trial. *Lancet, 356,* 1384–1391.

Beriwal, S., Singh, S., & Garcia-Young, J. A. (2002). Tumor lysis syndrome in extensive-stage small-cell lung cancer. *American Journal of Clinical Oncology, 25*(5), 474–475.

Blaylock, R. L. (1998). Neurodegeneration and aging of the central nervous system: Prevention and treatment by phytochemicals and metabolic nutrients. *Integrative Medicine; 1*(3), 117–133, 135–141.

Bradley, C. J., Given, C. W., & Roberts, C. (2001). Disparities in cancer diagnosis and survival. *Cancer, 91*(1), 178–188.

Bruce, S. (2001). Photodynamic therapy: Another option in cancer care. *Clinical Journal of Oncology Nursing, 5,* 95–99.

Cady, J. (2001). Understanding opioid tolerance in cancer pain. *Oncology Nursing Forum, 28,* 1561–1568.

Cairo, M. S., & Bishop, M. (2004). Tumour lysis syndrome: New therapeutic strategies and classification. *British Journal of Haematology, 127*(1), 3–11.

Cantril, C. A., & Haylock, P. J. (2004). Emergency. Tumor lysis syndrome. *American Journal of Nursing, 104*(4), 49–52.

Chapman, D., & Goodman, M. (2000). Breast cancer. In C. H. Yarbro, M. H. Frogge, M. Goodman, & S. L. Groenwald (Eds.), *Cancer nursing: Principles and practice* (5th ed., pp. 994–1047). Boston: Jones & Bartlett.

Cohen, G. L., & Falkson, C. I. (1998). Current treatment options for malignant melanoma. *Drugs, 55*(6), 791–799.

Dietrich, M., Block, G., Norkus, E. P., Hudes, M., Traber, M. G., Cross, C. E., et al. (2002). Smoking and exposure to environmental tobacco smoke decrease some plasma antioxidants and increase gamma-tocopherol *in vivo* after adjustment for dietary antioxidant intakes. *American Journal of Clinical Nutrition, 77*(1), 160–166.

Donahue, B. R., Wernz, J. C., & Cooper, J. S. (2000). HIV-associated malignancies. In J. D. Roseblatt, P. Okunieff, & J. V. Sitzmann (Eds.), *Clinical oncology: A multidisciplinary approach for physicians and students* (8th ed., pp. 199–207). Philadelphia: W. B. Saunders.

Dunlop R. J., & Campbell, C. W. (2000). Cytokines and advanced cancer. *Journal of Pain & Symptom Management, 20*(3), 214–232.

Farquhar, C., Marjoribanks, J., Basser, R., Hetrick, S., & Lethaby, A. (2006). High dose chemotherapy and autologous bone marrow or stem cell transplantation versus conventional chemotherapy for women with metastatic breast cancer. *Cochrane Breast Cancer Group Cochrane Database of Systematic Reviews (3).*

Ferrell, B. (2000). Article captures the essence and meaning of alopecia. *Oncology Nursing Forum, 27,* 17.

Ferrell, B., & McCaffery, M. (1997). Nurses' knowledge about equianalgesia and opioid dosing. *Cancer Nursing, 20,* 201–212.

Foltz, A. (2000). Nutritional disturbances. In C. H. Yarbro, M. H. Frogge, M. Goodman, & S. L. Groenwald (Eds.), *Cancer nursing: Principles and practice* (5th ed., pp. 754–775). Boston: Jones & Bartlett.

Fu, M. R. (2004). Post-breast cancer lymphedema and management. *Recent Advances: Research Updates, 5*(1), 125–138.

Fu, M. R. (2005). Breast cancer survivors' intentions of managing lymphedema. *Cancer Nursing, 28*(6), 446–457.

Fu, M. R., Anderson, C. M., McDaniel, R., & Armer, J. (2002). Patients' perception of fatigue in response to biochemotherapy as a treatment for metastatic melanoma. *Oncology Nursing Forum, 29*(6), 961–966.

Futreal, P. A., Kasprzyk, A., Birney, E., Mullikin, J. C., Wooster, R., & Stratton, M. R. (2001). Cancer and genomics. *Nature, 409*(6822), 850–852.

Haapoja, I. (2000). Paraneoplastic syndromes. In C. H. Yarbro, M. H. Frogge, M. Goodman, & S. L. Groenwald (Eds.), *Cancer nursing: Principles and practice* (5th ed., pp. 792–812). Boston: Jones & Bartlett.

Habib, G. S., & Saliba, W. R. (2002). Tumor lysis syndrome after hydrocortisone treatment in metastatic melanoma: A case report and review of the literature. *American Journal of the Medical Sciences, 323*(3), 155–157.

Hawkins, R. (2001). Mastering the intricate maze of metastasis. *Oncology Nursing Forum, 28*(6), 959–965.

Held-Warmkessel, J. (2000). Prostate cancer. In C. H. Yarbro, M. H. Frogge, M. Goodman, & S. L. Groenwald (Eds.), *Cancer nursing: Principles and practice* (5th ed., pp. 1427–1451). Boston: Jones & Bartlett.

Hill, R. P. (2001). The biology of cancer. In P. Rubin (Ed.), *Clinical oncology: A multidisciplinary approach for physicians and students* (pp. 32–45). Philadelphia: W. B. Saunders.

Holdsworth, M. T., & Nguyen, P. (2003). Role of i.v. allopurinol and rasburicase in tumor lysis syndrome. *American Journal of Health-System Pharmacy, 60*(21), 2213–2222.

Holland, J. (2001). New treatment modalities in radiation therapy. *Journal of Intravenous Nursing, 24,* 95–101.

Jasek, A. M., & Day, H. J. (1994). Acute spontaneous tumor lysis syndrome. *American Journal of Hematology, 47*(2), 129–131.

Karnofsky, D., Abelmann, W., Craver, L., & Burchenal, J. (1948). The use of nitrogen mustard in the palliative treatment of carcinoma. *Cancer, 1,* 634–656.

Katz, L. S., & Epstein, S. (2005). The relation of cancer-prone personality to exceptional recovery from cancer: A preliminary study. *Advances in Mind-Body Medicine, 21*(3/4), 6–20.

Kaye, J., Morton, J., Bowcutt, M., & Maupin, D. (2000). Stress, depression, and psychoneuroimmunology. *Journal of Neuroscience Nursing, 32,* 93–100.

Kee, J. L. (2002). *Laboratory and diagnostic tests with nursing implications* (6th ed.). Upper Saddle River, NJ: Prentice Hall Health.

Khalsa, J. H., Genser, S., Francis, H., & Martin, B. (2002). Clinical consequences of marijuana. *Journal of Clinical Pharmacology, 42*(11 Supplement), 7S–10S.

Legha, S., Ring, S., Eton, O., Bedikian, A., Buzaid, A. C., Plager, C., et al. (1998). Development of a biochemotherapy regiment with concurrent administration of cisplatin, vinblastine, dacarbazine, interferon alfa, and interleukin-2 for patients with metastatic melanoma. *Journal of Clinical Oncology, 16*(5), 1752–1759.

Li, C. I., Anderson, B. O., Daling, J. R., & Moe, R. E. (2002). Changing incidence of lobular carcinoma *in situ* of the breast. *Breast Cancer Research and Treatment, 75*(3), 259–268.

McDaniel, R., & Rhodes, V. (1998). Development of a sensory information videotape for women receiving chemotherapy for breast cancer. *Cancer Nursing, 21,* 143–148.

Misset, J., & Levi, F. (1995). Chronomodulated chemotherapy combining 5-fluorouracil, folinic acid, and oxaliplatin in advanced colorectal cancer: An overview of seven years of experience (Meeting abstract). *Cancer Investigation, 13*(Suppl 1), 49–50.

Mullan, F. (1985). Seasons of survival: Reflections of a physician with cancer. *New England Journal of Medicine, 313,* 270–273.

Neal, A., & Hoskin, P. (1997). *Clinical oncology: Basic principles and practice* (2nd ed.). New York: Oxford University Press.

Niederhuber, J. E. (2002). Surgical therapy. In M. D. Abeloff, J. O. Armitage, A. S. Lichter, & J. E. Niederhuber (Eds.), *Clinical oncology* (2nd ed., pp. 471–481). New York: Churchill Livingstone.

Oncology Nursing Society. (2006). Oncology Nursing Society position paper on quality cancer care. Retrieved May 11, 2006, from http://www.ons.org/publications/positions/QualityCancerCare.shtml

Pace, J. C. (2000). AIDS-related malignancies. In C. H. Yarbro, M. H. Frogge, M. Goodman, & S. L. Groenwald (Eds.), *Cancer nursing: Principles and practice* (5th ed., pp. 933–949). Boston: Jones & Bartlett.

Peto, R., Darby, S., Deo, H., Silcocks, P., Whitley, E., & Doll, R. (2000). Smoking, smoking cessation, and lung cancer in the UK since 1950: Combination of national statistics with two case-control studies. *BMJ, 321*(7257), 323–329.

Porth, C. (2005). *Pathophysiology: Concepts of altered health states* (7th ed.). Philadelphia: Lippincott.

Rahman, Z., Frye, D., Buzdar, A., Smith, T., Asmar, L., Champlin, R., et al. (1997). Impact of selection process on response rate and long-term survival of potential high-dose chemotherapy candidates treated with standard-dose doxorubicin-containing chemotherapy in patients with metastatic breast cancer. *Journal of Clinical Oncology, 15,* 3171–3177.

Rosenthal, D. (1998). Changing trends. *A Cancer Journal for Clinicians, 48*(1), 3–4.

Rossi, E. L. (2004). Stress-induced alternative gene splicing in mind-body medicine. *Advances in Mind-Body Medicine, 20*(2), 12–19.

Rubin, P., Williams, J. P., Okunieff, P., Rosenblatt, J. D., & Sitzmann, J. V. (2001). Statement of the clinical oncologic problem. In P. Rubin (Ed.), *Clinical oncology: A multidisciplinary approach for physicians and students* (pp. 1–31). Philadelphia: W. B. Saunders.

Scigliano, E., Vlachos, A., Najfeld, V., & Shank, B. (2001). The leukemias. In P. Rubin (Ed.), *Clinical oncology: A multidisciplinary approach for physicians and students* (pp. 565–614). Philadelphia: W. B. Saunders.

Selye, H. (1984). *The stress of life* (rev. 2nd ed.). New York: McGraw-Hill.

Sparber, A. (2001). State boards of nursing and scope of practice of registered nurses performing complementary therapies. *Online Journal of Issues in Nursing, 6*(2), 6–7.

Spitalnick, P. F., & diSant'Agnese, P. A. (2001). The pathology of cancer. In P. Rubin (Ed.), *Clinical oncology: A multidisciplinary approach for physicians and students* (pp. 47–61). Philadelphia: W. B. Saunders.

Stoves, J., Richardson, D., & Patel, H. (2001). Tumour lysis syndrome in a patient with metastatic melanoma treated with biochemotherapy. *Nephrology Dialysis Transplantation, 16*(1), 188–189.

Surbone, A. (2001). Ethical implications of genetic testing for breast cancer susceptibility. *Critical Reviews in Oncology-Hematology, 40*(2), 149–157.

Tanvetyanon, T., & Choudhury, A. M. (2004). Fatal acute tumor lysis syndrome, hepatic encephalopathy and flare phenomenon following combined androgen blockade. *Journal of Urology, 171*(4), 1627.

Teno, J. M., Clarridge, B., Casey, V., Edgman-Levitan, S., & Fowler, J. (2001). Validation of toolkit after-death bereaved family member interview. *Journal of Pain & Symptom Management, 22,* 752–758.

Weiss, R. B., Rifkin, R. M., Stewart, F. M., Theriault, R. L., Williams, L. A., Herman, A. A., & Beveridge, R. A. (2000). High dose chemotherapy for high-risk primary breast cancer: An on-site review of the Bezwoda study. *Lancet, 355,* 999–1003.

Williams, J., Wood, C., & Cunningham-Warburton, P. (1999). A narrative study of chemotherapy-induced alopecia. *Oncology Nursing Forum, 26,* 1463–1468.

Williams, M. D., & Sandler, A. B. (2001). The epidemiology of lung cancer. *Cancer Treatment & Research, 105,* 31–52.

Wu, T. Y., & Yu, M. Y. (2003). Reliability and validity of the mammography screening beliefs questionnaire among Chinese American women. *Cancer Nursing, 26*(2), 131–142.

Yarbro, J. (2005). Carcinogenesis. In C. H. Yarbro, M. H. Frogge, M. Goodman, & S. L. Groenwald (Eds.), *Cancer nursing: Principles and practice* (5th ed., pp. 48–57). Boston: Jones & Bartlett.

Zech, D., Grond, S., Lynch, J., Hertel, D., & Lehmann, K. (1995). Validation of World Health Organization Guidelines for cancer pain relief: A 10-year prospective study. *Pain, 63,* 65–76.

UNIT 3 BUILDING CLINICAL COMPETENCE
Pathophysiology and Patterns of Health

FUNCTIONAL HEALTH PATTERN: Health Perception-Health Management

In contrast to subsequent units of this text in which the conditions presented affect primarily one functional health pattern or body system, those discussed in this unit often affect multiple body systems and have a significant impact on several functional health patterns. In nearly all cases, however, the Health Perception-Health Management Pattern is affected. In some cases, a disruption in this pattern has led to the condition presented.

■ Think about clients with altered health perception or health management for whom you have cared in your clinical experiences.

- ■ What were the clients' major medical diagnoses? Did one of the conditions discussed in this unit *cause* the condition (e.g., a genetic disorder, trauma, infection, or altered immunity)? Or, did the condition discussed in this unit develop *secondarily* to the client's primary disorder (e.g., metabolic acidosis resulting from type 1 diabetes, pain related to cancer or surgery)? How did the condition affect the clients' healing and recovery?
- ■ How did the clients' health status affect their perceived health and well-being or their ability to manage their own health? Did the clients' healthcare behaviors interfere with their health?

■ The Health Perception-Health Management Pattern describes the client's perceived pattern of health and well-being and how they manage health. This pattern includes healthcare behaviors, such as health promotion and illness prevention activities, medical treatments, and follow-up care. Early intervention and health promotion–focused care can result in a higher level of wellness and often a longer and better quality of life. The client's perceived health and well-being and ability to manage health can be affected by factors within or beyond his or her ability to control them:

- ■ The individual has no control over his or her pattern of genetic inheritance. Genetic alterations may lead to a disorder directly linked to the pattern of genes, e.g., Huntington's disease (a single-gene autosomal dominant disorder), cystic fibrosis (an autosomal recessive disorder linked to a defect on chromosome 7), or classic hemophilia (a sex-linked recessive disorder). In other instances, the client's genetic makeup leads to an increased risk of developing a specific disorder such as cancer.
- ■ Factors and behaviors at least partially within the client's control also affect health and its management. Health and lifestyle behaviors affect the client's risk of developing and resisting infections and certain cancers. The risk for being affected by trauma often is fully or partially within the client's control.

■ The human body is continually threatened by foreign substances, infectious agents, and abnormal cells, resulting in alterations in well-being and the ability to manage health. The impact of these threats can lead to manifestations such as:

- ■ Pain (cellular damage or biochemicals released due to cell damage ► stimulation of pain receptors ► impulse transmission to thalamus and cerebral cortex ► perception of pain)
- ■ Fever (infectious or noninfectious disorder ► release of endogenous pyrogens from damaged host cells ► pyrogens increase thermoregulatory set point in the hypothalamus ► increased body temperature)
- ■ Inflammation (tissue damage due to trauma or entry of an antigen ► release of inflammatory mediators ► vasodilation, increased capillary permeability ► formation of fluid exudate ► tissue edema and increased numbers of WBCs in damaged tissue ► phagocytosis, trapping, and destruction of invading bacteria)
- ■ Tachycardia (blood or fluid loss, increased metabolic demands ► cardiac output inadequate to meet needs of body ► stimulation of sympathetic nervous system ► release of epinephrine and norepinephrine ► stimulation of sinus node ► increased heart rate)
- ■ Tachypnea (trauma, inflammation ► increased metabolic rate ► increased cellular demand for oxygen to support aerobic metabolism ► stimulation of respiratory centers in the brainstem ► increased respiratory rate).

■ Priority nursing diagnoses within the Health Perception-Health Management Pattern that may be appropriate for clients include:

- ■ *Risk for Infection* as evidenced by tissue trauma or impaired immune responses
- ■ *Ineffective Health Maintenance* as evidenced by lack of preventive care or health screening
- ■ *Ineffective Protection* as evidenced by impaired immunity related to cancer therapy or HIV disease
- ■ *Risk for Trauma* as evidenced by high-risk personal behaviors.

■ Nursing diagnoses from other functional health patterns often are of high priority for the client with conditions discussed in this unit:

- ■ *Acute Pain, Chronic Pain* (Cognitive-Perceptual)
- ■ *Disturbed Body Image* (Self-Perception-Self Concept)
- ■ *Impaired Tissue Integrity* (Nutritional-Metabolic)
- ■ *Risk for Post-Trauma Syndrome* (Coping Stress Tolerance)

Directions: Read the clinical scenario below and answer the questions that follow. To complete this exercise successfully, you will use not only knowledge of the content in this unit, but also principles related to setting priorities and maintaining client safety.

CLINICAL SCENARIO

You have been assigned to work with the following four patients for the 0700 shift on a medical-surgical unit. Significant data obtained during report are as follows:

- Allen Barber is a 55-year-old client with diabetes mellitus who is 4 days postoperative abdominal surgery with an inflammation of the incision site. Vital signs are T 101°F, P 94, R 24, BP 138/82. The abdominal incision appears red with warmth and edema around the incision. The client states his pain level is 8 on a pain scale of 1 to 10. Labs and wound cultures have been ordered.
- Tamra Sanders is a 22-year-old client with Down syndrome. She is admitted in sickle cell crisis with T of 102°F, P 90, R 30 and shallow, and BP of 110/84. She is complaining of severe chest pain with

shortness of breath. She states her pain scale level is 10 of 10. She has an order to begin morphine PCA.
- Mia Windham is a 26-year-old who was admitted yesterday with a maculopapular rash on the hands and feet that is spreading to the arms and legs. This morning she is complaining of abdominal pain, nausea, and bloody diarrhea. The client has a history of having a bone marrow transplant 3 months ago as treatment for leukemia.
- Harry Anderson is a 40-year-old in late stages of AIDS. He is confused, incontinent, and is very spastic. He is on seizure precautions. He needs to be turned every 2 hours to prevent pressure sores. He is currently yelling that he needs help.

Questions

1 In what order would you visit these patients after report?
1. _____
2. _____
3. _____
4. _____

2 What top two priority nursing diagnoses would you choose for each of the clients presented above? Can you explain, if asked, the rationale for your choices?

	Priority Nursing Diagnosis #1	Priority Nursing Diagnosis #2
Allen Barber		
Tamra Sanders		
Mia Windham		
Harry Anderson		

3 In which position does the nurse place the client with hypovolemic shock?
1. semi-Fowler's position with legs straight
2. Trendelenburg position with legs elevated 10 degrees
3. left lateral position with legs bent toward chest
4. supine position with legs elevated 20 degrees

4 The family of the client with sickle cell anemia asks the nurse how sickle cell anemia is transmitted from one family member to another. Which statement by the nurse is the correct response?
1. "The mother carries the gene for sickle cell anemia and passes it to the children."
2. "The father carries the gene for sickle cell anemia and passes it to the children."
3. "Both parents carry the gene for sickle cell anemia and children have a 25% chance of getting the disease process."
4. "One parent has the disease and one parent carries the affected gene, and they have a 50% chance of passing it to the children."

5 The client with HIV has experienced weight loss. The dietician teaches the client meal planning in which type of diet?
1. high protein, high fiber
2. high protein, high kilocalorie
3. low fiber, low protein
4. high carbohydrate, high vitamins

6 The nurse performs wound cleansing with which procedure?
1. Cleanse the wound with soap and water.
2. Use normal saline to cleanse the wound.
3. Cleanse the wound with povidone-iodine.
4. Hydrogen peroxide (half strength) is used to cleanse the wound.

7 Prior to administering cytotoxic agents, such as cyclophosphamide (Cytoxan), the nurse needs to notify the physician of which lab results?
1. hemoglobin of 10.8 g/dL, hematocrit of 35%
2. potassium of 3.4 mEq/L, sodium of 130 mEq/L
3. creatinine of 2 mg/dL, blood urea nitrogen of 30 mg/dL
4. white blood cell count of 3900 mm^3, platelets of 74,000 mm^3

8 Due to diarrhea, Ms. Windham's arterial blood gas results are pH, 7.30, Paco$_2$, 35 mmHg; PaO$_2$, 90 mmHg; HCO$_3^-$, 19 mEq/L. The nurse interprets these results as indicating the client has:
1. metabolic acidosis.
2. metabolic alkalosis.
3. respiratory acidosis.
4. respiratory alkalosis.

9 Which laboratory studies would you expect to draw on a client who is 4 days postoperative with an inflammation of the incision site?
1. white blood cell count/differential, erythrocyte sedimentation rate, C-reactive protein
2. troponins, metabolic panel for electrolytes, cultures of wound site
3. blood cultures, hematocrit and hemoglobin, blood glucose level
4. complete blood cell count, alkaline phosphatase, urine creatinine and blood urea nitrogen

10 The client is admitted to the emergency department for a severe anaphylactic reaction to aspirin. Which medication is ordered to be administered?
1. 0.5 mL of 1:1000 epinephrine subcutaneously
2. 0.3 mL of 1:10,000 epinephrine subcutaneously
3. intravenous infusion of 1:10,000 epinephrine
4. intravenous infusion of 1:100,000 epinephrine

11 When administering a blood transfusion, which manifestations indicate a hemolytic reaction to the blood being administered?
1. abdominal cramps and diarrhea
2. bradycardia and hypertension
3. dyspnea and hypotension
4. diaphoresis and tachycardia

12 The nurse teaches clients and families to decrease risk factors of cancer by following which cancer prevention recommendations? (Select all that apply.)
1. Avoid tobacco and excessive alcohol use.
2. Eat a diet low in fat and high in carbohydrates.
3. Increase intake of vitamins A, D, E, and K.
4. Limit exposure in sun from 11:00 A.M. to 4:00 P.M.
5. Increase vegetables and fruits in the diet.
6. Eat meats grilled over a charcoal fire instead of fried.

CASE STUDY

Mr. Johnson is a 60-year-old African American construction worker who is seen in the physician's office with complaints of dull chest pain, shortness of breath, swelling of his hands and feet, weight loss, fatigue, and weakness. On physical assessment, vital signs are temperature 99.8°F, pulse 84, respirations 24, blood pressure 168/92. His height is 5' 11" and weight is 175 pounds. Mr. Johnson states this is a loss of 35 pounds during the past 3 months. Wheezing is heard when breath sounds are auscultated. Coughing is noted with deep breathing. The remainder of the physical assessment is unremarkable. He has a medical history of high blood pressure for which he takes diltiazem and ramipril. He has a history of smoking one to two packs of cigarettes a day since he was 15 years old. He states he has been exposed to asbestos in his employment. Mr. Johnson's nutrition assessment indicates that his diet consists of fried meats (especially chicken), green vegetables cooked in fatback, eggs and bacon for breakfast, and at breaktime he eats doughnuts or cookies. His fluid intake consists of coffee for breakfast and breaktime, soda at lunch, and three to four beers at night.

Blood is drawn for a complete blood count, electrolytes, blood glucose, calcitonin, CEA, haptoglobulin, GGT, and creatinine. A sputum specimen is sent to the laboratory. A chest x-ray and CT scan are done. Based on the results of the chest x-ray, bronchoscopy and needle aspiration biopsies are performed to confirm the diagnosis of lung cancer. The oncologist recommends an initial treatment plan of radiation therapy followed by combination chemotherapy to reduce the tumor size followed by surgical resection of the tumor.

Based on Mr. Johnson's medical diagnosis and treatment plan, *Readiness for Enhanced Therapeutic Regimen Management* is identified as the priority nursing diagnosis at this time.

- Bronchial epithelial cell damage → cell mutation → progressive cell abnormalities → malignant cell forms clones which reproduce to form a tumor → tumor produces substances to support its growth → bronchial obstruction, replacement of normal lung tissue by tumor → cough and increasing dyspnea;

affects

Mr. J.
60 y.o. male
Lung cancer

leads to

assess

- C/o dull chest pain, SOB, peripheral edema, weight loss, fatigue and weakness.
- T 99.8° F, P 84, R 24, BP 168/92
- Ht 5' 11", wt 175 lb
- Wheezing and cough present
- Meds: diltiazem and ramipril for HTN
- 45-60 pack/year smoking history, consumes 3-4 beers/day, high fat diet
- Hx of occupational asbestos exposure

generates

- Ineffective Breathing Pattern as evidence by tachypnea
- Ineffective Airway Clearance as evidence by wheezing and cough
- Imbalanced Nutrition: Less than Body Requirements as evidenced by recent significant weight loss
- Ineffective Health Maintenance as evidenced by BP, smoking, alcohol and fat intake
- Readiness for Enhanced Coping related to new cancer diagnosis

generate nursing diagnosis

Readiness for Enhanced Management of Therapeutic Regimen

prioritized to

expected outcomes

- Actively participates in healthcare decisions, verbalizes understanding of planned treatment regimen
- Uses measures to reduce adverse effects of radiation and chemotherapy
- Joins smoking cessation program, enlisting family support for efforts to stop smoking.
- Takes antihypertensive medications as ordered, regularly monitors BP
- Discusses potential treatment outcomes and effects with family
- Meets, together with wife, with dietitian for menu planning to reduce fat and saturated fat intake

evaluate

Joins smoking cessation program with wife; asks family and friends to avoid smoking in their presence
- Skin and mucous membranes remain intact during radiation therapy
- Weight remains stable, BP 152/84, R 20, P 80
- Stops drinking, stating "It doesn't even taste good without a cigarette."
- Increased intake of fresh fruit, vegetables, and whole grains

Independent Interventions
- Assess knowledge and understanding of disease, contributory factors, and treatment plan
- Provide information and reinforce teaching as needed to promote understanding
- Involve family in teaching and discussions
- Teach measures to reduce/ manage adverse treatment effects
- Provide information about and referral to available smoking cessation programs
- Assist client to plan for the future by providing information about usual course of illness and treatment
- Facilitate communication among healthcare providers, client, and family
- Teach coping/stress management techniques
- Offer information about available community resources

Nutritional and Metabolic Patterns

Functional Health Patterns with Related Nursing Diagnoses

HEALTH PERCEPTION-HEALTH MANAGEMENT

- Perceived health status
- Perceived health management
- Healthcare behaviors: health promotion and illness prevention activities, medical treatments, follow-up care

NUTRITIONAL-METABOLIC

- Daily consumption of food and fluids
- Favorite foods
- Use of dietary supplements
- Skin lesions and ability to heal
- Condition of the integument
- Weight, height, temperature

ELIMINATION

- Patterns of bowel and urinary excretion
- Perceived regularity or irregularity of elimination
- Use of laxatives or routines
- Changes in time, modes, quality, or quantity of excretions
- Use of devices for control

ACTIVITY-EXERCISE

- Patterns of personally relevant exercise, activity, leisure, and recreation
- ADLs that require energy expenditure
- Factors that interfere with the desired pattern (e.g., illness or injury)

VALUE-BELIEF

- Values, goals, or beliefs (including spirituality) that guide choices or decisions
- Perceived conflicts in values, beliefs, or expectations that are health related

PART II NUTRITIONAL AND METABOLIC PATTERNS WITH RELATED NANDA NURSING DIAGNOSES

- Risk for Aspiration
- Risk for Imbalanced Body Temperature
- Impaired Dentition
- Feeding Self-Care Deficit
- Deficient Fluid Volume
- Fluid Volume Excess
- Risk for Deficient Fluid Volume
- Hyperthermia
- Hypothermia
- Risk for Infection
- Impaired Oral Mucous Membranes
- Nausea
- Imbalanced Nutrition: Less than Body Requirements
- Imbalanced Nutrition: More than Body Requirements
- Impaired Skin Integrity
- Risk for Impaired Skin Integrity
- Impaired Swallowing
- Ineffective Thermoregulation
- Impaired Tissue Integrity
- Risk for Trauma
- Adult Failure to Thrive

COPING-STRESS-TOLERANCE

- Capacity to resist challenges to self-integrity
- Methods of handling stress
- Support systems
- Perceived ability to control and manage situations

SEXUALITY-REPRODUCTIVE

- Satisfaction with sexuality or sexual relationships
- Reproductive pattern
- Female menstrual and perimenopausal history

ROLE-RELATIONSHIPS

- Perception of major roles, relationships, and responsibilities in current life situation
- Satisfaction with or disturbances in roles and relationships

SELF-PERCEPTION–SELF-CONCEPT

- Attitudes about self
- Perceived abilities, worth, self-image, emotions
- Body posture and movement, eye contact, voice and speech patterns

SLEEP-REST

- Patterns of sleep and rest-/relaxation in a 24-h period
- Perceptions of quality and quantity of sleep and rest
- Use of sleep aids and routines

COGNITIVE-PERCEPTUAL

- Adequacy of vision, hearing, taste, touch, smell
- Pain perception and management
- Language, judgment, memory, decisions

Responses to Altered Integumentary Structure and Function

UNIT
4

CHAPTER 15 Assessing Clients with Integumentary Disorders

LEARNING OUTCOMES

- Describe the anatomy, physiology, and functions of the skin, hair, and nails.
- Discuss factors that influence skin color.
- Identify specific topics for a health history interview of the client with problems involving the skin, hair, and nails.
- Explain techniques for assessing the skin, hair, and nails.
- Compare and contrast normal and abnormal findings when conducting an assessment of the integumentary system.
- Describe normal variations in assessment findings for the older client.
- Identify abnormal findings that may indicate impairment of the integumentary system.

CLINICAL COMPETENCIES

- Conduct and document a health history for clients who have or are at risk for alterations in the skin, hair, or nails.
- Conduct and document a physical assessment of the integumentary system.
- Monitor the results of diagnostic tests and report abnormal findings.

EQUIPMENT NEEDED

- Disposable gloves
- Ruler
- Flashlight

MEDIALINK

Resources for this chapter can be found on the Prentice Hall Nursing MediaLink DVD-ROM accompanying this textbook, and on the Companion Website at http://www.prenhall.com/lemone

The skin, the hair, and the nails make up the integumentary system. The skin, the largest organ of the body, provides an external covering for the body, separating and protecting the body's organs and tissues from the external environment. Functions of the skin, hair, and nails are summarized in Table 15–1.

Disorders of the integumentary structures may be caused by a variety of factors, including allergies, infection, infestation, cancer, and genetic influences.

ANATOMY, PHYSIOLOGY, AND FUNCTIONS OF THE INTEGUMENTARY SYSTEM

The Skin

The skin has a total surface area of 15 to 20 square feet and weighs about 9 pounds. It has been estimated that each square inch of skin contains 15 feet of blood vessels, 4 yards of nerves, 650 sweat glands, 100 oil glands, 1500 sensory receptors, and more than 3 million cells that are constantly dying and being replaced. The skin is composed of two regions: the epidermis and the dermis (Figure 15–1 ■).

The Epidermis

The epidermis, which is the surface or outermost part of the skin, consists of epithelial cells. The epidermis has either four or five layers, depending on its location; there are five layers over the palms of the hands and the soles of the feet, and four layers over the rest of the body.

The stratum basale is the deepest layer of the epidermis. It contains melanocytes, cells that produce the pigment **melanin**, and keratinocytes, which produce **keratin**. Melanin forms a protective shield to protect the keratinocytes and the nerve endings in the dermis from the damaging effects of ultraviolet light. Melanocyte activity probably accounts for the difference in skin color in humans. Keratin is a fibrous, water-repellent protein that gives the epidermis its tough, protective quality. As keratinocytes mature, they move upward through the epidermal layers, eventually becoming dead cells at the surface of the skin. Millions of these cells are worn off by abrasion each day, but millions are simultaneously produced in the stratum basale. The next layer of the epidermis is the stratum spinosum. Several cells thick, this layer contains abundant cells that arise from the bone marrow and migrate to the epidermis. Mitosis occurs at this layer, although not as abundantly as in the stratum basale.

The stratum granulosum is only two to three cells thick. The cells of the stratum granulosum contain a glycolipid that slows water loss across the epidermis. Keratinization, a thickening of the cells' plasma membranes, begins in the stratum granulosum. The stratum lucidum is present only in areas of thick skin. It is made up of flattened, dead keratinocytes.

The outermost layer of the epidermis, the stratum corneum, is also the thickest, making up about 75% of the epidermis's total thickness. It consists of about 20 to 30 sheets of dead cells filled with keratin fragments arranged in "shingles" that flake off as dry skin.

The Dermis

The dermis is the second, deeper layer of skin. Made of a flexible connective tissue, this layer is richly supplied with blood

TABLE 15–1 Functions of the Skin and Its Appendages

STRUCTURE	FUNCTIONS
Epidermis	Protects tissues from physical, chemical, and biologic damage. Prevents water loss and serves as a water-repellent layer. Stores melanin, which protects tissues from harmful effects of the ultraviolet radiation in sunlight. Converts cholesterol molecules to vitamin D when exposed to sunlight. Contains phagocytes, which prevent bacteria from penetrating the skin.
Dermis	Regulates body temperature by dilating and constricting capillaries. Transmits messages via nerve endings to the central nervous system.
Sebaceous (oil) glands	Secrete sebum, which lubricates skin and hair and plays a role in killing bacteria.
Eccrine sweat glands	Regulate body heat by excretion of perspiration.
Apocrine sweat glands	Remnant of sexual scent gland.
Hair	Cushions the scalp. Eyelashes and cilia protect the body from foreign particles. Provides insulation in cold weather.
Nails	Protect the fingers and toes, aid in grasping, and allow for various other activities, such as scratching the skin, picking up small items, peeling an orange, and so on.

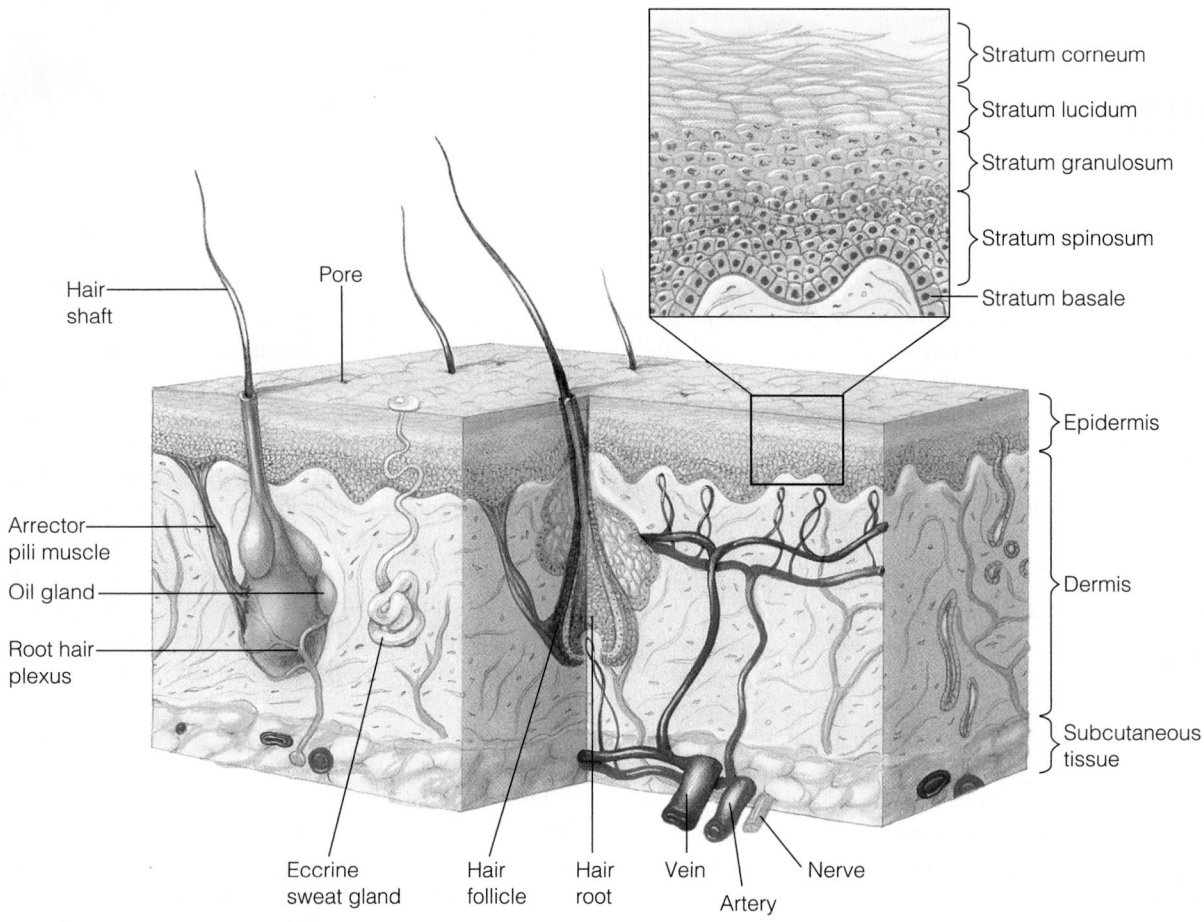

Figure 15–1 ■ Anatomy of the skin.

cells, nerve fibers, and lymphatic vessels. Most of the hair follicles, sebaceous glands, and sweat glands are located in the dermis. The dermis consists of a papillary and a reticular layer. The papillary layer contains ridges that indent the overlying epidermis. It also contains capillaries and receptors for pain and touch. The deeper, reticular layer contains blood vessels, sweat and sebaceous glands, deep pressure receptors, and dense bundles of collagen fibers. The regions between these bundles form lines of cleavage in the skin. Surgical incisions parallel to these lines of cleavage heal more easily and with less scarring than incisions or traumatic wounds across cleavage lines.

Superficial Fascia

A layer of subcutaneous tissue called the superficial fascia lies under the dermis. It consists primarily of adipose (fat) tissue and helps the skin adhere to underlying structures.

Glands of the Skin

The skin contains sebaceous (oil) glands, sudoriferous (sweat) glands, and ceruminous glands. Each of these glands has a different function.

Sebaceous glands are found all over the body except on the palms and soles. These glands secrete an oily substance called **sebum**, which usually is ducted into a hair follicle. Sebum softens and lubricates the skin and hair and also decreases wa-

ter loss from the skin in low humidity. Sebum also protects the body from infection by killing bacteria. The secretion of sebum is stimulated by hormones, especially androgens. If a sebaceous gland becomes blocked, a pimple or whitehead appears on the surface of the skin; as the material oxidizes and dries, it forms a blackhead. Acne vulgaris is an inflammation of the sebaceous glands.

There are two types of sweat glands: eccrine and apocrine. Eccrine sweat glands are more numerous on the forehead, palms, and soles. The gland itself is located in the dermis; the duct to the skin rises through the epidermis to open in a pore at the surface. Sweat, the secretion of the eccrine glands, is composed mostly of water but also contains sodium, antibodies, small amounts of metabolic wastes, lactic acid, and vitamin C. The production of sweat is regulated by the sympathetic nervous system and serves to maintain normal body temperature. Sweating also occurs in response to emotions.

Most apocrine sweat glands are located in the axillary, anal, and genital areas. The secretions from apocrine glands are similar to those of sweat glands, but they also contain fatty acids and proteins. Apocrine glands are a remnant of sexual scent glands. Ceruminous glands are modified apocrine sweat glands. Located in the skin of the external ear canal, they secrete yellow-brown waxy cerumen. This substance provides a sticky trap for foreign materials.

Skin Color

Skin color varies among individuals and among people of different races, ranging from a pinkish white to various shades of brown and black. Areas of the skin that are normally exposed to the sun and environment, such as the face and hands, may have a slightly different color from areas that are usually covered with clothing. Special care must be taken when assessing changes in skin color in people with dark skin, such as African Americans, Hispanics, Native Americans, Asians, people of Mediterranean descent, and Caucasians who are deeply suntanned.

The color of the skin is the result of varying levels of pigmentation. Melanin, a yellow-to-brown pigment, is darker and is produced in greater amounts in persons with dark skin color than in those with light skin. Exposure to the sun causes a buildup of melanin and a darkening or tanning of the skin in people with light skin. Carotene, a yellow-to-orange pigment, is found most in areas of the body where the stratum corneum is thickest, such as the palms of the hands. Carotene is more abundant in the skins of persons of Asian ancestry and, together with melanin, accounts for their golden skin tone. The epidermis in Caucasian skin has very little melanin and is almost transparent. Thus, the color of the hemoglobin found in red blood cells (RBCs) circulating through the dermis shows through, lending Caucasians a pinkish skin tone.

Skin color is influenced by emotions and illnesses. **Erythema**, a reddening of the skin, may occur with embarrassment (blushing), fever, hypertension, or inflammation. It may also result from a drug reaction, sunburn, acne rosacea, or other factors. A bluish discoloration of the skin and mucous membranes, called **cyanosis**, results from poor oxygenation of hemoglobin. **Pallor**, or paleness of skin, may occur with shock, fear, or anger or in anemia and hypoxia. **Jaundice** is a yellow-to-orange color visible in the skin and mucous membranes; it is most often the result of a hepatic disorder. Table 15–2 further defines these terms and compares and contrasts skin color changes in people with light and dark skin.

The Hair

Hair is distributed all over the body, except the lips, nipples, parts of the external genitals, the palms of the hands, and the

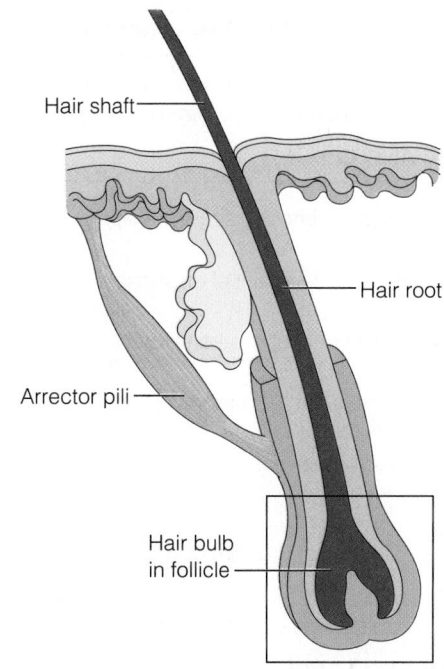

Figure 15–2 ■ Anatomy of a hair follicle.

soles of the feet. Hair is produced by a hair bulb, and its root is enclosed in a hair follicle (Figure 15–2 ■). The exposed part, called the shaft, consists mainly of dead cells. Hair follicles extend into the dermis and in some places, such as the scalp, below the dermis. Many factors, including nutrition and hormones, influence hair growth.

Hair in various parts of the body has protective functions: The eyebrows and eyelashes protect the eyes; hair in the nose helps keep foreign materials out of the upper respiratory tract; and hair on the head protects the scalp from heat loss and sunlight.

The Nails

A nail is a modified scalelike epidermal structure. Like hair, nails consist mainly of dead cells. They arise from the stratum germinativum of the epidermis. The body of the nail rests on the nail bed (Figure 15–3 ■). The nail matrix is the active,

Figure 15–3 ■ Anatomy of a nail (frontal and side views).

TABLE 15–2 Skin Color Assessment Variations in People with Light and Dark Skin

PALLOR: *A decrease or absence in skin color as the result of a decrease in tissue perfusion; a decrease in shape, size, or amount of RBCs; or absence of melanin (local or generalized).*

DISORDER AND CAUSE	CHANGE IN LIGHT SKIN	CHANGE IN DARK SKIN
Anemia (decreased or abnormal size and shape of RBCs)	Generalized paleness	Brown skin is dull and has a yellow cast; black skin is dull and has an ashen gray cast
Hemorrhage (decreased amount of circulating RBCs)	Generalized paleness	Brown skin is dull and has a yellow cast; black skin is dull and has an ashen gray cast
Shock (decreased amount of circulating RBCs or decreased perfusion)	Generalized paleness	Brown skin is dull and has a yellow cast; black skin is dull and has an ashen gray cast
Arterial insufficiency (trauma, acute arterial occlusion, or arteriosclerosis)	Local paleness	Dull, ashen gray
Vitiligo (patchy loss of melanocytes)	Patches of white spots, most often found over skin of the face, hands, or groin	Patches of white spots, most often found over skin of the face, hands, or groin
Albinism (total absence of melanin)	White/pink	Tan, cream, or white

CYANOSIS: *A bluish discoloration of the skin and mucous membranes resulting from a local or generalized excess of deoxygenated hemoglobin or a structural defect in the hemoglobin molecule.*

DISORDER AND CAUSE	CHANGE IN LIGHT SKIN	CHANGE IN DARK SKIN
Acute and chronic disorders of the structure and function of the heart and lungs (arterial insufficiency; exposure to cold, hypothermia)	Dusky blue (may be generalized or local, depending on cause)	Skin may appear darker, but will be dull; cyanosis is more readily assessed in the nail beds, oral mucous membranes, and conjunctivae

ERYTHEMA: *Redness of the skin or mucous membranes that is the result of dilatation and congestion of superficial capillaries.*

DISORDER AND CAUSE	CHANGE IN LIGHT SKIN	CHANGE IN DARK SKIN
Hyperemia (inflammation, increased body temperature, hot environmental temperature, embarrassment, alcohol ingestion)	Red or bright pink	Difficult to assess, skin may have dark red cast
Carbon monoxide poisoning (carbon monoxide displaces oxygen on the hemoglobin molecule, causing hypoxia, carboxyhemoglobinemia)	Cherry red in face and upper torso	Cherry red lips, oral mucous membranes, and nail beds
Venous stasis (inability of veins to return blood to heart; may result from edema, varicose veins, or pressure)	Dusky red	Difficult to assess

JAUNDICE: *Yellowish discoloration of the skin, mucous membranes, and sclerae of the eyes, caused by increased amounts of bilirubin or other pigments in the blood).*

DISORDER AND CAUSE	CHANGE IN LIGHT SKIN	CHANGE IN DARK SKIN
Increased serum bilirubin to >2–3 mg/100 mL (liver disease, pancreatic disease, gallbladder disease, hemolysis, such as following blood transfusion, severe burns or infections)	Yellowing of skin follows yellowing of sclerae and mucous membranes; may also be assessed in the fingernails and palms of the hands	Yellowing is best assessed at the junction of the hard palate and the soft palate or on the palms of the hands. Sclerae may be yellow near the limbus (do not confuse with normal yellow eye pigmentation)
Uremia (retained urochrome pigments in the blood)	Orange-green or gray cast to skin	Difficult to assess; may appear as yellowish-green color in the scleral of the eye

growing part of the nail. The proximal visible end of the nail has a white crescent, called a lunula. The sides of the nail are overlapped by skin, called nail folds. The proximal nail fold is thickened and is called the eponychium or cuticle. Nails form a protective coating over the dorsum of each digit on the fingers and toes.

ASSESSING THE INTEGUMENTARY SYSTEM

The functions of the integumentary system (skin, glands, hair, and nails) are assessed by findings from diagnostic tests, a health assessment interview to collect subjective data, and a physical assessment to collect objective data. See the box below for sample documentation of an assessment of the integument.

Diagnosis

The results of diagnostic tests of the structure and function of the integumentary system are used to support the diagnosis of a specific injury or disease, to provide information to identify or modify the appropriate medication or treatments used to treat the disease, and to help nurses monitor the clients' responses to nursing care interventions. Diagnostic tests to assess the integumentary system are described in the box on the following page and summarized in the following bulleted list. More information is included in the discussion of specific health problems, diseases, or injuries in Chapters 16 and 17 ∞.

- One of the most common diagnostic tests is a skin biopsy, used to differentiate a benign skin lesion from a skin cancer. Skin biopsies can be obtained by using a punch technique, incision, excision, or shaving.
- Cultures to identify infections may be conducted on tissue samples, drainage and exudate from lesions, and (if an illness is generalized), serum.
- Tests used to identify infections include immunofluorescent studies, Wood's lamp, potassium hydroxide, and the Tzanck test.
- Allergies may be determined through patch tests or scratch tests.

  Some studies are conducted to identify bacterial carriers. For example, if clients have repeated bacterial skin infections, or if a healthcare unit or agency experiences numerous bacterial infections of clients, nasal cultures may be performed to determine if the clients or the healthcare workers are carriers of the bacteria. Regardless of the type of diagnostic test, the nurse is responsible for explaining the procedure and any special preparation needed, for assessing for medication use that may affect the outcome of the tests, for supporting the client during the examination as necessary, for documenting the procedures as appropriate, and for monitoring the results of the tests.

Genetic Considerations

When conducting a health assessment interview and physical assessment, it is important for the nurse to consider genetic influences on health of the adult. During the health assessment interview, ask about integumentary disorders or abnormalities in immediate family members and also inquire about their gender. During the physical assessment, assess for any manifestations that indicate a genetic disorder (see Genetic Considerations: Integumentary System below). If data are found that indicate genetic risk factors or alterations, ask about genetic testing and refer for appropriate genetic counseling and evaluation. Chapter 8 ∞ provides further information about genetics in medical-surgical nursing.

Health Assessment Interview

A health assessment interview to determine problems with the integumentary system may be conducted as part of a health screening or total health assessment, or it may focus on a chief complaint (such as itching or a rash). If the client has a skin problem, analyze its onset, characteristics and course, severity, precipitating and relieving factors, and note the timing and circumstances of any associated symptoms. For example, ask the client:

- What type of itching have you experienced?
- When did you first notice a change in this mole?
- Did you change to any different kinds of shampoo or other hair products just before you started to lose your hair?

  Ask about any change in health, rashes, itching, color changes, dryness or oiliness, growth of or changes in warts or moles, and the presence of lesions. Precipitating causes, such as medications, the use of new soaps, skin care agents, cosmetics, pets, travel, stress, or dietary changes, must also be explored. In assessing hair problems, ask about any thinning or baldness, excessive hair loss, change in distribution of hair, use of hair care products, diet, and dieting. When assessing nail problems, ask about nail splitting or breakage, discoloration, infection, diet, and exposure to chemicals.

SAMPLE DOCUMENTATION
Assessment of the Integumentary System

A 50-year-old man with no history of skin lesions, hair loss, or disorders of the nails. Took antibiotic for respiratory infection approximately 10 days ago and reports having a fine, raised, red rash on trunk and arms that itched. Nurse practitioner prescribed antihistamine and rash cleared in 3 days. Skin light brown, warm, dry, and elastic. Patches of vitiligo present over dorsum of hands. No lesions or edema noted. Healed scar on lower left abdomen (appendectomy as a young adult). Hair dark brown with gray at the temples, clean. Nails are smooth, hard, and immobile.

GENETIC CONSIDERATIONS
Integumentary System

- Oculocutaneous albinism, an autosomal recessive inheritance disorder, causes hypopigmentation (albinism or absence of color) of the skin, hair, and eyes as a result of an inability to synthesize melanin.
- Keloids, which are elevated scars, have a familial tendency and are more commonly found in blacks. Vitiligo, the sudden appearance of white patches on the skin, has a familial tendency.
- Male pattern baldness (the most common cause of baldness in men) is genetically predetermined.
- Hirsutism (excessive hair in women) may be genetically predetermined.
- Blacks may have very dry scalps and dry, fragile hair of genetic origin.
- A family history of skin cancer is a risk factor.

DIAGNOSTIC TESTS of the Integumentary System

NAME OF TEST   Punch Skin Biopsy

PURPOSE AND DESCRIPTION   This biopsy is done to differentiate benign lesions from skin cancers. An instrument is used to remove a small section of dermis and subcutaneous fat. Depending on size, the incision may be sutured.

RELATED NURSING CARE   Explain the procedure to the client, and ensure a consent form is signed (if required). Assist with the procedure. Apply dressing and provide information about self-care and when to return for suture removal. Document the procedure and send the labeled specimen to the lab.

NAME OF TEST   Incisional Skin Biopsy

PURPOSE AND DESCRIPTION   This biopsy is done to differentiate benign lesions from skin cancers. An incision is

made and a *part* of the lesion or tumor is removed. The incision is closed with sutures.

RELATED NURSING CARE   See above.

NAME OF TEST   Excisional Skin Biopsy

PURPOSE AND DESCRIPTION   This biopsy is done to differentiate benign lesions from skin cancers. An incision is

made and the *entire* skin lesion or tumor is removed for analysis. The incision is closed with sutures.

RELATED NURSING CARE   See above.

NAME OF TEST   Shave Skin Biopsy

PURPOSE AND DESCRIPTION   This skin biopsy is done to shave off superficial lesions and to differentiate infectious

from inflammatory lesions. A single-edged razor is used for shaving.

RELATED NURSING CARE   See above.

NAME OF TEST   Culture

PURPOSE AND DESCRIPTION   A culture of scrapings from a lesion, from drainage, or of exudate is done to identify fungal, bacterial, or viral skin infections. Obtain the culture with a sterile Culturette swab and culture tubes.

RELATED NURSING CARE   Confirm physician's order. Explain the procedure to the client. Maintain strict asepsis while obtaining the culture. Document the procedure and send the labeled specimen to the lab.

NAME OF TEST   Oil Slides

PURPOSE AND DESCRIPTION   Oil slides are used to determine the type of skin infestation present. Scrapings of the lesion are placed on a slide with mineral oil and examined microscopically.

RELATED NURSING CARE   Explain the procedure to the client. Assist with or obtain the specimen and complete the slide. Document the procedure and send the labeled specimen to the lab.

NAME OF TEST   Immunofluorescent Slides

PURPOSE AND DESCRIPTION   Immunofluorescent studies of samples from skin and/or serum may be done to identify IgG antibodies (present in pemphigus vulgaris) and to identify

varicella in skin cells (for herpes zoster). Skin or blood samples are placed on a slide and examined microscopically.

RELATED NURSING CARE   See above.

NAME OF TEST   Wood's Lamp

PURPOSE AND DESCRIPTION   This test uses an ultraviolet light that causes certain organisms to fluoresce (such as

Pseudomonas organisms and fungi). The skin is examined under a special lamp.

RELATED NURSING CARE   Explain the procedure to the client. Document the procedure.

NAME OF TEST   Potassium Hydroxide (KOH)

PURPOSE AND DESCRIPTION   A specimen from hair or nails is examined for a fungal infection. The specimen is obtained by placing material from a scraping on a slide, adding a potassium hydroxide solution, and examining it microscopically.

RELATED NURSING CARE   Explain the procedure to the client. Assist with or obtain the specimen and complete the slide. Document the procedure and send the labeled specimen to the lab.

NAME OF TEST   Tzanck Test

PURPOSE AND DESCRIPTION   This test is used to diagnose herpes infections, but it does not differentiate herpes simplex from herpes zoster. Fluid and cells from the vesicles are obtained, put on a slide, stained, and examined microscopically.

RELATED NURSING CARE   Explain the procedure to the client. Use sterile procedure to assist with or obtain the specimen and complete the slide. Document the procedure and send the labeled specimen to the lab.

NAME OF TEST   Patch Test, Scratch Tests

PURPOSE AND DESCRIPTION   These tests are used to determine a specific allergen. In a patch test, a small amount of the suspected material is placed on the skin under an occlusive bandage. In a scratch test, a needle is used to "scratch" small amounts of potentially allergic materials on the skin surface.

RELATED NURSING CARE   Explain the procedure to the client, including the need to return in 48 hours to have the patched area or scratched areas evaluated. Document the procedure.

The client's medical history is important. Questions focus on previous problems, allergies, and lesions. Skin problems may be manifestations of other disorders, such as cardiovascular disease, endocrine disorders, hepatic disease, and hematologic disorders. Occupational and social history may provide cues to skin problems; ask the client about travel, exposure to toxic substances at work, use of alcohol, and responses to stress.

Assess the presence of risk factors for skin cancer carefully. These include male gender; age over 50; family history of skin cancer; extended exposure to sunlight; tendency to sunburn; history of sunburn or other skin trauma; light-colored hair or eyes; residence in high altitudes or near the equator; and exposure to radiation, x-rays, coal, tar, or petroleum products. (Risks for skin cancer are further discussed in Chapter 16 ∞.)

Also explore the risk factors for malignant melanoma. These include a large number of moles, the presence of atypical moles, a family history of melanoma, prior melanoma, repeated severe sunburns, ease of freckling and sunburning, or inability to tan.

See Functional Health Pattern Interview: Integumentary System below. Responses should be documented in the client's medical record.

Physical Assessment

Physical assessment of the skin, hair, and nails may be performed either as part of a total assessment or may be a

FUNCTIONAL HEALTH PATTERN INTERVIEW Integumentary System

Functional Health Pattern	Interview Questions and Leading Statements
Health Perception-Health Management	■ Describe any problems, injuries, or surgeries you have had. How were these treated? ■ Describe medications, herbs, and vitamins you currently are taking. ■ Describe your current problem. How long has it lasted? What have you done to treat it? ■ Do you have allergies to foods, plants, pets? ■ Describe what you do each day to care for your skin, hair, and nails.
Nutritional-Metabolic	■ Describe what you eat and how much and type of fluids you drink in a 24-hour period. ■ Do you have a history of food allergies? If so, describe what you are allergic to and how you respond. ■ Have you recently eaten any new foods? ■ Do you take any nutritional supplements, herbs, or vitamins? ■ How well do your cuts and scratches heal?
Elimination	■ Is your skin and scalp dry or oily? ■ Have you noticed swelling around your eyes or ankles? ■ Do you perspire a lot?
Activity-Exercise	■ Describe your physical activities in a typical day. ■ Do you bruise easily? ■ Do you use a sunscreen when you are outside? If so, what SPF? ■ Do you visit tanning salons?
Sleep-Rest	■ How many hours do you sleep each night? ■ Do you have trouble sleeping because of itching or sweating?
Cognitive-Perceptual	■ Do you have any of the following: pain, discomfort, itching, tingling, burning, tenderness, or numbness? If so, where?
Self-Perception-Self-Concept	■ How does this condition make you feel about yourself?
Role-Relationships	■ How does this condition affect your relationships with others? ■ Is there anything in your work environment that may have caused this condition?
Sexuality-Reproductive	■ Has this condition interfered with your usual sexual activities? ■ If you use a birth control method, could it have caused this condition?
Coping-Stress-Tolerance	■ Have you experienced any type of stress that may have worsened this condition? ■ Has this condition created stress for you? ■ Describe what you do when you feel stressed.
Value-Belief	■ Tell me how specific relationships or activities help you cope with this condition. ■ Describe specific cultural beliefs or practices that affect how you care for and feel about this condition. ■ Are there any specific treatments that you would not use to treat this condition?

focused assessment of the integument for clients with known or suspected problems. Physical assessment of the skin, hair, and nails is conducted by inspection and palpation. Assess the skin for color, presence of lesions (observable changes from normal skin structure), temperature, texture, moisture, turgor, and presence of edema. Characteristics of lesions to note include location and distribution, color, pattern, edges, size (measure with a ruler in centimeters), elevation, and type of exudate (if present). Common skin lesions of older adults are outlined in Box 15–1; see Table 15–3 for age-related integument changes. Examine the hair for color, texture, quality, and scalp lesions. Determine the shape, color, contour, and condition of the nails. Terminology of skin lesions with examples are outlined in Table 15–4.

The examination should be conducted in a warm, private room. The client removes all clothing and puts on a gown or drape. The areas to be examined should be fully exposed, but protect the client's modesty by keeping other areas covered. The client may be standing, sitting, or lying down at various times of the examination. Don disposable gloves when palpating open lesions, skin surfaces suspicious of infections or infestations, or discharge from lesions of the skin and mucous membranes. Standard precautions should be adhered to when conducting a skin assessment. A ruler is used to measure the size of lesions. A flashlight is used to better visualize lesions.

BOX 15–1 Common Skin Lesions of Older Adults

- *Skin tags:* soft brown or flesh-colored benign papules
- *Keratoses:* horny growth of keratinocytes, may be seborrheic (benign) or actinic (premalignant)
- *Lentigines ("liver spots"):* brown or black benign macule with a defined border
- *Angiomas (hemangioma):* benign vascular tumors with dilated blood vessels, found in the middle to upper dermis
- *Telangiectases:* single dilated blood vessels, capillaries, or terminal arteries
- *Venous lakes:* small, dark blue, slightly raised benign papules
- *Photoaging:* wrinkling, mottling, pigmented areas, loss of elasticity, benign or malignant lesions

---

TABLE 15–3 Age-Related Skin Changes

AGE-RELATED CHANGE	SIGNIFICANCE
Epidermis : ↓ thickness and miotic activity	■ Skin is more fragile and at greater risk for tears or injury ■ Delayed wound healing ■ Hyperkeratoses and skin cancers in sun-exposed areas are more evident
Epidermis: ↑ permeability, ↓ Langerhans cells	■ Increased risk of reactions to irritants ■ Decreased inflammatory response
Epidermis: ↓ number of active melanocytes	■ Increased susceptibility to sun exposure
Epidermis: hyperplasia of melanocytes, especially in sun-exposed areas	■ Small areas of hyperpigmentation ("liver spots") and hypopigmentation ("age spots"), especially on the hands
Epidermis: ↓ vitamin D production	■ Increased risk of osteomalacia, osteoporosis
Epidermis: dermal–epidermal junction flattens	■ Increased risk of skin tears, purpura, and pressure ulcers
Dermis: ↓ perfusion	■ More susceptible to dry skin ■ Decreased sensation (pain, touch, temperature, and peripheral vibration) ■ Increased risk of injury
Dermis: ↓ vasomotor response	■ Greater risk of hyperthermia and hypothermia
Dermis: elastic fibers degenerate	■ Decreased tone and elasticity, with wrinkle formation
Dermis: proliferation of capillaries	■ Cherry hemangiomas are common
Subcutaneous skin layer: thins	■ Greater risk of hypothermia ■ Increased risk of pressure ulcers
Subcutaneous skin layer: adipose tissue is redistributed	■ Cellulite forms ■ Bags over and under the eyes ■ Double chin forms ■ Abdominal fat increases ■ Breasts sag ■ Skin returns to normal more slowly when pinched (tenting)
Glands: ↓ eccrine and apocrine activity	■ Dry skin is common ■ Absent perspiration

TABLE 15–4 Terminology of Skin Lesions with Associated Disorders

LESION	EXAMPLES OF DISORDERS
Pigmented	Freckle, seborrheic keratosis, nevus, melanoma
Scaly	Psoriasis, dermatitis, xerosis, tinea, actinic keratoses
Pustular	Acne vulgaris, folliculitis, candidiasis
Vesicular	Herpes simplex, herpes zoster, scabies
Nodular	Warts, basal cell carcinoma, acne
Weepy, crusted	Acute contact allergic dermatitis, impetigo
Figurate (shaped) erythema	Urticaria, cellulitis
Bullous	Pemphigus, toxic epidermal necrolysis
Pruritic	Xerosis, scabies, pediculosis
Ulcerated	Pressure ulcer, skin cancer, herpes simplex

INTEGUMENTARY ASSESSMENTS

Technique/Normal Findings	Abnormal Findings
Inspect skin color and note any odors coming from the skin. *Skin color should be even, appropriate to the age and race of the client, without foul odors.*	■ A strong odor of perspiration may indicate poor hygiene and a need for client teaching. A foul odor may indicate a disorder of the sweat glands. ■ Pallor and/or cyanosis are seen with exposure to cold and with decreased perfusion and oxygenation. In cyanotic dark-skinned clients, skin loses glow and appears dull. Cyanosis may be more visible in the mucous membranes and nail beds of these clients. ■ In dark-skinned clients, jaundice may be most apparent in the sclerae of the eyes. ■ Redness, swelling, and pain are seen with various rashes, inflammations, infections, and burns. First-degree burns cause areas of painful erythema and swelling. Red, painful blisters appear in second-degree burns, whereas white or blackened areas are common in third-degree burns. ■ **Vitiligo**, an abnormal loss of melanin in patches, typically occurs over the face, hands, or groin. Vitiligo is thought to be an autoimmune disorder.
Inspect the skin for lesions and alterations, including calluses, scars, tattoos, and piercings. Include inspection of skin creases and folds. *Skin should be intact without abnormal lesions.*	Primary, secondary, and vascular lesions are described and shown in Tables 15–5 through 15–7. ■ Pearly edged nodules with a central ulcer are seen in basal cell carcinoma. ■ Scaly, red, fast-growing papules are seen in squamous cell carcinoma. ■ Dark, asymmetric, multicolored patches (sometimes moles) with irregular edges appear in malignant melanoma. ■ Circular lesions are usually present in ringworm and in tinea versicolor. ■ Grouped vesicles may be seen in contact dermatitis. ■ Linear lesions appear in poison ivy and herpes zoster. ■ **Urticaria** (hives) appears as patches of pale, itchy wheals in an erythematous area. ■ In psoriasis, scaly red patches appear on the scalp, knees, back, and genitals. ■ In herpes zoster, vesicles appear along sensory nerve paths, turn into pustules, and then crust over. ■ Bruises (**ecchymosis**) are raised bluish or yellowish vascular lesions. Multiple bruises in various stages of healing suggest trauma or abuse.
Palpate skin temperature. *Skin should be warm.*	■ Skin is warm and red in inflammation and is generally warm with elevated body temperature. ■ Decreased blood flow decreases the skin temperature; this may be generalized, as in shock, or localized, as in arteriosclerosis.
Palpate skin texture. *Skin should be smooth.*	■ Changes in the texture of the skin may indicate irritation or trauma. ■ The skin is soft and smooth in hyperthyroidism and coarse in hypothyroidism.

TABLE 15–5 **Primary Skin Lesions**

Macule, Patch

Flat, nonpalpable change in skin color. Macules are smaller than 1 cm, with a circumscribed border, and patches are larger than 1 cm and may have an irregular border.

Examples Macules: freckles, measles, and petechiae. Patches: Mongolian spots, port-wine stains, vitiligo, and chloasma.

Vesicle, Bulla

Elevated, fluid-filled, round or oval shaped, palpable mass with thin, translucent walls and circumscribed borders. Vesicles are smaller than 0.5 cm; bullae are larger than 0.5 cm.

Examples Vesicles: herpes simplex/zoster, early chickenpox, poison ivy, and small burn blisters. Bullae: contact dermatitis, friction blisters, and large burn blisters.

Papule, Plaque

Elevated, solid, palpable mass with circumscribed border. Papules are smaller than 0.5 cm; plaques are groups of papules that form lesions larger than 0.5 cm.

Examples Papules: elevated moles, warts, and lichen planus. Plaques: psoriasis, actinic keratosis, and also lichen planus.

Wheal

Elevated, often reddish area with irregular border caused by diffuse fluid in tissues rather than free fluid in a cavity, as in vesicles. Size varies.

Examples Insect bites and hives (extensive wheals).

Nodule, Tumor

Elevated, solid, hard or soft palpable mass extending deeper into the dermis than a papule. Nodules have circumscribed borders and are 0.5 to 2 cm; tumors may have irregular borders and are larger than 2 cm.

Examples Nodules: small lipoma, squamous cell carcinoma, fibroma, and intradermal nevi. Tumors: large lipoma, carcinoma, and hemangioma.

Pustule

Elevated, pus-filled vesicle or bulla with circumscribed border. Size varies.

Examples Acne, impetigo, and carbuncles (large boils).

Cyst

Elevated, encapsulated, fluid-filled or semisolid mass originating in the subcutaneous tissue or dermis, usually 1 cm or larger.

Examples Varieties include sebaceous cysts and epidermoid cysts.

TABLE 15–6 Secondary Skin Lesions

Atrophy

A translucent, dry, paper-like, sometimes wrinkled skin surface resulting from thinning or wasting of the skin due to loss of collagen and elastin.
Examples Striae, aged skin.

Ulcer

Deep, irregularly shaped area of skin loss extending into the dermis or subcutaneous tissue. May bleed. May leave scar.
Examples Decubitus ulcers (pressure sores), stasis ulcers, chancres.

Erosion

Wearing away of the superficial epidermis causing a moist, shallow depression. Because erosions do not extend into the dermis, they heal without scarring.
Examples Scratch marks, ruptured vesicles.

Fissure

Linear crack with sharp edges, extending into the dermis.
Examples Cracks at the corners of the mouth or in the hands, athlete's foot.

Lichenification

Rough, thickened, hardened area of epidermis resulting from chronic irritation such as scratching or rubbing.
Example Chronic dermatitis.

Scar

Flat, irregular area of connective tissue left after a lesion or wound has healed. New scars may be red or purple; older scars may be silvery or white.
Examples Healed surgical wound or injury, healed acne.

Scales

Shedding flakes of greasy, keratinized skin tissue. Color may be white, gray, or silver. Texture may vary from fine to thick.
Examples Dry skin, dandruff, psoriasis, and eczema.

Keloid

Elevated, irregular, darkened area of excess scar tissue caused by excessive collagen formation during healing. Extends beyond the site of the original injury. Higher incidence in people of African descent.
Examples Keloid from ear piercing or surgery.

Crust

Dry blood, serum, or pus left on the skin surface when vesicles or pustules burst. Can be red-brown, orange, or yellow. Large crusts that adhere to the skin surface are called scabs.
Examples Eczema, impetigo, herpes, or scabs following abrasion.

TABLE 15–7 Vascular Skin Lesions

Spider Angioma

Source: Custom Medical Stock Photo, Inc.

A flat, bright red dot with tiny radiating blood vessels ranging in size from a pinpoint to 2 cm. It blanches with pressure.

Cause A type of telangiectasis (vascular dilatation) caused by elevated estrogen levels, pregnancy, estrogen therapy, vitamin B deficiency, or liver disease, or may not be pathologic.

Localization/Distribution Most commonly appear on the upper half of the body.

Venous Star

Source: Phototake NYC

A flat blue lesion with radiating, cascading, or linear veins extending from the center. It ranges in size from 3 to 25 cm.

Cause A type of telangiectasis (vascular dilatation) caused by increased intravenous pressure in superficial veins.

Localization/Distribution Most commonly appear on the anterior chest and the lower legs near varicose veins.

Petechiae

Source: Custom Medical Stock Photo, Inc.

Flat red or purple rounded "freckles" approximately 1 to 3 mm in diameter. Difficult to detect in dark skin. Do not blanch.

Cause Minute hemorrhages resulting from fragile capillaries, petechiae are caused by septicemias, liver disease, or vitamin C or K deficiency. They may also be caused by anticoagulant therapy.

Localization/Distribution Most commonly appear on the dependent surfaces of the body (e.g., back, buttocks). In the client with dark skin, look for them in the oral mucosa and conjunctivae.

Purpura

Source: Custom Medical Stock Photo, Inc.

Flat, reddish blue, irregularly shaped extensive patches of varying size.

Cause Bleeding disorders, scurvy, and capillary fragility in the older adult (senile purpura).

Localization/Distribution May appear anywhere on the body, but are most noticeable on the legs, arms, and backs of hands.

Ecchymosis

Source: Photo Researchers, Inc.

A flat, irregularly shaped lesion of varying size with no pulsation. Does not blanch with pressure. In light skin, it begins as bluish purple mark that changes to greenish yellow. In brown skin, it varies from blue to deep purple. In black skin, it appears as a darkened area.

Cause Release of blood from superficial vessels into surrounding tissue due to trauma, hemophilia, liver disease, or deficiency of vitamin C or K.

Localization/Distribution Occurs anywhere on the body at the site of trauma or pressure.

Technique/Normal Findings	Abnormal Findings
Palpate skin moisture. *Skin should be dry.*	■ Excessively dry skin often is present in the elderly and clients with hypothyroidism. ■ Oily skin is common in adolescents and young adults. Oily skin may be a normal finding, or it may accompany a skin disorder such as acne vulgaris. ■ Excessive perspiration may be associated with shock, fever, increased activity, or anxiety.
Palpate skin turgor. *Skin fold should return rapidly to normal position.*	■ Pinch the client's skin gently over the back of the hand or collarbone. Tenting, in which the skin remains pinched for a few moments before resuming its normal position, is common in older clients who are thin (Figure 15–4 ■). ■ Skin turgor is decreased in dehydration. It is increased in edema and scleroderma.

Figure 15–4 ■ Tenting in an older client.

Assess for edema. *No edema should be present.*	■ Assess **edema** (accumulation of fluid in the body's tissues) by depressing the client's skin (Figure 15–5 ■). Record findings as follows: 1+ Slight pitting, no obvious distortion 2+ Deeper pit, no obvious distortion 3+ Pit is obvious; extremities are swollen 4+ Pit remains with obvious distortion ■ Edema is common in cardiovascular disorders, renal failure, and cirrhosis of the liver. It also may be a side effect of certain drugs.
Inspect distribution and quality of hair. *Hair should be evenly distributed for client's gender.*	■ A deviation in the normal hair distribution in the male or female genital area may indicate an endocrine disorder. **Hirsutism** (increased growth of coarse hair, usually on the face and trunk) is seen in Cushing's syndrome, acromegaly, and ovarian dysfunction. **Alopecia** (hair loss) may be related to changes in hormones, chemical or drug treatment, or radiation. In adult males whose hair loss follows the normal male pattern, the cause is usually genetic.

Slight pitting, no obvious distortion.   2mm   **1+**

Deeper pit, no obvious distortion.   4mm   **2+**

Pit is obvious; extremities are swollen.   6mm   **3+**

Pit remains with obvious distortion.   8mm   **4+**

A

B

Figure 15–5 ■ *A,* Degrees of pitting in edema. *B,* 4+ pitting.

Source: Dr. P. Marazzi/Science Photo Library/Photo Researchers, Inc.

Palpate hair texture. *Hair should be of even texture.*

- Some systemic diseases change the texture of the hair. For instance, hypothyroidism causes the hair to coarsen, whereas hyperthyroidism causes the hair to become fine.

Inspect the scalp for lesions. *There should be no lesions on the scalp.*

- Mild dandruff is normal, but excessive, greasy flakes indicate seborrhea requiring treatment.
- Hair loss, pustules, and scales appear on the scalp in tinea capitis (scalp ringworm).
- Red, swollen pustules appear around infected hair follicles and are called folliculitis.
- Head lice may be seen as oval nits (eggs) adhering to the base of the hair shaft. Head lice are usually accompanied by itching.

Inspect nail curvature. *Nails should not be excessively curved.*

- Clubbing (Figure 15–6 ■), in which the angle of the nail base is greater than 180 degrees, is seen in respiratory disorders, cardiovascular disorders, cirrhosis of the liver, colitis, and thyroid disease. The nail becomes thick, hard, shiny, and curved at the free end.

Flattened angle (180°)

Early clubbing

About 160°

A   Normal

B

Figure 15–6 ■ *A*, Assessing clubbing of the nails. *B*, Hand with nail clubbing.

Source: ISM/Phototake NYC.

Inspect the surface of the nails. *Nail surfaces should be smooth and nail folds firm, without redness.*

- The nail folds become inflamed and swollen and the nail loosens in paronychia, an infection of the nails.
- Inflammation and transverse rippling of the nail are associated with chronic paronychia and/or eczema.
- The nail plate may separate from the nail bed in trauma, psoriasis, and *Pseudomonas* and *Candida* infections. This separation is called oncolysis.
- Nail grooves may be caused by inflammation, by planus, or by nail biting.
- Nail pitting may be seen with psoriasis.
- A transverse groove (Beau's line) may be seen in trachoma and/or acute diseases.
- Thin spoon-shaped nails (Figure 15–7 ■) may be seen in anemia.

Figure 15–7 ■ Spoon-shaped nails.

Inspect nail color. *Nail color should be even.*

- The sudden appearance of a pigmented band may indicate melanoma in Caucasians. Pigmented bands are normally found in more than 90% of African Americans.
- Yellowish nails are seen in psoriasis and fungal infections.
- Dark nails occur with trauma, *Candida* infections, and hyperbilirubinemia.
- Blackish-green nails are apparent in injury and in *Pseudomonas* infection.
- Red splinter longitudinal hemorrhages may be seen in injury and/or psoriasis.

Inspect nail thickness. *Nails should not be excessively thick.*

- Trauma to the nails usually causes thickening. Other causes of thick nails include psoriasis, fungal infections, and decreased peripheral vascular blood supply.
- Thinning of the nails is seen in nutritional deficiencies.

EXPLORE MediaLink

Prentice Hall Nursing MediaLink DVD-ROM
Audio Glossary
NCLEX-RN® Review

COMPANION WEBSITE www.prenhall.com/lemone
Audio Glossary
NCLEX-RN® Review
Care Plan Activity: Integumentary Disorders
Case Studies
Assessing a Rash
Skin Assessment for a Client with a Bacterial Infection
MediaLink Applications
Moles
Skin Cancer
Links to Resources

TEST YOURSELF NCLEX-RN® REVIEW

1 Which layer of the skin contains most of the hair follicles, sebaceous glands, and sweat glands?
 1. epidermis
 2. dermis
 3. stratum basale
 4. stratum spinosum

2 What pigment is responsible for skin tanning?
 1. carotene
 2. red blood cells
 3. melanin
 4. sebum

3 Which of the four assessment techniques are used during assessment of the integumentary system? (Select all that apply.)
 1. inspection
 2. palpation
 3. percussion
 4. auscultation

4 What change in skin color is associated with an elevated body temperature?
 1. erythema
 2. jaundice
 3. pallor
 4. cyanosis

5 You are assessing a client who is complaining of severe itching. What would be an appropriate interview question?
 1. "Tell me how this itch feels."
 2. "Why do you keep scratching it?"
 3. "Have you used a new soap?"
 4. "Describe your daily fluid intake."

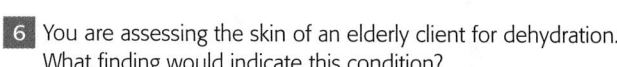

6 You are assessing the skin of an elderly client for dehydration. What finding would indicate this condition?
 1. decreased turgor
 2. increased moisture
 3. presence of lesions
 4. pallor or cyanosis

7 What part of the body would you palpate to assess edema?
 1. scalp
 2. fingers
 3. clavicle
 4. ankle/foot

8 You note that your client with chronic dermatitis has rough, thickened areas of skin. You document these areas as:
 1. ulcers.
 2. papules.
 3. atrophy.
 4. lichenification.

9 While making a home visit to an older woman, you notice multiple bruises on her arms and body. What might these indicate?
 1. high intake of vitamin A
 2. elder abuse
 3. caregiver strain
 4. aging skin

10 While assessing the hair of a family, you note small white eggs on the hair shaft. What type of infestation are you assessing?
 1. bacterial
 2. viral
 3. head lice
 4. head lichens

See Test Yourself answers in Appendix C.

BIBLIOGRAPHY

AARP. (2004). *Checkups and prevention: Skin cancer risks, treatments, and prevention.* Retrieved from http://www.aarp.org/health-prevention/Articles/a2004-07-07-skincancer.html

Amella, E. (2004). Presentation of illness in older adults: If you think you know what you're looking for, think again. *American Journal of Nursing, 104*(10), 40–51.

Bickley, L., & Szilagyi, P. (2005). *Bates' guide to physical examination and history taking* (9th ed.). Philadelphia: Lippincott.

Brinker, D., Hancox, J., & Bernardon, S. (2003). Assessment and intital treatment of lacerations, mammalian bites, and insect stings. *AACN Clinical Issues: Advanced Practice in Acute and Critical Care, 14*(4), 401–410.

Carter, K., Dufour, L., & Ballard, C. (2003). Wound & skin care: Identifying primary skin lesions. *Nursing, 33*(12), 58–69.

Finch, M. (2003). Assessment of skin in older people. *Nursing Older People, 15*(2), 29–30.

Fulmer, T. (2004). Try this: Best practices in nursing care to older adults from the Hartford Institute for Geriatric Nursing. Elder abuse and neglect assessment. *AAACN Viewpoint, 26*(2), 3–4.

Gray-Vickery, P. (2004). Combating elder abuse. *Nursing, 34*(10), 47–51.

Hayes, J. (2003). Are you assessing for melanoma? *RN, 66*(2), 36–41.

Jarvis, C. (2004). *Physical examination & health assessment.* St. Louis, MO: Mosby.

Kulkowski, K., & Ratliff, C. (2004). Wounds & skin care: Managing venous and neuropathic ulcers. *Nursing, 34*(8), 68.

Larson, K. (2003). Fluid balance in the elderly: Assessment and intervention—important role in community health and home care nursing. *Geriatric Nursing, 24*(5), 306–309.

McLeod, R. (2004). Lumps, bumps, and things that go itch in your office! *Journal of School Nursing, 20*(2), 115–116.

Oliviero, M. (2002). How to diagnose malignant melanoma. *Nursing Practitioner: American Journal of Primary Health Care, 27*(2), 26–27, 31–37.

Porth, C. (2005). *Pathophysiology: Concepts of altered health states* (7th ed.). Philadelphia: Lippincott.

Scanlon, E., & Stubbs, N. (2004). Pressure ulcer risk assessment in patients with darkly pigmented skin. *Professional Nurse, 19*(6), 339–341.

Stein, A. (2003). Aging is more than skin deep: Learn about the systemic effects and signs that may indicate abnormalities. *Nursing (Hospital Nursing), 33*(2), 32hn 7–8.

Weber, J., & Kelley, J. (2006). *Health assessment in nursing* (3rd ed.). Philadelphia: Lippincott-Williams Wilkins.

CHAPTER 16
Nursing Care of Clients with Integumentary Disorders

LEARNING OUTCOMES

- Describe the manifestations and nursing care of common skin problems and lesions.

- Compare and contrast the etiology, pathophysiology, interdisciplinary care, and nursing care of clients with infections and infestations, inflammatory disorders, and malignancies of the skin.

- Explain the risk factors for, pathophysiology of, and nursing interventions to prevent and care for pressure ulcers.

- Discuss surgical options for excision of neoplasms, reconstruction of facial or body structures, and cosmetic procedures.

- Explain the pathophysiology of selected disorders of the hair and nails.

- Discuss the effects and nursing implications of medications and treatments used to treat disorders of the integument.

CLINICAL COMPETENCIES

- Assess functional health status of clients with integumentary disorders, and monitor, document, and report abnormal manifestations.

- Use evidence-based research to plan and implement nursing care for clients with pressure ulcers.

- Determine priority nursing diagnoses, based on assessed data, to select and implement individualized nursing interventions for clients with integumentary disorders.

- Administer topical, oral, and injectable medications used to treat integumentary disorders knowledgeably and safely.

- Integrate interdisciplinary care into care of clients with integumentary disorders.

- Provide teaching appropriate for prevention and self-care of disorders of the integumentary system.

- Revise plan of care as needed to provide effective interventions to promote, maintain, or restore functional health status to clients with disorders of the integument.

The skin and its accessory structures (the integumentary system) enclose and cover the body, providing protection by serving as a barrier between the internal and external environments. As described in Chapter 15 ∞, the skin contains receptors for touch and sensation, helps regulate body temperature, and maintains fluid and electrolyte balance. The skin also provides cues to racial and ethnic background, and plays a major role in determining self-concept, roles, and relationships.

There are many disorders of the integument. Many of them are treated in an outpatient setting or by self-care. This chapter discusses disorders of the skin, hair, and nails; Chapter 17 ∞ discusses the client with burns. Primary and secondary skin lesions are described and illustrated in Tables 15–5 and 15–6. The terms from these tables are used throughout this and the next chapter.

COMMON SKIN PROBLEMS AND LESIONS

The disorders discussed in this section are those experienced by a large number of people. Although they are considered minor health problems in terms of health care, they may cause major problems for the person experiencing a high level of discomfort and/or chronicity.

THE CLIENT WITH PRURITUS

Pruritus is a subjective itching sensation that produces an urge to scratch. Pruritus may occur in a small, circumscribed area, or it may involve a widespread area; it may or may not be associated with a rash. Pruritus is believed to result from either stimulation of itch receptors in the skin or as a response to the stimulation of skin receptors for pain and touch. The central nervous system (CNS) interprets these stimuli as an itch through central summation (Porth, 2005).

Almost anything in the internal or external environment can cause pruritus. Insects, animals, plants, fabrics, metals, medications, allergies, and even emotional distress are among the most common causes. Pruritus also may occur as a secondary manifestation of systemic disorders, such as certain types of cancer, diabetes mellitus, hepatic disease, and renal failure. Although the exact physiology is unknown, it is known that heat and prostaglandins trigger pruritus and that histamine and morphine increase it.

The pathophysiologic response of pruritus to stimulation or irritation follows a similar pathway, regardless of cause. The irritating agent stimulates receptors in the junction between the epidermis and dermis, and may also trigger the release of his-

tamine and other chemical mediators that either further stimulate or mediate the itch response. The response of the person experiencing the itch is to scratch or rub the affected area. This may irritate the skin and cause further inflammation, which in turn sets off a cycle of increasingly intense itching and scratching, called the *itch–scratch–itch cycle.*

Secondary effects of pruritus include skin excoriation, erythema (redness), wheals, changes in pigmentation, and infections. Persistent pruritus may interrupt sleep patterns, because the itching sensation is often more intense at night. Long-term pruritus may be debilitating and increases the risk of infection as excoriation occurs.

Management of pruritus focuses on identifying and eliminating the cause and providing medications to relieve the itch. Antihistamines may relieve pruritus in some clients. Tranquilizers provide sedation, which may in turn relieve the emotional stress associated with pruritus; however, eliminating the stressors produces a more successful result. Systemic antibiotics are used to treat the infection resulting from the scratching and excoriation. Topical medications that contain corticosteroids are often used to relieve the pruritus and inflammation. Topical medications may also be administered through therapeutic baths or soaks with agents that relieve pruritus, such as cornstarch and baking soda or coal tar concentrates. Creams containing a topical anesthetic or antibiotic may also be used. Therapeutic baths are discussed in the Medication Administration box on the following page. Table 16–1 lists examples of topical agents used to treat skin disorders.

MEDICATION ADMINISTRATION Therapeutic Baths

AGENTS USED IN THERAPEUTIC BATHS
Saline or tap water
Antibacterial agents: potassium permanganate, acetic acid, hexachlorophene
Colloid substances: oatmeal (Aveeno), cornstarch, sodium bicarbonate
Coal tar derivatives: Balnetar, Zetar, Polytar
Emollients: Alpha Keri, Lubath, mineral oil.
Therapeutic baths have a variety of uses in treating skin disorders. Depending on the agent used, therapeutic baths soothe the skin, lower the skin bacteria count, clean and hydrate the skin, loosen scales, and relieve itching.

Nursing Responsibilities
- Ensure that the bath water is at a comfortable temperature that is neither too hot nor too cool, usually 110° to 115°F (45° to 46°C).
- Fill the tub one-third to one-half full.
- Mix the agent well with the water.

- Assist the client into and out of the tub to prevent falls.
- Dry the client by blotting with the towel.

Health Education for the Client and Family
- Use a bath mat in the tub, because the medications may cause the tub to become slippery.
- Keep the bathroom warm but adequately ventilated.
- Follow directions carefully for the amount of medication to use in the bath.
- Fill the bath one-third to one-half full of water that is at a comfortable temperature.
- Stay in the bath for 20 to 30 minutes, and immerse the areas to be treated.
- Do not get the bathwater in your eyes.
- Dry by blotting (not rubbing) with the towel.
- If the medications cause staining, use old towels or linens.
- If the itching is not relieved or the skin becomes excessively dry, call your healthcare provider.

THE CLIENT WITH DRY SKIN (XEROSIS)

Dry skin, also called **xerosis**, is most often a problem in the older adult. Xerosis commonly results, especially in the older adult, from a decrease in the activity of sebaceous and sweat glands, which reduces the skin's lubrication and moisture retention. However, dry skin may occur at any age from exposure to environmental heat and low humidity, sunlight, excessive bathing, and a decreased intake of liquids.

Two types of severe dry skin are xeroderma and ichthyosis. Xeroderma is a chronic skin condition characterized by dry, rough skin. Ichthyosis is an inherited dermatologic condition in which the skin is dry, fissured, and hyperkeratotic; the surface of the skin has the appearance of fish scales.

The primary manifestation of dry skin is pruritus. Other manifestations include visible flaking of surface skin and an observable pattern of fine lines over the area. If the skin has been excessively dry and pruritic for a long period, the client may have secondary skin lesions and lichenification (thickening).

Nursing care focuses on teaching the client and family how to reduce the dry skin and relieve the pruritus, as outlined in Box 16–1.

TABLE 16–1 Medications Used to Treat Skin Disorders

TYPE	USE	EXAMPLES
Creams	Moisturize the skin	Aquacare Curel Nutraderm
Ointments	Lubricate the skin Retard water loss	Aquaphor Vaseline
Lotions	Moisturize the skin Lubricate the skin	Alpha-Keri Dermassage Lubriderm
Anesthetics	Relieve itching	Xylocaine
Antibiotics	Treat infection	Bacitracin Polysporin Gentamicin Silvadene
Corticosteroids	Suppress inflammation Relieve itching	Dexamethasone Hydrocortisone Clocortolone Desonide

BOX 16–1 Teaching to Reduce Dry Skin and Relieve Pruritus

- Wash clothing in a mild detergent and rinse twice; do not use fabric softeners.
- Avoid using perfumes and lotions containing alcohol.
- Apply skin lubricants after a bath to help retain moisture.
- Soaps and hot water are drying. Clean the skin with tepid water and either a mild soap or cleansing creams. If soap is used, rinse it off carefully.
- It is not necessary to take a bath every day.
- If bath oils are used, add them to the bathwater at the end of the bath (the moist skin is more likely to retain the oil). Use care not to slip in the tub.
- Use a humidifier to humidify the air.
- Apply creams and lotions when the skin is slightly damp after bathing.
- Increase fluid intake.
- Keep nails trimmed short, wear loose clothing, and keep the environment cool.
- A brief application of pressure or cold may relieve pruritus.
- Cotton gloves may be worn at night if scratching during sleep causes skin excoriation.
- Distraction or relaxation techniques may prove helpful.

THE CLIENT WITH BENIGN SKIN LESIONS

The skin is subject to many different types and kinds of benign skin lesions, including cysts, keloids, nevi, angiomas, skin tags, and keratoses. Although these benign lesions are often considered more of a nuisance than an illness, they do require monitoring for an increase in size that interferes with the skin's appearance or function.

Most benign skin lesions do not require treatment, although excision or laser surgery may sometimes be desired or necessary. Cysts may enlarge, skin tags may become irritated and bleed, nevi may change in appearance, or any of the lesions may cause discomfort with appearance.

Cysts

Cysts of the skin are benign closed sacs in or under the skin surface that are lined with epithelium and contain fluid or a semisolid material. Epidermal inclusion cysts and pilar cysts are the most common types.

Epidermal inclusion cysts may occur anywhere on the body but are most often found on the head and trunk. Although they are painless, they may grow so large that they become irritated by contact with clothing (e.g., if located on the back of the neck) or cause obstruction (e.g., if located on the nose). The cysts contain a semisolid material composed mainly of keratin. Pilar cysts are found on the scalp and originate from sebaceous glands. They are also painless. Both types of cysts rarely require treatment unless they become large and bothersome.

Keloids

Keloids are elevated, irregularly shaped, progressively enlarging scars. They arise from excessive amounts of collagen in the stratum corneum during scar formation in connective tissue repair. These lesions are more common in young adults and appear within 1 year of the initial trauma.

This abnormal response most often occurs in people of African and Asian descent who sustain burns of the skin, but even seemingly minor trauma can result in keloid formation. There is a familial tendency to develop keloids. Other risk factors for keloid formation include excessive tension on a wound and poor alignment of skin edges following accidental or intentional skin trauma. Certain skin surfaces are also more likely to develop keloids: the chin, ears, shoulders, back, and lower legs.

The excessive scar formation is associated with increased metabolic activity of fibroblasts and increased type III collagen. The principal cells of the keloids are myofibroblasts, which have characteristics of both fibroblasts and smooth muscle cells. The swollen appearance of the keloids is the result of an excess of extracellular material.

The keloids first appear as red, firm, rubbery plaques that persist for several months after the initial trauma (Figure 16–1 ■). Uncontrolled overgrowth over time causes the keloids to extend beyond the original scar. Eventually, the keloid becomes smooth and hyperpigmented.

Nevi

Nevi, more commonly called *moles,* are flat or raised macules or papules with rounded, well-defined borders (Figure 16–2 ■).

Figure 16–1 ■ Keloids form as a result of deposits of excessive amounts of collagen during scar formation.
Source: Martin Rotker/Phototake NYC.

Nevi arise from melanocytes during early childhood, with the cells initially accumulating at the junction of the dermis and epidermis. Over time, the cluster of cells moves into the dermis, and the lesion becomes visible. Almost all adults have nevi.

Nevi range from flesh colored to black and occasionally contain hair. They can occur on any skin surface of the body and may arise as single lesions or in groups. Some pigmented nevi can transform into malignant lesions. Although the average adult has about 20 nevi, only 4 people out of 100,000 de-

Figure 16–2 ■ Nevi (moles) arise from melanocytes and are common in all adults.
Source: Stephen J. Krasemann/Photo Researchers, Inc.

velop a malignant melanoma (Porth, 2005). However, it is important to monitor nevi for changes in size, thickness, color, bleeding, or itching. If any of these changes occur, the person should seek immediate professional assessment.

Angiomas

Angiomas, also called *hemangiomas*, are benign vascular tumors. They appear in the adult in different forms:

- Nevus flammeus (port-wine stain) is a congenital vascular lesion that involves the capillaries. The lesions tend to occur on the upper body or face as macular patches that range from light red to dark purple. These lesions are present at birth and grow proportionately with the child into adulthood.
- Cherry angiomas are small, rounded papules that may occur at any age, but they most commonly arise in the 40s and gradually increase in number. The lesions range in color from bright red to purple. These lesions are often found on the trunk.
- Spider angiomas are dilated superficial arteries. They are common in pregnant women and in clients with hepatic disease. Spider angiomas occur most often on the face, neck, and upper chest. The lesions are usually small, bright red papules with radiating lines.
- Telangiectases are single dilated capillaries or terminal arteries that appear often on the cheeks and nose. These lesions are most common in older adults and result from photoaged skin. The lesions look like broken veins.
- Venous lakes are small, flat, blue blood vessels. They are seen on the exposed skin of the older adult: the ears, lips, and backs of the hands.

Skin Tags

Skin tags are soft papules on a pedicle. They can be as small as a pinhead or as large as a pea and are most often found on the front or side of the neck and in the axillae, as well as in areas where clothing (such as underwear) rubs the skin. These lesions have normal skin color and texture.

Keratoses

A **keratosis** is any skin condition in which there is a benign overgrowth and thickening of the cornified epithelium. These lesions most often appear in adults after age 50. *Seborrheic keratoses* appear as superficial flat, smooth, or warty-surfaced growths, 5 to 20 mm in diameter, most often on the face and trunk. The lesions may be tan, waxy yellow, dark brown, or flesh colored, and they often appear greasy. They are most often seen in the older adult and do not appear to be related to damage from sun exposure.

THE CLIENT WITH PSORIASIS

Psoriasis is a chronic immune skin disorder characterized by raised, reddened, round circumscribed plaques covered by silvery white scales (Figure 16–3 ■). The size of these lesions varies. The lesions may appear anywhere on the body, but they are most commonly found on the scalp, extensor surfaces of the arms and legs, elbows, knees, sacrum, and around the nails. As with any chronic illness, the skin manifestations may occur and disappear throughout life, with no discernible pattern to the recurrence.

Figure 16–3 ■ The characteristic lesions of psoriasis are raised, red, round plaques covered with thick, silvery white scales.
Source: NMSB/Custom Medical Stock Photo.

The incidence of psoriasis is lower in warm, sunny climates. Onset usually occurs in the 20s, but it may occur at any age. Psoriasis occurs more often in Caucasians; men and women are affected equally. Sunlight, stress, seasonal changes, hormone fluctuations, steroid withdrawal, and certain drugs (such as alcohol, corticosteroids, lithium, and chloroquine) appear to exacerbate the disorder. About one-third of clients have a family history of psoriasis. Trauma to the skin from such events as surgery, sunburn, or excoriation is also a common precipitating factor; lesions that result from trauma are called Köbner's reaction (Porth, 2005).

Pathophysiology

Normally, the keratinocyte (an epidermal cell making up 95% of the epidermis) migrates from the basal cell to the stratum corneum (the outer skin layer) in about 14 days and is sloughed off 14 days later. Psoriatic skin cells, by contrast, have a shorter cycle of growth, completing the journey to the stratum corneum in only 4 to 7 days, a condition called hyperkeratosis. These immature cells produce an abnormal keratin that forms thick, flaky scales at the surface of the skin. The more rapid cell metabolism stimulates increased vascularity, which contributes to the erythema of the lesions. As part of the abnormal process, certain immune cells become overactive and release proteins called cytokines. One of the cytokines is tumor necrosis factor (TNF); in psoriasis TNF causes inflammation, further contributing to plaque formation.

Psoriasis vulgaris is the most common form of psoriasis. The lesions can be found anywhere on the skin but most commonly involve the skin over the elbows, knees, and scalp. Initially, the lesions are papules that form into well-defined erythematous plaques with thick, silvery white scales. The plaques in darker skinned persons may appear purple.

Permanent remission of psoriasis is rare. The prognosis depends on the type, extent, and severity of the initial attack. The age of onset is also a factor; early onset disease is usually more severe.

Manifestations

The characteristic lesions in psoriasis are well-demarcated regions of erythematous plaques that shed thick, silvery white flakes. Pruritus is common over the psoriatic lesions. If the lesions are located in an intertriginous zone, such as between the toes, under the breasts, or in the perianal region, the psoriatic scales may soften, allowing painful fissures to form. When psoriasis affects the nails, pitting and a yellow or brown discoloration result. The nail may separate from the nail bed, thicken, and crumble. The involved nails, which are more often fingernails than toenails, are at high risk for infection. The client may also exhibit manifestations of psoriatic arthritis, seen most often in the distal interphalangeal joints, especially if the fingernails are involved.

INTERDISCIPLINARY CARE

Treatment is based on the type of psoriasis, the extent and location of the lesions, the age of the client, and the degree of disfigurement or disability.

Diagnosis

Skin biopsy may be done if the client presents with atypical manifestations or to differentiate psoriasis from other inflammatory or infectious skin disorders. In addition, an ultrasound may reveal typical psoriatic changes in the stratum corneum and inflammation of the dermis.

Medications

A variety of medications and treatments may be prescribed, including topical medications and photochemotherapy. Although there is no cure, treatment decreases the severity and pain of the lesions.

Topical medications are administered to decrease inflammation, prolong the maturity time of keratinocytes, and increase remission time. Corticosteroids, tar preparations, anthralin, and the retinoids are typically used. Box 16–2 outlines general guidelines for teaching clients to apply topical medications.

Topical corticosteroids decrease inflammation, suppress mitotic activity of psoriatic cells, and delay the movement of keratinocytes to the surface of the skin (thus giving them time to mature and decreasing hyperkeratosis). The most effective topical corticosteroids are potent preparations that are well absorbed through the skin and are used under an occlusive dressing. Cor-

ticosteroids may also be taken systemically or injected directly into the lesions. However, corticosteroids rarely cause a lasting remission and may cause the psoriasis to become unstable (McPhee et al., 2007). They are therefore used for repeated short periods of treatment and combined with other measures, such as tar preparations, occlusions, or a topical retinoid.

Tar preparations (such as Estar, Psorigel, and Fototar) suppress mitotic activity and are also anti-inflammatory. Their exact mechanism of action is unknown, but they are effective in removing scales and increasing remission time. Preparations made of coal tar are messy, cause staining, and have an unpleasant odor, but they are an effective form of treatment.

Topical anthralin (dithranol) inhibits the mitotic activity of epidermal cells and is effective in some cases of chronic, localized psoriasis that do not respond to other topical agents. The medication is applied to the plaque patches at bedtime and left in place for 8 to 12 hours. Clients should be tested for sensitivity to the drug before use, and it should not be applied to inflamed or open areas of skin.

Calcipotriene (Dovonex) (a vitamin D analog) has been effective and safe in both the short-term and long-term treatment of psoriasis. It inhibits cell proliferation in the epidermis and facilitates cell differentiation. Although a derivative of topical vitamin D, calcipotriene does not seem to affect bone or calcium metabolism. Although more irritating than calcipotriene, tazarotene gel (Avage, Tarorac) is a topical retinoid that may also be used to treat mild to moderate psoriasis. Etanercept (Enbrel), an anti-TNF receptor medication, may be given by injection to decrease inflammation, and is especially useful in treating psoriatic arthritis.

Treatments

Psoriasis that is generalized (i.e., involves more than 30% of the body surface) is difficult to treat with topical medications. Treatments for generalized psoriasis include ultraviolet light therapy and photochemotherapy.

ULTRAVIOLET LIGHT THERAPY Ultraviolet-B (UVB) light is the treatment of choice for generalized psoriasis (McPhee et al., 2007). UVB light decreases the growth rate of epidermal

---

BOX 16–2 General Guidelines for Applying Topical Medications

Each time a medication is applied, the skin surface must be clean and dry. Remove the medication from the previous application. Remove creams by washing the skin with tap water; remove ointments by washing the skin first with mineral oil and then with a mild soap and water.

- To apply gels, creams, and pastes: Squeeze about 1/2 to 1 inch of the gel or cream into the palm of the hand. Rub the hands together until they are covered. Apply gels and creams to the affected areas with long strokes until the skin is thinly covered. Differences from these general guidelines follow:
  a. Corticosteroids are usually applied two to three times a day in small amounts and rubbed directly onto the lesions. Apply the medication after a bath and cover with an occlusive dressing.

  b. Apply medications containing tar in the direction of hair growth. Do not apply these medications to the face, to the genitals, or in skin folds. If the tar is water based or oil based, it will stain clothing.
  c. Wear gloves when applying anthralin stains.
- To apply lotions: Shake the bottle of lotion well. Pour a small amount into the palm of the hand, and pat the medication onto the skin. If the lotion is thin, apply it with a gauze pad.
- To apply sprays: Hold the container about 6 inches from the skin, and apply the medication in a short spray.
- To apply medicated shampoo: Rinse out medication from the previous application. Apply the shampoo, massage into the hair and over the scalp carefully, and allow it to remain for the prescribed time. Rinse.
- To apply pastes: Use enough paste on an applicator (such as a wooden tongue depressor) to cover the lesion thinly.

cells, thereby decreasing hyperkeratosis. Mercury vapor lights or fluorescent UV tubes provide the UVB light; the latter are often arranged in a cabinet so the client can stand and expose psoriatic lesions more easily. These units may be purchased or constructed to be used in the client's home.

The light therapy is administered in gradually increasing exposure times, until the client experiences a mild erythema, like a mild sunburn. Treatments are given three times a week as an outpatient and are measured in seconds of exposure. The eyes are shielded during the treatment. The erythema response occurs in about 8 hours. Careful assessment is necessary to prevent more severe burning, which could exacerbate the psoriasis. In clients with extensive psoriasis, UVB treatments may be combined with tar preparations, which increase the photosensitivity of the skin.

PHOTOCHEMOTHERAPY In photochemotherapy, a light-activated form of the drug methoxsalen is used. This drug is an antimetabolite that inhibits DNA synthesis and thereby prevents cell mitosis, decreasing hyperkeratosis. Exposure to ultraviolet-A (UVA) rays activates methoxsalen; it is administered orally, and the client is exposed to UVA 2 hours later. The eyes are covered by dark glasses during the treatment. Treatments are administered 2 to 3 times a week; usually 10 to 20 total treatments are given over 1 to 2 months. Treatment causes tanning, and direct sunlight must be avoided for 8 to 12 hours thereafter. If the client exhibits erythema, the treatments are stopped until the redness and swelling resolve.

Photochemotherapy has had a high success rate in achieving remission of psoriasis, but it can accelerate aging of exposed skin, induce cataract development, alter immune function, and increase the risk of melanoma.

NURSING CARE

The client with psoriasis requires nursing care to meet physical and psychologic responses to the illness. The nurse provides teaching for self-care and emotional support through nonjudgmental acceptance.

Nursing Diagnoses and Interventions

The nursing interventions discussed in this section focus on common problems of impaired skin integrity and disturbed body image.

Impaired Skin Integrity

Psoriatic lesions range from several scales to large, open areas. Typical psoriatic skin lesions increase the risk of infection, which can further compromise healing. In addition, certain treatments (e.g., the use of UVA or retinoids) may cause erythema or peeling of the skin, further altering skin integrity.

- Teach methods to reduce injury to the skin when taking therapeutic baths or treatments:
  - Use warm, not hot, water.
  - Gently rub lesions with a soft washcloth, using a circular motion.
  - Dry the skin with a soft towel, using a blotting or patting motion.
  - Keep the skin lubricated at all times.

Hot water and dry skin increase pruritus, further stimulating the itch–scratch–itch cycle. Dry skin also worsens psoriasis. Washing or drying the skin with rough linens or pressure may excoriate the skin over the psoriatic lesions.

- Explain application of topical medications:
  - Apply the medication as prescribed in a thin layer, using hands (gloved, if appropriate), wooden tongue depressors, or a gauze pad.
  - Avoid getting medications in the eyes, on mucous membranes, or in skin folds.
  - Apply a covering (occlusive dressing) over the medicated areas as prescribed, especially when using corticosteroids. Usually, the covering is applied for only 8 hours, often during the evening and night hours. Choose some type of plastic wrap that covers the area well.

Applying a thin layer of medication more frequently is often more effective than applying a single thick layer of medication. The medications used to treat psoriasis may irritate the eyes and mucous membranes; when applied in skin folds, they may also cause maceration (skin breakdown due to prolonged exposure to moisture). Topical corticosteroids are often covered with occlusive dressings to increase absorption and thus facilitate treatment. However, constant occlusion may increase the effects of the medications to undesired levels and also increases the risk for infections.

- Teach manifestations of infection and how to contact the healthcare provider if these occur: elevated temperature, increased swelling, redness, pain, increase in drainage, and any change in the color of the drainage. *The client with skin lesions is at high risk for infection, as the skin is the body's first line of defense.*

- Teach manifestations of the complications of treatment: excoriation, increased erythema, increased peeling, and blister formation. *The topical medications or treatments may damage cells through chemical burns or excessive exposure to ultraviolet light. Times and methods of treatment need to be adjusted if these manifestations occur.*

Disturbed Body Image

The chronic skin lesions of psoriasis often cause clients to isolate themselves from social contacts, withdraw from normal roles and responsibilities, and feel helpless or powerless.

- Establish a trusting relationship by expressing acceptance of the client, both verbally and nonverbally. For example, touch the client during social communications, demonstrating that the lesions are not contagious or offensive. *One's body image is affected not only by self-perception but also by the responses of others. Nonjudgmental acceptance helps the client adapt to the change in body image. By touching the client during interactions, the nurse demonstrates that acceptance.*

- Encourage the client to verbalize feelings about self-perception in view of the chronic nature of psoriasis and to ask questions about the disease and treatment. *The client adapts to a changed body image through a process of recognition, acceptance, and resolution. Each person responds individually to disfigurement and loss.*

- Promote social interaction through family involvement in care, and referral to support groups of people with psoriasis or other chronic skin conditions. *Acceptance by others is critical to acceptance of self. Psoriasis treatment is lifelong, time consuming, and often unappealing. By becoming involved in care, the family communicates acceptance. Sharing experiences with others who have the same health problem is a source of strength in adjusting to a visible, chronic illness.*

Community-Based Care

Client and family teaching focuses on treatments and skin care needs. The following topics should be addressed:

- The chronic nature of the disease, factors that may precipitate an exacerbation, and methods to reduce stress
- Interventions for pruritus and dry skin, and specific care for psoriasis:
  - Expose the skin to sunlight, but avoid sunburn.
  - Avoid trauma to the skin (e.g., do not scrub off scales, and use only an electric razor).
  - Avoid exposure to contagious illnesses such as influenza and colds.
  - Discuss current medications with the healthcare provider. Certain drugs (such as indomethacin [Indocin], lithium, and beta-adrenergic blocking agents) are known to precipitate exacerbations of psoriasis.
- Suggest the National Psoriasis Foundation as a resource.

INFECTIONS AND INFESTATIONS OF THE SKIN

The skin's resistance to infections and infestations is provided by protective mechanisms, including skin flora, sebum, and the immune response. Although the skin is normally resistant to infections and infestations, these disorders may occur as a result of a break in the skin surface, a virulent agent, and/or decreased resistance due to a compromised immune system. This section discusses skin disorders resulting from bacterial infections, fungal infections, parasitic infestations, and viral infections.

THE CLIENT WITH A BACTERIAL INFECTION OF THE SKIN

A number of bacteria normally inhabit the skin and do not cause an infection. However, when a break in the skin allows invasion by pathogenic bacteria, an infection, called a *pyoderma*, may occur. The most common bacterial infections are caused by gram-positive *Staphylococcus aureus* and beta-hemolytic streptococci.

Bacterial infections of the skin may be primary or secondary. Primary infections are caused by a single pathogen and arise from normal skin; secondary infections develop in traumatized or diseased skin.

Most bacterial infections are treated by a primary care provider, and the client remains at home for care. If the infection becomes more serious, however, inpatient care may be required. In addition, nosocomial infections of wounds or open lesions in hospitalized clients are often the result of bacterial infections, especially by methicillin-resistant *Staphylococcus aureus* (MRSA).

Pathophysiology

Bacterial infections of the skin arise from the hair follicle, where bacteria can accumulate and grow and cause a localized infection. However, the bacteria also can invade deeper tissues and cause a systemic infection, a potentially life-threatening disorder. Various types of bacterial infections involve the skin, including folliculitis, furuncles, carbuncles, cellulitis, and erysipelas.

Folliculitis

Folliculitis is a bacterial infection of the hair follicle, most commonly caused by *Staphylococcus aureus*. The infection begins at the follicle opening and extends down into the follicle. The bacteria release enzymes and chemical agents that cause an inflammation. The lesions appear as pustules surrounded by an area of erythema on the surface of the skin (Figure 16–4 ■). The lesions are accompanied by discomfort ranging from slight burning to intense itching. A major complication is abscess formation. Folliculitis is found most often on the scalp and extremities. It is also often seen on the face of bearded men (called sycosis barbae), on the legs of women who shave, and on the eyelids (called a *stye*).

Although folliculitis may appear without any apparent cause, contributing factors include poor hygiene, poor nutrition, prolonged skin moisture, tight heavy fabrics on the upper legs, and trauma to the skin.

> **PRACTICE ALERT**
> A specific type of folliculitis, called "hot tub folliculitis," is caused by *Pseudomonas aeruginosa*, and is characterized by follicular or pustular lesions that occur 1 to 4 days after being in a hot tub, whirlpool, or public swimming pool.

Furuncles

Furuncles, often called *boils*, are also inflammations of the hair follicle. They often begin as folliculitis, but the infection spreads down the hair shaft, through the wall of the follicle, and into the

Figure 16–4 ■ The lesions of folliculitis are pustules surrounded by areas of erythema.

dermis. The causative organism is commonly *Staphylococcus aureus*. A furuncle is initially a deep, firm, red, painful nodule from 1 to 5 cm in diameter (Figure 16–5 ■). After a few days, the nodule changes into a large, painful cystic nodule. The cysts may drain substantial amounts of purulent drainage.

One or more furuncles may occur on any part of the body that has hair. Contributing factors include poor hygiene, trauma to the skin, areas of excessive moisture (including perspiration), and systemic diseases such as diabetes mellitus and hematologic malignancies.

Carbuncles

A **carbuncle** is a group of infected hair follicles. The lesion begins as a firm mass located in the subcutaneous tissue and the lower dermis. This mass becomes swollen and painful and has multiple openings to the skin surface. Carbuncles are most frequently found on the back of the neck, the upper back, and the lateral thighs. In addition to the local manifestations, the client may experience chills, fever, and malaise. The contributing factors for carbuncles are the same as for furuncles. Both infections are more common in hot, humid climates.

Cellulitis

Cellulitis is a localized infection of the dermis and subcutaneous tissue. Cellulitis can occur following a wound or skin ulcer or as an extension of furuncles or carbuncles. The infection spreads as a result of a substance produced by the causative organism, called spreading factor (hyaluronidase). This factor breaks down the fibrin network and other barriers that normally localize the infection. The area of cellulitis is red, swollen, and painful (Figure 16–6 ■). In some cases, vesicles may form over the area of cellulitis. The client may also experience fever, chills, malaise, headache, and swollen lymph glands.

Erysipelas

Erysipelas is an infection of the skin most often caused by group A streptococci. Chills, fever, and malaise are prodromal symptoms, occurring from 4 hours to 20 days before the skin lesion appears. The initial infection appears as firm red spots that enlarge and join to form a circumscribed, bright red, raised, hot lesion.

Figure 16–5 ■ A furuncle (boil) is a deep, firm, red, painful nodule.
Source: ISM/Phototake NYC.

Figure 16–6 ■ Cellulitis is a bacterial infection localized in the dermis and subcutaneous tissue. The involved area is red, swollen, and painful.
Source: Charles Stewart & Associates.

Vesicles may form over the surface of the erysipelas lesion. The area usually is painful, itches, and burns. Erysipelas most commonly appears on the face, ears, and lower legs.

INTERDISCIPLINARY CARE

The diagnosis of a bacterial infection of the skin is made by assessing the appearance of the lesion and by identifying the causative organism. Antibiotics specific to the organism are used in treatment.

Diagnosis

Drainage from a lesion or a blood culture may be ordered to identify the causative organism and target the most effective antibiotic. People who experience repeated bacterial skin infections or who provide care for others who exhibit infections may have a culture taken from the external nares to determine whether they are carriers of bacteria (e.g., MRSA) and are reinfecting themselves or others.

Medications

The primary treatment for bacterial infections of the skin is an antibiotic specific to the organism. The antibiotic is usually taken orally, but may also be applied topically. Multiple furuncles and carbuncles may be treated with cloxacillin (a penicillinase-resistant penicillin); the cephalosporins also are often effective.

NURSING CARE

Nursing care focuses on preventing the spread of infection and restoring normal skin integrity. Most clients provide self-care at home, but the incidence of secondary bacterial infections in the inpatient population is great enough to warrant their inclusion in planning and implementing care.

Nursing Diagnosis and Interventions
Risk for Infection

■ Practice good hand washing and teach its importance. *Careful hand washing is one of the most effective methods to reduce the spread of infection both in and out of the hospital setting. Healthcare providers must wash their hands with soap and water before and after client care and between each client contact. All clients, family members, and visitors (both in the home and hospital setting) should be taught the importance of hand washing, but it is even more important for the client with a bacterial infection.*

- Assess for and teach how to identify an increase in infection, which may be manifested systemically by fever, tachycardia, chills, and malaise. Local manifestations of the spread of the infection include an increase in erythema, the size of the lesion, and drainage. *This assessment is especially important for older, debilitated, or immunosuppressed clients, and for those who have large or dirty wounds.*

PRACTICE ALERT
If a client with a bacterial skin infection is hospitalized, place on isolation precautions to limit the spread of the organisms to other clients.

- Cover draining lesions with a sterile dressing, and handle soiled dressings or linens according to standard precautions. When changing dressings, always wear disposable gloves and masks. *These actions are necessary to prevent the spread of infection to other areas of the client's body, to other clients, to visitors, and to the nurse providing care.*

Community-Based Care

Client and family teaching focuses on facilitating tissue healing and eliminating the infection. Address the following topics:
- The importance of maintaining good nutrition
- The importance of maintaining cleanliness through careful hand washing and proper handling and disposal of dressings
- Preventing the spread of infection in the home by not sharing linens and towels and washing clothing and linens in hot water
- The importance of not squeezing or trying to open a bacterial lesion
- Avoiding plucking of nasal hair or picking nose
- The importance of taking the full course of prescribed antibiotics on a regular schedule until the prescribed supply is finished
- Bathing daily with an antibacterial soap (The client can gently wash off crusts during the bath. Warm compresses may be applied to the lesions two to three times a day to increase comfort and decrease swelling.)

THE CLIENT WITH A FUNGAL INFECTION

Fungi are free-living plantlike organisms that live in the soil, on animals, and on humans. The fungi that cause superficial skin infections are called dermatophytes. In humans, the dermatophytes live on keratin in the stratum corneum, hair, and nails. Fungal disorders are also called *mycoses*.

Pathophysiology

Fungal infections include dermatophytoses (tinea or ringworm) and candidiasis (yeast) infections.

Dermatophytoses (Tinea)

Superficial fungal infections of the skin are called **dermatophytoses** or, more commonly, *ringworm*. Fungal infections occur when a susceptible host comes in contact with the organism. The organism may be transmitted by direct contact with animals or other infected persons or by inanimate objects such as combs, pillowcases, towels, and hats. The most important factor in the development of the infection is moisture; the onset and spread of the fungal infection is greatest in areas where moisture content is high, such as within skin folds, between the toes, and in the mouth. Other factors that increase the risk of a fungal infection include the use of broad-spectrum antibiotics that kill off normal flora and allow the fungi to grow, diabetes mellitus, immunodeficiencies, nutritional deficiencies, pregnancy, increasing age, and iron deficiency. Fungal infections of the skin are more common in warm, humid climates. The dermatophyte infections are named by the body part affected, as follows:

- Tinea pedis is a fungal infection of the soles of the feet, the space between the toes, and/or the toenails (Figure 16–7 ■). More often called *athlete's foot*, this is the most common tinea infection. The lesions vary from mild scaliness to painful fissures with drainage, and they are usually accompanied by pruritus and a foul odor. The infection is often chronic, absent in winter but reappearing in hot weather when perspiring feet are encased in shoes.
- Tinea capitis is a fungal infection of the scalp. The primary lesions are gray, round, bald spots, often accompanied by erythema and crusting. The hair loss is usually temporary. Tinea capitis is seen more often in children than in adults.
- Tinea corporis is a fungal infection of the body. It can be caused by several different fungi, and the lesions vary according to the causative organism. The most common lesions are large circular patches with raised red borders of vesicles, papules, or pustules. Pruritus and erythema are also present.
- Tinea versicolor is a fungal infection of the upper chest, back, and sometimes the arms. The lesions are yellow, pink, or brown sheets of scaling skin. The patches do not have pigment and do not tan when exposed to ultraviolet light.

Figure 16–7 ■ Tinea pedis (athlete's foot) is a fungal infection that often occurs between the toes.
Source: SPL/Photo Researchers, Inc.

- Tinea cruris is a fungal infection of the groin that may extend to the inner thighs and buttocks. Often called "jock itch," it is often associated with tinea pedis and is more common in people who are physically active, are obese, and/or wear tight underclothing.

Candidiasis

Candidiasis infections are caused by *Candida albicans,* a yeastlike fungus. This fungus is normally found on mucous membranes, on the skin, in the vagina, and in the gastrointestinal tract. The fungus becomes a pathogen when the following factors encourage its growth:

- A local environment of moisture, warmth, or altered skin integrity
- The administration of systemic antibiotics
- Pregnancy
- The use of birth control pills
- Poor nutrition
- The presence of diabetes mellitus, Cushing's disease, or other chronic debilitating illnesses
- Immunosuppression
- Some malignancies of the blood.

Candidiasis affects the outer layers of the skin and mucous membranes of the mouth, vagina, uncircumcised penis, nails, and deep skin folds. The first sign of infection is a pustule that extends under the stratum corneum. The pustule has an inflamed base and often burns and itches. As the infection spreads, the accumulation of inflammatory cells and shedding of surface cells produce a white to yellow curdlike substance that covers the infected area (Figure 16–8). Satellite lesions (maculopapular areas found outside the clearly demarcated border of the original infection) are characteristic of candidiasis. The appearance of the infection differs by location, as summarized in Table 16–2.

INTERDISCIPLINARY CARE

Fungal infections are primarily diagnosed in outpatient settings and treated at home, but may also occur in hospitalized clients. The treatment is the same, regardless of the setting.

Figure 16–8 ■ *Candida albicans,* a fungus, causes a skin infection characterized by erythema, pustules, and a typical white substance covering the area.
Source: Stuart M. Levitz, M.D.

TABLE 16–2 Characteristics of Candidiasis Infections by Location

LOCATION	CHARACTERISTICS
Skin folds (under breasts, in groin, axillae, anus, umbilicus, and between toes or fingers)	Erythematous lesions that are either dry or moist. The lesions have clear borders, and satellite lesions are present.
Nails	Nail bed is red, swollen, and painful.
Mouth (thrush)	Mucous membranes are red and may be swollen; surface is covered with white, creamy material. Eroded areas may be present over the tongue and the oral cavity.
Penis (balanitis) (glans and shaft)	The penis is covered with small, red, clearly demarcated lesions that are painful and itch. The lesions may be covered with a white plaque.
Vagina	Red mucous membranes contain brighter red, demarcated, oozing lesions. The cervix may be covered with white plaque. A white, cheesy, foul-smelling vaginal discharge is present, accompanied by itching and burning. The vaginal and labial membranes may be swollen; the infection may extend to the anus and groin.

Diagnosis

Diagnostic tests are conducted to determine the causative fungi and may include cultures, microscopic examination using KOH, and examination of the skin with ultraviolet light (Wood's lamp). See Chapter 15 ∞ for further information.

Medications

Fungal infections of the skin are treated by topical or systemic antifungal medications. Nursing implications for the antifungal medications are described in the Medication Administration box on the following page.

- Tinea capitis is treated by shampooing the hair two to three times a week, applying a topical antifungal to inactivate organisms on the hair, and taking griseofulvin (Fulvicin), an antifungal agent, orally.
- Tinea pedis is treated by soaking the feet in Burrow's solution, potassium permanganate solution, or saline solution to remove crusts and scales. Topical antifungals are applied to the infected areas for several weeks.
- Mild cases of tinea cruris are treated with topical medications for 3 to 4 weeks. Over-the-counter (OTC) medications (such as miconazole, clotrimazole, butenafine, and terbinafine) are often less expensive and effective (McPhee et al., 2007). More severe cases may require oral griseofulvin.

Candidiasis infections are treated, depending on the location, with oral medication or with powder or vaginal suppositories.

MEDICATION ADMINISTRATION

ANTIFUNGAL AGENTS
Examples:

Butenafine (Mentax)   **Undecylenic acid (Desenex)**
Clotrimazole (Mycelex)   **Ketoconazole (Nizoral)**
Nystatin (Mycostatin, Nilstat)   **Fluconazole (Diflucan)**
Econazole (Spectazole)   **Amphotericin B (Fungizone)**
Oxiconazole (Oxistat)   **Griseofulvin (Fulvicin)**
Miconazole (Monistat)

Antifungal medications are prepared in a variety of forms, depending on the specific drug: powders, creams, shampoos, suspensions, troches, vaginal suppositories, and oral tablets. Some drugs interfere with the permeability of the fungal cell membrane, others interfere with DNA synthesis. Most of these medications are fungistatic but in large doses they may be fungicidal.

Nursing Responsibilities
- When taking the health history, ask about known hypersensitivity reactions to these agents; document carefully.
- Assess for side effects: skin rash, local irritation, gastrointestinal symptoms (if given PO), and mental status.
- Administer ketoconazole with food to minimize gastrointestinal irritation.
- Shake suspensions well before administration, and ask the client to swish them around the mouth before swallowing.
- Tell the client to allow oral tablets to dissolve in the mouth.

Health Education for the Client and Family
- Therapy usually continues over a long period of time, but regular use of medications for the recommended period is necessary. Do not miss doses, and complete the full treatment.
- For griseofulvin: Take with meals or foods high in fat (such as ice cream) to avoid stomach upset and help with absorption. Avoid alcohol (which may cause rapid pulse and flushing) and exposure to sunlight (this drug causes increased sensitivity).
- For nystatin: Dissolve lozenges completely in the mouth. Hold suspensions in the mouth and swish throughout the mouth as long as possible before swallowing. Insert intravaginal medication high in the vagina. Continue with intravaginal applications throughout the menses.
- For antifungal shampoo: Use two times a week for 4 weeks, allowing at least 3 days between each shampoo. Wet hair, apply shampoo to produce lather, leave in place for 1 minute, then rinse. Apply shampoo a second time, lather, leave in place for 3 minutes, then rinse thoroughly.
- For topical application: Rub well into the affected areas, but do not get the medication in your eyes.
- For vaginal candidiasis infections: During therapy, refrain from sexual intercourse or advise partner to use a condom.
- Your sexual partner will need to be treated at the same time so that you do not pass the infection back and forth to each other.

Nystatin (Mycostatin) is an antibiotic effective in controlling the infection. Fluconazole (Diflucan), an oral antifungal agent, is also effective.

NURSING CARE

Many people treat themselves with OTC antifungal medications. It is recommended, however, that the person be professionally diagnosed the first time the infection occurs. If symptoms reappear, self-treatment is usually satisfactory. The interventions discussed for nursing care of the client with a bacterial infection are also appropriate for the client with a fungal infection. Teaching topics specific to fungal infections are as follows:
- Fungal diseases are contagious. Do not share linens or personal items with others.
- Use a clean towel and washcloth each day.
- Carefully dry all skin folds, including those under the breasts, under the arms, and between the toes.
- Wear clean cotton underclothing each day.
- Fungi grow in moist environments, such as on sweaty feet. To prevent further infections:
  - Do not wear the same pair of shoes every day.
  - Wear socks that permit moisture to wick away from the skin surface.
  - Do not wear rubber- or plastic-soled shoes.
  - Use talcum powder or an OTC antifungal powder twice a day.
- For vaginal *Candida albicans* infection:
  - Avoid tight clothing, such as jeans and pantyhose.
  - Wear cotton or cotton-crotch underwear.
  - Bathe more frequently, and dry the genital area well.
  - Have your sexual partner treated at the same time to avoid passing the infection back and forth to each other.

PRACTICE ALERT
Recommend the client with repeated skin infections have a blood glucose test, because this may indicate diabetes mellitus.

THE CLIENT WITH A PARASITIC INFESTATION

Infestations of the skin by parasites are more common in developing countries but may occur in any geographic area of the world. They affect people of all social classes but are associated with crowded or unsanitary living conditions.

Pathophysiology

Two of the more common parasitic infestations of the skin are caused by lice and mites. These parasites do not normally live on the skin, but infest the skin through contact with an infested person or contact with clothing, linens, or objects infested with the parasites.

Pediculosis
Pediculosis is an infestation with lice, parasites that live on the blood of an animal or human host. The louse is a 2- to 4-mm oval organism with a stylet that pierces the skin; an anticoagulant in its saliva prevents host blood from clotting while it eats. The female louse lays its eggs (small pearl-gray or brown eggs, called nits) on hair shafts. The louse within the egg hatches, reaches the adult reproductive stage, and dies in 30 to 50 days (Porth, 2005).

There are three types of human pediculosis:

- Pediculosis corporis is an infestation with body lice. This type of infestation is more common in people who do not have access to facilities for bathing or washing clothes, such as the homeless. The lice live in clothing fibers and are transmitted primarily by contact with infested clothing and bed linens. The skin lesions occur at the site of a louse bite; macules appear initially, followed by wheals and papules. Pruritus is common, and scratching often results in linear excoriations. Secondary infections cause hyperpigmentation and scarring. The lesions are most often seen on the shoulders, trunk, and buttocks.
- Pediculosis pubis is an infestation with pubic lice (often called crabs). This infestation is spread through sexual activity with someone already infested or by contact with infested clothing or linens. The lice are found in the pubic region and occasionally spread to the axillae or men's beards. The lice cause skin irritation and intense itching.
- Pediculosis capitis is an infestation with head lice. The lice are most often found behind the ears and at the nape of the neck but may also spread to other hairy areas of the body: the eyebrows, pubic area, or beard. The lice are transmitted by contact with an infected person. Manifestations of head lice include pruritus, scratching, and erythema of the scalp. If untreated, the hair appears matted and crusted with a foul-smelling substance.

Scabies

Scabies is a parasitic infestation caused by a mite (*Sarcoptes scabiei*). The pregnant female mite burrows into the skin and lays two to three eggs each day for about a month. The eggs hatch in 3 to 5 days, and the larvae migrate to the surface but burrow into the skin for food or protection. The larvae develop, and the cycle repeats. Scabies infestation affects people of all socioeconomic classes. The infestation is found in webs between the fingers, the inner surfaces of the wrist and elbow, the axillae, the female nipple, the penis, the belt line, and the gluteal crease. The lesions are a small red-brown burrow, about 2 mm in length, sometimes covered with vesicles, which appears as a rash. Pruritus in response to the mite or its feces is common, especially at night, and excoriations may develop. The excoriations predispose the person to secondary bacterial infections.

INTERDISCIPLINARY CARE

Parasitic infestations are diagnosed by identifying the organism and are treated with medications that kill the lice or mites.

Diagnosis

When a client has manifestations of pediculosis, the hair shaft and the clothing are examined to identify the lice or the nits. Microscopic examination of the parasite provides a positive diagnosis. Scabies is diagnosed by skin scrapings and microscopic examination for the mites or their feces.

Medications

Lice are eradicated with agents that kill the parasite. Infestations of the body and pubic area are treated with topical medications that contain gamma benzene hexachloride, malathion (Prioderm lotion), or permethrin (NIX).

Infestations of the pubic hair are treated with shampoos containing lindane, such as Kwell. Head lice are treated with permethrin 1% cream (NIX). The medication is applied to the hair and left on for 30 minutes to 8 hours before being rinsed off. The treatment should be repeated in a week to kill newly hatched lice. A fine-toothed comb can be used to comb the dead nits off the hair shaft. Infestations of the eyebrows and eyelashes are treated by applying a thick covering of petroleum jelly twice a day for 8 days.

Scabies may be eradicated by a single treatment of lindane lotion or Kwell applied to the entire skin surface for 12 hours.

The associated itching is treated with systemic or topical medications, including corticosteroids. Secondary bacterial infections are treated with the appropriate antibiotic.

 ## NURSING CARE

Nursing care for clients with a parasite infestation most often focuses on teaching to prevent infestation or to eradicate an existing infestation. For a hospitalized client with pediculosis, isolation procedures are instituted until the client no longer has the infestation.

Client and family teaching is necessary to facilitate treatment at home, to prevent the spread of the infestation, and to dispel the myth that lice infest only people with poor hygiene or in dirty living conditions. Specific information includes the following:

- Wash clothing and linens in soap and hot water, or have them dry cleaned.
- Ironing the clothes kills any lice eggs.
- Personal care items, such as combs or brushes, may be boiled to kill the parasites.
- All family members and sexual partners must also be treated.
- Avoid using the combs, brushes, or hats of others.
- Lice and mites may infest anyone.

THE CLIENT WITH A VIRAL INFECTION

Viruses are pathogens that consist of an RNA or DNA core surrounded by a protein coat. They depend on live cells for reproduction and so are classified as intracellular pathogens. The viruses that cause skin lesions invade the keratinocyte, reproduce, and either increase cellular growth or cause cellular death.

An increase in the incidence of viral skin disorders has been attributed to a variety of causes. Some commonly used drugs, such as birth control medications and corticosteroids, are known to have immunosuppressive properties that allow the viruses to multiply. Other drugs, such as antibiotics, kill off normal skin bacteria that would otherwise serve as defense against viral infections.

Pathophysiology

Viral infections cause many different kinds of skin disorders, including warts, herpes simplex infections, and herpes zoster infections.

Warts

Warts, or *verrucae,* are lesions of the skin caused by the human papillomavirus (HPV). More than 60 types of HPVs have been found on the human skin and mucous membranes (Porth, 2005). Warts may be found on nongenital skin or genital skin and mucous membranes. Nongenital warts are benign lesions; genital warts may be precancerous. Warts are transmitted through skin contact. Wart lesions may be flat, fusiform (tapered at both ends), or round, but most are round and raised and have a rough, gray surface. There are many different types of warts; location and appearance of the warts depend on the causative virus. Those most common are as follows:

- A common wart (*verruca vulgaris*) may appear anywhere on the skin and mucous membranes of the body, but it most commonly appears on the fingers. Common warts grow above the skin surface and may be dome shaped with ragged borders (Figure 16–9 ■).
- Plantar warts occur at pressure points on the soles of the feet. The pressure of shoes and walking prevents these warts from growing outward, so they tend to extend deeper beneath the skin surface than do common warts. Plantar warts are often painful.
- A flat wart (*verruca plana*) is a small flat lesion, usually seen on the forehead or dorsum of the hand.
- Condylomata acuminata, also called HPV or venereal warts, occur in moist areas, along the glans of the penis, in the anal region, and on the vulva and cervix. They are usually cauliflower-like in appearance and have a pink or purple color.

Warts resolve spontaneously when immunity to the virus develops. This response may take up to 5 years.

Herpes Simplex

Herpes simplex (also called a *fever blister* or *cold sore*) virus infections of the skin and mucous membranes are caused by two types of herpesvirus: HSV-1 and HSV-2. Most infections above the waist are caused by HSV-1, with herpes simplex lesions most often found on the lips, face, and mouth. (Genital herpes infections, which result from either HSV-1 or HSV-2, are classified as sexually transmitted infections and are discussed in Chapter 52 ∞.) The virus may be transmitted by physical contact, oral sex, or kissing.

The infection begins with a burning or tingling sensation, followed by the development of erythema, vesicle formation, and pain (Figure 16–10 ■). The vesicles progress through pustules, ulcers, and crusting until healing occurs in 10 to 14 days.

Figure 16–9 ■ The common wart, caused by a virus, appears as a raised, dome-shaped lesion.

Figure 16–10 ■ Herpes simplex is a viral infection of the skin and mucous membranes.

The initial infection is often severe and accompanied by systemic manifestations, such as fever and sore throat; recurrences are more localized and less severe. The virus lives in nerve ganglia and may cause recurrent lesions in response to sunlight, menstruation, injury, or stress. Oral acyclovir may be used prophylactically to prevent reoccurrences and to treat recurrent outbreaks.

HERPES ZOSTER **Herpes zoster**, also called *shingles*, is a viral infection of a dermatome section of the skin caused by varicella zoster (the herpesvirus that also causes chickenpox). The infection is believed to result from reactivation of a varicella virus remaining in the sensory dorsal ganglia after a childhood infection of chickenpox. When reactivated, the virus travels from the ganglia to the corresponding skin dermatome area.

Herpes zoster most often affects adults over the age of 60 (Porth, 2005). Clients with Hodgkin's disease, certain types of leukemia, and lymphomas are more susceptible to an outbreak of the disease. Herpes zoster is more prevalent in immunocompromised people, such as those with human immunodeficiency virus (HIV) infections, those receiving radiation therapy or chemotherapy, and those who have had major organ transplants. The appearance of the lesions in people with HIV infections may be one of the first manifestations of immune compromise. The herpes eruption lasts for about 2 to 3 weeks and usually does not recur.

Herpes zoster lesions are vesicles with an erythematous base. The vesicles appear on the skin area supplied by the neurons of a single or associated group of dorsal root ganglia (although they may occur beyond this area in immunosuppressed people). The lesions usually appear unilaterally on the face, trunk, and thorax (Figure 16–11 ■). New lesions continue to erupt for 3 to 5 days, then crust and dry. Recovery occurs in 2 to 3 weeks. The client often experiences severe pain for up to 48 hours before and during eruption of the lesions. The pain may continue for weeks to months after the lesions have disappeared. The older adult is especially sensitive to the pain and often experiences more severe outbreaks of herpes zoster lesions.

Eruption of vesicles over a single dermatome usually only occurs one time. Generalized herpes zoster may indicate an associated immunocompromised disease, such as Hodgkin's disease or HIV infection. Clients infected with HIV are 20 times more likely to develop herpes zoster (McPhee et al., 2007).

Figure 16–11 ■ Herpes zoster is a viral infection of a dermatome section of the skin. The typical lesions are painful vesicles lying along the path of the nerve.
Source: Barts Medical Library/Phototake NYC.

Complications of herpes zoster include postherpetic neuralgia (a sharp, spasmodic pain along the course of one or more nerves) and visual loss. The neuralgia, described as burning or stabbing, results from inflammation of the root ganglia. This complication is more common in clients over the age of 55 (McPhee et al., 2007). Permanent loss of vision may follow occurrence of lesions that arise from the ophthalmic division of the trigeminal nerve. The disease may disseminate in immunocompromised clients, causing lesions beyond the dermatome, visceral lesions, and encephalitis. This serious complication may cause death.

INTERDISCIPLINARY CARE

The treatment for viral skin infections focuses on stopping viral replication and treating client responses, such as itching and pain.

Diagnosis

Although diagnosis is usually based on manifestations and appearance of the lesions, laboratory tests may be necessary to differentiate herpes zoster from impetigo, contact dermatitis, and herpes simplex. The laboratory tests include a Tzanck smear that identifies the herpes virus, but it does not distinguish herpes zoster from herpes simplex. Cultures of fluid from the vesicles and antibody tests are used to make the differential diagnosis of herpesvirus types. HIV testing should be considered if clients are under age 55 with a history of HIV risk factors.

Medications

Most viral skin disorders are treated with antiviral medications, and other types of medications are used to relieve pruritus and pain in clients with herpes zoster.

- *Warts.* Depending on their size, location, and any associated discomfort, warts may be treated with medications, cryotherapy, or electrodesiccation and curettage. A common method of wart removal is acid therapy, using a colloidal solution of 16% salicylic acid and 16% lactic acid. The solution is applied to the wart every 12 to 24 hours; the wart disappears in 2 to 3 weeks. Other methods of eradicating warts are cryosurgery, freezing

with liquid nitrogen, and electrodesiccation of the wart with an electric current followed by excision of the dead tissue. Venereal warts are further described in Chapter 52 ∞.

- *Herpes simplex.* Herpes simplex lesions are treated with topical acyclovir (Zovirax), an antifungal agent. Acyclovir shortens the time of symptoms and speeds healing.
- *Herpes zoster.* Antiviral drugs are used to treat herpes zoster infections. Acyclovir (Zovirax) interferes with viral synthesis and replication. Although it does not cure herpes infections, it does decrease the severity of the illness and also decreases pain. It may be administered topically, orally, or parenterally. It is more effective if administration begins within the first 1 to 2 days after the first vesicles appear. Other antiviral medications include famciclovir (Famvir) and valacyclovir (Valtrex). Nerve blocks may be needed to treat initial pain. Narcotic and nonnarcotic analgesics are prescribed for pain management, and antihistamines may be administered for relief of pruritus. Clients with eye involvement are treated with topical steroid ophthalmic ointments and mydriatics. Antivirals may sometimes be administered.

Zostavax, a shingles vaccine, is available to treat adults age 60 and over. The vaccine has been shown to prevent shingles approximately 50% of the time, thereby reducing incidence of the disease (WebMD, 2006).

 NURSING CARE

Clients with viral skin disorders require nursing care for infection, pruritus, and pain. They also require teaching about preventing the spread of the virus to others. Of the viral disorders, herpes zoster is the most painful and debilitating. See the following page for a Nursing Care Plan for the client with herpes zoster.

Nursing Diagnoses and Interventions

This section discusses care of the client with herpes zoster, focusing on the nursing diagnoses of acute pain, disturbed sleep patterns, and risk for infection.

Acute Pain

The client with herpes zoster often experiences severe pain over the entire dermatome supplied by the affected nerve root. The pain is described as burning, tearing, or stabbing. The client may avoid movement and does not want clothing or bed linens to touch the affected area.

- Monitor the location, duration, and intensity of the pain. *Accurate assessment of the client's perception and tolerance of pain is essential in facilitating pain management.*
- Explain the rationale for taking prescribed medications on a regular schedule. *Delaying medications may allow the pain to reach an intensity at which the medication is less effective in promoting relief.*
- Teach measures to relieve pruritus:
  - Take prescribed antipruritic medications.
  - Apply calamine lotion or wet compresses, if prescribed.
  - Keep the room temperature cool.
  - Use a bed cradle to keep sheets off affected areas of the body.
Pruritus is a common problem for clients with herpes zoster; scratching may excoriate the skin and increase the risk for

NURSING CARE PLAN A Client with Herpes Zoster

Jesus Rivera is a 34-year-old migrant farm worker who currently lives in temporary housing in a rural area of the southwestern United States. His family includes his wife, Marta, who is 3 months' pregnant, and two children, ages 3 and 5. He takes his wife to a medical clinic staffed by volunteer nurses, physicians, and students from a nearby university for a prenatal checkup. The clinic is open only on Saturday and provides care on a sliding fee scale or for free if the family is unable to pay. While Mrs. Rivera is being examined, Mr. Rivera asks the nurse to have someone look at some very painful blisters on his chest that developed about a week ago. He is afraid that exposure to pesticides has caused the sores.

ASSESSMENT

Mr. Rivera speaks Spanish and is able to communicate only slightly in English. The initial assessment of Mr. Rivera is performed by Anita Mendez, a student nurse fluent in Spanish. Mr. Rivera's history reveals problems with lower back pain but no significant past medical illnesses. He is not aware of any allergies and cannot remember having had chickenpox as a child. Two years ago, both children were sick and had blisters on their bodies, and a friend told them it was chickenpox. Mrs. Rivera thinks she had chickenpox as a child.

Because Mr. Rivera has not had any medical care for several years, baseline laboratory tests are ordered to screen for any other illnesses. The complete blood count (CBC), blood chemistry, and urinalysis are all within normal limits.

Mr. Rivera says that he did not feel well for several days before the blisters appeared, having experienced chills and general achiness. He had not taken his temperature because the family does not own a thermometer. Current vital signs are as follows: T 99°F (37.2°C), P 74, R 22, and BP 148/88.

Physical examination of the trunk reveals a bandlike pattern of lesions across the left thorax. Some of the lesions are vesicles filled with serous fluid; others are darker in color and are oozing a light yellow drainage. The skin around the lesions is red and inflamed. Mr. Rivera complains of a severe, burning pain with itching across his chest. He is diagnosed with herpes zoster.

DIAGNOSES

- *Risk for Infection* related to open oozing areas on the left thorax
- *Acute Pain* related to the presence of lesions and pruritus
- *Deficient Knowledge* of the cause of the skin disorder and recommended treatment
- *Anxiety* related to need to work in areas of pesticide application
- *Impaired Health Maintenance* related to limited access to health care due to transitory work conditions, and cultural and language barriers

EXPECTED OUTCOMES

- Skin lesions will heal without evidence of a secondary infection.
- Limit exposure (as much as possible) to his wife and children and to persons with debilitating illnesses to prevent the spread of the virus.
- Obtain relief of pain and pruritus with the proper use of medications.
- Verbalize an understanding of the disease process and participate in the treatment plan.

- Obtain follow-up care.
- Make an appointment for a referral for information about occupational hazards.

PLANNING AND IMPLEMENTATION

- Provide verbal and written instructions (in Spanish) for self-care:
  - Wear a clean cotton undershirt each day.
  - Trim the fingernails short, and keep the hands clean.
  - Wash the hands each time the area is touched.
  - Wash any soiled clothes or linens in hot water and soap.
  - Do not allow other family members to use your towels.
  - Take medications as prescribed for itching and pain.
  - Take the medicine for your sores every 4 hours, even during nighttime hours, for 7 days.
  - As much as possible, do not touch your wife and children until the sores are covered with scabs. Do not have sex with your wife while you have these sores.
- Teach how to take care of skin lesions:
  - Wear disposable gloves every time you do this treatment.
  - Wash the sores and the skin around them very gently with a soft washcloth and a mild soap.
  - Using your fingers, carefully rub the cream on the sores. Do this once every morning after breakfast and once every evening after supper.
  - Wash your hands carefully before and after each treatment.
- Make a follow-up appointment for the next week.
- Provide Mr. Rivera with the name and phone number of the Occupational Safety and Health Administration (OSHA) and recommend he call for an appointment to discuss his concerns about pesticides.

EVALUATION

Mrs. Rivera explains how she has taken care of her husband, and Mr. Rivera is careful to describe how he has followed the nurse's instructions. The skin lesions are dry and crusty, with no new blister formation. Mr. Rivera says he has not called OSHA and is not sure that he will, but he thanks Miss Mendez for the phone number. The nurses make an appointment in 1 month for a prenatal checkup for Mrs. Rivera and for follow-up of Mr. Rivera's herpes zoster. Mr. Rivera promises to return if they are still living close enough to keep the appointment.

CRITICAL THINKING IN THE NURSING PROCESS

1. Identify barriers to care present in this case study. How may nursing interventions promote healthcare delivery to disadvantaged populations?
2. Although most cases of herpes zoster are self-limiting, what further assessments and interventions might have been indicated had the lesions shown little improvement over time and/or the pain remained severe?
3. If Mr. Rivera is advised not to work until his lesions heal, the family may face economic and sociocultural hardships. Develop a plan of care for Mr. Rivera for the nursing diagnosis *Ineffective Role Performance.*

See *Evaluating Your Response* in Appendix C.

secondary infections. Pruritus may intensify the experience of pain. Lotions and cool, wet compresses are effective in decreasing the itch–scratch–itch cycle. Warmth and touch intensify pruritus.

■ Encourage the use of distraction (such as music) or a specific relaxation technique (such as progressive muscle relaxation or deep breathing). *Noninvasive methods to relieve pain not only help the client manage the pain experience but also increase the effectiveness of pain medications.*

Disturbed Sleep Pattern

The pain and pruritus of herpes zoster interfere with normal sleep patterns. Those responses often are more intense at night, probably as a result of decreased distraction.

■ Use appropriate measures to relieve pain and pruritus. *Pain and pruritus interfere with normal sleep. Analgesics and noninvasive methods of relief may be necessary before the client prepares for sleep.*

■ Maintain a cool environment and avoid heavy bed covering. *Heat and touch intensify pruritus. Pruritus stimulates scratching, which awakens the client. The client may then perceive the pain more acutely. A cycle is established that interferes with sleep.*

Risk for Infection

Clients with herpes zoster have impaired skin integrity and pruritus with scratching and possible excoriation; moreover, they may be immunocompromised. All of these factors contribute to a high risk for secondary bacterial infection. In addition, the client is contagious to others who did not have chickenpox as children.

■ Teach client the manifestations of infection:
  ■ Increased temperature
  ■ Increased redness, formation of pustules, and/or purulent drainage
■ Monitor white blood cell count
■ Assess lymph glands.
  Secondary bacterial infections may occur in any client with impaired skin integrity; if the client is immunocompromised, the risk is even greater. Fever, changes in lesions or drainage, an increased white blood cell count, and lymph gland enlargement are manifestations of an infection.

■ Teach interventions to decrease the itch–scratch–itch cycle, thereby decreasing the possibility of excoriation (see discussion about nursing care of clients with pruritus and psoriasis, earlier in this chapter). *Excoriation from scratching provides an avenue for bacterial invasion.*

■ Institute infection control procedures for clients who are hospitalized:
  ■ Maintain strict isolation for immunocompromised clients.
  ■ Wear gloves and gown if contact with lesions is likely.
  ■ Instruct pregnant women to avoid exposure until lesions have crusted over.
  Isolation procedures are instituted for the immunocompromised client to prevent client infection. Wear gloves and gown to prevent spreading the infection to self or others.

PRACTICE ALERT
Pregnant women must avoid exposure to people with herpes zoster because the herpesvirus can cross the placental barrier.

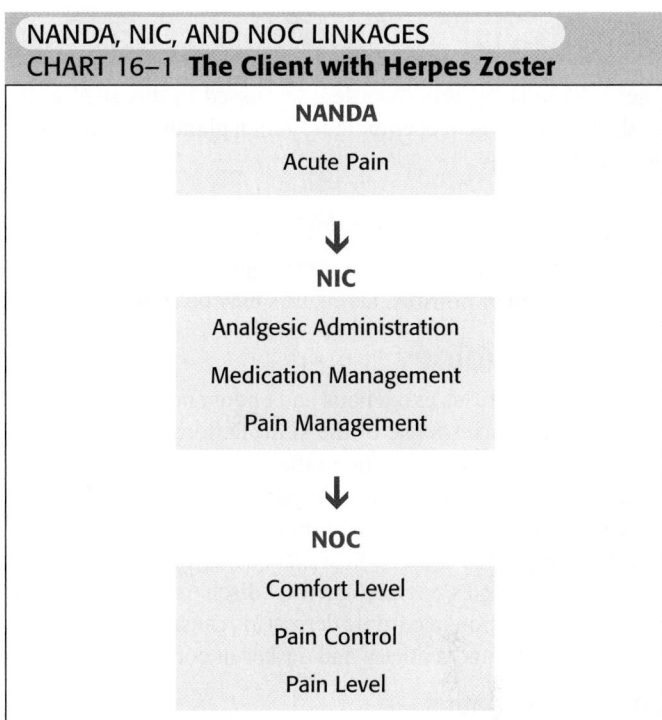

NANDA, NIC, AND NOC LINKAGES
CHART 16–1 The Client with Herpes Zoster

NANDA

Acute Pain

↓

NIC

Analgesic Administration

Medication Management

Pain Management

↓

NOC

Comfort Level

Pain Control

Pain Level

Data from *NANDA's Nursing Diagnoses: Definitions & Classification 2005–2006* by NANDA International (2005), Philadelphia; *Nursing Interventions Classification (NIC)* (4th ed.) by J. M. Dochterman & G. M. Bulechek (2004), St. Louis, MO: Mosby; and *Nursing Outcomes Classification (NOC)* (3rd ed.) by S. Moorhead, M. Johnson, and M. Maas (2004), St. Louis, MO: Mosby.

Using NANDA, NIC, and NOC

Chart 16–1 shows links between NANDA, NIC, and NOC when caring for the client with herpes zoster.

Community-Based Care

Because most clients with viral infections provide self-care at home, the nurse focuses on teaching the client and family how to provide the necessary care. With herpes zoster increasing in incidence in clients who are older or have a serious chronic illness, it may also be necessary to make a referral to a community health provider for continued support. Provide the following information and instructions:

■ The diseases are usually self-limiting and heal completely. Second occurrences of herpes zoster are rare.

■ Do not have social contact with children or pregnant women until crusts have formed over the blistered areas with herpes zoster, because the disease is contagious to people who have not had chickenpox.

■ Use pain medications regularly.

■ Follow suggestions to help reduce itching, scratching, and pain: Use medications as prescribed, wear lightweight cotton clothing, keep room temperatures cool, wear cotton gloves at night if scratching is a problem, and practice relaxation and distraction activities.

■ Report any increase in pain, fever, chills, drainage that smells bad and has pus, or a spread in the blisters to your healthcare provider.

INFLAMMATORY DISORDERS OF THE SKIN

The inflammatory skin disorders discussed in this section include dermatitis, acne, pemphigus, lichen planus, and toxic epidermal necrolysis.

THE CLIENT WITH DERMATITIS

Dermatitis is an inflammation of the skin characterized by erythema and pain or pruritus. Dermatitis may be acute or chronic.

Pathophysiology

In dermatitis, various exogenous and endogenous agents cause an inflammatory response of the skin. Different types of skin eruptions occur, often specific to the causative allergen, infection, or disease. The initial skin responses to these agents or illnesses include erythema, formation of vesicles and scales, and pruritus (Figure 16–12 ■). Subsequently, irritation from scratching promotes edema, a serous discharge, and crusting. Long-term irritation in chronic dermatitis causes the skin to become thickened and leathery and darker in color.

Contact Dermatitis

Contact dermatitis is a type of dermatitis caused by a hypersensitivity response or chemical irritation. The major sources known to cause contact dermatitis are dyes, perfumes, poison plants (ivy, oak, sumac), chemicals, and metals (Box 16–3). A contact dermatitis common in the healthcare field is latex (glove) dermatitis.

Figure 16–12 ■ Dermatitis may be a response to allergens, infections, or chemicals. This client has contact dermatitis resulting from the metal salts in a ring.
Source: Biophoto Associates/Photo Researchers, Inc.

Irritant contact dermatitis is an inflammation of the skin from irritants; it is not a hypersensitivity response. Common sources of irritant contact dermatitis include chemicals (such as acids), soaps, and detergents. The skin lesions are similar to those seen in allergic contact dermatitis.

Atopic Dermatitis

Atopic dermatitis is an inflammatory skin disorder that is also called *eczema*. The exact cause is unknown, but related factors include depressed cell-mediated immunity, elevated IgE levels, and increased histamine sensitivity. The disorder is seen more often in children, but chronic forms persist throughout life.

Clients with atopic dermatitis have a family history of hypersensitivity reactions, such as dry skin, eczema, asthma, and allergic rhinitis. Although up to one-third of clients with atopic dermatitis also have food allergies, a positive correlation has not been found.

The dermatitis results when mast cells, T lymphocytes, monocytes, and other inflammatory cells are activated and release histamine, lymphokines, and other inflammatory media-

FAST FACTS

Latex Allergy
■ The increased use of latex gloves among healthcare providers has resulted in increased reporting of latex allergies. It is estimated that 10% to 17% of healthcare providers are allergic to latex (Porth, 2005).
■ The most common type of allergic response to latex gloves is type IV, T-cell-mediated contact dermatitis.
■ Type I, IgE-mediated hypersensitivity, manifested by urticaria, rhinoconjunctivitis, asthma, or anaphylaxis, is far more serious than the T-cell-mediated type.
■ All clients with a latex allergy should be treated in a latex-free environment.
■ Healthcare providers with severe allergic responses to latex may have to seek a different type of employment.

Allergic contact dermatitis is a cell-mediated or delayed hypersensitivity to a wide variety of allergens. Sensitizing antigens include microorganisms, plants, chemicals, drugs, metals, or foreign proteins. On initial contact with the skin, the allergen binds to a carrier protein, forming a sensitizing antigen. The antigen is processed and carried to the T cells, which in turn become sensitized to the antigen. The first exposure is the sensitizing contact and the person does not experience manifestations, which then occur with subsequent exposures. The manifestations include erythema, swelling, and pruritic vesicles in the area of allergen contact. For example, a person hypersensitive to metal may have lesions under a ring or watch.

BOX 16–3 Common Causes of Contact Dermatitis

■ Acids
■ Alkalis: soaps, detergents, household ammonia, lye, cleaners
■ Bromide
■ Chlorine
■ Cosmetics: perfumes, dyes, oils
■ Dusts of lime, arsenic, wood
■ Hydrocarbons: crude petroleum, lubricating oil, mineral oil, paraffin, asphalt, tar

■ Iodine
■ Insecticides
■ Fabrics: wool, polyester, dyes, sizing
■ Metal salts: calcium chloride, zinc chloride, copper, mercury, nickel, silver
■ Plants: ragweed, poison oak, poison sumac, poison ivy, pine
■ Coloring agents
■ Rubber products
■ Soot

tors. The immune response interacts with the allergen to create a chronic inflammatory condition. In the adult form of atopic dermatitis, characteristic lesions include chronic lichenification, erythema, and scaling, the result of pruritus and scratching. The lesions are usually found on the hands, feet, or flexor surfaces of the arms and legs (Figure 16–13 ■). Scratching and excoriation increase the risk of secondary infections, as well as invasion of the skin by viruses such as herpes simplex. Serum studies may find elevated eosinophil and IgE levels.

Seborrheic Dermatitis

Seborrheic dermatitis is a chronic inflammatory disorder of the skin that involves the scalp, eyebrows, eyelids, ear canals, nasolabial folds, axillae, and trunk. The cause is unknown. This disorder is seen in all ages, from the very young (called "cradle cap") to the very old. Clients taking methyldopa (Aldomet) for hypertension occasionally develop this disorder, and it is a component of Parkinson's disease. Seborrheic dermatitis is also frequently seen in clients with AIDS.

The lesions are yellow or white plaques with scales and crusts. The scales are often yellow or orange and have a greasy appearance. Mild pruritus is also present. Diffuse dandruff with erythema of the scalp often accompanies the skin lesions.

Exfoliative Dermatitis

Exfoliative dermatitis is an inflammatory skin disorder characterized by excessive peeling or shedding of skin. The cause is unknown in about half of all cases, but a preexisting skin disorder (such as psoriasis, atopic dermatitis, contact dermatitis, or seborrheic dermatitis) is found in a majority of the cases (McPhee et al., 2007). Reactions to medications, such as sulfonamides, account for 20% to 40% of cases. Certain cancers (such as lymphoma) may also cause exfoliative dermatitis.

Both systemic and localized manifestations may appear. Systemic manifestations include weakness, malaise, fever, chills, and weight loss. Scaling, erythema, and pruritus may be localized or involve the entire body. In addition to peeling of skin, the client may lose the hair and nails. Generalized exfoliative dermatitis may cause debility and dehydration. The impairment of skin integrity increases the risk for local and systemic infections.

Figure 16–13 ■ Atopic dermatitis, or eczema, causes pruritus, resulting in lichenification, erythema, and scaling.
Source: NMSB/Custom Medical Stock Photo.

INTERDISCIPLINARY CARE

The client with dermatitis is treated primarily with topical medications and therapeutic baths. If the dermatitis is due to hypersensitivity to an allergen, the client avoids exposure to environmental irritants and suspected foods. The client also discontinues as many medications as possible to determine whether the dermatitis is the result of a drug allergy.

Diagnosis

The diagnosis is often based on the manifestations of the disorder, and on a history of exposure to a known allergen. Scratch tests and intradermal tests are used to identify a specific allergen.

Medications

The medications used depend on the cause of the dermatitis and the severity of the manifestations. Minor cases are treated with antipruritic medications, whereas more severe cases are treated with oral antihistamines, oral and/or topical corticosteroids, and wet dressings. Topical anti-infectives may be prescribed if necessary.

NURSING CARE

Nursing care of the client with dermatitis focuses primarily on providing information for self-care at home. The client is responsible for managing skin problems and requires education and support. Address the following topics:

■ Medications and treatments do not cure the disease; they only relieve the symptoms.
■ Dry skin increases pruritus, which stimulates scratching. Scratching may in turn cause excoriation, and excoriation increases the risk of infection.
■ It may be necessary to change the diet or environment to avoid contact with allergens.
■ When using steroid preparations, apply only a thin layer to slightly damp skin (e.g., after taking a bath).
■ If occlusive dressings are necessary, a plastic suit may be used.
■ When using oral corticosteroids, never abruptly stop taking the medication. Rather, follow instructions to taper the dosage gradually.
■ Antihistamines cause drowsiness. When using these medications, avoid alcohol and use caution when driving or working around machinery.

THE CLIENT WITH ACNE

Acne is a disorder of the pilosebaceous (hair and sebaceous gland) structure, which opens to the skin surface through a pore. The sebaceous glands, which empty directly into the hair follicle, produce sebum, a lipid substance. Sebaceous glands are present over the entire skin surface except the soles of the feet and the palms of the hands, but the largest glands are on the face, scalp, and scrotum. Sebum production is a response to direct hormonal stimulation by testicular androgens in men and adrenal and ovarian androgens in women.

Pathophysiology

Acne may be noninflammatory or inflammatory. Noninflammatory acne lesions are primarily **comedones**, more commonly called pimples, whiteheads, and blackheads. Whiteheads are pale, slightly elevated papules categorized as closed comedones. Blackheads are plugs of material that accumulate in the sebaceous glands. They are categorized as open comedones. The color is the result of the movement of melanin into the plug from surrounding epidermal cells. Inflammatory acne lesions include comedones, erythematous pustules, and cysts (Figure 16–14 ■). Inflammation close to the skin surface results in pustules; deeper inflammation results in cysts. The inflammation is believed to result from irritation from fatty acid constituents of the sebum and from substances produced by *Propionibacterium acnes* bacteria, both of which escape into the dermis when the follicular walls of closed comedones rupture.

Several forms of acne occur at different periods of the life span. The most common are acne vulgaris, acne rosacea, and acne conglobata.

Acne Vulgaris

Acne vulgaris is the form of acne common in adolescents and young to middle adults. The actual cause of acne vulgaris is unknown. Possible causes include androgenic influence on the sebaceous glands, increased sebum production, and proliferation of the organism *Propionibacterium acnes*. Many factors once thought to cause acne vulgaris, including high-fat diets, chocolate, infections, and cosmetics, have been disproved (Porth, 2005).

FAST FACTS
Acne Vulgaris
- Acne vulgaris is the most common of all skin conditions.
- Twelve percent of women and 3% of men over the age of 25 have acne vulgaris, and the rate does not begin to decrease until after age 44 (McPhee et al., 2007). Scarring may be a sequela of the disease, or may result from picking and manipulating the comedones by the client.

Mild cases may involve only a few scattered comedones, but severe cases are manifested by multiple lesions of all types. Most acne vulgaris lesions form on the face and neck, but they also occur on the back, chest, and shoulders. Women in their 30s and 40s, often with no prior acne, may develop papular le-

Figure 16–14 ■ Acne vulgaris lesions include comedones, erythematous pustules, and cysts.
Source: St. Bartholomew's Hospital/Photo Researchers, Inc.

sions on the chin and around the mouth. The lesions are usually mildly painful and may itch. The complications of acne vulgaris, especially in severe cases, are formation of cysts, pigment changes in persons with dark skin, severe scarring, and lowered self-concept from the skin eruptions.

Acne Rosacea

Acne rosacea is a chronic type of facial acne that occurs more often in middle and older adults. The cause is unknown. The lesions of acne rosacea begin with erythema over the cheeks and nose. Other skin lesions may appear. Over years of time, the skin color changes to dark red, and the pores over the area become enlarged. The soft tissue of the nose may exhibit rhinophyma, an irregular bullous thickening.

Acne Conglobata

Acne conglobata is a chronic type of acne of unknown cause that begins in middle adulthood. This type causes serious skin lesions. Comedones, papules, pustules, nodules, cysts, and scars occur primarily on the back, buttocks, and chest but may occur on other body surfaces. The comedones have multiple openings and a discharge that ranges from serous to purulent with a foul odor.

INTERDISCIPLINARY CARE

The management of acne is similar, regardless of type. Because acne vulgaris is most common, the discussions of interdisciplinary and nursing care focus on that type. Treatment is based on the type and severity of the lesions.

Diagnosis

The disease is diagnosed by the typical location and appearance of lesions. If the client has pustules, a culture of the drainage is performed to differentiate viral or bacterial dermatitis from acne.

Medications

The treatment of acne is tailored to the individual and is based on the severity of the lesions. For acne with comedones, tretinoin (retinoic acid, Retin-A) or benzoyl peroxide preparations are prescribed. Azelaic acid (Azelex) may also be used. The administration of these vitamin A analogues is discussed in the Medication Administration box on the following page. Benzoyl peroxide preparations are found in OTC medications such as Fostex, Acne-Dome, Desquam-X, Benzagel, Clear By Design, and Xerac BP. These products are keratolytic and loosen the comedones.

Mild forms of papular inflammatory acne are treated with topical clindamycin (Cleocin T), a bacteriostatic agent that decreases the amount of fatty acids on the skin surface. This medication may be combined with tretinoin therapy.

Moderate forms of papular inflammatory acne are treated with oral or topical antibiotics, such as tetracycline, erythromycin, and minocycline. These antiacne antibiotics are administered for 3 to 4 months; if the client's skin is clear, the dose is lowered gradually to a maintenance dose that will maintain clear skin.

Severe forms of papular inflammatory acne are treated with isotretinoin (Accutane). This drug is effective, but has serious side effects. Isotretinoin, with nursing responsibilities, is discussed in the Medication Administration box on the next page.

MEDICATION ADMINISTRATION Acne Medications

ANTIACNE RETINOIDS
Tretinoin (Retin-A)   Isotretinoin (Accutane)

Tretinoin is a vitamin A derivative classified as an acne agent. This topical agent acts as an irritant to decrease cohesiveness of follicular epithelial cells, thereby decreasing comedone formation while increasing the extrusion of comedones from the skin surface.

Isotretinoin is a vitamin A analogue classified as an acne product. It reduces the size of sebaceous glands, inhibits sebaceous gland differentiation to decrease sebum production, and alters sebum lipid composition.

Nursing Responsibilities
- Administer tretinoin with caution to pregnant women, because the effects of absorption on the developing fetus are not clearly defined.
- Isotretinoin is absolutely contraindicated for pregnant women or for women who want to become pregnant. The medication poses a high risk of major deformities in the infant if pregnancy occurs during use, even use that continues only for short periods.
- Do not administer to clients with eczema or to those who are hypersensitive to the sun.

Health Education for the Client and Family
Tretinoin
- Use the cream in a test area twice at night to test for sensitivity; if no reaction occurs, increase applications gradually to the prescribed frequency.
- A pea-sized amount of the cream is enough to cover the entire face.
- Apply the cream to clean, dry skin.
- Do not apply the cream to the eyes, mouth, angles of the nose, or mucous membranes.
- Wash your face no more than two to three times a day, using a mild soap. Do not use skin preparations (such as aftershave lotion or perfumes) that contain alcohol, menthol, spice, or lime; they may irritate your skin.
- The medication may cause a temporary stinging or warm sensation but should not cause pain.
- The skin where you apply the cream will be mildly red and may peel; if you experience a more severe reaction, consult your healthcare provider.
- The medication may cause increased sensitivity to sunlight, use sunscreens and wear protective clothing when outdoors.
- Your acne may become worse during the first 2 weeks of treatment; this is an expected response.

Isotretinoin
- Take the pills with food.
- Your acne may become worse during the initial period of treatment; this is an expected response.
- The medication causes dryness of the eyes, so you may have trouble wearing contact lenses during and after treatment.
- Do not take vitamin A supplements; they will increase the effects of the medication.
- Avoid prolonged exposure to sunlight; use sunscreen and protective clothing when in the sun.
- Notify the physician at once if you have abdominal pain, severe diarrhea, rectal bleeding, headache, nausea or vomiting, or visual disturbances.
- Do not drink alcohol while taking this medication (it causes an increase in triglycerides).
- Night vision may become worse; use caution when driving at night.
- Do not donate blood while, or for 1 month after, taking this medication.
- (For *female clients*) You must use two reliable forms of contraception simultaneously for at least 1 month before, during, and at least 1 month after therapy with this medication. The medication may cause deformities in a baby conceived at this time.

Treatments

Acne scars may alter the individual's self-concept. They may be removed by dermabrasion and laser treatment. Dermabrasion of inactive acne lesions can improve the client's appearance, especially if the scars are flat. (Dermabrasion is discussed in greater detail later in this chapter.) Laser excision of deep scars may also be performed.

NURSING CARE

Nursing care is individualized to the client's developmental needs and is conducted primarily through teaching in clinics or the home setting. Regardless of the client's age or gender, it is important to remember that almost all clients with acne are embarrassed by and self-conscious of their appearance. Prior to teaching, establish rapport with the client and clarify beliefs; for example, the client may believe the lesions result from poor hygiene, masturbation, use of cosmetics, eating the wrong types of foods, or lack of sexual activity. It is critical to teach the client about the causes of and factors involved in acne prior to teaching self-care.

The teaching plan for the client with acne includes general guidelines for skin care and health as well as specific guidelines for care of the acne lesions. The following topics should be addressed:
- Wash the skin with a mild soap and water at least twice a day to remove accumulated oils.
- Shampoo the hair often enough to prevent oiliness.
- Eat a regular, well-balanced diet. Foods do not cause or increase acne.
- Expose the skin to sunlight, but avoid sunburn.
- Get regular exercise and sleep.
- Try to avoid putting your hands on your face.
- Do not squeeze a pimple. Squeezing forces the material of the pimple deeper into the skin and may cause the pimple to become larger and infected.
- The treatment for acne lasts months, in some cases for the rest of one's life. It is very important to take the medications each day for the prescribed length of time.

THE CLIENT WITH PEMPHIGUS VULGARIS

Pemphigus vulgaris is a chronic disorder of the skin and oral mucous membranes characterized by blister formation. The disease is caused by autoantibodies that cause acantholysis (the separation of epidermal cells from one another). The disorder is associated with IgG antibodies and HLA-A10 antigen. Septicemia from an infection of *Staphylococcus aureus* is the most common cause of death.

The disease occurs in middle and older adults of all races and ethnic backgrounds. The disorder has been associated with other autoimmune disorders and with the administration of certain drugs, such as penicillamine and captopril.

The blisters that form in pemphigus vulgaris usually appear first in the mouth and scalp and then spread in crops or waves to involve large areas of the body, including the face, back, chest, umbilicus, and groin. Blisters in the mouth ulcerate. The blisters form in the epidermis and cause the epidermal cells to separate above the basal layer. These blisters rupture, leaving denuded skin, crusting, and oozing of fluid with a musty odor. The lesions are painful. Pressure on a blister causes it to spread to adjacent skin (Nikolsky's sign). The loss of fluid from the blisters may result in fluid and electrolyte imbalances. Secondary bacterial infections are a serious risk.

INTERDISCIPLINARY CARE

The goals of treatment are to control the severity of the disease, to prevent infection and loss of fluids, and to promote healing. Clients who experience severe attacks or secondary infections are usually hospitalized. Although the disease cannot be cured, the manifestations can be controlled.

Diagnosis

Pemphigus vulgaris is diagnosed by clinical manifestations and laboratory and diagnostic tests, including immunofluorescence microscopy, which is done to identify the presence of IgG antibodies in the epidermis and serum, and skin biopsy to determine the presence of acantholysis.

Medications

Early lesions are treated with highly potent topical corticosteroids. As the disease becomes more severe, systemic corticosteroids or immunosuppressive agents (such as azathioprine or methotrexate) are prescribed. Secondary infections are treated with topical and/or systemic antibiotics.

Treatments

Plasmapheresis is occasionally used to treat pemphigus. In this procedure, the plasma is selectively removed from whole blood and reinfused into the client. This decreases the serum level of antibodies for a period of time. Plasmapheresis with related nursing care is discussed in Chapter 46 .

NURSING CARE

The hospitalized client with pemphigus requires careful assessment of skin lesions and monitoring for manifestations of infection. Provide skin care through bathing and applying dressings to denuded areas, using aseptic technique to prevent infection. The client may be placed on reverse isolation as a protective measure. Monitor the client's hydration status to prevent fluid volume deficit and incorporate pain medications and noninvasive pain management techniques in the plan of care. Oral lesions often make eating difficult; the client requires meticulous oral hygiene and nonirritating foods. The client often is depressed and fearful; establishing a therapeutic relationship is essential, and referrals for counseling may be necessary.

Teaching the client and family how to provide care at home also involves skin care, oral care, diet, pain management, and prevention of infection. In addition, the nurse teaches the client and family how to take prescribed medications. A referral to a home health agency or local health department may be necessary.

THE CLIENT WITH LICHEN PLANUS

Lichen planus is an inflammatory disorder of the mucous membranes and skin. It has no known cause but has been associated with exposure to drugs or to film processing chemicals. The disease affects adults from 30 to 70 years of age.

The lesions first appear as violet papules, 2 to 10 mm in size, commonly occurring on the wrists, ankles, lower legs, and genitals. The lesions itch intensely. Over time, persistent lesions thicken and become dark red, forming hypertrophic lichen planus. Lesions on the oral mucous membranes appear as white lacy rings; lesions may also appear on the mucous membranes of the vagina and the penis. The nails become thin and may shed.

Lichen planus lesions are self-limiting but last for an average of 12 to 18 months. The disorder is diagnosed by clinical manifestations. Corticosteroids are used to control the inflammation, and antihistamines are used to control the pruritus.

THE CLIENT WITH TOXIC EPIDERMAL NECROLYSIS

Toxic epidermal necrolysis (TEN) is a rare, life-threatening disease in which the epidermis peels off the dermis in sheets, leaving large areas of denuded skin. Conjunctivitis and mucositis of the mouth, upper airway, esophagus, and sometimes the genitourinary tract are often associated with TEN. The client usually requires critical care, often in a burn center. The incidence of TEN has not been documented, but it is seen more often in men and in people of African descent. The mortality rate is decreasing because of current methods of care. The cause of death is almost always sepsis.

Pathophysiology

Although some cases have no known cause, most cases result from a drug reaction, and others are associated with a serious concomitant illness, such as cancer or AIDS. Drugs that have been associated with TEN are the sulfonamides, barbiturates, NSAIDs, phenytoin, allopurinol, and penicillin.

The pathophysiologic process in TEN is not completely understood, but the triggering mechanism is believed to be a hypersensitivity or immune response. TEN begins with a painful, localized erythema of the face and extremities, accompanied by fever, chills, muscle aches, and generalized malaise. A macular rash develops, followed by the formation of large, flaccid blisters over the body surface during the next 24 to 96 hours. The skin begins to slough, leaving the dermal surface exposed. Even in areas without blistering, the skin may peel off in layers. The skin sloughing continues over several days and can expose 95% or more of the dermal surface. Other manifestations include conjunctivitis, pharyngitis, stomatitis, and enlargement of lymph glands. Urethral slough is common, causing such painful voiding that the client voluntarily retains urine. The client is often disoriented, may be nearly comatose, and is seriously ill.

Complications

The loss of skin leads to fluid and electrolyte imbalances and secondary infections, as well as systemic effects on all other body systems. These complications may cause death. However, if the complications can be prevented, healing by epidermal regeneration occurs in about a month. The long-term complications of TEN include blindness, lacrimal duct occlusion, scarring and contractures, loss of nails, esophageal strictures, and glomerulonephritis.

INTERDISCIPLINARY CARE

The client is hospitalized and requires rapid diagnosis and treatment. Any medication in use by the client is stopped immediately. Interdisciplinary care involves fluid replacement, correction of electrolyte imbalances, prevention or management of infection, and pain control. The interdisciplinary and nursing care are essentially the same as for the client with burns, discussed in Chapter 17 ∞.

MALIGNANT SKIN DISORDERS

The skin is a common site for malignant lesions. Many of these lesions are found on skin surfaces that have undergone long-term exposure to the sun or the environment. Malignant skin tumors are the most common of all cancers.

THE CLIENT WITH ACTINIC KERATOSIS

Actinic keratosis, also called senile or solar keratosis, is an epidermal skin lesion directly related to chronic sun exposure and photodamage. The prevalence is highest in people with light-colored skin; these lesions are rare in people with dark skin. Actinic keratosis may progress to squamous cell carcinoma. Fewer than 1% of early lesions become malignant, but many of those that persist progress to malignancy (Porth, 2005). Because of this tendency, the lesions are classified as premalignant.

The lesions are erythematous rough macules a few millimeters in diameter. They are often shiny but may be scaly; if the scales are removed, the underlying skin bleeds. They occur in multiple patches, primarily on the face, dorsa of the hands, the forearms, and sometimes on the upper trunk (Figure 16–15 ■). Enlargement or ulceration of the lesions suggests transformation to malignancy.

THE CLIENT WITH NONMELANOMA SKIN CANCER

The skin, despite its ability to protect the internal body from external damage, is a fragile organ and is subject to damage from ultraviolet radiation and chemicals. Over time, this damage results in alterations in cellular structure and function, and malignancies of the skin occur. The nonmelanoma skin cancers are basal cell cancer and squamous cell cancer.

Incidence

Nonmelanoma skin cancer is the most common malignant neoplasm found in fair-skinned Americans. The American Cancer Society estimates that more than 1 million new cases of nonmelanoma skin cancer occur in the United States each year. Of that number 95% to 99% can be cured if detected and treated early. Men develop nonmelanoma skin cancer more often than do women, probably because of occupational exposures. Although nonmelanoma skin cancer can occur at any age, the incidence increases with each decade of life. Adults between the ages of 30 and 60 have the majority of these cancers.

Figure 16–15 ■ The effects of long-term sun exposure are illustrated in this epidermal skin lesion, called actinic keratosis.
Source: Medical-On-Line Ltd.

Risk Factors

Multiple etiologic factors are involved in the development of nonmelanoma skin cancer, including environmental factors and host factors.

FAST FACTS
Risk Factors for Nonmelanoma Skin Cancer
- Fair skin, freckles, blue or green eyes, and blond or red hair
- Family history of skin cancer
- Unprotected and/or excessive exposure to UV radiation (natural or artificial)
- Radiation treatment
- Occupational exposures to coal, tar, pitch, creosote, arsenic compounds, or radium
- Severe sunburns as a child

Environmental Factors

The environmental factors implicated in the nonmelanoma skin cancers are ultraviolet radiation, pollutants, chemicals, ionizing radiation, viruses, and physical trauma.

Ultraviolet radiation (UVR) from the sun is believed to be the cause of most nonmelanoma skin cancers. Sunlight contains both short-length rays (UVB) and long-length rays (UVA). UVB rays are absorbed by the top layer of skin and cause sunburn. UVA rays penetrate deeper into the skin layers, causing tissue damage. Both types of rays are believed to cause DNA alterations and also suppress T-cell and B-cell immunity. The amount of UVR reaching the earth is increasing, most likely from depletion of the ozone layer surrounding the planet. The U.S. Environmental Protection Agency predicts that for every 1% decrease in the ozone layer, a corresponding 1% to 3% increase in nonmelanoma skin cancer per year will occur.

Geographic, environmental, and lifestyle factors affect the amount of exposure to the sun and the risk for nonmelanoma skin cancer. People who live in latitudes close to the equator and those who live at higher altitudes receive greater ultraviolet radiation exposure. The amount of clothing worn, the time of day, and the amount of time in the sun also determine the amount of exposure. Exposure to ultraviolet radiation in tanning booths has also been implicated in the development of nonmelanoma skin cancer.

Certain chemicals have long been associated with nonmelanoma skin cancer. Polycyclic aromatic hydrocarbons, found in mixtures of coal, tar, asphalt, soot, and mineral oils, have been linked with skin cancers. Psoralens, used in conjunction with UVA for treatment of psoriasis and cutaneous T-cell lymphoma, increase the risk of squamous cell cancer.

Other factors associated with nonmelanoma skin cancer are the use of ionizing radiation, viruses, and physical trauma. X-ray therapy for tinea capitis and the use of radium to treat other malignancies are risk factors. Human papillomavirus is implicated in the development of squamous cell cancer, as is damage to the skin from burns.

Host Factors

Certain host factors increase the risk of nonmelanoma skin cancer. These include skin pigmentation as well as the presence of premalignant lesions.

Skin pigmentation is an important factor in the development of nonmelanoma skin cancer. The amount of melanin pigment produced by the melanocytes determines a person's skin color. The more melanin, the more the skin is protected from the damage produced by ultraviolet rays. Thus, African Americans, Asian Americans, and people of Mediterranean descent have a much lower incidence of nonmelanoma skin cancer than do people who have fair complexions and tend to freckle or sunburn easily, such as people of Irish, Scandinavian, or English ancestry.

Although most people have numerous pigmented lesions on their body, almost all of these are normal. However, a major risk factor in the development of nonmelanoma skin cancer is a change in an existing lesion or the presence of a premalignant lesion, such as actinic keratosis. Organ transplant recipients who undergo immunosuppression to prevent rejection are also at risk for the development of squamous cell cancer.

Pathophysiology

Basal cell cancer and squamous cell cancer arise from epithelial tissue but have different pathophysiology, classifications, and manifestations.

Basal Cell Cancer

Basal cell cancer is an epithelial tumor believed to originate either from the basal layer of the epidermis or from cells in the surrounding dermal structures. These tumors are characterized by an impaired ability of the basal cells of the epidermis to mature into keratinocytes, with mitotic division beyond the basal layer. This results in a bulky neoplasm that grows by direct extension and destroys surrounding tissue, including healthy skin, nerves, blood vessels, lymphatic tissue, cartilage, and bone. Basal cell cancer is the most common but least aggressive type of skin cancer, rarely metastasizing.

Basal cell cancers tend to recur. Tumors greater than 2 cm in diameter have a high recurrence rate. Predisposing factors for metastasis are the size of the tumor and the client's resistance to treatment with surgery or chemotherapy. Even though they rarely metastasize, untreated basal cell cancers invade surrounding tissue and may destroy body parts, such as the nose or eyelid.

Basal cell cancer is classified into different types: nodular, superficial, pigmented, morpheaform, and keratotic. These types are described below and are summarized in Table 16–3.

Nodular basal cell cancer, the most common type of basal cell cancer, most often appears on the face, neck, and head. The tumor is made up of masses of cells that resemble epidermal basal cells and grow in a bulky, nodular form from lack of keratinization. In early stages, the tumor is a papule that looks like a smooth pimple. It is often pruritic and continues to grow at a steady rate, doubling in size every 6 to 12 months. As the tumor grows, the epidermis thins, but it remains intact. The skin over

TABLE 16–3 Types and Characteristics of Basal Cell Cancers

TYPE	COMMON LOCATION	MANIFESTATION
Nodular	Face, neck, head	Small, firm papule; pearly, white, pink, or flesh colored; telangiectasis; enlarges; may ulcerate.
Superficial	Trunk, extremities	Papules or plaque that is flat, erythematous, or scaling; pink color; well-defined borders; may have shallow erosions and surface crusting.
Pigmented	Head, neck, face	Dark brown, blue, or black color; border is shiny and well defined.
Morpheaform	Head, neck	Looks like a flat scar; ivory or flesh colored.
Keratotic	Ear	Small, firm papule; pearly, white, pink, or flesh colored; may ulcerate.

the tumor is shiny, and either pearly white, pink, or flesh colored. Telangiectasis may be visible over the area of the tumor. As the tumor continues to increase in size, the center or periphery may ulcerate, and the tumor develops well-circumscribed borders. It bleeds easily from mild injury.

Superficial basal cell cancer, found most often on the trunk and extremities, is the second most common type of basal cell cancer. This tumor is a proliferating tissue that attaches to the undersurface of the epithelium. The tumor is a flat papule or plaque, often erythematous, with well-defined borders. The tumor may ulcerate and be covered with crusts or shallow erosions (Figure 16–16 ■).

Pigmented basal cell cancer, found on the head, neck, and face, is less common. This tumor concentrates melanin pigment in the center of the basal cancer cells, giving it a dark brown, blue, or black appearance. The border of the tumor is shiny and well defined.

Morpheaform basal cell cancer, the rarest form of basal cell cancer, usually develops on the head and neck. The tumor forms finger-like projections that extend in any direction along dermal tissue planes. The tumor resembles a flat ivory or flesh-colored scar. This form is more likely to extend into and destroy adjacent tissue, especially muscle, nerve, and bone. It is often more difficult to diagnose because of its appearance.

Keratotic basal cell cancer (basosquamous) is found on the preauricular and postauricular groove. It contains both basal cells and squamoid-appearing cells that keratinize. Its appearance is much like that of nodular basal cell cancer. This type of basal cell cancer tends to recur locally and also is the type most likely to metastasize.

Squamous Cell Cancer

Squamous cell cancer is a malignant tumor of the squamous epithelium of the skin or mucous membranes. It occurs most often on areas of skin exposed to ultraviolet rays and weather, such as the forehead, helix of the ear, top of the nose, lower lip, and back of the hands. Squamous cell cancer may also arise on skin that has been burned or has chronic inflammation. This is a much more aggressive cancer than basal cell cancer, with a faster growth rate and a much greater potential for metastasis if untreated.

Figure 16–16 ■ A superficial basal cell cancer is characterized by erythema, ulcerations, and well-defined borders.

Figure 16–17 ■ As a squamous cell cancer grows, it tends to invade surrounding tissue. It also ulcerates, may bleed, and is painful.

The tumors arise when the keratinizing cells of the squamous epithelium proliferate, producing a growth that eventually fills the epidermis and invades the dermal tissue planes. Keratinization of some cells is present, and the formation of keratin "pearls" is common. The keratin formation diminishes as the tumor grows. As the tumor grows, the tumor cells increase in number and rate of mitosis, forming odd shapes.

Squamous cell cancer begins as a small, firm red nodule. The tumor may be crusted with keratin products. As it grows, it may ulcerate, bleed, and become painful. As the tumor extends into the surrounding tissue and becomes a nodule, the area around the nodule becomes indurated (hardened) (Figure 16–17 ■).

Recurrent squamous cell cancer can be invasive, increasing the risk of metastasis. Invasive squamous cell cancer may arise from preexisting skin lesions, such as scars and actinic keratosis, and extend into the dermis (called intraepidermal squamous cell cancer). This form appears as a slightly raised erythematous plaque with well-defined borders. Metastasis occurs most often via the lymphatics. The degree of risk for metastasis depends on the size and depth of penetration of the tumor.

INTERDISCIPLINARY CARE

Treatment of nonmelanoma skin cancer focuses on removal of all malignant tissue using such methods as surgery, curettage and electrodesiccation, cryotherapy, or radiotherapy. These modalities offer a greater than 90% cure rate. After the malignant tissue is removed, the client should have regular examinations for recurrence.

Diagnosis

Nonmelanoma cancer is diagnosed by microscopic examination of tissue biopsied from the tumor. The biopsy is usually done as an office procedure under local anesthesia. The types of biopsy used are shave, punch, incisional, and excisional. See Chapter 15 ∞ for further information.

Treatments

Depending on the type, size, and location of a nonmelanoma cancer, it may be treated with surgical excision, Mohs surgery, curettage and electrodesiccation, or radiation.

SURGICAL EXCISION Both basal cell and squamous cell cancers are excised surgically. The surgery may be minor or major, depending on the size and location of the tumor. Surgery for small tumors is most often performed in the outpatient surgery department or in the surgeon's office. Surgical excision allows rapid healing and yields good cosmetic results, but, as with any surgery, carries the risk of infection.

The goal of surgical excision is to remove the tumor completely, so some surrounding tissue is excised along with the tumor. If the tumor is on the face, the incision is made along normal wrinkle or anatomic lines so that the scars will be less obvious. The incision is closed in layers to leave the smallest possible scar. A pressure dressing is usually applied over the incision to provide support.

If a large tumor is removed, a skin graft or skin flap may be performed to cover the excised area. If grafting is necessary, the client is hospitalized.

MOHS SURGERY In Mohs surgery, thin layers of the tumor are horizontally shaved off. A frozen section of the tissue is stained at each level to determine tumor margins. This method is the most accurate in assessing the extent of nonmelanoma skin cancer and the method that conserves the most normal tissue. It is often used in areas such as the nose, the nasolabial fold, the medial canthus, and the ear.

CURETTAGE AND ELECTRODESICCATION Curettage and electrodesiccation are used to treat basal cell cancers that are less than 2 cm in diameter, are superficial, or recur because of poor margin control. They may also be used for primary squamous cell cancers that are less than 1 cm in diameter and have distinct borders. This type of treatment is most successful for tumors on anatomic sites over a fixed underlying surface, such as the ear, chest, and temple.

Abnormal tissue is scraped away (curettage) within 1 to 2 mm of the margin and then a low-voltage electrode is used to abrade the tumor base (electrodesiccation). Tumor tissue is much softer and more friable than normal tissue. Therefore, curettage and electrodesiccation is not used for lesions where the dermis is thin (such as the eyelid) or where the tumor extends into the subcutaneous tissue.

Curettage and electrodesiccation provide good cosmetic results and preserve normal tissue. However, healing time is longer, and it is difficult to ensure that all tumor margins have been removed.

Instead of a low-voltage electrode, some physicians use a carbon dioxide laser to vaporize the tumor. When used in conjunction with curettage, this treatment is effective on superficial basal cell cancers. Carbon dioxide vaporization results in minimal thermal injury to adjacent cells, less pain, and quicker healing.

RADIATION THERAPY Radiation is most often used for lesions that are inoperable because of their location (such as tumors on the corner of the nose, the eyelid, the canthus, and the lip) or size (between 1 and 8 cm). Radiotherapy is also used for clients who are older or of poor surgical risk. Radiation is painless and can be used to treat areas surrounding the tumor if necessary. However, the treatment is given over 3 to 4 weeks in a clinical facility, does not allow control of tumor margins, and may itself cause skin cancer.

NURSING CARE

The increasing number of people with skin cancer means that nurses must be involved in prevention and early detection. Nurses have the opportunity to teach preventive behaviors in all settings, including the hospital, home, community, school, and clinic.

Nursing care for the client with nonmelanoma skin cancer depends on the treatment used. Surgical excision is the most common form of treatment; nursing care depends on the extent of the procedure. However, regardless of the type of treatment, the client will have impaired skin integrity, an increased risk for infection, and anxiety about the future following a diagnosis of cancer. Interventions with rationales for the client with any type of skin cancer are discussed in the following section on malignant melanoma.

Health Promotion

It is well known that cumulative sun exposure positively correlates with nonmelanoma skin cancers. Many skin cancers can be prevented by limiting exposure to risk factors. Primary prevention behaviors recommended by the American Cancer Society and the Skin Cancer Foundation are outlined in Box 16–4. Information about sunscreens is listed in Box 16–5.

Nurses also provide client and family education for early detection of nonmelanoma skin cancer. Numerous brochures describing the types of skin cancers, photographs of lesions, and prevention behaviors are available from the American Cancer Society, health education and support agencies, and pharmaceutical companies that manufacture sunscreen. Most of this literature is free.

The client or family at risk for or diagnosed with a skin cancer must be taught how to conduct a self-examination of the skin, described in Box 16–6, as well as the importance of conducting the examination on the same day of each month. Family members can help with areas that are hard to examine, such as the ears, scalp, and back.

BOX 16–4 Preventing Skin Cancer

- Minimize sun exposure between the hours of 10 A.M. and 3 P.M., when ultraviolet rays are the strongest.
- Cover up with a wide-brimmed hat, sunglasses, long-sleeved shirt, and long pants made of tightly woven materials when in the sun.
- Apply a waterproof or water-resistant sunscreen with an SPF of 15 or higher at least 30 minutes before every exposure to the sun. If swimming or sweating heavily, reapply every hour. Apply sunscreen not only on sunny days but also on cloudy days (when ultraviolet rays can penetrate 70% to 80% of the cloud cover).
- Use sunscreen and protective clothing when you are on or near sand, snow, concrete, or water (which can reflect more than 50% of the ultraviolet rays onto your skin).
- Avoid tanning booths; ultraviolet radiation emitted by tanning booths damages the deep skin layers.

BOX 16–5 Sunscreen Information

Types of Sunscreen

Chemical

Chemical sunscreens absorb ultraviolet light and act as a radiation filter. Examples follow:

- *p*-Aminobenzoic acid (PABA)
- Benzophenones
- Anthranilates
- Salicylates

Physical

Physical sunscreens reflect and scatter ultraviolet light. Examples follow:

- Zinc oxide
- Titanium dioxide
- Magnesium silicate
- Ferric chloride
- Kaolin
- Ichthyol

Adverse Reactions Associated with Sunscreens

Adverse reactions associated with sunscreens include contact and photocontact dermatitis. People with previous hypersensitivity reactions to benzocaine, procaine, sulfonamides, or para-phenylenediamine may develop hypersensitivity responses to PABA. People who are also taking systemic thiazide diuretics or sulfonamides may develop eczematous dermatitis.

Sunscreen Ratings

In the United States, the Food and Drug Administration rates commercial sunscreens according to their sun protection factor, or SPF. The SPF value is the ratio of the time required to produce minimal skin redness through a sunscreen product with the time required to produce the same degree of redness without the sunscreen. A person who can tolerate 1/2 hour of sun without a sunscreen should be able to tolerate 3 hours of sun when a sunscreen of SPF 6 is applied to the skin. SPF values of sunscreens range from 2 to 50.

Community-Based Care

Teach the client and family specific measures for self-care following surgery, including information about:

- How and when to change dressings
- The use of aseptic technique and careful hand washing when caring for the wound
- Symptoms to report (such as bleeding, fever, or signs of wound infection), and how to protect the operative site against trauma and irritations.

THE CLIENT WITH MALIGNANT MELANOMA

Malignant melanoma arises from melanocytes. This serious skin cancer is increasing in incidence each year. Melanoma accounts for about 4% of skin cancers, but it causes about 79% of skin cancer deaths (American Cancer Society, 2004b).

Incidence

This disease is more than 10 times more common in fair-skinned people than in dark-skinned people. As with the nonmelanoma skin cancers, an increase in the incidence of malignant melanoma is believed to be related to the thinning ozone layer and increased exposure to ultraviolet rays. The incidence is highest in Caucasian

BOX 16–6 Skin Self-Examination

1. Choose the same day each month (such as the first day) to do the examination.
2. The best time to do the examination is after you take a bath or shower. Examine yourself in a well-lighted room in front of a full-length mirror. Have a hand mirror, a chair, and a hair dryer available. If you have difficulty seeing your back and scalp (or any other parts of your body), ask someone to help you.
3. Follow the same pattern with each examination:

Examine head and face, using one or both mirrors. Use blow dryer to inspect scalp.

Check hands, including nails. In full-length mirror, examine elbows, arms, underarms.

Focus on neck, chest, torso. Women: Check under breasts.

With back to the mirror, use hand mirror to inspect back of neck and back including buttocks.

Sitting down, check legs and feet, including soles, heels, and nails. Use hand mirror to examine genitals.

upper-middle-class professionals who work indoors. This group of people often had severe sunburn with blistering during childhood and tend to vacation in areas of intense sun exposure. Malignant melanoma is also more common in people who live in sunny climates, burn easily, and patronize tanning parlors. However, malignant melanoma may arise from already present lesions or from skin normally covered with clothing.

Risk Factors

Although the exact cause of melanoma is unknown, it is known that certain risk factors are associated with the disease. The risk factors for melanoma are listed in Box 16–7.

Pathophysiology

Malignant melanomas arise from melanocytes, cells located at or near the basal layer (the deepest epidermal layer). These cells produce melanin, the dark skin pigment. Melanin is made in granules and transferred to keratinocytes, where it accumulates on the superficial side of each keratinocyte and forms a shield of pigment over the nucleus as protection against ultraviolet rays. Malignant melanomas can develop wherever there is pigment, but about one-third of them originate in existing nevi (moles).

Almost all malignant melanomas are more than 6 mm in diameter, are asymmetric, and initially develop within the epidermis over a long period. While they are still confined to the epidermis, the lesions (called malignant melanoma *in situ*) are flat and relatively benign. However, when they penetrate the dermis, they mingle with blood and lymph vessels and are capable of metastasizing. At this latter stage, the tumors develop a raised or nodular appearance and often have smaller nodules, called satellite lesions, around the periphery.

The prognosis for survival for people diagnosed with malignant melanoma is determined by several variables, including tumor thickness, ulceration, metastasis, site, age, and gender. Younger clients and women have a somewhat better chance of survival. Tumors on the hands, feet, and scalp have a poorer prognosis; tumors of the feet and scalp are less visible and may not be diagnosed until they grow into the dermis.

Precursor Lesions

The three specific precursor lesions for the development of malignant melanoma are congenital nevi, dysplastic nevi, and lentigo maligna. A precursor lesion is also called a premalignant lesion, a name that indicates that the lesion's risk of becoming malignant is greater than normal.

CONGENITAL NEVI Congenital nevi are present at birth. Some lesions are small; others are large enough to cover an entire body area. Their color can range from brown to black.

They are often slightly raised, with an irregular surface and a fairly regular border.

DYSPLASTIC NEVI Dysplastic nevi are also called atypical moles. Although dysplastic nevi are not present at birth, they appear as normal nevi during childhood and become dysplastic (having abnormal development) after puberty. A client with classic dysplastic nevi has more than 100 nevi, at least one of which is larger than 8 mm in diameter, and at least one has the characteristics of malignant melanoma (asymmetry, irregular border, color variegation, and a diameter greater than 6 mm). A familial tendency to dysplastic nevi increases the risk for the development of malignant melanoma. However, it is not known whether people with dysplastic nevi and no family history of melanoma face a higher risk of melanoma.

Dysplastic nevi most often appear on the face, trunk, and arms but also are seen on the scalp, female breast, groin, and buttocks. The pigmentation of the nevi is irregular, with mixtures of tan, brown, black, red, and pink. An area of lighter pigmentation is surrounded by a papular area of deeper pigmentation (described as a "fried egg appearance"). The borders of the nevi are irregular.

LENTIGO MALIGNA Lentigo maligna, also called Hutchinson's freckle, is a tan or black patch on the skin that looks like a freckle. It grows slowly, becoming mottled, dark, thick, and nodular. It is usually seen on one side of the face of an older adult who has had a large amount of sun exposure.

Classification

Malignant melanomas are classified into different types. The major types are superficial spreading melanoma, lentigo maligna melanoma, nodular melanoma, and acral lentiginous melanoma. Each of these tumors is characterized by a radial and/or vertical growth phase. During the initial radial phase, which may last from 1 to 25 years (depending on the type), the melanoma grows parallel to the skin surface. During this phase, the tumor rarely metastasizes and is often curable by surgical excision. However, during the vertical growth phase, atypical melanocytes rapidly penetrate into the dermis and subcutaneous tissue, greatly increasing the risk for metastasis and death.

SUPERFICIAL SPREADING MELANOMA Superficial spreading melanoma is the most common type, comprising about 70% of all melanomas (Porth, 2005). The lesions are usually flat and scaly or crusty and are about 2 cm in diameter. They often arise from a preexisting nevus. This type of melanoma is found on the trunk and back of men and on the legs of women. Superficial spreading melanomas occur more often in women than in men. The median age of occurrence is the 50s.

The radial growth phase lasts from 1 to 5 or more years. When the lesion enters the vertical growth phase, it grows rapidly, and its color changes from a mixture of tan, brown, and black to a characteristic red, white, and blue. The lesion also develops irregular borders and often has raised nodules and ulcerations (Figure 16–18 ■).

LENTIGO MALIGNA MELANOMA Lentigo maligna melanoma often arises from the precursor lesion, lentigo maligna. The lesions are large and tan with different shades of brown. This type

---

BOX 16–7 Risk Factors for Melanoma Skin Cancer

- A high number of moles, or large moles
- Fair skin, freckling, blond hair, or blue eyes
- Close relative with the disease
- Men with gene changes from a family history of breast or ovarian cancer
- Treatment with medications that suppress the immune system
- Too much exposure to UV radiation from sunlight, tanning lamps, or tanning booths
- Over age 50
- Xeroderma pigmentosus, a rare inherited disease in which people are less able to repair damage caused by sunlight
- Past history of melanoma

Figure 16–18 ■ Malignant melanoma is a serious skin cancer that arises from melanocytes.
Source: L. Solomon/Custom Medical Stock Photography.

of melanoma makes up 4% to 10% of malignant melanomas and is the least serious form (Porth, 2005). It occurs on skin that has had long-term sun exposure, such as the face, neck, and sometimes the dorsal surface of the hands and lower extremities. Lentigo maligna melanoma affects women more than men. It is typically diagnosed in people in their 60s and 70s.

Lentigo maligna melanoma is characterized by a proliferation of atypical melanocytes parallel to the basal layer of the epidermis. The radial growth phase may last from 10 to 25 years, with the lesion growing to as large as 10 cm. The lesion becomes malignant as soon as the melanocytes invade the dermis. In the vertical growth phase, raised nodules may appear on the surface of the lesion. The lesion tends to acquire a freckled or mottled appearance.

NODULAR MELANOMA Nodular melanoma lesions are raised, dome-shaped, blue-black or red nodules on areas of the head, neck, and trunk that may or may not have been exposed to the sun. The lesions may look like a blood blister, or they may ulcerate and bleed. The lesions arise from unaffected skin rather than from a preexisting lesion. This type makes up 15% to 30% of malignant melanomas and is often diagnosed in people in their 50s (Porth, 2005).

Nodular melanoma has only a vertical growth phase, but it grows aggressively during that phase. However, the absence of a radial growth phase makes this type more difficult to diagnose before it metastasizes.

ACRAL LENTIGINOUS MELANOMA Acral lentiginous melanoma, also called mucocutaneous melanoma, is less common in people with fair skin and more common in people with dark skin. The lesions progress from tan, brown, or black flat lesions to elevated nodules and are about 3 cm in diameter. The radial phase lasts from 2 to 5 years. They are found on the palms of the hands, soles of the feet, the mucous membranes, and the nail beds. Acral lentiginous melanoma affects both men and women equally and is most often diagnosed in people in their 50s and 60s.

INTERDISCIPLINARY CARE

The management of the client with malignant melanoma begins with identification, diagnosis, and tumor staging. If treat-able, the tumor is removed through surgical excision. Malignant melanoma is also treated with chemotherapy, immunotherapy, and radiation therapy. Other therapies used with success include biologic therapies with interleukin-2 and interferon and therapeutic vaccines containing melanoma antigens.

Identification

Malignant melanoma is most often found on the trunk of men and on the lower extremities of women. Nevertheless, it is important for the client to have a complete physical examination and total skin assessment. In addition to a visual examination of all skin surfaces, palpation of regional lymph nodes, the liver, and the spleen is essential to assess for metastasis when a melanoma is suspected or found.

A change in the color or size of a nevus is reported in 70% of people diagnosed with a malignant melanoma. The ABCD rule is used to assess suspicious lesions.

> ## FAST FACTS
> **The ABCD Rule**
> Using the ABCD rule to assess for melanoma:
> A = asymmetry (one half of the nevus does not match the other half)
> B = border irregularity (edges are ragged, blurred, or notched)
> C = color variation or dark black color
> D = diameter greater than 6 mm (size of a pencil eraser)

Diagnosis

In addition to biopsy of any suspicious lesion, diagnostic tests are conducted to determine whether the tumor has metastasized. Because malignant melanoma may metastasize to any organ or tissue of the body, a variety of tests may be conducted, including microscopic examination, biopsy, and tests for metastasis (liver function tests and computed tomography [CT] scan of the liver, a complete blood count, serum blood chemistry profile, chest x-ray, bone scan, and CT scan or magnetic resonance imaging of the brain).

Microstaging

The term *microstaging* describes the assessment of the level of invasion of a malignant melanoma and the maximum tumor thickness. In the Clark system of microstaging, the vertical growth of the lesion is measured from the epidermis to the subcutaneous tissue to determine the level of invasion (Figure 16–19 ■). However, variations in individual skin thicknesses and different anatomic sites can affect the accuracy of the measurement. In the Breslow system, an adaptation of the Clark system of assessment, the vertical thickness is measured from the granular level of the epidermis to the deepest level of tumor invasion. This determination is important, because as the thickness of the melanoma increases, survival rate decreases.

After the thickness and depth of the tumor are determined, a clinical stage is assigned. The traditional three-stage system is still used, although it does not include tumor thickness. The American Joint Committee on Cancer has adopted a four-stage system that includes tumor thickness, level of invasion, lymph node involvement, and evidence of metastasis.

Figure 16–19 ■ Clark's levels for staging measure the invasion of a melanoma from the epidermis to the subcutaneous tissue.

Treatments

Surgical excision is the preferred treatment for malignant melanoma. Other methods of treatment are chemotherapy, immunotherapy, and radiation therapy.

SURGERY If a biopsy identifies the lesion as a melanoma, a wide excision is performed that includes the full thickness of the skin and subcutaneous tissue. Because the risk of local recurrence for thin melanomas (those less than 0.76 mm) is quite low, margins of 0.5 to 1.0 cm of normal skin are excised around the tumor. Thick tumors require a 1- to 3-cm margin excision because they are at risk for local recurrence or satellite lesions.

Regional lymph nodes are the most common sites for metastasis of malignant melanoma. Standard surgical treatment for clinically suspicious lymph node involvement includes excision of the primary lesions as well as surgical dissection of the involved lymph nodes. Elective lymph node dissection (ELND) in the treatment of localized malignant melanoma remains controversial. Advocates of ELND believe that the procedure benefits clients with intermediate-thickness tumors because approximately 20% of people whose lymph nodes were clinically negative at diagnosis show some metastasis on removal of the nodes. Those opposed to ELND believe the risks associated with the procedure are too high for the 80% of people who have no evidence of metastasis after removal of the nodes.

Surgery also is indicated for palliative management of isolated metastasis. Removal of metastatic tumors in the brain, liver, lung, gastrointestinal tract, or subcutaneous tissue may relieve symptoms and prolong life.

IMMUNOTHERAPY Immunotherapy is a relatively new treatment modality for malignant melanoma. The role of the immunologic response initially was recognized because of the numerous spontaneous remissions seen in clients with melanoma—a higher occurrence than with any other adult tumor. In addition, researchers have recently identified tumor-specific antigen-antibodies in clients with melanoma. This also has stimulated an interest in immunotherapeutic interventions for the treatment of malignant melanoma.

Agents such as interferons, interleukins, monoclonal antibodies, bacille Calmette-Guérin, levamisole, transfer factors, and tumor vaccines have been used to treat melanoma, with varying response rates. The effectiveness of these agents, used either alone, in combination with chemotherapy, or in combination with each other, is under investigation.

RADIATION THERAPY Melanoma responds to higher dose radiation, especially if the tumor is small. Response rates to radiation therapy depend on the site of the tumor, the thickness of the tumor, the type of melanoma, and the client's general health, but may range from 0% to 71%. Radiation frequently is used for palliation of symptoms resulting from metastasis to the brain, bone, lymph nodes, gastrointestinal tract, skin, or subcutaneous tissue. Liver and lung metastases are not treated with radiation therapy because a loss of organ function may result.

NEW METHODS OF TREATMENT Melanoma skin cancer research is ongoing and directed toward more specific methods of diagnosis and treatment. Examples are as follows:

- *Gene therapy:* Clinical trials are in progress to test the effectiveness of adding certain genes to the malignant cells.
- *Melanoma DNA research:* Knowledge of how ultraviolet light harms DNA is increasing, providing support for referral for genetic counseling for people with a strong family history of melanoma.
- *Immune therapy:* Vaccines are being developed to make an individual immune to his or her melanoma cells, or to train the person's immune cells to fight the cancer.
- *Staging:* Very sensitive new tests can better detect the spread of melanoma to lymph nodes and can possibly better identify people who could be helped by a treatment such as immunotherapy after surgery.

NURSING CARE

Nurses have the opportunity to assess the skin of clients requiring care for many different health problems and may be the first healthcare provider to identify suspicious lesions. Wide excision and the high risk of metastasis from malignant melanoma usually require inpatient surgical treatment, with the nurse providing care and teaching. See the following page for a nursing care plan for a client with malignant melanoma.

Health Promotion

The most important aspect of preventing malignant melanoma is a health history and skin assessment. The American Cancer Society recommends that people between the ages of 20 and 40 see a skin specialist every 3 years and those over 40 have annual skin checkups. People with actinic keratoses should also have their skin checked regularly for any signs of change. Clients at risk (those with precancerous lesions and with personal risk factors), as well as those over age 40, should conduct a monthly skin self-examination (described earlier in Box 16–6). When self-assessing for melanoma, the client looks for a change in:

- Color, especially any lesion that becomes darker or variegated in shades of tan, brown, black, red, white, or blue
- Size, especially any lesion that becomes larger or spreads out

NURSING CARE PLAN   A Client with Malignant Melanoma

Geoff Sanders, age 69, is retired from the postal service. He has always been an avid participant in outdoor sports: When he was younger he played baseball and tennis, and for the last 10 years he has played golf at least twice a week. He now lives in Connecticut, but as a younger man he lived in Florida for almost 15 years. Mr. Sanders has a variety of warts and moles and rarely pays attention to them. However, after taking a shower one day he noticed that a mole on his left lower leg looked bigger and darker. Mr. Sanders had just seen a public announcement on television about the dangers of changes in moles, and he immediately called his primary HMO physician for an appointment at the dermatology clinic.

ASSESSMENT

On arriving at the clinic, Mr. Sanders is interviewed and examined by Tom Hall, a clinical nurse specialist. Following the assessment, Tom documents the following information.

Mr. Sanders has a family history of skin cancer; his father had several squamous cell cancers removed from his face. He has numerous nevi on his body; the one causing concern is located on the medial anterior left leg, 2 inches below the patella. Mr. Sanders states that the mole has been present for years but that he noticed just yesterday that it has become larger and darker. On further questioning, he states that the mole itches sometimes but has never hurt or bled. Mr. Sanders lived in Florida for 15 years and now experiences a sunburn early each summer before he tans. The sunburn involves the lower legs because Mr. Sanders wears shorts during his twice-weekly golf game.

A complete skin assessment reveals various freckles, warts, and nevi. With the exception of the nevus that prompted Mr. Sanders to come to the clinic, all lesions appear normal. The nevus in question is raised, 3 cm in diameter, with irregular borders and a nodular surface. It is variegated in color, with various shades of brown. The skin surrounding the nevus is slightly erythematous. Inguinal lymph nodes are not enlarged or painful. Tom Hall takes a photograph of the lesion with Mr. Sanders's permission.

Following the assessment, Mr. Sanders discusses the lesion with a surgeon, who recommends excision. They discuss the possibility of skin cancer and the importance of early detection and treatment. Mr. Sanders is scheduled for a biopsy of the nevus under a local anesthetic the following morning. Following the biopsy, histologic examination reveals lentigo maligna melanoma. Staging of the tumor reveals that it is a melanoma *in situ*, with no metastasis to regional lymph nodes. Mr. Sanders undergoes a wide excision of the lesion the following afternoon.

DIAGNOSES

- *Impaired Skin Integrity* related to excision of melanoma from the left lower leg
- *Risk for Infection* related to surgical wound on left lower leg
- *Acute Pain* related to wide excision of melanoma on left lower leg
- *Anxiety* related to diagnosis of skin cancer

EXPECTED OUTCOMES

- Demonstrate complete healing of the incision without manifestations of infection.
- Verbalize relief of pain by the time the incision is healed.
- Verbalize fears and concerns about his diagnosis.

PLANNING AND IMPLEMENTATION

- Make the first dressing change, but ensure that Mr. Sanders can safely change the dressing himself prior to discharge the day after surgery.
- On discharge, provide adequate dressings and tape for the first home dressing change; include in discharge instructions necessary information about where to buy supplies and how many dressing supplies will be needed.
- Review and provide written instruction for prescribed systemic antibiotic and pain medication.
- Provide written instructions for dressing change, manifestations of infection, and phone number of clinic; stress importance of calling if any abnormal symptoms occur.
- Teach how to protect the incision from bumps and to protect the site from irritants.
- Discuss diagnosis, positive outlook for treatment of melanoma *in situ*, and the client's concerns.
- Stress importance of lifelong regular healthcare evaluations to identify any recurrence or metastasis.

EVALUATION

Mr. Sanders returned to the dermatology clinic 1 week after his surgical incision. His incision is well approximated and shows no signs of infection. He is taking his antibiotic 4 times a day as prescribed and reports that his need for pain medications is decreasing. During his clinic visit the following week, Tom Hall removes the sutures and assesses the wound as healed. Mr. Sanders completed his antibiotics and no longer requires pain medications. He says he is still "scared to death" about having cancer, but he has decided to join a local cancer support group. He also says he had gotten a list of skin safety rules from the American Cancer Society and will be sure to cover up and use sunscreens when he plays golf. Mr. Sanders makes an appointment for follow-up care in 3 months.

CRITICAL THINKING IN THE NURSING PROCESS

1. Consider reasons why people who notice a change in a skin lesion put off seeking health care. What can nurses do to effect change?
2. Design a teaching plan for young adults for preventing skin cancers.
3. What would you say to Mr. Sanders if he called the clinic and said that the antibiotics were making him sick and he didn't think he needed them anyway?
4. Design a nursing care plan for Mr. Sanders for the diagnosis *Powerlessness*.

See Evaluating Your Response in Appendix C.

- Shape, especially any lesion that protrudes more from the skin or begins to have an irregular outline
- Appearance of a lesion, especially bleeding, drainage, oozing, ulceration, crusting, scaliness, or development of a mushrooming outward growth

- Consistency, especially any lesion that becomes softer or is more easily irritated
- Skin around a lesion, such as redness, swelling, or leaking of color from a lesion into the surrounding skin
- Sensation, such as itching or pain.

Assessment

Skin assessment is discussed in Chapter 15 ∞. Specific health history questions and assessments for skin cancer are outlined in Box 16–8.

Nursing Diagnoses and Interventions

Although many different nursing diagnoses may be appropriate for the client with a malignant melanoma, common responses are *Impaired Skin Integrity, Hopelessness,* and *Anxiety.*

Impaired Skin Integrity

Malignant melanomas not only destroy skin layers but also invade body structures. Certain types of melanomas may ulcerate prior to diagnosis, and treatment typically involves some type of surgical biopsy and excision. Any open lesion or incision increases the risk for secondary infection.

- Monitor for manifestations of infection: fever, tachycardia, malaise, incisional erythema, swelling, pain, or drainage that increases or becomes purulent. *Intact skin is the first line of defense against infection; impaired skin integrity increases the risk for infection. If infection is present, the client may have both systemic and local manifestations.*
- Keep the incision line clean and dry by changing dressings as necessary. *Moisture increases the risk of infection.*
- Follow principles of medical and surgical asepsis when caring for client's incision. Teach family members and visitors the importance of careful hand washing. Maintain standard precautions if drainage is present. Careful hand washing is essential in preventing the spread of infection. *Aseptic techniques are necessary when caring for any surgical incision to prevent infection.*

PRACTICE ALERT

Nurses must use standard precautions with blood and body fluids to protect themselves from exposure to HIV.

- Encourage and maintain adequate caloric and protein intake in the diet. Suggest a consultation with the dietitian if client does not want to eat. *Adequate kilocalories and protein are necessary for proper healing. The client with cancer has increased metabolic needs; if these needs are not met, nutritional problems that impair healing may result.*

Hopelessness

Hopelessness is an emotional state in which a person feels that there is no possibility that life will improve. Clients who experience hopelessness are often withdrawn, passive, and apathetic.

The diagnosis of malignant melanoma threatens the quality and quantity of life as the client faces the possibility or reality of metastasis; the possibility that the cancer may recur and cause death; and alterations in self-concept, roles, and relationships. Inspiring hope in clients during this health crisis is a legitimate nursing action.

- Provide an environment that encourages the client to identify and express feelings, concerns, and goals:
  - Use active listening, ask open-ended questions, and reflect on the client's statements.
  - Acknowledge and respect feelings of apathy and/or anger as expressions of distress.
  - Convey an empathetic understanding of the fears and concerns.
  - Provide opportunities to express positive emotions: hope, faith, a sense of purpose, and the will to live.

BOX 16–8 Nursing Assessment for Skin Cancer

Interview Questions

- Have any members of your family ever been treated for skin cancer?
- Have you had a skin cancer removed from any part of your body?
- Have you noticed any change in the size, shape, or color of a mole, wart, birthmark, or scar?
- Do you have any moles, warts, birthmarks, or scars that itch, are painful, have crusting, or bleed?
- In what parts of the country or world have you lived?
- Have you ever been badly sunburned?
- Do you visit tanning salons?
- Are you exposed to any hazardous chemicals in your job?
- Have you been taught how to examine your skin? If so, how do you do this examination? How often?

Physical Assessment

1. Ask the client to remove all clothing and put on an examination gown. Ensure good light; natural, bright light is best for inspection of lesions. The client may sit, stand, or lie down.
2. Inspect and palpate the skin. Stretching the skin tightly during assessment facilitates assessment of nodular and scaly lesions and lesions in the dermis. Assess for:
   a. Obvious lesions
   b. Visible swellings

c. Alterations in normal contour and borders of nevi
   d. Enlarged lymph glands
   e. Skin or mucosal discolorations
   f. Areas of ulceration, scaling, crusting, or erosion.
3. The order of assessment follows:
   a. Head and neck: entire scalp, eyelids, external ear, auditory canals, external surface of the nose, internal surface of the nose, the oral cavity, facial skin, the facial glands (parotid, submaxillary, sublingual)
   b. Thyroid and neck, including lymph glands
   c. Chest and abdomen, with special attention under pendulous breasts, in skin folds, and in areas covered with hair
   d. Back and buttocks, with special attention to the area between the buttocks
   e. Extremities, with special attention to the axillae, nail beds, webs between the fingers and toes, and soles of the feet
   f. External genitals, with special attention to skin folds, mucous membranes, and areas covered with hair.
4. Measure and record a description of all skin lesions on an anatomic chart. Take photographs (if possible) of any suspicious lesion, and include them in the client's record for future reference.

- Explore the client's perceptions, and modify or clarify them if necessary by providing information and correcting misconceptions.
- Encourage the client to identify support systems and sources of strength and coping in the past.

Verbalizing feelings, concerns, and goals allows others to validate or correct them, promotes a therapeutic nurse–client relationship, and fosters feelings of self-worth. Expressing positive emotions and calling on support systems and sources of strength that were effective in coping with past crises help the person resolve the crisis and develop hope.

- Encourage active participation in self-care as well as in mutual decision making and goal setting. *Meeting self-care needs and making decisions about care increase personal confidence in one's capacity for coping.*
- Encourage a focus not only on the present but also on the future: Review past occasions for hope, discuss the client's personal meaning of hope, establish and evaluate short-term goals with the client and family, and encourage them to express hope for the future. *The nurse mobilizes the client's resources to strengthen motivation, hope, and the will to live.*

Anxiety

The intensity of anxiety, aroused by a perceived threat, depends on the severity of the present situation and the client's ability to handle the threat. Anxiety is one of the most common psychosocial responses in clients with cancer. Anxiety increases at the time of diagnosis and remains a constant emotion throughout the course of treatment, regardless of treatment type or setting. Interventions center on helping the client recognize the manifestations of anxiety, determining whether the client wishes to do anything about the anxiety, and facilitating coping strategies.

- Provide reassurance and comfort:
  - Set aside time to sit quietly with the client.
  - Speak slowly and calmly.
  - Convey empathetic understanding by touch and supporting present coping mechanisms, such as crying and talking.
  - Do not make demands or expect the client to make decisions. *Coping behaviors differ from situation to situation and from person to person. Anxiety at moderate to severe levels narrows perceptions and the ability to function.*
- Decrease sensory stimuli by using short, simple sentences; focusing on the here and now; and providing concise information. *Higher levels of anxiety result in a focus on the present, inability to concentrate, and difficulty in understanding verbal communications.*
- Provide interventions that decrease anxiety levels and increase coping:
  - Provide accurate information about the illness, treatment, and expected length of recovery.
  - Encourage discussion of expected physical changes and ways to minimize disfigurement through cosmetics and clothing.
  - Include family members in teaching sessions.
  - Encourage participation in care. *Although the prognosis and treatment of melanoma depend on various factors, the prognosis of complete cure is decreased with metastasis. Surgical incisions include excision with wide margins, which may cause disfigurement. Active participation in care gives the client some control over the future and is often an effective means of coping with anxiety.*

Using NANDA, NIC, and NOC

Chart 16–2 shows links between NANDA, NIC, and NOC when caring for the client with malignant melanoma.

Community-Based Care

Health education for the client and family experiencing the diagnosis and treatment of malignant melanoma involves self-care and ongoing self-monitoring. Education for the client and family is specific to the type of treatment. In addition to wound care, clients who have had a lymph node dissection need instructions on how to protect the extremity from bleeding, trauma, and infection. Address the following topics:

- Schedule regular medical checkups every 3 months for the first 2 years, every 6 months for the next 5 years, and yearly thereafter.
- Proper self-care combined with regular medical care can help the client lead a fairly normal life.
- If assistance for home care is necessary, provide referrals to a community health agency or a home care agency. In addition, refer the client to a local cancer support group if desired. Other resources are:
- The American Cancer Society
- The Skin Cancer Foundation.

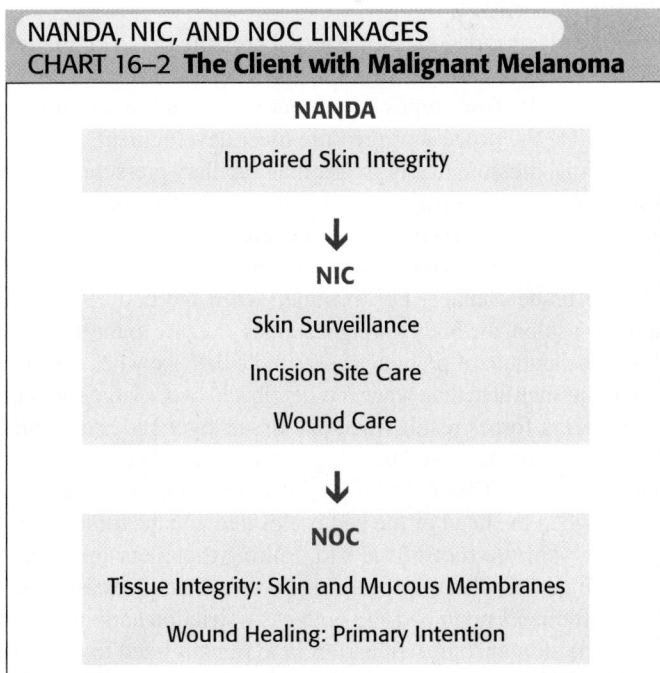

NANDA, NIC, AND NOC LINKAGES
CHART 16–2 The Client with Malignant Melanoma

NANDA

Impaired Skin Integrity

↓

NIC

Skin Surveillance

Incision Site Care

Wound Care

↓

NOC

Tissue Integrity: Skin and Mucous Membranes

Wound Healing: Primary Intention

Data from *NANDA's Nursing Diagnoses: Definitions & Classification 2005–2006* by NANDA International (2005), Philadelphia; *Nursing Interventions Classification (NIC)* (4th ed.) by J. M. Dochterman & G. M. Bulechek (2004), St. Louis, MO: Mosby; and *Nursing Outcomes Classification (NOC)* (3rd ed.) by S. Moorhead, M. Johnson, and M. Maas (2004), St. Louis, MO: Mosby.

MEDIALINK Cancer Support and Resources

SKIN TRAUMA

Trauma to the skin can be unintentional or intentional (as in the case of surgery). Chemicals, radiation, pressure, or thermal changes cause skin trauma. This section discusses pressure ulcers and frostbite, as well as intentional trauma from cutaneous and plastic surgery or treatment. Thermal injury (burns) is discussed in Chapter 17 ∞.

THE CLIENT WITH A PRESSURE ULCER

Pressure ulcers are ischemic lesions of the skin and underlying tissue caused by external pressure that impairs the flow of blood and lymph (Porth, 2005). The ischemia causes tissue necrosis and eventual ulceration. These ulcers, also called bed sores or decubitus ulcers, tend to develop over a bony prominence (such as the heels, greater trochanter, sacrum, and ischia), but they may appear on the skin of any part of the body subjected to external pressure, friction, or shearing forces.

Incidence

The incidence of pressure ulcers in hospitals, long-term care facilities, and home settings is high enough to warrant concern for healthcare providers. The incidence in hospitals has been reported as 8%, whereas the incidence in long-term care facilities is reported to range from 2.4% to 23% (Porth, 2005). Little research has been done to determine the extent of the problem in the home setting. However, with increasing numbers of clients (and especially older adult clients) being cared for in the home, it is probable that the incidence is great enough to warrant plans of care to prevent their occurrence.

Pathophysiology

Pressure ulcers develop from external pressure that compresses blood vessels or from friction and shearing forces that tear and injure vessels. Both types of pressure cause traumatic injury and initiate the process of pressure ulcer development.

External pressure that is greater than capillary pressure and arteriolar pressure interrupts blood flow in capillary beds. When pressure is applied to skin over a bony prominence for 2 hours, tissue ischemia and hypoxia from external pressure cause irreversible tissue damage. For example, when the body is in the supine position, the body's weight applies pressure to the sacrum. The same amount of pressure causes more damage when it is applied to a small area than when it is distributed over a large surface.

Shearing forces result when one tissue layer slides over another. The stretching and bending of blood vessels cause injury and thrombosis. Clients in hospital beds are subject to shearing forces when the head of the bed is elevated and the torso slides down toward the foot of the bed. Pulling the client up in bed also subjects the client to shearing forces. (For this reason, always lift clients up in bed.) In both cases, friction and moisture cause the skin and superficial fascia to remain fixed to the bed sheet, while the deep fascia and bony skeleton slides in the direction of body movement.

When a person lies or sits in one position for an extended length of time without moving, pressure on the tissue between a bony prominence and the external surface of the body distorts

capillaries and interferes with normal blood flow. If the pressure is relieved, blood flow to the area increases, and a brief period of reactive hyperemia occurs without permanent damage. However, if the pressure continues, platelets aggregate in the endothelial cells surrounding the capillaries and form microthrombi. These microthrombi impede blood flow, resulting in ischemia and hypoxia of tissues. Eventually, the cells and tissues of the immediate area of pressure and of the surrounding area die and become necrotic.

Alterations in the involved tissue depend on the depth of the injury. Injury to superficial layers of skin results in blister formation, whereas injury to deeper structures causes the pressure ulcer area to appear dark reddish-blue. As the tissues die, the ulcer becomes an open wound that may be deep enough to expose the bone. The necrotic tissue elicits an inflammatory response, and the client experiences increases in temperature, pain, and white blood cell count. Secondary bacterial invasion is common. Enzymes from bacteria and macrophages dissolve necrotic tissue, resulting in a foul-smelling drainage.

Pressure ulcers are graded or staged to classify the degree of damage. The stages are listed in Box 16–9.

RISK FACTORS Although a pressure ulcer may develop in an adult of any age who has an impairment in mobility, those most at risk are older adults with limited mobility, people with quadriplegia, and clients in the critical care setting (Porth, 2005). Other clients prone to develop pressure ulcers are those with fractures of large bones (e.g., hip or femur) or who have undergone orthopedic surgery or sustained spinal cord injury. In addition to deficits in mobility and activity, incontinence and nutritional deficit also increase the risk of pressure ulcer development. Clients with chronic illnesses, such as renal failure and anemia, and those with edema or infection are also at increased risk.

The older adult is at increased risk for the development of pressure ulcers because of age-related skin changes. The skin of the older adult has a thicker epidermis, a thinner dermis with decreased vascularity, decreased sebaceous gland activity, and decreased strength and elasticity. As a result, the more fragile and less nourished dermal layer is more prone to shear and friction problems. In addition, the skin of the older adult responds more slowly to inflammation, and wounds heal more slowly; when pressure ulcers occur, they are more difficult to reverse. See Nursing Care of the Older Adult on page 474 for information about preventing pressure ulcer development in older adults.

INTERDISCIPLINARY CARE

For the client at risk for pressure ulcers, the goal is prevention. Existing ulcers require interdisciplinary treatment to promote healing and restore skin integrity.

Diagnosis

Diagnostic tests are conducted to determine the presence of a secondary infection and to differentiate the cause of the ulcer. If the ulcer is deep or appears infected, drainage or biopsied tissue is cultured to determine the causative organism.

BOX 16–9 **Pressure Ulcer Staging**

STAGE I		Nonblanchable erythema of intact skin; the heralding lesion of skin ulceration. Identification of stage I pressure ulcers may be difficult in clients with darkly pigmented skin. *Note:* Reactive hyperemia can normally be expected to be present for one-half to three-fourths as long as the pressure occluded blood flow to the area. This should not be confused with stage I pressure ulcer.
STAGE II		Partial-thickness skin loss involving epidermis and/or dermis. The ulcer is superficial and presents clinically as an abrasion, blister, or shallow crater.
STAGE III		Full-thickness skin loss involving damage or necrosis of subcutaneous tissue that may extend down to, but not through, underlying fascia. The ulcer presents clinically as a deep crater with or without undermining of adjacent tissue.
STAGE IV		Full-thickness skin loss with extensive destruction, tissue necrosis, or damage to muscle, bone, or supporting structures (for example, tendon or joint capsule). Sinus tracts may also be associated with stage IV ulcers. *Note:* When eschar is present, accurate staging of the pressure ulcer is not possible until the eschar has sloughed or the wound has been debrided.

Source: Text is from *Pressure Ulcers in Adults: Prediction and Prevention* by the Agency for Health Care Policy and Research, 1992 Rockville, MD: U.S. Department of Health and Human Services. Photos courtesy of Karen Lou Kennedy, RN, FPN, www.kennedyterminalulcer.com.

Medications

Topical and systemic antibiotics specific to the infectious organism eradicate any infection present. Additionally, a variety of topical products promote healing. Examples are listed in Table 16–4.

Surgical Treatment

Surgical debridement may be necessary if the pressure ulcer is deep; if subcutaneous tissues are involved; or if an eschar (a scab or dry crust that forms over skin damaged by burns, infections, or excoriations) has formed over the ulcer, preventing healing by granulation. Large wounds may require skin grafting for complete closure.

NURSING CARE

The client with one or more pressure ulcers not only has impaired skin integrity but also is at increased risk for

NURSING CARE OF THE OLDER ADULT   Pressure Ulcer Prevention

Older adults are at a greater risk for developing pressure ulcers because of age related changes in the integumentary system. Cell renewal slows, resulting in skin that has decreased elasticity. The margin between the epidermis and the dermis separates more easily making the skin more prone to tearing. In addition, thinning subcutaneous tissue provides less cushioning over bony prominences. Water content decreases, and the skin becomes drier. These changes increase the older adult's susceptibility to skin trauma and prolong wound healing.

Chronic conditions associated with immobility and self-care deficit place older adults at risk of developing pressure ulcers. For example, bowel or bladder incontinence can produce regions of wet skin that are prone to infections and breakdown. Furthermore, sensory-perceptual alterations and impaired cognitive functioning may reduce the frequency with which the older adult shifts position when sitting or lying in bed. Finally, undernutrition, which is often seen in older adults, heightens the risk for developing pressure ulcers.

To prevent pressure ulcers, the skin of older adults should be kept clean, dry, and well hydrated. Moisturizers are recommended to keep the skin free of excessive dryness. Older adults should be taught to avoid bumping into furniture and to wear long skirts or pants to help protect the lower extremities from trauma.

When hospitalized, older adults should have a validated risk assessment for pressure ulcers completed on admission and as often as the tool suggests. A daily systematic skin inspection with particular attention to bony prominences should be completed.

Once pressure ulcers develop in older adults, the treatment is the same as for younger clients. However, additional steps may need to be taken. Because local perfusion to tissues is compromised, steps should be taken to prevent under- or overhydration. It is essential that optimal nutritional status be maintained. Also, keep in mind that it may take a longer time for the pressure ulcer to heal.

infection, pain, and decreased mobility. Pressure ulcers prolong treatment for other health problems, increase healthcare costs, and diminish the client's quality of life. See the Nursing Research box on the following page for information on evidence-based interventions.

Nursing Diagnoses and Interventions

The following interventions and rationales are adapted from the clinical guidelines developed by the Agency for Health Care Policy and Research (1992, 1994) in identifying adults at risk and treating those with stage I pressure ulcers.

Risk for Impaired Skin Integrity

- Identify at-risk individuals needing prevention and the specific factors placing them at risk.
- Assess bed- and chair-bound clients, as well as those who are unable to reposition themselves, for additional risk factors: immobility, incontinence, nutritional factors (such as inadequate dietary intake and impaired nutritional status), and altered level of consciousness.
- Assess clients on admission to acute care and rehabilitation hospitals, nursing homes, home care programs, and other healthcare facilities.

TABLE 16–4 Products Used to Treat Pressure Ulcers

STAGE	PRODUCT	PURPOSE
I	Skin Prep	Toughens intact skin and preserves skin integrity.
	Granulex	Prevents skin breakdown, increases blood supply, adds moisture, contains trypsin to aid in removal of necrotic tissue.
	Hydrocolloid dressing (e.g., DuoDerm)	Prevents skin breakdown and promotes healing without the formation of a crust over the ulcer. Is permeable to air and water vapor; prevents the growth of anaerobic organisms.
	Transparent dressing (e.g., Tegaderm)	Prevents skin breakdown; prevents entrance of moisture and bacteria but allows oxygen and moisture vapor permeability.
II	Transparent dressing	Enhances healing (see above).
	Hydrocolloid dressing	Enhances healing (see above). *Note*: If infection is present, these types of dressings are contraindicated. A sterile dressing should be applied instead.
III	Wet-to-dry gauze dressing with sterile normal saline	Allows necrotic material to soften and adhere to the gauze, so that the wound is debrided.
	Hydrocolloid dressing	Enhances healing (see above).
	Proteolytic enzymes (such as Elase)	Proteolytic enzymes serve as a debriding agent in inflamed and infected lesions.
IV	Wet-to-dry gauze dressing with sterile normal saline	Enhances healing (see above). *Note*: Transparent or hydrocolloid dressings or skin barriers are contraindicated.
	Vacuum-assisted closure (V.A.C.)	Creates a negative pressure to help reduce edema, increase blood supply and oxygenation, and decrease bacterial colonization. Also helps promote moist wound healing and the formation of granulation tissue.

NURSING RESEARCH   **Evidence-Based Practice for Treating Pressure Ulcers**

Despite advances in health care to extend life and improve functional status, older adults with chronic illnesses are at increased risk of developing pressure ulcers. The older adult, with age-related compromised cellular activity, is especially vulnerable to impaired healing of injured tissue such as pressure ulcers. This article (Frantz, 2004) describes an evidence-based protocol designed to enhance the healing of pressure ulcers in older clients by using evidence-based interventions. The following interventions are recommended:

- Assess all individuals admitted to a healthcare facility with a pressure ulcer for the risk of developing additional pressure ulcers by using a standardized risk assessment scale.
- Perform a complete history and physical examination, combined with a detailed assessment of the ulcer characteristics (location, stage, type of tissue, presence of tunneling or tracts, exudate, odor, and condition of skin around the ulcer).
- Remove necrotic tissue and debris from the ulcer to decrease the growth of bacteria and remove foreign materials, such as exudates and metabolic wastes.
- Provide a moist wound environment to promote reepithelialization and healing.
- Control bacterial levels in the wound by using cleansing and debridement, as well as systemic and topical antibiotics.
- Supply essential substrates for tissue repair, including protein, calories, vitamins, and minerals. Maintain a positive nitrogen balance.

- Manage tissue loads by positioning to avoid external force on the ulcer.

IMPLICATIONS FOR NURSING
The design and implementation of a pressure ulcer prevention and treatment plan is essential for any person at risk, including older adults, those with debilitating or multiple illnesses, and those with health problems limiting mobility. To effectively implement a plan, it is important to prepare providers to use a standard protocol through educational programs, and to monitor indicators of improvement or deterioration in the ulcer and presence or absence of new ulcers. These outcomes should be assessed and recorded on a weekly basis.

CRITICAL THINKING IN CLIENT CARE
1. Describe the differences and similarities in a pressure ulcer prevention plan of care you would develop for two clients: a 76-year-old man in a nursing home who has had a stroke that paralyzed his left side, and a 36-year-old man with a spinal cord injury from a motorcycle crash who cannot walk and lives at home.
2. Consider the activities to treat pressure ulcers. What would you do about the following:
   a. What level of healthcare provider would you delegate to care for the client?
   b. How much time in an 8-hour period would be needed for nursing care?
   c. What would you teach family caregivers about providing care at home?

Source: Franz, R. (2004). Treatment of pressure ulcers. *Journal of Gerontological Nursing, 30*(5), 4–10.

- Conduct a systematic risk assessment by using a validated risk assessment tool (such as the Braden scale).
- Document all assessments of risk. *Individuals at risk for pressure ulcers must be identified so that risk factors can be reduced through intervention. The primary risk factors for pressure ulcers are immobility and limited activity; therefore, assess clients who cannot reposition themselves or whose activity is limited to bed or chair. Validated tools ensure systematic evaluation of individual risk factors. The client requires periodic reassessment for pressure ulcers. Accurate and complete documentation of all risk assessments ensures continuity of care and may be used as a foundation for the skin care plan.*
- Conduct a systematic skin inspection at least once a day, paying particular attention to the bony prominences. Systematic, comprehensive, and routine skin care may decrease pressure ulcer incidence (although the exact role is unknown). Inspect the following to assess a pressure ulcer:
  - Location of any lesion or ulcer
  - Estimation of the stage
  - Dimensions of the ulcer: length, width, depth
  - Presence of any abnormal pathways in the wound:
    - Sinus tract: a cavity or channel underneath the wound
    - Tunneling: a passageway or opening that may be visible at skin level, but with most of the tunnel under the surface of the skin

- Undermining: areas of tissue destruction underneath intact skin along wound margins
- Visible necrotic tissue (Slough is necrotic tissue that is in the process of separating from viable tissue.)
- Presence of an exudate
- Presence or absence of granulation tissue

Skin inspection provides data the nurse uses in designing interventions to reduce risk and in evaluating outcomes of those interventions.

- Clean the skin at the time of soiling and at routine intervals, as frequently as the client's need or preference dictates. Avoid hot water, use a mild cleansing agent, and clean the skin gently, applying as little force and friction as possible. *Metabolic wastes and environmental contaminants accumulate on the skin; these potentially irritating substances should be removed frequently. Feces and urine cause chemical irritation and should be removed as soon as possible. Hot water may cause skin injury. Mild cleansing agents are less likely to remove the skin's natural barrier.*
- Minimize environmental factors leading to skin drying, such as low humidity and exposure to cold. Treat dry skin with moisturizers. *Well-hydrated skin resists mechanical trauma. Hydration decreases as the ambient air temperature decreases, especially when the air humidity is low. Poorly hydrated skin is less pliable, and severe dryness is associated with fissuring and cracking of the stratum corneum. Moisturizers reduce dry skin.*

- Avoid massage over bony prominences. *Although massage has been practiced for years, evidence now suggests that massage over bony prominences may lead to deep tissue trauma in clients at risk for, or with beginning, skin manifestations of a pressure ulcer.*
- Minimize skin exposure to moisture due to incontinence, perspiration, or wound drainage. When these sources of moisture cannot be controlled, use underpads or briefs made of materials that absorb moisture and present a quick-drying surface to the skin. Change underpads and briefs frequently. Do not place plastic directly against the skin. *Moisture from incontinence, perspiration, or wound drainage may contain factors that irritate the skin; moisture alone can increase the susceptibility of the skin to injury.*
- To minimize skin injury due to friction and shearing forces, use proper positioning, transferring, and turning techniques. Lubricants (such as cornstarch or creams), protective films (such as transparent dressings and skin sealants), protective dressings (such as hydrocolloids), and protective padding may also reduce friction injuries. *Shear injury occurs when skin remains stationary and the underlying tissue shifts. This shift diminishes the blood supply to the skin and results in ischemia and tissue damage. Proper positioning, however, can eliminate most shear injuries. Friction injuries to the skin occur when it moves across a coarse surface, such as bed linens. Most friction injuries can be avoided by using appropriate techniques to move clients so that their skin is never dragged across the linens. Any agent that eliminates contact or decreases the friction between the skin and the linens reduces the potential for injury.*
- Assess factors involved in inadequate dietary intake of protein or kilocalories. Offer nutritional supplements, and support the client during mealtimes. If dietary intake remains inadequate, consult with a dietitian about other dietary interventions. *The role nutrition plays in the development of (and to a lesser degree, the healing of) pressure ulcers is not understood, but poor dietary intake of kilocalories, protein, and iron has been associated with the development of pressure ulcers.*
- Maintain the client's current level of activity, mobility, and range of motion. *Frequent turning, repositioning, and movement are essential in reducing the risk of pressure ulcers.*
- For the client on bed rest or who is immobile, provide interventions against the adverse effects of external mechanical forces of pressure, friction, and shear:
  - Reposition all at-risk clients at least every 2 hours, using a written schedule for systematic turning and repositioning.
  - For clients on bed rest, use positioning devices, such as pillows or foam wedges, to protect bony prominences.
- For completely immobile clients, use devices to totally relieve pressure on the heels (the most common method is to raise the heels off the bed). Do not use donut-type devices.
- Avoid placing clients in the side-lying position directly on the trochanter.
- Maintain the head of the bed at the lowest degree of elevation consistent with the client's medical condition and other restrictions. Limit the amount of time the head of the bed is elevated.

- Use assistive devices, such as a trapeze or bed linen, to move clients in bed who cannot assist during transfers and position changes.
- Place any at-risk client on a pressure-reducing device, such as foam, static air, alternating air, gel, or water mattress. *Data indicate that the more spontaneous movements that bedridden, older adult clients make, the lower the incidence of pressure ulcers. Studies reveal that fewer pressure ulcers develop in at-risk clients who are turned every 2 to 3 hours. Proper positioning can reduce pressure on bony prominences. It is difficult to redistribute pressure under heels; suspending the heels is the best method. Do not use donut cushions, which are more likely to cause than to prevent pressure ulcers. Shearing forces are exerted on the body when the head of the bed is elevated. Lifting (rather than dragging) is less likely to cause injury from friction. Pressure-reducing devices and beds can decrease the incidence of pressure ulcers.*
- For chair-bound clients, use pressure-reducing devices. Consider postural alignment, distribution of weight, balance and stability, and pressure relief when positioning these clients. Avoid uninterrupted sitting in a chair or wheelchair. Reposition the client every hour. Teach clients who can do so to shift their weight every 15 minutes. Use a written plan for positioning, movement, and the use of positioning devices. Do not use donut devices. *Prolonged, uninterrupted mechanical pressure results in tissue breakdown. The client's weight should be shifted at least every hour.*

Community-Based Care

Client and family teaching for care of a pressure ulcer also focuses on prevention and includes much of the same information presented in the preceding section. Because many clients with pressure ulcers are older or have other serious illnesses, a caregiver may require teaching on such topics as the following:

- Definition and description of pressure ulcers
- Common locations of pressure ulcers
- Risk factors for the development of pressure ulcers
- Skin care
- Ways to avoid injury
- Diet.

Depending on the stage of the pressure ulcer, the nurse teaches the client or caregiver how to care for ulcers that are already present: how to change dressings, apply skin barriers, and avoid injury and infection. Referrals to a home health agency or community health department can help the family through the lengthy healing process.

THE CLIENT WITH FROSTBITE

Frostbite is an injury of the skin from freezing. If the exposure to freezing temperatures is limited, only the skin and subcutaneous tissues become involved. However, as exposure increases, deeper structures freeze. The skin freezes when the temperature drops to 14° to 24.8°F (210° to 24°C). Frostbite is most common on exposed or peripheral areas of the body, such as the nose, ears, feet, and hands.

As human tissues freeze, ice crystals form and increase intracellular sodium content. Small blood vessels initially vasoconstrict but then vasodilate and become more permeable, causing cellular and tissue swelling. With continued exposure, vasoconstriction and increased viscosity of the blood cause infarction and necrosis of the affected tissue.

Superficial frostbite causes numbness, itching, and prickling. The skin appears cyanotic, reddened, or white. Deeper frostbite causes stiffness and paresthesias. As the skin and tissues thaw, the skin becomes white or yellow and loses its elasticity. The client experiences burning pain. Edema, blisters, necrosis, and gangrene may appear.

Rapid thawing may significantly decrease tissue necrosis. General guidelines for rewarming areas of frostbite follow:

- If you are outdoors, treat superficial frostbite by applying firm pressure with a warm hand or by placing frostbitten hands in the axillae. If the feet are frostbitten, remove wet footwear, dry the feet, and put on dry footwear. Do not rub the areas with snow.
- In the hospital, rapidly rewarm affected areas in circulating warm water, 104° to 105°F (40° to 40.5°C) for 20 to 30 minutes. Do not rub or massage the areas.

Following rewarming, the client is kept on bed rest with the affected parts elevated. Pain medications and anti-inflammatory agents are administered. Blisters are debrided. Whirlpool therapy may be used to clean the skin and debride necrotic tissue. Recovery from frostbite is usually complete if the involved area has not become necrotic. Necrotic tissue may require amputation.

THE CLIENT UNDERGOING CUTANEOUS AND PLASTIC SURGERY

Although many skin disorders are so small and benign that no treatment is necessary, others require some type of surgery of the skin to remove the lesion. Other surgeries and treatments for skin lesions and deformities are used to restore function and change appearance. This section discusses both cutaneous and plastic surgery, as well as other types of treatment modalities used in the care of the client with a skin disorder.

Cutaneous Surgery and Procedures

The basic types of cutaneous surgery described here are excision, electrosurgery, cryosurgery, curettage, and laser surgery. Two nonsurgical procedures, chemical destruction and sclerotherapy, are also discussed. Most of these procedures are performed in the caregiver's office or outpatient clinic.

Fusiform Excision

Fusiform excision is the removal of a full thickness of the epidermis and dermis, usually with a thin layer of subcutaneous tissue. It is used to remove tissue for biopsies and for complete removal of benign and malignant lesions of the skin. Most fusiform excisions have a length-to-width ratio of 3 to 1.

Excision of small, superficial lesions is performed under a local anesthetic, and care is taken to place the incision in a way that will provide good cosmetic results. The incision line is usually closed with sutures, and the wound is covered with a dry dressing, an occlusive dressing, or a hydrocolloid dressing.

Electrosurgery

Electrosurgery involves the destruction or removal of tissue with high-frequency alternating current. A variety of surgical procedures may be performed, including *electrodesiccation* (which produces superficial skin destruction), *electrocoagulation* (which produces deeper tissue destruction), and *electrosection* (which can cut through skin and tissue). Electrodesiccation is used to remove benign surface lesions, such as skin tags, keratoses, warts, and angiomas. It is also used to produce hemostasis for capillary bleeding. Electrocoagulation is used to remove telangiectases, warts, and superficial nonmelanoma skin cancers. Electrosection is used to make incisions, excise tissue, and perform biopsies.

Cryosurgery

Cryosurgery is the destruction of tissue by cold or freezing with agents such as fluorocarbon sprays, carbon dioxide snow, nitrous oxide, and liquid nitrogen. Cryosurgery is used to treat many skin lesions (e.g., keratoses, lentigo maligna, venous lakes, nevi, keloids, and Kaposi's sarcoma). The freezing agents are applied topically to the lesion.

The effects of freezing depend on the degree of freeze. Light freezing causes damage to the epidermis with blistering or crusting that heals without scarring. Deeper freezes, used to treat malignant cells, cause edema, necrosis, and tissue slough. The effects of cryosurgery may not be obvious until 24 hours following treatment. Postoperatively, infection is prevented by applying a topical antibiotic and keeping the treated areas clean. Healing occurs in 2 to 3 weeks.

Curettage

Curettage is the removal of lesions with a curette (a semisharp cutting instrument). The design of the curette allows it to cut through soft or weak tissue, but not through normal tissue. It is used primarily to remove benign and malignant superficial epidermal lesions. Benign lesions removed by curettage include keratoses, nevi, and angiomas. Nonmelanoma skin lesions are removed by curettage if they are small, well-defined, primary tumors. Curettage is also used to remove specimens of tissue for biopsy.

Following curettage, the wound may be treated with electrodesiccation to destroy any remaining malignant cells and to provide hemostasis. These wounds are not closed; rather, they are left open to heal by second intention. Topical antibiotic ointments and dressings may be used in the postoperative period.

Laser Surgery

Laser surgery is used to treat clients with a wide variety of skin disorders, including port-wine stains, telangiectases, and venous lakes. A laser is an intense light that produces a thermal injury on contact with tissue. The injury causes coagulation, vaporization, excision, and ablation (removal of a growth). Argon, pulsed dye, carbon dioxide, and Nd:YAG lasers are used in cutaneous and plastic surgery. A local anesthetic may be used, although the pulsed dye laser causes minimal pain and rarely requires anesthesia.

The response differs by type of laser. Following treatment with the argon laser, the lesion appears from white to black in color, a blister forms, and the skin may peel. The area weeps, and an eschar forms; in 10 to 14 days, the eschar separates, revealing an underlying red area. The redness fades over a period of up to 1 year. However, pulsed dye laser treatment does not result in blistering or weeping; only rarely does it result in eschar.

Chemical Destruction

Chemical destruction is the application of a specific chemical to produce destruction of skin lesions. Chemical destruction is used to treat both benign and premalignant lesions. The chemical is applied to the lesion or is used to cause peeling. After application, the treated area forms a thin crust that sloughs off in about a week.

Sclerotherapy

Sclerotherapy is the removal of benign skin lesions with a sclerosing agent that causes inflammation with fibrosis of tissue. Agents that cause therapeutic sclerosis include aethoxysclerol (Sclerodex) and hypertonic sodium chloride. This type of treatment is used for telangiectases and superficial spider veins of the lower extremities. The solution is injected into the affected veins, causing a reaction that closes the lumen of the vein.

Plastic Surgery

Plastic surgery is the alteration, replacement, or restoration of visible portions of the body, performed to correct a structural or cosmetic defect. The word *plastic* comes from the Greek word *plastikos,* which means "able to be molded."

Many skin disorders discussed in this chapter cause changes in appearance. For example, acne may leave deep pitting scars, nevi and keloids are often disfiguring, and skin cancers may require wide excision and skin grafting. These scars, lesions, and wounds often cause embarrassment and alterations in body image. In addition, the removal of lesions may leave unsightly scars or areas of obviously missing tissue.

Cosmetic surgery, also called aesthetic surgery, is one of two fields within plastic surgery. Cosmetic surgery enhances the attractiveness of normal features. Almost 11.5 million surgical and nonsurgical cosmetic procedures were performed in 2005 (American Society for Aesthetic Plastic Surgery, 2005). The top five procedures are liposuction, breast augmentation, eyelid surgery, rhinoplasty, and "tummy tuck." The other field, reconstructive surgery, uses similar techniques; however, its purpose is to improve the function or appearance of parts of the body damaged by trauma, disease, or birth defects.

Many of the plastic surgeries permanently alter body image. To provide the client with a preview of what surgery will accomplish, some surgeons integrate computer imaging into preoperative teaching. The computer projects a photograph of the targeted area onto a monitor and uses graphics to demonstrate how the size and/or shape of the body part or area will change as a result of the surgery.

Skin Grafts and Flaps

Skin grafts and flaps are used to restore function while also maintaining an acceptable appearance. Both of these procedures involve the movement of skin from one part of the body to another part.

A **skin graft** is a surgical method of detaching skin from a donor site and placing it in a recipient site, where it develops a new blood supply from the base of the wound. Skin grafting is an effective way to cover wounds that have a good blood supply, are not infected, and in which bleeding can be controlled.

Skin grafts may be either split thickness or full thickness (Figure 16–20 ■). A *split-thickness graft* contains epidermis and only a portion of dermis of the donor site. Split-thickness grafts range in thickness from 0.010 inch to greater than 0.015 inch. A common donor site for a skin graft is the anterior thigh. Skin is removed in sheets from the donor site with a dermatome. Donor sites of split-thickness grafts heal by reepithelialization. A meshed graft is a type of split-thickness graft that is rolled under a special cutting machine to form a mesh pattern with perforations. The perforations allow drainage of serum and blood from under the graft. After healing, however, the skin has a rough appearance. A *full-thickness graft* contains both epidermis and dermis. These layers contain the greatest number of skin elements (sweat glands, sebaceous glands, or hair follicles) and are best able to withstand trauma. Areas of thin skin are the best donor sites for full-thickness skin grafts. The donor site must be surgically closed and will scar.

Other types of grafts are composite grafts and cultured epithelial grafts. Composite grafts are usually used on the face. They contain skin, subcutaneous tissue, cartilage, or other tissue. Cultured epithelial grafts are made from epithelial cells cultured *in vivo,* coalesced into sheets, and then used to cover full-thickness wounds. They are used primarily to treat burns.

Figure 16–20 ■ Skin depth of split-thickness and full-thickness grafts.

A *skin flap* is a piece of tissue whose free end is moved from a donor site to a recipient site while maintaining a continuous blood supply through its connection at the base or pedicle. Flaps carry their own blood supply and are therefore used to cover recipient sites that have a poor blood supply or have sustained a major tissue loss. They are often used for reconstruction or closure of large wounds. Microsurgical techniques, with anastomosis of small blood vessels and nerves, allow reconstruction with free flaps (in which the flap is completely removed from its donor site and moved to the recipient site).

Chemical Peeling

Chemical peeling is the application of a chemical to produce a controlled and predictable injury that alters the anatomy of the epidermis and superficial dermis. The result is skin that appears firmer, smoother, and less wrinkled. This form of cosmetic surgery is more useful in people who have fair, thin skin with fine wrinkling.

Chemical agents used for peeling include phenol, trichloroacetic acid (TCA), and alpha-hydroxy acids (AHAs). Phenol, a keratocoagulant, penetrates the epidermis and dermis; regeneration of the epithelium produces the desired results. After treatment, the entire surface of the face except the eyelids is covered with adhesive tape for 1 to 2 days. The adhesive is then removed, and the treated area forms a crust that heals in about a week. TCA has been used for years to obtain the desired effect. A light peel causes mild erythema followed by peeling (as from a mild sunburn) in 3 to 5 days. AHAs are organic acids used to produce light to moderate peeling to remove acne, fine lines, seborrheic keratosis, warts, and mild scarring. Both TCA and AHA treatments may be repeated weekly. One complication of chemical peeling is bleaching of the skin (due to removal of melanocytes).

Liposuction

Liposuction is a method of changing the contours of the body by aspirating fat from the subcutaneous layer of tissue. This treatment is used to remove excess fat from the buttocks, flanks, abdomen, thighs, upper arms, knees, ankles, and chin. It is not a cure for obesity and should not be used as a substitute for weight loss. The procedure is usually done for younger clients because their skin is more elastic. Liposuction may be performed on either an outpatient or inpatient basis.

To aspirate the fat, a small incision is made close to the area, and a suction cannula or curette is inserted and attached to a suction apparatus. The high vacuum pressure caused by the suction machine causes fat cells to emulsify, and they are aspirated out of the body. Following removal of the fat, a pressure dressing is applied to help the skin conform to the new tissue size.

Dermabrasion

Dermabrasion is a method of removing facial scars, severe acne, and pigment from unwanted tattoos. The area is sprayed with a chemical to cause light freezing and is then abraded with sandpaper or a revolving wire brush to remove the epidermis and a portion of the dermis.

Facial Cosmetic Surgery

Many different reconstructive surgeries may be performed to correct deformities or improve cosmetic appearance. Those discussed here are rhinoplasty, blepharoplasty, and rhytidectomy (facelift).

- A *rhinoplasty* is conducted to improve the appearance of the external nose. The nasal skeleton is reshaped, and the overlying skin and subcutaneous tissue are allowed to redrape over the new framework. A submucous resection of the nasal septum is often done at the same time; this surgery resects a segment of the septal cartilage to improve the nasal airway and also to alter the appearance of the nose. This surgery is done through incisions within the nose, so no visible scars remain after healing.

- A *blepharoplasty* is a cosmetic surgery in which loose skin and protruding periorbital fat is removed from the upper and lower eyelids. With aging, the eyelid skin sags, allowing the periorbital fat to bulge; the skin of the upper eyelid can be so lax that it partially obstructs vision. The procedure is performed under local anesthesia, and excess skin and fat are excised. The incision is made in the normal eyelid lines so that scars are not visible after healing.

- A *rhytidectomy,* or facelift, is a cosmetic surgery done to improve appearance by removing excess skin (and sometimes fat) from the face and neck. As one ages, the skin of the face and neck tends to become loose and wrinkled. The procedure is usually performed with local anesthesia. To perform the surgery, bilateral incisions are made from the scalp at the temple, in front of the ear in the natural skin line, around the ear lobe, and to the occipital scalp. The skin is then elevated, fat is removed or suctioned, and excess skin is excised. The incision lines are sutured, and a pressure dressing is applied.

NURSING CARE

Nursing care for the client having cutaneous or plastic surgery is highly individualized. It depends on the type of surgery or procedure performed, the type of deficit treated, the reason for the surgery or procedure, the expected results of the treatment, and the response of the client to the lesion or surgery. Although some surgeries, such as skin grafts and flaps, require in-hospital care, many of the surgeries are carried out in the primary care setting, and the client provides self-care at home following or between treatments.

Nursing Diagnoses and Interventions

Although a variety of nursing diagnoses may be appropriate for the client having cutaneous or plastic surgery or procedures, the most common are *Impaired Skin Integrity, Acute Pain,* and *Disturbed Body Image.*

Impaired Skin Integrity

The client having surgery of the skin has impaired skin integrity. Skin grafts and flaps are performed to repair large wounds, and it is necessary to inflict further wounds to collect the graft or flap from a donor site. Excisions and various cosmetic surgeries cause wounds. Skin is traumatized by freezing, chemicals, abrasion, sclerosing agents, electrical currents, and lasers. Although all of these treatment modalities are conducted to remove lesions, improve function, or improve appearance, they first impair the integrity of the skin. These impairments increase the risk for infection, which would further impair the skin integrity and may negate the benefits of surgery.

Nurses provide preoperative care and teaching, intraoperative assistance, and postoperative care and teaching; in each case, care and teaching are specific to the type of surgical treatment and the individual client. In all cases, the nurse provides appropriate preoperative interventions to prepare the client physically and emotionally for surgery and the postoperative period.

The following interventions are appropriate for the client having inpatient skin grafts or flaps:

- Monitor incisions and grafts, and flap donor and recipient sites, for manifestations of infection and necrosis:
  - Take and record vital signs every 4 hours.
  - Monitor all wounds for changes in color, consistency, amount, and odor of drainage every 4 to 8 hours.
  - Monitor wounds for increased swelling, redness, and pain every 4 to 8 hours.
  - Monitor and document assessment of graft every 4 hours.
  - Monitor and document temperature, turgor, color, dermal bleeding, and capillary refill of flaps every 4 hours.

  When bacterial infection is present, the inflammatory phase of wound healing is prolonged, retarding healing. Increased body temperature and tachycardia are manifestations of infection. The drainage in wounds that become infected is often increased in amount, purulent, thicker, and has a musty or foul odor. Tissue response to infection includes edema, increased erythema, and pain. Grafts and flaps that do not have adequate blood supply will appear black instead of the normal pink-red color.

- Provide care for the donor site:
  - Position the client to minimize pressure on the donor site.
  - Use a bed cradle to keep linens off the area.
  - If the donor site is left open and a heat lamp is to be applied to the area, place the lamp no closer than 2 feet from the wound.
  - Avoid moving the body part containing the donor site, if possible.
  - If the donor site is on the posterior portion of the body, place the client on a special bed (such as a low-pressure or fluidized bed) to decrease pressure and allow air circulation around the donor site.

  Minimizing trauma from pressure and movement facilitates healing of the donor site. Leaving the site open to the air and providing heat increase healing. Special beds minimize ischemia and allow donor sites on the posterior side of the body to dry.

- Encourage a diet high in protein, ascorbic acid, vitamins, and minerals. *An adequate protein intake is necessary to supply amino acids for tissue repair. Vitamin C is necessary for collagen formation and wound strength. Vitamins and minerals contribute to the healing process.*

- Change dressings as prescribed, or if the frequency is not indicated, as necessary. Determine which dressings are not to be removed during the healing process and which are to be changed, and whether the wound is to be kept dry or moist.
  - Use aseptic technique and follow standard precautions when changing dressings.

- Remove old dressings carefully and gently.
- Choose the appropriate dressing materials.

Donor sites may be covered with an adherent gauze dressing that is allowed to dry and remains adherent through the healing process. Aseptic techniques prevent secondary bacterial infections. Standard precautions protect the nurse from HIV infection. Unless care is taken, the removal of adherent old dressings may damage the wound by traumatizing granulation tissue or wound edges. The use of semipermeable transparent dressings provides an environment that optimizes wound healing by promoting collagen synthesis and the formation of granulation tissue; it also increases cell migration and epithelial resurfacing and prevents the formation of scabs, crusts, and eschar.

Acute Pain

The client having a graft or flap has two wounds; in fact, the donor site may be more painful than the recipient site. Cutaneous surgeries, dermabrasions, and chemical treatments result in blistering, swelling, and loss of epidermal tissue. The client having facial reconstructive surgery has edema, with resultant pain.

- Administer pain medications on a regular basis, following guidelines for controlling pain in clients having operative procedures (see Chapter 9 ∞). *Established, severe pain is difficult to control and has negative physical and psychologic consequences.*

- Use alternative pain relief measures as appropriate and prescribed, such as ice bags or cold compresses. *Cold reduces swelling, acts as a local anesthetic, and decreases pain.*

- Teach noninvasive methods of pain relief, such as deep breathing, relaxation, and guided imagery. *Noninvasive methods of pain relief increase the effectiveness of pain medications and also allow the client some control and self-management of pain.*

Disturbed Body Image

Cosmetic surgery is performed for a variety of reasons in adult clients of all ages. Changes in appearance, especially in a society that values youth and beauty, affect one's self-perception. Lesions or scars, especially of the face, may decrease self-esteem and cause a person to avoid social interactions and relationships. With aging, the skin becomes looser and wrinkles appear; this can be a source of anxiety and despair, especially to the woman who has always prided herself on her youthful appearance. Most clients cite one reason for having plastic surgery: to "feel better about myself."

- Provide preoperative teaching:
  - Explain that bruising and swelling will be present and that it will be several weeks before these responses to surgery disappear.
  - Explain that it may take a year for healing to complete and the final results to appear.

  Expectations differ; many people expect immediate results. Knowledge of postoperative responses is necessary for the client to adapt to change. The client may need to make arrangements to take time off from work during the initial healing stage.

- Provide time for the client to verbalize feelings and concerns. Be empathetic, and listen nonjudgmentally. *Such nurse–client interaction facilitates acceptance of changes in body image.*
- Refer to a consultant who can provide information on the use of cosmetics and apparel to enhance personal appearance. *Knowledgeable use of cosmetics and clothing can make scars much less noticeable. If the client feels better about appearance, body image is improved.*

Community-Based Care

The nurse teaches the client and family to provide self-care at home after cutaneous and plastic surgery and procedures. The nurse asks about the client's expectations and stresses that final results will not be seen for several months, providing written instructions about the following topics:

- Wound care, including application of topical medications and dressing changes. If the client is to return to the office or clinic for removal of tape or pressure dressings, or for dressing

changes in the first weeks after surgery, an appointment is made. For some procedures, the wound is left open to the air.
- Manifestations of wound infection, such as increased temperature, malaise, changes in the appearance of the wound, or changes in drainage. If any of these manifestations occur, the client should notify the healthcare provider immediately.
- Specific care for the type of surgery or procedure, such as type of oral care, avoiding blowing the nose, or limiting talking.
- Limitations on physical activity, especially lifting or straining.
- When to resume bathing or showering, shampooing the hair, and using cosmetics.
- The need to avoid picking at crusts or scabs. If the healing wound itches, the client should contact the healthcare provider for a topical medication.
- Use of a 15 (or higher) SPF sunblock when the client is outdoors. This may be prescribed for several months or for the rest of the client's life.

HAIR AND NAIL DISORDERS

Disorders of the hair and nails are not serious threats to health, but they may cause embarrassment and a negative body image. Changes in hair growth and pattern as in nail growth and character occur as secondary responses to other illnesses or treatments and are also a part of the aging process.

THE CLIENT WITH A DISORDER OF THE HAIR

Racial characteristics and gender influence the amount and type of hair. Caucasians typically have more facial and body hair than do Asians. People of Mongolian or Native American descent usually have straight hair, those of African descent have wavy to curly hair, and Caucasians have straight to curly hair. In addition, male hair growth characteristics (such as facial hair and hair on the lower extremities) are normal in certain women of some races and families. Women do not normally become bald.

The hair grows at various rates. Facial hair grows the most rapidly, followed by the hair of the scalp, axillae, thighs, and eyebrows. Normally, an adult's hair grows at a rate of 10 to 12 mm per month; however, the growth rate is influenced by both the person's state of health and the environment (hair grows faster in hot climates, more slowly in cold climates).

Pathophysiology

Hair color, growth, and pattern vary from person to person, and they are determined largely by genetic inheritance. However, changes do occur. For example, in some instances, hair loss recurs in successive generations of males in a family; in other cases, hair loss may be the result of chemotherapy. Excessive facial hair may be a response to certain endocrine disorders or to the loss of estrogen after menopause. These changes may seem minor, but they may create psychosocial problems for the person experiencing the changes.

Hirsutism

Hirsutism, also called hypertrichosis, is the appearance of excessive hair in normal and abnormal areas of the body in women. Hirsutism most often occurs in a male distribution (that is, on the upper lip, chin, abdomen, and chest) in women. The excess hair is primarily the result of an increase in androgen levels (especially testosterone), which may be due to any of the following:

- Familial predisposition (considered normal)
- Polycystic ovary syndrome
- Ovarian, adrenal, or pituitary tumors
- Cushing's syndrome
- Central nervous system disorders
- Medications, such as minoxidil, cyclosporine, phenytoin, certain progestins, and anabolic steroids.

The manifestations of hirsutism include increased male pattern hair growth, acne, and menstrual irregularities. If the androgen excess is great, defeminization (a decrease in breast size and loss of normal adipose tissue) and virilization (frontal balding, increased muscle mass, deepening of the voice, and enlargement of the clitoris) may occur. Virilization indicates the presence of an androgen-producing tumor.

Alopecia

Alopecia is loss of hair, or baldness (Figure 16–21 ■). Alopecia may result from scarring, various systemic diseases, or genetic predisposition. Scarring from trauma, radiation, and severe bacterial, fungal, or viral infections causes permanent and irreversible hair loss over the scarred area. Systemic diseases that may cause alopecia include systemic lupus erythematosus, thyroid disorders, and pituitary insufficiency. The hair loss from these disorders may be reversible. Hair loss from androgenic causes may also occur in the postmenopausal woman. Alopecia may be drug induced and is a side effect of a variety of medications (Box 16–10).

Figure 16–21 ■ Alopecia (baldness) may be the result of scarring, disease, or genetic predisposition.

Types of alopecia follow:

- Male pattern baldness is the most common cause of alopecia in men and is genetically predetermined. The hair loss begins at the temples, with recession of the hairline and baldness of the crown.
- Female pattern alopecia begins in women in their 20s and 30s, with progressive thinning and loss of hair over the central part of the scalp. Unlike men, women do not lose hair from the frontal hairline. Many of these women have elevated adrenal androgens.
- Alopecia areata is characterized by round or oval bald patches on the scalp as well as on other hairy parts of the body. The cause is unknown. This type of alopecia is usually self-limiting and reverses without treatment, although it often recurs.
- Alopecia totalis is the loss of all hair on the scalp. This rare condition is irreversible.
- Alopecia universalis is the total loss of hair on all parts of the body.

INTERDISCIPLINARY CARE

Alopecia is diagnosed by assessing the appearance of the hair and hair loss and by assessing the client for other systemic diseases and the use of medications that may cause hair loss. Various treatments are used to restore hair.

BOX 16–10 Medications Causing Alopecia

- Thallium
- Retinoids
- Anticoagulants
- Antimitotic agents
- Antithyroid drugs
- Oral contraceptives
- Trimethadione
- Excessive use of vitamin A
- Allopurinol
- Propranolol
- Indomethacin
- Amphetamines
- Salicylates
- Levodopa
- Gentamicin
- Chemotherapy

The client with hirsutism is examined for hormone levels and indications of other systemic illnesses. Hirsutism is treated by addressing the underlying systemic disorder and stopping medications that may be causing the problem.

Diagnosis

Diagnostic tests that may be ordered for the woman with hirsutism include serum testosterone levels and an adrenal CT scan. Testosterone levels are measured, and levels greater than 200 ng/dL indicate the need for further tests, such as a pelvic examination and tests of ovarian function. Adrenal tumors, a possible cause of hirsutism, are identified with an adrenal CT scan.

Medications

Hirsutism is treated with medications specific to the underlying cause. Oral contraceptives containing estrogen decrease ovarian androgen production and decrease free testosterone levels. Dexamethasone (Decadron) may be prescribed for people with high cortisol levels. Ketoconazole (Nizoral) inhibits androgen production. Antiandrogenic medications cause congenital abnormalities in male infants and are therefore given only to nonpregnant women, who are cautioned to avoid pregnancy while taking the medications.

Male pattern baldness has been successfully treated with topical minoxidil (Loniten) or Rogaine, a commercial product that contains minoxidil. These drugs, which are vasodilators, stimulate vertex hair growth, probably by stimulating the epithelium of the hair follicle. These agents have been most successful in clients who have a recent onset of alopecia or are less than 50 years old. About 40% of clients treated two times a day for a year will have moderate to dense regrowth of hair at the temples (McPhee et al., 2007).

Surgery

Hair transplant techniques are used to restore hair or reduce the size of areas of alopecia. Other types of surgical procedures include scalp reduction and flaps.

- Transplanting hairs as small hair plugs or single hairs taken from the back or sides of the scalp is an effective means of replacing hair to areas of alopecia. This procedure is done in an outpatient office or clinic.
- Scalp reduction is done by excising a portion of the affected scalp. In some cases, a tissue expander (such as a silicone balloon) is first implanted under the scalp to enlarge the hair-bearing scalp so that larger areas of alopecia can be removed.
- Flaps from hair-bearing areas of the scalp can be surgically transplanted from adjacent areas into areas of alopecia. This procedure may be done in stages.

NURSING CARE

The client with either hirsutism or alopecia is often self-conscious about appearance and tries a variety of OTC treatments before seeking medical care. Nursing care for the client with hair disorders focuses on teaching the client self-care and providing support during long-term care. Women with hirsutism are taught to use various means of removing unwanted hair, such as shaving, applying depilatories, waxing, undergoing electrolysis, or having laser treatments. Women with mild hirsutism may bleach facial hair to make it less obvious. Clients with alopecia may wear hair pieces or wigs.

THE CLIENT WITH A DISORDER OF THE NAILS

Nail disorders may be due to systemic diseases, trauma, allergies, or irritants. They may also be congenital or genetic. Nails may be discolored, multicolored, malformed, infected, or separated from underlying tissue.

Pathophysiology

The nail disorders discussed here are separation of the nail, infection, and ingrown toenails:

- *Onycholysis* is the separation of the distal nail plate from the nail bed. It occurs most often in the fingernails. This disorder may result from many different factors, including excessive or prolonged exposure to water, soaps, detergent, alkalies, and industrial keratolytic agents; *Candida* infections; nail hardeners; and thyroid disorders. Prolonged application of false fingernails may also cause this disorder.
- A **paronychia** is an infection of the cuticle of the fingernails or toenails. The disorder often follows a minor trauma and secondary infection with staphylococci, streptococci, or *Candida*. The acute form begins with a painful inflammation that may progress to an abscess. The chronic form is seen most often in people who have frequent exposure to water. In the chronic form, the skin around the nail is painful, edematous, and infected. The nail plate may become ridged and discolored.

- An *onychomycosis* is a fungal or dermatophyte infection of the nail plate. The nail plate elevates and becomes yellow or white. Psoriasis infections of the nail plate cause the nails to pit.
- An *ingrown toenail (unguis incarnatus)* results when the edge of the nail plate grows into the soft tissue of the toe. Pain and infection may occur. The infection, if untreated, may spread to the bone. This disorder is especially dangerous for the person with diabetes mellitus or peripheral vascular disease.

INTERDISCIPLINARY CARE

The treatments of disorders of the nail vary from pharmacologic treatment to surgical removal. Infections of the nails are treated, depending on the causative agent, with antifungal or antibiotic medications. If the causative agent is a fungus or chronic dermatologic disorder, treatment is difficult and may not be effective. Persistently painful and/or infected nails are in some cases surgically removed.

NURSING CARE

Nursing care of the client with a disorder of the nail focuses on teaching self-care. Clients with nail disorders that are caused by frequent exposure to water are taught to protect the hands or feet by wearing rubber gloves or boots and to keep the nails as clean and dry as possible. Clients with ingrown toenails are cautioned not to cut into the lateral nail bed, but rather to soak the nail twice a day and insert a piece of cotton or gauze under the softened nail until the nail has grown out enough to trim.

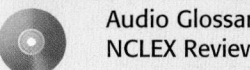

EXPLORE MEDIALINK

Prentice Hall Nursing MediaLink DVD-ROM
Audio Glossary
NCLEX Review

Animation/Video
Pressure Ulcers

COMPANION WEBSITE www.prenhall.com/lemone
Audio Glossary
NCLEX-RN® Review
Care Plan Activity: Pressure Ulcers
Case Study: Lesions and Pruritis
MediaLink Applications
Links to Resources

CHAPTER HIGHLIGHTS

- Pruritus (itching) accompanies dry skin (xerosis) and many skin disorders and may result in excoriation and infection as a result of scratching.
- Cysts, keloids, nevi, angiomas, skin tags, and keratoses are benign skin lesions. However, nevi should be monitored for changes indicating transformation into a malignant lesion.

- Psoriasis is a chronic immune skin disorder arising from keratinocytes. A variety of medications and treatments are used, with ultraviolet light therapy being most effective for generalized lesions.
- Skin disorders may be caused by a variety of bacterial infections, fungal infections, parasitic infestations, and viral infections.

The disorders are treated with a specific antibiotic, fungicide, antiviral agent, or agents that kill the parasites. Herpes zoster, believed to follow a childhood infection with chickenpox, causes acute pain.

- Inflammatory disorders of the skin range from mild dermatitis to potentially lethal toxic epidermal necrolysis. Acne, a disorder of the hair and sebaceous glands opening to the skin surface, is characterized by comedones, pustules, and cysts.
- Malignant skin disorders include actinic keratosis, nonmelanoma skin cancer (basal cell cancer and squamous cell cancer), and malignant melanoma skin cancer. Skin cancer is the most common malignancy found in fair-skinned Americans. Prevention by avoiding sunburn, using sunscreen, and maintaining monthly skin self-examination is critical in preventing loss of tissue or metastasis and death.
- Skin trauma may be intentional (as in the case of cutaneous and plastic surgery) or unintentional (as from trauma, frostbite, and pressure). Older adults with limited mobility, as well as clients who are unable to move or are in critical care units, are at greater risk for pressure ulcers. Prevention is the goal of both interdisciplinary and nursing care.
- Disorders of the hair include alopecia (loss of hair) and hirsutism (excess hair in women). Nails may be discolored, multicolored, malformed, infected, or separated from underlying tissue.

TEST YOURSELF NCLEX-RN® REVIEW

1 Your elderly client has severe xerosis. What topic should be included in your teaching plan?
   1. Take a hot bath every day.
   2. Use fabric softeners when laundering clothing.
   3. Apply skin lotions after a bath.
   4. Maintain a warm environment.

2 Which of the following common skin lesions has the potential of becoming malignant?
   1. nevi
   2. angiomas
   3. skin tags
   4. keloids

3 You have been asked to teach a woman with generalized psoriasis about ultraviolet light therapy (UVB). What should be included in teaching?
   1. "The exact effect of UVB is unknown, but it decreases severe itching."
   2. "When combined with hot baths, UVB is very effective."
   3. "Treatments with UVB have to be given in the hospital to be safe."
   4. "UVB slows the growth of epidermal cells and decreases keratosis."

4 Which of the following clients is at risk for the development of a candidiasis infection?
   1. an older adult with pruritus
   2. a young woman who is pregnant
   3. an older man with a premalignant skin condition
   4. a young man with multiple nevi

5 What question should be included in a health history of a client with a linear pattern of painful vesicles over the left thorax?
   1. Do you remember being sunburned as a child?
   2. Are you a regular patron of tanning booths?
   3. Have you ever been diagnosed with acne?
   4. Did you have chickenpox when you were young?

6 Which of the following statements is true of an infestation with lice?
   1. Only dirty people have lice.
   2. Anyone can have lice.
   3. Lice do not like to live on humans.
   4. Lice are a form of fungus.

7 Which assessments would indicate a greater risk to develop a nonmelanoma skin cancer?
   1. blond hair, freckles, fair skin
   2. alopecia, thin hair, itching
   3. dark hair, dark skin, dry skin
   4. tanned skin, dark hair, edema

8 Of the following, which is most significant to the development of a malignant melanoma?
   1. a change in the color or size of a nevus
   2. sexual contact with a person who has a herpes virus infection
   3. inadequate knowledge about infection prevention
   4. a dietary intake of high-calorie foods

9 The rationale for lifting, rather than pulling, a client up in bed is that:
   1. lifting a client allows a brief period of increased capillary circulation.
   2. lifting a client prevents tissue injury from shearing forces.
   3. pulling a client up in bed decreases tissue ischemia and hypoxia.
   4. pulling a client up in bed promotes capillary blood flow.

10 You are caring for a young adult with acne scars. He asks about treatment to reduce the scarring. Which of the following might you discuss?
   1. liposuction
   2. skin flap
   3. dermabrasion
   4. blepharoplasty

See Test Yourself answers in Appendix C.

BIBLIOGRAPHY

AARP. (2004). *Checkups and prevention. Skin cancer risks, treatments and prevention.* Retrieved from http://www.aarp.org/health-prevention/Articles/a2004-07-07-skincancer.html

Agency for Health Care Policy and Research. (1992). *Pressure ulcers in adults: Prediction and prevention.* Rockville, MD: USDHHS.

_____. (1994). *Treatment of pressure ulcers.* Rockville, MD: USDHHS.

Alexander, G. (2004). Selection of pressure relief mattresses for use in the home. *Journal of Community Nursing, 18*(6), 4, 6, 8.

American Academy of Dermatology. (2004). *2004 melanoma fact sheet.* Retrieved from http://www.aad.org/public/News/DermInfo/2004MelanomaFAQ.htm

American Cancer Society. (2003). *Skin cancer facts.* Retrieved from http://www.cancer.org/docroot/PED/content/ped_7_1_What_You_Need_To_Know_About_Skin_. . .

_____. (2004a). *Cancer facts and figures 2004.* Atlanta: Author.

_____. (2004b). *How many people get melanoma skin cancer?* Retrieved from http://www.cancer.org/docroot/CRI/content/CRI_2_2_IX_How_many_people_get_melanoma_ski. . .

_____. (2004c). *Radiation exposure and cancer.* Retrieved from http://www.cancer.org/docroot/PED/content/PED_1_3X_Radiation_Exposure_and_Cancer.asp?sit. . .

Baranoski, S. (2006). Pressure ulcers: A renewed awareness. *Nursing 2006, 36*(8), 36–42.

American Society for Aesthetic Plastic Surgery. (2005). *Cosmetic surgery quick facts: 2005 ASAPS statistics.* Retrieved from http://www.surgery.org/press/procedurefacts-asqf.php

Azziz, R. (2004). Women's health: Advances in the evaluation and treatment of unwanted hair growth. *Patient Care for the Nurse Practitioner, 38*(8), 23–28.

Barthel, D., & Crutchfield, C. (2004). Herpes zoster. *Dermatology Nursing, 16*(4), 362.

Bowman, J. (2004). Investigate all the options in skin care. *Professional Nurse, 19*(11), 43.

Brinker, D., Hancox, J., Bernardon, S., & Stull, D. (2003). Assessment and initial treatment of lacerations, mammalian bites, and insect stings. *AACN Clinical Issues: Advanced Practice in Acute and Critical Care, 14*(4), 401–410.

Britton, J. (2003). The use of emollients and their correct application. *Journal of Community Nursing, 17*(9), 22, 24–25.

Brown, J., Wimpenny, P., & Maughan, H. (2004). Skin problems in people with obesity. *Nursing Standard, 18*(35), 38–42.

Clark, A. (2003). The psychological impact of living with skin disease. *Professional Nurse, 18*(12), 689.

Dochterman, J., & Bulechek, G. (2004). *Nursing interventions classification (NIC)* (4th ed.). St. Louis, MO: Mosby.

FDA approves Enbrel to treat psoriasis. (2004). *Dermatology Nursing, 16*(5), 470–471.

Feller, A., Ariyan, S., & Heinrich, J. (2003). Skin cancer is on the rise: What you need to know about basal cell carcinoma, squamous cell carcinoma, and melanoma. *Surgical Physician Assistant, 9*(6), 9–18.

Frantz, R. (2004). Evidence-based protocol treatment of pressure ulcers. *Journal of Gerontological Nursing, 30*(5), 4–10.

Gorgos, D. (2004a). New laser therapy prevents acne from scarring. *Dermatology Nursing, 16*(5), 459.

_____. (2004b). Top 3 causes of hair disorders identified. *Dermatology Nursing, 16*(4), 367–368.

Gould, D., Goldstone, L., Kelly, D., & Gammon, J. (2004). Examining the validity of pressure ulcer risk scales: A replication study. *International Journal of Nursing Studies, 41*(3), 3331–3339.

Hainer, B., & Usatine, R. (2002). Electrosurgery for the skin. *American Family Physician, 66*(7), 1259–1266, 1147–1149.

Iyer, S., & Nunlely, J. (2003). Dermatologic look-alikes. Perplexing plaques. *Clinical Advisor, 6*(12), 81–83.

Jankowiak, B., Krajewska-Kulak, E., Van Damme-Ostapowicz, K., Wronska, I., Lukaszuk, C., Niczyporuk, W., et al. (2004). The need for health education among patients with psoriasis. *Dermatology Nursing, 16*(5), 439–444.

Kucera, K. (2004). Managing common skin problems in the elderly. *Clinical Advisor, 7*(6), 23–24, 27–30.

Lamanna, L. (2004). College students' knowledge and attitudes about cancer and perceived risk of developing skin cancer. *Dermatology Nursing, 16*(2), 161–164, 175–176.

Lapsley, P. (2003). The impact of skin diseases on people's lives. *Nurse2Nurse, 3*(10), 37–39.

McPhee, S., Papadakis, M., & Tierney, L. (2007). *Current medical diagnosis and treatment.* (46th ed.). New York: McGraw-Hill.

Moorhead, S., Johnson, M., & Maas, M. (2003). *Nursing outcomes classification (NOC)* (3rd ed.). St. Louis, MO: Mosby.

Norman, R. (2001). Causes and management of xerosis and pruritus in the elderly. *Annals of Long-Term Care, 9*(12), 35–40.

North American Nursing Diagnosis Association. (2005). *Nursing diagnoses: Definitions & classification 2005–2006.* Philadelphia: Author.

Peate, W. (2002). Occupational skin disease. *American Family Physician, 66*(6), 1025–1032, 1039–1040.

Porth, C. (2005). *Pathophysiology: Concepts of altered health states* (7th ed.). Philadelphia: Lippincott.

Price, L. (2004). Lentigo maligna melanoma. *Dermatology Nursing, 16*(5), 454.

Ravellla, P. (2004). Dry skin treatment. *Clinical Advisor, 7*(3), 86.

Rolewski, S. (2003). Topical retinoids. *Dermatology Nursing, 15*(5), 447–450, 459–465.

Seavolt, M., & Tomecki, K. (2003). Treatment of common cutaneous infections in the long-term care setting. *Annals of Long-Term Care, 11*(5), 48–52.

Sunscreen: From buying to applying. (2004). *Mayo Clinic Health Letter, 22*(5), 6.

Tan, H., & Goh, C. (2001). Parasitic skin infections in the elderly: Recognition and drug treatment. *Drugs & Aging, 18*(3), 165–176.

Thompson, H. (2004). Sun & skin cancer. *Practice Nurse, 28*(1), 40, 43–45.

Tinea types: Common dermatophyte infections. (2004) *Consultant, 44*(2), 217–218, 221–222, 225–226.

Tolmie, E., & Smith, L. (2002). A study of the prevention and management of pressure sores. *Clinical Effectiveness in Nursing, 6*(3), 111–120.

Tosanger, M., & Crutchfield, C. (2004a). Atrophic lichen planus. *Dermatology Nursing, 16*(1), 73–74.

_____. (2004b). Tinea corporis. *Dermatology Nursing, 16*(5), 453.

Trent, J., Federman, D., & Kirsner, R. (2003). Skin and wound biopsy: When, why, and how. *Advances in Skin & Wound Care, 16*(7), 372–375.

U.S. Preventive Services Task Force. (2004). Counseling to prevent skin cancer: Recommendations and rationale. *American Journal for Nurse Practitioners, 8*(3), 25–27, 31–32.

WebMD. (2006). FDA approves first shingles vaccine. Retrieved from http://www.webmd.com/content/Article/122/114846.htm.

Wilkinson, J. (2005). *Prentice Hall nursing diagnosis handbook with NIC interventions and NOC outcomes* (8th ed.). Upper Saddle River, NJ: Prentice Hall.

Wilson, B., Shannon, M., & Stang, C. (2005). *Prentice Hall nurse's drug guide 2005.* Upper Saddle River, NJ: Prentice Hall.

Wipke-Tevis, D., Williams, D., Rantz, M., Popejoy, L., Madsen, R., Petroski, G., et al. (2004). Nursing home quality and pressure ulcer prevention and management practices. *Journal of the American Geriatrics Society, 52*(4), 583–588.

Yarbo, C., Frogge, M, Goodman, M., & Groenwald, S. (Eds.). (2005). *Cancer nursing: Principles and practice* (6th ed.). Sudbury, MA: Jones & Bartlett.

Yosipovitch, G., & Hundley, J. (2004). Practical guidelines for relief of itch. *Dermatology Nursing, 16*(4), 325–328.

CHAPTER 17
Nursing Care of Clients with Burns

LEARNING OUTCOMES

- Discuss the types and causative agents of burns.
- Explain burn classification by depth and extent of injury.
- Describe the pathophysiology, interdisciplinary care, and nursing care for the client with a minor burn.
- Discuss the systemic pathophysiologic effects of a major burn and the stages of burn wound healing.
- Explain the interdisciplinary care and nursing implications necessary during the emergent/resuscitative stage, the acute stage, and the rehabilitative stage of a major burn.

CLINICAL COMPETENCIES

- Assess functional health status of clients with burns, and monitor, document, and report abnormal manifestations.
- Use evidence-based research to plan and implement nursing care for clients with burns.
- Determine priority nursing diagnoses, based on assessed data, to select and implement individualized nursing interventions for client with burns.
- Administer medications knowledgeably and safely to clients with burns.
- Integrate interdisciplinary care into care of clients with burns.
- Provide teaching appropriate for prevention of burns.
- Revise plan of care as needed to provide effective interventions to promote, maintain, or restore functional health status to clients with burns.

MEDIALINK

Resources for this chapter can be found on the Prentice Hall Nursing MediaLink DVD accompanying this textbook, and on the Companion Website at http://www.prenhall.com/lemone

A **burn** is an injury resulting from exposure to heat, chemicals, radiation, or electric current. A transfer of energy from a source of heat to the human body initiates a sequence of physiologic events that in the most severe cases leads to irreversible tissue destruction. Burns range in severity from a minor loss of small segments of the outermost layer of the skin to a complex injury involving all body systems. Treatments vary from simple application of a topical antiseptic agent in an outpatient clinic to an invasive, multisystem, interdisciplinary team approach in the aseptic environment of a burn center.

It is estimated that 1.1 million burn injuries that require medical intervention occur each year in the United States, and of those, about 45,000 require hospitalization with approximately 4500 of the burn injuries resulting in death (National Institute of General Medical Sciences, 2005). The home is the most common site for fire-related burns. Home fires cause 80% of all fire-related deaths, with about eight people dying in home fires each day. Most residential fires are caused by unattended cooking, which can lead to combustible grease catching fire and causing cabinets, wall coverings, curtains, paper or plastic bags, and other household items to burn. Smoking materials, including cigarettes, cigars, and pipes, are the leading cause of home fire deaths. Trash, followed by mattresses and upholstered furniture, are frequent ignited materials in the home.

FAST FACTS
Common Causes of Home Fires
- Cooking fires
- Smoking
- Heating equipment

Factors associated with deaths from burns are age (especially children under 5 and adults 65 and older), careless smoking, alcohol or drug intoxication, and physical and mental disabilities. A common source of burns in young children and older adults is from tap water scalds, whereas older children receive most burns from flame injuries. Older adults are more susceptible to deep burns from scalds because of their thinner skin. Fire injuries and deaths that occur among college-age students usually are due to alcohol use that impairs judgment and hampers escape (National Fire Protection Association, 2004). Occupations involving work with chemicals, gasoline, or electricity pose another risk factor. Abuse is suspected when scald burns show a clear line of demarcation, indicating deliberate immersion. The presence of small, circular burns may be from cigarette burns inflicted by an abuser.

Older adults are more vulnerable to fire and burn injury because of decreased visual acuity, depth perception, sense of smell, and hearing, in addition to impaired mobility. All of these factors increase the risk for accidentally starting a fire and diminish the ability to survive it.

FAST FACTS
Fire Deaths in Older Adults
- More than 1200 deaths in adults 65 and older occur each year.
- Leading causes of fire-related deaths are smoking, heating, and cooking.
- One-fifth of the deaths occur in bedridden or physically challenged older adults

Infants and older adults have a greater risk of mortality from burn injuries. Morbidity increases in clients with preexisting cardiac, pulmonary, or renal disorders, and diabetes mellitus. Clients who are alcoholics have lower survival rates of a major burn injury due to the development of more complications.

TYPES OF BURN INJURY

The four types of burn injury are thermal, chemical, electrical, and radiation. Although all four types can lead to generalized tissue damage and multisystem involvement, the causative agents and priority treatment measures are unique to each (Table 17–1).

Thermal Burns

Thermal burns result from exposure to dry heat (flames) or moist heat (steam and hot liquids). They are the most common burn injuries and occur most often in children and older adults. Direct exposure to the source of heat causes cellular destruction that can result in charring of vascular, bony, muscle, and nervous tissue.

Chemical Burns

Chemical burns are caused by direct skin contact with acids, alkaline agents, or organic compounds. More than 25,000 products found in the home or workplace can cause chemical burns. The chemical destroys tissue protein, leading to necrosis. Burns caused by alkalis (such as lye) are more difficult to neutralize

TABLE 17-1 Types, Causative Agents, and Priority Treatment Measures for Burns

TYPE	CAUSATIVE AGENT	PRIORITY TREATMENT
Thermal	Open flame Steam Hot liquids (water, grease, tar, metal)	Extinguish flame (stop, drop, and roll). Flush with cool water. Consult fire department.
Chemical	Acids Strong alkalis Organic compounds	Neutralize or dilute chemical. Remove clothing. Consult Poison Control Center.
Electrical	Direct current Alternating current Lightning	Disconnect source of current. Initiate CPR if necessary. Move to area of safety. Consult electrical experts.
Radiation	Solar (ultraviolet) X-rays Radioactive agents	Shield the skin appropriately. Limit time of exposure. Move the client away from the radiation source. Consult a radiation expert.

than are burns caused by acids. They also tend to have deeper penetration with a correspondingly more severe burn than from acid. Organic compound burns, such as by petroleum distillates, cause cutaneous damage through fat solvent action and may also cause renal and liver failure if absorbed.

Chemical agents are further classified according to the manner by which they structurally alter proteins. Oxidizing agents, such as household bleach, alter protein configuration through the chemical process of reduction. Corrosives, such as lye, cause extensive protein denaturation. Protoplasmic poisons, such as organic compounds, form salts with proteins, inhibiting calcium and other ions needed for cell viability. The severity of the chemical burn is related to the type of agent, the concentration of the agent, the mechanism of action, the duration of contact, and the amount of body surface area exposed. Box 17-1 lists household cleaning agents that may cause burns.

Electrical Burns

The severity of electrical burns depends on the type and duration of current, and amount of voltage. It is particularly difficult to assess the extent of the electrical burn injury, because the destructive processes initiated by the electrical insult are concealed and may persist for weeks beyond the time of the incident. It is challenging to assess the depth and extent of the burn, because electricity follows the path of least resistance, which in the human body tends to lie along muscles, bone, blood vessels, and nerves. Entry and exit wounds tend to be small, masking widespread tissue damage underneath the wound. Tissue necrosis results from impaired blood flow, secondary to blood coagulation at the site of the electrical injury. Because electrical burn wounds of the extremities often cause severe tissue necrosis, they frequently develop gangrene that necessitates amputation (Bishop, 2004).

Alternating current (AC), like that found in conventional households, produces repeated electrical surges that lead to tetanic muscle contractions. Such sustained muscle contractions inhibit respiratory efforts for the duration of contact and result in respiratory arrest. The contractions also cause the person to

BOX 17-1 Household Cleaning Agents That May Cause Burns

- Drain cleaners
- Lye
- Industrial-strength ammonia
- Household ammonia
- Oven cleaners
- Toilet bowl cleaners
- Dishwasher detergents
- Bleach

clamp down on the power source (such as an electrical cord) and thus may increase the duration of contact with the source. Direct current, as in injury from a lightning bolt, exposes the body to very high voltage for an instantaneous period of time. High-voltage (lightning) injury usually results in entry and exit wounds. The flashover effect, a phenomenon unique to lightning injury, actually saves the client from death. It is seen in those instances in which the current travels over the moist surface of the skin rather than through deeper structures. Cardiopulmonary arrest is the most common cause of death from lightning.

Radiation Burns

Radiation burns are usually associated with sunburn or radiation treatment for cancer. These kinds of burns tend to be superficial, involving only the outermost layers of the epidermis. All functions of the skin remain intact. Symptoms are limited to mild systemic reactions: headache, chills, local discomfort, nausea, and vomiting. More extensive exposure to radiation or radioactive substances, as in nuclear power accidents, leads to the same degree of tissue damage and multisystem involvement associated with other types of burns.

FACTORS AFFECTING BURN CLASSIFICATION

Tissue damage following a burn is determined primarily by two factors: depth of the burn (the layers of underlying tissue affected) and extent of the burn (the percentage of body surface area involved).

TABLE 17–2 **Characteristics of Burns by Depth**

CHARACTERISTIC	SUPERFICIAL	PARTIAL THICKNESS	FULL THICKNESS
Skin layers lost	Epidermis	Epidermis and dermis	Epidermis, dermis, and underlying tissues
Skin appearance over burn	Pink to red and dry; may have local edema	Fluid-filled blisters; bright pink or red with superficial partial-thickness burns	Waxy white; dry, leathery, charred
		Pale, mottled, waxy white with deep partial-thickness burns	
Skin function	Present	Absent	Absent
Pain sensation	Present	Present	Absent
Manifestations at the burn site	Pain; local edema	Severe pain; edema; weeping of fluid	Little pain; edema
Treatment	Regular cleaning	Regular cleaning	Regular cleaning
	Topical agent of choice	Topical agent of choice	Topical agent of choice
		May require skin grafting if deep partial-thickness burns present	Skin substitutes
			Excision of eschar
			Skin grafting
Scarring	None	May occur in deep burns	Of grafted area
Time to heal	3–6 days	14 to >21 days	Requires skin grafting to heal

Depth of the Burn

The depth of a burn injury is determined by the elements of the skin that have been damaged or destroyed. Burn depth results from a combination of the temperature of the burning agent and the length of contact. Burns are classified as either superficial, partial thickness, or full thickness. Characteristics of burns are described next, summarized in Table 17–2, and illustrated in Figure 17–1 ■.

Superficial Burns

A **superficial burn** involves only the epidermal layer of the skin. This type of burn most often results from damage from sunburn, ultraviolet light, minor flash injury (from a sudden ignition or explosion), or mild radiation burn associated with cancer treatment. Because the skin remains intact, this degree of burn is not calculated into the estimates of burn injury. The skin color ranges

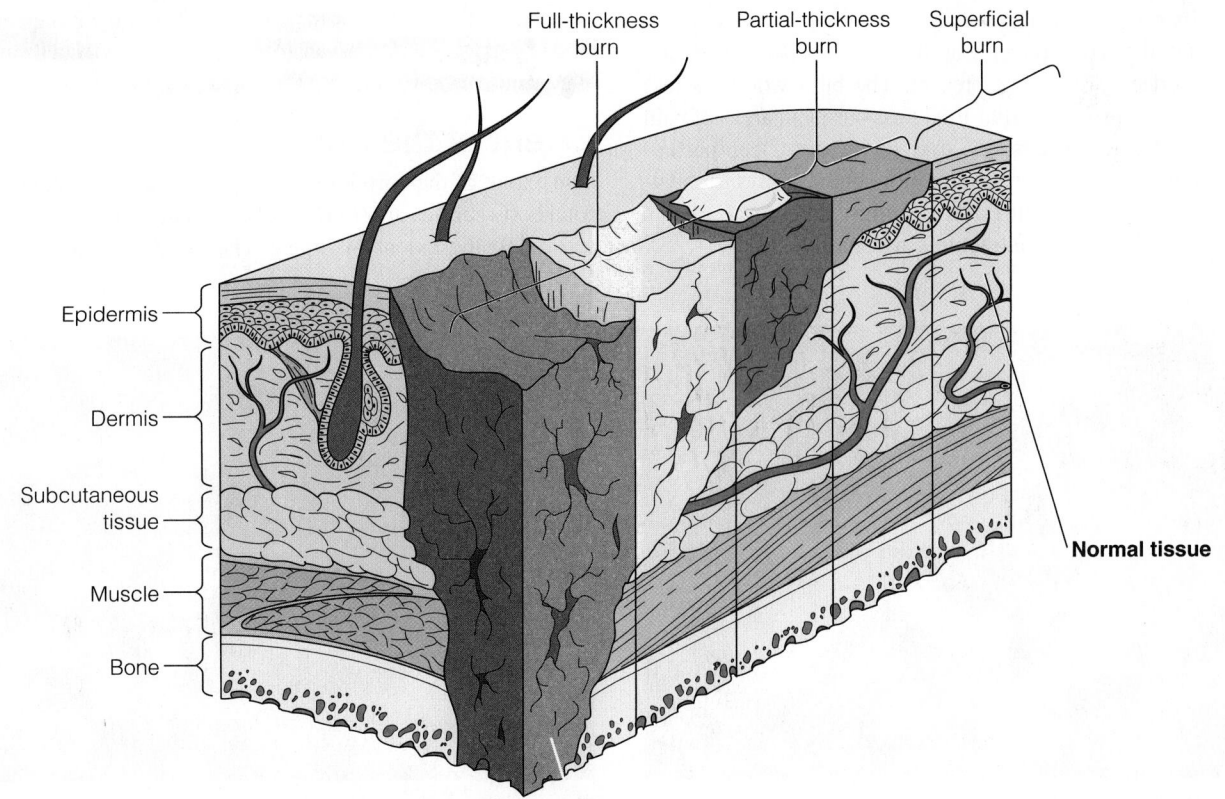

Figure 17–1 ■ Burn injury classification according to the depth of the burn.

from pink to bright red, and there may be slight edema over the burned area. Superficial burns involving large body surface areas may be manifested by chills, headache, nausea, and vomiting. The injury usually heals in 3 to 6 days, with dryness and peeling of the outer layer of skin. There is no scar formation. Superficial burns are treated with mild analgesics and the application of water-soluble lotions. Extensive superficial burns, especially in older adults, may require intravenous fluid treatment.

Partial-Thickness Burns

Partial-thickness burns may be subdivided into superficial partial-thickness and deep partial-thickness burns. The classification depends on the depth of the burn.

A *superficial partial-thickness burn* involves the entire dermis and the papillae of the dermis. Causes may include such injuries as brief exposure to a flash flame or dilute chemical agents, or contact with a hot surface. This burn is often bright red, but has a moist, glistening appearance with blister formation (Figure 17–2 ■). The burned area will blanch on pressure, and touch and pain sensation remain intact. Pain in response to temperature and air is usually severe. These injuries heal within 21 days with minimal or no scarring, but pigment changes are common. Analgesics are administered, and if large blistered areas are disrupted, skin substitutes may be used.

A *deep partial-thickness burn* also involves the entire dermis, but extends further into the dermis than a superficial partial-thickness burn. Hair follicles, sebaceous glands, and epidermal sweat glands remain intact (Porth, 2005). Hot liquids or solids, flash flame, direct flame, intense radiant energy, or chemical agents may cause this level of burn wound. The surface of the burn wound appears pale and waxy and may be moist or dry. Large, easily ruptured blisters may be present, or the blisters may look like flat, dry tissue paper. Capillary refill is decreased, and sensation to deep pressure is present. The burn wound is less painful than a superficial partial-thickness burn, but areas of pain and areas of decreased sensation may be present. Deep partial-thickness burn wounds often require more than 21 days for healing and may convert to a full-thickness injury if necrosis extends the depth of the wound. Contractures are possible, as are hyper-

Figure 17–3 ■ Burn contracture.
Courtesy of JPD/Custom Medical Stock Photo, Inc.

trophic scarring and functional impairment (Figure 17–3 ■). Excision and grafting may be necessary to decrease scarring and loss of function.

Full-Thickness Burns

A **full-thickness burn** involves all layers of the skin, including the epidermis, the dermis, and the epidermal appendages (Figure 17–4 ■). The burn wound may extend into the subcutaneous fat, connective tissue, muscle, and bone. Full-thickness burns are caused by prolonged contact with flames, steam, chemicals, or high-voltage electric current.

Depending on the cause of injury, the burn wound may appear pale, waxy, yellow, brown, mottled, charred, or non-blanching red. The wound surface is dry, leathery, and firm to the touch. Thrombosed blood vessels may be visible under the surface of the wound. There is no sensation of pain or light touch, because pain and touch receptors have been destroyed. Full-thickness burns require skin grafting to heal.

Extent of the Burn

The extent of the burn injury is expressed as a percentage of the total body surface area (TBSA). Several methods are used for determining the extent of injury. The "rule of nines" is a rapid

Figure 17–2 ■ Partial-thickness burn injury.
Courtesy of Dr. William Dominic, Valley Medical Center.

Figure 17–4 ■ Full-thickness burn injury.
Courtesy of Dr. William Dominic, Valley Medical Center.

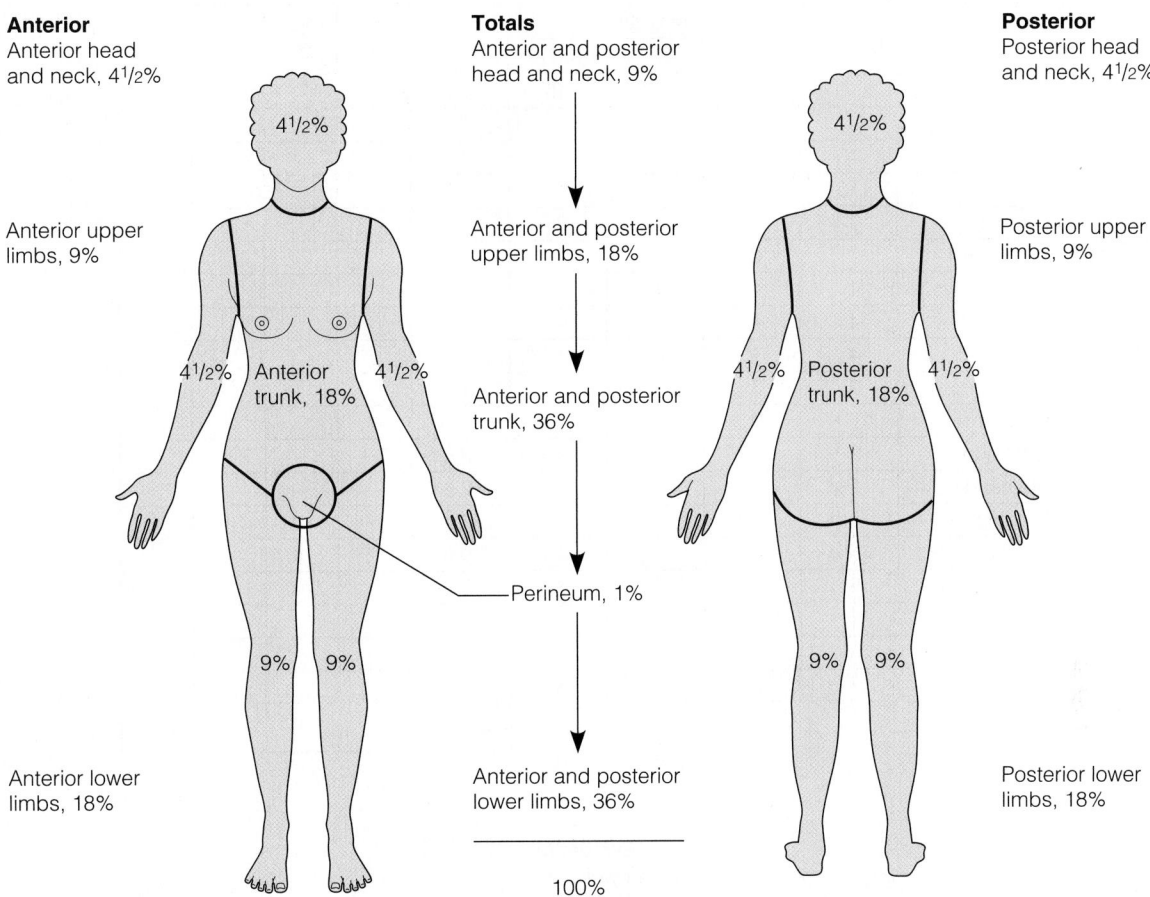

Figure 17–5 ■ The "rule of nines" is one method for quickly estimating the percentage of TBSA affected by a burn injury. Although useful in emergency care situations, the rule of nines is not accurate for estimating TBSA for adults who are short, obese, or very thin.

method of estimation used during the prehospital and emergency care phases. In this method, the body is divided into five surface areas—head, trunk, arms, legs, and perineum—and percentages that equal or total a sum of nines are assigned to each body area (Figure 17–5 ■). For example, a client with burns of the face, anterior right arm, and anterior trunk has burn injury involving 27% of the TBSA (in this example, face = 4.5%, arm = 4.5%, and trunk = 18% to total 27%). Only partial- and full-thickness burns are included in the estimation.

On the client's admission to the hospital, critical care area, or burn center, more accurate methods for estimating the extent of injury are employed. For example, the Lund and Browder method (Figure 17–6 ■) determines surface area measurements for each body part according to the age of the client.

A recognized system for describing a burn injury, developed by the American Burn Association, uses both the extent and depth of burn to classify burns as minor, moderate, or major (Table 17–3).

TABLE 17–3 American Burn Association Classification of Burn Injury

MINOR BURN INJURY	MODERATE BURN INJURY	MAJOR BURN INJURY
Excludes electrical injury, inhalation injury, complicated injuries (such as multiple trauma), and all clients who are considered to be at high risk (such as older adults and those with chronic illnesses)	Excludes electrical injury, inhalation injury, complicated injuries (such as multiple trauma), and all clients who are considered to be at high risk (such as older adults and those with chronic illnesses)	Includes all burns of the hands, face, eyes, ears, feet, and perineum; all electrical injuries, inhalation injuries, multiple-trauma injuries, and all clients who are considered to be at high risk
Partial-thickness burns of less than 15% of the TBSA in adults	Partial-thickness burns of 15% to 25% of the TBSA in adults	Partial-thickness burns of greater than 25% of the TBSA in adults
Full-thickness burns of less than 2% of the TBSA not involving special care areas (eyes, ears, face, hands, feet, joints, perineum)	Full-thickness burns of less than 10% of the TBSA not involving special care areas (eyes, ears, face, hands, feet, joints, perineum)	All full-thickness burns of 10% or greater of the TBSA

Note: Burn injuries described in this table (except minor burns) should be treated in a specialized burn center. These criteria have been established by the American Burn Association.

Area	Age (years)					% 1°	% 2°	% 3°	% Total
	0–1	1–4	5–9	10–15	Adult				
Head	19	17	13	10	7				
Neck	2	2	2	2	2				
Ant. trunk	13	13	13	13	13				
Post. trunk	13	13	13	13	13				
R. buttock	$2\frac{1}{2}$	$2\frac{1}{2}$	$2\frac{1}{2}$	$2\frac{1}{2}$	$2\frac{1}{2}$				
L. buttock	$2\frac{1}{2}$	$2\frac{1}{2}$	$2\frac{1}{2}$	$2\frac{1}{2}$	$2\frac{1}{2}$				
Genitalia	1	1	1	1	1				
R.U. arm	4	4	4	4	4				
L.U. arm	4	4	4	4	4				
R.L. arm	3	3	3	3	3				
L.L. arm	3	3	3	3	3				
R. hand	$2\frac{1}{2}$	$2\frac{1}{2}$	$2\frac{1}{2}$	$2\frac{1}{2}$	$2\frac{1}{2}$				
L. hand	$2\frac{1}{2}$	$2\frac{1}{2}$	$2\frac{1}{2}$	$2\frac{1}{2}$	$2\frac{1}{2}$				
R. thigh	$5\frac{1}{2}$	$6\frac{1}{2}$	$8\frac{1}{2}$	$8\frac{1}{2}$	$9\frac{1}{2}$				
L. thigh	$5\frac{1}{2}$	$6\frac{1}{2}$	$8\frac{1}{2}$	$8\frac{1}{2}$	$9\frac{1}{2}$				
R. leg	5	5	$5\frac{1}{2}$	6	7				
L. leg	5	5	$5\frac{1}{2}$	6	7				
R. foot	$3\frac{1}{2}$	$3\frac{1}{2}$	$3\frac{1}{2}$	$3\frac{1}{2}$	$3\frac{1}{2}$				
L. foot	$3\frac{1}{2}$	$3\frac{1}{2}$	$3\frac{1}{2}$	$3\frac{1}{2}$	$3\frac{1}{2}$				
					Total				

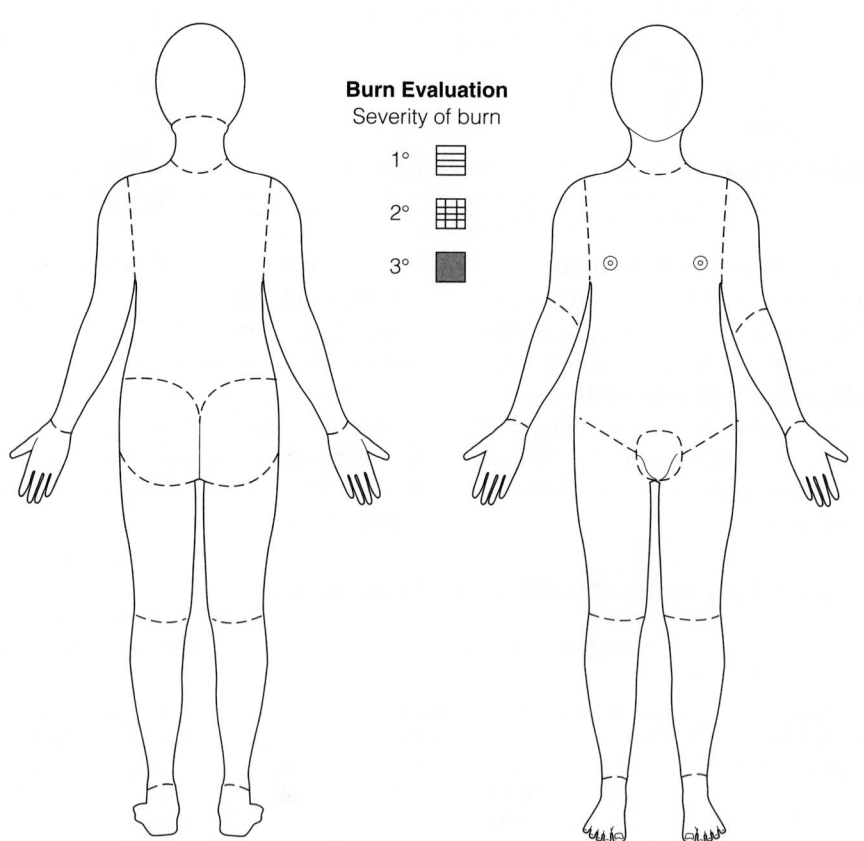

Burn Evaluation
Severity of burn

1°
2°
3°

Figure 17–6 ■ The Lund and Browder burn assessment chart. This method of estimating TBSA affected by a burn injury is more accurate than the "rule of nines" because it accounts for changes in body surface area across the life span.

BURN WOUND HEALING

Burns heal using the same processes as do other wounds, but the wound healing phases occur more slowly and last longer. The healing process involves three phases: inflammation, proliferation, and remodeling. The following physiologic events occur (Carrougher, 1998; Porth, 2005):

- *Inflammation.* Immediately following the injury, platelets coming in contact with the damaged tissue aggregate. Fibrin is deposited, trapping further platelets, and a thrombus is formed. The thrombus, combined with local vasoconstriction, leads to hemostasis, which walls off the wound from the systemic circulation.

  Local vasodilation and an increase in capillary permeability follow hemostasis. Neutrophils infiltrate the wound and peak in about 24 hours, and then monocytes predominate. The monocytes are converted into macrophages, which consume pathogens and dead tissue, and also secrete various growth factors. These growth factors stimulate the proliferation of fibroblasts and a deposit of a provisional wound matrix.

- *Proliferation.* Within 2 to 3 days postburn, fibroblasts are the major cell within the wound. Their number peaks at about 14 days after the injury. Granulation tissue begins to form, with complete reepithelialization occurring during this stage. Epithelial cells cover the wound as each cell stretches across the wound surface to join with other epithelial cell sheets or the other side of the wound. The proliferation phase lasts until complete reepithelialization occurs, by epithelial cell migration, surgical intervention, or a combination of the two.

- *Remodeling.* This phase may last for years. Collagen fibers, laid down during the proliferative phase, are reorganized into more compact areas. Scars contract and fade in color. In normal healing following a minor burn injury, the newly formed skin closely resembles its neighboring tissue. However, when a burn injury extends into the dermal layer of skin, two types of excessive scar may develop. A **hypertrophic scar** is an overgrowth of dermal tissue that remains within the boundaries of the wound. A **keloid** is a scar that extends beyond the boundaries of the original wound. People with dark skin are at greater risk for hypertrophic scars and keloids.

THE CLIENT WITH A MINOR BURN

Minor burn injuries consist of superficial burns that are not extensive, superficial partial-thickness burns that involve less than 15% of TBSA, and full-thickness burns that involve less than 2% of TBSA, excluding the special care areas (eyes, ears, face, hands, feet, perineum, and joints). Minor burn injuries are not associated with immunosuppression, hypermetabolism, or increased susceptibility to infection.

A minor burn injury is usually treated in an outpatient facility. The goal of therapy is to promote wound healing, eliminate discomfort, maintain mobility, and prevent infection.

Pathophysiology

Sunburn

Sunburns result from exposure to ultraviolet light. Such injuries, which tend to be superficial, are more commonly seen in clients with lighter skin. Because the skin remains intact, the manifestations in most cases are mild and are limited to pain, nausea, vomiting, skin redness, chills, and headache. Treatment is performed on an outpatient basis and generally consists of applying mild lotions, increasing liquid intake, administering mild analgesics, and maintaining warmth. Older adults should be monitored for evidence of dehydration. Proper use of sunscreen and limiting sun exposure to the less hazardous hours of the day (before 10 A.M. and after 3 P.M.) can prevent sunburn.

Scald Burn

Minor scald burns result from exposure to moist heat and involve superficial and superficial partial-thickness burns of less than 15% of TBSA. The goals of therapy are to prevent wound contamination and to promote healing. The nurse teaches the client to apply antibiotic solutions and light dressings and to maintain adequate nutritional intake. Mild analgesics may be ordered to help the client carry out activities of daily living. Tetanus toxoid is administered as appropriate.

INTERDISCIPLINARY CARE

In the outpatient facility, the wound may be washed with mild soap and water. Tetanus toxoid booster is recommended for all clients whose immunization histories are in doubt. Minor burns with blisters may be left intact, or debrided. Follow-up care for the minor burn injury includes twice daily wound cleansing with application of a topical ointment, range-of-motion exercises to affected joints, and weekly clinic appointments until the wound heals completely.

NURSING CARE

Although the nurse seldom treats the minor burn in the acute care environment, the burn treatment methods used in the outpatient setting follow the same standard approaches to care. General nursing measures include taking the history, estimating the extent and depth of the injury, cleansing the wound, applying topical agents, dressing the wound, controlling pain, and establishing follow-up care.

Community-Based Care

The nurse should address the following topics to facilitate self-care at home of minor burns.

- How to identify and report manifestations of impaired wound healing:
  - Change in healthy appearance of the wound (altered skin integrity, swelling, blister formation, erythema)
  - Signs of infection (fever, purulent drainage, foul odor)
- Wound care:
  - Daily cleansing with mild soap and water
  - Using sterile technique to change dressings
  - Correct application of ordered topical agents
- Pain management:
  - Use mild analgesics as ordered
  - Use alternative pain management therapies

THE CLIENT WITH A MAJOR BURN

A major burn involves serious injury to the underlying layers of skin and covers a large body surface area. The American Burn Association defines a major burn as one that involves:

- \>25% TBSA in adults less than 40 years of age
- \>20% TBSA in adults more than 40 years of age
- \>10% TBSA full-thickness burn
- Injuries to the face, eyes, ears, hands, feet, joints, or perineum
- High-voltage electrical injuries
- All burn injuries with inhalation injury or major trauma.

Pathophysiology

The pathophysiologic changes that result from major burn injuries involve all body systems. Extensive loss of skin (the body's protective barrier) can result in massive infection, fluid and electrolyte imbalances, and hypothermia. Often the person inhales the products of combustion, thus compromising respiratory function. Cardiac dysrhythmias and circulatory failure are common manifestations of serious burn injuries. A profound catabolic state dramatically increases caloric expenditure and nutritional deficiencies. An alteration in gastrointestinal motility predisposes the client to developing paralytic ileus, and hyperacidity leads to gastric and duodenal ulcerations. Dehydration slows glomerular filtration rates and renal clearance of toxic wastes and may lead to acute tubular necrosis and renal failure. Overall body metabolism may be profoundly altered. Systemic responses to burns are shown in Figure 17–7 ■ and discussed in the following sections.

Integumentary System

The loss of skin in burn injuries interrupts normal skin functions and its protective mechanisms (see Chapter 16 ∞). Key mechanisms lost in burn injuries include the prevention of evaporative water loss and bacteria entry, as well as the maintenance of body warmth.

Heat transfer to skin is a complex phenomenon. If the microcirculation of the skin remains intact during burning, it cools and protects the deeper portions of the skin and cools the outer surface once the heat source is removed. With extensive burn injury, the integrity of the microcirculation is lost, and the burning process continues even after the heat source is removed.

Burns have a characteristic skin surface appearance that resembles a bull's-eye, with the most severe burn located centrally and the lesser burns located along the peripheral wound edges. Depending on their intensity, burns consist of one, two, or three concentric three-dimensional zones closely corresponding on the skin surface to the depth of the burn (Figure 17–8 ■).

- The outer zone of hyperemia is unburned tissue, blanches on pressure, and heals in 2 to 7 days postburn.
- The medial zone of stasis is initially moist, red, and blistered and blanches on pressure. It may recover or become pale and necrotic on days 3 to 7 postburn due to decreased perfusion or infection.
- The inner zone of coagulation immediately appears leathery and coagulated. It may merge with the zone of stasis in 3 to 7 days postburn.

The overall thickness of the dermis and epidermis varies considerably from one area of the body to another. Similar temperatures produce different depths of injury to different body parts. For example, in the adult, skin covering the medial aspect of the forearm is thinner and more easily damaged than the skin covering the back of the same person. Skin dissipates heat maximally in areas of greatest vascularization. When heat absorption exceeds the rate of dissipation, cellular temperatures rise, and skin tissue is destroyed.

The burn injury results in the formation of necrotic skin and subcutaneous tissue. During the acute stage of the injury, a hard crust (**eschar**) forms, which covers the wound and harbors necrotic tissue. The eschar is characteristically leathery and rigid. Removal of the eschar facilitates healing.

Cardiovascular System

The effects of a major burn are manifested in all components of the vascular system, and include hypovolemic shock (burn shock), cardiac dysrhythmias (such as ventricular fibrillation), cardiac arrest, and vascular compromise.

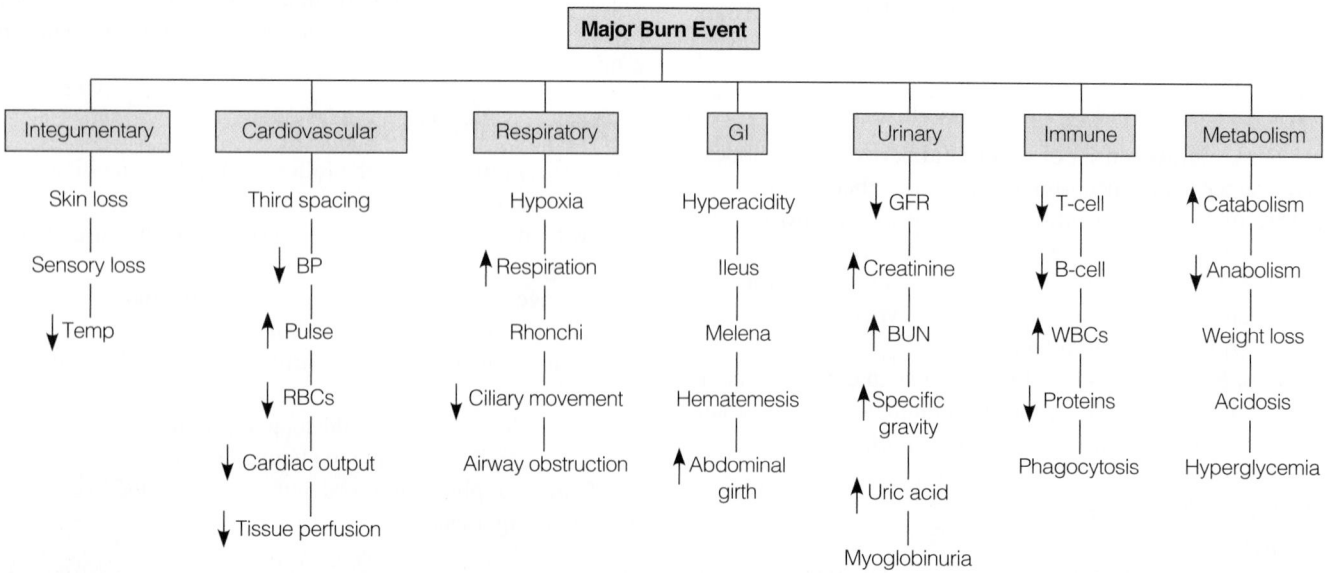

Figure 17–7 ■ Effects of a severe burn on major body systems and metabolism.

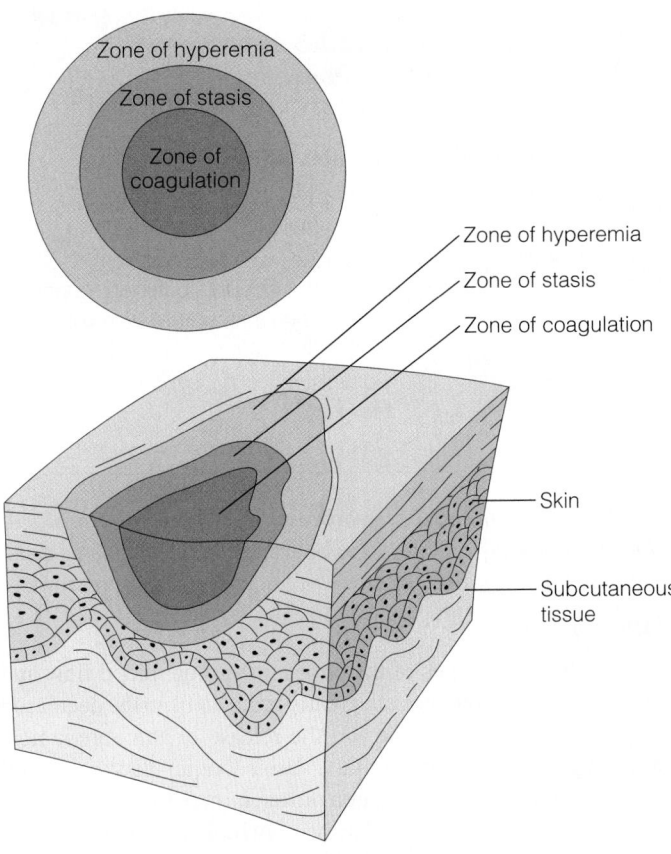

Figure 17–8 ■ The zones of injury.

HYPOVOLEMIC SHOCK (BURN SHOCK) Within minutes of the burn injury, a cascade of cellular events is initiated, and a massive amount of fluid shifts from the intracellular and intravascular compartments into the interstitium. This shift is a type of hypovolemic shock called **burn shock**, and it continues until capillary integrity is restored, usually within 24 to 36 hours of the injury. Although the pathophysiologic mechanisms of postburn vascular changes and fluid volume shifts are not clearly understood, three processes occur early in the postburn phase in clients with ≥40% TBSA:

- Increase in microvascular permeability at the burn wound site
- Generalized impairment of cell wall function, resulting in intracellular edema
- Increase in osmotic pressure of the burned tissue, leading to extensive fluid accumulation.

During burn shock, the shifting of fluid is the direct result of a loss of cell wall integrity at the site of injury and in the capillary bed. Fluid leaks from the capillaries into interstitial compartments located at the burn wound site and throughout the body, resulting in a decrease in fluid volume within the intravascular space. Plasma proteins and sodium escape into the interstitium, enhancing edema formation. Blood pressure falls as cardiac output diminishes.

Vasoconstriction results as the vascular system attempts to compensate for fluid loss. Abnormal platelet aggregation and white blood cell (WBC) accumulation result in ischemia in the deeper tissue below the burn, leading to eventual thrombosis. Red blood cells (RBCs) and WBCs remain in the circulation, producing an elevation in erythrocyte and leukocyte counts secondary to hemoconcentration.

The leakage of fluid into the interstitium compromises the lymphatic system, resulting in intravascular hypovolemia and edema at the burn wound site. Edematous body surfaces impair peripheral circulation and result in necrosis of the underlying tissue. During burn shock, potassium ions leave the intracellular compartment, predisposing the client to developing cardiac dysrhythmias. The process of burn shock continues until capillary integrity is restored, usually within 24 hours of the injury.

Burn shock reverses when fluid is reabsorbed from the interstitium into the intravascular compartment. The blood pressure rises as cardiac output increases, and urinary output improves. Diuresis continues from several days to 2 weeks postburn. During this phase, the extra cardiac workload may predispose the older client, or the client with cardiovascular disease, to fluid volume overload.

CARDIAC RHYTHM ALTERATIONS Burns of more than 40% TBSA cause significant myocardial dysfunction, with a decrease in myocardial contractibility and cardiac output. These changes, which occur prior to a decrease in plasma volume, are believed to be due to the release of substances and oxygen-free radicals from the burn wound and from ischemic myocardial cells. Electrical burns often result in cardiac dysrhythmias or cardiopulmonary arrest caused by heat damage to the myocardium or electrical interference with cardiac electrical activity.

PERIPHERAL VASCULAR COMPROMISE Direct heat damage to extremities, especially if circumferential burns are present, results in damage to blood vessels. Circulation to extremities may be further impaired by edema and by peripheral vasoconstriction that occurs during burn shock. In addition, **compartment syndrome** (in which the tissue pressure within a muscle compartment exceeds microvascular pressure, interrupting cellular perfusion) may result from circumferential burns and edema.

Respiratory System

Pulmonary damage may result from either direct inhalation injury or as part of the systemic response to the injury. Inhalation injury is a frequent and often lethal complication of burns. The injury may range from mild respiratory inflammation to massive pulmonary failure such as acute respiratory distress syndrome. Exposure to heat, asphyxiants, and smoke initiates the pathophysiologic process associated with inhalation injury.

Inflammation occurs at localized sites within the airway and is manifested as hyperemia. As a result, cells are destroyed and the bronchial cilia are rendered inactive. Because the mucociliary transport mechanism no longer functions, the client may develop bronchial congestion and infection.

Interstitial pulmonary edema develops secondary to the escape of fluid from the pulmonary vasculature into the interstitial compartment of the lung tissue. Surfactant is inactivated, resulting in atelectasis and alveolar collapse. Sloughing of the damaged and dead lung tissue occasionally produces debris that may lead to complete airway obstruction.

Upper airway (above the level of the glottis) thermal injury results from the inhalation of heated air or chemicals dissolved in water. Inhalation injury is suspected when the client has singed facial, scalp, or nasal hair. Physical findings include the presence of soot, charring, edema, blisters, and ulcerations along the mucosal lining of the oropharynx and larynx. The resulting edema in the airway peaks within the first 24 to 48 hours of injury. Ominous signs of hoarseness, labored breathing, or stridor indicate possible airway obstruction due to edema. Lower airway thermal injury is a rare occurrence. Because the lower airway is protected by laryngeal reflexes, thermal injury below the vocal cords is seldom seen. However, when it does occur, it is typically associated with the inhalation of steam or explosive gases or the aspiration of hot liquids. A classic finding is sputum containing soot or carbon particles (Sole et al., 2005).

Smoke poisoning results when toxic gases and particulate matter, the products of incomplete combustion, deposit directly onto the pulmonary mucosa. The composition of the products of combustion depends on the combustible material, the rate at which the temperature increases, and the amount of ambient oxygen present. Irritant gases and particulate matter have a direct cytotoxic effect. The degree of injury is determined by their solubility in water, duration of exposure, and the size of the particulate or aerosol droplet.

Carbon monoxide, a common asphyxiant, is a colorless, tasteless, odorless gas that has a 200 times greater affinity for hemoglobin than does oxygen. It displaces oxygen to bind with hemoglobin, forming carboxyhemoglobin. As a result, the decrease in arterial oxyhemoglobin produces tissue hypoxia. Carbon monoxide impairs both oxygen delivery and cellular oxygen use. The clinical manifestations of carbon monoxide poisoning range from mild visual impairment to coma and death (see the Manifestations box on this page).

Cyanide gas is released when plastics, polyurethane, nylon, or silk is burned. The resultant production of cyanide gas affects cellular respiration. The brain and heart are most vulnerable to cyanide poisoning.

FAST FACTS
Manifestations of Cyanide Poisoning
- Headache
- Dizziness
- Seizures
- Tachycardia
- Lethal dysrhythmias

Gastrointestinal System

Dysfunction of the gastrointestinal system is directly related to the size of the burn wound. Clients with ≥20% TBSA experience decreased peristalsis with resultant gastric distention and increased risk of aspiration. A decrease in or absence of bowel sounds is a manifestation of paralytic ileus (adynamic bowel) secondary to burn trauma. The resulting cessation of intestinal motility leads to gastric distention, nausea, vomiting, and hematemesis.

Stress ulcers (**Curling's ulcers**) are acute ulcerations of the stomach or duodenum that form following the burn injury. Abdominal pain, acidic gastric pH levels, hematemesis, and melena in the stool may indicate a gastric ulcer.

In addition, ischemia of the intestine from splanchnic vasoconstriction increases the intestinal mucosal permeability. As a result, normal intestinal bacteria move from the lumen of the

MANIFESTATIONS Carbon Monoxide Poisoning

Level of Carbon Monoxide	Manifestations
10% to 20%	Headache, dizziness, nausea, abdominal pain
21% to 40%	Headache, nausea, drowsiness, dizziness, irritability, confusion, stupor, hypotension, bradycardia, skin color ranging from pale to dark red
41% to 60%	Convulsion, coma, hypotension, tachycardia
>60%	Death

bowel to extraluminal sites, a process called *bacterial translocation*. This process is believed to be one of the mechanisms causing systemic sepsis and multiple organ dysfunction syndrome.

Urinary System

During the early stages of the burn injury, renal blood flow and glomerular filtration rates are greatly reduced from the decreased intravascular blood volume and the release of antidiuretic hormone by the posterior pituitary. Urine output decreases, and serum creatinine and blood urea nitrogen increase.

Dark brown concentrated urine may indicate myoglobinuria or hemoglobinuria, the result of underlying muscle damage or the release of large amounts of dead or damaged erythrocytes after a major burn injury. When large amounts of these pigments are released, the liver cannot keep pace with conjugation and the pigments pass through the glomeruli. The pigments can occlude the renal tubules and cause renal failure, especially when dehydration, acidosis, or shock is also present.

Immune System

The function of the immune system is to protect the human body from invasion by foreign microorganisms. The capillary leak that occurs in the early stages of the burn injury continues throughout the burn shock phase and impairs the active components of both the cell-mediated and humoral immune systems.

The humoral immune system relies on B cells to produce antibodies or immunoglobulins (see Chapter 13 ∞). In the burn client, the serum levels of all immunoglobulins are significantly diminished. Serum protein levels remain persistently low throughout the clinical course until wound closure is effected. A marked decrease in T-cell counts results in a reduction of cytotoxic activity and suppression of the cell-mediated immune system.

The compromise in the humoral and cell-mediated immune systems constitutes a state of acquired immunodeficiency, which places the burn client at risk for infection. The period of vulnerability is transient and may last from 1 to 4 weeks following the onset of the burn injury. During this time frame, opportunistic infections can be fatal despite aggressive antimicrobial therapy.

Metabolism

Two distinct phases characterize the body's metabolic response to the burn injury. The ebb phase, occurring during the first 3 days of the injury, is manifested by decreased oxygen consumption, fluid imbalance, shock, and inadequate circulating volume. These responses protect the body from the initial impact of the injury.

A second phase, the flow phase, occurs when adequate burn resuscitation has been accomplished. This phase is characterized by increases in cellular activity and protein catabolism, lipolysis, and gluconeogenesis. The basal metabolic rate (BMR) significantly increases, reaching twice the normal rate. Body weight and heat drop dramatically. Total energy expenditure may exceed 100% of normal BMR. Hypermetabolism persists until after wound closure has been accomplished and may reappear if complications occur.

INTERDISCIPLINARY CARE

The burn team is composed of an interdisciplinary group of healthcare professionals who together plan the care and treatment of the burn-injured client during the acute and rehabilitative stages. The burn team consists of the nurse, physician, physical therapist, dietitian, and social worker. The team members meet regularly to discuss client progress and to determine collaboratively the most effective regimen of care and psychosocial support.

Stages of Interdisciplinary Care

The clinical course of treatment for the burn client is divided into three stages: the emergent/resuscitative stage, the acute stage, and the rehabilitative stage. Although these stages are useful predictors of the clinical needs of the burn client, it is important to recognize that the process of burn injury is dynamic and that, in many cases, the clinical stage may not be clearly delineated. As-

sessment and management of the burn-injured client are ongoing processes determined by the clinical picture; they last throughout the course of treatment. Figure 17–9 ■ shows the burn client's progression through the healthcare system during each clinical stage of burn care. During each stage, different groups of nurses, physicians, and other healthcare specialists collaborate to manage the client's recovery.

THE EMERGENT/RESUSCITATIVE STAGE The emergent/resuscitative stage lasts from the onset of injury through successful fluid resuscitation. During this stage, healthcare workers estimate the extent of burn injury, institute first-aid measures, and implement fluid resuscitation therapies. The client is assessed for shock and evidence of respiratory distress. If indicated, intravenous lines are inserted, and the client may be prophylactically intubated. During this stage, healthcare workers determine whether the client is to be transported to a burn center for the complex intervention strategies of the professional, interdisciplinary burn team.

Although many burn injuries are treated in local tertiary care facilities, the American Burn Association has developed guidelines for determining whether the client should be transported to a burn center for interdisciplinary approaches to treatment and rehabilitation. Adult clients who should be treated at burn centers include those with:

■ Second- or third-degree burns >10% TBSA and older than 50 years of age
■ Second- or third-degree burns >20% TBSA in adults younger than 50
■ Third-degree burns >5% TBSA in adults of any age
■ Burns involving the hands, feet, face, eyes, ears, joints, or perineum

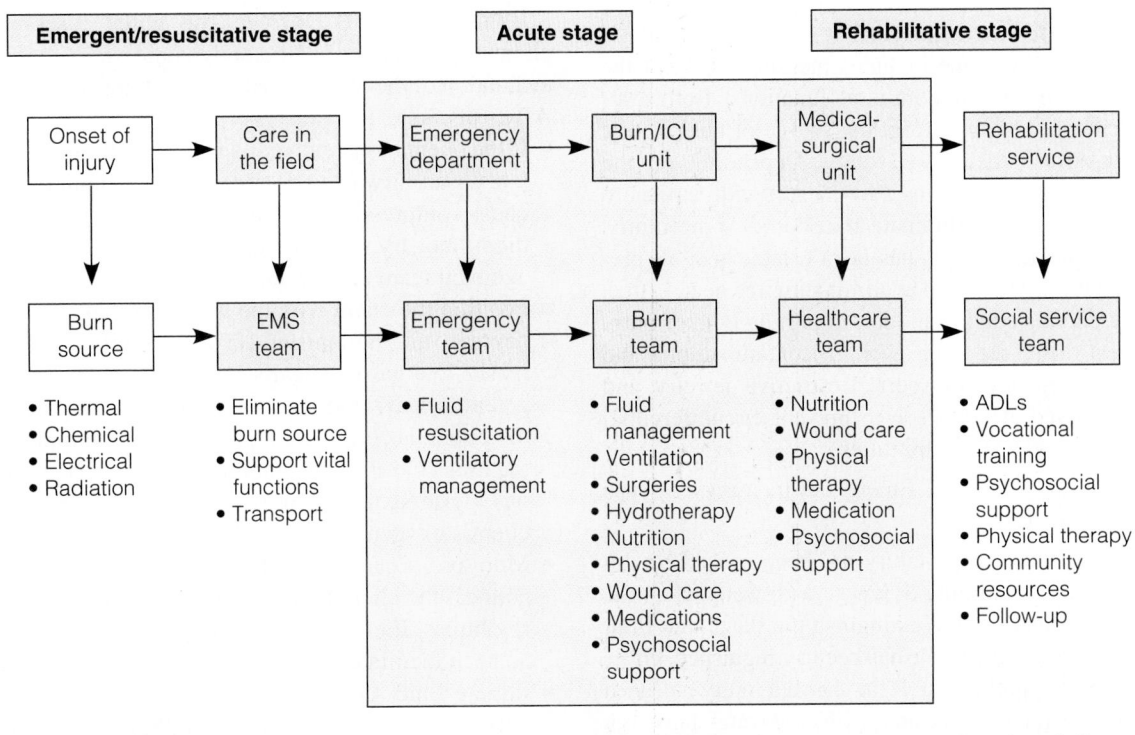

Figure 17–9 ■ The client's progression through the healthcare system during the emergent, acute, and rehabilitative stages of burn injury.

- Electrical (including lightning), chemical, and inhalation injuries
- Circumferential burns of the extremities and/or chest
- Any burn associated with extenuating problems, preexisting illness, fractures, or other trauma.

ACUTE STAGE The acute stage begins with the start of diuresis and ends with closure of the burn wound (either by natural healing or by using skin grafts). During this stage, wound care management, nutritional therapies, and measures to control infectious processes are initiated. Hydrotherapy and excision and grafting of full-thickness wounds are performed as soon as possible after injury. Enteral and parenteral nutritional interventions are started early in the treatment plan to address caloric needs resulting from extensive energy expenditure. Measures to combat infection are implemented during this stage, including the administration of topical and systemic antimicrobial agents. Pain management constitutes a significant segment of the nursing care plan throughout the clinical course of the burn-injured client. The administration of narcotic pharmaceutical agents must precede all invasive procedures to maximize client comfort and to reduce the anxieties associated with wound debridement and intensive physical therapy.

REHABILITATIVE STAGE The rehabilitative stage begins with wound closure and ends when the client returns to the highest level of health restoration, which may take years. During this stage, the primary focus is the biopsychosocial adjustment of the client, specifically the prevention of contractures and scars and the client's successful resumption of work, family, and social roles through physical, vocational, occupational, and psychosocial rehabilitation. The client is taught to perform range-of-motion exercises to enhance mobility and to support injured joints.

Prehospital Client Management

Treatment at the injury scene includes measures to limit the severity of the burn and support vital functions. Before attempting to remove the client from the source of burn injury, rescuers must ensure their own safety. Depending on the causative agent, rescuers may need to consult with experts to determine the best way to eliminate the source of the injury. Once the safety of the rescuers has been established, all prehospital interventions are aimed at eliminating the heat source, stabilizing the client's condition, identifying the type of burn, preventing heat loss, reducing wound contamination, and preparing for emergency transport. Restrictive jewelry and clothing are removed at the scene to prevent circumferential constriction of the torso and extremities.

STOP THE BURNING PROCESS Emergency measures, by type of injury, include the following.

Thermal Burns If the thermal injury has been caused by dry heat, smother inflamed clothing or lavage with water. Help the person "stop, drop, and roll" to extinguish the flame and limit the extent of burn. Once the flame has been extinguished, cover the body to prevent hypothermia. If the thermal injury has been caused by moist heat, lavage the area with cool water. Ice is not used for cooling because it causes vasoconstriction and may result in further injury. Tar and asphalt can be removed with min-

eral oil, petroleum ointments, Medisol (a citrus and petroleum distillate with hydrocarbon structure), or Crisco.

Chemical Burns For chemical burns, immediately remove the clothing and use a hose or shower to lavage the involved area thoroughly for a minimum of 20 minutes. Many chemicals are in powder form and as much dry chemical needs to be removed as possible before flushing the surface with water. Unusual chemicals may require consultation with a Poison Control Center about appropriate treatment. Protective clothing should be worn during this process to protect the rescuer from chemical exposure. Chemical splashes in or near the eye require immediate eye irrigation with clean, cool water or saline.

Electrical Burns Electrical injuries pose serious potential harm to both rescuer and burn victim. Ensure that the source of electrical current has been disconnected, or move the person to safety and away from the energy source using a nonconductive device such as an unpainted broomstick. If the person is unresponsive, assess for the presence of cardiac and respiratory function. If indicated, begin cardiopulmonary resuscitation (CPR). A spinal cord injury may be present secondary to the forceful contraction of the muscles of the neck and back during exposure to the current. If possible, place the person in a cervical collar and transport on a spinal board.

Radiation Burns Radiation injuries are usually minor and involve only the epidermal layer of skin. Treatment focuses on helping normal body mechanisms promote wound healing. For severe radiation burns, such as those that result from industrial radiation accidents, trained personnel may need to render the area safe for entry prior to rescue. All interventions are aimed at shielding, establishing distance, and limiting the time of exposure to the radioactive source.

SUPPORT VITAL FUNCTION The initial assessment of the client's respiratory and hemodynamic status begins with an evaluation of the client's airway, breathing, and circulation (the ABCs of care).

- If the client has no pulse and is not breathing, begin CPR. Establish an airway, and start mouth-to-mouth breathing and chest compressions. Continue CPR until spontaneous cardiopulmonary function returns or until the emergency management team takes over.
- Position the client with the head elevated at greater than 30 degrees, and administer 100% humidified oxygen by face mask. Use nasotracheal suction as necessary to maintain a patent airway. Endotracheal intubation may be necessary if the client has facial edema and inhalation injury. Auscultate the lungs often onsite to monitor respiratory status. Continuous pulse oximetry provides ongoing assessment of the client's oxygen saturation levels.
- Monitor for cardiac dysrhythmias or arrest. When available, connect the client to a cardiac monitor and observe for dysrhythmias. Elevate burned extremities above the level of the heart to facilitate circulation.
- Initiate fluid replacement therapy for burn wounds that involve more than 20% of the TBSA. Continuously assess heart and lung sounds and observe level of consciousness, cardiac rate and rhythm, blood pressure, and urine output.

- Cover the client to maintain body temperature and to prevent further wound contamination and tissue damage.

Emergency and Acute Care

Prehospital personnel report to the emergency department staff all findings and medical interventions that occurred at the scene of the injury. The nurse obtains a history of the injury, estimates the depth and extent of the burn, begins fluid resuscitation, and maintains ventilation according to protocol.

***FLUID RESUSCITATION* Fluid resuscitation** is the administration of intravenous fluids to restore the circulating blood volume during the acute period of increasing capillary permeability. To counteract the effects of burn shock, fluid resuscitation guidelines are used to replace the extensive fluid and electrolyte losses associated with major burn injuries. Fluid replacement is necessary in all burn wounds that involve ≥20% TBSA.

Crystalloid fluids are administered through two large-bore (14- to 16-gauge) catheters, preferably inserted through unburned skin. Warmed Ringer's lactate solution is the intravenous fluid most widely used during the first 24 hours after burn injury, because it most closely approximates the body's extracellular fluid composition. Several formulas may be used to replace fluid loss. Two commonly used formulas are as follows:

- Parkland formula, in which lactated Ringer's solution is administered 4 mL × kg × % TBSA burn
- ABLS Consensus formula, in which lactated Ringer's solution is administered 2 to 4 mL × kg × % TBSA burn (Ahrns, 2004).

These formulas specify the volume of fluid to be infused in the first 24 hours from the time of the burn injury, with 50% of the fluid to be infused during the first 8 hours, followed by the remaining 50% during the next 16 hours (25% per 8 hours). During the second 24 hours, fluids for clients with larger burns (such as more than 30% TBSA) are changed to a crystalloid solution of 5% dextrose in water titrated to maintain urine output (Sole et al., 2005).

Hourly urine output is often used as the indicator of effective fluid resuscitation, with 30 to 50 mL for an adult considered adequate. (With electrical burns, a urine output of 75 to 100 mL should be maintained.) Another indicator is heart rate; if fluid resuscitation is adequate, the rate should be less than 120 beats per minute or in the upper limits of normal for age. However, fear, anxiety, and pain that accompany burn injuries often increase heart rate (Ahrns, 2004). Blood pressure changes are less reliable because significant hypotension does not develop until volume losses exceed 30% due to the body's compensatory mechanisms. Assessment for narrowed pulse pressure, which indicates shock earlier, should be considered along with urine output, to monitor adequate fluid resuscitation (Sole et al., 2005).

During the fluid resuscitation stage, the client may require invasive hemodynamic monitoring (see Chapter 32 ∞). A pulmonary artery catheter can be used to monitor cardiac output, cardiac index, and pulmonary artery wedge pressures. All measurements must be maintained within normal limits to effect adequate fluid resuscitation.

RESPIRATORY MANAGEMENT Upon the client's admission to the emergency department, several baseline assessments of respiratory status must be obtained: chest x-ray study, arterial blood gases (ABGs), vital signs, and carboxyhemoglobin levels. Intubation is indicated for all clients with burns of the chest, face, or neck. The primary treatment plan is oriented toward preventing atelectasis and maintaining alveolar oxygen exchange. The following interventions should be initiated.

- Maintain the head of the bed at 30 degrees or greater to maximize the client's ventilatory efforts. Turn the client side to side every 2 hours to prevent hypostatic pneumonia.
- To keep airway passages clear, suction the client frequently, encourage the client to use incentive spirometry hourly, and help the client perform coughing and deep-breathing exercises every 2 hours.
- In the face of impending airway obstruction, the client will require immediate intubation. Nasotracheal tube placement is the preferred route because it seems to be better tolerated and can be more effectively secured. If the client has suffered nasolabial burns, however, the orotracheal route is preferred. Nasotracheal and orotracheal intubation are reserved for short-term ventilatory management. For long-term ventilatory management (i.e., greater than 3 weeks), a tracheostomy is performed.
- Humidification of either room air or oxygen helps prevent the drying of tracheal secretions. Ambient air or oxygen flow is based on ABG results. The client may be placed on a face mask, steam collar, T-piece, mechanical ventilation with positive end-expiratory pressure, pressure support ventilation, or high-frequency jet ventilation. The goal of all therapies is to maintain adequate tissue oxygenation with the least amount of inspired oxygen flow necessary.
- Medications to dilate constricted bronchial passages are administered intravenously and as inhalants to control bronchospasms and wheezing. Mucolytic agents liquefy tenacious sputum and aid in expectoration.
- An arterial line is placed in the client with major burn injury for continuous assessment of ABGs. Pulmonary artery pressure catheters may be inserted to measure pulmonary vascular resistance (PVR), pulmonary artery pressure (PAP), pulmonary artery wedge pressure (PAWP), and mixed venous oxygen saturation (SvO_2). The PVR and PAP rise in the presence of hypoxia. The SvO_2 is the average percentage of hemoglobin bound with oxygen in the venous blood and reflects overall tissue utilization of oxygen. Pulse oximetry monitors arterial oxygen saturation levels.
- In the presence of carbon monoxide (CO) poisoning, monitor carboxyhemoglobin (COHgb) levels. Pulse oximetry cannot distinguish between oxyhemoglobin and COHgb, thus a false normal or high pulse oximetry reading is seen. High-flow 100% oxygen is given immediately by nonrebreather mask. Clients with COHgb greater than 15% may require hyperbaric oxygen therapy to replace the CO.
- Pain medications are administered if the client is not in shock.

After stabilization in the emergency department, the client is transferred to the critical care unit or a specialized burn center (a facility that has a burn physician as director of a specialized nursing unit with dedicated burn beds). In both settings, continuous monitoring of diagnostic tests, administration of medications, pain control, wound management, and nutrition support therapies constitute the initial plan of care.

Diagnosis

The following diagnostic tests are used to evaluate the client's progress and to modify intervention strategies.

- *Urinalysis* indicates the adequacy of renal perfusion and the client's nutritional status. In catabolic states, nitrogen is excreted in large amounts into the urine. Nitrogen loss is measured through 24-hour urine collections for total nitrogen, urea nitrogen, and amino acid nitrogen. *Myoglobinuria,* which manifests as a dark brown, wine-colored urine, signals the development of acute tubular necrosis. Loss of plasma protein and dehydration lead to proteinuria and elevated urine specific gravity. Glycosuria is a transient development following major burn injury; it indicates a need to adjust the nutritional program.

- The *complete blood count* is monitored regularly. Hematocrit is elevated secondary to hemoconcentration and fluid shifts from the intravascular compartment. Hemoglobin is decreased secondary to hemolysis. WBCs are elevated if infection is present.

- *Serum electrolytes* are monitored regularly. Sodium levels are decreased secondary to massive fluid shifts into the interstitium. Potassium levels initially are elevated during burn shock, as a result of cell lysis and fluid shifts into the extracellular space. Potassium levels decrease after burn shock resolves, as fluid shifts back to intracellular and intravascular compartments.

- *Renal function* test results are closely monitored. Blood urea nitrogen (BUN) is elevated secondary to dehydration. Creatinine is elevated in the presence of renal insufficiency.

- *Total protein, albumin, transferrin, prealbumin, retinol binding protein, alpha one-acid glycoprotein,* and *C-reactive protein* indicate protein synthesis and nutritional status. Because of the fluid shifts that occur during the early stages of the burn injury, they are more useful markers during the rehabilitative phase of care.

- *Creatine phosphokinase (CPK)* is elevated following an electrical burn, secondary to extensive muscle damage. Blood glucose is transiently elevated after major burn injury.

- *Serial ABGs* indicate the presence of hypoxia and acid-base disturbances and indicate client responses to changes in oxygen therapies. The burn-injured client may demonstrate elevated or lowered pH, decreased P_{CO_2}, decreased P_{O_2}, and low-normal bicarbonate levels.

- *Pulse oximetry* allows continuous assessment of oxygen saturation levels. The burn-injured client may have saturation levels below 95%.

- *Serial chest x-ray studies* document changes within the first 24 to 48 hours that may reflect the presence of atelectasis, pulmonary edema, or acute respiratory distress syndrome (ARDS).

- *Serial 12-lead electrocardiograms (EKGs)* are necessary to monitor the development of dysrhythmias, especially those associated with hypokalemic and hyperkalemic states.

Medications

PAIN CONTROL Burns often cause excruciating pain. In the emergent stages of care, intravenously administered narcotics such as morphine, hydromorphone, or fentanyl are the best means of managing pain. Morphine is the drug of choice in a typical dosage of 3 to 5 mg intravenously every 5 to 10 minutes for an adult. Meperidine is avoided because of potential normeperidine accumulation, which can produce tremors and anxiety. Once the client has been stabilized, it is appropriate to administer narcotics, especially intravenous fentanyl, prior to initiating hydrotherapy or intensive exercising routines. Burn treatments can also produce high levels of anxiety, necessitating the use of anxiolytic agents such as midazolam and lorazepam (Montgomery, 2004). Anxiolytics are especially useful when administered 1 hour before wound care. During the acute stage, opioids are administered around the clock to decrease pain that occurs at rest. Patient-controlled analgesia enhances the client's ability to cope with pain. The oral, subcutaneous, or intramuscular route of administration should be avoided until hemodynamic stability and unimpaired tissue perfusion return.

As the client enters the rehabilitative stage of care, alternative therapies for pain control may be added to the plan of care. Distraction, self-hypnosis, guided imagery, and relaxation techniques are helpful adjuncts in managing pain and coping with loss. See Chapter 9 ∞ for a discussion of strategies for managing pain.

ANTIMICROBIAL AGENTS Systemic infection is a leading cause of death in major burn patients. Gram-positive organisms such as *Staphylococcus* and *Streptococcus* colonize the burn surface during the first week postburn; gram-negative enteric organisms become more common with longer periods of hospitalization. Diagnosing infection is best done through a burn wound biopsy (DeSanti, 2005). To eliminate infection on the surface of the burn wound, topical antimicrobial therapy is used, depending on protocol. Generally, topical antimicrobials are not applied until the client is admitted to a burn unit. Of the many antimicrobial agents available, the three most widely used are mafenide acetate (Sulfamylon) cream, silver nitrate 0.5% soaks, and sulfadiazine (Silvadene) cream. All three are broad-spectrum antibiotics. The choice of topical antibiotic is based on the extent of the burn wound, the presence of identified bacterial organisms, whether an open (exposing the wound to the air) or closed (using bulky dressings) method of treatment is used, and client response. Despite antimicrobial therapy, clients with major burn assault have a greater risk for sepsis and septic shock.

> ### FAST FACTS
> **Local Signs of Burn Wound Infection**
> - Increased sloughing of burn tissue
> - Increased edema around wound edges
> - Partial-thickness wound converting to full-thickness wound
> - Black or brown areas of discoloration

Clients with major burns are usually given prophylactic antibiotics. Systemic antimicrobial therapy is indicated in the immediate preoperative and postoperative period associated with excision and autografting. Postoperatively, the therapy is discontinued as soon as the client's hemodynamic status returns to normal, usually within the first 24 hours. In the long-term treatment of identified infectious processes, drug administration is limited to the least amount of time required to eradicate the infection. See the Medication Administration box for the nursing implications for topical antimicrobial therapy for the burn client.

MEDICATION ADMINISTRATION **Topical Burn Medications**

TOPICAL ANTIMICROBIAL AGENTS
Mafenide acetate (Sulfamylon)
Silver nitrate
Silver sulfadiazine (Silvadene)

Research shows that the most effective topical agents are those that (1) act against the major pathogens responsible for causing burn wound infection, (2) achieve levels of concentration sufficient to decrease microbial colonization, (3) are rapidly excreted or metabolized, (4) are nontoxic, and (5) are easy to use and inexpensive.

Mafenide Acetate

Mafenide is a synthetic antibiotic closely related chemically, but not pharmacologically, to the sulfonamides. Although the mechanism of action is unclear, the drug appears to interfere with the metabolism of bacterial cells. Mafenide is a bacteriostatic agent effective against many gram-positive and gram-negative organisms.

For topical administration, mafenide is used in an 8.5% cream in a water-miscible base. Following application, the drug is rapidly diffused through the burn eschar and absorbed systemically.

In the general circulation, mafenide metabolizes to a weak carbonic anhydrase inhibitor known as p-carboxybenzenesulfonamide, a substance that impairs the renal mechanisms involved in the buffering of blood. Bicarbonate excretion in the urine increases, and ammonia and chloride excretion decreases. To maintain normal acid-base balance, the pulmonary system effects a compensatory hyperventilatory state. If the compensatory hyperventilation is insufficient, the client develops metabolic acidosis.

Nursing Responsibilities

- Use mafenide with caution in clients with renal or pulmonary disease.
- Approximately 3% to 5% of clients develop a hypersensitivity to mafenide, resulting in a maculopapular rash on the unburned areas. Assess the client for the following:

Pruritus　　　　　　　**Urticaria**
Facial edema　　　　　**Blisters**
Swelling　　　　　　　**Eosinophilia**

If hypersensitivity reactions occur, discontinue the drug and administer antihistamines.
- Monitor the client for superinfection within the burn eschar, in the subeschar tissue, or in viable tissue adjacent to the wound.

Health Education for the Client and Family

- Expect intense pain, stinging, or a burning sensation following drug application. Take appropriate measures to control pain before applying the drug.
- Apply the drug to clean, debrided burn wounds once or twice daily. Continue applications until healing is apparent.
- If any signs of allergy develop, discontinue the drug and notify the physician.
- Report any sudden and prolonged increases in respiratory rate.

Silver Nitrate

Silver nitrate is a bacteriostatic agent that inhibits a wide variety of gram-positive and gram-negative organisms. Its antimicrobial effect is due to the actions of silver ions, which markedly alter the microbial cell wall and membrane. Additionally, the drug denatures bacterial protein, thereby inactivating and precipitating the microbes.

Nursing Responsibilities

- Silver nitrate is used as a 0.5% solution in distilled water. Apply the solution to bulky gauze dressings every 2 hours, and provide complete dressing changes twice daily.
- Silver nitrate has limited penetrating ability and is ineffective if used more than 72 hours following a burn injury.
- At the local tissue level, silver nitrate immediately interacts with chloride ions to form a black silver chloride precipitate that discolors both the burn wound and the adjacent tissues. The discoloration significantly hampers visual inspection of the wound.
- High concentrations of the drug result in cellular toxicity of surrounding healthy tissue.
- Because large amounts of water are systemically absorbed from the dressing site, the client may demonstrate a hypotonic state. Hyponatremia and hypochloremic alkalosis are common manifestations in burn-injured clients treated with silver nitrate.

Health Education for the Client and Family

- Watch for and report any signs and symptoms of hypotonicity: swelling, weight gain, difficulty in breathing.
- This drug causes a black discoloration on all skin surfaces and dressings with which it comes into contact.
- Because discoloration can conceal evidence of infection, watch for systemic manifestations of infection fever, malaise, rapid pulse rate, listlessness.
- Saturate the wound dressings every 2 hours with a 0.5% aqueous solution of the drug. Change the dressings completely twice daily.

Silver Sulfadiazine

Silver sulfadiazine, a sulfonamide, is the most commonly used topical agent. The drug acts on the cell membrane and cell wall of susceptible bacteria and binds to cellular DNA. The drug is bactericidal and effective against a wide variety of gram-negative and gram-positive organisms.

Nursing Responsibilities

- Many clients develop a marked leukopenia in response to this drug, which tends to improve spontaneously over the course of therapy. This finding does not contraindicate use of the drug.
- Hypersensitivity to silver sulfadiazine has been reported in a small number of cases. If the client develops hypersensitivity, administer antihistamine, and change the topical agent.
- If sulfa crystals form in the urine, keep the client well hydrated.
- Treatment with this drug can cause systemic uptake of propylene glycol, which results in an elevated serum osmolality and high urine specific gravity in the client who is not dehydrated. These findings tend to create confusion during the fluid resuscitative stage of care. Whenever the serum osmolality and urine specific gravity fail to correlate with a clinical picture that reflects fluid volume overload (elevated CVP/PCWP, rhonchi/wheezing, edema), suspect systemic propylene glycol uptake.

Health Education for the Client and Family

- Apply the drug to clean, debrided wounds once or twice daily, completely covering the burn wound at all times.
- Continue applying the drug until healing is apparent.
- If any signs of allergy develop, discontinue the drug and notify the physician.
- Watch for evidence of concentrated urine, and notify the physician.
- If not contraindicated, drink large amounts of fluids to prevent sulfa crystals from forming in the urine.

TETANUS PROPHYLAXIS If the client's immunization status is in doubt, tetanus toxoid is administered intramuscularly early in the acute phase of care to prevent *Clostridium tetani* infection.

PREVENTING GASTRIC HYPERACIDITY Hyperacidity must be controlled to prevent Curling's ulcer. A nasogastric tube is placed during the emergent phase of care, and gastric aspirant is obtained hourly. The gastric pH should be assessed and maintained at levels above 5. To control gastric acid secretion during the acute phase of care, histamine H_2 blockers (e.g., famotidine [Pepcid]) or proton pump inhibitors (e.g., pantoprazole [Protonix]) can be administered intravenously, either intermittently or as continuous infusions. As soon as bowel sounds become audible, the client is placed on an antacid regimen.

Treatments

SURGERY Three surgical interventions are commonly employed to manage the burn wound: escharotomy, surgical debridement, and autografting.

Escharotomy When the burn eschar forms circumferentially around the torso or extremities, it acts as a tourniquet, impairing circulation. Left unchecked, the affected body part becomes gangrenous.

To prevent circumferential constriction of the torso or extremity, an **escharotomy** is performed by the physician with a scalpel or by electrocautery (Figure 17–10 ■). A sterile surgical incision is made longitudinally along the extremity or the trunk to release taut skin and allow for expansion caused by edema formation. In the first 24 hours following the procedure, the incision should be gently packed with fine-mesh gauze. After 24 hours, the site may be treated with a direct application of a topical antimicrobial agent. See Box 17–2 for nursing implications for care of the client undergoing escharotomy.

Figure 17–10 ■ Escharotomy. The surgical procedure consists of removing the eschar formed on the skin and underlying tissue following severe burns. The procedure is particularly helpful in restoring circulation to the extremities of clients when scar tissue forms a tight, constrictive band around the circumference of a limb.
Courtesy of Dr. William Dominic, Valley Medical Center.

Surgical Debridement **Surgical debridement** refers to the process of excising the wound to the level of fascia (fascial excision) or sequentially removing thin slices of the burn wound to the level of viable tissue (tangential excision). Because **fascial excision**, or **fasciectomy**, sacrifices potentially viable fat and lymphatic tissue, its use is reserved for clients with extensive or full-thickness burns. The most common technique is electrocautery with cutting and coagulating current capabilities. Tangential excision is performed with the use of a dermatome. Shallow burns and some of moderate depth bleed briskly after one slice. If bleeding does not occur, the procedure is repeated until a viable bed of dermis or subcutaneous fat is reached. Following surgical debridement, the client is returned to the burn unit.

BOX 17–2 **Nursing Implications for Circumferential Wound Management**

Escharotomy

A circumferential burn wound increases the risk for impaired tissue perfusion of the involved area. To prevent arterial occlusion, an escharotomy is performed to release tension and permit unobstructed arterial blood flow. The nurse continuously assesses the involved area and notifies the physician of the need to perform this emergent procedure, which is done at the bedside. Because only the dead burn wound tissue is excised, the client experiences very little pain.

Nursing Responsibilities

- For circumferential burn wounds of the extremity, assess the extremity for absence of blood flow:
  a. Using a Doppler ultrasound stethoscope, check hourly for the presence of a pulse.
  b. Assess the extremity hourly for warmth, color, sensation, and capillary refill.
  c. Observe for evidence of numbness or tingling.
- For circumferential burn wounds of the torso, assess for evidence of respiratory distress:
  a. Obtain ABGs as needed.
  b. Auscultate lung sounds hourly.

  c. Observe for evidence of cyanosis, tachypnea, anxiety, or restlessness.
- For circumferential burn wounds of the neck, assess for evidence of respiratory distress. Prepare the client for prophylactic intubation.
- Monitor for excessive blood loss, and transfuse the client if indicated.
- Dress the open wound (escharotomy) with topical antimicrobial agents as ordered.

Health Education for the Client and Family

- Teach the client the importance of reporting any evidence of impaired circulation: numbness, tingling, blue color to the extremity, absence of sensation.
- Assure the client that the procedure will not be painful and will provide immediate relief.
- Teach the client the importance of protecting the open wound (escharotomy) from infection.
- Explain the rationale supporting prophylactic intubation for burn wounds involving the head and neck.
- Provide assurance that all blood loss will be replaced and that bleeding at the site will be controlled.

Figure 17–11 ■ Skin grafting procedure.
Courtesy of Dr. William Dominic, Valley Medical Center.

Autografting A procedure performed in the surgical suite, **autografting** is used to effect permanent skin coverage. Early burn wound excision and skin grafting decrease the hospital stay and enhance rehabilitation. Skin is removed from healthy tissue (donor site) of the burn-injured client and applied to the burn wound (Figure 17–11 ■ and Figure 17–12 ■). (Skin grafts and flaps are discussed in Chapter 16 ∞.) After the autograft is applied, the grafted area is immobilized. The site is assessed daily for evidence of adherence. The client resumes range-of-motion exercises 5 days postgraft. As the wound heals, the client may complain of itching, which can be treated with mild lotions.

Cultured epithelial autografting is a technique in which skin cells are removed from unburned sites on the client's body, then minced and placed in a culture medium for growth. Over a 5- to 7-day period, the cells expand 50 to 70 times the size of the initial biopsies. The cells are again separated out and placed in a new culture medium for continued growth. With this technique, enough skin can be grown over a period of 3 to 4 weeks to cover an entire human body. The cells are prepared in sheets

Figure 17–12 ■ Skin graft for burn injury (autograft).
Courtesy of Dr. William Dominic, Valley Medical Center.

and attached to petroleum jelly gauze backing, which is applied to the burn wound site. Problems with infection and lack of attachment have occurred.

BIOLOGIC AND BIOSYNTHETIC DRESSINGS The terms *biologic dressing* and *biosynthetic dressing* refer to any temporary material that rapidly adheres to the wound bed, promotes healing, and/or prepares the burn wound for permanent autograft coverage. Ideally, these kinds of dressings should be easy to apply and remove, inexpensive, nonantigenic, elastic, able to reduce pain, able to serve as a bacterial barrier, and able to enhance the natural healing process. The dressings are applied to the burn wound as soon as possible. Covering the wound eliminates the loss of water through evaporation, reduces infection, and promotes wound healing. Biologic and biosynthetic dressings that are currently in use include homograft (allograft), heterograft (xenograft), amnionic membranes, and synthetic materials.

Homograft, or **allograft**, is human skin that has been harvested from cadavers. It is stored in skin banks located throughout the nation. The development of methods to achieve prolonged storage of frozen, viable skin has increased the use of this dressing; however, its short supply and expense still pose problems. It is manufactured as strips cut to the pattern of the burn and applied using sterile technique. Under normal circumstances, a homograft is rejected within 14 to 21 days following application.

Heterograft, or **xenograft**, is skin obtained from an animal, usually a pig. Although fresh porcine heterograft is available at some centers, frozen heterograft is much more commonly used. Once applied, heterograft appears to undergo early softening and lysis from enzymatic action from the wound. As a result, frequent changes of the heterograft dressing are necessary. Because of the high infection rates associated with this dressing, silver-nitrate-treated porcine heterograft has been developed to retard microbial growth.

The multiple problems associated with the use of biologic dressings have driven the development of synthetic materials. One such material is Biobrane, a composite material consisting of nylon mesh bonded to silicone that has proved successful in the temporary coverage of second- and third-degree burns. Whereas Biobrane adheres well to moderately clean wounds, it cannot adhere to or lower bacterial counts in grossly contaminated wounds. Biobrane dressing is supplied in various sizes, cut to fit the wound site, and secured with tape or Steri-Strips. It spontaneously separates from the wound when the underlying tissue heals. Hydrocolloid dressings are another type of biosynthetic material. They are occlusive wafers of gumlike materials that provide a water-resistant outer layer for coverage of the donor site. They protect healing tissue from excessive drying, liquefy necrotic tissue, and absorb wound drainage.

If dermal thickness is lost in deep partial-thickness or full-thickness burns, several products can serve as a dermal replacement. Integra is a synthetic dermal substitute and Alloderm is human cadaver allograft dermis that is nonimmunogenic. These products are placed in the wound, and split-thickness autografts are then placed over the dermal replacement. These products are used to provide temporary wound coverage, reduce pain, and facilitate healing.

Two recent temporary skin substitutes are TransCyte and Apligraf. TransCyte is a bioengineered substance, derived from human fibroblast cells grown within mesh. As the cells grow, they secrete human dermal collagen, matrix proteins, and growth factors. The product is produced, extensively tested for any infectious agents, and then frozen. It is used as a temporary covering for surgically debrided full-thickness and deep partial-thickness burn wounds, and is an alternative to silver sulfadiazine and cadaver skin. TransCyte forms a transparent, protective barrier over the wound surface and is typically applied only once. The best results have been obtained when it was applied within 24 hours of injury. Apligraf is bilayered skin substitute cultured from neonatal foreskin.

The newest treatment method uses the vacuum-assisted closure (VAC) device (Figure 17–13 ■). VAC consists of a sponge placed over the wound with tubing that connects the sponge to a pump. An occlusive, adhesive dressing covers the wound and tubing, sealing the wound to create negative pressure. VAC is showing positive results in reducing wound edema, removing exudate, and improving wound healing in partial-thickness burns and deep hand burns (DeSanti, 2005).

WOUND MANAGEMENT The outcomes of care for the client with a major burn depend on the prevention and treatment of infection through daily topical wound care, wound monitoring, and wound excision and closure. The goals of wound management are as follows (Honari, 2004):

- Control microbial colonization and prevent wound infection.
- Prevent wound progression.
- Achieve wound coverage as early as possible.
- Promote function of healing skin.

Debriding the Wound Burned tissue releases chemical mediators that stimulate phagocytosis in an attempt to digest debris left by decaying necrotic tissue. Necrotic tissue that remains despite phagocytic action retards healing and prolongs inflammation. **Debridement** is the process of removing all loose tissue,

Figure 17–13 ■ Wound vacuum.
Courtesy of KCI Licensing, Inc.

wound debris, and eschar (dead tissue) from the wound. Three methods of debridement are employed: mechanical, enzymatic, and surgical (surgical debridement was previously discussed).

A nurse may perform mechanical debridement by applying and removing gauze dressings (wet-to-dry or wet-to-moist), hydrotherapy, irrigation, or scissors and tweezers. However, removal of gauze dressings can cause pain and possibly damage granulation tissue (Honari, 2004). During hydrotherapy (in an immersion tank, a shower, or on a spray table) the burn injury may be gently washed with a mild, nonperfumed, antimicrobial soap or wound cleanser solution to remove dead skin and separate eschar. The solution is then rinsed off with warm saline or tap water. Body hair (except for eyebrows) should be shaved within the burn and to within 2.5 cm of the wound edges. Blistered skin is grasped with a dry gauze and gently removed. The edges of blisters or eschar are trimmed with blunt scissors. The wound is then covered with a topical antimicrobial agent.

Enzymatic debridement involves the use of a topical agent to dissolve and remove necrotic tissue, as well as lift eschar. An enzyme (such as Accuzyme, collagenase [Santyl], or fibrinolysis-deoxyribonuclease [Elase]) is applied in a thin layer only within the wound area and covered with one layer of fine-mesh gauze. A topical antimicrobial agent is then applied and covered with a bulky wet dressing; the wound is immobilized with expandable mesh gauze. Enzymatic agents are discontinued once the eschar is removed and granulation tissue appears (Honari, 2004).

DRESSING THE WOUND Once the wound has been cleaned and debrided, it may be dressed using one of two methods. In the open method, the burn wound remains open to air, covered only by a topical antimicrobial agent. This method allows the wound to be easily assessed. Topical agents must be frequently reapplied because they tend to rub off onto the bedding. The open method also increases the risk for hypothermia (Sole et al., 2005).

In the closed method, a topical antimicrobial agent is applied to the wound site, which is covered with gauze or a nonadherent dressing and then gently wrapped with a gauze roll bandage (Figure 17–14 ■). With the closed method, burn wounds are usually dressed twice daily and as needed. Dressings are applied circumferentially in a distal-to-proximal manner. All fingers and toes are wrapped separately. Dressings are held in place with stockinettes rather than tape to prevent further skin injury. The closed method decreases heat loss but may impair range of motion (ROM).

Positioning, Splints, and Exercise **Contractures** are a common problem for clients with burn injuries. During therapy, the client must be maintained in positions that prevent contractures from forming. Because flexion is the natural resting position of joints and extremities, early physical therapy includes maintaining antideformity positions. Splints immobilize body parts and prevent contractures of the joints. They are applied as soon as possible after the injury and removed according to schedules established by the physical therapist.

Early in the acute phase of care, the physical therapist prescribes active and passive ROM exercises, which are performed every 2 hours at the bedside, most often by physical therapy. Ideally an exercise program is initiated on admission and con-

Figure 17–14 ■ Closed method of dressing a burn.
Courtesy of BSIP/Phototake NYC.

Figure 17–15 ■ The client may wear a custom-made elastic pressure garment for 6 months to a year postgraft.
Photo courtesy of Gottfried® Medical, Inc.

tinued until wounds are healed. Early ambulation is also part of the plan of care once the client's condition becomes stable.

Support Garments Applying uniform pressure can prevent or reduce hypertrophic scarring. Tubular support bandages are applied 5 to 7 days postgraft to maintain a tension ranging from 10 to 20 mmHg to control scarring. The client wears custom-made elastic pressure garments such as a Jobst garment for 6 months to a year postgraft (Figure 17–15 ■).

NUTRITIONAL SUPPORT The client with a major burn is in a hypermetabolic and catabolic state. The resting energy expenditure after severe burn injury can increase by as much as 100% above normal levels, depending on the extent of catabolism and the client's physical activity, size, age, and gender. This increase is believed due to heat loss from the burn wound, an increase in beta-adrenergic activity, pain, and infection. As a result, total caloric needs may be as great as 4000 to 6000 kcal/day.

Traditional dietary management based on oral intake seldom meets the kilocalorie requirements necessary to reverse negative nitrogen balance and begin the healing process. Enteral feedings with a nasointestinal feeding tube are therefore instituted within 24 to 48 hours of the burn injury to offset hypermetabolism, improve nitrogen balance, decrease sepsis, and decrease length of hospital stay. A nasointestinal feeding tube is placed under fluoroscopy, with the tip extending past the pylorus to prevent reflux and aspiration.

Although enteral feeding is the preferred nutritional therapy, it is contraindicated in Curling's ulcer, bowel obstruction, feeding intolerance, pancreatitis, or septic ileus. When the enteral route cannot be used, a central venous catheter is inserted via the subclavian or jugular vein for the administration of total parenteral nutrition.

NURSING CARE

The client with a major burn has complex, multisystem needs. Table 17–4 lists overall nursing interventions for the emergent, acute, and rehabilitative stages of burn injury. See the Nursing Care Plan on page 507.

Health Promotion

Although treatments have improved significantly during the last several decades, there is no cure for burns. Prevention remains the primary goal. With the public's increasing attention to health promotion and disease prevention, the nursing profession currently is well positioned to collaborate with other disciplines to develop initiatives to reduce the number of burn injuries. For example, as client advocates, nurses can alert political leaders to the need to pass legislation aimed at reducing the incidence of burns. Appropriate legislative themes might center on safety in the workplace (e.g., requirements for smoke alarms and sprinkler systems), on the highways (e.g., regulations regarding the transportation of flammable liquids), and in the home (e.g., requirements for safety devices for water heaters and wood-burning stoves, and for self-extinguishing cigarettes). As educators, nurses can develop teaching plans for families and communities to heighten awareness of the problem. As researchers, nurses can investigate conditions leading to burn injury and suggest methods to reduce its prevalence. Working together with healthcare policy makers and community leaders, nurses can join the effort to lower the number of annual burn cases.

Assessment

Nursing assessment is continuous from the initial contact with the client with a burn injury. This section describes the survey conducted when the client arrives at the emergency department. Once there, the staff must act quickly to obtain the client's history of the burn injury, including the time of injury, causative agents, early treatment, medical history, and client's age and body weight. In most cases, the client is awake and oriented and able to relate the information during the emergent phase of

TABLE 17–4 Interventions in Various Stages of Burn Injury

STAGE OF BURN INJURY	ONSET	END POINT	INTERVENTIONS
Emergent/resuscitative	Occurrence of burn injury	Successful fluid resuscitation	Remove client from heat source. Initiate first aid. Assess extent of burn injury. Prevent hypothermia. Assess for shock. Determine need for intubation. Determine need for intravenous therapy. Follow protocol for fluid resuscitation. Obtain history. Transport to tertiary care facility.
Acute	Diuresis	Wound closure	Begin hydrotherapy. Determine need for excision of burn wound. Control spread of infection. Institute wound care. Start nutrition support. Graft burn wound. Initiate physical therapy. Manage pain.
Rehabilitative	Wound closure	Return to highest level of health restoration	Prevent scar formation. Continue physical therapy. Address psychosocial, cultural, and spiritual needs. Consider occupational therapy. Consider vocational training. Assess home maintenance management.

care. Because changes in sensorium will become evident within the first few hours following a major burn injury, the nurse obtains as much information as is possible immediately on the client's arrival.

- *Time of injury.* In many cases, the client is admitted to the emergency department an hour or more after the injury occurred. The time of the burn injury must be documented as precisely as possible at the scene, because all fluid resuscitation calculations are based on the time of the burn injury, not on the client's time of arrival at the ER.
- *Cause of the injury.* Because the type of burn injury determines which nursing measures take priority, identify the specific causative agent to establish the appropriate plan of care.
- *First aid treatment.* Prior to the arrival of medical personnel, the client or family may have applied home remedies to treat the burn wound. It is important for the nurse to ascertain and document the nature of all home treatment interventions, including the application of neutralizing agents, liquids, and immobilizing devices used to splint associated injuries.
- *Past medical history.* Clients with histories of respiratory, cardiac, renal, metabolic, neurologic, gastrointestinal, or skin diseases; alcohol abuse; or altered immune states require more intense observation. Known allergies are obtained.
- *Age.* Older adults tend to require more supportive care (see the Meeting Individualized Needs box on page 508).
- *Medications.* Drugs, either prescribed or recreational, taken by the client prior to the burn injury may further complicate the treatment regimen. Drugs that affect any of the major

body systems or cause mood alterations will need to be factored into the treatment plan. As part of the early assessment, obtain and document blood levels of therapeutic pharmaceutical agents and mood-altering substances.
- *Body weight.* During the acute and rehabilitative phases of the burn injury, the client will lose as much as 20% of preburn weight. This fact will have significant implications for all clients, especially for those who are underweight or cachectic at the time of the injury.

Nursing Diagnoses and Interventions

A major burn affects virtually every body system, as well as social, cultural, economic, psychologic, and spiritual well-being. Immediate treatment in an intensive care setting is followed by years of rehabilitation and a lifetime of change in what was possible for an individual before the injury. Many nursing diagnoses are appropriate for the client with a major burn injury; those described here are *Impaired Skin Integrity, Deficient Fluid Volume, Acute Pain, Risk for Infection, Impaired Physical Mobility, Imbalanced Nutrition: Less than Body Requirements,* and *Powerlessness.*

Impaired Skin Integrity

The burn injury significantly impairs skin integrity. The severity of wounds varies according to the depth and extent of the burn. General treatment measures are designed to restore normal skin function as quickly as possible. Nursing care focuses on assessing and cleansing the wound and controlling infection.

NURSING CARE PLAN   A Client with a Major Burn

Craig Howard, a 39-year-old truck driver, is admitted to the hospital following an accident in which the cab of his truck caught on fire. He was freed from the truck by a passing motorist, who stayed with him until the rescue team arrived and transported him to a local ED. Mr. Howard's wife, Mary, and twin daughters, Jessica and Jane, age 10, have been notified.

ASSESSMENT

On his admission to the ED, Mr. Howard is diagnosed with deep partial-thickness and full-thickness burns of the anterior chest, arms, and hands. A quick assessment based on the rule of nines estimates the extent of his burn injury at 36% of TBSA. His vital signs are as follows: T 96.2°F (35.6°C), P 140, R 40, and BP 98/60. In the field, the paramedics had inserted a large-bore central line into Mr. Howard's right subclavian vein and started the rapid infusion of lactated Ringer's solution. Mr. Howard is receiving 40% humidified oxygen via face mask. Initial ABGs are: pH 7.49, Po_2 60 mmHg, Pco_2 32 mmHg, and bicarbonate 22 mEq/L. Lung sounds indicate inspiratory and expiratory wheezing, and a persistent cough reveals sooty sputum production. A Foley catheter is inserted and initially drains a moderate amount of dark, concentrated urine. A nasogastric tube is connected to low-intermittent suction. Mr. Howard is alert and oriented and complains of severe pain associated with the burn injuries. The burn unit is notified, and Mr. Howard is transferred there.

DIAGNOSIS

- *Risk for Ineffective Airway Clearance,* related to increasing lung congestion secondary to smoke inhalation
- *Deficient Fluid Volume,* related to abnormal fluid loss secondary to burn injury
- *Risk for Ineffective Tissue Perfusion* (peripheral), related to peripheral constriction secondary to circumferential burn wounds of the arms

EXPECTED OUTCOMES

- Demonstrate a patent airway, as evidenced by clear breath sounds; absence of cyanosis; and vital signs, chest X-ray findings, and ABGs within normal limits.
- Demonstrate adequate fluid volume and electrolyte balance, as evidenced by urine output, vital signs, mental status, and laboratory findings within normal limits.

- Demonstrate adequate tissue perfusion, as evidenced by palpable pulses, warm extremities, normal capillary refill, and absence of paresthesia.

PLANNING AND IMPLEMENTATION

- Prepare for prophylactic nasotracheal intubation to maintain airway patency.
- Initiate fluid resuscitation therapy using the Parkland formula to calculate intravenous fluid rate for the first 24 hours postburn.
- Assist the physician to perform escharotomies of both upper extremities.

EVALUATION

The nurse anesthetist inserted a nasotracheal tube and connected Mr. Howard to a T-piece delivering 40% oxygen. Vigorous respiratory toileting has significantly improved his ABGs. Bronchodilators have been parenterally administered and mucolytic agents added to his respiratory treatments. His tracheal secretions have begun to show evidence of clearing. Hourly urine outputs indicate adequate fluid resuscitation. Urine output has been maintained at 50 mL/h, and color and concentration have improved. CVP readings have been maintained at 6 cm H_2O, and blood pressure has increased to 100/64. The pulse rate has decreased to 100.

To improve tissue perfusion of both arms, the physician has performed bilateral escharotomies and the wounds are dressed, using sterile procedure. The extremities have demonstrated improved circulation.

CRITICAL THINKING IN THE NURSING PROCESS

1. Explain the rationale for the immediate insertion of a Foley catheter and nasogastric tube.
2. An escharotomy was performed on both arms. Why was this procedure necessary in Mr. Howard's case?
3. What is the rationale supporting the intravenous administration of narcotics to control Mr. Howard's pain?
4. Explain the sequence of events that led to a fluid and electrolyte shift during the first 24 to 48 hours after Mr. Howard sustained his injury.

See Evaluating Your Response in Appendix C.

- Estimate the extent and depth of the burn wound and recalculate extent of unhealed burns weekly. *The severity of the burn injury is the basis for determining which types of interventions are appropriate. Reassessment on a regular basis is necessary to monitor the healing process.*
- Provide daily wound care (including debridement method, dressing method, and medication administration) as prescribed *to remove dead tissue, control infection, and promote reepithelialization as soon as possible.*

PRACTICE ALERT

When cleansing wounds, avoid cross-contamination of the client's wounds.

- Elevate burned or newly skin grafted extremities at or above heart level *to increase venous return and to prevent edema formation.*
- Immobilize skin graft sites for 3 to 5 days or as ordered *to promote graft adherence and to prevent loss of newly grafted skin.*

PRACTICE ALERT

Move clients slowly and carefully across bed sheets to prevent shearing or dislodgement of the new skin grafts.

- Provide special skin care to sensitive body areas:
  - Clean burns involving the eyes with normal saline or sterile water *to prevent corneal and conjunctival drying and*

MEETING INDIVIDUALIZED NEEDS Burns in the Older Adult

Older adults are at greater risk for burns of all degrees of severity, with burns and fires being a major cause of death. Most burns are accidental, the result of slower reaction times, decreased mobility, visual deficits, a decreased sense of smell, forgetfulness, and impaired sensation. Many older adults are burned by stoves, hot water, hot food, irons, cookware, and heating pads. Older adults with cognitive impairments or dementias may start fires by leaving foods cooking unattended. The most common burns in this age group are the result of catching clothing on fire and scalding from tap water that is too hot.

The care of the older adult with burns often presents unique challenges. They may delay seeking treatment, thus increasing the risk of infection. Their care is often complicated by the pres-ence of other chronic illnesses. They may live alone, and have no one to care for them during rehabilitation. Even small burns have the potential to become lethal in older adults.

Burn prevention topics for older adults are as follows:
- Have a relative or neighbor routinely check for the odor of gas.
- Check the smoke detector battery once a month.
- Wear close-fitting clothing when cooking.
- Use a cooking timer with a loud alarm.
- Never lay anything over a heating device.
- Set the temperature of the hot water heater no higher than 120°F.
- Install antiscald devices in bathroom plumbing.
- Encourage no smoking in the house.

---

adherence. If contracture of the eyelid develops, apply drops or ointment to the eye *to prevent corneal abrasion.*
- Gently wipe burns of the lips with saline-soaked pads. Apply an antibiotic ointment as prescribed. Assess the mouth frequently, and perform mouth care routinely. If an oral endotracheal tube is in place, reposition it often *to prevent pressure ulcer formation.*
- Gently debride burns of the nose, and apply mafenide acetate (Sulfamylon) cream. Position nasogastric and nasotracheal tubes *to prevent excessive pressure.*
- Apply mafenide acetate (Sulfamylon) cream to burns of the ear. Gently debride and thoroughly clean the wound with a water spray. Do not cover ears with dressings. Do not use pillows; to reduce pressure to the area, use a foam doughnut instead. *Burns of the ears are prone to infection; special positioning devices are necessary to decrease pressure ulcer formation.*

Deficient Fluid Volume

Fluid resuscitation rates are adjusted periodically throughout the emergent stage of care. The nurse should be particularly aware of several situations that may warrant the administration of fluids at rates in excess of the calculations needed to maintain adequate urine output: initial underestimation of the burn size, sequestration of fluid into the lung tissue in inhalation injury, electrical injury (which tends to cause more extensive damage than is immediately visible), full-thickness burns, and inordinately delayed starts of fluid resuscitation.
- Assess blood pressure and heart rate frequently. *Vital signs rapidly deteriorate when fluid resuscitation is inadequate.*

PRACTICE ALERT

Tachycardia in the burn client is not considered until the heart rate is greater than 120 beats per minute.

- Monitor hemodynamic status, including central venous pressure (CVP) and pulmonary artery wedge pressure (PAWP). *Inadequate fluid resuscitation is manifested by a drop in the CVP and PAWP.*

- Follow prescribed protocols for intravenous fluid resuscitation. *Therapy for burn shock is aimed at supporting the client through the period of hypovolemic instability.*
- Monitor intake and output hourly. *Report urine outputs of less than 50 mL/h. Intake and output measurements indicate the adequacy of fluid resuscitation, and should range from 30 to 50 mL/h in an adult.*
- Weigh daily. *Body weight is used to calculate fluid requirements.*
- Test all stools and emesis for the presence of blood. *Occult blood in emesis or stool indicates gastrointestinal bleeding.*
- Maintain a warm environment. *Hypothermia leads to shivering and further loss of body fluid through increased energy expenditure and catabolism.*
- Monitor for fluid volume overload. *Older clients and those with underlying cardiac disease may demonstrate symptoms of heart failure during the fluid resuscitation stage.*

PRACTICE ALERT

Major burn clients receive 10 or more liters of fluid and will gain weight with the fluid shifts. When capillary membrane integrity resumes, clients have a high CVP and urine output that necessitates monitoring of urine electrolytes.

Acute Pain

The client experiences excruciating pain with extensive superficial and all partial-thickness burns. Intense pain is also experienced during wound care and physical therapy. In addition, increased levels of anxiety about treatments and outcomes may further increase the perception of pain.
- Measure the client's level of pain, using a consistent measurement tool. *Pain tolerance is the duration and intensity of pain that the client is able to endure. Pain tolerance differs from one client to the next and may vary in the same client in different situations.*
- Medicate before painful procedures and determine when PCA is appropriate. *The inability to manage pain results in feelings of despair and frustration.*

- Administer intravenous narcotic analgesics as prescribed. *Nurses' fears of precipitating addiction often make them reluctant to administer narcotics. During the acute stage of burn injury, however, invasive procedures and exposed neurosensory nerve endings dictate the need for narcotic pharmaceutical agents.*
- Explain all procedures and expected levels of discomfort. *Clients who are prepared for painful procedures and know beforehand the actual sensations they will feel experience less stress.*
- Use methods of nonnarcotic pain control in combination with medications for pain. *Noninvasive pain relief measures (e.g., relaxation, massage, distraction) can enhance the therapeutic effects of pain relief medications.*
- Allow the client to verbalize the pain experience. *Each person experiences and expresses pain in his or her own manner, using various sociocultural adaptation techniques.*

PRACTICE ALERT
Narcotics are always administered intravenously rather than orally, subcutaneously, or intramuscularly in the emergent or acute stage of a burn due to decreased circulation and absorption of medications.

Risk for Infection
From the onset of the burn injury, loss of the body's natural barrier to the external environment increases the risk of infection. Nursing interventions focus on controlling infectious processes. Monitor the results of diagnostic tests, maintain nutritional therapies, and apply antimicrobial agents to monitor and prevent the spread of infection, a major complication of the burn injury.

- Monitor daily for manifestations of wound infection. Remove topical medications and wound exudate and examine the entire wound. *Early manifestations of wound infection include swelling and inflammation in intact skin surrounding the wound; a change in the color, odor, or amount of exudate; increased pain; and loss of previously healed skin grafts.*

PRACTICE ALERT
An increased body temperature, without other manifestations of infection, is not indicative of infection in clients with large burn wounds (in which the hypermetabolic response resets the core temperature to a higher level).

- Monitor for positive blood cultures, *which indicate bacteremia.*
- Monitor for hyperemia, cough, chest pain, wheezing, rhonchi, decreased oxygen saturation, and purulent sputum, *which are manifestations of pneumonia.*
- Monitor for the presence of bacteria in the urine, fever, urgency, frequency, dysuria, and superpubic pain, *which are manifestations of urinary tract infections.*

PRACTICE ALERT
If the client has an indwelling catheter, assess the urine for cloudiness and a foul odor, and obtain a urine culture and sensitivity at least weekly.

- Obtain daily WBC counts. *Leukocyte counts are indicators of immune system function, and increase in the presence of infection.*
- Determine tetanus immunization status. *Burn clients are at risk for anaerobic infection caused by* Clostridium tetani.
- Maintain a high-kilocalorie intake. *Nutritional support provides the nutrients needed to maintain the body's defense mechanisms.*
- Maintain an aseptic environment, using standard precautions (including gloving, gowning, and sterile procedures). *Strict isolation technique deters the development of nosocomial infections.*
- Culture all wounds and body secretions per protocol. *Culture and sensitivity reports identify the presence of infectious microbes and indicate appropriate antimicrobial therapies.*
- Administer prescribed antimicrobial medications *to decrease invasive wound infections.*

Impaired Physical Mobility
As the burn wound heals and new skin tissue forms, the involved area tends to shrink. Contractures form at the site and significantly limit mobility, especially when a joint is involved. Physical therapy is important, beginning in the early stages of treatment. The nurse institutes ambulation and planned exercise regimens as soon as the client's condition stabilizes. See the Nursing Research box on page 510.

- Perform active or passive ROM exercises to all joints every 2 hours. Ambulate when stable. *Regular exercise prevents further loss of motion, restores movement, and improves functional status.*
- Apply splints as prescribed. Maintain antideformity positions, and reposition the client hourly. *Splinting and positioning retard the formation of contractures.*
- Maintain limbs in functional alignment *to preserve joint mobility.*
- Anticipate the need for analgesia. *Administering analgesics promotes the client's comfort during exercising sessions.*

PRACTICE ALERT
Assess all clients, but especially the older adult, for indications of pressure ulcer formation under a splint.

Imbalanced Nutrition: Less than Body Requirements
The burn injury initiates a complex series of events that have a profound effect on the body's use of nutrients and expenditure of energy. Daily kilocalorie requirements are determined by the dietitian, and as soon as possible, enteral feedings are initiated. Nasointestinal tubes are placed to enhance intestinal absorption and retard gastric reflux. Parenteral nutrition is reserved for instances in which enteral feedings are contraindicated. Nursing measures focus on assessing feeding tolerance and use of nutrients.

- Maintain nasogastric/nasointestinal tube placement. *Correct tube placement ensures appropriate absorption of nutrients and prevents aspiration.*

NURSING RESEARCH   Evidence-Based Practice: Client with a Major Burn

Clients with major burn injuries are at risk for pressure ulcers due to deficient fluid volume, inadequate nutrition, pain, and immobility. Healthy, intact skin can experience damage from friction and shearing forces, posing a second area of risk for pressure sores.

In an investigation of pressure sore prevention in burn patients (Gordon et al., 2004), a multidisciplinary team of burn care specialists reviewed and evaluated the current evidence of practice for preventing pressure sores. Pressure sores result from continuous, unrelieved pressure that causes reduced blood flow to vulnerable areas of the skin, resulting in tissue damage. Results of the study confirmed that contributing factors to the development of pressure sores in clients with burn injuries include inadequate dietary intake, malnutrition, decreased albumin levels, moisture and incontinence, reduced sensation, prolonged immobility, increased age, and altered level of consciousness.

IMPLICATIONS FOR NURSING

Nurses and all members of the burn team assume an integral role in preventing pressure ulcers. JCAHO has identified the prevention of healthcare-associated pressure ulcers as one of the new patient safety goals for 2006. To implement this goal, nurses must monitor constantly the client with major burn injuries for signs of pressure sores by using skin risk assessment scales on admission and weekly and by inspecting the skin daily. Frequent nutritional assessment is performed to meet the client's energy needs. Moisture accumulation can be decreased by keeping the skin clean and dry, applying skin barriers, and using a Foley catheter when incontinence exists. High-risk clients with burns should be considered candidates for the use of pressure-reducing beds. Healthcare team members must be knowledgeable about the proper techniques for positioning, transferring, and moving clients with burns. It is important to institute a multi-strategy approach in managing and preventing pressure sores for clients with major burns.

CRITICAL THINKING IN CLIENT CARE

1. The client's head must be elevated to 30 degrees when nasogastric tube feedings are implemented. What strategies would you recommend to prevent sacral pressure sores?
2. How could splints that are being used to prevent contractures be modified as the client's amount and extent of edema fluctuates?
3. Develop a teaching plan for instructing nursing assistants on how to move, position, and transfer clients in a burn center unit. Include in the teaching plan the proper technique for cleansing unburned skin.

- Maintain enteral/parenteral nutritional support as prescribed. Observe and report any evidence of feeding intolerance: diarrhea, vomiting, excessive gastric residual, abdominal distention, absent bowel sounds, and constipation. *The dietitian, in collaboration with the physician, selects and individualizes the feeding formula according to the client's daily energy expenditure requirements and feeding tolerance. Failure to maintain rates of infusion predisposes the client to continued catabolism and negative nitrogen balance.*
- Weigh the client daily. *Weight indicates the adequacy of nutritional support therapies.*
- Obtain daily laboratory values for protein, iron, CBC, glucose, and albumin. *Decreased serum values indicate inadequate nutritional intake.*

Powerlessness

Usually, the client with a major burn injury endures a lengthy hospital stay involving many treatments and care protocols that are beyond his or her control. During the early stages, much of the care regimen involves excruciating pain. Further, the foreign environment of the burn unit makes it difficult for the client to relate to the immediate surroundings. For example, the need to control infection in the burn unit requires hospital personnel and family members to don sterile clothing prior to coming to the client's bedside. Family members and nursing personnel appear radically different when they are masked and gowned, and their odd appearance can add to the burn-injured client's sense of alienation. The client's body image is often altered, depending on the extent and location of the burn injury.

- Allow the client as much control over the surroundings and daily routine as possible. For example, allow the client to choose times of dressing changes. *Powerlessness derives from the belief that one is unable to influence the outcome of a situation.*
- Keep needed items within reach, such as call bell, urinal, water pitcher, and tissues, *to reinforce the client's feelings of control.*
- Encourage the client to express feelings. *The nurse can help the client cope by therapeutically listening, displaying a caring presence, clarifying misconceptions, and providing positive feedback.*
- Set short-term, realistic goals (e.g., set a goal for the client to ambulate from bedside to chair twice daily). *Small incremental gains are easier to achieve and allow for frequent positive reinforcement.*

Using NANDA, NIC, and NOC

Chart 17–1 shows links between NANDA, NIC, and NOC when caring for the client with a major burn.

Community-Based Care

Client and family teaching is an important component of all phases of burn care. As treatment progresses, the nurse encourages family members to assume more responsibility in providing care. From admission to discharge, the nurse teaches the client and family to assess all findings, implement therapies, and evaluate progress. The following topics should be addressed when preparing the client and family for home care:

NANDA, NIC, AND NOC LINKAGES
CHART 17–1 **The Client with a Major Burn**

NANDA

Impaired Skin Integrity

↓

NIC

Skin Surveillance

Wound Care

Infection Protection

↓

NOC

Tissue Integrity: Skin

Wound Healing

Data from *NANDA's Nursing Diagnoses: Definitions & classification 2005–2006* by NANDA International (2003), Philadelphia; *Nursing Interventions Classification (NIC)* (4th ed.) by J. M. Dochterman & G. M. Bulechek (2004) St Louis, Mo: Mosby; and *Nursing Outcomes Classification (NOC)* (3rd ed.) by S. Moorhead, M. Johnson, and M. Maas (2004), St. Louis, MO: Mosby.

- The long-term goals of rehabilitation care: to prevent soft tissue deformity, protect skin grafts, maintain physiologic function, manage scars, and return the client to an optimal level of independence
- Avoiding exposure to people with colds or infections and following aseptic technique meticulously when caring for the wound
- The need for progressive physical activity
- How to apply splints, pressure support garments, and other assistive devices
- Dietary requirements with required kcalories
- Alternative pain control therapies, such as guided imagery, relaxation techniques, and diversional activities
- Care of the graft and donor sites
- Referral for occupational therapy, social service, clergy, and/or psychiatric services as appropriate
- Helpful resources:
  - American Burn Association
  - International Society for Burn Injuries
  - American Academy of Facial Plastic and Reconstructive Surgery
  - The Phoenix Society for Burn Survivors, Inc.

EXPLORE MEDIALINK

Prentice Hall Nursing MediaLink DVD-ROM
- Audio Glossary
- NCLEX-RN® Review

COMPANION WEBSITE www.prenhall.com/lemone
- Audio Glossary
- NCLEX-RN® Review
- Care Plan Activities
  - *A Client Having a Skin Graft*
  - *A Client with Burns*
  - *Inhalation Injury*
- Case Studies
- MediaLink Applications
- Links to Resources

CHAPTER HIGHLIGHTS

- Four types of burn injuries are thermal, chemical, electrical, and radiation. The depth of the burn injury determines whether it is classified as a superficial, partial-thickness, or full-thickness burn.
- The "rule of nines" is used to estimate the extent of a burn by assigning percentages to different parts of the body.
- Major burns involve multiorgan pathophysiologic alterations. Most critical is the fluid shift from the intracellular and intravascular compartments into the interstitium, resulting in a type of hypovolemic shock called burn shock. Other pathologic processes include an impaired immune system, disturbed functions of the skin, inhalation injury, gastrointestinal ulcerations and ileus, renal failure, and hypermetabolism.
- Interdisciplinary care focuses on managing the client during the emergent/resuscitative, acute, and rehabilitative stages. To counter the effects of burn shock, fluid resuscitation using guidelines such

as the Parkland formula are initiated to replace fluid and electrolyte losses.
- Additional management for the client with major burns includes preventing atelectasis, maintaining respiratory function, controlling pain, preventing infection and Curling's ulcer, promoting nutrition, and providing wound care.
- Extensive eschar of an extremity or the torso called circumferential wounds can potentially occlude arterial flow or decrease respiratory function. An escharotomy is used to release tension, preventing additional complications.
- Surgical management of burn wounds include debridement and skin grafting. Biologic and biosynthetic dressings provide temporary covering and prepare the wound for permanent autografts.
- Continual psychologic support of the client and family is essential throughout convalescence and rehabilitation.

TEST YOURSELF NCLEX-RN® REVIEW

1 During the emergent phase of burn management, what diagnostic test result should the nurse expect to find?
1. increased hematocrit
2. increased serum albumin
3. decreased serum potassium
4. decreased blood urea nitrogen (BUN)

2 A client is admitted with severe burns to the face and chest. The injured skin is dry and leathery, with no pain sensations present. The nurse recognizes that this burn is classified as:
1. superficial.
2. superficial partial thickness.
3. deep partial thickness.
4. full thickness.

3 Which of the following clients is at greatest risk for developing burn shock?
1. a 21-year-old with 90% superficial burn from a tanning bed
2. a 30-year-old with 10% TBSA from a gasoline explosion
3. a 39-year-old with radiation burns following treatment for cancer
4. a 48-year-old with >50% TBSA from a high-voltage electrical accident

4 A client with a major burn is receiving silver sulfadiazine (Silvadene) to treat the burns. What nursing action should be implemented when using this medication?
1. Premedicate for pain prior to application.
2. Monitor WBC count daily.
3. Observe for signs of dehydration.
4. Monitor serum electrolyte levels daily.

5 A client with full-thickness burns over 50% of the body arrives in the emergency department. The client weighs 70 kg. Using the Parkland formula, calculate the amount of fluid replacement that the nurse should deliver in the first 8 hours.
1. 3500 mL
2. 7000 mL
3. 10,500 mL
4. 14,000 mL

100 mL per Kg

6 For a client with a major burn, which of the following evaluation criteria indicate that fluid resuscitation is effective during the first 24 hours of care?
1. urine output of 30 to 50 mL/h
2. central venous pressure of 18
3. heart rate of 130 beats per minute
4. blood pressure 96/70

7 A client has deep partial-thickness burns to the entire left arm and left side of the back. What finding should be reported to the physician immediately?
1. fluid-filled vesicles on the left arm
2. pain in the left arm
3. blanching when pressure is applied to the left hand
4. decreased left radial pulse

8 A client received deep partial-thickness burns to the anterior trunk, perineum, and left arm anterior and posterior. Using the rule of nines, what is the percent of total body surface area (TBSA) that was burned?
1. 18%
2. 28%
3. 36%
4. 40%

9 Which of the following topics should be included in a presentation on burn prevention at a senior citizen center? (Select all that apply.)
1. Wear close-fitting clothing when cooking.
2. Use a solar-powered night-light.
3. Set the water heater no higher than 120°F.
4. Check smoke detectors annually.
5. Install antiscald devices in bathroom plumbing.
6. Have a neighbor routinely check for the odor of gas.

10 A client has possible carbon monoxide poisoning secondary to smoke inhalation. What manifestation should the nurse expect to find in a client with a 15% carbon monoxide level?
1. dark red skin color
2. drowsiness
3. dizziness
4. hypotension

BIBLIOGRAPHY

Abrams, A. C. (2004). *Clinical drug therapy* (7th ed.). Philadelphia: Lippincott Williams & Wilkins.

Ahrns, K. S. (2004). Trends in burn resuscitation: Shifting the focus from fluids to adequate endpoint monitoring, edema control, and adjuvant therapies. *Critical Care Nursing Clinics of North America, 16,* 75–98.

American Burn Association. (2003). Senior safety. Retrieved from http://www.ameriburn.org/Preven/2003Prevention/2003BurnAwareness.pdf

Badger, J. (2001). Burns: The psychological aspects. *American Journal of Nursing, 101*(11), 38–44.

Baird, M. S., Keen, J. H., & Swearingen, P. L. (2005). *Manual of critical care nursing* (5th ed.). St. Louis, MO: Elsevier Mosby.

Bishop, J. F. (2004). Burn wound assessment and surgical management. *Critical Care Nursing Clinics of North America, 16,* 145–177.

Carrougher, G. (1998). *Burn care and therapy,* St. Louis: Mosby.

Carrougher, G. J., Ptacek, J. T., Shareir, S. R., et al. (2003). Comparison of patient satisfaction and self-reports of pain in adult burn-injured patients. *Journal of Burn Care and Rehabilitation, 24*(1), 1–8.

DeSanti, L. (2005). Pathophysiology and current management of burn injury. *Advances in Skin and Wound Care, 18*(6), 323–332.

Dochterman, J., & Bulechek, G. (2004). *Nursing interventions classification (NIC)* (4th ed.). St. Louis, MO: Mosby.

Flynn, M. B. (2004). Nutritional support for the burn-injured patient. *Critical Care Nursing Clinics of North America, 16,* 139–144.

Gordon, M. D., Gottschlich, M. M., Helvig, E. I., Marvin, J. A., & Richard, R. L. (2004). Review of evidence-based practice for the prevention of pressure sores in burn patients. *Journal of Burn Care and Rehabilitation, 25*(5), 388–410.

Hall, B. (2005). Wound care for burn patients in acute rehabilitation settings. *Rehabilitation Nursing, 30*(3), 114–119.

Honari, S. (2004). Topical therapies and antimicrobials in the management of burn wounds. *Critical Care Nursing Clinics of North America, 16,* 1–11.

Joint Commission International Center for Patient Safety. (2005). *2006 Patient safety goals.* Retrieved from http://www.jcipatientsafety.org

Kee, J. L. (2005). *Laboratory and diagnostic tests with nursing implications* (7th ed.). Upper Saddle River, NJ: Prentice Hall.

Lehne, R. A. (2004). *Pharmacology for nursing care* (5th ed.). St. Louis, MO: Saunders.

McCance, K. L., & Huether, S. E. (2006). *Pathophysiology The biologic basis for disease in adults and children* (5th ed.). St. Louis, MO: Mosby.

Montgomery, R. K. (2004). Pain management in burn injury. *Critical Care Nursing Clinics of North America, 16,* 39–49.

Moorhead, S., Johnson, M., & Maas, M. (2003). *Nursing outcomes classification (NOC)* (3rd ed.). St. Louis, MO: Mosby.

National Fire Protection Association. (2004). *Leaving home: College fire safety and burn prevention campaign.* Quincy, MA: Author.

_____. (2005). *Smoking material-related fires.* Retrieved from http://www.nfpa.org/itemDetail.asp?categoryID=294&itemID19303&URL=Research%20&%20Reports/Fact%20sheets/Home%20safety/Smoking%20material-related%20fires

National Institute of General Medical Sciences. (2005). *Trauma, burn, shock, and injury: Facts and figures.* Retrieved from http://www.nigms.nih.gov/news/facts/traumaburnfactsfigures.html

North American Nursing Diagnosis Association. (2004). *Nursing diagnoses: Definitions & classification 2005–2006.* Philadelphia: Author.

Osborn, K. (2003). Nursing burn injuries. *Nursing Management, 34*(5), 49–56.

Porth, C. M. (2005). *Pathophysiology: Concepts of altered health states* (7th ed.). Philadelphia: Lippincott Williams & Wilkins.

Regojo, P. S. (2003). Burn care basics. *Nursing 2003, 33*(3), 50–53.

Sole, M. L., Klein, D. G., & Moseley, M. J. (2005). *Introduction to critical care nursing* (4th ed.). St. Louis, MO: Elsevier.

Supple, K. G. (2004). Physiologic response to burn injury. *Critical Care Nursing Clinics of North America, 16,* 119–126.

Wilson, B. A., Shannon, M. T., & Stang, C. L. (2006). *Nurse's drug guide 2006.* Upper Saddle River, NJ: Prentice Hall.

UNIT 4 BUILDING CLINICAL COMPETENCE
Responses to Altered Integumentary Structure and Function

FUNCTIONAL HEALTH PATTERN: Nutritional—Metabolic

■ Think about clients with altered nutrition or metabolic function for whom you have cared in your clinical experiences.

- What were the clients' major medical diagnoses (e.g., psoriasis, cysts, folliculitis, cellulitis, candidiasis, pediculosis, herpes zoster, seborrheic dermatitis, acne vulgaris, nonmelanoma skin cancer, malignant melanoma, basal cell carcinoma, pressure ulcers, or burn trauma)?
- What manifestations did each of these clients have? Were these manifestations similar or different?
- How did the clients' nutritional and metabolic status affect their integumentary system? What was their daily intake of foods and fluids? Were they gaining or losing weight? What medications or dietary supplements were they taking? What was the condition of their skin, hair, and nails? Did they complain of dry skin, itching, rashes, bruising, or hair loss? Did they note any changes in moles or warts? Did they have any pressure areas on the sacrum, hips, or ankles? Did they have any previous skin disorders and how were they treated? Did they use preventive measures to protect against temperature extremes?

■ The Nutritional-Metabolic Pattern includes food and fluid intake to maintain the nutritional and metabolic needs of the integumentary system. Breakdown of skin and its accessory structures leads to decreased protection between internal and external environments. Integumentary disorders are affected by nutritional and metabolic status in three primary ways:

- Lack of proper nutrients lowers the body's resistance to illness and can result in integumentary disorders such as infection (e.g., viral, bacterial) or skin breakdown (e.g., pressure ulcers).
- Exposure to extremes of cold or heat can result in trauma to the skin and accessory structures (e.g., frostbite, burn trauma).
- Use of certain medications, trauma, and medical disorders can result in hair distribution changes (e.g., hirsutism, alopecia).

■ Nutrients are used by the body to promote maintenance and repair of cells and tissues. Improper intake of nutrients affects the integumentary system's ability to maintain protection, regulate body temperature, and maintain fluid and electrolyte balance. Exposure to environmental extremes may alter the integrity of the skin, increasing the risk for infection and alterations of fluid/electrolye balance. Due to these factors, the client can develop skin, hair, and nail disorders, leading to manifestations such as:

- Skin ulcerations (external pressure impairs the flow of blood and lymph or friction and shearing from sliding tears and injures vessels ▶ tissue ischemia and hypoxia occur ▶ resulting in tissue death and necrosis)
- Infection (microorganisms invade tissue and replicate ▶ toxic by-products of microorganism metabolism, cell lysis, and immune response occur ▶ resulting in inflammation and tissue damage)
- Alopecia (scarring from trauma, infection, radiation, medications ▶ affects rapidly growing cells in hair follicles ▶ affected hair follicle cells slow down hair production ▶ resulting in loss of hair).

■ Priority nursing diagnoses within the Nutritional-Metabolic Pattern that may be appropriate for clients with integumentary disorders include:

- *Impaired Skin Integrity* as evidenced by open skin lesions, edema, delayed wound healing, itching, rashes
- *Risk for Infection* related to altered skin integrity, moisture, altered sensation, and obesity
- *Deficient Fluid Volume* as evidenced by dry skin and mucous membranes, decreased urine output, and elevated hemotocrit
- *Disturbed Body Image* as evidenced by verbalizations of altered body appearance and burn scars on face and arms.

■ Two nursing diagnoses from other functional health patterns often are of high priority for the client with integumentary disorders because the physiologic responses to these problems interfere with proper nutrition and metabolic functioning:

- *Acute Pain* (Cognitive-Perceptual)
- *Ineffective Protection* (Activity-Exercise)

CLINICAL SCENARIO

You have been assigned to work with the following four clients for the 0700 shift on a medical-surgical unit. Significant data obtained during report are as follows:

- Mr. Johnson is a 46-year-old who is hospitalized for surgery to release contractures at his elbows which resulted from a flash burn from a grill fire 3 years ago. He is scheduled for surgery at 0800 and needs vital signs, preoperative medication, and the preoperative checklist completed.
- Mrs. Carter is a 35-year-old who was hospitalized 2 days ago with cellulitis in the right calf. Vital signs are T 100.4°F, P 80, R 20, BP 116/76.

She is complaining of a headache and pain in the right calf. She was last medicated for pain at 0300.

- Mr. Jenkins is an 86-year-old with herpes zoster. He was admitted 4 days ago with lesions on his left neck and trunk. Vital signs are T 99°F, P 88, R 26, BP 158/90. He is complaining of burning pain across his back and is requesting a nurse to check his back for new lesions.
- Mr. Ugandi is a 34-year-old African male who has a history of AIDS. He was transferred from the burn ICU to the medical-surgical unit at 0600 after being treated for toxic epidermal necrolysis for the past month. He is ready to begin discharge teaching.

Questions

1 In what order would you visit these clients after report?

1. _____
2. _____
3. _____
4. _____

2 What top two priority nursing diagnoses would you choose for each of the clients presented above? Can you explain, if asked, the rationale for your choices?

	Priority Nursing Diagnosis #1	Priority Nursing Diagnosis #2
Mr. Johnson		
Mrs. Carter		
Mr. Jenkins		
Mr. Ugandi		

3 Mr. Johnson received partial-thickness and full-thickness flash burns on both anterior and posterior arms and his anterior trunk from a grill fire. Using the "rule of nines," what is the percentage of total body surface (TBSA) burned?

_____%

4 Morphine sulfate is the drug of choice for pain. Which manifestation requires immediate nursing intervention following morphine administration?

1. vomiting once after medication is administered
2. respiratory rate below 8 breaths per minute
3. blood pressure of 110/70 after a baseline blood pressure of 120/80
4. peripheral pulse of 68 after a baseline pulse of 78

5 A diet high in protein and iron may help prevent pressure ulcers on the client who is on prolonged bed rest. Which foods should the nurse encourage the client to eat to help prevent pressure ulcers?

1. eggs and chicken
2. broccoli and oranges
3. oatmeal and bananas
4. whole-grain bread and kidney beans

6 Mr. Jenkins is being discharged to home. Which statement does the nurse need to teach Mr. Jenkins about herpes zoster on discharge?

1. "Continue taking the antiviral medication to cure the herpes zoster."
2. "You can attend church functions because herpes zoster is not contagious."
3. "Use narcotic pain medications only for severe pain so you do not become addicted to the medication."
4. "Wear cotton clothing and keep room temperatures cool to decrease the pain and itching from the herpes zoster lesions."

7 Mrs. Carter was admitted with cellulitis in the right calf. Which manifestations would the nurse assess on admission?

1. redness, edema, and pain in the right calf
2. purulent drainage, pale skin, and pain in right calf
3. rash, redness, and swelling in right calf
4. itching, rash, and pain in right calf

8 The nurse applies mafenide acetate (Sulfamylon) to Mr. Ugandi's open skin wounds caused by toxic epidermal necrolysis. Which hypersensitivity reactions would require the nurse to discontinue the drug?

1. tachycardia and tachypnea
2. nausea and vomiting
3. facial edema and pruritis
4. diarrhea and *candidiasis*

9 Which serum laboratory values are decreased with inadequate nutritional intake, such as in a client with severe burns? Select all that apply.

1. protein
2. potassium
3. iron
4. complete blood cell count
5. glucose
6. calcium

10 When a client is admitted to the burn unit for treatment of severe burns, it is most important for the nurse to monitor the client for:

1. acute pain.
2. nausea and vomiting.
3. hypothermia.
4. fluid and electrolyte imbalance.

11 Which of these clients is most at risk for skin breakdown leading to pressure ulcers?

1. a 70-year-old who had a stroke with left-sided paralysis
2. a quadriplegic admitted to the hospital with pneumonia
3. a 56-year-old client on dialysis three times a week
4. an 84-year-old client in traction for a hip fracture

12 Health teaching for skin cancer includes which interventions? (Choose all that apply.)

1. Wear long-sleeved shirts and a wide-brimmed hat in the sun.
2. Apply sunscreen once a day.
3. Avoid tanning booths or prolonged exposure to the sun.
4. Minimize exposure to the sun between 1:00 P.M. and 4:00 P.M.
5. Apply sunscreen before and after swimming.

CASE STUDY

Ms. Rachel Chelen is a 23-year-old who is admitted to the medical-surgical unit for observation and treatment after being exposed to the sun for a prolonged period of time. On admission, Ms. Chelen stated she fell asleep lying on her stomach while sunbathing at the beach. Her vital signs are T 100.6°F, P 94, R, 26, BP 116/76. Her height is 5'2" and weight is 125 lbs. Assessment findings are that her back is red and slightly edematous with an area ~6 cm by 3 cm between the scapula that is beginning to develop blisters. The backs of her arms and legs, and soles of her feet are red and slightly edematous. She is complaining of pain on her back, arms, legs, and feet. She stated that she feels chilled, is nauseated, and has a headache. Blood is drawn for a complete blood count and electrolytes for baseline assessment. IV therapy is instituted to maintain hydration. The burn areas are washed with soap and water and an antibiotic ointment is applied. A mild analgesic is administered as ordered. The client is covered to prevent further chilling and to prevent burned areas from exposure to air.

She is diagnosed with superficial and superficial partial-thickness burns. Using the "rule of nines," the partial-thickness burn on her back is classified as approximately 5% total body surface area. The superficial burns over the rest of the reddened areas are not classified. Superficial burns involve the epidermis layer of the skin. Superficial partial-thickness burns involve the entire dermis and the papillae of the dermis. The pathophysiologic effects of the superficial and partial-thickness burns are the result of exposure to the sun for a prolonged time. An inflammatory response occurs in response to tissue injury. Platelets aggregate at the burn injury site, fibrin is deposited, and a thrombus is formed. The thrombus along with vasoconstriction walls off the burn injury site. Then vasodilation occurs with increased capillary permeability, which leads to redness and edema. Injury to the dermis results in a moist, glistening appearance as blisters form. The burned area will blanch on pressure. There is pain in response to touch and temperature changes. The burned area should heal within 14 to 21 days with minimal or no scarring, but may have pigment changes. Manifestations of superficial and superficial partial-thickness burns are skin redness, blister formation, local pain, headache, chills, nausea, and vomiting. Complications of superficial and superficial partial-thickness burns are infection, hypothermia, dehydration, and fluid and electrolyte imbalances.

Due to the severity of tissue injury from the burns, the priority nursing diagnosis of *Impaired Skin Integrity* is appropriate for guiding nursing care.

affects

- Inflammatory response to injury to dermis and epidermis
- Platelet aggregation and deposits of fibrin lead to hemostasis
- Fibroblasts are deposited and granulation tissue forms

Ms. C
23 y.o. female
Superficial and partial thickness burns

leads to

assess

- Partial thickness burns on back=5% TBS with redness and blistering
- Superficial burns with redness and blisters on posterior of arms, legs, and soles of feet
- Pain in burn areas

generates

- Acute Pain related to superficial and partial thickness burns
- Risk for Infection related to partial thickness burns
- Nausea related to effects of burns

generate nursing diagnosis

prioritized to

Impaired Skin Integrity

expected outcomes

- Burns heal within one month without manifestations of infection
- Provides wound care, including cleansing and application of topical medications
- Pain decreases to a 0 on a scale of 0 (least) to 10 (most) pain
- Verbalizes principles of safe sun exposure and risks of sunburn

evaluate

- Both superficial and partial thickness burns healed without infection
- Pain decreased within one week
- Verbalized understanding of safe sun exposure and risks of sunburn

Interdisciplinary Interventions
- Insert intravenous line and initiate fluids as prescribed
- Wash burn area and apply prescribed topical medications
- Administer prescribed analgesic for pain

Independent Interventions
- Explain reason for intravenous fluids, cleansing burn area, and applying topical medications
- Teach and request demonstration of wound care and application of topical medications (instruct client's housemate as burns are on her back)
- Teach effects, side effects, and times for taking analgesic for pain
- Teach manifestations of infection and need to notify healthcare provider if they occur
- Instruct in methods of safe sun exposure and risks of sunburn

UNIT 5

Responses to Altered Endocrine Function

CHAPTER 18 Assessing Clients with Endocrine Disorders

LEARNING OUTCOMES

- Describe the anatomy and physiology of the endocrine glands.
- Explain the functions of the hormones secreted by the endocrine glands.
- Identify specific topics to consider during a health history interview of the client with health problems involving endocrine function.
- Describe techniques for assessing the thyroid gland and the effects of altered endocrine function.
- Describe normal variations in assessment findings for the older adult.
- Identify abnormal findings that may indicate malfunction of the glands of the endocrine system.

CLINICAL COMPETENCIES

- Conduct and document a health history for clients who have or are at risk for alterations in the structure or function of the endocrine glands.
- Monitor the results of diagnostic tests and report abnormal findings.
- Conduct and document a physical assessment of the structure of the thyroid gland and the effects of altered endocrine function on other body structures and functions.

EQUIPMENT NEEDED

- Reflex hammer
- Safety pin, cotton ball, containers with hot and cold water, tuning fork
- Blood pressure cuff
- Stethoscope

The endocrine system is essential to regulate the body's internal environment. Through hormones secreted by its glands, the endocrine system regulates such varied functions as growth, reproduction, metabolism, fluid and electrolyte balance, and gender differentiation. It also helps the body adapt to constant alterations in the internal and external environment.

ANATOMY, PHYSIOLOGY, AND FUNCTIONS OF THE ENDOCRINE SYSTEM

The major endocrine organs are the pituitary gland, thyroid gland, parathyroid glands, adrenal glands, pancreas, and gonads (reproductive glands). The locations of these glands are illustrated in Figure 18–1 ■. Table 18–1 summarizes the functions of the endocrine organs and their hormones. Specific information about the ovaries and testes is found in Chapters 49 ∞ through 51 ∞.

Pituitary Gland

The pituitary gland (hypophysis) is located in the skull beneath the hypothalamus of the brain (Figure 18–2 ■). It often is called the "master gland" because its hormones regulate many body functions. The pituitary gland has two parts: the anterior pituitary

Figure 18–2 ■ Location of the pituitary gland.
Source: ISM/Phototake NYC.

(or adenohypophysis) and the posterior pituitary (or neurohypophysis). The anterior pituitary is glandular tissue, whereas the posterior pituitary is actually an extension of the hypothalamus.

Anterior Pituitary

The anterior pituitary has several types of endocrine cells and secretes at least six major hormones (Figure 18–3 ■).
- Somatotropic cells secrete growth hormone (GH) (also called somatotropin). GH stimulates growth of the body by signaling cells to increase protein production and by stimulating the epiphyseal plates of the long bones.
- Lactotropic cells secrete prolactin (PRL). Prolactin stimulates the production of breast milk.
- Thyrotropic cells secrete thyroid-stimulating hormone (TSH). TSH stimulates the synthesis and release of thyroid hormones from the thyroid gland.
- Corticotropic cells secrete adrenocorticotropic hormone (ACTH). ACTH stimulates release of hormones, especially glucocorticoids, from the adrenal cortex.
- Gonadotropic cells secrete the gonadotropin hormones, follicle-stimulating hormone (FSH), and luteinizing hormone (LH).

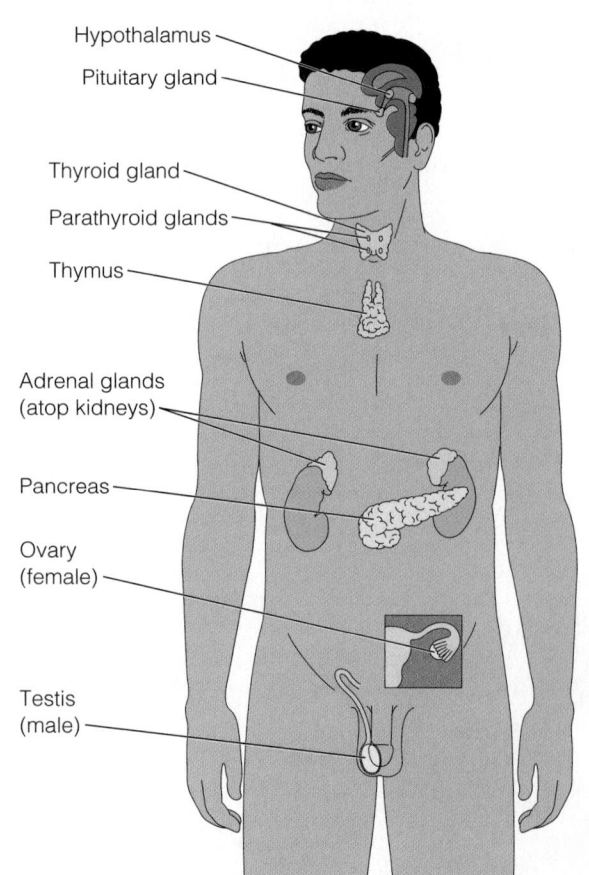

Hypothalamus
Pituitary gland
Thyroid gland
Parathyroid glands
Thymus
Adrenal glands (atop kidneys)
Pancreas
Ovary (female)
Testis (male)

Figure 18–1 ■ Location of the major endocrine glands.

TABLE 18–1 Organs, Hormones, Functions, and Feedback Mechanisms of the Endocrine System

ENDOCRINE ORGAN	HORMONE SECRETED	TARGET ORGAN AND FEEDBACK MECHANISM
Thyroid gland	Thyroid hormone (TH): thyroxine (T_4) is the major hormone secreted by the thyroid gland. It is converted to triiodothyronine (T_3) at the target tissues.	Maintains metabolic rate and growth and development of all tissues. T_3 and T_4 are secreted in response to thyroid-stimulating hormone (TSH).
	Calcitonin	Maintains serum calcium levels by decreasing bone resorption and decreasing resorption of calcium in the kidneys whenever levels of plasma calcium are elevated.
Parathyroid gland	Parathyroid hormone (PTH)	Maintains serum calcium levels by stimulating bone resorption and formation and by stimulating kidney resorption of calcium in response to falling levels of plasma calcium.
Adrenal cortex	Mineralocorticoids (e.g., aldosterone)	Promote kidney tubule reabsorption of sodium and water and excretion of potassium in response to elevated levels of potassium and low levels of sodium, thereby increasing blood pressure and blood volume.
	Glucocorticoids (e.g., cortisol)	Help regulate metabolism of carbohydrates, fats, and proteins. Activate anti-inflammatory responses to stressors. Low cortisol levels stimulate hypothalamic secretion of corticotropin-releasing hormone (CRH), which stimulates the anterior pituitary gland to release ACTH, which in turn stimulates the adrenal cortex to secrete cortisol.
	Gonadocorticoids (androgens and small amounts of estrogen and progesterone)	The quantity of sex hormones produced here is small, and the mechanism is not well understood.
Adrenal medulla	Catecholamines (epinephrine and norepinephrine)	Stimulate the heart, constrict blood vessels, inhibit visceral muscles, dilate bronchioles, increase respiration and metabolism, promote hyperglycemia. Secreted in response to physical or psychologic stress.
Anterior pituitary (adenohypophysis)	Growth hormone (GH)	Promotes growth of body tissues by enhancing protein synthesis and promoting use of fat for energy and thus conserving glucose. Release is stimulated by growth hormone releasing hormone (GHRH) in response to low GH levels, hypoglycemia, increased amino acids, low fatty acids, and stress.

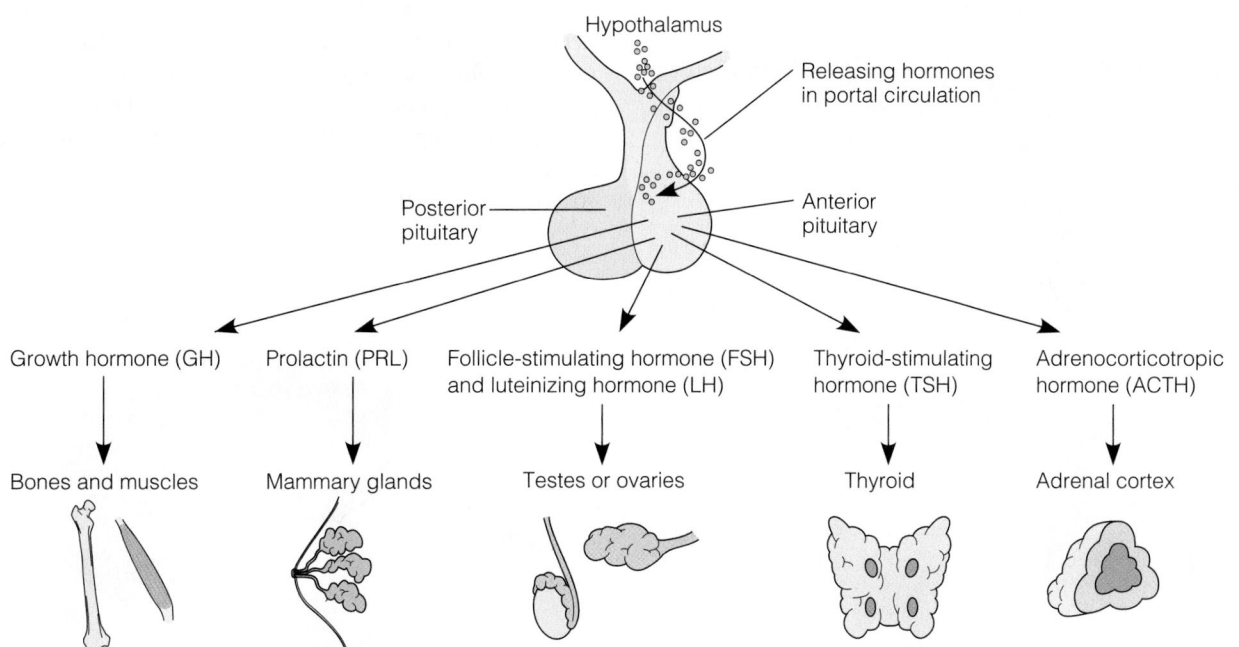

Figure 18–3 ■ Actions of the major hormones of the anterior pituitary.

These hormones stimulate the ovaries and testes (the gonads). In women, FSH stimulates the development of ovarian follicles and induces the secretion of estrogenic female sex hormones. Increasing levels of LH work together with FSH to lead to ovulation and the formation of the corpus luteum from an ovarian follicle. In men, FSH is involved in the development and maturation of sperm. LH in men is called the interstitial cell–stimulating hormone (ICSH), which stimulates the interstitial cells of the testes to produce male sex hormones.

Posterior Pituitary

The posterior pituitary is made of nervous tissue. Its primary function is to store and release antidiuretic hormone (ADH) and oxytocin, produced in the hypothalamus:

- ADH, also called vasopressin, decreases urine production by causing the renal tubules to reabsorb water from the urine and return it to the circulating blood.
- Oxytocin induces contraction of the smooth muscles in the reproductive organs. In women, oxytocin stimulates the myometrium of the uterus to contract during labor. It also induces milk ejection from the breasts.

Thyroid Gland

The thyroid gland (Figure 18–4 ■) is anterior to the upper part of the trachea and just inferior to the larynx. This butterfly-shaped gland has two lobes connected by a structure called the isthmus.

The glandular tissue consists of follicles filled with a jelly-like colloid substance called thyroglobin, a glycoprotein-iodine complex. Cells within the follicles secrete thyroid hormone (TH), a general name for two similar hormones: thyroxine (T_4) and triiodothyronine (T_3). The primary role of thyroid hormones in adults is to increase metabolism. TH secretion is initiated by the release of TSH by the pituitary gland and is dependent on an adequate supply of iodine.

The thyroid gland also secretes calcitonin, a hormone that decreases excessive levels of calcium in the blood by slowing the calcium-releasing activity of bone cells, serves as a marker for sepsis, and is believed to be a mediator of inflammatory responses. The functions of this hormone are not fully understood. When the thyroid gland is totally removed and thyroid hormone replaced, calcium homeostasis and bone density remain relatively unchanged without replacing calcitonin.

Parathyroid Glands

The parathyroid glands (usually four to six in number) are embedded on the posterior surface of the lobes of the thyroid gland. They secrete parathyroid hormone (PTH), or parathormone. When calcium levels in the plasma fall, PTH secretion increases. PTH also controls phosphate metabolism. It acts primarily by increasing renal excretion of phosphate in the urine, by decreasing the excretion of calcium, and by increasing bone reabsorption to cause the release of calcium from bones. Normal levels of vitamin D are necessary for PTH to exert these effects on bone and kidneys.

Adrenal Glands

The two adrenal glands are pyramid-shaped organs that sit on top of the kidneys (Figure 18–5 ■). Each gland consists of two parts, which are distinct organs: an inner medulla and an outer cortex.

The adrenal medulla produces two hormones (also called catecholamines): epinephrine (adrenaline) and norepinephrine (noradrenaline). These hormones are similar to substances released by the sympathetic nervous system and thus are not essential to life. Epinephrine increases blood glucose levels and stimulates the release of ACTH from the pituitary; ACTH in turn stimulates the adrenal cortex to release glucocorticoids. Epinephrine also increases the rate and force of cardiac contractions; constricts blood vessels in the skin, mucous membranes, and kidneys; and dilates blood vessels in the skeletal muscles, coronary arteries, and pulmonary arteries. Norepinephrine increases both heart rate and the force of cardiac contractions. It also vasoconstricts blood vessels throughout the body.

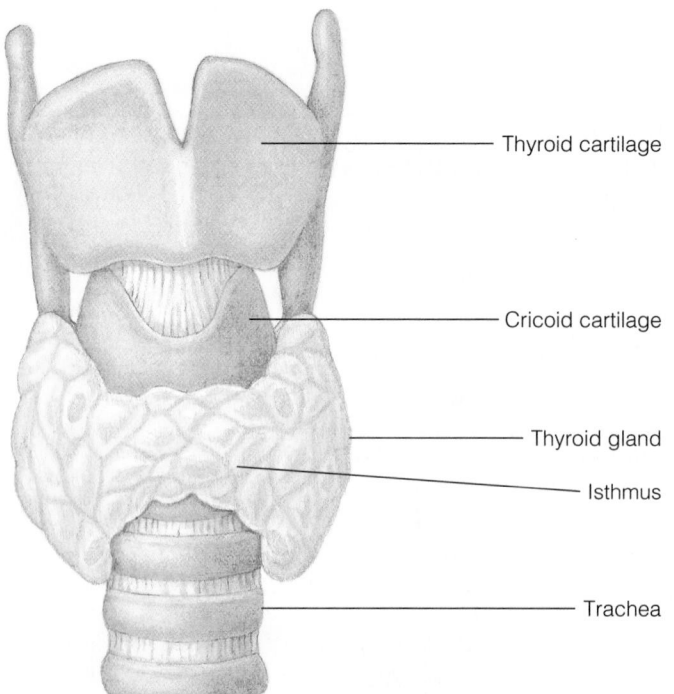

Thyroid cartilage

Cricoid cartilage

Thyroid gland

Isthmus

Trachea

Figure 18–4 ■ The thyroid gland.

Source: Dorling Kindersley Media Library.

Kidney

Adrenal gland

Figure 18–5 ■ Location of the adrenal glands.

Source: Dorling Kindersley Media Library.

The adrenal cortex secretes several hormones, all corticosteroids. They are classified into two groups: mineralocorticoids and glucocorticoids. These hormones are essential to life.

The release of the mineralocorticoids is controlled primarily by an enzyme called renin. When a decrease in blood pressure or sodium is detected, specialized kidney cells release renin to act on a substance called angiotensinogen, manufactured by the liver. Angiotensinogen is modified by renin and other enzymes to become angiotensin, which stimulates the release of aldosterone from the adrenal cortex. Aldosterone prompts the distal tubules of the kidneys to release increased amounts of water and sodium back into the circulating blood to increase circulating blood volume and pressure. This system (the rennin–angiotensin–aldosterone system) is illustrated in Chapter 10 ∞ with the discussion of body fluid regulation.

The glucocorticoids include cortisol and cortisone. These hormones affect carbohydrate metabolism by regulating glucose use in body tissues, mobilizing fatty acids from fatty tissue, and shifting the source of energy for muscle cells from glucose to fatty acids. Glucocorticoids are released in times of stress. An excess of glucocorticoids in the body depresses the inflammatory response and inhibits the effectiveness of the immune system.

Pancreas

The pancreas, located behind the stomach between the spleen and the duodenum, is both an endocrine gland (producing hormones) and an exocrine gland (producing digestive enzymes). The digestive enzymes produced by the pancreas are discussed in Chapter 21 ∞. The content in this chapter focuses on pancreatic hormones.

The endocrine cells of the pancreas produce hormones that regulate carbohydrate metabolism. They are clustered in bodies called pancreatic islets (or islets of Langerhans) scattered throughout the gland. Pancreatic islets have at least four different cell types:

- Alpha cells produce glucagon, which decreases glucose oxidation and promotes an increase in the blood glucose level by signaling the liver to release glucose from glycogen stores.
- Beta cells produce insulin, which facilitates the uptake and use of glucose by cells and prevents an excessive breakdown of glycogen in the liver and muscle. In this way, insulin decreases blood glucose levels. Insulin also facilitates lipid formation, inhibits the breakdown and mobilization of stored fat, and helps amino acids move into cells to promote protein synthesis. In general, the actions of glucagon and insulin oppose one another, helping to maintain a stable blood glucose level.
- Delta cells secrete somatostatin, which inhibits the secretion of glucagon and insulin by the alpha and beta cells.
- F cells secrete pancreatic polypeptide, which is believed to inhibit the exocrine activity of the pancreas.

Gonads

The gonads are the testes in men and the ovaries in women. These organs are the primary source of steroid sex hormones in the body. The hormones of the gonads are important in regulating body growth and promoting the onset of puberty.

In men, androgens (primarily testosterone) produced by the testes maintain reproductive functioning and secondary sex characteristics. Androgens also promote the production of sperm. In women, the ovaries secrete estrogens and progesterone to maintain reproductive functioning and secondary sex characteristics. Progesterone also promotes the growth of the lining of the uterus to prepare for implantation of a fertilized ovum. (The structure and functions of the gonads are discussed in Chapter 49 ∞ .)

AN OVERVIEW OF HORMONES

Hormones are chemical messengers secreted by the endocrine organs and transported throughout the body, where they exert their action on specific cells called target cells. Hormones do not cause reactions directly but rather regulate tissue responses. They may produce either generalized effects or local effects.

Hormones are transported from endocrine gland cells to target cells in the body in one of four ways:

- Endocrine glands release most hormones, including TH and insulin, into the bloodstream. Some hormones require a protein carrier.
- Neurons release some hormones, such as epinephrine, into the bloodstream. This is called the neuroendocrine route.
- The hypothalamus releases its hormones directly to target cells in the posterior pituitary by nerve cell extension.
- With the paracrine method, released messengers diffuse through the interstitial fluid. This method of transport involves a number of hormonal peptides that are released throughout various organs and cells and act locally. An example is endorphins, which act to relieve pain.

Hormones that are released into the bloodstream circulate as either free, unbound molecules or as hormones attached to transport carriers. Peptide and protein hormones (such as insulin) circulate unbound, while steroid and thyroid hormones are carried by specific transport carriers synthesized by the liver. Hormone receptors are complex molecular structures, located on or inside target cells. They act by binding to specific receptor sites located on the surfaces of the target cells. These receptors recognize a specific hormone and translate the message into a cellular response. The receptor sites are structured so that they respond only to a specific hormone; for example, receptors in the thyroid gland are responsive to TSH but not to LH. Drugs that compete with a hormone for binding with transport carrier molecules increase hormone action by increasing the availability of the free, unbound hormone. Hormone levels are controlled by the pituitary gland and by feedback mechanisms. Although most feedback mechanisms are negative, a few are positive. Negative feedback is controlled much as the thermostat in a house regulates temperature. Sensors in the endocrine system detect changes in hormone levels and adjust hormone secretion to maintain normal body levels. When the sensors detect a decrease in hormone levels, they begin actions to cause an increase in hormone levels; when hormone levels rise above normal, the sensors cause a decrease in hormone production and release. For example, when the hypothalamus or anterior pituitary gland senses increased blood levels of TH, it releases hormones, causing a reduction in the secretion of TSH, which in turn prompts a decrease in the output of TH by the thyroid gland. See Figure 18–6 ■.

In positive feedback mechanisms, increasing levels of one hormone cause another gland to release a hormone. For example, the increased production of estradiol (a female ovarian hormone) during the follicular stage of the menstrual cycle in turn stimulates increased FSH production by the anterior pituitary gland. Estradiol levels continue to increase until the ovarian follicle disappears, eliminating the source of the stimulation for FSH, which then decreases.

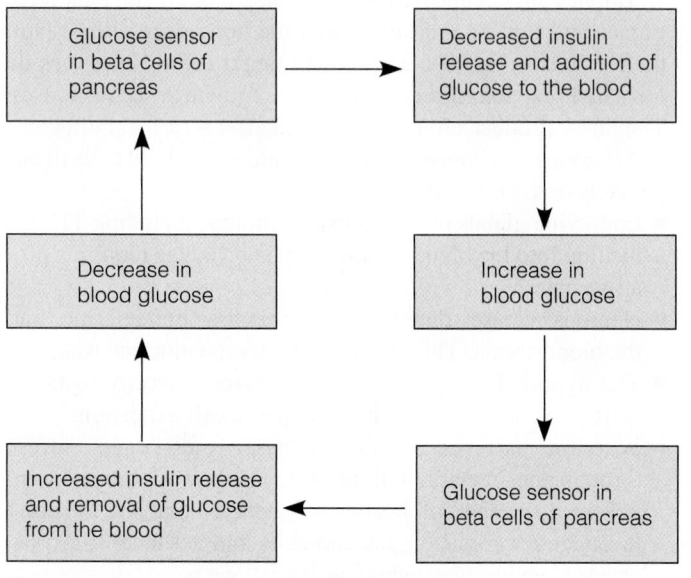

Figure 18–6 ■ Negative feedback.

Stimuli for hormone release may also be classified as hormonal, humoral, or neural (Figure 18–7 ■). In hormonal release, hypothalamic hormones stimulate the anterior pituitary to release hormones. Fluctuations in the serum level of these hormones in turn prompt other endocrine glands to release hormones. In humoral release, fluctuations in the serum levels of certain ions and nutrients stimulate specific endocrine glands to release hormones to bring these levels back to normal. In neural release, nerve fibers stimulate the release of hormones.

ASSESSING ENDOCRINE FUNCTION

The function of the endocrine glands is assessed by findings from diagnostic tests, a health assessment interview to collect subjective data, and a physical assessment to collect objective data. Hormones affect all body tissues and organs, and manifestations of dysfunction are often nonspecific, making assessment of endocrine function sometimes more difficult than assessment of other body systems.

Diagnostic Tests

The results of diagnostic tests of the endocrine system are used to support the diagnosis of a specific disease, to provide information to identify or modify the appropriate medication or therapy used to treat the disease, and to help nurses monitor the client's responses to treatment and nursing care interventions. Diagnostic tests to assess the structure and function of the glands of the endocrine system are described in the table on pages 523–526 and are summarized in the bulleted list that follows. More information is included in the discussion of specific disorders in Chapters 19 and 20 ∞ .

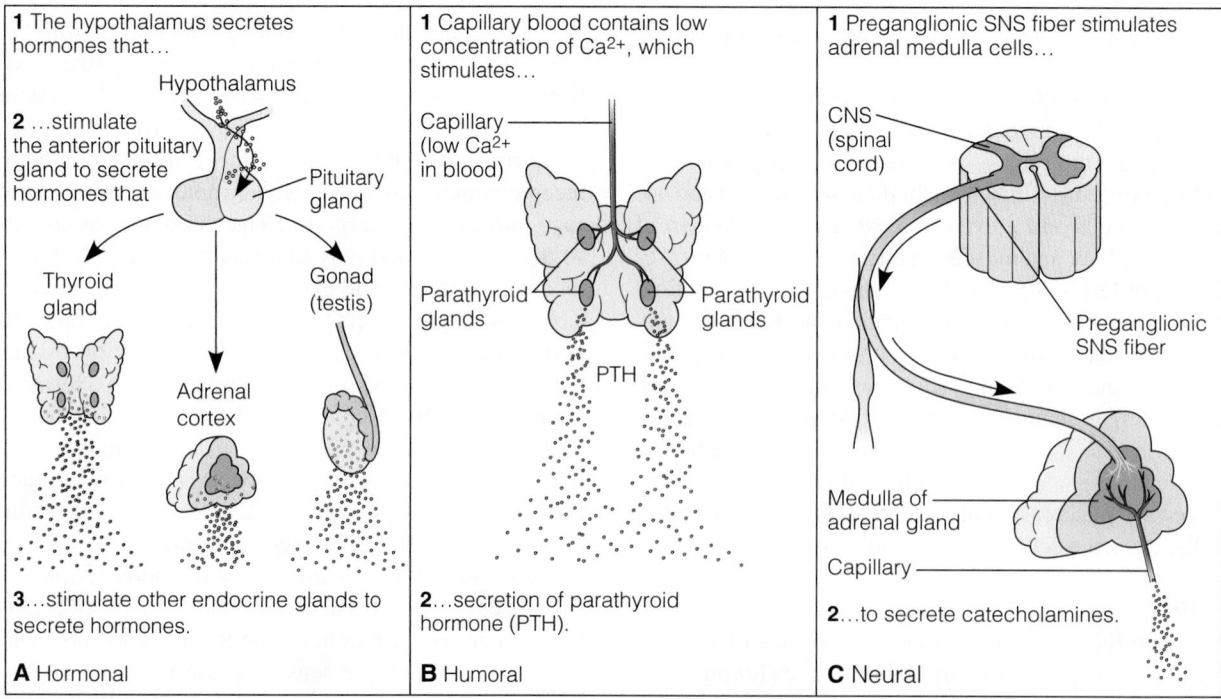

Figure 18–7 ■ Examples of three mechanisms of hormone release: *A*, hormonal; *B*, humoral; or *C*, neural.

DIAGNOSTIC TESTS of the Endocrine System

PITUITARY TESTS

NAME OF TEST   Growth Hormone (GH), Human Growth Hormone (hGH)

PURPOSE AND DESCRIPTION   In this serum test, GH levels (affected by food, stress, and activity) are measured to identify GH deficiency (dwarfism) or GH excess (gigantism, acromegaly).

Normal value:
Men: <5 ng/mL
Women: <10 ng/mL

RELATED NURSING CARE   Inform client not to eat or drink 8–10 hours prior to having blood drawn. Have client rest for 30 to 60 minutes before blood is drawn.

NAME OF TEST   Somatomedin C (Insulin-Like Growth Factor or IGF-1)

PURPOSE AND DESCRIPTION   The results of this serum test are used to evaluate secretion of growth factor and to identify GH deficiency or excess (as above).

Normal value:
125–250 ng/mL

RELATED NURSING CARE   None; overnight fasting is preferred but not necessary.

NAME OF TEST   Water Deprivation Test

PURPOSE AND DESCRIPTION   This combination blood and urine test is used to identify causes of polyuria (increased urine output), including central diabetes insipidus, neurogenic diabetes insipidus, syndrome of inappropriate antidiuretic hormone, and psychogenic polydipsia. ADH or vasopressin is given IM or subcutaneously. In clients without pathology, there is no change in urine and plasma osmolality.
Urine osmolality increases in central diabetes insipidus and decreases in nephrogenic diabetes insipidus.

RELATED NURSING CARE   Inform client not to smoke, eat, or drink after midnight, and that the test will take up to 8 hours. Every hour for ordered length of test: assess weight, take postural BP (lying and standing measures separated by 2 minutes), assess urine for volume and specific gravity, and send samples of urine to the lab for osmolality. Blood samples for osmolality are taken when urine samples are collected and when client demonstrates orthostatic hypotension.

NAME OF TEST   Magnetic Resonance Imaging (MRI)

PURPOSE AND DESCRIPTION   This radiographic study is done to identify tumors of the hypothalamus or pituitary gland.

RELATED NURSING CARE   Inform client of need to lie still during the examination. Assess for any metallic implants (such as pacemakers, body piercings, shrapnel). If present, test is not performed.

THYROID TESTS

NAME OF TEST   Thyroid-Stimulating Hormone (TSH)

PURPOSE AND DESCRIPTION   In this blood test, TSH and T_4 levels are measured to differentiate pituitary from thyroid causes of hypothyroidism. A decreased T_4 level and a normal or increased TSH level can indicate a thyroid disorder. A decreased T_4 level and a decreased TSH level can indicate a pituitary disorder.

Normal value:
<3 ng/mL

RELATED NURSING CARE   Inform clients to avoid shellfish for several days prior to the test. Evaluate medications: TSH value may be increased by aspirin, steroids, dopamine, and heparin; and decreased by lithium and potassium iodide.

NAME OF TEST   Thyroxine (T_4)

PURPOSE AND DESCRIPTION   This serum test is done to determine thyroid function and aid in the diagnosis of hyperthyroidism and hypothyroidism.
Normal value:
free T_4 1.0–2.3 ng/dL

RELATED NURSING CARE   Assess medications: Value may be decreased by cortisone, chlorpromazine (Thorazine), phenytoin (Dilantin), heparin, lithium, sulfonamides, reserpine (Serpasil), testosterone, propranolol (Inderal), tolbutamide (Orinase), and salicylates in high doses. Values may be increased by oral contraceptives, estrogen, clofibrate, and perphenazine (Trilafon).

NAME OF TEST   Triiodothyronine (T_3)

PURPOSE AND DESCRIPTION   This serum test is used to diagnose hyperthyroidism and to compare T_3 with T_4 for diagnosis of thyroid disorder.
Normal value:
80–200 ng/dL

RELATED NURSING CARE   Evaluate medications: Value can be decreased by propylthiouracil, methimazole (Tapazole), lithium, phenytoin (Dilantin), propranolol (Inderal), reserpine (Serpasil), large doses of aspirin, steroids, and sulfonamides. Value can be increased by estrogen, progestins, oral contraceptives, T_3, and methadone.

NAME OF TEST   Triiodothyronine Resin Uptake (T_3RU)

PURPOSE AND DESCRIPTION   This test is an indirect measure of free thyroxine (T_4). The client's blood is mixed with radioactive T_3 and synthetic resin, and the radioactive T_3 will bind with available thyroid-binding globulin sites. The unbound radioactive T_3 is added to resin for T_3 uptake. In hyperthyroidism there are few binding

sites left, more T_3 is taken up by the resin, and a high T_3 resin uptake results. The opposite occurs in hypothyroidism.
Normal value:
25–35% uptake

RELATED NURSING CARE   No special preparation is needed.

(continued)

DIAGNOSTIC TESTS of the Endocrine System (continued)

NAME OF TEST   Thyroid Antibodies (TA)

PURPOSE AND DESCRIPTION   A blood test used to identify thyroid immune disease (Graves' disease, chronic thyroiditis, Hashimoto's thyroiditis).

Normal values:
Antithyroglobulin: negative to titer <1:20
Antimicrosomal: negative to titer <1:100

RELATED NURSING CARE   Assess for family history of thyroid disease and ask about recent viral infection (which could trigger autoimmune disease).

NAME OF TEST   Radioactive Iodine Uptake (RIA)

PURPOSE AND DESCRIPTION   This test provides a direct measure of thyroid activity and is useful in evaluating the activity of solitary thyroid nodules. Based on the rationale that the thyroid gland takes up iodine in any form, radioactive iodine is given orally or intravenously, and the thyroid gland uptake is measured with a scanner at several hourly intervals and at 24 hours.

Normal value for uptake:
2–4 hours: 3–19%
24 hours: 11–30%

RELATED NURSING CARE   The client should not eat or drink for 6 to 8 hours before the test, but can have food 1 hour after the oral dose is given. Tell clients not to take supplemental iodine several weeks before the test and thyroid medications should be discontinued.

NAME OF TEST   Thyroid Scan

PURPOSE AND DESCRIPTION   This radiologic study evaluates thyroid nodules. Radioactive isotopes are given orally and a scanner is passed over the thyroid to make a graphic record of the radiation emitted. A normal thyroid scan has a

homogeneous pattern of radiation with symmetric lobes. Benign lesions appear as warm spots (take up more radiation); malignant tumors appear as cold spots (less radiation taken up).

RELATED NURSING CARE   No special preparation is needed.

PARATHYROID TESTS

NAME OF TEST   Parathyroid Hormone (PTH)

PURPOSE AND DESCRIPTION   A blood test done to identify hypoparathyroidism or hyperparathyroidism; also used to monitor response to PTH therapy.

Normal value:
Intact PTH: 11–54 pg/mL
C-terminal PTH: 50–330 pg/mL
N-terminal PTH: 8–24 pg/mL

RELATED NURSING CARE   Tell client not to eat or drink for 8 hours before the test.

NAME OF TEST   Calcium (Ca)

PURPOSE AND DESCRIPTION   This serum test is used to check for serum calcium excess or deficit in parathyroid and bone disorders; and to monitor calcium levels.

Normal value:
9.0–11.0 mg/dL, 4.5–5.5 mEq/L, or 2.3–2.8 mmol/L (SI units)

RELATED NURSING CARE   Assess for manifestations of tetany, including positive Chvostek's and Trousseau's signs, if hypocalcemia is present.

ADRENAL TESTS

NAME OF TEST   Cortisol

PURPOSE AND DESCRIPTION   A serum test is done to measure amount of total cortisol in the serum and evaluate adrenal cortex function. It is decreased in Addison's disease and hypothyroidism; increased in Cushing's syndrome and hyperthyroidism.

Normal value:
8 A.M.–10 A.M.: 138–635 nmol
4 P.M.–6 P.M.: 83–359 nmol

A 24-hour urine test may be conducted to measure free (unbound) cortisol

Normal value: <100 mcg/24 hours

RELATED NURSING CARE   Tell client not to eat or drink and to rest for 2 hours before the test. Evaluate medications: Cortisol is decreased by androgens, phenytoin (Dilantin), and increased by oral contraceptives, estrogen, spironolactone (Aldactone), and triparanol.

Instruct client how to save urine for 24-hour period, to eat a low-sodium diet before the test, and to avoid stressful situations and physical activity for at least 24 hours prior to the test. Assess medications; values may be increased by reserpine (Serpasil), diuretics, phenothiazines, and amphetamines.

DIAGNOSTIC TESTS of the Endocrine System (continued)

NAME OF TEST Aldosterone

PURPOSE AND DESCRIPTION This blood test is done to identify a deficit or an excess of aldosterone; and to compare blood and urine levels with other lab data to evaluate overhydration with increased sodium and adrenal malfunction.

Normal value: <16 mcg/dL (fasting)

A 24-hour urine test is considered a more reliable measure of aldosterone than a random aldosterone test.

Normal value: 6–25 mcg/24 hours

RELATED NURSING CARE Assess diet and lab results: Levels are increased by hyponatremia, hyperkalemia, and a low-salt diet. Assess medications: Values are increased by diuretics, hydralazine (Apresoline), diazoxide (Hyperstat), nitroprusside, and oral contraceptives.

Assess diet and lab results as for blood test. Assess medications: Urine aldosterone levels are increased by diuretics, lithium, and oral contraceptives.

NAME OF TEST Adrenocorticotropic Hormone (ACTH)

PURPOSE AND DESCRIPTION This serum test is done to determine if a decreased plasma level of cortisol is due to adrenal cortex hypofunction or pituitary hypofunction.

Normal value:
7 A.M.–10 A.M.: 8–80 pg/mL
4 P.M.: 5–30 pg/mL
10 P.M.–12 P.M.: <10 pg/mL

RELATED NURSING CARE Tell the client that food and fluids may be restricted, and to eat a low-carbohydrate diet for 24 hours prior to the test. Assess medications: ACTH values may be increased by metyrapone, vasopressin, and insulin; and decreased by steroids, estrogen amphetamines, and alcohol.

NAME OF TEST ACTH Stimulation

PURPOSE AND DESCRIPTION Done to check for pituitary hypofunction. The drug metyrapone (Metopirone) is given to block the production of cortisol, thus causing an increased ACTH

secretion. If the ACTH level does not increase, the problem is pituitary insufficiency.

RELATED NURSING CARE Assess medications as for ACTH test.

NAME OF TEST ACTH Suppression

PURPOSE AND DESCRIPTION Done to check for the origin of the condition. The drug dexamethasone (Decadron) is given to suppress ACTH production. If an extremely high dose is needed, the cause is of pituitary origin; if the plasma cortisol continues to be high with ACTH suppression, the cause could be adrenal cortex hyperfunction (Cushing's syndrome). Normally, the plasma cortisol level should double in 1 hour.

RELATED NURSING CARE Tell client to avoid tea, caffeinated coffee, and chocolates; no other food or fluid restriction is needed. Assess medications: False positives may be caused by phenytoin, barbiturates, meprobamate, and carbamazepine. If dexamethasone causes gastric irritation, milk or antacids may be required.

NAME OF TEST 17-Ketosteroids

PURPOSE AND DESCRIPTION This 24-hour urine test is done to measure metabolites in urine and evaluate adrenal cortex function.

Normal value:
Men: 5–25 mg in 24 hours
Women: 5–15 mg in 24 hours

RELATED NURSING CARE Instruct client how to save urine (urine must contain a preservative and be refrigerated). Assess medications and refer to information about the test: Levels are affected by a variety of drugs; if possible, these should be discontinued for 48 hours before the test. Women cannot have the test while menstruating because blood can cause a false-positive finding.

NAME OF TEST Computerized Tomography (CT) of the Abdomen

PURPOSE AND DESCRIPTION This radiologic study is used to assess the adrenal gland for tumors (including size and metastasis).

RELATED NURSING CARE Determine if contrast medium will be used; if so, assess client for allergy to iodine (shellfish).

PANCREATIC ENDOCRINE TESTS

NAME OF TEST Fasting Blood Sugar (FBS)

PURPOSE AND DESCRIPTION This test of serum or plasma is used to identify or confirm a diagnosis of diabetes mellitus. It is also used to monitor treatment of diabetes mellitus. A finding of greater than 125 mg/dL might indicate diabetes.

Normal value:
Serum/plasma: 70–100 mg/dL

RELATED NURSING CARE Tell the client not to eat or drink for 12 hours before the test. Do not administer insulin until blood specimen is taken. Assess medications: FBS may be increased by cortisone, diuretics, ACTH, levodopa, epinephrine, anesthetics, and phenytoin (Dilantin).

(continued)

DIAGNOSTIC TESTS of the Endocrine System (continued)

NAME OF TEST Oral Glucose Tolerance Test (OGTT)

PURPOSE AND DESCRIPTION Performed to diagnose diabetes mellitus if prior fasting blood sugar (FBS) findings are increased or inconsistent.

NURSING IMPLICATIONS FOR ORAL GLUCOSE TOLERANCE TEST

- The tests will not be done if client's FBS is consistently high (>200 mg/dL). The client drinks a solution of 75 to 100 grams of glucose and samples of blood and urine are taken immediately and at 30, 60, and 120 minutes (or it may extend from 3 to 6 hours).
  The reference values are:

Time	Serum (mg/dL)	Blood mg/dL
Fasting	70–110	60–100
0.5 hour	<160	<150
1 hour	<170	<160
2 hours	<125	<115
3 hours	Fasting level	Fasting level

NURSING IMPLICATIONS

- Tell the client not to eat or drink (except water) for 12 hours before the test.
- Tell the client that food, fluids (except water), and smoking are not allowed during the test.
- Assess medications: Drugs that may increase OGTT levels are steroids, oral contraceptives, estrogens, thiazide diuretics, and salicylates.
- Explain to the client that he or she may feel weak and may perspire during the test and these symptoms should be reported to the nurse. Although they usually are transitory, they may be manifestations of hyperinsulinism.

NAME OF TEST Glycosylated Hemoglobin (Hb A_1C)

PURPOSE AND DESCRIPTION This serum test is used to measure the effectiveness of treatment of diabetes mellitus. The results represent an average blood glucose level during a 1- to 4-month period; an elevated level indicates uncontrolled diabetes mellitus and increased risk for complications.

Normal value: 5.5–9% of total Hgb

RELATED NURSING CARE Monitor findings: Decreased levels can be caused by anemias, long-term blood loss, and chronic renal failure. Increased levels may result from hyperglycemia, alcohol ingestion, pregnancy, hemodialysis, and prolonged cortisone intake.

NAME OF TEST Computed Tomography (CT) of the Abdomen

PURPOSE AND DESCRIPTION This radiographic test is done to identify pancreatic tumors or cysts.

RELATED NURSING CARE If contrast medium is used, assess for allergy to iodine (shellfish).

- As a result of the many hormones produced by the pituitary gland and by the number of target organs for those hormones, many direct and indirect diagnostic tests are used to determine pituitary function. The diagnostic tests described in this chapter include those of growth hormone (GH), somatomedin C, causes of polyuria, and pituitary tumors.
- Although a substantial number of diagnostic tests are used to identify and monitor thyroid function, the most accurate is TSH. Other tests of thyroid structure and function include thyroxine, triiodothyronine, thyroid antibodies, radioactive iodine uptake, and thyroid scan.
- Diagnostic tests of the parathyroid hormone, which regulates serum calcium and phosphate levels, include PTH and serum calcium.
- Diagnostic tests for the adrenal glands assess the glucocorticoids, mineralocorticoids, and androgens through both blood

and 24-hour urine studies. The tests are of cortisol, aldosterone, ACTH, 17-ketosteroids, and CT of the abdomen to identify adrenal gland tumors.
- Diagnostic tests of the pancreas are performed primarily to identify, confirm, and monitor glucose levels in clients with diabetes mellitus. Those described are oral glucose tolerance test (OGTT), fasting blood sugar (FBS), glycosylated hemoglobin (Hb A_1C), and CT of the abdomen to identify pancreatic tumors or cysts.

Regardless of the type of diagnostic test, the nurse is responsible for explaining the procedure and any special preparation needed, for assessing for medication use that may affect the outcome of the tests, for supporting the client during the examination as necessary, for documenting the procedures as appropriate, and for monitoring the results of the tests.

Genetic Considerations

When conducting a health assessment interview and physical assessment, it is important for the nurse to consider genetic influences on health of the adult. During the health assessment interview, ask about endocrine disorders in immediate family members, including the family member's age of onset and gender. Ask the client about a family history of such diseases as diabetes mellitus, diabetes insipidus, thyroid disorders, growth problems, hypertension, and obesity. Ask women about problems with pregnancy, menstruation, and/or menopause.

During the physical assessment, assess for any manifestations that might indicate a genetic disorder (see box below). If data are found to indicate genetic risk factors or alterations, ask about genetic testing and refer for appropriate genetic counseling and evaluation. Chapter 8 ∞ provides further information about genetics in medical-surgical nursing.

Health Assessment Interview

A health assessment interview to determine problems with the endocrine system may be part of a health screening or total health assessment, or it may focus on a chief complaint (such as increased urination or changes in energy levels). If the client has a problem with endocrine function, the nurse analyzes its onset, characteristics and course, severity, precipitating and relieving factors, and any associated symptoms, noting the timing and circumstances. For example, the nurse may ask the client:

- Describe the swelling you noticed in the front of your neck. When did it begin? Have you noticed any changes in your energy level?
- When did you first notice that your hands and feet were getting larger?
- Have you noticed that your appetite has increased even though you have lost weight?

The health history includes information about the client's medical history, family history, and social and personal history. Ask the client about any changes in normal growth and development as well as in height and weight. Changes in the size of extremities can often be detected by asking whether the client has had to have rings enlarged or to buy increasingly larger gloves and shoes. Enlargement of the neck may be identified by asking whether the client has difficulty finding shirts or blouses with a collar that fits. Also explore changes such as difficulty swallowing; increased or decreased thirst, appetite, and/or urination; visual changes; sleep disturbances; altered patterns of hair distribution (such as increased facial hair in women); changes in menstruation; changes in memory or ability to concentrate; and changes in hair and skin texture. Ask the client about any blow to the head, as well as previous hospitalizations, chemotherapy, radiation (especially to the neck), and the use of medications (especially hormones or steroids).

The nurse also asks about the client's occupational and social history. Include questions about the client's satisfaction with occupation, personal relationships, and lifestyle. Other areas of assessment include the client's usual means of coping; use of alcohol, smoking, or drugs; diet (including weight gain or loss); exercise patterns; and sleep patterns. Although the client may not recognize changes in behavior, family members may be able to provide important information.

Interview questions categorized by functional health patterns are listed on page 528.

Physical Assessment

Physical assessment of the endocrine system may be performed as part of a total health assessment, or it may be a focused assessment of clients with known or suspected problems with endocrine function. Sample documentation of an assessment of the thyroid gland is included in the box below.

SAMPLE DOCUMENTATION
Assessment of the Thyroid Gland

A 37-year-old female presents at community clinic for complaints of "always feeling so hot," "always hungry but losing weight," and "can't sleep at night—too jittery." Weight 110 lb (loss of 12 pounds in last 3 months). BP 90/78 (averages 84/72), P 96. Skin very warm and moist. Anterior neck has diffuse enlargement. Thyroid gland enlarged bilaterally on palpation. Referral made to endocrine clinic for further evaluation.

The only endocrine organ that can be palpated is the thyroid gland; however, other assessments that provide information about endocrine problems include inspection of the skin, hair, nails, facial appearance, reflexes, and musculoskeletal system. Measuring and monitoring trends in height and weight and vital signs also provide clues to altered endocrine system function.

The client may sit during the examination. A reflex hammer is used to test deep tendon reflexes. Prior to the examination, the nurse collects the necessary equipment and explains the techniques to the client to decrease anxiety. Additional techniques for assessing hypocalcemic tetany, a complication of endocrine disorders or surgery, are included in the examination sequence. Normal age-related changes in assessment findings are described in Table 18–2.

GENETIC CONSIDERATIONS
Endocrine System

- Type 1 and type 2 diabetes mellitus are classified as multifactorial inheritance disorders because both genetic and environmental factors are necessary for onset of the disorder.
- Pendred syndrome is an inherited disorder in which people have hereditary deafness and a thyroid goiter.
- Hashimoto's disease (chronic thyroiditis) is believed to have a genetic component.
- Multiple endocrine neoplasia is a group of rare diseases caused by genetic defects leading to hyperplasia and hyperfunction of two or more components of the endocrine system (especially the parathyroid, pancreas, and pituitary glands).

MediaLink Case Study: Endocrine Assessment

FUNCTIONAL HEALTH PATTERN INTERVIEW Endocrine System

Functional Health Pattern	Interview Questions and Leading Statements
Health Perception-Health Management	■ Describe your overall state of health, rating it on a scale of 1 to 10 with 10 being the best health you have had. ■ Describe any problems you have had with an endocrine gland (pituitary, thyroid, parathyroid, adrenal, pancreas, ovaries, testes). ■ If you had a problem with any of these glands, how was it treated (medications, surgery, diet, hormone replacement)? ■ Do you smoke, drink alcohol, and/or use recreational drugs? If so, how much and what kind? ■ Have you ever been tested for high or low blood sugar?
Nutritional-Metabolic	■ Describe what you eat and how much (and type of) fluid you drink in a 24-hour period. ■ Do you take any nutritional supplements, herbs, or vitamins? ■ Have you noticed any change in your hunger or thirst? ■ Has your weight changed? If so, how many pounds and over what time period? ■ Have you noticed any change in your energy level? If so, explain. ■ Have you noticed any change in your ability to tolerate heat or cold? ■ Have you noticed any difficulty swallowing? Explain. ■ Have you noticed any change in the texture of your skin? If so, what were they?
Elimination	■ Have you noticed any change in the color, odor, amount, or frequency of urination? If so, describe it. ■ Have you ever had kidney stones? If so, how were they treated? ■ Has there been a change in your bowel elimination (such as diarrhea or constipation)? If so, explain the change.
Activity-Exercise	■ Describe your physical activities in a usual day. ■ Has your energy level increased or decreased? Explain. ■ Do some activities make you very tired? Explain how you feel.
Sleep-Rest	■ How many hours of sleep do you get each night? ■ Do you feel nervous and unable to rest? ■ Do you sweat at night?
Cognitive-Perceptual	■ Have you noticed any problem with your memory? ■ Do you feel restless, anxious, or confused? ■ Have you noticed any change in your voice? ■ Have you noticed any change in the color or condition of your skin and hair (color, dryness, oiliness, bruises)? ■ Have you had any headaches, memory loss, changes in sensation, depression? Describe them, if so. ■ Have you noticed any change in your vision? Describe them, if so. ■ Have you had any heart palpitations? ■ Have you had any abdominal pain? What is it like and where is it located? ■ Have you had any pain or stiffness in your muscles and joints?
Self Perception-Self-Concept	■ How does this condition make you feel about yourself? ■ How do you feel about taking medications?
Role-Relationships	■ How does this condition make you feel about yourself? How does this condition affect your relationships with others? ■ How does this condition make you feel about yourself? Does anyone in your family have an endocrine disorder? If so, when did it begin and how does it affect them? What family member is affected and at what age did it begin?
Sexuality-Reproductive	■ How does this condition make you feel about yourself? Has having this condition affected your usual sexual activities? ■ *For women:* Have you noticed any change in your menstrual periods? ■ *For women:* Have you had any problems becoming pregnant? ■ *For women:* If you have children, what were their weights at birth? ■ *For men:* Have you noticed any change in your ability to have an erection?
Coping-Stress-Tolerance	■ Does stress seem to make your condition worse? Explain. ■ Has this condition created stress for you? ■ Describe what you do when you feel stressed.
Value-Belief	■ Tell me how specific relationships or activities help you cope with this condition. ■ Describe specific cultural beliefs or practices that affect how you care for and feel about this condition. ■ Are there any specific treatments that you would not use to treat this condition?

TABLE 18–2 Age-Related Endocrine Changes

AGE-RELATED CHANGE	SIGNIFICANCE
Pituitary: ↓ production of ACTH , TSH, FSH	■ Decreased secretion of glucocorticoids, 17-ketosteroids, progesterone, androgen, and estrogen (and thus lower levels on diagnostic tests)
Thyroid: ↑ in fibrosis and nodularity, ↓ in gland activity	■ Lower basal metabolic rate ■ Increased incidence of hypothyroidism ■ Palpable nodules on palpation
Adrenal medulla: ↑ secretion and level of norepinephrine, ↓ beta-adrenergic response to norepinephrine	■ Decreased response to beta-adrenergic and receptor blockers (medications) ■ May contribute to increased incidence of hypertension
Pancreas: calcification of blood vessels and distention and dilation of pancreatic ducts	■ Decreased production of lipase with reduced fat absorption and digestion, leading to intolerance of fatty foods and indigestion ■ Decreased absorption of fat-soluble vitamins
Pancreas: delayed and decreased insulin release; believed accompanied by decreased sensitivity to circulating insulin	■ Decreased ability to metabolize glucose with higher and more prolonged blood glucose levels may contribute to increased incidence of type 2 diabetes mellitus with aging (however, higher than normal blood glucose levels are not unusual in nondiabetic older adults)

ENDOCRINE ASSESSMENTS

Technique/Normal Findings	Abnormal Findings

Skin Assessments with Abnormal Findings

Inspect skin color
Skin color should be even, and appropriate to age and race of the client.

- Hyperpigmentation may be seen in clients with Addison's disease or Cushing's syndrome.
- Hypopigmentation may be seen in diabetes mellitus, hyperthyroidism, or hypothyroidism.
- A yellowish cast to the skin might indicate hypothyroidism.
- Purple striae over the abdomen and bruising may be present in the client with Cushing's syndrome.

Palpate the skin, assessing texture, moisture, and the presence of lesions. *Skin should be appropriate to the client's race, smooth, warm, dry, and intact without abnormal lesions.*

- Rough, dry skin is often seen in clients with hypothyroidism, whereas smooth and flushed skin can be a sign of hyperthyroidism.
- Lesions (such as ulcerations) on the lower extremities might indicate diabetes mellitus.

Nails and Hair Assessment with Abnormal Findings

Assess texture, distribution, and condition of nails and hair. *Hair should be of normal texture, appropriately distributed for gender; nails surfaces should have even color with smooth surfaces.*

- Increased pigmentation of the nails is often seen in clients with Addison's disease.
- Dry, thick, brittle nails and hair may be apparent in hypothyroidism; thin, brittle nails and thin, soft hair may be apparent in hyperthyroidism.
- Hirsutism (excessive facial, chest, or abdominal hair) may be seen in Cushing's syndrome.

Facial Assessments with Abnormal Findings

Inspect the symmetry and form of the face. *Face should be bilaterally symmetrical.*

- Variations of form and structure may indicate growth abnormalities such as **acromegaly** (continued growth of bone from growth hormone hypersecretion).

Inspect position of eyes. *Eyes should be equal in position on both sides of the face. Eyelids should close over eyes.*

- **Exophthalmos** (protruding eyes) may be seen in hyperthyroidism.

Technique/Normal Findings	**Abnormal Findings**

Thyroid Gland Assessment with Abnormal Findings

Palpate the thyroid gland for size and consistency.
Stand behind the client, and place your fingers on either side of the trachea below the thyroid cartilage (Figure 18–8 ■). Ask the client to tilt the head to the right. Now ask the client to swallow. As the client swallows, displace the left lobe while palpating the right lobe. Repeat to palpate the left lobe. *Thyroid gland is not usually palpable. If it is, lobes should feel smooth, rubbery, and free of nodules.*

- The thyroid may be enlarged in clients with Graves' disease or a **goiter** (enlarged thyroid gland).
- Multiple nodules may be seen in metabolic disorders, whereas the presence of only one nodule may indicate a cyst or a benign or malignant tumor.
- One enlarged nodule suggests malignancy.

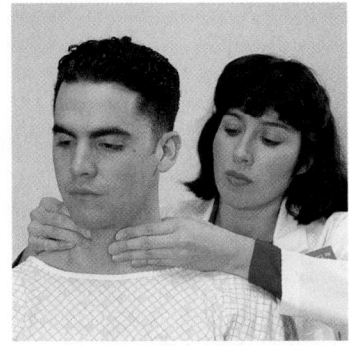

Figure 18–8 ■ Palpating the thyroid gland from behind the client.

Motor Function Assessment with Abnormal Findings

Assess the deep tendon reflexes. Deep tendon reflexes are assessed with the reflex hammer, and include the biceps reflex, brachioradialis reflex, triceps reflex, patellar reflex, and Achilles reflex. *Normal values range from 1+ (present, but decreased) to 2+ (normal) to 3+ (increased). See Chapter 43 ∞ for guidelines and illustrations of deep tendon reflex assessment.*

- Increased reflexes may be seen in hyperthyroidism; decreased reflexes may be seen in hypothyroidism.

Sensory Function Assessment with Abnormal Findings

Test the client's sensitivity to pain, temperature, vibration, light touch, and stereognosis (the ability to identify an object merely by touch). Compare symmetric areas on both sides of the body, and compare the distal to the proximal regions of the extremities. Ask the client to close his or her eyes.
Sensory function should be bilaterally intact.
- To test pain, use the blunt and sharp ends of a new safety pin. Discard the pin after use.
- To test temperature, use cups or other containers of cold and hot water.
- To test vibration, use a tuning fork over one of the client's finger or toe joints.
- To test light touch, use a cotton wisp.
- To test stereognosis, place in the client's hand a simple, familiar object, such as a rubber band, cotton ball, or button. Ask the client to identify the object.

- Peripheral neuropathy and paresthesias (altered sensations) may occur in diabetes, hypothyroidism, or acromegaly.

Technique/Normal Findings	Abnormal Findings

Musculoskeletal Assessment with Abnormal Findings

Inspect the size and proportions of the client's body structure. *Size and proportion of body structures should be bilaterally equal.*

- Extremely short stature may indicate **dwarfism**, which is caused by insufficient growth hormone.
- Extremely large bones may indicate acromegaly, which is caused by excessive growth hormone.

Assessing for Hypocalcemic Tetany

Assess for **Trousseau's sign** (a test for hypocalcemia) with resulting **tetany** (tonic muscle spasms) by inflating a blood pressure cuff above the antecubital space to a point greater than systolic blood pressure for 2–5 minutes. Trousseau's sign is discussed in relation to hypocalcemia in Chapter 10 ∞ . *A normal finding would be no carpal spasm in response to compression of the arm by the blood pressure cuff.*

- Decreased calcium levels cause the client's hand and fingers to contract (**carpal spasm**).

Assess for **Chvostek's sign** (a test for hypocalcemia) by tapping your finger in front of the client's ear at the angle of the jaw. A positive Chvostek's sign causes facial grimacing due to repeated contractions of the facial muscle. Chvostek's sign is discussed and illustrated in relation to hypocalcemia in Chapter 10 ∞ . *A normal finding would be no facial grimacing in response to tapping the client's face in front of the ear.*

- Decreased calcium levels cause the client's lateral facial muscles to contract.

EXPLORE MEDIALINK

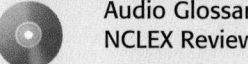

Prentice Hall Nursing MediaLink DVD-ROM
Audio Glossary
NCLEX Review

COMPANION WEBSITE www.prenhall.com/lemone
Audio Glossary
NCLEX-RN® Review
Care Plan Activity: Type 2 Diabetes
Case Studies
Assessing a Client for Hypocalcemia
Endocrine Assessment
MediaLink Application: Endocrine Hormones
Links to Resources

TEST YOURSELF NCLEX-RN® REVIEW

1 What physiologic response is expected if the pituitary produces an increased amount of ADH?
1. increased output of urine
2. decreased output of urine
3. increased facial hair growth in women
4. decreased production of testosterone

2 What assessment might be made to identify low calcium levels?
1. Save urine to measure 7-ketosteroids.
2. Palpate turgor of skin.
3. Conduct a Trousseau's sign test.
4. Observe color of skin.

3 Excessive amounts of glucocorticoids, produced by the adrenal cortex, result in what pathophysiologic health problem?
1. inhibited immune response
2. increased response to glucagon
3. delayed onset of puberty
4. decreased metabolic rate

4 When conducting a health history focused on the endocrine system, which of the following questions should be included?
1. "When did you first notice the pain in your abdomen?"
2. "Do your children have problems with urination?"
3. "Have you noticed a change in your thirst?"
4. "How did you get this scar on your leg?"

5 What assessments are made when palpating the thyroid gland?
1. edema and movement
2. size and consistency
3. character and texture
4. pain and pulse rate

6 Decreased calcium levels can be assessed with Chvostek's sign. To conduct this assessment, the nurse:

1. inflates a blood pressure cuff above the antecubital space.
2. taps the finger in front of the client's ear.
3. depresses the skin over the shin.
4. pinches a fold of skin over the sternum.

7 Which of the following tests is the most accurate indicator of thyroid function?
1. GH
2. FBS
3. aldosterone
4. TSH

8 Which is the only endocrine organ that can be palpated during physical assessment?
1. pancreas
2. liver
3. thyroid
4. pituitary

9 You are caring for a client with newly diagnosed hypothyroidism. What skin assessment might you find?
1. increased hair growth
2. rough, dry skin
3. smooth, flushed skin
4. cold and clammy skin

10 What endocrine disorder might be assessed by testing deep tendon reflexes?
1. Cushing's syndrome
2. acromegaly
3. tetany
4. hyperthyroidism

See Test Yourself answers in Appendix C.

BIBLIOGRAPHY

Amella, E. (2004). Presentation of illness in older adults: If you think you know what you're looking for, think again. *American Journal of Nursing, 104*(10), 40–52.

Are you missing serious illness in older patients? Improve assessment of geriatric patients. (2004). *Hospital Home Health, 21*(9), 105–106.

Bickley, L., & Szilagyi, P. (2007). *Bates' guide to physical examination and history taking* (9th ed.). Philadelphia: Lippincott.

Cosentino, B. (2004). Electrolyte imbalance: A matter of equilibrium. *Nursing Spectrum (New York/New Jersey Metro Edition), 16*(1), 4–6.

Eliopoulos, C. (2005). *Gerontological nursing.* (6th ed.). Philadelphia: Lippincott.

Kee, J. (2005). *Prentice Hall handbook of laboratory & diagnostic tests with nursing implications.* Upper Saddle River, NJ: Prentice Hall.

Kirk, L., Hash, R., Katner, H., & Jones T. (2000). Cushing's disease: Clinical manifestations and diagnostic evaluation. *American Family Physician, 62*(5), 945–948, 1119–1127, 1133–1134.

Kravitz, S., McGuire, J., & Shanahan, S. (2003). Physical assessment of the diabetic foot. *Advances in Skin and Wound Care, 16*(2), 68–77.

Kumrow, D., & Dahlen, R. (2002). Thyroidectomy: Understanding the potential for complications. *MEDSURG Nursing, 11*(5), 228–235.

Larson, K. (2003). Fluid balance in the elderly: Assessment and intervention—important role in community and home care nursing. *Geriatric Nursing, 24*(5), 306–309.

Levin, N., & Greer, K. (2004). Cutaneous manifestations of endocrine disorders. *Dermatology Nursing, 13*(3), 185–186, 189–196, 201–202.

MedlinePlus Medical Encyclopedia. (2005). *Lab tests online: Glucose.* Retrieved from http://www.labtestsonline.org/understanding/analytes/glucose/test.html

Murtagh, J. (2003). Fatigue—A general diagnostic approach. *Australian Family Physician, 32*(11), 873–876, 935–936.

National Institutes of Health. (2004). *Genes and diseases. Glands and hormones.* Retrieved from http://www.ncbi.nlm.nih.gov/books/bv.fcgi?rid=gnd.chapter8

Porth, C. (2005). *Pathophysiology: Concepts of altered health states* (7th ed.). Philadelphia: Lippincott.

Watson, R. (2001). Assessing endocrine system function in older people. *Nursing Older People, 12*(9), 27–28.

Weber, J., & Kelley, J. (2006). *Health assessment in nursing* (3rd ed.). Philadelphia: Lippincott.

CHAPTER 19
Nursing Care of Clients with Endocrine Disorders

LEARNING OUTCOMES

- Apply knowledge of normal anatomy, physiology, and assessments of the thyroid, parathyroid, adrenal, and pituitary glands when providing nursing care for clients with endocrine disorders.

- Compare and contrast the manifestations of disorders that result from hyperfunction and hypofunction of the thyroid, parathyroid, adrenal, and pituitary glands.

- Explain the nursing implications for medications prescribed to treat disorders of the thyroid and adrenal glands.

- Provide appropriate nursing care for the client before and after a subtotal thyroidectomy and an adrenalectomy.

- Use the nursing process as a framework for providing individualized care to clients with disorders of the thyroid, parathyroid, adrenal, and pituitary glands.

CLINICAL COMPETENCIES

- Assess functional health status of clients with endocrine disorders and monitor, document, and report abnormal manifestations.

- Use evidence-based research to provide appropriate teaching for self-medicating with thyroid hormone.

- Determine priority nursing diagnoses, based on assessed data, to select and implement individualized nursing interventions for clients with endocrine disorders.

- Teach clients that hormone replacement is lifelong, and how to take medications efficiently and effectively.

- Monitor respiratory function after thyroidectomy.

- Monitor for latent tetany following parathyroid removal, planned or inadvertent.

- Anticipate and recognize the effects of adrenal hormones.

- Revise plan of care as needed to provide effective interventions to promote, maintain, or restore functional health status to clients with endocrine disorders.

MEDIALINK

Resources for this chapter can be found on the Prentice Hall Nursing MediaLink DVD-ROM accompanying this textbook, and on the Companion Website at http://www.prenhall.com/lemone

The thyroid, parathyroid, adrenal, and pituitary glands are part of the endocrine system. Disorders of the structure and function of these glands alter normal hormone levels and the way body tissues use those hormones. When hormone production increases or decreases, people experience alterations in health.

Clients with disorders of the glands discussed in this chapter require nursing care for multiple problems. They often face exhausting diagnostic tests, changes in physical appearance and emotional responses, and permanent alterations in lifestyle. Nursing care is directed toward meeting physiologic needs, providing education, and ensuring psychologic support for the client and family. A holistic approach to the complex needs of clients with these endocrine disorders is an essential component of nursing care.

DISORDERS OF THE THYROID GLAND

Altered thyroid hormone (TH) production or use affects all major organ systems. In the adult, TH changes primarily affect metabolism, cardiovascular function, gastrointestinal function, and neuromuscular function. Thyroid disorders—both hyperthyroidism and hypothyroidism—are among the most common endocrine disorders.

THE CLIENT WITH HYPERTHYROIDISM

Hyperthyroidism (also called **thyrotoxicosis**) is a disorder caused by excessive delivery of TH to the peripheral tissues. Because the primary effect of TH is to increase metabolism and protein synthesis, hyperthyroidism affects all major organ systems of the body. The increase in metabolic rate and the alterations in cardiac output, peripheral blood flow, oxygen consumption, and body temperature are similar to those found in increased sympathetic nervous system activity (Porth, 2005).

The effects of hyperthyroidism are the result of increased circulating levels of TH. This hormonal excess increases the metabolic rate and heightens the sympathetic nervous system's physiologic response to stimulation. The sensitizing effect of abnormally elevated TH levels increases the cardiac rate and stroke volume. As a result, cardiac output and peripheral blood flow increase. Elevated TH levels also increase carbohydrate, protein, and lipid metabolism. Lipids are depleted, and glucose tolerance decreases. Protein degradation increases, resulting in a negative nitrogen balance. Over time, the hypermetabolic effects of excess TH result in caloric and nutritional deficiencies.

Pathophysiology and Manifestations

Hyperthyroidism results from many different factors, including autoimmune stimulation (as in Graves' disease), excess secretion of thyroid-stimulating hormone (TSH) by the pituitary gland, thyroiditis, neoplasms (such as toxic multinodular goiter), and an excessive intake of thyroid medications. The most common etiologies of hyperthyroidism are Graves' disease and toxic multinodular goiter.

The client with hyperthyroidism typically has an increased appetite, yet loses weight and may have hypermotile bowels and diarrhea. Additional manifestations related to hypermetabolism include heat intolerance, insomnia, palpitations, and increased sweating. The skin is smooth and warm, hair may become fine, and hair loss in the scalp, eyebrow, axillary, or pubic areas of the body is common. Emotional lability is common. The *Multisystem Effects of Hyperthyroidism* are shown on the following page.

Graves' Disease

Graves' disease, the most common cause of hyperthyroidism, is an autoimmune disorder, sometimes associated with the presence of other autoimmune disorders such as myasthenia gravis and pernicious anemia (Porth, 2005). The serum of more than 80% of clients with Graves' disease has an antibody that binds to thyroid-stimulating hormone (TSH) receptors in the thyroid follicles and causes the thyroid cells to hyperfunction (Tierney et al., 2005). When this antibody binds to the TSH receptors on the thyroid gland, it stimulates hormone synthesis and secretion, enlarging the gland. The cause is unknown, but there is a hereditary link.

Graves' disease is seen five times more often in women than in men and occurs most frequently between the ages of 20 and 40. It is seen worldwide, with the incidence often correlated with the amount of iodine in the diet. Increased iodine intake (such as from radiocontrast dyes used in diagnostic tests or from ingestion of kelp tablets) has been associated with an increased frequency of hyperthyroidism.

MULTISYSTEM EFFECTS OF **Hyperthyroidism**

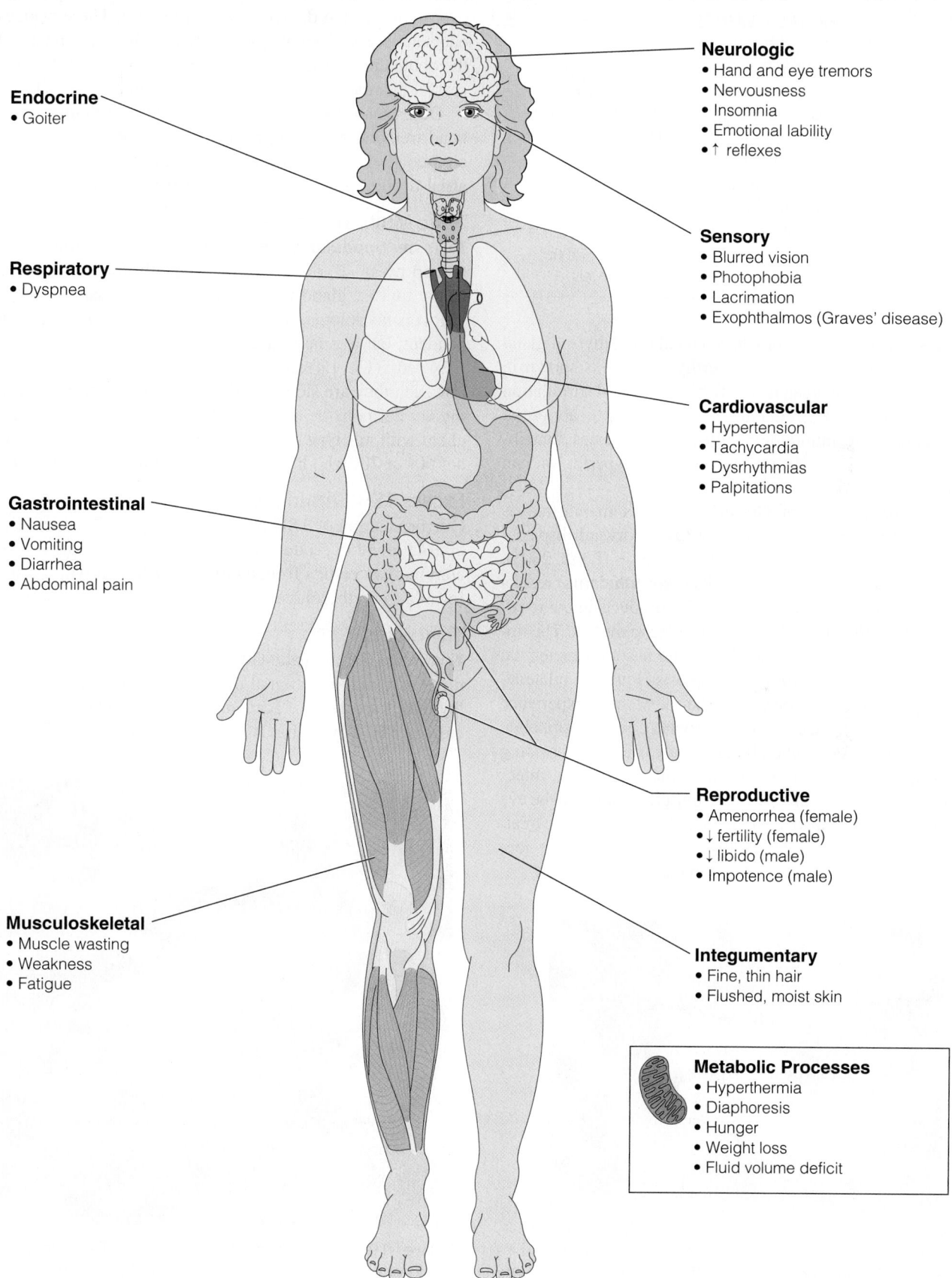

Neurologic
- Hand and eye tremors
- Nervousness
- Insomnia
- Emotional lability
- ↑ reflexes

Endocrine
- Goiter

Sensory
- Blurred vision
- Photophobia
- Lacrimation
- Exophthalmos (Graves' disease)

Respiratory
- Dyspnea

Cardiovascular
- Hypertension
- Tachycardia
- Dysrhythmias
- Palpitations

Gastrointestinal
- Nausea
- Vomiting
- Diarrhea
- Abdominal pain

Reproductive
- Amenorrhea (female)
- ↓ fertility (female)
- ↓ libido (male)
- Impotence (male)

Musculoskeletal
- Muscle wasting
- Weakness
- Fatigue

Integumentary
- Fine, thin hair
- Flushed, moist skin

Metabolic Processes
- Hyperthermia
- Diaphoresis
- Hunger
- Weight loss
- Fluid volume deficit

TABLE 19–1 Laboratory Findings in Hyperthyroidism

TEST	NORMAL VALUES	FINDINGS
Serum TA	Negative to 1:20	Increased
Serum TSH (sensitive assay)	2–10 mU/ml mU = microunits	Decreased in primary hyperthyroidism
Serum T_4	5 to 12 mcg/dL mcg = microgram	Increased
Serum T_3	80 to 200 ng/dL	Increased
T_3 uptake (T_3RU)	25 to 35 relative percentage	Increased
Thyroid suppression		Increased RAI uptake and T_4 levels

Clients with Graves' disease have an enlarged thyroid gland (**goiter**) and manifestations of hyperthyroidism (as shown in Table 19–1). The goiter can result from excess TSH stimulation (when the amount of circulating TH is deficient), abnormal growth-stimulating immunoglobulins, or substances that inhibit TH synthesis. A goiter may be present in hyperthyroidism or hypothyroidism.

The ophthalmopathy of Graves' disease is manifested as proptosis and visual dysfunction. **Proptosis** (forward displacement) of the eye occurs in about one-third of cases (Porth, 2005). The forward protrusion of the eyeballs (**exophthalmos**) results from an accumulation of inflammation by-products in the retro-orbital tissues. Often the sclera is visible above the iris. The upper lids are often retracted, and the person has a characteristic unblinking stare (Figure 19–1 ■). Proptosis is usually bilateral, but it may involve only one eye. The client may experience blurred vision, diplopia, eye pain, lacrimation, and photophobia. The inability to close the eyelids completely over the protruding eyeballs increases the risk of corneal dryness, irritation, infection, and ulceration. Infiltration of the muscles that move the eye and of the optic nerve lead to paralysis and vision loss. The treatment of Graves' disease may stabilize these symptoms but generally does not reverse these changes in the eyes.

A rare, characteristic dermopathy of Graves' disease is **pretibial myxedema**. Plaques and nodules develop bilaterally over the shins and dorsal surface of the feet. These plaques are edematous, erythematous, and sometimes hyperpigmented. Like the ophthalmopathy, the skin changes often persist despite successful treatment of Graves' disease (Levin & Greer, 2001).

Other manifestations include fatigue, difficulty sleeping, hand tremors, and changes in menstruation ranging from decreased flow to amenorrhea. Older clients may present with atrial fibrillation, angina, or congestive heart failure.

Toxic Multinodular Goiter

Toxic multinodular goiter (Figure 19–2 ■) is a tumor characterized by small, discrete, independently functioning nodules in the thyroid gland tissue that secrete excessive amounts of TH. It is not known how these nodules grow or become independent, but a genetic mutation of follicle cells is suspected. Elevated TH levels result in manifestations of hyperthyroidism; however, they are slower to develop and neither ophthalmopathy nor dermopathy develop (McCance & Huether, 2002). The client with this type of hyperthyroidism is usually a woman in her 60s or 70s who has had a goiter for a number of years.

Excess TSH Stimulation

Overproduction of TSH by the pituitary usually stimulates the thyroid gland to produce excess TH. The elevation in TSH secretion often results from a pituitary adenoma. This secondary form of hyperthyroidism is rare.

Thyroiditis

Thyroiditis (inflammation of the thyroid gland) is most often the result of a viral infection of the thyroid gland. The symptoms of thyroiditis are those of acute inflammation and the effects of increased TH. Thyroiditis is an acute disorder that may become

Figure 19–1 ■ Exophthalmos in a client with Graves' disease. The disease causes edema of fat deposits behind the eyes and inflammation of the extraocular muscles. The accumulating pressure forces the eyes outward from their orbits.

Source: University of Illinois, Custom Medical Stock Photo, Inc.

Figure 19–2 ■ Toxic multinodular goiter. The formation and growth of numerous nodules in the thyroid gland cause the characteristic massive enlargement of the neck.

Source: Custom Medical Stock Photo, Inc.

chronic, resulting in a hypothyroid state as repeated infections destroy gland tissue. See the discussion of Hashimoto's thyroiditis later in this chapter.

Thyroid Crisis

Thyroid storm (also called **thyroid crisis**) is an extreme state of hyperthyroidism that is rare today because of improved diagnosis and treatment methods (Porth, 2005). When it does occur, those affected are usually people with untreated hyperthyroidism (most often Graves' disease) and people with hyperthyroidism who have experienced a stressor, such as an infection, trauma, untreated diabetic ketoacidosis, or manipulation of the thyroid gland during surgery. Thyroid crisis is a life-threatening condition.

The rapid increase in metabolic rate that results from the excessive TH causes the manifestations of thyroid storm. The manifestations include hyperthermia, with body temperatures ranging from 102° to 106°F (39° to 41°C); tachycardia; systolic hypertension; and gastrointestinal symptoms (abdominal pain, vomiting, diarrhea). Agitation, restlessness, and tremors are common, progressing to confusion, psychosis, delirium, and seizures. The mortality rate is high. Rapid treatment of thyroid storm is essential to preserve life. Treatment includes cooling without aspirin (which increases free TH) or inducing shivering; replacing fluids, glucose, and electrolytes; relieving respiratory distress; stabilizing cardiovascular function; and reducing TH synthesis and secretion.

INTERDISCIPLINARY CARE

Treatment of hyperthyroidism focuses on reducing the production of TH by the thyroid gland, thus establishing a **euthyroid** (normal thyroid) state, and preventing or treating complications. Depending on the client's age and physical status, either medications, radioactive iodine therapy, or surgery may be used.

Diagnosis

Hyperthyroidism is diagnosed according to the manifestations of the specific disorders causing excessive TH, and by diagnostic test results. Elevated levels of TH (both T_3 and T_4) and increased radioactive iodine (RAI) uptake are diagnostic criteria of hyperthyroidism. Laboratory findings in hyperthyroidism were shown earlier in Table 19–1.

The following diagnostic tests may be ordered:

- *TA test.* Serum thyroid antibodies (TA) are measured to determine whether a thyroid autoimmune disease is causing the client's symptoms. TA is elevated in Graves' disease.
- *TSH test (sensitive assay).* Serum TSH levels are measured and compared with thyroxine (T_4) levels to differentiate pituitary from thyroid dysfunction. The best indicator of primary hyperthyroidism (such as in Graves' disease) is suppression of TSH below 0.1 mcg/mL. When the sensitive TSH is not suppressed, the hyperthyroidism is caused by a TSH-secreting pituitary tumor.
- *T_4 test.* Serum thyroxine levels are measured to determine TH concentration and to test thyroid gland function. T_4 levels are elevated in hyperthyroidism and in acute thyroiditis.

- *T_3 test.* Serum triiodothyronine (T_3) is measured by radioimmunoassay (T_3RIA), which measures bound and free forms of this hormone. This test is effective for the diagnosis of hyperthyroidism. T_3 levels may also be elevated in thyroiditis.
- *T_3 uptake test.* T_3 uptake (T_3RU) is measured by an *in vitro* test in which the client's blood is mixed with radioactive T_3; the results are elevated in hyperthyroidism.
- *RAI uptake test.* A radioactive iodine uptake test (thyroid scan) measures the absorption of ^{131}I or ^{123}I by the thyroid gland. A calculated dose of radioactive iodine is given orally or intravenously, and the thyroid is then scanned (often after 24 hours). The distribution of radioactivity in the gland is recorded (increased uptake of radioactive iodine is seen in Graves' disease). In addition, the scan reveals the size and shape of the gland.
- *Thyroid suppression test.* RAI and T_4 levels are measured first. The client then takes TH for 7 to 10 days, after which the tests are repeated. Failure of hormone therapy to suppress RAI and T_4 indicates hyperthyroidism.

Medications

Hyperthyroidism is treated by administering antithyroid medications that reduce TH production. Because these drugs do not affect the release or activity of hormone that is already formed, therapeutic effects may not be seen for several weeks. To rapidly decrease the cardiovascular symptoms associated with hyperthyroidism, propanolol (Inderal), a beta-blocker, is part of initial treatment. (See Chapter 31 ∞ for information on beta-blockers.) Some commonly prescribed drugs, their actions, and nursing implications are shown in the Medication Administration box on page 538.

Radioactive Iodine Therapy

Because the thyroid gland takes up iodine in any form, radioactive iodine (^{131}I) concentrates in the thyroid gland and damages or destroys thyroid cells so that they produce less TH. Radioactive iodine is given orally. Results typically occur in 6 to 8 weeks. In most instances, the client is not hospitalized during treatment and does not require radiation precautions. This type of therapy is contraindicated in pregnant women because radioactive iodine crosses the placenta and can have negative effects on the developing fetal thyroid gland. Because the amount of gland destroyed is not readily controllable, the client may become hypothyroid and require lifelong TH replacement. Adverse reactions include thyroiditis and cardiac instability due to liberation of stored thyroid hormone in the gland (Holcomb, 2006).

Surgery

Some hyperthyroid clients have such enlarged thyroid glands that pressure on the esophagus or trachea causes breathing or swallowing problems. In these cases, removal of all or part of the gland is indicated. A *subtotal thyroidectomy* is usually performed. This procedure leaves enough of the gland in place to produce an adequate amount of TH. A total **thyroidectomy** is performed to treat cancer of the thyroid; the client then requires lifelong hormone replacement (Kumrow & Dahlen, 2002).

MEDICATION ADMINISTRATION   Hyperthyroidism

IODINE SOURCES
Strong Iodine Solution (Lugol's Solution)
Potassium iodide (SSKI, Thyro-Block, Pima)
Large doses of iodine for a short term inhibit TH synthesis and re-lease. Iodine also makes the hyperplastic thyroid less vascular prior to surgery and hastens the ability of other antithyroid drugs to reduce natural hormone output. It is also used in thyroid storm. Potassium iodide is useful to protect the thyroid in radiation emergencies, blocking the uptake of radioactive iodine from nuclear fallout (Lehne, 2004).

Nursing Responsibilities
- Assess for hypersensitivity to iodine before giving medication; for example, ask client about allergies to shellfish.
- Dilute liquid iodine sources in water or orange juice to disguise bitter taste.
- Monitor for increased bleeding tendencies if the client is also taking anticoagulants; iodine increases their effect.

Health Education for the Client and Family
- The maximum effect of iodine in large doses usually occurs in 10 to 15 days.
- Long-term iodine therapy is not effective in controlling hyperthyroidism.

ANTITHYROID DRUGS
Methimazole (Tapazole)
Propylthiouracil (PTU, Propyl-Thyracil)
Antithyroid drugs inhibit TH production. They do not affect already formed hormones; thus, several weeks may elapse before the client experiences therapeutic effects. Methimazole can be taken in one daily dose; propylthiouracil must be taken in 3 doses daily; methimazole crosses the placenta and cannot be taken during pregnancy (Lehne, 2004).

Nursing Responsibilities
- Monitor for side effects: agranulocytosis, hypothyroidism, pruritus rash, elevated temperature, (for iodides) periorbital edema, anorexia, loss of taste, changes in menstruation.
- Administer drugs at the same time each day with meals to maintain stable blood levels.
- Monitor for symptoms of hypothyroidism: fatigue, weight gain.

Health Education for the Client and Family
- Watch for unusual bleeding, redness, swelling, nausea, loss of taste, or epigastric pain. Report any such symptoms to the physician.
- If you are also taking warfarin, report any signs of bleeding.
- If you are taking lithium, be aware of symptoms of hypothyroidism.
- It may take up to 12 weeks before you experience the full effects of the drugs. Take the medication regularly and exactly as prescribed. Do not discontinue abruptly.

Before surgery, the client should be in as nearly a euthyroid state as possible. The client may be given antithyroid drugs to reduce hormone levels and iodine preparations to decrease the vascularity and size of the gland (which also reduces the risk of hemorrhage during and after surgery). Nursing care of the client having a subtotal thyroidectomy is discussed in the box on the following page.

NURSING CARE

Health Promotion

Although hyperthyroidism is not preventable, it is important to teach clients the importance of regular healthcare provider visits and medication intake.

Assessment

The following data are collected through the health history and physical examination (see Chapter 18 ∞). Further focused assessments are described with nursing interventions.

- *Health history:* Other diseases, family history of thyroid disease, when symptoms began, severity of symptoms, intake of thyroid medications, menstrual history, changes in weight, bowel elimination.
- *Physical assessment:* Muscle strength, tremors, vital signs, cardiovascular and peripheral vascular systems, integument, size of thyroid, presence of bruit over thyroid, eyes and vision.

Nursing Diagnoses and Interventions

In planning and implementing nursing care for the client with hyperthyroidism, the nurse considers the client's responses to the systemic effects of the disorder. Although each client may have different needs, nursing diagnoses discussed in this section focus on the most common problems: cardiovascular problems, visual deficits, altered nutrition, and body image disturbance. See the accompanying Nursing Care Plan on page 540.

Risk for Decreased Cardiac Output

The client with hyperthyroidism is at risk for alterations in cardiac output. Excess TH directly affects the heart, resulting in increased rate and stroke volume. Increases in the metabolic demands and oxygen requirements of peripheral tissues increase the demands on the heart, and systolic hypertension, angina, arrhythmias, or cardiac failure may occur. The client often has palpitations and shortness of breath and is easily fatigued. The risk of complications is greater in clients with pre-existing cardiovascular disorders.

- Monitor blood pressure, pulse rate and rhythm, respiratory rate, and breath sounds. Assess for peripheral edema, jugular vein distention, and increased activity intolerance. *Increased TH increases cardiac rate, stroke volume, and tissue demand for oxygen, causing stress on the heart. This may result in hypertension, arrhythmias, tachycardia, and congestive heart failure.*

NURSING CARE OF THE CLIENT HAVING A Subtotal Thyroidectomy

PREOPERATIVE CARE

- Administer ordered antithyroid medications and iodine preparations, and monitor their effects. *Antithyroid drugs are given before surgery to promote a euthyroid state. Iodine preparations are given to the client before surgery to decrease vascularity of the gland, thereby decreasing the risk of hemorrhage.*
- Teach the client to support the neck by placing both hands behind the neck when sitting up in bed, while moving about, and while coughing. *Placing the hands behind the neck provides support for the suture line.*
- Answer questions, and allow time for the client to verbalize concerns. *Because the incision is made at the base of the throat, clients (especially women) are often concerned about their appearance after surgery. Explain that the scar will eventually be only a thin line and that jewelry or scarves may be used to cover the scar.*
- Teach the client to expect hoarseness due to generalized swelling at the suture line. *This is expected to diminish with healing and is not caused by laryngeal nerve damage.*

POSTOPERATIVE CARE

- Provide comfort measures: Administer analgesic pain medications as ordered, and monitor their effectiveness; place the client in a semi-Fowler's position after recovery from anesthesia; support head and neck with pillows. *Analgesic medications reduce the perception of pain and reduce physical stress during the postoperative period. Positioning the client in a semi-Fowler's position and supporting the head and neck decrease strain on the suture line.*
- Perform focused assessments to monitor for complications:
  a. Hemorrhage. Assess dressing (if present) and the area under the client's neck and shoulders for drainage. Monitor blood pressure and pulse for symptoms of hypovolemic shock. Assess tightness of dressing (if present). *The vascularity of the gland increases the risk of hemorrhage. The location of the incision and the position of the client may cause the drainage to run*

back and under the client. The danger of hemorrhage is greatest in the first 12 to 24 hours after surgery.
  b. Respiratory distress. Assess respiratory rate, rhythm, depth, and effort. Maintain humidification as ordered. Assist the client with coughing and deep breathing. Have suction equipment, oxygen, and a tracheostomy set available for immediate use. *Respiratory distress may result from hemorrhage and edema, which may compress the trachea; from tetany and laryngeal spasms resulting from decreased hormones due to removal or damage to the parathyroid glands; and from damage to the laryngeal nerve, causing spasms of the vocal cords. Stridor is heard in acute obstructions. This is a high-pitched, squeaky sound and is a sign of airway obstruction. Equipment must be immediately available if the client experiences respiratory distress that requires interventions and treatment.*
  c. Laryngeal nerve damage. Assess for the ability to speak aloud, noting quality and tone of voice. *The location of the laryngeal nerve increases the risk of damage during thyroid surgery. Although hoarseness may be due to edema or the endotracheal tube used during surgery and will subside, permanent hoarseness or loss of vocal volume is a potential danger.*
  d. Tetany. Assess for signs of latent tetany due to calcium deficiency, including tingling of toes, fingers, and lips; muscular twitches; positive Chvostek's and Trousseau's signs; and decreased serum calcium levels. Serum calcium levels will be monitored in the postoperative period. Keep calcium gluconate or calcium chloride available for immediate intravenous use, if necessary. *The parathyroid glands are located in and near the thyroid gland; surgery of the thyroid gland may injure or remove parathyroid glands, resulting in hypocalcemia and tetany. Tetany may occur in 1 to 7 days after thyroidectomy.*

- Suggest keeping the environment as cool and free of distraction as possible. Decrease stress by explaining interventions and teaching relaxation procedures. *A physically comfortable and psychologically calm environment can reduce stimuli and stressors. Stress increases circulating catecholamines, which further increase cardiac workload.*
- Encourage the client to balance activity with rest periods. *Rest periods decrease energy expenditure and tissue requirements for oxygen, decreasing demands on the heart by decreasing cardiac workload.*

Disturbed Sensory Perception: Visual

Visual changes that occur in clients with hyperthyroidism include difficulty in focusing, diplopia (double vision), or visual loss. If the client is unable to close the eyelids because of exophthalmos, the risk of corneal dryness with resultant infection or injury increases. Visual deficits may also result from

pressure on the optic nerve from retro-orbital edema and the shortening of eye muscles. Although treatment of hyperthyroidism may stop the progression of eye changes, not all symptoms are reversible.

- Monitor visual acuity, photophobia, integrity of the cornea, and lid closure. *The cornea is at risk for dryness, injury, conjunctivitis, and corneal infections. Injury and infection of the cornea can result in further loss of visual acuity.*
- Teach measures for protecting the eye from injury and maintaining visual acuity:
  - Use tinted glasses or shields as protection.
  - Use artificial tears to moisten the eyes.
  - Use cool, moist compresses to relieve irritation
  - Cover or tape eyelids shut at night if they do not close.
  - Elevate the head of the bed to 45 degrees to promote periorbital fluid decrease
  - Promptly report any pain or changes in vision.

NURSING CARE PLAN A Client with Graves' Disease

Mrs. Juanita Manuel is a 33-year-old mother of four small children. She is a second-year student at the local community college, within one semester of completing the requirements for an associate degree in child care. For the past 3 months, Juanita has been constantly hungry and has eaten more than usual, but she has still lost 15 lb (6.8 kg). She has repeated bouts of diarrhea and often feels nauseated. Her hands shake, she can feel her heart beating rapidly, and she finds herself laughing or crying for no apparent reason.

Mrs. Manuel makes an appointment with her family physician. The nurse at the office completes a health history and physical assessment. When asked how she has been feeling, Mrs. Manuel replies, "Well, I don't know what's wrong with me—but I keep losing weight and I cry at the drop of a hat. I am also just so hot all the time, and I've never had that problem before. I hope I find out what's wrong and it's nothing serious."

ASSESSMENT

The health history indicates that although her appetite has increased, Mrs. Manuel has lost 15 lb (6.8 kg). She states that she has had diarrhea, nausea, palpitations, heat intolerance, and mood changes. Physical assessment findings include the following: T 101°F (38.3°C), P 110, R 24, and BP 162/86. Her skin is moist and warm, her hair thin and fine. She has visible tremors in her hands. Her eyeballs protrude, and she is unable to close her eyelids completely. Her thyroid is enlarged and palpable. Diagnostic tests reveal the following abnormal results: T_3, 350 g/dL (normal range: 80 to 200 ng/dL), T_4, 15.1 mg/dL (normal range: 5 to 12 mg/dL). A thyroid scan demonstrates an enlarged thyroid with increased iodine uptake. After the medical diagnosis of Graves' disease is made, Mrs. Manuel is started on the antithyroid medication propylthiouracil, 150 mg orally every 8 hours.

DIAGNOSES

- *Risk for Imbalanced Nutrition: Less than Body Requirements* related to weight loss of 15 lb (6.8 kg), with present weight 10% less than normal for height
- *Diarrhea* related to increased peristalsis as evidenced by 8 to 10 liquid stools per day
- *Risk for Disturbed Sensory Perception: Visual* related to an inability to close the eyelids completely
- *Anxiety* related to a lack of knowledge about disease process

EXPECTED OUTCOMES

- Gain at least 1 lb (0.45 kg) every 2 weeks.
- Regain normal bowel elimination patterns.
- Maintain normal vision (with no evidence of corneal damage) and verbalize measures to protect her eyes.
- Verbalize medical treatment and self-care needs.
- Verbalize a decrease in anxiety.

PLANNING AND IMPLEMENTATION

- Request that she keep a record of daily weight.
- Discuss adopting a high-kilocalorie diet. Identify food likes and dislikes, as well as foods that increase diarrhea, before instituting a plan to increase food intake.
- Request that she keep a stool chart, noting the time, type, and precipitating factors for diarrhea stools. Teach comfort measures for irritated anal area (clean washcloth and soap, nonirritating ointment).
- Teach how to apply eyedrops (artificial tears).
- Explain the need to elevate the head of the bed to 45 degrees at night, and tape eye shields over eyes before sleep.
- Teach about Graves' disease, the medication's effects and side effects, and the need for continued medical care.

EVALUATION

By her next office visit, Mrs. Manuel has gained 1 lb (0.45 kg) and has discussed her dietary needs with the nurse and her husband. She is having diarrhea less often. She has safely applied the eyedrops and states that she uses the eye shields and elevates the head of her bed at night. The office nurse reviewed the written and verbal information about Graves' disease and the medication prescribed. Mrs. Manuel verbalizes her understanding, stating, "I'll always take my medicine—I never want to feel like that again!" She also says that she feels much less anxious now that she understands what has happened.

CRITICAL THINKING IN THE NURSING PROCESS

1. What is the pathophysiologic basis for Mrs. Manuel's abnormal vital signs?
2. What is the rationale for having the client with exophthalmos elevate the head of the bed at night?
3. Outline a teaching plan that could be given to clients for home care following a subtotal thyroidectomy.
See Evaluating Your Response in Appendix C.

PRACTICE ALERT
Teach the client to cover or tape the eyelids shut at night if they do not close and to sleep with the head of the bed elevated.

The measures outlined decrease the risk of injury, provide comfort, decrease periorbital edema that can further compromise vision, and ensure immediate care for problems, thereby minimizing the risk of further visual loss.

Imbalanced Nutrition: Less than Body Requirements

The hypermetabolic state that occurs in hyperthyroidism causes gastrointestinal hypermotility, with nausea, vomiting, diarrhea,

and abdominal pain. Although the client may have an increased appetite and eat more than usual, weight loss continues.

- Ask the client to weigh daily (at the same time each day), and keep a record of results. *The inability to meet metabolic demands results in loss of body weight. Regular monitoring detects continued weight loss.*
- In collaboration with a dietitian, teach the client the need for a diet high in carbohydrates and protein and including between-meal snacks. Six small meals a day may be more desirable than three large meals. Caloric intake may need to be increased to 4000 kcal/day if weight loss exceeds 10% to 17% for height and frame. *Increased nutrients as part of a well-balanced diet are necessary to meet metabolic*

demands. *Clients are often better able to increase food intake by eating frequent, small meals. A 1-lb weight gain requires approximately 3500 extra kilocalories.*

- Monitor nutritional status through results of laboratory data. Serum albumin, transferrin, and total lymphocyte counts are commonly lower than normal in nutritional deficits. *A negative nitrogen balance signifies a catabolic state in which protein is lost and metabolic demands are not being met.*

Disturbed Body Image

Physical changes common in hyperthyroidism include exophthalmos, goiter, tremors, hair loss, increased perspiration, loss of strength, fatigue, weight loss, and changes in reproductive and sexual function (amenorrhea in women, impotence in men, and increased libido in both men and women). In addition, the client often has mood changes and insomnia and is constantly nervous and anxious. There may even be periods of psychosis. These changes are frightening not only for the client but also for family members.

- Establish a trusting relationship; encourage the client to verbalize feelings about self and to ask questions about the illness and treatment. Provide reliable information and clarify misconceptions. *Establishing trust facilitates open sharing of feelings and perceptions.*

Community-Based Care

Clients with hyperthyroidism primarily provide self-care at home. Teaching is individualized to meet the client's needs. Address the following topics:

- The client taking oral medications must understand the need for lifelong treatment.
- The client who has a thyroidectomy requires information about postoperative wound care.
- The client having radioactive iodine therapy needs to know the symptoms of hypothyroidism.
- Depending on the age of the client and the support systems available, referral to community healthcare agencies may be necessary.
- In addition, suggest the following resources which are accessible via the Internet:
  - American Thyroid Association
  - Thyroid Foundation of Canada
  - Endocrine Society.

THE CLIENT WITH HYPOTHYROIDISM

Hypothyroidism is a disorder that results when the thyroid gland produces an insufficient amount of TH. Because a decrease in TH levels decreases metabolic rate and heat production, hypothyroidism affects all body systems (see the *Multisystem Effects of Hypothyroidism* on page 542). Hypothyroidism is common in women between ages 30 and 60; the incidence rises after age 50. However, the disorder can occur at any stage of life. Careful evaluation of symptoms is important in the older adult because manifestations of hypothyroidism are

often thought to be the result of aging instead of a pathologic process.

The hypothyroid state in adults is sometimes called **myxedema**. The term reflects the characteristic accumulation of nonpitting edema in the connective tissues throughout the body. The edema is the result of water retention in mucoprotein (hydrophilic proteoglycans) deposits in the interstitial spaces. The face of a client with myxedema appears puffy, the tongue is enlarged, and the voice is hoarse and husky (Porth, 2005).

Pathophysiology and Manifestations

Hypothyroidism may be either primary or secondary. Primary hypothyroidism (which is more common) may be caused by congenital defects in the gland, loss of thyroid tissue following treatment for hyperthyroidism with surgery or radiation, antithyroid medications, thyroiditis, or endemic iodine deficiency. The cardiac drug amiodarone (Cordarone), which contains 75 mg of iodine per 200 mg tablet, is increasingly being implicated in causing thyroid problems (Porth, 2005). Clofibrate, estrogens, methadone, amiodarone, and birth control pills increase T_4 measurement; anabolic steroids, androgens, lithium, phenytoin, propanolol, interferon alpha, and interleukin-2 decrease T_4 measurement in thyroid tests. Of course, the drugs propylthiouracil and methimazole, which are used to treat hyperthyroidism, decrease T_4 measurement (Medline Plus, 2006). Secondary hypothyroidism may result from pituitary TSH deficiency or peripheral resistance to thyroid hormones. Hypothyroidism has a slow onset, with manifestations occurring over months or even years. With treatment, the mental and physical symptoms rapidly reverse in clients of all ages.

When TH production decreases, the thyroid gland enlarges in a compensatory attempt to produce more hormone. The goiter that results is usually a simple or nontoxic form. People living in certain areas of the world where the soil is deficient in iodine, the substance necessary for TH synthesis and secretion, are more prone to become hypothyroid and develop simple goiter. (Iodine deficiency is discussed later.) Geriatric clients have a decrease in T_4 production of approximately 30% but serum levels are usually maintained because of the age-related decrease in T_4 degradation (Weissel, 2006).

Hypothyroid clients characteristically have the manifestations of goiter, fluid retention and edema, decreased appetite, weight gain, constipation, dry skin, dyspnea, pallor, hoarseness, and muscle stiffness. Many clients have a decreased sense of taste and smell, menstrual disorders, anemias, and cardiac enlargement. The pulse is typically slow. Deficient amounts of TH cause abnormalities in lipid metabolism, with elevated serum cholesterol and triglyceride levels. As a result, the client is at increased risk for atherosclerosis and cardiac disorders. Decreased renal blood flow and glomerular filtration rate reduce the kidney's ability to excrete water, which may cause hyponatremia. Sleep apnea is more common in clients with hypothyroidism. Factors that result in decreased TH (in addition to those described) include iodine deficiency and Hashimoto's thyroiditis. A severe state of hypothyroidism is

MULTISYSTEM EFFECTS OF **Hypothyroidism**

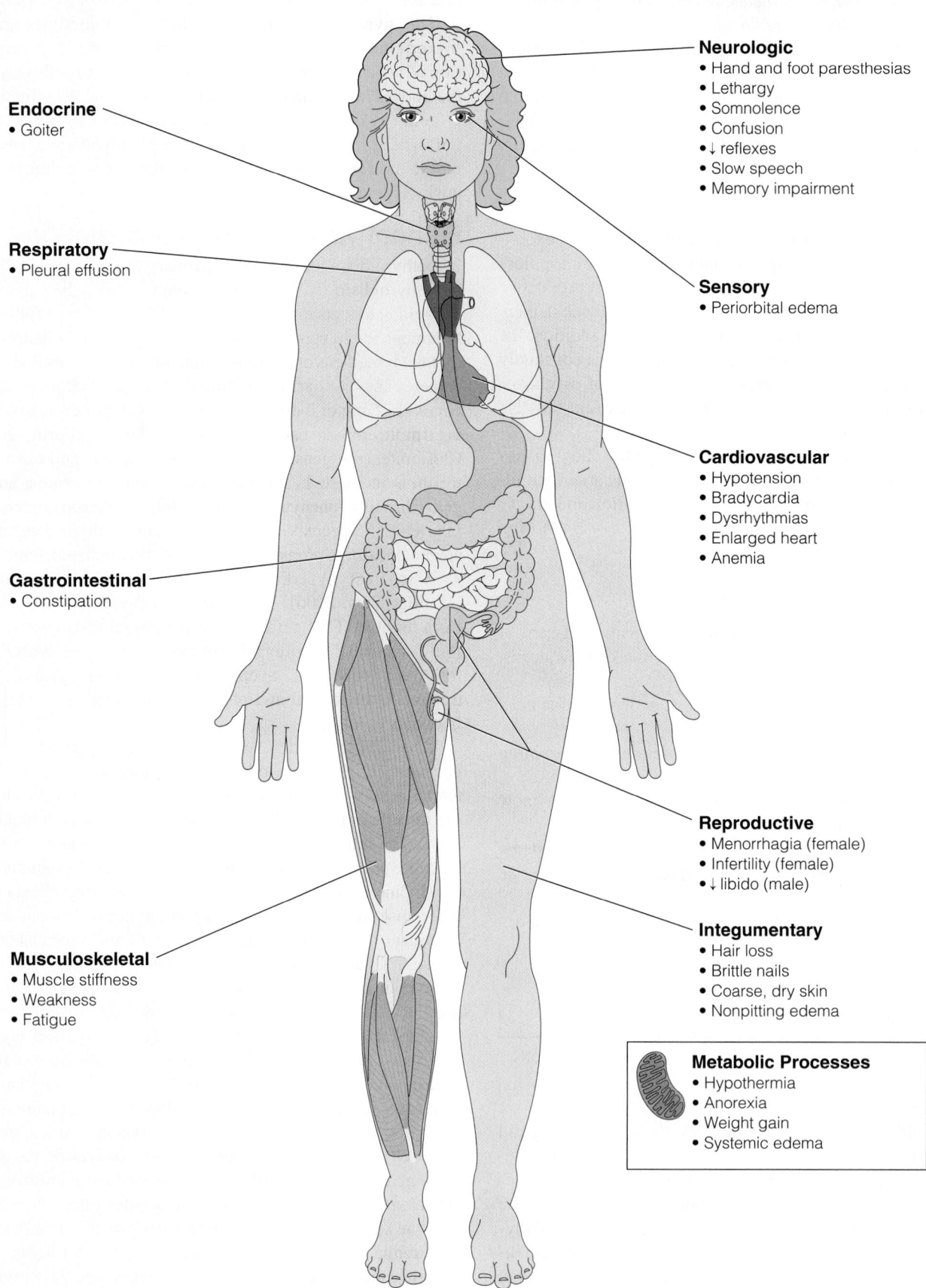

Endocrine
• Goiter

Respiratory
• Pleural effusion

Gastrointestinal
• Constipation

Musculoskeletal
• Muscle stiffness
• Weakness
• Fatigue

Neurologic
• Hand and foot paresthesias
• Lethargy
• Somnolence
• Confusion
• ↓ reflexes
• Slow speech
• Memory impairment

Sensory
• Periorbital edema

Cardiovascular
• Hypotension
• Bradycardia
• Dysrhythmias
• Enlarged heart
• Anemia

Reproductive
• Menorrhagia (female)
• Infertility (female)
• ↓ libido (male)

Integumentary
• Hair loss
• Brittle nails
• Coarse, dry skin
• Nonpitting edema

Metabolic Processes
• Hypothermia
• Anorexia
• Weight gain
• Systemic edema

called *myxedema coma* and is characterized by a shallow edema especially around the eyes, hands, and feet.

Iodine Deficiency

Iodine is necessary for TH synthesis and secretion. Iodine deficiency may result from certain goitrogenic drugs (which block TH synthesis); lithium carbonate, used to treat bipolar mental disorders; and antithyroid drugs. Goitrogenic compounds in foods such as turnips, rutabagas, and soybeans may also block TH synthesis if consumed in sufficient quantities. In areas of the world where the soil is deficient in iodine, dietary intake of iodine may be inadequate. However, the use of iodized salt has reduced this risk in the United States.

Hashimoto's Thyroiditis

Hashimoto's thyroiditis is the most common cause of goiter and primary hypothyroidism in adults and children. In this autoimmune disorder, antibodies develop that destroy thyroid tissue. Functional thyroid tissue is replaced with fibrous tissue, and TH levels decrease. In addition, decreasing levels of TH in the early stages of the disease prompt the gland to enlarge to compensate, causing a goiter. However, as the disease progresses, the thyroid gland becomes smaller. This disorder is more common in women and has a familial link.

Myxedema Coma

Myxedema coma is a life-threatening complication of long-standing, untreated hypothyroidism usually triggered by an acute illness or trauma (Tierney et al., 2005). It is characterized by severe metabolic disorders (hyponatremia, hypoglycemia, lactic acidosis), hypothermia, cardiovascular collapse, impaired mentation, and coma. Myxedema coma, although rare, most commonly occurs during the winter months in older women with chronic hypothyroidism (Porth, 2005).

Myxedema coma may be precipitated by trauma, infection, failure to take thyroid replacement medications, the use of central nervous system depressants, and exposure to cold temperatures (Porth, 2005). The treatment of myxedema coma addresses the precipitating factors and manifestations and involves maintaining a patent airway; maintaining fluid, electrolyte, and acid–base balance; maintaining cardiovascular status; increasing body temperature; and increasing TH levels. If untreated, the mortality rate is high (Tierney et al., 2005).

INTERDISCIPLINARY CARE

The treatment of the client with hypothyroidism focuses on diagnosis, prevention or treatment of complications, and replacement of the deficient TH. With early and continued treatment, both appearance and mental function return to normal.

Diagnosis

Hypothyroidism is diagnosed by the clinical manifestations and by a decrease in TH, especially T_4. See Table 19–2. TSH concentration often is increased, because the negative hormonal feedback from TH is lost. The same laboratory and diagnostic tests used to diagnose hyperthyroidism are also used to diagnose hypothyroidism, with opposite results in most cases.

TABLE 19–2 Laboratory Findings in Hypothyroidism

TEST	NORMAL VALUES	FINDINGS
Serum TA	None to 1:20	Normal
Serum TSH	2–10 mU/ml mU = microunit	Increased in primary hypothyroidism
Serum T_4	5 to 12 mcg/dL	Decreased
Serum T_3	80 to 200 ng/dL	Decreased
T_3 uptake (T_3RU)	25 to 35 relative percentage	Decreased
Thyroid suppression		No change in RAI uptake or T_4 levels

Medications

Hypothyroidism is treated with medications that replace TH. Levothyroxine (thyroxine, T_4) is the treatment of choice (Tierney et al., 2005). Medications commonly used to treat hypothyroidism and their nursing implications are shown in the Medication Administration box on page 544. In the geriatric clients, an age-related decrease in serum albumin and renal excretion can increase the amount of available drug and cause an exaggerated pharmacologic effect. Therefore, the older client may require less thyroid medication than a younger client.

Surgery

If the hypothyroid client has a goiter large enough to cause respiratory difficulties or dysphagia, a subtotal thyroidectomy may be performed (see page 539).

NURSING CARE

Health Promotion

One of the most critical factors in preventing hypothyroidism is education of the public about the necessity of an adequate dietary intake of iodine. The use of iodized salt meets the requirements for hormone production. It is important to teach clients the importance of regular healthcare provider visits and medication intake. See the Nursing Research box on page 545.

Assessment

Collect the following data through the health history and physical examination (see Chapter 18). Further focused assessments are described with nursing interventions below. When assessing the older client, be aware of normal changes with aging, outlined in the box on page 545.

- *Health history:* Pituitary diseases, when symptoms began, severity of symptoms, treatment of hyperthyroidism with medications or radioactive iodine, thyroid surgery, treatment of head or neck cancer with radiation, diet, use of iodized salt, bowel elimination, respiratory difficulties.
- *Physical assessment:* Muscle strength, deep tendon reflexes, vital signs, cardiovascular and peripheral vascular systems, integument, thyroid gland, weight.

MEDICATION ADMINISTRATION Hypothyroidism

THYROID PREPARATIONS

Levothyroxine sodium (T₄) (Levoxyl, Levothroid, Synthroid)

Liothyronine sodium (T₃) (Cytomel)

Liotrix (T₃–T₄) (Euthyroid, Thyrolar)

Thyroid preparations increase blood levels of TH, thus raising the client's metabolic rate. As a result, cardiac output, oxygen consumption, and body temperature increase. Levothyroxine speeds the elimination of vitamin K–dependent clotting factors enhancing the effects of warfarin (Coumadin). Patients are at increased risk of bleeding if warfarin dosages are appropriately reduced (Lehne, 2004). The dosage depends on the drug chosen and the client's degree of thyroid dysfunction, sensitivity to TH, age, body size, and health. The older adult may require lower doses.

Nursing Responsibilities

- Give 1 hour before meals or 2 hours after meals for best absorption.
- Thyroid preparations potentiate the effect of anticoagulant drugs. If the client is also receiving an anticoagulant, monitor for bruising, bleeding gums, and blood in the urine.
- Thyroid medications potentiate the effect of digitalis. If the client is also receiving a digitalis preparation, monitor for signs of digitalis toxicity.
- Monitor for symptoms of coronary insufficiency: chest pain, dyspnea, tachycardia.

- If the client has insulin-dependent diabetes, monitor the effects of insulin. The effect of the insulin may change as thyroid function increases.
- During dose adjustment, take pulse before administering drug. Report pulse >100.

Health Education for the Client and Family

- Do not substitute brands of drugs or use generic equivalents without the physician's approval.
- The medications must be taken for the rest of one's life.
- Report symptoms of excess thyroid hormone to the physician: excess weight loss, palpitations, leg cramps, nervousness, or insomnia.
- If you have diabetes and use insulin, monitor blood glucose levels closely; the thyroid medications may alter the amount of insulin required.
- Thyroid preparations increase the risk of iodine toxicity. Do not use iodized salt or over-the-counter drugs containing iodine.
- If you are also taking an anticoagulant, report any signs of bleeding.
- Report any changes in menstrual periods.
- Take the thyroid preparation each morning to decrease the possibility of insomnia.
- Closely monitor blood pressure and pulse (older clients).
- Avoid excessive intake of foods that are known to inhibit TH utilization such as turnips, cabbage, carrots, spinach, and peaches.

Nursing Diagnoses and Interventions

In planning and implementing care for clients with hypothyroidism, the nurse takes into account that the disorder affects all organ systems. Although many nursing diagnoses might be valid, this section focuses on client problems with cardiovascular function, elimination, and skin integrity. See the accompanying Nursing Care Plan on page 546.

Decreased Cardiac Output

A TH deficit causes a reduction in heart rate and stroke volume, resulting in decreased cardiac output. There may also be an accumulation of fluid in the pericardial sac (from the edema characteristic of hypothyroidism), and coronary artery disease may be present, further compromising cardiac function.

- Monitor blood pressure, rate and rhythm of apical and peripheral pulses, respiratory rate, and breath sounds. *Hypotension indicates decreasing peripheral blood. Fluid in the pericardial sac restricts cardiac function. Monopolysaccharide deposits in the respiratory system decrease vital capacity and cause hypoventilation.*
- Suggest the client avoid chilling; increase room temperature, use additional bed covers, and avoid drafts. *Chilling increases metabolic rate and puts increased stress on the heart.*
- Explain the need to alternate activity with rest periods. Ask the client to report any breathing difficulties, chest pain, heart palpitations, or dizziness. *Activity increases demands on the heart and should be balanced with rest. Symptoms of cardiac stress include dyspnea, chest pain, palpitations, and dizziness.*

Constipation

The hypothyroid client is likely to have a reduced appetite and decreased food intake, a diminished activity level because of muscle aches and weakness, and reduced peristalsis to the point that fecal impactions may occur.

- Encourage a fluid intake of up to 2000 mL per day. Discuss preferred liquids and the best times of day to drink fluids. If kilocalorie intake is restricted, ensure that liquids have no kilocalorie or are low in kilocalorie. *Sufficient fluid intake is necessary to promote proper stool consistency.*
- Discuss ways to maintain a high-fiber diet. *Diets high in fiber and fluid produce soft stools. Fiber that is not digested absorbs water, which adds bulk to the stool and assists in the movement of fecal material through the intestines.*
- Encourage activity as tolerated. *Activity influences bowel elimination by improving muscle tone and stimulating peristalsis.*

PRACTICE ALERT

High-fiber foods include beans, potatoes, fruits, breads, cereal, crackers, popcorn, and rice.

Risk for Impaired Skin Integrity

The client with hypothyroidism is at risk for impaired skin integrity related to the accumulation of fluid in the interstitial spaces and to dry, rough skin. Decreased peripheral circulation, decreased activity levels, and slow wound healing further in-

NURSING RESEARCH   Evidence-Based Practice: Self-Medicating with Thyroid Hormone

Michel, Neafsey, and Dzurec (2004) conducted a telephone survey of 38 women taking Neafsey levothyroxine for hypothyroidism. Clients taking levothyroxine have an increased risk of developing osteoporosis and are encouraged to take a calcium supplement to prevent bone loss. Prior research has shown that taking calcium carbonate within 4 hours of taking levothyroxine may decrease the absorption of the levothyroxine. The authors asked the subjects if they were taking calcium or multiple vitamin supplements and how they timed the ingestion of levothyroxine and the supplements. They also inquired about concurrent diseases and found that 13% had osteoporosis, 33% had hypertension, 27% had depression, 27% also had hyperlipidemia, and 24% had arthritis. Only 2 of the 38 subjects reported that calcium and levothyroxine should be administered separately. They learned this by patient information on pharmacy printouts. Those who were taking calcium (47%) reported taking it within 4 hours of taking levothyroxine; 17% took them together and 50% separated administration by 1 hour. Fifteen subjects taking calcium reported that a healthcare professional recommended it.

IMPLICATIONS FOR NURSING

Patient education about medication self-administration is within the scope of nursing practice. It is difficult to know the complex details about the vast number of medications and it is easy to overlook a supplement that is not prescribed by the healthcare provider. Nurses regularly review medication administration when clients are discharged from acute care facilities and levothyroxine is a common prescription. In fact, it is the second most commonly prescribed medication in the United States (Michel et al., 2004). Perhaps the best practice is to recommend clients read the pharmacy printout carefully for details about taking each medication and consult the pharmacist or healthcare provider if they have questions.

CRITICAL THINKING IN CLIENT CARE

1. How is hypothyroidism related to osteoporosis? What specific pathophysiologic processes increase the risk of osteoporosis? How does a calcium supplement prevent the development of osteoporosis?
2. What other factors contribute to the complexity of medication self-administration in the client with hypothyroidism?
3. What counsel about levothyroxine is important for clients with hypothyroidism? Should the client who has had the thyroid gland removed because of goiter or cancer receive the same counsel?

---

crease the risk. These interventions are outlined for the older client who is hospitalized for surgery or severe hypothyroidism.

- Monitor skin surfaces for redness or lesions, especially if the client's activity is greatly reduced. Use a pressure ulcer risk assessment scale to identify clients at risk. *Hypothyroidism causes dry, rough, edematous skin conditions that increase the risk of skin breakdown.*
- Provide or teach the immobile client measures to promote optimal circulation:
  - Use a turning schedule if the client is on bed rest, or teach the client to change position every 2 hours.
  - Limit the time for sitting in one position; shift weight or lift the body using arm rests every 20 to 30 minutes.
  - Use pillows, pads, or sheepskin or foam cushions for bed and/or chair.

- Teach and implement a schedule of range-of-motion exercises. *Prolonged pressure, especially in clients with edema and circulatory impairment, can occlude capillaries and cause hypoxic tissue damage.*
- Provide or teach the client measures to maintain skin integrity:
  - Take baths only as necessary; use warm (not hot) water.
  - Use gentle motions when washing and drying skin.
  - Use alcohol-free skin oils and lotions.
  Dry skin and edema increase the risk of skin breakdown. Hot water, rough massage, and alcohol-based preparations may increase skin dryness, further impairing the body's ability to maintain skin integrity.

PRACTICE ALERT

Lift the client up in bed to prevent tissue damage from shearing forces.

Community-Based Care

Clients with hypothyroidism require lifelong care, primarily at home. Address the following topics:

- The need to take medications for the rest of one's life
- The need for periodic dosage reassessments
- If the client is older or does not have a support system, helpful community resources
- Additional resources:
  - American Thyroid Association
  - Thyroid Foundation of Canada
  - Endocrine Society.

NURSING CARE OF THE OLDER ADULT
Variations in Assessment Findings—Hypothyroidism

Normal Changes with Aging

- The thyroid gland undergoes some degree of atrophy, fibrosis, and nodularity.
- Hair growth decreases.
- Nails are often thick, brittle, and yellow.
- Facial skin sags, and bones become more prominent.
- Deep tendon reflexes decrease.
- Response to questions may be slower.

MediaLink   Hypothyroidism Resources

NURSING CARE PLAN   A Client with Hypothyroidism

Jane Lee is a 60-year-old retired nurse living with her husband and daughter on a farm that has been in the family for four generations. Mrs. Lee has gained 10 lb (4.5 kg) in the past few months, even though she is rarely hungry and eats much less than normal. She is always tired and weak—so tired that she has not even been able to help with the chores on the farm or do housework. She is concerned about her appearance and the way she sounds when she talks. Her face is puffy, and her tongue always feels thick. Mr. Lee convinces his wife to make an appointment at a health center in a nearby town.

ASSESSMENT

Brian Henning, RN, completes the health assessment for Mrs. Lee at the health center. He finds that she now weighs 150 lb (68 kg), an increase of 10 lb (4.5 kg) over her weight at her last visit 6 months earlier. Mrs. Lee states that she always feels cold, tired, and weak. She also states that she is constipated, has difficulty remembering things, and looks different. Physical assessment findings include a palpable and bilaterally enlarged thyroid; dry, yellowish skin; nonpitting edema of the face and lower legs; and slow, slurred speech. Diagnostic tests revealed the following abnormal findings: T_3, 56 ng/dL (normal range: 80 to 200 ng/dL); T_4, 3.1 (normal range: 5 to 12 mg/dL); TSH increased. The medical diagnosis of hypothyroidism is made, and Mrs. Lee is started on levothyroxine 0.05 mg daily.

DIAGNOSES

- *Constipation* related to decreased peristalsis, as evidenced by hard, formed stools every 4 days
- *Impaired Verbal Communication* related to changes in speech patterns and enlarged tongue
- *Low Self-Esteem* related to changes in physical appearance and activity intolerance

EXPECTED OUTCOMES

- Regain normal bowel elimination patterns, having a soft, formed stool at least every other day.

- Experience improvement in verbal communication.
- Regain positive self-esteem as medication reduces physical changes and fatigue.

PLANNING AND IMPLEMENTATION

- Teach to increase fluids, bulk, and fiber in the diet to help regain a normal bowel elimination pattern of a soft, formed stool every other day.
- Take medication as prescribed and do not expect immediate reversal of symptoms affecting speech.
- Plan activities around rest periods. Encourage husband and daughter to help with housecleaning and cooking.

EVALUATION

On return to the health center 2 months later, Mrs. Lee reports that she is no longer constipated but that she is continuing to drink six glasses of water and eating oatmeal every day. She no longer feels cold, is regaining her normal energy, and even feels well enough to plant her garden. Her speech is clear and easy to understand. As she leaves the examining room, Mrs. Lee says, "It's hard to believe that I have changed so much—now I look and feel like the 'old' me!"

CRITICAL THINKING IN THE NURSING PROCESS

1. What physical changes that normally occur with aging are similar to the manifestations of hypothyroidism?
2. Describe the factors that put Mrs. Lee's safety at risk. What alterations in her home environment would you suggest to promote safety until the prescribed medication takes effect?
3. The client taking oral thyroid medications may become hyperthyroid. List the manifestations you would include in a teaching plan to signal this condition.
See Evaluating Your Response in Appendix C.

THE CLIENT WITH CANCER OF THE THYROID

Thyroid cancer is relatively rare, with an estimated rate of 25,690 new cases annually. Thyroid cancer accounts for approximately 1490 cancer deaths a year (American Cancer Society, 2005). The most consistent risk factor is exposure to ionizing radiation to the head and neck during childhood. For example, many adults in their 50s and 60s received x-ray treatments for colds and sinus infections during childhood.

Of the several types of thyroid cancer, the most common types are listed here:

- Papillary thyroid carcinoma is the most common thyroid malignancy. It is usually detected as a single nodule, but may arise from a multinodular goiter. The average age of diagnosis is 42, with 70% of cases occurring in women. Risks for the development of this form are exposure to external x-ray treatments to the head or neck as a child, childhood exposure to radioactive isotopes of iodine in nuclear fallout, and a family history. Papillary thyroid carcinoma is the least aggressive type, but does metastasize to the local and regional lymph nodes and lungs.

- Follicular thyroid cancer is the second most common thyroid malignancy. The average age of diagnosis is 50, with 75% of cases occurring in women. This form is more aggressive, with potential for vascular invasion and spread to lung and bone.

Thyroid cancer is manifested by a palpable, firm nontender nodule in the thyroid. If undetected, the tumor may grow and impinge on the esophagus or trachea, causing difficulty in swallowing or breathing. Most people with thyroid cancer do not have elevated thyroid hormone levels. The diagnosis is made by measuring thyroid hormones, performing thyroid scans, and by fine-needle biopsy of the nodule. The usual treatment is subtotal or total thyroidectomy. TSH suppression therapy with levothyroxine may be conducted prior to surgery. Radioactive iodine therapy (^{131}I) and chemotherapy are additional therapeutic options. The 5-year survival rate, if the tumor has not metastasized, is 97% (American Cancer Society, 2005). Nursing care for the client with cancer is discussed in Chapter 14 ∞ .

DISORDERS OF THE PARATHYROID GLANDS

Disorders of the parathyroid glands, hyperparathyroidism and hypoparathyroidism, are not as common as those of the thyroid gland. Hypercalcemia and hypocalcemia (the primary results of alterations in parathyroid function) are discussed in Chapter 10.

THE CLIENT WITH HYPERPARATHYROIDISM

Hyperparathyroidism results from an increase in the secretion of parathyroid hormone (PTH), which regulates normal serum levels of calcium. The increase in PTH affects the kidneys and bones, resulting in the following pathophysiologic changes:

- Increased resorption of calcium and excretion of phosphate by the kidneys, which increases the risk of hypercalcemia and hypophosphatemia
- Increased bicarbonate excretion and decreased acid excretion by the kidneys, which increases the risk of metabolic acidosis and hypokalemia
- Increased release of calcium and phosphorus by bones, with resultant bone decalcification
- Deposits of calcium in soft tissues and the formation of renal calculi.

Pathophysiology and Manifestations

Hyperparathyroidism occurs more often in older adults and is three times more common in women. The disorder itself is not common. The three types of hyperparathyroidism are as follows:

- Primary hyperparathyroidism occurs when there is hyperplasia or an adenoma in one of the parathyroid glands. These disorders interrupt the normal regulatory mechanism between serum calcium levels and PTH secretion and increase the absorption of calcium through the gastrointestinal tract.
- Secondary hyperparathyroidism is a compensatory response by the parathyroid glands to chronic hypocalcemia. It is characterized by an increased secretion of PTH.
- Tertiary hyperparathyroidism results from hyperplasia of the parathyroid glands and a loss of response to serum calcium levels. This disorder is most often seen in clients with chronic renal failure.

Many clients with hyperparathyroidism are asymptomatic. When symptoms occur, they are related to hypercalcemia and various musculoskeletal, renal, and gastrointestinal manifestations. Bone reabsorption results in pathologic fractures, while elevated calcium levels alter neural and muscular activity, leading to muscle weakness and atrophy. Proximal renal tubule function is altered, and metabolic acidosis, renal calculi formation, and polyuria occur.

Manifestations of the effect of hypercalcemia on the gastrointestinal tract include abdominal pain, constipation, anorexia, and peptic ulcer formation. Hypercalcemia also affects the cardiovascular system, causing arrhythmias, hypertension, and increased sensitivity to cardiotonic glycosides (e.g., digitalis preparations). The manifestations of hyperparathyroidism are summarized in the following box.

MANIFESTATIONS of Hyperparathyroidism

MUSCULOSKELETAL SYSTEM
- Bone pain (back, joints, shins)
- Pathologic fractures (women)
- Muscle weakness
- Muscle atrophy

RENAL EFFECTS
- Renal calculi
- Polyuria
- Polydipsia

GASTROINTESTINAL SYSTEM
- Abdominal pain
- Peptic ulcers
- Pancreatitis
- Nausea
- Constipation

CARDIOVASCULAR SYSTEM
- Arrhythmias
- Hypertension

CENTRAL NERVOUS SYSTEM
- Paresthesias
- Depression
- Psychosis

METABOLIC EFFECTS
- Acidosis
- Weight loss

INTERDISCIPLINARY CARE

Hyperparathyroidism is diagnosed by excluding all other possible causes of hypercalcemia; by at least a 6-month history of symptoms; and by laboratory analysis of levels of serum calcium and PTH levels (Tierney et al., 2005).

Treatment of hyperparathyroidism focuses on decreasing the elevated serum calcium levels. Clients with mild hypercalcemia are urged to drink fluids and keep active. They should avoid immobilization, thiazide diuretics, large doses of vitamins A and D, antacids containing calcium, and calcium supplements. Severe hypercalcemia requires hospitalization and intensive treatment with intravenous saline. Medications to inhibit bone resorption and reduce hypercalcemia, such as pamidronate (Aredia), alendronate (Fosamax), and zoledronate (Zometa), are used for short-term treatment and may relieve bone pain (Tierney et al., 2005). Calcitonin, a hormone produced by the thyroid gland, decreases plasma levels of calcium by inhibiting bone resorption and increasing calcium excretion by the kidney (Lehne, 2004). A form of calcitonin from salmon is available as a nasal spray or IM/SQ injection.

Surgical removal of the parathyroid glands affected by hyperplasia or adenoma treats primary hyperparathyroidism. The preoperative and postoperative nursing care of the client having surgery of the parathyroids is essentially the same as that for the client having a thyroidectomy (see page 539).

NURSING CARE

Nursing care of the client with hypercalcemia is discussed in Chapter 10 .

THE CLIENT WITH HYPOPARATHYROIDISM

Hypoparathyroidism results from abnormally low PTH levels. The most common cause is damage to or removal of the parathyroid glands during thyroidectomy. The lack of circulating PTH causes hypocalcemia and an elevated blood phosphate level.

Pathophysiology and Manifestations

Reduced levels of PTH result in impaired renal tubular regulation of calcium and phosphate. In addition, decreased activation of vitamin D results in decreased absorption of calcium by the intestines. The low calcium levels cause changes in neuromuscular activity, affecting peripheral motor and sensory nerves. Hypocalcemia lowers the threshold for nerve and muscle excitability; a slight stimulus anywhere along a nerve or muscle fiber initiates an impulse.

The neuromuscular manifestations that result include numbness and tingling around the mouth and in the fingertips, muscle spasms of the hands and feet, convulsions, and laryngeal spasms. Tetany, a continuous spasm of muscles, is the primary symptom of hypocalcemia. In severe cases of tetany, death may occur. Assessments for **tetany** include Chvostek's sign and Trousseau's sign (see Chapter 18 ∞). The manifestations of hypoparathyroidism are summarized in the box on this page.

INTERDISCIPLINARY CARE

Hypoparathyroidism is diagnosed by low serum calcium levels and high phosphorous levels in the absence of renal failure, an absorption disorder, or a nutritional disorder.

MANIFESTATIONS **of Hypoparathyroidism**

MUSCULOSKELETAL SYSTEM
- Muscle spasms
- Facial grimacing
- Carpopedal spasms
- Tetany or convulsions

INTEGUMENTARY SYSTEM
- Brittle nails
- Hair loss
- Dry, scaly skin

GASTROINTESTINAL SYSTEM
- Abdominal cramps
- Malabsorption

CARDIOVASCULAR SYSTEM
- Arrhythmias

CENTRAL NERVOUS SYSTEM
- Paresthesias (lips, hands, feet)
- Mood disorders (irritability, depression, anxiety)
- Hyperactive reflexes
- Psychosis
- Increased intracranial pressure

Treatment of hypoparathyroidism focuses on increasing calcium levels. Intravenous calcium gluconate is given immediately to reduce tetany. Long-term therapy includes supplemental calcium, increased dietary calcium, and vitamin D therapy.

NURSING CARE

Nursing care for the client with hypocalcemia is discussed in Chapter 10 ∞ .

DISORDERS OF THE ADRENAL GLANDS

Disorders of the adrenal cortex or adrenal medulla result in changes in the production of adrenocorticotropic hormone (ACTH). Hormones of the adrenal cortex are essential to life. They maintain homeostasis in response to stressors. Disorders of the adrenal cortex result in complex physical, psychologic, and metabolic alterations that are potentially life threatening. Hormones of the adrenal medulla are not essential to life, because the sympathetic nervous system produces similar body responses. The disorders that occur are hyperfunction and hypofunction of the adrenal cortex and hyperfunction of the adrenal medulla.

THE CLIENT WITH HYPERCORTISOLISM (CUSHING'S SYNDROME)

Cushing's syndrome is a chronic disorder in which hyperfunction of the adrenal cortex produces excessive amounts of circulating cortisol or ACTH. Cushing's syndrome is more common in women, with the average age of onset between 30 and 50 years (Figure 19–3 ■). However, the disorder may occur at any age, especially as the result of pharmacologic therapy. People who take steroids for long periods of time (e.g., for

Figure 19–3 ■ A woman before and after developing Cushing's syndrome. In the photo at right, notice the swollen facial features.
Courtesy of Dr. Charles Wilson, University of California, San Francisco.

the treatment of arthritis, after an organ transplant, or as an adjunct to chemotherapy) are at increased risk for developing the disorder.

Pathophysiology

Cushing's syndrome may be the result of various causes. The most common etiologies of the disorder are as follows (Porth, 2005):

- The pituitary form, with ACTH hypersecretion by a tumor of the pituitary (called *Cushing's disease*). This is most commonly caused by a small pituitary adenoma, with persistent but disorderly and random overproduction of ACTH. Forty-three percent of Cushing's disease is due to hypersecretion of ACTH by the pituitary.
- The ectopic form, caused by ACTH-secreting tumors (such as small-cell lung cancer). In this form, the ACTH is also random and episodic, but greater than in Cushing's disease.
- The adrenal form, resulting from excessive cortisol secretion by a benign or malignant adrenal tumor. The excess secretion suppresses pituitary ACTH production, resulting in atrophy of the uninvolved adrenal cortex. Thirty-two percent of Cushing's disease is due to excessive autonomous secretion of cortisol by the adrenal glands, independent of ACTH (Tierney et al., 2005).
- Iatrogenic Cushing's syndrome, resulting from long-term therapy with potent pharmacologic glucocorticoid preparations.

Manifestations

The manifestations of Cushing's syndrome result from the ACTH or cortisol excess, and manifest as exaggerated cortisol actions. Obesity and a redistribution of body fat result in fat deposits in the abdominal region (central obesity), fat pads under the clavicle, a "buffalo hump" over the upper back, and a round "moon" face. Changes in protein metabolism cause muscle weakness and wasting, especially in the extremities. Glucocorticoid excess inhibits fibroblasts, resulting in loss of collagen and connective tissue. Thinning of skin, abdominal striae (reddish purple "stretch marks"), easy bruising, poor wound healing, and frequent skin infections result. Glucose metabolism is altered in the majority of clients, and diabetes mellitus may occur. Electrolyte imbalances also occur with the increased hormone levels. Changes in calcium absorption result in osteoporosis, compression fractures of the vertebrae, fractures of the ribs, and renal calculi. Hypokalemia and hypertension occur as potassium is lost and sodium is retained. Inhibited immune responses increase the risk of infection, and increased gastric acid secretion increases the risk of peptic ulcers. Emotional changes range from depression to psychosis. In women, increasing androgen levels cause hirsutism (excessive facial hair in particular), acne, and menstrual irregularities. The manifestations and effects of Cushing's syndrome are grouped by body system in the box on this page.

The complications of untreated Cushing's syndrome include electrolyte imbalances (hyperglycemia, hypernatremia, and hypokalemia), hypertension, and emotional disturbances. Increased susceptibility to infections is also a factor. Compression fractures from osteoporosis and aseptic necrosis of

MANIFESTATIONS of Cushing's Syndrome

MUSCULOSKELETAL SYSTEM
- Weakness
- Muscle wasting
- Osteoporosis

INTEGUMENTARY SYSTEM
- Thin, easily bruised skin
- Skin infections
- Poor wound healing
- Eccyhmosis
- Purple striae (around thighs, breasts, abdomen)
- Hirsutism

CENTRAL NERVOUS SYSTEM
- Emotional lability
- Psychoses

GASTROINTESTINAL SYSTEM
- Peptic ulcers

CARDIOVASCULAR SYSTEM
- Hypertension

RENAL EFFECTS
- Renal calculi
- Polyuria
- Polydipsia
- Glycosuria

METABOLIC EFFECTS
- Hypokalemia
- Hypernatremia
- Truncal obesity

REPRODUCTIVE SYSTEM
- Oligomenorrhea or amenorrhea
- Impotence
- Decreased libido

the femoral head may result in serious disability. If the client undergoes a bilateral adrenalectomy as a treatment for Cushing's syndrome, an acute deficit of cortisol (Addisonian crisis) may result.

INTERDISCIPLINARY CARE

The treatment of Cushing's syndrome includes medications, radiation therapy, or surgery, depending on the etiologic origin of the disorder.

Diagnostic Tests

Cushing's syndrome is diagnosed through a variety of diagnostic tests. Findings are shown in Table 19–3 and in the following bulleted summary:

- *Plasma cortisol levels* are measured. If Cushing's disease is present, test results show a loss of the normal diurnal variations of higher levels in the morning and lower levels in the afternoon.
- *Plasma ACTH levels* are measured to determine the etiology of the syndrome. Normally, plasma ACTH levels are highest from 7 A.M. to 10 A.M. and lowest from 7 P.M. to 10 P.M. In secondary Cushing's syndrome, ACTH is elevated; in primary Cushing's syndrome, ACTH is decreased.
- *24-hour urine tests* (17-ketosteroids [17-KS] and *17-hydroxy-corticosteroids*) are conducted to measure free cortisol and androgens; these hormones are increased in Cushing's syndrome. Because synthesis and circulation of adrenal hormones are diurnal and episodic, 24-hour urine collections

TABLE 19-3 Laboratory Findings in Cushing's Syndrome

	TEST	NORMAL VALUES	FINDINGS
Serum	Cortisol	8 A.M. to 10 A.M.: 5 to 23 mcg/dL 4 P.M. to 6 P.M.: 3 to 13 mcg/dL	Increased
	Blood urea nitrogen (BUN)	5 to 25 mg/dL	Normal
	Sodium	135 to 145 mEq/L	Increased
	Potassium	3.5 to 5.0 mEq/L	Increased
	Glucose (serum)	70 to 100 mg/dL	Increased
Urine	17-KS	Male: 5 to 25 mg/24h Female: 5 to 15 mg/24h >Age 65: 4 to 8 mg/24h	Increased

more correctly reflect total hormone than serum levels drawn intermittently.

- *Serum potassium, calcium, and glucose levels* are measured to identify electrolyte imbalances.
- *ACTH suppression test* may be conducted to identify the cause of the disorder. A synthetic cortisol (dexamethasone) is given to suppress the production of ACTH, and plasma cortisol levels are measured. If an extremely high dose of cortisol is necessary to suppress ACTH, the primary disorder is adrenal cortex hyperplasia. If ACTH is not suppressed with the synthetic cortisol, an adrenal tumor is suspected (Kirk et al., 2002).

Medications

Cushing's syndrome that results from a pituitary tumor is treated by medications as an adjunct to surgery or radiation. Medications are also used for clients with inoperable pituitary or adrenal malignancies. Although the drugs control symptoms, they do not effect a cure. Examples of some commonly prescribed drugs follow:

- Mitotane directly suppresses activity of the adrenal cortex and decreases peripheral metabolism of corticosteroids. It is used to treat metastatic adrenal cancer.
- Aminogluthemide or ketoconazole (or both) inhibit cortisol synthesis by the adrenal cortex and may be administered to clients with ectopic ACTH-secreting tumors that cannot be surgically removed.
- Somatostatin analog (octreotide) suppresses ACTH secretion in some clients.

Surgery

When Cushing's syndrome is caused by an adrenal cortex tumor, an adrenalectomy may be performed to remove the tumor. Only one adrenal gland is usually involved; however, if an ACTH-producing ectopic tumor is involved, a bilateral adrenalectomy is performed. Lifelong hormone replacement is necessary if both adrenal glands are removed. Nursing care of the client having an adrenalectomy is discussed below.

Surgical removal of the pituitary gland (hypophysectomy) is indicated when Cushing's syndrome is the result of a pituitary disorder. The gland is removed either by a transsphenoidal route or by a craniotomy. Nursing care for the client having cranial surgery is discussed in Chapter 44 ∞.

 NURSING CARE

Health Promotion

Stress the risk of developing Cushing's syndrome for clients taking long-term steroids. The risk of abruptly discontinuing the medications is an essential component of teaching. For a review of glucocorticoid administration see Chapter 12 ∞.

NURSING CARE OF THE CLIENT HAVING AN Adrenalectomy

PREOPERATIVE CARE

- Request a dietary consultation to discuss with the client about a diet high in vitamins and proteins. If hypokalemia exists, include foods high in potassium. *Glucocorticoid excess increases catabolism. Vitamins and proteins are necessary for tissue repair and wound healing following surgery.*
- Use careful medical and surgical asepsis when providing care and treatments. *Cortisol excess increases the risk of infection.*
- Monitor the results of laboratory tests of electrolytes and glucose levels. *Electrolyte and glucose imbalances are corrected before the client has surgery.*
- Teach the client to turn, cough, and perform deep-breathing exercises. *Although they are important for all surgical clients, these activities are even more important for the client who is at risk for infection. Having the client practice and demonstrate the activities increases postoperative compliance.*

POSTOPERATIVE CARE

- Take and record vital signs, measure intake and output, and monitor electrolytes on a frequent schedule, especially during the first 48 hours after surgery. *Removal of an adrenal gland, especially a bilateral adrenalectomy, results in adrenal insufficiency. Addisonian crisis and hypovolemic shock may occur. Cortisol is often given on the day of surgery and in the postoperative period to replace inadequate hormone levels. Intravenous fluids are also administered.*
- Assess body temperature, WBC levels, and wound drainage. Change dressings using sterile technique. *Impaired wound healing increases the risk of infection in clients with adrenal disorders. Use aseptic technique to decrease this risk.*

Assessment

Collect the following data through the health history and physical examination (see Chapter 18 ∞). Further focused assessments are described with nursing interventions below.

■ *Health history:* History of pituitary, adrenal, pancreatic, or pulmonary tumor; frequent infections; gastrointestinal bleeding; stress fractures; pain, changes in weight distribution; change in height; fatigue; weakness; change in appearance; bruising; skin infections; menstrual history; sexual function.
■ *Physical assessment:* Vital signs, behavior, appearance, fat distribution, face, skin, hair quantity and distribution, muscle size and strength, gait.

Nursing Diagnoses and Interventions

The nurse caring for the client with Cushing's syndrome must take a holistic approach to plan and implement interventions for a wide variety of responses, including problems related to fluid and electrolyte balance, injury, infection, and body image. For additional information about clients with alterations in fluid and electrolyte balance, see Chapter 10. See accompanying Nursing Care Plan below.

Fluid Volume Excess

The excess cortisol, not mineralocorticoid, secretion associated with Cushing's syndrome results in sodium and water

---

NURSING CARE PLAN **A Client with Cushing's Syndrome**

Sara Domico is a 30-year-old lawyer living in a major metropolitan area. She has never been married, and she shares her life with her cat, Beau, and her parents, who live nearby. Her physician recently diagnosed Ms. Domico as having Cushing's syndrome and admits her to the hospital for surgery for an adrenal cortex tumor (adrenalectomy). She has been having increased muscle weakness, so much so that she has difficulty climbing the one flight of stairs to her apartment. She has also had difficulty sleeping, irregular menstrual periods, and hypertension. Ms. Domico is especially concerned about her protruding abdomen, round face, development of facial hair, and the numerous bruises that have appeared on her skin.

ASSESSMENT

When Ms. Domico arrives at the hospital the morning of surgery, she is admitted by her case manager, Ann Sprengel, RN, CNS. Ann completes a physical assessment that includes abnormal findings of thin lower extremities, an enlarged abdomen, purple striae over the abdomen and buttocks, a round face, and obvious facial hair. Her blood pressure is 160/96. Ms. Domico tells Ann that she is always tired and that sometimes it "just wears me out to walk from the bedroom to the kitchen." Diagnostic tests conducted prior to admission reveal the following abnormal findings (all except cortisol levels are corrected before surgery).

Glucose: 186 mg/dL (normal range: 70 to 110 mg/dL)
Sodium: 152 mEq/L (normal range: 135 to 145 mEq/L)
Potassium: 3.2 mEq/L (normal range: 3.5 to 5.0 mEq/L)
Calcium: 4.3 mEq/L (normal range: 4.5 to 5.5 mEq/L)
Cortisol: 35 mg/dL (normal for A.M.: 5 to 23 mg/dL)

DIAGNOSES

■ *Fluid Volume Excess* related to sodium retention causing edema and hypertension
■ *Risk for Injury* related to generalized fatigue and weakness
■ *Risk for Infection* related to impaired immune response and edema
■ *Disturbed Body Image* related to physical changes secondary to Cushing's syndrome

EXPECTED OUTCOMES

■ Regain a normal body fluid balance.
■ Remain free of injury.

■ Remain free of infection.
■ Verbalize understanding of the physical effects of the disease process and realistic expectations of desired changes in appearance.

PLANNING AND IMPLEMENTATION

■ Weigh each morning, using the same scale.
■ Maintain an accurate record of intake and output.
■ Ensure adequate lighting in the room, and wear glasses and shoes when getting out of bed.
■ Develop a written schedule of rest and activity periods.
■ If agreeable, provide a private room, and restrict visitors to parents at this time.
■ Use strict medical and surgical asepsis when providing care.
■ Provide time for discussion of the disease and treatment; encourage verbalization of feelings and identify successful coping mechanisms used in the past.
■ Encourage turning, coughing, and deep breathing and/or incentive spirometry every 2–4 hours.

EVALUATION

Ms. Domico states that she is "ready to have surgery and start feeling better." She has not fallen or injured herself, and she has remained free of infection. Although edema is still present, she has lost 8 lb (3.6 kg), and her blood pressure is decreased. Ms. Domico has openly discussed her concerns about the way she looks and feels; she understands that symptoms will improve following surgery. She has strong religious beliefs and family support, both of which provide strength and help her cope with the effects of the disorder and the need for any further treatment.

CRITICAL THINKING IN THE NURSING PROCESS

1. When Ms. Domico was admitted to the hospital, several of her test results were abnormal. Describe the pathophysiologic reason for those results.
2. List the assessments that nurses can make to determine body fluid balance.
3. Develop a plan of care for this client for the nursing diagnosis *Fatigue.*
See Evaluating Your Response in Appendix C.

reabsorption, causing fluid volume excess (Porth, 2005). The client will have weight gain, edema, and hypertension.

- Ask the client to weigh at the same time each day, and maintain a record of results. *Body weight is an accurate indicator of fluid status. One liter of fluid retention corresponds to about 2 lb (0.9 kg) of body weight.*
- Monitor blood pressure, rate and rhythm of pulse, respiratory rate, and breath sounds. Assess for peripheral edema and jugular vein distention. *Extracellular fluid volume excess resulting from sodium and water retention is manifested by hypertension and a bounding, rapid pulse. There may also be crackles and wheezes, dependent edema, and venous distention.*
- Teach the client and family the reasons for restricting fluid and the importance of limiting fluids if ordered. *Restricting fluid can help decrease the risk of fluid volume excess. Involving the client and family in the plan of care and teaching the rationale for interventions helps achieve goals.*

Risk for Injury

The client with Cushing's syndrome is at risk for injury from several causes. Excess cortisol causes increased absorption of calcium and demineralization of bones, resulting in risk of pathologic fractures. Muscle weakness and fatigue are common, increasing the potential for accidental falls.

- Teach the client and family to maintain a safe environment:
  - Keep unnecessary clutter and equipment out of the way and off the floor.
  - Ensure adequate lighting, especially at night.
  - Encourage the use of assistive devices for ambulation or to ask for help if needed.
  - If the client wears corrective lenses, be sure they are available and clean.
  - Encourage the use of nonskid slippers or shoes.
  - Monitor for signs of fatigue (increased pulse and respirations); plan rest periods.

  A well-lighted environment free of clutter decreases the risk of falls and injury. Sensory and motor deficits increase the risk of falls; corrective lenses, assistive devices, and nonslip footwear can decrease this risk. Rest relieves fatigue. To reduce energy expenditure, include alternating periods of rest and activity in daily schedules.

Risk for Infection

Elevated cortisol levels impair the immune response and put the client with Cushing's syndrome at increased risk for infection. Increased cortisol also affects protein synthesis, causing delayed wound healing, and inhibits collagen formation, which results in epidermal atrophy, further inhibiting resistance to infection. In addition, impaired blood flow to edematous tissue results in altered cellular nutrition, which increases the potential for infection. The following interventions are outlined for the client with Cushing's syndrome who is hospitalized:

- Place in a private room, and limit visitors. *The client must avoid exposure to environmental infection.*
- Monitor vital signs and verbalizations of subjective manifestations (e.g., the client's response to "How do you feel?") every 4 hours. *Increased body temperature and pulse are sys-

temic indicators of infection; however, because Cushing's syndrome impairs the normal inflammatory response, the usual indicators of inflammation may not be present.*

- Use principles of medical and sterile asepsis when caring for the client, conducting procedures, or providing wound care. *Impaired skin and tissues make aseptic techniques even more necessary to decrease the risk of infection. Intact skin is the first line of defense against infection; if invasive procedures are performed or a wound is present, this defense is lost.*
- If wounds are present, assess the color, odor, and consistency of wound drainage, and look for increased pain in and around the wound. *Cortisol excess delays wound healing and closure.*
- Teach the importance of increasing intake of protein and vitamins C and A. *Protein, vitamin C, and vitamin A are necessary to collagen formation; collagen helps support and repair body tissues.*

> **PRACTICE ALERT**
> A generalized feeling of malaise may be the primary manifestation of infection.

Disturbed Body Image

The client with Cushing's syndrome has obvious physical changes in appearance. The abnormal fat distribution, moon face, buffalo hump, striae, acne, and facial hair (in women) all contribute to disruptions in the way clients with this disorder perceive themselves.

- Encourage clients to express feelings and to ask questions about the disorder and its treatment. *The loss of one's normal body image may prompt feelings of hopelessness, powerlessness, anger, and depression. Understanding the disease and adapting to changes from that disease are the first steps in regaining control of one's own body.*
- Discuss strengths and previous coping strategies. Enlist the support of family or significant others in reaffirming the client's worth. *Disturbances in body image are often accompanied by low self-esteem. Self-esteem derives from one's perception of competence and from appraisals of others.*
- Discuss signs of progress in controlling symptoms; for example, decreased facial edema or increased activity tolerance. *Many physical changes from cortisol excess disappear with treatment. Clearly communicate this fact, because the client may believe changes are permanent.*

Using NANDA, NIC, and NOC

Chart 19–1 shows links between NANDA, NIC, and NOC when caring for the client with Cushing's syndrome.

Community-Based Care

The client with Cushing's syndrome requires education about self-care at home specific to the type of treatment given. Address the following topics:

- Safety measures to prevent falls if fatigue, weakness, and osteoporosis are present
- Taking medications as prescribed, with information about side effects. Clients often require medications for the rest of their lives, and dosage changes are highly likely

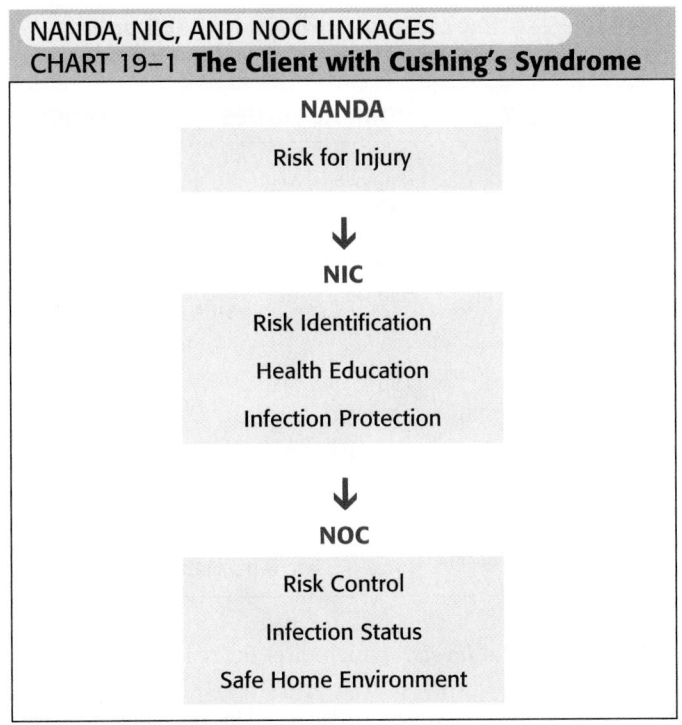

NANDA, NIC, AND NOC LINKAGES
CHART 19–1 The Client with Cushing's Syndrome

NANDA

Risk for Injury

↓

NIC

Risk Identification

Health Education

Infection Protection

↓

NOC

Risk Control

Infection Status

Safe Home Environment

Data from *NANDA's Nursing Diagnoses: Definitions & Classification 2005–2006* by NANDA International (2005), Philadelphia; *Nursing Interventions Classification (NIC)* (4th ed.) by J. M. Dochterman & G. M. Bulechek (2004), St. Louis, MO: Mosby; and *Nursing Outcomes Classification (NOC)* (3rd ed.) by S. Moorhead, M. Johnson, and M. Maas (2004), St. Louis, MO: Mosby.

- Having regular health assessments
- Wearing a medical ID indicating the client has Cushing's syndrome
- Helping the older client with referrals to social services or community health services because of the complexity of the treatment and care required
- Providing helpful resources:
  - American Association of Clinical Endocrinologists
  - Endocrine Society.

THE CLIENT WITH CHRONIC ADRENOCORTICAL INSUFFICIENCY (ADDISON'S DISEASE)

Addison's disease is a disorder resulting from destruction or dysfunction of the adrenal cortex. The result is chronic deficiency of cortisol, aldosterone, and adrenal androgens, accompanied by skin pigmentation. It can occur at any age, although it is more common in adults under the age of 60. Like many endocrine disorders, Addison's disease is more common in women.

Pathophysiology

There are many possible causes of Addison's disease. The etiologies include:

- Autoimmune destruction of the adrenals. This is the most common cause, accounting for about 80% of spontaneous cases (Holcomb, 2006; Tierney et al., 2005). It may occur alone, or as part of a polyglandular autoimmune syndrome (PGA). Type 2 PGA is seen in adults, often associated with autoimmune thy-

roid disease (usually hypothyroidism), type 1 diabetes, primary ovarian or testicular failure, and pernicious anemia.
- Clients who are taking anticoagulants, have major trauma, sepsis, or are having open heart surgery. Such clients may have bilateral adrenal hemorrhage.
- Adrenoleukodystrophy, an X-linked disorder characterized by an accumulation of very long chain fatty acids in the adrenal cortex, testes, brain, and spinal cord.
- ACTH deficit, resulting from pituitary tumors, pituitary surgery or irradiation, and the use of exogenous steroids.
- Clients who are abruptly withdrawn from long-term, high-dose steroid therapy. Other clients at risk are those with tuberculosis or acquired immune deficiency syndrome (AIDS); the pathogens responsible for either disease can infiltrate and destroy adrenal tissue.

Adrenocortical destruction initially causes a decrease in adrenal glucocorticoid reserve. Basal glucocorticoid secretion is normal, but does not increase in response to stress and surgery. Trauma or infection can precipitate an adrenal crisis. As the destruction of the adrenal cortex continues, even basal secretion of glucocorticoids and mineralocorticoids is deficient. Decreasing plasma cortisol reduces the feedback inhibition of pituitary ACTH and plasma ACTH rises.

Secondary adrenocortical insufficiency occurs when either large doses or prolonged therapy with glucocorticoids are given for their anti-inflammatory and immunosuppressive effects to treat diseases such as arthritis and asthma. If the steroid medications are suddenly discontinued, the hypothalamus and pituitary cannot respond normally to the reduced level of circulating glucocorticoids. The client may develop manifestations of chronic adrenocortical insufficiency or, if subjected to stress, adrenal crisis (Tierney et al., 2005).

Manifestations

The onset of Addison's disease is slow in most cases; the client experiences symptoms after about 90% of the function of the gland is lost. The primary manifestations are the result of elevated ACTH levels and decreased aldosterone and cortisol (see the box on page 554). Aldosterone deficiency affects the ability of the distal tubules of the nephron to conserve sodium. Sodium is lost, potassium is retained, extracellular fluid is depleted, and the blood volume is decreased. Postural hypotension and syncope are common, and hypovolemic shock may occur. Hyponatremia causes dizziness, confusion, and neuromuscular irritability. Hyperkalemia causes cardiac arrhythmias.

Cortisol insufficiency also causes decreased hepatic gluconeogenesis with hypoglycemia. The client tolerates stress poorly and experiences lethargy, weakness, anorexia, nausea, vomiting, and diarrhea. The increased ACTH levels stimulate hyperpigmentation in more than 90% of clients with Addison's disease (Porth, 2005). In Caucasian clients, the skin looks deeply suntanned or bronzed in both exposed and unexposed areas.

Addisonian Crisis

Addisonian crisis is a life-threatening response to acute adrenal insufficiency and occurs in about 25% of patients (Holcomb, 2006). Triggers include surgery, acute systemic illness,

MANIFESTATIONS of Addison's Disease

INTEGUMENTARY SYSTEM
- Delayed wound healing
- Hyperpigmentation

CARDIOVASCULAR SYSTEM
- Postural hypotension
- Tachycardia
- Arrhythmias

CENTRAL NERVOUS SYSTEM
- Lethargy
- Emotional lability
- Tremors
- Confusion

MUSCULOSKELETAL SYSTEM
- Weakness
- Joint pain
- Muscle wasting
- Muscle pain

GASTROINTESTINAL SYSTEM
- Anorexia
- Diarrhea
- Nausea and vomiting

REPRODUCTIVE SYSTEM
- Menstrual changes

METABOLIC EFFECTS
- Hyperkalemia
- Hypoglycemia
- Hyponatremia

TABLE 19–4 Laboratory Findings in Addison's Disease

	TEST	NORMAL VALUES	FINDINGS
Serum	Cortisol	8 A.M. to 10 A.M.: 5 to 23 mcg/dL 4 P.M. to 6 P.M.: 3 to 13 mcg/dL	Decreased
	Blood urea nitrogen (BUN)	5 to 25 mg/dL	Increased
	Sodium	135 to 145 mEq/L	Decreased
	Potassium	3.5 to 5.0 mEq/L	Increased
	Glucose (serum)	70 to 100 mg/dL	Decreased
Urine	17-KS	Male: 5 to 25 mg/24h Female: 5 to 15 mg/24h >Age 65: 4 to 8 mg/24h	Low/absent

- *Blood glucose levels,* which are decreased in adrenal insufficiency
- *Serum sodium levels,* which are decreased in adrenal insufficiency
- *Serum potassium levels,* which are increased in adrenal insufficiency
- *BUN levels,* which are increased in adrenal insufficiency
- *Urinary 17-hydroxycorticoids* and *17-KS levels,* which are decreased in adrenal insufficiency
- *Plasma ACTH levels,* which are increased in primary adrenal insufficiency but decreased in secondary adrenal insufficiency
- Possibly *ACTH stimulation test* (Cortisol levels rise with pituitary deficiency but do not rise in primary adrenal insufficiency.)
- *CT scans* of the head, which identify any intracranial lesion impinging on the pituitary gland.

Medications

The primary medical treatment of Addison's disease is replacement of corticosteroids and mineralocorticoids, accompanied by increased sodium in the diet. Hydrocortisone (Cortef) is given orally to replace cortisol; fludrocortisone (Florinef) is given orally to replace mineralocorticoids. Nursing implications in cortisol replacement are given in the box on the following page.

trauma, or abrupt withdrawal of long-term corticosteroid therapy. The disorder is chronic after the acute episode resolves.

This response can occur in any person with Addison's disease; however, it is most commonly precipitated by major stressors, especially if the disease is poorly controlled. Addisonian crisis may also occur in clients who are abruptly withdrawn from glucocorticoid medications or who have hemorrhage into the adrenal glands from either septicemia or anticoagulant therapy.

The client with Addisonian crisis may have any of the manifestations of Addison's disease, but the primary symptoms develop rapidly and are a high fever; weakness; severe, penetrating pain in the abdomen, lower back, and legs; severe vomiting; diarrhea; and hypotension; and circulatory collapse, shock, and coma.

Treatment of the crisis is rapid intravenous replacement of fluids and glucocorticoids. Fluid balance is usually restored in 4 to 6 hours.

INTERDISCIPLINARY CARE

The client with Addison's disease requires early diagnosis and treatment. Medical treatment includes cortisol replacement therapy.

Diagnostic Tests

Addison's disease is diagnosed through findings of decreased levels of cortisol, aldosterone, and urinary 17-KS. Dehydration may result in increased hematocrit and blood urea nitrogen (BUN). Blood glucose levels are decreased, and potassium is increased. A list of laboratory findings in Addison's disease is shown in Table 19–4. The following diagnostic tests are used:

- *Serum cortisol levels,* which are decreased in adrenal insufficiency

 ## NURSING CARE

Health Promotion

Health promotion interventions for the client with or at risk for Addison's disease focus on careful assessments during anticoagulant therapy, open heart surgery, and trauma treatment. If the disease is present, teaching to prevent or treat an Addisonian crisis is essential.

Assessment

Collect the following data through the health history and physical examination (see Chapter 18). Further focused assessments are described with nursing interventions in the following text.

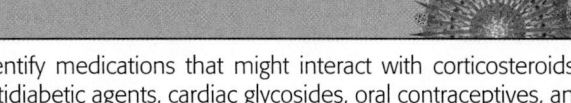

MEDICATION ADMINISTRATION   ADDISON'S DISEASE

CORTISOL REPLACEMENTS
Cortisone (Cortone, Cortogen)
Hydrocortisone (Cortisol, Hydrocortone, Cortef)
Fludrocortisone acetate (Florinef, F-Cortef)
Dexamethasone (Decadron, Hexadrol, Dexasone)
Prednisone (Meticorten, Deltasone, Orasone)
Prednisolone (Meticortelone)

NURSING ALERT
Prednisolone and predinsone are equivalent in potency; dexamethasone (Decadron) is four to five times more potent.

Methylprednisolone (Medrol, Solu-Medrol)
Adrenocorticosteroids are used for replacement therapy in acute and chronic adrenal insufficiency. These drugs have anti-inflammatory and immunosuppressant effects. They also facilitate coping with stress.

Because corticosteroids are immunosuppressants, their use is contraindicated when an infection is suspected because they mask the signs of infection. Immunizations with live vaccines should not be attempted. Corticosteroids are also contraindicated in many other disorders, including peptic ulcer, Cushing's syndrome, cardiac disease, hyperthyroidism, hypothyroidism, and tuberculosis. Concurrent use with NSAIDs is contraindicated because of the effect on the gastrointestinal tract.

When these drugs are administered in small doses for replacement therapy, side effects are uncommon. Large doses or prolonged therapy may cause a Cushing-like syndrome, with atrophy of the adrenal cortex. Older clients, especially postmenopausal women, are more prone to develop hypertension and osteoporosis when undergoing glucocorticoid therapy. These drugs are used with caution in children and the older adult and are not usually administered to pregnant women.

Nursing Responsibilities
- Establish baseline data, including mental status, neurologic function, vital signs, and weight.

- Identify medications that might interact with corticosteroids: antidiabetic agents, cardiac glycosides, oral contraceptives, anticoagulants, NSAIDs.
- Document and report increased blood pressure, edema or weight gain, bleeding or bruising, weakness, or manifestations of Cushing's syndrome.
- Administer oral forms of the drug with food to minimize its ulcerogenic effect.
- Monitor electrolyte levels for increased sodium and decreased potassium.
- Monitor capillary blood glucose for hyperglycemia in the diabetic client.

Health Education for the Client and Family
- Take medications with food or milk, and report any gastric distress or dark stools.
- Most people need to take the medications for the rest of their lives.
- Consume a diet that is low in potassium, and higher in sodium and protein.
- Weigh yourself each day at the same time, and report any consistent weight gain, which indicates fluid retention.
- Use safety measures in the home to prevent falls and injuries.
- Corticosteroids may impair the effectiveness of oral contraceptives.
- Take the medication regularly and continuously. *Abruptly discontinuing the medication is dangerous.*
- Obtain a Medic-Alert bracelet.
- Monitor for increased stressors (infection, dental work, personal crisis) and increase the dose as indicated by the physician.
- Anticoagulant drugs or insulin may decrease the effectiveness of corticosteroids.
- Report the following to the physician: dizziness on sitting or standing, nausea and vomiting, pain, thirst, feelings of anxiety, malaise, infections.

- *Health history:* Weight loss, changes in skin color, nausea and vomiting, anorexia, diarrhea, abdominal pain, weakness, amenorrhea, changes in sexual desire, confusion, intolerance of stress.
- *Physical assessment:* Height and weight, vital signs, skin, hair quality and distribution, muscle size and strength.

Nursing Diagnoses and Interventions
The client with Addison's disease requires nursing care for a wide variety of responses to the decrease in cortisol levels. Nursing diagnoses discussed in this section are directed toward problems with fluid and electrolyte balance and compliance with lifelong self-care. See the accompanying Nursing Care Plan on page 556.

Deficient Fluid Volume
Fluid volume deficit in the client with Addison's disease results from loss of water and sodium, as well as from vomiting and diarrhea. Extracellular fluid volume deficit, decreased cardiac

output, hypotension, and hypovolemic shock may occur, especially in crisis situations. Interventions for this diagnosis are outlined for the client who is hospitalized.

- Monitor intake and output, and assess for signs of dehydration: dry mucous membranes; thirst; poor skin turgor; sunken eyeballs; scanty, dark urine; increased urine specific gravity; weight loss; and increased hemoconcentration (increased hematocrit and BUN). *Glucocorticoid and mineralocorticoid depletion causes fluid volume deficit. Fluid volume deficit may reach crisis levels if undetected, causing altered tissue perfusion and hypovolemic shock.*
- Monitor cardiovascular status: Take and record vital signs, assess character of pulses, monitor potassium levels and ECGs. *Fluid volume deficit may lead to hypotension and a rapid, weak, or thready pulse. As aldosterone levels fall, renal excretion of potassium decreases, increasing blood levels of potassium.*

NURSING CARE PLAN A Client with Addison's Disease

A 51-year-old unemployed salesman, Mr. Don Sardoff, is brought to the emergency room by his wife, Ellen, at 8 A.M. Mrs. Sardoff tells the emergency room nurse that her husband has not been feeling well for the last week, but that when he got up this morning, he was so weak he couldn't dress himself and didn't know where he was. Mrs. Sardoff also tells the nurse that her husband has been taking a cortisone drug for treatment of his rheumatoid arthritis for the past 2 years, but notes, "We didn't have the money to buy it this month."

ASSESSMENT

On admission to the emergency room, Mr. Sardoff is dehydrated, with dry oral mucous membranes and tongue, poor skin turgor, and sunken eyeballs. His blood pressure is 94/44, and his pulse is rapid and thready. He is weak, dizzy, and disoriented about time and place. Diagnostic tests reveal the following abnormal findings at 8:30 A.M:

- EKG: widening QRS complex and increased PR interval
- Sodium: 129 mEq/L (normal range: 135 to 145 mEq/L)
- Glucose: 54 mg/dL (normal range: 70 to 110 mg/dL)
- Potassium: 5.3 mEq/L (normal range: 3.5 to 5 mEq/L)
- Cortisol: 2 mg/dL (normal for A.M.: 5 to 23 mg/dL)

The medical orders for Mr. Sardoff include intravenous administration of 5% dextrose in normal saline (D_5NS) at 250 mL/h and hydrocortisone (Solu-Cortef) 200 mg. After the fluids and medication are initiated, Mr. Sardoff is moved to an in-hospital medical bed.

DIAGNOSES

- *Deficient Fluid Volume* related to hypovolemia secondary to adrenal insufficiency
- *Ineffective Tissue Perfusion: Peripheral* related to fluid volume deficit
- *Anxiety* related to lack of knowledge about the effects and treatment of adrenal insufficiency

EXPECTED OUTCOMES

- Regain normal fluid balance.
- Regain normal peripheral perfusion with blood pressure within normal range.

- Verbalize knowledge of the causes and effects of adrenal insufficiency.

PLANNING AND IMPLEMENTATION

- Monitor intake and output closely.
- Take and record weight at the same time daily.
- Monitor blood pressure, pulses, and skin turgor every 2 hours until stable, then four times a day.
- Monitor electrolytes, and report abnormal results.
- Discuss a diet that is high in sodium, low in potassium, and has an increased fluid intake (3000 mL per day). Discuss the types of fluids desired and the best times for intake of increased fluids.
- Assist during activity to prevent falls.
- Provide verbal and written instructions, and encourage verbal feedback about the causes and effects of the disease, the effects of medications, the effects of not taking long-term cortisone drugs, the diet, and self-care at home.

EVALUATION

Following treatment for acute adrenal insufficiency, Mr. Sardoff is no longer dehydrated, and his blood pressure has returned to his normal reading of 132/88. He is alert and oriented, and anxious to learn to care for himself at home. After dietary instructions and teaching for self-care that included his wife, Mr. Sardoff verbalizes an understanding of his illness and the need to take his medication carefully and accurately. A referral is made to a social worker for assistance with costs of medications.

CRITICAL THINKING IN THE NURSING PROCESS

1. Adrenal insufficiency is often diagnosed only when the client becomes seriously ill in response to a stressor. Explain why this statement is or is not true.
2. Describe the physical assessments that are found in the severely dehydrated client.
3. Outline a teaching plan for Mr. Sardoff with foods for a high-sodium, low-potassium diet.

See Evaluating Your Response in Appendix C.

- Weigh the client daily at the same time and in the same clothing. *Dehydration is manifested by weight loss.*
- Encourage an oral fluid intake of 3000 mL per day and an increased salt intake. *Cortisol deficiency increases fluid loss, leading to extracellular fluid volume depletion. Oral fluid replacement is necessary to balance this loss. An increase in dietary sodium can decrease the hyponatremia characteristic of adrenal insufficiency.*
- Teach to sit and stand slowly, and provide assistance as necessary. *Extracellular fluid volume deficit causes orthostatic hypotension, dizziness, and possible loss of consciousness. These manifestations increase the risk of injury from falls.*

PRACTICE ALERT
Hyperkalemia causes changes in cardiac muscle function, which are reflected in ECG changes.

Risk for Ineffective Therapeutic Regimen Management

Clients with Addison's disease must learn to provide lifelong self-care that involves varied components: medications, diet, and recognizing and responding to responses to stress. Changes in lifestyle are difficult to maintain permanently.

- Teach the effects of illness and treatment. Discuss client and family concerns. *Lack of knowledge about the illness, as well as the possibility of complications from disregarding or altering the treatment, can negatively affect compliance.*
- Include the following in the teaching plan:
  - Self-administration of steroids
  - The importance of carrying at all times an emergency kit containing parenteral cortisone and a syringe/needle
  - Wearing a Medic-Alert bracelet that says "Adrenal insufficiency—takes hydrocortisone"
  - Increasing oral fluid intake

- Maintaining a diet high in sodium and low in potassium
- The necessity of altering the medication dose when experiencing emotional or physical stressors
- The importance of continuing health care.

One of the most important components of caring for the client with Addison's disease is teaching both the client and family to provide care. The length of treatment and the side effects of medications can discourage compliance.

Community-Based Care

The client with Addison's disease provides self-care at home. One of the most important components of caring for the client with Addison's disease is teaching both the client and family to provide care. Family stability, an awareness of the serious nature of the disease, and the effectiveness of treatment all promote compliance. The length of treatment and the side effects of medications, however, can discourage compliance. In addition to the information in the teaching topics included with nursing diagnoses and interventions, include the following topics:

- The importance of continuing health care
- Referral to social worker, if appropriate
- Referral to community agencies for continued education and support
- Helpful resources:
  - National Institute of Diabetes and Digestive and Kidney Diseases (Addison's disease)
  - Endocrine Society
  - American Association of Clinical Endocrinologists.

MediaLink Addison's Disease Resources

THE CLIENT WITH PHEOCHROMOCYTOMA

Pheochromocytomas are tumors of chromaffin tissues in the adrenal medulla. These tumors, which are usually benign, produce catecholamines (epinephrine or norepinephrine) that stimulate the sympathetic nervous system. Although many organs are affected, the most dangerous effects are peripheral vasoconstriction and increased cardiac rate and contractility with resultant paroxysmal hypertension. Systolic blood pressure may rise to 200 to 300 mmHg, the diastolic to 150 to 175 mmHg. Attacks are often precipitated by physical, emotional, or environmental stimuli. This condition is life threatening.

A pheochromocytoma is diagnosed by increased catecholamine levels in the blood or urine, by x-ray studies, and by surgical exploration. Vanillylmandelic acid is the end product of metabolism of all catecholamine substances and is collected in a 24-hour urine. Because catecholamine secretion is episodic, a 24-hour urine is a better surveillance method than serum catecholamines (Pagana & Pagana, 2002). Surgical removal of the tumor(s) by adrenalectomy is the treatment of choice.

DISORDERS OF THE PITUITARY GLAND

The pituitary gland produces hormones that affect multiple body systems through regulation of endocrine function. Target tissues include the thyroid, adrenal cortex, ovary, uterus, mammary glands, testes, and kidneys. Disorders result from an excess or deficiency of one or more of the pituitary hormones due to a pathologic condition within the gland itself or to hypothalamic dysfunction.

Although disorders of the pituitary cause diverse and serious problems, they are not as common as disorders of other endocrine glands. Hyperpituitarism and hypopituitarism are discussed in this section.

THE CLIENT WITH DISORDERS OF THE ANTERIOR PITUITARY GLAND

Hyperfunction of the anterior pituitary gland, characterized by excess production and secretion of one or more trophic hormones, is usually the result of a pituitary tumor or pituitary hyperplasia. The most common cause of hyperpituitarism is a benign adenoma. The manifestations result from pressure on the optic nerve causing visual changes or an excess of growth hormone (GH), prolactin (PRL), ACTH, or TSH. Typically, 70% to 90% of the anterior pituitary is damaged before clinical manifestations develop (Porth, 2005).

Hypofunction of the anterior pituitary gland results in a deficiency of one or more of the gland's hormones. Conditions causing hypopituitarism include pituitary tumors, surgical removal of the pituitary gland, radiation, and pituitary infarction, infection, or trauma.

Pathophysiology and Manifestations

Growth hormone (also called somatotropin) is produced by cells in the anterior pituitary throughout life. GH is necessary for growth and also contributes to metabolic regulation. GH stimulates all aspects of cartilage growth, and one of its major effects is to stimulate the growth of the epiphyseal cartilage plates of long bones. In addition, other body tissues respond to the metabolic effect of GH with increases in bone width and the growth of visceral and endocrine organs, skeletal and cardiac muscle, skin, and connective tissue. Gigantism and acromegaly (discussed next) result from overstimulation. Growth retardation and short stature result from deficient production of GH.

Hypersecretion of PRL affects reproductive and sexual function. Women may have irregular or absent menses, difficulty becoming pregnant, and decreased libido. Men may be impotent and have decreased libido. PRL deficiency in postpartal women causes a failure to lactate.

An excess secretion of ACTH overstimulates the adrenal cortex, which in turn increases secretion of adrenal hormones. The result is Cushing's syndrome. Deficiencies of TSH are uncommon, but cause hypothyroidism.

Gigantism

Gigantism occurs when GH hypersecretion begins before puberty and the closure of the epiphyseal plates. The person becomes abnormally tall, often exceeding 7 ft (213 cm) in height, but body proportions are relatively normal. Most often the result of a tumor, the condition is rare today as a result of improved diagnosis and treatment.

Acromegaly

Acromegaly, which literally means "enlarged extremities," occurs when sustained GH hypersecretion begins during adulthood, most commonly because of pituitary tumors. As a result of constant stimulation, bone and connective tissue continue to grow. The forehead enlarges, the maxilla lengthens, the tongue enlarges, and the voice deepens (Figure 19–4 ■). Overgrowth of bone and soft tissue in the hands and feet causes clients to buy increasingly larger rings, gloves, and shoes. This condition is different from Marfan's syndrome, a genetic disorder that results in elongated bones, optic changes, and severe cardiovascular effects. (See Chapter 32 for nursing care of clients with cardiovascular disorders.)

Other manifestations include peripheral nerve damage from entrapment of nerves, headache, hypertension, congestive heart failure, seizures, and visual disturbances. Impaired glucose tolerance and diabetes may also occur. Arthralgias develop secondary to the bone and connective tissue growth and may be relieved by treatment that halts excessive GH production (Lehne, 2004; Munzer & Fiebach, 2002).

INTERDISCIPLINARY CARE

Acromegaly is treated by surgical removal or irradiation of the pituitary tumor. A transsphenoidal or transfrontal surgical procedure is most commonly used. Octreotide (Sandostatin) suppresses the anterior pituitary gland and decreases GH levels. It is expensive and gastrointestinal side effects are common for the first couple of weeks. About 25% of patients develop cholesterol gallstones within a year (Lehne, 2004).

NURSING CARE

Clients with anterior pituitary disorders require interventions to help in coping with physical and emotional changes, as well as to prevent complications involving other organs and functions of the endocrine system. Nursing care for the client having cranial surgery is discussed in Chapter 44 ∞.

THE CLIENT WITH DISORDERS OF THE POSTERIOR PITUITARY GLAND

Disorders of the posterior pituitary are related primarily to excessive or deficient antidiuretic hormone (ADH) secretion. The disorders discussed here are the syndrome of inappropriate ADH secretion and diabetes insipidus.

Pathophysiology and Manifestations

Antidiuretic hormone is secreted in response to serum osmolality, which is monitored by osmoreceptors in the hypothalamus. When a condition of hyperosmolality occurs, ADH secretion increases, and renal water is reabsorbed. Hypoosmolality causes the suppression of ADH, and renal water excretion increases.

Syndrome of Inappropriate ADH Secretion

The **syndrome of inappropriate ADH secretion (SIADH)** is characterized by high levels of ADH in the absence of serum hypo-osmolality. This disorder is most often caused by the ectopic production of ADH by malignant tumors (e.g., oat cell carcinoma of the lung, pancreatic carcinoma, leukemia, and Hodgkin's disease). A transient form may follow a head injury, pituitary surgery, or the use of medications such as barbiturates, anesthetics, or diuretics.

Figure 19–4 ■ Manifestations of acromegaly. Progressive alterations in facial appearance include enlargement of the cheekbones and jaw along with thickening of soft-tissue structures such as the nose, lips, cheeks, and the flesh above the brows.

Courtesy of Clinical Pathological Conference, American Journal of Medicine.

Manifestations of SIADH occur as a result of water retention, hyponatremia, and serum hypo-osmolality. Blood volume expands, but the plasma is diluted. Aldosterone is suppressed; as a result, renal excretion of sodium increases. Water moves from the hypotonic plasma and the interstitial spaces into the cells.

Manifestations of SIADH (see Chapter 10) are usually nonspecific but are related to hyponatremia and water intoxication. Brain cells swell, causing neurologic symptoms including headache, changes in mental status or personality, lethargy, and irritability. Weight gain results from the retention of fluid (Held-Warmkessel, 2005). Usually no edema is present, because water is distributed between the intracellular and extracellular spaces.

Treatment addresses the low serum sodium and intracellular swelling. Besides keeping the client safe, nursing care involves teaching the client about restricting fluids to 1 L/day. Fluid restriction continues for 3 to 10 days until the malignant source of ADH is successfully destroyed. Demeclocycline (Declomycin) is a tetracycline antibiotic with the unique property of creating excessive urine flow. It is used as a treatment for SIADH (Lehne, 2004).

Diabetes Insipidus

Diabetes insipidus is the result of ADH insufficiency. The two types are as follows:

- *Neurogenic diabetes insipidus* can either result from a disruption of the hypothalamus and pituitary gland (as from trauma, irradiation, or cranial surgery) or be idiopathic.
- *Nephrogenic diabetes insipidus* is a disorder in which the renal tubules are not sensitive to ADH. This may be familial in origin or the result of renal failure.

Diabetes insipidus may result from brain tumors or infections, pituitary surgery, cerebral vascular accidents, and renal and organ failure. It is also a complication of closed-head trauma with increased intracranial pressure.

A deficit of ADH causes excretion of large amounts of dilute urine (*polyuria*), in some instances as much as 12 L/day. The client has extreme thirst and drinks large volumes of water (*polydipsia*). If unable to replace the water loss, the client becomes dehydrated and hypernatremic. Even though hyperosmolality is present, the urine is dilute and has a low specific gravity.

If this disorder is caused by cerebral injury, symptoms commonly appear 3 to 6 days after the initial injury and last for 7 to 10 days. If the increased intracranial pressure is relieved, symptoms of diabetes insipidus usually disappear. However, diabetes insipidus may also be a chronic illness requiring lifelong treatment and care. See Table 19–5 for a comparison of posterior pituitary gland disorders.

INTERDISCIPLINARY CARE

SIADH is treated by correcting underlying causes, treating the hyponatremia with intravenous hypertonic saline, and restricting oral fluids to less than 800 mL/day.

Diabetes insipidus is also treated by correcting underlying causes, if possible. Other medical interventions include administering intravenous hypotonic fluids, increasing oral fluids, and replacing ADH hormone. Desmopressin acetate, administered intranasally, orally, or parenterally, is the treatment of choice (Tierney et al., 2005).

NURSING CARE

Nursing care for the client with SIADH and diabetes insipidus focuses on client problems with fluid and electrolyte balance, as discussed in Chapter 10 ∞.

TABLE 19–5 Comparison of Posterior Pituitary Gland Disorders

SIADH	DIABETES INSIPIDUS
Excessive ADH	Deficient ADH
Fluid volume excess	Fluid volume deficit
Restrict fluid intake	Encourage fluid intake
Demeclocycline (Declomycin) (oral agent) causes excessive urination	Desmopressin (DDAVP) (nasal spray) causes increased water reabsorption

EXPLORE MediaLink

Prentice Hall Nursing MediaLink DVD-ROM
Audio Glossary
NCLEX-RN® Review

COMPANION WEBSITE www.prenhall.com/lemone
Audio Glossary
NCLEX-RN® Review
Care Plan Activity: Cushing's Syndrome
Case Studies
Compare and Contrast Endocrine Disorders
Hyperthyroidism
MediaLink Application: Exophthalmos
Links to Resources

CHAPTER HIGHLIGHTS

- Hormones regulate growth, development, and metabolism. Homeostasis is dependent on a balanced level of each type of hormone. Not only do hormones affect organ function, they interact and when excesses or deficits occur, signs and symptoms are manifested.
- The pituitary gland, in conjunction with the hypothalamus, is the master gland of the body. Fifteen hormones and regulatory factors are synthesized in the anterior pituitary and hypothalamus; many are trophic hormones that stimulate the release of other hormones.
- Thyroid disorders are the most common endocrine disorders. Occurring mainly among women, these diseases change body image and impose upsets to energy levels creating fatigue and exhaustion.
- Diagnostic tests and therapies are available to identify and treat thyroid disorders. Surgery, radiation therapy, and medications

support good quality of life, but the medications must be used throughout the lifetime.

- The parathyroid glands synthesize parathormone, which maintains serum calcium. Thyroid tissues surrounding the parathyroids synthesize a hormone, calcitonin, which decreases serum calcium to normal levels. These glands provide the proper level of serum calcium, which is vital for cardiac function, bone stability, nerve conduction, and muscle contraction.
- The adrenal glands regulate energy and fluid balance through corticosteroids and mineralocorticoids. Cushing's and Addison's disease are polar opposites and treatment eliminates the signs and symptoms of one and creates the manifestations of the other. Clients with these diseases require patient education until they fully grasp the significance of the condition and the importance of adhering to the treatment plan.

TEST YOURSELF NCLEX-RN® REVIEW

1. Graves' disease, the most common cause of hyperthyroidism, is categorized as what type of disorder?
   1. autoimmune
   2. infectious
   3. allergic
   4. genetic

2. What principle supports the treatment of hyperthyroidism with radioactive iodine?
   1. Radioactive iodine reduces the vascularity of the thyroid gland.
   2. Doses of radioactive iodine are too small to be hazardous to other body parts.
   3. The thyroid gland takes up iodine in any form.
   4. Irradiation of the thyroid gland decreases the risk of hypothyroidism.

3. You assess a client with newly diagnosed hypothyroidism as having an enlarged thyroid gland (goiter). What physiologic process causes this enlargement?
   1. an excess of TH stimulates thyroid follicles
   2. an increased dietary iodine intake
   3. a compensatory effort to produce more TH
   4. tissue hypertrophy in response to increased TH

4. Mrs. Jonah has taken cortisone for her rheumatoid arthritis for several years. What endocrine disorder is she most at risk for developing?
   1. hyperthyroidism
   2. hypothyroidism
   3. acromegaly
   4. Cushing's syndrome

5. Which statement illustrates that the client with Addison's disease understands your teaching?
   1. "I will be sure to stop taking my medications when I have an infection."
   2. "I have purchased an emergency kit and keep it with me all the time."
   3. "I know I should never alter my dose of medications."
   4. "I wonder why I look suntanned all the time."

6. Signs and symptoms of hyponatremia found in SIADH include:
   1. weight loss.
   2. irritability.
   3. hyperkalemia.
   4. constipation.

7. A home health nurse is caring for a client with hyperparathyroidism and osteoporosis. Which nursing diagnosis has priority with this client?
   1. *Risk for Fear*
   2. *Risk for Injury*
   3. *Risk for Isolation*
   4. *Risk for Chronic Low Self-Esteem*

8. A nurse is monitoring a client for signs of hypercalcemia. Which of the following is a sign of hypercalcemia?
   1. oliguria
   2. positive Chvostek's sign
   3. diminished bowel sounds
   4. hyperactive deep tendon reflexes

9. A client with increased ACTH levels and Addison's disease is likely to manifest:
   1. tremor.
   2. hair loss.
   3. gingival hyperplasia.
   4. dermal hyperpigmentation.

10. Clients treated with glucocorticoids are at risk for Addisonian crisis due to:
    1. rapid withdrawal of glucocorticoids.
    2. excessive ACTH.
    3. sodium retention.
    4. hypokalemia.

See Test Yourself answers in Appendix C.

BIBLIOGRAPHY

American Cancer Society. (2005). Cancer statistics. *CA: A Cancer Journal for Clinicians, 55*(1).

Cooper, D. S. (Ed.). (2001). *Medical management of thyroid disease.* New York: Marcel Dekker.

Dochterman, J., & Bulechek, G. (2004). *Nursing interventions classification (NIC)*(4th ed.). St. Louis, MO: Mosby.

Ginsberg, J. (2003). Diagnosis and management of Graves' disease. *Canadian Medical Association Journal, 168*(5), 575–585.

Goodman, M., & Wickham, R. (2005). Endocrine malignancies. In C. H. Yarbro, M. H. Frogge, & M. Goodman (Eds.), *Cancer nursing: Principles and practice* (6th ed.). Boston: Jones & Bartlett.

Held-Warmkessel, J. (2005). Managing 3 critical cancer complications. *Nursing, 35*(1), 58–64.

Holcomb, S. S. (2003). The lowdown on hypothyroidism. *Nursing Made Incredibly Easy!* September/October *1*(1), 44–48.

Holcomb, S. S. (2006). Hospital nursing: Do the clues add up to Addison's disease? *Nursing, 36*(3), 64hn1–64hn4.

Kirk, L. F., Jr., Hash, R. B., Katner, H. P., & Jones, T. (2002). Cushing's disease: Clinical manifestations and diagnostic evaluation. *American Family Physician, 62*(5),1119–1127, 1133–1134.

Kumrow, D., & Dahlen, R. (2002). Thyroidectomy: Understanding the potential for complications. *MEDSURG Nursing, 11(5)*, 228–235.

Lehne, R. A. (2004). *Pharmacology for nursing care* (4th ed.). St. Louis, MO: Saunders/Elsevier.

Levin, N.A., & Greer, K. E. (2001). Cutaneous manifestations of endocrine disorders. *Dermatology Nursing, 13*(3), 185–196.

McCance, K., & Huether, S. (2002). *Pathophysiology: The biologic basis for disease in adults and children* (4th ed.). St. Louis: Mosby.

McCloskey, J., & Bulechek, G. (Eds.). (2000). *Iowa intervention project: Nursing interventions classification (NIC)* (3rd ed.). St. Louis, MO: Mosby.

McPhee, S., Lingappa, V., Ganong, W., & Lange, J. (2000). *Pathophysiology of disease: An introduction to clinical medicine.* New York: Appleton & Lange.

Medline Plus. (2006). T4 tests. U.S. National Library of Medicine and the National Institutes of Health. Retrieved March 22, 2006, from http://www.nlm.nih.gov/medlineplus/ency/article/003517.htm

Michel, R. H., Neafsey, P. J., & Dzurec, L. C. (2004). Self medication practices among patients taking levothyroxine. *Internet Journal of Advanced Nursing Practice, 6*(2), 9p.

Moorhead, S., Johnson, M., & Maas, M. (2003). *Nursing outcomes classification (NOC)* (3rd ed.). St. Louis: Mosby.

Moorhead, S., Johnson, M., & Maas, M. (2004). *Nursing outcomes classification (NOC)* (3rd ed.). St. Louis, MO: Mosby.

Munzer, T., & Fiebach, N. (2002). Unmasking acromegaly in late life. *Journal of the American Geriatrics Society, 50*(5), 973–974.

Pagana, K. D., & Pagana, T. J. (2002). *Mosby's manual of diagnostic and laboratory tests* (2nd ed.) St. Louis, MO: Mosby.

Porth, C. (2005). *Pathophysiology: Concepts of altered health states* (7th ed.). Philadelphia: Lippincott.

Sheppard, M. (2001). Assessing fluid balance. *Nursing Times, 97*(6 Ntplus), XI–XII.

Skidmore-Roth, L. (2005). *Mosby's nursing drug reference*. St. Louis, MO: Elsevier Mosby.

Tierney, L. M., McPhee, S. J., & Papadakis, M. A. (Eds.). (2005). *Current medical diagnosis & treatment* (44th ed.). New York: Lange Medical Books/McGraw-Hill.

Weissel, M. (2006). Disturbances of thyroid function in the elderly. *The Middle European Journal of Medicine, 118*(1–2), 16–20.

Wilkinson, J. (2005). *Prentice Hall nursing diagnosis handbook with NIC interventions and NOC outcomes* (8th ed.). Upper Saddle River, NJ: Prentice Hall.

Yarbro, C., Frogge, M., Goodman, M., & Broenwald, S. (2001). *Cancer nursing: Principles and practice.* Sudbury, MA: Jones & Bartlett.

CHAPTER 20 Nursing Care of Clients with Diabetes Mellitus

LEARNING OUTCOMES

- Apply knowledge of normal endocrine anatomy, physiology, and assessments when providing nursing care for clients with diabetes mellitus.
- Describe the prevalence and incidence of diabetes mellitus.
- Explain the pathophysiology, risk factors, manifestations, and complications of type 1 and type 2 diabetes mellitus.
- Compare and contrast the manifestations and interdisciplinary care of hypoglycemia, diabetic ketoacidosis, and hyperosmolar hyperglycemic state.

- Identify the diagnostic tests used for screening, diagnosis, and monitoring of diabetes mellitus.
- Discuss the nursing implications for insulin and oral hypoglycemic agents used to treat clients with diabetes mellitus.
- Provide accurate information to clients with diabetes mellitus to facilitate self-management of medications, diet planning, exercise, and self-assessment, including foot care.
- Use the nursing process as a framework for providing individualized care to clients with diabetes mellitus.

CLINICAL COMPETENCIES

- Assess blood glucose levels and patterns of hyper- and hypoglycemia in clients with diabetes mellitus.
- Recognize the importance of early diagnosis and control of blood glucose to prevent complications.
- Determine priority nursing diagnoses, based on assessed data, to select and implement individualized nursing interventions for clients with type 1 and type 2 diabetes mellitus.
- Administer oral and injectable medications used to treat type 1 and type 2 diabetes mellitus knowledgeably and safely.
- Provide skilled care to clients with diabetic ketoacidosis and hyperosmolar hyperglycemic states.

- Integrate interdisciplinary care into care of clients with type 1 and type 2 diabetes mellitus, especially foot and eye care.
- Provide appropriate teaching to facilitate blood glucose monitoring, administration of oral and injectable hypoglycemic medications, diabetic diet, appropriate exercise, and foot care.
- Revise plan of care as needed to provide effective interventions to promote, maintain, or restore normal glucose levels.
- Teach the relationship of hygiene, neuropathy, and impaired microcirculation to infection; teach the principles and procedures of effective foot care.
- Assess clients' ability to read markings on syringes and to identify correct insulin and hypoglycemics.
- Relate insulin (endogenous and exogenous), dietary intake, and exercise to control of blood glucose.

Diabetes mellitus (DM) is a common chronic disease of adults requiring continuing medical supervision and client self-care education. However, depending on the type of diabetes and the age of the client, both client needs and nursing care may vary greatly. Consider the following examples:

- Cheryl Draheim is a 45-year-old schoolteacher. She developed diabetes at age 34 after an automobile accident caused severe pancreatic injuries. Cheryl has always been very careful about taking her insulin, following her diet, and exercising regularly. However, she is beginning to notice that her vision is getting worse and that she is having increasing pain in her legs, especially after standing for long periods of time. Cheryl says that sometimes she believes the disease controls her more than she controls it.

- Tom Chang is 53 years old. Early in his 40s, Tom was diagnosed with type 2 diabetes. Although Tom was taught about the disease and the importance of taking his oral medications, following his diet plan, and getting exercise, he rarely did more than take the medication. Five years ago, he was hospitalized for hyperglycemia and started taking insulin. Last year Tom had a stroke, leaving him unable to walk. He has now been admitted to the hospital for treatment of gangrene of the large toe on his left foot.

- Grace Staples is an independent 82-year-old woman who lives alone and happily takes care of her two cats. She is slightly overweight. Last year, during Grace's annual eye examination, eye changes typical for diabetes were found. She was referred to her family doctor, who diagnosed type 2 diabetes and started her on oral medications. Grace sticks to her diet, walks a mile every day, and plans to live to be 100.

As illustrated in these examples, diabetes mellitus is not a single disorder but a group of chronic disorders of the endocrine pancreas, all categorized under a broad diagnostic label. The condition is characterized by inappropriate hyperglycemia caused by a relative or absolute deficiency of insulin or by a cellular resistance to the action of insulin. Of the several classifications of diabetes, this chapter will focus on the two major types, type 1 and type 2. **Type 1 DM** is the result of pancreatic islet cell destruction and a total deficit of circulating insulin; **type 2 DM** results from insulin resistance with a defect in compensatory insulin secretion.

Diabetes mellitus has been recognized as a disease for centuries. *Diabetes* derives from a Greek word meaning "to siphon," referring to the increased output of urine. *Mellitus* derives from a Latin word meaning "sweet." The two words together identify the disease as an outpouring of sweet urine. It was not until 1921 that techniques were developed for extracting insulin from pancreatic tissue and for measuring blood glucose. At the same time, researchers discovered that insulin, when injected, produces a dramatic drop in blood glucose. This meant that diabetes was no longer a terminal illness because hyperglycemia could be controlled. Since that time, oral hypoglycemic drugs, human insulin products, insulin pumps, home blood glucose monitoring, and transplantation of the pancreas or of pancreatic islet or beta cells have advanced the treatment and care of people with diabetes.

Clients with DM face lifelong changes in lifestyle and health status. Nursing care is provided in many settings for the diagnosis and care of the disease and treatment of complications. A major role of the nurse is that of educator in both hospital and community settings.

INCIDENCE AND PREVALENCE

Approximately 1.3 million new cases of DM are diagnosed each year in the United States. This chronic illness affects an estimated 18.2 million people; of that number, 13 million have been diagnosed and an estimated 5.2 million are undiagnosed (National Institutes of Health [NIH], 2004). There is an increased prevalence of diabetes (especially type 2 diabetes) among older adults and in minority populations. See the Focus on Cultural Diversity box on page 564.

Diabetes is the sixth leading cause of death by disease in the United States, primarily because of the widespread cardiovascular effects that result in atherosclerosis, coronary artery disease, and stroke (Centers for Disease Control and Prevention [CDC], 2005). People with diabetes are two to four times more likely to have heart disease, and two to four times more likely to have a stroke than people who do not have diabetes. Diabetes is the leading cause of end-stage renal disease (kidney failure), and the major cause of newly diagnosed blindness in people ages 20 to 74. Diabetes

FOCUS ON CULTURAL DIVERSITY
Risk and Incidence of Diabetes Mellitus

- 13.1 million (8.7%) of all non-Hispanic whites aged 20 years or older have diabetes.
- 3.2 million (13.3%) of all non-Hispanic African Americans have diabetes, and are 1.8 times as likely to have diabetes as non-Hispanic whites of similar age. African Americans with type 2 diabetes have higher rates of coronary heart disease, CVA, and end-stage renal disease than do Caucasians with the disease.
- 2.5 million (9.5%) Hispanic/Latino Americans have diabetes, and are 1.7 times as likely to have diabetes as non-Hispanic whites of similar age. Mexican Americans are twice as likely to have diabetes as non-Hispanic whites of similar age.
- American Indians and Alaska Natives are 2.2 times more likely to have diabetes than non-Hispanic whites, and diabetes is especially prevalent in middle-aged and older American Indians. Diabetes mellitus is most common among Native Americans of the southern United States (27.8%) and least common among Alaska natives (8.1%) (CDC, 2005).

is also the most frequent cause of nontraumatic amputations with an estimated 82,000 amputations in 2002 in people with diabetes.

Americans with diabetes use a disproportionate share of the nation's healthcare services. They visit outpatient services and physicians' offices more often than people who do not have the disease, and they require more frequent hospitalizations with longer days of in-hospital treatment. The cost of illness and resulting loss of productivity for people with diabetes exceeds $132 billion per year, according to an estimate by the American Diabetes Association in 2002 (CDC, 2005).

OVERVIEW OF ENDOCRINE PANCREATIC HORMONES AND GLUCOSE HOMEOSTASIS

Hormones

The endocrine pancreas produces hormones necessary for the metabolism and cellular utilization of carbohydrates, proteins, and fats. The cells that produce these hormones are clustered in groups of cells called the islets of Langerhans. These islets have three different types of cells:

- Alpha cells produce the hormone *glucagon,* which stimulates the breakdown of glycogen in the liver, the formation of carbohydrates in the liver, and the breakdown of lipids in both the liver and adipose tissue. The primary function of glucagon is to decrease glucose oxidation and to increase blood glucose levels. Through **glycogenolysis** (the breakdown of liver glycogen) and **gluconeogenesis** (the formation of glucose from fats and proteins), glucagon prevents blood glucose from decreasing below a certain level when the body is fasting or in between meals. The action of glucagon is initiated in most people when blood glucose falls below about 70 mg/dL.

- Beta cells secrete the hormone **insulin**, which facilitates the movement of glucose across cell membranes into cells, decreasing blood glucose levels. Insulin prevents the excessive breakdown of glycogen in the liver and in muscle, facilitates lipid formation while inhibiting the breakdown of stored fats, and helps move amino acids into cells for protein synthesis. After secretion by the beta cells, insulin enters the portal circulation, travels directly to the liver, and is then released into the general circulation. Circulating insulin is rapidly bound to receptor sites on peripheral tissues (especially muscle and fat cells) or is destroyed by the liver or kidneys. Insulin release is regulated by blood glucose; it increases when blood glucose levels increase, and it decreases when blood glucose levels decrease. When a person eats food, insulin levels begin to rise in minutes, peak in 30 to 60 minutes, and return to baseline in 2 to 3 hours.

- Delta cells produce *somatostatin,* which is believed to be a neurotransmitter that inhibits the production of both glucagon and insulin.

Blood Glucose Homeostasis

All body tissues and organs require a constant supply of glucose; however, not all tissues require insulin for glucose uptake. The brain, liver, intestines, and renal tubules do not require insulin to transfer glucose into their cells. Skeletal muscle, cardiac muscle, and adipose tissue do require insulin for glucose movement into the cells.

Normal blood glucose is maintained in healthy people primarily through the actions of insulin and glucagon. Increased blood glucose levels, amino acids, and fatty acids stimulate pancreatic beta cells to produce insulin. As cells of cardiac muscle, skeletal muscle, and adipose tissue take up glucose, plasma levels of nutrients decrease, suppressing the stimulus to produce insulin. If blood glucose falls, glucagon is released to raise hepatic glucose output, raising glucose levels. Epinephrine, growth hormone, thyroxine, and glucocorticoids (often referred to as glucose counterregulatory hormones) also stimulate an increase in glucose in times of hypoglycemia, stress, growth, or increased metabolic demand. The regulation of blood glucose levels by insulin and glucagon is illustrated in Figure 20–1 ■.

PATHOPHYSIOLOGY OF DIABETES

DM is a group of metabolic diseases characterized by hyperglycemia resulting from defects in the secretion of insulin, the action of insulin, or both. There are four major types of DM. Type 1 diabetes (5% to 10% of diagnosed cases) was formerly called juvenile-onset diabetes or insulin-dependent diabetes mellitus (IDDM). Type 2 diabetes (90% to 95% of diagnosed cases) was formerly labeled non-insulin-dependent diabetes mellitus (NIDDM) or adult-onset diabetes. The other major types are gestational diabetes (2% to 5% of all pregnancies) and other specific types of diabetes (1% to 2% of diagnosed

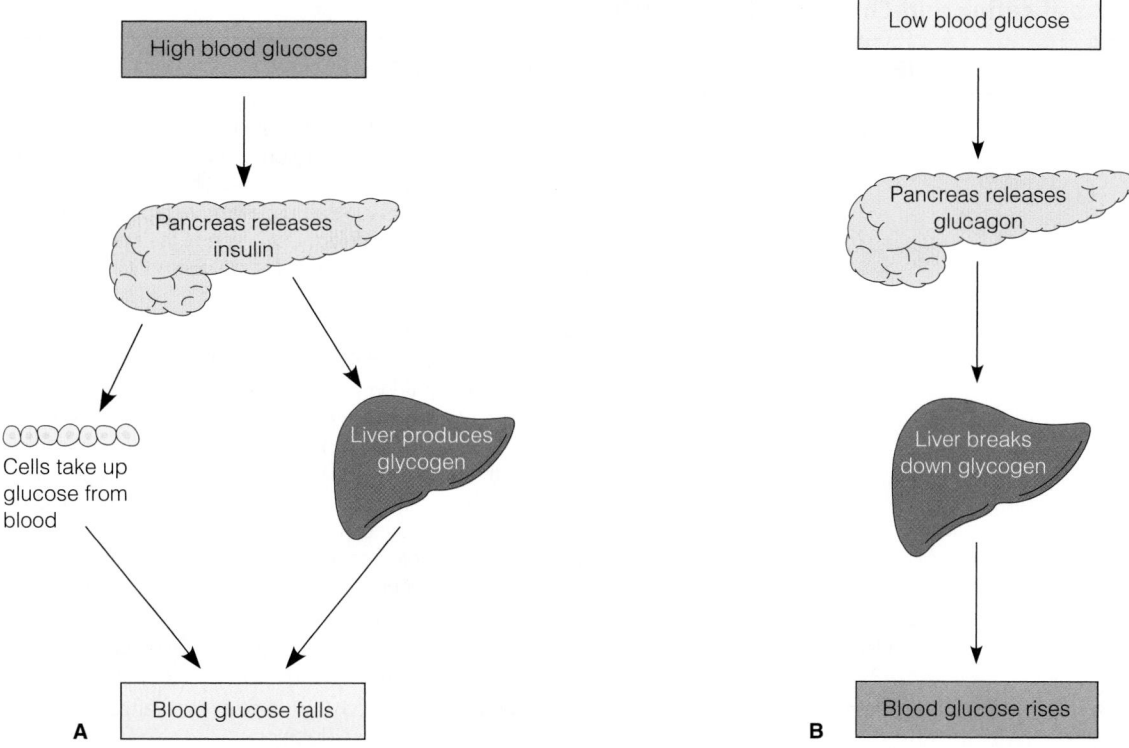

Figure 20–1 ■ Regulation (homeostasis) of blood glucose levels by insulin and glucagon. *A,* High blood glucose is lowered by insulin release. *B,* Low blood glucose is raised by glucagon release.

cases). The classification and characteristics of the four types are described in Table 20–1.

Type 1 Diabetes

Type 1 diabetes most often occurs in childhood and adolescence, but it may occur at any age, even in the 80s and 90s. This disorder is characterized by **hyperglycemia** (elevated blood glucose levels), a breakdown of body fats and proteins, and the development of **ketosis** (an accumulation of ketone bodies produced during the oxidation of fatty acids). Type 1 DM is the result of the destruction of the beta cells of the islets of Langerhans in the pancreas, the only cells in the body that make insulin. When beta cells are destroyed, insulin is no longer produced. Although type 1 DM may be classified as either an autoimmune or idiopathic disorder, 90% of the cases are immune mediated. The disorder begins with insulinitis, a chronic inflammatory process that occurs in response to the autoimmune destruction of islet cells. This process slowly destroys beta cell production of insulin, with the onset of hyperglycemia occurring when 80% to 90% of beta cell function is lost. This process usually occurs over a long preclinical period. It is believed that both alpha-cell and beta-cell functions are abnormal, with a lack of insulin and a relative excess of glucagon resulting in hyperglycemia.

Risk Factors
Genetic predisposition plays a role in the development of type 1 DM. Although the risk in the general population ranges from

1 in 400 to 1 in 1000, the child of a person with diabetes has a 1 in 20 to 1 in 50 risk. Genetic markers that determine immune responses—specifically, DR3 and DR4 antigens on chromosome 6 of the human leukocyte antigen (HLA) system—have been found in 95% of people diagnosed with type 1 DM. (HLAs are cell surface proteins, controlled by genes on chromosome 6.) Although the presence of these markers does not guarantee that the person will develop type 1 DM, they do indicate increased susceptibility (Porth, 2005).

Environmental factors are believed to trigger the development of type 1 DM. The trigger can be a viral infection (mumps, rubella, or coxsackievirus B4) or a chemical toxin, such as those found in smoked and cured meats. As a result of exposure to the virus or chemical, an abnormal autoimmune response occurs in which antibodies respond to normal islet beta cells as though they were foreign substances, destroying them. The manifestations of type 1 DM appear when approximately 90% of the beta cells are destroyed. However, manifestations may appear at any time during the loss of beta cells if an acute illness or stress increases the demand for insulin beyond the reserves of the damaged cells. The actual cause and exact sequence are not completely understood, but research continues to identify the genetic markers of this disorder and to investigate ways of altering the immune response to prevent or cure type 1 DM.

Manifestations
The manifestations of type 1 DM are the result of a lack of insulin to transport glucose across the cell membrane into the cells

TABLE 20–1 Classification and Characteristics of Diabetes

	CLASSIFICATION	CHARACTERISTICS
Type 1 Diabetes	Immune mediated	Beta cells are destroyed, usually leading to absolute insulin deficiency. Markers to the immune destruction of the beta cells include islet cell autoantibodies (ICAs) and insulin autoantibodies (IAAs). The rate of beta cell destruction is variable, usually more rapid in infants and children and slower in adults. Destruction of the beta cells has genetic predispositions and is also related to environmental factors as yet undefined.
	Idiopathic	Has no known etiologic causes. Most clients are of African or Asian descent. Is strongly inherited. Need for insulin may be intermittent.
Type 2 Diabetes		May range from predominantly insulin resistance with relative insulin deficiency to a predominantly secretory defect with insulin resistance. There is no immune destruction of beta cells. Initially, and in some cases for the entire life, insulin is not necessary. Most people with this form are obese, or have an increased amount of abdominal fat. Risks for development include increasing age, obesity, and a sedentary lifestyle. Occurs more frequently in women who have had gestational diabetes, and in people with lipid disorders or hypertension. There is a strong genetic predisposition.
Other Specific Types	Genetic defects of beta cell	Hyperglycemia occurs at an early age (usually before age 25). This type is referred to as maturity-onset diabetes of the young (MODY).
	Genetic defects in insulin action	Are genetically determined. Dysfunctions may range from hyperinsulinemia to severe diabetes.
	Diseases of the exocrine pancreas	Acquired processes causing diabetes include pancreatitis, trauma, infection, pancreatectomy, and pancreatic cancer. Severe forms of cystic fibrosis and hemochromatosis may also damage beta cells and impair insulin secretion.
	Endocrine disorders	Excess amount of hormones (e.g., growth hormone, cortisol, glucagon, and epinephrine) impair insulin secretion, resulting in diabetes in people with Cushing's syndrome, acromegaly, and pheochromocytoma.
	Drug or chemical induced	Many drugs impair insulin secretion, precipitating diabetes in people with predisposing insulin resistance. Examples are nicotinic acid, glucocorticoids, thyroid hormone, thiazides, and Dilantin.
	Infections	Certain viruses may cause beta cell destruction, including congenital measles, cytomegalovirus, adenovirus, and mumps.
Gestational Diabetes Mellitus (GDM)		Any degree of glucose intolerance with onset or first recognition during pregnancy.

(Figure 20–2 ■). Glucose molecules accumulate in the circulating blood, resulting in hyperglycemia. Hyperglycemia causes serum hyperosmolality, drawing water from the intracellular spaces into the general circulation. The increased blood volume increases renal blood flow, and the hyperglycemia acts as an osmotic diuretic. The resulting osmotic diuresis increases urine output. This condition is called **polyuria**. When the blood glucose level exceeds the renal threshold for glucose—usually about 180 mg/dL—glucose is excreted in the urine, a condition called **glucosuria**. The decrease in intracellular volume and the increased urinary output cause dehydration. The mouth becomes dry and thirst sensors are activated, causing the person to drink increased amounts of fluid (**polydipsia**).

Because glucose cannot enter the cell without insulin, energy production decreases. This decrease in energy stimulates hunger, and the person eats more food (**polyphagia**). Despite increased food intake, the person loses weight as the body loses

water and breaks down proteins and fats in an attempt to restore energy sources. Malaise and fatigue accompany the decrease in energy. Blurred vision is also common, resulting from osmotic effects that cause swelling of the lenses of the eyes.

Thus, the classic manifestations are polyuria, polydipsia, and polyphagia, accompanied by weight loss, malaise, and fatigue. Depending on the degree of insulin lack, the manifestations vary from slight to severe. People with type 1 DM require **exogenous insulin** to maintain life.

Type 2 Diabetes

Type 2 DM is a condition of fasting hyperglycemia that occurs despite the availability of **endogenous insulin**. Type 2 DM can occur at any age, but it is usually seen in middle-age and older people. Heredity plays a role in its transmission. The level of insulin produced varies in type 2 DM, and despite its availability, its

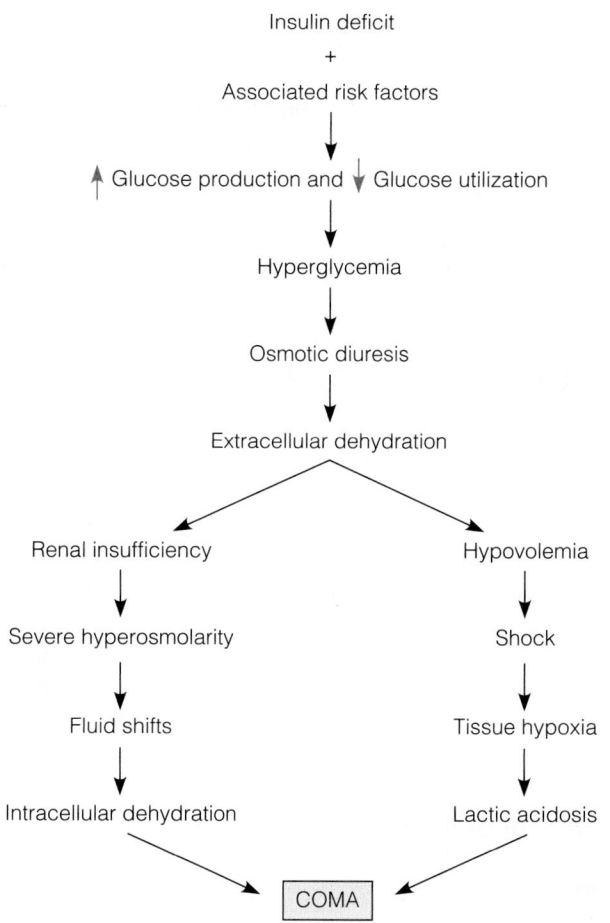

Insulin deficit

+

Associated risk factors

↑ Glucose production and ↓ Glucose utilization

Hyperglycemia

Osmotic diuresis

Extracellular dehydration

Renal insufficiency   Hypovolemia

Severe hyperosmolarity   Shock

Fluid shifts   Tissue hypoxia

Intracellular dehydration   Lactic acidosis

COMA

Figure 20–2 ■ Pathophysiologic results of type 1 DM.

function is impaired by insulin resistance. Insulin resistance forces the pancreas to work harder and produce more insulin, but when demand exceeds supply, DM results (Saudek & Margolis, 2005). Whatever the cause, there is sufficient insulin production to prevent the breakdown of fats with resultant ketosis; thus, type 2 DM is characterized as a nonketotic form of diabetes. However, the amount of insulin available is not sufficient to lower blood glucose levels through the uptake of glucose by muscle and fat cells. A major factor in the development of type 2 DM is cellular resistance to the effect of insulin. This resistance is increased by obesity, inactivity, illnesses, medications, and increasing age. In obesity, insulin has a decreased ability to influence glucose metabolism and uptake by the liver, skeletal muscles, and adipose tissue. Although the exact reason for this is not clear, it is known that weight loss and exercise may improve the mechanism responsible for insulin receptor binding or postreceptor activity (McCance & Huether, 2002). Type 2 diabetes has increased 33% in the past decade in the United States. Hyperglycemia increases gradually and may exist over a long time before diabetes is diagnosed, thus approximately half the newly diagnosed type 2 diabetics already have complications (Capriotti, 2005). Treatment usually begins with prescriptions for weight loss and increased activity. If these changes can be sustained, no further treatment will be necessary for many individuals. Hypoglycemic medications are begun

when lifestyle changes are insufficient. Often, a combination of insulin and hypoglycemic medication is used to achieve the best glycemic control in the client with type 2 DM.

Risk Factors

The major risk factors for type 2 DM are as follows:

- History of diabetes in parents or siblings. Although there is no identified HLA linkage, the children of a person with type 2 DM have a 15% chance of developing type 2 DM and a 30% risk of developing a glucose intolerance (the inability to metabolize carbohydrate normally).
- Obesity, defined as being at least 20% over desired body weight or having a body mass index of at least 27 kg/m². Obesity, especially of the upper body, decreases the number of available insulin receptor sites in cells of skeletal muscles and adipose tissues, a process called *peripheral insulin resistance*. In addition, obesity impairs the ability of the beta cells to release insulin in response to increasing glucose levels.
- Physical inactivity.
- Race/ethnicity (see the box on page 564).
- In women, a history of gestational DM, polycystic ovary syndrome, or delivering a baby weighing more than 9 lb.
- Hypertension (≥130/85 in adults), HDL cholesterol of ≥35 mg/dL, and/or a triglyceride level of ≥250 mg/dL
- Metabolic syndrome is a cluster of manifestations associated with type 2 DM and thought to link cardiovascular disease with insulin resistance (Larsen et al., 2003). Hypertension, abdominal obesity, dyslipidemia, elevated C-reactive protein, and a fasting blood glucose greater than 110 mg/dL increase the risk of DM, coronary heart disease, and stroke (Porth, 2005; Saudek & Margolis, 2005). This syndrome is thought to exist in more than half of Americans over 50 years old. Although there is widespread acknowledgment that these manifestations are associated, clinicians differ about appropriate treatment (Larsen et al., 2003; Tierney et al., 2005).

Manifestations

The person with type 2 DM experiences a slow onset of manifestations and is often unaware of the disease until seeking health care for some other problem. The hyperglycemia in type 2 is usually not as severe as in type 1, but similar symptoms occur, especially polyuria and polydipsia. Polyphagia is not often seen, and weight loss is uncommon. Other manifestations are also the result of hyperglycemia: blurred vision, fatigue, paresthesias, and skin infections. If available insulin decreases, especially in times of physical or emotional stress, the person with type 2 DM may develop diabetic ketoacidosis (DKA), but this occurrence is uncommon.

Diabetes in the Older Adult

Although the older adult may have either type 1 or type 2 DM, most have type 2. The National Institute of Diabetes and Kidney Disease estimates that nearly 11% of the U.S. population between the ages of 65 and 74 has diabetes. The prevalence of diabetes becomes greater with age, increasing from 8.2% with diagnosed diabetes in those age 20 years or older to 18.4% for those equal to or older than age 65 (American Diabetes Association [ADA],

2005). It is predicted that the number of older adults with diabetes will continue to increase, because the incidence of the disease increases with age and because the number of people over age 65 is increasing.

Although most older adults with diabetes have type 2 DM, the improved survival rates for people with diabetes have resulted in an increased number of older adults with type 1. The picture is complicated by the fact that blood glucose levels increase with age, beginning in the 50s. For this reason, it is more difficult to diagnose diabetes in the older adult; conversely, the older adult may be mistakenly diagnosed with the disease simply for exhibiting essentially normal age-related changes in glucose. The relationship between normal increases in glucose levels and the presence of diabetes is not yet understood.

The older adult with diabetes has multiple, complex healthcare problems and needs including risks for polypharmacy, depression, cognitive impairment, urinary incontinence, injurious falls, and persistent pain (ADA, 2005). The normal physiologic changes of aging may mask manifestations of the onset of diabetes. Signs and symptoms of diabetes in elders may not include the classic symptoms of polyuria and thirst. Conditions such as orthostatic hypotension, periodontal disease, infections, stroke, gastric hypotony, impotence, neuropathy, confu-sion, and glaucoma should be considered potential indicators of diabetes (Eliopoulos, 2005), and may also increase the potential for complications from the disease or its treatment. Table 20–2 presents common problems in the older adult that make the diagnosis and management of diabetes more difficult. The older adult with diabetes also has a longer recovery period after surgery or serious illness, often requiring insulin to maintain blood glucose levels. The benefits and risks of treatment to maintain glycemic control as well as blood pressure and lipid management must be carefully balanced.

INTERDISCIPLINARY CARE

The results of a 10-year Diabetes Control and Complications Trial, sponsored by the NIH, have significant implications for the management of type 1 DM. People in the study who kept their blood glucose levels close to normal by frequent monitoring, several daily insulin injections, and lifestyle changes that included exercise and a healthier diet reduced by 60% their risk for the development and progression of complications involving the eyes, the kidneys, and the nervous system. The DIGAMI study of 1995 stimulated interest in greater glycemic control in clients with type 2 DM (Cummings et al., 1999;

TABLE 20–2 Implications for Nursing Care of the Older Adult with Diabetes

HEALTH PROBLEM/COMPLICATION	IMPLICATIONS FOR NURSING CARE
Urinary incontinence	Polyuria, a classic manifestation of diabetes, often is ignored. This problem also often leads to social isolation.
Decreased thirst	Polydipsia, a classic manifestation of diabetes, often is ignored. This further increases the risk of dehydration and electrolyte imbalances.
Decreased hunger and weight loss	Polyphagia, a classic manifestation of diabetes, often is ignored. The aging process, medications, depression, or lack of socialization may decrease hunger. Weight loss may be gradual and go unnoticed.
Fatigue	Fatigue is a common symptom of diabetes but may be blamed on increased age.
Hypoglycemia	The older adult may have either very mild manifestations or none at all. As a result, hypoglycemia is often ignored until it causes serious effects.
Peripheral neuropathy	Manifestations may be thought to be due to arthritis, and over-the-counter drugs often are used to self-medicate. The risk of falls increases, as does the risk of gangrene and amputation.
Peripheral vascular disease	May go undetected if the person does not get enough exercise to cause claudication. May also impair abilities to climb stairs and walk.
Diabetic retinopathy	May be undetected if the person has cataracts. Diabetic clients also have an increased incidence of cataracts and glaucoma. Deficits in vision threaten independence, mobility, and social interactions. Yellowing of the lens with age makes it difficult to read colored test strips; numeric meters are preferable. Filling insulin syringes may be impossible for the client with macular degeneration or other causes of visual loss.
Hypertension	Treatment with diuretics may further impair glucose tolerance and result in electrolyte imbalances.
Arthritis	Older adults may believe the pain from arthritis to be more important than the diabetes management. Also, depression from chronic pain as well as inactivity and loss of appetite may interfere with diabetes self-care.
Parkinson's disease	The tremors and rigidity of this disease make self-care involving fine and gross motor skills difficult or impossible.
Medications	Older adults commonly take more than one type of medication and are at increased risk for problems relating to drug interactions.

Source: Adapted from "Diabetes Mellitus and the Older Adult" by M. M. Funnell and J. H. Merritt, pp. 755–830, in D. Haire-Joshu (Ed.), *Management of Diabetes Mellitus: Perspectives of Care Across the Lifespan* (2nd ed.), 1996, St. Louis, MO: Mosby; Eliopoulos, C., *Gerontological Nursing,* 2005, Philadelphia: Lippincott Williams & Wilkins.

Malmberg et al., 1995). Treatment of the client with diabetes focuses on maintaining blood glucose at levels as nearly normal as possible through medications, dietary management, and exercise. Type 2 DM benefits from similar levels of control.

Diagnosis

Diagnostic tests are conducted for screening purposes to diagnose diabetes, and ongoing laboratory tests are conducted to evaluate the effectiveness of diabetic management. Definitions of normal blood glucose levels vary in clinical practice, depending on the laboratory that performs the assay.

DIAGNOSTIC SCREENING Three diagnostic tests may be used to diagnose DM, and each must be confirmed, on a subsequent day, with one of the three tests. The following diagnostic criteria are recommended by the ADA (2005):

1. Symptoms of diabetes plus casual plasma glucose (PG) concentration > 200 mg/dL (11.1 mmol/L). Causal is defined as any time of day without regard to time since last meal.
2. Fasting plasma glucose (FPG) > 126 mg/dL (7.0 mmol/L). Fasting is defined as no caloric intake for 8 hours.
3. Two-hour PG > 200 mg/dL (11.1 mmol/L) during an oral glucose tolerance test (OGTT). The test should be performed with a glucose load containing the equivalent of 75 anhydrous glucose dissolved in water.

When using these criteria, the following levels are used for the FPG:

- Normal fasting glucose = 100 mg/dL (6.1 mmol/L)
- Impaired fasting glucose (IFG) > 100 (6.1 mmol/L) and <126 mg/dL (7.0 mmol/L)
- Diagnosis of diabetes > 126 mg/dL (7.0 mmol/L).

When using these criteria, the following levels are used for the OGTT:

- Normal glucose tolerance = 2-h PG < 140 mg/dL (7.8 mmol/L)
- Impaired glucose tolerance (IGT) = 2-h PG ≥ 140 (7.8 mmol/L) and < 200 mg/dL (11.1 mmol/L)
- Diagnosis of diabetes = 2-h PG ≥ 200 mg/dL (11.1 mmol/L). Note that although either method may be used to diagnose diabetes, in a clinical setting the FPG is the recommended screening test for nonpregnant adults (ADA, 2002).

Prediabetes *Prediabetes* is a term used to describe people who are at increased risk of developing diabetes. Prediabetes is characterized by blood sugar between 100 and 126 mg/dL after fasting overnight, which is high but not high enough to be classified as diabetes. In 2000, an estimated 41 million adults ages 40 to 74 had prediabetes. These test results indicate there is a risk for progression to diabetes, but it is not inevitable. Studies suggest that weight loss and increased physical activity among people with prediabetes prevent or delay diabetes and may return blood glucose levels to normal. People with prediabetes are already at increased risk for other adverse health outcomes such as heart disease and stroke (CDC, 2005).

DIAGNOSTIC TESTS TO MONITOR DIABETES MANAGEMENT The following diagnostic tests may be used to monitor diabetes management:

- *Fasting blood glucose (FBG).* This test is often ordered, especially if the client is experiencing symptoms of hypoglycemia or hyperglycemia. In most people, the normal range is 70 to 110 mg/dL.
- *Glycosylated hemoglobin (c) (A1c).* This test determines the average blood glucose level over approximately the previous 2 to 3 months. When glucose is elevated or control of glucose is erratic, glucose attaches to the hemoglobin molecule and remains attached for the life of the hemoglobin, which is about 120 days. The normal level depends on the type of assay done, but values above 7% to 9% are considered elevated. The ADA recommends that A1c be performed at the initial assessment, and then at regular intervals, individualized to the medical regimen used.
- *Urine glucose and ketone levels.* These are not as accurate in monitoring changes in blood glucose as blood levels. The presence of glucose in the urine indicates hyperglycemia. Most people have a renal threshold for glucose of 180 mg/dL; that is, when the blood glucose exceeds 180 mg/dL, glucose is not reabsorbed by the kidney and spills over into the urine. This number varies highly, however. **Ketonuria** (the presence of ketones in the urine) occurs with the breakdown of fats and is an indicator of DKA; however, fat breakdown and ketonuria also occur in states of less than normal nutrition.
- *Urine test* for the presence of protein as albumin (*albuminuria*). If albuminuria is present, a 24-hour urine test for creatinine clearance is used to detect the early onset of nephropathy.
- *Serum cholesterol and triglyceride levels.* These are indicators of atherosclerosis and an increased risk of cardiovascular impairments. The ADA (2005) recommends treatment goals to lower LDL cholesterol to <100 mg/dL, raise HDL cholesterol to >45 mg/dL, and lower triglycerides to <150 mg/dL.
- *Serum electrolytes.* Levels are measured in clients who have DKA or hyperosmolar hyperglycemic state (HHS) to determine imbalances.

Monitoring Blood Glucose

People with diabetes must monitor their condition daily by testing glucose levels. Two types of tests are available. The first type, long used prior to the development of devices to directly measure blood glucose, is urine testing for glucose and ketones. Urine testing is less commonly used today. The second type, direct measurement of blood glucose, is widely used in all types of healthcare settings and in the home.

URINE TESTING FOR KETONES AND GLUCOSE Urine testing for glucose and ketones was at one time the only available method for evaluating the management of diabetes. An inexpensive, noninvasive, and painless test, it has unpredictable results and cannot be used to detect or measure hypoglycemia. In the healthy state, glucose is not present in the urine because insulin maintains serum glucose below the renal threshold of 180 mg/dL. The accuracy of this measurement is not reliable in diabetes because the renal threshold may rise with aging or secondary to diabetes. Urine testing is recommended to monitor hyperglycemia and ketoacidosis in people with type 1 DM who have unexplained hyperglycemia during illness or pregnancy. Ketones may be detected through urine testing and reflect the presence of DKA. Urine testing may also be used by people who choose not to self-monitor blood glucose by other methods. (See Procedure 20–1: Testing Urine for Ketones and Glucose.)

SELF-MONITORING OF BLOOD GLUCOSE Self-monitoring of blood glucose (SMBG) allows the person with diabetes to monitor and achieve metabolic control and decrease the danger of hypoglycemia. The ADA recommends that all clients with diabetes must be taught some method of monitoring glycemic control. The timing of SMBG is highly individualized, depending on the person's diagnosis, general disease control, and physical state. SMBG is recommended three or more times a day for clients with type 1 DM; for clients with type 2 DM, testing should be sufficient to help them reach glucose goals. When adding or modifying therapy, clients with both types of DM should test more often than usual. SMBG is also useful when the person is ill or pregnant, or has symptoms of hypoglycemia or hyperglycemia (ADA, 2006).

The ADA annually publishes a comprehensive list of currently available blood glucose monitoring machines and strips with approximate prices in *Diabetes Forecast.* Most medical insurance policies cover the cost of these machines. A new technology for continuous blood glucose monitoring is now available and clients are learning to use these monitors, especially if they use insulin pumps. A new insulin pump receives transmitted data from a continuous glucose monitor (CGM) worn on the skin. Like the insulin pump, the CGM has a sensor that is inserted under the skin. This sensor continuously sends data to the transmitter, which sends the information to the pump by radio-frequency wireless technology. This data can warn of high or low glucose levels. Fingerstick measurements are required before making therapy adjustments (Medtronic MiniMed, 2006). The CGM is also used for diagnostic evaluation; clients wear the pump for 3 days under the supervision of physicians and nurses. The data reveal patterns of glycemic control useful for clinical recommendations.

Following is the equipment needed for SMBG:
- Some type of lancet device to perform a fingerstick for obtaining a drop of blood (such as an Autolet, Penlet, or Soft Touch).
- Chemically impregnated test strips that change color when they come into contact with glucose or that can be read by

machine (e.g., Glucostix and Chemstrip bG). The strip may also be read by comparing its color with a color chart on the side of the container or on an insert (Figure 20–3 ■).
- A blood glucose monitor (e.g., the Glucometer, the Accu-Chek, or the One Touch) if the most accurate measurement is desired or recommended. The manufacturer's instructions must be followed carefully. If the timing of the blood on the strip is not exact, the test will not be accurate. In addition, the machine must be cleaned according to the manufacturer's directions to ensure accuracy. Monitors that use no-wipe technology improve the accuracy of glucose measurement. Other monitors are computerized and/or include a memory of previous glucose readings to show a pattern of control. The stored information is useful for clinicians to review and determine therapeutic needs.

FACTORS THAT AFFECT GLUCOSE METER PERFORMANCE According to the U.S. Food and Drug Administration (FDA), several factors affect the accuracy of blood glucose test results. The quality of the meter and test strips, and training to use the meter contribute to the degree of accuracy. Other factors can create false positive or negative readings.

Figure 20–3 ■ Determination of blood glucose levels by visual reading. The color of the strip is compared with the color chart on the side of the container.

PROCEDURE 20-1 **TESTING URINE FOR KETONES AND GLUCOSE**

TO TEST THE URINE FOR KETONES

1. Ask the client to void, discard the urine, and drink a full glass of water.
2. Thirty minutes later, collect a urine sample.
3. For Acidtest tablets: Place the tablet on a white paper towel, place 1 drop of urine on the tablet, and wait 30 seconds. If the

tablet turns any shade from lavender to deep purple, the test is positive for ketones.

4. For Ketostix: Dip the reagent stick into the urine sample. Wait 15 seconds, and compare the color of the pad at the end of the stick to an accompanying color chart. Purple is indicative of ketones.

TO TEST THE URINE FOR GLUCOSE

1. Follow the same procedure to collect a urine sample.
2. Dip the reagent stick into the urine sample, and wait the time indicated. Compare the color of the pad on the end of the reagent

stick with an accompanying color chart. The glucose is expressed as a percentage (for example, 0.5%, 1%, 2%). Remember that normally no glucose is found in the urine, so the presence of glucose is an abnormal manifestation indicating hyperglycemia.

Hematocrit Clients with higher hematocrit values will usually test falsely low in blood glucose and clients with lower hematocrit will test falsely higher. Anemia and sickle cell anemia are two conditions that can affect hematocrit values.

Other Substances Overdoses of many medications will cause inaccurate results. Meters and supplies vary in sensitivity to medications. Uric acid (a natural substance in the body that can be more concentrated in some people with diabetes), glutathione (an antioxidant also called *GSH*), and ascorbic acid (vitamin C) are known to interfere. Check the package insert for each meter to find what substances might affect its testing accuracy (U.S. FDA, 2005).

Use of Correct Supplies and Sample Volume Be sure the test strips are compatible with the glucose meter and that they are not outdated or exposed to air and humidity, which can alter strip sensitivity. Insufficient amounts of blood on the testing strip cause inaccurate results. Although a meter may indicate a sufficient amount of blood on the test strip, it is best to observe that the receptacle is full of capillary blood. Yared et al. (2005) found that meters read significantly smaller than reference volumes and gave results varying 40% to 68% from the reference volume results. The erroneous results underestimated the true glucose value.

Medications

The pharmacologic treatment for diabetes mellitus depends on the type of diabetes. People with type 1 DM must have insulin; those with type 2 DM are usually able to control glucose levels with an oral hypoglycemic medication, but they may require insulin if control is inadequate.

INSULIN The person with type 1 DM requires a lifelong exogenous source of the insulin hormone to maintain life. Insulin is not a cure for diabetes; rather, it is a means of controlling hyperglycemia. Insulin is also necessary in other situations, such as these:

- People with diabetes who are unable to control glucose levels with oral antidiabetic drugs and/or diet. Introduced when beta cell function declines, insulin maintains glycemic control and prevents complications (Funnell, Kruger, & Spencer, 2004).

- People with diabetes who are experiencing physical stress (such as an infection or surgery) or who are taking corticosteroids.
- Women with gestational diabetes who are unable to control glucose with diet.
- People with DKA or HHS.
- People who are receiving high-calorie tube feedings or parenteral nutrition.

Sources of Insulin Preparations of insulin are derived from animal (pork pancreas) or synthesized in the laboratory from either an alteration of pork insulin or recombinant DNA technology, using strains of *E. coli* to form a biosynthetic human insulin. Insulin analogs have been developed by modifying the amino acid sequence of the insulin molecule. Although different types are prescribed on an individualized basis, it is standard practice to prescribe human insulin.

Insulin Preparations Insulins are available in rapid-acting, short-acting, intermediate-acting, and long-acting preparations. The trade names and times of onset, peak, and duration of action are listed in Table 20–3.

Insulin lispro (Humalog) is a human insulin analog that is derived from genetically altered *E. coli* that includes the gene for insulin lispro. It is classified as a rapid-acting or ultra-short-acting insulin. Compared to regular insulin, insulin lispro has a more rapid onset (<15 minutes), an earlier peak of glucose lowering (30 to 60 minutes), and a shorter duration of activity (3 to 4 hours). This means that lispro should be administered 15 minutes before a meal, rather than 30 to 60 minutes before as recommended for regular insulin. Clients with type 1 DM usually also require concurrent use of a longer acting insulin product. Lispro is much less likely than regular insulin to cause tissue changes and may lower the risk of nocturnal hypoglycemia in clients with type 1 DM.

Regular insulin is unmodified crystalline insulin, classified as a short-acting insulin. Regular insulin is clear in appearance and is the only insulin preparation that can be given by the intravenous route; the other types are suspensions and could be harmful if given by this route. Regular insulin is also used to treat DKA, to initiate treatment for newly diagnosed type 1

TABLE 20–3 Insulin Preparations

PREPARATION	NAME	ONSET (H)	PEAK (H)	DURATION (H)
Rapid acting	Lispro	0.25	1–1.5	3–4
	Aspart (NovoLog)	0.25	40–50 minutes	3–5
	Glulisine (Apidra)	0.25	1–1.5	3–5
Short acting	Regular (Novolin-R, Humulin-R)	0.5–1.0	2–3	4–6
Intermediate acting	NPH Humulin (N) NPH	2	6–8	12–16
Long acting	Lantus	2 (Onset and peak not defined)	16–20	24+ 24
Combinations	Humulin 50/50	0.5	3	22–24
	Humulin 70/30	0.5	4–8	24
	Novolin 70/30	0.5	4–8	24

DM, and in combination with intermediate-acting insulins to provide better glucose control.

The onset and peak and duration of action of insulin can be changed by adding acetate buffers and protamine. Zinc and protamine are added to NPH insulin to prolong their action, and they are classified as intermediate- or long-acting insulins. These preparations appear cloudy when properly mixed prior to injection. Protamine and zinc are foreign substances and may cause hypersensitivity reactions. As of July 6, 2005, Lilly discontinued manufacture of pork insulins and Humulin U and Humulin Lente insulin.

Insulin glargine (Lantus) is a 24-hour, long-acting rDNA human insulin analog that is given subcutaneously once a day, usually at bedtime, to treat clients with both type 1 and type 2 diabetes. It has a relatively constant effect (meaning it does not have a peak time of effect). It is not recommended for use in pregnancy. Do not mix this with other insulins; the pH is incompatible (Lehne, 2004; Tierney et al., 2005).

PRACTICE ALERT
Insulin glargine is clear unlike other intermediate or long-acting insulins. Do not mistake this for regular insulin. Do not mix with **any** other insulins. Do not inject intravenously, only subcutaneously.

Concentrations of Insulin Insulin is dispensed as 100 unit/mL (U-100) and 500 unit/mL (U-500) in the United States. U-100 is the standard insulin concentration used. U-500 insulin is only used in rare cases of insulin resistance when clients require very large doses. U-500 and the insulin analog lispro are the only insulins that require a prescription.

Insulin Administration Nursing implications for administering insulin are outlined in the Medication Administration box on the following page and further discussion follows in the chapter. The considerations for administering insulin include routes of administration, syringe and needle selection, preparing the injection, sites of injection, mixing insulins, and insulin regimens.

Routes of Administration. All insulins are given parenterally, although current research is investigating the development of a nasal spray and an oral preparation of insulin. Only regular insulin is given by both subcutaneous and intravenous routes; all others are given only subcutaneously. If the intravenous route is not available, regular insulin may also be administered intramuscularly in an emergency situation.

Continuous Subcutaneous Insulin Infusion. Regular or rapid-acting insulins are used in continuous subcutaneous insulin infusion (CSII) devices, often called *insulin pumps* (e.g., MiniMed and Disetronic pumps). CSII devices have a small pump that holds a syringe of insulin, connected to a subcutaneous needle by tubing. The pump is about the size of a pager and can be worn on a belt or tucked into a pocket. The needle is placed in the skin, usually in the abdomen, and is changed every 3 days. This device delivers a constant amount of programmed insulin throughout each 24-hour period. It also can be used to deliver a bolus of insulin manually (e.g., before meals).

Sliding Scale Insulin. Treatment of hospitalized type 1 and type 2 clients requires a medication regimen that is responsive to glycemic changes secondary to the admitting condition and its treatment, including surgery (Clement et al., 2004). Type 2 diabetics cannot manage with oral medications during hospitalization because of the risk of hypoglycemia from not eating and the slow response of these medications to correct hyperglycemia. There is growing acceptance of the need to achieve tighter control of blood sugar in individuals who are hospitalized with hyperglycemia, whether they are diagnosed with diabetes, have unrecognized diabetes, or have hospital-related diabetes (Clement et al., 2004; Magee, 2006). Researchers first recognized the benefit of normal blood sugars (80 to 110 mg/dL) maintained by intensive insulin therapy (intravenous regular insulin) in surgical ICU patients; the optimum degree of blood sugar control in medical ICU patients remains undetermined through research at this time although levels equal to or <180 mg/dL are generally accepted (Magee, 2006; Malmberg et al., 1995; Van den Berghe et al., 2006).

In a study of 1200 medical ICU patients, Van den Berghe et al. (2006) compared those receiving intensive insulin therapy with patients receiving conventional therapy (insulin administered when the blood glucose reached 215 mg/dL). Those in the intensively treated group who were in the ICU for 3 days or more had significantly reduced morbidity, slightly more incidents of hypoglycemia (although significantly less mortality related to hypoglycemia than those treated conventionally), and significantly reduced acquired kidney injury (defined as a serum creatinine level at least twice the admission level).

Maintaining normal blood glucose during hospitalization decreases the risk of postoperative infections and shortens hospital stays. Healing is impaired when hemoglobin is glycosylated (hemoglobin A_{1c}); glycosylated Hgb has increased affinity for oxygen, putting tissues at risk for ischemia (McCance & Huether, 2002). Further, diabetes leads to small-vessel disease, which impairs circulation and oxygenation of tissue for healing.

Intravenous insulin infusions are preferable for maintaining normal blood glucose during hospitalization, although their use is dependent on frequent blood glucose monitoring and intensive nursing care. Supplements of regular insulin following sliding scale prescriptions (relative to monitored blood glucose levels) are ineffective management protocols, risking both hyperglycemia and hypoglycemia. These supplements treat hyperglycemia after it has occurred rather than preventing it. When medical conditions lead to observable periods of hyperglycemia outside the ICU, it is preferable to provide a basal subcutaneous insulin such as insulin glargine or NPH and mealtime supplements with regular or aspart insulin. Correctional doses can be added to the mealtime doses

MEDICATION ADMINISTRATION   Insulin

Nursing Responsibilities

- Discard vials of insulin that have been open for several weeks or whose expiration date has passed.
- Refrigerate extra insulin vials not currently in use, but do not freeze them.
- Store insulin in a cool place, and avoid exposure to temperature extremes or sunlight.
- Store compatible mixtures of insulin for no longer than 1 month at room temperature or 3 months at 36° to 46°F (2° to 8°C).
- Discard any vials with discoloration, clumping, granules, or solid deposits on the sides.
- If breakfast is delayed, also delay the administration of rapid-acting insulin.
- Monitor and maintain a record of blood glucose readings 30 minutes before each meal and bedtime (or as prescribed).
- Monitor food intake, and notify the physician if food is not being consumed.
- Monitor electrolytes (especially potassium), blood urea nitrogen (BUN) levels, and creatinine.
- Observe injection sites for manifestations of hypersensitivity, lipodystrophy, and lipoatrophy.
- If symptoms of hypoglycemia occur, confirm by testing blood glucose level, and administer an oral source of a fast-acting carbohydrate, such as juice, milk, or crackers. Hypoglycemic symptoms may vary but commonly include feelings of shakiness, hunger, and/or nervousness accompanied by sweating, tachycardia, or palpitations.
- If symptoms of hyperglycemia occur, confirm by testing blood glucose level, and notify the physician.

Health Education for the Client and Family

- The manifestations of diabetes mellitus.
- Self-administration of insulin, with a return demonstration.
  a. Wash hands carefully.
  b. Have a vial of insulin, the insulin syringe with needle, and alcohol pads ready to use.
  c. Remove the cover from the needle.
  d. Fill the syringe with an amount of air equal to the number of units of insulin, and insert the needle into the vial.
  e. Push air into the vial, invert the vial, and withdraw the prescribed units of insulin.

  f. Replace the cover over the needle.
  g. Wipe the selected site with alcohol. The injection is less likely to be painful if the alcohol is allowed to dry.
  h. Pinch up a fold of skin, and insert the needle into the tissue at the recommended angle.
  i. Insert the insulin.
  j. Withdraw the needle; if desired, apply firm pressure to the site for a few seconds.
  k. Recap the needle. Many people with diabetes reuse disposable syringes with attached needles without adverse effects. The primary reason for discarding after several uses is that the needle becomes dull and makes the injection painful.
- Follow instructions for mixing insulins (refer to Box 20–3 on page 576).
- Always keep an extra vial of insulin available.
- Always have a vial of regular insulin available for emergencies.
- Be aware of the signs of hypersensitivity responses, hypoglycemia, and hyperglycemia.
- Keep candy or a sugar source available at all times to treat hypoglycemia, if it occurs. Eat within 15 minutes of injecting rapid-acting insulins.
- Vision may be blurred during the first 6 to 8 weeks of insulin therapy; this is the result of fluid changes in the eye and should clear up in 8 weeks.
- Avoid alcoholic beverages, which may cause hypoglycemia.
- Follow these guidelines for sick days:
  a. Never omit insulin.
  b. Always monitor blood glucose and/or urine ketones at least every 2 to 4 hours.
  c. Always drink plenty of fluids, try to drink at least one glass of water or other calorie-free, caffeine-free liquid each hour.
  d. Get as much rest as possible.
  e. Contact the physician if there is persistent fever, vomiting, shortness of breath, severe pain in the abdomen, dehydration, loss of vision, chest pain, persistent diarrhea, blood glucose levels above 250, or ketones in the urine.
- Establish a plan for rotating injection sites, and observe closely for changes in tissues such as hardness, dimpling, or sunken areas.

to keep serum glucose below 180 mg/dL (ADA, 2005; Clement et al., 2004).

See Box 20–1 for methods to calculate basal and bolus doses for hospitalized patients on scheduled subcutaneous insulin doses and patients with insulin pumps.

Programming the amount of insulin to be delivered with a pump is determined by frequent blood glucose monitoring. Several different pumps are available, and each has rechargeable batteries, a syringe, a programmable computer, and a motor and drive mechanism. The rapid-acting insulin analog lispro is an appropriate insulin for insulin pumps, and short-acting regular insulin may also be used. Lispro is not approved for use in pregnancy (Tierney et al., 2005).

Many people with diabetes believe the pump allows more normal regulation of blood glucose and provides greater lifestyle flexibility. Pumps are as safe as multiple-injection therapy when recommended procedures are followed. A potential complication is an undetected interruption in insulin delivery, which may result in a rapid onset of DKA. The needle site must be kept clean and changed on a regular basis (usually every 2 to 3 days) to prevent inflammation and infection. Although the client who chooses an insulin pump has much to learn, many are very satisfied with having more normal glucose control.

Syringe and Needle Selection. Insulin is administered in sterile, single-use, disposable insulin syringes, calibrated in units per

BOX 20–1 Insulin Total Daily Dose

1. The total amount of insulin that the patient administered daily by injection (rapid- or short-acting with intermediate- or long-acting); for example, 48 units (30 units NPH and 18 units regular insulin).
   OR
2. 0.5–1 unit/kg (normal kidney/liver function already on insulin), for example, 48 units for a 96-kg patient
   OR
3. 0.3–0.5 unit/kg (reduced kidney/liver function or initial insulin therapy).
   Test blood glucose with test strip AC and HS.

Basal Dose: 40% to 50% of the insulin total daily dose (ITDD).

1. *Insulin pump:* Multiply the ITDD by 50% (48.0 × 0.5 = 24 units). The basal insulin pump dose for this patient is 24 units. Divide the basal insulin pump dose by 24 to get the hourly basal pump dose and rate (24/24 = 1.0 unit/hour). Use rapid-acting or regular insulin.
2. *Subcutaneous insulin:* Multiply the ITDD by 50% (48.0 × 0.5 = 24 units. This will be administered as one insulin glargine SQ injection daily or NPH injections of 12 units each twice daily. These basal doses are made with long-acting or intermediate-acting insulins.

Mealtime Bolus Dose

1. *Insulin pump:* To calculate bolus doses, take the remaining 50% of insulin and divide it by four doses according to the patient's meal plan for the day. For example, the remaining 50% could be divided thus: 20% at breakfast = 10 units; 10% at lunch = 5 units; 15% at dinner = 8 units, and 5% with a bedtime snack = 2 units.

   To calculate the units for each of these four daily bolus doses, multiply the percent of each meal bolus times the total daily insulin pump dose. For example, for 48 units for a total daily dose:

Breakfast dose is

$$20\% \text{ (or 0.2)} \times 48 \text{ units} = 10 \text{ units}$$

Lunch dose is

$$10\% \text{ (or 0.1)} \times 48 \text{ units} = 5 \text{ units}$$

Dinner dose is

$$15\% \text{ (or 0.15)} \times 48 \text{ units} = 8 \text{ units}$$

Bedtime snack dose is

$$5\% \text{ (or 0.05)} \times 48 = 2 \text{ units. (Nursing, 2005).}$$

Correction doses may be needed if the client is hyperglycemic.

2. *Subcutaneous insulin mealtime dose:* Divide half of the ITDD into 3 mealtime doses.

$$\text{Breakfast} = 6 \text{ units; lunch} = 6 \text{ units; supper} = 6 \text{ units.}$$
$$\text{No bedtime dose is given.}$$

Rapid-acting insulin (regular or aspart) is given in conjunction with the meal.

Mealtime Correction Dose

This is different from sliding scale dosing because it is given with a scheduled insulin dose to prevent hyperglycemia after the meals. It is given with rapid-acting insulin combined with the mealtime dose.

1. Test blood glucose prior to each meal.
   If blood glucose mg/dL is:
   <80 or symptomatic for hypoglycemia
   Follow hypoglycemia protocol

81–100	No correction dose needed.
101–150	Add 1 or 2 units if mealtime dose is >20 units.
151–200	Add 2 or 3 units if mealtime dose is >20 units.
201–250	Add 3 or 4 units if mealtime dose is >20 units.
251–300	Add 4 or 5 units if mealtime dose is >20 units.
>300	Add 5 or 10 units if mealtime dose is >20 units.

Note: When correction doses are needed, the scheduled doses of rapid-acting insulin need to be reordered at higher doses.

milliliter. This means that in U-100 insulin, there are 100 units of insulin in 1 mL. Syringes for administering U-100 insulin can be purchased in either 0.3-mL (30-unit), 0.5-mL (50-unit), or 1.0-mL (100-unit) size. The advantage of the 0.3- and 0.5-mL sizes is that the distance between unit markings is greater, making it easier to measure the dose accurately. Although manufactured as "single-use," in the home environment clients may choose to reuse these syringes as long as the needles are sharp.

Most insulin syringes are manufactured with the needle permanently attached in a 25- to 27-gauge, 0.5-inch size. If this type of syringe is not available, an insulin syringe and a 25-gauge, 0.5-inch or 0.75-inch needle should be used.

Other special injection products are available for people with physical handicaps. These products include automatic injectors and jet spray injectors. Prefilled syringes are useful for people who are visually impaired or traveling. Prefilled syringes are stable for up to 30 days if stored in the refrigerator.

Preparing the Injection. The vial of insulin in use may be kept at room temperature for up to 4 weeks. Stored vials should be kept in the refrigerator and brought to room temperature prior to administration.

Regular insulin does not require mixing. If the solution is cloudy or discolored, the vial should be discarded. The other types of insulin must be mixed to disperse the particles evenly throughout the solution. Mix the vial by gently rolling it between the hands; vigorous shaking causes bubble formation and frothing, which makes the dose inaccurate. It is critical that no air bubbles remain in the prepared dose, because even a small bubble can displace several units of insulin.

Sites of Injection. Although in theory any area of the body with subcutaneous tissue can be used for injections of insulin, certain sites are recommended (Figure 20–4 ■). The rate of absorption and peak of action of insulin differ according to the site. The site

Figure 20–4 ■ Sites of insulin injection.

that allows the most rapid absorption is the abdomen, followed by the deltoid muscle, then the thigh, and then the hip. Because of the rapid absorption, the abdomen is the recommended site. See Box 20–2 for techniques to minimize painful injections.

When administering insulin, gently pinch a fold of skin and inject the needle at a 90-degree angle. If the person is very thin, a 45-degree angle may be required to avoid injecting into muscle. Routine aspiration to check for blood is not necessary. Do not massage the site after administering the injection, because this may interfere with absorption; pressure, however, may be applied for about 1 minute. Rotation of injection sites is recommended for clients using pork insulin; rotation within sites is recommended for those using human or purified pork insulin. The distance between injections should be about 1 inch (avoiding the area within a 2-inch radius around the umbilicus).

BOX 20–2 Techniques to Minimize Painful Injections

- Inject insulin that is at room temperature.
- Make sure no air bubbles remain in the syringe before the injection.
- Wait until alcohol on the skin completely dries before the injection.
- Relax muscles in the injection area.
- Penetrate the skin with the needle quickly.
- Don't change the direction of the needle during insertion or withdrawal.
- Don't reuse dull needles.

Source: Adapted from "Insulin Administration" by the American Diabetes Association, 1998, *Diabetes Care, 21* (Supplement 1), 572–575.

Insulin should not be injected into an area to be exercised (such as the thigh before a vigorous walk) or to which heat will be applied; exercise or heat may increase the rate of absorption and cause a more rapid onset and peak of action.

Lipodystrophy. **Lipodystrophy** (hypertrophy of subcutaneous tissue) or **lipoatrophy** (atrophy of subcutaneous tissue) may result if the same injection sites are used repeatedly, especially with pork and beef insulins. The tissues become hardened and have an orange-peel appearance. The use of refrigerated insulin may trigger the development of tissue atrophy or hypertrophy. These problems rarely occur with the use of human insulins. Lipodystrophy and lipoatrophy alter insulin absorption, delaying its onset or retaining the insulin in the tissue for a period of time instead of allowing it to be absorbed into the body. Lipodystrophy usually resolves if the area is unused for a minimum of 6 months.

Mixing Insulins. When a person with diabetes requires more than one type of insulin, mixing is recommended to avoid administering two injections per dose. Two different concentrations are administered, because a single dose of intermediate-acting or long-acting insulin rarely provides adequate control of blood glucose levels. The procedure for mixing insulins is described in Box 20–3. Following are some general guidelines:

- Commercially mixed insulins are recommended if the insulin ratio is appropriate for the requirements of the client.
- Regular insulin may be mixed with all types of insulin except glargine; it may be injected immediately after mixing or stored for future use.
- NPH insulin and PZI insulin may be mixed only with regular insulin.
- Do not mix human and animal insulins.
- Always withdraw regular insulin first to avoid contaminating the regular insulin with intermediate-acting insulin.

Insulin Regimens. The appropriate insulin dosage is individualized by achieving a balance among insulin, diet, and exercise. For most people with diabetes, the timing of insulin action requires two or more injections each day, often a mixture of rapid-acting and intermediate-acting insulins. Timing of the injections depends on blood glucose levels, food consumption, exercise, and types of insulin used. The objective is to avoid daytime hypoglycemia while achieving adequate blood glucose control overnight. Typical insulin regimens are discussed in Table 20–4.

HYPERSENSITIVITY RESPONSES When injected, insulin may cause local and systemic hypersensitivity responses. Manifestations of local reactions are a hardening and reddening of the area that develops over several hours. Local reactions result from a contaminant in the insulin and are more likely to occur when less purified insulin products are used.

Systemic reactions occur rapidly and are characterized by widespread red, intensely pruritic welts. Respiratory difficulty may occur if the respiratory system is involved. Systemic responses are due to an allergy to the insulin itself and are most common with beef insulin. The client can be desensitized by

BOX 20–3 Mixing Insulins: 10 Units of Regular and 20 Units of NPH

1. Wash hands.
2. Inspect regular insulin for clarity.
3. Gently rotate NPH insulin to mix well.
4. Wipe off the top of both vials with an alcohol pad.
5. Draw 20 units of air into the syringe, and inject air into the NPH vial (Figure A). Withdraw needle.
6. Draw 10 units of air into the syringe, and inject air into the regular vial (Figure B).
7. Invert the vial, and withdraw 10 units of regular insulin (Figure C). Withdraw the needle.
8. Insert the needle into the NPH vial, and carefully withdraw 20 units of NPH insulin (Figure D).
9. Administer the insulin.
10. Wash hands, and properly dispose of the syringe.

A Injecting air into the NPH vial.

B Injecting air into the regular insulin vial.

C Withdrawing regular insulin.

D Withdrawing NPH insulin.

administering small doses of purified pork or human insulin, followed by progressively larger doses.

HYPOGLYCEMIC AGENTS Hypoglycemic agents are used to treat people with type 2 DM. Nursing implications for this category of drugs are discussed in the Medication Administration box on page 578. These medications lower blood sugar by stimulating or increasing insulin secretion, preventing breakdown of glycogen to glucose by the liver, and increasing peripheral uptake of glucose by making cells less resistant to insulin. Peripheral uptake refers to uptake by muscles and fat in the arms and legs rather than in the trunk. Some hypoglycemics keep blood sugar low by blocking absorption of carbohydrates in the intestines. A new hypoglycemic that is not insulin but is only available as an injectable is exenatide (Byetta). It has several modes of action: (1) signals the pancreas to make insulin when nutrients are ingested and stop insulin release as blood sugar normalizes, (2) stops liver conversion of glycogen to glucose, and (3) decreases absorption of sugar from the intestines. The goal of therapy with these agents is to reduce glycosylated hemoglobin and lower fasting and postprandial glucose (Capriotti, 2005).

ASPIRIN THERAPY People with diabetes are up to four times more likely to die from cardiovascular disease. It is recommended that a once daily dose of 81 to 325 mg of enteric-coated aspirin be given to reduce atherosclerosis in clients with vascular disease or increased cardiovascular risk factors. Aspirin therapy is contraindicated for clients with aspirin allergy,

bleeding tendency, anticoagulant therapy, recent gastrointestinal bleeding, or active liver disease (ADA, 2003).

Nutrition

The management of diabetes requires a careful balance between the intake of nutrients, the expenditure of energy, and the dose and timing of insulin or oral antidiabetic agents. Although everyone has the same need for basic nutrition, the person with diabetes must eat a more structured diet to prevent hyperglycemia. The goals for dietary management for adults with diabetes, based on guidelines established by the ADA (2002), are as follows:

■ Maintain as near normal blood glucose levels as possible by balancing food intake with insulin or oral glucose.
■ Achieve optimal serum lipid levels.
■ Provide adequate calories to maintain or attain reasonable weights, and to recover from catabolic illness.
■ Prevent and treat the acute complications of insulin-treated DM, short-term illnesses, and exercise-related problems; or the long-term complications of diabetes.
■ Improve overall health through optimal nutrition, using Dietary Guidelines for Americans and the Food Guide Pyramid (see Chapter 2 ∞).

CARBOHYDRATES The ADA recommends that carbohydrates should be individualized to the client's needs, with recommended allowances of 45% to 65% of the daily diet. Carbohydrates contain 4 kcal per gram and intake should not be restricted to less than 130 g/day (Sheard et al., 2004). This group of nutrients consists

TABLE 20–4 Insulin Regimens

REGIMEN	INSULIN TYPE*	GENERAL INFORMATION
One injection per day *Insulin effect graph: Regular, NPH curves across Breakfast, Lunch, Dinner, Snack*	NPH or NPH/R before breakfast	One injection is used to cover all meals (see figure at left). This is a simple regimen, but it is often difficult to control FBG levels, and afternoon hypoglycemia may result from increases in NPH.
Two injections per day *Insulin effect graph: Regular, NPH, Regular, NPH curves across Breakfast, Lunch, Dinner, Snack*	NPH or NPH/R before breakfast and dinner	This regimen is the least complex of those aiming to mimic normal pancreatic function; the person must have a fairly rigid schedule of food intake and exercise.
Three or four injections per day *Insulin effect graph: Regular, Regular, Regular, NPH curves across Breakfast, Lunch, Dinner, Snack*	R before each meal; NPH at dinner or bedtime	This regimen more closely mimics normal pancreatic function; it allows greater choice in mealtimes and exercise (see figure at left). However, each prandial dose of R must be determined by blood glucose tests.

*Insulin types are abbreviated as follows: NPH = intermediate acting, R = regular, rapid acting.

of plant foods (grains, fruits, vegetables), milk, and some dairy products. Carbohydrates can be divided into simple sugars and complex carbohydrates. Glycemic index is the rate a food raises blood glucose and, thus, insulin. Proponents of low-carbohydrate diets use glycemic index as the scientific foundation for decreasing intake of foods with a high glycemic index. However, many factors affect the digestion of carbohydrates; to date research does not support using glycemic index as a basis for therapy. The ADA does not recommend reliance on glycemic index as a method to treat or prevent diabetes (ADA, 2006).

The use of sucrose as part of the total carbohydrate content in the diet does not impair blood glucose control in people with diabetes. Sucrose and sucrose-containing foods must be substi-

tuted for other carbohydrates gram for gram. Dietary fructose (from fruits and vegetables or from fructose-sweetened foods) produces a smaller rise in plasma glucose than sucrose and most starches, so it may offer an advantage as a sweetening agent. However, large amounts of fructose have potentially adverse effects on serum cholesterol and LDL cholesterol, so amounts used should be controlled.

PROTEIN The recommended daily protein intake is 15% to 20% of total daily kilocalorie intake. Protein has 4 kcal per gram. Sources of protein should be low in fat, low in saturated fat, and low in cholesterol. Although this amount of protein is much less than that which most people normally consume, it is

MEDICATION ADMINISTRATION Oral Hypoglycemic Agents

SULFONYLUREAS
Glimepiride (Amaryl)
Glipizide (Glucotrol, Glucotrol XL)
Glyburide (Diabeta, Micronase)
Tolazamide (Tolinase)
Tolbutamide (Orinase)

These drugs are used primarily to treat mild, nonketotic type 2 DM in people who are not obese. Glimepiride, glipizide, and glyburide, are 100 to 200 times more potent than tolbutamide. These clients cannot control the symptoms by diet alone, but they do not require insulin. The drugs act by stimulating the pancreatic cells to secrete more insulin and by increasing the sensitivity of peripheral tissues to insulin. Dose adjustments must be made gradually and therefore these drugs are not useful for meeting acute changes that occur in illness or surgery. The most common side effect is hypoglycemia and this is exacerbated by NPO status. These drugs are usually suspended during hospitalization (ADA, 2005).

MEGLITINIDES
Repaglinide (Prandin)

This drug lowers blood glucose levels by stimulating release of insulin from the pancreatic islet cells.

BIGUANIDES
Metformin (Glucophage)

Metformin reduces both the FBG and the degree of postprandial hyperglycemia in clients with type 2 DM. It primarily decreases the overproduction of glucose by the liver, and may also make insulin more effective in peripheral tissues. If renal insufficiency develops, metformin must be discontinued. It is used as an adjunct to diet, especially in clients who are obese or not responding to the sulfonylureas. Because of an increased risk of metformin-induced lactic acidosis, metformin is usually suspended during hospitalization. It should be discontinued temporarily before and after using contrast media for diagnostic imaging and anesthesia (Capriotti, 2005).

In recent studies, metformin has been successful in preventing diabetes. In the Diabetes Prevention Program, people treated with metformin reduced their risk of developing diabetes by 31% over 3 years. Treatment with metformin was most effective among younger, heavier people (those 25 to 40 years of age who were 50 to 80 pounds overweight) and less effective among older people and people who were not as overweight. Lifestyle changes including diet and regular moderate exercise were part of preventing or delaying the onset of diabetes.

ALPHA-GLUCOSIDE INHIBITORS
Acarbose (Precose)
Miglitol (Glyset)

These drugs work locally in the small intestine to slow carbohydrate digestion and delay glucose absorption. As a result, postprandial glucose and glycosylated hemoglobin are better controlled, reducing the risk of long-term complications. Like metformin, acarbose administered to those with prediabetes reduced the risk of developing diabetes by 25% over 3 years. In addition to preventing progression from IGT to diabetes, the combination of lifestyle changes and medications facilitated return to normal glucose tolerance (www.cdc.gov/diabetes/pubs/general.htm).

THIAZOLIDINEDIONES
Rosiglitazone (Avandia)
Pioglitazone (Actos)

This class of drugs acts by sensitizing peripheral tissue to insulin. Both drugs can be used alone or in combination with sulfonylureas, metformin, and insulin. These drugs increase intravascular volume and therefore create problems for anyone with acute coronary ischemia or CHF.

D-Phenylalanine (Amino Acid) Derivative
Nateglinide (Starlix)
Repaglinide (Prandin)

This is a new class of oral medications for treatment of type 2 diabetes. They stimulate rapid and short insulin secretion from the pancreatic beta cells to decrease spikes in glucose following meals and also reduce the overall blood glucose level. They should be taken shortly before meals; without a meal, hypoglycemia is a risk.

Nursing Responsibilities
- Assess clients taking oral hypoglycemic agents closely for the first 7 days to determine therapeutic response.
- Administer the drug with food.
- Teach the client the importance of maintaining a prescribed diet and exercise program.
- Monitor for hypoglycemia if the client is also taking nonsteroidal anti-inflammatory agents (NSAIDs), sulfonamide antibiotics, ranitidine, cimetidine, or beta blockers; these drugs intensify the action of sulfonylureas.
- Monitor for hyperglycemia if the client is also taking calcium channel blockers, oral contraceptives, glucocorticoids, phenothiazines, or thiazide diuretics; these drugs decrease the hypoglycemic responses to sulfonylureas.
- Do not administer these drugs to pregnant or lactating women.
- Assess for side effects: nausea, heartburn, diarrhea, dizziness, fever, headache, jaundice, skin rash, urticaria, photophobia, thrombocytopenia, leukopenia, or anemia.
- If the client is to have a thyroid test, determine whether the drug has been taken; sulfonylureas interfere with the uptake of radioactive iodine.
- Monitor for hypoglycemia with concurrent administration of an oral antidiabetic agent and insulin.
- Temporarily hold metformin for 2 days prior to injection of any radiocontrast agent to avoid potential lactic acidosis if renal failure occurs.
- Closely monitor liver function tests with administration of rosiglitazone and pioglitazone.

Health Education for the Client and Family
- Maintain prescribed diet and exercise regimen.
- You may need insulin if you have surgery, trauma, fever, or infection.
- Follow instructions to monitor blood glucose.
- Report illness or side effects to the healthcare provider.
- Undergo periodic laboratory evaluations as prescribed by your healthcare provider.
- Avoid alcohol intake, which may cause a reaction involving flushing, palpitations, and nausea.
- The medication interferes with the effectiveness of oral contraceptives; other birth control measures may be required.
- Mild symptoms of hyperglycemia may appear if a different agent is begun.
- Take medications as prescribed; for example, once a day at the same time each day. If you are taking acarbose, take the pill with the first bite of food at breakfast, lunch, and dinner.

recommended to help prevent or delay renal complications. To help the client accept the decrease in the amount of protein, the nurse may suggest a less severe restriction at diagnosis with a gradual decrease to take place over a period of years.

FATS Dietary fats should be low in saturated fat and cholesterol. Saturated fats should be no higher than 10% of the total kilocalories allowed per day, with dietary cholesterol less than 300 mg per day. Fat has 9 kcal per gram. Sources of the different types of fat include:

- *Saturated fat.* Sources are animal meats (meat and butter fats, lard, bacon), cocoa butter, coconut oil, palm oil, and hydrogenated oils.
- *Polyunsaturated fat.* Sources are oils of corn, safflower, sunflower, soybean, sesame seed, and cottonseed.
- *Monosaturated fat.* Sources are peanut oil, olive oil, and canola oil.

Limiting fat and cholesterol intake may help prevent or delay the onset of atherosclerosis, a common complication of diabetes.

FIBER Dietary fiber may be helpful in treating or preventing constipation and other gastrointestinal disorders, including colon cancer. It also helps provide a feeling of fullness, and large amounts of soluble fiber may be beneficial to serum lipids. Soluble fiber is found in dried beans, oats, barley, and in some vegetables and fruits (e.g., peas, corn, zucchini, cauliflower, broccoli, prunes, pears, apples, bananas, oranges). Insoluble fiber, which is found in wheat, corn, and in some vegetables and fruits (e.g., carrots, brussels sprouts, eggplant, green beans, pears, apples, strawberries), does facilitate intestinal motility and give a feeling of fullness.

The ideal level of fiber has not been determined, but an intake of 20 to 35 grams per day is recommended. An increase in fiber may cause nausea, diarrhea, or constipation, and increased flatulence, especially if the person does not also increase fluid intake. Fiber in the diet should therefore be increased gradually.

SODIUM Although the body requires sodium, most people consume much more than is needed each day, especially in processed foods. The recommended daily intake is 1000 mg of sodium per 1000 kcal, not to exceed 3000 mg. The primary concern with sodium is its association with hypertension, a common health problem in people with diabetes. It is suggested that table salt (which is 40% sodium) and processed foods high in sodium be avoided in the diabetes meal plan.

SWEETENERS The diet plan for people with diabetes restricts the amount of refined sugars. As a result, many people use noncaloric sweeteners and foods or drinks made with noncaloric sweeteners. Commercially produced nonnutritive sweeteners are approved for use by the FDA. Although questions have been raised about the safety of these substances in laboratory animal studies, they are considered safe for use by humans. Included in this category of sweeteners are saccharin (Sweet & Low), aspartame or neotame (Nutrasweet, Equal), sucralose (Splenda), and acesulfame potassium (Sunnette). The nonnutritive sweeteners have negligent amounts of or no kilocalories, do not produce dental caries, and produce very little or no changes in blood glucose levels.

People with diabetes also use nutritive sweeteners, including fructose, sorbitol, and xylitol. The kilocalorie content of these substances is similar to that of table sugar (sucrose), but they cause less elevation in blood glucose. They are often included in foods labeled as "sugar free." Sorbitol may cause flatulence and diarrhea.

Researchers are continuing to study the safety and effectiveness of the sweeteners. In addition, the FDA recommends that the food industry label products with the amount of each ingredient in milligrams per serving and the number of servings per container. When teaching clients about diet, the nurse should include information about the kilocalorie content of sweeteners and the meaning of such phrases as *sugar free* and *dietetic* on labels.

ALCOHOL Although drinking alcoholic beverages is not encouraged, neither is it totally prohibited for the client with diabetes. Alcohol consumption may potentiate the hypoglycemic effects of insulin and oral agents. The ADA recommends that men with diabetes consume no more than two drinks and women with diabetes no more than one drink per day. In the following list are guidelines for people who include alcohol in their diet plan:

- The signs of intoxication and hypoglycemia are similar; thus, the person with type 1 DM is at increased risk for an insulin reaction.
- Two oral hypoglycemic agents (chlorpropamide and tolbutamide) may interact with the alcohol, causing headache, flushing, and nausea.
- Liqueurs, sweet wines, wine coolers, and sweet mixes contain large amounts of carbohydrate.
- Light beer is the recommended alcoholic drink.
- Alcohol should be consumed with meals and added to the daily food intake. In most instances, the alcohol is substituted for fat in calculating the diet; a drink with 1.5 oz of alcohol is the equivalent of two fat exchanges (90 kcal). (Food exchanges are discussed below.)

MEAL PLANNING Several different systems for meal planning are available to the person with diabetes. These systems include a consistent-carbohydrate diabetes meal plan, exchange lists, point systems, food groups, carbohydrate counting, and calorie counting. No matter what system is used, however, it must take into account the person's individualized eating habits, diet history, food values, and special needs. Altering foods and meal patterns is often one of the most difficult parts of diabetes management; careful consideration of individualized preferences enhances compliance with the diet. Although the ADA recommends that a registered dietitian provide the nutrition prescription, nurses must know what is prescribed and be able to reinforce teaching and answer questions.

Consistent-Carbohydrate Diabetes Meal Plan The consistent-carbohydrate diabetes meal plan, which is replacing the traditional exchange list plan, focuses on carbohydrate content. The client eats a similar amount of carbohydrates at each meal or snack each day, based on an individual diet prescription and the Food Guide Pyramid. Carbohydrates in a meal have the most effect on postprandial (after meals) blood glucose levels. They also determine, to a greater extent than do proteins and fats, insulin requirements before meals. Clients should be taught to count carbohydrates so they can administer 1 unit of regular insulin or insulin lispro for each 10 or 15 g of carbohydrate eaten at a meal. This method provides a better connection between food, medications, and exercise.

The Exchange Lists The exchange list diet is based on the person's ideal (or reasonable) weight, activity level, age, and occupation. These factors determine the total kilocalories that the person may consume each day. After the calories have been determined, the proportions of carbohydrates, proteins, and fats are calculated, using guidelines established by the American Diabetes Association and the American Dietetic Association.

The distribution of foods throughout the day is based on exchange lists. The name and quantity of food that make up one exchange (or serving) are listed; standard household measurements are used. One food portion on the list can be substituted ("exchanged") for another with very little difference in calories or amount of carbohydrates, proteins, and fats. The meal plan prescribes how many exchanges are allowed for each food group per meal and snacks.

Diet Plan for Type 1 Diabetes Diet and insulin prescription must be integrated for optimal energy metabolism and the prevention of hyperglycemia or hypoglycemia. The goals of the diet plan are to achieve optimal glucose and lipid levels, improve overall health, and maintain reasonable body weight. To meet these goals, the following strategies must be implemented:

■ Glucose regulation requires correlating eating patterns with insulin onset and peak of action.
■ Meals, snacks, and insulin regimens should be based on the person's lifestyle.
■ Meal planning depends on the specific insulin regimen prescribed.
■ Snacks are an important consideration in relation to the amount and timing of exercise.
■ The diet plan must consider the availability of foods, based on occupational, financial, religious, and ethnic constraints.
■ Self-monitoring of blood glucose levels helps the client make adjustments for planned and unplanned changes in routines.

Diet Plan for Type 2 Diabetes The goals of the diet plan are to improve blood glucose levels, improve overall health, prevent or delay complications, and attain or maintain reasonable body weight. Because the majority of these clients are overweight, weight loss is important and facilitates achieving the other goals.

There are no specific guidelines for the type 2 diet, but in addition to decreasing kilocalories, it is recommended that the client consume three meals of equal size, evenly spaced approximately 4 to 5 hours apart, with one or two snacks. The person with type 2 DM should also decrease fat intake. If the exchange list is difficult to use, calorie counting or designing the diet by grams of fat may be more useful.

SICK-DAY MANAGEMENT When the person with diabetes is sick or has surgery, blood glucose levels increase, even though food intake decreases. The person often mistakenly alters or

omits the insulin dose, causing further problems. The guidelines for dietary management during illness focus on preventing dehydration and providing nutrition for promoting recovery. In general, sick-day management includes the following:

■ Monitoring blood glucose at least four times a day throughout an illness
■ Testing urine for ketones if blood glucose is greater than 240 mg/dL
■ Continuing to take the usual insulin dose or oral hypoglycemic agent
■ Sipping 8 to 12 oz of fluid each hour
■ Substituting easily digested liquids or soft foods if solid foods are not tolerated (The substituted liquids and foods should be carbohydrate equivalents, for example, 1/2 cup sweetened gelatin, 1/2 cup fruit juice, one Popsicle, 1/4 cup sherbet, and 1/2 cup regular soft drink.)
■ Calling the healthcare provider if the client is unable to eat for more than 24 hours or if vomiting and diarrhea last for more than 6 hours.

DIET PLAN FOR THE OLDER ADULT The majority of older adults have type 2 DM and should follow the general guidelines for that diet plan. However, special considerations for the older adult are important if the diet plan is to be followed, including:

■ Dietary likes and dislikes
■ Who prepares the meals
■ Age-related changes in taste perception
■ Dental health
■ Transportation to buy foods
■ Available income.

Other factors to consider in planning the diet for the older adult include the age-related decline in kilocalorie requirements, decline in physical activity due to age and/or chronic illnesses, and the onset or progression of other chronic illnesses. The older adult who is overweight should reduce kilocalorie intake to ensure weight loss, but at the same time, careful monitoring for malnutrition is necessary. It is possible for the older adult to revert to normal glucose tolerance if ideal body weight is regained.

Exercise

The third component of diabetes management is a regular exercise program. The benefits of exercise are the same for everyone, with or without diabetes: improved physical fitness, improved emotional state, weight control, and improved work capacity. In people with diabetes, exercise increases the uptake of glucose by muscle cells, potentially reducing the need for insulin. Exercise also decreases cholesterol and triglycerides, reducing the risk of cardiovascular disorders. People with diabetes should consult their primary healthcare provider before beginning or changing an exercise program. The ability to maintain an exercise program is affected by many different factors, including fatigue and glucose levels. It is as important to assess the person's usual lifestyle before establishing an exercise program as it is before planning a diet. Factors to consider include the client's usual exercise habits, living environment, and community programs. The exercise that the person enjoys most is probably the one that he or she will continue throughout life.

Use proper footwear, inspect the feet daily and after exercise, avoid exercise in extreme heat or cold, and avoid exercise during periods of poor glucose control. Stress EKG tests to detect ischemia are no longer recommended in asymptomatic individuals at low CAD risk (<10% risk of a cardiac event over 10 years) (Sigal, Kenny, Wasserman, & Castaneda-Sceppa, 2004).

TYPE 1 DIABETES In the person with type 1 DM, glycemic responses to exercise vary according to the type, intensity, and duration of the exercise. Other factors that influence responses include the timing of exercise in relation to meals and insulin injections, and the time of day of the activity. Unless these factors are integrated into the exercise program, the person with type 1 DM has an increased risk of hypoglycemia and hyperglycemia. Following are general guidelines for an exercise program:

- People who have frequent hyperglycemia or hypoglycemia should avoid prolonged exercise until glucose control improves.
- The risk of exercise-induced hypoglycemia is lowest before breakfast, when free-insulin levels tend to be lower than they are before meals later in the day or at bedtime.
- Low-impact aerobic exercises are encouraged.
- Exercise should be moderate and regular; brief, intense exercise tends to cause mild hyperglycemia, and prolonged exercise can lead to hypoglycemia.
- Exercising at a peak insulin action time may lead to hypoglycemia.
- Self-monitoring of blood glucose levels is essential both before and after exercise.
- Food intake may need to be increased to compensate for the activity.
- Fluid intake, especially water, is essential.

Young adults may continue participating in sports with some modifications in diet and insulin dosage. Athletes should begin training slowly, extend activity over a prolonged period, take a carbohydrate source (such as a drink consisting of 5% to 10% carbohydrate) after about 1 hour of exercise, and monitor blood glucose levels for possible adjustments. In addition, a snack should be available after the activity is completed. It may be necessary to omit the usual regular insulin dose prior to an athletic event; even if the athlete is hyperglycemic at the beginning of the event, blood glucose levels will fall to normal after the first 60 to 90 minutes of exercise.

TYPE 2 DIABETES An exercise program for the person with type 2 DM is especially important. The benefits of regular exercise include weight loss in those who are overweight, improved glycemic control, increased well-being, socialization with others, and a reduction of cardiovascular risk factors. A combination of diet, exercise, and weight loss often decreases the need for oral hypoglycemic agents. This decrease is due to an increased sensitivity to insulin, increased kilocalorie expenditure, and increased self-esteem. Regular exercise may prevent type 2 DM in high-risk individuals (Roberts & Barnard, 2005).

Following are general guidelines for an exercise program:
- Before beginning the program, have a medical screening for previously undiagnosed hypertension, neuropathy, retinopathy, and nephropathy.

- Begin the program with mild exercises, and gradually increase intensity and duration.
- Self-monitor blood glucose before and after exercise.
- Exercise at least three times a week or every other day, for at least 20 to 30 minutes.
- Include muscle-strengthening and low-impact aerobic exercises in the program.

Treatments

SURGERY Surgical management of diabetes involves replacing or transplanting the pancreas, pancreatic cells, or beta cells. Although it is still in the investigative stage, many researchers believe that transplantation of the tail of the pancreas is the most promising technique for achieving long-term disease control. Islet cell transplantation has had moderate success, and research is continuing. Other research is being conducted in the use of an internally implanted artificial pancreas, or closed-loop artificial beta cell.

Surgery is a stressor that often alters self-management and glycemic control in people with diabetes. In response to stress, levels of catecholamines, cortisol, glucagon, and growth hormones increase, as does insulin resistance. Hyperglycemia occurs, and protein stores are decreased. In addition, diet and activity patterns change, and medication types and dosages vary. As a result, surgical clients who have diabetes are at increased risk for postoperative infection, delayed wound healing, fluid and electrolyte imbalances, hypoglycemia, and DKA (Aragon et al., 2003).

Preoperatively, all clients should be in the best possible metabolic state. Screening for complications and regular blood glucose monitoring are part of preoperative preparation. Oral hypoglycemic agents may be withheld for 1 or 2 days before surgery, and regular insulin is often administered to the client with type 2 DM during the perioperative period. The client with type 1 DM follows a carefully prescribed insulin regimen individualized to specific needs.

The insulin regimen in the preoperative, intraoperative, and immediate postoperative periods is individualized and may involve any of the following:
- No intermediate- or long-acting insulin is given the day of surgery; regular insulin is given with intravenous glucose. When the client is NPO, short-acting insulin should not be given without intravenous glucose.
- Half of the usual intermediate- or long-acting insulin is given before surgery and the remaining half is given in the recovery room.
- The total daily dose of insulin is divided into four equal doses of regular insulin, and one dose is administered subcutaneously every 6 hours. An intravenous solution of 5% dextrose in 0.45% normal saline is administered for fluid replacement, and blood glucose monitoring precedes each insulin dose (Guthrie & Guthrie, 1997).
- Clients with type 1 DM or type 2 DM with preoperative blood glucose greater than 200 receive IV glucose and insulin infusion. The target blood glucose level during surgery is between 125 and 200 mg/dL. This avoids hypoglycemia,

which is difficult to detect under anesthesia, and prevents glycosuria, dehydration, and impaired wound healing. IV infusion of glucose, insulin, and added potassium is appropriate for all hyperglycemic patients undergoing surgery (Amiel & Alberti, 2005; Mabrey, 2004).

The surgical procedure should be scheduled for as early as possible in the morning to minimize the length of fasting. If there is no food intake after surgery, intravenous dextrose should be administered, accompanied by subcutaneous regular insulin every 6 hours. The dose can be adjusted to blood glucose levels. Although kilocalorie intake is decreased postoperatively, stress can increase insulin requirements. Glucose control is also affected postoperatively by nausea and vomiting, anorexia, and gastrointestinal suction.

During the postoperative period, the client with type 2 DM may continue to require insulin or may resume oral medications, depending on glucose control. The client with type 1 DM may require reduced insulin as healing progresses and stress diminishes. Regular blood glucose monitoring is essential, as are assessments for hypoglycemia.

COMPLICATIONS OF DIABETES

The person with DM, regardless of type, is at increased risk for complications involving many different body systems. Alterations in blood glucose levels, alterations in the cardiovascular system, neuropathies, an increased susceptibility to infection, and periodontal disease are common. In addition, the interaction of several complications can cause problems of the feet. The *Multisystem Effects of Diabetes Mellitus* illustration on the next page shows the progression from cardinal signs to acute and late complications for the client with diabetes. A discussion of each of these complications follows; related interdisciplinary care and nursing care are discussed later in the chapter.

Acute Complications: Alterations in Blood Glucose Levels

The following discussion provides additional information about hyperglycemia and hypoglycemia. Table 20–5 compares DKA, HHS, and hypoglycemia.

Hyperglycemia

The major problems resulting from hyperglycemia in the person with diabetes are DKA and HHS. Two other problems are the dawn phenomenon and the Somogyi phenomenon.

The **dawn phenomenon** is a rise in blood glucose between 4 A.M. and 8 A.M. that is not a response to hypoglycemia. This condition occurs in people with both type 1 and type 2 DM. The exact cause is unknown but is believed to be related to nocturnal increases in growth hormone, which decreases peripheral uptake of glucose. The **Somogyi phenomenon** is a combination of hypoglycemia during the night with a rebound morning rise in blood glucose to hyperglycemic levels. The hyperglycemia stimulates the counterregulatory hormones, which stimulate gluconeogenesis and glycogenolysis and also inhibit

peripheral glucose use. This may cause insulin resistance for 12 to 48 hours (McCance & Huether, 2002).

DIABETIC KETOACIDOSIS As the pathophysiology of untreated type 1 DM continues, the insulin deficit causes fat stores to break down, resulting in continued hyperglycemia and mobilization of fatty acids with a subsequent ketosis. **Diabetic ketoacidosis (DKA)** develops when there is an absolute deficiency of insulin and an increase in the insulin counterregulatory hormones. Glucose production by the liver increases, peripheral glucose use decreases, fat mobilization increases, and ketogenesis (ketone formation) is stimulated. Increased glucagon levels activate the gluconeogenic and ketogenic pathways in the liver. In the presence of insulin deficiency, hepatic overproduction of beta-hydroxybutyrate and acetoacetic acids (ketone bodies) causes increased ketone concentrations and an increased release of free fatty acids. As a result of a loss of bicarbonate (which occurs when the ketone is formed), bicarbonate buffering does not occur, and a metabolic acidosis occurs, called DKA. Depression of the central nervous system from the accumulation of ketones and the resulting acidosis may cause coma and death if left untreated (Porth, 2005). See Figure 20–5 ■.

DKA also may occur in a person with diagnosed diabetes when energy requirements increase during physical or emotional stress. Stress states initiate the release of gluconeogenic hormones, resulting in the formation of carbohydrates from protein or fat. The person who is sick, has an infection, or who decreases or omits insulin doses is at a greatly increased risk for developing DKA.

DKA involves four metabolic problems:

- Hyperosmolarity from hyperglycemia and dehydration
- Metabolic acidosis from an accumulation of ketoacids
- Extracellular volume depletion from osmotic diuresis
- Electrolyte imbalances (such as loss of potassium and sodium) from osmotic diuresis.

Manifestations of DKA result from severe dehydration and acidosis. These manifestations are summarized in the box on page 585. Laboratory findings include the following:

- Blood glucose levels higher than 250 mg/dL
- Plasma pH less than 7.3
- Plasma bicarbonate less than 15 mEq/L
- Presence of serum ketones
- Presence of urine ketones and glucose
- Abnormal levels of serum sodium, potassium, and chloride.

Treatment of DKA DKA requires immediate medical attention. Admission to the hospital is appropriate when the person has a blood glucose of greater than 250 mg/dL, a decreasing pH, and ketones in the urine. If the client is alert and conscious, fluids may be replaced orally. In the first 12 hours of treatment, adults usually require 8 to 10 L of fluid to replace losses from polyuria and vomiting (Lehne, 2004). However, alterations in level of consciousness, vomiting, and acidosis are common, necessitating intravenous fluid replacement. The initial fluid replacement may be accomplished by administering 0.9% saline solution at a rate of 500 to 1000 mL/h. After 2 to 3 hours

MULTISYSTEM EFFECTS OF Diabetes Mellitus

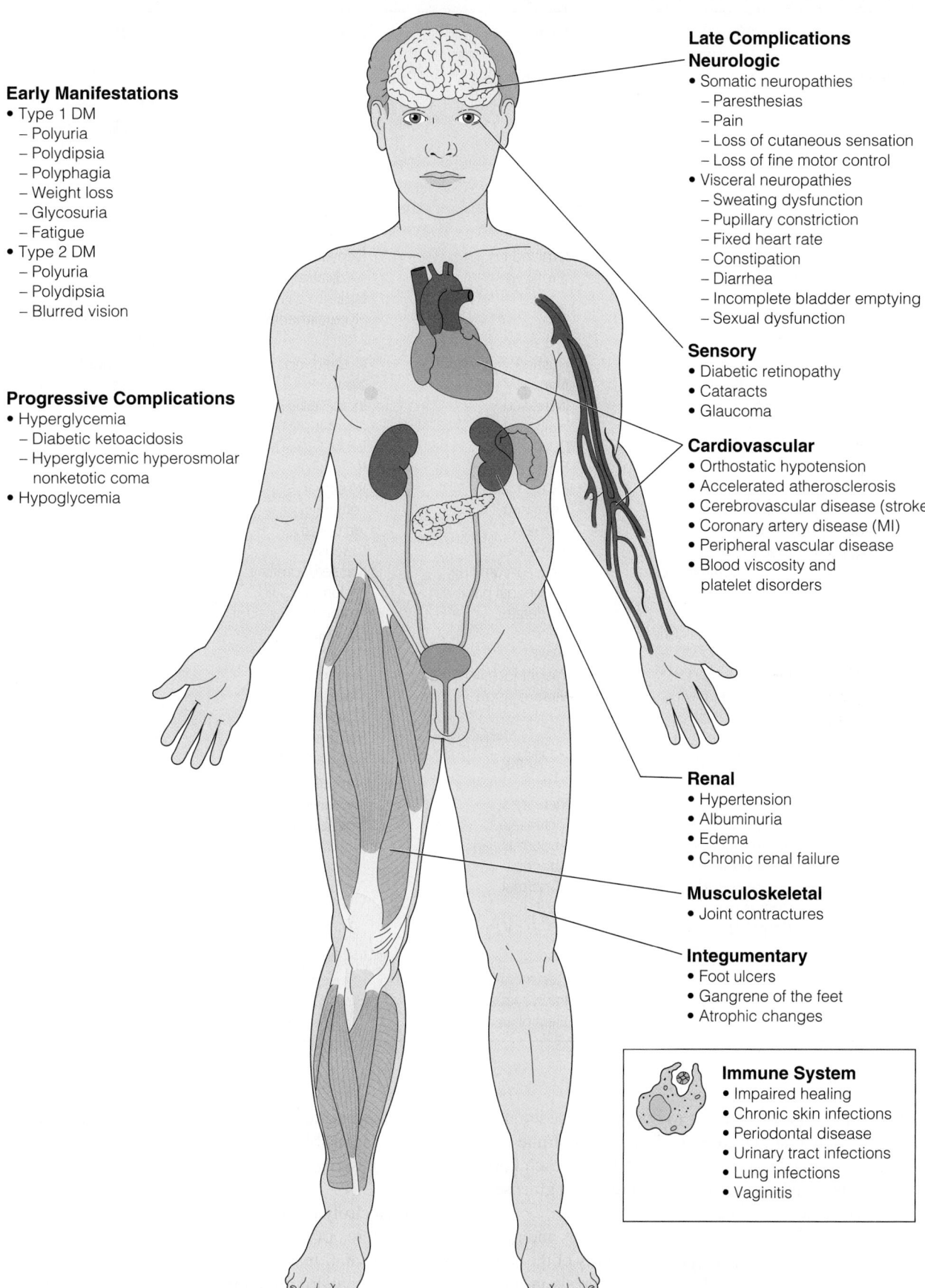

Early Manifestations
- Type 1 DM
  - Polyuria
  - Polydipsia
  - Polyphagia
  - Weight loss
  - Glycosuria
  - Fatigue
- Type 2 DM
  - Polyuria
  - Polydipsia
  - Blurred vision

Progressive Complications
- Hyperglycemia
  - Diabetic ketoacidosis
  - Hyperglycemic hyperosmolar nonketotic coma
- Hypoglycemia

Late Complications

Neurologic
- Somatic neuropathies
  - Paresthesias
  - Pain
  - Loss of cutaneous sensation
  - Loss of fine motor control
- Visceral neuropathies
  - Sweating dysfunction
  - Pupillary constriction
  - Fixed heart rate
  - Constipation
  - Diarrhea
  - Incomplete bladder emptying
  - Sexual dysfunction

Sensory
- Diabetic retinopathy
- Cataracts
- Glaucoma

Cardiovascular
- Orthostatic hypotension
- Accelerated atherosclerosis
- Cerebrovascular disease (stroke)
- Coronary artery disease (MI)
- Peripheral vascular disease
- Blood viscosity and platelet disorders

Renal
- Hypertension
- Albuminuria
- Edema
- Chronic renal failure

Musculoskeletal
- Joint contractures

Integumentary
- Foot ulcers
- Gangrene of the feet
- Atrophic changes

Immune System
- Impaired healing
- Chronic skin infections
- Periodontal disease
- Urinary tract infections
- Lung infections
- Vaginitis

TABLE 20–5 DKA, HHS, and Hypoglycemia Comparison

		DKA	HHS	HYPOGLYCEMIA
Diabetes Type		Primary type 1	Type 2	Both
Onset		Slow	Slow	Rapid
Cause		↓ Insulin	↓ Insulin	↑ Insulin
		Infection	Older age	Omitted meal/snack
				Error in insulin dose
Risk Factors		Surgery	Surgery	Surgery
		Trauma	Trauma	Trauma
		Illness	Illness	Illness
		Omitted insulin	Dehydration	Exercise
		Stress	Medications	Medications
			Dialysis	Lipodystrophy
			Hyperalimentation	Renal failure
				Alcohol intake
Assessments	Skin	Flushed; dry; warm	Flushed; dry; warm	Pallor; moist; cool
	Perspiration	None	None	Profuse
	Thirst	Increased	Increased	Normal
	Breath	Fruity	Normal	Normal
	Vital signs	BP ↓	BP ↓	BP ↓
		P ↑	P ↑	P ↑
		R Kussmaul's	R normal	R normal
	Mental status	Confused	Lethargic	Anxious; restless
	Thirst	Increased	Increased	Normal
	Fluid intake	Increased	Increased	Normal
	Gastrointestinal effects	Nausea/vomiting; abdominal pain	Nausea/vomiting; abdominal pain	Hunger
	Fluid loss	Moderate	Profound	Normal
	Level of consciousness	Decreasing	Decreasing	Decreasing
	Energy level	Weak	Weak	Fatigue
	Other	Weight loss	Weight loss	Headache
		Blurred vision	Malaise	Altered vision
			Extreme thirst	Mood changes
			Seizures	Seizures
Laboratory Findings	Blood glucose	>300 mg/dL	>600 mg/dL	<50 mg/dL
	Plasma ketones	Increased	Normal	Normal
	Urine glucose	Increased	Increased	Normal
	Urine ketones	Increased	Normal	Normal
	Serum potassium	Abnormal	Abnormal	Normal
	Serum sodium	Abnormal	Abnormal	Normal
	Serum chloride	Abnormal	Abnormal	Normal
	Plasma pH	<7.3	Normal	Normal
	Osmolality	>340 mOsm/L	>340 mOsm/L	Normal
Treatment		Insulin	Insulin	Glucagon
		Treatment	Intravenous fluids	Rapid-acting carbohydrate
		Intravenous fluids	Electrolytes	Intravenous solution of
		Electrolytes		50% glucose

(or when blood pressure is returning to normal), the administration of 0.45% saline at 200 to 500 mL/h may continue for several more hours. When the blood glucose levels reach 250 mg/dL, dextrose is added to prevent rapid decreases in glucose; hypoglycemia could result in fatal cerebral edema.

Regular insulin is used in the management of DKA and may be given by various routes, depending on the severity of the condition. Mild ketosis may be treated with subcutaneous insulin,

whereas severe ketosis requires intravenous insulin infusion. Nursing responsibilities for the client receiving intravenous insulin are described in the Medication Administration box on page 586.

The electrolyte imbalance of primary concern is depletion of body stores of potassium. Initially, serum potassium levels may be normal, but they decrease during treatment. In DKA (and from rehydration), the body loses potassium from in-

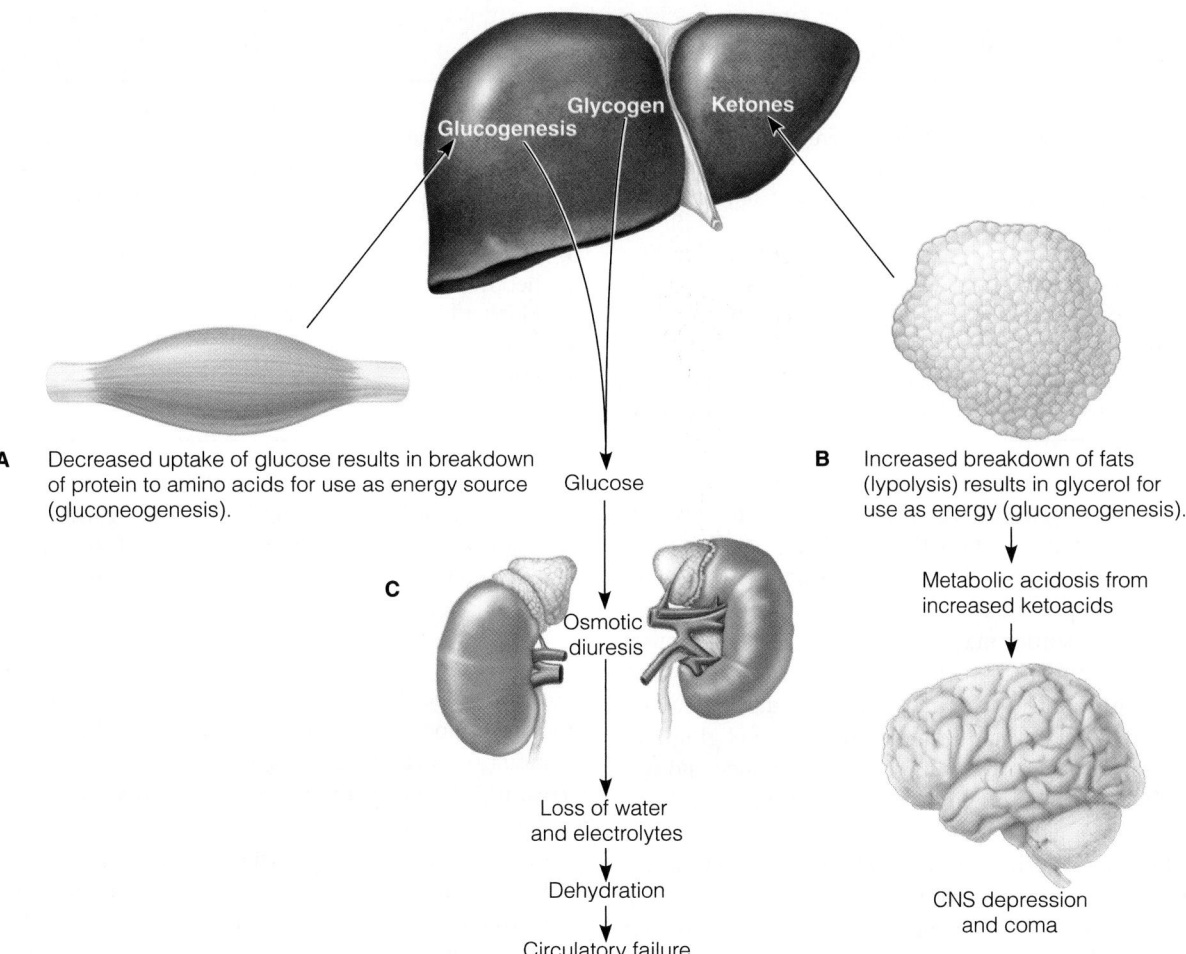

A Decreased uptake of glucose results in breakdown of protein to amino acids for use as energy source (gluconeogenesis).

Glucogenesis Glycogen Ketones

Glucose

B Increased breakdown of fats (lypolysis) results in glycerol for use as energy (gluconeogenesis).

Metabolic acidosis from increased ketoacids

C

Osmotic diuresis

Loss of water and electrolytes

Dehydration

Circulatory failure

CNS depression and coma

Figure 20–5 ■ In Type I diabetes mellitus, without adequate insulin, muscle (a) and fat (b) cells are metabolized to provide sources of energy. Amino acids from skeletal muscle are converted to glucose in the liver; glycerol from fat cells is converted to glucose and fatty acids (ketoacids) which cause CNS depression and coma. Increased glucose (c) causes osmotic diuresis leading to dehydration and decreased circulatory volume. These processes create the symptoms of diabetic ketoacidosis (DKA). The symptoms can be reversed with intravenous insulin to lower blood glucose. Blood pressure is raised to prevent circulatory failure by administering intravenous fluids; electrolytes are monitored and corrected.

MANIFESTATIONS of Diabetic Ketoacidosis (DKA)

DEHYDRATION (FROM HYPERGLYCEMIA)
- Thirst
- Warm, dry skin with poor turgor
- Soft eyeballs
- Dry mucous membranes
- Weakness
- Malaise
- Rapid, weak pulse
- Hypotension

METABOLIC ACIDOSIS (FROM KETOSIS)
- Nausea and vomiting
- Ketone (fruity, alcohol-like) breath odor
- Lethargy
- Coma

OTHER MANIFESTATIONS
- Abdominal pain (cause unknown)
- Kussmaul's respirations (increased rate and depth of respirations, with a longer expiration; a compensatory response to prevent a further decrease in pH)

creased urinary output, acidosis, catabolic state, and vomiting or diarrhea. Potassium replacement is begun early in the course of treatment, usually by adding potassium to the rehydration fluids. Replacement is essential for preventing cardiac dysrhythmias secondary to hypokalemia. Cardiac rhythms and potassium levels must be monitored every 2 to 4 hours.

HYPEROSMOLAR HYPERGLYCEMIC STATE (HHS) The metabolic problem called **hyperosmolar hyperglycemic state (HHS)** occurs in people who have type 2 DM. HHS is characterized by a plasma osmolarity of 340 mOsm/L or greater (the normal range is 280 to 300 mOsm/L), greatly elevated blood glucose levels (over 600 mg/dL and often 1000 to 2000 mg/dL), and altered levels of consciousness. HHS is a serious, life-threatening medical emergency and has a higher mortality rate than DKA. Mortality is high not only because the metabolic changes are serious but also because people with diabetes are usually older and have other medical problems that either

---

MEDICATION ADMINISTRATION **Intravenous Insulin**

GENERAL GUIDELINES

- Regular insulin may be given undiluted directly into the vein or through a Y-tube or three-way stopcock.
- Insulin is usually diluted in 0.9% saline or 0.45% saline solution for infusion.
- The glass or plastic infusion container and plastic tubing may reduce insulin potency by at least 20% and possibly by up to 80% before the insulin reaches the venous system.

Nursing Responsibilities

- Monitor blood glucose levels hourly.
- Infuse the insulin solution separately from the hydration solution.

- Flush the intravenous tubing with 50 mL of insulin mixed with normal saline solution to saturate binding sites on the tubing before administering the insulin to the client; this step increases the amount of insulin delivered over the first few hours.
- Do not discontinue the intravenous infusion until subcutaneous administration of insulin is resumed.
- Monitor for manifestations of hypoglycemia.
- Ensure that glucagons and D_{50} is readily available as an antidote for insulin overdose.

---

cause or are caused by HHS. The precipitating factors associated with HHS include infection, therapeutic agents, therapeutic procedures, acute illness, and chronic illness (Box 20–4). The most common precipitating factor is infection. The manifestations of this disorder may be slow to appear, with onset ranging from 24 hours to 2 weeks. The manifestations are initiated by hyperglycemia, which causes increased urine output. With increased output, plasma volume decreases and glomerular filtration rate drops. As a result, glucose is retained and water is lost. Glucose and sodium accumulate in the blood and increase serum osmolarity.

Serum hyperosmolarity results in severe dehydration, reducing intracellular water in all tissues, including the brain. The person has dry skin and mucous membranes, extreme thirst, and altered levels of consciousness (progressing from lethargy to coma). Neurologic deficits may include hyperthermia, motor and sensory impairment, positive Babinski's sign, and seizures. *Metabolic acidosis is not part of the pathology; despite elevated blood glucose, sufficient insulin is present to prevent metabolism of fats with the resulting fatty acids and ketones of DKA.* Treatment is directed toward correcting fluid and electrolyte imbalances, lowering blood glucose levels with insulin, and treating underlying conditions.

Treatment of HHS HHS is a serious, life-threatening metabolic condition. The client admitted to the ICU for treatment typically manifests blood glucose levels over 700 mg/dL, increased serum osmolarity, and altered levels of consciousness or seizures. Treatment is similar to that of DKA: correcting fluid and electrolyte imbalances and providing insulin to lower hyperglycemia. In general, treatment modalities include the following:

- Establishing and maintaining adequate ventilation
- Correcting shock with adequate intravenous fluids
- Instituting nasogastric suction if comatose to prevent aspiration
- Maintaining fluid volume with intravenous isotonic or colloid solutions
- Administering potassium intravenously to replace losses
- Administering insulin to reduce blood glucose, usually discontinuing administration when blood glucose levels reach 250 mg/dL (Because ketosis is not present, there is no need to continue insulin, as with DKA.)

Hypoglycemia

Hypoglycemia (low blood glucose levels) is common in people with type 1 DM and occasionally occurs in people with type 2 DM who are treated with oral hypoglycemic agents. This condition is often called insulin shock, **insulin reaction**, or "the lows" in clients with type 1 DM. Hypoglycemia results primarily from a mismatch between insulin intake (e.g., an error in insulin dose), physical activity, and carbohydrate availability (e.g., omitting a meal). The intake of alcohol and drugs such as chloramphenicol (Chloromycetin), Coumadin, monoamine oxidase inhibitors, probenecid (Benemid), salicylates, and sulfonamides can also cause hypoglycemia.

The manifestations of hypoglycemia (see the box on the next page) result from a compensatory autonomic nervous system (ANS) response and from impaired cerebral function due to a decrease in glucose available for use by the brain. The manifestations vary, particularly in older adults. The onset is sudden, and blood glucose is usually less than 45 to 60 mg/dL. Severe hypoglycemia may cause death.

BOX 20–4 Factors Associated with Hyperosmolar Hyperglycemic State

Therapeutic Agents
- Glucocorticoids
- Diuretics
- Beta-adrenergic blocking agents
- Immunosuppressants
- Chlorpromazine
- Diazoxide

Acute Illness
- Infection
- Gangrene
- Urinary infection
- Burns
- Gastrointestinal bleeding
- Myocardial infarction
- Pancreatitis
- Stroke

Therapeutic Procedures
- Peritoneal dialysis
- Hemodialysis
- Hyperosmolar alimentation (oral or parenteral)
- Surgery

Chronic Illness
- Renal disease
- Cardiac disease
- Hypertension
- Previous stroke
- Alcoholism

MANIFESTATIONS of Hypoglycemia

MANIFESTATIONS CAUSED BY RESPONSES OF THE AUTONOMIC NERVOUS SYSTEM

- Hunger
- Nausea
- Anxiety
- Pale, cool skin
- Sweating
- Shakiness
- Irritability
- Rapid pulse
- Hypotension

MANIFESTATIONS CAUSED BY IMPAIRED CEREBRAL FUNCTION

- Strange or unusual feelings
- Headache
- Difficulty in thinking
- Inability to concentrate
- Change in emotional behavior
- Slurred speech
- Blurred vision
- Decreasing levels of consciousness
- Seizures
- Coma

People who have type 1 DM for 4 or 5 years fail to secrete glucagon in response to a decrease in blood glucose. They then depend on epinephrine to serve as a counterregulatory response to hypoglycemia. However, this compensatory response can become absent or blunted. The person then develops a syndrome called *hypoglycemia unawareness*. The person does not experience symptoms of hypoglycemia, even though it is present. Because treatment is not initiated in the absence of symptoms, the person is likely to have episodes of severe hypoglycemia.

***TREATMENT OF HYPOGLYCEMIA* Mild Hypoglycemia** When mild hypoglycemia occurs, immediate treatment is necessary. People experiencing hypoglycemia should take about 15 g of a rapid-acting sugar. This amount of sugar is found, for example, in three glucose tablets, 1/2 cup of fruit juice or regular soda, 8 oz of skim milk, five Life Savers candies, three large marshmallows, or 3 tsp of sugar or honey. Sugar should not be added to fruit juice. Adding sugar to the fruit sugar already in the juice could cause a rapid rise in blood glucose, with persistent hyperglycemia.

If the manifestations continue, the 15/15 rule should be followed: Wait 15 minutes, monitor blood glucose, and, if it is low, eat another 15 g of carbohydrate. This procedure can be repeated until blood glucose levels return to normal (Haire-Joshu, 1996). People with diabetes should have some source of carbohydrate readily available at all times so that hypoglycemic symptoms can be quickly reversed. If hypoglycemia occurs more than two or three times a week, the diabetes management plan should be adjusted.

Severe Hypoglycemia People with diabetes who have severe hypoglycemia are often hospitalized. The criteria for hospitalization are one or more of the following:

- Blood glucose is less than 50 mg/dL, and the prompt treatment of hypoglycemia has not resulted in recovery of sensorium.
- The client has coma, seizures, or altered behavior.
- The hypoglycemia has been treated, but a responsible adult cannot be with the client for the following 12 hours.
- The hypoglycemia was caused by a sulfonylurea drug.

If the client is conscious and alert, 10 to 15 g of an oral carbohydrate may be given. If the client has altered levels of consciousness, parenteral glucose or glucagon is administered.

Glucose is administered intravenously as a 25% to 50% solution, usually at a rate of 10 mL over 1 minute by intravenous push, followed by intravenous infusion of 5% dextrose in water (D_5W) at 5 to 10 g/h (Haire-Joshu, 1996). This is the most rapid method of increasing blood glucose levels.

Glucagon is an antihypoglycemic agent that raises blood glucose by promoting the conversion of hepatic glycogen to glucose. It is used in severe insulin-induced hypoglycemia and may be given in the recommended dose of 1 mg by the subcutaneous, intramuscular, or intravenous route. Glucagon has a short period of action; an oral (if the client is conscious) or intravenous carbohydrate should be administered following the glucagon to prevent a recurrence of hypoglycemia. If the client has been unconscious, glucagon may cause vomiting when consciousness returns.

Chronic Complications

Alterations in the Cardiovascular System

The macrocirculation (large blood vessels) in people with diabetes undergoes changes due to atherosclerosis; abnormalities in platelets, red blood cells, and clotting factors; and changes in arterial walls. It has been established that atherosclerosis has an increased incidence and earlier age of onset in people with diabetes (although the reason is unknown). Other risk factors that contribute to the development of macrovascular disease of diabetes are hypertension, hyperlipidemia, cigarette smoking, and obesity. Alterations in the vascular system increase the risk of the long-term complications of coronary artery disease, cerebral vascular disease, and peripheral vascular disease.

Alterations in the microcirculation in the person with diabetes involve structural defects in the basement membrane of smaller blood vessels and capillaries. (The basement membrane is the structure that supports and serves as the boundary around the space occupied by epithelial cells.) These defects cause the capillary basement membrane to thicken, eventually resulting in decreased tissue perfusion. Changes in basement membranes are believed to be due to one or more of the following: the presence of increased amounts of sorbitol (a substance formed as an intermediate step in the conversion of glucose to fructose), the formation of abnormal glycoproteins, or problems in the release of oxygen from hemoglobin (Porth, 2005). The effects of alterations in the microcirculation affect all body tissues but are seen primarily in the eyes and the kidneys.

CORONARY ARTERY DISEASE Coronary artery disease is a major risk factor in the development of myocardial infarction in people with diabetes, especially in the middle to older adult with type 2 DM. Coronary artery disease is the most common cause of death in people with diabetes (NIH, 2004). People with diabetes who have myocardial infarction are more prone to develop congestive heart failure as a complication of the infarction and are also less likely to survive in the period immediately following the infarction. (Myocardial infarction is discussed in Chapter 31 ∞.)

HYPERTENSION Hypertension (blood pressure ≥140/90 mmHg) is a common complication of DM. It affects 20% to 60% of all people with diabetes, and is a major risk factor for cardiovascular disease and microvascular complications such as retinopathy and nephropathy. Hypertension may be reduced by weight loss, exercise, and decreasing sodium intake and alcohol consumption. If these methods are not effective, treatment with antihypertensive medications is necessary.

STROKE (CEREBROVASCULAR ACCIDENT) People with diabetes, especially older adults with type 2 DM, are 2 to 6 times more likely to have a stroke. Although the exact relationship between diabetes and cerebral vascular disease is unknown, hypertension (a risk factor for stroke) is a common health problem in those who have diabetes. In addition, atherosclerosis of the cerebral vessels develops at an earlier age and is more extensive in people with diabetes (Porth, 2005).

The manifestations of impaired cerebral circulation are often similar to those of hypoglycemia or HHS: blurred vision, slurred speech, weakness, and dizziness. People with these manifestations have potentially life-threatening health problems and require constant medical attention.

PERIPHERAL VASCULAR DISEASE Peripheral vascular disease of the lower extremities accompanies both types of DM, but the incidence is greater in people with type 2 DM. Atherosclerosis of vessels in the legs of people with diabetes begins at an earlier age, advances more rapidly, and is equally common in both men and women. Impaired peripheral vascular circulation leads to peripheral vascular insufficiency with intermittent claudication (pain) in the lower legs and ulcerations of the feet. Occlusion and thrombosis of large vessels and small arteries and arterioles, as well as alterations in neurologic function and infection, result in gangrene (necrosis, or the death of tissue). Gangrene from diabetes is the most common cause of nontraumatic amputations of the lower leg. In people with diabetes, dry gangrene is most common, manifested by cold, dry, shriveled, and black tissues of the toes and feet. The gangrene usually begins in the toes and moves proximally into the foot.

DIABETIC RETINOPATHY Diabetic retinopathy is the name for the changes in the retina that occur in the person with diabetes. The retinal capillary structure undergoes alterations in blood flow, leading to retinal ischemia and a breakdown in the blood–retinal barrier. Diabetic retinopathy is the leading cause of blindness in people between ages 20 and 74 (NIH, 2004). Retinopathy has three stages:

- Stage I: nonproliferative retinopathy. Dilated veins, microaneurysms, edema of the macula, and the presence of exudates characterize this stage.
- Stage II: preproliferative retinopathy. Retinal ischemia causes infarcts of the nerve fiber layer, with characteristic "cotton wool" patches on the retina. Shunts form between occluded and patent vessels.

- Stage III: proliferative retinopathy. As fibrous tissue and new vessels form in the retina or optic disc, traction on the vitreous humor may cause hemorrhage or retinal detachment.

After 20 years of diabetes, almost all clients with type 1 DM and more than 70% of clients with type 2 DM will have some degree of retinopathy, in most cases without vision loss (Saudek & Margolis, 2005). If exudate, edema, hemorrhage, or ischemia occurs near the fovea, the person experiences visual impairment at any stage. In addition, the person with diabetes is at increased risk for developing cataracts (opacity of the lens) as a result of increased glucose levels within the lens itself. Screening for retinopathy is important, as laser photocoagulation surgery has proven beneficial in preventing loss of vision.

DIABETIC NEPHROPATHY Diabetic nephropathy is a disease of the kidneys characterized by the presence of albumin in the urine, hypertension, edema, and progressive renal insufficiency. This disorder accounts for 44% of new cases of end-stage renal disease requiring dialysis or transplantation in the United States. Nephropathy occurs in 30%–40% of people with type 1 DM and 20% of those with type 2 (Saudek & Margolis, 2005).

Despite research, the exact pathologic origin of diabetic nephropathy is unknown; it has been established, however, that thickening of the basement membrane of the glomeruli eventually impairs renal function. It has been suggested that an increased intracellular concentration of glucose supports the formation of abnormal glycoproteins in the basement membrane and mesangium. The accumulation of these large proteins stimulates glomerulosclerosis (fibrosis of the glomerular tissue). Glomerulosclerosis thickens the basement membrane and simultaneously makes it functionally leaky allowing large molecules such as protein to be lost in the urine. Kimmelstiel-Wilson syndrome is a type of glomerulosclerosis found only in people with diabetes. In advanced nephropathy, tubular atrophy occurs, and end-stage renal disease results. (Renal failure is discussed in Chapter 29 ∞.)

The first indication of nephropathy is microalbuminuria, a low but abnormal level of albumin in the urine. Without specific interventions, people with type 1 DM with sustained microalbuminuria will develop overt nephropathy, accompanied by hypertension, over a period of 10 to 15 years. People with type 2 DM often have microalbuminuria and overt nephropathy shortly after diagnosis, because the diabetes has often been present but undiagnosed for many years. Because the hypertension accelerates the progress of diabetic nephropathy, aggressive antihypertensive management should be instituted. Management includes control of hypertension with ACE inhibitors such as captopril (Capoten), weight loss, reduced salt intake, and exercise.

Alterations in the Peripheral and Autonomic Nervous Systems

Peripheral and visceral neuropathies are disorders of the peripheral nerves and the autonomic nervous system. In people with diabetes, these disorders are often called diabetic neuropathies. The etiology of diabetic neuropathies involves (1) a thickening of the walls of the blood vessels that supply nerves, causing a decrease in nutrients; (2) demyelination of the Schwann cells that surround and insulate nerves, slowing nerve conduction; and (3) the formation and accumulation of sorbitol within the Schwann cells, impairing nerve conduction. The manifestations depend on the locations of the lesions.

The peripheral neuropathies (also called *somatic neuropathies*) include polyneuropathies and mononeuropathies. *Polyneuropathies,* the most common type of neuropathy associated with diabetes, are bilateral sensory disorders. The manifestations appear first in the toes and feet and progress upward. The fingers and hands may also be involved, but usually only in later stages of diabetes. The manifestations of polyneuropathy depend on the nerve fibers involved.

The person with polyneuropathy commonly has distal paresthesias (a subjective feeling of a change in sensation, such as numbness or tingling); pain described as aching, burning, or shooting; and feelings of cold feet. Other manifestations may include impaired sensations of pain, temperature, light touch, two-point discrimination, and vibration. There is no specific treatment for polyneuropathy.

Mononeuropathies are isolated peripheral neuropathies that affect a single nerve. Depending on the nerve involved, manifestations may include the following:

- Palsy of the third cranial (oculomotor) nerve, with headache, eye pain, and an inability to move the eye up, down, or medially
- Radiculopathy, with pain over a dermatome and loss of cutaneous sensation, most often located in the chest
- Diabetic femoral neuropathy, with motor and sensory deficits (pain, weakness, areflexia) in the anterior thigh and medial calf
- Entrapment or compression of the medial nerve at the wrist, resulting in carpal tunnel syndrome with pain and weakness of the hand; the ulnar nerve at the elbow, with weakness and loss of sensation over the palmar surface of the fourth and fifth fingers; and the peroneal nerve at the head of the fibula, with foot drop.

VISCERAL NEUROPATHIES The visceral neuropathies (also called *autonomic neuropathies*) cause various manifestations, depending on the area of the ANS involved. These neuropathies may include the following:

- Sweating dysfunction, with an absence of sweating (*anhydrosis*) on the hands and feet and increased sweating on the face or trunk
- Abnormal pupillary function, most commonly seen as constricted pupils that dilate slowly in the dark
- Cardiovascular dysfunction, resulting in such abnormalities as a fixed cardiac rate that does not change with exercise, postural hypotension, and a failure to increase cardiac output or vascular tone with exercise
- Gastrointestinal dysfunction, with changes in upper gastrointestinal motility (*gastroparesis*) resulting in dysphagia, anorexia, heartburn, nausea, and vomiting and altered blood glucose control. Constipation is one of the most common gastrointestinal symptoms associated with diabetes, possibly a result of hypomotility of the bowel. Diabetic diarrhea is not

as common, but it does occur and is often associated with fecal incontinence during sleep due to a defect in internal sphincter function.

- Genitourinary dysfunction, resulting in changes in bladder function and sexual function. Bladder function changes include an inability to empty the bladder completely, loss of sensation of bladder fullness, and an increased risk of urinary tract infections. Sexual dysfunctions in men include ejaculatory changes and impotence. Sexual dysfunctions in women include changes in arousal patterns, vaginal lubrication, and orgasm. Alterations in sexual function in people with diabetes are the result of both neurologic and vascular changes.

Mood Alterations

Persons with DM, both type 1 and type 2, endure the chronic strains of living with complex self-care and are at a somewhat increased risk for depression, which can negatively affect management of DM. Treating depression has been associated with better control of serum glucose so screening for depression is an important part of assessing the individual's ability to manage the disease. Tests to identify the scope of depression are available (Harper-Jacques, 2004).

Interventions for helping clients with depression include a combination of antidepressant medications and psychotherapy, focused on restoring logical thinking and problem-solving skills (Williams et al., 2004). Nurses can assist depressed clients by correcting misconceptions about depression, identifying individual strengths in managing diabetes, acknowledging negative feelings that may be expressed, and suggesting problem-solving behaviors to better manage the disease.

Increased Susceptibility to Infection

The person with diabetes has an increased risk of developing infections. The exact relationship between infection and diabetes is not clear, but many dysfunctions that result from diabetic complications predispose the person to develop an infection (Aragon et al., 2003). Vascular and neurologic impairments, hyperglycemia, and altered neutrophil function are believed to be responsible (Porth, 2005).

The person with diabetes may have sensory deficits resulting in inattention to trauma, and vascular deficits that decrease circulation to the injured area; as a result, the normal inflammatory response is diminished and healing is slowed. Nephrosclerosis and inadequate bladder emptying with retention of urine predispose the person with diabetes to pyelonephritis and urinary tract infections. Bacterial and fungal infections of the skin, nails, and mucous membranes are common. Tuberculosis is more prevalent in people with diabetes than in the general population. Hospitalized clients with a blood glucose value greater than 220 mg/dL have higher infection rates (ADA, 2005).

Periodontal Disease

Although periodontal disease does not occur more often in people with diabetes, it does progress more rapidly, especially if the diabetes is poorly controlled. It is believed to be caused by microangiopathy, with changes in vascularization of the gums. As a result, gingivitis (inflammation of the gums) and periodontitis (inflammation of the bone underlying the gums) occur.

Complications Involving the Feet

The high incidence of both amputations and problems with the feet in people with diabetes is the result of angiopathy, neuropathy, and infection. People with diabetes are at high risk for amputation of a lower extremity, with increased risk in those who have had DM for more than 10 years, are male, have poor glucose control, or have cardiovascular, retinal, or renal complications.

Vascular changes in the lower extremities of the person with diabetes result in arteriosclerosis. Diabetes-induced arteriosclerosis tends to occur at an earlier age, occurs equally in men and women, is usually bilateral, and progresses more rapidly. The blood vessels most often affected are located below the knee. Blockages form in the large, medium, and small arteries of the lower legs and feet. Multiple occlusions with decreased blood flow result in the manifestations of peripheral vascular disease (see the box on this page). Peripheral vascular disease is discussed in Chapters 33 and 35 ∞.

Diabetic neuropathy of the foot produces multiple problems. Because the sense of touch and perception of pain are absent, the person with diabetes may have some type of foot trauma without being aware of it. The person thus is at increased risk for trauma to tissues of the feet, leading to ulcer development. Infections commonly occur in traumatized or ulcerated tissue (Figure 20–6 ■).

Despite the many potential sources of foot trauma in the person with diabetes, the most common are cracks and fissures caused by dry skin or infections such as athlete's foot, blisters caused by improperly fitting shoes, pressure from stockings or

Figure 20–6 ■ Ulceration following trauma in the foot of the person with diabetes.

Source: Harry Przekop, Medichrome/The Stock Shop, Inc.

MANIFESTATIONS of Peripheral Vascular Disease

- Loss of hair on lower leg, feet, and toes
- Atrophic skin changes: shininess and thinning
- Cold feet
- Feet and ankles darker than leg
- Dependent rubor, blanching on elevation
- Thick toenails
- Diminished or absent pulses
- Nocturnal pain
- Pain at rest, relieved by standing or walking
- Intermittent claudication
- Patchy areas of gangrene on feet and toes

---

shoes, ingrown toenails, and direct trauma (cuts, bruises, or burns). It is important to remember that the person with diabetic neuropathy who has lost the perception of pain may not be aware that these injuries have occurred. In addition, when a part of the body loses sensation, the person tends to dissociate from or ignore the part, so that an injury may go unattended for days or weeks. The injury may even be forgotten entirely.

Foot lesions usually begin as a superficial skin ulcer. In time, the ulcer extends deeper into muscles and bone, leading to abscess or osteomyelitis. Gangrene can develop on one or more toes; if untreated, the whole foot eventually becomes gangrenous. (Care of the feet, an essential part of client and family education, is discussed later in the chapter.)

NURSING CARE

The responses of the person with diabetes to the illness are often complex and individual, involving multiple body systems. Assessments, planning, and implementation differ for the person with newly diagnosed diabetes, the person with long-term diabetes, and the person with acute complications of diabetes. The plan of care and content of teaching also differ according to the type of diabetes, the person's age and culture, and the person's intellectual, psychologic, and social resources. However, nursing care often focuses on teaching the client to manage the illness. The Nursing Research box on the following page describes a study of quality of life in people with diabetes.

Health Promotion

Health promotion activities primarily focus on preventing the complications of diabetes. The prevention of the disease has not been determined, although it is recommended that all people should prevent or decrease excess weight, follow a sensible and well-balanced diet, and maintain a regular physical exercise program. Blood glucose screening at 3-year intervals beginning at age 45 is recommended for those in the high-risk groups. These same activities, when combined with medications and self-monitoring, are also beneficial in reducing the onset of complications.

NURSING RESEARCH | **Evidence-Based Practice: Balancing Quality of Life and Living with Diabetes**

Adaptation to and management of a chronic illness such as diabetes are simultaneous and interdependent as the person comes to terms with the illness, gains support from caregivers, creates relationships with others, and learns about the illness and its management. Learning about diabetes comes from many sources and in varied settings. Learning in group settings is efficient for the teacher but may not meet the needs of the learner. Printed information may seem impersonal and not applicable to specific needs. Recognizing the need to improve individual understanding and care, Corbett (2003) evaluated individualized educational interventions about foot care for 40 home healthcare clients with type 2 diabetes.

The method was to evaluate and then educate. A systematic assessment of each participant was made for (1) foot ulceration risk, (2) knowledge of appropriate foot self-care, (3) reported foot care practices, and (4) confidence in performing effective foot care (self-efficacy). Following the assessment, feedback was given regarding individual foot ulcer risk, instructions both written and in-person on proper foot care, demonstrated foot care techniques such as toenail care, and addressed concerns of each client. The risk assessments were repeated at entry, at week 6, and at week 12. Individualized education was provided at week 6 in the intervention group. Clients in the control group of the study received only the foot care education at week 12.

A high risk for lower extremity ulceration was found; 70% of participants had sensory loss in their feet, 67% had impaired lower extremity circulation, 61% had inappropriate toenail length, 50% had foot deformity such as bunions or hammer toes, and 49% wore worn-out shoes, wore only socks around the house, or walked barefoot. Fifty percent of the subjects had more than one of these risks. The clients who received the individualized intervention had statistically significant improvements in knowledge, reported practices, and self-efficacy. The control group clients had no significant change in foot care knowledge, reported practices, and self-efficacy. The individually focused interventions led to improved knowledge, self-care skill, and confidence for performing foot care.

Corbett (2003) observed that clients who had individualized education in their homes are able to make significant, satisfying changes in their routines. The interventions were brief and could be performed by home health nurses on routine visits. The home is an ideal setting for diabetic clients to learn how to manage specific cares and involve those who assist and support them.

IMPLICATIONS FOR NURSING

All teaching plans should be individualized and developed in collaboration with the client. Nurses often focus on diabetes management and control, especially compliance with prescribed regimens. Although clients are sometimes termed "noncompliant," this term conveys judgment about dependence. A focus on individualized education based on assessment of individual needs facilitates higher levels of compliance and improved self-care. It is important to also understand that self-control behaviors can change with variations in life and the disease itself, and that each person with diabetes responds uniquely to situations and interventions. Respecting and valuing what a person has learned from living with diabetes is critical to providing effective care.

CRITICAL THINKING IN CLIENT CARE

1. You are caring for two clients with diabetes who are receiving home care for complications of long-term diabetes. One client follows the medical regimen faithfully, the other adapts it to his own schedule and needs. What differences can you identify in your own reaction to these two different clients? How would these reactions affect your relationship with the clients?
2. Imagine you have just been diagnosed with type 1 diabetes. Make a list of the questions you would have and the areas that would cause you the most difficulty in complying with your medical care.
3. How would you respond if your client tells you, "Sometimes I eat whatever I want to for several days." What do you think this behavior indicates?

Assessment

The following data are collected through the health history and physical examination (see Chapter 18 ∞). Further focused assessments are described with nursing interventions in the following text. When assessing the older client, be aware of normal aging changes in all body systems that may alter interpretation of findings.

- *Health history:* Family history of diabetes; history of hypertension or other cardiovascular problems; history of any change in vision (e.g., blurring) or speech, dizziness, numbness or tingling in hands or feet; pain when walking; frequent voiding; change in weight, appetite, infections, and healing; problems with gastrointestinal function or urination; or altered sexual function.
- *Physical assessment:* Height/weight ratio, vital signs, visual acuity, cranial nerves, sensory ability (touch, hot/cold, vibration) of extremities, peripheral pulses, skin and mucous membranes (hair loss, appearance, lesions, rash, itching, vaginal discharge).

Nursing Diagnoses and Interventions

Although many different nursing diagnoses are appropriate for the person with diabetes, those discussed in this section address problems with skin integrity, infection, injury, sexuality, coping, and health maintenance. The goals of care are to maintain function, prevent complications, and teach self-management. See the accompanying Nursing Care Plan for more information.

Risk for Impaired Skin Integrity

The person with diabetes is at increased risk for altered skin integrity as a result of decreased or absent sensation from neuropathies, decreased tissue perfusion from cardiovascular complications, and infection. In addition, poor vision increases the risk of trauma, and an open lesion is more prone to infection and delayed healing. Impaired skin and tissue integrity, with resultant gangrene, is especially common in the feet and lower extremities.

MᴇᴅɪᴀLɪɴᴋ Care Plan Activity: DM Type 2

Conduct baseline and ongoing assessments of the feet, including:

- Musculoskeletal assessment that includes foot and ankle joint range of motion, bone abnormalities (bunions, hammertoes, overlapping digits), gait patterns, use of assistive devices for walking, and abnormal wear patterns on shoes.
- Neurologic assessment that includes sensations of touch and position, pain, and temperature.
- Vascular examination that includes assessment of lower-extremity pulses, capillary refill, color and temperature of skin, lesions, and edema.
- Hydration status, including dryness or excessive perspiration.
- Lesions, fissures between toes, corns, calluses, plantar warts, ingrown or overgrown toenails, redness over pressure points, blisters, cellulitis, or gangrene.

People with diabetes are at significant risk for lower-extremity gangrene. Peripheral neuropathies may result in alterations in the perception of pain, loss of deep tendon reflexes, loss of cutaneous pressure and position sensation, foot drop, changes in the shape of the foot, and changes in bones and joints. Peripheral vascular disease may cause intermittent claudication, absent pulses, delayed venous filling on elevation, dependent rubor, and gangrene. Injuries, lesions, and changes in skin hydration potentiate infections, delayed healing, and tissue loss in the person with diabetes mellitus.

PRACTICE ALERT
Teach the person with diabetes to always test the water temperature in the shower or bath before stepping in.

- Teach foot hygiene. Wash the feet daily with lukewarm water and mild hand soap; pat dry, and dry well between the toes. Apply a very thin coat of lubricating cream if dryness is present (but not between the toes). *Proper hygiene decreases the chance of infection. Temperature receptors may be impaired, so the water should always be tested before use.*
- Discuss the importance of not smoking if client smokes. *Nicotine in tobacco causes vasoconstriction, further decreasing the blood supply to the feet.*
- Discuss the importance of maintaining blood glucose levels through prescribed diet, medication, and exercise. *Hyperglycemia promotes the growth of microorganisms.*
- Conduct foot care teaching sessions as often as necessary (see the box on page 594). Include information about proper shoe fit and composition, avoiding clothing or activities that decrease circulation to the feet, foot inspections, the care of toenails, and the importance of obtaining medical care for lesions. If the person has visual deficits, is obese, or cannot reach the feet, teach the caregiver how to inspect and care for the feet. Feet should be inspected daily. *Foot care is a priority in diabetes management to prevent serious problems. Many people with diabetes are unaware of lesions or injury until infection and compromised circulation are far advanced. The hows and whys of each component must be included in teaching. A variety of methods may be used, including demonstration, return demonstra-*

tion, audiovisual aids, and written lists. If the person is wearing shoes and socks, ask him or her to remove them to practice foot care effectively.

PRACTICE ALERT
Suggest the use of a hand mirror to check the bottom of the feet and the back of the heel.

Risk for Infection
The person with diabetes is at increased risk for infection. The risk of infection is believed to be due to vascular insufficiency that limits the inflammatory response, neurologic abnormalities that limit the awareness of trauma, and a predisposition to bacterial and fungal infections.

- Use and teach meticulous hand washing. *Hand washing is the single most effective method for preventing the spread of infection.*
- Monitor for manifestations of infection: increased temperature, pain, malaise, swelling, redness, discharge, cough. *Early diagnosis and treatment of infections can control their severity and decrease complications.*
- Discuss the importance of skin care. Keep the skin clean and dry, using lukewarm water and mild soap. *People with diabetes are more prone to develop furuncles and carbuncles; the infection often increases the need for insulin. Clean, intact skin and mucous membranes are the first line of defense against infection.*
- Teach dental health measures:
  - Obtain a dental examination every 4 to 6 months.
  - Maintain careful oral hygiene, which includes brushing the teeth with a soft toothbrush and fluoridated toothpaste at least twice a day and flossing as recommended.
  - Be aware of the symptoms requiring dental care: bad breath; unpleasant taste in the mouth; bleeding, red, or sore gums; and tooth pain.
  - If dental surgery is necessary, monitor for need to make adjustments in insulin. *All people with diabetes need to be taught proper oral hygiene, the risk of periodontal disease, and the importance of obtaining dental care for symptoms of oral or dental problems.*
- Teach women with diabetes the symptoms and preventive measures for vaginitis caused by *Candida albicans*. The symptoms are an odorless, white or yellow cheeselike discharge and itching. Sexual transmission is unlikely, but discomfort may cause the client to avoid sexual activity. *Diabetes is a predisposing factor for* Candida albicans *vaginitis, the most common form of vaginitis. Poor personal hygiene and wearing clothing that keeps the vaginal area warm and moist increase the risk of vaginitis. The infection may spread to the urinary tract, resulting in urinary tract infections; preventing and treating vaginitis decrease this risk.*

PRACTICE ALERT
Teach women with DM to take preventive measures by maintaining good personal hygiene, wiping front to back after voiding, wearing cotton underwear, avoiding tight jeans and nylon pantyhose, and avoiding douching.

NURSING CARE PLAN   A Client with Type 1 Diabetes

Jim Meligrito, age 24, is a third-year nursing student at a large mid-western university. Mr. Meligrito also works 20 hours a week as a campus student security guard. His working hours are 8 P.M. to midnight, five nights a week. He lives with his father, who is also a student. Neither of the two men likes to cook, and they usually eat "whatever is handy." Mr. Meligrito has smoked 8 to 10 ciga-rettes a day for 5 years. He was diagnosed with type 1 diabetes mellitus at age 12. Although his insulin dosage has varied, he cur-rently takes a total of 32 units of insulin each day, 10 units of NPH and 6 units of regular insulin each morning and evening. He mon-itors his blood glucose about three times a week. He feels that he is too busy for a regular exercise program and that he gets enough exercise in clinicals and in weekend sports activities. He has not seen a healthcare provider for over a year.

One day during a 6-hour clinical laboratory in pediatrics, Mr. Meligrito notices that he is urinating frequently, is thirsty, and has blurred vision. He also is very tired but blames all his symptoms on drinking a couple of beers and having had only 4 hours of sleep the night before while studying for an examination, and the stress he has been under lately from school and work. When he remembers that he had forgotten to take his insulin that morning, he realizes he must have hyperglycemia but decides that he will be all right until he gets home in the afternoon. Around noon, he begins having abdominal pain, feels weak, has a rapid pulse, and vomits. When he reports his physical symptoms to his clinical in-structor, she sends him immediately to the hospital emergency department, accompanied by another student.

ASSESSMENT

As soon as Mr. Meligrito arrives at the emergency room, his blood glucose level is measured at 300 mg/dL. Urine samples and ad-ditional blood samples are sent to the laboratory for analysis. Blood glucose is 330 mg/dL, HgbA1c is 9.5%, urine shows the presence of ketones, electrolytes are normal, and pH is 7.1. His vital signs are as follows: T 99°F (37.2°C), P 140, R 28, and BP 102/52. An intravenous infusion of 1000 mL normal (0.9%) saline with 40 mEq of KCl is started at a rate of 400 mL/h. Intra-venous regular insulin at 5 unit/h (diluted in 0.9% saline) is be-gun. Hourly blood glucose monitoring is initiated. Mr. Meligrito is nauseated and lethargic but remains oriented. Three hours later, he has a blood glucose level of 160, and his pulse and blood pressure are normal. He is dismissed from the emergency de-partment after making an appointment for the next morning with the hospital's diabetes nurse educator. When he meets with the diabetes educator, he says that he no longer feels in control of the diabetes or his future goal to become a nurse anesthetist.

DIAGNOSES

- *Powerlessness* related to a perceived lack of control of dia-betes due to present demands on time
- *Deficient Knowledge* of self-management of diabetes
- *Risk for Ineffective Role Performance* related to uncertainty about capacity to achieve desired role as registered nurse

EXPECTED OUTCOMES

- Identify those aspects of diabetes that can be controlled and participate in making decisions about self-managing care.

- Demonstrate an understanding of diabetes self-management through planned medication, diet, exercise, and blood glucose self-monitoring activities.
- Explore and clarify Mr. Meligrito's perceptions of his role as a student nurse, verbalizing his ability to meet his expectations.

PLANNING AND IMPLEMENTATION

- Mutually establish specific and individualized short-term and long-term goals for self-management to control blood glucose.
- Provide opportunities to express his feelings about himself and his illness.
- Explore perceptions of his own ability to control his illness and his future, and clarify these perceptions by providing informa-tion about resources and support groups.
- Facilitate decision-making abilities in self-managing his pre-scribed treatment regimen.
- Provide positive reinforcement for increasing involvement in self-care activities.
- Provide relevant learning activities about insulin administra-tion, dietary management, exercise, self-monitoring of blood glucose, and healthy lifestyle.

EVALUATION

After taking an active part in the weekly educational meetings for 2 months, Mr. Meligrito has greatly enhanced his under-standing of and compliance with self-management of his dia-betes. He states that he finally understands how insulin, food, and exercise affect his body, having previously thought they were "just things I should do when I wanted to." He decides to perform self-management activities 1 week at a time, rather than think too far into (and thereby feel overwhelmed by) the future. Both son and father have developed a workable meal schedule and weekly grocery list, and they have begun eating breakfast and dinner together. Jim and a friend have arranged to walk 2 to 3 miles three times a week on a community hik-ing trail. To gain a sense of control over his illness, he has also worked out a schedule that allows time for school, health care, and himself.

CRITICAL THINKING IN THE NURSING PROCESS

1. What is the pathophysiologic basis for the changes in temper-ature, pulse, respirations, and blood pressure that occurred on Mr. Meligrito's admission to the hospital emergency depart-ment?
2. How can smoking and poor self-management of diabetes in-crease the risk of long-term complications?
3. Is powerlessness a common response to a chronic illness? Why or why not?
4. Consider that you are teaching Mr. Meligrito and another client, Mr. McDaniel (age 75, newly diagnosed with type 2 DM). What components of your teaching plan would be the same and what components would be different?
5. What does the HgbA1c of 9.5% suggest about Mr. Meligrito's control of his diabetes?

See Evaluating Your Response in Appendix C.

MEETING INDIVIDUALIZED NEEDS Foot Care Teaching Session

BUYING AND WEARING SHOES AND STOCKINGS

- Shoes that allow 1/2 to 3/4 inch of toe room are best; there should be room for toes to spread out and wiggle. The lining and inside stitching should be smooth, and the insole soft. The sole should be flexible and cushion the foot. The heel should fit snugly, and the arch support should give good support.
- Do not wear open-toed shoes, sandals, high heels, or thongs; they increase the risk of trauma.
- Buy shoes late in the afternoon, when feet are at their largest; always buy shoes that feel comfortable and do not need to be "broken in."
- Shoes made of natural fibers (leather, canvas) allow perspiration to escape.
- Check the shoes before each wearing for foreign objects, wrinkled insoles, and cracks that might cause lesions.
- Stockings made of wool or cotton allow perspiration to dry.
- Do not wear garters, knee stockings, or pantyhose; they may interfere with circulation.
- Wear insulated boots in the winter.

INSPECTING THE FEET

- Check the feet daily for red areas, cuts, blisters, corns, calluses, or cracks in the skin. Check between the toes for cracks or reddened areas.
- Check the skin of the feet for dry or damp areas.
- Use a mirror to check each sole and the back of each heel.

- If you are unable to inspect the feet daily, be sure that someone else does so.

CARE OF TOENAILS

- Cut the toenails after washing, when they are softer and easier to trim.
- Cut the nails straight across with a clipper, and smooth edges and corners with an emery board.
- Do not use razor blades to trim the toenails.
- If you are unable to see well or to reach the feet easily, have someone else trim the nails. If the nails are very thick or ingrown, if the toes overlap, or if circulation is poor, get professional care from a podiatrist.

GENERAL INFORMATION

- Never go barefoot. Wear slippers when leaving the bed during the night.
- Do not use commercial corn medicines or pads, chemicals (such as boric acid, iodine, or hydrogen peroxide), or over-the-counter cortisone medications on the feet.
- Do not put heating pads, hot water bottles, or ice packs on the feet. If the feet become cold at night, wear socks or use extra blankets.
- Do not allow the feet to become sunburned.
- Do not put tape on the feet.
- Do not sit with the legs crossed at the knees or ankles.

Risk for Injury

The person with diabetes is at risk for injury from multiple factors. Neuropathies may alter sensation, gait, and muscle control. Cataracts or retinopathy may cause visual deficits. Hyperglycemia often causes osmotic changes in the lenses of the eye, resulting in blurred vision. In addition, changes in blood glucose alter levels of consciousness and may cause seizures. The impaired mobility, sensory deficits, and neurologic effects of complications of diabetes increase the risk of accidents, burns, falls, and trauma.

- Assess for the presence of contributing or causative factors that increase the risk of injury: blurred vision, cataracts, decreased adaptation to dark, decreased tactile sensitivity, hypoglycemia, hyperglycemia, hypovolemia, joint immobility, unstable gait. *A knowledge base is necessary to develop an individualized plan of care. The risk of injury increases with the number of factors identified.*
- Reduce environmental hazards in the healthcare facility, and teach the client about safety in the home and in the community.

IN THE HEALTHCARE FACILITY

- Orient the client to new surroundings on admission.
- Keep the bed at the lowest level.
- Keep the floors free of objects.
- Use a night-light.
- Check the temperature of the bath or shower water before the client uses it.
- Instruct the client to wear shoes or slippers when out of bed.

- Monitor blood glucose levels regularly.
- Monitor for side effects of prescribed medications, such as dizziness or drowsiness.

IN THE HOME AND COMMUNITY

- Use a night-light, preferably one with a soft, nonglare bulb.
- Turn the head away when switching on a bright light.
- Avoid directly looking into headlights when driving at night.
- Test the temperature of the bath or shower water before use.
- Conduct a daily foot inspection.
- Wear shoes and slippers with nonskid soles.
- Do not use throw rugs.
- Install hand grips in the tub and shower and next to the toilet.
- Wear a seat belt when driving or riding in a car.
  Strange environments and the presence of hazardous environmental factors increase the risk of falls or other accidents. Glare is often responsible for falls in people with visual deficits. The nurse can reduce factors that increase the risk of injury by implementing care and teaching safe practices during the activities of daily life.

PRACTICE ALERT

Make frequent assessments to monitor for symptoms of HHS in the older adult who has had major surgery.

- Monitor for and teach the client and family to recognize and seek care for the manifestations of DKA in the client with type 1 DM: hyperglycemia, thirst, headaches, nausea and vomiting, increased urine output, ketonuria, dehydration, and decreasing level of consciousness. *Blood glucose levels increase if the insulin need is unmet or insufficiently met; the cellular use of fats for fuel results in ketosis. Osmotic diuresis increases urinary output, resulting in thirst and dehydration.*

- Monitor for and teach the client and family to recognize and seek care for the manifestations of HHS in the client with type 2 DM: extreme hyperglycemia, increased urinary output, thirst, dehydration, hypotension, seizures, and decreasing level of consciousness. *HHS is a life-threatening condition requiring recognition and treatment.*
- Monitor for and teach the client and family to recognize and treat the manifestations of hypoglycemia: low blood glucose, anxiety, headache, uncoordinated movements, sweating, rapid pulse, drowsiness, and visual changes. Teach client and family to carry some form of rapid-acting sugar source at all times. *Severe hypoglycemia causes a decrease in the level of consciousness. The decrease in blood glucose most often results from too much insulin, too little food, or too much exercise.*
- Recommend that the client wear a Medic-Alert bracelet or necklace identifying self as a person with diabetes. *In case of sudden, severe illness or accident, a Medic-Alert bracelet can allow immediate medical attention for diabetes to be instituted.*

Sexual Dysfunction

Sexuality is a complex and inseparable part of every person. It involves not only physical sexual activities but also a person's self-perception as male or female, roles and relationships, and attractiveness and desirability. Changes in sexual function and in sexuality have been identified in both men and women with diabetes.

Alterations in erectile ability occur in approximately 50% of all men with diabetes. The incidence of impotence increases with the duration of the diabetes and is often associated with peripheral neuropathy. Libido is usually unaffected, even when impotence is present.

PRACTICE ALERT
Sexual function is a private matter, and clients rarely share concerns unless the nurse initiates the discussion.

Women with diabetes also have alterations in sexual function, although the reason is less clear. The problems reported by women involve decreased desire and decreased vaginal lubrication. Women with diabetes are also at increased risk for vaginitis and may avoid sexual intercourse in order to avoid pain.

- Include a sexual history as a part of the initial and ongoing assessment of the client with diabetes. A specific history form may be used that addresses sexual development, personal and family values, current sexual practices and concerns, and changes desired. Ask a nonthreatening, open-ended question to elicit information, such as "Tell me about your experience with sexual function since you have been diagnosed with diabetes." *Obtaining accurate information to assess the sexual health of a client is necessary before counseling can begin or referrals can be made.*
- Provide information about the actual and potential physical effects of diabetes on sexual function. Include the effect of

poor control of blood glucose on sexual function as part of any teaching plan. *Clients benefit from basic information about male and female anatomy and the sexual response cycle, and how diabetes can affect this part of the body. Changes in blood glucose levels not only may cause changes in desire and physical response but also may alter sexual responses as a result of depression, anxiety, and fatigue.*

- Provide counseling or make referrals as appropriate. The nurse is responsible for knowing about sexuality and sexual health throughout the life span and provides information based on knowledge of the effects of illness and treatment on sexual function. For example, men who are impotent may regain the ability to have sexual intercourse through penile implants, suction apparatus, the use of sildenafil citrate (Viagra), or injections of medications (such as yohimbine, an alpha-2 adrenergic blocker) that increase vascular blood flow into the corpus of the penis. Women with decreased vaginal lubrication can decrease painful intercourse by using vaginal lubricants (such as K-Y Jelly) or estrogen creams.
The nurse may make specific suggestions to facilitate positive sexual functioning, referring the client to the appropriate health care provider as necessary for intensive therapy.

Ineffective Coping

Coping is the process of responding to internal or environmental stressors or potential stressors. When coping responses are ineffective, the stressors exceed the individual's available resources for responding. The person diagnosed with diabetes is faced with lifelong changes in many parts of his or her life. Diet, exercise habits, and medications must be integrated into the person's lifestyle and be carefully controlled. Daily injections may be a reality. Fear of potential complications and of negative effects on the future is common.

If the person is unable to cope successfully with these changes, emotional stress can interfere with glycemic control. In addition, unsuccessful coping often results in noncompliance with prescribed treatment modalities, further impairing glycemic control and increasing the potential for acute and chronic complications.

- Assess the client's psychosocial resources, including emotional resources, support resources, lifestyle, and communication skills. *Chronic illness affects all dimensions of a person's life, as well as the lives of family members and significant others. A comprehensive assessment of strengths and weaknesses is the first step in developing an individualized plan of care to facilitate coping.*
- Explore with the client and family the effects (actual and perceived) of the diagnosis and treatment of diabetes on finances, occupation, energy levels, and relationships. *Common frustrations associated with diabetes are the disease itself, the treatment modalities, and the healthcare system. Effective coping involves maintaining a healthy self-concept and satisfying relationships, emotional balance, and handling emotional stress.*
- Teach constructive problem-solving techniques. *Problem-focused behaviors include setting attainable and realistic goals, learning about all aspects of the problem, learning*

new procedures or skills that increase self-esteem, and reaching out to others for support.

- Provide information about support groups and resources, such as suppliers of products, journals, books, and cookbooks for people with diabetes. *Sharing with others who have similar problems provides opportunities for mutual support and problem solving. Using available resources improves the ability to cope.*

Using NANDA, NIC, and NOC

Chart 20–1 shows links between NANDA, NIC, and NOC when caring for the client with diabetes.

Community-Based Care

Teaching the client and family to self-manage diabetes is a nursing responsibility. Even if a formal teaching plan is developed and implemented by advanced practice nurses, all nurses must be able to reinforce knowledge and answer questions. Teaching is necessary for both the person who is newly diagnosed and for the person who has had diabetes for years. In fact, the latter may need almost as much teaching as the newly diagnosed person. Products for diabetes care, especially insulins, have changed dramatically and knowledge about risk reduction to prevent complications has increased.

The American Diabetes Association recommends that teaching be carried out on three levels. The first level focuses on sur-

vival skills, with the person learning basic knowledge and skills to be able to provide diabetes management for the first week or two while he or she adjusts to the idea of having the disease. The second level focuses on home management, emphasizing self-reliance and independence in the daily management of diabetes. The third level aims at improving lifestyle and educating clients to individualize self-management of the illness.

For the hospitalized client with diabetes, teaching should begin on admission. Prior to designing the teaching plan, the nurse makes an initial assessment of the client's and family's knowledge and learning needs, outlining past diabetes management practices and identifying physical, emotional, and sociocultural needs. Educational level, preferred learning methods and style, life experiences, and support systems are also assessed. Paterson (2001) investigated the self-care decision making of clients with long-standing type 1 diabetes, examining their degree of empowerment as equal partners with their healthcare providers. These clients revealed that despite invitations and verbal assurances that clients are equal partners with the provider, accountable for and capable of making self-care decisions, interactions concerning management of the disease frequently included discounting the clients' experiential knowledge of diabetes over time and failure to provide resources necessary to make informed decisions. Nurses must be cautious about adopting an overly hierarchic approach of telling clients how to manage and withholding resources they need to participate in decision making (Larsen et al., 2003).

It is important that the nurse and client mutually establish goals based on the assessment data. It is equally important that family members understand that the responsibility for daily management lies with the client and that the primary role of the family is supportive. The client is the person with the disease, and it is the client who each day must take medications or inject insulin, test blood or urine, calculate and balance foods, exercise, adjust medications, inspect the body for injury, and determine whether and when medical assistance is needed. However, family members require the same knowledge so that they can provide emotional support as well as physical care if necessary.

The following should be included in teaching the client and family about care at home.

- Information about normal metabolism, diabetes mellitus, and how diabetes changes metabolism
- Diet plan: how diet helps keep blood glucose in normal range; number of kcal required and why; amount of carbohydrates, meats, and fats allowed and why; and how to calculate the diet, integrating personal food preferences
- Exercise: how it helps lower blood glucose; the importance of a regular program; types of exercise; integrating personal exercise preferences; how to handle increased activity
- Self-monitoring of blood glucose: how to perform the tests accurately, how to care for equipment, what to do for high or low blood glucose
- Medications:
  - *Insulin:* type, dosage, mixing instructions (if necessary), times of onset and peak actions, how to get and care for equipment, how to give injections, where to give injections

---

NANDA, NIC, AND NOC LINKAGES
CHART 20–1 The Client with Type 1 DM

NANDA

Deficient Knowledge: Self-Management of DM

↓

NIC

Teaching: Individual

Teaching: Disease Process

Teaching: Foot Care

Teaching: Prescribed Diet

↓

NOC

Knowledge: Diabetes Management

Knowledge: Disease Process

Knowledge: Treatment Regimen

Knowledge: Health Promotion

Data from *NANDA's Nursing Diagnoses: Definitions & Classification 2005–2006* by NANDA International (2005), Philadelphia; *Nursing Interventions Classification* (NIC) (4th ed.) by J. M. Dochterman & G. M. Bulechek (2004), St. Louis, MO: Mosby; and *Nursing Outcomes Classification (NOC)* (3rd ed.) by S. Moorhead, M. Johnson, and M. Mass (2004), St. Louis, MO: Mosby.

- *Insulin: Oral agents:* type, dosage, side effects, interaction with other drugs
- Manifestations of acute complications of hypoglycemia and hyperglycemia; what to do when they occur
- Hygiene: skin care, dental care, foot care
- Sick days: what to do about food, fluids, and medications
- Helpful resources:
  - The American Diabetes Association
  - The American Dietetic Association
  - National Diabetes Information Clearinghouse
  - Department of Veterans Affairs
  - Indian Health Service
  - National Council of La Raza

Teaching may have to be adapted to the special needs of the older adult. Because 40% of all people with diabetes are over the age of 65, considering the special needs of this population is essential. Uncontrolled diabetes in the older adult increases the potential for functional loss, social disengagement, and increased morbidity and mortality. Education for self-care allows the older adult to be more actively involved in his or her diabetes management and decreases the potential for acute and long-term complications from the disease. Considerations for teaching the older adult with diabetes include the following:

- Changes in diet may be difficult to implement for many reasons. Favorite foods are difficult to give up. Balanced meals at regular intervals may not have been part of the client's lifestyle. Purchasing, storing, and preparing foods may be a problem. Dentures may not fit well. Changes in taste sensation often cause the client to increase the use of salt and sugar.
- Exercise of any type may not have been part of the activities of daily living. Exercise must be individualized for any physical limitations imposed by other chronic illnesses, such as arthritis, Parkinson's disease, chronic respiratory diseases, and/or cardiovascular diseases.
- The diagnosis of a chronic illness threatens independence and self-worth. After years of taking care of self, the older adult with diabetes may now have to depend on others for help in meeting self-care needs. This in turn often leads to withdrawal from social interactions with others.
- Money to purchase medications and supplies often must be taken out of a fixed income.
- Visual deficits make insulin administration difficult or impossible. Visual deficits also interfere with blood glucose monitoring, food preparation, exercises, and foot care.

EXPLORE MEDIALINK

Prentice Hall Nursing MediaLink DVD-ROM
    Audio Glossary
    NCLEX-RN® Review

    Animations
        Glipizide
        Responding to Hypoglycemia

COMPANION WEBSITE www.prenhall.com/lemone
    Audio Glossary
    NCLEX-RN® Review
    Care Plan Activity: Diabetes Mellitus Type 2
    Case Studies
        Compare and Contrast SIADH and DI
        Diabetes Mellitus Type 1
    MediaLink Applications
        Diabetes and Nutrition
        Diabetes Foot Care
        Diabetic Neuropathy
    Links to Resources

CHAPTER HIGHLIGHTS

- The incidence of type 2 DM is increasing in epidemic proportions in all racial and ethnic groups in the United States.
- Approximately 1.3 million new cases of DM are diagnosed each year in the United States. Diabetes is the sixth leading cause of death by disease in the United States, primarily due to widespread cardiovascular effects.
- Type 2 DM has a hereditary link and is characterized by obesity and sedentary lifestyles. Unlike type 1 DM, in which the onset

is often sudden, the development of symptoms that bring clients to their healthcare providers for evaluation is slow; it is estimated that 50% of newly diagnosed type 2 DM clients have already developed complications secondary to hyperglycemia.

- The risk factors for acute and chronic complications are known, but clinical practice has not integrated these factors thoroughly into assessment and planning.

- Tighter, more intensive glycemic control is increasingly the focus of care for hospitalized clients with hyperglycemia. Correcting hyperglycemia is considered a benefit to diabetics and nondiabetics alike.
- New products for clients with DM include insulins, noninsulin hypoglycemics, and blood glucose monitoring devices. Nurses must be familiar with these products and help clients become proficient in their use.

- Motivation for self-care by the client with diabetes continues to be a challenge because treatment commonly includes lifestyle changes. Through education and support, clients can achieve control of DM and avoid complications.

TEST YOURSELF NCLEX-RN® REVIEW

1 Increased susceptibility to the development of type 1 diabetes is indicated by which of the following?
  1. genetic markers that determine immune response
  2. persistent obesity throughout the adolescent years
  3. delivery of a baby that weighs less than 6 lb
  4. excessive amounts of plasma glucagon

2 Diabetic ketoacidosis is the result of which pathologic process?
  1. An excess amount of insulin drives all glucose into the cells.
  2. A decreased amount of glucagon causes low protein levels.
  3. A deficit of insulin causes fat stores to be used as an energy source.
  4. An increase occurs in the breakdown of glucose molecules with hypoglycemia.

3 Which of the following clients would be most at risk for the development of type 2 DM?
  1. young adult who is a professional basketball player
  2. middle-age man who maintains normal weight
  3. middle-age woman who is the sole caretaker of her parents
  4. woman over age 70 who is overweight and sedentary

4 You note that your assigned client has a nursing diagnosis of *Peripheral Neurovascular Dysfunction* involving both feet. Which of the following assessments would support this diagnosis?
  1. normal sensation to touch
  2. loss of normal reflexes
  3. states "I can't feel my feet anymore."
  4. states "I have been having chest pain."

5 Which of the following statements would indicate your client understands teaching about foot care at home?
  1. "I will walk barefooted as long as I am in the house."
  2. "I always buy my shoes as soon as the stores open."
  3. "I will check my feet for cuts and bruises every night."
  4. "If I get a blister, I just put alcohol on it and bandage it."

6 Lantus insulin, a long-acting insulin, has a unique insulin characteristic that increases the risk for administration error. The nurse understands that this long-acting insulin is:
  1. combined with glucose to raise energy levels.
  2. subject to being inactivated by light.
  3. a clear solution like regular insulin, unlike intermediate and long-acting insulins.
  4. activated by vigorous agitation.

7 The nurse is preparing an insulin infusion for a client in diabetic ketoacidosis (DKA). She is careful to select the only type of insulin that can be administered intravenously, which is:
  1. Lantus.
  2. NPH.
  3. regular.
  4. Humalog.

8 Glycosylated hemoglobin (HgbA1c) is useful for evaluating the degree of blood glucose control the client with diabetes has been maintaining for the previous 2 to 3 months. The ADA recommended goal for HgbA1c in the general population with diabetes is:
  1. >10%.
  2. <8%.
  3. <6%.
  4. <3%.

9 When the insulin-dependent client is NPO on the day of surgery, short-acting regular insulin should be:
  1. given intravenously.
  2. chilled to slow absorption.
  3. given with intravenous glucose.
  4. combined with long-acting insulin.

10 Subcutaneous injections of insulin can be made in several locations in the body. The nurse teaches the client that the most rapid absorption occurs in the:
  1. hip.
  2. thigh.
  3. deltoid.
  4. abdomen.

See Test Yourself answers in Appendix C.

BIBLIOGRAPHY

American Diabetes Association. (2002). Evidence-based nutrition principles and recommendations for the treatment and prevention of diabetes and related complications. *Diabetes Care, 25,* 202–212.

American Diabetes Association. (2003). Aspirin therapy in diabetes. *Diabetes Care, 26*(S1), S87–S88.

_____. (2005). Standards of medical care in diabetes. *Diabetes Care, 28*(S1) S4–S36.

American Diabetes Association. (2006). Diagnosis and classification of diabetes mellitus. *Diabetes Care, 29* (1), S43–S48.

American Diabetes Association. (2006). Standards of medical care in diabetes–2006. *Diabetes Care, 29* (1), S6–S42.

Amiel, S. A., & Alberti, K. G. (2005). Diabetes and surgery. In S. Inzucchi, D. Porte, R. S. Sherwin, & A. Baron (Eds.), *The diabetes mellitus manual: A primary care companion to Ellenberg & Rifkin's* (6th ed., pp. 231–242). New York: McGraw-Hill.

Aragon, D., Ring, C. A., & Covelli, M. (2003). The influence of diabetes mellitus on postoperative infections. *Critical Care Nursing Clinics of North America, 15,* 125–135.

Batts, M., Gary, T., Huss, K., Hill, M., Bone, L., & Brancatt, F. (2001). Patient priorities and needs for diabetes care among urban African American adults. *Diabetes Educator, 27*(3), 405–412.

Bohannon, N. (1998). Treatment of vulvovaginal candidiasis in patients with diabetes. *Diabetes Care, 21*(3), 451–456. (This is the best information to date.)

Burke, D. (2001). Diabetes education for the Native American Population. *Diabetes Educator, 27*(2), 181–189.

Cameron, B. (2002). Making diabetes management routine. *American Journal of Nursing, 102*(2), 26–33.

Capriotti, T. (2005). Type 2 diabetes epidemic increases use of oral anti-diabetic agents. *MEDSURG Nursing, 14*(5), 341–347.

Carter, J., Gilliland, S., Perez, G., Levin, S., Broussand, B., Valdez, L., et al. (1997). Tool chest. Native American Diabetes Project: Designing culturally relevant education materials. *Diabetes Educator, 23*(2), 133–134.

Centers for Disease Control. (2005). National Diabetes Fact Sheet. http://www.cdc.gov/diabetes/pubs/factsheet05.htm

Chodosh, J., Morton, S. C., Mojica, W., Maglione, M., Suttorp, M. J., Hilton, L., et al. (2005). Improving patient care. Meta-analysis: Chronic disease self-management programs for older adults. *Annals of Internal Medicine, 143*(6), 427–438.

Clement, S., Braithwaite, S. S., Magee, M. F., Ahmann, A., Smith, E. P., Schafer, R. G., & Hirsch, I. R., on behalf of the diabetes in hospitals writing committee. (2004). Management of diabetes and hyperglycemia in hospitals. *Diabetes Care, 27,* 553–591.

Clifford, R. M., Davis, W. A., Batty, K. T., & Davis, T. M. E. (2005). Effect of a pharmaceutical care program on vascular risk factors in type 2 diabetes: The Fremantle Diabetes Study. *Diabetes Care, 28*(4), 771–776.

Corbett, C. F. (2003). A randomized pilot study of improving foot care in home health patients with diabetes. *Diabetes Educator, 29*(2), 273–282.

Cummings, J., Mineo, K., Levy, R., & Josephson, R. (1999). A review of the DIGAMI Study: Intensive insulin therapy during and after myocardial infarctions in diabetic patients. *Diabetes Spectrum, 12*(2), 84–88.

Dochterman, J., & Bulechek, G. (2004). *Nursing interventions classification (NIC)* (4th ed.). St. Louis, MO: Mosby.

Dutton, G. R., Johnson, J., Whitehead, D., Bodenlos, J. S., & Brantley, P. J. (2005). Barriers to physical activity among predominantly low-income African-American patients with type 2 diabetes. *Diabetes Care, 28*(5), 1209–1210.

Eli Lilly and Company. (2006). *Product discontinuation information.* Retrieved April 22, 2006, from http://www.lillydiabetes.com

Eliopoulos, C. (2005). *Gerontological nursing* (6th ed.). Philadelphia: Lippincott Williams & Wilkins.

Fain, J. A. (2004). Blood glucose meters: Different strokes for different folks. *Nursing, 34*(11), 48–51.

Fanning, E. L., Larme, A. C., Selwyn, B. M., & DeFronzo, R. A. (2004). Improving efficacy of diabetes management using treatment algorithms in a mainly Hispanic population. *Diabetes Care, 27*(7), 1638–1646.

Funnell, M. M., Kruger, D. F., & Spencer, M. (2004). Self-management support for insulin therapy in type 2 diabetes. *The Diabetes Educator, 30*(2), 274–280.

Goldberg, J. M. (2001). *Nutrition and exercise. RN, 64*(7), 34–39.

Guthrie, D., & Guthrie, R. (1997). *Nursing management of diabetes mellitus* (4th ed.). New York: Springer.

Haire-Joshu, D. (Ed.). (1996). *Management of diabetes mellitus: Perspectives of care across the life span* (2nd ed.). St. Louis: Mosby.

Hanna, K., & Guthrie, D. (2001). Health-compromising behavior and diabetes mismanagement among adolescents and young adults. *Diabetes Educator, 27*(2), 223–230.

Harper-Jacques, S. (2004). Diabetes and depression: Addressing the depression can improve glycemic control. *American Journal of Nursing, 104*(9), 56–59.

Herman, W. H., Hoerger, T. J., Brandle, M., Hicks, K., Sorensen, S., Zhang P., et al. (2005). The cost-effectiveness of lifestyle modification or metformin in preventing type 2 diabetes in adults with impaired glucose tolerance. *Annals of Internal Medicine, 142*(5), 323–332, I-28.

Hernandez, D. (1998). Microvascular complications of diabetes: Nursing assessment and intervention. *American Journal of Nursing, 98*(6), 26–31.

Johnson, M., & Maas, M. (Eds.). (1997). *Nursing outcomes classification (NOC).* St. Louis, MO: Mosby.

Larsen, P. R., Kronenberg, H. M., Melmed, S., & Polonsky, K. S. (2003). *Williams textbook of endocrinology* (10th ed.). Philadelphia: Saunders.

Lehne, R. A. (2004). *Pharmacology for nursing care* (4th ed.). St. Louis, MO: Saunders/Elsevier.

Ludwig, D. S. (2002). The glycemic index: Physiological mechanisms relating to obesity, diabetes, and cardiovascular disease. *Journal of the American Medical Association, 287*(18), 2414–2423.

Mabrey, M. E. (2004). Using insulin to prevent hyperglycemia in surgical patients. *Nursing, 34*(10), 22.

Magee, M. (2006). Insulin therapy for intensive glycemic control in hospital patients. *Hospital Physician, 42*(4), 17–27, 38.

Malmberg, K., Ryden, L., Hamsten, A., Herlitz, J., Waldenstrom, A., Wedel, H., et al. (1995). Randomized trial of insulin-glucose infusion followed by subcutaneous insulin treatment in diabetic patients with acute myocardial infarction (DIGAMI study): Effects on mortality at 1 year. *Journal of the American College of Cardiology, 26,* 56–65.

McCance, K., & Huether, S. (2002). *Pathophysiology: The biologic basis for disease in adults and children* (4th ed.). St. Louis, MO: Mosby.

McCloskey, J. C., & Bulechek, G. M. (Eds.). (2000). *Nursing interventions classification (NIC).* St. Louis, MO: Mosby.

Medtronic MiniMed, Inc. (2006). MiniMed Paradigm® REAL-Time Insulin Pump and Continuous Glucose Monitoring System. Retrieved April 24, 2006, from http://www.minimed.com/products/insulinpumps/realtime/index.html

Moorhead, S., Johnson, M., & Maas, M. (2003). *Nursing outcomes classification (NOC)* (3rd ed.). St. Louis, MO: Mosby.

National Institutes of Health. (2004). *Diabetes statistics in the United States.* Retrieved from http://diabetes.niddk.nih.gov/dm/pubs/statistics/

North American Nursing Diagnosis Association. (2001). *Nursing diagnoses: Definitions & classification 2001–2002.* Philadelphia: Author.

Nutrition Sub-committee of the Diabetes Care Advisory Committee of Diabetes UK. (2003). The dietitian's challenge: The implementation of nutritional advice for people with diabetes. *Journal of Human Nutrition and Dietetics, 16*(6), 421–456.

Oswald, G., Kinch, A., & Ruddy, E. (2004). Transfer to a patient centered, carbohydrate counting and insulin matching programme in a shortened time frame: A structured education programme for type 1 diabetes incorporating intensified conventional therapy and CSII. *Practical Diabetes International, 21*(9), 334–338.

Pagana, K. D., & Pagana, T. J. (2002). *Mosby's manual of diagnostic and laboratory tests* (2nd ed.). St. Louis, MO: Mosby.

Paterson, B. (2001). Myth of empowerment in chronic illness. *Journal of Advanced Nursing, 34*(5), 574–581.

Pattillo, M. M. (2004). Therapeutic and healing foot care: A healthy feet clinic for older adults. *Journal of Gerontological Nursing, 30*(12), 25–32, 50–51.

Porth, C. (2005). *Pathophysiology: Concepts of altered health states* (7th ed.). Philadelphia: Lippincott.

Roberts, C. K., & Barnard, R. J. (2005). Effects of exercise and diet on chronic disease. *Journal of Applied Physiology, 98,* 3–30.

Saudek, C. D., & Margolis, S. (2005). *Diabetes. The Johns Hopkins White Papers.* Baltimore, MD; Johns Hopkins Medicine.

Sen, M. (2005). Continuing education needs of currently practicing nurses toward the self-care management of patients with type 2 diabetes. *Journal for Nurses in Staff Development, 21*(1), 31–36.

Sheard, N. F., Clark, N. G., Brand-Miller, J. C., Franz, M. J., Pi-Sunyer, F. X., Mayer-Davis, E., et al. (2004). Dietary carbohydrate (amount and type) in the prevention and management of diabetes: ADA statement. *Diabetes Care, 27,* 2266–2271.

Sigal, R. J., Kenny, G. P., Wasserman, D. H., & Castaneda-Sceppa, C. (2004). Physical activity/exercise and type 2 diabetes. *Diabetes Care, 27,* 2518–2539.

Solowiejczyk, J. (2004). The family approach to diabetes management: Theory into practice toward the development of a new paradigm. *Diabetes Spectrum, 17*(1), 31–36.

Struther, R., Schanche Hodge, F., Geishirt-Cantrell, B., & DeCora, L. (2003). Participant experiences of Talking Circles on Type 2 diabetes in two northern plains American Indian tribes. *Qualitative Health Research, 13*(8), 1094–1115.

Tierney, L., McPhee, S., & Papadakis, M. (Eds.). (2005). *Current medical diagnosis & treatment* (44th ed.). Stamford, CT: Appleton & Lange.

Tkacs, N. (2002). Hypoglycemia unawarenesss. *American Journal of Nursing, 102*(2), 34–41.

U.S. Food and Drug Administration. (2005). *Diabetes information: Glucose meters and diabetes management.* Retrieved April 24, 2006, from http://www.fda.gov/diabetes/glucose.html#8

Van den Berghe, G., Wilmer, A., Hermans, G., Meersseman, W., Wouters, P. J., Milants, I., Van Wijngaerden, E., Bobbaers, H., & Bouillon, R. (2006). Intensive insulin therapy in the medical ICU. *The New England Journal of Medicine, 354*(5), 449–461.

Whittemore, R. (2000). Strategies to facilitate lifestyle change associated with diabetes mellitus. *Journal of Nursing Scholarship, 32*(3), 225–232.

Williams, J. W., Katon, W., Lin, E., Nöel, P., Worchel, J., Cornell, J., et al. (2004). The effectiveness of depression care management on diabetes-related outcomes in older patients. *Annals of Internal Medicine, 140*(12), 1015–1024.

Yared, Z., Aljaberi, K., Renouf, N., & Yale, J. (2005). The effect of blood sample volume on 11 glucose monitoring systems. *Diabetes Care, 28,* 1836–1837.

Zulkowski, K. R., & Ratliff, C. R. (2004). Managing venous and neuropathic ulcers. *Nursing, 34*(8), 68.

FUNCTIONAL HEALTH PATTERN: Nutritional-Metabolic

■ Think about clients with altered nutritional or metabolic function for whom you have cared in your clinical experiences.

- What were the clients' major medical diagnoses (e.g., Graves' disease, myxedema, thyroid cancer, Cushing's syndrome, Addison's disease, pheochromocytoma, syndrome of inappropriate antidiuretic hormone secretion, or diabetes mellitus)?
- What manifestations did each of these clients have? Were these manifestations similar or different?
- How did the clients' endocrine problems interfere with their nutritional and metabolic status? Were they on a prescribed diet? What was their daily intake of foods and fluids? Did they have an increased appetite with loss of weight? Did they notice their hands and feet getting larger? Did they have difficulty swallowing or notice swelling in the front of their neck? Did they note an increase or decrease in urination? Did they note a change in energy levels? Did they notice any visual changes? Did they complain of sleep disturbances? Did they have any changes in hair distribution, such as facial hair or changes in skin texture? Was there a change in memory or the ability to concentrate? Did the clients use hormones or steroids? Was there a family history of diabetes mellitus, thyroid problems, hypertension, or obesity?

■ The Nutritional-Metabolic Pattern includes metabolism, which is the biochemical processes that take place in the body in response to hormones produced and released by the endocrine glands. These processes include the distribution of nutrients after digestion of carbohydrates, proteins, and fats. The endocrine system regulates growth, reproduction, metabolism, fluid and electrolyte balance, and gender differentiation. Endocrine disorders affect metabolic status in two primary ways:

- A deficit of hormones may result in disorders of the thyroid gland (e.g., hypothyroidism), disorders of the parathyroid gland (e.g., hypoparathyroidism), disorders of the adrenal gland (e.g., chronic adrenocortical insufficiency), disorders of the pituitary gland (e.g., hypopituitarism, diabetes insipidus), or disorders of the pancreas (e.g., hypoglycemia).
- Excess hormones may result in disorders of the thyroid gland (e.g., hyperthyroidism), disorders of the parathyroid gland (e.g., hyperparathyroidism), disorders of the adrenal gland (e.g., hypercortisolism), disorders of the pituitary gland (e.g., hyperpituitarism, SIADH), or disorders of the pancreas (e.g., hyperglycemia).

■ Hormones are chemical substances, secreted by the endocrine glands, which initiate or regulate functioning of a target organ by binding to a receptor site located on the surface of the target organ. They are regulated by a negative or positive feedback system in which decreased or increased hormone levels signal the release of hormones to maintain homeostasis of the body's internal environment. Imbalance of hormones can result in endocrine disorders, leading to manifestations such as:

- Weight loss (associated with varying disorders, including increased thyroid hormones which cause increased metabolism of carbohydrates, proteins, and lipids ► resulting in caloric and nutritional deficiencies)
- Blurred vision (for example, a lack of insulin production by the beta cells of the islets of Langerhans of the pancreas ► causes osmotic effects in the eye tissue ► resulting in swelling of the lenses of the eyes)
- Increased urination (common to several endocrine disorders, including a deficit of antidiuretic hormones ► which results in the excretion of large amounts of urine ► resulting in dehydration).

■ Priority nursing diagnoses within the Nutritional-Metabolic Pattern that may be appropriate for clients with endocrine disorders include:

- *Imbalanced Nutrition: Less than Body Requirements* as evidenced by increased food intake with weight loss
- *Deficient Fluid Volume* as evidenced by dry mucous membranes, thirst, and decreased urine output
- *Hyperthermia* as evidenced by body temperatures ranging from 102°F (39°C) to 106°F (41°C)
- *Impaired Skin Integrity* as evidenced by dry, rough, reddened, and edematous skin.

■ Two nursing diagnoses from other functional health patterns often are of high priority for the client with endocrine disorders because the physiologic responses to these problems interfere with proper metabolism:

- *Disturbed Body Image* (Self-Perception-Self-Concept)
- *Ineffective Therapeutic Regimen Management* (Health Perception, Health Management)

Directions: Read the clinical scenario below and answer the questions that follow. To complete this exercise successfully, you will use not only knowledge of the content in this unit, but also principles related to setting priorities and maintaining client safety.

CLINICAL SCENARIO

You have been assigned to work with the following four clients for the 0700 shift on a medical-surgical unit. Significant data obtained during report are as follows:

- Mr. Blew is a 54-year-old who is admitted with complaints of poly-dipsia, polyuria, and polyphagia. There is a fruity odor to his breath and he seems confused at times. Vital signs on admission are T 99°F, P 90, R 30 and deep, BP 110/68. His blood glucose is 650 on admission at 0630.
- Mrs. Rant is a 65-year-old who is admitted with severe back pain in the flank area on the right side, nausea, and vomiting. She is being evaluated for treatment of renal calculi. She has a history of hyper-parathyroidism. Vital signs are T 97.6°F with clammy skin, P 100,

R 24, and BP of 168/94. She is requesting pain medication for the back pain.
- Mrs. Fox is an 86-year-old who was transferred from the medical ICU yesterday. She was admitted after being found unconscious by her daughter. On admission her blood sugar was 45, serum sodium was 128, T 96.6°F, and P 50. Vital signs this A.M. are T 98.4°F, P 78, R 18, BP 140/86. She is scheduled to have blood drawn for electrolytes at 0730.
- Mr. Rite is a 56-year-old who was admitted 4 days ago after falling from a ladder and hitting his head. He is complaining of a headache and thirst even after drinking 2000 mL of fluids during the night. Vital signs are T 100°F, P 98, R 14, BP 114/84.

Questions

1 In what order would you visit these clients after report?

1. _____
2. _____
3. _____
4. _____

2 What top two priority nursing diagnoses would you choose for each of the clients presented above? Can you explain, if asked, the rationale for your choices?

	Priority Nursing Diagnosis #1	Priority Nursing Diagnosis #2
Mr. Blew		
Mrs. Rant		
Mrs. Fox		
Mr. Rite		

3 If Mr. Blew's blood glucose drops to 50, which manifestations might he exhibit?

1. bradycardia, nausea, vomiting
2. tachycardia, hypotension, shakiness
3. thirst, diarrhea, fatigue
4. hypertension, edema, dyspnea

4 Mr. Blew understands diabetic teaching done by the nurse when he states:

1. "I will check my blood glucose before every meal."
2. "If I follow my prescribed diet, I will not have to check my blood sugar."
3. "If my blood glucose drops below 60, I can drink juice or milk to raise it."
4. "If my blood sugar is over 200, I can eat graham crackers to lower it."

5 The nurse explains to Mrs. Rant the dietary treatment for hyper-parathyroidism. Which is the appropriate dietary teaching for this client?

1. Increase fluids in the diet and avoid taking vitamin D supplements.
2. Increase potassium in the diet and avoid taking vitamin C supplements.
3. Decrease sodium in the diet and take vitamin B_6 supplements.
4. Decrease phosphorus in the diet and take vitamin A supplements.

6 The nurse assessing a client with hyperthyroidism may find which manifestations?

1. diaphoresis, diarrhea, alopecia, weight loss
2. dry skin, constipation, hirsutism, obesity
3. hypertension, abdominal pain, constipation, anorexia
4. dry skin, numbness around mouth, tetany

7 Based on the manifestations of headache and excessive thirst that Mr. Rite is exhibiting 4 days after his fall, the nurse should monitor for symptoms of what complication?

1. migraine headache
2. hypertensive crisis
3. increased intracranial pressure
4. infection

8 A prescription for levothyroxine sodium (Synthroid) is given to Mrs. Fox after she is diagnosed with hypothyroidism. The client voices understanding of how to take the medication when she states:

1. "I must take the medication with meals."
2. "I must take my pulse before taking the medication and report to the doctor a pulse below 100."
3. "I will only need to take this medication until my thyroid blood levels are back to normal."
4. "I can eat any food I choose because foods do not interfere with the medications."

9 Which laboratory studies would be conducted for Mr. Blew to monitor his diabetes management? (Select all that apply.)

1. fasting blood glucose
2. glycosylated hemoglobin
3. urinalysis
4. complete blood cell count
5. serum electrolytes
6. serum cholesterol and triglyceride levels

10 In postoperative thyroidectomy nursing care, it is *most* important for the nurse to monitor the client for which of these complications?

1. hyperthermia
2. laryngeal nerve damage
3. tetany
4. respiratory distress

11 Metabolic syndrome is a cluster of clinical manifestations associated with type 2 diabetes mellitus. Which clinical manifestations are indicative of metabolic syndrome?

1. hypertension, abdominal obesity, blood glucose > 110 mg/dL
2. tachycardia, weight gain, blood glucose < 110 mg/dL
3. hypotension, weight loss, blood glucose > 150 mg/dL
4. bradycardia, stomach obesity, blood glucose < 100 mg/dL

12 Which of the following laboratory value results may be seen in a client with untreated Cushing's syndrome?

1. serum sodium 150 mEq/L, serum potassium 2.8 mEq/L
2. blood glucose 68 mg/dL, blood urea nitrogen 28 mg/dL
3. serum calcium 9.0 mg/dL, serum sodium 130 mEq/L
4. blood glucose 350 mg/dL, serum potassium 5.2 mEq/L

CASE STUDY

Mr. Gregg is a 65-year-old African American male who was admitted with health problems of increased urination, increased thirst, fatigue, blurred vision, and numbness in his feet. He states that he retired 9 months ago after 45 years as a construction worker. He now leads a sedentary lifestyle and doesn't have as much energy as he used to have. He has gained 30 pounds since retirement. Upon assessment, Mr. Gregg weighs 255 pounds and is 5'11" tall. Vital signs are T 98.8°F, P 88, R 20, and BP 150/90. Decreased pulses are palpated in dorsal pedalis and posterior tibial pulses. Both feet are cool to touch with slow capillary refill in toes. The following laboratory studies are ordered to confirm the diagnosis of type 2 diabetes mellitus: plasma glucose concentration, fasting blood glucose, and oral glucose tolerance test.

Type 2 diabetes mellitus is a disease of fasting hyperglycemia despite the production of some insulin by the beta cells of the pancreas. The level of insulin production varies, affecting the amount available cellular metabolism.

With increased age, sedentary lifestyle, and obesity, cells become resistant to insulin. The uptake of glucose by muscle and fat cells is not sufficient to lower the blood glucose. In obesity, insulin has a decreased ability to influence glucose metabolism and affect the uptake of glucose by cells in the liver, skeletal muscles, and adipose tissue, resulting in a high blood glucose level.

The manifestations of type 2 diabetes mellitus include polyuria, polydipsia, blurred vision, fatigue, paresthesias, and skin infections. In times of physical or emotional stress, the client may develop a hyperosmolar hyperglycemic state (HHS). Complications of type 2 diabetes mellitus include coronary heart disease (myocardial infarction), hypertension, stroke, peripheral vascular disease (atherosclerosis, vascular insufficiency, amputations), end-stage renal disease (nephropathy), and blindness (retinopathy).

Based on Mr. Gregg's manifestations and weight gain, a priority nursing diagnosis of *Imbalanced Nutrition: More than Body Requirements* is appropriate for guiding nursing care on this client.

- Beta cells decrease insulin production; cells become less sensitive to insulin
- Glucose accumulates in blood; chronic hyperglycemia affects function of cells and tissues

affects

Mr. G
65 y.o. male
Type 2 diabetes mellitus

leads to

assess

- Ht: 5', 11", Wt: 255
- Retired, sedentary lifestyle
- States he has gained 30 pounds in 9 months
- Lab findings of hyperglycemia

generates

- Ineffective Tissue Perfusion related to effects of chronic hyperglycemia
- Deficient Knowledge: Cause and effects of Type 2 DM
- Deficient Knowledge: Self-care of Type 2 DM

generate nursing diagnosis

prioritized to

Imbalanced Nutrition: More Than Body Requirements

expected outcomes

- Loses 2 pounds per week for the next month
- Takes part in exercise program at local fitness center
- Walks each day for a minimum of 30 minutes
- Discusses diet requirements with dietitian
- Verbalizes importance of a balance of diet, exercise, and medications for type 2 diabetes mellitus

evaluate

- Verbalized cause and effects of DM
- Enrolled in both fitness class and support group
- Has lost 15 pounds in 8 weeks
- Walks briskly for 45 minutes each day

Interdisciplinary Interventions
- Make referral to dietitian to discuss appropriate diet

Independent Interventions
- Discuss understanding of balance of diet, exercise, and medications in controlling illness
- Suggest enrollment in senior wellness activities at community recreation center
- Encourage to weigh self at least every 2 days and maintain record of weights
- Teach pathophysiology, manifestations, and complications of type 2 diabetes mellitus
- Teach effects and guidelines for taking oral hypoglycemic medications

Responses to Altered Nutrition

CHAPTER 21 Assessing Clients with Nutritional and Gastrointestinal Disorders

LEARNING OUTCOMES

- Describe the sources of nutrients, and their functions in the human body.

- Describe the anatomy, physiology, and functions of the gastrointestinal system.

- Explain the processes of carbohydrate, fat, and protein metabolism.

- Identify specific topics to consider during a health history assessment interview of the client with nutritional and gastrointestinal disorders.

- Explain techniques used for assessing nutritional and gastrointestinal status.

- Describe normal variations in assessment findings for the older adult.

- Identify abnormal findings that may indicate alterations in gastrointestinal function.

CLINICAL COMPETENCIES

- Conduct and document a health history for clients who have or are at risk for alterations in nutrition and gastrointestinal function.

- Conduct and document a physical assessment of nutritional status and the gastrointestinal system.

- Monitor the results of diagnostic tests and report abnormal findings.

EQUIPMENT NEEDED

- Stethoscope

- Balance scale with height measuring attachment

- Tape measure

- Skin fold calipers

MEDIALINK

Resources for this chapter can be found on the Prentice Hall Nursing MediaLink DVD-ROM accompanying this textbook, and on the Companion Website at http://www.prenhall.com/lemone

KEY TERMS

bile, *612*
borborygmus, *624*
bruit, *624*
cheilosis, *622*

gingivitis, *623*
glossitis, *622*
leukoplakia, *623*
metabolism, *613*

nutrition, *605*
peristalsis, *610*
striae, *624*

Nutrition is the process by which the body ingests, absorbs, transports, uses, and eliminates nutrients in food. The digestive organs responsible for these processes are the gastrointestinal tract (also called the alimentary canal) and the accessory digestive organs. The gastrointestinal tract consists of the mouth, pharynx, esophagus, stomach, small intestine, and large intestine. The accessory digestive organs include the liver, gallbladder, and pancreas (Figure 21–1 ■). This chapter discusses the assessment of these organs except the large intestine. Assessment of the large intestine, which is primarily responsible for elimination, is discussed in Chapter 25 ∞.

NUTRIENTS

Nutrients are substances found in food and are used by the body to promote growth, maintenance, and repair. The categories of nutrients are carbohydrates, proteins, fats, vitamins, minerals, and water. Dietary guidelines for Americans specific to nutrients are summarized in Table 21–1. (See Chapter 2 ∞ for the

Oral cavity
Tongue
Esophagus
Liver
Gallbladder
Pancreas
Small intestine
Cecum
Vermiform appendix
Anus

Salivary glands
Pharynx
Spleen
Stomach
Transverse colon
Ascending colon
Descending colon
Large intestine
Sigmoid colon
Rectum

Figure 21–1 ■ Organs of the gastrointestinal tract and accessory digestive organs.

TABLE 21–1 Recommended Dietary Guidelines for Americans 2005

CATEGORY	RECOMMENDATION
General dietary guidelines	■ Consume a variety of nutrient-dense foods and beverages within and among the basic food groups while choosing foods that limit the intake of saturated and *trans* fats, cholesterol, added sugars, salt, and alcohol. ■ Meet recommended intakes by adopting a balanced eating pattern, such as that provided by the USDA Food Guide Pyramid. ■ Balance calories from foods and beverages with calories expended to maintain body weight. ■ Over time, make small decreases in food and beverage calories and increase physical activity to prevent gradual weight gain.
Food groups	■ For a 2000-calorie diet, consume 2 cups of fruit and 2 1/2 cups of vegetables per day (increase or decrease amounts depending on calorie level). ■ Select from all five vegetable subgroups (dark green, orange, legumes, starchy vegetables, other vegetables) several times a week. ■ Consume 3 or more ounce equivalents of whole-grain products each day, with the rest of recommended grains coming from enriched or whole-grain products. In general, at least half of the grains should be from whole grains. ■ Consume 3 cups per day of fat-free or low-fat milk or equivalent milk products.
Carbohydrates	■ Choose fiber-rich foods, vegetables, and whole grains often. ■ Choose and prepare foods with little added sugars or caloric sweeteners.
Fats	■ Consume less than 10% of calories from saturated fatty acids and less than 300 mg/day of cholesterol; keep *trans* fatty acid consumption as low as possible. ■ Keep total fat intake between 20% and 35% of calories, with most fats coming from sources of polyunsaturated and monounsaturated fatty acids, such as fish, nuts, and vegetable oil. ■ When selecting and preparing meats, poultry, dry beans, and milk or milk products, make choices that are lean, low fat, or fat free.
Sodium and potassium	■ Consume less than 2300 mg (about 1 teaspoon of salt) of sodium each day. ■ Choose and prepare foods with little salt. ■ Consume potassium-rich foods, such as fruits and vegetables.

Source: United States Department of Agriculture. (2005). *Dietary guidelines for Americans 2005. Key recommendations for the general population*. Available http://www.health.gov/dietaryguidelines/dga2005/recommendations.htm

new USDA Food Guide Pyramid, which is useful for planning and teaching about nutritional intake.)

Carbohydrates

The primary sources of carbohydrates (which include sugars and starches) are plant foods. Monosaccharides and disaccharides come from milk, sugar cane, sugar beets, honey, and fruits. Polysaccharide starch is found in grains, legumes, and root vegetables. Following ingestion, digestion, and metabolism, carbohydrates are converted primarily to glucose, the molecule body cells use to make adenosine triphosphate (ATP). Excess glucose in the healthy person is converted to glycogen or fat. Glycogen is stored in the liver and muscles; fat is stored as adipose tissue. Carbohydrate use by the body is shown in Figure 21–2A ■.

Regardless of the source, all carbohydrates supply 4 kcal per gram. The minimum necessary daily carbohydrate intake is unknown, but the recommended daily intake is 125 to 175 g, most of which should be complex carbohydrates (such as milk, potatoes, and whole grains). Excess intake of carbohydrates over time can result in obesity, dental caries, and elevated plasma triglycerides. Over extended periods of time, carbohydrate deficiencies lead to tissue wasting from protein breakdown and metabolic acidosis from an excess of ketones as a by-product of fat breakdown.

Proteins

Proteins are classified as either complete or incomplete. Complete proteins are found in animal products such as eggs, milk, milk products, and meat. They contain the greatest amount of amino acids and meet the body's amino acid requirements for tissue growth and maintenance. Incomplete proteins are found in legumes, nuts, grains, cereals, and vegetables. These sources are low in or lack one or more of the amino acids essential for building complete proteins.

The body uses proteins to build many different structures, including skin keratin, the collagen and elastin in connective tissues, and muscles. They also are used to make enzymes, hemoglobin, plasma proteins, and some hormones. Protein use by the body is shown in Figure 21–2B.

Proteins provide 4 kcal per gram. The recommended daily intake of protein is 56 g for men and 45 g for women. Healthy people with adequate caloric intake have an equal rate of protein synthesis and protein breakdown and loss, reflected as nitrogen balance. If the breakdown and loss of proteins exceed intake, a negative nitrogen balance results. This may be due to starvation, altered physical states (e.g., from injury or illness), and altered emotional states (such as depression or anxiety). A positive nitrogen balance, which results when protein intake exceeds breakdown, is normal during growth, tissue repair, and pregnancy.

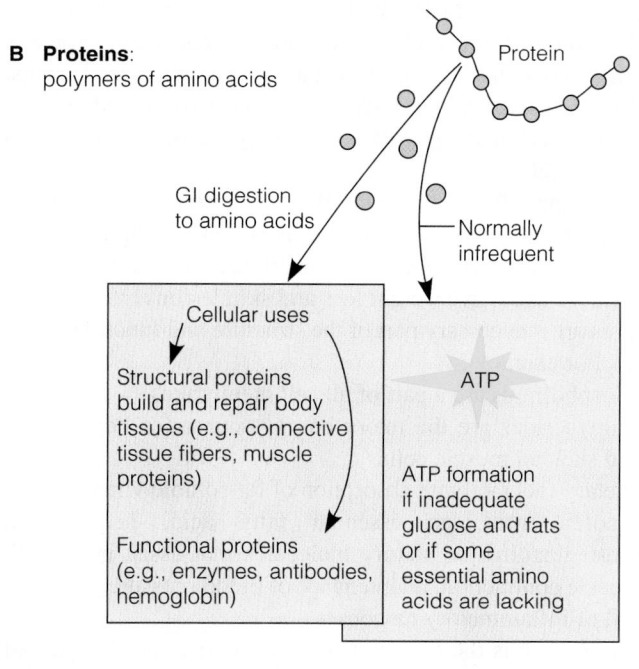

A **Carbohydrates**: composed of simple sugars (monosaccharides)

Polysaccharide

Monosaccharides

GI digestion to glucose

Cellular uses

ATP

Excesses stored as glycogen or fat

Glycogen and fat broken down for ATP formation

Monosaccharides

To capillary

Broken down to glucose and released to blood

B **Proteins**: polymers of amino acids

Protein

GI digestion to amino acids

Normally infrequent

Cellular uses

Structural proteins build and repair body tissues (e.g., connective tissue fibers, muscle proteins)

Functional proteins (e.g., enzymes, antibodies, hemoglobin)

ATP

ATP formation if inadequate glucose and fats or if some essential amino acids are lacking

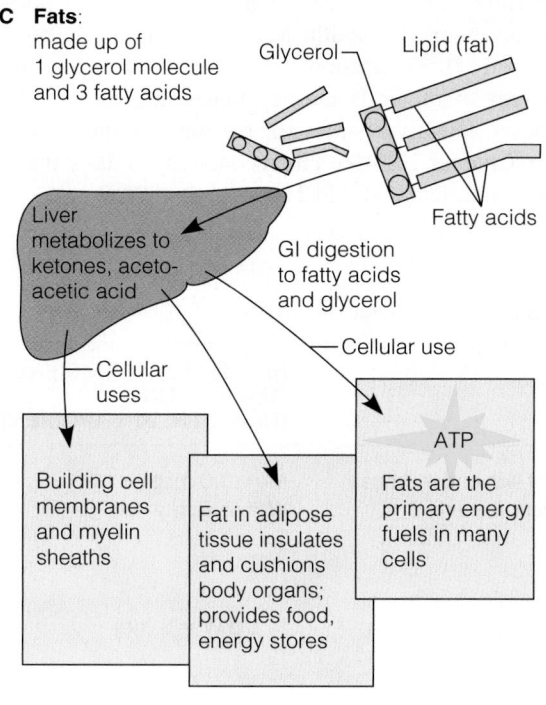

C **Fats**: made up of 1 glycerol molecule and 3 fatty acids

Glycerol

Lipid (fat)

Fatty acids

Liver metabolizes to ketones, aceto-acetic acid

GI digestion to fatty acids and glycerol

Cellular uses

Cellular use

Building cell membranes and myelin sheaths

Fat in adipose tissue insulates and cushions body organs; provides food, energy stores

ATP

Fats are the primary energy fuels in many cells

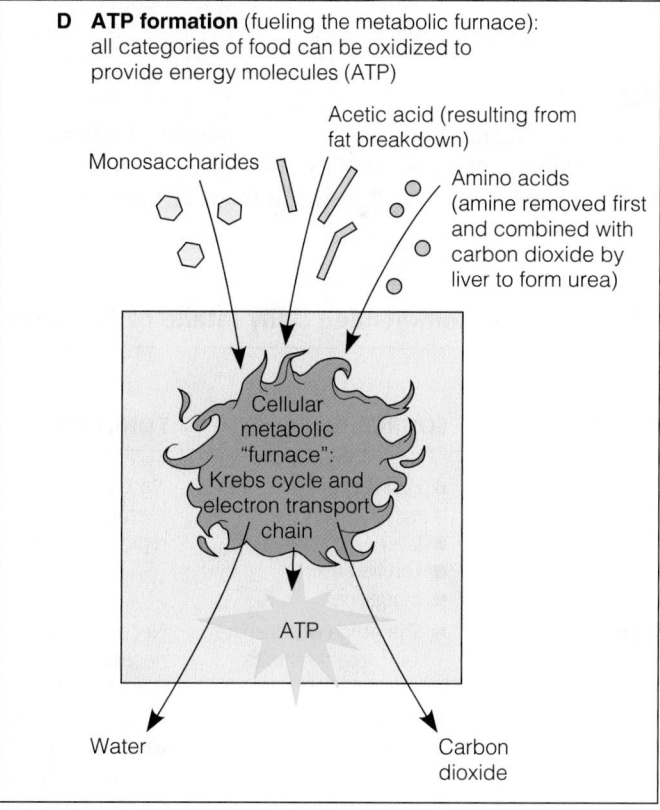

D **ATP formation** (fueling the metabolic furnace): all categories of food can be oxidized to provide energy molecules (ATP)

Monosaccharides

Acetic acid (resulting from fat breakdown)

Amino acids (amine removed first and combined with carbon dioxide by liver to form urea)

Cellular metabolic "furnace": Krebs cycle and electron transport chain

ATP

Water

Carbon dioxide

Figure 21–2 ■ A schematic overview of nutrient use by body cells, including *A,* carbohydrates; *B,* proteins; *C,* fats; and *D,* ATP formation.

Anabolic steroids affect the rate of protein use; for example, the adrenal corticosteroids are released in times of stress to increase protein breakdown and conversion of amino acids to glucose. Excessive intake of proteins may lead to obesity, whereas deficits cause weight loss and tissue wasting, edema, and anemia.

Fats (Lipids)

Fats, or lipids, include phospholipids; steroids, such as cholesterol; and neutral fats, more commonly known as triglycerides. Neutral fats are the most abundant fats in the diet. They may be either saturated or unsaturated. Saturated fats are found in animal products (milk and meats) and in some plant products (such as coconut). Unsaturated fats are found in seeds, nuts, and most vegetable oils. Sources of cholesterol include meats, milk products, and egg yolks. Fat use by the body is shown in Figure 21–2C.

Fats supply 9 kcal per gram. When a person consumes more than the body requires, the excess is stored as adipose tissue, increasing the risk of obesity and heart disease. A deficit of fats may cause excessive weight loss and skin lesions.

Fats are a necessary part of the structure and function of the body. For example:

■ Phospholipids are a part of all cell membranes.
■ Triglycerides are the major energy source for hepatocytes and skeletal muscle cells.
■ Dietary fats facilitate absorption of fat-soluble vitamins.
■ Linoleic acid, an essential fatty acid, helps form prostaglandins, regulatory molecules that assist in smooth muscle contraction, maintenance of blood pressure, and control of inflammatory responses.
■ Cholesterol is the essential component of bile salts, steroid hormones, and vitamin D.
■ Adipose tissue serves as a protection around body organs, as a layer of insulation under the skin, and as a concentrated source of fuel for cellular energy.

Vitamins

Vitamins are organic compounds that facilitate the body's use of carbohydrates, proteins, and fats. All of the vitamins except vitamins D and K must be ingested in foods or taken as supplements. Vitamin D is made by ultraviolet irradiation of cholesterol molecules in the skin, and vitamin K is synthesized by bacteria in the intestine.

Vitamins are categorized as either fat soluble or water soluble. The fat-soluble vitamins (A, D, E, and K) bind to ingested fats and are absorbed as the fats are absorbed. Water-soluble vitamins (the B complex and C) are absorbed with water in the GI tract (however, vitamin B_{12} must become attached to intrinsic factor to be absorbed). Fat-soluble vitamins are stored in the body, and excesses may cause toxicity; water-soluble vitamins in excess of body requirements are excreted in the urine.

The recommended amounts of vitamins, previously labeled recommended daily allowances (RDAs), are now labeled by the National Academy of Sciences as dietary reference intakes (DRIs) per day. The source, function, and minimum daily recommended intake levels are provided for each vitamin in Tables 21–2 and Table 21–3.

Minerals

Minerals work with other nutrients to maintain the structure and function of the body. An adequate supply of calcium, phosphorus, potassium, sulfur, sodium, chloride, and magnesium—as well as other trace elements such as iron, iodine, copper, and zinc—is necessary to health. Most minerals in the body are found in body fluids or are bound to organic compounds. The best sources of minerals are vegetables, legumes, milk, and some meats. Dietary sources for the major minerals are discussed in Chapter 10 ∞ . The recommended daily intake for minerals is outlined in Table 21–4.

TABLE 21–2 Recommended Daily Intake of Fat-Soluble Vitamins

NAME	SOURCE	FUNCTION	MINIMUM RECOMMENDED DAILY INTAKE (M = MEN, W = WOMEN)
Vitamin A (retinol)	■ Fish liver oils ■ Egg yolk ■ Liver ■ Fortified milk ■ Margarine	Necessary for vision, integrity of skin and mucous membranes, cell membrane function, and reproductive function	M = 900 mcg W = 700 mcg
Vitamin D	■ The action of sunshine on cholesterol in the skin	Necessary for blood calcium homeostasis (in turn necessary for blood clotting), bone formation, and neuromuscular function	M and W = 5 mcg
Vitamin E	■ Vegetable oils ■ Margarine ■ Whole grains ■ Dark green leafy vegetables	As an antioxidant, helps prevent the oxidation of vitamins A and C in the intestines and decreases the oxidation of unsaturated fatty acids to facilitate cell membrane integrity	M and W = 15 mcg
Vitamin K	■ Synthesized by coliform bacteria in the large intestine ■ Green, leafy vegetables ■ Cabbage ■ Cauliflower ■ Pork	Essential for the formation of clotting proteins in the liver	M = 120 mcg W = 90 mcg

TABLE 21–3 Recommended Daily Intake of Water-Soluble Vitamins

NAME	SOURCE	FUNCTION	MINIMUM RECOMMENDED DAILY INTAKE (M = MEN, W = WOMEN)
Vitamin B$_1$ (thiamin)	■ Lean meats ■ Liver ■ Eggs ■ Green leafy vegetables ■ Legumes ■ Whole grains	An essential coenzyme for carbohydrate metabolism and use; also for healthy function of nerves, muscles, and the heart	M = 1.2 mg W = 1.1 mg
Vitamin B$_2$ (riboflavin)	■ Liver ■ Egg white ■ Whole grains ■ Meat ■ Poultry ■ Fish ■ Milk	Involved in the catabolism and use of carbohydrates, fats, and proteins; the use of other B vitamins; and is important for the production of adrenal hormones	M = 1.3 mg W = 1.1 mg
Vitamin B$_6$ (pyridoxine)	■ Meat ■ Poultry ■ Fish ■ Potatoes ■ Tomatoes ■ Sweet potatoes ■ Spinach	Necessary for amino acid metabolism, formation of antibodies, and formation of hemoglobin	M and W < age 51 = 1.3 M > age 51 = 1.7 mg W > age 51 = 1.5 mg
Vitamin B$_{12}$ (cyanocobalamin)	■ Liver ■ Meat ■ Poultry ■ Dairy foods (except butter) ■ Eggs	Essential for the production of nucleic acids and red blood cells in the bone marrow; also plays an important role in the use of folic acid and carbohydrates, and in healthy function of the nervous system.	M and W = 2.4 mcg
Vitamin C (ascorbic acid)	■ Citrus fruits ■ Potatoes ■ Tomatoes ■ Green leafy vegetables	Acts as an antioxidant and vasoconstrictor; also serves in the formation of connective tissue, conversion for cholesterol to bile salts, iron absorption and use, and conversion of folic acid to an active form	M = 90 mg W = 75 mg
Vitamin B$_3$ niacin (nicotinamide)	■ Meat ■ Poultry ■ Fish ■ Liver ■ Peanuts ■ Green leafy vegetables	Plays an important role in the metabolism of carbohydrates and fats; inhibits cholesterol synthesis; important for integumentary, nervous, and digestive system health; assists in the manufacture of reproductive hormones	M and W = 35 mg
Biotin	■ Liver ■ Eggs ■ Nuts ■ Legumes	Essential for the catabolism of fatty acids and carbohydrates, and helps dispose of the waste products of protein catabolism	M and W = 30 mcg
Pantothenic acid	■ Meats ■ Whole grains ■ Egg yolk ■ Liver ■ Yeast ■ Legumes	Assists in the synthesis of steroids and of the heme in hemoglobin; is essential for the metabolism of carbohydrates and fats, and for the manufacture of reproductive hormones	M and W = 5 mg
Folic acid (folate)	■ Liver ■ Dark green vegetables ■ Lean beef ■ Eggs ■ Veal ■ Whole grains ■ Synthesized by bacteria in the intestine	The basis of a coenzyme necessary to the manufacture of nucleic acids and so is essential for the formation of red blood cells, growth and development, and nervous system health	M and W = 400 mcg

MediaLink Case Study: Counseling a College Student about Vitamins

TABLE 21–4 **Recommended Daily Intake of Minerals**	
NAME	**MINIMUM RECOMMENDED DAILY INTAKE (M = MEN, W = WOMEN)**
Calcium	M and W = 1000 mg W > menopause = 1200 mg
Phosphorus	M and W = 1000 mg
Iron	M and W = 18 mg
Zinc	M and W = 15 mg
Manganese	M = 2.3 mg W = 1.8 mg
Molybdenum	M and W = 75 mcg
Chromium	M and W = 120 mcg
Iodine	M and W = 150 mcg
Selenium	M and W = 70 mcg
Magnesium	M and W = 400 mg
Copper	M and W = 2.0 mg
Chloride	M and W = 3400 mg

ANATOMY, PHYSIOLOGY, AND FUNCTIONS OF THE GASTROINTESTINAL SYSTEM

The gastrointestinal tract is a continuous hollow tube, extending from the mouth to the anus. Once foods are placed in the mouth, they are subjected to a variety of processes that move them and break them down into end products that can be absorbed from the lumen of the small intestine into the blood or lymph. These digestive processes are as follows:

- Ingestion of food
- Movement of food and wastes
- Secretion of mucus, water, and enzymes
- Mechanical digestion of food
- Chemical digestion of food
- Absorption of digested food.

The Mouth

The mouth, also called the oral or buccal cavity, is lined with mucous membranes and is enclosed by the lips, cheeks, palate, and tongue (Figure 21–3 ■).

The lips and cheeks are skeletal muscle covered externally by skin. Their function is to keep food in the mouth during chewing. The palate consists of two regions: the hard palate and the soft palate. The hard palate covers bone in the roof of the mouth and provides a hard surface against which the tongue forces food. The soft palate, extending from the hard palate and ending at the back of the mouth as a fold called the uvula, is primarily muscle. When food is swallowed, the soft palate rises as a reflex to close off the oropharynx.

The tongue, composed of skeletal muscle and connective tissue, is located in the floor of the mouth. It contains mucous and serous glands, taste buds, and papillae. The tongue mixes food with saliva during chewing, forms the food into a mass (called a *bolus*), and initiates swallowing. Some papillae pro-

vide surface roughness to facilitate licking and moving food; other papillae house the taste buds.

Saliva moistens food so it can be made into a bolus, dissolves food chemicals so they can be tasted, and provides enzymes (such as amylase) that begin the chemical breakdown of starches. Saliva is produced by salivary glands, most of which lie superior or inferior to the mouth and drain into it. The salivary glands include the parotid, the submaxillary, and the sublingual glands.

The teeth chew (masticate) and grind food to break it down into smaller parts. As the food is masticated, it is mixed with saliva. Adults have 32 permanent teeth. The teeth are embedded in the gingiva (gums), with the crown of each tooth visible above the gingiva.

The Pharynx

The pharynx consists of the oropharynx and the laryngopharynx (see Figure 21–3). Both structures provide passageways for food, fluids, and air. The pharynx is made of skeletal muscles and is lined with mucous membranes. The skeletal muscles move food to the esophagus via the pharynx through **peristalsis** (alternating waves of contraction and relaxation of involuntary muscle). The mucosa of the pharynx contains mucous-producing glands that provide fluid to facilitate the passage of the bolus of food as it is swallowed.

The Esophagus

The esophagus, a muscular tube about 10 inches (25 cm) long, serves as a passageway for food from the pharynx to the stomach (see Figures 21–1 and 21–3). The epiglottis, a flap of cartilage over the top of the larynx, keeps food out of the larynx

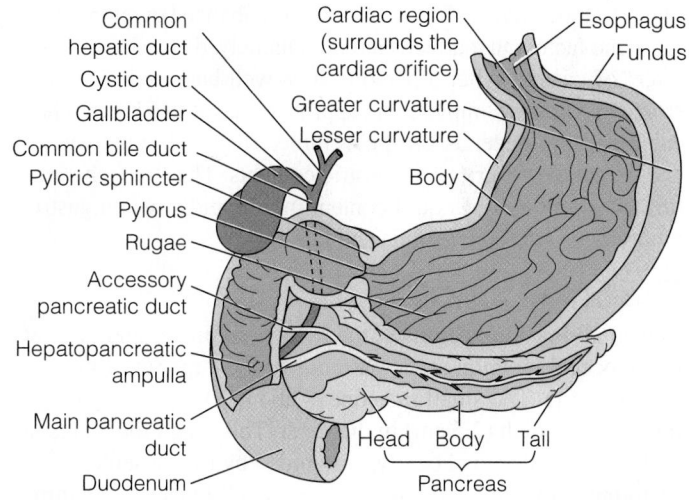

Figure 21–3 ■ Structures of the mouth, the pharynx, and the esophagus.

during swallowing. The esophagus descends through the thorax and diaphragm, entering the stomach at the cardiac orifice. The gastroesophageal sphincter surrounds this opening. This sphincter, along with the diaphragm, keeps the orifice closed when food is not being swallowed.

For most of its length, the esophagus is lined with stratified squamous epithelium; simple columnar epithelium lines the esophagus where it joins the stomach. The mucosa and submucosa of the esophagus lie in longitudinal folds when the esophagus is empty.

The Stomach

The stomach, located high on the left side of the abdominal cavity, is connected to the esophagus at the upper end and to the small intestine at the lower end (Figure 21–4 ■). Normally about 10 inches (25 cm) long, the stomach is a distensible organ that can expand to hold up to 4 L of food and fluid. The concave surface of the stomach is called the lesser curvature; the convex surface is called the greater curvature. The stomach may be divided into regions extending from the distal end of the esophagus to the opening into the small intestine. These regions are the cardiac region, fundus, body, and pylorus (see Figure 21–4). The pyloric sphincter controls emptying of the stomach into the duodenal portion of the small intestine. The stomach is a storage reservoir for food, continues the mechanical breakdown of food, begins the process of protein digestion, and mixes the food with gastric juices into a thick fluid called chyme.

The stomach is lined with columnar epithelial, mucous-producing cells. Millions of openings in the lining lead to gastric glands that can produce 4 to 5 L of gastric juice each day. The gastric glands contain a variety of secretory cells, including the following:

Figure 21–4 ■ The internal anatomic structures of the stomach, including the pancreatic, cystic, and hepatic ducts; the pancreas; and the gallbladder.

- Mucous cells produce alkaline mucus that clings to the lining of the stomach and protects it from being digested by gastric juice.
- Zymogenic cells produce pepsinogen (an inactive form of pepsin, a protein-digesting enzyme).
- Parietal cells secrete hydrochloric acid and intrinsic factor. Hydrochloric acid activates and increases the activity of protein-digesting cells and also is bactericidal. Intrinsic factor is necessary for the absorption of vitamin B_{12} in the small intestine.
- Enteroendocrine cells secrete gastrin, histamine, endorphins, serotonin, and somatostatin. These hormones or hormone-like

substances diffuse into the blood. Gastrin is important in regulating secretion and motility of the stomach.

The secretion of gastric juice is under both neural and endocrine control. Stimulation of the parasympathetic vagus nerve increases secretory activity; in contrast, stimulation of sympathetic nerves decreases secretions. The three phases of secretory activity are the cephalic phase, the gastric phase, and the intestinal phase.

- The cephalic phase prepares for digestion and is triggered by the sight, odor, taste, or thought of food. During this initial phase, motor impulses are transmitted via the vagus nerve to the stomach.
- The gastric phase begins when food enters the stomach. Stomach distention (stimulating stretch receptors) and chemical stimuli from partially digested proteins initiate this phase. Gastrin-secreting cells produce gastrin, which in turn stimulates the gastric glands (especially the parietal cells) to produce more gastric juice. Histamine also stimulates hydrochloric acid secretion.
- The intestinal phase is initiated when partially digested food begins to enter the small intestine, stimulating mucous cells of the intestine to release a hormone that promotes continued gastric secretion.

Mechanical digestion in the stomach is accomplished by peristaltic movements that churn and mix the food with the gastric juices to form chyme. Gastric motility is enhanced or retarded by the same factors that affect secretion, namely, distention and the effect of gastrin. After a person eats a well-balanced meal, the stomach empties completely in approximately 4 to 6 hours. Gastric emptying depends on the volume, chemical composition, and osmotic pressure of the gastric contents. The stomach empties large volumes of liquid content more rapidly, while gastric emptying is slowed by solids and fats.

The Small Intestine

The small intestine begins at the pyloric sphincter and ends at the ileocecal junction at the entrance of the large intestine (see Figure 21–1). The small intestine is about 20 ft (6 m) long but only about 1 inch (2.5 cm) in diameter. This long tube hangs in coils in the abdominal cavity, suspended by the mesentery and surrounded by the large intestine. The small intestine has three regions: the duodenum, the jejunum, and the ileum. The duodenum begins at the pyloric sphincter and extends around the head of the pancreas for about 10 inches (25 cm). Both pancreatic enzymes and bile from the liver enter the small intestine at the duodenum. The jejunum, the middle region of the small intestine, extends for about 8 ft (2.4 m). The ileum, the terminal end of the small intestine, is approximately 12 ft (3.6 m) long and meets the large intestine at the ileocecal valve.

Food is chemically digested, and most of it absorbed, as it moves through the small intestine. Circular folds (deep folds of the mucosa and submucosa layers), villi (finger-like projections of the mucosa cells), and microvilli (tiny projections of the mucosa cells) increase the surface area of the small intestine to enhance absorption of food. Although up to 10 L of food, liquids, and secretions enter the GI tract each day, less than 1 L reaches the large intestine.

Enzymes in the small intestine break down carbohydrates, proteins, lipids, and nucleic acids. Pancreatic amylase acts on starches, converting them to maltose, dextrins, and oligosaccharides; the intestinal enzymes dextrinase, glucoamylase, maltase, sucrase, and lactase further break down these products into monosaccharides. Pancreatic enzymes (trypsin and chymotrypsin) and intestinal enzymes continue to break down proteins into peptides. Pancreatic lipases digest lipids in the small intestine. Triglycerides enter as fat globules and are coated by bile salts and emulsified. Nucleic acids are hydrolyzed by pancreatic enzymes and then broken apart by intestinal enzymes. Both pancreatic enzymes and bile are excreted into the duodenum in response to the secretion of secretin and cholecystokinin, hormones produced by the intestinal mucosa cells when chyme enters the small intestine.

Nutrients are absorbed through the mucosa of the intestinal villi into the blood or lymph by active transport, facilitated transport, and passive diffusion. Almost all food products and water, as well as vitamins and most electrolytes, are absorbed in the small intestine, leaving only indigestible fibers, some water, and bacteria to enter the large intestine. (The large intestine is discussed in Chapter 25 ∞.)

The Accessory Digestive Organs

The liver, gallbladder, and exocrine pancreas secrete substances necessary for the digestion of chyme. The liver produces bile, necessary for fat digestion and absorption, and stores it in the gallbladder. The liver also receives nutrients absorbed by the small intestine and metabolizes or synthesizes these nutrients so they are in a form that can be used by the cells of the body. The exocrine pancreas produces enzymes necessary for digestion of fats, proteins, and carbohydrates.

The Liver and Gallbladder

The liver weighs about 3 lb (1.4 kg) in the average-size adult. It is located in the right side of the abdomen, inferior to the diaphragm and anterior to the stomach (see Figure 21–1). The liver has four lobes: right, left, caudate, and quadrate. A mesenteric ligament separates the right and left lobes and suspends the liver from the diaphragm and anterior abdominal wall. The liver is encased in a fibroelastic capsule, called the Glisson capsule. This capsule contains blood vessels, lymphatics, and nerves. When the liver is diseased or swollen, distention causes pain and the lymphatics may ooze fluid into the peritoneal cavity.

Liver tissue consists of units called lobules, which are composed of plates of hepatocytes (liver cells). A branch of the hepatic artery, a branch of the hepatic portal vein, and a bile duct communicate with each lobule. Sinusoids, blood-filled spaces within the lobules, are lined with Kupffer cells. These phagocytic cells remove debris from the blood.

Bile production is the liver's primary digestive function. **Bile** is a greenish, watery solution containing bile salts, cholesterol, bilirubin, electrolytes, water, and phospholipids. These substances are necessary to emulsify and promote the absorption of fats. Liver cells make from 700 to 1200 mL of bile daily. When bile is not needed for digestion, the sphincter of Oddi (located at the point at which bile enters the duodenum) is closed, and the bile backs up the cystic duct into the gallbladder for storage.

Bile is concentrated and stored in the gallbladder, a small sac cupped in the inferior surface of the liver. When food containing fats enters the duodenum, hormones stimulate the gallbladder to secrete bile into the cystic duct. The cystic duct joins the hepatic duct to form the common bile duct, from which bile enters into the duodenum (see Figure 21–4).

The major digestive and metabolic functions of the liver are outlined in Box 21–1. These functions require a large amount of blood, with the liver receiving blood from both venous and arterial blood vessels. The hepatic artery, branching from the abdominal aorta, provides oxygenated blood at the rate of 400 to 500 mL/min. The hepatic portal vein delivers about 1000 to 1200 mL/min of deoxygenated blood to the liver from the inferior and superior mesenteric veins and the splenic vein.

The Exocrine Pancreas

The pancreas, a gland located between the stomach and small intestine, is the primary enzyme-producing organ of the digestive system. It is a triangular gland extending across the abdomen, with its tail next to the spleen and its head next to the duodenum (see Figure 21–4). The body and tail of the pancreas are retroperitoneal, lying behind the greater curvature of the stomach. The pancreas is actually two organs in one, having both exocrine and endocrine structures and functions. The exocrine portion of the pancreas, through secretory units called acini, secretes alkaline pancreatic juice containing many different enzymes. The acini, clusters of secretory cells surrounding ducts, drain into the pancreatic duct. The pancreatic duct joins with the common bile duct just before it enters the duodenum (so that pancreatic juice and bile from the liver enter the small intestine together). The pancreas also has endocrine functions, discussed in Chapter 18 ∞.

The pancreas produces from 1 to 1.5 L of pancreatic juice daily. Pancreatic juice is clear and has high bicarbonate content. This alkaline fluid neutralizes the acidic chyme as it enters the duodenum, optimizing the pH for intestinal and pancreatic enzyme activity. The secretion of pancreatic juice is controlled by the vagus nerve and the intestinal hormones secretin and cholecystokinin. Pancreatic juice contains enzymes that aid in the digestion of all categories of foods: lipase promotes fat breakdown and absorption; amylase completes starch digestion; and trypsin, chymotrypsin, and carboxypeptidase are responsible for half of all protein digestion. Nucleases break down nucleic acids.

METABOLISM

After nutrients (carbohydrates, fats, and proteins) are ingested, digested, absorbed, and transported across cell membranes, they must be metabolized to produce and provide energy to maintain life. **Metabolism** is the process of biochemical reactions occurring in the body's cells. Metabolic processes are either catabolic or anabolic. Catabolism involves the breakdown of complex structures into simpler forms, for example, the breakdown of carbohydrates to produce ATP, an energy molecule that fuels cellular activity. In the process of anabolism, simpler molecules combine to build more complex structures, for example, amino acids bond to form proteins.

The biochemical reactions of metabolism produce water, carbon dioxide, and ATP (see Figure 21–2D on page 607). The energy value of foods is measured in kilocalories (kcal). A kilocalorie is defined as the amount of heat energy needed to raise the temperature of 1 kilogram (kg) of water 1 degree centigrade.

ASSESSING NUTRITIONAL STATUS AND GASTROINTESTINAL FUNCTION

Nutritional status and the function of the gastrointestinal system are assessed by findings from diagnostic tests, a health assessment interview to collect subjective data, and a physical assessment to collect objective data. See the box below for sample documentation of a nutritional status assessment.

SAMPLE DOCUMENTATION
Assessment of Nutritional Status

22-year-old female visiting health clinic for regular check-up. Height 5 feet, 5 inches (165 cm); Weight 128 pounds (58 kg). BMI: 24. MAC: 28 cm. Waist-to-hip ratio: 0.6. Skin is warm, moist and smooth without lesions other than well-healed scar on RLQ of abdomen from appendectomy, age 15. Oral mucosa and tongue pink and moist. No breath odor. All teeth present with evidence of dental care. Abdomen slightly concave when lying on back, bowel sounds present in all four quadrants, liver nonpalpable, tympany over lower abdomen on percussion.

BOX 21–1 **Major Metabolic and Digestive Functions of the Liver**

- Secretes bile.
- Stores fat-soluble vitamins (A, D, E, and K).
- Metabolizes bilirubin.
- Stores blood and releases blood into the general circulation during hemorrhage.
- Synthesizes plasma proteins to maintain plasma oncotic pressure.
- Synthesizes prothrombin, fibrinogen, and factors I, II, VII, IX, and X, which are necessary for blood clotting.
- Synthesizes fats from carbohydrates and proteins to be either used for energy or stored as adipose tissue.

- Synthesizes phospholipids and cholesterol necessary for the production of bile salts, steroid hormones, and plasma membranes.
- Converts amino acids to carbohydrates through deamination.
- Releases glucose during times of hypoglycemia.
- Takes up glucose during times of hyperglycemia and stores it as glycogen or converts it to fat.
- Alters chemicals, foreign molecules, and hormones to make them less toxic.
- Stores iron as ferritin, which is released as needed for the production of red blood cells.

Diagnostic Tests

The results of diagnostic tests of nutritional status and gastrointestinal function are used to support the diagnosis of a specific disease, to provide information to identify or modify the appropriate medication or therapy used to treat the disease, and to help nurses monitor the client's responses to treatment and nursing care interventions. Diagnostic tests to assess nutritional status and function of the gastrointestinal tract and the accessory organs are described on pages 615–617 and summarized in the list that follows. More information, including specific laboratory tests, is included in the discussion of disorders in Chapters 22, 23, and 24 ∞.

- Diagnostic tests of the esophagus and stomach include tests of esophageal pressure and acidity, x-rays of the esophagus and stomach using barium (Figure 21–5 ■), direct visualization with an endoscope, CT, MRI, and analysis of gastric secretions and emptying. These tests are used to evaluate chronic acid reflux, esophageal varices, inflammation, ulceration, hernia, foreign bodies, polyps, diverticula, tumors, and GI bleeding.
- Gallbladder and pancreatic tissue and duct structure and function are evaluated with ultrasound, x-ray series with a contrast medium, fluoroscopy, MRI, CT, and direct visualization. In addition to evaluating structure and function, the tests are used to identify tumors, cysts, ascites, gallstones, and obstructions; and to retrieve gallstones, dilate structures, and biopsy tumors. Blood serum lipase and amylase tests assess pancreatic function, with alterations in serum amylase being highly diagnostic of acute pancreatitis.
- Liver biopsy is used to rule out metastatic cancer, or to detect a liver cyst or cirrhosis. Other laboratory tests used to diagnose and monitor liver disorders are included in Chapter 24 ∞ with discussions of interdisciplinary care.

Regardless of the type of diagnostic test, the nurse is responsible for explaining the procedure and any special preparation needed, for supporting the client during the examination as necessary, for documenting the procedure as appropriate, and for monitoring the results of the test.

Figure 21–5 ■ A barium x-ray of a healthy stomach.

Source: Biophoto Associates/Photo Researchers, Inc.

Genetic Considerations

When conducting a health assessment interview and physical assessment, it is important for the nurse to consider genetic influences on health of the adult. During the health assessment interview, ask about family members with known abnormalities of copper accumulation in the body, hypercholesteremia, abnormal cholesterol or fat metabolism, obesity, or cancer of the pancreas. During the physical assessment, assess for any manifestations that might indicate a genetic disorder (see the Genetic Considerations box below). If data are found to indicate genetic risk factors or alterations, ask about genetic testing and refer for appropriate genetic counseling and evaluation. Chapter 8 ∞ provides further information about genetics in medical-surgical nursing.

Health Assessment Interview

A health assessment interview to determine problems with nutrition and digestion may be conducted during a health screening, may focus on a chief complaint (such as nausea or unexplained weight loss), or may be part of a total health assessment. If the client has a health problem involving nutrition and digestion, analyze its onset, characteristics and course, severity, precipitating and relieving factors, and any associated symptoms, noting the timing and circumstances. For example, the nurse may ask the client:

- Have you had any episodes of indigestion, nausea, vomiting, diarrhea, or constipation? If so, describe the appearance of what was vomited or the stools and anything that makes these problems better or worse. How long have you had these problems?
- What is your usual dietary intake pattern during a 24-hour period?
- Describe what you believe to be a "healthy" diet.

When collecting information about the client's current health status, ask about any changes in weight, appetite, and the ability to taste, chew, or swallow. What is the client's perception of the role of nutrition in maintaining health? Who buys and prepares the food? What medications (prescribed, over-the-counter, or

---

GENETIC CONSIDERATIONS
Nutritional and Gastrointestinal System

- Cleft lip and/or palate are influenced by genetic factors.
- An autosomal recessive disorder, Wilson's disease is an abnormality of copper transport, resulting in copper accumulation and toxicity to the liver and grain. Neurologic disease results in adults.
- Tangier disease is a disease of cholesterol transport, leading to characteristic orange tonsils, very low levels of high-density lipoprotein, and an enlarged liver and spleen.
- Hypercholesterolemia has a familial tendency.
- About 90% of human pancreatic cancers show a chromosome defect.
- Obesity is believed to result from a variety of factors, including genetics.
- Gaucher disease, more common in descendants of Jewish people from Eastern Europe, results in lack of an enzyme to break down fats. Fats accumulate in the liver, spleen, and bone marrow, causing pain, fatigue, jaundice, bone damage, anemia, and even death.

DIAGNOSTIC TESTS of Gastrointestinal Disorders

ESOPHAGEAL AND STOMACH TESTS

NAME OF TEST Esophageal Acidity, Esophageal Manometry, Acid Perfusion (Bernstein Test)

PURPOSE AND DESCRIPTION Esophageal acidity is measured to diagnose problems of the lower esophageal sphincter and chronic reflux esophagitis. A catheter with a pH electrode is inserted into the esophagus through the mouth. The measurement may be one time, or over a 24-hour period.

Esophageal manometry is done to measure esophageal sphincter pressure and peristaltic contractions for diagnosis of esophageal motility problems, such as achalasia. A manometric catheter with a pressure transducer is inserted into the esophagus through the mouth and esophageal pressure is measured before and after swallowing.

Acid perfusion (Bernstein test) tests are done to distinguish between gastric acid reflux and cardiac involvement. A catheter is inserted through the nose into the esophagus. A saline solution, followed by a HCL solution, is dripped into the catheter and the client is asked to indicate when pain occurs. Normal esophageal pH is 5 to 6.

RELATED NURSING CARE Advise the client to be NPO and to avoid alcohol intake for 8 to 12 hours prior to the exam. Assess medications: Results of the tests may be affected by antacids, anticholinergics, and cimetidine-like drugs, which increase the pH, reducing acidity and causing false test results.

NAME OF TEST Barium Swallow or Upper GI Series

PURPOSE AND DESCRIPTION To diagnose esophageal varices, inflammation, ulcerations, hiatal hernia, foreign bodies, polyps, diverticula, and tumors of the esophagus, stomach, and duodenal bulb. These radiologic studies are done by observing the movement of a contrast medium with a fluoroscope.

RELATED NURSING CARE Advise the client to be NPO and avoid smoking for 8–12 hours before the exam; client will drink 16–20 ounces of a chalky liquid (barium sulfate or meglumine diatrizoate [Gastrografin]) before the exam. Withhold medications for 8 hours before the exam. Following the exam, ensure the client eliminates the barium by giving laxatives and forcing fluids as appropriate.

NAME OF TEST Upper GI Endoscopy (Esophagogastroduodenoscopy [EGD])

PURPOSE AND DESCRIPTION To directly visualize mucous membrane lining of the esophagus, stomach, and duodenum. A flexible fiber-optic endoscope is used to visualize inflammations, ulcerations, tumors, or varices; and video imaging may illustrate gastric motility. May also be combined with an ultrasound examination by attaching an ultrasound transducer to the endoscope.

CLIENT PREPARATION

- Schedule at least 2 days after barium swallow or upper gastrointestinal series.
- Ensure the informed consent is signed prior to premedication.
- Encourage questions, and provide answers and support.
- Withhold food and fluids for 6 to 8 hours before the procedure.
- Remove dentures and eyewear.

HEALTH EDUCATION FOR THE CLIENT AND FAMILY

- Do not eat or drink anything for 6 to 8 hours before the procedure.
- The procedure is somewhat uncomfortable but requires only 20 to 30 minutes to complete.
- A local anesthetic will be used in your throat and you will be given a sedative during the procedure.
- After the procedure, you will be allowed to eat and drink as soon as your gag reflex returns and you are able to swallow.
- You may experience mild bloating, belching, or flatulence following the procedure.
- Contact your physician immediately if you develop any of the following: difficulty swallowing; epigastric, substernal or shoulder pain; vomiting blood or black tarry stools; or fever.

NAME OF TEST Magnetic Resonance Imaging (MRI)

PURPOSE AND DESCRIPTION To identify source of gastric bleeding.

RELATED NURSING CARE Assess for metal implants or pregnancy (will not do the exam if present). Explain need to be NPO for at least 6 hours prior to the exam.

NAME OF TEST Gastroscopy

PURPOSE AND DESCRIPTION See Upper GI Endoscopy.

RELATED NURSING CARE See Upper GI Endoscopy.

NAME OF TEST Gastric Analysis

PURPOSE AND DESCRIPTION To evaluate gastric secretions and detect an increase or decrease of free hydrochloric acid. To conduct the gastric analysis, a nasogastric tube is inserted into the stomach and specimens are aspirated to evaluate gastric acidity. A stimulation gastric analysis may follow, with a gastric stimulant (such as Histalog or pentagastrin) administered and several gastric samples aspirated.

Normal values:
Fasting: 1.0–5.0 mEq/L/per hour
Stimulation: 10–25 mEq/L/per hour

RELATED NURSING CARE Advise client to remain NPO with no smoking for 8 to 12 hours prior to the exam. Assess medications and fluid intake: Anticholinergics, cholinergics, adrenergic blockers, antacids, steroids, alcohol, and coffee can alter results. Remove loose dentures. Insert nasogastric tube. Aspirate gastric contents at 15- to 20-minute intervals as ordered.

(continued)

DIAGNOSTIC TESTS of Gastrointestinal Disorders (continued)

NAME OF TEST Gastric Emptying Studies

PURPOSE AND DESCRIPTION To evaluate the ability of the stomach to empty liquids or solids. In this nuclear imaging study, the client is asked to eat a cooked egg containing Tc-^{99m} (solids) or to drink orange juice with Tc^{99m} (liquids). Sequential images are recorded with a gamma camera every 2 minutes for up to an hour.

RELATED NURSING CARE Explain to client that the substances contain only very small amounts of radioactivity and are not hazardous.

GALLBLADDER AND PANCREAS TESTS

NAME OF TEST Abdominal Ultrasound, Hepatobiliary Ultrasound, Gallbladder Ultrasound

PURPOSE AND DESCRIPTION Abdominal ultrasound is used to detect abdominal tumors, cysts, and ascites.

Hepatobiliary ultrasound is used to visualize the biliary ducts, and to detect subphrenic abscesses, cysts, tumors, and cirrhosis of the liver.

Gallbladder ultrasound is used to detect gallstones.

These noninvasive procedures record ultrasound waves as they are reflected off body structures. A conductive gel is applied to the skin and a transducer placed on the area.

RELATED NURSING CARE Advise the client to remain NPO for 8 to 12 hours prior to the test.

NAME OF TEST Cholecystography (Oral) (GB Series)

If the GB cannot be visualized with an oral contrast substance, an IV cholangiography may be ordered. *If the client is also having GI x-rays with barium, the GB tests should be done first, because barium would interfere with the test.*

PURPOSE AND DESCRIPTION To detect gallbladder stones, inflammation or tumors, and obstruction of the cystic duct. Evening before the test, radiopaque tablets (for example, iopanoic acid [Telepaque], sodium ipodate [Oragrafin], iodoal-phionic acid [Priodax], or iodipamide meglumine [Cholografin]) are given, the following morning x-rays are taken. A high-fat meal may be given after the fasting x-rays are completed and further x-rays taken to determine how fast the GB expels the dye.

RELATED NURSING CARE Advise client to eat a fat-free diet 24 hours prior to test. No food or fluids except sips of water should be taken 12 hours before the test. Assess client for allergy to iodine, seafood, or x-ray dye (many contain iodine).

NAME OF TEST Cholangiography

• Percutaneous Transhepatic Cholangiogram (PTC)

• Surgical Cholangiogram

PURPOSE AND DESCRIPTION A PTC is done to evaluate filling of the hepatic and biliary ducts. Using local anesthesia, the liver and bile duct is entered with a long needle (using fluoroscopy), bile is withdrawn, and a contrast medium is injected into the bile duct.

During a surgical cholangiogram with general anesthesia, contrast medium is injected into the common bile duct to evaluate filling of the common bile duct.

RELATED NURSING CARE Assess client for allergy to iodine, seafood, or x-ray dye (many contain iodine). Monitor for bile leakage or hemorrhage following the tests.

NAME OF TEST Magnetic Resonance Cholangiopancreatography (MRCP)

PURPOSE AND DESCRIPTION This noninvasive MRI study is done to evaluate the biliary and pancreatic ducts

RELATED NURSING CARE Assess for metal implants or pregnancy (will not do the exam if present).

NAME OF TEST Computed Tomography (CT)

PURPOSE AND DESCRIPTION A noninvasive procedure, using radio-frequency waves and a magnetic field; used to evaluate disorders of the GB, pancreas, biliary tract, and liver.

RELATED NURSING CARE No special preparation is needed.

NAME OF TEST Endoscopic Retrograde Cholangiopancreatography (ERCP)

PURPOSE AND DESCRIPTION To directly visualize gastrointestinal structures, and to retrieve gallstones from the distal common bile duct, dilate structures, and biopsy tumors. A fiberoptic endoscope is inserted (under fluoroscopy) through the mouth through the esophagus, stomach, and descending duodenum, and the common bile ducts and pancreatic ducts are cannulated. Contrast medium is injected into the ducts and structures are visualized.

RELATED NURSING CARE Advise the client to be NPO for 8 hours before the test. Following the test, assess vital signs and gag reflex, and monitor for complications (pancreatitis is the most common).

NAME OF TEST Serum Lipase

PURPOSE AND DESCRIPTION This blood test is used to measure the secretion of lipase by the pancreas.

Normal value: 0–160 Unit/L

RELATED NURSING CARE No special preparation is needed.

DIAGNOSTIC TESTS **of Gastrointestinal Disorders (continued)**

NAME OF TEST   Serum Amylase

PURPOSE AND DESCRIPTION   This blood test is used to measure the secretion of amylase by the pancreas. It is used to diagnose acute pancreatitis, when amylase level peaks in 24 h and then drops to normal in 48 to 72 h.

Normal value: 0–130 Unit/L

RELATED NURSING CARE   No special preparation is needed.

LIVER TESTS

NAME OF TEST   Liver Biopsy

PURPOSE AND DESCRIPTION   To rule out metastatic cancer or to detect a cyst or cirrhosis of the liver. Using ultrasound, a biopsy needle is inserted into the liver and guided to the pathologic site. See Figure 21–6 ■.

RELATED NURSING CARE   Related nursing care of the client having a liver biopsy is described below.

PREPARATION OF CLIENT

- Review chart for signed consent form.
- Withhold food and fluids per policy, usually 4 to 6 hours preprocedure.
- Assess and record baseline vital signs.
- Review prothrombin time (PT) and platelet count; administer vitamin K as ordered.
- Instruct to empty bladder immediately before the biopsy.
- Place in supine position on far right side of bed; turn head to left and extend right arm above head to improve access to the biopsy site.

HEALTH EDUCATION FOR THE CLIENT AND FAMILY

- Discuss preparation for the biopsy and expected sensations during the procedure.
- Hold your breath following expiration during needle insertion to keep diaphragm and liver high and stabilized in the abdominal cavity.
- Obtaining the tissue sample usually requires only 10 to 15 seconds; there may be some pain or discomfort during this time.
- Direct pressure is applied to the site immediately after the needle is removed; you will be placed on your right side to maintain site pressure.
- You may develop pain in the right shoulder as the anesthetic loses effect.

Figure 21–6 ■ Liver biopsy. *A.* The client exhales completely, then holds his or her breath. This brings the liver and diaphragm to their highest position. *B.* The biopsy needle is inserted into the liver. *C.* Approximately 1 mL of saline is injected to clear the needle of blood and tissue. *D.* The needle is advanced, and a tissue sample is aspirated. Pressure is applied to the site immediately after the needle is withdrawn. The specimen is sent to the laboratory for analysis.

- You will be monitored for bleeding after the procedure.
- Food and fluids are withheld for 2 hours after the biopsy; you then can resume your usual diet.
- Avoid coughing, lifting, or straining for 1 to 2 weeks.

Note: A wide variety of blood tests are used to diagnose and monitor liver disease. These are discussed in appropriate interdisciplinary care sections in Chapter 24 ∞.

vitamins) is the client currently taking? Does the client take any vitamins, herbal supplements, or other "health food" items? Does the client consume alcohol (how much and type)? If the client has experienced nausea or vomiting, ask whether the vomitus contains bright red blood, dark (old) blood, bile, or fecal material. If the client is very thin or verbalizes concerns about body size incongruent with the ratio of height to weight, ask whether the client induces vomiting or uses laxatives to control weight. Ask whether the client has appliances such as braces, bridges, or dentures, and what self-care measures are used for such appliances, as well as oral hygiene practices and frequency of dental visits.

Ask the client to describe any heartburn, indigestion, abdominal discomfort, or pain. Explore the location of the pain, the type of pain, the time it occurs, foods that aggravate or relieve it, and how it is relieved. Abdominal pain is often referred to other sites (see Chapter 9 ∞). For example, a client with a liver disorder may experience pain over the right shoulder (Kehr's sign). Epigastric (middle upper abdominal) pain is experienced in cases of acute gastritis, obstruction of the small intestine, and acute pancreatitis. Pain in the right upper quadrant is associated with cholecystitis. Pain in the left upper quadrant may be related to a gastric ulcer.

The health history should include questions about any prior surgeries or trauma of the GI tract. Explore the past history of any medical condition that may affect the client's ingestion, digestion, and/or metabolism (for example, Crohn's disease, diabetes mellitus, irritable bowel syndrome, peptic ulcers, or pancreatitis).

Other areas significant to assessment of nutritional status and the gastrointestinal system are food allergies (especially to milk, which is evidenced as lactose intolerance with abdominal cramping, excessive flatus, and loose stools) and a family history that may provide clues to increased risk for health problems.

FUNCTIONAL HEALTH PATTERN INTERVIEW Nutritional Status and Gastrointestinal System

Functional Health Pattern	Interview Questions and Leading Statements
Health Perception–Health Management	■ Have you had any illness or surgery that affects your nutrition and digestion? If so, how were these treated? ■ Describe your current problem; how long has it lasted; what have you done to treat it? ■ What medications do you take? Do you take antacids? If so, what do you use them for and how often do you take them? ■ Do you have allergies to foods? What are they and how do you react? ■ Do you have tooth or gum pain that interferes with your ability to eat? ■ When was your last dental examination? ■ Describe what you do each day to take care of your teeth.
Nutritional–Metabolic	■ Describe what you eat and how much (and type) of fluids you drink in a 24-hour period. ■ Describe herbs, vitamins, and dietary supplements you currently are taking. ■ Have you noticed any change in your appetite? Explain. ■ What is your current weight? What do you feel your ideal weight would be? Have you had a recent gain or loss? Explain. ■ Describe your food likes and dislikes. ■ Do you have any of the following: indigestion, belching, nausea, vomiting, difficulty swallowing? If so, what causes this and how do you treat it? ■ Do you drink alcohol? If so, what type? Describe your average number of drinks each day. ■ Questions specific to the client's culture and ethnic group would be included in this functional health pattern area, such as what types of food are preferred or not eaten, what types of foods are never eaten together, and what types of foods are eaten to remain healthy.
Elimination	■ Are your bowel movements affected by what you eat? Explain. ■ Have you noticed any change in the color of your urine or bowel movements? Explain. ■ Have you ever used laxatives or made yourself vomit to control your weight? Explain.
Activity-Exercise	■ Describe your activities on a typical day. ■ What type of exercise do you get and how often? ■ Do you smoke? If so, what and how many cigarettes per day?
Sleep-Rest	■ Do you wake up hungry during the night? ■ Does abdominal pain, cramping, nausea, or diarrhea ever interfere with your sleep? Explain.
Cognitive-Perceptual	■ Describe the amount and type of foods you should eat each day. ■ Rate your ability to taste and smell foods on a scale of 1 to 10 (with 10 being excellent). ■ Describe any pain you have had in your mouth, stomach, or abdomen. What type of pain was it (dull, crampy, achy, burning)? What seems to cause it? What do you do to relieve it?
Self-Perception–Self-Concept	■ Are you satisfied with your appearance in terms of weight? If no, why? ■ Have you been successful in the past in gaining or losing weight? ■ How does this condition make you feel about yourself?
Role-Relationships	■ How does this condition affect your relationships with others? ■ Do you eat with others regularly? If so, who.
Sexuality-Reproductive	■ Has this condition interfered with your usual sexual activities?
Coping-Stress-Tolerance	■ Have you experienced any type of stress that may have worsened this condition? ■ Has having this condition created stress for you? ■ Describe what you do when you feel stressed.
Value-Belief	■ Tell me how specific relationships or activities help you cope with this problem. ■ Describe specific cultural beliefs or practices that affect how you care for and feel about this condition. ■ Are there any specific treatments that you would not use to treat this condition?

In addition to other factors assessed in the health history, culture and ethnicity are important components of nutritional status and gastrointestinal health. Nutritional diversity is common among cultural and ethnic groups and questions should be included to identify specific customs, food likes and dislikes, and how foods are prepared and served. In some ethnic groups, for example, dietary substances are used to protect health, such as eating raw garlic or onions (Spector, 2004). In other cultures, dietary balance is believed to be necessary to keep the body in balance or harmony. It is therefore necessary for nurses to be cognizant of specific culturally related nutritional values and practices, and ask questions to identify health-related concerns specific to individualized dietary intake.

Interview questions categorized by functional health patterns are listed in the box on the previous page.

Physical Assessment

Physical assessment of gastrointestinal and nutritional status may be performed as part of a total health assessment, as a focused assessment of clients with known or suspected health problems, in combination with assessment of the urinary and reproductive systems (problems that may cause manifestations similar to those of the gastrointestinal system), or alone for clients with known or suspected health problems. The techniques of inspection, auscultation, percussion, and palpation are used. Palpation is the last method used in assessing the abdomen.

PRACTICE ALERT
When assessing the abdomen, use palpation last, because pressure on the abdominal wall and contents may interfere with bowel sounds and cause pain, ending the examination.

Collect objective data by obtaining anthropometric measurements (height, weight, triceps skin folds, and midarm circumference) and by examining the mouth and abdomen. Prior to the examination, collect all necessary equipment and explain techniques to the client to decrease anxiety. The client may be seated during assessment of the mouth, but is supine during the abdominal assessment.

Physical assessment of the integumentary system, nervous system, musculoskeletal system, cardiovascular system, and respiratory system may also reflect the client's nutritional status. Table 21–5 summarizes abnormal nutritional assessment findings related to these body systems. Normal age-related findings for the older adult are summarized in Table 21–6.

TABLE 21–5 Assessment Findings Due to Malnutrition

BODY SYSTEM	ASSESSMENT FINDINGS
Nails	Soft and spoon shaped in iron deficiency. Splinter hemorrhages in vitamin C deficiency.
Hair	Dry, dull, and scarce in zinc, protein, and linoleic acid deficiencies.
Skin	Flaky and dry in vitamin A, vitamin B, and/or linoleic acid deficiency. Cracks and/or hyperpigmentation in niacin deficiency. Bruising in vitamin C or vitamin K deficiency.
Eyes	Eyes become dry and soft with decrease in vitamin A. Conjunctiva is pale with a decrease in iron, and red with a decrease in riboflavin.
Nervous system	Reflexes are decreased and client may have peripheral neuropathies with thiamine deficiency. Client may be irritable and/or disoriented with thiamine deficiency.
Musculoskeletal system	Muscle wasting is seen with deficits in protein, carbohydrate, and fat metabolism. Calf pain occurs with thiamine deficiency; joint pain may occur with vitamin C deficiency.
Cardiovascular system	Heart size and rate may increase with thiamine deficiency. Diastolic blood pressure may be increased with a high intake of fat. Lowered cardiac output and decreased blood pressure may occur with caloric deficiencies over a long time period.
Gastrointestinal system	Cheilosis (sores at corner of mouth) seen in vitamin B-complex deficiencies, especially riboflavin. Stomatitis and spongy, bleeding gums may also be seen in malnutrition.

TABLE 21–6 Age-Related Gastrointestinal Changes

AGE-RELATED CHANGE	SIGNIFICANCE
Teeth: ↑ number of root cavities and cavities around existing dental work; tooth enamel harder and more brittle; dentin is more fibrous; tooth cusps flatten; root pulp shrinks; ↑ loss of bone supporting teeth	Increase in periodontal disease and tooth loss Increase in fractures of teeth Increased incidence of dentures
Gums: Gingiva retracts	Increase in periodontal disease
Taste: Less acute as tongue atrophies, especially for sweet sensations	Excessive seasoning of foods
Saliva: ↓ amount is produced (1/3 of that produced in younger years)	Decreased ability to break down starches Swallowing may take longer
Esophageal motility: ↓ intensity of propulsive waves and slower emptying time, weaker gag reflex	Discomfort when swallowing food Increased risk of aspiration
Stomach: Mucosa atrophies, ↓ production of hydrochloric acid and pepsin leading to higher pH in stomach	Increase in incidence of gastric irritation
Liver: Less efficient handling of cholesterol	Increased incidence of gallstones

NUTRITIONAL AND GASTROINTESTINAL ASSESSMENTS

Technique/Normal Findings	Abnormal Findings

Anthropometric Assessment with Abnormal Findings

Weigh the client and measure the client's height. Compare the client's actual weight to ideal body weight (IBW) (Table 21–7). *Weight should be appropriate to height as indicated on a standardized table.*

- A weight 10% to 20% less than ideal body weight indicates malnutrition.
- A weight 10% above ideal body weight is considered overweight.
- A weight 20% above ideal body weight is considered obese.

TABLE 21–7 Example of a Height and Weight Table

	HEIGHT		WEIGHT*		
	FEET	INCHES	SMALL FRAME	MEDIUM FRAME	LARGE FRAME
Men (ages 25–29)	5	2	128–134	131–134	138–150
	5	3	130–136	133–143	140–153
	5	4	132–138	135–145	142–156
	5	5	134–140	137–148	144–160
	5	6	136–142	139–151	146–164
	5	7	138–145	142–154	149–168
	5	8	140–148	145–157	152–172
	5	9	142–151	148–160	155–176
	5	10	144–154	151–163	158–180
	5	11	146–157	154–166	161–184
	6	0	149–160	157–170	164–188
	6	1	152–164	160–174	168–192
	6	2	155–168	164–178	172–197
	6	3	158–172	167–182	176–202
	6	4	162–176	171–187	181–207
Women (ages 25–29)	4	10	102–111	109–121	118–131
	4	11	103–113	111–123	120–134
	5	0	104–115	113–126	122–137
	5	1	106–118	115–129	125–140
	5	2	108–121	118–132	128–143
	5	3	111–124	121–135	131–147
	5	4	114–127	124–138	134–151
	5	5	117–130	127–141	137–155
	5	6	120–133	130–144	140–159
	5	7	123–136	133–147	143–163
	5	8	126–139	136–150	146–167
	5	9	129–142	139–153	149–170
	5	10	132–145	142–156	152–173
	5	11	135–148	145–159	155–176
	6	0	138–151	148–162	158–179

Calculate the client's percentage of ideal body weight (%IBW). Use the formula in Table 21–8 to determine the presence of obesity and/or malnutrition based on percentage of ideal body weight). *Ideal body weight should be within normal range.*

TABLE 21–8 Indications of Nutritional Status by Body Weight

%IBW	%UBW	NUTRITIONAL STATUS
>120	—	Obese
110–120	—	Overweight
80–90	85–95	Mildly undernourished
70–79	75–84	Moderately undernourished
<70	<75	Severely undernourished

UBW = usual body weight

Technique/Normal Findings	Abnormal Findings

Calculate the client's percentage of usual body weight (% UBW) to determine weight change, using this formula:

Refer to Table 21–8 to determine nutritional status based on %UBW.

- Using %IBW may result in overlooking malnutrition in a very obese client.

$$\frac{\text{Current weight}}{\text{Usual weight}} \times 100$$

Measure body mass index (BMI). Determine BMI by using one of the following formulas. *BMI should be between 20 and 25.*

- A BMI of 25 to 29.9 kg/m² indicates overweight.
- A BMI of 30 kg/m² indicates obesity.

$$\frac{\text{Weight in kilograms}}{\text{Height in meters}^2} = \text{BMI}$$

$$\frac{\text{Weight in pounds} \times 705}{\text{Height in inches}^2} = \text{BMI}$$

Measure triceps skinfold thickness (TSF). Find the midpoint between the client's olecranon and acromion processes. Grasp the skin and fat, and pull it away from the muscle. Apply skinfold calipers for 3 seconds, and record reading (Figure 21–7 ■). Repeat three times, and average the three readings. Compare the client's reading to the standard values shown in Table 21–9. *TSF should be within normal range as compared to standard values.*

- Triceps readings are 10% or more below standards in malnutrition and 10% or more above standards in obesity or overnutrition.

Figure 21–7 ■ Measuring MAC with calipers.

TABLE 21–9 Values for Anthropometric Measurements

	STANDARD VALUE	
MEASUREMENT	MALE	FEMALE
Triceps skinfold thickness	12.5 mm	16.5 mm
Midarm circumference	29.3 cm	28.5 cm
Midarm muscle circumference	25.3 cm	23.2 cm

Measure midarm circumference (MAC). Find the midpoint between the client's olecranon and acromion processes. Wind tape measure around arm (Figure 21–8 ■). Compare the client's reading to the standard values shown in Table 21–9. *MAC should be within normal range as compared to standard values.*

- MAC decreases with malnutrition and increases with obesity.

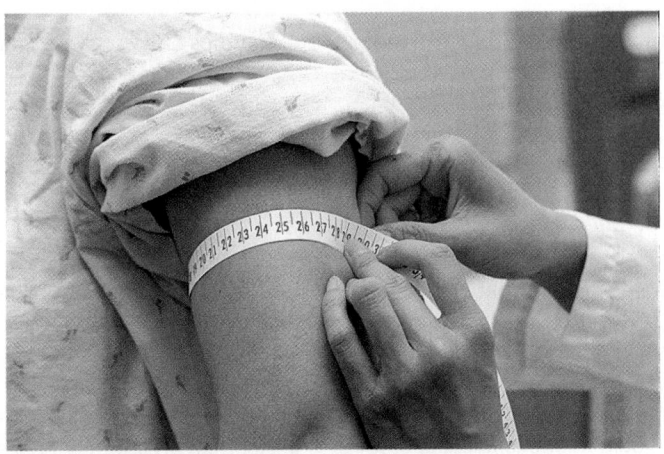

Figure 21–8 ■ Measuring MAC with a tape measure.

Technique/Normal Findings	Abnormal Findings
Calculate midarm muscle circumference (MAMC). Use the client's triceps skinfold measurement and midarm circumference readings to calculate the client's MAMC: Compare the result to the standard values shown in Table 21–9. *MAMC should be within normal range as compared to standard values.*	■ In mild malnutrition, the MAMC is 90% of the standard; in moderate malnutrition, 60% to 90%. In severe malnutrition (muscle wasting), the MAMC is less than 60% of the standard. $$\boxed{MAMC = MAC - (0.314 \times TSF)}$$
Determine waist-to-hip ratio. With the client standing measure the waist, and then measure the hips midway between the iliac crest and the greater trochanter. Use the formula below to calculate the waist-to-hip ratio. *Normal findings: females, waist ratio less than or equal to 0.80; males, waist ratio less than or equal to 1.0.*	■ Females with a ratio greater than 0.80 and males with a ratio greater than 1.0 have a three to five times greater risk for having a heart attack or stroke (Weber & Kelley, 2003). $$\boxed{\frac{Waist\ circumference}{Hip\ circumference} = \text{waist-to-hip ratio}}$$

Oral Assessment with Abnormal Findings

Inspect and palpate the lips. *Lips should be of normal color for race without lesions.*	■ **Cheilosis** (painful lesions at corners of mouth) is seen with riboflavin and/or niacin deficiency. ■ Cold sores or clear vesicles with a red base are seen in herpes simplex 1.

> **PRACTICE ALERT**
> Always wear gloves when assessing the oral cavity.

Inspect and palpate the tongue. *Tongue should be pink, smooth, and have good turgor.*	■ Atrophic smooth **glossitis** is characterized by a bright red tongue. It is seen in B_{12}, folic acid, and iron deficiencies. ■ Vertical fissures are seen in dehydration. ■ A black, hairy tongue may be seen following antibiotic therapy.
Inspect and palpate the buccal mucosa. *Mucosa should be moist, without lesions and of appropriate color.*	■ **Leukoplakia** (small white patches) may be a sign of a premalignant condition. ■ A reddened, dry, swollen mucosa may be seen in stomatitis. ■ Candidiases (white cheesy patches that bleed when scraped) may be seen in immune-suppressed clients receiving antibiotics or chemotherapy and in terminally ill clients.
Inspect and palpate the teeth. *Teeth should be in a state of good hygiene without caries.*	■ Cavities and excessive plaque are seen with poor nutrition and/or poor oral hygiene.
Inspect and palpate the gums. *Gums should be of even color without swelling.*	■ Swollen, red gums that bleed easily (**gingivitis**) are seen in periodontal disease, vitamin C deficiencies, or with hormonal changes.
Inspect the throat and tonsils. *Tonsils (if present) should be of appropriate color and size.*	■ In acute infections, tonsils are red and swollen and may have white spots.
Note the client's breath. *Breath should not have unusual or foul odors.*	■ Sweet, fruity breath is noted in diabetic ketoacidosis. ■ Acetone breath may be a sign of uremia. ■ Foul breath may result from liver disease, respiratory infections, and poor oral hygiene.

Technique/Normal Findings   **Abnormal Findings**

Abdominal Assessment with Abnormal Findings

The quadrants of the abdomen, with related internal structures, are illustrated in Figure 21–9 ■. Box 21–2 provides guidelines for abdominal assessment.

Midline
Aorta
Bladder
Uterus

◯ = Umbilicus

Right Upper Quadrant
Liver and gallbladder
Pylorus
Duodenum
Head of pancreas
Right adrenal gland
Portion of right kidney
Hepatic flexure of colon
Portions of ascending and
  transverse colon

Left Upper Quadrant
Left lobe of liver
Spleen
Stomach
Body of pancreas
Left adrenal gland
Portion of left kidney
Splenic flexure of colon
Portions of transverse and
  descending colon

Right Lower Quadrant
Lower pole of right kidney
Cecum and appendix
Portion of ascending colon
Bladder (if distended)
Right ovary and salpinx
Right spermatic cord
Right ureter

Left Lower Quadrant
Lower pole of left kidney
Sigmoid colon
Portion of descending colon
Bladder (if distended)
Left ovary and salpinx
Uterus (if enlarged)
Left spermatic cord
Left ureter

Figure 21–9 ■ The four quadrants of the abdomen, with anatomic location of organs within each quadrant.

BOX 21–2 Guidelines for Assessing the Abdomen

Ask the client to empty the bladder before beginning the examination. Assist the client to the dorsal recumbent (supine) position, with a small pillow under the head, a pillow under the knees (if desired), and the arms at the sides of the body. Warm the stethoscope before applying it to the client's skin. Ask the client to point to areas that are painful, and explain that those areas will be examined last. Expose the abdomen from below the breasts to the pubic symphysis, and drape the client's thoracic and genital areas. When you document your findings, specify the location by abdominal quadrant.

General guidelines for abdominal assessment are as follows:

1. Inspect the abdomen under a good light source that is shining across the abdomen. Sit at the right side of the client, and note symmetry, distention, masses, visible peristalsis, and respiratory movements. If masses are detected, ask the client to take a deep breath, which decreases the size of the abdominal cavity and makes any abnormality more visible.

2. Auscultate each quadrant of the abdomen, using the diaphragm of the stethoscope Listen for bowel sounds, arterial bruits, venous hums, and friction rubs.

3. Percuss several areas within each quadrant of the abdomen, using a systematic path. (For example, always begin in the lower left quadrant, then proceed to the lower right quadrant, upper right quadrant, and upper left quadrant, respectively). The predominant percussion tones for the entire abdomen are tympany and dullness. Tympany is present over gas-filled intestines. Dullness is present over the liver, the spleen, an enlarged kidney, or a full stomach. Percuss for fluid, gaseous distention, and masses.

4. Palpate each quadrant of the abdomen for shape, position, mobility, size, consistency, and tenderness of the major abdominal organs. Begin this part of the assessment with light palpation, and increase the depth of palpation to elicit tenderness or better identify organ size and shape. Deep palpation should be conducted only by nurses with considerable experience. Remember to palpate areas of indicated tenderness last and to use gentle pressure. Palpation may be difficult or impossible if the client exhibits muscle guarding from pain or is ticklish. The gallbladder and the spleen are normally not palpable

---

Inspect abdominal contour, skin integrity, venous pattern, and aortic pulsation. *Abdomen should be slightly concave or rounded with intact skin. There should not be distended veins or obvious aortic pulsations.*

- Generalized abdominal distention may be seen in gas retention or obesity.
- Lower abdominal distention is seen in bladder distention, pregnancy, or ovarian mass.
- General distention and an everted umbilicus are seen with ascites and/or tumors.
- A scaphoid (sunken) abdomen is seen in malnutrition or when fat is replaced with muscle.
- **Striae** (whitish-silver stretch marks) are seen in obesity and during or after pregnancy.
- Spider angiomas may be seen in liver disease.
- Dilated veins are prominent in cirrhosis of the liver, ascites, portal hypertension, or venocaval obstruction.
- Pulsation is increased in aortic aneurysm.

Technique/Normal Findings

Abnormal Findings

Auscultate all four quadrants of the abdomen with the diaphragm of the stethoscope (Figure 21–10 ■). Begin in the lower right quadrant, where bowel sounds are almost always present. *Normal bowel sounds (gurgling or clicking) occur every 5 to 15 seconds. Listen for at least 5 minutes in each of the four quadrants to confirm the absence of bowel sounds.*

- **Borborygmus** (hyperactive high-pitched, tinkling, rushing, or growling bowel sounds) is heard in diarrhea or at the onset of bowel obstruction.
- Bowel sounds may be absent later in bowel obstruction, with an inflamed peritoneum, and/or following surgery of the abdomen.

Figure 21–10 ■ Auscultating the abdomen with the diaphragm of the stethoscope.

Auscultate the abdomen for vascular sounds with the bell of the stethoscope (Figure 21–11 ■). *No sounds (bruits, venous hum, or friction rub) other than bowel sounds should be auscultated.*

- **Bruits** (blowing sound due to restriction of blood flow through vessels) may be heard over constricted arteries. A bruit over the liver may be heard in hepatic carcinoma.
- A venous hum (continuous medium-pitched sound) may be heard over a cirrhotic liver.
- Friction rubs (rough grating sounds) may be heard over an inflamed liver or spleen.

Figure 21–11 ■ Location of placement of the stethoscope for auscultation of arteries of the abdomen.

Percuss the abdomen in all four quadrants (Figure 21–12 ■). *Normally, tympany is heard over the stomach and gas-filled bowels.*

- Dullness is heard when the bowel is displaced with fluid or tumors or filled with a fecal mass.

Figure 21–12 ■ Location of sites for systematic percussion of all four quadrants.

Technique/Normal Findings	Abnormal Findings
Percuss the liver (see Box 21–3 for guidelines for liver percussion and palpation; see Figure 21–13 ■ for landmarks). *The lower border of liver dullness is located at the costal margin to 1 to 2 cm below.*	■ In cirrhosis and/or hepatitis, the liver is greater than 6 to 10 cm in the MCL and greater than 4 to 8 cm in the midsternal line (MSL).

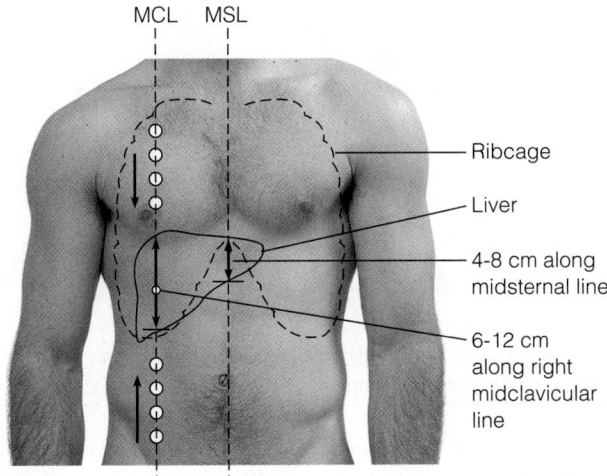

Figure 21–13 ■ Anatomic location of the liver, with the midclavicular line (MCL) and midsternal line (MSL) superimposed. The normal liver span is 6 to 12 cm.

BOX 21–3 Guidelines for Percussing and Palpating the Liver

The size of the liver may be determined by percussion and palpation, as follows:

1. Percuss, in the midclavicular line (MCL), beginning below the umbilicus (see Figure 21–13). Begin to percuss over a region of tympany, and move upward. The first dull percussion tone occurs at the lower border of the liver. Determine the upper liver border by beginning percussion over an area of lung resonance (in the MCL) and percussing downward to the first dull tone. Usually at the 5th to 7th interspace. Mark each of these locations, and measure the distance from one mark to the other to determine liver size. The normal liver size is 6 to 12 cm in the MCL; however, men have larger livers than women.

2. Conduct bimanual palpation of the liver by placing your left hand under the client at the level of the 11th to 12th ribs and applying upward pressure. Place your right hand below the costal margin, ask the client to take a deep breath, and palpate for the liver border. The liver is not normally palpable in a healthy adult, although it may be in very thin people.

Percuss the spleen for dullness posterior to the midaxillary line at the level of the 6th to 11th rib (Figure 21–14 ■). *The spleen is percussed as an oval area of dullness approximately 7 cm wide near the left 10th rib and slightly posterior to the midaxillary line.*	■ A large area of dullness that extends to the left anterior axillary line on inspiration is associated with an enlarged spleen and may be related to trauma, infection, or mononucleosis.

Figure 21–14 ■ Percussing the spleen.

Technique/Normal Findings	Abnormal Findings

Percuss for shifting dullness (Figure 21–15 ■). *If ascites is not present, the borders between tympany and dullness remain relatively constant despite position changes.*

- In a client with ascites, the level of dullness increases when the client turns to the side.

Figure 21–15 ■ Percussing for shifting dullness in ascites. *A,* Common percussion tones when the client is lying supine; *B,* changes in percussion tones (shifting dullness) when the client turns to the side.

Palpate the abdomen in all four quadrants. *There should be no abdominal masses or pain on palpation.*

Use a circular motion to move the abdominal wall over underlying structures (Figure 21–16 ■). Feel for masses and note any tenderness or pain the client may have during this part of the exam. Palpate lightly at first (0.5 to 0.75 inch), then deeply (1.5 to 2 inches) with caution. If a mass is palpated, ask the client to raise head and shoulders. A mass in the abdomen may become more prominent with this maneuver, as will a ventral abdominal wall hernia. If the mass is no longer palpable, it is deeper in the abdomen.

- In cases of peritoneal inflammation, palpation causes abdominal pain and involuntary muscle spasms.
- Abnormal masses include aortic aneurysms, neoplastic tumors of the colon or uterus, and a distended bladder or distended bowel due to obstruction.
- A rigid, boardlike abdomen may be palpated when the client has a perforated duodenal ulcer.

PRACTICE ALERT

Never use deep palpation in a client who has had a pulsatile abdominal mass, renal transplant, polycystic kidneys, or is at risk for hemorrhage.

Figure 21–16 ■ Light to moderate palpation of the abdomen. *A,* In light palpation, the examiner, keeping the fingers approximated, gently depresses the abdominal wall about 1 cm to assess for large masses, slight tenderness, and muscle guarding. *B,* The examiner performs moderate palpation by using the palm or the side of the hand to depress the abdominal wall to a slightly greater depth than in light palpation. This technique is useful for assessing abdominal organs that move with respiration (such as the liver and the spleen).

Technique/Normal Findings	Abnormal Findings

Palpate for rebound tenderness. Press the fingers into the abdomen slowly and release the pressure quickly. *Releasing pressure should not cause or increase pain.*

- In peritoneal inflammation, pain occurs when the fingers are withdrawn.
- Right upper quadrant pain occurs with acute cholecystitis.
- Upper middle abdominal pain occurs with acute pancreatitis.
- Right lower quadrant pain occurs with acute appendicitis.
- Left lower quadrant pain is seen in acute diverticulitis.

Palpate the liver (Figure 21–17 ■). Note whether the client guards the abdomen or reports any sharp pain, especially on inspiration. *The abdomen should be nontender, and the liver is usually nonpalpable.*

- An enlarged liver with a smooth, tender edge may indicate hepatitis or venous congestion.
- An enlarged, nontender liver may be felt in malignant condition.
- The client with inflammation of the gallbladder feels sharp pain on inspiration and stops inspiring. This is called Murphy's sign.

Figure 21–17 ■ Palpating the liver with the bimanual method.

EXPLORE MediaLink

Prentice Hall Nursing MediaLink DVD-ROM
Audio Glossary
NCLEX-RN® Review

Animation
GI A&P

COMPANION WEBSITE www.prenhall.com/lemone
Audio Glossary
NCLEX-RN® Review
Care Plan Activity: Gallstones
Case Studies
Assessing Dietary Intake
Counseling a College Student about Vitamins
Teaching Plan: Regular Dental Check-Ups and Older Adults
MediaLink Application: Nursing Tools for Assessing the
Nutritional Status of Clients
Links to Resources

TEST YOURSELF NCLEX-RN® REVIEW

1 What is the digestive function of the liver?
  1. to secrete bile
  2. to release glucose
  3. to synthesize plasma proteins
  4. to store iron as ferritin

2 The breakdown of carbohydrates to produce ATP is an example of:
  1. metabolism.
  2. anabolism.
  3. catabolism.
  4. lipidism.

3 Your client asks you what type of foods are complete proteins. What would be your best response?
  1. none
  2. eggs and milk
  3. fruits and vegetables
  4. butter and oils

4 A client who is deficient in vitamin K may have what type of problem with minor surgery?
  1. infection
  2. blood clotting
  3. keloid formation
  4. slow peristalsis

5 During a health history for nutritional problems, it is important to ask the client to describe:
1. the type, amount, and character of pain experienced.
2. the odor and color of urine.
3. the ability to put joints through full range of motion.
4. the usual food and fluid intake for a 24-hour period.

6 On monitoring a client's lab results, you notice a greatly elevated serum amylase level. What disease does this indicate?
1. cheilosis
2. gastric reflux
3. gallstones
4. acute pancreatitis

7 While assessing an older adult, you notice her teeth have obvious caries and she has difficulty swallowing. She says, "My mouth is so dry." What health problem might result from these findings?
1. nutritional deficit
2. acute pain
3. altered elimination
4. risk for infection

8 Which quadrant of the abdomen would you palpate to assess the liver border?
1. right upper
2. right lower
3. left upper
4. left lower

9 Clients with ascites are assessed for changes in what type of percussion sounds?
1. inaudible bowel sounds
2. resonance
3. alternating amplitude
4. shifting dullness

10 When assessing the abdomen, what assessment technique is used last?
1. observation
2. auscultation
3. palpation
4. percussion

See Test Yourself answers in Appendix C.

BIBLIOGRAPHY

Amella, E. (2004). Presentation of illness in older adults: If you think you know what you're looking for, think again. *American Journal of Nursing, 104*(10), 40–51.

Are you missing serious illness in older patients? Improve assessment of geriatric patients. *Hospital Home Health, 21*(9), 105–106.

Balance your nutrition: Update on recommended daily intakes-1. (2004). Retrieved from http://www.balanceyournutrition.com/BYN_updateRDA.htm

Bartz, S. (2003). Gastrointestinal disorders in the elderly. *Annals of Long-Term Care, 11*(7), 33–39.

Blackwood, H. (2004). Obesity: A rapidly expanding challenge. *Nursing Management, 35*(5), 27–36.

Cromling, T. (2003). Use these tips to assess and treat ingestions. *ED Nursing, 6*(8), 97–98.

DeKruif, J., & Vos, A. (2003). An algorithm for the clinical assessment of nutritional status in hospitalized patients. *British Journal of Nutrition, 90*(4), 829–836.

Eliopoulos, C. (2005). *Gerontological nursing* (6th ed). Philadelphia: Lippincott.

Hanson, C. (2004). Mouth care — how important is it? *Journal of Community Nursing, 18*(8), 4–6, 8.

Jarvis, C. (2004). *Physical examination & health assessment.* St. Louis, MO: Mosby.

Kee, J. (2005). *Prentice Hall handbook of laboratory & diagnostic tests with nursing implications.* Upper Saddle River, NJ: Prentice Hall.

McCormick, S., & Clarke, C. (2004). Prevention and management of overweight/obesity in the community. *Nutrition Bulletin, 29*(3), 274–279.

Mehta, M. (2003). Assessing the abdomen: Use sight, sound and touch to screen for abnormalities. *Nursing, 33*(5), 54–55.

National Institutes of Health. (2003). *Genes and disease: Nutritional and metabolic diseases.* Retrieved from http://www.ncbi.nlm.nih.gov/books/bv.fcgi?rid=gnd.section.239

Porth, C. (2005). *Pathophysiology: Concepts of altered health states* (7th ed.). Philadelphia: Lippincott.

Pullen, R. (2004). Clinical do's & don'ts: Measuring gastric residual volume. *Nursing, 34*(4), 18.

Spector, R. (2004). *Cultural diversity in health and illness* (6th ed.). Upper Saddle River, NJ: Prentice Hall.

U.S. Department of Health. (2005). *Dietary guidelines for Americans 2005. Key recommendations for the general population.* Retrieved from http://www.health.gov/dietaryguidelines/dga2005/recommendations.htm

Walker, B. (2004). Assessing gastrointestinal infections. *Nursing, 34*(5), 48–52.

Weber, J., & Kelley, J. (2006). *Health assessment in nursing* (3rd ed.). Philadelphia: Lippincott Williams Wilkins .

Woodrow, P. (2003). Assessing blood results in older people: Haematology and liver function tests. *Nursing Older People, 15*(3), 29–31.

CHAPTER 22 Nursing Care of Clients with Nutritional Disorders

LEARNING OUTCOMES

- Compare and contrast the pathophysiology and manifestations of nutritional disorders.
- Identify causes and predict effects of nutritional disorders on client health status.
- Explain interdisciplinary care for clients with nutritional disorders.
- Develop strategies to promote nutrition for client populations.

CLINICAL COMPETENCIES

- Assess the functional health status of clients with nutritional disorders.
- Monitor nutritional status and responses to care; document and report abnormal or unexpected responses.
- Use assessed data to determine priority nursing diagnoses and select and implement nursing interventions.
- Administer medications and enteral and parenteral nutrition knowledgeably and safely.
- Integrate interdisciplinary care in the plan of care.
- Adapt cultural values and variations into the plan of care for clients with nutritional disorders.
- Plan and provide client and family teaching to restore, promote, and maintain functional health status.
- Evaluate responses to care and use data to revise plan of care as needed.

MEDIALINK

Resources for this chapter can be found on the Prentice Hall Nursing MediaLink DVD-ROM accompanying this textbook, and on the Companion Website at http://www.prenhall.com/lemone

Obesity and malnutrition, the major nutritional disorders in the world today, affect many systems and organs. They often cause serious health problems, such as hypertension, heart disease, fluid and electrolyte imbalances, disability, and even death.

Clients with nutritional disorders require complex, skilled nursing care. Developmental, sociocultural, psychologic, and physiologic factors may play a role in these disorders: A holistic approach to nursing care is vital. Nursing care focuses on identifying causes, meeting nutritional and physiologic needs, providing client education, and meeting the psychologic needs of clients and families. Before proceeding with the discussion of obesity and malnutrition, review the sections on metabolism and nutrients in Chapter 21 ∞ .

THE CLIENT WITH OBESITY

Obesity, an excess of adipose tissue, is one of the most prevalent, preventable health problems in the United States. Obesity has serious physiologic and psychologic consequences, and is associated with increased morbidity and mortality. It contributes to poor health-related quality of life to a greater extent than smoking, excess alcohol use, or poverty. It will soon replace smoking as the leading preventable cause of death in the United States if current trends continue (Uphold & Graham, 2003). Health-related problems associated with obesity are listed in Table 22–1.

While obesity is often defined by weight, it is more accurately defined by the **body mass index (BMI)**, an indirect measure of the amount of body fat, or adipose tissue. Adipose tissue is created when energy consumption exceeds energy expenditure. A BMI of 25 to 29.9 kg/m^2 is classified as *overweight*; obesity is a BMI of 30 kg/m^2 or greater (National Institutes of Health [NIH], 2004). The terms *overweight* and *obese* are not mutually exclusive; a client who is obese also is overweight.

Incidence and Prevalence

More than 30% of the adult population in the United States is obese; nearly two-thirds of all adults in the United States are overweight. The incidence of obesity is higher in women, in blacks, and in economically disadvantaged people of all races (Kasper et al., 2005; Tierney et al., 2005). While the prevalence of overweight has been increasing since 1960, the prevalence of obesity is increasing to a greater extent, particularly during the past 10 to 15 years (National Heart, Lung, and Blood Institute [NHLBI], 2000). Of particular concern is the increasing incidence of obesity in children and young adults. The incidence

TABLE 22–1 Health-Related Problems Associated with Obesity

BODY SYSTEM	OBESITY-RELATED PROBLEMS
Cardiovascular	Atherosclerosis, hypercholesterolemia Coronary heart disease Heart failure Hypertension Stroke Varicosities Venous thrombosis
Respiratory	Sleep disorders Sleep apnea
Gastrointestinal	Gallbladder disease Hiatal hernia Colon cancer
Genitourinary	Cancers of the breast, uterus, prostate, and colon Complications of pregnancy Stress incontinence
Musculoskeletal	Low back pain Muscle strains and sprains Osteoarthritis
Endocrine and Reproductive	Diabetes mellitus, type 2 Endometrial cancer Polycystic ovarian syndrome
Other	Depression Binge-eating disorder Postoperative complications

of overweight and obesity varies among ethnic and cultural groups. Adults of Asian heritage generally have a lower incidence of overweight and obesity. See the Focus on Cultural Diversity box that follows.

FAST FACTS

Prevalence of overweight and obesity in the United States:

- Women
  - Black: 77.3%
  - Hispanic: 71.9%
  - White: 57.3%
- Men
  - Black: 60.7%
  - Hispanic: 74.7%
  - White: 67.4%

Risk Factors

Many factors contribute to obesity, including genetic, physiologic, psychologic, environmental, and sociocultural factors. Heredity may contribute as much as 25% to 40% of the risk for obesity (NHLBI, 1998). The inheritance of obesity does not usually follow a clear Mendelian pattern, and it is difficult to separate the role of environment from genetic factors. However, there is a strong correlation between the weight of adopted children and their biologic parents. Identical twins tend to have similar BMIs, whether raised together or apart, providing further evidence of a genetic link to obesity. While several genes that contribute to appetite and fat deposition have been identified, obesity as a purely genetic condition is rare (Kasper et al., 2005).

Physical inactivity is probably the most important factor contributing to obesity. Inactive people may consume fewer calories than active people and continue to gain weight due to lack of energy expenditure. Cultural and environmental factors such as labor-saving devices, reliance on the automobile for transportation, and increased time spent using the computer contribute to decreased energy expenditure among adults in the United States. Increased time spent watching television is seen as a major contributing factor to the increased incidence of obesity among children and adolescents (Kasper et al., 2005).

Environmental influences, such as an abundant and readily accessible food supply, fast-food restaurants, advertising, and vending machines, contribute to increased food intake. Sociocultural influences that contribute to obesity include overeating at family meals, rewarding behavior with food, religious and family gatherings that promote food intake, and sedentary lifestyles. Socioeconomic status also tends to correlate with the risk for overweight and obesity: In the United States, women with low incomes or low educational levels are more likely to be obese than those of higher socioeconomic status (NHLBI, 1998). The association between socioeconomic status and obesity is less clear in men.

Psychologic factors, such as low self-esteem, also play a role in obesity. Low self-esteem may precipitate unhealthy eating behaviors, and the resulting weight gain in turn may diminish self-image even further. A person may overeat as a result of anxiety, depression, guilt, or boredom or as a means of getting attention. Some experts characterize overeating as a food addiction and as a coping mechanism for stressful life events.

Overview of Normal Physiology

All body activities require energy, including activities of daily living, as well as those necessary to maintain cell and tissue function. **Nutrients** in food (or enteral or parenteral feedings) provide this energy and are the building blocks for growth and tissue repair. The body stores excess nutrients and energy (measured as kilocalories) to meet the body's needs when required nutrients are unavailable. This ability to store and release energy is important to maintaining body function. More than 70% of the energy expended each day goes to maintaining the **basal metabolic rate (BMR)**, essentially the "cost" (in kilocalories) of being alive. Physical activity accounts for only 5% to 10% of the energy spent daily.

Energy is primarily stored as fat in adipose tissue. Although mature fat cells (adipocytes) do not multiply, the immature cells in adipose tissue can multiply, particularly when exposed to estrogen during puberty, in late adolescence, during breast-feeding, and in middle-aged adults who are overweight. Fat cells store excess energy as **triglycerides**, formed from dietary fats and carbohydrates. The body breaks down the triglycerides in fat cells when needed to provide energy (Porth, 2005).

Pathophysiology

Obesity occurs when excess calories are stored as fat. It can result from excess energy intake, decreased energy expenditure, or a combination of both. The etiology of obesity is not, however, as simple as excess kilocalorie intake in relation to energy expenditure. The systems that regulate food intake, energy storage, and energy expenditure are complex and not fully understood.

Appetite, which affects food intake, is regulated by the central nervous system and by emotional factors. The hunger center in the hypothalamus stimulates appetite in response to stimuli such as hypoglycemia. As nutrient levels rise, the satiety center (also in the hypothalamus) sends the message to stop eating. Gastrointestinal filling and hormonal factors also signal *satiety* (a sensation of fullness). Appetite may have little relationship to hunger: People may eat to relieve depression or anxiety.

Several hormones are involved in regulating obesity, including thyroid hormone, insulin, and leptin (a peptide produced by fatty tissue that suppresses appetite and increases energy expenditure). Some studies suggest that leptin resistance is a cause of obesity. Insulin is associated with body fat distribution. The two major types of body fat distribution are upper body and lower body obesity.

Upper body obesity (also called *central obesity*) is identified by a waist-to-hip ratio of greater than 1 in men or 0.8 in women. (See Chapter 21 ∞ for a method to calculate the waist-to-hip ratio.) People with upper body obesity tend to have more intra-abdominal fat and higher levels of circulating free fatty acids (Porth, 2005). As a result, upper body obesity is associated with a greater risk of complications such as hypertension, abnormal blood lipid levels, heart disease, stroke, and elevated insulin levels. Men tend to have more intra-abdominal fat than women, although women develop a central fat distribution pattern after menopause.

Lower body obesity (also known as *peripheral obesity*), in which the waist-to-hip ratio is less than 0.8, is more commonly seen in women. The risk for hyperinsulinemia, abnormal lipids, and heart disease is lower in people with lower body obesity than in those with upper body obesity. Lower body obesity may be more difficult to treat, however.

Complications of Obesity

As obesity increases, adverse consequences of obesity increase. Individuals with **morbid obesity** (greater than 200% ideal body weight) have a risk of dying that is 12 times that of people who are not obese (Kasper et al., 2005).

Obesity is a significant risk factor for cardiovascular disease, including hypertension, coronary heart disease (CHD), and heart failure. The prevalence of hypertension in obese men and women is approximately twice that in people with a BMI of less than 25 (NHLBI, 1998). The increases in blood pressure seen with obesity increase the risk for CHD and stroke. Approximately 60% of obese individuals have *metabolic syndrome,* including three or more of the following: increased waist circumference, hypertension, elevated blood triglycerides and fasting blood glucose, and low HDL cholesterol (Tierney et al., 2005). The metabolic syndrome is an identified risk factor for atherosclerosis and CHD. The Nurses' Health Study showed that the relative risk for CHD in women increases with a BMI of 25 or higher (NHLBI, 1998). Obesity also increases the risk for developing heart failure. Left ventricular muscle mass increases, and the ventricle dilates in obese individuals, possibly related to increased blood volume and cardiac output. Obesity-associated obstructive sleep apnea also contributes to the risk for heart failure.

Obesity increases the risk of insulin resistance and type 2 diabetes. Both weight gain in adulthood and abdominal (central) obesity are positively correlated with the risk for developing type 2 diabetes (NHLBI, 1998). It affects reproductive function in both men and women. Androgen (male sex hormone) levels are reduced in obese men; menstrual irregularities and polycystic ovarian syndrome (PCOS) are more common in obese women. PCOS is an additional risk factor for hyperinsulinemia and insulin resistance. Increased weight also increases the risk for developing gallstones in both men and women. The risk for developing several types of cancer, including colon, breast, and endometrial, increases in obesity. Increased weight places abnormal stress on joints, increasing the prevalence of joint pain and osteoarthritis, particularly in weight-bearing joints (especially the knee joints). Other health-related problems associated with obesity are listed in Table 22–1.

INTERDISCIPLINARY CARE

Because obesity has many contributing factors, its treatment is far more complex than just reducing the amount of food consumed. Treatment is an ongoing process requiring a number of strategies. Most experts recommend an individualized program of exercise, diet, and behavior modification designed to meet the client's specific needs.

Diagnosis

Although body weight may be used to identify obesity, measures of body fat are more accurate. Males at ideal body weight have 10% to 20% body fat, whereas females at ideal body weight have 20% to 30% body fat.

- *Body mass index* is used to identify excess adipose tissue. BMI is calculated by dividing the weight (in kilograms) by the height in meters squared (m^2). See Box 22–1. BMI calculations may not as accurately reflect the extent of adipose tissue in people who are highly muscular (e.g., body builders) or in those who have lost muscle mass (e.g., older adults). Table 22–2 provides a tool for determining BMIs between 19 and 35.
- *Anthropometry* includes measurements of height, weight, bone size, and skinfold measurements to estimate subcutaneous fat. See Chapter 21 ∞ for more information about anthropometric measurements.
- *Underwater weighing (hydrodensitometry)* is considered the most accurate way to determine body fat. This technique involves submerging the whole body and then measuring the amount of displaced water.
- *Bioelectrical impedance* uses a low-energy electrical impulse to determine the percentage of body fat by measuring the electrical resistance of the body.
- *Waist circumference* is measured to determine body fat distribution. Men with a waist measurement of 40 inches (102 cm) or greater and women with a waist measurement of 35 inches (88 cm) or greater have a higher risk for complications of obesity.

Other diagnostic tests may be done to help identify a physiologic cause of obesity, as well as complications of obesity.

- A *thyroid profile,* including a T_3 total and T_3 uptake, T_4 free (FT_4) and T_4 total, free thyroxine index (FTI), and TSH, is done to rule out thyroid disease (see Chapter 18 ∞).
- *Serum glucose* is measured to identify coexisting diabetes mellitus.
- *Serum cholesterol* is measured to assess for elevated levels.
- A *lipid profile* is ordered; high-density lipoprotein (HDL) levels may be reduced in obese clients, whereas low-density lipoprotein (LDL) levels are elevated.
- An *electrocardiogram (ECG)* is performed to detect effects of obesity on the heart, such as rate or rhythm disruptions, myocardial infarction, or heart enlargement.

BOX 22–1 Calculating Body Mass Index (BMI)

BMI = weight (kg)/height^2 (m^2)
Normal = BMI 18.5−24.9 kg/m^2
Overweight = BMI 25−29.9 kg/m^2
Obese = BMI > 30 kg/m^2
Extreme obesity = BMI > 40 kg/m^2

TABLE 22–2 Body Mass Index Table for BMIs 19 to 35

BMI	NORMAL						OVERWEIGHT						OBESE				
	19	20	21	22	23	24	25	26	27	28	29	30	31	32	33	34	35
HEIGHT (INCHES)	BODY WEIGHT (POUNDS)																
58	91	96	100	105	110	115	119	124	129	134	138	143	148	153	158	162	167
59	94	99	104	109	114	119	124	128	133	138	143	148	153	158	163	168	173
60	97	102	107	112	118	123	128	133	138	143	148	153	158	163	168	174	179
61	100	106	111	116	122	127	132	137	143	148	153	158	164	169	174	180	185
62	104	109	115	120	126	131	136	142	147	153	158	164	169	175	180	186	191
63	107	113	118	124	130	135	141	146	152	158	163	169	175	180	186	191	197
64	110	116	122	128	134	140	145	151	157	163	169	174	180	186	192	197	204
65	114	120	126	132	136	144	150	156	162	168	174	180	186	192	198	204	210
66	118	124	130	136	142	148	155	161	167	173	179	186	192	198	204	210	216
67	121	127	134	140	146	153	159	166	172	178	185	191	198	204	211	217	223
68	125	131	138	144	151	158	164	171	177	184	190	197	203	210	216	223	230
69	128	135	142	149	155	162	169	176	182	189	196	203	209	216	223	230	236
70	132	139	146	153	160	167	174	181	188	195	202	209	216	222	229	236	243
71	136	143	150	157	165	172	179	186	193	200	208	215	222	229	236	243	250
72	140	147	154	162	169	177	184	191	199	206	213	221	228	235	242	250	258
73	144	151	159	166	174	182	189	197	204	212	219	227	235	242	250	257	265
74	148	155	163	171	179	186	194	202	210	218	225	233	241	249	256	264	272
75	152	160	168	176	184	192	200	208	216	224	232	240	248	256	264	272	279
76	156	164	172	180	189	197	205	213	221	230	238	246	254	263	271	279	287

Source: National Institutes of Health, National Heart, Lung, and Blood Institute, North American Association for the Study of Obesity. (2000). *The Practical Guide: Identification, Evaluation, and Treatment of Overweight and Obesity in Adults.* Bethesda, MD: NIH.

Medications

Many prescription and over-the-counter drugs have been used to help people lose weight. When used in combination with diet and exercise, drugs can help promote weight loss. Their long-term efficacy, however, is questionable; rebound weight gain following the cessation of drug use is common. In addition, tolerance, addiction, and side effects may occur. These products are usually recommended only as an adjunct to therapy and only when traditional therapies have been unsuccessful.

Amphetamines (which have a high potential for abuse) and nonamphetamine appetite suppressants (such as phentermine) may be used for a short time to promote weight loss. Phentermine is believed to act directly on the appetite control center in the central nervous system (CNS). As with amphetamines, nonamphetamine appetite suppressants stimulate the CNS, with resulting increased alertness, nervousness, and insomnia. They reduce fatigue, and can interfere with sleep. They are used with caution in clients with preexisting heart disease, because they can increase blood pressure and heart rate and cause anginal pain.

Sibutramine (Meridia) is an appetite suppressant that acts on the CNS. Sibutramine also may increase the metabolic rate, promoting weight loss. It has the additional benefit of lowering cholesterol and triglyceride levels. Sibutramine increases both the pulse rate and blood pressure, potentially limiting its ap-

propriateness for use in clients with hypertension, CHD, or heart failure.

Orlistat (Xenical) has a different mechanism of action: It inhibits fat absorption from the GI tract, leading to weight loss. It has the added benefit of lowering blood glucose and cholesterol. The adverse effects of orlistat relate to its inhibition of fat absorption: oily stools, flatulence, and fecal urgency. These effects tend to diminish when dietary fat intake is limited. See the Medication Administration box on page 634 for the nursing implications of these drugs.

Over-the-counter products such as phenylpropanolamine, benzocaine, and bulk-forming agents are commonly used in weight management efforts. Phenylpropanolamine (Acutrim, Dexatrim) is an adrenergic agent that suppresses appetite. This product is contraindicated in clients with hypertension, CHD, diabetes mellitus, and thyroid disease. Methylcellulose and other bulk-forming products may decrease appetite by producing a sensation of fullness. Clients taking these products may experience flatulence or diarrhea and may need to increase fluid intake.

Treatments

Successful treatment of obesity (sustained achievement of normal body weight without adverse consequences) is rarely achieved. Treatment focuses on reducing the health risks associated with

MEDICATION ADMINISTRATION   Drugs to Treat Obesity

APPETITE SUPPRESSANTS

- Phentermine (Adipex-P, Fastin, Ionamin, Obestin-30, Oby-Trim, others)
- Sibutramine (Meridia)

Phentermine acts directly on the appetite-control center in the CNS to suppress the appetite and reduce hunger. Sibutramine reduces hunger and increases sensations of satiety by inhibiting the uptake of serotonin, norepinephrine, and dopamine. These drugs may be used to treat obesity in clients with a BMI of >30 kg/m^2 and obese clients who have risk factors such as diabetes or hypertension.

Nursing Responsibilities

- Assess for contraindications, such as pregnancy or lactation, use of other appetite suppressants, impaired liver or kidney function, history of CHD, or alcohol abuse.
- Regularly monitor blood pressure and heart rate during treatment. Increases may indicate need to reduce dose or discontinue treatment.

Health Education for the Client and Family

- Take as directed; do not exceed recommended dose. Do not take if you may be pregnant or are nursing.
- Take your last dose no later than 4 P.M. to avoid insomnia.
- You may experience difficulty sleeping, nervousness, or palpitations while taking this drug.

- Increase your fluid intake to reduce possible side effects of dry mouth and constipation.
- This drug does not replace diet and exercise for weight loss; continue to follow your prescribed regimen.

LIPASE INHIBITOR

- Orlistat (Xenical)

Orlistat inhibits lipases necessary for the breakdown and absorption of fat, thus decreasing the absorption of dietary fat. Its action is primarily local, within the GI tract, with few systemic effects.

Nursing Responsibilities

- Administer with meals or up to 1 hour following a meal.
- Provide a fat-soluble vitamin supplement (A, D, E, and K) daily. Separate administration time from orlistat by at least 2 hours.

Health Education for the Client and Family

- Take as directed; do not increase dose. You may skip a dose if you do not consume a meal.
- Use in conjunction with a low-calorie, low-fat diet.
- Common gastrointestinal side effects include oily or fatty stools, flatulence, oily discharge, or frequent stools with difficulty controlling defecation. These side effects may diminish with time or increase if a meal high in fat is consumed.
- Notify your healthcare provider if you become pregnant while taking this medication.

---

obesity by changing both eating and exercise habits. A pound of body fat is equivalent to 3500 kcal. To lose 1 pound, therefore, a person must reduce daily caloric intake by 500 kcal for 7 days or increase activity enough to burn the equivalent kilocalories. A weight loss goal of 1 to 2 pounds per week and a 10% reduction in body weight in 6 months of therapy is recommended (NHLBI, 2000). A combination of physical activity, dietary therapy, behavior modification, pharmacology, and, in some cases, surgery is required to achieve and maintain weight loss (Table 22–3).

EXERCISE Exercise is a critical element in weight loss and maintenance. Physical activity increases energy consumption and pro-

motes weight loss while preserving lean body mass. Physical activity improves physical fitness, decreases appetite, promotes self-esteem, and increases the basal metabolic rate. An exercise or activity program should reflect the client's physical condition, interest, lifestyle, and abilities. Evaluation by a healthcare practitioner is important before beginning an exercise program. The practitioner instructs the client to increase the duration and intensity of activity and to stop exercising and report symptoms if chest pain or shortness of breath occurs. An aerobic exercise program of 30 to 40 minutes of exercise five or more days a week promotes weight loss while reducing adipose tissue, increasing lean body mass, and promoting long-term weight control. Table 22–4 presents examples of moderate activities, that when performed at the

---

TABLE 22–3 Treatment Recommendations for Overweight and Obesity

TREATMENT	BMI				
	25–26.9	27–29.9	30–34.9	35–39.9	≥40
Diet, exercise, and behavior modification	With two or more comorbidities[1]	With two or more comorbidities[1]	Yes	Yes	Yes
Pharmacotherapy[2]		With two or more comorbidities[1]	Yes	Yes	Yes
Surgery			With 2 or more comorbidities[1]		

[1]For example, hypertension, hyperlipidemia, diabetes, and other obesity-related complications.
[2]Considered when 6 months of combined therapy has not produced a loss of 1 pound per week.
Source: Adapted from National Institutes of Health, National Heart, Lung, and Blood Institute, North American Association for the Study of Obesity. (2000). *The Practical Guide: Identification, Evaluation, and Treatment of Overweight and Obesity in Adults.* Bethesda, MD: NIH.

TABLE 22–4 Moderate Physical Activites to Use Approximately 150 kcal/day

COMMON CHORES	SPORTS & RECREATION	
Washing and waxing a car: 45–60 min	Playing volleyball: 45–60 min	Less vigorous, more time
Washing windows or floors: 45–60 min	Playing touch football: 45 min	
Gardening: 45–60 min	Walking 1¾ miles: 35 min	
Wheeling self in wheelchair: 30–40 min	Bicycling 5 miles: 30 min	
Pushing a stroller 1½ miles: 30 min	Dancing fast (social): 30 min	
Raking leaves: 30 min	Swimming laps: 20 min	
Walking 2 miles: 30 min	Playing basketball: 15–30 min	
Shoveling snow: 15 min	Jumping rope: 15 min	
Stairwalking: 15 min	Running 1½ miles: 15 min	More vigorous, less time

Source: National Institutes of Health, National Heart, Lung, and Blood Institute, North American Association for the Study of Obesity. (2000). *The Practical Guide: Identification, Evaluation, and Treatment of Overweight and Obesity in Adults.* Bethesda, MD: NIH.

identified intensity and duration, will use approximately 150 kcal per day or about 1000 kcal per week.

NUTRITION The diet is planned to create a daily 500- to 1000-kcal deficit. Ideally, the diet should be low in kilocalories and fat and contain adequate nutrients, minerals, and fiber. The client should eat regular meals with small servings. A gradual, slow weight loss of no more than 1 to 2 pounds per week is recommended. For most people, this means a diet of 1000 to 1200 kcal/day for most women, and 1200 to 1600 kcal/day for men. Fewer than 1200 kcal each day may lead to loss of lean tissue and nutritional deficiencies. The recommended diet generally is low in fat and high in dietary fiber (Table 22–5). Excessive calorie restrictions can lead to failure to follow the prescribed diet, feelings of guilt, and overeating. "Yo-yo" dieting (repeated cycles of weight loss and gain) may lead to a metabolic deficiency that makes subsequent weight loss efforts increasingly difficult. Therefore, it is critical that dieters take any weight loss effort seriously and include plans for long-term maintenance. The best approach is to modify dietary intake without severe restrictions, eating a well-balanced, low-fat diet

and developing improved eating habits. Table 22–6 provides sample daily menus for a reduced kcal diet.

Very low calorie diets (VLCDs) are generally reserved for clients who have a BMI greater than 30 (Weight-Control Information Network [WIN], 2003b). This type of program offers a protein-sparing modified fast (400 to 800 kcal/day or less) under close medical supervision. In a typical program, the client consumes 45 to 70 g of high-quality protein, 30 to 50 g of carbohydrate, and about 2 g of fat per day for a 1- to 2-month period. Exercise, nutrition, and behavior modification counseling should accompany the diet. The client generally experiences a dramatic and rapid weight loss while maintaining lean body mass. Suppression of hunger brought on by ketone production associated with fat metabolism is an added benefit of the diet. Complications generally are minor, and the benefits include decreased blood pressure, blood glucose, and cholesterol and triglyceride levels, along with improved exercise tolerance (Kasper et al., 2005). VLCDs may not be appropriate for use in people over age 50 due to normal loss of lean body mass and adverse effects of the diet. Adverse effects generally are minor, but could include fatigue, constipation, nausea, diarrhea, and gallstone formation (WIN, 2003b).

TABLE 22–5 Recommended Nutrient Intake for Weight Loss

NUTRIENT	RECOMMENDED INTAKE
Calories	1000 to 1600 per day or approximately 500 to 1000 less than usual daily intake
Total fat	30% or less of total calories
Saturated fats	10% or less of total calories
Cholesterol	< 300 mg/day
Protein (from plant and lean animal sources)	Approximately 15% of total calories
Carbohydrate (complex carbohydrates from vegetables, fruits, and whole grains)	55% or more of total calories
Fiber (e.g., oat bran, legumes, barley, most fruits and vegetables)	20 to 30 g/day
Sodium chloride	< 2.4 g sodium or 6 g sodium chloride/day
Calcium	1000 to 1500 mg/day

Source: Adapted from National Institutes of Health, National Heart, Lung, and Blood Institute, North American Association for the Study of Obesity. (2000). *The Practical Guide: Identification, Evaluation, and Treatment of Overweight and Obesity in Adults.* Bethesda, MD: NIH.

TABLE 22–6 Sample Menus for a Reduced Kilocalorie Diet

	TRADITIONAL AMERICAN	REDUCED CARBOHYDRATE	SOUTHERN CUISINE	ASIAN AMERICAN	MEXICAN AMERICAN
Breakfast	Whole-wheat toast with jelly, 1 slice High-fiber cereal, 1 cup Milk 1%, 1 cup Orange juice, 6 oz Coffee	Whole-wheat toast with low-fat cream cheese Egg substitute, ½ cup, scrambled Vegetable juice, 1 cup Coffee	Oatmeal, ½ cup, prepared with 1% milk Milk 1%, ½ cup English muffin with low-fat cream cheese Orange juice, 6 oz Coffee	Banana, 1 small Whole-wheat toast with soft margarine, 2 slices Milk 1%, 1 cup Orange juice, 6 oz Tea	Farina, ½ cup prepared with 1% milk White toast with soft margarine and jelly Cantaloupe, 1 cup Orange juice, 1 cup Coffee
Lunch	Roast beef sandwich: 2 slices whole-wheat bread, 2 oz lean roast beef, lettuce, tomato, and low-kilocalorie mayonnaise Apple, 1 medium Water	Salad greens with 2 oz sliced turkey, 1 oz low-fat cheese, and 1 oz low-fat salad dressing Apple, 1 medium Water	Baked chicken, no skin, 2 oz Mixed vegetable salad with 2 tsp oil and vinegar dressing White rice, ½ cup Baking powder biscuit, 1 small with soft margarine Water	Beef broth, ½ cup Chinese noodle and beef salad: 3 oz roast beef, 1 tsp peanut oil, low-sodium soy sauce, carrots, zucchini, onion, and ¼ soft Chinese noodles Apple, 1 medium Tea	Beef enchilada: 2 corn tortillas, 2½ oz lean roast beef, onion, tomato, lettuce, chili peppers, and ¼ cup refried beans (prepared with vegetable oil) Carrots, celery Milk 1%, ½ cup Water
Dinner	Salmon, 3 oz Baked potato, ¾ medium Soft margarine, 1 tsp Green beans, ½ cup Carrots, ½ cup White dinner roll, 1 medium Ice milk, ½ cup Iced tea, unsweetened Water	Salmon, 3 oz Baked sweet potato, 1 small Soft margarine, 1 tsp Green beans, 1 cup Orange, 1 medium Ricotta cheese, ¼ cup, with artificial sweetener and ¼ tsp flavoring extract Iced tea, unsweetened Water	Lean roast beef, 3 oz Beef gravy (water-based), 1 Tbsp Turnip greens Baked sweet potato, 1 small, with soft margarine, ground cinnamon, and 1 tsp brown sugar Corn bread, ½ medium slice Honeydew melon, ¼ medium Sweetened iced tea	Pork stir-fry with vegetables: 2 oz pork cutlet, 1 tsp peanut oil, low-sodium soy sauce, broccoli, carrots, mushrooms Steamed white rice, 1 cup Tea, unsweetened	Chicken taco: 1 corn tortilla, 2 oz chicken breast without skin, 1 oz low-fat cheddar cheese, 2 Tbsp guacamole, and salsa Corn, ½ cup Spanish rice without meat, ½ cup Banana Coffee
Snack	Popcorn, 2½ cups with ½ tsp margarine	Apple, 1 small Low-fat cheese stick, 1	Saltine crackers, unsalted tops, 4 Mozzarella cheese, part skim, 1 oz	Almond cookies, 2 Milk 1%, ¾ cup	

BEHAVIOR MODIFICATION Behavior modification is a critical component of successful weight management. Strategies such as keeping food records, eliminating cues that precipitate eating, and changing the act of eating are often helpful.

Recording food intake, amount, location of eating, and situations that induce eating often help the dieter gain self-control. These strategies are often most effective when used in combination with other behavior modification approaches.

Researchers have found that most overweight people are stimulated to eat by external cues, such as the proximity to food and the time of day. In contrast, hunger and satiety are the cues that regulate eating in adults of normal weight. Strategies to control food cues include keeping food out of view, eliminating snack foods, and eating only in designated areas. See Box 22–2 for a list of behavior modification strategies.

Other behavior modification approaches focus on helping clients examine factors that affect eating behaviors. Examining lifestyle, personality, and environment helps the client understand eating behaviors and their consequences. The goal is to empower the person who is stimulated to eat to choose activities that are not related to food.

Social support and group programs such as Weight Watchers, Overeaters Anonymous, and Take Off Pounds Sensibly (TOPS) promote weight loss success through peer support. Most organized programs require participants to pay a fee, which may improve compliance.

SURGERY Surgical treatment of obesity (*bariatric surgery*) generally is limited to morbidly obese clients (BMI of over 40 kg/m² or 200% ideal body weight) who are unable to lose weight through diet and exercise or who have serious obesity-related problems such as metabolic syndrome, hypertension, or heart disease (WIN, 2004). In addition, clients must be able to tolerate surgery and be free of addiction to alcohol or other

---

BOX 22–2 Behavioral Change Strategies for the Obese Client

Controlling the Environment
- Purchase low-calorie foods.
- Shop from a prepared list and on a full stomach.
- Keep all foods in the kitchen.
- Store all foods in the refrigerator or in the cabinets in opaque containers.
- Prepare exact portions of food to eliminate leftovers.
- Eat all foods in the same place, avoid eating in the kitchen.
- Avoid eating when watching television or reading.
- Reduce frequency of eating out at restaurants, parties, and picnics.

Controlling Physiologic Responses to Food
- Eat slowly by taking small bites, allowing 20 minutes for a meal.
- Eat a salad or drink a hot beverage before a meal.

- Chew each bite thoroughly and slowly.
- Put eating utensils or food down between bites.
- Concentrate on the eating process, savor the food.
- Stop eating with the first feelings of fullness.

Controlling Psychologic Responses to Food
- Appreciate the aesthetic experience of eating.
- Use attractive dinnerware, and prepare a formal setting for eating.
- Use small plates and cups to make servings of food look larger.
- Concentrate on conversations and socialization during the meal.
- Use nonfood rewards for meeting a goal.
- Acknowledge small successes and improvements in all behavior.
- Substitute other activities for eating (e.g., reading, exercise, hobbies).

---

drugs. A thorough psychologic evaluation is done before surgery. The benefits of surgery include major weight loss and improved blood pressure, plus a reduced risk of diabetes, sleep apnea, angina, heart failure, blood lipid levels, and venous disease (Kasper et al., 2005). Bariatric surgery, however, is not without risk, and the decision to undergo surgery is a significant one.

The most common bariatric surgical procedures used in the United States restrict stomach capacity, limiting food intake, and bypass a portion of the small intestine to restrict absorption of calories and nutrients. In the Roux-en-Y gastric bypass (RGB, Figure 22–1A ■), a small stomach pouch is created to restrict food intake. A Y-shaped section of the jejunum is then attached to the pouch to allow food to bypass the lower stomach and duodenum. As a result, calorie and nutrient absorption is limited. A more complex procedure, the biliopancreatic diversion (BPD), carries a higher risk of nutritional deficiencies and is used less frequently. In BPD, a portion of the stomach is removed to reduce its capacity. The duodenum and jejunum are bypassed by connecting the ileum directly to the stomach pouch or just distal to the pyloric valve.

These combined restrictive/malabsorptive surgeries have the advantage of resulting in rapid weight loss that is maintained over time. Many clients maintain a 60% to 70% weight

loss for 10 years or more following RGB surgery (WIN, 2004). They also help improve obesity-associated health problems such as type 2 diabetes, hypertension, and sleep apnea. Because these procedures allow food to bypass the duodenum and jejunum, nutrient deficiencies are common, particularly of iron, calcium, vitamin B_{12}, and, possibly, the fat-soluble vitamins.

Restrictive procedures, which are safer but generally less effective in the long term, include adjustable gastric banding (AGB) and the vertical banded gastroplasty (VBG). In AGB (Figure 22–1B), a hollow band of silicone rubber is placed around the upper (proximal) portion of the stomach. The band is inflated with saline solution to create a small stomach pouch with a narrow passage through to the rest of the stomach. The amount of band inflation can be adjusted using a port implanted under the skin. The VBG (Figure 22–1C) uses both a band and staples to create a small stomach pouch. Both procedures may be performed laparoscopically and can be reversed if necessary. Few nutritional deficiencies are associated with restrictive bariatric procedures. Vomiting is a common postoperative risk with restrictive procedures. The band may slip or break, necessitating a return to surgery. About 15% to 20% of clients undergoing VBG procedures may require a second procedure. Because of this and

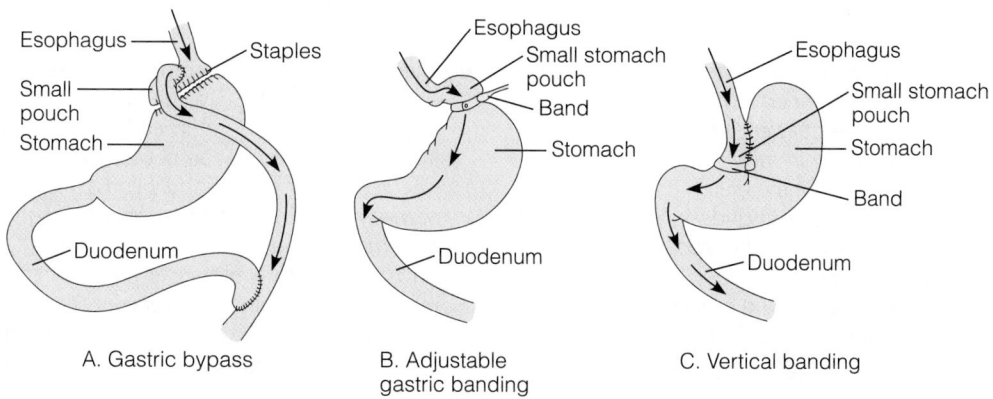

A. Gastric bypass   B. Adjustable gastric banding   C. Vertical banding

Figure 22–1 ■ Types of surgical procedures to treat obesity. *A.* Roux-en-Y gastric bypass surgery; *B.* Adjustable gastric banding. *C.* Vertical banded gastroplasty.

the increased complexity of this procedure, it is performed less commonly than AGB (WIN, 2004). While clients typically lose about 50% of their excess body weight within the first year after these procedures, less than one-quarter maintain that weight loss over a 10-year period (WIN, 2004).

Although the risk for postoperative complications is high, the mortality rate for bariatric procedures is low (less than 1% for restrictive surgeries and up to 5% for combination procedures). Possible postoperative complications include anastomosis leak with peritonitis, abdominal wall hernia, gallstones, wound infections, deep venous thrombosis, nutritional deficiencies, and gastrointestinal symptoms (Tierney et al., 2005). Dumping syndrome, which can be precipitated by a meal high in simple carbohydrates, may develop following combined bariatric surgeries such as RGB and BPD. In dumping syndrome, stomach contents move rapidly through the small intestine, drawing fluid into the intestine by osmosis. The client experiences nausea, bloating, abdominal pain, weakness, sweating, and possibly syncope. See Chapter 23 ∞ for more information about dumping syndrome.

Nursing care for the client who has undergone bariatric surgery is substantially the same as for a client who has undergone a gastric resection. See Chapter 23 ∞ for more information about gastric resection and associated nursing care. Bariatric surgery clients, however, have some additional nursing care needs related to the effects of the surgery on gastrointestinal function. See the box below.

Maintaining Weight Loss

Losing weight and maintaining that loss are two separate but related issues. Most experts agree that the majority of dieters regain lost weight within a 2-year period. The potential risks associated

with regaining weight make maintenance a critical issue. Clients are encouraged to continue exercise, self-monitoring, and treatment support. Long-term weight loss and maintenance mean a lifelong commitment to significant lifestyle changes, including food and eating habits, activity and exercise routines, and behavior modification. Failure to maintain weight loss can lead to feelings of inadequacy, powerlessness, and hopelessness.

NURSING CARE

Health Promotion

Maintaining a healthy weight throughout the life span begins in childhood. Obese children and teenagers become obese adults. Promote healthy eating, including a diet rich in whole grains, fruits, and vegetables and low in fat. The USDA Food Guide Pyramid (Chapter 2 ∞) and the Healthy Eating Pyramid provide visual guidance for appropriate food choices to maintain a healthy, well-balanced diet. Encourage all children and adults to maintain an active lifestyle, engaging in at least 30 minutes of aerobic activity daily. Encourage parents to limit time children spend watching television, using the computer, and playing video games. Discuss the effects of smoking and excess alcohol use on nutrition and activity.

Adults commonly gain about 20 pounds between early and middle adulthood. Encourage clients to reduce the amount of calories consumed as energy needs change.

Assessment

Collect the following data through the health history and physical examination (see Chapter 21 ∞):

MEETING INDIVIDUALIZED NEEDS Recommended Diet Following Bariatric Surgery

Clients undergoing bariatric surgery to restrict stomach capacity and/or nutrient absorption have unique learning needs to prevent discomfort and nutritional complications after surgery:

- A liquid diet generally is prescribed in the initial postoperative period. Fruit juices and other concentrated sugars are avoided. *The client is at risk for developing dumping syndrome in the early postoperative period; simple carbohydrates increase the risk.*

- When clear liquids are tolerated, nonfat or low-fat milk is added to the diet. Soy milk may be used if milk intake results in bloating and gas. *Milk provides a protein source. Fat-free milk or nonfat milk is recommended to reduce the risk of diarrhea. People with a lactase deficiency may not be able to digest the natural lactose sugar in milk.*

- Pureed foods are introduced into the diet in approximately 1 to 2 weeks, and it is advanced to include soft foods within about 1 month after surgery. *Gradual increases in food textures allow the restricted stomach to adapt.*

- Increasing fluid intake and maintaining protein intake are priorities during the healing process. *Fluid intake is necessary to maintain fluid balance, proteins for nitrogen balance and tissue healing.*

- Instruct clients who have undergone restrictive surgery to chew food very well and slow their pace of eating. *Failure to thoroughly chew food and eat slowly can lead to vomiting and abdominal discomfort. Without behavior modification, protein-calorie malnutrition can develop.*

- Advise the client to take an adult multiple vitamin and mineral supplement after restrictive surgery. *Because the overall quantity of food consumed is reduced, the client may develop a micronutrient deficiency.*

- Clients who have had combination restrictive/malabsorptive surgery generally require supplements of folate, sublingual vitamin B_{12}, and calcium, in addition to an adult multivitamin. Iron supplement may be necessary if anemia develops (see Chapter 34 ∞). *Intestinal bypass interferes with absorption of many vitamins and minerals usually absorbed in the duodenum or jejunum.*

- Advise clients to avoid sugar and concentrated sweets (fruit juice, sugar-containing beverages, honey) and to separate consumption of solid foods and liquids by at least 30 minutes. *Concentrated sugars can precipitate dumping syndrome.*

Source: Adapted from Nutritional Considerations after Bariatric Surgery (2003), by K. Elliot, *Critical Care Nursing Quarterly, 26*(2), 133–138.

- *Health history:* Risk factors; current and usual weight; recent weight gains or losses; perception of weight and effect on health; usual diet and food intake; exercise/activity patterns; prior weight loss efforts and results; current medications; co-existing disorders such as cardiovascular disease and diabetes; tobacco use; family history of overweight, diabetes, and weight-related morbidity.
- *Physical examination:* Vital signs; weight and height; skinfold measurements; waist-to-hip ratio; BMI; inspect skin under the breasts and abdominal folds.

PRACTICE ALERT
Use of an inappropriate size sphygmomanometer is a common source of error in measuring blood pressure in obese clients. Choose a cuff on which the width of the bladder is 40% of the circumference of the arm and the length of the bladder is sufficient to cover at least 65% of the arm circumference.

Nursing Diagnoses and Interventions

Nursing care for overweight and obese clients is community based and holistic, focusing on both physiologic and psycho-logic responses to weight and appearance. See below for a Nursing Care Plan for the client with obesity.

Imbalanced Nutrition: More than Body Requirements

Although many factors contribute to obesity, it always involves an imbalance of kcal consumption to energy expenditure.

- Encourage the client to identify the factors that contribute to excess food intake. *Identification of cues to eating helps the client eliminate or reduce these cues.*
- Establish realistic weight loss goals and exercise/activity objectives. *Small, reasonable goals, such as loss of 1 to 2 pounds per week, increase the likelihood of success.*
- Assess the client's knowledge and discuss well-balanced diet plans. Provide necessary teaching about diet. *Knowledge empowers the client to participate and make appropriate diet choices.*
- Discuss behavior modification strategies, such as self-monitoring and environmental management. *Behavior modification, diet, and exercise are critical to promoting successful, long-term weight loss.*

NURSING CARE PLAN   A Client with Obesity

Sam Elliott, age 57, has gained 30 pounds since his retirement 2 years ago. The most active thing he does each day is "puttering around" and "walking to the end of the driveway to get the mail." His diet includes juice, oatmeal, muffin, and coffee with cream for breakfast; donuts and coffee with friends midmorning; a bologna-and-cheese sandwich with chips and a root beer for lunch; and cheese, crackers, and wine before a dinner of meat, potatoes, vegetables, and dessert. He tells the nurse, "I have never had to diet. I just don't know how to get this weight off."

ASSESSMENT
Mr. Elliott is 5′ 8″ (173 cm) tall and weighs 201 lb (91.2 kg). His BMI is 30.1 kg/m². His cholesterol is 240 mg/dL (normal 150 to 200 mg/dL) with an HDL of 37 mg/dL (normal male value > 45 mg/dL) and an LDL of 180 mg/dL (normal <130 mg/dL). His BP is 138/90. His fasting blood glucose is normal at 103 mg/dL. His ECG shows normal sinus rhythm. He reports fatigue and shortness of breath with activity. His healthcare provider has advised a weight loss of 30 pounds and a regular exercise program.

DIAGNOSES
- *Imbalanced Nutrition: More than Body Requirements* related to food intake in excess of energy expenditure
- *Risk for Ineffective Therapeutic Regimen Management* related to knowledge deficit
- *Activity Intolerance* related to sedentary lifestyle

EXPECTED OUTCOMES
- Lose 1 pound each week.
- Walk 30 minutes 5 days each week.
- Verbalize an understanding of the relationship between weight loss, weight control, and exercise.
- Identify behavior modification strategies to avoid overeating.
- Identify support systems for behavior modification.

PLANNING AND IMPLEMENTATION
- Assess weight and blood pressure once or twice each week.
- Discuss current eating habits and strategies to reduce fat and calorie intake.
- Discuss cues that promote eating. Identify strategies to eliminate or reduce eating cues.
- Teach to keep a food diary to examine and change eating habits.
- Discuss the role of regular exercise in weight loss and weight control. Instruct to maintain an exercise record to track the intensity and duration of activity.
- Discuss lifestyle and behavior modification strategies to promote successful weight loss and control.

EVALUATION
Two weeks after changing his diet and beginning to exercise, Mr. Elliott has lost 2 pounds. He has maintained a food diary. He has identified boredom as a cue to eating. In light of that fact, he has started volunteering at the local hospital, where he is working with children. He is walking for 30 minutes 5 days a week. He plans to increase his activity periods to 45 minutes. He verbalizes commitment to a lifelong plan of exercising and eating a low-fat diet. His BP has ranged from 132/76 to 136/84. He plans to have the employee health nurse at the hospital check his weight and BP each week and to join Weight Watchers for ongoing support.

CRITICAL THINKING IN THE NURSING PROCESS
1. What are some possible pathophysiologic bases for Mr. Elliott's abnormal cholesterol, HDL, and LDL levels?
2. Develop a teaching plan for a group of overweight men and women.
3. Identify potential barriers to losing weight and strategies to reduce or eliminate these barriers.
See Evaluating Your Response in Appendix C.

- Monitor weight loss, blood pressure, and laboratory data, including blood glucose and lipid levels. *Continuing assessment not only is important to evaluate the safety of weight loss strategies, but also to reinforce positive benefits of weight loss.*

Activity Intolerance

Obese clients may experience excess fatigue, tachycardia, and shortness of breath with activity due to the physiologic effects of excess weight as well as a sedentary lifestyle. A medical evaluation may be needed before beginning an exercise program.

- Assess current activity level and tolerance of that activity. Assess vital signs. *This provides baseline information to plan an activity program and assess response to that activity.*
- After medical clearance, plan with the client a program of regular, gradually increasing exercise. Consider a consultation with an exercise physiologist. *An individualized exercise program promotes activities within the client's physical capabilities.*

Ineffective Therapeutic Regimen Management

Most overweight or obese clients experience some difficulty integrating all the components of a weight loss program into a daily routine. For a weight loss and maintenance program to be successful, the overweight client must modify dietary intake in a world of daily temptations. There may be many obstacles to exercise, including a busy schedule, activity intolerance, impaired physical mobility, lack of equipment, and the embarrassment of being fat.

- Discuss ability and willingness to incorporate changes into daily patterns of diet, exercise, and lifestyle. *This provides data from which to set realistic goals with the client.*
- Help the client identify behavior modification strategies and support systems for weight loss and maintenance. *Weight loss and maintenance are most successful if the client establishes lifestyle patterns that promote interest and motivation and thus exercise and diet management. Family and social support is critical to successful adherence to the therapeutic regime.*
- Have the client establish strategies for dealing with "stress" eating or interruptions in the therapeutic regime. *A sense of failure associated with overeating or lack of exercise can lead to further overeating. Identifying positive strategies to deal with these situations promotes self-acceptance and limits self-punishment through overeating.*

Chronic Low Self-Esteem

Although many obese clients may have accepted their weight and body appearance on some level, most overweight and obese individuals verbalize the experience of "fat prejudice" in their family, workplace, or community. Obese clients may experience ridicule, prejudice, and health problems attributed to being "fat." These experiences, coupled with day-to-day problems such as finding attractive clothing or a chair large enough to sit on can affect self-esteem. Many clients report that "fat" jokes or comments contribute to a sense of negative self-worth.

- Encourage the client to verbalize the experience of being overweight, and validate the client's experience. *This provides baseline data to use in developing individualized interventions to address self-esteem issues.*

- Set small goals with the client and offer positive feedback and encouragement. *Small goals provide more opportunities for success. Positive feedback and encouragement provide a comfortable environment in which to develop self-esteem.*
- Refer for counseling as appropriate. *Many clients benefit from counseling for issues related to self-esteem.*

Using NANDA, NIC, and NOC

Chart 22–1 shows links between NANDA nursing diagnoses, NIC, and NOC for obese clients.

Community-Based Care

Weight reduction usually occurs in community-based settings. Weight loss and maintenance require a long-term commitment by the client, family, and support systems. Address the following topics with the client and family:

- Lifestyle changes are more effective than diets. Fad diets promote rapid weight loss but often are not nutritionally sound or may be difficult to maintain for a lifetime.
- All household members should consume a diet that is nutritionally sound, low in fat, and high in fiber.
- Establish realistic weight loss goals and a system of nonfood rewards for achieving each goal.

NANDA, NIC, AND NOC LINKAGES
CHART 22–1 The Client with Obesity

NANDA

Imbalanced Nutrition: More than Body Requirements

↓

NIC

Nutrition Management

Weight Reduction Assistance

Behavior Modification

Body Image Enhancement

Self-Esteem Enhancement

↓

NOC

Nutritional Status

Nutrient Intake

Weight Control

Body Image

Self-Esteem

Data from *NANDA's Nursing Diagnoses: Definitions & Classification 2005–2006* by NANDA International (2005), Philadelphia; *Nursing Interventions Classification (NIC)* (4th ed.) by J. M. Dochterman & G. M. Bulechek (2004), St. Louis, MO: Mosby; and *Nursing Outcomes Classification (NOC)* (3rd ed.) by S. Moorhead, M. Johnson, and M. Maas (2004), St. Louis, MO: Mosby.

- Identify an "exercise buddy" or support system to promote continued physical activity.
- Expect occasional failures. Resume prescribed diet and exercise routine as soon as possible; the goal is long-term weight management.
- Community resources such as Weight Watchers, TOPS, or healthcare-based programs provide information, strategies, and support for successful weight management.

THE CLIENT WITH MALNUTRITION

Malnutrition results from inadequate intake of nutrients. There may be a lack of major nutrients (calories, carbohydrates, proteins, and fats) or micronutrients such as vitamins and minerals. Malnutrition may be caused by inadequate nutrient intake; impaired absorption and use of nutrients; loss of nutrients due to diarrhea, hemorrhage, or renal failure; or increased metabolic needs (e.g., infection or physiologic stressors).

Incidence and Prevalence

Malnutrition is a widespread cause of disease and mortality throughout the world. It is endemic in regions affected by famine. Groups at risk for malnutrition in the United States include the young, poor, elderly, homeless, low-income women, and ethnic minorities. Even when food is plentiful, clients may be undernourished because of poor food choices.

It is estimated that approximately half of all hospitalized clients are malnourished (Kasper et al., 2005). Malnutrition may be present on admission or develop as a result of surgery or serious illness. Malnutrition increases both mortality and the incidence of complications in both medical and surgical clients. The incidence of malnutrition is even higher in long-term care residents, where up to 85% of residents may be malnourished (DiMaria-Ghalili & Amella, 2005). See Box 22–3 for conditions commonly associated with malnutrition.

Risk Factors

Risk factors for malnutrition include the following:
- Age—older adults are at greater risk for malnutrition due to a variety of factors (see the Meeting Individualized Needs box on page 642)
- Poverty, homelessness, inadequate food storage and preparation facilities
- Functional health problems that limit mobility or vision
- History of weight loss of more than 20% of usual weight

BOX 22–3 Conditions Associated with Malnutrition

■ Acute respiratory failure	■ Eating disorders
■ Aging	■ Gastrointestinal disorders
■ AIDS	■ Neurologic disorders
■ Alcoholism	■ Renal disease
■ Burns	■ Short bowel syndrome
■ COPD	■ Surgery
■ Dementia	■ Trauma

- Oral or gastrointestinal problems that affect food intake, digestion, and absorption
- Inability to eat for 5 or more days
- Chronic pain or chronic diseases such as pulmonary, cardiovascular, renal, or endocrine disorders, or cancer
- Dementia, mental health disorders
- Medications or treatments that affect appetite
- Alcohol or drug addition
- Acute problems such as infection, surgery, or trauma

Pathophysiology

Carbohydrates and fats in the diet are the body's primary energy source. Approximately 15% to 25% of the body is fat, the body's energy reservoir. The remainder (muscles, bones, other body tissues and organs) is lean body mass, metabolically active tissue. Proteins in the diet primarily are used to maintain this tissue. Glycogen and proteins in this lean body mass also act as energy stores.

When dietary intake of nutrients does not meet the body's energy needs, the body uses glycogen, body proteins, and lipids (fats) to support metabolism. In **starvation** (inadequate dietary intake), glycogen initially is used to provide energy. After the first 24 hours of starvation, gluconeogenesis (formation of glucose from proteins) is the major source of energy. As starvation continues, the body breaks down fats into free fatty acids and ketones, which provide energy for the brain. The size of all body compartments is reduced as body fats and muscle proteins are used to meet energy needs. As lean body mass is reduced, metabolically active tissue is lost, and energy expenditure decreases.

The stress of acute illness or trauma produces a different response. The acute stress response produces a state of hypermetabolism and **catabolism** (cell and tissue breakdown). This hypermetabolic state increases energy expenditure and nutrient needs. Lean body mass is broken down to meet these needs. If untreated, up to half of the body's protein stores can be used within 3 weeks.

Many hospitalized clients are malnourished (starved) on admission. Surgery or illness promote a stress response, resulting in **protein-calorie malnutrition (PCM)**. In PCM, both protein and calories are deficient. Chronic protein deficiency with adequate calories to meet energy needs is called *kwashiorkor*. When both proteins and calories are insufficient to meet the body's needs, PCM is known as *marasmus*.

Manifestations

The manifestations of malnutrition may vary among clients. Weight loss is the most apparent manifestation of malnutrition. The malnourished client may have a body weight of less than 90% of ideal. Body mass also is reduced (see Box 22–1), as is skinfold thickness. Other manifestations include a wasted appearance, dry and brittle hair, and pale mucous membranes. Peripheral or abdominal edema may be present. Older adults may present with general symptoms of frailty, including weakness, slow walking speed, low physical activity level, unintentional weight loss, and exhaustion (DiMaria-Ghalili & Amella, 2005). Manifestations of specific nutrient deficiencies may be present (see box on page 642). See page 643 for the *Multisystem Effects of Malnutrition*.

MEETING INDIVIDUALIZED NEEDS Nutrition for the Older Adult

Older adults are at greater risk for malnutrition. Age-related changes that contribute to this problem include changes in taste and smell, a higher incidence of gastrointestinal disease, poor oral health, loss of teeth or ill-fitting dentures, anorexia caused by medications, and functional limitations that impair the ability to shop and cook. Psychosocial issues also contribute to the problem. Older adults living on fixed incomes, many at the poverty level, may not be able to afford well-balanced meals. Loss of appetite is a problem commonly seen with depression. Social isolation and loneliness contribute to the problem. Eating is a social event, and older adults who eat alone may not eat as well as those who share meals with companions, and may consume too few, or too many, calories.

Conduct a thorough assessment to determine nutritional status. Assess psychologic factors that influence eating habits, such as loneliness, isolation, and depression. Note the client's general appearance and obtain a diet history, including information about foods and nutrients the client consumes, and recent weight loss or gain. Review laboratory values, including complete blood count, total protein, and albumin.

TEACHING FOR HOME CARE

To maintain nutritional status, the older client should be advised to:

- Eat a well-balanced diet.
- Eat fresh fruits and vegetables.
- Shop wisely to get the most value for the money.
- Avoid processed foods.
- Avoid foods high in fat.
- Drink adequate fluids.
- Exercise regularly.
- Contact local agencies for the availability of congregate meals (e.g., at local senior centers) or home-delivered meals (e.g., Meals-on-Wheels).

Subcutaneous fat and muscle proteins are broken down in PCM, impairing mobility and increasing the risk for skin and tissue breakdown (pressure ulcers). Protein synthesis is inhibited and wound healing delayed. Serum albumin levels fall, leading to abdominal edema, diarrhea, and impaired nutrient absorption. Immune function is impaired, increasing the risk of infection. Cardiac output falls, and the risk for postural hypotension increases.

INTERDISCIPLINARY CARE

The goal of treatment for the malnourished client is to restore ideal body weight while replacing and restoring depleted nutrients and minerals. The client's age, severity of malnutrition, and coexisting health problems help determine interventions. Treatment may include oral supplementation, tube feedings, or total parenteral nutrition.

Diagnosis

A nutrition screening tool such as the one in Box 22–4 can help identify clients at risk for malnutrition. As with obesity, the standard measurements to assess for malnutrition include height, weight, calculation of BMI, and skinfold measurements. A BMI of less than 18 to 20 kg/m² may indicate malnutrition. The following laboratory studies also may be ordered:

- *Serum albumin* is reduced in PCM, and may be below 3.0 g/dL.
- *Prealbumin* (also known as *transthyretin*) should be measured for any client at risk for malnutrition and anyone with a serum albumin of less than 2.8 g/dL. Prealbumin, which has a short (2-day) half-life, is a better measure of nutritional status than albumin because it is sensitive to acute changes in nutritional status and less influenced by liver disease (Kuszajewski & Clontz, 2005). See Table 22–7 for normal prealbumin levels and the implications of reduced prealbumin levels.
- The *total lymphocyte count* is evaluated by multiplying the WBC by the percentage of lymphocytes. The total lymphocyte count is reduced in PCM.

MANIFESTATIONS of Specific Nutrient Deficiencies

DEFICIENCY	ASSESSMENT DATA
Calorie	Weight loss Weakness, listlessness Loss of subcutaneous fat Muscle wasting
Protein	Thin or sparse hair Flaking skin Hepatomegaly
Vitamin A	Night blindness Altered taste and smell Dry, scaling, rough skin
Thiamine	Confusion, apathy Cardiomegaly, dyspnea Muscle cramping and wasting Paresthesias, neuropathy Ataxia
Riboflavin	Cheilosis, stomatitis Neuropathy, glossitis
Vitamin C	Swollen, bleeding gums Delayed wound healing Weakness, depression Easy bruising
Iron	Smooth tongue Listlessness, fatigue Dyspnea

- *Serum electrolytes* are measured. Potassium levels are low in severe malnutrition.

The following specialized procedures to evaluate the extent of malnutrition may be ordered:

- *Bioelectric impedance analysis* measures body fat and total body water. Differences in the conductivity of a weak current

MULTISYSTEM EFFECTS OF **Malnutrition**

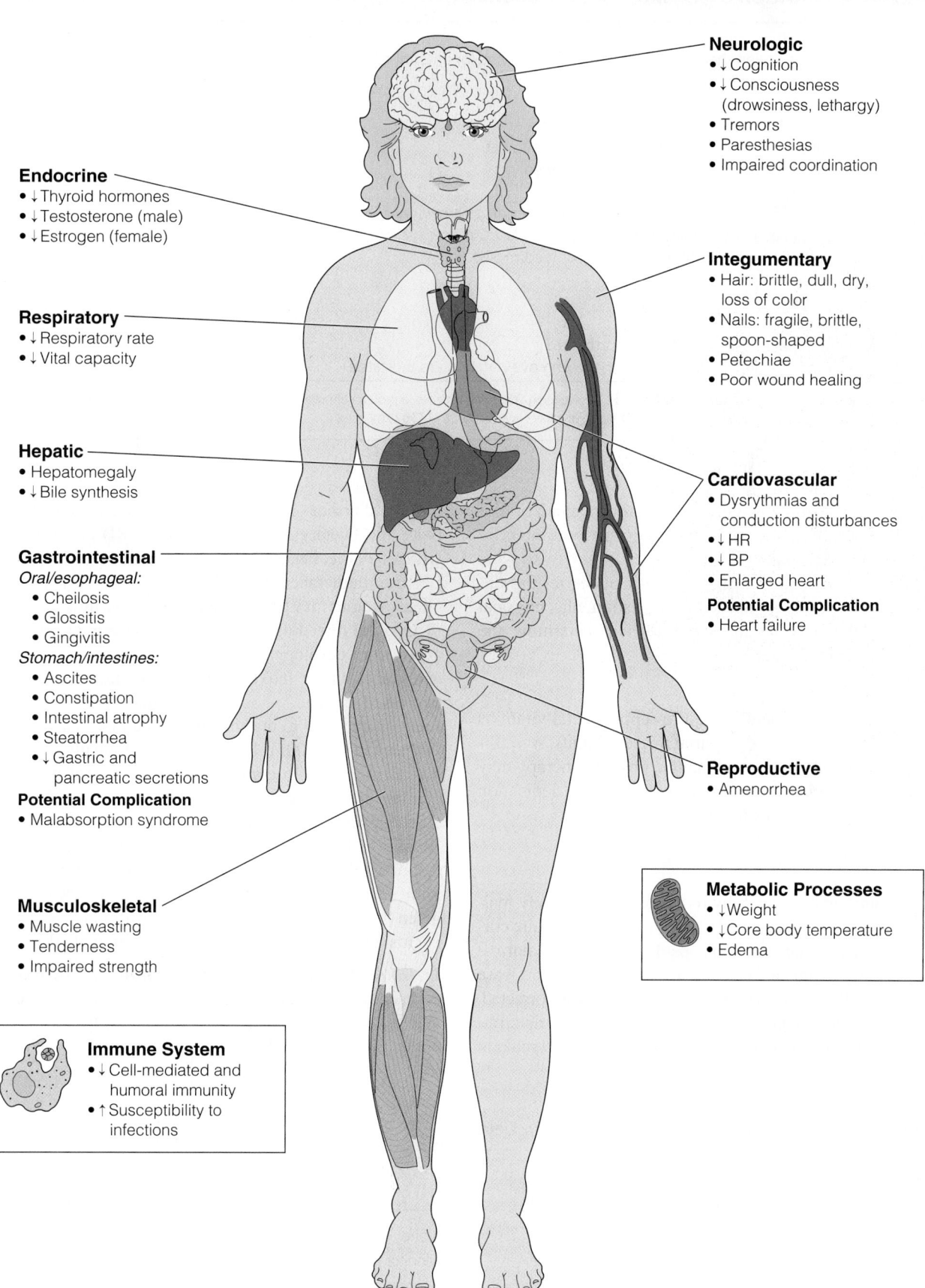

Neurologic
- ↓ Cognition
- ↓ Consciousness (drowsiness, lethargy)
- Tremors
- Paresthesias
- Impaired coordination

Endocrine
- ↓ Thyroid hormones
- ↓ Testosterone (male)
- ↓ Estrogen (female)

Respiratory
- ↓ Respiratory rate
- ↓ Vital capacity

Hepatic
- Hepatomegaly
- ↓ Bile synthesis

Gastrointestinal
Oral/esophageal:
- Cheilosis
- Glossitis
- Gingivitis
Stomach/intestines:
- Ascites
- Constipation
- Intestinal atrophy
- Steatorrhea
- ↓ Gastric and pancreatic secretions

Potential Complication
- Malabsorption syndrome

Musculoskeletal
- Muscle wasting
- Tenderness
- Impaired strength

Integumentary
- Hair: brittle, dull, dry, loss of color
- Nails: fragile, brittle, spoon-shaped
- Petechiae
- Poor wound healing

Cardiovascular
- Dysrythmias and conduction disturbances
- ↓ HR
- ↓ BP
- Enlarged heart

Potential Complication
- Heart failure

Reproductive
- Amenorrhea

Metabolic Processes
- ↓ Weight
- ↓ Core body temperature
- Edema

Immune System
- ↓ Cell-mediated and humoral immunity
- ↑ Susceptibility to infections

BOX 22–4 A Nutrition Screening Tool for Clients

	Yes (points)
■ I have an illness or condition that made me change the kind and/or amount of food I eat.	2
■ I eat fewer than two meals per day.	3
■ I eat few fruits or vegetable or milk products.	2
■ I have three or more drinks of beer, liquor, or wine almost every day.	2
■ I have tooth or mouth problems that make it hard for me to eat.	2
■ I don't always have enough money to buy the food I need.	4
■ I eat alone most of the time.	1
■ I take three or more different prescribed or over-the-counter drugs a day.	1
■ Without wanting to, I have lost or gained 10 pounds in the last 6 months.	2
■ I am not always physically able to shop, cook, and/or feed myself.	2
TOTAL	

If the total score is:

0–2   Minimal nutritional risk

3–5   Moderate nutritional risk; recheck in 3 months

6 or more   High nutritional risk; interventions to improve nutrition are indicated

Source: Adapted from *Determine Your Nutritional Health,* by The Nutrition Screening Initiative, a product of American Academy of Family Physicians, The American Dietetic Association, and The National Council on the Aging, Inc. Available at http://www.aafp.org/x17367.xml

(measured between the hands and feet) allow calculation of body fat and water (current flows more slowly through fat tissue than through water).

- *Total daily energy expenditure* (which includes resting energy expenditure, energy needed for digestion, plus physical activity needs) may be measured to help determine the client's calorie intake needs.

Medications

Malnourished clients generally require supplemental vitamins and minerals to restore these essential micronutrients. A multivitamin and mineral supplement may be given, or therapy may be tailored to correct specific deficiencies. See the Medication Administration box on page 645 for nursing implications of vitamin and mineral supplements.

Nutrition

Fluids and nutrients are carefully reintroduced in severely malnourished clients. First, fluid and electrolyte imbalances are corrected, with particular attention paid to restoring normal potassium, magnesium, and calcium levels, as well as acid–base balance. Once fluid and electrolyte imbalances are corrected, protein and calories are gradually reintroduced into the diet. Initial feedings are limited amounts (100 mL) of liquid formula to

prevent diarrhea. Vitamin and mineral supplements at about twice the Dietary Reference Intake (DRI) are provided along with refeeding. Fat and lactose are reintroduced into the diet last. Lactose intolerance may develop in severely malnourished clients; yogurt may be tolerated better than a milk-based formula.

Gradual refeeding is necessary to prevent electrolyte imbalances from developing as potassium, magnesium, phosphorus, and glucose move into the cells. Heart failure may occur due to depressed cardiac function. Abnormalities in gastrointestinal function can lead to malabsorption and diarrhea with refeeding (Tierney et al., 2005). Food intake is gradually increased until the client is able to consume about 5000 kcal per day, and is gaining 3 to 5 pounds (1.5 to 2.0 kg) weekly. Commercially available nutritional supplements (such as Carnation Instant Breakfast, Ensure, and Sustacal) may supplement protein and calorie intake. Administering 2 ounces of nutritional supplement with each medication given (unless the medication must be given on an empty stomach) may be an effective way to increase clients' calorie and protein intake (Bender et al., 2000).

ENTERAL NUTRITION **Enteral nutrition**, or tube feeding, may be used to meet calorie and protein requirements in clients unable to consume adequate food. Indications for tube feedings include difficulty swallowing, unresponsiveness, oral or neck

TABLE 22–7 Normal and High Risk Prealbumin Levels

PREALBUMIN LEVEL	IMPLICATIONS	SUGGESTED INTERVENTIONS
15–35 mg/dL	Within normal limits	None
11–14.9 mg/dL	High risk for nutritional deficit	Monitor level biweekly
5–10.9 mg/dL	Significant risk for malnutrition	Aggressive nutritional support (e.g., enteral feedings or total parenteral
≤5mg/dL	Malnourished	nutrition)

MEDICATION ADMINISTRATION Vitamin and Mineral Supplements

FAT-SOLUBLE VITAMINS
Vitamin A
Vitamin D
Vitamin E
Vitamin K
The fat-soluble vitamins are absorbed in the gastrointestinal tract. Vitamins A and D are stored in the liver.

All fat-soluble vitamins may become toxic if taken in excess amounts.

Nursing Responsibilities
- Monitor for manifestations of vitamin excess as well as for adverse effects from vitamin administration.
- Monitor carefully for hypersensitivity reactions during the parenteral administration. Have emergency equipment available.
- Administer vitamin A with food.
- Do not administer vitamin K intravenously.

Health Education for the Client and Family
- Teach the importance of eating a well-balanced diet. If indicated, provide lists of foods high in specific vitamins.
- Caution that excessive intake of these vitamins may lead to vitamin toxicity.

WATER-SOLUBLE VITAMINS
Vitamin C (ascorbic acid)
Vitamin B complex:
    Thiamine (B₁)
    Riboflavin (B₂)
    Niacin (nicotinic acid)
    Pyridoxine hydrochloride (B₆)
    Pantothenic acid
    Biotin
These vitamins are used to prevent or treat deficiency problems. If the diet is deficient in one vitamin, it is usually deficient in other vitamins as well; therefore, multivitamin preparations are often

administered. Most of these vitamins are well absorbed from the gastrointestinal tract.

Nursing Responsibilities
- Monitor for responses to replacement therapy.
- Monitor for hypersensitivity reactions from parenteral administration. Have emergency equipment available.

Health Education for the Client and Family
- Do not exceed the recommended daily allowances for the specific vitamin.

MINERALS

Sodium	**Copper**	**Manganese**
Potassium	**Fluoride**	**Chromium**
Magnesium	**Iodine**	**Selenium**
Calcium	**Zinc**	

Minerals are inorganic chemicals that are vital to a variety of physiologic functions. Also called trace elements, these minerals are part of a balanced diet. Recommended daily intakes have not been established for all mineral substances. The dosage of prescribed minerals depends on the specific deficiency, route of administration, and the client's general health.

Nursing Responsibilities
- Monitor for manifestations of mineral imbalance.
- Prior to administration, dilute oral mineral preparations.
- Prior to the administration, of iodine, assess for history of hypersensitivity to iodine or seafood; if hypersensitive notify the physician.

Health Education for the Client and Family
- Encourage the client to avoid exceeding the known recommended daily intake of the mineral.
- Instruct the client to take minerals other than fluoride and zinc with or after meals.

---

surgery or trauma, anorexia, or serious illness. Tube feedings may provide part or all of a client's nutritional needs. Recent evidence supports using the enteral route for nutritional support whenever possible. Enteral feedings provide nutrients directly to the gut and other digestive organs, reduce the incidence of enteric pathogens, promote blood flow to the gut, and support other functions of the GI tract such as the release of hormones and epidermal growth factor (Kasper et al., 2005).

Tube feedings are usually administered through a soft, small-caliber nasogastric or nasoduodenal tube with a weighted mercury tip (Figure 22–2 ■). They also can be administered through a gastrostomy or jejunostomy tube. Small-bore feeding tubes are easily displaced; appropriate tube placement should be periodically checked by aspirating the tube and checking the pH of aspirated contents. A pH of < 4 indicates placement in the stomach; pH > 6 indicates the tube is in the jejunum. See Box 22–5 and the Nursing Research box on page 647.

Most tube feeding formulas provide 1 kcal/mL with approximately 14% of the calories from protein, 60% from carbohydrates, and 25% to 30% from fat. Administering 1500 mL per day provides the recommended daily intake of all vitamins

Figure 22–2 ■ A nasoduodenal tube and a jejunostomy tube.
Courtesy of Michal Heron/Pearson Education/PH College

and minerals. Formulas that provide more calories per milliliter, more grams of protein, added fiber, or lower fat also are available (Table 22–8). Commercial products provide instructions for initiating therapy. Enteral feedings may initially be

BOX 22–5 Measures to Verify Feeding Tube Placement

After inserting the feeding tube and verifying appropriate placement through pH of the aspirate and an x-ray, mark the feeding tube position with indelible marker. Prior to each feeding (or every 8 to 12 hours if continuous feedings are being administered), assess the abdomen and tube placement. Use the following steps to assess tube placement:

■ Assess the abdomen for distention, bowel sounds, and tenderness using the sequence of inspection, auscultation, percussion, and palpation.

■ Assess tube condition and placement by verifying that the indelible mark remains at the same position. Ask the client to open the mouth, and inspect the position of the tube in the oropharynx. Do not administer a feeding if the client is having difficulty speaking or is coughing.

■ Using a 60-mL syringe, inject 30 mL of air into the feeding tube, then aspirate a small amount of stomach contents and check the pH of the aspirate.

Reassess tube placement if the client vomits or retches, requires oropharyngeal suctioning, complains of discomfort or reflux into the mouth, or develops signs of respiratory distress (Best, 2005).

Figure 22–3 ■ The nurse secures the feeding tube of a client receiving a continuous enteral feeding.
Courtesy of Michal Heron/Pearson Education/PH College

ach. To avoid aspiration, the nurse elevates the head of the bed at least 30 degrees during feeding and for at least 1 hour after feeding. Dual-lumen tubes that allow gastric suction with simultaneous instillation of an enteral feeding into the jejunum also reduce the risk for aspiration. Formulas that contain fiber can reduce the incidence of diarrhea. Fluid and electrolyte status is monitored carefully, and additional water is administered as needed.

PARENTERAL NUTRITION **Total parenteral nutrition (TPN),** also known as *hyperalimentation*, is the intravenous administration of carbohydrates (high concentrations of dextrose), protein (amino acids), electrolytes, vitamins, minerals, and fat emulsions. These hypertonic solutions usually are administered through a central vein, such as the subclavian vein (Figure 22–4 ■). A peripherally inserted central catheter

started with smaller volumes to prevent diarrhea, with the volume gradually increased to provide the required calories for maintenance and healing. Formulas may be administered as a bolus feeding or as a continuous-drip feeding regulated by a feeding pump (Figure 22–3 ■).

Aspiration and diarrhea are the most common complications of enteral feedings. Continuous infusion of the formula reduces the risk of aspiration. The risk also is reduced by placing the feeding tube in the jejunum rather than the stom-

TABLE 22–8 Selected Enteral Feeding Formulas

FORMULA TYPE	CONTAINS	EXAMPLES
Complete—suitable for most clients requiring enteral feedings	■ 1 kcal/mL ■ Protein: ~14% total kcal ■ Fat: ~ 30% total kcal ■ Carbohydrate: ~ 60% total kcal ■ Recommended daily intake of all minerals and vitamins is 1500 mL/day	Compleat, Ensure, Isocal, Nutren, Isolan, Sustacal, Resource
High-calorie complete—appropriate for clients on fluid restriction	As above; provides 1.5 to 2 kcal/mL	Ensure Plus, Sustacal HC, Comply, Nutren 1.5, Resource Plus, Isocal HCN, Magnacal, TwoCal HN
Complete lactose-free, high-residue—used to prevent/treat diarrhea, constipation	As above; provides fiber	Jevity, Profiber, Nutren 1.0 with fiber, Fiberlan, Sustacal with fiber, Ultracal, Ensure with fiber, Fibersource, Accupep HPF, Reabfin, others
Disease-specific formulas:		
Renal failure	Contain essential amino acids	Amin-Aid, Travasorb Renal, Aminess
Respiratory failure	Fat: > 50% total kcal	Pulmocare, NutriVent
Liver failure with hepatic encephalopathy	High amounts of branched-chain amino acids	Hepatic-Acid II, Travasorb Hepatic

NURSING RESEARCH Evidence-Based Practice: Determining Feeding Tube Placement

The auscultatory method of determining the location for feeding tubes on initial placement and prior to initiating feeding is commonly recommended in nursing textbooks and is frequently used. The premise is that injecting a small amount of air into the tube will produce a distinctive sound if the tube is correctly located, presumably in the stomach. Sounds produced by tubes located in the esophagus, intestines, and respiratory tract are presumed to be different enough to alert the nurse to the improper location. However, based on a series of studies (Metheny et al., 1998), the auscultatory method for determining placement is not reliable. This is especially true for small-bore feeding tubes. Testing the pH level of aspirates from newly inserted feeding tubes and of tubes from clients receiving intermittent feedings can help distinguish gastric from respiratory and intestinal placement. Based on the pH of a large number of samples of aspirates from feeding tubes, a pH between 0 and 4 suggests gastric placement and a pH of 7 or greater indicates respiratory placement. As the tube advances through the stomach into the intestine, pH levels increase and the color of the aspirate changes. If placement in the small intestine is required, a confirmatory x-ray should be taken. These researchers recommend that the pH method be used rather than the auscultatory method and that protocols be updated to reflect current information.

IMPLICATIONS FOR NURSING

With the advent of small-bore nasogastric and nasointestinal feeding tubes and the increasing use of gastrostomy and jejunostomy feeding tubes, more and more clients are receiving enteral feedings. Nurses need to use alternative methods to auscultation to determine correct initial and continued placement of these tubes. Aspiration of contents and pH testing is more effective for determining tube placement.

CRITICAL THINKING IN CLIENT CARE

1. This study investigated differences in auscultatory sounds through small-lumen feeding tubes. Would the sound be more noticeably different with the larger bore tubes used for gastric lavage and drainage?
2. What other methods for determining tube placement are recommended in fundamentals and skills texts?
3. Compare the normal pH of aspirates obtained from the respiratory tract, esophagus, stomach, duodenum, and jejunum.
4. Develop a teaching plan for the client being discharged with a gastrostomy or jejunostomy feeding tube.

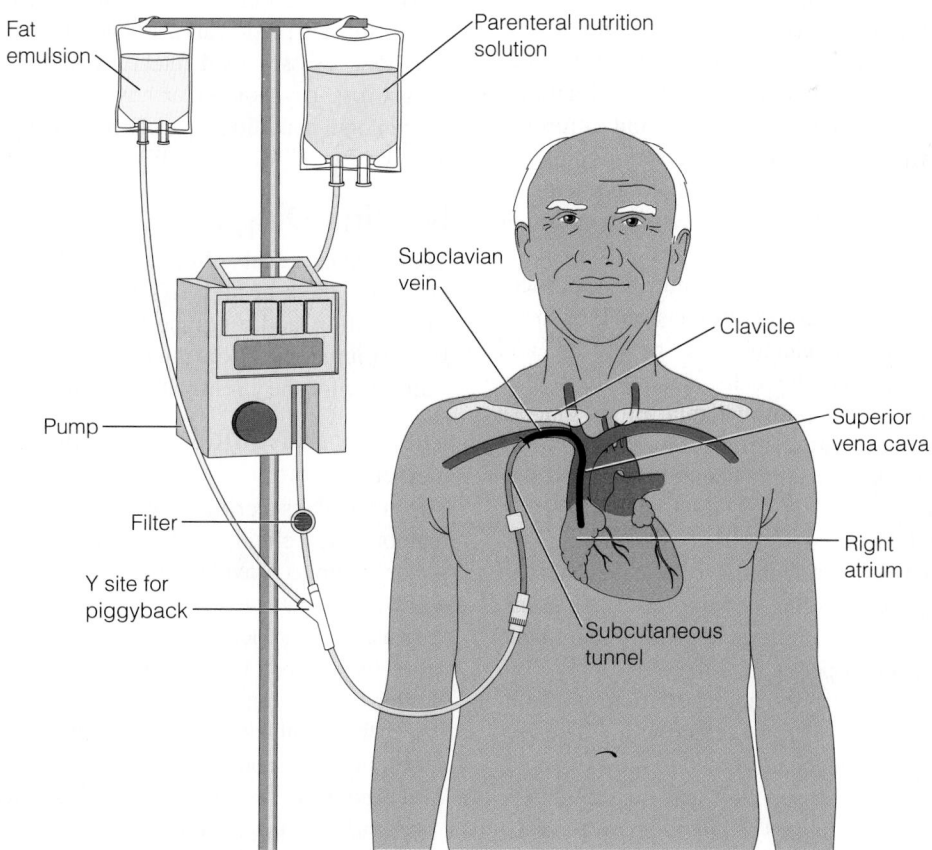

Figure 22–4 ■ Total parenteral nutrition through a catheter in the right subclavian vein.

(PICC) line may be used for short-term TPN. *Partial parenteral nutrition* (used to support the client who is able to consume some nutrients or in conjunction with enteral feeding) may be given through a peripheral vein.

TPN is initiated when a client's nutritional requirements cannot be met through diet, enteral feedings, or peripheral vein infusions. Clients who have undergone major surgery or trauma or are seriously undernourished are often candidates for TPN. TPN is used for both short- and long-term management of nutritional deficiencies, and many clients are discharged to home with TPN and monitored by home health nurses.

To begin therapy, the physician inserts the central venous catheter under aseptic conditions. The location of the catheter tip is confirmed by x-ray. A triple-lumen catheter is most commonly used. This type of catheter permits administration of medications, intralipids, or blood through other lumens. Parenteral nutrition solutions are mixed in the pharmacy using sterile technique under a laminar-flow-air hood. A commonly used solution includes 500 mL of 50% dextrose, 500 mL of an 8.5% amino acid solution, electrolytes, minerals, and vitamins. The sterility of the solution is maintained, and no medication, other than intralipids, is added to the solution after it is mixed or to the lumen through which the TPN is being administered. Most hospitals have specific policies and procedures for changing the tubing and the dressing at the insertion site as well as for hanging new containers. TPN solutions are always administered with an infusion pump to ensure the correct rate of infusion.

The client receiving parenteral nutrition is at risk for mechanical, metabolic, and infectious complications. Pneumothorax, hemothorax, brachial plexus injury, and improper position are possible complications of central venous catheter insertion. Once in place, the catheter may dislodge, leak, or break and become an embolus. Clots also may form within or around the catheter.

Fluid overload is a risk with parenteral nutrition, particularly in older adults. The high-glucose formulas can lead to osmotic diuresis or shifts of electrolytes, potassium and phosphorus in particular, into the cells, leading to hyperglycemia, hypokalemia, or hypophosphatemia. Blood glucose and serum electrolyte levels are carefully monitored during treatment. In addition to electrolyte imbalances, acid–base disturbances may develop, as well as refeeding edema or heart failure (Kasper et al., 2005). Long-term use of parenteral nutrition can lead to gallstone formation and liver disease. Nutrient deficiencies may develop, including deficiencies of vitamins, iron, and other minerals when parenteral nutrition is continued for three or more months (Kasper et al., 2005).

Disruption of the skin barrier and administration of a solution high in glucose presents a risk for infection in clients receiving TPN. Infection may be local, limited to the exit site or surrounding a tunneled catheter, or may lead to sepsis. The temperature and other manifestations of infection are carefully monitored. Meticulous sterile technique is used for site and catheter care and bag and tubing changes.

 NURSING CARE

Health Promotion

Aggressive nursing assessment and interventions can help prevent malnutrition associated with hospitalization or long-term care. In hospitalized clients, carefully monitor food intake. When the client is placed on NPO status for surgery or tests, ask the care provider to restore diet orders as soon as possible. If allowed, encourage family members to provide favorite foods to promote intake. In long-term care settings, promote socialization during meals. Assess food likes and dislikes for clients, and provide foods they are likely to eat.

Assessment

Collect nutritional assessment data on admission and periodically (once or twice a week) during long-term institutionalization.

- *Health history:* Usual daily dietary pattern (type and amount of foods consumed); usual weight and recent changes; appetite and food tolerance; specific food likes and dislikes; difficulty swallowing; problems such as anorexia, nausea, diarrhea, or constipation; history of surgery and/or chronic diseases (e.g., chronic lung disease) and medications.
- *Physical examination:* Height, weight, skinfold thickness, BMI; vital signs; general appearance, muscle wasting, mobility; skin and mucous membranes; bowel sounds; laboratory studies.

Use of a nutritional assessment tool can help identify clients (older adults in particular) at risk for malnutrition (see Box 22–4). This tool assesses food intake, mobility, and BMI, as well as weight loss, psychologic or physiologic stress, and dementia or psychologic conditions to determine the presence of or risk for malnutrition (DiMaria-Ghalili & Amella, 2005).

Nursing Diagnoses and Interventions

The complex effects of malnutrition on multiple body systems place the client at high risk for a number of other problems. This section addresses problems with nutrition, infections, fluid volume, and skin integrity. See page 649 for a Nursing Care Plan for the client with malnutrition.

Imbalanced Nutrition: Less than Body Requirements

The nurse plays a critical role in the ongoing assessment of the malnourished client, while collaborating with the multidisciplinary team to provide nutritional therapies.

- If the client is able to eat, provide an environment and nursing measures that encourage eating. Eliminate foul odors, provide oral hygiene before and after meals, make meals appetizing, and offer frequent, small meals including preferred foods. Consult with the nutrition support team to provide adequate protein, calories, minerals, and vitamins. *Oral hygiene and a pleasant environment make food more appetizing. Small, frequent meals are generally more appealing and less overwhelming to a client with anorexia. Many clients require complicated nutritional therapy such as enteral or parenteral therapy to meet nutritional needs.*

NURSING CARE PLAN   A Client with Malnutrition

Rose Chow is an 88-year-old widow who lives alone. She typically rises early and has a cup of tea before spending her morning puttering in her garden. She consumes her main meal of the day at lunch, which usually includes rice and some vegetables. For dinner, she generally eats a bowl of rice with "whatever seems to be in the refrigerator." She admits to little interest in cooking or eating since her husband died 10 years ago and her group of friends has been "dying off too."

ASSESSMENT

Mrs. Chow weighs 95 lb (43.1 kg) and is 5'3" (160 cm) tall, for a BMI of 16.8. She reports weighing 118 lb (53.5 kg) 5 years ago. Her triceps skinfold thickness measurement is 11 mm (normal values for a female: >13 mm). Her skin is pale, and she appears thin and wasted. Her temperature is 97°F (36.1°C). Diagnostic test results include serum albumin 2.9 g/dL (normal 3.4 to 4.8 g/dL) and serum cholesterol 130 mg/dL (normal 150 to 200 mg/dL). A diagnosis of protein-calorie malnutrition is made, and a 1500-calorie per day diet is recommended.

DIAGNOSES

- *Imbalanced Nutrition: Less than Body Requirements* related to lack of knowledge and inadequate food intake
- *Risk for Infection* related to protein-calorie malnutrition
- *Impaired Social Interaction* related to widowhood and reduced social support group

EXPECTED OUTCOMES

- Gain at least 1 pound per week.
- Verbalize understanding of nutritional requirements and identify strategies to incorporate requirements into daily diet after discharge.
- Remain infection free, evidenced by normal vital signs.

- Identify strategies to increase social interaction, such as participating in senior citizens' lunches at local senior center.

PLANNING AND IMPLEMENTATION

- Weigh weekly at a consistent time of day.
- Refer to dietitian for evaluation of nutritional needs.
- Teach about nutritional requirements, and plan an eating program that includes high-calorie, high-protein foods and supplements and reflects her food preferences. Encourage small, frequent meals.
- Encourage to keep a food intake diary.
- Teach strategies to reduce risks for infection.
- Provide information about communal meals available to seniors in the community, and help Mrs. Chow develop a plan to participate.

EVALUATION

One month later, Mrs. Chow has gained 3 pounds and reports feeling "more energetic." A friend is helping her shop to ensure that she purchases foods to maintain her protein, calorie, and nutrient intake. She has begun attending senior lunches twice a week, and is enjoying "being around people again." Although she still doesn't enjoy cooking like she used to, she is using prepared foods and supplements to maintain her nutrient intake.

CRITICAL THINKING IN THE NURSING PROCESS

1. What is the physiologic basis for Mrs. Chow's low albumin and cholesterol levels?
2. Mrs. Chow asks, "Can I get better by just taking more vitamins?" How will you respond?
3. Design a teaching plan for a Hispanic client with protein-calorie malnutrition.
   See Evaluating Your Response in Appendix C.

- Provide a rest period before and after meals. *Eating requires energy, and the malnourished client may have decreased physical strength and energy.*
- Assess knowledge and provide appropriate teaching. *Lack of knowledge often contributes to undernutrition. Education empowers the client to make healthy choices.*

Risk for Infection

Malnourished clients have a much higher risk for infection than well-nourished people. Malnutrition affects many components of the immune system, including the skin, mucous membranes, and lymph tissue and cells.

- Monitor temperature and assess for manifestations of infection every 4 hours. *Although the baseline temperature may be subnormal in malnourished clients, any elevation from baseline may indicate infection. Manifestations of infection may include chills, malaise, erythema, and leukocytosis. Early detection of infection may prevent complications.*
- Maintain medical asepsis when providing care and surgical asepsis when carrying out procedures. *Hand washing is the best strategy to prevent the spread of pathogens. Sterile tech-*

nique is required for procedures such as inserting central lines and changing dressings.
- Teach the signs and symptoms of infection, good hand washing technique, and factors that increase the risk for infection. *Knowledge empowers the client to participate in self-care, thus reducing exposure to infectious pathogens.*

Risk for Deficient Fluid Volume

The client with malnutrition may also have a fluid volume deficit. Difficulty swallowing food and fluids or administration of hyperosmolar nutritional solutions may lead to dehydration or electrolyte disturbances.

- Monitor oral mucous membranes, urine specific gravity, level of consciousness, and laboratory findings every 4 to 8 hours. *Dry mucous membranes, increased urine specific gravity, decreased level of consciousness, and electrolyte imbalances may indicate dehydration.*
- Weigh daily and monitor intake and output. *Daily weights and intake and output measurements help monitor fluid balance.*
- If allowed, offer fluids frequently in small amounts, considering the client's preferences. *Frequent, small amounts of fluids are better tolerated and promote adequate intake.*

Risk for Impaired Skin Integrity

Skin integrity depends on adequate nutrition. Loss of subcutaneous tissue and muscle increase the risk of pressure ulcers. In addition, healing is impaired in malnourished clients.

- Assess skin every 4 hours. *Baseline and ongoing assessments allow prompt identification of early manifestations of skin breakdown.*
- Turn and position at least every 2 hours. Encourage passive and active range-of-motion exercises. *These measures reduce pressure and promote oxygenation of cells.*
- Keep skin dry and clean, and minimize shearing forces. Keep linens smooth, clean, and dry. Provide therapeutic beds, mattresses, or pads. *These nursing measures promote comfort and reduce the risk of skin breakdown.*

Using NANDA, NIC, and NOC

Chart 22–2 shows links between NANDA nursing diagnoses, NIC, and NOC for the client with malnutrition.

Community-Based Care

Clients with malnutrition may be cared for at home or in the hospital with diet, enteral, or parenteral therapy. Each year, it is more common to see clients managing tube feeding or TPN at home. Teaching for the client and family includes the following topics:

- Diet recommendations and use of nutritional supplements
- Where to obtain recommended foods and nutritional supplements

---

NANDA, NIC, AND NOC LINKAGES
CHART 22–2 The Client with Malnutrition

NANDA

Imbalanced Nutrition: Less than Body Requirements

↓

NIC

Weight Gain Assistance

Fluid Monitoring

Nutrition Therapy

Infection Protection

↓

NOC

Nutritional Status

Nutritional Status: Nutrient Intake

Immune Status

Data from *NANDA's Nursing Diagnoses: Definitions & Classification 2005–2006* by NANDA International (2005), Philadelphia; *Nursing Interventions Classification (NIC)* (4th ed.) by J. M. Dochterman & G. M. Bulechek (2004), St. Louis, MO: Mosby; and *Nursing Outcomes Classification (NOC)* (3rd ed.) by S. Moorhead, M. Johnson, and M. Maas (2004), St. Louis, MO: Mosby.

- If continuing enteral or parenteral nutrition, how to (1) prepare and/or handle solutions, (2) add them to either the feeding tube or central line, (3) manage infusion pumps, (4) care for the feeding tube or central catheter, (5) recognize and manage problems and complications, and (6) how and when to notify the healthcare provider of problems.

THE CLIENT WITH AN EATING DISORDER

Eating disorders are characterized by severely disturbed eating behavior and weight management. Eating disorders are more common in affluent societies where food is plentiful. Women are much more commonly affected than men. **Anorexia nervosa** is characterized by a body weight less than 85% of expected for age and height and an intense fear of gaining weight or of loss of control over food intake. Anorexia nervosa affects about 0.5% to 3.7% of women in the United States at some time in their lives (NIH, 2001). **Bulimia nervosa**, which affects 1% to 4% of women in the United States, is characterized by recurring episodes of binge eating followed by purge behaviors such as self-induced vomiting, use of laxatives or diuretics, fasting, or excessive exercise. A third eating disorder, **binge-eating disorder**, is believed to affect many more people than either anorexia or bulimia. Binge-eating disorder is characterized by recurrent episodes of binge eating—eating an excessive amount of food during a defined period of time and a sense of lack of control over eating during binge episodes (NIH, 2001).

Anorexia Nervosa

Anorexia nervosa typically begins during adolescence. Clients with anorexia nervosa have a distorted body image and irrational fear of gaining weight. Refusal to maintain body weight at or above a minimally normal level for height and body type is a common manifestation of anorexia nervosa. Clients maintain weight loss by restricted calorie intake, often accompanied by excessive exercise. Some may exhibit binge–purge behavior. Although its cause is unknown, a number of risk factors, both biologic and psychosocial, have been identified for anorexia nervosa. Abnormal levels of neurotransmitters and other hormones may play a role. Current research suggests genetic factors in the development of eating disorders as well (National Eating Disorders Association, 2004). Women who develop anorexia nervosa tend to be obsessive and perfectionistic, and often feel inadequate or unable to maintain control in their lives. Family, social, or occupational (e.g., a career in modeling or ballet) pressures to maintain low body weight also contribute. Clients with anorexia often experience depression or anxiety.

The manifestations and complications of anorexia nervosa are listed in the box on page 651. Clients who engage in binge–purge behavior have a higher risk for complications.

Bulimia Nervosa

Bulimia nervosa develops in late adolescence or early adulthood, often following failed attempts to lose weight through dieting. Some studies suggest that bulimia may affect as many as

MANIFESTATIONS AND COMPLICATIONS of Eating Disorders

Disorder	Manifestations	Complications
Anorexia Nervosa	■ Weight < 85% of normal, muscle wasting ■ Fear of weight gain, refusal to eat ■ Disturbed body image, excessive exercise ■ Amenorrhea ■ Skin and hair changes ■ Hypotension, bradycardia ■ Hypothermia ■ Constipation ■ Insomnia	■ Electrolyte and acid–base disturbances ■ Reduced cardiac muscle mass, low cardiac output, dysrhythmias ■ Anemia ■ Hypoglycemia, elevated serum uric acid levels ■ Osteoporosis ■ Enlarged salivary glands ■ Delayed gastric emptying ■ Abnormal liver function
Bulimia Nervosa	■ Weight often normal; may be slightly overweight ■ Binge–purge behavior ■ Oligomenorrhea or amenorrhea ■ Lacerations of palate; callous on fingers or dorsum of hand	■ Enlarged salivary glands ■ Stomatitis, loss of dental enamel ■ Fluid, electrolyte, and acid–base imbalances ■ Dysrhythmias ■ Esophageal tears, stomach rupture
Binge-Eating Disorder	■ Usually overweight or obese ■ Recurrent episodes of binge eating (2 or more days a week for 6 months) ■ Episodes characterized by: 　■ Eating more rapidly than usual 　■ Eating until uncomfortably full 　■ Eating large amounts of food when not physically hungry 　■ Eating alone due to embarrassment over quantity 　■ Disgust, depression, or guilt following a binge episode ■ Marked distress about binging behavior	■ Type 2 diabetes ■ Hypertension, hyperlipidemia ■ Coronary heart disease, heart failure ■ Gallbladder disease ■ Depression, social isolation

19% of college-age women (Tierney et al., 2005). The client with bulimia typically reports binge eating followed by purging 5 to 10 times per week (Kasper et al., 2005). Foods consumed during a binge often are high calorie, high fat, and sweet. After binge eating, the client induces vomiting (usually by stimulating the gag reflex), or may take excessive quantities of laxatives or diuretics. In contrast to anorexia, the client's weight often is normal. Fluid and electrolyte balance, in contrast, may be severely disrupted by loss of fluid and gastrointestinal secretions. The complications of bulimia nervosa (see the box above) primarily result from the purging behavior.

Binge-Eating Disorder

Binge-eating disorder (BED) was identified as a distinct condition in 1992 (Eating Disorders Association, 2004). While many of the characteristics of bulimia and binge-eating disorder are similar, clients with BED do not purge. BED commonly affects middle-aged adults and is slightly more common in women than in men. It affects blacks and whites equally. People with BED usually are overweight or obese, often morbidly obese (NIH, 2004). The cause of BED is unknown, although genetics may play a role in its development. Psychosocial factors contribute; up to half of people with BED either are depressed or have experienced depression in the past. Alcohol abuse and impulsivity are common behavioral traits in clients with BED (NIH, 2004).

People with BED consume an excessive amount of food during binging episodes, eating even when not hungry and continuing to eat until uncomfortably full. Binging often occurs when the person is alone. After overeating, the client may feel disgusted or guilty about the amount of food consumed, and depressed about the inability to control eating.

INTERDISCIPLINARY CARE

Eating disorders, anorexia nervosa in particular, are difficult to effectively treat. Because of the intense fear of weight gain and the distorted body image of clients with anorexia, they strongly resist increasing food intake. While community-based care is appropriate for most clients with an eating disorder, complications of the disorder or resistance to treatment may necessitate hospitalization for some clients. In all cases, a comprehensive treatment plan for eating disorders includes medical care and monitoring, psychosocial interventions, and nutrition counseling (NIH, 2001).

Diagnosis

There is no specific diagnostic test for anorexia, bulimia, or binge-eating disorder. Laboratory studies in clients with anorexia or bulimia may show anemia and leukopenia on CBC, abnormal serum electrolyte levels, and elevated BUN and serum creatinine. In clients with BED, the blood glucose and lipid levels may be elevated. The BMI usually is above the normal range, and may identify the client as obese or morbidly obese.

A mental health evaluation is indicated for clients with eating disorders to identify contributing factors and help direct treatment.

Treatment

Clients with anorexia nervosa may require hospitalization, particularly if their weight is less than 75% of normal. Refeeding is gradually introduced to avoid complications such as heart failure. Meals must be supervised and a firm but empathetic attitude conveyed about the importance of adequate food intake. Intravenous feeding may be required in some cases. Psychologic treatment, initiated when malnutrition has been corrected and weight gain begun, focuses on providing emotional support during weight gain and helping clients base their self-esteem on factors other than weight (e.g., personal relationships, satisfaction with achieving occupational goals) (Kasper et al., 2005). Cognitive-behavioral or psychotherapy may be used; families may be included in the treatment program. A selective serotonin reuptake inhibitor (SSRI) such as fluoxetine (Prozac) or sertraline (Zoloft) may be prescribed to facilitate weight maintenance and reduce anxiety.

The goal of bulimia treatment is to reduce or eliminate binge eating and purging behavior. A combination of nutritional counseling and therapy, psychosocial interventions, and medications may be used. Nutritional counseling is directed at establishing a regular meal pattern and encouraging an appropriate amount of regular exercise. An antidepressant drug such as fluoxetine (Prozac) may benefit the client with bulimia nervosa and help prevent relapse. Cognitive-behavioral therapy also is used to treat bulimia, focusing on excessive concerns about weight, persistent dieting, and binge–purge behaviors.

Treatment for clients with binge-eating disorder focuses on establishing healthy eating patterns, psychosocial therapy (including cognitive-behavioral therapy and group counseling) to address underlying issues, and management of obesity and its complications. Clients with BED also may benefit from an SSRI or other antidepressant drug.

NURSING CARE

Nurses can be instrumental in identifying clients with eating disorders and referring them for treatment. It is particu-

larly important to identify these disorders early to prevent adverse effects on growth and increase the success of treatment.

The nurse is an integral part of the eating disorders treatment team. *Imbalanced Nutrition: Less than Body Requirements* is a primary nursing diagnosis for clients with anorexia or bulimia, and *Imbalanced Nutrition: More than Body Requirements* is a priority nursing diagnosis for clients with binge-eating disorder. The following nursing diagnoses also should be considered:

- *Ineffective Sexuality Patterns*
- *Chronic Low Self-Esteem*
- *Disturbed Body Image*
- *Ineffective Therapeutic Regimen Management: Family*
- *Powerlessness.*

When planning and implementing care, consider the following nursing activities.

- Regularly monitor weight, using standard conditions. *Weight gain or loss provides information about the effectiveness of care, as well as the client's risk for complications.*
- Monitor food intake during meals, recording percentage of meal and snack consumed. Maintain close observation for at least 1 hour following meals; do not allow client alone in bathroom. *Observing the client during and after meals helps prevent disposal of food and purging behavior after eating. Recording actual food intake allows accurate calculation of calorie intake.*
- Serve balanced meals, including all nutrient groups. Increase serving size gradually. *The client may find "normal" food servings overwhelming, reducing the desire to eat. Calorie intake is initially limited to prevent complications associated with refeeding, then gradually increased.*
- Serve frequent, small feedings of cold or room temperature foods. *Cool foods reduce sensations of early satiety, promoting greater food intake at a meal or snack.*
- Administer a multivitamin and mineral supplement to replace losses.

Clients with eating disorders require extended treatment of the disorder. Involvement of the family and social support persons is vital to success. Encourage family members to participate in teaching and nutritional counseling sessions. Discuss the value of family therapy to address issues that have contributed to the disorder. Emphasize the need to provide consistent messages of support for healthy eating habits. Discuss using rewards for food and calorie intake rather than weight gain. Provide referrals to a dietitian, nutritional support team, counseling, and support groups for people with eating disorders.

EXPLORE MediaLink

CHAPTER HIGHLIGHTS

- Nutritional disorders are common, affecting people worldwide, and contributing significantly to mortality and morbidity. While malnutrition is a serious problem in underdeveloped nations, obesity and its consequences are more prevalent in the United States and other industrialized societies.

- Obesity, defined as excess adipose tissue and a BMI greater than 30 kg/m², is linked with many disorders, including type 2 diabetes, coronary heart disease, gallbladder disease, and osteoarthritis.

- Exercise and reduced kilocalorie intake are the mainstays of obesity treatment. Drugs that suppress the appetite or interfere with fat absorption in the gut may be used to facilitate weight loss in clients with multiple risk factors for obesity complications or people who have had difficulty achieving weight loss through diet and exercise.

- Bariatric surgery is a treatment option for morbidly obese clients. The primary types of bariatric surgery used in the United States are restrictive procedures that limit stomach capacity and food consumption, and combination restrictive/malabsorptive procedures that limit both capacity and nutrient absorption.

- Nursing care for obese clients focuses on health promotion, education, and support of the prescribed treatment plan.

- In the United States, protein-calorie malnutrition is a common problem among hospitalized clients. Malnutrition increases the risk for complications and impairs healing. Early identification and prevention are the primary focuses of treatment; nurses can be instrumental in identifying at-risk clients (e.g., the elderly, clients living alone, people on extended NPO status).

- Refeeding of malnourished clients is a gradual process. Enteral feedings (oral or by feeding tube) are preferred whenever possible. Total parenteral nutrition may be required when enteral feeding is not possible or not tolerated by the client.

- Eating disorders, including anorexia nervosa, bulimia nervosa, and binge-eating disorder, can be difficult to effectively treat and maintain in remission. While clients with anorexia typically are underweight and malnourished, resisting efforts to achieve a normal weight, clients with bulimia are more likely to be of normal weight and those with binge-eating disorder to be overweight or obese.

- Treatment for eating disorders is multifaceted, including physical care to restore electrolyte balance and treat complications, nutritional counseling and therapy, psychosocial therapy, family support, and possibly medications.

TEST YOURSELF NCLEX-RN® REVIEW

1 Of the following noted in a client's history, which does the nurse identify as the greatest risk factor for obesity?
1. adopted at 2 months of age
2. usual diet includes "fast-food" lunches twice a week
3. does not engage in regular activity
4. allergic to chocolate and strawberries

2 A client on a reduced-calorie diet asks the nurse what she can do to lose weight faster, because most weeks she loses no more than 0.5 lb. "At this rate, it will take me years to get to my goal!" The most appropriate response by the nurse would be:

1. "Let's reevaluate your long-term goal. Perhaps it was set too low for you."
2. "A pound of body fat equals 3500 calories. Let's reevaluate your diet and exercise plan for calorie intake and expenditure."
3. "Perhaps we should look into a diet supplement since you are unable to stick with your prescribed diet plan."
4. "You sound frustrated. Would you like to take some time off from your diet and exercise plan?"

3 An expected finding in a client admitted with a diagnosis of protein-calorie malnutrition would be:
1. recent 5-lb weight loss.
2. increased skinfold thickness measurements.
3. hyperactive bowel sounds.
4. anxiety and agitation.

4 Before administering an intermittent enteral feeding, the nurse confirms placement of the small-bore feeding tube in the stomach by:
1. instilling water and listening for the gastric gurgle.
2. withdrawing the tube slightly, then reinserting it.
3. aspirating gastric contents and checking for a pH of <4.
4. obtaining a flat-plate x-ray of the stomach.

5 The nurse identifies which of the following as a realistic goal for a client with anorexia nervosa?
1. Will consume 100% of a 2500-calorie diet.
2. Will gain 2 pounds per week.
3. Will rest alone in room following meals.
4. Will participate in family counseling.

6 The nurse identifies which nursing diagnosis as high priority for a client with a BMI of 30.4 kg/m^2 and a waist-hip ratio of 1.1?
1. *Health-Seeking Behaviors: Weight Loss*
2. *Risk for Impaired Tissue Perfusion: Cardiovascular*
3. *Ineffective Coping*
4. *Deficient Knowledge: Diet*

7 The nurse teaching a client about sibutramine (Meridia) includes which of the following instructions? (Select all that apply.)
1. You may skip a dose of the drug if you skip a meal.
2. Do not consume alcohol while taking this drug.
3. Do not drive while taking this drug because the drug may increase sleepiness.
4. Increase your intake of water and other fluids while taking this drug.
5. Continue to follow your prescribed diet while taking this drug.

8 The nurse caring for a home-bound older adult who is losing 1 to 2 pounds monthly plans for which of the following? (Select all that apply.)
1. Meals-on-Wheels deliveries
2. Ensure nutritional supplements
3. placement in a residential care facility
4. transportation to congregate senior meals
5. follow-up by primary care physician
6. referral for diagnostic studies

9 Which of the following is a high-priority nursing intervention to prevent malnutrition in the surgical client?
1. aggressive pain management
2. daily weights
3. maintaining intravenous flow
4. requesting early restoration of oral intake

10 Three days after gastric bypass surgery, the client complains of increasing abdominal pain. Bowel sounds are absent; the abdomen is firm and very tender. The nurse should:
1. report findings to the surgeon.
2. ambulate the client to promote peristalsis.
3. chart assessment data and continue to monitor.
4. evaluate the effectiveness of analgesia.

See Test Yourself answers in Appendix C.

BIBLIOGRAPHY

American Obesity Association. (2002). AOA fact sheets. *Obesity in minority populations.* Retrieved from http://www.obesity.org/subs/fastfacts/Obesity_Minority_Pop.shtml

Barry, D. (2004). An emerging model of behavior change in women maintaining weight loss. *Nursing Science Quarterly, 17*(3), 242–252.

Bender, S., Pusateri, M., Cook, A., Ferguson, M., & Hall, J. C. (2000). Malnutrition: Role of the TwoCal® HN med pass program. *MEDSURG Nursing, 9*(6), 284–295.

Best, C. (2005). Caring for the patient with a nasogastric tube. *Nursing Standard, 20*(3), 59–65.

Candela, L., & Meiner, S. E. (2004). Vitamin B$_{12}$ deficiency: Issues in nursing care. *MEDSURG Nursing, 13*(4), 247–252.

Conner, T. M., & Carver, D. (2005). The role of gastric pH testing with small-bore feeding tubes in the intensive care unit. *Dimensions of Critical Care Nursing, 24*(5), 210–214.

Copstead, L. C., & Banasik, J. L. (2005). *Pathophysiology* (3rd ed.). St. Louis, MO: Elsevier/Saunders.

Crouch. J. (2005). Adult obesity in the United States. A call to arms. *Advance for Nurse Practitioners, 13*(1), 57–60.

DiMaria-Ghalili , R. A., & Amella, E. (2005). Nutrition in older adults. *American Journal of Nursing, 105*(3), 40–50.

Eating Disorders Association. (2004). *Binge eating and other eating disorders.* Retrieved from January 3, 2006, http://www.edauk.com/sub_what_are_binge.htm

Eberhardie, C. (2004). Assessment and management of eating skills in the older adult. *Professional Nurse, 19*(6), 318–322.

Elliot, K. (2003). Nutritional considerations after bariatric surgery. *Critical Care Nursing Quarterly, 26*(2), 133–138.

Foster, D., Parr, J., & Wright, L. (2005). Applied leadership. Tackling malnutrition. *Nursing Management, 12*(5), 28–30.

Green, S., & McDougall, T. (2002). Screening and assessing the nutritional status of older people. *Nursing Older People, 14*(6), 31–32.

Johnson, R. W., & Broadnax, P. A. (2003, May/June). A perspective on obesity. *ABNF Journal,* 69–70.

Kasper, D. L., Braunwald, E. , Fauci, A. S., Hauser, S. L., Longo, D. L., & Jameson, J. L. (Eds.). (2005). *Harrison's principles of internal medicine* (16th ed.). New York: McGraw-Hill.

Keele-Smith, R., & Leon, T. (2003). Evaluation of individually tailored interventions on exercise adherence. *Western Journal of Nursing Research, 25*(6), 623–640.

Kuszajewski, M. L., & Clontz, A. S. (2005). Eye on diagnostics. Prealbumin is best for nutritional monitoring. *Nursing, 35*(5), 70–71.

Lee, V. K. (2004). Problems with eating and nutrition: Geriatric self-learning module. *MEDSURG Nursing, 13*(6), 405–408.

Leininger, S. M. (2002). The role of nutrition in wound healing. *Critical Care Nursing Quarterly, 25*(1), 13–21.

Metheny, N. A., Dahms, T. E., Stewart, B. J., Stone, K. S., Frank, P. A., & Clouse, R. E. (2005). Verification of inefficacy of the glucose method in detecting aspiration associated with tube feedings. *MEDSURG Nursing, 14*(2), 112–121.

_____ , & Titler, M. G. (2001). Assessing placement of feeding tubes. *American Journal of Nursing, 101*(5), 36–45.

_____ , Wehrle, M., Wiersema, L., & Clark, J. (1998). pH, color, and feeding tubes. *RN, 61*(1), 25–27.

National Eating Disorders Association. (2004). *What causes eating disorders?* Retrieved January, 3, 2006, from http://www.NationalEatingDisorders.org

National Heart, Lung, and Blood Institute. (1998). *Clinical guidelines on the identification, evaluation, and treatment of overweight and obesity in adults: The evidence report* (National Institutes of Health: Publication No. 98-4083). Retrieved from http://www.nhlbi.nih.gov

_____. (2000). *The practical guide. Identification, evaluation, and treatment of overweight and obesity in adults* (NIH Publication No. 00-4084). Retrieved from http://www.nhlbi.nih.gov

National Institute for Clinical Excellence. (2004). *Quick reference guide. Eating disorders. Core interventions in the treatment and management of anorexia nervosa, bulimia nervosa and related eating disorders.* London: Author. Retrieved from http://www.nice.org.uk

National Institutes of Health. (2001). *Eating disorders. Facts about eating disorders and the search for solutions.* (NIH Publication No. 01-4901).

_____. (2004). *Statistics related to overweight and obesity.* Retrieved from http://www.niddk.nih.gov/win

North American Nursing Diagnosis Association. (2005). *NANDA nursing diagnoses: Definitions & classification 2005–2006.* Philadelphia: Author.

Orbanic, S. (2001). Understanding bulimia. *American Journal of Nursing, 101*(3), 35–41.

Padula, C. A., Kenny, A., Planchon, C., & Lamoureax, C. (2004). Enteral feedings: What the evidence says. *American Journal of Nursing, 104*(7), 62–69.

Porth, C. M. (2005). *Pathophysiology: Concepts of altered health states* (7th ed.). Philadelphia: Lippincott.

Reid, M. B., & Allard-Gould, P. (2004). Malnutrition and the critically ill elderly patient. *Critical Care Nursing Clinics of North America, 16*(4), 531–536.

Reising, D. L., & Neal, R. S. (2005). Enteral tube flushing. *American Journal of Nursing, 105*(3), 58–63.

Sabol, V. K. (2004). Nutrition assessment of the critically ill adult. *AACN Clinical Issues, 15*(4), 595–606.

Sammons, D. (2002). Roux-en-Y gastric bypass. *American Journal of Nursing, 102*(10), 24A–24D.

Shuttleworth, A. (2003). Managing obesity in children and adults. *Professional Nurse, 19*(3), 165.

Sweeney, J. (2005). Clinical queries. How do I verify NG tube placement? *Nursing, 35*(8), 25.

Tierney, L. M., McPhee, S. J., & Papadakis, M. A. (2005). *Current medical diagnosis & treatment* (44th ed.). New York: Lange Medical Books/McGraw-Hill.

Timmerman, G. M., & Gregg, E. K. (2003). Dieting, perceived deprivation, and preoccupation with food. *Western Journal of Nursing Research, 25*(4), 405–418.

Uphold, C. R., & Graham, M. V. (2003). *Clinical guidelines in adult health* (3rd ed.). Gainesville, FL: Barmarrae Books.

U.S. Preventive Services Task Force. (2003). Behavioral counseling in primary care to promote a healthy diet: Recommendations and rationale. *American Journal of Nursing, 103*(8), 81–82, 85–86, 89–90.

_____. (2004). Screening for obesity in adults: Recommendations and rationale. *American Journal of Nursing, 104*(5), 94–95, 97–98, 100.

Weight-control Information Network. (2003a). *Medical care for obese patients* (NIH Publication No. 03-5335). Bethesda, MD: National Institutes of Health.

_____. (2003b). *Very-low-calorie diets* (NIH Publication No. 03-3894). Bethesda, MD: National Institutes of Health.

_____. (2004). *Gastrointestinal surgery for severe obesity.* (NIH Publication No. 04-4006). Bethesda, MD: National Institutes of Health.

CHAPTER 23 Nursing Care of Clients with Upper Gastrointestinal Disorders

LEARNING OUTCOMES

- Describe the pathophysiology of common disorders of the mouth, esophagus, and stomach.

- Relate manifestations and diagnostic test results to the pathophysiologic processes involved in upper gastrointestinal disorders.

- Explain interdisciplinary care for clients with upper gastrointestinal disorders.

- Describe the role of the nurse in interdisciplinary care of clients with upper gastrointestinal disorders.

CLINICAL COMPETENCIES

- Assess the functional health status of clients with upper gastrointestinal disorders.

- Monitor, document, and, as needed, report manifestations of upper gastrointestinal disorders and their complications.

- Plan nursing care using evidence-based research.

- Determine priority nursing diagnoses and interventions based on assessed data.

- Administer medications and prescribed care knowledgeably and safely.

- Coordinate and integrate interdisciplinary care into plan of care.

- Construct and revise individualized plans of care considering the culture and values of the client.

- Plan and provide client and family teaching to promote, maintain, and restore functional health.

MEDIALINK

Resources for this chapter can be found on the Prentice Hall Nursing MediaLink DVD-ROM accompanying this textbook, and on the Companion Website at http://www.prenhall.com/lemone

achalasia, *668*
acute gastritis, *677*
anorexia, *677*
cachectic, *689*
chronic gastritis, *677*
Curling's ulcers, *677*
Cushing's ulcers, *677*
diffuse esophageal spasm, *668*
dumping syndrome, *689*
duodenal ulcers, *680*
dysphagia, *668*
erosive (stress-induced) gastritis, *677*
esophagojejunostomy, *689*

gastric lavage, *675*
gastric mucosal barrier, *671*
gastric outlet obstruction, *684*
gastric ulcers, *680*
gastritis, *677*
gastroduodenostomy (Billroth I), *689*
gastroesophageal reflux, *663*
gastroesophageal reflux disease (GERD), *663*
gastrojejunostomy (Billroth II), *689*
hematemesis, *674*
hematochezia, *674*
hemorrhage, *681*

hiatal hernia, *667*
melena, *674*
nausea, *671*
occult bleeding, *674*
partial gastrectomy, *689*
peptic ulcer disease (PUD), *680*
peptic ulcers, *680*
perforation, *684*
steatorrhea, *684*
stomatitis, *656*
total gastrectomy, *689*
ulcer, *680*
vomiting, *671*
Zollinger-Ellison syndrome, *684*

The upper gastrointestinal tract includes the mouth, esophagus, stomach, and proximal small intestine. Food and fluids, ingested through the mouth, move through the esophagus to the stomach. The stomach and upper intestinal tract (duodenum and jejunum) are responsible for the majority of food digestion. When an acute or chronic disease process interferes with the function of this portion of the gastrointestinal (GI) tract, nutritional status can be affected and the client may experience symptoms that interfere with lifestyle.

Nurses provide both acute care for the hospitalized client and teaching about the skills and knowledge needed to manage these conditions at home.

DISORDERS OF THE MOUTH

Inflammations, infections, and neoplastic lesions of the mouth affect food ingestion and nutrition. Oral lesions may have a variety of causes, including infection, mechanical trauma, irritants such as alcohol, and hypersensitivity. Appropriate treatment of the disorder, any underlying factors, and associated symptoms is essential.

THE CLIENT WITH STOMATITIS

Stomatitis, inflammation of the oral mucosa, is a common disorder of the mouth. It may be caused by viral (herpes simplex) or fungal (*Candida albicans*) infections, mechanical trauma (e.g., cheek biting), and irritants such as tobacco or chemotherapeutic agents. Stomatitis is commonly seen in people who are immunocompromised (e.g., clients with HIV disease), people with cancer, frail older adults, and at the end of life (Dahlin, 2004). Box 23–1 lists common risk factors for stomatitis.

FAST FACTS

- Up to 75% of people undergoing chemotherapy to treat cancer experience *oral mucositis*, a type of stomatitis.
- Oral mucositis tends to affect younger clients, women, and people receiving fluorouracil (5FU) more frequently than others.
- Clients who also use alcohol and tobacco have a greater risk of developing oral mucositis.
- 100% of clients undergoing radiation therapy of the head and neck develop oral mucositis.
- Nearly 90% of clients treated with stem cell transplant develop oral mucositis (Cawley & Benson, 2005).

BOX 23–1 Risk Factors for Stomatitis

- Age > 65 years
- Impaired immune status (HIV disease, cancer, diabetes)
- Chronic renal failure or heart failure
- Chemotherapy, radiation therapy, stem cell transplant
- Oxygen therapy, mouth breathing
- Medications (antibiotics, phenytoin, anticholinergics, corticosteroids)
- Poor oral hygiene, ill-fitting dentures
- Tobacco or alcohol use

Pathophysiology and Manifestations

The oral mucosa, which lines the oral cavity, is a relatively thin, fragile layer of stratified squamous epithelial cells. The blood supply to the oral mucosa is rich. As epithelial cells slough, stem cells in the submucosa develop into epithelial cells to replace those that are lost. The health and integrity of the oral mucosa are, therefore, dependent on the ability of stem cells to continuously reproduce (Cawley & Benson, 2005).

Frequent exposure to the environment, a rich blood supply, and the oral mucosa's delicate nature increase the risk of infection or inflammation, reaction to toxins, and trauma. Stomatitis results from persistent damage to oral mucosal cells. Damage is initially superficial, progressing to ulceration and involvement of the entire epithelium. Finally, healing begins within 2 to 4 weeks (Dahlin, 2004).

The pathophysiology of oral mucositis has only recently been fully understood. Radiotherapy and chemotherapy damage the DNA of epithelial cells, resulting in necrosis and death of some cells. This stimulates the release of inflammatory mediators that further damage tissues, causing additional epithelial cells to die. As a result, the oral mucosa thins. Tumor necrosis factor alpha (TNF-α) is released, which activates additional inflammatory cytokines. Tissues below the mucosa are damaged as well. In the ulcerative stage of oral mucositis, irregular ulcers that extend from the epithelium into the submucosa develop. As nerve endings are exposed, this stage is accompanied by significant pain. Although healing begins within 2 to 3 weeks, the oral mucosa does not fully recover, and remains vulnerable to damage or inflammation (Cawley & Benson, 2005).

The clinical manifestations of stomatitis vary according to its cause. Table 23–1 outlines common causes of stomatitis with their manifestations and treatment. Chemotherapy or chemical irritation may result in initial generalized redness and swelling, followed by development of deep, irregular ulcerations. Ulcers may be covered with pseudomembranes. Oral pain and pseudomembranes can interfere with the ability to eat, drink, and swallow normally (Cawley & Benson, 2005).

Stomatitis can lead to malnutrition, fluid and electrolyte imbalance, and other complications such as sepsis and bacterial endocarditis.

INTERDISCIPLINARY CARE

Stomatitis is diagnosed by direct physical examination and, if indicated, cultures, smears, and evaluation for systemic illness. Treatment addresses both the underlying cause and any coexisting illnesses. An undiagnosed oral lesion present for more than 1 week and that does not respond to therapy must be evaluated for malignancy.

Direct smears and cultures of lesions may be obtained to identify causative organisms. If systemic illness is suspected, a variety of diagnostic tests may be ordered to identify the underlying cause.

General treatment measures include providing meticulous oral hygiene, with brushing and flossing (as tolerated). A solution of saline, sodium bicarbonate, or a combination of saline/bicarbonate promotes comfort and healing when used after and between meals.

Medications

Using a topical anesthetic, such as 2% viscous lidocaine, diphenhydramine (Benadryl) solution, or benzocaine spray or gel can promote comfort and the ability to consume oral food and fluids. Lidocaine solution is not swallowed to avoid impairment of the swallowing mechanism. Orabase, a protective paste, may be applied to oral ulcers to promote comfort. Triamcinolone acetonide

TABLE 23–1 Manifestations and Treatment of Common Stomatitis Conditions

TYPE	CAUSE	MANIFESTATIONS	TREATMENT
Cold sore, fever blister	Herpes simplex virus	■ Initial burning at site ■ Clustered vesicular lesions on lip or oral mucosa	■ Self-limiting ■ Acyclovir, valacyclovir to shorten course
Aphthous ulcer (canker sore, ulcerative stomatitis)	Unknown; may be type of herpes virus	■ Well-circumscribed, shallow erosions with white or yellow center encircled by red ring ■ Less than 1 cm in diameter ■ Painful	■ Topical steroid ointment ■ Amlexanox oral paste (Aphthasol) ■ Oral prednisone
Candidiasis (thrush)	*Candida albicans*	■ Creamy white, curdlike patches ■ Red, erythematous mucosa	■ Fluconazole (Diflucan) ■ Ketoconazole (Nizoral) ■ Clotrimazole troches ■ Nystatin vaginal troches (dissolved orally) or mouth rinse
Necrotizing ulcerative gingivitis (trench mouth, Vincent's infection)	Infection with spirochetes and bacilli or systemic infection	■ Acute gingival inflammation and necrosis ■ Bleeding, halitosis ■ Fever ■ Cervical lymphadenopathy	■ Correct any underlying disorders ■ Warm, half-strength peroxide mouthwashes ■ Oral penicillin
Oral mucositis	Damage to epithelial cells and stem cells in the submucosa caused by chemotherapy or radiation therapy	■ Erythema and inflammation of oral mucosa ■ Painful, irregularly shaped ulcerations, initially superficial, progressing to deep ulcers that may be confluent (overlapping with one another) ■ Pseudomembranes covering ulcers ■ Tissue necrosis with spontaneous bleeding, potential sepsis	■ Regular oral hygiene with brushing and flossing ■ Saline or sodium bicarbonate solution mouth rinses after and between meals ■ Gelclair mouth rinse before meals for analgesia ■ Palifermin, an epithelial cell growth factor ■ Low-level laser therapy

may be mixed in Orabase to reduce inflammation and promote healing. Other coating agents include Amphojel or Kaopectate. Sodium bicarbonate mouthwashes may provide relief and promote cleansing, whereas alcohol-based mouthwashes may cause pain and burning and should be avoided. Agents that form a film over exposed nerve endings and deep ulcerations (e.g., Zilactin, Gelclair) may be used in clients with oral mucositis.

Fungal infections often are treated with a nystatin oral suspension; clients "swish and swallow" the solution. Clotrimazole lozenges also treat oral fungal infections. If the infection does not resolve, oral antifungal medications such as fluconazole or ketoconazole may be used. Antifungals are usually continued for at least 3 days after symptoms disappear.

Herpetic lesions may be treated with topical or oral acyclovir or valacyclovir (Valtrex). Acyclovir ointment provides comfort and lubrication while limiting the spread of the virus. Acyclovir capsules reduce the severity of symptoms and the duration of the lesions.

Bacterial infections are treated with antibiotics based on cultures and smears. Oral penicillin is the treatment of choice if the client is not allergic and the cultured bacteria are sensitive. Nursing implications for selected drugs used to treat stomatitis are outlined below.

An epithelial cell growth-stimulating factor, Palifermin, has been approved to reduce the incidence and duration of oral mucositis in clients undergoing high-dose chemotherapy with or without radiation therapy in preparation for bone marrow or stem cell transplant (National Cancer Institute, 2005). See the Medication Administration box below.

 ## NURSING CARE

Health Promotion

Nurses can help prevent stomatitis by identifying clients at risk and suggesting measures to reduce the likelihood that stomatitis will develop. Teach and encourage all clients to regularly perform mouth care, including teeth brushing and flossing. Provide frequent mouth care with nondrying agents for clients who are unable to provide self-care. Encourage clients with ill-fitting dentures or other dental prostheses (such as partial plates) to see a qualified dentist or denturist. Suggest clients taking an extended course of antibiotic therapy or who have impaired immune function consume 8 oz. of yogurt containing live bacterial cultures or 8 oz of buttermilk daily unless contraindicated. Discuss dietary modifications, such as limiting consumption of highly spiced or acidic foods and avoiding very hot beverages. Clients undergoing chemotherapy or radiation therapy should avoid use of alcohol and tobacco because these substances further damage oral mucosa, increasing the risk for oral mucositis.

Assessment

Oral assessment is important not only for clients who have been diagnosed with stomatitis, but also for those with risk factors,

---

MEDICATION ADMINISTRATION **Drugs Used to Treat Stomatitis**

TOPICAL ORAL ANESTHETICS
Orajel
Viscous lidocaine
Anbesol
Triamcinolone acetonide
These drugs reduce the pain associated with mucous membrane lesions or stomatitis. They provide temporary relief of pain. Any oral lesion that persists longer than 1 week should be evaluated by an oral surgeon.

Nursing Responsibilities
- Instruct the client to seek medical attention for any oral lesion that does not heal within 1 week.
- Monitor for local hypersensitivity reactions, and discontinue use if they occur.

Health Education for the Client and Family
- Apply every 1 to 2 hours as needed.
- Perform oral hygiene after meals and at bedtime.

TOPICAL ANTIFUNGAL AGENTS
Clotrimazole
Nystatin
These products help in the topical treatment of candidiasis. Their effects are primarily local rather than systemic.

Nursing Responsibilities
- Instruct the client to dissolve lozenges in the mouth.

- Instruct the client to rinse mouth with oral suspension for at least 2 minutes and expectorate or swallow as directed.
- These drugs are contraindicated in pregnancy.

Health Education for the Client and Family
- Take medication as prescribed.
- Do not eat or drink 30 minutes after medication.
- Contact physician if symptoms worsen.
- Perform good oral hygiene after meals and at bedtime; remove dentures at bedtime.

ANTIVIRAL AGENTS
Acyclovir (Zovirax)
Valacyclovir (Valtrex)
Acyclovir and valacyclovir are useful in the treatment of oral herpes simplex virus. They help reduce the severity and frequency of infections. These antiviral agents interfere with the DNA synthesis of herpes simplex virus.

Nursing Responsibilities
- Start therapy as soon as herpetic lesions are noted.
- Administer with food or on an empty stomach.

Health Education for the Client and Family
- The virus remains latent and can recur during stressful events, fever, trauma, sunlight exposure, and treatment with immunosuppressive drugs.
- Take the medication as ordered, and contact the physician if symptoms worsen.

manifestations, or evidence of possible complications (e.g., recent weight loss).

- *Health history:* Complaints of mouth pain, altered taste, lack of appetite, malaise; presence of dentures, regularity of dental care; current health status including chronic diseases; current medications; use of alcohol or tobacco.
- *Physical examination:* Inspect lips, gums, teeth, interior cheeks, tongue and base of tongue, soft and hard palate; tonsils, and oral pharynx. Observe and assess general health status including temperature, weight.
- *Diagnostic tests:* WBC, sedimentation rate, serum albumin.

Nursing Diagnoses and Interventions

Nursing care for the client with stomatitis or oral mucositis focuses not only on the oral inflammation, but also on any underlying systemic diseases and the effects of the condition on the client's comfort and nutrition.

Impaired Oral Mucous Membrane

Stomatitis and oral mucositis disrupt the integrity of the oral mucous membrane. Regardless of cause, the pain and symptoms must be relieved to promote comfort as well as food and fluid intake.

- Assess and document oral mucous membranes and the character of any lesions every 4 to 8 hours. *Baseline and ongoing assessment data provide the basis for evaluation.*
- Assist with thorough mouth care after meals, at bedtime, and every 2 to 4 hours while awake. If unable to tolerate a toothbrush, offer sponge or gauze toothettes. Avoid using alcohol-based mouthwashes or lemon-glycerin swabs. Provide saline or sodium bicarbonate rinse or a combined saline/sodium bicarbonate rinse after every meal and between meals. *Mouth care promotes hygiene, comfort, and healing. Alcohol-based mouthwashes and lemon-glycerin swabs may dry and irritate mucous membranes, causing pain and further tissue damage, whereas saline or bicarbonate rinses promote comfort and healing (Cawley & Benson, 2005).*
- Assess knowledge and teach about condition, mouth care, and treatments. Instruct to avoid alcohol, tobacco, and spicy or irritating foods. *Knowledge promotes client participation in the plan of care and compliance. Alcohol, tobacco, and hot, spicy, or rough foods may injure the inflamed mucous membranes.*

Imbalanced Nutrition: Less than Body Requirements

Oral lesions and pain may limit oral intake, which may in turn lead to nutritional deficits. Anorexia and general malaise may also contribute to decreased intake.

- Assess food intake as well as the client's ability to chew and swallow. Weigh daily. Provide appropriate assistive devices such as straws or feeding syringes. *Adequate nutrition is essential for healing. Daily weights allow monitoring of the adequacy of food intake. Assistive devices may allow food intake while avoiding irritation of ulcerations or lesions.*
- Encourage a high-calorie, high-protein diet considerate of food preferences. Offer soft, lukewarm, or cool foods or liquids such as eggnogs, milk shakes, nutritional supplements, popsicles, and puddings frequently in small amounts. Obtain nutritional con-

sultation. *Oral intake may be limited, and enriched foods and liquids enhance nutrition. A nutritional consultation can help ensure an adequate diet and assist in meeting nutritional needs.*

- Provide analgesics for pain relief as needed. *Significant pain associated with stomatitis or oral mucositis can interfere with effective mouth care and food and fluid intake. Pain management is a vital part of nursing care.*

Using NANDA, NIC, and NOC

Chart 23–1 shows links between NANDA nursing diagnoses, NIC, and NOC when caring for the client with stomatitis.

Community-Based Care

Clients with mild stomatitis generally provide self-care. While clients with cancer treatment–related oral mucositis may require more aggressive therapy, the client and caregivers often are able to manage the regimen in home or community-based settings. Include the following topics in teaching for home care:

- Managing any underlying health conditions and ongoing treatments such as chemotherapy
- The recommended diet and oral hygiene regime, including foods and substances (e.g., alcohol, tobacco products) to avoid
- Nutritional supplements to help meet nutritional requirements
- Prescribed medication, its route, side effects, frequency of administration, and signs and symptoms to report

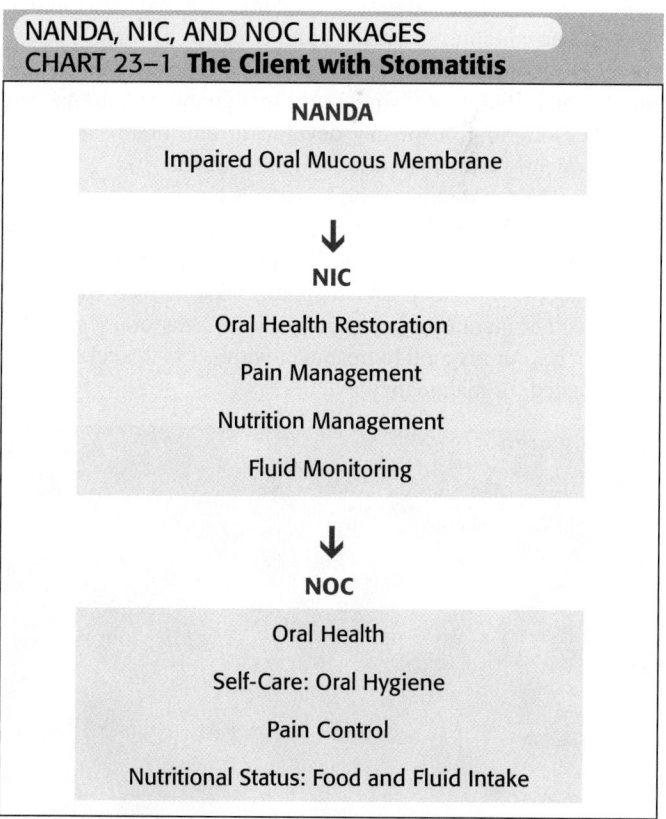

NANDA, NIC, AND NOC LINKAGES
CHART 23–1 The Client with Stomatitis

NANDA

Impaired Oral Mucous Membrane

↓

NIC

Oral Health Restoration

Pain Management

Nutrition Management

Fluid Monitoring

↓

NOC

Oral Health

Self-Care: Oral Hygiene

Pain Control

Nutritional Status: Food and Fluid Intake

Data from *NANDA's Nursing Diagnoses: Definitions & Classification 2005–2006* by NANDA International (2005), Philadelphia; *Nursing Interventions Classification (NIC)* (4th ed.) by J. M. Dochterman & G. M. Bulechek (2004), St. Louis, MO: Mosby; and *Nursing Outcomes Classification (NOC)* (3rd ed.) by S. Moorhead, M. Johnson, and M. Maas (2004), St. Louis, MO: Mosby.

■ The importance of completing the full course of antibiotic, antiviral, or antifungal treatment

■ Manifestations to report and the importance of follow-up care.

THE CLIENT WITH ORAL CANCER

Oral cancer, malignancy of the oral mucosa, may develop on the lips, tongue, floor of the mouth, or other oral tissues. It is uncommon, accounting for only 5% of all cancers. It has, however, a high rate of morbidity and mortality. The incidence of this type of head and neck cancer is twice as high in men as in women, and it is seen more often in men over age 40. The stage of an oral cancer determines the prognosis, treatment, and degree of disability. The primary risk factors for oral cancer are smoking, drinking alcohol, and chewing tobacco. Marijuana use, occupational exposures to chemicals, and viruses such as human papilloma virus (HPV) also may contribute to the risk for oral cancer.

Pathophysiology and Manifestations

Oral cancer is usually a squamous cell carcinoma. Although a cancerous lesion can develop in any area of the mouth, the most common sites are the lower lip, tongue, and floor of the mouth. Most early cancers present as inflamed areas with irregular, ill-defined borders. These lesions typically are not painful. More advanced cancers appear as deep ulcers that are fixed to deeper tissues. Early lesions involve the mucosa or submucosa, whereas more advanced tumors may invade and destroy underlying tissues, including muscles and bones of the face. Tumors frequently metastasize to regional lymph nodes. Other cancerous lesions, including lymphoma, malignant melanoma, and Kaposi's sarcoma, also may develop in the mouth, although less frequently than squamous cell carcinoma.

The earliest symptom of oral cancer is a painless oral ulceration or lesion (Figure 23–1 ■). Later symptoms vary and may include difficulty speaking, swallowing, or chewing; swollen lymph nodes; and blood-tinged sputum. See the accompanying box for other manifestations of oral cancer. Any oral lesion that does not heal or respond to treatment within 1 to 2 weeks should be evaluated for malignancy.

Figure 23–1 ■ Oral cancer.

Source: Biophoto Associates/Photo Researchers, Inc.

MANIFESTATIONS of Oral Cancer

■ White patches (leukoplakia)
■ Red patches (erythroplakia)
■ Ulcers
■ Masses
■ Pigmented areas (brownish or black)
■ Fissures
■ Asymmetry of the head, face, jaws, or neck

INTERDISCIPLINARY CARE

The first component of treatment is eliminating any causative factors such as chewing tobacco, smoking, or drinking alcohol. Tumor staging then determines therapy. The TNM (tumor, nodes, metastasis) classification is used to stage oral cancer. See Box 23–2. A biopsy of the oral lesion allows direct visualization of cells to determine the presence or absence of cancerous cells. Staging may require additional diagnostic studies such as computed tomography (CT) scans or magnetic resonance imaging (MRI).

Radiation and chemotherapy may be considered based on the client's age, tumor stage, general condition, and preferences. Radiation therapy may be used preoperatively to "shrink" the tumor or postoperatively to limit the risks of metastasis. Chemotherapy may be indicated depending on the stage of the tumor. See Chapter 14 ∞ for more information about radiation and chemotherapy to treat cancer.

Following the biopsy and staging of the tumor, surgery is generally indicated, although an advanced or extensive tumor may be considered unresectable. If the tumor involves surrounding tissues, the cosmetic effects of surgery are important considerations. The goal of surgery is removal of the lesion and potentially cancerous surrounding tissue or lymph nodes. Advanced carcinomas may require extensive excision or a *radical neck dissection,* a potentially disfiguring procedure in which the lymph nodes and muscles of the neck are removed. A tracheostomy is performed at the time of surgery. The tracheostomy may be temporary, but often is permanent. See Chapter 37 ∞ for more information about caring for a client following radical neck dissection and a tracheostomy.

BOX 23–2 Oral Cancer Staging

Stage	
Stage 0	Carcinoma *in situ*
Stage I	Tumor ≤ 2 cm; no regional node involvement
Stage II	Tumor > 2 cm to ≤ 4 cm; no regional node involvement
Stage III	Tumor ≤ 2 cm to > 4 cm; one involved lymph node
Stage IVA & B	Tumor may invade adjacent structures; one or more nodes involved
Stage IVC	Distant metastasis present

NURSING CARE

Health Promotion

Reducing or eliminating tobacco use (smoking and smokeless tobacco) and excess alcohol consumption can significantly reduce the incidence of oral cancer. Teach children and adolescents about the dangers of using tobacco and alcohol. Emphasize the relationship between smokeless tobacco and oral cancer. Discuss strategies to deal with peer pressure to use tobacco and alcohol.

To promote early identification of and intervention for oral cancer, teach clients about the risk factors for and manifestations of the disease. This is a particularly important nursing strategy in older men who have the highest incidence, and in populations in whom the disease often is advanced when detected (people of lower socioeconomic status, people who rarely see a dentist, and African American men) (Powe & Finnie, 2004).

Assessment

Early precancerous oral lesions are very treatable. Unfortunately, these lesions usually are painless, so diagnosis and treatment often is delayed. Assess the oral cavity of all clients, particularly those with risk factors for oral cancer.

- *Health history:* Complaints of oral lesions that fail to heal; use (current or past) of tobacco products or excess alcohol.
- *Physical examination:* Inspect and palpate lips and oral mucosa (including tongue and floor of mouth under the tongue) for tumors or lesions. Lesions may appear as velvety red or white patches that do not scrape off, or as ulcers or areas of necrosis.

Nursing Diagnoses and Interventions

The mouth allows food ingestion, and the lips are integral to verbal and nonverbal expression. The head, mouth, and lips are important to self-perception and body image. Nursing diagnoses discussed in this section consider such problems as airway clearance, nutrition, communication, and body image. See the accompanying Nursing Care Plan below.

NURSING CARE PLAN A Client with Oral Cancer

Juan Chavez, a married 44-year-old farmer, has two adult children. He and his wife raise and sell fruits and vegetables. Two months ago, Mr. Chavez developed a sore on his tongue that would not heal. Mr. Chavez tells his admission nurse, Sara Bucklin, "The doctor says he will have to remove part of my tongue," and anxiously asks, "Will I ever look the same? How will I be able to talk?"

ASSESSMENT

Mr. Chavez's admission history reveals that he has been healthy, but has smoked two packs of cigarettes a day for more than 20 years, and usually drinks two to four beers per day. He admits to being anxious and fearful of surgery and its outcomes. He says he quit smoking and drinking 2 weeks ago. The biopsy report is positive for squamous cell carcinoma of the tongue. Mr. Chavez has no enlarged cervical nodes and says he has no bloody sputum or saliva, difficulty swallowing, chewing, or talking. His weight is in the normal range for his height. A wide excision of the oral lesion is planned.

DIAGNOSES

- *Risk for Ineffective Airway Clearance* related to oral surgery
- *Risk for Imbalanced Nutrition: Less than Body Requirements* related to oral surgery
- *Impaired Verbal Communication* related to excision of a portion of the tongue
- *Disturbed Body Image* related to surgical excision of the tongue

EXPECTED OUTCOMES

- Maintain a patent airway and remain free of respiratory distress.
- Maintain a stable weight and level of hydration.
- Effectively communicate with staff and family using a magic slate and flash cards.
- Communicate an increased ability to accept changes in body image.

PLANNING AND IMPLEMENTATION

- Assess airway patency and respiratory status every hour until stable.

- Maintain semi-Fowler's position, supporting arms. Encourage to turn, cough, and deep breathe every 2 to 4 hours.
- Teach the importance of activity, turning, coughing, and deep breathing.
- Monitor daily weights.
- Consult with dietitian to assess calorie needs and plan appropriate enteral feeding. Assess response to enteral feedings.
- Demonstrate and allow to practice using magic slate and flash cards prior to surgery.
- Allow adequate time for communication efforts.
- Keep emergency call system in reach at all times and answer light promptly. Alert all staff of inability to respond verbally.
- Encourage expression of feelings regarding perceived and actual changes.
- Provide emotional support and encourage self-care and participation in decision making.

EVALUATION

At the time of discharge, Mr. Chavez has maintained his weight and has started on oral liquids, including supplements and enriched liquids. His airway has remained clear, and he is effectively coughing and deep breathing. He has used the magic slate to communicate throughout his hospital stay. He is regaining use of his tongue, and can speak a few words. Although initially distressed, he is communicating an increased ability to cope with loss of part of his tongue. He and his wife say they understand his discharge instructions, including diet, activity, follow-up care, and signs and symptoms to report.

CRITICAL THINKING IN THE NURSING PROCESS

1. What measures can you, as a nurse, implement to reduce the incidence of oral cancer?
2. Plan a health education program for young athletes who chew tobacco.
3. Mr. Chavez's wife calls you 2 weeks after discharge. She tells you that he refuses to try to talk and is relying on his magic slate to communicate. How will you respond?
See Evaluating Your Response in Appendix C.

Risk for Ineffective Airway Clearance

The location and the extent of an oral cancer and its excision may compromise the airway. Swelling of adjacent tissues, increased oral secretions, or difficulty swallowing may contribute to respiratory distress. If extensive surgery is performed, a tracheostomy usually is performed to maintain airway patency.

PRACTICE ALERT

In the initial postoperative period, assess airway patency and respiratory status at least hourly. A patent airway is vital to maintain respirations and oxygenation of tissues. Frequent assessment allows early identification of possible airway compromise.

- Unless contraindicated, place in Fowler's position, supporting arms. Assist the client to turn, cough, and deep breathe at least every 2 to 4 hours. *Fowler's position promotes lung expansion. Turning, coughing, and deep breathing help maintain a patent airway by preventing pooling of secretions.*
- Maintain adequate hydration (2000 to 3000 mL per day unless contraindicated) and humidity of inspired air. *Adequate hydration helps thin and loosen secretions.*

Imbalanced Nutrition: Less than Body Requirements

Surgery affects oral food and fluid intake. Enteral feedings or total parenteral nutrition may be required. A gastrostomy tube usually is inserted during surgery to maintain nutrition. If an oral diet is permitted, anorexia or pain may affect intake.

- Weigh daily. Assess oral intake for adequacy of protein, calories, and nutrients. *Daily weights and nutritional assessments provide information about the adequacy of diet.*

- Offer soft, bland foods with supplements as indicated. Provide small, frequent feedings, making mealtimes pleasant. *Soft, bland foods may be better tolerated following oral surgery. Large meals may be overwhelming; small, frequent meals promote food and nutrient intake.*
- Provide enteral feedings per gastrostomy tube as ordered. Elevate the head of the bed 30 to 40 degrees. *Enteral feedings maintain nutritional status in the client who is unable to consume foods orally. Elevating the head of the bed reduces the risk of regurgitation and aspiration of gastric contents.*
- Assess for gastric residual volume per facility protocol for the type of feeding (intermittent or continuous). See the Nursing Research box below. Notify the physician of volumes greater than 200 mL or 50% of previous feeding if feeding is intermittent. *Excess residual volume may increase the risk for aspiration.*
- Consider a nutritional consultation to assess diet and plan appropriate supplements. *A registered dietitian can calculate energy requirements and develop an individualized diet plan to meet nutritional requirements.*

Impaired Verbal Communication

Oral surgery can interfere with communication. Effective communication is vital to postoperative recovery and prevention of complications.

- Before surgery, establish and practice a communication plan such as using a magic slate or flash cards. *Practicing communication techniques reduces fear and anxiety while promoting communication.*

NURSING RESEARCH   Evidence-Based Practice for Clients with Enteral Feeding Tubes

Practices and protocols for assessing gastric residual volume in clients with nasogastric or gastrostomy feeding tubes are inconsistent. Researchers have come to varying conclusions about the amount of gastric residual volume that is safe and does not increase gastric distention and the risk for aspiration. In one study, while more than 30% of the clients had residual volumes greater than 150 mL, only 4% had evidence of formula in their airways. In an extensive review of the literature regarding measurement of gastric residual volume, Edwards and Metheny (2000) also found that nursing practice often was inconsistent with hospital protocols. These researchers, together with Schallom (Metheny et al., 2004), went on to study the effect of feeding site on the risk for aspiration. This literature review led to the conclusion that despite differences in feeding tube location (stomach, duodenum, jejunum), evaluation of gastric emptying through measurement of gastric residual volume is the preferred predictor of risk for aspiration in clients with feeding tubes.

IMPLICATIONS FOR NURSING

Gastric motility slows following surgery or trauma, in diabetes, sepsis, or electrolyte imbalance, and with medications such as narcotic analgesics. Excessive gastric distention appears to increase the risk for aspiration of gastric contents. However, when enteral feedings are withheld unnecessarily, the nutritional status of the client is at risk. Impaired nutrition affects healing and recovery.

The authors suggest a protocol for enteral infusions that includes (1) checking residual volume every 4 hours; (2) assessing the client and contacting the physician if the residual volume is greater than 200 mL or 50% of the previous bolus feeding; and (3) withholding the feeding only when directed to do so by the physician (Edwards & Metheny, 2000, Metheny et al., 2004).

CRITICAL THINKING IN CLIENT CARE

1. What factors might influence the accuracy of residual volume measurements? What measures can be taken to obtain accurate measurements?
2. What would be the effect of withholding one bolus feeding of 240 mL of a standard enteral formula? If this is repeated daily for a week, what is the cumulative effect?
3. One reason frequently cited for avoiding checking residual volume is the risk of plugging the feeding tube. Identify measures to prevent this potential problem.

- Provide ample time for communication efforts and do not answer for the client. Be alert for nonverbal communications. Use yes/no questions and simple phrases. *Providing adequate time allows the client opportunity to express ideas and thoughts. Nonverbal communication provides cues regarding comfort or other needs. Simple yes/no questions are easily answered nonverbally.*
- If indicated, refer to or consult with a speech therapist. *A speech therapist can help promote or restore effective communication.*

PRACTICE ALERT
Provide an emergency call system and respond promptly. Make all staff aware that the client cannot respond over an intercom system by posting an alert on the intercom. Nonverbal clients rely on an emergency call system to summon help. Answering promptly reduces fear and anxiety and maintains safety.

Disturbed Body Image
Radical surgery of the head or neck seriously affects body image. An altered speech pattern and any disfigurement affect the ability to feel attractive or effective in work or social roles. Clients may defer lifesaving surgery to postpone disfiguring interventions or therapies.

- Assess coping style, self-perception, and responses to altered appearance or function. *This information can be used to identify appropriate interventions and care.*
- Encourage verbalization of feelings regarding perceived and actual changes. *Nonjudgmental acceptance of feelings and fears helps establish trust.*
- Provide emotional support, encourage self-care, and provide decision-making opportunities. *Self-care promotes self-acceptance and independence. Giving choices empowers the client to participate in care.*

Community-Based Care
Discharge planning for the client with oral cancer depends on the type of treatment planned and surgery performed. Depending on the client's age, condition, and availability of support systems, referral to community healthcare agencies may be an essential component of care. Visits from home care nurses can assist in meeting healthcare needs.

Discuss the following topics with the client and family members or care providers:
- Diagnosis and prescribed care
- Monitoring for new lesions or recurrences
- Diet, nutrition, and activity
- Pain management
- Airway management, care of incision, and signs and symptoms to report.

DISORDERS OF THE ESOPHAGUS

The esophagus plays an essential role in the ingestion of food and liquids. Disorders of the esophagus can be inflammatory, mechanical, or cancerous. Because of its location and neighboring organs, the symptoms of esophageal disorders may mimic those of a variety of other illnesses.

THE CLIENT WITH GASTROESOPHAGEAL REFLUX DISEASE

Gastroesophageal reflux is the backward flowing of gastric contents into the esophagus. When this occurs, the client experiences heartburn. Many people with gastroesophageal reflux have few symptoms, while others develop inflammatory esophagitis as a result of exposure to gastric juices. **Gastroesophageal reflux disease (GERD)** is a common gastrointestinal disorder.

FAST FACTS
- GERD affects 15% to 20% of adults.
- Up to 7% of people experience daily symptoms such as heartburn, regurgitation, and indigestion, and as many as 15% have symptoms weekly (Kasper et al., 2005; Tierney et al., 2005).

Pathophysiology
Normally, the lower esophageal sphincter remains closed except during swallowing. Reflux (backflow) of gastric contents into the esophagus is prevented by pressure differences between the stomach and the lower esophagus. The diaphragm, the lower esophageal sphincter, and the location of the gastroesophageal junction below the diaphragm help maintain this pressure difference (Figure 23–2 ■).

Gastroesophageal reflux may result from transient relaxation of the lower esophageal sphincter, an incompetent lower esophageal sphincter, and/or increased pressure within the stomach (Figure 23–3 ■). Factors contributing to gastroesophageal reflux include increased gastric volume (e.g., after meals), positioning that allows gastric contents to remain close to the gastroesophageal junction (e.g., bending over, lying down), and increased gastric pressure (e.g., obesity or wearing tight clothing). A hiatal hernia may contribute to GERD.

Gastric juices contain acid, pepsin, and bile, which are corrosive substances. Esophageal peristalsis and bicarbonate in salivary secretions normally clear and neutralize gastric juices in the esophagus. During sleep, however, and in clients with impaired esophageal peristalsis or salivation, the esophageal mucosa is damaged by gastric juices, causing an inflammatory response. With prolonged exposure, esophagitis develops. Superficial ulcers develop, and the mucosa becomes red, friable (easily torn), and may bleed. If untreated, scarring and esophageal stricture may develop.

Manifestations
GERD causes heartburn, usually after meals, with bending over, or when reclining. Regurgitation of sour material into the mouth, or difficulty and pain with swallowing may develop.

MediaLink   Case Study: GERD

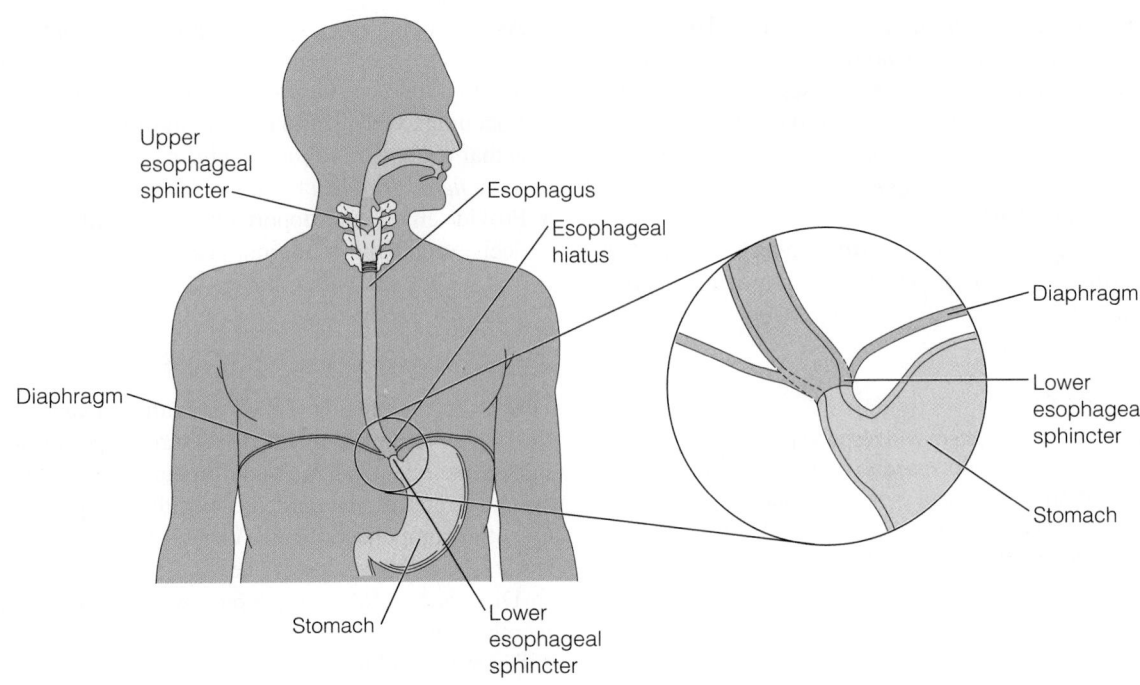

Figure 23–2 ■ The esophagus. The inset shows a closer view of the lower esophageal sphincter.

Other manifestations may include atypical chest pain, sore throat, and hoarseness. See the Manifestations box below. Aspiration of gastric contents can cause hoarseness or respiratory symptoms.

Complications include esophageal strictures and Barrett's esophagus. Strictures can lead to dysphagia. Barrett's esophagus is characterized by changes in the cells lining the esopha-

gus and an increased risk of developing esophageal cancer (Porth, 2005).

INTERDISCIPLINARY CARE

Often the diagnosis of GERD is made by the history of symptoms and predisposing factors. Interdisciplinary care focuses on lifestyle changes, diet modification, and for more severe cases, drug therapy. Surgery is reserved for clients who develop serious complications.

Diagnosis

Diagnostic tests that may be ordered for clients with manifestations of GERD include:

■ *Barium swallow* to evaluate the esophagus, stomach, and upper small intestine.

MANIFESTATIONS of **GERD**

- Heartburn
- Dysphagia
- Regurgitation
- Chest pain
- Pain after eating
- Belching

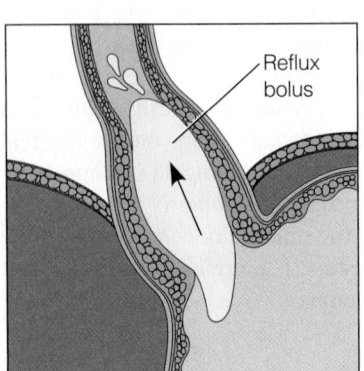

Transient lower esophageal
sphincter relaxation

Incompetent lower esophageal
sphincter

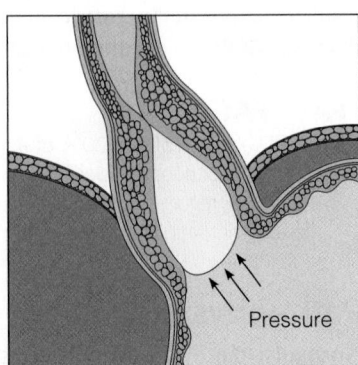

Increased intragastric pressure

Figure 23–3 ■ Mechanisms of gastroesophageal reflux.

- *Upper endoscopy* to permit direct visualization of the esophagus. Tissue may be obtained for biopsy to establish the diagnosis and rule out malignancy. See Chapter 21 ∞ for nursing care of the client undergoing an upper endoscopy.
- *24-hour ambulatory pH monitoring* may be performed to establish the diagnosis of GERD. For this test, a small tube with a pH electrode is inserted through the nose into the esophagus. The electrode is attached to a small box worn on the belt that records the data. The data are later analyzed by computer.
- *Esophageal manometry* measures pressures of the esophageal sphincters and esophageal peristalsis.

Medications

Antacids, such as Mylanta or Maalox, relieve mild or moderate symptoms by neutralizing stomach acid. Gaviscon, which forms a floating barrier between the gastric contents and the esophageal mucosa when the client is upright, may also be used.

Omeprazole (Prilosec), lansoprazole (Prevacid), pantoprazole (Protonix), and rabeprazole (Aciphex) are proton-pump inhibitors (PPIs) that reduce gastric secretions. PPIs promote healing of erosive esophagitis and also relieve symptoms. An 8-week course of treatment is initially prescribed, although some clients may require 3 to 6 months of therapy.

Histamine$_2$-receptor (H$_2$-receptor) blockers reduce gastric acid production and are effective in treating GERD symptoms. When treating GERD, H$_2$-receptor blockers are usually given twice a day or more frequently for a prolonged period of time. Cimetidine, ranitidine, famotidine, and nizatidine are all approved by the FDA for the treatment of GERD and are available over the counter.

A promotility agent, such as metoclopramide (Reglan), may be ordered to enhance esophageal clearance and gastric emptying. Metoclopramide is used to treat clients with regurgitation, symptoms of indigestion, and nighttime symptoms. However, it is not recommended for long-time use. See the Medication Administration box below for the nursing implications of drugs used to treat GERD.

MEDICATION ADMINISTRATION Drugs Used to Treat GERD, Gastritis, and Peptic Ulcer Disease

PROTON-PUMP INHIBITORS
Esomeprazole (Nexium)
Lansoprazole (Prevacid)
Omeprazole (Prilosec)
Pantoprazole (Protonix)
Rabeprazole (Aciphex)
Proton-pump inhibitors are the drugs of choice for severe GERD. PPIs inhibit the hydrogen-potassium-ATP pump, reducing gastric acid secretion. Initially, the PPI may be given twice a day, with the dose reduced to once daily (at bedtime) after 8 weeks.

Nursing Responsibilities
- Administer before breakfast and at bedtime if ordered twice a day; at bedtime if once a day.
- Do not crush tablets.
- Monitor liver function tests for possible abnormal values, including increased AST, ALT, alkaline phosphatase, and bilirubin levels.

Health Education for the Client and Family
- Take the drug as ordered for the full course of therapy, even if symptoms are relieved.
- Do not crush, break, or chew tablets.
- Avoid cigarette smoking, alcohol, aspirin, and NSAIDs while taking this drug because these substances may interfere with healing.
- Report black tarry stools, diarrhea, or abdominal pain to your primary care provider.

H$_2$-RECEPTOR BLOCKERS

Cimetidine (Tagamet)	**Ranitidine (Zantac)**
Famotidine (Pepcid)	**Nizatidine (Axid)**

H$_2$-receptor blockers reduce acidity of gastric juices by blocking the ability of histamine to stimulate acid secretion by the gastric parietal cells. As a result, both the volume and concentration of hydrochloric acid in gastric juice are reduced. H$_2$-receptor blockers are given orally or intravenously. Both prescription and over-the-counter preparations are available.

Nursing Responsibilities
- To ensure absorption, do not give an antacid within 1 hour before or after giving an H$_2$-receptor blocker.
- When administered intravenously, do not mix with other drugs. Administer in 20 to 100 mL of solution over 15 to 30 minutes. Rapid intravenous injection as a bolus may cause dysrhythmias and hypotension.
- Monitor for interaction with such drugs as oral anticoagulants, beta-blockers, benzodiazepines, tricyclic antidepressants, and others. H$_2$-receptor blockers may inhibit the metabolism of other drugs, increasing the risk of toxicity.

Health Education for the Client and Family
- Take the drug as directed, even if pain and gastric discomfort are relieved early in the course of therapy.
- Take at bedtime if once-a-day dosing is ordered. If spaced through the day, take before meals. Avoid taking antacids for 1 hour before and 1 hour after taking this drug.
- To promote healing, avoid cigarette smoking (which increases gastric acid secretion) and gastric mucosal irritants such as alcohol, aspirin, and NSAIDs.
- Long-term use of these drugs can lead to gynecomastia (breast enlargement) and impotence in men and breast tenderness in women. Discontinuing the drug will reverse these effects.
- Report possible adverse effects such as diarrhea, confusion, rash, fatigue, malaise, or bruising to your care provider.

ANTIULCER AGENT
Sucralfate (Carafate)
Sucralfate reacts with gastric acid to form a thick paste that adheres to damaged gastric mucosal tissue. It protects gastric mucosa and promotes healing through this local action.

(continued)

MEDICATION ADMINISTRATION Drugs Used to Treat GERD, Gastritis, and Peptic Ulcer Disease (continued)

Nursing Responsibilities
- Administer on an empty stomach, 1 hour before meals and at bedtime.
- Do not crush tablets.
- Separate administration time from antacids by at least 30 minutes.

Health Education for the Client and Family
- Take as directed, even after symptoms have been relieved.
- Do not crush or chew tablets; shake suspension well.
- Increase your intake of fluids and dietary fiber to prevent constipation.

ANTACIDS

Maalox   Gaviscon   Gelusil   Tums
Mylanta   Aludrox   Riopan   Amphojel

Antacids buffer or neutralize gastric acid, usually acting locally. Antacids are used in GERD, gastritis, and peptic ulcer disease to relieve pain and prevent further damage to esophageal and gastric mucosa.

Nursing Responsibilities
- Antacids interfere with the absorption of many drugs given orally; separate administration times by at least 2 hours.
- Monitor for constipation or diarrhea resulting from antacid therapy. Notify the physician should either develop; a different antacid may be ordered.
- Although most antacids have little systemic effect, electrolyte imbalances can develop. Monitor serum electrolytes, particularly sodium, calcium, and magnesium levels.

Health Education for the Client and Family
- Take your antacid frequently as prescribed, 1 to 3 hours after meals and at bedtime. To be effective, the antacid must be in your stomach.
- Avoid taking an antacid for approximately 2 hours before and 1 hour after taking another medication.

- Shake suspensions well prior to administration.
- Chew tablets thoroughly, and follow with 4 to 6 ounces of water.
- Report worsening symptoms, diarrhea, or constipation to your primary care provider.
- Continue taking the antacid for the duration prescribed. Although pain and discomfort often are relieved soon after treatment begins, healing takes 6 to 8 weeks.

PROMOTILITY AGENT
Metoclopramide (Reglan)
By acting on the central nervous system, metoclopramide stimulates upper gastrointestinal motility and gastric emptying. As a result, nausea, vomiting, and symptoms of GERD are reduced.

Nursing Implications
- Do not administer this drug to clients with possible gastrointestinal obstruction or bleeding, or a history of seizure disorders, pheochromocytoma, or Parkinson's disease.
- Monitor for extrapyramidal side effects (e.g., difficulty speaking or swallowing, loss of balance, gait disruptions, twitching or twisting movements, weakness of arms or legs) or manifestations of tardive dyskinesia (uncontrolled rhythmic facial movement, lip-smacking, tongue rolling). Report immediately.
- Give oral doses 30 minutes before meals and at bedtime.
- May be given by direct intravenous push over 1 to 2 minutes, or diluted by slow infusion over 15 to 30 minutes.

Health Education for the Client and Family
- Take this drug as directed. If you miss a dose, take as soon as you remember unless it is close to time for the next dose.
- Do not drive or engage in other activities that require alertness if this drug makes you drowsy.
- Avoid using alcohol or other CNS depressants while you are taking this drug.
- Immediately contact your healthcare provider if you develop involuntary movements of your eyes, face, or limbs.

Nutrition and Lifestyle Management

GERD is a chronic condition. Dietary and lifestyle changes are important to reduce symptoms and long-term effects of the disorder. Acidic foods such as tomato products, citrus fruits, spicy foods, and coffee are eliminated from the diet. Fatty foods, chocolate, peppermint, and alcohol relax the lower esophageal sphincter or delay gastric emptying, so they should be avoided. The client is advised to maintain ideal body weight, eat smaller meals, refrain from eating for 3 hours before bedtime, and stay upright for 2 hours after meals. Elevating the head of the bed on 6- to 8-inch blocks often is beneficial. Stopping smoking is a necessary lifestyle change. Avoiding tight clothing and avoiding bending may help to relieve symptoms.

Surgery

Surgery may be used for clients who do not respond to pharmacologic and lifestyle management. Antireflux surgeries increase pressure in the lower esophagus, inhibiting gastric content reflux. Laparoscopic fundoplication, a procedure in which the gastric fundus is wrapped around the distal esopha-

gus, is the treatment of choice for GERD. An open surgical procedure known as Nissen fundoplication also may be done (Figure 23–4 ■). Other laparoscopic procedures to tighten the lower esophageal sphincter may include use of an endoscopic suturing system or burning spots on the muscle surrounding the sphincter to create scar tissue. Surgery or ablation therapy also is recommended to reduce the risk of esophageal cancer in clients with persistent cell changes in the distal esophagus.

NURSING CARE

Assessment

Assessment data related to GERD include the following:
- *Health history:* Manifestations such as frequent heartburn; intolerance of foods that are acidic, spicy, or fatty; regurgitation of acidic gastric juice; increased symptoms when bending over, lying down, or wearing tight clothing; difficulty swallowing.
- *Physical assessment:* Epigastric tenderness.

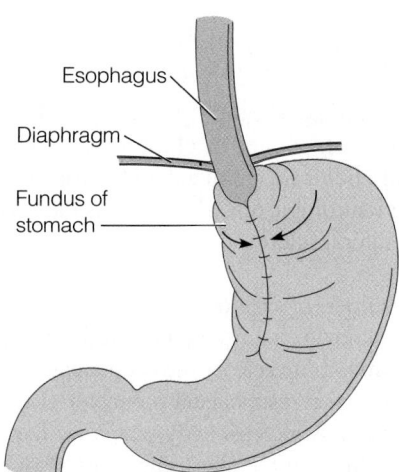

Figure 23–4 ■ Nissen fundoplication. The fundus of the stomach is wrapped around the lower esophagus and the edges are sutured together.

Nursing Diagnoses and Interventions

Relieving the discomfort associated with GERD is the priority of nursing care. Teaching focuses on preventing symptoms and long-term consequences of the disorder.

Pain

The epigastric pain associated with GERD can be severe, interfering with rest and causing anxiety.

- Provide small, frequent meals. Restrict intake of fat, acidic foods, coffee, and alcohol. *Limiting the size of meals reduces pressure in the stomach, reducing esophageal reflux. Fatty, acidic foods, coffee, and alcohol increase gastric acidity and interfere with gastric emptying, increasing the incidence of gastroesophageal reflux.*
- Instruct to stop smoking. Refer to a smoking cessation clinic or program as needed. *Cigarette smoking increases gastric acidity and interferes with healing of damaged mucosa.*
- Administer antacids, H₂-receptor blockers, and PPIs as ordered. Instruct client to continue therapy as prescribed, even after symptoms have been relieved. *These drugs neutralize or reduce gastric acid secretion, relieving symptoms and promoting healing.*
- Discuss the long-term nature of GERD and its management. *Lifestyle changes need to be continued after healing and symptom relief to manage the long-term effects of GERD.*

Using NANDA, NIC, and NOC

Chart 23–2 shows links between NANDA nursing diagnoses, NIC, and NOC when caring for a client with GERD.

Community-Based Care

GERD is a lifelong condition best managed by the client. Teach the client and family about continuing management strategies, including dietary changes, remaining upright after meals, and avoiding eating for at least 3 hours before bedtime. Suggest elevating the head of the bed on 6- to 8-inch wooden blocks placed under the legs. Discuss the need for continued gastric acid reduction using

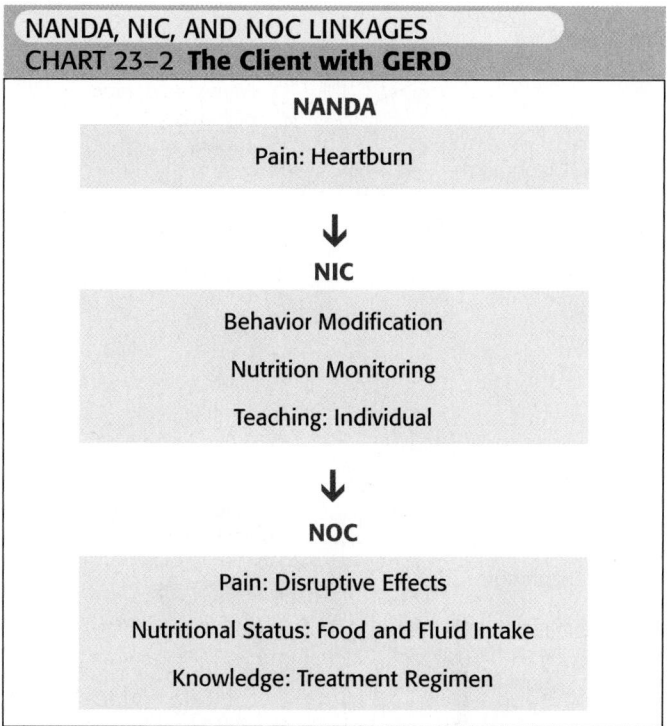

NANDA, NIC, AND NOC LINKAGES
CHART 23–2 The Client with GERD

NANDA

Pain: Heartburn

↓

NIC

Behavior Modification

Nutrition Monitoring

Teaching: Individual

↓

NOC

Pain: Disruptive Effects

Nutritional Status: Food and Fluid Intake

Knowledge: Treatment Regimen

Data from *NANDA's Nursing Diagnoses: Definitions & Classification 2005–2006* by NANDA International (2005), Philadelphia; *Nursing Interventions Classification (NIC)* (4th ed.) by J. M. Dochterman & G. M. Bulechek (2004), St. Louis, MO: Mosby; and *Nursing Outcomes Classification (NOC)* (3rd ed.) by S. Moorhead, M. Johnson, and M. Mass (2004), St. Louis, MO: Mosby.

antacids, H₂-receptor blockers, or PPIs. All are effective to reduce the acidity of gastric juices. Antacids, the most cost-effective measure, require frequent doses to neutralize gastric acid. H₂-receptor blockers, also available over the counter, are a cost-effective management strategy that require only twice-a-day dosing.

THE CLIENT WITH HIATAL HERNIA

A **hiatal hernia** occurs when part of the stomach protrudes through the esophageal hiatus of the diaphragm into the thoracic cavity. Although hiatal hernia is thought to be a common problem, most affected individuals are asymptomatic. The incidence of hiatal hernia increases with age.

In a *sliding hiatal hernia,* the gastroesophageal junction and the fundus of the stomach slide upward through the esophageal hiatus (Figure 23–5A ■). Several factors may contribute to a sliding hiatal hernia, including weakened gastroesophageal-diaphragmatic anchors, shortening of the esophagus, or increased intra-abdominal pressure. Small sliding hiatal hernias produce few symptoms.

In a *paraesophageal hiatal hernia,* the junction between the esophagus and stomach remains in its normal position below the diaphragm while a part of the stomach herniates through the esophageal hiatus (Figure 23–5B). A paraesophageal hernia can become incarcerated (constricted) and strangulate, impairing blood flow to the herniated tissue. Clients with paraesophageal hernia may develop gastritis, or chronic or acute gastrointestinal bleeding. The manifestations of hiatal hernias are listed in the box on the following page.

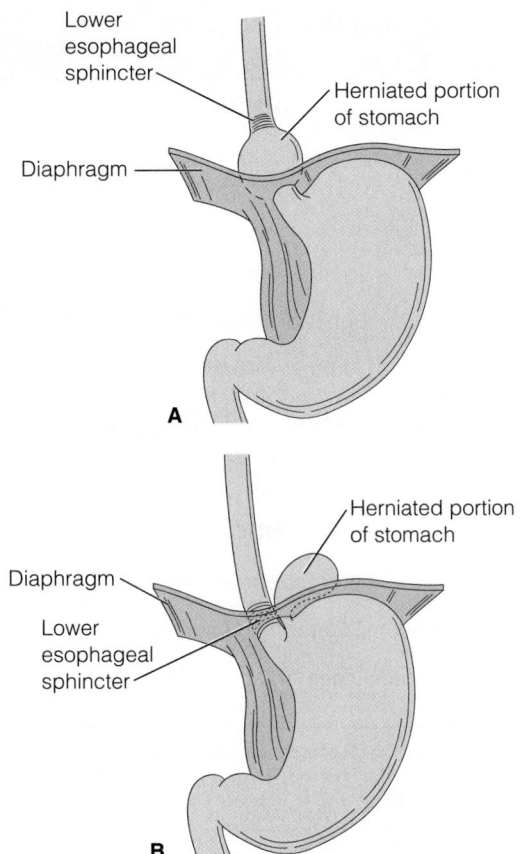

Figure 23–5 ■ Hiatal hernias. *A*, Sliding hiatal hernia. *B*, Paraesophageal hiatal hernia.

A barium swallow or an upper endoscopy may be done to diagnose hiatal hernia. Many clients with hiatal hernia require no treatment. If symptoms are present, treatment measures such as those for clients with GERD may be ordered. If medical management is ineffective or the hernia becomes incarcerated, surgery may be required. The most common surgical procedure is the Nissen fundoplication (see Figure 23–4). This surgery, which may be done laparoscopically, prevents the gastroesophageal junction from slipping into the thoracic cavity.

Nursing care for the client with a hiatal hernia is similar to that for the client with GERD. If surgery is performed, nursing care is similar to that for clients undergoing gastric or thoracic surgery (see Chapter 4 ∞).

MANIFESTATIONS   of Hiatal Hernia

- Reflux, heartburn
- Feeling of fullness
- Substernal chest pain
- Dysphagia
- Occult bleeding
- Belching, indigestion

THE CLIENT WITH IMPAIRED ESOPHAGEAL MOTILITY

Disorders of esophageal motility can cause **dysphagia** (difficult or painful swallowing) or chest pain. It is estimated that nearly 75% of clients hospitalized with stroke experience dysphagia. Other neurologic disorders such as Parkinson's disease, amyotrophic lateral sclerosis, and Alzheimer's disease also can cause dysphagia.

Primary disorders of swallowing are less common. **Achalasia**, a disorder of unknown etiology, is characterized by impaired peristalsis of the smooth muscle of the esophagus and impaired relaxation of the lower esophageal sphincter (LES). The client experiences gradually increasing dysphagia with both solid foods and liquids. Fullness in the chest during meals, chest pain, and nighttime cough are additional manifestations. Other clients may experience **diffuse esophageal spasm** that causes nonperistaltic contraction of esophageal smooth muscle. This disorder causes chest pain and/or dysphagia. The chest pain can be severe, and usually occurs at rest.

Treatment of achalasia may include endoscopically guided injection of botulinum toxin into the lower esophageal sphincter or balloon dilation of the LES. Botulinum toxin injection lowers LES pressure, but may need to be repeated every 6 to 9 months. Balloon dilation tears muscle fibers in the LES, reducing its pressure (Figure 23–6 ■). A laparoscopic myotomy (in-

Figure 23–6 ■ Balloon dilation of the lower esophageal sphincter.

cision into the circular muscle layer of the LES) also reduces pressure and relieves symptoms.

THE CLIENT WITH ESOPHAGEAL CANCER

Cancer of the esophagus is a relatively uncommon malignancy in the United States. It does, however, have a high mortality rate, primarily because symptoms often are not recognized until late in the course of the disease.

FAST FACTS

- Esophageal cancer is the sixth leading cause of death in men.
- It accounted for an estimated 13,570 deaths in 2005.
- 10,530 deaths attributed to esophageal cancer in 2005 were in men.
- Esophageal cancer affects African Americans about 50% more frequently than Caucasians (American Cancer Society, 2005)
- Most esophageal tumors develop in the lower third of the esophagus.

Pathophysiology

There are two types of esophageal tumors, adenocarcinoma and squamous cell carcinoma. Over the past two decades, the incidence of squamous cell tumors of the esophagus has been decreasing, whereas the incidence of adenocarcinoma has increased dramatically, particularly among white males (Kasper et al., 2005). Cigarette smoking and chronic alcohol use are strong risk factors for squamous cell esophageal tumors, and also appear to contribute to the risk of developing adenocarcinoma. Box 23–3 lists major identified risk factors for esophageal cancer.

Only about 15% of esophageal tumors develop in the upper portion of the esophagus; about 35% develop in the midportion. The lower third of the esophagus is the most common site, accounting for about 50% of tumors. Adenocarcinomas tend to develop in dysplastic (abnormal) columnar epithelium in the distal esophagus. It is commonly associated with Barrett's esophagus, a possible complication of chronic GERD and achalasia.

The disease usually spreads to adjacent and supraclavicular lymph nodes, the liver, lungs, and the pleura.

BOX 23–3 Risk Factors for Esophageal Cancer

- Excess alcohol consumption
- Cigarette smoking
- Ingested carcinogens such as nitrates and industrial chemicals
- Smoked opiates
- Physical mucosal damage (e.g., lye ingestion, radiation damage, chronic achalasia)
- Congenital disorders
- Chronic gastric reflux

MANIFESTATIONS of Esophageal Cancer

■ Dysphagia	■ Regurgitation
■ Anemia	■ Anorexia
■ Weight loss	■ Chest pain
■ GERD-like symptoms	■ Persistent cough

Manifestations

The most common symptoms of esophageal carcinoma are progressive dysphagia and recent weight loss. Other manifestations are listed in the box above. The cancer often is advanced and incurable by the time the disease is diagnosed, because symptoms such as difficulty swallowing don't develop until more than 60% of the circumference of the esophagus is affected by tumor (Kasper et al., 2005).

Tracheoesophageal fistulas may develop as the disease progresses, leading to aspiration and pneumonia. Paraneoplastic symptoms such as hypercalcemia also may accompany advanced esophageal cancer.

INTERDISCIPLINARY CARE

Controlling dysphagia and maintaining nutritional status are essential goals of therapy for clients with esophageal cancer, regardless of the stage of the disease. Treatment may involve surgery, radiation therapy, and/or chemotherapy.

Diagnosis

Diagnostic and staging procedures for esophageal cancer may include esophagography, bronchoscopy, and scans to detect metastasis. The following diagnostic tests may be performed (see Chapter 21 ∞):

- *Barium swallow* to identify irregular mucosal patterns or narrowing of the lumen, which suggests esophageal cancer.
- *Esophagoscopy* to allow direct visualization of the tumor and obtain tissue for biopsy.
- *Chest x-ray, CT scans,* or *MRI* to identify possible tumor metastases to other organs or tissues.
- *Complete blood count (CBC)* may indicate anemia due to chronic blood loss. *Serum albumin levels* may be low due to malnutrition, and *liver function tests (ALT, alkaline phosphatase, AST,* and *bilirubin)* are elevated if liver metastases are present.

Treatments

The treatment of esophageal cancer depends on the stage of the disease, as well as factors such as the client's condition and preference.

Clients with early, "curable" esophageal cancer may be treated with surgery alone. Surgery involves resection of the affected portion of the esophagus (*esophagectomy*) and possible anastomosis of the stomach to the remaining esophagus. Mediastinal lymph nodes may be resected at the time of surgery. Esophagectomy is not without risk; potential surgical complications include anastomosis leak, respiratory complications such as pneumonia or acute respiratory distress syndrome, gastric necrosis or bleeding, cardiac dysrhythmias, and infection and sepsis. Intensive nursing care is required postoperatively to prevent and rapidly identify and treat complications that do develop (Mackenzie et al., 2004).

Other approaches to early esophageal cancer include combined radiation and chemotherapy, or a combination of radiation therapy and chemotherapy prior to surgical resection of the tumor. Complications associated with radiation therapy to the esophagus include perforation, hemorrhage, and strictures. When the tumor has spread locally or to distant sites, palliative therapy relieves dysphagia and pain (Tierney et al., 2005). Palliative therapy may include surgical resection, radiation therapy, or local treatments such as wire stents or laser therapy to keep the esophagus patent.

 NURSING CARE

Health Promotion

Health promotion measures to reduce the risk for and incidence of esophageal cancer include educating people (especially young people) about the dangers of cigarette smoking and excess alcohol use. Refer to smoking cessation and alcohol treatment programs as indicated. Educate clients with GERD about the relationship between chronic damage to the esophagus due to reflux and esophageal cancer, and stress the importance of effective disease management.

Assessment

Early diagnosis and treatment of esophageal cancer can make a difference in the client's prognosis. Collect the following assessment data related to esophageal cancer:
- *Health history:* Current symptoms such as chest pain, dysphagia, odynophagia (pain with swallowing), coughing or hoarseness; duration of symptoms; recent weight loss; smoking history; current and past patterns of alcohol consumption.
- *Physical examination:* weight; general health status; skin color; supraclavicular and cervical lymph nodes for lymphadenopathy.

Nursing Diagnoses and Interventions

Disruption of the integrity and function of the esophagus and the discomfort associated with swallowing in clients with esophageal cancer affect the client's ability to maintain adequate nutritional status, and, potentially, a patent airway.

Imbalanced Nutrition: Less than Body Requirements

The client diagnosed with esophageal cancer may already suffer from some degree of malnutrition because of difficulty and pain with swallowing. Enteral nutrition via nasogastric feeding tube or gastrostomy tube or parenteral nutrition maintain nutritional status after surgery or if the tumor is inoperable and obstruction occurs. See Chapter 21 ∞ for nursing interventions related to enteral and parenteral feedings.

Risk for Ineffective Airway Clearance

After surgery for esophageal cancer, the client is at high risk for aspiration and difficulty maintaining a patent airway due to disruption of the esophagus and incision into the thoracic cavity.
- Assess mental and respiratory status (including rate, depth, breath sounds, and oxygen saturation levels) at least every hour during the initial postoperative period. *Altered mental status increases the risk for aspiration. An increased respiratory rate, dyspnea, diminished breath sounds, or decreased oxygen saturation levels may indicate impaired airway clearance or possible aspiration pneumonia.*
- Provide aggressive pulmonary hygiene measures, including endotracheal suctioning and chest physiotherapy as indicated or ordered. Following extubation, encourage frequent coughing, deep breathing, and use of the incentive spirometer. *Respiratory complications are a frequent complication of esophagectomy. Aggressive nursing care helps mobilize secretions and prevent atelectasis and possible pneumonia.*
- If present, monitor chest tube function and drainage. Promptly report drainage that is bright red and excessive in amount (> 70 mL/h) or purulent. Maintain patency of chest tubes per unit protocol or physician's order. *If a thoracic incision has been used, chest tubes are placed to promote lung reinflation. Proper chest tube function is necessary to prevent pneumothorax and impaired lung inflation.*
- Monitor cardiopulmonary status and hemodynamic pressures. Administer intravenous fluids and fluid boluses as ordered. *Fluid volume imbalances that compromise cardiopulmonary status may develop following esophagectomy. Maintaining adequate fluid intake and preventing fluid overload are important postoperatively. The client also is at risk for acute respiratory distress syndrome, a critical complication that can further compromise ventilation, gas exchange, and circulation.*
- Do not move or manipulate the nasogastric tube. Maintain low gastric suction as ordered. *Manipulating or moving the nasogastric tube may disrupt suture lines, resulting in a leak into the mediastinum.*
- Verify enteral tube feeding placement by checking the pH of gastric aspirate (see Chapter 22 ∞). Stop enteral feedings if feelings of fullness or nausea occur. Suction gastrointestinal contents as needed, positioning the client on the side. *Overdistention of the stomach or delayed gastric emptying may result in regurgitation of stomach contents. Nausea or a feeling of fullness may indicate stomach overdistention. Suctioning and positioning limit the risk of aspiration.*

Anticipatory Grieving

Upon a diagnosis of cancer, the client and family may experience a grief reaction. The pessimistic prognosis associated with esophageal cancer and the disruptions in relationships may result in an intense sense of loss. Chapter 5 ∞ discusses care of client experiencing grief and loss.

Community-Based Care

Most care for clients with esophageal cancer is provided in community-based and home settings. Include the following topics in client and family teaching for home care:

- Planned treatment options including the risks, benefits, and potential adverse effects of each
- Wound and follow-up care following surgery
- Prevention and manifestations of complications such as wound or chest infection, anastomosis leak, deep venous thrombosis

- How to prepare, implement, and care for tube feedings or home parenteral nutrition.

Based on the client's needs and prognosis, referral to a home health agency and/or hospice may be appropriate.

DISORDERS OF THE STOMACH AND DUODENUM

The stomach and upper small intestine (duodenum and jejunum) are responsible for the majority of food digestion. The major disorders that affect digestion are nausea and vomiting, gastritis, peptic ulcer disease, and cancer of the stomach. Nursing roles in managing these disorders include both acute care for the hospitalized client and teaching to give the client the skills and knowledge to manage these conditions at home.

OVERVIEW OF NORMAL PHYSIOLOGY

Normally, the stomach is protected from the digestive substances it secretes—namely, hydrochloric acid and pepsin—by the **gastric mucosal barrier**. The gastric mucosal barrier includes:

- An impermeable hydrophobic lipid layer that covers gastric epithelial cells. This lipid layer prevents diffusion of water-soluble molecules, but substances such as aspirin and alcohol can diffuse through it.
- Bicarbonate ions secreted in response to hydrochloric acid secretion by the parietal cells of the stomach. When bicarbonate (HCO_3^-) secretion is equal to hydrogen ion (H^+) secretion, the gastric mucosa remains intact. Prostaglandins, chemical messengers involved in the inflammatory response, support bicarbonate production and blood flow to the gastric mucosa.
- Mucous gel that protects the surface of the stomach lining from the damaging effects of pepsin and traps bicarbonate to neutralize hydrochloric acid. This gel also acts as a lubricant, preventing mechanical damage to the stomach lining from its contents.

When an acute or chronic irritant disrupts the mucosal barrier, or when disease alters the processes that maintain the barrier, the gastric mucosa becomes irritated and inflamed. Lipid-soluble substances such as aspirin and alcohol penetrate the gastric mucosal barrier, leading to irritation and possible inflammation. Bile acids also break down the lipids in the mucosal barrier, increasing the potential for irritation (Porth, 2005). In addition, aspirin and other nonsteroidal anti-inflammatory drugs (NSAIDs) inhibit prostaglandins. Aspirin and NSAIDs also alter the nature of gastric mucus, affecting its protective function.

THE CLIENT WITH NAUSEA AND VOMITING

Nausea and vomiting are common gastrointestinal symptoms. **Nausea** is a vague, but unpleasant sensation of sickness or queasiness. It may or may not be accompanied by (and possibly relieved by) vomiting. **Vomiting** is the forceful expulsion of the contents of the upper gastrointestinal tract resulting from contraction of muscles in the gut and abdominal wall. Nausea and vomiting without abdominal pain are commonly associated with food poisoning, infectious gastroenteritis (discussed in Chapter 26 ∞), gallbladder disease, or ingestion of toxins (such as drugs or alcohol). When associated with severe abdominal pain, they may indicate a serious disorder such as peritonitis, acute gastrointestinal obstruction, or pancreatitis.

Pathophysiology

Nausea, an unpleasant subjective sensation, occurs when the vomiting center in the medulla of the brain is stimulated. Distention of the duodenum is a common stimulus for nausea. The vomiting center can be stimulated by input from several different sources:

- The gastrointestinal tract produced by distention, irritation, or infection
- The vestibular system of the ear
- Higher central nervous system centers in response to certain sights, smells, or emotional experiences
- Chemoreceptors outside the blood–brain barrier that are stimulated by drugs, chemotherapeutic agents, toxins, systemic disorders, and pregnancy
- Disorders such as acute myocardial infarction and heart failure commonly produce nausea and vomiting, possibly due to direct stimulation of the vomiting center by hypoxia
- Increased intracranial pressure (e.g., due to intracranial bleeding or a tumor) produces vomiting that may or may not be accompanied by nausea.

Anorexia, loss of appetite, commonly precedes nausea, just as nausea frequently precedes vomiting. Vomiting, a response that requires coordinated movements of the thorax and abdominal wall, the gut, the pharynx, and muscles of the mouth and face, is coordinated by the brainstem. *Emesis* (or *vomitus*) is produced when inspiratory muscles of the thorax (including the diaphragm) and abdomen contract, increasing intrathoracic and intra-abdominal pressures. The gastroesophageal sphincter relaxes, and the larynx moves upward to facilitate oral expulsion of gastric contents.

In addition to the subjective sensation of queasiness, nausea frequently is accompanied by autonomic nervous system manifestations such as pallor, sweating, tachycardia, and increased salivation. Vomiting, which stimulates the vagus nerve and parasympathetic nervous system, may be accompanied by dizziness, light-headedness, hypotension, and bradycardia.

Potential complications of vomiting include dehydration, hypokalemia, metabolic alkalosis (from loss of hydrochloric acid from the stomach), aspiration with resulting pneumonia, and rupture or tears of the esophagus.

INTERDISCIPLINARY CARE

In most cases, nausea and vomiting are self-limited and require no treatment. If vomiting is severe or accompanied by other symptoms, acute care may be required to determine the underlying problem and prevent or treat complications.

Diagnostic tests may include serum electrolytes; pregnancy testing if indicated; liver, pancreatic, and renal function studies; and imaging studies (flat plate of the abdomen, abdominal CT scan) to detect gastrointestinal obstruction. An upper endoscopy may be performed (see Chapter 21 ∞ for nursing care of the client undergoing upper endoscopy). CT scan or MRI of the head may be ordered if an intracranial problem is suspected as the cause. Specialized testing such as gastrointestinal motility studies may be indicated when other diagnostic studies are negative for an anatomic cause of nausea and vomiting.

Food is initially withheld, although clear liquids in small quantities are encouraged to prevent dehydration. Dry foods such as soda crackers also may reduce nausea and promote comfort.

Medications

Unless vomiting is associated with pregnancy, antiemetic medications may be prescribed to prevent or control nausea and vomiting. These drugs fall into several different classes, and often are more effective when given in combination.

- Serotonin receptor antagonists are the most effective drugs available for clients experiencing nausea and vomiting due to chemotherapy. They are effective when given only once or twice a day, an additional advantage. Drugs within this class include ondansetron (Zofran), granisetron (Kytril), and dolasetron (Anzemet).
- Dopamine antagonists include the phenothiazines (e.g., prochlorperazine [Compazine], promethazine [Phenergan], thiethylperazine [Torcan]), butyrophenones (haloperidol [Haldol] and droperidol [Inapsine]), and other drugs such as metoclopramide (Reglan). These drugs, while effective, can produce extrapyramidal symptoms, sedation, and hypotension.
- Antihistamines such as meclizine (Antivert), hydroxyzine (Vistaril, Atarax), and dimenhydrinate (Dramamine) are primarily used to treat nausea and vomiting arising from vestibular center stimuli (e.g., motion sickness).
- Two drugs classed as cannabinoids, related to marijuana, are approved to treat nausea and vomiting associated with chemotherapy. These drugs, dronabinol (Marinol) and nabilone (Cesamet), may produce unpleasant psychiatric effects such as dissociation and dysphoria, and are contraindicated for clients with psychiatric disorders. They also may produce tachycardia and hypotension.
- While corticosteroids are not approved as a class for treating nausea and vomiting, two drugs in this class, methylprednisolone (Solu-Medrol) and dexamethasone (Decadron), may be used in combination to treat vomiting associated with cancer treatment.
- Lorazepam (Ativan) is a benzodiazepine drug approved for use as an antiemetic. It produces a degree of sedation, but can suppress anticipatory vomiting (e.g., before chemotherapy).

It also helps control extrapyramidal symptoms associated with the phenothiazine antiemetics (dopamine antagonists).

Nursing responsibilities and client education for antiemetic drugs are outlined in the accompanying Medication Administration box.

Complementary and Alternative Medicine

Mind–body interventions such as biofeedback, guided imagery, music therapy, and hypnosis may be effective for some clients with nausea. Biofeedback uses machinery to translate physiologic processes into audible or visible signals to teach the client to exert conscious control over those processes. In guided imagery, the client uses imagination to invoke specific images to modify physiologic responses. Music therapy employs creating or listening to music to affect physiologic and psychologic responses. In hypnosis, an altered mind state is induced to make the client receptive to suggestions.

Ginger, an aromatic root frequently used in cooking, may also be helpful in relieving nausea and vomiting, particularly when due to motion sickness (Fontaine, 2005; Spencer & Jacobs, 2003). In limited clinical trials, it also has been shown to be safe for reducing nausea associated with pregnancy. It may also help relieve nausea associated with cancer chemotherapy. Ginger can inhibit platelet aggregation, and may increase the risk of bleeding in clients taking antiplatelet or anticoagulant drugs (Lehne, 2004).

NURSING CARE

Assessment of the client is vital to help determine the cause of nausea and vomiting, and to rule out underlying systemic disease or acute conditions that require immediate care (e.g., bowel obstruction). When the cause is known or no other acute symptoms are present, nursing interventions can promote comfort and prevent complications.

Nausea

The nursing diagnosis of nausea is defined as a subjective, unpleasant, wavelike sensation in the throat, epigastric region, or abdomen that may lead to vomiting (Wilkinson, 2005).

- Monitor subjective complaints of nausea. *Nausea is a subjective sensation best described by the client.*
- Monitor vital signs, skin turgor and condition, and weight. Maintain accurate intake and output records. Monitor amount, color, and specific gravity of urine. *Nausea can cause aversion to food and fluids, leading to dehydration even when it is not accompanied by vomiting.*
- Administer antiemetic medication as ordered, prior to meals and before treatments or procedures known to stimulate nausea. *Preventing nausea is particularly important for clients receiving chemotherapy, to avoid the association between the treatment and nausea.*
- Instruct to deep breathe to voluntarily suppress the vomiting reflex. *Controlling vomiting helps prevent dehydration and other complications associated with prolonged or severe vomiting.*
- Instruct to consume small quantities of clear fluids and dry foods at separate times. *Separating the intake of dry foods and fluids helps reduce the nausea stimulus.*

MEDICATION ADMINISTRATION **Drugs Used to Prevent and Treat Nausea and Vomiting**

SEROTONIN RECEPTOR ANTAGONISTS
Ondansetron (Zofran)
Granisetron (Kytril)
Dolasetron (Anzemet)
The serotonin receptor antagonists suppress nausea and vomiting by blocking the effect of serotonin on vagal afferent nerves that stimulate the vomiting center. Their primary uses are to prevent vomiting associated with chemotherapy, radiation therapy, and surgery.

Nursing Responsibilities
- Administer 30 to 60 minutes prior to chemotherapy or surgery as directed.
- May be given orally or intravenously (push or infusion; follow directions specific to the drug used).
- Monitor liver function and clotting studies; report abnormal levels to the physician.

Health Education for the Client and Family
- Take this drug exactly as directed.
- This drug may be taken without regard to food intake.
- Headache is a common side effect of these drugs, use acetaminophen or another mild analgesic as directed by your physician.

DOPAMINE ANTAGONISTS
Prochlorperazine (Compazine)
Promethazine (Phenergan)
Thiethylperazine (Torcan)
Haloperidol (Haldol)
Droperidol (Inapsine)
Metoclopramide (Reglan)
These drugs act by blocking dopamine receptors in the chemoreceptor trigger zone (CTZ). Their primary uses are to suppress nausea and vomiting associated with surgery, cancer chemotherapy, and toxins. The major adverse effects associated with these drugs are sedation, hypotension, and extrapyramidal reactions. Older adults are more sensitive to the effects of these drugs; a lower dose often is indicated.

Nursing Responsibilities
- Administer orally or parenterally as ordered before surgery or before meals and procedures known to produce nausea and vomiting.
- These drugs may interact with a number of other medications, often increasing their sedative and hypotensive effects.
- Administer with caution to older adults, closely monitoring for adverse effects such as confusion, agitation, changes in vital signs.
- Monitor for evidence of extrapyramidal symptoms, including tremor, restlessness, hyperactivity, anxiety, impaired coordination; notify physician if symptoms develop.

Health Education for the Client and Family
- Use the drug as ordered; do not increase your dose without consulting your primary care provider.
- These drugs may cause drowsiness. Avoid using other central nervous system (CNS) depressants such as alcohol while taking these drugs.
- Change positions from lying to sitting and sitting to standing slowly because these drugs can cause light-headedness or dizziness.

- Promptly report changes in coordination, tremors, difficulty speaking or swallowing, or weakness to your physician.

ANTIHISTAMINES
Meclizine (Antivert)
Hydroxyzine (Vistaril, Atarax)
Dimenhydrinate (Dramamine)
Antihistamines are primarily used to treat nausea and vomiting associated with motion sickness. They act by blocking histamine and acetylcholine (muscarinic) receptors in the neural pathway from the inner ear to the vomiting center in the brainstem.

Nursing Responsibilities
- Do not administer these drugs to clients for whom anticholinergic drugs are contraindicated: people with narrow-angle glaucoma, urinary retention, bowel obstruction.
- May be administered orally, parenterally, or rectally, depending on the preparation and the client's ability to tolerate oral preparations.
- Use with caution in clients who are taking other CNS depressants or antihistamine preparations, tricyclic antidepressants, or monoamine oxidase inhibitors.

Health Education for the Client and Family
- These drugs frequently cause drowsiness. Use caution when operating machinery or performing tasks requiring mental alertness.
- Avoid using alcohol or other substances that cause drowsiness or sedation while taking these drugs.
- The medication may cause dry mouth. Sips of water, ice chips, hard candies, and sugarless gum can be used for comfort.
- Use sunscreen and protective clothing to protect from sunburn while using these drugs.

CANNABINOIDS
Dronabinol (Marinol)
Nabilone (Cesamet)
Drugs in this class, which contain the same active ingredient as marijuana, are reserved for use to relieve nausea and vomiting associated with cancer chemotherapy in clients who have not responded to treatment with other antiemetics. Their action is thought to result from inhibition of the vomiting center in the medulla.

Nursing Responsibilities
- Use with caution in older adults and people with a history of cardiovascular disease or substance abuse. These drugs are contraindicated for clients with a history of psychiatric disorders.
- Monitor for adverse effects such as dizziness, tachycardia, hypotension, impaired thinking and judgment, incoordination, irritability, depersonalization, distorted vision, and hallucinations.

Health Education for the Client and Family
- Take the drug 1 to 3 hours before chemotherapy.
- Change positions slowly after taking this drug to prevent dizziness.
- You may experience distorted thinking, visual disturbances, confusion, and other mental symptoms while taking this drug.
- Keep this and all drugs out of the reach of children. Do not share this drug with anyone else.

Community-Based Care

Instruct the client to restrict intake to small quantities of clear liquids (tea, apple juice, broth, Jell-O) and dry foods such as soda crackers to help reduce nausea and prevent vomiting. Teach to avoid food-preparation odors if they produce nausea. Advise to restrict fluid intake for 1 hour before and after meals. Stress the need to maintain fluid intake to prevent dehydration and the importance of seeking additional medical help if unable to take in fluids or keep food down. Provide information about electrolyte replacement solutions such as sports drinks and commercially available electrolyte replacement solutions.

THE CLIENT WITH GASTROINTESTINAL BLEEDING

Because of its constant exposure to the environment, the gastrointestinal tract can be subjected to trauma, exposure to toxins, infection with pathogens such as *Helicobacter pylori*, inflammatory processes, and insults such as ischemia due to systemic diseases. While the mucosal lining of the GI tract is remarkably able to withstand these insults and heal rapidly, its rich supply of blood can result in significant bleeding when a vessel is eroded or abnormally distended (*varices*). Gastrointestinal hemorrhage is a relatively common admitting diagnosis and complication of critical illnesses. It is a medical emergency requiring aggressive medical and nursing care.

Although bleeding and hemorrhage can occur anywhere in the GI tract, the upper portion of the tract is more commonly affected. The three primary disorders leading to upper (UGI) hemorrhage are erosive gastritis, peptic ulcer disease, and esophageal varices. Erosive gastritis and peptic ulcer disease are discussed in the following sections of this chapter; esophageal varices, usually seen as a complication of cirrhosis of the liver, are discussed in Chapter 24 ∞.

FAST FACTS

- About 50% of UGI bleeds are due to peptic ulcer disease.
- Erosive gastritis is the second leading cause of UGI hemorrhage, responsible for about 20% of bleeds.
- The third leading cause, esophageal varices, has the highest mortality rate, between 40% and 70% (Urden et al., 2006).

Pathophysiology

Blood in the GI tract has several effects. It is irritating to the stomach, and typically leads to nausea and vomiting (**hematemasis**, vomiting blood). If the blood has been present in the stomach for a period of time and is partially digested, it may have a "coffee-grounds" appearance, rather than presenting as bright red blood. The accumulation of blood in the GI tract stimulates peristasis, leading to hyperactive bowel sounds and diarrhea. Stools may be black and tarry (**melena**) or frankly bloody (**hematochezia**); stool containing partially digested blood has a characteristic odor. With significant upper GI bleeding, digestion of blood proteins increases blood urea nitrogen (BUN) levels.

Physiologic responses to an upper GI bleed depend on the rapidity and magnitude of the blood loss. GI bleeding resulting from erosion of a small vessel typically is slow, and may not be identified until the client presents with manifestations of blood loss anemia due to depletion of iron stores. (See Chapter 34 ∞ for further discussion of blood loss anemia.) Although no visible blood may be present in the stool, **occult** (or hidden) **bleeding** may be detected by chemical means.

GI hemorrhage, with loss of a significant amount of blood within a few hours, rapidly depletes blood volume, producing manifestations of decreased cardiac output: tachycardia, hypotension, pallor, and decreased urine output. Peripheral blood vessels constrict to maintain perfusion of vital organs. Unless the blood volume is restored, hypovolemic shock progresses, leading to acidosis, renal failure, bowel infarction, acute coronary syndrome, coma, and death. See Chapter 11 ∞ for more information about shock and its management.

INTERDISCIPLINARY CARE

The acuity of the bleed and the client's condition dictate the timing and extent of diagnostic testing and interventions. A client with a massive GI hemorrhage is admitted to the critical care unit and aggressively treated to stem bleeding, restore blood volume, and stabilize the cardiovascular system. Identifying the cause of the bleeding is postponed in many cases until the client's condition has been stabilized.

When the bleeding is slow or chronic, diagnostic testing and treatment may be managed in a community-based setting.

Diagnosis

Diagnostic testing focuses on determining the extent and effects of the bleed, as well as its cause.

- A *complete blood count with hemoglobin and hematocrit* are obtained. In an acute bleed, the CBC, hemoglobin, and hematocrit may not initially indicate the extent of blood loss because plasma is lost along with blood cells.
- *Blood type and crossmatch* are performed to prepare for transfusion as necessary.
- *Serum electrolytes, osmolality*, and *BUN* are obtained to determine the effects of the blood loss and protein digestion on blood chemistries.
- *Liver function studies* and a *coagulation profile* may be obtained to help determine the cause of the bleeding.
- An *upper endoscopy* is performed as soon as possible to identify and, if possible, treat the source of bleeding. See Chapter 21 ∞ for nursing care of the client undergoing upper endoscopy.

Treatments

In acute GI hemorrhage, initial treatment focuses on stemming the bleeding and restoring cardiovascular stability. Intravenous fluids such as normal saline or a balanced electrolyte solution are administered through a large-bore intravenous catheter. Fresh whole blood, which contains clotting factors, is administered to restore blood volume and components in an acute hemorrhage. In less acute situations, packed red cells may be administered to restore the oxygen-carrying capacity of the blood.

Hemostasis is achieved using upper endoscopy whenever possible. A sclerosing agent may be injected into the bleeding vessel, or the vessel may be sealed using a heated probe, electrocautery, or laser. Rarely, emergency surgery is required to stop hemorrhage.

GASTRIC LAVAGE **Gastric lavage**, washing out of stomach contents, may be done in clients with upper GI hemorrhage to remove blood from the GI tract, prevent vomiting, and prepare for upper endoscopy. See Procedure 23–1 for nursing responsibilities related to gastric lavage.

 # NURSING CARE

Health Promotion

Preventing gastrointestinal bleeding is the most important step in reducing the mortality and morbidity associated with an acute GI hemorrhage. Identifying clients at risk and instituting regular gastric pH monitoring and maintenance of drug therapy to reduce gastric acidity are important preventive measures. All critically ill clients should be considered to be at risk for stress-related erosive gastritis.

Assessment

Assessment of the client experiencing an acute GI hemorrhage is very focused on the immediate crisis. The ability to obtain subjective information may be limited; however, it is important to identify possible contributing factors such as use of aspirin, other platelet inhibitors, or anticoagulant medications and the presence of any acute or chronic conditions that may contribute to bleeding (e.g., hypertension, a clotting disorder, peptic ulcer disease, chronic hepatitis, or cirrhosis of the liver). If possible, identify all current medications and their purpose, as well as any allergies to medications or other substances.

Physical examination focuses on the effect of the bleeding on cardiovascular status. Obtain vital signs and orthostatic vital signs (an early sign of hypovolemia). Place the acutely ill client on a cardiac monitor and obtain a rhythm strip. Obtain oxygen saturation level. Assess peripheral pulse strength, as well as color, temperature, and capillary refill of extremities. Evaluate mental status, including level of consciousness and orientation. An indwelling catheter may be inserted to evaluate urine output.

Nursing Diagnoses and Interventions

Nursing care priorities for the client with an acute GI bleed focus on restoring and maintaining an effective cardiac output and tissue perfusion, and on stopping the hemorrhage and preventing further bleeding.

Decreased Cardiac Output

Significant amounts of blood may be lost in a very short time with an acute GI hemorrhage. Because some of the blood enters the bowel, it may be difficult to accurately estimate the amount of blood lost by measuring emesis, gastric suction return, and blood expelled as feces. As blood volume drops, venous return decreases. The heart rate increases to maintain the cardiac output, and peripheral blood vessels constrict to improve venous return and cardiac output.

- Frequently assess and document vital signs, including blood pressure, pulse rate and cardiac rhythm, respiratory rate, and oxygen saturation levels. Obtain hemodynamic pressure measurements as ordered, reporting trends and changes. *The vital signs, oxygen saturation levels, and hemodynamic pressure values provide indicators of the effectiveness of peripheral tissue perfusion, oxygenation, and fluid replacement.*
- Monitor for and report changes in skin color, temperature, and moisture, or slow capillary refill. *Peripheral vasoconstriction and activation of the sympathetic nervous system typically cause pale, cool, and moist or diaphoretic skin. Development of cyanosis or mottling indicates a further decrease in tissue perfusion and oxygenation.*
- Insert an indwelling urinary catheter and measure urine output hourly. Report an output of less than 30 mL for two consecutive hours. *A fall in urine output may indicate further reduction in cardiac output. As cardiac output falls, the kidneys become ischemic and acute renal failure may develop.*
- Unless contraindicated, insert a nasogastric tube and connect to low suction. Measure gastric output hourly unless otherwise directed. *Measuring gastric output provides information about the amount of blood and fluid lost. This information helps determine fluid and blood replacement needs.*
- Maintain two peripheral intravenous lines with large-bore catheters or a central venous catheter for fluid and blood administration as ordered. Frequently monitor vital signs, respiratory status, and hemodynamic pressure measurements, reporting changes in status. *Rapid administration of isotonic intravenous fluids, blood, and blood products can lead to fluid overload and potential heart failure.*
- Replace gastric drainage with balanced electrolyte intravenous solutions as ordered. *GI losses are replaced in addition to fluids given to meet daily requirements to prevent fluid volume deficiency.*

Impaired Tissue Integrity: Gastrointestinal

- Maintain gastric suction and drainage and patency of nasogastric tube. *Blood is irritating to the GI tract, precipitating vomiting and stimulating peristalsis, leading to diarrhea. In addition, digested blood can increase BUN levels, potentially leading to confusion and altered mental status.*
- Irrigate the nasogastric tube with room temperature saline or tap water as ordered. Calculate intake and output, subtracting the amount of irrigant from gastric output. *Irrigation of the nasogastric tube helps remove irritating blood from the gut and produces a degree of vasoconstriction in stomach mucosa, slowing bleeding.*
- Prepare for upper endoscopy or surgery as planned. *Endoscopy or emergency surgery may be performed to repair the bleeding site or sclerose bleeding vessels.*
- Following an acute bleed and in clients at risk for GI bleeding, monitor gastric pH as ordered and check vomitus and feces for the presence of occult blood. Maintain infusions of drugs to reduce gastric acidity as ordered. *The client remains*

PROCEDURE 23-1 GASTRIC LAVAGE

When it is important to remove or dilute gastric contents rapidly, gastric lavage (irrigation or washing out of the stomach) may be indicated. In acute poisoning or ingestion of a caustic substance, a large-bore 30- to 36-Fre. nasogastric tube is inserted, and lavage performed. An 18-Fr. nasogastric tube may be used when the procedure is performed to remove blood from the upper GI tract. Because the GI tract is not sterile, clean technique is appropriate for use, although the solution used will generally be sterile.

- Obtain baseline assessment, including vital signs, abdominal inspection, girth, and bowel sounds. *It is important to have assessment data documented prior to instituting the procedure for comparison.*
- Explain the procedure, answering questions and clarifying perceptions. Instruct to report any pain, difficulty breathing, or other problems during the procedure. *A client who is able to understand and cooperate with the procedure will tolerate lavage better. The client may be aware of symptoms of complications such as perforation or tube displacement before they are evident to the nurse.*
- Place in semi-Fowler's or Fowler's position. If unable to tolerate elevation of the head of the bed because of hypotension, place in left side-lying position. *Elevating of the head of the bed or side-lying position will minimize the risk of aspiration.*
- Insert a nasogastric tube if one is not already in place. Verify tube placement by aspirating gastric contents and test pH of aspirate. *Proper placement is vital to prevent aspiration or overdistention of the small bowel with irrigating solution.*
- Irrigate the stomach, using either a closed or an open system technique.

CLOSED-SYSTEM IRRIGATION

- Wearing clean gloves, connect bag or bottle of normal saline irrigating solution to nasogastric tube using a Y connector. Attach drainage or suction tube to other arm of connector (Figure 23–7 ■). Empty the stomach, clamp drain tube or turn off suction, and allow 50 to 200 mL of solution to run into stomach by gravity. Stop solution and

allow to drain or suction out. Repeat until ordered amount has been used or desired results are obtained, for example, no further clots and solution returns clear or light pink. Measure the amount of drainage, subtracting the amount of irrigant instilled, to obtain gastric output. *The closed system minimizes the risk of contact with body fluids for the nurse. Measuring gastric output is important in monitoring fluid balance.*

INTERMITTENT OPEN SYSTEM

- Wearing clean gloves and other personal protective equipment as necessary (gown and face protection), empty the stomach using suction or a 50-mL catheter-tip syringe. Measure and discard the aspirate. Using the syringe, draw up approximately 50 mL of irrigation solution, and instill it using gentle pressure. Aspirate the nasogastric tube, and discard the solution into a measuring container. Continue this procedure until the desired amount of irrigant or desired results have been obtained. *Manual irrigation with a catheter-tip syringe may be more effective than gravity flow in removing clots from the stomach and nasogastric tube.*
- Continue to monitor vital signs (including temperature), tolerance of the procedure, and other assessment data. *The client may be unstable and require continuous reevaluation. Gastric lavage may cause hypothermia; therefore, monitor temperature and indications of hypothermia, such as lethargy and changes in cardiac rate and rhythm.*
- If the aspirate has not cleared to light pink or pink tinged after 20 to 30 minutes of lavage or if the client is unable to tolerate the procedure, notify the physician. *Medical or surgical intervention may be necessary to stop hemorrhage in some instances.*
- On completion of lavage, provide mouth and nares care. Continue to monitor vital signs, abdominal status, and other assessment data.
- Document the procedure, including the amount and type of irrigant used, gastric output character and amount, and the client's condition and tolerance of the procedure.

Figure 23–7 ■ The client with a closed-system gastric lavage.

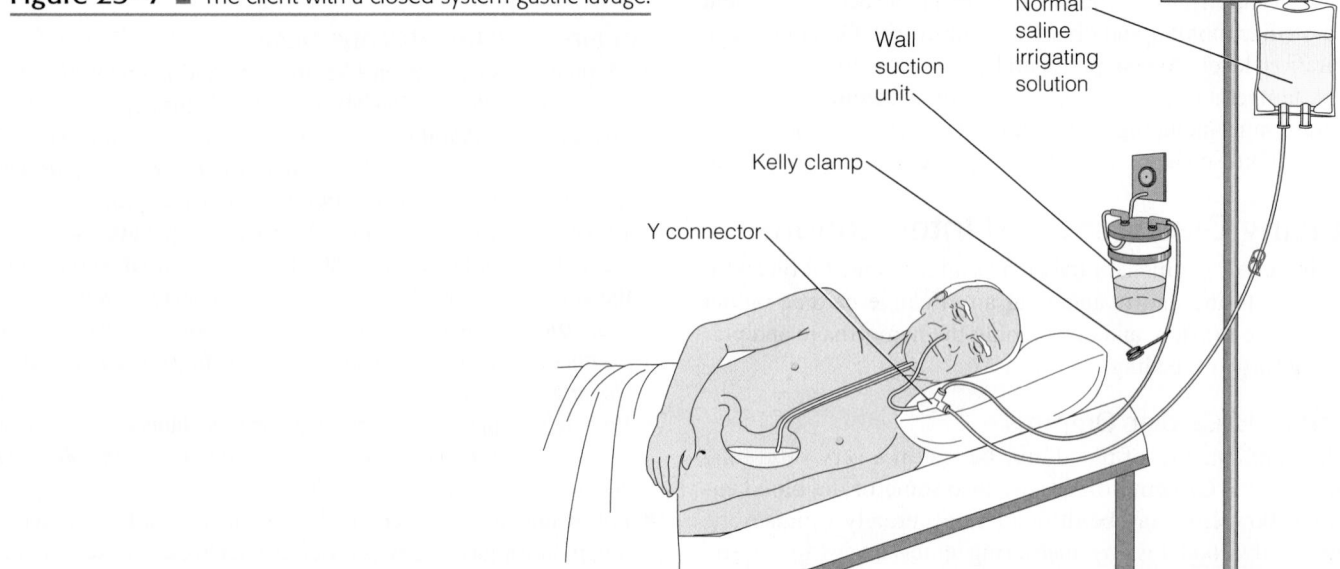

Normal saline irrigating solution

Wall suction unit

Kelly clamp

Y connector

at risk for GI bleeding. Monitoring for occult blood helps identify slow bleeding or recurrent hemorrhage. Reducing the acidity of gastric secretions reduces irritation of the gastric mucosa, reducing the risk of bleeding.

Community-Based Care

Following an acute GI hemorrhage, continuing care focuses on resolving the underlying disease process if possible and preventing future episodes of GI bleeding. If a bleeding gastric ulcer was identified, testing for *H. pylori* infection will be done, and a treatment regimen prescribed to eradicate the infection (see the section on peptic ulcer disease later in this chapter). The client who experienced an episode of erosive stress gastritis will often be discharged with instructions to continue taking a gastric acid–reducing medication and avoid known gastric irritants such as aspirin and alcohol. The client with esophageal varices due to cirrhosis or chronic hepatitis needs additional instructions. See Chapter 24 ∞.

Clients with minor or slow GI bleeding often are managed in the community. Provide teaching about the cause of the bleeding and measures to prevent future episodes. Provide verbal and written instructions for prescribed medications such as acid reducers and oral iron supplements. Discuss appropriate nutrition; while a special diet to "soothe the stomach" rarely is indicated, foods rich in iron may be recommended to treat the resulting anemia.

Discuss indicators of GI bleeding to be reported to the physician. If the source of bleeding has not been identified, provide instructions about prescribed follow-up diagnostic testing.

THE CLIENT WITH GASTRITIS

Gastritis, inflammation of the stomach lining, results from irritation of the gastric mucosa. Gastritis is common, and may be caused by a variety of factors. The most common form of gastritis, **acute gastritis**, is generally a benign, self-limiting disorder associated with the ingestion of gastric irritants such as aspirin, alcohol, caffeine, or foods contaminated with certain bacteria. Manifestations of acute gastritis may range from asymptomatic to mild heartburn to severe gastric distress, vomiting, and bleeding with hematemesis (vomiting blood).

Chronic gastritis is a separate group of disorders characterized by progressive and irreversible changes in the gastric mucosa (Porth, 2005). Chronic gastritis is more common in the elderly, chronic alcoholics, and cigarette smokers. When symptoms of chronic gastritis occur, they are often vague, ranging from a feeling of heaviness in the epigastric region after meals to gnawing, burning, ulcer-like epigastric pain unrelieved by antacids.

Pathophysiology

Acute Gastritis

Acute gastritis is characterized by disruption of the mucosal barrier by a local irritant. This disruption allows hydrochloric acid and pepsin to come into contact with the gastric tissue, resulting in irritation, inflammation, and superficial erosions. The gastric mucosa rapidly regenerates, generally making acute gastritis a self-limiting disorder, with resolution and healing occurring within several days.

The ingestion of aspirin or other NSAIDs, corticosteroids, alcohol, and caffeine is commonly associated with the development of acute gastritis. Accidental or purposeful ingestion of a corrosive alkali (such as ammonia, lye, Lysol, and other cleaning agents) or acid leads to severe inflammation and possible necrosis of the stomach. Gastric perforation, hemorrhage, and peritonitis are possible results. Iatrogenic causes of acute gastritis include radiation therapy and administration of certain chemotherapeutic agents.

Erosive Gastritis

A severe form of acute gastritis, **erosive** or **stress-induced gastritis**, occurs as a complication of other life-threatening conditions such as shock, severe trauma, major surgery, sepsis, burns, or head injury. When these erosions follow a major burn, they are called **Curling's ulcers**, after Thomas Curling, a British physician, who first described them in 1842. When stress ulcers occur following head injury or CNS surgery, they are referred to as **Cushing's ulcers**, after Harvey Cushing, a U.S. surgeon.

The primary mechanisms leading to erosive gastritis appear to be ischemia of the gastric mucosa resulting from sympathetic vasoconstriction, and tissue injury due to gastric acid. As a result, multiple superficial erosions of the gastric mucosa develop. Maintaining the gastric pH at greater than 3.5 and inhibiting gastric acid secretion with medications help prevent erosive gastritis.

MANIFESTATIONS The client with acute gastritis may have mild symptoms such as **anorexia** (loss of appetite), or mild epigastric discomfort relieved by belching or defecating. More severe manifestations include abdominal pain, nausea, and vomiting. Gastric bleeding may occur, with hematemesis or melena (black, tarry stool that contains blood). Erosive gastritis is not typically associated with pain. The initial symptom often is painless gastric bleeding occurring 2 or more days after the initial stressor. Bleeding typically is minimal, but can be massive. Corrosive gastritis can cause severe bleeding, signs of shock, and an *acute abdomen* (severely painful, rigid, boardlike abdomen) if perforation occurs. See the Manifestations box below.

MANIFESTATIONS of Acute and Chronic Gastritis

ACUTE GASTRITIS

Gastrointestinal
- Anorexia
- Nausea and vomiting
- Hematemesis
- Melena
- Abdominal pain

Systemic
- Possible shock

CHRONIC GASTRITIS

Gastrointestinal
- Vague discomfort after eating; may be asymptomatic

Systemic
- Anemia
- Fatigue

Chronic Gastritis

Unrelated to acute gastritis, chronic gastritis is a progressive disorder that begins with superficial inflammation and gradually leads to atrophy of gastric tissues. The initial stage is characterized by superficial changes in the gastric mucosa and a decrease in mucus. As the disease evolves, glands of the gastric mucosa are disrupted and destroyed. The inflammatory process involves deep portions of the mucosa, which thins and atrophies. There appear to be at least two different forms of chronic gastritis, classified as type A and type B.

Type A gastritis, the less common form of chronic gastritis, usually affects people of Northern European heritage. This type of gastritis is thought to have an autoimmune component. In type A or autoimmune gastritis, the body produces antibodies to parietal cells and to intrinsic factor. These antibodies destroy gastric mucosal cells, resulting in tissue atrophy and the loss of hydrochloric acid and pepsin secretion. Because intrinsic factor is required for the absorption of vitamin B_{12}, this immune response also results in pernicious anemia. For further discussion of pernicious anemia, see Chapter 34 ∞.

Type B gastritis is the more common form of chronic gastritis. Its incidence increases with age, reaching nearly 100% in people over the age of 70. Type B gastritis is caused by chronic infection of the gastric mucosa by *H. pylori,* a gram-negative spiral bacterium. *H. pylori* infection causes inflammation of the gastric mucosa, with infiltration by neutrophils and lymphocytes. The outermost layer of gastric mucosa thins and atrophies, providing a less effective barrier against the autodigestive properties of hydrochloric acid and pepsin.

Infection with *H. pylori* also is associated with an increased risk for peptic ulcer disease. *H. pylori* infection significantly increases the risk of developing gastric cancer. See the sections that follow for more information about these disorders.

MANIFESTATIONS Chronic gastritis is often asymptomatic until atrophy is sufficiently advanced to interfere with digestion and gastric emptying. The client may complain of vague gastric distress, epigastric heaviness after meals, or ulcer-like symptoms. These symptoms typically are not relieved by antacids. In addition, the client may experience fatigue and other symptoms of anemia. If intrinsic factor is lacking, paresthesias and other neurologic manifestations of vitamin B_{12} deficiency may be present. See the Manifestations box on previous page.

INTERDISCIPLINARY CARE

Acute gastritis is usually diagnosed by the history and clinical presentation. In contrast, the vague symptoms of chronic gastritis may require more extensive diagnostic testing.

Clients with acute and chronic gastritis are generally managed in community settings. The client requires acute care only when nausea and vomiting are severe enough to interfere with normal fluid and electrolyte balance and nutritional status. If hemorrhage results, surgical intervention may be required.

Diagnosis

Diagnostic tests that may be ordered for the client with gastritis include the following:

- *Gastric analysis* to assess hydrochloric acid secretion. A nasogastric tube is passed into the stomach, and pentagastrin is injected subcutaneously to stimulate gastric secretion of hydrochloric acid. Secretion may be decreased in clients with chronic gastritis.
- *Hemoglobin, hematocrit,* and *red blood cell (RBC) indices* are evaluated for evidence of anemia. The client with gastritis may develop pernicious anemia because of parietal cell destruction, or iron-deficiency anemia because of chronic blood loss.
- *Serum vitamin B_{12} levels* are measured to evaluate for possible pernicious anemia. Normal values for vitamin B_{12} are 200 to 1000 pg/mL, with lower levels seen in older adults.
- *Upper endoscopy* may be done to inspect the gastric mucosa for changes, identify areas of bleeding, and obtain tissue for biopsy. Bleeding sites may be treated with electro- or laser coagulation or injected with a sclerosing agent during the procedure. See the Diagnostic Tests box on page 615 in Chapter 21 ∞ for client preparation and teaching related to an upper endoscopy.

Medications

Drugs such as a PPI, H_2-receptor blocker, or sucralfate may be ordered to prevent or treat acute stress gastritis. PPIs and H_2-receptor blockers reduce the amount or effects of hydrochloric acid on the gastric mucosa. Lansoprazole (Prevacid), esomeprazole (Nexium), and omeprazole (Prilosec) are examples of PPIs. H_2-receptor blockers include cimetidine (Tagamet), ranitidine (Zantac), famotidine (Pepcid), and nizatidine (Axid). These drugs also are available in nonprescription strength. Sucralfate (Carafate) works locally to prevent the damaging effects of acid and pepsin on gastric tissue. It does not neutralize or reduce acid secretion. Nursing implications for drugs commonly used in managing gastritis are included in the Medication Administration box on pages 665–666.

The client with type B chronic gastritis may be treated to eradicate the *H. pylori* infection. This generally involves combination therapy consisting of two antibiotics (such as metronidazole and clarithromycin or tetracycline) and a PPI. In some cases, eradication of the infection is not warranted, and the client is treated symptomatically.

Treatments

In acute gastritis, gastrointestinal tract rest is provided by 6 to 12 hours of NPO status, then slow reintroduction of clear liquids (broth, tea, gelatin, carbonated beverages), followed by ingestion of heavier liquids (cream soups, puddings, milk), and finally a gradual reintroduction of solid food.

If nausea and vomiting threaten fluid and electrolyte balance, intravenous fluids and electrolytes are ordered.

GASTRIC LAVAGE Acute gastritis resulting from ingestion of a poisonous or corrosive substance (acid or strong alkali) is treated with immediate dilution and removal of the substance.

Vomiting is not induced because it might further damage the esophagus and possibly the trachea; instead, gastric lavage, washing out of the stomach contents, is performed. See Procedure 23–1.

COMPLEMENTARY THERAPIES Complementary therapies such as herbal remedies or aromatherapy may be appropriate to recommend for clients with gastritis. Refer the client to a healthcare provider trained in natural and herbal remedies or to an aromatherapist for an individualized treatment plan. Recommendations may include:

- Chamomile tea or the essential oil used in aromatherapy
- Garlic; one clove chopped fine and taken daily at bedtime
- Ginger, powdered or in capsules or made into a tea taken before or after meals
- Mint oil aromatherapy via a diffuser, in a bath, or diluted with a carrier oil and used for a soothing massage.

NURSING CARE

Health Promotion

Teach all clients and community members about measures to prevent acute gastritis. Food contaminated with bacteria is a significant cause of acute gastritis. Discuss food safety measures such as fully cooking meats and egg products, and promptly refrigerating foods after cooking to avoid bacterial growth. Stress that food contaminated with potential pathogens often looks, smells, and tastes good, making it difficult to identify. Teach clients to abstain from eating or drinking anything during an acute episode of vomiting, then reintroduce clear liquids gradually once vomiting has stopped (2 to 4 hours after the last episode of vomiting). Suggest using liquids such as Pedialyte or a sport drink to replace lost electrolytes and fluid. Instruct clients to avoid milk and milk products until they easily tolerate clear liquids and solid foods such as dry toast or saltine crackers.

Assessment

Assessment data to collect for clients with acute or chronic gastritis include the following:

- *Health history:* Current symptoms and their duration; relieving and aggravating factors; history of ingestion of toxins, contaminated food, alcohol, aspirin, or NSAIDs; other medications.
- *Physical examination:* Vital signs including orthostatic vitals if indicated; peripheral pulses; general appearance; abdominal assessment including appearance, bowel sounds, and tenderness.

Nursing Diagnoses and Interventions

In planning and implementing nursing care for the client with acute or chronic gastritis, consider both the direct effects of the disorder on the gastrointestinal system and nutritional status as well as its effects on lifestyle and psychosocial integrity. This section focuses on problems of fluid balance and nutrition.

Deficient Fluid Volume

Nausea, vomiting, and abdominal distress are the primary manifestations of acute gastritis. The risk for fluid and electrolyte imbalance is high because of inadequate intake of food and fluids, and abnormal losses of fluids and electrolytes with vomiting.

- Monitor and record vital signs at least every 2 hours until stable, then every 4 hours. Check for orthostatic hypotension.

> **PRACTICE ALERT**
> Tachycardia, tachypnea, and hypotension, especially orthostatic hypotension, may indicate fluid volume deficit. Electrolyte or acid–base imbalances resulting from vomiting may cause cardiac dysrhythmias or changes in respirations.

- Weigh daily. Monitor and record intake and output; record urine output every 1 to 4 hours as indicated. *Daily weights are an accurate indicator of fluid volume. Urine output of less than 30 mL per hour indicates decreased cardiac output and a need for prompt fluid replacement.*
- Monitor skin turgor, color, and condition and status of oral mucous membranes frequently. Provide skin and mouth care frequently. *Skin turgor and mucous membrane assessments indicate hydration status. Good skin and mouth care are necessary to maintain skin and mucous membrane integrity.*
- Monitor laboratory values for electrolytes and acid–base balance. Report significant changes or deviations from normal. *Electrolytes are lost through vomiting, increasing the risk of electrolyte and acid–base imbalances. These imbalances, in turn, affect multiple body systems.*
- Administer oral or parenteral fluids as ordered. *Oral fluids may be withheld until vomiting has ceased, then gradually reintroduced. Intravenous fluids restore or maintain hydration until adequate oral intake is resumed.*
- Administer antiemetic and other drugs as ordered to relieve vomiting and facilitate oral feeding. Encourage fluids as soon as feasible. *The oral route is preferred for fluid and nutrient intake; medications may be used to allow earlier resumption of feeding.*

> **PRACTICE ALERT**
> Ensure safety: Place call light within reach, put up the side rails, instruct client to avoid getting up without assistance. Orthostatic hypotension may lead to syncope and to falls if the client attempts to get up without assistance.

Imbalanced Nutrition: Less than Body Requirements

Manifestations of chronic gastritis may lead to reduced food intake and malnutrition. The client often associates these unpleasant sensations with eating, and may gradually reduce food intake. Associated anorexia also contributes to poor food intake.

- Monitor and record food and fluid intake and any abnormal losses (such as vomiting). *Careful monitoring can help in developing a dietary plan to meet the caloric needs of the client.*

- Monitor weight and laboratory studies such as serum albumin, hemoglobin, and RBC indices. *Weights and laboratory values provide data regarding nutritional status and the effectiveness of interventions.*
- Arrange for dietary consultation to determine caloric and nutrient needs and develop a dietary plan. Consider food preferences and tolerances in menu planning. *A diet high in protein, vitamins, and minerals may be prescribed to meet nutritional needs of the client with chronic gastritis. In addition, specific food intolerances may need to be considered. Planning to include preferred foods in the diet helps ensure consumption of the prescribed diet.*
- Provide nutritional supplements between meals or frequent small feedings as needed. *Many clients with chronic gastritis tolerate small, frequent feedings better than three large meals per day.*
- Maintain tube feedings or parenteral nutrition as ordered. Refer to Chapter 22 ∞ for further information on enteral and parenteral feedings.

Community-Based Care

Because acute or chronic gastritis is usually managed in community-based settings, teaching is vital. For the client with acute gastritis, teaching focuses on managing acute symptoms, reintroducing fluids and solid foods, identifying indicators of possible complications (e.g., continued vomiting, signs of fluid and electrolyte imbalance), and preventing future episodes.

Provide the following information for clients with chronic gastritis:

- Maintaining optimal nutrition
- Helpful dietary modifications
- Using prescribed medications
- Avoiding known gastric irritants, such as aspirin, alcohol, and cigarette smoking.

Referral to smoking cessation classes or programs to treat alcohol abuse may be necessary.

THE CLIENT WITH PEPTIC ULCER DISEASE

Peptic ulcer disease (PUD), a break in the mucous lining of the gastrointestinal tract where it comes in contact with gastric juice, is a chronic health problem. PUD affects approximately 10% of the population or 4 million people in the United States every year (Kasper et al., 2005; Tierney et al., 2005).

Peptic ulcers occur in any area of the gastrointestinal tract exposed to acid-pepsin secretions, including the esophagus, stomach, or duodenum. **Duodenal ulcers** are the most common. They usually develop between the ages of 30 and 55, and are more common in men than women. **Gastric ulcers** more often affect older clients, between the ages of 55 and 70. Ulcers are more common in people who smoke and who are chronic users of NSAIDs. Alcohol and dietary intake do not seem to cause PUD, and the role of stress is uncertain. Although the incidence of PUD has dramatically decreased, the incidence of gastric ulcers is increasing, believed due to the widespread use of NSAIDs (Tierney et al., 2005).

Risk Factors

Chronic *H. pylori* infection and use of aspirin and NSAIDs are the major risk factors for PUD. Contributing risk factors are listed in Box 23–4. Overall, an estimated one in six clients infected with *H. pylori* develops PUD. Of the NSAIDs, aspirin is the most ulcerogenic. A strong familial pattern suggests a genetic factor in the development of PUD. Cigarette smoking is a significant risk factor, doubling the risk of PUD. Cigarette smoking inhibits the secretion of bicarbonate by the pancreas and possibly causes more rapid transit of gastric acid into the duodenum.

Pathophysiology

The innermost layer of the stomach wall, the gastric mucosa, consists of columnar epithelial cells, supported by a middle layer of blood vessels and glands, and a thin outer layer of smooth muscle. The mucosal barrier of the stomach, a thin coating of mucous gel and bicarbonate, protects the gastric mucosa. The mucosal barrier is maintained by bicarbonate secreted by the epithelial cells, by mucous gel production stimulated by prostaglandins, and by an adequate blood supply to the mucosa (see the overview of normal physiology on page 671).

An **ulcer**, or break in the gastrointestinal mucosa, develops when the mucosal barrier is unable to protect the mucosa from damage by hydrochloric acid and pepsin, the gastric digestive juices. See the accompanying *Pathophysiology Illustrated: Peptic Ulcer Disease* on pages 682–683.

H. pylori infection, found in about 70% of people who have PUD, is unique in colonizing the stomach. It is spread person to person (oral–oral or fecal–oral), and contributes to ulcer formation in several ways. The bacteria produce enzymes that reduce the efficacy of mucous gel in protecting the gastric mucosa. In addition, the host's inflammatory response to *H. pylori* contributes to gastric epithelial cell damage without producing immunity to the infection. Although the gastric mucosa is the usual site for *H. pylori* infection, this infection also contributes to duodenal ulcers. This is possibly related to increased gastric acid production associated with *H. pylori* infection.

NSAIDs contribute to PUD through both systemic and topical mechanisms. Prostaglandins are necessary for maintaining the gastric mucosal barrier. NSAIDs interrupt prostaglandin

---

BOX 23–4 Risk Factors for Peptic Ulcer Disease

- *H. pylori* infection
  - Low socioeconomic status
  - Crowded, unsanitary living conditions
  - Unclean food or water
- Use of NSAIDs
- Advanced age
- History of ulcer
- Concurrent use of other drugs such as glucocorticoids or other NSAIDs
- Cigarette smoking
- Family history of PUD

MediaLink Case Study: Peptic Ulcer Disease

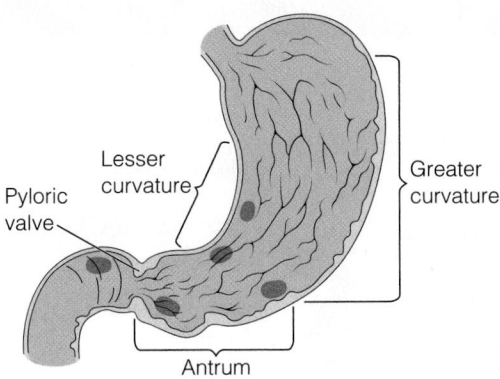

Figure 23–8 ■ Common sites affected by peptic ulcer disease.

synthesis by disrupting the action of the enzyme cyclooxygenase (COX). The two forms of this enzyme are COX-1 and COX-2. The COX-1 enzyme is necessary to maintain the integrity of the gastric mucosa, but the anti-inflammatory effects of NSAIDs are due to their ability to inhibit the COX-2 enzyme. The COX-2–selective NSAIDs may be less damaging to the gastric mucosa because they have less effect on the COX-1 enzyme. In addition to their systemic effect, aspirin and many NSAIDs cross the lipid membranes of gastric epithelial cells, damaging the cells themselves.

The ulcers of PUD may affect the esophagus, stomach, or duodenum. They may be superficial or deep, affecting all layers of the mucosa (see *Pathophysiology Illustrated: Peptic Ulcer Disease*). Duodenal ulcers, the most common, usually develop in the proximal portion of the duodenum, close to the pylorus (Figure 23–8 ■). They are sharply demarcated and usually less than 1 cm in diameter (Figure 23–9 ■). Gastric ulcers often are found on the lesser curvature and the area immediately proximal to the pylorus. Gastric ulcers are associated with an increased incidence of gastric cancer.

Peptic ulcer disease may be chronic, with spontaneous remissions and exacerbations. Exacerbations of the disease may be associated with trauma, infection, or other physical or psychologic stressors.

Figure 23–9 ■ A superficial peptic ulcer.
Source: SPL/Photo Researchers, Inc.

Manifestations

Pain is the classic symptom of peptic ulcer disease. The pain is typically described as gnawing, burning, aching, or hunger-like and is experienced in the epigastric region, sometimes radiating to the back. The pain occurs when the stomach is empty (2 to 3 hours after meals and in the middle of the night) and is relieved by eating with a classic "pain–food–relief" pattern. The client may complain of heartburn or regurgitation and may vomit.

The presentation of peptic ulcer disease in the older adult is often less clear, with vague and poorly localized discomfort, perhaps chest pain or dysphagia, weight loss, or anemia. In the older adult, a complication of PUD such as upper GI hemorrhage or perforation of the stomach or duodenum may be the presenting symptom.

Complications

The complications associated with peptic ulcers include hemorrhage, obstruction, and perforation. See the box below for the manifestations of these complications.

Among people with PUD, 10% to 20% experience **hemorrhage** as a result of ulceration and erosion into the blood vessels of the gastric mucosa. In the older adult, bleeding is the most frequent complication. When small blood vessels erode, blood loss may be slow and insidious, with occult blood in the stool the only initial sign. If bleeding continues, the client becomes anemic and experiences symptoms of weakness, fatigue, dizziness, and orthostatic hypotension. Erosion into a larger vessel can lead to sudden and severe bleeding with hematemesis, melena, or hematochezia (blood in the stool), and signs of hypovolemic shock.

MANIFESTATIONS of PUD Complications

HEMORRHAGE
- Occult or obvious blood in the stool
- Hematemesis
- Fatigue
- Weakness, dizziness
- Orthostatic hypotension
- Hypovolemic shock

OBSTRUCTION
- Sensations of epigastric fullness
- Nausea and vomiting
- Electrolyte imbalances
- Metabolic alkalosis

PERFORATION
- Severe upper abdominal pain, radiating to the shoulder
- Rigid, boardlike abdomen
- Absence of bowel sounds
- Diaphoresis
- Tachycardia
- Rapid, shallow respirations
- Fever

Peptic Ulcer Disease

Normal gastric mucosa

In the stomach and duodenum, the mucosal barrier protects the gastric mucosa (including the epithelial, vascular, and smooth muscle layers) from damage. Specialized mucous cells throughout the gastric mucosa produce a mucus (a mixture of water, lipids, and glycoproteins) that serves as a barrier to the diffusion of ions (such as hydrogen ion) and molecules (such as pepsin). A thin layer of bicarbonate, secreted by surface epithelial cells, forms between the mucus and cell membranes. Blood flow to the gastric mucosa is vital to maintain this barrier. Prostaglandins and nitric oxide stimulate mucus and bicarbonate production, helping maintain it as well. The mucosal barrier constantly bathes surfaces of the gastric epithelial lining.

Disruption of mucosal barrier

The mucosal barrier can be disrupted by a number of factors. Ischemia of the gastric mucosa (e.g., due to hemorrhage, hypotension, or shock) impairs mucous production, increasing the risk of damage to the mucosa. Aspirin disrupts the mucosal barrier, and, along with other nonsteroidal anti-inflammatory drugs, inhibits prostaglandins which are necessary to maintain mucous production. Alcohol and bile acids also damage the mucous barrier. *Helicobacter pylori*, a common pathogen to infect the gastric mucosa, disrupts the mucosal barrier.

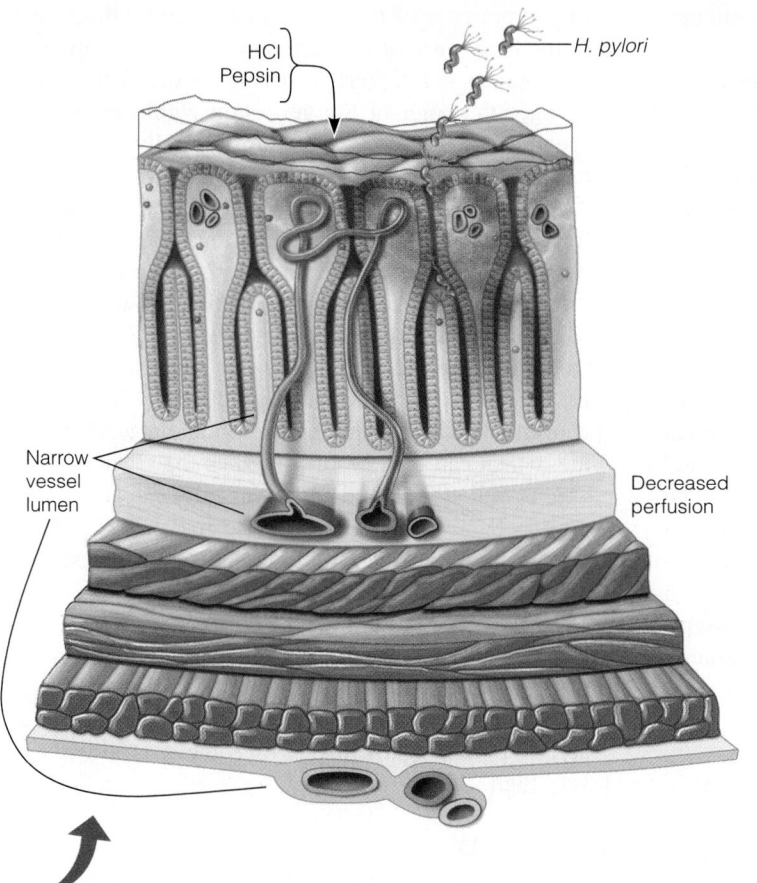

HCl Pepsin

H. pylori

Narrow vessel lumen

Decreased perfusion

Inflammatory process

When the mucosal barrier is damaged, gastric acid and digestive juices disrupt the epithelial cell membranes, allowing acid to diffuse into cell walls. An acute inflammatory process results. Gastric epithelial cells migrate to the damaged area, a process known as restitution. Adequate blood flow and an alkaline environment are necessary for this repair process. Prostaglandins play an important role in epithelial repair. In the presence of *H. pylori* infection, excess acid production, inadequate blood flow, inhibition of prostaglandins, and other factors that are less clear, the inflammatory process further damages gastric and duodenal epithelial cells, leading to ulceration of the mucosa.

Erosion and ulcer formation

Superficial ulcers (erosions) erode the mucosa, but do not penetrate the muscularis mucosae. True ulcers extend through the muscularis mucosae and into deeper layers of the gastrointestinal wall, damaging blood vessels and potentially penetrating the entire wall. Hemorrhage and peritonitis are potential acute complications of peptic ulcers.

Acute ulcer   Erosion   Chronic ulcer

Mucosal barrier

Muscularis mucosae

Gastric mucosa

Scarring

Serosa

Gastric outlet obstruction may result from edema surrounding the ulcer, smooth muscle spasm, or scar tissue. Generally, obstruction is a gradual rather than an acute process. Symptoms include a feeling of epigastric fullness, accentuated ulcer symptoms, and nausea. If the obstruction becomes complete, vomiting occurs. Hydrochloric acid, sodium, and potassium are lost in vomitus, potentially leading to fluid and electrolyte imbalance and metabolic alkalosis.

The most lethal complication of PUD is **perforation** of the ulcer through the mucosal wall. When perforation occurs, gastric or duodenal contents enter the peritoneum, causing an inflammatory process and peritonitis. Chemical peritonitis from the hydrochloric acid, pepsin, bile, and pancreatic fluid is immediate; bacterial peritonitis follows within 6 to 12 hours from gastric contaminants entering the normally sterile peritoneal cavity. When an ulcer perforates, the client has immediate, severe upper abdominal pain, radiating throughout the abdomen and possibly to the shoulder. The abdomen becomes rigid and boardlike, with absent bowel sounds. Signs of shock may be present, including diaphoresis, tachycardia, and rapid, shallow respirations. Classic symptoms of perforation may not be present in an older adult. The older adult may instead present with mental confusion and other nonspecific symptoms. This atypical presentation can lead to delays in diagnosis and treatment, increasing the associated mortality rate.

Zollinger-Ellison Syndrome

Zollinger-Ellison syndrome is peptic ulcer disease caused by a gastrinoma, or gastrin-secreting tumor of the pancreas, stomach, or intestines. Gastrinomas may be benign, although 50% to 70% are malignant tumors. Gastrin is a hormone that stimulates the secretion of pepsin and hydrochloric acid. The increased gastrin levels associated with these tumors result in hypersecretion of gastric acid, which in turn causes mucosal ulceration.

The peptic ulcers of Zollinger-Ellison syndrome may affect any portion of the stomach or duodenum, as well as the esophagus or jejunum. Characteristic ulcer-like pain is common. The high levels of hydrochloric acid entering the duodenum may also cause diarrhea and **steatorrhea** (excess fat in the feces) from impaired fat digestion and absorption. Complications of bleeding and perforation are often seen with Zollinger-Ellison syndrome. Fluid and electrolyte imbalances may also result from persistent diarrhea with resultant losses of potassium and sodium in particular.

INTERDISCIPLINARY CARE

Treatment for PUD focuses on eradicating *H. pylori* infection and treating or preventing ulcers related to use of NSAIDs.

Diagnosis

- *Upper GI series* using barium as a contrast medium can detect 80% to 90% of peptic ulcers. It commonly is the diagnostic procedure chosen first; it is less costly and less invasive than gastroscopy. Small or very superficial ulcers may be missed, however.
- *Gastroscopy* allows visualization of the esophageal, gastric, and duodenal mucosa and direct inspection of ulcers. Tissue also can be obtained for biopsy. Nursing care of the client undergoing a gastroscopy is outlined in Chapter 21 ∞.
- Biopsy specimens obtained during a gastroscopy can be tested for the presence of *H. pylori* using several different methods. In the *biopsy urease test,* the specimen is put into a gel containing urea. If *H. pylori* is present, the urease that it produces changes the color of the gel, often within minutes. Biopsy specimen cells also can be microscopically examined or cultured for evidence of *H. pylori.* Although these tests are highly specific for *H. pylori* infection, their invasiveness, cost, and lack of availability in some areas limits their usefulness.
- Noninvasive methods of detecting *H. pylori* infection include *serologic testing* (to detect IgG antibodies through ELISA), fecal antigen immunoassays (to detect antigens to *H. pylori* in the feces), and the *urea breath test.* In this test, radiolabeled urea is given orally. The urease produced by *H. pylori* bacteria converts the urea to ammonia and radiolabeled carbon dioxide, which can then be measured as the client exhales. This test, as well as fecal antigen testing, also can be used to evaluate the effectiveness of treatment to eradicate *H. pylori.* Treatment with PPIs interferes with urea breath test and fecal antigen test results, so these drugs should be discontinued for 1 to 2 weeks prior to testing (Tierney et al., 2005).
- If Zollinger-Ellison syndrome is suspected, *gastric analysis* may be performed to evaluate gastric acid secretion. Stomach contents are aspirated through a nasogastric tube and analyzed. In Zollinger-Ellison syndrome, gastric acid levels are very high.

Medications

The medications used to treat PUD include agents to eradicate *H. pylori,* drugs to decrease gastric acid content, and agents that protect the mucosa. Nursing responsibilities related to selected drugs to treat GERD, gastritis, and PUD are found in the Medication Administration box on pages 665–666.

Eradication of *H. pylori* is often difficult. Combination therapies that use two antibiotics with a proton-pump inhibitor (e.g., combinations of a PPI, clarithromycin, and amoxicillin, or a PPI, bismuth subsalicylate, tetracycline, and metronidazole) are necessary. With complete eradication of *H. pylori,* reinfection rates are less than 0.5% per year.

In clients who have NSAID-induced ulcers, the NSAID in use should be discontinued if at all possible. If this is not possible, twice-daily PPIs enable ulcer healing.

Medications that decrease gastric acid content include PPIs and the H_2-receptor antagonists.

- Proton-pump inhibitors bind the acid-secreting enzyme (H^+, K^+ ATPase) that functions as the proton pump, disabling it for up to 24 hours. These drugs are very effective, resulting in more than 90% ulcer healing after 4 weeks. Compared to the H_2-receptor blockers, the PPIs provide faster pain relief and more rapid ulcer healing.
- Histamine$_2$-receptor blockers inhibit histamine binding to the receptors on the gastric parietal cells to reduce acid secretion. These drugs are very well tolerated and have few serious side effects; however, drug interactions can occur. These drugs must be continued for 8 weeks or longer for ulcer healing.

Agents that protect the mucosa include sucralfate, bismuth, antacids, and prostaglandin analogs.

- Sucralfate binds to proteins in the ulcer base, forming a protective barrier against acid, bile, and pepsin. Sucralfate also stimulates the secretion of mucus, bicarbonate, and prostaglandin.
- Bismuth compounds (Pepto-Bismol) stimulate mucosal bicarbonate and prostaglandin production to promote ulcer healing. In addition, bismuth has an antibacterial action against *H. pylori*. There are very few side effects, other than a harmless darkening of stools.
- Antacids stimulate gastric mucosal defenses, thereby aiding in ulcer healing. They provide rapid relief of ulcer symptoms, and are often used as needed to supplement other antiulcer medications. Antacids are inexpensive, but clients often have difficulty with a regular regimen because the drugs must be taken frequently and may cause either constipation (from the aluminum-type antacids) or diarrhea (from the magnesium-based antacids). Antacids also interfere with the absorption of iron, digoxin, some antibiotics, and other drugs.
- Prostaglandin analogs (misoprostol) promote ulcer healing by stimulating mucus and bicarbonate secretions and by inhibiting acid secretion. Although not as effective as the other drugs discussed, misoprostol is used to prevent NSAID-induced ulcers.

Treatments

NUTRITION In addition to pharmacologic treatment, clients are encouraged to maintain good nutrition, consuming balanced meals at regular intervals. It is important to teach clients that bland or restrictive diets are no longer necessary. Mild alcohol intake is not harmful. Smoking should be discouraged, because it slows the rate of healing and increases the frequency of relapses.

SURGERY The identification of *H. pylori* as a cause of PUD and the availability of drugs to treat the infection and heal peptic ulcers has all but eliminated surgery as a treatment option for peptic ulcer disease. Older clients, however, may have undergone gastric resection surgery for PUD, and may have long-term complications related to the surgery. See the section on gastric cancer for more information about gastric surgery and its potential complications.

Treatment of Complications

The client hospitalized with a complication of PUD such as bleeding, gastrointestinal obstruction, or perforation and peritonitis requires additional interventions to restore homeostasis.

In hemorrhage associated with PUD, initial interventions focus on restoring and maintaining circulation. Normal saline, lactated Ringer's, or other balanced electrolyte solutions are administered intravenously to restore intravascular volume if signs of shock (tachycardia, hypotension, pallor, low urine output, and anxiety) are present. Whole blood or packed red blood cells may be administered to restore hemoglobin and hematocrit levels. A nasogastric tube is inserted to prevent aspiration of vomited gastric contents.

Gastroscopy with direct injection of a clotting or sclerosing agent into the bleeding vessel may be performed. Laser photocoagulation, using light energy, or electrocoagulation, which

uses electric current to generate heat, can also be done via gastroscopy to seal bleeding vessels.

The client is kept NPO until bleeding is controlled. Proton-pump inhibitors are administered intravenously (e.g., 40 mg of pantoprazole [Protonix] per intravenous push or admixture daily) to reduce the risk of rebleeding. Surgery may be necessary if medical measures are ineffective in controlling bleeding. Older adults who experience bleeding as a complication of PUD are more likely to rebleed or require surgery to control the hemorrhage. See page 690 for nursing care of the client having gastric surgery.

Repeated inflammation, healing, scarring, edema, and muscle spasm can lead to gastric outlet (pyloric) obstruction. Initial treatment includes gastric decompression with nasogastric suction and administration of intravenous normal saline and potassium chloride to correct fluid and electrolyte imbalance. H_2-receptor blockers are given intravenously as well. Balloon dilation of the gastric outlet may be done via upper endoscopy. If these measures are unsuccessful in relieving obstruction, surgery may be required.

Gastric or duodenal perforation resulting in contamination of the peritoneum with gastrointestinal contents often requires immediate intervention to restore homeostasis and minimize peritonitis. Intravenous fluids maintain fluid and electrolyte balance. Nasogastric suction removes gastric contents and minimizes peritoneal contamination. Placing the client in Fowler's or semi-Fowler's position allows peritoneal contaminants to pool in the pelvis. Intravenous antibiotics aggressively treat bacterial infection from intestinal flora. Laparoscopic surgery or an open laparotomy may close the perforation.

 NURSING CARE

Health Promotion

Although it is difficult to predict which clients will develop peptic ulcer disease, promote health by advising clients to avoid risk factors such as excessive aspirin or NSAID use and cigarette smoking. In addition, encourage clients to seek treatment for manifestations of GERD or chronic gastritis, both of which also are associated with *H. pylori* infection.

Assessment

Collect the following subjective and objective data when assessing the client with peptic ulcer disease:

- *Health history:* Complaints of epigastric or left upper quadrant pain, heartburn, or discomfort; its character, severity, timing and relationship to eating; measures used for relief; nausea or vomiting, presence of bright blood or "coffee-grounds" appearing material in vomitus; current medications including use of aspirin or other NSAIDs; cigarette smoking and use of alcohol or other drugs.
- *Physical examination:* General appearance including height and weight relationship; vital signs including orthostatic measurements; abdominal examination including shape and contour, bowel sounds, and tenderness to palpation; presence of obvious or occult blood in vomitus and stool.

Nursing Diagnoses and Interventions

The priorities of nursing care for the client with peptic ulcer disease are reducing discomfort, maintaining nutritional status, and preventing or rapidly identifying and intervening for potential complications. See the accompanying Nursing Care Plan below.

Pain

The pain of peptic ulcer disease is often predictable and preventable. Pain is typically experienced 2 to 4 hours after eating, as high levels of gastric acid and pepsin irritate the exposed mucosa. Measures to neutralize the acid, minimize its production, or protect the mucosa often relieve this pain, minimizing the need for analgesics.

- Assess pain, including location, type, severity, frequency, and duration, and its relationship to food intake or other contributing factors.

PRACTICE ALERT

Avoid making assumptions about pain. Acute pain may indicate a complication, such as perforation (often heralded by sudden, severe epigastric pain and a rigid, boardlike abdomen) or it may be totally unrelated to PUD (e.g., angina, gallbladder disease, or pancreatitis).

- Administer PPIs, H_2-receptor antagonists, antacids, or mucosal protective agents as ordered. Monitor for effectiveness and side effects or adverse reactions. *The pain associated with*

NURSING CARE PLAN   A Client with Peptic Ulcer Disease

Sean O'Donnell is a 47-year-old police officer who lives and works in a metropolitan area. Mr. O'Donnell has had "heartburn" and abdominal discomfort for years, but thought it went along with his job. Last year, after becoming weak, light-headed, and short of breath, he was found to be anemic and was diagnosed as having a duodenal ulcer. He took omeprazole (Prilosec) and ferrous sulfate for 3 months before stopping both, saying he had "never felt better in his life." Mr. O'Donnell has now been admitted to the hospital with active upper GI bleeding.

ASSESSMENT

Rachel Clark is Mr. O'Donnell's admitting nurse and case manager. On initial assessment, Mr. O'Donnell is alert and oriented, though very apprehensive about his condition. Skin pale and cool; BP 136/78, P 98; abdomen distended and tender with hyperactive bowel sounds; 200 mL bright red blood obtained on nasogastric tube insertion. Hemoglobin 8.2 g/dL and hematocrit 23% on admission. Mr. O'Donnell is taken to the endoscopy lab where his bleeding is controlled using laser photocoagulation. On his return to the nursing unit, he receives two units of packed RBCs and intravenous fluids to restore blood volume. A 5-day course of high-dose oral omeprazole (40 mg bid) is ordered to prevent rebleeding, and Mr. O'Donnell is allowed to begin a clear liquid diet 24 hours after his endoscopy. Tissue biopsy obtained during endoscopy confirms the presence of *H. pylori* infection.

DIAGNOSES

- *Deficient Fluid Volume* related to acutely bleeding duodenal ulcer
- *Risk for Injury* related to acute blood loss
- *Fear* related to threat to well-being
- *Ineffective Therapeutic Regimen Management* related to lack of knowledge regarding PUD and its treatment

EXPECTED OUTCOMES

- Maintains normal blood pressure, pulse, and urine output (>30 mL/h).
- Remains free of injury.
- Seeks information to reduce fear.
- Identifies and uses coping strategies to manage fear.
- Describes prescribed therapeutic regimen.
- Verbalizes ability to manage prescribed regimen.

PLANNING AND IMPLEMENTATION

- Place call light within reach and encourage to ask for help when getting up or ambulating. Remind to rise slowly from lying to sitting and sitting to standing.
- Discuss situation and provide information about all procedures and treatments.
- Reassure about the effectiveness of treatment in reducing the risk for further bleeding.
- Discuss current and planned treatment measures; stress the importance of completing the prescribed treatment to reduce the risk of further ulcer development.
- Encourage to avoid using aspirin or NSAIDs in the future; suggest alternative medications such as acetaminophen.
- Discuss stress reduction techniques and refer for stress reduction counseling or workshops as indicated.

EVALUATION

Mr. O'Donnell is discharged 48 hours after admission. He has had no further evidence of bleeding, and has resumed a regular diet. His hemoglobin and hematocrit remain low, and he has a prescription for ferrous sulfate. He will complete the prescribed high-dose omeprazole regimen at home, then begin treatment with omeprazole, amoxicillin, and clarithromycin (Biaxin) to eradicate the *H. pylori* infection detected during endoscopy. After 2 weeks of this regimen, he will continue taking omeprazole at bedtime for 4 to 8 weeks. He verbalizes a good understanding of his treatment and the importance of completing the entire regimen. Mr. O'Donnell expresses concern about his ability to "keep his cool on the inside" when under stress. Ms. Clark, his case manager, gives him the names of several resources to help with stress management in case he wants help.

CRITICAL THINKING IN THE NURSING PROCESS

1. How does *H. pylori* infection contribute to the development of peptic ulcers?
2. Describe the physiologic responses to fear and anxiety. Why is it important to alleviate fear and its physical consequences in clients with PUD?
3. What suggestions can you make to help Mr. O'Donnell manage his complex treatment regimen during the next 3 months?
4. Develop a teaching plan that includes stress reduction techniques Mr. O'Donnell can use while performing his duties as a police officer.

See Evaluating Your Response in Appendix C.

PUD is generally caused by the effect of gastric juices on exposed mucosal tissue. These medications reduce pain and promote healing by reducing acid production, neutralizing acid, or providing a barrier for the damaged mucosa.

- Teach relaxation, stress reduction, and lifestyle management techniques. Refer for stress management counseling or classes as indicated. *Although there is no clear relationship between stress and PUD, measures to relieve stress and promote physical and emotional rest help reduce the perception of pain and may reduce ulcer genesis.*

Disturbed Sleep Pattern

Nighttime ulcer pain, which typically occurs between 1:00 and 3:00 A.M., may disrupt the sleep cycle and result in inadequate rest. Anticipation of pain may lead to insomnia or other sleep disruptions.

- Stress the importance of taking medications as prescribed. *The bedtime dose of PPI or H_2-receptor blocker minimizes hydrochloric acid production during the night, reducing nighttime pain.*
- Instruct to limit food intake after the evening meal, eliminating any bedtime snack. *Eating before bed can stimulate the production of gastric acid and pepsin, increasing the likelihood of nighttime pain.*
- Encourage use of relaxation techniques and comfort measures such as soft music as needed to promote sleep. *Once the pain associated with PUD has been controlled, these measures help reduce anxiety and reestablish a normal sleep pattern.*

Imbalanced Nutrition: Less than Body Requirements

In an attempt to avoid discomfort, the client with peptic ulcer disease may gradually reduce food intake, sometimes jeopardizing nutritional status. Anorexia and early satiety are additional problems associated with PUD.

- Assess current diet, including pattern of food intake, eating schedule, and foods that precipitate pain or are being avoided in anticipation of pain. *The client may not realize the extent of self-imposed dietary limitations, especially if symptoms have persisted for an extended time. Assessment increases awareness and also helps identify the adequacy of nutrient intake.*
- Refer to a dietitian for meal planning to minimize PUD symptoms and meet nutritional needs. Consider normal eating patterns and preferences in meal planning. *Although no specific diet is recommended for PUD, clients should avoid foods that increase pain. Six small meals per day often help increase food tolerance and decrease postprandial discomfort.*
- Monitor for complaints of anorexia, fullness, nausea, and vomiting. Adjust dietary intake or medication schedule as indicated. *PUD and resultant scarring can lead to impaired gastric emptying, necessitating a treatment change.*

> **PRACTICE ALERT**
> Advise the client to report increasing or persistent symptoms of anorexia, nausea and vomiting, or fullness to the healthcare provider.

- Monitor laboratory values for indications of anemia or other nutritional deficits. Monitor for therapeutic and side effects of treatment measures such as oral iron replacement. Instruct the client taking oral iron replacement to avoid using an antacid within 1 to 2 hours of taking the iron preparation. *Anemia can result from poor nutrient absorption or chronic blood loss in clients with PUD. Oral iron supplements may cause GI distress, nausea, and vomiting; if these side effects are intolerable, notify the physician for a possible change of therapy. Antacids bind with oral iron preparations, blocking absorption.*

Deficient Fluid Volume

Erosion of a blood vessel with resultant hemorrhage is a significant risk for the client with peptic ulcer disease. Acute bleeding can lead to hypovolemia and fluid volume deficit, which can lead to a decrease in cardiac output and impaired tissue perfusion.

> **PRACTICE ALERT**
> Monitor and record blood pressure and apical pulse every 15 to 30 minutes until stable; monitor central venous pressure or pulmonary artery pressure as indicated. Insert a Foley catheter and monitor urinary output hourly. Weigh daily. Continuous monitoring of cardiac output parameters is essential in clients with an acute hemorrhage to identify possible shock and intervene at an early stage.

- Monitor stools and gastric drainage for overt and occult blood. Assess gastric drainage (vomitus or from a nasogastric tube) to estimate the amount and rapidity of hemorrhage. *Drainage is bright red with possible clots in acute hemorrhage; dark red or the color of coffee grounds when blood has been in the stomach for a period of time. Hematochezia (stool containing red blood and clots) is present in acute hemorrhage; melena (black, tarry stool) is an indicator of less acute bleeding. When small vessels are disrupted, bleeding may be slow and not overtly evident. With chronic or slow gastrointestinal bleeding, the risk of a fluid volume deficit is minimal; anemia and activity intolerance are more likely.*
- Maintain intravenous therapy with fluid volume and electrolyte replacement solutions; administer whole blood or packed cells as ordered. *Both fluids and electrolytes are lost through vomiting, nasogastric drainage, and diarrhea in an episode of acute bleeding. To prevent shock, it is essential to maintain a blood volume and cardiac output sufficient to perfuse body tissues. Whole blood and packed cells replace both blood volume and red blood cells, providing additional oxygen-carrying capacity to meet cell needs.*
- Insert a nasogastric tube and maintain its position and patency. Initially, measure and record gastric output every hour, then every 4 to 8 hours. *Nasogastric suction removes blood from the gastrointestinal tract, preventing vomiting and possible aspiration. Gastric output is replaced milliliter for milliliter with a balanced electrolyte solution to maintain homeostasis.*
- Monitor hemoglobin and hematocrit, serum electrolytes, BUN, and creatinine values. Report abnormal findings. *Hemoglobin and hematocrit are lower than normal with acute or chronic GI bleeding. In acute hemorrhage, initial results may be within*

normal range because both cells and plasma are lost. Loss of fluids and electrolytes with gastric drainage and diarrhea will alter normal levels. Digestion and absorption of blood in the GI tract may result in elevated BUN and creatinine levels.

- Assess abdomen, including bowel sounds, distention, girth, and tenderness every 4 hours and record findings. *Borborygmi or hyperactive bowel sounds with abdominal tenderness are common with acute GI bleeding. Increased distention, increasing abdominal girth, absent bowel sounds, or extreme tenderness with a rigid, boardlike abdomen may indicate perforation.*

- Maintain bed rest with the head of the bed elevated. Ensure safety. *Loss of blood volume may cause orthostatic hypotension with resultant syncope or dizziness upon standing.*

Using NANDA, NIC, and NOC

Chart 23–3 shows links between NANDA nursing diagnoses, NIC, and NOC when caring for a client with peptic ulcer disease.

Community-Based Care

Peptic ulcer disease is managed in home and community-based settings; only its complications typically require treatment in an acute care setting. Provide the following information when preparing the client for home care:

- Prescribed medication regimen, including desired and potential adverse effects

NANDA, NIC, AND NOC LINKAGES
CHART 23–3 The Client with Peptic Ulcer Disease

NANDA

Ineffective Health Maintenance

↓

NIC

Medication Management

Nausea Management

Fluid/Electrolyte Management

Teaching: Disease Process

↓

NOC

Comfort Level

Nutritional Status: Food and Fluid Intake

Hydration

Knowledge Status: Treatment Regimen

Data from *NANDA's Nursing Diagnoses: Definitions & Classification 2005–2006* by NANDA International (2005), Philadelphia; *Nursing Interventions Classification (NIC)* (4th ed.) by J. M. Dochterman & G. M. Bulechek (2004), St. Louis, MO: Mosby; and *Nursing Outcomes Classification (NOC)* (3rd ed.) by S. Moorhead, M. Johnson, and M. Mass (2004), St. Louis, MO: Mosby.

- Importance of continuing therapy even when symptoms are relieved

- Relationship between peptic ulcers and factors such as NSAID use and smoking. If indicated, refer to a smoking cessation clinic or program.

- Importance of avoiding aspirin and other NSAIDs; stress the necessity of reading the labels of over-the-counter medications for possible aspirin content

- Manifestations of complications that should be reported to the care provider, including increased abdominal pain or distention, vomiting, black or tarry stools, light-headedness, or fainting

- Stress and lifestyle management techniques that may help prevent exacerbation. Refer to resources for stress management, such as classes, counseling, and formal or informal groups.

THE CLIENT WITH CANCER OF THE STOMACH

Worldwide, cancer of the stomach is the most common cancer (after skin cancer), but it is less common in the United States.

FAST FACTS

- An estimated 21,800 new cases of stomach cancer are diagnosed annually in the United States (ACS, 2005).
- Its incidence is highest in Hispanics, African Americans, and Asian Americans.
- Men are affected twice as often as women.

Older adults are more likely to develop gastric cancer: The mean age at time of diagnosis is 63. People in lower socioeconomic groups are more often affected by gastric cancer.

Risk Factors

H. pylori infection is a major risk factor for cancer of the distal portion of the stomach; from 35% to 89% of cases can be attributed to this infection. Other risk factors are a genetic predisposition, chronic gastritis, pernicious anemia, gastric polyps, and carcinogenic factors in the diet (such as smoked foods and nitrates). Achlorhydria, a lack of hydrochloric acid in the stomach, is a known risk factor. The risk for gastric cancer also is increased in people who have had a partial gastric resection.

Pathophysiology

Adenocarcinoma, which involves the mucous-producing cells of the stomach, is the most common form of gastric cancer. These carcinomas may arise anywhere on the mucosal surface of the stomach but are most frequently found in the distal portion. Half of all gastric cancers occur in the antrum or pyloric region (Porth, 2005). Gastric cancer begins as a localized lesion (*in situ*), then progresses to involve the mucosa or submucosa (early gastric carcinoma). Lesions may spread by direct extension to tissues surrounding the stomach, the liver in particular. The lesion may ulcerate or appear as a polypoid (polyp-like) mass (Figure 23–10 ■). Lymph node involvement and metastasis occur early due to the rich blood and lymphatic supply to the stomach. Metastatic lesions are often found in the liver, lungs, ovaries, and peritoneum.

Figure 23–10 ■ The spread and forms (polypoid and ulcerating) of gastric cancer.

Source: Robert Margulies/Phototake NYC.

Manifestations

Few symptoms are associated with gastric cancer. Unfortunately, the disease is often quite advanced and metastases are usually present at the time of diagnosis. Early symptoms are vague, including feelings of early satiety, anorexia, indigestion, and possibly vomiting. The client may experience ulcer-like pain unrelieved by antacids, typically occurring after meals. As the disease progresses, weight loss occurs, and the client may be **cachectic** (in very poor health and malnourished) at the time of diagnosis. An abdominal mass may be palpable, and occult blood may be present in the stool, indicating gastrointestinal bleeding.

INTERDISCIPLINARY CARE

Diagnosis

Anemia detected by a CBC often is the first indication of gastric cancer. An upper GI x-ray with barium swallow is useful to identify lesions, and ultrasound or other radiologic techniques may identify a mass. Upper endoscopy with visualization and biopsy of the lesion provides the definitive diagnosis.

Surgery

When gastric cancer is identified prior to the development of metastasis, surgical removal of part or all of the stomach and regional lymph nodes is the treatment of choice. **Partial gastrectomy** involves removal of a portion of the stomach, usually the distal half to two-thirds. In partial gastrectomy, the surgeon constructs an anastomosis from the remainder of the stomach directly to the duodenum or to the proximal jejunum. The **gastroduodenostomy**, or **Billroth I**, and the **gastrojejunostomy**, or **Billroth II**, are commonly used partial gastrectomy procedures (Figures 23–11A ■ and B).

A **total gastrectomy**, removal of the entire stomach, may be done for diffuse cancer that is spread throughout the gastric mucosa but limited to the stomach. In a total gastrectomy, the surgeon constructs an anastomosis from the esophagus to the duodenum or jejunum. Total gastrectomy with **esophagojejunostomy** is illustrated in Figure 23–11C.

Nursing care of the client who has undergone gastric surgery is outlined in the box on the following page.

Complications

Several long-term complications may develop following gastrectomy procedures. **Dumping syndrome** is the most common problem. It may follow a partial gastrectomy with duodenal or jejunal anastomosis. When the pylorus has been resected or bypassed, a hypertonic, undigested food bolus may rapidly enter the duodenum or jejunum. Water is pulled into the lumen of the intestine by the hyperosmolar character of the chyme, resulting

Figure 23–11 ■ Partial and total gastrectomy procedures. *A,* Partial gastrectomy with anastomosis to the duodenum. *B,* Partial gastrectomy with anastomosis to the jejunum. *C,* Total gastrectomy with anastomosis of the esophagus to the jejunum.

NURSING CARE OF THE CLIENT HAVING Gastric Surgery

PREOPERATIVE NURSING CARE
- See Chapter 4 ∞ for routine preoperative care and teaching.
- Insert a nasogastric tube if ordered preoperatively. *Although it is often inserted in the surgical suite just prior to surgery, the nasogastric tube may be placed preoperatively to remove secretions and empty stomach contents.*

POSTOPERATIVE NURSING CARE
- Provide routine care for the surgical client as outlined in Chapter 4 ∞.
- Assess position and patency of nasogastric tube, connecting it to low suction. Gently irrigate with sterile normal saline if tube becomes clogged. *The nasogastric tube will be placed in surgery to avoid disruption of the gastric suture lines and should be well secured. If repositioning or tube replacement is needed, notify the surgeon. Patency must be maintained to keep the stomach decompressed, reducing pressure on sutures.*
- Assess color, amount, and odor of gastric drainage, noting any changes in these parameters or the presence of clots or bright bleeding. *Initial drainage is bright red. It becomes dark, then clear or greenish-yellow over the first 2 to 3 days. A change in the color, amount, or odor may indicate a complication such as hemorrhage, intestinal obstruction, or infection.*
- Maintain intravenous fluids while nasogastric suction is in place. *The client on nasogastric suction is not only unable to take oral food and fluids but also is losing electrolyte-rich fluid through the nasogastric tube. If replacement fluid and electrolytes are not maintained, the client is at risk for dehydration, imbalances of sodium, potassium, and chloride; and metabolic alkalosis.*

- Provide antiulcer and antibiotic therapy as ordered. *These medications may be ordered for the postoperative client, depending on the procedure performed. Antibiotic therapy is a common preventive measure for infection that may result from contamination of the abdominal cavity with gastric contents.*
- Monitor bowel sounds and abdominal distention. *Bowel sounds indicate resumption of peristalsis. Increasing distention may indicate third spacing, obstruction or infection.*
- Resume oral food and fluids as ordered. Initial feedings are clear liquids, progressing to full liquids and then frequent small feedings of regular foods. Monitor bowel sounds and for abdominal distention frequently during this period. *Oral feedings are reintroduced slowly to minimize trauma to the suture lines by possible gastric distension.*
- Encourage ambulation. *Ambulation stimulates peristalsis.*
- Begin discharge planning and teaching. Consult with a dietitian for diet instructions and menu planning; reinforce teaching. Teach the client about potential postoperative complications, such as abdominal abscess, dumping syndrome, postprandial hypoglycemia, or pernicious anemia. Also, teach the client to recognize signs and symptoms and preventive measures. *The client's gastric capacity is reduced after partial gastrectomy, necessitating a corresponding reduction in meal size. Changes in gastric emptying and reduction in gastric secretions may change the client's tolerance for many foods, requiring slow reintroduction of these foods. Dumping syndrome, postprandial hypoglycemia, and pernicious anemia are possible long-term complications of partial gastrectomy. For most clients, dietary modifications can control both dumping syndrome and postprandial hypoglycemia.*

in decreased blood volume and intestinal dilation. Peristalsis is stimulated, and intestinal motility is increased.

Early symptoms of dumping syndrome occur within 5 to 30 minutes after eating. These symptoms result from intestinal dilation, peristaltic stimulation, and hypovolemia caused by undigested food in the proximal small intestine. Manifestations include nausea with possible vomiting, epigastric pain with cramping and borborygmi (loud, hyperactive bowel sounds), and diarrhea. Systemic symptoms from the hypovolemia and reflex sympathetic stimulation include tachycardia, orthostatic hypotension, dizziness, flushing, and diaphoresis.

The entry of hyperosmolar chyme into the jejunum also causes a rapid rise in the blood glucose. This stimulates the release of an excessive amount of insulin, leading to hypoglycemic symptoms 2 to 3 hours after the meal. The pathogenesis and clinical manifestations of dumping syndrome are represented in Figure 23–12 ■. Dumping syndrome is typically self-limiting, lasting 6 to 12 months after surgery; however, a small percentage of people continue to experience long-term symptoms.

Dumping syndrome is managed primarily by a dietary pattern that delays gastric emptying and allows smaller boluses of undigested food to enter the intestine. Meals should be small and more frequent. Liquids and solids are taken at separate times instead of together during a meal. The amount of

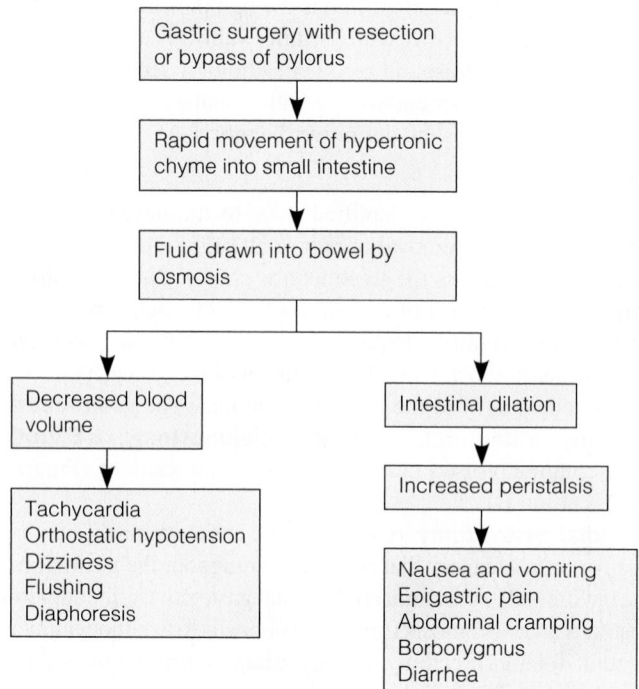

Figure 23–12 ■ The pathogenesis and manifestations of dumping syndrome.

proteins and fats in the diet is increased, because they exit the stomach more slowly than carbohydrates. Carbohydrates, especially simple sugars, are reduced. The client is instructed to rest in a recumbent or semirecumbent position for 30 to 60 minutes after meals. Anticholinergics, sedatives, and antispasmodics may be prescribed.

Anemia may be a chronic problem after a major gastric resection. Iron is absorbed primarily in the duodenum and proximal jejunum; rapid gastric emptying or a gastrojejunostomy may interfere with adequate absorption.

The cells of the stomach produce intrinsic factor, required for the absorption of vitamin B_{12}. Vitamin B_{12} deficiency leads to pernicious anemia. Because of hepatic stores of vitamin B_{12}, symptoms of anemia may not be seen for 1 to 2 years after surgery. Vitamin B_{12} levels are routinely monitored following extensive gastric resections.

Other nutritional problems seen following surgery include folic acid deficiency and decreased absorption of calcium and vitamin D. Poor absorption of nutrients, combined with the inability to eat large meals, puts the client at risk for weight loss in addition to the more specific nutrient deficiencies. Nearly 50% of clients who have gastric surgery experience significant weight loss, primarily because of insufficient calorie intake. Factors contributing to insufficient intake of calories include early satiety (feeling of fullness), decreased stomach size, and altered emptying patterns.

Other Therapies

Radiation or chemotherapy may be used to eliminate any lymphatic or metastatic spread. For the client with more advanced disease, treatment is palliative and may include surgery and chemotherapy. These clients may require a gastrostomy or jejunostomy feeding tube (Figure 23–13 ■). See the box on page 692 for nursing care of the client with a gastrostomy or jejunostomy tube.

Because gastric cancer is generally advanced by the time of diagnosis, the prognosis is poor. The 5-year survival rate of all clients treated for gastric carcinoma is 10%.

 ## NURSING CARE

Health Promotion

Although the exact causes of gastric cancer are unknown, contributing factors such as *H. pylori* infection and consumption of foods preserved with nitrates have been identified. To reduce their risk of developing gastric cancer, encourage clients with known *H. pylori* infection to complete the prescribed course of treatment and verify that it has eradicated the infection. With all clients, discuss the relationship between gastric cancer and consumption of foods preserved with nitrates (such as bacon and other processed meats), and encourage limited consumption of these products.

Assessment

Assessment data related to gastric cancer include the following:

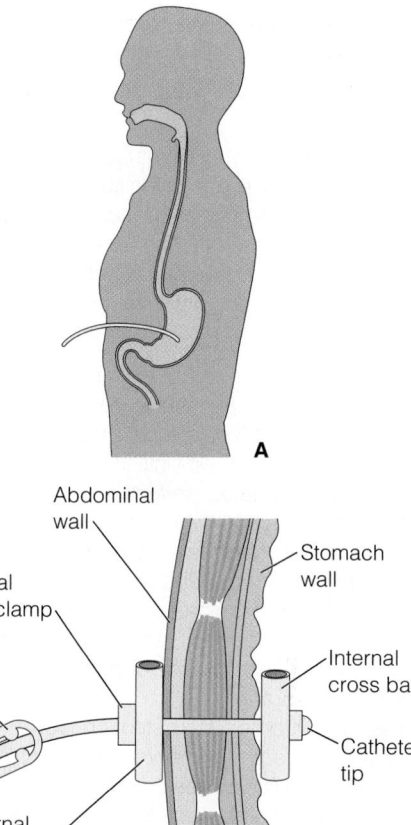

Figure 23–13 ■ Gastrostomy. *A,* Gastrostomy tube placement. *B,* The tube is fixed against both the abdomen and stomach walls by cross bars.

- *Health history:* Manifestations such as anorexia, early satiety, indigestion, or vomiting; epigastric pain after meals; recent unintentional weight loss.
- *Physical assessment:* General appearance, weight for height; abdominal distention or a palpable upper abdominal mass; occult blood in stool or vomitus.

Nursing Diagnoses and Interventions

Priorities of nursing care for the client with gastric cancer focus on effects of the disease and its treatment on nutritional status, and on the effects of a potentially fatal disease on the client and family. See the accompanying Nursing Care Plan on pages 692–693.

Imbalanced Nutrition: Less than Body Requirements

The client with gastric cancer may be malnourished because of anorexia, early satiety, and increased metabolic needs related to the tumor. Extensive gastric resection also makes it difficult to consume an adequate diet. Malnourishment, in turn, impairs healing and the client's ability to tolerate cancer treatment.

Clients who have had extensive gastric surgery or who require long-term enteral feedings to maintain nutrition may have a gastrostomy or jejunostomy tube inserted.

PROCEDURE

Gastrostomy tubes are surgically placed in the stomach, with the stoma in the epigastric region of the abdomen (see Figure 23–13). Jejunostomy tubes are placed in the proximal jejunum. Immediately following the procedure, the tube may be connected to low suction or plugged. If the client has been receiving tube feedings, these may be reinitiated shortly after tube placement.

NURSING CARE

- Assess tube placement by aspirating stomach contents and checking the pH of aspirate to determine gastric or intestinal placement. A pH of 5 or less indicates gastric placement; the pH is generally 7 or higher with intestinal placement. *Recent studies show auscultation to be ineffective in determining feeding tube placement. Measuring the pH of aspirate from the tube is more reliable as a means of determining tube placement.*
- Inspect the skin surrounding the insertion site for healing, redness, swelling, and the presence of any drainage. If drainage is present, note the color, amount, consistency, and odor. *Changes in the insertion site, drainage, or lack of healing may indicate an infection.*
- Assess the abdomen for distention, bowel sounds, and tenderness *to evaluate functioning of the gastrointestinal tract.*
- Until the stoma is well healed, use sterile technique for dressing changes and site care. Clean technique is appropriate for use once healing is complete. *Sterile technique reduces the risk of wound contamination by pathogens that can lead to infection. Once healing has occurred, clean technique is ac-*ceptable because the gastrointestinal tract is not a sterile body cavity.
- Wearing clean gloves, remove old dressing. Cleanse the site with saline or soap and water, and rinse as appropriate. A well-healed stoma may be cleansed in the shower with the tube clamped or plugged. Pat dry with 4 × 4 gauze pads, and allow to air dry. Apply Stomahesive, karaya, or other protective agents around tube as needed to protect the skin. *Gastric acid and other wound drainage is irritating to the skin. Meticulous care is important to maintain the integrity of the skin surrounding the stoma.*
- Redress the wound using a stoma dressing or folded 4 × 4 gauze pads. *Do not cut gauze pads, because threads may enter the wound, causing irritation and increasing the risk of inflammation.*
- Irrigate the tube with 30 to 50 mL of water, and clean the tube inside and out as indicated or ordered. Soft gastric tubes may require cleaning of the inner lumen with a special brush to maintain patency. *Tube feeding formulas may coat the inside of the gastrostomy tube and eventually cause it to become occluded. Regular irrigation with water and brushing as indicated maintain tube patency.*
- Provide mouth care or remind the client to do so. *When feedings are not being taken orally, the usual stimulus to do mouth care is lost. In addition, salivary fluids may not be as abundant, and oral mucous membranes may become dry and cracked.*
- If indicated, teach the client and family how to care for the tube and feedings. Refer to a home health agency or visiting nurse for support and reinforcement of learning. *Gastrostomy tubes are often in place long term. When the client and family are able to assume care, independence and self-image are enhanced.*

NURSING CARE PLAN   A Client with Gastric Cancer

George Harvey is a 61-year-old estate attorney who lives with his wife, Harriet. For the last 3 months, Mr. Harvey has had increasing anorexia and difficulty eating. He has lost 10 pounds. His physician has diagnosed gastric cancer, and Mr. Harvey is admitted for a partial gastrectomy and gastrojejunostomy. The oncologist has recommended postoperative chemotherapy and radiation. Mr. Harvey reports that the doctor told him "that will give me the best chance for cure."

ASSESSMENT

On admission before surgery, Mr. Harvey tells his nurse, Lauren Walsh, that he has eaten very little in the past few weeks. He asks, "What will happen to my wife if something happens to me? I'm afraid this cancer will get me." Mr. Harvey weighs 147 lb (67 kg) and is 72 inches (183 cm) tall. He is pale and thin; his vital signs are BP 148/86, P 92, R 18, and T 97.8°F PO. A firm mass is palpable in the left epigastric region. The rest of his physical assessment data are within normal limits. Mr. Harvey's hemoglobin is 12.8 g/dL, hematocrit is 39%, and serum albumin level is 3.2 g/dL, indicating that he is mildly malnourished. All other preoperative laboratory and diagnostic studies are within normal limits.

DIAGNOSES

- *Imbalanced Nutrition: Less than Body Requirements* related to anorexia and difficulty eating

- *Acute Pain* related to surgical incision and manipulation of abdominal organs
- *Risk for Ineffective Airway Clearance* related to upper abdominal surgery
- *Anticipatory Grieving* related to recent diagnosis of cancer

EXPECTED OUTCOMES

- Maintain present weight during hospitalization.
- Resume a high-calorie, high-protein diet by time of discharge.
- Verbalize effective pain management, maintaining a reported pain level of 3 or less on a scale of 1 to 10.
- Maintain a patent airway and clear breath sounds.
- Verbalize feelings regarding diagnosis and participate in decision making.

PLANNING AND IMPLEMENTATION

- Weigh daily.
- Maintain nasogastric tube placement, patency, and suction as ordered.
- Maintain intravenous fluids and total parenteral nutrition as ordered until oral food intake is resumed.
- Arrange for diet teaching, including strategies to prevent dumping syndrome, before discharge.
- Maintain patient-controlled analgesia until able to take oral analgesics.

(continued)

NURSING CARE PLAN **A Client with Gastric Cancer (continued)**

- Assess respiratory status including rate, depth, and breath sounds every hour initially, then every 4 hours.
- Assist to cough, deep breathe, and use inspirometer every 2 to 4 hours and as needed. Splint abdomen during coughing.
- Encourage verbalization of feelings about diagnosis and perceived losses.
- Encourage participation in decision making.

EVALUATION

Mr. Harvey's weight remained stable through his hospitalization. On discharge he is taking a high-protein, high-calorie diet in six small feedings per day. He and his wife have reviewed his diet with the dietitian and are planning on using some dietary supplements at home to meet protein needs. He verbalizes an understanding of measures to prevent dumping syndrome, including separating his intake of solid foods and liquids. Mr. Harvey is using oral analgesics in the morning and at bedtime to control his

pain. He and his wife have begun to discuss the meaning of his diagnosis. Mrs. Harvey tells the discharge nurse, "We are going to go to a support group called 'Coping with Cancer' when George is stronger."

CRITICAL THINKING IN THE NURSING PROCESS

1. What is the rationale for maintaining nasogastric suction after gastrojejunostomy?
2. Develop a preoperative teaching plan for a client undergoing a partial gastrectomy.
3. Mr. Harvey calls you just before the initial dose of chemotherapy and says, "Everyone tells me that chemotherapy will cause vomiting, and I don't think I can take being sick again." How would you respond?
4. Design interventions to ensure adequate nutrition for people with advanced gastric cancer.

See Evaluating Your Response in Appendix C.

- Consult with dietitian for a complete nutrition assessment and diet planning. *The client is at risk for protein-calorie malnutrition, which impairs the ability to heal and recover from extensive surgery.*
- Weigh daily. Monitor laboratory values such as hemoglobin, hematocrit, and serum albumin levels. *Daily weights are a valuable measurement of both fluid and nutritional status. Laboratory values provide further evidence of nutritional status.*
- Provide preferred foods; have family prepare meals when possible. Provide supplemental feedings between meals. *Small, frequent feedings and preferred foods encourage intake of nutrients.*

PRACTICE ALERT
Assess ability to consume adequate nutrients. Nausea and feelings of early satiety may impair nutrient consumption, indicating a need to institute enteral or parenteral feedings.

- Arrange for visitors to be present during meals. *Eating is a social function as well as a physiologic one. Companionship often improves food intake.*
- Administer pain and antiemetic medications as needed before meals. *Pain and nausea suppress the appetite; relief promotes food intake.*

Anticipatory Grieving
- Encourage family members to spend as much time as possible with the client. *The family may feel helpless and ineffectual. Supporting family members' presence can encourage this vital interaction.*
- Do not negate denial if present. *Denial is a coping mechanism that protects the client from hopelessness.*
- Allow clients to talk openly if desired about their condition and the prognosis. *Acceptance of the clients' fears helps reduce anxiety and promote coping behaviors.*

- Actively listen to the client's and family's expressions of grieving. Avoid interrupting or offering meaningless words of consolation. *Being present and listening actively are often the most effective interventions for the grieving client.*

Using NANDA, NIC, and NOC

Chart 23–4 shows links between NANDA nursing diagnoses, NIC, and NOC when caring for a client with gastric cancer.

NANDA, NIC, AND NOC LINKAGES
CHART 23–4 The Client with Gastric Cancer

NANDA

Imbalanced Nutrition: Less than Body Requirements

NIC

Diet Staging

Nutrition Management

Weight Gain Assistance

NOC

Nutritional Status: Nutrient Intake

Weight Control

Data from *NANDA's Nursing Diagnoses: Definitions & Classification 2005–2006* by NANDA International (2005), Philadelphia; *Nursing Interventions Classification (NIC)* (4th ed.) by J. M. Dochterman & G. M. Bulechek (2004), St. Louis, MO: Mosby; and *Nursing Outcomes Classification (NOC)* (3rd ed.) by S. Moorhead, M. Johnson, and M. Mass (2004), St. Louis, MO: Mosby.

Community-Based Care

Although the client with gastric cancer may be hospitalized for surgery, most care is provided in the home and community-based settings such as hospice care. When preparing the client and family for home care, discuss the following topics:

■ Care of incision and feeding tube (if present) or central venous line

■ Maintaining nutrition and preventing complications of surgery such as dumping syndrome
■ Pain management
■ Provide referrals to home care agencies, hospice, and cancer support groups as appropriate.
■ Provide information about services available through the local chapter of the American Cancer Society.

EXPLORE MediaLink

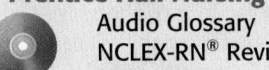

Prentice Hall Nursing MediaLink DVD-ROM
Audio Glossary
NCLEX-RN® Review

Animation
Ranitidine

COMPANION WEBSITE www.prenhall.com/lemone
Audio Glossary
NCLEX-RN® Review
Care Plan Activity: Peptic Ulcer Disease and Pain
Case Studies
GERD
Peptic Ulcer Disease
MediaLink Applications
Oral Cancer
Reflux Dyspareunia
Links to Resources

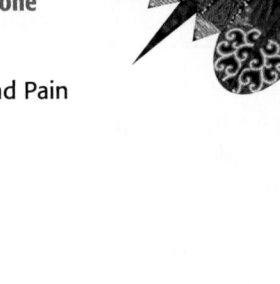

CHAPTER HIGHLIGHTS

■ Nausea and vomiting, common GI symptoms, may be indicative of disorders affecting many organ systems, including the GI tract, inner ear, CNS, or heart. Complications such as dehydration, electrolyte imbalance, and aspiration of gastric contents are primary concerns in treating nausea and vomiting.

■ Stomatitis and oral mucositis are common disorders of the mouth, potentially having a significant effect on comfort and nutrition.

■ Tobacco and alcohol use contribute to a number of upper GI disorders, including GERD, oral and esophageal cancers, and peptic ulcer disease. Encourage all clients to stop smoking or using smokeless tobacco and to consume alcohol in moderate amounts if at all to reduce their risk or these disorders.

■ Gastroesophageal reflux disease (GERD) is common. While it often is considered to be a benign condition, prolonged exposure of the lower esophagus to gastric juices can lead to esophagitis, hemorrhage, and scarring.

■ Both esophageal and gastric cancer often are diagnosed late in the disease because their symptoms may be vague. Encourage clients with complaints of dyphagia, a sensation of gastric fullness, or

heartburn to seek medical evaluation. Surgical resection of the cancerous portion of the esophagus or stomach is the treatment of choice when the tumor is diagnosed early.

■ Upper gastrointestinal bleeding can lead to significant blood loss and shock. Peptic ulcer disease accounts for the majority of UGI hemorrhage, although erosive gastritis and esophageal varices also are common causes.

■ Acute gastritis, often associated with aspirin or NSAID use, is generally benign and self-limited. Erosive gastritis, a complication of critical conditions such as shock, trauma, a major burn, or head injury, can lead to unexpected gastric hemorrhage. Chronic gastritis is an unrelated disorder associated with *H. pylori* infection.

■ *H. pylori* infection also is a major risk factor for peptic ulcer disease and gastric cancer. Effectively treating the infection can reduce or eliminate the risk of future exacerbations of PUD.

■ An acute change in the nature of abdominal pain in a client with PUD, especially when accompanied by vomiting, guarding of the abdomen, or a change in bowel sounds, could indicate an obstruction or perforation and release of gastric contents into the peritoneal cavity.

TEST YOURSELF NCLEX-RN® REVIEW

1 The nurse assessing for oral cancer risk factors in a client with a persistent sore on his tongue asks about:
   1. consumption of highly spiced foods.
   2. thumb sucking or pacifier use as a child.
   3. regular use of dental floss.
   4. tobacco use in any form.

2 The nurse teaching a client with gastroesophageal reflux disease includes which of the following instructions? (Select all that apply.)

   1. This is a benign disease requiring no treatment.
   2. Elevate the head of the bed on 6- to 8-inch blocks.
   3. Stop taking the prescribed proton-pump inhibitor once symptoms are relieved.
   4. Peppermint and chocolate candies can help relieve symptoms.
   5. Avoid lying down for several hours after eating.

3 The nurse evaluates his teaching of a client with acute stress gastritis as effective when the client states that she will:
1. avoid using aspirin or NSAIDs for routine pain relief.
2. consume only bland foods.
3. return for yearly upper endoscopy exams.
4. fully cook all meat, poultry, and egg products.

4 The nurse identifies which of the following nursing diagnoses as highest priority for the client admitted with peptic ulcer disease and possible perforation?
1. *Acute Pain*
2. *Ineffective Health Maintenance*
3. *Nausea*
4. *Impaired Tissue Integrity: Gastrointestinal*

5 Following a partial gastrectomy for gastric cancer, a client complains of nausea, abdominal pain and cramping, and diarrhea after eating. Recognizing manifestations of dumping syndrome, the nurse recommends:
1. fasting for a period of 6 to 12 hours before meals.
2. decreasing the protein content of meals.
3. frequent small meals that contain solid foods or liquids, but not both.
4. a diet rich in carbohydrates to maintain blood glucose levels.

6 The nurse caring for a client with esophageal cancer affecting the middle portion of the esophagus would immediately report which of the following?
1. crackles in the base of the right lung
2. bright bleeding from the mouth
3. weight loss
4. difficulty swallowing solid foods

7 The physician has ordered omeprazole 20 mg twice daily, clarithromycin 500 mg twice daily, and amoxicillin 1 g daily for a client with peptic ulcer disease. It is most important for the nurse to instruct the client to:
1. stop the drugs immediately and notify the physician if a rash, hives, or itching develop.
2. consume 8 oz. of yogurt or buttermilk daily while taking these drugs.
3. take the drugs on an empty stomach, 1 hour before breakfast and at least 2 hours after dinner.
4. take the drugs with a full glass of water.

8 When planning care for a client with stomatitis, the nurse identifies which of the following as a priority intervention?
1. Assist to cleanse mouth with mouthwash following meals.
2. Allow client to select appealing foods from a menu.
3. Provide viscous lidocaine to relieve mouth pain before meals.
4. Refer the client to a smoking cessation program.

9 The evening following a gastric resection, the nurse notes that there has been no drainage from the nasogastric tube for the past 3 hours. The nurse should:
1. chart the finding.
2. reposition the nasogastric tube.
3. gently irrigate the tube with normal saline.
4. notify the surgeon.

10 A client with a history of peptic ulcer disease suddenly begins to complain of severe abdominal pain. The nurse should: (Select all that apply.)
1. administer the prescribed proton-pump inhibitor.
2. obtain an order for a narcotic analgesic.
3. withhold oral food and fluids.
4. place the client in Fowler's position.
5. notify the physician.

See Test Yourself answers in Appendix C.

BIBLIOGRAPHY

Aiken, K. (2004). Managing tissue necrosis associated with oral carcinoma. *Clinical Journal of Oncology Nursing, 8*(4), 408–409.

American Cancer Society. (2005). *Cancer facts and figures 2005*. Atlanta: Author.

Brooks-Brunn, J. A. (2000). Esophageal cancer: An overview. *MEDSURG Nursing, 9*(5), 248–254.

Carlson, D. S., & Pfadt, E. (2004). Perforated peptic ulcer. *Nursing, 34*(12), 88.

Cawley, M. M., & Benson, L. M. (2005). Current trends in managing oral mucositis. *Clinical Journal of Oncology Nursing, 9*(5), 584–594.

Copstead, L. C., & Banasik, J. L. (2005). *Pathophysiology* (3rd ed.). St. Louis, MO: Elsevier/Saunders.

Dahlin, C. (2004). Oral complications at the end of life. *American Journal of Nursing, 104*(7), 40–47.

Dorey, E. (2004). Bug and guts. *Gastrointestinal Nursing, 2*(6), 10–13.

Edwards, S. J., & Metheny, N. A. (2000). Measurement of gastric residual volume: state of the science. *MEDSURG Nursing, 9*(3), 125–128.

Fontaine, K. L. (2005). *Healing practices: Alternative therapies for nursing* (2nd ed.). Upper Saddle River, NJ: Prentice Hall Health.

Gunter, D. A. (2004). A nursing guide to the assessment of GERD in long term care. *Director, 12*(4), 221, 223–227.

Hanson, C. (2004). Mouth care—How important is it? *Journal of Community Nursing, 18*(8), 4–6, 8.

Kasper, D. L., Braunwald, E., Fauci, A. S., Hauser, S. L., Longo, D. L., & Jameson, J. L. (2005). *Harrison's principles of internal medicine* (16th ed.). New York: McGraw-Hill.

Knudtson, M., & Davis, R. H. Jr. (2005). Frequent heartburn: An evidence-based approach to cost-effective management. *American Journal for Nurse Practitioners, 9*(1), 137–144.

Lehne, R. A. (2004). *Pharmacology for nursing care* (5th ed.). St. Louis, MO: Elsevier.

Levy, R. A., Stamm, L., & Meiner, S. E. (2002). Conservative management of GERD: A case study. *MEDSURG Nursing, 11*(4), 169–175, 182.

Mackenzie, D. J., Popplewell, P. K., & Billingsley, K. G. (2004). Care of patients after esophagectomy. *Critical Care Nurse, 24*(1), 16, 18–31.

Mattonen, M. C. (2001). Managing heartburn in adults. *MEDSURG Nursing, 10*(5), 269–276.

McCancer, K. L., & Huether, S. E. (2006). *Pathophysiology* (5th ed.). St. Louis, MO: Mosby.

McGinley, S. R. (2003). The other tobacco threat. Smokeless does not mean harmless. *Advance for Nurse Practitioners, 11*(4), 29–30, 34, 90.

Meeker, M. H., & Rothrock, J. C. (1999). *Alexander's care of the patient in surgery* (11th ed.). St. Louis, MO: Mosby.

Metheny, N. A., Schallom, M. E., & Edwards, S. J. (2004). Effect of gastrointestinal motility and feeding tube site on aspiration risk in critically ill patients: A review. *Heart & Lung, 33*(3), 131–145.

_____, & Titler, M. G. (2001). Assessing placement of feeding tubes. *American Journal of Nursing, 101*(5), 36–45.

National Cancer Institute. (2005). *Oral complications of chemotherapy and head/neck radiation (PDQ®)*. Bethesda, MD: National Institutes of Health.

Neafsey, P. J. (2004). Double trouble: Acetaminophen increases the risk of upper GI complications for people taking NSAIDS. *Home Healthcare Nurse, 22*(9), 641–642.

North American Nursing Diagnosis Association. (2005). *NANDA nursing diagnoses: Definitions & classification 2005–2006*. Philadelphia: Author.

Porth, C. M. (2005). *Pathophysiology: Concepts of altered health states* (7th ed.). Philadelphia: Lippincott.

Powe, B. D., & Finnie, R. (2004). Knowledge of oral cancer risk factors among African Americans: Do nurses have a role? *Oncology Nursing Forum, 31*(4), 785–792.

Rayhorn, N. (2004). Gastroesophageal reflux disease (GERD). *Nursing, 34*(7), 54–55.

Reavis, C. (2005). Rural health alert: *Helicobacter pylori* in well water. *Journal of the American Academy of Nurse Practitioners, 17*(7), 283–289.

Resto, M. A. (2000). Hospital extra. Gastroesophageal reflux disease. *American Journal of Nursing, 100*(9), 24D, 24F, 24H.

Rothrock, J. C. (2003). *Alexander's care of the patient in surgery* (12th ed.). St. Louis, MO: Mosby.

Slyk, M. P. (2004). Pathophysiology and management challenges of GERD in seniors. *Director, 12*(3), 147–153.

Smith, G. (2004). Gastritis. *Gastrointestinal Nursing, 2*(8), 33–40.

_____. (2004). The management of acute upper gastrointestinal bleeding. *Nursing Times, 100*(26), 40–43.

Spencer, J. W., & Jacobs, J. J. (2003). *Complementary and alternative medicine: An evidence-based approach* (2nd ed.). St. Louis, MO: Mosby.

Terrado, M., Russell, C., & Bowman, J. B. (2001). Dysphagia: An overview. *MEDSURG Nursing, 10*(5), 233–248.

Tierney, L. M., McPhee, S. J., & Papadakis, M. A. (2005). *Current medical diagnosis & treatment* (44th ed.). New York: Lange Medical Books/McGraw-Hill.

Uphold, C. R., & Graham, M. V. (2003). *Clinical guidelines in adult health* (3rd ed.). Gainesville, FL: Barmarrae Books.

Urden, L. D., Stacy, K. M., & Lough, M. E. (2006). *Thelan's critical care nursing* (5th ed.). St. Louis, MO: Mosby.

Use evidence-based clinical guidelines to prevent and treat oral mucositis. *ONS News, 20*(2), 7.

Walton, J. C., Miller, J., & Tordecilla, L. (2001). Elder oral assessment and care. *MEDSURG Nursing, 10*(1), 37–44.

Way, L. W., & Doherty, G. M. (2003). *Current surgical diagnosis & treatment* (11th ed.). New York: McGraw-Hill.

Wilkinson, J. M. (2005). *Nursing diagnosis handbook with NIC interventions and NOC outcomes* (8th ed.). Upper Saddle River, NJ: Prentice Hall Health.

Williams, J. L. (2003). Gastroesophageal reflux disease in the elderly. *Director, 11*(3), 107–109.

Wollner, T. (2004). Eradicate *H. pylori* with effective treatment regimens. *Nurse Practitioner: American Journal of Primary Health Care, 29*(6), 40–41, 43–44.

CHAPTER 24 Nursing Care of Clients with Gallbladder, Liver, and Pancreatic Disorders

LEARNING OUTCOMES

- Describe the pathophysiology of commonly occurring disorders of the gallbladder, liver, and exocrine pancreas.

- Use knowledge of normal anatomy and physiology to understand the manifestations and effects of biliary, hepatic, and pancreatic disorders.

- Relate changes in normal assessment data to the pathophysiology and manifestations of gallbladder, liver, and exocrine pancreatic disorders.

CLINICAL COMPETENCIES

- Assess functional health status of clients with gallbladder, liver, or pancreatic disease.

- Monitor for, document, and report expected and unexpected manifestations in clients with gallbladder, liver, or pancreatic disease.

- Prepare clients for and understand the purpose and significance of diagnostic tests for gallbladder, liver, and pancreatic disorders.

- Integrate appropriate dietary, pharmacologic, and other interdisciplinary measures into nursing care and teaching of the client with a gallbladder, liver, or pancreatic disorder.

- Provide appropriate nursing care for the client who has surgery of the gallbladder, liver, or pancreas.

- Integrate psychosocial, cultural, and spiritual considerations into the plan of care for a client with a gallbladder, liver, or pancreatic disorder.

- Use evidence-based practice to develop, implement, evaluate, and, as needed, revise the plan of care for clients with disorders of the gallbladder, liver, or pancreas.

- Provide appropriate client and family teaching to promote, maintain, and restore functional health status for clients with gallbladder, liver, and pancreatic disorders.

MEDIALINK

Resources for this chapter can be found on the Prentice Hall Nursing MediaLink DVD-ROM accompanying this textbook, and on the Companion Website at http://www.prenhall.com/lemone

KEY TERMS

alcoholic cirrhosis, *710*
ascites, *704*
balloon tamponade, *718*
biliary colic, *698*
cholecystitis, *698*
cholelithiasis, *697*
chronic hepatitis, *706*
cirrhosis, *710*
esophageal varices, *704*

fulminant hepatitis, *706*
gastric lavage, *718*
hematochezia, *722*
hepatitis, *705*
hepatorenal syndrome, *704*
jaundice, *704*
laparoscopic cholecystectomy, *699*
liver transplantation, *719*
pancreatitis, *726*

paracentesis, *717*
portal hypertension, *704*
**portal systemic
   encephalopathy,** *704*
steatorrhea, *727*
**transjugular intrahepatic
   portosystemic shunt (TIPS),** *719*

Gallbladder, liver, and exocrine pancreatic disorders may occur as primary disorders, or develop secondarily to other disease processes. One organ's functioning frequently affects that of another. Duct inflammation or obstruction, and changes in the multiple functions of these organs, can cause significant health effects.

Clients with a gallbladder, liver, or pancreatic disorder may experience pain, multiple metabolic and nutritional disturbances, and altered body image. Nursing care addresses physiologic and psychosocial needs of the client and family.

GALLBLADDER DISORDERS

Altered bile flow through the hepatic, cystic, or common bile duct is a common problem. It often leads to inflammation and other complications. Gallstones are the most common cause of obstructed flow. Tumors and abscesses also can obstruct bile flow.

THE CLIENT WITH GALLSTONES

Cholelithiasis is the formation of stones (*calculi* or *gallstones*) within the gallbladder or biliary duct system. Cholelithiasis is a common problem in the United States, affecting more than 10% of men and 20% of women by age 65 (Tierney et al., 2005). Box 24–1 lists risk factors for gallstones. The incidence of gallstones varies among people of different ethnic backgrounds; see the accompanying Focus on Cultural Diversity box.

Physiology Review

Normally, bile is formed by the liver and stored in the gallbladder. Bile contains bile salts, bilirubin, water, electrolytes, cholesterol, fatty acids, and lecithin. In the gallbladder, some of the water and electrolytes are absorbed, further concentrating the bile. Food entering the intestine stimulates the gallbladder

FOCUS ON CULTURAL DIVERSITY
Gallstones

Native Americans in both the Northern and Southern Hemispheres, and those of the Pima tribe in particular, have a higher incidence of gallstones than do Caucasians of American or European heritage. This is thought to result from genes that promote efficient calorie use and fat storage—a beneficial trait when the availability of adequate food varies over time. Gallstones composed of cholesterol are less common in African Americans, and Asians have a low incidence of the disease (Tierney et al., 2005).

to contract and release bile through the common bile duct and sphincter of Oddi into the intestine. The bile salts in bile increase the solubility and absorption of dietary fats.

Pathophysiology and Manifestations
Cholelithiasis

Gallstones form when several factors interact: abnormal bile composition, biliary stasis, and inflammation of the gallbladder. Most gallstones (80%) consist primarily of cholesterol; the rest contain a mixture of bile components. Excess cholesterol in bile is associated with obesity, a high-calorie, high-cholesterol diet, and drugs that lower serum cholesterol levels. When bile is supersaturated with cholesterol, it can precipitate out to form stones. Biliary stasis, or slowed emptying of the gallbladder, contributes to cholelithiasis. Stones do not form when the gallbladder empties completely in response to hormonal stimulation. Slowed or incomplete emptying allows cholesterol to concentrate and increases the risk of stone formation. Finally, inflammation of the gallbladder allows excess water and bile salt reabsorption, increasing the risk for lithiasis.

BOX 24–1 Risk Factors for Gallstones

- Age
- Family history of gallstones
- Race or ethnicity: Native American (either Northern or Southern Hemisphere); Northern European heritage
- Obesity, hyperlipidemia
- Rapid weight loss
- Female gender; use of oral contraceptives
- Biliary stasis: pregnancy, fasting, prolonged parenteral nutrition
- Diseases or conditions: cirrhosis; ileal disease or resection; sickle cell anemia; glucose intolerance

PRACTICE ALERT
Certain very-low-calorie diets are associated with a high risk of cholelithiasis. Increased cholesterol concentration in the bile and decreased gallbladder contractions associated with fasting increase the risk of gallstone formation.

Most gallstones are formed in the gallbladder. They then may migrate into the ducts (Figure 24–1 ■), leading to *cholangitis* (duct inflammation). Although some people with cholelithiasis are asymptomatic, many develop manifestations. Early manifestations of gallstones may be vague: epigastric fullness or mild gastric distress after eating a large or fatty meal. Stones that obstruct the cystic duct or common bile duct lead to distention and increased pressure behind the stone. This causes **biliary colic**, a severe, steady pain in the epigastric region or right upper quadrant of the abdomen. The pain may radiate to the back, right scapula, or shoulder. The pain often begins suddenly following a meal, and may last as long as 5 hours. It often is accompanied by nausea and vomiting.

Obstruction of the common bile duct may cause bile reflux into the liver, leading to jaundice, pain, and possible liver damage. If the common duct is obstructed, pancreatic enzymes will be unable to enter the small intestine, and pancreatitis (discussed later in this chapter) becomes a potential complication.

Cholecystitis
Cholecystitis is inflammation of the gallbladder. *Acute cholecystitis* usually follows obstruction of the cystic duct by a stone. The obstruction increases pressure within the gallbladder, leading to ischemia of the gallbladder wall and mucosa. Chemical and bacterial inflammation often follow. The ischemia can lead to necrosis and perforation of the gallbladder wall.

Acute cholecystitis usually begins with an attack of biliary colic. The pain involves the entire right upper quadrant (RUQ), and may radiate to the back, right scapula, or shoulder. Movement or deep breathing may aggravate the pain. The pain usually lasts longer than biliary colic, continuing for 12 to 18 hours. Anorexia, nausea, and vomiting are common. Fever of-

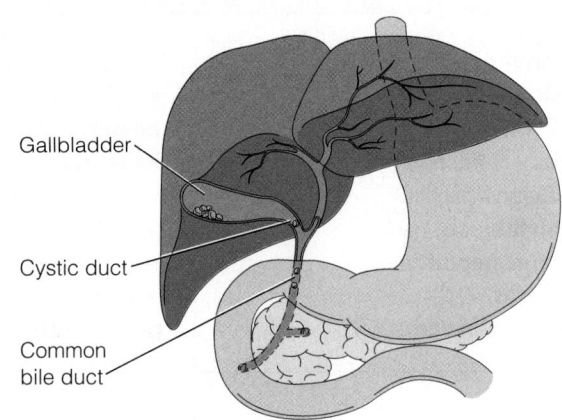

Figure 24–1 ■ Common locations of gallstones.

ten is present, and may be accompanied by chills. The RUQ is tender to palpation.

Chronic cholecystitis may result from repeated bouts of acute cholecystitis or from persistent irritation of the gallbladder wall by stones. Bacteria may be present in the bile as well. Chronic cholecystitis often is asymptomatic.

Complications of cholecystitis include *empyema*, a collection of infected fluid within the gallbladder; gangrene and perforation with resulting peritonitis or abscess formation; formation of a fistula into an adjacent organ (such as the duodenum, colon, or stomach); or obstruction of the small intestine by a large gallstone (*gallstone ileus*). Table 24–1 compares the manifestations and complications of acute cholelithiasis with those of cholecystitis.

INTERDISCIPLINARY CARE

Treatment of the client with cholelithiasis or cholecystitis depends of the acuity of the condition and the client's overall health status. When gallstones are present but asymptomatic and the client has a low risk for complications, conservative treatment is indicated. However, when the client experiences frequent symp-

TABLE 24–1 Manifestations and Complications of Cholelithiasis and Cholecystitis

MANIFESTATIONS	CHOLELITHIASIS	CHOLECYSTITIS
Pain	■ Abrupt onset ■ Severe, steady ■ Localized to epigastrium and RUQ of abdomen ■ May radiate to back, right scapula, and shoulder ■ Lasts 30 minutes to 5 hours	■ Abrupt onset ■ Severe, steady ■ Generalized in RUQ of abdomen ■ May radiate to back, right scapula, and shoulder ■ Lasts 12 to 18 hours ■ Aggravated by movement, breathing
Associated symptoms	■ Nausea, vomiting	■ Anorexia, nausea, vomiting ■ RUQ tenderness and guarding ■ Chills and fever
Complications	■ Cholecystitis ■ Common bile duct obstruction with possible jaundice and liver damage ■ Common duct obstruction with pancreatitis	■ Gangrene and perforation with peritonitis ■ Chronic cholecystitis ■ Empyema ■ Fistula formation ■ Gallstone ileus

toms, has acute cholecystitis, or has very large stones, the gallbladder and stones are usually surgically removed.

Diagnosis

Diagnostic tests are ordered to identify the presence and location of stones, identify possible complications, and help differentiate gallbladder disease from other disorders.

- *Serum bilirubin* is measured. Elevated direct (conjugated) bilirubin may indicate obstructed bile flow in the biliary duct system (Box 24–2).
- *Complete blood count (CBC)* may indicate infection and inflammation if the WBC count is elevated.
- *Serum amylase* and *lipase* are measured to identify possible pancreatitis related to common duct obstruction.
- *Abdominal x-ray* (flat plate of the abdomen) may show gallstones that have a high calcium content.
- *Ultrasonography of the gallbladder* is a noninvasive exam that can accurately diagnose cholelithiasis. It also can be used to assess emptying of the gallbladder.
- *Oral cholecystogram* is performed using a dye administered orally to assess the gallbladder's ability to concentrate and excrete bile.
- *Gallbladder scans* use an intravenous radioactive solution that is rapidly extracted from the blood and excreted into the biliary tree to diagnose cystic duct obstruction and acute or chronic cholecystitis.

See Chapter 21 ∞ for more information about and the nursing implications of these diagnostic tests.

Medications

Clients who refuse surgery or for whom surgery is inappropriate may be treated with a drug to dissolve the gallstones. Urso-

diol (Actigall) and chenodiol (Chenix) reduce the cholesterol content of gallstones, leading to their gradual dissolution. These drugs act by reducing cholesterol production in the liver, thus reducing the cholesterol content of bile. Consequently, these drugs are most effective in treating stones with high cholesterol content. They are less effective in treating radiopaque stones with high calcium salt content. Ursodiol is generally well tolerated with few side effects, whereas chenodiol has a high incidence of diarrhea at therapeutic doses. It also is hepatotoxic, so periodic liver function studies are required during therapy.

The primary disadvantages of pharmacologic treatment for gallstones include its cost, long duration (2 years or more), and the high incidence of recurrent stone formation when treatment is discontinued. If infection is suspected, antibiotics may be ordered to cure the infection and reduce associated inflammation and edema. Clients with pruritus (itching) due to severe obstructive jaundice and an accumulation of bile salts on the skin may be given cholestyramine (Questran). This drug binds with bile salts to promote their excretion in the feces. A narcotic analgesic such as morphine may be required for pain relief during an acute attack of cholecystitis.

Treatments

SURGERY **Laparoscopic cholecystectomy** (removal of the gallbladder) is the treatment of choice for symptomatic cholelithiasis or cholecystitis. This minimally invasive procedure has a low risk of complications and generally requires a hospital stay of less than 24 hours. Not all clients are candidates for laparoscopic cholecystectomy, and there is a risk that a laparoscopic cholecystectomy may be converted to a *laparotomy* (surgical opening into the abdomen) during the procedure. See the following page for nursing care for a client having a laparoscopic cholecystectomy. The Nursing Research box on page 700 discusses evidence-based practice for managing pain in clients undergoing laparoscopic cholecystectomy.

When stones are lodged within the ducts, a cholecystectomy with common bile duct exploration may be done. A T-tube (Figure 24–2 ■) is inserted to maintain patency of the

---

BOX 24–2 Sorting Out Total, Direct, and Indirect Bilirubin Levels

When serum bilirubin levels are drawn, the results usually are reported as the total bilirubin, direct bilirubin, and indirect bilirubin levels. Most bilirubin is formed from hemoglobin, as aging or abnormal RBCs are removed from circulation and destroyed. It is then bound to protein and transported to the liver. This protein-bound bilirubin is called *indirect* or *unconjugated* bilirubin. Once in the liver, bilirubin is separated from the protein and converted to a soluble form, *direct* or *conjugated* bilirubin. Conjugated bilirubin is then excreted in the bile.

- **Total** (serum) **bilirubin,** the total bilirubin in the blood, includes both indirect and direct forms. In adults, the normal total bilirubin is 0.3 to 1.2 mg/dL. Total bilirubin levels increase when more is being produced (e.g., RBC hemolysis), or when its metabolism or excretion are impaired (e.g., liver disease or biliary obstruction).
- **Direct** (conjugated) **bilirubin** levels, normally 0 to 0.2 mg/dL in adults, rise when its excretion is impaired by obstruction within the liver (e.g., in cirrhosis, hepatitis, exposure to hepatotoxins) or in the biliary system.
- **Indirect** (unconjugated) **bilirubin** levels, normally <1.1 mg/dL in adults, rise in RBC hemolysis (e.g., sickle cell disease or transfusion reaction).

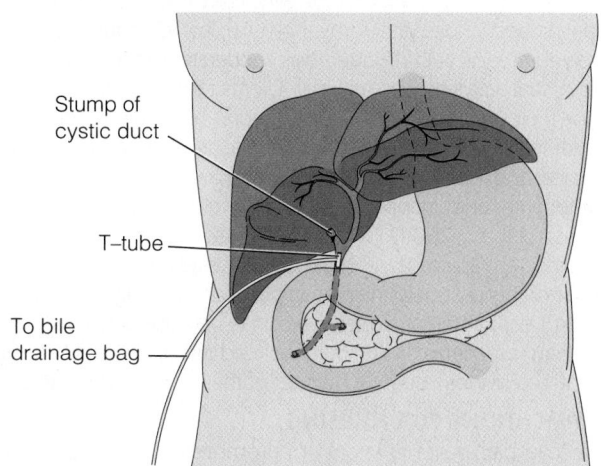

Figure 24–2 ■ T-tube placement in the common bile duct. Bile fluid flows with gravity into a drainage collection device below the level of the common bile duct.

NURSING CARE OF THE CLIENT HAVING Laparoscopic Cholecystectomy

PREOPERATIVE CARE

- Provide routine preoperative care as ordered (see Chapter 4 ∞).
- Reinforce teaching about the procedure and postoperative expectations, including pain management, deep breathing, and mobilization. *Preoperative teaching reduces anxiety and promotes rapid postoperative recovery.*

POSTOPERATIVE CARE

- Provide routine postoperative recovery care as outlined in Chapter 4 ∞.
- Assist to chair at bedside as allowed. *Early mobilization promotes lung ventilation and circulation, reducing the potential for postoperative complications.*

- Advance oral intake from ice chips to regular diet as tolerated. *Oral intake can be rapidly resumed due to minimal disruption of the gastrointestinal tract during surgery.*
- Provide and reinforce teaching: pain management, incision care, activity level, postoperative follow-up appointments. *With early discharge, the client and family assume responsibility for the majority of postoperative care. A clear understanding of this care and expected needs reduces anxiety and the risk of postoperative complications.*
- Initiate follow-up contact 24 to 48 hours after discharge to evaluate adequacy of pain control, incision management, and discharge understanding. *Contact following discharge provides an opportunity to evaluate care and reinforce teaching.*

duct and promote bile passage while the edema decreases. Excess bile is collected in a drainage bag secured below the surgical site. If it is suspected that a stone has been retained following surgery, a postoperative cholangiogram via the T-tube or direct visualization of the duct with an endoscope may be performed. See the box on page 701 for nursing care for a client with a T-tube.

Some clients who are poor surgical risks and for whom laparoscopic cholecystectomy is inappropriate may have either a *cholecystostomy* to drain the gallbladder, or a *choledochostomy* to remove stones and position a T-tube in the common bile duct.

NUTRITION Food intake may be eliminated during an acute attack of cholecystitis, and a nasogastric tube inserted to relieve nausea and vomiting. Dietary fat intake may be limited, especially if the client is obese. If bile flow is obstructed, fat-soluble vitamins (A, D, E, and K) and bile salts may need to be administered.

OTHER THERAPIES In some cases, shock wave lithotripsy may be used with drug therapy to dissolve large gallstones. In *extracorporeal shock wave lithotripsy*, ultrasound is used to align the stones with the source of shock waves and the com-

NURSING RESEARCH   Evidence-Based Practice: Client Undergoing Laparoscopic Cholecystectomy

Following ambulatory surgery procedures such as laparoscopic cholecystectomy, clients must self-manage their pain after discharge. In a study of pain severity and management among ambulatory surgery clients, Watt-Watson, Chung, Chan, and McGillion (2004) found that while the most severe pain was experienced within the first 72 hours, some clients reported severe pain episodes up to a week after surgery. For most clients undergoing laparoscopic cholecystectomy, however, by 72 hours postoperatively the worst pain reported was moderate and the interference with usual activities was minimal. Clients tended to significantly reduce their use of analgesics by 72 hours after surgery, perhaps because many experienced adverse effects such as constipation, nausea, and/or drowsiness. Overall, analgesic use was found to be inadequate and inappropriate among study participants (Watt-Watson et al., 2004). Most clients used acetaminophen with codeine, an analgesic with known dose-related adverse effects. Some clients did not fill their prescription for the analgesic or stopped taking it early in the postoperative course because of nausea or constipation experiences. Preoperative teaching about pain management was inadequate for a number of the participants in this study.

IMPLICATIONS FOR NURSING

Effective pain relief is known to promote healing and immune function following surgery. This study indicates a crucial need to

carefully prepare clients undergoing ambulatory surgery, including laparoscopic cholecystectomy, for pain management strategies. Effective postoperative pain management requires a combination of good preoperative education, discharge planning related to the client's expectations of pain, and postoperative pain management.

CRITICAL THINKING IN CLIENT CARE

1. Some clients in this study reported purposely not filling their analgesic prescription due to anticipated adverse effects of the drug. How can the nurse intervene to prevent this and promote effective postoperative pain management? What teaching could you provide to help clients manage adverse effects of the prescribed drug?
2. Few clients in this study reported use of adjunctive pain relief measures (nonsteroidal anti-inflammatory drugs, application of heat or cold, etc.). What adjunctive pain relief measures would be appropriate for the nurse to teach clients undergoing laparoscopic cholecystectomy?
3. Some clients in this study expressed concern about becoming addicted to opioid analgesics, citing this as a reason to discontinue their use within 48 to 72 hours after surgery. How would you respond to a client who expresses this as a concern?

Source: Data from Pain management following discharge after ambulatory same-day surgery, by Judy Watt-Watson, Frances Chung, Vincent W. S. Chan, and Michael McGillion (2004). *Journal of Pain Management, 12*(3), 153–161.

NURSING CARE OF THE CLIENT WITH A T-Tube

- Ensure that the T-tube is properly connected to a sterile container; keep the tube below the level of the surgical wound. *This position promotes the flow of bile and prevents backflow or seepage of caustic bile onto the skin. The tube itself decreases biliary tree pressure.*
- Monitor drainage from the T-tube for color and consistency; record as output. Normally, the tube may drain up to 500 mL in the first 24 hours after surgery; drainage decreases to less than 200 mL in 2 to 3 days, and is minimal thereafter. Drainage may be blood tinged initially, changing to green-brown. Report excessive drainage immediately (after 48 hours, drainage greater than 500 mL is considered excessive). *Stones or edema and inflammation can obstruct ducts below the tube, requiring treatment.*

- Place in Fowler's position. *This promotes gravity drainage of bile.*
- Assess skin for bile leakage during dressing changes. *Bile irritates the skin; it may be necessary to apply skin protection with karaya or another barrier product.*
- Teach client how to manage the tube when turning, ambulating, and performing activities of daily living. *Direct pulling or traction on the tube must be avoided.*
- If indicated, teach care of the T-tube, how to clamp it, and signs of infection. *Clients may be discharged home with the tube in place. Reporting early signs of infection facilitates prompt treatment.*

---

puterized lithotripter. Positioning is of prime importance throughout the procedure, which usually takes an hour. Mild sedation may be given during the procedure. Nursing care after the procedure includes monitoring for biliary colic, which can result from the gallbladder contracting to remove stone fragments; nausea; and transient hematuria. *Percutaneous cholecystostomy,* ultrasound-guided drainage of the gallbladder, may be done in high-risk clients to postpone or even eliminate the need for surgery.

COMPLEMENTARY THERAPIES The herb goldenseal has been used in treating cholecystitis. One of the active ingredients in goldenseal, berberine, stimulates secretion of bile and bilirubin. It also inhibits the growth of many common pathogens, including those known to infect the gallbladder. A study of the effectiveness of berberine in clients with cholecystitis demonstrated relief of all symptoms. Goldenseal can stimulate the uterus, so it is contraindicated for use during pregnancy. It also should not be used by nursing mothers.

NURSING CARE

In addition to the nursing care discussed in this section, a Nursing Care Plan for a client with cholelithiasis is found on page 702.

Health Promotion

Although most risk factors for cholelithiasis cannot be controlled or modified, several can. Modifiable risk factors include obesity, hyperlipidemia, extremely low-calorie diets, and diets high in cholesterol. Encourage clients who are obese to increase their activity level and follow a low-carbohydrate, low-fat, low-cholesterol diet to promote weight loss and reduce their risk for developing gallstones. Discuss the dangers of "yo-yo" dieting, with cycles of weight loss followed by weight gain, and of extremely low-calorie diets. Encourage clients with high serum cholesterol levels to discuss using cholesterol-lowering drugs with their primary care provider.

Assessment

Assessment data related to cholelithiasis and cholecystitis include the following:
- *Health history:* Current manifestations, including RUQ pain, its character and relationship to meals, duration, and radiation, nausea and vomiting, or other symptoms; duration of symptoms; risk factors or previous history of symptoms; chronic diseases such as diabetes, cirrhosis, or inflammatory bowel disease; current diet; use of oral contraceptives or possibility of pregnancy.
- *Physical assessment:* Current weight; color of skin and sclera; abdominal assessment including light palpation for tenderness; color of urine and stool.
- *Diagnostic tests:* Monitor results of WBC, serum bilirubin, liver enzymes, and pancreatic enzymes (amylase and lipase).

Nursing Diagnoses and Interventions

Priority nursing diagnoses for the client with cholelithiasis or cholecystitis often include pain related to biliary colic or surgery, imbalanced nutrition related to the effects of altered bile flow and to nausea and anorexia, and risk for infection related to potential rupture of an acutely inflamed gallbladder. Nursing interventions for the client who has undergone a laparoscopic or open cholecystectomy are similar to those for other clients having abdominal surgery. See Chapter 4 ∞ .

Pain

The pain associated with cholelithiasis can be severe. Sometimes a combination of interventions is indicated.
- Discuss the relationship between fat intake and the pain. Teach ways to reduce fat intake (Box 24–3). *Fat entering the duodenum initiates gallbladder contractions, causing pain when gallstones are present in the ducts.*
- Withhold oral food and fluids during episodes of acute pain. Insert nasogastric tube and connect to low suction if ordered. *Emptying the stomach reduces the amount of chyme entering the duodenum and the stimulus for gallbladder contractions, thus reducing pain.*

NURSING CARE PLAN | A Client with Cholelithiasis

Joyce Red Wing is a 44-year-old married mother of three children. A member of the Chickasaw tribe, she is active in tribal activities and works part time as a cook at a community kitchen. Recently Mrs. Red Wing has noticed a dull pain in her upper abdomen that gets worse after eating fatty foods; nausea and sometimes vomiting accompany the pain. She had a similar pain after the birth of her last child. She is diagnosed with cholelithiasis, and is admitted for a laparoscopic cholecystectomy.

ASSESSMENT

David Corbin, RN, takes Mrs. Red Wing's admission history. It includes intolerance to fatty foods and intermittent "stabbing" abdominal pain that radiates to her back. Her usual diet includes tacos or fried bread and biscuits with gravy for breakfast. She reports "not wanting to eat much of anything lately." She states she has never had surgery before and hopes "everything goes well." Physical assessment includes T 100°F (37.7°C), P 88, R 20, and BP 130/84. She has had a recent 5 lb weight loss, currently weighing 130 lb (59 kg). She is 63 inches (160 cm) tall. Abdominal examination elicits tenderness in the right upper abdominal quadrant. She has no jaundice, chills, or evidence of complications.

DIAGNOSES

- *Imbalanced Nutrition: Less than Body Requirements* related to anorexia and recent weight loss
- *Pain* related to inflamed gallbladder and surgical incisions
- *Risk for Infection* related to potential bacterial contamination of abdominal cavity
- *Anxiety* related to lack of information about perioperative experience

EXPECTED OUTCOMES

- Maintain present weight within 5 lb (2.3 kg) over the next 3 weeks.
- Resume regular diet, decreasing intake of foods high in fat.

- Verbalize adequate pain control after surgery and with activity resumption.
- Remain free of infection.
- Verbalize a decrease in anxiety before surgery.

PLANNING AND IMPLEMENTATION

- Teach about the gallbladder and the function of bile.
- Discuss pre- and postoperative care, including self-care following discharge.
- Promote mobility as soon as allowed after surgery.
- Teach home care of incisions and recognition of signs of infection.
- Review specific high-fat foods to avoid and ways to maintain her weight.
- Provide analgesia as needed postoperatively. Teach appropriate analgesic use after discharge.

EVALUATION

Mrs. Red Wing is discharged the morning after her surgery. She is afebrile, has no signs of infection, and is able to appropriately care for her incisions. She identifies signs of infection and talks about ways to reduce her fat intake while keeping her weight stable. She verbalizes understanding of initial activity restrictions and resumption of normal activities. Mrs. Red Wing states, "It wasn't as bad as I thought it would be at first." She has an appointment to see her surgeon in 1 week.

CRITICAL THINKING IN THE NURSING PROCESS

1. What is the rationale for a low-fat diet with cholelithiasis? Discuss nutritional practices as they relate to the medical problem and Mrs. Red Wing's culture.
2. How would your discharge teaching for Mrs. Red Wing differ if she had had an open cholecystectomy instead of a laparoscopic cholecystectomy?
3. Design a nursing care plan for Mrs. Red Wing for the nursing diagnosis *Fatigue*.
   See Evaluating Your Response in Appendix C.

BOX 24–3 Examples of High-Fat Foods

- Whole-milk products (e.g., cream, ice cream, cheese)
- Doughnuts, deep-fried
- Avocados
- Sausage, bacon, hot dogs
- Gravies with fat, cream
- Most nuts (e.g., pecans, cashews)
- Corn chips and potato chips
- Butter and cooking oils
- Fried foods (e.g., cheeseburgers, hamburgers, french fries)
- Peanut butter
- Chocolate candies

- For severe pain, administer morphine, meperidine, or other narcotic analgesia as ordered. *Recent research indicates that morphine is no more likely to cause spasms of the sphincter of Oddi than meperidine.*

- Place in Fowler's position. *Fowler's position decreases pressure on the inflamed gallbladder.*
- Monitor vital signs, including temperature, at least every 4 hours. *Bacterial infection often is present in acute cholecystitis, and may cause an elevated temperature and respiratory rate.*

Imbalanced Nutrition: Less than Body Requirements

The client with severe gallbladder disease may develop nutritional imbalances related to anorexia, pain, and nausea following meals, and impaired bile flow that alters absorption of fat and fat-soluble vitamins (A, D, E, and K) from the gut.

- Assess nutritional status, including diet history, height and weight, and skinfold measurements (see Chapters 21 and 22 ∞). *Even though often obese, clients with gallbladder disease may have an imbalanced diet or may have specific vitamin deficiencies, particularly of the fat-soluble vitamins.*
- Evaluate laboratory results, including serum bilirubin, albumin, glucose, and cholesterol levels. Report abnormal results

to the primary care provider. *Elevated serum bilirubin may indicate impaired bilirubin excretion due to obstructed bile flow. A low serum albumin may indicate poor nutritional status. Glucose intolerance and hypercholesterolemia are risk factors for cholelithiasis.*

- Refer to a dietitian or nutritionist for diet counseling to promote healthy weight loss and reduce pain episodes. *A low-carbohydrate, low-fat, higher protein diet reduces symptoms of cholecystitis. While fasting and very-low-calorie diets are contraindicated, a moderate reduction in calorie intake and increased activity levels promote weight loss.*
- Administer vitamin supplements as ordered. *Clients who do not absorb fat well due to obstructed bile flow may require supplements of the fat-soluble vitamins.*

Risk for Infection

An acutely inflamed gallbladder may become necrotic and rupture, releasing its contents into the abdominal cavity. While the resulting infection often remains localized, peritonitis can result from chemical irritation and bacterial contamination of the peritoneal cavity.

> **PRACTICE ALERT**
> Rupture of an acutely inflamed gallbladder may be heralded by abrupt but transient pain relief as contents are released from the distended gallbladder into the abdomen. Promptly report this change to the physician.

Following open cholecystectomy (*laparotomy*), the risk for pulmonary infection is significant due to the high abdominal incision.

- Monitor vital signs including temperature every 4 hours. Promptly report vital sign changes or temperature elevation. *Tachycardia, increased respiratory rate, or an elevated temperature may indicate an infectious process.*
- Assess abdomen every 4 hours and as indicated (e.g., when pain level changes abruptly). *Increasing abdominal tenderness or a rigid, boardlike abdomen may indicate rupture of the gallbladder with peritonitis.*
- Assist to cough and deep breathe or use incentive spirometer every 1 to 2 hours while awake. Splint abdominal incision with a blanket or pillow during coughing. *The high abdominal incision of an open cholecystectomy interferes with effective coughing and deep breathing, increasing the risk of atelectasis and respiratory infections such as pneumonia.*
- Place in Fowler's position and encourage ambulation as allowed. *Fowler's position and ambulating promote lung expansion and airway clearance, reducing the risk of respiratory infections.*
- Administer antibiotics as ordered. *Antibiotics may be given preoperatively to reduce the risk of infection from infected gallbladder contents, and may be continued postoperatively to prevent infection.*

Community-Based Care

Teaching varies, depending on the choice of treatment options for cholelithiasis and cholecystitis. If surgery is not an option, teach about medications that dissolve stones, their use and adverse effects (diarrhea is a common side effect), and maintaining a low-fat, low-carbohydrate diet if indicated. Include an explanation about the role of bile and the function of the gallbladder in terms that the client and family can understand.

Provide appropriate preoperative teaching for the planned procedure. Discuss the possibility of open cholecystectomy even when a laparoscopic procedure is planned. Teach postoperative self-care measures to manage pain and prevent complications. If the client will be discharged with a T-tube, provide instructions about its care (see the Nursing Care box on page 701). Discuss manifestations of complications to report to the physician. Stress the importance of follow-up appointments.

Following cholecystectomy, a low-fat diet may be initially recommended. Refer the client and food preparer to a dietitian to review low-fat foods. (See Box 24–3 for examples of high-fat foods to avoid.) Higher fat foods may be gradually added to the diet as tolerated.

THE CLIENT WITH CANCER OF THE GALLBLADDER

Gallbladder cancer is rare, primarily affecting people over age 65. Women are more likely to develop the disorder. Manifestations of gallbladder cancer include intense pain and a palpable mass in the RUQ of the abdomen. Jaundice and weight loss are common. Gallbladder cancers spread by direct extension to the liver, and metastasize via the blood and lymph system.

At the time of diagnosis, the cancer usually is too advanced to treat surgically. Ninety-five percent of clients with primary cancer of the gallbladder die within 1 year. Radical and extensive surgical interventions may be performed, but the prognosis is poor regardless of treatment (Tierney et al., 2005). Nursing care is palliative, focusing on maintaining comfort and independence to the extent possible.

LIVER DISORDERS

The liver is a complex organ with multiple metabolic and regulatory functions. Optimal liver function is essential to health. Because of the significant amount of blood in the liver at all times, it is exposed to the effects of pathogens, drugs, toxins, and possibly malignant cells. As a result, liver cells may become inflamed or damaged, or cancerous tumors may develop.

Physiology Review

The essential functions of the liver include the metabolism of proteins, carbohydrates, and fats. It also is responsible for the metabolism of steroid hormones and most drugs. It synthesizes essential blood proteins, including albumin and clotting factors in particular. The liver detoxifies alcohol and other toxic substances. Ammonia, a toxic by-product of protein metabolism, is converted to urea in the liver for elimination by the kidneys. The liver produces bile, an essential substance for absorbing fats and eliminating bilirubin from the body. Minerals and fat-soluble vitamins are stored in the liver, as is glycogen (stored carbohydrate for energy reserves). The Kupffer cells that line the sinusoids phagocytize foreign cells and damaged blood cells. See Chapter 21 ∞ for more information about the liver.

Common Manifestations of Liver Disorders

Although many different disorders can disrupt liver function, their manifestations relate to three primary effects: disrupted liver cell function, impaired bilirubin conversion and excretion leading to jaundice, and disrupted blood flow through the liver, with resulting portal hypertension.

Hepatocellular Failure

The liver is vital to digestion and metabolism of nutrients; the production of plasma proteins, including those involved in clotting; and the metabolism and excretion of compounds such as bilirubin, steroid hormones, and ammonia, as well as toxins (such as alcohol) and drugs. Impaired function of liver cells has multiple effects, including:

- Impaired protein metabolism with decreased production of albumin and clotting factors. Low albumin levels contribute to edema in peripheral tissues and **ascites**, accumulation of fluid in the abdomen, as plasma oncotic pressure is reduced. Impaired clotting factor production increases the risk for bleeding.
- Disrupted glucose metabolism and storage with resulting alterations in blood glucose levels (either hyperglycemia or hypoglycemia).
- Reduced bile production that impairs the absorption of lipids and fat-soluble vitamins. Inadequate vitamin K, a fat-soluble vitamin, affects the production of clotting factors, leading to a bleeding tendency.
- Impaired metabolism of steroid hormones (including estrogen and testosterone) leads to feminization in men and irregular menses in women.

Jaundice

Disrupted metabolism and excretion of bilirubin allows it to accumulate in tissues, leading to **jaundice**, yellow staining of tissues. Jaundice (also called *icterus*) often is first noticeable in the sclera of the eyes, then the skin.

When RBCs are destroyed (due to cell aging or disease), hemoglobin is released. The hemoglobin molecule breaks up into globin, a protein, and heme, the iron-containing portion of the molecule. In this process, biliverdin, later converted to fat-soluble bilirubin (*unconjugated bilirubin*), is released. The bilirubin binds with albumin to be transported to the liver. In the liver, it is converted to a water-soluble form (*conjugated bilirubin*) to be excreted in the bile. See Box 24–2 for more information about bilirubin metabolism.

Jaundice can result from disruptions at any point in the production and metabolism of bilirubin:

- *Hemolytic jaundice* develops when excess RBC destruction (hemolysis) releases more bilirubin into circulation than the liver is able to process. High blood levels of unconjugated bilirubin are seen.
- *Hepatic jaundice* occurs when impaired liver cell (*hepatocyte*) function disrupts the conversion and excretion of bilirubin. Blood levels of both conjugated and unconjugated bilirubin may be elevated. Stools may appear normal or clay colored, and urine is dark because the conjugated bilirubin is excreted by the kidneys.
- Obstruction of bile flow within the biliary system (the gallbladder and bile ducts) impairs bilirubin excretion, leading to *obstructive jaundice*. Levels of conjugated bilirubin are elevated. Stools are light or clay colored due to lack of bile pigment; and urine is dark because the kidneys excrete bilirubin.

Portal Hypertension

Impaired blood flow through the liver increases pressure in the portal venous system that drains the gastrointestinal tract, the spleen, and surface veins of the abdomen. **Portal hypertension**, increased pressure in the portal system, has several effects when it is prolonged:

- Dilation of veins in the gastrointestinal tract and the abdominal wall. This congestion tends to suppress the appetite, and lead to formation of collateral vessels in the distal esophagus, stomach, and rectum. The dilated, congested vessels in the esophagus are known as **esophageal varices**; in the rectum, they lead to the development of hemorrhoids. In advanced liver failure, superficial varices may develop around the umbilicus, a feature known as *caput medusae*.
- Splenomegaly, or enlargement of the spleen.
- Ascites, accumulation of fluid in the peritoneal cavity. Increased hydrostatic pressure in abdominal vessels forces fluid out of the vessels and into the peritoneal cavity. Low serum albumin levels (*hypoalbuminemia*) contribute to fluid accumulation by reducing the osmotic draw of fluid back into vessels.
- **Portal systemic encephalopathy** (or hepatic *encephalopathy*), impaired consciousness and mental status due to the accumulation of toxic waste products in the blood (ammonia in particular) as blood bypasses the congested liver. It appears that factors other than elevated ammonia levels contribute, including toxic fatty acids, altered neurotransmitters, and an imbalance of plasma amino acid ratios. Cerebral edema develops late in the course of liver failure, resulting from both the accumulation of toxins and vascular mechanisms. As cerebral edema progresses, intracranial pressure increases, cerebral perfusion decreases, and brain cells become hypoxic.
- **Hepatorenal syndrome** is acute renal failure due to disrupted blood flow to the kidneys. See Chapter 29 ∞ for more information about renal failure.

See the section of this chapter on cirrhosis for more information about the effects and complications associated with portal hypertension.

THE CLIENT WITH HEPATITIS

Hepatitis is inflammation of the liver. It is usually caused by a virus, although it may result from exposure to alcohol, drugs and toxins, or other pathogens. Hepatitis may be acute or chronic in nature. Cirrhosis, discussed in the next section, is a potential consequence of severe hepatocellular damage. Chronic hepatitis also increases the risk for developing liver cancer.

Pathophysiology and Manifestations

The inflammatory process of hepatitis, whether caused by a virus, toxin, or other mechanism, damages hepatic cells and disrupts liver function. Cell-mediated immune responses damage hepatocytes and Kupffer cells, leading to hyperplasia, necrosis, and cellular regeneration. The flow of bile through bile canaliculi and into the biliary system can be impaired by the inflammatory process, leading to jaundice. When the inflammatory process is mild (e.g., hepatitis A), the liver parenchyma is not significantly damaged. The inflammatory processes associated with hepatitis B and hepatitis C, however, can lead to severe liver damage. The metabolism of nutrients, drugs, alcohol, and toxins and the process of bile elimination are disrupted by the inflammation of hepatitis. See Chapter 21 ∞ for more information about the liver, and the preceding section for more information about the effects of disrupted liver function.

Viral Hepatitis

At least five viruses are known to cause hepatitis: hepatitis A virus (HAV), hepatitis B virus (HBV), hepatitis C virus (HCV), the hepatitis B–associated delta virus (HDV), and hepatitis E virus (HEV). With the exception of HBV, all of the hepatitis viruses are RNA viruses; HBV is a DNA virus. The viruses differ from one another in mode of transmission, incubation period, the severity and type of liver damage they cause, and their ability to become chronic or develop a carrier (asymptomatic) state. The illnesses they cause, however, are clinically very similar. Table 24–2 identifies unique features of the primary hepatitis viruses.

FAST FACTS

In the United States, hepatitis A, hepatitis B, and hepatitis C dominate.

- Hepatitis A is slightly more common than hepatitis B, with a reported 7,653 cases in 2003. The rate of hepatitis A infections per 100,000 population has fallen steadily since 1971, when it peaked at 28.9, to a rate of 2.6 in 2003.
- There were 7,526 reported cases of hepatitis B in 2003. In 1966, the rate of reported hepatitis B infections was 0.8 per 100,000 population. It peaked at 11.5 in 1985, since then falling to 2.6.
- In 2003, 891 cases of hepatitis C were reported, for a rate of 0.4 per 100,000 population (Centers for Disease Control and Prevention [CDC], 2006).
- The estimated number of actual cases of viral hepatitis is significantly higher than the number of reported cases for all three types of viral hepatitis.

Hepatitis viruses replicate in the liver, damaging liver cells (hepatocytes). The viruses provoke an immune response that causes inflammation and necrosis of hepatocytes as well. Although the extent of damage and the immune response vary among the different hepatitis viruses, the disease itself usually follows a predictable pattern.

No manifestations are present during the incubation period after exposure to the virus. The *prodromal* or *preicteric* (before jaundice) *phase* may begin abruptly or insidiously, with general malaise, anorexia, fatigue, and muscle and body aches. These manifestations often are mistaken for the flu. Nausea, vomiting, diarrhea, or constipation may develop, as well as mild RUQ abdominal pain. Chills and fever may be present.

The *icteric* (jaundiced) *phase* usually begins 5 to 10 days after the onset of symptoms. It is heralded by jaundice of the sclera, skin, and mucous membranes. Inflammation of the liver and bile ducts prevents bilirubin from being excreted into the small intestine. As a result, the serum bilirubin levels are elevated, causing yellowing of the skin and mucous membranes. Pruritus may develop due to deposition of bile salts on the skin.

TABLE 24–2 Comparison of Types of Viral Hepatitis

VIRUS	HEPATITIS A (HAV)	HEPATITIS B (HBV)	HEPATITIS C (HCV)	HEPATITIS D (HDV)	HEPATITIS E (HEV)
Mode of transmission	Fecal–oral	Blood and body fluids; perinatal	Blood and body fluids	Blood and body fluids; perinatal	Fecal–oral
Incubation (in weeks)	2–6	6–24	5–12	3–13	3–6
Onset	Abrupt	Slow	Slow	Abrupt	Abrupt
Carrier state	No	Yes	Yes	Yes	Yes
Possible complications	Rare	Chronic hepatitis Cirrhosis Liver cancer	Chronic hepatitis Cirrhosis Liver cancer	Chronic hepatitis Cirrhosis Fulminant hepatitis	May be severe in pregnant women
Laboratory findings	Anti-HAV antibodies present	Positive HBsAg (HBV surface antigen); anti-HBV antibodies present	Anti-HCV antibodies present	Positive HDVAg (delta antigen) early; anti-HDV antibodies later	Anti-HEV antibodies present

The stools are light brown or clay colored because bile pigment is not excreted through the normal fecal pathway. Instead, the pigment is excreted by the kidneys, causing the urine to turn brown. Whereas clients with acute hepatitis A or B are likely to develop jaundice, many people with hepatitis C do not develop jaundice. As a result, the infection may go undiagnosed for an extended period of time.

During the icteric phase, the initial prodromal manifestations usually diminish even though the serum bilirubin increases. The appetite increases, and the temperature returns to normal. When uncomplicated, spontaneous recovery usually begins within 2 weeks of the onset of jaundice.

The *convalescent phase* follows jaundice and lasts several weeks. During this time, manifestations gradually improve: Serum enzymes decrease, liver pain decreases, and gastrointestinal symptoms and weakness subside. See the box on this page for the manifestations of each phase of hepatitis.

HEPATITIS A Hepatitis A, or *infectious hepatitis,* often occurs in either sporadic attacks or mild epidemics. It is transmitted by the fecal–oral route via contaminated food, water, shellfish, and direct contact with an infected person. The virus is in the stool of infected persons up to 2 weeks before symptoms develop. Once jaundice develops, the amount of virus in the stool and the risk of spreading the disease decrease significantly (Kasper et al., 2005). Although hepatitis A usually has an abrupt onset, it is typically a benign and self-limited disease with few long-term consequences. Symptoms last up to 2 months.

HEPATITIS B Hepatitis B can cause acute hepatitis, chronic hepatitis, *fulminant* (rapidly progressive) hepatitis, or a carrier state. In a *carrier state,* the person harbors the active virus and is capable of spreading it to others, even though there are no discernible manifestations of the disease. This virus is spread through contact with infected blood and body fluids. Healthcare workers are at risk through exposure to blood and needle-stick injuries. Other high-risk groups for hepatitis B include injection drug users, people with multiple sex partners, men who have sex with other men, and people frequently exposed to blood products (such as people on hemodialysis). Hepatitis B is a major risk factor for primary liver cancer.

In hepatitis B, liver cells are damaged by the immune response to this antigen. Damage may affect only portions or the majority of the liver. The liver shows evidence of injury and scarring, regeneration, and proliferation of inflammatory cells. During the prodromal period, clients with HBV may experience such immune-mediated manifestations as urticaria and other rashes, arthralgias, serum sickness, or glomerulonephritis (Copstead & Banasik, 2005). The disease itself may be asymptomatic.

HEPATITIS C Hepatitis C, formerly known as non-A, non-B hepatitis, is the primary worldwide cause of chronic hepatitis, cirrhosis, and liver cancer (Porth, 2005). It is transmitted through infected blood and body fluids. Injection drug use is the primary risk factor for HCV infection. Acute hepatitis C usually is asymptomatic; if symptoms do develop, they often are mild and nonspecific. The disease often is recognized long after exposure occurred, when secondary effects of the disease (such as chronic hepatitis or cirrhosis) develop. Hepatitis C is unique, in that it does not produce lasting immunity to reinfection (Kasper et al., 2005). Only about 15% of acute infections completely resolve; most progress to chronic active hepatitis (Copstead & Banasik, 2005).

HEPATITIS DELTA Hepatitis delta only causes infection in people who also are infected with hepatitis B. It can cause acute or chronic infection, and can increase the severity of HBV infection (Porth, 2005). It is transmitted in the same manner as HBV. Because of its dependence on HBV, recovery from hepatitis B results in concurrent recovery from hepatitis delta.

HEPATITIS E Hepatitis E is rare in the United States. It is transmitted by fecal contamination of water supplies in developing areas such as southeast Asia, parts of Africa, and Central America. It primarily affects young adults. It can cause fulminant, fatal hepatitis in pregnant women.

Chronic Hepatitis

Chronic hepatitis is chronic infection of the liver. Although it may cause few symptoms, it is the primary cause of liver damage leading to cirrhosis, liver cancer, and liver transplantation. Three of the known hepatitis viruses cause chronic hepatitis: HBV, HCV, and HDV. Manifestations of chronic hepatitis include malaise, fatigue, and hepatomegaly. Occasional icteric (jaundiced) periods may occur. Liver enzymes, particularly serum aminotransferase levels, typically are elevated.

In *chronic active hepatitis*, inflammation extends to involve entire hepatic lobules. Chronic active hepatitis usually leads to cirrhosis and end-stage liver failure.

Fulminant Hepatitis

Fulminant hepatitis is a rapidly progressive disease, with liver failure developing within 2 to 3 weeks after the onset of symptoms. Although uncommon, it is usually related to HBV with concurrent HDV infection.

MANIFESTATIONS of Acute Hepatitis

PREICTERIC PHASE
- "Flulike" symptoms: malaise, fatigue, fever
- Gastrointestinal: anorexia, nausea, vomiting, diarrhea, constipation
- Muscle aches, polyarthritis
- Mild right upper abdominal pain and tenderness

ICTERIC PHASE
- Jaundice
- Pruritus
- Clay-colored stools
- Brown urine
- Decrease in preicteric phase symptoms (e.g., appetite improves; no fever)

POSTICTERIC/CONVALESCENT PHASE
- Serum bilirubin and enzymes return to normal levels
- Energy level increases
- Pain subsides
- Gastrointestinal: minimal to absent

Toxic Hepatitis

Many substances, including alcohol, certain drugs, and other toxins, can directly damage liver cells. Alcoholic hepatitis can result from chronic alcohol abuse or from an acute toxic reaction to alcohol. Alcoholic hepatitis causes necrosis of hepatocytes and inflammation of the liver parenchyma (functional tissue). Unless alcohol intake is avoided, progression to cirrhosis is common.

Other potential hepatotoxins include acetaminophen, benzene, carbon tetrachloride, halothane, chloroform, and poisonous mushrooms. These substances directly damage liver cells, leading to necrosis. The degree of damage often depends on age and the extent of exposure (dose) to the hepatotoxin. Acetaminophen is a common cause of hepatocellular damage.

Hepatobiliary Hepatitis

Hepatobiliary hepatitis is due to cholestasis, the interruption of the normal flow of bile. Cholestasis may result from obstruction of the hepatic duct with stones or inflammation secondary to cholelithiasis. Other agents, such as oral contraceptives and allopurinol (a drug used to lower uric acid levels), also can cause cholestasis. When bile flow is disrupted, the liver parenchyma may become inflamed. Reestablishing bile flow by removing the stone or other causative agent is the treatment for hepatobiliary hepatitis.

INTERDISCIPLINARY CARE

Management of hepatitis focuses on determining its cause, providing appropriate treatment and support, and teaching strategies to prevent further liver damage. Effective management begins with thorough assessment of diagnostic and laboratory data.

Diagnosis

Liver function tests, such as blood levels of bilirubin and enzymes commonly released when liver cells are damaged, are obtained. These include the following:

- *Alanine aminotransferase (ALT)* is an enzyme contained within each liver cell. When liver cells are damaged, ALT is released into the blood. Levels may exceed 1000 U/L or more in acute hepatitis.
- *Aspartate aminotransferase (AST)* is an enzyme found predominantly in heart and liver cells. AST levels rise when liver cells are damaged; with severe damage, blood levels may be 20 to 100 times normal values.
- *Alkaline phosphatase (ALP)* is an enzyme present in liver cells and bone. Serum ALP levels often are elevated in hepatitis.
- *Gamma-glutamyltransferase (GGT)* is an enzyme present in cell membranes. Its blood levels rise in hepatitis and obstructive biliary disease, and remain elevated until function is restored.
- *Lactic dehydrogenase (LDH)*, an enzyme present in many body tissues, is a nonspecific indicator of tissue damage. Its isoenzyme, LDH5, is a specific indicator of liver damage.
- *Serum bilirubin* levels, including *conjugated* and *unconjugated*, are elevated in viral hepatitis due to impaired bilirubin metabolism and obstruction of the hepatobiliary ducts by inflammation

and edema. The bilirubin level decreases as inflammation and edema subside.
- Laboratory tests for viral antigens and their specific antibodies may be done to identify the infecting virus and its state of activity. These tests are summarized in Table 24–2.
- A *liver biopsy* may be done to detect and evaluate chronic hepatitis. (Nursing implications for this test are outlined in the box on page 617.)

See Chapter 21 ∞ for more information about diagnostic tests and their nursing implications.

Medications

PREVENTION Hepatitis A and hepatitis B are preventable diseases. Vaccines are available, as are preparations to prevent the disease following known or suspected exposure.

Vaccines Hepatitis A vaccine provides long-term protection against HAV infection. It is an inactivated whole-virus vaccine available in pediatric and adult formulations. Although more than 95% of adults achieve immunity after one dose of the vaccine, two doses are recommended for full protection. See Table 24–3.

Three doses of hepatitis B vaccine provide immunity to HBV infection in 90% of healthy adults. Because the hepatitis delta virus requires the presence of the hepatitis B virus, hepatitis B vaccine also protects against HDV. Hepatitis B vaccine is a recombinant vaccine. Vaccines produced by different manufacturers may be used interchangeably, although their dosages differ. Older adults are less likely to achieve immunity than younger adults. Clients on hemodialysis and people who are immunocompromised may need larger or more doses of the vaccine to achieve adequate protection. Serologic testing for immunity is recommended on completion of the series for people in these high-risk groups.

A combined hepatitis A and hepatitis B vaccine is available for use. It is recommended for the same high-risk populations as the single vaccines. Three doses are given: the initial dose, followed by doses no sooner than 4 weeks and 6 months later.

Postexposure Prophylaxis Postexposure prophylaxis may be recommended for household or sexual contacts of people with HAV or HBV and other people who are known to have been exposed to these viruses. It is not necessary if the exposed person has been vaccinated and is known to be immune.

Hepatitis A prophylaxis is provided by a single dose of immune globulin (IG) given within 2 weeks after exposure. IG is recommended for all people with household or sexual contact with a person known to be infected with hepatitis A. See Table 24–3 for further recommendations.

Hepatitis B postexposure prophylaxis is indicated for people exposed to the hepatitis B virus. Hepatitis B immune globulin (HBIG) is given to provide for short-term immunity. HBV vaccine may be given concurrently. Candidates for postexposure prophylaxis include those with known or suspected percutaneous or permucosal contact with infected blood, sexual partners of clients with acute HBV or who are HBV carriers, and household contacts of clients with acute HBV infection (National Immunization Program, 2005).

TABLE 24–3 CDC Recommendations for Hepatitis Prevention in Adults

DISEASE/STRATEGY	IMMUNIZATION	ADVERSE REACTIONS	POPULATION RECOMMENDATIONS
Hepatitis A			
Prevention	Hepatitis A vaccine (Havrix; VAQTA), 2 doses (initial dose with booster in 6–12 months) IM into deltoid muscle Combined hepatitis A and hepatitis B vaccine (Twinrix), 3 doses (initial dose followed by doses 4 weeks and 6 months later) given IM into deltoid muscle	Pain at injection site	■ Children > 2 yr ■ International travelers ■ Men who have sex with men ■ Drug users ■ Persons with clotting-factor disorders, chronic liver disease, hepatitis C ■ Persons with occupational risk
Postexposure prophylaxis	Standard immune globulin IM into large muscle mass within 2 weeks of exposure	Rare; risk of anaphylaxis in people with IgA deficiency	■ Close contacts of people with known hepatitis A ■ People potentially exposed to hepatitis A at child care center or restaurant with infected food handler
Hepatitis B			
Prevention	Recombinant hepatitis B vaccine (Recombivax HB; Engerix-B), 3 doses (initial dose followed by doses at 4 weeks and 5 months later) given IM into deltoid muscle Combined hepatitis A and hepatitis B vaccine (Twinrix), 3 doses (initial dose followed by doses 4 weeks and 6 months later) given IM into deltoid muscle	Pain at injection site; fatigue, headache	■ Infants and adolescents ■ Adults with increased risk of HBV ■ Men who have sex with men ■ Prostitutes; heterosexuals with multiple sexual partners ■ People with an STI ■ Injection drug users ■ Long-term male prisoners ■ People on hemodialysis ■ Healthcare workers
Postexposure prophylaxis	Hepatitis B immune globulin (HBIG) given IM into large muscle mass within 24 hours to 7 days of exposure, second dose 28 to 30 days after exposure; concurrent initiation of hepatitis B vaccine series	Infrequent; muscle stiffness, pain	■ Infants born to women with HBV infection ■ Percutaneous or permucosal exposure to HBV when unvaccinated or antibody response is negative or unknown

Source: From *Epidemiology and Prevention of Vaccine-Preventable Diseases* (8th ed.) by Centers for Disease Control and Prevention, January 2005, Atlanta: Department of Health and Human Services.

Treatments

In most cases of acute viral hepatitis, pharmacologic treatment of the infection is not indicated. Acute hepatitis C generally is treated with interferon alpha, an antiviral agent, to reduce the risk of chronic hepatitis C. While treatment with interferon alpha alone is common, it may be combined with the antiviral drug ribavirin (Rebetol, Virazole).

Interferon alpha is used to treat both chronic hepatitis B and chronic hepatitis C. Interferon α interferes with viral replication, reducing the viral load. It is given by intramuscular or subcutaneous injection. Virtually all clients treated with interferon alpha develop a flulike syndrome with fever, fatigue, muscle aches, headache, and chills. Acetaminophen helps alleviate some of these adverse effects. Depression also is a common adverse effect of this drug.

An alternate drug for treating chronic hepatitis B is lamivudine (Epivir HBV), an antiviral drug that can reduce liver inflammation and fibrosis. Although it has minimal side effects, clients may become resistant to the beneficial effects of lamivudine.

The treatment of choice for chronic hepatitis C is combination therapy of interferon alpha with ribavirin, an oral antiviral drug. This combination therapy improves the response rate over either drug used alone. Ribavirin has two major adverse effects: hemolytic anemia and birth defects. Blood counts are obtained before and during treatment to detect early signs of hemolytic anemia. Because of the risk for birth defects, this drug is contraindicated for use during pregnancy, and two reliable methods of birth control must be used by women taking the drug and female sexual partners of men taking the drug.

Treatment of acute hepatitis also includes as-needed bed rest, adequate nutrition as tolerated, and avoidance of strenuous activity, alcohol, and agents that are toxic to the liver. In most cases, clinical recovery takes 3 to 16 weeks.

COMPLEMENTARY THERAPIES Milk thistle, with its active ingredient silymarin, has been used by herbalists to treat liver disease for over 2000 years. Clinical studies have demonstrated that treatment with silymarin promotes recovery and reduces complications in clients with viral hepatitis (Agency for Healthcare Research and Quality, 2000; National Center for Complementary and Alternative Medicine, 2004). It also is beneficial for clients who have liver damage due to toxins, cirrhosis, and alcoholic liver disease. Silymarin's beneficial effects are attributed to its ability to promote liver cell growth, block toxins from entering and damaging liver cells, and reduce liver inflammation. It also is a powerful antioxidant.

Herbalists also may use licorice root to treat hepatitis. It has both antiviral and anti-inflammatory effects. Long-term use of licorice root, however, can lead to hypertension and affect fluid and electrolyte balance.

Herbal preparations also may be used to relieve the adverse effects of interferon alpha. Ginger can help relieve nausea, and St. John's wort is used for the depression associated with interferon alpha.

NURSING CARE

Health Promotion

Nurses play an instrumental role in preventing the spread of hepatitis. Stress the importance of hygiene measures such as hand washing after toileting and before all food handling. Discuss the dangers of injection drug use and, with drug users, of sharing needles or other equipment. Encourage all sexually active clients to use safer sexual practices such as abstinence, mutual monogamy, and barrier protection (such as male or female condoms).

Discuss recommendations for hepatitis A and hepatitis B vaccine with people in high or moderate risk groups for these infections. Ensure that nurses and other healthcare workers at risk for exposure to blood and body fluids are effectively vaccinated against hepatitis A and B. Encourage all people with known or probable exposure to HAV or HBV to obtain postexposure prophylaxis.

Assessment

Collect assessment data related to hepatitis, such as the following:
- *Health history:* Current manifestations, including anorexia, nausea, vomiting, abdominal discomfort, changes in bowel elimination or color of stools; muscle or joint pain, fatigue; changes in color of skin or sclera; duration of symptoms; known exposure to hepatitis; high-risk behaviors such as injection drug use or multiple sexual partners; previous history of liver disorders; current medications, prescription and over the counter.
- *Physical assessment:* Vital signs including temperature; color of sclera and mucous membranes; skin color and condition; abdominal contour and tenderness; color of stool and urine.
- *Diagnostic tests:* Serum bilirubin, liver function tests, serologic antibody–antigen levels.

Nursing Diagnoses and Interventions

Clients with acute or chronic hepatitis usually are treated in community settings; rarely is hospitalization required. Nursing care focuses on preventing spread of the infection to others and promoting the client's comfort and ability to provide self-care.

Risk for Infection (Transmission)

An important goal when caring for clients with acute viral hepatitis is preventing spread of the infection.
- Use standard precautions. Practice meticulous hand washing. *The hepatitis viruses are spread by direct contact with feces or blood and body fluids. Standard precautions and good hand washing protect both healthcare workers and other clients from exposure to the virus.*
- For clients with HAV or HEV, use standard precautions and contact isolation if fecal incontinence is present. *The fecal–oral route is the primary mode of transmission of these viruses. Other hepatitis viruses are transmitted through blood and other body fluids.*
- Encourage prophylactic treatment of all members of household and intimate sexual contacts. *Prophylactic treatment of people in close contact with the client decreases their risk of contacting the disease or, if already infected, the severity of the disease.*

> **PRACTICE ALERT**
> If the client diagnosed with hepatitis A is employed as a food handler or child care worker, contact the local health department to report possible exposure of patrons. Maintain confidentiality. Prophylactic treatment of people who have possibly been exposed to the virus can prevent a local epidemic of the disease.

Fatigue

Fatigue and possible weakness are common in acute hepatitis. Although bed rest is rarely indicated, adequate rest periods and limitation of activities may be necessary. Many clients with acute hepatitis may be unable to resume normal activity levels for 4 or more weeks.
- Encourage planned rest periods throughout the day. *Adequate rest is necessary for optimal immune function.*
- Assist to identify essential activities and those that can be deferred or delegated to others. *Identifying essential and nonessential activities promotes the client's sense of control.*
- Suggest using level of fatigue to determine activity level, with gradual resumption of activities as fatigue and sense of well-being improves. *Fatigue associated with activity is an indicator of appropriate and inappropriate activity levels. As recovery progresses, increasing activity levels are tolerated with less fatigue.*

Imbalanced Nutrition: Less than Body Requirements

Adequate nutrition is important for immune function and healing in clients with acute or chronic hepatitis.
- Help plan a diet of appealing foods that provides a high-kilocalorie intake of approximately 16 carbohydrate kilocalories per kilogram of ideal body weight. *Sufficient energy is required for healing; adequate carbohydrate intake can spare protein.*

MediaLINK Care Plan Activity: A Client with Hepatitis A

- Encourage planning food intake according to symptoms of the disease. Discuss eating smaller meals and using between-meal snacks to maintain nutrient and calorie intake. *Clients with acute hepatitis often are more anorexic and nauseated in the afternoon and evening; planning the majority of calorie intake in the morning helps maintain adequate intake. Limiting fat intake and the size of meals may reduce the incidence of nausea.*
- Instruct to avoid alcohol intake and diet drinks. *Alcohol avoidance is vital to prevent further liver damage and promote healing. Diet drinks (e.g., diet sodas or juice drinks) provide few calories when an increased calorie intake is needed for healing.*
- Encourage use of nutritional supplements such as Ensure or instant breakfast drinks to maintain calorie and nutrient intake. *Nutritional supplement drinks are an additional source of concentrated calories and nutrients.*

Disturbed Body Image

Jaundice and associated rashes and itching can affect the client's body image. Nursing measures to prevent skin breakdown and address body image are discussed in the following section on cirrhosis.

Using NANDA, NIC, and NOC

Chart 24–1 shows linkages between NANDA nursing diagnosis, NIC, and NOC for the client with viral hepatitis.

Community-Based Care

Provide discharge teaching to clients and their families for home care. Include the following topics:

- Recommended prophylactic treatment
- Infection control measures such as frequent hand washing, not sharing eating utensils, avoiding food handling or prepa-

ration activities by the client with hepatitis A; abstaining from sexual relations during acute infection and using barrier protection if a carrier or for chronic infection
- Managing fatigue and limited activity
- Managing pruritus and maintaining skin integrity: use warm, not hot water when bathing, use mild or no soap, limit duration of baths and showers; pat dry, do not rub, apply an alcohol-free lotion soon after bathing to retain skin moisture; wear loose cotton garments that allow moisture to evaporate from skin; reduce room temperature, especially at night, to prevent overheating; keep fingernails short, and wear cotton mittens or gloves as needed to prevent scratching during sleep
- Promoting nutrient intake
- Avoiding hepatic toxins such as alcohol, acetaminophen, and selected other drugs; encourage to alert all care providers to presence of infection
- Recommended follow-up.

If chronic hepatitis B or C is being treated with medications, teach how to administer the drug, its dosing schedule, precautions, and management of adverse effects. Stress the importance of keeping follow-up appointments, including recommended laboratory testing.

THE CLIENT WITH CIRRHOSIS

Cirrhosis is the end stage of chronic liver disease. It is a progressive, irreversible disorder, eventually leading to liver failure.

FAST FACTS
- Cirrhosis is the 12th leading cause of death in the United States overall.
- In adults ages 25 to 64 years, however, cirrhosis/chronic liver disease is the 6th leading cause of death.
- Overall, the death rate due to cirrhosis and chronic liver disease in men is twice that of women (National Center for Health Statistics [NCHS], 2005).

Alcoholic or *Laënnec's* **cirrhosis** is the most common type of cirrhosis in North America and many parts of Europe and South America (Kasper et al., 2005). Cirrhosis also may result from chronic hepatitis B or C; prolonged obstruction of the biliary (bile drainage) system; long-term, severe right heart failure, and other uncommon liver disorders. The incidence and mortality attributable to cirrhosis and chronic liver disease vary significantly among populations. See the accompanying Focus on Cultural Diversity box.

Pathophysiology

In cirrhosis, functional liver tissue is gradually destroyed and replaced by fibrous scar tissue. As hepatocytes and liver lobules are destroyed, the metabolic functions of the liver are lost. Structurally abnormal nodules encircled by connective tissue form. This fibrous connective tissue forms constrictive bands that disrupt blood and bile flow within liver lobules. Blood no longer flows freely through the liver to the inferior vena cava.

> **NANDA, NIC, AND NOC LINKAGES**
> **CHART 24–1 The Client with Viral Hepatitis**
>
> **NANDA**
>
> Imbalanced Nutrition: Less than Body Requirements
>
> ↓
>
> **NIC**
>
> Energy Management
>
> Nutrition Management
>
> ↓
>
> **NOC**
>
> Energy Conservation
>
> Nutritional Status: Nutrient Intake

Data from *NANDA's Nursing Diagnoses: Definitions & Classification 2005–2006* by NANDA International (2005), Philadelphia; *Nursing Interventions Classification (NIC)* (4th ed.) by J. M. Dochterman & G. M. Bulechek (2004), St. Louis, MO: Mosby; and *Nursing Outcomes Classification (NOC)* (3rd ed.) by S. Moorhead, M. Johnson, and M. Maas (2004), St. Louis, MO: Mosby.

FOCUS ON CULTURAL DIVERSITY
Cirrhosis

- Although cirrhosis/chronic liver disease is the 12th leading cause of death overall in the United States, it is the 6th leading cause of death for people of Native American (including Alaska Natives) and Hispanic (or Latino) origin.
- Native American men have the highest incidence and mortality rate from cirrhosis and chronic liver disease, followed by Native American women, Hispanic men, and women of Hispanic or Latino origin (NCHS, 2005).
- At this time, there is no clear explanation for these differences. Contributory factors may include:
  - Socioeconomic factors that lead to greater stress and alcohol consumption among certain populations
  - Patterns of alcohol consumption (e.g., consuming alcohol without food calories)
  - Variations in alcohol metabolism among populations (Mann et al., 2003).

This restricted blood flow leads to portal hypertension, increased pressure in the portal venous system.

Alcoholic Cirrhosis

Alcoholic or Laënnec's cirrhosis is the end result of alcoholic liver disease. Its development is directly related to alcohol consumption: total amount of alcohol consumed, number of years of excessive alcohol consumption, and blood alcohol levels. Women develop cirrhosis at lower overall levels of alcohol use than men. This may relate to less effective metabolism of alcohol in women, resulting in higher blood alcohol levels (Mann et al., 2003).

Alcohol causes metabolic changes in the liver: Triglyceride and fatty acid synthesis increases, and the formation and release of lipoproteins decrease, leading to fatty infiltration of hepatocytes (fatty liver). At this stage, abstinence from alcohol can allow the liver to heal. With continued alcohol abuse, the disease progresses. Inflammatory cells infiltrate the liver (alcoholic hepatitis), causing necrosis, fibrosis, and destruction of functional liver tissue. In the final stage of alcoholic cirrhosis, regenerative nodules form, and the liver shrinks and develops a nodular appearance. Malnutrition commonly accompanies alcoholic cirrhosis. See *Pathophysiology Illustrated: Cirrhosis and Portal Hypertenseion* on the following pages.

Biliary Cirrhosis

When bile flow is obstructed within the liver or in the biliary system, retained bile damages and destroys liver cells close to the interlobular bile ducts. This leads to inflammation, fibrosis, and formation of regenerative nodules.

Posthepatic Cirrhosis

Advanced progressive liver disease resulting from chronic hepatitis B or C or from an unknown cause is known as posthepatic or postnecrotic cirrhosis. Chronic viral hepatitis appears to be the leading cause of posthepatic cirrhosis in the United States (Kasper et al., 2005). The liver is shrunken and nodular, with extensive liver cell loss and fibrosis.

Manifestations and Complications

Early in the course of cirrhosis, few manifestations may be present. The liver usually is enlarged and may be tender. A dull, aching pain in the RUQ may be present. Other early signs include weight loss, weakness, and anorexia. Bowel function is disrupted with diarrhea or constipation (Porth, 2005).

As the disease progresses, manifestations related to liver cell failure and portal hypertension develop. Impaired metabolism causes such manifestations as bleeding, ascites, gynecomastia (breast enlargement) in men and infertility in women, jaundice, and neurologic changes. Portal hypertension accounts from such manifestations as ascites, peripheral edema, anemia, and low WBC and platelet counts. See *Multisystem Effects of Cirrhosis* on page 714.

Portal Hypertension

Portal hypertension causes blood to be rerouted to adjoining lower pressure vessels. This *shunting* of blood involves collateral vessels. Affected veins, which become engorged and congested, are located in the esophagus, rectum, and abdomen. Portal hypertension increases the hydrostatic pressure in vessels of the portal system. Increased hydrostatic pressure in the capillaries pushes fluid out, contributing to ascites formation.

Splenomegaly

The spleen enlarges (splenomegaly) because portal hypertension causes blood to be shunted into the splenic vein. Splenomegaly increases the rate at which red and white blood cells and platelets are removed from circulation and destroyed. This increased blood cell destruction leads to anemia, leukopenia, and thrombocytopenia (Porth, 2005).

Ascites

Ascites is the accumulation of plasma-rich fluid in the abdominal cavity. Although portal hypertension is the primary cause of ascites, decreased serum proteins and increased aldosterone also contribute to the fluid accumulation. *Hypoalbuminemia,* low serum albumin, decreases the colloidal osmotic pressure of plasma. This pressure normally holds fluid in the intravascular compartment; when plasma colloidal osmotic pressure decreases, fluid escapes into extravascular compartments. *Hyperaldosteronism,* an increase in aldosterone, causes sodium and water retention, contributing to ascites and generalized edema. See the box on page 715 for selected manifestations of cirrhosis and their underlying pathophysiology.

Esophageal Varices

Esophageal varices are enlarged, thin-walled veins that form in the submucosa of the esophagus. These collateral vessels form when blood is shunted from the portal system due to portal hypertension. The thin-walled varices may rupture, causing massive hemorrhage; even eating high-roughage foods can precipitate bleeding. Thrombocytopenia, platelet deficiency, and impaired production of clotting factors by the liver contribute to the risk for hemorrhage.

Normal liver

The liver contains multiple lobules made up of plates of hepatocytes, the functional cells of the liver, surrounded by small capillaries called sinusoids. These sinusoids receive a mixture of venous and arterial blood from branches of the portal vein and hepatic artery. Blood from the sinusoids drains into the central vein of the lobule. Hepatocytes produce bile, which drains outward to bile ducts.

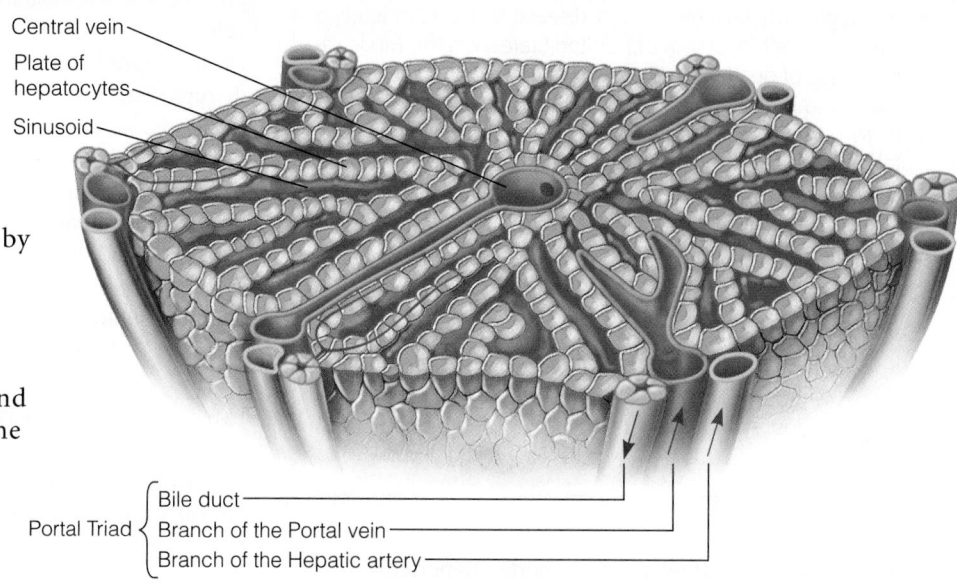

Central vein
Plate of hepatocytes
Sinusoid

Portal Triad
Bile duct
Branch of the Portal vein
Branch of the Hepatic artery

Fatty liver

Ingested alcohol is primarily metabolized in the liver. Acetaldehyde, formed when alcohol is metabolized, damages hepatocytes and impairs the oxidation of fatty acids. As a result, fat accumulates within hepatocytes and liver lobules. Other alcohol metabolism byproducts, including oxygen free radicals, promote inflammation and may stimulate autoantibody production.

◆ Auto-antibodies

▲ Free radicals

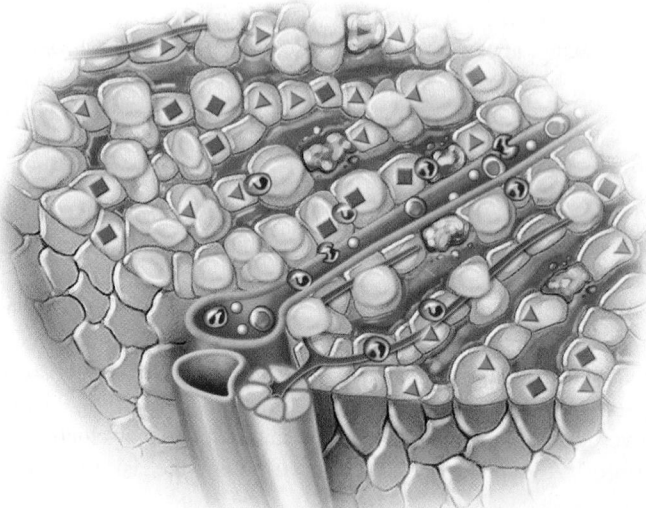

Alcoholic hepatitis

With continued alcohol intake, liver cells degenerate and spotty cellular necrosis occurs. Inflammatory cells such as polymorphonuclear leukocytes and lymphocytes infiltrate the lobule.

Alcoholic cirrhosis

Cellular necrosis and inflammation transform some liver cells into fibroblasts that produce and deposit collagen. Weblike bands of connective tissue develop around the portal triads and central vein, eventually connecting with one another. Small islands of liver cells continue to regenerate, forming nodules. Hepatocyte destruction outpaces regeneration. As a result of cell loss, fibrosis and scarring, the liver shrinks and becomes hard and nodular.

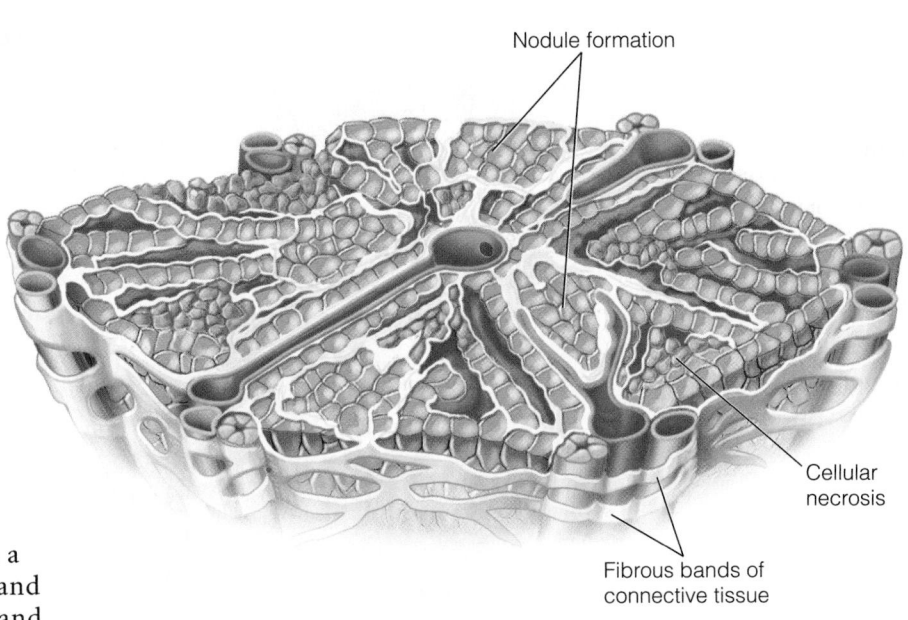

Nodule formation

Cellular necrosis

Fibrous bands of connective tissue

Portal hypertension

Bands of fibrotic scar tissue obstruct the sinusoids and blood flow from the portal vein to the hepatic vein. Pressure in the portal venous system, which drains the gastrointestinal tract, pancreas, and spleen, increases. This increased pressure opens collateral vessels in the esophagus, anterior abdominal wall, and rectum, allowing blood to bypass the obstructed portal vessels. Prolonged portal hypertension leads to the development of (1) varices (fragile, distended veins) in the lower esophagus, stomach, and rectum; (2) splenomegaly (an enlarged spleen); (3) ascites (accumulation of fluid in the abdomen); and (4) hepatic encephalopathy (disrupted CNS function with altered consciousness).

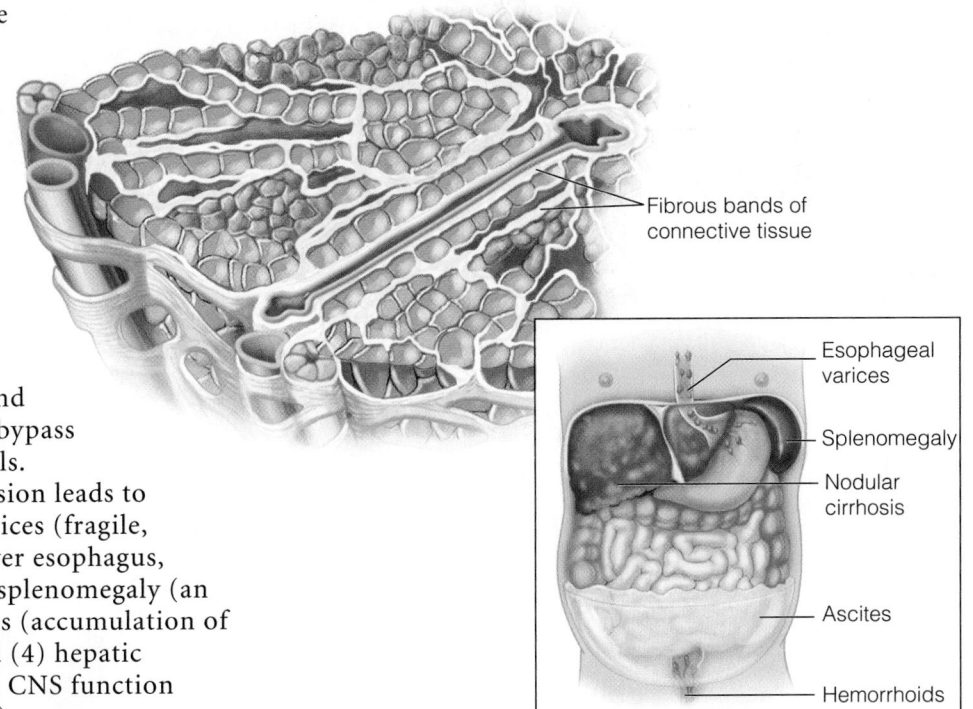

Fibrous bands of connective tissue

Esophageal varices

Splenomegaly

Nodular cirrhosis

Ascites

Hemorrhoids

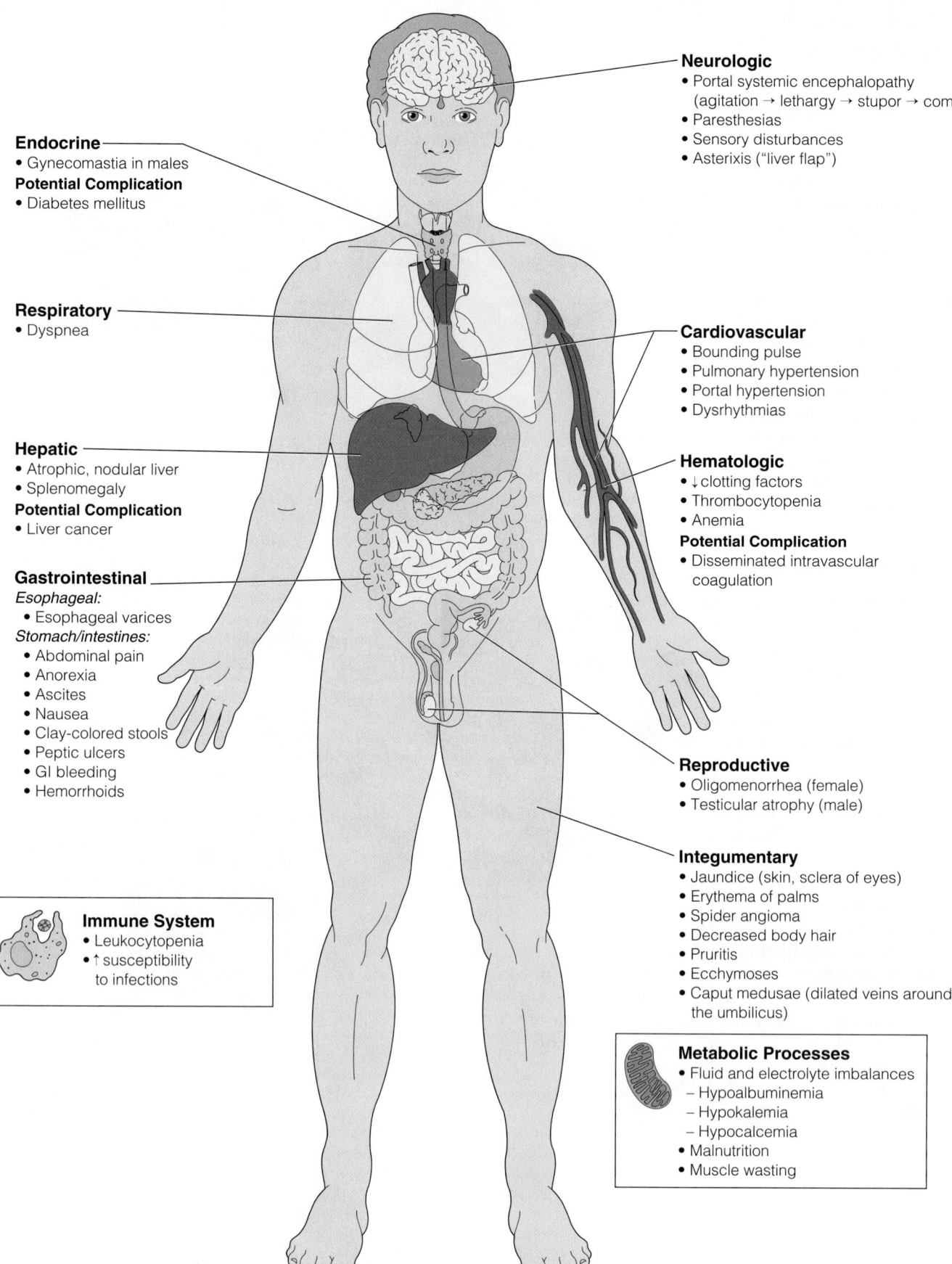

Neurologic
- Portal systemic encephalopathy (agitation → lethargy → stupor → coma)
- Paresthesias
- Sensory disturbances
- Asterixis ("liver flap")

Endocrine
- Gynecomastia in males

Potential Complication
- Diabetes mellitus

Respiratory
- Dyspnea

Cardiovascular
- Bounding pulse
- Pulmonary hypertension
- Portal hypertension
- Dysrhythmias

Hepatic
- Atrophic, nodular liver
- Splenomegaly

Potential Complication
- Liver cancer

Hematologic
- ↓ clotting factors
- Thrombocytopenia
- Anemia

Potential Complication
- Disseminated intravascular coagulation

Gastrointestinal
Esophageal:
- Esophageal varices

Stomach/intestines:
- Abdominal pain
- Anorexia
- Ascites
- Nausea
- Clay-colored stools
- Peptic ulcers
- GI bleeding
- Hemorrhoids

Reproductive
- Oligomenorrhea (female)
- Testicular atrophy (male)

Integumentary
- Jaundice (skin, sclera of eyes)
- Erythema of palms
- Spider angioma
- Decreased body hair
- Pruritis
- Ecchymoses
- Caput medusae (dilated veins around the umbilicus)

Immune System
- Leukocytopenia
- ↑ susceptibility to infections

Metabolic Processes
- Fluid and electrolyte imbalances
  - Hypoalbuminemia
  - Hypokalemia
  - Hypocalcemia
- Malnutrition
- Muscle wasting

MANIFESTATIONS of Cirrhosis with Underlying Cause

MANIFESTATION	UNDERLYING PATHOPHYSIOLOGY
Edema, ascites	■ Impaired plasma protein synthesis (hypoalbuminemia) ■ Disrupted hormone balance and fluid retention ■ Increased pressure in portal venous system
Bleeding, bruising	■ Decreased clotting factor synthesis ■ Increased platelet destruction by enlarged spleen ■ Impaired vitamin K absorption and storage
Esophageal varices, hemorrhoids	■ Increased pressure in portal venous system with collateral vessel development
Gastritis, anorexia, diarrhea	■ Engorged veins in gastrointestinal system ■ Alcohol ingestion ■ Impaired bile synthesis and fat absorption
Abdominal wall vein distention (caput medusae)	■ Portal hypertension
Jaundice	■ Impaired bilirubin metabolism and excretion
Malnutrition, muscle wasting	■ Impaired nutrient metabolism ■ Impaired fat absorption ■ Impaired hormone metabolism
Anemia, leukopenia, increased risk for infection	■ Bleeding ■ Increased blood cell destruction by spleen
Asterixis, encephalopathy	■ Accumulated metabolic toxins ■ Impaired ammonia metabolism and excretion
Gynecomastia, infertility, impotence	■ Altered sex hormone metabolism

Portal Systemic Encephalopathy

Portal systemic encephalopathy (*hepatic encephalopathy*) results from accumulation of neurotoxins in the blood and cerebral edema. Ammonia, a by-product of protein metabolism, contributes to hepatic encephalopathy. Ammonium ion is produced as proteins and amino acids are broken down by bacteria in the intestinal tract. Normally, the ammonia produced is then converted by the liver to urea before entering the general circulation. As functional liver tissue is destroyed, ammonia can no longer be converted to urea, and it accumulates in the blood. Other nervous system depressants, such as narcotics and tranquilizers, also can contribute to hepatic encephalopathy. Box 24–4 lists selected precipitating factors for hepatic encephalopathy. Accumulation of other metabolic toxins are thought to contribute as well.

Asterixis (liver flap), a muscle tremor that interferes with the ability to maintain a fixed position of the extremities and causes involuntary jerking movements, is an early sign of portal systemic encephalopathy. Asterixis primarily affects the upper extremities, but also may affect the tongue and feet. Asterixis is elicited by instructing the client to extend the arms and dorsiflex the wrists. If present, asterixis causes a downward flapping of the hands (Figure 24–3 ■). Changes in personality and mentation develop; agitation, restlessness, impaired judgment, and slurred speech also are early manifestations of hepatic encephalopathy. As it progresses, confusion, disorientation, and incoherence develop. Cerebral edema that leads to increased intracranial pressure and cerebral hypoxia is the leading cause of death in people with portal systemic encephalopathy and liver failure.

BOX 24–4 Factors Precipitating Portal Systemic Encephalopathy

■ High serum ammonia level
■ Constipation
■ Blood transfusions
■ Gastrointestinal bleeding
■ Medications: sedatives, tranquilizers, narcotic analgesics, anesthetics
■ Hypoxia
■ High-protein diet
■ Severe infection
■ Surgery

Figure 24–3 ■ Asterixis. Note the downward tremor of the hand on dorsiflexion of the wrist.

Hepatorenal Syndrome

Although the cause is unclear, renal failure with azotemia (excess nitrogenous waste products in the blood), sodium retention, oliguria, and hypotension may develop in clients with advanced cirrhosis and ascites. Hepatorenal syndrome appears to be the result of imbalanced blood flow, leading to constriction of vessels leading to and within the kidneys. The syndrome may be precipitated by gastrointestinal bleeding, aggressive diuretic therapy, or by an unknown cause.

SPONTANEOUS BACTERIAL PERITONITIS Clients with cirrhosis and ascites may develop bacterial peritonitis, even in the absence of known contamination of the peritoneal cavity or other specific risk factors (e.g., paracentesis). The inflammatory response to peritonitis worsens ascites by increasing the permeability of capillaries in the mesentery. The manifestations of spontaneous bacterial peritonitis may be subtle, with increased abdominal discomfort or pain, fever, increasing ascites, worsening encephalopathy, and an overall decline in condition.

INTERDISCIPLINARY CARE

Care for the client with cirrhosis is holistic, addressing physiologic, psychosocial, and spiritual needs. The importance of including the family in the plan of care cannot be overemphasized, particularly if alcohol abuse is identified as the cause. Treatment includes medications to help regulate protein metabolism, maintenance of fluid and electrolyte balance, and supportive therapies, including treatment of underlying problems, such as malnutrition, anemia, bleeding, encephalopathy, renal failure, and infections.

Diagnosis

Studies to confirm the diagnosis of cirrhosis and identify its cause and effects are performed. Diagnostic tests may include the following:

- *Liver function studies* include *ALT, AST, ALP,* and *GGT.* All may be elevated in cirrhosis, but usually not as severely as in acute hepatitis. Elevations in these enzymes may not correlate well with the extent of liver damage in cirrhosis.
- *CBC with platelets* is done. A low RBC count, hemoglobin, and hematocrit demonstrate anemia related to bone marrow suppression, increased RBC destruction, bleeding, and deficiencies of folic acid and vitamin B_{12}. Platelets are low, related to increased destruction by the spleen. Leukopenia (low WBC count) also relates to splenomegaly.
- *Coagulation studies* show a prolonged prothrombin time due to impaired production of coagulation proteins and lack of vitamin K.
- *Serum electrolytes* are measured. Hyponatremia is common, due to hemodilution. Hypokalemia, hypophosphatemia, and hypomagnesemia also are frequently seen, related to malnutrition and altered renal excretion of these electrolytes.
- *Bilirubin* levels are usually elevated in severe cirrhosis, including both direct (conjugated) and indirect (unconjugated) bilirubin.
- *Serum albumin* levels show hypoalbuminemia due to impaired liver production.
- *Serum ammonia* levels are elevated, because the liver fails to effectively convert ammonia to urea for renal excretion.

- *Serum glucose* and *cholesterol* levels frequently are abnormal in clients with cirrhosis.
- *Abdominal ultrasound* is performed to evaluate liver size, detect ascites, and identify liver nodules. Ultrasound may be used in conjunction with *Doppler studies* to evaluate blood flow through the liver and spleen (Tierney et al., 2005).
- *Esophagoscopy* (upper endoscopy) may be done to determine the presence of esophageal varices.
- *Liver biopsy* is not always necessary to diagnose cirrhosis, but may be done to distinguish cirrhosis from other forms of liver disease. See the box on page 617 for nursing implications for a client having a liver biopsy. Figure 21–7 shows the site and position for liver biopsy. Biopsy may be deferred if the bleeding time is prolonged (such as a prothrombin time [PT] greater than 3 seconds over the control).

See Chapter 21 ∞ for more information about and the nursing implications of the above diagnostic tests.

Medications

Medications are used to treat the complications and effects of cirrhosis; they do not reverse or slow the process of cirrhosis itself. Known hepatotoxic drugs and alcohol are avoided, as are drugs metabolized by the liver (e.g., barbiturates, sedatives, hypnotics, and acetaminophen). Several groups of drugs are commonly prescribed. See the Medication Administration box on page 717 for nursing responsibilities and client teaching for commonly used drugs in clients with cirrhosis.

- Diuretics reduce fluid retention and ascites. Spironolactone (Aldactone) is frequently the drug of first choice because it addresses one of the causes of ascites—increased aldosterone levels. If additional diuresis is necessary, a loop diuretic such as furosemide (Lasix) may be added to the regimen.
- Medications to reduce the nitrogenous load and lower serum ammonia levels are added when manifestations of hepatic encephalopathy develop. Two commonly administered medications are lactulose and neomycin. Both exert their effects locally, in the bowel. Lactulose reduces the number of ammonia-forming organisms in the bowel and increases the acidity of colon contents, converting ammonia into ammonium ion. Ammonium ion is not absorbable, and is excreted in the feces. Neomycin sulfate is a locally acting antibiotic that also reduces the number of ammonia-forming bacteria in the bowel.
- The beta-blocker nadolol (Corgard) may be given together with isosorbide mononitrate (Ismo, Imdur, Monoket) to prevent rebleeding of esophageal varices. This drug combination also lowers hepatic venous pressure.
- Ferrous sulfate and folic acid are given as indicated to treat anemia. Vitamin K may be ordered to reduce the risk of bleeding. When bleeding is acute, packed RBCs, fresh frozen plasma, or platelets may be administered to restore blood components and promote hemostasis.
- Antacids are prescribed as indicated. A drug regimen to treat *H. pylori* infection may also be effective (see Chapter 23 ∞).
- Oxazepam (Serax), a benzodiazepine antianxiety/sedative drug, is not metabolized by the liver, and may be used to treat acute agitation.

MEDICATION ADMINISTRATION   The Client with Cirrhosis

DIURETICS

Spironolactone (Aldactone)   Furosemide (Lasix)

Spironolactone is a potassium-sparing diuretic that competes with aldosterone. It reduces ascites by increasing renal excretion of fluid and decreasing aldosterone levels. Furosemide is a loop diuretic that promotes the excretion of potassium. Drugs may be given in combination if serum potassium level permits.

Nursing Responsibilities
- Monitor ECG, serum potassium, BUN, creatinine levels, and hydration status.
- Weigh daily.
- Carefully monitor intake and output.
- Monitor for signs of hyperkalemia if taking spironolactone alone: bradycardia; widening QRS, spiking T waves, or ST segment depression on ECG, diarrhea; and muscle twitching.
- Assess for hyponatremia: confusion, lethargy, apprehension.

Health Education for the Client and Family
- Maintain diet and fluid restrictions as prescribed.
- Report increases in weight or edema.
- Immediately report signs of hyponatremia, hyperkalemia, or hypokalemia (see Chapter 10 ∞).
- Expect increased urinary output; take medications in morning hours to avoid nocturia.

LAXATIVES

Lactulose (Cephulac, Chronulac)

Lactulose is a disaccharide laxative that is not absorbed by the gastrointestinal tract. It reduces the number of ammonia-producing bacteria and lowers the pH in the colon. The lower pH (increased acidity) converts ammonia to ammonium ion, a nonabsorbable form that is excreted in the feces. Lactulose also pulls water into the bowel lumen, increasing the number of daily stools.

Nursing Responsibilities
- Assess bowel sounds and abdominal girth.
- Maintain accurate stool chart.
- Adjust dose to achieve two to four soft stools per day.
- Monitor electrolytes and hydration.

Health Education for the Client and Family
- Drink adequate fluids.
- Report diarrhea; if present, decrease dose. You should have an average of two to four stools per day.
- This drug may cause nausea. Continue taking the drug; taking it with crackers or a soft drink may reduce nausea.

ANTI-INFECTIVE AGENTS

Neomycin sulfate (Neo Tabs)

Neomycin sulfate is a nonsystemic aminoglycoside antibiotic that reduces intestinal bacteria and decreases ammonia production in the bowel lumen. The drug may be administered as an oral or rectal preparation.

Nursing Responsibilities
- Monitor hearing, renal, and neurologic functions. Drug is ototoxic, nephrotoxic, and neurotoxic.
- Prior to administration, check for previous hypersensitivity reaction.
- Monitor intake and output.
- Monitor BUN and creatinine levels.
- If the client is taking digitalis, monitor levels; oral neomycin interferes with its absorption.

Health Education for the Client and Family
- Report dizziness, tinnitus (ringing in ears), hearing loss, headaches, tremors, or vision changes immediately.
- Keep follow-up appointments.
- Maintain fluids, avoid dehydration. (Teach signs of dehydration.)

Treatments

Treatment of cirrhosis is supportive, directed at slowing the progression to liver failure and reducing complications.

NUTRITION Dietary support is an essential part of care for the client with cirrhosis. Dietary needs change as hepatic function fluctuates.

- Sodium intake is restricted to under 2 g/day, and fluids are restricted as necessary to reduce ascites and generalized edema. Fluids are often limited to 1500 mL/day. Fluid needs are calculated based on response to diuretic therapy, urine output, and serum electrolyte values.
- Unless serum ammonia levels are high, a palatable diet with adequate calories and protein is recommended. If hepatic encephalopathy is acute, protein may initially be eliminated from the diet; for chronic hepatic encephalopathy, protein generally is restricted to 60 g/day (Kasper et al., 2005). When encephalopathy resolves and serum ammonia levels stabilize, protein intake is allowed as tolerated. The diet is high in calories and includes moderate fat intake to promote healing. See Table 24–4 for examples of protein-restricted menus. Parenteral nutrition is used as needed to maintain nutritional status when food intake is limited.
- Vitamin and mineral supplements are ordered based on laboratory values. Deficiencies in the B-complex vitamins, particularly thiamin, folate, and B_{12}, and the fat-soluble vitamins A, D, and E are common. These vitamins may need to be administered in a water-soluble form. Clients with alcohol-induced cirrhosis are at high risk for magnesium deficiency, which needs to be replaced.

COMPLICATION MANAGEMENT **Paracentesis**, aspiration of fluid from the peritoneal cavity, may be a diagnostic or a therapeutic procedure. It may be done therapeutically to relieve severe ascites that does not respond to diuretic therapy. The goal of paracentesis is to relieve respiratory distress caused by excess fluid in the abdomen. Ascites fluid may be withdrawn in moderate amounts of 500 mL to 1 L daily to reduce the risk of fluid and electrolyte imbalances. Large-volume paracentesis, withdrawal of 4 to 6 L of fluid at one time, may be used. Albumin is often administered intravenously during large-volume paracentesis to maintain intravascular volume as the pressure of the ascites fluid in the abdomen is relieved. Nursing implications for the client undergoing paracentesis are listed in Box 24–5. Figure 24–4 ∎ shows insertion sites and client positioning during paracentesis.

TABLE 24–4 Sample Menus for Protein-Restricted Diets

	SEVERE RESTRICTION	MODERATE RESTRICTION	MILD RESTRICTION
Breakfast	1 orange ½ cup rice or creamed cereal with sugar 1 slice whole-wheat bread with butter or margarine and jam ½ cup milk 1 egg or 1 Tbsp peanut butter Coffee or tea	1 orange ½ to 1 cup cooked oatmeal with 1 cup milk and sugar 1 slice whole-wheat toast with butter or margarine and jam Coffee or tea	1 orange 1 egg or 1 Tbsp peanut butter ½ to ¾ cup cooked oatmeal with 1 cup milk and sugar 1 slice whole-wheat toast with butter or margarine and jam Coffee or tea
Lunch	1 oz lean fish, poultry, meat, or 1 small piece soft tofu or 3 Tbsp cottage cheese 1 slice whole-wheat bread with butter or margarine and jelly Cooked green vegetable Green salad with oil and vinegar dressing Fresh fruit Coffee or tea	3 oz lean fish, poultry, meat, or 1 large piece soft tofu or ⅓ cup cottage cheese 1 slice whole-wheat bread with butter or margarine and jelly Cooked green vegetable Starch such as potato, squash, or corn Fresh fruit Coffee or tea	4 oz lean fish, poultry, meat, or 1 large piece soft tofu or ½ cup cottage cheese 2 slices whole-wheat bread with butter or margarine and jelly Cooked green vegetable Starch such as potato, squash, or corn Fresh fruit 1 cup milk Coffee or tea
Afternoon snack	Apple juice Soda crackers with margarine or butter and jelly	½ cup milk Graham crackers with margarine or butter and jelly	1 cup milk Graham crackers with margarine or butter and jelly
Dinner	1 oz lean fish, poultry, meat, or 1 small piece soft tofu or 3 Tbsp cottage cheese 1 whole-wheat dinner roll with butter or margarine and jelly Cooked green vegetable Baked potato Fresh or canned fruit ⅓ cup sherbet Coffee or tea	3 oz lean fish, poultry, meat, or 1 large piece soft tofu or ⅓ cup cottage cheese 1 whole-wheat dinner roll with butter or margarine and jelly Cooked green vegetable Baked potato Fresh or canned fruit ⅓ cup sherbet Coffee or tea	4 oz lean fish, poultry, meat, or 1 large piece soft tofu or ½ c cottage cheese 2 whole-wheat dinner rolls with butter or margarine and jelly Cooked green vegetable Baked potato Fresh or canned fruit 1 cup or ⅓ cup ice cream Coffee or tea
Evening snack	1 banana	1 banana	1 banana with ½ cup milk

BOX 24–5 Nursing Implications for Diagnostic Tests

Abdominal Paracentesis

Client Preparation

- Verify presence of an informed consent.
- Weigh prior to paracentesis.
- Assess vital signs for baseline.
- Have client void immediately prior to the test to avoid bladder puncture.
- Position seated, either on the side of the bed or in a chair, with feet supported.

Health Education for the Client and Family

- Describe what to expect during and following paracentesis, blood pressure is monitored during the procedure.
- Following cleansing and local anesthesia, a small incision may be made and a needle or trocar inserted to withdraw fluid. The trocar is connected to tubing and a collection bottle; specimens may be sent to laboratory.
- A small dressing is placed over the puncture site after the needle is withdrawn. There may be some fluid leakage from the site.
- Salt-poor albumin may be given after the procedure to replace lost protein.

Bleeding esophageal varices are life threatening and require intensive care management. Restoration of hemodynamic stability is the first priority. A central line is inserted and central venous and pulmonary artery pressures are monitored (see Chapter 32 ∞). Blood is given to restore blood volume, and fresh frozen plasma may be administered to restore clotting factors. Somatostatin or octreotide, drugs that constrict blood vessels in the gut, are given intravenously to reduce blood flow in the portal venous system. Vasopressin, a drug that produces generalized vasoconstriction, also may be used.

When the blood pressure and cardiac output have stabilized, upper endoscopy is performed to evaluate and treat the varices. A large nasogastric tube is inserted prior to endoscopy, and **gastric lavage** (irrigation of the stomach with large quantities of normal saline) is performed to improve visualization. During endoscopy, the varices may be banded or sclerosed to reduce the risk of recurrent bleeding. In *banding* (*variceal ligation*), small rubber bands are placed on varices to occlude blood flow. *Endoscopic sclerosis* involves injecting a sclerosing agent directly into the varices to induce inflammation and clotting. See Chapter 21 ∞ for the nursing implications of endoscopy.

Balloon tamponade of bleeding varices may be used if bleeding cannot be controlled through vasoconstriction or if

Figure 24–4 ■ Sites and position for paracentesis. *A,* Potential sites of needle or trocar insertion to avoid abdominal organ damage. *B,* The client sits comfortably; in this position, the intestines float back and away from the insertion site.

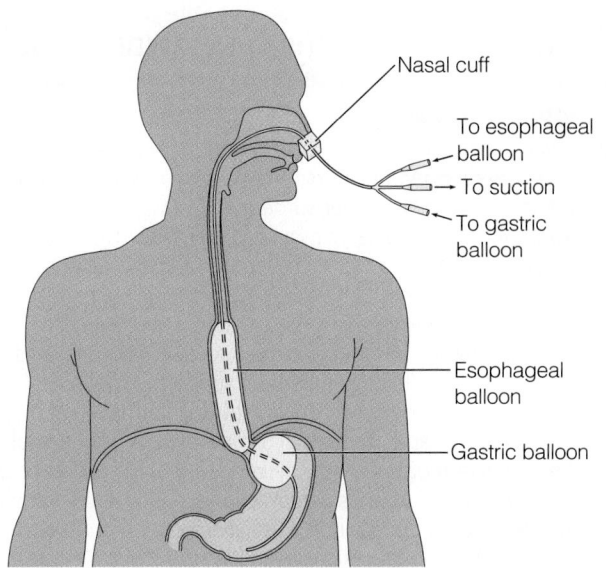

Figure 24–5 ■ Triple-lumen nasogastric tube (Sengstaken-Blakemore) used to control bleeding esophageal varices.

endoscopy is unavailable. A multiple-lumen nasogastric (NG) tube (such as a Sengstaken-Blakemore tube or a Minnesota tube) is inserted, and the gastric and esophageal balloons are inflated to apply direct pressure on the bleeding varices (Figure 24–5 ■). Tension is applied to the tube to further compress the varices. Balloon tamponade carries a number of risks, including aspiration, airway obstruction, and tissue ischemia and necrosis. An endotracheal tube is inserted prior to nasogastric intubation to support the airway and reduce the risk of aspiration. This short-term measure is used only until more definitive treatment can be done.

PRACTICE ALERT
When caring for a client with a multiple-lumen NG tube, always deflate the esophageal balloon before the gastric balloon. This practice prevents the balloon from becoming misplaced and occluding the airway. Always keep an appropriate syringe at the bedside to deflate the esophageal balloon should the client develop respiratory distress.

Transjugular intrahepatic portosystemic shunt (TIPS) is used to relieve portal hypertension and its complications of esophageal varices and ascites. A channel is created through the liver tissue using a needle inserted transcutaneously (Figure 24–6 ■). An expandable metal stent is inserted into this channel to allow blood to flow directly from the portal vein into the hepatic vein, bypassing the cirrhotic liver. The shunt relieves pressure in esophageal varices and allows better control of fluid retention with diuretic therapy. Stenosis and occlusion of the shunt are frequent complications. TIPS also increases the risk of developing hepatic encephalopathy (due to decreased perfusion of the liver and impaired ammonia metabolism) and may reduce long-term survival. It generally is used as a short-term measure until liver transplant is performed.

SURGERY **Liver transplantation** is indicated for some clients with irreversible, progressive cirrhosis. A decline in functional status, increasing bilirubin levels, falling albumin levels, and increasing problems with complications that respond poorly to treatment are indications for liver transplantation. Malignancy,

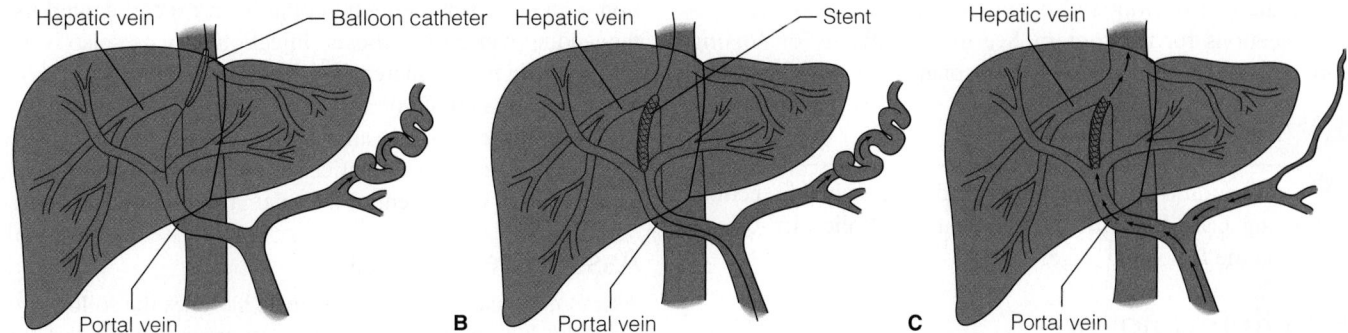

Figure 24–6 ■ Transjugular intrahepatic portosystemic shunt (TIPS). *A,* Guided by angiography, a balloon catheter inserted via the jugular vein is advanced to the hepatic veins and through the substance of the liver to create a portacaval (portal vein-to-vena cava) channel. *B,* A metal stent is positioned into the channel, and expanded by inflating the balloon. *C,* The stent remains in place after the catheter is removed, creating a shunt for blood to flow directly from the portal vein into the hepatic vein.

NURSING CARE OF THE CLIENT UNDERGOING Liver Transplantation

PREOPERATIVE CARE

- Obtain a complete nursing history and physical examination. *A complete preoperative nursing assessment provides baseline data for comparison after surgery.*
- Provide routine preoperative care as ordered (see Chapter 4 ∞). *Preoperative care is similar to that provided for other clients undergoing major surgery.*
- Discuss preoperative and postoperative expectations with the client and family. Introduce to the intensive care unit, and discuss anticipated drainage tubes and supportive measures in the immediate postoperative period. Provide information about visiting policies and family accommodations (if available). *Preoperative teaching helps relieve anxiety in the client and family members. Clients return from surgery to an intensive care or specialized care unit. Restrictions on the number of visitors and the time they may spend with the client are common.*
- Once a donor liver is located, check for evidence of infection; if no infection is present, begin preoperative antibiotics as ordered. *An acute or chronic infection may contraindicate liver transplantation as drugs given postoperatively to suppress rejection of the transplanted organ also impair the ability to fight infection.*

POSTOPERATIVE CARE

- Provide routine postoperative care as outlined in Chapter 4 ∞.
- Maintain airway and ventilatory support until awake and alert. *Until the new liver clears the anesthesia, the client requires measures to support respirations and ventilation.*
- Monitor temperature and implement rewarming measures (such as warming blankets, heating lamps, and head covers) as indicated. *The client often is hypothermic after liver transplant, necessitating careful rewarming while maintaining hemodynamic stability.*
- Frequently monitor hemodynamic pressures, including arterial blood pressure, central venous pressure, and pulmonary artery pressures. *Postoperative fluid volume status may be difficult to determine without careful pressure measurements. The rate and type of fluids administered are determined by hemodynamic status.*
- Monitor urine output hourly; maintain careful intake and output records. Weigh daily. *Urine output and weight provide ad-*

ditional information about fluid volume status. In addition, renal function may be altered after liver transplant; acute renal failure is a significant risk. See Chapter 29 ∞ for more information about acute renal failure and its management.

- Monitor for signs of active bleeding, including excess drainage, increasing abdominal girth, bloody nasogastric drainage, black tarry stools, tachypnea, tachycardia, diminished peripheral pulses, or pallor. Report immediately. *Altered coagulation in the early postoperative period increases the risk for bleeding. Blood products to replace volume and clotting factors may be necessary.*
- Monitor serum electrolytes and laboratory values related to blood coagulation, liver function, and renal function. Report abnormal results or significant changes immediately. *Electrolyte imbalances are common postoperatively. Altered liver or renal function tests may indicate rejection of the transplanted liver or acute renal failure. Other early signs of transplant rejection include fever, a drop in bile output, or a change in bile color and viscosity (Urden, Stacy, & Lough, 2006).*
- Monitor neurologic status. *With good function of the transplanted organ, mental status should clear within days of the transplant.*
- Provide discharge teaching:
  a. Teach how to reduce risk of infection, and signs of infection to report.
  b. Instruct to recognize and report signs of organ rejection.
  c. Discuss all medications, including their purpose, schedule, adverse effects, and potential long-term effects. Stress the importance of complying with all prescribed medications and postoperative precautions for the remainder of the client's life.
  d. Discuss possible changes in body image and psychologic responses to receiving a transplanted organ. Refer to a counselor or support group as indicated.
  e. Refer for home health services for continued assessment and teaching.
  f. Stress importance of continued follow-up with transplant team and primary care provider.

---

active alcohol or drug abuse, and poor surgical risk are contraindications for the surgery. See the box above for nursing care of the client having a liver transplant.

NURSING CARE

In addition to the nursing care discussed in this section, a Nursing Care Plan for a client with alcoholic cirrhosis is found on the following page.

Health Promotion

For most clients, high-risk behaviors are the risk factors for cirrhosis. With all clients (including children and young adults), stress the relationship between alcohol and drug abuse and liver disorders. While many clients tolerate alcohol use in modera-

tion with no adverse effects on the liver, excess alcohol use is the leading cause of cirrhosis. Injection drug use also is a significant risk factor, increasing the risk for contracting bloodborne hepatitis (B, C, or D). These types of viral hepatitis can lead to chronic hepatitis and, ultimately, to cirrhosis. Discuss abstinence or safer sex practices as another measure to prevent viral hepatitis and potential liver damage.

Assessment

Assessment data related to cirrhosis includes the following:
- *Health history:* Current manifestations, including abdominal pain or discomfort, recent weight loss, weakness, and anorexia; altered bowel elimination; excess bleeding or bruising; abdominal distention; jaundice, pruritus; altered libido or impotence; duration of symptoms; history of liver or gallbladder disease;

NURSING CARE PLAN   A Client with Alcoholic Cirrhosis

Richard Wright is a 48-year-old divorced father of two teenagers. Mr. Wright has been admitted to the community hospital with ascites and malnutrition. He has had three previous hospital stays for cirrhosis, the most recent 6 months ago.

ASSESSMENT

Mr. Wright is lethargic but responds appropriately to verbal stimuli. He complains of "spitting up blood the past week or so" and says, "I'm just not hungry." He has lost 20 lb (9 kg) since his previous admission. He is jaundiced and has petechiae and ecchymoses on his arms and legs. Liz Mowdi, Mr. Wright's nurse, notes pitting pretibial edema. Abdominal assessment reveals a tight, protuberant abdomen with caput medusae. The liver margin is not palpable; the spleen is enlarged. Vital signs are T 100°F (37.7°C), P 110, R 24, and BP 110/70.

Abnormal laboratory results include WBC 3700/mm³ (normal 4300 to 10,800/mm³); RBC 4.0 million/mm³ (normal 4.6 to 5.9 million/mm³); platelets 75,000/mm³ (normal 150,000 to 350,000/mm³); serum ammonia 105 μm/dL (normal 35 to 65 μm/dL); total bilirubin 4.9 mcg/dL (normal 0.1 to 1.0 mcg/dL); and serum sodium 150 mEq/L (normal 135 to 145 mEq/L). Potassium, hemoglobin, hematocrit, total protein, and albumin levels are markedly decreased. Hepatic enzymes are elevated. Blood urea nitrogen and creatinine levels are marginally elevated. Oxygen saturation (O₂ sat) is 88% (normal range: 96% to 100%) per pulse oximetry.

Endoscopy shows bleeding from gastric ulcer, and the diagnosis of alcoholic cirrhosis with gastritis is made. Mr. Wright is started on Aldactone, 25 mg PO q8h; Riopan, 30 mL 2 h p.c. and hs; lactulose, 30 mL qh until onset of diarrhea, then 15 mL tid; and low-protein, 800 mg sodium diet; fluid restriction of 1500 mL/day.

DIAGNOSES

- *Impaired Gas Exchange* related to pressure of ascites fluid on the diaphragm as manifested by tachypnea and decreased oxygen saturation
- *Excess Fluid Volume* related to electrolyte imbalance and hypoalbuminemia as manifested by ascites and peripheral edema
- *Imbalanced Nutrition: Less than Body Requirements* related to anorexia and possible alcohol abuse as manifested by weight loss and low serum protein levels
- *Disturbed Thought Processes* related to effects of high ammonia levels as manifested by lethargy
- *Ineffective Protection* related to impaired platelet formation and malnutrition

EXPECTED OUTCOMES

- Respiratory rate and O₂ sats will be within normal limits.
- Abdominal girth will decrease by 1 to 2 cm per day; peripheral edema will decrease.

- Will gain 1 lb (0.45 kg) per week without evidence of increased fluid retention. Serum albumin levels will return to normal range.
- Will be alert and oriented; serum ammonia levels are within normal range.
- Will demonstrate no further evidence of active bleeding.
- Will verbalize willingness to join a community support group.

PLANNING AND IMPLEMENTATION

- Weigh daily.
- Provide high-calorie, low-salt, low-protein diet with between-meal snacks.
- Maintain stool chart.
- Assign same nurses to care as much as possible to facilitate evaluation of mental status. Promptly report changes in status or laboratory values.
- Measure abdominal girth every 8 h, marking level of measurement.
- Institute bleeding precautions.
- Elevate head of bed; assist to chair with legs elevated tid as tolerated.
- Include significant others in care and teaching; refer to community agencies for discharge follow-up.

EVALUATION

A week after admission, Mr. Wright's ascites has decreased and no further active bleeding is noted. His serum protein levels have increased, and his laboratory values are improving. No further bruising is noted during hospitalization. Although he shows a 5-lb weight loss as excess water is eliminated, he is consuming 100% of his diet. His serum ammonia levels have returned to normal. On discharge, O₂ sat is 96%; respirations are 18. Lactulose will be continued on discharge.

Ms. Mowdi provides both written and verbal information about the medication and cirrhosis, including measures to prevent complications. Mr. Wright and his children express interest in Alcoholics Anonymous and Al-Anon and are referred to those agencies. Prior to discharge, follow-up appointments are made with a psychiatric social worker and a primary caregiver.

CRITICAL THINKING IN THE NURSING PROCESS

1. Describe the relationship between portal hypertension, liver dysfunction, and ascites.
2. Outline a 1-day menu for a low-protein, low-sodium high-calorie diet.
3. What is the pathophysiologic basis for hepatic encephalopathy? What are the nursing responsibilities related to lactulose and neomycin?
4. Design a nursing care plan for Mr. Wright for the diagnosis *Ineffective Coping.*
   See Evaluating Your Response in Appendix C.

---

pattern and extent of alcohol or injection drug use; use of other prescription and nonprescription drugs.

- *Physical assessment:* Vital signs; mental status; color and condition of skin and mucous membranes; peripheral pulses and presence of peripheral edema; abdominal assessment including appearance, shape and contour, bowel sounds, ab-

dominal girth, percussion for liver borders, and palpation for tenderness and liver size.

Nursing Diagnoses and Interventions

Nursing care of the client with cirrhosis presents many challenges because liver function affects all body systems. The nurse is responsible for coordinating care among care providers. Many nursing diagnoses may apply. The diagnoses discussed in this section focus on problems with fluid and electrolyte balance, disturbed thought processes, risk for bleeding, skin integrity, and nutrition.

Excess Fluid Volume

Cirrhosis affects water and salt regulation due to portal hypertension, hypoalbuminemia, and hyperaldosteronism. Signs of fluid volume overload and portal hypertension may develop: ascites, peripheral edema, internal hemorrhoids and varices, and prominent abdominal wall veins. Careful monitoring is necessary, because treatment measures can lead to further fluid and electrolyte imbalances.

- Weigh daily. Assess for jugular vein distention, measure abdominal girth daily, and check for peripheral edema. Monitor intake and output. *Careful assessment is important to detect fluid shifts.*
- Assess urine specific gravity. *Specific gravity measures the concentration of urine, an indicator of hydration.*

PRACTICE ALERT

Monitor the client with cirrhosis for signs of impaired renal function, such as oliguria, a fixed specific gravity of about 1.012, central edema (around the eyes and of the face), and increasing serum creatinine and BUN levels. Such signs may indicate hepatorenal syndrome or acute renal failure from another cause.

- Provide a low-sodium diet (500 to 2000 mg/day) and restrict fluids as ordered. *Excess sodium leads to water retention, and can increase fluid volume, ascites, and portal hypertension.*

Disturbed Thought Processes

Accumulated nitrogenous waste products and other metabolites affect mental status and thought processes. Effects of hepatic encephalopathy can range from mild confusion to agitation to coma.

- Assess neurologic status, including level of consciousness and mental status. Observe for signs of early encephalopathy: changes in handwriting, speech, and asterixis. *Early identification of evidence of encephalopathy allows prompt intervention—subtle changes in neurologic functioning are important!*

PRACTICE ALERT

Closely monitor clients who have experienced gastrointestinal bleeding for signs of hepatic encephalopathy. Blood in the intestinal tract is digested as a protein, increasing serum ammonia levels and the risk for hepatic encephalopathy.

- Avoid factors that may precipitate hepatic encephalopathy. Avoid hepatotoxic medications and CNS depressant drugs. *Cautious use of medications and close monitoring can eliminate iatrogenic causes of encephalopathy.*
- If possible, plan for consistent nursing care assignments. *Consistent care providers facilitate early identification of subtle neurologic changes indicative of hepatic encephalopathy.*

- Provide low-protein diet as prescribed; teach the family the importance of maintaining diet restrictions. *Nitrogenous byproducts from dietary protein increase serum ammonia levels.*
- Administer medications or enemas as ordered to reduce nitrogenous products. Monitor bowel function and provide measures to promote regular elimination and prevent constipation. *Oral or rectally administered (per enema) medications are ordered to reduce intestinal bacteria and the ammonia they produce. Regular bowel elimination promotes protein and ammonia elimination in the feces.*
- Orient to surroundings, person, and place; provide simple explanations and reassurance. *Modification of verbal interactions to level of understanding and mental status may reduce anxiety and agitation.*

Ineffective Protection

Impaired coagulation, esophageal varices, and possible acute gastritis place the client with cirrhosis at significant risk for hemorrhage. Clotting is altered by vitamin K deficiency; impaired manufacture of coagulation Factors II, VII, IX, and X; and increased platelet destruction due to splenomegaly.

- Monitor vital signs; report tachycardia or hypotension. *Increased pulse and decreasing blood pressure may indicate hypovolemia due to hemorrhage.*
- Institute bleeding precautions (Box 24–6). *Preventive measures can decrease the risk for active bleeding.*
- Monitor coagulation studies and platelet count. Report abnormal results. *Coagulation studies help determine the risk for bleeding and the need for treatment.*
- Carefully monitor the client who has had bleeding esophageal varices for evidence of rebleeding: hematemesis, **hematochezia** (bright blood in the stool) or tarry stools, signs of hypovolemia or shock. *Rebleeding is common following variceal hemorrhage, especially within the first week.*

PRACTICE ALERT

Carefully monitor the respiratory status of the client with a Sengstaken-Blakemore or Minnesota tube. Displacement of the tube can obstruct the airway unless an endotracheal tube is in place. The esophageal balloon prevents the client from swallowing oral secretions, increasing the risk for aspiration. Keep the head of the bed elevated to 45 degrees to reduce the risk of aspiration and promote gas exchange.

BOX 24–6 Bleeding Precautions

- Prevent constipation.
- Avoid rectal temperatures or enemas.
- Avoid injections; if needed, use small-gauge needle and apply gentle pressure.
- Monitor platelet count, PT, and aPPT.
- Assess for ecchymotic areas and areas of purpura.
- Apply pressure to bleeding sites. After venipuncture, apply direct pressure for at least 5 minutes.
- Use only a soft toothbrush.
- Avoid blowing nose.
- Assess oral cavity for bleeding gums.

Impaired Skin Integrity

Severe jaundice with bile salt deposits on the skin may cause pruritus. Scratching related to the pruritus damages the skin and impairs its integrity. Malnutrition, particularly protein deficiency, and edema also increase the risk for tissue breakdown and impaired skin integrity.

- Use warm water rather than hot water when bathing. *Hot water increases pruritus.*
- Use measures to prevent dry skin: Apply an emollient or lubricant as needed to keep skin moist, avoid soap or preparations with alcohol, and do not rub the skin. *Dry skin contributes to pruritus.*
- If indicated, apply mittens to the hands to prevent scratching. *Clients with encephalopathy may not understand the need to refrain from scratching.*
- Institute measures to prevent skin and tissue breakdown: Turn at least every 2 hours, use an alternating pressure mattress, and frequently assess skin condition. *Frequent position changes relieve pressure and promote circulation and tissue oxygenation.*
- Administer prescribed antihistamine (to relieve pruritus) cautiously. *Decreased liver function increases the risk for altered drug responses.*

Imbalanced Nutrition: Less than Body Requirements

The client with cirrhosis is at risk for malnutrition for a number of reasons: possible chronic alcohol use, anorexia, impaired vitamin and mineral absorption, and impaired protein metabolism. In addition, salt and protein restrictions may make the diet less palatable and appealing to the client.

- Weigh daily. Instruct to weigh at least weekly at home. *Weight is a good indicator of both nutritional status and fluid balance. Short-term weight fluctuations tend to reflect fluid balance, while longer term changes in weight are more reflective of nutritional status.*
- Provide small meals with between-meal snacks. *A small meal is more appealing for an anorexic client. Between-meal snacks help maintain adequate calorie and nutrient intake.*
- Unless protein is restricted due to impending hepatic encephalopathy, promote protein and nutrient intake by providing nutritional supplements such as Ensure or instant breakfasts. *The sodium and protein content of all meals and snacks must be calculated when maintaining restrictions of these nutrients.*
- Arrange for consultation with a dietitian for diet planning while hospitalized and at home. *The dietitian can provide detailed instructions, sample menus, and suggestions for improving the palatability of the diet and promoting intake.*

Using NANDA, NIC, and NOC

Chart 24–2 shows links between NANDA nursing diagnoses, NIC, and NOC for the client with cirrhosis.

Community-Based Care

Cirrhosis is a chronic, progressive disease. As such, the client and family assume major roles in managing the disease and its

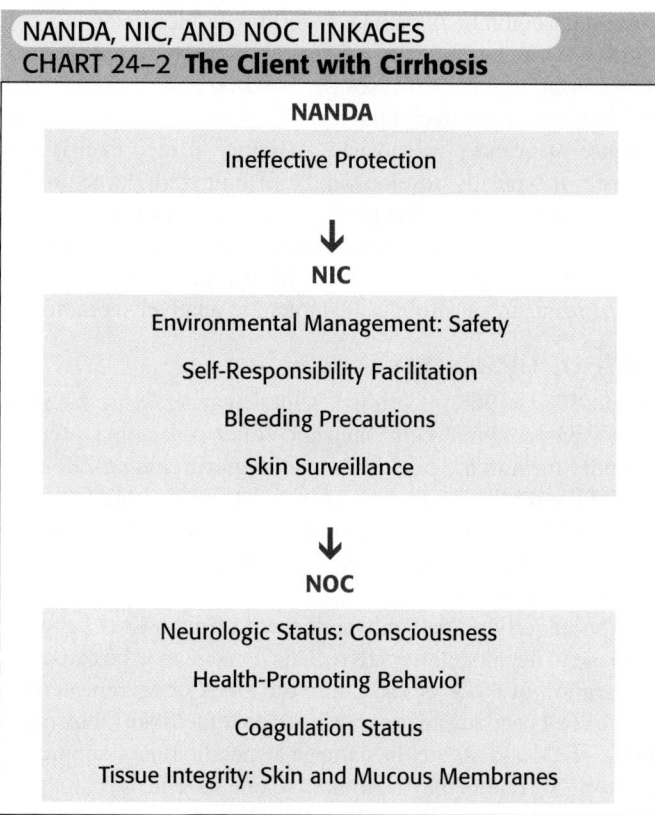

NANDA, NIC, AND NOC LINKAGES
CHART 24–2 The Client with Cirrhosis

NANDA

Ineffective Protection

↓

NIC

Environmental Management: Safety

Self-Responsibility Facilitation

Bleeding Precautions

Skin Surveillance

↓

NOC

Neurologic Status: Consciousness

Health-Promoting Behavior

Coagulation Status

Tissue Integrity: Skin and Mucous Membranes

Data from *NANDA's Nursing Diagnoses: Definitions & Classification 2005–2006* by NANDA International (2005), Philadelphia; *Nursing Interventions Classification (NIC)* (4th ed.) by J. M. Dochterman & G. M. Bulechek (2004), St. Louis, MO: Mosby; and *Nursing Outcomes Classification (NOC)* (3rd ed.) by S. Moorhead, M. Johnson, and M. Maas (2004), St. Louis, MO: Mosby.

manifestations and in preventing complications. Teaching topics for home care include:

- The absolute necessity of avoiding alcohol and other hepatotoxic drugs. Suggest inpatient or community-based alcohol treatment programs and Alcoholics Anonymous as indicated.
- Diet and fluid intake restrictions and recommendations. Include suggestions to promote nutritional intake and increase the flavor of food when sodium is restricted.
- Prescribed medications; their timing, intended and adverse effects, and manifestations to report to the primary care provider.
- Bleeding precautions (see Box 24–6).
- Manifestations of potential complications to be reported to the primary care provider. Stress the importance of promptly reporting evidence of gastrointestinal bleeding for prompt intervention for potential hemorrhage.
- Skin care techniques to reduce pruritus and the risk of damage.
- Ways to manage fatigue and conserve energy.

Provide referrals for home health services, dietary consultation, social services, and counseling as needed by the client and family. Suggest local support groups where available. If appropriate, suggest hospice services for the client with end-stage liver disease.

THE CLIENT WITH CANCER OF THE LIVER

Primary liver cancer is uncommon in the United States, accounting for only 0.5% to 2% of all cancers (Porth, 2005). It is, however, a common malignancy worldwide. Hepatocellular carcinoma is common in parts of Asia and Africa, where the incidence is as high as 500 cases per 100,000 people. This higher incidence is linked to chronic hepatitis B or C infection. The incidence of primary liver cancer is higher in men than it is in women. It typically develops in the fifth or sixth decade of life (Kasper et al., 2005). The prognosis for primary liver cancer is poor, in part because the disease often is advanced at the time of diagnosis. Metastasis to the liver from primary tumors of the lung, breast, and gastrointestinal tract are relatively common.

Pathophysiology

About 80% to 90% of primary hepatic cancers arise from the liver's parenchymal cells (hepatocellular carcinoma); the remainder form in the bile ducts (cholangiocarcinoma). Regardless of the origin, the progress of the disease is similar. Several etiologic factors have been identified (Box 24–7). Most primary liver cancer in the United States is related to alcoholic cirrhosis, HBV, or HCV.

The underlying pathophysiology of primary liver cancer is damage to hepatocellular DNA. This damage may be caused by integration of HBV or HCV into the DNA or by repeated cycles of cell necrosis and regeneration that facilitate DNA mutations. HBV and aflatoxins damage a specific tumor suppressor gene, p53. Tumors may be limited to one specific area, may occur as nodules throughout the liver, or may develop as surface infiltrates. The tumor interferes with normal hepatic function, leading to biliary obstruction and jaundice, portal hypertension, and metabolic disruptions (hypoalbuminemia, hypoglycemia, and bleeding disorders). It also may secrete bile products and produce hormones (paraneoplastic syndrome) that may lead to polycythemia, hypoglycemia, and hypercalcemia. Tumors usually grow rapidly and metastasize early.

Manifestations

Initial manifestations of liver cancer develop insidiously and often are masked by the presence of cirrhosis or chronic hepatitis. Weakness, anorexia, weight loss, fatigue, and malaise are common early manifestations. Abdominal pain and a palpable mass in the right upper quadrant are common presenting symptoms. See the following box for manifestations of primary liver cancer. Ascites and jaundice may be present at diagnosis. Signs of liver failure with portal hypertension, splenomegaly, and altered metabolism develop as the tumor progresses. Most clients die within 6 months of the diagnosis (Porth, 2005).

BOX 24–7 Suspected Causes of Primary Liver Cancer

- Chronic hepatitis C infection
- Chronic hepatitis B infection
- Cirrhosis, regardless of type
- Chronic aflatoxin (a toxin produced by *Aspergillus* molds) exposure
- Arsenic-contaminated water
- Carcinogens in food
- Possible hormonal factors (e.g., long-term use of androgens)

MANIFESTATIONS of Primary Liver Cancer

- Malaise
- Anorexia
- Lethargy
- Weight loss
- Fever of unknown origin
- Jaundice
- Feeling of abdominal fullness
- Painful right upper quadrant mass
- Manifestations of liver failure

INTERDISCIPLINARY CARE

Liver tumors are identified by CT scans and MRI. A liver biopsy may be done to confirm the diagnosis and identify the tumor type or origin. See the box on page 617 for the nursing implications of liver biopsy. Serum alpha-fetoprotein (AFP) levels, normally low in nonpregnant adults, rise in most clients with hepatocellular cancer.

Small, localized tumors may be surgically resected, offering the only viable chance for cure. Most tumors, however, have spread extensively or have distant metastasis at the time of diagnosis, so this is frequently not an option. Liver transplantation may be done; however, the tumor may recur in the transplanted organ.

Radiation therapy is used to shrink the tumor, decreasing pressure on surrounding organs and reducing pain. Chemotherapy may be used as primary treatment or adjunctive therapy. Direct continuous hepatic arterial infusion with an implanted pump has shown promise in prolonging survival rates. See Chapter 14 ∞ for nursing care for clients receiving radiation therapy or chemotherapy.

NURSING CARE

Encourage clients with risk factors for primary liver cancer to avoid alcohol and other substances that may further damage the liver. Urge them to discuss regular screening for liver tumors (such as serum AFP levels) with their primary care physician.

Both the client and the family need extensive nursing support. Controlling pain is a priority. Because of the poor prognosis, early referral for hospice services may be appropriate.

Nursing diagnoses, interventions, and teaching for the client with liver cancer are similar to those for clients with cirrhosis; see pages 721–723.

THE CLIENT WITH LIVER TRAUMA

Blunt or penetrating trauma to the abdomen can damage the liver. Liver trauma is frequently seen in combination with injuries to other abdominal organs. Motor vehicle crashes, stab or gunshot wounds, and iatrogenic sources such as liver biopsy are among the causes of these injuries.

Pathophysiology and Manifestations

Liver trauma generally causes bleeding due to the vascularity of the organ. Liver injury may cause a surface hematoma, hematoma within the liver parenchyma, laceration of liver tissue, or disruption of vessels leading to or from the liver. Severe bleeding can rapidly disrupt hemodynamic stability and lead to shock.

PRACTICE ALERT

Bleeding due to liver trauma may not be immediately apparent. Instruct the client with apparent or potential liver trauma to immediately report light-headedness, rapid heart rate, shortness of breath, thirst, or increasing abdominal pain.

INTERDISCIPLINARY CARE

Diagnostic peritoneal lavage is often used along with CT scan to diagnose liver trauma. The procedure is performed by making a small abdominal incision into the peritoneum (after the bladder has been emptied), and inserting a small catheter into the peritoneal cavity. If blood is immediately detected, the client is taken directly to surgery for abdominal exploration. If frank bleeding is not apparent, a liter of isotonic fluid is instilled into the abdomen, then drained and sent for laboratory analysis.

Intravenous fluids, fresh frozen plasma, platelets, and other clotting factors are administered to restore blood volume and promote hemostasis. Hemodynamic status is closely monitored; continued instability may indicate a need for surgical intervention to control hemorrhage. Postoperative nursing care focuses on preventing pulmonary complications, such as atelectasis, and detecting and preventing infection.

NURSING CARE

Nursing care of the client with liver trauma focuses on fluid management and other supportive care related to shock. Keeping family members informed is an important aspect of care, especially during the period of client instability. Diagnoses include the following:

- *Deficient Fluid Volume* related to hemorrhage
- *Risk for Infection* related to wound or abdominal contamination
- *Ineffective Protection* related to impaired coagulation.

THE CLIENT WITH LIVER ABSCESS

Liver abscesses usually are bacterial or amoebic (protozoal) in origin. Bacterial abscesses may follow trauma or surgical procedures, including biopsy. Multiple or single abscesses occur most commonly in the right lobe. Amoebic abscesses most frequently occur following infestation of the liver by *Entamoeba histolytica*. Amoebic infestation is associated with poor hygiene, unsafe sexual practices, or travel in areas where drinking water is contaminated.

Pathophysiology and Manifestations

Following bacterial or amoebic invasion of the liver, healthy tissue is destroyed, leaving an area of necrosis, inflammatory exudate, and blood. This damaged region becomes walled off from the healthy liver tissue. Pyogenic (bacterial) liver abscess may be caused by cholangitis, or distant or intra-abdominal infections, such as peritonitis or diverticulitis. *Escherichia coli* is the most frequently identified causative organism. The onset of pyogenic abscess is usually sudden, causing acute symptoms such as fever, malaise, vomiting, hyperbilirubinemia, and pain in the right upper abdomen.

The infection pathway for amoebic hepatic abscesses usually is the portal venous circulation from the right colon. Generally, the onset of amoebic abscess is insidious.

INTERDISCIPLINARY CARE

Hepatic abscess is diagnosed through biopsy, hepatic aspirate, blood and fecal cultures, and CT scan and ultrasound studies. Therapy is based on identifying the causative organism through laboratory cultures. Pyogenic abscesses are treated with antibiotics to which the causative organism is sensitive.

Pharmacologic agents used for amebic hepatic abscess are the same as those used for intestinal amebic infestation (see Chapter 26 ∞); combination therapy is commonly used. Two commonly used drugs for treating amebic liver abscesses are metronidazole (Flagyl) and iodoquinol (Diquinol). Both medications can cause gastrointestinal symptoms. Bone marrow suppression is a risk with metronidazole.

If the abscess does not respond to antibiotic therapy, percutaneous aspiration or surgical drainage may be done. In these procedures, a *percutaneous closed-catheter drain* is placed in the abscess to promote drainage of purulent material.

NURSING CARE

A major aspect of nursing care is prevention; teaching clients to avoid contaminated water and foods is especially important. Nursing interventions include teaching hikers to treat water and food handlers to wash hands thoroughly.

Clients who have a liver abscess require supportive care to prevent dehydration from the accompanying fever, nausea, vomiting, and anorexia. Careful monitoring of fluid and electrolyte status is indicated, as are comfort measures for abdominal pain. Possible nursing diagnoses include the following:

- *Risk for Deficient Fluid Volume* related to effects of prolonged fever and vomiting
- *Deficient Knowledge* related to transmission of amebic abscess
- *Activity Intolerance* related to pain and weakness.

EXOCRINE PANCREAS DISORDERS

The pancreas is both an exocrine and an endocrine gland. It is made up of two basic cell types, each having different functions. The exocrine cells produce enzymes that empty through ducts into the small intestine, whereas the endocrine cells produce hormones that enter the bloodstream directly. Disorders of the exocrine pancreas affect the secretion and glandular control of digestive enzymes, whereas disorders of the endocrine pancreas affect the production of hormones necessary for normal carbohydrate, protein, and fat metabolism. Disorders of the exocrine pancreas are discussed in this section of the chapter; diabetes mellitus, a disorder of the endocrine pancreas, is discussed in Chapter 20 ∞ .

THE CLIENT WITH PANCREATITIS

Pancreatitis, or inflammation of the pancreas, is characterized by release of pancreatic enzymes into the tissue of the pancreas itself, leading to hemorrhage and necrosis. Pancreatitis may be either acute or chronic. About 5000 new cases of acute pancreatitis are diagnosed every year in the United States. It is a serious disease, with a mortality rate of approximately 10% (Kasper et al., 2005). Alcoholism and gallstones are the primary risk factors for acute pancreatitis.

The incidence of chronic pancreatitis is less clear, because many people with chronic pancreatitis do not have classic manifestations of the disease. Clients with pancreatitis may have long-term effects of the disease, with chronic changes in enzyme and hormone production.

Physiology Review

Knowledge of the normal structure and functions of the exocrine pancreas is important to understand how inflammation affects it and the client. The exocrine pancreas consists of lobules of acinar cells. The acinar cells secrete digestive enzymes and fluids (pancreatic juices) into ducts that empty into the main pancreatic duct (the duct of Wirsung). The pancreatic duct joins the common bile duct and empties into the duodenum through the ampulla of Vater (in some people the main pancreatic duct empties directly into the duodenum). The epithelial lining of the pancreatic ducts secretes water and bicarbonate to modify the composition of the pancreatic secretions. Pancreatic enzymes are secreted primarily in an inactive form and are activated in the intestine, a modification that prevents digestion of pancreatic tissue by its own enzymes (Porth, 2005). The pancreatic enzymes, with related functions, are as follows:

- Proteolytic enzymes, including trypsin, chymotrypsin, carboxypolypeptidase, ribonuclease, and deoxyribonuclease, which break down dietary proteins
- Pancreatic amylase, which breaks down starch
- Lipase, which breaks down fats into glycerol and fatty acids.

Pathophysiology

Acute Pancreatitis

Acute pancreatitis is an inflammatory disorder that involves self-destruction of the pancreas by its own enzymes through autodigestion. The milder form of acute pancreatitis, *interstitial edematous pancreatitis*, leads to inflammation and edema of pancreatic tissue. It often is self-limiting. The more severe form, *necrotizing pancreatitis*, is characterized by inflammation, hemorrhage, and ultimately necrosis of pancreatic tissue.

Acute pancreatitis is more common in middle adults; its incidence is higher in men than in women. Acute pancreatitis is usually associated with gallstones in women and with alco-holism in men. Some clients recover completely, others experience recurring attacks, and still others develop chronic pancreatitis. The mortality and symptoms depend on the severity and type of pancreatitis: With mild pancreatic edema, mortality is low (6%); with severe necrotic pancreatitis, the mortality rate is high (23%) (Porth, 2005).

Although the exact cause of pancreatitis is not known, the following factors may activate pancreatic enzymes within the pancreas, leading to autodigestion, inflammation, edema, and/or necrosis.

- Gallstones may obstruct the pancreatic duct or cause bile reflux, activating pancreatic enzymes in the pancreatic duct system.
- Alcohol causes duodenal edema, and may increase pressure and spasm in the sphincter of Oddi, obstructing pancreatic outflow. It also stimulates pancreatic enzyme production, thus raising pressure within the pancreas.

Other factors associated with acute pancreatitis include tissue ischemia or anoxia, trauma or surgery, pancreatic tumors, third-trimester pregnancy, infectious agents (viral, bacterial, or parasitic), elevated calcium levels, and hyperlipidemia. Some medications have been linked with this disorder, including thiazide diuretics, estrogen, steroids, salicylates, and NSAIDs.

Regardless of the precipitating factor, the pathophysiologic process begins with the release of activated pancreatic enzymes into pancreatic tissue. Activated proteolytic enzymes, trypsin in particular, digest pancreatic tissue and activate other enzymes such as phospholipase A, which digests cell membrane phospholipids, and elastase, which digests the elastic tissue of blood vessel walls. This leads to proteolysis, edema, vascular damage and hemorrhage, and necrosis of parenchymal cells. Cellular damage and necrosis release activated enzymes and vasoactive substances that produce vasodilation, increase vascular permeability, and cause edema. A large volume of fluid may shift from circulating blood into the retroperitoneal space, the peripancreatic spaces, and the abdominal cavity.

MANIFESTATIONS Acute pancreatitis develops suddenly, with an abrupt onset of continuous severe epigastric and abdominal pain. This pain commonly radiates to the back and is relieved somewhat by sitting up and leaning forward. The pain often is initiated by a fatty meal or excessive alcohol intake.

Other manifestations include nausea and vomiting; abdominal distention and rigidity; decreased bowel sounds; tachycardia; hypotension; elevated temperature; and cold, clammy skin. Within 24 hours, mild jaundice may appear. Retroperitoneal bleeding may occur 3 to 6 days after the onset of acute pancreatitis; signs of bleeding include bruising in the flanks (Turner's sign) or around the umbilicus (Cullen's sign). See the Manifestations box on the following page.

COMPLICATIONS Systemic complications of acute pancreatitis include intravascular volume depletion with acute tubular necrosis and renal failure (see Chapter 29 ∞ for more information about acute renal failure), and acute respiratory distress syndrome (ARDS). Acute renal failure usually develops within 24 hours after the onset of acute pancreatitis. Manifestations of ARDS may be seen 3 to 7 days after its onset, particularly in

MANIFESTATIONS of Acute and Chronic Pancreatitis

ACUTE PANCREATITIS
- Abrupt onset of severe epigastric and left upper quadrant pain, may radiate to back
- Nausea, vomiting; fever
- Decreased bowel sounds; abdominal distention and rigidity
- Tachycardia, hypotension; cold, clammy skin
- Possible jaundice
- Positive Turner's sign (flank ecchymosis) or Cullen's sign (periumbilical ecchymosis)

CHRONIC PANCREATITIS
- Recurrent epigastric and LUQ pain, radiates to back
- Anorexia, nausea and vomiting, weight loss
- Flatulence, constipation
- Steatorrhea

clients who have experienced severe volume depletion. See Chapter 39 ∞ for more information about ARDS.

Localized complications include pancreatic necrosis, abscess, pseudocysts, and pancreatic ascites. Pancreatic necrosis causes an inflammatory mass that may be infected. It may lead to shock and multiple organ failure. A pancreatic abscess may form late in the course of the disease (6 or more weeks after its onset), causing an epigastric mass and tenderness (Tierney et al., 2005). Pancreatic pseudocysts, encapsulated collections of fluid, may develop both within the pancreas itself and in the abdominal cavity. They may impinge on other structures, or may rupture, causing generalized peritonitis. Rupture of a pseudocyst or of the pancreatic duct can lead to pancreatic ascites. Pancreatic ascites is recognized by gradually increasing abdominal girth and persistent elevation of the serum amylase level without abdominal pain.

Chronic Pancreatitis

Chronic pancreatitis is characterized by gradual destruction of functional pancreatic tissue. In contrast to acute pancreatitis, which may completely resolve with no long-term effects, chronic pancreatitis is an irreversible process that eventually leads to pancreatic insufficiency. Alcoholism is the primary risk factor for chronic pancreatitis in the United States. Malnutrition is a major worldwide risk factor. About 10% to 20% of chronic pancreatitis is idiopathic, with no identified cause. A genetic mutation on a gene associated with cystic fibrosis may play a role in these cases. Children or young adults with cystic fibrosis may develop chronic pancreatitis as well.

In chronic pancreatitis related to alcoholism, pancreatic secretions have an increased concentration of insoluble proteins. These proteins calcify, forming plugs that block pancreatic ducts and the flow of pancreatic juices. This blockage leads to inflammation and fibrosis of pancreatic tissue. In other cases, a stricture or stone may block pancreatic outflow, causing chronic obstructive pancreatitis. In chronic pancreatitis, recurrent episodes of inflammation eventually lead to fibrotic changes in the parenchyma of the pancreas, with loss of ex-

ocrine function. This leads to malabsorption from pancreatic insufficiency. If endocrine function is disrupted as well, clinical diabetes mellitus may develop.

MANIFESTATIONS Chronic pancreatitis typically causes recurrent episodes of epigastric and left upper abdominal pain that radiates to the back. This pain may last for days to weeks. As the disease progresses, the interval between episodes of pain becomes shorter. Other manifestations include anorexia, nausea and vomiting, weight loss, flatulence, constipation, and **steatorrhea** (fatty, frothy, foul-smelling stools caused by a decrease in pancreatic enzyme secretion).

COMPLICATIONS Complications of chronic pancreatitis include malabsorption, malnutrition, and possible peptic ulcer disease. Pancreatic pseudocyst or abscess may form, or stricture of the common bile duct may develop. Diabetes mellitus may develop, and there is an increased risk for pancreatic cancer. Narcotic addiction related to frequent, severe pain episodes is common.

INTERDISCIPLINARY CARE

Acute pancreatitis often is a mild, self-limiting disease. Treatment focuses on reducing pancreatic secretions and providing supportive care. Treatment to eliminate the causative factor is begun after the acute inflammatory process resolves. Severe necrotizing pancreatitis may require intensive care management. Treatment for chronic pancreatitis often focuses on managing pain and treating malabsorption and malnutrition.

Diagnosis

The laboratory tests that may be ordered when pancreatitis is suspected are summarized in Table 24–5. Diagnostic studies include the following:
- *Ultrasonography* can identify gallstones, a pancreatic mass, or pseudocyst.
- *CT scan* may be ordered to identify pancreatic enlargement, fluid collections in or around the pancreas, and perfusion deficits in areas of necrosis.
- *Endoscopic retrograde cholangiopancreatography (ERCP)* may be performed to diagnose chronic pancreatitis and to differentiate inflammation and fibrosis from carcinoma.
- *Endoscopic ultrasonography* can detect changes indicative of chronic pancreatitis in the pancreatic duct and parenchyma.
- *Percutaneous fine-needle aspiration biopsy* may be performed to differentiate chronic pancreatitis from cancer of the pancreas; the cells that are aspirated are examined for malignancy.

More information about these tests and their nursing implications can be found in Chapter 21 ∞.

Medications

The treatment of acute pancreatitis is largely supportive. Narcotic analgesics such as morphine sulfate are used to control pain. Antibiotics often are prescribed to prevent or treat infection.

Clients with chronic pancreatitis also require analgesics, but are closely monitored to prevent drug dependence. Narcotics are avoided when possible. Pancreatic enzyme supplements are given to reduce steatorrhea (see the Medication Administration

TABLE 24–5 Laboratory Tests in Exocrine Pancreatic Disorders

TEST	NORMAL VALUE	SIGNIFICANCE
Serum amylase	0–130 Unit/L	Rises within 2 to 12 hours of onset of acute pancreatitis to two to three times normal. Returns to normal in 3 to 4 days.
Serum lipase	0–160 Unit/L	Levels rise in acute pancreatitis; remain elevated for 7 to 14 days.
Serum trypsinogen	<80 mcg/L	Elevated in acute pancreatitis; may be decreased in chronic pancreatitis.
Urine amylase	4 to 37 Unit/L/2h	Urine amylase levels rise in acute pancreatitis.
Serum glucose	70 to 110 mg/dL	May be transient elevation in acute pancreatitis.
Serum bilirubin	0.1 to 1.0 mg/dL	Compression of the common duct may increase bilirubin levels in acute pancreatitis.
Serum alkaline phosphatase	30 to 95 Unit/L	Compression of the common duct may increase levels in acute pancreatitis.
Serum calcium	8.9 to 10.3 mg/dL or 4.5 to 5.5 mEq/L	Hypocalcemia develops in up to 25% of clients with acute pancreatitis.
White blood cells	4500/mm^3 to 10,000/mm^3	Leukocytosis indicates inflammation and is usually present in acute pancreatitis.

box below). Clients with chronic pancreatitis may need to remain on pancreatic enzyme supplements for life. H$_2$ blockers such as cimetidine (Tagamet) and ranitidine (Zantac), and proton-pump inhibitors such as omeprazole (Prilosec) may be given to neutralize or decrease gastric secretions. Octreotide (Sandostatin), a synthetic hormone, suppresses pancreatic enzyme secretion and may be used to relieve pain in chronic pancreatitis.

Treatments

NUTRITION Oral food and fluids are withheld during acute episodes of pancreatitis to reduce pancreatic secretions and promote rest of the organ. A nasogastric tube may be inserted and connected to suction. Intravenous fluids are administered to maintain vascular volume, and total parenteral nutrition (TPN) is initiated. Oral food and fluids are begun once the serum amylase levels have returned to normal, bowel sounds are present, and pain disappears. A low-fat diet is ordered, and alcohol intake is strictly prohibited.

SURGERY If the pancreatitis is the result of a gallstone lodged in the sphincter of Oddi, an *endoscopic transduodenal sphinc-* *terotomy* may be performed to remove the stone. When cholelithiasis is identified as a causative factor, a cholecystectomy is performed once the acute pancreatitis has resolved. Surgical procedures to promote drainage of pancreatic enzymes into the duodenum or resection of all or part of the pancreas may be done to provide pain relief in clients with chronic pancreatitis. Large pancreatic pseudocysts may be drained endoscopically or surgically.

COMPLEMENTARY THERAPIES Several complementary therapies may be used in conjunction with traditional treatments for clients with acute or chronic pancreatitis. Fasting or use of low-salt, low-fat vegetarian diets may reduce episodes of recurrent pain. Qigong, a system of gentle exercise, meditation, and controlled breathing, is believed to balance the flow of qi (a vital life force) through the body. Qigong lowers the metabolic rate, and may reduce the stimulation of pancreatic enzyme secretion. Magnetic field therapy also may be employed for clients with pancreatitis. All complementary therapies should be prescribed by a trained and competent practitioner.

MEDICATION ADMINISTRATION The Client with Chronic Pancreatitis

PANCREATIC ENZYME REPLACEMENT
Pancrelipase (Lipancreatin)
Pancrelipase enhances the digestion of starches and fats in the gastrointestinal tract by supplying an exogenous source of the enzymes protease, amylase, and lipase. The drug promotes nutrition and decreases the number of bowel movements.

Nursing Responsibilities
- Assess for allergy to pork protein.
- Monitor frequency and consistency of stools.
- Weigh every other day. Record weights.
- Give with meals; if not enteric coated, H$_2$ antagonists or antacids may be given concurrently to prevent destruction of the enzymes by hydrochloric acid.

- Monitor for side effects: rash, hives, respiratory difficulty, hematuria, hyperuricemia, or joint pain.

Health Education for the Client and Family
- Take with meals or snacks.
- If medicine is enteric coated, do not crush, chew, or mix with alkaline foods (e.g., milk, ice cream)
- Be sure to follow prescribed diet.
- Continue taking this drug until or unless advised by physician that it is no longer necessary.

NURSING CARE

In addition to the nursing care discussed in this section, a Nursing Care Plan for a client with acute pancreatitis is found below.

Health Promotion

Teach clients who abuse alcohol about the risk for developing pancreatitis. Advise abstinence to reduce this risk, and refer to an alcohol treatment program or Alcoholics Anonymous.

Assessment

Assessment data related to acute or chronic pancreatitis include the following:

■ *Health history:* Current manifestations; abdominal pain (location, nature, onset and duration, identified precipitating factors); anorexia, nausea or vomiting; flatulence, diarrhea, constipation, or stool changes; recent weight loss; history of previous episodes or gallstones; alcohol use (extent and duration); current medications.

NURSING CARE PLAN   A Client with Acute Pancreatitis

Rose Schliefer is a 59-year-old wife, mother of three, and grandmother of four. She has been hospitalized for the past 6 weeks for acute hemorrhagic pancreatitis and pseudocyst. The pancreatitis was caused by gallstones. Mrs. Schliefer spent 3 weeks in intensive care, and then underwent surgery to remove the gallstones and to insert drains into the pseudocyst. Prior to discharge, she had progressed to a soft, high-carbohydrate, low-fat diet; had all drains removed; and was able to walk in the hall. Mrs. Schliefer was referred to a community health agency in her home town for continued follow-up.

ASSESSMENT

Lee Quinn, the community health nurse, assesses Mrs. Schliefer at home after discharge. Mrs. Schliefer is thin and appears anxious and tired. She states that she lost 30 lb (13.6 kg) in the hospital and now weighs only 102 lb (46 kg). She is 66 inches (168 cm) tall. Her vital signs are within normal limits. Mrs. Schliefer has a well-healed upper abdominal scar and two small wounds (from drains) on each side of her abdomen. The wounds are closed but still have scabs. Her skin is cool and dry, and turgor is poor. She is alert and oriented and responds appropriately to questions. Blood glucose levels are normal. Mrs. Schliefer states that her main problems are lack of energy and lack of appetite for the low-fat diet that has been ordered. Mrs. Schliefer's husband and daughters express concern about their ability to provide care. Although they have been taught all about the disease and how to provide care, they still are not sure they know exactly what should be done now that Mrs. Schliefer is at home.

DIAGNOSES

■ *Fatigue* related to decreased metabolic energy production
■ *Imbalanced Nutrition: Less than Body Requirements* related to prolonged hospitalization, dietary restrictions, and impaired digestion
■ *Bathing/Hygiene Self-Care Deficit* (Level II: requires help of another person, supervision, and teaching) related to decreased strength and endurance
■ *Risk for Caregiver Role Strain* related to inexperience with caregiving tasks

EXPECTED OUTCOMES

■ Set priorities for daily and weekly activities, and incorporate a rest period into daily activity.
■ Gain 1 to 2 lbs per week.
■ Bathe and maintain personal hygiene without assistance.
■ Family members will verbalize comfort with providing necessary care.

PLANNING AND IMPLEMENTATION

■ Explain causes of fatigue. Review effects of pancreatitis, surgery, and acute illness on energy levels.

■ Develop activity goals, incorporating small, incremental steps toward achieving goals. Mrs. Schliefer indicates that she wants to cook a meal for the whole family. To reach this goal, she will:
  a. Schedule the meal when her energy level is highest.
  b. List actions necessary to prepare the meal and delegate difficult tasks to family members.
  c. Ask daughters to reorganize the kitchen to avoid unnecessary steps.
  d. Plan the meal no sooner than the third week after being home.
■ Instruct to:
  a. Rest in bed each day from 1:00 P.M. to 3:00 P.M.
  b. Eat six small meals a day with family members or friends.
  c. Sit and rest quietly for 15 minutes before eating.
■ Discuss dietary restrictions and how to adapt them to usual diet.
■ Advise to use shower chair and develop self-care goals for bathing and hygiene in small steps. Add self-care tasks gradually as tolerated.
■ Discuss division of responsibilities for physical care, home maintenance, and medical care with family members.
■ Encourage family discussion of concerns about future; acknowledge family strengths.

EVALUATION

One month after discharge, Mrs. Schliefer and her family have established new routines based on her energy levels. Mrs. Schliefer now fixes lunch because she feels best during midday. She and her husband share this time together without interruption. Mrs. Schliefer still rests during the day but can now provide self-care. She has gained only 2 lb, but states that she is getting used to the new diet and that "things are even starting to taste good without butter." She also says that sitting quietly before meals is helpful and that she prefers eating six small meals a day. Mr. and Mrs. Schliefer and their daughters agree that their initial worries about Mrs. Schliefer's care have been resolved; now they all know what they must do, and the future looks much brighter.

CRITICAL THINKING IN THE NURSING PROCESS

1. Your client with acute pancreatitis is also an alcoholic. Describe assessments that indicate the beginnings of withdrawal.
2. Discuss the pathophysiologic basis of hypovolemic shock in acute necrotic pancreatitis.
3. Outline a teaching plan that includes specific foods to omit and to include in a high-carbohydrate, low-protein, low-fat diet.
4. Develop a plan of care for the nursing diagnosis *Impaired Home Maintenance*.
See Evaluating Your Response in Appendix C.

- *Physical assessment:* Vital signs including orthostatic vitals and peripheral pulses; temperature; skin temperature and color, presence of any flank or periumbilical ecchymoses; abdominal assessment including bowel sounds, presence of distention, tenderness, or guarding.

Nursing Diagnoses and Interventions

Nursing care for the client with acute pancreatitis focuses on managing pain, nutrition, and maintaining fluid balance.

Pain

Obstruction of pancreatic ducts and inflammation, edema, and swelling of the pancreas caused by pancreatic autodigestion cause severe epigastric, left upper abdominal, or midscapular back pain. The pain often is accompanied by nausea and vomiting, abdominal tenderness, and muscle guarding.

- Using a standard pain scale (see Chapter 9 ∞), assess pain, including location, radiation, duration, and character. Note nonverbal cues of pain: restlessness or remaining rigidly still; tense facial features; clenched fists; rapid, shallow respirations; tachycardia; and diaphoresis. Administer analgesics on a regular schedule. *Pain assessment before and after analgesic administration measures its effectiveness. Administering analgesics on a regular schedule prevents pain from becoming established, severe, and difficult to control. Unrelieved pain has negative consequences; for example, pain, anxiety, and restlessness may increase pancreatic enzyme secretion.*

PRACTICE ALERT
Regularly assess respiratory status (at least every 4 to 8 hours), including respiratory rate, depth, and pattern; breath sounds; oxygen saturation and arterial blood gas results. Report tachypnea, adventitious or absent breath sounds, oxygen saturation levels below 92%, $PaO_2 < 70$ mmHg or $PaCO_2 > 45$ mmHg. Severe abdominal pain causes shallow respirations and hypoventilation, and suppresses cough effectiveness, which can lead to pooling of secretions, atelectasis, and pneumonia.

- Maintain NPO status and nasogastric tube patency as ordered. *Gastric secretions stimulate hormones that stimulate pancreatic secretion, aggravating pain. Eliminating oral intake and maintaining gastric suction reduce gastric secretions. Nasogastric suction also decreases nausea, vomiting, and intestinal distention.*
- Maintain bed rest in a calm, quiet environment. Encourage use of nonpharmacologic pain management techniques such as meditation and guided imagery. *Decreasing physical movement and mental stimulation decreases metabolic rate, gastrointestinal secretion, pancreatic secretions, and resulting pain. Adjunctive pain relief measures enhance the effectiveness of analgesics (see Chapter 9 ∞).*
- Assist to a comfortable position, such as a side-lying position with knees flexed and head elevated 45 degrees. *Sitting up, leaning forward, or lying in a fetal position tends to decrease pain caused by stretching of the peritoneum by edema and swelling.*
- Remind family and visitors to avoid bringing food into the client's room. *The sight or smell of food may stimulate secretory activity of the pancreas through the cephalic phase of digestion.*

Imbalanced Nutrition: Less than Body Requirements

The effects of pancreatitis and its treatment may result in malnutrition. Inflammation increases metabolic demand and frequently causes nausea, vomiting, and diarrhea. At a time of increased metabolic demand, NPO status and gastric suction further decrease available nutrients. In the client with chronic pancreatitis, loss of digestive enzymes affects the digestion and use of nutrients.

- Monitor laboratory values: serum albumin, serum transferrin, hemoglobin, and hematocrit. *Serum albumin, serum transferrin (which transports iron in the blood), hemoglobin, and hematocrit levels are decreased in malnutrition. Decreased pancreatic enzymes affect protein catabolism and absorption; decreased transferrin affects iron absorption and transport, thereby decreasing hematocrit and hemoglobin levels.*
- Weigh daily or every other day. *Short-term weight changes (over hours to days) accurately reflect fluid balance, whereas weight changes over days to weeks reflect nutritional status.*
- Maintain stool chart; note frequency, color, odor, and consistency of stools. *Protein and fat metabolism are impaired in pancreatitis; undigested fats are excreted in the stool. Steatorrhea indicates impaired digestion and, possibly, an increase in the severity of pancreatitis.*
- Monitor bowel sounds. *The return of bowel sounds indicates return of peristalsis; nasogastric suction usually is discontinued within 24 to 48 hours thereafter.*
- Administer prescribed intravenous fluids and/or TPN. *Intravenous fluids are given to maintain hydration. TPN is used to provide fluids, electrolytes, and kilocalories when fasting is prolonged (more than 2 to 3 days).*
- Provide oral and nasal care every 1 to 2 hours. *Fasting and nasogastric suction increase the risk for mucous membrane irritation and breakdown.*
- When oral intake resumes, offer small, frequent feedings. Provide oral hygiene before and after meals. *Oral hygiene decreases oral microorganisms that can cause foul odor and taste, decreasing appetite. Small, frequent feedings reduce pancreatic enzyme secretion and are more easily digested and absorbed.*

Risk for Deficient Fluid Volume

Acute pancreatitis can lead to a fluid shift from the intravascular space into the abdominal cavity (third spacing). Third spacing of fluid may cause hypovolemic shock, affecting cardiovascular function, respiratory function, renal function, and mental status.

- Assess cardiovascular status every 4 hours or as indicated, including vital signs, cardiac rhythm, hemodynamic parameters (central venous and pulmonary artery pressures); peripheral pulses and capillary refill; skin color, temperature, moisture, and turgor. *These measurements are indicative of fluid volume status and are used to monitor response to treatment. Stable values are as follows: heart rate less than 100; blood pressure within 10 mmHg of baseline; central venous pressure 0 to 8 mmHg; pulmonary wedge pressure 8 to 12 mmHg; cardiac output approximately 5 L/min; and skin warm, dry, with good turgor and color. (See Chapter 11 ∞ for a full discussion of hypovolemic shock.)*

- Monitor renal function. Obtain hourly urine output; report if less than 30 mL per hour. Weigh daily. *Urine output of less than 30 mL per hour indicates decreased renal perfusion or acute renal failure, a major complication of acute pancreatitis. Weight changes are an effective indicator of fluid volume status.*
- Monitor neurologic function, including mental status, level of consciousness, and behavior. *Hypotension and hypoxemia may decrease cerebral perfusion, causing changes in mental status, decreased level of consciousness, and changes in behavior. In addition, alcohol withdrawal is a risk in the client with acute pancreatitis.*

Using NANDA, NIC, and NOC

Chart 24–3 shows linkages between NANDA nursing diagnosis, NIC, and NOC for the client with pancreatitis.

Community-Based Care

The client with pancreatitis is often acutely ill and, along with family members, needs information about both hospital procedures and self-care at home following discharge. During the acute stage, keep explanations brief and simple.

Prior to discharge, teach the client and family about the disease and how to prevent further attacks of inflammation. Include the following topics as appropriate:

- Alcohol can cause stones to form, blocking pancreatic ducts and the outflow of pancreatic juice. Continued alcohol intake is likely to cause further inflammation and destruction of the pancreas. Avoid alcohol entirely.
- Smoking and stress stimulate the pancreas and should be avoided.
- If pancreatic function has been severely impaired, discuss appropriate use of pancreatic enzymes, including timing, dose, potential side effects, and monitoring of effectiveness.

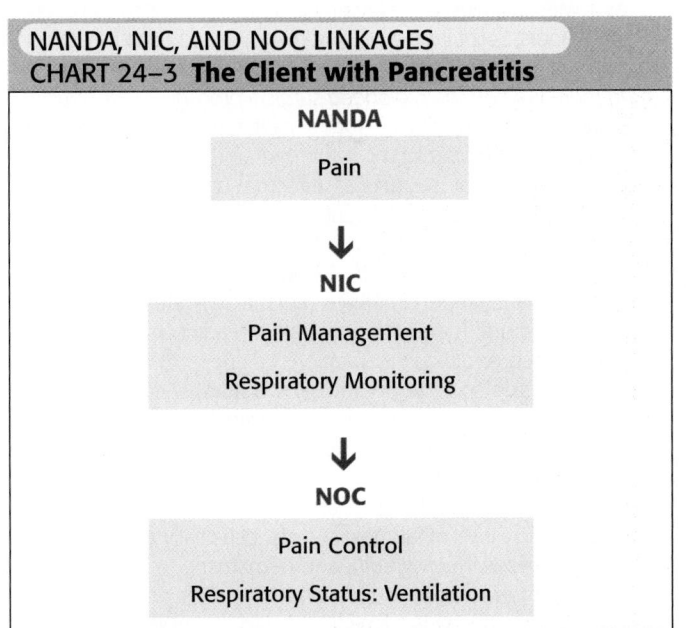

NANDA, NIC, AND NOC LINKAGES
CHART 24–3 The Client with Pancreatitis

NANDA

Pain

↓

NIC

Pain Management

Respiratory Monitoring

↓

NOC

Pain Control

Respiratory Status: Ventilation

Data from *NANDA's Nursing Diagnoses: Definitions & Classification 2005–2006* by NANDA International (2005), Philadelphia; *Nursing Interventions Classification (NIC)* (4th ed.) by J. M. Dochterman & G. M. Bulechek (2004), St. Louis, MO: Mosby; and *Nursing Outcomes Classification (NOC)* (3rd ed.) by S. Moorhead, M. Johnson, & M. Maas (2004), St. Louis, MO: Mosby.

- A low-fat diet is recommended. Provide a list of high-fat foods to avoid. Crash dieting and binge eating also should be avoided as they may sometimes precipitate attacks. Spicy foods, coffee, tea, or colas, and gas-forming foods stimulate gastric and pancreatic secretions and may precipitate pain. Avoid them if this occurs.
- Report symptoms of infection (fever of 102°F [38.8°C] or more, pain, rapid pulse, malaise) because a pancreatic abscess can develop after initial recovery.

Refer to a dietitian or nutritionist for diet teaching as needed. If appropriate, refer to community agencies, such as Alcoholics Anonymous, or to an alcohol treatment program. Provide referrals to community or home health agencies as needed for continued monitoring and teaching at home.

THE CLIENT WITH PANCREATIC CANCER

Cancer of the pancreas accounts for approximately 2% of all cancers. It is, however, one of the most lethal cancers: More than 98% of people with pancreatic cancer die. An estimated 32,180 new cases occurred in the United States in 2005, with approximately 31,800 deaths from cancer of the pancreas occurring the same year (American Cancer Society, 2005). The incidence of pancreatic cancer increases after age 50. The incidence is slightly higher in women than men, and is higher in blacks than in whites.

FAST FACTS

Identified risk factors for pancreatic cancer include:
- Cigarette smoking—the incidence is twice as high in smokers as in nonsmokers
- Exposure to industrial chemicals or environmental toxins
- Chronic pancreatitis
- Diabetes mellitus
- Obesity, high-fat diet.

In contrast to acute and chronic pancreatitis, alcohol abuse and gallstones are not identified risk factors for pancreatic cancer.

Pathophysiology and Manifestations

Most cancers of the pancreas occur in the exocrine pancreas, are adenocarcinomas, and cause death within 1 to 3 years after diagnosis.

Cancer of the pancreas has a slow onset, with manifestations of anorexia, nausea, weight loss, flatulence, and dull epigastric pain. The pain increases in severity as the tumor grows. Other manifestations depend on the location of the tumor. Cancer of the head of the pancreas, which is the most common site, often obstructs bile flow through the common bile duct and the ampulla of Vater, resulting in jaundice, clay-colored stools, dark urine, and pruritus. Cancer of the body of the pancreas presses on the celiac ganglion, causing pain that increases when the person eats or lies supine. Cancer of the tail of the pancreas often causes no symptoms until it has metastasized. Other late manifestations include a palpable abdominal mass and ascites. Because the manifestations are nonspecific, up to 85% of

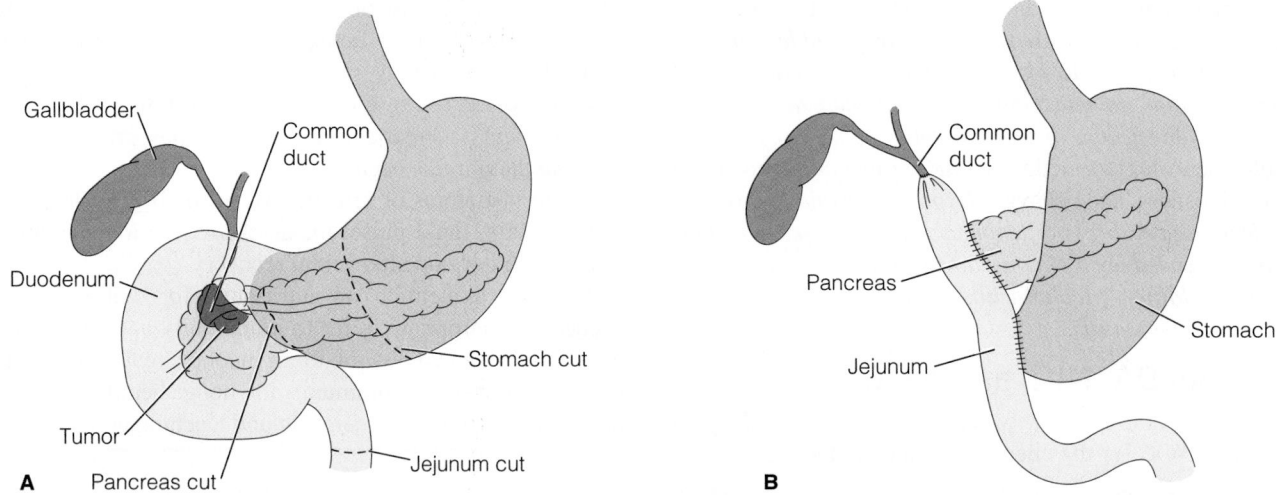

Figure 24–7 ■ Pancreatoduodenectomy (Whipple's procedure). *A,* areas of resection; *B,* appearance following resection.

clients with cancer of the pancreas do not seek health care until the cancer becomes too far advanced for a cure.

INTERDISCIPLINARY CARE

Early cancers of the head of the pancreas may be resectable. A pancreatoduodenectomy (commonly called Whipple's procedure) is performed to remove the head of the pancreas, the entire duodenum, the distal third of the stomach, a portion of the jejunum, and the lower half of the common bile duct. The common bile duct is then sutured to the end of the jejunum, and the remaining pancreas and stomach are sutured to the side of the jejunum (Figure 24–7 ■). Radiation and chemotherapy are often used in addition to surgery.

NURSING CARE OF THE CLIENT UNDERGOING   Whipple's Procedure

PREOPERATIVE CARE
- Provide routine preoperative nursing care as outlined in Chapter 4 ∞.
- Clarify teaching and learning as needed. Provide psychologic support for client and family. *The client and family faced with a diagnosis of pancreatic cancer may require reinforcement of teaching as anxiety, fear, and possible denial can interfere with learning.*

POSTOPERATIVE CARE
- Provide postoperative care as outlined in Chapter 4 ∞.
- Maintain in semi-Fowler's position. *Semi-Fowler's position facilitates lung expansion and reduces stress on the anastomosis and suture line.*
- Maintain low gastrointestinal suction. If drainage is not adequate, obtain an order to irrigate, using minimal pressure. Do not reposition nasogastric tube. *Pressure within the operative area from retained secretions increases intraluminal pressure and places stress on the suture line. Forceful irrigations and repositioning of the nasogastric tube may disrupt the suture line.*
- Maintain pain control using analgesics as prescribed (PCA, infusion, or given on a regular basis). Assess effectiveness of pain management. *Doses higher than normal may be required if narcotic analgesics have been used prior to surgery to manage pain.*
  Increased pain may indicate complications such as disruption of suture line, leakage from anastomosis, or peritonitis. Adequate pain management increases resistance to stress, facilitates

healing, and increases the ability to cough, deep breathe, and change position.
- Assist with coughing, deep breathing, and changing position every 1 to 2 hours. Splint incision during coughing and deep breathing. *The location of the incision makes coughing and deep breathing more painful. The prolonged surgical procedure, anesthesia, location of incision, and immobility increase the risk of retained secretions, atelectasis, and pneumonia. Changing position facilitates drainage of secretions; effective coughing and deep breathing remove secretions and open distal alveoli.*
- Monitor for complications:
  a. Take vital signs every 2 to 4 hours or as indicated; immediately report changes (such as elevated temperature; hypotension; weak, thready pulse; increased or difficult respirations).
  b. Assess skin color, temperature, moisture, and turgor.
  c. Measure urinary output, gastrointestinal output, and drainage from any other tubes; monitor amount and type of wound drainage.
  d. Assess level of consciousness.
  e. Monitor results of laboratory tests, especially arterial blood gases, hemoglobin, and hematocrit.
  The major complications following Whipple's procedure are hemorrhage, hypovolemic shock, and hepatorenal failure. The assessments listed provide information about the client's status and alert the nurse to abnormal findings that signal the onset of these complications.

Postoperative nursing care of the client undergoing Whipple's procedure is outlined on page 732. Immediate postoperative care is often provided in the intensive care unit.

The client with pancreatic cancer has multiple problems requiring nursing care. Chapter 14 ∞ provides a discussion of care of the client with cancer; the nursing diagnoses and interventions discussed for the client with pancreatitis are also appropriate for the client with pancreatic cancer.

EXPLORE MediaLink

DVD-ROM
Audio Glossary
NCLEX-RN® Review

Animation/Video
Cirrhosis

COMPANION WEBSITE www.prenhall.com/lemone
Audio Glossary
NCLEX-RN® Review
Care Plan Activity: A Client with Hepatitis A
Case Studies
  Hepatitis B
  Traditional Native American Diet and Gallbladder
    Disease
MediaLink Applications
  GI Disorders and Gall Bladder Disease
  Treatment of Liver Cancer
Links to Resources

CHAPTER HIGHLIGHTS

- Gallstones (cholelithiasis) are common and often unrecognized until the client develops manifestations of biliary colic or acute cholecystitis. Laparoscopic cholecystectomy is the treatment of choice for symptomatic gallbladder disease.
- Hepatitis, inflammation of functional liver tissue, usually is a viral disease and therefore cannot be cured at this time. Preventing the spread of hepatitis through use of standard and body substance precautions is an important nursing responsibility.
- Hepatitis A, commonly transmitted via the fecal-oral route, generally is a self-limiting disease with few long-term sequelae. Some types of viral hepatitis, most notably hepatitis B and C, can become chronic and ultimately lead to liver failure and an increased risk for liver cancer. Hepatitis B and C can result in a carrier state in which the infected client has no symptoms of the disease, but can spread it to others.
- Alcohol abuse is a significant risk factor for liver and pancreatic disorders. Prevention, early identification, and treatment of alcohol abuse reduces the risk of these disorders. Absolute abstinence from alcohol is an important part of the treatment plan for clients with liver and pancreatic disorders.
- Cirrhosis leads to portal hypertension and liver failure, which, in turn, account for most of the manifestations and complications of the disorder. Complications such as ascites, splenomegaly, esophageal varices, and hepatic encephalopathy affect multiple body systems and significantly contribute to mortality and morbidity associated with cirrhosis.
- Bleeding from esophageal varices may be massive, resulting in a medical emergency and requiring prompt control to maintain cardiac output.
- Acute pancreatitis often develops as a complication of gallstones. Acute pancreatitis often resolves with no long term consequences. Chronic pancreatitis is more frequently related to alcohol abuse and can lead to continuing pain and digestive disruptions.

TEST YOURSELF NCLEX-RN® REVIEW

1 When assessing the client admitted for a laparoscopic cholecystectomy, the nurse would expect to find:
  1. a history of intermittent episodes of right upper quadrant pain.
  2. significant jaundice of the sclera and skin.
  3. complaints of recurrent heartburn and acid reflux.
  4. ascites and peripheral edema.

2 Which of the following does the nurse include in her teaching for a client with acute cholecystitis? (Select all that apply.)

  1. Avoid consumption of foods high in fat such as gravies and peanut butter.
  2. Limit your intake to dry crackers and clear liquids during episodes of acute pain.
  3. A low-carbohydrate diet such as the Atkins diet is recommended for weight loss.
  4. Call your doctor if you develop severe abdominal pain and a temperature.
  5. Surgery for gallstones is optional; they pose little risk when fat intake is minimal.

3 During an outbreak of hepatitis A traced to a food handler at a local restaurant, the nurse teaches staff at the restaurant that the most cost-effective means of protecting customers from further outbreaks is to:
1. insist that all food handlers be immunized against hepatitis A.
2. test all new employees for hepatitis A antigen.
3. wash hands thoroughly before handling food and after using the bathroom.
4. use gloves for handling food if any cuts or scrapes are on hands.

4 The nurse would evaluate teaching as effective when a client with chronic hepatitis C states which of the following?
1. "I will reduce my alcohol intake and use only acetaminophen for pain relief."
2. "I understand that I must return to the doctor every year for a follow-up liver biopsy."
3. "Even though no treatment is available for this disease, I plan to live a long life."
4. "I will avoid donating blood and will use barrier protection during sex."

5 When evaluating for people possibly exposed to hepatitis A by a recently diagnosed client, the nurse inquires about
1. sexual partners within the past 6 months.
2. close household contacts within the past 4 weeks.
3. food preparation activities since the development of jaundice.
4. immunization status of the client.

6 A client hospitalized with cirrhosis, ascites, and mild hepatic encephalopathy suddenly vomits 200 mL of bright red blood. Which of the following should the nurse do first?
1. Insert a nasogastric tube.
2. Place in Fowler's position.
3. Contact the physician.
4. Check stool for occult blood.

7 The nurse caring for a client scheduled for an abdominal paracentesis instructs the client to
1. avoid eating or drinking fluid for 6 hours prior to the procedure.
2. scrub the abdomen with antiseptic soap before the procedure.
3. empty the bladder before the procedure.
4. report excess flatus following the procedure to the physician.

8 A client hospitalized with severe ascites due to cirrhosis develops a fever and confusion. The nurse should
1. auscultate bowel sounds and palpate for abdominal tenderness.
2. inquire about headache and check for nuchal rigidity.
3. observe for neck vein distention and auscultate lung sounds.
4. measure abdominal girth and percuss for shifting dullness.

9 A 54-year-old woman admitted with acute pancreatitis says, "I don't understand how I got this disease. I thought alcoholics got pancreatitis—I never drink." Which of the following is the most appropriate response by the nurse?
1. "Was there a time in your life that you did drink heavily?"
2. "It also is prevalent in smokers; do you smoke cigarettes?"
3. "Gallstones also are a risk factor. We'll evaluate for them."
4. "Intravenous drug use is a risk factor. Do you use drugs by injection?"

10 The nurse caring for a client returning to the unit following Whipple's procedure identifies which of the following as of highest priority in the plan of care?
1. referral to a smoking cessation program
2. frequent turning, coughing, and deep breathing exercises
3. early mobilization including ambulation as tolerated
4. maintaining patency of the nasogastric tube

See Test Yourself answers in Appendix C.

BIBLIOGRAPHY

Agency for Healthcare Research and Quality. (2000). *Milk thistle: Effects on liver disease and cirrhosis and clinical adverse effects. Summary, evidence report/technology assessment* (AHRQ Pub. No. 01-E024). Retrieved from http://www.ahrq.gov/clinic/epcsums/milktsum.htm

Allen, G. (2004). Evidence for practice. Hepatitis B vaccination schedules. *AORN Journal 79*(6), 1322–1323.

_____. (2005). Evidence for practice. Conversion from laparoscopic to open cholecystectomy. *AORN Journal, 81*(3), 690, 693.

American Cancer Society. (2005). *Cancer facts and figures 2005*. Atlanta: Author.

Atassi, K. A. (2002). Bleeding esophageal varices. *Nursing, 32*(4), 96.

Barthelsson, C., Lutzen, K., Anderberg, B., & Nordstrom, G. (2003). Patients' experiences of laparoscopic cholecystectomy in day surgery. *Journal of Clinical Nursing, 12*(2), 253–259.

Binnekade, J. M. (2005). Review: Enteral nutrition reduces infections, need for surgical intervention, and length of hospital stay more than parenteral nutrition in acute pancreatitis. *Evidence-Based Nursing, 8*(1), 19.

Burruss, N., & Holz, S. (2005). Understanding acute pancreatitis. *Nursing, 35*(3), 32hn2, 32hn4.

Centers for Disease Control and Prevention. (2006). *Reported cases of acute viral hepatitis, by type and year, United States, 1966–2003.* Retrieved from http://www.cdc.gov/ncidod/diseases/hepatitis/resource/PDFs/surv_table.pdf

Cole, L. (2002). Unraveling the mystery of acute pancreatitis. *Dimensions of Critical Care Nursing, 26*(6), 86–89.

Copstead, L. C., & Banasick, J. L. (2005). *Pathophysiology* (3rd ed.). St. Louis, MO: Elsevier/Saunders.

Despins, L. A., Kivlahan, C., & Cox K. R. (2005). Emergency. Acute pancreatitis: Diagnosis and treatment of a potentially fatal condition. *American Journal of Nursing, 105*(11), 54–57.

Durston, S. (2005). What you need to know about viral hepatitis. *Nursing, 35*(8), 36–42.

Fontaine, K. L. (2000). *Healing practices: Alternative therapies for nursing.* Upper Saddle River, NJ: Prentice Hall Health.

Glacken, M., Coates, V., Kernohan, G., & Hegarty, J. (2003). The experience of fatigue for people living with hepatitis C. *Journal of Clinical Nursing, 12*(2), 244–252.

Hainsworth, T. (2005). NT clinical. Improving identification and awareness of hepatitis C. *Nursing Times, 101*(42), 23–24.

Jarrett, M., & Cox, P. (2004). Hepatitis C virus. *Nursing Clinics of North America, 39*(1), 219–229.

Kasper, D. L., Braunwald, E., Fauci, A. S., Hauser, S. L., Longo, D. L., & Jameson, J. L. (Eds.). (2005). *Harrison's principles of internal medicine* (16th ed.). New York: McGraw-Hill.

Knight, J. A. (2005). Liver function tests: Their role in the diagnosis of hepatobiliary diseases. *Journal of Infusion Nursing, 28*(2), 108–117.

Lee, J. M., Botteman, M. F., Xanthakos, N., & Nicklasson, L. (2005). Needlestick injuries in the United States: Epidemiologic, economic, and quality of life issues. *AAOHM Journal, 53*(3), 117–133.

Mann, R. E., Smart, R. G., & Govoni, R. (2003). The epidemiology of alcoholic liver disease. *Alcohol Research & Health, 27*(3), 209–219.

McCance, K. L., & Huether, S. E. (2002). *Pathophysiology: The biologic basis for disease in adults & children* (4th ed.). St. Louis, MO: Mosby.

Medical Encyclopedia: Diet – liver disease. (2005). Retrieved from http://www.nlm.nih.gov/medlineplus/ency/article/oo2441.htm.

Meeker, M. H., & Rothrock, J. C. (1999). *Alexander's care of the patient in surgery* (11th ed.). St. Louis, MO: Mosby.

NANDA International. (2005). *NANDA nursing diagnoses: Definitions & classification 2005–2006.* Philadelphia: Author.

National Center for Complementary and Alternative Medicine, National Institutes of Health. (2004). *Research report. Hepatitis C and complementary and alternative medicine: 2003 update* (NCCAM Pub. No. D004). Retrieved from http://www.nccam.nih.gov/health/hepatitisc/

National Center for Health Statistics. (2005). *Health, United States, 2005, with chartbook on trends in the health of Americans.* Hyattsville, MD: Author.

National Immunization Program. (2005). *Epidemiology and prevention of vaccine-preventable diseases* (8th ed.). Atlanta: Centers for Disease Control and Prevention.

Porth, C. M. (2005). *Pathophysiology: Concepts of altered health states* (7th ed.). Philadelphia: Lippincott.

Smith, D. R., & Leggat, P. A. (2005). Needlestick and sharps injuries among nursing students. *Journal of Advanced Nursing, 51*(5), 449–455.

Stevenson, L., Faucher, Y., Hewlett, S., Klemm, K., & Nelson, D. (2004). Chronic hepatitis C virus and the Hispanic community: Cultural factors impacting care. *Gastroenterology Nursing, 27*(5), 230–238.

Tierney, L. M., McPhee, S. J., & Papadakis, M. A. (2005). *Current medical diagnosis & treatment* (44th ed.). New York: Lange Medical Books/McGraw-Hill.

Urden, L. D., Stacy, K. M., & Lough, M. E. (2006). *Thelan's critical care nursing: Diagnosis and management* (5th ed.). St. Louis, MO: Mosby.

Watt-Watson, J., Chung, F., Chan, V. W. S., & McGillion, M. (2004). Pain management following discharge after ambulatory same-day surgery. *Journal of Nursing Management, 12*(3), 153–161.

Wilkinson, J. M. (2005). *Nursing diagnosis handbook with NIC interventions and NOC outcomes* (8th ed.). Upper Saddle River, NJ: Prentice Hall Health.

Wilson, T. R. (2005). The ABCs of hepatitis. *Nurse Practitioner, 30*(6), 12–15, 18, 20–23.

UNIT 6 BUILDING CLINICAL COMPETENCE
Responses to Altered Nutrition

FUNCTIONAL HEALTH PATTERN: Nutritional—Metabolic

■ Think about clients with altered nutrition for whom you have cared in your clinical experiences.

- What were the clients' major medical diagnoses (e.g., gastroesophageal reflux disease, cholelithiasis and cholecystitis, hepatitis, pancreatitis)?
- What kinds of manifestations did each of these clients have? Were these manifestations similar or different?
- How did the clients' nutritional problems interfere with their health status? How was their appetite? Were they on a prescribed diet? What was their daily intake of foods and fluids? Did the clients add salt to foods or eat processed foods? What types of fluids were they consuming, including caffeinated beverages? Did they use dietary supplements? Did they have difficulty chewing or swallowing? Were they gaining or losing weight? Did the clients' nutritional disorders affect healing or their immune status?

■ The Nutritional-Metabolic Health Pattern encompasses those activities and processes involved in taking in, assimilating, and using nutrients to produce energy and to maintain and repair body tissues. Disorders of nutritional intake and disorders of the organ systems involved in consuming, digesting, absorbing, and metabolizing nutrients can disrupt the Nutritional-Metabolic Pattern in several ways:

- Inability to consume and metabolize required nutrients can result in nutritional disorders (e.g., malnutrition) and impaired tissue repair.
- Insufficient nutrient intake can result from functional disorders (e.g., lack of access to appropriate foods), structural disorders (e.g., oral or esophageal cancer, hiatal hernia), inflammatory responses (e.g., cholecystitis, gastritis, hepatitis), or eating disorders (e.g., anorexia nervosa, bulimia nervosa).
- Disorders such as pancreatitis and cirrhosis affect the ability to absorb and metabolize nutrients consumed, impairing nutritional status.
- Excess intake of nutrients, particularly when combined with decreased energy expenditure, can result in nutritional disorders (e.g., obesity, alcoholic cirrhosis).

■ Nutrients are used by the body to promote growth, maintenance, and repair. Categories of nutrients include proteins, carbohydrates, fats, vitamins, and minerals. Improper intake of these nutrients affects the body's ability to maintain itself, leading to manifestations such as:

- Nausea (unpleasant, wave-like sensations in the stomach ► feelings of urge or need to vomit)
- Heartburn (backflow of gastric contents into esophagus ► high acidity of stomach contents causes inflammatory response ► pain and irritation of mucosa lining the esophagus)
- Pain (viral or bacterial infection, tissue inflammation, obstruction ► tissue damage, ischemia, and/or edema ► stimulate pain receptors ► transmit pain impulses to the brain).

■ Priority nursing diagnoses within the Nutritional-Metabolic Pattern that may be appropriate for clients with nutritional disorders or disorders of the upper gastrointestinal tract and accessory organs include:

- *Imbalanced Nutrition: Less than Body Requirements* as evidenced by decreased food intake, weight loss 20% or more of ideal body weight, dry and brittle hair, weakness, impaired tissue healing
- *Deficient Fluid Volume* as evidenced by dry mucous membranes, poor skin turgor, thirst, increased body temperature
- *Nausea* as evidenced by complaints of stomach discomfort, increased salivation, tachycardia, and cold and clammy skin
- *Impaired Skin Integrity* as evidenced by disruption of skin surface, pain, itching.

■ Two nursing diagnoses from other functional health patterns often are of high priority for the client with gastrointestinal disorders because the physiologic responses to these problems interfere with proper nutrition:

- *Acute Pain* (Cognitive-Perceptual)
- *Diarrhea* (Elimination)

CLINICAL SCENARIO

You have been assigned to work with the following four patients for the 0700 shift. Significant data obtained during report are as follows:

- Thomas Jones, age 56, was transferred to your unit yesterday after treatment in the ICU for esophageal varices. Significant history includes alcohol consumption (6 to 12 beers or a pint of liquor daily for several years) and smoking (2 packs per day for the past 30 years). Current vital signs are T 100°F, P 96, R 28, BP 150/90. He complains of abdominal tenderness and dyspnea. He appears anxious and irritable.

- Ruth Green, age 35, was admitted with right upper quadrant pain radiating to the left shoulder and a feeling of abdominal fullness. She has a history of cholelithiasis and cholecystitis. Her assessment reveals T 99.6°F, P 90, R 24, BP 140/84, with pallor, diaphoresis, and complaints of nausea. She is scheduled for a cholecystectomy at 9:00 A.M.

- Tonya Cooper, age 21, was admitted with dehydration, weakness, fainting. Her weight is 90 lb (40.9 kg) and height is 5'5". Her vital signs are T 97°F, P 70, R 26, BP 90/56 mmHg with orthostatic BP 70/48 mmHg. She has a 3-year history of anorexia nervosa and laxative use. She has an IV of 0.9% NaCl with KCl infusing. She is to be monitored for food intake and watched for 1 hour after meals. She is ringing her call light to get up to the bathroom.

- Joseph Brown, age 82, was admitted 1 hour ago with acute gastritis. He relates a 2-day history of nausea, vomiting, and diarrhea. He has a history of hypertension and angina pectoris. Current vital signs are T 101.6°F, P 102, R 20, BP 130/70. He is pale and listless. His abdomen is distended and tender with decreased bowel sounds. He is requesting medication for nausea.

Questions

1 In what order would you visit these patients after report?

1. _____
2. _____
3. _____
4. _____

2 What top two priority nursing diagnoses would you choose for each of the clients presented above? Can you explain, if asked, the rationale for your choices?

	Priority Nursing Diagnosis #1	Priority Nursing Diagnosis #2
Thomas Jones		
Ruth Green		
Tonya Cooper		
Joseph Brown		

3 You need to complete preoperative preparation on Mrs. Green. Which of the following do you need to do?

1. Complete preoperative checklist, witness signed consent, and administer preoperative medication when requested.
2. Explain the procedure, obtain informed consent, and complete the preoperative checklist.
3. Sign the operative consent, explain complications of the procedure, and take vital signs on call.
4. Obtain signed consent, discuss with the family the surgical procedure, and have the client void prior to going to the OR.

4 Mrs. Green understands the postoperative teaching done by the nurse when she states:

1. "I will be on bed rest for two days after surgery."
2. "I will need to cough and deep breathe while splinting my incision."
3. "I will be able to begin eating when I return from surgery."
4. "I will be medicated for pain without having to request it."

5 The nurse explains a diet of low-fat foods to Mrs. Green. She understands this diet when she picks which meal plan?

1. eggs, sausage, and toast
2. turkey, mashed potatoes and gravy, and corn
3. grilled chicken, tossed salad, peaches
4. hamburger with lettuce and tomato, french fries

6 The priority nursing diagnosis for Mr. Brown with acute gastritis is:

1. *Sleep Disturbance*
2. *Acute Pain*
3. *Nausea*
4. *Imbalanced Nutrition: Less than Body Requirements*

7 Which assessment findings on Mr. Brown would be suggestive of dehydration?

1. hypertension, bradycardia, skin taut and dry
2. hypotension, tachycardia, poor skin turgor, dry mucous membranes
3. decreased body temperature, thirst, weakness
4. increased body temperature, slow thready pulse, listless

8 Mr. Brown voices understanding of how to take lansoprazole (Prevacid) after discharge when he states:

1. "I will take it after breakfast to protect my stomach."
2. "I will take it with grapefruit juice at breakfast."
3. "I can stop taking it when my nausea is gone."
4. "I will take it before breakfast to help my stomach feel better."

9 Which of the following laboratory results would be expected findings for Mr. Jones? (Select all that apply.)

1. AST 123 U/L
2. cardiac troponin T 0.8 mcg/L
3. ALP 431 U/L
4. Hct 47%
5. LDH 250 U/L
6. ALT 45 U/L

10 To prepare Mr. Jones for an esophagoscopy, the nurse institutes the following interventions:

1. Explain that it is not a painful procedure but he will be medicated for pain.
2. Keep the client NPO for 12 hours prior to the procedure.
3. Remove dentures and provide mouth care.
4. Place in a supine position with the head slightly hyperextended.

11 With Ms. Cooper's history of anorexia for 3 years, which is a priority nursing intervention in the plan of care for her?

1. Monitor for cardiac dysrhythmias due to electrolyte imbalances.
2. Monitor weight for loss or gain to determine effectiveness of nursing care.
3. Maintain close observation for at least 1 hour after meals.
4. Serve small, frequent meals, increasing serving size gradually.

12 In planning discharge for Ms. Cooper, the family and client participate in teaching and diet counseling sessions. Which is the priority item for the family and Ms. Cooper to follow after discharge?

1. Monitor weight regularly to determine further weight loss.
2. Use rewards for food and caloric intake rather than weight gain.
3. Gradually increase the amount of food taken at meals.
4. Attend support groups for people with eating disorders.

CASE STUDY

Louis Haches, an 82-year-old white male, has a history of hypertension, degenerative arthritis, and angina pectoris for which he takes furosemide, atenolol, extra-strength aspirin, and Nitrostat. He states that his blood pressure is controlled when he takes his medications as prescribed. Lately, he has been having some financial difficulties and does not take his medications as often as he should. He lives with his 80-year-old wife, who also has health problems. He does the cooking and grocery shopping. He has a son who lives nearby who looks in on them every couple of days.

Mr. Haches feels that he cooked some outdated food that made him ill. He states he has been trying to stretch their grocery budget by reducing their serving sizes and shopping less frequently. He says he has had nausea and loose, dark stools for the past 2 days. This morning, he is weak and dizzy, and states he nearly fainted in the shower. He also states he has not been able to take his medications for the past 2 days and feels that his heart is beating too fast. His son brought him to the hospital because he was weak, confused, and very pale when he checked on him prior to going to work in the morning.

Based on Mr. Haches's medical diagnosis and treatment plan, *Imbalanced Nutrition: Less than Body Requirements* is identified as the priority nursing diagnosis at this time.

- Local irritant (e.g. aspirin) disrupts mucosal barrier
- Hydrochloric acid and pepsin contact gastric tissue, leading to irritation, inflammation, superficial erosions and bleeding

    affects   leads to

Mr. H.
82 y.o. male
Acute gastritiss

    assess

- 5' 10" tall
- 150 lbs - states usual weight is 165 lbs.
- T 101.6°F, P 102, R 20
- BP 110/60
- Pallor, skin cool and dry
- Listless, complaints of nausea
- Abdomen flat, slightly tender, decreased bowel sounds
- Stool guiac positive

    generates

- Deficient fluid volume as evidenced by low food pressure, tachycardia
- Nausea as evidenced by complaints of discomfort in stomach
- Risk for injury related to lightheadedness and confusion secondary to decreased blood volume

generate nursing diagnosis   prioritized to

Imbalanced Nutrition: Less than Body Requirements

expected outcomes

- Consumes 100% of preferred diet and high-calorie snacks
- Consumes adequate fluids without nausea and vomiting
- Gains 1 to 1.5 lb per week
- Urine output greater than 30mL/hr
- Hgb, hct, and serum albumin within normal ranges
- Skin intact
- Able to explain relationship of aspirin intake to acute gastritis
- Identifies alternate medications to manage chronic arthritis pain
- Uses community resources such as Meals-on-Wheels to maintain adequate food intake

    evaluate

- Evaluation (at discharge 2 days p adm)
- Weight 155 lbs; intake 2400 ml / output 1500 mL past 24 hr
- Serum electrolytes, hgb, hct WNL
- Can explain relationship between aspirin, gastritis, and GI bleeding
- Met with social services; states he will contact local food bank and Meals-on-Wheels
- States he will try acetaminophen and heat to relieve arthritis pain

Interdisciplinary Interventions
- Weigh daily, and monitor intake, output, and calorie consumption
- Reintroduce food intake with clear liquids, gradually increasing to 6 small, high-calorie meals/day
- Analyze laboratory results, including serum electrolytes and albumin, hgb and hct

Independent Interventions
- Discuss effects of aspirin and other irritants on gastric mucosa
- Discuss alternate analgesics and measures to control pain of chronic arthritis
- Refer to social services for food assistance

PART III

Elimination Patterns

Functional Health Patterns with Related Nursing Diagnoses

HEALTH PERCEPTION-HEALTH MANAGEMENT

- Perceived health status
- Perceived health management
- Healthcare behaviors: health promotion and illness prevention activities, medical treatments, follow-up care

VALUE-BELIEF

- Values, goals, or beliefs (including spirituality) that guide choices or decisions
- Perceived conflicts in values, beliefs, or expectations that are health related

COPING-STRESS-TOLERANCE

- Capacity to resist challenges to self-integrity
- Methods of handling stress
- Support systems
- Perceived ability to control and manage situations

NUTRITIONAL-METABOLIC

- Daily consumption of food and fluids
- Favorite foods
- Use of dietary supplements
- Skin lesions and ability to heal
- Condition of the integument
- Weight, height, temperature

PART III ELIMINATION PATTERNS NANDA NURSING DIAGNOSES

- Bowel Incontinence
- Constipation
- Perceived Constipation
- Risk for Constipation
- Diarrhea
- Impaired Urinary Elimination
- Functional Urinary Incontinence
- Reflex Urinary Incontinence
- Stress Urinary Incontinence
- Total Urinary Incontinence
- Urge Urinary Incontinence
- Risk for Urge Urinary Incontinence
- Urinary Retention
- Toileting: Self-Care Deficit

SEXUALITY-REPRODUCTIVE

- Satisfaction with sexuality or sexual relationships
- Reproductive pattern
- Female menstrual and perimenopausal history

ELIMINATION

- Patterns of bowel and urinary excretion
- Perceived regularity or irregularity of elimination
- Use of laxatives or routines
- Changes in time, modes, quality, or quantity of excretions
- Use of devices for control

ROLE-RELATIONSHIPS

- Perception of major roles, relationships, and responsibilities in current life situation
- Satisfaction with or disturbances in roles and relationships

ACTIVITY-EXERCISE

- Patterns of personally relevant exercise, activity, leisure, and recreation
- ADLs that require energy expenditure
- Factors that interfere with the desired pattern (e.g., illness or injury)

SELF-PERCEPTION–SELF-CONCEPT

- Attitudes about self
- Perceived abilities, worth, self-image, emotions
- Body posture and movement, eye contact, voice and speech patterns

SLEEP-REST

- Patterns of sleep and rest-/relaxation in a 24-h period
- Perceptions of quality and quantity of sleep and rest
- Use of sleep aids and routines

COGNITIVE-PERCEPTUAL

- Adequacy of vision, hearing, taste, touch, smell
- Pain perception and management
- Language, judgment, memory, decisions

UNIT 7

Responses to Altered Bowel Elimination

CHAPTER 25
Assessing Clients with Bowel Elimination Disorders

LEARNING OUTCOMES

- Describe the anatomy, physiology, and functions of the intestines.
- Explain the physiologic processes involved in bowel elimination.
- Identify specific topics to consider during a health history assessment interview of the client with problems of bowel elimination.

- Describe techniques used to assess bowel integrity and function.
- Describe normal variations in assessment findings for the older adult.
- Identify manifestations of altered intestinal function.

CLINICAL COMPETENCIES

- Conduct and document a health history for clients who have or are at risk for alterations in bowel elimination.
- Conduct and document a physical assessment of the intestinal system.

- Monitor the results of diagnostic tests and report abnormal findings.

EQUIPMENT NEEDED

- Water-soluble lubricant
- Occult blood test kit, such as Occultest or Hemoccult II

- Disposable gloves
- Stethoscope

MEDIALINK

Resources for this chapter can be found on the Prentice Hall Nursing MediaLink DVD accompanying this textbook, and on the Companion Website at http://www.prenhall.com/lemone

After foods are eaten and broken down into usable elements, nutrients are absorbed and indigestible materials are eliminated. Bowel elimination is the end process in digestion. This chapter describes the structure and function of the large intestine, including the rectosigmoid region and the anus, as well as the assessment of bowel function. The anatomy and physiology of the small intestine are discussed in relation to nutrition in Chapter 21 ∞; the information in this chapter is provided as a base for understanding health problems from altered bowel function. In addition, this chapter discusses the function of the small intestine in the absorption of digested end products. Malabsorption (impaired absorption of nutrients) is discussed fully in Chapter 26 ∞.

ANATOMY, PHYSIOLOGY, AND FUNCTIONS OF THE INTESTINES

The small and large intestines provide structures to absorb nutrients and vitamins and to eliminate wastes from food ingested and processed in the upper gastrointestinal (GI) tract.

The Small Intestine

The small intestine begins at the pyloric sphincter and ends at the ileocecal junction at the entrance of the large intestine. The small intestine is about 20 feet (6 m) long, but only about 1 inch (2.5 cm) in diameter. This long tube hangs in coils in the abdominal cavity, suspended by the mesentery and surrounded by the large intestine.

The small intestine has three regions: the duodenum, the jejunum, and the ileum. The duodenum begins at the pyloric sphincter and extends around the head of the pancreas for about 10 inches (25 cm). Both pancreatic enzymes and bile from the liver enter the small intestine at the duodenum. The jejunum is the middle region of the small intestine. It extends for about 8 feet (2.4 m). The ileum, the terminal end of the small intestine, is approximately 12 feet (3.6 m) long and meets the large intestine at the ileocecal valve.

Food is chemically digested and mostly absorbed as it moves through the small intestine. Circular folds (deep folds of the mucosa and submucosa layers), villi (finger-like projections of the mucosa cells), and microvilli (tiny projections of the mucosa cells) all increase the surface area of the small intestine to enhance absorption of food. Although up to 10 L of food, liquids, and secretions enter the gastrointestinal tract each day, most is digested and absorbed in the small intestine; less than 1 L reaches the large intestine.

Enzymes in the small intestine break down carbohydrates, proteins, lipids, and nucleic acids as follows:

- Pancreatic amylase acts on starches, converting them to maltose, dextrins, and oligosaccharides; the intestinal enzymes dextrinase, glucoamylase, maltase, sucrase, and lactase further break down these products into monosaccharides.
- Proteins are broken down into peptides by the pancreatic enzymes trypsin and chymotrypsin and by intestinal enzymes. Pancreatic enzymes (trypsin and chymotrypsin) and intestinal enzymes continue to break down proteins into peptides.

- Pancreatic lipases break down lipids.
- Triglycerides enter as fat globules, and are then coated by bile salts and emulsified.
- Nucleic acids are hydrolyzed by pancreatic enzymes, then broken apart by intestinal enzymes.

Both pancreatic enzymes and bile are excreted into the duodenum in response to the secretion of secretin and cholecystokinin, hormones produced by the intestinal mucosa cells when chyme enters the small intestine.

Nutrients are absorbed through the mucosa of the intestinal villi into the blood or lymph by active transport, facilitated transport, and passive diffusion. Almost all food products and water, as well as vitamins and most electrolytes, are absorbed in the small intestine, leaving only indigestible fibers, some water, and bacteria to enter the large intestine.

The Large Intestine

The large intestine, or colon, begins at the ileocecal valve and terminates at the anus (Figure 25–1 ■). It is about 5 feet (1.5 m) long. The large intestine frames the small intestine on three sides and includes the cecum, the appendix, the colon, the rectum, and the anal canal.

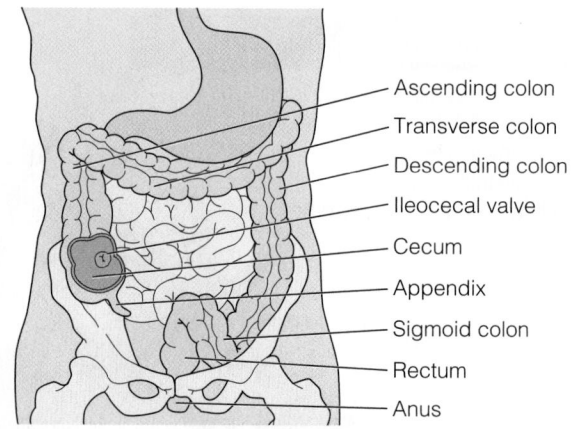

Ascending colon
Transverse colon
Descending colon
Ileocecal valve
Cecum
Appendix
Sigmoid colon
Rectum
Anus

Figure 25–1 ■ Anatomy of the large intestine.

The first section of the large intestine is the cecum. The appendix is attached to its surface as an extension. The appendix, a twisted structure in which bacteria can accumulate, may become inflamed.

The colon is divided into ascending, transverse, and descending segments. The ascending colon extends along the right side of the abdomen to the hepatic flexure, where it makes a right-angle turn. The next segment, called the transverse colon, crosses the abdomen to the splenic flexure. At this juncture, the descending colon descends down the left side of the abdomen and ends at the S-shaped sigmoid colon. The sigmoid colon terminates at the rectum.

The rectum is a mucosa-lined tube approximately 12 cm in length (Figure 25–2 ■). The rectum has three transverse folds (valves of Houston) that retain feces yet allow flatus to be passed through the anus. The rectum ends at the anal canal, which terminates at the anus.

The anus, a hairless, dark-skinned area, is the end of the digestive tract. It has both an internal involuntary sphincter and an external voluntary sphincter. The sphincters are usually open only during defecation. The anorectal junction separates the rectum from the anal canal and may be the site of internal hemorrhoids (clusters of dilated veins in swollen anal tissue).

The major function of the large intestine is to eliminate indigestible food residue from the body. The large intestine absorbs water, salts, and vitamins formed by the food residue and bacteria. The semiliquid chyme that passes through the ileocecal valve is formed into feces as it moves through the large intestine. Feces are moved along the intestine by **peristalsis**, waves of alternating contraction and relaxation. Goblet cells lining the large intestine secrete mucous that facilitates the lubrication and passage of feces.

The defecation reflex is initiated when feces enter the rectum and stretch the rectal wall. This spinal cord reflex causes the walls of the sigmoid colon to contract and the anal sphincters to relax. This reflex can be suppressed by voluntary control of the external sphincter. Closing the glottis and contracting the diaphragm and abdominal muscles to increase intra-abdominal pressure **(Valsalva's maneuver)** facilitates expulsion of feces. Prolonged suppression of defecation can result in a weakened reflex that may in turn lead to **constipation** (infrequent and often uncomfortable passage of hard, dry stool). Frequent bouts of constipation may lead to external hemorrhoids at the area of the external hemorrhoidal plexus.

ASSESSING BOWEL FUNCTION

Bowel elimination and the function of the intestines are assessed by findings from diagnostic tests, a health assessment interview to collect subjective data, and a physical assessment to collect objective data. See sample documentation of an abdominal assessment below.

SAMPLE DOCUMENTATION
Abdominal Assessment

72-year-old female, currently a resident in an extended care facility, states she had not had a bowel movement for a week, and normally has one every other day. She also says she has lost her appetite and "just feels terrible." Abdominal assessment reveals a firm, slightly distended abdomen. Bowel sounds are active with gurgles in all 4 quadrants. Slight dullness to percussion in LLQ (sigmoid colon). States she has some generalized abdominal discomfort with moderate palpation. Hard stool present in rectum. Stool negative for occult blood.

Diagnostic Tests

The results of diagnostic tests of intestinal function are used to support the diagnosis of a specific disease, to provide information to identify or modify the appropriate medication or therapy used to treat the disease, and to help nurses monitor the client's responses to treatment and nursing care interventions. Diagnostic tests to assess the structures and function of the intestines are described on pages 744–745 and summarized in the bulleted list that follows. More information about diagnostic tests for specific disorders is included in Chapter 26 ∞.

- Stool specimens are examined grossly for volume, water, color, blood, pus, mucus, and fat; and microscopically for white blood cells (WBCs), unabsorbed fat, and parasites.
- Both the small bowel (small-bowel series) and the large bowel (barium enema) are examined by using a contrast medium and examining the intestinal tract under radiologic fluoroscopy. These tests are done to identify structural abnormalities.
- An abdominal ultrasound and/or an MRI may be used to identify sources of GI bleeding, abdominal masses, ascites, and disorders of the appendix. An MRI is often used to stage colon cancer.
- Direct visualization of the anus, rectum, sigmoid colon (sigmoidoscopy), and of the entire large intestine (colonoscopy) is accomplished by using a flexible tube. These tests are done to identify tumors, polyps, infections, inflammations, bleeding

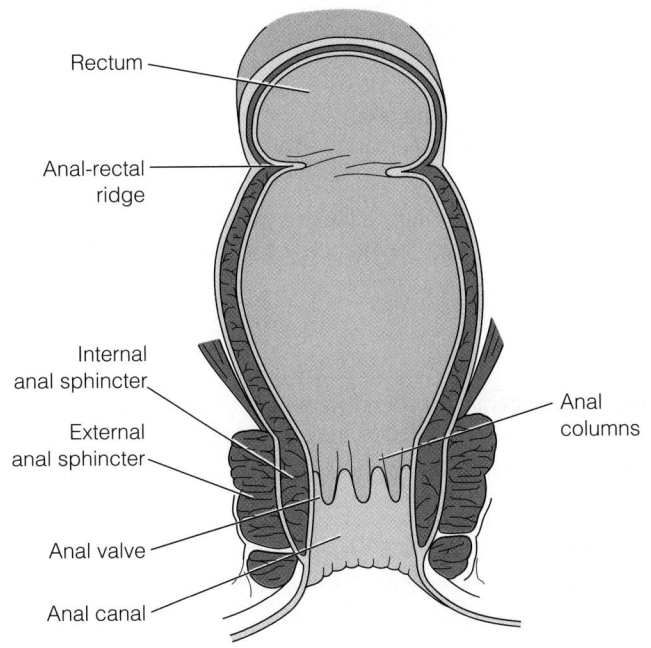

Figure 25–2 ■ Structure of the rectum and anus.

Rectum

Anal-rectal ridge

Internal anal sphincter

External anal sphincter

Anal valve

Anal canal

Anal columns

DIAGNOSTIC TESTS of Intestinal Disorders

NAME OF TEST Stool Specimen, Stool Culture

PURPOSE AND DESCRIPTION A sample of stool is collected for gross and microscopic examination, as well as for form, consistency, and color. Gross examination includes volume and water content, and the presence of any blood, pus, mucus, or excess fat. Microscopic examination identifies the presence of WBCs, unabsorbed fat, and parasites. When an enteric pathogen is suspected, a stool culture is done.

RELATED NURSING CARE Ask client to provide a fresh stool sample. A sterile container should be used to collect a stool sample for a culture. Ask women of childbearing age if they are having their menstrual period; if so, note this on the laboratory request.

NAME OF TEST Test for **Occult Blood** (Hidden Blood)

PURPOSE AND DESCRIPTION A stool specimen may be sent to the laboratory, or the test may be done with a commercial kit such as Hemoccult II or Occultest.

RELATED NURSING CARE When testing for occult blood with a commercial kit following a rectal examination, place a smear of stool on the designated area and drop the reagent on the area. A blue color that develops in response to the reagent indicates the presence of blood.

NAME OF TEST Small-Bowel Series

PURPOSE AND DESCRIPTION This radiologic examination is done to diagnose abnormalities of the small intestine. The client drinks a contrast medium and films are taken every 20 minutes until the medium reaches the terminal ileum. It may also be done in conjunction with an upper GI series or barium swallow.

CLIENT PREPARATION

- Ensure the presence of a signed informed consent for the procedure.
- A low-residue diet may be ordered for 48 hours preceding the examination, and a tap-water enema or cathartic may be given the evening before.
- Instruct to withhold all food for 8 hours and water for 4 hours before the examination.

- Withhold medications affecting bowel motility for 24 hours prior to examination if possible (unless prescribed as part of the preparation procedure).

HEALTH EDUCATION FOR THE CLIENT AND FAMILY

- Although the test is not uncomfortable, it requires several hours to complete. Bring reading material, paperwork, or crafts along to occupy time.
- For a small-bowel exam, the barium may be administered orally, or instilled through a weighted tube inserted into the small bowel, or endoscopically.
- Increase intake of fluids for at least 24 hours after the procedure to facilitate evacuation of the barium. A laxative or cathartic may be prescribed.
- Stool will be chalky white for up to 72 hours after the exam. Normal stool color will return on complete evacuation of barium.

NAME OF TEST Barium Enema (Ba Enema)

PURPOSE AND DESCRIPTION To identify structural abnormalities of the rectum and colon.

This fluoroscopic radiologic examination of the colon is done by administering a contrast medium rectally. Double-contrast or air-contrast studies are the examination of choice, with air being infused after the barium is evacuated.

CLIENT PREPARATION

- Ensure presence of a signed informed consent for the procedure.
- Provide or instruct to follow a clear liquid diet for 24 hours prior to the test. All food and fluids may be withheld for 8 hours prior to the test.
- Administer or instruct to use laxatives, enemas, or suppositories as ordered the evening prior to the procedure. Additional bowel preparation may be ordered for the morning just prior to the procedure.

HEALTH EDUCATION FOR THE CLIENT AND FAMILY

Before Procedure

- The procedure takes approximately 1 hour.
- The barium will be instilled through a lubricated tube inserted into your rectum. You will experience a sensation of fullness, and may feel the need to defecate.
- You will be positioned on the left side, on your back, and prone during this procedure.
- A fluoroscope will be used to follow the progress of the barium, and x-rays will be taken.
- You will expel the barium in the bathroom.

After Procedure

- Following the procedure, a laxative will be given.
- Stools may be white for the next 1 to 2 days.

NAME OF TEST Abdominal Ultrasound

PURPOSE AND DESCRIPTION Used to identify abdominal masses, ascites, and disorders of the appendix. A lubricant gel is applied to the skin and a transducer is placed over the area of interest. High-frequency sound waves pass through the body structures and are recorded as they are reflected.

RELATED NURSING CARE Tell client not to eat or drink for 8 to 12 hours prior to the examination.

NAME OF TEST Magnetic Resonance Imaging (MRI)

PURPOSE AND DESCRIPTION May be done to identify sources of GI bleeding and to stage colon cancer.

RELATED NURSING CARE Ask if client is pregnant or has a metal implant (examination will be canceled).

DIAGNOSTIC TESTS of Intestinal Disorders (continued)

NAME OF TEST Sigmoidoscopy

PURPOSE AND DESCRIPTION A visual examination of the anus, rectum, and sigmoid colon to identify tumors, polyps, infections, inflammations, hemorrhoids, and fissures. Test is done by using a flexible sigmoidoscope. Specimens are obtained and polyps removed during the procedure.

CLIENT PREPARATION

- Ensure the presence of a signed informed consent form.
- Generally, clear liquid or a light diet is ordered for the evening before the procedure.
- Instruct to take a laxative.
- Administer an enema or rectal suppository before the procedure as ordered.

HEALTH EDUCATION FOR THE CLIENT AND FAMILY

Before Procedure

- The procedure takes approximately 15 minutes.

- A mild sedative or tranquilizer may be given during the procedure.
- You may be positioned on your left side or in the knee–chest position.
- The scope will be inserted through the anus into the sigmoid colon.
- Feces may be suctioned.
- A biopsy may be taken. Polyps may be removed.
- Taking deep breaths when you feel discomfort may help you relax.

After Procedure

- Sit up slowly to avoid dizziness or lightheadedness.
- You may pass large amounts of flatus if air was instilled into the bowel.
- Report any abdominal pain, fever, chills, or rectal bleeding.
- If a polyp is removed, avoid heavy lifting for 7 days, and avoid high-fiber foods for 1 to 2 days.

NAME OF TEST Colonoscopy

PURPOSE AND DESCRIPTION A visual examination of the entire colon to the ileocecal valve to identify tumors, polyps, and inflammatory bowel disease and to dilate strictures. A flexible endoscope is inserted anally and advanced through the colon. Polyps are removed during the procedure to prevent them from becoming malignant.

CLIENT PREPARATION

- Ensure presence of a signed informed consent for the procedure.
- A liquid diet may be prescribed for 2 days prior to the procedure, and the client is usually NPO for 8 hours just before the procedure.
- Administer or instruct the client in bowel preparation procedures such as taking citrate of magnesia or polyethylene glycol the evening before.
- Sedation is usually given during the procedure.

HEALTH EDUCATION FOR THE CLIENT AND FAMILY

Before Procedure

- Explain dietary restrictions and their purpose.
- The procedure takes 30 minutes to 1 hour.
- The scope is inserted through the anus and advanced to the cecum.
- A biopsy may be taken, and polyps may be removed.
- Discomfort is minimal.
- Arrange for transportation as you may not be allowed to drive for 24 hours after the procedure.

After Procedure

- You may have increased flatus as air is instilled into the bowel during the procedure.
- Report any abdominal pain, chills, fever, rectal bleeding, or mucopurulent discharge.
- If a polyp has been removed, avoid heavy lifting for 7 days, and avoid high-fiber food for 1 to 2 days.

---

sites, hemorrhoids, and fissures. During the examination, specimens may be obtained, strictures dilated, and polyps removed. These tests are conducted for diagnosis, but are also part of the American Cancer Society recommendations for cancer screening for adults over age 50.

Regardless of the type of diagnostic test, the nurse is responsible for explaining the procedure and any special preparation needed, for assessing for any medication use that might affect the outcome of the tests, for supporting the client during the examination as necessary, for documenting the procedures as appropriate, and for monitoring the results of the tests.

Genetic Considerations

When conducting a health assessment interview and physical assessment, it is important for the nurse to consider genetic influences on health of the adult. During the health assessment interview, ask about family members with inflammatory bowel disorders, celiac disease, colon polyps, and/or colon cancer. During the physical assessment, assess for any manifestations that might indicate a genetic disorder (see page 746 for genetic considerations). If data are found to indicate genetic risk factors or alterations, ask about genetic testing and refer for appropriate genetic counseling and evaluation. Chapter 8 ∞ provides further information about genetics in medical-surgical nursing.

Health Assessment Interview

A health assessment interview to determine problems with bowel structure and function may be conducted during a health screening, may focus on a chief complaint (such as abdominal pain or change in bowel patterns), or may be part of a total health assessment. The assessment of bowel sounds is a common part of routine assessments. Clients may feel embarrassed to talk about bowel elimination patterns. To promote effective rapport, ask about less personal information first.

GENETIC CONSIDERATIONS
Intestinal Tract

- Familial adenomatous polyposis (FAP) and hereditary non-polyposis colorectal cancer (HNPCC) are inherited disorders in which there is progressive development of colorectal adenomas. Unless treated, colorectal cancer inevitably occurs by the fourth or fifth decade of life.
- In about 20% of cases, Crohn's disease (an inflammatory bowel disease) appears to be familial in origin.
- Colon cancer is one of the most common inherited cancer syndromes.
- Celiac disease (CD) is a genetic, inheritable disease responsible for the malabsorption of nutrients resulting in malnutrition. If people with CD eat certain types of proteins (glutens, found in wheat, barley, rye, and oats) an autoimmune response causes damage to the small intestine, so that nutrients are not absorbed.

If the client has a health problem involving bowel function, analyze its onset, characteristics and course, severity, precipitating and relieving factors, and any associated symptoms, noting the timing and circumstances. For example, ask the client:

- Can you describe the type of cramping and abdominal pain you are experiencing?
- Have you ever had bleeding from your rectum?
- Have you noticed increased constipation since your surgery?

Begin the interview by inquiring about any medical conditions that may influence the client's bowel elimination pattern, such as a stroke or spinal cord impairment, inflammatory gastrointestinal diseases, endocrine disorders, and allergies. Note any recent travel to other countries. Information about the client's psychosocial history is also important. Assess the client's lifestyle for any patterns of psychologic stress and/or depression, which may alter bowel elimination. Depression may be associated with constipation, whereas **diarrhea** (frequent passage of loose, watery stools) may occur in situations of high stress and anxiety. Explore the client's activities of daily living (ADLs), including exercise, sleep–rest patterns, and dietary and fluid intake. Changes in ADLs can influence bowel elimination patterns.

Determine whether the client has had any lower abdominal pain or rectal pain, which may be associated with a distended colon filled with gas or fluid. Crampy, colicky pains occur with

diarrhea and/or constipation. Sudden onset of lower abdominal cramping occurs in obstruction of the colon. Left lower abdominal pain is associated with diverticulitis. Rectal pain may occur with stool retention and/or hemorrhoids. See Chapter 9 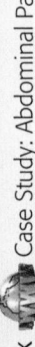 for further information about a pain assessment.

Ask the client to describe the frequency and character of the stools. Ask about any history of diarrhea, constipation, or bleeding from the rectum, and collect information about the use of laxatives, suppositories, or enemas. Anticholinergic drugs, antihistamines, tranquilizers, or narcotics may cause constipation.

If the client has an **ostomy** (surgical opening into the bowel), ask about skin care problems, consistency of stool, foods that cause problems with diarrhea or **flatus** (intestinal gas), the number of times that the client empties the appliance bag each day, and irrigation habits. It is also important to explore the client's feelings about the appliance.

To obtain information about the client's nutritional status, ask about changes in weight, appetite, food preferences, food intolerances, special diets, and any cultural or ethnic influences on dietary intake. Ask whether the client is experiencing nausea and vomiting; if so, determine any relation to food intake, and ask the client to describe the character of the emesis. In addition, ask about indigestion, the use of antacids or other over-the-counter medications, herbal preparations, and episodes of diarrhea and its character.

Explore any family history of colon cancer, colitis, gallbladder disease, or malabsorption syndromes, such as lactose intolerance and celiac sprue. Assess the client's risk factors for cancer, including age greater than 50; family member with colon cancer; history of endometrial, ovarian, or breast cancer; and previous diagnoses of colon inflammation, polyps, or cancer.

Interview questions categorized by functional health patterns are listed on the following page.

Physical Assessment

The function of the bowels is assessed by inspecting the abdomen, auscultating bowel sounds, and performing a rectal examination, an anal examination, an examination for inguinal hernia, and examination of the client's stool. Normal age-related findings for the older adult are summarized in Table 25–1.

Physical assessment of the abdomen may be performed as part of a total health assessment, in combination with assessment of the urinary and reproductive systems (problems which may cause clinical manifestations similar to those of the gastroin-

TABLE 25–1 Age-Related Intestinal Changes

AGE-RELATED CHANGE	SIGNIFICANCE
Small intestine: ↓ number of absorbing cells on intestinal wall, slowed fat absorption, faulty absorption of vitamin B$_{12}$, vitamin D, calcium, and iron.	■ Decreased ability to absorb vitamins A, D, E, and K ■ Increased risk of osteoporosis and fractures (↓ calcium and vitamin D) ■ Increased risk of iron-deficiency anemia (weakness, lassitude, pallor) (↓ iron) ■ Increased risk of pernicious anemia (weakness, dyspnea, glossitis, numbness, dementia, depression) (↓ vitamin B$_{12}$)
Large intestine: ↓ mucous secretion and elasticity of the wall of the rectum, loss of tone in internal sphincter with decreased awareness of need to defecate.	■ Increased tendency for constipation

FUNCTIONAL HEALTH PATTERN INTERVIEW Intestinal Tract

Functional Health Pattern	Interview Questions and Leading Statements
Health Perception-Health Management	■ Have you had any illnesses or surgery that would affect your bowel elimination patterns? If so, describe how it was treated. ■ *Depending on age:* Have you had your colon screened for cancer (such as a colonoscopy)? ■ Do you use any medications to prevent or treat constipation or diarrhea? What do you use and how often? ■ Do you use any treatment for hemorrhoids? Describe.
Nutritional-Metabolic	■ Do you have any food intolerances or food allergies? What type of reaction do you have (such as indigestion, nausea, vomiting, diarrhea, excess gas, abdominal pain)? ■ What do you normally eat and drink in a 24-hour period? ■ Does your bowel problem prevent you from eating specific foods? What are they? ■ *If client has an ostomy:* Do certain foods cause elimination problems such as gas or diarrhea? Describe. Do you have skin irritation around your stoma?
Elimination	■ How often do you have a bowel movement? ■ Describe the color and consistency of your bowel movements. ■ Have your bowel habits changed recently? If so, how? ■ Do you have to strain excessively to have a bowel movement? ■ Have you ever noticed bright red blood on your bowel movement or on the paper after you wiped? ■ *If the client has an ostomy:* How often do you irrigate your ostomy? How often do you have to empty your ostomy bag?
Activity-Exercise	■ Describe your activities in a usual day. ■ Does your bowel elimination pattern interfere with your usual activities? Explain.
Sleep-Rest	■ Does your bowel elimination pattern interfere with your ability to rest and sleep? Explain. ■ Does abdominal cramping or pain interfere with your ability to rest and sleep? Explain.
Cognitive-Perceptual	■ Describe the bowel elimination pattern that is normal for you. ■ Do you have abdominal or rectal pain? Where is it located? What brings it on or relieves it?
Self-Perception-Self-Concept	■ How does having this condition make you feel about yourself?
Role-Relationships	■ How does having this condition affect your relationships with others?
Sexuality-Reproductive	■ Has this condition interfered with your usual sexual activity?
Coping-Stress-Tolerance	■ Has having this condition created stress for you? ■ Have you experienced any kind of stress that makes this condition worse? Explain. ■ Describe what you do when you feel stressed.
Value-Belief	■ Describe how specific relationships or activities help you cope with this problem. ■ Describe specific cultural beliefs or practices that affect how you care for and feel about this problem. ■ Are there any specific treatments that you would not use to treat this condition?

testinal system), or alone for clients with known or suspected health problems. The techniques of inspection, auscultation, percussion, and palpation are used. Figure 25–3 ■ illustrates the four quadrants of the abdomen. A list of organs in each quadrant, as well as photographs of abdominal assessment techniques, are found in Chapter 21 ∞. Box 25–1 provides guidelines for abdominal assessment.

PRACTICE ALERT
Palpation is the last method used in assessing the abdomen, because pressure on the abdominal wall and contents may interfere with bowel sounds and cause pain, ending the examination. Follow standard precautions when palpating the inguinal, perianal, and rectal areas.

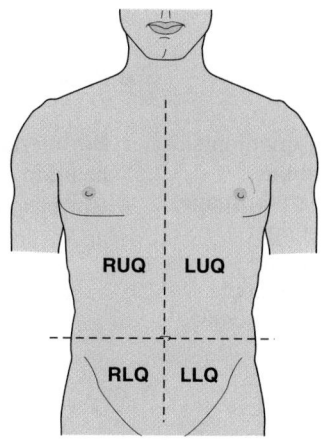

Figure 25–3 ■ The four quadrants of the abdomen.

BOX 25–1 Guidelines for Assessing the Abdomen

Ask the client to empty the bladder before beginning the examination. Assist the client to the dorsal recumbent (supine) position, with a small pillow under the head, a pillow under the knees (if desired), and the arms at the sides of the body. Warm the stethoscope before applying it to the client's skin. Ask the client to point to areas that are painful, and explain that those areas will be examined last. Expose the abdomen from below the breasts to the pubic symphysis, and drape the client's thoracic and genital areas. When you document your findings, specify the location by abdominal quadrant.

General guidelines for abdominal assessment are as follows:

1. Inspect the abdomen under a good light source that is shining across the abdomen. Sit at the right side of the client, and note symmetry, distention, masses, visible peristalsis, and respiratory movements. If masses are detected, ask the client to take a deep breath, which decreases the size of the abdominal cavity and makes any abnormality more visible.

2. Auscultate each quadrant of the abdomen, using the diaphragm of the stethoscope. Listen for bowel sounds, arterial bruits, venous hums, and friction rubs.

3. Percuss several areas within each quadrant of the abdomen, using a systematic path. (For example, always begin in the lower left quadrant, then proceed to the lower right quadrant, upper right quadrant, and upper left quadrant, respectively). The predominant percussion tones for the entire abdomen are tympany and dullness. Tympany is present over gas-filled intestines. Dullness is present over the liver, the spleen, an enlarged kidney, or a full stomach. Percuss for fluid, gaseous distention, and masses.

4. Palpate each quadrant of the abdomen for shape, position, mobility, size, consistency, and tenderness of the major abdominal organs. Begin this part of the assessment with light palpation, and increase the depth of palpation to elicit tenderness or better identify organ size and shape. Deep palpation should be conducted only by nurses with considerable experience. Remember to palpate areas of indicated tenderness last and to use gentle pressure. Palpation may be difficult or impossible if the client exhibits muscle guarding from pain or is ticklish. The gallbladder and the spleen are normally not palpable.

Ask the client to empty the bladder before the examination and lie in the supine position for the abdominal and rectal assessments. Have the client turn to the left lateral (Sims') position for the rectal examination. The older client or the client with limited mobility may need assistance in assuming this position. The client should be standing to assess for an inguinal hernia.

Explain what will happen during the examination, and encourage the client to take deep, regular breaths to increase relaxation. Explain that during the examination, it may feel as though the client is about to have a bowel movement and that sometimes flatus ("gas") is passed. Assure the client that this is normal. Ensure that the examination area is private and the client is draped properly to prevent unnecessary exposure.

BOWEL ASSESSMENT

Technique/Normal Findings	Abnormal Findings

Abdominal Assessment

Inspect abdominal contour, skin integrity, venous pattern, and aortic pulsation. *Abdomen should be slightly concave with intact skin. There should not be distended veins or obvious aortic pulsations.*

- Generalized abdominal distention may be seen in gas retention or obesity.
- Lower abdominal distention is seen in bladder distention, pregnancy, or ovarian mass.
- General distention and an everted umbilicus are seen with ascites and/or tumors.
- A scaphoid (sunken) abdomen is seen in malnutrition or when fat is replaced with muscle.
- **Striae** (whitish-silver stretch marks) are seen in obesity and during or after pregnancy.
- Spider angiomas may be seen in liver disease.
- Dilated veins are prominent in cirrhosis of the liver, ascites, portal hypertension, or venocaval obstruction.
- Pulsation is increased in aortic aneurysm.

Auscultate all four quadrants of the abdomen with the diaphragm of the stethoscope. Begin in the lower right quadrant, where bowel sounds are almost always present. *Normal bowel sounds (gurgling or clicking) occur every 5 to 15 seconds. Listen for at least 5 minutes in each of the four quadrants to confirm the absence of bowel sounds.*

- **Borborygmus** (hyperactive high-pitched, tinkling, rushing, or growling bowel sounds) is heard in diarrhea or at the onset of bowel obstruction.
- Bowel sounds may be absent later in bowel obstruction, with an inflamed peritoneum, and/or following surgery of the abdomen.

Technique/Normal Findings	Abnormal Findings
Auscultate the abdomen for vascular sounds with the bell of the stethoscope. *No sounds (bruits, venous hum, or friction rub) other than bowel sounds should be auscultated.*	■ **Bruits** (blowing sound due to restriction of blood flow through vessels) may be heard over constricted arteries. A bruit over the liver may be heard in hepatic carcinoma. ■ A venous hum (continuous medium-pitched sound) may be heard over a cirrhotic liver. ■ Friction rubs (rough grating sounds) may be heard over an inflamed liver or spleen.
Percuss the abdomen in all four quadrants (see Figure 25–3). *Normally, tympany is heard over the stomach and gas-filled bowels.*	■ Dullness is heard when the bowel is displaced with fluid or tumors or filled with a fecal mass.
Palpate the abdomen in all four quadrants. Use a circular motion to move the abdominal wall over underlying structures. Feel for masses and note any tenderness or pain the client may have during this part of the exam. Palpate lightly at first (0.5 to 0.75 inch), then more deeply (1.5 to 2 inches) with caution. If a mass is palpated, ask the client to raise head and shoulders. *There should be no abdominal masses or pain on palpation.*	■ A mass in the abdomen may become more prominent when the head and shoulders are raised, as will a ventral abdominal wall hernia. If the mass is no longer palpable, it is deeper in the abdomen. **PRACTICE ALERT** Never use deep palpation in a client who has had a pulsatile abdominal mass, renal transplant, polycystic kidneys, or is at risk for hemorrhage. ■ In cases of peritoneal inflammation, palpation causes abdominal pain and involuntary muscle spasms. ■ Abnormal masses include aortic aneurysms, neoplastic tumors of the colon or uterus, and a distended bladder or distended bowel due to obstruction. ■ A rigid, boardlike abdomen may be palpated when the client has a perforated duodenal ulcer.
Palpate for rebound tenderness. Press the fingers into the abdomen slowly and release the pressure quickly. *Releasing pressure should not cause or increase pain.*	■ In peritoneal inflammation, pain occurs when the fingers are withdrawn. ■ Right upper quadrant pain occurs with acute cholecystitis. ■ Upper middle abdominal pain occurs with acute pancreatitis. ■ Right lower quadrant pain at McBurney's point occurs with acute appendicitis. ■ Left lower quadrant pain is seen in acute diverticulitis.

Inguinal Area Assessment

Inspect the inguinal area for bulges after asking the client to bear down. *The inguinal area is normally free of bulges.*	■ Bulges that appear in the inguinal area when the client bears down may indicate a **hernia** (a defect in the abdominal wall that allows abdominal contents to protrude outward).
Palpate the inguinal area with the gloved hand. Ask the client to shift weight to the left to palpate the right inguinal area and vice versa. Place your right index finger upward into the inguinal area and ask the client to bear down or cough. *Bulging or masses are normally not palpable.*	■ A bulge or mass may indicate a hernia.

Technique/Normal Findings	Abnormal Findings

Perianal Assessment

Inspect the perianal area. Wearing gloves, spread the client's buttocks apart. Observe the area, and ask client to bear down as if trying to have a bowel movement. *The perianal area should be intact, without obvious lesions.*

- Swollen, painful, longitudinal breaks in the anal area may appear in clients with anal fissures. (These are caused by the passing of large, hard stools or by diarrhea.)
- Dilated anal veins appear with hemorrhoids.
- A red mass may appear with prolapsed internal hemorrhoids.
- Doughnut-shaped red tissue at the anal area may appear with a prolapsed rectum.

Palpate the anus and rectum. Lubricate the gloved index finger and ask the client to bear down. Touch the tip of your finger to the client's anal opening. Flex the index finger, and slowly insert it into the anus, pointing the finger toward the umbilicus (Figure 25–4 ■). Rotate the finger in both directions to palpate any lesions or masses. *There should be no masses in the anus or rectum.*

- Movable, soft masses may be polyps.
- Hard, firm, irregular embedded masses may indicate carcinoma.

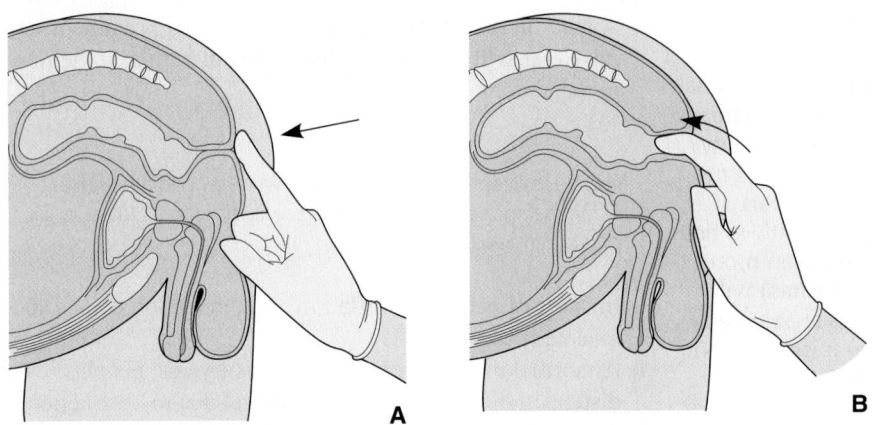

Figure 25–4 ■ Digital examination of the *A*, anus; and *B*, rectum.

Fecal Assessment

Inspect the client's feces. After palpating the rectum, withdraw your finger gently. Inspect any feces on the glove. Note color and/or presence of blood. Also use gloved fingers to note consistency. *Stool should be soft with no blood present, either on the stool or as occult blood.*

- See Box 25–2 for information about stool characteristics.

BOX 25–2 Assessing Stool Characteristics

Inspect feces for color, odor, and consistency after the rectal exam or after defecation. Both hands are gloved.

Color
- Blood *on* the stool results from bleeding from the sigmoid colon, anus, or rectum. Blood *within* the stool indicates bleeding from the colon due to ulcerative colitis, diverticulosis, or tumors. Black, tarry stools, called **melena,** occur with upper gastrointestinal bleeding. Oral iron may turn stools black and mask melena.
- Grayish or whitish stools can result from biliary tract obstruction due to lack of bile in stool.
- Greasy, frothy, yellow stools, called **steatorrhea**, may appear with fat malabsorption.

Odor
- Distinct, foul odors may be noted with stools containing blood or extra fat or in cases of colon cancer.

Consistency
- Hard stools or long, flat stools may result from a spastic colon or bowel obstruction due to a tumor or hemorrhoids. Hard stools may also result from ingestion of oral iron.
- Mucousy, slimy feces may indicate inflammation and occur in irritable bowel syndrome.
- Watery, diarrhea stools appear with malabsorption problems, irritable bowel syndrome, emotional or psychologic stress, ingestion of spoiled foods, or lactose intolerance.

Technique/Normal Findings	Abnormal Findings
Test the feces for occult blood. Use a testing kit such as Occultest or Hemoccult II. *There should be no blood in the feces.*	■ A positive occult blood test requires further testing for colon cancer or gastrointestinal bleeding due to peptic ulcers, ulcerative colitis, or diverticulosis.
Note the odor of the feces. *No distinctly foul odors should be present.*	■ Distinctly foul odors may be noted with stools containing blood or extra fat or in cases of colon cancer.

EXPLORE MediaLink

Prentice Hall Nursing MediaLink DVD-ROM

Audio Glossary
NCLEX-RN® Review

COMPANION WEBSITE www.prenhall.com/lemone
Audio Glossary
NCLEX-RN® Review
Care Plan Activity: Bowel Elimination Disorder
Case Studies
  Abdominal Pain
  Post-Op Complications
MediaLink Application: Chronic Constipation
Links to Resources

TEST YOURSELF NCLEX-RN® REVIEW

1 In which part of the intestinal tract are most nutrients and vitamins absorbed?
1. pancreas
2. small intestine
3. large intestine
4. rectum

2 What is the major function of the large intestine?
1. to produce hormones necessary to digest food
2. to break down lipids, proteins, and carbohydrates
3. to secrete bile into the small intestine
4. to eliminate undigested food residue

3 The appendix is attached to the surface of what segment of the large intestine?
1. cecum
2. ascending colon
3. transverse colon
4. rectum

4 A client asks you to tell her what internal hemorrhoids are. What would you say?
1. "They are part of the arteries of the body."
2. "They are just bits of tissue that occur for no reason."
3. "They are swollen veins in the anal canal."
4. "They are part of the lymphatic system."

5 Which of the following questions or statements would be appropriate for the client with an ostomy?
1. "Have you had any bleeding from your hemorrhoids?"
2. "Has your appetite changed lately?"
3. "Tell me about your family."
4. "Describe the consistency of your stools."

6 Which diagnostic tests would be most appropriate to detect intestinal parasites?

1. colonoscopy
2. CT of the abdomen
3. barium enema
4. stool specimen

7 Why is removal of polyps from the colon important?
1. to identify genetic disorders
2. to prevent the development of cancer
3. to facilitate further examination of the bowel
4. to decrease future problems with constipation

8 What assessment technique is used to assess bowel sounds?
1. inspection
2. palpation
3. percussion
4. auscultation

9 What term is used to describe black, tarry stools?
1. occult blood
2. hematemesis
3. melena
4. steatorrhea

10 You are caring for a client the first day following bowel surgery. You do not hear bowel sounds during your initial assessment. What would you do?
1. Immediately call the physician and report this abnormal finding.
2. Repeat the assessment in 30 minutes to ensure accuracy of findings.
3. Document the assessment as normal following abdominal surgery.
4. Ask another nurse to check your assessment before reporting it.

See Test Yourself answers in Appendix C.

BIBLIOGRAPHY

Amella, E. (2004). Presentation of illness in older adults: If you think you know what you're looking for, think again. *American Journal of Nursing, 104*(10), 40–52.

Bickley, L., & Szilagyi, P. (2007). *Bates' guide to physical examination and history taking* (9th ed.). Philadelphia: Lippincott, Williams & Wilkins.

Bland-Reid, C. (2004). Abdominal trauma: Dealing with the damage. *Nursing, 34*(9), 36–42.

Celiac Sprue Association. (2004). *What is celiac disease?* Retrieved form http://www.csaceliacs.org/celiac_defined.php

Eliopoulos, C. (2005). *Gerontological nursing* (6th ed.). Philadelphia: Lippincott Williams & Wilkins.

Irwin, K. (2003). Back to basics 1: Assessment of bowel dysfunction. *Journal of Community Nursing, 17*(11), 26, 28, 30–32.

Jarvis, C. (2004). *Physical examination & health assessment.* St. Louis, MO: Mosby.

Kee, J. (2005). *Prentice Hall handbook of laboratory & diagnostic tests with nursing implications.* Upper Saddle River, NJ: Prentice Hall.

McCormick, S., & Clarke, C. (2004). Prevention and management of overweight/obesity in the community. *Nutrition Bulletin, 29*(3), 274–279.

Mehta, M. (2003). Assessing the abdomen: Use sight, sound and touch to screen for abnormalities. *Nursing, 33*(5), 54–55.

Nathan, A. (2004). Acute & chronic diarrhoea. *Practice Nurse, 28*(5), 44–45, 47.

National Institutes of Health. (2003). *Genes and disease: The digestive system.* Retrieved from http://www.ncbi.nlm.nih.gov/books/bv.fcgi?rid=gnd.section.115

Norton, C., & Chelvanayagam, S. (2000). A nursing assessment tool for adults with fecal incontinence. *Journal of WOCN, 27*(5), 279–291.

Perform abdominal assessment, or risk missing life-threatening trauma injury: Don't allow "invisible" injuries to escape detection in your ED. (2004). *ED Nursing, 7*(7), 73–75.

Porth, C. (2005). *Pathophysiology: Concepts of altered health states* (7th ed.). Philadelphia: Lippincott.

Walker, B. (2004). Assessing gastrointestinal infections. *Nursing, 34*(5), 48–52.

Watson, R. (2001). Assessing the gastrointestinal tract in older people. 2: The lower GI tract. *Nursing Older People, 13*(1), 27–28.

Weber, J., & Kelley, J. (2006). *Health assessment in nursing* (3rd ed.). Philadelphia: Lippincott.

CHAPTER 26 Nursing Care of Clients with Bowel Disorders

LEARNING OUTCOMES

- Compare and contrast the causes, pathophysiology, manifestations, interdisciplinary care and nursing care of clients with diarrhea, constipation, irritable bowel syndrome, and fecal incontinence.

- Explain the pathophysiology, manifestations, complications, interdisciplinary care, and nursing care of clients with acute inflammatory and infectious bowel disorders, chronic inflammatory bowel disorders, malabsorption syndromes, neoplastic disorders, structural and obstructive bowel disorders, and anorectal disorders.

- Discuss the purposes, nursing implications, and health education for the client and family of medications used to treat bowel disorders.

- Explain the rationale for using selected diets, including those for diarrhea and constipation and low-residue, gluten-free, and high-fiber diets.

- Describe the surgical procedures of the bowel, including colectomy, colostomy, ileostomy, and perianal surgery.

CLINICAL COMPETENCIES

- Assess the functional status of clients with bowel disorders, and monitor, document, and report abnormal manifestations.

- Use evidence-based research to prevent aspiration in critically ill clients with enteral feedings, and to make accurate assessments of fecal incontinence in older adults.

- Determine priority nursing diagnoses, based on assessed data, to select and implement individualized nursing interventions for clients with bowel disorders.

- Administer medications used to treat bowel disorders knowledgeably and safely.

- Provide skilled care to clients having an ileostomy, colostomy, or perianal surgery.

- Integrate interdisciplinary care into care of clients with bowel disorders.

- Provide appropriate teaching to promote nutrition, prevent infectious and helminthic infestations, encourage preventive screening for colon cancer, and facilitate community-based care for healthcare needs resulting from bowel disorders.

- Revise plan of care as needed to provide effective interventions to promote, maintain, or restore functional health status to clients with bowel disorders.

MEDIALINK

Resources for this chapter can be found on the Prentice Hall Nursing MediaLink DVD-ROM accompanying this textbook, and on the Companion Website at http://www.prenhall.com/lemone

Disorders of intestinal absorption and bowel elimination can affect not only functional elimination status, but also other functional health patterns including but not limited to health perception-health management, nutritional-metabolic, activity-exercise, self-perception-self-concept, and sexuality-reproductive. Bowel function can be affected by inflammations, infections, tumors, obstructions, or changes in structure.

Clients with intestinal disorders often face extensive diagnostic testing, surgery, and permanent changes in physical appearance and lifestyle. Nursing care is directed toward meeting the client's physiologic needs, providing emotional support, and educating the client to adapt to changes in lifestyle.

DISORDERS OF INTESTINAL MOTILITY

Few body functions respond as readily to internal and external influences as the process of defecation. Factors affecting the gastrointestinal (GI) tract directly, such as food intake and bacterial population, affect the number and consistency of stools. Indirect factors, such as psychologic stress or voluntary postponement of defecation, also affect elimination.

In modern society, "normal" bowel elimination patterns vary widely. For some clients, two to three stools per day is the usual pattern. Others may normally have as few as three stools per week. It is important to evaluate each client's bowel elimination against his or her own normal pattern.

THE CLIENT WITH DIARRHEA

Diarrhea is an increase in the frequency, volume, and fluid content of the stool. In diarrhea, the water content of feces is increased, usually due to either malabsorption or water secretion in the bowel. It is a manifestation rather than a primary disorder.

Diarrhea may be acute or chronic. Acute diarrhea, which lasts less than a week, is usually due to an infectious agent. Chronic diarrhea (diarrhea that persists longer than 3 to 4 weeks) may be caused by inflammatory bowel disorders, malabsorption, or endocrine disorders.

Pathophysiology

About 1500 mL of digested material enters the large intestine daily. Normally, most of the water and some of the solutes are reabsorbed in the bowel, leaving only about 200 mL of feces to be eliminated.

Large-volume diarrhea, characterized by both increased numbers and volume of stools, is caused by increased water content of the stool. This increased water content may result from either osmotic or secretory processes. Water may be pulled into the bowel lumen by osmosis when the feces contain osmotically active molecules. Some stool softeners and laxatives work on this principle.

When the lactose in milk is not broken down and absorbed, the lactose molecules exert an osmotic pull, causing diarrhea. The diarrhea associated with cholera and *Escherichia coli* infection is caused by increased water secretion in the small and large intestines. Unabsorbed dietary fat, some cathartics and other drugs, and other factors can cause secretory diarrhea.

Small-volume diarrhea, characterized by frequent small stools, is usually caused by inflammation or disease of the colon. Diseases that affect the intestinal mucosa, such as inflammatory bowel disease, cause an exudative diarrhea. The mucosal inflammation causes plasma, serum proteins, blood, and mucus to accumulate in the bowel, increasing fecal bulk and fluidity. An increased rate of propulsion within the bowel can also decrease the amount of water normally absorbed from the chyme, leading to diarrhea. For this reason, laxatives that increase bowel motility and bowel resection or bypass can lead to diarrhea.

Manifestations

The manifestations of diarrhea depend on its cause, duration, and severity, as well as the area of bowel affected and the client's general health. Diarrhea can present as several large, watery stools daily, or very frequent small stools that contain blood, mucus, or exudate.

Complications

Diarrhea can have devastating effects. Water and electrolytes are lost in diarrheal stool. This can lead to dehydration, particularly in the very young, the older adult, or the debilitated client unable to respond to thirst. With severe diarrhea, vascular collapse and hypovolemic shock may occur. Potassium and magnesium are lost, potentially leading to hypokalemia and hypomagnesemia. The loss of bicarbonate in the stool can lead to metabolic acidosis. See Chapter 10 ∞ for further discussion of the effects of these imbalances.

INTERDISCIPLINARY CARE

Management of diarrhea focuses on identifying and treating the underlying cause. In addition, the diarrhea itself may need to be treated to promote comfort and to prevent complications. The history (including the onset and associated circumstances of the diarrhea) and physical examination often provide enough information to identify its cause.

Diagnosis

Diagnostic tests that may be ordered to help identify the cause of diarrhea include a stool specimen analysis and culture. A sigmoidoscopy may be conducted to directly visualize the bowel mucosa. (See Chapter 25 ∞ for further information on diagnostic tests.) Tissue biopsy may be performed to identify chronic inflammatory processes, infection, and other causes of diarrhea. In addition, laboratory tests of serum electrolytes, serum osmolality, and arterial blood gases (ABGs) may be ordered to assess for adverse effects of diarrhea. Increased serum osmolality indicates water loss and dehydration.

Medications

Antidiarrheal medications are used sparingly or not at all until the cause of diarrhea has been identified. In diarrhea associated with botulism or bacillary dysentery, giving an antidiarrheal agent can worsen or prolong the disease by slowing elimination of the toxin from the bowel. Once the underlying cause for diarrhea has been established, specific medications may be ordered to treat the underlying cause. Antibiotics are used with caution because they alter the normal bacterial population of the bowel and may actually worsen diarrhea. A balanced electrolyte solution may be required to replace fluid losses. Intravenous or oral potassium preparations may also be prescribed.

Opium and some of its derivatives, anticholinergics, absorbants, and demulcents are commonly used as antidiarrheal preparations. Specific preparations, their method of action, and the nursing implications for these medications are outlined in the Medication Administration box on page 756.

Nutrition

Fluid replacement is of primary importance in managing the client with diarrhea. If the client is able to tolerate oral fluids (i.e., if the client is not experiencing nausea and vomiting), an oral glucose/balanced electrolyte solution provides the best fluid replacement. Commercial preparations such as Gatorade and other sports drinks are available, as are pediatric solutions (e.g., Pedialyte), which can be used for adults as well as children. A solution of 5 mL (1 teaspoon) each of table salt and baking soda and 4 teaspoons (20 mL) of granulated sugar added with desired flavoring (such as lemon extract or juice) to 1 quart (1 L) of water can be made at home to replace water and electrolytes.

Solid food is withheld in the first 24 hours of acute diarrhea to rest the bowel. After that time, frequent, small, soft feedings can be added. Milk and milk products are added last, because the lactose they contain frequently aggravates the diarrhea. Raw fruits and vegetables, fried foods, bran, whole-grain cereals, condiments, spices, coffee, and alcoholic beverages are avoided during the recovery period.

Clients with chronic diarrhea may benefit by eliminating specific foods from the diet. Foods and nonfood substances that may aggravate diarrhea are outlined in Table 26–1. The diet should be high in calories and nutritional value. Vitamin supplements may be necessary, particularly the fat-soluble vitamins (A, D, E, and K). Clients with severe chronic diarrhea may require parenteral nutrition (see Chapter 21 ∞).

Complementary and Alternative Therapies

Herbal or homeopathic therapies may be used to help relieve diarrhea. Clients who are lactose intolerant (discussed later in the chapter) should take 1 to 2 lactase enzymes with each meal (Balch & Stengler, 2004). Herbal treatments may include a strong tea of black pepper, chamomile, coriander, rosemary, sandalwood, or thyme. Ginger in the form of tea or capsules can be helpful in reducing intestinal inflammation and lessens the effects of food poisoning. Homeopathic practitioners may use podophyllum tablets when there is a rumbling, gurgling, and cramping in the abdomen, followed by diarrhea (Balch & Stengler, 2004). Refer the client to a qualified practitioner for more information about using complementary and alternative therapies to treat diarrhea.

NURSING CARE

Health Promotion

Teach all clients about the importance of hand washing as a measure to prevent the spread of infectious diseases, including those that cause diarrhea. Teach safe food handling techniques to prevent bacterial contamination, and discuss measures to ensure safe drinking water. For clients planning to travel outside

TABLE 26–1 Foods That May Aggravate Chronic Diarrhea

FOODS	REASON
Milk, ice cream, yogurt, soft cheeses, cottage cheese	Contain lactose; not tolerated by clients with lactase deficiency who cannot digest lactose.
Apple juice, pear juice, grapes, honey, dates, nuts, figs, fruit-flavored soft drinks	Contain fructose; when consumed in large quantities, fructose may not be totally absorbed, causing an osmotic pull of fluid into the bowel.
Table sugar	Contains sucrose; not tolerated by clients with sucrase deficiency.
Apple juice, pear juice, sugarless gums and mints	May contain sorbitol or mannitol, sugars that are not absorbed and can cause osmotic draw.
Antacids	Magnesium-containing antacids decrease bowel transit time and contain poorly absorbed salts that can exert an osmotic draw.
Coffee, tea, cola drinks, over-the-counter analgesics	Contain caffeine, which can decrease bowel transit time.

MEDICATION ADMINISTRATION Antidiarrheal Preparations

ABSORBANTS AND PROTECTANTS
Kaolin and pectin (Kaopectate, Donnagel-MB)
Bismuth subsalicylate (Pepto-Bismol)
Absorbant preparations act locally in the intestines to bind substances that can cause diarrhea. Absorbants are safe and are generally available over the counter. Their efficacy has not been proved, although bismuth subsalicylate has been shown to be somewhat effective in preventing and managing traveler's diarrhea, usually related to contaminated water supplies. Bismuth salts also have a protective and antimicrobial effect.

Nursing Responsibilities
- Assess for contraindications to antidiarrheal therapy, such as some infections or chronic inflammatory bowel disease, including ulcerative colitis.
- If fever is present, check with physician before giving the medication.
- Administer these medications at least 1 hour before or 2 hours after other oral medications; they may interfere with the absorption of other drugs.
- Observe the client's response to the medication. Constipation is a potential problem.

Health Education for the Client and Family
- Take the recommended dosage at the onset of diarrhea and after each loose stool.
- Do not take any of these preparations for more than 48 hours. If diarrhea persists, notify the physician.
- Do not give antidiarrheal medications to debilitated older clients without physician supervision.
- Chew bismuth subsalicylate tablets, rather than swallowing them whole, for maximal effectiveness. This medication may cause harmless darkening of the tongue and stool.
- If you are allergic to aspirin, use bismuth subsalicylate with caution; as a general rule, avoid taking aspirin while taking bismuth subsalicylate.

OPIUM AND OPIUM DERIVATIVES
Camphorated tincture of opium (Paregoric)
Tincture of opium (laudanum, opium tincture)
Difenoxin (Motofen)
Diphenoxylate (Lomotil, Lotrol, others)
Loperamide hydrochloride (Imodium)
Opium and its derivatives act on the central nervous system (CNS) to decrease the motility of the ileum and colon, slowing transit time and promoting more water absorption. They also decrease the sensation of a full rectum and increase anal sphincter tone. Paregoric and tincture of opium have a greater potential for abuse and are prescription drugs subject to controls under the federal Controlled Substance Act of 1970. Difenoxin, diphenoxylate, and loperamide are derivatives of opium with few analgesic, euphoric, or abuse-promoting effects and are in more common use today.

Nursing Responsibilities
- Assess for contraindications to antidiarrheal or narcotic medications prior to giving these drugs.
- Administer paregoric undiluted with water.
- Do not administer difenoxin and diphenoxylate to clients receiving monoamine oxidase inhibitors (MAOIs); hypertensive crises may occur.
- Observe closely for increased effects of other CNS depressants, such as alcohol, narcotic analgesics, or barbiturate sedatives.
- Observe for abdominal distention; toxic megacolon may occur if these drugs are given to the client with ulcerative colitis.

Health Education for the Client and Family
- Take the medication as recommended at the onset of diarrhea and after each loose stool.
- These drugs may be habit forming; use for no more than 48 hours.
- Avoid using alcohol and over-the-counter cold preparations while taking these drugs.
- These preparations may cause drowsiness, avoid driving or operating machinery while taking them.

ANTICHOLINERGICS
Atropine
Belladonna alkaloids (Donnagel, Donnatal)
Anticholinergic medications reduce bowel spasticity and acid secretion in the stomach. They are used to treat diarrhea that is associated with peptic ulcer disease and irritable bowel syndrome. These are nonspecific drugs; their systemic effects are their major drawback.

Nursing Responsibilities
- Assess for contraindications to atropine and other anticholinergic medications: glaucoma, prostatic hypertrophy, and gastrointestinal or genitourinary obstruction.
- Observe for side effects, such as eye pain, impaired urination, or constipation.

Health Education for the Client and Family
- Take only as directed, stop the drug and notify the physician if you develop eye pain, impaired urination, constipation.
- Do not operate machinery while taking this medication; drowsiness may occur.
- Hard candies help relieve oral dryness associated with these preparations.

the United States or to wilderness areas, teach measures to purify water for drinking and cooking.

Assessment

The nursing assessment can help identify the cause of the client's diarrhea, as well as early signs of complications. Collect the following assessment data:

- *Health history:* Duration and extent of diarrhea; associated manifestations; dietary intake; recent travel out of the country or to wilderness areas; previous history of diarrhea; chronic diseases; prescription and nonprescription medications.
- *Physical examination:* Vital signs (including orthostatic blood pressure); peripheral pulses; skin temperature, moisture, turgor; color and moisture of mucous membranes; abdominal

contour and girth; bowel sounds; stool for obvious or occult blood, pus, mucus, or **steatorrhea** (bulky, foul-smelling stool).

Nursing Diagnoses and Interventions

Nursing care of the client with diarrhea focuses on identifying the cause, relieving the manifestations, preventing complications, and preventing the potential spread of infection to others.

Diarrhea

Nursing interventions for diarrhea are provided to help the client recover a normal elimination pattern without adverse consequences.

- Monitor and record the frequency and characteristics of bowel movements *to provide a measure of the effectiveness of treatment.*
- Measure abdominal girth and auscultate bowel sounds every 8 hours as indicated. Loud, rushing bowel sounds (**borborygmi**) indicate increased peristalsis, and may be heard in clients with acute diarrhea. *Diminished or absent bowel sounds may indicate a complication of treatment, such as constipation or toxic megacolon.*
- Use standard precautions, including gloves and hand washing. *Standard precautions help prevent the spread of infection to others.*
- Provide ready access to bathroom, commode, or bedpan. *The client may have little warning of the need to defecate. Easily accessed toileting facilities reduce the risk for soiling or injury.*
- Administer antidiarrheal medications as prescribed *to promote comfort and prevent excess fluid loss.*
- Limit food intake if the diarrhea is acute, reintroducing solid foods slowly, in small amounts, *to allow the bowel to rest and mucosa to heal in acute diarrhea states.*

Risk for Deficient Fluid Volume

The increased water content of diarrheal stool places the client at risk for fluid deficit.

- Record intake and output; weigh daily; assess skin turgor, mucous membranes, and urine specific gravity every 8 hours. *These assessments are used to monitor fluid volume status.*

> **PRACTICE ALERT**
> Assess skin turgor over the sternum in the older adult. Loss of subcutaneous fat associated with aging makes skin turgor assessment on the arms or hands less reliable.

- Monitor vital signs, including orthostatic blood pressures. *Orthostatic hypotension is identified by a drop in BP of more than 10 mmHg and pulse increase of 10 beats per minute (bpm) when changing from a lying to a sitting position or from a sitting to a standing position. It is an indicator of fluid volume deficit.*

> **PRACTICE ALERT**
> Institute safety precautions such as providing assistance when ambulating the client with orthostatic hypotension. The fall in blood pressure with position changes can cause light-headedness and syncope.

- Provide fluid and electrolyte replacement solutions as indicated. Ensure ready access to fluids; assist the debilitated client with fluid intake. Notify the care provider if the client is unable to tolerate oral fluids. *Oral fluids are encouraged as tolerated to prevent dehydration. Intravenous fluids are necessary if oral fluids are not tolerated. An intake of 3000 mL/day or more is often needed to replace fluid losses.*

Risk for Impaired Skin Integrity

Decreased extracellular fluid volume and the irritating effects of diarrheal stool increase the risk for skin breakdown.

- Assist with cleaning the perianal area as needed. Use warm water, a gentle cleanser, and soft cloths. *Cleansing removes irritating substances in the stool. Gentle cleansing helps maintain integrity of dehydrated skin.*
- Apply protective ointment to the perianal area. *Moisture-barrier ointments or creams protect the skin from excoriation and help prevent tissue breakdown.*

Using NANDA, NIC, and NOC

Chart 26–1 shows links between NANDA nursing diagnoses, NIC, and NOC for the client with diarrhea.

NANDA, NIC, AND NOC LINKAGES
CHART 26–1 The Client with Altered Bowel Motility

NANDA

Diarrhea

↓

NIC

Diarrhea Management

Electrolyte Monitoring

Fluid Management

Medication Management

Perineal Care

↓

NOC

Bowel Continence

Electrolyte & Acid–Base Management

Fluid Balance

Medication Response

Symptom Severity

Data from *NANDA's Nursing Diagnoses: Definitions & Classification 2005–2006* by NANDA International (2005), Philadelphia; *Nursing Interventions Classification (NIC)* (4th ed.) by J. M. Dochterman & G. M. Bulechek (2004), St. Louis, MO: Mosby; and *Nursing Outcomes Classification (NOC)* (3rd ed.) by S. Moorhead, M. Johnson, and M. Maas (2004), St. Louis, MO: Mosby.

Community-Based Care

Acute and chronic diarrhea generally are managed by the client in the home. Teach the client and family members about the following subjects:

- Causes of diarrhea (as directed by the diagnosis)
- Importance of hand washing and hygiene measures
- Importance of maintaining adequate fluid intake to replace lost water and electrolytes
- Use of a balanced electrolyte solution such as Gatorade or a similar product (purchased or home prepared) for fluid replacement
- Recommendations to limit food intake during acute diarrhea, and resume gradually with small feedings of foods that have a constipating effect: applesauce, bananas, crackers, rice, potatoes
- To avoid foods high in fiber, milk products, and caffeine
- Ways to maintain nutrition if chronic diarrhea is a problem: frequent small meals, nutritional supplements, vitamin supplements
- Precautions and limitations of antidiarrheal preparations
- Importance of seeking medical intervention if diarrhea continues or recurs.

THE CLIENT WITH CONSTIPATION

Constipation is defined as the infrequent (two or fewer bowel movements weekly) or difficult passage of stools. Constipation affects older adults more frequently than younger people. Recent studies indicate that approximately 20% to 35% of people over age 65 report recurrent constipation and laxative use. Although fecal transit in the large intestine slows with aging, the increased incidence of constipation is thought to relate more to impaired general health status, increased medication use, and decreased physical activity in the older adult.

Pathophysiology

Constipation may be a primary problem or a manifestation of another disease or condition. Acute constipation, a definite change in the bowel elimination pattern, often is caused by an organic process. A change in bowel patterns that persists or becomes more frequent or severe may be due to a tumor or other partial bowel obstruction. With chronic constipation, functional causes that impair storage, transport, and evacuation mechanisms impede the normal passage of stools. Common causes of constipation are listed in Table 26–2.

Psychogenic factors are the most frequent causes of chronic constipation. These factors include postponing defecation when the urge is felt, and the perception of satisfaction with defecation. Clients often use laxatives and enemas to stimulate a bowel movement when constipation is perceived. Overuse of these measures can lead to real intestinal problems that worsen the condition. For example, *cathartic colon* (impaired colonic motility and changes in bowel structure) mimics ulcerative colitis in that the normal pouchlike or saccular appearance of the colon is lost. *Melanosis coli* is a brownish-black discoloration of the colon mucosa. Both conditions may be caused by long-term laxative use.

TABLE 26–2 **Selected Causes of Constipation**	
FACTOR	**RELATED CAUSE**
Activity	Lack of exercise: bed rest
Dietary	Highly refined, low-fiber foods; inadequate fluid intake
Drugs	Antacids containing aluminum or calcium salts; narcotic analgesics; anticholinergics; many antidepressants, tranquilizers, and sedatives; antihypertensives, such as ganglionic blockers, calcium-channel blockers, beta-adrenergic blockers, and diuretics; iron salts
Large bowel	Diverticular disease, inflammatory disease, tumor, obstruction; changes in rectal or anal structure or function
Psychogenic	Voluntary suppression of urge; perceived need to defecate on schedule; depression
Systemic	Advanced age; pregnancy; neurologic conditions (trauma, multiple sclerosis, tumors, cerebrovascular accident, Parkinsonism); endocrine and metabolic disorders (hypothyroidism, hypercalcemia, uremia, porphyria)
Other	Chronic laxative or enema use

Manifestations

The manifestations of constipation include having bowel movements less often than the usual pattern, frequent flatus, abdominal discomfort, anorexia, straining to have a bowel movement, and the passage of hard, dry stools.

With significant constipation or long-term dependence on laxatives or enemas, **fecal impaction** may develop. Impaction may also occur following barium administration for radiologic exam. The impaction is felt as a rock-hard or putty-like mass of feces in the rectum. Abdominal cramping and a full sensation in the rectal area may be manifestations of impaction. Watery mucus or foul-smelling liquid stool may be passed around the impaction, causing the client to complain of diarrhea.

INTERDISCIPLINARY CARE

Initial evaluation of constipation is based on the history and physical examination. The abdomen may appear somewhat distended, and bowel sounds may be reduced. If an impaction is present, digital examination of the rectum reveals a palpable, hard or putty-like fecal mass.

Simple or chronic constipation is treated with education (a daily bowel movement is not necessary for health), and modification of diet and exercise routines. If the problem is acute or does not resolve, further diagnostic examination may be ordered.

Diagnosis

A barium enema may be ordered to identify bowel structure, tumors, or diverticula. If the problem is acute, a sigmoidoscopy or colonoscopy may be used for evaluation and biopsy. (See Chapter 25 ∞ for nursing implications of these tests.)

Medications

Laxative and cathartic preparations are used to promote stool evacuation. Milder preparations are generally known as laxatives; cathartics have a stronger effect. Most laxatives are appropriate only for short-term use. Cathartics and enemas interfere with normal bowel reflexes and should not be used for simple constipation. Laxatives should never be given if a client has an undiagnosed intestinal obstruction, abdominal pain, fecal impaction, rectal fissures, ulcerated hemorrhoids, Crohn's disease, ulcerative colitis, or chronic inflammatory bowel disease (Peate, 2003). When the bowel is obstructed, laxatives or cathartics may cause serious mechanical damage and perforate the bowel.

The only laxatives that are appropriate and safe for long-term use are bulking agents, such as psyllium seed, calcium polycarbophil, and methylcellulose. These agents act by increasing the bulk of the feces and drawing water into the bowel to soften it. Commonly prescribed laxatives and cathartics are discussed in the Medication Administration box on this page.

Nutrition

Foods that have a high fiber content are recommended. Vegetable fiber is largely indigestible and unabsorbable, so it increases stool bulk. Fiber also helps draw water into the fecal mass, softening the stool and making defecation easier. Raw fruits and vegetables are good sources of dietary fiber, as is cereal bran. Use 2 to 3 teaspoons of unprocessed bran with meals (sprinkled on fruit or cereal) or up to 1/4 cup daily to supply adequate fiber.

Fluids are also important to maintain bowel motility and soft stools. The client should drink 6 to 8 glasses of fluid per day. It is important to advise the client to increase fluid intake when dietary fiber is initially increased to decrease flatus and help maintain softer stools.

In older adults, constipation may be due to inadequate food intake. Carefully evaluate diet history and usual daily intake.

Enemas

Significant or chronic constipation or a fecal impaction may require the administration of an enema. As a general rule, enemas should be used only in acute situations and only on a short-term basis. They may also be ordered to prepare the bowel for diagnostic testing or examination. The following types of enemas may be prescribed:

- A *saline enema* using 500 to 2000 mL of warmed physiologic saline solution is the least irritating to the bowel.
- *Tap-water enemas* use 500 to 1000 mL of water to soften feces and irritate the bowel mucosa, stimulating peristalsis and evacuation.
- *Soap-suds enemas* consist of a tap-water solution to which soap is added as a further irritant.
- *Phosphate enemas* (e.g., Fleet) use a hypertonic saline solution to draw fluid into the bowel and irritate the mucosa, leading to evacuation.
- *Oil retention enemas* instill mineral or vegetable oil into the bowel to soften the fecal mass. The instilled oil is retained overnight or for several hours before evacuation.

The repeated use of enemas can lead not only to impaired bowel function, but also to fluid and electrolyte imbalances. Tap-water and phosphate enemas are particularly likely to cause these problems. In acute conditions with risk of bowel obstruction, perforation, ulceration, or other problem, enemas should not be administered until their safe use can be established.

Complementary and Alternative Therapies

Herbal or homeopathic therapies may be used to help relieve constipation. Flaxseed oil lubricates the colon for easier passage of stool. Clients are instructed to take 1 to 2 tablespoons daily. Flax seeds are a lesser known but a highly concentrated source of fiber, and 1 to 2 tablespoons of ground flaxseeds can be sprinkled on cereals or salads daily, followed by 10 ounces of water. Acupressure, massage, reflexology, aromatherapy, and stress management therapies can also be very beneficial in relieving constipation (Balch & Stengler, 2004). Other recommendations include exercise to stimulate intestinal contractions.

 NURSING CARE

Health Promotion

Education can prevent constipation. Teach clients the importance of maintaining a diet high in natural fiber. Foods such as fresh fruits, vegetables, whole-grain products, and bran provide natural fiber. Encourage reducing consumption of meats and refined foods, which are low in fiber and can be constipating. Emphasize the need to maintain a high fluid intake every day, particularly during hot weather and exercise. Discuss the relationship between exercise and bowel regularity. Encourage clients to engage in some form of exercise, such as walking daily.

Discuss normal bowel habits, and explain that a daily bowel movement is not the norm for all people. Encourage clients to respond to the urge to defecate when it occurs. Suggest setting aside a time, usually following a meal, for elimination.

Assessment

To assess the client with real or perceived constipation, collect the following data:

- *Health history:* Usual and current pattern of defecation, including time of day, amount, and stool consistency; usual diet, fluid intake, and activity pattern; possible contributing factors such as narcotic analgesics, activity limitations, painful hemorrhoids, perianal surgery; chronic diseases such as endocrine or neurologic disorders; prescribed and nonprescription medications.
- *Physical examination:* Abdominal girth and shape, bowel sounds, tenderness, and percussion tone; digital exam of the rectum if impaction is suspected.

For discussion of constipation in the older adult see Meeting Individualized Needs on page 761.

Nursing Diagnoses and Interventions

Nursing interventions for the client with constipation focus chiefly on education.

MEDICATION ADMINISTRATION Laxatives and Cathartics

BULK-FORMING AGENTS
Bran
Calcium polycarbophil (Fibercon)
Methylcellulose (Citrucel)
Psyllium hydrophilic mucilloid (Metamucil, Effer-Syllium)
Bulk-forming agents are the only safe laxatives for long-term use. They contain vegetable fiber, which is not digested or absorbed in the gut. This natural fiber creates bulk and draws water into the intestine, softening the stool mass.

Nursing Responsibilities
- Mix the agent with a full glass of cool liquid just prior to administering.
- Do not administer to clients with possible stool impaction or bowel obstruction.

Health Education for the Client and Family
- Drink at least 6 to 8 full glasses of nonalcoholic fluid per day. Adequate hydration is necessary to produce the drug's laxative effect.
- These agents may be mixed with water, milk, or fruit juice.
- Take the drug in the morning or with meals. To reduce the risk of impaction, do not take at bedtime.
- Because of the increased risk of impaction, check with the physician before increasing dietary fiber while you are taking these agents.

WETTING AGENTS
Docusate (Colace, Surfak, Doxidan, others)
Wetting agents reduce stool surface tension and form an emulsion of fat and water, softening the stool. They are used primarily to prevent straining and reduce the discomfort of expelling hard stools.

Nursing Responsibilities
- Administer with ample fluids to promote softening effect.
- Wetting agents may alter the absorption of other drugs. Do not administer within 1 hour of other oral medications.
- Do not attempt to crush or open caplets; a liquid form is available for clients who cannot swallow pills or capsules.

Health Education for the Client and Family
- Do not use for more than 1 week or less unless specifically recommended by the physician.
- Take the medication in the morning or evening, but avoid taking it with other medications.
- Adequate fluid is necessary to obtain the beneficial effect of the drug. Drink 6 to 8 glasses of nonalcoholic fluid per day.

OSMOTIC AND SALINE LAXATIVES/CATHARTICS
Lactulose (Rhodialose)
Sorbitol
Magnesium hydroxide (Milk of Magnesia)
Magnesium citrate
Polyethylene glycol (Klean-Prep)
Laxatives in this group contain poorly absorbed salts or carbohydrates that remain in the bowel, increasing osmotic pressure and drawing water into the intestine. Stool volume increases, consistency decreases, and peristalsis is stimulated. Many of these agents also have an irritant effect on the bowel, further stimulating peristalsis. They are used to stimulate rapid or complete bowel

evacuation to relieve constipation and to prepare the bowel for diagnostic and surgical procedures. They should be limited to acute, short-term use; chronic use may suppress normal bowel reflexes.

Nursing Responsibilities
- Assess for possible contraindications to osmotic or saline laxatives, including bowel ulceration or obstruction, dehydration, electrolyte imbalances, heart failure (which may be aggravated by the sodium content), or renal failure.
- Administer with a full glass of liquid, preferably in the morning to avoid sleep disturbance.
- Monitor fluid and electrolyte status: skin turgor, mucous membranes, intake and output; daily weight, and laboratory studies, such as hemoglobin and hematocrit levels, serum osmolality and electrolytes, and urine specific gravity.

Health Education for the Client and Family
- Do not use these agents on a routine basis to treat or prevent constipation.
- Chill the solution to increase its palatability.
- Expect some abdominal cramping.
- Use only as directed. Increase fluid intake to at least 6 to 8 glasses of nonalcoholic fluid.
- Notify the physician if adverse effects occur, including abdominal pain, bloody stool, excessive skin or mucous membrane dryness, rapid weight loss, dizziness, or other unusual symptoms.
- These agents work in 3 to 6 hours; take them in the morning or early evening to avoid sleep disturbance.

IRRITANT OR STIMULANT LAXATIVES
Bisacodyl (Dulcolax, Bisco-Lax, Carter's Liver Pills, Codylax, others)
Phenolphthalein (Evac-U-Gen, Evac-U-Lax, Feen-A-Mint, Phenolax, others)
Cascara sagrada
Senna (Senna laxative, Fletcher's Castoria)
Castor oil
Stimulant laxatives work by stimulating the motility and secretion of intestinal mucosa. Their use results in watery stool, often accompanied by abdominal cramping and pain. They are used to relieve constipation, although they should not be used as the initial treatment. Stimulant laxatives are also used for preparing the bowel for diagnostic testing.

Nursing Responsibilities
- Assess for potential contraindications to these laxatives, including abdominal pain and cramping, nausea and vomiting, anal or rectal fissures.
- Administer on an empty stomach to minimize the effects of food on its dissolution and absorption.
- Do not crush enteric-coated bisacodyl tablets or administer with alkaline products. This may hasten their dissolution in the stomach, leading to gastric distress.

Health Education for the Client and Family
- Discourage the use of this type of laxative, even in over-the-counter preparations, for the initial or continuing relief of constipation.
- Do not use the laxative for more than 1 week; chronic use can be habit forming and may suppress normal bowel reflexes.
- These laxatives are excreted in breast milk and should not be used by lactating women.

(continued)

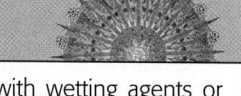

MEDICATION ADMINISTRATION   Laxatives and Cathartics (continued)

- Phenolphthalein-containing products may discolor the urine pink or red. Report possible hypersensitivity manifestations, such as difficulty breathing, dizziness or light-headedness, or skin rashes, to the primary care provider, and stop taking the medication.

LUBRICANTS
Mineral oil
Mineral oil is the only lubricant laxative available. It acts by forming an oily coat on the fecal mass, preventing the reabsorption of water, and resulting in softer stool. Problems associated with the use of mineral oil as a laxative include reduced absorption of the fat-soluble vitamins A, D, E, and K; possible damage to the liver and spleen due to systemic absorption; and potential pneumonitis from aspiration of oil droplets into the lungs.

Nursing Responsibilities
- Assess for possible contraindications to use of mineral oil, including advanced age, preexisting lung disease, and hemorrhoids or other rectal lesions.

- Do not give mineral oil concurrently with wetting agents or stool softeners, because these increase the potential for systemic absorption and increase the effects of the mineral oil.
- Administer mineral oil in the evening before bedtime to reduce the effect on the absorption of fat-soluble vitamins and minimize the risk of aspiration.
- Assess for manifestations of vitamin deficiency. Monitor the client taking oral anticoagulants for evidence of increased bleeding, such as bleeding gums, easy bruising, or melena.

Health Education for the Client and Family
- Long-term use of mineral oil is not recommended because of its risks and adverse effects.
- Do not use mineral oil if hemorrhoids or rectal lesions are present; leakage of the oil through the anal sphincter may cause itching and interfere with healing.
- Suck on a lemon or orange slice after taking oral mineral oil to reduce the oily aftertaste.

Constipation
Whether real or perceived, constipation is disruptive to the client's activities of daily living (ADLs) and life satisfaction.

- Monitor pattern of defecation and stool consistency. *This information helps establish the client's usual pattern of defecation and differentiate between actual and perceived constipation.*
- Provide additional fluids to maintain an intake of at least 2500 mL per day. *A generous fluid intake helps maintain soft stool consistency and promote intestinal motility.*
- Encourage drinking a glass of warm water before breakfast. Provide time and privacy following breakfast for bowel elimination. *This helps develop a pattern of natural elimination; the warm water provides mild stimulation of bowel peristalsis.*

- Consult with the dietitian to provide a diet high in natural fiber unless contraindicated. Provide foods such as natural bran, prunes, or prune juice. *Natural fiber adds bulk to the stool and has a mild stimulant effect.*
- Encourage activities such as ambulation or chair exercises (e.g., range of motion, stretching, wheelchair lifts) as tolerated. *Activity stimulates peristalsis and strengthens abdominal muscles, facilitating elimination.*
- If indicated, consult with primary care provider about the use of bulk laxatives, stool softeners, or other laxatives as needed. *Laxatives may be necessary to relieve acute constipation. Clients with long-term activity or diet restrictions or impaired abdominal muscle strength may need a bulk-forming laxative to maintain normal elimination patterns and prevent constipation.*

Community-Based Care
Include the following topics when teaching self-care measures to prevent and treat constipation:

- Increasing dietary fiber intake by including fresh fruits and vegetables, whole grains, high-fiber breakfast cereals, and unprocessed bran in the diet (Bran can be sprinkled on cereals, mixed into bread or muffin recipes, or mixed with fruit juice to increase its palatability.)
- Maintaining fluid intake of 6 to 8 glasses of water per day (unless contraindicated)
- Suggestions for remaining physically active to promote bowel function and maintain muscle tone
- Responding to the urge to defecate when perceived
- Appropriate use of laxatives:
  - Do not use laxatives, suppositories, or enemas on a regular basis.
  - Bulk-forming agents provide insoluble fiber, and are safe for long-term use; it is important to drink at least 6 to 8 glasses of water daily when using these (or any) laxatives.

- Other laxatives such as milk of magnesia, docusate (Colace, DSS), bisacodyl (Dulcolax), cascara, or castor oil should be used only occasionally to relieve constipation.
- Reporting any change in bowel habits such as new or persistent constipation or diarrhea, abdominal pain, black or bloody stools, nausea or anorexia, weakness, or unexplained weight loss to the primary care provider.

THE CLIENT WITH IRRITABLE BOWEL SYNDROME

Irritable bowel syndrome (IBS), also known as spastic bowel or functional colitis, is a motility disorder of the lower GI tract. It is a functional disorder with no identifiable organic cause. IBS is often characterized by abdominal pain with constipation, diarrhea, or both.

Irritable bowel syndrome is common, affecting up to 20% of people in Western civilization. It usually affects young people, although it may also occur in older adults. Reduced pain perception is offered as one explanation for lower diagnosis in older adults (Ehrenpreis, 2005). There is a higher prevalence of IBS in women than in men (Hungin et al., 2005).

Pathophysiology

In IBS, it appears that CNS regulation of the motor and sensory functions of the bowel is altered. Clients with IBS often experience increased motor reactivity of the small bowel and colon in response to stimuli such as food intake, hormonal influences, and physiologic or psychologic stress. IBS is characterized by visceral hypersensitivity and hyperactivity of the GI tract. Hypersecretion of colonic mucus is a common feature of the syndrome.

A lower visceral pain threshold is often found in clients with IBS. Clients may complain of pain, bloating, and distention when intestinal gas levels are normal.

Psychologic factors such as depression or anxiety have been linked to IBS; however, they have not been identified as causes of the disorder. Clients may respond to counseling or stress management techniques; however, it is important to emphasize that these methods are designed to cope with a chronic uncomfortable condition and do not suggest a psychiatric illness (Kupecz & Beradinelli, 2003). Recent research does indicate a correlation between emotional, physical, and sexual abuse and IBS.

Manifestations

Irritable bowel syndrome is characterized by abdominal pain that often is relieved by defecation and a change in bowel habits (see the Manifestations box on this page). The pain may be either colicky, occurring in spasms, or dull and continuous. Altered patterns of defecation may include:

- A change in frequency
- Abnormal stool form (hard or lumpy, loose or watery)
- Altered stool passage (straining, urgency, or a sensation of incomplete evacuation)
- Passage of mucous.

The client may also complain of abdominal bloating and excess gas. Other manifestations include nausea, vomiting, and anorexia;

MANIFESTATIONS of Irritable Bowel Syndrome

- Abdominal pain
  - May be relieved by defecation
  - May be intermittent and colicky or dull and continuous
- Altered bowel elimination
  - Constipation
  - Diarrhea
  - Mucous stools
- Abdominal bloating and flatulence
- Abdominal tenderness, especially over sigmoid colon
- Possible nausea, vomiting

fatigue, headache, depression, or anxiety. The abdomen is often tender to palpation, particularly over the sigmoid colon.

INTERDISCIPLINARY CARE

Irritable bowel syndrome is diagnosed based on the presence of abdominal pain or discomfort that has two of the following three characteristics: (1) relieved by defecation; (2) associated with a change in frequency of elimination; (3) associated with a change in stool form (Tierney et al., 2005). Management is directed toward relieving manifestations and reducing or eliminating precipitating factors. Stress reduction measures, exercises, or dietary education may benefit the client.

Diagnosis

The primary purpose of diagnostic testing is to rule out other causes of abdominal pain and altered fecal elimination. The stools may be examined for occult blood, ova and parasites, and WBCs. A sigmoidoscopy, colonoscopy, and/or a small-bowel series (upper GI series with small-bowel follow-through) and barium enema may be performed to visually examine the bowel mucosa, measure intraluminal pressures, and biopsy suspicious lesions. Nursing care for these procedures is outlined in Chapter 25 ∞. Laboratory tests include a complete blood count (CBC) with differential and erythrocyte sedimentation rate to evaluate for anemia from bleeding or a possible tumor. Increased WBCs indicate a bacterial infection.

Medications

Although not curative, medications may be prescribed to manage the manifestations of IBS. Bulk-forming laxatives (such as bran, methylcellulose, or psyllium) may help reduce bowel spasm and normalize the number and form of bowel movements. An anticholinergic drug such as dicyclomine (Antispas, Bentyl) or hyoscyamine (Anaspaz) may be ordered to inhibit bowel motility by interfering with parasympathetic stimulation of the gastrointestinal tract. It relieves postprandial abdominal pain when given 30 to 60 minutes before meals. In clients with diarrhea, loperamide (Imodium) or diphenoxylate (Lomotil) may be used prophylactically to prevent diarrhea in selected situations. Tegaserod mesylate (Zelnorm) is a 5-HT$_4$-receptor agonist that is used for short-term treatment of IBS when the primary manifestation is constipation. It increases the number of bowel movements and facilitates stool formation.

Antidepressant drugs, including tricyclics and selective serotonin reuptake inhibitors (SSRIs), may help relieve abdominal pain associated with IBS. Although the anticholinergic side effects of the tricyclics (such as desipramine [Norpramin] and imipramine [Tofranil]) may help decrease diarrhea, they have more adverse effects than SSRIs such as sertraline (Zoloft) and fluoxetine (Prozac).

Nutrition

Many clients with IBS benefit from additional dietary fiber. Adding bran to meals provides added bulk and water content to the stool, reducing the incidence of both loose diarrheal stools and hard, constipated stools. Other dietary changes are specific to individual triggers for IBS manifestations. Some clients may benefit from limiting lactose, fructose, or sorbitol intake (see Table 26–1). When excess gas and flatulence are problems, reducing the intake of gas-forming foods, such as beans, cabbage, apple and grape juices, nuts, and raisins, may be helpful. Caffeinated drinks, such as coffee, tea, and soft drinks, act as gastrointestinal stimulants; limiting intake of these fluids may also prove beneficial.

Complementary and Alternative Therapies

Herbal preparations may provide some benefit for clients with IBS. Herbs with an antispasmodic effect, such as anise, chamomile, peppermint, and sage, may be used to reduce the manifestations of IBS. Ginger root can also be consumed as a tea or capsule to assist with reduction of gas, bloating, and diarrhea and to improve the functioning of the stomach (Balch & Stengler, 2004).

NURSING CARE

Clients with irritable bowel syndrome rarely require acute care for IBS as a primary problem. However, nurses frequently interact with these clients in clinics and other community settings.

Assessment

Careful assessment is important to help identify the effects of IBS on the client. Collect the following assessment data:

- *Health history:* Current manifestations, their onset and duration; current treatment measures; effect of manifestations on lifestyle; careful exploration of history of emotional, physical, or sexual abuse.
- *Physical examination:* Apparent general state of health; abdominal shape and contour, bowel sounds, tenderness.

Nursing Diagnoses and Interventions

The primary nursing responsibility is education; providing referrals and counseling are additional nursing responsibilities to clients who have irritable bowel syndrome. See the previous sections on diarrhea and constipation for selected nursing interventions.

Community-Based Care

Include the following topics in teaching for the client with irritable bowel syndrome:

- The nature of the disorder and the reality of the client's manifestations
- The relationship between IBS and stress, anxiety, and depression
- Stress and anxiety reduction techniques, such as meditation, visualization, exercise, "time-out," and progressive relaxation
- Dietary influences that may contribute to IBS and suggested dietary changes, such as additional fiber and water intake
- The use and role of prescribed medications, their adverse effects, and when to contact the physician
- The importance of routine follow-up appointments and of notifying the primary care provider if manifestations change (such as blood in the stool, significant constipation or diarrhea, increasing abdominal pain, or weight loss).

If needed, refer the client to a counselor or other mental health professional for assistance in dealing with psychologic factors.

THE CLIENT WITH FECAL INCONTINENCE

Fecal incontinence, the loss of voluntary control of defecation, occurs less frequently than urinary incontinence but is no less distressing to the client. Multiple factors contribute to fecal incontinence, including both physiologic and psychologic conditions (Box 26–1). Bowel incontinence is usually considered a manifestation of a disorder rather than a disorder unto itself. Clients often do not reveal fecal incontinence in discussing health concerns. Little information is available about its incidence and prevalence. Because many of the etiologic factors

---

BOX 26–1 Selected Causes of Fecal Incontinence

Neurologic Causes
- Spinal cord injury or disease
- Head injury, stroke, or brain tumor
- Degenerative neurologic disease, such as multiple sclerosis, amyotrophic lateral sclerosis (ALS), dementia
- Diabetic neuropathy

Local Trauma
- Obstetric tears
- Anorectal injury
- Anorectal surgery with sphincter damage

Inflammatory Processes
- Infection
- Radiation

Other Physiologic Causes
- Diarrhea
- Stool impaction
- Pelvic floor relaxation or loss of sphincter tone
- Tumors

Psychologic Causes
- Depression
- Confusion and disorientation

are more prevalent in the older adult, older clients are more often affected (see the Nursing Research box below).

Pathophysiology

To understand the pathophysiology of fecal incontinence, it is necessary to understand the normal mechanisms of defecation. The rectum is normally empty. When it is distended by feces entering from the sigmoid colon, the defecation reflex is stimulated. This reflex causes involuntary relaxation of the internal sphincter and stimulates the urge to defecate. When the external sphincter, which is under both somatic (voluntary) and autonomic (involuntary) control, relaxes, defecation occurs. Adults normally can override the defecation reflex by voluntary contraction of the external sphincter and pelvic floor muscles. The wall of the rectum gradually relaxes, and the urge to defecate subsides.

The most common causes of fecal incontinence are those that interfere with either sensory or motor control of the rectum and anal sphincters. If the external sphincter is paralyzed as a result of spinal cord injury or disease, defecation occurs automatically when the internal sphincter relaxes with the defecation reflex. If sphincter muscles have been damaged or excessive pelvic floor relaxation has occurred, it may not be possible to override the defecation reflex with voluntary control.

Age-related changes in anal sphincter tone and response to rectal distention increase the risk for fecal incontinence in older adults. Resting and maximal anal sphincter pressures are decreased, particularly in older women. In addition, less rectal distension is needed to produce sustained relaxation of the anal sphincter in older females.

INTERDISCIPLINARY CARE

The diagnosis of fecal incontinence is based on the client's history. Physical examination of the pelvic floor and anus is performed to evaluate muscle tone and rule out a fecal impaction. Impaired sphincter muscle may be palpable on digital exam. Anorectal manometry or a rectal motility test may be used to evaluate the functional ability of the sphincter muscles. In this test, a small, flexible balloon catheter is introduced into the rectum, and pressures are measured in the rectum and internal and external sphincters. Normally, rectal dilation causes the internal sphincter to relax and the external sphincter to contract. Sigmoidoscopy also may be used to examine the rectum and anal canal.

Management of fecal incontinence is directed toward the identified cause. Medications to relieve diarrhea or constipation may be prescribed. A high-fiber diet, ample fluids, and regular exercise are helpful for many clients. Exercises to improve sphincter and pelvic floor muscle tone (Kegel exercises) may be of long-term benefit. See Chapter 28 ∞ for more information about Kegel exercises.

Clients also may benefit from using loperamide before meals and prophylactically before running errands or leaving the house (Tierney et al., 2005). Biofeedback therapy may be used for

---

NURSING RESEARCH | **Evidence-Based Practice: Fecal Incontinence**

When fecal incontinence occurs at any age, it is highly distressing to the individual. Little is known about how older adults living in the community manage this problem in their daily lives. This study was conducted to survey older men and women about self-care practices and factors that affected both the number of self-care practices and the reporting of fecal incontinence to healthcare providers (Bliss et al., 2005).

Of the 1352 subjects, 18% had fecal incontinence several times a year or more. These men and women used one or more self-care practices. The practices most commonly used were changing diet (such as avoiding certain foods); wearing a sanitary panty liner, pad, or brief; and reducing activity or exercise. The type of practice used depended on the severity of the incontinence. For example, those who soiled their outer clothing were more likely to change their diet than those who soiled only their undergarments. Women were more likely to use self-care methods than were men, and less than half of the subjects reported the problem to their healthcare provider.

IMPLICATIONS FOR NURSING
The major implication of the findings from this study is that nurses who care for older adults living in the community need to include questions about the occurrence of fecal incontinence when conducting a health history and physical assessment. In most in-

stances, the older adult will not voluntarily report this problem because it is considered embarrassing. If fecal incontinence is identified, further questions should be asked about self-care measures, including sanitary pads or briefs, diet and exercise, and use of antidiarrheal medications. Education should be carried out to assure older adults that incontinence of any type (urinary or fecal) is not an inevitable part of aging, but may rather be an indication of some other health problem. In addition, evaluation of the older adult's ability to carry out self-care measures if indicated is an important component of nursing care.

CRITICAL THINKING IN CLIENT CARE
1. Although you observe evidence of fecal incontinence when providing home care to an elderly man, he denies this problem when you ask about it. What would you do next?
2. Fecal incontinence often results in skin irritation and discomfort around the rectum. What would you recommend if a client asks you how to relieve this problem?
3. One of your home care clients is an 85-year-old woman, living on a small and limited income. She has fecal incontinence, and says to you, "I don't know what to do about this. I am so embarrassed. I guess I just need to go to a nursing home and let them keep me clean." How would you respond? What type of referrals might you make?

mentally alert clients with intact sphincter muscles but low muscle tone. With motivation and reinforcement, clients achieve improved sphincter control in response to a stimulus. The goal of biofeedback is to improve sensation, coordination, and strength of the sphincter muscle (Halverson, 2005).

When damage to the sphincter or rectal prolapse (protrusion of rectal mucous membrane through the anus) is the cause of fecal incontinence, surgical repair is the treatment of choice. Surgery may also be indicated when conservative measures have not been effective. Permanent colostomy, the creation of an opening from the large bowel on the abdominal wall, is a last choice option for some clients, but it can control fecal output when other measures fail.

 NURSING CARE

Health Promotion

A bowel training program to establish a regular pattern of elimination often is effective in relieving fecal incontinence. Teach the client to establish a regular time of day for elimination, usually 15 to 30 minutes after breakfast. A stimulant, such as a cup of coffee, a rectal suppository, or even a phosphate enema, may be given to prompt defecation. Clients with neurologic incontinence may learn to stimulate the anal canal digitally to initiate defecation.

Dietary changes may be useful in managing fecal incontinence. If incontinence occurs only with mild loose or liquid stools, increasing dietary fiber or using a bulking agent to increase stool bulk and solidity may be effective. The majority of the fiber should come from a fiber-rich diet because fiber supplements provide only a limited amount of additional fiber (Halverson, 2005). When incontinence of solid stool occurs, a low-residue diet of foods that are easily digested and absorbed may be prescribed to reduce the frequency of defecation.

Assessment

- *Health history:* Extent, onset, and duration of incontinence; identified contributing factors; history of spinal cord or anorectal injury or surgery; chronic diseases such as diabetes, multiple sclerosis, or other neurologic disorders.
- *Physical examination:* Mental status; general health; examination of perianal tissues; digital rectal examination.

Nursing Diagnoses and Interventions
Bowel Incontinence

Nurses are often responsible for instituting bowel training programs and other measures to manage fecal incontinence.

- Teach caregivers to place the client on a toilet or commode and provide for privacy at a certain time of day. *Placing the client in a normal position to defecate at a consistent time of day stimulates the defecation reflex and helps reestablish a pattern of stool evacuation.*
- If necessary, insert a glycerin or bisacodyl (Dulcolax) suppository 15 to 20 minutes before positioning on the toilet or commode. *This helps to stimulate evacuation. Once a regular elimination pattern is established, it may be possible to discontinue suppository use.*

- Maintain a caring, nonjudgmental manner in providing care. *This promotes a feeling of acceptance when the client may feel unacceptable.*

> **PRACTICE ALERT**
> Provide room odor control with deodorizer tablets, sprays, or other devices. Controlling odor is important to preserve the client's self-esteem.

Risk for Impaired Skin Integrity

Good skin care is vital for the client with fecal incontinence. Stool contains enzymes and other irritating substances that promote skin breakdown when they are not promptly removed. This can lead to pressure ulcers, particularly when a neurologic disorder (such as spinal cord injury, dementia, or stroke) impairs mobility.

- Clean the skin thoroughly with mild soap and water after each bowel movement. *Toilet tissue may be more irritating to the skin and less effective in removing fecal material.*
- Apply a skin barrier cream or ointment after each bowel movement. *These help protect the skin from irritating substances in the feces.*
- If incontinence pads or briefs are used, check frequently for soiling and change when feces is noted. *Although these help protect bedding and clothing from soiling, they can contribute to skin breakdown if they are not checked and changed frequently.*

Community-Based Care

Managing fecal incontinence is a challenging problem for the client and family caregivers. For the client with intact cognition, it can be psychologically devastating. The client may become socially isolated from fear of odor or soiling clothing. Self-esteem may suffer from a sense of lost control over body functions and the inability to provide self-care. It is important to stress that incontinence is never normal (i.e., aging alone is not a cause of incontinence) and often is treatable. Encourage the client to seek medical evaluation of the problem.

Topics of client and family education include:

- Recommended dietary measures such as consuming a high-fiber diet and ample fluids to maintain soft, formed stool, or a low-residue diet to reduce the number of stools.
- Suggestions for regular exercise to stimulate bowel peristalsis and regular evacuation.
- Use of bulk-forming laxatives, such as psyllium seed (Metamucil), to provide stool bulk and reduce the number of small, liquid stools.
- Prescribed medications (such as loperamide to reduce the number of stools), their appropriate use, and management of adverse effects (such as constipation).
- Bowel training program instructions, including techniques for digital anal stimulation, inserting suppositories, or administering enemas as recommended. For digital anal simulation, teach to insert a lubricated gloved finger through the anal sphincter into the rectum 1.5 to 2 inches while seated on the toilet or

commode, then use a circular side-to-side movement to gently stretch the rectal wall until the internal sphincter relaxes.
■ The importance of good skin care, particularly if neurologic impairment is present.

■ The potential benefits and associated risks of biofeedback and surgical treatment, if recommended.
■ Provide referrals for home care or community health services as indicated.

ACUTE INFLAMMATORY AND INFECTIOUS BOWEL DISORDERS

The GI tract is particularly vulnerable to inflammation and infection because of its continual exposure to the external environment. Although most pathogens affecting the GI tract are ingested in food or water, infection also may be spread by direct contact, possibly by the respiratory route. Pathogens may also be transmitted sexually through anal intercourse.

Acute disease of the GI tract may be caused by the pathogen itself or by a bacterial or other toxin. Acute inflammatory disorders such as appendicitis and peritonitis result from contamination of damaged or normally sterile tissue by the client's own endogenous or resident bacteria.

THE CLIENT WITH APPENDICITIS

Appendicitis, inflammation of the vermiform appendix, is a common cause of acute abdominal pain. It is the most common reason for emergency abdominal surgery, affecting 10% of the population (Tierney et al., 2005). Appendicitis can occur at any age, but is more common in adolescents and young adults and slightly more common in males than females.

Pathophysiology

The appendix is a tubelike pouch attached to the cecum just below the ileocecal valve. It is usually located in the right iliac region, at an area designated as McBurney's point (Figure 26–1A ■). The function of the appendix is not fully understood, although it regularly fills with and empties digested food.

Obstruction of the proximal lumen of the appendix is apparent in most acutely inflamed appendices. The obstruction is often caused by a *fecalith*, or hard mass of feces. Other obstructive causes include a calculus or stone, a foreign body, inflammation, a tumor, parasites (e.g., pinworms), or edema of lymphoid tissue. Following obstruction, the appendix becomes distended with fluid secreted by its mucosa. Pressure within the lumen of the appendix increases, impairing its blood supply and leading to inflammation, edema, ulceration, and infection. Purulent exudate forms, further distending the appendix. Within 24 to 36 hours, tissue necrosis and gangrene result, leading to perforation if treatment is not initiated. Perforation results in bacterial peritonitis.

Appendicitis can be classified as simple, gangrenous, or perforated, depending on the stage of the process. In *simple appendicitis,* the appendix is inflamed but intact. When areas of tissue necrosis and microscopic perforations are present in the appendix, the disorder is called gangrenous appendicitis. A perforated appendix shows evidence of gross perforation and contamination of the peritoneal cavity.

Manifestations

Continuous mild generalized or upper abdominal pain is the initial characteristic manifestation of acute appendicitis. Over

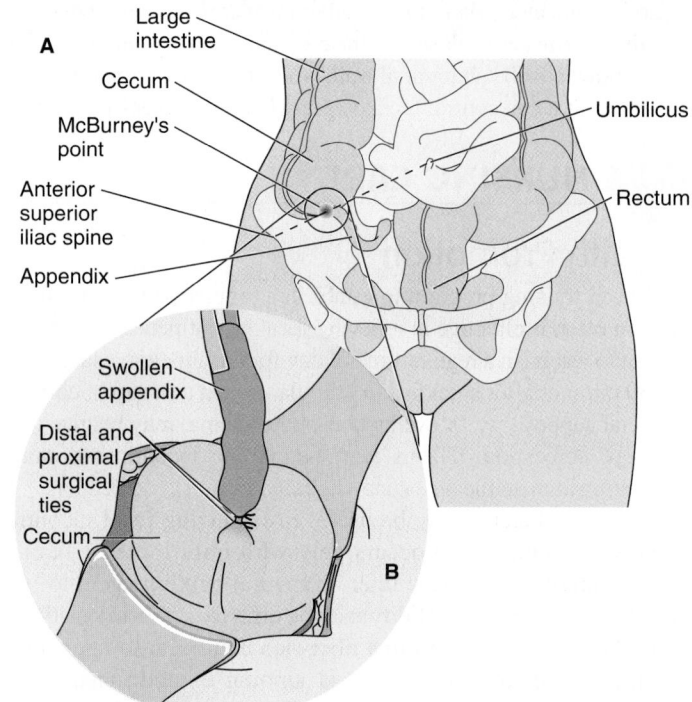

Figure 26–1 ■ *A,* McBurney's point, located midway between the umbilicus and the anterior iliac crest in the right lower quadrant. It is the usual site for localized pain and rebound tenderness due to appendicitis. *B,* In an appendectomy, the appendix and cecum are brought through the incision to the surface of the abdomen. The base of the appendix is clamped and ligated; the appendix is then removed.

the next 4 hours, the pain intensifies and localizes in the right lower quadrant of the abdomen. It is aggravated by moving, walking, or coughing. On palpation, localized and rebound tenderness are noted at McBurney's point. Rebound tenderness is demonstrated by relief of pain with direct palpation of McBurney's point followed by pain on release of pressure. Extension or internal rotation of the right hip increases the pain. In addition to pain, a low-grade temperature, anorexia, nausea, and vomiting are often present.

Pain and local tenderness may be less acute in older adults, delaying the diagnosis, and leading to a 15% mortality of perforated appendicitis in the older adult (Tierney et al., 2005). This can present a significant problem; the course of acute appendicitis in older adults is more virulent and complications develop sooner. Pregnant women may develop right lower quadrant, periumbilical, or right subcostal (under the rib cage) pain due to possible displacement of the appendix by the distended uterus.

Complications

Perforation, peritonitis, and abscess are possible complications of acute appendicitis. Perforation is manifested by increased pain and a high fever. It can lead to a small, localized abscess, local peritonitis, or significant generalized peritonitis. (Peritonitis is discussed in the next section of this chapter.)

A less common disorder is chronic appendicitis, characterized by chronic abdominal pain and recurrent acute attacks at intervals of several months or more. Other conditions, such as inflammatory bowel disease and renal disorders, often cause manifestations attributed to chronic appendicitis.

INTERDISCIPLINARY CARE

The acutely inflamed appendix can perforate within 24 hours, so rapid diagnosis and treatment are important. Because of this urgency and the low incidence of surgical complications, diagnostic testing and preoperative treatment are limited. The client is admitted to the hospital, and intravenous fluids are initiated. Oral food and fluids are withheld until a diagnosis is confirmed. Once the diagnosis is established, an appendectomy is performed.

Diagnosis

Diagnostic and laboratory tests are used to help confirm the diagnosis and rule out other possible causes for the manifestations. Abdominal ultrasound is the most effective test for diagnosing acute appendicitis. Ultrasound examination has reduced the incidence of exploratory surgery and is particularly useful with clients with atypical symptoms, such as older adults. Other diagnostic tests used to accurately diagnose appendicitis include abdominal x-rays, an intravenous pyelogram, a urinalysis, and a pelvic examination. In addition, a WBC count with differential is obtained. With appendicitis, the total white count is elevated (10,000 to 20,000/mm³), with an increased number of immature WBC (bands).

Medications

Prior to surgery, intravenous fluids are given to restore or maintain vascular volume and prevent electrolyte imbalance. Antibiotic therapy with a third-generation cephalosporin effective against many gram-negative bacteria, such as cefoperazone (Cefobid), cefotaxime (Claforan), ceftazidime (Fortaz), or ceftriaxone (Rocephin), is initiated prior to surgery. The antibiotic is repeated during surgery and continued for at least 48 hours postoperatively. (The nursing implications for cephalosporin antibiotics are discussed in Chapter 12 ∞.) Pain medications are administered as prescribed.

Surgery

The treatment of choice for acute appendicitis is an *appendectomy*, surgical removal of the appendix. Either a laparoscopic approach (insertion of an endoscope to view abdominal contents) or laparotomy (surgical opening of the abdomen) may be used for appendectomy. Laparoscopic appendectomy requires a very small incision through which the laparoscope is inserted. This procedure has several advantages: (1) Direct visualization of the appendix allows definitive diagnosis without laparotomy; (2) postoperative hospitalization is short; (3) postoperative complications are infrequent; and (4) recovery and resumption of normal activities is rapid.

An open appendectomy is performed by laparotomy. A small transverse incision is made at McBurney's point (Figure 26–1A); the appendix is isolated and ligated (tied off) to prevent contamination of the site with bowel contents, and then removed (Figure 26–1B). Laparotomy generally is used when the appendix has ruptured. It allows removal of contaminants from the peritoneal cavity by irrigation with sterile normal saline. Occasionally the wound may be left unsutured for periodic irrigation. Recovery is generally uneventful. Refer to Chapter 4 ∞ for discussion of preoperative and postoperative nursing care.

NURSING CARE

A Nursing Care Plan for a client with appendicitis is included on page 768.

Assessment

Because appendicitis can rapidly progress from inflammation to perforation, prompt assessment is vital. Obtain the following assessment data:

- *Health history:* Current manifestations, including onset, duration, progression, and aggravating or relieving factors; most recent food or fluid intake; known medication or other allergies; current medications; history of chronic diseases.
- *Physical examination:* Vital signs including temperature; apparent general health; abdominal shape and contour, bowel sounds, tenderness to light palpation.

Nursing Diagnoses and Interventions

Preoperative nursing care is directed toward preparing the client physically and psychologically for emergency surgery. Limited time is available for preoperative teaching.

> **PRACTICE ALERT**
> Keep the client with suspected appendicitis NPO, and do not administer laxatives or enemas, which may cause perforation of the appendix. No heat should be applied to the abdomen; this may increase circulation to the appendix and also cause perforation.

Risk for Infection

Preventing complications during the preoperative and postoperative periods is a primary nursing care goal. Perforation and peritonitis are the most likely preoperative complications; postoperative complications include wound infection, abscess, and possible peritonitis.

> **PRACTICE ALERT**
> Assess abdominal status frequently, including distention, bowel sounds, and tenderness. Increasing generalized pain, a rigid, boardlike abdomen, and abdominal distention may indicate developing peritonitis.

NURSING CARE PLAN A Client with Acute Appendicitis

Jamie Lynn is a 19-year-old college student majoring in physical therapy. Ms. Lynn arrives at the emergency department at 1:00 A.M. complaining of general lower abdominal pain that had started the previous evening. By midnight, the pain was more localized over the right lower quadrant. She also reports nausea and vomiting.

ASSESSMENT

Sue Grady, RN, completes the admission assessment in the emergency department. Ms. Lynn is complaining of nausea and severe abdominal pain, stating, "Walking makes my stomach hurt worse." Physical assessment findings include T 100.2°F (37.8°C), P 84, R 16, and BP 110/70; skin warm to touch; abdomen flat and guarded, with marked tenderness in right lower quadrant. Ms. Lynn's CBC shows WBC 14,000/mm³; neutrophils 81.1%; lymphocytes 12.5%. The diagnosis of acute appendicitis is made, and Ms. Lynn is transferred to surgery for a laparoscopic appendectomy.

DIAGNOSES

- *Impaired Skin Integrity* related to surgical incision
- *Acute Pain* related to surgical intervention
- *Anxiety* related to situational crisis

EXPECTED OUTCOMES

- Incision will heal without infection or complications.
- Will verbalize adequate pain relief.
- Will verbalize decreased anxiety.
- Will return to preoperative activities.

PLANNING AND IMPLEMENTATION

- Assess pain using a pain scale; provide analgesics as needed.
- Teach pain management following discharge.
- Teach abdominal splinting during coughing, turning, or ambulating as needed.
- Teach home care of incision.
- Discuss activity limitations as ordered.
- Instruct to report fever or warmth, redness, or drainage from the incision.

EVALUATION

On discharge the following evening, Ms. Lynn is fully ambulatory. Her appetite has returned, and she is tolerating food and fluids well. Her temperature is normal. The nurse provides Ms. Lynn with written and verbal information on postoperative care following an appendectomy.

CRITICAL THINKING IN THE NURSING PROCESS

1. What is the pathophysiologic basis for Ms. Lynn's elevated WBC?
2. How would Ms. Lynn's postoperative care and teaching differ if she had undergone a laparotomy instead of a laparoscopic appendectomy?
3. Outline a teaching plan to give to clients for home care following an appendectomy.
4. Develop a care plan for Ms. Lynn for the nursing diagnosis, *Anxiety* related to a situational crisis.
   See Evaluating Your Response in Appendix C.

- Monitor vital signs, including temperature. *Tachycardia and rapid shallow respirations may indicate perforation of the appendix with resulting peritonitis. Fever may develop as well, and the blood pressure may fall if sepsis is present.*
- Maintain intravenous infusion until oral intake is adequate. *Intravenous fluids are given to maintain vascular volume and to provide a route for antibiotic administration.*
- Assess wound, abdominal girth, and postoperative pain. *Swelling of the wound, increased abdominal girth, or an increase in pain may indicate infection or peritonitis.*

Acute Pain

The client with appendicitis experiences pain before and after surgery. Analgesia is limited until the diagnosis is established. Postoperative pain is controlled by narcotic or nonnarcotic analgesics.

- Assess pain, including its character, location, severity, and duration. Report any unexpected changes in the nature of pain. *Both preoperatively and postoperatively, the client's pain provides important clues about the diagnosis and possible complications such as rupture of the appendix or peritonitis.*

PRACTICE ALERT

Sudden relief of preoperative pain may signal rupture of the distended and edematous appendix.

- Administer analgesics as ordered. *Preoperatively, pain medication can be given after a diagnosis is established. Postoperatively, provide analgesics to maintain comfort and enhance mobility.*
- Assess effectiveness of medication 30 minutes after administration. Report unrelieved pain. *Pain unrelieved by prescribed analgesic may indicate a complication or the need for further assessment. For example, continued abdominal discomfort and distention may indicate excess intestinal gas that may be better relieved by ambulation.*

Using NANDA, NIC, and NOC

Chart 26–2 shows links between NANDA nursing diagnoses, NIC, and NOC for the client with appendicitis.

Community-Based Care

Preoperative teaching may be limited by pain and the emergent nature of surgery. Explain why food and fluids are not permitted during this time. If time allows, teach postoperative turning, coughing, deep breathing, and pain management.

With uncomplicated appendectomy, the client often is discharged either the day of surgery or the day following surgery. Postoperative teaching includes:

- Wound or incision care, including hand washing and dressing change procedures as indicated

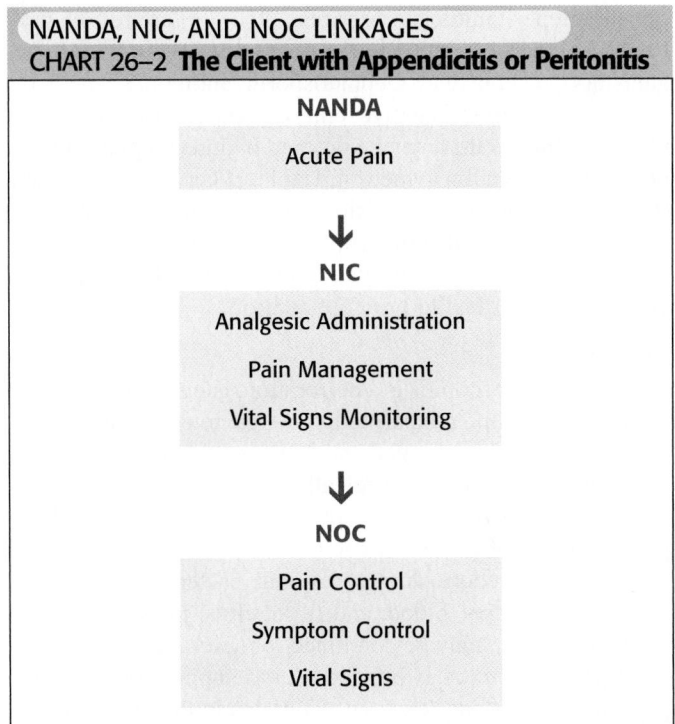

- Instructions to report fever, increased abdominal pain, swelling, redness, drainage, bleeding, or warmth of the operative site to the physician
- Activity limitations (e.g., lifting, driving), if any
- Returning to work if appropriate.

THE CLIENT WITH PERITONITIS

Peritonitis, inflammation of the peritoneum, is a serious complication of many acute abdominal disorders. It is usually caused by enteric bacteria entering the peritoneal cavity through a perforated ulcer, ruptured appendix, perforated diverticulum (discussed later in this chapter), necrotic bowel, or during abdominal surgery. Pelvic inflammatory disease, gallbladder rupture, abdominal trauma, or peritoneal dialysis can also lead to peritonitis.

Pathophysiology

The peritoneum is a double-layered serous membrane lining the walls (parietal peritoneum) and organs (visceral peritoneum) of the abdominal cavity. There is a potential space between the parietal and visceral layers of the peritoneum that contains a small amount of serous fluid. This space, the peritoneal cavity, normally is sterile.

Peritonitis results from contamination of the normally sterile peritoneal cavity by infection or a chemical irritant. Chemical peritonitis often precedes bacterial peritonitis. Perforation of a peptic ulcer or rupture of the gallbladder releases gastric juices (hydrochloric acid and pepsin) or bile into the peritoneal cavity, causing an acute inflammatory response.

Bacterial peritonitis usually is caused by infection by *Escherichia coli, Klebsiella, Proteus,* or *Pseudomonas* bacteria, which normally inhabit the bowel. Inflammatory and immune defense mechanisms are activated when bacteria enter the peritoneal space. These defenses can effectively eliminate small numbers of bacteria, but may be overwhelmed by massive or continued contamination. When this occurs, mast cells release histamine and other vasoactive substances, causing local vasodilation and increased capillary permeability. Polymorphonuclear leukocytes (a type of WBC) infiltrate the peritoneum to phagocytize bacteria and foreign matter. Fibrinogen-rich plasma exudate promotes bacterial destruction and forms fibrin clots to seal off and segregate the bacteria. This process helps limit and localize the infection, allowing host defenses to eradicate it. Continued contamination, however, leads to generalized inflammation of the peritoneal cavity. The inflammatory process causes fluid to shift into the peritoneal space (third spacing). Circulating blood volume is depleted, leading to hypovolemia. *Septicemia,* a systemic disease caused by pathogens or their toxins in the blood, may follow.

Manifestations

Manifestations of peritonitis depend on the severity and extent of the infection, as well as the age and general health of the client. Both local and systemic manifestations are present (see the box below). The client often presents with evidence of an *acute abdomen,* an abrupt onset of diffuse, severe abdominal pain. The pain may localize and intensify near the area of infection. Movement may intensify the pain. The entire abdomen is tender, with guarding or rigidity of abdominal muscles. The acute abdomen is often described as boardlike. Rebound tenderness may be present over the area of inflammation. Peritoneal inflammation inhibits peristalsis, resulting in a paralytic ileus. (Paralytic ileus is discussed in a later section of this chapter.) Bowel sounds are

---

MANIFESTATIONS of Peritonitis

Abdominal/Gastrointestinal Manifestations
- Diffuse or localized pain
- Tenderness with rebound
- Boardlike rigidity
- Diminished or absent bowel sounds
- Distention
- Anorexia, nausea, and vomiting

Systemic Manifestations
- Fever
- Malaise
- Tachycardia
- Tachypnea
- Restlessness
- Confusion or disorientation
- Oliguria

markedly diminished or absent, and progressive abdominal distention is noted. Pooling of GI secretions may cause nausea and vomiting. Systemic manifestations of peritonitis include fever, malaise, tachycardia and tachypnea, restlessness, and possible disorientation. The client may be oliguric (having little urine output) and show signs of dehydration and shock.

The older, chronically debilitated, or immunosuppressed client may present with few of the classic signs of peritonitis. Increased confusion and restlessness, decreased urinary output, and vague abdominal complaints may be the only manifestations present. These clients are at increased risk for delayed diagnosis, contributing to a higher mortality rate.

Complications

Complications of peritonitis may be life threatening. Abscess formation is common. The very defense mechanisms designed to isolate and localize the infection can protect it from immune responses and systemic antibiotics. Fibrous adhesions in the abdominal cavity are a late complication and may lead to subsequent obstruction.

Without prompt and effective treatment, septicemia and septic shock can develop. Fluid loss into the abdominal cavity may also lead to hypovolemic shock. These potentially lethal complications require immediate, aggressive intervention to prevent multiple organ failure and death. Shock and its management are discussed in Chapter 11 ∞.

FAST FACTS
Mortality from Peritonitis
- The overall mortality rate associated with peritonitis is about 40%.
- Clients with other medical conditions, older clients, and those with greater bacterial contamination have a higher risk of dying.
- Young people with perforated ulcers or appendicitis, those with less extensive bacterial contamination, and those who receive early surgical intervention have mortality rates of less than 10%.

INTERDISCIPLINARY CARE

Care of the client with peritonitis focuses on establishing the diagnosis and identifying and treating its cause as well as the peritonitis. Preventing complications is an important aspect of care.

Diagnosis

Diagnostic tests are performed to establish the diagnosis of peritonitis, rule out other disorders, and help identify the cause. The tests that may be ordered include a WBC count (elevated to approximately 20,000/mm^3 in peritonitis), blood cultures, abdominal x-rays, liver and renal function studies, serum electrolytes, and a paracentesis (in peritonitis, peritoneal fluid will contain increased protein and WBCs). Increased numbers of immature blood cells are present as the bone marrow releases them in response to the infection.

Medications

Until the infecting organism has been identified, a broad-spectrum antibiotic effective against organisms commonly im-

plicated in peritonitis is prescribed. Once culture results have been obtained, antibiotic therapy is modified to the specific organism(s) responsible. Cephalosporin antibiotics are often prescribed if gram-negative enteric bacteria are suspected. Other antibiotics that may be ordered include ampicillin (e.g., Omnipen, Polycillin), metronidazole (Flagyl), clindamycin (Cleocin), or an aminoglycoside antibiotic such as gentamicin (Garamycin) or amikacin (Amikin). Nursing implications for antibiotic therapy are discussed in Chapter 12 ∞. Analgesics are prescribed to promote comfort.

Surgery

If the cause of peritonitis is a perforation, gangrenous bowel, or inflamed appendix, a laparotomy is done to close the perforation or remove the damaged and inflamed tissue. If an abscess is present, it also may be surgically drained or removed.

Peritoneal lavage, washing of the peritoneal cavity with copious amounts of warm isotonic fluid, may be done during surgery. This procedure dilutes residual bacteria and removes gross contaminants, blood, and fibrin clots. In rare instances, peritoneal lavage may be continued for several days following surgery. The solution is infused into the upper portion of the peritoneal cavity and removed via drains in the pelvic cul-de-sac. Careful attention to fluid and electrolyte status and strict aseptic technique are necessary.

Clients who have had laparotomy for peritonitis often return from surgery with either Penrose or closed drain systems such as a Jackson-Pratt drain. In some cases, the incision may be left unsutured. With severe and long-standing peritonitis, the abdomen may be closed temporarily with polypropylene mesh containing a nylon zipper or Velcro to allow repeated exploration of the abdomen and drainage of infectious sites.

Nutrition

Intravenous fluids and electrolyte replacements are administered to maintain vascular volume and fluid and electrolyte balance. Parenteral nutrition is given until adequate oral intake resumes.

OTHER TREATMENTS The client is placed on bed rest in Fowler's position to help localize the infection and promote lung ventilation. Oxygen is often ordered to facilitate cellular metabolism and healing.

INTESTINAL DECOMPRESSION The inflammatory process of peritonitis often draws large amounts of fluid into the abdominal cavity and the bowel. In addition, peristaltic activity of the bowel is slowed or halted by the inflammation, causing **paralytic ileus** (or *ileus*), impaired propulsion or forward movement of bowel contents. Intestinal decompression is used to relieve abdominal distention, facilitate closure, and minimize postoperative respiratory problems. A nasogastric or long intestinal tube is inserted and connected to continuous drainage (Figure 26–2 ■). If prolonged intestinal decompression is anticipated, a jejunostomy may be performed for comfort. Suction is maintained until peristalsis resumes, bowel sounds are present, and the client is passing flatus. Food and fluids are withheld until intestinal motility has returned and suction is discontinued.

Weighted Balloon

Figure 26–2 ■ The weighted tip or inflated balloon at the end of an intestinal tube is drawn into the intestine by gravity and peristalsis.

NURSING CARE

Peritonitis is a serious illness. Early recognition and treatment are important to minimize the risk of complications.

Assessment

- *Health history:* Pain, its onset, character, severity, location, aggravating and relieving factors; associated symptoms such as anorexia, nausea, vomiting; current and previous history of peptic ulcer disease, gallbladder disease, chronic diseases; current medications.
- *Physical examination:* Vital signs including temperature; level of consciousness; skin color, temperature, warmth, capillary refill and turgor; abdominal shape, contour, bowel sounds, tenderness, tympany, and guarding.

Nursing Diagnoses and Interventions

Clients with peritonitis require intensive nursing and medical care to prevent complications and recover fully. Nursing care priorities include interventions to manage pain; altered fluid balance; altered protection due to infection; and anxiety.

Acute Pain

Abdominal distention and acute inflammation contribute to the pain associated with peritonitis. Surgery further disrupts abdominal muscles and other tissues, causing pain. Effective pain management promotes immune function, healing, mobility, and recovery.

- Assess pain, including its location, severity (using a standard pain scale), and type. Monitor analgesic effectiveness. Report changes to the primary care provider.

PRACTICE ALERT
Unrelieved pain or a change in the location, severity, or type of pain may indicate spread of infection, abscess formation, or other complications of peritonitis.

- Place in Fowler's or semi-Fowler's position with the knees and feet elevated. *This position reduces stress on abdominal structures and facilitates respirations, promoting comfort.*
- Administer analgesics as ordered on a routine basis or using patient-controlled analgesia (PCA). *Routine analgesic administration maintains a therapeutic blood level and helps maintain comfort, facilitating healing and movement.*
- Teach and assist with adjunctive pain management techniques such as meditation, visualization, massage, and progressive relaxation. *Adjunctive measures augment analgesics and help promote a sense of control over pain.*

Deficient Fluid Volume

In peritonitis, significant amounts of fluid are drawn into the abdominal cavity and bowel, reducing vascular volume and cardiac output. This fluid also may be lost from the body by intestinal suction or through drains placed in the abdomen during surgery. An unsutured incision causes additional significant fluid loss.

- Maintain accurate intake and output records. Measure urine output every 1 to 2 hours; report output of less than 30 mL/h. Measure gastrointestinal output at least every 4 hours. *Intake and output records provide valuable information about fluid volume status.*

PRACTICE ALERT
Urine output of less than 30 mL/hr may indicate hypovolemia, decreased cardiac output, and impaired tissue perfusion.

- Monitor vital signs and hemodynamic parameters such as central venous pressure, cardiac output, and pulmonary artery pressures every hour or as indicated. *These measurements provide important information about fluid and vascular volumes as well as cardiovascular status.*
- Weigh daily. *Weight is an accurate indicator of fluid status. Rapid weight gains or losses reflect changes in fluid volume.*
- Assess skin turgor, color, temperature, and mucous membranes at least every 8 hours. *Warm, dry skin with poor turgor and dry, shiny mucous membranes indicate dehydration.*
- Measure or estimate fluid losses through abdominal drains and on dressings. *Significant amounts of exudative fluid may be lost.*
- Monitor laboratory values, including hemoglobin and hematocrit, urine specific gravity, serum osmolality and electrolytes, and ABGs. Report changes to the physician. *Laboratory results provide information about fluid and electrolyte status and acid–base balance.*
- Administer intravenous fluids and electrolytes as ordered. Gastrointestinal drainage may be replaced milliliter for milliliter with a balanced electrolyte solution. *Intravenous fluids are necessary to meet daily fluid intake needs, as well as replace continuing losses of water and electrolytes.*

- Provide good skin care and frequent oral hygiene. *Fluid deficit increases the risk of skin breakdown and ulceration of mucous membranes.*

Ineffective Protection

Repeated surgeries, an unsutured incision, and the presence of drains interrupt skin integrity and the body's first line of defense against microorganisms. In addition, immune defenses are stressed by the infection and potential malnutrition. As a result, the risk for impaired healing and further infection is increased.

- Monitor temperature, pulse rate, and for localized signs of infection such as redness and swelling around incisions and drain sites, increased or purulent drainage, and cloudy or malodorous urine. *Impaired defenses increase the risk for extension of the infection or unrelated infections.*
- Obtain cultures of purulent drainage from any site. *Early identification of any additional infection allows timely intervention.*
- Monitor WBC and differential, serum protein, and albumin. *An increased WBC with a higher percentage of immature cells present in the blood is an indicator of infection and normal immune response. Serum albumin and protein levels are indicators of nutritional status as well as immune function.*
- Practice meticulous hand washing and use standard precautions at all times. *Hand washing reduces transient bacteria on the skin and remains the most important method of controlling infection. Standard precautions reduce the risk of spreading infection to or from the client.*

- Use strict aseptic technique for dressing changes, wound care, and irrigations. *Disruption of the protective barrier of the skin increases the risk of contamination and further infection.*
- Maintain fluid balance and nutritional status through enteral or parenteral feedings, as indicated. See the research box below for evidence-based recommendations for care of enterally fed clients. *Adequate nutrition and fluid balance are necessary for optimal immune system function.*

PRACTICE ALERT

An acute infection such as peritonitis causes a stress response with excess energy expenditure and loss of body proteins and cell mass. Glycogen stores are rapidly depleted, and body proteins are used to meet energy needs. Withholding food further complicates this process, leading to rapid development of protein-calorie malnutrition (PCM). PCM impairs the immune response and slows healing.

Anxiety

The severity and potential threat to life associated with peritonitis present a situational crisis for the client and family. Anxiety is a common response.

- Assess the client's and family's anxiety level and present coping skills. *Interventions need to be tailored to the needs and strengths of the client and family.*
- Present a calm, reassuring manner. Encourage expression of concerns; listen carefully, and acknowledge their validity. *This helps establish trust.*

NURSING RESEARCH   Evidence-Based Practice: Enterally Fed, Critically Ill Client

A vital component of the treatment and care of critically ill clients (such as those with peritonitis) is providing nutritional support, primarily through enteral feedings. Although this remains the method of choice for this population, and has many advantages, enteral feeding also comes with the risk of bronchopulmonary aspiration as a complication. Aspiration occurs in as many as 40% of clients and up to 50% to 75% of clients who have an endotracheal tube in place. Several methods are currently used to detect aspiration, but not as much information has been published about how to prevent aspiration in enterally fed clients. This study (Sanko, 2004) was conducted to review and synthesize current research in order to make recommendations to improve the quality and safety of administering enteral nutrition to critically ill clients. Recommended prevention techniques included the following:

- Preventing aspiration with feeding tube placement by verifying placement with an x-ray. After verifying the placement, the tube should be securely taped and the external tube length should be measured, noted, and marked on the tube as a reference point for further tube placement checks. If the position of the tube is questioned, the x-ray should be repeated.
- Maintaining the head of the bed at an angle of at least 30 degrees, with 45% being ideal, and stopping feedings 30 to 60 minutes before placing the client in the supine position.
- Maintaining cuff pressure in clients with artificial airways at 20 to 30 cm H_2O.

Based on publishing findings, there is not sufficient evidence to support placement of feeding tubes beyond the pylorus or using small-bore tubes to prevent aspiration.

IMPLICATIONS FOR NURSING

Based on this review of the relevant research, it is obvious that more research is needed in this area of care. However, daily assessments of the client and the feeding tube with multiple methods (including X-ray, external length marking, pH testing, aspirate characteristics, or trypsin/pepsin levels) should be conducted by caregivers who have the knowledge to accurately interpret the results.

CRITICAL THINKING IN CLIENT CARE

1. Aspiration is defined as the inhalation of oropharyngeal or gastric contents into the larynx and lower respiratory tract. The result is usually aspiration pneumonitis or aspiration pneumonia. What assessments would you conduct and monitor to identify these complications?
2. You are on a committee that is evaluating the practice of adding blue dye to feeding solutions in order to better detect aspiration. The literature does not support this method. How and what would you do to convince the committee that this practice should not be continued?
3. What principle supports elevating the head of the bed to prevent aspiration? (Consider gravity and the placement of internal organs with the client in this position.)

- Maintain consistent caregiver assignments. *Consistency of nursing care and care providers helps reduce anxiety. Complex wound care and irrigation procedures are best performed by people who are very familiar with prescribed techniques.*
- Explain all treatments, procedures, tests, and examinations. *An increased understanding of what is being done can reduce anxiety.*
- Reinforce and clarify information as needed. *This improves understanding and promotes acceptance.*
- Teach and assist with relaxation techniques such as meditation, visualization, and progressive relaxation. *These measures promote positive coping skills and reduce physical manifestations of anxiety.*

Using NANDA, NIC, and NOC

Linkages between NANDA nursing diagnoses, NIC, and NOC for the client with peritonitis are illustrated in Chart 26–2 in the preceding section.

Community-Based Care

Teaching for home care includes the following topics:

- Wound care procedures, including dressing changes or irrigations. Provide verbal and written instructions on how to change dressings or do irrigations as well as where to obtain supplies, and allow opportunities to practice and demonstrate the procedure prior to discharge.
- Prescribed medications, including name and purpose of the drug, potential adverse effects, and their management.
- Manifestations of further infection (redness, heat, swelling, purulent drainage, chills, and fever) and potential complications to be reported to the care provider.
- Prescribed activity restrictions.
- Instructions for a high-calorie, high-protein diet for healing and optimal immune function.

Provide a referral to home health services for assessment, wound care, and further teaching, as needed.

THE CLIENT WITH GASTROENTERITIS

Gastroenteritis, or *enteritis,* is an inflammation of the stomach and small intestine. Enteritis may be caused by bacteria, viruses, parasites, or toxins. Upper GI manifestations such as anorexia, nausea, and vomiting are common. Diarrhea of varying intensity and abdominal discomfort are nearly universal features of gastroenteritis.

The infectious organism usually enters the body in contaminated water or food. For this reason, gastroenteritis often is called "food poisoning." Viruses commonly cause acute diarrheal illness. Diarrhea due to rotaviruses or the Norwalk virus occurs year-round in both adults and children. These illnesses are generally mild and self-limited, but can have severe consequences in the very young, the very old, or in people with impaired immune function.

Pathophysiology

Bacterial or viral infection of the GI tract produces inflammation, tissue damage, and manifestations by two primary mechanisms:

- *The production of exotoxins.* A number of bacteria produce and excrete an exotoxin that enters the surrounding environment (intestinal lumen), causing damage and inflammation. Exotoxins in the GI tract are often referred to as *enterotoxins.* They impair intestinal absorption and can cause secretion of significant amounts of electrolytes and water into the bowel, resulting in diarrhea and fluid loss. Common bacterial enterotoxins include those produced by *Staphylococcus, Clostridium perfringens, Clostridium botulinum,* some strains of *Escherichia coli, Vibrio cholera,* and *C. difficile.*
- *Invasion and ulceration of the mucosa.* Other bacteria, including some *Shigella, Salmonella,* and *E. coli* species, damage tissue more directly. They invade the intestinal mucosa of the small bowel or colon, producing microscopic ulceration, bleeding, fluid exudate, and water and electrolyte secretion.

In some cases, the mechanism of injury is unclear. It may be a combination of direct and toxic damage. For example, the Norwalk virus damages the mucosa of the jejunum, with fluid and electrolyte secretion.

Manifestations

Although the manifestations of bacterial and viral enteritis vary according to the organism involved, several features are common (see the Manifestations box below). Anorexia, nausea, and vomiting are caused by distention of the upper GI tract by unabsorbed chyme and excess water. Bowel distention, along with irritation of the bowel mucosa and gas production due to fermentation of undigested food, lead to abdominal pain and cramping. Borborygmi, excessively loud and hyperactive bowel sounds, are another result. The abdomen is often distended and tender.

Diarrhea is usually predominant with enteritis. Fluid is secreted into the bowel lumen, and the unabsorbed chyme and electrolytes create an osmotic pull of fluid into the bowel. Motility is stimulated, and stools become watery and frequent. Loss of fluids and electrolytes through diarrhea can lead to the most serious manifestations of enteritis. Fluid volume can be rapidly depleted, leading to dehydration and hypovolemia. Orthostatic hypotension and fever may be noted initially. If fluid loss continues, hypovolemic shock may develop.

MANIFESTATIONS   **of Gastroenteritis**

Gastrointestinal Effects
- Anorexia, nausea, and vomiting
- Abdominal pain and cramping
- Borborygmi
- Diarrhea

General Effects
- Malaise, weakness, and muscle aches
- Headache
- Dry skin and mucous membranes
- Poor skin turgor
- Orthostatic hypotension, tachycardia
- Fever

Complications

Electrolyte and acid–base imbalances may result from gastroenteritis. Extensive vomiting can lead to metabolic alkalosis due to the loss of hydrochloric acid from the stomach. When diarrhea predominates, metabolic acidosis is more likely. Potassium is lost in either case, leading to hypokalemia. Hyponatremia may develop if fluids are replaced with pure water. Headache, cardiac irregularities, changes in respiratory rate and pattern, malaise and weakness, muscle aching, and signs of neuromuscular irritability are the possible manifestations of these disturbances in homeostasis.

Specific Types of Gastrointestinal Infections

Several gastrointestinal infections produce specific effects that are discussed below and summarized in Table 26–3.

TRAVELER'S DIARRHEA People traveling to another country frequently develop diarrhea within 2 to 10 days, particularly

TABLE 26–3 Selected Bacterial Infections of the Bowel

DISEASE AND ORGANISM	INCUBATION	PATHOGENESIS	MANIFESTATIONS	MANAGEMENT
Traveler's diarrhea: *Escherichia coli*	24 to 72 hours	Enterotoxin causes hypersecretion of the small intestine.	Abrupt onset of diarrhea; vomiting rare	Prophylactic bismuth subsalicylate; antidiarrheals such as loperamide or diphenoxylate; 3- to 5-day course of norfloxacin, ciprofloxacin, or trimethoprim-sulfamethoxazole
Staphylococcal food poisoning	2 to 8 hours	Enterotoxin impairs intestinal absorption and affects vomiting centers in the brain.	Severe nausea and vomiting; abdominal cramping and diarrhea; headache and fever	Fluid and electrolyte replacement as needed
Cholera: *Vibrio cholerae*	1 to 3 days	Enterotoxin affects entire small intestine, causing secretion of water and electrolytes into bowel lumen.	Severe diarrhea with "rice water stool," gray, cloudy, odorless, with no blood or pus; vomiting; thirst, oliguria, muscle cramps, weakness; dehydration and vascular collapse	Oral or intravenous rehydration; possible antimicrobial therapy with ampicillin, tetracycline, trimethoprim-sulfamethoxazole, others
Hemorrhagic colitis: *E. coli*	1 to 3 days	Enterotoxin causes direct mucosal damage in large intestine; also toxic to vascular endothelial cells.	Severe abdominal cramping, watery diarrhea that becomes grossly bloody; fever; possible complications: hemolytic uremic syndrome and thrombotic thrombocytopenic purpura	Supportive care with fluid replacement and bland diet; may require dialysis or plasmapheresis for complications
Salmonellosis: *Salmonella*	8 to 48 hours	Superficial infection of the GI tract without invasion or production of toxins.	Diarrhea with abdominal cramping, nausea, and vomiting; low-grade fever, chills, weakness	Treatment of symptoms; trimethoprim-sulfamethoxazole, ampicillin, or ciprofloxacin for severe illness
Shigellosis (bacillary dysentery): *Shigella*	1 to 4 days	Local tissue invasion, primarily involving large intestine and distal ileum; endotoxin causes fluid and electrolyte secretion into bowel lumen.	Watery diarrhea with severe abdominal cramping and tenesmus; lethargy	Fluid and electrolyte replacement; correction of acidosis; antibiotic therapy with trimethoprim-sulfamethoxazole, ciprofloxacin, or ampicillin
Clostridium Difficile Colitis (*C. difficile*)	1 to 2 weeks	Antibiotic therapy interferes with normal protective bacteria in the colon; *C. difficile* colonizes and releases toxins that cause mucosal inflammation and damage	Diarrhea, abdominal cramps, malaise, fever, anorexia.	Cessation of the causative antibiotic; antibiotic therapy with vancomycin or metronidazole (specific for *C. difficile*)

when there is a significant difference in climate, sanitation standards, or food and drink. Strains of enterotoxin-producing *E. coli, Shigella* species, *Salmonella,* and *Campylobacter* are the most frequent causes of traveler's diarrhea (Yates, 2005). Other bacteria and viruses also may cause traveler's diarrhea.

Up to 10 or more loose stools per day and abdominal cramping are common manifestations. Nausea and vomiting are less frequent; fever is rare. Manifestations usually resolve within 2 to 5 days. Complications are rare.

STAPHYLOCOCCAL FOOD POISONING

Certain foods provide an excellent medium for staphylococcal growth when contaminated and left at room temperature. Examples include meats and fish, dairy products (e.g., custards), and bakery products (e.g., cream-filled pastries). The organism itself does not affect the bowel; the toxin it produces, however, impairs intestinal absorption and acts on receptors in the gut, stimulating the medullary center to produce vomiting.

The onset of staphylococcal food poisoning is abrupt, occurring within 2 to 8 hours after consuming the contaminated food. Nausea and vomiting are severe. Manifestations typically last 3 to 6 hours, and include abdominal cramping, diarrhea, headache, and fever. Complications such as fluid and electrolyte imbalances are rare, but may develop in older adults and people with underlying chronic disease processes.

CHOLERA

Cholera is an acute diarrheal illness caused by strains of *Vibrio cholerae*. It is endemic in parts of Asia, the Middle East, and Africa. Epidemics occur periodically. Cholera is spread by the fecal–oral route through contaminated water or food. The organism produces an enterotoxin, enzymes, and other substances that affect the entire small intestine. Water and electrolytes are secreted into the bowel lumen in response to the toxin. The enzymes and other substances produced by the bacteria may affect mucous protection of bowel endothelium.

Cholera ranges in severity from very mild, with few or no manifestations, to acute and fulminant. Its onset is typically abrupt, with severe, frequent, watery diarrhea. Up to 1 L of stool may be passed in an hour, rapidly depleting fluid volume. Stool is often described as "rice water stool" and is characteristically gray and cloudy, with no fecal odor, blood, or pus. Vomiting may accompany the diarrhea. Other manifestations relate to the loss of fluid and electrolytes: thirst, oliguria, muscle cramps, weakness, and significant signs of dehydration. Metabolic acidosis and hypokalemia develop. If untreated, circulatory collapse and acute renal failure may occur.

Recovery from cholera usually occurs spontaneously within 3 to 6 days. With prompt and adequate fluid replacement, mortality is less than 1%.

ESCHERICHIA COLI HEMORRHAGIC COLITIS

Most pathologic forms of *E. coli* bacteria cause little more than common traveler's diarrhea. However, some strains, such as serotype 0157:H7, produce a potent enterotoxin in the large intestine after being ingested. This toxin damages bowel mucosa and the endothelial cells of blood vessels in the GI tract. If absorbed, the toxin can damage other blood vessels as well, such as those of the kidney.

Cattle provide the reservoir for *E. coli* 0157:H7. It is usually spread through undercooked beef (hamburger in particular) and unpasteurized milk or apple juice. It may also be spread by direct contact via the fecal–oral route. The onset of hemorrhagic colitis is abrupt, with severe abdominal cramping and watery diarrhea that becomes grossly bloody within 24 hours. Fever may be present.

Hemolytic uremic syndrome and thrombotic thrombocytopenic purpura are significant complications of *E. coli* hemorrhagic colitis, affecting about 5% of people with the disease. Older adults have the highest risk for developing complications.

CLOSTRIDIUM DIFFICILE COLITIS

Clostridium difficile colitis (*C. difficile* colitis) is associated with antibiotic therapy. Treatment with antibiotics (especially broad-spectrum antibiotics) predisposes to interference with the normal protective bacteria of the colon, leading to colonization by *C. difficile* by the oral–fecal route. Subsequent release of toxins by the bacteria causes mucous damage and inflammation. This is primarily a problem in hospitalized clients, causing diarrhea and abdominal cramping. These manifestations commonly begin within 1 to 2 weeks of antibiotic treatment. It is also being seen in the community in healthy adults. The bacteria can be identified in the stool.

SALMONELLOSIS

Salmonellosis is food poisoning caused by ingesting raw or improperly cooked meat, poultry, eggs, and dairy products contaminated with *Salmonella* bacteria. These bacteria cause superficial infection of the GI tract, rarely invading further. They do not produce a toxin.

Manifestations develop 8 to 48 hours after ingesting the bacteria. Diarrhea may be violent with abdominal cramping, nausea, and vomiting. A low-grade fever, chills, and weakness may accompany GI manifestations. The disease usually is self-limited, resolving within 3 to 5 days, although bacteremia may develop.

SHIGELLOSIS (BACILLARY DYSENTERY)

Shigellosis (or bacillary dysentery) occurs worldwide, accounting for up to 5% to 10% of diarrheal illness in some regions. It may be endemic or occur in epidemics. Humans are the reservoir for *Shigella* organisms, which are spread directly via the fecal–oral route or indirectly through contaminated food, fomites (such as inanimate objects), and vectors (such as fleas). The incubation period for shigellosis is 1 to 4 days.

Shigella organisms infect the lower intestine, and sometimes the distal ilium. They invade the tissue, causing inflammation, and they produce an enterotoxin. The result is watery diarrhea containing blood, mucus, and inflammatory exudate. The onset of diarrhea is abrupt, with severe abdominal cramping, and *tenesmus,* a sensation of urgent and continuing need to defecate. Lethargy is common; rarely, neurologic manifestations occur.

In adults, shigellosis is usually mild and self-limiting. Older adults and debilitated clients are at risk for volume depletion and electrolyte imbalances. Secondary infection is another potential complication, as is acute blood loss from mucosal ulcerations.

INTERDISCIPLINARY CARE

The goals of care for gastroenteritis are to manage the manifestations, prevent complications, identify the cause of the infection, and prevent its spread. The history and manifestations provide valuable cues about the cause. Diagnostic testing is used to identify the pathogen and evaluate its effects. In most cases, treatment is supportive, directed toward relieving manifestations, restoring fluid and electrolyte balance, and maintaining function.

Diagnosis

If manifestations are severe or do not resolve within about 48 hours, laboratory testing is used to identify the causative organism and to assess fluid, electrolyte, and acid–base balance. A stool specimen for culture, ova and parasites, and fecal leukocytes usually reveals the infective organism, but may require up to 6 weeks to identify some bacteria. In infections such as botulism, the toxin itself may be isolated in the stool. Contamination of the stool by urine or treatment with antibiotics, bismuth subsalicylate (Pepto-Bismol), or mineral oil may interfere with pathogen growth, altering stool culture results. Use a clean bedpan or collection device to obtain the stool specimen, and instruct the client to avoid mixing the stool with urine or toilet tissue.

A sigmoidoscopy may be done to differentiate inflammatory bowel disease from infectious processes. It does not replace stool cultures, because the lesions associated with some infectious processes are indistinguishable from those of ulcerative colitis. (Nursing care of the client having a sigmoidoscopy is discussed in Chapter 25 ∞ .)

Serum osmolality and electrolytes and ABGs are done to assess and monitor fluid, electrolyte, and acid–base balance. Common imbalances associated with enteritis and diarrhea are outlined in Table 26–4.

Medications

Acute enteritis usually resolves spontaneously, and no drug treatment is required. If the client is severely ill and manifestations are prolonged, medications may be prescribed.

Antibiotic therapy specific to the organism may be used to treat bacterial colitis, cholera, salmonellosis, or shigellosis. Trimethoprim-sulfamethoxazole (Septra, Bactrim), ciprofloxacin (Cipro), ampicillin (Ampicin, Omnipen, Polycillin-N), or another antibiotic may be prescribed. Stool culture is obtained prior to starting antibiotics, but treatment may begin before culture results are available. A presumptive diagnosis based on history and presenting manifestations guides the choice of antibiotic.

An antidiarrheal drug may be prescribed to promote comfort and reduce fluid loss. Nursing measures related to antidiarrheal medications are outlined in the Medication Administration box on page 756.

Nutrition and Fluids

Replacing lost fluids and electrolytes is vital when vomiting and/or diarrhea are severe or prolonged. In many cases of enteritis, fluid and electrolyte replacement are all that is required until the infection resolves.

Oral rehydration is preferred for replacing physiologic fluids. An oral glucose-electrolyte solution is often well tolerated in sips, even when vomiting is present. Commercial preparations such as Gatorade, All-Sport, and Pedialyte are available.

TABLE 26–4 Laboratory Values Associated with Enteritis and Diarrhea

TEST	NORMAL VALUE	CHANGE WITH SIGNIFICANT DIARRHEA
Serum osmolality	275 to 295 mOsm/kg	Increased; levels above 320 mOsm/kg indicate significant dehydration.
Serum potassium	3.5 to 5.0 mEq/L	Decreased due to loss through stool and vomitus; levels below 2.5 mEq/L are critical.
Serum sodium	136 to 148 mEq/L	Decreased due to loss through stool and vomitus; may be significant when fluid losses are replaced with pure water; levels below 120 mEq/L may be critical.
Serum chloride	96 to 106 mEq/L	Increased when sodium loss is greater than chloride loss; decreased with severe diarrhea and with vomiting; possible critical values are below 80 mEq/L or above 115 mEq/L.
Blood gases		
■ pH	Arterial: 7.35 to 7.45	Decreased in metabolic acidosis, a possible result of severe diarrhea; increased in metabolic alkalosis, a possible result of severe vomiting and chloride loss; values below 7.25 or above 7.55 are critical.
■ P_{CO_2}	Arterial: 35 to 45 mmHg	Typically decreased in metabolic acidosis as the body attempts to eliminate excess acid by "blowing off" CO_2; increased with metabolic alkalosis as the body retains CO_2 in an attempt to normalize pH.
■ Bicarbonate	22 to 26 mEq/L	Decreased in metabolic acidosis; increased in metabolic alkalosis.
Hematocrit	Males: 40% to 50% Females: 37% to 47%	Increased with dehydration and hypovolemia as a result of concentration of blood cells.
Urine specific gravity	1.010 to 1.025	Increased with dehydration and hypovolemia as kidneys attempt to conserve fluid.

A solution of 5 mL (1 teaspoon) table salt, 5 mL baking soda, 20 mL (4 teaspoons) granulated sugar, and flavoring (such as lemon extract or juice) to 1 L (1 quart) of water also is effective.

Intravenous rehydration may be necessary with severe diarrhea and fluid loss. In some cases, a combination of oral and intravenous fluids may be used to replace lost fluids and maintain vascular volume. Balanced electrolyte solutions, such as glucose in normal saline and Ringer's solution, are used. Lactated Ringer's solution or another alkalinizing solution may be ordered if metabolic acidosis is present.

Gastric Lavage

Gastric lavage and catharsis—in effect, "washing out" the stomach and intestines—may be performed to remove unabsorbed toxin from the GI tract if botulism is suspected. The client with botulism is closely observed for signs of respiratory distress. Respiratory support with endotracheal intubation or tracheostomy and mechanical ventilation may be required (see Chapter 36 ∞).

Plasmapheresis

Plasmapheresis (plasma exchange therapy) may be performed to remove circulating toxins for hemorrhagic colitis caused by *E. coli*. See Chapter 46 ∞ for the nursing care of a client having this procedure. Potential complications include those associated with intravenous catheters, shifts in fluid balance, and altered blood clotting.

Dialysis

Acute tubular necrosis and renal failure associated with hemorrhagic colitis may necessitate dialysis to remove wastes and prevent severe fluid and electrolyte imbalances and metabolic acidosis. Although acute renal failure often resolves spontaneously and renal function resumes, dialysis can be lifesaving. Either hemodialysis or peritoneal dialysis may be used, generally as a temporary measure. Nursing care related to acute renal failure and dialysis is discussed in Chapter 29 ∞ .

NURSING CARE

Although *C. difficile* colitis bacterial infections are hospital acquired, few clients with acute enteritis require hospitalization. Most are treated in community settings. Assessment, education, and support of self-care measures are major nursing responsibilities.

Health Promotion

Nurses play a significant role in preventing enteritis as educators, community health providers, and advocates for environmental safety.

Teach the importance of proper food handling and maintaining appropriate temperatures. Adequate cooking of meat products is vital to prevent disorders such as staphylococcal food poisoning, *E. coli* hemorrhagic colitis, and salmonellosis. Emphasize the importance of not consuming raw meat products, and cooking hamburger, in particular, to the point that no redness is noted in the meat. The highly pathogenic *E. coli* serotype 0157:H7 is present in the gut of infected animals. Meats from the animal may be contaminated with bowel contents. The organism is readily destroyed by heat, so cuts of meat such as steaks or roasts are less likely to cause infection, since the organism is on the outside of the meat. However, the process of grinding hamburger allows *E. coli* to be mixed throughout the meat. Thorough cooking destroys the organism. This pathogen (and others) may also be spread through unpasteurized milk. Discuss the dangers of consuming milk that has not been pasteurized and encourage clients to avoid it.

Dairy products, eggs, and egg products left at room temperature provide a good growth medium for bacteria. Discuss the importance of prompt refrigeration of meats and these products to minimize this risk. Many gastrointestinal infections are spread through contaminated water. Encourage travelers to consume only bottled water unless local water supplies are clearly safe. Water purification tablets are available for hikers and campers, and may also be used when traveling abroad.

Assessment

- *Health history:* Onset, duration, and severity of manifestations; recent activities such as attending a picnic or potluck, international travel, or camping; other affected members of the household; measures taken to relieve manifestations or replace fluids.
- *Physical examination:* Vital signs including temperature and orthostatic blood pressure; skin color, temperature, moisture, and turgor; peripheral pulses and capillary refill; abdominal shape, contour, bowel sounds, tenderness.

Nursing Diagnoses and Interventions

Diarrhea and fluid volume deficit are priority nursing diagnoses. See the earlier section of this chapter on diarrhea for specific nursing interventions related to these diagnoses.

Community-Based Care

Discuss the following topics with the client for self-care:
- The importance of good hand washing, particularly before handling food and after each bowel movement
- The need to wash clothing and linens contaminated with feces separately in hot water and detergent
- Oral solutions to replace lost fluids and electrolytes
- Appropriate use of antidiarrheal medications if recommended
- Manifestations of complications to report to the healthcare provider.

THE CLIENT WITH A PROTOZOAL BOWEL INFECTION

Parasites live within, on, or at the expense of other organisms. Parasitic intestinal infections are common in developing countries. They include both protozoal and helminthic (parasitic worms) infections. Parasites that infect the bowel usually enter the GI tract through the mouth by the fecal–oral route; some are spread by direct contact or through sexual activity.

Of the protozoal bowel infections, only giardiasis is common in the United States. Amebiasis is found chiefly in the tropics and where sanitation is poor. Cryptosporidiosis, a form of coccidiosis, is an important worldwide cause of sporadic mild diarrhea, traveler's diarrhea, and severe diarrhea in people who are immunocompromised.

Pathophysiology and Manifestations

The most common protozoal infections of the bowel are discussed below and summarized in Table 26–5.

Giardiasis

Giardiasis is a protozoal infection of the upper small intestine caused by *Giardia lamblia*. It is the most common intestinal protozoal pathogen in the United States. Humans are the reservoir for *Giardia*. It is spread by the fecal–oral route, usually in contaminated food or water. It is also spread by direct contact. When the cyst form of the organism is ingested, trophozoites emerge in the duodenum and jejunum, attaching themselves to the intestinal mucosa. This leads to superficial invasion, inflammation, and destruction of the mucosa of the small intestine.

Giardiasis may be asymptomatic, although manifestations may develop suddenly or insidiously. Diarrhea is common. It is usually mild, with one or more large, loose stools per day. Diarrhea may be severe, however, with frequent, copious, frothy, malodorous, and greasy stools. Other manifestations include weight loss and weakness; anorexia, nausea, and vomiting; epi-gastric pain, abdominal cramping and distention, flatulence, and belching. Malabsorption may develop.

Amebiasis

Amebiasis (amebic dysentery) is caused by the protozoon *Entamoeba histolytica*. Several strains of the protozoon have been identified. Tropical strains tend to be more virulent and pathogenic than those found in temperate climates. Humans are the host for this parasite. It usually is transmitted through food or water contaminated by feces and by person-to-person contact. The parasite enters the intestines, where it may live without causing disease, or it may invade the intestinal wall to cause ulceration and inflammation. The cecum, appendix, ascending colon, sigmoid colon, and rectum are most often affected. Ulcers may spread to cause hemorrhage, edema, and mucosal sloughing. The infection may spread via the blood to the liver, lungs, or brain.

Amebiasis is usually asymptomatic. Mild manifestations include abdominal cramps, flatulence, and intermittent diarrhea containing blood and mucus. Severe manifestations of amebic dysentery include frequent watery stools containing blood, mucous, and necrotic tissue; colic, tenesmus, and abdominal tenderness; nausea and vomiting; and fever. The liver may be enlarged and tender to palpation.

Complications are rare, but may include appendicitis, bowel perforation with peritonitis, and fulminating colitis.

TABLE 26–5 Common Protozoal Infections of the Bowel

DISEASE AND ORGANISM	INCUBATION	PATHOGENESIS	MANIFESTATIONS	MANAGEMENT
Giardiasis: *Giardia lamblia*	1 to 3 weeks or more	Trophozoite attaches to mucosa in duodenum and jejunum, causing superficial invasion, inflammation, and tissue destruction.	Diarrhea, mild or severe, daily or intermittent; anorexia, nausea, vomiting; epigastric pain, cramping, distention; flatulence and belching; may be asymptomatic	Metronidazole quinacrine, furazolidone
Amebiasis: *Entamoeba histolytica*	2 to 4 weeks	Organisms may reside in large intestine without causing disease or can invade colon wall, causing ulceration; may be carried via blood to liver to produce abscess.	Usually asymptomatic; diarrhea may be mild, with few semiformed mucous-containing stools per day, or severe, with 10 to 20 blood-streaked liquid stools per day; abdominal cramps and flatulence; colic, tenesmus, vomiting, tenderness; fatigue, weight loss; prostration and toxicity	Metronidazole and diloxanide furoate or iodoquinol; chloroquine for hepatic abscess
Cryptosporidiosis: *Cryptosporidium*	2 to 10 days	Organisms attach to epithelial surface of small bowel (jejunum), causing villous atrophy and mild inflammatory changes; may secrete enterotoxin.	In immunocompetent clients: asymptomatic to profuse, watery diarrhea of sudden onset, abdominal cramping; malaise, fever; anorexia, nausea, vomiting. In immunodeficient clients: profuse watery diarrhea with loss of up to 15 to 20 L/ day; severe malabsorption, electrolyte imbalance; weight loss; lymphadenopathy	Self-limiting in immuno-competent clients. For immunodeficient clients: spiramycin, zidovudine (AZT), paromomycin (Humatin), octreotide, eflornithine; fluid and electrolyte replacement; parenteral nutrition as needed

Cryptosporidiosis (Coccidiosis)

Cryptosporidiosis causes sporadic mild diarrhea and traveler's diarrhea in all age groups. In people with impaired immune function, such as those with human immunodeficiency virus (HIV) disease, it causes severe diarrhea, malabsorption, and significant weight loss.

This organism is transmitted by the fecal–oral route. Contaminated water is a frequent source of infection. The organism attaches to bowel epithelium, causing surface damage and inflammation. It does not invade the tissues, but secretes an enterotoxin that causes characteristic watery diarrhea. The disease is self-limited in people with competent immune systems. Watery diarrhea may be accompanied by low-grade fever, nausea, vomiting, abdominal cramps, and general malaise.

Immunocompromised clients develop profuse watery diarrhea with significant fluid and electrolyte losses and severe malabsorption. Lymphadenopathy (enlarged lymph nodes) also may develop.

INTERDISCIPLINARY CARE

Management of protozoal bowel infections includes identifying the causative organism and administering medications.

Diagnosis

Diagnostic testing may include a stool examination for ova and parasites. Many protozoa are shed intermittently rather than continuously; stools are collected sequentially (e.g., every other day for a total of three specimens). A sigmoidoscopy may be performed to examine the bowel mucosa and collect a stool specimen for examination (in this case, no bowel prep is done prior to the test). When giardiasis is suspected, a duodenal string test (Entero-Test), duodenal aspiration, or duodenal biopsy may be conducted. Duodenal aspirate is stained and examined microscopically for the protozoa. Small bowel biopsy can identify *Cryptosporidium* infection.

Medications

Pharmacologic treatment includes both local and systemic antiparasitic drugs, such as iodoquinol (Amebaquine), paromomycin (Humatin), metronidazole (Flagyl), furazolidone (Furoxone), or albendazole (Albenza). Treatment is usually provided on an outclient basis. Severe amebic dysentery may require hospitalization for intravenous fluid and electrolyte replacements. Nursing care related to common antiprotozoal drugs is outlined in the Medication Administration box on page 780.

NURSING CARE

Nursing assessment, diagnoses, and interventions for the client with a protozoal GI infection are similar to those indicated for clients with bacterial or viral infections. *Diarrhea* and *Risk for Deficient Fluid Volume* are priority nursing diagnoses. See previous sections of this chapter for specific nursing interventions related to these diagnoses.

Nurses need to teach the public how parasitic diseases are transmitted and how to avoid spreading the infection. Prevention of amebiasis and giardiasis involves:

- Provision of safe water supplies
- Appropriate disposal of human feces
- Safe food storage, handling, and preparation
- Adequate hand washing after defecating and before handling food

Instruct people living in high-risk areas (e.g., tropical climates, areas with untreated water supplies) to boil, filter, or treat water supplies with iodine to eliminate protozoal contamination. Instruct them to avoid foods that cannot be peeled or cooked. Teach the manifestations of protozoal infections and where to obtain treatment.

Emphasize the importance of keeping toilet areas clean and maintaining good personal hygiene. Advise the client to avoid rectal contact during sexual activity. Other household members should also have stool specimens examined for parasites.

THE CLIENT WITH A HELMINTHIC DISORDER

Helminths are parasitic worms, capable of causing infectious diseases in humans. Helminths are subclassified as round worms (nematodes), flukes (trematodes), or tapeworms (cestodes).

Pathophysiology

Although all helminths can infect humans, the definitive host and intermediate hosts vary with each organism. In nearly all instances of helminthic disorders, the organism enters the body through the GI tract in contaminated and inadequately cooked foods. Some of these organisms remain in the intestinal tract; others migrate to infect the liver, lungs, or other structures. Table 26–6 summarizes the most common helminths and their effects.

INTERDISCIPLINARY CARE

The management of helminthic disorders includes diagnostic testing and medications.

Diagnosis

The primary means of diagnosing helminthic disorders is examination of the stool for ova and parasites. Enterobiasis is diagnosed by the presence of the parasite's eggs on the perianal skin or on cellulose tape placed over the anus. A CBC may also be ordered. Anemia may be present, particularly with hookworm disease. *Eosinophilia* (an increased percentage of eosinophils in the blood) is common in helminthic disorders. With trichinosis, serum muscle enzymes such as the creatinine kinase (CK) and aspartate aminotransferase (AST) are typically elevated. Serologic testing for antibodies to the worm may also be performed. Blood, duodenal washings, and cerebrospinal fluid (CSF) may be examined for the presence of the trichinosis larvae. Inflamed muscle may be biopsied.

Medications

Helminthic infections often are treated with a single oral dose or 3-day course of pyrantel pamoate (Antiminth) or mebendazole (Vermox). Doses may need to be repeated every 2 weeks for clients with heavy infections. These drugs are generally

MEDICATION ADMINISTRATION   Antiprotozoal Agents

LOCAL (GASTROINTESTINAL) AGENTS
Iodoquinol (Yodoxin, Amebaquine)
Paromomycin (Humatin)

These drugs exert a local amebicidal effect in the intestines and are poorly absorbed when administered orally. Local agents have the advantage of provoking fewer side effects than systemically active agents.

Nursing Responsibilities
- Assess for potential contraindications:
  a. Hypersensitivity to the drug or drug class.
  b. Iodoquinol: malnutrition, thyroid disorders; hepatic or renal impairment, optic neuropathy, or hypersensitivity to iodine.
  c. Paromomycin: ulcerative bowel lesions; hypersensitivity to aminoglycoside antibiotics, impaired renal function, intestinal obstruction.
- Observe for adverse effects: anorexia, nausea, vomiting, abdominal cramping, diarrhea, and increased flatulence; report skin rash, visual disturbances, or changes in blood work to primary care provider.

Health Education for the Client and Family
- Take as prescribed for the full course of therapy.
- Take with food to reduce gastrointestinal effects.
- Keep follow-up appointments as recommended to evaluate the effects of treatment.
- Report adverse effects to the physician.
  a. Any change in vision
  b. Numbness, tingling, or pain in extremities
  c. Chills, fever, skin rash or boils
  d. A change in urination or character of urine
  e. Diminished hearing or tinnitus
  f. Weight loss, diarrhea, fatty stools
  g. Candidiasis of the mouth or vagina.
- Practice good hand washing, particularly after using the toilet, to prevent spreading the disease to others.

SYSTEMIC AGENTS
Metronidazole (Flagyl, Satric, Metzol, others)
Furazolidone (Furoxone), Albendazole (Albenza)

Clients with symptomatic protozoal infections are generally treated with a systemic antiprotozoal agent. Metronidazole is the most widely used of these antiprotozoal agents and is the drug of choice for treating amebiasis.

Nursing Responsibilities
- Assess for possible contraindications to therapy:
  a. Hypersensitivity to the prescribed agent or related drugs
  b. Liver dysfunction or blood dyscrasias
  c. Concurrent use of alcohol or an MAOI
  d. Pregnancy.
- Administer as ordered.
  a. Metronidazole may be given orally after meals or as a continuous or intermittent intravenous infusion.
  b. Administer furazolidone and albendazole orally with meals to minimize gastric distress.
- Observe for possible adverse effects; notify the physician if significant. Gastrointestinal effects are common.
  a. Peripheral neuropathy and CNS effects may occur with metronidazole.
  b. Blood dyscrasias may develop with furazolidone or albendazole; monitor CBC and report abnormal results.
  c. Furazolidone can cause hypoglycemia; carefully monitor blood glucose in diabetic clients.
  d. Report abnormal liver function test results.
- Monitor the character and number of stools; obtain specimens as ordered to evaluate the effectiveness of therapy.

Health Education for the Client and Family
- Take the drug as prescribed for the full duration of the prescription.
- Taking oral preparations after meals helps minimize gastrointestinal side effects. Notify the physician if nausea and vomiting continue.
- Do not use alcohol while taking these drugs. An Antabuse-type response with severe headache, flushing, and vomiting may occur.
- Report adverse effects to the physician, including dizziness and other nervous system changes, sore throats, fatigue, bruising, or infection.
- Candidiasis of the mouth or vagina may occur with metronidazole therapy. Report symptoms to the physician.
- A harmless change in urine color to deep yellow (quinacrine) or rust or brown (metronidazole or chloroquine) may occur while taking these drugs.
- If you are diabetic taking furazolidone, carefully monitor blood glucose levels because hypoglycemia may develop.
- Practice good hand washing, particularly after using the toilet, to prevent transmitting the protozoa to others.

safe, requiring few precautions. Giving the drug after meals minimizes GI side effects. Treatment is followed by a stool culture at 2 weeks to evaluate effectiveness. If necessary, an additional course of the drug is prescribed. Other members of the household are generally also treated.

Most clients with trichinosis recover spontaneously without long-term effects. The intestinal phase of the disease is treated with albendazole, taken twice daily for as long as 60 days, or a 13-day course of mebendazole. Hospitalization may be required during the muscle invasion phase of the disease if the infection is severe. Corticosteroids may be used to reduce the inflammation and manage the manifestations.

NURSING CARE

Because many clients with these disorders are asymptomatic, nurses need to be alert for histories that indicate risk and subtle manifestations of the disorder. Use standard precautions to minimize the risk of spreading these infections to other clients. Wear gloves and gowns as necessary to prevent fecal contamination of hands and clothing. On rare occasions, parasites may be present in the sputum or vomitus, so handle these secretions with care. Disinfect toilets, toilet seats, and commodes after use. Teach the client the importance of washing hands after using the toilet and before handling food to prevent reinfection.

TABLE 26–6 Selected Helminthic Diseases

	INFECTION	HOST	AREA	PATHOGENESIS	MANIFESTATIONS
Nematode infections	Ascariasis	Humans	Worldwide, cosmopolitan; warm, moist climates	Eggs are ingested in fecally contaminated food and drink; motile larvae migrate to lungs and back to small intestine, where they mature to produce more eggs.	Pulmonary: low-grade fever, cough, blood-tinged sputum, wheezing, dyspnea, substernal chest pain. GI: ulcer-like epigastric pain, vomiting, abdominal distention
	Enterobiasis (pinworm infection)	Humans	Worldwide, cosmopolitan	Infect cecum; eggs deposit on perianal skin, organisms may be transmitted to others or reinfect host by oral ingestion.	Nocturnal perianal and perineal pruritus; insomnia, irritability, restlessness
	Hookworm disease	Humans	Tropics and subtropics	Larvae enter through skin or by ingestion and migrate to lungs, up bronchial tree, and down esophagus to mature in upper small bowel, where they attach and suck blood.	Skin: pruritic dermatitis at site of entry Pulmonary: dry cough, wheezing, blood-tinged sputum GI: anorexia, diarrhea, abdominal pain Systemic: anemia, pallor, cardiac insufficiency
	Trichinosis	Pigs, dogs, cats, rats, many wild animals	Temperate areas where pork is consumed	Larvae are ingested in undercooked meat; adult female burrows into mucosa of small intestine to produce larvae that disseminate via blood and lymphatic system to body tissues and become encysted in striated muscle.	GI: diarrhea, abdominal cramps, malaise Muscle: fever; muscle pain, tenderness, edema, and spasm Systemic: periorbital and facial edema, sweating; photophobia and conjunctivitis; manifestations of inflammation in tissues invaded by larvae
Cestode infections	Fasciolopsiasis (intestinal fluke) Tapeworm	Humans; other mammals and fish	Worldwide	Organism is ingested by eating uncooked fish or meat containing embryo cysts, by fecal contamination, or by swallowing infected intermediate hosts, such as arthropods, fleas, or lice; head (scolex) of adult worm attaches in upper small intestine, and eggs form in individual segments.	Large tapeworms: often asymptomatic; infection may cause mild nausea, diarrhea, abdominal pain; anemia, thrombocytopenia, and mild leukopenia Small tapeworms: may be asymptomatic; diarrhea, abdominal pain, anorexia, vomiting, weight loss, and irritability

Discuss measures to prevent spread of the disease in the household. Emphasize the importance of hygiene measures including changing bedding, daily cleaning of toilets with disinfectant, and hand washing.

Many helminthic disorders are acquired by consuming food that has been fecally contaminated or contains larvae of the organism. Explain the importance of not fertilizing food or grain crops with fecal material, particularly human feces. Teach clients to cook all meats and fish adequately to destroy possible larvae. In general, pickled or salt-preserved meats and fish are no safer than raw. Smoking, another means of preserving fish and meat, may not achieve temperatures high enough to destroy the organ-

isms. Vegetables grown in soil that may be contaminated with eggs or larvae should be peeled or cooked prior to eating.

Emphasize the importance of safe water supplies. Encourage people traveling to areas in which water supplies are questionable to drink only bottled water or carry purification tablets. Work with clients who have private water systems to protect water from fecal contamination by either humans or animals.

The client with a helminthic disorder may feel dirty or be ashamed of the disease. Emphasize the prevalence of these disorders, and assure the client that infection can occur despite good health practices when the eggs or larva of the organism are prevalent.

CHRONIC INFLAMMATORY BOWEL DISORDERS

THE CLIENT WITH INFLAMMATORY BOWEL DISEASE

Chronic **inflammatory bowel disease (IBD)** includes two separate but closely related conditions: ulcerative colitis and Crohn's disease. These conditions have a number of similarities. The etiology of both illnesses is unknown, but both have a geographic distribution and a genetic component. IBD occurs more frequently in the United States and northern European nations than it does in southern Europe and countries in the Southern Hemisphere. IBD affects certain ethnic groups more than others, as outlined in the Focus on Cultural Diversity box on this page. As many as 1 million Americans have IBD, with that number divided about equally between ulcerative colitis and Crohn's disease (Crohn's & Colitis Foundation of America [CCFA], 2005). It tends to run in families, with 20% to 25% of clients having a close relative with one of the types of IBD (CCFA, 2005). Factors such as an infectious agent and altered immune responses are thought to play a role in the development of IBD. Autoimmunity is thought to play a role (see Chapter 13 ∞), and lifestyle factors (such as smoking) may also affect its development.

The peak incidence of IBD is in adolescents and young adults between the ages of 15 and 35 years but it can also affect older adults (Porth, 2005). IBD is a chronic and recurrent disease process. Responses to physiologic or psychologic stresses do not cause IBD, but often play a role in exacerbations of the disease.

Despite the similarities, ulcerative colitis and Crohn's disease have distinct differences. Ulcerative colitis primarily affects the large bowel in a continuous pattern, progressing distally to proximally. In Crohn's disease, a patchy pattern of involvement is seen, affecting primarily the small intestine. Ulcerative colitis shows mainly mucosal involvement; in Crohn's disease, the submucosal layers of the bowel are affected. A comparison of ulcerative colitis and Crohn's disease is found in Table 26–7. The *Multisystem Effects of Inflammatory Bowel Disease* are illustrated on page 783.

FOCUS ON CULTURAL DIVERSITY
Incidence and Prevalence of IBD

- American Jews of European descent are four to five times more likely to develop IBD than the general population.
- There has been a steady increase of IBD in African Americans.
- The prevalence rates of IBD for Asians and Hispanics are lower than those for whites and African Americans.

TABLE 26–7 Characteristics of Ulcerative Colitis and Crohn's Disease

	CHARACTERISTIC	ULCERATIVE COLITIS	CROHN'S DISEASE
Clinical	Gender	Equal	Equal
	Age at onset	15 to 35 years; secondary peak between 50 and 70 years	10 to 30 years
	Course of disease	Typically chronic and intermittent	Slowly progressive, relapsing
	Diarrhea	5 to 30 stools per day with blood and mucous	Common, usually less severe than colitis, with no obvious blood or mucous in stool
	Abdominal pain	Cramping in left lower quadrant; relieved by defecation	Cramping or steady right lower quadrant or periumbilical pain; tenderness and mass noted in right lower quadrant
	Nutritional deficit	Common; involves anemia, hypoalbuminemia, and weight loss	Common and significant: involves anemia, weight loss, and multiple vitamin and mineral deficits
	Constitutional manifestations	Fever rare; may have associated arthritic, skin, or other organ involvement, such as erythema nodosum or uveitis	Fever, malaise, fatigue; may have some associated conditions plus urinary complications
Pathologic	Depth of involvement	Mucosa and submucosa	Transmural (entire bowel wall)
	Portion of bowel involved	Typically rectum and sigmoid colon; may extend to involve entire large bowel	Any portion of GI tract; terminal ileum and ascending colon involvement predominates
	Distribution	Continuous from rectum	Patchy; skip lesions
	Appearance of mucosa	Granular, dull, hyperemic, friable; disease uniform in affected bowel; pseudopolyps may be seen	Cobblestone appearance, with areas of normal tissue surrounded by ulceration and fissures
Complications	Acute	Toxic megacolon, perforation, massive hemorrhage	Obstruction, fistulization, abscess formation, malabsorption
	Long term	Colorectal cancer	Colon cancer

MULTISYSTEM EFFECTS OF Inflammatory Bowel Disease

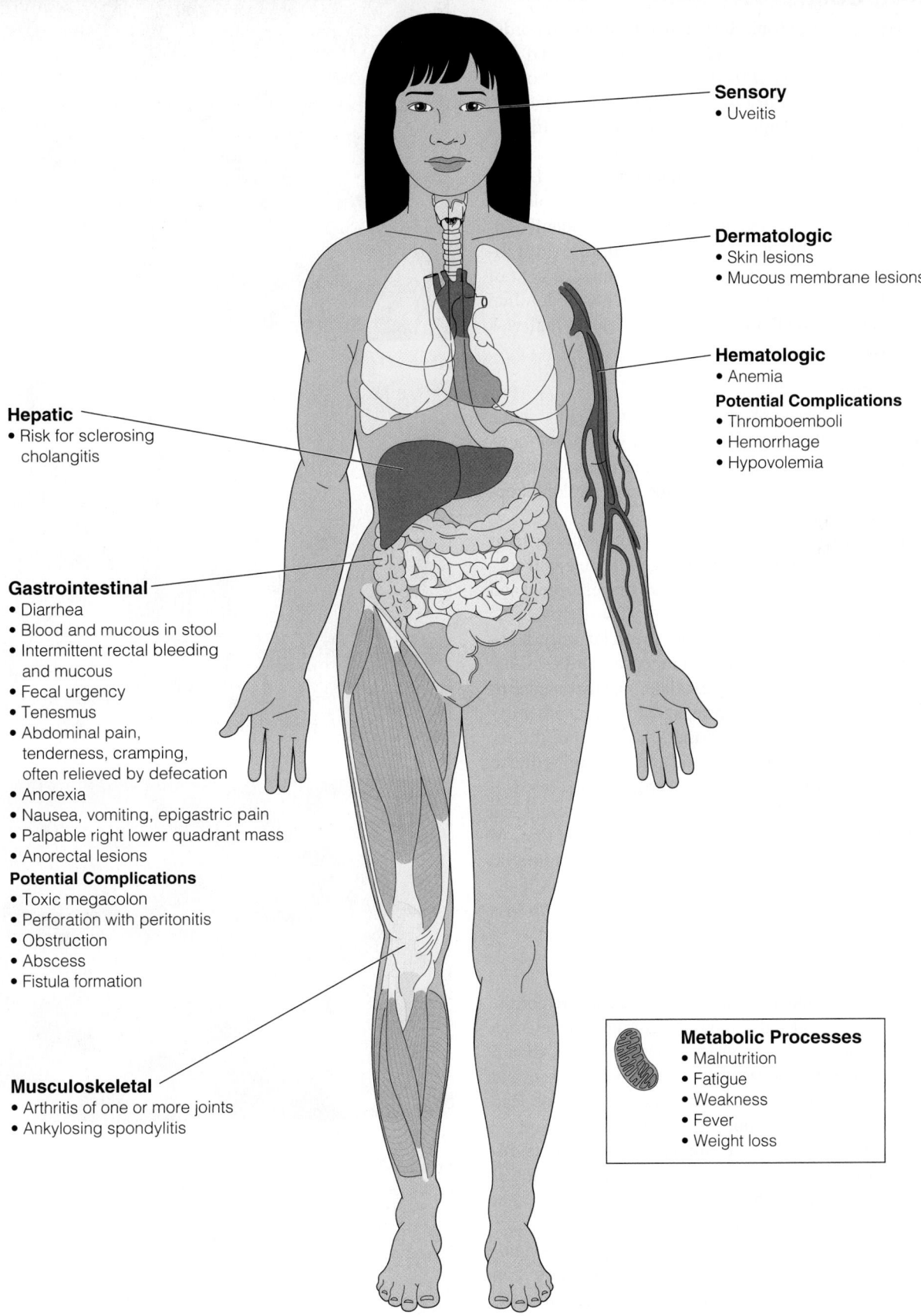

Sensory
- Uveitis

Dermatologic
- Skin lesions
- Mucous membrane lesions

Hematologic
- Anemia

Potential Complications
- Thromboemboli
- Hemorrhage
- Hypovolemia

Hepatic
- Risk for sclerosing cholangitis

Gastrointestinal
- Diarrhea
- Blood and mucous in stool
- Intermittent rectal bleeding and mucous
- Fecal urgency
- Tenesmus
- Abdominal pain, tenderness, cramping, often relieved by defecation
- Anorexia
- Nausea, vomiting, epigastric pain
- Palpable right lower quadrant mass
- Anorectal lesions

Potential Complications
- Toxic megacolon
- Perforation with peritonitis
- Obstruction
- Abscess
- Fistula formation

Musculoskeletal
- Arthritis of one or more joints
- Ankylosing spondylitis

Metabolic Processes
- Malnutrition
- Fatigue
- Weakness
- Fever
- Weight loss

Ulcerative Colitis

Ulcerative colitis is a chronic inflammatory bowel disorder that affects the mucosa and submucosa of the colon and rectum. *Chronic intermittent colitis* (recurrent ulcerative colitis) is the most common form of the disease and affects 250,000 to 500,000 people in the United States each year, resulting in steep hospital and drug costs as well as lost work (Hellekson, 2005). Its onset is insidious, with attacks that last 1 to 3 months occurring at intervals of months to years. Typically, only the distal colon is affected, with few systemic manifestations of the disease. Approximately 15% of people with ulcerative colitis develop *fulminant colitis*, with involvement of the entire colon, severe bloody diarrhea, acute abdominal pain, and fever. Clients with fulminant disease are at high risk for complications.

Pathophysiology

The inflammatory process of ulcerative colitis begins at the rectosigmoid area of the anal canal and progresses proximally. In most clients, the disease is confined to the rectum and sigmoid colon. It may progress to involve the entire colon, stopping at the ileocecal junction.

Ulcerative colitis begins with inflammation at the base of the crypts of Lieberkühn in the distal large intestine and rectum. Microscopic, pinpoint mucosal hemorrhages occur, and crypt abscesses develop (Figure 26–3 ■). These abscesses penetrate the superficial submucosa and spread laterally, leading to necrosis and sloughing of bowel mucosa. Further tissue damage is caused by inflammatory exudates and the release of inflammatory mediators, such as prostaglandins and other cytokines (see Chapter 12 ∞ for further discussion of the inflammatory process). The mucosa is red and edematous due to vascular congestion, friable (easily broken), and ulcerated. It bleeds easily, and hemorrhage is common. Edema creates a granular appearance. Pseudopolyps, tonguelike projections of bowel mucosa into the lumen, may develop as the epithelial lining of the bowel regenerates. Chronic inflammation leads to atrophy, narrowing, and shortening of the colon, with loss of its normal haustra.

Manifestations

Diarrhea is the predominant manifestation of ulcerative colitis. Stools contain both blood and mucous. Nocturnal diarrhea may occur. Mild ulcerative colitis is characterized by fewer than 5 stools per day, intermittent rectal bleeding and mucous, and few systemic manifestations. Severe ulcerative colitis can lead to more than 6 to 10 bloody stools per day, extensive colon involvement, anemia, hypovolemia, and malnutrition. Rectal inflammation causes fecal urgency and tenesmus. Left lower quadrant cramping relieved by defecation is common. Other manifestations include fatigue, anorexia, and weakness.

Clients with severe disease may also have systemic manifestations such as arthritis involving one or several joints, skin and mucous membrane lesions, or *uveitis* (inflammation of the uvea, the vascular layer of the eye, which may also involve the sclera and cornea). Some clients develop thromboemboli, with blood vessel obstruction due to clots carried from the site of

A

B

C

Figure 26–3 ■ *A,* Photomicrograph of the mucosa of the large intestine showing the entrances to the crypts of Lieberkühn. The crypts are the focal points for, *B,* ulcerative colitis and, *C,* Crohn's disease.

Source: B, Dr. E. Walker/Photo Researchers, Inc., C, Javier Domingo/Photo Researchers, Inc.

their formation. Sclerosing cholangitis (inflammation and scarring of the bile ducts) may occur, more often in men than women, and most commonly in the third to fifth decade of life (Porth, 2005).

Complications

Acute complications of ulcerative colitis include hemorrhage, toxic megacolon, and colon perforation. Massive hemorrhage may occur with severe attacks of the disease. *Toxic megacolon,* a condition characterized by acute motor paralysis and dilation of the colon to greater than 6 cm, may affect part or all of the colon. The transverse segment of the bowel is most often affected. Toxic megacolon may be triggered by the use of laxatives, narcotics, and anticholinergic drugs and the presence of hypokalemia (Porth, 2005). Manifestations of toxic megacolon include fever, tachycardia, hypotension, dehydration, abdominal tenderness and cramping, and a change in the number of stools per day. Perforation is rare, but the risk of this dangerous complication is increased with toxic megacolon. Perforation leads to peritonitis.

The risk for colorectal cancer is increased in clients with ulcerative colitis. Beginning 8 to 10 years after the diagnosis, yearly colonoscopies with biopsy to detect masses or cell dysplasia are recommended for clients who have extensive ulcerative colitis (Hellekson, 2005).

Crohn's Disease

Like ulcerative colitis, **Crohn's disease**, also known as regional enteritis, is a chronic, relapsing inflammatory disorder affecting the gastrointestinal tract. Crohn's disease can affect any portion of the GI tract from the mouth to the anus, but usually affects the terminal ileum and ascending colon. Only the small bowel is involved in about 30% to 40% of clients with Crohn's disease. The disease is limited to the colon only in 15% to 20% of those affected. Both the small and large intestine are involved in the majority of clients (Porth, 2005).

Pathophysiology

Crohn's disease typically begins as a small inflammatory *aphthoid lesion* (shallow ulcers with a white base and elevated margin, similar to a canker sore) of the mucosa and submucosa of the bowel. These initial lesions may regress, or the inflammatory process can progress to involve all layers of the intestinal wall. Deeper ulcerations, granulomatous lesions, and fissures (knifelike clefts that extend deeply into the bowel wall) develop. The inflammatory process involves the entire bowel wall (transmural).

The lumen of the affected bowel assumes a "cobblestone appearance" as fissures and ulcers surround islands of intact mucosa over edematous submucosa. The inflammatory lesions of Crohn's disease are not continuous; rather, they often occur as "skip" lesions with intervening areas of normal-appearing bowel. Some evidence suggests that despite its normal appearance, the entire bowel is affected by this disorder.

As the disease progresses, fibrotic changes in the bowel wall cause it to thicken and lose flexibility, taking on an appearance that has been likened to a rubber hose. The inflammation, edema, and fibrosis can lead to local obstruction, abscess development, and the formation of fistulas between loops of bowel or bowel and other organs (Figure 26–4 ■). Fistulas between loops of bowel are known as enteroenteric fistulas; those that occur between bowel and bladder are known as enterovesical fistulas; and fistulas that occur between bowel and skin are known as enterocutaneous fistulas. Perineal fistulas are relatively common, originating in the ileum.

Depending on the severity and extent of the disease, malabsorption and malnutrition may develop as the ulcers prevent absorption of nutrients. When the jejunum and ileum are affected, the absorption of multiple nutrients may be impaired, including carbohydrates, proteins, fats, vitamins, and folate.

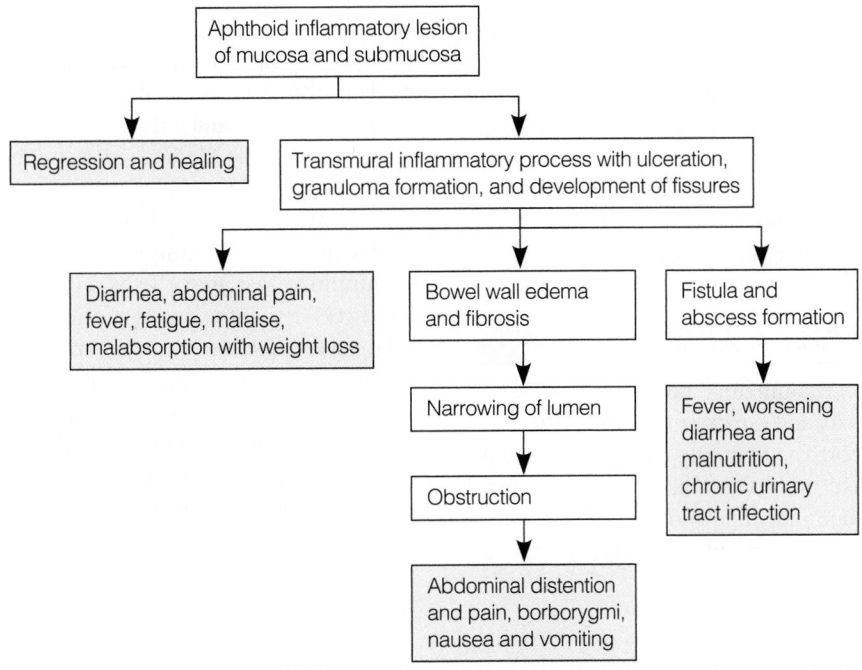

Figure 26–4 ■ The progression of Crohn's disease.

Disease in the terminal ileum can lead to vitamin B_{12} malabsorption and bile salt reabsorption. The ulcerations can also lead to protein loss and chronic, slow blood loss with consequent anemia.

Manifestations

Because the GI system involvement in Crohn's disease can be so diverse, manifestations vary among clients. The majority of people with Crohn's disease experience persistent diarrhea. Stools are liquid or semiformed and typically do not contain blood, although blood may be passed if the colon is involved. Abdominal pain and tenderness are also common. The pain may be located in the right lower quadrant and relieved by defecation. A palpable right lower quadrant mass is often present. Systemic manifestations such as fever, fatigue, malaise, weight loss, and anemia are common. Anorectal lesions such as fissures, ulcers, fistulas, and abscesses also are common and may occur years before intestinal disease is apparent. If the stomach and duodenum are involved, nausea, vomiting, and epigastric pain may occur.

Complications

Certain complications of Crohn's disease (e.g., intestinal obstruction, abscess, and fistula) are so common that they are considered part of the disease process. For many clients, the disease initially presents with one of these complications. Intestinal obstruction is a common complication caused by repeated inflammation and scarring of the bowel that leads to fibrosis and stricture. Obstruction of the bowel lumen causes abdominal distention, cramping pain, and borborygmi. Nausea and vomiting may occur.

Fistulas may be asymptomatic, particularly if they occur between loops of small bowel. When fistulization causes an abscess, chills and fever, a tender abdominal mass, and leukocytosis develop. A fistula between the small bowel and colon may exacerbate diarrhea, weight loss, and malnutrition. When the bladder is involved, recurrent urinary tract infections occur.

Perforation of the bowel is uncommon, but can lead to generalized peritonitis. Massive hemorrhage also is an uncommon complication of Crohn's disease. Long-standing Crohn's disease increases the risk of cancer of the small intestine or colon by 5 to 6 times. This cancer risk, however, is significantly lower than the risk associated with ulcerative colitis.

INTERDISCIPLINARY CARE

Interdisciplinary care for inflammatory bowel disease begins by establishing the diagnosis and the extent and severity of the disease. Treatment is supportive, including medications and dietary measures to decrease inflammation, promote intestinal rest and healing, and reduce intestinal motility. Many clients with IBD require surgery at some point to manage the disease or its complications.

Diagnosis

Diagnostic testing is used to establish the diagnosis of IBD, assess the extent of the disease, and evaluate the effects of the disorder. A sigmoidoscopy, colonoscopy, or a barium upper and lower x-ray series is performed to inspect the bowel mucosa for characteristic changes of IBD. (Nursing implications for these diagnostic tests are outlined in Chapter 25 ∞).

Laboratory tests to differentiate IBD and to identify effects and complications of the disease include a stool examination for blood and mucous, and stool cultures to rule out infectious causes of bowel inflammation and diarrhea. CBC with hemoglobin and hematocrit shows anemia from chronic inflammation, blood loss, and malnutrition, and leukocytosis due to inflammation and possible abscess formation. The sedimentation rate is typically elevated during periods of acute inflammation. Serum albumin may be decreased because of malabsorption, malnutrition, protein loss through intestinal lesions, and chronic inflammation. Folic acid and serum levels of most vitamins, including A, B complex, C, and the fat-soluble vitamins, often are decreased due to malabsorption; and liver function tests may show elevated liver enzymes (such as ALT, alkaline phosphatase, AST, GGTP, and LDH) and bilirubin levels if sclerosing cholangitis is present.

Medications

The ultimate goal of care is to terminate acute attacks as quickly as possible and reduce the incidence of relapse. Drug therapy plays a key role in achieving this goal. Locally acting and systemic anti-inflammatory drugs are the primary medications used to manage mild to moderate IBD. Drugs to suppress the immune response may be used to treat clients with severe disease.

Sulfasalazine (Azulfidine) is a sulfonamide antibiotic that is poorly absorbed from the gastrointestinal tract and acts topically on the colonic mucosa to inhibit the inflammatory process. The active anti-inflammatory ingredient in sulfasalazine, 5-aminosalicylic acid, also is available in preparations that do not contain sulfa, such as olsalazine and mesalamine. They have the advantage of causing fewer adverse effects than sulfasalazine. Azo compounds, such as balsalazide and olsalazine, are 5-aminosalicylic acid compounds that are released in the colon and are especially useful to treat ulcerative colitis. Specific preparations, their method of action, and nursing implications for these medications are outlined in the Medication Administration box on page 787.

For acute exacerbations of IBD, corticosteroids are given to reduce inflammation and induce remission. For ulcerative colitis, the drug may be administered rectally for its local effect and to minimize systemic effects. Hydrocortisone can be administered rectally. Intravenous corticosteroids may be required to treat severe disease; oral preparations are used for less severe manifestations and long-term therapy. Many clients are unable to withdraw from steroid therapy without experiencing relapse and may need chronic low-dose therapy.

Mercaptopurine (6-MP, Purinethol) and other immunosuppressive agents such as azathioprine (Imuran) and cyclosporine (Sandimmune) can be used to treat clients who have not responded to other treatments or who require chronic steroid therapy. These drugs may allow withdrawal from corticosteroids, maintain remission, and facilitate healing. Long-term therapy may be required to produce a beneficial effect. For more information about immunosuppressive drugs, see Chapter 13 ∞ .

MEDICATION ADMINISTRATION Inflammatory Bowel Disease

SULFASALAZINE (AZULFIDINE)

Sulfasalazine is an anti-inflammatory drug used for its local effect on the intestinal mucosa in inflammatory bowel disease. The active part of the drug is 5-aminosalicylic acid, which inhibits prostaglandin production in the bowel. Prostaglandin is an important mediator of the inflammatory process; blocking its production reduces inflammation.

Nursing Responsibilities

- Assess for contraindications, including pregnancy or a history of hypersensitivity to sulfonamides or salicylates.
- Assess baseline values for renal function tests (serum creatinine, BUN, urinalysis), liver function tests, and CBC.
- Administer as ordered. Suppositories or retention enemas may be administered at bedtime. Administer oral forms with a full glass of water.
- Have resuscitation equipment available; anaphylactic responses may occur.
- Evaluate for therapeutic response, including reduced number of stools, reduced mucus and blood, and improved stool consistency.
- Monitor for possible adverse responses:
    a. Skin rash, dermatitis, urticaria, or pruritus
    b. Evidence of blood dyscrasias, such as bleeding, easy bruising, fever
    c. Leukopenia, thrombocytopenia, hemolytic anemia, or angranulocytosis
    d. Changes in urinary output or renal function studies
    e. Evidence of hepatitis or myocarditis.

Health Education for the Client and Family

- Take oral preparations after meals to decrease gastric distress.
- Drink at least 2 quarts of fluid per day to reduce the risk of kidney damage.
- Use sunscreen to prevent burns; this drug increases sensitivity to sun.
- Do not take aspirin, vitamin C, or any other over-the-counter medications containing aspirin or vitamin C without consulting your doctor.
- This medication may interfere with the effectiveness of oral contraceptives; use alternative methods of contraception.
- Notify your doctor if you develop skin rash or hives, sore throat or mouth, bleeding gums, joint pain, easy bruising, or fever.

MESALAMINE (ASACOL ROWASA) AND OLSALAZINE (DIPENTUM)

Mesalamine and olsalazine contain the same active ingredient, 5-aminosalicylic acid, as sulfasalazine, but cause fewer adverse effects. Their mechanism of action is the same as that of sulfasalazine. These drugs are available as suppositories, suspension for enema, or oral tablets.

Nursing Responsibilities

- Assess for possible contraindications such as pregnancy, lactation, or hypersensitivity to these drugs or aspirin.
- Administer as ordered. If more than one dose per day is ordered, space doses evenly over the 24-hour period.
- Evaluate for desired effects (as for sulfasalazine) and potential adverse effects.
    a. Nausea, diarrhea, abdominal cramps, or flatulence
    b. CNS effects including headache, dizziness, insomnia, weakness, or fatigue

    c. Rash or itching
    d. Flulike symptoms, general malaise.

Health Education for the Client and Family

- Teach the recommended method of administration, including how to insert rectal suppositories or administer a retention enema.
- Shake suspension forms well prior to using.
- Diarrhea is the most common side effect of these drugs. Notify your doctor if adverse effects occur.

CORTICOSTEROIDS
Methylprednisolone (Medrol, Solu-Medrol)
Prednisolone (Delta-Cortel) Prednisone

Glucocorticoids are hormones produced by the adrenal cortex. These hormones are necessary for the stress response. Cortisol, the main glucocorticoid, has potent anti-inflammatory effects. Corticosteroids are used to treat acute episodes of IBD. Because of their multiple and significant side effects, they are not used to maintain remission.

Nursing Responsibilities

- Assess for conditions that may be adversely affected by corticosteroid drugs: peptic ulcer disease, glaucoma or cataracts, diabetes, or psychiatric disorders.
- Obtain baseline vital signs and weight; monitor both routinely during therapy. Hypertension and weight gain may result from salt and water retention.
- Monitor for edema.
- Administer as ordered. For daily or alternate-day dosing, administer in the morning, when physiologic glucocorticoid levels are highest, to reduce adrenal cortisone suppression.
- Administer oral preparations with food to decrease gastrointestinal side effects. Antacids or histamine H_2-receptor blocking agents, such as cimetidine (Tagamet), may be prescribed during corticosteroid therapy.
- Monitor for desired effects: reduced diarrhea, less blood and mucous in the stool, and less abdominal cramping.
- Monitor for adverse effects:
    a. Increased susceptibility to infection and masking of early signs of infection
    b. Hyperglycemia
    c. Hypokalemia, as manifested by muscle weakness, nausea, vomiting, and cardiac rhythm disturbances
    d. Edema, hypertension, and signs of heart failure
    e. Peptic ulcer formation and possible gastrointestinal hemorrhage (abdominal pain, black or tarry stools, and signs of bleeding)
    f. Changes in mental status, including depression, euphoria, aggression, and behavioral changes
    g. With long-term use, Cushingoid effects, such as abnormal fat deposits in the face (moon faces) and trunk (buffalo hump), muscle wasting and thin extremities, thinning of the skin, and osteoporosis.

Health Education for the Client and Family

- Take as prescribed; do not change the dose or time of day. Do not stop the medication abruptly. The dose will be tapered down gradually when the drug is discontinued.

(continued)

MEDICATION ADMINISTRATION **Inflammatory Bowel Disease (continued)**

- Notify the physician if adverse or Cushingoid effects occur.
- Take with food or at mealtimes to decrease the gastrointestinal effects.
- Monitor weight. If a gain of more than 5 pounds is noted, notify the physician.

- Moderate salt intake and avoid foods and snacks high in sodium, such as processed meats and potato chips. Increase intake of foods high in potassium, such as fruits, vegetables, and lean meats.
- Carry a card or wear a bracelet or tag at all times identifying corticosteroid use.

Newer treatments for IBD employ other immune response modifiers, such as the monoclonal antibody infliximab (Remicade) to suppress tumor necrosis factor (TNF, an inflammatory mediator substance) in clients who have not responded to standard therapies. Mesalamine (Canasa, Rowasa) is an orally or rectally administered anti-inflammatory medication that provides topical anti-inflammatory action in the colon of clients with ulcerative colitis.

Although antibiotic therapy generally is not indicated in IBD, metronidazole (Flagyl) has active anti-inflammatory effects. It may be prescribed to help prevent remission after ileal resection in Crohn's disease. Ciprofloxacin (Cipro) is an alternative to metronidazole.

Antidiarrheal agents, such as loperamide and diphenoxylate, may be given to slow gastrointestinal motility and reduce diarrhea. These drugs are safe for clients with mild, chronic manifestations, but they are not given during acute attacks because they may precipitate toxic dilation of the colon.

Nutrition

Antigens in the diet may stimulate the immune response in the bowel, exacerbating IBD. As a result, dietary management for inflammatory bowel disease is individualized. Some clients benefit from eliminating all milk and milk products from the diet. Increased dietary fiber may help reduce diarrhea and relieve rectal manifestations, but is contraindicated for clients with intestinal strictures caused by repeated inflammation and scarring.

All food may be withheld to promote bowel rest during an acute exacerbation of Crohn's disease. Nutritional status is maintained using enteral or total parenteral nutrition (TPN). See Chapter 22 ∞ for more information about enteral feedings and TPN. TPN carries a higher risk of complications than does enteral nutrition. An elemental diet such as Ensure, which contains all essential nutrients in a residue-free formula, may be prescribed. Enteral diets provide essential nutrients to the small intestine to support cell growth, but are not always palatable.

Surgery

Surgical interventions for IBD differ, depending on the primary disease process and the portion of the bowel affected. Generally, surgery is performed only when necessitated by complications of the disease or failure of conservative treatment measures.

Bowel obstruction is the leading indication for surgery in Crohn's disease. Other complications that may require surgical intervention include perforation, internal or external fistula, abscess, and perianal complications. Resection of the affected portion of bowel with an end-to-end anastomosis to preserve as much bowel as possible is the usual treatment. The disease process tends to recur in other areas following removal of affected bowel segments. There is an increased risk of fistula formation following surgery. Bowel strictures may be treated with a strictureplasty. In this procedure, longitudinal incisions are made in the narrowed segment to relieve the stricture while preserving bowel.

COLECTOMY Clients with extensive chronic ulcerative colitis may require a total **colectomy** (surgical resection and removal of the colon) to treat the disease itself; for complications such as toxic megacolon, perforation, or hemorrhage; or as a prophylactic measure due to the high colon cancer risk associated with extensive ulcerative colitis.

The surgical procedure of choice for extensive ulcerative colitis is a *total colectomy with an ileal pouch-anal anastomosis (IPAA)*. In this procedure, the entire colon and rectum are removed; a pouch is formed from the terminal ileum; and the pouch is brought into the pelvis and anastomosed to the anal canal (Figure 26–5 ■). A temporary or loop ileostomy (described in the next section) is generally performed at the same time and is maintained for 2 to 3 months to allow the anal anastomosis to heal. When the healing is complete, the ileostomy is closed, and the client has six to eight daily bowel movements through the anus. Advanced age, obesity, or other factors may

Figure 26–5 ■ Ileal pouch-anal anastomosis (IPAA).

preclude an IPAA. For these clients, a permanent ileostomy or continent ileostomy may be created.

OSTOMY An intestinal ostomy is a surgically created opening between the intestine and the abdominal wall that allows the passage of fecal material. The surface opening is called a **stoma** (Figure 26–6 ■). The precise name of the ostomy depends on the location of the stoma. An **ileostomy** is an ostomy made in the ileum of the small intestine. In an ileostomy, the colon, rectum, and anus are usually completely removed (*total proctocolectomy with permanent ileostomy*). The anal canal is closed, and the end of the terminal ileum is brought to the body surface through the right abdominal wall to form the stoma. A temporary or *loop ileostomy* may be formed to eliminate feces and allow tissue healing for 2 to 3 months following an IPAA. A loop of ileum is brought to the body surface to

form a stoma and allow stool drainage into an external pouch. When the ileostomy is no longer necessary, a second surgery is performed to close the stoma and repair the bowel, restoring fecal elimination through the anus.

In a *continent ileostomy* (Figure 26–7 ■), an intra-abdominal reservoir is constructed and a nipple valve formed (the ileum folded back on itself) from the terminal ileum, before it is brought to the surface of the abdominal wall. Stool collects in the internal pouch; the nipple valve prevents it from leaking through the stoma. A catheter is inserted into the pouch to drain the stool.

Nursing care of the client with an ileostomy is outlined in the box below. Procedure 26–1 on page 791 describes how to apply one- and two-piece drainable ostomy pouches.

Figure 26–6 ■ A healthy-appearing stoma.
Courtesy of Carol Williams, RN, BS, UC Davis Medical Center.

Figure 26–7 ■ Continent (Kock's) ileostomy.

NURSING CARE OF THE CLIENT HAVING AN Ileostomy

PREOPERATIVE CARE
- Provide routine preoperative care and teaching as outlined in Chapter 4 ∞.
- Refer to an enterostomal therapist for marking and teaching about the stoma location, ostomy care, and options for ostomy appliances. *It is important to begin teaching prior to surgery to facilitate learning and acceptance of the ostomy postoperatively.*
- Discuss the availability of a local United Ostomy Association chapter, and provide a referral as necessary or desired. *Local chapters often have members with ostomies who are willing to provide both preoperative and postoperative teaching, listening, and support.*
- Provide preoperative bowel preparation as ordered. *Cathartics, enemas, and preoperative antibiotics are often ordered to reduce the risk of abdominal contamination and infection after surgery.*

POSTOPERATIVE CARE
- Provide routine postoperative care and teaching as outlined in Chapter 4 ∞.
- Apply an ostomy pouch over the stoma. (See Procedure 26–1.) *Stool from an ileostomy is expressed continuously or irregularly,*

and it is liquid in nature; continuous use of a pouch to collect the drainage is necessary.
- Assess frequently for bleeding, stoma viability, and function. In the early postoperative period, small amounts of blood in the pouch are expected. A healthy stoma appears pink or red and moist as a result of mucous production (Figure 26–6). It should protrude approximately 2 cm from the abdominal wall. *Frequent assessment is particularly important in the initial postoperative period to ensure stoma health and monitor for possible complications. A dusky, brown, black, or white stoma indicates circulatory compromise. Other possible stoma complications include retraction (indentation or loss of the external portion of the stoma) or prolapse (outward telescoping of the stoma, that is, an abnormally long stoma).*
- As the stoma starts to function, empty the pouch, explaining the procedure to the client. Initial drainage is dark green, viscid, and usually odorless. Drainage gradually thickens and becomes yellow-brown. Empty the pouch when it is one-third full. Measure drainage, and include it as output on intake and output records. Rinse the pouch and reapply the clamp. *Emptying the pouch when it is no more than one-third full helps prevent the skin seal from breaking as a result of the*

(continued)

NURSING CARE OF THE CLIENT HAVING AN   Ileostomy (continued)

weight of the pouch. Because of the potential for excess fluid loss through ileostomy drainage, it is important to include it as fluid output.

- Assess the peristomal skin. Skin around the stoma should remain clean and pink and free of irritation, rashes, inflammation, or excoriation. *Skin complications may arise from appliance irritation or hypersensitivity, excoriation from a leaking appliance, or Candida albicans, a yeast infection.*
- Protect peristomal skin from enzymes and bile salts in the ileostomy effluent. Using a skin barrier on the pouch is essential. Change the pouch if leakage occurs or if the client complains of burning or itching skin. *Enzymes and bile salts normally reabsorbed in the large intestine are irritating to the skin. Excoriation of skin surrounding the stoma impairs the first line of defense against microorganisms and can interfere with the ability to achieve a tight skin seal and prevent pouch leakage.*
- Report the following abnormal assessment findings to the physician:
  a. Allergic or contact dermatitis. *A rash may result from contact with fecal drainage or indicate sensitivity to pouch, paste, tape, or sealant.*
  b. Purulent ulcerated areas surrounding the stoma. *Disruption of the protective barrier of the skin allows bacterial entry.*
  c. A red, bumpy, itchy rash or white-coated area. *This is a manifestation of Candida albicans, a yeast infection.*
  d. Bulging around the stoma. *This finding may indicate herniation, caused by loops of intestine protruding through the abdominal wall.*
- Apply protective ointments to the perirectal area of clients with newly functioning ileoanal reservoirs and anastomoses. *This helps protect the skin from the initial stools. As stools thicken and become fewer per day, the client experiences less perirectal irritation.*

Health Education for the Client and Family

- While caring for the ostomy, explain procedures to the client. *Teaching is immediate and ongoing to facilitate acceptance of the ostomy and self-care.*
- Teach to manage the pouch clamp, to empty, rinse, and perform pouch changes. *Self-care is vital to independence and self-esteem.*
- Instruct now to use an electric razor to shave the peristomal hair if necessary. *An electric razor prevents accidental cutting of the stoma with a razor blade.*
- Teach to check the stoma and peristomal skin with each pouch change. *Ongoing assessment is important for optimal health and function of the stoma and surrounding skin. Stripping of tape or excessively frequent pouch removal may cause mechanical trauma to peristomal skin. Chronic skin irritation by ileostomy effluent may lead to pseudoveracous lesions, or wartlike nodules.*
- Instruct to report abnormal appearance of the stoma or surrounding skin (as noted previously and below) to the physician:
  a. Narrowing of the stoma lumen. *This indicates stenosis and may interfere with fecal elimination.*

  b. Lacerations or cuts in the stoma. *The stoma contains no nerves, so trauma may occur without pain.*
  c. Separation of the stoma from the abdominal surface. This potential complication may require surgical repair.
- Emphasize the importance of adequate fluid and salt intake; the risk for dehydration and hyponatremia is increased particularly during hot weather, when fluid is lost through perspiration as well as ileostomy drainage. Water intake should be sufficient to maintain pale urine and an output of at least 1 quart per day. When exercising in hot weather, the client should consume extra water and salt. High-potassium foods, such as bananas and oranges, may also be recommended. *Loss of the reabsorptive surface of the large bowel increases the amount of water and sodium loss in the stool. If the ileostomy is high (more proximal in the ileum), additional potassium losses may also occur.*
- Discuss manifestations of fluid and electrolyte imbalances:
  a. Extreme thirst
  b. Dry skin and oral mucous membrane
  c. Decreased urine output
  d. Weakness, fatigue
  e. Muscle cramps
  f. Abdominal cramps, nausea, vomiting
  g. Shortness of breath
  h. Orthostatic hypotension (feeling faint when suddenly changing positions).
- Discuss dietary concerns. A low-residue diet is recommended initially (see Table 26–8). Foods that may cause excessive odor or gas are typically avoided as well. *Because food blockage is a potential problem, high-fiber foods are limited, and foods that may cause blockage, such as popcorn, corn, nuts, cucumbers, celery, fresh tomatoes, figs, strawberries, blackberries, and caraway seeds, are avoided. Symptoms of food blockage include abdominal cramping, swelling of the stoma, and absence of ileostomy output for over 4 to 6 hours.*
- Teach self-care measures to relieve food blockage:
  a. Take a warm shower or tub bath. *This can help relax the abdominal muscles.*
  b. Assume a knee–chest position. *The knee–chest position reduces intra-abdominal pressure.*
  c. Drink warm fluids or grape juice if not vomiting. *This provides a mild cathartic effect.*
  d. Massage peristomal area. *Massage may stimulate peristalsis and fecal elimination.*
  e. Remove pouch if the stoma is swollen, and apply a pouch with a larger opening. *If the stoma swells, the pouch may create a mechanical obstruction to output.*
- Notify the physician or enterostomal therapy nurse if:
  a. The above measures fail to relieve the obstruction.
  b. Signs of a partial obstruction persist including high-volume odorous fluid output, abdominal cramps, nausea, and vomiting.
  c. There is no ileostomy output for 4 to 6 hours.
  d. Signs of fluid and electrolyte imbalance occur, such as weakness, dizziness, lightheadedness, or headache.

Should self-care measures not succeed in breaking up a blockage, ileostomy lavage, as described in Procedure 26–2, may be required.

PROCEDURE 26–1 CHANGING A ONE- OR TWO-PIECE DRAINABLE OSTOMY POUCH

GATHER SUPPLIES

- Disposable gloves
- One- or two-piece pouch
- Skin barrier paste
- Skin prep
- Clamp
- Pouch deodorant
- Measuring guide
- Adhesive remover
- Skin cleanser
- Washcloths
- Plastic bag

BEFORE THE PROCEDURE

Explain the procedure and provide for privacy.
Follow standard precautions. Don gloves.

PROCEDURE

1. Remove soiled pouch (and the flange if a two-piece pouch) by gently pulling on the pouch or flange and pushing on skin. Use adhesive remover to remove skin barrier paste.
2. Empty pouch, discarding it and the flange (if applicable) in a plastic bag. Save the tail closure clamp. The pouch from a two-piece system may be cleaned out and reused.
3. Cleanse skin and stoma with warm water and skin cleanser or mild soap. Rinse skin and stoma, and pat dry.
4. Note stoma color and peristomal skin condition.
5. If necessary, clip or shave peristomal hair.
6. Use measuring guide or previous pattern to check size of stoma.
   a. Presized pouch: check to verify that size is correct.
   b. Cut-to-fit pouch or flange: Trace the correct size of the stoma onto the back of the flange, and cut the opening to match the pattern. The opening should be no more than 1/8 inch larger than stoma.
7. Apply skin prep to skin covered by a wafer, pouch, or tape. Allow to dry.
8. Remove backings from pouch or flange.
9. Apply a bead of skin barrier paste around the stoma base or around the opening of the pouch or flange. Allow the paste to air-dry for 1 to 2 minutes.
10. Center the pouch or flange over the stoma, and press to adhere.
11. For a two-piece pouch, snap the pouch onto skin barrier flange.
12. Place deodorizing tablets or a few drops of liquid pouch deodorizer (in some cases, antiseptic mouthwash may be used) in the pouch. Apply the clamp.
13. "Picture frame" the pouch with tape to provide extra security.

TABLE 26–8 Low-Residue Diet

FOOD GROUP	ALLOWED	AVOID
Beverages	Coffee, teas, juices, carbonated beverages; milk limited to 2 cups per day	Alcohol, prune juice
Breads and cereals	Products made from refined flours (white bread, crackers) or finely milled grains (e.g., corn flakes, crisp rice cereal, puffed wheat)	Whole-grain breads, rolls, or cereal; breads or rolls with seeds, nuts, or bran
Desserts	Gelatins, tapioca, plain custards, or puddings; angel-food or sponge cake; ice cream or frozen desserts without fruit or nuts	Any desserts containing dried fruits, nuts, seeds, or coconut; rich pastries, pies
Fruits	Fruit juices and strained fruits; cooked or canned apples, apricots, cherries, peaches, pears; bananas	All other raw or cooked fruits
Meats and other protein sources	Roasted, baked, or broiled tender or ground beef, veal, pork, lamb, poultry, or fish; smooth peanut butter; cottage, cream, American, or mild cheddar cheeses in small amounts	Tough or spiced meats and those prepared by frying; highly flavored cheeses; nuts
Potatoes, rice, and pasta	Peeled potatoes; white rice; most pasta products	Potato skins, potato chips, or fried potatoes; brown rice; whole-grain pasta products
Sweets	Sugar, honey, jelly, hard candy and gumdrops, plain chocolates	Jam, marmalade; candy made with seeds, nuts, coconut
Vegetables	Vegetable juices and strained vegetables; cooked or canned vegetables	Raw or whole cooked vegetables
Other	Salt, ground seasonings; cream sauce and plain gravy	Chili sauce, horseradish; popcorn, seeds of any kind; whole spices, olives, vinegar

PROCEDURE 26–2 ILEOSTOMY LAVAGE

GATHER SUPPLIES

- Disposable gloves
- Disposable irrigation sleeve
- 60 mL catheter-tipped syringe
- #14 Fr. catheter
- Water-soluble lubricant
- Normal saline for irrigation
- Bedpan
- Clean ostomy pouch

BEFORE THE PROCEDURE

Explain the procedure and provide for privacy.
Follow standard precautions. Don gloves.

PROCEDURE

1. Remove the pouch. Apply disposable irrigation sleeve.
2. Clamp the bottom of the sleeve, or place it into the bedpan.
3. Gently examine stoma digitally to break up any fecal mass proximal to stoma and determine direction of the bowel.
4. Lubricate catheter, and insert into stoma until blockage is reached. If the catheter does not reach the blockage after 8 to 10 cm, notify the physician. This may indicate a more proximal obstruction.
5. Instill 30 to 50 mL normal saline.
6. Remove catheter. Allow stoma to drain.
7. Repeat the procedure until the mass is removed.
8. When the blockage is removed, remove the irrigation sleeve.
9. Clean peristomal skin.
10. Apply pouch and clamp.

AFTER THE PROCEDURE

1. Document the procedure, amount of solution used, consistency of results, and the client's tolerance of the procedure.
2. Discuss dietary intake to help determine cause of blockage.

Complementary and Alternative Therapies

The chronic nature of inflammatory bowel disease and adverse effects of many prescribed treatments lead many clients with IBD to seek or use complementary and alternative therapies. Chiropractic care, megavitamin therapy, dietary supplements, and herbal medicine have been reported as common complementary and alternative therapies for IBD (Heuschkel et al., 2002; Verhoef et al., 2002). A study by Langmead et al. (2002) concluded that herbal remedies such as slippery elm, fenugreek, devil's claw, Mexican yam, termentil, and wei tong ning have antioxidant effects and may provide an effect similar to that of 5-aminosalicylic acid preparations. Peppermint tea is an excellent tonic for reducing nausea, relieving abdominal pain, and providing a calming effect. Chamomile tea helps to reduce intestinal inflammation (Balch & Stengler, 2004). Many complementary and alternative therapies for IBD may interact with prescribed medications; instruct the client to discuss all potential therapies with the primary care provider. Accupressure, body massage, reflexology, aromatherapy, and stress reduction therapies can also aid in reducing manifestations of IBD.

NURSING CARE

Health Promotion

Although inflammatory bowel disease cannot, at this time, be predicted or prevented, effective management may help the client avoid complications of the disease. Stress the importance of complying with the prescribed treatment regimen and promptly reporting manifestations of exacerbations to the physician.

Assessment

Assessment data related to inflammatory bowel disease includes the following subjective and objective data:

- *Health history:* Current manifestations, including onset, duration, severity (number of stools per day, presence of blood or mucous in stool, abdominal pain or cramping, tenesmus); usual diet, ability to maintain weight and nutrition, food intolerances; associated manifestations such as arthralgias, fatigue, malaise; current medications; previous treatment and diagnostic tests.
- *Physical examination:* General appearance; weight; vital signs including orthostatic vitals and temperature; abdominal assessment including shape, contour, bowel sounds, palpation for tenderness and masses, presence of stoma or scars.

Nursing Diagnoses and Interventions

When planning nursing care for the client with inflammatory bowel disease, it is vital to consider the chronic, recurrent nature of the disorder. Teaching is a major aspect of care. Diarrhea and disturbed body image are significant nursing care problems for the client with IBD. With severe disease, impaired nutrition must be considered a priority problem as well. A Nursing Care Plan for a client with ulcerative colitis is included on the following page.

Diarrhea

During an acute exacerbation of IBD, diarrhea can be frequent and painful. The frequency of defecation and associated abdominal pain and cramping may interfere with ADLs and increase the risk for fluid volume deficit and impaired skin integrity.

- Record the frequency, amount, and color of stools using a stool chart. Measure and record liquid stool as output. *The severity of diarrhea is an indicator of the severity of the disease and helps determine the need for fluid replacement.*

NURSING CARE PLAN   A Client with Ulcerative Colitis

Cortez Lewis is a 42-year-old real estate agent and mother of three school-age children. She has had ulcerative colitis for 18 years and has been treated with prednisone and sulfasalazine. Over the past 4 months she has been having abdominal pain and cramping and frequent bloody diarrhea stools. During the same period, she has lost 20 lb (9 kg); and has had difficulty maintaining her career. She recently developed several lesions of the lower leg identified as erythema nodosum. A recent colonoscopy revealed extensive involvement of the entire colon. On admission, Mrs. Lewis states, "I'm tired of fighting this disease. I am a prisoner in my home because of the diarrhea." She is admitted for a total proctocolectomy and ileal pouch-anal anastomosis.

ASSESSMENT

Janet Wheeler, RN, completes the admission assessment. Mrs. Lewis now weighs 115 lb (52.2 kg). She complains of abdominal cramping, pain, and frequent bloody diarrhea stools. Several reddened lesions are noted on her lower legs. Physical assessment findings include T 98°F (36.6°C), P 72, R 20, and BP 104/72. Skin cool and pale. Abnormal laboratory findings include hemoglobin 7.3 g/dL (normal 11.7 to 15.7 g/dL); hematocrit 23.3% (normal 35% to 47%); WBC 15,580/mm³ (normal 3500 to 11,000/mm³); platelet count 995,000/mm³ (normal 150,000 to 450,000/mm³); serum protein 4.6 g/dL (normal 6 to 8 g/dL); serum albumin 2.4 g/dL (normal 3.5 to 5 g/dL). Preparation for surgery is begun.

DIAGNOSES

- *Imbalanced Nutrition: Less than Body Requirements* related to impaired absorption
- *Diarrhea* related to inflammation of bowel
- *Risk for Deficient Fluid Volume* related to abnormal fluid loss
- *Risk for Impaired Tissue Integrity* related to drainage from temporary ileostomy
- *Acute Pain* related to surgical intervention
- *Risk for Sexual Dysfunction* related to temporary ileostomy.

EXPECTED OUTCOMES

- Resume prescribed diet within 5 days after surgery.
- Demonstrate normal fecal elimination through the temporary ileostomy.
- Maintain adequate fluid balance.

- Demonstrate appropriate ostomy care prior to discharge.
- Report a tolerable level of discomfort.
- Verbalize feelings about sexuality and acknowledge importance of discussing sexual issues with husband.

PLANNING AND IMPLEMENTATION

- Discuss dietary modifications related to nutritional status and presence of ileostomy. Provide referral to dietitian for diet planning and teaching.
- Teach importance of maintaining a high fluid intake and manifestations of dehydration.
- Teach to empty and change ostomy, pouch of choice.
- Teach stoma and peristomal skin assessment with each pouch change.
- Teach food blockage management.
- Refer to local United Ostomy Association.
- Provide list of local medical suppliers for ostomy appliances.

EVALUATION

On discharge, Mrs. Lewis is caring for her ileostomy by demonstrating her ability to empty, rinse, and change the pouch. The ET nurse has provided written and verbal instructions on ileostomy care. Mrs. Lewis verbalizes her understanding of the recommended diet and the need to limit high-fiber food intake and avoid enteric-coated and timed-release medications. The ET nurse has discussed sexual aspects of having an ileostomy and has given Mrs. Lewis a booklet, "Sex and the Female Ostomate," available through the United Ostomy Association. Mrs. Lewis is looking forward to the planned surgery to close the temporary ileostomy.

CRITICAL THINKING IN THE NURSING PROCESS

1. Why is the client with an ileostomy at risk for dehydration? How can Mrs. Lewis monitor her fluid status at home?
2. Why were Mrs. Lewis's hemoglobin and hematocrit low on admission? If her hemoglobin had been low but her hematocrit normal on admission, what might be the explanation?
3. Outline a teaching plan that could be given to clients for home care of an ileostomy.
4. Develop a care plan for Mrs. Lewis for the nursing diagnosis *Risk for Impaired Skin Integrity.*
   See Evaluating Your Response in Appendix C.

PRACTICE ALERT

Observe stools for obvious blood and test for occult blood as indicated. Report grossly bloody stools (**hematochezia**), which may indicate hemorrhage and necessitate emergency surgery.

- Monitor vital signs every 4 hours. *Tachycardia, tachypnea, and fever may be indicators of fluid volume deficit.*
- Weigh daily and record. *Rapid weight loss (over days to a week) usually indicates fluid loss, whereas weight loss over weeks to months may indicate malnutrition.*
- Assess for other indications of fluid deficit: warm, dry skin, poor skin turgor, dry shiny mucous membranes, weakness, lethargy, complaints of thirst. *The extent of fluid loss may not*

be readily evident with diarrhea, particularly if the client uses the bathroom without assistance. Systemic manifestations of fluid volume deficit may be the first indicators of the problem.

- Maintain bowel rest by keeping NPO or limiting oral intake to elemental feedings as indicated. *Bowel rest during an acute exacerbation of IBD promotes healing and reduces diarrhea and other manifestations.*
- Administer prescribed anti-inflammatory and antidiarrheal medications as indicated. *Anti-inflammatory medications reduce the extent of bowel inflammation and diarrhea. Unless contraindicated, antidiarrheal medications help reduce fluid loss and increase comfort.*

- Maintain fluid intake by mouth or intravenously as indicated. *The client with IBD requires fluid to replace ongoing losses, as well as fluid to meet the usual daily needs of the body. If an elemental diet or total parenteral nutrition is prescribed, additional fluids may be required to meet fluid intake needs.*
- Provide good skin care. *Fluid deficit and tissue dehydration increase the risk for skin excoriations or breakdown.*
- Assess perianal area for irritation or denuded skin from the diarrhea. Use gentle cleansing agents, such as Peri-Wash or Tucks, diaper wipes, or cotton balls saturated with witch hazel. Apply a protective cream, such as zinc oxide–based preparations, to protect skin from the irritating effects of diarrheal stool. *Digestive enzymes in the stool are very corrosive, increasing the risk of skin breakdown where exposed to diarrheal stool.*

Disturbed Body Image

The client with IBD may experience frustration at not being able to control, or even predict, fecal elimination, particularly when the disease is severe. Diarrhea can interfere with the ability to complete tasks, maintain employment or engage in social activities, and even meet basic needs such as eating, sleeping, and sexual activity. Body image can suffer as a result. Treatment of IBD, be it total colectomy with ileal pouch-anal anastomosis, ileostomy, or chronic corticosteroid therapy, also can affect the view of self.

- Accept feelings and perception of self. *Negating or denying the reality of the client's perception impairs trust.*
- Encourage discussion of physical changes and their consequences as they relate to self-concept. *This demonstrates acceptance and provides an opportunity to express the impact of the disease and its treatment on the client's life.*
- Encourage discussion about concerns regarding the effect of the disease or treatment on close personal relationships. *This demonstrates understanding and provides an opportunity for the client to express feelings about the impact of the disease on relationships and significant others.*
- Encourage the client to make choices and decisions regarding care. *This increases the client's sense of control over the disease and his or her future.*
- Discuss possible treatment options and their effects openly and honestly. *Open discussion allows more informed decisions.*
- Involve the client in care, teaching and demonstrating as needed. *This encourages and facilitates independence and decision making.*
- Provide care in an accepting, nonjudgmental manner. *Acceptance of the client despite potential embarrassment about odors or diarrhea enhances self-esteem.*
- Arrange for interaction with other clients or groups of people with IBD or ostomies. *The client may feel that no one who has not experienced a similar problem can understand his or her feelings.*

- Teach coping strategies (odor control, dietary modifications, and so on), and support their use. *This facilitates healthy adaptation to the disease.*

Imbalanced Nutrition: Less than Body Requirements

Crohn's disease can significantly alter the bowel's ability to absorb nutrients. In both forms of IBD, blood and protein-rich fluid may be lost in diarrheal stools. With malabsorption and continuing nutrient losses, multiple nutrient deficits can develop, affecting growth and development, healing, muscle mass, bone density, and electrolyte balances.

- Monitor laboratory results, including hemoglobin and hematocrit, serum electrolytes, and total serum protein and albumin levels. *These studies provide an indicator of nutritional status.*
- Provide the prescribed diet: high-kilocalorie, high-protein, low-fat diet with restricted milk and milk products if lactose intolerance is present. *Calories and protein are important to replace lost nutrients. Fat restriction helps reduce diarrhea and nutrient loss, particularly when significant portions of the terminal ileum have been resected.*
- Provide parenteral nutrition as necessary if the client is unable to absorb enteral nutrients. *Parenteral nutrition can help reverse nutritional deficits and promote weight gain and healing in the client with acute manifestations.*
- Arrange for dietary consultation. Consider food preferences as allowed. *Providing preferred foods in the prescribed diet increases intake and supports nutritional status.*
- Provide or administer elemental enteral nutrition and supplements as ordered. *Elemental enteral nutritional supplements support healing while providing for bowel rest. They can replace losses and improve nutritional status more rapidly than diet alone.*
- Include family members, the primary food preparer in particular, in teaching and dietary discussions. *Families can reinforce teaching and help the client maintain required restrictions or kilocalorie intake.*

Using NANDA, NIC, and NOC

Chart 26–3 shows links between NANDA nursing diagnoses, NIC, and NOC when caring for the client with inflammatory bowel disease.

Community-Based Care

Inflammatory bowel disease is a chronic condition for which the client provides daily self-management. For this reason, teaching is a vital component of care. Teach the client and family about the following topics:

- The type of inflammatory bowel disease affecting the client, including the disease process, short- and long-term effects, the relationship of stress to disease exacerbations, and the manifestations of complications
- Prescribed medications, including drug names, desired effects, schedules for tapering the doses if ordered (as with corticosteroids), and possible side effects or adverse reactions and their management
- The recommended diet and the rationale for any specific restrictions

NANDA, NIC, AND NOC LINKAGES
CHART 26–3 The Client with Inflammatory Bowel Disease

NANDA

Ineffective Coping

↓

NIC

Coping Enhancement

Decision-Making Support

Emotional Support

Teaching: Individual

↓

NOC

Acceptance of Health Status

Adaptation to Physical Disability

Decision Making

Knowledge: Health Resources

Data from *NANDA's Nursing Diagnoses: Definitions & Classification 2005–2006* by NANDA International (2005), Philadelphia; *Nursing Interventions Classification (NIC)* (4th ed.) by J. M. Dochterman & G. M. Bulechek (2004), St. Louis, MO: Mosby; and *Nursing Outcomes Classification (NOC)* (3rd ed.) by S. Moorhead, M. Johnson, and M. Maas (2004), St. Louis, MO: Mosby.

- Use of nutritional supplements such as Ensure to maintain weight and nutritional status
- Indicators of malabsorption and impaired nutrition; recommendations for self-care and when to seek medical intervention
- If discharged with a central catheter and home parenteral nutrition, written and verbal instructions on catheter care, troubleshooting, and TPN administration (Have the client and a family member demonstrate catheter care and TPN maintenance.)
- The importance of maintaining a fluid intake of at least 2 to 3 quarts per day, increasing fluid intake during warm weather, exercise, or strenuous work, and when fever is present
- The increased risk for colorectal cancer and importance of regular bowel exams
- Risks and benefits of various treatment options

If surgery is planned or has been done, include the following topics in home care instructions:

- Ileal pouch-anal anastomosis or ileostomy care as indicated
- Where to obtain ostomy supplies
- Use of nonprescription drugs, such as enteric-coated and timed-release capsules that may not be adequately absorbed before elimination through the ileostomy
- Community and national ostomy support groups (see below).

Provide referrals to a dietary consultant or nutritionist, a community healthcare agency, home care services, and home intravenous care services as indicated. In addition, suggest the following resources:

- Crohn's and Colitis Foundation of America, Inc.
- The Israel Foundation for Crohn's Disease and Ulcerative Colitis
- United Ostomy Association, Inc.

MALABSORPTION SYNDROMES

Malabsorption is a condition in which the intestinal mucosa ineffectively absorbs nutrients—including carbohydrates, proteins, fats, water, electrolytes, minerals, and vitamins—resulting in their excretion in the stool. Multiple different bowel disorders can lead to malabsorption.

Diseases of the small intestine often cause malabsorption. Other medical and/or surgical conditions can result in malabsorption if they affect digestion or the intestinal mucosa. Primary diseases of the small-bowel mucosa, such as sprue, Crohn's disease, and acute infections, can lead to malabsorption. It can also result from *maldigestion,* inadequate preparation of chyme for absorption. For example, major gastric resections, pancreatic disorders with impaired pancreatic enzyme secretion, and biliary disorders that affect bile secretion can impair digestion and absorption of chyme. Selected causes of impaired absorption and digestion are listed in Table 26–9.

Regardless of the cause, malabsorption causes common manifestations resulting from impaired absorption of chyme and the nutrients it contains (Table 26–10). Predominant GI manifestations include anorexia; abdominal bloating; diarrhea with loose,

TABLE 26–9 Selected Causes of Malabsorption

CAUSE	RELATED FACTORS OR CONDITIONS
Impaired absorption	Sprue
	Short bowel syndrome
	Acute enteritis and other bowel infections or infestations
	AIDS-related opportunistic infections and Kaposi's sarcoma
	Celiac disease
	Crohn's disease
	Intestinal ischemia or infarction
	Scleroderma
Impaired digestion	Lactose intolerance
	Gastrectomy
	Chronic pancreatitis, cancer of the pancreas
	Cystic fibrosis
	Biliary obstruction
	Cirrhosis, hepatitis, or liver failure
	Zollinger-Ellison syndrome

TABLE 26–10 Local and Systemic Manifestations of Malabsorption

CATEGORY	MANIFESTATION	CAUSE
Local (GI)	Diarrhea	Impaired absorption of fluid and electrolytes, leading to excess water in the stool
	Abdominal distention	Gas formation from fermentation of undigested carbohydrates
	Steatorrhea	Impaired fat absorption leading to excess fat in feces
Systemic	Weight loss	Carbohydrate, protein, and fat deficit
	Weakness and malaise	Kilocalorie deficit, anemia, fluid, and electrolyte losses
	Anemia	Vitamin B_{12}, folic acid, and iron deficits
	Bone pain	Calcium and vitamin D deficits
	Muscle cramps, paresthesias	Protein wasting, vitamin B_{12} and electrolyte deficits
	Easy bruising and bleeding	Vitamin K deficit
	Glossitis, cheilosis	Iron, folic acid, and vitamin B_{12} deficits

bulky, foul-smelling stools; and steatorrhea (fatty stools). Weight loss, weakness, general malaise, muscle cramps, bone pain, abnormal bleeding, and anemia are common systemic manifestations of malabsorption. These manifestations result from malnutrition and fluid loss due to poor absorption.

Three common malabsorption disorders in adults are sprue, lactose intolerance, and short bowel syndrome.

THE CLIENT WITH SPRUE

Sprue is a chronic primary disorder of the small intestine in which the absorption of nutrients, particularly fats, is impaired. The severity of the disease depends on the extent of mucosal involvement in the intestine and the duration of the disease. Two major forms of sprue are celiac disease (celiac sprue) and tropical sprue.

Pathophysiology

Most absorption of nutrients occurs in the small intestine. The mucosa of the small intestine is arranged in microscopic folds, which in turn contain even smaller finger-like projections called villi. The cells of the villi are covered with microscopic hairs, microvilli, projecting from the cell membrane. The folds, villi, and microvilli of the intestinal mucosa provide a huge surface area for nutrient absorption. Cells of the intestines are specialized to absorb different nutrients. Readily digested nutrients are absorbed in the proximal intestine; others are absorbed more distally in the intestines. Nutrients are absorbed by the processes of simple diffusion (water and small lipids), facilitated diffusion (water-soluble vitamins), and active transport (glucose and amino acids). Once absorbed into the cells of the villi, nutrients enter the blood or lymph for systemic distribution.

Sprue is characterized by flattening of the intestinal mucosa with a loss of villi and microvilli. With the loss of villi, intestinal absorptive surface is lost, and digestive enzyme production, including disaccharidase and particularly lactase, is reduced.

Celiac Sprue

Celiac sprue, also known as celiac disease or nontropical sprue, is a chronic malabsorption disorder characterized by sensitivity to the gliadin fraction of gluten, a cereal protein. Gluten is found in wheat, rye, barley, and oats. It is also used as a filler in many prepared foods and in medications. The cause of celiac sprue is unknown; however, genetic, environmental, and immune factors are known to play a role in its development. Caucasians of European descent are most commonly affected (Tierney et al., 2005). Manifestations of celiac sprue often develop in childhood, but may develop at any age.

In celiac sprue, it appears that the intestinal mucosa is damaged by an immunologic response. Gliadin acts as an antigen (a substance that induces the formation of antibodies that interact specifically with it), prompting the formation of antibodies and immune complexes. These complexes may deposit in the intestinal mucosa, prompting an inflammatory response and loss of villi. Gluten also may directly damage the villi, causing cell loss, inflammation, and edema. The villi shorten and atrophy, resulting in loss of intestinal folds and absorptive surface.

MANIFESTATIONS Manifestations of celiac sprue may develop at any age. Local manifestations include abdominal bloating and cramps, diarrhea, and steatorrhea. Systemic manifestations result from the effects of malabsorption and resulting deficiencies. Anemia is common. Clients with celiac disease are often small in stature, and may have delayed maturity. Other signs of nutrient deficiencies include tetany, vitamin deficiencies, muscle wasting, and rickets (impaired bone development). When gluten is removed from the diet, the manifestations resolve.

Gastrointestinal malignancies and intestinal lymphoma are potential complications of celiac sprue. Other complications include intestinal ulceration and development of refractory sprue, or disease that no longer responds to a gluten-free diet.

Tropical Sprue

Tropical sprue is a chronic disease of unknown cause, although bacterial infection or toxins are thought to contribute. Tropical sprue occurs chiefly in the Caribbean, south India, and southeast Asia. Its onset may be abrupt or insidious. The pathophysiologic changes in bowel mucosa closely resemble those of celiac sprue, although gluten intake has no effect on this condition.

MANIFESTATIONS Manifestations of tropical sprue include sore tongue, diarrhea, and weight loss. Initially, diarrhea may be explosive and watery; as the disease progresses, stools become fewer in number and more solid with obvious steatorrhea. Folic acid deficiency is common. Vitamin B_{12} and iron deficiencies may occur, resulting in glossitis; stomatitis; dry, rough skin; and anemia.

INTERDISCIPLINARY CARE

With any malabsorptive disorder, the initial focus of management is to identify the cause. Once this has been determined, specific therapy can be prescribed.

Diagnosis

Laboratory and diagnostic testing are used to make the differential diagnosis for various causes of malabsorption syndromes and to determine the severity of nutrient deficiencies.

An enteroscopy permits direct examination of intestinal mucosa and collection of a tissue specimen for biopsy. Upper GI series with small-bowel follow-through may be done to evaluate the structures of the upper GI tract. With sprue, the typical "feathery" pattern of barium in the small bowel is lost, and the barium may precipitate and clump. Nursing implications of diagnostic tests are included in Chapter 25 ∞.

Laboratory tests are used to identify pathophysiologic effects and monitor compliance with the prescribed diet. Fecal fat is measured to document the presence of steatorrhea. The expected result is less than 10 g of fat per 24 hours (Tierney et al., 2005). The fat content of stool is increased in many malabsorptive disorders, including celiac and tropical sprue. Serologic testing for IgA endomysial antibodies, and IgG and IgA antigliadin antibodies is used to diagnose celiac sprue and evaluate compliance with the prescribed gluten-free diet. Serum levels of protein, albumin, cholesterol, electrolytes, and iron may be ordered to evaluate for nutrient deficiencies. The hemoglobin, hematocrit, and RBC indices are used to evaluate anemia. Prothrombin time is increased in vitamin K deficiency.

Medications

Clients with severe nutritional deficits may require vitamin and mineral supplements, as well as iron and folic acid to correct anemia. Vitamin K may be administered parenterally if the prothrombin time is prolonged. In clients whose disease fails to respond to dietary management, corticosteroids may be ordered to suppress the inflammatory response.

Tropical sprue is treated with a combination of folic acid and tetracycline. This regimen is continued for 1 to 2 months.

Nutrition

The client with celiac sprue is placed on a gluten-free diet. This treatment is generally successful, as long as the client avoids gluten totally. Gluten is so widely used in prepared foods that this may be no easy task. Consultation with a dietitian and detailed dietary instructions are necessary. Clients need to become aware of hidden sources of gluten and to analyze dietary labels. Common sources of gluten and foods to be avoided are indicated in Table 26–11.

The prescribed diet is high in calories and protein to correct nutrient deficits. Fat content is restricted to minimize steatorrhea. Initially, the diet usually is restricted in lactose as well to compensate for the loss of lactase-containing microvilli. Foods containing lactose may be reintroduced once remission has occurred (Tierney et al., 2005).

NURSING CARE

Nursing care for the client with sprue focuses on the effects of the disorder on health and nutrition, as well as the client's ability to manage the disease.

Assessment

- *Health history:* Onset, duration, and severity of manifestations; number and character of stools; history of travel to the Caribbean or southeast Asia; previous teaching related to disorder; current treatment and diet.
- *Physical examination:* Vital signs; abdominal shape, contour, bowel sounds; manifestations of malnutrition (e.g., anemia, small stature, muscle wasting, signs of other nutrient deficiencies).

Nursing Diagnoses and Interventions

Diarrhea and malnutrition are significant problems for the client with sprue and the priority foci for nursing intervention.

Diarrhea

Steatorrhea and diarrhea typically occur with sprue because fat, water, and other nutrients are poorly absorbed, remaining in the

TABLE 26–11 Dietary Sources of Gluten

FOOD GROUP	CONTAINS GLUTEN	MAY CONTAIN GLUTEN
Cereals, grains, and grain products	Bread, crackers, cereal, and pasta containing wheat, rye, or barley grain or flour	Seasoned rice and potato mixes
Beverages	Malt, Postum, Ovaltine, beers, and ales	Commercial chocolate milk, cocoa, and other beverage mixes, such as instant tea mix, dietary supplements
Desserts	Cakes, cookies, and pastries made with wheat, rye, or barley flour	Commercial ice cream and sherbet
Meats and other protein sources		Meat loaf, cold cuts and prepared meats, breaded meats; cheese products; soy protein meat substitutes; commercial egg products
Fruits and vegetables		Commercial seasoned vegetable mixes or vegetables with sauce; canned baked beans; commercial pie fillings
Miscellaneous		Commercial salad dressings and mayonnaise; ketchup and prepared mustard; gravy, white sauce; nondairy creamer; syrups; commercial pickles

bowel to be eliminated in the stool. Diarrhea can interfere with lifestyle, ADLs, skin integrity, and fluid and electrolyte balance.

- Assess and document the frequency and nature of stools. *Bowel elimination reflects the severity of the disease and efficacy of treatment. With effective treatment, stools become less frequent and more normal in color and appearance.*
- Weigh daily, monitor intake and output, and assess skin turgor and mucous membranes for indications of fluid balance. *Diarrhea increases the risk for hypovolemia and dehydration resulting from excess fluid loss in the stool.*
- Assess and document perianal skin condition. *Frequent defecation can irritate skin and mucous membranes, increasing the risk of breakdown.*
- Encourage a liberal fluid intake. *Oral fluids help replace fluid lost through diarrheal stool.*

Imbalanced Nutrition:
Less than Body Requirements

Celiac sprue is a chronic condition. With continuing malabsorption, multiple nutrient deficits may occur, resulting in impaired growth and development, impaired healing, muscle wasting, bone disease, and electrolyte imbalances.

- Maintain accurate dietary intake records. *Assessment of dietary intake provides information about compliance with the prescribed diet as well as the adequacy of nutrient intake.*
- Monitor laboratory results, including hemoglobin and hematocrit, serum electrolytes, total serum protein, and albumin levels. *These studies provide information about nutritional status.*
- Arrange for dietary consultation. Provide for food preferences as allowed. *An individualized diet developed to address the client's food preferences as well as nutrient needs will promote appetite and food intake.*
- Provide the prescribed high-kilocalorie, high-protein, low-fat, gluten-free diet for the client with celiac sprue. Restrict lactose (dairy product) intake as indicated. *Calories and protein are important to replace lost nutrients. Fat restriction helps reduce diarrhea and nutrient loss. Lactose may be restricted during initial treatment, then slowly reintroduced into the diet as the gut heals and its normal structure is restored.*
- Provide parenteral nutrition as ordered if the client is unable to absorb enteral nutrients. *Parenteral nutrition can help reverse nutritional deficits and promote weight gain when manifestations are acute.*
- Encourage nutritional supplements. *Nutritional supplements often are necessary to replace losses and restore nutrient levels to normal more rapidly than diet alone can achieve.*
- Include family members, the primary food preparer in particular, in teaching and dietary discussions. *Families can reinforce teaching and help the client maintain required restrictions or kilocalorie intake.*

Community-Based Care

Although tropical sprue can be treated with antibiotic and folic acid therapy, the client with celiac sprue has a chronic condition that requires continuing dietary management.

Provide a detailed list of foods that contain gluten and need to be eliminated from the diet, as well as foods that are allowed.

Teach the client and family how to identify gluten-containing commercial products by reading labels and lists of ingredients. Encourage the purchase and use of a gluten-free cookbook.

If corticosteroids have been prescribed, stress the importance of taking the medication as ordered. Emphasize the need to avoid stopping the medication abruptly and to notify all caregivers that a corticosteroid is part of the client's medication regimen. Instruct to frequently monitor weight. A weight gain of 5 lb (2.3 kg) or more in less than a week usually reflects fluid gain, a possible adverse effect of corticosteroids. Other potential effects include decreased resistance to infection, an impaired inflammatory response, and changes in the metabolism of carbohydrates, proteins, and fats.

THE CLIENT WITH LACTASE DEFICIENCY

For carbohydrates to be absorbed from the small intestine, they first must be broken down into simple sugars, or monosaccharides. Lactose is the primary carbohydrate in milk and milk products. It is a disaccharide, requiring the enzyme lactase for digestion and absorption. Lactase deficiency can lead to **lactose intolerance** and manifestations of malabsorption. Lactase deficiency usually is genetic in origin, but also occurs secondarily to celiac sprue, Crohn's disease, and other disorders affecting the mucosa of the small intestine. There is a racial/ethnic component to the disorder, as described in the Focus on Cultural Diversity box below.

Manifestations

Many people with lactase deficiency are asymptomatic. Small to moderate amounts of milk (one to two 8-ounce glasses) may be well tolerated. Manifestations of lactose intolerance include lower abdominal cramping, pain, and diarrhea following milk ingestion. Undigested lactose ferments in the intestine, forming gases that contribute to bloating and flatus. Lactic and fatty acids produced by this fermentation irritate the bowel, leading to increased motility and abdominal cramping. The undigested lactose draws water into the intestine, which contributes to increased motility and diarrhea. The diarrhea associated with lactose intolerance may be explosive.

INTERDISCIPLINARY CARE

The diagnosis of lactose intolerance usually is based on a history of intolerance to milk and milk products, and a trial of a

---

FOCUS ON CULTURAL DIVERSITY
Lactase Deficiency

- Lactase deficiency affects up to 90% of Asians and Native Americans.
- Lactase deficiency affects approximately 70% of African Americans.
- Lactase deficiency is common among Jewish Americans and Hispanics.
- Less than 25% of Caucasians are affected.

lactose-free diet. If manifestations resolve when lactose intake is eliminated, the diagnosis of lactose intolerance is confirmed.

Diagnosis

The lactose breath test is a noninvasive test that may be used to diagnose lactose intolerance. Expired hydrogen gas (H_2) is measured following oral administration of 50 g of lactose. If lactose is digested and absorbed normally, then little change occurs in the amount of exhaled H_2 from fasting to postlactose administration. With lactose intolerance, exhaled H_2 increases following lactose administration as the sugar ferments in the bowel.

For the lactose tolerance test, 100 g of lactose solution is orally administered, followed by measurement of blood glucose levels at intervals of 30, 60, and 120 minutes. If lactose is digested and absorbed normally, the blood glucose rises more than 20 mg/dL. The expected blood glucose elevation does not occur in lactose intolerance.

Nutrition

A lactose-free or reduced lactose diet relieves the manifestations of the disorder. Some clients require total elimination of milk and milk products from the diet. Many can tolerate limited amounts of lactose. Milk pretreated with lactase is readily available. Nonprescription lactase enzyme preparations are available to improve milk tolerance. Yogurt containing bacterial lactases may be well tolerated. Calcium supplements are often recommended, particularly for women on a reduced-lactose or lactose-free diet.

NURSING CARE

Nursing care for the client with lactose intolerance focuses on providing education and support. Discuss sources of lactose: Milk, ice cream, and cottage cheese are high in lactose; aged cheese and yogurt contain much smaller amounts. Potential hidden sources of lactose include sherbets, desserts made from milk and milk chocolate, sauces and gravies, and cream soups. Suggest a trial of lactase-treated milk or lactase enzyme supplements. Emphasize the importance of obtaining nutrients contained in dairy products from other sources. Proteins may be obtained from meats, eggs, legumes, and grains. Other sources of calcium include sardines, oysters, and salmon, as well as plant sources such as beans, cauliflower, rhubarb, and green leafy vegetables.

THE CLIENT WITH SHORT BOWEL SYNDROME

The small bowel may be resected due to tumors, infarction of bowel mucosa, incarcerated hernias, Crohn's disease, trauma, and enteropathy resulting from radiation therapy. Resection of significant portions of the small intestine may result in a condition known as *short bowel syndrome*. The severity of the disorder depends on the total amount of bowel resected, as well as the portions of bowel removed. Removal of the proximal portions, including the duodenum, jejunum, and proximal ileum, and the distal portion of the ileum is associated with more severe malabsorption and manifestations than is resection of midportions of the ileum.

Resection of the small intestine affects the absorption of water, nutrients, vitamins, and minerals. Transit time of ingested foods and fluids is reduced, and digestive processes are impaired. The bowel undergoes an adaptive process in which the remaining villi enlarge and lengthen to increase absorptive surface following resection. For many clients, absorption and bowel function return to preoperative or near-normal levels. Others have continued significant impairment of digestion and absorption, leading to nutrient deficiencies, weight loss, and diarrhea.

INTERDISCIPLINARY CARE

Management of short bowel syndrome focuses on alleviating manifestations. Clients often simply require frequent, small, high-kilocalorie, high-protein feedings.

Diagnosis

Laboratory and diagnostic studies are used to evaluate nutrient deficiencies. Total serum proteins and albumin are reduced, as are serum levels of folate, iron, vitamins, minerals, and electrolytes. Anemia and a prolonged prothrombin time (indicative of vitamin K deficiency) may develop.

Medications

Multivitamin and mineral supplementation is also frequently necessary. Antidiarrheal medications are used to reduce bowel motility, allowing a greater amount of time for nutrient absorption. Some clients are affected by gastric hypersecretion following bowel resection. For these clients, a proton-pump inhibitor such as omeprazole (Prilosec) may be ordered. Clients with severe manifestations of short bowel syndrome may require TPN.

NURSING CARE

Nursing care for the client with short bowel syndrome focuses on the problems of potential fluid volume deficit, malnutrition, and diarrhea.

Fluid losses are generally greatest in the initial periods following surgery, warranting the closest attention at that time. Close monitoring of vital signs, intake and output, daily weights, skin turgor, and condition of mucous membranes is vital. It is important to remember that the risk also is high when other abnormal fluid losses occur through, for example, fever, draining wounds, or excess perspiration.

Document nutritional status, including weight, anthropometric measurements, laboratory values, and kilocalorie intake. Provide nutritional supplementation with enteral feedings as needed. Maintain central lines and TPN, using aseptic technique.

For diarrhea, document the number and character of stools. Administer antidiarrheal medications as ordered. If the client is lactose intolerant, limit intake of milk and milk products. Provide good skin care of the perianal region to prevent breakdown from frequent bowel movements. Refer to the discussion of nursing care for the client with sprue for other measures for altered nutrition and diarrhea.

The client and family affected by this condition require extensive education. Because there is no way to cure or replace the lost bowel at this time, the client must manage the disorder on a day-to-day basis. Provide instructions about the recommended diet and medication regimen. Emphasize the importance of maintaining an adequate fluid intake, particularly in hot weather or during strenuous exercise. Teach the client to monitor his or her weight frequently and report changes. Include teaching about possible manifestations of dehydration and nutrient deficiencies that should be reported to the physician. Referring the client to a dietitian or counselor can help the person cope with what may be a lifelong problem.

NEOPLASTIC DISORDERS

Cancer remains the second leading cause of death in the United States, preceded only by heart disease. Although cancer may affect any portion of the digestive tract, the large intestine and rectum are the most common sites. Malignant neoplasms of the lower bowel are the second leading cause of death from cancer (after lung cancer), making this a significant healthcare concern.

THE CLIENT WITH POLYPS

A *polyp* is a mass of tissue that arises from the bowel wall and protrudes into the lumen. Polyps may develop in any portion of the bowel, but they occur most often in the sigmoid colon and rectum. They vary considerably in size and may be single or multiple. It is estimated that approximately 30% of people over the age of 50 have polyps. Although most polyps are benign, some have the potential to become malignant.

Pathophysiology

Polyps are identified by their structure and tissue type. Most polyps are adenomas, benign epithelial tumors that are considered premalignant lesions. Greater than 95% of adenocarcinomas arise from adenomas. Of polyps that are removed during colonoscopy, more than 70% are adenomatous (Tierney et al., 2005).

Adenomatous polyps represent disruption of the normal process of cell proliferation to replace epithelial cells lining the intestine. Cells are constantly being reproduced to replace those shed as feces move through the colon. Disruption of the normal process of cell division and maturation can lead to formation of a polyp composed of tightly packed epithelial cells. The cells may appear grossly normal or show signs of dysplasia. Polyps may develop as tubular, villous, or tubulovillous adenomas. Polyps may be named by the way they are attached to the bowel wall as either sessile (raised nodules) or pedunculated (attached by a stalk) (Figure 26–8 ■).

Tubular adenomas (also called pedunculated polyps) are more common than sessile polyps and account for about 65% of benign polyps of the large intestine (Porth, 2005). A tubular adenoma is a globelike structure attached to the intestinal wall by a thin, stalk-like stem. The incidence of this type of polyp increases with age, although it occurs in all age groups and in both genders. Most are small, 1 cm or less in diameter, although they may be as large as 4 to 5 cm. The malignant potential of these polyps seems to be related to their size. Small adenomas less than 1 cm have a low risk of being malignant, and larger adenomas greater than 1 cm have a much higher risk of harboring malignancy or a high-grade dysplasia. Adenomatous polyps are present in 35% of adults greater than 50 years of age (Tierney et al., 2005).

Villous adenomas (also called sessile polyps) have a broad base and an elevated, cauliflower-like surface (Figure 26–8B). They typically develop in the rectosigmoid colon. This type of polyp is often larger than tubular adenomas, usually more than 5 cm. Villous adenomas are not common, accounting for about 10% of colon polyps. They have a higher malignant potential than tubular adenomas. Some adenomatous polyps contain both tubular epithelium and villi and are known as *tubulovillous adenomas*.

Figure 26–8 ■ *A*, Tubular (or pedunculated) polyps; and *B*, villous (or sessile) polyps.

Source: ISM/Phototake NYC

Manifestations

Most polyps are asymptomatic, found coincidentally during routine examination or diagnostic testing. Intermittent painless rectal bleeding, bright or dark red, is the most common presenting complaint. A large polyp may cause abdominal cramping, pain, or manifestations of obstruction. Diarrhea and mucous discharge may be associated with a large villous adenoma.

INTERDISCIPLINARY CARE

The diagnosis of intestinal polyps is generally based on diagnostic studies such as sigmoidoscopy or colonoscopy. A rectal polyp may be palpable on digital examination, but further studies are necessary to determine its size and type and the extent of colon involvement, and to assess for malignancy.

Once identified, polyps are removed because of the risk of malignancy. Pedunculated polyps and small villous lesions may be removed during colonoscopy using an electrocautery snare or hot biopsy forceps passed through the scope. This relatively safe procedure has less than a 2% risk of complications such as perforation or hemorrhage. Large villous adenomas are completely excised and examined histologically for evidence of malignancy. In some cases, the colon segment containing the polyp is resected; a total colectomy with ileorectal anastomosis may be performed for multiple polyps in different anatomic parts of the colon.

Treatment following polypectomy depends on histologic examination of the excised tissue. Because polyps tend to recur, follow-up colonoscopy is recommended in 3 years and then every 5 years if no further polyps are detected. When the polyp is found to be malignant, follow-up care is determined by the tissue type and degree of invasion.

NURSING CARE

Health Promotion

The incidence of intestinal polyps increases with age. They affect men and women equally. It is believed that an adenomatous polyp requires more than 5 years of growth to become significant in size and malignant potential. Advise all clients to have a screening for colorectal cancer (with a colonoscopy being the "gold standard" for diagnosis) at age 50 and as recommended thereafter for early detection of polyps (American Cancer Society [ACS], 2005a).

Assessment

Polyps are a "silent" disease, with few or no manifestations.
- *Health history:* Rectal bleeding; personal or family history of intestinal polyps or colorectal cancer.

Nursing Diagnoses and Interventions

Nursing care for the client with polyps focuses on education and assisting the client through diagnostic testing and polyp removal. Before and after colonoscopy and polypectomy, provide direct care and teaching about the procedure, expected sensations during the procedure, and anticipated postoperative care. Cathartics are prescribed prior to colonoscopy; cleansing enemas also may be ordered. Observe for evidence of fluid and electrolyte imbalance during preoperative preparation. If enemas are ordered, use normal saline (not tap water) to reduce the risk of electrolyte imbalances. Following polypectomy, observe closely for possible complications such as hemorrhage.

Community-Based Care

Include the following topics when teaching for home care:
- The significance of polyps and their relationship to colorectal cancer
- The importance of keeping follow-up appointments and undergoing repeat colonoscopy as recommended: at 3 years following polypectomy, then every 5 to 10 years unless additional polyps are found
- Manifestations to report to the physician, such as diarrhea, pain, rectal bleeding, light-headedness, or other indications of possible blood loss.

THE CLIENT WITH COLORECTAL CANCER

Colorectal cancer (cancer of the colon or rectum) is the third most common cancer diagnosed in the United States. In the United States, about 145,290 new cases of colorectal cancer were diagnosed in 2005, and is expected to cause about 56,290 deaths (28,540 men and 27,750 women) during 2005 (ACS, 2005b). Earlier diagnosis and improved treatment have improved the survival rate for colorectal cancer. Its incidence, which is nearly equal among men and women, has been declining in the United States for the past 15 years. Colorectal cancer occurs most frequently after age 50. The incidence continues to rise with increasing age. With early diagnosis and treatment, the 5-year survival rate for colorectal cancer is 90%; however, only 39% of colorectal cancers are diagnosed at this early stage.

Although the specific cause of colorectal cancer is unknown, a number of risk factors have been identified (Box 26–2). Genetic factors are strongly linked to the risk for colorectal cancer. Up to 20% of people who develop colorectal cancer have a family history of the disease (ACS, 2005c). Persons with familial adenomatous polyposis inevitably will develop colon cancer unless the colon is removed. Hereditary nonpolyposis colorectal cancer (also known as Lynch syndrome) is an autosomal dominant disorder that significantly increases the risk for developing colorectal and other cancers. Tumors associated with Lynch

---

BOX 26–2 Risk Factors for Colorectal Cancer

- Age over 50 years
- Polyps of the colon and/or rectum
- Family history of colorectal cancer
- Inflammatory bowel disease
- Exposure to radiation
- Diet: high animal fat and kilocalorie intake

syndrome often affect the ascending colon, and tend to occur at an earlier age. Inflammatory bowel diseases also increase the risk of colorectal cancer.

Diet plays a role in the development of colorectal cancer. The disease is prevalent in economically prosperous countries where people consume diets high in calories, meat proteins, and fats. This dietary pattern, common in the United States, is thought to increase the population of anaerobic bacteria in the gut. These anaerobes convert bile acids into carcinogens. Diets high in fruits and vegetables, folic acid, and calcium appear to reduce the risk of colorectal cancer. Cereal fiber, once thought to reduce colorectal cancer risk, does not now appear to play a role either way in its development. Other factors that may reduce the risk of colorectal cancer include regular exercise, taking a daily multivitamin, and the use of aspirin and other NSAIDs.

Pathophysiology

Nearly all colorectal cancers are adenocarcinomas that begin as adenomatous polyps. Most tumors develop in the rectum and sigmoid colon, although any portion of the colon may be affected (Figure 26–9 ■). The tumor typically grows undetected, producing few manifestations. By the time manifestations occur, the disease may have spread into deeper layers of the bowel tissue and adjacent organs. Colorectal cancer spreads by direct extension to involve the entire bowel circumference, the submucosa, and outer bowel wall layers. Neighboring structures such as the liver, greater curvature of the stomach, duodenum, small intestine, pancreas, spleen, genitourinary tract, and abdominal wall also may be involved by direct extension. Metastasis to regional lymph nodes is the most common form of tumor spread. This is not always an orderly process; distal nodes may contain cancer cells while regional nodes remain normal. Cancerous cells from the primary tumor may also spread by way of the lymphatic system or circulatory system to secondary sites such as the liver, lungs, brain, bones, and kidneys. "Seeding" of the tumor to other areas of the peritoneal cavity can occur when the tumor extends through the serosa or during surgical resection.

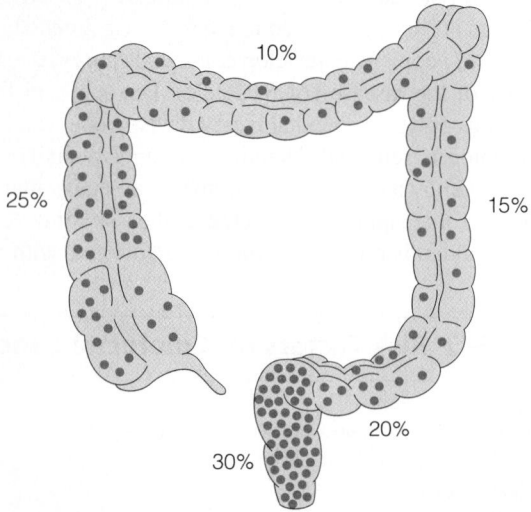

Figure 26–9 ■ The distribution and frequency of cancer of the colon and rectum.

Manifestations

Bowel cancer often produces no manifestations until it is advanced. Because it grows slowly, 5 to 15 years of growth may occur before manifestations develop. The manifestations depend on its location, type and extent, and complications. Rectal bleeding is often the initial manifestation that prompts clients to seek medical care. Other common early manifestations include a change in bowel habits, either diarrhea or constipation. Pain, anorexia, and weight loss are characteristic in advanced disease. A palpable abdominal or rectal mass may be present. Occasionally the client presents with anemia from occult bleeding.

Complications

The primary complications associated with colorectal cancer are (1) bowel obstruction due to narrowing of the bowel lumen by the lesion; (2) perforation of the bowel wall by the tumor, allowing contamination of the peritoneal cavity by bowel contents; and (3) direct extension of the tumor to involve adjacent organs.

Most recurrences of colorectal cancer after tumor removal occur within the first 4 years. The size of the primary tumor does not necessarily relate to long-term survival. The number of involved lymph nodes, penetration of the tumor through the bowel wall, and tumor adherence to adjacent organs are better predictors of the prognosis for the disease.

INTERDISCIPLINARY CARE

The focus of interdisciplinary care for colorectal cancer is prevention, early detection, and intervention. Colorectal cancer is always treated by surgical resection, with chemotherapy and radiation therapy used as adjuncts.

Prevention

Measures to prevent colon cancer that are considered to be effective and safe include oral supplements of calcium and folic acid, diets high in fruits and vegetables and low in saturated fat and red meat, regular exercise, avoiding obesity, and quitting smoking. Although considered safe, these measures are the subject of further research to demonstrate conclusive proof of effectiveness (MedicineNet.com, 2005).

Screening

The American Cancer Society (2005c) recommends one of the following testing schedules for the early detection of colorectal cancer, beginning at age 50. These options are acceptable choices for average-risk adults.

- Yearly fecal occult blood test (FOBT) or fecal immunochemical test (FIT). (For FOBT, the take-home multiple sample method should be used.)
- Flexible sigmoidoscopy every 5 years.
- Yearly FOBT or FIT plus flexible sigmoidoscopy every 5 years.
- Double-contrast barium enema every 5 years.
- Colonoscopy every 10 years.

Diagnosis

Diagnostic and laboratory tests are used for screening, diagnosis, and monitoring purposes. Diagnostic tests include a sigmoidoscopy or colonoscopy as the primary diagnostic test used to detect and visualize tumors. While flexible sigmoidoscopy can detect 50% to 65% of colorectal cancers, many clinicians recommend colonoscopy. Tissue for biopsy is obtained at the time of endoscopy to confirm cancerous tissue and evaluate cell differentiation (see Chapter 14 ∞). Current staging methods primarily use the TNM system, as outlined in Table 26–12. Radiologic examinations may include a chest x-ray to detect tumor metastasis to the lung, and computed tomography (CT) scan, magnetic resonance imaging (MRI), or ultrasonic examination may be used to assess tumor depth and involvement of other organs by direct extension or metastasis.

Laboratory tests used are a fecal occult blood (by guaiac or hemocult testing) to detect blood in the feces, a CBC to detect anemia resulting from chronic blood loss and tumor growth, and a carcinoembryonic antigen (CEA) level, which is a tumor marker that can be detected in the blood of clients with colorectal cancer. CEA levels are used to estimate prognosis, monitor treatment, and detect cancer recurrence.

Laser Photocoagulation

Laser photocoagulation uses a very small, intense beam of light to generate heat in tissues toward which it is directed. The heat generated by the laser beam can be used to destroy small tumors. It is also used for palliative surgery of advanced tumors to remove obstruction. Laser photocoagulation can be performed endoscopically and is useful for clients who cannot tolerate major surgery.

Surgery

Surgical resection of the tumor, adjacent colon, and regional lymph nodes is the treatment of choice for colorectal cancer. Options for surgical treatment vary from destruction of the tumor by laser photocoagulation performed during endoscopy to abdominoperineal resection with permanent colostomy. When possible, the anal sphincter is preserved and colostomy avoided.

Other surgical treatment options for small, localized tumors include local excision and fulguration. These procedures also may be performed during endoscopy, eliminating the need for abdominal surgery. Local excision may be used to remove a disk of rectum containing a tumor in clients with a small, well-differentiated, mobile polypoid lesion. *Fulguration* or electrocoagulation is used to reduce the size of some large tumors for clients who are poor surgical risks. This procedure requires general anesthesia and may need to be repeated at intervals.

Most clients with colorectal cancer undergo surgical resection of the colon with anastomosis of remaining bowel as a curative procedure. The distribution of regional lymph nodes determines the extent of resection because these may contain metastatic lesions. Most tumors of the ascending, transverse, descending, and sigmoid colon can be resected.

Tumors of the rectum usually are treated with an abdominoperineal resection in which the sigmoid colon, rectum, and anus are removed through both abdominal and perineal incisions. A permanent sigmoid colostomy is performed to provide for elimination of feces. Nursing care of the client having bowel surgery is outlined on page 804.

COLOSTOMY Surgical resection of the bowel may be accompanied by a colostomy for diversion of fecal contents. A **colostomy** is an ostomy made in the colon. It may be created if the bowel is obstructed by the tumor, as a temporary measure to promote healing of anastomoses, or as a permanent means of fecal evacuation when the distal colon and rectum are removed. Colostomies take the name of the portion of the colon from which they are formed: ascending colostomy,

TABLE 26–12 The TNM Classification for Colorectal Cancer

STAGE	PRIMARY TUMOR (T)	REGIONAL LYMPH NODES (N)	DISTANT METASTASIS (M)
	TX—Primary tumor cannot be assessed T0—No evidence of primary tumor	NX—Regional lymph node cannot be assessed	MX—Presence of distant metastasis cannot be assessed
Stage 0	Tis—Carcinoma *in situ*	N0—No regional lymph node metastasis	M0—No distant metastasis
Stage I	T1—Tumor invades submucosa T2—Tumor invades muscularis propria		
Stage II	T3—Tumor invades through muscularis propria into subserosa or into non-peritonealized pericolic or perirectal tissues		
	T4—Tumor perforates visceral peritoneum or directly invades other organs or structures		
Stage III	Any T	N1—Metastasis in 1 to 3 pericolic or perirectal lymph nodes	
		N2—Metastasis in 4 or more pericolic or perirectal lymph nodes	
		N3—Metastasis in any lymph node along course of a major named vascular trunk	
Stage IV	Any T	Any N	M1—Distant metastasis

NURSING CARE OF THE CLIENT HAVING Bowel Surgery

PREOPERATIVE NURSING CARE

- Provide routine preoperative care for the surgical client as outlined in Chapter 4 ∞.
- Arrange for consultation with enterostomal therapy (ET) specialist if appropriate. *The ET nurse is trained to identify and mark an appropriate stoma location, taking into consideration the level of ostomy, skinfolds, and the client's clothing preferences. Initial ostomy care teaching also is provided by the ET nurse during the preoperative visit.*
- Insert a nasogastric tube if ordered. *Although it is often inserted in the surgical suite just prior to surgery, the nasogastric tube may be placed preoperatively to remove secretions and empty stomach contents.*
- Perform bowel preparation procedures as ordered. *Oral and parenteral antibiotics as well as cathartics and enemas may be prescribed preoperatively to clean the bowel and reduce the risk of peritoneal contamination by bowel contents during surgery.*

POSTOPERATIVE NURSING CARE

- Provide routine care for the surgical client (Chapter 4 ∞).
- Monitor bowel sounds and degree of abdominal distention. *Surgical manipulation of the bowel disrupts peristalsis, resulting in an initial ileus. Bowel sounds and the passage of flatus indicate a return of peristalsis.*
- Assess the position and patency of the nasogastric tube, connecting it to low suction. If the tube becomes clogged, gently irrigate with sterile normal saline. *A nasogastric or gastrostomy tube is used postoperatively to provide gastrointestinal decompression and facilitate healing of the anastomosis. Ensuring its patency is important for comfort and healing.*
- Assess color amount, and odor of drainage from surgical drains and the colostomy (if present), noting any changes or the presence of clots or bright bleeding. *Initial drainage may be bright red and then become dark and finally clear or greenish yellow over the first 2 to 3 days. A change in the color, amount, or odor of the drainage may indicate a complication such as hemorrhage, intestinal obstruction, or infection.*
- Alert all personnel caring for the client with an abdominoperineal resection to avoid rectal temperatures, suppositories, or other rectal procedures. *These procedures could disrupt the anal suture line, causing bleeding, infection, or impaired healing.*
- Maintain intravenous fluids while nasogastric suction is in place. *The client on nasogastric suction is unable to take oral food and fluids and, moreover, is losing electrolyte-rich fluid through the nasogastric tube. If replacement fluid and electrolytes are not maintained, the client is at risk for dehydration, sodium, potassium, and chloride imbalance, and metabolic alkalosis.*
- Provide antacids, histamine$_2$ receptor antagonists, and antibiotic therapy as ordered. *The above medications may be ordered for the postoperative client, depending on the procedure performed. Antibiotic therapy is a common measure to prevent infection resulting from contamination of the abdominal cavity with gastric contents.*
- Resume oral food and fluids as ordered. Initial feedings may be clear liquids, progressing to full liquids, and then frequent small feedings of regular foods. Monitor bowel sounds and monitor for abdominal distention frequently during this period. *Oral feedings are reintroduced slowly to minimize abdominal distention and trauma to the suture lines.*
- Begin discharge planning and teaching. Consult with a dietitian for instructions and menu planning; reinforce teaching. Teach about potential postoperative complications such as abdominal abscess, or bowel obstruction, their signs and symptoms, and preventive measures.

---

transverse colostomy, descending colostomy, and sigmoid colostomy (Figure 26–10 ■).

A *sigmoid colostomy* is the most common permanent colostomy performed, particularly for cancer of the rectum. It

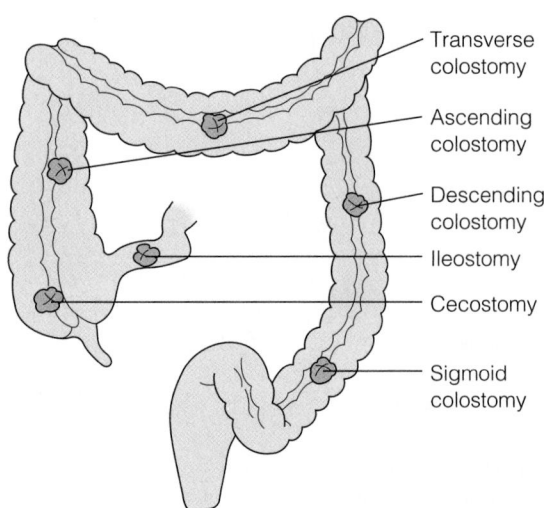

Figure 26–10 ■ Various ostomy levels and sites.

Transverse colostomy
Ascending colostomy
Descending colostomy
Ileostomy
Cecostomy
Sigmoid colostomy

is usually created during an abdominoperineal resection. This procedure involves the removal of the sigmoid colon, rectum, and anus through abdominal and perineal incisions. The anal canal is closed, and a stoma formed from the proximal sigmoid colon. The stoma usually is located on the lower left quadrant of the abdomen.

When a *double-barrel colostomy* is performed, two separate stomas are created (Figure 26–11 ■). The distal colon is not removed, but bypassed. The proximal stoma, which is functional, diverts feces to the abdominal wall. The distal stoma, also called the mucous fistula, expels mucus from the distal colon. It may be pouched or dressed with a 4 × 4 gauze dressing. A double-barrel colostomy may be created for cases of trauma, tumor, or inflammation, and it may be temporary or permanent.

An emergency procedure used to relieve an intestinal obstruction or perforation is called a *transverse loop colostomy*. During this procedure, a loop of the transverse colon is brought out from the abdominal wall and suspended over a plastic rod or bridge, which prevents the loop from slipping back into the abdominal cavity. The loop stoma may be opened at the time of surgery or a few days later at the client's bedside. The bridge may be removed in 1 to 2 weeks. Transverse loop colostomies are typically temporary.

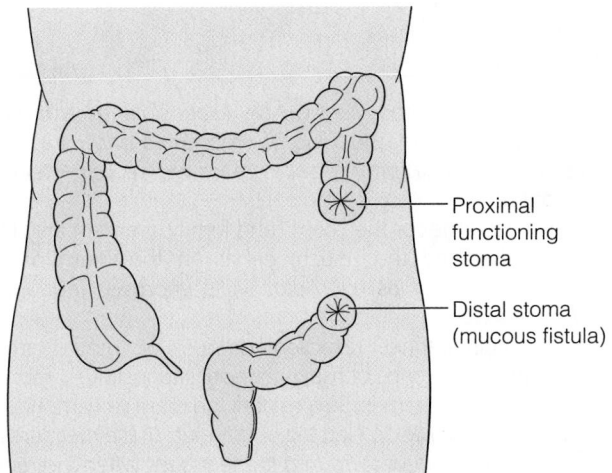

- Proximal functioning stoma
- Distal stoma (mucous fistula)

Figure 26–11 ■ A double-barrel colostomy. The proximal stoma is the functioning stoma; the distal stoma expels mucus from the distal colon.

In a *Hartmann procedure,* a common temporary colostomy procedure, the distal portion of the colon is left in place and is oversewn for closure. A temporary colostomy may be done to allow bowel rest or healing, such as following tumor resection or inflammation of the bowel. It also may be created following traumatic injury to the colon, such as a gunshot wound. Anastomosis of the severed portions of the colon is delayed because bacterial colonization of the colon would prevent proper healing of the anastomosis. About 3 to 6 months following a temporary colostomy, the colostomy is closed and the colon is reconnected. Clients with temporary colostomies require the same care as clients with permanent colostomies. See nursing care for a client with a colostomy on page 806.

Radiation Therapy

Although radiation therapy is not used as a primary treatment for colon cancer, it is used with surgical resection for treating rectal tumors. Small rectal cancers may be treated with intracavitary, external, or implantation radiation. Rectal cancer has a high rate of regional recurrence following complete surgical resection, particularly when the tumor has invaded tissues outside the bowel wall or regional lymph nodes. Pre- or postoperative radiation therapy reduces the recurrence of pelvic tumors, although the effect of radiation therapy on long-term survival is less clear. Radiation therapy also is used preoperatively to shrink large rectal tumors enough to permit surgical removal of the tumor.

Chemotherapy

Chemotherapeutic agents, such as intravenous fluorouracil (5-FU) and folinic acid (leucovorin), are also used postoperatively as adjunctive therapy for colorectal cancer. When combined with radiation therapy, chemotherapy reduces the rate of tumor recurrence and prolongs survival for clients with stage II and stage III rectal tumors. The benefit for colon cancers is less clear, but chemotherapy may be used to reduce its spread to the liver and prevent recurrence. Irinotecan (CPT-11) or oxaliplatin also may be used in chemotherapy regimens for colorectal can-

cer. Further discussion about chemotherapy and nursing implications is included in Chapter 14 .

NURSING CARE

Health Promotion

Primary prevention of colorectal cancer is a significant nursing care issue. Teach clients about dietary recommendations provided by the American Cancer Society for the prevention of colorectal cancer. These recommendations include decreasing the amount of fat, refined sugar, and red meats in the diet while increasing intake of dietary fiber. Foods that contain high amounts of fiber include raw fruits and vegetables, legumes, and whole-grain products.

Stress the importance of regular health examinations, including digital rectal exams. Discuss recommendations for regular hemoccult testing of stool after age 40. Include the importance of seeking medical treatment if blood is noted in or on the stool. Teach clients the warning signs for cancer, including those specific to bowel cancer, such as a change in bowel habits.

Assessment

- *Health history:* Usual bowel patterns and any recent changes; weight loss, fatigue, decreased activity tolerance; presence of blood in the stool; pain with defecation, abdominal discomfort, perineal pain; usual diet; family history of colon cancer, other specific risk factors such as inflammatory bowel disease or colon polyps.
- *Physical examination:* General appearance; weight; abdominal shape, contour; bowel sounds, abdominal tenderness; stool hemoccult or guaiac.

Nursing Diagnoses and Interventions

In planning and implementing care, consider both physical care needs and emotional response to the diagnosis. Because colorectal cancer is often advanced at the time of diagnosis, the prognosis, even with treatment, may be poor. Denial and anger are common. Extensive abdominal surgery and potentially a colostomy may be necessary, and the effects of chemotherapy and radiation therapy can leave the client fatigued and discouraged. A nursing care plan for a client with colorectal cancer is included on page 807.

Nursing care includes providing emotional support, teaching, and direct care before and after diagnostic procedures and surgery and during adjunctive treatments. Priority nursing diagnoses include *Acute Pain, Imbalanced Nutrition,* and *Anticipatory Grieving. Risk for Sexual Dysfunction* should be considered as a priority diagnosis if a colostomy has been created.

> **PRACTICE ALERT**
> If an abdominoperineal resection has been performed, alert all care personnel to avoid rectal temperatures, suppository use, or other procedures that could damage sutures.

NURSING CARE OF THE CLIENT WITH A Colostomy

- Assess the location of the stoma and the type of colostomy performed. *Stoma location is an indicator of the section of bowel in which it is located and a predictor of the type of fecal drainage to expect.*
- Assess stoma appearance and surrounding skin condition frequently (see the box page 789). *Assessment of stoma and skin condition is particularly important in the early postoperative period, when complications are most likely to occur and most treatable.*
- Position a collection bag or drainable pouch over the stoma. *Initial drainage may contain more mucus and serosanguineous fluid than fecal material. As the bowel starts to resume function, drainage becomes fecal in nature. The consistency of drainage depends on the stoma location in the bowel.*
- If ordered, irrigate the colostomy, instilling water into the colon similar to an enema procedure. *The water stimulates the colon to empty.*
- When a colostomy irrigation is ordered for a client with a double-barrel or loop colostomy, irrigate the proximal stoma. Digital assessment of the bowel direction from the stoma can assist in determining which is the proximal stoma. *The distal bowel carries no fecal contents and does not need irrigation. It may be irrigated for cleansing just prior to reanastomosis.*
- Empty a drainable pouch or replace the colostomy bag as needed or when it is no more than one-third full. *If the pouch is allowed to overfill, its weight may impair the seal and cause leakage.*
- Provide stomal and skin care for the client with a colostomy as for the client with an ileostomy (see the box on page 789). *Good skin and stoma care is important to maintain skin integrity and function as the first line of defense against infection.*
- Use caulking agents, such as Stomahesive or karaya paste, and a skin barrier wafer as needed to maintain a secure ostomy pouch. This may be particularly important for the client with a loop colostomy. *The main challenge for a client with a transverse loop colostomy is to maintain a secure ostomy pouch over the plastic bridge.*
- A small needle hole high on the colostomy pouch will allow flatus to escape. This hole may be closed with a Band-Aid and opened only while the client is in the bathroom for odor control. *Ostomy bags may "balloon" out, disrupting the skin seal, if excess gas collects.*

Health Education for the Client and Family
- Prior to discharge, provide written, verbal, and psychomotor instruction on colostomy care, pouch management, skin care, and irrigation for the client. *Whether the colostomy is tempo-*

rary or permanent, the client will be responsible for its management. Good understanding of procedures and care enhances the ability to provide self-care, as well as self-esteem and control.
- Allow ample time for the client (and family, if necessary) to practice changing the pouch, either on the client or a model. *Practice of psychomotor skills improves learning and confidence.*
- If an abdominoperineal resection has been performed, emphasize the importance of using no rectal suppositories, rectal temperatures, or enemas. Suggest that the client carry medical identification or a Medic-Alert tag or bracelet. *These measures are important to prevent trauma to the tissues when the rectum has been removed.*
- The diet for a client with a colostomy is individualized and may require no alteration from that consumed preoperatively. Dietary teaching should, however, include information on foods that cause stool odor and gas and foods that thicken and loosen stools. Foods that cause these effects on ostomy output are listed below.

Foods That Increase Stool Odor
- Asparagus
- Beans
- Cabbage
- Eggs
- Fish
- Garlic
- Onions
- Some spices

Foods That Increase Intestinal Gas
- Beer
- Broccoli
- Brussels sprouts
- Cabbage
- Carbonated drinks
- Cauliflower
- Corn
- Cucumbers
- Dairy products
- Dried beans
- Peas
- Radishes
- Spinach

Foods That Thicken Stools
- Applesauce
- Bananas
- Bread
- Cheese
- Yogurt
- Pasta
- Pretzels
- Rice
- Tapioca
- Creamy peanut butter

Foods That Loosen Stools
- Chocolate
- Dried beans
- Fried foods
- Greasy foods
- Highly spiced foods
- Leafy green vegetables
- Raw fruits and juices
- Raw vegetables

Foods That Color Stools
- Beets
- Red gelatin

Acute Pain

The client with colorectal cancer may experience pain related to preparatory procedures, diagnostic examinations, and surgery. Following an abdominoperineal resection, "phantom" rectal pain related to the severing of nerves during the wide excision of the rectum may develop. Finally, the primary tumor it-

self and, potentially, metastatic tumors may impinge on nerves and other organs, causing pain. In the early postoperative period, an epidural infusion or PCA often is used to manage pain. PCA, routine administration of ordered analgesics, or a continuous analgesia delivery (CAD) system also may be used for pain management when the tumor is far enough advanced to

NURSING CARE PLAN   A Client with Colorectal Cancer

William Cunningham is a 65-year-old retired railroad employee, husband, and father of three grown children. For the past 3 months, Mr. Cunningham has noticed small amounts of blood and occasional mucous in his stools. He has a sensation of pressure in the rectum, and notices that his stools are smaller in diameter, about the size of pencil. After palpating a mass on digital examination of the rectum, the physician orders a colonoscopy. A large sessile lesion is found in the rectum and biopsied. The pathology report shows the lesion to be adenocarcinoma. Mr. Cunningham is scheduled for an abdominoperineal resection and sigmoid colostomy.

ASSESSMENT

Madonna Hart, RN, completes the admission assessment. Mr. Cunningham states that his bowel habits have recently changed, but denies pain or other symptoms. Physical assessment findings include T 98.4°F (36.9°C), P 82, R 18, and BP 118/78. He is 70 inches (178 cm) tall and weighs 185 lb (84 kg). Laboratory findings are normal except for the previous pathology report of adenocarcinoma of rectal lesion.

Mr. Cunningham states, "I really don't want a colostomy, but if that is what it takes to get rid of this, I'm ready to get it over with."

DIAGNOSES

- *Acute Pain* related to surgical intervention
- *Risk for Impaired Skin Integrity (Peristomal)* related to fecal drainage and pouch adhesive
- *Risk for Constipation/Diarrhea* related to effects of surgery on bowel function
- *Disturbed Body Image* related to colostomy
- *Risk for Sexual Dysfunction* related to wide rectal incision, radiation therapy, and colostomy

EXPECTED OUTCOMES

- Report pain within an acceptable range that allows ease of movement and ambulation.

- Perform colostomy care using correct technique.
- Demonstrate willingness to discuss changes in sexual function.
- Wear clothing to enhance physical and emotional self-esteem.

PLANNING AND IMPLEMENTATION

- Provide analgesia as ordered, evaluating its effectiveness.
- Discuss foods that cause odor and gas.
- Teach colostomy care.
- Maintain consistent nursing personnel assignment to facilitate trust.
- Refer to the local United Ostomy Association.
- Provide a list of local medical supply companies for ostomy supplies.
- Provide for privacy when teaching and discussing concerns about ostomy.

EVALUATION

On discharge, Mr. Cunningham is able to empty and rinse out his colostomy pouch. He is changing the pouch and caring for surrounding skin appropriately. Ms. Hart has given him verbal and written instructions on colostomy care. He verbalizes understanding of phantom rectal pain, and the importance of avoiding rectal suppositories. He expresses an understanding of the need to avoid heavy lifting, and the importance of follow-up care. Ms. Hart has referred Mr. Cunningham to a home health agency in his community for further questions and follow-up care.

CRITICAL THINKING IN THE NURSING PROCESS

1. What is the cause of phantom rectal pain?
2. Why is it important to discuss dietary concerns with a client with a colostomy, especially odor- and gas-forming foods?
3. Outline a plan to teach Mr. Cunningham how to irrigate a colostomy.
4. Develop a care plan for Mr. Cunningham for the nursing diagnosis *Disturbed Body Image*.

See Evaluating Your Response in Appendix C.

---

preclude surgical resection. See Chapter 9 ∞ for more information on caring for clients with pain.

- Monitor for adequate pain relief. Use subjective and objective information, including the location, intensity, and character of the pain, as well as nonverbal signs, such as grimacing; muscle tension; apparent dozing; changes in pulse or blood pressure; rapid, shallow respirations. *The client may assume that pain is to be expected or tolerated or may fear becoming addicted to analgesic medications. Careful questioning and assessment can provide accurate information about pain status, allowing better control of discomfort.*

- Ask client to rate pain using a 0 to 10 pain scale. Document the level of pain. *Pain is a subjective experience. Clients perceive and respond to pain differently. Religion and ethnic background may affect the response to pain.*

- Monitor analgesic effectiveness 30 minutes after administration. Monitor for pain relief and adverse effects. *The method of delivery, dosage, or medication itself may need to be adjusted to provide adequate pain relief.*

- Assess the incision for inflammation or swelling; assess drainage catheters and tubes for patency. *Poorly controlled pain or pain that changes may be related to organ distention from an obstructed nasogastric tube, urinary catheter, or wound drain, or may indicate an infection.*

- Assess the abdomen for distention, tenderness, and bowel sounds. *Intra-abdominal bleeding, peritonitis, or paralytic ileus can cause pain that may be confused with incisional pain.*

- Administer analgesia prior to an activity or procedure. *Adequate pain relief reduces muscle tension, allowing for more comfortable participation in activities.*

- Assist with adjunctive comfort measures, such as positioning, diversional activities, management of environmental stimuli, guided imagery, and teaching relaxation techniques. *These measures enhance the effects of analgesia by reducing muscle tension.*

- Splint incision with a pillow, and teach the client how to self-splint when coughing and deep breathing *to prevent respiratory complications related to fear of pain.*

Imbalanced Nutrition: Less than Body Requirements

Bowel preparation for diagnostic procedures, surgery, radiation therapy, and chemotherapy place the client with colorectal cancer at risk for nutritional deficiencies. Fluid and electrolyte replacement is provided following surgery, along with possible TPN (see Chapter 22 ∞). Adequate kilocalorie and nutrient intake are necessary for healing after surgery. Additionally, if the tumor is advanced, metabolic needs may be increased and the appetite decreased.

- Assess nutritional status, using data such as height and weight, skinfold measurements, body mass index (BMI) calculation (see Chapter 21 ∞), and laboratory data including serum albumin level. Refer to dietitian or nutritionist for dietary management. *The client who is malnourished before beginning aggressive cancer treatment requires more vigorous nutrition management to promote healing.*
- Assess readiness for resumption of oral intake after surgery or procedures using data such as statements of hunger, presence of bowel sounds, passage of flatus, and minimal abdominal distention. *Manipulation of the bowel interrupts peristalsis of the GI tract. It is important to ensure that peristalsis has resumed prior to resumption of oral intake.*
- Monitor and document food and fluid intake. *Documentation helps identify the adequacy of kilocalories and other nutrient intake.*
- Weigh daily. *Weight fluctuation may indicate adequate or inadequate dietary intake.*
- Maintain TPN and central intravenous lines as ordered. *Parenteral nutrition prevents tissue catabolism and promotes healing when food intake is disrupted for more than 2 to 3 days.*
- When oral intake resumes, help the client develop a meal plan that incorporates food preferences and considers the client's schedule and environment. *Consideration of likes, dislikes, and circumstances in meal planning promotes adequate intake.*

Anticipatory Grieving

When a bowel resection is performed for colorectal cancer, the client needs to adjust to the loss of a major body part as well as to the diagnosis of cancer. Even when the prognosis for recovery is good, many people perceive cancer as fatal. Supporting the client and family during the initial stages of grieving can improve physical recovery as well as psychologic coping and eventual adaptation.

- Work to develop a trusting relationship with the client and family. *This increases the nurse's effectiveness in helping them work through the grieving process.*
- Listen actively, encouraging the client and family to express their fears and concerns. Assist to identify strengths, past experiences, and support systems:
  - Demonstrate respect for cultural, spiritual, and religious values and beliefs; encourage use of these resources to cope with losses.
  - Encourage discussion of the potential impact of loss on individual family members, family structure, and family

function. Assist family members to share concerns with one another.
  - Refer to cancer support groups, social services, or counseling as appropriate.
  These resources can be used throughout the grieving process.

Risk for Sexual Dysfunction

Colorectal cancer and ostomy surgery increase the risk for sexual dysfunction, defined as a change in sexual function so that it becomes unsatisfying, unrewarding, or inadequate (NANDA, 2005). Physical factors that can lead to sexual dysfunction include disruption of nerves and blood vessels that supply the genitals, radiation therapy, chemotherapy, and other medications prescribed after surgery.

Psychologically, an *ostomate* (client with an ostomy) experiences an altered body image and may develop low self-esteem. The client may feel undesirable and fear rejection. He or she may be concerned about odors or pouch leakage during sexual activity. This emotional stress can also contribute to sexual dysfunction.

- Provide opportunities for the client and family to express feelings about the cancer diagnosis, ostomy, and effects of other treatments. *Encouraging verbalization of feelings about the diagnosis, ostomy, and treatments provides an opportunity to validate that feelings of anger and depression are normal responses to the diagnosis and change in body function.*
- Provide consistent colostomy care. *An accepting attitude and consistent care that provides a secure appliance and controls odor and leakage instill a sense of confidence in the client.*
- Encourage expression of sexual concerns. Provide privacy and caregivers who have established trust with the client and family and are comfortable with discussions about sexual concerns. *Sexuality is a very private concern to most people. The client and family are not likely to express their concerns openly unless trust has been established.*
- Reassure the client and significant other that the effect of physical illness and prescribed interventions on sexuality usually is temporary. *The client and partner may misinterpret an initial decrease in libido as evidence that sexual activity will not be possible or resume following recovery.*
- Refer the client and partner to social services or a family counselor for further interventions. *Clients are often discharged from acute care settings well before concerns about sexual activity surface. Ongoing counseling provides a continuing resource.*
- Arrange for a visit from a member of the United Ostomy Association. *People who are living and coping with an ostomy can provide information and support, helping the new ostomate overcome feelings of isolation and rejection.*

Using NANDA, NIC, and NOC

Chart 26–4 shows links between NANDA nursing diagnoses, NIC, and NOC when caring for the client with colorectal cancer.

Community-Based Care

During the diagnostic and preoperative periods, provide instruction about the following topics:

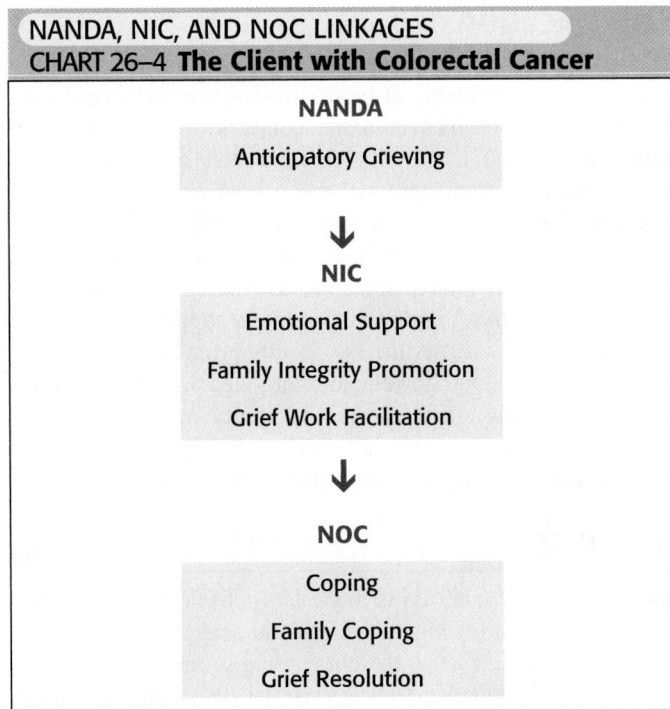

NANDA, NIC, AND NOC LINKAGES
CHART 26–4 The Client with Colorectal Cancer

NANDA

Anticipatory Grieving

↓

NIC

Emotional Support

Family Integrity Promotion

Grief Work Facilitation

↓

NOC

Coping

Family Coping

Grief Resolution

Data from *NANDA's Nursing Diagnoses: Definitions & Classification 2005–2006* by NANDA International (2005), Philadelphia; *Nursing Interventions Classification (NIC)* (4th ed.) by J. M. Dochterman & G. M. Bulechek (2004), St. Louis, MO: Mosby; and *Nursing Outcomes Classification (NOC)* (3rd ed.) by S. Moorhead, M. Johnson, and M. Maas (2004), St. Louis, MO: Mosby.

- Tests to be performed and preparatory procedures, including dietary restrictions, laxatives, enemas, and food and fluid restrictions just prior to the procedure
- Recommended postprocedure care and potential adverse effects to report
- Preoperative care, such as intestinal preparation and food and fluid restrictions

If a colostomy is planned, refer to an enterostomal therapist for stoma placement and initial teaching.

Once treatment has been initiated, include the following topics (as appropriate) in teaching for home care:

- Pain management
- Skin care and management of potential adverse effects of radiation therapy and/or chemotherapy (Refer to Chapter 14 ∞ for further discussion of teaching needs related to these therapies.)
- Incision and ostomy care
- Recommended diet
- Follow-up appointments and care.

If the tumor is inoperable or a cure is not anticipated, provide information about pain and symptom management. Discuss the hospice philosophy and available services. Provide a referral to a local hospice or home health department.

STRUCTURAL AND OBSTRUCTIVE BOWEL DISORDERS

Any portion of the intestines may be affected by a structural or obstructive disorder. When the structural defect is in the bowel wall, the intestine may be directly affected, as is the case with diverticula. Defects in the abdominal wall may allow intra-abdominal contents (such as loops of bowel) to protrude, indirectly affecting bowel function. Likewise, obstructions may result from disease of the bowel itself or from obstruction of the bowel lumen by an external force.

THE CLIENT WITH A HERNIA

A **hernia** is a defect in the abdominal wall that allows abdominal contents to protrude out of the abdominal cavity. Trauma, surgery, and increased intra-abdominal pressure caused by such conditions as pregnancy, obesity, weight lifting, or tumors are risk factors for hernia formation.

Pathophysiology

Hernias are classified by location (Figure 26–12 ■), and may be congenital or acquired. Most hernias occur in the groin (inguinal or femoral hernias). Inguinal hernias often are congenital, caused by improper closure of the tract that develops as the testes descend into the scrotum during fetal development. Groin hernias may be acquired, resulting from weakness of fascia in a region called Hesselbach's area or from dilation of the femoral ring (e.g., during pregnancy and childbirth). Ventral or incisional hernias of the abdominal wall generally are acquired, caused by weakening of nor-

Ventral (Incisional) hernia

Inguinal hernia

Figure 26–12 ■ An abdominal wall (ventral or incisional) hernia and an inguinal hernia.

mal abdominal wall musculature. Umbilical hernias also are congenital, and usually are detected in infancy. Hiatal hernias develop in the diaphragm (see Chapter 23 ∞).

Inguinal Hernia

Inguinal hernias usually affect males, and may be classified as indirect or direct inguinal hernias. *Indirect inguinal hernias* are caused by improper closure of the tract that develops as the testes descend into the scrotum before birth. A sac of abdominal contents protrudes through the internal inguinal ring into the inguinal canal. It often descends into the scrotum. Although indirect inguinal hernias are congenital defects, they often are not evident until adulthood, when increased intra-abdominal pressure and dilation of the inguinal ring allow abdominal contents to enter the channel.

Direct inguinal hernias are acquired defects that result from weakness of the posterior inguinal wall. Direct inguinal hernias usually affect older adults. *Femoral hernias* are also acquired defects in which a peritoneal sac protrudes through the femoral ring. These hernias usually affect obese or pregnant women.

Inguinal hernias may produce no manifestations and are discovered during routine physical examination. They may cause a lump, swelling, or bulge in the groin, particularly with lifting or straining. An inguinal hernia may cause sharp pain or a dull ache that radiates into the scrotum. A palpable mass may be present in the groin, although it may be felt only with increased intra-abdominal pressure (as occurs during coughing) and invagination of the scrotum toward the inguinal ring.

Umbilical Hernia

Pregnancy and obesity contribute to the development of umbilical hernias in adults. *Umbilical hernias* may be congenital and evident during infancy, or acquired as the tissue closing the umbilical ring weakens, allowing protrusion of abdominal contents. These hernias are more common in women. Other predisposing factors include multiple pregnancies with prolonged labor, ascites, and large intra-abdominal tumors.

Umbilical hernias tend to enlarge steadily and contain omentum, although they may also contain small or large bowel. The hernia may cause sharp pain on coughing or straining or a dull, aching sensation. Strangulation is a common complication of umbilical hernias.

Incisional or Ventral Hernia

Incisional or *ventral hernias* occur at a previous surgical incision or following abdominal muscle tears. Inadequate healing of the incision or tear can lead to hernia development. Contributing factors include poor wound closure, postoperative infection, age or debility, obesity, inadequate nutrition, and excess incisional stress caused by vigorous coughing.

Ventral hernias are characterized by a bulge at the incisional site, often noted when the client pulls to a sitting position from a lying position. Ventral hernias often are asymptomatic, and the risk of incarceration is low because of the size of the defect.

Manifestations

Abdominal contents (peritoneum, bowel, and other abdominal organs) can protrude through the abdominal wall to form a sac covered by skin and subcutaneous tissues. In most cases, abdominal contents move into the sac when intra-abdominal pressure increases, then return to the abdominal cavity when pressure returns to normal or when manual pressure is placed on the bulging sac. This is known as a *reducible hernia*.

Complications

The risk for complications is low with a reducible hernia. If the contents of a hernia cannot be returned to the abdominal cavity, it is said to be *incarcerated*. Contents of an incarcerated hernia are trapped, usually by a narrow neck or opening to the hernia. Incarceration increases the risk of complications, including obstruction and strangulation. Obstruction occurs when the lumen of the bowel contained within the hernia becomes occluded, much like the crimping of a hose. A *strangulated hernia* develops when blood supply to bowel and other tissues in the hernia sac is compromised, leading to necrosis. The affected bowel can infarct, leading to perforation with contamination of the peritoneal cavity. Manifestations of a strangulated hernia include severe abdominal pain and distention, nausea, vomiting, tachycardia, and fever.

INTERDISCIPLINARY CARE

The diagnosis of a hernia is made by a physical examination. The client is examined in a supine or standing position. A bulge may be seen or felt when the client coughs or bears down. No laboratory or diagnostic testing is usually required, unless bowel obstruction or strangulation is suspected.

Surgical repair, or *herniorrhaphy,* is the usual treatment of hernia. Surgery is generally well tolerated by people of all ages and carries a much lower risk than the complications of incarceration, obstruction, and strangulation. Emergency surgery is indicated for a hernia that is incarcerated, painful, or tender. In a herniorrhaphy, the abdominal wall defect is closed by suturing or with wire or mesh over the defect. If incarceration has occurred or strangulation is suspected, the abdomen is explored at the time of surgery and any infarcted bowel resected. Heavy lifting and heavy manual labor are restricted for approximately 3 weeks after surgery.

When surgery is contraindicated, the client may be taught to reduce the hernia by lying down and gently pushing against the mass. A binder or truss may be worn to prevent or control the protrusion. An incarcerated hernia should not be reduced by the client.

NURSING CARE

Assessment

- *Health history:* Manifestations of hernia, such as bulging in the groin or of the abdominal wall when coughing, straining, or moving from lying to standing; pain (abdominal, groin, or scrotal); history of hernia or abdominal surgery.
- *Physical examination:* Observe for bulging of the abdominal wall or around the umbilicus when raising head and shoulders from supine position; wearing gloves, palpate inguinal region for bulges when the client coughs or bears down (Valsalva maneuver) while standing.

Nursing Diagnoses and Interventions

Herniorrhaphy is generally an uncomplicated procedure, usually performed as same-day surgery. Preoperative assessment and teaching and immediate postoperative care are the primary nursing care needs. Care is similar to that provided for a client with an appendectomy.

Risk for Ineffective Tissue Perfusion: Gastrointestinal

When providing care for a client with a known hernia, the possibility of obstruction and strangulation must be considered throughout nursing assessments. Although nursing interventions may not be able to prevent these complications, rapid identification of the problem allows timely surgical treatment. Prompt treatment may prevent major complications related to infection and peritoneal contamination by bowel contents.

■ Assess bowel sounds and abdominal distention at least every 8 hours. *A change in bowel sounds—either cessation of sounds or an onset of hyperactive, high-pitched sounds—may indicate obstruction. With obstruction, abdominal girth may increase.*

PRACTICE ALERT
Promptly report any acute increase in abdominal, groin, perineal, or scrotal pain. An abrupt increase in the intensity of pain may indicate bowel ischemia due to strangulation.

■ Notify primary care provider if the hernia becomes painful or tender. *Pain and tenderness may indicate incarceration and increased risk for strangulation.*
■ If signs of possible obstruction or strangulation occur, notify the physician. Place client in supine position with the hips elevated and knees slightly bent. Withhold all food and fluids (NPO), and begin preparations for surgery. *This position helps relax abdominal muscles and may facilitate reduction of the hernia. Strangulation or obstruction require immediate surgical intervention.*

Community-Based Care

Include the following topics when teaching clients about hernias and home care:

■ Rationale for examining the groin and abdomen for bulges
■ The nature of hernia, risk factors, and manifestations
■ Surgical intervention for hernia
■ How to reduce a hernia if necessary
■ The importance of seeking immediate medical intervention for signs of strangulation or obstruction
■ The need to notify the physician if upper respiratory infection and cough develop preoperatively (forceful coughing is not recommended postoperatively)
■ Postoperative pain management and activity restrictions.

THE CLIENT WITH INTESTINAL OBSTRUCTION

Intestinal obstruction is failure of intestinal contents to move through the bowel lumen. Intestinal obstructions may affect either the large or small bowel. The small intestine is more commonly affected; however, bowel obstructions may also occur in the large intestine. Obstruction is the most common reason for small-bowel surgery.

Pathophysiology

Intestinal obstructions may be either mechanical or functional in nature. *Mechanical* obstructions may be caused by (1) problems outside the intestine, such as bands of scar tissue or hernias; (2) problems within the intestine, such as tumors or inflammatory bowel disease; or (3) obstruction of the intestinal lumen. The obstruction may be partial or complete. *Functional* obstruction occurs when peristalsis fails to propel intestinal contents although there is no mechanical obstruction. *Adynamic ileus* (also known as *paralytic ileus* or simply *ileus*) is the most common functional obstruction after abdominal surgery, and probably accounts for most intestinal obstructions altogether (Porth, 2005). Obstructions are further classified by the portion of intestine affected.

When the intestine is obstructed, gas and fluid accumulate proximal to and within the obstructed segment, distending the bowel. Swallowed air accounts for most of the gas. Ingested fluid, saliva, gastric juice, and pancreatic secretions contribute to accumulated fluid. Water and sodium are drawn into the bowel lumen, contributing to fluid accumulation, distention, and vascular fluid losses.

In some mechanical obstructions, such as a strangulated hernia, blood supply to the affected portion of bowel also is impaired, leading to necrosis and bacterial peritonitis.

Significant bowel distention, vomiting, and third spacing of fluids in the bowel and peritoneal cavity can lead to massive loss of fluids and electrolytes with resulting hypovolemia, hypokalemia, renal insufficiency, and shock.

Small-Bowel Obstruction

Adhesions, or bands of scar tissue, and hernias account for most mechanical small bowel obstructions. In adults, adhesions develop following abdominal surgery or inflammatory processes. Adhesions usually produce a *simple obstruction,* or single blockage in one portion of the intestine (Figure 26–13A ■). The obstruction produced by an incarcerated hernia is a *closed-loop obstruction,* with two different portions of the bowel lumen obstructed (Figure 26–13B).

Tumors, either intrinsic (of the bowel itself) or extrinsic (of another organ but affecting the bowel because of their size), can progressively occlude the bowel lumen and eventually obstruct it (Figure 26–13C). Other, less common causes of bowel obstruction include intussusception (rare in adults) (Figure 26–13D); volvulus, which is the rotation of loops of bowel about a fixed point (Figure 26–13E); foreign bodies; stricture; and inflammatory bowel disease.

Both volvulus and an incarcerated hernia can cause a *strangulated obstruction.* In a strangulated obstruction, not only is the lumen of the bowel obstructed, but the blood supply to the affected portion is also compromised.

In a functional obstruction or adynamic ileus, peristalsis stops due to either neurogenic or muscular impairment. The bowel lumen remains patent, but contents are not propelled forward. Temporary ileus commonly follows gastrointestinal surgery. It may also result from tissue anoxia or peritoneal irritation due to hemorrhage, peritonitis, or perforation of an organ. Other conditions that can precipitate paralytic ileus include renal colic, spinal cord injuries, uremia, and electrolyte

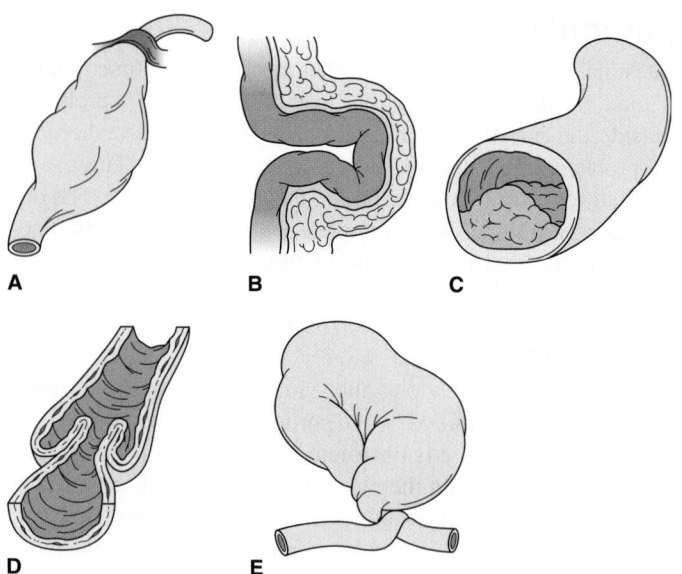

Figure 26–13 ■ Selected causes of mechanical obstruction. *A,* Adhesions; *B,* incarcerated hernia; *C,* tumor; *D,* intussusception; and *E,* volvulus.

imbalances, hypokalemia in particular. In addition, the effects of some narcotics, anticholinergic drugs, and antidiarrheal medications such as diphenoxylate can produce a functional obstruction.

MANIFESTATIONS The manifestations of a small-bowel obstruction vary, depending on the level of obstruction and how rapidly it develops. Cramping or colicky abdominal pain that may be intermittent or increasing in intensity is common. Vomiting is common, particularly in high or proximal obstructions, because distention of the lumen stimulates the vomiting center. As bacterial fermentation occurs, vomitus often contains fecal matter, particularly with a low or distal obstruction. Flatus and feces already present in the lower bowel may be expelled early in the obstructive process, but this expulsion ceases as the obstruction continues.

Early in the course of a mechanical obstruction, borborygmi and high-pitched tinkling bowel sounds are present, as the intestine attempts to propel contents past the obstruction. Visible peristaltic waves may be noted in the distended loops of bowel in thin clients. In the later stages, the bowel becomes silent. With a paralytic ileus, bowel sounds are greatly diminished or absent throughout the process. Abdominal distention is minimal with proximal obstructions, but may be pronounced with distal obstruction and paralytic ileus. The abdomen may be tender to palpation as well.

In addition to abdominal and gastrointestinal manifestations, signs of fluid and electrolyte imbalance develop. Hypovolemia can develop rapidly as extracellular fluid is sequestered in the bowel and vomiting occurs. Although early vital signs may be normal, changes are noted as dehydration and hypovolemia develop. The client becomes tachycardic and tachypneic, and blood pressure falls. Temperature may be elevated. Urine output drops, and signs of hypovolemic shock may be seen.

COMPLICATIONS Hypovolemia and hypovolemic shock with multiple organ dysfunction is a significant complication of bowel obstruction and can lead to death. Renal insufficiency from hypovolemia can lead to acute renal failure. Pulmonary ventilation may be impaired because abdominal distention elevates the diaphragm and interferes with respiratory processes.

Strangulation associated with incarcerated hernia or volvulus impairs the blood supply to the bowel. Gangrene may rapidly result, causing bleeding into the bowel lumen and peritoneal cavity and eventual perforation. With perforation, bacteria and toxins from the strangulated intestine enter the peritoneum and, potentially, the circulation, resulting in peritonitis and possible septic shock. Strangulation greatly increases the risk of mortality.

Large-Bowel Obstruction

Obstruction of the large intestine occurs much less frequently than small-bowel obstruction. Although any portion of the colon may be affected, obstruction usually occurs in the sigmoid segment. Cancer of the bowel is the most common cause; other causes include volvulus, diverticular disease, inflammatory disorders, and fecal impaction.

MANIFESTATIONS Constipation and colicky abdominal pain are usual manifestations of large-bowel obstruction. The pain is often deep and cramping; severe, continuous pain may signal bowel ischemia and possible perforation. Vomiting is a late sign, if it occurs at all. The abdomen is distended, with high-pitched, tinkling bowel sounds with rushes and gurgles. On palpation, localized tenderness or a mass may be noted.

COMPLICATIONS If the ileocecal valve between the small and large intestines is competent, distention proximal to the obstruction is limited to the colon itself. This is known as a *closed-loop obstruction.* It can lead to massive colon dilation as the ileum continues to empty gas and fluid into the colon. Increasing pressure within the obstructed colon impairs circulation to the bowel wall. Gangrene and perforation are potential complications.

INTERDISCIPLINARY CARE

The management of a bowel obstruction focuses on relieving the pressure and obstruction, and providing supportive care. The intestine is decompressed, and fluid and electrolyte balance is restored. Surgery may be necessary to relieve a mechanical obstruction or if strangulation is suspected.

Diagnosis

Radiologic studies (x-rays and CT scan) are used to confirm the diagnosis of bowel obstruction. Laboratory testing is used to evaluate for the presence of infection and fluid and electrolyte imbalances.

An abdominal x-ray often shows distended loops of intestine with fluid and gas in a small-bowel obstruction. Free air under the diaphragm indicates a perforation. X-ray or CT scan with contrast media may be required to confirm a mechanical obstruction and assess the completeness of the obstruction. Meglumine diatrizoate (Gastrografin) is often used to provide contrast rather than barium when a bowel obstruction is suspected. Barium enema may be used to confirm the diagnosis of large-bowel obstruction and determine its location, unless perforation is suspected.

Laboratory tests used are WBC, serum amylase, serum osmolality, electrolytes, and arterial blood gases. These tests will show the following results with a bowel obstruction:

- *WBC* often shows mild leukocytosis due to an inflammatory response to changes within the obstructed bowel lumen. With strangulation, leukocytosis is marked.
- *Serum amylase levels* may be elevated, particularly when strangulation is present.
- *Serum osmolality* and *electrolyte levels* are affected by fluid and electrolyte losses from vomiting and fluid sequestering in the bowel lumen. With hypovolemia, the serum osmolality and urine specific gravity increase. Potassium and chloride are lost through vomiting, leading to hypokalemia and hypochloremia.
- ABGs may reveal metabolic alkalosis (pH > 7.45, bicarbonate > 26 mEq/L, P_{CO_2} > 45 mmHg) with small-bowel obstruction due to loss of hydrochloric acid from the stomach.

Gastrointestinal Decompression

Most partial small-bowel obstructions are successfully treated with gastrointestinal decompression using a nasogastric or long intestinal tube. Functional obstructions respond to treatment with bowel rest and intestinal decompression as well. Intestinal tubes (see Figure 26–2) may be inserted through the nares or via gastrostomy. A balloon or weighted tip draws the tube from the stomach into the intestine and to the area of obstruction. Collected fluid and gas are removed using low suction until peristalsis resumes or the obstruction is relieved.

Surgery

Surgical intervention is required for complete mechanical obstructions as well as for strangulated or incarcerated obstructions of the small intestine. Clients with incomplete mechanical obstruction may also require surgery if the obstruction persists.

Prior to surgery, a nasogastric tube is inserted to relieve vomiting and abdominal distention and to prevent aspiration of intestinal contents. Fluid and electrolyte balance must be restored before surgery. Isotonic intravenous fluids, such as normal (physiologic) saline, Ringer's solution, or other balanced electrolyte solutions, are used. Additional electrolytes may be added to the solution to correct low levels. It is particularly important to correct hypokalemia prior to surgery. Acid–base imbalances are also addressed, often using intravenous acidifiers or alkalinizing agents. If strangulation has occurred, the client may require plasma or blood replacement. Intravenous broad-spectrum antibiotics are administered prophylactically (see the section on peritonitis).

A laparotomy usually is performed to allow inspection of the small intestine and removal of infarcted or gangrenous tissue. If the obstruction was caused by adhesions, they are removed or lysed. Obstructing tumors are resected, and foreign bodies are removed. Any bowel that appears to be gangrenous is resected, usually followed by an end-to-end anastomosis of remaining intestine. If a large tumor mass or dense adhesions are found, the area of obstruction may be bypassed by anasto-

mosis of proximal small bowel to small or large intestine distal to the obstruction. Nursing care of the client having bowel surgery is included in the box on page 804.

Obstructions of the large intestine usually necessitate surgery. The primary goal is to relieve colonic distention and prevent perforation; the secondary goal is to remove the obstructing lesion. In some cases, colonoscopy may be used to relieve the distention. If the client's condition prohibits major surgery or the obstructing tumor is advanced, laser photocoagulation may be used to enlarge the bowel lumen. Removal of the obstructing lesion is the preferred treatment. The proximal and distal bowel segments may be anastomosed, or a permanent colostomy or ileostomy may be required.

NURSING CARE

Health Promotion

Teach health promotion activities, such as increasing dietary fiber intake, maintaining a generous fluid intake, and exercising daily to help prevent constipation and possible large-bowel obstruction, particularly in the older adult. Stress the importance of complying with dietary restrictions (such as avoiding popcorn) for clients who experience repeated small-bowel obstructions.

Assessment

Nurses may be instrumental in the early identification of intestinal obstructions in older adults, the homebound client, or the institutionalized client. Early identification and intervention significantly reduce morbidity from bowel obstruction.

- *Health history:* Complaints of abdominal pain and bloating, constipation; previous history of bowel obstruction or risk factors such as hernia, inflammatory bowel disease, diverticulosis, or previous abdominal surgery; current medications.
- *Physical examination:* Vital signs including orthostatic blood pressure, temperature; skin color, temperature, texture, and turgor; color and moisture of mucous membranes; abdominal shape, contour, bowel sounds, presence of tenderness or masses on palpation.

Nursing Diagnoses and Interventions

In clients with a suspected or confirmed bowel obstruction, frequent assessment for complications such as fluid and electrolyte imbalance, acid–base imbalances, hypovolemic shock, perforation, and peritonitis is necessary.

Deficient Fluid Volume

Because of the large collection of fluid in the bowel proximal to an obstruction, the accompanying vomiting, and nasogastric suction, the client with an intestinal obstruction often has a fluid volume deficit. If not corrected promptly, hypovolemic shock, acute renal failure, and multiple organ system dysfunction from poor tissue perfusion may result.

- Monitor vital signs, pulmonary artery pressures, cardiac output (CO), and central venous pressure (CVP) hourly. *A decrease in blood pressure, tachycardia, and tachypnea may indicate hypovolemia. Although invasive, hemodynamic parameters such as pulmonary artery pressures, CO, and CVP allow accurate assessment of fluid volume status.*

- Measure urinary output hourly and nasogastric drainage every 2 to 4 hours. *A urinary output of 30 mL per hour or more usually indicates an adequate glomerular filtration rate (GFR), another indicator of fluid volume. Nasogastric output provides a tool for evaluating fluid replacement needs.*

PRACTICE ALERT
Promptly report urine output of less than 30 mL per hour. This often indicates hypovolemia and an increased risk for shock and acute renal failure.

- Maintain intravenous fluids and blood volume expanders as ordered. The amount of fluid administered is calculated to meet ongoing fluid needs and replace previous and current losses. *Restoration and maintenance of blood volume are necessary to maintain cardiac output and tissue and organ perfusion.*
- Measure abdominal girth every 4 to 8 hours. Mark the level of measurement on the abdomen. *A reference mark allows consistent, accurate measurements. An increase in abdominal girth indicates increasing intestinal distention.*
- Notify the physician of changes in status. *Changes in vital signs, pain, and signs of increasing distention can indicate the need for immediate surgical intervention.*

Ineffective Tissue Perfusion: Gastrointestinal

Perfusion of the intestinal wall and mucosa may be impaired by the obstructive process itself (e.g., strangulation or volvulus) or by significant intestinal distention. The goal is to maintain tissue perfusion and promote normal peristalsis and bowel elimination.

- Monitor vital signs hourly. Assess peripheral pulses, skin color, temperature, and capillary refill. *Cardiovascular assessment is vital to detect early signs of hypovolemic shock resulting from sequestering large volumes of fluid in the intestines. Hypovolemia and shock can convert mild bowel ischemia to infarction as the blood supply to the tissue falls.*
- Monitor urine output hourly. Report output of less than 30 mL per hour. *Urine output is a good indicator of the GFR and tissue perfusion. The urine output often falls before vital sign changes are apparent in hypovolemia.*
- Monitor temperature at least every 4 hours. *An elevated temperature may be an early indication of sepsis from bowel perforation as a result of gangrene.*
- Frequently assess pain. *A change in the character of pain or a rapid increase in its intensity may signal bowel infarction or perforation.*
- Maintain NPO status until peristalsis resumes. *Enteral food or fluids may increase distention and bowel ischemia. They also are restricted until the possibility of perforation is eliminated.*

Ineffective Breathing Pattern

Significant abdominal distention from a bowel obstruction can cause the diaphragm to flatten, impairing pulmonary ventilation. Following surgery, splinting of abdominal muscles to avoid pain can lead to shallow respirations. These factors, plus the risk of aspiration of gastrointestinal contents during vomit-

ing, place the client at high risk for respiratory complications, particularly with a small-bowel obstruction.

- Assess respiratory rate, pattern, and lung sounds at least every 2 to 4 hours. *Tachypnea, shortness of breath, or apparent dyspnea may be early signs of respiratory compromise. Diminished breath sounds, particularly in the bases of the lungs, or crackles indicate poor lung expansion and possible impaired ventilation.*
- Monitor ABG results for possible effects of altered respiratory status. *Tachypnea may lead to respiratory alkalosis as excess carbon dioxide is eliminated. Conversely, impaired chest expansion can lead to respiratory acidosis because of alveolar hypoventilation.*
- Elevate the head of the bed. *Elevating the head of the bed reduces the work of breathing and improves alveolar ventilation by reducing the pressure of abdominal distention on the diaphragm.*
- Provide a pillow or folded bath blanket to use in splinting the abdomen while coughing postoperatively. *Splinting abdominal muscles and incisions improves the ease and effectiveness of coughing postoperatively.*
- Maintain nasogastric or intestinal tube patency. *Maintaining gastrointestinal suction helps reduce abdominal distention and prevent aspiration associated with vomiting.*
- Encourage use of incentive spirometer or other assistive device hourly. *These devices encourage deep breathing, opening distal airways and preventing atelectasis.*
- Contact respiratory therapy as indicated. *The respiratory therapist may suggest or perform additional measures to maintain effective pulmonary ventilation.*
- Provide good oral care at least every 4 hours. *Dehydration and nasogastric suction dry the mucous membranes of the mouth and throat, increasing the risk of bacterial growth. Many respiratory infections result from aspirated organisms.*

Using NANDA, NIC, and NOC

Linkages between NANDA, NIC, and NOC when caring for the client with intestinal obstruction are similar to those for clients with appendicitis. (See Chart 26–2.)

Community-Based Care

Include the following topics when teaching the client with intestinal obstruction in preparation for home care:

- Wound care
- Activity level, return to work, and any other recommended restrictions
- Recommended follow-up care
- Care of temporary colostomy (if appropriate) and planned reanastomosis
- For recurrent obstructions, their cause, early identification of manifestations, and possible preventive measures.

THE CLIENT WITH DIVERTICULAR DISEASE

Diverticula are small (0.5- to 1.0-cm) outpouchings of the colon that occur in rows (Figure 26–14 ■). Diverticula may oc-

Figure 26–14 ■ Diverticula of the colon.

cur anywhere in the intestinal tract, excluding the rectum. The vast majority, however, affect the large intestine, with 90% occurring in the sigmoid colon (Welch & Cohen, 2004).

FAST FACTS
Diverticular Disease
- People in the United States, Australia, the United Kingdom, and France have high and increasing incidence rates of diverticular disease. The incidence of diverticula increases with age, with 5% to 10% of the population older than 45 years of age and almost 80% of those older than 85 years of age experiencing it.
- Most of the people diagnosed with diverticular disease remain asymptomatic.
- Men and women are equally affected.

Cultural factors, diet in particular, are thought to play an important role in the development of diverticula. A diet consisting of highly refined and fiber-deficient foods is believed to be the major factor contributing to the disease. Decreased activity levels and delaying defecation have been suggested as contributing factors. The increasing incidence of diverticula with aging suggests that dietary factors (lack of fiber), a decrease in physical activity, poor bowel habits (neglecting the urge to defecate), and the effects of aging contribute to development of the disease (Porth, 2005).

Pathophysiology

Diverticula form when increased pressure within the bowel lumen causes bowel mucosa to herniate through defects in the colon wall. The circular and longitudinal muscles often thicken or hypertrophy in the area affected by diverticula. This narrows the bowel lumen, increasing intraluminal pressure. Deficient dietary fiber and a lack of fecal bulk contribute to muscle hypertrophy and narrowing of the bowel. Contraction of the muscles in response to normal stimuli such as meals may occlude the narrowed lumen, further increasing intraluminal pressure. The high pressure causes mucosa to herniate through the mus-

cle wall, forming a diverticulum. Areas where nutrient blood vessels penetrate the circular muscle layer are the most common sites for diverticula formation.

Diverticulosis

Diverticulosis indicates the presence of diverticula. More than two-thirds of clients with diverticulosis are asymptomatic. When manifestations such as episodic pain (usually left-sided), constipation, and diarrhea occur, they often can be attributed to irritable bowel syndrome, which commonly accompanies diverticular disease. (Irritable bowel syndrome is discussed earlier in this chapter.) As the disease progresses, abdominal cramping, narrow stools (decrease in caliber), increased constipation, bleeding in the stools, weakness, and fatigue may develop.

Complications of diverticulosis include hemorrhage and diverticulitis. A diverticulum may bleed, whether it is inflamed or not, possibly due to erosion of an adjacent blood vessel by a fecalith (hard mass) in the diverticulum.

Diverticulitis

Diverticulitis is inflammation in and around the diverticular sac. It typically affects only one diverticulum, usually in the sigmoid colon. Undigested food and bacteria collect in the diverticula, forming a hard mass that impairs the mucosal blood supply, allowing bacterial invasion. Mucosal ischemia leads to perforation. With microscopic perforation, inflammation is localized. Gross perforation of a diverticulum results in more extensive bacterial contamination and can lead to abscess formation or peritonitis.

MANIFESTATIONS Pain is a common manifestation of diverticulitis. It is usually left-sided and may be mild to severe and either steady or cramping. The client may also experience either constipation or increased frequency of defecation. Depending on the location and severity of the inflammation, nausea, vomiting, and a low-grade fever may occur. On examination, the abdomen may be distended, with tenderness and a palpable mass in the left lower quadrant resulting from the inflammatory response.

The older adult may have less specific manifestations, complaining of vague abdominal pain. A palpable mass and signs of a large bowel obstruction may be present.

COMPLICATIONS Complications associated with diverticulitis (in addition to peritonitis and abscess formation) include bowel obstruction, fistula formation, and hemorrhage. Severe or repeated episodes of diverticulitis may lead to scarring and fibrosis of the bowel wall, further narrowing the bowel lumen. This increases the risk for obstruction of the large bowel. Acutely inflamed tissue may adhere to the small bowel, increasing the potential for small-bowel obstruction as well. Fistulas may form, usually between the sigmoid colon and the bladder. Urinary tract infection is the usual sign of a colovesical fistula. Fistulas may also perforate into the small intestine, ureter, vagina, perineum, or abdominal wall. Bleeding from perforation of a vessel wall can occur with diverticulitis. Although it may be significant, bleeding usually stops spontaneously.

INTERDISCIPLINARY CARE

Management of diverticular disease varies from no prescribed treatment to surgical resection of affected colon, depending on the severity of the disease and its complications.

Diagnosis

Diagnostic testing is used to identify diverticular disease when the disease is symptomatic or complications develop. In addition to illustrating diverticula, a barium enema and X-rays can reveal segmental spasm and muscular thickening with a narrowed bowel lumen. Flexible sigmoidoscopy or colonoscopy may be done to detect diverticulosis, assess for strictures or bleeding, and rule out tumor as the cause of the client's manifestations. Abdominal X-ray films may show free abdominal air associated with diverticulitis and perforation. CT scan may be done with or without contrast media to assess inflammation and detect an abscess or fistula.

Laboratory tests include hemoccult or guaiac testing of stool to identify the presence of occult blood, and a WBC count, which may show leukocytosis with a left shift (an increased number of immature WBCs) due to inflammation in diverticulitis.

Medications

Systemic broad-spectrum antibiotics effective against usual bowel flora are prescribed to treat acute diverticulitis. Oral antibiotics such as metronidazole (Flagyl) and ciprofloxacin (Cipro) or trimethoprim-sulfamethoxazole (Septra, Bactrim) may be prescribed if manifestations are mild. Severe, acute attacks often necessitate hospitalization and treatment with intravenous fluids and antibiotics effective against anaerobic and gram-negative bacteria. Therapy may include a second-generation cephalosporin such as cefoxitin (Mefoxin), or another antibiotic such as piperacillin-tazobactam (Zosyn) or ticarcillin-clavulanate (Timentin). Antibiotics and their nursing implications are discussed in Chapter 12 .

Pentazocine (Talwin) may be prescribed for relief of pain associated with diverticulitis. This analgesic causes less increase in colonic pressure than morphine or meperidine (Demerol).

Although a stool softener such as docusate sodium (Colace) may be prescribed, it is important to note that laxatives (which can further increase intraluminal pressure in the colon) are avoided for the client with diverticular disease.

Nutrition

Dietary modification is central to the management of diverticular disease. It appears that dietary changes can reduce the risk of complications of diverticulosis. A high-fiber diet is recommended; it increases stool bulk, decreases intraluminal pressures, and may reduce spasm (Table 26–13). Bran is a low-cost fiber supplement that can be added to cereal, soups, salads, or other foods. Commercial bulk-forming products, such as psyllium seed (Metamucil) or methylcellulose also may be recommended. These products are discussed in the Medication Administration box on pages 759–760. The client may be advised to avoid foods with small seeds (such as popcorn, caraway seeds, figs, or berries), which could obstruct diverticula.

Bowel rest is prescribed during an acute episode of diverticulitis. The client initially may be NPO with intravenous fluids and possibly TPN. Feeding is resumed gradually. Initially, a clear liquid diet is prescribed with gradual advancement to a soft, low-roughage diet (i.e., a diet low in insoluble fiber) with daily added psyllium seed to soften stool and increase its bulk. Among the foods the client should avoid are wheat and corn bran, vegetable and fruit skins, nuts, and dry beans. The high-fiber diet is resumed following full recovery.

Surgery

Clients with acute diverticulitis may require surgery, usually to treat generalized peritonitis or an abscess that fails to respond to medical treatment. Hemorrhage that recurs or cannot be controlled may also necessitate surgery. Elective surgery may be performed for recurrent episodes of diverticulitis or persistent diverticulitis with continuing pain, tenderness, and a palpable mass.

The affected bowel segment is resected, and if possible an anastomosis of the proximal and distal portions is performed. When an acute infection and diverticulitis are present, a two-stage Hartmann procedure is required. A temporary colostomy

TABLE 26–13 **Foods Recommended in a High-Fiber, High-Residue Diet**	
FOOD GROUP	**RECOMMENDED FOODS**
Cereals and grains	Wheat or oat bran; cooked cereals, such as oatmeal; dry cereals, such as bran buds or flakes, corn flakes, shredded wheat; whole-grain breads or crackers; brown rice; popcorn
Fruits	Unpeeled raw apples, peaches, and pears; blackberries, raspberries, strawberries; oranges
Vegetables	Dried beans (navy, kidney, pinto), lima beans; broccoli; peas; corn; squash; raw vegetables, such as carrots, celery, and tomatoes; potatoes (with skins)

is created and anastomosis delayed until the inflammation has subsided. A second surgery is performed 2 to 3 months later to reconnect the bowel and close the temporary colostomy.

NURSING CARE

Health Promotion

Teaching clients about the benefits of a high-fiber diet is important primary prevention for diverticular disease. Nurses working with groups and individuals in the community should emphasize the importance of a high-fiber diet and its benefits in preventing diverticular disease and other disorders. In facilities such as residential settings, the nurse can work with dietary staff and care providers to increase the amount of fiber in residents' diets, unless this is contraindicated by a preexisting condition.

Assessment

Because most clients with diverticular disease have few or no manifestations, nursing assessment focuses on manifestations of complications.

- *Health history:* Abdominal pain or cramping, chronic constipation or irregular bowel habits; nausea and vomiting; history of diverticular disease or irritable bowel syndrome.
- *Physical examination:* Bowel sounds, presence of abdominal tenderness of masses and location; stool for occult blood.

Nursing Diagnoses and Interventions

Clients with acute diverticulitis are acutely ill and have multiple nursing care needs. Priority nursing diagnoses include *Impaired Tissue Integrity, Acute Pain,* and *Anxiety* related to the possibility of a significant complication or possible surgery.

Impaired Tissue Integrity: Gastrointestinal

During an acute attack of diverticulitis, inflammation and mucosal ischemia place the client at risk for perforation and peritonitis. In addition to maintaining bowel rest to reduce the risk of perforation, the nurse monitors for manifestations of perforation and possible sepsis.

- Monitor vital signs including temperature at least every 4 hours. *Tachycardia and tachypnea may be early indications of increased inflammation and resulting fluid shift. Fever greater than 101°F (38.3°C) may indicate increased inflammation or spread of inflammation. Note, however, that little temperature elevation may occur in the older client. A change in behavior or increasing lethargy may be subtle indications of infection in the older adult.*
- Assess abdomen every 4 to 8 hours or more often as indicated, including measuring abdominal girth, auscultating bowel sounds, and palpating for tenderness. Promptly report significant changes to the physician. *Increasing abdominal distention, a decrease or change in the quality of bowel sounds, and/or increasing tenderness or guarding may indicate spread of the infectious process or peritonitis.*
- Assess for evidence of lower intestinal bleeding by visual examination and guaiac testing of stools for occult blood. *Perforation of a diverticulum may produce either intestinal or intra-abdominal bleeding and require immediate treatment such as surgery.*
- Maintain intravenous fluids, TPN, and accurate intake and output records. *During acute diverticulitis, oral intake is usually prohibited or restricted. Intravenous fluids are given to maintain fluid and electrolyte balance; TPN is used to maintain nutritional status, facilitating healing and recovery.*

Acute Pain

Pain is a common manifestation of acute diverticulitis. It results from inflammation of the bowel and edema of affected tissues. If surgery is required, postoperative pain is managed with narcotic analgesics.

- Ask the client to rate pain using a 0 to 10 pain scale. Document the level of pain, and note any changes in location or character of pain. *The perception and response to pain is individual and is affected by past experiences, culture, ethnic background, and many other factors. A change in the character or intensity of the pain may indicate a complication such as perforation or abscess formation.*
- Administer prescribed analgesic or maintain PCA as ordered. Assess analgesic effectiveness. Avoid administering morphine. Provide adjunctive medications as ordered, and encourage use of adjunctive techniques, such as relaxation, positioning, and distraction. Notify the physician if pain management is inadequate. *If client has not obtained adequate pain relief, further assessment and intervention are required.*
- Maintain bowel rest and total body rest (bed rest with limited activity). *Rest helps reduce inflammation and promote healing, increasing comfort.*
- Reintroduce oral foods and fluids slowly, providing a soft, low-fiber diet with bulk-forming agents. *This allows continued healing of the affected bowel while promoting soft, easily expelled stools.*

Anxiety

The client with acute diverticulitis faces not only hospitalization, but also potential serious complications such as peritonitis and hemorrhage. Surgery and formation of a temporary colostomy may be necessary. Furthermore, episodes of acute diverticulitis are often recurrent, and the client may fear future problems.

- Assess and document level of anxiety. *Severe anxiety or panic states can interfere with the ability to respond to instructions and assist with care. Low to moderate anxiety levels enhance learning and compliance with prescribed interventions.*
- Demonstrate empathy and awareness of the perceived threat to health. *It is important to recognize and respect the client's feelings and perceptions as reality.*
- Attend to physical care needs. *This provides reassurance that these needs will be met and relieves concerns about them.*
- Spend as much time as possible with the client. *Presence of a caring nurse helps relieve fears of abandonment or that help will not be available if needed. It also enhances trust and provides opportunity for expression of fears or concerns.*
- Assess level of understanding about disease and condition. *This allows misperceptions that may contribute to anxiety to be corrected.*

- Encourage supportive family and friends to remain with the client as much as possible. *This provides a supportive environment for the client and also distracts from physical concerns.*
- Assist the client to identify and use appropriate coping mechanisms. *Coping mechanisms provide immediate relief of anxiety while the client adapts to the situation.*
- Involve the client and family (as appropriate) in care decisions. *This increases the client's sense of control over the situation.*

Community-Based Care

The client with diverticular disease is responsible for self-care. Discuss the following topics for home care:

- Prescribed high-fiber diet and the need to maintain the diet for life to reduce the incidence of complications, including ways to increase dietary fiber
- Complications of diverticular disease and its manifestations. Provide a referral to a dietitian for teaching as indicated.

Prior to discharge of the client with acute diverticulitis, discuss the following:

- Food and fluid limitations, including recommendations for a low-residue diet during the initial period of healing
- Colostomy management (if a temporary colostomy has been created), including where to obtain supplies and dietary management
- Planned procedure to reanastomose the colon and revise the colostomy. Refer to community healthcare agencies as indicated.

ANORECTAL DISORDERS

Anorectal lesions include hemorrhoids, a normal condition common to all adults that may become enlarged and painful; anal fissure; anorectal abscess; anorectal fistulas; and pilonidal disease.

THE CLIENT WITH HEMORRHOIDS

The anus and anal canal contain two superficial venous plexuses with the hemorrhoidal veins. When pressure on these veins is increased or venous return impeded, they can develop *varices,* or varicosities, becoming weak and distended. This condition is commonly known as **hemorrhoids**, or "piles." When asymptomatic, hemorrhoids are considered to be a normal condition found in all adults.

Pathophysiology and Manifestations

Hemorrhoids develop when venous return from the anal canal is impaired. Straining to defecate increases venous pressure and is the most common cause of distended hemorrhoids. Pregnancy increases intra-abdominal pressure, raising venous pressure, and is another cause of hemorrhoids. Other factors that may contribute to symptomatic hemorrhoids include prolonged sitting, obesity, chronic constipation, and a low-fiber diet.

Hemorrhoids are classed as either internal or external. *Internal* hemorrhoids affect the venous plexus above the mucocutaneous junction of the anus (Figure 26–15 ■). Internal hemorrhoids rarely cause pain, usually presenting with bleeding. Bleeding from internal hemorrhoids is bright red and unmixed with the stool. It can vary in quantity from streaks on toilet tissue to enough to color the water in the toilet. Recurrent bleeding of internal hemorrhoids may be sufficient to cause anemia. Mucous discharge and a feeling of incomplete evacuation of stool also may be manifestations of internal hemorrhoids.

External hemorrhoids affect the inferior hemorrhoidal plexus below the mucocutaneous junction. Bleeding is rare with external hemorrhoids. Anal irritation, a feeling of pressure, and difficulty cleaning the anal region may be manifestations of external hemorrhoids.

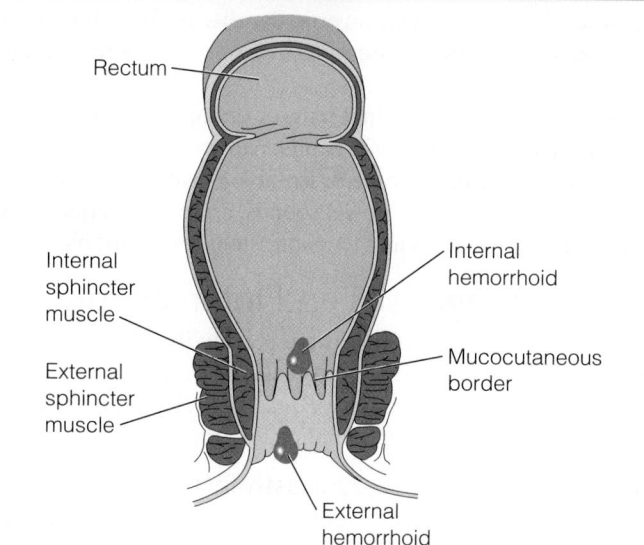

Figure 26–15 ■ The location of internal and external hemorrhoids.

As they enlarge, hemorrhoids may prolapse or protrude through the anus. Initially, prolapse occurs only with defecation and the hemorrhoids spontaneously regress back into the anal canal. Eventually, the client may need to manually replace internal hemorrhoids after defecation, or they may become permanently prolapsed, in which case replacement is not possible. Manifestations of permanently prolapsed hemorrhoids include mucous discharge and clothing soilage.

"Normal" hemorrhoids are not painful. Prolapsed hemorrhoids may become strangulated as a result of congestion and edema, leading to thrombosis. Hemorrhoidal thrombosis causes extreme pain and may lead to infarction of skin and mucosa overlying the hemorrhoid. Internal hemorrhoids associated with portal hypertension in liver disease may bleed profusely if ruptured. (See Chapter 24 ∞ for further discussion of portal hypertension.)

A *thrombosed external hemorrhoid* is a thrombosis of the subcutaneous external hemorrhoidal veins of the anal canal, rather than a true hemorrhoid. It appears as a painful bluish hematoma beneath the skin and typically occurs following a sudden increase in venous pressure, for example, heavy lifting, coughing, or straining. Pain is significant at onset but gradually subsides. Spontaneous rupture with bleeding may occur. Thrombosed external hemorrhoids resolve without intervention.

INTERDISCIPLINARY CARE

Because hemorrhoids are a normal condition, management is conservative unless complications such as permanent prolapse or thrombosis occur.

Diagnosis

Hemorrhoids are diagnosed by the client's history and by examination of the anorectal area. External hemorrhoids can be seen on visual inspection, especially if thrombosed. The client is asked to strain (Valsalva's maneuver) during the examination to detect prolapse. Internal hemorrhoids are usually not palpable or tender on digital examination of the rectum. Anoscopic examination is used to detect and evaluate internal hemorrhoids. For this exam, a speculum or endoscope is introduced into the anus to provide visual inspection of the tissues. Additional diagnostic examinations include testing of stool for occult blood and sigmoidoscopy, performed to rule out cancer of the colon or rectum, which may aggravate hemorrhoidal manifestations or produce similar manifestations. If liver disease with portal hypertension is suspected, liver function studies are ordered.

Medications

Bulk-forming laxatives such as psyllium seed (Metamucil) or stool softeners such as docusate sodium (Colace) may be prescribed to improve constipation and reduce straining as well. Suppositories and local ointments such as Preparation H or Nupercaine have an anesthetic and astringent effect, reducing discomfort and irritation of surrounding tissues. They have little or no effect on the hemorrhoid itself. Warm sitz baths, bed rest, and local astringent compresses may be recommended to reduce the swelling of edematous prolapsed hemorrhoids after digital reduction.

Nutrition

Hemorrhoids that are not permanently prolapsed or acutely thrombosed generally are treated conservatively. A high-fiber diet and increased water intake to increase stool bulk, improve its softness, and reduce straining is effective for most clients with internal or external hemorrhoids.

Sclerotherapy

Hemorrhoids that are permanently prolapsed, are thrombosed, or produce significant manifestations may be treated more aggressively. *Sclerotherapy* involves injecting a chemical irritant into tissues surrounding the hemorrhoid to induce inflammation and eventual fibrosis and scarring. It is used to treat recurrent bleeding and early prolapse of internal hemorrhoids. The treatment produces minimal pain. Enlarged or prolapsing hemorrhoids also may be treated with rubber band ligation. A rubber band is placed snugly around the hemorrhoidal plexus and sur-

rounding mucosa, causing the tissue to necrose and slough within 7 to 10 days. Treatment is limited to one hemorrhoidal complex at a time, so repeat treatments may be necessary. Pain should be minimal if the band is placed appropriately; persistent pain following band ligation may signal an infection. Bleeding can occur as the hemorrhoid sloughs. Other procedures used to treat hemorrhoids include cryosurgery, in which hemorrhoids are necrosed by freezing with a cryoprobe; infrared photocoagulation; or electrocoagulation.

Hemorrhoidectomy

Clients with chronic manifestations, permanent prolapse, chronic bleeding and anemia, or painful thrombosed hemorrhoids may be treated surgically with a *hemorrhoidectomy*. In this procedure, hemorrhoids are surgically excised, leaving normal skin and surrounding tissues. This procedure may use conventional techniques or a laser to remove both internal and external hemorrhoids. Few complications are associated with hemorrhoidectomy.

NURSING CARE

Primary prevention of symptomatic hemorrhoids involves education of clients of all ages. Stress the importance of maintaining an adequate intake of dietary fiber, a liberal fluid intake, and regular exercise to maintain stool bulk, softness, and regularity. Discuss the need to respond to the urge to defecate rather than postponing defecation. Teach appropriate constipation management, including the use of bulk-forming laxatives.

Most clients with hemorrhoids are treated in community settings where the primary nursing focus is educational. Discuss the appropriate use of over-the-counter preparations and sitz baths for the relief of minor hemorrhoidal manifestations. If necessary, teach clients how to reduce prolapsed hemorrhoids digitally.

Teach manifestations of possible hemorrhoidal complications, such as chronic bleeding, prolapse, and thrombosis. Stress the need to seek medical evaluation if manifestations persist. Discuss the link between manifestations of hemorrhoids and colorectal cancer, and urge the client to seek medical intervention for persistent, unresolved, or progressive manifestations.

When a hemorrhoidectomy is performed, the client requires more direct nursing intervention. Postoperative care of the client with perianal surgery is outlined in Box 26–3. Anal packing may be in place for the first 24 hours following the procedure. When removed, observe the client closely for bleeding. Pain is a common postoperative problem. Although the operative procedure is minor, postoperative discomfort can be significant because the anal region is richly innervated and muscle spasms may occur. In addition to systemic analgesics, sitz baths usually are ordered. These not only help promote relaxation and reduce discomfort but also clean the anal area. Use of a rubber ring or donut device minimizes pressure on the surgical site while the client sits in the bath.

The client may remain hospitalized until after the first postoperative bowel movement. Stool softeners, adequate fluids,

---

BOX 26–3 Perianal Postoperative Care

Assessment

- Monitor vital signs every 4 hours for 24 hours.
- Inspect rectal dressing every 2 to 3 hours for 24 hours.
- Monitor urinary output.

Pain Control

- Assist to position of comfort, usually side-lying.
- Provide analgesics as prescribed.
- Keep fresh ice packs over the rectal dressing as ordered.
- Assist with sitz bath three to four times per day.
- Provide a flotation pad for use when sitting.

Elimination

- Give stool softeners as prescribed.
- Give an analgesic before the first postoperative bowel movement if possible.
- When tolerated, encourage fluid intake of at least 2000 mL per day.

Client and Family Teaching

- Take sitz bath after each bowel movement for 1 to 2 weeks after surgery.
- Drink at least 2 quarts of fluid per day.
- Eat adequate dietary fiber, and exercise moderately.
- Take stool softeners as prescribed.
- Report to the physician the following symptoms: rectal bleeding, continued pain on defecation, fever greater than 101°F (38.3°C), purulent rectal drainage.

---

and analgesia before defecation can reduce anxiety and discomfort. Adequate cleaning following defecation, usually with a sitz bath, is vital.

Whether caring for a client with hemorrhoids or a hemorrhoidectomy, consider the following nursing diagnoses:

- Acute or Chronic *Pain* related to inflamed anal tissues
- *Constipation* related to dietary habits and/or delay of defecation
- *Risk for Infection* related to disruption of anal tissue.

THE CLIENT WITH AN ANORECTAL LESION

Unlike the rectum, which is relatively insensitive to pain, the anal canal is richly supplied with sensory nerves and highly sensitive to painful stimuli. Lesions of the anorectal area may cause significant pain, particularly with defecation. Infection is a potential complication of anorectal lesions because of contamination by fecal bacteria. The superior boundary of the anal canal (the anorectal juncture or pectinate line) contains 8 to 12 anal crypts where anorectal abscesses or fistulas can form. Lesions of the anorectal area include fissures, abscesses, fistulas, and pilonidal disease.

Anal Fissure

Anal fissures or ulcers occur when the epithelium of the anal canal over the internal sphincter becomes denuded or abraded. Irritating diarrheal stools and tightening of the anal canal with increased sphincter tension are frequent causes of anal fissures. Other factors that may contribute to their development include childbirth trauma, habitual cathartic use, laceration by a foreign body, and anal intercourse. Chronic inflammation and infection of surrounding tissues accompanies an anal fissure.

Clients with anal fissures typically have periods of exacerbation and remission. Because they occur below the mucocutaneous line, anal fissures are painful. The pain occurs with defecation and may be described as tearing, burning, or cutting. Bright red bleeding is noted with a bowel movement. Bleeding is typically minor and noted on toilet tissue. Because of fear of defecation, the client may develop constipation, which further disrupts normal bowel habits and aggravates manifestations.

The diagnosis of anal fissure is made on gentle digital examination of the anal canal and anoscopy using a small anoscope. Treatment is usually conservative, involving dietary changes to increase fiber intake and stool bulk, increased fluid intake, and use of bulk-forming laxatives. A topical agent such as hydrocortisone cream may be prescribed. Surgical intervention with an internal sphincterotomy, an incision into the internal sphincter to increase its diameter, is considered when the fissure does not heal with medical intervention.

Anorectal Abscess

Invasion of the pararectal spaces by pathogenic bacteria can lead to an *anorectal abscess*. Commonly caused by infection that extends from the anal crypt into a pararectal space, the abscess may appear small but often contains a large amount of pus. Multiple pathogens may be present, including *Escherichia coli, Proteus,* streptococci, and staphylococci. Other factors that may contribute to the development of an anorectal abscess include infection of a hair follicle, sebaceous gland, or sweat gland, and abrasions, fissures, or anal trauma. The incidence of anorectal abscess is higher in men.

Pain is the primary manifestation of an anorectal abscess. Sitting or walking may aggravate the pain, but it is unrelated to defecation. External swelling, redness, heat, and tenderness are apparent on examination. With a deeper abscess, swelling may not be visible, but the abscess is palpable on digital examination.

If the abscess either does not drain spontaneously or is not drained surgically, adjacent anatomic spaces will be affected. Systemic sepsis is also a potential complication.

Incision and drainage is the treatment of choice for an anorectal abscess because it rarely resolves with antibiotic therapy alone. This treatment often leads to a persistent fistula, which is surgically closed after the infection has cleared.

Anorectal Fistula

A fistula is a tunnel or tubelike tract with openings at each end. *Anorectal fistulas* have one opening in the anal canal with the other usually found in perianal skin. Most occur spontaneously or as a result of anorectal abscess drainage. Crohn's disease is also a predisposing factor to fistula development.

The primary manifestation of an anorectal fistula is intermittent or constant drainage or discharge, which may be purulent. This may be accompanied by local itching, tenderness, and pain associated with defecation.

Digital and anoscopic examination with gentle probing of the fistula tract are used to establish the diagnosis. Although some fistulas may heal spontaneously, the treatment of choice is a fistulotomy. The primary opening of the fistula is removed, and the tract is opened to allow it to heal by secondary intention, from the inside outward. If the sphincter is involved, a two-stage operation may be done to preserve the muscle and prevent fecal incontinence.

Pilonidal Disease

The client with *pilonidal disease* has an acute abscess or chronic draining sinus in the sacrococcygeal area. Underlying the abscess or sinus is a cyst with granulation tissue, fibrosis, and, often, hair tufts. This disease usually affects young hirsute (hairy) males and is probably due to hair entrapment in deep tissues of the sacrococcygeal area. Some researchers, however, believe that it is a congenital disorder.

The lesion of pilonidal disease is generally asymptomatic unless it becomes acutely infected. Manifestations of acute inflammation accompany infection, including pain, tenderness, redness, heat, and swelling of the affected area. Purulent discharge may be noted from one or more sinuses or openings in the midline.

The preferred treatment option for pilonidal disease is incision and drainage. The sinus tract and underlying cyst are excised and closed by either primary- or secondary-intention healing. The client may be instructed to remove hair from the area routinely by shaving or using a depilatory to prevent further hair entrapment and recurrence of the problem.

NURSING CARE

Clients with anorectal disorders are often treated in the community, and the primary nursing responsibility is education. Teach the importance of maintaining a high-fiber diet and liberal fluid intake to increase stool bulk and softness and thereby decrease discomfort with defecation. Stress the importance of responding to the urge to defecate to prevent constipation.

Following surgical treatment of any of these disorders, teach the client to keep the perianal region clean and dry. If a dressing is in place, instruct to avoid soiling it with urine or feces during elimination. Following removal of the dressing, teach to clean the area gently with soap and water following a bowel movement. Discuss the use of sitz baths for cleaning and comfort. Suggest taking an analgesic if necessary prior to defecation, but caution that some analgesics may promote constipation. Teach signs and manifestations of infection or other possible complications to report to the physician. If an antibiotic has been prescribed, provide written and verbal instructions about its use, its desired and possible adverse effects, and their management.

EXPLORE MediaLink

Prentice Hall Nursing MediaLink DVD-ROM
  Audio Glossary
  NCLEX-RN® Review

COMPANION WEBSITE www.prenhall.com/lemone
  Audio Glossary
  NCLEX-RN® Review
  Care Plan Activity: Irritable Bowel Syndrome
  Case Studies
    Enteral Tube Complications
    Irritable Bowel Syndrome
  Teaching Plan: Colon Cancer
  MediaLink Applications
    Crohn's Disease and Ulcerative Colitis
    Crohn's Disease Teaching Sheet

CHAPTER HIGHLIGHTS

- Disorders of intestinal motility include diarrhea, constipation, irritable bowel syndrome, and fecal incontinence. Diarrhea is a manifestation of many other bowel disorders, including lactose intolerance, infections with bacteria, and inflammatory diseases of the bowel. Constipation may be a primary problem (especially for the older adult) or a manifestation of another disorder. Irritable bowel syndrome (IBS) is a functional disorder without any identifiable organic cause. Fecal incontinence is usually considered to be the manifestation of a disorder rather than a disorder itself.
- Appendicitis is an acute inflammation of the vermiform appendix, manifested by abdominal pain that localizes in the right lower

quadrant of the abdomen. On palpation, localized and rebound tenderness is present at McBurney's point. It is treated most often with an appendectomy.
- Peritonitis (inflammation of the peritoneum from infection or chemical irritant) is a serious complication of a wide variety of acute abdominal disorders, including perforated ulcer, ruptured appendix, abdominal trauma or surgery, or necrotic bowel. Complications may be life threatening; without prompt and effective treatment, septicemia and septic shock may occur.
- Gastroenteritis, which may result from bacterial or viral infections, parasites, or toxins, is often the result of consuming contaminated

water or food. Manifestations include nausea and vomiting, diarrhea, and abdominal discomfort.

■ Nurses provide education to help prevent protozoal infections (such as giardiasis, amebiasis, and coccidiosis) and helminthic infestations (by roundworms, flukes, or tapeworms). Both types of bowel disorders are treated with medications.

■ Chronic inflammatory bowel disease (IBD) includes two separate but closely related conditions: ulcerative colitis and Crohn's disease. Ulcerative colitis affects the mucosa and submucosa of the colon and rectum. Crohn's disease can affect any part of the GI tract, but usually involves the terminal ilium and ascending colon. Diarrhea is common to both disorders. A colectomy (removal of the large colon) may be performed to treat ulcerative colitis; an ileostomy (artificial opening from the abdomen to the ileum) may be performed to treat Crohn's disease.

■ Malabsorption syndromes, in which the intestinal mucosa ineffectively absorbs nutrients, may be caused by a wide variety of diseases. However, three common malabsorption disorders in adults are sprue (a primary disorder of the small intestine, there are two types: celiac and tropical), lactose intolerance of milk and milk products (resulting from a lactase deficiency), and short bowel syndrome (a condition that can develop following resection of the small bowel).

■ Malignant tumors of the lower bowel are the second leading cause of death from cancer. The risk of colon cancer may be reduced through health-related screenings and a diet high in fruits, vegetables, folic acid, and calcium. Rectal bleeding is the most common initial manifestation but may not occur until the cancer is well advanced. Surgical treatment is through surgical resection of the bowel, accompanied by a colostomy for diversion of fecal contents.

■ A hernia is a defect in the abdominal wall that allows intra-abdominal contents to protrude out of the abdominal cavity. Hernias may follow trauma, surgery, and increased intra-abdominal pressure (as from pregnancy or obesity). Hernias may be congenital or acquired, and may be inguinal, umbilical, incisional, or ventral.

■ Intestinal obstructions occur when intestinal contents cannot move through the lumen of the bowel. They may occur in either the large or small intestine, may be partial or complete, and are caused by many factors, ranging from surgical ileus following abdominal surgery to adhesions or tumors.

■ Diverticula are saclike projections of mucosa through the muscular layer of the colon. When these sacs become inflamed, the condition is labeled diverticulitis. A diet high in fiber is recommended for self-care.

■ Anorectal disorders include hemorrhoids, anorectal lesions (fissures, abscess, and fistula), and pilonidal disease. These disorders are painful and pose a risk for bleeding and infection.

TEST YOURSELF NCLEX-RN® REVIEW

1 A client presents at the urgent care clinic with complaints of diarrhea for the past week. The nurse should first:
1. advise the client to abstain from all food intake until the diarrhea subsides.
2. ask the client to describe the number and character of daily stools.
3. question the client about possible exposure to an enterotoxin or protozoal infection.
4. recommend an over-the-counter antidiarrheal preparation such as Pepto-Bismol.

2 The nurse caring for a client admitted with possible appendicitis appropriately plans which of the following?
1. Initiate bowel preparation for a barium enema.
2. Restrict intake to clear liquids.
3. Prepare for possible immediate appendectomy.
4. Insert saline lock for intravenous antibiotic therapy.

3 When teaching a client with inflammatory bowel disease about prescribed sulfasalazine, the nurse instructs the client to:
1. use a sunscreen while taking the drug.
2. take the drug on an empty stomach.
3. limit fluid intake to 1500 mL per day or less.
4. take vitamin C while on this drug.

4 A client reports frequent large, fatty, foul-smelling stools. The nurse recognizes this as:
1. hematochezia, a manifestation of GI bleeding.
2. characteristic of inflammatory bowel disease.
3. a common early manifestation of colorectal cancer.
4. steatorrhea, a manifestation of malabsorption.

5 A client tells the nurse that both his father and grandfather died of colon cancer, and he is worried that he is going to die from "the same horrible disease." Which of the following does the nurse include in her recommendations?
1. There is no genetic link seen in colon cancer, so his risk is equal to that of people with no family history of the disease.
2. He should plan for annual digital rectal exams and periodic colonoscopy for early identification of possible tumors.
3. He should have annual CEA levels drawn to screen for early tumor development.
4. It is imperative that he change his diet immediately, significantly increasing his intake of dietary fiber.

6 A client has a nasogastric tube in place to maintain gastric decompression. Which nursing actions are important in monitoring responses to *Deficient Fluid Volume* when caring for this client? (Select all that apply.)
1. Low suction is used to decompress the stomach.
2. Give the client as much water as he or she wants to drink.
3. Listen to bowel sounds prior to checking the placement of the NG tube.
4. Document the amount and color of NG tube drainage every shift.
5. Keep an accurate record of intake and output every 2 to 4 hours.
6. Listen to bowel sounds after palpating the stomach for tenderness.
7. Measure abdominal girth every 4 to 8 hours.

7 A client has developed a paralytic ileus following a recent abdominal surgery. What is the most important nursing consideration when caring for this client?
  1. Ensure that the client is able to eat a clear liquid diet.
  2. Maintain the client on strict bedrest.
  3. Monitor bowel sounds every hour.
  4. Ensure nasogastric tube is functioning.

8 Mrs. Jones has a history of diverticulosis and has been having abdominal pain recently. When educating Mrs. Jones about her diet prior to discharge from the hospital, what type of foods should be excluded from Mrs. Jones diet?
  1. whole-wheat bread
  2. popcorn
  3. soup
  4. apples

9 Your 85-year-old client Mr. Allen was admitted with a diagnosis of constipation. Which of the following is important in your discharge education for this client? (Select all that apply.)
  1. Eat plenty of fresh fruits and vegetables daily.
  2. Take a bisacodyl (Dulcolax) daily.
  3. Drink 6 to 8 glasses of nonalcoholic fluid daily.
  4. Take docusate (Colace) at nighttime only.
  5. Eat whole-wheat bread instead of white bread.
  6. Eat a bran cereal for breakfast.

10 A small-bowel obstruction can occur due to:
  1. eating extra fiber in the diet.
  2. abdominal adhesions.
  3. drinking too much water.
  4. a nasogastric tube.

See Test Yourself answers in Appendix C.

BIBLIOGRAPHY

American Cancer Society. (2005a). Can colorectal cancer be prevented? Retrieved from http://www.cancer.org/docroot/CRI/content/CRI_2_4_2X_Can_colon_and_rectum_cancer_be_prevented . . .

_____. (2005b). *Cancer facts & figures 2005.* Atlanta: Author.

_____. (2005c). What are the risk factors for colorectal cancer? Retrieved from http://www.cancer.org/docroot/CRI/content/CRI_2_4_2X_What_are_the_risk_factors_for_colon_and_rec . . .

Balch, J. F., & Stengler, M. (2004). *Prescription for natural cures: A self-care guide for treating health problems with natural remedies including diet and nutrition, nutritional supplements, bodywork, and more.* Hoboken, NJ: Wiley & Sons.

Bliss, D., Fischer, L., & Savik, K. (2005). Managing fecal incontinence: Self-care practices of older adults. *Journal of Gerontological Nursing, 31*(7), 35–44.

Centers for Disease Control and Prevention. (2004). *Escherichia coli O157:H7.* Retrieved from http://www.cdc.gov/ncidod/dbmd/diseaseinfo/escherichiacoli_g.htm

Corbett, J. V. (2004). *Laboratory tests and diagnostic procedures with nursing diagnosis* (6th ed.). Upper Saddle River, NJ: Prentice Hall.

Crohn's & Colitis Foundation of America. (2005). *About Crohn's disease.* Retrieved from http://www.ccfa.org/info/about/crohns

Dochterman, J., & Bulechek, G. (2004). *Nursing interventions classification (NIC)* (4th ed.). St. Louis, MO: Mosby.

Eberhardie, C. (2003). Constipation: Identifying the problem. *Nursing Older People, 15*(9), 22–26.

Ehrenpreis, E. D. (2005). Irritable bowel syndrome: 10% to 20% of older adults have symptoms consistent with diagnosis. *Geriatrics, 60*(1), 25–28.

Farrekkm, H., & Friedman, L. (2005). The management of lower gastrointestinal bleeding. *Alimentary Pharmacology & Therapeutics, 21*(11), 1281–1298.

Halverson, A. L. (2005). Nonoperative management of fecal incontinence. *Clinics in Colon and Rectal Surgery, 16*(1), 17–20.

Heitkemper, M., & Jarrett, M. (2005). Overlapping conditions in women with irritable bowel syndrome. *Urologic Nursing, 25*(1), 25–31.

Hellekson, K. (2005). ACG releases updated practice guidelines for ulcerative colitis in adults. *American Family Physician, 71*(3), 604–606.

Heuschkel, R., Afzal, N., Wuerth, A., Zurakowski, D., Leichtner, A., Kemper, K., et al. (2002). Complementary medicine use in children and young adults with inflammatory bowel disease. *American Journal of Gastroenterology, 97*(2), 382–388.

Hungin, A. P. S., Chang, L., Locke, G. R., Dennis, E. H., & Barghout, V. (2005). Irritable bowel syndrome in the United States: Prevalence, symptom patterns and impact. *Alimentary Pharmacologic Therapy, 21,* 1365–1375.

Kee, J. (2004). *Handbook of laboratory and diagnostic tests with nursing implications* (5th ed.). Upper Saddle River, NJ: Prentice Hall.

Kupecz, D., & Beradinelli, C. (2003). New therapy for women with irritable bowel syndrome. *Nurse Practitioner, 28*(4), 48–50.

Langmead, L., Dawson, C., Hawkins, C., Banna, N., Loo, S., & Rampton, D. S. (2002). Antioxidant effects of herbal therapies used by clients with inflammatory bowel disease: An *in vitro* study. *Alimentary Pharmacologic Therapy, 16*(2), 197–205.

MedicineNet.com. (2005). *Colon cancer prevention information.* Retrieved from http://www.MedicineNet.com/colon_cancer_prevention/page3.htm

Moorhead, S., Johnson, M., & Maas, M. (2004). *Nursing outcomes classification (NOC)* (3rd ed.). St. Louis, MO: Mosby.

NANDA International. (2005). *Nursing diagnoses: Definitions & classification 2005–2006.* Philadelphia: Author.

Peate, I., (2003). Nursing role in the management of constipation: Use of laxatives. *British Journal of Nursing, 12*(19), 1130–1136.

Porth, C. M. (2005). *Pathophysiology: Concepts of altered health states* (7th ed.). Philadelphia: Lippincott.

Pountney, D. (2005). In control of incontinence. *Gastrointestinal Nursing, 3*(4), 14–15.

Roberson, C. M. (2004). Lactose intolerance. *Alabama Nurse, 31*(4), 23–24.

Sanko, J. (2004). Aspiration assessment and prevention in critically ill enterally fed clients: Evidence-based recommendations for practice. *Gastroenterology Nursing, 27*(6), 279–285.

Stein, P. (2004). Ulcerative colitis—diagnosis and surgical treatment. *AORN Journal, 80*(2), 242–253, 255–256, 258.

Tierney, L., McPhee, S., & Papadakis, M. (Eds.). (2005). *Current medical diagnosis & treatment* (44th ed.). Stamford, CT: Appleton & Lange.

Verhoef, M. J., Rapchuk, I., Liew, T., Weir, V., & Hilsden, R. J. (2002). Complementary practitioners' views of treatment for inflammatory bowel disease. *Canadian Journal of Gastroenterology, 16*(2), 95–100.

Welch, J., & Cohen, J. (2004). *Section 5 Chapter 12 Diverticulitis.* Retrieved from http://www.acssurgery.com/acsonline/chapters/ch0512.htm

Wilkinson, J. (2005). *Prentice Hall nursing diagnosis handbook with NIC interventions and NOC outcomes* (8th ed.). Upper Saddle River, NJ: Prentice Hall.

Wilson, B., Shannon, M., & Stang, C. (2005). *Prentice Hall nurse's drug guide 2005.* Upper Saddle River, NJ: Prentice Hall.

Yarbo, C., Frogge, M., & Goodman, M. (2005). *Cancer nursing: Principles and practice* (6th ed.). Sudbury, MA: Jones & Bartlett.

Yates, J., (2005). Traveler's diarrhea. *American Family Physician, 71*(11), 2095–2100.

FUNCTIONAL HEALTH PATTERN: Elimination

■ **Think about clients with altered bowel elimination for whom you have cared in your clinical experiences.**

■ What were the clients' major medical diagnoses (e.g., irritable bowel syndrome, appendicitis, peritonitis, gastroenteritis, inflammatory bowel disorder, sprue, short bowel syndrome, polyps, colorectal cancer, hernia, intestinal obstruction, diverticular disease, or hemorrhoids)?

■ What manifestations did each of these clients have? Were these manifestations similar or different?

■ How did the clients' bowel elimination problems interfere with their elimination pattern? How often did they have a bowel movement? Had the bowel routine changed recently? If so, how? Could they describe the color and consistency of the stool? Were their bowel movements loose or did they strain excessively to have a bowel movement? Did they use laxatives? If so, how often and what type? Did they notice any bleeding with the bowel movement or on the paper after wiping? Could they describe the type of cramping or abdominal pain they were experiencing? Did they use any medications that affect bowel movements? Did they have any illnesses or surgery that affects bowel movements? Did they have any food intolerances or were they on a special diet? Had they had a colonoscopy or other diagnostic tests of the rectum or colon? Do they have any ostomy? How often did they empty the ostomy bag? How often do they irrigate the ostomy?

■ **The Elimination Pattern includes patterns of elimination, changes in elimination characteristics, use of laxatives or bowel routines, and use of an ostomy for bowel elimination. Bowel function can be affected by inflammation, infection, tumors, obstructions, or changes in structure. Bowel disorders affect elimination status in two primary ways:**

■ Direct factors that affect the consistency of stools are food and fluid intake (e.g., constipation or diarrhea), food poisoning or bacterial infections (e.g., diarrhea), surgical procedures (e.g., diarrhea or constipation), medical conditions such as spinal cord injury (e.g., constipation), medication intake such as narcotics (e.g., constipation), or herbal preparations (e.g., diarrhea).

■ Indirect factors that affect the consistency of stools are psychologic stress (e.g., diarrhea), depression (e.g., constipation), voluntary postponement of defecation (e.g., constipation), or decreased exercise activity (e.g., constipation).

■ **Bowel elimination is the end process of digestion. Nutrients are absorbed during digestion and indigestible materials are eliminated from the body through the gastrointestinal tract. Bowel elimination disorders interrupt normal patterns of bowel elimination, leading to manifestations such as:**

■ Diarrhea (mucosal inflammation ▶ causes plasma, serum protein, blood and mucus to increase fluidity and bulk of stool ▶ resulting in increased rate of propulsion of loose, watery stool)

■ Constipation (decreased motility, denial of urge to defecate, or decreased fluid intake ▶ causes hard, dry stool ▶ resulting in difficulty passing stool)

■ Flatus (excessive amount of air or gas in the intestines ▶ causes distention of the intestines with mild to moderate pain ▶ resulting in rectal passage of excessive air or gas).

■ **Priority nursing diagnoses within the Elimination Pattern that may be appropriate for clients with bowel disorders include:**

■ *Bowel Incontinence* as evidenced by urgency, inability to delay defecation, or fecal staining of clothing

■ *Diarrhea* as evidenced by abdominal cramping, hyperactive bowel sounds, or at least three loose and liquid stools per day

■ *Constipation* as evidenced by hard stool, distended abdomen, or flatus.

■ **Two nursing diagnoses from other functional health patterns often are of high priority for clients with bowel elimination disorders because of the physiologic responses to these disorders:**

■ *Acute Pain* (Cognitive-Perceptual)

■ *Imbalanced Nutrition: Less than Body Requirements* (Nutritional-Metabolic)

CLINICAL SCENARIO

You have been assigned to work with the following four clients for the 0700 shift on a medical-surgical unit. Significant data obtained during report are as follows:

■ Jason Phillips is a 23-year-old who was admitted 1 hour ago with right lower quadrant pain. On admission to the medical-surgical unit his vital signs were T 100°F, P 98, R 22 and shallow, BP 130/84. He complains of nausea and pain of 8 on a scale of 1 to 10. He calls the nurse's station stating his pain has stopped and he wants to be discharged.

■ Mary Joslin, age 56 years, has been hospitalized for 2 days for treatment with antibiotics for pneumonia. Her last vital signs were T 99°F, P 88, R 16, BP 120/82. She suddenly develops severe diarrhea and abdominal cramping.

■ Grace Freeman is a 36-year-old who had a temporary colostomy placed 5 days ago due to an abdominal injury from a motor vehicle crash. Vital signs at 0400 were T 98.6°F, P 78, R 14, BP 112/78. She put on her call light for assistance because her colostomy bag is full and she needs help emptying it.

■ Paul Bruner, age 86 years, was admitted the previous evening with sharp lower abdominal pain. During the admission assessment, a mass was palpated in his abdomen. His vital signs on admission were T 100.4°F, P 88, R 26, BP 150/86. He is to be prepped for surgery this morning.

Questions

1 In what order would you visit these clients after report?

1. _____
2. _____
3. _____
4. _____

2 What top two priority nursing diagnoses would you choose for each of the clients presented above? Can you explain, if asked, the rationale for your choices?

	Priority Nursing Diagnosis #1	Priority Nursing Diagnosis #2
Jason Phillips		
Mary Joslin		
Grace Freeman		
Paul Bruner		

3 Which is an appropriate nursing intervention for the client with suspected appendicitis?

1. Administer an enema to cleanse the bowel for surgery.
2. Apply heat to the abdomen to reduce pain.
3. Administer narcotics while diagnostic tests are being conducted.
4. Assess the abdomen frequently for distention and bowel sounds.

4 Mrs. Joslin asks the nurse why she has suddenly developed diarrhea. Which response by the nurse is accurate?

1. "Diarrhea is an adverse effect from taking antibiotics because the antibiotics decrease the normal bacterial count in the intestines."
2. "Antibiotics lower your resistance to fighting off infections while you are hospitalized."
3. "You must have been exposed to someone with diarrhea during your hospital stay."
4. "Have any of your visitors developed diarrhea or any other illnesses after visiting you?"

5 Which discharge instructions will the nurse teach Mrs. Freeman regarding how to take care of the colostomy?

1. "The types of foods you eat will not affect the colostomy output."
2. "Empty the colostomy pouch or replace the bag when it is half full."
3. "Irrigate the colostomy with water to stimulate the colon to empty."
4. "Cleanse the area around the stoma with deodorant soap to decrease odor."

6 Which is the most common initial manifestation of malignant tumors of the lower bowel?

1. rectal bleeding
2. diarrhea
3. rectal pain
4. constipation

7 Teaching appropriate constipation management includes which actions? (Select all that apply.)

1. Decrease dietary fiber.
2. Increase fluid intake.
3. Increase exercise activity.
4. Use bulk-forming laxatives.
5. Use enemas daily.

8 Clients with celiac disease are placed on a gluten-free diet. The client understands dietary instructions when choosing which meal?

1. corned beef sandwich on rye bread
2. tossed green salad with oatmeal raisin cookie
3. eggs and bacon with whole wheat toast
4. tomato soup with cornbread

9 Clients with severe diarrhea may develop metabolic acidosis. Which arterial blood gases indicate metabolic acidosis?

1. pH 7.45, Paco$_2$ 40 mmHg, bicarbonate 25 mEq/L
2. pH 7.28, Paco$_2$ 30 mmHg, bicarbonate 19 mEq/L
3. pH 7.55, Paco$_2$ 50 mmHg, bicarbonate 30 mEq/L
4. pH 7.33, Paco$_2$ 36 mmHg, bicarbonate 24 mEq/L

10 To prepare a client for a colonoscopy, the nurse teaches the client to implement which interventions?

1. Maintain a liquid diet for 4 days prior to the procedure.
2. Remain NPO for 4 hours prior to the procedure.
3. Take prescribed bowel preparation the evening before the procedure.
4. Administer a cleansing enema the evening before the procedure.

11 When assessing a client with a large bowel obstruction, which manifestations are typically noted on assessment?

1. tachycardia and diarrhea
2. colicky abdominal pain and constipation
3. severe abdominal cramping and vomiting
4. dull bowel sounds and nausea

12 Antidiarrheal medications, such as kaolin and pectin (Kaopectate), may interfere with the absorption of other medications. What is the best way to administer Kaopectate?

1. at bedtime after other medications are administered
2. at mealtimes to prevent stomach upset with other medications
3. one hour before and 2 hours after taking other medications
4. before lunch so as not to interfere with medications taken at breakfast

CASE STUDY

Janet Simpson is a 45-year-old married white female who came to the emergency department with complaints of abdominal cramping, pain, and frequent bloody diarrhea-type stools. Vital signs on admission are T 98°F, P 72, R 20, BP 104/72. Her skin is cool and pale. On the admission assessment it is noted that she has several reddened lesions on her lower legs. Her weight is 115 pounds. Blood is drawn for a CBC, serum protein, folic acid and serum vitamin levels, and liver function tests. Abnormal laboratory results are hemoglobin, 7.3; hematocrit, 23.3; and a serum protein of 4.6. A colonoscopy was performed, with findings of edema, inflammation, pus, abscesses, and bleeding.

Based on the assessment and laboratory studies, the diagnosis of ulcerative colitis is determined. The pathophysiology of ulcerative colitis begins at the rectosigmoid section of the anal canal and progresses proximally. The initial lesions are at the base of the crypts of Lieberkühn. Microscopic hemorrhages occur in the mucosa and abscesses form in the crypts. The abscesses lead to necrosis and sloughing of bowel mucosa. Further tissue damage is caused by inflammatory exudates and the release of prostaglandins and other cytokines. The mucosa is red and edematous due to vascular congestion, friable (easily damaged), and ulcerated. It bleeds easily. Chronic inflammation leads to atrophy, narrowing, and shortening of the colon. Manifestations of ulcerative colitis are diarrhea, stool with blood and mucus, fecal urgency, tenesmus, left lower quadrant cramping, fatigue, anorexia, nausea and vomiting, weakness, skin and mucous membrane lesions, uveitis, and arthritis in joints. Complications of ulcerative colitis include hemorrhage, toxic megacolon, colon perforation, and the risk for colorectal cancer.

Based on the medical diagnosis of ulcerative colitis and the manifestations she has, the nursing diagnosis of *Diarrhea* is appropriate for guiding nursing care for Mrs. Simpson.

- Inflammation of large intestine and rectum
- Mucosa sloughs, ulcerates
- Hemorrhages, abscesses, and necrosis of mucosa occur

affects →

Mrs. S.
45 y.o. female
Ulcerative colitis

leads to

assess →

- Abdominal cramping and pain (6 on 1-10 scale) and rectal discomfort
- Frequent (7-8) loose stools containing blood per day
- Hgb=7.3, Hct=23.3, Serum protein=4.6

generates →

- Risk for Deficient Fluid Volume related to frequent diarrhea
- Acute Pain related to effects of disease process
- Disturbed Body Image related to frequent diarrhea

generate nursing diagnosis

prioritized to

Diarrhea

expected outcomes

- Lab values within normal limits
- Abdominal pain decreases to at least a 2 on a scale of 0 (least) to 10 (most) pain
- Decreased rectal discomfort
- Number of stools per day decrease
- Identifies foods that aggravate diarrhea

evaluate →

- Lab values show trend to normal
- Abdominal pain decreasing, still a 4; rectal discomfort much improved
- Met with dietitian and verbalizes diet instructions to increase fiber and eliminate milk
- Number of stools decreased to 3-4 per day

Interdisciplinary Interventions
- Monitor results of lab tests and report abnormal findings to the physician
- Administer prescribed anti-inflammatory and antibiotic medications
- Maintain bowel rest by keeping NPO as ordered
- Make referral to dietitian to discuss diet

Independent Interventions
- Teach effects, side effects, and any special instruction for prescribed medications
- Post NPO sign over head of bed and explain rationale to client and her family
- Provide oral care q 4 hours
- Use comfort measure to decrease rectal discomfort (cleanse gently, apply protective cream)

Responses to Altered Urinary Elimination

UNIT
8

CHAPTER 27
Assessing Clients with Urinary Elimination Disorders

LEARNING OUTCOMES

- Describe the anatomy, physiology, and functions of the urinary system.

- Explain the role of the urinary system in maintaining homeostasis.

- Identify specific topics for consideration during a health history assessment interview of the client with health problems involving the urinary system.

- Describe techniques used to assess the integrity and function of the urinary system.

- Describe normal variations in assessment findings for the older adult.

- Identify manifestations of impairment of the urinary system.

CLINICAL COMPETENCIES

- Conduct and document a health history for clients who have or are at risk for alterations in urinary elimination.

- Conduct and document a physical assessment of the urinary system.

- Monitor the results of diagnostic tests and report abnormal findings.

EQUIPMENT NEEDED

- Urine specimen cup

- Disposable gloves

- Stethoscope

MEDIALINK

Resources for this chapter can be found on
the Prentice Hall Nursing MediaLink DVD-ROM
accompanying this textbook, and
on the Companion Website at
http://www.prenhall.com/lemone

calculi, *838*
dysuria, *839*
glomerular filtration rate (GFR),
    831

hematuria, *839*
micturition, *834*
nocturia, *839*
oliguria, *839*

polyuria, *839*
pyuria, *839*
urea, *834*

The functions of the urinary system (also called the renal system) are to regulate body fluids, to filter metabolic wastes from the bloodstream, to reabsorb needed substances and water into the bloodstream, and to eliminate metabolic wastes and water as urine. Any alteration in the structure or function of the urinary system affects the whole body. In turn, healthy urinary system function depends on the health of other body systems, especially the circulatory, endocrine, and nervous systems.

ANATOMY, PHYSIOLOGY, AND FUNCTIONS OF THE URINARY SYSTEM

The organs of the urinary system are the paired kidneys, the paired ureters, the urinary bladder, and the urethra (Figure 27–1 ■). Each structure is essential to the total functioning of the urinary system.

The Kidneys

The two kidneys are located outside the peritoneal cavity and on either side of the vertebral column at the levels of T_{12}

Hepatic veins (cut) Esophagus (cut)

Inferior
vena cava

Adrenal
gland

Renal vein

Kidney

Ureter

Uterus

Urinary
bladder

Urethra

Renal artery

Renal hilum

Aorta

Iliac crest

Rectum
(cut)

T_{12}

Kidney

Ureter

L_5

Bladder

Urethra

A

B

Figure 27–1 ■ The urinary system. *A,* Anterior view of the urinary system in a female. *B,* The kidneys are shown in relation to the vertebrae and ribs.

through L₃. These highly vascular, bean-shaped organs are approximately 4.5 inches (11.4 cm) long and 2.5 inches (6.4 cm) wide. The lateral surface of the kidney is convex; the medial surface is concave and forms a vertical cleft, the hilum. The ureter, renal artery, renal vein, lymphatic vessels, and nerves enter or exit the kidney at the level of the hilum.

The kidney is supported by three layers of connective tissue: the outer renal fascia, the middle adipose capsule, and the inner renal capsule. The renal fascia, made up of dense connective tissue, surrounds the kidney (and the adrenal gland, a discrete organ that sits on top of each kidney) and anchors it to surrounding structures. The middle adipose capsule is a fatty mass that holds the kidney in place and also cushions it against trauma. The inner renal capsule provides a barrier against infection and helps protect the kidney from trauma.

Internally, each kidney has three distinct regions: the cortex, medulla, and pelvis. The outer region, or renal cortex, is light in color and has a granular appearance (Figure 27–2 ■). This region of the kidney contains the glomeruli, small clusters of capillaries. The glomeruli bring blood to and carry waste products from the nephrons, the functional units of the kidney.

The renal medulla, just below the cortex, contains cone-shaped tissue masses called renal pyramids, formed almost entirely of bundles of collecting tubules. Areas of lighter colored tissue called renal columns are extensions of the cortex and serve to separate the pyramids. The collecting tubules that make up the pyramids channel urine into the innermost region, the renal pelvis.

The renal pelvis is continuous with the ureter as it leaves the hilum. Branches of the pelvis known as the major and minor calyces extend toward the medulla and serve to collect urine and empty it into the pelvis. From the pelvis, urine is channeled through the ureter and into the bladder for storage. The walls of the calyces, the renal pelvis, and the ureter contain smooth muscle that moves urine along by peristalsis.

Each kidney contains approximately 1 million nephrons, which process the blood to make urine (Figure 27–3 ■). Each nephron contains a tuft of capillaries called the glomerulus, which is completely surrounded by the glomerular capsule (or Bowman's space). Together, the glomerulus and its surrounding capsule are called the renal corpuscle. The endothelium of the glomerulus allows capillaries to be extremely porous. Thus, large amounts of solute-rich fluid pass from the capillaries into the capsule.

This fluid, called the filtrate, is the raw material of urine. Filtrate leaves the capsule and is channeled into the proximal convoluted tubule (PCT) of the nephron. Microvilli on the tubular cells increase the surface area for reabsorption of substances from the filtrate into plasma in the peritubular capillaries. Substances moved by active transport include glucose, sodium, potassium, amino acids, proteins, and vitamins. About 70% of the water in the filtrate, as well as chloride and bicarbonate, are reabsorbed by passive transport.

The filtrate then moves into the U-shaped loop of Henle and is concentrated. The descending limb of the U is relatively thin and freely permeable to water, whereas the ascending segment is thick and thereby less permeable. The distal convoluted tubule (DCT) receives filtrate from the loop of Henle. Although this segment is structurally similar to the PCT, it lacks microvilli and is more involved with secreting solutes into the filtrate than in reabsorbing substances from it. The collecting duct receives the newly formed urine from many nephrons and channels urine through the minor and major calyces of the renal pelvis and into the ureter.

Figure 27–2 ■ Internal anatomy of the kidney.

Labels in figure:
Capsule
Renal cortex
Renal medulla (pyramid)
Major calyx
Renal column
Minor calyx
Renal artery
Renal vein
Renal pelvis
Ureter

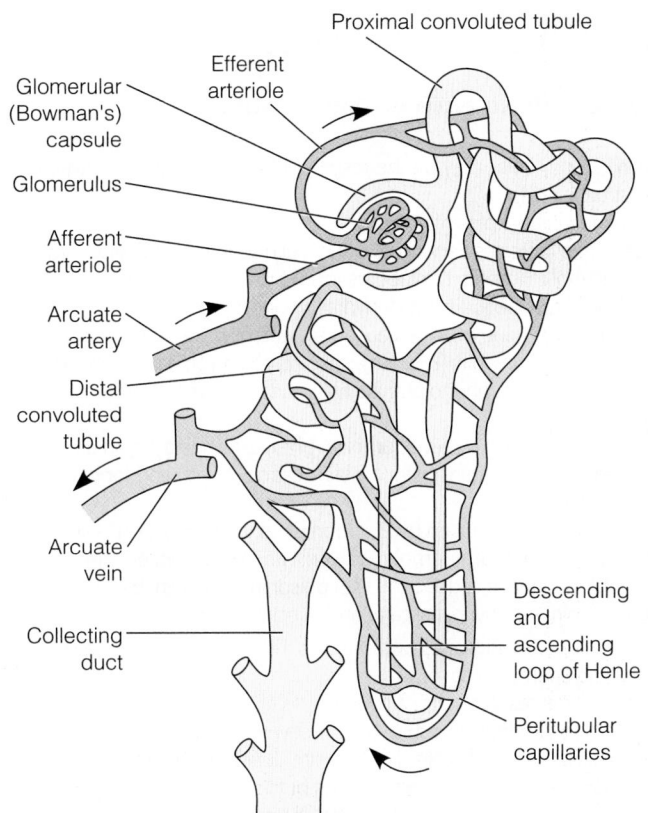

Figure 27–3 ■ The structure of a nephron, showing the glomerulus within the glomerular capsule.

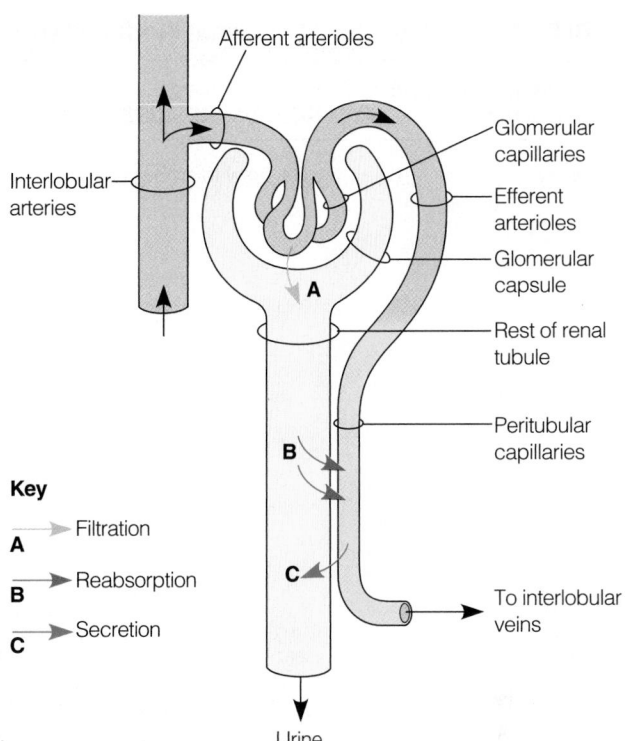

Figure 27–4 ■ Schematic view of the three major mechanisms by which the kidneys adjust to the composition of plasma: *A,* glomerular filtration; *B,* tubular reabsorption; and *C,* tubular secretion.

The functions of the kidney are to:

- Form urine.
- Balance solute and water transport.
- Excrete metabolic waste products.
- Conserve nutrients.
- Regulate acid–base balance.
- Secrete hormones to help regulate blood pressure, erythrocyte production, and calcium metabolism.

Formation of Urine

The complex structures of the kidneys process about 180 L (47 gal) of blood-derived fluid each day. Of this amount, only 1% is excreted as urine; the rest is returned to the circulation. (Normal and abnormal findings of urine on laboratory analysis are listed in Table 27–1.) Urine formation is accomplished entirely by the nephron through three processes: glomerular filtration, tubular reabsorption, and tubular secretion (Figure 27–4 ■).

GLOMERULAR FILTRATION Glomerular filtration is a passive, nonselective process in which hydrostatic pressure forces fluid and solutes through a membrane. The amount of fluid filtered from the blood into the capsule per minute is called the **glomerular filtration rate (GFR)**. Three factors influence this rate: the total surface area available for filtration, the permeability of the filtration membrane, and the net filtration pressure.

The glomerulus is a far more efficient filter than most capillary beds, because the filtration membrane of the glomerulus is much more permeable to water and solutes than are other cap-

illary membranes. In addition, the glomerular blood pressure is much higher, resulting in higher net filtration pressure.

Net filtration pressure is responsible for the formation of filtrate and is determined by two forces: hydrostatic pressure ("push") and osmotic pressure ("pull"). The glomerular hydrostatic pressure pushes water and solutes across the membrane. This pressure is opposed by the osmotic pressure in the glomerulus (primarily the colloid osmotic pressure of plasma proteins in the glomerular blood) and the capsular hydrostatic pressure exerted by fluids within the glomerular capsule. The difference between these forces determines the net filtration pressure, which is directly proportional to the GFR.

The normal GFR in both kidneys is 120 to 125 mL/min in adults. This rate is held constant under normal conditions by intrinsic controls (or renal autoregulation). The myogenic mechanism, which responds to pressure changes in the renal blood vessels, controls the diameter of the afferent arterioles, thereby achieving autoregulation. An increase in systemic blood pressure causes the renal vessels to constrict, whereas a decline in blood pressure causes the afferent arterioles to dilate. These changes adjust the glomerular hydrostatic pressure and, indirectly, maintain the glomerular filtration rate.

Another intrinsic control of the GFR is the result of the rennin–angiotensin mechanism at work in the kidneys. Special cells known as the juxtaglomerular apparatus are located in the distal tubules and respond to slow filtrate flow by releasing chemicals that cause intense vasodilation of the afferent arterioles. Conversely, an increase in the flow of filtrate promotes vasoconstriction, decreasing the GFR. A drop in systemic

TABLE 27–1 Normal and Abnormal Findings: Urinalysis

CHARACTERISTIC OR COMPONENT	NORMAL RESULTS	ABNORMAL FINDING WITH POSSIBLE CAUSE
Color	Light straw to amber yellow	■ Red, dark, smoky color may be the result of blood in the urine (hematuria or menstrual blood). ■ Cloudy urine occurs from infection. ■ Colorless urine indicates very dilute urine, such as in overhydration, kidney disease, alcohol ingestion, or diabetes insipidus. ■ Very dark yellow urine indicates dehydration and/or fever. ■ Red or red brown urine may be caused by sulfisoxazole-phenazopyridine (Azo Gantrisin), phenytoin (Dilantin), cascara, chlorpromazine (Thorazine), docusate calcium and phenolphthalein (Doxidan); and by carrots, rhubarb, and food coloring. ■ Orange urine is caused by fever, urobilin, phenazopyridine (Pyridium), amidopyrine, nitrofurantoin, sulfonamides, carrots, beets, and food coloring. ■ Blue or green urine is caused by *Pseudomonas*, amitriptyline (Elavil), methylene blue, methocarbamol (Robaxin), and yeast concentrate. ■ Brown or black urine is caused by Lysol poisoning, melanin, bilirubin, methemoglobin, porphyrin, cascara, and injectable iron.
Appearance	Clear	■ Hazy or cloudy urine indicates bacteria, pus, RBCs, WBCs, phosphates, prostatic fluid spermatozoa, or urates. ■ Milky urine is the result of fats or pyuria. ■ Yellow foam results from bilirubin, bile, or severe cirrhosis of the liver. ■ A dark yellow to brownish color is seen with deficient fluid volume.
Odor	Aromatic	■ Ammonia smell increases as urine stands outside the body. ■ Urinary tract infection (UTI) causes a foul or unpleasant odor, depending on the causative organism. ■ Asparagus causes a distinctive odor. ■ Mousy odors result from phenylketonuria. ■ Sweet or fruity odors occur in starvation and diabetic ketoacidosis.
pH	4.5–8.0	■ <4.5: metabolic acidosis, respiratory acidosis, diet high in meat protein, ammonium chloride and mandelic acid. ■ >8.0: bacteriuria, UTI, antibiotics (neomycin, kanamycin), sulfonamides, sodium bicarbonate, acetazolamide (Diamox), potassium citrate.
Specific gravity	1.005–1.030	■ <1.005: diabetes insipidus, overhydration, renal disease, severe potassium deficit. ■ >1.030: dehydration, fever, diabetes mellitus, vomiting, diarrhea, contrast media.
Protein	2–8 mg/dL	■ >8 mg/dL: proteinuria, exercise, fever, stress, acute infection, kidney disease, lupus erythematosus, leukemia, multiple myeloma, cardiac disease, toxemia of pregnancy, septicemia, lead, mercury, neomycin, barbiturates, sulfonamides.
Glucose	Negative	■ >15 mg/dL or +4: diabetes mellitus, stroke, Cushing's syndrome, anesthesia, glucose infusions, severe stress, infections, ascorbic acid, aspirin, cephalosporins, and epinephrine.
Ketones	Negative	■ +1 to +3: ketoacidosis, starvation, high-protein diet.
RBCs	Rare	■ >2 per low-power field: kidney trauma, kidney diseases, renal calculi, cystitis, excess aspirin, anticoagulants, sulfonamides, menstrual contamination.
WBCs	3–4	■ >4 per low-power field: UTI, fever, strenuous exercise, kidney diseases.
Casts	Occasional hyaline	■ Fever, kidney diseases, heart failure.

blood pressure often triggers the juxtaglomerular cells to release renin. Rennin acts on a plasma globulin, angiotensinogen, to release angiotensin I, which is in turn converted to angiotensin II. As a vasoconstrictor, angiotensin II activates vascular smooth muscle throughout the body, causing systemic blood pressure to rise. Thus, the rennin–angiotensin mechanism is a factor in renal autoregulation, even though its main purpose is the control of systemic blood pressure.

Glomerular filtration is also under an extrinsic control mechanism through the sympathetic nervous system. During periods of extreme stress or emergency, sympathetic nervous system stimulation causes strong constriction of the afferent arterioles and inhibits filtrate formation. The sympathetic nervous system also stimulates the juxtaglomerular cells to release renin, increasing systemic blood pressure.

TUBULAR REABSORPTION Tubular reabsorption is a transepithelial process that begins as the filtrate enters the proximal tubules. In healthy kidneys, virtually all organic nutrients such as glucose and amino acids are reabsorbed. However, the tubules constantly regulate and adjust the rate and degree of water and ion reabsorption in response to hormonal signals. Reabsorption may be active or passive. Substances reclaimed through active tubular reabsorption are usually moving against electrical and/or chemical gradients. These substances, including glucose, amino acids, lactate, vitamins, and most ions, require an ATP-dependent carrier to be transported into the interstitial space. In passive tubular reabsorption, which includes diffusion and osmosis, substances move along their gradient without expenditure of energy.

TUBULAR SECRETION The final process in urine formation is tubular secretion, which is essentially reabsorption in reverse. Substances such as hydrogen and potassium ions, creatinine, ammonia, and organic acids move from the blood of the peritubular capillaries into the tubules themselves as filtrate. Thus, urine consists of both filtered and secreted substances. Tubular secretion is important for disposing of substances not already in the filtrate, such as medications. This process eliminates undesirable substances that have been reabsorbed by passive processes and rids the body of excessive potassium ions. It is also a vital force in the regulation of blood pH.

Maintaining Normal Composition and Volume of Urine

Maintaining the normal composition and volume of urine involves a countercurrent exchange system. In this system, fluid flows in opposite directions through the parallel tubes of the loop of Henle and the vasa recta, tiny capillaries that run along the loop of Henle. Fluid is exchanged across these parallel membranes in response to a concentration gradient (Figure 27–5 ■). When the filtrate enters the proximal convoluted tubule, its osmolality (at 300 mOsm/kg) is essentially the same as that of the plasma and the interstitial fluid of the renal cortex. Note the following steps in the process:

1. The descending loop of Henle is highly permeable to water and allows chloride and sodium to enter the loop through diffusion. The hyperosmotic interstitium causes

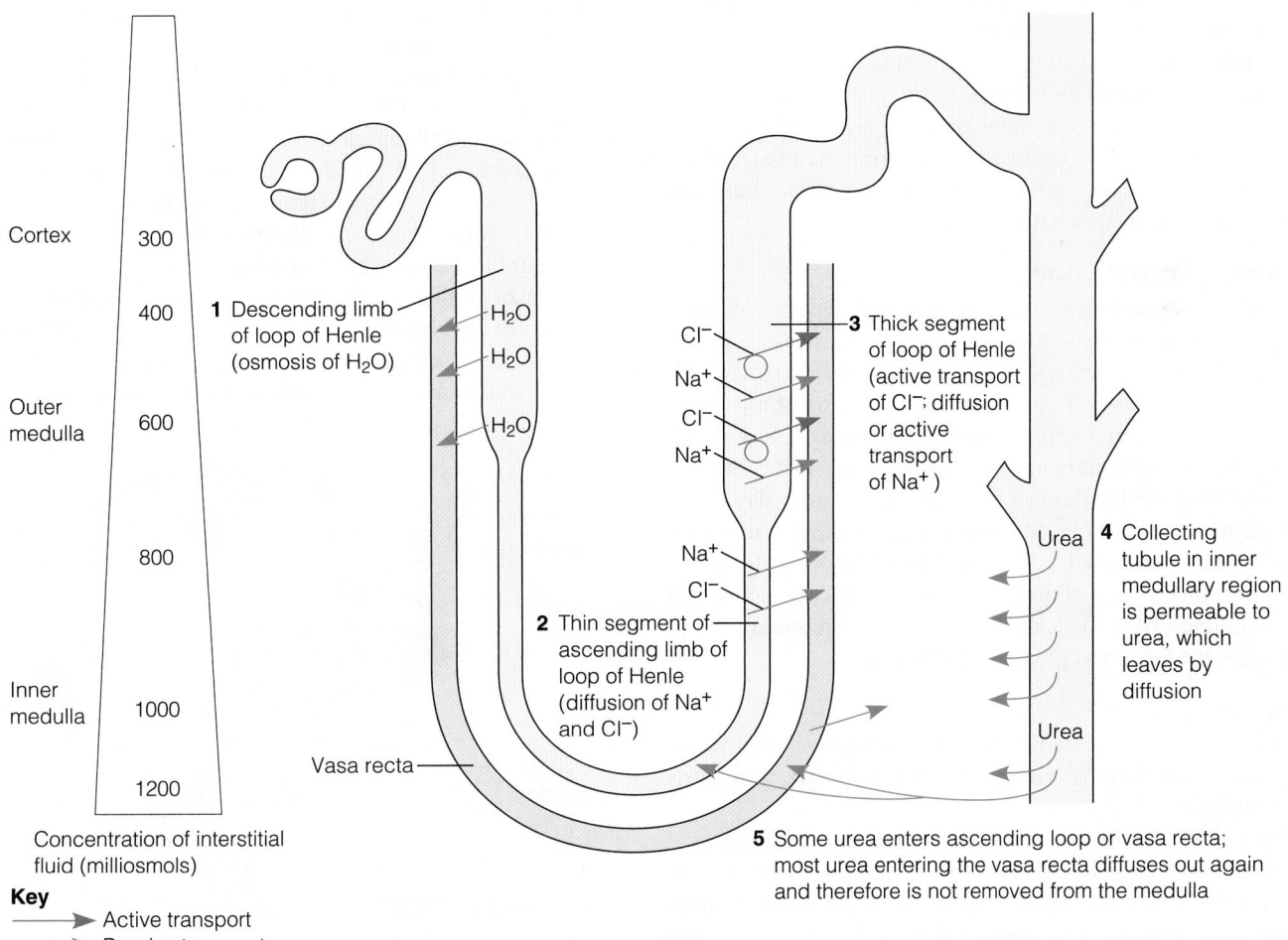

Figure 27–5 ■ The countercurrent exchange system is responsible for establishing and maintaining an osmotic gradient necessary to the composition, volume, and pH of urine.

water to move out of the descending loop, so that the remaining filtrate becomes increasingly concentrated.

2. The lumen of the ascending loop of Henle is impermeable to water but allows chloride and sodium to move out into the interstitium of the medulla. As a result, the filtrate in the ascending loop becomes hypoosmotic, and the medullary interstitium becomes hyperosmotic.

3. As the filtrate progresses through the ascending limb of the loop of Henle and enters the distal convoluted tubule, sodium and chloride are removed and water is retained. Thus, the filtrate becomes more dilute.

4. As the filtrate passes through the deep medullary regions, urea (an end product of protein metabolism and, along with water, the main constituent of urine) begins to diffuse out from the collecting tubules into the interstitial space and establishes a concentration gradient to facilitate water movement.

5. Some urea enters the ascending loop of Henle. Urea entering the vasa recta typically diffuses out again.

The dilution or concentration of urine is largely determined by the action of antidiuretic hormone (ADH), which is secreted by the posterior pituitary gland. ADH causes the pores of the collecting tubules to enlarge, so that increased amounts of water move into the interstitial space. As the end result, water is reabsorbed and urine is more highly concentrated. When ADH is not secreted, the filtrate passes through the system without further water reabsorption, so that the urine is more dilute.

Urine is composed, by volume, of about 95% water and 5% solutes. The largest component of urine by weight is urea. Other solutes normally excreted in the urine include sodium, potassium, phosphate, sulfate, creatinine, uric acid, calcium, magnesium, and bicarbonate.

Clearing Waste Products

The kidneys excrete water-soluble waste products and other chemicals or substances from the body. This process is called renal plasma clearance, which refers to the ability of the kidneys to clear (cleanse) a given amount of plasma of a particular substance in a given time (usually 1 minute). The kidneys clear 25 to 30 g of **urea** (a nitrogenous waste product formed in the liver from the breakdown of amino acids) each day. They also clear creatinine (an end product of creatine phosphate, found in skeletal muscle), uric acid (a metabolite of nucleic acid metabolism), and ammonia as well as bacterial toxins and water-soluble drugs. Tests of renal clearance are often used to determine the GFR and glomerular damage.

Renal Hormones

Hormones either activated or synthesized by the kidneys include the active form of vitamin D, erythropoietin, and natriuretic hormone.

Vitamin D is necessary for the absorption of calcium and phosphate by the small intestine. In an inactive form, vitamin D enters the body either by dietary intake or through the action of ultraviolet rays on cholesterol in the skin. Activation occurs in two steps, the first in the liver and the second in the kidneys. The renal step is stimulated by parathyroid hormone, which in turn responds to a decreased plasma calcium level.

Erythropoietin stimulates the bone marrow to produce red blood cells in response to tissue hypoxia. The stimulus for the production of erythropoietin by the kidneys is decreased oxygen delivery to kidney cells.

The right atria of the heart releases natriuretic hormone in response to increased volume and stretch, as occurs in increased extracellular volume. This hormone inhibits ADH secretion, so that the collecting tubules are less porous and a large amount of dilute urine is produced.

The Ureters

The ureters are bilateral tubes approximately 10 to 12 inches (26 to 30 cm) long. They transport urine from the kidney to the bladder through peristaltic waves originating in the renal pelvis. The wall of the ureter has three layers: an inner epithelial mucosa, a middle layer of smooth muscle, and an outer layer of fibrous connective tissue.

The Urinary Bladder

The urinary bladder is posterior to the symphysis pubis and serves as a storage site for urine. In males, the bladder lies immediately in front of the rectum; in females, the bladder lies in front of the vagina and the uterus. Openings for the ureters and the urethra are inside the bladder: The trigone is the smooth triangular portion of the base of the bladder outlined by these three openings (Figure 27–6 ■).

The layers of the bladder wall (from internal to external) are the epithelial mucosa lining the inside, the connective tissue submucosa, the smooth muscle layer, and the fibrous outer layer. The muscle layer, called the detrusor muscle, consists of fibers arranged in inner and outer longitudinal layers and in a middle circular layer. This arrangement allows the bladder to expand or contract according to the amount of urine it holds.

The size of the bladder varies with the amount of urine it contains. In healthy adults, the bladder holds about 300 to 500 mL of urine before internal pressure rises and signals the need to empty the bladder through **micturition** (also called urination

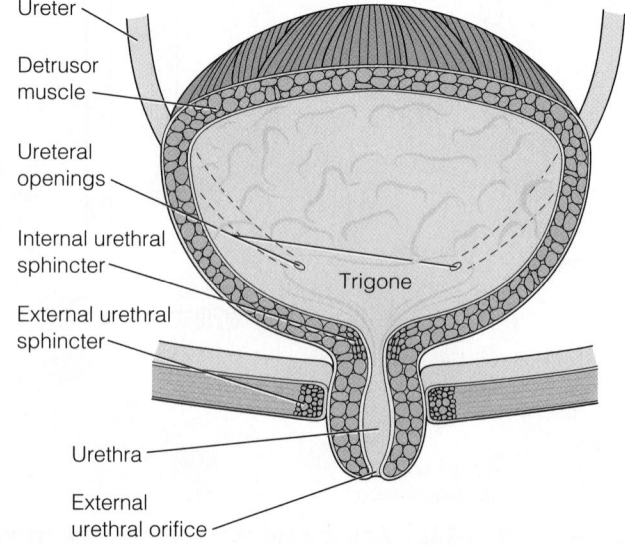

Figure 27–6 ■ Internal view of the urinary bladder and trigone.

or voiding). However, the bladder can hold more than twice that amount if necessary. The bladder has an internal urethral sphincter that relaxes in response to a full bladder and signals the need to urinate. A second external urethral sphincter is formed by skeletal muscle and is under voluntary control.

The Urethra

The urethra is a thin-walled muscular tube that channels urine to the outside of the body. It extends from the base of the bladder to the external urinary meatus. In females, the urethra is approximately 1.5 inches (3 to 5 cm) long, and the urinary meatus is anterior to the vaginal orifice. In males, the urethra is approximately 8 inches (20 cm) long and serves as a channel for semen as well as urine. The prostate gland encircles the urethra at the base of the bladder in males. The male urinary meatus is located at the end of the glans penis.

ASSESSING URINARY SYSTEM FUNCTION

Urinary system function is assessed by findings from diagnostic tests, a health assessment interview to collect subjective data, and a physical assessment to collect objective data. Sample documentation of an assessment of urinary system function is included in the box on this page.

> **SAMPLE DOCUMENTATION**
> **Assessment of Urinary System Function**
>
> *Home visit made to 66-year-old woman with end-stage chronic kidney failure. Skin pale and oral mucous membranes dry. 4+ edema in ankles and feet. Eyelids swollen. Skin tight and shiny over abdomen and bilateral lower extremities. Abdomen distended and tender on light palpation; further palpation deferred. Urinary bladder not palpable. Urine output for past 24 hours is 15 mL.*

Diagnostic Tests

The results of diagnostic tests of urinary system function are used to support the diagnosis of a specific disease, to provide information to identify or modify the appropriate medication or therapy used to treat the disease, and to help nurses monitor the client's responses to treatment and nursing care interventions. Diagnostic tests to assess the structures and functions of the urinary system are described in the box below and summarized in the bulleted list that follows. More information is included in the discussion of specific disorders in Chapters 28 ∞ and 29 ∞.

DIAGNOSTIC TESTS of Urinary System Disorders

NAME OF TEST   Blood urea nitrogen (BUN)

PURPOSE AND DESCRIPTION   This blood test measures urea, the end product of protein metabolism. Increased levels may result from dehydration, vomiting, diarrhea, digested blood, or prerenal/renal failure.

Normal values: 5–25 mg/dL

RELATED NURSING CARE   No special preparation is needed. If values are increased in a client who is dehydrated, they should return to normal with hydration. If not, this is an indicator of kidney disease.

NAME OF TEST   Serum creatinine

PURPOSE AND DESCRIPTION   This blood test is used to diagnose kidney dysfunction. Creatinine is a by-product of the breakdown of muscle and is excreted by the kidneys. When 50% or more nephrons are destroyed, serum creatinine levels rise.

Normal value: Serum: 0.5–1.5 mg/dL.

(Older adults may have decreased values due to decreased muscle mass.)

RELATED NURSING CARE   No special preparation is needed. Values may be increased by antibiotics, ascorbic acid, L-dopa, methyldopa, and lithium carbonate. Value is not affected by hydration status.

NAME OF TEST   Routine urinalysis (UA)

PURPOSE AND DESCRIPTION   An examination of the constituents of a sample of urine to establish a baseline, to provide data for diagnosis, or to monitor results of treatment. Normal findings and abnormal findings with causes are outlined in Table 27–1.

RELATED NURSING CARE   Provide a clean specimen cup for a sample of urine. Note if client is menstruating. Assess medications, fluid status, and foods that might affect urinalysis results.

NAME OF TEST   Urine culture (midstream, clean-catch)

PURPOSE AND DESCRIPTION   A culture of a urine sample to identify the causative organism of a UTI.

Normal value: <10,000 organisms/mL (urine is sterile but urethra contains bacteria and a few WBCs).

Values of >100,000 organisms/mL indicate UTI.

RELATED NURSING CARE   Provide client with sterile container. Ask women to separate labia with one hand and clean labia with other hand, using sterile cotton sponges saturated with a cleansing solution, and wiping three times front to back. Ask men to retract the foreskin and cleanse glans with three cotton sponges saturated with a cleansing solution, using a circular motion. After cleaning, tell client to begin voiding and then collect specimen in the container (initial voiding will contain urethral contaminants). If client is unable to void, it may be necessary to obtain a specimen with a urinary catheterization.

(continued)

NAME OF TEST   Residual urine (postvoiding residual urine)

PURPOSE AND DESCRIPTION   Conducted to measure amount of urine left in the bladder after voiding.

Normal value: ≤50 mL

RELATED NURSING CARE   Ask client to void in a collection device and measure the amount. Immediately after voiding, catheterize using aseptic technique and a straight catheter. Drain bladder completely. Document time, amount voided, amount obtained on catheterization, color, clarity, odor, and any other significant data. Report amount of residual urine if it is more than 100 mL. Document voiding amount and residual amount.

NAME OF TEST   Portable ultrasonic bladder scan

PURPOSE AND DESCRIPTION   Used to obtain information about residual urine. Warmed ultrasound gel is applied over the lower abdomen, and the ultrasound probe is placed just above the pubic bone. The scanner shows an outline of the bladder and displays the amount of urine in the bladder in milliliters. Obtain several readings and use the largest (the most accurate).

Print the information, place it on the client's chart, and document the residual urine amount.

RELATED NURSING CARE   No special preparation is needed, but the test is usually not used for pregnant women. Report a residual amount more than 100 mL.

NAME OF TEST   Creatinine clearance

PURPOSE AND DESCRIPTION   A 24-hour urine test to identify renal dysfunction and to monitor renal function.

Normal value: 85–135/min

Women and older adults may have slightly lower values.

RELATED NURSING CARE   Assess medications: Phenacetin, steroids, and thiazides may decrease creatinine clearance; ascorbic acid, steroids, L-dopa, methyldopa (Aldomet), and cefoxitin may increase creatinine clearance. Levels of creatinine are elevated in hypothyroidism, hypertension, pregnancy, and exercise. Obtain appropriate specimen container. Ask client to void and discard first voiding. Instruct client, family, and staff to then save all urine for a clearly designated 24-hour period, maintaining the specimen in the container on ice or in the refrigerator.

NAME OF TEST   Uroflowmetry

PURPOSE AND DESCRIPTION   This test measures the volume of urine voided per second.

RELATED NURSING CARE   Ask client to increase fluid intake and refrain from voiding for several hours before the test to ensure a full bladder and a strong urge to void during testing. Tell the client he or she will be asked to urinate into a funnel.

NAME OF TEST   Cystometrogram (CMG) (voiding cystogram)

PURPOSE AND DESCRIPTION   Conducted to evaluate bladder capacity and neuromuscular functions of the bladder, urethral pressures, and causes of bladder dysfunction. A measured quantity of fluid is instilled into the bladder, and the filling capacity and voiding pressures are measured.

Normal value: Urine stream strong and uninterrupted, normal filling pattern and sensation of fullness; bladder capacity: 300–600 mL; urge to void: >150 mL; fullness felt: 300 mL.

RELATED NURSING CARE   Tell client that the bladder will be filled and during filling he or she will be asked to describe the first urge to void, and the sensation of being unable to delay urination any longer.

NAME OF TEST   Intravenous pyelogram (IVP)

PURPOSE AND DESCRIPTION   This radiologic examination is done to visualize the entire urinary tract to identify abnormal size, shape, and function of the kidneys or to detect renal calculi (stones), tumors, or cysts. A radiopaque substance is injected IV and a series of x-rays taken.

CLIENT PREPARATION

- Assess knowledge and understanding of procedure, clarifying information as needed.
- Schedule IVP prior to any ordered barium test or gallbladder studies using contrast material.
- Ask about allergy to seafood, iodine, or radiologic contrast dye. Notify physician or radiologist if allergies are known.
- Verify the presence of a signed consent for the procedure.
- Assess renal and fluid status, including serum osmolality, creatinine, and blood urea nitrogen (BUN) levels. Notify the physician of any abnormal values.
- Instruct the client to complete ordered pretest bowel preparation, including prescribed laxative or cathartic the evening before the test, and an enema or suppository the morning of the test. Withhold food for 8 hours prior to the test; clear liquids are allowed.
- Obtain baseline vital signs and record.

After the Test

- Monitor vital signs and urine output.
- Report manifestations of delayed reaction to the contrast media such as dyspnea, tachycardia, itching, hives, or flushing.

HEALTH EDUCATION FOR THE CLIENT AND FAMILY

- X-rays and a dye that is rapidly excreted in the urine are used to show the structures of the kidney, ureters, and bladder. The test takes about 30 minutes.
- A laxative and possibly an enema or suppository are used before the test to clear the bowel of feces and gas. Do not eat after the ordered time the evening before the test; you may drink clear fluids such as water, coffee, or tea (without creamer).
- As the dye is injected, you may feel a transient flushing or burning sensation, along with possible nausea and a metallic taste.
- Notify your doctor immediately if you develop a rash, difficulty breathing, rapid heart rate, or hives during or after the test.
- Increase fluid intake after the test is completed.

NAME OF TEST Retrograde pyelogram

PURPOSE AND DESCRIPTION This radiologic test is done to evaluate the structures of the ureters and kidney pelvis. It may be performed alone or in conjunction with a cystoscopy. A contrast dye is injected through a catheter into the ureters and kidney pelvis and x-rays are taken.

RELATED NURSING CARE Nursing care for the client having a retrograde pyelogram is the same as that for clients having an IVP.

NAME OF TEST Renal arteriogram or angiogram

PURPOSE AND DESCRIPTION This radiologic test is done to visualize renal blood vessels in order to detect renal artery stenosis, renal thrombosis or embolism, tumors, cysts, or aneurysm; to determine the causative factor for hypertension; and to evaluate renal circulation. A contrast medium is injected into the femoral artery.

RELATED NURSING CARE Assess for allergy to iodine, seafood, or other contrast dye from other x-ray procedures. A laxative or cleansing enema is usually given the night before, and the client should be NPO for 8–12 hours prior to the test. Anticoagulants should be discontinued. Results may be affected by feces, gas, and barium sulfate. After the test, monitor for bleeding from the femoral artery, restrict activity for a day, assess peripheral pulses, and monitor urine output.

NAME OF TEST Cystoscopy (cystogram), cystography

PURPOSE AND DESCRIPTION Direct visualization of the bladder wall and urethra is accomplished by using a cystoscope. During the procedure small renal calculi can be removed from the ureter, bladder, or urethra, and tissue biopsy can be done. It also permits determination of the cause of hematuria or UTI. A stent may be inserted during the procedure to facilitate urinary drainage past an obstruction. A retrograde pyelogram may be done during the cystoscopy. By instilling a contrast dye into the bladder (*cystography*), neurogenic bladder, fistulas, tumors, or ruptures can be identified.

CLIENT PREPARATION

- Assess knowledge and understanding of the procedure, clarifying information as needed.
- Verify the presence of a signed consent for the procedure.
- Instruct in pretest preparation as ordered, including prescribed laxatives the evening prior to the test and any ordered food or fluid restrictions.
- Administer sedation and other medications as ordered prior to the test.

HEALTH EDUCATION FOR THE CLIENT AND FAMILY

- Cystoscopy is performed in a special cystoscopy room, using local or general anesthesia. You may feel some pressure or a need to urinate as the scope is inserted through the urethra into the bladder. The procedure takes approximately 30 to 45 minutes.
- Do not attempt to stand without assistance immediately after the procedure because you may feel dizzy or faint.
- Burning on urination for a day or two after the procedure is to be expected.
- Immediately notify the physician if your urine remains bloody for more than three voidings after the procedure, or if you develop bright bleeding, low urine output, abdominal or flank pain, chills, or fever.
- Warm sitz baths, analgesic agents, and antispasmodic medications may relieve discomfort after the procedure.
- Increase fluid intake to decrease pain and difficulty voiding and reduce the risk of infection.
- Laxatives may be ordered after the procedure to prevent constipation and straining, which may cause urinary tract bleeding.

NAME OF TEST Renal ultrasound

PURPOSE AND DESCRIPTION This noninvasive test is conducted to detect renal or perirenal masses, identify obstructions, and diagnose renal cysts and solid masses. It is done by applying a conductive gel to the skin and placing a small external ultrasound probe on the client's skin. Sound waves are recorded on a computer as they are reflected off tissues.

RELATED NURSING CARE No special preparation is indicated.

NAME OF TEST CT scan of kidneys

PURPOSE AND DESCRIPTION The CT scan allows evaluation of kidney size, tumors, abscesses, suprarenal masses, and obstructions. A contrast dye is injected IV, allowing increased visualization of the density of renal tissue and masses in comparison to an ultrasound.

RELATED NURSING CARE Assess the client for allergies to iodine, x-ray contrast dye, and seafood. Tell the client to remain NPO for 4 hours prior to the test, and that laxatives or enemas may be ordered to remove gas or fecal material from the bowel.

NAME OF TEST MRI of the kidneys

PURPOSE AND DESCRIPTION An MRI is used to visualize the kidneys by assessing computer-generated films of radiofrequency waves and changes in magnetic fields.

RELATED NURSING CARE Ask client to remove all metal objects. Assess for metal implants. (Test will not be conducted if present.)

NAME OF TEST Renal scan

PURPOSE AND DESCRIPTION This test is done to evaluate kidney blood flow, location, size, and shape; and to assess kidney perfusion and urine production. Radioactive isotopes are injected IV and radiation detector probes are placed over the kidneys to monitor activity in the kidneys. Radioisotope distribution in the kidneys is scanned and graphed. Nonfunctioning tissue, such as in tumors and cysts, appears as cold spots.

RELATED NURSING CARE Ask client to drink several glasses of water prior to the test. Obtain weight and have client void. After the procedure, increase fluid intake.

(continued)

DIAGNOSTIC TESTS of Urinary System Disorders (continued)

NAME OF TEST Renal biopsy

PURPOSE AND DESCRIPTION A renal biopsy is done to obtain tissue to diagnose or monitor kidney disease. The test is usually done by inserting a needle through the skin into the lower lobe of the kidney. It can also be done with CT or ultrasound guidance.

CLIENT PREPARATION

- Informed consent is required for a kidney biopsy. Answer questions and provide additional information as needed.
- Maintain NPO status from midnight before the procedure.
- Note hemoglobin and hematocrit prior to the procedure.
- If the procedure is to be performed at the bedside, obtain biopsy tray and other necessary supplies.
- Following procedure, apply a pressure dressing and position supine to help maintain pressure on the biopsy site.
- Monitor closely for bleeding during the first 24 hours after the procedure:
  a. Check vital signs frequently. Notify the physician of tachycardia, hypotension, or other signs of shock.
  b. Monitor biopsy site for bleeding.
  c. Check hemoglobin and hematocrit, comparing with pre-procedure values.
  d. Observe for and report complaints of flank or back pain, shoulder pain (caused by diaphragmatic irritation if hemorrhage occurs), pallor, light-headedness.
  e. Monitor urine output for quantity and hematuria. Initial hematuria should clear within 24 hours.
- Monitor for other potential complications such as inadvertent penetration of the liver or bowel. Report abdominal pain, guarding, and decreased bowel sounds.
- Encourage fluids during the initial postprocedure period.

HEALTH EDUCATION FOR THE CLIENT AND FAMILY

- Local anesthesia is used at the injection site. The procedure may be uncomfortable but should not be painful.
- When the needle is inserted, you will be instructed not to breathe to prevent kidney motion.
- The entire procedure takes approximately 10 minutes.
- Avoid coughing during the first 24 hours after the procedure. Strenuous activity such as heavy lifting may be prohibited for approximately 2 weeks after the procedure.
- Report any manifestations of complications, such as hemorrhage or urinary tract infection, to the physician.

- Urine may be tested for characteristics and components through routine analysis, a urine culture, a postvoiding residual urine, and a 24-hour collection for creatinine. Results of these tests include findings to serve as baseline data, to support diagnosis of various health problems, to evaluate the ability to empty the bladder of urine, and to evaluate renal function.
- The ability to empty the urinary bladder of urine may be evaluated by an ultrasonic bladder scan to evaluate for residual urine, uroflowmetry to measure the volume of urine voided per second, and a cystometrogram (CMG) to evaluate bladder capacity, neuromuscular functions of the bladder, urethral pressures, and causes of bladder dysfunction.
- Radiologic examinations include an intravenous pyelogram, a retrograde pyelogram, and a renal arteriogram or angiogram. These examinations are useful in visualizing (via x-ray film) the urinary tract to identify abnormal size, shape, and function of the kidneys, the kidney pelvis, and ureters; and to detect renal **calculi** (stones), tumors, or cysts.
- A cystoscopy allows direct visualization of the bladder wall and urethra. During the procedure small stones can be removed, a sample of tissue may be taken for biopsy, and a retrograde pyelogram may be done at the same time. If a contrast dye is instilled in the bladder, fistulas, tumors, or ruptures can be identified.
- Noninvasive tests include a renal ultrasound, computed tomography (CT) scan, magnetic resonance imaging (MRI), and renal scan. These tests are used to identify and evaluate kidney size and structure, as well as renal or perirenal masses and obstructions. In addition, a renal scan may be used to evaluate kidney blood flow, perfusion, and urine production.
- A kidney biopsy is done to obtain tissue to diagnose or monitor kidney disease.

Regardless of the type of diagnostic test, the nurse is responsible for explaining the procedure and any special preparation needed, assessing for medication use that may affect the outcome of the tests, supporting the client during the examination as necessary, documenting the procedures as appropriate, and monitoring the results of the tests.

Genetic Considerations

When conducting a health assessment interview and physical assessment, it is important for the nurse to consider genetic influences on adult health. During the health assessment interview, ask about family members with health problems affecting kidney function, or of family members diagnosed with polycystic disease or diabetes mellitus. During the physical assessment, assess for any manifestations that might indicate a genetic disorder (see Genetic Considerations on the next page). If data are found to indicate genetic risk factors or alterations, ask about genetic testing and refer for appropriate genetic counseling and evaluation. Chapter 8 ∞ provides further information about genetics in medical-surgical nursing.

Health Assessment Interview

A health assessment interview to determine problems with urinary structure and function may be conducted during a health screening, may focus on a chief complaint (such as burning on urination or difficulty starting the stream when urinating), or may be part of a total health assessment. As with alterations in bowel function, clients with problems with urinary system func-

Genetic Considerations
Urinary System

- Adult polycystic kidney disease (APKD) is linked to a familial chromosome 16 disorder. The disease is characterized by large cysts in one or both kidneys and a gradual loss of kidney tissue with resultant chronic renal failure.
- Chronic renal failure may be a complication of type 1 and type 2 diabetes mellitus (DM), but is seen more often in clients with type 1 DM. Type 1 and type 2 DM are classified as multifactorial inheritance disorders because both genetic and environmental factors are necessary for onset of the disorder.

tion may be embarrassed to talk about urinary elimination patterns. It is often helpful to discuss less personal information first.

Current urinary status should include the following data.

- Color, odor, and amount of urine
- Difficulty initiating a stream of urine
- Frequency of urination
- Painful urination (**dysuria**)
- Excessive urination at night (**nocturia**)
- Blood in the urine (**hematuria**)
- Voiding scant amounts of urine (**oliguria**)
- Voiding excessive amounts of urine (**polyuria**)
- Discharge
- Flank pain.

If you identify a problem with urinary elimination, analyze its onset, characteristics and course, severity, precipitating and relieving factors, and any associated symptoms, noting the timing and circumstances. For example, you may ask the following questions:

- Have you noticed any burning when you urinate?
- Do you have difficulty starting to urinate?
- When did you first notice that you were unable to control the loss of urine from your bladder?

Further explore any abnormalities in the client's current urinary status. Focus questions on changes in patterns of urination, changes in the urine, and pain.

Assess changes in patterns of urination by asking the client: How many times a day do you urinate? Do you feel that you empty your bladder each time? How many times do you get up at night to urinate? Do you experience a very strong desire to urinate and feel that you just cannot wait? Have you noticed that you urinate small amounts of dark, strong-smelling urine?

Changes in the urine that should be explored include the presence of blood or a cloudy appearance of the urine. If the client has noticed blood, explore the use of medications (such as anticoagulants or dye-containing drugs) and other bleeding problems. Women may not understand that blood in the toilet or on toilet tissue after urination is normal during menstruation. Cloudy, foul-smelling urine often indicates infection (**pyuria**); ask the client about temperature elevations, chills, and general malaise. Cloudy urine in men may result from retrograde ejaculation (when semen is discharged into the bladder instead of from the penis) during intercourse.

If the client reports pain, explore its location, duration, and intensity. Kidney pain is experienced in the back and the costovertebral angle (the angle between the lower ribs and adjacent vertebrae) and may spread toward the umbilicus. Renal colic (pain in response to renal calculi moving through the ureter) is severe, sharp, stabbing, and excruciating; often it is felt in the flank, bladder, urethra, testes, or ovaries. Bladder and urethral pain is usually dull and continuous but may be experienced as spasms. The client with a distended bladder experiences constant pain increased by any pressure over the bladder.

Information about surgeries or other treatment of previous urinary problems is essential to the health history, as is a family history of altered structure or function. A family history of renal problems may be the first clue to abnormalities in the client's urinary function. Explore information regarding family occurrence of end-stage renal disease, renal calculi, and frequent infections as well as related problems such as hypertension and diabetes mellitus.

Questions about lifestyle, diet, and work history should explore cigarette smoking and/or exposure to toxic chemicals (to identify risks for cancer), usual fluid intake, type of fluid intake, and self-care measures to replace fluids lost during work or physical activity in hot temperatures.

Interview questions categorized by functional health patterns are listed in the box on the next page.

Physical Assessment

The structure and function of the urinary system is assessed by examination of the skin, abdomen, kidneys, bladder, and urinary meatus. Guidelines for abdominal assessment are outlined in both Chapters 21 ∞ and 25 ∞. Normal age-related findings for the older adult are summarized in Table 27–2.

Physical assessment of the urinary system may be performed as part of a total health assessment, as part of an abdominal assessment, or as part of the back examination (for the kidneys). The techniques of inspection, auscultation, palpation, and percussion are used.

PRACTICE ALERT
Auscultate immediately after inspection because percussion or palpation may increase bowel motility and interfere with sound transmission during auscultation.

Before beginning the assessment, ask the client to provide a clean-catch urine specimen and give the client a specimen cup. Assess the specimen for color, odor, and clarity before you send it to the laboratory.

At the beginning of the assessment, the client may be sitting or lying supine. Prior to the examination, collect all necessary equipment and explain the techniques to the client to decrease anxiety. Because the examination involves exposure of the genital area, give the client a gown and drape the client appropriately to minimize exposure.

Guidelines for percussion and palpation of the kidneys are outlined in Box 27–1.

FUNCTIONAL HEALTH PATTERN INTERVIEW Urinary System

Functional Health Pattern	Interview Questions and Leading Statements
Health Perception-Health Management	■ Have you ever had a bladder or kidney disease, injury, or surgery? Describe. ■ If so, how was the problem treated? ■ Describe your usual intake of fluids for a 24-hour period. What type of fluids do you drink? ■ Have you ever smoked? If so, how many cigarettes per day? ■ Describe the problem you are having with your kidneys or bladder. ■ Are you taking medications for this or any other health problem? If so, what do you take and how often? ■ *For women:* Describe how you care for yourself when you urinate (for example, direction of wiping with tissue). ■ If you have a surgical diversion of urine, describe how you care for yourself (what skin and appliance care do you do, how often do you empty the bag?). ■ Do you wear or have you ever worn an external catheter, indwelling catheter, or incontinence briefs? Explain. ■ Have you ever done self-catheterization? If so, why and how often?
Nutritional-Metabolic	■ How much coffee, tea, or alcohol do you drink in a 24-hour period? ■ Have you ever limited your fluid intake? Explain. ■ Do you limit the amount of salt you eat? Explain. ■ Do you have swelling in your ankles? If so, what do you do?
Elimination	■ How many times a day do you urinate? Do you have to get up at night to urinate? Has there been a change in your usual pattern of urination? ■ Do you experience a sudden urge to urinate? ■ Has there been a change in your urine, such as a change in amount, color, or odor? Have you ever noticed blood in your urine or on the tissue after you wipe? ■ Is it difficult for you to begin or end your flow of urine? ■ Have you ever had problems controlling your urine when you laugh, sneeze, or cough? ■ Do you have any discharge from your urethra? Explain.
Activity-Exercise	■ Do your urinary problems interfere with your activities of daily living? Explain. ■ Describe your usual energy level. Has there been a change? Explain. ■ Have you ever been taught to do Kegel exercises to help you control your urination? If so, how often do you practice these?
Sleep-Rest	■ Does a problem with urination interfere with your ability to sleep and rest? Explain. ■ Has there been a change in the number of times you wake up at night to urinate? Explain.
Cognitive-Perceptual	■ Do you have any pain or burning when you urinate? ■ Have you experienced any tenderness or pain over the lower sides of your back or severe pain that spreads over your lower abdomen? If so, describe its location, intensity, aggravating factors, and duration.
Self-Perception-Self-Concept	■ How does having this condition make you feel about yourself?
Role-Relationships	■ How does having this condition affect your relationships with others?
Sexuality-Reproductive	■ Has this condition interfered with your usual sexual activity?
Coping-Stress-Tolerance	■ Has having this condition created stress for you? ■ Have you experienced any kind of stress that makes this condition worse? Explain. ■ Describe what you do when you feel stressed.
Value-Belief	■ Describe how specific relationships or activities help you cope with this problem. ■ Describe specific cultural beliefs or practices that affect how you care for and feel about this problem. ■ Are there any specific treatments that you would not use to treat this condition?

TABLE 27–2 Age-Related Urinary System Changes

AGE-RELATED CHANGE	SIGNIFICANCE
Kidneys: ↓ size of renal cortex and number of nephrons, ↓ growth of renal tissue, ↑ risk of atherosclerosis, all of which may result in atrophy of the kidneys.	■ Decreased renal blood flow. ■ Decreased GFR by about 50% between ages 20 and 90.
Renal tubules: ↓ function, with less effective exchange of substances, water and sodium conservation and suppression of ADH secretion in presence of hypoosmolality.	■ Risk of hyponatremia and nocturia. ■ Effects of medications may be altered (with decreased filtration). ■ Decreased reabsorption of glucose may result in 1+ proteinuria and glycosuria, which are **not** of major clinical significance.
Bladder: ■ Muscles weaken and bladder capacity decreases. ■ More difficult to empty bladder. ■ Delayed micturition reflex.	■ Urinary retention is more common. ■ Urinary frequency, urgency, and nocturia are more common with aging. ■ Larger amounts of residual urine present after voiding. ■ Some stress incontinence may occur, especially in women who have had several children. ■ Urinary incontinence is not a normal outcome of aging.

BOX 27–1 Guidelines for Physical Assessment of the Kidneys

Percussion of the Kidneys

Percussion of the kidneys helps assess pain or tenderness. Assist the client to a sitting position, and stand behind the client. For indirect percussion, place the palm of your nondominant hand over the costovertebral angle (see Figure A). Strike this area with the ulnar surface of your dominant hand, curled into a fist (see Figure B). For direct percussion, also strike the area over the costovertebral angle with the ulnar surface of your dominant hand, curled into a fist. Repeat the technique for the other kidney.

You should do percussion of the kidneys with only enough force so the client feels a gentle thud. Percussion is usually done at the end of the assessment.

Palpation of the Kidneys

Although the technique of palpation of the kidneys is outlined here, this technique is best performed by an advanced practitioner, be-cause it involves deep palpation. In addition, the kidneys are difficult to palpate.

Assist the client to the supine position and stand at the right side of the client. To palpate the left kidney, reach across the client and place your left hand under the client's left flank with your palm upward. Elevate the left flank with your fingers, displacing the kidney upward. Ask the client to take a deep breath and use the palmer surface of your right hand to palpate the kidney (Figure C). Repeat the technique for the right kidney.

B Percussing the kidney.

C Palpating the left kidney.

—12th rib

Costovertebral angle

A Location of the kidneys and the costovertebral angle.

URINARY ASSESSMENTS

Technique/Normal Findings	Abnormal Findings

Skin Assessment

Inspect the skin and mucous membranes, noting color, turgor, and excretions. *The color of skin and mucous membranes should be even and appropriate to the age and race of the client; skin should be dry with no visible excretions.*

- Pallor of the skin and mucous membranes may indicate kidney disease with resultant anemia.
- Decreased turgor of the skin may indicate dehydration.
- Edema (generalized or in the lower extremities) may indicate fluid volume excess. (Changes in skin turgor may indicate renal insufficiency with either excess fluid loss or retention.)
- An accumulation of uric acid crystals, called uremic frost, may be seen on the skin of the client with late-stage renal failure.

Abdominal Assessment

Inspect the abdomen, noting size, symmetry, masses or lumps, swelling, distention, glistening, or skin tightness. *The abdomen should be slightly concave, symmetric, without distention or masses.*

- Enlargements or asymmetry may indicate a hernia or superficial mass.
- If the urinary bladder is distended, it rises above the symphysis pubis as a rounded mass.
- Distention, glistening, or skin tightness may be associated with fluid retention.
- Ascites is an accumulation of fluid in the peritoneal cavity.

Urinary Meatus Assessment

This technique is not part of a routine assessment, but it is an important component in clients with health problems of the urinary system. Further discussion is included in Chapter 49 ∞.

For the male client: With the client in a sitting or standing position, compress the tip of the glans penis with your gloved hand to open the urinary meatus (Figure 27–7 ■).

For the female client: With the client in the dorsal lithotomy position, spread the labia with your gloved hand to expose the urinary meatus.

The urinary meatus should be midline and free of redness, lesions, or discharge.

- Increased redness, swelling, or discharge from the urinary meatus may indicate infection or sexually transmitted infection.
- Ulceration of the urinary meatus may indicate a sexually transmitted infection.
- Hypospadias is displacement of the urinary meatus to the ventral surface of the penis.
- Epispadias is displacement of the urinary meatus to the dorsal surface of the penis.

Figure 27–7 ■ Inspecting the urinary meatus of the male.

Kidney Assessment

See Box 27–1 for assessment guidelines for percussion and palpation of the kidneys.

Auscultate the renal arteries by placing the bell of the stethoscope lightly in the areas of the renal arteries, located in the left and right upper abdominal quadrants. *Bruits are not normally heard over the renal arteries.*

- Systolic bruits ("whooshing" sounds) may indicate renal artery stenosis.

Technique/Normal Findings	Abnormal Findings
Percuss the kidneys for tenderness or pain. *No tenderness or pain should be elicited.*	■ Tenderness and pain on percussion of the costovertebral angle suggest glomerulonephritis or glomerulonephrosis.
Palpate the kidneys. The lower pole of the right kidney may be palpable with deep palpation; the remaining right kidney and the left kidney are normally not palpable. *If palpable, they should be nontender, bilaterally of appropriate size and density, without palpable masses.*	■ A mass or lump may indicate a tumor or cyst. ■ Tenderness or pain on palpation may suggest an inflammatory process. ■ A soft kidney that feels spongy may indicate chronic renal disease. ■ Bilaterally enlarged kidneys may suggest polycystic kidney disease. ■ Unequal kidney size may indicate hydronephrosis.

Bladder Assessment

Percuss the bladder for tone and position. *The bladder should be midline without dullness.*	■ A dull percussion tone over the bladder of a client who has just urinated may indicate urinary retention.
Palpate the bladder (over the symphysis pubis and abdomen) for distention. *The bladder is normally not palpable.*	■ A distended bladder may be palpated at any point from the symphysis pubis to the umbilicus and is felt as a firm, rounded organ. It indicates urinary retention.

EXPLORE MEDIALINK

Prentice Hall Nursing MediaLink DVD-ROM
   Audio Glossary
   NCLEX-RN® Review

   Animation
   The Kidney

COMPANION WEBSITE www.prenhall.com/lemone
   Audio Glossary
   NCLEX-RN® Review
   Care Plan Activity: Urinary System Disorder
   Case Studies
      Urinary Calculi
      Urine Characteristics
   MediaLink Applications
      Renal Function
      Urinary Diversions
   Links to Resources

TEST YOURSELF NCLEX-RN® REVIEW

1 What part of the kidney processes the blood to make urine?
   1. ureter
   2. medulla
   3. pyramids
   4. nephrons

2 A client has been vomiting for 4 hours. What hormone is increased as a result?
   1. thyroxine
   2. renin
   3. aldosterone
   4. ADH

3 What diagnostic test can be used to determine GFR as well as glomerular damage?
1. routine urinalysis
2. renal scan
3. creatinine clearance
4. renal biopsy

4 What gland encircles the male urethra at the base of the bladder?
1. spleen
2. pancreas
3. prostate
4. adrenal

5 Your client tells you of having to get up to void several times a night. You record this finding as:
1. polyuria.
2. nocturia.
3. dysuria.
4. hematuria.

6 What question would you ask a client prior to an IVP?
1. "Are you allergic to shellfish?"
2. "Do you have burning on urination?"
3. "Have you ever had kidney stones?"
4. "Why are you having this test?"

7 Before beginning the physical assessment of the urinary system, you should ask the client to:
1. empty the bladder.
2. take several deep breaths.
3. provide a urine specimen.
4. drink several glasses of water.

8 Following surgery, your client has not voided for 12 hours. What assessment should you make?
1. Palpate for bladder distention.
2. Auscultate for bowel sounds.
3. Inspect for edema of the urethra.
4. Percuss for gastric tympany.

9 Of the following health problems an older woman may have, which is not normally a part of aging of the urinary system?
1. increased risk for hematuria
2. decreased risk for infection
3. urine that is darker in color
4. urinary incontinence

10 What assessment would you use to assess hydration status of a client?
1. auscultation of renal arteries
2. palpation for skin turgor
3. percussion for dullness over bladder
4. palpation of both kidneys

See Test Yourself answers in Appendix C.

BIBLIOGRAPHY

Amella, E. (2004). Presentation of illness in older adults: If you think you know what you're looking for, think again. *American Journal of Nursing, 104*(10), 40–52.

Bickley, L., & Szilagyi, P. (2005). *Bates' guide to physical examination and history taking* (9th ed.). Philadelphia: Lippincott.

Bland-Reid, C. (2004). Abdominal trauma: Dealing with the damage. *Nursing, 34*(9), 36–42.

Consentino, B. (2004, January 12). Electrolyte imbalance: A matter of equilibrium. *Nursing Spectrum (New York/New Jersey Metro Edition),* pp. 4–6.

Cooper, G., & Watt, E. (2003). An exploration of acute care nurses' approach to assessment and management of people with urinary incontinence. *Journal of WOCN, 30*(6), 305–313.

Dowling-Castronovo, A. (2004). Try this: Best practices in nursing care to older adults from the Hartford Institute for Geriatric Nursing. Urinary incontinence assessment. *Dermatology Nursing, 16*(1), 97–98.

Eliopoulos, C. (2005). *Gerontological nursing* (6th ed.). Philadelphia: Lippincott Williams & Wilkins.

Enriquez, E. (2004). A nursing analysis of the causes of and approaches for urinary incontinence among elderly women in nursing homes. *Ostomy/Wound Management, 50*(6), 24–26, 28, 30.

Hunt, S. (2002). Making sense of assessment data—continence charts. *ACCNS Journal for Community Nurses, 7*(1), 17.

Jarvis, C. (2004). *Physical examination & health assessment.* St. Louis, MO: Mosby.

Kee, J. (2005). *Prentice Hall handbook of laboratory & diagnostic tests with nursing implications.* Upper Saddle River, NJ: Prentice Hall.

Kershen, R., & Appell, R. (2004). Voiding dysfunction: Evaluation and treatment after anti-incontinence surgery. *Contemporary Urology, 16*(3), 31–32, 35–38, 41–43.

Lekan-Rutledge, D. (2004). Urinary incontinence strategies for frail elderly women. *Urologic Nursing, 24*(4), 281–283, 287–302.

Mehta, M. (2003). Assessing the abdomen: Use sight, sound and touch to screen for abnormalities. *Nursing, 33*(5), 54–55.

Midthun, S. (2004). Criteria for urinary tract infection in the elderly: Variables that challenge nursing assessment. *Urologic Nursing, 24*(3), 157–162, 166–170, 186.

National Institutes of Health. (2003). *Genes and disease: Cancers.* Retrieved from http://www.ncbi.nlm.nih.gov/books/bv.fcgi?rid=gnd.section.109

Palmer, M. (2004). Physiologic and psychologic age-related changes that affect urologic clients. *Urologic Nursing, 24*(4), 247–252, 257.

Perform abdominal assessment, or risk missing life-threatening trauma injury: Don't allow 'invisible' injuries to escape detection in your ED. (2004). *ED Nursing, 7*(7), 73–75.

Porth, C. (2005). *Pathophysiology: Concepts of altered health states* (7th ed.). Philadelphia: Lippincott.

Weber, J., & Kelley, J. (2006). *Health assessment in nursing* (3rd ed.). Philadelphia: Lippincott.

CHAPTER 28 Nursing Care of Clients with Urinary Tract Disorders

LEARNING OUTCOMES

- Explain the pathophysiology of common urinary tract disorders.
- Describe the manifestations of urinary tract disorders, relating manifestations to the pathophysiology of the disorder.
- Discuss tests used to diagnose disorders affecting the urinary tract with their nursing implications.
- Discuss the nursing implications of medications and treatments prescribed for clients with urinary tract disorders.
- Describe surgical procedures used in treating urinary tract disorders.

CLINICAL COMPETENCIES

- Assess the functional health status of clients with urinary tract disorders, using data to determine priority nursing diagnoses and select individualized nursing interventions.
- Identify, report, and document abnormal or unexpected assessments, monitoring client status.
- Use evidence-based research to plan and implement nursing care for clients with urinary tract disorders.
- Integrate the interdisciplinary plan of care into care for clients with urinary tract disorders.
- Knowledgeably and safely administer prescribed medications and treatments for clients with urinary tract disorders.
- Provide effective nursing care for clients undergoing surgery of the urinary tract.
- Plan and provide appropriate teaching for prevention of and self-care of urinary tract disorders.
- Evaluate client responses, revising plan of care as needed to promote, maintain, or restore functional health of clients with urinary tract disorders.

MEDIALINK

Resources for this chapter can be found on the Prentice Hall Nursing MediaLink DVD-ROM accompanying this textbook, and on the Companion Website at http://www.prenhall.com/lemone

The urinary system includes the kidneys, ureters, urinary bladder, and urethra. This organ system can be affected by a variety of disorders, including congenital malformations, infections, obstructions, trauma, tumors, and neurologic conditions. Any portion of the system—from the kidney through the urethra—can be affected with serious or even life-threatening consequences unless the problem is appropriately diagnosed and treated. Kidney disorders can affect urine production and waste elimination directly, and are discussed in the next chapter. Disorders of the **urinary drainage system** (the kidney pelvis, ureters, bladder, and urethra) may obstruct urine flow or spread to the kidneys, affecting urine production and elimination. The anatomy and physiology and nursing assessment related to the urinary tract is presented in Chapter 27 ∞.

When caring for clients with urinary tract disorders, it is important to consider the client's modesty in voiding, possible difficulty in discussing the genitals, embarrassment about being exposed for examination and testing, and fear of changes in body image or function. These psychosocial issues may interfere with the client's willingness to seek help, discuss treatment, and learn about preventive measures.

Nursing interventions for clients with urinary tract disorders are directed toward primary prevention, early detection, and management of the disorder through health teaching and nursing care.

THE CLIENT WITH A URINARY TRACT INFECTION

Bacterial infections of the urinary tract are a common reason for seeking health services, second only to upper respiratory infections. More than 8 million people are treated annually for urinary tract infection (UTI) (Porth, 2005). Community-acquired UTIs are common in young women, and unusual in men under the age of 50.

Most community-acquired UTIs are caused by *Escherichia coli*, a common gram-negative enteral bacteria. About 10% to 15% of symptomatic UTIs are caused by *Staphylococcus saprophyticus*, a gram-positive organism. Catheter-associated UTIs often involve other gram-negative bacteria such as *Proteus*, *Klebsiella*, *Serratia*, and *Pseudomonas*.

Risk Factors for UTI

Clients can be predisposed to UTI by a variety of factors (Box 28–1). Some risk factors cannot be changed (e.g., aging and the short urethra of the female). In women, sexual activity in-

creases the risk for UTI, because bacteria can be introduced into the bladder via the urethra during sexual intercourse. Use of spermicidal compounds with a diaphragm, cervical cap, or condom alters the normal bacterial flora of the vagina and perineal tissues and further increases the risk for UTI. Some females lack a normally protective mucosal enzyme and have decreased levels of cervicovaginal antibodies to enterobacteria, further increasing their risk. Prostatic hypertrophy and bacterial prostatitis are risk factors among males. Circumcision appears to have a protective effect. Anal intercourse also is a risk factor for men. Congenital or acquired factors contributing to the risk of infection include urinary tract obstruction by tumors or calculi, structural abnormalities such as strictures, impaired bladder innervation, bowel incontinence, and chronic diseases such as diabetes mellitus. Instrumentation of the urinary tract (e.g., catheterization or cystoscopy) is a major risk factor for UTI. Even when performed under strict aseptic conditions, catheterization can result in bladder infection. Recent research indicates that the risk for catheter-associated UTI is reduced when anesthetic lubricating gels are inserted into the urethra prior to catheter insertion (Bardsley, 2005). The placement of the catheter prevents the flushing action of voiding, and bacteria may as-

---

BOX 28–1 Risk Factors for UTI

Female
- Short, straight urethra
- Proximity of urinary meatus to vagina and anus
- Sexual intercourse
- Use of diaphragm and spermicidal compounds for birth control
- Pregnancy

Male
- Uncircumcised
- Prostatic hypertrophy
- Anal intercourse

Both
- Aging
- Urinary tract obstruction
- Neurogenic bladder dysfunction
- Vesicoureteral reflux
- Genetic factors
- Catheterization

cend to the bladder either through the catheter lumen or via exudate between the urethral mucosa and the catheter.

> **FAST FACTS**
> - Up to three UTIs annually is considered to be within normal limits for sexually active women and does not usually warrant additional diagnostic tests beyond urine culture.
> - In healthy adult men, however, UTIs are unusual and may prompt additional diagnostic testing.

Older clients have an increased incidence of UTI. The greatest degree of increase is seen in men, as the ratio of female-to-male UTI in older adults changes from 50:1 to less than 5:1. An increased risk of urinary stasis, chronic disease states (such as diabetes mellitus), and an impaired immune response contribute to the higher incidence of UTI in the older adult. In men, the prostate typically hypertrophies with aging, potentially resulting in urinary retention as the urethra narrows. Prostatic secretions are lessened, diminishing their protective, antibacterial effect. In older women, loss of tissue elasticity and weakening of perineal muscles often contribute to the development of a cystocele or rectocele. Resulting changes in bladder and urethral position increase the risk of incomplete bladder emptying.

Physiology Review

The urinary tract is normally sterile above the urethra. Adequate urine volume, a free flow from the kidneys through the urinary meatus, and complete bladder emptying are the most important mechanisms maintaining sterility. Pathogens that enter and contaminate the distal urethra are washed out during voiding. Other defenses for maintaining sterile urine include its normal acidity and bacteriostatic properties of the bladder and urethral cells. The peristaltic activity of the ureters and a competent vesicoureteral junction help maintain sterility of the upper urinary tract. As the ureter enters the bladder, its distal portion tunnels between the mucosa and muscle layers of the bladder wall (Figure 28–1 ■). During voiding, increased *intravesicular* (within the bladder) pressure compresses the ureter, preventing **reflux**, or backflow of urine toward the kidneys. In males, a long urethra and the antibacterial effect of zinc in prostatic fluid also help prevent contamination of this normally sterile environment.

Pathophysiology and Manifestations

Pathogens usually enter the urinary tract by ascending from the mucous membranes of the perineal area into the lower urinary tract. Bacteria that have colonized the urethra, vagina, or perineal tissues are the usual source of infection (Porth, 2005). From the bladder, bacteria may continue to ascend the urinary tract, eventually infecting the *parenchyma* (functional tissue) of the kidneys (Kasper et al., 2005). Hematogenous spread of infection to the urinary tract is rare. Infections introduced in this manner are usually associated with previous damage or scarring of the urinary tract. Bacteria introduced into the urinary tract may cause asymptomatic bacteriuria or an inflammatory response with manifestations of UTI.

Urinary tract infections can be categorized in several ways. Anatomically, UTIs may affect the lower or the upper urinary tract. Lower urinary tract infections include *urethritis*, inflammation of the urethra; *prostatitis*, inflammation of the prostate gland (discussed in Chapter 49 ∞); and **cystitis**, inflammation of the urinary bladder. The most common upper urinary tract infection is **pyelonephritis**, inflammation of the kidney and renal pelvis. The infection may involve superficial tissues such as the bladder mucosa, or may invade other tissues such as prostate or renal tissues. Epidemiologically, UTIs are identified as community acquired or **nosocomial**, associated with catheterization.

Cystitis

Cystitis, inflammation of the urinary bladder, is the most common UTI. The infection tends to remain superficial, involving the bladder mucosa. The mucosa becomes hyperemic (red) and may hemorrhage (Figure 28–2 ■). The inflammatory response causes pus to form. This process causes the classic manifestations associated with cystitis. Typical presenting symptoms of cystitis include **dysuria** (painful or difficult urination), urinary frequency and **urgency** (a sudden, compelling need to urinate), and **nocturia** (voiding two or more times at night). In addition,

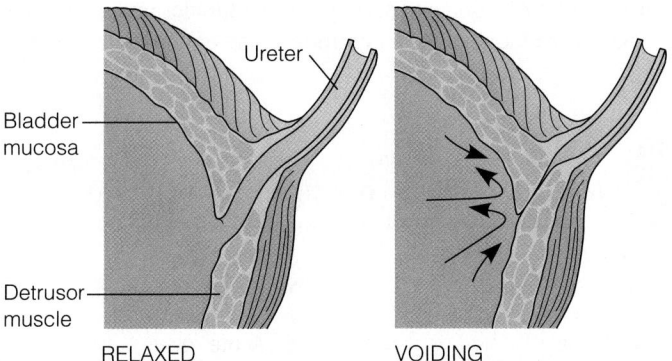

Figure 28–1 ■ A competent vesicoureteral junction. Note how increased intravesicular pressure during voiding occludes the distal portion of the ureter, preventing reflux.

Figure 28–2 ■ Appearance of the bladder wall affected by cystitis.
Source: Craig Zuckerman/Phototake NYC

the urine may have a foul odor and appear cloudy (*pyuria*) or bloody (**hematuria**) because of mucus, excess white cells in the urine, and bleeding of the inflamed bladder wall. Suprapubic pain and tenderness also may be present. See the box below for manifestations of cystitis.

Cystitis occurs most frequently in adult females, usually because of colonization of the bladder by bacteria normally found in the lower gastrointestinal tract. These bacteria gain entry by ascending the short, straight female urethra. In addition to the risk factors listed on page 846, personal hygiene practices and voluntary urinary retention can contribute to the risk for UTI in women.

Older clients may not experience the classic symptoms of cystitis. Instead, they often present with nonspecific manifestations such as nocturia, incontinence, confusion, behavior change, lethargy, anorexia, or "just not feeling right." Fever may be present; however, hypothermia also may develop in an older adult.

Although the bacteriostatic effect of prostatic fluid and a longer urethra provide an effective barrier to bladder infection for adult males, the prostatic hypertrophy commonly associated with aging increases the risk of cystitis in elderly males. An enlarged prostate can impede urine flow, leading to incomplete bladder emptying and urinary stasis. Bacteria are not completely flushed with voiding, allowing colonization of the bladder.

Cystitis is usually uncomplicated and readily responds to treatment. When left untreated, the infection can ascend to involve the kidneys. Severe or prolonged infection may lead to sloughing of bladder mucosa and ulcer formation. Chronic cystitis can lead to bladder stones (discussed later in this chapter).

Catheter-Associated UTI

At least 10% to 15% of hospitalized clients with indwelling urinary catheters develop bacteriuria. The longer the catheter remains in place, the greater the risk for infection. Bacteria, including *E. coli, Proteus, Pseudomonas,* and *Klebsiella,* reach the bladder by either migrating through the column of urine within the catheter or by moving up the mucous sheath of the urethra outside the catheter (Kasper et al., 2005). Bacteria enter the catheter system at the connection between the catheter and drainage system or through the emptying tube of the drainage bag. Colonization of perineal skin by bowel flora is a common source of infection in catheterized women.

Catheter-associated UTIs often are asymptomatic. Gram-negative bacteremia is the most significant complication associated with these UTIs. Most catheter-associated UTIs resolve quickly when the catheter is removed and a short course of antibiotic is administered. Intermittent catheterization carries a lower risk of infection than does an indwelling catheter, and is preferred for clients who are unable to empty their bladder by voiding.

Instillation of anesthetic lubricating gel into the urethra prior to catheter insertion further reduces the risk by dilating the urethra and reducing trauma to fragile urethral tissues (Bardsley, 2005).

Pyelonephritis

Pyelonephritis is inflammation of the renal pelvis and parenchyma, the functional kidney tissue. *Acute pyelonephritis* is a bacterial infection of the kidney; *chronic pyelonephritis* is associated with nonbacterial infections and inflammatory processes that may be metabolic, chemical, or immunologic in origin.

ACUTE PYELONEPHRITIS Acute pyelonephritis usually results from an infection that ascends to the kidney from the lower urinary tract. Asymptomatic bacteriuria or cystitis can lead to acute pyelonephritis. Risk factors include pregnancy (because of slowed ureteral peristalsis), urinary tract obstruction, and congenital malformation. Urinary tract trauma, scarring, calculi (stones), kidney disorders such as polycystic or hypertensive kidney disease, and chronic diseases such as diabetes may also contribute to pyelonephritis. *Vesicoureteral reflux,* a condition in which urine moves from the bladder back toward the kidney, is a common risk factor in children who develop pyelonephritis and is also seen in adults when bladder outflow is obstructed.

The infection spreads from the renal pelvis to the renal cortex. The pelvis, calyces, and medulla of the kidney are primarily affected, with white blood cell (WBC) infiltration and inflammation. The kidney becomes grossly edematous. Localized abscesses may develop on the cortical surface of the kidney. As with cystitis, *E. coli* is the organism responsible for 85% of the cases of acute pyelonephritis. Other organisms commonly found include *Proteus* and *Klebsiella,* bacteria that normally inhabit the intestinal tract.

The onset of acute pyelonephritis is typically rapid, with chills and fever, malaise, vomiting, flank pain, costovertebral tenderness, urinary frequency, and dysuria (see the Manifestations box below). Symptoms of cystitis also may be present. The older adult may present with a change in behavior, acute confusion, incontinence, or a general deterioration in condition.

CHRONIC PYELONEPHRITIS Chronic pyelonephritis involves chronic inflammation and scarring of the tubules and interstitial tissues of the kidney. It is a common cause of chronic renal fail-

---

MANIFESTATIONS of Cystitis

- Dysuria
- Frequency
- Urgency
- Nocturia
- Pyuria
- Hematuria
- Suprapubic discomfort

MANIFESTATIONS of Acute Pyelonephritis

URINARY	SYSTEMIC
■ Urinary frequency	■ Vomiting
■ Dysuria	■ Diarrhea
■ Pyuria	■ Acute fever
■ Hematuria	■ Shaking chills
■ Flank pain	■ Malaise
■ Costovertebral tenderness	

ure. It may develop as a result of UTIs or other conditions that damage the kidneys, such as hypertension or vascular conditions, severe vesicoureteral reflux, or obstruction of the urinary tract.

The client with chronic pyelonephritis may be asymptomatic or have mild manifestations such as urinary frequency, dysuria, and flank pain. Hypertension can develop as kidney tissue is destroyed.

FAST FACTS

- The most common route of entry for a urinary tract infection is ascending, from colonization of the perineal tissues by fecal bacteria (usually *E. coli*), through the urethra, into the bladder (cystitis) and possibly kidney tissue (pyelonephritis).

INTERDISCIPLINARY CARE

Treatment of UTI focuses on eliminating the causative organism, preventing relapse or reinfection, and identifying and correcting any contributing factors. Drug treatment with antibiotics and urinary anti-infectives is commonly used. In some cases, surgery may be indicated to correct contributing factors.

Diagnosis

Laboratory testing for UTI includes:

- *Urinalysis* to assess for pyuria, bacteria, and blood cells in the urine. A bacteria count greater than 100,000 (10^5) per milliliter is indicative of infection. Rapid tests for bacteria in the urine include using a *nitrite dipstick* (which turns pink in the presence of bacteria) and the *leukocyte esterase test,* an indirect method of detecting bacteria by identifying lysed or intact WBCs in the urine.

  Urine should be a midstream clean-catch specimen; if necessary, straight catheterization or "mini-cath," with strict aseptic technique, may be used. Catheterization is avoided if possible to reduce the risk of further infection. See the Diagnostic Tests table beginning on page 835 for nursing care related to collecting a urinalysis specimen.
- *Gram stain of the urine* may be done to identify the infecting organism by shape and characteristic (gram-positive or gram-negative).
- *Urine culture and sensitivity* tests may be ordered to identify the infecting organism and the most effective antibiotic. Culture requires 24 to 72 hours, so treatment to eliminate the most common organisms often is initiated without culture.
- *WBC with differential* may be done to detect typical changes associated with infection, such as *leukocytosis* (elevated WBC) and increased numbers of neutrophils.

In men and in adult women with recurrent infections or persistent bacteriuria, additional diagnostic testing may be ordered to evaluate for structural abnormalities and other contributing factors:

- *Intravenous pyelography (IVP),* also known as *excretory urography,* is used to evaluate the structure and excretory function of the kidneys, ureters, and bladder. As the kidneys clear an intravenously injected contrast medium from the blood, the size and shape of the kidneys, their calyces and pelvises, the ureters, and the bladder can be evaluated, and

structural or functional abnormalities, such as vesicoureteral reflux, may be detected.

- *Voiding cystourethrography* involves instilling contrast medium into the bladder, then using x-rays to assess the bladder and urethra when filled and during voiding. This study can detect structural or functional abnormalities of the bladder and urethral strictures. This test has a lower risk of allergic response to the contrast dye than IVP.
- *Cystoscopy,* direct visualization of the urethra and bladder through a cystoscope, may be used to diagnose conditions such as prostatic hypertrophy, urethral strictures, bladder calculi, tumors, polyps or diverticula, and congenital abnormalities. A tissue biopsy may be obtained during the procedure, and other interventions performed (e.g., stone removal or stricture dilation).
- *Manual pelvic* or *prostate examinations* are done to assess for structural changes of the genitourinary tract, such as prostatic enlargement, cystocele, or rectocele.

Nursing implications for these diagnostic procedures are presented in Chapter 27 ∞ .

Medications

Most uncomplicated infections of the lower urinary tract can be treated with a short course of antibiotic therapy. Upper urinary tract infections, in contrast, usually require longer treatment (2 or more weeks) to eradicate the infecting organism.

Short-course therapy (either a single antibiotic dose or a 3-day course of treatment) reduces treatment cost, increases compliance, and has a lower rate of side effects. Single-dose therapy is associated with a higher rate of recurrent infection and continued vaginal colonization with *E. coli,* making a 3-day course of treatment the preferred option for uncomplicated cystitis. Oral trimethoprim-sulfamethoxazole (TMP-SMZ), TMP, or a quinolone antibiotic such as ciprofloxacin (Cipro) or enoxacin (Penetrex) may be ordered.

Men and women with pyelonephritis, urinary tract abnormalities or stones, or a history of previous infections with antibiotic-resistant infections require a 7- to 10-day course of TMP-SMZ, ciprofloxacin, ofloxacin (Floxin), or an alternate antibiotic. The client with severe illness may need hospitalization. Intravenous ciprofloxacin, gentamicin, ceftriaxone (Rocephin), or ampicillin may be prescribed for severe illness or sepsis associated with UTI. See Chapter 12 ∞ for the nursing implications for antibiotic therapy.

The outcome of treatment for UTI is determined by follow-up urinalysis and culture. *Cure,* as evidenced by no pathogens present in the urine, is the desired outcome. When therapy fails to eradicate bacteria in the urine, it is known as *unresolved bacteriuria. Persistent bacteriuria* or *relapse* occurs when a persistent source of infection causes repeated infection after initial cure. *Reinfection* is the development of a new infection with a different pathogen following successful UTI treatment (Tierney et al., 2005).

PRACTICE ALERT

Follow-up urine culture is scheduled 10 days to 2 weeks following completion of antibiotic therapy for UTI to ensure that bacteria have been eradicated from the urinary tract.

Clients who experience frequent symptomatic UTIs may be treated with prophylactic antibiotic therapy with a drug such as TMP-SMZ, TMP, or nitrofurantoin (Furadantin, Macrodantin, Macrobid). TMP and nitrofurantoin do not achieve effective plasma concentrations at recommended doses, but do reach effective concentrations in the urine. Nitrofurantoin also may be used to treat UTI in pregnant women. Nursing implications for these urinary anti-infectives and for phenazopyridine (Pyridium), a urinary analgesic, are outlined in the Medication Administration box below.

Antibiotics and urinary anti-infectives are not generally recommended to treat asymptomatic bacteriuria in catheterized clients. The preferred treatment for catheter-associated UTI is removal of the indwelling catheter followed by a 10- to 14-day course of antibiotic therapy to eliminate the infection.

Surgery

Surgery may be indicated for recurrent UTI if diagnostic testing indicates calculi, structural anomalies, or strictures that contribute to the risk of infection. Table 28–1 lists major causes of urinary tract obstruction that may contribute to UTI.

Stones, or *calculi*, in the renal pelvis or in the bladder are an irritant and provide a matrix for bacterial colonization. Treatment may include surgical removal of a large calculus from the renal

---

MEDICATION ADMINISTRATION **Urinary Anti-Infectives and Analgesics**

URINARY ANTI-INFECTIVES
Nitrofurantoin (Furadantin, Macrodantin, Macrobid)
Trimethoprim (Proloprim, Trimpex)
Urinary anti-infectives are usually used prophylactically to prevent recurrence of UTI in clients with frequent symptomatic infections. Nitrofurantoin also may be used to treat UTI in pregnant women.

Nursing Responsibilities
- Ensure adequate fluid intake (1500 to 2000 mL/day) to maintain a urine output of at least 1500 mL of urine per 24 hours. Do not overhydrate.
- Administer with meals to minimize GI side effects, such as nausea, gastric upset, and abdominal cramping.
- Trimethoprim is contraindicated for use in clients with renal or hepatic impairment; nitrofurantoin is contraindicated for clients with impaired renal function. Report abnormal laboratory values such as elevated creatinine or BUN, bilirubin, alanine aminotransferase (ALT), aspartate aminotransferase (AST), and lactic dehydrogenase (LDH).
- Use with caution in older or chronically ill clients. Monitor closely for adverse effects.
- Do not administer trimethoprim to pregnant women because of possible adverse effects on the fetus.
- Monitor the client taking nitrofurantoin for an acute or chronic pulmonary reaction with manifestations of dyspnea, cough, chills, fever, and chest pain. Discontinue the drug and notify the physician.
- Nitrofurantoin may cause peripheral neuropathy, especially in older clients and adult diabetics. Notify the physician if symptoms develop.
- Nitrofurantoin oral suspension may stain the teeth; have the client rinse the mouth thoroughly after administering.
- Monitor for signs of phenytoin toxicity (sedation, ataxia, and increased blood levels) if trimethoprim is given concurrently. Phenytoin doses may need to be reduced.

Health Education for the Client and Family
- These drugs are used along with hygiene practices to prevent recurrent UTI. Take as directed, even when no symptoms are present.
- Drink six to eight glasses of water or fluid per day while taking these drugs.
- Take the drug with meals or food to reduce gastric effects; however, avoid milk products because they may interfere with absorption.

- Trimethoprim should not be taken during pregnancy. Contact your physician before attempting to become pregnant.
- Contact your doctor if you develop any of the following: chest pain, difficulty breathing, cough, chills, and fever; numbness and tingling or weakness of the extremities; rash or pruritus (itching).
- If you are taking an oral suspension of nitrofurantoin, rinse your mouth thoroughly after each dose to avoid staining the teeth.
- Nitrofurantoin turns the urine brown. This is not harmful and subsides when the drug is discontinued.
- If you are taking trimethoprim along with phenytoin (Dilantin) or a related anticonvulsant, contact your doctor if you become sedated or begin to stagger.

URINARY ANALGESIC
Phenazopyridine (Pyridium)
Phenazopyridine is a urinary tract analgesic that may be used for symptomatic relief of the pain, burning, frequency, and urgency associated with UTI during the first 24 to 48 hours of therapy. Its use is somewhat controversial, because it does not treat the infection and may delay effective treatment in the client with recurrent UTI who saves a dose or two "for the next time."

Nursing Responsibilities
- Monitor renal function (urine output, weight, serum creatinine, and BUN) during treatment; report changes.
- Stop the drug and contact the physician if sclera or skin become yellow, tinged. This may indicate reduced excretion and toxicity.

Health Education for the Client and Family
- Take with meals to minimize gastric upset.
- Consume 2 to 3 quarts of fluid daily while taking this drug.
- If you are a diabetic, check your blood sugars regularly while taking this drug.
- This drug turns urine orange or red. Protect your clothing from staining.
- Contact lenses may become stained if worn while taking this drug.
- Promptly contact your doctor if symptoms of UTI recur; do not take phenazopyridine before you seek medical treatment.
- If you develop itching or notice a yellow tinge to your skin or eyes, stop taking the drug and notify the physician.

TABLE 28–1	**Major Causes of Urinary Tract Obstruction by Location**
LOCATION	**OBSTRUCTIVE PROCESS**
Kidney pelvis	Calculi (stones)
	Polycystic kidney disease
	Infection and scarring
Ureters	Calculi
	Scarring and stricture
	Congenital defects or strictures
	External processes such as pregnancy, tumors, lymph node enlargement
Bladder	Neurogenic bladder
	Tumors
	Calculi and other foreign bodies
Urethra	Benign prostatic hypertrophy
	Tumors
	Scarring and stricture
	Trauma

pelvis or cystoscopic removal of bladder calculi. *Percutaneous ultrasonic pyelolithotomy* or *extracorporeal shock wave lithotripsy* (described in the next section of this chapter) may be used instead of surgery to crush and remove stones. (See the Diagnostic Tests box on page 837 for nursing care related to cystoscopy.)

Ureteroplasty, surgical repair of a ureter, may be indicated for structural abnormality or stricture of a ureter. This may be combined with a ureteral reimplantation if vesicoureteral reflux is present. The client returns from these surgeries with an indwelling urinary catheter (Foley or suprapubic) and a **ureteral stent** (a thin catheter inserted into the ureter to provide for urine flow and ureteral support), which remains in place for 3 to 5 days. Care of the client with a ureteral stent is outlined in the box below.

COMPLEMENTARY THERAPIES Complementary therapies such as aromatherapy or herbal preparations may be used in conjunction with antibiotics to treat UTI. Low-sugar cranberry juice or extract and blueberry juice also are commonly used to prevent and treat UTI. Adding bergamot, sandalwood, lavender, or juniper oil to bath water helps relieve the discomfort of UTI. Herbal supplements such as saw palmetto have a urinary antiseptic effect, and may be beneficial in treating or preventing UTI. Consult a qualified herbologist for recommended doses and appropriate use.

NURSING CARE

Health Promotion

Teach measures to prevent UTI to all clients, particularly to young, sexually active women. Encourage clients to maintain a generous fluid intake of 2.0 to 2.5 quarts per day, increasing

NURSING CARE OF THE CLIENT WITH A   Ureteral Stent

Ureteral stents are used to maintain patency and promote healing of the ureters (see figure below). A stent may be temporary, used during and after a surgical procedure, or it may be used for longer periods in clients with ureteral obstruction due to tumors, strictures, or other causes.

Stents may be positioned during surgery or cystoscopy. They are made of a nontoxic material such as silicone or polyurethane, with

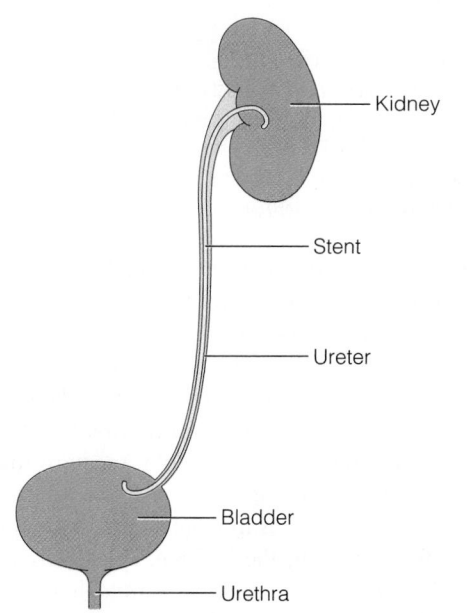

side drainage holes placed along the length of the stent. Stents are radiopaque for easy radiographic identification. One or both ends of the stent may be pigtail or J shaped to prevent migration.

- Label all drainage tubes including stents for easy identification. Attach each catheter and stent to a separate closed drainage system. *Careful labeling allows close monitoring of output from all sources and reservoirs. Separate drainage systems minimize the risk of infection.*
- If the stent has been brought to the surface, secure it and maintain its position. *The stent is usually placed in the renal pelvis. It is important to secure it well to prevent trauma to the kidney, inadvertent removal of the stent, and ureter obstruction.*
- Monitor urine output, including color, consistency, and odor. Monitor for signs of infection or bleeding: fever, tachycardia, pain, hematuria, and cloudy or malodorous urine. *The stent facilitates urine flow but may become obstructed because of bleeding, calculi, or sediment. Obstruction may result in hydronephrosis and kidney damage. The stent itself is a foreign body in the urinary tract and can increase the risk of UTI.*
- Maintain fluid intake, encouraging fluids that acidify urine, such as low-sugar apple, cranberry, and blueberry juice. *The stent can precipitate calculus formation as well as UTI. Increasing fluid intake and acidifying the urine help prevent these complications.*
- For an indwelling stent, stress the need for regular follow-up to monitor for and prevent complications such as UTI and calculi. *The client with an indwelling stent may tend to forget that the stent is in place and become lax in compliance with follow-up and preventive measures.*

intake during hot weather or strenuous activity. Discuss the need to avoid voluntary urinary retention, emptying the bladder every 3 to 4 hours. Instruct women to cleanse the perineal area from front to back after voiding and defecating. Teach to void before and after sexual intercourse to flush out bacteria introduced into the urethra and bladder. Teach measures to maintain the integrity of perineal tissues: Avoid bubble baths, feminine hygiene sprays, and vaginal douches; wear cotton briefs, avoid synthetic materials; if postmenopausal, use hormone replacement therapy or estrogen cream. Unless contraindicated, suggest measures to maintain acid urine: Drink two glasses of low-sugar cranberry juice daily; take ascorbic acid (vitamin C), and avoid excess intake of milk and milk products, other fruit juices, and sodium bicarbonate (baking soda).

Assessment

Focused assessment data for the client with a UTI includes the following:

- *Health history:* Current symptoms, including frequency, urgency, burning on urination, voidings per night; color, clarity, and odor of urine; other manifestations such as lower abdominal, back, or flank pain, nausea or vomiting, fever; duration of symptoms and any treatment attempted; history of previous UTIs and their frequency; possibility of pregnancy and type of birth control used; chronic diseases such as diabetes; current medications and any known allergies.
- *Physical examination:* General health; vital signs including temperature; abdominal shape, contour, tenderness to palpation (especially suprapubic); percuss for costovertebral tenderness (see Box 27–1).

See Chapter 27 ∞ for complete nursing assessment of the urinary system.

Nursing Diagnoses and Interventions

The client's general health, abilities for self-care, and risk factors that may contribute to UTI are considered when planning and implementing nursing care for the client with a UTI. Priority nursing diagnoses focus on comfort, urinary elimination, and teaching/learning needs. A nursing care plan for the client with cystitis can be found on page 853.

Pain

Pain is a common manifestation of both lower and upper UTI. Urinary tract pain is caused primarily by distention and increased pressure within the tract. The severity of the pain is related to the rate at which inflammation and distention develop, not their degree.

In cystitis, inflammation causes a sensation of fullness; dull, constant suprapubic pain; and possibly low back pain. The inflamed bladder wall and urethra cause dysuria, pain, and burning on urination. Bladder spasms may develop, causing periodic severe, stabbing discomfort. Pain associated with pyelonephritis is often steady and dull, localized to the outer abdomen or flank region. Urologic disorders rarely cause central abdominal pain.

- Assess pain: timing, quality, intensity, location, duration, and aggravating and alleviating factors. *A change in the nature,*

location, or intensity of the pain could indicate an extension of the infection or a related but separate problem.

> ### PRACTICE ALERT
> The older adult with a UTI may not complain of dysuria with a UTI. Be alert for other manifestations of UTI such as incontinence or cloudy or malodorous urine. Inflammatory and immune responses tend to diminish with aging, reducing the irritative symptoms of UTI.

- Teach or provide comfort measures such as warm sitz baths, warm packs or heating pads, and balanced rest and activity. Systemic analgesics, urinary analgesics, or antispasmodic medication may be used as ordered. *Warmth relaxes muscles, relieves spasms, and increases local blood supply. Because pain can stimulate a stress response and delay healing, it should be relieved when possible.*
- Increase fluid intake unless contraindicated. *Increased fluid dilutes urine, reducing irritation of the inflamed bladder and urethral mucosa.*
- Instruct to notify primary care provider if pain and discomfort continue or intensify after therapy is initiated. *Pain and discomfort in voiding typically are relieved within 24 hours of the initiation of antibiotic therapy. Continued discomfort may indicate a complicated UTI or other urinary tract disorder.*

Impaired Urinary Elimination

Inflammation of the bladder and urethral mucosa affects the normal process and patterns of voiding, causing frequency, urgency, and burning on urination, as well as nocturia. Urine may be blood tinged, cloudy, and malodorous. The client with short- or long-term urinary retention (see the section on urinary retention later in this chapter) requires additional measures to assess for and prevent UTI.

- Monitor (or instruct the client to monitor) color, clarity, and odor of urine. *Urine should return to clear yellow within 48 hours, unless drug therapy causes a change in the color of urine. If clarity does not return, further investigation may be necessary.*

> ### PRACTICE ALERT
> Provide for easy access to a bedpan, urinal, commode, or bathroom. Make sure that lighting is adequate and that pathways are free of obstacles. Frequency, urgency, and nocturia increase the risk of urinary incontinence and of injury due to falls, particularly in the older or debilitated client.

- Instruct to avoid caffeinated drinks, including coffee, tea, and cola; citrus juices; drinks containing artificial sweeteners; and alcoholic beverages. *Caffeine, citrus juices, and artificial sweeteners irritate bladder mucosa and the detrusor muscle, and can increase urgency and bladder spasms.*
- Use strict aseptic technique and a closed urinary drainage system when inserting a straight or indwelling urinary catheter. Insert indwelling catheters to the full recommended length (4 or more inches in women and to the bifurcation in men) before inflating the balloon. *Bacteria colonizing the perineal tissues or on the nurse's hands can be introduced into the bladder during catheterization. Aseptic technique*

NURSING CARE PLAN   A Client with Cystitis

Miija Waisanen is a 25-year-old second-year nursing student. She was recently married, and she and her husband live in an apartment near the college she attends. Mrs. Waisanen has never been pregnant, and she is using a diaphragm for birth control. She presents at the local urgent care clinic complaining of low back pain, frequency, urgency, and burning on urination that began the day before.

ASSESSMENT

Patrice Ramiros, RN, admits Mrs. Waisanen to the clinic. Mrs. Waisanen denies having had similar symptoms in the past or ever having been diagnosed with a urinary tract infection. She describes her pain as a constant, dull ache that does not change with movement. She feels the need to urinate almost constantly, but experiences difficulty in starting her stream, and burning pain and cramping when voiding. She reports getting up four times the night before to urinate. She denies painful intercourse and states that her last menstrual period began only 2 weeks ago. Physical examination reveals: BP 112/68; P 90 and regular, afebrile. Suprapubic tenderness noted but no flank or costovertebral angle tenderness. Clean-catch urine specimen shows hematuria, multiple WBCs, and a bacteria count greater than 10^5 per milliliter.

The nurse practitioner prescribes trimethoprim-sulfamethoxazole (TMP-SMZ) 160 mg/800 mg PO bid for 3 days, and aspirin or acetaminophen gr × PO every 4 hours as needed for pain. Mrs. Waisanen is instructed to return to the clinic in 7 days for a follow-up urine culture, or sooner if her symptoms do not improve.

DIAGNOSES

- *Pain* related to infection and inflammatory process in the urinary tract
- *Impaired Urinary Elimination* related to inflammation as evidenced by frequency, urgency, nocturia, and dysuria
- *Deficient Knowledge* related to lack of information about risk factors for UTI

EXPECTED OUTCOMES

- Report relief of low back pain and burning on urination.
- Regain a normal voiding pattern without frequency, urgency, nocturia, and abnormal urine characteristics.

- Verbalize understanding of the disease process, related risk factors, follow-up instructions, and symptoms of recurrence indicating the need for medical attention.

PLANNING AND IMPLEMENTATION

- Teach comfort measures: warm sitz baths, a heating pad on low heat applied to her lower back or abdomen, rest, increased fluid intake, avoiding caffeinated beverages, and aspirin or acetaminophen as ordered.
- Advise to refrain from sexual intercourse until infection and inflammation have cleared to avoid further irritation of inflamed tissues.
- Discuss the possible relationship between using a diaphragm for birth control and UTI in women.
- Discuss dietary and hygiene practices to prevent UTI, symptoms indicating the need for further intervention, and the risks of undertreatment.

EVALUATION

Six months later, Mrs. Waisanen rotates through the urgent care clinic for her community-based nursing experience. Ms. Ramiros asks how she is doing. Mrs. Waisanen reports that her symptoms and urine cleared within about a day after starting the antibiotic and she has had no further problems. She has seen her women's healthcare nurse practitioner to change her birth control to oral contraceptives, increased her intake of fluid and vitamin C, and no longer puts off urinating until she "has time to go!"

CRITICAL THINKING IN THE NURSING PROCESS

1. What physiologic and psychosocial factors put Mrs. Waisanen at risk for developing a UTI?
2. Compare and contrast the benefits and drawbacks to short-course therapy versus conventional therapy for UTI.
3. Why was it appropriate for the nurse practitioner to use short-course therapy with the advice to return if symptoms did not clear?
4. Develop a care plan for Mrs. Waisanen for the nursing diagnosis *Ineffective Health Maintenance*.

See Evaluating Your Response in Appendix C.

---

reduces this risk. Inflation of the balloon while in the urethra damages urethral tissues and can cause significant discomfort for the client. See page 854 for evidence-based practice for male catheterization.

PRACTICE ALERT

Unless contraindicated, instillation of an anesthetic lubricating gel into the urethra (10 mL for a male and 6 mL for a female) promotes comfort during the procedure, protects fragile urethral tissues from trauma, and reduces the risk for catheter-associated UTI (Bardsley, 2005).

- When possible, use intermittent straight catheterization to relieve urinary retention. Remove indwelling urinary catheters as soon as possible. *Using intermittent straight catheterization allows the bladder to fill and completely empty in a more nor-*

mal manner, maintaining physiologic function. The risk of infection associated with an indwelling catheter is about 3% to 5% per day of catheterization (Kasper et al., 2005).

- Maintain the closed urinary drainage system, and use aseptic technique when emptying the catheter drainage bag. Maintain gravity flow, preventing reflux of urine into the bladder from the drainage system. *Bacteria can enter the drainage system when its integrity is interrupted (e.g., disconnecting the catheter from the drainage system) or during emptying of the drainage bag. These bacteria can ascend the column of urine to the bladder, causing UTI.*
- Provide perineal care on a regular basis and following defecation. Use antiseptic preparations only as ordered. *Regular cleansing of perineal tissues reduces the risk of colonization by bowel or other bacteria. While antiseptic solutions may be ordered for catheter care, they can dry perineal tissues and*

NURSING RESEARCH   Evidence-Based Practice: Male Catheterization

Insertion of an indwelling (retention) catheter is a commonly performed procedure in hospitals and long-term care facilities. While the location of the female urethral meatus presents a challenge to maintaining catheter sterility during insertion, the anatomy of the male urethra presents a different set of challenges. Little research is available to support evidence-based practice for male urethral catheterization. In addition, reports of urethral injury in men related to catheter insertion and balloon inflation are not uncommon. A multidisciplinary team of researchers at University of Colorado Hospital conducted a study to determine the correct urethral catheter placement in male adults (Daneshgari et al., 2002). Their research showed that inserting the catheter to the bifurcation (attachment of the arm for balloon inflation) always placed the retention balloon well within the urinary bladder prior to its inflation. Insertion to any lesser distance was inadequate to ensure safe balloon inflation without potential damage to the urethra.

IMPLICATIONS FOR NURSING

Nursing fundamentals and skills texts recommend inserting the catheter from 6 to 8 or 10 inches into the male urethra before inflating the balloon of a retention catheter. Some texts recommend inserting the catheter 1 to 2 inches beyond the point at which urine is obtained before inflating the balloon. This study (Daneshgari et al., 2002) showed that these recommendations could result in an attempt to inflate the balloon while that portion of the catheter is still in the urethra, not fully into the bladder. To ensure safe practice and reduce the risk for injury and discomfort, insert a retention catheter to the bifurcation before inflating the balloon.

CRITICAL THINKING IN CLIENT CARE

1. Why is insertion of a urinary catheter frequently a more uncomfortable and difficult procedure for a male client than a female client? What nursing measures or techniques can be used to reduce this discomfort?
2. Sterile technique generally is used when catheterizing clients in acute care settings. However, clients who require intermittent catheterization to empty their bladder typically use clean technique. Would clean technique be appropriate in an acute or long-term care setting? Why or why not?

Source: From "Evidence-Based Multidisciplinary Practice: Improving the Safety and Standards of Male Bladder Catheterization" by F. Daneshgari, M. Krugman, A. Bahn, and R. S. Lee, 2002, *Medsurg Nursing, 11*(5), 236–241, 246.

---

reduce normal flora, increasing the risk of colonization by pathogens, and should not routinely be used.

Ineffective Health Maintenance

The client with a urinary tract infection is at an increased risk for future UTI and needs to understand the disease process, risk factors, measures to prevent recurrent infection, diagnostic procedures, and home care. In addition, once the manifestations of UTI are relieved, motivation to continue the treatment plan declines. Failure to complete the full course of therapy and recommended follow-up can lead to continued bacteriuria and recurrent infections.

- Teach how to obtain a midstream clean-catch urine specimen. *Cleansing of the urinary meatus and perineal area reduces contamination of the specimen by external cells and bacteria. Ninety percent of urethral bacteria are cleared in the first 10 mL of voided urine; a midstream specimen is representative of urine in the bladder.*
- Assess knowledge about the disease process, risk factors, and preventive measures. *The client may have little understanding of UTI, its causes, and contributing factors.*
- Discuss the prescribed treatment plan and the importance of taking all prescribed antibiotics.

PRACTICE ALERT

Symptoms are largely relieved within 24 to 48 hours of starting antibiotic therapy; however, bacteria may remain in the urinary tract. Completing the prescribed regime is important to prevent recurrent infections and resistant bacteria.

- Help the client develop a plan for taking medications, such as taking them with meals (unless contraindicated) or setting out all doses for the day in the morning. *Missed doses of antibiotic can result in subtherapeutic blood levels and reduced effectiveness. Taking medication in association with a regular daily activity such as meals helps clients remember doses.*
- Instruct to keep appointments for follow-up and urine culture. *Follow-up urine culture, often scheduled 7 to 14 days after completion of antibiotic therapy, is vital to ensure complete eradication of bacteria and prevent relapse or recurrence.*
- Teach measures to prevent future UTI (see the preceding Health Promotion section). *Keeping urine dilute and acidic and voiding regularly flush bacteria out of the bladder and urethra. The proximity of the female urethral meatus to the vagina and anus increases the risk of bacterial contamination, especially during intercourse. Bubble baths, feminine hygiene sprays, synthetic fibers, and douches may dry and irritate perineal tissues, promoting bacterial growth.*

Community-Based Care

Because both upper and lower urinary tract infections are usually managed in the community, teaching is the most important nursing intervention. Provide instruction on the following topics:

- Risk factors for UTI and how to minimize or eliminate these factors through increased fluid intake, regular elimination, and personal hygiene measures
- Early manifestations of UTI and the importance of seeking medical intervention promptly
- Maintaining optimal immune system function by attending to physical and psychosocial stressors, such as lack of adequate rest, poor nutrition, and high levels of emotional stress
- The importance of completing the prescribed treatment and keeping follow-up appointments

- Minimizing the risk of UTI when an indwelling urinary catheter is necessary:
  a. Use alternatives to an indwelling catheter when possible. For urinary incontinence, try scheduled toileting, incontinence pads or diapers, and external catheters if possible. For urinary retention, teach the client or a family member to perform straight catheterization every 3 to 4 hours using clean technique.
  b. Teach care measures such as perineal care, managing and emptying the collection chamber, maintaining a closed system, and bladder irrigation or flushing if ordered when an indwelling catheter is necessary.

THE CLIENT WITH URINARY CALCULI

Urinary calculi, stones in the urinary tract, are the most common cause of upper urinary tract obstruction (Porth, 2005). The term **lithiasis** means "stone formation"; when the stones form in the kidney, it is known as *nephrolithiasis;* when they form elsewhere in the urinary tract (for example, the bladder), it is called *urolithiasis.* Stones may form and obstruct the urinary tract at any point (Figure 28–3 ■). In the United States and other industrialized countries, renal or kidney stones are the most common.

Incidence and Risk Factors

Urolithiasis affects up to 720,000 people annually in the United States (Tierney et al., 2005). In the United States, the incidence varies by region, with the highest frequency in southern and midwestern states. Males are affected two or three times more often than females (Porth, 2005). Calculi are more common among whites than blacks. Most people affected are in young or middle adulthood.

Although the majority of stones are idiopathic (having no demonstrable cause), a number of risk factors have been identified. The greatest risk factor for stone formation is a prior personal or family history of urinary calculi. A genetic predisposition toward the accumulation of certain mineral substances in the urine or a congenital lack of protective factors may explain the familial link. Other identified risk factors include dehydration with resultant increased urine concentration, immobility, and excess dietary intake of calcium, oxalate, or proteins. Gout, hyperparathyroidism, and urinary stasis or repeated infections also contribute to calculus formation.

Physiology Review

Normally, a balance exists in the kidneys between the need to conserve water and to eliminate poorly soluble materials such as calcium salts. This balance is affected by factors such as diet, environmental temperature, and activity. Protective inorganic and organic substances in the urine, such as pyrophosphate, citrate, and glycoproteins, normally inhibit stone formation.

Pathophysiology

Three factors contribute to urolithiasis: supersaturation, nucleation, and lack of inhibitory substances in the urine.

When the concentration of an insoluble salt in the urine is very high, that is, when the urine is supersaturated, crystals may form. Usually, these crystals disperse and are eliminated because the bonds holding them together are weak. However, a nucleus of crystals may develop stable bonds to form a stone. More often, crystals form around an organic matrix or mucoprotein nucleus to become a stone. The stimulus required to initiate crystallization in supersaturated urine may be minimal. Ingesting a meal high in insoluble salt, or decreased fluid intake as occurs

Figure 28–3 ■ Development and location of calculi within the urinary tract.

Source: Dr. E. Walker/Photo Researchers, Inc.

during sleep, allows the concentration to increase to the point where precipitation occurs and stones are formed and grow. When fluid intake is adequate, no stone growth occurs. The acidity or alkalinity of the urine and the presence or absence of calculus-inhibiting compounds also affect lithiasis.

Most (75% to 80%) kidney stones are *calcium stones*, composed of calcium oxalate and/or calcium phosphate. These stones are generally associated with high concentrations of calcium in the blood or urine. *Uric acid stones* develop when the urine concentration of uric acid is high. They are more common in men, and may be associated with gout. Genetic factors contribute to the development of uric acid stones and calcium stones. *Struvite stones* are associated with UTI caused by urease-producing bacteria such as *Proteus*. These stones can grow to become very large, filling the renal pelvis and calyces. They often are called *staghorn stones* because of their shape. *Cystine stones* are rare, and are associated with a genetic defect. The types of renal calculi, contributing factors, and recommended dietary modifications are listed in Table 28–2.

FAST FACTS
- Most urinary stones form in the renal pelvis and are composed primarily of calcium salts.
- Loss of calcium from the bones (e.g., due to immobility) and dehydration are major risk factors for urinary stones.

Manifestations

The symptoms caused by urinary calculi vary with their size and location (see the Manifestations box on this page). Manifestations develop as a result of obstructed urine flow with resulting distention, and tissue trauma caused by passage of the rough-edged, crystalline stone.

Calculi affecting the kidney calyces and pelvis may cause few symptoms. If the stone has gradually or partially obstructed urinary flow, dull, aching flank pain may be present,

---

MANIFESTATIONS of Urinary Calculi

KIDNEY STONES
- Often asymptomatic
- Dull, aching flank pain
- Microscopic hematuria
- Manifestations of UTI

URETERAL STONES
- Renal colic
  - Acute, severe flank pain on affected side
  - Often radiates to suprapubic region, groin, and external genitals
- Nausea, vomiting, pallor, and cool, clammy skin

BLADDER STONES
- May be asymptomatic
- Dull suprapubic pain, possibly associated with exercise or voiding
- Gross or microscopic hematuria
- Manifestations of UTI

---

but renal calculi often are silent, without symptoms. Bladder calculi may cause few symptoms other than dull suprapubic pain with exercise or after voiding.

Renal colic, acute, severe flank pain on the affected side, develops when a stone obstructs the ureter, causing ureteral spasm. The pain of renal colic may radiate to the suprapubic region, groin, and external genitals (the scrotum or labia). The severity of the pain often causes a sympathetic response with associated nausea, vomiting, pallor, and cool, clammy skin.

Manifestations of UTI, including chills and fever, frequency, urgency, and dysuria, may accompany urinary calculi at any level. Trauma to the urinary tract by the calculi may cause gross or microscopic hematuria. Gross hematuria is often the only sign of bladder stones.

TABLE 28–2 Risk Factors and Interventions for Renal Calculi

STONE TYPE AND INCIDENCE	RISK FACTORS	MANAGEMENT
Calcium phosphate and/or oxalate 75–80%	Hypercalciuria and hypercalcemia: hyperparathyroidism, immobility, bone disease, vitamin D intoxication, multiple myeloma, renal tubular acidosis, prolonged steroid intake Alkaline urine Dehydration Inflammatory bowel disease	Pharmacology: Thiazide diuretics, phosphates, calcium-binding agents Dietary: Limit foods high in calcium and oxalate, increase foods that acidify urine Other: Increase hydration, exercise
Struvite 15–20%	UTIs, especially *Proteus* infections	Pharmacology: Antibiotic therapy for UTI Other: Surgical intervention or lithotripsy to remove stone
Uric acid 5–10%	Gout, increased purine intake, acid urine	Pharmacology: Potassium citrate, allopurinol Dietary: Low purine diet Other: Increase hydration
Cystine (uncommon)	Genetic defect, acid urine	Pharmacology: Penicillamine, sodium bicarbonate Dietary: Sodium restriction Other: Increase hydration

Complications

Urinary stones may obstruct urine flow at any point of the urinary tract, leading to complications such as hydronephrosis and urinary stasis with subsequent infection.

Obstruction

Stones can obstruct the urinary tract at any point from the calyces of the kidney to the distal urethra, impeding the outflow of urine. If the obstruction develops slowly, there may be few or no symptoms, whereas sudden obstruction (e.g., blockage of a ureter by a passing stone) may cause severe manifestations. Urinary tract obstruction can ultimately lead to renal failure. The degree of obstruction, its location, and the duration of impaired urine flow determine the effect on renal function.

HYDRONEPHROSIS The kidneys continue to produce urine, causing increased pressure and distention of the urinary tract behind the obstruction. **Hydronephrosis**, distention of the renal pelvis and calyces, and *hydroureter,* distention of the ureter, are possible results. If the pressure is unrelieved, the collecting tubules, proximal tubules, and glomeruli of the kidney are damaged, causing a gradual loss of renal function.

Acute hydronephrosis typically causes colicky pain on the affected side. The pain may radiate into the groin. Chronic hydronephrosis develops slowly, and may have few manifestations other than dull, aching back or flank pain. When hydronephrosis is significant, a palpable mass may be felt in the flank region. Hematuria and signs of UTI such as pyuria, fever, and discomfort may occur. Gastrointestinal symptoms such as nausea, vomiting, and abdominal pain may accompany hydronephrosis (see the Manifestations box below).

INFECTION The urinary stasis associated with partial or complete obstruction increases the risk of urinary tract infection. Either upper or lower UTI may develop.

INTERDISCIPLINARY CARE

Management of urinary calculi focuses on relieving acute symptoms, destroying or removing stones, and preventing fur-

ther stone formation. Asymptomatic stones (those not causing pain, infection, or obstruction) are treated conservatively.

Diagnosis

Laboratory and diagnostic tests that may be ordered when urinary calculi are suspected include the following:

- *Urinalysis* to assess for hematuria and the possible presence of WBCs and crystal fragments. The urine pH is helpful in identifying the type of stone.
- *Chemical analysis* of any stones passed in the urine determines the type of stone and suggests measures to prevent further stone formation. Retrieving stones or teaching the client to do so is a nursing responsibility. All urine is strained and may be saved. Any visible stones or sediment is sent for analysis.
- *Urine calcium, uric acid,* and *oxalate* levels measure the amount of these substances excreted over a 24-hour period, and may be assessed to help identify possible causes of lithiasis. Elevated calcium levels occur in hyperparathyroidism, Cushing's syndrome, and osteoporosis, all of which may contribute to lithiasis. Uric acid levels may be elevated in clients with gout and those at risk for forming uric acid calculi. Urine oxalate excretion may help to differentiate calcium oxalate from calcium phosphate stones.
- *Serum calcium, phosphorus,* and *uric acid* levels may be obtained to help identify factors contributing to calculus formation.
- *KUB* (kidneys, ureters, and bladder) is a flat-plate X-ray of the lower abdomen that requires no special preparation. Calculi may be identified as opacities in the kidneys, ureters, and bladder.
- *Renal ultrasonography* is a noninvasive test that uses reflected sound waves to detect stones and evaluate the kidneys for possible hydronephrosis.
- *Computed tomography (CT) scan* of the kidney, with or without contrast medium, uses x-rays directed at the kidney from many angles to provide a computer-generated photograph that shows calculi, ureteral obstruction, and other renal disorders.
- *IVP* may be done to visualize the kidneys, ureters, and bladder after injection of a contrast medium. IVP may be done when KUB, renal ultrasonography, and CT scan fail to demonstrate clear evidence of urinary calculi. (See nursing care of the client undergoing an IVP.)
- *Cystoscopy* is used to visualize and possibly remove calculi from the urinary bladder and distal ureters.

Nursing implications and care for clients undergoing these tests and procedures is outlined in Chapter 27 ∞.

Medications

An acute episode of renal colic is treated with analgesia and hydration. A narcotic analgesic such as morphine sulfate is given, often intravenously, to relieve pain and reduce ureteral spasm. Indomethacin, a nonsteroidal anti-inflammatory drug (NSAID), given as a suppository, may reduce the amount of narcotic analgesia required for acute renal colic. Oral or intravenous fluids reduce the risk of further stone formation and promote urine output.

MANIFESTATIONS of Acute and Chronic Hydronephrosis

ACUTE
- Acute, colicky pain; may radiate into groin
- Hematuria, pyuria
- Fever
- Nausea, vomiting, abdominal pain

CHRONIC
- Dull, aching flank pain
- Hematuria, pyuria
- Fever
- Palpable flank mass

After analysis of the calculus, various medications may be ordered to inhibit or prevent further lithiasis. A thiazide diuretic, frequently prescribed for calcium calculi, acts to reduce urinary calcium excretion and is very effective in preventing further stones. Potassium citrate alkalinizes urine (raises the pH), and is often prescribed to prevent stones that tend to form in acidic urine (uric acid, cystine, and some forms of calcium stones). See Table 28–2 for other preparations related to types of stones. Nursing responsibilities focus on teaching the client about the prescribed medication, its importance in preventing further stone formation, and potential adverse effects.

Nutrition and Fluid Management

Diet modifications are often prescribed to change the character of the urine and prevent further lithiasis.

Increased fluid intake of 2.5 to 3.0 L per day is recommended, regardless of stone composition. A fluid intake to ensure the production of approximately 2.0 to 2.5 L of urine a day prevents the stone-forming salts from becoming concentrated enough to precipitate. Fluid intake should be spaced throughout the day and evening. Some authorities recommend that clients drink one to two glasses of water at night to prevent concentration of urine during sleep.

Recommended dietary changes may include reduced intake of the primary substance forming the calculi. For calcium stones, dietary calcium and vitamin D–enriched foods are limited. Limiting vitamin D inhibits the absorption of calcium from the GI tract. Calcium stones may be either a calcium phosphate salt, calcium oxalate, or a combination of both; therefore, phosphorus and/or oxalate may also be limited in the diet.

The client with uric acid stones requires a diet low in purines. Organ meats, sardines, and other high-purine foods are eliminated from the diet. Foods with moderate levels of purines, such as red and white meats and some seafoods, may be limited.

In addition to limiting certain foods, the diet may be modified to maintain a urinary pH that does not promote lithiasis. Uric acid and cystine stones tend to form in acid urine. Foods that tend to alkalinize the urine may be recommended. Because alkaline urine promotes formation of calcium stones and urinary tract infections, the diet may be modified to lower the pH of the urine. Foods that affect urinary pH and foods high in various stone components are summarized in Table 28–3.

Surgery

Treatment of existing calculi depends on the location of the stone, the extent of obstruction, renal function, the presence or absence of UTI, and the client's general state of health. In general, the stone is removed if it is causing severe obstruction, infection, unrelieved pain, or serious bleeding (Kasper et al., 2005).

Lithotripsy, using sound or shock waves to crush a stone, is the preferred treatment for urinary calculi. Several techniques are available. **Extracorporeal shock wave lithotripsy (ESWL)** is a noninvasive technique for fragmenting kidney stones using shock waves generated outside the body. Acoustic shock waves are aimed under fluoroscopic guidance at the stone (Figure 28–4 ■). These shock waves travel through soft tissue without causing damage, but shatter the stone as its greater density

TABLE 28–3 Teaching Clients with Urolithiasis: Possible Food and Fluid Modifications

Foods high in calcium	Beans and lentils, chocolate and cocoa, dried fruits, canned or smoked fish except tuna, flour, milk and milk products
Foods high in oxalate	Asparagus, beer and colas, beets, cabbage, celery, chocolate and cocoa, fruits, green beans, nuts, tea, tomatoes
Purine-rich foods	Goose, organ meats, sardines and herring, venison; moderate in beef, chicken, crab, pork, salmon, veal
Acidifying foods	Cheese, cranberries, eggs, grapes, meat and poultry, plums and prunes, tomatoes, whole grains
Alkalinizing foods	Green vegetables, fruit (except as noted above), legumes, milk and milk products, rhubarb

stops their progress. Repeated shock waves pulverize the stone into fragments small enough to be eliminated in the urine. The procedure may require 30 minutes to 2 hours to complete. Intravenous sedation generally is adequate to maintain comfort during the procedure (Way & Doherty, 2003). See the box on the next page for nursing care of the client undergoing a lithotripsy procedure.

Lithotripsy also may be performed using a percutaneous ultrasonic or laser technique. *Percutaneous ultrasonic lithotripsy* uses a nephroscope inserted into the kidney pelvis through a small flank incision (Figure 28–5 ■). The stone is fragmented using a small ultrasonic transducer, and the fragments are removed through the nephroscope. *Laser lithotripsy* is an alternative to ultrasonic lithotripsy. Laser beams are used to disintegrate the stone, without damaging soft tissue. A nephroscope or a ureteroscope (passed up the ureter from the bladder

Figure 28–4 ■ Extracorporeal shock-wave lithotripsy. Acoustic shock waves generated by the shock wave generator travel through soft tissue to shatter the urinary stone into fragments, which are then eliminated in the urine.

Source: Visuals Unlimited

NURSING CARE OF THE CLIENT HAVING Lithotripsy

PREOPERATIVE CARE

- Assess knowledge and understanding of the procedure, providing information as needed. *Anxiety is reduced, and recovery is enhanced and hastened when the client is fully prepared for surgery.*
- Follow directions from the radiology department, physician, or anesthetist for withholding food and fluids and for bowel preparation prior to surgery. *Conscious sedation, general anesthesia, or spinal anesthesia may be required, depending on the procedure. Fecal material in the bowel may impede fluoroscopic visualization of the kidney and stone.*

POSTOPERATIVE CARE

- In the initial period, monitor vital signs frequently. *The kidney is highly vascular; therefore, hemorrhage and resulting shock are potential complications of lithotripsy. Bleeding may be internal or retroperitoneal and difficult to detect.*
- Monitor amount, color, and clarity of urine output. *Urine is often bright red initially, but bleeding should diminish within 48*

to 72 hours. Cloudy urine may indicate the presence of an infection.
- Maintain placement and patency of urinary catheters. Anchor ureteral catheters or nephrostomy tubes securely. Irrigate gently if ordered. *A kinked or plugged catheter may result in hydroureter, hydronephrosis, and kidney damage. Decreased urinary output and flank pain are possible symptoms of obstructed urine flow. Excessive force in irrigation may cause trauma and bleeding.*
- Prepare for discharge by teaching care of the indwelling catheter, urine-collection device, and incision site (if present). Teach signs and symptoms to report: urine leakage from incision for more than 4 days, symptoms of infection, pain, bright hematuria. *Many clients are discharged with dressings and catheters in place. The client and family need necessary information to provide self-care.*
- Teach measures to reduce the risk of further lithiasis. *Many clients have repeated episodes of lithiasis and renal colic. Prevention of stone formation is important to preserve renal function.*

during cystoscopy) is used to guide the laser probe into direct contact with the stone.

A double J stent may be inserted into the affected ureter to maintain its patency following ESWL or other lithotripsy procedures. (See the box on page 851 for nursing care of the client with a ureteral stent.)

Figure 28–5 ■ Percutaneous ultrasonic lithotripsy. A nephroscope is inserted into the renal pelvis, and ultrasonic waves are used to fragment the stone. The fragments then are removed through the nephroscope.

On rare occasions, surgical intervention is necessary to remove a calculus in the renal pelvis or ureter. *Ureterolithotomy* is incision in the affected ureter to remove a calculus. *Pyelolithotomy* is incision into and removal of a stone from the kidney pelvis. A staghorn calculus that invades the calyces and renal parenchyma may require a *nephrolithotomy* for removal. See Chapter 4 ∞ for care of the surgical client.

Bladder stones may be removed using an instrument passed through a cystoscope to crush the stones. The remaining stone fragments are then irrigated out of the bladder using an acid solution to counteract the alkalinity that precipitated stone formation.

NURSING CARE

Nursing care for the client with urolithiasis is directed at providing for comfort during acute renal colic, assisting with diagnostic procedures, ensuring adequate urinary output, and teaching the client information necessary to prevent future stone formation.

Health Promotion

Discuss the importance of maintaining an adequate fluid intake with all clients. Stress the need to increase fluid intake during warm weather and strenuous exercise or physical labor. Discuss the relationship between weight-bearing activity and retention of calcium in the bones. Encourage all clients to remain as physically active as possible to prevent bone resorption (loss) and possible hypercalciuria.

Instruct clients with known gout to maintain a generous fluid intake so as to produce at least 2 L of urine every day. Discuss the risk of lithiasis with clients who have frequent UTIs, and teach measures to reduce the incidence of UTI and the risk for lithiasis.

Assessment

Obtain subjective and objective assessment data specific to urolithiasis:

- *Health history:* Complaints of flank, back, or abdominal pain, radiation, characteristics and timing, aggravating or relieving factors; other symptoms such as nausea and vomiting; possible contributing factors such as dehydration; previous or family history of kidney stones; current or previous treatment measures.
- *Physical examination:* General appearance including position, vital signs; skin color, temperature, moisture, turgor; abdominal, flank, or costovertebral tenderness; amount, color, and characteristics of urine (presence of hematuria, bacteria, pyuria, pH).

Nursing Diagnoses and Interventions

See the Nursing Care Plan that follows this section for additional nursing diagnoses and interventions.

Acute Pain

Pain is the primary outward manifestation of urolithiasis, particularly when a stone lodges within a ureter, causing acute obstruction and distention. Invasive and noninvasive procedures to remove or crush stones also may be painful. Clients undergoing surgery also experience incisional pain.

PRACTICE ALERT

The intensity of renal colic pain can cause a vasovagal response with resulting hypotension and syncope. Always provide for the client's safety.

- Assess pain using a standard pain scale and its characteristics. Administer analgesia as ordered and monitor its effectiveness. *The intensity, type of pain, and its responsiveness to analgesia provide valuable clues as to its cause. Regular administration of prescribed analgesics controls pain more effectively than waiting until pain becomes intolerable. Administering an ordered NSAID on a routine schedule may significantly reduce the need for narcotic analgesia in clients with renal colic.*
- Unless contraindicated, encourage fluid intake and ambulation in the client with renal colic. *Increased fluids and ambulation increase urinary output, facilitating movement of the calculus through the ureter and decreasing pain.*
- Use nonpharmacologic measures such as positioning, moist heat, relaxation techniques, guided imagery, and diversion as adjunctive therapy for pain relief. *Adjunctive pain relief measures can enhance the effectiveness of analgesics and other prescribed treatment.*
- If surgery has been performed, monitor urinary output, catheters, incision, and wound drainage. *Pain may be a symptom of proximal distention due to a blocked catheter. Infection or hematoma at the surgical site can significantly increase perceived pain.*

Impaired Urinary Elimination

Obstruction of the urinary tract is the primary problem associated with urolithiasis. Obstruction can ultimately lead to stasis, infection, or irreversible renal damage.

- Monitor amount and character of urine output. If catheterized, measure output hourly. Document any hematuria, dysuria, frequency, urgency, and pyuria. Strain all urine for stones, saving any recovered stones for laboratory analysis. *The amount of urine output helps determine possible urinary tract obstruction and adequacy of hydration. Hematuria, gross or microscopic, is often associated with calculi and with procedures used to remove stones, such as cystoscopy or lithotripsy. A change in the amount of hematuria may indicate stone passage or a complication. Dysuria, frequency, urgency, and cloudy urine are symptoms of UTI, often associated with urolithiasis. Antibiotic therapy may be required. Analysis of stones recovered from the urine can direct measures to prevent further lithiasis.*

PRACTICE ALERT

A stone that completely obstructs the ureter can lead to hydronephrosis and kidney damage on the affected side. Report symptoms of hydronephrosis such as dull flank pain or aching and changes in renal function studies (BUN and serum creatinine). Because the other kidney continues to function, urine output may not fall significantly with obstruction of one ureter. A rising BUN and serum creatinine may be early signs of renal failure.

- Maintain patency and integrity of all catheter systems. Secure catheters well, label as indicated, and use sterile technique for all ordered irrigations or other procedures. *A kinked or plugged catheter, particularly a ureteral catheter or nephrostomy tube, may damage the urinary system. Labeling catheters can prevent mistakes, such as inappropriate irrigation or clamping. Any catheter increases the risk of infection; aseptic technique in all procedures reduces this risk.*

Deficient Knowledge

The client with urolithiasis has multiple learning needs. These include information about the disease and its possible consequences, any diagnostic or therapeutic procedures performed, and strategies to prevent future lithiasis.

- Assess understanding and previous learning. *Relating information to previously learned material enhances retention and understanding.*
- Present all material in a manner appropriate to knowledge base, developmental and educational level, and current needs. *Learning is an active process that requires the client's participation. Tailoring teaching to the individual increases involvement.*
- Teach about all diagnostic and treatment procedures. *Knowing what to expect reduces anxiety, enhances compliance, and hastens recovery.*
- If the client will be managed in the community, teach to:
  a. Collect and strain all urine, saving any stones.
  b. Report stone passage to the physician and bring the stone in for analysis.
  c. Report any changes in the amount or character of urine output to physician.

When pain can be managed with oral analgesics, urinary stones are managed in the community. The client needs to know how and why to collect the calculus and indicators of

NURSING CARE PLAN · A Client with Urinary Calculi

Richard Leton, age 44, owns a small business. He is admitted to the medical unit from the emergency department after awakening at 4:00 A.M. with severe right-sided pain. His CBC is normal, and urinalysis reveals microscopic hematuria, but no protein or bacteria. A renal ultrasound shows a 4- to 5-mm stone partially obstructing the right ureter.

Stephen Phillips, Mr. Leton's admitting nurse, notes that he is pale, diaphoretic, and very anxious. He complains of nausea and asks for an emesis basin. Mr. Leton received 4 mg of intravenous morphine sulphate shortly after admission to the ED, approximately 2.5 hours ago. He denies pain at this time, but says, "I'm scared to death that it'll come back—I couldn't even move, it hurt so bad."

ASSESSMENT

Mr. Leton's history reveals no previous episodes of renal calculi. He felt well until the pain awakened him during the night. He admits that he has been working under a deadline to complete a construction project and that he probably has not been drinking enough fluids "considering how hot it's been." Physical assessment findings include T 100.4°F (38.0°C) PO, P 98, R 24, and BP 160/86. Color is pale to ashen, skin cool and moist. Abdomen firm with moderate tenderness in the right upper outer quadrant. The ED physician orders an IV of 5% dextrose in 1/2 normal saline at 200 mL/h until nausea relieved, then PO fluids of at least 3000 mL/24 h; morphine sulfate (MS) 2 to 10 mg IV prn severe pain; indomethacin (Indocin) 50 mg per rectal suppository q8h; promethazine (Phenergan) 25 mg PO or per suppository q6h prn nausea; activity to tolerance; and strain all urine, sending recovered stones for analysis.

DIAGNOSES

- *Anxiety* related to anticipation of recurrent severe pain
- *Risk for Imbalanced Nutrition: Less than Body Requirements* related to nausea
- *Acute Pain* related to partial obstruction of right ureter by calculus
- *Impaired Urinary Elimination* related to partial obstruction of ureter by calculus
- *Deficient Knowledge* related to lack of information about disease process, contributing factors, and management

EXPECTED OUTCOMES

- Demonstrate reduced anxiety by relaxed facial expression, vital signs within his normal range, and ability to rest when not disturbed.
- Consume at least 50% of diet and 100% of ordered fluids without nausea or vomiting.
- Request analgesia as needed at onset of pain; report effective pain relief.

- Maintain urine output of 2500 mL/24 h with no signs of infection or obstruction (such as increased pain, dysuria, pyuria, or hematuria).
- Relate an understanding of the process of urolithiasis and contributing factors.
- Verbalize dietary, fluid intake, and other measures to reduce risk of future stone formation.

PLANNING AND IMPLEMENTATION

- Reassure that measures to prevent further episodes of renal colic are being implemented, and that medication is available to relieve pain promptly.
- Assess the effectiveness of analgesia and its adverse effects, especially nausea.
- Maintain IV as ordered until oral fluid intake exceeds 200 mL of fluid per hour while awake.
- Measure and strain all urine. Assess urine for color, clarity, and odor.
- Teach about urolithiasis and its risk factors, especially as they relate to Mr. Leton.
- Teach the importance of maintaining a high fluid intake, especially when working outdoors in hot weather; recommended dietary modifications and their rationale; ordered medications and their effects; how to identify and prevent UTI; and symptoms that should be reported to the physician.

EVALUATION

Mr. Leton passed the obstructing stone the evening after admission and is discharged the following day. On discharge, he denies pain or nausea, his urine is clear and pale yellow, and urinalysis is normal. Laboratory analysis shows that the calculus was calcium. Mr. Leton is able to state the importance of continuing a high fluid intake. He verbalizes that he will reduce his intake of calcium-rich foods, such as milk and milk products, and that he will increase his intake of foods to acidify his urine. He is able to list foods to include in his diet. He states, "You'd better believe I'll follow my diet, drink my water, and make sure I don't get an infection. I hope to never feel pain like that again!"

CRITICAL THINKING IN THE NURSING PROCESS

1. What factors contributed to the onset and timing of Mr. Leton's ureteral colic?
2. What is the rationale for administering indomethacin, an NSAID, to a client with ureteral colic?
3. Why did Mr. Phillips include a nursing intervention to assess for a relationship between Mr. Leton's nausea, his pain, and the ordered analgesic agent?

See Evaluating Your Response in Appendix C.

---

complications, *such as reduced urine output and cloudy or bloody urine.*

- Teach measures to prevent further urolithiasis:
  a. Increase fluid intake to 2500 to 3500 mL per day.
  b. Follow recommended dietary guidelines.
  c. Maintain activity level to prevent urinary stasis and bone resorption.
  d. Take medications as prescribed.

The risk of recurrent lithiasis is approximately 50%; however, this risk can be reduced by measures to prevent conditions favoring stone formation.

- Teach about the relationship between urinary calculi and UTI, emphasizing preventive measures and the importance of prompt treatment. *Urinary tract infection promotes urolithiasis and thus requires prompt treatment to reduce this risk.*

Community-Based Care

The client with urinary calculi needs to know how to manage existing stones and what to do to reduce the risk of future stone formation. Discuss the following topics to prepare the client and family for home care:

- Importance of maintaining a fluid intake adequate to produce 2.0 to 2.5 quarts of urine per day
- Prescribed medications, their management, and potential adverse effects
- Dietary recommendations
- Prevention, recognition, and management of UTI
- Any further diagnostic or treatment measures planned.

When the client is to be discharged with dressings, a nephrostomy tube, or a catheter, teach the client and family about the following:

- How to change dressings, maintaining aseptic technique
- Assessment of the wound and skin for healing and possible complications such as infection or skin breakdown
- How to manage drainage systems and maintain their patency
- Emptying drainage bags and assessing urine output
- When to contact the physician and recommendations for follow-up care.

THE CLIENT WITH A URINARY TRACT TUMOR

A malignancy can develop in any part of the urinary tract; however, 90% develop in the bladder, about 8% develop in the renal pelvis, and only 2% in the ureter or urethra (Kasper et al., 2005). When diagnosed early, the 5-year survival rate for bladder cancer is 94% (American Cancer Society [ACS], 2005).

Incidence and Risk Factors

An estimated 63,210 new cases of bladder cancer were diagnosed in the United States in 2005, and 13,180 people died as a result of the disease. The incidence of bladder cancer is about 4 times higher in men than it is in women, and about twice as high in whites as it is in blacks (ACS, 2005). Most people who develop bladder cancer are over age 60.

Two major factors are implicated in the development of bladder cancer: the presence of carcinogens in the urine and chronic inflammation or infection of bladder mucosa. Cigarette smoking is the primary risk factor for bladder cancer. The risk in smokers is twice that of nonsmokers (ACS, 2005). The chemicals and dyes used in the plastics, rubber, and cable industries; substances in the work environment of textile workers, leather finishers, spray painters, and petroleum workers; and the chronic use of phenacetin-containing analgesic agents also are associated with a higher risk. Additional risk factors for bladder cancer include residence in an urban area, chronic UTIs, and bladder calculi. The parasite *Schistosoma haematobium,* endemic to Egypt and the Sudan, also increases the risk for bladder cancer (Porth, 2005). The risk for bladder cancer appears to be reduced by increasing the intake of fluids and vegetables (ACS, 2005).

FAST FACTS

The major risk factors for bladder cancer are:

- Male gender, age >60, residence in urban area
- Cigarette smoking
- Occupational exposure to dyes or solvents
- Chronic phenacetin ingestion
- Chronic UTI or bladder calculi.

Pathophysiology

Most urinary tract malignancies arise from epithelial tissue. Transitional epithelium lines the entire tract from the renal pelvis through the urethra. Carcinogenic breakdown products of certain chemicals and from cigarette smoke are excreted in the urine and stored in the bladder, possibly causing a local influence on abnormal cell development. Squamous cell carcinoma of the urinary tract occurs less frequently than transitional epithelial cell tumors.

Urinary tract tumors begin as nonspecific cellular alterations that develop into either flat or papillary lesions. These lesions may be either superficial or invasive. About 75% of bladder tumors are papillary lesions (*papillomas*), a polyp-like structure attached by a stalk to the bladder mucosa (Figure 28–6 ■). Papillomas are generally superficial, noninvasive tumors that bleed easily and frequently recur (Kasper et al., 2005). They rarely progress to become invasive, and the prognosis for recovery is good.

Carcinoma *in situ* (CIS), which occurs less frequently, is a poorly differentiated flat tumor that invades directly and is associated with a poorer prognosis. Bladder tumors are rated by their cell type and grade. Grade I tumors are highly differentiated and

Figure 28–6 ■ Papillary transitional cell carcinoma of the urinary bladder.

Source: Custom Medical Stock Photo, Inc.

rarely progress to become invasive, whereas grade III tumors are poorly differentiated and usually progress (Kasper et al., 2005). The staging of bladder tumors is outlined in Table 28–4. See Chapter 14 for more information about tumor grading and staging. When metastasis occurs, the pelvic lymph nodes, lungs, bones, and liver are most commonly involved.

Manifestations

Painless hematuria is the presenting sign in 75% of urinary tract tumors. Hematuria may be gross or microscopic and is often intermittent, causing delay in seeking treatment (Porth, 2005). Inflammation surrounding the tumor occasionally causes manifestations of a urinary tract infection, including frequency, urgency, and dysuria. Ureteral tumors may cause colicky pain from obstruction. Tumors of the urinary tract typically cause few outward signs and may not be discovered until obstructed urine flow causes flank pain or renal failure.

PRACTICE ALERT
Intermittent painless hematuria is the most common presenting symptom of bladder cancer. Instruct all clients with painless hematuria to contact their physician for follow-up testing.

INTERDISCIPLINARY CARE

Treatment of the client with a tumor of the urinary tract focuses on removing or destroying the cancerous tissue, preventing further invasion or metastasis, and maintaining renal and urinary function.

Diagnosis

When a urinary tract tumor is suspected, the following diagnostic tests may be ordered:

- *Urinalysis* is done to evaluate for hematuria. Gross or microscopic hematuria is often the first indicator of a neoplasm in the urinary tract.
- *Urine cytology,* microscopic examination of cells in the urine, is performed to identify abnormal cells (tumor or pretumor cells). Periodic urine cytology is recommended for clients at high risk for bladder cancer or its recurrence due to carcinogen exposure.
- *Ultrasound of the bladder* is a noninvasive test to detect bladder tumors. No dye is required, and the client is not exposed to radiation.

- *Intravenous pyelography* is used to evaluate the structure and function of the kidneys, ureters, and bladder. IVP may reveal a rigid deformity of the bladder wall, obstruction of urine flow at the point of the tumor, or bladder filling or emptying defects.
- *Cystoscopy* and *ureteroscopy* allow direct visualization, assessment, and biopsy of lesions of the urethra, bladder, or ureters using a lighted scope inserted through the urethra. Cystoscopy or ureteroscopy with biopsy allows definitive diagnosis of urinary tract tumors.
- *CT scan* or *MRI* is primarily used to evaluate tumor invasion or metastasis.

See Chapter 27 for nursing care related to these diagnostic tests.

Medications

Immunologic or chemotherapeutic agents administered by intravesical instillation (into the bladder) may be used either as the primary treatment for bladder cancer when multiple early lesions are present or to prevent recurrence following endoscopic tumor removal. Bacille Calmette-Guérin (BCG; BCGLive, TheraCys) is a suspension of attenuated *Mycobacterium bovis* used to treat CIS and recurrent bladder tumors. Instillation into the bladder causes a local inflammatory reaction that eliminates or reduces superficial tumors. Systemic mycobacterial infection is a rare complication of intravesical BCG therapy that may require antituberculin treatment (Tierney et al., 2005). Other chemotherapeutic agents also may be administered intravesically, including doxorubicin, mitomycin C, and interferon. Bladder irritation, frequency, dysuria, and contact dermatitis are possible adverse reactions to intravesical chemotherapy. Suppression of bone marrow function also can occur as a result of intravesical treatment.

Radiation Therapy

Radiation is another adjunctive therapy used in the treatment of urinary tumors. Although radiation alone is not curative, it can reduce tumor size prior to surgery and is used as palliative treatment for inoperable tumors and clients who cannot tolerate surgery. Radiation therapy also is used in combination with systemic chemotherapy to improve local and distant relapse rates (Tierney et al., 2005) (see Chapter 14).

TABLE 28–4 Bladder Tumor Staging

DEPTH OF INVOLVEMENT	TNM (TUMOR, NODE, METASTASIS) STAGE	TUMOR INVOLVEMENT
Superficial	T_a	Limited to the bladder mucosa
	T_1	Involvement of the bladder mucosa and submucosal layers
Invasive	T_2	Invasion of superficial muscle of bladder wall
	T_{3a}	Deep muscle invasion
	T_{3b}	Involvement of perivesicular fat
	$T_{3-4}N_+$	Regional (pelvic) lymph node involvement
	$T_{3-4}M_1$	Metastasis to distant lymph nodes or organs

TABLE 28–5 Surgical Procedures to Treat Bladder Tumors

PROCEDURE	INDICATIONS	NURSING IMPLICATIONS
Transurethral resection of bladder tumor	Diagnose and treat superficial bladder tumors having low rate of recurrence; control bleeding	Maintain continuous bladder irrigation postoperatively; monitor for excessive bleeding; ensure catheter patency. Increase fluids to 2500–3000 mL/day. Give stool softeners to prevent straining.
Partial cystectomy	Resect solitary, isolated tumor at stage T_2 or T_3 not involving trigone	Maintain patency of urethral and/or suprapubic catheter to make sure suture lines are free of pressure; monitor for excess bleeding.
Complete or radical cystectomy	Remove large, invasive tumors; involvement of trigone	Permanent urinary diversion is required. Maintain patency and position of stents; urethral catheter may be in place to drain pelvic cavity.

Surgery

A number of surgical procedures, ranging from simple resection of noninvasive tumors to removal of the bladder and surrounding structures, are used to treat urinary tract tumors. Indications for each procedure and specific nursing implications are outlined in Table 28–5.

Transurethral tumor resection may be performed by excision, *fulguration* (destruction of tissue using electric sparks generated by high-frequency current), or *laser photocoagulation* (use of light energy to destroy abnormal tissue). Laser surgery carries the lowest risk of bleeding and perforation of the bladder wall. Following cystoscopic tumor resection, clients are followed at 3-month intervals for tumor recurrence. Recurrences may develop anywhere in the urinary tract, including the renal pelvis, ureter, or urethra (Kasper et al., 2005).

Cystectomy, surgical removal of the bladder, is necessary to treat invasive cancers. Partial cystectomy may be done to remove a solitary lesion; however, radical cystectomy is the standard treatment for invasive tumors. The bladder and adjacent muscles and tissues are removed. In men, the prostate and seminal vessels are also removed, resulting in impotence. In women, a total hysterectomy and bilateral salpingo-oophorectomy (removal of the uterus, fallopian tubes, and ovaries) accompanies the procedure, causing sterility. At the time of surgery, a **urinary diversion** is created to provide for urine collection and drainage. Either an *ileal conduit* (Figure 28–7A ■) or a *continent urinary diversion* (Figure 28–7B) is created to collect and drain urine. Table 28–6 describes the most frequently used urinary diversion techniques.

Surgical procedures to remove tumors involving other portions of the urinary tract vary according to the site and stage of the tumor. When the distal ureter is involved, the tumor may be resected and the ureter implanted into the opposite ureter to provide for drainage. A proximal ureteral tumor necessitates removal of the ureter and kidney on the affected side.

See the box on page 866 for nursing care of the client undergoing tumor resection and a urinary diversion.

A

B

Figure 28–7 ■ Common urinary diversion procedures. *A,* Ileal conduit. A segment of ileum is separated from the small intestine and formed into a tubular pouch with the open end brought to the skin surface to form a stoma. The ureters are connected to the pouch. *B,* A continent urinary diversion. A segment of ileum is separated from the small intestine and formed into a pouch. Nipple valves are formed at each end of the pouch by intussuscepting tissue backward into the reservoir to prevent leakage.

TABLE 28–6 Urinary Diversion Procedures

PROCEDURE	DESCRIPTION	NURSING CONSIDERATIONS
Ileal conduit	Portion of ileum is isolated from small intestine, leaving vascular, lymphatic, and neural connections intact; ileum is formed into pouch with open end brought to surface to form a stoma; ureters are inserted into pouch.	Most common urinary diversion. Continuous urine drainage necessitates appliance. Postoperative edema may interfere with urine output. Risk of infection is less than for cutaneous ureterostomy, but potential for reflux is high. Good skin care vital because of constant contact with urine.
Continent internal ileal reservoir or continent ileal bladder conduit (Kock pouch)	Pouch is created as for ileal conduit but nipple valves are formed by intussuscepting tissue backward into a reservoir to connect pouch to the skin and the ureters to the pouch; filling pressure closes valves, preventing leakage and reflux.	Drainage collection device not necessary. Client must be willing and able to perform clean intermittent self-catheterization every 2 to 4 hours. Continence valve mechanism may fail, requiring surgery for revision.
Indiana continent urinary reservoir	A portion of the terminal ileum, ascending colon, and cecum is isolated from the bowel with vascular and neural connections intact. Reservoir is formed from colon and cecum; portion of the ileum is brought to the surface to form nipple valve and stoma or is attached to urethral stump.	As for Kock pouch. Client must be able and motivated to manage self-catheterization. Reservoir may absorb urea and electrolytes, resulting in imbalances. Significant portion of bowel is required to form pouch and stoma.
Ileocystoplasty or Camey procedure	Section of the ileum is isolated and formed into U shape. Ureters are implanted in upper portion of the U. Urethra is anastomosed to central section.	Appropriate for men only because urethra is removed with cystectomy in women. Allows client to void by relaxing pelvic muscles and using Valsalva maneuver.

NURSING CARE

The client who undergoes treatment for a tumor of the urinary tract has many nursing care needs because of alterations in the functional health patterns of elimination, health perception-health management, cognitive-perceptual, self-perception-self-concept, role-relationships, and coping-stress-tolerance.

Health Promotion

Encourage all clients not to smoke. Provide referral to smoking cessation programs or clinics for clients who wish to quit smoking. Encourage clients at high risk for developing bladder cancer (see page 862) to have periodic examinations, including urinalysis and possible urine cytology.

Assessment

Nursing assessment related to urinary tract cancer includes both subjective and objective information:
- *Health history:* Risk factors; history of hematuria or manifestations of UTI (dysuria, frequency, urgency, pyuria); lower abdominal discomfort or flank pain.
- *Physical examination:* General health; abdominal tenderness; urine for analysis.

Nursing Diagnoses and Interventions

Maintaining urinary output is the priority nursing care focus for the client with a bladder tumor. For additional potential nursing diagnoses and interventions for the client with a bladder tumor, see the Nursing Care Plan that follows.

Impaired Urinary Elimination

Whether the client has undergone transurethral resection of a bladder tumor or radical cystectomy with urinary diversion, urinary elimination is altered at least temporarily.
- Monitor urine output from all catheters, stents, and tubes for amount, color, and clarity hourly for the first 24 hours postoperatively, then every 4 to 8 hours. *Decreased urine output may indicate impaired catheter or drainage system patency. Prompt intervention is necessary to prevent hydronephrosis. A change in color or clarity may indicate a complication such as hemorrhage or infection.*

PRACTICE ALERT

Promptly report urine output of less than 30 mL per hour, which may indicate low vascular volume or renal insufficiency. Prompt intervention is vital to restore cardiac output and prevent acute renal failure.

- Label all catheters, stents, and their drainage containers. Maintain separate closed gravity drainage systems for each. *Clear identification of each tube can prevent errors in irrigating and calculating outputs. Separate closed systems minimize the risk and extent of potential bacterial contamination and resultant infection.*

PRACTICE ALERT

Use aseptic techniques and strictly follow guidelines for irrigating catheters. Catheters placed in the kidney pelvis are irrigated using gentle pressure and small amounts of fluid (10 to 15 mL) to avoid damaging renal tissues.

NURSING CARE OF THE CLIENT HAVING A Cystectomy and Urinary Diversion

PREOPERATIVE CARE

■ Provide routine preoperative care as outlined in Chapter 4 ∞.

■ Assess knowledge of the proposed surgery and its long-term implications, clarifying misunderstandings and discussing concerns. *Clients having surgery for cancer of the urinary tract are trying to cope with diagnosis of cancer and may not fully understand the surgery and its potential effects. Open discussion can facilitate postoperative recovery and adjustment.*

■ Begin teaching about postoperative tubes and drains, self-care of stoma, and control of drainage and odor. *Postoperative physiologic and psychologic stressors may interfere with learning. A basic understanding of what to expect in the way of tubes, drains, and procedures reduces stress in the immediate postoperative period. Preoperative teaching can enhance recall and postoperative learning.*

■ Assist in identifying stoma site, avoiding folds of skin, bones, scar tissue, and the waistline or belt area. Be sure to consider the client's occupation and style of clothing. The site should be visible to the client and accessible for manipulation. *Stoma placement is a vital component of adjustment and self-care. Care is taken to place the stoma away from areas of constant irritation by clothing or movement. It should be located so that the client can cover and disguise the collecting device, maintain the seal to prevent leakage, and effectively cleanse and maintain the site.*

■ Perform bowel-preparation activities as ordered. *Bowel preparation is done to prevent fecal contamination of the peritoneal cavity and to decompress the bowel during surgery.*

POSTOPERATIVE CARE

■ Provide routine postoperative care (See Chapter 4 ∞).

■ Monitor intake and output carefully, assessing urine output every hour for the first 24 hours, then every 4 hours or as ordered. Call the physician if urine output is less than 30 mL per hour. *Tissue edema and bleeding may interfere with urinary output from stoma, catheters, or drains. Maintenance of urine*

outflow is vital to prevent hydronephrosis and possible renal damage. A urine output of at least 30 mL per hour is necessary for effective renal function.

■ Assess color and consistency of urine. Expect pink or bright red urine fading to pink and then clearing by the third postoperative day. Urine may be cloudy due to mucous production by bowel mucosa. *Bright red blood in the urine from a urinary diversion may indicate hemorrhage, necessitating further surgery. Excessive cloudiness or malodorous urine may indicate infection.*

■ Assess size, color, and condition of the stoma and surrounding skin every 2 hours for the first 24 hours, then every 4 hours for 48 to 72 hours. Expect the stoma to appear bright red and slightly edematous initially. Slight bleeding during cleansing is normal. *Compromised circulation causes the stoma to appear pale, gray, or cyanotic or blanch when touched. Other complications, such as infection or impaired healing, may be evidenced by a change in the appearance of the stoma or incision.*

■ Irrigate the ileal diversion catheter with 30 to 60 mL of normal saline every 4 hours or as ordered. *Mucus produced by the bowel wall may accumulate in the newly devised reservoir or obstruct catheters.*

■ Monitor serum electrolyte values, acid–base balance, and renal function tests such as BUN and serum creatinine. *Reabsorption of electrolytes from reservoirs created by portions of bowel may result in electrolyte imbalance and metabolic acidosis. Optimal renal function is necessary to maintain a normal state of homeostasis.*

■ Teach the client and family about stoma and urinary diversion care, including odor management, skin care, increased fluid intake, pouch application and leakage prevention, self-catheterization for clients with continent reservoirs, and signs of infection and other complications. *The ability to provide self-care is a significant factor in the adjustment to a changed body image. Teaching family members facilitates acceptance and adjustment. The family also needs this knowledge in case illness or disability interferes with the self-care capacity.*

■ Secure ureteral catheters and stents with tape; prevent kinking or occlusion; and maintain gravity flow by keeping drainage bag below level of kidneys. *Impaired urine flow can lead to urinary retention and distention of the bladder, a newly created reservoir, or the renal pelvis (hydronephrosis).*

■ Encourage fluid intake of 3000 mL per day. *Increased fluid intake maintains a high urinary output, reducing the risk of infection. Dilute urine is less irritating to the skin surrounding the stoma site. Electrolyte reabsorption from reservoirs may increase risk of calculi; high fluid intake and urine output reduce this risk.*

PRACTICE ALERT

Monitor urine output closely for first 24 hours after stents or ureteral catheters are removed. Edema or stricture of ureters may impede output, leading to hydronephrosis and kidney damage.

■ Encourage activity to tolerance. *Ambulation promotes drainage of urine from reservoirs and helps prevent calcium loss from bones, which could precipitate calculus formation.*

Risk for Impaired Skin Integrity

The skin surrounding the stoma site of an ileal conduit is at risk for irritation and breakdown. Because urine is acidic and contains high concentrations of electrolytes, it has a corrosive effect on skin. In addition, adhesives and sealants used to prevent pouch leakage may irritate the skin.

■ Assess peristomal skin for redness, excoriation, or signs of breakdown. Assess for urine leakage from catheters, stents, or drains. Keep the skin clean and dry. Change wet dressings. *Intact skin is the first line of defense against infection. Impaired skin integrity may lead to local or systemic infection and impaired healing.*

NURSING CARE PLAN A Client with a Bladder Tumor

Ben Hussain is a 61-year-old automobile salesman. He is married and has five children, all of whom are grown and living away from home. One week ago, Mr. Hussain became alarmed when his urine became bright red. Even though he had no other symptoms, he called his physician. The physician ordered a urinalysis and urine cytology, revealing gross hematuria and poorly differentiated abnormal cells. Cystoscopy and tissue biopsy confirm a stage C tumor involving the bladder trigone. Mr. Hussain is admitted for a radical cystectomy and continent urinary diversion.

ASSESSMENT

Mr. Hussain's admission history, obtained by Tara Mills, RN, his primary nurse, indicates that he has lost 10 to 15 pounds during the last few months. He smoked two to three packs of cigarettes per day for 40 years, but cut back to a pack a day about a year ago. He says he could not quit smoking entirely. He drinks five to six cups of coffee daily and consumes a moderate amount of alcohol, averaging three to four drinks a day. Mr. Hussain says that he is "a little nervous about surgery and what they're going to find." Ms. Mills notes that he fidgets and talks rapidly throughout their interview. He also expresses concern about how he will handle the pain after surgery, because he has never been hospitalized before his cystoscopy. Physical assessment findings include T 98.2°F (36.7°C) PO, P 84, R 18, and BP 154/86. Examinations of the skin, neuromuscular, and cardiac systems are within normal limits. Scattered expiratory crackles are noted on auscultation of lung fields. Bowel sounds are very active; Mr. Hussain explains that he began taking his bowel-preparation laxative the day before admission. Slight tenderness is noted in the suprapubic region. Mr. Hussain's urine is clear and bright pink. CBC and chemistry screening results are within normal limits. Surgery is planned for 9:00 A.M. the following day.

DIAGNOSES

- *Anxiety* related to undetermined extent of disease and fear of pain
- *Deficient Knowledge* related to care and management of continent urinary diversion
- *Impaired Urinary Elimination* related to cystectomy and urinary diversion
- *Risk for Impaired Gas Exchange* related to smoking history and effects of anesthesia

EXPECTED OUTCOMES

- Verbalize decreased feelings of anxiety.
- Demonstrate appropriate postoperative pain relief through subjective reports of pain severity and objective findings.
- Be able to care for urinary diversion and surrounding skin, prior to discharge.
- Demonstrate self-catheterization of stoma using appropriate technique prior to discharge.

- Maintain normal urine output with acceptable color and clarity and no signs of infection.
- Maintain adequate gas exchange as evidenced by good skin color, O_2 saturation greater than 95%, and clear lung sounds on auscultation.

PLANNING AND IMPLEMENTATION

- Spend as much time as possible with Mr. Hussain and his family preoperatively, answering questions fully and encouraging expression of fears.
- Provide written and verbal explanations when feasible.
- Administer analgesia on a regular basis for the first 48 to 72 hours. Monitor for objective signs of unrelieved pain.
- Explain all procedures related to stoma and diversion care as they are being performed.
- Encourage Mr. Hussain to look at stoma and touch it when ready.
- Teach stoma and skin care, as well as self-catheterization, emphasizing measures to prevent skin irritation and urinary tract infection.
- Monitor urine output, color, clarity, and consistency every hour for first 24 hours, then every 4 hours for 24 hours, then every 8 hours. Report output of less than 30 mL per hour, bright bleeding, excessively cloudy or malodorous urine.
- Assist with use of incentive spirometer every hour while awake. Ambulate as soon as possible. Assess lung sounds every 4 hours, reporting increased crackles or diminished breath sounds.
- Refer Mr. and Mrs. Hussain to local stoma group on discharge.

EVALUATION

On discharge, Mr. Hussain has performed self-catheterization and stoma and skin care several times. His wife also is able to catheterize the stoma and demonstrate skin care. His urine is pale yellow and slightly cloudy. Mr. Hussain is ambulating independently and using oxycodone (Percocet) twice a day for pain relief. His lungs are clear, and he is very proud of having "survived" 7 days without a cigarette. He says, "Now I'm going to shoot for 7 weeks, then 7 months, then 7 years without a smoke!" A home health referral is made to continue teaching Mr. Hussain to care for his diversion and appliance.

CRITICAL THINKING IN THE NURSING PROCESS

1. How does cigarette smoking contribute to the increased risk of urinary tract tumors?
2. Suppose Mr. Hussain had become confused, disoriented, and tremorous and had begun to experience visual hallucinations 2 to 3 days postoperatively. What would you suspect the cause to be? What would be the appropriate response?
3. Develop a care plan for Mr. Hussain for the nursing diagnosis *Risk for Sexual Dysfunction.*
   See Evaluating Your Response in Appendix C.

- Ensure gravity drainage of urine collection device or empty bag every 2 hours. *Overfilling of the collection bag may damage the seal, allowing leakage and contact of urine with skin.*

- Change urine collection appliance as needed, removing any mucus from stoma. See Box 28–2 for care of a urinary drainage stoma. *Meticulous care and protection of skin surrounding stoma can maintain integrity and prevent breakdown.*

BOX 28–2 Urinary Stoma Care

- Gather all supplies: a clean, disposable pouch; liquid skin barrier or barrier ring; 4-by-4 gauze squares; stoma guide; adhesive solvent; clean gloves; and a clean washcloth.
- Assess knowledge, learning needs, and ability and willingness to assist with procedure. Explain the procedure as needed.
- Use standard precautions.
- Remove old pouch, pulling gently away from skin. Warm water or adhesive solvent may be used to loosen the seal if necessary.
- Assess stoma. Normally the stoma is bright red and appears moist. Report a dark purple, black, or very pale stoma to the physician. Slight bleeding with cleansing is normal, especially in the immediate postoperative period.
- Prevent urine flow during cleaning by placing a rolled gauze square or tampon over the stoma opening.
- Cleanse skin around the stoma with soap and water, rinse, and pat or air dry.
- Use the stoma guide to determine correct size for the bag opening and/or protective ring seal. Trim the bag or seal as needed.
- Apply skin barrier; allow to dry.
- Apply the bag with an opening no more than 1 to 2 mm wider than outside of stoma. Allow no wrinkles or creases where the bag contacts the skin.
- Connect bag to the urine-collection device. Dispose of old pouch, used supplies, and gloves appropriately. Wash hands.
- Chart procedure, including stoma appearance and response of the client.

Disturbed Body Image

A radical cystectomy and urinary diversion affect the client's body image. In most cases, an abdominal stoma is created, requiring either a drainage appliance or regular catheterization of the stoma to drain urine. Removal of the prostate and seminal vesicles or the uterus and ovaries leaves the client sterile. If radiation or chemotherapy is planned as adjunctive therapy, the client may experience hair loss, stomatitis, nausea and vomiting, or other disturbing side effects of therapy.

- Use therapeutic communication techniques, actively listening and responding to the client's and family's concerns. *Clients must know their feelings and concerns are respected and valued. Denial, anger, guilt, bargaining, or depression are common during grieving and normal for a client undergoing a significant change in body image.*
- Recognize and accept behaviors that indicate use of coping mechanisms, encouraging adaptive mechanisms. *The client may initially use defensive coping mechanisms such as denial, minimization, and dissociation from the immediate situation to reduce anxiety and maintain psychologic integrity. Adaptive mechanisms include learning as much as possible about the surgery and its effects, practicing procedures, setting realistic goals, and rehearsing various alternative outcomes.*
- Encourage looking at, touching, and caring for the stoma and appliance as soon as possible. Allow the client to proceed gradually, providing support and encouragement. *Accepting the stoma as part of the self is vital to adapting to the changed body image and is indicated by a willingness to provide self-care.*
- Discuss concerns about returning to usual activities, perceived relationship changes, and resumption of sexual relations. Provide referral to support group or provide for contact with someone who has successfully adjusted to a urinary diversion. *Clients and families may be reluctant to discuss topics of concern. An atmosphere of openness and acceptance facilitates expression of concerns and anxieties related to the changed body image.*

Risk for Infection

Diagnostic instrumentation procedures, surgical manipulation, and disruption of normal urinary tract defense mechanisms increase the risk of ascending urinary tract infection. When an ileal conduit or artificial bladder is created using bowel tissue, the normal bacteriostatic activity of bladder mucosa is lost. In addition, the peristaltic action of the ureters may be disrupted, and the vesicoureteral junction no longer prevents urine reflux. Adjunctive chemotherapy or radiation treatments may impair normal immune function and further increase the risk of infection.

- Maintain separate closed drainage systems, keeping drainage bags lower than the kidney, and prevent loops or kinks in drainage tubing, which impede urine flow. *Although urine is sterile when it leaves the kidney, bacteria grow rapidly in urine. Prevention of urine reflux is essential to preventing UTI.*
- Monitor for signs of infection: elevated temperature, cloudy or foul-smelling urine, hematuria, general malaise, back or abdominal pain, and nausea and vomiting. *Infection undermines the healing process. Early detection and treatment help prevent long-term consequences such as chronic pyelonephritis.*

PRACTICE ALERT

Impaired immune function (due to aging or the effects of chemotherapy) and urine cloudiness (related to the effects of urine on ileal mucosa) can mask usual signs of UTI such as fever and altered urine clarity. Be alert for more generalized manifestations such as increased fatigue and malaise.

- Teach signs and symptoms of infection and self-care measures to prevent UTI. *The client with a cystectomy and ileal diversion, urostomy, or continent reservoir is at risk of UTI for life because of impaired urinary defense mechanisms. Using clean or aseptic technique in providing care, increasing fluid intake, and using measures to acidify urine minimize this risk to a certain degree but do not eliminate it.*

Community-Based Care

The need for individual and family teaching for the client who has had surgery to treat a urinary tract tumor is significant. For many clients, surgery means a lifelong change in urinary elimination. Even the client who has undergone transurethral excision of bladder tumors requires follow-up cystoscopy on a regular basis and needs to be alert for signs of tumor recurrence.

The client who has had a urinary diversion needs teaching about care of the stoma and surrounding skin, prevention of urine reflux and infection, signs and symptoms of UTI and renal calculi, and, in some cases, self-catheterization using clean technique.

THE CLIENT WITH URINARY RETENTION

Urinary retention, incomplete emptying of the bladder, can lead to overdistention of the bladder, poor detrusor muscle contractility, and inability to urinate. If the problem persists, hydroureter and hydronephrosis can result.

Physiology Review

Normally, bladder emptying is controlled by the interaction of muscle tone and the autonomic nervous system. The sympathetic nervous system (SNS) relaxes the detrusor muscle, allowing the bladder to fill with urine. The internal sphincter, a continuation of the detrusor muscle, remains closed during filling. Pressures within the bladder remain low during filling, in contrast to high sphincter and urethral pressures. Voluntary muscles of the external sphincter and pelvic floor help maintain these high pressures. When the bladder contains 150 to 300 mL of urine, signals from stretch receptors in the bladder wall are transmitted to the spinal cord and cerebral cortex. Reflexive bladder emptying can be consciously inhibited. During *micturition* (bladder emptying), parasympathetic stimulation causes the detrusor muscle of the bladder fundus to contract, opening the internal sphincter. The external sphincter then relaxes, allowing urine to flow out.

Pathophysiology

Either mechanical obstruction of the bladder outlet or a functional problem can cause urinary retention. *Benign prostatic hypertrophy (BPH)* is a common cause; difficulty initiating and maintaining urine flow is often the presenting complaint in men with BPH. Acute inflammation associated with infection or trauma of the bladder, urethra, or perineal tissues may also interfere with micturition. Scarring due to repeated urinary tract infection can lead to urethral stricture and a mechanical obstruction. Bladder calculi may also obstruct the urethral opening from the bladder.

Surgery, particularly abdominal or pelvic surgery, may disrupt detrusor muscle function, leading to urine retention. Drugs also may interfere with its function. Anticholinergic medications such as atropine, glycopyrrolate (Robinul), propantheline bromide (Pro-Banthine), scopolamine hydrochloride (Transderm-Scop), and others can lead to acute urinary retention and bladder distention. Many other drug groups have anticholinergic side effects and may cause urinary retention. Among these are antianxiety agents such as diazepam (Valium), antidepressant and tricyclic drugs such as imipramine (Tofranil), antiparkinsonian drugs, antipsychotic agents, and some sedative/hypnotic drugs. In addition, antihistamines common in over-the-counter cough, cold, allergy, and sleep-promoting drugs have anticholinergic effects and may interfere with bladder emptying. Diphenhydramine (Benadryl) is an example of a nonprescription antihistamine.

Voluntary urinary retention (particularly common among nurses!) may lead to overfilling of the bladder and a loss of detrusor muscle tone.

Manifestations

The client with urinary retention is unable to empty the bladder completely. Overflow voiding or incontinence may occur, with 25 to 50 mL of urine eliminated at frequent intervals. Assessment reveals a firm, distended bladder that may be displaced to one side of midline. Percussion of the lower abdomen reveals a dull tone, reflective of fluid in the bladder.

Severe urinary retention with resulting bladder distention impairs the ability of the vesicoureteral junction to prevent backflow of urine into the ureters (see Figure 28–1 on page 847). Reflux of urine from the distended bladder distends the ureters (hydroureter) and kidneys (hydronephrosis). Hydronephrosis impairs renal function, and acute renal failure can result. See Chapter 29 ∞ for more information about acute renal failure.

INTERDISCIPLINARY CARE

Urinary retention is confirmed using a bladder scan or by inserting a urinary catheter (if possible) and measuring the urine output. Use of a bladder scan is preferred to reduce the risk of UTI (Teng et al., 2005).

An indwelling urinary catheter or intermittent straight catheterization can prevent urinary retention and overdistention of the bladder. Cholinergic medications such as bethanechol chloride (Urecholine), which promote detrusor muscle contraction and bladder emptying, may be used. A medication with no anticholinergic side effects may be substituted when urinary retention is related to drug therapy.

Mechanical obstructions are treated by removing or repairing the obstruction when possible. Resection of the prostate gland may be done for urinary retention related to BPH. Bladder calculi are removed, and measures to prevent their formation are instituted.

NURSING CARE

Health promotion measures to prevent urinary retention include monitoring urine output in at-risk clients and evaluating drug regimens for medications known to interfere with detrusor muscle function. Pay particular attention to elimination when these drugs are ordered for (or used by) a client with BPH or other mechanical obstruction of urine flow.

Impaired Urinary Elimination

Nursing measures to promote urination include placing the client in normal voiding position and providing for privacy. Additional measures include running water, placing the client's hands in warm water, pouring warm water over the perineum, or taking a warm sitz bath.

In acute urinary retention, catheterization may be necessary to relieve bladder distention and prevent hydronephrosis. Use a relatively small catheter (16 Fr. for a man, 14 Fr. for a woman). A coudé-tipped catheter is passed more easily in the older man with an enlarged prostate. Using 2% lidocaine gel (10 mL injected into the male urethra or 6 mL injected into the female urethra) reduces discomfort during catheterization and the risk of catheter-associated infection and promotes pelvic muscle relaxation (Bardsley, 2005). Carefully observe the client as the distended bladder drains.

PRACTICE ALERT

Some clients may experience a vasovagal response, becoming pale, sweaty, and hypotensive if the bladder is rapidly drained. Draining urine in 500-mL increments and clamping the catheter for 5 to 10 minutes between increments may prevent this response. Hematuria also may occur with rapid bladder decompression. Promptly notify the physician if hematuria develops.

Home care for the client with urinary retention varies, depending on the cause. Some clients may be taught intermittent self-catheterization. Instruct all clients who have experienced urinary retention to avoid over-the-counter drugs that affect micturition, especially those with an anticholinergic effect (allergy and cold medications, many nonprescription sleep aids). Other home care measures include double-voiding (urinate, remain on the toilet for 2 to 5 minutes, then urinate again), scheduled voiding, or, when other measures fail, an indwelling catheter. When an indwelling catheter is necessary, teach the client and family to use clean technique when changing from overnight bag to leg bag, and to promptly report signs of UTI to the primary care provider.

THE CLIENT WITH NEUROGENIC BLADDER

The neurologic connections influencing bladder filling, the perception of fullness and the need to void, and bladder emptying are complex. Disruption of the central or peripheral nervous systems may interfere with normal mechanisms, causing **neurogenic bladder**.

Pathophysiology

As noted in the physiology section on urinary retention, bladder filling and emptying are controlled by the central nervous system (CNS). This neurologic control can be disrupted at any level: the cerebral cortex (voluntary impulses), the micturition center of the midbrain, the spinal cord tracts, or the peripheral nerves of the bladder itself.

Spastic Bladder Dysfunction

A simple reflex arc exists between the bladder and the spinal cord at levels S_2 through S_4. The stimulus of more than 400 mL of urine in the bladder causes reflex contraction of the detrusor muscle and bladder emptying unless voluntary control (cerebral input) is used to suppress it. Disruption of CNS transmission above the sacral spinal cord segment typically leads to *spastic neurogenic bladder*. Both sensory and voluntary control of urination are interrupted partially or totally, while the sacral reflex arc remains intact. The stimuli generated by bladder filling cause frequent spontaneous detrusor muscle contraction and involuntary bladder emptying. Spinal cord injury above the sacral segment is the most common cause of a spastic bladder.

Other causes include stroke, multiple sclerosis, and other CNS lesions (Porth, 2005).

Flaccid Bladder Dysfunction

Damage to the sacral spinal cord at the level of the reflex arc, the cauda equina, or the sacral nerve roots causes loss of detrusor muscle tone and a *flaccid neurogenic bladder*. The perception of bladder fullness is lost, and the bladder becomes overdistended, with weak and ineffective detrusor muscle contractions. Flaccid neurogenic bladder is seen with myelomeningocele and during the spinal shock phase of a spinal cord injury above the sacral region. During the spinal shock phase, all reflex activity below the level of spinal cord injury is suppressed.

Peripheral neuropathies may also cause bladder atony and overfilling. Either sensory or motor pathways (or both) may be disrupted, leading to incomplete bladder emptying and large residual volumes after voiding (Porth, 2005). Diabetes mellitus is the most common cause of peripheral bladder neuropathy. Other causes include multiple sclerosis, chronic alcoholism, and prolonged overdistention of the bladder.

INTERDISCIPLINARY CARE

Management of neurogenic bladder focuses on maintaining continence and avoiding complications associated with overfilling or incomplete emptying of the bladder. Because self-care is the goal, teaching is a primary intervention for the healthcare team.

Diagnosis

The following diagnostic tests may be ordered for the client with a neurogenic bladder:

- *Urine culture* to detect possible urinary tract infection related to impaired bladder function.
- *Urinalysis* and *serum creatinine* and *BUN* to evaluate renal function. See the diagnostic tests table on page 835 for normal BUN and creatinine levels. Ascending infection or hydronephrosis resulting from bladder overfilling and vesicoureteral reflux can damage the kidneys. Impaired renal function may lead to blood cells or protein in the urine, and elevated BUN and creatinine levels.
- *Postvoid catheterization* to measure residual urine. Amounts greater than 50 mL may indicate ineffective detrusor muscle contractions, common in neurogenic bladder.
- *Cystometrography* to evaluate bladder filling and the detrusor muscle tone and function. See page 836 for nursing care of the client undergoing cystometrography.

Medications

Medications may be prescribed to increase or decrease the contractility of the detrusor muscle, to increase or decrease the tone of the internal sphincter, or to relax the external urethral sphincter.

Bethanechol, a cholinergic drug, stimulates detrusor muscle contraction in flaccid neurogenic bladder. It is generally used to manage short-term urinary retention (e.g., following surgery or childbirth). It may used in combination with bladder-training techniques to promote complete emptying of a neurogenic bladder. Anticholinesterase drugs such as neostigmine (Prostigmin) and pyridostigmine (Mestinon) also may be used to increase detrusor muscle tone.

Anticholinergic drugs (parasympathetic blockers) relax the detrusor muscle and contract the internal sphincter, increasing bladder capacity in clients with spastic bladder dysfunction. Oxybutynin (Ditropan) and tolterodine (Detrol) inhibit the muscarinic effects of acetylcholine on smooth muscle, reducing detrusor muscle spasticity and promoting bladder filling. Other anticholinergic drugs also may be used, including propantheline (Pro-Banthine) or flavoxate (Urispas). Dry mouth, blurred vision, and constipation are potential adverse effects of anticholinergic medications. See the Medication Administration box below for drugs used to modify detrusor muscle activity.

Nutrition

Dietary measures to reduce the risk for UTI and urinary calculi may be suggested for the client with neurogenic bladder. A moderate to high fluid intake and a diet that acidifies the urine are helpful. Cranberry juice is recommended to maintain urine acidity. See Table 28–3 for additional foods to include or avoid in the diet to help prevent UTI and urolithiasis. The timing of fluid intake may be regulated to promote continence.

Bladder Retraining

Clients with spastic neurogenic bladder may use measures to stimulate reflex voiding, allowing scheduled toileting. Techniques include using trigger points, for example, stroking or pinching the abdomen, inner thigh, or glans penis. Pulling pubic hairs, tapping the suprapubic region, or inserting a gloved finger into the rectum and gently stretching the anal sphincter can also stimulate urination.

The *Credé's method* (applying pressure to the suprapubic region with the fingers of one or both hands), manual pressure on the abdomen, and the Valsalva maneuver (bearing down while holding one's breath) promote bladder emptying for the client with a spastic or flaccid bladder.

PRACTICE ALERT

Increasing lower abdominal and bladder pressure with the Credé's method can stimulate autonomic dysreflexia in some clients with spinal cord injuries. Autonomic dysreflexia is a medical emergency in which the blood pressure rises rapidly due to SNS stimulation.

See Chapter 45 ∞ for a discussion of autonomic dysreflexia.

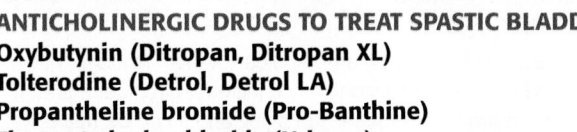

MEDICATION ADMINISTRATION The Client with Neurogenic Bladder

ANTICHOLINERGIC DRUGS TO TREAT SPASTIC BLADDER
Oxybutynin (Ditropan, Ditropan XL)
Tolterodine (Detrol, Detrol LA)
Propantheline bromide (Pro-Banthine)
Flavoxate hydrochloride (Urispas)

Anticholinergic drugs inhibit the response to acetylcholine, relaxing the detrusor muscle and increasing internal sphincter tone. The combination of detrusor relaxation and internal sphincter contraction increases the bladder capacity of clients with spastic or hyperreflexive neurogenic bladder. Of these medications, tolterodine has the most specific effects on the detrusor muscle with fewer anticholinergic side effects.

Nursing Responsibilities
- Assess for contraindications, such as glaucoma, gastrointestinal or urinary tract obstruction, severe ulcerative colitis or toxic megacolon, unstable cardiovascular status, or myasthenia gravis.
- Observe for the desired effect of increased bladder capacity with decreased incontinence and spasm.
- Monitor for possible interaction with other drugs such as narcotic analgesics, antidysrhythmic medications, antihistamines, antidepressants, or psychoactive drugs.
- Monitor heart rate and blood pressure, especially when given to clients with known cardiovascular disease.
- Assess for adverse effects such as urinary hesitancy or retention, dysrhythmias, mental status changes, and gastrointestinal disturbances.

Health Education for the Client and Family
- Promptly report eye pain, rapid heart beat, difficulty breathing, rash or hives, or changes in mental function to your primary care provider.
- These drugs may cause drowsiness or blurred vision. Use caution when driving, operating machinery, or performing other tasks requiring mental acuity.

- Hard candies help relieve dry mouth associated with these drugs.
- Do not use alcohol or nonprescription antihistamines while taking these drugs.

CHOLINERGIC DRUGS TO STIMULATE MICTURITION
Bethanechol chloride (Urecholine)

Bethanechol stimulates the parasympathetic nervous system, increasing detrusor muscle tone and producing a contraction strong enough to initiate micturition. It is used primarily to treat acute postoperative and postpartum urinary retention.

Nursing Responsibilities
- Assess for contraindications, including hypersensitivity, hyperthyroidism, peptic ulcer disease, asthma, significant bradycardia or hypotension, coronary heart disease, epilepsy, and parkinsonism.
- Do not give to clients who have had recent gastrointestinal or bladder surgery or those with possible gastrointestinal or urinary tract obstruction.
- Give oral forms on an empty stomach to reduce the risk of nausea and vomiting.
- Administer parenteral bethanechol subcutaneously. Keep atropine, the antidote for bethanechol overdose or toxicity, available.
- Observe for desired effect within 30 to 60 minutes after oral administration, 5 to 15 minutes after injection.
- Assess for adverse effects such as malaise, headache, abdominal cramping, nausea, hypotension with reflex tachycardia, wheezing, and dyspnea.

Health Education for the Client and Family
- Take the medication 1 hour before or 2 hours after meals.
- Use caution when rising from a recumbent or sitting position; you may feel dizzy or light-headed.

The client with a flaccid bladder may require catheterization to completely empty the bladder. An indwelling catheter may be used initially, but intermittent catheterization is preferred. Clean intermittent self-catheterization is performed every 3 to 4 hours to prevent overdistention of the bladder (see Procedure 45–1 ∞).

Surgery

Surgery may be required when urination cannot be effectively managed using more conservative measures. *Rhizotomy,* or destruction of the nerve supply to the detrusor muscle or the external sphincter, may be used for clients with hyperreflexia or spasticity. Urinary diversion is another surgical technique used when conservative management fails. Implantation of an artificial sphincter may be useful for some clients with neurogenic bladder. See Table 28–6 for urinary diversion techniques and page 866 for nursing care of the client undergoing a urinary diversion.

NURSING CARE

Nursing care of the client with a neurogenic bladder is directed toward promoting urinary drainage and continence, preventing complications, and teaching the client and family self-care techniques.

Assessment

Nursing assessment for neurogenic bladder includes obtaining a complete nursing history, focusing on information related to CNS or spinal cord injury or disease, as well as disorders that affect the peripheral nervous system (e.g., diabetes). Ask about measures used to stimulate or control urination. Inspect and palpate the lower abdomen and suprapubic region for tenderness or bladder distention. Percuss the suprapubic region for a dull percussion tone indicative of a full bladder. Dullness up to the level of the umbilicus indicates at least 500 mL of urine in the bladder (Gray, 2000). Assess urine for color, clarity, and odor. Collect a specimen for analysis as indicated.

Nursing Diagnoses and Interventions

Although each client has individual nursing care needs, examples of nursing diagnoses appropriate for the client with a neurogenic bladder include the following:
- *Impaired Urinary Elimination* related to impaired bladder innervation
- *Self-Care Deficit: Toileting* related to neurologic injury
- *Risk for Impaired Skin Integrity* related to urinary incontinence
- *Risk for Infection* related to impaired urination reflex.

Community-Based Care

Include the following in teaching for the client with neurogenic bladder and family members:
- Measures to stimulate reflex voiding and promote bladder emptying
- Use of prescribed medications, including desired and adverse effects, and interactions with other drugs
- Manifestations of UTI or urolithiasis, and measures to reduce the risk of these complications.

THE CLIENT WITH URINARY INCONTINENCE

The most common manifestation of impaired bladder control is **urinary incontinence (UI)**, or involuntary urination. UI can have a significant impact on clients, leading to physical problems such as skin breakdown, infection, and rashes. Psychosocial consequences include embarrassment, isolation and withdrawal, feelings of worthlessness and helplessness, and depression.

Incidence and Prevalence

Approximately 17 million people in the United States have some degree of urinary incontinence (Mason et al., 2003). The estimated cost of managing UI is $10 billion yearly. UI is especially common among older clients (see the box on the following page). An estimated 30% or more of older women living in the community experience UI. In long-term care, foster care, and homebound populations, the incidence is about 50% (Mason et al., 2003; Tierney et al., 2005). The actual prevalence of urinary incontinence is nearly impossible to determine. Embarrassment and the availability of products to protect clothing and prevent detection contribute to clients' not seeking evaluation of and treatment for incontinence.

FAST FACTS
- UI is especially common among older clients. Although the prevalence of urinary incontinence increases in older adults, it is *not* a normal consequence of aging and it *can* be treated.
- An estimated 30% or more of older women living in the community experience UI.
- In long-term care, foster care, and homebound populations, the incidence is about 50% (Mason et al., 2003; Tierney et al., 2005).

Pathophysiology

Urinary continence requires a bladder able to expand and contract and sphincters that can maintain a urethral pressure higher than that in the bladder. Incontinence results when the pressure within the urinary bladder exceeds urethral resistance, allowing urine to escape. Any condition causing higher than normal bladder pressures or reduced urethral resistance can potentially result in incontinence. Relaxation of the pelvic musculature, disruption of cerebral and nervous system control, and disturbances of the bladder and its musculature are common contributing factors.

Incontinence may be an acute, self-limited disorder, or it may be chronic. The causes may be congenital or acquired, reversible or irreversible. Congenital disorders associated with incontinence include *epispadias* (absence of the upper wall of the urethra), and *meningomyelocele* (a neural tube defect in which a portion of the spinal cord and its surrounding meninges protrude through the vertebral column). CNS or spinal cord trauma, stroke, and chronic neurologic disorders such as multiple sclerosis and Parkinson's disease are examples of acquired, irreversible causes of incontinence. Reversible causes

NURSING CARE OF THE OLDER ADULT   Minimizing the Risk for UTI and UI

Older adults have a higher incidence of two common urinary tract disorders: urinary tract infection and urinary incontinence.

Urinary Tract Infection

Aging affects normal protective mechanisms to prevent UTI. The pH of urine increases with aging, allowing bacteria to grow and multiply more readily. Glucosuria, more common in older adults due to the higher incidence of diabetes, facilitates bacterial growth. Incomplete bladder emptying and urinary retention are more common due to problems such as prostatic hypertrophy in men, bladder prolapse in women, and neurogenic bladder in both sexes. Changes in vaginal pH in women and decreased prostatic secretions in men may also contribute to an increased incidence of UTI.

While many UTIs in older adults are asymptomatic and self-limited, infections can lead to bacteremia, sepsis, and shock. Manifestations of UTI in the elderly include dysuria, urgency, frequency, incontinence, occasional hematuria, and confusion. Symptoms such as fever, chills, and flank pain and tenderness may be absent. Dementia may make diagnosis more difficult.

Urinary Incontinence

Urinary incontinence, the involuntary loss of urine, is a common problem in older adults. While incontinence should never be considered a *normal* consequence of aging, age-related changes contribute to its development. Bladder capacity tends to decline with age and involuntary bladder muscle contractions are more common. In women, decreased estrogen levels and pelvic muscle relaxation decrease bladder outlet and urethral resistance pressures. Decreased estrogen also causes atrophic vaginitis and urethritis, with manifestations of dysuria and urgency. Other risk factors for UI in older adults include impaired mobility and chronic degenerative diseases, impaired cognition, medications, low fluid intake, diabetes, and stroke.

Assessing for Home Care

Assessment for urinary problems in the older adult focuses on risk factors, the extent and manifestations of the disorder, and contributing factors. Using clear language, ask about problems with urine loss, its frequency, and any contributing factors. Inquire about frequency, urgency, and burning on urination. Identify current medications and the time of day each is taken. Assess patterns of fluid intake and output. Assess the abdomen for evidence of bladder distention or tenderness. Perform a mental status examination if indicated.

Assess the home environment (whether in the community or a residential living facility) for possible barriers to urinary elimination:

- Inadequate lighting, particularly at night
- Narrow doorways that may interfere with access to the toilet
- Inadequate toilet facilities
- The need for mobility aids such as safety bars, a raised toilet seat, or a bedside commode.

Teaching for Home Care

Discuss the following points to help prevent UTI and UI in the older adult:

- Maintain a generous fluid intake. Reduce or eliminate fluid intake after the evening meal to reduce nocturia.
- Wear comfortable clothing that is easy to remove for toileting.
- Maintain good hygiene, but do not bathe more often than necessary; frequent bathing and feminine hygiene sprays or douches may dry perineal tissues, increasing the risk of UTI or UI.
- Perform pelvic muscle exercises (Kegel exercises) several times a day to increase perineal muscle tone.
- Reduce consumption of caffeine-containing beverages (coffee, tea, colas), citrus juices, and artificially sweetened beverages containing Nutra-Sweet.
- Use behavioral techniques such as scheduled toileting, habit training, and bladder training to reduce the frequency of incontinence. *Scheduled toileting* is toileting at regular intervals (e.g., every 2 to 4 hours). *Habit training* is toileting the client on a schedule that corresponds with the normal pattern. *Bladder training* gradually increases the bladder capacity by increasing the intervals between voidings and resisting the urge to void.
- See your primary care provider regularly for a pelvic or prostate exam.
- For women, discuss possible benefits and risks of hormone replacement therapy, physical therapy, or surgery to treat incontinence.
- Report a change in urine color, odor, or clarity or symptoms such as burning, frequency, or urgency to your primary care provider.

Resources for Home Care

National Association for Continence
P.O. Box 1019
Charleston, SC 29402-1019
1-800-BLADDER (252-3357)
Website: www.nafc.org

---

include acute confusion, medications such as diuretics or sedatives, prostatic enlargement, vaginal and urethral atrophy, UTI, and fecal impaction.

Incontinence is commonly categorized as stress incontinence, urge incontinence (also known as overactive bladder), overflow incontinence, and functional incontinence. Table 28–7 summarizes each type with its physiologic cause and associated factors. *Mixed incontinence,* with elements of both stress and urge incontinence, is common. *Total incontinence* is loss of all voluntary control over urination, with urine loss occurring without stimulus and in all positions.

Incontinence is associated with an increased risk for falls, fractures, pressure ulcers, urinary tract infection, and depression. It contributes to the stress of caregivers, and may be a factor in institutionalizing the client.

INTERDISCIPLINARY CARE

Urinary incontinence management is directed at identifying and correcting the cause if possible. If the underlying disorder cannot be corrected, techniques to manage urine output can often be taught.

TABLE 28–7 Types of Urinary Incontinence

	DESCRIPTION	PATHOPHYSIOLOGY	CONTRIBUTING FACTORS
Stress	Loss of urine associated with increased intra-abdominal pressure during sneezing, coughing, lifting. Quantity of urine lost is usually small	Relaxation of pelvic musculature and weakness of urethra and surrounding muscles and tissues leads to decreased urethral resistance	■ Multiple pregnancies ■ Decreased estrogen levels ■ Short urethra, change in angle between bladder and urethra ■ Abdominal wall weakness ■ Prostate surgery ■ Increased intra-abdominal pressure due to tumor, ascites, obesity
Urge	Involuntary loss of urine associated with a strong urge to void	Hypertonic or overactive detrusor muscle leads to increased pressure within bladder and inability to inhibit voiding	■ Neurologic disorders such as stroke, Parkinson's disease, multiple sclerosis; peripheral nervous system disorders ■ Detrusor muscle overactivity associated with bladder outlet obstruction, aging, or disorders such as diabetes
Overflow	Inability to empty bladder, resulting in overdistention and frequent loss of small amounts of urine	Outlet obstruction or lack of normal detrusor activity leads to overfilling of bladder and increased pressure	■ Spinal cord injuries below S_2 ■ Diabetic neuropathy ■ Prostatic hypertrophy ■ Fecal impaction ■ Drugs, especially those with anticholinergic effect
Functional	Incontinence resulting from physical, environmental, or psychosocial causes	Ability to respond to the need to urinate is impaired	■ Confusion or dementia ■ Physical disability or impaired mobility ■ Diuretic therapy or sedation ■ Depression ■ Regression

Evaluation for incontinence begins with a complete history, including the duration, frequency, volume, and associated circumstances of urine loss. A voiding diary (Figure 28–8 ■) is often used to collect detailed information. The history also includes information about chronic or acute illnesses, previous surgeries, and current medication use, both prescription and over the counter.

Physical assessment includes abdominal, rectal, and pelvic assessment as well as evaluation of mental and neurologic status, mobility, and dexterity. Findings often associated with incontinence in women include weak abdominal and pelvic muscle tone, cystocele or urethrocele, and atrophic vaginitis. In men, an enlarged prostate gland is the physical finding most commonly associated with incontinence.

See the Nursing Research feature on page 876 on evidence-based practice for diagnosing urge incontinence using specific client assessment data.

Diagnosis

- *Urinalysis* and *urine culture* using a clean-catch specimen are done to rule out infection and other acute causes of incontinence.
- *Postvoiding residual (PVR) volume* is measured to determine how completely the bladder empties with voiding. Less than 50 mL PVR is expected; when 100 mL or more is obtained, further testing is indicated.
- *Cystometrography* is used to assess neuromuscular function of the bladder by evaluating detrusor muscle function, pres-

sure within the bladder, and the filling pattern of the bladder. The client describes sensations and any urge to void as sterile water or saline is instilled into the bladder. Normally, the urge to void is perceived at 150 to 450 mL, and the bladder feels full at 300 to 500 mL. Bladder pressure and volume are recorded on a graph. When the bladder is full, the client voids, and intravesical pressure is noted during voiding.

- *Uroflowmetry* is a noninvasive test used to evaluate voiding patterns. The uroflowmeter, contained in a funnel, measures the rate of urine flow, the continuous flow time, and the total voiding time.
- *IVP* may be ordered to evaluate structure and function of the upper and lower urinary tract.
- *Cystoscopy* or *ultrasonography* may be ordered to identify structural disorders contributing to incontinence, such as an enlarged prostate or a tumor.

Nursing implications for the specialized studies for urinary incontinence are outlined in Chapter 27 ∞.

Medications

Both stress and urge incontinence may improve with drug treatment.

Drugs that contract the smooth muscles of the bladder neck may reduce episodes of mild stress incontinence. Phenylpropanolamine (Acutrim, Allerest, Contac, others), a commonly used decongestant and nonprescription diet aid, is an effective preparation. Adverse effects such as hypertension, palpitations, and nervousness may limit its use.

Your Daily Voiding Diary   Date _____

This diary will help you and your healthcare team identify factors causing bladder control problems. Choose a 24-hour period when you can record your fluid intake (type and amount), urine output and episodes of urine leakage, any strong urge to void just prior to leaking, and your activity when leak episodes occur. The line below illustrates how to use your diary.

Time	Fluid Intake		Urine Output			Leaks			Urge		Activity
	Amount	Type							Yes	No	
7 am	2 cups	coffee	sm	(med)	lg	(sm)	med	lg	Yes		walking
			sm	med	lg	sm	med	lg			
			sm	med	lg	sm	med	lg			
			sm	med	lg	sm	med	lg			
			sm	med	lg	sm	med	lg			
			sm	med	lg	sm	med	lg			
			sm	med	lg	sm	med	lg			
			sm	med	lg	sm	med	lg			
			sm	med	lg	sm	med	lg			
			sm	med	lg	sm	med	lg			
			sm	med	lg	sm	med	lg			
			sm	med	lg	sm	med	lg			
			sm	med	lg	sm	med	lg			
			sm	med	lg	sm	med	lg			
			sm	med	lg	sm	med	lg			
			sm	med	lg	sm	med	lg			
			sm	med	lg	sm	med	lg			
			sm	med	lg	sm	med	lg			

I used ___ pads today. I used ___ diapers today.

Questions to ask my health care team: _____

_____

_____

Figure 28–8 ■ A sample voiding diary.

Source: Adapted from *Your Daily Bladder Diary,* National Kidney and Urologic Diseases Information Center, National Institute of Diabetes and Digestive and Kidney Disease (NIDDK), National Institutes of Health.

When incontinence is associated with postmenopausal atrophic vaginitis, estrogen therapy may be effective. Both systemic estrogens and local creams are used.

Clients with urge incontinence may be treated with preparations that increase bladder capacity. The primary drugs used to inhibit detrusor muscle contractions and increase bladder capacity include oxybutynin (Ditropan and the extended-release form, Ditropan XL), an anticholinergic drug, and tolterodine (Detrol and its longer acting form, Detrol LA), a more specific antimuscarinic agent. These drugs can be taken once or twice a day, and have fewer side effects than less specific anticholinergic drugs. Drugs with anticholinergic effects are contraindicated for the client with acute glaucoma. Urinary retention is a potential side effect that must be considered when these drugs are used (see the Medication Administration box on page 871).

Surgery

Surgery may be used to treat stress incontinence associated with cystocele or urethrocele and overflow incontinence associated with an enlarged prostate gland.

Suspension of the bladder neck, a technique that brings the angle between the bladder and urethra closer to normal, is effective in treating stress incontinence associated with urethrocele in 80% to 95% of clients. A laparoscopic, vaginal, or abdominal approach may be used to perform this surgery. Care of the client with a bladder neck suspension is outlined on page 876.

Prostatectomy, using either the transurethral or suprapubic approach, is indicated for the client who is experiencing overflow incontinence as a result of an enlarged prostate gland and urethral obstruction. Care of the client with a prostatectomy is outlined in Chapter 50 ∞.

Other surgical procedures of potential benefit in the treatment of incontinence include implantation of an artificial sphincter, formation of a urethral sling to elevate and compress the urethra, and augmentation of the bladder with bowel segments to increase bladder capacity.

Complementary Therapies

Biofeedback and relaxation techniques may help reduce episodes of urinary incontinence. Biofeedback uses electronic monitors to teach conscious control over physiologic responses

NURSING RESEARCH   Evidence-Based Practice: Urinary Incontinence

While an accurate diagnosis of stress urinary incontinence often is made based on clinical data, motor urge incontinence has been more difficult to accurately diagnose without urodynamic testing. This presents difficulty for nurses and nurse practitioners planning care for incontinent clients when urologic testing is not feasible or readily available. A model developed by Gray et al., (2001) may be useful to address this problem in cognitively intact adults. By comparing client data with urodynamic testing results, this team of researchers identified factors predictive of motor urge incontinence. These factors included age, gender, and three key symptoms: diurnal frequency (urinating more often than every 2 hours while awake), nocturia (awakening with urge to urinate more than once per night if under age 65, twice per night if over age 65), and urge incontinence (urine loss associated with a strong desire to urinate). The presence of all three symptoms was more than 92% predictive of motor urge incontinence in study participants of all ages (range 18 to 89; median 61) and both genders.

IMPLICATIONS FOR NURSING
Asking specific questions about urinary tract symptoms can facilitate accurate identification of the nursing diagnosis *Urge Urinary*

Incontinence. Accurate diagnosis is vital to planning and implementing appropriate care measures, and achieving the desired outcome of continence. Successful treatment promotes self-esteem and provides positive reinforcement for continuing planned strategies.

CRITICAL THINKING IN CLIENT CARE
1. What nursing care measures and client teaching will you provide for the client with stress incontinence that may not be appropriate or necessary for the client with urge incontinence? For the client with urge incontinence but not stress incontinence?
2. Identify circumstances in which it may not be possible or feasible to have the client undergo urodynamic testing to differentiate stress, urge, or mixed (stress and urge) incontinence.
3. The clients in this study lived independently in the community and were cognitively intact. Can the data in this study be generalized to clients residing in a long-term care facility? Can the results be applied to all types of incontinence? Why or why not?

Source: From "A Model for Predicting Motor Urge Urinary Incontinence" by M. Gray et al., 2001, *Nursing Research, 50*(2), p. 116–122.

of which the individual is not normally aware. Developing awareness of perceptible information allows the client to gain voluntary control over urination. Biofeedback is widely used to manage urinary incontinence.

NURSING CARE

Health Promotion
Although urinary incontinence rarely causes serious physical effects, it frequently has significant psychosocial effects, and can lead to lowered self-esteem, social isolation, and even institution-

alization (Lauver et al., 2004). Get the word out—inform all clients that UI is not a normal consequence of aging and that treatments are available. To reduce the incidence of UI, teach all women to perform pelvic floor muscle (Kegel) exercises (Box 28–3) to improve perineal muscle tone. Advise women to seek advice from their women's healthcare or primary care practitioner about using topical or systemic hormone therapy during menopause to maintain perineal tissue integrity. Advise older men to have routine prostate examinations to prevent urethral obstruction and overflow incontinence. Pelvic floor muscle exercises also may benefit men who experience UI following prostatectomy, but evidence supporting this is limited (Moore & Gray, 2004).

NURSING CARE OF THE CLIENT HAVING A   Bladder Neck Suspension

PREOPERATIVE CARE
- Provide routine preoperative care and teaching as outlined in Chapter 4 ∞.
- Discuss the need to avoid straining and the Valsalva maneuver postoperatively. Suggest measures such as increasing fluid and fiber intake and using a stool softener to prevent postoperative constipation. *Straining and increased abdominal pressure during the Valsalva maneuver may place excessive stress on suture lines and interfere with healing.*

POSTOPERATIVE CARE
- Provide routine postoperative care as outlined in Chapter 4 ∞.
- Monitor urine output, including quantity, color, and clarity. Expect urine to be pink initially, gradually clearing. *Bright red urine, excessive vaginal drainage, or incisional bleeding may indicate hemorrhage. Instrumentation of the urinary*

tract increases the potential for UTI; cloudy urine may be an early sign.
- Maintain stability and patency of suprapubic and/or urethral catheters. Secure catheters in position. *Maintaining bladder decompression eliminates pressure on suture lines. Preventing movement or pulling on catheters reduces the risk for resultant pressure on surgical incisions.*
- Carefully monitor urine output after catheter removal. *Difficulty voiding is common following catheter removal. Early intervention to prevent bladder distention is important to prevent pressure on suture lines.*
- If the urethral or suprapubic catheter will remain in place on discharge, teach proper care to the client and family members as needed. *Appropriate self-care and early recognition of problems reduce the risk for significant complications.*

BOX 28–3 Pelvic Floor Muscle (Kegel) Exercises

- Identify the pelvic muscles with these techniques:
  a. Stop the flow of urine during voiding and hold for a few seconds.
  b. Tighten the muscles at the vaginal entrance around a gloved finger or tampon.
  c. Tighten the muscles around the anus as though resisting defecation.
- Perform exercises by tightening pelvic muscles, holding for 10 seconds, and relaxing for 10 to 15 seconds. Continue the sequence (tighten, hold, relax) for 10 repetitions.
- Keep abdominal muscles and breathing relaxed while performing exercises.
- Initially, exercises should be performed twice per day, working up to four times a day.
- Encourage exercising at a specific time each day or in conjunction with another daily activity (such as bathing or watching the news). Establish a routine because these exercises should be continued for life.
- Assistive devices, such as vaginal cones and biofeedback, may be useful for clients who have difficulty identifying appropriate muscle groups.

Assessment

Nursing assessment for the client with urinary incontinence includes both subjective and objective data:

- *Health history:* Voiding diary; frequency of incontinent episodes, amount of urine loss and activities associated with incontinence; methods used to deal with incontinence; use of Kegel exercises or medications; any chronic diseases, related surgeries, etc.; effects of incontinence on usual activities, including social activities.
- *Physical examination:* Physical and mental status, including any physical limitations or impaired cognition; inspect, palpate, and percuss abdomen for bladder distention; inspect perineal tissues for redness, irritation, or tissue breakdown; observe for bulging of bladder into vagina when bearing down; assess pelvic muscle tone as indicated.

Nursing Diagnoses and Interventions

In planning nursing care, consider the client's mental status, mobility, and motivation. Behavioral techniques can be effective, but require long-term commitment and the physical and mental capability to use them.

Nursing care and modification of routines can restore continence fully or partially even in the institutionalized client. Scheduled toileting, bladder training, and prompted voiding combined with positive reinforcement such as praise can reduce the need for diapers, incontinence pads, and indwelling catheters.

See the Nursing Care Plan that follows for additional nursing diagnoses and interventions for the client with urinary incontinence.

Urinary Incontinence: Stress and/or Urge

Exercises to strengthen pelvic floor muscles, dietary modifications, and bladder training programs often are effective to restore and maintain continence.

- Instruct to keep a voiding diary, recording the time and amount of all fluid intake and urinary output, status at the time of voiding (dry or wet) and on arising from sleep, and activities. *Voiding diaries provide valuable information for identifying the type of incontinence and possible measures to reduce or eliminate incontinent episodes.*
- Teach pelvic floor muscle exercises (see Box 28–3). Instruct to consciously tighten pelvic muscles when the need to void is perceived and to relax the abdomen while walking to the bathroom. *Improved pelvic muscle strength helps retain urine and prevent stress incontinence by increasing urethral pressure. Exercises also decrease abnormal detrusor muscle contractions, decreasing pressure within the bladder.*

PRACTICE ALERT
Do not advise clients who have difficulty emptying the bladder completely to stop urine flow while voiding to identify pelvic floor muscles. Repeated interruption of micturition can interfere with complete bladder emptying and increase the risk for UTI.

- Using the client's voiding diary, suggest dietary and fluid intake modifications to reduce stress and urge incontinence. Include limiting caffeine, alcohol, citrus juice, and artificial sweetener consumption; limiting fluid intake to no less than 1.5 to 2.0 L per day; and limiting evening fluid intake. *Caffeine, alcohol, and citrus juices are bladder irritants and tend to promote detrusor instability, increasing the risk of urge incontinence. Artificial sweeteners may also irritate the bladder. Fluid intake of 1.5 to 2.0 L per day is adequate to maintain health for most clients; excess fluid may increase stress incontinence if bathroom facilities are not readily available.*

PRACTICE ALERT
Limiting total fluid intake to less than 1.5 to 2.0 L per day is not recommended for clients with urinary incontinence. Inadequate fluid increases urine concentration, leading to bladder wall irritation and possibly increasing problems of urge incontinence.

Self-Care Deficit: Toileting

Functional incontinence may be the predominant problem in an institutionalized older adult. Limited mobility, impaired vision, dementia, lack of access to facilities and privacy, and tight staffing patterns increase the risk for incontinence in previously continent residents. The primary problem in functional incontinence is an outside factor that interferes with the ability to respond normally to the urge to void. An immobilized client may wet the bed if a call light is not within reach; a client with Alzheimer's disease may perceive the urge to void but be unable to interpret its meaning or respond by seeking a bathroom. For these clients, self-care deficit in toileting is a primary problem.

NURSING CARE PLAN · A Client with Urinary Incontinence

Anna Giovanni, a 76-year-old retired teacher, has been widowed for 10 years and lives alone. Mrs. Giovanni's eldest daughter expresses concern that her mother seems increasingly reluctant to leave her apartment to visit friends and family. She reports a strong odor of urine throughout her mother's apartment and that her mother's bed is often wet. She expresses worry about needing to place her mother in a nursing home if she cannot continue to live independently.

ASSESSMENT

Jane Oberle, RN, a nurse practitioner, examines Mrs. Giovanni who admits that she has problems with urine leakage when laughing and coughing, and a strong urge to void on hearing the sound of running water. At night, her urge to void is so strong that she often cannot reach the bathroom in time. Mrs. Giovanni denies a history of UTIs, neurologic disorders, or difficulty with her bowels. She had a hysterectomy at age 52 and was on hormone replacement therapy for about 10 years afterward. She is taking digoxin 0.125 mg daily, furosemide 40 mg twice daily, and potassium chloride 20 mEq three times daily for mild heart failure.

Physical assessment reveals a moderate cystourethrocele and atrophy of vaginal and vulvar tissues. Moderate perineal dermatitis is noted. Pelvic floor strength is weak. Urinalysis is within normal limits, and postvoiding residual urine is 5 mL.

Analysis of Mrs. Giovanni's voiding diary shows moderate consumption of tea and juices throughout the day, nine daytime voidings and four night voidings with an average volume of about 250 mL per void. She notices urine leakage most often in the late afternoon and at night. Ms. Oberle identifies a diagnosis of stress incontinence with an urgency component and decides to try a conservative approach before referring Mrs. Giovanni for further testing and possible cystourethrocele repair. She prescribes estrogen cream, tolterodine (Detrol), and a barrier cream to treat Mrs. Giovanni's vulvitis.

DIAGNOSES

- *Stress Urinary Incontinence* related to weak pelvic floor musculature and tissue atrophy
- *Urge Urinary Incontinence* related to excess intake of caffeine and citrus juices
- *Impaired Skin Integrity* related to constant contact of urine with perineal tissues
- *Ineffective Coping* related to inability to control urine leakage

EXPECTED OUTCOMES

- Remain dry between voidings and at night.
- Demonstrate improved perineal muscle strength.
- Regain and maintain perineal skin integrity.
- Return to her previous level of social activity.

PLANNING AND IMPLEMENTATION

- Teach how to identify pelvic floor muscles and how to perform Kegel exercises.
- Suggest drinking decaffeinated tea and noncitrus fruit juices (grape, apple, and cranberry).
- Encourage to minimize fluid intake after evening meal.
- Change afternoon dose of furosemide from 9:00 P.M. to 3:00 P.M.
- Instruct to void by the clock, gradually increasing intervals from every 45 to 60 minutes to every 2 to 2.5 hours. Advise to maintain shorter voiding intervals for 2 to 3 hours after furosemide doses.
- Teach to cleanse perineal area, wiping front to back, after each voiding or incident of urine leakage.
- Introduce commercial products available for clothing and furniture protection, encouraging experimentation to identify the most helpful product(s).
- Provide a commode for bedside at night and adequate lighting to prevent injury.
- Schedule follow-up visits and evaluations to reinforce teaching.

EVALUATION

Three months after her initial visit, Mrs. Giovanni states that she is doing very well, experiencing only occasional leakage of small amounts of urine, primarily when sneezing, coughing, or laughing. She finds a minipad adequate for protection and is often able to remain dry all day. She has had no further problems with enuresis since changing her evening furosemide dose to late afternoon and limiting her fluids after dinner. She can make it to the bathroom and no longer needs the bedside commode. Her perineal tissue is intact, and she demonstrates improved muscle strength. Anna's daughter says her mother is beginning to resume her normal social activities, and that she is no longer worried about her mother's ability to care for herself independently.

CRITICAL THINKING IN THE NURSING PROCESS

1. What factors in Mrs. Giovanni's past medical history and current medication regimen contributed to her nighttime incontinence?
2. What is the rationale for including an intervention to teach Mrs. Giovanni about perineal cleansing as part of her care plan?
3. Develop a care plan for Mrs. Giovanni for the nursing diagnosis *Situational Low Self-Esteem* related to urinary incontinence.

See Evaluating Your Response in Appendix C.

- **Assess physical and mental abilities and limitations, usual voiding pattern, and ability to assist with toileting.** *A thorough assessment allows planned interventions to address specific needs and promote independence.*
- **Provide assistive devices as needed to facilitate independence, such as raised toilet seats, grab bars, a bedside commode, or night-lights.** *Fostering independence in toileting bolsters self-concept and maintains a positive body image.*
- **Plan a toileting schedule based on the client's normal elimination patterns to achieve approximately 300 mL of urine** output with each voiding. *Allowing the bladder to fill to a point at which the urge to void is experienced and then emptying it completely helps maintain normal bladder capacity and bacteriostatic functions.*
- **Position for ease of voiding—sitting for females, standing for males—and provide privacy.** *Normal positioning, usual toileting facilities, and privacy enhance the ability to void on schedule and empty the bladder completely.*
- **Adjust fluid intake so that the majority of fluids are consumed during times of the day when the client is most able to remain**

continent. Unless fluids are restricted, maintain a fluid intake of at least 1.5 to 2.0 L per day. *An adequate fluid intake is vital to promote hydration and urinary function. Overly concentrated urine can irritate the bladder, increasing incontinence.*

- Assist with clothing that is easily removed (e.g., elastic-waist pants or loose dresses). Velcro and zipper fasteners may be easier to use than snaps and buttons. *Clothing that is difficult to remove can increase the risk of incontinence in the client with mobility problems or impaired dexterity.*

Social Isolation

Urinary incontinence increases the risk for social isolation due to embarrassment, fear of not having ready access to a bathroom, body odor, or other factors. Social isolation, in turn, can increase problems of incontinence, because normal cues and relationships are lost, and the need to remain dry is less strongly felt.

- Assess reasons for and extent of social isolation. Verify the degree of social isolation with the client or significant other. *Do not assume that social isolation is only related to urinary incontinence. Other problems frequently associated with aging (such as a hearing deficit) may be primary or contributing factors.*
- Refer client for urologic examination and incontinence evaluation. *Clients who assume that urinary incontinence is a normal part of the aging process may not be aware of treatment options.*
- Explore alternative coping strategies with client, significant other, staff, and other healthcare team members. *Protective pads or shields, good perineal hygiene, scheduled voiding, and clothing that does not interfere with toileting can enhance continence.*

Linking NANDA, NIC, and NOC

Chart 28–1 shows links between NANDA nursing diagnoses, NIC, and NOC when caring for the client with urinary incontinence.

NANDA, NIC, AND NOC LINKAGES
CHART 28–1 The Client with Urinary Incontinence

NANDA

Stress Urinary Incontinence

↓

NIC

Pelvic Muscle Exercise

Urinary Incontinence Care

Weight Management

↓

NOC

Urinary Continence

Data from *NANDA's Nursing Diagnoses: Definitions & Classification 2005–2006* by NANDA International (2005), Philadelphia; *Nursing Interventions Classification (NIC)* (4th ed.) by J. M. Dochterman & G. M. Bulechek (2004), St. Louis, MO: Mosby; and *Nursing Outcomes Classification (NOC)* (3rd ed.) by S. Moorhead, M. Johnson, and M. Maas (2004), St. Louis, MO: Mosby.

Community-Based Care

Because urinary incontinence is a contributing factor in the institutionalization of many older people, client and family teaching can have a significant impact on maintaining independence and residence in the community. Address possible causes of incontinence and appropriate treatment measures. Refer for urologic examination if not already completed. Discuss fluid intake management, perineal care, and products for clothing protection.

EXPLORE MEDIALINK

DVD-ROM
Audio Glossary
NCLEX-RN® Review

COMPANION WEBSITE www.prenhall.com/lemone
Audio Glossary
NCLEX RN® Review
Care Plan Activity: Urinary Tract Infection
Case Studies
  Bladder Cancer
  Urinary Tract Infection
Concept Map: Bladder Cancer
MediaLink Applications
  Bladder Training
  Urinary Tract Disorders
Links to Resources

CHAPTER HIGHLIGHTS

- Urinary tract infections are very common and are a leading complication among hospitalized clients. Short-course antibiotic therapy is appropriate for uncomplicated infections of the lower urinary tract that are not associated with the presence of an indwelling urinary catheter.
- Teach clients about perineal hygiene and the importance of maintaining adequate fluid intake as measures to help prevent UTI.
- Urinary stones (most commonly kidney stones in the United States) can obstruct the urinary tract at any level, and cause significant pain as they move from the kidney through the ureter. Instruct clients who have had a kidney stone to maintain a generous fluid intake, particularly during exercise and warm weather, to reduce the risk of further stone formation.
- The risk for bladder cancer is greater among men than women, and cigarette smoking is the most significant risk factor for bladder cancer. Most tumors can be resected transurethrally if diagnosed early, before spreading to deeper layers of the bladder wall, the lymph nodes, and adjacent tissue.

- When resection of the urinary bladder is necessary, a urinary diversion is created to collect urine. A collection appliance must be worn constantly on an ileal conduit; when a continent urinary diversion is created, the pouch is emptied by intermittent catheterization of the stoma.
- Urinary retention may occur as a result of some medications, neurologic damage or disease, or obstruction (e.g., an enlarged prostate gland). If the underlying condition cannot be treated, medications or intermittent catheterization are used to promote bladder emptying.
- Older adults in particular are at risk for urinary incontinence, a treatable condition. A health history, voiding diary, and diagnostic testing are used to establish the type of urinary incontinence and direct treatments such as surgery, pelvic floor muscle exercises, medications, and scheduled toileting.

TEST YOURSELF NCLEX-RN® REVIEW

1 A 23-year-old woman presents to the urgency clinic with symptoms of a urinary tract infection. The nursing history reveals that the client was treated 3 months previously for a UTI. Additional questions the nurse should ask include:
1. "Did you complete your antibiotic prescription for your first UTI?"
2. "What form of birth control are you using?"
3. "Does your partner have similar symptoms?"
4. "How much fluid do you drink each day?"

2 A 58-year-old woman presents at her primary care provider's office with symptoms of frequency, urgency, nocturia, dysuria, and cloudy, rust-colored urine for the third time in the past 2 years. The nurse should plan to include which of the following in her teaching for this client? (Select all that apply.)
1. return to the office in 10 days for follow-up culture
2. preprocedure instruction for an IVP
3. the potential benefits of estrogen vaginal cream
4. recommendations for perineal cleansing
5. recommendations for screening cystoscopy

3 Recognizing the risk for urolithiasis in the immobilized client, the nurse appropriately plans to:
1. administer a calcium supplement.
2. regularly monitor urine pH.
3. maintain an indwelling urinary catheter.
4. increase fluid intake to 3000 mL per day.

4 A client admitted with possible kidney stones develops sudden complaints of acute crampy pain on the left side that radiates into the groin. He is nauseated, and vomits clear fluid. On voiding, his urine is pink. The nurse should:
1. obtain a bladder scan to assess for residual urine.
2. administer the prescribed narcotic analgesic.
3. notify the physician.
4. strain all urine.

5 The nurse teaching a group of community members about wellness and disease prevention includes which of the following as a measure to reduce the risk for bladder cancer?
1. Do not start smoking; if you smoke, stop.
2. Avoid using hair dyes and pesticides in the home.
3. Limit your intake of coffee and other caffeinated beverages.
4. Empty your bladder every 2 hours.

6 At a local health fair, a man remarks to the nurse that his urine occasionally appears pink. He wonders if this is anything to be concerned about. The nurse should
1. instruct the man to notify his physician if he develops pain or difficulty voiding.
2. advise the man to make an appointment to see his physician.
3. instruct the man to track the relationship between urine color and his activities.
4. tell the man to increase his fluid intake to 2 1/2 to 3 quarts per day.

7 The nurse evaluates her teaching as effective when the client with a newly created continent ileal diversion is able to:
1. demonstrate care for the collection device.
2. state the importance of promptly reporting cloudy urine to the physician.
3. demonstrate self-catheterization of the stoma.
4. identify factors contributing to his risk for bladder cancer.

8 The nurse identifies which of the following as a high-priority goal for a client with stress incontinence?
1. Can identify products for protecting clothing and furniture.
2. States chronic and benign nature of the disorder.
3. Performs pelvic floor muscle exercises as taught at least twice a day.
4. Limits intake of beverages containing artificial sweeteners.

9 A client tells the nurse that she has difficulty getting to the bathroom in time to prevent urine leaks once she feels the need to void. The nurse instructs the client to:

1. limit intake of caffeine-containing beverages, particularly in the evening.
2. establish a voiding schedule, emptying her bladder at least every 2 hours.
3. discuss potential benefits of bladder suspension surgery with her physician.
4. wear clothing that is easily removed for toileting.

10 The nurse caring for a client in the spinal shock phase following spinal cord injury appropriately plans to:

1. insert a Foley catheter to accurately measure output.
2. stimulate voiding using Credé's method.
3. assess for urinary retention following each voiding.
4. catheterize with straight catheter every 3 to 4 hours.

See Test Yourself answers in Appendix C.

BIBLIOGRAPHY

American Cancer Society. (2005). *Cancer facts and figures 2005.* Atlanta: Author.

Bardsley, A. (2005). Use of lubricant gels in urinary catheterization. *Nursing Standard, 20*(8), 41–46.

Baumgartner, R. G., Wells, N., Chang, S. S., Cookson, M. S., & Smith, J. A., Jr. (2002). Causes of increased length of stay following radical cystectomy. *Urology Nursing, 22*(5), 319–323, 339.

Bissett, L. (2004). The control of urinary tract infection in hospitalised older people. *Nursing Times, 100*(8), 54–56.

Blais, D. (2004). Urinary tract infections among the institutionalized older adult. *Perspectives, 28*(2), 23–27, 29–34.

Boyd, L. A. (2003). Intravesical bacillus Calmette-Guérin for treating bladder cancer. *Urology Nursing, 23*(3), 189–191, 199.

Copstead, L. C., & Banasik, J. L. (2005). *Pathophysiology* (3rd ed.). St. Louis, MO: Elsevier/Saunders.

Daneshgari, F., Krugman, M., Bahn, A., & Lee, R. S. (2002). Evidence-based multidisciplinary practice: Improving the safety and standards of male bladder catheterization. *Medsurg Nursing, 11*(5), 236–241, 246.

Engberg, S., Kincade, J., & Thompson, D. (2004). Future directions for incontinence research with frail elders. *Nursing Research, 53*(6S), S22–S29.

Fontaine, K. L. (2005). *Complementary & alternative therapies for nursing practice* (2nd ed.). Upper Saddle River, NJ: Prentice Hall.

Frerick, J. (2004). Gerontologic nurse practitioner care guidelines: Urinary tract infection. *Geriatric Nursing, 24*(3), 185–187.

Gray, M. (2000). Urinary retention: Management in the acute care setting. *American Journal of Nursing, 100*(7), 40–47.

Gray, M., McClain, R., Peruggia, M., Patrie, J., & Steers, W. D. (2001). A model for predicting motor urge urinary incontinence. *Nursing Research, 50*(2), 116–122.

Kasper, D. L., Braunwald, E., Fauci, A. S., Hauser, S. L., Longo, D. L., & Jameson, J. L. (Eds.). (2005). *Harrison's principles of internal medicine* (16th ed.). New York: McGraw-Hill.

Lauver, D. R., Gross, J., Ruff, C., & Wells, T. J. (2004). Patient-centered interventions: Implications for incontinence. *Nursing Research, 53*(6S), S30–S35.

Maloney, C. (2002). Estrogen & recurrent UTI in postmenopausal women. *American Journal of Nursing, 102*(8), 44–52.

Mason, D.J., Newman, D.K., & Palmer, M. H. (2003). Changing UI practice. *American Journal of Nursing, 103*(3) Supplement, 2–3.

McCance, K. L., & Huether, S. E. (2006). *Pathophysiology: The biologic basis for disease in adults & children* (5th ed.). St. Louis, MO: Mosby.

McLoughlin, C. (2004). Antimuscarinic drugs. *Professional Nurse, 20*(1), 50–51.

Moore, K. N., & Gray, M. (2004). Urinary incontinence in men. *Nursing Research, 53*(6S), S36–S41.

Naish, W. (2003). Intermittent self-catheterisation for managing urinary problems. *Professional Nurse, 18*(10), 585–587.

Newman, D. K., & Palmer, M. H. (Eds.). (2003). The state of the science on urinary incontinence. *American Journal of Nursing, 103*(3 Suppl), 1–58.

Nicolle, L. E. (2001). Urinary tract infections in long-term care facilities. *Infection Control & Hospital Epidemiology, 22*(3), 167–175.

Palmer, M. H., & Newman, D. K. (2004). Bladder matters: Urinary incontinence in nursing homes. *American Journal of Nursing, 104*(11), 57–59.

Pashos, C. L., Botteman, M. F., Laskin, B. L., & Redaelli, A. (2002). Bladder cancer: Epidemiology, diagnosis, and management. *Cancer Practitioner, 10*(6), 311–322.

Porth, C. M. (2005). *Pathophysiology: Concepts of altered health states* (7th ed.). Philadelphia: Lippincott.

Prieto-Fingerhut, T., Banovac, K., & Lynne, C. M. (1997). A study comparing sterile and nonsterile urethral catheterization in patients with spinal cord injury. *Rehabilitation Nursing, 22*(6), 299–302.

Rothrock, J. C. (2003). *Alexander's care of the patient in surgery* (12th ed.). St. Louis, MO: Mosby.

Sampselle, C. M., Palmer, M. H., Boyington, A. R., O'Dell, K. K., & Wooldridge, L. (2004). Prevention of urinary incontinence in adults: Population-based strategies. *Nursing Research, 53*(6S), S61–S67.

Simmons, R. (2005). Conservative and surgical approaches to the treatment of overactive bladder. *Professional Nurse, 20*(6), 31–33.

Spencer, J. W., & Jacobs, J. J. (2003). *Complementary and alternative medicine: An evidence-based approach* (2nd ed.). St. Louis, MO: Mosby.

Suchinski, G. A., Piano, M. R., Rosenberg, N., & Zerwic, J. J. (1999). Treating urinary tract infections in the elderly. *Dimensions of Critical Care Nursing, 18*(1), 21–27.

Teng, C. H., Huang, Y. H., Kuo, B. J., & Bih, L. I. (2005). Application of portable ultrasound scanners in the measurement of post-void residual urine. *Journal of Nursing Research, 13*(3), 216–223.

Tierney, L. M., Jr., McPhee, S. J., & Papadakis, M. A. (Eds.). (2005). *Current medical diagnosis & treatment* (44th ed.). New York: McGraw-Hill.

Uphold, C. R., & Graham, M. V. (2003). *Clinical guidelines in adult health* (3rd ed.). Gainesville, FL: Barmarrae Books.

Vinsnes, A. G., Harkless, G. E., Haltbakk, J., Bohm, J., & Hunskaar, S. (2001). Healthcare personnel's attitudes towards patients with urinary incontinence. *Journal of Clinical Nursing, 10*(4), 455–462.

Wareing, M. (2003). Urinary retention: Issues of management and care. *Emergency Nursing, 11*(8), 24–27.

Way, L. W., & Doherty, G. M. (2003). *Current surgical diagnosis & treatment* (11th ed.). New York: McGraw-Hill.

Wilkinson, J. M. (2005). *Nursing diagnosis handbook* (8th ed.). Upper Saddle River, NJ: Prentice Hall.

Woods, A. (2005). Managing UTIs in older adults. *Nursing, 35*(3), 12.

CHAPTER 29 Nursing Care of Clients with Kidney Disorders

LEARNING OUTCOMES

- Describe the pathophysiology of common kidney disorders, relating pathophysiology to normal physiology and manifestations of the disorder.

- Discuss risk factors for kidney disorders and nursing care to reduce these risks.

- Explain diagnostic studies used to identify disorders of the kidneys and their effects.

- Discuss the effects and nursing implications for medications and treatments used for clients with kidney disorders.

- Compare and contrast dialysis procedures used to manage acute and chronic renal failure.

CLINICAL COMPETENCIES

- Assess the functional health status of clients with kidney disorders.

- Monitor, document, and report unexpected or abnormal manifestations in clients with kidney disorders.

- Provide appropriate and effective nursing care for clients undergoing dialysis, surgery involving the kidneys, or renal transplant.

- Based on assessment data, determine priority nursing diagnoses and interventions for clients with renal disorders.

- Plan and implement evidence-based nursing care for clients with renal disorders using research and best practices.

- Collaborate with the client and other members of the interdisciplinary team to prioritize and implement care.

- Provide teaching appropriate to the client and situation for clients with kidney disorders.

- Evaluate client responses to care, revising the plan of care as needed to promote, maintain, or restore functional health status for clients with renal disorders.

MEDIALINK

Resources for this chapter can be found on the Prentice Hall Nursing MediaLink DVD-ROM accompanying this textbook, and on the Companion Website at http://www.prenhall.com/lemone

The internal environment of the body normally remains in a relatively constant or *homeostatic* state. The kidneys help maintain homeostasis by regulating the composition and volume of extracellular fluid. They excrete excess water and solutes and also can conserve water and solutes when deficits occur. In addition, the kidneys help regulate acid–base balance and they excrete metabolic wastes. Regulation of blood pressure is also a key function of the kidneys.

Both primary kidney disorders (such as glomerulonephritis) and systemic diseases (such as diabetes mellitus) can affect renal function. In North America, more than 20 million people are affected by kidney and urinary tract diseases (National Kidney and Urologic Diseases Information Clearinghouse [NKUDIC], 2004). Every year, approximately 1 in every 1000 people in the United States develops end-stage renal disease (ESRD), the final phase of chronic renal failure in which little or no kidney function remains. Chronic renal disease accounts for about 80,000 deaths per year and is a major cause of lost work time and wages (U.S. Renal Data System [USRDS], 2005). Ironically, the increased prevalence of chronic renal disease in recent years is partially related to the success of dialysis and transplantation.

AGE-RELATED CHANGES IN KIDNEY FUNCTION

Glomeruli in the renal cortex (see Chapter 27 ∞ for a review of normal kidney structure and function) are lost with aging, reducing kidney mass. Because of the large functional reserve of the kidneys, however, renal function remains adequate unless additional stressors affect the renal system. The **glomerular filtration rate (GFR)**, the amount of filtrate made by the kidneys per minute, declines due to age-related factors affecting the renovascular system (such as arteriosclerosis, decreased renal vascularity, and decreased cardiac output). By age 80, the GFR may be less than half of what it was at age 30.

Age-related changes in renal function have significant implications. The kidneys are less able to concentrate urine and compensate for increased or decreased salt intake. When combined with diminished effectiveness of antidiuretic hormone (ADH) and a reduced thirst response, both common in aging, this decreased ability to concentrate urine increases the risk for dehydration. Potassium excretion may be decreased because of lower aldosterone levels. As a result, fluid and electrolyte imbalances are more common and potentially critical in the older client.

Decreased GFR in the older adult also reduces the clearance of drugs excreted through the kidneys. This reduced clearance prolongs the half-life of drugs and may necessitate lower drug doses and longer dosing intervals. Common medications affected by decreased GFR include:

- Cardiac drugs: digoxin, procainamide
- Antibiotics: aminoglycosides, tetracyclines, cephalosporins
- Histamine H_2 antagonists: cimetidine
- Antidiabetic agents: chlorpropamide.

When caring for older adults, it is especially important to monitor drugs that are toxic to the renal tubules. Radiologic dyes and aminoglycoside, tetracycline, and the cephalosporin antibiotics are part of this group.

Age-related changes in renal function and related nursing implications are summarized in Table 29–1.

THE CLIENT WITH A CONGENITAL KIDNEY MALFORMATION

Congenital kidney disorders can affect the form and/or function of the kidney. Functional congenital kidney disorders are usually identified in childhood or adolescence. If function is not affected, congenital malformations may be detected only coincidentally. Malformations include agenesis, hypoplasia, alterations in kidney position, and horseshoe kidney.

Agenesis, absence of the kidney, and *hypoplasia,* underdevelopment of the kidney, typically affect only one of these paired organs. Renal function remains normal unless the unaffected kidney is compromised. Abnormal kidney position affects the ureters and urine flow, potentially leading to urinary stasis, increased risk of urinary tract infection (UTI), and lithiasis, or stone formation (see Chapter 28 ∞).

One in every 500 to 1000 people has *horseshoe kidney,* making it one of the most common renal malformations (Porth, 2005). Failure of the embryonic kidneys to ascend normally can result in a single, horseshoe-shaped organ. The two kidneys are fused at either the upper or lower pole (usually the lower). This malformation does not typically affect renal function; however, because the ureters cross the fused poles, there is an increased risk for *hydronephrosis,* or distention of the renal pelvis and

TABLE 29–1 Nursing Implications of Age-Related Changes in Kidney Function

FUNCTIONAL CHANGE	EFFECT	IMPLICATIONS
Decreased GFR	Decreased clearance of drugs excreted primarily through the kidneys increases drug half-life and blood levels, and risk of drug toxicity.	Monitor carefully for signs of toxicity, especially when administering digoxin, aminoglycoside antibiotics, tetracycline, vancomycin, chlorpropamide, procainamide, cimetidine, and cephalosporin antibiotics.
Decreased number of functional nephrons; lower levels of aldosterone; increased resistance to ADH	Decreased ability to conserve water and sodium; impaired potassium excretion; and decreased hydrogen ion excretion, resulting in reduced ability to compensate for acidosis.	Monitor for dehydration and hyponatremia; maintain fluid intake of 1500 to 2500 mL/day unless contraindicated; monitor for hyperkalemia, especially if taking a potassium-sparing diuretic, heparin, angiotensin-converting enzyme (ACE) inhibitor, beta-blocker, or NSAID; increased risk for acidosis.
Reduced numbers of functional nephrons	Decreased renal reserve with increased risk of failure.	Avoid giving nephrotoxic drugs if possible; monitor urine output and blood chemistries for early signs of renal failure.

calyces with urine (see Chapter 28 ∞). Recurrent UTI and renal calculi are also common in clients with horseshoe kidney.

Renal ultrasonography and intravenous pyelography are used to diagnose horseshoe kidney. Correction of the abnormality is rarely necessary, although surgical resection of the isthmus (connection between the kidneys) may be done to relieve ureteral obstruction or allow access to the abdominal aorta, which lies behind it.

Nursing care for clients with horseshoe kidney or other congenital malformations is primarily educational. Because abnormal kidney shape or position increases the risk of infection and stone formation, teach the client to maintain a fluid intake of at least 2500 mL per day. Emphasize the importance of avoiding dehydration by increasing fluids during hot weather and strenuous exercise. Teach hygiene practices such as perineal cleansing and voiding before and after intercourse to help prevent UTI. Teach the early manifestations of UTI and instruct to seek treatment promptly to prevent infection of the kidney. See Chapter 28 ∞.

THE CLIENT WITH POLYCYSTIC KIDNEY DISEASE

Polycystic kidney disease, a hereditary disease characterized by cyst formation and massive kidney enlargement, affects both children and adults. This disease has two forms: The autosomal dominant form affects adults; the autosomal recessive form is present at birth (Porth, 2005). Autosomal recessive polycystic kidney disease is rare. It usually is diagnosed prenatally or in infancy. Renal failure generally develops during childhood, necessitating kidney transplant or dialysis. Autosomal dominant polycystic kidney disease is relatively common, affecting 1 in every 300 to 1000 people and accounting for approximately 4% of clients with ESRD in the United States (Kasper et al., 2005). See the genetics box on this page. This section focuses on autosomal dominant polycystic kidney disease, the more common, adult form of the disorder.

GENETIC CONSIDERATIONS
Adult Polycystic Kidney Disease

- Approximately 90% of cases are inherited as an autosomal dominant trait; the remaining 10% are due to spontaneous mutations.
- Type 1, due to mutation of a gene on chromosome 16, accounts for approximately 85% of cases. It tends to have an earlier onset of symptoms and renal failure.
- Type 2, due to gene mutation on chromosome 4, is responsible for most remaining cases. The onset of manifestations and renal failure is later with type 2 polycystic kidney disease (Kasper et al., 2005).
- In both types, the genetic mutation affects production of *polycystin* membrane proteins and tubular epithelial cell growth and differentiation (Porth, 2005).

Pathophysiology

Renal cysts are fluid-filled sacs affecting the nephron, the functional unit of the kidneys. The cysts may range in size from microscopic to several centimeters in diameter and affect the renal cortex and medulla of both kidneys. As the cysts fill, enlarge, and multiply, the kidneys also enlarge. Renal blood vessels and nephrons are compressed and obstructed, and functional tissue destroyed (Figure 29–1 ■). The renal parenchyma atrophies and becomes fibrotic and scarred (Kasper et al., 2005).

People affected by polycystic kidney disease often develop cysts elsewhere in the body, including the liver, spleen, pancreas, and other organs. Diverticular disease of the colon is common, and may lead to perforation of the bowel (Kasper et al., 2005). Up to 10% of people affected experience subarachnoid hemorrhage from a type of congenital intracranial aneurysm. About 25% of people with polycystic kidney disease have mitral valve prolapse ("floppy" mitral valves). There also is an increased incidence of aortic and tricuspid valve insufficiency in people with polycystic kidney disease (Kasper et al., 2005).

Figure 29–1 ■ A polycystic kidney. The functional tissue of the kidneys is gradually destroyed and replaced with fluid-filled cysts.

Source: A. Glauberman/Photo Researchers, Inc.

Manifestations

Polycystic kidney disease is slowly progressive. Symptoms usually develop by age 40 to 50. Common manifestations include flank pain, microscopic or gross **hematuria** (blood in the urine), **proteinuria** (proteins in the urine), and *polyuria* and *nocturia,* as the concentrating ability of the kidney is impaired. Urinary tract infection and renal calculi are common, as cysts interfere with normal urine drainage. Most clients develop hypertension from disruption of renal vessels. The kidneys become palpable, enlarged, and knobby. Symptoms of renal insufficiency and chronic renal failure typically develop by age 60 to 70. The progression to ESRD tends to occur more rapidly in men than in women.

INTERDISCIPLINARY CARE

Diagnostic tests used to determine the extent of polycystic kidney disease include the following:

- *Renal ultrasonography* is the diagnostic procedure of choice for polycystic kidney disease.
- *Intravenous pyelography (IVP)* is used to detect cysts, evaluate their size, and determine the extent of kidney involvement.
- *Computed tomography (CT) scan* of the kidney is used to detect and differentiate renal masses such as cystic disease or tumors.

See the Diagnostic Tests table in Chapter 27 ∞ for the nursing implications of these tests.

Management of adult polycystic kidney disease is largely supportive. Care is taken to avoid further renal damage by nephrotoxic substances, UTI, obstruction, or hypertension. A fluid intake of 2000 to 2500 mL per day is encouraged to help prevent UTI and lithiasis. Hypertension associated with polycystic disease is generally controlled using angiotensin-converting enzyme (ACE) inhibitors or other antihypertensive agents (see Chapter 35 ∞). Ultimately, dialysis or renal transplantation is required. Clients with polycystic kidney disease are typically good candidates for transplantation because of the absence of associated systemic disease.

NURSING CARE

For those with adult polycystic kidney disease, an autosomal dominant disorder, discuss genetic counseling and screening of family members for evidence of the disease. This is particularly important if renal transplantation is contemplated and family members are potential donors. Consider the following nursing diagnoses when planning care for the client with polycystic kidney disease:

- *Excess Fluid Volume* related to impaired renal function
- *Anticipatory Grieving* related to potential loss of kidney function
- *Deficient Knowledge* regarding measures to help preserve kidney function
- *Risk for Ineffective Coping* related to potential genetic transmission of the disorder to offspring.

Teach the client with polycystic kidney disease about the disease, its genetic nature, and usual course. Discuss measures to maintain optimal renal function. Instruct to maintain a fluid intake of at least 2500 mL per day. Include additional information about preventing UTI (such as hygiene measures) and early manifestations of UTI. Stress the importance of seeking treatment to prevent further kidney damage. Advise to avoid drugs that are potentially toxic to the kidneys and to check with the primary care provider before taking any new drug. Discuss the potential benefits of genetic counseling with the client and family.

THE CLIENT WITH A GLOMERULAR DISORDER

Disorders and diseases involving the glomerulus are the leading cause of chronic renal failure in the United States. They are the underlying disease process for more than half of those people needing dialysis and result in a significant number of deaths per year (NKUDIC, 2004).

Glomerular disorders may be either primary, involving mainly the kidney, or secondary to a multisystem disease or hereditary condition. Primary glomerular disease is often immunologic or idiopathic in origin. Diabetes mellitus, systemic lupus erythematosus (SLE), and Goodpasture's syndrome are frequently implicated in secondary glomerular disorders.

FAST FACTS

- Glomerular disorders and diseases are the leading cause of chronic renal failure in the United States.
- Hematuria, proteinuria, and hypertension often are early manifestations of glomerular disorders.
- Acute poststreptococcal glomerulonephritis (also called acute proliferative glomerulonephritis) is the most common primary glomerular disorder.
- Diabetes mellitus and SLE are common causes of secondary glomerulonephritis.

Physiology Review

The glomerulus is a tuft of capillaries surrounded by a thin, double-walled capsule (Bowman's capsule). (See Figure 27–3.)

About 20% of the resting cardiac output flows through the glomeruli of the kidneys, forming approximately 180 L of plasma ultrafiltrate. More than 99% of this filtrate is reabsorbed in the renal tubules. The rate of glomerular filtration is controlled by opposing forces: The pressure and amount of blood flowing through the glomeruli promote filtration, and the pressure in Bowman's capsule and colloid osmotic (*oncotic*) pressure of the blood oppose it. The total surface area of glomerular capillaries also affects the GFR. The glomerular capillary membrane has three layers: the capillary endothelial layer, the basement membrane, and the capsule epithelial layer. Water and the smallest solutes (such as electrolytes) pass freely across this membrane, whereas larger molecules (such as plasma proteins) are retained in the blood.

Pathophysiology

Glomerular disease affects both the structure and function of the glomerulus, disrupting glomerular filtration. The capillary membrane becomes more permeable to plasma proteins and blood cells. This increased permeability in the glomerulus causes the manifestations common to glomerular disorders: hematuria, proteinuria, and edema. The GFR falls, leading to **azotemia** (increased blood levels of nitrogenous waste products) and hypertension. Glomerular involvement may be diffuse, involving all glomeruli, or focal, involving some glomeruli while others remain essentially normal.

Both hematuria and proteinuria are caused by glomerular capillary membrane damage, which allows blood cells and proteins to escape from the blood into the glomerular filtrate. Hematuria may be either gross or microscopic. Proteinuria is considered to be the most important indicator of glomerular injury, because it increases progressively with increased glomerular damage. Loss of plasma proteins leads to *hypoalbuminemia* (low serum albumin levels), which in turn reduces the plasma oncotic pressure (osmotic pressure created by plasma proteins), leading to edema.

As plasma proteins are lost, the forces opposing filtration diminish, and the amount of filtrate increases. The increased flow of filtrate stimulates the renin–angiotensin–aldosterone mechanism (see Chapter 27 ∞), producing vasoconstriction and a fall in GFR. Increased aldosterone production causes salt and water retention, which further contribute to edema. As the GFR falls, filtration and elimination of nitrogenous wastes, including urea, decrease, causing azotemia. **Oliguria**, urine output of less than 400 mL in 24 hours, may result from the decreased GFR. Hypertension results from fluid retention and disruption of the renin–angiotensin system, a key regulator of blood pressure.

The major primary glomerular disorders include acute glomerulonephritis, rapidly progressive glomerulonephritis, nephrotic syndrome, and chronic glomerulonephritis. Diabetic nephropathy and lupus nephritis are the most common secondary forms of glomerular disease.

Acute Proliferative Glomerulonephritis
Glomerulonephritis is inflammation of the glomerular capillary membrane. Acute glomerulonephritis can result from sys-

temic diseases or primary glomerular diseases, but acute post-streptococcal glomerulonephritis (also known as acute proliferative glomerulonephritis) is the most common form. Infection of the pharynx or skin with group A beta-hemolytic streptococcus is the usual initiating event for this disorder. Staphylococcal or viral infections, such as hepatitis B, mumps, or varicella (chickenpox), can lead to a similar postinfectious acute glomerulonephritis (Porth, 2005). This primarily childhood disease also can affect adults.

In acute glomerulonephritis, circulating antigen–antibody immune complexes formed during the primary infection become trapped in the glomerular membrane, leading to an inflammatory response. The complement system is activated, and vasoactive substances and inflammatory mediators are released. Endothelial cells proliferate, and the glomerular membrane swells and becomes permeable to plasma proteins and blood cells (Figure 29–2 ■). Renal involvement is diffuse, spread throughout the kidneys. See *Pathophysiology Illustrated: Acute Glomerulonephritis* on the next page.

MANIFESTATIONS AND COMPLICATIONS Acute proliferative glomerulonephritis is characterized by an abrupt onset of hematuria, proteinuria, salt and water retention, and evidence of azotemia occurring 10 to 14 days after the initial infection. The urine often appears brown or cola-colored. Salt and water retention increase extracellular fluid volume, leading to hypertension and edema. The edema is primarily noted in the face, particularly around the eyes (*periorbital* edema). Dependent edema, affecting the hands and upper extremities in particular, may also be noted. Other manifestations may include fatigue, anorexia, nausea

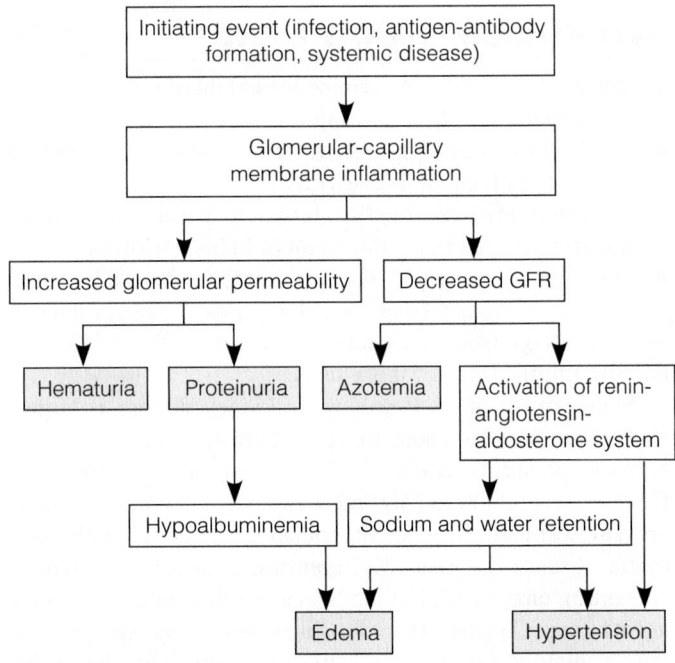

Figure 29–2 ■ The pathogenesis of glomerulonephritis.

Acute Glomerulonephritis

Infection from group A beta-hemolytic Streptococcus causes an immune response that causes inflammation and damage to the glomeruli. Protein and red blood cells are allowed to pass through the glomeruli. Blood flow to the glomeruli is reduced due to obstruction with damaged cells and renal insufficiency results, leading to the retention of sodium, water, and waste.

Kidney

Glomerulus

INFECTION

IMMUNE RESPONSE
Antigen–antibody complexes are deposited into the glomerular capillary filtration membrane

Monocyte (leukocyte)

Membrane

IgG (ab-antigen)

Inflammation and attack on the glomerular membrane occurs by neutrophils and monocytes

Coagulation system may be activated, leading to a proliferation of cells in the glomerular membrane

Enzymes are released that damage glomerular cell walls

Subepithelial deposits of gamma globulins (immune complex)

Neutrophil

Endothelial cell proliferation

Mesangial cell proliferation

Increased membrane permeability permits the passage of protein and red blood cells into the urine

RBC

Protein

Leukocyte

RBCs and leukocytes leak into capsular space causing edema

Capillary lumen occluded with proliferating cells and leukocytes

Renal blood flow and glomerular filtration are decreased

Renal insufficiency; retention of sodium, water, and waste

and vomiting, and headache (see the Manifestations box on the next page).

The older adult may have less apparent symptoms. Nausea, malaise, arthralgias, and proteinuria are common manifestations; hypertension and edema are seen less often. Pulmonary infiltrates may occur early in the disorder, often due to worsening of a preexisting condition such as heart failure.

The prognosis for adults with acute glomerulonephritis is less favorable than it is for children. The symptoms may re-solve spontaneously within 10 to 14 days. Full recovery is usual in children, whereas 60% or more affected adults recover completely. The remainder have persistent symptoms, and some have permanent kidney damage (Porth, 2005).

Rapidly Progressive Glomerulonephritis

Rapidly progressive glomerulonephritis (RPGN) is charac-terized by manifestations of severe glomerular injury with-out a specific, identifiable cause. This type of

---

MANIFESTATIONS of Acute Glomerulonephritis

- Hematuria, cola-colored urine
- Proteinuria
- Salt and water retention
- Edema, periorbital and facial, dependent
- Hypertension
- Azotemia
- Fatigue
- Anorexia, nausea, and vomiting
- Headache

---

glomerulonephritis often progresses to renal failure within months. It may be idiopathic (primary), or secondary to a systemic disorder such as SLE or Goodpasture's syndrome. It affects people of all ages.

In RPGN, glomerular cells proliferate and, together with macrophages, form crescent-shaped lesions that obliterate Bowman's space (Porth, 2005). Glomerular damage is diffuse, leading to a rapid, progressive decline in renal function. Irreversible renal failure often develops over weeks to months (Kasper et al., 2005).

Clients with RPGN typically present with complaints of weakness, nausea, and vomiting. Some may relate a history of a flulike illness preceding the onset of the glomerulonephritis. Other symptoms include oliguria and abdominal or flank pain. Moderate hypertension may develop. On urinalysis, hematuria and massive proteinuria are noted.

GOODPASTURE'S SYNDROME *Goodpasture's syndrome* is a rare autoimmune disorder of unknown etiology. It is characterized by formation of antibodies to the glomerular basement membrane. These antibodies also may bind to alveolar basement membranes, damaging alveoli and causing pulmonary hemorrhage. Goodpasture's syndrome usually affects young men between ages 18 and 35, although it can occur at any age and affect women as well.

Although the glomeruli may be nearly normal in appearance and function in Goodpasture's syndrome, extensive cell proliferation and crescent formation characteristic of rapidly progressive glomerulonephritis are more common. Renal manifestations include hematuria, proteinuria, and edema. Rapid progression to renal failure may occur. Alveolar membrane damage can lead to mild or life-threatening pulmonary hemorrhage. Cough, shortness of breath, and hemoptysis (bloody sputum) are early respiratory manifestations.

Nephrotic Syndrome

Nephrotic syndrome is a group of clinical findings as opposed to a specific disorder. It is characterized by massive proteinuria, hypoalbuminemia, hyperlipidemia, and edema. A number of disorders can affect the glomerular capillary membrane, changing its porosity and allowing plasma proteins to escape into the urine.

Minimal change disease (MCD) is the most common cause of nephrotic syndrome in children and accounts for 20% of

adults with nephrotic syndrome (Kasper et al., 2005). In MCD, the size and form of glomeruli appear normal by light microscopy. The prognosis for MCD is good.

In adults, *membranous glomerulonephropathy* is the most common cause of idiopathic nephrotic syndrome. The glomerular basement membrane thickens, although no inflammation is present. This form of nephrotic syndrome also occurs with some systemic diseases such as SLE and hepatitis B, and with drugs such as gold or penicillamine. *Focal sclerosis,* in which scarring (sclerosis) of glomeruli occurs, and *membranoproliferative glomerulonephritis,* caused by thickening and proliferation of glomerular basement membrane cells, are additional forms of nephrotic syndrome.

With plasma protein loss in the urine and resulting hypoalbuminemia, the oncotic pressure of the plasma falls. Fluid shifts from the vascular compartment to interstitial spaces, causing the edema characteristic of nephrotic syndrome. Salt and water retention, possibly due to activation of the renin–angiotensin system, contribute to the edema. Edema may be severe, affecting the face and periorbital area as well as dependent tissues (Figure 29–3 ■).

Loss of plasma proteins stimulates the liver to increase albumin production and lipoprotein synthesis. As a result, serum triglyceride and low-density lipoprotein (LDL) levels increase, as do urine lipids (*lipiduria*). Hyperlipidemia increases the risk for atherosclerosis in clients with nephrotic syndrome.

Thromboemboli (mobilized blood clots) are a relatively common complication of nephrotic syndrome. Loss of clotting and anticlotting factors along with plasma proteins are thought to disrupt the coagulation system, increasing the risk for renal venous thrombosis, deep venous thrombosis, and pulmonary embolism. Renal venous thrombosis can cause flank or groin pain on one or both sides, gross hematuria, and a reduced GFR (Porth, 2005).

Nephrotic syndrome usually resolves without long-term effects in children. The prognosis for adults is less optimistic because the syndrome often occurs secondarily to another disorder. Many adults do not recover completely, experiencing persistent proteinuria and potentially, progressive renal impairment.

Chronic Glomerulonephritis

Chronic glomerulonephritis is typically the end stage of other glomerular disorders such as RPGN, lupus nephritis, or diabetic nephropathy. In many cases, however, no previous glomerular disease has been identified.

Slow, progressive destruction of the glomeruli and a gradual decline in renal function are characteristic of chronic glomerulonephritis. The kidneys decrease in size symmetrically, and their surfaces become granular or roughened. Eventually, entire nephrons are lost.

Symptoms develop insidiously, and the disease is often not recognized until signs of renal failure develop. Chronic glomerulonephritis may also be diagnosed when hypertension and impaired renal function are found coincidentally during a routine physical examination or treatment for an unrelated disorder. Viral

Figure 29–3 ■ Severe edema characteristic of nephrotic syndrome.

Source: Science Photo Library/Library Researcher, Inc.

or bacterial infectious diseases can exacerbate the disorder, prompting its diagnosis.

The course of chronic glomerulonephritis varies, with years to decades between the diagnosis and the development of end-stage renal failure.

Diabetic Nephropathy

Diabetic nephropathy, kidney disease common in the later stages of diabetes mellitus (DM), is the leading cause of ESRD in North America. Thirty percent of clients with type 1 DM and about 20% of type 2 diabetic clients develop nephropathy. ESRD resulting from diabetic nephropathy is seen more frequently in blacks with type 2 DM and in whites with type 1 DM (Kasper et al., 2005).

Initial evidence of microproteinuria indicating renal damage is typically seen within 10 to 15 years after the onset of diabetes. Overt proteinuria and nephropathy generally develop within 15 to 20 years of the initial diagnosis.

The characteristic lesion of diabetic nephropathy is glomerulosclerosis and thickening of the glomerular basement membrane. As the disease progresses, the glomerular capillary lumen narrows, reducing the surface area for glomerular filtration. Arteriosclerosis, a common feature of long-term diabetes and hypertension, contributes to the disease, as do nephritis and tubular lesions. Pyelonephritis, inflammation of the kidney, is also implicated in the development of diabetic nephropathy. A further discussion is found in Chapter 20 ∞.

Lupus Nephritis

Systemic lupus erythematosus (SLE) is an inflammatory autoimmune disorder affecting the connective tissue of the body. Between 40% and 85% of clients with SLE develop manifestations of nephritis (Kasper et al., 2005). Immune complexes that form within the glomerular capillary wall are the usual trigger for glomerular injury in SLE. Manifestations of lupus nephritis range from microscopic hematuria to massive proteinuria. Its progression may be slow and chronic or *fulminant,* with a sudden onset and the rapid development

of renal failure. Most clients with minimal or mild lesions survive for at least 10 years. Improved management of the underlying disease, immunotherapy, dialysis, and renal transplantation have significantly improved the prognosis in recent years.

INTERDISCIPLINARY CARE

Management of all types of glomerulonephritis, acute and chronic, primary and secondary, focuses on identifying the underlying disease process and preserving kidney function. In most glomerular disorders, there is no specific treatment to achieve a cure. Treatment goals are to maintain renal function, prevent complications, and support the healing process.

Diagnosis

Laboratory and diagnostic testing are valuable to identify the cause of glomerulonephritis and evaluate kidney function.

The following studies may be ordered to help identify the underlying cause or etiology:

- *Throat or skin cultures* detect infection by group A beta-hemolytic streptococci. Although poststreptococcal glomerulonephritis typically follows the acute infection by 1 to 2 weeks, treatment to eradicate any remaining organisms is initiated to minimize antibody production.
- *Antistreptolysin O (ASO) titer* and other tests detect streptococcal *exoenzymes* (bacterial enzymes that stimulate the immune response in acute poststreptococcal glomerulonephritis). Other titers such as antistreptokinase (ASK) or antideoxyribonuclease B (ADNAase B) may be obtained as well.
- *Erythrocyte sedimentation rate (ESR)* is a general indicator of inflammatory response. It may be elevated in acute poststreptococcal glomerulonephritis and in lupus nephritis.
- *KUB* (kidney, ureter, bladder) *abdominal x-ray* may be done to evaluate kidney size and rule out other causes of the client's manifestations. The kidneys may be enlarged in acute glomerulonephritis, whereas bilateral small kidneys are typical of late chronic glomerulonephritis.
- *Kidney scan,* a nuclear medicine procedure, allows visualization of the kidney after intravenous administration of a radioisotope. In glomerular diseases, the uptake and excretion of the radioactive material are delayed.
- *Biopsy,* microscopic examination of kidney tissue, is the most reliable diagnostic procedure for glomerular disorders. Biopsy helps determine the type of glomerulonephritis, the prognosis, and appropriate treatment. Renal biopsy is usually done percutaneously, by inserting a biopsy needle through the skin into the kidney to obtain a tissue sample. Open biopsy, which requires surgery, may also be done.

See Chapter 27 ∞ for the nursing implications of diagnostic tests used to evaluate glomerular disorders.

The following studies are used to evaluate kidney function:

- *Blood urea nitrogen (BUN)* measures urea nitrogen, the end product of protein metabolism. It is created by the breakdown and metabolism of both dietary and body proteins. Urea is eliminated from the body by filtration in the glomerulus; minimal amounts are reabsorbed in the renal tubules. Glomerular diseases interfere with filtration and elimination of urea nitrogen, causing blood levels to rise. Increased protein catabolism (destruction), which may occur with GI bleeding or tissue breakdown, can also raise the BUN. Normal BUN values are listed in Table 29–2. Levels up to 50 mg/dL or 17.7 mmol/L indicate mild azotemia, and levels higher than 100 mg/dL or 35.7 mmol/L indicate severe renal impairment.

■ *Serum creatinine* measures the amount of creatinine in the blood. Creatinine is also a metabolic by-product, produced in relatively constant amounts by skeletal muscles. It is excreted entirely by the kidneys, making the serum creatinine a good indicator of kidney function. Normal values (see Table 29–2) are lower in the older adult because of decreased muscle mass. Levels greater than 4 mg/dL indicate serious impairment of renal function.

■ *Urine creatinine* also is an indicator of renal function and the GFR. Urine creatinine levels decrease when renal function is impaired because it is not effectively eliminated from the body.

■ *Creatinine clearance* is a specific indicator of renal function used to evaluate the GFR. The *clearance,* or amount of blood cleared of creatinine in 1 minute, depends on the amount and pressure of blood being filtered and the filtering ability of the glomeruli. Levels normally decline with aging as the GFR decreases in the older adult. Disorders such as glomerulonephritis affect glomerular filtration, decreasing the creatinine clearance.

■ *Serum electrolytes* are evaluated because impaired kidney function alters their excretion. Monitoring serum electrolytes is particularly important to prevent complications associated with imbalances.

■ *Urinalysis* often shows red blood cells (RBCs) and proteins in the urine of clients with a glomerular disorder. These substances, normally too large to enter glomerular filtrate, escape due to increased porosity of glomerular capillaries in glomerular disorders. A 24-hour urine specimen is used to determine the amount of protein in the urine.

Medications

Although no drugs are available to cure glomerular disorders, medications are used to treat underlying disorders, reduce inflammation, and manage the symptoms.

Antibiotics are prescribed for the client with poststreptococcal glomerulonephritis to eradicate any remaining bacteria, removing the stimulus for antibody production. Nephrotoxic antibiotics, such as the aminoglycoside antibiotics, streptomycin, and some cephalosporins, are avoided.

Aggressive immunosuppressive therapy is used to treat acute inflammatory processes such as rapidly progressive glomerulonephritis, Goodpasture's syndrome, and exacerbations of SLE. When begun early, immunosuppressive therapy significantly reduces the risk of end-stage renal disease and renal failure. Prednisone, a glucocorticoid, is prescribed in relatively large doses of 1 mg per kilogram of body weight per day (e.g., a 160-pound man would receive 70 to 75 mg per day). Other immunosuppressive agents such as cyclophosphamide (Cytoxan) or azathioprine (Imuran) are prescribed in

TABLE 29–2 Changes in Laboratory Values Associated with Kidney Disease

TEST	NORMAL VALUE	VALUE IN RENAL DISEASE
Blood urea nitrogen (BUN)	5–20 mg/dL Slightly higher in older adult	20–50 mg/dL or higher
Creatinine, serum	Female: 0.5–1.1 mg/dL Male: 0.6–1.2 mg/dL Slightly lower in older adult	Elevated; levels >4 mg/dL indicate severe impairment of renal function
Creatinine clearance	Female: 88–128 mL/min Male: 97–137 mL/min Values decline in older adult	Reduced renal reserve: 32.5–90.0 mL/min Renal insufficiency: 6.5–32.5 mL/min Renal failure: <6.5 mL/min
Serum albumin	3.2–5 g/dL; 3.2–4.8 g/dL in older adult	Decreased in nephrotic syndrome
Serum electrolytes	Potassium: 3.5–5.0 mEq/L Sodium: 136–145 mEq/L Calcium: 4.5–5.5 mEq/L or 8.2–10.5 mg/dL Phosphorus: 3.0–4.5 mg/dL	Increased in renal insufficiency Decreased in nephrotic syndrome Decreased in renal failure Increased in renal failure
Red blood cell count	Female: 4.0–5.5 million/mm^3 Male: 4.5–6.2 million/mm^3	Decreased in chronic renal failure
Urine creatinine	Female: 600–1800 mg/24 hours Male: 800–2000 mg/24 hours	Decreased in disorders of impaired renal function
Urine protein	Resting: 50–80 mg/24 hours Ambulatory: <150–250 mg/24 hours	Increased in disorders of impaired renal function
Urine red blood cells	<2–3/HPF; no RBC casts	Present in glomerular disorders

conjunction with corticosteroids. Corticosteroid use in post-streptococcal glomerulonephritis may actually worsen the condition, so it is avoided.

Oral glucocorticoids such as prednisone also are used in high doses to induce remission of nephrotic syndrome. When glucocorticoids alone are ineffective, other immunosuppressive agents such as cyclophosphamide or chlorambucil (Leukeran) may be used to induce or maintain remission. See Chapter 13 ∞ for more information about corticosteroids and other immunosuppressive drugs.

ACE inhibitors may be ordered to reduce protein loss associated with nephrotic syndrome. These drugs reduce proteinuria and slow the progression of renal failure. They have a protective effect on the kidney in clients with diabetic nephropathy. Nonsteroidal anti-inflammatory drugs (NSAIDs) also reduce proteinuria in some clients, but can increase salt and water retention (Kasper et al., 2005).

Antihypertensives may be prescribed to maintain the blood pressure within normal levels. Blood pressure management is important because systemic and renal hypertension are associated with a poorer prognosis in clients with glomerular disorders.

Treatments

Bed rest may be ordered during the acute phase of poststreptococcal glomerulonephritis. When the edema of nephrotic syndrome is significant or the client is hypertensive, sodium intake may be restricted to 1 to 2 g per day. Dietary protein may be restricted if azotemia is present. When proteins are restricted, those included in the diet should be complete or high-value proteins. Complete proteins supply the essential amino acids required for growth and tissue maintenance. Complete and incomplete proteins are compared in Table 29–3.

Plasma exchange therapy (**plasmapheresis**), a procedure to remove damaging antibodies from the plasma, is used in conjunction with immunosuppressive therapy to treat RPGN and Goodpasture's syndrome. Plasma and glomerular-damaging antibodies are removed using a blood cell separator. The RBCs are then returned to the client along with albumin or human plasma to replace the plasma removed. This procedure is usually done in a series of treatments. It is not without risk, and informed consent is required. Potential complications of plasma

exchange therapy include those associated with intravenous catheters, fluid volume shifts, and altered coagulation.

Renal failure resulting from a glomerular disorder may necessitate dialysis to restore fluid and electrolyte balance and remove waste products from the body. Dialysis procedures and related nursing care are explained in the acute renal failure section later in this chapter.

 NURSING CARE

Health Promotion

Discuss the importance of effectively treating streptococcal infections in all age groups to help reduce the risk for acute glomerulonephritis. Stress the importance of completing the full course of antibiotic therapy to eradicate the infecting bacteria. Teach clients with diabetes mellitus and SLE about potential renal effects of their disease. Discuss measures to reduce the risk of associated nephritis, such as effectively managing the disease, treating hypertension, and avoiding drugs and substances that are potentially toxic to the kidneys.

Assessment

Review Chapter 27 ∞ for complete assessment of the renal and urinary systems. Focused assessment data related to glomerular disorders include the following:
- *Health history:* Complaints of facial or peripheral edema or weight gain, fatigue, nausea and vomiting, headache, general malaise, abdominal or flank pain; cough or shortness of breath; changes in amount, color, or character of urine (e.g., frothy urine); history of skin or pharyngeal streptococcal infection, diabetes, SLE, or kidney disease; current medications.
- *Physical examination:* General appearance; vital signs; weight; presence of periorbital, facial, or peripheral edema; skin for lesions, infection; inspect throat, obtain culture as indicated; urine specimen for color, character, odor.

Nursing Diagnoses and Interventions

Nursing care is supportive and educational. Monitoring renal function and fluid volume status are key components of care, as is protecting the client from infection. Both manifestations of glomerular disorders and their treatment can interfere with a client's ability to maintain usual roles and responsibilities. For additional potential nursing diagnoses and interventions, see the Nursing Care Plan that follows.

Excess Fluid Volume

Excess fluid volume and resulting edema are common manifestations of glomerular disorders. When proteins are lost in the urine, the oncotic pressure of plasma falls, and fluid shifts into the interstitial spaces. The body responds to this fluid shift by retaining sodium and water to maintain intravascular volume, leading to excess fluid volume.

TABLE 29–3 **Complete and Incomplete Protein Sources**		
	COMPLETE PROTEINS	**INCOMPLETE PROTEINS**
Definition	Provide all essential amino acids needed for growth and tissue maintenance	Lack one or more essential amino acids or contain inadequate proportions
Examples	Milk, eggs, cheese, meats, poultry, fish, and soy	Vegetables, breads, cereals and grains, legumes, seeds, and nuts

NURSING CARE PLAN A Client with Acute Glomerulonephritis

Jung-Lin Chang is a 23-year-old graduate student in biology. He presents at the university health center with brown and foamy urine. The physician there admits him to the infirmary and orders a throat culture, ASO titer, CBC, BUN, serum creatinine, and urinalysis.

ASSESSMENT

Connie King, the nurse admitting Mr. Chang, notes that his history is essentially negative for past kidney or urinary problems. He relates having had a "pretty bad" sore throat a couple of weeks before admission. However, it was during midterms, so he took a few antibiotics he had from a previous bout of strep throat, increased his fluids, and did not see a doctor. The sore throat resolved, and he felt well until noticing the change in his urine. He admits that his eyes seemed a little puffy, but he thought this was due to lack of sleep and fatigue. He has eaten little the past 2 days, but was not alarmed because his food intake is irregular most of the time.

Physical assessment findings include T 98.8°F (37.1°C) PO, P 98, R 18, and BP 136/90. Weight 165 pounds (75 kg), up from his normal of 160 (72.5 kg). Moderate periorbital edema and edema of hands and fingers noted.

Throat culture is negative, but the ASO titer is high. CBC essentially normal. BUN 42 mg/dL, serum creatinine 2.1 mg/dL. Urinalysis reveals the presence of protein, red blood cells, and RBC casts. A subsequent 24-hour urine protein analysis shows 1025 mg of protein (normal 30 to 150 mg/24 hours).

The physician diagnoses acute poststreptococcal glomerulonephritis and places Mr. Chang on bed rest with bathroom privileges. He orders fluid restriction (1200 mL/day) and a restricted sodium and protein diet.

DIAGNOSES

- *Excess Fluid Volume* related to plasma protein deficit and sodium and water retention
- *Risk for Imbalanced Nutrition: Less than Body Requirements* related to anorexia
- *Anxiety* related to prescribed activity restriction
- *Risk for Ineffective Therapeutic Regimen Management* related to lack of information about glomerulonephritis and treatment

EXPECTED OUTCOMES

- Maintain blood pressure within normal limits.
- Return to usual weight with no evidence of edema.
- Consume adequate calories following prescribed dietary limitations.
- Verbalize reduced anxiety regarding ability to continue studies.

- Demonstrate an understanding of acute glomerulonephritis and prescribed treatment regimen.

PLANNING AND IMPLEMENTATION

- Vital signs every 4 hours; notify physician of significant changes.
- Weigh daily; intake and output every 8 hours.
- Schedule fluids allowing 650 mL on day shift, 450 mL on evening shift, and 100 mL on night shift.
- Arrange dietary consultation to plan a diet that includes preferred foods as allowed.
- Provide small meals with high-carbohydrate between-meal snacks.
- Encourage Mr. Chang to talk about his condition and its potential effects.
- Assist with problem solving and exploring options for maintaining studies.
- Enlist friends and family to listen and provide support.
- Teach Mr. Chang and his family about acute glomerulonephritis and prescribed treatment.
- Instruct in appropriate antibiotic use.

EVALUATION

Mr. Chang is released from the infirmary after 4 days. He decides to return to his parents' home for the 6 to 12 weeks of convalescence prescribed by his doctor. Mr. Chang's renal function gradually returns to normal with no further azotemia and minimal proteinuria after 4 months. He verbalizes understanding of the relationship between the strep throat, his inappropriate use of antibiotics, and the glomerulonephritis. He says, "I may not always remember to take every pill on time in the future, but I sure won't save them for the next time again!"

CRITICAL THINKING IN THE NURSING PROCESS

1. How did Mr. Chang's use of "a few" previously prescribed antibiotics to treat his sore throat affect his risk for developing poststreptococcal glomerulonephritis?
2. What additional risk factors did Mr. Chang have for developing glomerulonephritis?
3. The initial manifestations of acute poststreptococcal glomerulonephritis and rapidly progressive glomerulonephritis are very similar. What diagnostic test would the physician use to make the differential diagnosis? Develop a plan of care for a client undergoing this examination.

See Evaluating Your Response in Appendix C.

- Monitor vital signs, including blood pressure, apical pulse, respirations, and breath sounds, at least every 4 hours. Report significant changes. *Excess fluid increases the cardiac workload and the blood pressure. Tachycardia may result. Associated electrolyte imbalances can cause dysrhythmias. Increased pulmonary vascular pressure can lead to pulmonary edema, tachypnea, dyspnea, and crackles (rales) in the lungs.*

- Record intake and output every 4 to 8 hours, or more frequently as indicated. *Accurate intake and output records help determine fluid volume status.*

PRACTICE ALERT

Weigh daily, using consistent technique (time of day, scale, and clothing). Accurate daily weights are the best indicator of approximate fluid balance (Wise et al., 2000).

- Monitor serum electrolytes, hemoglobin and hematocrit, BUN, and creatinine. *Glomerular disorders affect fluid balance and may alter electrolyte balance as well, potentially leading to complications such as cardiac dysrhythmias (see Chapter 10 ∞). Increased intravascular volume can result in low hemoglobin and hematocrit values. BUN and creatinine provide information about renal function.*
- Maintain fluid restriction as ordered. Offer ice chips (in limited and measured amounts) and frequent mouth care to relieve thirst. With the client, develop a fluid intake schedule. *Fluids may be restricted to reduce fluid overload, edema, and hypertension. Ice chips and frequent mouth care moisten mucous membranes and help relieve thirst while maintaining oral tissue integrity. Including the client in planning fluid intake promotes a sense of control and understanding of the treatment regimen.*

PRACTICE ALERT
Carefully monitor and regulate intravenous infusions; include fluid used to dilute IV medications as intake. Significant "hidden" fluid intake can occur with intravenous medication administration.

- Arrange dietary consultation regarding sodium or protein-restricted diets. *Including the client and dietitian in planning allows individualization of the diet to client preferences. The glomerular disorder may reduce appetite; considering food preferences can help maintain adequate nutrition.*
- Monitor for desired and adverse effects of prescribed medications. *Diuretic therapy helps reduce excess fluid volume; however, glomerular disorders can affect the client's response to treatment. In addition, diuretics can exacerbate the electrolyte imbalances and muscle weakness often associated with glomerular disorders.*
- Provide frequent position changes and good skin care. *Perfusion may be altered by tissue edema, increasing the risk of breakdown.*

Fatigue
Fatigue is a common manifestation of glomerular disorders. Anemia, loss of plasma proteins, headache, anorexia, and nausea compound this fatigue. The ability to maintain usual physical and mental activities may be impaired.

- Document energy level. *As glomerular function improves, fatigue begins to resolve, and energy increases.*
- Schedule activities and procedures to provide adequate rest and energy conservation. Prevent unnecessary fatigue. *Adequate rest and energy conservation reduce fatigue and improve the client's ability to tolerate and cope with required treatments and activities.*
- Assist with ADLs as needed. *The goal is to conserve limited energy reserves.*
- Discuss the relationship between fatigue and the disease process with client and family. *Understanding the nature of the disease and associated fatigue helps the client and fam-*

ily cope with reduced energy and comply with prescribed rest.
- Reduce energy demands with frequent, small meals and short periods of activity. Limit the number of visitors and visit length. *Small, frequent meals reduce the energy needed for eating and digestion. Limiting visitors and visit length helps conserve energy. In addition, nurses can assist the fatigued client who may be reluctant to ask visitors to leave.*

Ineffective Protection
The effects of both the glomerular disorder and treatment with anti-inflammatory and cytotoxic drugs can depress the immune system, increasing the risk for infection. The anti-inflammatory effect of corticosteroids may also mask early manifestations of infection.

PRACTICE ALERT
Monitor vital signs, temperature, and mental status every 4 hours. An elevated temperature may indicate infection; anti-inflammatory drugs may moderate this response, however. Tachycardia, increasing lethargy, or confusion may be the initial signs of infection.

- Assess frequently for other signs of infection such as purulent wound drainage, productive cough, adventitious breath sounds, and red or inflamed lesions. Monitor for manifestations of UTI, such as dysuria, frequency and urgency, and cloudy, foul-smelling urine. *Early identification and treatment of infection is important to prevent systemic complications in the susceptible client.*
- Monitor CBC, focusing on the WBC and differential. *An elevated WBC and increased numbers of immature WBCs in the blood (left shift) may be early indicators of infection.*
- Use good hand washing technique. Protect from cross-infection by providing a private room and restricting ill visitors. *Clients with decreased resistance to infection need increased protection.*
- Avoid or minimize invasive procedures. *Maintaining the protective skin barrier is especially important for the client with altered immune status.*
- If catheterization is required, use sterile intermittent straight catheterization or maintain a closed drainage system for an indwelling catheter. Prevent urine reflux from the drainage system to the bladder or the bladder to the kidneys by ensuring a patent, gravity flow system. *The urinary tract is a frequent entry point for infection, particularly in the hospitalized or institutionalized client. Maintaining strict asepsis during catheterization is vital. Intermittent catheterization is associated with a lower risk of UTI than an indwelling catheter.*
- Provide a nutritionally sound diet with complete proteins. *A well-balanced, nutritionally sound diet is important to maintain nutritional status and support immune function.*
- Teach measures to prevent infection. *Care often is provided in the home, requiring the client and family to use appropriate infection control measures.*

Ineffective Role Performance

The manifestations and treatment of glomerular disorders can affect the ability to maintain usual roles and activities. Fatigue and muscle weakness may limit physical and social activities. Bed rest or activity limitations may be ordered to minimize the degree of proteinuria. If azotemia is present, malaise, nausea, and mental status changes can interfere with role function. Facial and periorbital edema affect the client's self-esteem and may lead to isolation.

- Establish a strong therapeutic relationship. *It is important to gain the client's trust and confidence.*
- Encourage self-care and participation in decision making. *Increased autonomy helps restore self-confidence and reduce powerlessness.*
- Provide time for verbalization of thoughts and feelings; listen actively, acknowledging and accepting fears and concerns. *Adequate time and active listening encourage expression of concerns and the effect of the disease or treatments on daily life. This helps the client deal with the illness, its treatment, and associated losses.*
- Support coping skills, helping the client identify personal strengths. *This support helps the client gain confidence.*
- When possible, enlist the support of family, other clients, and friends. *These people can provide physical, psychologic, emotional, and social support.*
- Discuss the effect of the disease and treatments on roles and relationships, helping identify potential changes in roles, relationships, and lifestyle. Help the client and family develop a plan for alternative behaviors and relationships, encouraging the client to maintain usual roles to the extent possible. *Developing a plan helps reduce the strain of role changes and maintain a sense of dignity and control.*
- Provide accurate and optimistic information about the disorder and its short- and long-term effects. *The client and family need accurate information to plan for the future.*
- Evaluate the need for additional support and social services for the client and family. Provide referrals as indicated. *Depending on client and family strengths, the severity of the disorder, and its treatment and prognosis, ongoing social support services may be necessary to facilitate coping and adaptation.*

Community-Based Care

Glomerular disorders may be self-limited or progressive. In either case, the course is lengthy, ranging from months to years. Self-management is essential. Provide instructions for the client and family, including the following topics:

- Information about the disease and the prognosis
- Prescribed treatment, including activity and diet restrictions; the use and potential effects, both beneficial and adverse, of all medications
- Risks, manifestations, prevention, and management of complications such as edema and infection
- Signs, symptoms, and implications of improving or declining renal function
- Measures to prevent further kidney damage, such as nephrotoxic drugs to avoid
- Community resources, such as home care providers and support groups.

THE CLIENT WITH A VASCULAR KIDNEY DISORDER

Renal function is dependent on an adequate supply of blood. Blood supports renal cell metabolism and is vital to kidney function, the nephron in particular. The kidney can regulate fluid, electrolyte, and acid–base balance and serve as a major organ of excretion only when its blood supply is sufficient. Vascular disorders, therefore, can have a significant impact on renal function.

Hypertension

Hypertension, sustained elevation of the systemic blood pressure, can result from or cause kidney disease.

Prolonged hypertension damages the walls of arterioles and accelerates the process of atherosclerosis. This damage primarily affects the heart, brain, kidneys, eyes, and major blood vessels. In the kidney, arteriosclerotic lesions develop in the *afferent* (leading into) and *efferent* (going out of) arterioles and the glomerular capillaries. The glomerular filtration rate declines and tubular function is affected, resulting in proteinuria and microscopic hematuria. Approximately 10% of deaths attributed to hypertension result from renal failure (Kasper et al., 2005).

Malignant hypertension is a rapidly progressive form of hypertension that can develop in clients with untreated primary hypertension. The diastolic pressure is in excess of 120 mmHg and may be as high as 150 to 170 mmHg. Malignant hypertension affects less than 1% of hypertensive clients; it is more common in African Americans than in people of European ancestry. Untreated, malignant hypertension causes a rapid decline in renal function due to vessel changes, renal ischemia, and infarction.

Approximately 5% to 10% of hypertensive clients have *secondary hypertension,* which is actually a manifestation of an underlying disease. Renal vascular disease and diseases of the renal parenchyma, such as diabetic nephropathy, are commonly associated with secondary hypertension.

Management of hypertension to maintain the blood pressure within normal limits is vital to prevent kidney damage. When hypertension is secondary to kidney disease, adequate blood pressure control can slow the decline in renal function. Hypertension and its management is discussed in depth in Chapter 35 ∞.

Renal Artery Occlusion

Renal arteries can be occluded by either a primary process affecting the renal vessels or by emboli, clots, or other foreign material. Risk factors for *acute renal artery thrombosis* (formation of a blood clot in the renal artery) include severe abdominal trauma, vessel trauma from surgery or angiography, aortic or renal artery aneurysms, and severe aortic or renal artery atherosclerosis. Emboli from the left side of the heart can travel via the aorta to occlude the renal artery. Emboli may form as a result of atrial fibrillation (irregular and uncoordinated electrical activity of the atria), following myocardial infarction, as vegetative growths on heart valves associated with bacterial endocarditis, or from fatty plaque in the aorta.

Renal arterial occlusion may be asymptomatic when the occlusion develops slowly and the affected vessels are small.

Acute occlusion leading to ischemia and infarction typically causes sudden, severe localized flank pain, nausea and vomiting, fever, and hypertension. Hematuria and oliguria may occur. In the older client, the new onset of hypertension or worsening of previously controlled hypertension may signal renal artery thrombosis.

Laboratory studies reveal leukocytosis (elevated WBC), and elevated renal enzyme levels, including aspartate transaminase (AST) and lactic dehydrogenase (LDH). These enzymes, normally present in renal cells, are released into the circulation when cells necrose and die. With bilateral arterial occlusion and infarction, renal function deteriorates rapidly, leading to acute renal failure (Kasper et al., 2005).

Surgery to restore blood flow to the affected kidney may be indicated for acute occlusion. Management usually is more conservative, using anticoagulant therapy, hypertension control, and supportive treatment.

Renal Vein Occlusion

A thrombus (clot) formed in a renal vein can occlude the vessel. The cause of the thrombus often is unclear. In adults, renal venous thrombosis usually occurs with nephrotic syndrome. Other predisposing factors include pregnancy, oral contraceptive use, and certain malignancies.

Gradual or acute deterioration of renal function may be the only manifestation of renal vein occlusion. If the thrombus breaks loose, it can become a pulmonary embolism. The definitive diagnosis is made by visualizing the thrombus through renal venography.

Thrombolytic drugs such as streptokinase or tissue plasminogen activator (tPA) may be given to dissolve or break up the thrombus. Anticoagulant therapy also is used to prevent further clotting and pulmonary emboli. Renal function often improves with treatment.

Renal Artery Stenosis

Renal artery stenosis (narrowing) causes 2% to 5% of all cases of hypertension (Kasper et al., 2005). It can affect one or both kidneys.

Atherosclerosis with gradual occlusion of the renal artery lumen by plaque is the primary cause of renal artery stenosis in men. In younger women, the most common cause is fibromuscular dysplasia, structural abnormalities involving the intimal, medial, or adventitial layers of the arterial wall.

Renal artery stenosis is suspected when hypertension develops before age 30 or after age 50 with no prior history of high blood pressure. An epigastric bruit (murmur) and other manifestations of vascular insufficiency may also be present. The affected kidney appears small and atrophied on renal ultrasound. The captopril test for renin activity and renal angiography are used to confirm the diagnosis. Clients with renovascular hypertension show higher levels of renin activity following administration of captopril, an ACE inhibitor drug (see Chapter 35 ∞), than clients with essential or primary hypertension (Kasper et al., 2005). Renal angiography uses radiologic contrast dye injected into the renal arteries to allow visualization of renal blood vessels.

The preferred treatment for renal artery stenosis is dilation of the stenotic vessel by percutaneous transluminal angioplasty. In this procedure, a balloon-tipped catheter is inserted via the femoral artery and aorta to dilate the renal artery. It relieves symptoms immediately in 90% of clients with fibromuscular dysplasia. One year after treatment, 60% remain symptom free. Some clients require a bypass graft of the renal artery. A section of saphenous vein or hypogastric artery is grafted from the aorta to the renal artery beyond the stenosis. The blood pressure may not return to normal following treatment, but is more easily managed using medications.

THE CLIENT WITH KIDNEY TRAUMA

The kidneys are relatively well protected by the rib cage and back muscles, but trauma due to blunt force or penetrating injury may inflict damage. Many renal injuries heal uneventfully, but prompt diagnosis and immediate treatment can be lifesaving in the event of major damage.

Pathophysiology and Manifestations

Blunt force is the most common cause of kidney injury. Falls, motor vehicle accidents, and sports injuries can damage the kidney. The injury may be minor, causing a contusion or small hematoma, or more serious, resulting in laceration or other damage. The kidney may fragment or "shatter," causing significant blood loss and urine extravasation. Tearing of the renal artery or vein may cause rapid hemorrhage, with shock and possible death.

Gunshot wounds, knife wounds, impalement injuries, and fractured ribs can penetrate the kidney. Minor penetrating injuries may lacerate the capsule or renal cortex. Major injuries include laceration or destruction of renal parenchyma or the vascular supply. Renal artery, renal vein, and renal pelvis lacerations are critical injuries.

The primary manifestations of kidney trauma are hematuria (gross or microscopic), flank or abdominal pain, and oliguria or anuria. There may be localized swelling, tenderness, or ecchymoses in the flank region. Retroperitoneal bleeding from the kidney may cause Turner's sign, a bluish discoloration of the flank. Signs of shock may be present, including hypotension, tachycardia, tachypnea, cool and pale skin, and an altered level of consciousness.

INTERDISCIPLINARY CARE

Hemoglobin and hematocrit levels fall in significant renal injury with hemorrhage. Hematuria is typically noted on urinalysis. AST levels rise within 12 hours of significant renal trauma. Renal ultrasonography is used to diagnose bleeding and kidney damage. A CT scan and IVP to visualize renal structures may be done to establish a definitive diagnosis. Renal arteriography is used when major injury is suspected and surgery is anticipated.

Treatment of minor kidney injuries is generally conservative, including bed rest and observation. In these injuries, bleeding is typically minor and self-limiting. With major or critical trauma, immediate treatment focuses on controlling hemorrhage and treating or preventing shock. Surgery or percutaneous arterial embolization during angiography may be required to stop the bleeding. Major lacerations may require surgical repair, partial nephrectomy, or total **nephrectomy** (removal) of the affected kidney.

NURSING CARE

Nursing care for the client who has experienced renal trauma focuses on timely and accurate assessment and appropriate intervention to preserve life and prevent complications. Obtain a urine specimen for analysis when kidney trauma is suspected. Monitor level of consciousness, vital signs, skin color and temperature, and urine output for possible signs of shock. See Chapter 11 ∞ for additional nursing care measures for the client who has had a traumatic injury or who develops shock.

THE CLIENT WITH A RENAL TUMOR

Renal tumors may be either benign or malignant, primary or metastatic. Benign renal tumors are infrequent and are often found only on autopsy. Primary renal malignancies account for about 2% of adult cancers and approximately 12,600 deaths per year (American Cancer Society, 2005). Most primary renal tumors arise from renal cells; a primary tumor also may develop in the renal pelvis, although less frequently. Metastatic lesions to the kidney are associated with lung and breast cancer, melanoma, and malignant lymphoma.

Males are affected by renal cancer more than females by a 2:1 ratio. The highest incidence is seen in people over the age of 55 years. Smoking and obesity are risk factors; chronic irritation associated with renal calculi may also contribute. Some renal cancers are associated with genetic factors. Clients with ESRD also may develop renal cancer.

Pathophysiology and Manifestations

Most (85% to 95%) primary renal tumors are renal cell carcinomas (Kasper et al., 2005; Porth, 2005). These tumors arise from tubular epithelium and can occur anywhere in the kidney. The tumor, which can range in size up to several centimeters, has clearly defined margins and contains areas of ischemia, necrosis, and hemorrhage. Renal tumors tend to invade the renal vein, and often have metastasized when first identified. Metastases tend to occur in the lungs, bone, lymph nodes, liver, and brain.

Renal tumors are often silent, with few manifestations. The classic triad of symptoms, gross hematuria, flank pain, and a palpable abdominal mass, is seen in only about 10% of people with renal cell carcinoma. Hematuria, often microscopic, is the most consistent symptom. Systemic manifestations include fever without infection, fatigue, and weight loss. See the box on this page.

The tumor may produce hormones or hormone-like substances, including parathyroid hormone, prostaglandins, prolactin, renin, gonadotropins, and glucocorticoids. These substances produce *paraneoplastic syndromes,* with additional manifestations such as hypercalcemia, hypertension, and hyperglycemia. The progression of renal cell carcinomas varies from prolonged periods of stable disease to very aggressive. Table 29–4 outlines the staging and prognosis for renal cell cancers.

INTERDISCIPLINARY CARE

Hematuria is often the only initial manifestation of renal cancer; its presence indicates a need for further diagnostic studies, including:

- *Renal ultrasonography* to detect renal masses and differentiate cystic kidney disease from renal carcinoma
- *CT scan* to determine tumor density, local extension of the tumor, and regional lymph node or vascular involvement
- *IVP* and *magnetic resonance imaging* (MRI) may be done to evaluate renal structure and function
- *Renal angiography, aortography,* and *inferior venacavography* may be used to evaluate the extent of vascular involvement prior to surgery
- *Chest x-ray, bone scan,* and *liver function studies* to identify potential metastases.

Radical nephrectomy is the treatment of choice for kidney tumors. In a radical nephrectomy, the adrenal gland, upper ureter, fat and fascia surrounding the kidney, as well as the entire kidney, are removed. Regional lymph nodes may also be resected. Although nephrectomy can be done using a laparoscopic approach, laparotomy primarily is used for radi-

MANIFESTATIONS of Renal Tumors

- Microscopic or gross hematuria
- Flank pain
- Palpable abdominal mass
- Fever
- Fatigue
- Weight loss
- Anemia or polycythemia

TABLE 29–4 Renal Cell Cancer Staging

STAGE	EXTENT OF TUMOR	PROGNOSIS
I	Confined to the kidney capsule	66% 5-year survival
II	Invasion through the capsule but confined to local fascia	64% 5-year survival
III	Regional lymph node, ipsilateral renal vein, or inferior vena cava involvement	42% 5-year survival
IV	Locally invasive or distant metastases	11% or less 5-year survival

Source: Adapted from *Harrison's Principles of Internal Medicine* (16th ed.) by D. L. Kasper et al. (Eds.), 2005, New York: McGraw-Hill.

cal nephrectomy. Nursing care for the client having a nephrectomy is summarized in the box below.

No effective treatment is available for advanced renal carcinoma with metastases. Biologic therapies such as interferon or interleukin-2 have been used, but rarely achieve a durable effect. No chemotherapy drug consistently causes tumor regression in more than 20% of clients (Kasper et al., 2005).

NURSING CARE

Nursing Diagnoses and Interventions

Nursing care for the client with renal cancer focuses on needs related to the cancer diagnosis and to the surgical intervention. Postoperative pain may be significant and the risk for respiratory complications is high. The remaining kidney must be protected from damage to preserve renal function. Psychologically, the client may grieve the loss of a major organ and the diagnosis of cancer.

Pain

The size and location of the incision used for a radical nephrectomy (Figure 29–4 ■) make pain management a challenge. Intercostal blocks, patient-controlled analgesia (PCA), or routine analgesic administration can effectively relieve the discomfort.

Nursing care focuses on assessing pain relief, providing supportive measures to enhance analgesia, and ensuring that pain or the fear of pain does not lead to respiratory complications.

■ Assess frequently for adequate pain relief. Use a standard pain scale and nonverbal signs such as grimacing, tense body position, apparent dozing, elevated pulse, change of blood pressure, or rapid, shallow respirations. Notify the physician of inadequate pain relief. *The client may assume that pain is to be expected or may fear becoming addicted to analgesics. Careful questioning and assessment allow effective pain management. Responses to analgesics are individual, and the prescribed dose may need to be adjusted.*

■ Assess the incision for inflammation or swelling and drainage catheters and tubes for patency. *An obstructed catheter can lead to hydronephrosis, hematoma, or abscess, increasing incisional pain.*

PRACTICE ALERT
Assess for abdominal distention, tenderness, and bowel sounds. Intra-abdominal bleeding, peritonitis, or paralytic ileus can cause pain that may be confused with incisional pain.

■ Use adjunctive pain relief measures such as positioning, diversional activities, management of environmental stimuli,

---

NURSING CARE OF THE CLIENT HAVING A   Nephrectomy

PREOPERATIVE CARE
■ Provide routine preoperative care as outlined in Chapter 4 ∞.
■ Report abnormal laboratory values to the surgeon. *Bacteriuria, blood coagulation abnormalities, or other significant abnormal values may affect surgery and postoperative care.*
■ Discuss operative and postoperative expectations as indicated, including the location of the incision (Figure 29–4) and anticipated tubes, stents, and drains. *Preoperative teaching about postoperative expectations reduces anxiety for the client and family during the early postoperative period.*

POSTOPERATIVE CARE
■ Provide routine postoperative care as described in Chapter 4 ∞.
■ Frequently assess urine color, amount, and character, noting any hematuria, pyuria, or sediment. Promptly report oliguria or anuria, as well as changes in urine color or clarity. *Preserving function of the remaining kidney is critical; frequent assessment allows early intervention for potential problems.*
■ Note the placement, status, and drainage from ureteral catheters, stents, nephrostomy tubes, or drains. Label each clearly. Maintain gravity drainage; irrigate only as ordered. *Maintaining drainage tube patency is vital to prevent potential hydronephrosis. Bright bleeding or unexpected drainage may indicate a surgical complication.*
■ Support the grieving process and adjustment to the loss of a kidney. *Loss of a major organ leads to a body image change and grief response. When renal cancer is the underlying diagnosis, the client may also grieve the loss of health and potential loss of life.*

■ Provide the following home care instructions for the client and family:
  a. The importance of protecting the remaining kidney by preventing UTI, renal calculi, and trauma. See Chapter 28 ∞ for measures to prevent UTI and calculi. *Damage to the remaining kidney by UTI, renal calculi, or trauma can lead to renal failure.*
  b. Maintain a fluid intake of 2000 to 2500 mL per day. *This important measure helps prevent dehydration and maintain good urine flow.*
  c. Gradually increase exercise to tolerance, avoiding heavy lifting for a year after surgery. Participation in contact sports is not recommended to reduce the risk of injury to the remaining kidney. *Lifting is avoided to allow full tissue healing. Trauma to the remaining kidney could seriously jeopardize renal function.*
  d. Care of the incision and any remaining drainage tubes, catheters, or stents. *This routine postoperative instruction is vital to prepare the client for self-care and prevent complications.*
  e. Report signs and symptoms to the physician, including manifestations of UTI (dysuria, frequency, urgency, nocturia, cloudy, malodorous urine) or systemic infection (fever, general malaise, fatigue), redness, swelling, pain, or drainage from the incision or any catheter or drain tube site. *Prompt treatment of postoperative infection is vital to allow continued healing and prevent compromise of the remaining kidney.*

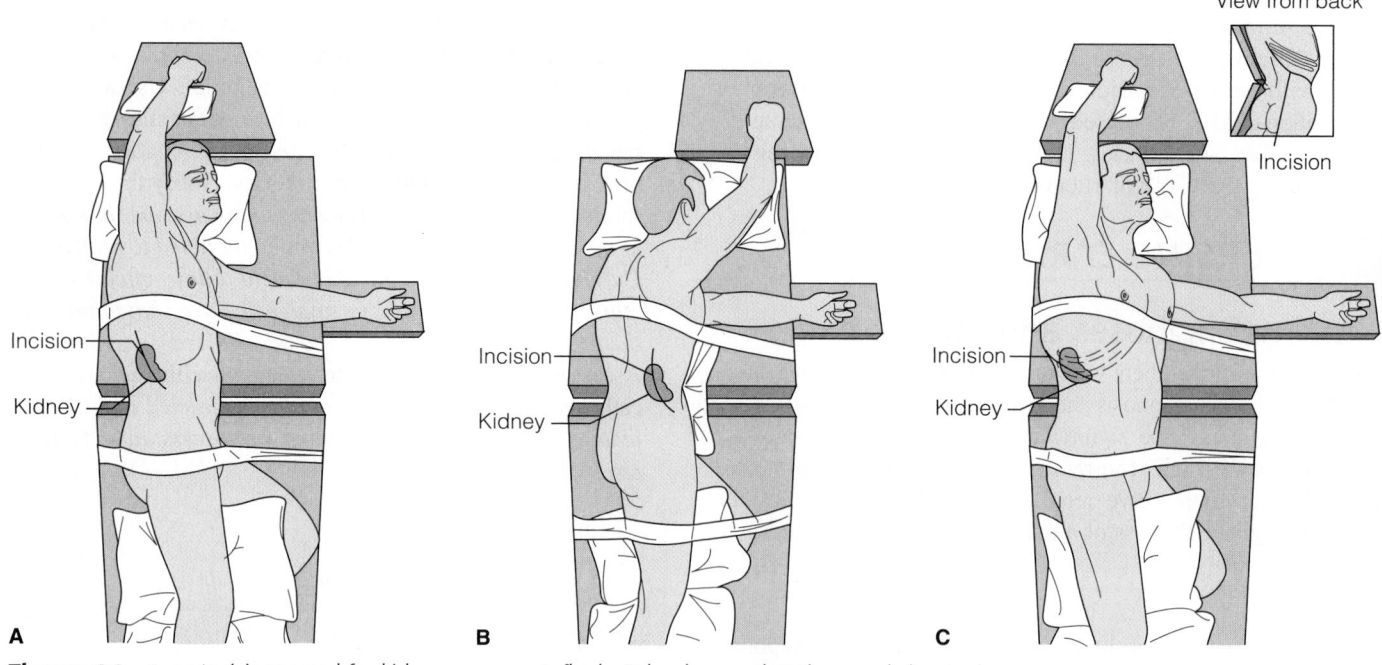

Figure 29–4 ■ Incisions used for kidney surgery: *A,* flank; *B,* lumbar; and *C,* thoracoabdominal.

guided imagery, and relaxation techniques. *These can enhance the effects of analgesia.*

Ineffective Breathing Pattern

The location of the incision combined with the respiratory depressant effects of narcotic analgesics increases the risk for respiratory complications in the client who has had a nephrectomy.

- Position to promote respiratory excursion, using semi-Fowler's position and side-lying positions as allowed and tolerated. *Lung expansion is improved in semi-Fowler's and Fowler's positions.*

PRACTICE ALERT
Assess respiratory status frequently, including rate and depth, cough, breath sounds, oxygen saturation, and temperature. Pneumothorax on the operative side is common. Early identification and intervention can prevent major respiratory complications.

- Change position frequently, ambulate as soon as possible. *These measures promote lung expansion and the movement of mucus out of airways.*
- Encourage frequent (every 1 to 2 hours) deep breathing, spirometer use, and coughing. Assist to splint the incision. *These measures promote alveolar ventilation, gas exchange, and airway clearance.*

Risk for Impaired Urinary Elimination

Surgery involving the urinary tract increases the risk for altered renal function and urine elimination. In addition, removal of one kidney dictates extra caution to maintain renal circulation, a sterile urinary tract, and free urine flow.

- Monitor vital signs, CVP, and urine output every 1 to 2 hours initially, then every 4 hours. *Hypovolemia due to hemorrhage,*

diuresis, or fluid sequestering (third spacing) reduces blood flow to the kidney and increases the risk of renal ischemia with possible acute tubular necrosis and acute renal failure.

- Frequently assess the amount and nature of drainage on surgical dressings and from drainage tubes, stents, and catheters. Measure and record output from each drain or catheter separately. *Frequent and accurate assessment of drainage helps to identify excess bleeding, abnormal fluid loss, infection, or other potential surgical complications.*

PRACTICE ALERT
Prevent kinking, twisting, or tension on drains and tubes. Do not clamp. Irrigate carefully and only with a physician's order. Notify the physician immediately if any tube becomes dislodged. It is vital to maintain the patency of drains, particularly any affecting the remaining kidney, to prevent the excess pressure of hydronephrosis.

- Maintain fluid intake with intravenous fluids until oral intake is resumed. Encourage an intake of 2000 to 2500 mL per day as soon as the client tolerates oral liquids. *A liberal fluid intake prevents dehydration, helps to dilute any nephrotoxic substances, and promotes good urinary output.*
- Use strict aseptic technique in caring for all urinary catheters, tubes, stents, drains, and incisions. *Asepsis is vital to prevent infection and possible compromise of the remaining kidney.*
- Following catheter removal, assess frequently for urinary retention. Notify the physician if the client is unable to void within 4 to 6 hours or if manifestations of retention (distended bladder, discomfort, urinary dribbling) develop. *Maintenance of urine output is vital to prevent stasis and possible complications such as infection and hydronephrosis.*
- Monitor laboratory results, including urinalysis, BUN, serum creatinine, and serum electrolytes. Report abnormal findings

to the physician. *Abnormal values may indicate early acute renal failure; prompt intervention is necessary to preserve renal function.*

Anticipatory Grieving

The client having a radical nephrectomy for renal cancer not only loses a major organ but also has to adjust to the diagnosis of cancer. Although the prognosis for recovery may be good, many people perceive cancer as always fatal. Providing support for the client and family during the initial stages of grieving can improve physical recovery, psychologic coping, and eventual adaptation.

- Work to develop a trusting relationship with the client and family. *Trust increases the nurse's effectiveness in helping them work through the process of grieving.*
- Listen actively, encouraging the client and family to express fears and concerns. *As they begin to express their concerns, client and family can begin to deal more effectively with them.*
- Assist the client and family to identify strengths, past experiences, and support systems. *These resources can be employed in working through the grieving process.*
- Demonstrate respect for cultural, spiritual, and religious values and beliefs; encourage use of these resources to cope with losses. *Value and belief systems can provide a structure and form for dealing with the grieving process.*
- Encourage discussion of the potential impact of loss on the client and the family structure and function. Assist family members to share concerns with one another. *Sharing of fears and concerns among family members promotes involvement and support of the entire family unit so that the individual is not left to cope alone.*
- Refer to cancer support groups, social services, or counseling as appropriate. *Support groups and counseling services provide additional resources for coping.*

Community-Based Care

If renal cancer was detected at an early stage and cure is anticipated, teaching for home care focuses on protecting the remaining kidney. Include the following measures to prevent infection, renal calculi, hydronephrosis, and trauma:

- Maintain a fluid intake of 2000 to 2500 mL per day, increasing the amount during hot weather or strenuous exercise.
- Urinate when the urge is perceived, and before and after sexual intercourse.
- Properly clean the perineal area.
- Watch for manifestations of UTI, and understand the importance of early and appropriate evaluation and intervention.
- If the client is an older adult male, he should watch for manifestations of prostatic hypertrophy, a major cause of urinary tract obstruction. Stress the importance of routine screening examinations.
- Avoid contact sports such as football or hockey; use measures to prevent motor vehicle accidents and falls, which could damage the kidney.

RENAL FAILURE

Renal failure is a condition in which the kidneys are unable to remove accumulated metabolites from the blood, leading to altered fluid, electrolyte, and acid–base balance. The cause may be a primary kidney disorder, or renal failure may be secondary to a systemic disease or other urologic defects. Renal failure may be either acute or chronic. **Acute renal failure** has an abrupt onset and with prompt intervention is often reversible. **Chronic renal failure** is a silent disease, developing slowly and insidiously, with few symptoms until the kidneys are severely damaged and unable to meet the excretory needs of the body. Both forms of renal failure are characterized by azotemia, increased levels of nitrogenous wastes in the blood.

FAST FACTS

- Acute renal failure has an abrupt onset and often is reversible with prompt treatment.
- Chronic renal failure is the end stage of long-term kidney disease. It is irreversible; renal replacement therapies (transplant or dialysis) are necessary to sustain life.
- Both acute and chronic renal failure are characterized by azotemia, accumulation of nitrogenous (protein) waste products in the blood.

Renal failure is common and costly. In 2001, more than 93,000 new clients began receiving treatment for **end-stage renal disease (ESRD)**. Annually, nearly 287,500 clients with ESRD undergo dialysis, about 15,300 have kidney transplants, and another 59,000 are awaiting kidney transplants. The annual cost of ESRD treatment (in 2001 dollars) is $22.8 billion. The cost is also measured in lives and lifestyle. The 5-year survival rate for clients undergoing dialysis is 31.9% (NKUDIC, 2004). Although many clients report satisfaction with their quality of life, often clients on dialysis are unable to work, and the family structure may disintegrate under the strain of treatment.

THE CLIENT WITH ACUTE RENAL FAILURE

Acute renal failure (ARF) is a rapid decline in renal function with azotemia and fluid and electrolyte imbalances. The most common causes of acute renal failure are ischemia and nephrotoxins. The kidney is particularly vulnerable to both because of the amount of blood that passes through it. A fall in blood pressure or volume can cause ischemia of kidney tissues. Nephrotoxins in the blood damage renal tissue directly.

Incidence and Risk Factors

Approximately 5% of all hospitalized clients develop ARF; the incidence jumps to as much as 30% in critical and special care units (Kasper et al., 2005). The mortality rate for ARF in seriously ill clients is up to 75%. This high death rate is probably more related to the populations affected by ARF—

older clients and the critically ill—than to the disorder itself (Porth, 2005).

Major trauma or surgery, infection, hemorrhage, severe heart failure, severe liver disease, and lower urinary tract obstruction are risk factors for ARF. Drugs and radiologic contrast media that are toxic to the kidney (*nephrotoxic*) also increase the risk for ARF. Older adults develop ARF more frequently due to their higher incidence of serious illness, hypotension, major surgeries, diagnostic procedures, and treatment with nephrotoxic drugs. The older adult also may have some degree of preexisting renal insufficiency associated with aging.

Physiology Review

The functional unit of the kidneys, the nephron (see Figure 27–3 ∞), produces urine through three processes: glomerular filtration, tubular reabsorption, and tubular secretion. In the *glomerulus,* a filtrate of water and small solutes is formed. The solute concentration of this filtrate is equal to that of plasma, with the exception of large molecules such as plasma proteins and blood cells. The GFR, the amount of filtrate formed per minute, is affected by blood volume and pressure, the autonomic nervous system, and other factors. From the glomerulus, the filtrate flows into the *tubules,* where its composition is changed by the processes of *tubular reabsorption* and *tubular secretion.* Most water and many filtered solutes such as electrolytes and glucose are reabsorbed. Metabolic waste products such as urea, hydrogen ion, ammonia, and some creatinine are secreted into the tubule for elimination. By the time urine exits the collecting duct into the renal pelvis, 99% of the filtrate has been reabsorbed.

Pathophysiology

The causes and pathophysiology of acute renal failure are commonly categorized as prerenal, intrinsic, and postrenal ARF. Prerenal ARF is the most common, accounting for about 55% of the total. In *prerenal ARF,* hypoperfusion leads to

acute renal failure without directly affecting the integrity of kidney tissues. *Intrinsic* (or *intrarenal*) *ARF*, due to direct damage to functional kidney tissue, is responsible for another 40%. Urinary tract obstruction with resulting kidney damage is the precipitating factor for *postrenal ARF*, the least common form (~5%). Table 29–5 summarizes the causes of acute renal failure. See *Pathophysiology Illustrated: Acute Renal Failure* on the next page.

Prerenal ARF

Prerenal ARF results from conditions that affect renal blood flow and perfusion. Any disorder that significantly decreases vascular volume, cardiac output, or systemic vascular resistance can affect renal blood flow. The kidneys normally receive 20% to 25% of the cardiac output to maintain the GFR. A drop in renal blood flow to less than 20% of normal causes the GFR to fall. As the filtration of substances by the glomeruli is reduced, less reabsorption of substances in the tubule is required. As a result, kidney cells require less energy and oxygen, and their metabolism slows. Prerenal ARF is rapidly reversed when blood flow is restored, and the renal parenchyma remains undamaged. Continued ischemia can lead to tubular cell necrosis and significant nephron damage (Kasper et al., 2005; Porth, 2005). Intrinsic ARF due to ischemic injury may result.

FAST FACTS

- Prerenal ARF is common, particularly in trauma, surgical, and critically ill clients.
- Restoration of blood pressure and blood flow to the kidneys rapidly reverses prerenal ARF.
- If not promptly identified and treated, prerenal ARF leads to ischemic acute tubular necrosis and intrarenal or intrinsic ARF.

Postrenal ARF

Obstructive causes of acute renal failure are classified as postrenal. Any condition that prevents urine excretion can lead to postrenal ARF. Benign prostatic hypertrophy is the most

TABLE 29–5 Causes of Acute Renal Failure

	CAUSE	EXAMPLES
Prerenal	Hypovolemia	Hemorrhage, dehydration, excess fluid loss from GI tract, burns, wounds
	Low cardiac output	Heart failure, cardiogenic shock
	Altered vascular resistance	Sepsis, anaphylaxis, vasoactive drugs
Intrarenal	Glomerular/microvascular injury	Glomerulonephritis, DIC, vasculitis, hypertension, toxemia of pregnancy, hemolytic uremic syndrome
	Acute tubular necrosis	Ischemia due to conditions associated with prerenal failure; toxins such as drugs, heavy metals; hemolysis, rhabdomyolysis (muscle cell breakdown)
	Interstitial nephritis	Acute pyelonephritis, toxins, metabolic imbalances, idiopathic
Postrenal	Ureteral obstruction	Calculi, cancer, external compression
	Urethral obstruction	Prostatic enlargement, calculi, cancer, stricture, blood clot

Acute Renal Failure

The initial kidney injury is usually associated with an acute condition such as sepsis, trauma, and hypotension, or the result of treatment for an acute condition with a nephrotoxic medication. Injury to the kidney can occur because of glomerular injury, vasoconstriction of capillaries, or tubular injury. All consequences of injury lead to decreased glomerular filtration and oliguria.

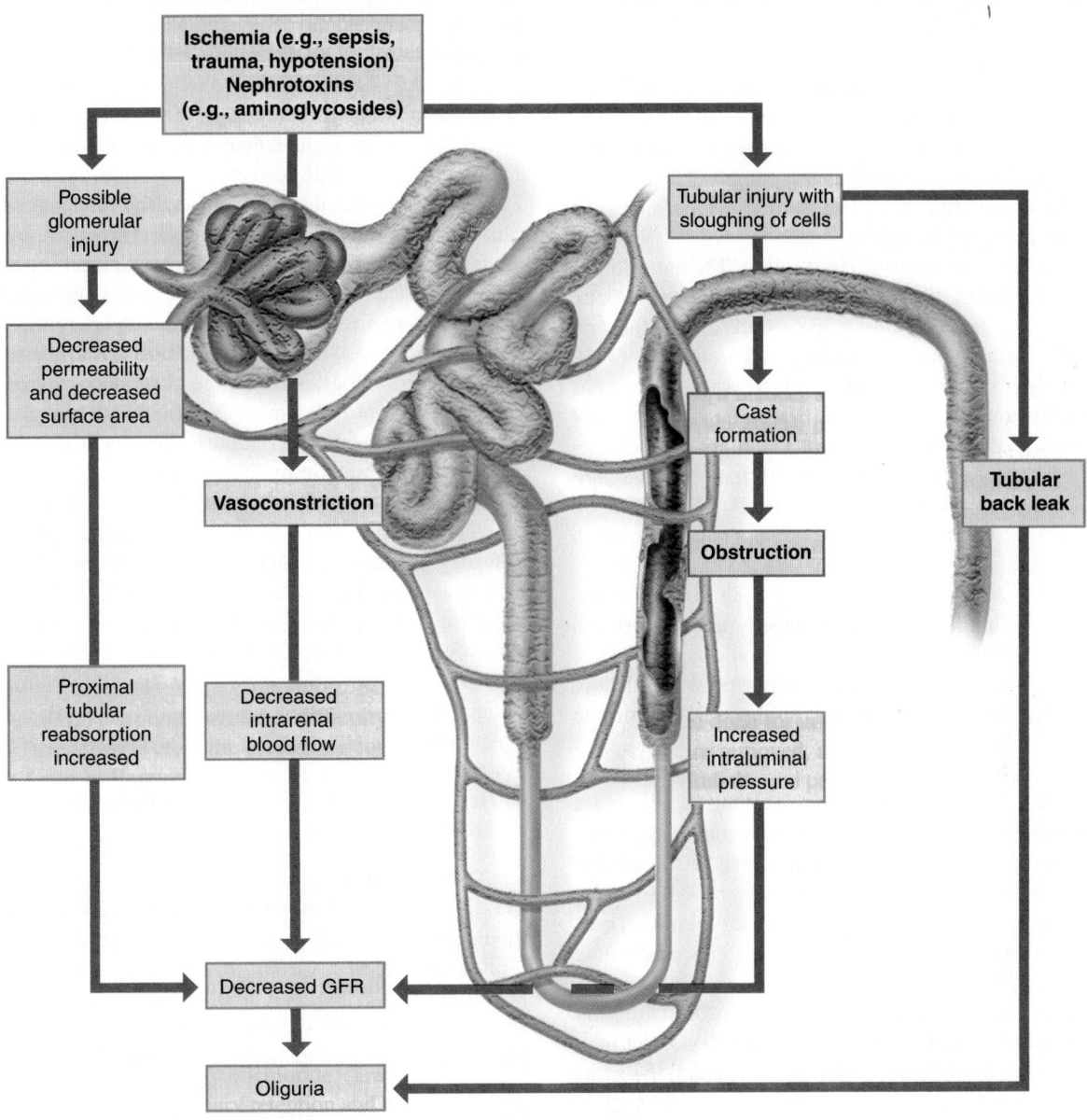

common precipitating factor. Others include renal or urinary tract calculi and tumors. See Chapter 28 ∞ for further discussion of urinary tract obstruction.

Intrinsic (Intrarenal) ARF

Intrinsic or intrarenal failure is characterized by acute damage to the renal parenchyma and nephrons. Intrarenal causes include diseases of the kidney itself and acute tubular necrosis, the most common intrarenal cause of ARF.

In acute glomerulonephritis, glomerular inflammation can reduce renal blood flow and cause ARF. Vascular disorders affecting the kidney, such as vasculitis (inflammation of the blood vessels), malignant hypertension, and arterial or venous occlusion, can damage nephrons sufficiently to result in acute renal failure.

ACUTE TUBULAR NECROSIS Nephrons are especially susceptible to injury from ischemia or exposure to nephrotoxins. **Acute tubular necrosis (ATN)**, destruction of tubular epithelial cells, causes an abrupt and progressive decline of renal function. Prolonged ischemia is the primary cause of ATN. When ischemia and nephrotoxin exposure occur concurrently, the risk for ATN and tubular dysfunction is especially high. See Figure 29–5 ■ for the pathogenesis of acute renal failure due to ATN. Risk factors for ischemic ATN include major surgery, severe hypovolemia, sepsis, trauma, and burns. The impact of ischemia resulting from vasodilation and fluid loss in sepsis, trauma, and burns often is compounded by toxins released by bacteria or from damaged tissue.

Ischemia lasting more than 2 hours causes severe and irreversible damage to kidney tubules with patchy cellular necrosis and sloughing. The GFR is significantly reduced as a result of (1) ischemia, (2) activation of the renin–angiotensin system, and (3) tubular obstruction by cellular debris, which raises the pressure in the glomerular capsule.

Common nephrotoxins associated with ATN include the aminoglycoside antibiotics and radiologic contrast media. Many other drugs (e.g., NSAIDs and some chemotherapy drugs), heavy metals such as mercury and gold, and some common chemicals such as ethylene glycol (antifreeze) are also potentially toxic to the renal tubule. The risk for ATN is higher when nephrotoxic drugs are given to older clients or clients with preexisting renal insufficiency, and when used in combination with other nephrotoxins. Dehydration increases the risk by increasing the toxin concentration in nephrons.

Nephrotoxins destroy tubular cells by both direct and indirect effects. As tubular cells are damaged and lost through necrosis and sloughing, the tubule becomes more permeable. This increased permeability results in filtrate reabsorption, further reducing the ability of the nephron to eliminate wastes.

Rhabdomyolysis may account for 7% to 15% of all cases of ARF (Criddle, 2003; Russell, 2005). It is caused by release of excess myoglobin from injured skeletal muscles. Myoglobin is a protein that acts as the oxygen reservoir for muscle fibers, much as hemoglobin does for the blood. Muscle trauma, strenuous exercise, hyperthermia or hypothermia, drug overdose, infection, and other factors can precipitate rhabdomyolysis. The myoglobin clogs renal tubules causing ischemic injury, and contains an iron pigment that directly damages the tubules. *Hemolysis,* red blood cell destruction, releases hemoglobin into the circulation, with much the same effect as rhabdomyolysis.

Course and Manifestations

The course of acute renal failure due to ATN typically includes three phases: initiation, maintenance, and recovery.

Initiation Phase

The *initiation phase* may last hours to days. It begins with the initiating event (e.g., hemorrhage) and ends when tubular injury occurs. If ARF is recognized and the initiating event is effectively treated during this phase, the prognosis is good. The initiation phase of ARF has few manifestations; in fact, it is often identified only when manifestations of the maintenance phase develop.

Maintenance Phase

The *maintenance phase* of ARF is characterized by a significant fall in GFR and tubular necrosis. Oliguria may develop, although many clients continue to produce normal or near-normal amounts of urine (nonoliguric ARF). Even though urine may be produced, the kidney cannot efficiently eliminate metabolic wastes, water, electrolytes, and acids from the body during the maintenance phase of ARF. Azotemia, fluid retention, electrolyte imbalances, and metabolic acidosis develop. These abnormalities are more severe in the oliguric client than in the nonoliguric one, leading to a poorer prognosis with oliguria.

During the maintenance phase, salt and water retention cause edema, increasing the risk for heart failure and pulmonary edema. Impaired potassium excretion leads to hyperkalemia. When the serum potassium level is greater than 6.0 to 6.5 mEq/L, manifestations of its effect on neuromuscular function develop. These include muscle weakness, nausea and diarrhea, electrocardiographic changes, and possible cardiac arrest. Other electrolyte imbalances include hyperphosphatemia and hypocalcemia. Metabolic acidosis results from impaired hydrogen ion elimination by the kidneys.

Anemia develops after several days of ARF due to suppressed erythropoietin secretion by the kidneys. Immune function may be impaired, increasing the risk for infection. Other manifestations of the maintenance phase include:
- Edema and hypertension due to salt and water retention
- Confusion, disorientation, agitation or lethargy, hyperreflexia, and possible seizures or coma due to azotemia and electrolyte and acid–base imbalances
- Anorexia, nausea, vomiting, and decreased or absent bowel sounds
- Uremic syndrome if ARF is prolonged (see the section on chronic renal failure that follows).

Recovery Phase

The recovery phase of ARF is characterized by a process of tubule cell repair and regeneration and gradual return of the GFR to normal or pre-ARF levels. Diuresis may occur as the nephrons and GFR recover, and retained salt, water, and solutes are excreted. Serum creatinine, BUN, potassium, and phosphate levels remain high and may continue to rise in spite of increasing urine output. Renal function improves rapidly during the first 5 to 25 days of the recovery phase, and continues to improve for up to 1 year.

INTERDISCIPLINARY CARE

Preventing acute renal failure is a goal in caring for all clients, especially those in high-risk groups. Maintaining an adequate vascular volume, cardiac output, and blood pressure is vital to preserve kidney perfusion. Nephrotoxic drugs are avoided if possible. When a nephrotoxic drug or substance must be used, the risk of ARF can be reduced by us-

A Ischemic injury. Severe hypotension, hypovolemia, and shock lead to ischemia of tubular epithelium. Renal tubular cells are very sensitive to anoxia. Cellular ATP is depleted, calcium accumulates within the cells, and free radicals damage cell membranes. Ischemia causes patchy necrosis and rupture of the basement membrane in the proximal convoluted tubule and ascending limb of the loop of Henle.

B Toxic injury. Nephrotoxins damage tubular cells by their direct effects on the cell itself, or by indirect effect (e.g., vasoconstriction and ischemia). Nephrotoxic damage primarily affects the proximal tubule in a uniform pattern. It frequently is less severe than ischemic damage.

C Injured tubular cells release intracellular debris, which combines with proteins within the tubules to form casts. These casts, together with sloughed necrotic cells, occlude the tubular lumen, increasing tubular pressure and disrupting the flow of glomerular filtrate. Glomerular filtration slows. The increased pressure pushes filtrate out of the damaged tubule into interstitial tissues (back leak). Renal blood flow and glomerular filtration may be further reduced by intrarenal angiotension II release and vasoconstriction.

Figure 29–5 ■ Acute tubular necrosis. In ATN, tubular epithelial cells are destroyed by either ischemic or toxic injury.

ing the minimum effective dose, maintaining hydration, and eliminating other known nephrotoxins from the medication regimen.

Treatment goals for acute renal failure are to (1) identify and correct the underlying cause, (2) prevent additional kidney damage, (3) restore the urine output and kidney function, and

(4) compensate for renal impairment until kidney function is restored. Fluid and electrolyte balance is a key component in managing ARF.

The client's history and physical assessment can provide clues about the initiating event for ARF. Impaired perfusion for as few as 30 minutes may cause significant renal ischemia.

Diagnosis

Diagnostic tests are used to identify the cause of acute renal failure and monitor its effects on homeostasis:

- *Urinalysis* often shows the following abnormal findings in acute renal failure:
  a. A fixed specific gravity of 1.010 (equal to the specific gravity of plasma) because the tubules are unable to concentrate the filtrate
  b. Proteinuria if glomerular damage is the cause of ARF
  c. The presence of RBCs (due to glomerular dysfunction), WBCs (related to inflammation), and renal tubular epithelial cells (indicating ATN)
  d. Cell casts, which are protein and cellular debris molded in the shape of the tubular lumen (in ARF, RBCs, WBCs, and renal tubular epithelial casts may be present. Brownish pigmented casts and positive tests for occult blood indicate hemoglobinuria or myoglobinuria.)
- *Serum creatinine* and *BUN* are used to evaluate renal function. In ARF, serum creatinine levels increase rapidly, within 24 to 48 hours of the onset. Creatinine levels generally peak within 5 to 10 days. Creatinine and BUN levels tend to increase more slowly when urine output is maintained. The onset of recovery is marked by a halt in the rise of the serum creatinine and BUN.
- *Serum electrolytes* are monitored to evaluate the fluid and electrolyte status. The serum potassium rises at a moderate rate and is often used to indicate the need for dialysis. Hyponatremia is common, due to the water excess associated with ARF.
- *Arterial blood gases* often show a metabolic acidosis due to the kidneys' inability to adequately eliminate metabolic wastes and hydrogen ions (see Chapter 10 ∞).
- *CBC* shows reduced RBCs, moderate anemia, and a low hematocrit. ARF affects erythropoietin secretion and RBC production. Iron and folate absorption may also be impaired, further contributing to anemia.

Laboratory findings associated with kidney disease are summarized in Table 29–2.

- *Renal ultrasonography* is used to identify obstructive causes of renal failure, and to differentiate acute renal failure from end-stage chronic renal failure. In ARF, the kidneys may be enlarged, whereas they typically appear small and shrunken in chronic renal failure.
- *CT scan* also may be done to evaluate kidney size and identify possible obstructions.
- *IVP, retrograde pyelography,* or *antegrade pyelography* may also be used to evaluate kidney structure and function. Radiologic contrast media are used with extreme caution because of their potential nephrotoxicity. Retrograde pyelography, in which contrast dye is injected into the ureters, and antegrade pyelography, in which the contrast medium is injected per-

cutaneously into the renal pelvis, are preferred because they have fewer nephrotoxic effects than IVP.
- *Renal biopsy* may be necessary to differentiate between acute and chronic renal failure.

See Chapter 27 ∞ for nursing implications of tests used to identify causes of renal failure.

Medications

The primary focus in drug management for acute renal failure is to restore and maintain renal perfusion and to eliminate drugs that are nephrotoxic from the treatment regimen.

Intravenous fluids and blood volume expanders are given as needed to restore renal perfusion. Dopamine (Intropin), administered in low doses by intravenous infusion, increases renal blood flow. Dopamine is a sympathetic neurotransmitter that improves cardiac output and dilates blood vessels of the mesentery and kidneys when given in low therapeutic doses.

If restoration of renal blood flow does not improve urinary output, a potent loop diuretic such as furosemide (Lasix) or an osmotic diuretic such as mannitol may be given with intravenous fluids. The purpose is twofold. First, if nephrotoxins are present, the combination of fluids and potent diuretics may, in effect, "wash out" the nephrons, reducing toxin concentration. Second, establishing urine output may prevent oliguria, and reduce the degree of azotemia and fluid and electrolyte imbalances. Furosemide also may be used to manage salt and water retention associated with ARF.

Aggressive hypertension management limits renal injury when ARF is associated with disorders such as toxemia and pregnancy-induced hypertension. ACE inhibitors or other antihypertensive medications are used to control arterial pressures.

All drugs that are either directly nephrotoxic or that may interfere with renal perfusion (such as potent vasoconstrictors) are discontinued. NSAIDs, nephrotoxic antibiotics, and other potentially harmful drugs are avoided throughout the course of acute renal failure.

The client in acute renal failure has an increased risk of gastrointestinal bleeding, probably related to the stress response and impaired platelet function. Regular doses of antacids, histamine H_2-receptor antagonists (e.g., famotidine or ranitidine), or a proton-pump inhibitor such as omeprazole (Prilosec) are often ordered to prevent GI hemorrhage.

Hyperkalemia may require active intervention as well as restricted potassium intake. Serum levels of greater than 6.5 mEq/L are treated to prevent cardiac effects of hyperkalemia. With significant hyperkalemia, calcium chloride, bicarbonate, and insulin and glucose may be given intravenously to reduce serum potassium levels by moving potassium into the cells. A potassium-binding exchange resin such as sodium polystyrene sulfonate (Kayexalate, SPS Suspension) may be given orally or by enema. This agent removes potassium from the body by exchanging sodium for potassium, primarily in the large intestine. When given orally, it is often combined with sorbitol to prevent constipation. Rectally, it is instilled as a retention enema, allowed to remain in the bowel for approximately 30 to 60 minutes, and then irrigated out using a tap-water enema.

Aluminum hydroxide (AlternaGEL, Amphojel, Nephrox), an antacid, is used to control hyperphosphatemia in renal failure. It binds with phosphates in the GI tract, which are then excreted in the feces.

Because many drugs are eliminated from the body by the kidney, drug dosages may need to be adjusted. Doses within the usual range can lead to potentially toxic blood levels, because their elimination is slowed and half-life prolonged. Nursing implications for medications commonly prescribed for the client in ARF are summarized in the Medication Administration box below.

Fluid Management

Once vascular volume and renal perfusion are restored, fluid intake is usually restricted. The allowed daily fluid intake is calculated by allowing 500 mL for insensible losses (respiration, perspiration, bowel losses) and adding the amount excreted as urine (or lost in vomitus) during the previous 24 hours. For example, if a client with ARF excretes 325 mL of urine in 24 hours, the client is allowed a fluid intake (including oral and intravenous fluids) of 825 mL for the next 24 hours. Fluid balance is carefully monitored, using accurate weight measurements and the serum sodium as the primary indicators.

MEDICATION ADMINISTRATION   **The Client with Acute Renal Failure**

LOOP DIURETICS
Bumetanide (Bumex)
Ethacrynic acid (Edecrin)
Furosemide (Lasix)
Torsemide (Demadex)

The loop diuretics, named for their primary site of action in the loop of Henle, are *high-ceiling diuretics:* The response increases with increasing doses. These are highly effective diuretics used in early ARF to reestablish urine flow and convert oliguric renal failure to nonoliguric renal failure. Loop diuretics may be given with intravenous dopamine to promote renal blood flow. In ATN due to a nephrotoxin, loop diuretics are used to clear the toxin from the nephrons more rapidly. Loop diuretics cause potassium wasting, which is generally not a concern in ARF because renal failure impairs normal potassium elimination.

Nursing Responsibilities
- Assess weight and vital signs for baseline data.
- Monitor intake and output, daily weight (or more frequently as ordered), vital signs, skin turgor, and other indicators of fluid volume status frequently.
- Assess for orthostatic hypotension because these potent diuretics can lead to hypovolemia.
- Monitor laboratory results, especially serum electrolyte, glucose, BUN, and creatinine levels.
- Administer by mouth or, if ordered, by intravenous injection:
  a. Furosemide undiluted at a rate of no more than 20 mg per minute
  b. Ethacrynic acid 50 mg diluted with 50 mL of normal saline at a rate of no more than 10 mg per minute
  c. Bumetanide undiluted over at least 1 minute or diluted in lactated Ringer's solution, normal saline, or 5% dextrose in water for infusion
  d. Torsemide undiluted over at least 2 minutes.
- Assess response. Urine output typically increases within 10 minutes after intravenous administration.
- Monitor hearing and for complaints such as tinnitus. High doses of loop diuretics increase the risk of ototoxicity, especially with ethacrynic acid. These effects may be reversible if detected early and the drug is discontinued.
- Avoid administering concurrently with other ototoxic agents, such as aminoglycoside antibiotics and cisplatin.

Health Education for the Client and Family
- Unless contraindicated, maintain a fluid intake of 2 to 3 quarts per day.

- Rise slowly from lying or sitting positions, because a fall in blood pressure may cause light-headedness.
- Take in the morning and, if ordered twice a day, late afternoon to avoid sleep disturbance.
- Take with food or milk to prevent gastric distress.
- NSAIDs interfere with the effectiveness of loop diuretics and should be avoided.

OSMOTIC DIURETICS
Mannitol (Osmitrol, Isotol)
Urea (Ureaphil)

The osmotic diuretics act by increasing the osmotic draw in the blood and urine. In the blood, the effect is to pull extracellular water into the vascular system, increasing the GFR. These substances are then freely filtered in the glomerulus and increase the osmotic draw of the urine, inhibiting water reabsorption. The effect is to increase urine volume and flow. In addition, osmotic diuretics dilute waste products in the urine, decreasing the risk of renal damage due to excess concentrations.

Nursing Responsibilities
- Assess urine output. Osmotic diuretics are used in early renal failure to maintain urine output but are contraindicated in anuria. A test dose may be administered; urine output of 30 mL per hour following the test dose shows an adequate response.
- Do not give these diuretics to clients who have heart failure or who are severely dehydrated. They increase vascular volume and may worsen heart failure. These drugs are not effective unless extracellular volume is adequate.
- Administer mannitol intravenously, diluting before use if indicated. Check solution for crystallization. Dissolve crystals by warming the solution slightly. Infuse 15% to 25% mannitol solutions through a filter over 30 to 90 minutes.
- Administer urea intravenously, diluting in 100 mL of 5% or 10% dextrose in water for every 30 g of urea. Administer no faster than 4 mL per minute through a filter.
- Monitor vital signs, breath sounds, and urinary output.
- Discontinue the drug if signs of heart failure or pulmonary edema develop or if renal function continues to decline.

Health Education for the Client and Family
- Report shortness of breath, headache, chest pain, or dizziness immediately.

ELECTROLYTES AND ELECTROLYTE MODIFIERS
Calcium chloride
Calcium gluconate

(continued)

MEDICATION ADMINISTRATION The Client with Acute Renal Failure (continued)

Sodium bicarbonate
Sodium polystyrene sulfonate (Kayexalate)

Calcium chloride or gluconate and sodium bicarbonate are administered intravenously in the initial management of hyperkalemia. Calcium is also administered to correct hypocalcemia and reduce hyperphosphatemia (calcium and phosphate have a reciprocal relationship in the body; as the level of one rises, the level of the other falls). Sodium bicarbonate helps correct acidosis and move potassium back into the intracellular space. Sodium polystyrene sulfonate is not used to replace an electrolyte, but to remove excess potassium from the body by exchanging sodium for potassium in the large intestine.

Nursing Responsibilities

- Assess serum electrolyte levels prior to and during therapy. Report rapid shifts or adverse responses to the physician.
- Administer as appropriate:
  a. Intravenous calcium chloride at less than 1 mL per minute; intravenous calcium gluconate at 0.5 mL per minute. Inject

into a large vein through a small-bore needle; avoid infiltration because extravasation of intravenous solution will cause tissue necrosis.
  b. Intravenous sodium bicarbonate infusion over 4 to 8 hours; oral tablets as prescribed.
  c. Sodium polystyrene sulfonate as an oral solution mixed with sorbitol to prevent constipation, or as a retention enema mixed with warm water. Leave in the bowel for 30 to 60 minutes, irrigate using a small tap-water enema.
- Monitor for adverse reactions, such as dysrhythmias, electrolyte imbalances, and metabolic alkalosis.

Health Education for the Client and Family

- Intravenous calcium may make you light-headed; remain in bed for at least 30 minutes after administration.
- Chew sodium bicarbonate tablets and follow with 8 ounces of water. Do not take with milk.
- Retain the sodium polystyrene sulfonate enema as long as possible.

Nutrition

Renal insufficiency and the underlying disease process increase the rate of *catabolism* (the breakdown of body proteins) and decrease the rate of *anabolism* (body tissue repair). The client with ARF needs adequate nutrients and calories to prevent catabolism. Proteins are limited to 0.6 g per kilogram of body weight per day to minimize the degree of azotemia. Dietary proteins should be of high biologic value (rich in essential amino acids). Carbohydrates are increased to maintain adequate calorie intake and provide a protein-sparing effect.

Parenteral nutrition providing amino acids, concentrated carbohydrates, and fats may be instituted when the client cannot consume an adequate diet (e.g., due to nausea, vomiting, or underlying critical illness). The disadvantages of parenteral nutrition in the client with ARF are the high volume of fluid required and the risk for infection through the venous line.

Renal Replacement Therapy: Dialysis

Manifestations of **uremia**, organ dysfunction due to accumulated metabolic wastes, severe fluid overload, hyperkalemia, or metabolic acidosis in a client with renal failure, indicate a need to replace renal function. **Dialysis** is the diffusion of solute molecules across a semipermeable membrane from an area of higher solute concentration to one of lower concentration. It is used to remove excess fluid and metabolic waste products in renal failure. Early use of dialysis can reduce the rate of complications. Dialysis may also be used to rapidly remove nephrotoxins in acute tubular necrosis. While dialysis compensates for lost renal elimination functions, it does not replace lost erythropoietin production. Anemia is a continuing problem for the client receiving dialysis.

In dialysis, blood is separated from a dialysis solution (**dialysate**) by a semipermeable membrane. Either **hemodialysis**, a procedure in which blood passes through a semipermeable membrane filter outside the body, or **peritoneal dialysis**, which uses the peritoneum surrounding the abdominal cavity as the dialyzing membrane, may be used for the client with

ARF. **Continuous renal replacement therapy (CRRT)**, in which blood is continuously circulated through a highly porous hemofilter from artery to vein or vein to vein, is a newer form of dialysis that may be used to treat ARF.

HEMODIALYSIS Hemodialysis uses the principles of diffusion and ultrafiltration to remove electrolytes, waste products, and excess water from the body. Blood is taken from the client via a vascular access and pumped to the dialyzer (Figure 29–6 ■). The porous membranes of the dialyzer unit allow small molecules such as water, glucose, and electrolytes to pass through, but block larger molecules such as serum proteins and blood cells. The dialysate, a solution of approximately the same composition and temperature as normal extracellular fluid, passes along the other side of the membrane. Small solute molecules move freely across the membrane by diffusion. The direction of movement for any substance is determined by the concentrations of that substance in the blood and the dialysate. Electrolytes and waste products such as urea and creatinine diffuse from the blood into the dialysate. If it is necessary to add something to the blood, such as calcium to replace depleted stores, it can be added to the dialysate to diffuse into the blood. Excess water is removed by creating a higher hydrostatic pressure of the blood moving through the dialyzer than of the dialysate, which flows in the opposite direction. This process is known as **ultrafiltration**.

Initially, clients with ARF typically undergo daily hemodialysis, then three to four sessions per week as indicated. Hemodialysis is not used if the client is hemodynamically unstable (e.g., with hypotension or low cardiac output). Following are complications associated with hemodialysis:

- Hypotension, the most frequent complication during hemodialysis, is related to changes in serum osmolality, rapid removal of fluid from the vascular compartment, vasodilation, and other factors.
- Bleeding is related to altered platelet function associated with uremia and the use of heparin during dialysis.

Figure 29–6 ■ *A,* The components of a hemodialysis system. *B,* A woman receiving kidney dialysis.

■ Infection (local or systemic) is related to WBC damage and immune system suppression. *Staphylococcus aureus* septicemia is commonly associated with contamination of the vascular access site. Clients on chronic hemodialysis have higher rates of hepatitis B, hepatitis C, cytomegalovirus, and HIV infection than the general population.

See the box on the next page for nursing care for the client undergoing hemodialysis.

CONTINUOUS RENAL REPLACEMENT THERAPY Clients with acute renal failure may be unable to tolerate hemodialysis and rapid fluid removal if their cardiovascular status is unstable

(e.g., due to trauma, major surgery, heart failure). Continuous renal replacement therapy, which allows more gradual fluid and solute removal, often is used for these clients. In CRRT, blood is continuously circulated from an artery to a vein or a vein to a vein through a highly porous hemofilter for a period of 12 or more hours. Excess water and solutes such as electrolytes, urea, creatinine, uric acid, and glucose drain into a collection device. Fluid may be replaced with normal saline or a balanced electrolyte solution as needed during CRRT. This slower process helps maintain hemodynamic stability and avoid complications associated with rapid changes in ECF composition. The most common CRRT techniques are outlined in Table 29–6.

TABLE 29–6 Continuous Renal Replacement Therapies

TYPE	INDICATIONS	DESCRIPTION
Continuous arteriovenous hemofiltration (CAVH)	Remove fluid and some solutes	Arterial blood circulates through a hemofilter, then returns to client through venous line; ultrafiltrate collects in a drainage bag.
Continuous arteriovenous hemodialysis (CAVHD)	Remove fluid and waste products	Arterial blood circulates through a hemofilter surrounded by dialysate, then returns to client through venous line; ultrafiltrate collects in a drainage bag.
Continuous venovenous hemodialysis (CVVHD)	Remove fluid and waste products	Venous blood circulates through a hemofilter surrounded by dialysate, then returns to client through double-lumen venous catheter; ultrafiltrate collects in a drainage bag.

NURSING CARE OF THE CLIENT UNDERGOING Hemodialysis

PREDIALYSIS CARE

- Assess vital signs, including orthostatic blood pressures (lying, sitting, and standing), apical pulse, respirations, and lung sounds. *These data provide baseline information to help evaluate the effects of hemodialysis. Hypertension may indicate excess fluid volume. The client who is hypotensive may not tolerate rapid fluid volume changes during dialysis. Abnormal heart sounds (e.g., a gallop or murmur) and changes in heart rate or rhythm may indicate excess fluid volume or electrolyte imbalance. Fluid overload may also cause dyspnea, tachypnea, and rales or crackles in the lungs.*
- Record weight. *Weight changes are an effective indicator of fluid volume.*
- Assess vascular access site for a palpable pulsation or vibration and an audible bruit and for inflammation. *Infection and thrombus formation are the most common problems affecting the access site in hemodialysis clients.*
- Alert all personnel to avoid using the extremity with the vascular access site (or the nondominant arm, if long-term access has not been established) for blood pressures or venipuncture. *These procedures may damage vessels and lead to failure of the arteriovenous fistula.*

POSTDIALYSIS CARE

- Assess and document vital signs, weight, and vascular access site condition. *Rapid fluid and solute removal during dialysis may lead to orthostatic hypotension, cardiopulmonary changes, and weight loss.*
- Monitor BUN, serum creatinine, serum electrolyte, and hematocrit levels between dialysis treatments. *These values help determine the effectiveness of the treatment, the need for fluid and diet restrictions, and the timing of future dialysis sessions. The anemia associated with renal failure does not improve with dialysis, and iron and folate supplements or periodic blood transfusions may be needed.*

- Assess for dialysis disequilibrium syndrome, with headache, nausea and vomiting, altered level of consciousness; and hypertension. *Rapid changes in BUN, pH, and electrolyte levels during dialysis may lead to cerebral edema and increased intracranial pressure.*
- Assess for other adverse responses to dialysis, such as dehydration, nausea and vomiting, muscle cramps, or seizure activity. Treat as ordered. *Excess fluid removal and rapid changes in electrolyte balance can cause fluid deficit, nausea, vomiting, and seizure activity.*
- Assess for bleeding at the access site or elsewhere. Use standard precautions at all times. *Renal failure and heparinization during dialysis increase the risk for bleeding. Frequent exposure to blood and blood products increase the risk for hepatitis B or C or other bloodborne diseases.*
- If a transfusion is given during dialysis, monitor for possible transfusion reaction (e.g., chills and fever; dyspnea; chest, back, or arm pain; and urticaria or itching). *Clients in renal failure may receive multiple transfusions, increasing the risk of transfusion reaction. Close monitoring during and after the transfusion is important to identify early signs of a reaction.*
- Provide psychologic support and listen actively. Address concerns and accept responses such as anger, depression, and noncompliance. Reinforce client and family strengths in coping with renal failure and hemodialysis. *Grieving is a normal response to loss of organ function. The client may feel hopeless or helpless and resent dependence on a machine. The nurse can help the client and family work through these responses and focus on positive aspects of living.*
- Refer to social services and counseling as indicated. *Clients with renal failure may need additional support services to help them adapt to and live with their disease.*

CRRT is typically performed in an intensive care unit or specialized nephrology unit. Both arterial and venous lines are required for some types of CRRT (Figure 29–7 ■); for others, a double-lumen venous catheter is used. Strict aseptic technique is vital in caring for vascular access sites to reduce the risk of infection.

VASCULAR ACCESS Acute or temporary vascular access for hemodialysis or CRRT usually is gained by inserting a double-lumen catheter into the subclavian, jugular, or femoral vein. The double-lumen catheter has a central partition separating the blood withdrawal side of the catheter from the return side. Blood is drawn into the catheter through small openings in the proximal portion of the catheter, and returned to the circulation through an opening in the distal end of the catheter to avoid withdrawing the blood that has just been dialyzed.

For longer term vascular access, an *arteriovenous (AV) fistula* (Figure 29–8 ■) is created. In preparation for fistula formation, the nondominant arm is not used for venipuncture or blood pressure measurement during renal failure. The fis-

tula is created by surgical anastomosis of an artery and vein, usually the radial artery and cephalic vein. It takes about a month for the fistula to mature so that it can be used for taking and replacing blood during dialysis. A functional AV fistula has a palpable pulsation and a bruit on auscultation. Venipunctures and blood pressures are avoided on the arm with the fistula.

In chronic renal failure, an *arteriovenous graft* is most often used for vascular access. The graft, a tube made of Gortex, is surgically implanted and connects the artery and the vein. Blood flows through the graft from the artery to the vein. Occasionally, an *external AV shunt* connecting a peripheral artery with a peripheral vein is used for vascular access.

The rate of complications and mortality associated with catheter access is higher than with AV fistulas or grafts. Ideally, an AV fistula or graft is created as soon as the potential need for long-term renal replacement therapies is identified (Dinwiddie, 2004). Localized AV fistula, graft, or shunt problems can occur, however. Infection and clotting or thrombosis are the most common shunt problems. Aneurysms may also

Figure 29–7 ■ Continuous arteriovenous hemofiltration (CAVH).

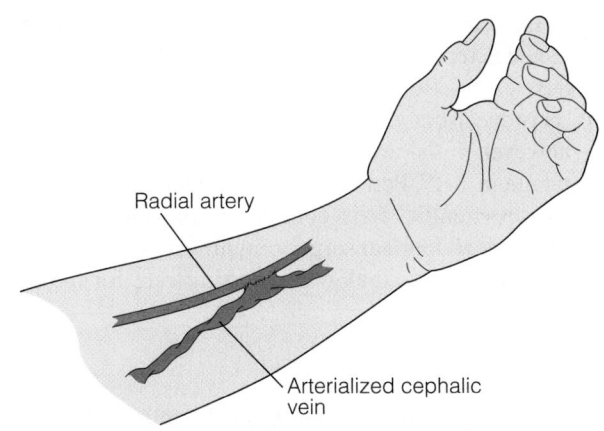

Figure 29–8 ■ An arteriovenous fistula.

develop. Both infection and thrombosis can lead to systemic manifestations such as septicemia and embolization. These local complications may cause the fistula or graft to fail, necessitating development of a new site. The psychologic impact of AV fistula or graft failure is significant, often causing depression and low self-esteem.

PERITONEAL DIALYSIS In peritoneal dialysis, the highly vascular peritoneal membrane serves as the dialyzing surface (Figure 29–9 ■). Warmed sterile dialysate is instilled into the peritoneal cavity through a catheter inserted into the peritoneal cavity. Metabolic waste products and excess electrolytes diffuse into the dialysate while it remains in the abdomen. Water movement is controlled using dextrose as an osmotic agent to draw it into the dialysate. The fluid is then drained by gravity out of the peritoneal cavity into a sterile bag. This process of

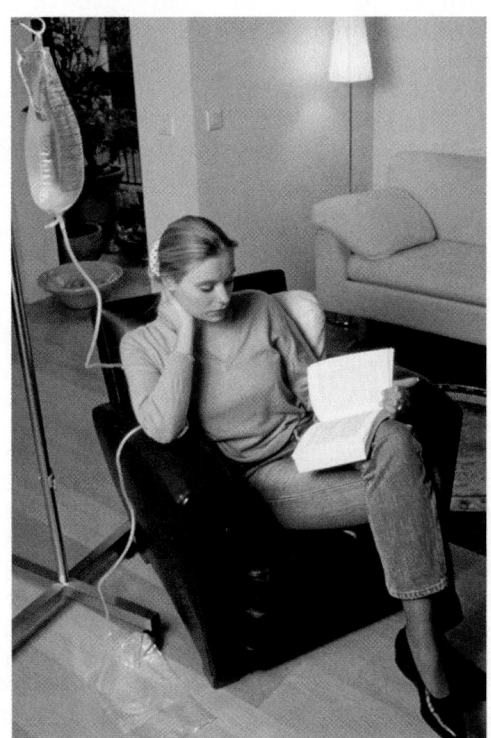

Figure 29–9 ■ *A,* Peritoneal dialysis. *B,* Woman receiving peritoneal dialysis.

dialysate infusion, dwell time of the solution in the abdomen, and drainage is repeated at prescribed intervals.

Because excess fluid and solutes are removed more gradually in peritoneal dialysis, it poses less risk for the unstable client; however, this slower rate of metabolite removal can be a disadvantage in ARF. Peritoneal dialysis increases the risk for developing peritonitis. It is contraindicated for clients who have had recent abdominal surgery, significant lung disease, or peritonitis. See the box below for nursing care for the client having peritoneal dialysis.

 NURSING CARE

Health Promotion

Acute renal failure often can be prevented by measures that maintain fluid volume and cardiac output and reduce the risk of exposure to nephrotoxins. Carefully monitor critically ill, post-operative, and other at-risk clients for early signs of hypovolemia (low urine output, altered mental status, changes in vital signs, skin color or temperature). Promptly report a fall in

---

 NURSING CARE OF THE CLIENT UNDERGOING Peritoneal Dialysis

PREDIALYSIS CARE

- Document vital signs including temperature, orthostatic blood pressures (lying, sitting, and standing), apical pulse, respirations, and lung sounds. *These baseline data help assess fluid volume status and tolerance of the dialysis procedure. Hypertension, abnormal heart or lung sounds, or dyspnea may indicate excess fluid volume. Poor respiratory function may affect the ability to tolerate peritoneal dialysis. Temperature measurement is vital, because infection is the most common complication of peritoneal dialysis.*
- Weigh daily or between dialysis runs as indicated. *Weight is an accurate indicator of fluid volume status.*
- Note BUN, serum electrolyte, creatinine, pH, and hematocrit levels prior to peritoneal dialysis and periodically during the procedure. *These values are used to assess the efficacy of treatment.*
- Measure and record abdominal girth. *Increasing abdominal girth may indicate retained dialysate, excess fluid volume, or early peritonitis.*
- Maintain fluid and dietary restrictions as ordered. *Fluid and diet restrictions help reduce hypervolemia and control azotemia.*
- Have the client empty the bladder prior to catheter insertion. *Emptying the bladder reduces the risk of inadvertent puncture.*
- Warm the prescribed dialysate solution to body temperature (98.6°F or 37°C) using a warm water bath or heating pad on low setting. *Dialysate is warmed to prevent hypothermia.*
- Explain all procedures and expected sensations. *Knowledge helps reduce anxiety and elicit cooperation.*

INTRADIALYSIS CARE

- Use strict aseptic technique during the dialysis procedure and when caring for the peritoneal catheter. *Peritonitis is a common complication of peritoneal dialysis; sterile technique reduces the risk.*
- Add prescribed medications to the dialysate; prime the tubing with solution and connect it to the peritoneal catheter, taping connections securely and avoiding kinks. *This allows dialysate to flow freely into the abdominal cavity and prevents leaking or contamination.*
- Instill dialysate into the abdominal cavity over a period of approximately 10 minutes. Clamp tubing and allow the dialysate to remain in the abdomen for the prescribed dwell time. Keep drainage tubing clamped at all times during instillation and dwell time. *Dialysate should flow freely into the abdomen if the peritoneal catheter is patent. Dialysis, the exchange of*

solutes and water between the blood and dialysate, occurs across the peritoneal membrane during the dwell time.
- During instillation and dwell time, observe closely for signs of respiratory distress, such as dyspnea, tachypnea, or crackles. Place in Fowler's or semi-Fowler's position and slow the rate of instillation slightly to relieve respiratory distress if it develops. *Respiratory compromise may result from overly rapid filling or overfilling of the abdomen or from a diaphragmatic defect that allows fluid to enter the thoracic cavity.*
- After prescribed dwell time, open drainage tubing clamps and allow dialysate to drain by gravity into a sterile container. Note the clarity, color, and odor of returned dialysate. *Blood or feces in the dialysate may indicate organ or bowel perforation; cloudy or malodorous dialysate may indicate an infection.*
- Accurately record amount and type of dialysate instilled (including any added medications), dwell time, and amount and character of the drainage. *When more dialysate drains than has been instilled, excess fluid has been lost (output). If less dialysate is returned than has been instilled, a fluid gain has occurred (intake).*
- Monitor BUN, serum electrolyte, and creatinine levels. *These values are used to assess the effectiveness of dialysis.*
- Troubleshoot for possible problems during dialysis:
  a. Slow dialysate instillation. Increase the height of the container and reposition the client. Check tubing and catheter for kinks. Check abdominal dressing for wetness, indicating leakage around the catheter. *Slow dialysate flow may be related to a partially obstructed tube or catheter.*
  b. Excess dwell time. *Prolonged dwell time may lead to water depletion or hyperglycemia.*
  c. Poor dialysate drainage. Lower the drainage container, reposition, check for tubing kinks. Check abdominal dressing. *Tubing or catheter obstruction can also interfere with dialysate drainage.*

POSTDIALYSIS CARE

- Assess vital signs, including temperature. *Comparison of pre- and postdialysis vital signs helps identify beneficial and adverse effects of the procedure.*
- Time meals to correspond with dialysis outflow. *Scheduling meals while the abdomen is empty of dialysate enhances intake and reduces nausea.*
- Teach the client and family about the procedure. *The client may elect to use peritoneal dialysis at home to manage end-stage renal disease and prevent uremia.*

urine output to less than 30 mL per hour and other evidence of decreased cardiac output. Maintain intravenous fluids as ordered. Alert the physician if the client is receiving more than one nephrotoxic drug or if a nephrotoxic drug is ordered for a dehydrated client. Closely observe clients receiving blood or blood cells for early signs of transfusion reaction and intervene appropriately.

Assessment

Both subjective and objective data are useful when assessing the client with acute renal failure:

- *Health history:* Complaints of anorexia, nausea, weight gain, or edema; recent exposure to a nephrotoxin such as an aminoglycoside antibiotic or radiologic procedure using an injected contrast medium; previous transfusion reaction; chronic diseases such as diabetes, heart failure, or kidney disease.
- *Physical examination:* Vital signs including temperature; urine output (amount, color, clarity, specific gravity, presence of blood cells or protein); weight; skin color, peripheral pulses; presence of edema (periorbital or dependent); lung sounds, heart sounds, and bowel tones.

Nursing Diagnoses and Interventions

The client with acute renal failure has numerous nursing care needs related not only to the renal failure but also to the underlying condition that precipitated it. Priority nursing care needs relate to fluid volume alterations, appetite and nutrition, and teaching/learning. For additional nursing diagnoses and interventions, see the Nursing Care Plan on the next page.

Excess Fluid Volume

In acute renal failure, the kidneys often cannot excrete adequate urine to maintain a normal extracellular fluid balance. Fluid retention is greater in oliguric renal failure than in non-oliguric failure. Rapid weight gain and edema indicate fluid retention. In addition, heart failure and pulmonary edema may develop. In the older adult or severely debilitated client, fluid retention can present a significant management problem.

- Maintain hourly intake and output records. *Accurate intake and output records help guide therapy, especially fluid restrictions.*
- Weigh daily or more frequently, as ordered. Use standard technique (same scale, clothing, or coverings) to ensure accuracy. *Rapid weight changes are an accurate indicator of fluid volume status, particularly in the oliguric client.*
- Assess vital signs at least every 4 hours. *Hypertension, tachycardia, and tachypnea may indicate excess fluid volume.*

PRACTICE ALERT
Frequently assess breath and heart sounds, neck veins for distention, and back and extremities for edema. Report abnormal findings. Adventitious breath sounds (crackles), abnormal heart sounds such as an S_3 or S_4 gallop, distended neck veins, and peripheral edema may indicate hypervolemia, heart failure, or pulmonary edema.

- If not contraindicated, place in semi-Fowler's position *to enhance cardiac and respiratory function.*
- Report abnormal serum electrolyte values and manifestations of electrolyte imbalance. The client with ARF is at particular risk for the following electrolyte imbalances:
  a. *Hyperkalemia* due to impaired potassium excretion. Manifestations include irritability, nausea, diarrhea, abdominal cramping, cardiac dysrhythmias, and ECG changes.
  b. *Hyponatremia* due to water retention. Manifestations include nausea, vomiting, and headache, with possible central nervous system (CNS) manifestations of lethargy, confusion, seizures, and coma.
  c. *Hyperphosphatemia* due to decreased phosphate excretion. Manifestations include hyperreflexia, paresthesias, and possible tetany.
  ARF impairs electrolyte and water excretion, causing multiple electrolyte imbalances.
- Restrict fluids as ordered. Provide frequent mouth care and encourage using hard candies to decrease thirst. If ice chips are allowed, include the water content (approximately one-half of the total volume) as intake. *Fluids are restricted to minimize fluid retention and complications of fluid volume excess.*
- Administer medications with meals. *Giving oral medications with meals minimizes ingestion of excess fluids.*
- Turn frequently and provide good skin care. *Edema decreases tissue perfusion and increases the risk of skin breakdown, especially in the older or debilitated client.*

Imbalanced Nutrition: Less than Body Requirements

Anorexia and nausea associated with renal failure often interfere with food intake and nutrition. In addition, the disease process leading to ARF may contribute to increased nutritional needs for healing and decreased food intake.

- Monitor and record food intake, including the amount and type of food consumed. *A detailed intake record helps guide decisions about nutritional status and necessary supplements.*
- Weigh daily. *Weight changes over time (days to weeks) reflect nutritional status, while rapid weight changes are more reflective of fluid volume status. In ARF, weight may remain stable or increase due to fluid retention even though tissue mass is being lost.*
- Arrange for dietary consultation to plan meals within prescribed limitations that consider the client's food preferences. *Diets restricted in protein, salt, and potassium can be unpalatable; intake and appetite improve when preferred foods are included as allowed.*
- Engage the client in planning daily menus. *Participation in meal planning increases the client's sense of control and autonomy.*
- Allow family members to prepare meals within dietary restrictions. Encourage family members to eat with the client. *Familiar foods and social interaction encourage eating and increase enjoyment of meals.*
- Provide frequent, small meals or between-meal snacks. *These measures promote food intake in the fatigued or anorectic client.*

NURSING CARE PLAN A Client with Acute Renal Failure

Judy Devak is driving home late one evening when she loses control of her car trying to avoid hitting a deer in the road. Her car strikes a tree and rolls into a deep ditch beside the road, out of sight of passing cars. The wreck is not discovered until 2 hours later. On arrival at the accident scene, the paramedics find Ms. Devak hypotensive: BP 90/60, P 120, and R 24. She is alert and in severe pain, with a fractured right femur. After immobilizing Ms. Devak's neck and back and extricating her from the car, they apply a traction splint to her leg and transport her to the local hospital.

ASSESSMENT

Katie Leaper, RN, obtains a nursing history on Ms. Devak's admission to the intensive care unit. Ms. Devak indicates that she has been healthy, having experienced only minor illnesses and chickenpox as a child. She has never been hospitalized, and knows of no allergies to medications. Ms. Devak is not currently taking prescription or nonprescription drugs. Physical assessment findings include T 97.4°F (36.3°C) PO, P 100, R 18, and BP 124/68. Skin pale, cool, and dry, with multiple scrapes, minor abrasions, and bruises on face and extremities. A linear bruise is noted on her chest and abdomen from the seat belt. Lung sounds clear, heart tones normal, and abdomen tender but soft to palpation. Right leg alignment maintained with skeletal traction. One unit of whole blood was infused prior to ICU admission, a second unit is currently infusing. An indwelling urinary catheter and a nasogastric tube are in place.

During the first few hours after admission, Ms. Leaper notes that Ms. Devak's hourly output has dropped from 55 mL to 45 to 28 mL of clear yellow urine. The physician orders a 500-mL intravenous fluid challenge, STAT urinalysis, BUN, and serum creatinine. The fluid challenge elicits only a slight increase in urine output. Urinalysis results show a specific gravity of 1.010 and the presence of WBCs, red and white cell casts, and tubular epithelial cells in the sediment. Ms. Devak's BUN is 28 mg/dL; her serum creatinine, 1.5 mg/dL. The physician diagnoses probable acute renal failure and orders a nephrology consultation. In addition, the physician orders aluminum hydroxide, 10 mL every 2 hours per nasogastric tube, and ranitidine 50 mg intravenously every 8 hours.

DIAGNOSES

- *Acute Pain* related to injuries sustained in accident
- *Anxiety* related to being in the intensive care unit
- *Risk for Excess Fluid Volume* related to impaired renal function
- *Impaired Physical Mobility* related to skeletal traction
- *Ineffective Protection* related to injuries and invasive procedures

EXPECTED OUTCOMES

- Report adequate pain control.
- Verbalize reduced anxiety.
- Maintain stable weight and vital signs within normal range.

- Maintain skin integrity.
- Use the trapeze appropriately to adjust position in bed while maintaining body alignment.
- Remain free of infection, bleeding, or respiratory distress.

PLANNING AND IMPLEMENTATION

- Maintain PCA.
- Assess frequently for pain control and response to analgesia.
- Encourage expression of thoughts, feelings, and fears about condition and placement in ICU.
- Document vital signs and heart and lung sounds at least every 4 hours.
- Weigh every 12 hours.
- Document hourly intake and output.
- Restrict fluids as ordered, including diluent for all intravenous medications as intake.
- Assist with mouth care every 3 to 4 hours; allow frequent rinsing of mouth and ice chips as allowed.
- Assist with position changes at least every 2 hours; teach use of the overhead trapeze.
- Monitor frequently for signs of infection, bleeding, or respiratory distress.

EVALUATION

After just over 3 days of oliguria, Ms. Devak's urine output increases. By the end of the fourth day she is excreting 60 to 80 mL/h of urine. Although her BUN, serum creatinine, and potassium levels remain high, they never reach a critical point, and dialysis is not required. She is transferred from the ICU on the fifth day after admission. When Ms. Devak is able to begin eating, she is placed on a low-potassium diet, restricted to 50 g of protein. Her renal function gradually improves. By discharge, results of her renal function studies, including BUN and serum creatinine, are nearly normal. Ms. Devak verbalizes an understanding of the need to avoid nephrotoxins such as NSAIDs until allowed by her physician.

CRITICAL THINKING IN THE NURSING PROCESS

1. What was the most likely specific precipitating factor for Ms. Devak's acute renal failure? Did anything else contribute to her risk?
2. Why did the physician prescribe aluminum hydroxide and ranitidine? Consider both the acute renal failure and Ms. Devak's placement in the intensive care unit.
3. Ms. Devak is at risk for respiratory distress related to potential fluid volume excess. How does her fractured femur further contribute to risk for respiratory distress?
4. Develop a care plan for Ms. Devak for the nursing diagnosis of *Deficient Diversional Activity.*
See Evaluating Your Response in Appendix C.

- Administer antiemetics as ordered and provide mouth care prior to meals. *Nausea and a metallic taste in the mouth, common manifestations of uremia, can decrease food intake.*
- Administer parenteral nutrition as ordered if the client is unable to eat or tolerate enteral nutrition. *Preventing or slowing tissue catabolism is important for the client with ARF.*

PRACTICE ALERT

Intravenous lines and parenteral nutrition solutions can increase the risk for infection. Monitor sites carefully for signs of infection or inflammation.

Deficient Knowledge

The client with ARF has multiple learning needs. These include information about ARF, diagnostic and laboratory studies, management strategies, and implications for the recovery period.

- Assess anxiety level and ability to comprehend instruction. Tailor information and presentation to developmental level and physical, mental, and emotional status. *The client with ARF may be critically ill or have uremic effects that hinder learning. During the initial stages of ARF it may be necessary to limit information to immediate concerns.*
- Assess knowledge and understanding. *To enhance understanding and retention, relate information presented to previous learning.*
- Teach about diagnostic tests and therapeutic procedures. *Teaching reduces anxiety and improves understanding and cooperation.*
- Discuss dietary and fluid restrictions. *These measures may be continued after discharge.*
- If the client is discharged prior to the recovery phase of ARF, teach the signs and symptoms of complications, such as fluid volume excess or deficit, heart failure, and electrolyte imbalances. *As kidney function returns, urine output increases, but the concentrating ability of the nephrons and electrolyte excretion remain impaired. This impaired function increases the risk of excess fluid loss, possible dehydration, orthostatic hypotension, and electrolyte imbalance.*
- Teach how to monitor weight, blood pressure, and pulse. *These are important means of assessing fluid status.*
- Instruct to avoid nephrotoxic drugs and chemicals for up to 1 year following an episode of ARF. *During recovery, nephrons are vulnerable to damage by nephrotoxins such as NSAIDs, some antibiotics, radiologic contrast media, and heavy metals. Because alcohol can increase the nephrotoxicity of some materials, discourage alcohol ingestion.*

Linking NANDA, NIC, and NOC

Chart 29–1 shows links between NANDA nursing diagnoses, NIC, and NOC for the client with ARF.

Community-Based Care

Often the client is critically ill when ARF develops. Critical illness and the resulting state of client and family crisis can impair learning and retention of information. Include family members in teaching during the initial stages to promote understanding of what is happening and the reasons for specific treatment measures. Inclusion of the family reduces their anxiety, and provides a valuable resource for reinforcing client teaching about care after discharge.

Client teaching needs for home care include:

- Avoiding exposure to nephrotoxins, particularly those in over-the-counter products
- Preventing infection and other major stressors that can slow healing
- Monitoring weight, blood pressure, and pulse
- Manifestations of relapse

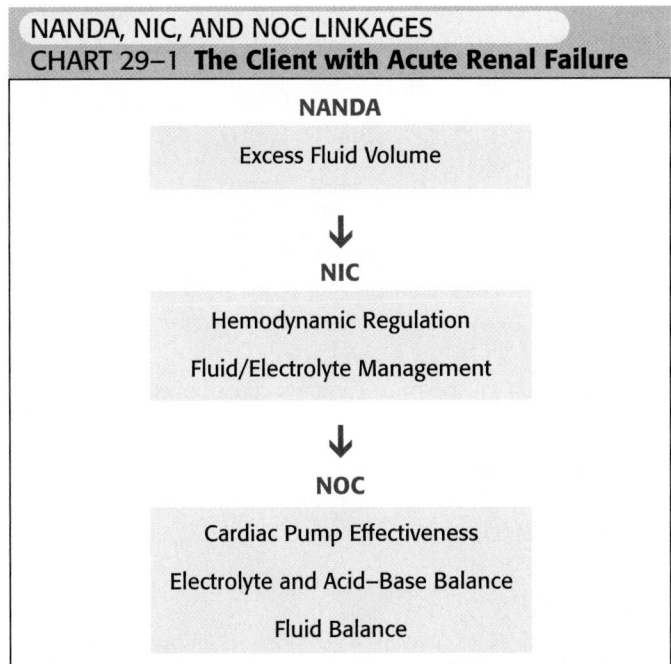

NANDA, NIC, AND NOC LINKAGES
CHART 29–1 The Client with Acute Renal Failure

Data from *NANDA's Nursing Diagnoses: Definitions & Classification 2005–2006* by NANDA International (2005), Philadelphia; *Nursing Interventions Classification (NIC)* (4th ed.) by J. M. Dochterman & G. M. Bulechek (2004), St. Louis, MO: Mosby; and *Nursing Outcomes Classification (NOC)* (3rd ed.) by S. Moorhead, M. Johnson, and M. Maas (2004), St. Louis, MO: Mosby.

- Continuing dietary restrictions
- Knowing when to contact the physician.

See the box on the next page for home care assessment of the older adult with ARF.

THE CLIENT WITH CHRONIC RENAL FAILURE

Although the kidneys usually recover from acute injury, many chronic conditions can lead to progressive renal tissue destruction and loss of function. Nephron units are lost and renal mass decreases, with progressive deterioration of glomerular filtration, tubular secretion, and reabsorption. This process of chronic renal failure (CRF) may progress slowly for many years without being recognized. Eventually, the kidneys are unable to excrete metabolic wastes and regulate fluid and electrolyte balance adequately, a condition known as end-stage renal disease, the final stage of CRF.

The incidence of ESRD is increasing, particularly in older adults. In 2001, more than 93,000 people started treatment for ESRD for a total of about 392,000 people undergoing ESRD treatment (NKUDIC, 2004). African Americans have the highest incidence of ESRD, followed by Native Americans, Asians, and European Americans (USRDS, 2005).

Conditions causing CRF typically involve diffuse, bilateral disease of the kidneys with progressive destruction and scarring of the entire nephron. As indicated in Figure 29–10 ■, diabetes is the leading cause of ESRD in all population groups

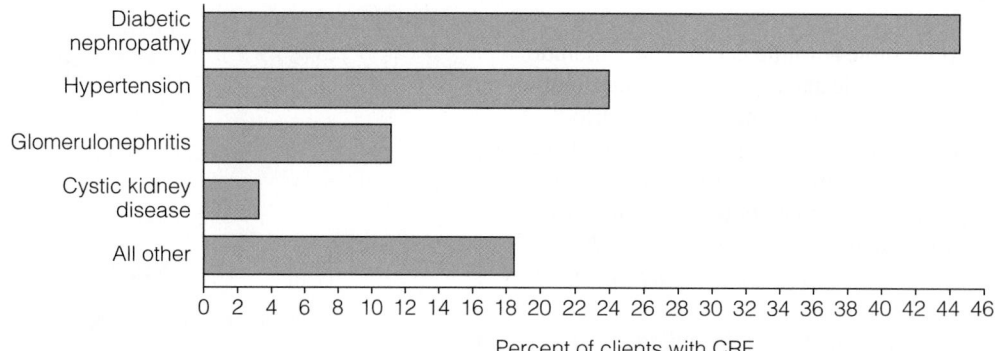

Figure 29–10 ■ The most common causes of chronic renal failure (USRDS, 2005).

in the United States. Hypertension closely follows diabetes as a major cause of ESRD; in many clients, these disorders coexist (USRDS, 2005).

FAST FACTS
- Acute renal failure develops abruptly and often can be reversed with appropriate treatment.
- Chronic renal failure is the end stage of progressive destruction of the kidneys and cannot be reversed.
- Diabetes is the leading cause of chronic renal failure, followed by hypertension, glomerulonephritis, cystic kidney disease, and all other causes.

Pathophysiology

The pathophysiology of CRF involves a gradual loss of entire nephron units. In the early stages, as nephrons are destroyed, remaining functional nephrons hypertrophy. Glomerular capillary flow and pressure increase in these nephrons, and more solute particles are filtered to compensate for lost renal mass. This increased demand predisposes the remaining nephrons to glomerular sclerosis (scarring), resulting in their eventual destruction. This process of continued loss of nephron function may continue even after the initial disease process has resolved (Kasper et al., 2005). Table 29–7 outlines common pathologic processes leading to nephron destruction and ESRD.

NURSING CARE OF THE OLDER ADULT   Renal Failure

Structural and functional changes occur in the aging kidney. Structurally, the number of nephrons decreases. The GFR decreases, resulting in decreased renal clearance of drugs. Urine-concentrating ability decreases, and the kidney is less able to conserve sodium. Renal compensation for acid–base imbalances takes longer. Despite these changes, the kidney retains its ability to regulate fluid and electrolyte homeostasis remarkably well unless additional stresses are added. Any additional stressors such as hypotension, exposure to nephrotoxic drugs, or an inflammatory process such as glomerulonephritis may precipitate renal failure in the older adult.

The manifestations of renal failure often are missed in aging clients (e.g., edema may be attributed to heart failure or high blood pressure to preexisting hypertension). Serum creatinine levels may rise slowly. Because older adults have less muscle mass, they produce less creatinine, a by-product of muscle cell metabolism. Likewise, the BUN may remain within normal limits.

The same measures are used to treat renal failure in older adults as in younger people. Hemodialysis, peritoneal dialysis, and renal transplantation are appropriate if necessary. Treatment options (including conservative treatment or no treatment) and their potential benefits and ramifications should be clearly explained.

Assessing for Home Care

A number of factors should be considered in assessing the older adult's ability to manage treatment such as dialysis at home:

- Does the client have reasonable access to a dialysis center or outpatient unit? Is transportation available?
- Would home hemodialysis be appropriate? Is a caregiver available to be trained to manage dialysis? Does the client's home have appropriate electrical and plumbing fixtures?
- Would continuous ambulatory peritoneal dialysis be appropriate? Does the client have the manual dexterity, will, and cognitive ability to manage dialysis infusions? If not, would intermittent peritoneal dialysis using a dialyzing machine be more appropriate?
- Are family members or other support persons available to provide assistance to the client as needed?

Resources for Home Care

The following resources may be useful for clients with kidney disease:

- American Association of Kidney Patients
  800-749-2257
  813-636-8100
  www.aakp.org
- American Kidney Fund
  800-638-8299
  866-300-2900 (Spanish help line)
  www.kidneyfund.org
- National Kidney Foundation
  800-622-9010
  www.kidney.org

TABLE 29–7 Pathophysiology of Chronic Renal Failure

CAUSE	EXAMPLES
Diabetic nephropathy	Changes in the glomerular basement membrane, chronic pyelonephritis, and ischemia lead to sclerosis of the glomerulus and gradual destruction of the nephron.
Hypertensive nephrosclerosis	Long-standing hypertension leads to renal arteriosclerosis and ischemia resulting in glomerular destruction and tubular atrophy.
Chronic glomerulonephritis	Bilateral inflammatory process of the glomeruli leads to ischemia, nephron loss, and shrinkage of the kidney.
Chronic pyelonephritis	Chronic infection commonly associated with an obstructive or neurologic process and vesicoureteral reflux leads to reflux nephropathy (renal scarring, atrophy, and dilated calyces).
Polycystic kidney disease	Multiple bilateral cysts gradually destroy normal renal tissue by compression.
Systemic lupus erythematosus	Basement membrane damage by circulating immune complexes leads to focal, local, or diffuse glomerulonephritis.

The course of CRF is variable, progressing over a period of months to many years. In the early stage, known as *decreased renal reserve,* unaffected nephrons compensate for the lost nephrons. The GFR is about 50% of normal, and the client is asymptomatic with normal BUN and serum creatinine levels. As the disease progresses and the GFR falls to 20% to 50% of normal, azotemia and some manifestations of *renal insufficiency* may be seen. Any further insult to the kidneys at this stage (such as infection, dehydration, exposure to nephrotoxins, or urinary tract obstruction) can further reduce function and precipitate the onset of *renal failure* or overt uremia. This stage is characterized by a GFR of less than 20% of normal. The serum creatinine and BUN levels rise sharply (Figure 29–11 ■), the client becomes oliguric, and manifestations of uremia are seen. In ESRD, the final stage of CRF, the GFR is less than 5% of normal and renal replacement therapy is necessary to sustain life (Kasper et al., 2005; Porth, 2005). Table 29–8 summarizes the stages of chronic renal failure.

Manifestations and Complications

Chronic renal failure often is not identified until its final, uremic stage is reached. **Uremia,** which literally means "urine in the blood," refers to the syndrome or group of symptoms associated with ESRD. In uremia, fluid and electrolyte balance is altered, the regulatory and endocrine functions of the kidney are impaired, and accumulated metabolic waste products affect essentially every other organ system (Kasper et al., 2005; Porth, 2005).

Early manifestations of uremia include nausea, apathy, weakness, and fatigue, symptoms that are dismissed as a viral infection or influenza. As the condition progresses, frequent vomiting, increasing weakness, lethargy, and confusion develop (Porth, 2005). The *Multisystem Effects of Uremia* are illustrated on page 917.

Fluid and Electrolyte Effects

Loss of functional kidney tissue impairs its ability to regulate fluid, electrolyte, and acid–base balance. In the early stages of

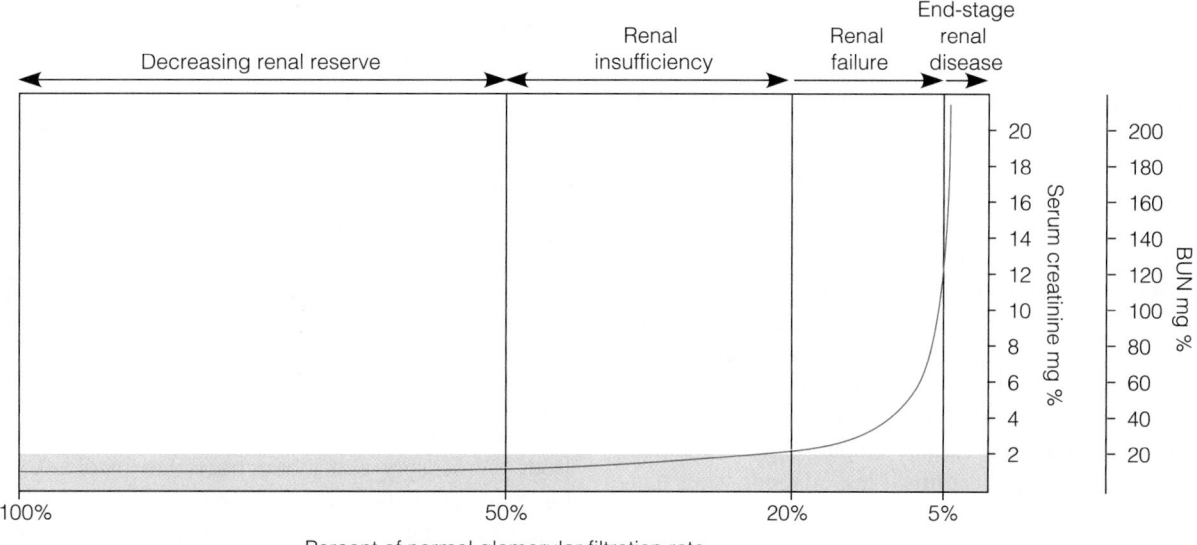

Figure 29–11 ■ The relationship of renal function to BUN and serum creatinine values through the course of chronic renal failure.

TABLE 29–8 Stages of Chronic Renal Failure

STAGE	GLOMERULAR FILTRATION RATE	MANIFESTATIONS
Decreased renal reserve	Approximately 50% of normal	None; normal BUN and creatinine
Renal insufficiency	20% to 50% of normal	Polyuria with low, fixed specific gravity; azotemia; anemia; hypertension
Renal failure	< 20% of normal	Increasing azotemia; edema, metabolic acidosis, hypercalcemia; possible uremia
End-stage renal disease	< 5% of normal	Kidney atrophy and fibrosis; overt uremia

CRF, impaired filtration and reabsorption lead to proteinuria, hematuria, and decreased urine-concentrating ability. Salt and water are poorly conserved, and risk for dehydration increases. Polyuria, nocturia, and a fixed specific gravity of 1.008 to 1.012 are common (Porth, 2005). As the GFR decreases and renal function deteriorates further, sodium and water retention are common, necessitating salt and water restrictions.

Hyperkalemia develops as renal failure progresses. Manifestations of hyperkalemia, such as muscle weakness, paresthesias, and ECG changes, are not usually seen until the GFR is less than 5 mL/min. Phosphate excretion is also impaired, leading to hyperphosphatemia and hypocalcemia. Reduced calcium absorption due to impaired vitamin D activation also contributes to hypocalcemia. Hypermagnesemia develops with advancing renal failure; magnesium-containing antacids are avoided for this reason.

As renal failure advances, hydrogen-ion excretion and buffer production are impaired, leading to metabolic acidosis. Respiratory rate and depth increase (Kussmaul's respirations) to compensate for metabolic acidosis. Although metabolic acidosis is often asymptomatic, other possible manifestations include general malaise, weakness, headache, nausea and vomiting, and abdominal pain (see Chapter 10 ∞).

Cardiovascular Effects

Cardiovascular disease is a common cause of death in ESRD, and results from accelerated atherosclerosis. Hypertension, hyperlipidemia, and glucose intolerance all contribute to the process. Cerebral and peripheral vascular manifestations of atherosclerosis are also seen.

Systemic hypertension is a common complication of ESRD. Hypertension results from excess fluid volume, increased renin–angiotensin activity, increased peripheral vascular resistance, and decreased prostaglandins. Increased extracellular fluid volume also can lead to edema and heart failure. Pulmonary edema may result from heart failure and increased permeability of the alveolar capillary membrane.

Retained metabolic toxins can irritate the pericardial sac, causing an inflammatory response and signs of pericarditis. *Cardiac tamponade,* a potential complication of pericarditis, occurs when inflammatory fluid in the pericardial sac interferes with ventricular filling and cardiac output. Once a common complication of uremia, pericarditis is less common when dialysis is initiated early.

Hematologic Effects

Anemia is common in uremia, caused by multiple factors. The kidneys produce erythropoietin, a hormone that controls RBC production. In renal failure, erythropoietin production declines. Retained metabolic toxins further suppress RBC production, and contribute to a shortened RBC life span. Nutritional deficiencies (iron and folate) and increased risk for blood loss from the GI tract also contribute to anemia.

Anemia contributes to manifestations such as fatigue, weakness, depression, and impaired cognition. It also affects cardiovascular function, and may be a major contributing factor to coronary heart disease and heart failure associated with ESRD (Porth, 2005).

Renal failure impairs platelet function, increasing the risk of bleeding disorders such as epistaxis and GI bleeding. The mechanism of impaired platelet function associated with renal failure is poorly understood.

Immune System Effects

Uremia increases the risk for infection. High levels of urea and retained metabolic wastes impair all aspects of inflammation and immune function. The WBC declines, humoral and cell-mediated immunity are impaired, and phagocyte function is defective. Both the acute inflammatory response and delayed hypersensitivity responses are affected (Porth, 2005). Fever is suppressed, often delaying the diagnosis of infection.

Gastrointestinal Effects

Anorexia, nausea, and vomiting are the most common early symptoms of uremia. Hiccups also are commonly experienced. Gastroenteritis is frequent. Ulcerations may affect any level of the GI tract and contribute to an increased risk of GI bleeding. Peptic ulcer disease is particularly common in uremic clients. *Uremic fetor,* a urine-like breath odor often associated with a metallic taste in the mouth, may develop. Uremic fetor can further contribute to anorexia.

Neurologic Effects

Uremia alters both central and peripheral nervous system function. CNS manifestations occur early and include changes in mentation, difficulty concentrating, fatigue, and insomnia. Psychotic symptoms, seizures, and coma are associated with advanced uremic encephalopathy.

Peripheral neuropathy is also common in advanced uremia. Both the sensory and motor tracts are involved. The lower limbs are initially affected. "Restless leg syndrome," sensations of crawling or creeping, prickling, or itching of the lower legs with frequent leg movement, increases during rest. Paresthesias and sensory loss typically occur in a "stocking-glove" pattern. As uremia progresses, motor function is also impaired,

MULTISYSTEM EFFECTS OF Uremia

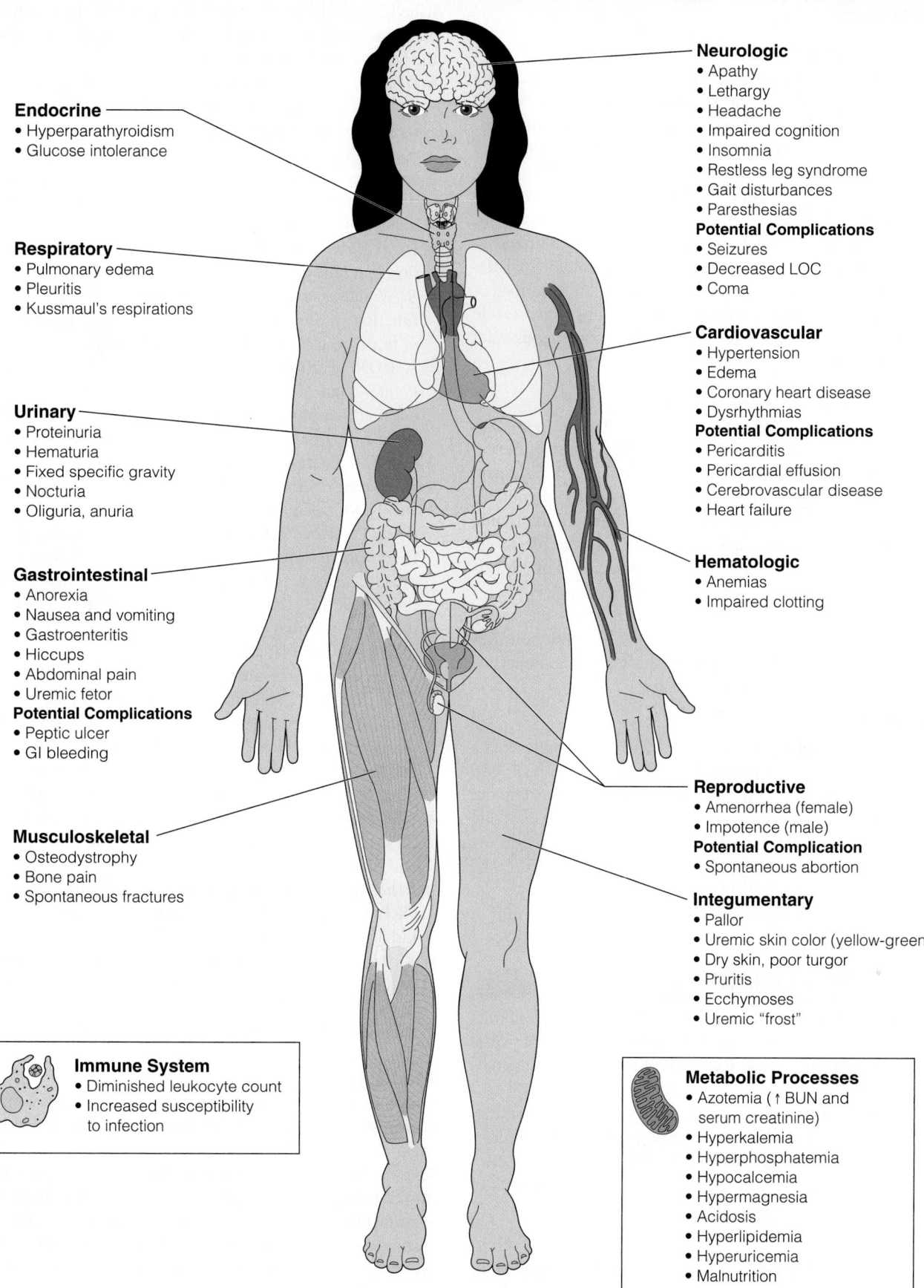

Endocrine
- Hyperparathyroidism
- Glucose intolerance

Respiratory
- Pulmonary edema
- Pleuritis
- Kussmaul's respirations

Urinary
- Proteinuria
- Hematuria
- Fixed specific gravity
- Nocturia
- Oliguria, anuria

Gastrointestinal
- Anorexia
- Nausea and vomiting
- Gastroenteritis
- Hiccups
- Abdominal pain
- Uremic fetor
Potential Complications
- Peptic ulcer
- GI bleeding

Musculoskeletal
- Osteodystrophy
- Bone pain
- Spontaneous fractures

Immune System
- Diminished leukocyte count
- Increased susceptibility to infection

Neurologic
- Apathy
- Lethargy
- Headache
- Impaired cognition
- Insomnia
- Restless leg syndrome
- Gait disturbances
- Paresthesias
Potential Complications
- Seizures
- Decreased LOC
- Coma

Cardiovascular
- Hypertension
- Edema
- Coronary heart disease
- Dysrhythmias
Potential Complications
- Pericarditis
- Pericardial effusion
- Cerebrovascular disease
- Heart failure

Hematologic
- Anemias
- Impaired clotting

Reproductive
- Amenorrhea (female)
- Impotence (male)
Potential Complication
- Spontaneous abortion

Integumentary
- Pallor
- Uremic skin color (yellow-green)
- Dry skin, poor turgor
- Pruritis
- Ecchymoses
- Uremic "frost"

Metabolic Processes
- Azotemia (↑ BUN and serum creatinine)
- Hyperkalemia
- Hyperphosphatemia
- Hypocalcemia
- Hypermagnesia
- Acidosis
- Hyperlipidemia
- Hyperuricemia
- Malnutrition

causing muscle weakness, decreased deep tendon reflexes, and gait disturbances.

Musculoskeletal Effects

Hyperphosphatemia and hypocalcemia associated with uremia stimulate parathyroid hormone secretion. Parathyroid hormone causes increased calcium resorption from bone. In addition, osteoblast (bone-forming) and osteoclast (bone-destructing) cell activity is affected. This bone resorption and remodeling, combined with decreased vitamin D synthesis and decreased calcium absorption from the GI tract, lead to *renal osteodystrophy,* also known as renal rickets. Osteodystrophy is characterized by *osteomalacia,* softening of the bones, and *osteoporosis,* decreased bone mass. Bone cysts may develop. Manifestations of osteodystrophy include bone tenderness, pain, and muscle weakness. The client is at increased risk for spontaneous fractures (Porth, 2005).

Endocrine and Metabolic Effects

Accumulated waste products of protein metabolism are a primary factor involved in the effects and manifestations of uremia. Serum creatinine and BUN levels are significantly elevated. Uric acid levels are increased, contributing to an increased risk of gout.

Tissues become resistant to the effects of insulin in uremia, leading to glucose intolerance. High blood triglyceride levels and lower than normal high-density lipoprotein (HDL) levels contribute to the accelerated atherosclerotic process.

Reproductive function is affected. Pregnancies are rarely carried to term, and menstrual irregularities are common. Reduced testosterone levels, low sperm counts, and impotence affect the male client with ESRD.

Dermatologic Effects

Anemia and retained pigmented metabolites cause pallor and a yellowish hue to the skin in uremia. Dry skin with poor turgor, a result of dehydration and sweat gland atrophy, is common. Bruising and excoriations are frequently seen. Metabolic wastes not eliminated by the kidneys may be deposited in the skin, contributing to itching or pruritus. In advanced uremia, high levels of urea in the sweat may result in *uremic frost,* crystallized deposits of urea on the skin.

INTERDISCIPLINARY CARE

Early management of CRF focuses on eliminating factors that may further decrease renal function and measures to slow the progression of the disease to ESRD. Additional treatment goals are to:

- Maintain nutritional status while minimizing the accumulation of toxic waste products and manifestations of uremia.
- Identify and treat complications of CRF.
- Prepare for renal replacement therapies such as dialysis or renal transplant.

Diagnosis

Diagnostic testing is used both to identify CRF and to monitor kidney function. A number of tests may be performed to deter-

mine the underlying renal disorder. Once the diagnosis is established, renal function is monitored primarily through blood levels of metabolic wastes and electrolytes. See Chapter 27 ∞ for the nursing implications of selected tests.

- *Urinalysis* is done to measure urine specific gravity and detect abnormal urine components. In CRF, the specific gravity may be fixed at approximately 1.010, equivalent to that of plasma. This fixed specific gravity is due to impaired tubular secretion, reabsorption, and urine concentrating ability. Abnormal proteins, blood cells, and cellular casts may also be noted in the urine.
- *Urine culture* is ordered to identify any urinary tract infection that may hasten the progress of CRF.
- *BUN* and *serum creatinine* are obtained to evaluate kidney function in eliminating nitrogenous waste products. Levels of both are monitored to assess the progress of renal failure. A BUN of 20 to 50 mg/dL signals mild azotemia; levels greater than 100 mg/dL indicate severe renal impairment. Uremic symptoms are seen when the BUN is around 200 mg/dL or higher. Serum creatinine levels of greater than 4 mg/dL indicate serious renal impairment.
- *Creatinine clearance* evaluates the GFR and renal function. In early CRF (renal insufficiency), the GFR is more than 20% of normal and the creatinine clearance 30 mL/min or greater. As the disease progresses and the stage of renal failure is reached, the GFR is reduced to less than 20% of normal and the creatinine clearance to 15 to 29 mL/min. In ESRD, the GFR is less than 5% of normal and the creatinine clearance is less than 15 mL/min (Kasper et al., 2005).
- *Serum electrolytes* are monitored throughout the course of CRF. The serum sodium may be within normal limits or low because of water retention. Potassium levels are elevated but usually remain below 6.5 mEq/L. Serum phosphate is elevated, and the calcium level is decreased. Metabolic acidosis is identified by a low pH, low CO_2, and low bicarbonate levels.
- *CBC* reveals moderately severe anemia with a hematocrit of 20% to 30% and a low hemoglobin. The number of RBCs and platelets is reduced.
- *Renal ultrasonography* is done to evaluate kidney size. In CRF, kidney size decreases as nephrons are destroyed and kidney mass is reduced.
- *Kidney biopsy* may be done to identify the underlying disease process if this is unclear. It is also used to differentiate acute from chronic failure. Kidney biopsy may be performed in surgery or done percutaneously using needle biopsy.

Medications

Chronic renal failure affects both the pharmacokinetic and pharmacodynamic effects of drug therapy. Most medications are excreted primarily by the kidney. The half-life and plasma levels of many drugs increase in chronic renal failure. Drug absorption may be decreased when phosphate-binding agents are administered concurrently. Proteinuria can significantly reduce plasma protein levels, leading to manifestations of toxicity when highly protein-bound drugs are given. In addition, any potentially nephrotoxic agent is avoided or used with extreme caution. Drugs such as meperidine, metformin (Glucophage), and other oral hypoglycemic agents eliminated by the kidney are avoided entirely (Kasper et al., 2005).

Diuretics such as furosemide or other loop diuretics may be prescribed to reduce extracellular fluid volume and edema. Diuretic therapy also can reduce hypertension and cause potassium wasting, lowering serum potassium levels. Other antihypertensive agents are used to maintain the blood pressure within normal levels, slow the progress of renal failure, and prevent complications of coronary heart disease and cerebral vascular disease. ACE inhibitors are preferred, although any class of antihypertensive agent may be prescribed (see Chapter 35 ∞).

Other drugs may be used to manage electrolyte imbalances and acidosis. Sodium bicarbonate or calcium carbonate may be used to correct mild acidosis. Oral phosphorus binding agents such as calcium carbonate or calcium acetate are given to lower serum phosphate levels and normalize serum calcium levels. Aluminum hydroxide may be used in acute treatment of hyperphosphatemia. Its use is limited to short term by complications such as encephalopathy and osteodystrophy associated with long-term administration of aluminum-containing preparations (Tierney et al., 2005). Vitamin D supplements may be given to improve calcium absorption.

If the serum potassium rises to dangerously high levels, a combination of bicarbonate, insulin, and glucose may be given intravenously to promote potassium movement into the cells. Sodium polystyrene sulfonate (Kayexalate), a potassium-ion exchange resin, can be given either orally or rectally (as an enema).

Folic acid and iron supplements are given to combat anemia associated with chronic renal failure. A multiple vitamin preparation is also often prescribed, because anorexia, nausea, and dietary restrictions may limit nutrient intake.

Nutrition and Fluid Management

As renal function declines, the elimination of water, solutes, and metabolic wastes is impaired. Accumulation of these wastes in the body leads to uremic symptoms. Instituted early in the course of CRF, dietary modifications can slow the progress of nephron destruction, reduce uremic symptoms, and help prevent complications.

Unlike carbohydrates and fats, the body is unable to store excess proteins. Unused dietary proteins are degraded into urea and other nitrogenous wastes, which are then eliminated by the kidneys. Protein-rich foods also contain inorganic ions such as hydrogen ion, phosphate, and sulfites that are eliminated by the kidneys. Research has shown that restricting dietary protein intake slows the progression of CRF and reduces uremic symptoms (Kasper et al., 2005). A daily protein intake of 0.6 g/kg of body weight, or approximately 40 g/day for an average male client, provides the amino acids necessary for tissue repair. Proteins should be of high biologic value, rich in the essential amino acids. Carbohydrate intake is increased to maintain energy requirements and provide approximately 35 kcal/kg per day.

Water and sodium intake are regulated to maintain the extracellular fluid volume at normal levels. Water intake of 1 to 2 L per day is generally recommended to maintain water balance.

Sodium is restricted to 2 g per day initially. More stringent water and sodium restrictions may be necessary as renal failure progresses. The client is instructed to monitor weight daily and report any weight gain in excess of 5 pounds over a 2-day period.

When the GFR falls to less than 10 to 20 mL/min, potassium and phosphorous intake are also restricted. Potassium intake is limited to less than 60 to 70 mEq/day (normal intake is about 100 mEq/day) (Tierney et al., 2005). The client is cautioned to avoid using salt substitutes, which typically contain high levels of potassium chloride. Foods high in phosphorus include eggs, dairy products, and meat.

Renal Replacement Therapies

When pharmacologic and dietary management strategies are no longer effective to maintain fluid and electrolyte balance and prevent uremia, dialysis or kidney transplantation is considered.

A number of considerations affect the choice of long-term treatment. Hemodialysis and peritoneal dialysis each have advantages and disadvantages. Establishing vascular access for hemodialysis may take several months. Planning ahead to develop the access before dialysis is necessary can ease the transition to dialysis. Established access is not a consideration for peritoneal dialysis. The peritoneal catheter can be placed and treatment initiated as soon as it is indicated. When dialysis treatments will be performed at home, initiating instruction before it is required can result in more effective learning. If a family member will serve as a dialysis helper, training begins prior to the onset of uremia.

If transplantation is considered, tissue typing and identification of potential living related donors can be done prior to the onset of ESRD. To make an informed decision, both the client and the potential donor need to understand the risks, benefits, and options available. If the decision for transplant is made early, dialysis can potentially be avoided. The client's age, concurrent health problems, donor availability, and personal preference influence the choice of renal replacement therapy.

DIALYSIS Approximately 80% of all people being treated for ESRD in the United States are receiving dialysis at an average maintenance cost of about $65,000 per year (USRDS, 2005). For the client who is not a candidate for renal transplantation or who has had a transplant failure, dialysis is life sustaining.

The most common therapies for ESRD in the United States are hemodialysis performed in a dialysis center, followed by peritoneal dialysis and kidney transplant (NKUDIC, 2004). Both hemodialysis and peritoneal dialysis can be done in the home, but few clients use home hemodialysis. Of the two, peritoneal dialysis is typically the choice for at-home treatment. Because the morbidity and mortality for each are comparable, factors such as the desire and ability to manage home care, employment, and availability of a dialysis center become the primary factors influencing the choice of hemodialysis or peritoneal dialysis.

Clients on long-term dialysis have a higher risk for complications and death than the general population. Many have other severe diseases along with ESRD. Infection and cardiovascular disease are common causes of illness and death. The 1-year survival rate for clients receiving dialysis is nearly 78%; long-term survival, however, falls to 32% at 5 years and about 9% at 10 years (NKUDIC, 2004).

The decision to initiate dialysis is not easy. Like insulin therapy for the diabetic, dialysis manages the symptoms of ESRD but does not cure it. Dialysis is a constant factor of life, requiring thinking and planning ahead at all times. Clients on dialysis may not be able to maintain a job. Families often fall apart with the day-to-day stress. Even with dialysis, the client may have constant flulike symptoms, never feeling truly well. Clients on hemodialysis may feel powerless because of their dependence on others for treatment. On the other hand, home peritoneal dialysis places a continuing burden on the client to maintain treatment. In the end, the client may choose to discontinue treatment, preferring death over continued dialysis.

Hemodialysis for ESRD typically is done three times a week for a total of 9 to 12 hours. The amount of dialysis needed (or *dialysis dose*) is individually determined by factors such as body size and residual renal function, dietary intake, and concurrent illness. Hypotension and muscle cramps are common complications during hemodialysis treatments. Infection and vascular access problems are common long-term complications of hemodialysis. Cardiovascular disease is the leading cause of death for clients receiving hemodialysis. The death rate from cardiovascular disease is higher in clients on hemodialysis than those on peritoneal dialysis or who have had a kidney transplant for reasons that are unclear (Kasper et al., 2005). See the previous section on ARF and the box on page 908 for more information about hemodialysis and related nursing care.

Peritoneal dialysis is currently used by approximately 10% of people who require long-term dialysis in the United States. In Canada and Europe, 35% to 45% of clients with ESRD are treated with peritoneal dialysis. In Third World countries, peritoneal dialysis is used to treat the majority of clients with ESRD.

Continuous ambulatory peritoneal dialysis (CAPD) is the most common form of peritoneal dialysis used. Dialysate (2 L) is instilled into the peritoneal cavity, and the catheter is sealed. The client can then continue normal daily activities, emptying the peritoneal cavity and replacing the dialysate every 4 to 6 hours. No special equipment is needed. A variation of CAPD is *continuous cyclic peritoneal dialysis (CCPD)*, which uses a delivery device during nighttime hours and a continuous dwell during the day. CAPD can be performed anywhere, and CCPD allows for home treatment at night, leaving the client free during the day.

Peritoneal dialysis has several advantages over hemodialysis. Heparinization and vascular complications associated with an AV fistula are avoided. The clearance of metabolic wastes is slower but more continuous, avoiding rapid fluctuations in extracellular fluid composition and associated symptoms. More liberal intake of fluids and nutrients is often allowed for the client on CAPD. While glucose absorbed from dialysate can increase blood glucose levels in the diabetic, regular insulin can be added to the infusion to manage hyperglycemia. The client on peritoneal dialysis is better able to self-manage the treatment regimen, reducing feelings of helplessness.

The major disadvantages of peritoneal dialysis include less effective metabolite elimination and risk of infection (peritonitis). Peritoneal dialysis may not be effective for large clients with no residual kidney function. Serum triglyceride levels increase with peritoneal dialysis. Finally, the presence of an indwelling peritoneal catheter may cause a body image disturbance. See the previous section of this chapter and the box on page 910 for more information about dialysis and nursing care for the client undergoing peritoneal dialysis.

KIDNEY TRANSPLANT Kidney transplant has become the treatment of choice for many clients with ESRD. Kidneys are the solid organ most commonly transplanted, and to date kidney transplantation is the most successful of transplantation procedures. The first kidney transplant was performed in 1954; the donor and recipient were identical twins. Kidney transplant as a treatment for ESRD is limited primarily by availability of organs. In 2004, more than 16,000 people received a kidney transplant; however, there currently are nearly 62,000 awaiting a transplant (Organ Procurement and Transplantation Network, 2005; United Network for Organ Sharing, 2005).

Kidney transplant improves both survival and quality of life for the client with ESRD. The client on dialysis has a 62.9% probability of surviving after 2 years of dialysis; the transplant recipient has a greater than 91.6% probability of survival after 2 years. At 5 years, the difference is even greater: 31.9% for dialysis compared with 80.6% for transplant (NKUDIC, 2004). The transplant client is no longer tethered to a dialysis catheter, machine, or center. Dietary and fluid restrictions are reduced, and the body image is more "whole."

Most transplanted kidneys are obtained from cadavers; however, transplants from living donors are increasing. In 2004, of transplanted kidneys, 41.5% came from living donors, most of whom were related to the recipient (UNOS, 2005). With both cadaver and living donor transplants, a close match between blood and tissue type is desired. Human leukocyte antigens (HLAs) are compared between the donor and recipient; six antigens in common is considered to be a "perfect" match. The success of well-matched living-donor transplants is better than for cadaver organ transplants, with a 1-year graft survival of 97.6% compared to 93.7% for cadaver transplants (NKUDIC, 2004). Close tissue matching probably accounts for the better outcome with living donors. People with normal kidneys who are in good physical health may donate a kidney. Predonation counseling is vital: Nephrectomy is major surgery and involves a risk of trauma or disease damaging the remaining kidney in the future. If the transplant fails, the psychologic impact on the donor can be significant. Nursing care of the client having a nephrectomy is summarized in the box on page 897.

Cadaver kidneys are obtained from people who meet the criteria for brain death, are less than 65 years old, and are free of systemic disease, malignancy, or infection, including HIV and hepatitis B or C. Kidneys are removed after brain death has been determined, and are preserved by hypothermia or a technique called continuous hypothermic pulsatile perfusion. A kidney preserved by hypothermia is transplanted within 24 to 48 hours. Continuous pulsatile perfusion allows up to 3 days

BOX 29–1 **How Cadaver Kidneys Are Allocated for Transplant**

The scarcity of organs for transplant raises questions about how cadaver kidneys are allocated—who receives a kidney and who does not. Past inequities in the allocation process (e.g., more men than women, more Caucasians than people of color, more rich than poor, and more young than old) led to the development of the United Network for Organ Sharing (UNOS) in 1986. UNOS has policies for organ distribution, including kidneys, hearts, livers, and other transplanted organs.

UNOS maintains national, regional, and local lists of clients awaiting transplants. When an organ becomes available, donor information is entered into the UNOS computer. The computer then runs a match program, generating a list of clients ranked by criteria such as blood and tissue type, organ size, and medical urgency of the client. Factors such as time on the waiting list and distance between the donor and the transplant center also are considered. A candidate with a perfect match (six HLAs in common) and compatible blood type gets priority for the kidney, regardless of region or geographic area. Otherwise, the list of clients in the local area is checked first, then the regional list of clients awaiting transplant. If no match is found in the region, the organ becomes available to clients nationwide.

The UNOS allocation system, standardized fees, and Medicare coverage for transplantation have done much to ensure equitable access to available kidneys. Still, controversy exists. Clients with resources for travel may register in several different regions for an organ. Up to 10% of clients receiving a transplant in any center may be foreign nationals competing with U.S. citizens for scarce organ resources. A transplant center can accept or reject a candidate for transplant who has lost a kidney because of noncompliance.

As long as the demand for kidneys exceeds the supply of donor organs, it is likely that controversy will exist regarding their allocation. Nurses can help by identifying potential donors and contacting the transplant coordinator. In addition, nurses can inform the public about organ donation and the allocation system, and encourage donation.

---

before transplantation. The system used to allocate cadaver kidneys for transplantation is outlined in Box 29–1.

The donor kidney is placed in the lower abdominal cavity of the recipient, and the renal artery, vein, and ureter are anastomosed (Figure 29–12 ■). The renal artery of the donor kidney is connected to the hypogastric artery, and the renal vein to the iliac vein. The ureter is connected to one of the recipient's ureters or directly to the bladder, using a tunnel technique to prevent reflux. Nursing care for the client having a kidney transplant is outlined in the box on the next page.

Unless the donor and recipient are identical twins, the grafted organ stimulates an immune response to reject the transplanted organ. Immunosuppressive drugs minimize this response. Azathioprine or mycophenolate mofetil are commonly used, often in combination with prednisone, a corticosteroid. Cyclosporine, a potent immunosuppressive, also may be used. These drugs suppress a portion of the immune system and the inflammatory response, increasing the risk for infections and cancers with long-term therapy. The nursing implications of immunosuppressive therapy are outlined in Chapter 13 ∞.

Glucocorticoids such as prednisone and methylprednisolone are used for both maintenance immunosuppression and to treat acute rejection episodes. Side effects of long-term corticosteroid use include impaired wound healing, emotional disturbances, osteoporosis, and cushingoid effects on glucose, protein, and fat metabolism.

Azathioprine inhibits both cellular and humoral immunity. Because this drug is rapidly metabolized by the liver, the dose may not need to be altered in the presence of renal failure. Bone marrow suppression, abnormalities of liver function, and alopecia are the primary significant adverse effects for azathioprine. The action of mycophenolate mofetil is similar to that of azathioprine. Its advantages are minimal bone marrow suppression and increased potency in preventing or reversing rejection of the transplanted organ (Kasper et al., 2005).

Cyclosporine primarily affects cellular immunity, the helper T cells in particular. Among its many adverse effects, which in-

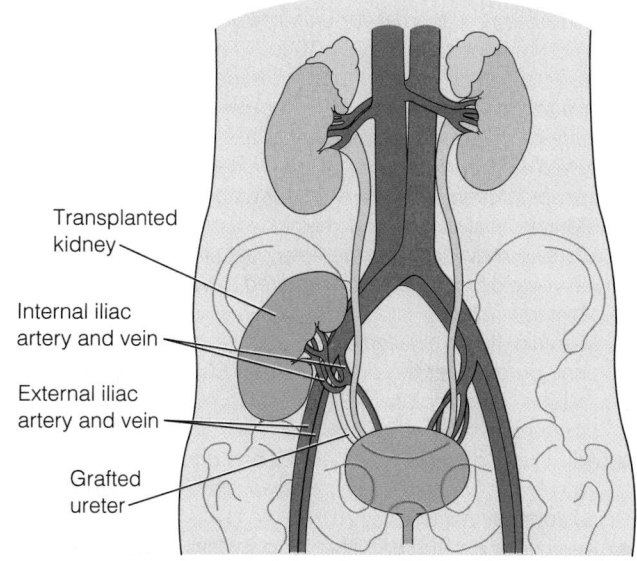

Internal iliac artery and vein

External iliac artery and vein

Transplanted kidney

Grafted ureter

Figure 29–12 ■ Placement of a transplanted kidney in the iliac fossa with anastomosis to the hypogastric artery, iliac vein, and bladder.

clude hepatotoxicity and hirsutism, nephrotoxicity is a primary concern for the kidney transplant client.

Even with immunosuppressive therapy, the transplanted kidney can be rejected at any time. Either acute or chronic rejection may develop. *Acute rejection* develops within months of the transplant. It is caused by a cellular immune response with T-lymphocyte proliferation (Porth, 2005). Few manifestations may be apparent other than a rise in serum creatinine and possible oliguria. Methylprednisolone, a glucocorticoid, and OKT3 monoclonal antibody (see Chapter 13 ∞) are used to manage acute rejection episodes. OKT3 can cause severe systemic reactions, including chills, fever, hypotension, headache, and possible pulmonary edema (Kasper et al., 2005). *Chronic rejection,* which may develop months to years following the transplant, is a major

MediaLink Case Study: Kidney Transplant

NURSING CARE OF THE CLIENT HAVING A KIDNEY TRANSPLANT

PREOPERATIVE CARE

- Provide routine preoperative care as outlined in Chapter 4 ∞.
- Assess knowledge and feelings about the procedure, answering questions and clarifying information as needed. Listen and address concerns about surgery, the source of the donor organ, and possible complications. *Addressing concerns and reducing preoperative anxiety improve postoperative recovery.*
- Continue dialysis as ordered. *Continued renal replacement therapy is necessary to manage fluid and electrolyte balance and prevent uremia prior to surgery.*
- Administer immunosuppressive drugs as ordered before surgery. *Immunosuppression is initiated before transplantation to prevent immediate graft rejection.*

POSTOPERATIVE CARE

- Provide routine postoperative care as outlined in Chapter 4 ∞.
- Maintain urinary catheter patency and a closed system. *Catheter patency is vital to keep the bladder decompressed and prevent pressure on suture lines. A closed drainage system minimizes the risk for urinary tract infection.*
- Measure urine output every 30 to 60 minutes initially. *Careful assessment of urine output helps determine fluid balance and transplant function. Acute tubular necrosis is a common early complication, usually due to tissue ischemia during the period between removal of the kidney from the donor and transplantation. Oliguria is an early sign.*
- Monitor vital signs and hemodynamic pressures closely. *Diuresis may occur immediately, resulting in hypovolemia, low cardiac output, and impaired perfusion of the transplanted kidney.*
- Maintain fluid replacement, generally calculated to replace urine output over the previous 30 or 60 minutes, milliliter for milliliter. *Fluid replacement is vital to maintain vascular volume and tissue perfusion.*
- Administer diuretics as ordered. *Loop and/or osmotic diuretics such as furosemide or mannitol may be used to promote postoperative diuresis.*
- Remove the catheter within 2 to 3 days or as ordered. Encourage to void every 1 to 2 hours and assess frequently for signs of urinary retention following catheter removal. *The bladder may have atrophied prior to surgery, reducing its capacity. Urinary retention places stress on suture lines and increases the risk of infection.*
- Monitor serum electrolytes and renal function tests. *These tests are used to monitor graft function and fluid and electrolyte status. Electrolyte imbalances may develop as the transplanted kidney begins to function and diuresis occurs. Elevated serum creatinine and BUN levels may be early signs of rejection or graft failure.*

- Monitor for possible complications:
  a. *Hemorrhage* from an arterial or venous anastomosis can be either acute or insidious. Indicators include swelling at the operative site, increased abdominal girth, and signs of shock, including changes in vital signs and level of consciousness. *Hemorrhage is a surgical emergency, requiring prompt recognition and treatment to preserve the graft.*
  b. *Ureteral anastomosis failure* causes urine leakage into the peritoneal cavity. It may be marked by decreased urine output with abdominal swelling and tenderness. *Failure of the ureteral anastomosis requires surgical intervention.*
  c. *Renal artery thrombosis* is characterized by an abrupt onset of hypertension and reduced GFR. *Renal artery thrombosis can result in transplant failure.*
  d. *Infection* due to immunosuppression is an immediate and continuing risk. The inflammatory response is blunted, and infection may not significantly elevate the temperature. Monitor for signs such as change in level of consciousness, cloudy or malodorous urine, or purulent drainage from the incision. *Prevention and prompt treatment of infections is particularly important in the immunosuppressed client.*
- Include the following in predischarge teaching for the client and family:
  a. The use and effects of prescribed medications, including antihypertensive medications, immunosuppressive agents, prophylactic antibiotics, and others as ordered.
  b. Monitoring vital signs (including temperature) and weight.
  c. Manifestations of organ rejection, such as swelling and tenderness over the graft site, fever, joint aching, weight gain, and decreased urinary output. Stress the importance of promptly reporting signs and symptoms to the physician.
  d. Ordered or recommended dietary restrictions such as restricted carbohydrate and sodium intake, and increased protein intake.
  e. Measures to prevent infection, such as avoiding crowds and obviously ill individuals.
  The client and family will manage care after discharge, and therefore need a good understanding of what to expect, how to monitor graft status, and measures to reduce the adverse effects of medications.
- Provide psychologic support, address concerns, and provide information as needed. *The client knows that transplant success is not guaranteed. In addition, the client has often been managing a chronic disease independently and is used to having a degree of control. Providing information and allowing the client to retain control relieves anxiety and improves recovery.*

cause of graft loss. Both humoral and cellular immune responses are involved in chronic rejection. It does not respond to increased immunosuppression. The presenting manifestations of chronic rejection—progressive azotemia, proteinuria, and hypertension—are those of progressive renal failure.

Hypertension is a possible complication of kidney transplant, resulting from graft rejection, renal artery stenosis, or re-

nal vasoconstriction. Clients may develop glomerular lesions and manifestations of nephrosis. Hypertension and altered blood lipids (increased LDLs and decreased HDLs) increase the risk of death from myocardial infarction and stroke following transplant (Kasper et al., 2005).

Long-term immunosuppression has adverse effects as well. Infection is a continuing threat. Bacterial and viral infections may develop, as well as fungal infections of the blood, lungs, and CNS. Tumors are also common, with carcinoma *in situ* of the cervix, lymphomas, and skin cancers most prevalent. The risk of congenital anomalies is increased in infants whose mothers have undergone immunosuppressive therapy. Corticosteroid use may lead to bone problems, gastrointestinal disorders such as peptic ulcer disease, and cataract formation.

 NURSING CARE

Health Promotion

Measures to reduce the risk of CRF focus on preventing kidney disease and appropriately managing diabetes and hypertension. Promote early and effective treatment of all infections, particularly skin and pharyngeal infections caused by streptococcal bacteria. Discuss measures to reduce the risk for urinary tract infections, and stress the importance of prompt treatment to eradicate the infecting organism. Discuss the relationship between diabetes, hypertension, and kidney disease. Emphasize that maintaining blood glucose levels and the blood pressure within the recommended ranges reduces the risk of adverse effects on the kidneys. Ensure that all clients with less than optimal renal function are well hydrated, particularly when a nephrotoxic drug is prescribed or anticipated. Finally, encourage the client with ESRD to investigate options for early transplantation to avoid long-term dialysis.

Assessment

Both subjective and objective data are used to assess the client with CRF:
- *Health history:* Complaints of anorexia, nausea, weight gain, or edema; current treatment (if any), including type and frequency of dialysis or previous kidney transplant; chronic diseases such as diabetes, heart failure, or kidney disease.
- *Physical examination:* Mental status; vital signs including temperature, heart and lung sounds, and peripheral pulses; urine output (if any); weight; skin color, moisture, condition; presence of edema (periorbital or dependent); bowel tones; presence and location of an AV fistula, shunt, or graft, or peritoneal catheter.

See the box on page 914 ∞ for assessment of the older adult with ESRD.

Nursing Diagnoses and Interventions

Whether the client with ESRD is facing long-term dialysis or renal transplantation, a number of nursing care needs can be identified. This section focuses on nursing care related to impaired renal function, nutritional deficits due to dietary restrictions and nausea, increased risk for infection, and changes in body image. Also see the Nursing Care Plan on the next page for additional potential nursing diagnoses and interventions for the client with chronic renal failure.

Ineffective Tissue Perfusion: Renal

Capillaries are an integral part of the nephron. As nephrons are destroyed, kidney perfusion progressively declines. As renal perfusion and nephron function fall, the kidney is less able to maintain fluid and electrolyte balance and eliminate waste products from the body.
- Monitor intake and output, vital signs including orthostatic blood pressures, and weight. *These provide important data to identify changes in fluid volume.*

> **PRACTICE ALERT**
> Weight changes are a more accurate indicator of fluid volume status in the oliguric or anuric client than intake and output measurements.

- Restrict fluids as ordered. *As renal function declines, the ability to eliminate excess fluid is impaired.*
- Monitor respiratory status, including lung sounds, every 4 to 8 hours. *Fluid volume overload may lead to heart failure and possible pulmonary edema.*
- Monitor BUN, serum creatinine, pH, electrolytes, and CBC. Report significant changes. *As renal function declines, progressive azotemia with increasing BUN and serum creatinine is seen. Metabolic acidosis develops as the kidney is unable to eliminate hydrogen ions and conserve bicarbonate. Hyponatremia, hyperkalemia, hyperphosphatemia, and hypocalcemia are associated with renal failure. The RBC count, hemoglobin, and hematocrit decline due to deficient erythropoietin to stimulate cell production in the bone marrow. An acute fall in hemoglobin and hematocrit may indicate GI bleeding, a risk in clients with ESRD.*
- Report manifestations of electrolyte imbalances, such as cardiac dysrhythmias and other ECG changes, muscle tremors and possible tetany, and Kussmaul's respirations. *Manifestations of electrolyte imbalance may indicate the need for intervention.*
- Administer medications to treat electrolyte imbalances as ordered. *Medications may be prescribed to help maintain electrolyte and acid–base balance and prevent adverse effects of imbalances.*

> **PRACTICE ALERT**
> Monitor carefully for desired and adverse effects of all medications. Impaired renal function affects drug elimination and increases the risk for toxic effects.

- Administer antihypertensive medications as ordered. *Hypertension management is an important factor in slowing the progression of CRF.*
- Time activities and procedures to allow rest periods. *The anemia associated with CRF may cause significant fatigue and activity intolerance.*

Imbalanced Nutrition: Less than Body Requirements

Anorexia, nausea, and vomiting are common manifestations of ESRD and uremia. The client often has a metallic taste and bad breath, which also diminish appetite. A diet restricted in protein and sodium will compound these problems. Food intake may be insufficient to meet metabolic needs. Catabolism, the breakdown of body proteins to meet energy needs, exacerbates azotemia and uremia.

NURSING CARE PLAN   A Client with End-Stage Renal Disease

Walter Cohen, 45 years old, is the print shop manager at a local community college. He has been a type 1 diabetic since the age of 20, and was diagnosed with diabetic nephropathy 10 years ago. Despite blood pressure control with antihypertensive medications and frequent blood glucose monitoring with insulin coverage, he developed overt proteinuria 5 years ago and has now progressed to end-stage renal disease. He enters the nephrology unit for temporary hemodialysis to relieve uremic symptoms. While there, a CAPD catheter will be inserted. Mr. Cohen's desire to continue working is the primary factor in his choice of CAPD over hemodialysis.

ASSESSMENT

Richard Gonzalez, Mr. Cohen's care manager, obtains a nursing assessment. Mr. Cohen states that his diabetes has always been difficult to control. He has had numerous hypoglycemic episodes and has been hospitalized "four or five times" for ketoacidosis. Recently he has developed symptoms of peripheral neuropathy and increasing retinopathy. He attributed his lack of appetite, nausea, vomiting, and fatigue over the past month to "a touch of the flu." His weight remained stable, so he did not worry about not eating much.

Physical assessment findings include T 97.8°F (36.5°C) PO, P 96, R 20, and BP 178/100. Skin cool and dry, with minor excoriations on forearms and lower legs. Breath odor fetid. Scattered fine rales noted in bilateral lung bases. Soft S_3 gallop noted at cardiac apex. Bilateral pitting edema of lower extremities to just below the knees; fingers and hands also edematous. Abdominal assessment essentially normal, with hypoactive bowel sounds. Urinalysis shows a specific gravity of 1.011, gross proteinuria, and multiple cell casts. CBC results: RBC 2.9 million/mm³; hemoglobin 9.4 g/dL; hematocrit 28%. Blood chemistry abnormalities include BUN 198 mg/dL; creatinine 18.5 mg/dL; sodium 125 mEq/L; potassium 5.7 mEq/L; calcium 7.1 mg/dL; phosphate 6.8 mg/dL. A temporary jugular venous catheter will be placed for hemodialysis the next day, followed by peritoneal catheter insertion later in the week.

DIAGNOSES

- *Excess Fluid Volume* related to failure of kidneys to eliminate excess body fluid
- *Imbalanced Nutrition: Less than Body Requirements* related to effects of uremia
- *Impaired Skin Integrity* of lower extremities related to dry skin and itching
- *Risk for Infection* related to invasive catheters and impaired immune function

EXPECTED OUTCOMES

- Adhere to the prescribed fluid restriction of 750 mL per day.
- Demonstrate reduced extracellular fluid volume by weight loss, decreased peripheral edema, clear lung sounds, and normal heart sounds.
- Consume and retain 100% of prescribed diet, including snacks.

- Demonstrate healing of lower extremity skin lesions.
- Remain free of infection.
- Demonstrate appropriate peritoneal catheter care and CAPD.

PLANNING AND IMPLEMENTATION

- Space fluids, allowing 400 mL from 0700 to 1500, 200 mL from 1500 to 2300, and 100 mL from 2300 to 0700.
- Provide mouth care at least every 4 hours and before every meal.
- Keep sugarless hard candy and ice chips at the bedside; include ice consumed as fluid intake.
- Weigh daily before breakfast; monitor vital signs, and heart and lung sounds, every 4 hours.
- Document intake and output every 4 hours.
- Arrange dietary consultation for menu planning.
- Administer prescribed antiemetic 1 hour before meals.
- Monitor food intake, noting percentage and types of food consumed.
- Clean lesions on lower extremities every 8 hours and assess healing.
- Teach CAPD procedure and peritoneal catheter care.
- Assist to identify strengths and needs in health regimen management.

EVALUATION

Mr. Cohen was hospitalized for 2 weeks, undergoing four hemodialysis sessions to reduce uremic symptoms. An arteriovenous fistula has been created in his left arm in case he should need hemodialysis in the future. He begins peritoneal dialysis the second week, and by discharge he is able to manage the catheter care and dialysis runs with the help of his wife. His heart and lung sounds are normal, and he has minimal peripheral edema on discharge. The excoriations on his legs have healed. His temperature is normal, and no evidence of infection is noted. Mr. Cohen remains anorectic and slightly nauseated, but is eating most of his prescribed diet and snacks. He has lost 10 pounds with excess fluid removal by dialysis, but his weight remains stable during the second week. Mr. Cohen and his wife have been introduced to another client who has been on CAPD for several years and promises to help them with problem solving.

CRITICAL THINKING IN THE NURSING PROCESS

1. How does diabetes mellitus damage the kidneys and lead to ESRD? Why is this more significant for a client with type 1 diabetes than for someone with type 2 diabetes (see Chapter 20∞)?
2. Why do high levels of urea in the blood often cause changes in cognition and mental status? What manifestations of encephalopathy would you expect to see?
3. How might Mr. Cohen's insulin dosage and diet need to be changed with the institution of peritoneal dialysis? Why?
4. Develop a care plan for the nursing diagnosis *Disturbed Body Image*.

See Evaluating Your Response in Appendix C.

Directions: Read the clinical scenario below and answer the questions that follow. To complete this exercise successfully, you will use not only knowledge of the content in this unit, but also principles related to setting priorities and maintaining client safety.

CLINICAL SCENARIO

You have been assigned to work with the following four clients for the 0700 shift on a renal medical-surgical unit. Significant data obtained during report are as follows:

- Phillip Connor is a 45-year-old who was admitted 2 days ago after a fall from a deer hunting stand. He experienced a bruised right kidney and numerous ecchymotic areas on his right side from the fall. His vital signs are T 99°F, P 98, R 28, BP 110/68. He is complaining of abdominal pain and difficulty urinating.
- Agnes Gibson is an 84-year-old who was admitted 2 hours ago with manifestations of urinary incontinence, anorexia, confusion, and lethargy. Her vital signs on admission were T 97°F, P 88, R 20, BP 148/90. The physician ordered trimethoprim-sulfamethoxazole (Bactrim) to be started as soon as possible.
- Joseph Rouse is a 45-year-old who is to undergo surgery for removal of uric acid stones after having a failed lithotripsy. His vital signs are T 99.6°F, P 94, R 24, BP 112/68. His skin is pale, cool, and clammy. He is complaining of nausea, severe left-sided flank pain with spasms, and light-headedness.
- Angela Baldwin is a 34-year-old who has a medical history of systemic lupus erythematosus. She was admitted with complaints of left flank pain and generalized edema. Urinalysis results indicate hematuria and proteinuria. Vital signs are T 100°F, P 88, R 26, BP 144/90. She is admitted for aggressive immunosuppressive therapy.

Questions

1 In what order would you visit these patients after report?

1. _____
2. _____
3. _____
4. _____

2 What top two priority nursing diagnoses would you choose for each of the clients presented above? Can you explain, if asked, the rationale for your choices?

	Priority Nursing Diagnosis #1	Priority Nursing Diagnosis #2
Phillip Connor		
Agnes Gibson		
Joseph Rouse		
Angela Baldwin		

3 The physician ordered trimethoprim-sulfamethoxazole (Bactrim) for Agnes Gibson's uncomplicated cystitis. Mrs. Smith understands the length of antibiotic therapy when she verbalizes which statement?

1. "I should be able to return home after three days of antibiotics."
2. "I can be discharged after five days of antibiotics."
3. "I need to stay in the hospital for one week to finish the antibiotics."
4. "I can stay in the hospital for five days of antibiotics and take five days of antibiotics at home."

4 The physician orders phenazopyridine (Pyridium) for relief of pain and burning with cystitis. Which does the nurse teach the client about the use of this medication?

1. Take the medication with antacids to prevent stomach upset.
2. Drink less fluid to allow the drug to concentrate in the bladder.
3. Wear a sanitary pad to protect your clothing from stains while taking this drug.
4. Stop taking the drug if nausea and diarrhea occur.

5 The client diagnosed with uric acid stones is ordered to follow a diet low in purines. Which is the meal plan lowest in purines?

1. liver with onions and potatoes
2. chicken sandwich with french fries
3. spaghetti with ground beef meat sauce
4. macaroni and cheese with stewed tomatoes

6 When assessing a client with glomerulonephritis, which manifestations are indicative of an early disease process?

1. pyuria, leukocytosis, and hyperthermia
2. hematuria, proteinuria, and hypertension
3. dysuria, hyperglycemia, and hypertension
4. oliguria, flank pain, and hypotension

7 Which are risk factors of urinary tract infections? (Select all that apply.)

1. circumcision in males
2. decreased cervicovaginal antibodies
3. sexual intercourse in women
4. short urethra in men
5. aging in men
6. urinary catheterization

8 Which is the most accurate indicator of fluid volume status in the oliguric or anuric client?

1. intake and output
2. weight changes
3. restricted fluids
4. BUN and creatinine levels

9 The most reliable diagnostic procedure to determine glomerular disorders is which diagnostic test?

1. kidney scan
2. antistreptolysin O titer
3. kidney biopsy
4. blood urea nitrogen

10 A new postoperative client is complaining of inability to void. A bladder ultrasound indicates that there is a significant amount of urine in the bladder. Which interventions does the nurse perform?

1. Insert a urinary catheter and completely drain the bladder at once.
2. Insert a urinary catheter and drain urine in 500-mL increments.
3. Ambulate client to the bathroom to try to void and run water in the sink.
4. Give the client a glass of water to drink to encourage voiding.

11 Which nursing actions are instituted for the client with kidney trauma?

1. Monitor level of consciousness and urine output.
2. Monitor vital signs for hypotension and bradycardia.
3. Observe for hypertension and check urine for hematuria.
4. Observe urine for oliguria and proteinuria.

12 After a client has returned from surgery, the nurse needs to report which urinary output?

1. 20 mL per hour
2. 40 mL per hour
3. 300 mL per 8 hours
4. 400 mL per 8 hours

FUNCTIONAL HEALTH PATTERN: Elimination

■ Think about clients with altered urinary elimination for whom you have cared in your clinical experiences.

- What were the clients' major medical diagnoses (e.g., urinary tract infection, kidney stones, bladder cancer, acute glomerulonephritis, acute or chronic renal failure)?
- What manifestations did each of these clients have? Was the appearance or odor of their urine affected? Did the clients complain of pain or discomfort? Were other body systems affected by their primary diagnosis (e.g., neurologic or cardiovascular)? How were their manifestations similar or different?
- How did the clients' urinary tract problems interfere with their elimination status? How many times did they urinate during the day and at night? Was their ability to control urination and completely empty their bladder affected?
- Did these clients have difficulty talking about urination or the effects of their condition on social interactions? What measures did you use to assist the clients in openly expressing their concerns?

■ The Elimination Pattern describes the client's patterns of excretory function, including urinary and bowel elimination and perspiration. Urinary system disorders disrupt the elimination pattern because they affect urine production and elimination.

   The urinary system is responsible for regulating body fluids, filtering metabolic wastes from the bloodstream, reabsorbing needed substances and water back into the bloodstream from the filtrate, and eliminating metabolic wastes and water as urine. Any alteration in the structure and function of the urinary system can potentially affect the whole body, leading to manifestations such as:

- Hematuria (inflamed or infected urinary tract tissue ▶ local release of inflammatory mediators ▶ vasodilation and increased capillary permeability ▶ escape of WBCs and RBCs into tissue, filtrate, and urine; tumor growth and tissue invasion ▶ blood vessel damage and growth of new, fragile vessels into tumor ▶ vessel rupture and bleeding into urine)
- Proteinuria (inflammation ▶ increased glomerular capillary permeability ▶ proteins escape from the bloodstream across the capillary membrane into the filtrate ▶ presence of protein in the urine)
- Pyuria (breakdown of local defense mechanisms in urinary tract mucosa ▶ bacteria invade mucosa and multiply ▶ activation of immune responses and formation of immune complexes ▶ phagocytosis of immune complexes by neutrophils and macrophages ▶ pus formation)

■ Priority nursing diagnoses within the Elimination Pattern that may be appropriate for clients with urinary disorders include:

- *Impaired Urinary Elimination* as evidenced by frequency, urgency, hesitancy, dysuria, and nocturia
- *Urge Urinary Incontinence* as evidenced by frequency, urgency, loss of urine before reaching toilet, and voiding in small or large amounts
- *Urinary Retention* as evidenced by sensation of bladder fullness, dribbling urine, dysuria, and bladder distention
- *Stress Urinary Incontinence* as evidenced by dribbling urine with increased abdominal pressure, urinary urgency, and urinary frequency.

■ Two nursing diagnoses from other functional health patterns often are of high priority for the client with urinary elimination disorders. The first nursing diagnosis is important because of the client's need to actively manage many urinary elimination disorders. Physiologic responses to the second problem can interfere with urinary elimination:

- *Ineffective Health Maintenance* (Health Perception-Health Management)
- *Acute Pain* (Cognitive-Perceptual)

- Monitor food and nutrient intake as well as episodes of vomiting. *Careful monitoring helps determine the adequacy of intake.*
- Weigh daily before breakfast. *This provides the most accurate measurement. Remember that a gain of 2 pounds or more over a 24-hour period is more likely to reflect fluid retention than a gain in body mass.*
- Administer antiemetic agents 30 to 60 minutes before eating. *Antiemetics reduce nausea and the risk of vomiting with food intake.*
- Assist with mouth care prior to meals and at bedtime. *Mouth care improves taste, stimulates the appetite, and maintains the integrity of oral mucous membranes.*
- Serve small meals and provide between-meal snacks. *Small meals are less likely to prompt nausea and help improve food intake.*
- Arrange for a dietary consultation. Provide preferred foods to the extent possible, and involve the client in planning daily menus. Encourage family members to bring food as dietary restrictions allow. *Providing preferred foods within restrictions promotes intake.*
- Monitor nutritional status by tracking weight, laboratory values such as serum albumin and BUN, and anthropometric measurements (see Chapters 21 ∞ and 22 ∞). *Indicators of impaired nutrition develop gradually and may be subtle. Careful assessment is important.*
- Administer parenteral nutrition as prescribed. Routinely monitor blood glucose levels, and use strict aseptic technique when handling the solution and venous access site. *Parenteral nutrition may be necessary to prevent catabolism and increasing azotemia. Hyperglycemia and infection are risks associated with parenteral nutrition (see Chapter 22 ∞). Immune system suppression associated with renal failure further increases the risk for infection.*

Risk for Infection

Chronic renal failure affects the immune system and leukocyte function, increasing susceptibility to infection. Invasive devices required for hemodialysis or peritoneal dialysis add to this risk. The client who has had a kidney transplant remains on immunosuppressive therapy for life, further depressing the immune system and increasing the risk for infection.

- Use standard precautions and good hand washing technique at all times. *Hand washing is a primary means of preventing the transfer of organisms. Clients who are on hemodialysis or who have had multiple blood transfusions to treat anemia have an increased risk for hepatitis B, hepatitis C, and HIV infection.*

PRACTICE ALERT

Use strict aseptic technique when managing ports, catheters, and incisions, to reduce the risk of introducing infectious organisms when immune responses are impaired.

- Monitor temperature and vital signs at least every 4 hours. *A low-grade fever or increased pulse rate may indicate an infection in the immunosuppressed client.*

- Monitor WBC count and differential. *Increased WBCs may indicate a bacterial infection; decreased WBCs may indicate viral infection. A shift in the differential showing more immature WBCs (bands) in circulation is another indicator of infection.*
- Culture urine, peritoneal dialysis fluid, and other drainage as indicated. *Culture is done to verify the presence of pathogens.*

PRACTICE ALERT

Monitor clarity of dialysate return. Dialysate should return clear in the client undergoing peritoneal dialysis. Cloudy dialysate may indicate peritonitis, the most common complication of peritoneal dialysis, and should be reported and cultured.

- Provide good respiratory hygiene including position changes, coughing, and deep breathing. *These measures improve clearance of respiratory secretions, reducing the risk for infection.*
- Restrict visits from obviously ill people. Teach the client and family about the risk for infection and measures to reduce the spread of infection. *The client's resistance to infection is impaired, necessitating extra caution in preventing unnecessary exposures.*

Disturbed Body Image

Chronic disease and impaired kidney function can affect the client's body image. Hemodialysis requires an arteriovenous fistula or shunt; a permanent peritoneal catheter is required for peritoneal dialysis. While kidney transplant can restore an image of wholeness, a visible scar remains and the organ may be perceived as "foreign."

- Involve the client in care, including meal planning, dialysis, and catheter, port, or incision care to the extent possible. *Involvement improves acceptance and stimulates discussion about the effect of the disease and treatment measures on the client's life.* See the Nursing Research box on the next page.
- Encourage expression of feelings and concerns, accepting perceptions and feelings without criticism. *Self-expression enhances the client's self-worth and acceptance.*
- Include the client in decision making and encourage self-care. *Increased autonomy enhances the client's sense of control, independence, and self-worth.*
- Support positive gains, but do not support denial. *The client may have difficulty accepting the renal failure, but adaptation to the loss is important.*
- Help the client develop and achieve realistic goals. *Realistic goals allow the client to see progress.*
- Provide positive reinforcement and feedback. *These measures support growth and adaptation.*
- Reinforce effective coping strategies. *Reinforcement helps the client develop positive versus negative strategies for coping.*
- Facilitate contact with a support group or other community members affected by renal failure. *The client benefits by providing and receiving support in a group of people going through similar circumstances.*
- Refer for mental health counseling as indicated or desired. *Counseling can help the client develop effective coping and adaptation strategies.*

NURSING RESEARCH   Evidence-Based Practice: Client on Hemodialysis

In a study of clients undergoing hemodialysis for CRF, researchers in Sweden looked at suffering on three levels: related to sickness and treatment, related to care provided, and related to the client's unique life experience and existence (Hagren et al., 2001). The study included 15 clients between ages 50 and 86.

The researchers identified dependence on the hemodialysis machine and dependence on caregivers as the primary sources of suffering in these clients. This dependence and the loss of freedom associated with hemodialysis affected marital and family relationships and social lives of the sufferers. Accepting dependence on the hemodialysis machine and being seen as an individual by caregivers, thus promoting autonomy, relieved clients' suffering.

IMPLICATIONS FOR NURSING

Treating all clients with ESRD holistically, respecting their individual and unique characteristics and experience, is vital to promote acceptance and autonomy. Listen carefully, responding to each person's concerns. Discuss the effects of the disease and its treatment on the client's life, marital and family relationships, and socialization. Suggest strategies to maintain independence and provide relief for caregivers. When appropriate, discuss alternatives to hemodialysis for treating ESRD, such as kidney transplant or peritoneal dialysis. Peritoneal dialysis may be managed independently by the client, reducing dependence on others and time spent in treatment.

CRITICAL THINKING IN CLIENT CARE

1. Identify assessment tools and data you could use to evaluate degree of suffering in the client receiving long-term hemodialysis.
2. In addition to the above, what interventions can you, as the nurse, implement to promote autonomy and acceptance of hemodialysis in the client with ESRD?
3. Develop a teaching plan for families and significant others to help them promote acceptance and autonomy in the client undergoing long-term hemodialysis.

Community-Based Care

Chronic renal failure and ESRD are long-term processes that require client management. No matter what treatment option is chosen (hemodialysis, peritoneal dialysis, or renal transplantation), day-to-day management falls to the client and family. Teaching for home care includes the following topics:

- Nature of the kidney disease and renal failure, including expected progression and effects
- Monitoring weight, vital signs, and temperature
- Prescribed dietary and fluid restrictions (Involve the client, a dietitian, and the family member usually responsible for cooking. Include strategies to manage nausea and relieve thirst within allowed fluid limits.)
- How to assess and protect a fistula or shunt for hemodialysis (or the extremity to be used if one is anticipated)

- Peritoneal catheter care and the procedure for peritoneal dialysis as indicated (Include a family member or significant other, in case the client is unable to perform the procedure independently at some time.)
- Following kidney transplant, prescribed medications, adverse effects and their management, infection prevention, graft protection, and manifestations of organ rejection.

Refer to a dietitian for diet planning and counseling. If home hemodialysis is planned, refer the designated dialysis helper for formal training. Both the National Kidney Foundation and the American Association of Kidney Patients may be able to provide support and educational materials for the client with ESRD (see the box on page 914). Local and state chapters of these organizations can provide additional support.

EXPLORE MEDIALINK

Prentice Hall Nursing MediaLink DVD-ROM
Audio Glossary
NCLEX-RN® Review

Animation/Video
Furosemide
The Kidney

COMPANION WEBSITE www.prenhall.com/lemone
Audio Glossary
NCLEX-RN® Review
Care Plan Activity: Acute Glomerulonephritis
Case Studies
Acute Glomerulonephritis
Kidney Transplant
MediaLink Applications
Kidney Disorders
Renal Insufficiency
Links to Resources

CHAPTER HIGHLIGHTS

- Congenital and acquired disorders of the kidneys can profoundly affect urinary elimination and ultimately all body systems.
- Glomerulonephritis, inflammation of the glomerulus of the kidney, leads to loss of proteins and blood cells in the urine, a decrease in the glomerular filtration rate, and severe edema.
- The renal and cardiovascular systems are closely interrelated. Vascular disorders, such as hypertension, renal artery stenosis, or obstruction of the renal artery or vein, can have serious consequences in terms of renal function.
- Renal cell malignancies, while uncommon, often are not evident until the cancer is advanced and has metastasized to other sites.

- Acute renal failure is a frequent complication of critical illnesses, typically occurring in people with no prior history of kidney disorders. Ischemic and nephrotoxic damage to the kidney are the most common precipitating factors for ARF.
- Chronic renal failure is the end stage of numerous systemic and kidney disorders, such as diabetes mellitus, systemic lupus erythematosus, and chronic glomerulonephritis.
- When the kidneys fail, renal replacement therapies are necessary to eliminate metabolic waste products and sustain life. Dialysis and kidney transplant are the primary renal replacement therapies used.

TEST YOURSELF NCLEX-RN® REVIEW

1 The physician orders digoxin 0.125 mg three times per week for an 82-year-old client with heart failure. The nurse should:
1. question the order because older clients frequently require larger doses of the drug due to impaired ability of the kidneys to concentrate urine.
2. administer the drug as ordered, monitoring the client for manifestations of toxicity.
3. assess the client's urine specific gravity and pH before administering the drug at this dose.
4. use 0.25-mg digoxin tablets, cutting the tablet in half to save money for the client.

2 A client newly diagnosed with polycystic kidney disease asks if there is anything his children need to know about their risk for getting the disorder. The appropriate response by the nurse is:
1. because the condition was just diagnosed, it is due to a new genetic mutation, and there is no risk of passing the condition on to his children.
2. when his children prepare to marry, they and their potential partners should undergo genetic testing to determine if their children will be at risk.
3. the adult form of this disorder is transmitted as a dominant gene; each child has a 50% risk of having inherited the defective gene.
4. his children would have developed symptoms of the disorder *in utero* or shortly after birth if they had inherited the defective gene.

3 In obtaining a nursing history from a 22-year-old client admitted with a diagnosis of acute glomerulonephritis, the nurse specifically asks the client about a recent history of which of the following?
1. urinary tract infection
2. strep throat
3. x-ray using contrast media
4. illicit drug use

4 The nurse evaluates his teaching for a client with acute glomerulonephritis as effective when the client:
1. chooses soy or animal proteins for allowed grams of protein in diet.
2. states the need to remain on bed rest until his urine returns to clear yellow.
3. demonstrates care for the vascular shunt or peritoneal catheter.
4. limits fluid intake to less than 1500 mL per day.

5 Appropriate postoperative nursing interventions for the client who has had a partial or total nephrectomy include:

1. connecting all catheters and drains to a single collection device.
2. routine irrigation of all catheters with sterile normal saline.
3. administering cough suppressant medication as needed.
4. labeling and securing all catheters, tubes, and drains.

6 Important nursing interventions to prevent acute renal failure in the critically ill client include:
1. maintaining fluid volume and cardiac output.
2. avoiding all potentially nephrotoxic drugs.
3. administering antihypertensive drugs.
4. assessing for a history of diabetes or systemic lupus erythematosus.

7 The nurse evaluates her teaching as effective when the client recovering from acute renal failure states that he will:
1. limit his fluid intake to 1500 mL or less per day.
2. consume only vegetable proteins.
3. avoid taking drugs that may be nephrotoxic.
4. self-catheterize for residual urine at least once a week.

8 The nurse caring for a client preparing to undergo hemodialysis includes which of the following in the plan of care? (Select all that apply.)
1. Obtain weight and orthostatic vital signs.
2. Assess blood pressure of extremity where fistula has been created.
3. Monitor serum creatinine, BUN, and hematocrit levels.
4. Determine urine specific gravity and pH.
5. Restrict fluid and protein intake.

9 An appropriate goal of nursing care for a client with end-stage renal disease is the client will be able to:
1. identify a live-in caregiver.
2. state the advantages and disadvantages of hemodialysis, peritoneal dialysis, and kidney transplant as renal replacement therapies.
3. demonstrate the ability to independently perform hemodialysis in the home.
4. relate the hospice philosophy and identify indicators of the need for hospice care.

10 Following a kidney transplant, the nurse notes that the client's urine is cloudy. The most appropriate response by the nurse is to:
1. record the finding.
2. increase the intravenous flow rate.
3. irrigate the urinary catheter.
4. notify the physician.

BIBLIOGRAPHY

American Cancer Society. (2005). *Cancer facts and figures 2005.* Atlanta: Author.

Barone, C. P., Martin-Watson, A. L., & Barone, G. W. (2004). The postoperative care of the adult renal transplant recipient. *Medsurg Nursing, 13*(5), 296–302.

Bartucci, M. R. (1999). Kidney transplantation: State of the art. *AACN Clinical Issues: Advanced Practice in Acute and Critical Care, 10*(2), 153–163.

Burrows-Hudson, S. (2005). Chronic kidney disease: An overview. *American Journal of Nursing, 105*(2), 40–49.

Campoy, S., & Elwell, R. (2005). Pharmacology & CKD: How chronic kidney disease and its complications alter drug response. *American Journal of Nursing, 105*(9), 60–72.

Cannon, J. D. (2004). Recognizing chronic renal failure . . . the sooner, the better. *Nursing, 34*(1), 50–53.

Compton, A. (2004). Chronic kidney disease. Avoiding the point of no return. *Advance for Nurse Practitioners, 12*(6), 75–78.

Copstead, L. C., & Banasik, J. L. (2005). *Pathophysiology* (3rd ed.). St. Louis, MO: Elsevier/Saunders.

Criddle, L. M. (2003). Rhabdomyolysis. Pathophysiology, recognition, and management. *Critical Care Nurse, 23*(6), 14–22, 24–26, 28+.

Cross, J. (2003). Renal transplantation—demystifying the process. *CANNT Journal, 13*(3), 40–59.

Curtin, R. B., Johnson, H. K., & Schatell, D. (2004). The peritoneal dialysis experience: Insights from long-term patients. *Nephrology Nursing Journal, 31*(6), 615–625.

Daines, P. A. (2004). Pain management at the end of life in a patient with renal failure. *CANNT Journal, 14*(2), 20–23, 26–29.

Dinwiddie, L. C. (2004). Managing catheter dysfunction for better patient outcomes: A team approach. *Nephrology Nursing Journal, 31*(6), 653–660, 661–662, 671.

Dochterman, J., & Bulechek, G. (2004). *Nursing interventions classification (NIC)* (4th ed.). St. Louis, MO: Mosby.

Fischbach, F. (2002). *Nurses' quick reference to common laboratory and diagnostic tests* (3rd ed.). Philadelphia: Lippincott.

Fox, H. L., & Swann, D. (2001). Goodpasture syndrome: Pathophysiology, diagnosis, and management. *Nephrology Nursing Journal, 28*(3), 305–312.

Hagren, B., Petterson, I. M., Severinsson, E., Lutzon, K., & Clyne, N. (2001). The haemodialysis machine as a lifeline: Experiences of suffering from end-stage renal disease. *Journal of Advanced Nursing, 34*(2), 196–202.

Harwood, L., Locking-Cusolito, H., Spittal, J., Wilson, B., & White, S. (2005). Preparing for hemodialysis: Patient stressors and responses. *Nephrology Nursing Journal, 32*(3), 295–303.

Harriston, S. (2004). A review of rhabdomyolysis. *Dimensions of Critical Care Nursing, 23*(4), 155–161.

Holcomb, S. S. (2005). Evaluating chronic kidney disease risk. *Nurse Practitioner: American Journal of Primary Health Care, 30*(4), 12–14, 17–18, 23–27.

Kaplow, R., & Barry, R. (2002). Continuous renal replacement therapies. *American Journal of Nursing, 102*(11), 26–33.

Kasper, D. L., Braunwald, E., Fauci, A. S., Hauser, S. L., Longo, D. L., & Jameson, J. L. (Eds.). (2005). *Harrison's principles of internal medicine* (16th ed.). New York: McGraw-Hill.

Kelley, K. T. (2004). How peritoneal dialysis works. *Nephrology Nursing Journal, 31*(5), 481–482, 488–491.

Kostadaras, A. (2001). Erythropoietin for the anemia of chronic renal failure. *Home Health Care Consultant, 8*(7), 27–31.

Kring, D. (2005). Outmuscling rhabdomyolysis. *Nursing Management, Critical Care Choices 2005,* 24, 26, 29.

Krishnan, M., & Adams, E. (2004). Managing the anemia of end-stage renal disease after hospitalization. *Nephrology Nursing Journal, 31*(5), 541–544.

Lang, M. M., & Towers, C. (2001). Identifying poststreptococcal glomerulonephritis. *Nurse Practitioner: American Journal of Primary Health Care, 26*(8), 34, 37–38, 40–42+.

Legg, V. (2005). Complications of chronic kidney disease. *American Journal of Nursing, 105*(6), 40–49.

Lindqvist, R., Carlsson, M., & Sjödén, P. (2004). Coping strategies of people with kidney transplants. *Journal of Advanced Nursing, 45*(1), 47–52.

Maaz, D. E. (2004). Troubleshooting non-infectious peritoneal dialysis issues. *Nephrology Nursing Journal, 31*(5), 521–533, 545.

McCance, K. L., & Huether, S. E. (2002). *Pathophysiology: The biologic basis for disease in adults & children* (4th ed.). St. Louis, MO: Mosby.

McCarley, P. B., & Salai, P. B. (2005). Cardiovascular disease in chronic kidney disease. *American Journal of Nursing, 105*(4), 40–52.

McCarthy, M. (2004). Issues in renal nutrition: Focus on nutritional care for nephrology patients. The chronic kidney disease epidemic: Nutrition intervention and control. *Nephrology Nursing Journal, 31*(1), 83–84.

Meister, J., & Reddy, K. (2002). Rhabdomyolysis: An overview. *American Journal of Nursing, 102*(2), 75, 77, 79.

Moorhead, S., Johnson, M., & Maas, M. (2004). *Nursing outcomes classification (NOC)* (3rd ed.) St. Louis, MO: Mosby.

Munshi, S. K., Bell, S. L., Vigayskumar, N., & Warwick, G. (2003). Ageism in renal replacement therapy. *Nursing of Older People, 15*(9), 14–16.

Myhre, M. J. (2000). Herbal remedies, nephropathies, and renal disease. *Nephrology Nursing Journal, 27*(5), 473–480.

NANDA International. (2005). *Nursing diagnoses: Definitions and classification 2005–2006.* Philadelphia: Author.

National Kidney and Urologic Diseases Information Clearinghouse. (2004). *Kidney and urologic disease statistics for the United States* (NIH Publication No. 04-3895). Retrieved from http://www.niddk.nih.gov/kudiseases/kidney/pubs/kustats

Organ Procurement and Transplantation Network. (2005). Transplants by donor type. Retrieved from http://www.optn.org/latestData/rptData.asp

Paton, M. (2003). Continuous renal replacement therapy: Slow but steady. *Nursing, 33*(6), 48–50.

Porth, C. M. (2005). *Pathophysiology: Concepts of altered health states* (7th ed.). Philadelphia: Lippincott.

Russell, T. R. (2005). Acute renal failure related to rhabdomyolysis: Pathophysiology, diagnosis, and collaborative management. *Nephrology Nursing Journal, 32*(4), 409–417.

Schneider, R. A. (2004). Chronic renal failure: Assessing the Fatigue Severity Scale for use among caregivers. *Journal of Clinical Nursing, 13,* 219–225.

Seaton-Mills, D. (1999). Acute renal failure: Causes and considerations in the critically ill patient. *Nursing in Critical Care, 4*(6), 293–297.

Small, K. R., & McMullen, M. (2005). When clear becomes cloudy: A review of acute tubular necrosis, a form of renal failure. *American Journal of Nursing, 105*(1), Critical Care Extra: 72AA–BB, 72EE, 72GG.

Sofer, D. (2003). Chronic kidney disease: The emerging epidemic. *American Journal of Nursing, 103*(12), 23.

Spencer, J. W., & Jacobs, J. J. (2003). *Complementary and alternative medicine: An evidence-based approach* (2nd ed.). St. Louis, MO: Mosby.

Tierney, L. M., Jr., McPhee, S. J., & Papadakis, M. A. (Eds.). (2005). *Current medical diagnosis & treatment* (44th ed.). New York: McGraw-Hill.

Tritt, L. (2004). Nutritional assessment and support of kidney transplant recipients. *Journal of Infusion Nursing, 27*(1), 45–51.

United Network for Organ Sharing: Organ Donation and Transplantation. (2005). U.S. Transplantation Data. Retrieved from http://www.unos.org/data/default.asp?display Type=usData

Urden, L. D., Stacy, K. M., & Lough, M. E. (2002). *Thelan's critical care nursing: Diagnosis and management* (4th ed.). St. Louis, MO: Mosby.

U.S. Renal Data System. (2005). *2005 annual data report: Atlas of end-stage renal disease in the United States.* Bethesda, MD: National Institutes of Health, National Institute of Diabetes and Digestive and Kidney Diseases.

Wallace, L. S. (2001). Rhabdomyolysis: A case study. *Medsurg Nursing, 10*(3), 113–120.

Wallace, M. A. (2003). What is new with renal transplantation? *AORN Journal, 77*(5), 946–966.

Way, L. W., & Doherty, G. M. (2003). *Current surgical diagnosis and treatment* (11th ed.). New York: McGraw-Hill.

Wilkinson, J. M. (2005). *Nursing diagnosis handbook* (8th ed.). Upper Saddle River, NJ: Prentice Hall.

Wise, L. C., Mersch, J., Racioppi, J., Crosier, J., & Thompson, C. (2000). Evaluating the reliability and utility of cumulative intake and output. *Journal of Nursing Care Quality, 14*(3), 37–42.

Zabat, E. (2003). When your patient needs peritoneal dialysis. Brush up on this necessary but infrequently used skill that you may need if your patient has chronic renal failure. *Nursing, 33*(8), 52–54.

CASE STUDY

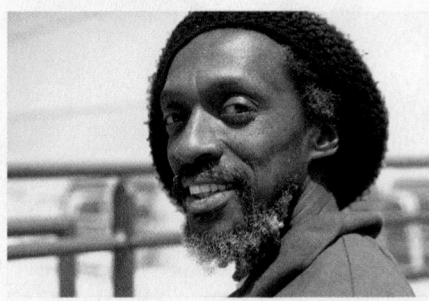

Joe Jenkins is a 45-year-old black male who has been a truck driver for the past 20 years. He is admitted to the hospital with complaints of nausea for several weeks, weakness, fatigue, and loss of appetite. He has been feeling very depressed. He has a past medical history of type 1 diabetes mellitus, hypertension, and diabetic nephropathy. On admission, his vital signs are temperature 98.7°F, P 96, R 20, BP 170/110. He has bilateral pitting edema of the lower extremities. His fingers and hands are also edematous. He complains of dry and itching skin. His urine is dark, frothy, and scanty. A specimen is collected for a urinalysis and blood work is drawn and sent to the laboratory. Results returned with the urinalysis show a specific gravity of 1.011, gross hematuria, and 3+ protein. His blood work reveals a BUN of 198 mg/dL and creatinine of 12.5 mg/dL. Based on his past medical history of diabetes, hypertension, and diabetic nephropathy, and the current findings, a medical diagnosis of chronic renal failure is established.

Based on Mr. Jenkins' assessment and past medical history, the nursing diagnosis of *Impaired Urinary Elimination* is identified as the highest priority for planning nursing care.

- Glomerulosclerosis, thickening of glomerular asement membrane → glomerular capillary lumen arrows → reduced surface area for glomerular filtration gradual loss of nephron units → eventual renal insufficiency and failure

affects

Mr. J.J.
45 y.o. male
Chronic renal failure

leads to

assess

- C/o nausea, weakness, fatigue, anorexia
- States "feeling depressed"
- T 98.7°F, P 96, R 20, BP 170/110
- Bilateral pitting edema of hands, fingers, & lower extremities
- Skin dry, excoriated
- Scanty output of dark, frothy urine; sp grav 1.011, gross hematuria, 3+ protein
- BUN 198 mg/dL, serum creatinine 18.5 mg/dL

generates

- Excess Fluid Volume as evidenced by peripheral edema
- Nausea as evidenced by subjective complaints and anorexia
- Impaired Skin Integrity as evidenced by dry, excoriated skin
- Powerlessness as evidenced by complaints of feeling depressed

generate nursing diagnosis

prioritized to

Impaired Urinary Elimination

expected outcomes

- Adheres to prescribed fluid and dietary restrictions
- Demonstrates reduced extracellular fluid volume: weight loss, reduced edema, clear lung sounds
- Verbalizes understanding of renal replacement options and select preferred option from those presented by nephrologist
- Demonstrates ability to effectively manage diabetes and maintain blood glucose WNL

evaluate

- 5 days after admission:
- Weight down 6 lb
- BP 150/88, P 82, R 18
- Peripheral edema 1 + or less to ankles
- Has undergone 2 hemodialysis sessions; preparing for peritoneal catheter placement
- Met with dietitian and diabetic educator X 3

Interdisciplinary Interventions
- Space fluid intake, considering total allowed intake and client preferences.
- Request dietary consult to plan palatable menus within prescribed restrictions of proteins and simple carbohydrates.
- Weigh q12h under standard conditions.
- Administer diuretics and antihypertensives as ordered.

Independent Interventions
- Discuss renal replacement therapy options with client and family, assisting them to determine the most feasible.
- Refer to diabetic educator for teaching and management of treatment regimen.

PART
IV

Activity and Exercise Patterns

Functional Health Patterns with Related Nursing Diagnoses

HEALTH PERCEPTION-HEALTH MANAGEMENT

- Perceived health status
- Perceived health management
- Healthcare behaviors: health promotion and illness prevention activities, medical treatments, follow-up care

VALUE-BELIEF

- Values, goals, or beliefs (including spirituality) that guide choices or decisions
- Perceived conflicts in values, beliefs, or expectations that are health related

COPING-STRESS-TOLERANCE

- Capacity to resist challenges to self-integrity
- Methods of handling stress
- Support systems
- Perceived ability to control and manage situations

NUTRITIONAL-METABOLIC

- Daily consumption of food and fluids
- Favorite foods
- Use of dietary supplements
- Skin lesions and ability to heal
- Condition of the integument
- Weight, height, temperature

PART IV
ACTIVITY-EXERCISE PATTERNS
NANDA NURSING DIAGNOSES

- Activity Intolerance
- Risk for Activity Intolerance
- Bathing/Hygiene Self-Care Deficit
- Dressing/Grooming Self-Care Deficit
- Impaired Bed Mobility
- Risk for Disuse Syndrome
- Deficient Diversional Activity
- Fatigue
- Risk for Falls
- Impaired Home Maintenance
- Impaired Physical Mobility
- Impaired Wheelchair Mobility
- Impaired Transfer Ability
- Impaired Walking
- Delayed Surgical Recovery
- Decreased Cardiac Output
- Ineffective Breathing Pattern
- Ineffective Airway Clearance
- Impaired Gas Exchange
- Risk for Peripheral Neurovascular Dysfunction
- Impaired Tissue Integrity
- Ineffective Tissue Perfusion
- Impaired Spontaneous Ventilation
- Dysfunctional Ventilatory Weaning Response

SEXUALITY-REPRODUCTIVE

- Satisfaction with sexuality or sexual relationships
- Reproductive pattern
- Female menstrual and perimenopausal history

ROLE-RELATIONSHIPS

- Perception of major roles, relationships, and responsibilities in current life situation
- Satisfaction with or disturbances in roles and relationships

ELIMINATION

- Patterns of bowel and urinary excretion
- Perceived regularity or irregularity of elimination
- Use of laxatives or routines
- Changes in time, modes, quality, or quantity of excretions
- Use of devices for control

ACTIVITY-EXERCISE

- Patterns of personally relevant exercise, activity, leisure, and recreation
- ADLs that require energy expenditure
- Factors that interfere with the desired pattern (e.g., illness or injury)

SELF-PERCEPTION–SELF-CONCEPT

- Attitudes about self
- Perceived abilities, worth, self-image, emotions
- Body posture and movement, eye contact, voice and speech patterns

SLEEP-REST

- Patterns of sleep and rest/relaxation in a 24-h period
- Perceptions of quality and quantity of sleep and rest
- Use of sleep aids and routines

COGNITIVE-PERCEPTUAL

- Adequacy of vision, hearing, taste, touch, smell
- Pain perception and management
- Language, judgment, memory, decisions

UNIT
9

Responses to Altered Cardiac Function

CHAPTER 30 Assessing Clients with Cardiac Disorders

LEARNING OUTCOMES

- Describe the anatomy, physiology, and functions of the heart.
- Trace the circulation of blood through the heart and coronary vessels.
- Identify normal heart sounds and relate them to the corresponding events in the cardiac cycle.
- Explain cardiac output and the influence of various factors in its regulation.
- Describe normal variations in assessment findings for the older adult.
- Identify manifestations of impaired cardiac structure and functions.

CLINICAL COMPETENCIES

- Assess an ECG strip and identify normal and abnormal cardiac rhythm.
- Conduct and document a health history for clients having or at risk for having alterations in the structure and functions of the heart.
- Conduct and document a physical assessment of cardiac status.
- Monitor the results of diagnostic tests and report abnormal findings.

EQUIPMENT NEEDED

- Stethoscope with a diaphragm and a bell
- Good light source
- Watch with a second hand
- Centimeter ruler

MEDIALINK

Resources for this chapter can be found on the Prentice Hall Nursing MediaLink DVD accompanying this textbook, and on the Companion Website at http://www.prenhall.com/lemone

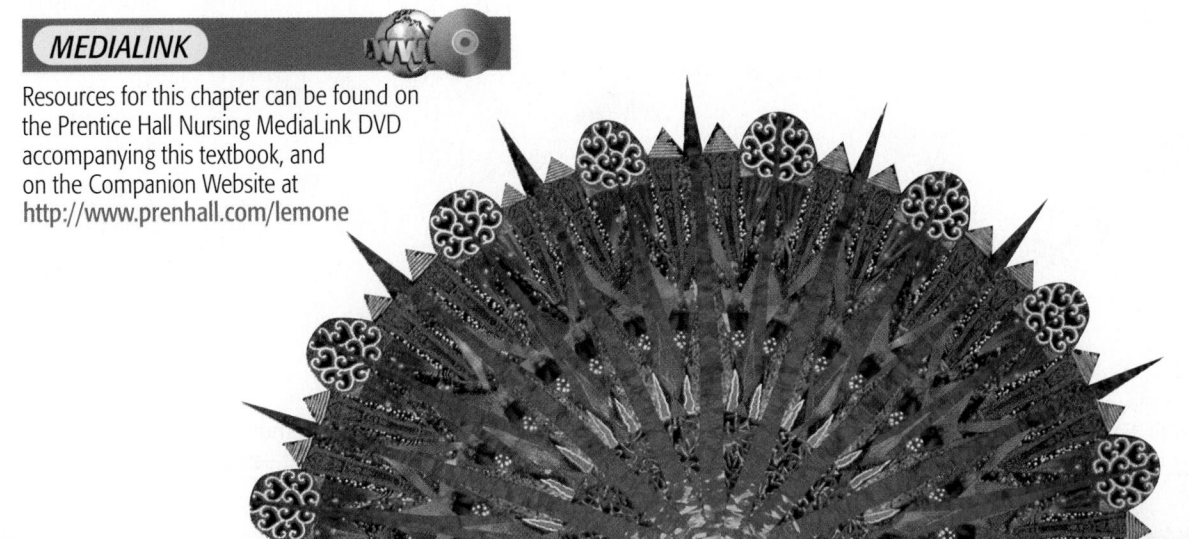

The heart, a muscular pump, beats an average of 70 times per minute, or once every 0.86 second, every minute of a person's life. This continuous pumping moves blood through the body, nourishing tissue cells and removing wastes. Deficits in the structure or function of the heart affect all body tissues.

Changes in cardiac rate, rhythm, or output may limit almost all human functions, including self-care, mobility, and the ability to maintain fluid volume status, respirations, tissue perfusion, and comfort. Cardiac changes may also affect self-concept, sexuality, and role performance.

ANATOMY, PHYSIOLOGY, AND FUNCTIONS OF THE HEART

The heart is a hollow, cone-shaped organ approximately the size of an adult's fist, weighing less than 1 lb. It is located in the mediastinum of the thoracic cavity, between the vertebral column and the sternum, and is flanked laterally by the lungs. Two-thirds of the heart mass lies to the left of the sternum; the upper base lies beneath the second rib, and the pointed apex is approximate with the fifth intercostal space, midpoint to the clavicle (Figure 30–1 ■).

The Pericardium

The heart is covered by the pericardium, a double layer of fibroserous membrane (Figure 30–2 ■). The pericardium encases the heart and anchors it to surrounding structures, forming the pericardial sac. The snug fit of the pericardium prevents the heart from overfilling with blood. The outermost layer is the parietal pericardium, and the visceral pericardium

Figure 30–1 ■ Location of the heart in the mediastinum of the thorax. *A,* Relationship of the heart to the sternum, ribs, and diaphragm. *B,* Cross-sectional view showing relative position of the heart in the thorax. *C,* Relationship of the heart and great vessels to the lungs.

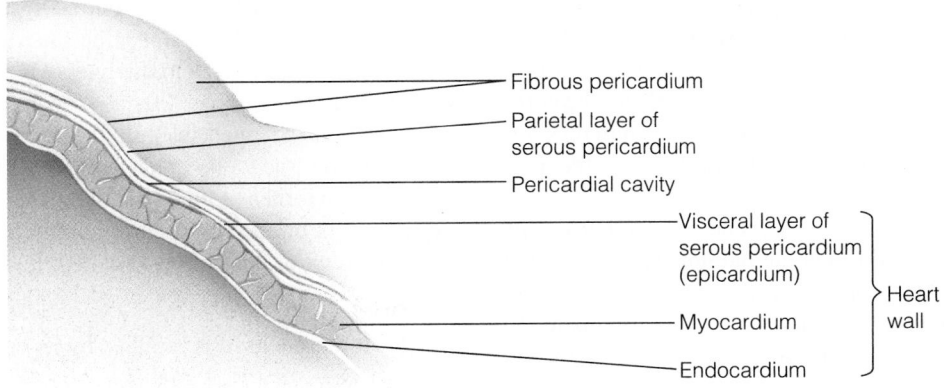

Figure 30–2 ■ Coverings and layers of the heart.

(or epicardium) adheres to the heart surface. The small space between the visceral and parietal layers of the pericardium is called the pericardial cavity. A serous lubricating fluid produced in this space cushions the heart as it beats.

Layers of the Heart Wall

The heart wall consists of three layers of tissue: the epicardium, the myocardium, and the endocardium (see Figure 30–2). The epicardium covers the entire heart and great vessels, and then folds over to form the parietal layer that lines the pericardium and adheres to the heart surface. The myocardium, which is the middle layer of the heart wall, consists of specialized cardiac muscle cells (myofibrils) that provide the bulk of contractile heart muscle. The endocardium, which is the innermost layer, is a thin membrane composed of three layers; the innermost layer is made up of smooth endothelial cells that line the inside of the heart's chambers and great vessels.

Chambers and Valves of the Heart

The heart has four hollow chambers, two upper atria and two lower ventricles. They are separated longitudinally by the interventricular septum (Figure 30–3 ■).

Figure 30–3 ■ The internal anatomy of the heart, frontal section.

The right atrium receives deoxygenated blood from the veins of the body: The superior vena cava returns blood from the body area above the diaphragm, the inferior vena cava returns blood from the body below the diaphragm, and the coronary sinus drains blood from the heart. The left atrium receives freshly oxygenated blood from the lungs through the pulmonary veins.

The right ventricle receives deoxygenated blood from the right atrium and pumps it through the pulmonary artery to the pulmonary capillary bed for oxygenation. The newly oxygenated blood then travels through the pulmonary veins to the left atrium. Blood enters the left atrium and crosses the mitral (bicuspid) valve into the left ventricle. Blood is then pumped out of the aorta to the arterial circulation.

Each of the heart's chambers is separated by a valve that allows unidirectional blood flow to the next chamber or great vessel (see Figure 30–3). The atria are separated from the ventricles by the two atrioventricular (AV) valves; the tricuspid valve is on the right side, and the bicuspid (or mitral) valve is on the left. The flaps of each of these valves are anchored to the papillary muscles of the ventricles by the chordae tendineae. These structures control the movement of the AV valves to prevent backflow of blood. The ventricles are connected to their great vessels by the semilunar valves. On the right, the pulmonary (pulmonic) valve joins the right ventricle with the pulmonary artery. On the left, the aortic valve joins the left ventricle to the aorta.

Closure of the AV valves at the onset of contraction (systole) produces the first heart sound, or S_1 (characterized by the syllable "lub"); closure of the semilunar valves at the onset of relaxation (diastole) produces the second heart sound, or S_2 (characterized by the syllable "dub").

Systemic, Pulmonary, and Coronary Circulation

Because each side of the heart both receives and ejects blood, the heart is often described as a double pump. Blood enters the right atrium and moves to the pulmonary bed at almost the exact same time that blood is entering the left atrium. The circulatory system has two parts: the pulmonary circulation (moving blood through the capillary bed surrounding the lungs to link with the gas exchange system of the lungs), and the systemic circulation, which supplies blood to all other body tissues. In addition, the heart muscle itself is supplied with blood via the coronary circulation.

Systemic Circulation

The systemic circulation consists of the left side of the heart, the aorta and its branches, the capillaries that supply the brain and peripheral tissues, the systemic venous system, and the vena cava. The systemic system, which must move blood to peripheral areas of the body, is a high-pressure system.

Pulmonary Circulation

The pulmonary circulation consists of the right side of the heart, the pulmonary artery, the pulmonary capillaries, and the pulmonary vein. Because it is located in the thorax near the heart, the pulmonary circulation is a low-pressure system. Pulmonary circulation begins with the right side of the heart. De-

oxygenated blood from the venous system enters the right atrium through two large veins, the superior and inferior venae cavae, and is transported to the lungs via the pulmonary artery and its branches (Figure 30–4 ■). After oxygen and carbon dioxide are exchanged in the pulmonary capillaries, oxygen-rich blood returns to the left atrium through several pulmonary veins. Blood is then pumped out of the left ventricle through the aorta and its major branches to supply all body tissues. This second circuit of blood flow is called the systemic circulation.

Coronary Circulation

The heart muscle itself is supplied by its own network of vessels through the coronary circulation. The left and right coronary arteries originate at the base of the aorta and branch out to encircle the myocardium (Figure 30–5A ■), supplying blood, oxygen, and

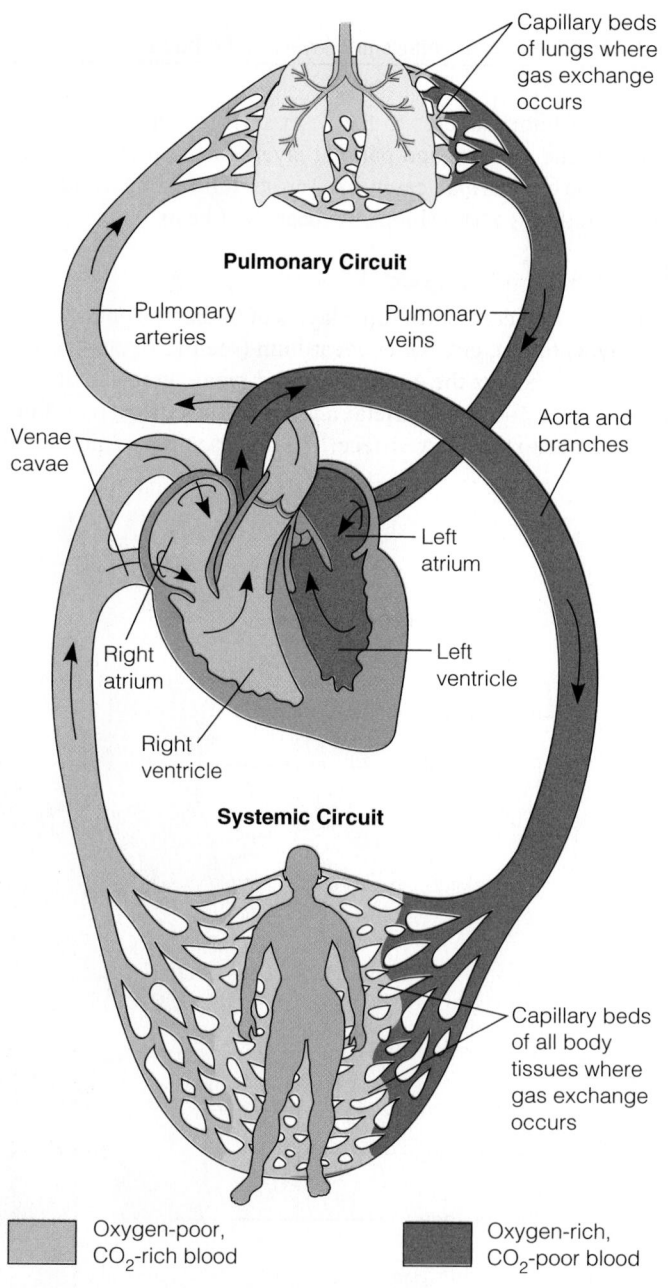

Figure 30–4 ■ Pulmonary and systemic circulation.

Figure 30–5 ■ Coronary circulation. *A,* Coronary arteries; *B,* coronary veins.

nutrients to the myocardium. The left main coronary artery divides to form the anterior descending and circumflex arteries. The anterior descending artery supplies the anterior interventricular septum and the left ventricle. The circumflex branch supplies the left lateral wall of the left ventricle. The right coronary artery supplies the right ventricle and forms the posterior descending artery. The posterior descending artery supplies the posterior portion of the heart. While ventricular contraction delivers blood through the pulmonary circulation and the systemic circulation, it is during ventricular relaxation that the coronary arteries fill with oxygen-rich blood. After the blood perfuses the heart muscle, the cardiac veins drain the blood into the coronary sinus, which empties into the right atrium of the heart (Figure 30–5B).

Blood flow through the coronary arteries is regulated by several factors. Aortic pressure is the primary factor. Other factors include the heart rate (most flow occurs during diastole, when the muscle is relaxed), metabolic activity of the heart, and blood vessel tone (constriction).

The Cardiac Cycle and Cardiac Output

The contraction and relaxation of the heart constitutes one heartbeat and is called the cardiac cycle (Figure 30–6 ■). Ventricular filling is followed by ventricular systole, a phase during which the ventricles contract and eject blood into the pulmonary and systemic circuits. Systole is followed by a relaxation phase known as diastole, during which the ventricles refill, the atria contract, and the myocardium is perfused. Normally, the complete cardiac cycle occurs about 70 to 80 times per minute, measured as the heart rate (HR).

During diastole, the volume in the ventricles is increased to about 120 mL (the end-diastolic volume), and at the end of systole, about 50 mL of blood remains in the ventricles (the

Figure 30–6 ■ The cardiac cycle has three events: (1) ventricular filling in mid-to-late diastole, (2) ventricular systole, and (3) isovolumetric relaxation in early diastole.

end-systolic volume). The difference between the end-diastolic volume and the end-systolic volume is called the **stroke volume (SV)**. Stroke volume ranges from 60 to 100 mL/beat and averages about 70 mL/beat in an adult. The **cardiac output (CO)** is the amount of blood pumped by the ventricles into the pulmonary and systemic circulations in 1 minute. Multiplying the stroke volume (SV) by the heart rate (HR) determines the cardiac output: CO × HR = SV. The **ejection fraction** is the stroke volume divided by the end-diastolic volume and represents the fraction or percent of the diastolic volume that is ejected from the heart during systole (Porth, 2005). For example, an end-diastolic volume of 120 mL divided by a stroke volume of 80 mL equals an ejection fraction of 66%. The normal ejection fraction ranges from 50% to 70%.

The average adult cardiac output ranges from 4 to 8 L/min. Cardiac output is an indicator of how well the heart is functioning as a pump. If the heart cannot pump effectively, cardiac output and tissue perfusion are decreased. Body tissues that do not receive enough blood and oxygen (carried in the blood on hemoglobin) become **ischemic** (deprived of oxygen). If the tissues do not receive enough blood flow to maintain the functions of the cells, the cells die (cellular death results in necrosis or infarction).

Activity level, metabolic rate, physiologic and psychologic stress responses, age, and body size all influence cardiac output. In addition, cardiac output is determined by the interaction of four major factors: heart rate, preload, afterload, and contractility. Changes in each of these variables influence cardiac output intrinsically, and each also can be manipulated to affect cardiac output. The heart's ability to respond to the body's changing need for cardiac output is called **cardiac reserve**.

Heart Rate

Heart rate is affected by both direct and indirect autonomic nervous system stimulation. Direct stimulation is accomplished through the innervation of the heart muscle by sympathetic and parasympathetic nerves. The sympathetic nervous system increases the heart rate, whereas the parasympathetic vagal tone slows the heart rate. Reflex regulation of the heart rate in response to systemic blood pressure also occurs through activation of sensory receptors known as baroreceptors or pressure receptors located in the carotid sinus, aortic arch, venae cavae, and pulmonary veins.

If heart rate increases, cardiac output increases (up to a point) even if there is no change in stroke volume. However, rapid heart rates decrease the amount of time available for ventricular filling during diastole. Cardiac output then falls because decreased filling time decreases stroke volume. Coronary artery perfusion also decreases because the coronary arteries fill primarily during diastole. Cardiac output decreases during bradycardia if stroke volume stays the same, because the number of cardiac cycles is decreased.

Contractility

Contractility is the inherent capability of the cardiac muscle fibers to shorten. Poor contractility of the heart muscle reduces the forward flow of blood from the heart, increases the ventricu-

lar pressures from accumulation of blood volume, and reduces cardiac output. Increased contractility may stress the heart.

Preload

Preload is the amount of cardiac muscle fiber tension, or stretch, that exists at the end of diastole, just before contraction of the ventricles. Preload is influenced by venous return and the compliance of the ventricles. It is related to the total volume of blood in the ventricles: The greater the volume, the greater the stretch of the cardiac muscle fibers, and the greater the force with which the fibers contract to accomplish emptying. This principle is called Starling's law of the heart.

This mechanism has a physiologic limit. Just as continuous overstretching of a rubber band causes the band to relax and lose its ability to recoil, overstretching of the cardiac muscle fibers eventually results in ineffective contraction. Disorders such as renal disease and congestive heart failure result in sodium and water retention and increased preload. Vasoconstriction also increases venous return and preload.

Too little circulating blood volume results in a decreased venous return and therefore a decreased preload. A decreased preload reduces stroke volume and thus cardiac output. Decreased preload may result from hemorrhage or maldistribution of blood volume, as occurs in third spacing (see Chapter 10 ∞).

Afterload

Afterload is the force the ventricles must overcome to eject their blood volume. It is the pressure in the arterial system ahead of the ventricles. The right ventricle must generate enough tension to open the pulmonary valve and eject its volume into the low-pressure pulmonary arteries. Right ventricle afterload is measured as pulmonary vascular resistance (PVR). The left ventricle, in contrast, ejects its load by overcoming the pressure behind the aortic valve. Afterload of the left ventricle is measured as systemic vascular resistance (SVR). Arterial pressures are much higher than pulmonary pressures; thus, the left ventricle has to work much harder than the right ventricle.

Alterations in vascular tone affect afterload and ventricular work. As the pulmonary or arterial blood pressure increases (e.g., through vasoconstriction), PVR and/or SVR increases, and the work of the ventricles increases. As workload increases, consumption of myocardial oxygen also increases. A compromised heart cannot effectively meet this increased oxygen demand, and a vicious cycle ensues. By contrast, a very low afterload decreases the forward flow of blood into the systemic circulation and the coronary arteries.

Clinical Indicators of Cardiac Output

For many critically ill clients, invasive hemodynamic monitoring catheters are used to measure cardiac output in quantifiable numbers. However, advanced technology is not the only way to identify and assess compromised blood flow. Because cardiac output perfuses the body's tissues, clinical indicators of low cardiac output may be manifested by changes in organ function that result from compromised blood flow. For example, a decrease in blood flow to the brain presents as a change in level of consciousness. Other manifestations of decreased cardiac output are discussed in Chapters 10 and 31 ∞ .

Cardiac index (CI) is the cardiac output adjusted for the client's body size, also called the client's body surface area (BSA). Because it takes into account the client's BSA, the cardiac index provides more meaningful data about the heart's ability to perfuse the tissues and therefore is a more accurate indicator of the effectiveness of the circulation.

BSA is stated in square meters (m^2), and cardiac index is calculated as CO divided by BSA. Cardiac measurements are considered adequate when they fall within the range of 2.5 to 4.2 $L/min/m^2$. For example, two clients are determined to have a cardiac output of 4 L/min. This parameter is within normal limits. However, one client is 5 feet, 2 inches (157 cm) tall and weighs 120 lb (54.5 kg), with a BSA of 1.54 m^2. This client's cardiac index is $4 \div 1.54$, or 2.6 $L/min/m^2$. The second client is 6 feet, 2 inches (188 cm) tall and weighs 280 lb (81.7 kg), with a BSA of 2.52 m^2. This client's cardiac index is $4 \div 2.52$, or 1.6 $L/min/m^2$. The cardiac index results show that the same cardiac output of 4 L/min is adequate for the first client but grossly inadequate for the second client.

The Conduction System of the Heart

The cardiac cycle is perpetuated by a complex electrical circuit commonly known as the intrinsic conduction system of the heart. Cardiac muscle cells possess an inherent characteristic of self-excitation, which enables them to initiate and transmit impulses independent of a stimulus. However, specialized areas of myocardial cells typically exert a controlling influence in this electrical pathway.

One of these specialized areas is the sinoatrial (SA) node, located at the junction of the superior vena cava and right atrium (Figure 30–7 ■). The SA node acts as the normal "pacemaker" of the heart, usually generating an impulse 60 to 100 times per minute. This impulse travels across the atria via internodal pathways to the atrioventricular (AV) node, in the floor of the interatrial septum. The very small junctional fibers of the AV node slow the impulse, slightly delaying its transmission to the ventricles. It then passes through the bundle of His at the atrioventricular junction and continues down the interventricular septum through the right and left bundle branches and out to the Purkinje fibers in the ventricular muscle walls.

This path of electrical transmission produces a series of changes in ion concentration across the membrane of each cardiac muscle cell. The electrical stimulus increases the permeability of the cell membrane, creating an action potential (electrical potential). The result is an exchange of sodium, potassium, and calcium ions across the cell membrane, which changes the intracellular electrical charge to a positive state. This process of depolarization results in myocardial contraction. As the ion exchange reverses and the cell returns to its resting state of electronegativity, the cell is repolarized, and cardiac muscle relaxes. The cellular action potential serves as the basis for electrocardiography (ECG), a diagnostic test of cardiac function.

The Action Potential

Movement of ions across cell membranes causes the electrical impulse that stimulates muscle contraction. This electrical activity, called the *action potential,* produces the waveforms represented on ECG strips.

In the resting state, positive and negative ions align on either side of the cell membrane, producing a relatively negative charge within the cell and a positive extracellular charge (Figure 30–8 ■). The cell is said to be polarized. The negative resting membrane

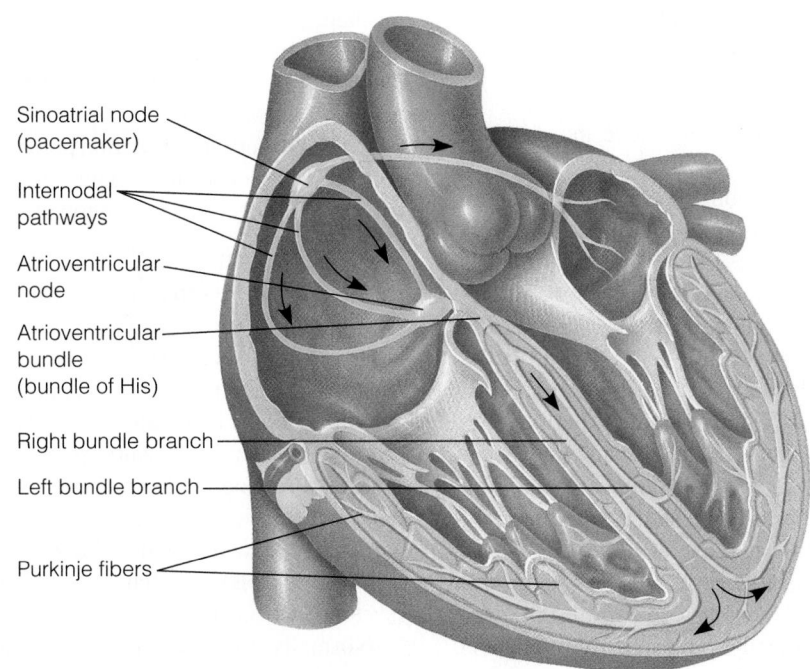

Sinoatrial node (pacemaker)

Internodal pathways

Atrioventricular node

Atrioventricular bundle (bundle of His)

Right bundle branch

Left bundle branch

Purkinje fibers

Figure 30–7 ■ The intrinsic conduction system of the heart.

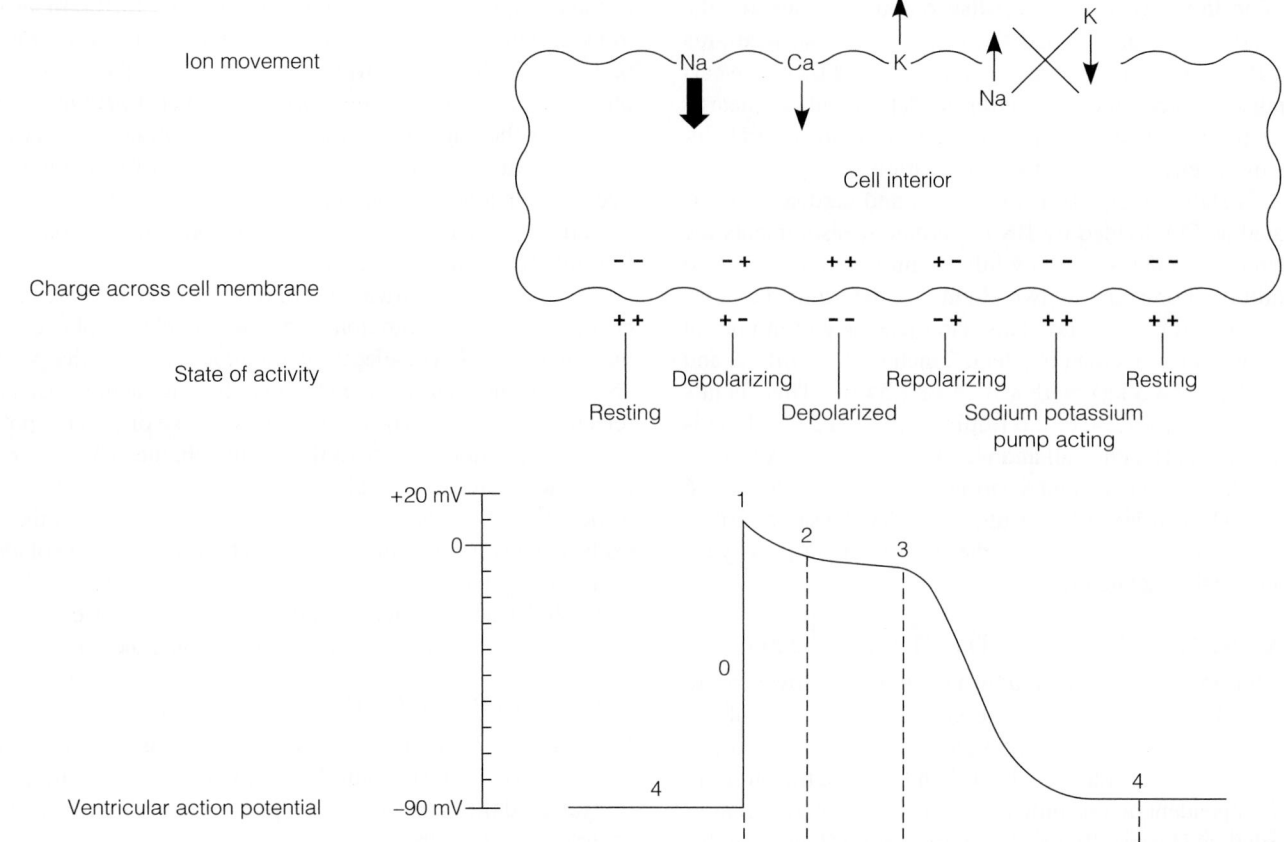

Figure 30–8 ■ Action potential of a cardiac muscle cell. In the resting state (phase 4), the cell membrane is polarized; the cell's interior has a negative charge compared to that of extracellular fluid. On depolarization (phase 0), sodium ions diffuse rapidly across the cell membrane into the cell, and calcium channels open. In the fully depolarized state (phase 1), the cell's interior has a net positive charge compared to its exterior. During the plateau period (phase 2), calcium moves into the cell and potassium diffusion slows, prolonging the action potential. In phase 3, calcium channels close, the sodium-potassium pump removes sodium from the cell, and the cell membrane again becomes polarized with a net negative charge.

potential is maintained at about −90 millivolts (mV) by the sodium-potassium pump in the cell membrane.

Depolarization

Two types of ion channels function to produce the electrical changes that occur during the depolarization phase: the fast sodium channels and the slow calcium channels. A fast action potential occurs in atrial and ventricular muscle cells and the Purkinje conduction system and uses the fast sodium channels. The slow type occurs in the SA and AV nodes, which use the slow calcium channels. The action potential for contraction of the heart is initiated in the SA node. When a resting cell is stimulated by an electrical charge from a neighboring cell or by a spontaneous event, its cell membrane permeability changes. Sodium ions enter the cell, and the membrane becomes less permeable to potassium ions. Addition of positively charged ions to intracellular fluid changes the membrane potential from negative to slightly positive at +20 to +30 mV. This change in the electrical charge across the cell membrane is called depolarization.

As the cell becomes more positive, it reaches a point called the threshold potential. When the threshold potential is

reached, an action potential is generated. The response to the action potential in the myocardial muscle cells causes a chemical reaction of calcium within the cell. This, in turn, causes actin and myosin filaments to slide together, producing cardiac muscle contraction. The action potential spreads to surrounding cells, causing a coordinated muscle contraction. As soon as the myocardium is completely depolarized, repolarization begins.

Repolarization

Repolarization returns the cell to its resting, polarized state. During rapid repolarization, fast sodium channels close abruptly, and the cell begins to regain its negative charge. During the plateau phase, muscle contraction is prolonged as slow calcium-sodium channels remain open. When these channels close, the sodium-potassium pump restores ion concentration to normal resting levels. The cell membrane is then polarized, ready for the cycle to start again. Each heartbeat represents one cardiac cycle, with one depolarization and repolarization cycle and one complete cardiac muscle contraction and relaxation (systole and diastole).

Normally, only pacemaker cells demonstrate automaticity. Pacemaker cells have a resting potential that is much less negative (−70 to −50 mV) than other cardiac muscle cells. Their threshold potential also is lower than that of other myocardial cells. These differences result from constant leakage of sodium and potassium ions into the cell.

Myocardial cells have a unique protective property, the refractory period, during which they resist stimulation. This property protects cardiac muscle from spasm and tetany. During the absolute refractory period, depolarization will not occur no matter how strongly the cell is stimulated. It is followed by the relative refractory period, during which a greater than normal stimulus is required to generate another action potential. During the supernormal period that follows, a mild stimulus will cause depolarization. Many cardiac dysrhythmias are triggered during the relative refractory and supernormal periods.

ASSESSING CARDIAC FUNCTION

Cardiac function is assessed by findings from diagnostic tests, a health assessment interview to collect subjective data, and a physical assessment to collect objective data. Sample documentation of an assessment of cardiac function is included in the box below.

Diagnostic Tests

The results of diagnostic tests of cardiac function are used to support the diagnosis of a specific disease, to provide information to identify or modify the appropriate medications or therapy used to treat the disease, and to help nurses monitor the client's responses to treatment and nursing care interventions. Diagnostic tests to assess the structures and functions of the heart are described on pages 944–946 and summarized in the following bulleted list. More information is included in the discussion of specific disorders in Chapters 31 and 32 ∞.

- The primary test used to identify the risk of coronary artery disease (CAD) or to monitor treatment for alterations in lipid levels is a measurement of lipid components of cholesterol, triglycerides, and lipolipids in the blood.
- Noninvasive tests of cardiac structure and function include a chest x-ray and stress/exercise tests. The treadmill test is the most basic exercise test, with diagnostic ability to measure cardiac perfusion enhanced by administering IV ra-

dioisotopes during the test. A treadmill exercise test is often combined with other tests to evaluate cardiac function under stress. The exercise thallium or technetium test is probably the most useful noninvasive test to monitor and diagnose CAD.

- Abnormal areas of the heart may be identified and evaluated by an MRI to locate areas of myocardial infarction, a CT scan to quantify calcium deposits in coronary arteries, or a PET test to evaluate myocardial perfusion and myocardial metabolic function.
- Echocardiograms are conducted in conjunction with Dopplers and color flow imaging to produce audio and graphic data about the motion, wall thickness, and chamber size of the heart and of the blood flow and velocity.
- A transesophageal echocardiogram (TEE) allows visualization of structures adjacent to the esophagus to visualize cardiac and extracardiac structures, including mitral valve and aortic valve pathology, left atrium intracardiac thrombosis, acute dissection of the aorta, endocarditis, and ventricular function during and after surgery.
- A cardiac catheterization with either coronary angiography or coronary arteriography may be performed to identify CAD or cardiac valvular disease, to determine pulmonary artery or heart chamber pressures, to obtain a myocardial biopsy, to evaluate artificial valves, or to do angioplasty or stent of an area of CAD.
- Pericardiocentesis is a procedure done to remove fluid from the pericardial sac for diagnostic or therapeutic purposes. It may also be an emergency procedure to treat cardiac tamponade.

Regardless of the type of diagnostic test, the nurse is responsible for explaining the procedure and any special preparation needed, for assessing for medication use that may affect the outcome of the tests, for supporting the client during the examination as necessary, for documenting the procedures as appropriate, and for monitoring the results of the tests.

Genetic Considerations

When conducting a health assessment interview and physical assessment, it is important for the nurse to consider genetic influences on health of the adult. During the health assessment interview, ask about family members with health problems affecting cardiac function, or of a family history of high cholesterol levels or early onset coronary artery disease. During the physical assessment, assess for any manifestations that might indicate a genetic disorder (see the box on page 950). If data are found to indicate genetic risk factors or alterations, ask about genetic testing and refer for appropriate genetic counseling and evaluation. Chapter 8 ∞ provides further information about genetics in medical-surgical nursing.

The Health Assessment Interview

A health assessment interview to determine problems with cardiac structure and function may be conducted during a health screening, may focus on a chief complaint (such as

---

SAMPLE DOCUMENTATION
Assessment of Cardiac Function

56-year-old male admitted to cardiac critical care unit from ED to rule out myocardial infarction. States he has pain in the middle of his chest that is "like a heavy pressure"; 6 on a 10-point scale. Skin cool, slightly moist. BP 190/94 right arm and 186/92 left arm (both reclining). Apical pulse 92, regular and strong. No pulse deficit. Respirations 28. Apical impulse nonpalpable, no visible heaves or thrusts. S₁ and S₂ auscultated without murmurs or clicks. S₄ noted.

DIAGNOSTIC TESTS   of Cardiac Disorders

NAME OF TEST   Lipids

PURPOSE AND DESCRIPTION   Blood lipids are cholesterol, triglycerides, and phospholipids. They circulate bound to proteins, and so are known as lipoproteins. Lipids are measured to evaluate risk for CAD and to monitor effectiveness of anti-cholesterol medications.

Normal values:
Cholesterol: 140–200 mg/dL
Triglycerides: 40–190 mg/dL

HDL: Men=37–70 mg/dL
Women=40–88 mg/dL
LDL: <130 mg/dL
(*Note:* Normal values may vary by laboratory.)

RELATED NURSING CARE   Cholesterol levels alone may be measured at any time of the day, regardless of food or fluid intake. When measuring triglycerides and lipoproteins (HDL and LDL), fasting for 12 hours (except for water) with no alcohol intake for 24 hours prior to the test is recommended.

NAME OF TEST   Electrocardiogram (ECG)

PURPOSE AND DESCRIPTION   See Boxes 30–1 and 30–2.

RELATED NURSING CARE   No special preparation is needed.

NAME OF TEST   Chest x-ray

PURPOSE AND DESCRIPTION   An x-ray of the thorax can illustrate the contours, placement, and chambers of the heart. It may be done to identify heart displacement or hypertrophy, or fluid in the pericardial sac.

RELATED NURSING CARE   No special preparation is needed.

NAME OF TEST   Stress/exercise tests
- Treadmill test

PURPOSE AND DESCRIPTION   Stress testing is based on the theory that CAD results in depression of the ST segment with exercise. Depression of the ST segment and depression or inversion of the T wave indicates myocardial ischemia. When the client is walking on a treadmill machine, the work rate of the heart is changed every 3 minutes for 15 minutes by increasing the speed and degree of incline by 3% each time. Clients exercise until they are fatigued, develop symptoms, or reach their maximum predicted heart rate.

RELATED NURSING CARE   *For all stress/exercise tests:* Ask the client to wear comfortable shoes, and to avoid food, fluids, and smoking for 2 to 3 hours before the test, assess for events that contraindicate the tests: recent myocardial infarction; severe, unstable angina; controlled dysrhythmias; congestive heart failure; or recent pulmonary embolism.

NAME OF TEST   Thallium/technetium stress test (myocardial imaging perfusion test, cardiac blood pool imaging)

PURPOSE AND DESCRIPTION   *Thallium stress test:* Thallium-201, a radioisotope that accumulates in myocardial cells, is used during the stress test to evaluate myocardial perfusion. Second scans are done 2 to 3 hours later when the heart is at rest; this is to differentiate between an ischemic area and an infarcted or scarred area of myocardium.

Exercise technetium perfusion test: Technetium 99m-laced compounds are administered and a scan is done to evaluate cardiac perfusion, wall motion, and ejection fraction. This is probably the most useful noninvasive test to diagnose and monitor CAD.

RELATED NURSING CARE   Assess medications; those that affect the blood pressure or heart rate should be discontinued for 24 to 36 hours prior to the test (unless the test is being done to monitor the effectiveness of the medications).

NAME OF TEST   Nuclear persantine [dipyridamole] stress test

PURPOSE AND DESCRIPTION   This test is used when the client is not physically able to walk on the treadmill. Persantine, given IV, dilates the coronary arteries and increases myocardial blood flow. Coronary arteries that are narrowed from CAD cannot dilate to increase myocardial perfusion.

RELATED NURSING CARE   Client is NPO after midnight except for water. Food, fluids, and drugs that contain caffeine should be avoided for 24 hours prior to the test, as should decaffeinated fluids. Some drugs, such as theophylline preparations, are discontinued for 36 hours prior to the test.

NAME OF TEST   Nuclear dobutamine stress test

PURPOSE AND DESCRIPTION   Dobutamine is an adrenergic drug that increases myocardial contractility, heart rate, and systolic blood pressure, which increases coronary oxygen consumption and thus increases coronary blood flow.

RELATED NURSING CARE   Client is NPO after midnight except for water. Discontinue beta-blockers, calcium channel blockers, and ACE inhibitors for 36 hours prior to the test. Do not administer nitrates for 6 hours prior to the test.

NAME OF TEST   Magnetic resonance imaging (MRI)

PURPOSE AND DESCRIPTION   An MRI may be used to identify and locate areas of myocardial infarction.

RELATED NURSING CARE   Assess for any metallic implants (such as pacemaker, body piercing, or artificial joint), which would contraindicate the test.

DIAGNOSTIC TESTS of Cardiac Disorders (continued)

NAME OF TEST Computed tomography (CT) scan

PURPOSE AND DESCRIPTION A CT scan may be conducted to quantify calcium deposits in coronary arteries.

RELATED NURSING CARE Assess for allergy to iodine or seafood if contrast medium is to be administered.

NAME OF TEST Cardiolite scan

PURPOSE AND DESCRIPTION Used to evaluate blood flow in different parts of the heart. Cardiolite (technetium 99m sestamibi) is injected IV. In a dipyridamole cardiolite scan, dipyridamole (Persantine) is injected to increase blood flow to coronary arteries. These scans may be done in conjunction with a treadmill test.

RELATED NURSING CARE See information in this table for treadmill test. Instruct the client to avoid intake of caffeine for 12 hours before having a test with dipyridamole cardiolite.

NAME OF TEST Positron emission tomography (PET)

PURPOSE AND DESCRIPTION Two scans are performed following injection of radionuclides, and the resulting images compared for myocardial perfusion and myocardial metabolic function. A stress test (treadmill) may be a part of the test. If the myocardium is ischemic or damaged, the images will be different. Normally, the images will be the same.

RELATED NURSING CARE Assess client's blood glucose: For accurate metabolic activity images, the blood glucose level must be between 60 and 140 mg/dL. If exercise is included in the test, the client will need to be NPO and avoid smoking and caffeine for 24 hours prior to the test.

NAME OF TEST Blood pool imaging

PURPOSE AND DESCRIPTION Following intravenous injection of technetium 99m pertechnetate, sequential evaluation of the heart can be performed for several hours. Useful for evaluation of cardiac status following myocardial infarction and congestive heart failure and effectiveness of cardiac medications. Can be done at the client's bedside.

RELATED NURSING CARE No special preparation is needed.

NAME OF TEST Echocardiogram

- M-mode
- Two-dimensional (2-D)
- Cardiac Doppler
- Color Doppler
- Stress echocardiogram

PURPOSE AND DESCRIPTION Echocardiograms use a transducer to record waves that are bounced off the heart, and to record the direction and flow of blood through the heart in audio and graphic data. An *M(motion)-mode echocardiogram* records the motion, wall thickness, and chamber size of the heart. A *2-D echocardiogram* provides a cross-sectional view of the heart. *Color flow imaging* combines 2-D echocardiography and Doppler technology to evaluate the speed and direction of blood flow through the heart, which can identify pathology such as leaky valves. *Stress echocardiography* combines a treadmill test with ultrasound images to evaluate segmental function and wall motion. If the client is not physically able to exercise, IV dobutamine may be administered and ultrasound images takes.

RELATED NURSING CARE No special preparation is needed; see related nursing care for the client having a treadmill test for a stress echocardiogram.

NAME OF TEST Transesophageal echocardiography (TEE)

PURPOSE AND DESCRIPTION Allows visualization of adjacent cardiac and extracardiac structures to identify or monitor mitral and aortic valve pathology, left atrium intracardiac thrombus, acute dissection of the aorta, endocarditis, perioperative left ventricular function, and intracardiac repairs during surgery. A transducer (probe) attached to an endoscope is inserted into the esophagus, and images are taken. Concurrent IV contrast medium, Doppler ultrasound, and color flow imaging may be used.

NAME OF TEST Cardiac catheterization (coronary angiography, coronary arteriography)

PURPOSE AND DESCRIPTION A cardiac catheterization may be performed to identify CAD or cardiac valvular disease, to determine pulmonary artery or heart chamber pressures, to obtain a myocardial biopsy, to evaluate artificial valves, or to perform angioplasty or stent an area of CAD. The test is performed by inserting a long catheter into a vein or artery (depending on whether the right side or the left side of the heart is being examined) in the arm or leg. Using fluoroscopy, the catheter is then threaded to the heart chambers or coronary arteries or both. Contrast dye is injected and heart structures are visualized and heart activity is filmed. The test is done for diagnosis and before heart surgery.

Right cardiac catheterization: The catheter is inserted into the femoral vein or antecubital vein and then threaded through the inferior vena cava into the right atrium to the pulmonary artery. Pressures are measured at each site and blood samples can be obtained for the right side of the heart. The functions of the tricuspid and pulmonary valves can be observed.

Left cardiac catheterization: The catheter is inserted into the brachial or femoral artery and advanced retrograde through the aorta to the coronary arteries and/or left ventricle. The patency of the coronary arteries and/or functions of the aortic and mitral valves and left ventricle can be observed.

NURSING CARE: CARDIAC CATHETERIZATION

Before the Procedure

- Explain the procedure to the client.
- No food or fluids are allowed for 6 to 8 hours before the test.

(continued)

DIAGNOSTIC TESTS of Cardiac Disorders (continued)

- Assess for allergies to seafood, iodine, or iodine contrast dyes (if previous tests have been done). If an allergic response to the dye is possible, antihistamines (such as Benadryl) or steroids may be administered the evening before and the morning of the test.
- Assess for use of aspirin or NSAIDs (risk of bleeding), Viagra (risk of heart problems), or history of kidney disease (dye used may be toxic to the kidneys).
- Discontinue oral anticoagulant medications. Heparin may be ordered to prevent thrombi.
- An IV of 5% D$_5$W is started at a keep-vein-open rate (to be available if emergency drugs have to be administered).
- Establish baseline of peripheral pulses.
- Take and record baseline vital signs.

Procedure

- Client is positioned on a padded table that tilts. A local anesthetic is used at the site of catheter insertion. ECG leads are applied and vital signs are monitored during the procedure.

The client lies supine and is asked to cough and deep breathe frequently. The procedure takes 1/2 to 3 hours.
- Tell the client that a hot, flushing sensation may be felt for a minute or two when the dye is injected.

After the Procedure

- Monitor vital signs every 15 minutes for the first hour and then every 30 minutes until stable. Assess cardiac rhythm and rate for alterations. Assess peripheral pulses distal to the insertion site.
- Assess client for complaints of chest heaviness, shortness of breath, and abdominal or groin pain.
- Monitor catheter insertion site for bleeding or hematoma.
- Administer pain medications as prescribed.
- Instruct client to remain on bed rest for 6 to 12 hours (or as ordered). If a collagen-like plug was inserted after removal of the catheter, only a 2- to 3-hour bed rest is necessary.
- Encourage oral fluids unless contraindicated (i.e., if the client has congestive heart failure).

NAME OF TEST Pericardiocentesis

PURPOSE AND DESCRIPTION This procedure is performed to remove fluid from the pericardial sac for diagnostic or therapeutic purposes. It may also be done as an emergency procedure for the client with cardiac tamponade (which may result in death). A large-gauge (16 to 18) needle is inserted to the left of the xiphoid process into the pericardial sac and excess fluid is withdrawn (see Figure 30–9 ■). The needle is attached to an ECG lead to help determine if the needle is touching the epicardial surface, thus preventing piercing of the myocardium.

NURSING CARE: PERICARDIOCENTESIS

Before the Procedure

- Gather all supplies:
  a. Pericardiocentesis tray
  b. ECG machine and electrode patches
  c. Emergency cart with defibrillator
  d. Dressing
  e. Culture bottles (if indicated)
- Reinforce teaching and answer questions about the procedure or associated care. Provide emotional support.
- Ensure that informed consent has been obtained.
- Provide for privacy.
- Obtain and document baseline vital signs.
- Connect the client to a cardiac monitor; obtain a baseline rhythm strip for comparison during and after the procedure.
- Connect the precordial ECG lead of the hub of the aspiration needle using an alligator clamp.

During the Procedure

- Follow standard precautions.
- Position seated at a 45- to 60-degree angle. Place a dry towel under the rib cage to catch blood or fluid leakage.
- Observe the ST segment for elevation and the ECG monitor for signs of myocardial irritability (PVCs) during the procedure. These indicate that the needle is touching the myocardium and should be withdrawn slightly.

Myocardium

Pericardial sac

Figure 30–9 ■ Pericardiocentesis.

- Notify the physician of changes in cardiac rhythm, blood pressure, heart rate, level of consciousness, and urine output. These may indicate cardiac complications.
- Monitor central venous pressure (CVP) and blood pressure closely. As the effusion is relieved, CVP will decrease, and BP will increase.

After the Procedure

- Document the procedure and the client's response to and tolerance of the procedure.
- Continue to monitor vital signs and cardiac rhythm every 15 min during the first hour, every 30 min during the next hour, every hour for the next 24 hours.
- Record the amount of fluid removed as output on the intake and output record.
- If indicated, send a sample of aspirated fluid for culture and sensitivity and laboratory analysis.
- Assess heart and breath sounds.

BOX 30–1 Electrocardiogram

The electrocardiogram (ECG) is a graphic record of the heart's activity. Electrodes applied to the body surface are used to obtain a graphic representation of cardiac electrical activity. These electrodes detect the magnitude and direction of electrical currents produced in the heart. They attach to the electrocardiograph by an insulated wire called a lead. The electrocardiograph converts the electrical impulses it receives into a series of waveforms that represent cardiac depolarization and repolarization. Placement of electrodes on different parts of the body allows different views of this electrical activity, much like turning the head while holding a camera provides different views of the scenery. ECG waveforms and patterns are examined to detect dysrhythmias as well as myocardial damage, the effects of drugs, and electrolyte imbalances.

ECG waveforms reflect the direction of electrical flow in relation to a positive electrode. Current flowing toward the positive electrode produces an upward (positive) waveform; current flowing away from the positive electrode produces a downward (negative) waveform. Current flowing perpendicular to the positive pole produces a biphasic (both positive and negative) waveform. Absence of electrical activity is represented by a straight line called the isoelectric line.

ECG waveforms are recorded by a heated stylus on heat-sensitive paper. The paper is marked at standard intervals that represent time and voltage or amplitude (see Figure 1). Each small box is 1 mm². The recording speed of the standard ECG is 25 mm/second, so each small box represents 0.04 second. Five small boxes horizontally and vertically make one large box, equivalent to 0.20 second. Five large boxes represent 1 full second. Measured vertically, each small box represents 0.1 mV.

Both bipolar and unipolar leads are used in recording the ECG. A bipolar lead uses two electrodes of opposite polarity (negative and positive). In a *unipolar* lead, one positive electrode and a negative reference point at the center of the heart are used. The electrical potential between the two monitoring points is graphically recorded as the ECG waveform.

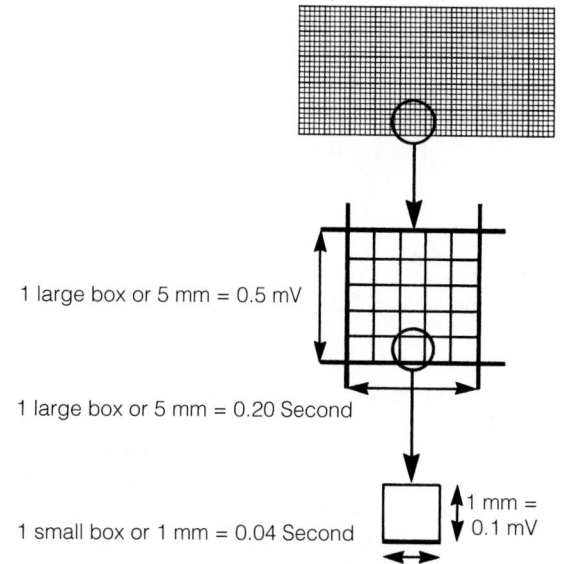

1) Time and voltage measurements on ECG paper at a recording speed of 25 mm/second.

The heart can be viewed from both the frontal plane and the horizontal plane (see Figure 2). Each plane provides a unique perspective of the heart muscle. The frontal plane is an imaginary cut through the body that views the heart from top to bottom (superior–inferior) and side to side (right–left). This perspective of the heart is analogous to a paper doll cutout. It provides information about the inferior and lateral walls of the heart. The horizontal plane is a cross-sectional view of the heart from front to back (anterior–posterior) and side to side (right–left). Information regarding the anterior, septal, and lateral walls of the heart, as well as the posterior wall, are obtained from this view.

A

Frontal plane

B

Horizontal plane

2) Planes of the heart. *A,* Frontal plane, *B,* horizontal plane.

(continued)

BOX 30–1 Electrocardiogram (continued)

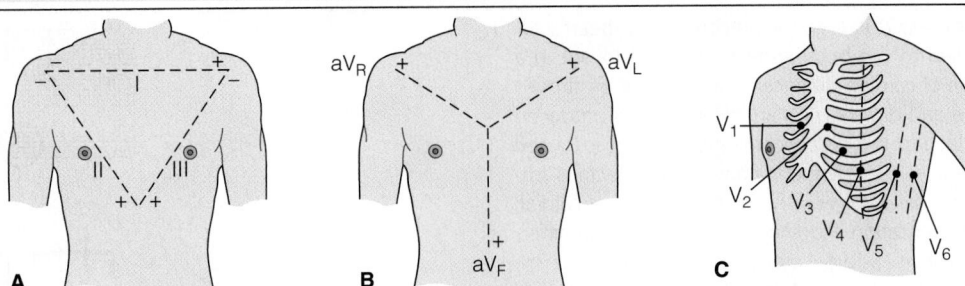

A   **B**   **C**

3) Leads of the 12-lead ECG. *A,* Bipolar limb leads I, II, III; *B,* Unipolar limb leads aV$_R$, aV$_L$, aV$_F$; *C,* Unipolar precordial leads V$_1$ to V$_6$.

A standard 12-lead ECG provides a simultaneous recording of six limb leads and six precordial leads (see Figure 3). The limb leads provide information about the heart in the frontal plane and include three bipolar leads (I, II, III) and three unipolar leads (aV$_R$, aV$_L$, and aV$_F$). The bipolar limb leads measure electrical activity between a negative lead on one extremity and a positive lead on another. The unipolar limb leads (called augmented leads) measure the electrical activity between a single positive electrode on a limb (right arm [R], left arm [L], or left leg [F for foot]), and the center of the heart.

The precordial leads, also known as chest leads or V leads, view the heart in the horizontal plane. They include six unipolar leads (V$_1$, V$_2$, V$_3$, V$_4$, V$_5$, and V$_6$), which measure electrical activity between the center of the heart and a positive electrode on the chest wall.

The cardiac cycle is depicted as a series of waveforms, the P, Q, R, S, and T waves (see Figure 4).

■ The *P wave* represents atrial depolarization and contraction. The impulse is from the sinus node. The P wave precedes the QRS complex and is normally smooth, round, and upright. P waves may be absent when the SA node is not acting as the pacemaker. Atrial repolarization occurs during ventricular depolarization and usually is not seen on the ECG.

■ The *PR interval* represents the time required for the sinus impulse to travel to the AV node and into the Purkinje fibers. This interval is measured from beginning of P wave to beginning of QRS complex. If no Q wave is seen, the beginning of the R wave is used. The PR interval is normally 0.12 to 0.20 second (up to 0.24 second is considered normal in clients over age 65). PR intervals greater than 0.20 second indicate a delay in conduction from the SA node to the ventricles.

■ The *QRS complex* represents ventricular depolarization and contraction. The QRS complex includes three separate waves: The Q wave is the first negative deflection, the R wave is the positive or upright deflection, and the S wave is the first negative deflection after the R wave. Not all QRS complexes have all three waves; nonetheless, the complex is called a QRS complex. The normal duration of a QRS complex is from 0.06 to 0.10 second. QRS complexes greater than 0.10 second indicate delays in transmitting the impulse through the ventricular conduction system.

■ The *ST segment* signifies the beginning of ventricular repolarization. The ST segment, the period from the end of the QRS complex to the beginning of the T wave, should be isoelectric. An abnormal ST segment is displaced (elevated or depressed) from the isoelectric line.

■ The *T wave* represents ventricular repolarization. It normally has a smooth, rounded shape that is usually less than 10 mm tall. It usually points in the same direction as the QRS complex. Abnormalities of the T wave may indicate myocardial ischemia or injury, or electrolyte imbalances.

■ The *QT interval* is measured from the beginning of the QRS complex to the end of the T wave. It represents the total time of ventricular depolarization and repolarization. Its duration varies with gender, age, and heart rate; usually, it is 0.32 to 0.44 second long. Prolonged QT intervals indicate a prolonged relative refractory period and a greater risk of dysrhythmias. Shortened QT intervals may result from medications or electrolyte imbalances.

■ The *U wave* is not normally seen. It is thought to signify repolarization of the terminal Purkinje fibers. If present, the U wave follows the same direction as the T wave. It is most commonly seen in hypokalemia.

Sinoatrial node

Atrioventricular node

QRS complex

R

Ventricular depolarization

Ventricular repolarization

Atrial depolarization

P

T

PR Interval

Q

S

ST Segment

Time(s)   0   0.2   0.4   0.6   0.8

QT Interval

4) Normal ECG waveform and intervals.

BOX 30–2 Interpreting an ECG

Interpreting an ECG strip to determine the cardiac rhythm is a skill that takes practice to learn and master. Many methods are used to analyze ECGs. It is important to use a consistent method for ECG analysis. Identifying and interpreting complex dysrhythmias requires advanced skills and knowledge obtained through further training. One method follows:

■ *Step 1: Determine rate.* Assess heart rate. Use P waves to determine the atrial rate and R waves for the ventricular rate. Several approaches can determine the heart rate.

  ■ Count the number of complexes in a 6-second rhythm strip (the top margin of ECG paper is marked at 3-second intervals), and multiply by 10. This provides an estimate of the rate and is particularly valuable if rhythms are irregular.

  ■ Count the number of large boxes between two consecutive complexes, and divide 300 (the number of large boxes in 1 minute) by this number. For example, there are 6 large boxes between two R waves; 300 divided by 6 equals a ventricular rate of 50 bpm. Memorize the following sequence for rapid rate determination: 300, 150, 100, 75, 60, 50, 43. One large box between complexes equals a rate of 300; two, a rate of 150; three, a rate of 100; and so on.

  ■ Count the number of small boxes between two consecutive complexes, and divide 1500 (the number of small boxes in 1 minute) by this number. For example, there are 19 small boxes between two R waves; 1500 divided by 19 equals a ventricular rate of 79 bpm. This is the most precise measurement of heart rate.

■ *Step 2: Determine regularity.* Regularity is the consistency with which the P waves or QRS complexes occur. In a regular rhythm, all waves occur at a consistent rate. Rhythm regularity is determined by measuring the interval between consecutive waves. Place one point of an ECG caliper (a measuring device) on the peak of the P wave (for atrial rhythm) or the R wave (for ventricular rhythm). Adjust the other point to the peak of the next wave, P to P or R to R (see the figure in this box). Keeping the calipers set at this distance, evaluate intervals between consecutive waves. The rhythm is *regular* if all caliper points fall on succeeding wave peaks. Alternately, use a strip of blank paper on top of the ECG strip, marking the peaks of two or three consecutive waves. Then move the paper along the strip to consecutive waves. Wave peaks that vary by more than one to three small boxes (depending on the rate) are *irregular*. Irregular rhythms may be *irregularly irregular* (if the intervals have no pattern) or *regularly irregular* (if a consistent pattern to the irregularity can be identified).

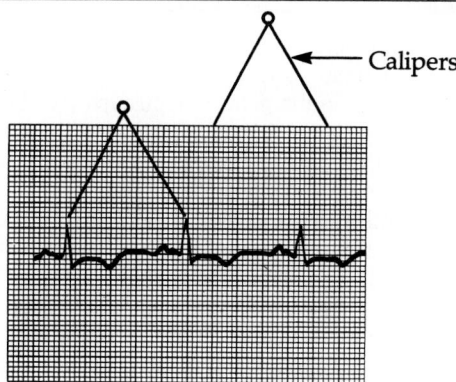

Calipers

■ *Step 3: Assess P wave.* The presence or absence of P waves helps determine origin of the rhythm. All the P waves should be alike in size and shape (*morphology*). If P waves are not seen or they differ in shape, the rhythm may not originate in the sinus node.

■ *Step 4: Assess P to QRS relationship.* Determine the relationship between P waves and QRS complexes. There should be one and only one P wave for every QRS complex, because the normal stimulus for ventricular contraction originates in the sinus node.

■ *Step 5: Determine interval durations.* To evaluate impulse transmission through the cardiac conduction system, measure the PR interval, QRS duration, and QT interval. To measure, count the number of small boxes from the beginning of the interval to the end, and multiply by 0.04 second. Then determine whether the interval duration is within its normal limits. For example, the PR interval is 3.5 small boxes wide, or 0.14 second. This is within the normal limits of 0.12 to 0.20 second. This interval should be consistent, not varying from beat to beat. A PR interval greater than 0.20 second or one that varies from beat to beat is abnormal.

The QRS complex duration is normally between 0.06 and 0.10 second. A QRS complex greater than 0.12 second indicates delayed ventricular conduction.

The QT interval is normally 0.32 to 0.44 second. It varies inversely with the heart rate: The faster the heart rate, the shorter the QT interval. As a general rule, the QT interval should be no more than half the previous R–R interval. A prolonged QT interval indicates a prolonged relative refractory period of the heart.

■ *Step 6: Identify abnormalities.* Note the presence and frequency of *ectopic* (extra) beats, deviation of the ST segment above or below the baseline, and abnormalities in waveform shape and duration.

chest pain), or may be part of a total health assessment. If the client has a problem with cardiac function, analyze its onset, characteristics, course, severity, precipitating and relieving factors, and any associated symptoms, noting the timing and circumstances. For example, ask the client:

■ What is the location of the chest pain you experienced? Did it move up to your jaw or into your left arm?

■ Describe the type of activity that brings on your chest pain.

■ Have you noticed any changes in your energy level?

■ Have you felt light-headed during the times your heart is racing?

The interview begins by exploring the client's chief complaint (e.g., chest pain, palpitations, or shortness of breath). Describe the client's chest pain in terms of location, quality or character, timing, setting or precipitating factors, severity, aggravating and relieving factors, and associated symptoms (Table 30–1).

Explore the client's history for heart disorders such as angina, heart attack, congestive heart failure (CHF), hypertension

GENETIC CONSIDERATIONS
Cardiac Disorders

- Familial hypercholesterolemia is a single gene disorder that results in atherosclerosis and CAD, which may occur at an earlier age than in the general population (i.e., before age 55 in men and age 65 in women). However, increased cholesterol levels may also be inherited and are a risk factor for CAD in both men and women.

- Marfan's syndrome is an autosomal-dominant inherited disorder that affects the skeleton, the eyes, and the cardiovascular system. The cardiovascular effects are a dilatation of the proximal aorta and aortic dissection associated with degeneration of the elastic fibers in the tunica media of the aorta. There may also be thoracic aortic aneurysms.

- Supraventricular aortic stenosis (SVAS) is a genetic vascular disorder resulting in an hourglass-shaped stenosis of the ascending aorta. It may also affect other major arteries, including the pulmonary, carotid, cerebral, renal, and coronary arteries.

- Hypertropic cardiomyopathy, a disease of sarcomere proteins, has a genetic transmission.

- Williams syndrome is a rare genetic disorder characterized by characteristic "elfin-like" features and heart and blood vessel problems (as well as other physical problems).

- Long QT syndrome (LQTS) is an inherited genetic disorder that results from structural abnormalities of the potassium channels in the heart, leading to dysrhythmias. This can result in unconsciousness, and may cause sudden cardiac death in teenagers and young adults when exposed to stressors ranging from exercise to loud sounds.

TABLE 30–1 Assessing Chest Pain

CHARACTERISTIC	EXAMPLES
Location	Substernal, precordial, jaw, back Localized or diffuse Radiation to neck, jaw, shoulder, arm
Character/quality	Pressure; tightness; crushing, burning, or aching quality; heaviness; dullness; "heartburn" or indigestion
Timing: onset, duration, and frequency	Onset: Sudden or gradual? Duration: How many minutes does the pain last? Frequency: Is the pain continuous or periodic?
Setting/precipitating factors	Awake, at rest, sleep interrupted? With activity? With eating, exertion, exercise, elimination, emotional upset?
Intensity/severity	Can range from 0 (no pain) to 10 (worst pain ever felt)
Aggravating factors	Activity, breathing, temperature
Relieving factors	Medication (nitroglycerin, antacid), rest; there may be no relieving factors
Associated symptoms	Fatigue, shortness of breath, palpitations, nausea and vomiting, sweating, anxiety, light-headedness or dizziness

(HTN), and valvular disease. Ask the client about previous heart surgery or illnesses, such as rheumatic fever, scarlet fever, or recurrent streptococcal throat infections. Also ask about the presence and treatment of other chronic illnesses such as diabetes mellitus, bleeding disorders, or endocrine disorders. Review the client's family history for CAD, HTN, stroke, hyperlipidemia, diabetes, congenital heart disease, or sudden death.

Ask the client about past or present occurrence of various cardiac symptoms, such as chest pain, shortness of breath, difficulty breathing, cough, palpitations, fatigue, light-headedness or dizziness, fainting, heart **murmur**, blood clots, or swelling. Because cardiac function affects all other body systems, a full history may need to explore other related systems, such as respiratory function and/or peripheral vascular function.

Review the client's personal habits and nutritional history, including body weight; eating patterns; dietary intake of fats, salt, fluids; dietary restrictions; hypersensitivities or intolerances to food or medication; and the use of caffeine and alcohol. If the client uses tobacco products, ask about type (cigarettes, pipe, cigars, snuff), duration, amount, and efforts to quit. If the client uses street drugs, ask about type, method of intake (e.g., inhaled or injected), duration of use, and efforts to quit. Include questions about the client's activity level and tolerance, recreational activities, and relaxation

habits. Assess the client's sleep patterns for interruptions in sleep due to dyspnea, cough, discomfort, urination, or stress. Ask how many pillows the client uses when sleeping. Also consider psychosocial factors that may affect the client's stress level: What is the client's marital status, family composition, and role within the family? Have there been any changes? What is the client's occupation, level of education, and socioeconomic level? Are resources for support available? What is the client's emotional disposition and personality type? How does the client perceive his or her state of health or illness, and how able is the client to comply with treatment?

Interview questions categorized by functional health patterns are listed in the table on the next page.

Physical Assessment

Physical assessment of cardiac function may be performed either as part of a total assessment or alone for clients with suspected or known problems with cardiac function. Assess the heart through inspection, palpation, and auscultation over the precordium (the area of the chest wall overlying the heart). Normal age-related findings for the older adult are summarized in Table 30–2. Before beginning the assessment, collect all required equipment and explain the techniques to the client to decrease anxiety. A quiet environment is essential to hear and assess heart sounds accurately.

The client may sit or lie in the supine position. Movements over the precordium may be more easily seen with tangential

FUNCTIONAL HEALTH PATTERN INTERVIEW The Cardiac System

Functional Health Pattern	Interview Questions and Leading Statements
Health Perception–Health Management	■ Have you ever had any problems with your heart, such as angina (pain), heart attack, or disease of the valves? If so, describe. What was used to treat these problems? ■ Have you been diagnosed with high blood pressure? If so, how is it treated? ■ Do you have a history of rheumatic fever, scarlet fever, or strep throat infections? If so, describe them and their treatment. ■ Have you had your cholesterol checked recently? What is it? If you have high cholesterol, how is it treated? ■ Have you ever had tests to check the function of your heart? Describe them if so. ■ Do you take any medications to make your heart function more effectively, such as aspirin, those to control your heart rate, anticoagulants, or diuretics? How often do you take them? ■ Do you have a pacemaker? At what age and for what problem? How do you check the batteries? ■ Do you smoke, chew tobacco, or use snuff? If so, how often and how much? ■ Do you drink alcohol? If so, what type, how much, and for how long? ■ Are you able to manage your activities of daily living and work independently? Explain.
Nutritional-Metabolic	■ Describe your food and liquid intake in a 24-hour period. How often do you eat fried foods, fast foods, or meat? ■ How much salt do you use on food? ■ Do you eat high-fiber foods? If so, what are they and how often? ■ Have you had a recent weight gain or loss? Explain. ■ Have you noticed any change in color of your skin; for example, pale or dusky or flushed? If so, do you know what causes this? ■ Have you had any swelling in your feet or legs? Where and how much? What do you do to relieve it? ■ Do you feel tired during the day? What do you do when you are tired?
Elimination	■ Has a heart problem interfered with your usual bowel and bladder elimination? Explain.
Activity-Exercise	■ Describe your usual activity in a 24-hour period. ■ Has there been any change in your ability, energy, or strength to perform your usual activities (such as bathing, cleaning house, yard work, shopping)? If so, explain. ■ Do you ever have to stop and rest while doing daily activities? Explain. ■ Do you notice shortness of breath with certain activities? If so, what are they? How long does this last? What do you do to breathe better? ■ Describe any cough you have had. Was it dry or wet? Do you cough up mucus? If so, what color is it? How long have you had the cough? ■ Have you experienced any numbness or tingling, dizziness or light-headedness, or palpitations? Describe if so. ■ Have you ever used oxygen?
Sleep-Rest	■ How long do you sleep each night? Do you feel rested after you sleep? ■ Does your heart problem interfere with your ability to sleep and rest? Explain. ■ How many pillows do you use at night? ■ Where do you sleep at night (e.g., in a recliner to breathe more easily)? ■ Do you ever feel short of breath while you are resting or sleeping? Does this wake you up if so? Explain.
Cognitive-Perceptual	■ Describe any chest pain you have experienced. When did it occur? Where was it located? On a scale of 0 to 10, with 10 being the worst pain you have ever had, rate the pain and describe it (for example, burning, crushing, stabbing, squeezing, heavy, tight). ■ What were you doing when the pain began, for example, were you working or resting? Did it begin suddenly or gradually? How long did it last? ■ Did you have any other symptoms with the pain, such as nausea or vomiting, sweating, racing heart, pale skin, palpitations? ■ What made the pain worse? What did you do to try to relieve the pain? Did that work?
Self-Perception–Self-Concept	■ How does having this condition make you feel about yourself?
Role-Relationships	■ How does this condition affect your relationships with others? ■ Has having this condition interfered with your ability to work? Explain.

(continued)

FUNCTIONAL HEALTH PATTERN INTERVIEW The Cardiac System (continued)

Functional Health Pattern	Interview Questions and Leading Statements
Sexuality-Reproductive	■ Has this condition interfered with your usual sexual activity? ■ Have you ever had chest pain during sexual activity? What do you do for it? ■ Do you use a slower pace or different positions that are less stressful for you during sexual activities? Does this help?
Coping-Stress-Tolerance	■ Has having this condition created stress for you? ■ Have you experienced any kind of stress that makes this condition worse? Explain. ■ Describe what you do when you feel stressed.
Value-Belief	■ Describe how specific relationships or activities help you cope with this problem. ■ Describe specific cultural beliefs or practices that affect how you care for and feel about this problem. ■ Are there any specific treatments that you would not use to treat this problem?

lighting (in which the light is directed at a right angle to the area being observed, producing shadows). Assess the following types of movements:

■ The **apical impulse** is a normal, visible pulsation (**thrust**) in the area of the midclavicular line in the left fifth intercostal space. It can be seen on inspection in about half of the adult population. (The apical impulse was previously called the point of maximal impulse [PMI] but this is no longer used because a maximal impulse may occur in other areas of the precordium as a result of abnormal conditions.)

■ **Retraction** is a pulling in of the tissue of the precordium; a slight retraction just medial to the midclavicular line at the area of the apical impulse is normal and is more likely to be visible in thin clients.

■ **Pulsations** (other than the normal apical pulsations), which may be called **heaves** or **lifts**, are considered abnormal. They may occur as the result of an enlarged ventricle.

TABLE 30–2 Age-Related Cardiac Changes

AGE-RELATED CHANGE	SIGNIFICANCE
Myocardium: ↓ efficiency and contractibility. Sinus node: ↑ in thickness of shell surrounding the node, and a ↓ in the number of pacemaker cells	■ Decreased cardiac output when under physiologic stress with resulting tachycardia that lasts longer. The person may require rest time between physical activities.
Left ventricle: Slight hypertrophy, prolonged isometric contraction phase and relaxation time; ↑ time for diastolic filling and systolic emptying cycle.	■ Stroke volume may increase to compensate for tachycardia, leading to increased blood pressure.
Valves and blood vessels: Aorta is elongated and dilated, valves are thicker and more rigid, and resistance to peripheral blood flow increases by 1% per year.	■ Blood pressure increases to compensate for increased peripheral resistance and decreased cardiac output.

CARDIAC ASSESSMENTS

Technique/Normal Findings	Abnormal Findings

Apical Impulse Assessment

| First using the palmar surface and then repeating with finger pads, palpate the precordium for symmetry of movement | ■ An enlarged or displaced heart is associated with an apical impulse lateral to the midclavicular line (MCL) or below the fifth left intercostal space (ICS).
■ Increased size, amplitude, and duration of the apical impulse are associated with left ventricular volume overload (increased afterload) in conditions such as HTN and aortic |

Technique/Normal Findings	Abnormal Findings

and the apical impulse for location, size, amplitude, and duration. The sequence for palpation is shown in Figure 30–10 ■. To locate the apical impulse, ask the client to assume a left lateral recumbent position. Simultaneous palpation of the carotid pulse may also be helpful. *The apical impulse is not palpable in all clients. The apical impulse may be palpated in the mitral area, and has only a brief small amplitude.*

stenosis, and with pressure overload (increased preload) in conditions such as aortic or mitral regurgitation.

- Increased amplitude alone may occur with hyperkinetic states, such as anxiety, hyperthyroidism, and anemia.
- Decreased amplitude is associated with a dilated heart in cardiomyopathy.
- Displacement alone may also occur with dextrocardia, diaphragmatic hernia, gastric distention, or chronic lung disease.

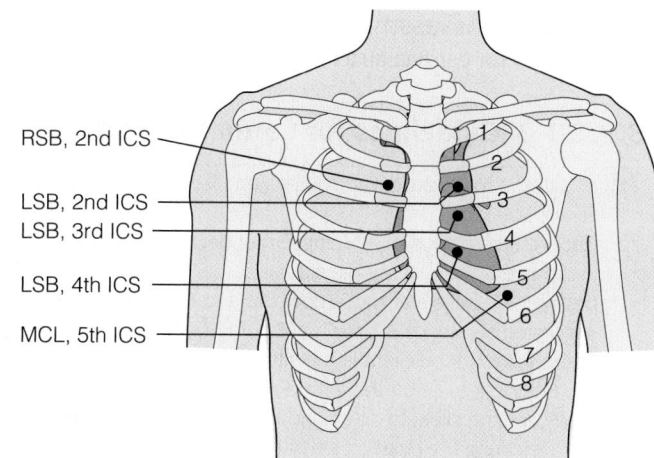

RSB, 2nd ICS
LSB, 2nd ICS
LSB, 3rd ICS
LSB, 4th ICS
MCL, 5th ICS

Figure 30–10 ■ Areas for inspection and palpation of the precordium, indicating the sequence for palpation.

- A **thrill** (a palpable vibration over the precordium or an artery) may accompany severe valve stenosis.
- A marked increase in amplitude of the apical impulse at the right ventricular area occurs with right ventricular volume overload in atrial septal defect.
- An increase in amplitude and duration occurs with right ventricular pressure overload in pulmonic stenosis and pulmonary hypertension. A lift or heave may also be seen in these conditions (and in chronic lung disease).
- A palpable thrill in this area occurs with ventricular septal defect.

Palpate the subxiphoid area with the index and middle finger. *No pulsations or vibrations should be palpated.*

- Right ventricular enlargement may produce a downward pulsation against the fingertips.
- An accentuated pulsation at the pulmonary area may be present in hyperkinetic states.
- A prominent pulsation reflects increased flow or dilation of the pulmonary artery.
- A thrill may be associated with aortic or pulmonary stenosis, aortic stenosis, pulmonary HTN, or atrial septal defect.
- Increased pulsation at the aortic area may suggest aortic aneurysm.
- A palpable second heart sound (S_2) may be noted with systemic HTN.

Cardiac Rate and Rhythm Assessment

Auscultate heart rate. *The heart rate should be 60 to 100 beats per minute with regular rhythm.*

- A heart rate exceeding 100 beats per minute (beats/min) is tachycardia. A heart rate less than 60 beats/min is bradycardia.

Simultaneously palpate the radial pulse while listening to the apical pulse. *The radial and apical pulses should be equal.*

- If the radial pulse falls behind the apical rate, the client has a pulse deficit, indicating weak, ineffective contractions of the left ventricle.

Auscultate heart rhythm. *The heart rhythm should be regular.*

- **Dysrhythmias** (abnormal heart rate or rhythm) may be regular or irregular in rhythm; their rates may be slow or fast. Irregular rhythms may occur in a pattern (e.g., an early beat every second beat, called bigeminy), sporadically, or with frequency and disorganization (e.g., atrial fibrillation). A pattern of gradual increase and decrease in heart rate that is within normal heart rate and that correlates with inspiration and expiration is called sinus arrhythmia.

MediaLink

Dysrhythmia Animation

Technique/Normal Findings   **Abnormal Findings**

Heart Sounds Assessment

See guidelines for cardiac auscultation in Box 30–3.

BOX 30–3 Guidelines for Cardiac Auscultation

1. Locate the major auscultatory areas on the precordium (see Figure 30–11).
2. Choose a sequence of listening. Either begin from the apex and move upward along the sternal border to the base, or begin at the base and move downward to the apex. One suggested sequence is shown in Figure 30–11.
3. Listen first with the client in the sitting or supine position. Then ask the client to lie on the left side, and focus on the apex. Lastly, ask the client to sit up and lean forward. These position changes bring the heart closer to the chest wall and enhance

auscultation. Carry out the following steps when the client assumes each of these positions:

a. First, auscultate each area with the diaphragm of the stethoscope to listen for high-pitched sounds: S_1, S_2, murmurs, pericardial friction rubs.
b. Next, auscultate each area with the bell of the stethoscope to listen for lower pitched sounds: S_3, S_4, murmurs.
c. Listen for the effect of respirations on each sound; while the client is sitting up and leaning forward, ask the client to exhale and hold the breath while you listen to heart sounds.

Identify S_1 (first heart sound) and note its intensity. At each auscultatory area, listen for several cardiac cycles. See Figure 30–11 ■ for auscultation areas. *S_1 is loudest at the apex of the heart.*

- An accentuated S_1 occurs with tachycardia, states in which cardiac output is high (fever, anxiety, exercise, anemia, hyperthyroidism), complete heart block, and mitral stenosis.
- A diminished S_1 occurs with first-degree heart block, mitral regurgitation, CHF, CAD, and pulmonary or systemic HTN. The intensity is also decreased with obesity, emphysema, and pericardial effusion. Varying intensity of S_1 occurs with complete heart block and grossly irregular rhythms.

Figure 30–11 ■ Areas for auscultation of the heart.

Listen for splitting of S_1. *Splitting of S_1 may occur during inspiration.*

- Abnormal splitting of S_1 may be heard with right bundle branch block and premature ventricular contractions.

Identify S_2 (second heart sound) and note its intensity. *S_2 immediately follows S_1 and is loudest at the base of the heart.*

An accentuated S_2 may be heard with HTN, exercise, excitement, and conditions of pulmonary HTN such as CHF and cor pulmonale.
- A diminished S_2 occurs with aortic stenosis, a fall in systolic blood pressure (shock), and increased anteroposterior chest diameter.

Listen for splitting of S_2. *No splitting of S_2 should be heard.*

- Wide splitting of S_2 is associated with delayed emptying of the right ventricle, resulting in delayed pulmonary valve closure (e.g., mitral regurgitation, pulmonary stenosis, and right bundle branch block).
- Fixed splitting occurs when right ventricular output is greater than left ventricular output and pulmonary valve closure is delayed (e.g., with atrial septal defect and right ventricular failure).
- Paradoxical splitting occurs when closure of the aortic valve is delayed (e.g., left bundle branch block).

Identify extra heart sounds in systole. *Extra heart sounds are not present.*

- Ejection sounds (or clicks) result from the opening of deformed semilunar valves (e.g., aortic and pulmonary stenosis).
- A midsystolic click is heard with mitral valve prolapse (MVP).

MEDIALINK | Heart Sounds Animation

Technique/Normal Findings	Abnormal Findings
Identify the presence of extra heart sounds in diastole. *Extra heart sounds are not present in diastole.*	■ An opening snap results from the opening sound of a stenotic mitral valve. ■ A pathologic S_3 (a third heart sound that immediately follows S_2, called a ventricular gallop) results from myocardial failure and ventricular volume overload (e.g., CHF, mitral or tricuspid regurgitation). ■ An S_4 (a fourth heart sound that immediately precedes S_1, called an atrial gallop) results from increased resistance to ventricular filling after atrial contraction (e.g., HTN, CAD, aortic stenosis, and cardiomyopathy). ■ A combined S_3 and S_4 is called a summation gallop and occurs with severe CHF.
Identify extra heart sounds in both systole and diastole. *No extra heart sounds should be heard during systole and diastole.*	■ A pericardial friction rub results from inflammation of the pericardial sac, as with pericarditis.

Murmur Assessment

Identify any murmurs. Note location, timing, presence during systole or diastole, and intensity. Use the following scale to grade murmurs: I = Barely heard II = Quietly heard III = Clearly heard IV = Loud V = Very loud VI = Loudest; may be heard with stethoscope off the chest. A thrill may accompany murmurs of grade IV to grade VI. Note pitch (low, medium, high), and quality (harsh, blowing, or musical). Note pattern/shape, crescendo, decrescendo, and radiation/transmission (to axilla, neck). *No murmurs should be heard.*	■ Midsystolic murmurs are heard with semilunar valve disease (e.g., aortic and pulmonary stenosis) and with hypertrophic cardiomyopathy. ■ Pansystolic (holosystolic) murmurs are heard with AV valve disease (e.g., mitral and tricuspid regurgitation, ventricular septal defect). ■ A late systolic murmur is heard with MVP. ■ Early diastolic murmurs occur with regurgitant flow across incompetent semilunar valves (e.g., aortic regurgitation). ■ Middiastolic and presystolic murmurs, such as with mitral stenosis, occur with turbulent flow across the AV valves. ■ Continuous murmurs throughout systole and all or part of diastole occur with patent ductus arteriosus.

EXPLORE MediaLink

Prentice Hall Nursing MediaLink DVD-ROM
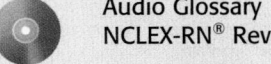
Audio Glossary
NCLEX-RN® Review

Animation/Videos
Cardiac A&P
Dysrhythmias
Heart Sounds
Hemodynamics
Oxygen Transport

COMPANION WEBSITE www.prenhall.com/lemone
Audio Glossary
NCLEX-RN® Review
Care Plan Activity: Cardiac Catheterization
Case Study: Chest Pain
MediaLink Application: Heart Sounds
Links to Resources

TEST YOURSELF NCLEX-RN® REVIEW

1 Which circulatory process supplies the heart with blood?
1. the systemic circulation
2. the pulmonary circulation
3. the coronary circulation
4. the hepatic circulation

2 The amount of blood pumped by the ventricles in 1 minute is known as:
1. heart rate.
2. ventricular contraction.
3. stroke volume.
4. cardiac output.

3 During what part of the cardiac cycle is the myocardium perfused?
1. prior to atrial filling
2. prior to ventricular relaxation
3. during diastole
4. during pulmonary perfusion

4 A client who is hemorrhaging has decreased preload. What physiologic event will follow?
1. increased afterload
2. increased ejection fraction
3. decreased cardiac output
4. decreased action potential

5 What physiologic process is responsible for the electrical impulse that stimulates myocardial contraction?
1. action potential
2. cardiac reserve
3. cardiac potential
4. ventricular contraction

6 The intensity of chest pain may be assessed by asking which question?
1. "Did the pain move into your left arm?"
2. "Was your pain relieved by resting or worse when you were busy?"
3. "On a scale of 0 (no pain) to 10 (worst pain), what number was your pain?"
4. "Was the pain a pressure, a burning, or a tightness?"

7 Which of the following is the most basic exercise stress test?
1. treadmill test
2. lipid profile
3. echocardiogram
4. cardiac catheterization

8 At what anatomic location would you assess the apical impulse?
1. left midclavicular, fifth intercostal space
2. left substernal, sixth intercostal space
3. right midaxillary, second intercostal space
4. right nipple line, any intercostal space

9 Your client's pulse rate is 50. You would document this as:
1. tachycardia.
2. bradycardia.
3. hypertension.
4. hypotension.

10 When auscultating heart sounds, where would S_1 be heard most loudly?
1. over the clavicles
2. at the apex of the heart
3. at the carotid pulse
4. at the base of the heart

See Test Yourself answers in Appendix C.

BIBLIOGRAPHY

Amella, E. (2004). Presentation of illness in older adults: If you think you know what you're looking for, think again. *American Journal of Nursing, 104*(10), 40–52.

Bench, S. (2004). Clinical skills: Assessing and treating shock. A nursing perspective. *British Journal of Nursing, 13*(12), 715–721.

Bickley, L., & Szilagyi, P. (2007). *Bates' guide to physical examination and history taking* (9th ed.). Philadelphia: Lippincott.

Burger, C. (2004). Emergency: Hypokalemia. Averting crisis with early recognition and intervention. *American Journal of Nursing, 104*(11), 61–65.

Coviello, J. (2004). Cardiac assessment 101: A new look at the guidelines for cardiac homecare patients. *Home Healthcare Nurse, 22*(2), 116–123.

Dulak, S. (2004). Hands-on help assessing heart sounds. *RN, 67*(8), 24ac1–4.

Eliopoulos, E. (2005). *Gerontological nursing* (6th ed.). Philadelphia: Lippincott Williams & Wilkins.

Harvey, S. (2004). Coronary heart disease. The nursing assessment and management of patients with angina. *British Journal of Nursing, 13*(10), 598–601.

Hayes, D. (2004). Bradycardia: Slow heart rate. Think fast! *Critical Care Choices, 4*(10), 12, 15.

Jarvis, C. (2004). *Physical examination & health assessment*. St. Louis, MO: Mosby.

Kee, J. (2005). *Prentice Hall handbook of laboratory & diagnostic tests with nursing implications*. Upper Saddle River, NJ: Prentice Hall.

Lindsey, J. (2005). Heart sounds: Do you hear what I see? *Journal of Emergency Medical Services, 30*(4), 104, 106.

MedlinePlus Medical Encyclopedia. (2004). *Cardiac catheterization*. Retrieved from http://www.nlm.nih.gov/medlineplus/ency/article/003419.htm.

Milewixz, D., & Seidman, C. (2000). Genetics of cardiovascular disease. *Circulation, 102* (Supplement 4), IV–103.

Murdaugh, J. (2003). Fatigue—a general diagnostic approach. *Australian Family Physician, 32*(11), 873–876, 935–936.

National Institutes of Health. (2003). *Genes and disease: The heart and blood vessels*. Retrieved from http://www.ncbi.nlm.nih.gov/books/bv.fcgi?rid=gnd.section.239

Porth, C. (2005). *Pathophysiology: Concepts of altered health states* (7th ed.). Philadelphia: Lippincott.

Tanabe, P., Steinmann, R., Kippenhan, M., Stehman, C., & Beach, C. (2004). Undiagnosed hypertension in the ED setting—an unrecognized opportunity by emergency nurses. *Journal of Emergency Nursing, 30*(3), 225–229, 292–297.

Weber, J., & Kelley, J. (2006). *Health assessment in nursing* (3rd ed.). Philadelphia: Lippincott.

CHAPTER 31
Nursing Care of Clients with Coronary Heart Disease

LEARNING OUTCOMES

- Discuss the coronary circulation and electrical properties of the heart.

- Compare and contrast the pathophysiology and manifestations of coronary heart disease and common cardiac dysrhythmias.

- Describe interdisciplinary and nursing care for clients with coronary heart disease and/or cardiac dysrhythmias.

- Relate the outcomes of diagnostic tests and procedures to the pathophysiology of cardiac disorders and implications for client responses to the disorder.

- Discuss nursing implications for medications and treatments used to prevent and treat coronary heart disease and dysrhythmias.

- Describe nursing care for the client undergoing diagnostic testing, an interventional procedure, or surgery for coronary heart disease or a dysrhythmia.

CLINICAL COMPETENCIES

- Assess functional health status of clients with coronary heart disease and/or a dysrhythmia, including the impact of the disorder on the client's ability to perform activities of daily living and usual tasks.

- Use knowledge of the normal anatomy and physiology of the heart in caring for clients with coronary heart disease.

- Monitor clients with coronary heart disease or dysrhythmias for expected and unexpected manifestations, reporting and recording findings as indicated.

- Use assessed data to select nursing diagnoses, determine priorities of care, and develop and implement individualized nursing interventions for clients with coronary heart disease and dysrhythmias.

- Administer medications and treatments for clients with coronary heart disease and dysrhythmias safely and knowledgeably.

- Integrate interdisciplinary care into nursing care planning and implementation for clients with coronary heart disease and dysrhythmias.

- Provide appropriate teaching for prevention, health promotion, and self-care related to coronary heart disease and dysrhythmias.

- Evaluate the effectiveness of nursing interventions, revising or modifying the plan of care as needed to promote, maintain, or restore functional health for clients with coronary heart disease or dysrhythmias.

Impaired blood flow to the myocardium, changes in the conduction of electrical impulses through the heart, and structural changes in the heart itself affect the heart's ability to fulfill its major purpose: to pump enough blood to meet the body's demand for oxygen and nutrients. Impaired cardiac function, no matter what the underlying cause, affects the client's ability to participate in exercise and activities and to fulfill life roles. Disruptions in cardiac function affect other organ systems as well, potentially leading to organ system failure and death.

Cardiovascular disease (CVD) is a generic term for disorders of the heart and blood vessels. CVD is the leading cause of death and disability in the United States. Over 64 million people have some type of cardiovascular disease. The economic costs of CVD, both direct and indirect, to the nation are estimated at $368 billion annually (National Heart, Lung, and Blood Institute [NHLBI], 2004).

On an encouraging note, however, the incidence of new CVD cases per year is decreasing. Public education aimed at reducing fat intake, increasing exercise, and lowering cholesterol levels

FAST FACTS
- Heart disease accounts for nearly 696,000 deaths annually in the United States.
- Although heart disease is primarily thought of as a disease affecting older adults, it is the third leading killer of adults ages 25 to 44 (behind accidents and cancer), and the second leading cause of death in adults ages 45 to 64 (behind only cancer).

have made people more aware of risk factors associated with CVD. The mortality rate from heart disease peaked in 1963 and has shown a slow but steady decline since that time.

This chapter focuses on disorders of myocardial blood flow (coronary heart disease) and cardiac rhythm. Disorders of cardiac structure and function are discussed in Chapter 32 ∞. Review the normal anatomy and physiology and nursing assessment of the heart in Chapter 30 ∞ before proceeding with this chapter.

DISORDERS OF MYOCARDIAL PERFUSION

THE CLIENT WITH CORONARY HEART DISEASE

Coronary heart disease (CHD), or *coronary artery disease (CAD)*, affects 13.2 million people in the United States and causes more than 500,000 deaths annually (NHLBI, 2004). CHD is caused by impaired blood flow to the myocardium. Accumulation of atherosclerotic plaque in the coronary arteries is the usual cause. Coronary heart disease may be asymptomatic, or may lead to angina pectoris, acute coronary syndrome, myocardial infarction (MI or heart attack), dysrhythmias, heart failure, and even sudden death.

Incidence and Prevalence

Many risk factors for CHD can be controlled through lifestyle modification. In fact, with increased public awareness of risk factors related to CHD, mortality rates are declining by about 3.3% per year. Nevertheless, CHD remains a major public health problem. Heart disease is the leading cause of death for all U.S. ethnic groups except Asian females (NHLBI, 2004). See the accompanying box. Nurses are in a prime position to encourage and support positive lifestyle changes by teaching

FOCUS ON CULTURAL DIVERSITY
Heart Disease

- Native Americans (American Indians and Alaska Natives) have the highest prevalence of coronary heart disease, followed by whites, African Americans, Mexican Americans and native Hawaiians, and Asian Americans.
- People with less than a high school diploma have the highest rate of CHD; people with a bachelor's degree or higher have the lowest.
- Economic status is a factor; the rate of CHD in people with a family income of less than $35,000 per year have a significantly higher rate than those with incomes greater than $75,000 per year.
- Regionally, the rate of CHD is highest in the South and lowest in the West.

and promoting healthy living practices. Individual choices can and do affect health.

The highest incidence of CHD is in the Western world, mainly in white males age 45 and older. Both men and women are affected by coronary heart disease; in women, however, the onset is about 10 years later because of the heart-protective effects of estrogen. After menopause, women's risk is equal to that of men.

Physiology Review

The two main coronary arteries, the left and the right, supply blood, oxygen, and nutrients to the myocardium. They originate in the root of the aorta, just outside the aortic valve. The *left main coronary artery* divides to form the anterior descending and circumflex arteries. The *anterior descending* artery supplies the anterior interventricular septum and the left ventricle, including the apex of the heart. The *circumflex* branch supplies the lateral wall of the left ventricle. The *right coronary artery* supplies the right ventricle and forms the posterior descending artery. The *posterior descending* artery supplies the posterior portion of the heart (see Figure 30–5).

Blood flow through the coronary arteries is regulated by several factors. Aortic pressure is the primary factor. Other factors include the heart rate (most flow occurs during diastole, when the muscle is relaxed), metabolic activity of the heart, blood vessel tone (constriction), and collateral circulation. Although there are no connections between the large coronary arteries, small arteries are joined by **collateral channels**. If large vessels are gradually occluded, these channels enlarge, providing alternative routes for blood flow (Porth, 2005).

Pathophysiology

Coronary atherosclerosis is the most common cause of reduced coronary blood flow.

Atherosclerosis

Atherosclerosis is a progressive disease characterized by *atheroma* (plaque) formation, which affects the intimal and medial layers of large and midsize arteries. See *Pathophysiology Illustrated: Coronary Heart Disease* on pages 960–961.

Atherosclerosis is initiated by unknown precipitating factors that cause lipoproteins and fibrous tissue to accumulate in the arterial wall. Although the precise mechanisms are unknown, abnormal lipid metabolism and injury to or inflammation of endothelial cells lining the artery appear to be key to its development.

In the bloodstream, lipids are transported attached to proteins called apoproteins. High levels of certain *lipoproteins*, a type of apoprotein, increase the risk of atherosclerosis. *Low-density lipoproteins*, which are high in cholesterol, carry cholesterol to peripheral tissues where some of it is released to be taken up and incorporated into cells for use in producing energy. *Very-low-density lipoproteins*, large molecules primarily composed of triglycerides and cholesterol, carry triglycerides to muscle and fat cells. When the triglycerides are released into these tissues, the remainder of the molecule is a low-density lipoprotein. *High-density lipoproteins*, in contrast, attract cholesterol, returning it from peripheral tissues to the liver.

Hyperlipidemia itself may damage arterial endothelium. Other potential mechanisms of vessel injury include excessive pressures within the arterial system (hypertension), toxins found in cigarette smoke, infections, and inflammation (Copstead & Banasik, 2005). Endothelial damage promotes platelet adhesion and aggregation, and attracts leukocytes to the area.

At the site of injury, *atherogenic* (atherosclerosis-promoting) lipoproteins collect in the intimal lining of the artery. These lipoproteins appear to actually bind with the extracellular portion of the vessel endothelium. Macrophages migrate to the injured site as part of the inflammatory process. Contact with platelets, cholesterol, and other blood components stimulates smooth muscle cells and connective tissue within the vessel wall to proliferate abnormally. Although blood flow is not affected at this stage, this early lesion appears as a yellowish fatty streak on the inner lining of the artery. Fibrous plaque develops as smooth muscle cells enlarge, collagen fibers proliferate, and blood lipids accumulate. The lesion protrudes into the arterial lumen and is fixed to the inner wall of the intima. It may invade the muscular media layer of the vessel as well. The developing plaque not only gradually occludes the vessel lumen but also impairs the vessel's ability to dilate in response to increased oxygen demands. Fibrous plaque lesions often develop at arterial bifurcations or curves or in areas of narrowing. As the plaque expands, it can produce severe stenosis or total occlusion of the artery.

The final stage of the process is the development of *atheromas,* complex lesions consisting of lipids, fibrous tissue, collagen, calcium, cellular debris, and capillaries. These calcified lesions can ulcerate or rupture, stimulating thrombosis. The vessel lumen may be rapidly occluded by the thrombus, or it may embolize to occlude a distal vessel.

Plaque formation may be *eccentric,* located in a specific, asymmetric region of the vessel wall, or *concentric,* involving the entire vessel circumference. Manifestations of the process usually do not appear until about 75% of the arterial lumen has been occluded.

Atherosclerosis tends to develop where arteries *bifurcate* or branch. Certain vessels have a higher likelihood of being affected, including the coronary arteries (the left anterior descending artery in particular), the renal arteries, the bifurcation of the carotid arteries, and branching sections of peripheral arteries. In addition to obstructing or occluding blood flow, atherosclerosis weakens arterial walls, and is a major cause of aneurysm in vessels such as the aorta and iliac arteries.

Myocardial Ischemia

Myocardial cells become ischemic when the oxygen supply is inadequate to meet metabolic demands. The critical factors in meeting metabolic demands of cardiac cells are coronary perfusion and myocardial workload. Coronary perfusion can be affected by several different mechanisms:

- One or more vessels may be partially occluded by large, stable areas of plaque.
- Platelets can aggregate in narrowed vessels, forming a thrombus.
- Normal or already narrowed vessels may spasm.
- A drop in blood pressure may lead to inadequate flow through coronary vessels.
- Normal autoregulatory mechanisms that increase flow to working muscles may fail (Copstead & Banasik, 2005).

Coronary Heart Disease

Coronary heart disease usually is due to *athero-sclerosis*, occlusion of the coronary arteries by fibrous, fatty plaque. Coronary heart disease is manifested by *angina pectoris, acute coronary syndrome,* and/or *myocardial infarction*. Risk factors for coronary heart disease include age (over 50 years), heredity, smoking, obesity, high serum cholesterol levels, hypertension, and diabetes mellitus. Other factors, such as diet and lack of exercise, also contribute to the risk of CHD.

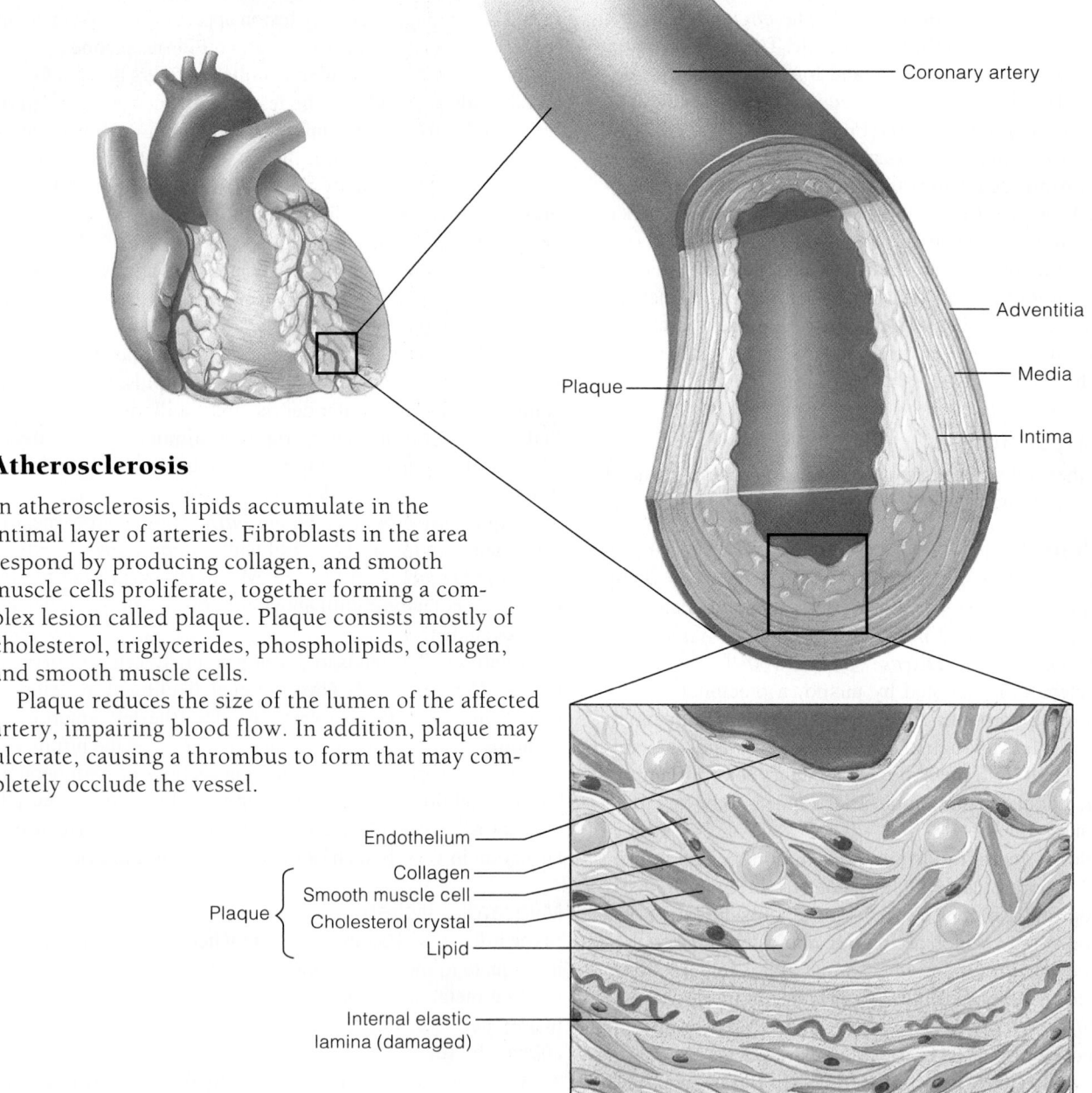

Coronary artery

Adventitia

Media

Intima

Plaque

Atherosclerosis

In atherosclerosis, lipids accumulate in the intimal layer of arteries. Fibroblasts in the area respond by producing collagen, and smooth muscle cells proliferate, together forming a complex lesion called plaque. Plaque consists mostly of cholesterol, triglycerides, phospholipids, collagen, and smooth muscle cells.

Plaque reduces the size of the lumen of the affected artery, impairing blood flow. In addition, plaque may ulcerate, causing a thrombus to form that may completely occlude the vessel.

Endothelium

Collagen

Smooth muscle cell

Plaque {

Cholesterol crystal

Lipid

Internal elastic lamina (damaged)

Fibrosis

Angina Pectoris

Angina is characterized by episodes of chest pain, usually precipitated by exercise and relieved by rest. When myocardial oxygen needs are greater than partially occluded vessels can supply, myocardial cells become ischemic and shift to anaerobic metabolism. Anaerobic metabolism produces lactic acid that stimulates nerve endings in the muscle, causing pain. The pain subsides when the oxygen supply again meets myocardial demand.

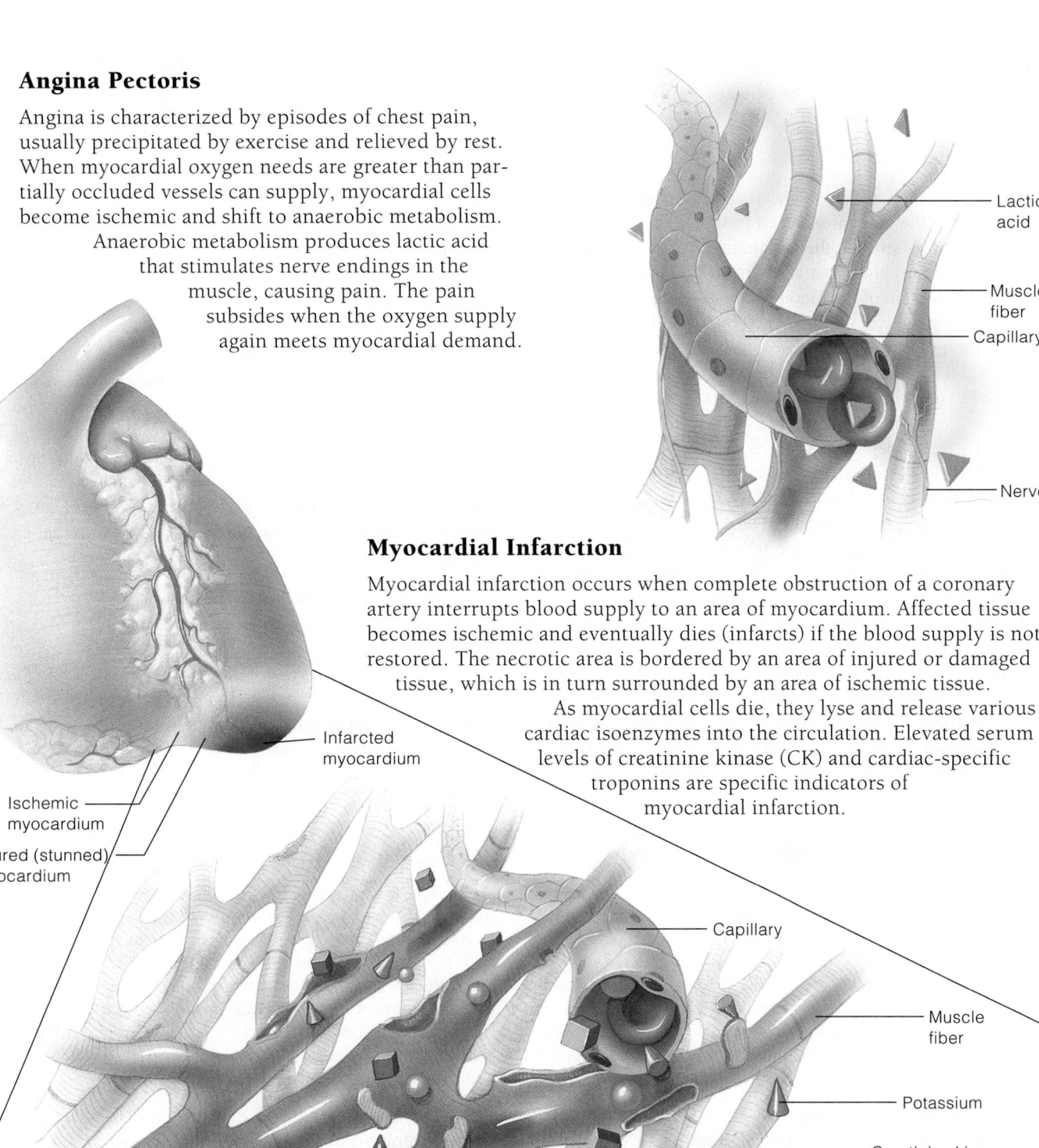

Lactic acid

Muscle fiber

Capillary

Nerve

Infarcted myocardium

Ischemic myocardium

Injured (stunned) myocardium

Myocardial Infarction

Myocardial infarction occurs when complete obstruction of a coronary artery interrupts blood supply to an area of myocardium. Affected tissue becomes ischemic and eventually dies (infarcts) if the blood supply is not restored. The necrotic area is bordered by an area of injured or damaged tissue, which is in turn surrounded by an area of ischemic tissue.

As myocardial cells die, they lyse and release various cardiac isoenzymes into the circulation. Elevated serum levels of creatinine kinase (CK) and cardiac-specific troponins are specific indicators of myocardial infarction.

Capillary

Muscle fiber

Potassium

Creatinine kinase isoenzyme (CK)

Lactic dehydrogenase isoenzyme (LDH)

TABLE 31–1 Factors Contributing to Myocardial Ischemia

CORONARY PERFUSION	MYOCARDIAL WORKLOAD	BLOOD OXYGEN CONTENT
■ Atherosclerosis	■ Rapid heart rate	■ Reduced atmospheric oxygen pressure
■ Thrombosis	■ Increased preload, afterload, or contractility	■ Impaired gas exchange
■ Vasospasm	■ Increased metabolic demands (e.g., hyperthyroidism)	■ Low red blood cells and hemoglobin content
■ Poor perfusion pressure		

Workload is affected by the heart rate, myocardial contractility, preload (the amount of blood in the ventricles just prior to systole), and afterload (the peripheral pressure that must be overcome to move blood out of the heart into the circulation). The oxygen content of the blood and hematocrit are contributing factors to myocardial ischemia. Table 31–1 lists factors that may lead to myocardial ischemia.

Myocardial cells have limited supplies of adenosine triphosphate (ATP) for energy storage. When myocardial workload increases or the supply of blood and oxygen falls, cellular ATP stores are quickly depleted, affecting their contractility. Cellular metabolism switches from an efficient aerobic process to anaerobic metabolism. Lactic acid accumulates, and cells are damaged. If blood flow is restored within 20 minutes, aerobic metabolism and contractility are restored, and cellular repair begins (McCance & Huether, 2006). Continued ischemia results in cell necrosis and death (infarction).

Coronary heart disease is generally divided into two categories, chronic ischemic heart disease and acute coronary syndromes. *Chronic ischemic heart disease* includes stable and vasospastic angina, and silent myocardial ischemia. In women, angina is the most common presenting symptom of CHD. *Acute coronary syndromes* range from unstable angina to myocardial infarction (Porth, 2005). Acute coronary syndromes and myocardial infarction are the most common presenting symptoms of CHD in men. These disorders are discussed in the following sections of this chapter.

Risk Factors

The causes of atherosclerosis are not known, but certain risk factors have been linked with the development of atherosclerotic plaques. The Framingham Heart Study provided vital research into the relationship between risk factors and the development of heart disease (Box 31–1). Research into CHD is ongoing, looking at causative factors, manifestations, and protective measures for many populations. Risk factors for CHD are frequently classified as *nonmodifiable,* factors that cannot be changed, and *modifiable,* those factors that can be changed (Table 31–2).

Nonmodifiable Risk Factors

Age is a nonmodifiable risk factor. More than 50% of heart attack victims are 65 or older; 80% of deaths due to myocardial infarction occur in this age group. *Gender* and *genetic factors* also are nonmodifiable risk factors for CHD. Men are affected by CHD at an earlier age than women. A family history of CHD in a male first-degree relative younger than age 55 or a female first-degree relative younger than 65 years is identified as a risk

BOX 31–1 The Framingham Heart Study

The Framingham Heart Study (FHS) is an ongoing, significant clinical research study that has provided data about cardiovascular disease for over 50 years. The study was initiated in 1948 with an original study group of 5209 participants in the town of Framingham, Massachusetts. Every 2 years, this original group is evaluated for cardiovascular "events" via their medical history, physical findings, and diagnostic testing. Children of the original group have also been studied as part of the Framingham Offspring Study. It was in reports of the Framingham study that the term "risk factor" first appeared.

Implications for Nursing

The data collected from both the Framingham Heart Study and the Framingham Offspring Study provide a rich database from which to develop evidence-based approaches for clients with heart disease. A major application of these research findings to practice is in primary preventive education, for example, through community cardiovascular health programs. As noted in the text, although research shows that increased public awareness of cardiovascular risk factors has lowered morbidity and mortality from heart disease, heart disease remains the number-one killer in the United States. Education about the effects of lifestyle on the cardiovascular system must begin in the early school years and be reinforced throughout the formative years. When healthy choices become habit, cardiac disease will be reduced.

A second application of these findings is in interdisciplinary treatment. Nurses should keep up to date on the latest strategies for medical treatment so that they can provide accurate rationales to clients and formulate effective nursing treatment plans that complement medical management strategies. The result is better communication, a sense of collegiality and teamwork, and positive client outcomes.

Critical Thinking in Client Care

1. What kinds of strategies can be used in elementary school settings to teach cardiovascular health in a fun, informative manner?
2. Which healthcare providers should be included in a multidisciplinary effort to encourage clients to modify their lifestyles?
3. What changes do you need to make in your lifestyle to role model heart healthy living?

TABLE 31–2 Risk Factors for Coronary Heart Disease

NONMODIFIABLE	MODIFIABLE	
	Pathophysiologic	Lifestyle

Age
  Men ≥45 years
  Women ≥55 years
Gender
Heredity
	Hyperlipidemia
	  Elevated LDL cholesterol
	  Elevated triglycerides
	  Low HDL cholesterol
	Hypertension
	Diabetes mellitus
	Women only: premature menopause
	Emerging risk factors:
	  Elevated homocysteine levels
	  Thrombogenic factors
	  Inflammatory factors
	  Impaired fasting glucose
		Cigarette smoking
		Obesity
		Physical inactivity
		Atherogenic diet
		Women only: use of oral contraceptives,
		hormone replacement therapy

factor for CHD (National Cholesterol Education Program [NCEP], 2002).

Modifiable Risk Factors

Modifiable risk factors include lifestyle factors and pathologic conditions that predispose the client to developing CHD. Disease conditions that contribute to CHD include hypertension, diabetes mellitus, and hyperlipidemia. Although these conditions are not a matter of choice, they are modifiable risk factors that can often be controlled through medication, weight control, diet, and exercise.

Behavioral or lifestyle factors can be controlled or completely eliminated. Lifestyle changes require significant commitment by the client; ongoing support from the healthcare team is vital for success.

HYPERTENSION Hypertension is consistent blood pressure readings greater than 140 mmHg systolic or 90 mmHg diastolic. Hypertension is common, affecting more than one-third of people over age 50 in the United States. Its prevalence is higher in African Americans than in Hispanics, and higher in Hispanics than in white Americans. Hypertension damages the endothelial cells of arteries, possibly by excess pressure and altered characteristics of blood flow. This damage can stimulate the development of atherosclerotic plaque.

DIABETES Diabetes mellitus contributes to CHD in several ways. Diabetes is associated with higher blood lipid levels, a higher incidence of hypertension, and obesity—all risk factors in their own right. In addition, diabetes affects the endothelium of blood vessels, contributing to the process of atherosclerosis. Hyperglycemia and hyperinsulinemia, altered platelet function, elevated fibrinogen levels, and inflammation also are thought to play a role in the development of atherosclerosis in people with diabetes.

ABNORMAL BLOOD LIPIDS Hyperlipidemia is an abnormally high level of blood lipids and lipoproteins. Lipoproteins carry cholesterol in the blood. Low-density lipoproteins (LDLs) are the primary carriers of cholesterol. High levels of LDL (memory cue: LDLs = **l**ess **d**esirable **l**ipoproteins) promote atherosclerosis because LDL deposits cholesterol on artery walls. Table 31–3 lists desirable and high-risk levels for total and LDL cholesterol. In contrast, high-density lipoproteins (HDLs = **h**ighly **d**esirable **l**ipoproteins) help clear cholesterol from the arteries, transporting it to the liver for excretion. HDL levels above 35 mg/dL have a protective effect, reducing the risk of CHD; in contrast, HDL levels lower than 35 mg/dL are associated with an increased risk for CHD. Triglycerides, compounds of fatty acids bound to glycerol and used for fat storage by the body, are carried on very low-density lipoprotein

TABLE 31–3 Classification of Serum Cholesterol and Triglyceride Values*

	TOTAL CHOLESTEROL (MG/DL)	LDL CHOLESTEROL (MG/DL)	TRIGLYCERIDE (MG/DL)
Optimal		Less than 100	
Desirable	Under 200	100–129	<150
Borderline high	200 to 239	130 to 159	150 to 199
High	240 or higher	160 to 189	200 to 499
Very high		≥190	≥500

*As defined by the National Blood, Lung, and Heart Institute's National Cholesterol Education Program.

(VLDL) molecules. Elevated triglycerides also contribute to the risk for CHD.

CIGARETTE SMOKING *Cigarette smoking* is an independent risk factor for CHD, responsible for more deaths from CHD than from lung cancer or pulmonary disease (Woods et al., 2004). The effects of smoking on the cardiovascular system are dose dependent (NCEP, 2002). The male cigarette smoker has two to three times the risk of developing heart disease of the nonsmoker; the female who smokes has up to four times the risk. For both men and women who stop smoking, the risk of mortality from CHD is reduced by half. Second-hand (or environmental) tobacco smoke also increases the risk of death from CHD, by as much as 30% (Woods et al., 2004). Tobacco smoke promotes CHD in several ways. Carbon monoxide damages vascular endothelium, promoting cholesterol deposition. Nicotine stimulates catecholamine release, increasing blood pressure, heart rate, and myocardial oxygen use. Nicotine also constricts arteries, limiting tissue perfusion (blood flow and oxygen delivery). Further, nicotine reduces HDL levels and increases platelet aggregation, increasing the risk of thrombus formation.

FAST FACTS

■ Cigarette smoking is the leading independent risk factor for coronary heart disease and a primary target of risk factor management.

OBESITY *Obesity* (excess adipose tissue), generally defined as a body mass index (BMI) of 30 kg/m^2 or greater, and fat distribution affect the risk for CHD. Obese people have higher rates of hypertension, diabetes, and hyperlipidemia. In the Framingham study, obese men over age 50 had twice the incidence of CHD and acute myocardial infarction (MI) of those who were within 10% of their ideal weight. Central obesity, or intra-abdominal fat, is associated with an increased risk for CHD. The best indicator of central obesity is the waist circumference. A waist-to-hip ratio of greater than 0.8 (women) or 0.9 (men) increases the risk for CHD.

PHYSICAL INACTIVITY *Physical inactivity* is associated with a higher risk of CHD. Research data indicate that people who maintain a regular program of physical activity are less prone to developing CHD than sedentary people. Cardiovascular benefits of exercise include increased availability of oxygen to the heart muscle, decreased oxygen demand and cardiac workload, and increased myocardial function and electrical stability. Other positive effects of regular physical activity include decreased blood pressure, blood lipids, insulin levels, platelet aggregation, and weight.

DIET *Diet* is a risk factor for CHD, independent of fat and cholesterol intake. Diets high in fruits, vegetables, whole grains, and unsaturated fatty acids appear to have a protective effect. The underlying factors are not clear, but probably relate to nutrients such as antioxidants, folic acid, other B vitamins, omega-3 fatty acids, and other unidentified micronutrients (NCEP, 2002).

EMERGING RISK FACTORS Recent research demonstrates a link between elevated serum *homocysteine levels* and CHD.

Until menopause, women have lower homocysteine levels than men, which may partially explain their lower risk for CHD. Homocysteine levels are negatively correlated with serum folate and dietary folate intake; that is, increasing folate intake lowers homocysteine levels.

Based on evidence that aspirin and antiplatelet therapies reduce the risk for MI, *clot-promoting factors* are identified as CHD risk factors. *Inflammation* also has recently been identified as a risk factor. Inflammatory processes may increase the development of atherosclerotic plaque, and are implicated in plaque rupture (NCEP, 2002). Inflammation also promotes clot formation at the site of ruptured plaque. Although identified as risk factors, it is not generally recommended that clients routinely be tested for these factors.

METABOLIC SYNDROME The *metabolic syndrome,* a group of metabolic risk factors occurring in an individual, is a strong risk factor for CHD (Box 31–2). The metabolic syndrome has emerged as a risk factor for premature CHD that is equal to cigarette smoking. Three underlying causes of metabolic syndrome have been identified: overweight/obesity, physical inactivity, and genetic factors. It is closely associated with *insulin resistance,* impaired tissue responses to insulin. Genetic factors play a role in insulin resistance, as do the acquired factors of abdominal obesity and physical inactivity (NCEP, 2002).

RISK FACTORS UNIQUE TO WOMEN Risk factors unique to women include *premature menopause, oral contraceptive use,* and *hormone replacement therapy (HRT).* At menopause, serum HDL levels drop and LDL levels rise, increasing the risk of CHD. Early menopause (natural or surgically induced) increases the risk of CHD and MI. Women who have bilateral oophorectomy before age 35 without hormone replacement are eight times more likely to have an MI than women experiencing natural menopause. Estrogen replacement therapy reduces the risk of CHD and MI in these women. Oral contraceptives, by contrast, increase the risk for myocardial infarction, particularly in women who also smoke. This increased risk is due to the tendency of oral contraceptives to promote clotting, and their effects on blood pressure, serum lipids, and glucose tolerance (Woods et al., 2004). The Women's Health Initiative randomized trial of HRT showed an increased risk for CHD in previously healthy women taking a commonly prescribed combination of estrogen and progestin (Writing Group, 2002). This well-controlled research study (see the box on the next page) was terminated early when it showed a small but significant increased risk for CHD, stroke, pulmonary embolism, and invasive breast cancer in women taking HRT.

BOX 31–2 Characteristics of the Metabolic Syndrome

■ Abdominal obesity
■ Abnormal blood lipids (low HDL, high triglycerides)
■ Hypertension
■ Elevated fasting blood glucose
■ Clotting tendency
■ Inflammatory factors

NURSING RESEARCH **Evidence-Based Practice: Postmenopausal Women**

The Women's Health Initiative (WHI) is studying the risks and benefits of strategies to reduce the incidence of heart disease, breast and colorectal cancer, and fractures in postmenopausal women (Writing Group, 2002). A group of 161,809 postmenopausal women between ages 50 and 79 were originally enrolled in WHI trials. Of these women, a subgroup of 16,608 women with intact uteri became part of a randomized trial to assess the risks and benefits of HRT, using the most frequently prescribed combined hormone (estrogen and progestin [Prempro]) replacement in the United States.

After a mean of 5.2 years of follow-up, this study was stopped due to convincing evidence that the risk for invasive breast cancer exceeded the benefits of HRT. The study also demonstrated increased risks for coronary heart disease, stroke, deep vein thrombosis, and pulmonary embolism, although overall mortality was not affected. HRT reduced the risk for colorectal cancer and hip fracture in this study group. The risk for CHD appears to be independent of other CHD risk factors such as age, ethnicity, hypertension, diabetes, smoking, obesity, and other identified risk factors.

IMPLICATIONS FOR NURSING

Nurses often are in the position of advising women about menopause, its manifestations, and hormone replacement ther-apy. While HRT does reduce unpleasant menopausal effects such as night sweats and hot flashes, and it reduces the risk of osteoporosis and subsequent fractures, it carries associated risks. Advise each client about the risks and benefits of HRT, clearly presenting the evidence. Suggest alternative strategies to reduce menopausal symptoms, such as complementary medicines (see Chapter 51 ∞). Encourage measures such as weight-bearing exercise, calcium supplements, and a diet high in fiber and antioxidants to reduce the risks for osteoporosis, fracture, and colorectal cancer. Ultimately, each client will make her own decision about postmenopausal HRT.

CRITICAL THINKING IN CLIENT CARE

1. What factors might you suggest that a client consider when deciding whether to use HRT for menopausal manifestations and risks?
2. In this study, the increased risk for CHD was not related to the duration of time taking HRT, whereas the increased risk for stroke and invasive breast cancer emerged more than 1 year after randomization (stroke in the second through fifth year of the study, breast cancer within several years following randomization). Will this data affect your advice to menopausal women inquiring about HRT? If so, how?

FAST FACTS

- Risk factors for coronary heart disease are those factors that promote atherosclerosis and plaque development.
- Angina pectoris, acute coronary syndromes, and myocardial infarction are the manifestations of myocardial ischemia and coronary heart disease due to atherosclerosis.
- Atherosclerosis also is the primary underlying cause of stroke and peripheral vascular disease; therefore, the risk factors for atherosclerosis also are the risk factors for coronary heart disease, including angina, acute coronary syndromes, and myocardial infarction.

INTERDISCIPLINARY CARE

Care of clients with coronary heart disease focuses on aggressive risk factor management to slow the atherosclerotic process and maintain myocardial perfusion. Until manifestations of chronic or acute ischemia are experienced, the diagnosis often is presumptive, based on history and the presence of risk factors.

Diagnosis

Laboratory testing is used to assess for risk factors such as an abnormal blood lipid profile (elevated triglyceride and LDL levels and decreased HDL levels).

- *Total serum cholesterol* is elevated in hyperlipidemia. A *lipid profile* includes triglyceride, HDL, and LDL levels as well, and enables calculation of the ratio of HDL to total cholesterol. The ratio should be at least 1:5, with 1:3 being the ideal ratio. Elevated lipid levels are associated with an increased risk of atherosclerosis (see Table 31–3). In clients with a strong family history of premature CHD or familial hypercholesterolemia, *lipoprotein (a)* also may be measured. Elevated levels of Lp(a) may independently increase the risk of CHD. Other subsets of blood lipids may also be measured in selected clients. See Chapter 30 ∞ for nursing care related to lipid profile studies.

Diagnostic tests to identify subclinical (asymptomatic) CHD may be indicated when multiple risk factors are present.

- *C-reactive protein* is a serum protein associated with inflammatory processes. Recent evidence suggests that elevated blood levels of this protein may be predictive of CHD.
- The *ankle-brachial blood pressure index (ABI)* is an inexpensive, noninvasive test for peripheral vascular disease that may be predictive of CHD. The systolic blood pressure in the brachial, posterior tibial, and dorsalis pedis arteries is measured by Doppler. An ABI of <0.9 in either leg indicates the presence of peripheral arterial disease and a significant risk for CHD.
- *Exercise ECG testing* may be performed. ECGs are used to assess the response to increased cardiac workload induced by exercise. The test is considered "positive" for CHD if myocardial ischemia is detected on the ECG (depression of the ST segment by greater than 3 mm; see Figure 31–1), the client develops chest pain, or the test is stopped due to excess fatigue, dysrhythmias, or other symptoms before the predicted maximal heart rate is achieved.
- *Electron beam computed tomography (EBCT)* creates a three-dimensional image of the heart and coronary arteries that can reveal plaque and other abnormalities. This noninvasive test requires no special preparation, and can identify clients at risk for developing myocardial ischemia.

■ *Myocardial perfusion imaging* (see the section on angina that follows) may be used to evaluate myocardial blood flow and perfusion, both at rest and during stress testing (exercise or mental stress). These diagnostic tests are further explained in Chapter 30 ∞ and the section on angina. Perfusion imaging studies are costly, and therefore not recommended for routine CHD risk assessment.

Risk Factor Management

Conservative management of CHD focuses on risk factor modification, including smoking, diet, exercise, and management of contributing conditions.

SMOKING Smoking cessation reduces the risk for CHD within months after quitting and improves cardiovascular status. People who quit reduce their risk by 50%, regardless of how long they smoked before quitting. For women, the risk becomes equivalent to a nonsmoker within 3 to 5 years of smoking cessation (Woods et al., 2004). In addition, stopping smoking improves HDL levels, lowers LDL levels, and reduces blood viscosity. All smokers are advised to quit. Health promotion activities focus on preventing children, teenagers, and adults from starting to smoke.

DIET Dietary recommendations by the National Cholesterol Education Program (2002) include reduced saturated fat and cholesterol intake, and strategies to lower LDL levels (Table 31–4). Most fats are a mixture of saturated and unsaturated fatty acids. The highest proportions of saturated fat are found in whole-milk products, red meats, and coconut oil. Nonfat dairy products, fish, and poultry as primary protein sources are recommended. Solidified vegetable fats (e.g., margarine, shortening) contain *trans* fatty acids, which behave more like saturated fats. Soft margarines and vegetable oil spreads contain low levels of *trans* fatty acids, and should be used instead of butter, stick margarine, and shortening. Monounsaturated fats, found in olive, canola, and peanut oils, actually lower LDL and cholesterol levels. Certain

TABLE 31–4 Dietary Recommendations to Reduce Total Cholesterol, LDL Levels, and CHD Risk

NUTRIENT	RECOMMENDATION
Calories	Adjusted to attain/maintain desirable body weight
Total fat	25%–35% of total calories
■ Saturated fats	■ <7% of total calories
■ Polyunsaturated fat	■ Up to 10% of total calories
■ Monounsaturated fat	■ Up to 20% of total calories
■ Cholesterol	■ <200 mg/day
Carbohydrate (primarily complex carbohydrates, such as whole grains, fruits, and vegetables)	50%–60% of total calories
Dietary fiber	20–30 g/day
Protein	About 15% of total calories

Source: Compiled from *Adult Treatment Panel III Final Report by the National Cholesterol Education Program, 2002.*

cold-water fish, such as tuna, salmon, and mackerel, contain high levels of omega-3 fatty acids, which help raise HDL levels, and decrease serum triglycerides, total serum cholesterol, and blood pressure.

In addition, increased intake of soluble fiber (found in oats, psyllium, pectin-rich fruit, and beans) and insoluble fiber (found in whole grains, vegetables, and fruit) is recommended. Folic acid and vitamins B_6 and B_{12} affect homocysteine metabolism, reducing serum levels. Leafy green vegetables (e.g., spinach and broccoli) and legumes (e.g., black-eyed peas, dried beans, and lentils) are rich sources of folate. Meat, fish, and poultry are rich in vitamins B_6 and B_{12}. Vitamin B_6 also is found in soy products; B_{12} is in fortified cereals. Increased intake of antioxidant nutrients (vitamin E, in particular) and foods rich in antioxidants (fruits and vegetables) appears to increase HDL levels and have a protective effect on CHD.

In middle-aged and older adults, moderate alcohol intake may reduce the risk for CHD (NCEP, 2002). Consumption of no more than two drinks per day for men or one drink per day for women is recommended. A drink is 5 ounces of wine, 12 ounces of beer, or 1.5 ounces of whiskey. People who do not drink alcohol, however, should not be encouraged to start consuming it as a heart-protective measure.

People who are overweight or obese are encouraged to lose weight through a combination of reduced calorie intake (maintaining a nutritionally sound diet) and increased exercise. High-protein, high-fat weight loss programs are not recommended for weight reduction.

EXERCISE Regular physical exercise reduces the risk for CHD in several ways. It lowers VLDL, LDL, and triglyceride levels, and raises HDL levels. Regular exercise reduces the blood pressure and insulin resistance. Unless contraindicated, all clients are encouraged to participate in at least 30 minutes of moderate intensity physical activity 5 to 6 days each week. To achieve weight loss and prevent weight gain, 60 to 90 minutes of moderate intensity exercise daily is recommended (U.S. Department of Health and Human Services, 2005).

HYPERTENSION Although hypertension often cannot be prevented or cured, it can be controlled. Hypertension control (maintaining a blood pressure lower than 140/90 mmHg) is vital to reduce its atherosclerosis-promoting effects and to reduce the workload of the heart. Management strategies include reducing sodium intake, increasing calcium intake, regular exercise, stress management, and medications. Hypertension management is discussed in Chapter 35 ∞.

DIABETES Diabetes increases the risk of CHD by accelerating the atherosclerotic process. Weight loss (if appropriate), reduced fat intake, and exercise are particularly important for the diabetic client. Because hyperglycemia apparently also contributes to atherosclerosis, consistent blood glucose management is vital. See Chapter 20 ∞ for a detailed discussion about diabetes and blood glucose management.

Medications

Drug therapy to lower total serum cholesterol and LDL levels and to raise HDL levels now is an integral part of CHD management. It is used in conjunction with diet and other lifestyle changes, and is based on the client's overall risk for CHD.

Drugs used to treat hyperlipidemia act specifically by lowering LDL levels. The goal of treatment is to achieve an LDL level of <130 mg/dL (NCEP, 2002). Medications to treat hyperlipidemia are not inexpensive; the cost–benefit ra-

tio needs to be considered, because long-term treatment may be required. The four major classes of cholesterol-lowering drugs are statins, bile acid sequestrants, nicotinic acid, and fibrates. The nursing implications and client teaching for these drug classes are outlined in the Medication Administration box below.

MEDICATION ADMINISTRATION Cholesterol-Lowering Drugs

STATINS
Lovastatin (Mevacor)
Pravastatin (Pravachol)
Simvastatin (Zocor)
Fluvastatin (Lescol)
Atorvastatin (Lipitor)
Statins inhibit the enzyme HMG-CoA reductase in the liver, lowering LDL synthesis and serum levels. The statins are first-line treatment for elevated LDL, used in conjunction with diet and lifestyle changes. Although their side effects are minimal, they may cause increased serum liver enzyme levels and myopathy.

Nursing Responsibilities
- Monitor serum cholesterol and liver enzyme levels before and during therapy. Report elevated liver enzyme levels.
- Assess for muscle pain and tenderness. Monitor CPK level if present.
- If taking digoxin concurrently, monitor for and report digoxin toxicity.

Health Education for the Client and Family
- Promptly report muscle pain, tenderness, or weakness; skin rash or hives, or changes in skin color; abdominal pain, nausea, or vomiting.
- Do not use these drugs if you are pregnant or plan to become pregnant.
- Inform your doctor if you are taking any other medications concurrently.

BILE ACID SEQUESTRANTS
Cholestyramine (Questran)
Colestipol (Colestid)
Colesevelam (Welchol)
Bile acid sequestrants lower LDL levels by binding bile acids in the intestine, reducing its reabsorption and cholesterol production in the liver. They are used in combination therapy regimens and for women who are considering pregnancy. Their primary disadvantages are inconvenience of administration due to bulk and gastrointestinal side effects such as constipation.

Nursing Responsibilities
- Mix cholestyramine and colestipol powders with 4 to 6 oz of water or juice; administer once or twice a day as ordered with meals.
- Store in a tightly closed container.

Health Education for the Client and Family
- Promptly report constipation, severe gastric distress with nausea and vomiting, unexplained weight loss, black or bloody stools, or sudden back pain to your doctor.
- Drinking ample amounts of fluid while taking these drugs reduces problems of constipation and bloating.
- Do not omit doses as this may affect the absorption of other drugs you are taking.

NICOTINIC ACID
Niacin (Nicobid, Nicolar, Niaspan, others)
Nicotinic acid in both prescription and nonprescription forms lowers total and LDL cholesterol and triglyceride levels. The crystalline form and Niaspan, a prescription extended release tablet, also raise HDL levels. Because the doses required to achieve significant cholesterol-lowering effects are associated with multiple side effects, nicotinic acid generally is used in combination therapy, particularly with the statin drugs.

Nursing Responsibilities
- Give oral preparations with meals and accompanied by a cold beverage to minimize GI effects.
- Administer with caution to clients with active liver disease, peptic ulcer disease, gout, or type 2 diabetes.
- Monitor blood glucose, uric acid levels, and liver function tests during treatment.

Health Education for the Client and Family
- Flushing of face, neck, and ears may occur within 2 hours following dose; these effects generally subside as treatment continues. Alcohol use during nicotinic acid therapy may worsen this effect.
- Report weakness or dizziness with changes in posture (lying to sitting; sitting to standing) to your doctor. Change positions slowly to reduce the risk of injury.

FIBRIC ACID DERIVATIVES
Gemfibrozil (Lopid)
Fenofibrate (Tricor)
Clofibrate (Atromid-S)
The fibrates are used to lower serum triglyceride levels; they have only a slight to modest effect on LDL. They affect lipid regulation by blocking triglyceride synthesis. They are used to treat very high triglyceride levels, and may be used in combination with statins.

Nursing Responsibilities
- Monitor serum LDL and VLDL levels, electrolytes, glucose, liver enzymes, renal function tests, and CBC during therapy. Report abnormal values.
- Up to 2 months of treatment may be required to achieve a therapeutic effect; rebound, with decreasing benefit, may occur in the second or third month of treatment.

Health Education for the Client and Family
- Take with meals if the drug causes gastric distress.
- Promptly report flulike symptoms (fatigue, muscle aching, soreness, or weakness) to your doctor.
- Do not use this drug if you are pregnant or plan to become pregnant. Use reliable birth control measures while taking this drug.
- Contact your doctor before stopping this drug and before taking any over-the-counter preparations.

The statins, including lovastatin (Mevacor), pravastatin (Pravachol), simvastatin (Zocor), and others, are first-line drugs for treating hyperlipidemia. They effectively lower LDL levels and may also increase HDL levels. The statins can cause myopathy; all clients are instructed to report muscle pain and weakness or brown urine. Liver function tests are monitored during therapy, because these drugs may increase liver enzyme levels.

The other cholesterol-lowering drugs, such as the bile acid sequestrants, nicotinic acid, and fibrates, are primarily used when combination therapy is required to effectively lower serum cholesterol levels. They also may be used for selected clients, such as younger adults, women who wish to become pregnant, or to specifically lower triglyceride levels.

Clients at high risk for MI are often started on prophylactic low-dose aspirin therapy. The dose ranges from 80 to 325 mg/day (Tierney et al., 2005). In women, the benefit of low-dose aspirin in reducing the risk for CHD is not clear prior to age 65 (NHLBI, 2005). Aspirin is contraindicated for clients who have a history of aspirin sensitivity, bleeding disorders, or active peptic ulcer disease. Angiotensin-converting enzyme (ACE) inhibitors or angiotensin receptor blockers also may be prescribed for high-risk clients, including diabetics with other CHD risk factors.

Complementary Therapies

Diet and exercise programs that emphasize physical conditioning and a low-fat diet rich in antioxidants have been shown to be effective in managing CHD (Box 31–3). Supplements of vitamins C, E, B_6, B_{12}, and folic acid may be beneficial. Other potentially helpful complementary therapies include herbals such as ginkgo biloba, garlic, curcumin, and green tea; and consumption of red wine, foods containing bioflavonoids, and nuts. Emphasize the need for clients to talk to their physician prior to taking any herbal preparations, as interactions with prescribed drugs are common. Behavioral therapies of benefit for clients with CHD include relaxation and stress management, guided imagery, treatment of depression, anger/hostility management, and meditation, tai chi, and yoga.

BOX 31–3 **Complementary Therapies: Diet for CHD**

Two diet programs have been shown to have a beneficial effect on CHD. The *Pritikin diet* is basically vegetarian, high in complex carbohydrates and fiber, low in cholesterol, and extremely low in fat (<10% of daily calories). Egg whites and limited amounts of nonfat dairy or soy products are allowed. The Pritikin program requires 45 minutes of walking daily and recommends multivitamin supplements, including vitamins C and E and folate.

The *Ornish diet* also is vegetarian, although egg whites and a cup of nonfat milk or yogurt per day are allowed. No oil or fat is permitted, even for cooking. Two ounces of alcohol a day are permitted. The Ornish program also calls for stress reduction, emotional social support systems, daily stretching, and walking for 1 hour three times a week.

NURSING CARE

Nurses are instrumental in educating adults about their risk for coronary heart disease, promoting participation in screening programs to identify that risk, and teaching all clients measures to reduce their risk for CHD.

Health Promotion

Present information about healthy lifestyle habits to community and religious groups, school children (grades K through 12), and through the print media. In promoting healthy lifestyle habits, nurses can positively affect the incidence, morbidity, and mortality from CHD.

Strongly encourage all clients to avoid smoking in the first place, and to stop all forms of tobacco use. Discuss the adverse effects of smoking and the benefits of quitting. Provide information about dietary recommendations to maintain a healthy weight and optimal cholesterol levels. Discuss the benefits and importance of regular exercise. Finally, encourage clients with cardiovascular risk factors to undergo regular screening for hypertension, diabetes, and abnormal blood lipids.

Assessment

Nursing assessment for CHD focuses on identifying risk factors.

- *Health history:* Current manifestations such as chest pain or heaviness, shortness of breath, weakness; current diet, exercise patterns, and medications; smoking history and pattern of alcohol intake; history of heart disease, hypertension, or diabetes; family history of CHD or other cardiac problems.
- *Physical examination:* Current weight and its appropriateness for height; body mass index; waist-to-hip ratio; blood pressure; strength and equality of peripheral pulses.

Nursing Diagnoses and Interventions

Imbalanced Nutrition:
More than Body Requirements

This nursing diagnosis may be appropriate for clients who are obese, have a waist-to-hip ratio greater than 0.8 (female) or 0.9 (male), or whose diet history or serum cholesterol levels indicate a need to reduce fat and cholesterol intake. See Chapters 21 ∞ and 22 for more information about assessing obesity.

- Encourage assessment of food intake and eating patterns to help identify areas that can be improved. *Clients often are unaware of their fat and cholesterol intake, particularly when many meals are eaten away from home. Careful assessment increases awareness and allows the client to make conscious changes.*
- Discuss American Heart Association and therapeutic lifestyle change (TLC) dietary recommendations, emphasizing the role of diet in heart disease. Provide guidance regarding specific food choices with healthy alternatives. *Specific diet information and suggestions help the client make better food choices.*
- Refer to a clinical dietitian for diet planning and further teaching. Suggest cookbooks that offer low-fat recipes to encourage healthier eating, and provide American Heart Association and American Cancer Society recipe pamphlets and information

on low-fat eating. *These resources provide tools for the client to use as eating patterns change.*

- Encourage gradual but progressive dietary changes. *Drastic changes in eating patterns may cause frustration and discourage the client from maintaining a healthy diet over the long term.*

- Discourage use of high-fat, low-carbohydrate, or other fad diets for weight loss. *These diets may adversely affect serum cholesterol and triglyceride levels, and often are too drastic to maintain over the long term.*

- Encourage reasonable goals for weight loss (e.g., 1.0 to 1.5 lb per week and a 10% weight loss over 6 months). Provide information about weight loss programs and support groups such as Weight Watchers and Take Off Pounds Sensibly (TOPS). *Gradual but steady weight loss is more likely to be sustained. Recognized programs that emphasize healthy eating provide support and incentive for making lifetime dietary changes.*

Ineffective Health Maintenance

Clients with risk factors for CHD may be unable to identify or independently manage their risk factors.

- Discuss risk factors for CHD, stressing that changing or managing those factors that can be modified reduces the client's overall risk for the disease. *Clients with significant nonmodifiable risk factors may be discouraged, reducing their ability to eliminate or control modifiable risk factors.*

- Discuss the immediate benefits of smoking cessation. Provide resource materials from the American Heart Association, the American Lung Association, and the American Cancer Society. Refer to a structured smoking cessation program to increase the likelihood of success in quitting. *Long-time smokers may assume that the damage from smoking has already been done, and quitting would not be "worth the price."*

- Help the client identify specific sources of psychosocial and physical support for smoking cessation, dietary, and lifestyle changes. *Support persons, groups, and aids such as nicotine patches help the client achieve success and provide encouragement during difficult times (such as withdrawal symptoms).*

- Discuss the benefits of regular exercise for cardiovascular health and weight loss. Help identify favorite forms of exercise or physical activity. Encourage planning for 30 minutes of continuous aerobic activity (i.e., walking, running, bicycling, swimming) four to five times a week. Encourage identification of an "exercise buddy" to help maintain motivation. *Engaging in preferred activities with a partner maintains motivation and increases the likelihood of maintaining an exercise program. Encourage continuation of the plan, even when days are missed. Exercise is cumulative, so increasing the duration of exercise on subsequent days can "make up" for a lost day.*

- Provide information and teaching about prescribed medications such as cholesterol-lowering drugs. Discuss the relationship between hypertension, diabetes, and CHD. *Teaching is important to promote understanding of and compliance with the prescribed drug regimen.*

Community-Based Care

Encourage participation in some form of cardiac rehabilitation program. Formal programs provide comprehensive assessment of, interventions for, and teaching of clients with cardiac disease. Monitored exercise and information about risk factors help clients identify ways to lower their risk for CHD.

Because clients themselves are primarily responsible for maintaining the lifestyle changes necessary to reduce the risk of CHD, provide teaching and support as outlined in the previous section. Assist the client to make healthy choices and reinforce positive changes. Emphasize the importance of regular follow-up appointments to monitor progress.

THE CLIENT WITH ANGINA PECTORIS

Angina pectoris, or *angina,* is chest pain resulting from reduced coronary blood flow, which causes a temporary imbalance between myocardial blood supply and demand. The imbalance may be due to coronary heart disease, atherosclerosis, or vessel constriction that impairs myocardial blood supply. Hypermetabolic conditions such as exercise, thyrotoxicosis, stimulant abuse (e.g., cocaine), hyperthyroidism, and emotional stress can increase myocardial oxygen demand, precipitating angina. Anemia, heart failure, ventricular hypertrophy, or pulmonary diseases may affect blood and oxygen supplies as well, causing angina.

Pathophysiology

The imbalance between myocardial blood supply and demand causes temporary and reversible myocardial ischemia. **Ischemia,** deficient blood flow to tissue, may be caused by partial obstruction of a coronary artery, coronary artery spasm, or a thrombus. Obstruction of a coronary artery deprives cells in the region of the heart normally supplied by that vessel of oxygen and nutrients needed for metabolic processes. Cellular processes are compromised as ATP stores are depleted. Reduced oxygen causes cells to switch from aerobic metabolism to anaerobic metabolism. Anaerobic metabolism causes lactic acid to build up in the cells. It also affects cell membrane permeability, releasing substances such as histamine, kinins, and specific enzymes that stimulate terminal nerve fibers in the cardiac muscle and send pain impulses to the central nervous system. The pain radiates to the upper body because the heart shares the same dermatome as this region. Return of adequate circulation provides the nutrients needed by cells, and clears the waste products. More than 30 minutes of ischemia irreversibly damages myocardial cells (necrosis).

Three types of angina have been identified:

- *Stable angina* is the most common and predictable form of angina. It occurs with a predictable amount of activity or stress, and is a common manifestation of CHD. Stable angina usually occurs when the work of the heart is increased by physical exertion, exposure to cold, or by stress. Stable angina is relieved by rest and nitrates.

- *Prinzmetal's (variant) angina* is atypical angina that occurs unpredictably (unrelated to activity), and often at night. It is caused by coronary artery spasm with or without an atherosclerotic lesion. The exact mechanism of coronary artery spasm is unknown. It may result from hyperactive sympathetic nervous system responses, altered calcium flow in smooth muscle, or reduced prostaglandins that promote vasodilation.

- *Unstable angina* occurs with increasing frequency, severity, and duration. Pain is unpredictable and occurs with decreasing levels of activity or stress and may occur at rest. Clients with unstable angina are at risk for myocardial infarction. Unstable angina is discussed further in the section on acute coronary syndromes that follows.

Silent myocardial ischemia, or asymptomatic ischemia, is thought to be common in people with CHD. Silent ischemia may occur with either activity or with mental stress. Mental stress increases the heart rate and blood pressure, increasing myocardial oxygen demand (McCance & Huether, 2006). Like symptomatic angina, silent myocardial ischemia is associated with an increased chance of myocardial infarction and death (Kasper et al., 2005).

FAST FACTS
- Stable angina occurs with a predictable amount of activity or stress.
- Unstable angina occurs with increasing frequency and severity; it may occur at times unrelated to activity or stress.
- Prinzmetal's angina is the only type of angina not necessarily related to coronary heart disease and atherosclerosis, developing due to coronary artery spasm.

Course and Manifestations

The cardinal manifestation of angina is chest pain. The pain typically is precipitated by an identifiable event, such as physical activity, strong emotion, stress, eating a heavy meal, or exposure to cold. The classic sequence of angina is activity–pain, rest–relief. The client may describe the pain as a tight, squeezing, heavy pressure, or constricting sensation. It characteristically begins beneath the sternum and may radiate to the jaw, neck, shoulder, or arm. Less characteristically, the pain may be felt in the jaw, epigastric region, or back. Anginal pain usually occurs in a *crescendo–decrescendo* pattern (increasing to a peak, then gradually decreasing) and typically lasts 2 to 5 minutes. It generally is relieved by rest. Additional manifestations of angina include dyspnea, pallor, tachycardia, and great anxiety and fear.

Women frequently present with atypical symptoms of angina, including indigestion or nausea, vomiting, and upper back pain. The manifestations of angina are summarized in the accompanying box.

The severity of angina can be graded by the degree to which it limits the client's activities. Class I angina does not occur with ordinary physical activities. It is prompted by strenuous, rapid, or prolonged physical exertion. Class II angina may develop with rapid or prolonged walking or stair climbing, whereas Class III angina significantly limits ordinary physical activities. The client with Class IV angina may have angina at rest, as well as with any physical activity (Kasper et al., 2005).

MANIFESTATIONS   of Angina

- Chest pain: Substernal or precordial (across the chest wall); may radiate to neck, arms, shoulders, or jaw
- Quality: Tight, squeezing, constricting, or heavy sensation; may also be described as burning, aching, choking, dull, or constant
- Associated manifestations: Dyspnea, pallor, tachycardia, anxiety, and fear
- Atypical manifestations: Indigestion, nausea, vomiting, upper back pain
- Precipitating factors: Exercise or activity, strong emotion, stress, cold, heavy meal
- Relieving factors: Rest, position change; nitroglycerin

INTERDISCIPLINARY CARE

The management of stable angina focuses on maintaining coronary blood flow and cardiac function. Stable angina often can be managed by medical therapy. Measures to restore coronary blood flow are discussed in the section on acute coronary syndrome. As for CHD, risk factor management is a vital component of care for the client with angina (see the preceding section of this chapter).

Diagnosis

The diagnosis of angina is based on past medical history and family history, a comprehensive description of the chest pain, and physical assessment findings. Laboratory tests may confirm the presence of risk factors, such as an abnormal blood lipid profile and elevated blood glucose. Diagnostic tests provide information about overall cardiac function.

Common diagnostic tests to assess for coronary heart disease and angina include electrocardiography, stress testing, nuclear medicine studies, echocardiography (ultrasound), and coronary angiography.

ELECTROCARDIOGRAPHY A resting ECG may be normal, may show nonspecific changes in the ST segment and T wave, or may show evidence of previous myocardial infarction. Characteristic ECG changes are seen during anginal episodes. During periods of ischemia, the ST segment is depressed or downsloping, and the T wave may flatten or invert (Figure 31–1 ■). These changes reverse when ischemia is relieved. For more details about the ECG, its waveforms, and its uses, see Box 30–1 in Chapter 30 ∞.

STRESS ELECTROCARDIOGRAPHY Stress electrocardiography (exercise stress test) uses ECGs to monitor the cardiac response to an increased workload during progressive exercise. See the Diagnostic Tests box in the previous chapter for more information about exercise stress tests.

RADIONUCLIDE TESTING Radionuclide testing is a safe, noninvasive technique to evaluate myocardial perfusion and left ventricular function. The amount of radioisotope injected is very small; no special radiation precautions are required during or after the scan. Thallium-201 or a technetium-based radiocompound is injected intravenously, and the heart is scanned with a radiation detector. Ischemic or infarcted cells of the

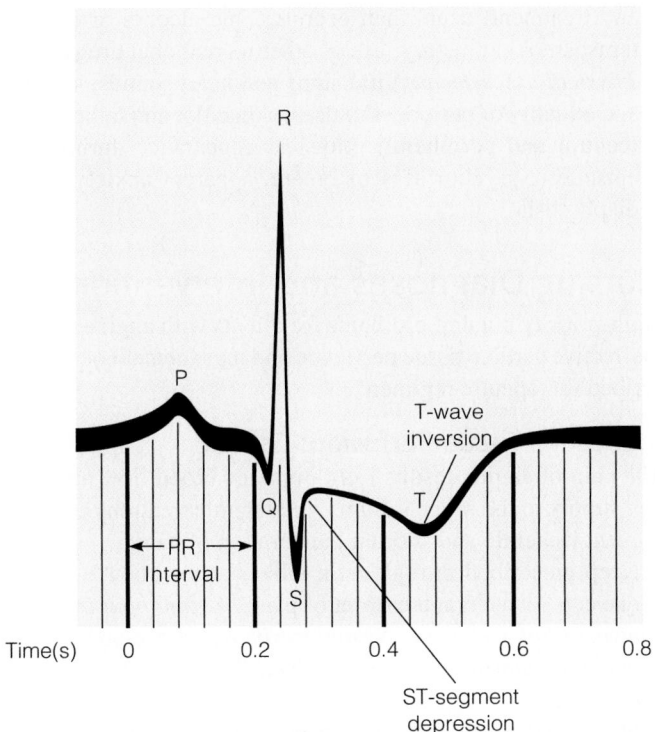

Figure 31–1 ■ ECG changes during an episode of angina. Note characteristic T-wave inversion and ST-segment depression of myocardial ischemia.

myocardium do not take up the substance normally, appearing as a "cold spot" on the scan. If the ischemia is transient, these spots gradually fill in, indicating the reversibility of the process. With severe ischemia or a myocardial infarction, these areas may remain devoid of radioactivity.

Left ventricular function can also be evaluated. Whereas the ejection fraction, or portion of blood ejected from the left ventricle during systole, normally increases during exercise, it may actually decrease in coronary heart disease and stress-induced ischemia.

Radionuclide testing may be combined with pharmacologic stress testing for clients who are physically unable to exercise or to detect subclinical myocardial ischemia. A vasodilator is injected to induce the same ischemic changes that occur with exercise in the diseased heart. Coronary arteries unaffected by atherosclerosis dilate in response to the drugs, increasing blood flow to already well-perfused tissue. This reduces flow to ischemic muscle, called *myocardial steal syndrome*.

ECHOCARDIOGRAPHY Echocardiography is a noninvasive test that uses ultrasound to evaluate cardiac structure and function. It may be done at rest, during supine exercise, or immediately following upright exercise to evaluate movement of the myocardial wall and assess for possible ischemia or infarction.

Transesophageal echocardiography (TEE) uses ultrasound to identify abnormal blood flow patterns as well as cardiac structures. In TEE, the probe is on the tip of an endoscope inserted into the esophagus, positioning it close to the posterior heart (especially the left atrium and the aorta). It avoids interference by breasts, ribs, or lungs. See the Diagnostic Tests box

in Chapter 30 ∞ for more information about and the nursing care for clients undergoing these tests.

CORONARY ANGIOGRAPHY Coronary angiography is the gold standard for evaluating the coronary arteries. Guided by fluoroscopy, a catheter introduced into the femoral or brachial artery is threaded into the coronary artery. Dye is injected into each coronary opening, allowing visualization of the main coronary branches and any abnormalities, such as stenosis or obstruction. Narrowing of the vessel lumen by more than 50% is considered significant; most lesions that cause symptoms involve more than 70% narrowing. Vessel obstructions are noted on a coronary artery "map" that provides a guide for tracking disease progression and for elective treatment with angioplasty or cardiac surgery. During angiogram, the drug ergonovine maleate may be injected to induce coronary artery spasm and diagnose Prinzmetal's angina. See the Diagnostic Tests box in Chapter 30 for nursing care of clients undergoing coronary angiography.

Medications

Drugs may be used for both acute and long-term relief of angina. The goal of drug treatment is to reduce oxygen demand and increase oxygen supply to the myocardium. Three main classes of drugs are used to treat angina: nitrates, beta blockers, and calcium channel blockers.

NITRATES Nitrates, including nitroglycerin and longer-acting nitrate preparations, are used to treat acute anginal attacks and prevent angina.

Sublingual nitroglycerin is the drug of choice to treat acute angina. It acts within 1 to 2 minutes, decreasing myocardial work and oxygen demand through venous and arterial dilation, which in turn reduce preload and afterload. It may also improve myocardial oxygen supply by dilating collateral blood vessels and reducing stenosis. Rapid-acting nitroglycerin is also available as a buccal spray in a metered system. For some clients, this may be easier to handle than small nitroglycerin tablets.

> **PRACTICE ALERT**
> ■ Sublingual nitroglycerin tablets and nitroglycerin spray are the only medications appropriate to treat an acute anginal attack.

Longer-acting nitroglycerin preparations (oral tablets, ointment, or transdermal patches) are used to prevent attacks of angina, not to treat an acute attack. The primary problem with long-term nitrate use is the development of *tolerance*, a decreasing effect from the same dose of medication. Tolerance can be limited by a dosing schedule that allows a nitrate-free period of at least 8 to 10 hours daily. This is usually scheduled at night, when angina is less likely to occur.

Headache is a common side effect of nitrates, and may limit their usefulness. Nausea, dizziness, and hypotension are also common effects of therapy.

BETA BLOCKERS Beta blockers, including propranolol, metoprolol, nadolol, and atenolol, are considered first-line drugs to treat stable angina. They block the cardiac-stimulating effects of norepinephrine and epinephrine, preventing anginal attacks by reducing heart rate, myocardial contractility, and blood pressure, thus reducing myocardial oxygen demand. Beta blockers may be used alone or with other medications to prevent angina.

Beta blockers are contraindicated for clients with asthma or severe COPD (see Chapter 39 ∞) because they may cause severe bronchospasm. They are not used in clients with significant bradycardia, or AV conduction blocks, and are used cautiously in heart failure. Beta blockers are not used to treat Prinzmetal's angina because they may make it worse.

CALCIUM CHANNEL BLOCKERS Calcium channel blockers reduce myocardial oxygen demand and increase myocardial blood and oxygen supply. These drugs, which include verapamil, diltiazem, and nifedipine, lower blood pressure, reduce myocardial contractility, and, in some cases, lower the heart rate, decreasing myocardial oxygen demand. They are also potent coronary vasodilators, effectively increasing oxygen supply. Like beta blockers, calcium channel blockers act too slowly to effectively treat an acute attack of angina; they are used for long-term prophylaxis. Because they may actually increase ischemia and mortality in clients with heart failure or left ventricular dysfunction, these drugs are not usually prescribed in the initial treatment of angina. They are used cautiously in clients with dysrhythmias, heart failure, or hypotension.

The nursing implications of antianginal medications are summarized in the Medication Administration box on the next page.

ASPIRIN The client with angina, particularly unstable angina, is at risk for myocardial infarction because of significant narrowing of the coronary arteries. Low-dose aspirin (80 to 325 mg/day) is often prescribed to reduce the risk of platelet aggregation and thrombus formation.

NURSING CARE

The focus of nursing care for clients with angina is similar to the interdisciplinary care focus: to reduce myocardial oxygen demand and improve the oxygen supply. Angina usually is treated in community settings; the primary nursing focus is education.

Health Promotion

In addition to health promotion measures identified for CHD, emphasize the importance of active CHD risk factor management to slow progression of the disease. Encourage clients to stop smoking. Discuss the use of cholesterol-lowering drug therapy with clients who have hypercholesterolemia. Encourage regular aerobic exercise and a diet based on American Heart Association or National Cholesterol Education Program guidelines.

Assessment

Focused assessment data for the client with angina includes the following:

- *Health history:* Chest pain, including type, intensity, duration, frequency, aggravating factors, and relief measures; associated symptoms; history of other cardiovascular disorders, peripheral vascular disease, or stroke; current medications

and treatment; usual diet, exercise, and alcohol intake patterns; smoking history; use of other recreational drugs.
- *Physical assessment:* Vital signs and heart sounds; strength and equality of peripheral pulses; skin color and temperature (central and peripheral); physical appearance during pain episode (e.g., shortness of breath, apparent anxiety, color, diaphoresis).

Nursing Diagnoses and Interventions

High-priority nursing problems for clients with angina include ineffective cardiac tissue perfusion and management of the prescribed therapeutic regimen.

Ineffective Tissue Perfusion: Cardiac

The pain of angina results from impaired blood flow and oxygen supply to the myocardium. Nursing interventions can both prevent ischemia and shorten the duration of pain.

- Keep prescribed nitroglycerin tablets at the client's side so one can be taken at the onset of pain. *Anginal pain indicates myocardial ischemia. Nitroglycerin reduces cardiac work and may improve myocardial blood flow, relieving ischemia and pain.*
- Start oxygen at 4 to 6 L/min per nasal cannula or as prescribed. *Supplemental oxygen reduces myocardial hypoxia.*
- Space activities to allow rest between them. *Activity increases cardiac work and may precipitate angina. Spacing of activities allows the heart to recover.*
- Teach about prescribed medications to maintain myocardial perfusion and reduce cardiac work. Emphasize that long-acting nitrates, beta blockers, and calcium channel blockers are used to *prevent* anginal attacks, not to *treat* an acute attack. *It is important for the client to understand the purpose and use of prescribed drugs to maintain optimal myocardial perfusion.*
- Instruct to take sublingual nitroglycerin before engaging in activities that precipitate angina (e.g., climbing stairs, sexual intercourse). *This prophylactic dose of nitroglycerin helps maintain cardiac perfusion when increased work is anticipated, preventing ischemia and chest pain.*
- Encourage to implement and maintain a progressive exercise program under the supervision of the primary care provider or a cardiac rehabilitation professional. *Exercise slows the atherosclerotic process and helps develop collateral circulation to the heart muscle.*
- Refer to a smoking cessation program as indicated. *Nicotine causes vasoconstriction and increases the heart rate, decreasing myocardial perfusion and increasing cardiac workload.*

Risk for Ineffective Therapeutic Regimen Management

Denial may be strong in the client with angina pectoris. Because many people think of the heart as the locus of life itself, problems such as angina remind people of their mortality, an uncomfortable fact. Denial may lead to "forgetting" to take prescribed medications or to attempting activities that will precipitate angina. Some clients, by contrast, may become "cardiac cripples," afraid

MEDICATION ADMINISTRATION   Antianginal Medications

ORGANIC NITRATES
Nitroglycerin (Nitropaste, Nitro-Dur, Nitro-Bid, Nitrol, Transderm-Nitro, Nitrogard, Nitrodisc, Tridil)
Isosorbide dinitrate (Isordil)
Isosorbide mononitrate (ISMO)
Amyl nitrite

Nitrates dilate both arterial and venous vessels, depending on the dose. Coronary artery vasodilation increases blood flow and myocardial oxygen supply. Venous dilation allows peripheral blood pooling, reducing venous return, preload, and cardiac work. Arterial dilation reduces vascular resistance and afterload, also reducing cardiac work. Sublingual nitroglycerin (NTG) tablets are used to treat and prevent acute anginal attacks (when taken prophylactically before activity). Nitrates are administered sublingually, by buccal spray, or intravenously for immediate effect; or orally or topically for sustained effect.

Nursing Responsibilities
■ Dilute intravenous nitroglycerin before infusing; use only glass bottles for the mixture. Nitroglycerin adheres to PVC bags and tubing, affecting the amount of drug that is delivered. Use non-PVC infusion tubing.
■ Wear gloves when applying nitroglycerin paste or ointment to prevent absorbing the drug through the skin. Measure dose carefully and spread evenly in a 2- by 3-inch area.
■ Remove nitroglycerin patches or ointment at night to help prevent tolerance.

Health Education for the Client and Family
■ Use only the sublingual, buccal, and spray forms of nitrates to treat acute angina.
■ If the first nitrate dose does not relieve angina within 5 minutes, take a second dose. After 5 more minutes, you may take a third dose if needed. If the pain is unrelieved or lasts for 20 minutes or longer, seek medical assistance immediately.
■ Carry a supply of nitroglycerin tablets with you. Dissolve sublingual nitroglycerin tablets under the tongue or between the upper lip and gum. Do not eat, drink, or smoke until the tablet is completely dissolved.
■ Keep sublingual tablets in their original amber glass bottle to protect them from heat, light, and moisture. Replace your supply every 6 months.
■ You may experience a burning or tingling sensation under the tongue and develop a transient headache when you take the drug. These are expected; the headache will diminish over time.
■ Use caution when standing from a sitting position; nitroglycerin may make you light-headed.
■ Rotate ointment or transdermal patch application sites. Apply to a hairless area; spread ointment evenly without rubbing or massaging. Remove the patch or residual ointment at bedtime daily. Apply a fresh dose in the morning.
■ If you are using a long-acting nitrate, keep a supply of immediate-acting nitrates to treat acute angina.

BETA BLOCKERS
Atenolol (Tenormin)
Metoprolol (Lopressor)
Propranolol (Inderal)
Nadolol (Corgard)

Beta blockers decrease cardiac workload by blocking beta receptors on the heart muscle, decreasing heart rate, contractility, myocardial oxygen consumption, and blood pressure. Beta blockers also reduce *reflex tachycardia* (an increased heart rate in response to stimuli such as increased SNS activity or vasodilation), which may develop with other antianginal drugs. Beta blockers are frequently prescribed as antianginal and antihypertensive agents.

Nursing Responsibilities
■ Document heart rate and blood pressure before administering the medication. Withhold drug if the heart rate is below 50 bpm or the blood pressure is below prescribed limits. Notify the physician.
■ Assess for and report possible contraindications to therapy, including heart failure, bradycardia, AV block, asthma, or COPD.
■ Concurrent use of beta blockers and calcium channel blockers increases the risk for heart failure; notify the physician if these drugs are prescribed together.
■ Do not abruptly discontinue these drugs after long-term therapy, as this can increase heart rate, contractility, and blood pressure, and cause fatal dysrhythmia, myocardial infarction, or stroke.

Health Education for the Client and Family
■ Beta blockers help prevent angina but will not relieve an acute attack. Keep a supply of fast-acting nitrates on hand for acute anginal attacks.
■ Do not suddenly stop taking this medication. Discuss discontinuing this medication with your doctor.
■ Take your pulse daily. Do not take the drug, and contact your doctor, if your heart rate is below 50 bpm. Check your blood pressure frequently.
■ Report a slow or irregular pulse, swelling or weight gain, or difficulty breathing to your doctor.

CALCIUM CHANNEL BLOCKERS
Nifedipine (Adalat, Procardia)
Diltiazem (Cardizem)
Verapamil (Isoptin, Calan)
Bepridil (Vascor)
Felodipine (Plendil)
Isradipine (DynaCirc)
Nicardipine (Cardene)
Nimodipine (Nimotop)

Calcium channel blockers are used to control angina, hypertension, and dysrhythmias. By blocking the entry of calcium into cells, these drugs reduce contractility, slow the heart rate and conduction, and cause vasodilation. Calcium channel blockers increase myocardial oxygen supply by dilating the coronary arteries; they decrease the workload of the heart by lowering vascular resistance and oxygen demand. Calcium channel blockers are often prescribed for clients with coronary artery spasm (Prinzmetal's angina).

Nursing Responsibilities
■ Do not mix verapamil in any solution containing sodium bicarbonate. Administer IV push verapamil over 2 to 3 minutes.
■ Document blood pressure and heart rate before administering the drug. Withhold the drug if the heart rate is below 50 bpm. Notify the physician.

(continued)

to engage in activities because of anticipated chest pain. Their inactivity may actually hasten the atherosclerotic process and inhibit collateral circulation development, worsening angina.

- Assess knowledge and understanding of angina. *Assessment allows tailoring of teaching and interventions to the needs of the client.*
- Teach about angina and atherosclerosis as needed, building on current knowledge base. *This can help the client understand that angina is a manageable disease and that pain can usually be controlled and the disease progress slowed.*
- Provide written and verbal instructions about prescribed medications and their use. *Written instructions reinforce teaching and are available to the client for future reference.*
- Stress the importance of taking chest pains seriously while maintaining a positive attitude. *Although it is vital to recognize the significance of chest pain and deal with it appropriately, it is also important to maintain a positive outlook.*
- Refer to a cardiac rehabilitation program or other organized activities and support groups for clients with coronary heart disease. *Programs such as these help the client develop risk factor management strategies, maintain a program of supervised activity, and gain coping skills.*

Community-Based Care

Many clients with stable angina manage their pain effectively, continuing to live active and productive lives. To promote effective management of this disorder, include the following topics in teaching for home care:

- Coronary heart disease and the processes that cause chest pain, including the relationship between the pain and reduced blood flow to the heart muscle
- Use and effects (desired and adverse) of prescribed medications; importance of not discontinuing medications abruptly
- Nitroglycerin use for acute angina: always carry several tablets (not the entire supply); prophylactic use before activities that often cause chest pain; take tablet at first indication of pain rather than waiting to see if the pain develops; seek immediate medical assistance if three nitroglycerin tablets over 15 to 20 minutes do not relieve the pain
- The importance of calling 911 or going to the emergency department immediately for unrelieved chest pain

- Appropriate storage of nitroglycerin: This unstable compound needs to be stored in a cool, dry, dark place; no more than a 6-month supply should be kept on hand.

For the client who has undergone cardiac surgery, also include the following:

- Respiratory care, activity, and pain management
- The importance of actively participating in rehabilitation
- Manifestations of infection or other potential complications and their management.

THE CLIENT WITH ACUTE CORONARY SYNDROME

Acute coronary syndrome (ACS) is a condition of unstable cardiac ischemia. ACS includes unstable angina and acute myocardial ischemia with or without significant injury of myocardial tissue. Although the term ACS may, in some cases, be applied to acute myocardial infarction (myocardial tissue death), myocardial infarction is discussed separately in the next section of this chapter. An estimated 1.4 million Americans are admitted to the hospital annually with ACS (Kasper et al., 2005).

FAST FACTS
- Acute coronary syndrome (severe cardiac ischemia), a common cause of hospital admission, includes unstable angina and acute myocardial infarction.
- Unstable angina is characterized by injury to myocardial cells; with prompt restoration of blood flow, muscle tissue recovers.
- Myocardial infarction is characterized by necrosis and death of myocardial cells; scar tissue forms and functional muscle is lost.
- ACS is the most common identified cause of sudden cardiac death (American Heart Association [AHA], 2005a).

Pathophysiology

ACS is a dynamic state in which coronary blood flow is acutely reduced, but not fully occluded. Myocardial cells are injured by the acute ischemia that results. Most people affected by ACS have significant stenosis of one or more coronary arteries.

ACS is precipitated by one or more of the following processes: (1) rupture or erosion of atherosclerotic plaque with formation of a blood clot that does not fully occlude the vessel; (2) coronary artery spasm (e.g., Prinzmetal's angina); (3) progressive vessel obstruction by atherosclerotic plaque or restenosis following a percutaneous revascularization (PCR) procedure; (4) inflammation of a coronary artery; or (5) increased myocardial oxygen demand and/or decreased supply (e.g., acute blood loss or anemia) (Braunwald et al., 2002). Of these, ruptured or eroded plaque is the predominant pathophysiology underlying ACS (AHA, 2005a). Plaque rupture often is triggered by hemodynamic factors such as increased heart rate, blood flow, and blood pressure in response to a surge of sympathetic nervous system (SNS) activity. Increased SNS activity also is thought to contribute to the higher incidence of plaque rupture within the first hour of arising from bed in the morning (Porth, 2005).

When atherosclerotic plaque ruptures or erodes, the exposed lipid core of the plaque stimulates platelet aggregation and the extrinsic clotting pathway. Thrombin is generated and fibrin is deposited, forming a clot that severely impairs or obstructs blood flow to tissue distal to the area of plaque rupture. As a result, these cells become ischemic.

Injured myocardial cells contract less effectively, potentially reducing cardiac output if a large area of myocardium is affected. Lactic acid released from ischemic cells stimulates pain receptors, causing chest pain. Ischemia and injury affect electrical impulse conduction, producing inversion of the T wave and possibly elevation of the ST segment on the ECG.

Manifestations

The cardinal manifestation of ACS is chest pain, usually substernal or epigastric. The pain often radiates to the neck, left shoulder, and/or left arm. The pain may occur at rest and typically lasts longer than 10 to 20 minutes. In ACS, the chest pain is more severe and prolonged than that previously experienced by the client. It may be a new onset of pain, or may represent a pattern of increasing frequency and severity of anginal pain. Dyspnea, diaphoresis, pallor, and cool skin may be present. Tachycardia and hypotension may occur. The client may be nauseated or feel light-headed. Table 31–5 compares the features of stable angina, ACS, and acute myocardial infarction.

INTERDISCIPLINARY CARE

The client with ACS generally presents at the emergency department or physician's office with complaints of severe chest pain. The pain may be unrelieved by nitroglycerin or may be more severe and of longer duration than previous anginal episodes. The ECG is used in conjunction with blood levels of cardiac markers to differentiate between unstable angina and acute myocardial infarction. Clients with unstable angina generally are admitted to the acute care unit on bed rest with cardiac monitoring for 12 to 24 hours. Coronary revascularization procedures may be performed within 48 hours if significant CHD is identified.

Diagnosis

The ECG and serum cardiac markers are the primary tests used to establish the diagnosis of ACS. Serum cardiac markers, proteins released from injured and necrotic heart muscle, can be measured. (See the following section on acute myocardial infarction and Table 31–6 for more information about serum cardiac markers.)

- Cardiac muscle troponins, *cardiac-specific troponin T (cT_nT)* and *cardiac-specific troponin I (cT_nI)*, are sensitive indicators of myocardial damage. Troponins may be elevated in

TABLE 31–5 Comparing Stable Angina, Acute Coronary Syndrome, and Acute Myocardial Infarction

	STABLE ANGINA	ACUTE CORONARY SYNDROME	ACUTE MYOCARDIAL INFARCTION
Pathophysiology	Myocardial ischemia occurs with increased workload (e.g., during exercise) due to stable atherosclerotic plaque narrowing the coronary arteries.	Coronary artery spasm or partial occlusion results from unstable plaque and thrombus formation with increasing myocardial ischemia.	Obstruction of a coronary artery by a thrombus blocks blood supply to a portion of myocardium, resulting in necrosis.
Chest Pain	Stable and predictable, occurring with exertion or emotion Crescendo–decrescendo pattern May radiate to neck, shoulder, arms Usually lasts 2 to 5 minutes, relieved by rest	Occurs at rest; increasing frequency and severity Lasts 10 minutes or longer Radiates to neck, left shoulder, and arm	Begins abruptly, unrelated to rest or exercise Severe, "crushing" Unrelieved by rest or nitroglycerin Radiates to arms, neck, jaw
Other Manifestations	Indigestion, nausea Possible shortness of breath Anxiety	Epigastric pain Dyspnea Tachycardia, hypotension Cool, pale skin	Epigastric pain, nausea Dyspnea Pallor, diaphoresis Tachycardia or bradycardia, hyper- or hypotension
Diagnosis	ECG: T-wave inversion during anginal episodes Cardiac markers: within normal range	ECG: ST-segment depression, T-wave inversion Cardiac markers: within normal range or transient elevation	ECG: ST-segment elevation, possible Q wave Cardiac markers: elevated

ACS or may be within normal limits if chest pain is due to unstable angina.

- Creatine kinase (CK) and CK-MB (specific to myocardial muscle) levels are likely to be within normal limits or demonstrate transient elevation, returning to normal levels within 12 to 24 hours.

The ECG, particularly when done during the acute episode of chest pain, is a valuable diagnostic tool for ACS. ST-segment changes (elevation or depression) during chest pain that resolve when the pain abates usually indicate acute myocardial ischemia and severe underlying CHD.

Medications

Medications include drugs to reduce myocardial ischemia and those to reduce the risk for blood clotting. Fibrinolytic drugs (that is, drugs that break down the fibrin in blood clots) may be given prior to or on admission to the emergency department. These drugs restore blood flow to ischemic cardiac muscle and can prevent permanent damage. See the section on myocardial infarction for more information about fibrinolytic drugs and their nursing implications.

Nitrates and beta blockers are used to restore blood flow to the ischemic myocardium and reduce the workload of the heart. Nitroglycerin is given by sublingual tablet or buccal spray. If chest pain is unrelieved after three doses 5 minutes apart, an intravenous nitroglycerin infusion is initiated. The infusion may be continued until the chest pain is relieved or for 12 to 24 hours. Topical or oral nitrates are then initiated. Beta-adrenergic blockers are initially given intravenously, followed by oral beta-blockers. See the Medication Administration box on page 973 for the nursing implications of these drugs.

Aspirin, other antiplatelet drugs, and heparin are given to inhibit blood clotting and reduce the risk of thrombus formation. Aspirin and clopidogrel (Plavix) are given to clients with ACS who do not have an excessive bleeding risk. Aspirin and clopidogrel suppress platelet aggregation, interrupting the process of forming a stable blood clot. Both increase the risk of serious hemorrhage; for most clients, however, the benefit outweighs the risk. Intravenous antiplatelet drugs such as abciximab (ReoPro), eptifibatide (Integrilin), or tirofiban (Aggrastat) may be used when an invasive coronary revascularization procedure is anticipated in the immediate or near future. Nursing implications for the antiplatelet drugs are outlined in the Medication Administration box below.

Revascularization Procedures

Several procedures may be used to restore blood flow and oxygen to ischemic tissue. Nonsurgical techniques include translu-

---

MEDICATION ADMINISTRATION   Antiplatelet Drugs

ORAL ANTIPLATELET DRUGS
Aspirin
Clopidogrel (Plavix)

Antiplatelet drugs suppress platelet aggregation in arteries, preventing the development of an arterial thrombus. Aspirin and clopidogrel block different platelet activation pathways to inhibit platelet aggregation and clot formation. The dose of aspirin given to achieve antiplatelet effects is low, typically 80 to 325 mg/day.

Nursing Responsibilities
- Inquire about a history of intracranial hemorrhage, upper gastrointestinal bleeding, peptic ulcer disease, or known bleeding tendency.
- Observe for and report increased bruising, petechiae, purpura, apparent or occult bleeding (e.g., melena, hematemesis).
- Do not administer concurrently with warfarin (Coumadin).

Health Education for the Client and Family
- Take as directed. Take aspirin with food or milk; clopidogrel may be taken at any time of day.
- Do not use NSAIDs or other over-the-counter drugs that may contain aspirin or an NSAID unless prescribed by your physician.
- Check with your physician before taking any herbal remedies such as evening primrose oil, feverfew, garlic, ginkgo biloba, or grapeseed extract while taking these medications.
- Report unusual bruising or excessive bleeding.
- Inform all care providers (including dental professionals) of use of these drugs.

INTRAVENOUS ANTIPLATELET DRUGS
Abciximab (ReoPro)
Eptifibatide (Integrelin)
Tirofiban (Aggrastat)

The intravenously administered antiplatelet drugs, abciximab, epifibatide, and tirofiban, block the final common pathway of platelet activation, and thus are more effective. However, the risk of bleeding is greater than with the orally administered antiplatelet drugs.

Nursing Responsibilities
- Determine history of bleeding disorders, intracranial hemorrhage, recent trauma or surgery.
- Inquire about recent use of oral antiplatelet or anticoagulant drugs.
- Monitor CBC including hemoglobin, hematocrit, and platelet count; clotting studies, including PT, INR, PTT; vital signs; and ECG during therapy.
- Maintain a separate intravenous line for blood draws and administration of other drugs during infusion.
- Closely observe for and immediately report anaphylaxis or bleeding uncontrolled by pressure. Keep resuscitation equipment readily available.
- Maintain bed rest during infusion.

Health Education for the Client and Family
- This drug is given to reduce the risk of clotting and myocardial infarction. It helps maintain blood flow through the affected vessel following angioplasty and stent placement.
- Immediately report any chest tightness, difficulty breathing, shortness of breath, or itching that develops during the infusion.
- Your risk of bleeding should return to normal within about 2 days following the infusion.
- Immediately report any unusual bruising or bleeding to your doctor.

minal coronary angioplasty, laser angioplasty, coronary atherectomy, and intracoronary stents. Coronary artery bypass grafting (CABG) is a surgical procedure that may be used.

PERCUTANEOUS CORONARY REVASCULARIZATION *Percutaneous coronary revascularization (PCR)* procedures are used to restore blood flow to the ischemic myocardium in clients with CHD. Approximately 600,000 PCR procedures are done annually in the United States. PCR is used to treat clients with:

- Moderately severe, chronic stable angina unrelieved by medical therapy
- Unstable angina
- Acute myocardial infarction
- Significant stenosis of the left anterior descending coronary artery
- Stenosis of a CABG (Kasper et al., 2005; Tierney et al., 2005).

PCR procedures are similar to the procedure used for coronary angiography. A catheter introduced into the arterial circulation is guided into the opening of the narrowed coronary artery. A flexible guidewire is inserted through the catheter lumen into the affected vessel. The guidewire is then used to thread an angioplasty balloon, arterial stent, or other therapeutic device into the narrowed segment of the artery. The procedure is performed in the cardiac catheterization laboratory using local anesthesia. The hospital stay is short (1 to 2 days), minimizing costs.

In a *percutaneous transluminal coronary angioplasty (PTCA)*, a balloon-tipped catheter is threaded over the guidewire, with the balloon positioned across the area of narrowing (Figure 31–2 ■). The balloon is inflated in a step-by-step fashion for about 30 seconds to 2 minutes to compress the plaque against the arterial wall, with a goal of reducing the vessel obstruction to less than 50% of the arterial lumen. PTCA typically is accompanied by placement of a stent. *Intracoronary stents* are metallic scaffolds used to maintain an open arterial lumen. Stents reduce the rate of restenosis following angioplasty by about one-third, and are now used in the majority of all PCR procedures (Kasper et al., 2005). The stent is placed over a balloon catheter, guided into position, and expanded as the balloon is inflated. It then remains in the artery as a prop after the balloon is removed. Endothelial cells will completely line the inner wall of the stent to produce a smooth inner lining. Antiplatelet medications (aspirin and ticlopidine) are given following stent insertion to reduce the risk of thrombus formation at the site.

In contrast to stent procedures, which enlarge the artery by displacing plaque, *atherectomy* procedures remove plaque from the identified lesion. The directional atherectomy catheter shaves the plaque off vessel walls using a rotary cutting head, retaining the fragments in its housing and removing them from the vessel. Rotational atherectomy catheters pulverize plaque into particles small enough to pass through the coronary microcirculation. Laser atherectomy devices use laser energy to remove plaque.

Complications following PCR procedures include hematoma at the catheter insertion site, pseudoaneurysm, embolism, hypersensitivity to contrast dye, dysrhythmias, bleeding, vessel perforation, and restenosis, or reocclusion of the treated vessel.

Nursing care of the client undergoing PCR is outlined in the box on the next page.

CORONARY ARTERY BYPASS GRAFTING Surgery for coronary heart disease involves using a section of a vein or an artery to create a connection (or bypass) between the aorta and the coronary artery beyond the obstruction (Figure 31–3 ■). This then allows blood to perfuse the ischemic portion of the heart. The internal mammary artery in the chest and the saphenous vein from the leg are the vessels most commonly used for CABG.

Bypass grafts are safe and effective. Angina is totally relieved or significantly reduced in 90% of clients who undergo

Figure 31–2 ■ Percutaneous coronary revascularization. *A,* The balloon catheter with the stent is threaded into the affected coronary artery. *B, C,* The stent is positioned across the blockage and expanded. *D,* The balloon is deflated and removed, leaving the stent in place.

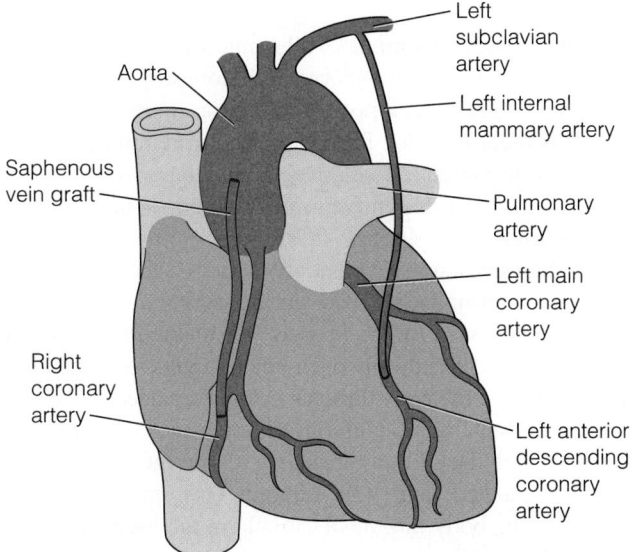

Figure 31–3 ■ Coronary artery bypass grafting using the internal mammary artery and a saphenous vein graft.

NURSING CARE OF THE CLIENT HAVING PCR

BEFORE THE PROCEDURE

- Assess knowledge of the procedure and expectations of treatment. *This allows information to be tailored to the client's needs and provides an opportunity to clarify misconceptions.*
- Describe the cardiac catheterization laboratory and the planned PCR procedure, including:
  - Preoperative preparation (see Chapter 4 ∞)
  - Planned anesthesia or sedation to be used.
  - Drugs that may be given during the procedure, such as anticoagulants to reduce the risk of thrombus formation, and intravenous nitroglycerin and a calcium channel blocker to dilate coronary arteries and prevent anginal pain.
- Discuss possible sensations during the procedure, including flushing or warmth and a metallic taste in the mouth as the contrast dye is injected, and a feeling of pressure or chest pain during balloon inflation. *Advanced preparation for expected sensations reduces anxiety and improves outcomes.*
- Perform a comprehensive assessment, including hydration status (skin and mucous membrane moisture, turgor) and peripheral circulation (color, warmth, sensation, pulses, and capillary refill).

AFTER THE PROCEDURE

- Complete a head-to-toe assessment. Note any complaints of chest pain, or evidence of decreased cardiac output or myocardial infarction. *Assessment provides a baseline for subsequent assessments and allows early identification of possible complications.*
- Monitor vital signs and cardiac rhythm continuously. Treat dysrhythmias as ordered. Obtain a 12-lead ECG if signs of ischemia develop, and notify physician. *Vital signs reflect cardiac output. Dysrhythmias may develop with reperfusion of the ischemic myocardium. ECG changes may indicate infarction or restenosis of the affected vessel.*
- Maintain intravenous nitroglycerin infusion. Administer anticoagulant and antiplatelet medications, nitrates, and calcium channel blockers as ordered. *These drugs decrease oxygen demand and increase oxygen supply by dilating the coronary arteries and systemic vasculature. They also reduce the risk of thrombus formation.*
- Monitor for and treat or report chest pain as indicated. *Chest pain may indicate ischemia and possible myocardial infarction.*
- Maintain bed rest as ordered with the head of the bed at 30 degrees or less. Prevent flexion of the leg on the affected side. Following sheath removal, follow protocol for pressure dressing or device or sandbag placement. *A large puncture wound occurs at the insertion site. Immobilization allows the wound to seal; a pressure dressing helps prevent bleeding.*
- Monitor distal pulses, color, movement, sensation, and temperature of the affected leg, and insertion site every 15 minutes for the first hour, every 30 minutes for the next hour, every hour for the next 8 hours, then every 4 hours. *A clot may form at the site, reducing perfusion of the affected leg. The site and dressing are monitored for excessive bleeding, hematoma formation, or pseudoaneurysm. Pseudoaneurysm occurs as a result of inadequate hemostasis after catheter removal.*
- Monitor intake and output, serum electrolytes, blood urea nitrogen (BUN), creatinine, complete blood count (CBC), partial thromboplastin time (PTT), and cardiac enzymes. Report abnormal results to the physician. *Contrast dye causes osmotic diuresis and may cause renal damage or a hypersensitivity reaction. Electrolyte imbalances increase the risk of dysrhythmias. Cardiac enzymes are monitored for indications of possible myocardial damage during the procedure. The PTT monitors the effectiveness of heparin therapy.*
- Monitor for bradycardia, light-headedness, hypotension, diaphoresis, and loss of consciousness during sheath removal. Keep atropine at bedside during sheath removal. *Bradycardia and signs of decreased cardiac output may occur during sheath removal because of a vasovagal reaction. Atropine decreases vagal tone and increases heart rate.*

---

complete revascularization. While anginal pain may recur within 3 years, it rarely is as severe as before surgery. Coronary artery bypass graft has a positive effect on mortality in many cases. It is recommended for clients who have multiple vessel disease and impaired left ventricular function or diabetes, and for clients who have significant obstruction of the left main coronary artery (Kasper et al., 2005).

A median sternotomy commonly is used to access the heart. The heart is usually stopped during surgery. The *cardiopulmonary bypass (CPB) pump* is used to maintain perfusion to the rest of the organs during open-heart surgery. Venous blood is removed from the body through a cannula placed in the right atrium or the superior and inferior venae cavae. Blood then circulates through the CPB pump, where it is oxygenated, its temperature regulated, and it is filtered. Oxygenated blood is returned to the body through a cannula in the ascending aorta (Figure 31–4 ■). Cardiopulmonary bypass enables surgeons to operate on a quiet heart and a relatively bloodless field. Hypothermia can be maintained to reduce the metabolic rate and decrease oxygen demand during surgery.

Newer techniques have been developed that allow surgeons to perform CABG without cardioplegia (stopping the heart) and CPB. Off-pump coronary artery bypass (OPCAB) allows use of a smaller incision for access. Although cardiopulmonary bypass is employed for the majority of coronary artery bypass procedures, OPCAB is a promising alternative. Controlled studies demonstrate lower mortality and morbidity rates and faster recovery for clients undergoing OPCAB as compared to CABG with cardiopulmonary bypass (Eagle et al., 2004).

When the saphenous vein is used, it is excised from its normal attachments in the leg, flushed with a cold heparinized saline solution, and then reversed so that its valves do not interfere with blood flow. When appropriate, a laparoscopic approach may be used to remove the vein. The vein is

Figure 31-4 ■ A diagrammatic representation of cardiopulmonary bypass. A cannula in the superior and inferior venae cavae removes venous blood, which is then pumped through an oxygenator and heat exchanger. After filtering, oxygenated blood is returned to the ascending aorta.

anastomosed (grafted) to the aorta and the coronary artery, distal to the occlusion (see Figure 31–3). This provides a bridge or conduit for blood flow past the obstruction. If the internal mammary artery (IMA) is used, its distal end is excised and anastomosed to the coronary artery distal to the obstruction. The IMA often is used to revascularize the left coronary artery because of the greater oxygen demand of the left ventricle.

Once grafting is completed, cardiopulmonary bypass is discontinued and the client is rewarmed. Rewarming stimulates the heart to resume beating. Temporary pacing wires are sutured in place and passed through the chest wall in case temporary pacing is necessary. Chest tubes are placed in the pleural space and mediastinum to drain blood and reestablish negative pressure in the thoracic cavity. The sternum is closed using heavy wires and bone wax, the skin is closed with sutures or staples, and sterile dressings are applied over sternal and leg incisions.

Pre- and postoperative nursing care and teaching for the client having a coronary artery bypass graft or other open-heart surgery are outlined on pages 980–982.

MINIMALLY INVASIVE CORONARY ARTERY SURGERY *Minimally invasive coronary artery surgery* is a potential future alternative to CABG. Two approaches may be used: *Port-access coronary artery bypass* uses several small holes, or "ports," in the chest wall to access vessels for connection to the CPB pump and the surgical site. Alternatively, the femoral artery and femoral vein may be used for CPB (Eagle et al., 2004). CPB is avoided altogether using the *minimally invasive direct coronary artery bypass (MIDCAB)* approach. With MIDCAB, a small surgical incision and several chest wall ports are used to graft a chest wall artery to the affected coronary vessel while the heart continues to beat.

TRANSMYOCARDIAL LASER REVASCULARIZATION A new development in myocardial revascularization techniques is called *transmyocardial laser revascularization (TMLR)*. In this procedure, a laser is used to drill tiny holes into the myocardial muscle itself to provide collateral blood flow to ischemic muscle. Clients whose coronary artery obstructions are too diffuse to bypass are candidates for this new surgical treatment.

NURSING CARE

Health promotion, assessment, nursing diagnoses and interventions for the client with ACS are similar to those identified for clients with angina and with acute myocardial infarction. See the preceding and subsequent sections of this chapter for specific nursing care activities, as well as the Nursing Care Plan that follows.

NURSING CARE OF THE CLIENT HAVING A Coronary Artery Bypass Graft

PREOPERATIVE CARE

- Provide routine preoperative care and teaching as outlined in Chapter 4 ∞.
- Verify presence of laboratory and diagnostic test results in the chart, including CBC, coagulation profile, urinalysis, chest x-ray, and coronary angiogram. *These baseline data are important for comparison of postoperative results and values.*
- Type and crossmatch four or more units of blood as ordered. *Blood is made available for use during and after surgery as needed.*
- Provide specific client and family teaching related to procedure and postoperative care. Include the following topics.
  - Cardiac recovery unit; sensory stimuli, personnel; noise and alarms; visiting policies
  - Tubes, drains, and general appearance
  - Monitoring equipment, including cardiac and hemodynamic monitoring systems
  - Respiratory support: ventilator, endotracheal tube, suctioning; communication while intubated
  - Incisions and dressings
  - Pain management

Preoperative teaching reduces anxiety and prepares the client and family for the postoperative environment and expected sensations.

POSTOPERATIVE CARE

- Provide routine postoperative care as outlined in Chapter 4 ∞. In addition to the care needs of all clients having major surgery, the cardiac surgery client has specific care needs related to open-heart and thoracic surgery. These are outlined under the nursing diagnoses identified below.

Decreased Cardiac Output

Cardiac output may be compromised postoperatively due to bleeding and fluid loss; depression of myocardial function by drugs, hypothermia, and surgical manipulation; dysrhythmias; increased vascular resistance; and a potential complication, *cardiac tamponade*, compression of the heart due to collected blood or fluid in the pericardium.

- Monitor vital signs, oxygen saturation, and hemodynamic parameters every 15 minutes. Note trends and report significant changes to the physician. *Initial hypothermia and bradycardia are expected; the heart rate should return to the normal range with rewarming. The blood pressure may fall during rewarming as vasodilation occurs. Hypotension and tachycardia, however, may indicate low cardiac output. Pulmonary artery pressure (PAP), pulmonary artery wedge pressure (PAWP), cardiac output, and oxygen saturation are monitored to evaluate fluid volume, cardiac function, and gas exchange. Hemodynamic monitoring is further discussed in Chapter 32 ∞.*
- Auscultate heart and breath sounds on admission and at least every 4 hours. *A ventricular gallop, or S₃, is an early sign of heart failure; an S₄ may indicate decreased ventricular compliance. Muffled heart sounds may be an early indication of cardiac tamponade. Adventitious breath sounds (wheezes, crackles, or rales) may be a manifestation of heart failure or respiratory compromise.*
- Assess skin color and temperature, peripheral pulses, and level of consciousness with vital signs. *Pale, mottled, or cyanotic coloring, cool and clammy skin, and diminished pulse amplitude are indicators of decreased cardiac output.*
- Continuously monitor and document cardiac rhythm. *Dysrhythmias are common, and may interfere with cardiac filling and contractility, decreasing the cardiac output.*
- Measure intake and output hourly. Report urine output less than 30 mL/h for 2 consecutive hours. *Intake and output measurements help evaluate fluid volume status. A fall in urine output may be an early indicator of decreased cardiac output.*
- Record chest tube output hourly. *Chest tube drainage greater than 70 mL/h or that is warm, red, and free flowing indicates hemorrhage and may necessitate a return to surgery. A sudden drop in chest tube output may indicate impending cardiac tamponade.*
- Monitor hemoglobin, hematocrit, and serum electrolytes. *A drop in hemoglobin and hematocrit may indicate hemorrhage that is not otherwise obvious. Electrolyte imbalances, potassium, calcium, and magnesium in particular, affect cardiac rhythm and contractility.*
- Administer intravenous fluids, fluid boluses, and blood transfusions as ordered. *Fluid and blood replacement helps ensure adequate blood volume and oxygen-carrying capacity.*
- Administer medications as ordered. *Medications ordered in the early postoperative period to maintain the cardiac output include inotropic drugs (e.g., dopamine, dobutamine) to increase the force of myocardial contractions; vasodilators (e.g., nitroprusside or nitroglycerin) to decrease vascular resistance and after-load; and antidysrhythmics to correct dysrhythmias that affect cardiac output.*
- Keep a temporary pacemaker at the bedside; initiate pacing as indicated. *Temporary pacing may be needed to maintain the cardiac output with bradydysrhythmias, such as high-level AV blocks.*

PRACTICE ALERT

Assess for signs of cardiac tamponade: increased heart rate, decreased BP, decreased urine output, increased central venous pressure, a sudden decrease in chest tube output, muffled/distant heart sounds, and diminished peripheral pulses. Notify physician immediately. Cardiac tamponade is a life-threatening complication that may develop postoperatively. Cardiac tamponade interferes with ventricular filling and contraction, decreasing cardiac output. Untreated, cardiac tamponade leads to cardiogenic shock and possible cardiac arrest.

Hypothermia

Hypothermia is maintained during cardiac surgery to reduce the metabolic rate and protect vital organs from ischemic damage. Although rewarming is instituted on completion of the surgery, the client often remains hypothermic on admission to cardiac recovery. Gradual rewarming is necessary to prevent peripheral vasodilation and hypotension.

- Monitor core body temperature (e.g., tympanic membrane, pulmonary artery, bladder) for the first 8 hours following surgery. *Oral and rectal temperature measurements are not reliable indicators of core body temperature during this period.*

NURSING CARE OF THE CLIENT HAVING A **Coronary Artery Bypass Graft (continued)**

- Institute rewarming measures (e.g., warmed intravenous solutions or blood transfusion, warm blankets, warm inspired gases, radiant heat lamps) as needed to maintain a temperature above 96.8°F (36°C). Administer Thorazine, morphine, or diltiazem as ordered to relieve shivering. *Low body temperature may cause shivering, increasing oxygen demand and consumption. Hypothermia also increases the risk for hypoxia, metabolic acidosis, vasoconstriction and increased cardiac work, altered clotting, and dysrhythmias.*

Acute Pain

Following a CABG, pain is experienced due to both the thoracic incision and removal of the saphenous vein from the leg. Dissection of the internal mammary artery (usually the left IMA) from the chest wall also causes chest pain on the affected side. Chest tube sites are also uncomfortable. The leg from which the saphenous vein graft was obtained may be more painful than the chest incision.

- Frequently assess for pain, including its location and character. Document its intensity using a standard pain scale. Assess for verbal and nonverbal indicators of pain. Validate pain cues with the client. *Pain is subjective, and differs among individuals. Incisional pain is expected; however, anginal pain also may develop. It is important to differentiate the type of pain.*

PRACTICE ALERT

Promptly report anginal or cardiac pain. Cardiac pain may indicate a perioperative or postoperative myocardial infarction.

- Administer analgesics on a scheduled basis, by PCA, or by continuous infusion for the first 24 to 48 hours. *Research demonstrates that adequate pain management in the immediate postoperative period reduces complications from sympathetic stimulation and allows faster recovery. Pain causes muscle tension and vasoconstriction, impairing circulation and tissue perfusion, slowing wound healing, and increasing cardiac work.*
- Premedicate 30 minutes before activities or planned procedures. *Premedication and the subsequent reduction of pain improves client participation and cooperation with care.*

Ineffective Airway Clearance/Impaired Gas Exchange

Atelectasis due to impaired ventilation and airway clearance is a common pulmonary complication of cardiac surgery. Gas exchange may also be affected by blood loss and decreased oxygen-carrying capacity following surgery. Phrenic nerve paralysis is a potential complication of cardiac surgery which may also contribute to impaired ventilation and gas exchange.

- Evaluate respiratory rate, depth, effort, symmetry of chest expansion, and breath sounds frequently. *Pain, anxiety, excess fluid volume, surgical injury, narcotics and anesthesia, and altered homeostasis can affect respiratory rate, depth, and effort postoperatively. Decreased chest expansion or asymmetrical movement may indicate impaired ventilation of one lung, and needs further evaluation.*

- Note endotracheal tube (ETT) placement on chest x-ray. Mark tube position and secure in place. Insert an oral airway if an oral ETT is used. *The chest x-ray documents correct ETT placement above the bifurcation to the right and left mainstem bronchus. Marking its appropriate placement allows evaluation of potential tube movement. Secure the tube firmly in place to prevent slippage or inadvertent removal. An oral airway helps prevent obstruction of an oral ETT by biting.*
- Maintain ventilator settings as ordered. Monitor arterial blood gases (ABGs) as ordered. *Mechanical ventilation promotes optimal lung expansion and oxygenation postoperatively. ABGs are used to evaluate oxygenation and acid–base balance.*
- Suction as needed. *Suctioning is performed only as indicated to clear airway secretions.*
- Prepare for ventilator weaning and extubation, as appropriate. *The client is removed from the ventilator and extubated as soon as possible to reduce complications associated with mechanical ventilation and intubation.*
- After extubation, teach use of the incentive spirometer, and encourage use every 2 hours. Encourage deep breathing; advise against vigorous coughing. Teach use of a "cough pillow" to splint chest incision and decrease pain. Frequently turn and encourage movement. Dangle on postoperative day 1. *Deep breathing, controlled coughing, and position changes improve ventilation and airway clearance and help prevent complications. Vigorous coughing may excessively increase intrathoracic pressure and cause sternal instability.*

Risk for Infection

Following an open chest procedure, a sternal infection may develop that can progress to involve the mediastinum. Incisions for removal of the saphenous vein also may become infected. Clients with IMA grafts, who are diabetic, older, or malnourished, are at high risk: Harvesting of IMA disrupts blood supply to the sternum, and these clients have impaired immune responses and healing.

- Assess sternal incision and leg wounds every shift. Document redness, warmth, swelling, and/or drainage from the site. Note wound approximation. *These assessments provide indicators of inflammation and healing.*
- Maintain a sterile dressing for the first 48 hours, then leave the incision open to air. Use Steri-Strips as needed to maintain approximation of the wound edges. *The sterile dressing prevents early contamination of the wound, whereas exposing the incision after 48 hours promotes healing.*
- Report signs of wound infection: a swollen, reddened area that is hot and painful to the touch; drainage from the wound; impaired healing, or healed areas that reopen. *Evidence of infection or impaired healing requires further evaluation and treatment.*
- Culture wound drainage as indicated. *Identifying the infective organism facilitates appropriate antibiotic therapy.*
- Collaborate with the dietitian to promote nutrition and fluid intake. *Good nutritional status is vital to healing and immune function.*

(continued)

NURSING CARE OF THE CLIENT HAVING A   Coronary Artery Bypass Graft (continued)

Disturbed Thought Processes

Many factors affect neuropsychologic function after CABG, including the length of cardiopulmonary bypass, age, presurgery organic brain dysfunction, severity of illness, and decreased cardiac output. Sensory overload and deprivation, sleep disruption, and numerous drugs also affect thinking and mental clarity.

- Frequently reorient during initial recovery period. State that surgery is over and that the client is in the recovery area. *Frequent reorientation provides emotional support and reality checks.*
- Explain all procedures before performing them. Speak in a clear, calm voice. Encourage questions, and give honest answers. *These measures provide information, decrease anxiety, and establish trust.*
- Secure all intravenous lines and invasive catheters/tubes (e.g., ETT, Foley catheter, nasogastric tube). *Disoriented clients may tug or pull at invasive equipment, disrupting them and increasing the risk of injury.*
- Note verbal responses to questions. Correct misconceptions immediately (e.g., "Mr. Snow, look at all the special equipment in this room. Does this room look like your bedroom at home?"). *Helping the client recognize differences in the hospital environment offers a basis for continual reality checks.*
- Maintain a calendar and clock within the client's view. *This provides current information regarding day, date, and time.*
- Involve family members in providing reorientation. Place familiar objects and photographs within view. Encourage family presence. *The family provides reassurance and contact with the familiar, assisting with orientation.*
- Promote client participation in care and decision making as appropriate. *This allows the client to maintain a degree of power and control and enables the client to take an active role in recovery.*
- Report signs of hallucinations, delusions, depression, or agitation. *These may indicate progressive deterioration of mental status.*
- Administer sedatives cautiously. *Mild sedation may help prevent injury. Some sedatives may, however, have adverse effects, increasing confusion and disorientation.*
- Reevaluate neurologic status every shift. *These data allow evaluation of the effect of interventions.*

THE CLIENT WITH ACUTE MYOCARDIAL INFARCTION

An **acute myocardial infarction (AMI)**, necrosis (death) of myocardial cells, is a life-threatening event. If circulation to the affected myocardium is not promptly restored, loss of functional myocardium affects the heart's ability to maintain an effective cardiac output. This may ultimately lead to cardiogenic shock and death.

Heart disease remains the leading cause of death in the United States. Of the major heart diseases, myocardial infarction or *heart attack,* and other forms of ischemic heart disease cause the majority of deaths. Annually, approximately 700,000 people in the United States experience their first MI; another 500,000 suffer an MI subsequent to the initial one. Nearly 492,000 people died of coronary heart disease in 2002, with most of these deaths related to MI (NHLBI, 2004).

The majority of deaths from MI occur during the initial period after symptoms begin: approximately 60% within the first hour, and 40% prior to hospitalization. Heightening public awareness of the manifestations of MI, the importance of seeking immediate medical assistance, and training in cardiopulmonary resuscitation (CPR) techniques are vital to decrease deaths due to MI.

Myocardial infarction rarely occurs in clients without preexisting coronary heart disease. While no specific cause has been identified, the risk factors for MI are those for coronary heart disease: age, gender, heredity, race; smoking, obesity, hyperlipidemia, hypertension, diabetes, sedentary lifestyle, diet, and others. See the previous section of this chapter on coronary heart disease for further discussion of these risk factors.

Pathophysiology

Atherosclerotic plaque may form stable or unstable lesions. *Stable* lesions progress by gradually occluding the vessel lumen, whereas *unstable* (or *complicated*) lesions are prone to rupture and thrombus formation. Stable lesions often cause angina (discussed in the previous sections); unstable lesions often lead to acute coronary syndromes, or acute ischemic heart diseases. Acute coronary syndromes include unstable angina, myocardial infarction, and sudden cardiac death (Braunwald et al., 2002).

Myocardial infarction occurs when blood flow to a portion of cardiac muscle is completely blocked, resulting in prolonged tissue ischemia and irreversible cell damage. Coronary occlusion is usually caused by ulceration or rupture of a complicated atherosclerotic lesion. When an atherosclerotic lesion ruptures or ulcerates, substances are released that stimulate platelet aggregation, thrombin generation, and local vasomotor tone. As a result, the vessel constricts and a thrombus (clot) forms, occluding the vessel and interrupting blood flow to the myocardium distal to the obstruction.

Cellular injury occurs when the cells are denied adequate oxygen and nutrients. When ischemia is prolonged, lasting more than 20 to 45 minutes, irreversible hypoxemic damage causes cellular death and tissue necrosis. Oxygen, glycogen, and ATP stores of ischemic cells are rapidly depleted. Cellular metabolism shifts to an anaerobic process, producing hydrogen ions and lactic acid. Cellular acidosis increases cells' vulnerability to further damage. Intracellular enzymes are released through damaged cell membranes into interstitial spaces.

Cellular acidosis, electrolyte imbalances, and hormones released in response to cellular ischemia affect impulse conduction and myocardial contractility. The risk for dysrhythmias increases, and myocardial contractility decreases, reducing stroke volume, cardiac output, blood pressure, and tissue perfusion.

The subendocardium suffers the initial damage, within 20 minutes of injury, because this area is the most susceptible to

NURSING CARE PLAN **A Client with Coronary Artery Bypass Surgery**

Six weeks ago, John Clements, age 50, was discharged from the hospital after emergency triple bypass surgery. Despite having emergency surgery, his postoperative recovery was uneventful, and he was discharged 6 days after admission. He returns to the clinic for a postoperative stress test and to discuss his cardiac rehabilitation program. Anne Wagner, RN, CNS, a cardiac clinical nurse specialist and the program coordinator, meets Mr. Clements to obtain specific information regarding his medical status.

ASSESSMENT

Mr. Clements's medical history reveals significant CHD, an anterior wall myocardial infarction that led to his emergency triple bypass, and hyperlipidemia. Current medications include Cardizem, Isordil, Ecotrin, and Transderm-Nitro 5. The ECG reveals sinus rhythm with some ST segment and T wave flattening. Resting heart rate 68, and blood pressure 136/84.

Mr. Clements has a strong family history of CHD. He does not smoke and uses alcohol occasionally in social situations. He enjoys "good Southern-style cooking" and watching television. Mr. Clements states his only regular exercise used to be an evening of dancing with his wife and friends about once a month, "But I get short of breath walking around the block now, so I guess I can't go dancing anymore!"

Mr. Clements owns his own contracting business and states that he typically works about 50 to 60 hours per week. He tells Ms. Wagner, "I don't know what this program is supposed to do for me. I have got to get back to work! You just can't sit around in my business—you have to make sure that the work is getting done on time, and you have to check on supplies and equipment and the like. But I feel like a weakling—I need to get my energy back!"

DIAGNOSES

- *Activity Intolerance* related to general weakness and fatigue
- *Ineffective Role Performance* related to health crisis

EXPECTED OUTCOMES

- Verbalize an understanding of the definition and components of his structured cardiac rehabilitation program.
- Verbalize a desire to make lifestyle changes.
- Identify resources available in the community to assist with lifestyle changes.
- Participate in his activity program without suffering any complications.
- Verbalize an increase in energy after 6 weeks on the program.
- Accept the reality of the temporary change in his usual work responsibilities.

PLANNING AND IMPLEMENTATION

- Define the purpose and components of a cardiac rehabilitation program.
- Enroll in "heart health" classes, including cardiac anatomy, physiology, and coronary heart disease; exercise and activity prescriptions; lifestyle modifications, including diet counseling and stress management; emotional reactions to CAD; sexual activity; use of cardiac medications; and self-responsibility for health.
- Plan an exercise program based on stress test results, physical examination, and interview.
- Encourage to schedule rest periods before and after activity/exercise.
- Review signs and symptoms of overexertion.
- Provide information about community resources for emotional and educational support.
- Assist to identify strategies for dealing with concerns about his business role.

EVALUATION

Mr. Clements decides to "give the rehab program a try." Ms. Wagner and an exercise physiologist work with him to plan an individualized exercise/activity program. A registered dietitian provides dietary counseling. Ms. Wagner emphasizes stress management strategies. Mr. Clements is able to list manifestations of overexertion and states that he realizes the need for gradual activity progression.

After 6 weeks, Mr. Clements has reported a significant increase in energy and strength. "I am feeling much stronger, and have been sleeping better. Mary and I are taking evening walks around the neighborhood. My chest soreness is also gone." He has completed the 12-week cardiac rehabilitation program, and another stress test indicates that his cardiac function is adequate. Mr. Clements has joined the local Mended Hearts support group and states that he is now incorporating "heart-healthy" considerations into his daily routines.

CRITICAL THINKING IN THE NURSING PROCESS

1. Develop a personalized risk factor reduction plan for Mr. Clements.
2. How might denial affect Mr. Clements's ability to (a) accept the need for cardiac rehabilitation, (b) comply with the proposed lifestyle changes, and (c) make permanent adjustments to his daily life?
3. How does spousal support influence a client's compliance with a structured cardiac rehabilitation program?
4. Mr. Clements tells you that since the surgery, his wife has been afraid that sexual activity will induce another heart attack. How would you respond to these concerns?

See Evaluating Your Response in Appendix C.

---

changes in coronary blood flow. If blood flow is restored at this point, the infarction is limited to subendocardial tissue (a *subendocardial* or *non-Q-wave infarction*). The damage progresses to the epicardium within 1 to 6 hours. When all layers of the myocardium are affected, it is known as a *transmural infarction*. A significant Q wave develops with a transmural infarction, so this also may be called a *Q-wave MI.*

Complications such as heart failure are more frequently associated with Q-wave MIs; however, clients with non-Q-wave MIs frequently experience recurrent ischemia or subsequent MI within weeks or months of the event (Woods et al., 2004).

The necrotic, infarcted tissue is surrounded by regions of injured and ischemic tissues. Tissue in this ischemic area is potentially viable; restoration of blood flow minimizes the amount of tissue lost. This surrounding tissue also undergoes metabolic changes. It may be *stunned*, its contractility impaired for hours to days following reperfusion, or *hibernating*, a process that protects myocytes until perfusion is restored. *Myocardial remodeling* also may occur, with cellular hypertrophy and loss of contractility in regions distant from the infarction. Rapid restoration of blood flow limits these changes (McCance & Huether, 2006).

When a larger artery is compromised, *collateral vessels* connecting smaller arteries in the coronary system dilate to maintain blood flow to the cardiac muscle. The degree of collateral circulation helps determine the extent of myocardial damage from ischemia. Acute occlusion of a coronary artery without any collateral flow results in massive tissue damage and possible death. Progressive narrowing of the larger coronary arteries allows collateral vessels to develop and enlarge, meeting the demand for blood flow. Good collateral circulation can limit the size of an MI.

Myocardial infarctions are described by the damaged area of the heart. The coronary artery that is occluded determines the area of damage. Myocardial infarction usually affects the left ventricle because it is the major "workhorse" of the heart; its muscle mass is greater, as are its oxygen demands. Occlusion of the left anterior descending (LAD) artery affects blood flow to the anterior wall of the left ventricle (an *anterior MI*) and part of the interventricular septum. Occlusion of the left circumflex artery (LCA) causes a *lateral MI*. *Right ventricular, inferior,* and *posterior infarcts* involve occlusions of the right coronary artery (RCA) and posterior descending artery (PDA). Occlusion of the left main coronary artery is the most devastating, causing ischemia of the entire left ventricle, and a grave prognosis. Identifying the infarct site helps predict possible complications and determine appropriate therapy.

Cocaine-Induced MI

Acute myocardial infarction may develop due to cocaine intoxication. Cocaine increases sympathetic nervous system activity by both increasing the release of catecholamines from central and peripheral stores and interfering with the reuptake of catecholamines. This increased catecholamine concentration stimulates the heart rate and increases its contractility, increases the automaticity of cardiac tissues and the risk of dysrhythmias, and causes vasoconstriction and hypertension. The client with cocaine-induced MI may present with an altered level of consciousness, confusion and restlessness, seizure activity, tachycardia, hypotension, increased respiratory rate, and respiratory crackles.

Manifestations

Pain is a classic manifestation of myocardial infarction. Chest pain due to MI is more severe than anginal pain. However, it is not the intensity of the chest pain that distinguishes MI from angina or acute coronary syndrome, but its duration and its continuous nature. The onset of pain is sudden and usually is not associated with activity. In fact, most MIs occur in the early morning. Clients with a history of angina may have more frequent anginal attacks in the days or weeks prior to an MI (unstable angina or ACS). Chest pain may be described as crushing and severe; as a pressure, heavy, or squeezing sensation; or as chest tightness or burning. The pain often begins in the center of the chest (*substernal*), and may radiate to the shoulders, neck, jaw, or arms. It lasts more than 15 to 20 minutes and is not relieved by rest or nitroglycerin.

Women and older adults often experience atypical chest pain, presenting with complaints of indigestion, heartburn, nausea, and vomiting (see the box below). Up to 25% of clients with acute MI deny chest discomfort (Woods et al., 2004).

Compensatory mechanisms cause many of the other symptoms of MI. Sympathetic nervous system stimulation causes anxiety, tachycardia, and vasoconstriction. This results in cool, clammy, mottled skin. Pain and blood chemistry changes stimulate the respiratory center, causing tachypnea. The client often has a sense of impending doom and death. Tissue necrosis causes an inflammatory reaction that increases the white blood cell count and elevates the temperature. Serum cardiac enzyme levels rise as enzymes are released from necrotic cardiac cells.

MEETING INDIVIDUALIZED NEEDS **Recognizing Acute Myocardial Infarction in Women and Older Adults**

Women and older adults often present with atypical manifestations of MI. However, heart disease is the number one cause of death in both groups, making early recognition and aggressive treatment vital.

Women are more likely than men to have a "silent" or unrecognized heart attack, or to present in cardiac arrest or with cardiogenic shock. Women often experience epigastric pain and nausea, causing them to blame their discomfort on heartburn. Shortness of breath is common, as is fatigue and weakness of the shoulders and upper arms.

Older people often seek treatment for vague complaints of difficulty breathing, confusion, fainting, dizziness, abdominal pain, or cough. They often attribute their symptoms to a stroke. The prevalence of silent ischemia is greater in older adults.

Stress the importance of seeking medical help promptly for atypical manifestations of MI. Prompt diagnosis and intervention reduces the mortality and morbidity of MI in women and older adults, just as it does in men. Despite this fact, both women and older adults are more likely to delay seeking treatment and are less likely to be accurately diagnosed and aggressively treated for CHD. Younger women are a particularly important group to reach; their mortality rate when MI occurs is twice that of men (Kasper et al., 2005).

Other manifestations may vary, depending on the location and amount of infarcted tissue. Hypertension, hypotension, or signs of heart failure may develop. Vagal stimulation may cause nausea and vomiting, bradycardia, and hypotension. Hiccuping may develop due to diaphragmatic irritation. If a large vessel is occluded, the first sign of MI may be sudden death. Typical manifestations of MI are listed in the box below.

Complications

The risk of complications associated with myocardial infarction is related to the size and location of the MI.

Dysrhythmias

Dysrhythmias, disturbances or irregularities of heart rhythm, are the most frequent complication of MI. Dysrhythmias are discussed in detail in the next section of this chapter.

Infarcted tissue is *arrhythmogenic;* that is, it affects the generation and conduction of electrical impulses in the heart, increasing the risk of dysrhythmias. Premature ventricular contractions (PVCs) are common following an MI, developing in more than 90% of clients with an acute MI. While not dangerous in themselves, they may be predictive of more dangerous dysrhythmias such as ventricular tachycardia or ventricular fibrillation (Woods et al., 2004). The risk of ventricular fibrillation is greatest the first hour after MI; it is a frequent cause of sudden cardiac death associated with acute MI. Its incidence declines with time. If the infarct affects a conduction pathway, electrical conduction may be affected. Any degree of atrioventricular (AV) block may occur following MI, especially when the anterior wall is infarcted. First-degree and Mobitz I (Wenckebach) blocks are most common, although complete heart block may develop. Bradydysrhythmias (abnormal slow rhythms) also may develop, particularly when the inferior wall of the ventricle is affected.

Pump Failure

Myocardial infarction reduces myocardial contractility, ventricular wall motion, and compliance. Impaired contractility and filling may produce heart failure. The risk of heart failure is greatest when large portions of the left ventricle are infarcted. Heart failure may be more severe with an anterior infarction. Loss of 20% to 30% of the left ventricular muscle mass may cause manifestations of left-sided heart failure, including dyspnea, fatigue, weakness, and respiratory crackles on auscultation. Inferior or right ventricular MI may lead to right-sided heart failure with manifestations such as neck vein distention and peripheral edema. Hemodynamic monitoring is often initiated for clients with evidence of heart failure. Heart failure and its manifestations are discussed in greater depth in Chapter 32 ∞ .

CARDIOGENIC SHOCK *Cardiogenic shock,* impaired tissue perfusion due to pump failure, results when functioning myocardial muscle mass decreases by more than 40%. The heart is unable to pump enough blood to meet the needs of the body and maintain organ function. Low cardiac output due to cardiogenic shock also impairs perfusion of the coronary arteries and myocardium, further increasing tissue damage. Mortality from cardiogenic shock is greater than 70%, although this can be reduced by prompt intervention with revascularization procedures. See Chapter 11 ∞ for a more extensive discussion of cardiogenic shock.

Infarct Extension

Approximately 10% of clients experience extension or reinfarction in the area of the original infarction during the first 10 to 14 days after an MI. *Extension* of the MI is characterized by increased myocardial necrosis from continued blood flow impairment and ongoing injury. *Expansion* of the MI is described as a permanent expansion of the infarcted area from thinning and dilation of the muscle. Infarct extension and expansion may cause manifestations such as continuing chest pain, hemodynamic compromise, and worsening heart failure.

Structural Defects

Necrotic muscle is replaced by scar tissue that is thinner than the ventricular muscle mass. This can lead to such complications as ventricular aneurysm, rupture of the interventricular septum or papillary muscle, and myocardial rupture. A *ventricular aneurysm* is an outpouching of the ventricular wall. It may develop when a large section of the ventricle is replaced by scar tissue. Because it does not contract during systole, stroke volume decreases. Blood may pool within the aneurysm, causing clots to form. Ischemia of the papillary muscle or chordae tendineae may cause structural damage leading to papillary muscle dysfunction or rupture. This affects AV valve function (usually the mitral valve), causing *regurgitation,* backflow of blood into the atria during systole. The interventricular septum may perforate or rupture due to ischemia and infarction. Myocardial rupture is a risk between days 4 and 7 after MI, when the injured tissue is soft and weak. This potential complication of MI is often fatal.

Pericarditis

Tissue necrosis prompts an inflammatory response. *Pericarditis,* inflammation of the pericardial tissue surrounding the heart, may

---

MANIFESTATIONS **of Acute Myocardial Infarction**

- Chest pain: substernal or precordial (across the entire chest wall); may radiate to neck, jaw, shoulder(s), or left arm
- Tachycardia, tachypnea
- Dyspnea, shortness of breath
- Nausea and vomiting
- Anxiety, sense of impending doom
- Diaphoresis
- Cool, mottled skin; diminished peripheral pulses
- Hypotension or hypertension
- Palpitations, dysrhythmias
- Signs of left heart failure
- Decreased level of consciousness

complicate AMI, usually within 2 to 3 days. Pericarditis causes chest pain that may be aching or sharp and stabbing, aggravated by movement or deep breathing. A *pericardial friction rub* may be heard on auscultation of heart sounds.

Dressler's syndrome, thought to be a hypersensitivity response to necrotic tissue or an autoimmune disorder, may develop days to weeks after AMI. It is a symptom complex characterized by fever, chest pain, and dyspnea. Dressler's syndrome may spontaneously resolve or recur over several months, causing significant discomfort and distress.

> **FAST FACTS**
> ■ Dysrhythmias are the most common complication of AMI.
> ■ Heart failure also is a common complication or consequence of myocardial infarction, developing due to loss of functional muscle tissue.

INTERDISCIPLINARY CARE

Immediate treatment goals for the MI client are to:
■ Relieve chest pain.
■ Reduce the extent of myocardial damage.
■ Maintain cardiovascular stability.
■ Decrease cardiac workload.
■ Prevent complications.
Slowing the process of coronary heart disease and reducing the risk of future MI is a major long-term management goal for the client.

Rapid assessment and early diagnosis is important in treating AMI. "Time is muscle" is a medical truism for the client with AMI. The evolution of an AMI is dynamic: The quicker the artery is reopened (medically, surgically, or spontaneously), the more myocardium can be salvaged. Survival and long-term outcomes following AMI are improved by rapidly restoring blood flow to the "stunned" myocardium surrounding the infarcted tissue, reducing myocardial oxygen demand and limiting the accumulation of toxic by-products of necrosis and reperfusion (Kasper et al., 2005). The AHA recommends initiation of definitive treatment within 1 hour of entry into the healthcare system. A recent study by De Luca et al. (2004) showed that every minute of delay in treating clients with AMI affects the mortality risk during the first year.

The major problem interfering with timely reperfusion is delay in seeking medical care following the onset of symptoms. Up to 44% of clients with symptoms of chest discomfort or pain wait more than 4 hours before seeking treatment. Many factors are cited as reasons for treatment delay, including advanced age, the perception of the seriousness of symptoms, denial, access to medical care, the availability of an emergency response system, and in-hospital delays. Immediate evaluation of the client presenting with manifestations of myocardial infarction is essential to early diagnosis and treatment.

Diagnosis

Diagnostic testing is used to establish the diagnosis of AMI.

Serum cardiac markers are proteins released from necrotic heart muscle. The proteins most specific for diagnosis of MI are the creatine kinase (CK, or creatine phosphokinase, CPK) and cardiac-specific troponins (Table 31–6).

■ *Creatine kinase* is an important enzyme for cellular function found principally in cardiac and skeletal muscle and the brain. CK levels rise rapidly with damage to these tissues, appearing in the serum 4 to 6 hours after AMI, peaking within 12 to 24 hours, and then declining over the next 48 to 72 hours. The CK level correlates with the size of the infarction; the greater the amount of infarcted tissue, the higher the serum CK level.

■ *CK-MB* (also called MB-bands) is a subset of CK specific to cardiac muscle. This isoenzyme of CK is considered the most sensitive indicator of MI. Elevated CK alone is not specific for MI; elevated CK-MB greater than 5% is considered a positive indicator of MI. CK-MB levels do not normally rise with chest pain from angina or causes other than MI.

■ Cardiac muscle troponins, *cardiac-specific troponin T (cT_nT) and cardiac-specific troponin I (cT_nI),* are proteins released during myocardial infarction that are sensitive indicators of myocardial damage. These proteins are part of the actin-myoclin unit in cardiac muscle and normally are not detectable in the blood. With necrosis of cardiac muscle, troponins are released and blood levels rise. The specificity of cT_nT and cT_nI to cardiac muscle necrosis makes these markers particularly useful when skeletal muscle trauma contributes to elevated CK levels (e.g., when CPR has been performed or traumatic injury occurred at the time of the MI). They are sensitive enough to detect very small infarctions that do not cause significant CK elevation. Both cT_nT and cT_nI remain in the blood for 10 to 14 days after an MI, making them useful to diagnose MI when medical treatment is delayed.

Serum levels of cardiac markers are ordered on admission and for 3 succeeding days. Serial blood levels help establish the diagnosis and determine the extent of myocardial damage.

Other laboratory tests may include the following:
■ *Myoglobin* is one of the first cardiac markers to be detectable in the blood after an MI. It is released within a few hours of symptom onset. Its lack of specificity to cardiac muscle and rapid excretion (blood levels return to normal within 24 hours) limit its use, however (Kasper et al., 2005).

■ *Complete blood count (CBC)* shows an elevated white blood cell (WBC) count due to inflammation of the injured myocardium. The *erythrocyte sedimentation rate (ESR)* also rises because of inflammation.

■ *Arterial blood gases (ABGs)* may be ordered to assess blood oxygen levels and acid–base balance.

Electrocardiography, echocardiography, and myocardial nuclear scans are the most common diagnostic tests performed when AMI is suspected. With the exception of the ECG, the timing of these tests depends on the client's immediate condition. Hemodynamic monitoring may be initiated in the unstable client following MI.

■ The *electrocardiogram* reflects changes in conduction due to myocardial ischemia and necrosis. Classic ECG changes

TABLE 31-6 Cardiac Markers

MARKER	NORMAL LEVEL	PRIMARY TISSUE LOCATION	SIGNIFICANCE OF ELEVATION	Changes Occurring with MI		
				APPEARS	PEAKS	DURATION
CK (CPK)	Male: 12 to 80 unit/L Female: 10 to 70 unit/L	Cardiac muscle, skeletal muscle, brain	Injury to muscle cells	3 to 6 hours	12 to 24 hours	24 to 48 hours
CK-MB	0% to 3% of total CK	Cardiac muscle	MI, cardiac ischemia, myocarditis, cardiac contusion, defibrillation	4 to 8 hours	18 to 24 hours	72 hours
cT_nT	<0.2 mcg/L	Cardiac muscle	Acute MI, unstable angina	2 to 4 hours	24 to 36 hours	10 to 14 days
cT_nI	<3.1 mcg/L	Cardiac muscle	Acute MI, unstable angina	2 to 4 hours	24 to 36 hours	7 to 10 days

seen in AMI include T-wave inversion, ST-segment elevation, and formation of a Q wave. Ischemic changes in the heart are seen as depression of the ST segment or inversion of the T wave (see Figure 31–2). With myocardial injury, elevation of the ST segment occurs (Figure 31–5A ■). Significant Q-wave development (Figure 31–5B) indicates a transmural, or full-thickness infarction. Myocardial damage can be localized using the 12-lead ECG. See Chapter 30 ∞ for more information about ECGs.

■ *Echocardiography* is done to evaluate cardiac wall motion and left ventricular function. Stunned and infarcted tissue does not contract as effectively (if at all) as healthy myocardium.

■ *Radionuclide imaging* may be done to evaluate myocardial perfusion. These studies cannot differentiate between an acute MI and old scar tissue, but do help identify the specific area of myocardial ischemia and damage.

■ *Hemodynamic monitoring* may be initiated when AMI significantly affects cardiac output and hemodynamic status. These invasive procedures are described in Chapter 32 ∞.

Medications

Aspirin, a platelet inhibitor, is now considered an essential part of treating AMI. A 160- to 325-mg aspirin tablet is given by emergency personnel, with the instruction that it is to be chewed (for buccal absorption). This initial dose is followed by a daily oral dose of 160 to 325 mg of aspirin.

Fibrinolytic agents, analgesics, and antidysrhythmic agents are among the principal classes of drugs used in treating AMI.

ANALGESIA Pain relief is vital in treating the client with AMI. Pain stimulates the sympathetic nervous system, increasing the heart rate and blood pressure and, in turn, myocardial workload. Sublingual nitroglycerin may be given (up to three 0.4-mg doses at 5-minute intervals). Intravenous nitroglycerin may be continued for the first 24 to 48 hours to reduce myocardial work. In addition to pain relief, nitroglycerin decreases myocardial oxygen demand and may increase the supply of oxygen to the myocardium. Nitroglycerin is a peripheral and arterial vasodilator that reduces afterload. It dilates coronary arteries and collateral channels in the heart, increasing coronary blood flow to save myocardial tissue at risk. Nitrates may, however, cause reflex tachycardia or excessive hypotension, so close monitoring is necessary during administration. It also is important to ask the client about use of sildenafil (Viagra) within the previous 24 hours before administering nitroglycerin, as the combination can precipitate a significant drop in blood pressure. See the Medication Administration box on page 973 for the nursing implications of nitroglycerin and other drugs given to reduce myocardial work following AMI.

Morphine sulfate is the drug of choice for pain unrelieved by nitroglycerin and for sedation. Following an initial intravenous dose of 4 to 8 mg, small doses (2 to 4 mg) may be repeated intravenously every 5 minutes until pain is relieved. It is important to assess frequently for pain relief and possible adverse effects of analgesia, such as excessive sedation. Pain unrelieved by expected or usual doses should be reported to the physician as it may indicate a complication such as extension of the infarct. See Chapter 9 ∞ for more details about morphine administration. Antianxiety agents such as diazepam (Valium) may also be administered to promote rest.

FIBRINOLYTIC THERAPY Fibrinolytic agents, drugs that dissolve or break up blood clots, are first-line drugs used to treat acute MI when access to a cardiac catheterization lab for revascularization procedures is not immediately available. Fibrinolytic drugs activate the fibrinolytic system to *lyse* or destroy the clot, restoring blood flow to the obstructed artery. Early fibrinolytic administration (within the first 6 hours of MI onset) limits infarct size, reduces heart damage, and improves outcomes. Activation of the fibrinolytic system can cause multiple complications; approximately 0.5% to 5% of clients receiving fibrinolytic drugs experience serious bleeding complications. Not every client is a candidate for fibrinolytic therapy; for example, it is contraindicated in clients

Figure 31–5 ■ ECG changes characteristic of MI. *A*, ST-segment elevation characteristic of myocardial injury. *B*, Clinically significant Q-wave characteristic of a transmural infarction.

with known bleeding disorders, history of cerebrovascular disease, uncontrolled hypertension, pregnancy, or recent trauma or surgery of the head or spine (Tierney et al., 2005).

Several fibrinolytic agents are commonly used today. Among these, little difference in effectiveness has been demonstrated; there are, however, big differences in cost. Streptokinase, a biologic agent derived from group C *Streptococcus* organisms, is the least expensive of the drugs. Its primary drawback is the risk of a severe hypersensitivity reaction, including anaphylaxis. Streptokinase is administered by intravenous infusion. Anisoylated plasminogen streptokinase activator complex (APSAC) is a related drug that can be administered by bolus over 2 to 5 minutes. It has many of the same effects as streptokinase, but is considerably more expensive. Tissue plasminogen activator (t-PA), tenecteplase (TNK), and reteplase (rPA) are more effective in reestablishing myocardial perfusion, especially when the pain developed more than 3 hours previously. These drugs, however, are the most expensive. Nursing care of the client receiving a fibrinolytic agent is outlined on the next page.

ANTIDYSRHYTHMICS Dysrhythmias are a common complication of AMI, particularly in the first 12 to 24 hours. Antidysrhythmic medications are used as needed to treat dysrhythmias. They also may be given prophylactically to prevent dysrhythmias. Ventricular dysrhythmias are treated with a class I or class III antidysrhythmic drug (see the Medication Administration box on page 1006). Symptomatic bradycardia (bradycardia with associated hypotension and other signs of low cardiac output) is treated with intravenous atropine, 0.5 to 1 mg. Intra-

venous verapamil or the short-acting beta blocker esmolol (Brevibloc) may be ordered to treat atrial fibrillation or other supraventricular tachydysrhythmias.

OTHER MEDICATIONS Beta blockers such as propranolol (Inderal), atenolol (Tenormin), and metoprolol (Lopressor) reduce pain, limit infarct size, and decrease the incidence of serious ventricular dysrhythmias in AMI. These drugs decrease the heart rate, reducing cardiac work and myocardial oxygen demand. Initial doses are given intravenously. Oral beta blocker therapy is continued to reduce the risk of reinfarction and death related to cardiovascular causes (Kasper et al., 2005).

ACE inhibitors also reduce mortality associated with AMI. These drugs reduce ventricular remodeling following an MI, reducing the risk for subsequent heart failure. They also may reduce the risk of reinfarction (Kasper et al., 2002).

Anticoagulants and antiplatelet medications often are prescribed to maintain coronary artery patency following thrombolysis or a revascularization procedure. Abciximab (ReoPro) suppresses platelet aggregation and reduces the risk of reocclusion following angioplasty. It also improves vessel opening with fibrinolytic therapy, permitting lower doses of fibrinolytic drugs. Standard or low-molecular-weight heparin preparations often are given to clients with AMI. Heparin helps establish and maintain patency of the affected coronary artery. It also is used, along with long-term warfarin, to prevent systemic or pulmonary embolism in clients with significant left ventricular impairment or atrial fibrillation following AMI. See the Medication Administration box on page 976 for the nursing implications of an-

NURSING CARE OF THE CLIENT RECEIVING Fibrinolytic Therapy

PREINFUSION CARE

- Obtain nursing history, and perform a physical assessment. *Information obtained from the history and physical exam helps determine whether fibrinolytic therapy is appropriate. The goal is to initiate fibrinolytic therapy within 30 minutes of arrival.*
- Evaluate for contraindications to fibrinolytic therapy: recent surgery or trauma (including prolonged CPR), bleeding disorders or active bleeding, cerebral vascular accident, neurosurgery within the last 2 months, gastrointestinal ulcers, diabetic hemorrhagic retinopathy, and uncontrolled hypertension. *Fibrinolytic agents dissolve clots and therefore may precipitate intracranial, internal, or peripheral bleeding.*
- Inform the client of the purpose of the therapy. Discuss the risk of bleeding and the need to keep the extremity immobile during and after the infusion. *Minimal movement of the extremity is necessary to prevent bleeding from the infusion site.*

DURING THE INFUSION

- Assess and record vital signs and the infusion site for hematoma or bleeding every 15 minutes for the first hour, every 30 minutes for the next 2 hours, and then hourly until the intravenous catheter is discontinued. Assess pulses, color, sensation, and temperature of both extremities with each vital sign check. *Vital signs and the site are frequently assessed to detect possible complications.*
- Remind the client to keep the extremity still and straight. Do not elevate head of bed above 15 degrees. *Extremity immobilization helps prevent infusion site trauma and bleeding. Hypotension may develop; keeping the bed flat helps maintain cerebral perfusion.*
- Maintain continuous cardiac monitoring during the infusion. Keep antidysrhythmic drugs and the emergency cart readily available for treatment of significant dysrhythmias. *Ventricular dysrhythmias commonly occur with reperfusion of the ischemic myocardium.*

POSTINFUSION CARE

- Assess vital signs, distal pulses, and infusion site frequently as needed. *The client remains at high risk for bleeding following fibrinolytic therapy.*
- Evaluate response to therapy: normalization of ST segment, relief of chest pain, reperfusion dysrhythmias, early peaking of the CK and CK-MB. *These are signs that the clot has been dissolved and the myocardium is being reperfused.*
- Maintain bed rest for 6 hours. Keep the head of the bed at or below 15 degrees. Reinforce the need to keep the extremity straight and immobile. Avoid any injections for 24 hours after catheter removal. *Precautions such as these are important to prevent bleeding.*
- Assess puncture sites for bleeding. On catheter removal hold direct pressure over the site for at least 30 minutes. Apply a pressure dressing to any venous or arterial sites as needed. Perform routine care in a gentle manner to avoid bruising or injury. *Fibrinolytic therapy disrupts normal coagulation. Peripheral bleeding may occur at puncture sites, and there may not be sufficient fibrin to form a clot. Direct or indirect pressure may be needed to control the bleeding.*
- Assess body fluids, including urine, vomitus, and feces, for evidence of bleeding; frequently assess for changes in level of consciousness and manifestations of increased intracranial pressure, which may indicate intracranial bleeding. Assess surgical sites for bleeding. Monitor hemoglobin and hematocrit levels, prothrombin time (PT), and partial thromboplastin time (PTT). *These provide additional means of assessing for bleeding.*
- Administer platelet-modifying drugs (e.g., aspirin, dipyridamole) as ordered. *Platelet inhibitors decrease platelet aggregation and adhesion and are used to prevent reocclusion of the artery.*
- Report manifestations of reocclusion, including changes in the ST segment, chest pain, or dysrhythmias. *Early recognition of reocclusion is vital to save myocardial tissue.*

tiplatelet drugs, and Chapter 34 ∞ for more information about anticoagulant therapy.

Clients with pump failure and hypotension may receive intravenous dopamine, a vasopressor. At low doses (less than 5 mg/kg/min), it improves blood flow to the kidneys, preventing renal ischemia and possible acute renal failure (see Chapter 29 ∞). With increasing doses, dopamine increases myocardial contractility and causes vasoconstriction, improving blood pressure and cardiac output.

Antilipemic agents are used for the client with hyperlipidemia. A stool softener such as docusate sodium is prescribed to maintain normal bowel function and reduce straining.

Treatments

The client with a suspected or confirmed MI is monitored continuously. Care is provided in the intensive coronary care unit for the first 24 to 48 hours, after which time less intensive monitoring (e.g., telemetry) may be required. An intra-

venous line is established to allow rapid administration of emergency medications.

Bed rest is prescribed for the first 12 hours to reduce the cardiac workload. The bedside commode generally is allowed; studies have shown this to be less stressful than using a bedpan. If the client's condition is stable, sitting in a chair at the bedside is permitted after 12 hours. Activities are gradually increased as tolerated. A quiet, calm environment with limited outside stimuli is preferred. Visitors are limited to promote rest. Oxygen is administered by nasal cannula at 2 to 5 L/min to improve oxygenation of the myocardium and other tissues.

A liquid diet may be prescribed for the first 4 to 12 hours to reduce gastric distention and myocardial work. Following that, a low-fat, low-cholesterol, reduced-sodium diet is allowed. Sodium restrictions may be lifted after 2 to 3 days if no evidence of heart failure is present. Small, frequent feedings are often recommended. Drinks containing caffeine, and very hot and cold foods, may also be limited.

Revascularization Procedures

Many clients with AMI are treated with immediate or early per-cutaneous coronary revascularization such as angioplasty and stent placement. PCR may follow fibrinolytic therapy or be used in place of fibrinolytic therapy to restore blood flow to is-chemic myocardium. When compared with fibrinolytic ther-apy, prompt PCR reduces hospital mortality (Kasper et al., 2005). In some cases, CABG surgery may be performed. The choice of procedure depends on the client's age and immediate condition, the time elapsed from the onset of manifestations, and the extent of myocardial disease and damage. These pro-cedures and related nursing care are covered in more depth in the preceding section on acute coronary syndrome.

Other Invasive Procedures

For clients with large MIs and evidence of pump failure, inva-sive devices may be used to temporarily take over the function of the heart, allowing the injured myocardium to heal. The intra-aortic balloon pump is widely used to augment cardiac output. Ventricular assist devices are indicated for clients requiring more or longer term artificial support than the intra-aortic balloon pump provides.

INTRA-AORTIC BALLOON PUMP The *intra-aortic balloon pump (IABP)*, also called intra-aortic balloon counterpulsation, is a mechanical circulatory support device that may be used af-ter cardiac surgery or to treat cardiogenic shock following AMI. The IABP temporarily supports cardiac function, allow-ing the heart gradually to recover by decreasing myocardial workload and oxygen demand and increasing perfusion of the coronary arteries.

A catheter with a 30- to 40-mL balloon is introduced into the aorta, usually via the femoral artery. The balloon catheter is connected to a console that regulates the inflation and deflation of the balloon. The IABP catheter inflates during diastole, in-creasing perfusion of the coronary and renal arteries, and de-flates just prior to systole, decreasing afterload and cardiac workload (Figure 31–6 ■). The inflation–deflation sequence is triggered by the ECG pattern. During the most acute period, the balloon inflates and deflates with each heartbeat (1:1 ratio), providing maximal assistance to the heart. As the client's con-dition improves, the IABP is weaned to inflate–deflate at vary-ing intervals (e.g., 1:2, 1:4, 1:8). This provides a continually decreasing amount of support as the heart muscle recovers. When mechanical assistance is no longer required, the IABP catheter is removed.

VENTRICULAR ASSIST DEVICES Use of *ventricular assist de-vices (VADs)* to aid the failing heart is becoming more com-mon with advances in technology. Whereas the IABP can supplement cardiac output by approximately 10% to 15%, the VAD temporarily takes partial or complete control of cardiac function, depending on the type of device used. VADs may be used as temporary or complete assist in AMI and cardiogenic shock when there is a chance for recovery of normal heart function after a period of cardiac rest. The device also may be

A Diastole   **B** Systole

Figure 31–6 ■ The intra-aortic balloon pump. *A,* When inflated during diastole, the balloon supports cerebral, renal, and coronary artery perfusion. *B,* The balloon deflates during systole, so cardiac output is unimpeded.

used as a bridge to heart transplant. Nursing care for the client with a VAD is supportive and includes assessing hemody-namic status and for complications associated with the de-vice. Clients with VAD are at considerable risk for infection; strict aseptic technique is used with all invasive catheters and dressing changes. Pneumonia also is a risk due to immobility and ventilatory support. Mechanical failure of the VAD is a life-threatening event that requires immediate intervention (Urden et al., 2006).

Cardiac Rehabilitation

Cardiac rehabilitation is a long-term program of medical evaluation, exercise, risk factor modification, education, and counseling designed to limit the physical and psychologic effects of cardiac illness and improve the client's quality of life (Woods et al., 2004). Cardiac rehabilitation begins with admission for a cardiac event such as AMI or a revasculariza-tion procedure. Phase 1 of the program is the inpatient phase. A thorough assessment of the client's history, current status, risk factors, and motivation is obtained. During this phase, ac-tivity progresses from bed rest to independent performance of activities of daily living (ADLs) and ambulation within the fa-cility. Both subjective and objective responses to increasing activity levels are evaluated. Excess fatigue, shortness of breath, chest pain, tachypnea, tachycardia, or cool, clammy skin indicate activity intolerance. Phase 2, immediate outpa-tient cardiac rehabilitation, begins within 3 weeks of the car-diac event. The goals for the outpatient program are to increase activity level, participation, and capacity; improve psychosocial status and treat anxiety or depression; and pro-vide education and support for risk factor reduction. Contin-uation programs, phase 3 of cardiac rehabilitation, are directed at providing a transition to independent exercise and exercise maintenance. During this final phase, the client may "check in" every 3 months to evaluate risk factors, quality of life, and exercise habits (Woods et al., 2004).

NURSING CARE

Nursing care of the client with an acute myocardial infarction focuses on reducing cardiac work, identifying and treating complications in a timely manner, and preparing the client for rehabilitation. See the following Nursing Care Plan for a client with an AMI.

Health Promotion

Health promotion activities to prevent acute myocardial infarction are those outlined for coronary heart disease and angina in previous sections of this chapter. In addition, discuss risk factor management, use of prescribed medications, and cardiac rehabilitation to reduce the risk of complications or future infarctions.

NURSING CARE PLAN | A Client with Acute Myocardial Infarction

Betty Williams, a 62-year-old psychologist, is admitted to the emergency department with complaints of severe substernal chest pain. Mrs. Williams states that the pain began after lunch, about 4 hours ago. She initially attributed the pain to indigestion. She described the pain, which now radiates to her jaw and left arm, as "really severe heartburn." It is accompanied by a "choking feeling," severe shortness of breath, and diaphoresis. The pain is unrelieved by rest, antacids, or three sublingual nitroglycerin tablets (0.4 mg).

Oxygen is started per nasal cannula at 5 L/min. Central and peripheral intravenous lines are inserted. A 12-lead ECG and the following labwork are obtained: cardiac troponins, CK and CK isoenzymes, ABGs, CBC, and a chemistry panel. Morphine sulfate relieves Mrs. Williams's pain.

Mrs. Williams's medical history includes type 2 diabetes, angina, and hypertension. She has a 45-year history of cigarette smoking, averaging 1.5 to 2 packs per day. Family history reveals that Mrs. Williams's father died at age 42 of AMI, and her paternal grandfather died at age 65 of AMI. Mrs. Williams is taking the following medications: tolbutamide (Orinase), hydrochlorothiazide, and isosorbide (Isordil).

Based on ECG changes and cardiac markers, an acute anterior MI is diagnosed. Mrs. Williams has no contraindications to fibrinolytic therapy and is deemed a good candidate. Intravenous alteplase (t-PA, Activase) is given by bolus followed by intravenous infusions of alteplase and heparin. She is transferred to the coronary care unit (CCU).

ASSESSMENT

Dan Morales, RN, is Mrs. Williams's primary care nurse. Mrs. Williams is alert and oriented to person, place, and time. Vital signs are T 99.6°F (37.5°C), P 118, R 24 with adequate depth, and BP 172/92. Auscultation reveals an S_4 and fine crackles in the bases of both lungs. The ECG shows sinus tachycardia with occasional PVCs. Her skin is cool and slightly diaphoretic. Capillary refill is less than 3 seconds, and peripheral pulses are strong and equal. Her nail beds are pink.

A triple-lumen central line is in place. Nitroglycerin is infusing at 200 mcg/min in the distal lumen; the alteplase infusion is in the middle lumen; and a heparin infusion is in the proximal lumen. The peripheral intravenous line has a saline lock. Mrs. Williams states, "The pain is better since the nurse in the ER gave me a shot. But it has been coming and going. I would rate it a 4 right now, but it was terrible before. The doctor told me that this drug I'm getting will quickly open up the artery that is blocked. I hope it works! Do many people get this drug?"

DIAGNOSES

- *Acute Pain* related to ischemic myocardial tissue
- *Anxiety* and *Fear* related to change in health status
- *Ineffective Protection* related to the risk of bleeding secondary to fibrinolytic therapy
- *Risk for Decreased Cardiac Output* related to altered cardiac rate and rhythm

EXPECTED OUTCOMES

- Rate chest pain as 2 or lower on a pain scale of 0 to 10.
- Verbalize reduced anxiety and fear.
- Demonstrate no signs of internal or external bleeding.
- Maintain an adequate cardiac output during and following reperfusion therapy.

PLANNING AND IMPLEMENTATION

The following interventions are planned and implemented during the immediate phase of Mrs. Williams's hospitalization.

- Instruct to report all chest pain. Monitor and evaluate pain using a scale of 0 to 10. Titrate intravenous nitroglycerin infusion for chest pain; stop infusion if systolic BP is below 100 mmHg. Administer 2 to 4 mg morphine intravenously for chest pain unrelieved by nitroglycerin infusion.
- Encourage verbalization of fears and concerns. Respond honestly, and correct misconceptions about the disease, therapeutic interventions, or prognosis.
- Assess knowledge of CHD. Explain the purpose of fibrinolytic therapy to dissolve the fresh clot and reperfuse the heart muscle, limiting heart damage.
- Explain the need for frequent monitoring of vital signs and potential bleeding.
- Assess for manifestations of internal or intracranial bleeding: complaints of back or abdominal pain, headache, decreased level of consciousness, dizziness, bloody secretions or excretions, or pallor. Test all stools, urine, and vomitus for occult blood. Notify physician immediately of any abnormal findings.
- Monitor for signs of reperfusion: decreased chest pain, return of ST segment to baseline, reperfusion dysrhythmias (e.g., PVCs, bradycardia, and heart block).
- Continuously monitor ECG for changes in cardiac rate, rhythm, and conduction. Assess vital signs.
- Treat dangerous dysrhythmias or other cardiac events per protocol. Notify the physician.
- Discuss continuing cardiac care and rehabilitation.

(continued)

NURSING CARE PLAN A Client with Acute Myocardial Infarction (continued)

EVALUATION

The initial morphine dose reduces Mrs. Williams's chest pain from a rating of 8 to 4. The nitroglycerin infusion and fibrinolytic therapy further reduce her pain to 2. The nitroglycerin infusion is gradually discontinued after 24 hours. As her pain subsides, Mrs. Williams states that she feels "much better now that the pain is gone. I was afraid it would just get worse." She verbalizes an understanding of fibrinolytic therapy to limit myocardial damage. No indication of bleeding problems are noted. Reperfusion is indicated by relief of chest pain, return of the ST segment to baseline on the ECG, early peaking of CK levels, and increased frequency of PVCs but no significant dysrhythmias. Mrs. Williams remains in CCU for 36 hours and is transferred to the floor.

CRITICAL THINKING IN THE NURSING PROCESS

1. How would the initial plan of care have changed if Mrs. Williams were not a candidate for fibrinolytic therapy?
2. Two days after her initial therapy, Mrs. Williams complains of palpitations. You notice frequent PVCs on the ECG monitor. What do you do?
3. What health promotion topics would you teach Mrs. Williams before discharge?
4. Mrs. Williams states, "I've been smoking for over 45 years, and I'm not going to stop now! Besides, it calms me down when I'm anxious." How would you respond to this statement?
See Evaluating Your Response in Appendix C.

Assessment

Nursing assessment for the client with AMI must be both timely and ongoing. Assessment data related to AMI include the following:

- *Health history:* Complaints of chest pain, including its location, intensity, character, radiation, and timing; associated symptoms such as nausea, heartburn, shortness of breath, and anxiety; treatment measures taken since onset of pain; past medical history, especially cardiac related; chronic diseases; current medications and any known allergies to medications; smoking history and use of recreational drugs and alcohol.
- *Physical examination:* General appearance including obvious signs of distress; vital signs; peripheral pulses; skin color, temperature, moisture; level of consciousness; heart and breath sounds; cardiac rhythm (on beside monitor); bowel sounds, abdominal tenderness.

Nursing Diagnoses and Interventions

Priorities of nursing care include relieving chest pain, reducing cardiac work, and promoting oxygenation. Psychosocial support is especially important, because an acute myocardial infarction can be devastating, bringing the client face to face with his or her own mortality for the first time.

Acute Pain

Chest pain occurs when the oxygen supply to the heart muscle does not meet the demand. Myocardial ischemia and infarction cause pain, as does reperfusion of an ischemic area following fibrinolytic therapy or emergent PTCA. Pain stimulates the sympathetic nervous system, increasing cardiac work. Pain relief is a priority of care for the client with AMI.

- Assess for verbal and nonverbal signs of pain. Document characteristics and the intensity of the pain, using a standard pain scale. Verify nonverbal indicators of pain with the client. *Frequent, careful pain assessment allows early intervention to reduce the risk of further damage. Pain is a subjective experience; its expression may vary with location and intensity, previous experiences, and cultural and social background.*

Pain scales provide an objective tool for measuring pain and a way to assess pain relief or reduction.

- Administer oxygen at 2 to 5 L/min per nasal cannula. *Supplemental oxygen increases oxygen supply to the myocardium, decreasing ischemia and pain.*
- Promote physical and psychologic rest. Provide information and emotional support. *Rest decreases cardiac workload and sympathetic nervous system stimulation, promoting comfort. Information and emotional support help decrease anxiety and provide psychologic rest.*
- Titrate intravenous nitroglycerin as ordered to relieve chest pain, maintaining a systolic blood pressure greater than 100 mmHg. *Nitroglycerin decreases chest pain by dilating peripheral vessels, reducing cardiac work, and dilating coronary vessels, including collateral channels, improving blood flow to ischemic tissue.*

PRACTICE ALERT

Intravenous nitroglycerin causes peripheral vasodilation, which may lead to hypotension, reduced coronary blood flow, and tachycardia. Reduce the nitro flow rate and notify the physician if this occurs.

- Administer 2 to 4 mg morphine by intravenous push for chest pain as needed. *Morphine is an effective narcotic analgesic for chest pain. It decreases pain and anxiety, acts as a venodilator, and decreases the respiratory rate. The resulting reduction in preload and sympathetic nervous system stimulation reduces cardiac work and oxygen consumption.*

PRACTICE ALERT

Reassess for relief of chest pain. The goal of care is to achieve pain relief, not simply a reduction in pain to a "manageable" level.

Ineffective Tissue Perfusion

Cardiac muscle damage affects compliance, contractility, and cardiac output. The extent of the effect on tissue perfusion depends on the location and amount of damage. Anterior wall infarcts have a greater effect on cardiac output than do right ventricular infarcts. Infarcted muscle also increases the risk for cardiac dysrhythmias, which can also affect the delivery of blood and oxygen to the tissues.

- Assess and document vital signs. Report increases in heart rate and changes in rhythm, blood pressure, and respiratory rate. *Decreased cardiac output activates compensatory mechanisms that may cause tachycardia and vasoconstriction, increasing cardiac work.*
- Assess for changes in level of consciousness (LOC); decreased urine output; moist, cool, pale, mottled, or cyanotic skin; dusky or cyanotic mucous membranes and nail beds; diminished to absent peripheral pulses; delayed capillary refill. *These are manifestations of impaired tissue perfusion. A change in LOC is often the first manifestation of altered perfusion because brain tissue and cerebral function depend on a continuous supply of oxygen.*
- Auscultate heart and breath sounds. Note abnormal heart sounds (e.g., an S_3 or S_4 gallop or a murmur) or adventitious lung sounds. *Abnormal heart sounds or adventitious lung sounds may indicate impaired cardiac filling or output, increasing the risk for decreased tissue perfusion.*
- Monitor ECG rhythm continuously. *Dysrhythmias can further impair cardiac output and tissue perfusion.*

PRACTICE ALERT
Obtain a 12-lead ECG to assess complaints of chest pain. Report marked changes to the physician. Continued or unrelieved chest pain may indicate further myocardial ischemia and extension of the infarct; an ECG during episodes of chest pain provides a valuable diagnostic tool to assess myocardial perfusion.

- Monitor oxygen saturation levels. Administer oxygen as ordered. Obtain and assess ABGs as indicated. *Oxygen saturation is an indicator of gas exchange, tissue perfusion, and the effectiveness of oxygen administration. ABGs provide a more precise measurement of blood oxygen levels and allow assessment of acid–base balance.*
- Administer antidysrhythmic medications as needed. *Dysrhythmias affect tissue perfusion by altering cardiac output.*
- Obtain serial CK, isoenzyme, and troponin levels as ordered. *Levels of cardiac markers, CK isoenzymes in particular, correlate with the extent of myocardial damage.*
- Plan for invasive hemodynamic monitoring. *Hemodynamic monitoring facilitates AMI management and treatment evaluation by providing a means of assessing pressures in the systemic and pulmonary arteries, the relationship between oxygen supply and demand, cardiac output, and cardiac index.*

PRACTICE ALERT
Continuously evaluate the response to interventions such as fibrinolytic therapy, drugs to improve cardiac output and tissue perfusion, and drugs to reduce cardiac work. Adverse effects of therapy may reduce the effectiveness of treatment. Bleeding due to fibrinolytic therapy may affect vascular volume and cardiac output; reperfusion dysrhythmias also may affect cardiac output. Drugs used to improve cardiac output may also increase cardiac work, whereas those given to reduce cardiac work may significantly affect contractility and cardiac output.

Ineffective Coping
Coping mechanisms help a person deal with a life-threatening event or with acute changes in health. However, certain coping mechanisms may be detrimental to restoring health, particularly if the client relies on them for a prolonged period. Denial, for example, is a common coping mechanism among post–MI clients. In the initial stages, denial can reduce anxiety. Continued denial, however, can interfere with learning and compliance with treatment.

- Establish an environment of caring and trust. Encourage the client to express feelings. *Establishing a trusting nurse–client relationship provides a safe environment for the client to discuss feelings of helplessness, powerlessness, anxiety, and hopelessness. The nurse may then be able to provide additional resources to meet the client's needs.*
- Accept denial as a coping mechanism, but do not reinforce it. *Denial may initially help by diminishing the psychologic threat to health, decreasing anxiety. However, its prolonged use can interfere with acceptance of reality and cooperation, possibly delaying treatment and hindering recovery.*
- Note aggressive behaviors, hostility, or anger. Document any failure to comply with treatments. *These signs can indicate anxiety and denial.*
- Help the client identify positive coping skills used in the past (e.g., problem-solving skills, verbalization of feelings, asking for help, prayer). Reinforce use of positive coping behaviors. *Coping behaviors that have been successful in the past can help the client deal with the current situation. These familiar methods can decrease feelings of powerlessness.*
- Provide opportunities for the client to make decisions about the plan of care, as possible. *This promotes self-confidence and independence. Participating in care planning gives the client a sense of control and the opportunity to use positive coping skills.*
- Provide privacy for the client and significant other to share their questions and concerns. *Privacy provides an opportunity for the client and partner to share their feelings and fears, offer support and encouragement to one another, relieve anxiety, and establish effective coping methods.*

Fear
The fear of death and disability can be a paralyzing emotion that adversely affects the client's recovery from acute myocardial infarction.

- Identify the client's level of fear, noting verbal and nonverbal signs. *This information enables the nurse to plan appropriate interventions. Clients may not voice concerns; attention to nonverbal indicators is important. Controlling fear helps decrease sympathetic nervous system responses and catecholamine release that may increase feelings of fear and anxiety.*
- Acknowledge the client's perception of the situation. Allow to verbalize concerns. *A sudden change in health status causes anxiety and fear of the unknown. Verbalizing these fears may help the client cope with change and allow the healthcare team to provide information and correct misconceptions.*
- Encourage questions and provide consistent, factual answers. Repeat information as needed. *Accurate and consistent information can reduce fear. Honest explanations help*

strengthen the client–nurse relationship and help the client develop realistic expectations. Anxiety and fear decrease the ability to concentrate and retain information; therefore, information may need to be repeated.

- Encourage self-care. Allow the client to make decisions regarding the plan of care. *This promotes personal responsibility for health and allows some control over the situation. Clients' confidence increases as their dependence decreases.*

- Administer antianxiety medications as ordered. *These medications promote rest and relaxation and decrease feelings of anxiety, which may act as barriers to health restoration.*

- Teach nonpharmacologic methods of stress reduction (e.g., relaxation techniques, mental imagery, music therapy, breathing exercises, meditation, massage). *Stress management techniques can help reduce tension and anxiety, provide a sense of control, and enhance coping skills.*

NANDA, NIC, and NOC Linkages

Chart 31–1 shows links between NANDA nursing diagnoses, NIC, and NOC for the client with acute myocardial infarction.

Community-Based Care

Cardiac rehabilitation begins with admission to the healthcare facility and continues through the inpatient stay and after discharge into the rehabilitative period. The emphasis is on realistic application of information to maintain lifestyle changes.

Assessing readiness to learn is an important first step in preparing for home care. The client in strong denial may not identify any relevance to the information being taught. Evaluate ability to learn, assessing physiologic and psychologic health, beliefs regarding personal responsibility for health, and expectations of the healthcare system. Also assess developmental level, ability to perform psychomotor skills, cognitive function, learning disabilities, existing knowledge base, and the influence of previous learning experiences. Provide written material to supplement teaching and encourage questions.

Include the following topics in teaching for home care:

- The normal anatomy and physiology of the heart, and the specific area of heart damage
- The process of CHD and implications of MI
- Purposes and side effects of prescribed medications
- The importance of complying with the medical regimen and cardiac rehabilitation program and of keeping follow-up appointments

---

NANDA, NIC, AND NOC LINKAGES
CHART 31–1 The Client with Acute Myocardial Infarction

NANDA

Ineffective Tissue Perfusion: Cardiopulmonary

NIC

Cardiac Care: Acute

Hemodynamic Regulation

Bleeding Precautions

Dysrhythmia Management

Cardiac Care: Rehabilitative

NOC

Cardiac Pump Effectiveness

Circulation Status

Tissue Perfusion: Cardiac

Tissue Perfusion: Peripheral

Data from *NANDA's Nursing Diagnoses: Definitions & classification 2005–2006* by NANDA International (2005), Philadelphia; *Nursing Interventions Classification (NIC)* (4th ed.) by J. M. Dochterman & G. M. Bulecheck (2004), St. Louis, MO: Mosby; and *Nursing Outcomes Classification (NOC)* (3rd ed.) by S. Moorhead, M. Johnson, and M. Maas (2004), St. Louis, MO: Mosby.

- Information about community resources, such as the local chapter of the American Heart Association.

After discharge, follow up by telephone within 1 week and periodically thereafter during the recovery period. Provide telephone numbers of resource personnel who are available to respond to questions and concerns after discharge. Research demonstrates the value of motivational and social support in adopting healthier behaviors after AMI (see the research box on the next page).

Because the client who has had an MI is at high risk for sudden cardiac death; encourage family members to learn CPR and provide information about community resources for CPR training.

CARDIAC RHYTHM DISORDERS

Heart muscle contracts in response to electrical stimulation. In the normal heart, electrical stimulation produces a synchronized, rhythmic heart muscle contraction that propels blood into the vascular system. Changes in cardiac rhythm affect this synchronized activity and the heart's ability to effectively pump blood to body tissues.

THE CLIENT WITH A CARDIAC DYSRHYTHMIA

A cardiac dysrhythmia is a disturbance or irregularity in the electrical system of the heart. Cardiac dysrhythmias may be benign or have lethal consequences. Prompt recognition of a lethal dysrhythmia and quick action can be lifesaving.

NURSING RESEARCH Evidence-Based Practice: Women Following Myocardial Infarction

Coronary heart disease is the leading killer of women in the United States. The risk of death and disability resulting from acute myocardial infarction is higher in women than in men. Although clients often can significantly reduce their risk for subsequent cardiac events by making behavioral changes, the success of efforts to promote these changes has been limited.

In a study of behavioral changes in women following AMI, McSweeney and Coon (2004) identified six inhibitors and four facilitators to change. Financial concerns presented the major barrier to the desired behavior changes, from taking prescribed medications and complying with recommendations for follow-up care, to eating a low-fat diet, exercise, and smoking cessation. Environmental factors and physical problems or symptoms also presented major barriers to dietary changes, exercise, and smoking cessation. Other inhibitors included social support, reduced quality of life, and motivation. Many of the same factors identified as barriers for some women were perceived as enablers of change by others. Social support and financial stability or support were the major factors enabling change, along with motivators and environmental factors.

IMPLICATIONS FOR NURSING

The nurse needs to look holistically at women when addressing lifestyle changes following AMI. Because the very same factors were perceived as barriers by some women and facilitators by others, it is important for the nurse to work collaboratively with the client to develop successful strategies for behavior change.

Nurses are in a unique position to advocate for the client when medication samples or lower cost alternative drugs can help the client adhere to prescribed treatment, and to suggest referral to cardiac rehabilitation when a structured exercise program will benefit the client (e.g., when the client lives in an area in which she does not feel safe walking). Nurses also often are much more aware of the unique stressors in the woman's life, such as caring for grandchildren, aging parents, or a disabled spouse. Tailoring strategies for change to the individual and his or her circumstances increases the probability of success and continuation of the adopted healthy lifestyle habit.

CRITICAL THINKING IN CLIENT CARE

1. Why might the same factors (finances, social support, environment, and motivation) be perceived as barriers to changing eating, exercise, and smoking behaviors in some women and as facilitators of change in others?
2. Identify some questions the nurse might ask to help ascertain both barriers to and facilitators of change related to smoking cessation, exercise, and eating habits.
3. How would you intervene when a woman tells you she is not taking the beta blocker and cholesterol-lowering statin prescribed by her physician?
4. Identify some strategies for incorporating daily exercise into the life of a woman who is raising her two pre-teen grandchildren and caring for her aging mother who has Alzheimer's disease.

Source: Adapted from "Women's Inhibitors and Facilitators Associated with Making Behavioral Changes after Myocardial Infarction," by J. C. McSweeney & S. Coon (2004), *Medsurg Nursing, 13*(1), 49–56.

Dysrhythmias develop for many reasons. Not all are pathologic; some alterations in cardiac rhythm occur in response to events such as exercise or fear. For example, a rapid heart rate due to exercise, fever, or excitement is a normal response to the body's demand for oxygen or to stimulation of the sympathetic nervous system. Slow heart rates also may be normal. *Athletic heart syndrome,* which results from long-term training on the heart muscle, allows the heart to beat more slowly and forcefully while maintaining cardiac output and tissue perfusion. Many athletes have a heart rate of less than 60 beats per minute. Aging affects cardiac rhythm as well (see the box on page 996).

Regardless of cause, a dysrhythmia can significantly affect cardiac performance, depending on heart muscle health. The client's response to the dysrhythmia is key in determining the urgency and type of treatment needed.

Physiology Review

The unique properties of cardiac cells allow effective heart function. Four properties are electrical; the fifth is cardiac muscle's mechanical response to electrical stimulation.

- *Automaticity* is the ability of pacemaker cells to spontaneously initiate an electrical impulse (action potential). The SA node is the dominant pacemaker, generating impulses at 60 to 100 times a minute. Myocardial muscle cells do not possess this ability.

- *Excitability* is the ability of myocardial cells to respond to stimuli generated by pacemaker cells.

- *Conductivity* is the ability to transmit an impulse from cell to cell. When one cell is stimulated, the impulse rapidly spreads throughout the heart muscle.

- *Refractoriness* is the inability of cardiac cells to respond to additional stimuli immediately following depolarization. In the absolute refractory period, depolarization will not occur in response to any stimulus. A stronger than normal stimulus is required to initiate depolarization during the relative refractory period. This is followed by the supernormal period, during which a mild stimulus will cause depolarization.

- *Contractility* is the ability of myocardial fibers to shorten in response to a stimulus. Heart muscle responds in an *all-or-nothing* manner: Stimulation of one muscle fiber causes the entire muscle mass to contract to its fullest extent as one unit.

Electrical activity of the heart is normally controlled by the cardiac conduction system (see Figure 30–7). The sinoatrial (SA) node, the primary pacemaker of the heart, usually generates impulses at a regular rate of 60 to 100 beats/min. The impulse spreads through the atria, is briefly delayed at the AV node, then spreads through conduction pathways of the ventricles and to ventricular muscle. The AV nodal delay allows the

NURSING CARE OF THE OLDER ADULT Cardiac Dysrhythmias

Aging affects the heart and the cardiac conduction system, increasing the incidence of dysrhythmias and conduction defects. Older adults may experience dysrhythmias even when no evidence of heart disease is found.

Older adults have a higher incidence of both ventricular and supraventricular dysrhythmias without detrimental effects than younger people. Ectopic beats, including short runs of ventricular tachycardia, occur more commonly during exercise in older adults. These dysrhythmias do not affect cardiac morbidity or mortality. Fibrosis of the bundle branches can lead to atrioventricular blocks; a prolonged PR interval is common in clients over the age of 65. Older adults also have a higher incidence of diseases that may affect heart rhythm. An elderly client with hyperthyroidism, for example, may present with atrial fibrillation, syncope, and confusion instead of the usual manifestations of goiter, tremor, and exophthalmos.

Assessing for Home Care

Assessing older adults for problems related to cardiac dysrhythmias focuses on the effect of the dysrhythmia on functional health status.

- Ask about a history of cardiovascular disease and current medications.
- Inquire about symptoms such as episodes of dizziness, lightheadedness, fainting, palpitations, chest pain, or shortness of breath.

- Ask about relationship of symptoms such as palpitations to intake of certain foods and caffeine-containing beverages.
- Evaluate for other contributing factors such as smoking or alcohol intake.
- Inquire about a history of falls, particularly those occurring without apparent reason.

Teaching for Home Care

Teach measures to reduce the risk of cardiac dysrhythmias and potential adverse consequences of dysrhythmias.

- Emphasize the importance of taking medications as prescribed. Discuss possible effects of over-the-counter medications on the heart.
- Encourage reducing or eliminating caffeine intake. Caffeine increases the risk of ectopic beats and rapid heart rates.
- Encourage participation in a smoking cessation program and to reduce or eliminate alcohol intake if appropriate.
- Encourage engaging in regular exercise. Discuss the beneficial effects of exercise to maintain muscle mass, including cardiac muscle, and cardiovascular health.
- Instruct to contact primary care provider for evaluation of symptoms such as dizziness, fainting, frequent palpitations, shortness of breath, unexplained falls, or chest pain.

---

atria to contract, delivering an extra bolus of blood to the ventricles before they contract (the **atrial kick**). The AV node also controls the number of impulses that reach the ventricles, preventing extremely rapid heart rates.

Pathophysiology

Dysrhythmias arise through disruption of the very properties that stimulate and control the heartbeat: automaticity, excitability, conductivity, and refractoriness.

Dysrhythmias due to altered impulse formation include changes in rate and rhythm and the development of ectopic beats. This category includes *tachydysrhythmias* (rapid heart rates), *bradydysrhythmias* (slow heart rates), and ectopic rhythms. These dysrhythmias result from a change in the automaticity of cardiac cells. The rate of impulse formation may abnormally increase or decrease. Aberrant (abnormal) impulses may originate outside normal conduction pathways, causing **ectopic beats**. Ectopic beats interrupt the normal conduction sequence and may not initiate a normal muscle contraction. Depending on the site and timing of abnormal impulses, they may have little effect on the client or pose a significant threat.

Ischemia, injury, and infarction of myocardial tissue affect its excitability and ability to conduct and respond to an electrical stimulus. Conduction abnormalities cause varying degrees of **heart block**, a block in the normal conduction pathways. Myocardial injury or infarction can obstruct or delay impulse conduction. Bundle branch blocks are common in acute myocardial infarction.

The *reentry phenomenon*, a phenomenon of normal and slow conduction, is a major cause of tachydysrhythmias. A stimulus such as an ectopic beat triggers the reentry phenomenon. The impulse is delayed in one area of the heart (e.g., an area of ischemia or injury) but conducted normally through the rest. Muscle that has been depolarized by the normally conducted impulse is repolarized by the time the impulse traveling through the area of slow conduction reaches it, thus initiating another cycle of depolarization (Porth, 2005). The result is a dysrhythmia that propagates itself.

Several forms of reentry may occur. The impulse may travel through a set pathway to reenter repolarized tissue. Many atrial dysrhythmias follow this pattern, including atrial flutter. In functional reentry, local differences in the conduction of an impulse interrupt the normal wave of depolarization, sending it back upon itself in a spiral pattern and setting up a permanent rotation. This type of pattern suppresses normal pacemaker activity and can lead to atrial fibrillation (Porth, 2005).

Cardiac rhythms are classified according to the site of impulse formation or the site and degree of conduction block. *Supraventricular rhythms* arise above the ventricles. These rhythms usually produce a QRS complex within the normal range. Sinus rhythms, atrial rhythms, and junctional (arising from the AV junction) rhythms are all supraventricular rhythms. *Ventricular rhythms* originate in the ventricles and may prove fatal if left untreated. *AV conduction blocks* result from a defect in impulse transmission from the atria to the ventricles. The major normal and abnormal cardiac rhythms are summarized in Table 31–7.

TABLE 31–7 **Characteristics of Selected Cardiac Rhythms and Dysrhythmias**

RHYTHM/ECG APPEARANCE	ECG CHARACTERISTICS	MANAGEMENT
Supraventricular Rhythms		
Normal sinus rhythm (NSR) 	Rate: 60 to 100 beats/min Rhythm: Regular P:QRS: 1:1 PR interval: 0.12 to 0.20 sec QRS complex: 0.6 to 0.10 sec	None; normal heart rhythm.
Sinus arrhythmia 	Rate: 60 to 100 beats/min Rhythm: Irregular, varying with respirations P:QRS: 1:1 PR interval: 0.12 to 0.20 sec QRS complex: 0.6 to 0.10 sec	Generally none; considered a normal rhythm in the very young and very old.
Sinus tachycardia 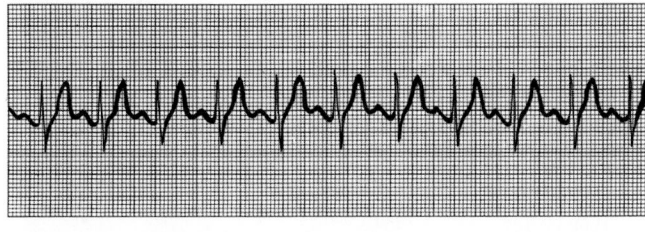	Rate: 101 to 150 beats/min Rhythm: Regular P:QRS: 1:1 (With very fast rates, P wave may be hidden in preceding T wave) PR interval: 0.12 to 0.20 sec QRS complex: 0.6 to 0.10 sec	Treated only if symptomatic or client is at risk for myocardial damage. Treat underlying cause (e.g., hypovolemia, fever, pain). Beta blockers or verapamil may be used.
Sinus bradycardia 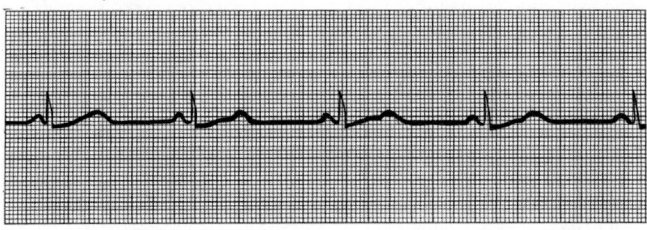	Rate: < 60 beats/min Rhythm: Regular P:QRS: 1:1 PR interval: 0.12 to 0.20 sec QRS complex: 0.6 to 0.10 sec	Treated only if symptomatic. Intravenous atropine or isoproterenol, and/or pacemaker therapy may be used.
Premature atrial contractions (PAC) 	Rate: Variable Rhythm: Irregular, with normal rhythm interrupted by early beats arising in the atria P:QRS: 1:1 PR interval: 0.12 to 0.20 sec, but may be prolonged QRS complex: 0.6 to 0.10 sec	Usually require no treatment. Advise to reduce alcohol and caffeine intake, to reduce stress, and to stop smoking. Beta blocker may be prescribed
Paroxysmal supraventricular tachycardia (PSVT) 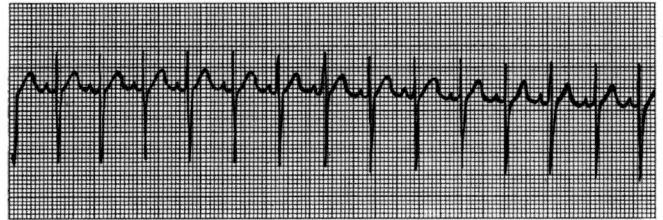	Rate: 100 to 280 beats/min (usually 150 to 200 beats/min) Rhythm: Regular P:QRS: P waves often not identifiable PR interval: Not measured QRS complex: 0.6 to 0.10 sec	Treat if symptomatic. Treatment may include vagal maneuvers (Valsalva, carotid sinus massage); oxygen therapy; adenosine or a beta blocker; temporary pacing, or synchronized cardioversion.

(continued)

TABLE 31–7 Characteristics of Selected Cardiac Rhythms and Dysrhythmias (continued)

RHYTHM/ECG APPEARANCE	ECG CHARACTERISTICS	MANAGEMENT
Atrial flutter 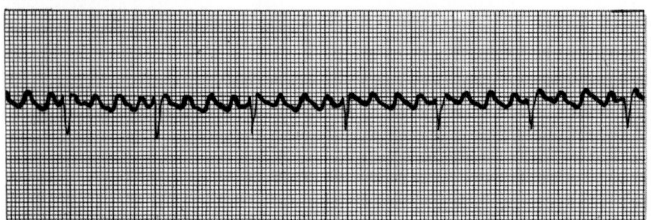	Rate: Atrial 240 to 360 beats/min, ventricular rate depends on degree of AV block and usually is <150 beats/min Rhythm: Atrial regular; ventricular usually regular P:QRS: 2:1, 4:1, 6:1; may vary PR interval: Not measured QRS complex: 0.6 to 0.10 sec	Synchronized cardioversion; medications to slow ventricular response such as a beta blocker or calcium channel blocker, followed by a class I antidysrhythmic agent or amiodarone.
Atrial fibrillation	Rate: Atrial 300 to 600 beats/min (too rapid to count); ventricular 100 to 180 beats/min in untreated clients Rhythm: Irregularly irregular P:QRS: Variable PR interval: Not measured QRS complex: 0.06 to 0.10 sec	Synchronized cardioversion; medications to reduce ventricular response rate: metaprolol, diltiazem, or digoxin; anticoagulant therapy to reduce risk of clot formation and stroke.
Junctional escape rhythm 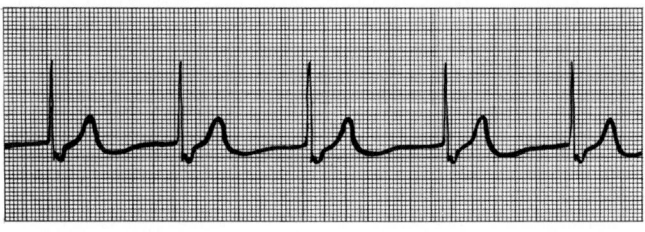	Rate: 40 to 60 beats/min; junctional tachycardia 60 to 140 BPM Rhythm: Regular P:QRS: P waves may be absent, inverted and immediately preceding or succeeding QRS complex, or hidden in QRS complex PR interval: <0.10 sec QRS complex: 0.06 to 0.10 sec	Treat cause if symptomatic.

Ventricular Rhythms

RHYTHM/ECG APPEARANCE	ECG CHARACTERISTICS	MANAGEMENT
Premature ventricular contractions (PVC) 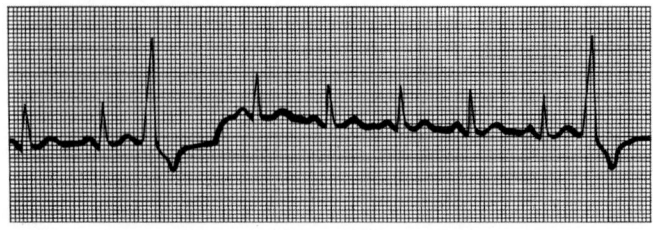	Rate: Variable Rhythm: Irregular, with PVC interrupting underlying rhythm and followed by a compensatory pause P:QRS: No P wave noted before PVC PR interval: Absent with PVC QRS complex: Wide (>0.12 sec) and bizarre in appearance; differs from normal QRS complex	Treat if symptomatic or in presence of severe heart disease. Advise against stimulant use (caffeine, nicotine). Beta blockers, or class I or III antidysrhythmic agents (see the box on page 1006) may be used in clients with severe heart disease who are symptomatic
Ventricular tachycardia (VT, V tach)	Rate: 100 to 250 beats/min Rhythm: Regular P:QRS: P waves usually not identifiable PR interval: Not measured QRS complex: 0.12 sec or greater; bizarre shape	Treat if VT is sustained, symptomatic, or associated with organic heart disease. Treatment includes DC cardioversion or intravenous procainamide, lidocaine, or a class III antidysrhythmic agent if hemodynamic instability accompanies. Surgical ablation or antitachycardia pacing with an implanted cardioverter/defibrillator (ICD) for repeated episodes.

TABLE 31–7 Characteristics of Selected Cardiac Rhythms and Dysrhythmias (continued)

RHYTHM/ECG APPEARANCE	ECG CHARACTERISTICS	MANAGEMENT
Ventricular fibrillation (VF, V fib) 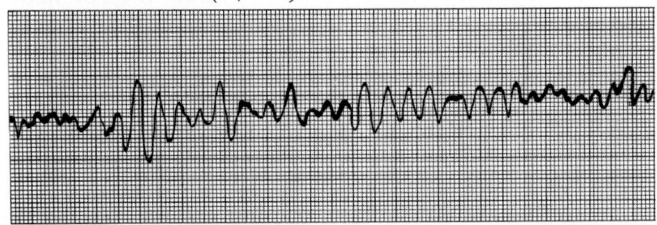	Rate: Too rapid to count Rhythm: Grossly irregular P:QRS: No identifiable P waves PR interval: None QRS: Bizarre, varying in shape and direction	Immediate cardioversion/defibrillation.
Atrioventricular Conduction Blocks *First-degree AV block* 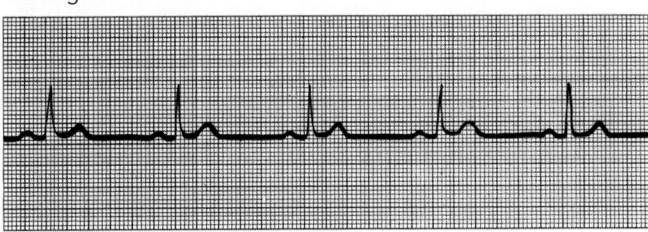	Rate: Usually 60 to 100 beats/min Rhythm: Regular P:QRS: 1:1 PR interval: >0.21 sec QRS complex: 0.06 to 0.10 sec	None required.
Second-degree AV block, type I (Mobitz I, Wenckebach) 	Rate: 60 to 100 beats/min Rhythm: Atrial regular; ventricular irregular P:QRS: 1:1 until P wave blocked with no subsequent QRS complex PR interval: Progressively lengthens in a regular pattern QRS complex: 0.06 to 0.10 sec; sudden absence of QRS complex	Monitoring and observation; rarely progresses to a higher degree of block or requires treatment.
Second-degree AV block, type II (Mobitz II) 	Rate: Atrial 60 to 100 beats/min; Ventricular <60 beats/min Rhythm: Atrial regular; ventricular irregular P:QRS: Typically 2:1, may vary PR interval: Constant PR interval for each conducted QRS complex QRS complex: 0.06 to 0.10 sec	Atropine or isoproterenol; pacemaker therapy.
Third-degree AV block (Complete heart block) 	Rate: Atrial 60 to 100 beats/min; ventricular 15 to 60 beats/min Rhythm: Atrial regular; ventricular regular P:QRS: No relationship between P waves and QRS complexes; independent rhythms PR interval: Not measured QRS complex: 0.06 to 0.10 sec if junctional escape rhythm; >0.12 sec if ventricular escape rhythm	Immediate pacemaker therapy.

FAST FACTS

- The normal sinus rate is 60 to 100 beats per minute. Each complex includes a P wave, QRS, and T wave.
- Supraventricular dysrhythmias arise in the sinus node or the atria. A P wave may be present; the QRS appears normal, and a T wave may be seen.
- Junctional dysrhythmias arise in tissue just above or just below the AV node. The P wave may be inverted, and may precede, follow, or be buried in the QRS complex. The QRS usually appears normal and is followed by a T wave.
- Ventricular dysrhythmias arise in ventricular myocardium. They do not reset the SA node or activate the atria. QRS complexes are wide and bizarre.

Supraventricular Rhythms

NORMAL SINUS RHYTHM **Normal sinus rhythm (NSR)** is the normal heart rhythm, in which impulses originate in the SA (sinus) node and travel through all normal conduction pathways without delay. All waveforms are of normal configuration, look alike, and have consistent (fixed) durations. The rate is between 60 and 100 bpm.

SINUS NODE DYSRHYTHMIAS Sinus node dysrhythmias may occur as a normal compensatory response (e.g., to exercise) or because of altered automaticity. In these rhythms, as in NSR, the initiating impulse is from the sinus node. They differ from NSR in rate or regularity of the rhythm. Sinus dysrhythmias include sinus arrhythmia, sinus tachycardia, and sinus bradycardia.

Sinus Arrhythmia *Sinus arrhythmia* is a sinus rhythm in which the rate varies with respirations, causing an irregular rhythm. The rate increases during inspiration and decreases with expiration. Sinus arrhythmia is common in the very young and the very old. It can be caused by an increase in vagal tone, by digitalis toxicity, or by morphine administration.

Sinus Tachycardia *Sinus tachycardia* has all of the characteristics of NSR, except that the rate is greater than 100 bpm. Tachycardia arises from enhanced automaticity in response to changes in the internal environment. Sympathetic nervous system stimulation or blocked vagal (parasympathetic) activity increases the heart rate. Tachycardia is a normal response to any condition or event that increases the body's demand for oxygen and nutrients, such as exercise or hypoxia. In the client on bed rest, tachycardia is an ominous sign. Sinus tachycardia may be an early sign of cardiac dysfunction, such as heart failure. Tachycardia is detrimental in clients with cardiac disease because it increases cardiac work and oxygen use.

Common causes of sinus tachycardia include exercise, excitement, anxiety, pain, fever, hypoxia, hypovolemia, anemia, hyperthyroidism, myocardial infarction, heart failure, cardiogenic shock, pulmonary embolism, caffeine intake, and certain drugs, such as atropine, epinephrine (Adrenalin), or isoproterenol (Isuprel).

Manifestations of sinus tachycardia include a rapid pulse rate. The client may complain of feeling that the heart is "racing," shortness of breath, and dizziness. In the presence of heart disease, sinus tachycardia may precipitate chest pain.

Sinus Bradycardia *Sinus bradycardia* has all of the characteristics of NSR, but the rate is less than 60 beats/min. Sinus bradycardia may result from increased vagal (parasympathetic) activity or from depressed automaticity due to injury or ischemia to the sinus node. Sinus bradycardia may be normal (e.g., in clients with athletic heart syndrome). The heart rate also normally slows during sleep because the parasympathetic nervous system is dominant at this time. Other causes of sinus bradycardia include pain, increased intracranial pressure, sinus node disease, AMI (especially with inferior wall damage), hypothermia, acidosis, and certain drugs.

Sinus bradycardia may be asymptomatic; it is important to assess the client before treating the rhythm. Manifestations of decreased cardiac output, such as decreased level of consciousness, syncope (faintness), or hypotension, indicate a need for intervention.

Sick Sinus Syndrome *Sick sinus syndrome (SSS)* results from sinus node disease or dysfunction that causes problems with impulse formation, transmission, and conduction. Sick sinus syndrome is often found in older adults. It may be caused by direct injury to sinus tissue, fibrosis of conduction fibers associated with aging, and such drugs as digitalis, beta blockers, and calcium channel blockers.

ECG characteristics of SSS include sinus bradycardia, sinus arrhythmia, sinus pauses or arrest, and atrial tachydysrhythmias such as atrial fibrillation, atrial flutter, or atrial tachycardia. Bradycardia-tachycardia syndrome, characterized either by **paroxysmal** (abrupt onset and termination) atrial tachycardia followed by prolonged sinus pauses or alternating periods of bradycardia and tachycardia also may indicate sinus node dysfunction.

Manifestations of sinus node dysfunction often are intermittent, related to a drop in cardiac output caused by the irregular rhythm. Fatigue, dizziness, light-headedness, and syncope are common. The heart rate may not increase in response to stressors such as exercise or fever.

SUPRAVENTRICULAR DYSRHYTHMIAS When an action potential originates in atrial tissue outside the sinus node, the resulting rhythm is classified as a *supraventricular rhythm*. In these dysrhythmias, an ectopic pacemaker takes over, or overrides, the SA node. They may also occur when the SA node fails; an *escape rhythm* develops as a fail-safe mechanism to maintain the heart rate. The most common supraventricular dysrhythmias are premature atrial contractions, paroxysmal supraventricular tachycardia, atrial flutter, and atrial fibrillation. These rhythms may be paroxysmal, that is, occur in bursts with an abrupt beginning and end.

Premature Atrial Contractions A *premature atrial contraction (PAC)* is an ectopic atrial beat that occurs earlier than the next expected sinus beat. PACs can arise anywhere in the atria. They are usually asymptomatic and benign, but they may initiate paroxysmal supraventricular tachycardia in susceptible individuals. PACs are common in older adults, often occurring without an obvious cause. Strong emotions, excessive alcohol intake, tobacco, and stimulants such as caffeine can precipitate PACs. They also may be associated with myocardial infarction, heart failure and other cardiac disorders, hypoxemia, pulmonary embolism, digitalis toxicity, and electrolyte or acid–base imbalances. In clients with underlying heart disease, PACs may precede a more serious dysrhythmia.

The ECG tracing shows interruption of the underlying rhythm by a premature complex that looks similar to the underlying beats. The ectopic impulse of the PAC is usually conducted normally, leading to depolarization of cardiac muscle and a normal QRS complex. Because the impulse arises above the ventricles, it follows normal conduction pathways through the ventricles. The QRS complex is narrow or matches those of the underlying rhythm. The shape of the P wave of a PAC differs from normal P waves because its impulse arises outside the sinus node. A *noncompensatory pause* usually follows, as the PAC resets the SA node rhythm. Occasionally, the ectopic impulse may not be conducted through the heart, resulting in a lone P wave without a QRS, or a nonconducted PAC.

PACs cause few manifestations. If frequent, they may cause palpitations or a fluttering sensation in the chest. Early beats may be noted on auscultating or palpating the pulse.

Paroxysmal Supraventricular Tachycardia *Paroxysmal supraventricular tachycardia (PSVT)* is tachycardia of sudden onset and termination. PSVT is usually initiated by a reentry loop in or around the AV node; that is, an impulse reenters the same section of tissue over and over, causing repeated depolarizations.

PSVT occurs more frequently in women. Sympathetic nervous system stimulation and stressors such as fever, sepsis, and hyperthyroidism may precipitate PSVT. It also may be associated with heart diseases such as CHD, myocardial infarction, rheumatic heart disease, myocarditis, or acute pericarditis. Abnormal conduction pathways associated with Wolff-Parkinson-White (WPW) syndrome may account for PSVT.

PSVT affects ventricular filling and cardiac output, and decreases coronary artery perfusion. Its manifestations include complaints of palpitations and a "racing" heart, anxiety, dizziness, dyspnea, anginal pain, diaphoresis, extreme fatigue, and polyuria (urine output may reach up to 3 L in the first few hours after PSVT onset).

Atrial Flutter *Atrial flutter* is a rapid and regular atrial rhythm thought to result from an intra-atrial reentry mechanism. Causes include sympathetic nervous system stimulation due to anxiety or caffeine and alcohol intake; thyrotoxicosis; coronary heart disease or myocardial infarction; pulmonary embolism; and abnormal conduction syndromes, such as WPW syndrome. Older persons with rheumatic heart disease and/or valvular disease are especially vulnerable.

Two types of atrial flutter have been identified. Type I atrial flutter has an atrial rate of 240 to 340 beats per minute. It develops due to a reentry mechanism in the right atrium. The mechanism leading to type II atrial flutter has not been identified. In this type of flutter, the atrial rate is faster, to 350 beats per minute.

Clients with atrial flutter may complain of palpitations or a fluttering sensation in the chest or throat. If the ventricular rate is rapid, manifestations of decreased cardiac output, such as decreased level of consciousness, hypotension, decreased urinary output, and cool clammy skin, may be noted. The atrial kick

(additional ventricular filling with atrial contraction) is lost because of inadequate atrial filling.

ECG characteristics include a "sawtooth" or "picket fence" appearance of P waves, which are labeled flutter (F) waves. The atrial rate is rapid, often around 300 beats/min. As a protective mechanism, many impulses are blocked at the AV node, and the ventricular rate is rarely greater than 150 to 170 beats/min. Usually, atrial impulses are evenly conducted through the AV node, for example, two impulses to one QRS complex (2:1), four impulses to one QRS complex (4:1), or six impulses to one QRS complex (6:1). A constant conduction ratio results in a regular ventricular rhythm; the ventricular rhythm is irregular if the conduction ratio varies. The ventricular rate usually ranges from 150 to 170 beats/min in 2:1 conduction and 60 to 75 beats/min for lower conduction ratios. The T wave is usually hidden by overriding F waves; some F waves may be hidden in the QRS complex.

Atrial Fibrillation *Atrial fibrillation* is a common dysrhythmia characterized by disorganized atrial activity without discrete atrial contractions. Multiple small reentry circuits develop in the atria. Atrial cells cannot repolarize in time to respond to the next stimulus (Porth, 2005). Extremely rapid atrial impulses bombard the AV node, resulting in an irregularly irregular ventricular response. Atrial fibrillation may occur suddenly and recur, or it may persist as a chronic dysrhythmia. Atrial fibrillation is commonly associated with heart failure, rheumatic heart disease, coronary heart disease, hypertension, and hyperthyroidism.

Manifestations of atrial fibrillation relate to the rate of the ventricular response. With rapid response rates, manifestations of decreased cardiac output such as hypotension, shortness of breath, fatigue, and angina may develop. Clients with extensive heart disease may develop syncope or heart failure. Peripheral pulses are irregular and of variable amplitude (strength).

The specific ECG characteristics of atrial fibrillation include an irregularly irregular rhythm and the absence of identifiable P waves. The atrial rate is so rapid that it is not measurable. The ventricular rate varies.

Atrial fibrillation increases the risk for formation of thromboemboli. Organ infarction may occur as a result; the incidence of stroke is high.

Junctional Dysrhythmias

Rhythms that originate in AV nodal tissue are termed *junctional*. The AV junction includes the AV node and the bundle of His, which branches into the right and left bundle branches. An impulse arising from the AV junction may occur in response to failure of higher pacemakers, as in a *junctional escape rhythm,* or it may result from an abnormal mechanism, such as altered automaticity. An impulse arising from the AV junction may or may not be conducted back up to the atria. This conduction against the normal flow or pattern is called *retrograde conduction.* The resulting atrial wave, called a P′ wave, may be found before, during, or after the QRS complex, depending on the speed of conduction. The P′ wave is inverted in some ECG leads because the impulse moves from the AV node up to the atria instead of from the SA node down toward the AV node. In addition, the P'R interval is shorter than normal (less than 0.12 sec). The QRS complex is typically narrow.

A junctional rhythm may be due to drug toxicity (e.g., digitalis, beta blockers, or calcium channel blockers) or other causes such as hypoxemia, hyperkalemia, increased vagal tone or damage to the AV node, myocardial infarction, and heart failure. Loss of synchronized atrial contraction and the atrial kick may affect cardiac output, leading to manifestations of decreased cardiac output and impaired myocardial tissue perfusion. Heart failure may develop.

Premature junctional contractions (PJCs) occur before the next expected beat of the underlying rhythm. Isolated PJCs may occur in healthy people and are insignificant. *Junctional tachycardia* is a junctional rhythm with a rate greater than 60 beats/min. It is caused by increased automaticity of AV nodal tissue. The ventricular rate is usually less than 140 beats/min. Both rhythms are most commonly associated with digitalis toxicity, hypoxia, ischemia, or electrolyte imbalances.

Ventricular Dysrhythmias

Ventricular dysrhythmias originate in the ventricles. Because the ventricles pump blood into the pulmonary and systemic vasculature, any disruption of their rhythm can affect cardiac output and tissue perfusion. A wide and bizarre QRS complex (greater than 0.12 sec) is a characteristic feature of ventricular dysrhythmias. This occurs because ventricular ectopic impulses begin and travel outside normal conduction pathways. Other characteristics include no relationship of the QRS complex to a P wave, increased amplitude of the QRS complex, an abnormal ST segment, and a T wave deflected in the opposite direction from the QRS complex.

PREMATURE VENTRICULAR CONTRACTIONS *Premature ventricular contractions (PVCs)* are ectopic ventricular beats that occur before the next expected beat of the underlying rhythm. They usually do not reset the atrial rhythm and are followed by a full compensatory pause. PVCs often have no significance in people without heart disease. Frequent, recurrent, or multifocal PVCs may be associated with an increased risk for lethal dysrhythmias. PVCs result from either enhanced automaticity or a reentry phenomenon. They may be triggered by anxiety or stress; tobacco, alcohol, or caffeine use; hypoxia, acidosis, and electrolyte imbalances; sympathomimetic drugs; coronary heart disease; heart failure; and mechanical stimulation of the heart (e.g., the insertion of a cardiac catheter); or reperfusion after fibrinolytic therapy. The incidence and significance of PVCs is greatest after myocardial infarction.

PVCs may be isolated or occur in a specific pattern. Two PVCs in a row are called a *couplet* or *paired* PVCs. Three consecutive PVCs (a *triplet* or *salvo*) is a short run of ventricular tachycardia. *Ventricular bigeminy* is characterized by a PVC following each normal beat; a PVC noted every third beat is called *ventricular trigeminy*. When the ventricular impulse arises from one ectopic site, all PVCs look the same (*monomorphic*) and are called *unifocal* PVCs. *Multifocal* PVCs arise from different ectopic sites and appear different from one another on the ECG (*polymorphic*).

The frequency and patterns of PVCs can be indicative of myocardial irritability and the risk for a lethal dysrhythmia.

The following are considered warning signs in the client with acute heart disease (e.g., an acute MI).

- PVCs that develop within the first 4 hours of an MI
- Frequent PVCs (six or more per minute)
- Couplets or triplets
- Multifocal PVCs
- R-on-T phenomenon (PVCs falling on the T wave).

In people without heart disease, isolated PVCs usually are insignificant and do not require treatment. Clients may complain of feeling their hearts "skip a beat" or of palpitations. In clients with preexisting heart disease, PVCs may indicate a drug toxicity or an increased risk for lethal dysrhythmias and cardiac arrest. The risk is greatest following acute MI.

VENTRICULAR TACHYCARDIA *Ventricular tachycardia (VT, V tach)* is a rapid ventricular rhythm defined as three or more consecutive PVCs. Ventricular tachycardia may occur in short bursts, or "runs," or may persist for more than 30 seconds (sustained ventricular tachycardia). The rate is greater than 100 beats/min, and the rhythm is usually regular. Reentry is the usual electrophysiologic mechanism responsible for VT. Myocardial ischemia and infarction are the most common predisposing factors for VT. It also is associated with cardiac structural disorders such as valvular disease, rheumatic heart disease, or cardiomyopathy. It may occur in the absence of heart disease, and with anorexia nervosa, metabolic disorders, and drug toxicity.

Nonsustained VT may occur paroxysmally and convert back to an effective rhythm spontaneously. The client may experience a fluttering sensation in the chest or complain of palpitations and brief shortness of breath. Clients in sustained VT generally develop signs and symptoms of decreased cardiac output and hemodynamic instability, including severe hypotension, a weak or nonpalpable pulse, and loss of consciousness. Allowed to continue, VT can deteriorate into ventricular fibrillation. Sustained ventricular tachycardia is a medical emergency that requires immediate intervention, particularly in clients with cardiac disease.

Toursades de pointes is a type of ventricular tachycardia associated with *long QT syndrome,* a prolongation of the QT interval. Long QT syndrome may be genetic or acquired, occurring secondarily to electrolyte disruptions, myocardial infarction, cocaine use, liquid protein diets, medications, or other conditions. In toursades de pointes, the QRS complexes vary in size, shape, and amplitude (Figure 31–7 ■). Clients with toursades de pointes may have multiple bursts or episodes of ventricular tachycardia or may develop ventricular fibrillation and sudden cardiac death (Kasper et al., 2005; Porth, 2005).

VENTRICULAR FIBRILLATION *Ventricular fibrillation (VF, V fib)* is extremely rapid, chaotic ventricular depolarization causing the ventricles to quiver and cease contracting; the heart does not pump. This is known as **cardiac arrest**; it is a medical emergency requiring immediate intervention with cardiopulmonary resuscitation (CPR). Death will follow the onset of VF within 4 minutes if the rhythm is not recognized and terminated and an effective perfusing rhythm reestablished.

Ventricular fibrillation is usually triggered by severe myocardial ischemia or infarction. It occurs without warning 50%

Figure 31–7 ■ Toursades de pointes. Note the wide and bizarre QRS complexes of varying size, shape (morphology), and amplitude.

of the time. It is the terminal event in many disease processes or traumatic conditions. Ventricular fibrillation may be precipitated by a single PVC or may follow VT. Other causes of VF include digitalis toxicity, reperfusion therapy, antidysrhythmic drugs, hypokalemia and hyperkalemia, hypothermia, metabolic acidosis, mechanical stimulation (as with the insertion of cardiac catheters or pacing wires), and electric shock.

Clinically, loss of ventricular contractions results in absence of a palpable or audible pulse. The client loses consciousness and stops breathing as perfusion ceases. The ECG shows grossly irregular, bizarre complexes with no discernible rate or rhythm.

Atrioventricular Conduction Blocks

Conduction defects that delay or block transmission of the sinus impulse through the AV node are called *atrioventricular conduction blocks*. Impaired conduction may result from tissue injury or disease, increased vagal (parasympathetic) tone, drug effects, or a congenital defect. AV conduction blocks vary in severity from benign to severe.

> **FAST FACTS**
> - First-degree AV block = delayed conduction through the AV node and a long PR interval.
> - Second-degree AV block = complete blockage of *some* impulses through the AV node; some P waves are not followed by a QRS complex.
> - Third-degree AV block = complete blockage of *all* impulses through the AV node; no relationship between P waves and QRS complexes.

FIRST-DEGREE AV BLOCK *First-degree AV block* is a benign conduction delay that generally poses no threat, has no symptoms, and requires no treatment. Impulse conduction through the AV node is slowed, but all atrial impulses are conducted to the ventricles. It may result from injury or infarct of the AV node, other cardiac diseases, or drug effects. The ECG shows all characteristics of NSR, except the PR interval is greater than 0.20 second.

SECOND-DEGREE AV BLOCK *Second-degree AV block* is characterized by failure to conduct one or more impulses from the atria to the ventricles. Two patterns of second-degree AV block are seen, identified as type I and type II.

Second-Degree AV Block—Type I *Type I second-degree AV block (Mobitz type I* or *Wenckebach phenomenon)* is characterized by a repeating pattern of increasing AV conduction delays until an impulse fails to conduct to the ventricles. On the ECG, PR intervals progressively lengthen until one QRS complex is not conducted, or dropped. The ventricular rate remains adequate to maintain cardiac output, and the client usually is asymptomatic. Mobitz type I AV block usually is transient, associated with acute MI or drug intoxication (e.g., digitalis, beta blockers, or calcium channel blockers). It rarely progresses to complete heart block.

Second-Degree AV Block—Type II *Type II second-degree AV block (Mobitz type II)* involves intermittent failure of the AV node to conduct an impulse to the ventricles without preceding delays in conduction. The PR interval remains constant, but not all P waves are followed by QRS complexes (e.g., there may be two P waves for every QRS). Conduction through the His-Purkinje system usually is delayed as well, causing a widened QRS complex (Braunwald et al., 2002). Mobitz type II block is frequently associated with acute anterior wall MI and a high rate of mortality (Porth, 2005). Manifestations of Mobitz type II block depend on the ventricular rate. Pacemaker therapy may be required to maintain the cardiac output.

THIRD-DEGREE AV BLOCK *Third-degree AV block (complete heart block)* occurs when atrial impulses are completely blocked at the AV node, and fail to reach the ventricles. As a result, the atria and ventricles are controlled by different and independent pacemakers, with separate rates and rhythms. The ventricular impulse arises from either junctional fibers (with a rate of 40 to 60 beats/min) or a ventricular pacemaker at a rate of less than 40 beats/min. The width of the QRS complex depends on the location of the escape pacemaker. The QRS is wide and the rate is slow when the rhythm arises distal to the bundle of His.

Third-degree block is frequently associated with an inferior or anteroseptal myocardial infarction. Other causes include congenital conditions, acute or degenerative cardiac disease or damage, drug effects, and electrolyte imbalances. The slow escape rhythm significantly affects cardiac output, causing manifestations such as syncope (known as a *Stokes-Adams attack*), dizziness, fatigue, exercise intolerance, and heart failure. Third-degree AV block is life threatening and requires immediate intervention to maintain adequate cardiac output.

AV DISSOCIATION Complete dissociation of atrial and ventricular rhythms can occur in conditions other than third-degree AV block. The two primary factors leading to AV dissociation are severe sinus bradycardia and a lower pacemaker (junctional or ventricular) that competes with or exceeds the normal sinus rhythm (Braunwald et al., 2002). AV dissociation may result from acute myocardial ischemia or infarction, cardiac surgery, or drug effects. The ECG shows separate and competing atrial (P waves) and ventricular (QRS complexes) rhythms.

Intraventricular Conduction Blocks

Once the impulse enters the ventricles, its conduction through the right and left bundle branches may be impaired (*bundle branch block*). As a result, the impulse is conducted more slowly than normal through the ventricles. On the ECG, the QRS complex is prolonged. Its appearance varies, depending on the affected bundle (right or left). Typically, no clinical manifestations are associated with bundle branch block unless it occurs in conjunction with an AV block.

INTERDISCIPLINARY CARE

Cardiac dysrhythmias may be either benign or critical: Recognizing lethal dysrhythmias is a matter of life and death. Major goals of care include identifying the dysrhythmia, evaluating its effect on physical and psychosocial well-being, and treating underlying causes. This may involve correcting fluid and electrolyte or acid–base imbalances; treating hypoxia, pain, or anxiety; administering antidysrhythmic medications; or mechanical and surgical interventions.

Diagnosis

Diagnostic tests for dysrhythmias include the electrocardiogram, cardiac monitoring, and electrophysiology studies. Laboratory tests such as serum electrolytes, drug levels, and ABGs may be done to help identify the cause of the dysrhythmia.

ELECTROCARDIOGRAM The 12-lead ECG may be required to accurately diagnose a dysrhythmia. It also provides information about underlying disease processes, such as myocardial infarction or other cardiac disease. The ECG may also be used to monitor the effects of treatment. See Chapter 30 ∞ for more information about the 12-lead ECG.

CARDIAC MONITORING Cardiac monitoring allows continuous observation of the cardiac rhythm. It is used in many different circumstances (Box 31–4). Different types of ECG monitoring are employed for different situations.

Continuous Cardiac Monitoring Continuous monitoring of the cardiac rhythm is provided by bedside and central monitoring stations. Electrodes placed on the client's chest attach to cables connected to a monitor. The heart rate and rhythm is visually displayed on a bedside monitor connected to a central monitoring station. The central station allows simultaneous monitoring of multiple clients within a nursing unit. Alarms on both bedside and central monitors warn of potential problems such as very rapid or very slow heart rates. Alarm limits are preset by the nurse for the individual client. Procedure 31–1 describes how to place a client on cardiac monitoring.

Telemetry may be used in acute care settings when the client is ambulatory. Chest electrodes are connected to a portable transmitter worn around the neck or waist; the ECG is transmitted electronically to a central monitoring station for continuous monitoring.

Home Monitoring Clients often complain of palpitations or other heart symptoms but are asymptomatic during evaluation in a hospital or community-based setting. Ambulatory or Holter monitoring may be used to identify intermittent dys-

---

BOX 31–4 Indications for Cardiac Monitoring

- Perioperative monitoring of heart rate and rhythm
- Detecting and identifying dysrhythmias
- Monitoring the effects of cardiac and noncardiac diseases on the heart
- Monitoring clients with potentially life-threatening conditions:
  a. Major trauma (especially cardiac trauma)
  b. Dissecting aneurysm
  c. Acute myocardial infarction
  d. Heart failure
  e. Shock
  f. Other emergency conditions
- Evaluating responses to procedures and interventions:
  a. Drug therapies
  b. Diagnostic procedures
  c. Ablative techniques
  d. Angioplasty or cardiac catheterization
  e. Cardiac surgery
  f. Pacemaker function
  g. Automatic implantable cardioverter-defibrillator function

---

rhythmias, to detect silent ischemia, to monitor the effects of treatment, and to assess pacemaker or automatic cardioverter-defibrillator function. Electrodes are applied and the leads attached to the portable telemetry monitor that records and stores all electrical activity. Clients are instructed to leave the electrode pads in place during monitoring, record any cardiac symptoms or events in a journal (such as chest pain, palpitations, syncope), and are told when to return to the clinic. After the prescribed period, usually 48 to 72 hours, the client returns and the monitor is removed. Diary entries are compared to the recorded heart rhythms to identify the effects of dysrhythmias.

ELECTROPHYSIOLOGY STUDIES Diagnostic cardiac *electrophysiology (EP) procedures* are used to identify dysrhythmias and their causes. EP studies are used to analyze components of the conduction system, identify sites of ectopic stimulation, and evaluate the effectiveness of treatment. EP procedures can be used for both diagnosis and as a therapeutic intervention.

In the electrophysiology laboratory, electrode catheters are guided by fluoroscopy into the heart through the femoral or brachial vein. The timing and sequence of electrical activation during normal and abnormal (aberrant) rhythms is observed and measured. Electrical stimulation may be used to induce dysrhythmias similar to the client's clinical dysrhythmia (Woods et al., 2004). Following diagnosis, an EP procedure may be used to treat the dysrhythmia, for example, by overdrive pacing (stimulating the client's heart rate to a rate faster than that of the tachydysrhythmia) to break the dysrhythmia's cycle, or to perform ablative therapy to destroy the ectopic site. See the section on ablative techniques for further information.

Nursing care for the client undergoing an EP procedure is similar to that for a percutaneous coronary revascularization (see the box on page 978). The procedure and expected sensations are explained. The client remains awake during the procedure; antianxiety medications or sedatives are given to reduce

PROCEDURE 31–1 **INITIATING CARDIAC MONITORING**

GATHER SUPPLIES

- Bedside monitor and cable or telemetry unit with fresh battery
- Electrodes—self-adherent, pregelled, disposable
- Lead wires
- Washcloth, soap, and towel
- Alcohol prep pads
- Dry gauze pads or ECG prep pads

BEFORE THE PROCEDURE

Explain the reason for ECG monitoring. Reassure client that changes in heart rhythm can be noted and immediately treated if necessary. Explain that loose or disconnected lead wires, poor electrode contact, excessive movement, electrical interference, or equipment malfunc- tion may trigger alarms and alert the staff, allowing correction of the problem. Reassure that movement is allowed, within activity restric- tions, while on the monitor. Explain skin preparation procedure. Pro- vide for privacy, and drape appropriately.

PROCEDURE

1. Follow standard precautions.
2. Check equipment for damage (i.e., fraying, bent, or broken wires). Connect lead wires to cable, and secure connections.
3. Select electrode sites on the chest wall, avoiding areas of ex- cessive movement, joints, skin creases, scar tissue, or other lesions.
4. Clean sites with soap and water, and dry thoroughly. Alcohol may be used to remove skin oils; allow the skin to dry for 60 seconds after use.
5. Gently rub the site with a dry gauze pad or ECG prep pad to re- move dead skin cells, debris, and residue.
6. Open the electrode package; peel the backing from the elec- trode, and check to ensure that the center of the pad is moist with conductive gel.
7. Apply electrode pads, pressing firmly to ensure contact (see figure).
8. Attach leads and position cable with sufficient slack for com- fort. Place the telemetry unit (if used) in gown pouch or pocket.
9. Assess ECG tracing on the monitor, adjusting settings as needed.

10. Set monitor alarm limits typically at 20 bpm higher and lower than the client's baseline rate. Turn alarms on, and leave on at all times. Assess immediately if an alarm is triggered.
11. Time and date pads with every change.

AFTER THE PROCEDURE

Monitor periodically for comfort. Assess electrode and lead wire connections as needed. Remove and apply new pads every 24 to 48 hours or whenever the pad becomes dislodged or nonadher- ent. Clean gel residue from previous site, and document skin con- dition under the pads. Choose an alternative site if the skin appears irritated or blistered. Document ECG strips according to unit policy and/or physician's order, as well when the cardiac rhythm or the client's condition changes (especially with com- plaints of chest pain, decreased level of consciousness, or changes in vital signs). Note the date, time, client identification, monitor lead, duration of PR and QT intervals, and rhythm inter- pretation on each ECG strip.

---

apprehension. Intravenous heparin may be given during the pro- cedure to reduce the risk of thromboembolism.

Complications of EP procedures are infrequent, but include fatal ventricular fibrillation, cardiac perforation, and major ve- nous thrombosis (Woods et al., 2004). Careful postprocedure monitoring is vital.

Medications

The goal of drug therapy is to suppress dysrhythmia formation. No drug has been found to be completely safe and effective. Antidysrhythmic drugs are primarily used for acute treatment of dysrhythmias, although they may also be used to manage chronic conditions. The overall goal of therapy is to maintain an effective cardiac output by stabilizing cardiac rhythm.

It is important to remember that virtually all antidysrhyth- mic drugs also have *prodysrhythmic* effects; that is, they can worsen existing dysrhythmias and precipitate new ones. Be- cause of this tendency, studies that demonstrate higher mortal- ity rates in clients receiving antidysrhythmic medications, and the increasing safety and availability of interventional tech- niques, antidysrhythmic medications are used sparingly.

Most antidysrhythmic drugs are classified by their effects on the cardiac action potential. Most are class I drugs, or fast sodium channel blockers. By blocking sodium channels, these drugs slow impulse conduction in the atria and ventricles. This class is further divided into subclasses A, B, and C. Class II drugs are beta blockers, which decrease SA node automaticity, AV conduction velocity, and myocardial contractility. Class III agents block potassium channels, delaying repolarization and prolonging the relative refractory period. Class IV drugs are calcium channel blockers. Their effect is similar to that of beta blockers. Adenosine and digoxin do not fit within the major classes. Both drugs reduce SA node automaticity and slow AV conduction. Ibutilide and magnesium also fall outside the major classes, but are used to treat dysrhythmias. The Medication Administration box below identifies common antidysrhythmic drugs within each class and the nursing implications in caring for clients receiving these drugs.

Drugs that affect the autonomic nervous system may also be used to treat dysrhythmias. Sympathomimetics, such as epinephrine, stimulate the heart, increasing both heart rate and contractility. Anticholinergic agents such as atropine are used

---

MEDICATION ADMINISTRATION — Antidysrhythmic Drugs

CLASS I DRUGS: SODIUM CHANNEL BLOCKERS

Class IA
Quinidine (Cardioquin, Quinidex, Quinaglute)
Procainamide (Pronestyl, Procan SR)
Disopyramide (Norpace, Norpace CR)
Moricizine (Ethmozine)
Class IA drugs decrease the flow of sodium into the cell and prolong the action potential. This decreases automaticity, slows the rate of impulse conduction, and prolongs refractoriness. They are used to treat both supraventricular and ventricular tachycardias.

Class IB
Lidocaine (Xylocaine)   **Tocainide (Tonocard)**
Mexiletine (Mexitil)   **Phenytoin (Dilantin)**
Class IB, or lidocaine-like, drugs decrease the refractory period but have little effect on automaticity. Drugs in this class are used primarily to treat ventricular dysrhythmias, including PVCs and ventricular tachycardia.

Class IC
Flecainide (Tambocor)   **Propafenone (Rythmol)**
Class IC drugs slow impulse conduction velocity but have little effect on refractoriness. They are used to reduce or eliminate tachydysrhythmias associated with reentry. Their significant prodysrhythmic effects limit their usefulness, but they may be used to treat supraventricular tachycardia.

CLASS II DRUGS: BETA-BLOCKERS
Esmolol (Brevibloc)
Propranolol (Inderal)
Metoprolol (Toprol)
Class II drugs are beta blockers that decrease automaticity and conduction through the AV node. They also reduce the heart rate and myocardial contractility. They are used to treat supraventricular tachycardia and to slow the ventricular response rate to atrial fibrillation. These drugs may cause bronchospasm and are contraindicated for clients with asthma, chronic obstructive pulmonary disease (COPD), or other restrictive or obstructive lung diseases.

CLASS III DRUGS: POTASSIUM CHANNEL BLOCKERS
Sotalol (Betapace)   **Bretylium (Bretylol)**
Amiodarone (Cordarone)   **Ibutilide (Corvert)**
Dofetilide (Tikosyn)
Class III drugs block potassium channels, prolonging repolarization and the refractory period. Drugs in this class are used primarily to treat ventricular tachycardia and ventricular fibrillation. Amiodarone may also be used for supraventricular tachycardias.

CLASS IV DRUGS: CALCIUM CHANNEL BLOCKERS
Verapamil (Calan, Isoptin, Verelan)
Diltiazem (Cardizem, Dilacor XR)
Calcium channel blockers decrease automaticity and AV nodal conduction. They are used to manage supraventricular tachycardias. Like the beta blockers, calcium channel blockers reduce myocardial contractility.

OTHER DRUGS
Adenosine (Adenocard)   Digoxin
Adenosine and digoxin decrease conduction through the AV node and are used to treat supraventricular tachycardias.

Nursing Responsibilities
- Obtain baseline data including vital signs, cardiac rhythm (including rate, PR and QT intervals, and QRS duration), and physical assessment (especially cardiac, neurologic, and respiratory status).
- Assess medication regimen to identify drugs that may interfere with antidysrhythmic therapy.
- Monitor ECG to evaluate the effectiveness of therapy and to assess for possible dysrhythmias precipitated by treatment.
- Immediately report manifestations of drug toxicity:
  - Procainamide—signs of heart failure; conduction delays or ventricular dysrhythmias; skin rash, myalgias or arthralgias, flulike symptoms.
  - Disopyramide—urinary retention, heart failure, eye pain
  - Lidocaine—changes in neurologic status, such as agitation, confusion, dizziness, nervousness
  - Amiodarone—pulmonary fibrosis (increasing dyspnea, cough, hepatic dysfunction—changes in liver function tests, jaundice); vision changes, photosensitivity
  - Digoxin—anorexia, nausea, vomiting; blurred or double vision; yellow green halos; new-onset dysrhythmias
- Use an infusion pump to administer intravenous infusions. Monitor the dose and assess its appropriateness (in mg/min or mcg/kg/min).

Health Education for the Client and Family
- Take the drug exactly as prescribed. Do not skip or double doses. Check with your physician if a dose is missed.
- Take your pulse and record the rate daily before rising. Count the pulse for 1 full minute. Bring the record with you to each office or clinic visit
- Report the following to the physician: irregular pulse rate or rhythm, dizziness, eye pain, changes in vision, skin rashes or color changes, wheezing or other respiratory problems, changes in behavior.

to decrease vagal tone and increase the heart rate. Magnesium sulfate is an unclassified drug that has been shown to be safe and effective in treating ventricular tachycardias.

Countershock

Countershock is used to interrupt cardiac rhythms that compromise cardiac output and the client's welfare. Delivery of a direct current charge depolarizes all cardiac cells at the same time. This simultaneous depolarization may stop a tachydysrhythmia and allow the sinus node to recover control of impulse formation. There are two types of countershock: synchronized cardioversion and defibrillation.

SYNCHRONIZED CARDIOVERSION *Synchronized cardioversion* delivers direct electrical current synchronized with the client's heart rhythm. Synchronization of the shock with the QRS complex prevents ventricular fibrillation by avoiding current delivery during the vulnerable period of repolarization.

Cardioversion is usually done as an elective procedure to treat supraventricular tachycardia, atrial fibrillation, atrial flutter, or hemodynamically stable ventricular tachycardia.

The nurse assists with cardioversion by preparing the client before the procedure; obtaining any laboratory tests ordered; obtaining and documenting ECG strips prior to, during, and after treatment; setting up the equipment; and monitoring the client's response. Procedure 31–2 describes synchronized cardioversion.

Clients in atrial fibrillation are at high risk for thromboembolism following cardioversion. Loss of atrial contractions with atrial fibrillation leads to blood pooling in the atria, increasing the risk of clot formation. When the atria begin to contract following successful cardioversion, clots may be dislodged, embolizing to the pulmonary or systemic circulation. If possible, anticoagulants are given for several weeks before cardioversion is attempted.

PROCEDURE 31–2 ELECTIVE SYNCHRONIZED CARDIOVERSION

GATHER SUPPLIES

- Cardioverter-defibrillator with ECG cable and monitor
- Conductive gel pads or paste
- Dry gauze pads
- Emergency drug kit and resuscitation equipment
- IV supplies (catheter, solution, administration set)

BEFORE THE PROCEDURE

Explain the purpose of the procedure (to restore an effective cardiac rhythm). Describe the procedure in simple, nonthreatening terms. Advise that some discomfort may be felt with each countershock, but a sedative will be given to minimize discomfort. Witness the signature on an informed consent form for this procedure. Document preprocedure rhythm on an ECG strip. Ensure a patent intravenous access site for emergency drug administration. Keep NPO as specified prior to the procedure. Assess acid-base and electrolyte levels (especially potassium, magnesium, and calcium) and drug levels if appropriate. Report abnormalities to the physician prior to the procedure. Document vital signs, level of consciousness, and peripheral pulses. Administer the prescribed sedative, and provide for safety. Remove any medication patches from the chest and all metallic objects. Place in supine position, and provide for privacy.

PROCEDURE

1. Use standard precautions.
2. Turn on the cardioverter-defibrillator and ECG monitor.
3. Connect the client's ECG cable to the cardioverter. Select a lead with prominent R waves for monitoring.
4. Set cardioverter to "synchronize" mode. Observe the ECG waveform on the monitor for indications of synchronization, such as a flashing bold line or a blip. Many units also display the message "synchronized mode" on the monitor.
5. Place conductive pads on the chest below the right clavicle to the right of the sternum and in the midaxillary line on the left. If using conductive paste, spread it evenly on the defibrillator paddles.
6. Turn on the ECG recording strip for a continuous printout during the procedure.

7. Charge the paddles to the prescribed energy dose. The machine will beep to indicate that the selected energy level has been reached and that the paddles are ready for discharge.
8. The paddles are applied firmly to the chest over the conductive pads by the physician.
9. Turn oxygen off and remove it.
10. Ensure that no one is touching the client or the bed prior to discharge of the electrical shock. There may be a slight delay in shock delivery as the machine synchronizes with the R wave.
11. Assess client status and ECG rhythm. Assure a patent airway and the presence of a pulse.
12. The procedure may be repeated if unsuccessful. The energy level may be increased with each attempt.
13. Remove conductive pads. Using a dry gauze pad, clean paste from the chest and the paddles.

AFTER THE PROCEDURE

Assess client for return of consciousness from sedative or cardioversion. Evaluate neurologic, cardiovascular, and respiratory status. Assess for possible complications, including emboli (especially cerebral), respiratory depression, and dysrhythmias. Document postcardioversion rhythm strip. Assess skin for burns. Document the procedure and the client's response in the medical record.

DEFIBRILLATION Unlike carefully synchronized cardioversion, *defibrillation* is an emergency procedure that delivers direct current without regard to the cardiac cycle. Ventricular fibrillation is immediately treated as soon as the dysrhythmia is recognized. Early defibrillation has been shown to improve survival in clients experiencing VF.

Defibrillation can be delivered by external or internal paddles or pads. Conductive gel pads or paste is applied, and external paddles or pads are placed on the chest wall at the apex and base of the heart (Figure 31–8 ■). Internal paddles are applied directly on the heart, and may be used in surgery, the emergency department, or critical care. Internal defibrillation is done only by a physician; external defibrillation may be performed by any healthcare provider who has been trained in the procedure. Automatic external defibrillators (AEDs) are available on most hospital units to allow early defibrillation for cardiac arrest. (See Procedure 31–3.)

Pacemaker Therapy

A **pacemaker** is a pulse generator used to provide an electrical stimulus to the heart when the heart fails to generate or conduct its own at a rate that maintains the cardiac output. The pulse generator is connected to *leads* (insulated wires) passed intravenously into the heart or sutured directly to the epicardium. The leads sense intrinsic electrical activity of the heart and provide an electrical stimulus to the heart when necessary (pacing).

Figure 31–8 ■ Placement of paddles for defibrillation.
Source: Floyd Jackson

Pacemakers are used to treat both acute and chronic conduction defects such as third-degree AV block. They also may be used to treat bradydysrhythmias and tachydysrhythmias.

Temporary pacemakers use an external pulse generator (Figure 31–9 ■) attached to a lead threaded intravenously into the right ventricle, to temporary pacing wires implanted during cardiac surgery, or to external conductive pads placed on the chest wall for emergency pacing.

PROCEDURE 31-3 EMERGENCY EXTERNAL DEFIBRILLATION

GATHER SUPPLIES

- Automatic external defibrillator or defibrillator with ECG cable and monitor
- Conductive gel pads or paste
- Dry gauze pads
- Emergency medications and cart with pacemaker, airway management equipment, and oxygen supplies.

BEFORE THE PROCEDURE

Verify the lethal dysrhythmia, such as pulseless VT, VF, or asystole. Initiate the cardiac arrest (code) procedure, and obtain the defibrillator. If one is not immediately available, begin CPR until the emergency cart and defibrillator are brought to the bedside. Place client in supine position on a firm surface.

PROCEDURE

1. Turn on the defibrillator. Set it in *defibrillation* mode.
2. Turn ECG recording on for a continuous printout of events during the procedure.
3. Set the energy level and charge the paddles. Initial defibrillation is usually performed at 200 joules.
4. Place conductive pads on the chest, or spread conductive paste evenly on the paddles.
5. Position the paddles, holding them firmly on the chest wall.
6. **Ensure that no one is touching the client or the bed. State, "All clear."**
7. Depress the button on each paddle simultaneously to discharge the energy.
8. Immediately resume CPR.
9. Evaluate cardiac rhythm and for a pulse after approximately 2 minutes.
10. If the first attempt is unsuccessful, repeat the procedure, increasing the energy level to 300 joules and 360 joules for successive attempts. Reapply conductive paste as necessary.
11. Implement ACLS protocols.

AFTER THE PROCEDURE

If the dysrhythmia is successfully converted, evaluate and support neurologic, cardiovascular, and respiratory status. Monitor and titrate any intravenous infusions as ordered. Maintain ventilatory support as needed. Evaluate skin for burns. Obtain blood for laboratory analysis as ordered. Monitor vital signs and ECG continuously. Transfer to the intensive care unit (ICU) as indicated. Provide support and information to the client and family.

Figure 31–9 ■ Programmable settings on a temporary pacemaker.
Courtesy of Medtronics, Inc.

Permanent pacemakers use an internal pulse generator placed in a subcutaneous pocket in the subclavian space or abdominal wall. The generator connects to leads sewn directly onto the heart (*epicardial*) or passed transvenously into the heart (*endocardial*). Epicardial pacemakers (Figure 31–10 ■) require surgical exposure of the heart. Leads may be placed during cardiac surgery, or using a small subxiphoid incision to expose on the heart. Transvenous pacemaker leads are positioned in the right heart via the cephalic, subclavian, or jugular vein (Figure 31–11 ■). Local anesthesia can be used for permanent pacemaker insertion.

Pacemakers are programmed to stimulate the atria or the ventricles (*single-chamber pacing*), or both (*dual-chamber pacing*). Table 31–8 defines terms used to describe pacemaker modes and functions. The most commonly used pacemakers either (1) sense activity in and pace the ventricles only; or (2) sense activity in and pace both the atria and the ventricles. Dual-chamber or *atrioventricular sequential pacing* stimulates both chambers of the heart in sequence. AV pacing imitates the normal sequence of atrial contraction followed by ventricular contraction, improving cardiac output.

Pacing is detected on the ECG strip by the presence of pacing artifact (Figure 31–12 ■). A sharp spike is noted before the P wave with atrial pacing, and before the QRS complex with ventricular pacing. Pacing spikes are seen before both the P wave and QRS complex in AV sequential pacing. Capture is noted if there is a contraction of the chamber immediately following the pacer spike. Problems in sensing, pacing, and capture are noted in Table 31–9.

Care of the client with a temporary or permanent pacemaker focuses on monitoring for pacemaker malfunctioning, maintaining safety (Box 31–5), and preventing infection and postoperative complications. Nursing care for the client having a pacemaker implant is outlined on page 1012.

Implantable Cardioverter-Defibrillator

Sudden cardiac death claims more than 300,000 lives per year in the United States (Woods et al., 2004). The *implantable cardioverter-defibrillator (ICD)* detects life-threatening changes in the cardiac rhythm and automatically delivers an electric shock to convert the dysrhythmia back into a normal

Figure 31–10 ■ A permanent epicardial pacemaker. The pulse generator may be placed in subcutaneous pockets in the subclavian or abdominal regions.

Figure 31–11 ■ A permanent transvenous (endocardial) pacemaker with the lead placed in the right ventricle via the subclavian vein.
Source: Phototake NYC

TABLE 31–8 **Terms Used to Describe Pacemaker Functions**

TERM	DEFINITION
Asynchronous pacing	Pacemaker delivers a pacing stimulus at a set rate regardless of intrinsic cardiac activity.
Base rate	Rate at which the pacemaker paces when no cardiac activity is sensed.
Capture	The ability of the pacing stimulus to generate a cardiac depolarization.
Demand pacing	Pacemaker delivers a pacing stimulus only when the intrinsic rate falls below the pacemaker's base rate.
Dual-chamber pacing	Allows both the atria and the ventricles to be paced; most frequently used permanent pacing mode.
Lead	An insulated wire that senses intrinsic cardiac activity and delivers a pacing stimulus as programmed.
Output	The electrical stimulus delivered by the pulse generator.
Pacing spike	A small vertical spike noted on the ECG with every pacemaker stimulus.
Sensing	The pacemaker's ability to identify and respond to intrinsic cardiac activity.
Single-chamber pacing	Pacing of only the atria or the ventricles, not both; most common temporary pacing mode used.

Source: Adapted from *Cardiac Nursing* (5th ed.) by S. L. Woods, E. S. Froelicher, S. A. Motzer, & E. Bridges, 2004, Philadelphia: Lippincott.

rhythm. ICDs are used for sudden death survivors, clients with recurrent ventricular tachycardia, and clients with demonstrated risk factors for sudden death. ICDs can deliver a shock as needed, provide pacing on demand, and can store ECG records of tachycardic episodes (Woods et al., 2004).

A pulse generator connected to lead electrodes for rhythm detection and current delivery is implanted in the left pectoral region. The lead is threaded transvenously to the apex of the right ventricle. The ICD is programmed to sense a change in heart rate or rhythm. When it detects a potentially lethal rhythm, it shocks the heart to convert the rhythm. The device can be programmed or reprogrammed at the bedside as necessary. The ICD may be tested prior to discharge.

Local or general anesthesia is used, and the client may be discharged within 24 hours. The lithium-powered battery must be surgically replaced every 5 years. Complications and nursing care are similar to that for a client having a permanent pacemaker implant (see the Nursing Care box on page 1012).

The client may briefly lose consciousness before the device discharges, typically regaining consciousness quickly after the episode. Some clients report significant discomfort with ICD

A

B

C

Figure 31–12 ■ Pacing artifacts. *A,* Atrial pacing and ventricular sensing. Note the pacer spike preceding the P wave. *B,* Ventricular demand pacing. Note the absence of pacer spikes when the client's natural rhythm predominates. *C,* Atrioventricular pacing. Note the pacer spikes preceding both P waves and QRS complexes.

BOX 31–5 **Safety for Clients with a Temporary Pacemaker**

- Ensure that all electrical equipment in use has a grounded plug; do not use adapters or extension cords.
- Encourage the use of battery-powered equipment (e.g., electric razor).
- Remove any damaged electrical equipment from the unit, including equipment that
  a. Has been abused (e.g., has been dropped or in which liquid has been spilled).
  b. Has given anyone a shock.
  c. Has frayed, worn, or otherwise damaged electrical cords or plugs.
  d. Has other evidence of impaired function, such as a hot smell during use or control knobs that are loose or do not consistently produce the expected response.
- Wear gloves when handling the pacemaker electrodes or wires.
- Insulate pacemaker terminals and pacing wires with nonconductive, moistureproof material (e.g., a rubber glove).
- Test the pacemaker battery prior to use.
- Keep a spare pacemaker, cable, batteries, and battery tester available at all times.
- Immediately report any apparent deviation from expected pacemaker function.

TABLE 31–9 Potential Pacemaker Problems and Corrective Strategies

PROBLEM	POSSIBLE CAUSES	CORRECTIVE MEASURES
Undersensing Device fails to detect existing cardiac depolarizations, therefore competes with the native rhythms. 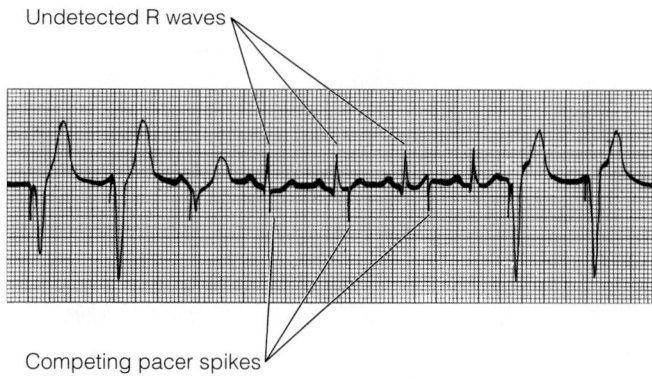 Undetected R waves Competing pacer spikes	Lead disconnected from pacer or from viable myocardium. Sensitivity set too low. Lead fracture. Low battery.	Check connection of lead to pacer. Increase sensitivity. Reposition or change lead. Change battery.
Oversensing Device detects noncardiac electrical events and interprets them as cardiac depolarizations, therefore is wrongly inhibited from pacing. When artifact ceases, pacing resumes Pacer interprets artifact as cardiac activity and fails to fire	Sensitivity set too high. Interference from electrical sources (ungrounded equipment, short circuits) is detected and misinterpreted by the device. Lead disconnected from pacer or from viable myocardium.	Decrease sensitivity (turn sensing control to a LARGER number). Remove all ungrounded electrical equipment or have it evaluated by hospital engineers. Check connection of lead to pacer.
Noncapture Device emits stimuli that fail to depolarize the myocardium. Pacer stimuli that fail to initiate myocardial depolarization	Output set too low in the noncaptured chamber. Lead fracture. High pacing threshold due to medication or metabolic changes. Low battery.	Increase output in the noncaptured chamber. Reposition or change lead. Alter medication regimen, correct metabolic changes. Change battery.

Source: From "Cardiac Rhythm Control Devices" (p. 92) by C. L. Witherell, 1994, *Critical Care Nursing Clinics of North America, 6*(1).

NURSING CARE OF THE CLIENT HAVING A Permanent Pacemaker Implant

Preoperative Care

- Provide routine preoperative care and teaching as outlined in Chapter 4 ∞.
- Assess knowledge and understanding of the procedure, clarifying and expanding on existing knowledge as needed. *Clarifying knowledge, providing information, and conveying emotional support reduces anxiety and fear and allows the client to develop a realistic outlook regarding pacer therapy.*
- Place ECG monitor electrodes away from potential incision sites. *This helps preserve skin integrity.*
- Teach range-of-motion (ROM) exercises for the affected side. *ROM exercises of the affected arm and shoulder prevent stiffness and impaired function following pacemaker insertion.*

Postoperative Care

- Provide postoperative monitoring, analgesia, and care as outlined in Chapter 4 ∞.
- Obtain a chest x-ray as ordered. *A postoperative chest x-ray is used to identify lead location and detect possible complications, such as pneumothorax or pleural effusion.*
- Position for comfort. Minimize movement of the affected arm and shoulder during the initial postoperative period. *Restricting movement minimizes discomfort on the operative side and allows the leads to become anchored, reducing the risk of dislodging.*
- Assist with gentle ROM exercises at least three times daily, beginning 24 hours after pacemaker implantation. *ROM exercises help restore normal shoulder movement and prevent contractures on the affected side.*
- Monitor pacemaker function with cardiac monitoring or intermittent ECGs. Report pacemaker problems to the physician:
  - Failure to pace. *This may indicate battery depletion, damage or dislodgement of pacer wires, or inappropriate sensing.*
  - Failure to capture (the pacemaker stimulus is not followed by ventricular depolarization). *The electrical output of the pacemaker may not be adequate, or the lead may be dislodged.*
  - Improper sensing (the pacemaker is firing or not firing, regardless of the intrinsic rate). *This increases the risk for decreased cardiac output and dysrhythmias.*
  - Runaway pacemaker (a pacemaker firing at a rapid rate). *This may be due to generator malfunction or problems with sensing.*
  - Hiccups. *A lead positioned near the diaphragm can stimulate it, causing hiccups. Hiccups may occur in extremely thin clients or may indicate a medical emergency with perforation of the right ventricle by the pacing electrode tip.*
- Assess for dysrhythmias and treat as indicated. *Until the catheter is "seated" or adheres to the myocardium, its move-*

ment may cause myocardial irritability and dysrhythmias. Fibrotic tissue develops within 2 to 3 days.
- Document the date of pacemaker insertion, the model and type, and settings. *This information is important for future reference.*
- Immediately report signs of potential complications, including myocardial perforation, cardiac tamponade, pneumothorax or hemothorax, emboli, skin breakdown, bleeding, infection, endocarditis, or poor wound healing (see Chapter 32 ∞ for more information about cardiac tamponade and endocarditis, and Chapter 38 ∞ for pneumothorax and hemothorax). *Early identification of complications allows for aggressive intervention.*
- Provide a pacemaker identification card including the manufacturer's name, model number, mode of operation, rate parameters, and expected battery life. *This card provides a reference for the client and future healthcare providers.*

Home Care

Provide appropriate teaching for the client and family about:
- Placement of the pacemaker generator and leads in relation to the heart.
- How the pacemaker works and the rate at which it is set.
- Battery replacement. Most pacemaker batteries last 6 to 12 years. Replacement requires an outpatient surgery to open the subcutaneous pocket and replace the battery.
- How to take and record the pulse rate. Instruct to assess pulse daily before arising and notify the physician if 5 or more bpm slower than the preset pacemaker rate.
- Incision care and signs of infection. Bruising may be present following surgery.
- Signs of pacemaker malfunction to report, including dizziness, fainting, fatigue, weakness, chest pain, or palpitations.
- Activity restrictions as ordered. This usually is limited to contact sports (which may damage the generator) and avoiding heavy lifting for 2 months after surgery.
- Resume sexual activity as recommended by the physician. Avoid positions that cause pressure on the site.
- Avoid tight-fitting clothing over the pacemaker site to reduce irritation and avoid skin breakdown.
- Carry the pacemaker identification card at all times, and wear a Medic-Alert bracelet or tag.
- Notify all care providers of the pacemaker.
- Do not hold or use certain electrical devices over the pacemaker site, including household appliances or tools, garage door openers, antitheft devices, or burglar alarms. Pacemaker will set off airport security detectors; notify security officials of its presence.
- Maintain follow-up care with the physician as recommended.

discharge (like a "blow to the chest"). A person in direct contact with the client when the device discharges may experience a tingling sensation.

Cardiac Mapping and Catheter Ablation

Cardiac mapping and catheter ablation are used to locate and destroy an ectopic focus. These diagnostic and therapeutic measures use electrophysiology techniques, and can be per-

formed in the cardiac catheterization laboratory. *Cardiac mapping* is used to identify the site of earliest impulse formation in the atria or the ventricles. Intracardiac and extracardiac catheter electrodes and computer technology are used to pinpoint the ectopic site on a map of the heart. These same catheters can be used to deliver the ablative intervention.

Ablation destroys, removes, or isolates an ectopic focus. In most instances, radio-frequency energy produced by high-frequency alternating current is used to create heat as it passes through tissue. Catheter ablation is used to treat supraventricular tachycardias, atrial fibrillation and flutter, and, in some cases, paroxysmal ventricular tachycardia (Woods et al., 2004).

Anticoagulant therapy may be started after catheter ablation to reduce the risk of clot formation at the ablation site.

Other Therapies

In addition to medications and interventional techniques, other measures may be used to treat selected dysrhythmias. Vagal maneuvers that stimulate the parasympathetic nervous system may be used to slow the heart rate in supraventricular tachycardias. These maneuvers include *carotid sinus massage* and the *Valsalva maneuver*. Carotid sinus massage is performed only by a physi-

cian during continuous cardiac monitoring. Excessive slowing of the heart rate may result. The Valsalva maneuver, forced exhalation against a closed glottis (e.g., bearing down), increases intrathoracic pressure and vagal tone, slowing the pulse rate.

NURSING CARE

Caring for the client with cardiac dysrhythmias requires the ability to recognize, identify, and, in some cases, promptly treat the dysrhythmia. The urgency of intervention is determined by the effects of the dysrhythmia on the client. Nursing care focuses on maintaining cardiac output, monitoring the response to therapy, and teaching. Also see the Nursing Care Plan for a client with a dysrhythmia.

NURSING CARE PLAN   A Client with Supraventricular Tachycardia

Elisa Vasquez, 53 years old, is admitted to the cardiac unit with complaints of palpitations, light-headedness, and shortness of breath. Her history reveals rheumatic fever at age 12 with subsequent rheumatic heart disease and mitral stenosis. An intravenous line is in place and she is receiving oxygen. Marcia Lewin, RN, is assigned to Ms. Vasquez.

ASSESSMENT

Ms. Lewin's assessment reveals that Ms. Vasquez is moderately anxious. Her ECG shows supraventricular tachycardia (SVT) with a rate of 154. Vital signs: T 98.8°F (37.1°C), R 26, BP 95/60. Peripheral pulses weak but equal, mucous membranes pale pink, skin cool and dry. Fine crackles noted in both lung bases. A loud S_3 gallop and a diastolic murmur are noted. Ms. Vasquez is still complaining of palpitations and tells Ms. Lewin, "I feel so nervous and weak and dizzy." Ms. Vasquez's cardiologist orders 2.5 mg of verapamil to be given slowly via intravenous push and tells Ms. Lewin to prepare to assist with synchronized cardioversion if drug therapy does not control the ventricular rate.

DIAGNOSES

- *Decreased Cardiac Output* related to inadequate ventricular filling associated with rapid tachycardia
- *Ineffective Tissue Perfusion: Cerebral/Cardiopulmonary/ Peripheral* related to decreased cardiac output
- *Anxiety* related to unknown outcome of altered health state

EXPECTED OUTCOMES

- Maintain adequate cardiac output and tissue perfusion.
- Demonstrate a ventricular rate within normal limits and stable vital signs.
- Verbalize reduced anxiety.
- Verbalize an understanding of the rationale for the treatment measures to control the heart rate.

PLANNING AND IMPLEMENTATION

- Provide oxygen per nasal cannula at 4 L/min.
- Continuously monitor ECG for rate, rhythm, and conduction. Assess vital signs and associated symptoms with changes in ECG. Report findings to physician.
- Explain the importance of rapidly reducing the heart rate. Explain the cardioversion procedure and encourage questions.

- Encourage verbalization of fears and concerns. Answer questions honestly, correcting misconceptions about the disease process, treatment, or prognosis.
- Administer intravenous diazepam as ordered before cardioversion.
- Document pretreatment vital signs, level of consciousness, and peripheral pulses.
- Place emergency cart with drugs and airway management supplies in client unit.
- Assist with cardioversion as indicated.
- Assess LOC, level of sedation, cardiovascular and respiratory status, and skin condition following cardioversion.
- Document procedure and postcardioversion rhythm, and response to intervention.

EVALUATION

Intravenous verapamil lowers Ms. Vasquez's heart rate to 138 for a short time, after which it increases to 164 with BP of 82/64. Her cardiologist, Dr. Mullins, performs carotid sinus massage. The ventricular rate slows to 126 for 2 minutes, revealing atrial flutter waves, and then returns to a rate of 150. Dr. Mullins explains the treatment options, including synchronized cardioversion. Ms. Vasquez agrees to the procedure.

Ms. Vasquez is lightly sedated and synchronized cardioversion is performed. One countershock converts Ms. Vasquez to regular sinus rhythm at 96 beats/min with BP 112/60.

Ms. Vasquez is sleepy from the sedation but recovers without incident. She states that she feels "much better," and her vital signs return to her normal levels. She remains in NSR with a rate of 86 to 92 for the remainder of her hospital stay. Dr. Mullins places Ms. Vasquez on furosemide to treat manifestations of mild heart failure.

CRITICAL THINKING IN THE NURSING PROCESS

1. What is the scientific basis for using carotid massage to treat supraventricular tachycardias? Was this an appropriate maneuver in the case of Ms. Vasquez?
2. What other treatment options might the physician have used to treat Ms. Vasquez's supraventricular tachycardia if she had been asymptomatic with stable vital signs?
3. Develop a teaching plan for Ms. Vasquez related to her prescription for furosemide.

See Evaluating Your Response in Appendix C.

Health Promotion

Health promotion measures to prevent coronary heart disease also reduce the risk for dysrhythmias. In most cases, dysrhythmias develop as a result of ischemic or structural changes in the heart, rather than in isolation. Advise clients who are at risk or who complain of occasional palpitations or "flutters" in their chest to reduce their intake of caffeine and other sympathetic nervous system stimulants, such as excess chocolate.

Assessment

Assessment is vital before treating any suspected dysrhythmia. What appears to be ventricular tachycardia on the monitor may be the client scratching or brushing the teeth. Apparent asystole on the monitor may be due to a loose electrode patch. Similarly, a heart rate of 52 beats/min may not affect the overall cardiac output in some clients. Review Chapter 30 ∞ for complete assessment of the client with a cardiac problem.

- *Health history:* Complaints of palpitations (ask for further definition of palpitations), "fluttering" sensations, or a sensation of the heart racing; episodes of dizziness, lightheadedness, or syncope (fainting); timing (duration, time of day); correlation with food or beverage intake, activity; presence of chest pain, shortness of breath, or other associated symptoms; history of heart or endocrine disease (such as hyperthyroidism); current medications.
- *Physical examination:* LOC; vital signs, including apical pulse for a full minute; regularity and amplitude of peripheral pulses; color; presence of dyspnea, adventitious lung sounds; ECG rhythm analysis; oxygen saturation levels.

Nursing Diagnoses and Interventions

The effect of the dysrhythmia on cardiac output is the priority of nursing care. Other potential nursing diagnoses related to dysrhythmias may include *Ineffective Tissue Perfusion, Activity Intolerance,* and *Fear* or *Anxiety.*

Decreased Cardiac Output

Dysrhythmias can affect cardiac output. Bradycardias decrease cardiac output if the stroke volume does not increase to compensate for the slow heart rate. Tachycardia reduces diastolic filling time, affecting stroke volume and coronary artery perfusion. Loss of the atrial kick in junctional rhythms, atrial fibrillation, and AV blocks also decreases ventricular filling and cardiac output. In ventricular fibrillation, loss of ventricular contractions causes cardiac arrest and no cardiac output.

> **PRACTICE ALERT**
> Before treating any dysrhythmia, assess the client, not just the monitor! Loose electrode pads, disconnected leads or cables, and muscle movement can simulate critical dysrhythmias. The client's condition is the best indicator of the need for treatment.

- Assess for decreased cardiac output: decreased LOC; tachycardia; tachypnea; hypotension; low oxygen saturation; diaphoresis; low urine output; cool, clammy, mottled skin; pallor or cyanosis; diminished peripheral pulses. *Initial signs of decreased cardiac output may be subtle, such as decreased*

LOC. Early recognition of the dysrhythmia's effect on cardiac output facilitates appropriate treatment and may prevent further adverse effects.

- Monitor ECG; post ECG strip every shift and when rhythm changes occur. *Documenting cardiac rhythm provides a record of disease progression and treatment effectiveness.*

> **PRACTICE ALERT**
> Assess vital signs, ECG, and oxygen saturation every 5 to 15 minutes during acute dysrhythmic episodes and during antidysrhythmic drug infusions. These data provide a record of cardiac output during the dysrhythmia. Antidysrhythmic drugs can adversely affect heart rate, rhythm, and blood pressure, further decreasing cardiac output.

- Assess for underlying causes of dysrhythmias, such as hypovolemia, hypoxia, anemia, vagal stimulation, or medications. *Sinus tachycardia often develops in response to tissue hypoxia. Vagal stimulation (such as the Valsalva maneuver) can precipitate bradycardia.*
- Assess serum electrolytes (especially potassium, calcium, and magnesium) and digitalis and antidysrhythmic drug levels as indicated. Report abnormal values. *Electrolyte imbalances affect cardiac depolarization and repolarization and may cause dysrhythmias. Toxic levels of digitalis and antidysrhythmic drugs can precipitate further dysrhythmias. Impaired renal or hepatic function increases the risk for toxicity, as does aging.*
- Be prepared to administer antidysrhythmic medications as indicated. Implement advanced cardiac life support (ACLS) protocols as needed. *Emergency drugs should be readily available, especially on units with high-risk clients. See Table 31–7 and the Medication Administration box on page 1006 for drugs used to treat common dysrhythmias that may affect cardiac output.*
- If appropriate, instruct to perform the Valsalva maneuver (bear down as if straining or coughing) for supraventricular tachycardia or ventricular tachycardia without angina. *Vagal maneuvers stimulate the parasympathetic system and may terminate some dysrhythmias. The Valsalva maneuver is contraindicated if chest pain occurs with the dysrhythmia.*
- Prepare to assist with cardioversion. Prepare the client per orders or hospital protocol (see Procedure 31–2). Explain the procedure to reduce anxiety. Have emergency equipment readily available. *Elective or emergency cardioversion is a treatment of choice for certain dysrhythmias.*

> **PRACTICE ALERT**
> On recognizing ventricular fibrillation and cardiac arrest, begin emergency procedures. Call for help. Obtain defibrillator and immediately defibrillate. If the defibrillator will be brought by another healthcare provider, begin CPR. Initiate ACLS protocols and assist with resuscitation measures as directed. Cardiac output ceases with ventricular fibrillation. Immediate or early defibrillation has been shown to have the greatest impact on survival following cardiac arrest.

- After cardiac arrest, transfer to critical care. Perform and document head-to-toe assessment; obtain laboratory tests,

12-lead ECG, and chest X-ray as ordered; monitor and maintain oxygenation and intravenous infusions; and monitor vital signs and cardiac rhythm. *The period following resuscitation is critical, necessitating careful monitoring. Postarrest assessment allows comparison of the client's condition with prearrest status and may identify CPR-related injuries. Correcting electrolyte disturbances, hypoxia, and acid–base imbalances is important to prevent further dysrhythmias and potential adverse effects on cardiac output. Intravenous access is crucial to maintain drug infusions. Hemodynamic monitoring may be instituted. The 12-lead ECG documents myocardial status, and the chest X-ray provides information about pulmonary status and possible thoracic injury due to CPR.*

■ Notify the family of significant changes in the client's condition or cardiac arrest, providing up-to-date information. Prepare family members prior to visits by explaining interventions (such as invasive tubes, a ventilator, or additional equipment) implemented since the last visit. *Concern for the family and significant others is part of holistic nursing. Researchers studying the needs of families have found that one of the most important needs was information about their loved one's condition. Clients and families need and appreciate honest communication and compassionate care. Preparing the family for critical changes in the client's condition and plan of care helps them to cope with a situational crisis.*

Community-Based Care

Dysrhythmias have a significant physical and psychologic impact on the client and all family members. Many of these clients and their families are under a great deal of stress from frequent hospitalizations, experimentation with therapies, frustration, and the fear of sudden cardiac death. A major teaching effort focuses on coping strategies and lifestyle changes, as well as specific management of prescribed therapies. Include the following topics as appropriate when teaching the client and family for home care:

■ Function, maintenance, precautions, and signs of malfunction or complications of any implanted device such as a pacemaker or ICD
■ Monitoring pulse rate and rhythm
■ Activity or dietary restrictions, and any potential effects of the dysrhythmia or its treatment on lifestyle
■ Medication management to reduce the risk of dysrhythmias, including the desired and potential adverse effects of antidysrhythmic drugs
■ Specific instructions related to planned diagnostic tests or procedures
■ The importance of follow-up visits with the cardiologist
■ The importance of and where to obtain CPR training for the client and family members.

In addition, discuss fears related to treatment or implanted devices, such as that of shocking a significant other during close contact or sexual activity. Explain that if a shock occurs, the partner may feel a slight buzz or tingling but should not be harmed. Refer to and encourage the client and family to attend a peer support group for the specific condition.

THE CLIENT WITH SUDDEN CARDIAC DEATH

Sudden cardiac death (SCD) is defined as unexpected death occurring within 1 hour of the onset of cardiovascular symptoms. It usually is caused by ventricular fibrillation and cardiac arrest. *Cardiac arrest* is the sudden collapse, loss of consciousness, and cessation of effective circulation that precedes biologic death. Worldwide, less than 6% of out-of-hospital cardiac arrest victims survive. In communities of North America that have organized lay rescuer and automated external defibrillator (AED) programs, the survival rate is significantly better, ranging from 49% to 74% when a witnessed arrest due to ventricular fibrillation occurs (AHA, 2005a).

Almost 50% of all deaths due to coronary heart disease are attributed to SCD. Coronary heart disease causes up to 80% of all sudden cardiac deaths in the United States. Other cardiac pathologies such as cardiomyopathy and valvular disorders also may lead to SCD. Noncardiac causes of sudden death include electrocution, pulmonary embolism, and rapid blood loss from a ruptured aortic aneurysm.

Ventricular fibrillation is the most common dysrhythmia associated with sudden cardiac death, accounting for 65% to 80% of cardiac arrests. Sustained severe bradydysrhythmias, *asystole* or cardiac standstill, and pulseless electrical activity (organized cardiac electrical activity without a mechanical response) are responsible for most remaining SCDs (Kasper et al., 2005). Selected cardiac and noncardiac causes of sudden cardiac death are listed in Box 31–6.

Risk factors for SCD are those associated with coronary heart disease (see the first section of this chapter). Advancing age and male gender are powerful risk factors. After age 65, the gap between male and female incidence of SCD narrows (Kasper et al., 2005). Clients with dysrhythmias such as recurrent VT may have a higher risk of SCD. Women with acute myocardial infarction, however, are more likely to present with

---

BOX 31–6 Selected Causes of Sudden Cardiac Death

Cardiac Causes
■ Coronary heart disease
■ Reperfusion following ischemia
■ Myocardial hypertrophy
■ Cardiomyopathy
■ Inflammatory myocardial disorders
■ Valve disorders
■ Primary electrical disorders
■ Dissecting or ruptured aortic or ventricular aneurysm
■ Cardiac drug toxicity

Noncardiac Causes
■ Pulmonary embolism
■ Cerebral hemorrhage
■ Autonomic dysfunction
■ Choking
■ Electrical shock
■ Electrolyte and acid–base imbalances

cardiac arrest and cardiogenic shock than with ventricular tachycardia (Kasper et al., 2005).

Pathophysiology

Evidence of coronary heart disease with significant atherosclerosis and narrowing of two or more major coronary arteries is found in 75% of SCD victims. Although most have had prior myocardial infarction, only 20% to 30% have recent acute myocardial infarction. An acute change in cardiovascular status precedes cardiac arrest by up to 1 hour; however, often the onset is instantaneous or abrupt. Tachycardia develops, and the number of PVCs increases. This is followed by a run of ventricular tachycardia that deteriorates into ventricular fibrillation (Kasper et al., 2005).

Abnormalities of myocardial structure or function also contribute. Structural abnormalities include infarction, hypertrophy, myopathy, and electrical anomalies. Functional deviations are caused by such factors as ischemia followed by reperfusion, altered homeostasis, autonomic nervous system and hormone interactions, and toxic effects. The interactions of the two cause myocardial instability and may precipitate fatal dysrhythmias.

Manifestations

SCD may be preceded by typical manifestations of acute coronary syndrome or myocardial infarction, including severe chest pain, dyspnea or orthopnea, and palpitations or light-headedness. The event itself is abrupt, with complete loss of consciousness and death within minutes. If ventricular tachycardia precedes cardiac arrest, consciousness and mentation may be impaired prior to collapse and loss of consciousness.

INTERDISCIPLINARY CARE

The goal of care is to restore cardiac output and tissue perfusion. Treatment measures are initiated as soon as clinical cardiac arrest is verified by the absence of respirations and carotid or femoral pulses. Basic and ACLS measures must be instituted within 2 to 4 minutes of cardiac arrest to prevent permanent neurologic damage and ischemic injury to other organs.

Basic Life Support

Basic life support (BLS) begins with identification of the cardiac arrest and initiation of an emergency response.

Providers trained in use of the *AED* should immediately defibrillate the client in VF. Self-adhesive conductive pads attached to connecting cables are positioned on the chest (Figure 31–13). The AED analyzes the rhythm, and advises the provider to charge the device if VF is detected. After warning all personnel to stand clear, the shock button is depressed to deliver a shock. Following the shock, CPR is immediately initiated. After approximately 2 minutes or five cycles of CPR, the rhythm is evaluated and circulation checked. The sequence of analysis, shock, CPR is continued and ACLS protocols are initiated (AHA, 2005a).

Cardiopulmonary resuscitation is a mechanical attempt to maintain tissue perfusion and oxygenation using oral resuscitation and external cardiac compressions. All healthcare providers need to be proficient in CPR. The technique should be performed according to AHA guidelines and hospital protocol. (See Box 31–7.) Research demonstrates clear benefit from sustained, effective chest compressions, yet compressions often are interrupted for ventilation, assessment of pulses, and other measures. Many clients are excessively ventilated and underperfused during CPR (Sanders & Ewy, 2005). The AHA 2005 guidelines for CPR reflect this research (AHA, 2005a).

CPR carries a high risk for both cardiac and noncardiac trauma. CPR-related complications include injuries to the skin, thorax, upper airway, abdomen, lungs, heart, and great vessels. These complications can be minimized by adhering to accepted CPR techniques.

Advanced Life Support

Advanced life support (ALS), provided by specially trained healthcare personnel, includes advanced airway support (inser-

Figure 31–13 ■ Schematic of an automated external defibrillator (AED) attached to a client.

BOX 31-7 Cardiopulmonary Resuscitation

1. Assess for responsiveness; shake the client and shout.
2. Call for help. Dial 911 (if outside the healthcare facility) or initiate the institutional code or cardiac arrest procedure.
3. Open the airway using the head-tilt/chin-lift maneuver. Simultaneously press down on the forehead with one hand while lifting the chin upward with the other (part A of the accompanying figure).
4. Check for breathing; look and listen. Inspect the chest for rise and fall with respirations; listen and feel for air movement through the nose or mouth. This step should take no more than 10 seconds.
5. If not breathing, begin rescue breathing using a pocket mask, mouth shield, or bag-valve mask (see part A of the figure). Administer two breaths (1 second per breath), observing for rise of the chest with each breath.
6. Check the carotid or femoral artery for a pulse (≤10 second).
7. If a pulse is present, continue rescue breathing, administering 8 to 10 breaths per minute, until help arrives or spontaneous respirations resume. Recheck the carotid pulse every 2 minutes.
8. If no pulse is present, analyze rhythm and defibrillate or, if unwitnessed arrest or AED unavailable, initiate external cardiac compressions. Place on a firm surface. Position the heel of one hand in the center of the chest between the nipples (child and adult), with the other hand on top and the fingers either interlocked or extended (see part B of the figure).
9. Initiate hard and fast cardiac compressions, pressing straight down to depress the sternum 1.5 to 2 inches, keeping the elbows locked and positioning the shoulders directly over the hands (part C of the figure). Release pressure completely between compressions but do not lift the hands from the chest.
10. Compress the chest at a rate of approximately 100 times per minute. With one- or two-rescuer CPR, provide two breaths after each 30 compressions. Assess the pulse after five complete cycles of 30 compressions and two breaths; continue CPR until help arrives.

A

B

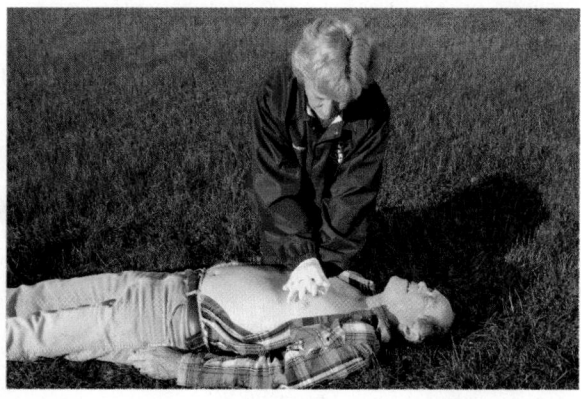

C

A, Head-tilt/chin-lift maneuver and using a bag-valve mask.
B, Placement of hands on the sternum between the nipples.
C, Arm, hand, and shoulder position for cardiac massage.

tion of a laryngeal mask airway, esophageal-tracheal Combitube, or endotracheal intubation) to maintain the airway and oxygenation, use of intravenous drugs following specific protocols, and additional interventions such as repeated defibrillation procedures and cardiac pacing. Epinephrine, vasopressin, sodium bicarbonate, and antidysrhythmic drugs such as amiodarone, bretylium, lidocaine, procainamide, magnesium sulfate, and atropine are used to attempt to restore and maintain an effective cardiac rhythm.

Postresuscitation Care

Clients who experience sudden cardiac death associated with ventricular fibrillation and acute MI have the best prognosis (Kasper et al., 2005). The client is transferred to a coronary care unit and MI treatment measures are instituted. Antidysrhythmic drugs may be continued for 24 to 48 hours to reduce the risk of subsequent episodes of VF.

Because the risk for recurrent SCD is significant in survivors, extensive diagnostic testing and interventions such as angioplasty or surgical revascularization of the myocardium, ablation, or an implantable cardioverter-defibrillator may be indicated.

NURSING CARE

Nursing care of the client experiencing sudden cardiac death requires prompt recognition of the event and immediate initiation of BLS and ALS protocols. As noted before, fast and effective cardiac compressions and early defibrillation of unstable VT and VF are the most important keys to survival of cardiac arrest victims. Important concepts of emergency cardiac care follow:

- Treat the client, not the monitor. Recognize signs and symptoms of cardiac compromise early.
- Activate the emergency medical services system (i.e., call a code or call 911).
- Begin and continue basic cardiac life support principles throughout the resuscitation effort.
- Continually assess the effectiveness of emergency interventions.
- Defibrillate pulseless VT or VF as soon as possible.
- Initiate ALS protocols early.

The family is not forgotten during resuscitation. If the family is present, they are usually offered a private consultation room in which to await the outcome. If the family is not present, they are notified that their family member is not doing well and asked to come to the hospital as soon as possible. The situation is presented in a careful manner to prevent the family from racing to the hospital, precipitating an automobile crash. Pastoral care or the family's choice of spiritual support is offered to help during this difficult time. Attendance of family members during resuscitation efforts is controversial, and depends on institutional protocols and family desires.

After successful resuscitation, the nurse provides care specific to the client's underlying disease processes and needs. Intravenous infusions such as lidocaine, bretylium, or dopamine may be ordered to prevent further dysrhythmias and maintain hemodynamic stability.

If the client does not survive the arrest, the nurse provides postmortem care and emotional and spiritual support to the family.

Nursing diagnoses to consider for the client experiencing SCD include the following:

- *Ineffective Tissue Perfusion: Cerebral* related to ineffective cardiac output
- *Impaired Spontaneous Ventilation* related to cardiac arrest
- *Spiritual Distress* related to unexplained sudden cardiac death
- *Disturbed Thought Processes* related to compromised cerebral circulation
- *Fear* related to risk for future episodes of sudden cardiac death.

The risk for a future episode of sudden cardiac death requires careful and effective teaching for home care prior to discharge. Discuss the following topics with the client and family:

- Risk factor reduction for coronary heart disease
- Planned diagnostic studies to identify the cause of SCD and possible interventions
- The risks and benefits of an ICD if appropriate
- The importance of carrying a card at all times listing all current medications and the healthcare provider
- Early manifestations or warning signs of cardiac arrest
- The importance of CPR training and maintaining proficiency in performing CPR (Provide referral to local CPR training providers or scheduled classes through the AHA or American Red Cross.)

Nurses can impact death rates from cardiac arrest through community teaching as well. Survival rates from sudden cardiac death improve in communities in which a significant portion of the population is trained in CPR and early response by EMS agencies is stressed. Work with community groups and individuals can help create a population of people able to perform effective CPR.

EXPLORE MediaLink

Prentice Hall Nursing MediaLink DVD-ROM
Audio Glossary
NCLEX-RN® Review

Animation/Video
Automated External Defibrillation
Coronary Heart Disease
Dysrhythmias
Nifedipine
Propranolol

COMPANION WEBSITE www.prenhall.com/lemone
Audio Glossary
NCLEX-RN® Review
Care Plan Activity: Perioperative Pacemaker Care
Case Study: Myocardial Infarction
Exercise: Match the Rhythm
MediaLink Applications
Links to Resources

CHAPTER HIGHLIGHTS

- Atherosclerosis is the primary underlying process in coronary heart disease, impaired perfusion of myocardial tissue.
- The risk factors for coronary heart disease are those for atherosclerosis: age, gender, and genetic factors; hypertension, diabetes, abnormal blood lipids; cigarette smoking, obesity, physical inactivity, and diet; and emerging risk factors such as the metabolic syndrome and homocysteine levels.
- Smoking cessation, exercise, diet modification, weight loss, medications to achieve desired blood lipid values, and effective hypertension and diabetes management are the primary treatment measures for coronary heart disease.
- Atherosclerosis of coronary vessels impairs the supply of blood, oxygen, and nutrients to the myocardium. Myocardial ischemia results in the manifestations of coronary heart disease: angina pectoris, acute coronary syndrome, and myocardial infarction.
- Stable angina develops with a predictable amount of activity or stress, and typically follows an activity–pain, rest–relief pattern. Stable angina often can be managed effectively by medications and risk factor modification. The nursing focus is on education.
- Acute coronary syndrome or unstable angina is characterized by increasingly severe chest pain that occurs unpredictably. Acute coronary syndrome often requires aggressive interventions such as percutaneous coronary revascularization or coronary artery bypass surgery.
- Myocardial infarction, necrosis of myocardial tissue, results from complete blockage of a coronary artery, usually due to atherosclerotic plaque rupture and thrombus formation. Prompt restoration of blood flow through a revascularization procedure or administration of a fibrinolytic drug to dissolve the blood clot is necessary to preserve functional muscle tissue.
- The nursing focus for clients with acute coronary syndrome and myocardial infarction is on reducing myocardial work through measures such as pain relief and activity limitation, promoting blood flow and oxygenation through medication and oxygen administration and positioning, and early recognition and treatment of complications.
- Cardiac dysrhythmias may arise anywhere in conductive tissue of the myocardium. Dysrhythmias may be either benign or fatal, depending on their effect on cardiac output.
- Tachycardias increase the workload of the heart and may interfere with cardiac output if ventricular filling is impaired by the rapid rate.
- Bradycardias can affect cardiac output when the rate is too slow to meet the metabolic needs of the body.
- Atrial fibrillation is a common dysrhythmia that can lead to formation of blood clots within the heart and subsequent stroke if these clots lodge in cerebral blood vessels.
- Frequent ventricular dysrhythmias may indicate an increased risk for ventricular fibrillation and cardiac arrest.
- AV conduction blocks interfere with conduction of the sinus or atrial impulse through the AV node and to the ventricles.
- Although many antidysrhythmic medications are available, all increase the risk of dysrhythmia development, so they are used sparingly.
- The nurse's role in caring for clients with cardiac dysrhythmias focuses on prompt identification of the rhythm disruption, assessment of its effect on the client, administration of medications and other treatment measures, and institution of life support procedures as indicated.

TEST YOURSELF NCLEX-RN® REVIEW

1 The nurse evaluates her teaching as effective when a client identifies which of the following modifiable risk factors for coronary heart disease (CHD) as contributing to the greatest extent?
1. obesity
2. diet
3. smoking
4. stress

2 When teaching a client about lovastatin (Mevacor), the nurse instructs the client to:
1. promptly report muscle pain or tenderness to the physician.
2. consume a diet that includes no more than 20% of calories from saturated fat.
3. abstain from alcohol use while taking this drug.
4. take the drug with meals to minimize gastric distress.

3 When assessing a client with stable angina, the nurse would expect to find:
1. persistent ECG changes.
2. correlation between activity level and pain.
3. increasing nocturnal pain.
4. evidence of impaired cardiac output such as weak peripheral pulses.

4 The nurse caring for a client with acute coronary syndrome identifies which of the following nursing diagnoses to be of highest priority?
1. *Anxiety* related to unknown outcome of disorder
2. *Ineffective Health Maintenance* related to lack of knowledge about coronary heart disease
3. *Decreased Cardiac Output* related to myocardial ischemia
4. *Ineffective Tissue Perfusion: Cardiopulmonary* related to underlying coronary heart disease

5 The nurse caring for a client returning from a coronary angioplasty with stent placement plans which of the following interventions?
1. securing chest tubes to bedding
2. maintaining leg extension on the affected side
3. discontinuing intravenous lines when taking oral fluids
4. treating chest pain with intravenous morphine as needed

6 In planning care for the client with acute myocardial infarction (AMI), the nurse identifies the highest priority goal of care as:
1. stable ECG rhythm.
2. ability to verbalize causes and effects of CHD.
3. compliance with prescribed bed rest.
4. relief of pain.

7 Which of the following nursing diagnoses is of highest priority for the client undergoing fibrinolytic therapy?
1. *Ineffective Protection*
2. *Ineffective Health Maintenance*
3. *Risk for Powerlessness*
4. *Anxiety*

8 In reviewing laboratory results for a client admitted with acute chest pain, the nurse is most concerned about which of the following?
1. hematocrit 35%
2. AST 65 unit/L
3. CK 320 unit/L
4. APTT 35 seconds

9 The nurse recognizes second-degree AV block, type II (Mobitz II), and intervenes appropriately when he:
1. records the finding in the chart.
2. prepares for temporary pacemaker insertion.
3. administers a class IB antidysrhythmic drug.
4. places the client in Fowler's position.

10 On identifying sinus bradycardia at a rate of 45 bpm, the nurse should:
1. assess mental status and blood pressure.
2. assess peripheral pulses on all four extremities.
3. determine if an apical-radial pulse deficit is present.
4. prepare to administer intravenous atropine.

See Test Yourself answers in Appendix C.

BIBLIOGRAPHY

Alber, C. M., Chae, C. U., Grodstein, F., Rose, L. M., Rexrode, K. M., Ruskin, J. N., et al. (2003). Prospective study of sudden cardiac death among women in the United States. *Circulation, 2003*(207), 2096–2101. Retrieved from http://www.circulationaha.org

American Heart Association. (2005a). 2005 Guidelines for CPR and ECC. *Circulation, 112*, IV1–IV205. Retrieved from www.circulationaha.org

_____. (2005b). *Heart disease and stroke statistics– 2005 update.* Dallas, TX: Author.

Artinian, N. T. (2001). Perceived benefits and barriers of eating heart healthy. *Medsurg Nursing, 10*(3), 129–138.

Aschcraft, A. S. (2004). Differentiating between pre-arrest and failure-to-rescue. *Medsurg Nursing, 13*(4), 211–215.

Ayers, D. M. M. (2002). EBCT: Beaming in on coronary artery disease. *Nursing, 32*(4), 81.

Blumenthal, R. S., & Margolis, S. (2005). *The Johns Hopkins white papers. Heart attack prevention.* Redding, CT: Medletter Associates.

Braunwald, E., Antman, E. M., Beasley, J. W., Califf, R. M., Cheitlin, M. D., Hochman, J. S., et al. (2002). *ACC/AHA 2002 guideline update for the management of patients with unstable angina and non-ST-segment elevation myocardial infarction: A report of the American College of Cardiology/American Heart Association Task Force on Practice Guidelines (Committee on the Management of Patients with Unstable Angina).* Retrieved from www.acc.org/clinical/guidelines/unstable/unstable.pdf

Chan, D. S., Chan, J. P., & Chang, A. M. (2005). Acute coronary syndromes: Cardiac rehabilitation programmes and quality of life. *Journal of Advanced Nursing, 49*(6), 591–599.

Copstead, L. C., & Banasik, J. L. (2005). *Pathophysiology* (3rd ed.). St. Louis, MO: Saunders.

Crane, P. B., & McSweeney, J. C. (2003). Exploring older women's lifestyle changes after myocardial infarction. *Medsurg Nursing, 12*(3), 170–176.

De Luca, G., Suryapranata, H., Ottervanger, J. P., & Antman, E. M. (2004). Time delay to treatment and mortality in primary angioplasty for acute myocardial infarction: Every minute of delay counts. *Circulation, March 16, 2004.* Retrieved from www.circulationaha.org

DeVon, H. A., & Zerwic, J. J. (2004). Differences in the symptoms associated with unstable angina and myocardial infarction. *Progress in Cardiovascular Nursing, 19*(1) 6–11.

Dochterman, J., & Bulechek, G. (2004). *Nursing Interventions Classification (NIC)* (4th ed.). St. Louis, MO: Mosby.

Eagle, K. A., Guyton, R. A., Davidoff, R., Edwards, F. H., Ewy, G. A., Gardner, T. J., et al. (2004). *ACC/AHA 2004 guideline update for coronary artery bypass graft surgery: A report of the American College of Cardiology/American Heart Association Task Force on Practice Guidelines.* Retrieved from www.acc.org/clinical/guidelines/cabg/cabg.pdf

Engler, M. B. (2004). Familial hypercholesterolemia: Genetic predisposition to atherosclerosis. *Medsurg Nursing, 13*(4), 253–257.

Foley, S. (2005). Update on risk factors for atherosclerosis: The role of inflammation and apolipoprotein E. *Medsurg Nursing, 14*(1), 43–50.

Glessner, T. M., & Walker, M. K. (2001). Standardized measures: Documenting processes and outcomes of care for patients undergoing coronary artery bypass grafting. *Medsurg Nursing, 10*(1), 23–29.

Granger, B. B., & Miller, C. M. (2001). Acute coronary syndrome. *Nursing, 31*(11), 36–43.

Granot, M., Goldstein-Ferber, S., & Azzam, A. S. (2004). Gender differences in the perception of chest pain. *Journal of Pain and Symptom Management, 27*(2), 149–155.

Hart, P. L. (2005). Women's perceptions of coronary heart disease: An integrative review. *Journal of Cardiovascular Nursing, 20*(3), 170–176.

Hummard, J. (2004). Management of atrial fibrillation. *Nursing Times, 100*(6), 42–44.

Kasper, D. L., Braunwald, E., Fauci, A. S., Hauser, S. L., Longo, D. L., & Jameson, J. L. (2005). *Harrison's principles of internal medicine* (16th ed.). New York: McGraw-Hill.

Kellen, J. C. (2004) Implications for nursing care of patients with atrial fibrillation: Lessons learned from the AFFIRM and RACE studies. *Journal of Cardiovascular Nursing, 19*(2), 128–137.

McCance, K. L., & Huether, S. E. (2006). *Pathophysiology: The biologic basis for disease in adults and children* (5th ed.). St. Louis, MO: Mosby.

McSweeney, J. C., & Coon, S. (2004). Women's inhibitors and facilitators associated with making behavioral changes after myocardial infarction. *Medsurg Nursing, 13*(1), 49–56.

Meeker, M. H., & Rothrock, J. C. (1999). *Alexander's care of the patient in surgery* (11th ed.). St. Louis, MO: Mosby.

Miller, K. H., & Grindel, C. G. (2004). Comparison of symptoms of younger and older patients undergoing coronary artery bypass surgery. *Clinical Nursing Research, 13*(3), 179–193.

Milner, K. A., Funk, M., Richards, S., Vaccarino, V., & Krumholz, H. M. (2001). Symptom predictors of acute coronary syndromes in younger and older patients. *Nursing Research, 50*(4), 233–241.

Moorhead, S., Johnson, M., & Maas, M. (2004). *Nursing outcomes classification (NOC)* (3rd ed.). St. Louis, MO: Mosby.

NANDA International. (2005). *NANDA's nursing diagnoses: Definitions & classification 2005–2006.* Philadelphia: Author.

National Cholesterol Education Program. (2002). *Third report of the National Cholesterol Education Program (NCEP) Expert Panel on detection, evaluation, and treatment of high blood cholesterol in adults (Adult Treatment Panel III). Final report.* Bethesda, MD: National Institutes of Health.

National Heart, Lung, and Blood Institute (NHLBI). (2004). *Morbidity & mortality: 2004 chart book of cardiovascular, lung, and blood diseases.* Bethesda, MD: National Institutes of Health.

_____. (2005). Statement from Elizabeth G. Nabel, M.D., director of the National Heart, Lung and Blood Institute of the National Institutes of Health on the findings of the Women's Health Study. *NIH News, March 7.* Retrieved from www.nhlbi.hih.gov

National High Blood Pressure Education Program. (2004). *The seventh report of the Joint National Committee on Prevention, Detection, Evaluation, and Treatment of High Blood Pressure.* Bethesda, MD: National Heart, Lung, and Blood Institute, National Institutes of Health.

Nicholls, C., & Sani, M. (2004). Antiplatelet therapy. *Nursing of Older People, 16*(8), 35–36.

Obias-Manno, D., & Wijetunga, M. (2004). Risk stratification and primary prevention of sudden cardiac death: Sudden death prevention. *AACN Clinical Issues, 15*(3), 404–418.

Palatnik, A. M. (2001). Critical care. Acute coronary syndrome: New advances and nursing strategies. *Nursing, 31*(5), 32cc1–32cc2, 32cc4, 32cc6.

Paparella, S. (2004). Fibrinolytic therapy: No room for error. *Journal of Emergency Nursing, 30*(4), 348–350.

Pelter, M. M., & Adams, M. G. (2004). Premature beats. *American Journal of Critical Care, 13*(6), 519–520.

Porth, C. M. (2005). *Pathophysiology: Concepts of altered health states* (7th ed.). Philadelphia: Lippincott.

Quigley, M. P. (2004). Promoting cardiac rehabilitation. *Nursing, 34*(8), 24.

Ridker, P. M., Cook, N. R., Lee, I, Gordon, D., Gaziano, J. M., Manson, J. E., et al. (2005). A randomized trial of low-dose aspirin in the primary prevention of cardiovascular disease in women. *New England Journal of Medicine, 352.* Retrieved from http://content.nejm.org/cgi/content/full/352/13/1293

Rosenfeld, A. G. (2004). Treatment-seeking delay among women with acute myocardial infarction: Decision trajectories and their predictors. *Nursing Research, 53*(4), 225–236.

Ryan, C. J., DeVon, H. A., & Zerwic, J. J. (2005). Typical and atypical symptoms: Diagnosing acute coronary syndromes accurately. *American Journal of Nursing, 105*(2), 34–36.

Sanders, A. B., & Ewy, G. A. (2005). Cardiopulmonary resuscitation in the real world: When will the guidelines get the message? *JAMA, 293*(3), 363–365.

Shaffer, R. S. (2002). ICD therapy: The patient's perspective. *American Journal of Nursing, 102*(2), 46–49.

Stewart, S. (2004). Epidemiology and economic impact of atrial fibrillation. *Journal of Cardiovascular Nursing, 19*(2), 94–102.

Tierney, L. M., McPhee, S. J., & Papadakis, M. A. (2005). *Current medical diagnosis & treatment* (44th ed.). New York: McGraw-Hill.

Urden, L. D., Stacy, K. M., & Lough, M. E. (2006). *Thelan's critical care nursing: Diagnosis and management* (5th ed.). St. Louis, MO: Mosby.

U.S. Department of Health & Human Services. (2005). *Dietary guidelines for Americans 2005.* Washington, DC: U.S. Department of Agriculture. Retrieved from www.healthierus.gov/dietaryguidelines

U.S. Preventive Services Task Force. (2002a). Aspirin for the primary prevention of cardiovascular events: Recommendations and rationale. *American Journal of Nursing, 102*(3), 67, 69–70.

_____. (2002b). Screening for lipid disorders in adults: Recommendations and rationale. *American Journal of Nursing, 102*(6), 91, 93, 95.

Way, L. W., & Doherty, G. M. (2003). *Current surgical diagnosis and treatment* (11th ed.). New York: McGraw-Hill.

Wilkinson, J. M. (2005). *Nursing diagnosis handbook with NIC interventions and NOC outcomes* (8th ed.). Upper Saddle River, NJ: Prentice Hall Health.

Wolf, Z. R., Miller, P. A., & Devine, M. (2003). Relationship between nurse caring and patient satisfaction in patients undergoing invasive cardiac procedures. *Medsurg Nursing, 12*(3), 391–396.

Woods, S. L., Froelicher, E. S., Motzer, S. A., & Bridges, E. (2004). *Cardiac nursing* (5th ed.). Philadelphia: Lippincott.

Writing Group for the Women's Health Initiative Investigators. (2002). Risks and benefits of estrogen plus progestin in healthy postmenopausal women. [On-line]. *JAMA, 288*(3). Retrieved from http://jama.ama-assn.org/issues/v288n3/fffull/joc21036.html

Wung, S. (2002). Genetic advances in coronary artery disease. *Medsurg Nursing, 11*(6), 296–300.

Zerwic, J. J., & Ryan, C. J. (2004). Delays in seeking MI treatment. *American Journal of Nursing, 104*(1), 81–83.

CHAPTER 32 Nursing Care of Clients with Cardiac Disorders

LEARNING OUTCOMES

- Compare and contrast the etiology, pathophysiology, and manifestations of common cardiac disorders, including heart failure, structural disorders, and inflammatory disorders.
- Explain risk factors and preventive measures for cardiac disorders such as heart failure, inflammatory disorders, and valve disorders.

- Discuss indications for and management of clients undergoing hemodynamic monitoring.
- Discuss the effects and nursing implications for medications commonly prescribed for clients with cardiac disorders.
- Describe nursing care for the client undergoing cardiac surgery or cardiac transplant.

CLINICAL COMPETENCIES

- Apply knowledge of normal cardiac anatomy and physiology and assessment techniques in caring for clients with cardiac disorders.
- Assess functional health status of clients with cardiac disorders, documenting and reporting deviations for expected findings.
- Based on client assessment and knowledge of the disorder, determine priority nursing diagnoses.
- Plan, prioritize, and provide evidence-based, individualized care for clients with cardiac disorders.

- Safely and knowledgeably administer prescribed medications and treatments to clients with cardiac disorders.
- Actively participate in planning and coordinating interdisciplinary care for clients with cardiac disorders.
- Provide appropriate teaching and community-based care for clients with cardiac disorders and their families.
- Evaluate the effectiveness of nursing care, revising the plan of care as needed to promote, maintain, or restore functional health status of clients with cardiac disorders.

Cardiac disorders affect the structure and/or function of the heart. These disorders interfere with the heart's primary purpose: to pump enough blood to meet the body's demand for oxygen and nutrients. Disruptions in cardiac function affect the functioning of other organs and tissues, potentially leading to organ system failure and death.

Heart failure is the most common cardiac disorder. Other cardiac disorders discussed in this chapter include structural cardiac disorders, such as valve disorders and cardiomyopathy, and inflammatory cardiac disorders, such as endocarditis and pericarditis. Before continuing with this chapter, please review the heart's anatomy and physiology, nursing assessment, and diagnostic tests in Chapter 30 ∞.

HEART FAILURE

Heart failure is a complex syndrome resulting from cardiac disorders that impair the ventricles' ability to fill with and effectively pump blood (Hunt et al., 2005). In heart failure, the heart is unable to pump enough blood to meet the metabolic demands of the body. It is the end result of many conditions. Frequently, it is a long-term effect of coronary heart disease (CHD) and myocardial infarction (MI) when left ventricular damage is extensive enough to impair cardiac output (see Chapter 31 ∞). Other diseases of the heart also may cause heart failure, including structural and inflammatory disorders. In normal hearts, failure can result from excessive demands placed on the heart. Heart failure may be acute or chronic.

THE CLIENT WITH HEART FAILURE

As mentioned, heart failure develops when the heart cannot effectively fill or contract with adequate strength to function as a pump to meet the needs of the body. As a result, cardiac output falls, leading to decreased tissue perfusion. The body initially adjusts to reduced cardiac output by activating inherent compensatory mechanisms to restore tissue perfusion. These normal mechanisms may result in vascular congestion—hence, the commonly used term *congestive heart failure (CHF)*. As these mechanisms are exhausted, heart failure ensues, with increased morbidity and mortality.

Heart failure is a disorder of cardiac function. It frequently is due to *impaired myocardial contraction,* which may result from CHD and myocardial ischemia or infarct or from a primary cardiac muscle disorder such as cardiomyopathy or myocarditis. Structural cardiac disorders, such as valve disorders or congenital heart defects, and hypertension also can lead to heart failure when the heart muscle is damaged by the long-standing *excessive workload* associated with these conditions. Other clients without a primary abnormality of myocardial function may present with manifestations of heart failure due to *acute excess demands* placed on the myocardium, such as volume overload, hyperthyroidism, and massive pulmonary embolus (Table 32–1). Hypertension and coronary heart disease are the leading causes of heart failure in the United States. The high prevalence of hypertension in African Americans contributes significantly to their risk for and incidence of heart failure.

Incidence, Prevalence, and Risk Factors

Nearly 5 million people in the United States are currently living with heart failure; approximately 550,000 new cases of heart failure are diagnosed annually (American Heart Associa-

TABLE 32–1 Selected Causes of Heart Failure

IMPAIRED MYOCARDIAL FUNCTION	INCREASED CARDIAC WORKLOAD	ACUTE NONCARDIAC CONDITIONS
■ Coronary heart disease	■ Hypertension	■ Volume overload
■ Cardiomyopathies	■ Valve disorders	■ Hyperthyroidism
■ Rheumatic fever	■ Anemias	■ Fever, infection
■ Infective endocarditis	■ Congenital heart defects	■ Massive pulmonary embolus

tion [AHA], 2005). Its incidence and prevalence increase with age: Less than 5% of people between ages 55 and 64 have heart failure, whereas 6% to 10% of people older than 65 are affected (see the box below) (AHA, 2005). The prevalence and mortality rate for heart failure is higher in African Americans than in whites. See the accompanying Cultural Diversity box.

Ischemic heart disease (coronary heart disease) is the leading risk factor for heart failure. Cardiomyopathies are the second leading cause of heart failure. Other, less common causes of heart failure are hypertension and congenital and valvular heart disease (Kasper et al., 2005).

The prognosis for a client with heart failure depends on its underlying cause and how effectively precipitating factors can be treated. Most clients with heart failure die within 8 years of the diagnosis. The risk for sudden cardiac death is dramatically increased, occurring at a rate six to nine times that of the general population (AHA, 2005).

Physiology Review

The mechanical pumping action of cardiac muscle propels the blood it receives to the pulmonary and systemic vascular systems for reoxygenation and delivery to the tissues. *Cardiac output (CO)* is the amount of blood pumped from the ventricles in 1 minute. Cardiac output is used to assess cardiac performance, especially left ventricular function. Effective cardiac output depends on adequate functional muscle mass and the ability of the ventricles to work together. Cardiac output normally is regulated by the oxygen needs of the body: As oxygen use increases, cardiac output increases to maintain cellular function. *Cardiac reserve* is the ability of the heart to increase CO to meet metabolic demand. Ventricular damage reduces the cardiac reserve.

Cardiac output is a product of heart rate and stroke volume. *Heart rate (HR)* affects cardiac output by controlling the number of ventricular contractions per minute. It is influenced by the autonomic nervous system, catecholamines, and thyroid hormones. Activation of a stress response (e.g., hypovolemia or fear) stimulates the sympathetic nervous system, increasing the heart rate and its contractility. Elevated heart rates increase cardiac output. Very rapid heart rates, however, shorten ventricular filling time (diastole), reducing stroke volume and cardiac output. On the other hand, a slow heart rate reduces cardiac output simply because of fewer cardiac cycles.

Stroke volume, the volume of blood ejected with each heartbeat, is determined by preload, afterload, and myocardial contractility. *Preload* is the volume of blood in the ventricles at end diastole (just prior to contraction). The blood in the ventricles exerts pressure on the ventricle walls, stretching muscle fibers. The greater the blood volume, the greater the force with which the ventricle contracts to expel the blood. End diastolic volume depends on the amount of blood returning to the ventricles (*venous return*) and the distensibility or stiffness of the ventricles (*compliance*). See Box 32–1.

Afterload is the force needed to eject blood into the circulation. This force must be great enough to overcome arterial pressures

FOCUS ON CULTURAL DIVERSITY

- Up to 5 million Americans have heart failure; of these, about 725,000 (15%) are African Americans.
- In African Americans:
  - Manifestations of heart failure develop at an earlier age.
  - The disease progresses more rapidly.
  - More hospital visits are attributed to heart failure.
  - The mortality rate is higher than in white men and women.

NURSING CARE OF THE OLDER ADULT   Heart Failure

Heart failure is common in older adults, affecting nearly 10% of people over the age of 75 years.

Aging affects cardiac function. Diastolic filling is impaired by decreased ventricular compliance. With aging, the heart is less responsive to sympathetic nervous system stimulation. As a result, maximal heart rate, cardiac reserve, and exercise tolerance are reduced. Concurrent health problems such as arthritis that affect stamina or mobility often contribute to a more sedentary lifestyle, further decreasing the heart's ability to respond to increased stress.

Assessing for Home Care

The older adult with heart failure may not be dyspneic, instead presenting with weakness and fatigue, somnolence, confusion, disorientation, or worsening dementia. Dependent edema and respiratory crackles may or may not indicate heart failure in older adults.

Assess the diet of the older adult. Decreased taste may lead to increased use of salt to bring out food flavors. Limited mobility or visual acuity may cause the older adult to rely on prepared foods that are high in sodium such as canned soups and frozen meals. Discuss normal daily activities and assess sleep and rest patterns. It is also important to assess the environment for:

- Safe roads or neighborhoods for walking
- Access to pharmacy, medical care, and assistive services such as a cardiac rehabilitation program or structured exercise programs designed for older adults.

Health Education for the Client and Family

Teaching for the older adult with heart failure focuses on maintaining function and promptly identifying and treating episodes of heart failure. Teach clients how to adapt to changes in cardiovascular function associated with aging, such as:

- Allowing longer warm-up and cool-down periods during exercise
- Engaging in regular exercise such as walking five or more times a week
- Resting with feet elevated (e.g., in a recliner) when fatigued
- Maintaining adequate fluid intake
- Preventing infection through pneumococcal and influenza immunizations.

BOX 32–1 Explaining Physiologic Terms Using Practical Examples

The concepts of preload, the Frank-Starling mechanism, compliance, and afterload can be difficult to understand and to explain to clients. Use common analogies to make these concepts easier to understand.

- *Preload:* Think about a new rubber band. As you stretch the rubber band further, it snaps back into shape with greater force.
- *Frank-Starling mechanism:* When you repeatedly stretch that rubber band beyond a certain limit, it loses some elasticity and fails to return to its original shape and size.
- *Compliance:* Use a new rubber balloon to illustrate this concept. A new balloon is not very compliant—it takes a lot of work (force) to inflate it. As the balloon is repeatedly inflated and stretched, it becomes more compliant, expanding easily with less force.
- *Afterload:* When a hose is crimped or plugged, more force is required to eject a stream of water out its end.

within the pulmonary and systemic vascular systems. The right ventricle must generate enough force to open the pulmonary valve and eject its blood into the pulmonary artery. The left ventricle ejects its blood into the systemic circulation by overcoming the arterial resistance behind the aortic valve. Increased systemic vascular resistance (e.g., hypertension) increases afterload, impairing stroke volume and increasing myocardial work.

Contractility is the natural ability of cardiac muscle fibers to shorten during systole. Contractility is necessary to overcome arterial pressures and eject blood during systole. Impaired contractility affects cardiac output by reducing stroke volume. The *ejection fraction (EF)* is the percentage of blood in the ventricle that is ejected during systole. A normal ejection fraction is approximately 60%.

Pathophysiology

When the heart begins to fail, mechanisms are activated to compensate for the impaired function and maintain the cardiac output. The primary compensatory mechanisms are (1) the Frank-Starling mechanism, (2) neuroendocrine responses including activation of the sympathetic nervous system and the renin–angiotensin system, and (3) myocardial hypertrophy. These mechanisms and their effects are summarized in Table 32–2.

Decreased cardiac output initially stimulates aortic baroreceptors, which in turn stimulate the sympathetic nervous system (SNS). SNS stimulation produces both cardiac and vascular responses through the release of norepinephrine. Norepinephrine increases heart rate and contractility by stimulating cardiac beta-receptors. Cardiac output improves as both heart rate and stroke volume increase. Norepinephrine also causes arterial and venous vasoconstriction, increasing venous return to

TABLE 32–2 Compensatory Mechanisms Activated in Heart Failure

MECHANISM	PHYSIOLOGY	EFFECT ON BODY SYSTEMS	COMPLICATIONS
Frank-Starling mechanism	The greater the stretch of cardiac muscle fibers, the greater the force of contraction.	■ Increased contractile force leading to increased CO	■ Increased myocardial oxygen demand ■ Limited by overstretching
Neuroendocrine response	Decreased CO stimulates the sympathetic nervous system and catecholamine release.	■ Increased HR, BP, and contractility ■ Increased vascular resistance ■ Increased venous return	■ Tachycardia with decreased filling time and decreased CO ■ Increased vascular resistance ■ Increased myocardial work and oxygen demand
	Decreased CO and decreased renal perfusion stimulate renin–angiotensin system.	■ Vasoconstriction and increased BP	■ Increased myocardial work ■ Renal vasoconstriction and decreased renal perfusion
	Angiotensin stimulates aldosterone release from adrenal cortex.	■ Salt and water retention by the kidneys ■ Increased vascular volume	■ Increased preload and afterload ■ Pulmonary congestion
	ADH is released from posterior pituitary.	■ Water excretion inhibited	■ Fluid retention and increased preload and afterload ■ Pulmonary congestion
	Atrial natriuretic peptide and brain natriuretic peptide are released.	■ Increased sodium excretion ■ Diuresis ■ Vasodilation	
	Blood flow is redistributed to vital organs (heart and brain).	■ Decreased perfusion of other organ systems ■ Decreased perfusion of skin and muscles	■ Renal failure ■ Anaerobic metabolism and lactic acidosis
Ventricular hypertrophy	Increased cardiac workload causes myocardial muscle to hypertrophy and ventricles to dilate.	■ Increased contractile force to maintain CO	■ Increased myocardial oxygen demand ■ Cellular enlargement

the heart. Increased venous return increases ventricular filling and myocardial stretch, increasing the force of contraction (the Frank-Starling mechanism). Overstretching the muscle fibers past their physiologic limit results in an ineffective contraction.

Blood flow is redistributed to the brain and the heart to maintain perfusion of these vital organs. Decreased renal perfusion causes renin to be released from the kidneys. Activation of the renin–angiotensin system produces additional vasoconstriction and stimulates the adrenal cortex to produce aldosterone and the posterior pituitary to release antidiuretic hormone (ADH). Aldosterone stimulates sodium reabsorption in renal tubules, promoting water retention. ADH acts on the distal tubule to inhibit water excretion and also causes vasoconstriction. The effect of these hormones is significant vasoconstriction and salt and water retention, with a resulting increase in vascular volume. Increased ventricular filling increases the force of contraction, improving cardiac output. The effects of the renin–angiotensin–aldosterone system and ADH release are counterbalanced to a certain extent by two additional hormones. The increased vascular volume and venous return prompted by vasoconstriction and sodium and water retention increase the volume and pressures in the heart. Stimulation of stretch receptors in the atria and ventricles lead to the release of *atrial natriuretic peptide (ANP)* and *brain natriuretic peptide (BNP)* from stores in the atria (ANP and BNP) and ventricles (BNP). These hormones promote sodium and water excretion and inhibit the release of norepinephrine, renin, and ADH, with resulting vasodilation. Although beneficial, the effects of these hormones are too weak to completely counteract the vasoconstriction and sodium and water retention that occurs in heart failure.

Ventricular remodeling occurs as the heart chambers and myocardium adapt to fluid volume and pressure increases. The chambers dilate to accommodate excess fluid resulting from increased vascular volume and incomplete emptying. Initially, this additional stretch causes more effective contractions. *Ventricular hypertrophy* occurs as existing cardiac muscle cells enlarge, increasing their contractile elements (actin and myosin) and force of contraction.

Although these responses may help in the short-term regulation of cardiac output, it is now recognized that they hasten the deterioration of cardiac function. The onset of heart failure is heralded by *decompensation,* the loss of effective compensation. Heart failure progresses due to the very mechanisms that initially maintained circulatory stability.

The rapid heart rate shortens diastolic filling time, compromises coronary artery perfusion, and increases myocardial oxygen demand. Resulting ischemia further impairs cardiac output. Beta-receptors in the heart become less sensitive to continued SNS stimulation, decreasing heart rate and contractility. As the beta-receptors become less sensitive, norepinephrine stores in the cardiac muscle become depleted. In contrast, alpha-receptors on peripheral blood vessels become increasingly sensitive to persistent stimulation, promoting vasoconstriction and increasing afterload and cardiac work.

Initially, ventricular hypertrophy and dilation increase cardiac output, but chronic distention causes the ventricular wall eventu-

ally to thin and degenerate. The purpose of hypertrophy is thus defeated. In addition, chronic overloading of the dilated ventricle eventually stretches the fibers beyond the optimal point for effective contraction. The ventricles continue to dilate to accommodate the excess fluid, but the heart loses the ability to contract forcefully. The heart muscle may eventually become so large that the coronary blood supply is inadequate, causing ischemia.

Chronic distention exhausts stores of ANP and BNP. The effects of norepinephrine, renin, and ADH prevail, and the renin–angiotensin pathway is continually stimulated. This mechanism ultimately raises the hemodynamic stress on the heart by increasing both preload and afterload. As heart function deteriorates, less blood is delivered to the tissues and to the heart itself. Ischemia and necrosis of the myocardium further weaken the already failing heart, and the cycle repeats.

In normal hearts, the cardiac reserve allows the heart to adjust its output to meet metabolic needs of the body, increasing the cardiac output by up to five times the basal level during exercise. Clients with heart failure have minimal to no cardiac reserve. At rest, they may be unaffected; however, any stressor (e.g., exercise, illness) taxes their ability to meet the demand for oxygen and nutrients. Manifestations of activity intolerance when the person is at rest indicate a critical level of cardiac decompensation.

Classifications and Manifestations of Heart Failure

Heart failure is commonly classified in several different ways, depending on the underlying pathology. Classifications include systolic versus diastolic failure, left-sided versus right-sided failure, high-output versus low-output failure, and acute versus chronic failure.

FAST FACTS

Terms used to describe or classify heart failure:
- Systolic or diastolic failure
- Left ventricular (or sided) or right ventricular (or sided) failure
- Low-output or high-output failure
- Acute or chronic failure
- Forward or backward effects.

Systolic versus Diastolic Failure

Systolic failure occurs when the ventricle fails to contract adequately to eject a sufficient blood volume into the arterial system. Systolic function is affected by loss of myocardial cells due to ischemia and infarction, cardiomyopathy, or inflammation. The manifestations of systolic failure are those of decreased cardiac output: weakness, fatigue, and decreased exercise tolerance.

Diastolic failure results when the heart cannot completely relax in diastole, disrupting normal filling. Passive diastolic filling decreases, increasing the importance of atrial contraction to preload. Diastolic dysfunction results from decreased ventricular compliance due to hypertrophic and cellular changes and impaired relaxation of the heart muscle. Its manifestations result from increased pressure and congestion behind the ventricle:

shortness of breath, tachypnea, and respiratory crackles if the left ventricle is affected; distended neck veins, liver enlargement, anorexia, and nausea if the right ventricle is affected. Many clients have components of both systolic and diastolic failure.

Left-Sided versus Right-Sided Failure

Depending on the pathophysiology involved, either the left or the right ventricle may be primarily affected. In chronic heart failure, however, both ventricles typically are impaired to some degree. Coronary heart disease and hypertension are common causes of *left-sided heart failure,* whereas *right-sided heart failure* often is caused by conditions that restrict blood flow to the lungs, such as acute or chronic pulmonary disease. Left-sided heart failure also can lead to right-sided failure as pressures in the pulmonary vascular system increase with congestion behind the failing left ventricle.

As left ventricular function fails, cardiac output falls. Pressures in the left ventricle and atrium increase as the amount of blood remaining in the ventricle after systole increases. These increased pressures impair filling, causing congestion and increased pressures in the pulmonary vascular system. Increased pressures in this normally low-pressure system increase fluid movement from the blood vessels into interstitial tissues and the alveoli (Figure 32–1 ■).

The manifestations of left-sided heart failure result from pulmonary congestion (*backward effects*) and decreased cardiac output (*forward effects*). Fatigue and activity intolerance are common early manifestations. Dizziness and syncope also may result from decreased cardiac output. Pulmonary congestion causes dyspnea, shortness of breath, and cough. The client may develop **orthopnea** (difficulty breathing while lying down), prompting use of two or three pillows or a recliner for sleeping. Cyanosis from impaired gas exchange may be noted. On auscultation of the lungs, inspiratory crackles (rales) and wheezes may be heard in lung bases. An S_3 gallop may be present, reflecting the heart's attempts to fill an already distended ventricle.

In right-sided heart failure, increased pressures in the pulmonary vasculature or right ventricular muscle damage impair the right ventricle's ability to pump blood into the pulmonary circulation. The right ventricle and atrium become distended, and blood accumulates in the systemic venous system. Increased venous pressures cause abdominal organs to become congested and peripheral tissue edema to develop (Figure 32–2 ■).

Dependent tissues tend to be affected because of the effects of gravity; edema develops in the feet and legs, or if the client

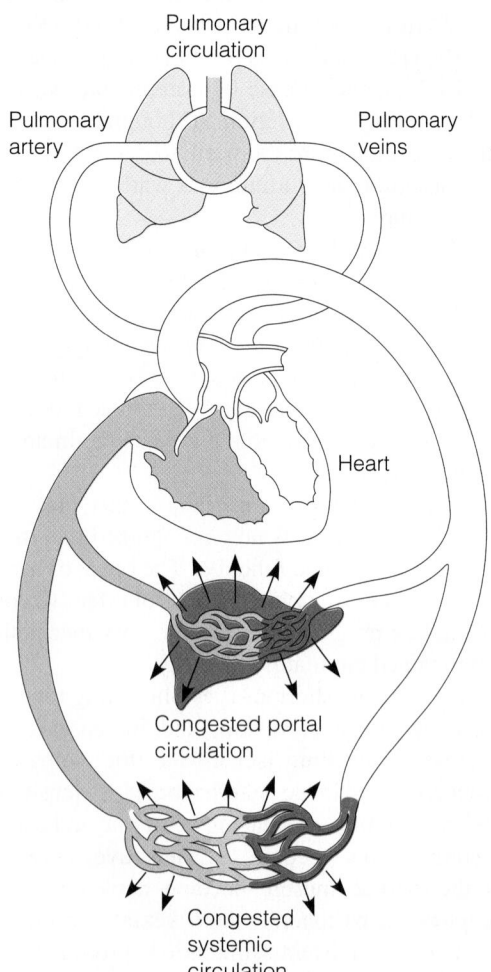

Figure 32–1 ■ The hemodynamic effects of left-sided heart failure.

Figure 32–2 ■ The hemodynamic effects of right-sided heart failure.

is bedridden, in the sacrum. Congestion of gastrointestinal tract vessels causes anorexia and nausea. Right upper quadrant pain may result from liver engorgement. Neck veins distend and become visible even when the client is upright, due to increased venous pressure.

Low-Output versus High-Output Failure

Clients with heart failure due to coronary heart disease, hypertension, cardiomyopathy, and other primary cardiac disorders develop *low-output failure* and manifestations such as those previously described. Clients in hypermetabolic states (e.g., hyperthyroidism, infection, anemia, or pregnancy) require increased cardiac output to maintain blood flow and oxygen to the tissues. If the increased blood flow cannot meet the oxygen demands of the tissues, compensatory mechanisms are activated to further increase cardiac output, which in turn further increases oxygen demand. Thus, even though cardiac output is high, the heart is unable to meet increased oxygen demands. This condition is known as *high-output failure.*

Acute versus Chronic Failure

Acute failure is the abrupt onset of a myocardial injury (such as a massive MI) resulting in suddenly decreased cardiac function and signs of decreased cardiac output. *Chronic failure* is a progressive deterioration of the heart muscle due to cardiomyopathies, valvular disease, or CHD.

Other Manifestations

In addition to the previous manifestations for the various classifications of heart failure, other signs and symptoms commonly are seen.

A fall in cardiac output activates mechanisms that cause increased salt and water retention. This causes weight gain and further increases pressures in the capillaries, resulting in edema. *Nocturia,* voiding more than one time at night, develops as edema fluid from dependent tissues is reabsorbed while the client is supine. **Paroxysmal nocturnal dyspnea (PND),** a frightening condition in which the client awakens at night acutely short of breath, also may develop. Paroxysmal nocturnal dyspnea occurs when edema fluid that has accumulated during the day is reabsorbed into the circulation at night, causing fluid overload and pulmonary congestion. Severe heart failure may cause dyspnea at rest as well as with activity, signifying little or no cardiac reserve. Both an S_3 and an S_4 gallop may be heard on auscultation.

See page 1028 for the *Multisystem Effects of Heart Failure.*

Complications

The compensatory mechanisms initiated in heart failure can lead to complications in other body systems. Congestive hepatomegaly and splenomegaly caused by engorgement of the portal venous system result in increased abdominal pressure, ascites, and gastrointestinal problems. With prolonged right-sided heart failure, liver function may be impaired. Myocardial distention can precipitate dysrhythmias, further impairing cardiac output. Pleural effusions and other pulmonary problems may develop. Major complications of severe heart failure are cardiogenic shock (described in Chapter 11 ∞) and acute

pulmonary edema, a medical emergency described in the next section of this chapter.

INTERDISCIPLINARY CARE

The main goals for care of heart failure are to slow its progression, reduce cardiac workload, improve cardiac function, and control fluid retention. Treatment strategies are based on the evolution and progression of heart failure (Table 32–3).

Diagnosis

Diagnosis of heart failure is based on the history, physical examination, and diagnostic findings.

- *Atrial natriuretic peptide (ANP),* also called *atrial natriuretic hormone (ANH),* and *brain natriuretic peptide (BNP)* are hormones released by the heart muscle in response to changes in blood volume. Blood levels of these hormones increase in heart failure. BNP levels, in particular, have been shown to positively correlate with pressures in the left ventricle and the pulmonary vascular system. As the severity of left ventricular failure increases, BNP levels increase (White, 2005). It is important to remember, however, that BNP levels may be elevated in women and in people over age 60 who do not have heart failure. Therefore, an elevated BNP cannot be used alone to diagnosis heart failure (Hunt et al., 2005).
- *Serum electrolytes* are measured to evaluate fluid and electrolyte status. Serum osmolarity may be low due to fluid retention. Sodium, potassium, and chloride levels provide a baseline for evaluating the effects of treatment; serum calcium and magnesium are measured as well.
- *Urinalysis, blood urea nitrogen (BUN),* and *serum creatinine* are obtained to evaluate renal function.
- *Liver function tests* including ALT, AST, LDH, serum bilirubin, and total protein and albumin levels are obtained to evaluate possible effects of heart failure on liver function.
- Thyroid function tests, including TSH and TH levels, are obtained because both hyperthyroidism and hypothyroidism can be either a primary or a contributing cause of heart failure (Hunt et al., 2005).
- In acute heart failure, *arterial blood gases (ABGs)* are drawn to evaluate gas exchange in the lungs and tissues.
- *Chest x-ray* may show pulmonary vascular congestion and cardiomegaly in heart failure.
- *Electrocardiography* is used to identify ECG changes associated with ventricular enlargement and to detect dysrhythmias, myocardial ischemia, or infarction.
- *Echocardiography with Doppler flow studies* are performed to evaluate left ventricular function. Either *transthoracic echocardiography* or *transesophageal echocardiography* may be used. See Chapter 30 ∞ for more information and the nursing implications of these tests.
- *Radionuclide imaging* is used to evaluate ventricular function and size (see Chapter 30 ∞).

Hemodynamic Monitoring

Hemodynamics is the study of forces involved in blood circulation. Hemodynamic monitoring is used to assess cardiovascular function in the critically ill or unstable client. The main

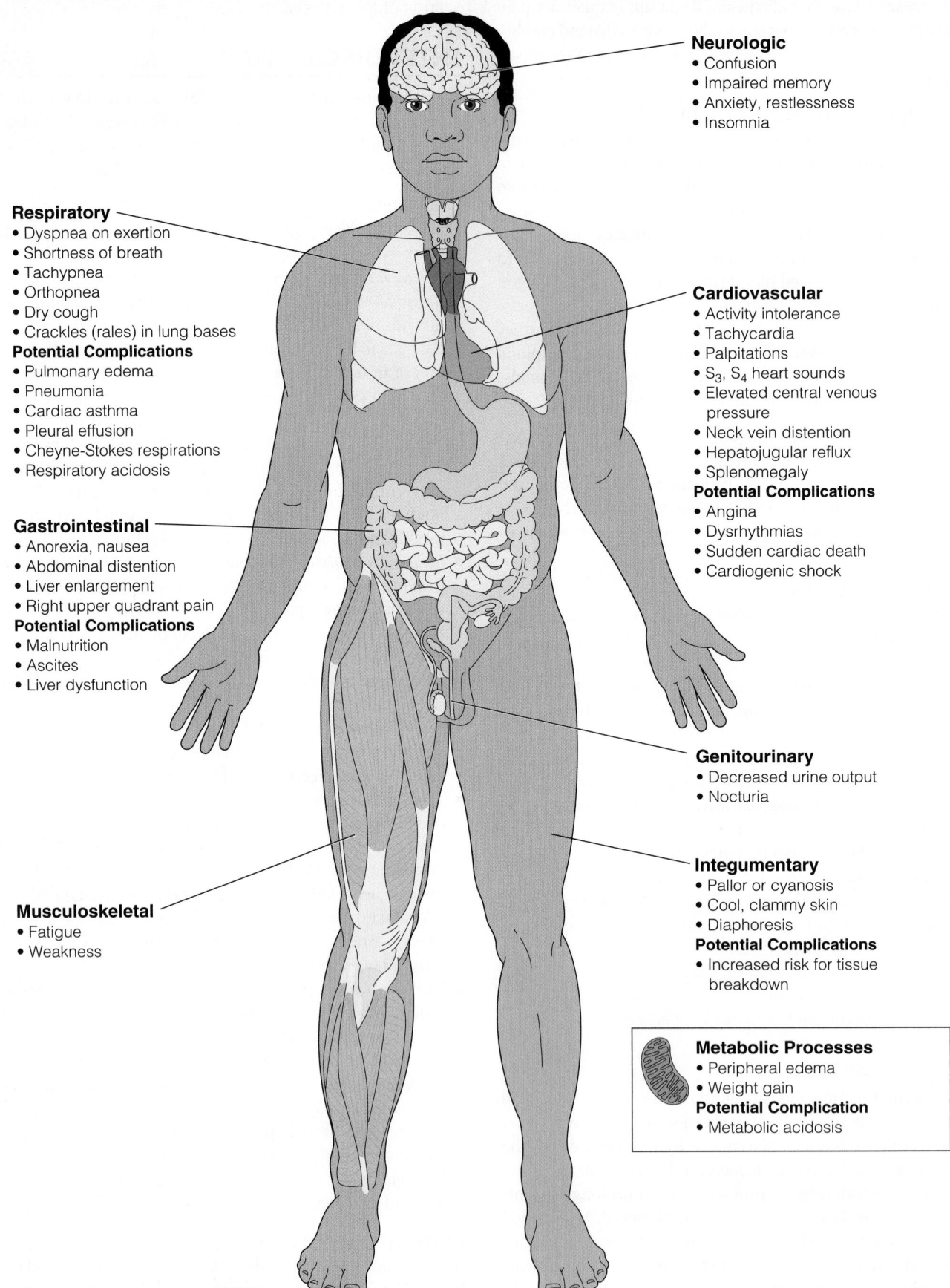

MULTISYSTEM EFFECTS OF **Heart Failure**

Neurologic
- Confusion
- Impaired memory
- Anxiety, restlessness
- Insomnia

Respiratory
- Dyspnea on exertion
- Shortness of breath
- Tachypnea
- Orthopnea
- Dry cough
- Crackles (rales) in lung bases

Potential Complications
- Pulmonary edema
- Pneumonia
- Cardiac asthma
- Pleural effusion
- Cheyne-Stokes respirations
- Respiratory acidosis

Cardiovascular
- Activity intolerance
- Tachycardia
- Palpitations
- S_3, S_4 heart sounds
- Elevated central venous pressure
- Neck vein distention
- Hepatojugular reflux
- Splenomegaly

Potential Complications
- Angina
- Dysrhythmias
- Sudden cardiac death
- Cardiogenic shock

Gastrointestinal
- Anorexia, nausea
- Abdominal distention
- Liver enlargement
- Right upper quadrant pain

Potential Complications
- Malnutrition
- Ascites
- Liver dysfunction

Genitourinary
- Decreased urine output
- Nocturia

Integumentary
- Pallor or cyanosis
- Cool, clammy skin
- Diaphoresis

Potential Complications
- Increased risk for tissue breakdown

Musculoskeletal
- Fatigue
- Weakness

Metabolic Processes
- Peripheral edema
- Weight gain

Potential Complication
- Metabolic acidosis

TABLE 32–3 Stages of Heart Failure

STAGE	DESCRIPTION	RECOMMENDED TREATMENT MEASURES
A	Clients at high risk for developing heart failure, but without structural heart disease or symptoms of heart failure (clients with hypertension, CHD, diabetes, obesity, metabolic syndrome, or who have a family history of cardiomyopathy, or who are taking cardiotoxic drugs)	Treat underlying risk factors (e.g., hypertension) including lipid disorders ACE inhibitor or angiotensin-receptor blocker (ARB) therapy as appropriate Exercise Salt restriction Smoking cessation Discourage alcohol, illicit drug use Control blood glucose in clients with metabolic syndrome
B	Clients with structural heart disease but no manifestations of heart failure (clients with previous MI, asymptomatic valve disease, or left ventricular dysfunction)	As for stage A ACE inhibitor or ARB therapy as appropriate Beta-blocker therapy if indicated
C	Clients with structural heart disease and current or prior symptoms of heart failure (shortness of breath, fatigue, decreased exercise tolerance)	As for stages A and B Drug therapy with a diuretic, ACE inhibitor, and/or beta-blocker Additional drugs as indicated, such as an aldosterone antagonist, ARB, digitalis, hydralazine, nitrates Ventricular pacing or an implantable defibrillator (ICD) as indicated
D	Refractory heart failure (clients with manifestations of heart failure at rest despite aggressive treatment)	As for stages A, B, and C as appropriate Hospice care Hemodynamic monitoring Continual infusion of positive inotropic agents Valve replacement, cardiac transplant as indicated Permanent mechanical support; experimental surgery or drug therapy

Source: Adapted from "ACC/AHA 2005 Guideline Update for the Diagnosis and Management of Chronic Heart Failure in the Adult: Executive Summary: A Report of the American College of Cardiology/American Heart Association Task Force on Practice Guidelines (Writing Committee to Update the 2001 Guidelines for the Evaluation and Management of Heart Failure)" by S. A. Hunt, W. T. Abraham, M. H. Chin, A. M. Feldman, G. S. Francis, T. G. Ganiats, M. Jessup, M. A. Konstam, D. M. Mancini, K. Michl, M. A. Silver, L. W. Stevenson, and C. W. Yancy, 2005, American College of Cardiology Web Site. Available at http://www.acc.org/clinical/guidlines/failure/index/pdf

goals of invasive hemodynamic monitoring are to evaluate cardiac and circulatory function and the response to interventions.

Hemodynamic parameters include heart rate, arterial blood pressure, central venous or right atrial pressure, pulmonary pressures, and cardiac output. *Direct* hemodynamic parameters are obtained straight from the monitoring device (e.g., heart rate, arterial and venous pressures). *Indirect* or *derived* measurements are calculated using the direct data (e.g., the cardiac index, mean arterial blood pressure, and stroke volume). Invasive hemodynamic monitoring is routinely used in critical care units.

Hemodynamic monitoring systems measure the pressure within a vessel and convert this signal into an electrical waveform that is amplified and displayed. The electrical signal may be graphically recorded on graph paper and displayed digitally on the monitor. System components include an invasive catheter threaded into an artery or vein connected to a transducer by stiff, high-pressure tubing. The pressure transducer translates pressures into an electrical signal that is relayed to the monitor. Additional components of the system include stopcocks and a continuous flush system with normal saline or heparinized saline and an infusion pressure bag to prevent clots from forming in the catheter. Figure 32–3 ■ illustrates a pressure transducer and typical hemodynamic monitoring system.

Hemodynamic pressure monitoring may be used to measure peripheral arterial pressures, or central pressures, such as central venous pressure or right atrial pressure and pulmonary artery pressure. Although the information obtained from invasive monitoring is valuable, the procedure is not without risk. Nursing care of the client undergoing hemodynamic monitoring is outlined on page 1031. Box 32–2 lists potential complications of central pressure monitoring.

INTRA-ARTERIAL PRESSURE MONITORING Intra-arterial pressure monitoring is commonly used in intensive and coronary care units. An indwelling arterial line, commonly called an *art line* or an *A line*, allows direct and continuous monitoring of systolic,

---

BOX 32–2 Potential Complications of Central Catheters

- Bleeding
- Hematoma
- Pneumothorax
- Hemothorax
- Arterial puncture
- Dysrhythmias
- Venospasm
- Infection
- Air embolism
- Thromboembolism
- Brachial nerve injury
- Thoracic duct injury

Figure 32–3 ■ A hemodynamic monitoring setup.

diastolic, and mean arterial blood pressure and provides easy access for arterial blood sampling. Arterial lines are used to assess blood volume, to monitor the effects of vasoactive drugs, and to obtain frequent ABG determinations. Because the invasive catheter is inserted directly into the artery, it offers immediate access for blood gas measurements and blood testing.

The arterial blood pressure reflects the cardiac output and the resistance to blood flow created by the elastic arterial walls (*systemic vascular resistance, SVR*). Cardiac output is determined by the blood volume and the ability of the ventricles to fill and effectively pump that blood. Systemic vascular resistance is primarily determined by vessel diameter and distensibility (compliance). Factors such as SNS input, circulating hormones (e.g., epinephrine, norepinephrine, ANP, and vasopressin), and the renin–angiotensin system affect SVR.

The systolic blood pressure, normally about 120 mmHg in healthy adults, reflects the pressure generated during ventricular systole. During diastole, elastic arterial walls keep a minimum pressure within the vessel (diastolic blood pressure) to maintain blood flow through the capillary beds. The average diastolic pressure in a healthy adult is 80 mmHg. The **mean arterial pressure (MAP)** is the average pressure in the arterial circulation throughout the cardiac cycle. It reflects the driving pressure, or perfusion pressure, an indicator of tissue perfusion. The formula MAP = CO × SVR often is used to show the relationships between factors determining the blood pressure. Mean arterial pressure can be calculated by adding one-third of the pulse pressure (PP) to the diastolic pressure (MAP = DBP + PP/3). For example, a blood pressure of 120/80 results in a MAP of 93. Mean arterial pressures of 70 to 90 mmHg are desirable. Perfusion to vital organs is severely jeopardized at MAPs of 50 or less; MAPs greater than 105 mmHg may indicate hypertension or vasoconstriction.

VENOUS PRESSURE MONITORING *Central venous pressure (CVP)* and *right atrial pressure (RAP)* are measures of blood volume and venous return. They also reflect right heart filling pressures. Pressures are elevated in right-sided heart failure. CVP and RAP are primarily used to monitor fluid volume status. To measure venous and atrial pressures, a catheter is inserted in the internal jugular or subclavian vein. The distal tip of the catheter is positioned in the superior vena cava just above or just inside the right atrium. CVP may be measured in either centimeters of water (cm H_2O) or in millimeters of mercury (mmHg). A water manometer is a clear tube with calibrated markings that is attached between a central catheter and the intravenous fluid bag. Pressure in the venous system causes fluid in the manometer to rise or fall. The CVP is recorded by noting the fluid level in the manometer. If the central line is connected to a pressure transducer, venous pressure is displayed digitally in millimeters of mercury.

The normal range for CVP is 2 to 8 cm H_2O or 2 to 6 mmHg, but CVP varies in individual clients. Hypovolemia and shock decrease the CVP; fluid overload, vasoconstriction, and cardiac tamponade increase CVP.

PULMONARY ARTERY PRESSURE MONITORING The pulmonary artery (PA) catheter is a flow-directed, balloon-tipped catheter first used in the early 1970s. The PA catheter is often called a *Swan-Ganz catheter,* after the physicians who developed it. The PA catheter is used to evaluate left ventricular and overall cardiac function. The PA catheter is inserted into a central vein, usually the internal jugular or subclavian vein, and threaded into the right atrium. A small balloon at the tip of the catheter allows the catheter to be drawn into the right ventricle and from there into the pulmonary artery (Figure 32–4 ■). The inflated balloon carries the catheter forward until the balloon wedges in a small branch of pulmonary vasculature. Once in

NURSING CARE OF THE CLIENT UNDERGOING Hemodynamic Monitoring

- Calibrate and level the system at least once a shift using the right atrium as a constant reference level. Relevel the transducer after a change in position. Mark the right atrial position (at the fourth intercostal space, midaxillary line) on the chest wall, and use this as a reference point for all readings. *Calibration and leveling ensure that accurate pressures are recorded. Marking the right atrial level provides a consistent reference point for all caregivers.*
- Measure all pressures between breaths. *This ensures that intrathoracic pressure does not influence pressure readings.*
- Maintain 300 mmHg of pressure on the flush solution at all times. *This ensures a continuous flow of flush solution through the pressure tubing and catheter to prevent clot formation and catheter occlusion.*
- Monitor pressure trends rather than individual readings. *Individual readings may not reflect the client's true status. Trends in pressure readings along with clinical observations provide a better overall picture of the client's status.*
- Obtain a chest x-ray before infusing intravenous fluid into any newly placed central line. *Chest x-ray verifies the location of the catheter and helps prevent pulmonary complications of incorrect catheter placement such as pneumothorax.*
- Set alarm limits for monitored hemodynamic variables. Turn alarms on. *Alarms warn of hemodynamic instability. Always investigate alarms. They may be temporarily silenced to change tubing or draw blood but should never be turned off.*
- Use aseptic technique during catheter insertion and site care. *Aseptic technique is important to prevent infection.*
- Assess and document appearance of the insertion site at least every shift; observe for signs of infiltration, infection, or

phlebitis. *Frequent assessment allows early detection and prompt treatment of complications.*
- Change intravenous solutions every 24 hours, site dressing every 48 hours, and tubing to the insertion site every 72 hours. Label solution, tubing, and dressing with date and time of change. *These measures help prevent infection.*
- Thoroughly flush stopcock ports after drawing blood samples from the pressure line. *Flushing prevents colonization of bacteria and occlusion of the catheter.*
- Assess pulse and perfusion distal to the monitoring site. *Frequent assessment is vital to ensure perfusion of the distal extremity.*
- When discontinuing the pressure line, apply manual pressure to the insertion site as soon as the catheter tip is out. Hold pressure for 5 to 15 minutes or until the bleeding stops. *This is particularly important for arterial lines to prevent bleeding and hematoma formation.*
- Secure all connections and stopcocks. *This is done to prevent disconnection of the invasive line and potential hemorrhage.*
- Ensure that electrical equipment is grounded, intact, and operating as expected. *This helps prevent electrical injury.*
- Loosely restrain the affected extremity if the client pulls on the catheter or connections. *Restraints may be necessary to prevent injury from accidental or intentional disconnection or discontinuation of invasive lines (i.e., if the client has dementia or is agitated).*
- Keep tubing free of kinks and tension. *This prevents the catheter from becoming clotted or inadvertently dislodged.*

place, the balloon is deflated, and multiple lumens of the catheter allow measurement of pressures in the right atrium, pulmonary artery, and left ventricle. The normal PA pressure is around 25/10 mmHg; normal mean pulmonary artery pressure is about 15 mmHg (Figure 32–5A ■). Pulmonary artery pressure is increased in left-sided heart failure.

Inflation of the balloon effectively blocks pressure from behind the balloon and allows measurement of pressures generated by the left ventricle. This is known as pulmonary artery wedge pressure (PAWP or PWP) and is used to assess left ventricular function. The normal PAWP is 8 to 12 mmHg (Figure 32–5B). PAWP is increased in left ventricular failure and pericardial tamponade, and decreased in hypovolemia.

Cardiac output also can be measured with the PA catheter using a technique called *thermodilution*. Cardiac output and the cardiac index are used to assess the heart's ability to meet the body's oxygen demands. Because body size affects overall cardiac output, the cardiac index is a more precise measure of heart function. The *cardiac index* is a calculation of cardiac output per square meter of body surface area. The normal cardiac index is 2.8 to 4.2 L/min/m^2.

Medications

Clients with heart failure often receive multiple medications to reduce cardiac work and improve cardiac function. The main drug classes used to treat heart failure are the angiotensin-converting enzyme (ACE) inhibitors, angiotensin II receptor blockers (ARBs), beta-blockers, diuretics, inotropic medications (including digitalis, sympathomimetic agents, and phosphodiesterase inhibitors), direct vasodilators, and antidysrhythmic drugs. Nursing implications for ACE inhibitors and ARBs,

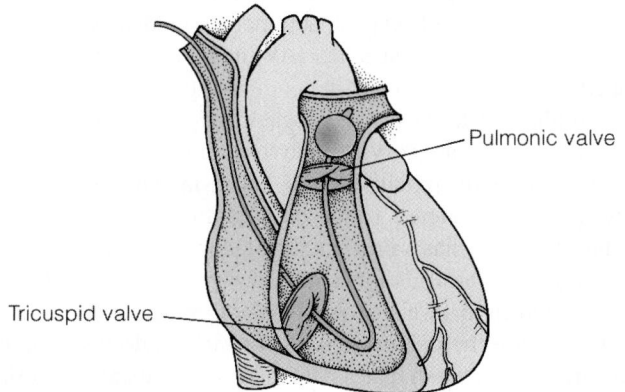

Figure 32–4 ■ Inflation of the balloon on the flow-directed catheter allows it to be carried through the pulmonic valve into the pulmonary artery.

Pulmonary Artery Pressure (PAP)

Pulmonary Capillary Wedge Pressure (PCWP)

Figure 32–5 ■ Typical waveforms seen when measuring (*A*) pulmonary artery pressure and (*B*) pulmonary wedge pressure.

diuretics, and inotropic medications are found in the Medication Administration box on the following page.

ACE inhibitors, ARBs, and beta-blockers interfere with the neurohormonal mechanisms of sympathetic activation and the renin–angiotensin system. ACE inhibitors interrupt the conversion of angiotensin I to angiotensin II by inhibiting the enzyme that mediates the conversion (angiotensin-converting enzyme). Angiotensin II causes intense vasoconstriction, increasing afterload and ventricular wall stress and increasing preload and ventricular dilation. It also stimulates aldosterone and ADH production, causing fluid retention. ACE inhibitors block this renin–angiotensin system activity, decreasing cardiac work and increasing cardiac output. They reduce the progression and manifestations of heart failure, thus reducing the number and frequency of hospital admissions, decreasing mortality rates, and preventing cardiac complications (Kasper et al., 2005).

In contrast to ACE inhibitors, ARBs do not block the production of angiotensin II; instead, they block its action. The pharmacologic effect is similar, and they also are used in heart failure to slow its progression, reduce manifestations, and prevent cardiac complications.

Beta-blockers improve cardiac function in heart failure by inhibiting SNS activity. This prevents the long-term deleterious effects of sympathetic stimulation. Because beta-blockers reduce the force of myocardial contraction and may actually worsen symptoms, they are used in low doses. The combination of ACE inhibitors and beta-blockers improves client outcomes. Beta-blockers are discussed on pages 973–974.

Clients with symptomatic heart failure often are treated with diuretics as well. Diuretics relieve symptoms related to fluid retention. They may, however, cause significant electrolyte imbal-

ances and rapid fluid loss. Clients with severe heart failure are often treated with a loop, or high-ceiling, diuretic such as furosemide (Lasix), bumetanide (Bumex), torsemide (Demadex), or ethacrynic acid (Edecrin). These drugs have a rapid onset of action, inhibiting chloride reabsorption in the ascending loop of Henle, prompting sodium and water excretion. Their major drawback is their efficacy in promoting diuresis; loss of vascular volume can stimulate the SNS. Thiazide diuretics may be used for clients with less severe manifestations of heart failure. These agents promote fluid excretion by blocking sodium reabsorption in the terminal loop of Henle and the distal tubule.

Vasodilators relax smooth muscle in blood vessels, causing dilation. Arterial dilation reduces peripheral vascular resistance and afterload, reducing myocardial work. Venous dilation reduces venous return and preload. Pulmonary vascular relaxation reduces pulmonary capillary pressure, allowing reabsorption of fluid from interstitial tissues and the alveoli. Vasodilators include nitrates, hydralazine, and prazosin, an alpha-adrenergic blocker. See Chapter 35 ∞ for more information about vasodilators.

Nitrates produce both arterial and venous vasodilation. They may be given by nasal spray or the sublingual, oral, or intravenous route. Sodium nitroprusside is a potent vasodilator that may be used to treat acute heart failure. It can cause excessive hypotension, so it is often given along with dopamine or dobutamine to maintain the blood pressure. Isosorbide or nitroglycerin ointment may be used in long-term management of heart failure. See pages 973–974.

In 2005, the U.S. Food and Drug Administration (FDA) approved a new drug for treatment of heart failure in African Americans. This drug, known as BiDil, is a combination of two vasodilators, hydralazine and isosorbide, in fixed doses. In a study of African Americans with severe heart failure, BiDil improved symptoms and significantly reduced the number of hospitalizations and deaths attributed to heart failure (U.S. FDA, 2005). The Cultural Diversity box on page 1035 discusses the nursing implications for BiDil.

Digitalis glycosides are used judiciously in symptomatic heart failure. Digitalis has a *positive inotropic effect* on the heart, increasing the strength of myocardial contraction by increasing the intracellular calcium concentrations. Digitalis also decreases sinoatrial (SA) node automaticity and slows conduction through the atrioventricular (AV) node, increasing ventricular filling time.

Digitalis has a narrow therapeutic index; in other words, therapeutic levels are very close to toxic levels. Early manifestations of digitalis toxicity include anorexia, nausea and vomiting, headache, altered vision, and confusion. A number of cardiac dysrhythmias are also associated with digitalis toxicity, including sinus arrest, supraventricular and ventricular tachycardias, and high levels of AV block. Low serum potassium levels increase the risk of digitalis toxicity, as do low magnesium and high calcium levels. Older adults are at particular risk for digitalis toxicity.

Digitalis levels may be affected by a number of other drugs; check for potential interactions.

MEDICATION ADMINISTRATION Heart Failure

ANGIOTENSIN-CONVERTING ENZYME (ACE) INHIBITORS

Enalapril (Vasotec) Lisinopril (Prinivil, Zestril)
Captopril (Capoten) Fosinopril (Monopril)
Moexipril (Univasc) Quinapril (Accupril)
Ramipril (Altace) Trandolapril (Mavik)

ANGIOTENSIN II RECEPTOR BLOCKERS (ARBS)

Candesartan (Atacand) Irbesartan (Avapro)
Losartan (Cozaar) Telmisartan (Micardis)
Valsartan (Diovan)

ACE inhibitors and ARBs prevent acute coronary events and reduce mortality in heart failure. ACE inhibitors interfere with production of angiotensin II, resulting in vasodilation, reduced blood volume, and prevention of its effects in the heart and blood vessels. In heart failure, ACE inhibitors reduce afterload and improve cardiac output and renal blood flow. They also reduce pulmonary congestion and peripheral edema. ACE inhibitors suppress myocyte growth and reduce ventricular remodeling in heart failure. While the pharmacologic effect of ARBs is similar, they block the action of angiotensin II at the receptor rather than interfering with its production.

Nursing Responsibilities

- Do not give these drugs to women in the second and third trimesters of pregnancy.
- Carefully monitor clients who are volume depleted or who have impaired renal function.
- Use an infusion pump when administering ACE inhibitors intravenously.
- Monitor blood pressure closely for 2 hours following first dose and as indicated thereafter.
- Monitor serum potassium levels; ACE inhibitors can cause hyperkalemia (this is less of a concern with ARBs).
- Monitor white blood cell (WBC) count for potential neutropenia. Report to the physician.

Health Education for the Client and Family

- Take the drug at the same time every day to ensure a stable blood level.
- Monitor your blood pressure and weight weekly. Report significant changes to your doctor.
- Avoid making sudden position changes; for example, rise from bed slowly. Lie down if you become dizzy or light-headed, particularly after the first dose.
- Report any signs of easy bruising and bleeding, sore throat or fever, edema, or skin rash. Immediately report swelling of the face, lips, or eyelids, and itching or breathing problems.
- A persistent, dry cough may develop if you are taking an ACE inhibitor. Contact your doctor if this becomes a problem.
- Take captopril or moexipril 1 hour before meals.

DIURETICS

Chlorothiazide (Diuril) Spironolactone (Aldactone)
Furosemide (Lasix) Triamterene (Dyrenium)
Ethacrynic acid (Edecrin) Amiloride (Midamor)
Bumetanide (Bumex) Acetazolamide (Diamox)
Hydrochlorothiazide (HydroDIURIL)

Diuretics act on different portions of the kidney tubule to inhibit the reabsorption of sodium and water and promote their excretion. With the exception of the potassium-sparing diuretics—spironolactone, triamterene, and amiloride—diuretics also promote potassium excretion, increasing the risk of hypokalemia. Spironolactone, an al-

dosterone receptor blocker, reduces symptoms and slows progression of heart failure. Aldosterone receptors in the heart and blood vessels promote myocardial remodeling and fibrosis, activate the sympathetic nervous system, and promote vascular fibrosis (which decreases compliance) and baroreceptor dysfunction.

Nursing Responsibilities

- Obtain baseline weight and vital signs.
- Monitor blood pressure, intake and output, weight, skin turgor, and edema as indicators of fluid volume status.
- Assess for volume depletion, particularly with loop diuretics (furosemide, ethacrynic acid, and bumetanide): dizziness, orthostatic hypotension, tachycardia, muscle cramping.
- Report abnormal serum electrolyte levels to the physician. Replace electrolytes as indicated.
- Do not administer potassium replacements to clients receiving a potassium-sparing diuretic.
- Evaluate renal function by assessing urine output, BUN, and serum creatinine.
- Administer intravenous furosemide slowly, no faster than 20 mg/minute. Evaluate for signs of ototoxicity. Do not administer this drug or ethacrynic acid concurrently with aminoglycoside antibiotics (e.g., gentamicin), which are also ototoxic.

Health Education for the Client and Family

- Drink at least 6 to 8 glasses of water per day.
- Take your diuretic at times that will be the least disruptive to your lifestyle, usually in the morning and early afternoon if a second dose is ordered. Take with meals to decrease gastric upset.
- Monitor your blood pressure, pulse, and weight weekly. Report significant weight changes to your doctor.
- Report any of the following to your doctor: severe abdominal pain, jaundice, dark urine, abnormal bleeding or bruising, flu-like symptoms, signs of hypokalemia, hyponatremia, and dehydration (thirst, salt craving, dizziness, weakness, rapid pulse). See Chapter 10 ∞ for manifestations of electrolyte imbalances.
- Avoid sudden position changes. You may experience dizziness, light-headedness, or feelings of faintness.
- Unless you are taking a potassium-sparing diuretic, integrate foods rich in potassium into your diet (see Chapter 10 ∞). Limit sodium use.

POSITIVE INOTROPIC AGENTS

Digitalis Glycosides
Digoxin (Lanoxin)

Digitalis improves myocardial contractility by interfering with ATPase in the myocardial cell membrane and increasing the amount of calcium available for contraction. The increased force of contraction causes the heart to empty more completely, increasing stroke volume and cardiac output. Improved cardiac output improves renal perfusion, decreasing renin secretion. This decreases preload and afterload, reducing cardiac work. Digitalis also has electrophysiologic effects, slowing conduction through the AV node. This decreases the heart rate and reduces oxygen consumption.

Nursing Responsibilities

- Assess apical pulse before administering. Withhold digitalis and notify the physician if heart rate is below 60 bpm and/or

(continued)

MEDICATION ADMINISTRATION Heart Failure (continued)

manifestations of decreased cardiac output are noted. Record apical rate on medication record.

- Evaluate ECG for scooped (spoon-shaped) ST segment, AV block, bradycardia, and other dysrhythmias (especially PVCs and atrial tachycardias).
- Report manifestations of digitalis toxicity: anorexia, nausea, vomiting, abdominal pain, weakness, vision changes (diplopia, blurred vision, yellow-green or white halos seen around objects), and new-onset dysrhythmias.
- Assess potassium, magnesium, calcium, and serum digoxin levels before giving digitalis. Hypokalemia can precipitate toxicity even when the serum digitalis level is in the "normal" range.
- Monitor clients with renal insufficiency or renal failure and older adults carefully for digitalis toxicity.
- Prepare to administer digoxin immune fab (Digibind) for digoxin toxicity.

Health Education for the Client and Family

- Take your pulse daily before taking your digoxin. Do not take the digoxin if your pulse is below 60 bpm or if you are weak, fatigued, light-headed, dizzy, short of breath, or having chest pain. Notify your physician immediately.
- Contact your doctor if you develop manifestations of digitalis toxicity: palpitations, weakness, loss of appetite, nausea, vomiting, abdominal pain, blurred or colored vision, double vision.
- Avoid using antacids and laxatives; they decrease digoxin absorption.
- Notify your physician immediately if you develop manifestations of potassium deficiency: weakness, lethargy, thirst, depression, muscle cramps, or vomiting.
- Incorporate foods high in potassium into your diet: fresh orange or tomato juice, bananas, raisins, dates, figs, prunes, apricots, spinach, cauliflower, and potatoes.

Sympathomimetic Agents
Dopamine (Inotropin)
Dobutamine (Dobutrex)

Sympathomimetic agents stimulate the heart, improving the force of contraction. Dobutamine is preferred in managing heart failure because it does not increase the heart rate as much as dopamine, and it has a mild vasodilatory effect. These drugs are given by intravenous infusion and may be titrated to obtain their optimal effects.

Phosphodiesterase Inhibitors
Amrinone (Inocor)
Milrinone (Primacor)

Phosphodiesterase inhibitors are used in treating acute heart failure to increase myocardial contractility and cause vasodilation. The net effects are an increase in cardiac output and a decrease in afterload.

Nursing Responsibilities

- Use an infusion pump to administer these agents. Monitor hemodynamic parameters carefully.
- Avoid discontinuing these drugs abruptly.
- Change solutions and tubing every 24 hours.
- Amrinone is given as an intravenous bolus over 2 to 3 minutes, followed by an infusion of 5 to 10 mg/kg/min.
- Amrinone may be infused full strength or diluted in normal saline or half-strength saline. Do not mix this drug with dextrose solutions. After dilution, amrinone can be piggybacked into a line containing a dextrose solution.
- Monitor liver function and platelet counts; amrinone may cause hepatotoxicity and thrombocytopenia.

Health Education for the Client and Family

- Notify the nursing staff if you experience abdominal pain or notice a skin rash or bruising.

Dysrhythmias are common in clients with heart failure. Although premature ventricular contractions (PVCs) may be frequent, they are often not associated with an increased risk of ventricular tachycardia and fibrillation. Because many antidysrhythmic medications depress left ventricular function, PVCs are frequently left untreated in heart failure. Amiodarone is the drug of choice to treat nonsustained ventricular tachycardia, which is associated with a poor prognosis. See page 1006.

Nutrition and Activity

A sodium-restricted diet is recommended to minimize sodium and water retention. Intake is generally limited to 1.5 to 2 g of sodium per day, a moderate restriction. Box 10–4 lists high-sodium foods to avoid; Box 10–5 includes client teaching regarding sodium-restricted diet.

Exercise intolerance, decreased ability to participate in activities using large skeletal muscles due to fatigue or dyspnea, is a common early manifestation of heart failure. Activity may be restricted to bed rest during acute episodes of heart failure to reduce cardiac workload and allow the heart to recompen-

sate. Prolonged bed rest and continued activity limitations, however, are not recommended. A moderate, progressive activity program is prescribed to improve myocardial function. Exercise should be performed 3 to 5 days per week, and each session should include a 10- to 15-minute warm-up period, 20 to 30 minutes of exercise at the recommended intensity, and a cool-down period. Walking is encouraged on nontraining days (Piña et al., 2003).

Other Treatments

In end-stage heart failure, devices to provide circulatory assistance or surgery may be required. Surgery may be used to treat the underlying cause of failure (e.g., replacement of diseased valves) or to improve quality of life. Valve replacement is discussed later in this chapter. Heart transplant is currently the only clearly effective surgical treatment for end-stage heart failure; its use is limited by the availability of donor hearts.

CIRCULATORY ASSISTANCE Devices such as the intra-aortic balloon pump or a left-ventricular assist device may be used when the client is expected to recover or as a bridge to trans-

FOCUS ON CULTURAL DIVERSITY   BiDil for Treating Heart Failure in African Americans

BiDil, a fixed-dose combination of two vasodilators (hydralazine and isosorbide), is indicated as an adjunctive treatment in African Americans with heart failure. It has been shown to reduce symptoms, decrease the number of hospitalizations, and prolong life in blacks. The recommended dose is 1 to 2 tablets three times per day, although the dose may be as low as 1/2 tablet three times a day if side effects are intolerable.

Nursing Implications
- Assess vital signs and fluid volume status before administering this drug, because hypotension (orthostatic hypotension in particular) is a common effect.
- Notify the physician if manifestations of systemic lupus erythematosus, glomerulonephritis, or peripheral neuropathy develop.
- Use caution when administering concurrently with monoamine oxidase inhibitors.
- Closely monitor for hypotension when administered concurrently with any potent parenteral antihypertensive agent.

Health Education for the Client and Family
- Take this drug as prescribed.
- Headache is a common adverse effect of this drug, particularly when first starting therapy. Headaches tend to subside with continued treatment.
- Notify your doctor if headaches continue after the first few weeks of therapy, or if you develop chest pain or palpitations while taking this drug.
- This drug can cause a drop in blood pressure, particularly when changing positions from lying to sitting or sitting to standing. Change positions slowly and use caution to prevent falls.
- Do not use drugs such as sildenafil (Viagra, Revatio), vardenafil (Levitra), or tadalafil (Cialis) while taking this medication because the combination may cause an extreme drop in blood pressure leading to fainting, chest pain, or a heart attack.

---

plant. (See Chapter 31 ∞.) Newer devices that will allow longer term support outside the hospital are in the developmental stages. These devices will serve either as a bridge to transplant or allow the myocardium to heal over an extended period of time.

CARDIAC TRANSPLANTATION Heart transplant is the treatment of choice for end-stage heart disease. Survival rates are good: 83% at 1 year and 76% at 3 years. More than 90% of clients return to normal, unrestricted functional abilities following transplant (Kasper et al., 2005). The most frequently used transplant procedure leaves posterior walls of the atria, the superior and inferior venae cavae, and pulmonary veins of the recipient intact (Figure 32–6A ■). The atrial walls of the donor heart are then anastomosed to the recipient's atria (Figure 32–6B). The donor pulmonary artery and aorta are anastomosed to the recipient vessels (Figure 32–6C). Care is taken to avoid damaging the sinus node of the donor heart and to ensure integrity of the suture line to prevent postoperative bleeding. Donor organs typically are obtained from young accident victims with no evidence of cardiac trauma.

Nursing care of the heart transplant client is similar to care of any cardiac surgery client (see pages 980–982). Bleeding is a major concern in the early postoperative period. Chest tube drainage is frequently monitored (initially every 15 minutes), as are the cardiac output, pulmonary artery pressures, and CVP. Cardiac tamponade (compression of the heart) can develop, presenting as either a sudden event or a gradual process. Chest tubes are gently milked (not stripped) as needed to maintain patency. Atrial dysrhythmias are relatively common following cardiac transplant. Temporary pacing wires are placed during surgery as the conduction system may be disrupted by surgical manipulation or postoperative swelling. Hypothermia is induced during surgery; postoperatively, the client is gradually rewarmed over a 1- to 2-hour period. Prevention of rapid rewarming and shivering are important to maintain hemodynamic stability and reduce oxygen consumption. Cardiac function is impaired in up to 50% of transplanted hearts during

Figure 32–6 ■ Cardiac transplantation. *A,* The heart is removed, leaving the posterior walls of the atria intact. The donor heart is anastomosed to the atria, *B,* and the great vessels, *C.*

the early postoperative period. Inotropic agents such as low-dose dopamine, dobutamine, or milrinone may be required to support cardiac function and circulation (Wade et al., 2004).

Infection and rejection are major postoperative concerns; these are the chief causes of mortality in transplant clients. Rejection may develop immediately after transplant (a rare occurence), within weeks to months, or years after the transplant. Acute rejection usually presents within weeks of the transplant, developing when the transplanted organ is recognized by the immune system as foreign. Lymphocytes infiltrate the organ, and myocardial cell necrosis can be detected on biopsy. Acute rejection often can be treated using immunosuppressive drugs (Wade et al., 2004). These drugs also are given to prevent rejection of the transplanted organ, even when the tissue match is good (see Chapter 13 ∞). Although immunosuppressive medications help prevent organ rejection, they impair the client's defenses against infection. Early postoperative infections commonly are bacterial or fungal (*candida*). Multiple invasive lines, prolonged ventilator support, and immunosuppressive therapy contribute to the transplant recipient's risk for infection. Aggressive nursing care directed at prevention of infection is vital: limiting visitors with communicable diseases, pulmonary hygiene measures, early ambulation, and strict aseptic technique (Wade et al., 2004).

The donor heart is denervated during the transplant procedure. Lack of innervation by the autonomic nervous system affects the heart rate (usually between 90 and 110 bpm in transplanted hearts), its response to position changes, stress, exercise, and certain drugs.

OTHER PROCEDURES Other surgical procedures such as cardiomyoplasty and ventricular reduction surgery do not improve the prognosis or quality of life in clients with end-stage heart failure. *Cardiomyoplasty* involves wrapping the latissimus dorsi muscle around the heart to support the failing myocardium. The muscle is stimulated in synchrony with the heart, providing a more forceful contraction and increasing cardiac output. In ventricular reduction surgery (or *partial ventriculectomy*), a portion of the anterolateral left ventricular wall is resected to improve cardiac function (Tierney et al., 2005).

Complementary Therapies

Strong evidence supports the use of several complementary therapies for heart failure. Hawthorn, a shrubby tree, contains natural cardiotonic ingredients in its blossoms, leaves, and fruit. It increases the force of myocardial contraction, dilates blood vessels, and has a natural ACE inhibitor. Hawthorn should never be used without consulting an experienced herb practitioner and advising the physician (Fontaine, 2005). Nutritional supplements of coenzyme Q10, magnesium, and thiamine may be used in conjunction with other treatments. Coenzyme Q10 improves mitochondria function and energy production.

End-of-Life Care

Unless a cardiac transplant is performed, chronic heart failure is ultimately a terminal disease. The client and family need honest discussions about the anticipated course of the disease and treatment options. It is important to discuss advance directives such as the living will and medical power of attorney, differentiating

potential acute events from which recovery would be anticipated (e.g., reversible exacerbation of heart failure, sudden cardiac arrest) from prolonged life support without reasonable expectation of functional recovery. Hospice services are available for clients with heart failure, and should be offered when appropriate. Severe dyspnea is common in the final stages of the disease. It may be managed with narcotic analgesics or with frequent intravenous diuretics and continuous infusion of a positive inotropic agent (Hunt et al., 2005).

 # NURSING CARE

Health Promotion

Health promotion activities to reduce the risk for and incidence of heart failure are directed at the risk factors. Teach clients about coronary heart disease, the primary underlying cause of heart failure. Discuss CHD risk factors and ways to reduce those risk factors (see Chapter 31 ∞).

Hypertension also is a major cause of heart failure. Routinely screen clients for elevated blood pressure, and refer clients to a primary care provider as indicated. Discuss the importance of effectively managing hypertension to reduce the future risk for heart failure. Likewise, stress the relationship between effective diabetes management and reduced risk of heart failure.

Assessment

Obtain both subjective and objective data when assessing the client with heart failure:
- *Health history:* Complaints of increasing shortness of breath, dyspnea with exertion, decreasing activity tolerance, or paroxysmal nocturnal dyspnea; number of pillows used for sleeping; recent weight gain; presence of a cough; chest or abdominal pain; anorexia or nausea; history of cardiac disease, previous episodes of heart failure; other risk factors such as hypertension or diabetes; current medications; usual diet and activity and recent changes.
- *Physical examination:* General appearance; ease of breathing, conversing, changing positions; apparent anxiety; vital signs including apical pulse; color of skin and mucous membranes; neck vein distention, peripheral pulses, capillary refill, presence and degree of edema; heart and breath sounds; abdominal contour, bowel sounds, tenderness; right upper abdominal tenderness, liver enlargement.
- *Diagnostic tests:* BNP, serum electrolyte, BUN, creatinine, and digitalis levels; ABG results; ECG, echocardiogram, and chest x-ray reports.

Nursing Diagnoses and Interventions

Heart failure impacts quality of life, interfering with such daily activities as self-care and role performance. Reducing the oxygen demand of the heart is a major nursing care goal for the client in acute heart failure. This includes providing rest and carrying out prescribed treatment measures to reduce cardiac work, improve contractility, and manage symptoms. See also the accompanying Nursing Care Plan for additional nursing diagnoses and interventions for the client with heart failure.

NURSING CARE PLAN A Client with Heart Failure

One year ago, Arthur Jackson, 67 years old, had a large anterior wall MI and underwent subsequent coronary artery bypass surgery. On discharge, he was started on a regimen of enalapril (Vasotec), digoxin, furosemide (Lasix), warfarin (Coumadin), and a potassium chloride supplement. He is now in the cardiac unit complaining of severe shortness of breath, hemoptysis, and poor appetite for 1 week. He is diagnosed with acute heart failure.

ASSESSMENT

Mr. Jackson refuses to settle in bed, preferring to sit in the bedside recliner in high Fowler's position. He states, "Lately, this is the only way I can breathe." Mr. Jackson states that he has not been able to work in his garden without getting short of breath. He complains of his shoes and belt being too tight.

When Ms. Takashi, RN, Mr. Jackson's nurse, obtains his nursing history, Mr. Jackson insists that he takes his medications regularly. He states that he normally works in his garden for light exercise. In his diet history, Mr. Jackson admits fondness for bacon and Chinese food and sheepishly admits to snacking between meals "even though I need to lose weight."

Mr. Jackson's vital signs are: BP 95/72 mmHg, HR 124 and irregular, R 28 and labored, and T 97.5°F (36.5°C). The cardiac monitor shows atrial fibrillation. An S_3 is noted on auscultation; the cardiac impulse is left of the midclavicular line. He has crackles and diminished breath sounds in the bases of both lungs. Significant jugular venous distention, 3+ pitting edema of feet and ankles, and abdominal distention are noted. Liver size is within normal limits by percussion. Skin cool and diaphoretic. Chest x-ray shows cardiomegaly and pulmonary infiltrates.

DIAGNOSES

- *Excess Fluid Volume* related to impaired cardiac pump and salt and water retention
- *Activity Intolerance* related to impaired cardiac output
- *Impaired Health Maintenance* related to lack of knowledge about diet restrictions

EXPECTED OUTCOMES

- Demonstrate loss of excess fluid by weight loss and decreases in edema, jugular venous distention, and abdominal distention.
- Demonstrate improved activity tolerance.
- Verbalize understanding of diet restrictions.

PLANNING AND IMPLEMENTATION

- Hourly vital signs and hemodynamic pressure measurements.
- Administer and monitor effects of prescribed diuretics and vasodilators.
- Weigh daily; strict intake and output.
- Enforce fluid restriction of 1500 mL/24 hours: 600 mL day shift, 600 mL evening shift, 300 mL at night.

- Auscultate heart and breath sounds every 4 hours and as indicated.
- Administer oxygen per nasal cannula at 2 L/min. Monitor oxygen saturation continuously. Notify physician if less than 94%.
- High Fowler's or position of comfort.
- Notify physician of significant changes in laboratory values.
- Teach about all medications and how to take and record pulse. Provide information about anticoagulant therapy and signs of bleeding.
- Design an activity plan with Mr. Jackson that incorporates preferred activities and scheduled rest periods.
- Instruct about sodium-restricted diet. Allow meal choices within allowed limits.
- Consult dietitian for planning and teaching Mr. and Mrs. Jackson about low-sodium diet.

EVALUATION

Mr. Jackson is discharged after 3 days in the cardiac unit. He has lost 8 pounds during his stay and states it is much easier to breathe and his shoes fit better. He is able to sleep in semi-Fowler's position with only one pillow. His peripheral edema has resolved. Mr. and Mrs. Jackson met with the dietitian, who helped them develop a realistic eating plan to limit sodium, sugar, and fats. The dietitian also provided a list of high-sodium foods to avoid. Mr. Jackson is relieved to know that he can still enjoy Chinese food prepared without monosodium glutamate (MSG) or added salt. Ms. Takashi and the physical therapist designed a progressive activity plan with Mr. Jackson that he will continue at home. He remains in atrial fibrillation, a chronic condition. His knowledge of digoxin and Coumadin has been assessed and reinforced. Ms. Takashi confirms that he is able to accurately check his pulse and can list signs of digoxin toxicity and excessive bleeding.

CRITICAL THINKING IN THE NURSING PROCESS

1. Mr. Jackson's medication regimen remains the same after discharge. What specific teaching does he need related to potential interactions of these drugs?
2. Mr. Jackson tells you, "Talk to my wife about my medications—she's Tarzan and I'm Jane now." How would you respond?
3. Design an exercise plan for Mr. Jackson to prevent deconditioning and conserve energy.
4. Mr. Jackson tells you, "Sometimes I forget whether I have taken my aspirin, so I'll take another just to be sure. After all, they are only baby aspirin. One or two extra a day shouldn't hurt, right?" What is your response?
5. Mr. Jackson is admitted to the neuro unit 6 months later with a cerebral vascular accident (CVA). What is the probable cause of his stroke?

See Evaluating Your Response in Appendix C.

Decreased Cardiac Output

As the heart fails as a pump, stroke volume and tissue perfusion decrease.

- Monitor vital signs and oxygen saturation as indicated. *Decreased cardiac output stimulates the SNS to increase the heart rate in an attempt to restore CO. Tachycardia at rest is*

common. Diastolic blood pressure may initially be elevated because of vasoconstriction; in late stages, compensatory mechanisms fail, and BP falls. Oxygen saturation levels provide a measure of gas exchange and tissue perfusion.

- Monitor BNP levels, reporting trends. *BNP levels indicate the severity of heart failure: as the cardiac index decreases and left ventricular pressures increase, BNP levels increase. Noting trends provides additional information about cardiac output and effectiveness of the cardiac pump.*

- Auscultate heart and breath sounds regularly. S_1 *and* S_2 *may be diminished if cardiac function is poor. A ventricular gallop* (S_3) *is an early sign of heart failure; atrial gallop* (S_4) *may also be present. Crackles are often heard in the lung bases; increasing crackles, dyspnea, and shortness of breath indicate worsening failure.*

PRACTICE ALERT
Report manifestations of decreased cardiac output and tissue perfusion: changes in mentation; decreased urine output; cool, clammy skin; diminished pulses; pallor or cyanosis; dysrhythmias. These are manifestations of decreased tissue perfusion to organ systems.

- Administer supplemental oxygen as needed. *This improves oxygenation of the blood, decreasing the effects of hypoxia and ischemia.*
- Administer prescribed medications as ordered. *Drugs are used to decrease the cardiac workload and increase the effectiveness of contractions.*
- Encourage rest, explaining the rationale. Elevate the head of the bed to reduce the work of breathing. Provide a bedside commode, and assist with activities of daily living (ADLs). Instruct to avoid the Valsalva maneuver. *These measures reduce cardiac workload.*

PRACTICE ALERT
Promote psychologic rest and decrease anxiety. Maintain a quiet environment, and encourage expression of fears and feelings. Explain care measures and their purpose. Psychologic rest decreases oxygen consumption and improves cardiac function.

Excess Fluid Volume

As cardiac output falls, compensatory mechanisms cause salt and water retention, increasing blood volume. This increased fluid volume places additional stress on the already failing ventricles, making them work harder to move the fluid load.

- Assess respiratory status and auscultate lung sounds at least every 4 hours. Notify the physician of significant changes in condition. *Declining respiratory status indicates worsening left heart failure.*

PRACTICE ALERT
Immediately notify the physician if the client develops air hunger, an overwhelming sense of impending doom or panic, tachypnea, severe orthopnea, or a cough productive of large amounts of pink, frothy sputum. Acute pulmonary edema, a medical emergency, can develop rapidly, necessitating immediate intervention to preserve life.

- Monitor intake and output. Notify the physician if urine output is less than 30 mL/h. Weigh daily. *Careful monitoring of fluid volume is important during treatment of heart failure. Diuretics may reduce circulating volume, producing hypo-*

volemia despite persistent peripheral edema. A fall in urine output may indicate significantly reduced cardiac output and renal ischemia. Weight is an objective measure of fluid status: 1 L of fluid is equal to 2.2 lb of weight.

- Record abdominal girth every shift. Note complaints of a loss of appetite, abdominal discomfort, or nausea. *Venous congestion can lead to ascites and may affect gastrointestinal function and nutritional status.*
- Monitor and record hemodynamic measurements. Report significant changes and negative trends. *Hemodynamic measurements provide a means of monitoring condition and response to treatment.*
- Restrict fluids as ordered. Allow choices of fluid type and timing of intake, scheduling most fluid intake during morning and afternoon hours. Offer ice chips and frequent mouth care; provide hard candies if allowed. *Providing choices increases the client's sense of control. Ice chips, hard candies, and mouth care relieve dry mouth and thirst and promote comfort.*

Activity Intolerance

Clients with heart failure have little or no cardiac reserve to meet increased oxygen demands. As the disease progresses and cardiac function is further compromised, activity intolerance increases. The low cardiac output and inability to participate in activities may hinder self-care.

PRACTICE ALERT
Monitor vital signs and cardiac rhythm during and after activities. Tachycardia, dysrhythmias, increasing dyspnea, changes in blood pressure, diaphoresis, pallor, complaints of chest pain, excessive fatigue, or palpitations indicate activity intolerance. Instruct to rest if manifestations are noted. The failing heart is unable to increase cardiac output to meet increased oxygen demands associated with activity. Assessing response to activities helps evaluate cardiac function. Decreasing activity tolerance may signal deterioration of cardiac function, not overexertion.

- Organize nursing care to allow rest periods. *Grouping activities together allows adequate time to "recharge."*
- Assist with ADLs as needed. Encourage independence within prescribed limits. *Assisting with ADLs helps ensure that care needs are met while reducing cardiac workload. Involving the client promotes a sense of control and reduces helplessness.*
- Plan and implement progressive activities. Use passive and active range-of-motion (ROM) exercises as appropriate. Consult with physical therapist on activity plan. *Progressive activity slowly increases exercise capacity by strengthening and improving cardiac function without strain. Activity also helps prevent skeletal muscle atrophy. ROM exercises prevent complications of immobility in severely compromised clients.*
- Provide written and verbal information about activity after discharge. *Written information provides a reference for important information. Verbal information allows clarification and validation of the material.*

Deficient Knowledge: Low-Sodium Diet

Diet is an important part of long-term management of heart failure to manage fluid retention.

- Discuss the rationale for sodium restrictions. *Understanding fosters compliance with the prescribed diet.*
- Consult with dietitian to plan and teach a low-sodium and, if necessary for weight control, low-kilocalorie diet. Provide a list of high-sodium, high-fat, high-cholesterol foods to avoid. Provide American Heart Association materials. *Dietary planning and teaching increase the client's sense of control and participation in disease management. Food lists are useful memory aids.*

> ### PRACTICE ALERT
> Teach how to read food labels for nutritional information. Many processed foods contain "hidden" sodium, which can be identified by careful label reading.

- Assist the client to construct a 2-day meal plan choosing foods low in sodium. *This allows learning assessment, clarification of misunderstandings, and reinforcement of teaching.*
- Encourage small, frequent meals rather than three heavy meals per day. *Small, frequent meals provide continuing energy resources and decrease the work required to digest a large meal.*

NANDA, NIC, and NOC Linkages

Chart 32–1 shows links between NANDA nursing diagnoses, NIC, and NOC for the client with heart failure.

Community-Based Care

Heart failure is a chronic condition requiring active participation by the client and family for effective management. In teaching for home care, include the following topics:
- The disease process and its effects on the client's life
- Warning signals of cardiac decompensation that require treatment
- Desired and adverse effects of prescribed drugs; monitoring for effects; importance of compliance with drug regimen to prevent acute and long-term complications of heart failure
- Prescribed diet and sodium restriction; practical suggestions for reducing salt intake; recommend American Heart Association materials and recipes
- Exercise recommendations to strengthen the heart muscle and improve aerobic capacity (Box 32–3)
- The importance of keeping scheduled follow-up appointments to monitor disease progression and effects of therapy.

  Provide referrals for home health care and household assistance (shopping, transportation, personal needs, and housekeeping) as indicated. Referrals to community agencies, such as local cardiac rehabilitation programs, heart support groups, or the AHA, can provide the client and family with additional materials and psychosocial support.

THE CLIENT WITH PULMONARY EDEMA

Pulmonary edema is an abnormal accumulation of fluid in the interstitial tissue and alveoli of the lung. Both cardiac and noncardiac disorders can cause pulmonary edema. Cardiac causes

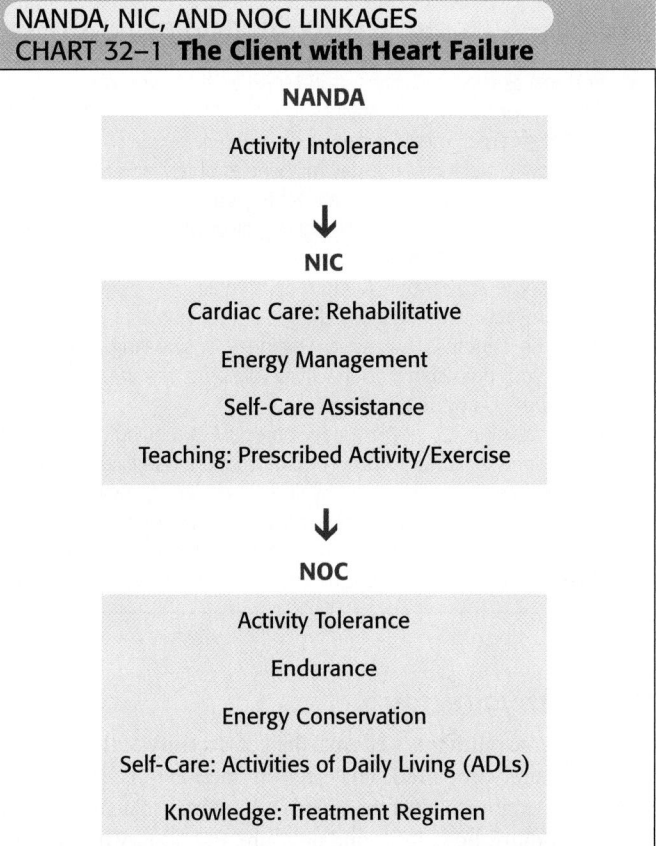

NANDA, NIC, AND NOC LINKAGES
CHART 32–1 **The Client with Heart Failure**

NANDA

Activity Intolerance

↓

NIC

Cardiac Care: Rehabilitative

Energy Management

Self-Care Assistance

Teaching: Prescribed Activity/Exercise

↓

NOC

Activity Tolerance

Endurance

Energy Conservation

Self-Care: Activities of Daily Living (ADLs)

Knowledge: Treatment Regimen

Data from *NANDA's Nursing Diagnoses: Definitions & Classification 2005–2006* by NANDA International (2005), Philadelphia; *Nursing Interventions Classification (NIC)* (4th ed.) by J. M. Dochterman & G. M. Bulechek (2004), St. Louis, MO: Mosby; and *Nursing Outcomes Classification (NOC)* (3rd ed.) by S. Moorhead, M. Johnson, and M. Maas (2004), St. Louis, MO: Mosby.

include acute myocardial infarction, acute heart failure, and valvular disease. *Cardiogenic pulmonary edema*, the focus of this section, is a sign of severe cardiac decompensation. Noncardiac causes of pulmonary edema include primary pulmonary disorders, such as acute respiratory distress syndrome (ARDS), trauma, sepsis, drug overdose, or neurologic sequelae. Pulmonary edema due to ARDS is discussed in Chapter 39 ∞.

> ### FAST FACTS
> - Cardiogenic pulmonary edema is a severe form of heart failure. Risk factors are those associated with heart failure, and treatment focuses on maintaining oxygenation and improving cardiac function.
> - Noncardiogenic pulmonary edema is a primary or secondary lung disorder. It usually occurs secondarily to a critical event such as major trauma, shock, or disseminated intravascular coagulation (DIC). Treatment focuses on maintaining oxygenation and the primary, underlying disorder.

Pulmonary edema is a medical emergency: The client is literally drowning in the fluid in the alveolar and interstitial pulmonary spaces. Its onset may be acute or gradual, progressing to severe respiratory distress. Immediate treatment is necessary.

BOX 32–3 Home Activity Guidelines for the Client with Heart Failure

- Perform as many activities as independently as you can.
- Space your meals and activities.
  a. Eat six small meals a day.
  b. Allow time during the day for periods of rest and relaxation.
- Perform all activities at a comfortable pace.
  a. If you get tired during any activity, stop what you are doing and rest for 15 minutes.
  b. Resume activity only if you feel up to it.
- Stop any activity that causes chest pain, shortness of breath, dizziness, faintness, excessive weakness, or sweating. Rest. Notify your physician if your activity tolerance changes and if symptoms continue after rest.
- Avoid straining. Do not lift heavy objects. Eat a high-fiber diet and drink plenty of water to prevent constipation. Use laxatives or stool softeners, as approved by your physician, to avoid constipation and straining during bowel movements.
- Begin a graded exercise program. Walking is good exercise that does not require any special equipment (except a good pair of

walking shoes). Plan to walk twice a day at a comfortable, slow pace for the first couple of weeks at home, and then gradually increase the distance and pace. Below is a suggested schedule—but progress at your own speed. Take your time. Aim for walking at least 3 times per week (every other day).

Week 1	200 to 400 ft	Twice a day, slow leisurely pace
Week 2	1/4 mile	15 min, minimum of 3 times per week
Weeks 2 to 3	1/2 mile	30 min, minimum of 3 times per week
Weeks 3 to 4	1 mile	30 min, minimum of 3 times per week
Weeks 4 to 5	1 1/2 mile	30 min, minimum of 3 times per week
Weeks 5 to 6	2 miles	40 min, minimum of 3 times per week

Pathophysiology

In cardiogenic pulmonary edema, the contractility of the left ventricle is severely impaired. The ejection fraction falls because the ventricle is unable to eject the blood that enters it, causing a sharp rise in end-diastolic volume and pressure. Pulmonary hydrostatic pressures rise, ultimately exceeding the osmotic pressure of the blood. As a result, fluid leaking from the pulmonary capillaries congests interstitial tissues, decreasing lung compliance and interfering with gas exchange. As capillary and interstitial pressures increase further, the tight junctions of the alveolar walls are disrupted, and the fluid enters the alveoli, along with large red blood cells (RBCs) and protein molecules. Ventilation and gas exchange are severely disrupted, and hypoxia worsens.

Manifestations

The client with acute pulmonary edema presents with classic manifestations (see box below). Dyspnea, shortness of breath, and labored respirations are acute and severe, accompanied by orthopnea (inability to breathe when lying down). Cyanosis is present, and the skin is cool, clammy, and diaphoretic. A productive cough with pink, frothy sputum develops due to fluid, RBCs, and plasma proteins in the alveoli and airways. Crackles are heard throughout the lung fields on auscultation. As the condition worsens, lung sounds become harsher. The client often is restless and highly anxious, although severe hypoxia may cause confusion or lethargy.

As noted earlier, pulmonary edema is a medical emergency. Without rapid and effective intervention, severe tissue hypoxia and acidosis will lead to organ system failure and death.

INTERDISCIPLINARY CARE

Immediate treatment for acute pulmonary edema focuses on restoring effective gas exchange and reducing fluid and pressure in the pulmonary vascular system. The client is placed in

an upright sitting position with the legs dangling to reduce venous return by trapping some excess fluid in the lower extremities. This position also facilitates breathing.

Diagnostic testing is limited to assessment of the acute situation. *ABGs* are drawn to assess gas exchange and acid–base balance. Oxygen tension (PaO_2) is usually low. Initially, carbon dioxide levels ($PaCO_2$) may also be reduced because of rapid respirations. As the condition progresses, the $PaCO_2$ rises and respiratory acidosis develops (see Chapter 10 ∞). *Oxygen saturation* levels also are continuously monitored. The *chest x-ray* shows pulmonary vascular congestion and alveolar edema. Provided the client's condition allows, *hemodynamic monitoring* is instituted. In cardiogenic pulmonary edema, the PAWP is elevated, usually over 25 mmHg. Cardiac output may be decreased.

Morphine is administered intravenously to relieve anxiety and improve the efficacy of breathing. It also is a vasodilator that reduces venous return and lowers left atrial pressure. Although morphine is very effective for clients with cardiogenic

MANIFESTATIONS of Pulmonary Edema

RESPIRATORY
- Tachypnea
- Labored respirations
- Dyspnea
- Orthopnea
- Paroxysmal nocturnal dyspnea
- Cough productive of frothy, pink sputum
- Crackles, wheezes

CARDIOVASCULAR
- Tachycardia
- Hypotension
- Cyanosis
- Cool, clammy skin
- Hypoxemia
- Ventricular gallop

NEUROLOGIC
- Restlessness
- Anxiety
- Feeling of impending doom

pulmonary edema, naloxone, its antidote, is kept readily available in case respiratory depression occurs.

Oxygen is administered using a positive pressure system that can achieve a 100% oxygen concentration. A continuous positive airway pressure (CPAP) mask system may be used, or the client may be intubated and mechanical ventilation employed (see Chapter 39 ∞). Positive pressure increases alveolar pressures and gas exchange while decreasing fluid diffusion into the alveoli.

Potent loop diuretics such as furosemide, ethacrynic acid, or bumetanide are administered intravenously to promote rapid diuresis. Furosemide is also a venous dilator, reducing venous return to the heart. Vasodilators such as intravenous nitroprusside are given to improve cardiac output by reducing afterload. Dopamine or dobutamine and possibly digoxin are administered to improve the myocardial contractility and cardiac output. Intravenous aminophylline may be used cautiously to reduce bronchospasm and decrease wheezing.

When the client's condition has stabilized, further diagnostic tests may be done to determine the underlying cause of pulmonary edema, and specific treatment measures directed at the cause instituted.

NURSING CARE

Nursing care of the client with acute pulmonary edema focuses on relieving the pulmonary effects of the disorder. Interventions are directed toward improving oxygenation, reducing fluid volume, and providing emotional support.

The nurse often is instrumental in recognizing early manifestations of pulmonary edema and initiating treatment. As with many critical conditions, emergent care is directed toward the ABCs: airway, breathing, and circulation.

Nursing Diagnoses and Interventions

Promoting effective gas exchange and restoring an effective cardiac output are the priorities for nursing and interdisciplinary care of the client with cardiogenic pulmonary edema. The experience of acute dyspnea and shortness of breath is terrifying for the client; the nurse is instrumental in providing emotional support and reassurance.

Impaired Gas Exchange

Accumulated fluid in the alveoli and airways interferes with ventilation of the lungs. As a result, alveolar oxygen levels fall and carbon dioxide levels may rise. Reduced alveolar oxygen decreases diffusion of the gas into pulmonary capillaries. In addition, pulmonary edema increases the distance over which gases must diffuse to cross the alveolar–capillary membrane, further reducing oxygen levels in the blood and oxygen delivery to the tissues.

- Ensure airway patency. *A patent airway is absolutely vital for pulmonary function, including ventilation and gas exchange.*

PRACTICE ALERT
Assess the effectiveness of respiratory efforts and airway clearance. Pulmonary edema increases the work of breathing. This increased effort can lead to fatigue and decreased respiratory effort.

- Assess respiratory status frequently, including rate, effort, use of accessory muscles, sputum characteristics, lung sounds, and skin color. *The status of a client in acute pulmonary edema can change rapidly for the better or worse.*
- Place in high-Fowler's position with the legs dangling. *The upright position facilitates breathing and decreases venous return.*
- Administer oxygen as ordered by mask, CPAP mask, or ventilator. *Supplemental oxygen promotes gas exchange; positive pressure increases the pressure within the alveoli, airways, and thoracic cavity, decreasing venous return, pulmonary capillary pressure, and fluid leak into the alveoli.*
- Encourage to cough up secretions; provide nasotracheal suctioning if necessary. *Coughing moves secretions from smaller airways into larger airways where they can be suctioned out if necessary.*

PRACTICE ALERT
Have emergency equipment readily available in case of respiratory arrest. Be prepared to assist with intubation and initiation of mechanical ventilation. Fatigue, impaired gas exchange, and respiratory acidosis can lead to respiratory and cardiac arrest.

Decreased Cardiac Output

Cardiogenic pulmonary edema usually is caused by either an acute decrease in myocardial contractility or increased workload that exceeds the ability of the left ventricle. The significant decrease in cardiac output increases pressure within the pulmonary vascular system and triggers compensatory mechanisms that increase the heart rate and blood volume. These compensatory mechanisms further increase the workload of the failing heart.

- Monitor vital signs, hemodynamic status, and rhythm continuously. *Acute pulmonary edema is a critical condition, and cardiovascular status can change rapidly.*
- Assess heart sounds for possible S_3, S_4, or murmurs. *These abnormal heart sounds may be due to excess work or may indicate the cause of the acute pulmonary edema.*
- Initiate an intravenous line for medication administration. Administer morphine, diuretics, vasodilators, bronchodilators, and positive inotropic medications (e.g., digoxin) as ordered. *These drugs reduce cardiac work and improve contractility.*

PRACTICE ALERT
Insert an indwelling catheter; record output hourly. Urine output of less than 30 mL/h indicates impaired renal perfusion due to severely impaired cardiac output and a risk for renal failure or other complications.

- Keep accurate intake and output records. Restrict fluids as ordered. *Fluids may be restricted to reduce vascular volume and cardiac work.*

Fear

Acute pulmonary edema is a very frightening experience for everyone (including the nurse).

- Provide emotional support for the client and family members. *Fear and anxiety stimulate the sympathetic nervous system, which can lead to ineffective respiratory patterns and interfere with cooperation with care measures.*
- Explain all procedures and the reasons they are performed to the client and family members. Keep information brief and to the point. Use short sentences and a reassuring tone. *Anxiety and fear interfere with the ability to assimilate information; brief, factual information and reassurance reduce anxiety and fear.*
- Maintain close contact with the client and family, providing reassurance that recovery from acute pulmonary edema is often as dramatic as its onset.

- Answer questions, and provide accurate information in a caring manner. *Knowledge reduces anxiety and psychologic stress associated with this critical condition.*

Community-Based Care

During the acute period, teaching is limited to immediate care measures. Once the acute episode of pulmonary edema has resolved, teach the client and family about its underlying cause and prevention of future episodes. If pulmonary edema follows an acute MI, include information related to CHD and the acute AMI, as well as information related to heart failure. Review the teaching and home care for clients with these disorders for further information.

INFLAMMATORY HEART DISORDERS

Any layer of cardiac tissue—the endocardium, myocardium, or pericardium—can become inflamed, thus damaging the heart valves, heart muscle, or pericardial lining. Manifestations of inflammatory heart disorders range from very mild to life threatening. This section discusses the causes and management of rheumatic heart disease, endocarditis, myocarditis, and pericarditis.

THE CLIENT WITH RHEUMATIC FEVER AND RHEUMATIC HEART DISEASE

Rheumatic fever is a systemic inflammatory disease caused by an abnormal immune response to pharyngeal infection by group A beta-hemolytic streptococci. Rheumatic fever usually is a self-limiting disorder, although it may become recurrent or chronic. Although the heart commonly is involved in the acute inflammatory process, only about 10% of people with rheumatic fever develop rheumatic heart disease (Porth, 2005). Rheumatic heart disease frequently damages the heart valves and is a major cause of mitral and aortic valve disorders discussed in the next section of this chapter.

Incidence, Prevalence, and Risk Factors

In the United States and other industrialized nations, rheumatic fever and its sequelae are rare. The peak incidence of rheumatic fever is between ages 5 and 15; although it is rare after age 40, it may affect people of any age. About 3% of people with untreated group A streptococcal pharyngitis develop rheumatic fever (Kasper et al., 2005). Rheumatic fever and rheumatic heart disease remain significant public health problems in many developing countries. Highly virulent strains of group A streptococci have caused scattered outbreaks in the United States in recent years (McCance & Huether, 2006).

Risk factors for streptococcal infections of the pharynx include environmental and economic factors such as crowded living conditions, malnutrition, immunodeficiency, and poor access to health care. Evidence also suggests an unknown genetic factor in susceptibility to rheumatic fever.

FAST FACTS
- The peak incidence of rheumatic fever is in children ages 5 to 15.
- Young adults (in late adolescence and the early 20s) are the primary adult population affected by rheumatic fever.
- People past age 40 rarely develop the disease, unless it is a case of recurrent rheumatic fever.
- Although crowded living conditions and lower socioeconomic status are risk factors, a relatively recent outbreak in the United States occurred in people with ready access to health care. Mucoid strains of *streptococcus pyogenes* have been associated with this outbreak (Veasy et al, 2004).

Pathophysiology

The pathophysiology of rheumatic fever is not yet totally understood. It is thought to result from an abnormal immune response to M proteins on group A beta-hemolytic streptococcal bacteria. These antigens can bind to cells in the heart, muscles, and brain. They also bind with receptors in synovial joints, provoking an autoimmune response (McCance & Huether, 2006). The resulting immune response to the bacteria also leads to inflammation in tissues containing these M proteins. Inflammatory lesions develop in connective tissues on the heart, joints, and skin. The antibodies may remain in the serum for up to 6 months following the initiating event. See Chapters 12 ∞ and 13 ∞ for more information about the immune system and inflammatory response.

Carditis, inflammation of the heart, develops in about 50% of people with rheumatic fever. The inflammatory process usually involves all three layers of the heart—the pericardium, myocardium, and endocardium. *Aschoff bodies,* localized areas of tissue necrosis surrounded by immune cells, develop in cardiac tissues. Pericardial and myocardial inflammation tends to be mild and self-limiting. Endocardial inflammation, however, causes swelling and erythema of valve structures and small vegetative lesions on valve leaflets. As the inflammatory process resolves, fibrous scarring occurs, causing deformity.

Rheumatic heart disease (RHD) is a slowly progressive valvular deformity that may follow acute or repeated attacks of rheumatic fever. Valve leaflets become rigid and deformed; commissures (openings) fuse, and the chordae tendineae fibrose and shorten. This results in stenosis or regurgitation of the valve. In **stenosis**, a narrowed fused valve obstructs forward blood flow. **Regurgitation** occurs when the valve fails to close properly (an *incompetent* valve), allowing blood to flow back through it. Valves on the left side of the heart are usually affected; the mitral valve is most frequently involved.

Manifestations

Manifestations of rheumatic fever typically follow the initial streptococcal infection by about 2 to 3 weeks. Fever and migratory joint pain are often initial manifestations. The knees, ankles, hips, and elbows are common sites of swelling and inflammation. *Erythema marginatum* is a temporary nonpruritic skin rash characterized by red lesions with clear borders and blanched centers usually found on the trunk and proximal extremities. Neurologic symptoms of rheumatic fever, although rare in adults, may range from irritability and an inability to concentrate to clumsiness and involuntary muscle spasms.

Manifestations of carditis include chest pain, tachycardia, a pericardial friction rub, or evidence of heart failure. On auscultation, an S_3, S_4, or a heart murmur may be heard. Cardiomegaly or pericardial effusion may develop. Other manifestations of rheumatic fever are listed in the box below.

INTERDISCIPLINARY CARE

Management of the client with rheumatic heart disease (RHD) focuses on eradicating the streptococcal infection and managing the manifestations of the disease. Carditis and resulting heart failure are treated with measures to reduce the inflammatory process and manage the heart failure. Activities are limited, but bed rest is not generally ordered.

MANIFESTATIONS of Rheumatic Fever

CARDIAC
- Chest pain
- Friction rub
- Heart murmur

MUSCULOSKELETAL
- *Migratory polyarthritis:* redness, heat, swelling, pain, and tenderness of more than one joint
- Usually affects large joints of extremities

SKIN
- *Erythema marginatum:* transitory pink, nonpruritic, macular lesions on trunk or inner aspect of upper arms or thighs
- *Subcutaneous nodules* over extensors of wrist, elbow, ankle, and knee joints

NEUROLOGIC
- *Sydenham's chorea:* irritability, behavior changes; sudden, jerky, involuntary movements

---

Diagnosis

In addition to the history and physical examination, a number of laboratory and diagnostic tests may be ordered for the client with suspected rheumatic fever. Table 32–4 identifies tests and values indicative of carditis associated with rheumatic fever.

- *Complete blood count (CBC)* and *erythrocyte sedimentation rate (ESR)* are indicators of the inflammatory process. The WBC count is elevated, and the number of RBCs may be low due to the inflammatory inhibition of erythropoiesis. The ESR, a general indicator of inflammation, is elevated.
- *C-reactive protein (CRP)* is positive in an active inflammatory process.
- *Antistreptolysin (ASO) titer* is a test for streptococcal antibodies. It rises within 2 months of the onset and is positive in most clients with rheumatic fever.
- Throat culture is positive for group A beta-hemolytic streptococcus in only 25% to 40% of clients with acute rheumatic fever (Kasper et al., 2005).

Medications

As soon as rheumatic fever is diagnosed, antibiotics are started to eliminate the streptococcal infection. Penicillin is the antibiotic of choice to treat group A streptococci. Antibiotics are prescribed for at least 10 days. Erythromycin or clindamycin is used if the client is allergic to penicillin. Prophylactic antibiotic therapy is continued for 5 to 10 years to prevent recurrences. Recurrences after 5 years or age 25 are rare (Tierney et al., 2005). Penicillin G, 1.2 million units injected intramuscularly every 3 to 4 weeks, is the prophylaxis of choice. Oral penicillin, amoxicillin, sulfadiazine, or erythromycin may also be used.

TABLE 32–4 Diagnostic Tests for Rheumatic Heart Disease

TEST	VALUES CHARACTERISTIC OF RHEUMATIC HEART DISEASE
White blood cell (WBC) count	Greater than 10,000/mm^3
Red blood cell (RBC) count	Less than 4 million/mm^3
Erythrocyte sedimentation rate (ESR)	More than 20 mm/h
C-reactive protein	Positive
Antistreptolysin (ASO) titer	Above 250 international unit/mL
Throat culture	Usually positive for group A beta-hemolytic streptococci
Cardiac enzymes	Elevated in severe carditis
ECG changes	Prolonged PR interval
Chest x-ray	May show cardiac enlargement
Echocardiogram	May show valvular damage, enlarged chambers, decreased ventricular function, or pericardial effusion

Joint pain and fever are treated with salicylates (e.g., aspirin), ibuprofen, or another nonsteroidal anti-inflammatory drug (NSAID); corticosteroids may be used for severe pain due to inflammation or carditis. See Chapter 13 ∞ for information about the use of these anti-inflammatory medications.

 NURSING CARE

Health Promotion

Rheumatic fever is preventable. Prompt identification and treatment of streptococcal throat infections help decrease spread of the pathogen and the risk for rheumatic fever. Characteristics of streptococcal sore throat; include a red, fiery-looking throat; pain with swallowing; enlarged and tender cervical lymph nodes; fever range of 101° to 104°F (38.3° to 40.0°C); and headache. Emphasize the importance of finishing the complete course of medication to eradicate the pathogen.

Assessment

Assess clients at risk for rheumatic fever (prolonged, untreated, or recurrent pharyngitis) for possible manifestations.

- *Health history:* Complaints of recent sore throat with fever, difficulty swallowing, and general malaise; treatment measures; previous history of strep throat or rheumatic fever; history of heart murmur or other cardiac problems; current medications.
- *Physical examination:* Vital signs including temperature; skin color, presence of rash on trunk or proximal extremities; mental status; evidence of inflamed joints; heart and lung sounds.
- *Diagnostic tests:* WBC and differential, ESR, CRP results; ASO titer and throat culture results; ECG and echocardiogram reports.

Nursing Diagnoses and Interventions

The nursing care focus for the client with RHD is on providing supportive care and preventing complications. Teaching to prevent recurrence of rheumatic fever is extremely important. *Pain* and *Activity Intolerance* are priority nursing diagnoses for the client with rheumatic fever and RHD.

Acute Pain

Joint and chest pain due to acute inflammation is common in rheumatic fever. Pain and inflammation may interfere with rest and healing.

- Administer anti-inflammatory drugs as ordered. Promptly report manifestations of aspirin toxicity, including tinnitus, vomiting, and gastrointestinal bleeding. Give aspirin and other NSAIDs with food, milk, or antacids to minimize gastric irritation. *Joint pain and fever may be treated with anti-inflammatory agents such as aspirin and NSAIDs. When used for its anti-inflammatory effect, aspirin doses may be high, and it is given around the clock (e.g., every 4 hours). Steroids may be prescribed for severe carditis.*

- Provide warm, moist compresses for local pain relief of acutely inflamed joints. *Moist heat helps relieve pain associated with inflamed joints by reducing inflammation.*
- Auscultate heart sounds as indicated (every shift or each home visit). Notify the physician if a pericardial friction rub or a new murmur develops. *A friction rub is produced as inflamed pericardial surfaces rub against each other. This also stimulates pain receptors, and may increase discomfort.*

Activity Intolerance

The client with acute carditis or RHD may develop heart failure if the heart is unable to supply enough oxygen to meet the body's demand. Manifestations of fatigue, weakness, and dyspnea on exertion may result.

- Explain the importance of activity limitations and reinforce teaching as needed. *Activities are limited during the acute phase of carditis to reduce the workload of the heart. Understanding the rationale improves cooperation with the limitations.*
- Encourage social and diversional activities such as visits with friends and family, reading, playing cards or board games, watching television, and listening to music or talking books. *Diversional activities provide a focus for the client whose physical activities must be limited.*
- Encourage gradual increases in activity, monitoring for evidence of intolerance or heart failure. Consult a cardiac rehabilitation specialist to help design an activity progression schedule. *Gradual activity progression is encouraged as the client's condition improves. Activity tolerance is monitored and activities modified as needed.*

Community-Based Care

Most clients with rheumatic fever and carditis do not require hospitalization. Teaching for home care focuses on both acute care and preventing recurrences and further tissue damage. Include the following topics:

- The importance of completing the full course of antibiotic therapy and continuing antibiotic prophylaxis as prescribed. For the client with chronic RHD, include the importance of antibiotic prophylaxis for invasive procedures (e.g., dental care, endoscopy, or surgery) to prevent bacterial endocarditis. Pamphlets on endocarditis prevention are helpful reminders, and are available from the American Heart Association.
- Preventive dental care and good oral hygiene to maintain oral health and prevent gingival infections, which can lead to recurrence of the disease.
- Early recognition of streptococcal sore throat and appropriate treatment for both the client and family members.
- Early manifestations of heart failure to report to the physician.
- Prescribed medications, including their dosage, route, intended and potential adverse effects, and manifestations to report to the physician.
- Dietary sodium restriction if ordered or recommended. A high-carbohydrate, high-protein diet may be recommended to facilitate healing and combat fatigue.

Refer for home health services or household assistance as indicated.

THE CLIENT WITH INFECTIVE ENDOCARDITIS

Endocarditis, inflammation of the endocardium, can involve any portion of the endothelial lining of the heart. The valves usually are affected. Endocarditis is usually infectious in nature, characterized by colonization or invasion of the endocardium and heart valves by a pathogen.

> **FAST FACTS**
> - Subacute bacterial endocarditis develops more slowly and usually occurs in people with previous heart valve damage.
> - Acute bacterial endocarditis has an abrupt onset and typically affects people with no previous history of heart problems.

Figure 32–7 ■ A vegetative lesion of bacterial endocarditis.
Source: M. English/Custom Medical Stock Photo, Inc.

Incidence and Risk Factors

Endocarditis is relatively uncommon, with an incidence of 1.5 to 6.2 cases per 100,000 people in developed countries (Kasper et al., 2005). The greatest risk factor for endocarditis is previous heart damage. Lesions develop on deformed valves, on valve prostheses, or in areas of tissue damage due to congenital deformities or ischemic disease. The left side of the heart, the mitral valve in particular, is usually affected. Intravenous drug use also is a significant risk factor. The right side of the heart usually is affected in these clients. Other risk factors include invasive catheters (e.g., a central venous catheter, hemodynamic monitoring, or an indwelling urinary catheter), dental procedures or poor dental health, and recent heart surgery.

Prosthetic valve endocarditis (PVE) may occur in clients with a mechanical or tissue valve replacement. This infection may develop in the early postoperative period (within 2 months after surgery) or late. Prosthetic valve endocarditis accounts for 10% to 20% of endocarditis cases. It usually affects males over the age of 60, and is more frequently associated with aortic valve prostheses than with mitral valve replacements. Early PVE is usually due to prosthetic valve contamination during surgery or perioperative bacteremia. Its course often is rapid, and mortality is high. Late-onset PVE more closely resembles subacute endocarditis.

Pathophysiology

Entry of pathogens into the bloodstream is required for infective endocarditis to develop. Bacteria may enter through oral lesions, during dental work or invasive procedures, such as intravenous catheter insertion, surgery, or urinary catheterization; during intravenous drug use; or as a result of infectious processes such as urinary tract or upper respiratory infection.

The initial lesion is a sterile platelet-fibrin vegetation formed on damaged endothelium (Figure 32–7 ■). In acute infective endocarditis, these lesions develop on healthy valve structures, although the mechanism is unknown. In subacute endocarditis, they usually develop on already damaged valves or in endocardial tissue that has been damaged by abnormal pressures or blood flow within the heart.

Organisms that have invaded the blood colonize these vegetations. The vegetation enlarges as more platelets and fibrin are attracted to the site and cover the infecting organism. This covering "protects" the bacteria from quick removal by immune defenses such as phagocytosis by neutrophils, antibodies, and complement. Vegetations may be singular or multiple. They expand while loosely attached to edges of the valve. Friable vegetations can break or shear off, embolizing and traveling through the bloodstream to other organ systems. When they lodge in small vessels, they may cause hemorrhages, infarcts, or abscesses. Ultimately, the vegetations scar and deform the valves and cause turbulence of blood flowing through the heart. Heart valve function is affected, either obstructing forward blood flow, or closing incompletely.

Endocarditis is classified by its acuity and disease course (Table 32–5). *Acute infective endocarditis* has an abrupt onset and is a rapidly progressive, severe disease. Although almost any organism can cause infective endocarditis, virulent organisms such as *Staphylococcus aureus* cause a more abrupt onset and destructive course. *S. aureus* is commonly the infective organism in acute endocarditis. In contrast, *subacute infective endocarditis* has a more gradual onset, with predominant systemic manifestations. It is more likely to occur in clients with preexisting heart disease. *Streptococcus viridans,* enterococci, other gram-negative and gram-positive bacilli, yeasts, and fungi tend to cause the subacute forms of endocarditis (Porth, 2005).

Manifestations

The manifestations of infective endocarditis often are nonspecific (see the box on page 1046). A temperature above 101.5°F (39.4°C) and flulike symptoms develop, accompanied by cough, shortness of breath, and joint pain. The presentation of acute staphylococcal endocarditis is more severe, with a sudden onset, chills, and a high fever. Heart murmurs are heard in 90% of persons with infective endocarditis. An existing murmur may worsen, or a new murmur may develop.

Splenomegaly is common in chronic disease. Peripheral manifestations of infective endocarditis result from microemboli or circulating immune complexes. These manifestations include:

- *Petechiae:* small, purplish-red hemorrhagic spots on the trunk, conjunctiva, and mucous membranes

TABLE 32–5 Classifications of Infective Endocarditis

	ACUTE INFECTIVE ENDOCARDITIS	SUBACUTE INFECTIVE ENDOCARDITIS
Onset	Sudden	Gradual
Usual organism	*Staphylococcus aureus*	*Streptococcus viridans*, enterococci, gram-negative and gram-positive bacilli, fungi, yeasts
Risk factors	Usually occurs in previously normal heart; intravenous drug use, infected intravenous sites	Usually occurs in damaged or deformed hearts; dental work, invasive procedures, and infections
Pathologic process	Rapid valve destruction	Valve destruction leading to regurgitation; embolization of friable vegetations
Presentation	Abrupt onset with spiking fever and chills; manifestations of heart failure	Gradual onset of febrile illness with cough, dyspnea, arthralgias, abdominal pain

MANIFESTATIONS of Infective Endocarditis

- Chills and fever
- General malaise, fatigue
- Arthralgias
- Cough, dyspnea
- Heart murmur
- Anorexia, abdominal pain
- Petechiae, splinter hemorrhages
- Splenomegaly

- *Splinter hemorrhages:* hemorrhagic streaks under the fingernails or toenails
- *Osler's nodes:* small, reddened, painful raised growths on finger and toe pads
- *Janeway lesions:* small, nontender, purplish-red macular lesions on the palms of the hands and soles of the feet
- *Roth's spots:* small, whitish spots (cotton-wool spots) seen on the retina.

Complications

Embolization of vegetative fragments may affect any organ system, particularly the lungs, brain, kidneys, and the skin and mucous membranes, with resulting organ infarction. Other common complications of infective endocarditis include heart failure, abscess, and aneurysms due to infiltration of the arterial wall by organisms. Without treatment, endocarditis is almost universally fatal; fortunately, antibiotic therapy is usually effective to treat this disease.

INTERDISCIPLINARY CARE

Eradicating the infecting organism and minimizing valve damage and other adverse consequences of infective endocarditis are the priorities of care.

Diagnosis

There are no definitive tests for infective endocarditis, but diagnostic tests help establish the diagnosis.

- *Blood cultures* usually are positive for bacteria or other pathogens. Blood cultures are considered positive when a typical infecting organism is identified from two or more separate blood cultures (drawn from different sites and/or at different times, e.g., 12-hour intervals).
- *Echocardiography* (either transthoracic or transesophageal) to visualize vegetations can be diagnostic for infective endocarditis when combined with positive blood cultures. See Chapter 30 ∞ for more information about echocardiography.
- *Serologic immune testing* for circulating antigens to typical infective organisms may be done.

Other diagnostic tests may include the CBC, ESR, serum creatinine, chest x-ray, and an electrocardiogram.

Medications

Preventing endocarditis in clients at high risk is important. Antibiotics are commonly prescribed for clients with preexisting valve damage or heart disease prior to high-risk procedures (Table 32–6).

Antibiotic therapy effectively treats infective endocarditis in most cases. The goal of therapy is to eradicate the infecting organism from the blood and vegetative lesions in the heart. The fibrin covering that protects colonies of organisms from immune defenses also protects them from antibiotic therapy. Therefore, an extended course of multiple intravenous antibiotics is required.

Following blood cultures, antibiotic therapy is initiated with drugs known to be effective against the most common infecting organisms: staphylococci, streptococci, and enterococci. The initial regimen may include nafcillin or oxacillin, penicillin or ampicillin, and gentamicin. Once the organism has been identified, therapy is tailored to that organism. Streptococcal and enterococcal infections are treated with a combination of penicillin and gentamicin. If the client is allergic to penicillin, ceftriaxone, cefazolin, or vancomycin may be used. Staphylococcal infections are treated with nafcillin or oxacillin and gentamicin; cefazolin or vancomycin may be used if penicillin allergy is present. Intravenous drug therapy is continued for 2 to 8 weeks, depending on the infecting organism, the drugs used, and the results of repeat blood cultures. See Chapter 12 ∞ for the nursing implications for antibiotic therapy.

The client with prosthetic valve endocarditis requires extended treatment, usually 6 to 8 weeks. Combination therapy

TABLE 32-6 Antibiotic Prophylaxis for Infective Endocarditis

INDICATIONS FOR PROPHYLAXIS	SELECTED PROCEDURES FOR WHICH PROPHYLAXIS IS RECOMMENDED	SUGGESTED ANTIBIOTICS
Prosthetic valves	Dental procedures in which bleeding is likely, including cleaning	Amoxicillin
Previous episode(s) of infective endocarditis		Erythromycin
Rheumatic heart disease	Most surgeries	Ampicillin
Hypertrophic cardiomyopathy	Bronchoscopy	Clindamycin
Mitral valve prolapse with regurgitation and murmur	Cystoscopy	Vancomycin
	Urinary catheterization when infection is present	(*Note:* Choice of antibiotic depends on procedure.)
Sclerotic aortic valve	Incision and drainage of infected tissue	
Most congenital heart malformations	Vaginal delivery if infection is present	

using vancomycin, rifampin, and gentamicin is used to treat these resistant infections.

Surgery

Some clients with infective endocarditis require surgery to:
- Replace severely damaged valves.
- Remove large vegetations at risk for embolization.
- Remove a valve that is a continuing source of infection that does not respond to antibiotic therapy.

The most common indication for surgery is valvular regurgitation that causes heart failure and does not respond to medical therapy. When the infection has not responded to antibiotic therapy within 7 to 10 days, the infected valve may be replaced to facilitate eradication of the organism. Clients with fungal endocarditis usually require surgical intervention. More information on valve replacement surgery is provided in the section on valve disorders.

 NURSING CARE

Health Promotion

Prevention of endocarditis is vital in susceptible people. Education is a key part of prevention. Use every opportunity to educate individuals and the public about the risks of intravenous drug use, including endocarditis. Discuss preventive measures with all clients with specific risk factors, such as a heart murmur or known heart disease.

Assessment

Assessment related to ineffective endocarditis includes identifying risk factors and manifestations of the disease.
- *Health history:* Complaints of persistent flulike symptoms, fatigue, shortness of breath, and activity intolerance; history of recent dental work or other invasive procedures; known heart murmur, valve or other heart disorder; recent intravenous drug use.
- *Physical examination:* Vital signs including temperature; apical pulse and heart sounds; rate and ease of respirations, lung sounds; skin color, temperature, and presence of petechiae or splinter hemorrhages.
- *Diagnostic tests:* WBC and differential, ESR; blood culture and sensitivity results; echocardiogram reports.

Nursing Diagnoses and Interventions

Nursing care focuses on managing the manifestations of endocarditis, administering antibiotics, and teaching the client and family members about the disorder. In addition to the diagnoses identified below, nursing diagnoses and interventions for heart failure also may be appropriate for clients with infective endocarditis.

Risk for Imbalanced Body Temperature

Fever is common in clients with infective endocarditis. It may be acutely elevated and accompanied by chills, particularly with acute infective endocarditis. The inflammatory process initiates a cycle of events that affects the regulation of temperature and causes discomfort.
- Record temperature every 2 to 4 hours. Report temperature above 101.5°F (39.4°C). Assess for complaints of discomfort. *Fever is usually low grade (below 101.5°F [39.4°C]) in infective endocarditis; higher temperatures may cause discomfort. The temperature usually returns to normal within 1 week after initiation of antibiotic therapy. Continued fever may indicate a need to modify the treatment regimen.*
- Obtain blood cultures as ordered, before initial antibiotic dose. *Initial blood cultures are obtained before antibiotic therapy is started to obtain adequate organisms to culture and identify. Follow-up cultures are used to assess the effectiveness of therapy.*
- Provide anti-inflammatory or antipyretic agents as prescribed. *Fever may be treated with anti-inflammatory or antipyretic agents such as aspirin, ibuprofen, or acetaminophen.*
- Administer antibiotics as ordered; obtain peak and trough drug levels as indicated. *Intravenous antibiotics are given to eradicate the pathogen. Peak and trough levels are used to evaluate the dose effectiveness in maintaining a therapeutic blood level.*

Risk for Ineffective Tissue Perfusion

Embolization of vegetative lesions can threaten tissue and organ perfusion. Vegetations from the left heart may lodge in arterioles or capillaries of the brain, kidneys, or peripheral tissues, causing infarction or abscess. A large embolism can cause manifestations of stroke or transient ischemic attack, renal failure, or tissue ischemia. Emboli from the right side of the heart become entrapped in pulmonary vasculature, causing manifestations of pulmonary embolism.

- Assess for, document, and report manifestations of decreased organ system perfusion:
  a. *Neurologic:* changes in level of consciousness, numbness or tingling in extremities, hemiplegia, visual disturbances, or manifestations of stroke
  b. *Renal:* decreased urine output, hematuria, elevated BUN or creatinine
  c. *Pulmonary:* dyspnea, hemoptysis, shortness of breath, diminished breath sounds, restlessness, sudden chest or shoulder pain
  d. *Cardiovascular:* chest pain radiating to jaw or arms, tachycardia, anxiety, tachypnea, hypotension.
  All major organs and tissues, and the microcirculation, may be affected by emboli when vegetations break off due to turbulent blood flow. Emboli may cause manifestations of organ dysfunction. The most devastating effects of emboli are in the brain and the myocardium, with resulting infarctions. Intravenous drug users have a high risk of pulmonary emboli as a result of right-sided endocardial fragments.
- Assess and document skin color and temperature, quality of peripheral pulses, and capillary refill. *Peripheral emboli affect tissue perfusion, with a risk for tissue necrosis and possible extremity loss.*

Ineffective Health Maintenance

The client with endocarditis often is treated in the community. Teaching about disease management and prevention of possible recurrences of endocarditis is vital.

- Demonstrate intravenous catheter site care and intermittent antibiotic administration if the client and family will manage therapy. Have the client and/or significant other redemonstrate appropriate techniques. *Intermittent antibiotic infusions may be managed by the client or family members, or the client may go to an outpatient facility to receive the infusions. Appropriate site care is necessary to reduce the risk of trauma and infection.*
- Explain the actions, doses, administration, and desired and adverse effects of prescribed drugs. Identify manifestations to be reported to the physician. Provide practical information about measures to reduce the risk of superinfection (e.g., consuming 8 oz of yogurt or buttermilk containing live bacterial cultures daily). *Careful compliance with prescribed drug therapy is vital to eradicate the infecting organism. Antibiotic therapy can, however, cause superinfections such as candidiasis due to elimination of normal body flora.*
- Teach about the function of heart valves and the effects of endocarditis on heart function. Include a simple definition of endocarditis, and explain the risk for its recurrence. *Information helps the client and family understand endocarditis, its treatment, and its effects. Understanding increases compliance.*
- Describe the manifestations of heart failure to be reported to the physician. *Evidence of heart failure may necessitate modification of the treatment regimen or replacement of infected valves.*

PRACTICE ALERT

Stress the importance of notifying all care providers of valve disease, heart murmur, or valve replacement before undergoing invasive procedures. Invasive procedures provide a portal of entry for bacteria. A history of valve disease increases the risk for the development or recurrence of endocarditis.

- Encourage good dental hygiene and mouth care and regular dental checkups. Teach how to prevent bleeding from the gums and avoid developing mouth ulcers (e.g., gentle toothbrushing, ensuring that dentures fit properly, and avoiding toothpicks, dental floss, and high-flow water devices). *The oropharynx harbors streptococci, which are common causes of endocarditis. Bleeding gums offer an opportunity for bacteria to enter the bloodstream.*
- Encourage the client to avoid people with upper respiratory infections. *Streptococci are normal pathogens in the upper respiratory tract; exposure to people with upper respiratory infections may increase the risk of infection.*
- If anticoagulant therapy is ordered, explain its actions, administration, and major side effects. Identify manifestations of bleeding to be promptly reported to the physician. *Clients with valve disease or a prosthetic valve following infective endocarditis may require continued anticoagulant therapy to prevent thrombi and emboli. Knowledge is vital for appropriate management of anticoagulant therapy and prevention of complications.*

Community-Based Care

When preparing the client with infective endocarditis for home care, provide teaching as outlined for the nursing diagnosis *Ineffective Health Maintenance.* In addition, discuss the following topics:

- Although serious and frightening, infective endocarditis can usually be treated effectively with intravenous antibiotics.
- The importance of promptly reporting any unusual manifestation, such as a change in vision, sudden pain, or weakness, so that interventions to control complications can be promptly implemented.
- The rationale for all treatments and procedures.
- Preventing recurrences of infective endocarditis.
- The importance of maintaining contact with the physician for follow-up care and monitoring for long-term effects such as progressive valve damage and dysfunction.
- If appropriate, explain the risks associated with intravenous drug use.

Provide educational materials on infective endocarditis from the American Heart Association. Refer as appropriate to home health or home intravenous therapy services. Refer the client and family members or significant others as appropriate to a drug or substance abuse treatment program or facility. Provide follow-up care to ensure compliance with the referral and treatment plan.

THE CLIENT WITH MYOCARDITIS

Myocarditis is inflammation of the heart muscle. It usually results from an infectious process, but also may occur as an immunologic response, or due to the effects of radiation, toxins, or drugs. In the United States, myocarditis is usually viral, caused by coxsackievirus B. Approximately 10% of people with HIV disease develop myocarditis due to infiltration of the myocardium by the virus. Bacterial myocarditis, much less common, may be associated with endocarditis caused by *S. aureus,* or with diphtheria. Parasitic infections caused by *Trypanosoma cruzi* (Chagas' disease) are common in Central and South America (Kasper et al., 2005).

Incidence and Risk Factors

Myocarditis may occur at any age, and it is more common in men than women. Factors that alter immune response (e.g., malnutrition, alcohol use, immunosuppressive drugs, exposure to radiation, stress, and advanced age) increase the risk for myocarditis. It also is a common complication of rheumatic fever and pericarditis.

Pathophysiology

In myocarditis, myocardial cells are damaged by an inflammatory process that causes local or diffuse swelling and damage. Infectious agents infiltrate interstitial tissues, forming abscesses. Autoimmune injury may occur when the immune system destroys not only the invading pathogen but also myocardial cells. The extent of damage to cardiac muscle ultimately determines the long-term outcome of the disease. Viral myocarditis usually is self-limited; it may progress, however, to become chronic, leading to dilated cardiomyopathy (see the section of this chapter that follows). Severe myocarditis may lead to heart failure.

Manifestations

The manifestations of myocarditis depend on the degree of myocardial damage. The client may be asymptomatic. Nonspecific manifestations of inflammation such as fever, fatigue, general malaise, dyspnea, palpitations, and arthralgias may be present. A nonspecific febrile illness or upper respiratory infection often precedes the onset of myocarditis symptoms. Abnormal heart sounds such as muffled S_1, an S_3, murmur, and pericardial friction rub may be heard. In some cases, manifestations of myocardial infarction, including chest pain, may occur.

INTERDISCIPLINARY CARE

Myocarditis treatment focuses on resolving the inflammatory process to prevent further damage to the myocardium.

Diagnostic studies may be ordered to help diagnose myocarditis:

- *Electrocardiography* may show transient ST-segment and T-wave changes, as well as dysrhythmias and possible heart block.
- *Cardiac markers,* such as the creatinine kinase, troponin T, and troponin I, may be elevated, indicating myocardial cell damage.
- *Endomyocardial biopsy* to examine myocardial cells is necessary to establish a definitive diagnosis; patchy cell necrosis and the inflammatory process can be identified.

If appropriate, antimicrobial therapy is used to eradicate the infecting organism. Antiviral therapy with interferon alpha may be instituted. Immunosuppressive therapy with corticosteroids or other immunosuppressive agents (see Chapter 13 ∞) may be used to minimize the inflammatory response. Heart failure is treated as needed, using ACE inhibitors and drugs. Clients with myocarditis often are particularly sensitive to the effects of digitalis, so it is used with caution. Other medications used in treating myocarditis include antidysrhythmic agents to control dysrhythmias and anticoagulants to prevent emboli.

Bed rest and activity restrictions are ordered during the acute inflammatory process to reduce myocardial work and prevent myocardial damage. Activities may be limited for as long as 6 months to a year (Porth, 2005).

 NURSING CARE

Nursing care is directed at decreasing myocardial work and maintaining cardiac output. Both physical and emotional rest are indicated, because anxiety increases myocardial oxygen demand. Hemodynamic parameters and the ECG are monitored closely, especially during the acute phase of the illness. Activity tolerance, urine output, and heart and breath sounds are frequently assessed for manifestations of heart failure. Consider the following nursing diagnoses for the client with myocarditis:

- *Activity Intolerance* related to impaired cardiac muscle function
- *Decreased Cardiac Output* related to myocardial inflammation
- *Fatigue* related to inflammation and impaired cardiac output
- *Anxiety* related to possible long-term effects of the disorder
- *Excess Fluid Volume* related to compensatory mechanisms for decreased cardiac output.

Community-Based Care

Include the following topics when preparing the client with myocarditis for home care:

- Activity restrictions and other prescribed measures to reduce cardiac workload
- Early manifestations of heart failure to report to the physician
- The importance of following the prescribed treatment regimen
- Any recommended dietary modifications (such as a low-sodium diet for heart failure)
- Prescribed medications, their purpose, doses, and possible adverse effects
- The importance of adhering to the treatment plan and recommended follow-up appointments to reduce the risk of long-term consequences such as cardiomyopathy.

THE CLIENT WITH PERICARDITIS

The pericardium is the outermost layer of the heart. It is a two-layered membranous sac with a thin layer of serous fluid (normally no more than 30 to 50 mL) separating the layers. It protects and cushions the heart and the great vessels, provides a barrier to infectious processes in adjacent structures, prevents displacement of the myocardium and blood vessels, and prevents sudden distention of the heart.

Pericarditis is the inflammation of the pericardium. Pericarditis may be a primary disorder or develop secondarily to another cardiac or systemic disorder. Some possible causes of pericarditis are listed in Box 32–4. Acute pericarditis is usually viral and affects men (usually under the age of 50) more frequently than women (Tierney et al., 2005). Pericarditis affects 40% to 50% of clients with end-stage renal disease and uremia. Postmyocardial infarction pericarditis and postcardiotomy (following open-heart surgery) pericarditis also are common.

Pathophysiology

Pericardial tissue damage triggers an inflammatory response. Inflammatory mediators released from the injured tissue cause vasodilation, hyperemia, and edema. Capillary permeability increases, allowing plasma proteins, including fibrinogen, to escape into the pericardial space. White blood cells amass at the site of injury to destroy the causative agent. Exudate is formed, usually fibrinous or serofibrinous (a mixture of serous fluid and fibrinous exudate). In some cases, the exudate may contain red blood cells or, if infectious, purulent material. The inflammatory process may resolve without long-term effects, or scar tissue and adhesions may form between the pericardial layers.

Fibrosis and scarring of the pericardium may restrict cardiac function. Pericardial effusions may develop as serous or purulent exudate (depending on the causative agent) collects in the pericardial sac. Pericardial effusion may be recurrent. Chronic inflammation causes the pericardium to become rigid.

Manifestations

Classic manifestations of acute pericarditis include chest pain, a pericardial friction rub, and fever. Chest pain, the most common symptom, has an abrupt onset. It is caused by inflammation of nerve fibers in the lower parietal pericardium and pleura covering the diaphragm. The pain is usually sharp, may be steady or intermittent, and may radiate to the back or neck. The pain can mimic myocardial ischemia; careful assessment is important to rule out myocardial infarction. Pericardial pain is aggravated by respiratory movements (i.e., deep inspiration and/or coughing), changes in body position, or swallowing. Sitting upright and leaning forward reduces the discomfort by moving the heart away from the diaphragmatic side of the lung pleura.

Although not always present, a *pericardial friction rub* is the characteristic sign of pericarditis. A pericardial friction rub is a leathery, grating sound produced by the inflamed pericardial layers rubbing against the chest wall or pleura. It is heard most clearly at the left lower sternal border with the client sitting up or leaning forward. The rub is usually heard on expiration and may be constant or intermittent.

A low-grade fever (below 100°F [38.4°C]) often develops due to the inflammatory process. Dyspnea and tachycardia are common.

Complications

Pericardial effusion, cardiac tamponade, and constrictive pericarditis are possible complications of acute pericarditis.

Pericardial Effusion

A *pericardial effusion* is an abnormal collection of fluid between the pericardial layers that threatens normal cardiac function. The fluid may consist of pus, blood, serum, lymph, or a combination. The manifestations of a pericardial effusion depend on the rate at which the fluid collects. Although the pericardium normally contains about 30 to 50 mL of fluid, the sac can stretch to accommodate a gradual accumulation of fluid. Over time, the pericardial sac can accommodate up to 2 L of fluid without immediate adverse effects. Conversely, a rapid buildup of pericardial fluid (as little as 100 mL) does not allow the sac to stretch and can compress the heart, interfering with myocardial function. This compression of the heart is known as **cardiac tamponade**. Slowly developing pericardial effusion is often painless and has few manifestations. Heart sounds may be distant or muffled. The client may have a cough or mild dyspnea.

Cardiac Tamponade

Cardiac tamponade is a medical emergency that must be aggressively treated to preserve life. Cardiac tamponade may result from pericardial effusion, trauma, cardiac rupture, or hemorrhage. Rapid collection of fluid in the pericardial sac interferes with ventricular filling and pumping, critically reducing cardiac output.

Classic manifestations of cardiac tamponade result from rising intracardiac pressures, decreased diastolic filling, and decreased cardiac output. A hallmark of cardiac tamponade is a paradoxical pulse, or *pulsus paradoxus*. A paradoxical pulse markedly decreases in amplitude during inspiration. Intrathoracic pressure normally drops during inspiration, enhancing venous return to the right heart. This draws more blood into the right side of the heart than the left, causing the interventricular septum to bulge slightly into the left ventricle. When ventricular filling is impaired by excess fluid in the pericardial sac, this bulging of the interventricular septum decreases cardiac output during inspiration (see Figure 32–8). On palpation of the carotid or femoral artery, the pulse is diminished or absent during inspiration. A drop in systolic blood pressure of more than 10 mmHg during inspiration also indicates pulsus paradoxus.

Other manifestations of cardiac tamponade include muffled heart sounds, dyspnea and tachypnea, tachycardia, a nar-

BOX 32–4 Selected Causes of Pericarditis

Infectious
- Viruses
- Bacteria
- Tuberculosis
- Fungi
- Syphilis
- Parasites

Noninfectious
- Myocardial and pericardial injury
- Uremia
- Neoplasms
- Radiation
- Trauma or surgery
- Myxedema
- Autoimmune disorders
- Rheumatic fever
- Connective tissue diseases
- Prescription and nonprescription drugs
- Postcardiac injury

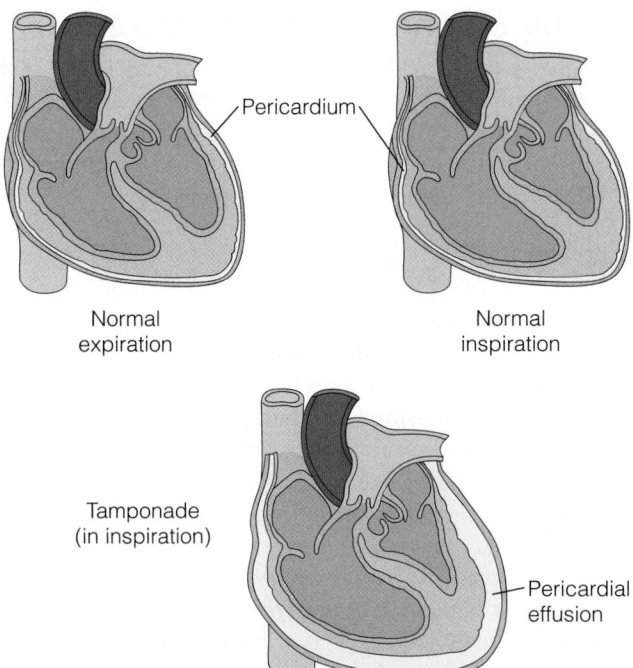

Figure 32-8 ■ Cardiac tamponade. Note increased volume in the right ventricle during inspiration in both the normal heart and the heart affected by a pericardial effusion. In tamponade, fluid in the pericardial sac and the distended right ventricle restrict filling of the left ventricle and consequently, cardiac output.

Figure 32-9 ■ Constrictive pericarditis.
Source: Custom Medical Stock Photo, Inc.

rowed pulse pressure, and distended neck veins (see the box below).

Chronic Constrictive Pericarditis

Chronic pericardial inflammation can lead to scar tissue formation between the pericardial layers. This scar tissue eventually contracts, restricting diastolic filling and elevating venous pressure. Constrictive pericarditis may follow viral infection, radiation therapy, or heart surgery. Its manifestations include progressive dyspnea, fatigue, and weakness. Ascites is common; peripheral edema may develop. Neck veins are distended, and may be particularly noticeable during inspiration (*Kussmaul's sign*). This occurs because the right atrium is unable to dilate to accommodate increased venous return during inspiration. See Figure 32-9 ■.

MANIFESTATIONS of Cardiac Tamponade

- Paradoxical pulse
- Narrowed pulse pressure, hypotension
- Tachycardia
- Weak peripheral pulses
- Distant, muffled heart sounds
- Jugular venous distention
- High central venous pressure
- Decreased level of consciousness
- Low urine output
- Cool, mottled skin

INTERDISCIPLINARY CARE

Care for the client with pericarditis focuses on identifying its cause if possible, reducing inflammation, relieving symptoms, and preventing complications. The client is closely monitored for early manifestations of cardiac tamponade so that it can be treated promptly.

Diagnosis

There are no specific laboratory tests to diagnose pericarditis, but tests are often performed to differentiate pericarditis from myocardial infarction.

- *CBC* shows elevated WBCs and an ESR greater than 20 mm/h, indicating acute inflammation.
- *Cardiac enzymes* may be slightly elevated because the inflammatory process extends to involve the epicardial surface of the heart. Cardiac enzymes are typically much lower in pericarditis than in myocardial infarction.
- *Electrocardiography* shows typical changes associated with pericarditis, such as diffuse ST-segment elevation in all leads. This resolves more quickly than changes of acute MI and is not associated with the QRS-complex and T-wave changes typically seen in MI. With a large pericardial effusion, the QRS amplitude may be decreased. Atrial dysrhythmias may occur in acute pericarditis.
- *Echocardiography* is used to assess heart motion, for pericardial effusion, and the extent of restriction.
- *Hemodynamic monitoring* may be used in acute pericarditis or pericardial effusion to assess pressures and cardiac output. Elevated pulmonary artery pressures and venous pressures occur with impaired filling due to pericardial effusion or constrictive pericarditis.
- *Chest x-ray* may show cardiac enlargement if a pericardial effusion is present.

- *Computed tomography (CT) scan* or *magnetic resonance imaging (MRI)* may be used to identify pericardial effusion or constrictive pericarditis.

Medications

Drug treatment for pericarditis addresses its manifestations. Aspirin and acetaminophen may be used to reduce fever. NSAIDs are used to reduce inflammation and promote comfort. In severe cases or with recurrent pericarditis, corticosteroids may be given to suppress the inflammatory response.

Pericardiocentesis

Pericardiocentesis may be done to remove fluid from the pericardial sac for diagnostic or therapeutic purposes (see Figure 30–15 ∞). The physician inserts a large (16- to 18-gauge) needle into the pericardial sac and withdraws excess fluid. The needle is attached to an ECG monitoring lead to help determine if the needle is touching the epicardial surface, which helps prevent piercing the myocardium. Pericardiocentesis may be an emergency procedure for the client with cardiac tamponade. Nursing implications for pericardiocentesis are outlined in Chapter 30 ∞.

Surgery

For recurrent pericarditis or recurrent pericardial effusion, a rectangular piece of the pericardium, or "window," may be excised to allow collected fluid to drain into the pleural space. Constrictive pericarditis may necessitate a partial or total *pericardiectomy,* removal of part or all of the pericardium, to relieve the ventricular compression and allow adequate filling.

 ## NURSING CARE

Health Promotion

While it may not yet be possible to identify many clients at risk for and to prevent acute pericarditis, early identification and treatment of the disorder can reduce the risk of complications. Promptly report a pericardial friction rub or other manifestations of pericarditis in clients with recent acute AMI, cardiac surgery, or systemic diseases associated with a risk for pericarditis.

Assessment

Assessment data to collect from the client with suspected pericarditis includes:

- *Health history:* Complaints of acute substernal or precordial chest pain, effect of movement and breathing on discomfort, pain radiation, associated symptoms; recent acute AMI, heart surgery, or other cardiac disorder; current medications; chronic conditions such as renal failure or a connective tissue or autoimmune disorder.
- *Physical examination:* Vital signs including temperature, variation in systolic BP with respirations; strength of peripheral pulses, variations with respiratory movement; apical pulse, clarity, changes with respiratory movement, presence of a friction rub; neck vein distention; level of consciousness, skin color, and other indicators of cardiac output.
- *Diagnostic tests:* WBC and differential, ESR; cardiac enzyme levels; ECG and echocardiogram reports.

Nursing Diagnoses and Interventions

Nursing care for the client with pericarditis may occur in the acute or community setting. Closely observe for early manifestations of increasing effusion or cardiac tamponade. Priority nursing diagnoses relate to comfort, the risk for tamponade, and effects of the acute inflammatory process.

Acute Pain

Inflamed pericardial layers rubbing against each other and the lung pleura stimulate phrenic nerve pain fibers in the lower portion of the parietal pericardium. Pain is usually acute and may be severe until inflammation resolves.

- Assess chest pain using a standard pain scale and noting the quality and radiation of the pain. Note nonverbal cues of pain (grimacing, guarding behaviors), and validate with the client. *Careful assessment helps identify the cause of pain. The pain of pericarditis may radiate to the neck or back and is aggravated by movement, coughing, or deep breathing. A pain scale allows evaluation of the effectiveness of interventions.*
- Auscultate heart sounds every 4 hours. *Presence of a pericardial friction rub often correlates with the location and severity of the pain.*
- Administer NSAIDs on a regular basis as prescribed with food. Document effectiveness. *NSAIDs reduce fever, inflammation, and pericardial pain. They are most effective when administered around the clock on a consistent basis. Administering the medications with food helps decrease gastric distress.*
- Maintain a quiet, calm environment, and position of comfort. Offer back rubs, heat/cold therapy, diversional activity, and emotional support. *Supportive interventions enhance the effects of the medication, may decrease pain perception, and convey a sense of caring.*

Ineffective Breathing Pattern

Respiratory movement intensifies pericardial pain. In an effort to decrease pain, the client often breathes shallowly, increasing the risk for pulmonary complications.

> **PRACTICE ALERT**
> Document respiratory rate, effort, and breath sounds every 2 to 4 hours. Report adventitious or diminished breath sounds. Shallow, guarded respirations may lead to increased respiratory rate and effort. Poor ventilation of peripheral alveoli may lead to congestion or atelectasis.

- Encourage deep breathing and use of the incentive spirometer. Provide pain medication before respiratory therapy, as needed. *Deep breathing and an incentive spirometer promote alveolar ventilation and prevent atelectasis. Administration of analgesia prior to respiratory treatments improves their effectiveness by decreasing guarding.*
- Administer oxygen as needed. *Supplementary oxygen promotes optimal gas exchange and tissue oxygenation.*
- Place in Fowler's or high-Fowler's position. Assist to a position of comfort. *Appropriate positioning reduces the work of breathing and decreases chest pain due to pericarditis.*

Risk for Decreased Cardiac Output

The acute inflammatory process of pericarditis can lead to significant pericardial effusion and cardiac tamponade. This potentially fatal complication can also occur with chronic pericardial effusion if the amount of fluid exceeds the ability of the pericardial sac to expand. Constrictive pericarditis increases the risk for decreased cardiac output because of restricted cardiac filling.

- Document vital signs hourly during the acute inflammatory processes. *Frequent assessment allows early recognition of manifestations of decreased cardiac output, such as tachycardia, hypotension, or changes in pulse pressure.*

PRACTICE ALERT
Assess heart sounds and peripheral pulses, and observe for neck vein distention and paradoxical pulse hourly. Promptly report distant, muffled heart sounds, new murmurs or extra heart sounds, decreasing quality of peripheral pulses, and distended neck veins. Acute pericardial effusion interferes with normal cardiac filling and pumping, causing venous congestion and decreased cardiac output. As the amount of fluid increases in the pericardial sac, heart sounds are obscured. A drop in systolic blood pressure of more than 10 mmHg on inspiration signifies an abnormal response to changes in intrathoracic pressure.

- Report significant changes or trends in hemodynamic parameters and dysrhythmias. *Compression of the heart interferes with venous return, increasing CVP and right atrial pressures; dysrhythmias may also occur.*
- Promptly report other signs of decreased cardiac output: decreased level of consciousness; decreased urine output; cold, clammy, mottled skin; delayed capillary refill; and weak peripheral pulses. *These signs of decreased organ and tissue perfusion indicate a significant drop in cardiac output.*
- Maintain at least one patent intravenous access site. *The client in cardiac tamponade may require rapid intravenous fluid infusion to restore blood volume and administration of emergency drugs to support the circulation.*
- Prepare for emergency pericardiocentesis and/or surgery as necessary. Provide appropriate explanations and reassurance. Observe for adverse responses during pericardiocentesis. *Excess pericardial fluid must be rapidly evacuated to prevent further compromise of cardiac output and death. Emotional support and explanations reduce the client's and family's anxiety and promote a caring atmosphere.*

Activity Intolerance

In chronic constrictive pericarditis, pericardial adhesions and scarring restrict pericardial compliance, restricting heart filling and movement. Restricted filling and ineffective cardiac contraction decrease the cardiac output. The heart cannot compen-

sate for increased metabolic demands by increasing cardiac output, and cardiac reserve falls significantly.

- Document vital signs, cardiac rhythm, skin color, and temperature before and after activity. Note any subjective complaints of fatigue, shortness of breath, chest pain, palpitations, or other symptoms with activity. *These parameters help determine the response to increased cardiac work. Increased heart rate and respiratory rate and effort, decreased blood pressure, and dysrhythmias are indicators of activity intolerance. Pallor or cyanosis and cool, clammy, mottled skin are signs of decreased tissue perfusion. Complaints of weakness, shortness of breath, fatigue, dizziness, or palpitations are further evidence of activity intolerance.*
- Work with the client and physical therapist to develop a realistic, progressive activity plan. Monitor response. Encourage independence, but provide assistance as needed. *Client involvement in planning increases the likelihood of success, as well as the client's self-esteem and sense of control. Promoting self-care provides additional control and independence and enhances self-image. Activity that significantly increases the heart rate (more than 20 beats/min over resting) should be stopped and reassessed for intensity.*
- Plan interventions and care activities to allow uninterrupted rest and sleep. *This supports healing and restoration of physical and emotional health.*

Community-Based Care

Include the following topics when teaching the client and family in preparation for home care:

- The importance of continuing anti-inflammatory medications as ordered. Advise to take NSAIDs with food, milk, or antacids to minimize gastric distress, and to notify the physician if unable to tolerate the drug. Instruct to avoid aspirin or preparations containing aspirin while taking NSAIDs because it may interfere with activity.
- Prescribed medications, including dose, desired and possible adverse effects, and interactions with other drugs or food.
- Monitoring weight twice weekly because NSAIDs may cause fluid retention.
- Maintaining fluid intake of at least 2500 mL/day to minimize the risk of renal toxicity due to NSAID use.
- Measures to maintain activity restriction if ordered. Activity will be gradually increased once the inflammatory process has resolved.
- Manifestations of recurrent pericarditis, and the importance of reporting these manifestations promptly to the physician.

DISORDERS OF CARDIAC STRUCTURE

THE CLIENT WITH VALVULAR HEART DISEASE

Proper heart valve function ensures one-way blood flow through the heart and vascular system. **Valvular heart disease** interferes with blood flow to and from the heart. Acquired valvular disorders can result from acute conditions, such as infective endocarditis, or from chronic conditions, such as rheumatic heart disease. Rheumatic heart disease is the most common cause of valvular disease (McCance & Huether,

2006). Acute myocardial infarction also can damage heart valves, causing tearing, ischemia, or damage to the papillary muscles that affects valve leaflet function. Congenital heart defects may affect the heart valves, often with no manifestations until adulthood. Aging affects heart structure and function, and also increases the risk for valvular disease.

Physiology Review

The heart valves direct blood flow within and out of the heart. The valves are fibroelastic tissue supported by a ring of fibrous tissue (the annulus) that provides support.

The AV valves, the **mitral** (or *bicuspid*) **valve** on the left and the **tricuspid valve** on the right, separate the atria from the ventricles. These valves normally are fully open during diastole, allowing blood to flow freely from the atria into the ventricles. Rising pressure within the ventricles at the onset of systole (contraction) closes the AV valves, creating the S_1 heart sound ("lub"). The leaflets of the AV valves are connected to ventricular papillary muscles by fibrous *chordae tendineae*. The chordae tendineae prevent the valve leaflets from bulging back into the atria during systole.

The semilunar valves, the **aortic** and **pulmonic valves**, separate the ventricles from the great vessels. They open during systole, allowing blood to flow out of the heart with ventricular contraction. As the ventricle relaxes and intraventricular pressure falls at the beginning of diastole, the higher pressure within the great vessels (the aorta and pulmonary artery) closes these valves, creating the S_2 heart sound ("dup").

Pathophysiology

Valvular heart disease occurs as two major types of disorders: stenosis and regurgitation. Stenosis occurs when valve leaflets fuse together and cannot fully open or close. The valve opening narrows and becomes rigid (Figure 32–10A ■). Scarring of the valves from endocarditis or infarction, and calcium deposits can lead to stenosis. Stenotic valves impede the forward flow of blood, decreasing cardiac output because of impaired ventricular filling or ejection and stroke volume. Because stenotic

valves also do not close completely, some backflow of blood occurs when the valve should be fully closed.

Regurgitant valves (also called *insufficient* or *incompetent* valves) do not close completely (Figure 32–10B). This allows regurgitation, or backflow of blood, through the valve into the area it just left. Regurgitation can result from deformity or erosion of valve cusps caused by the vegetative lesions of bacterial endocarditis, by scarring or tearing from myocardial infarction, or by cardiac dilation. As the heart enlarges, the valve *annulus* (supporting ring of the valve) is stretched, and the valve edges no longer meet to allow complete closure.

Valvular disease causes hemodynamic changes both in front of and behind the affected valve. Blood volume and pressures are reduced in front of the valve, because flow is obstructed through a stenotic valve and backflow occurs through a regurgitant valve. By contrast, volumes and pressures characteristically increase behind the diseased valve. These hemodynamic changes may lead to pulmonary complications or heart failure. Higher pressures and compensatory changes to maintain cardiac output lead to remodeling and hypertrophy of the heart muscle.

Stenosis increases the work of the chamber behind the affected valve as the heart attempts to move blood through the narrowed opening. Excess blood volume behind regurgitant valves causes dilation of the chamber. In mitral stenosis, for example, the left atrium hypertrophies to generate enough pressure to open and deliver its blood through the narrowed mitral valve. Not all of the blood is delivered before the valve closes, leaving blood to accumulate in the left atrium. This chamber dilates to accommodate the excess volume.

Eventually, cardiac output falls as compensatory mechanisms become less effective. The normal balance of oxygen supply and demand is upset, and the heart begins to fail. Increased muscle mass and size increase myocardial oxygen consumption. The size and workload of the heart exceed its blood supply, causing ischemia and chest pain. Eventually, necrosis occurs and functional muscle is lost. Contractile force, stroke volume, and cardiac output decrease. High pressures on the left side of the heart are reflected backward into the pulmonary system, causing pulmonary edema, pulmonary hypertension, and, eventually, right ventricular failure.

Valvular disorders interfere with the smooth flow of blood through the heart. The flow becomes turbulent, causing a **murmur**, a characteristic manifestation of valvular disease. Table 32–7 describes the murmurs associated with various types of valvular disorders.

Blood forced through the narrowed opening of a stenotic valve or regurgitated from a higher pressure chamber through an incompetent valve creates a jet stream effect (much like water spurting out of a partially occluded hose opening). The physical force of this jet stream damages the endocardium of the receiving chamber, increasing the risk for infective endocarditis.

The higher pressures on the left side of the heart subject its valves (the mitral and aortic valves) to more stress and damage than those on the right side of the heart (the tricuspid and pulmonic). Pulmonic valve disease is the least common of the valvular disorders.

 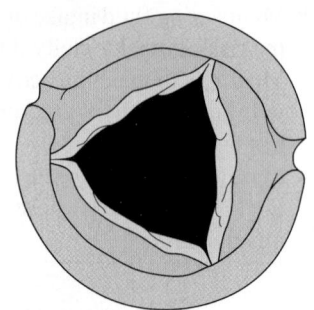

A. Thickened and stenotic valve leaflets

B. Retracted fibrosed valve openings

Figure 32–10 ■ Valvular heart disorders. *A,* Stenosis of a heart valve. *B,* An incompetent or regurgitant heart valve.

TABLE 32–7 Heart Murmur Timing and Characteristics

MURMUR	CARDIAC CYCLE TIMING	AUSCULTATION SITE	CONFIGURATION OF SOUND	CONTINUITY
Mitral stenosis	Diastole	Apical	S_2 ⟶ S_1	Rumble that increases in sound toward the end, continuous
Mitral regurgitation	Systole	Apex	S_1 ⟶ S_2	Holosystolic (occurs throughout systole), continuous
Aortic stenosis	Midsystolic	Right sternal border (RSB) 2nd intercostal space (ICS)	S_1 ⟶ S_2	Crescendo–decrescendo, continuous
Aortic regurgitation	Diastole (early)	3rd ICS, left sternal border (LSB)	S_2 ⟶ S_1	Decrescendo, continuous
Tricuspid stenosis	Diastole	Lower LSB	S_2 ⟶ S_1	Rumble that increases in sound toward the end, continuous
Tricuspid regurgitation	Systole	4th ICS, LSB	S_1 ⟶ S_2	Holosystolic, continuous

Mitral Stenosis

Mitral stenosis narrows the mitral valve, obstructing blood flow from the left atrium into the left ventricle during diastole. It is usually caused by rheumatic heart disease or bacterial endocarditis; it rarely results from congenital defects. It affects females more frequently (66%) than males (Kasper et al., 2005). Mitral stenosis is chronic and progressive.

In mitral valve stenosis, fibrous tissue replaces normal valve tissue, causing valve leaflets to stiffen and fuse. Resulting changes in blood flow through the valve lead to calcification of the valve leaflets. As calcium is deposited in and on the valve, the leaflets become more rigid and narrow the opening further. As the valve leaflets become less mobile, the chordae tendineae fuse, thicken, and shorten. Thromboemboli may form on the calcified leaflets.

The narrowed mitral opening impairs blood flow into the left ventricle, reducing end-diastolic volume and pressure, and decreasing stroke volume. The narrowed opening also forces the left atrium to generate higher pressure to deliver blood to the left ventricle. This leads to left atrial hypertrophy. The left atrium also dilates as obstructed blood flow increases its volume. As the resistance to blood flow increases, high atrial pressures are reflected back into the pulmonary vessels, increasing pulmonary pressures (Figure 32–11 ■). Pulmonary hypertension increases the workload of the right ventricle, causing it to dilate and hypertrophy. Eventually, heart failure occurs.

MANIFESTATIONS Mitral stenosis may be asymptomatic or cause severe impairment. Its manifestations depend on cardiac output and pulmonary vascular pressures. Dyspnea on exertion is typically the earliest manifestation. Others include cough, hemoptysis, frequent pulmonary infections such as bronchitis and pneumonia, paroxysmal nocturnal dyspnea, orthopnea, weakness, fatigue, and palpitations. As the stenosis worsens, manifestations of right heart failure, including jugular venous distention, hepatomegaly, ascites, and peripheral edema, develop. Crackles may be heard in the lung bases. In severe mitral stenosis, cyanosis of the face and extremities may be noted. Chest pain is rare but may occur.

On auscultation, a loud S_1, a split S_2, and a mitral opening snap may be heard. The opening snap reflects high left atrial pressure. The murmur of mitral stenosis occurs during diastole, and is typically low pitched, rumbling, crescendo–decrescendo. It is heard best with the bell of the stethoscope in the apical region. It may be accompanied by a palpable thrill (vibration).

COMPLICATIONS Atrial dysrhythmias, particularly atrial fibrillation, are common due to chronic atrial distention. Thrombi may form and subsequently embolize to the brain, coronary arteries, kidneys, spleen, and extremities—potentially devastating complications.

Women with mitral stenosis may be asymptomatic until pregnancy. As the heart tries to compensate for increased circulating volume (30% more in pregnancy) by increasing cardiac output,

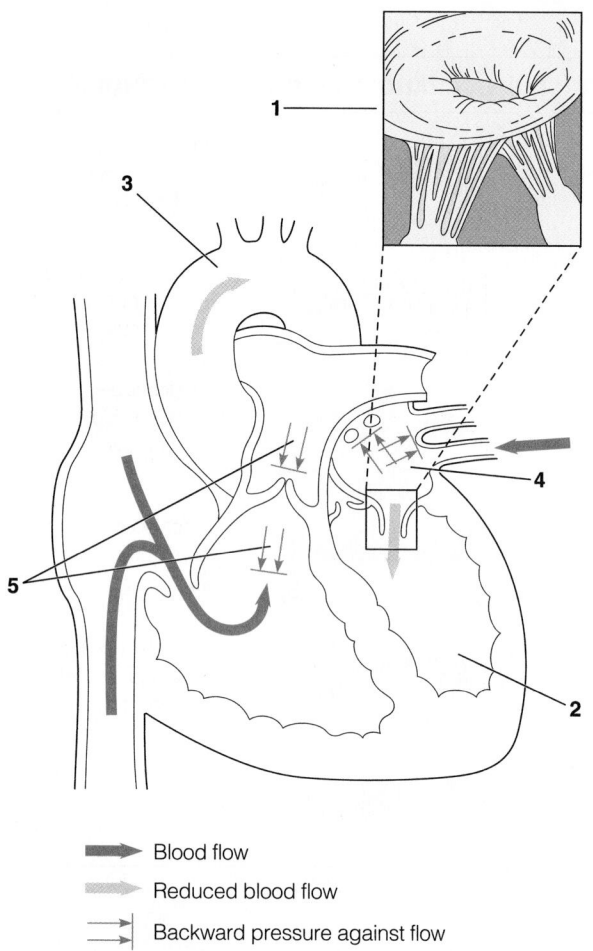

	Blood flow
	Reduced blood flow
	Backward pressure against flow

Figure 32–11 ■ Mitral stenosis. Narrowing of the mitral valve orifice *(1)* reduces blood volume to left ventricle *(2)* reducing cardiac output *(3)*. Rising pressure in the left atrium *(4)* causes left atrial hypertrophy and pulmonary congestion. Increased pressure in pulmonary vessels *(5)* causes hypertrophy of the right ventricle and right atrium.

left atrial pressures rise, tachycardia reduces ventricular filling and stroke volume, and pulmonary pressures increase. Sudden pulmonary edema and heart failure may threaten the lives of the mother and fetus.

Mitral Regurgitation

Mitral regurgitation or *insufficiency* allows blood to flow back into the left atrium during systole because the valve does not close fully. Rheumatic heart disease is a common cause of mitral regurgitation. Men develop mitral regurgitation more frequently than women. Degenerative calcification of the mitral annulus may cause mitral regurgitation in older women. Processes that dilate the mitral annulus or affect the supporting structures, papillary muscles, or the chordae tendineae may cause mitral regurgitation (e.g., left ventricular hypertrophy and MI). Congenital defects also may cause mitral regurgitation.

In mitral regurgitation, blood flows into both the systemic circulation and back into the left atrium through the deformed valve during systole. This increases left atrial volume (Figure 32–12 ■). The left atrium dilates to accommodate its extra volume, pulling

the posterior valve leaflet further away from the valve opening and worsening the defect. The left ventricle dilates to accommodate its increased preload and low cardiac output, further aggravating the problem.

MANIFESTATIONS Mitral regurgitation may be asymptomatic or cause symptoms such as fatigue, weakness, exertional dyspnea, and orthopnea. In severe or acute regurgitation, manifestations of left-sided heart failure develop, including pulmonary congestion and edema. High pulmonary pressures may lead to manifestations of right-sided heart failure.

The murmur of mitral regurgitation is usually loud, high pitched, rumbling, and holosystolic (occurring throughout systole). It is often accompanied by a palpable thrill and is heard most clearly at the cardiac apex. It may be characterized as a cooing or gull-like sound or have a musical quality (Kasper et al., 2005).

MITRAL VALVE PROLAPSE *Mitral valve prolapse (MVP)* is a type of mitral insufficiency that occurs when one or both mitral valve cusps billow into the atrium during ventricular systole.

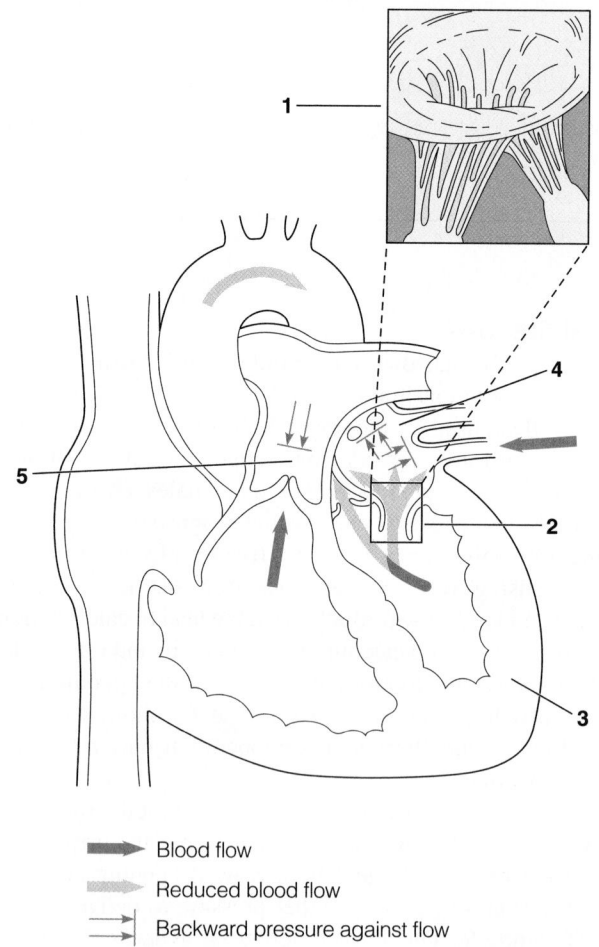

	Blood flow
	Reduced blood flow
	Backward pressure against flow

Figure 32–12 ■ Mitral regurgitation. The mitral valve closes incompletely *(1)*, allowing blood to regurgitate during systole from the left ventricle to the left atrium *(2)*. Cardiac output falls; to compensate, the left ventricle hypertrophies *(3)*. Rising left atrial pressure *(4)* causes left atrial hypertrophy and pulmonary congestion. Elevated pulmonary artery pressure *(5)* causes slight enlargement of the right ventricle.

MVP is more common in young women between ages 14 and 30; its incidence declines with age. Its cause often is unclear. It also can result from acute or chronic rheumatic damage, ischemic heart disease, or other cardiac disorders. It commonly affects people with inherited connective tissue disorders such as Marfan syndrome (see the Genetic Considerations box below). Mitral valve prolapse usually is benign, but about 0.01% to 0.02% of people with MVP have thickened mitral leaflets and a significant risk of morbidity and sudden death.

Excess collagen tissue in the valve leaflets and elongated chordae tendineae impair closure of the mitral valve, allowing the leaflets to billow into the left atrium during systole. Some ventricular blood volume regurgitates into the left atrium (Figure 32–13 ■).

MANIFESTATIONS AND COMPLICATIONS Mitral valve prolapse usually is asymptomatic. A midsystolic ejection click or murmur may be audible. A high-pitched late systolic murmur, sometimes described as a "whoop" or "honk," due to the regurgitation of blood through the valve, may develop in MVP. Atypical chest pain is the most common symptom of MVP. It may be left sided or substernal and is frequently related to fatigue, not exertion. Tachydysrhythmias may develop with MVP, causing palpitations, light-headedness, and syncope. Increased sympathetic nervous system tone may cause a sense of anxiety (Woods et al., 2004).

Mitral valve prolapse increases the risk for bacterial endocarditis. Progressive worsening of regurgitation can lead to heart failure. Thrombi may form on prolapsed valve leaflets; embolization may cause transient ischemic attacks (TIAs).

Aortic Stenosis

Aortic stenosis obstructs blood flow from the left ventricle into the aorta during systole. Aortic stenosis is more common in males (80%) than females (Kasper et al., 2005). Aortic stenosis may be idiopathic, or due to a congenital defect, rheumatic damage, or degenerative changes. When rheumatic heart disease is the cause, mitral valve deformity is also often present. RHD destroys aortic valve leaflets, with fibrosis and calcification causing rigidity and scarring. In the older adult, calcific aortic stenosis may result from degenerative changes associ-

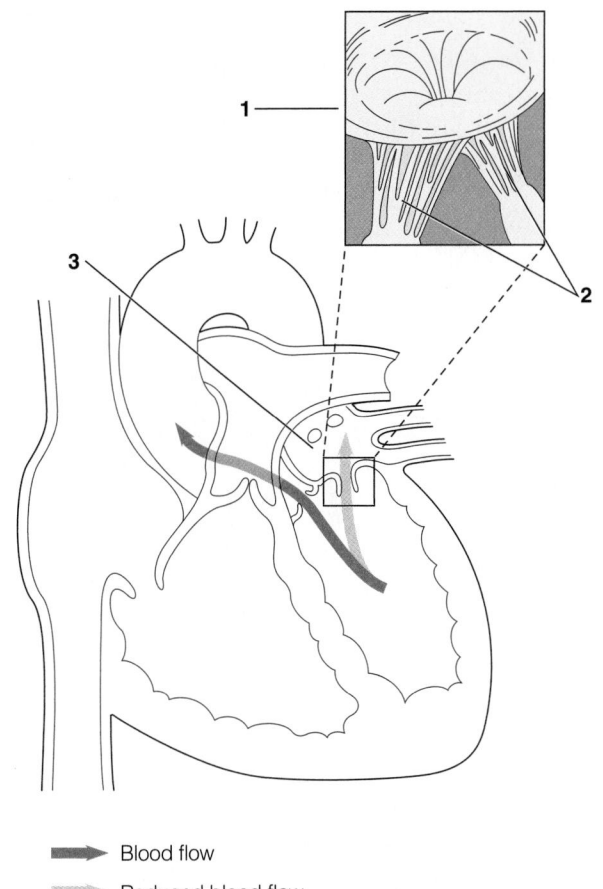

Blood flow

Reduced blood flow

Figure 32–13 ■ Mitral valve prolapse. Excess tissue in the valve leaflets *(1)* and elongated chordae tendineae *(2)* impair mitral valve closure during systole. Some ventricular blood regurgitates into the left atrium *(3)*.

ated with aging. Constant "wear and tear" on this valve can lead to fibrosis and calcification. Idiopathic calcific stenosis generally is mild and does not impair cardiac output.

As aortic stenosis progresses, the valve annulus decreases in size, increasing the work of the left ventricle to eject its volume through the narrowed opening into the aorta. To compensate, the ventricle hypertrophies to maintain an adequate stroke volume and cardiac output (Figure 32–14 ■). Left ventricular compliance also decreases. The additional workload increases myocardial oxygen consumption, which can precipitate myocardial ischemia. Coronary blood flow may also decrease in aortic stenosis. As left ventricular end-diastolic pressure increases because of reduced stroke volume, left atrial pressures increase. These pressures also affect the pulmonary vascular system; pulmonary vascular congestion and pulmonary edema may result.

COURSE AND MANIFESTATIONS Aortic stenosis may be asymptomatic for many years. As the disease progresses and compensation fails, usually between age 50 and 70 years, obstructed cardiac output causes manifestations of left ventricular failure. Dyspnea on exertion, angina pectoris, and exertional syncope are classic manifestations of aortic stenosis. Pulse pressure, an indicator of stroke volume, narrows to 30 mmHg

---

GENETIC CONSIDERATIONS
Clients with Marfan Syndrome

Marfan syndrome is a genetic (autosomal dominant) connective tissue disorder that affects the skeleton, eyes, and cardiovascular system. Skeletal characteristics include a long, thin body, with long extremities and long, tapering fingers, sometimes called *arachnodactyly* (spider fingers) (Copstead & Banasik, 2005). Joints are hyperextensible, and skeletal deformities such as kyphosis, scoliosis, pigeon chest, or pectus excavatum are common. The potentially life-threatening cardiovascular effects of Marfan syndrome include mitral valve prolapse, progressive dilation of the aortic valve ring, and weakness of arterial walls. People with Marfan syndrome frequently die young, between 30 and 40 years, often due to dissection and rupture of the aorta (Porth, 2005).

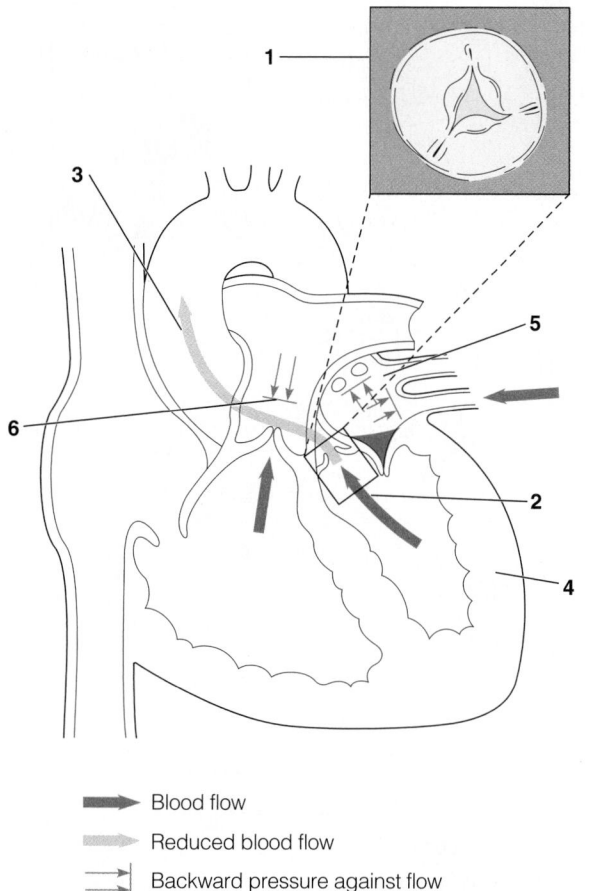

Blood flow

Reduced blood flow

Backward pressure against flow

Figure 32–14 ■ Aortic stenosis. The narrowed aortic valve orifice *(1)* decreases the left ventricular ejection fraction during systole *(2)* and cardiac output *(3)*. The left ventricle hypertrophies *(4)*. Incomplete emptying of the left atrium *(5)* causes backward pressure through pulmonary veins and pulmonary hypertension. Elevated pulmonary artery pressure *(6)* causes right ventricular strain.

or less. Hemodynamic monitors show increased left atrial pressure and pulmonary artery wedge pressure, as well as decreased stroke volume and cardiac output.

Aortic stenosis produces a harsh systolic murmur best heard in the second intercostal space to the right of the sternum. This crescendo–decrescendo murmur is produced by turbulence of blood entering the aorta through the stenotic valve. A palpable thrill is often felt. The murmur may radiate to the carotid arteries. Ventricular hypertrophy displaces the cardiac impulse to the left of the midclavicular line. As aortic stenosis progresses, S_3 and S_4 heart sounds may be heard, indicating heart failure and reduced left ventricular compliance.

As cardiac output falls, tissue perfusion decreases. Late in the disease, pulmonary hypertension and right ventricular failure develop. Untreated, symptomatic aortic stenosis has a poor prognosis; 10% to 20% of these clients experience sudden cardiac death (Kasper et al., 2005).

Aortic Regurgitation

Aortic regurgitation, also called *aortic insufficiency,* allows blood to flow back into the left ventricle from the aorta during diastole.

It is more common in males (75%) in its "pure" form; in females, it is commonly associated with coexisting mitral valve disease. Most aortic regurgitation (67%) results from rheumatic heart disease (Kasper et al., 2005). Other causes include congenital disorders, infective endocarditis, blunt chest trauma, aortic aneurysm, syphilis, Marfan syndrome, and chronic hypertension.

In aortic regurgitation, thickened and contracted valve cusps, scarring, fibrosis, and calcification impede complete valve closure. Chronic hypertension and aortic aneurysm may dilate and stretch the aortic valve opening, increasing the degree of regurgitation.

In aortic regurgitation, volume overload affects the left ventricle as blood from the aorta adds to blood received from the atrium during diastole. This increases diastolic left ventricular pressure. Increased preload causes more forceful contractions and a high stroke volume (Figure 32–15 ■). With time, muscle cells hypertrophy to compensate for increased cardiac work and afterload; eventually this hypertrophy compromises cardiac output and increases regurgitation.

High left-ventricular pressures increase left atrial workload and pressure. This pressure is transmitted to the pulmonary vessels, causing pulmonary congestion. The workload of the right

Blood flow

Reduced blood flow

Backward pressure against flow

Figure 32–15 ■ Aortic regurgitation. The cusps of the aortic valve widen and fail to close during diastole *(1)*. Blood regurgitates from the aorta into the left ventricle *(2)*, increasing left ventricular volume and decreasing cardiac output *(3)*. The left ventricle dilates and hypertrophies *(4)* in response to the increase in blood volume and workload.

ventricle increases as a result, and right-sided heart failure may develop. Acute aortic regurgitation from traumatic injury or infective endocarditis causes a rapid decline in hemodynamic status from acute heart failure and pulmonary edema, because compensatory mechanisms do not have time to develop.

MANIFESTATIONS Aortic regurgitation may be asymptomatic for many years, even when severe. The increased stroke volume may cause complaints of persistent palpitations, especially when recumbent. A throbbing pulse may be visible in arteries of the neck; the force of contraction may cause a characteristic head bob (Musset's sign) and shake the whole body. Other symptoms include dizziness and exercise intolerance.

Fatigue, exertional dyspnea, orthopnea, and paroxysmal nocturnal dyspnea are common in aortic regurgitation. Anginal pain may result from excessive cardiac work and decreased coronary perfusion. Unlike CHD, angina often occurs at night and may not respond to conventional therapy.

The murmur of aortic regurgitation is heard during diastole as blood flows back into the left ventricle from the aorta. It is a "blowing," high-pitched sound heard most clearly at the third left intercostal space. A palpable thrill and ventricular heave may be noted. An S_3 and S_4 may be heard as the heart fails and ventricular compliance diminishes. The apical impulse is displaced to the left.

High systolic and low diastolic pressures cause a widened pulse pressure. The arterial pressure waveform has a rapid upstroke and quickly collapsing downstroke, known as a *water-hammer pulse*. It is caused by the force of rapid and early delivery of the stroke volume into the aorta.

Tricuspid Valve Disorders

Tricuspid stenosis obstructs blood flow from the right atrium to the right ventricle. It usually results from rheumatic heart disease; mitral stenosis often occurs concurrently with tricuspid stenosis.

Fibrosed, retracted tricuspid valve cusps and fused leaflets narrow the valve orifice and prevent complete closure. Right ventricular filling is impaired during diastole, and during systole, some blood regurgitates back into the right atrium. Pressure in the right atrium increases, and it enlarges in response to the increased pressure and workload. This increased right atrial pressure is reflected backward into the systemic circulation. Right ventricular stroke volume decreases, reducing the volume delivered to the pulmonary system and left heart. Stroke volume, cardiac output, and tissue perfusion fall.

Manifestations of tricuspid stenosis relate to systemic congestion and right-sided heart failure. They include increased CVP, jugular venous distention, ascites, hepatomegaly, and peripheral edema. Low cardiac output causes fatigue and weakness. The low-pitched, rumbling diastolic murmur of tricuspid stenosis is most clearly heard in the fourth intercostal space at the left sternal border or over the xiphoid process.

Tricuspid regurgitation usually occurs secondarily to right ventricular dilation. Stretching distorts the valve and its supporting structures, preventing complete valve closure. Left ventricular failure is the usual cause of right ventricular overload; pulmonary hypertension is another cause. The valve may also be damaged by rheumatic heart disease, infective endocarditis, inferior MI, trauma, or other conditions.

Tricuspid regurgitation allows blood to flow back into the right atrium during systole, increasing right atrial pressures. Increased right atrial pressure causes manifestations of right-sided heart failure, including systemic venous congestion and low cardiac output. Atrial fibrillation due to atrial distention is common. The retrograde flow of blood over the deformed tricuspid valve causes a high-pitched, blowing systolic murmur heard over the tricuspid or xiphoid area.

Pulmonic Valve Disorders

Pulmonic stenosis obstructs blood flow from the right ventricle into the pulmonary system. It usually is a congenital disorder, although rheumatic heart disease or cancer also may cause pulmonic stenosis. The right ventricle hypertrophies to generate the pressure needed to pump blood into the pulmonary system. The right atrium also hypertrophies to overcome the high pressures generated in the right ventricle. Right-sided heart failure occurs when the ventricle can no longer generate adequate pressure to force blood past the narrowed valve opening.

Pulmonic stenosis typically is asymptomatic unless severe. Dyspnea on exertion and fatigue are early signs. As the condition progresses, right-sided heart failure develops, with peripheral edema, ascites, hepatomegaly, and increased venous pressures. Turbulent blood flow caused by the narrowed valve generates a harsh, systolic crescendo–decrescendo murmur heard in the pulmonic area, the second left intercostal space.

Pulmonic regurgitation is more common than pulmonary stenosis. It is a complication of pulmonary hypertension, which stretches and dilates the pulmonary orifice, causing incomplete valve closure. Infective endocarditis, pulmonary artery aneurysm, and syphilis also may cause pulmonic regurgitation.

Incomplete valve closure allows blood to flow back into the right ventricle during diastole, decreasing blood flow to the pulmonary circuit. The extra blood increases right ventricular end-diastolic volume. When the ventricle can no longer compensate for the increased volume, right-sided heart failure develops. The murmur of pulmonic regurgitation is a high-pitched, decrescendo, blowing sound heard along the left sternal border during diastole.

INTERDISCIPLINARY CARE

A heart murmur identified during routine physical examination often is the initial indication of valvular disease. If no symptoms are present, close observation for disease progression and prophylactic therapy to prevent infection of the diseased heart may be the only treatment.

Manifestations of heart failure are treated with diet and medications (see the preceding section on heart failure). When medical management is no longer effective, surgery is considered.

Diagnosis

The following diagnostic tests help to identify and diagnose valvular disease. See Chapter 30 ∞ for more information about these tests and related nursing care.

- *Echocardiography* is used routinely to diagnose valvular disease. Thickened valve leaflets, vegetations or growths on valve leaflets, myocardial function, and chamber size can be determined, and pressure gradients across valves and pulmonary artery pressures can be estimated. Either transthoracic or transesophageal echocardiography may be used.
- *Chest x-ray* can identify cardiac hypertrophy, chamber and great vessel enlargement, and dilation of the pulmonary vasculature. Calcification of the valve leaflets and annular openings may also be visible.
- *Electrocardiography* can demonstrate atrial and ventricular hypertrophy, conduction defects, and dysrhythmias associated with valvular disease.
- *Cardiac catheterization* may be used to assess contractility and to determine the pressure gradients across the heart valves, in the heart chambers, and in the pulmonary system.

Medications

Heart failure resulting from valvular disease is treated with diuretics, ACE inhibitors, vasodilators, and possibly digitalis glycosides. Digitalis increases the force of myocardial contraction to maintain cardiac output. Diuretics, ACE inhibitors, and vasodilators reduce preload and afterload. (See the Medication Administration box on pages 1033–1034.)

In clients with valvular disorders, atrial distention often causes atrial fibrillation. Digitalis or small doses of beta-blockers are given to slow the ventricular response. (See Chapter 31 ∞ for more information about atrial fibrillation and its treatment.) Anticoagulant therapy is added to prevent clot and embolus formation, a common complication of atrial fibrillation as blood pools in the noncontracting atria. Anticoagulant therapy also is required following insertion of a mechanical heart valve. See Chapter 35 ∞ for more information about anticoagulant therapy.

Valvular damage increases the risk for infective endocarditis as altered blood flow allows bacterial colonization. Antibiotics are prescribed prophylactically prior to any dental work, invasive procedures, or surgery to minimize the risk of bacteremia (bacteria in the blood) and subsequent endocarditis.

Percutaneous Balloon Valvuloplasty

Percutaneous balloon valvuloplasty is an invasive procedure performed in the cardiac catheterization laboratory. A balloon catheter similar to that used in coronary angioplasty procedures is inserted into the femoral vein or artery. Guided by fluoroscopy, the catheter is advanced into the heart and positioned with the balloon straddling the stenotic valve. The balloon is then inflated for approximately 90 seconds to divide the fused leaflets and enlarge the valve orifice (Figure 32–16 ■). Balloon valvuloplasty is the treatment of choice for symptomatic mitral valve stenosis. It is used to treat children and young adults with aortic stenosis, and may be indicated for older adults who are poor surgical risks, and as a "bridge to surgery" when heart function is severely compromised (Kasper et al., 2005). Nursing care of the client with a balloon valvuloplasty is similar to that of the client following percutaneous coronary revascularization (see page 978).

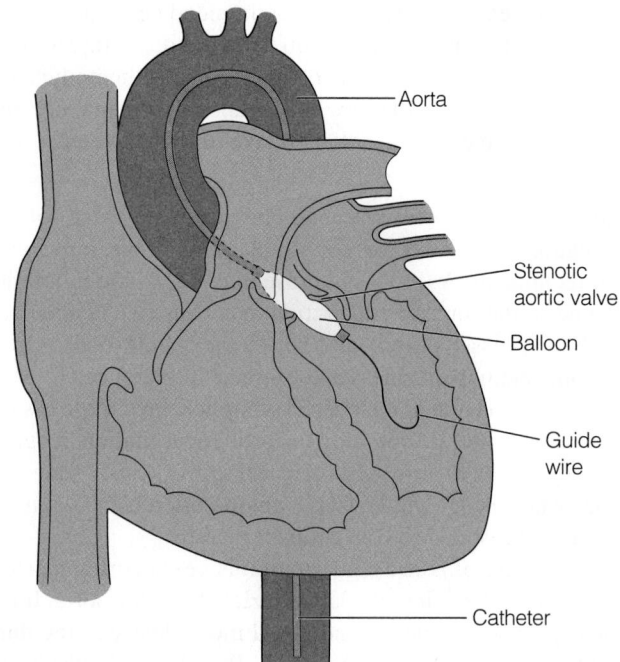

Figure 32–16 ■ Balloon valvuloplasty. The balloon catheter is guided into position straddling the stenosed valve. The balloon is then inflated to increase the size of the valve opening.

Labels: Aorta; Stenotic aortic valve; Balloon; Guide wire; Catheter

Surgery

Surgery to repair or replace the diseased valve may be done to restore valve function, alleviate symptoms, and prevent complications and death. Ideally, diseased valves are repaired or replaced before cardiopulmonary function is severely compromised. The diseased valve is repaired when possible, because the risk for surgical mortality and complications is lower than with valve replacement.

RECONSTRUCTIVE SURGERY *Valvuloplasty* is a general term for reconstruction or repair of a heart valve. Methods include "patching" the perforated portion of the leaflet, resecting excess tissue, debriding vegetations or calcification, and other techniques. Valvuloplasty may be used for stenotic or regurgitant mitral and tricuspid valves, mitral valve prolapse, and aortic stenosis. Common valvuloplasty procedures include the following:

- *Open commissurotomy,* surgical division of fused valve leaflets, is done to open stenotic valves. Fused commissures (junctions between valve leaflets or cusps) are incised, and calcium deposits are debrided as needed.
- *Annuloplasty* repairs a narrowed or an enlarged or dilated valve annulus, the supporting ring of the valve. A prosthetic ring may be used to resize the opening, or stitches and purse-string sutures may be used to reduce and gather excess tissue. Annuloplasty may be used for either stenotic or regurgitant valves.

VALVE REPLACEMENT Valve replacement is indicated when manifestations of valve dysfunction develop, preferably before left heart function is seriously impaired. In general, three factors determine the outcome of valve replacement surgery: (1) heart function at the time of surgery, (2) intraoperative and

TABLE 32–8 Advantages and Disadvantages of Prosthetic Heart Valves

CATEGORY	TYPES	ADVANTAGES	DISADVANTAGES
Mechanical valves	Ball-and-cage Tilting disk	Long-term durability Good hemodynamics	Lifetime anticoagulation Audible click Risk of thromboembolism Infections are harder to treat
Biologic tissue valves	Porcine heterograft Bovine heterograft Human aortic homograft	Low incidence of thromboembolism No long-term anticoagulation Good hemodynamics Quiet Infections are easier to treat	Prone to deterioration Frequent replacement is required

postoperative care, and (3) characteristics and durability of the replacement valve.

Many different prosthetic heart valves are available, including mechanical and biologic tissue valves. Selection depends on the valve hemodynamics, resistance to clot formation, ease of insertion, anatomic suitability, and client acceptance (Rothrock, 2003). The client's age, underlying condition, and contraindications to anticoagulation (such as a desire to become pregnant) also are considered in selecting the appropriate prosthesis. Table 32–8 lists the advantages and disadvantages of biologic and mechanical valves.

Biologic tissue valves may be *heterografts,* excised from a pig (Figure 32–17A ■) or made of calf pericardium, or *homografts* from a human (obtained from a cadaver or during heart transplant). Biologic valves allow more normal blood flow and have a low risk of thrombus formation. As a result, long-term anticoagulation rarely is necessary. They are less durable, however, than mechanical valves. Up to 50% of biologic valves must be replaced by 15 years.

Mechanical prosthetic valves have the major advantage of long-term durability. These valves are frequently used when life expectancy exceeds 10 years. Their major disadvantage is the need for lifetime anticoagulation to prevent the development of clots on the valve.

Most mechanical valves are either a tilting-disk (Figure 32–17B) or a ball-and-cage design. The tilting-disk valve designs are frequently used because they have a lower profile than the caged-ball types, allowing blood to flow through the valve with less obstruction. The St. Jude bileaflet design has good hemodynamics and low risk for clot formation. Both biologic and mechanical valves increase the risk of endocarditis, although its incidence is fairly low.

 NURSING CARE

Health Promotion

Preventing rheumatic heart disease is a key element in preventing heart valve disorders. Rheumatic heart disease is a consequence of rheumatic fever (see the previous section of this chapter), an immune process that may be a sequela to beta-hemolytic streptococcal infection of the pharynx (strep throat). Early treatment of strep throat prevents rheumatic fever. Teach individual clients, families, and communities

A   B

Figure 32–17 ■ Prosthetic heart valves. *A,* Mosaic tissue valve. *B,* Medtronic Hall Prosthetic valve.

about the importance of timely and effective treatment of strep throat. Emphasize the importance of completing the full prescription of antibiotics to prevent development of resistant bacteria. Prophylactic antibiotic therapy before invasive procedures to prevent infectious endocarditis is an important health promotion measure for clients with preexisting heart disease.

Assessment

Assessment data related to valvular heart disease include the following:

- *Health history:* Complaints of decreasing exercise tolerance, dyspnea on exertion, palpitations; history of frequent respiratory infections; previous history of rheumatic heart disease, endocarditis, or a heart murmur.
- *Physical examination:* Vital signs; skin color and temperature, evidence of clubbing or peripheral edema; neck vein distention; breath sounds; heart sounds and presence of S_3, S_4, or murmur; timing, grade, and characteristics of any murmur; palpate for cardiac heave and thrills; abdominal contour, liver and spleen size.
- *Diagnostic tests:* Echocardiogram and cardiac catheterization reports; cardiac index and cardiac output.

Nursing Diagnoses and Interventions

Nursing priorities include maintaining cardiac output, managing manifestations of the disorder, teaching about the disease process and its management, and preventing complications. Nursing care of the client undergoing valve surgery is similar to that of the client having other types of open-heart surgery, with increased attention to anticoagulation and preventing endocarditis.

Decreased Cardiac Output

Nearly all valve disorders affect ventricular filling and/or emptying, reducing cardiac output. Stenosis of the AV valves impairs ventricular filling and increases atrial pressures. Regurgitation of these valves reduces cardiac output as a portion of the blood in the ventricle regurgitates into the atria during systole. Stenosis of the semilunar valves obstructs ventricular outflow to the great vessels; regurgitation allows blood to flow back into the ventricles, creating higher filling pressures. When compensatory measures fail, heart failure develops.

- Monitor vital signs and hemodynamic parameters, reporting changes from the baseline. *A fall in systolic blood pressure and tachycardia may indicate decreased cardiac output. Increasing pulmonary artery and pulmonary wedge pressures may also indicate decreased cardiac output, causing increased congestion and pressure in the pulmonary vascular system.*

PRACTICE ALERT
Promptly report changes in level of consciousness; distended neck veins; dyspnea or respiratory crackles; urine output less than 30 mL/h; cool, clammy, or cyanotic skin; diminished peripheral pulses; or slow capillary refill. These findings indicate decreased cardiac output and impaired tissue and organ perfusion.

- Monitor intake and output; weigh daily. Report weight gain of 3 to 5 lb within 24 hours. *Fluid retention is a compensatory mechanism that occurs when cardiac output decreases; 2.2 lb (1 kg) of weight equals 1 L of fluid.*
- Restrict fluids as ordered. *Fluid intake may be restricted to reduce cardiac workload and pressures within the heart and pulmonary circuit.*
- Monitor oxygen saturation continuously and arterial blood gases as ordered. Report oxygen saturation less than 95% (or as specified) and abnormal ABG results. *Oxygen saturation levels and ABGs allow assessment of oxygenation.*
- Elevate the head of the bed. Administer supplemental oxygen as ordered. *These measures improve alveolar ventilation and oxygenation.*
- Provide for physical, emotional, and mental rest. *Physical and psychologic rest decrease the cardiac workload.*
- Administer prescribed medications as ordered to reduce cardiac workload. *Diuretics, ACE inhibitors, and direct vasodilators may be prescribed to reduce fluid volume and afterload, reducing cardiac work.*

Activity Intolerance

Altered blood flow through the heart impairs delivery of oxygen and nutrients to the tissues. As the heart muscle fails and is unable to compensate for altered blood flow, tissue perfusion is further compromised. Dyspnea on exertion is often an early symptom of valvular disease.

- Monitor vital signs before and during activities. *A change in heart rate of more than 20 bpm, a change of 20 mmHg or more in systolic BP, and complaints of dyspnea, shortness of breath, excessive fatigue, chest pain, diaphoresis, dizziness, or syncope may indicate activity intolerance.*
- Encourage self-care and gradually increasing activities as allowed and tolerated. Provide for rest periods, uninterrupted sleep, and adequate nutritional intake. *Gradual progression of activities avoids excessive cardiac stress. Encouraging self-care increases the client's self-esteem and sense of power. Adequate rest and nutrition facilitate healing, decrease fatigue, and increase energy reserves.*
- Provide assistance as needed. Suggest use of a shower chair, sitting while brushing hair or teeth, and other energy-saving measures. *Reducing energy expenditure helps maintain a balance of oxygen supply and demand.*
- Consult with cardiac rehabilitation specialist or physical therapist for in-bed exercises and an activity plan. *In-bed exercises may help improve strength.*
- Discuss ways to conserve energy at home. *Information provides practical ways to deal with activity limitations and empowers the client to manage these limitations.*

Risk for Infection

Damaged and deformed valve leaflets and turbulent blood flow through the heart significantly increase the risk of infective endocarditis. Invasive diagnostic and monitoring lines (e.g., cardiac catheterization, hemodynamic monitoring) and disrupted skin with surgery also increase the risk of infection.

- Use aseptic technique for all invasive procedures. *Invasive procedures breach the body's protective mechanisms, poten-*

tially allowing bacteria to enter. Aseptic technique reduces this risk.

> **PRACTICE ALERT**
> Record temperature every 4 hours; notify physician if temperature exceeds 100.5°F (38.5°C). Fever may be an early indication of infection.

- Assess wounds and catheter sites for redness, swelling, warmth, pain, or evidence of drainage. *These signs of inflammation may signal infection.*
- Administer antibiotics as ordered. Ensure completion of the full course. *Antibiotics are used to prevent and treat infection. Completion of the full course of therapy prevents drug-resistant organisms from multiplying.*
- Monitor WBC and differential. Notify physician of leukocytosis or leukopenia. *A high WBC count and increased percentage of immature WBCs (bands) may indicate bacterial infection; a low WBC count may indicate an impaired immune response and increased susceptibility to infection.*

Ineffective Protection

Anticoagulant therapy commonly is prescribed for clients with chronic atrial fibrillation, a history of emboli, and following valve replacement surgery. Although chronic anticoagulant therapy decreases the risk of clots and emboli, it increases the risk for bleeding and hemorrhage.

> **PRACTICE ALERT**
> Monitor the International Normalized Ratio (INR) or prothrombin time (PT or protime). Report an INR > 3.5 or a PT > 2.5 times the normal to the physician. An excessively high INR or PT indicate excessive anticoagulation and an increased risk for bleeding.

- Test stools and vomitus for occult blood. *Bleeding due to excessive anticoagulation may not be apparent.*
- Instruct to avoid using aspirin or other NSAIDs. Encourage reading ingredient labels on over-the-counter drugs; many contain aspirin. *Aspirin and other NSAIDs interfere with clotting and may potentiate the effects of the anticoagulant therapy.*
- Advise using a soft-bristled toothbrush, electric razor, and gentle touch when cleaning fragile skin. *These measures decrease the risk of skin or gum trauma and bleeding.*

> **PRACTICE ALERT**
> Monitor hemoglobin, hematocrit, and platelet count as ordered. Notify the physician of decreasing hemoglobin and hematocrit levels or if the platelet count falls below 50,000/mm³. Low hemoglobin and hematocrit indicate blood loss. Platelet counts below 50,000/mm³ significantly increase the risk of bleeding.

Community-Based Care

For most clients, valvular disease is a chronic condition. The client has the primary responsibility for managing effects of the disorder. To prepare the client and family for home care, discuss the following topics:

- Management of symptoms, including any necessary activity restrictions or lifestyle changes
- The importance of adequate rest to prevent fatigue
- Diet restrictions to reduce fluid retention and symptoms of heart failure
- Information about prescribed medications, including purpose, desired and possible adverse effects, scheduling, and possible interactions with other drugs
- The importance of keeping follow-up appointments to monitor the disease and its treatment
- Notifying all healthcare providers about valve disease or surgery to facilitate prescription of prophylactic antibiotics before invasive procedures or dental work
- Manifestations to immediately report to the healthcare provider: increasing severity of symptoms, especially of worsening heart failure or pulmonary edema; signs of transient ischemic attacks or other embolic events; evidence of bleeding, such as joint pain, easy bruising, black and tarry stools, bleeding gums, or blood in the urine or sputum.

Provide referrals to community resources such as home maintenance services, home health services, and structured cardiac rehabilitation programs. Refer the client and family (especially the primary food preparer) to a dietitian or nutritionist for teaching and assistance with menu planning. See the accompanying Nursing Care Plan for additional nursing care and teaching for a client with mitral valve prolapse.

THE CLIENT WITH CARDIOMYOPATHY

The **cardiomyopathies** are disorders that affect the heart muscle itself. They are a diverse group of disorders that affect both systolic and diastolic functions. Cardiomyopathies may be either primary or secondary in origin. Primary cardiomyopathies are idiopathic; their cause is unknown. Secondary cardiomyopathies occur as a result of other processes, such as ischemia, infectious disease, exposure to toxins, connective tissue disorders, metabolic disorders, or nutritional deficiencies. In many cases, the cause of cardiomyopathy is unknown. Close to 27,000 deaths annually are directly attributed to cardiomyopathy. Mortality associated with cardiomyopathy is higher in older adults, men, and African Americans (AHA, 2005).

Pathophysiology

The cardiomyopathies are categorized by their pathophysiology and presentation into three groups: dilated, hypertrophic, and restrictive. Table 32–9 compares the causes, pathophysiology, manifestations, and management of the cardiomyopathies.

Dilated Cardiomyopathy

Dilated cardiomyopathy is the most common type of cardiomyopathy, accounting for 87% of cases (AHA, 2005). Dilated cardiomyopathy also is a common cause of heart failure, accounting for about one in three cases. It is primarily a disease of middle age males; African American males have a higher risk than whites (Kasper et al., 2005).

NURSING CARE PLAN   A Client with Mitral Valve Prolapse

Julie Snow, a 22-year-old college student, sees a nurse practitioner at the college health clinic for a physical examination after experiencing palpitations, fatigue, and a headache during midterm examinations. Ms. Snow tells Lakisha Johnson, FNP, "I'm scared that something is wrong with me."

Over the last few months, Ms. Snow has had occasional palpitations that she describes as "feeling like my heart is doing flip-flops." Rarely, these palpitations have been accompanied by a sharp, stabbing pain in her chest that lasts only a few seconds. She initially attributed her symptoms to stress, but she is increasingly concerned because the "attacks" are becoming more frequent. Ms. Snow states that she has "always been healthy," does not smoke, uses alcohol socially, and exercises, albeit intermittently. Ms. Snow admits that she has been drinking a lot of coffee and cola and eating a lot of "junk food" lately.

ASSESSMENT

Ms. Johnson's assessment of Ms. Snow documents the following: height 66 in. (168 cm), weight 140 lb (63.6 kg), T 99.3, BP 118/64, P 82, and R 18. Slightly anxious but in no acute distress. Systolic click and soft crescendo murmur grade II/VI noted on auscultation. Apical impulse at fifth ICS left MCL. Lungs clear to auscultation. Review of remaining systems reveals no apparent abnormalities. An ECG shows sinus rhythm with occasional PACs. Based on the admission history, manifestations, and physical assessment, Ms. Johnson suspects mitral valve prolapse (MVP).

DIAGNOSES

- *Anxiety* related to fear of heart disease and implications for lifestyle
- *Powerlessness* related to unpredictability of symptoms
- *Risk of Infection (Endocarditis)* related to altered valve function

EXPECTED OUTCOMES

- Verbalize an understanding of MVP and its management.
- Discuss ways to decrease or relieve MVP symptoms.
- Acknowledge the risk for endocarditis and identify precautions to prevent it.

PLANNING AND IMPLEMENTATION

- Consult with and refer to cardiologist for continued monitoring and follow-up.
- Teach about MVP, including heart valve anatomy, physiology, and function, common manifestations of MVP, and treatment rationale.
- Discuss symptoms of progressive mitral regurgitation, and the need to report these to the cardiologist.
- Discuss recommended follow-up care and its rationale.

- Allow to verbalize feelings and share concerns about MVP. Encourage to attend an MVP support group meeting.
- Discuss the prognosis for MVP, emphasizing that most clients live normal lives using diet and lifestyle management.
- Instruct to keep a weekly record of symptoms and their frequency for 1 month.
- Discuss lifestyle changes to manage symptoms: aerobic exercise with warm-up and cooldown periods; maintaining adequate fluid intake, especially during hot weather or exercise; relaxation techniques (e.g., meditation, deep-breathing exercises, music therapy, yoga, guided imagery, heat therapy, or progressive muscle relaxation) to perform daily; avoiding caffeine and crash diets; forming healthy eating habits.
- Teach about infective endocarditis risk and prevention with prophylactic antibiotics. Encourage notifying dentist and other healthcare providers of MVP before dental or any invasive procedure.

EVALUATION

After several educational sessions at the college health clinic, Ms. Snow verbalizes an understanding of MVP by explaining heart valve function, listing common manifestations of MVP, and describing indications of deteriorating heart function. She states she will report these manifestations to her cardiologist if they occur. She is given a booklet on MVP for additional reading. She also verbalizes understanding of the risk of endocarditis, and states that she will notify her doctors of her MVP and the need for antibiotics before invasive procedures. Ms. Snow is attending a monthly MVP support group (led by a cardiology clinical nurse specialist) on campus and states, "I am so glad to know I'm not alone! It really helps to know that others are living well with MVP." Her weekly symptom log shows her symptoms are associated with late-night studying and drinking large amounts of coffee and cola. Ms. Snow has moderated her caffeine intake and increased her fluids, relieving her symptoms. In addition, Ms. Snow is taking a relaxation music therapy class. Ms. Snow states that she realizes that she has "the ability to control my life through the choices I make."

CRITICAL THINKING IN THE NURSING PROCESS

1. Develop an action plan for Ms. Snow that outlines specific activities she can use to manage symptoms of MVP.
2. Why are clients with symptomatic MVP encouraged to include regular exercise in their health habits?
3. How does the support of family, friends, and other people with MVP assist MVP clients in managing their condition?
4. What manifestations would indicate a progressive worsening of Ms. Snow's mitral regurgitation?

See Evaluating Your Response in Appendix C.

The cause of dilated cardiomyopathy is unknown, although it appears to frequently result from toxins, metabolic conditions, or infection. Reversible dilated cardiomyopathy may develop due to alcohol and cocaine abuse, chemotherapeutic drugs, pregnancy, and systemic hypertension. Up to 20% of cases of dilated cardiomyopathy may be genetic in origin, most commonly transmitted in an autosomal dominant pattern, although autosomal recessive, X-linked, and mitochondrial

patterns of inheritance also are seen (Kasper et al., 2005; Porth, 2005).

In dilated cardiomyopathy, heart chambers dilate and ventricular contraction is impaired. Both end-diastolic and end-systolic volumes increase, and the left ventricular ejection fraction is substantially reduced, decreasing cardiac output. Left ventricular dilation is prominent; left ventricular hypertrophy is usually minimal. The right ventricle also may be enlarged. Ex-

TABLE 32–9 Classifications of Cardiomyopathy

	DILATED	HYPERTROPHIC	RESTRICTIVE
Causes	Usually idiopathic; may be secondary to chronic alcoholism or myocarditis	Hereditary; may be secondary to chronic hypertension	Usually secondary to amyloidosis, radiation, or myocardial fibrosis
Pathophysiology	Scarring and atrophy of myocardial cells Thickening of ventricular wall Dilation of heart chambers Impaired ventricular pumping Increased end-diastolic and end-systolic volumes Mural thrombi common	Hypertrophy of ventricular muscle mass Small left ventricular volume Septal hypertrophy may obstruct left ventricular outflow Left atrial dilation	Excess rigidity of ventricular walls restricts filling Myocardial contractility remains relatively normal
Manifestations	Heart failure Cardiomegaly Dysrhythmias S_3 and S_4 gallop; murmur of mitral regurgitation	Dyspnea, anginal pain, syncope Left ventricular hypertrophy Dysrhythmias Loud S_4 Sudden death	Dyspnea, fatigue Right-sided heart failure Mild to moderate cardiomegaly S_3 and S_4 Mitral regurgitation murmur
Management	Management of heart failure Implantable cardioverter-defibrillator (ICD) as needed Cardiac transplantation	Beta-blockers Calcium channel blockers Antidysrhythmic agents ICD, dual-chamber pacing Surgical excision of part of the ventricular septum	Management of heart failure Exercise restriction

tensive interstitial fibrosis (scarring) is evident; necrotic myocardial cells also may be seen (Kasper et al., 2005).

MANIFESTATIONS AND COURSE Manifestations of dilated cardiomyopathy develop gradually. Heart failure often presents years after the onset of dilation and pump failure. Both right- and left-sided failure occur, with dyspnea on exertion, orthopnea, paroxysmal nocturnal dyspnea, weakness, fatigue, peripheral edema, and ascites. Both S_3 and S_4 heart sounds are commonly heard, as well as an AV regurgitation murmur. Dysrhythmias are common, including supraventricular tachycardias, atrial fibrillation, and complex ventricular tachycardias. Untreated dysrhythmias can lead to sudden death (Porth, 2005). Mural thrombi (blood clots in the heart wall) may form in the left ventricular apex and embolize to other parts of the body.

The prognosis of dilated cardiomyopathy is grim; most clients get progressively worse and 50% die within 5 years after the diagnosis; 75% die within 10 years (AHA, 2005).

Hypertrophic Cardiomyopathy

Hypertrophic cardiomyopathy is characterized by decreased compliance of the left ventricle and hypertrophy of the ventricular muscle mass. This impairs ventricular filling, leading to small end-diastolic volumes and low cardiac output. About half of all clients with hypertrophic cardiomyopathy have a family history of the disease. It is genetically transmitted in an autosomal dominant pattern (Kasper et al., 2005).

The pattern of left ventricular hypertrophy is unique in that the muscle may not hypertrophy "equally." In a majority of clients, the interventricular septal mass, especially the upper portion, increases to a greater extent than the free wall of the ventricle. The enlarged upper septum narrows the passageway of blood into the aorta, impairing ventricular outflow. For this reason, this disorder is also known as *idiopathic hypertrophic subaortic stenosis (IHSS)* or *hypertrophic obstructive cardiomyopathy (HOCM)*.

MANIFESTATIONS AND COURSE Hypertrophic cardiomyopathy may be asymptomatic for many years. Symptoms typically occur when increased oxygen demand causes increased ventricular contractility. They may develop suddenly during or after physical activity; in children and young adults, sudden cardiac death may be the first sign of the disorder. Hypertrophic cardiomyopathy is the probable or definite cause of death in 36% of young athletes who die suddenly (AHA, 2005). It is hypothesized that sudden cardiac death is due to ventricular dysrhythmias or hemodynamic factors. Predictors of sudden cardiac death in this population include age of less than 30 years, a family history of sudden death, syncopal episodes, severe ventricular hypertrophy, and ventricular tachycardia seen on ambulatory ECG monitoring (Kasper et al., 2005). (For a brief synopsis of a nursing research study regarding family presence during CPR and invasive procedures, see the box below.)

The usual manifestations of hypertrophic cardiomyopathy are dyspnea, angina, and syncope. Angina may result from ischemia due to overgrowth of the ventricular muscle, coronary artery abnormalities, or decreased coronary artery perfusion. Syncope may occur when the outflow tract obstruction severely decreases cardiac output and blood flow to the brain. Ventricular dysrhythmias are common; atrial fibrillation also may develop. Other manifestations of hypertrophic cardiomyopathy include fatigue, dizziness, and palpitations. A harsh, crescendo–decrescendo systolic murmur of variable intensity heard best at the lower left sternal border and apex is characteristic in hypertrophic cardiomyopathy. An S_4 may also be noted on auscultation.

Restrictive Cardiomyopathy

The least common form of cardiomyopathy, *restrictive cardiomyopathy*, is characterized by rigid ventricular walls that impair diastolic filling. Causes of restrictive cardiomyopathy include myocardial fibrosis and infiltrative processes, such as amyloidosis. Fibrosis of the myocardium and endocardium causes excessive stiffness and rigidity of the ventricles. Decreased ventricular compliance impairs filling, with decreased ventricular size, elevated end-diastolic pressures, and decreased cardiac output. Contractility is unaffected, and the ejection fraction is normal.

MANIFESTATIONS AND COURSE The manifestations of restrictive cardiomyopathy are those of heart failure and decreased tissue perfusion. Dyspnea on exertion and exercise intolerance are common. Jugular venous pressure is elevated, and S_3 and S_4 are common. The prognosis for restrictive cardiomyopathy is poor. Most clients die within 3 years, and the systemic nature of the underlying disease process precludes effective treatment.

INTERDISCIPLINARY CARE

With the exception of treating an underlying cause, little can be done to treat either dilated or restrictive cardiomyopathies. For these disorders, treatment focuses on managing heart failure and treating dysrhythmias. Refer to the section of this chapter

---

NURSING RESEARCH **Evidence-Based Practice: Sudden Cardiac Death**

When cardiac arrest occurs or invasive procedures are performed, family members typically are asked to leave the client's care unit. The traditional rationale for this practice is fear of disrupted clinical interventions, trauma of the witnesses, and risk for increased hospital liability. However, in 1995, the Emergency Nurses Association (ENA) adopted a position supporting family presence during invasive procedures, including resuscitation efforts (CPR), as a means of "preserving the wholeness, dignity, and integrity of the family unit from birth to death" (Myers et al., 2000, p. 33). This study evaluated the responses of families, nurses, and physicians to family presence during invasive procedures and CPR.

Results of the study showed that families saw their presence as a positive experience and their right. They viewed themselves as active care partners, and being present met their needs for information and providing comfort and connection with the client. Nurses overwhelmingly supported family presence; attending physicians also demonstrated a positive response. Physician residents were the least supportive of family presence.

IMPLICATIONS FOR NURSING

Family members often are asked to leave the client's side during invasive procedures and CPR with the intention of protecting them from the trauma of witnessing painful or distressing events.

This study clearly showed being present as a positive experience, even when the ultimate outcome was the client's death.

Offering the opportunity to be present and providing information as well as psychologic and emotional support to an appropriate family member during invasive procedures and CPR supports the family unit and the client during times of crisis. Screening is important: People who are combative, emotionally unstable, or have altered mental status (e.g., dementia, alcohol intoxication) probably are not appropriate. It also is important to allow families to decline the invitation without guilt.

CRITICAL THINKING IN CLIENT CARE

1. Identify procedures and situations in which family members are often asked to leave the client's side. When would it be appropriate to allow at least one significant other to remain with the client?
2. How would you present the option and prepare a family member for being present during a traumatic event such as CPR following the sudden death of a young adult with undiagnosed hypertrophic cardiomyopathy?
3. You support family presence during traumatic events and procedures, but your charge nurse does not. What steps might you use to effect a change in policy on your unit?

on heart failure and Chapter 31 ∞ for specific treatment strategies. Treatment of hypertrophic cardiomyopathy focuses on reducing contractility and preventing sudden cardiac death. Strenuous physical exertion is restricted, because it may precipitate dysrhythmias or sudden cardiac death. Dietary and sodium restrictions may help diminish the manifestations.

Diagnosis

Diagnosis begins with a history and physical assessment to rule out known causes of heart failure. Other tests may include the following:

- *Echocardiography* is done to assess chamber size and thickness, ventricular wall motion, valvular function, and systolic and diastolic function of the heart.
- *Electrocardiography* and *ambulatory ECG monitoring* demonstrate cardiac enlargement and detect dysrhythmias.
- *Chest x-ray* shows cardiomegaly, enlargement of the heart, and any pulmonary congestion or edema.
- *Hemodynamic studies* are used to assess cardiac output and pressures in the cardiac chambers and pulmonary vascular system.
- *Radionuclear scans* help identify changes in ventricular volume and mass, as well as perfusion deficits.
- *Cardiac catheterization* and *coronary angiography* may be done to evaluate coronary perfusion, the cardiac chambers, valves, and great vessels for function and structure, pressure relationships, and cardiac output.
- *Myocardial biopsy* uses the transvenous route to obtain myocardial tissue for biopsy. The cells are examined for infiltration, fibrosis, or inflammation.

Medications

The drug regimen used to treat heart failure also is used for dilated or restrictive cardiomyopathy. This includes ACE inhibitors, vasodilators, and digitalis (see the previous section of this chapter). Beta-blockers also may be used with caution in clients with dilated cardiomyopathy. Anticoagulants are given to reduce the risk of thrombus formation and embolization. Antidysrhythmic drugs are avoided if possible due to their tendency to precipitate further dysrhythmias (Kasper et al., 2005).

Beta-blockers are the drugs of choice to reduce anginal symptoms and syncopal episodes associated with hypertrophic cardiomyopathy. The negative inotropic effects of beta-blockers and calcium channel blockers decrease the myocardial contractility, decreasing obstruction of the outflow tract. Beta-blockers also decrease heart rate and increase ventricular compliance, increasing diastolic filling time and cardiac output. Vasodilators, digitalis, nitrates, and diuretics are contraindicated. Amiodarone may be used to treat ventricular dysrhythmias (Kasper et al., 2005).

Surgery

Without definitive treatment, clients with cardiomyopathy develop end-stage heart failure. Cardiac transplant is the definitive treatment for dilated cardiomyopathy. Ventricular assist devices may be used to support cardiac output until a donor heart is available. Transplantation is not a viable option for restrictive cardiomyopathy, because transplantation does not eliminate the underlying process causing infiltration or fibrosis, and eventually the transplanted organ is affected as well. See the section on heart failure for more information about cardiac transplantation.

In severely symptomatic clients with obstructive hypertrophic cardiomyopathy, excess muscle may be surgically resected from the aortic valve outflow tract. The septum is incised, and tissue is removed. This procedure provides lasting improvement in about 75% of clients (Kasper et al., 2005).

An implantable cardioverter-defibrillator (ICD) often is inserted to treat potentially lethal dysrhythmias, reducing the need for antidysrhythmic medications. A dual-chamber pacemaker also may be used to treat hypertrophic cardiomyopathy.

NURSING CARE

Nursing assessment and care for clients with dilated and restrictive cardiomyopathy are similar to those for clients with heart failure. Teaching about the disease process and its management is vital. Some degree of activity restriction often is necessary; assist to conserve energy while encouraging self-care. Support coping skills and adaptation to required lifestyle changes. Provide information and support for decision making about cardiac transplantation if that is an option. Discuss the toxic and vasodilator effects of alcohol, and encourage abstinence. See the nursing care section for heart failure for nursing diagnoses and suggested interventions.

The client with hypertrophic cardiomyopathy requires care similar to that provided for myocardial ischemia; nitrates and other vasodilators, however, are avoided. If surgery is performed, nursing care is similar to that for any client undergoing open-heart surgery or cardiac transplant. Discuss the genetic transmission of hypertrophic cardiomyopathy, and suggest screening of close relatives (parents and siblings).

Provide pre- and postoperative care and teaching as appropriate for clients undergoing invasive procedures or surgery for cardiomyopathy.

Nursing diagnoses that may be appropriate for clients with cardiomyopathy include:

- *Decreased Cardiac Output* related to impaired left ventricular filling, contractility, or outflow obstruction
- *Fatigue* related to decreased cardiac output
- *Ineffective Breathing Pattern* related to heart failure
- *Fear* related to risk for sudden cardiac death
- *Ineffective Role Performance* related to decreasing cardiac function and activity restrictions
- *Anticipatory Grieving* related to poor prognosis.

Community-Based Care

Cardiomyopathies are chronic, progressive disorders generally managed in home and community care settings unless surgery or transplant is planned or end-stage heart failure develops. When teaching the client and family for home care, include the following topics:

- Activity restrictions and dietary changes to reduce manifestations and prevent complications

- Prescribed drug regimen, its rationale, intended and possible adverse effects
- The disease process, its expected ultimate outcome, and treatment options
- Cardiac transplantation, including the procedure, the need for lifetime immunosuppression to prevent transplant rejection, and the risks of postoperative infection and long-term immunosuppression

- Symptoms to report to the physician or for which immediate care is needed.
- Cardiopulmonary resuscitation procedures and available training sites.

Refer the client and family for home and social services and counseling as indicated. Provide community resources such as support groups or the AHA.

EXPLORE MEDIALINK

Prentice Hall Nursing MediaLink DVD-ROM
    Audio Glossary
    NCLEX-RN® Review

    Animations
      Digoxin
      Hemodynamics

COMPANION WEBSITE www.prenhall.com/lemone
    Audio Glossary
    NCLEX-RN® Review
    Care Plan Activity: Acute Pulmonary Edema
    Case Study: Rheumatic Fever
    MediaLink Applications
      Beta Blockers
      Heart Failure
    Links to Resources

CHAPTER HIGHLIGHTS

- All of the disorders discussed in this chapter can lead to heart failure, a condition in which the heart is unable to pump effectively to meet the body's needs for blood and oxygen to the tissues.
- Coronary heart disease (myocardial ischemia) and cardiomyopathies are the leading causes of heart failure.
- When the heart starts to fail, compensatory mechanisms are activated to help maintain tissue perfusion. While these mechanisms, including increased contractile force, vasoconstriction, sodium and water retention, and remodeling of the heart, effectively maintain cardiac output in the short term, in the long term they hasten deterioration of heart function.
- The goals of heart failure management are to reduce the workload of the heart and improve its function. Medical management includes administration of drugs such as ACE inhibitors, beta blockers, diuretics, and vasodilators to reduce the workload of the heart, and inotropic medications such as digitalis to improve the strength of cardiac muscle contraction.
- Nursing care of the client with heart failure is primarily supportive and educative, providing the client and family with necessary knowledge and resources to manage this chronic condition.
- Cardiogenic pulmonary edema, a manifestation of severe cardiac decompensation, is a medical emergency, requiring immediate and effective treatment to preserve life. The nurse's role in managing pulmonary edema focuses on supporting respiratory

and cardiac function, administering prescribed medications, and providing reassurance to the client and family.
- Inflammatory and infectious processes, such as rheumatic fever, endocarditis, myocarditis, and pericarditis, can affect any layer of the heart. While some, such as myocarditis and pericarditis, typically are mild and self-limiting, others can have long-term effects on cardiac structure and function.
- Processes such as rheumatic heart disease, endocarditis, and congenital conditions can affect the structure and function of the heart valves, resulting in either stenosis (narrowing) of the valve and restricted flow through it, or regurgitation, backflow of blood through a valve that does not fully close. The mitral and aortic valves are commonly affected due to the higher pressures and increased workload of the left side of the heart.
- Valve disorders may be mild, producing a heart murmur but no functional impairment for the client, or severe, causing symptoms of heart failure even at rest. Repair or replacement of the valve may ultimately be required.
- Cardiomyopathies affect the heart muscle and its ability to stretch during filling and contract effectively. Dilated cardiomyopathy, the most common type, is progressive, ultimately necessitating heart transplant. Hypertrophic cardiomyopathy affects both ventricular filling and outflow through the aortic valve. Surgical resection of excess tissue may relieve its manifestations.

TEST YOURSELF NCLEX-RN® REVIEW

1 In reviewing the physician's admitting notes for a client with heart failure, the nurse notes that the client has an ejection fraction of 25%. The nurse recognizes this as meaning:
1. ventricular function is severely impaired.
2. the amount of blood being ejected from the ventricles is within normal limits.
3. 25% of the blood entering the ventricle remains in the ventricle after systole.
4. cardiac output is greater than normal, overtaxing the heart.

2 In assessing a client admitted 24 hours previously with heart failure, the nurse notes that the client has lost 2.5 lb (1 kg) of weight, his heart rate is 88 (HR was 105 on admission), and he now has crackles in the bases of his lung fields only. The nurse correctly interprets these data as indicating:
1. the client's condition is unchanged from admission.
2. a need for more aggressive treatment.
3. the treatment regimen is achieving the desired effect.
4. no further treatment is required at this time as the failure has resolved.

3 The nurse assessing a client admitted with left ventricular failure would recognize which of the following findings as consistent with the diagnosis? (Select all that apply.)
1. 5 cm jugular vein distention at 30°
2. complaints of shortness of breath with minimal exertion
3. substernal chest pain during exercise
4. bilateral inspiratory crackles to midscapula
5. fatigue

4 The nurse caring for a client undergoing pulmonary artery pressure monitoring provides appropriate care when he
1. secures the intravenous line to the bed linens.
2. maintains flush solution flow by gravity.
3. reports waveform dampening during wedge pressure measurements.
4. calibrates and levels the system every shift.

5 Morphine 2 to 5 mg IV as needed for pain and dyspnea is ordered for a client in acute pulmonary edema. The nurse appropriately:
1. questions this order because no time intervals have been specified.
2. administers the drug as ordered, monitoring respiratory status.
3. withholds the drug until the client's respiratory status improves.
4. administers the drug only when the client complains of chest pain.

6 The nurse notes a grating heart sound when auscultating the apical pulse of a client with pericarditis. The most appropriate response is to

1. note the finding in the client's medical record.
2. obtain an electrocardiogram.
3. immediately notify the physician.
4. initiate resuscitation measures.

7 An appropriate goal of nursing care for the client with acute infective endocarditis would be:
1. "Will resume usual activities within 1 week of treatment."
2. "Will relate the benign and self-limiting nature of the disease."
3. "Will consider cardiac transplantation as a viable treatment option."
4. "Will state the importance of continuing intravenous antibiotic therapy as ordered."

8 An expected assessment finding in a client with mitral stenosis being admitted for a valve replacement would be:
1. muffled heart sounds.
2. S_3 and S_4 heart sounds.
3. diastolic murmur heard at the apex.
4. cardiac heave.

9 A client facing heart valve replacement asks the nurse which type of valve is the best, biologic or mechanical. An appropriate response would be:
1. the need to take drugs to prevent rejection of biologic tissue is a major consideration.
2. clotting is a risk with mechanical valves, necessitating anticoagulant drug therapy after insertion.
3. biologic valves tend to be more durable than mechanical valves.
4. endocarditis is a risk following valve replacement; it is more easily treated with mechanical valves.

10 The parents of a young athlete who collapsed and died due to hypertrophic cardiomyopathy ask the nurse how it is possible that their son had no symptoms of this disorder before experiencing sudden cardiac death. The nurse responds:
1. "Exercise causes the heart to contract more forcefully, and can lead to changes in the heart's rhythm or the outflow of blood from the heart in people with hypertrophic cardiomyopathy."
2. "It is likely that your son had symptoms of the disorder before he died, but he may not have thought them important enough to tell someone about."
3. "In this type of cardiomyopathy, the ventricle does not fill normally. During exercise, the heart may not be able to meet the body's needs for blood and oxygen."
4. "Cardiomyopathy results in destruction and scarring of cardiac muscle cells. As a result, the ventricle may rupture during strenuous exercise, leading to sudden death."

See Test Yourself answers in Appendix C.

BIBLIOGRAPHY

Albert, N. M. (2004a). A "current" choice for hemodynamic monitoring. *Nursing, 34*(10), 58–60.

Albert, N. M. (2004b). Ventricular dysrhythmias in heart failure. *Journal of Cardiovascular Nursing, 19*(6S), S11–S26.

Aldred, H., Gott, M., & Gariballa, S. (2005). Advanced heart failure: Impact on older patients and informal carers. *Journal of Advanced Nursing, 49*(2), 116–124.

American Heart Association. (2005). *Heart disease and stroke statistics–2005 update.* Dallas, TX: Author.

Artinian, N. T. (2003). The psychosocial aspects of heart failure. *American Journal of Nursing, 103*(12), 32–42.

Benton, M. J. (2005). Safety and efficacy of resistance training in patients with chronic heart failure: Research-based evidence. *Progressive Cardiovascular Nursing, 20*(1), 17–23.

Bixby, M. (2005). Turn back the tide of cardiogenic pulmonary edema. *Nursing, 35*(5), 56–61.

Bolton, M. M., & Wilson, B. A. (2005). The influence of race on heart failure in African-American women. *Medsurg Nursing, 14*(1), 8–15.

Bond, A. E., Nelson, K., Germany, C. L., & Smart, A. N. (2003). The left ventricular assist device. *American Journal of Nursing, 103*(1), 32–40.

Brodie, D. A., & Inoue, A. (2005). Motivational interviewing to promote physical activity for people with chronic heart failure. *Journal of Advanced Nursing, 50*(5), 518–527.

Brown, H. (2005). Action stat. Cardiac tamponade. *Nursing, 35*(3), 88.

Brown, P. A., Launius, B. K., Mancini, M. C., & Cush, E. M. (2004). Depression and anxiety in the heart transplant patient: A case study. *Critical Care Nursing Quarterly, 27*(1), 92–95.

Bruce, J. (2005). Getting to the heart of cardiomyopathies. *Nursing, 35*(8), 44–47.

Carter, T., & Brooks, C. A. (2005). Pericarditis: Inflammation or infarction? *Journal of Cardiovascular Nursing, 20*(4), 239–244.

Chronic heart failure: Patient teaching saves lives and money. (2005). *Nursing, 35*(4), 33–34.

Clark, J. C., & Lan, V. M. (2004). Heart failure patient learning needs after hospital discharge. *Applied Nursing Research, 17*(3), 150–157.

Copstead, L. C., & Banasik, J. L. (2005). *Pathophysiology* (3rd ed.). St. Louis, MO: Elsevier/Saunders.

Deaton, C., Bennett, J. A., & Riegel, B. (2004). State of the science for care of older adults with heart disease. *Nursing Clinics of North America, 39*(3), 495–528.

Dochterman, J., & Bulechek, G. (2004). *Nursing interventions classification (NIC)* (4th ed.). St. Louis, MO: Mosby.

Dunbar, S. B., Clark, P. C., Deaton, C., Smith, A. L., De, A. K., & O'Brien, M. C. (2005). Family education and support interventions in heart failure: A pilot study. *Nursing Research, 54*(3), 158–166.

Fischbach, F. (2005). *Nurses' quick reference to common laboratory and diagnostic tests* (4th ed.). Philadelphia: Lippincott.

Fontaine, K. L. (2005). *Healing practices: Alternative therapies for nursing* (2nd ed.). Upper Saddle River, NJ: Prentice Hall Health.

Goldrick, B. A. (2003). Emerging infections. Endocarditis associated with body piercing. *American Journal of Nursing, 103*(1), 26–27.

Graham-Cryzn, M. A., Rowe, G., Hathaway, L., Biddle, S., Tripodi, D., & Fananapazir, L. (2004). Obstructive hypertrophic cardiomyopathy. *Progressive Cardiovascular Nursing, 19*(4), 133–140.

Hamner, J. B., & Ellison, K. J. (2005). Predictors of hospital readmission after discharge in patients with congestive heart failure. *Heart & Lung, 34*(4), 231–239.

Holcomb, S. S. (2004). Recognizing and managing endocarditis. *Nursing, 34*(2), Critical Care 32cc1–32cc2, 32cc5.

Hunt, S. A., Abraham, W. T., Chin, M. H., Feldman, A. M., Francis, G. S., Ganiats, T. G., et al. (2005). ACC/AHA 2005 guideline update for the diagnosis and management of chronic heart failure in the adult: A report of the American College of Cardiology/American Heart Association Task Force on Practice Guidelines (Writing Committee to Update the 2001 Guidelines for the Evaluation and Management of Heart Failure). American College of Cardiology Web site. Retrieved from http://www.acc.org/clinical/guidelines/failure/index/pdf

Hussey, L. C., & Hardin, S. (2005). Comparison of characteristics of heart failure by race and gender. *Dimensions of Critical Care Nursing, 24*(1), 41–46.

Kasper, D. L., Braunwald, E., Fauci, A. S., Hauser, S. L., Longo, D. L., & Jameson, J. L. (Eds.). (2005). *Harrison's principles of internal medicine* (16th ed.). New York: McGraw-Hill.

King, J. E. (2004). How to classify heart failure. *Nursing, 34*(5), 15.

Konick-McMahan, J., Bixby, B., & McKenna, C. (2003). Heart failure in older adults. Providing nursing care to improve outcomes. *Journal of Gerontology Nursing, 29*(12), 35–41.

Luggen, A. S., & Parton, A. (2004). Gerontologic nurse practitioner care guidelines: Early management of heart failure. *Geriatric Nursing, 25*(4), 251–253.

Martinen, M., & Freundl, M. (2004). Managing congestive heart failure in long-term care: Development of an interdisciplinary protocol. *Journal of Gerontology Nursing, 30*(12), 5–12.

McCance, K. L., & Huether, S. E. (2006). *Pathophysiology: The biologic basis for disease in adults and children* (5th ed.). St. Louis, MO: Mosby.

Moorhead, S., Johnson, M., & Maas, M. (2004). *Nursing outcomes classification (NOC)* (3rd ed.). St. Louis, MO: Mosby.

Munson, B. L. (2005). Myths and facts . . . About infective endocarditis. *Nursing, 35*(2), 71.

Myers, T. A., Eichhorn, D. J., Guzzetta, C. E., Clark, A. P., Klein, J. D., Taliaferro, E., et al. (2000). Family presence during invasive procedures and resuscitation: The experience of family members, nurses, and physicians. *American Journal of Nursing, 100*(2), 32–42.

NANDA International. (2005). *Nursing diagnoses: Definitions and classification 2005–2006.* Philadelphia: Author.

National Heart, Lung, and Blood Institute. National Institutes of Health. (2004). *Morbidity & mortality: 2004 chart book of cardiovascular, lung, and blood diseases.* Bethesda, MD: Author.

Pericardiocentesis: A lifesaving procedure. (2004). *RN, 67*(5), 40.

Phillips, L., Harrison, T., & Houck, P. (2005). Return to work and the person with heart failure. *Heart & Lung, 34*(2), 79–88.

Piano, M. R. (2005). Beats & breaths. The cardiovascular effects of alcohol: The good and the bad. *American Journal of Nursing, 105*(7), 87, 89–91.

Piña, I. L., Apstein, C. S., Balady, G. J., Belardinelli, R., Chaitman, B. R., Duscha, B. D., et al. (2003). *AHA scientific statement: Exercise and heart failure.* American Heart Association. Retrieved from http://www.circulationaha.org

Porth, C. M. (2005). *Pathophysiology: Concepts of altered health states* (7th ed.). Philadelphia: Lippincott.

Quillen, T. F. (2005). Myths & facts...About mitral valve prolapse. *Nursing, 35*(9), 71.

Rock-Prior, P. (2004). Variables predictive of poor postdischarge outcomes for hospitalized elders in heart failure. *Western Journal of Nursing Research, 26*(5), 533–546.

Rothrock, J. C. (2003). *Alexander's care of the patient in surgery* (12th ed.). St. Louis, MO: Mosby.

Sauls, J. L., & Rone, T. (2005). Emerging trends in the management of heart failure: Beta blocker therapy. *Nursing Clinics of North America, 40*(1), 135–148.

Scott, L. D., Setter-Kline, K., & Britton, A. S. (2004). The effects of nursing interventions to enhance mental health and quality of life among individuals with heart failure. *Applied Nursing Research, 17*(4), 248–256.

Shatzer, M., & Castor, A. (2004). Eye on diagnostics. How transthoracic echocardiography detects cardiac tamponade. *Nursing, 34*(3), 73–74.

Spencer, J. W., & Jacobs, J. J. (2003). *Complementary and alternative medicine: An evidence-based approach* (2nd ed.). St. Louis, MO: Mosby.

Steinbis, S. (2003). Hypertrophic obstructive cardiomyopathy and septal ablation. *Critical Care Nurse, 23*(3), 47–50.

Tierney, L. M., Jr., McPhee, S. J., & Papadakis, M. A. (Eds.). (2005). *Current medical diagnosis & treatment* (44th ed.). New York: McGraw-Hill.

Understanding cardiomyopathies. (2004). *Nursing, 34*(4), 62–63.

U.S. Food and Drug Administration, Center for Drug Evaluation and Research. (2005). BiDil. Retrieved from: www.fda.gov/cdev/cdev/foi/label/2005/020727lbl.pdf

Veasy, L. G., Tani, L. Y., Daly, J. A., Korgenski, K., Miner, L., Bale, J., et al. (2004). Temporal association of the appearance of mucoid strains of *Streptococcus pyogenes* with a continuing high incidence of rheumatic fever in Utah. *Pediatrics, 113*(3), e168–e172.

Wadas, T. M. (2005). The implantable hemodynamic monitoring system. *Critical Care Nurse, 25*(5), 14–16, 18–20, 22–24, 26.

Wade, C. R., Reith, K. K., Sikora, J. H., & Augustine, S. M. (2004). Postoperative nursing care of the cardiac transplant recipient. *Critical Care Nursing Quarterly, 27*(1), 17–28.

Way, L. W., & Doherty, G. M. (2003). *Current surgical diagnosis & treatment* (11th ed.). New York: Lange Medical/McGraw-Hill.

Wheeler, E. C., Klemm, P., Hardic, T., Plowfield, L., Birney, M., Polek, C., et al. (2004). Racial disparities in hospitalized elderly patients with chronic heart failure. *Journal of Transcultural Nursing, 15*(4), 291–297.

White, R. M. (2005). The role of brain natriuretic peptide in systolic heart failure. *Dimensions of Critical Care Nursing, 24*(4), 171–174.

Wiegand, D. L. (2003). Advances in cardiac surgery: Valve repair. *Critical Care Nurse, 23*(2), 72–91.

Wilkinson, J. M. (2005). *Nursing diagnosis handbook* (8th ed.). Upper Saddle River, NJ: Prentice Hall.

Woods, S. L., Froelicher, E. S., Motzer, S. A., & Bridges, E. (2004). *Cardiac nursing* (5th ed.). Philadelphia: Lippincott.

Yee, C. A. (2005). Endocarditis: The infected heart. *Nursing Management, 36*(2), 25–30.

FUNCTIONAL HEALTH PATTERN: Activity-Exercise

■ Think about clients with cardiac disorders and altered activity and/or exercise patterns for whom you have cared in your clinical experiences.

- What were the clients' major pathophysiologic conditions (medical diagnoses) (e.g., myocardial infarction, heart failure, valvular heart disease)?
- What manifestations did each of these clients have? Were these manifestations similar or different?
- How did each of these clients respond to activities such as talking, eating, completing activities of daily living (ADLs), moving from bed to chair or bathroom, ambulating? Did their heart rates increase or decrease? How about their respiratory rates and effort? Did any of your clients become light-headed or develop chest pain during activity? Did their oxygen saturation levels remain stable or drop during activity?

■ The Activity-Exercise Pattern includes ADLs and patterns of exercise and activity—all of which require the expenditure of energy. The heart functions as a pump to deliver fuel for energy production to the cells. Cardiac disorders affect the heart's pumping ability in two primary ways:

- The heart muscle is directly damaged by ischemic processes (e.g., coronary heart disease), inflammatory responses (e.g., rheumatic carditis, endocarditis), or a primary cardiac muscle disorder (cardiomyopathy).
- Excessive cardiac work (e.g., resulting from hypertension, valve disorders, or congenital defects) prompts compensatory mechanisms to meet cellular needs for fuel; over time, these compensatory mechanisms damage the heart muscle.

■ When the cardiac pump fails, less fuel is delivered to the cells and energy production falls. This in turn affects the client's ability to exercise and maintain ADLs, leading to manifestations such as:

- Fatigue (decreased oxygen and glucose delivery to cells ► decreased ATP production)
- Shortness of breath, dyspnea (decreased cardiac output ► decreased pulmonary blood flow ► carbon dioxide retention stimulates the respiratory center; decreased cellular oxygen ► shift to anaerobic cellular metabolism ► increased production of nonvolatile acids and stimulation of the respiratory center)
- Tachycardia (decreased stroke volume ► decreased cardiac output ► catecholamine release ► increased heart rate and contractility ► increased cardiac work)

■ Priority nursing diagnoses within the Activity-Exercise Pattern that may be appropriate for clients with cardiac disease include:

- *Decreased Cardiac Output* as evidenced by increased heart rate, fatigue, shortness of breath, decreased urine output, impaired mental processing, decreased level of consciousness
- *Activity Intolerance* as evidenced by prolonged heart rate increases following activity, shortness of breath with exercise, activity-related chest pain, fatigue
- *Fatigue* as evidenced by inability to consume a full meal without resting, frequent napping or dozing, expressions of tiredness, weakness
- *Ineffective Tissue Perfusion* as evidenced by cool, dusky skin, decreased urine output, chest pain.

■ Two nursing diagnoses from other functional health patterns often are of high priority for the client with heart disease because the physiologic responses to these problems increase cardiac work:

- *Acute Pain* (Cognitive-Perceptual)
- *Anxiety* (Coping-Stress-Tolerance)

Directions: Read the clinical scenario below and answer the questions that follow. To complete this exercise successfully, you will use not only knowledge of the content in this unit, but also principles related to setting priorities and maintaining client safety.

CLINICAL SCENARIO

You have been assigned to work with the following four clients for the shift on a cardiac telemetry unit. Significant data obtained during report is as follows:

- Betty Williams, age 62, was admitted with acute anterior MI and had successful fibrinolytic therapy 3 days ago. Significant history includes type 2 diabetes, angina, hypertension, and a history of smoking (1.5 to 2 packs per day for 45 years). Her CCU course was uneventful. Current vital signs are T 98.8°F, P 76, R 16, BP 148/88. Cardiac monitor shows normal sinus rhythm with no ectopy. She has been pain free since her nitroglycerin drip was titrated off in the CCU 2 days ago. Lungs sounds are clear.
- Arnold Markus, age 71, was admitted with acute heart failure 2 days ago, treated and stabilized in the CCU, and transferred to the cardiac telemetry unit. Current vital signs are T 98.4°F, P 88, R 18, BP 112/74. Cardiac monitor shows normal sinus rhythm with new iso-

lated premature ventricular contractions (PVCs). Lung sounds are clear in upper lobes with crackles in the left base, and he was able to sleep intermittently during the night using 2 pillows.
- Sandra Thomas, age 53, was admitted for mitral valve replacement 4 days ago (mechanical valve) to treat mitral regurgitation secondary to rheumatic heart disease. Her surgical course was uneventful, but she continues to experience sternal incision pain requiring medication every 4 to 6 hours. Current vital signs are T 99.6°F, P 78, R 20, BP 136/84. Cardiac monitor shows normal sinus rhythm. Lung sounds are diminished at the bases with poor cough effort due to pain. She was last medicated an hour before intershift report with good effect.
- Randall Stevens, age 34, was admitted with infective endocarditis 4 hours ago. Current vital signs are T 102.2°F, P 104, R 18, BP 128/72. Monitor shows sinus tachycardia. He reports chills and generalized weakness.

Questions

1 In what order would you visit these clients after report?
1. _____
2. _____
3. _____
4. _____

2 What top two priority nursing diagnoses would you choose for each of the clients presented above? Can you explain, if asked, the rationale for your choices?

	Priority Nursing Diagnosis #1	Priority Nursing Diagnosis #2
Betty Williams		
Arnold Markus		
Sandra Thomas		
Randall Stevens		

3 You plan to do client teaching with Ms. Williams later in the day. What are the top three priority items to include in the teaching session for today?
1. signs of MI, smoking cessation, and age as a risk factor
2. smoking cessation, age, and benefits of a cardiac rehabilitation program
3. controlling hypertension and diabetes, and smoking cessation
4. all modifiable and nonmodifiable risk factors for recurrent MI

4 You are completing a beginning-of-shift assessment with Mr. Markus. Which of the following items would take priority?
1. rhythm strip analysis
2. lung sounds
3. oxygen saturation
4. heart sounds

5 After conducting a baseline assessment, which of the following should be a priority item to review with Ms. Thomas?
1. calling for pain medication whenever pain is a 4 or higher on a scale of 1 to 10
2. getting out of bed and ambulating to improve breath sounds
3. care of leg incisions
4. splinting of incision to cough and deep breathe

6 A telephone laboratory report is received for Mr. Stevens. You are most interested in the results for which of the following studies? (Select all that apply.)
1. serum potassium
2. white blood cell count
3. erythrocyte sedimentation rate
4. blood urea nitrogen
5. troponins
6. LDH

7 The charge nurse tells you that the monitor at the nursing station shows that Mr. Markus is having an increase in PVCs. You would be most concerned after reviewing a rhythm strip if the PVCs had which of the following characteristics?
1. had a frequency of 4 per minute
2. could be felt by the patient
3. were unifocal in morphology
4. fell on the T wave of the preceding beat

8 Ms. Williams rings the call bell and tells you that she is having pressure in her chest. On assessment, she rates it as a 5. Which of the following nursing actions should take priority?
1. Obtain a full symptom assessment.
2. Administer a prn nitroglycerin tablet SL.
3. Call for an electrocardiogram.
4. Notify the physician.

9 Which additional piece of cardiac assessment data is the priority for Mr. Stevens at this time?
1. heart sounds to detect murmurs
2. peripheral pulses to determine adequacy of cardiac output
3. point of maximal impulse to detect cardiac enlargement
4. jugular vein filling to determine right heart failure

10 Considering the mitral valve replacement surgery that Ms. Thomas underwent, the nurse would be most concerned about possible risks to medication therapy if she had a history of which of the following disorders listed in the medical record?
1. glaucoma
2. gout
3. duodenal ulcer
4. osteoarthritis

11 A priority item when planning discharge teaching for Mr. Stevens and his family would be which of the following?
1. home administration of antibiotic therapy
2. avoid going to malls or any crowded places
3. expect intermittent shortness of breath indefinitely
4. need for future antibiotic prophylaxis before invasive procedures

12 The physician prescribes captopril (Capoten) for Mr. Markus to reduce his risk for future episodes of acute heart failure. The nurse includes which of the following instructions in her teaching about this drug?
1. Take the drug after meals to prevent gastric upset.
2. Edema of the face and ankles are expected initially; they will clear with time.
3. Change positions slowly, as this drug may cause dizziness or light-headedness.
4. Monitor your pulse daily. Do not take the drug and notify your physician if it is less than 60 bpm.

CASE STUDY

Fritz Matthews, age 72, has had uncontrolled hypertension for the past 2 years. His healthcare provider has tried different antihypertensives to control his disease. Mr. Matthews has been admitted to the hospital four times in the last 6 months. This is his fourth admission with acute heart failure. The physician explained to Mr. Matthews that hypertension that is not controlled can cause an excessive workload to the heart, thus decreasing the heart's ability to pump efficiently.

Mr. Matthews has recently lost his wife and is living alone. He states that he forgets to take his medication at the prescribed times. He also eats a lot of frozen dinners and does not have the energy to cook his meals. Mr. Matthews has gained 10 pounds since his last admission. He has had difficulty sleeping at night and uses two pillows due to shortness of breath. He also reports that he frequently gets up at night, at least twice to urinate. Mr. Matthews complains of fatigue during the day and is unable to even walk to his mailbox. He also tells the nurse that he is tired even on rising in the morning.

Based on Mr. Matthews' physical assessment and complaints of fatigue and orthopnea, *Decreased Cardiac Output* is identified as the highest priority nursing diagnosis.

- ↓ CO → SNS stimulation → ↑ HR, contractility, vasoconstriction → ↑ cardiac work
- ↓ CO → ↓ renal perfusion → renin released → vasoconstriction; ADH and aldosterone release → Na+ & water retention → ↑ cardiac work
- ↑ fluid volume and pressure → ventricular remodeling and hypertrophy → ↓ pump effectiveness

Mr. M
72 y.o. male
Heart failure

affects   *leads to*

assess

- 5' 8" tall, 242 lbs.
- T 98.4°, P. 88, R 18
- BP 172/74
- ECG normal sinus rhythm with new isolated PVCs
- Crackles in lung bases bilaterally
- Dyspnea noted with activity
- Dozing frequently, c/o fatigue
- Moderate edema to mid calf bilaterally and of sacral region
- BNP 500 pg/mL

generates

- *Excess Fluid Volume* as evidenced by increased heart rate, respiratory crackles, and edema
- *Activity Intolerance* as evidenced by DOE
- *Fatigue* as evidenced by expressions of tiredness

generate nursing diagnosis   *prioritized to*

Decreased Cardiac Output

expected outcomes

- Lose 1-2 pounds per week.
- Attend formal cardiac rehab program 3 X/week as prescribed.
- Take antihypertensive medications as prescribed; have BP checked weekly.
- Report increased activity tolerance and decreased fatigue with ADLs.

evaluate

Two days after admission:
- BP 146/79, P 84, R 20; lungs clear; heart rhythm: Isolated PVC's
- BNP 250
- Weight 231 lbs.
- Attended a heart healthy diet program while on cardiac telemetry
- Worked with the dietitian to establish a food chart and plan home meals
- Relates importance of taking medications as ordered; will buy pill-minder box and fill weekly
- Enrolled in cardiac rehab program as prescribed; states he is looking forward to meeting other people "in as bad shape as I am"

Independent Interventions
- Discuss strategies for improved medication management.
- Teach to weigh self at same time daily.
- Instruct how to read food labels and select low-sodium, low-fat foods.
- Discuss manifestations to report to primary care provider.
- Discuss benefits of cardiac rehab program and assist to plan ways to incorporate increasing activities into daily regimen.

UNIT 10

Responses to Altered Peripheral Tissue Perfusion

CHAPTER 33 Assessing Clients with Hematologic, Peripheral Vascular, and Lymphatic Disorders

LEARNING OUTCOMES

- Describe the anatomy, physiology, and functions of the hematologic, peripheral vascular, and lymphatic systems.

- Explain the physiologic dynamics of blood flow, peripheral resistance, and blood pressure.

- Compare and contrast the major factors influencing arterial blood pressure.

- Describe normal variations in assessment findings for the older adult.

- Identify manifestations of impairment in the function of the hematologic, peripheral vascular, and lymphatic systems.

CLINICAL COMPETENCIES

- Conduct and document a health history for clients having or at risk for alterations in the hematologic, peripheral vascular, and lymphatic systems.

- Conduct and document a physical assessment of hematologic, peripheral vascular, and lymphatic status.

- Monitor the results of diagnostic tests and report abnormal findings.

EQUIPMENT NEEDED

- Stethoscope

- Blood pressure cuff

- Tape measure

- Metric ruler

- Doppler ultrasound device (if unable to auscultate blood pressure or palpate pulse)

- Transducer gel for Doppler device

MEDIALINK

Resources for this chapter can be found on the Prentice Hall Nursing MediaLink DVD-ROM accompanying this textbook, and on the Companion Website at
http://www.prenhall.com/lemone

As the heart ejects blood with each beat, a closed system of blood vessels transports oxygenated blood to all body organs and tissues and then returns deoxygenated blood to the heart for reoxygenation in the lungs. The blood components are the hematologic system, and the branching network of vessels is the peripheral vascular system: the arteries, veins, and capillaries. The lymphatic system is a special vascular system that helps maintain sufficient blood volume in the cardiovascular system by picking up excess tissue fluid and returning it to the bloodstream.

ANATOMY, PHYSIOLOGY, AND FUNCTIONS OF THE HEMATOLOGIC SYSTEM

Blood is an exchange medium between the external environment and the body's cells. Blood consists of plasma, solutes (e.g., proteins, electrolytes, and organic constituents), red blood cells, white blood cells, and platelets (which are fragments of cells). The hematopoietic (blood-forming) system includes the bone marrow (myeloid) tissues, where blood cells form, and the lymphoid tissues of the lymph nodes, where white blood cells mature and circulate. All blood cells originate from cells in the bone marrow called stem cells, or hemocytoblasts. The origin of the cellular components of blood is illustrated in Figure 33–1 ■.

Regulatory mechanisms cause stem cells to differentiate into families of parent cells, each of which gives rise to one of the formed elements of the blood (red blood cells, platelets, and white blood cells). The functions of blood include transporting oxygen, nutrients, hormones, and metabolic wastes; protecting against invasion of pathogens; maintaining blood coagulation; and regulating fluids, electrolytes, acids, bases, and body temperature.

Red Blood Cells

Red blood cells (RBCs, erythrocytes) and the hemoglobin molecules they contain are required to transport oxygen to body tissues. Hemoglobin also binds with some carbon dioxide, carrying it to the lungs for excretion. Abnormal numbers of RBCs, changes in their size and shape, or altered hemoglobin content or structure can adversely affect health. **Anemia**, the most common RBC disorder, is an abnormally low RBC count or reduced hemoglobin content. **Polycythemia** is an abnormally high RBC count.

The red blood cell is shaped like a biconcave disk (Figure 33–2 ■). This unique shape increases the surface area of the cell and allows the cell to pass through very small capillaries without disrupting the cell membrane. RBCs are the most common type of blood cell.

Hemoglobin is the oxygen-carrying protein within RBCs. It consists of the heme molecule and globin, a protein molecule. Globin is made of four polypeptide chains—two alpha chains and two beta chains (Figure 33–3 ■). Each of the four polypeptide chains contains a heme unit containing an iron atom. The iron atom binds reversibly with oxygen, allowing it to transport oxygen as *oxyhemoglobin* to the cells. Hemoglobin is synthesized within the RBC. The rate of synthesis depends on the availability of iron (Porth, 2005).

Normal adult laboratory values for red blood cells are defined and identified in Table 33–1. The size, color, and shape of stained RBCs also may be analyzed. RBCs may be normocytic (normal size), smaller than normal (microcytic), or larger than normal (macrocytic). Their color may be normal (normochromic) or diminished (hypochromic).

Red Blood Cell Production and Regulation

In adults, RBC production (**erythropoiesis**) (Figure 33–4 ■) begins in red bone marrow of the vertebrae, sternum, ribs, and pelvis, and is completed in the blood or spleen. Erythroblasts begin forming hemoglobin while they are in the bone marrow, a process that continues throughout the RBC life span. Erythroblasts differentiate into normoblasts. As these slightly smaller cells mature, their nucleus and most organelles are ejected, eventually causing normoblasts to collapse inward and assume the characteristic biconcave shape of RBCs. The cells enter the circulation as reticulocytes, which fully mature in about 48 hours. The complete sequence from stem cell to RBC takes 3 to 5 days.

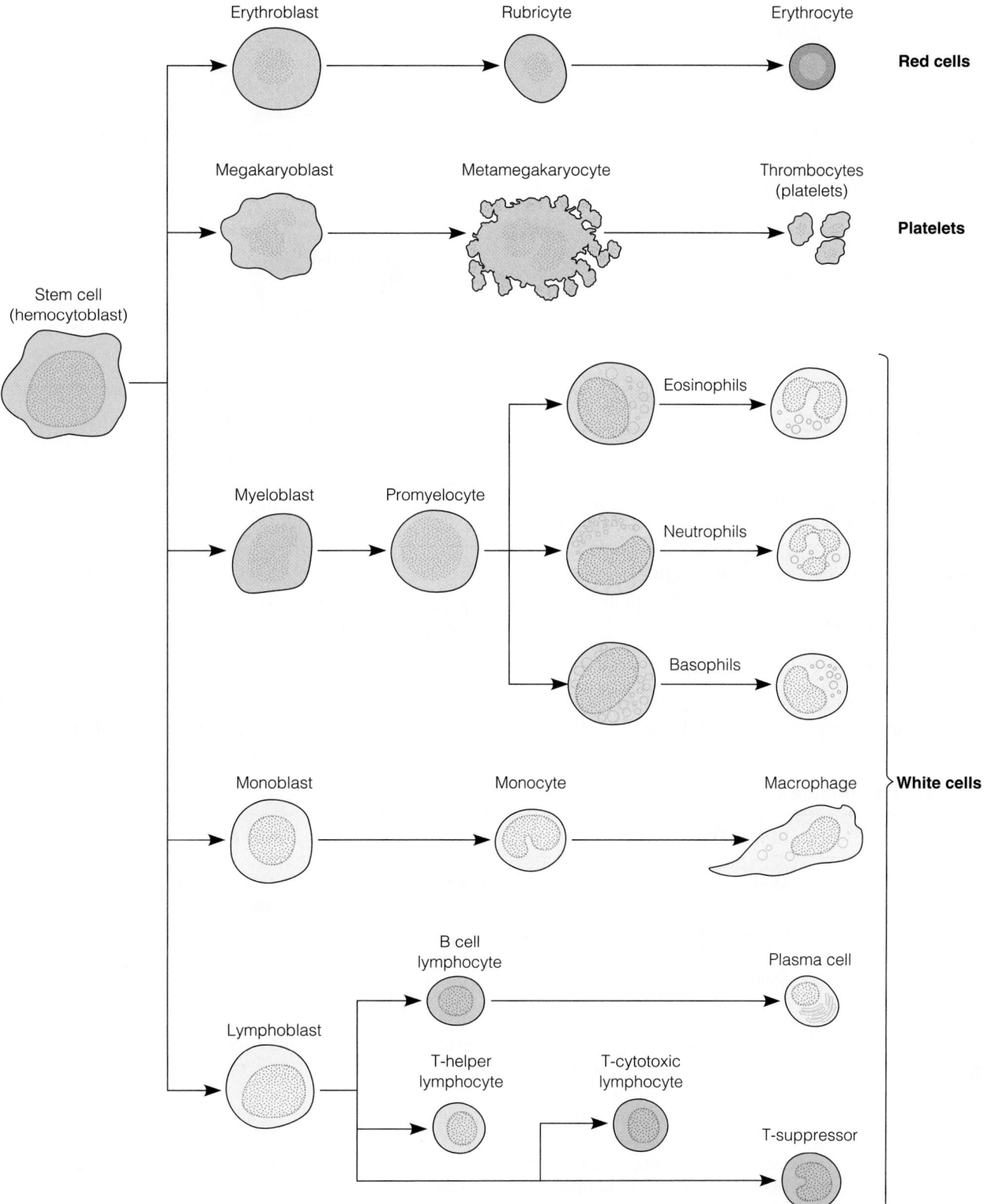

Figure 33–1 ■ Blood cell formation from stem cells. Regulatory factors control the differentiation of stem cells into blasts. Each of the five kinds of blasts is committed to producing one type of mature blood cell. Erythroblasts, for example, can differentiate only into RBCs; megakaryoblasts can differentiate only into platelets.

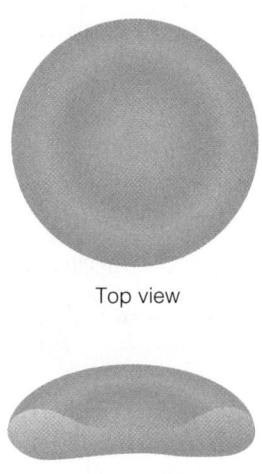

Top view

Side view

Figure 33–2 ■ Top and side view of a red blood cell (erythrocyte). Note the distinctive biconcave shape.

Figure 33–3 ■ The hemoglobin molecule includes globin (a protein) and heme, which contains iron. Globin is made of four subunits, two alpha and two beta polypeptide chains. A heme disk containing an iron atom (red dot) nests within the folds of each protein subunit. The iron atoms combine reversibly with oxygen, transporting it to the cells.

The stimulus for RBC production is tissue hypoxia. The hormone erythropoietin is released by the kidneys in response to hypoxia. It stimulates the bone marrow to produce RBCs. However, the process of RBC production takes about 5 days to maximize. During periods of increased RBC production, the percentage of reticulocytes (immature RBCs) in the blood exceeds that of mature cells.

Red Blood Cell Destruction

RBCs have a life span of about 120 days. Old or damaged RBCs are lysed (destroyed) by phagocytes in the spleen, liver, bone marrow, and lymph nodes. The process of RBC destruction is called **hemolysis**. Phagocytes save and reuse amino acids and iron from heme units in the lysed RBCs. Most of the heme unit is converted to bilirubin, an orange-yellow pigment that is removed from the blood by the liver and excreted in the bile. During disease processes causing increased hemolysis or impaired

TABLE 33–1   Complete Blood Count (CBC)

COMPONENT	PURPOSE	NORMAL VALUES
Hemoglobin (Hb)	Measures the capacity of the hemoglobin to carry gases	Women: 12–16 g/dL Men: 13.5–18 g/dL
Hematocrit (Hct)	Measures packed cell volume of RBCs, expressed as a % of the total blood volume	Women: 38%–47% Men: 40%–54%
Total RBC count	Counts number of circulating RBCs	Women: $4–5 \times 10^6/\mu L$ Men: $4.5–6 \times 10^6/\mu L$
Red cell indices: MCV	Determines relative size of MCV (mean corpuscular volume)	82–98 fl
10^6MCH	Measures average weight of Hb/RBC (MCH = mean corpuscular hemoglobin)	27–33 pg
MCHC	Evaluates RBC saturation with Hb (MCHC = mean corpuscular hemoglobin concentration)	32%–36%
WBC count	Measures total number of leukocytes (total count) and whether each kind of WBC is present in proper proportion (differential)	Total WBC count: 4000–11,000/ μL $(4–11 \times 10^9/L)$ WBC differential: Neutrophils: 50%–70% Eosinophils: 2%–4% Basophils: 0%–2% Lymphocytes: 20%–40% Monocytes: 4%–8%
Platelets	Measures number of platelets available to maintain clotting functions	150,000–400,000/μL $(15–400 \times 10^9/L)$

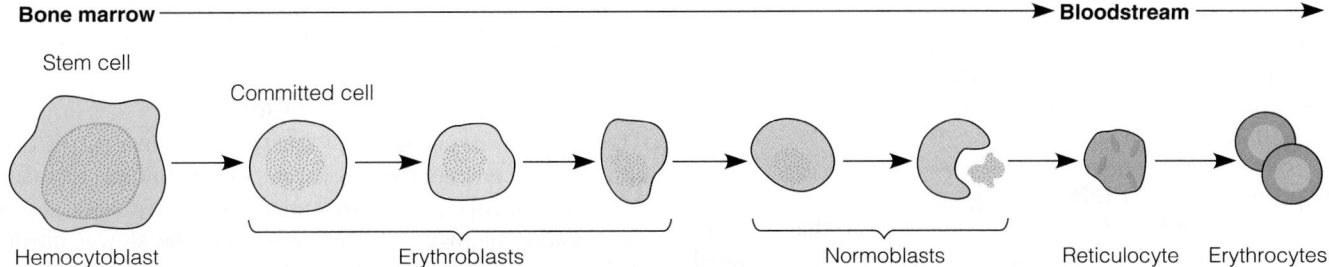

Figure 33–4 ■ Erythropoiesis. RBCs begin as erythroblasts within the bone marrow, maturing into normoblasts, which eventually eject their nucleus and organellas to become reticulocytes. Reticulocytes mature within the blood or spleen to become erythrocytes.

liver function, bilirubin accumulates in the serum, causing a yellowish appearance of the skin and sclera (jaundice).

White Blood Cells

White blood cells (WBCs, leukocytes) are a part of the body's defense against microorganisms. On average, there are 5000 to 10,000 WBCs per microliter of blood, accounting for about 1% of total blood volume. **Leukocytosis** is a higher than normal WBC count; **leukopenia** is a WBC count that is lower than normal.

WBCs originate from hemopoietic stem cells in the bone marrow. These stem cells differentiate into the various types of white blood cells (see Figure 33–1).

The two basic types of WBCs are granular leukocytes (or granulocytes) and nongranular leukocytes. Granulocytes have horseshoe-shaped nuclei and contain large granules in the cytoplasm. Stimulated by granulocyte-macrophage colony-stimulating factor (GM-CSF) and granulocyte colony-stimulating factor (G-CSF), granulocytes mature fully in the bone marrow before being released into the bloodstream. The three types of granulocytes are as follows:

- Neutrophils (also called polymorphonuclear [*PMN*] or segmented [*segs*] leukocytes) comprise 60% to 70% of the total circulating WBCs. Their nuclei are divided into three to five lobes. Neutrophils are active phagocytes, the first cells to arrive at a site of injury. Their numbers increase during inflammation. Immature forms of neutrophils (bands) are released during inflammation or infections, and are referred to as having a shift to the left (so named because immature cell frequencies appear on the left side of the graph) on a differential blood count. Neutrophils have a life span of only about 10 hours and are constantly being replaced.
- Eosinophils comprise 1% to 3% of circulating WBCs, but are found in large numbers in the mucosa of the intestines and lungs. Their numbers increase during allergic reactions and parasitic infestations.
- Basophils, which comprise less than 1% of the WBC count, contain histamine, heparin, and other inflammatory mediators. Basophils increase in numbers during allergic and inflammatory reactions.

Nongranular WBCs (agranulocytes) include the monocytes and lymphocytes. They enter the bloodstream before final maturation.

- Monocytes are the largest of the WBCs. They comprise approximately 3% to 8% of the total WBC count. Monocytes contain powerful bactericidal substances and proteolytic enzymes. They are phagocytic cells that mature into macrophages. Macrophages dispose of foreign and waste material, especially in inflammation. They are an active part of the immune response.
- Lymphocytes comprise 20% to 30% of the WBC count. Lymphocytes mature in lymphoid tissue into B cells and T cells. B cells are involved in the humoral immune response and antibody formation, whereas T cells take part in the cell-mediated immunity process (see Chapter 13 ∞). Plasma cells (which arise from B cells) are lymphoid cells found in bone marrow and connective tissue; they also are involved in immune reactions.

Platelets

Platelets (thrombocytes) are cell fragments that have no nucleus and cannot replicate. They are metabolically active, however, producing ATP and releasing mediators required for clotting. Platelets are formed in the bone marrow as pinched-off portions of large megakaryocytes (see Figure 33–1). Platelet production is controlled by thrombopoietin, a protein produced by the liver, kidney, smooth muscle, and bone marrow. The number of circulating platelets controls thrombopoietin release. Once released from the bone marrow, platelets remain in the spleen for about 8 hours before entering the circulation. Platelets live up to 10 days in circulation. There are about 250,000 to 400,000 platelets in each microliter of blood. An excess of platelets is *thrombocytosis*. A deficit of platelets is *thrombocytopenia*.

Hemostasis

Platelet and coagulation disorders affect **hemostasis**, control of bleeding. Hemostasis is a series of complex interactions between platelets and clotting mechanisms that maintains a relatively steady state of blood volume, blood pressure, and blood flow through injured vessels. The five stages of hemostasis are (1) vessel spasm, (2) formation of the platelet plug, (3) development of an insoluble fibrin clot, (4) clot retraction, and (5) clot dissolution.

Vessel Spasm

When a blood vessel is damaged, thromboxane A_2 (TXA_2) is released from platelets and cells, causing vessel spasm. This spasm constricts the damaged vessel for about 1 minute, reducing blood flow.

Formation of the Platelet Plug

Platelets attracted to the damaged vessel wall change from smooth disks to spiny spheres. Receptors on the activated platelets bind with von Willebrand's factor, a protein molecule, and exposed collagen fibers at the site of injury to form the platelet plug (Figure 33–5 ■). The platelets release adenosine diphosphate (ADP) and TXA_2 to activate nearby platelets, adhering them to the developing plug. Activation of the clotting pathway on the platelet surface converts fibrinogen to fibrin.

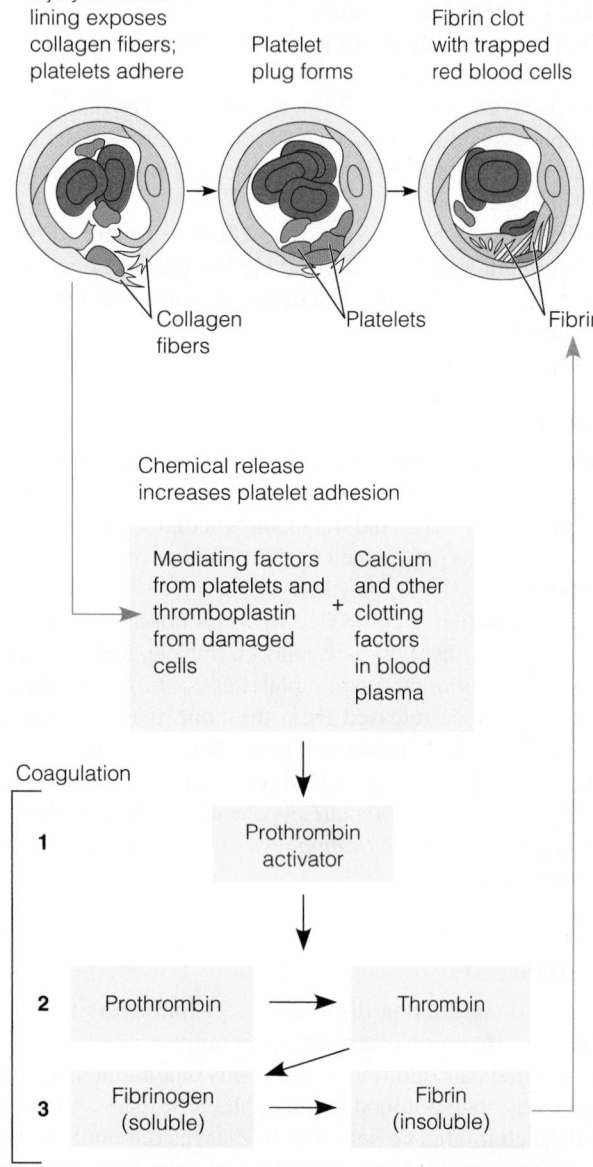

Figure 33–5 ■ Platelet plug formation and blood clotting. The flow diagram summarizes the events leading to fibrin clot formation.

Fibrin, in turn, forms a meshwork that binds the platelets and other blood cells to form a stable plug (Figure 33–6 ■).

Development of the Fibrin Clot

The process of coagulation creates a meshwork of fibrin strands that cements the blood components to form an insoluble clot. Coagulation requires many interactive reactions and two clotting pathways (Figure 33–7 ■). The slower intrinsic pathway is activated when blood contacts collagen in the injured vessel wall; the faster extrinsic pathway is activated when blood is exposed to tissues. The final outcome of both pathways is fibrin clot formation. Each procoagulation substance is activated in sequence; the activation of one coagulation factor activates another in turn. Table 33–2 lists known factors, their origin, and their function or pathway. A deficiency of one or more factors or inappropriate inactivation of any factor alters normal coagulation.

Clot Retraction

After the clot is stabilized (within about 30 minutes), trapped platelets contract, much like muscle cells. Platelet contraction squeezes the fibrin strands, pulling the broken portions of the ruptured blood vessel closer together. Growth factors released by the platelets stimulate cell division and tissue repair of the damaged vessel.

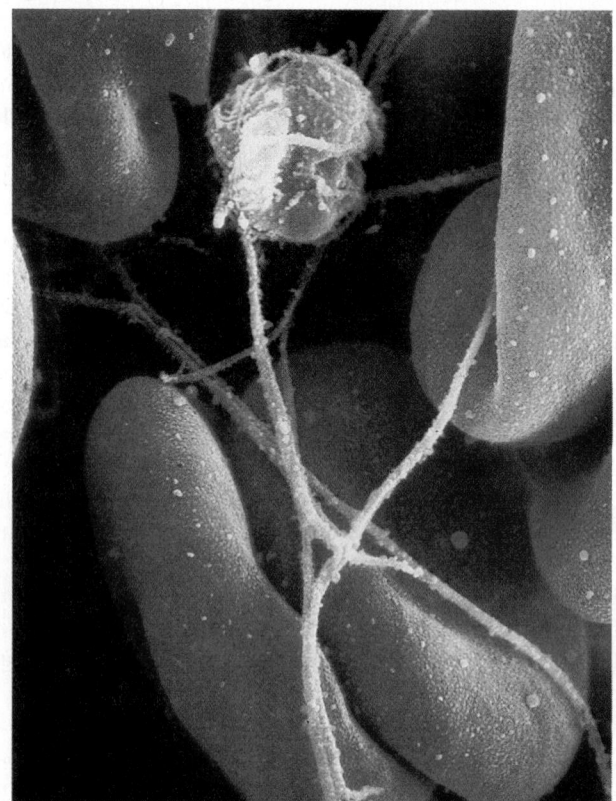

Figure 33–6 ■ Scanning electron micrograph of a RBC trapped in a fibrin mesh. The spherical gray object at top is a platelet.

Source: Copyright © Boehniger Ingelheim; photo Lennart Nilsson, Albert Bonniers Förlog AB.

Figure 33-7 ■ Clot formation. Both the slower intrinsic pathway and the more rapid extrinsic pathway activate factor X. Factor X then combines with other factors to form prothrombin activator. Prothrombin activator transforms prothrombin into thrombin, which then transforms fibrinogen into long fibrin strands. Thrombin also activates Factor XIII, which draws the fibrin strands together into a dense meshwork. The complete process of clot formation occurs within 3 to 6 minutes after blood vessel damage.

Clot Dissolution

Fibrinolysis, the process of clot dissolution, begins shortly after the clot has formed, restoring blood flow and promoting tissue repair. Like coagulation, fibrinolysis requires a sequence of interactions between activator and inhibitor substances. Plasminogen, an enzyme that promotes fibrinolysis, is converted into plasmin, its active form, by chemical mediators released from vessel walls and the liver. Plasmin dissolves the clot's fibrin strands and certain coagulation factors. Stimuli such as exercise, fever, and vasoactive drugs promote plasminogen activator release. The liver and endothelium also produce fibrinolytic inhibitors.

TABLE 33–2 Blood Coagulation Factors

FACTOR	NAME	FUNCTION OR PATHWAY
I	Fibrinogen	Converted to fibrin strands
II	Prothrombin	Converted to thrombin
III	Thromboplastin	Catalyzes conversion of thrombin
IV	Calcium ions	Needed for all steps of coagulation
V	Proaccelerin	Extrinsic/intrinsic pathways
VII	Serum prothrombin conversion accelerator	Extrinsic pathway
VIII	Antihemophilic factor	Intrinsic pathway
IX	Plasma prothrombin component	Intrinsic pathway
X	Stuart factor	Extrinsic/intrinsic pathways
XI	Plasma prothrombin antecedent	Intrinsic pathway
XII	Hageman factor	Intrinsic pathway
XIII	Fibrin stabilizing factor	Cross-links fibrin strands to form insoluble clot

ANATOMY, PHYSIOLOGY, AND FUNCTIONS OF THE PERIPHERAL VASCULAR SYSTEM

The two main components of the peripheral vascular system are the arterial network and the venous network. The arterial network begins with the major arteries that branch from the aorta. The major arteries of the systemic circulation are illustrated in Figure 33–8 ■. These major arteries branch into successively smaller arteries, which in turn subdivide into the smallest of the arterial vessels, called *arterioles*. The smallest arterioles feed into beds of hairlike capillaries in the body's organs and tissues.

In the capillary beds, oxygen and nutrients are exchanged for metabolic wastes, and deoxygenated blood begins its journey back to the heart through venules, the smallest vessels of the venous network. Venules join the smallest of veins, which in turn join larger and larger veins. The blood transported by the veins empties into the superior and inferior venae cavae entering the right side of the heart. The major veins of the systemic circulation are shown in Figure 33–9 ■.

Structure of Blood Vessels

The structure of blood vessels reflects their different functions within the circulatory system (Figure 33–10 ■). Except for the tiniest vessels, blood vessel walls have three layers: the tunica intima, the tunica media, and the tunica adventitia. The tunica intima, the innermost layer, is made of simple squamous epithelium (the endothelium); this provides a slick surface to facilitate the flow of blood. In arteries, the middle layer, or tunica media, is made of smooth muscle and is thicker than the tunica media of veins. This makes arteries more elastic than veins and allows the arteries to alternately expand and recoil as the heart contracts and relaxes with each beat, producing a pressure wave, which can be felt as a **pulse** over an artery. The smaller arterioles are less elastic than arteries but contain more smooth muscle, which promotes their constriction (narrowing) and dilation (widening). In fact, arterioles exert the major control over arterial blood pressure. The tunica adventitia, or outermost layer, is made of connective tissue and serves to protect

and anchor the vessel. Veins have a thicker tunica adventitia than do arteries.

Blood in the veins travels at a much lower pressure than blood in the arteries. Veins have thinner walls, a larger lumen, and greater capacity, and many are supplied with valves that help blood flow against gravity back to the heart (see Figure 33–10). The "milking" action of skeletal muscle contraction (called the muscular pump) also supports venous return. When skeletal muscles contract against veins, the valves proximal to the contraction open, and blood is propelled toward the heart. The abdominal and thoracic pressure changes that occur with breathing (called the respiratory pump) also propel blood toward the heart.

The tiny capillaries, which connect the arterioles and venules, contain only one thin layer of tunica intima that is permeable to the gases and molecules exchanged between blood and tissue cells. Capillaries typically are found in interwoven networks. They filter and shunt blood from precapillary arterioles to postcapillary venules.

Physiology of Arterial Circulation

The factors that affect arterial circulation are blood flow, peripheral vascular resistance, and blood pressure. **Blood flow** refers to the volume of blood transported in a vessel, in an organ, or throughout the entire circulation over a given period of time. It is commonly expressed as liters or milliliters per minute or cubic centimeters per second.

Peripheral vascular resistance (PVR) refers to the opposing forces or impedance to blood flow as the arterial channels become more and more distant from the heart. Peripheral vascular resistance is determined by three factors:

- *Blood viscosity:* The greater the viscosity, or thickness, of the blood, the greater its resistance to moving and flowing.
- *Length of the vessel:* The longer the vessel, the greater the resistance to blood flow.

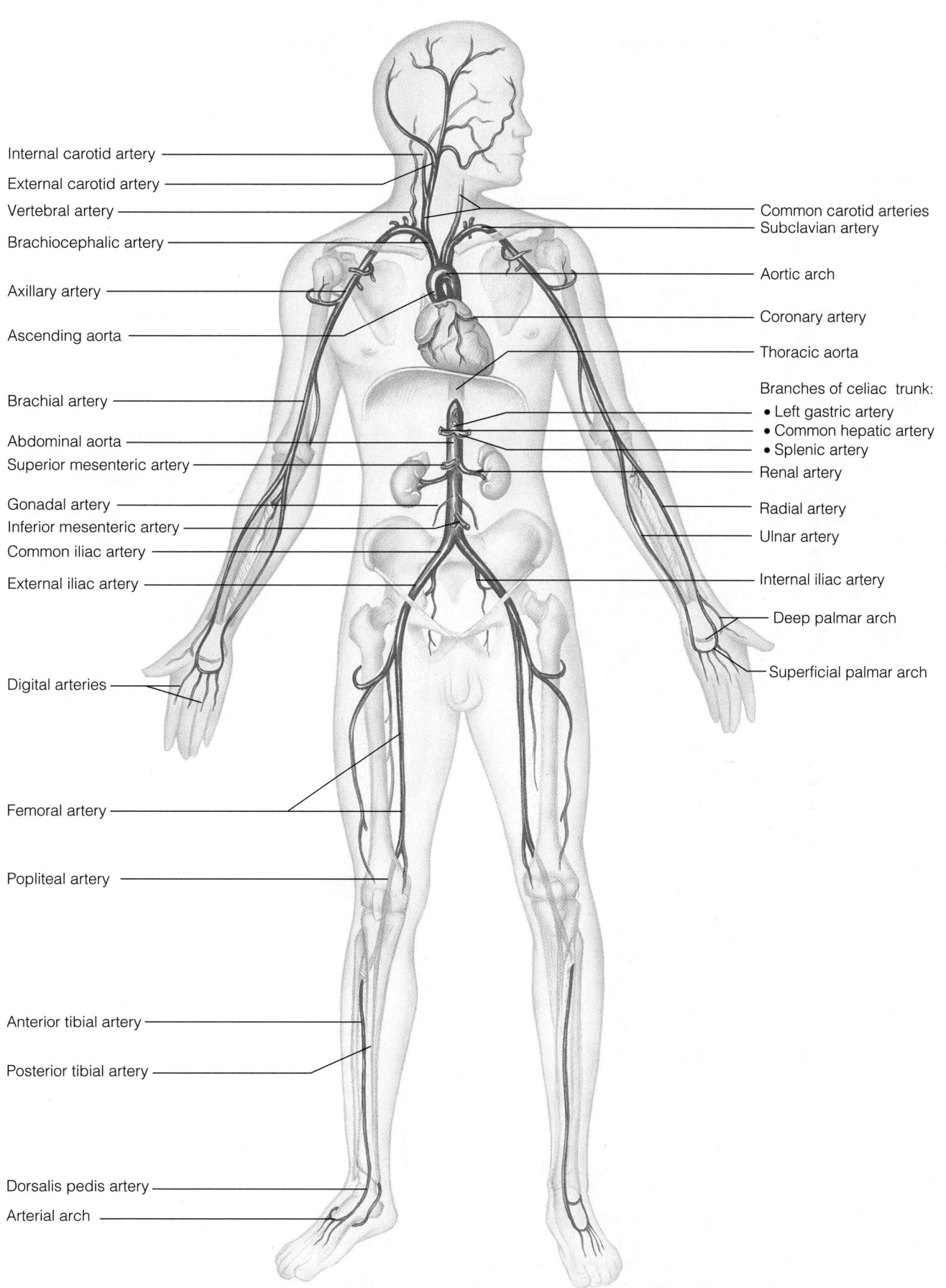

Internal carotid artery

External carotid artery

Vertebral artery

Brachiocephalic artery

Axillary artery

Ascending aorta

Brachial artery

Abdominal aorta

Superior mesenteric artery

Gonadal artery

Inferior mesenteric artery

Common iliac artery

External iliac artery

Digital arteries

Femoral artery

Popliteal artery

Anterior tibial artery

Posterior tibial artery

Dorsalis pedis artery

Arterial arch

Common carotid arteries

Subclavian artery

Aortic arch

Coronary artery

Thoracic aorta

Branches of celiac trunk:
• Left gastric artery
• Common hepatic artery
• Splenic artery

Renal artery

Radial artery

Ulnar artery

Internal iliac artery

Deep palmar arch

Superficial palmar arch

Figure 33–8 ■ Major arteries of the systemic circulation.

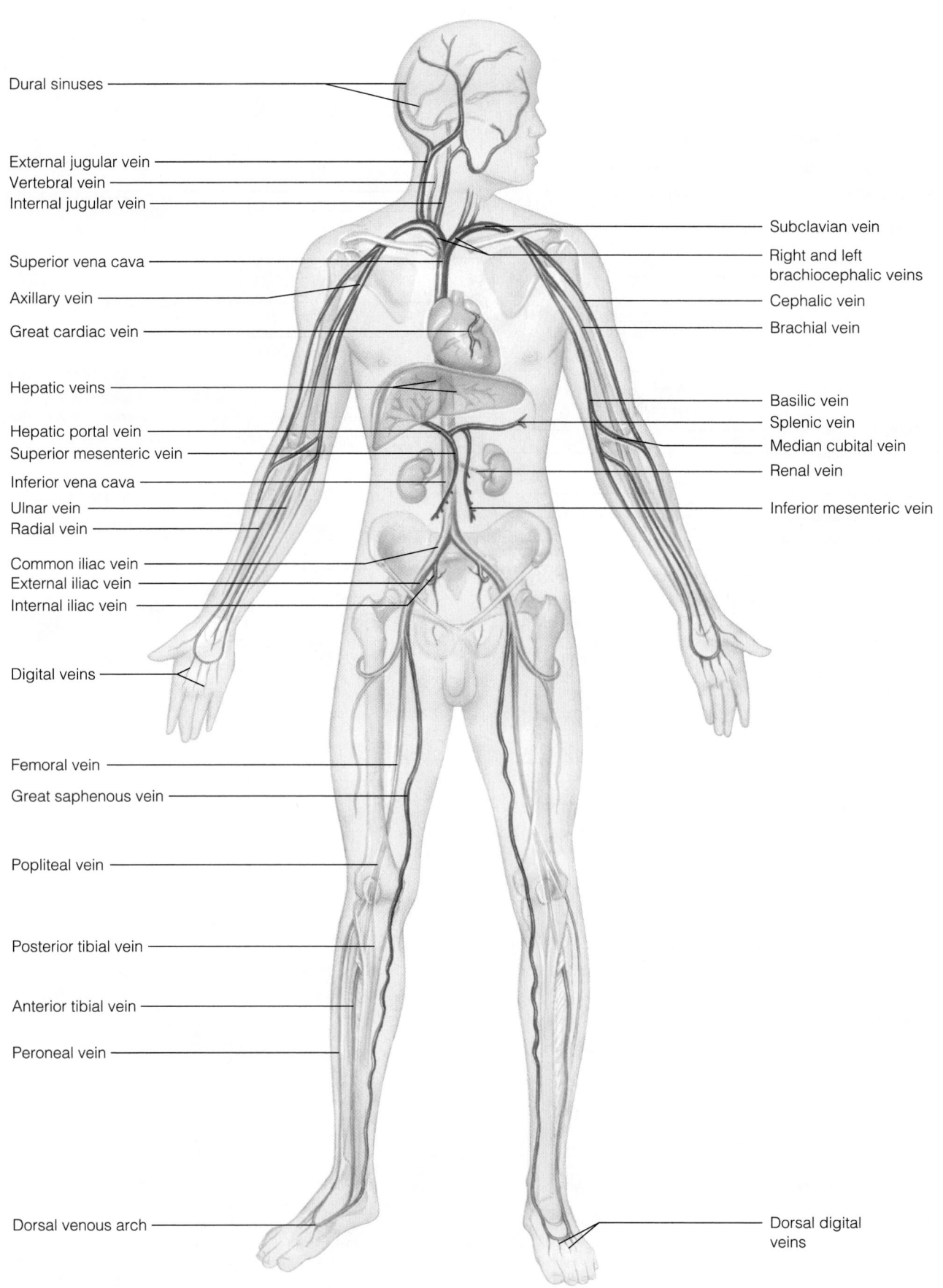

Figure 33–9 ■ Major veins of the systemic circulation.

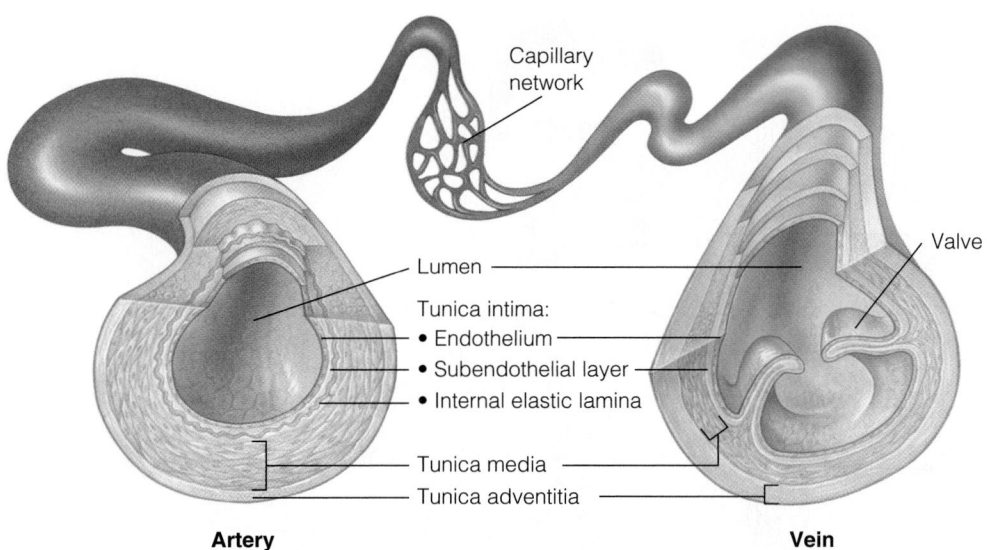

Figure 33–10 ■ Structure of arteries, veins, and capillaries. Capillaries are composed of only a fine tunica intima. Notice that the tunica media is thicker in arteries than in veins.

■ *Diameter of the vessel:* The smaller the diameter of a vessel, the greater the friction against the walls of the vessel and, thus, the greater the impedance to blood flow.

Blood pressure is the force exerted against the walls of the arteries by the blood as it is pumped from the heart. It is most accurately referred to as **mean arterial pressure (MAP)**. The highest pressure exerted against the arterial walls at the peak of ventricular contraction (systole) is called the systolic blood pressure. The lowest pressure exerted during ventricular relaxation (diastole) is the diastolic blood pressure.

Mean arterial blood pressure is regulated mainly by cardiac output (CO) and peripheral vascular resistance (PVR), as represented in this formula: $MAP = CO \times PVR$. For clinical use, the MAP may be estimated by calculating the diastolic blood pressure plus one-third of the pulse pressure (the difference between the systolic and diastolic blood pressure).

Factors Influencing Arterial Blood Pressure

Blood flow, peripheral vascular resistance, and blood pressure, which influence arterial circulation, are in turn influenced by various factors, as follows:

■ The sympathetic and parasympathetic nervous systems are the primary mechanisms that regulate blood pressure. Stimulation of the sympathetic nervous system exerts a major effect on peripheral resistance by causing vasoconstriction of the arterioles, thereby increasing blood pressure. Parasympathetic stimulation causes vasodilation of the arterioles, lowering blood pressure.

■ Baroreceptors and chemoreceptors in the aortic arch, carotid sinus, and other large vessels are sensitive to pressure and

chemical changes and cause reflex sympathetic stimulation, resulting in vasoconstriction, increased heart rate, and increased blood pressure.

■ The kidneys help maintain blood pressure by excreting or conserving sodium and water. When blood pressure decreases, the kidneys initiate the renin–angiotensin mechanism. This stimulates vasoconstriction, resulting in the release of the hormone aldosterone from the adrenal cortex, increasing sodium ion reabsorption and water retention. In addition, pituitary release of antidiuretic hormone (ADH) promotes renal reabsorption of water. The net result is an increase in blood volume and a consequent increase in cardiac output and blood pressure.

■ Temperatures may also affect peripheral resistance: Cold causes vasoconstriction, whereas warmth produces vasodilation. Many chemicals, hormones, and drugs influence blood pressure by affecting CO and/or PVR. For example, epinephrine causes vasoconstriction and increased heart rate; prostaglandins dilate blood vessel diameter (by relaxing vascular smooth muscle); endothelin, a chemical released by the inner lining of vessels, is a potent vasoconstrictor; nicotine causes vasoconstriction; and alcohol and histamine cause vasodilation.

■ Dietary factors, such as intake of salt, saturated fats, and cholesterol elevate blood pressure by affecting blood volume and vessel diameter.

■ Race, gender, age, weight, time of day, position, exercise, and emotional state may also affect blood pressure. These factors influence the arterial pressure. Systemic venous pressure, though it is much lower, is also influenced by such factors as blood volume, venous tone, and right atrial pressure.

ANATOMY, PHYSIOLOGY, AND FUNCTIONS OF THE LYMPHATIC SYSTEM

The structures of the lymphatic system include the lymphatic vessels and several lymphoid organs (Figure 33–11 ■). The organs of the lymphatic system are the lymph nodes, the

spleen, the thymus, the tonsils, and the Peyer's patches of the small intestine. Lymph nodes are small aggregates of specialized cells that assist the immune system by removing foreign

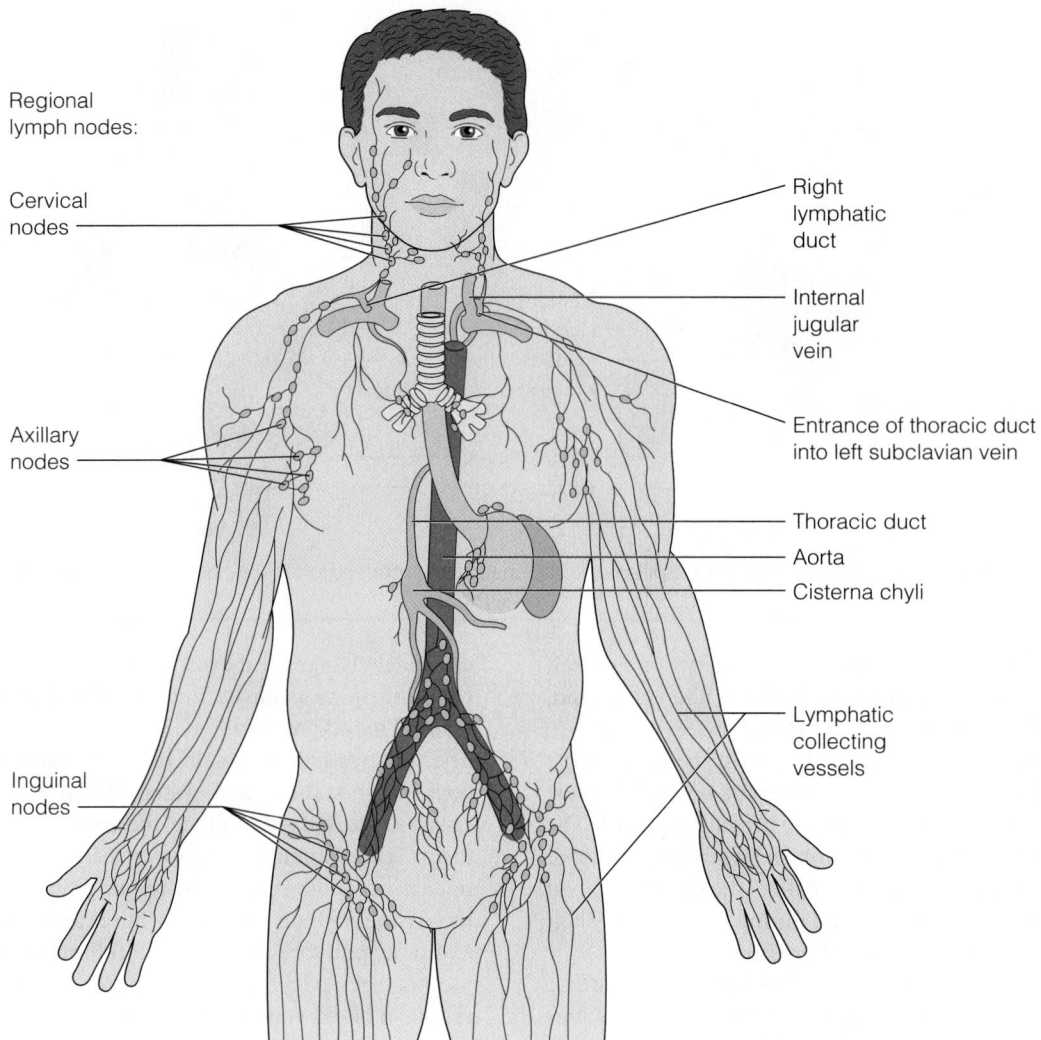

Figure 33–11 ■ The lymphatic system.

material, infectious organisms, and tumor cells from lymph. Lymph nodes are distributed along the lymphatic vessels, forming clusters in certain body regions such as the neck, axilla, and groin (see Figure 33–11). The spleen, the largest lymphoid organ, is in the upper left quadrant of the abdomen under the thorax. The main function of the spleen is to filter the blood by breaking down old red blood cells and storing or releasing to the liver their by-products (such as iron). The spleen also synthesizes lymphocytes, stores platelets for blood clotting, and serves as a reservoir of blood. The thymus gland is in the lower throat and is most active in childhood, producing hormones (such as thymosin) that facilitate the immune action of lymphocytes. The tonsils of the pharynx and Peyer's patches of the small intestine are lymphoid organs that protect the upper respiratory and digestive tracts from foreign pathogens.

The lymphatic vessels, or lymphatics, form a network around the arterial and venous channels and interweave at the capillary beds. They collect and drain excess tissue fluid, called *lymph*, that "leaks" from the cardiovascular system

and accumulates at the venous end of the capillary bed. The lymphatics return this fluid to the heart through a one-way system of lymphatic venules and veins that eventually drain into the right lymphatic duct and left thoracic duct, both of which empty into their respective subclavian veins. Lymphatics are a low-pressure system without a pump; their fluid transport depends on the rhythmic contraction of their smooth muscle and the muscular and respiratory pumps that assist venous circulation.

ASSESSING HEMATOLOGIC, PERIPHERAL VASCULAR, AND LYMPHATIC FUNCTION

Hematologic, peripheral vascular, and lymphatic function are assessed by findings from diagnostic tests, a health assessment interview to collect subjective data, and a physical assessment to collect objective data. Sample documentation of an assessment for peripheral vascular function is included in the box on the next page.

SAMPLE DOCUMENTATION
Assessment of the Peripheral Vascular System

57-year-old male with medical history of type 1 diabetes for 15 years. Client states he has smoked cigars for 20 years (1/day), but "knows he shouldn't." Reports he can't walk more than 20 steps without pain in his legs and sometimes has pain in his feet at night. Pulses in lower extremities (dorsalis pedis, posterior tibial, and popliteal): regular but weak. No bruits auscultated over femoral arteries. When legs elevated and then lowered, the skin was pale on elevation and dusky red when dependent in the sitting position with lower legs dangling. Skin on both lower extremities from knees to toes is cool, shiny, and hairless. Capillary refill of toenails (which are thickened) on great toe is 6 seconds bilaterally. No ankle or tibial edema assessed.

Diagnostic Tests

The results of diagnostic tests of hematologic, peripheral vascular, and lymphatic function are used to support the diagnosis of a specific disease, to provide information to identify or modify the appropriate medications or therapy used to treat the disease, and to help nurses monitor the client's responses to treatment and nursing care interventions. Diagnostic tests to assess the structures and functions of the hematologic, peripheral vascular, and lymphatic systems are described in the Diagnostic Tests table below and summarized in the bulleted list that follows. More information is included in the discussion of specific disorders in Chapters 34 ∞ and 35.

- Tests to evaluate the structure, function, and adequacy of the blood and blood-forming organs include a complete blood count (CBC), erythrocyte sedimentation rate (ESR), and a bone marrow examination.

DIAGNOSTIC TESTS   of Hematologic, Peripheral Vascular, and Lymphatic Disorders

HEMATOLOGIC DISORDERS

NAME OF TEST   Complete blood count (CBC)

PURPOSE AND DESCRIPTION   This is a blood test involving several measurements of blood components. See Table 33–1.

RELATED NURSING CARE   None

NAME OF TEST   Erythrocyte sedimentation rate (ESR)

PURPOSE AND DESCRIPTION   This blood test is done as a measure of inflammation, and is increased in many illnesses, including cancer, heart disease, and kidney disease.

Normal values:
Women: 1–20 mm in 1 hour
Men: 1–15 mm in 1 hour

RELATED NURSING CARE   None

NAME OF TEST   Bone marrow

PURPOSE AND DESCRIPTION   Conducted to evaluate blood-forming tissue; to diagnose multiple myeloma, leukemia, and some lymphomas; and to assess effectiveness of therapy for leukemia. Bone marrow is removed from a site such as the posterior iliac crest with needle aspiration.

NURSING CARE: BONE MARROW STUDIES

Bone marrow specimens are obtained by either aspiration or biopsy. The preferred site for bone marrow aspiration is the posterior iliac crest; the sternum may also be used. The procedure is performed by inserting a needle into the bone and drawing out a sample of the blood in the marrow. A bone marrow biopsy is performed by making a small incision over the bone and screwing a core biopsy instrument into the bone to obtain a specimen. Bone marrow studies are used to diagnose leukemias, metastatic cancer, lymphoma, aplastic anemia, and Hodgkin's disease.

Preparation of the Client

- Explain the purpose and procedure of the test.
- Record vital signs. Assure presence of a signed consent for the procedure.
- Ask the client to void.

- Place in supine position if the specimen will be obtained from the sternum or anterior iliac crest; prone position if the posterior iliac crest will be used.
- Assist in remaining still during the procedure.

After the Procedure

- Apply pressure to the puncture site for 5 to 10 minutes.
- Assess vital signs, and compare results to preprocedure readings.
- Apply a dressing to the puncture site, and monitor for bleeding and infection for 24 hours.

Health Education for the Client and Family

- The procedure (either aspiration or biopsy) takes about 20 minutes.
- A sedative may be given prior to the procedure.
- It is important to remain very still during the procedure to prevent accidental injury.
- Although the area will be anesthetized with a local anesthetic, insertion of the needle will be painful for a short time. Taking deep breaths may make this part of the procedure less painful.
- The aspiration site may ache for 1 or 2 days.
- Report any unusual bleeding immediately.

(continued)

DIAGNOSTIC TESTS of Hematologic, Peripheral Vascular, and Lymphatic Disorders (continued)

NAME OF TEST Magnetic resonance angiography (MRA)

PURPOSE AND DESCRIPTION Used to visualize vascular occlusive disease and aneurysms of the abdominal aorta. The procedure is done by using a non-iodine-based contrast medium injected IV.

RELATED NURSING CARE Assess for any metallic implants, such as a pacemaker or body piercings (if present, test is not performed).

NAME OF TEST Magnetic resonance imaging (MRI)

PURPOSE AND DESCRIPTION A radiologic study used to visualize liver, spleen, and lymph nodes. Does not require injection of contrast medium.

RELATED NURSING CARE Assess for any metallic implants, such as a pacemaker or body piercings. If present, the test will not be performed.

NAME OF TEST CT scan

PURPOSE AND DESCRIPTION A radiologic study used to evaluate the lymph nodes. Contrast medium may be used when assessing the nodes of the abdomen.

RELATED NURSING CARE Assess for allergy to iodine (such as shellfish).

NAME OF TEST Liver and/or spleen scan

PURPOSE AND DESCRIPTION A radiologic study used to assess the liver and/or spleen. A radioisotope is injected IV prior to the scan.

NAME OF TEST Lymphangiography (lymphangiogram)

PURPOSE AND DESCRIPTION This is an x-ray examination of the lymphatic vessels and lymph nodes, used to assess metastasis of the lymph nodes, to identify malignant lymphoma, and to identify the cause of lymphedema. An iodine contrast substance is injected at various sites and fluoroscopy is used to visualize lymphatic filling.

RELATED NURSING CARE Ask the client about allergies to seafood, iodine, or contrast medium used in a previous x-ray test. Tell the client that the blue contrast dye discolors the urine and possibly the skin for a few days.

NAME OF TEST Lymph node biopsy

PURPOSE AND DESCRIPTION Done to obtain tissue for histologic examination for diagnosis and treatment. May be

open (performed in the operating room) or closed (needle) by needle aspiration of tissue from a lymph node.

RELATED NURSING CARE Use sterile technique when changing dressings.

- Disorders of the arteries and veins are diagnosed by various noninvasive examinations, including several discussed in Chapter 30 ∞ (transesophageal echocardiography [TEE], ultrasound, and Doppler studies). A magnetic resonance angiography (MRA) may be done to visualize vascular occlusive disease and abdominal aorta aneurysms.
- Tests of the lymphatic system, including a lymphangiogram and a lymph node biopsy, may be done to identify malignancies, assess metastasis of cancer to lymph nodes, identify the causes of lymphedema, and obtain tissue for diagnosis and treatment.

Regardless of the type of diagnostic test, the nurse is responsible for explaining the procedure and any special preparation needed, assessing for medication use that may affect the outcome of the tests, supporting the client during the examination as necessary, documenting the procedures as appropriate, and monitoring the results of the tests.

Genetic Considerations

When conducting a health assessment interview and a physical assessment, it is important for the nurse to consider genetic in-

fluences on the health of the adult. During the health assessment interview, ask about family members with health problems affecting hematologic, peripheral vascular, or lymphatic function. In addition, ask about a family history of high blood pressure, hemophilia, chronic myeloid leukemia, porphyria, and/or atherosclerosis. Depending on the racial and ethnic background of the client, ask about any family members with sickle cell anemia or thalassemia. During the physical assessment, assess for any manifestations that might indicate a genetic disorder (see the Genetics box on the next page). If data are found to indicate genetic risk factors or alterations, ask about genetic testing and refer for appropriate genetic counseling and evaluation. Chapter 8 ∞ provides further information about genetics in medical-surgical nursing.

Health Assessment Interview

A health assessment interview to determine problems with the structure and functions of the hematologic, peripheral vascular, and/or lymphatic systems may be conducted during a health screening, may focus on a chief complaint (such as fatigue and bleeding), or may be part of a total health assess-

GENETIC CONSIDERATIONS
Hematologic, Peripheral Vascular, and Lymphatic Disorders

- There is a genetic link in 30% to 40% of clients with primary hypertension.
- Sickle cell anemia is the most common inherited blood disorder in the United States, affecting 1 in 500 African Americans. It is characterized by episodes of pain, chronic hemolytic anemia, and severe infections.
- Gaucher disease, more common in descendants of Eastern European Jewish people, is an inherited illness caused by a gene mutation. The gene is responsible for an enzyme that breaks down a specific fat. When the fat is not broken down, it accumulates in the liver, spleen, and bone marrow, causing pain, fatigue, jaundice, bone damage, anemia, and even death.
- Hemophilia A is a hereditary blood disorder, primarily affecting males, characterized by a deficiency of the blood clotting factor named Factor VIII. Abnormal bleeding results.
- Chronic myeloid leukemia (CML), a cancer of blood cells, is characterized by replacement of bone marrow with malignant, leukemic cells. Leukemic cells also circulate in the blood, causing enlargement of the spleen, liver, and other organs. This leukemia is the result of chromosomal abnormality called the Philadelphia chromosome.
- Porphyria is a group of genetic blood diseases in which heme production is disrupted. When heme production is disrupted, porphyrins (a part of heme) are overproduced and cause illnesses; they also give urine a reddish-purple color.
- Thalassemia, an inherited disease of faulty hemoglobin synthesis, is more often found in descendants of people living near the Mediterranean Sea, Africa, the Middle East, and Asia. It comprises a group of disorders that range from very mild blood abnormalities to severe or fatal anemia.
- Atherosclerosis is characterized by narrowing of arteries by cholesterol-rich plaques of immune system cells. Risk factors may be genetic and/or environmental. Although it may affect people at any age, it usually does not cause health problems until people are in their 40s and 50s.

---

ment. Interview questions categorized by functional health patterns are listed in the Functional Health Pattern Interview on the next page.

Peripheral Vascular System

If the client has problems involving the peripheral vascular system, analyze its onset, characteristics and course, severity, precipitating and relieving factors, and any associated symptoms, noting the timing and circumstances. For example, ask the client the following:

- Does the leg pain occur only with activities such as walking, or also during rest?
- Do your ankles swell at the end of the day, after sitting for prolonged periods, or after sleeping all night?
- Does temperature or the position of your body affect the symptoms?

Explore the client's medical and family history for any cardiovascular disorders, such as heart disease, arteriosclerosis, peripheral vascular disease (PVD), stroke, hypertension (HTN), hyperlipidemia (elevated fat in blood) and blood clots, or other chronic illnesses (e.g., diabetes). Ask about past surgery of the heart or blood vessels or tests to evaluate their function and about any medications that affect circulation or blood pressure.

Ask the client about past or present pain, burning, numbness, or tingling in the limbs or digits; leg fatigue or cramps; changes in skin color or temperature, texture of hair, ulcers or skin irritation, varicose veins, phlebitis (inflamed veins) or edema (swelling). Explore the client's nutritional history for intake of protein, vitamins and minerals, salt, fats, and fluid. Quantify any consumption of caffeine and alcohol and history of smoking (packs per day for how many years) or other tobacco use. Assess the client's activity level for exercise habits and tolerance.

It is important to consider socioeconomic factors that may precipitate or aggravate circulatory problems (e.g., inadequate clothing, shoes, or shelter) and occupational factors, such as prolonged standing or sitting or exposure to temperature extremes. Also assess psychosocial factors that may affect the client's stress level and emotional state.

Lymphatic System

The health assessment of the lymphatic system includes a review of specific problems, such as lymph node enlargement or swollen glands, as well as other more general complaints about infection or impaired immunity, such as fever, fatigue, or weight loss. If a health problem exists, analyze its onset, characteristics, severity, and precipitating and relieving factors, noting the timing and circumstances. For example, ask the client the following:

- Did you notice that the glands in your neck became swollen after an infection?
- Have you noticed increased fatigue or weakness?
- Have you ever been exposed to radiation?

Explore the client's history for chronic illnesses (e.g., cardiovascular disease, renal disease, cancer, tuberculosis, HIV infection), predisposing factors (e.g., surgery, trauma, infection, blood transfusions, intravenous drug use), and environmental exposure (e.g., radiation, toxic chemicals, travel-related infectious disease). Review the family history for any incidence of cancer, anemia, or blood dyscrasias. Ask the client about past or present bleeding (e.g., from the nose, gums, or mouth; from vomiting; from the rectum; bruising) and associated symptoms (e.g., pallor, dizziness, fatigue, difficulty breathing); lymph node changes (e.g., enlargement, pain or tenderness, itching, warmth); swelling of extremities; and recurrent irritations or infections. Lastly, an assessment

FUNCTIONAL HEALTH PATTERN INTERVIEW   Hematologic, Peripheral Vascular, and Lymphatic Systems

Functional Health Pattern	Interview Questions and Leading Statements
Health Perception-Health Management	■ Describe any problems you have had with bleeding, bruising, swollen glands, and circulation (for example, heart disease, hardening of the arteries, high blood pressure, stroke, clots, high cholesterol). ■ Have you ever been diagnosed with a health problem involving the blood, heart, blood vessels, or lymph glands? If so, what were they and how were they treated? ■ Is there a family history of bleeding, cancer, or anemia? Explain. ■ What medications, vitamins, dietary supplements, or over-the-counter drugs do you take now? ■ Do you or have you ever smoked? If so, what, for how long, and how many a day?
Nutritional-Metabolic	■ Describe your usual intake of food and fluids in a 24-hour period. ■ Do you drink liquids with caffeine? If so, how much? ■ Do you drink alcohol? If so, what type, how much, and how often? ■ Describe how much salt you use on your food. ■ Describe what type of fatty foods you eat. How often? ■ Have you noticed any change in the color, temperature, or appearance of the skin on your arms, hands, legs, or feet? If so, what were they? ■ Have you noticed any glands that are sore and swollen? What do you think causes this? ■ Have you noticed an increase in the time it takes your blood to clot or how easily you bruise? ■ Have you noticed loss of hair, bulging veins, sores that will not heal on your legs, or thicker toenails? Have you ever worn support stockings? ■ Do your feet ever swell or your shoes feel tight? If so, when does this happen and what do you do to decrease the swelling?
Elimination	■ Have you noticed any blood in your urine or bowel movements? ■ Have your bowel movements been a dark black color?
Activity-Exercise	■ Describe your activities in a typical day. ■ Do you exercise regularly? Describe what you do when you exercise. ■ Have your activities or exercise abilities changed? If so, explain. ■ Do you have leg pain when you walk? If so, where is it located? How far do you walk before you have pain? Describe the pain. What do you do to relieve it? ■ Do you feel tired even after sleep and rest? Describe the feeling.
Sleep-Rest	■ How much rest and sleep do you get each day? ■ Do leg cramps ever wake you at night? If so, describe the pain and what you do to relieve it.
Cognitive-Perceptual	■ Do you have any of these sensations in your legs or feet: pain, cramps, burning, numbness, tingling? ■ If you have these sensations, when do they occur, how long do they last, and what do you do to relieve them?
Self-Perception-Self-Concept	■ How does having this condition make you feel about yourself?
Role-Relationships	■ How has having this condition affected your relationships with others? ■ Has having this condition interfered with your ability to work? Explain. ■ Does your work environment bring you into contact with any chemicals? Describe them.
Sexuality-Reproductive	■ Has this condition interfered with your usual sexual activity? ■ For women: Have you noticed any changes in your menstrual flow? If so, describe them.
Coping-Stress-Tolerance	■ Has having this condition created stress for you? ■ Have you experienced any kind of stress that makes the condition worse? Explain. ■ Describe what you do when you feel stressed.
Value-Belief	■ Describe how specific relationships or activities help you cope with this problem. ■ Describe specific cultural beliefs or practices that affect how you care for and feel about this problem. ■ Are there any specific treatments (such as blood transfusions) that you would not use to treat this problem?

of the client's socioeconomic status, lifestyle, intravenous drug use, and sexual practices may be significant in determining risk for diseases associated with impaired lymphatic function.

Physical Assessment

Physical assessment of the hematologic, peripheral vascular, and lymphatic systems can be performed either as part of a total assessment or alone for clients with suspected or known problems with function of these systems, either from disease or from surgery or immobility. The techniques used to assess these systems include inspection of the skin for such changes as edema, ulcerations, or alterations in color and temperature; auscultation of blood pressure; and palpation of the major pulse points of the body (Figure 33–12 ■) and lymph nodes. The client may be assessed in the supine, sitting, and standing positions. Normal age-related findings for the older adult are summarized in Table 33–3.

Physical assessment of the lymphatic system is usually integrated into the assessment of other body systems. For example, the tonsils are inspected with the pharynx during the head and neck assessment; the regional lymph nodes are evaluated with corresponding body regions (e.g., occipital, auricular, and cervical nodes are evaluated with assessment of the head and neck, axillary nodes with assessment of the breast or thorax, epitrochlear node with assessment of the peripheral vascular

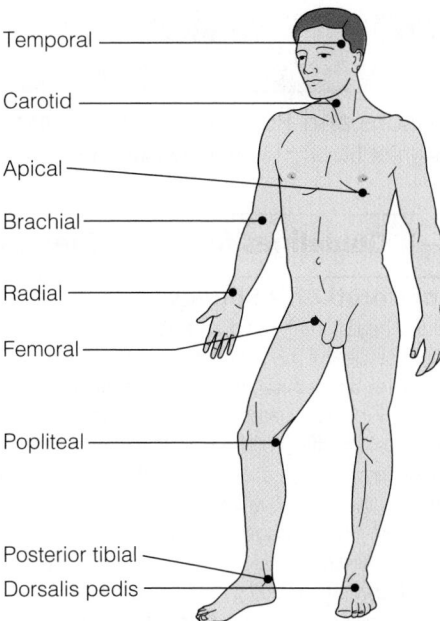

Figure 33–12 ■ Body sites at which peripheral pulses are most easily palpated.

exam of the arms, and inguinal nodes with assessment of the abdomen); the spleen can be palpated during the abdominal assessment. The techniques of inspection and palpation are used for the lymphatic examination.

TABLE 33–3 Age-Related Changes in the Hematologic, Peripheral Vascular, and Lymphatic Systems

AGE-RELATED CHANGE	SIGNIFICANCE
Bone marrow: ↓ ability of bone marrow to respond to need for increased RBCs, WBCs, and platelets.	■ Anemia may result.
Blood vessels: ■ *Tunica intima*: fibrosis, calcium and lipid accumulation, cellular proliferation. ■ *Tunica media*: thins, elastin fibers calcify; increase in calcium results in stiffening. Baroreceptor function is impaired and peripheral resistance increases. ■ *Tunica adventicia*: no change.	■ As a result of age-related changes, the systolic blood pressure rises. Decreased arterial elasticity results in vascular changes in the heart, kidneys, and pituitary gland. Decreased baroreceptor function results in postural hypotension. Vessels in the head, neck, and extremities are more prominent. ■ Inefficient vasoconstriction, decreased cardiac output, and reduced muscle mass and subcutaneous tissue lead to a reduced ability to respond to cold temperatures. ■ With a decrease in blood pressure and changes in blood vessel walls, tissue perfusion may be inadequate, leading to edema, inflammation, pressure ulcers, and changes in effects of medications.
Immune system: ■ Impaired function of B and T lymphocytes. ■ ↓ production of antibodies. ■ Unable to distinguish "self" from "non-self." ■ Phagocytic immune response delayed.	■ Increased risk for infection, with decreased manifestations of an actual infection. ■ Increased incidence of cancers. ■ Altered response to antigens (such as PPD test). ■ May have reactivation of TB.

HEMATOLOGIC, PERIPHERAL VASCULAR, AND LYMPHATIC ASSESSMENTS

Blood Pressure and Pulse Pressure Assessment

See Box 33–1 for blood pressure measurement guidelines.

BOX 33–1 Guidelines for Blood Pressure Assessment

Review of Korotkoff's Sounds

The first sound heard is the systolic pressure; at least two consecutive sounds should be clear. If the sound disappears and then is heard again 10 to 15 mm later, an auscultatory gap is present; this may be a normal variant, or it may be associated with hypertension. The first diastolic sound is heard as a muffling of the Korotkoff's sound and is considered the best approximation of the true diastolic pressure. The second diastolic sound is the level at which sounds are no longer heard.

The American Heart Association recommends documenting all three readings when measuring blood pressure, for example, 120/72/64. If only two readings are documented, the systolic and the second diastolic pressure are taken, for example, 120/64.

Technique Reminders

- Choose a cuff of an appropriate size: The cuff should snugly cover two-thirds of the upper arm, and the bladder should completely encircle the arm. The bladder should be centered over the brachial artery, with the lower edge 2 to 3 cm above the antecubital space.
- The client's arm should be slightly flexed and supported (on a table or by the examiner) at heart level.
- To determine how high to inflate the cuff, palpate the brachial pulse, and inflate the cuff to the point on the manometer at which the pulse is no longer felt; then, add 30 mmHg to this reading, and use the sum as the target for inflation. Wait 15 seconds before reinflating the cuff to auscultate the BP.
- To recheck a BP, wait at least 30 seconds before attempting another inflation.
- Always inflate the cuff completely, then deflate it. Once deflation begins, allow it to continue; do not try to reinflate the cuff if the first systolic sound is not heard or if the cuff inadvertently deflates.
- The bell of the stethoscope more effectively transmits the low-pitched sounds of BP.

Sources of Error

- Falsely high readings can occur if the cuff is too small, too loose, or if the client supports his or her own arm.
- Falsely low readings can occur if a standard cuff is used on a client with thin arms.

- Inadequate inflation may result in underestimation of the systolic pressure or overestimation of the diastolic pressure if an auscultatory gap is present.
- Rapid deflation and repeated or slow inflations (causing venous congestion) can lead to underestimation of the systolic BP and overestimation of the diastolic BP.

Factors Altering Blood Pressure

- A change from the horizontal to upright position causes a slight decrease (5 to 10 mm) in systolic BP; the diastolic BP remains unchanged or rises slightly.
- BP taken in the arm is lower when the client is standing.
- If the BP is taken with the client in the lateral recumbent position, a lower BP reading may be obtained in both arms; this is especially apparent in the right arm with the client in the left lateral position.
- Factors that increase BP include exercise, caffeine, cold environment, eating a large meal, painful stimuli, and emotions.
- Factors that lower BP include sleep (by 20 mmHg) and very fast, slow, or irregular heart rates.
- BP tends to be higher in taller or heavier clients.

Alternative Methods of Blood Pressure Measurement

- The palpatory method may be necessary if severe hypotension is present and the BP is inaudible. Palpate the brachial pulse, and inflate the cuff 30 mm above the point where the pulse disappears; deflate the cuff, and note the point on the manometer where the pulse becomes palpable again. Record this as the palpatory systolic BP.
- Leg BP measurement may be needed when there is injury of the arms or to rule out coarctation of the aorta or aortic insufficiency when arm diastolic BP is over 90 mmHg. Place the client in the prone or supine position with the leg slightly flexed. Place a large leg cuff on the thigh with the bladder centered over the popliteal artery. Place the bell of the stethoscope over the popliteal space. Normal leg systolic BP is higher than arm BP; diastolic BP should be equal to or lower than arm BP. Abnormally low leg BP occurs with aortic insufficiency and coarctation of the aorta.

Technique/Normal Findings	Abnormal Findings
Auscultate blood pressure in each arm with the client seated. *The normal blood pressure is considered to be <120/<80, with readings of 120–139/80–89 diagnosed as prehypertension.*	<ul><li>Consistent BP readings over 140/90 in adults under age 40 is considered hypertension.</li><li>BP under 90/60 is considered hypotension.</li><li>An **auscultatory gap**—a temporary disappearance of sound between the systolic and diastolic BP—may be a normal variation, or it may be associated with systolic HTN or a drop in diastolic BP due to aortic stenosis.</li><li>**Korotkoff's sounds** (see Box 33–1) may be heard down to zero with cardiac valve replacements, hyperkinetic states, thyrotoxicosis, and severe anemia, as well as after vigorous exercise.</li><li>The sounds of aortic regurgitation may obscure the diastolic BP.</li><li>A difference of over 10 mmHg between arms suggests arterial compression on the side of the lower reading, aortic dissection, or coarctation of the aorta.</li></ul>

Technique/Normal Findings	Abnormal Findings
Auscultate blood pressure in each arm with the client standing. If orthostatic changes occur, measure the BP with the client supine, legs dangling, and again with the client standing, 1 to 3 minutes apart. *A decrease of systolic BP is expected, but should be <10 mmHg; diastolic BP should not drop on standing.*	■ A decrease in systolic BP of over 10 to 15 mmHg and a drop in diastolic BP on standing is called **orthostatic hypotension**. Causes include antihypertensive medications, volume depletion, PVD, prolonged bed rest, and aging.
Observe the pulse pressure. The **pulse pressure** is the difference between the systolic and diastolic BP. For example, if the BP is 140/80, the pulse pressure is 60. *A normal pulse pressure is one-third the systolic measurement.*	■ A widened pulse pressure with an elevated systolic BP occurs with exercise, arteriosclerosis, severe anemia, thyrotoxicosis, and increased intracranial pressure. ■ A narrowed pulse pressure with a decreased systolic BP occurs with shock, cardiac failure, and pulmonary embolus.

PRACTICE ALERT

If unable to auscultate blood pressure or palpate pulses, a Doppler ultrasound device may be used to evaluate blood flow. Apply a dime-sized amount of gel over the blood vessel to be assessed and lightly place the probe over the gel. Listen for a whooshing (artery) or rushing (vein) sound.

Skin Assessment Inspect the color of the skin. *The skin color should be appropriate to the client's age and race.*	■ Pallor reflects constriction of peripheral blood flow (e.g., due to syncope or shock) or decreased circulating oxyhemoglobin (e.g., due to hemorrhage or anemia). ■ Central cyanosis of the lips, earlobes, oral mucosa, and tongue suggests chronic cardiopulmonary disease. (See Box 33–2 for abnormal findings associated with peripheral vascular and lymphatic assessment.)
Inspect the skin of the extremities and over the regional lymph nodes, noting any edema, erythema, red streaks, or skin lesions. *There should be no edema, redness, or lesions over the regional lymph nodes.*	■ Lymphangitis (inflammation of a lymphatic vessel) may produce a red streak with induration (hardness) following the course of the lymphatic collecting duct; infected skin lesions may be present, particularly between the digits. ■ **Lymphedema** (swelling due to lymphatic obstruction) occurs with congenital lymphatic anomaly (Milroy's disease) or with trauma to the regional lymphatic ducts from surgery or metastasis (e.g., arm lymphedema after radical mastectomy with axillary node removal). ■ Edema of lymphatic origin is usually not pitting, and the skin may be thickened; one example is the taut swelling of the face and body that occurs with myxedema, associated with hypothyroidism.

BOX 33–2 Abnormal Findings Associated with Peripheral Vascular and Lymphatic Assessment

- *Pallor* is an absence of color of the skin. The degree of pallor depends on the client's normal skin color and health status. Dark skin may appear ashen or have a yellowish tinge.
- *Cyanosis* is a bluish discoloration of the skin and mucous membranes in people with light skin. In people with dark skin, cyanosis may be difficult to observe. Inspect the nail beds and conjunctiva.
- *Edema* is an abnormal accumulation of fluid in the interstitial spaces of body tissues. It is often most apparent in the lower extremities.
- *Varicose veins* are tortuous and dilated veins that have incompetent valves. The saphenous veins of the legs are most commonly affected.
- *Enlarged lymph nodes* result from infection or malignancy.

- *Atrophic changes* are changes in size or activity of body tissues as the result of pathology or injury. Decreased blood flow and oxygenation of the lower extremities often cause atrophic changes of loss of hair, thickened toe nails, changes in pigmentation, and ulcerations.
- *Gangrene* is the necrosis (or death) of tissue, most often the result of loss of blood supply and infection. Gangrene often begins in the most distal of the tissues of the extremities.
- *Pressure ulcers*, also called decubitus ulcers or bed sores, are the result of ischemia and hypoxia of tissue following prolonged pressure. These ulcers often are located over bony prominences. If untreated, the tissue changes proceed from red skin to deep, crater-like ulcers.

Technique/Normal Findings	Abnormal Findings

Artery and Vein Assessment

Palpate the temporal arteries. *There should be no redness, swelling, nodules, or variations in pulse amplitude.*

- Redness, swelling, nodularity, and variations in pulse amplitude may occur with temporal arteritis.

Inspect and palpate the carotid arteries. Note symmetry, the pulse rate, rhythm, volume, and amplitude. *Note any variation with respiration. Describe all pulses as increased, normal, diminished, or absent. Scales ranging from 0 to 4+ are sometimes used as follows:*

0 = Absent
1+ = Diminished
2+ = Normal
3+ = Increased
4+ = Bounding

Pulse waveforms are shown in Box 33–3. *The carotid pulses should be bilaterally equal in rate, rhythm, volume, and amplitude.*

- A unilateral pulsating bulge is seen with a tortuous or kinked carotid artery.
- Alterations in pulse rate or rhythm are due to cardiac dysrhythmias.
- An absent pulse indicates arterial occlusion.
- A hypokinetic (weak) pulse is associated with decreased stroke volume (Box 33–3B). This may be due to congestive heart failure (CHF), aortic stenosis, or hypovolemia; to increased peripheral resistance, which may result from cold temperatures; or to arterial narrowing, commonly found with atherosclerosis.
- A hyperkinetic (bounding) pulse occurs with increased stroke volume and/or decreased peripheral resistance (Box 33–3C). This may result from states in which cardiac output is high or from aortic regurgitation. It also may occur with anemia, hyperthyroidism, bradycardia, or reduced compliance, as with atherosclerosis.
- A bigeminal pulse is marked by decreased amplitude of every second beat (Box 33–3D). This may be due to premature contractions (usually ventricular).
- Pulsus alternans is a regular pulse with alternating strong and weak beats (Box 33–3E). This may be due to left ventricular failure and severe HTN.

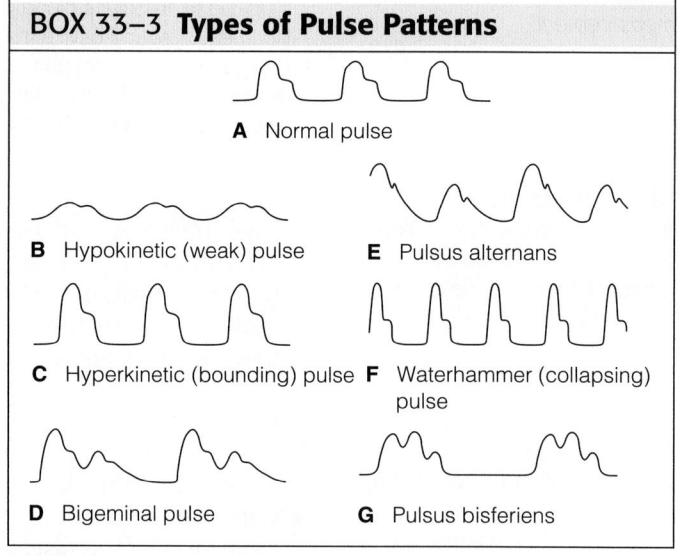

BOX 33–3 Types of Pulse Patterns

A Normal pulse

B Hypokinetic (weak) pulse

C Hyperkinetic (bounding) pulse

D Bigeminal pulse

E Pulsus alternans

F Waterhammer (collapsing) pulse

G Pulsus bisferiens

Auscultate the carotid arteries, using the bell of the stethoscope. *No bruits should be heard.*

- A murmuring or blowing sound heard over stenosed peripheral vessels is known as a *bruit*. A bruit heard over the middle to upper carotid artery suggests atherosclerosis.

Inspect and palpate the internal and external jugular veins for venous pressure. *See Box 33–4 for guidelines for assessing jugular venous pressure (JVP).*

- An increase in jugular venous pressure (JVP) over 3 cm and located above the sternal angle reflects increased right atrial pressure. This occurs with right ventricular failure or, less commonly, with constrictive pericarditis, tricuspid stenosis, and superior venae cavae obstruction.

Technique/Normal Findings   **Abnormal Findings**

BOX 33–4 Assessing Jugular Venous Pressure

When a client with normal venous pressure lies in the supine position, full neck veins are normally visible, but as the head of the bed is elevated, the pulsations disappear. In the client with greatly elevated venous pressure, visible pulsations of the jugular vein are present even in the upright position. To conduct the inspection:

1. Remove clothing from the client's neck and chest. Elevate the head of the bed 30 to 45 degrees, and turn the client's head to the opposite side. Shine a light tangentially across the neck to increase shadows. If the external jugular veins are distended, they will be visible vertically between the mandible and outer clavicle.

2. If jugular distention is present, assess the JVP by measuring from the highest point of visible distention to the sternal angle (the point at which the clavicles meet) on both sides of the neck (see the accompanying figure). Bilateral measurements above 3 cm are considered elevated and indicate increased venous pressure; distention on only one side may indicate obstruction.

Assessment of the highest point of jugular vein distention.

If venous pressure is elevated, assess the hepatojugular reflex. (Compress the liver in the right upper abdominal quadrant with the palm of the hand for 30 to 60 seconds while observing the jugular veins.)

- A decrease in venous pressure reflects reduced left ventricular output or blood volume.
- Unilateral neck vein distention suggests local compression or anatomic anomaly.
- A rise in the column of neck vein distention over 1 cm with liver compression indicates right heart failure.

Upper Extremity Assessment

Inspect and palpate the arms and hands, noting size and symmetry, skin color, and temperature. *Arms and hands should be symmetrical in size and shape, warm, and of appropriate skin color.*

- Unilateral swelling with venous prominence occurs with venous obstruction.
- Extreme localized pallor of the fingers is seen with Raynaud's disease.
- Cyanosis of the nail beds reflects chronic cardiopulmonary disease.
- Cold temperature of the hands and fingers occurs with vasoconstriction.

Palpate the nail beds for capillary refill. (Apply pressure to the client's fingertips. Watch for blanching of the nail beds. Release the pressure. Note the time it takes for capillary refill, indicated by the return of pink color on release of the pressure.) *Capillary refill should be less than 2 seconds (i.e., immediate).*

- Capillary refill that takes more than 2 seconds reflects circulatory compromise, such as hypovolemia or anemia.

Assess venous pattern and pressure. (Elevate one of the client's arms over the head for a few seconds. Slowly lower the arm. Observe the filling of the client's hand veins.) *Hand veins should fill equally and immediately.*

- Distention of hand veins at elevations over 9 cm above heart level reflects an increase in systemic venous pressure.

Technique/Normal Findings	Abnormal Findings
Palpate the radial and brachial pulses. Note rate, rhythm, volume amplitude, symmetry, variations with respiration. (See Box 33–3 for pulse patterns.) *Radial and brachial pulses should have equal and normal rate, be strong, and not vary with respirations.*	■ Alterations in pulse rate or rhythm are due to cardiac dysrhythmias (such as atrial fibrillation, atrial flutter, and premature ventricular contractions). A pulse rate over 100 bpm is tachycardia; a pulse rate below 60 bpm is bradycardia. ■ A pulse deficit (slower radial rate than apical rate) occurs with dysrhythmias and CHF. ■ Irregularities of rhythm produce early beats and pauses (skipped beats) in the pulse, which may be regular in pattern, sporadic, or grossly irregular. ■ Diminished or absent radial pulses may be due to thromboangiitis obliterans (Buerger's disease) or acute arterial occlusion. ■ A weak and thready pulse, often with tachycardia, reflects decreased cardiac output. ■ A bounding pulse occurs with hyperkinetic states and atherosclerosis. ■ Unequal pulses between extremities suggest arterial narrowing or obstruction on one side. ■ In sinus dysrhythmia (a normal variant, especially in young adults), the pulse rate increases with inspiration and decreases with expiration.
If arterial insufficiency is suspected, palpate the ulnar pulse and perform the Allen test: ■ Have the client make a tight fist. ■ Compress both the radial and ulnar arteries. ■ Have the client open the hand to a slightly flexed position. ■ Observe for pallor and manifestations of pain. ■ Release the ulnar artery and observe for the return of pink color within 3 to 5 seconds. ■ Repeat the procedure on the radial artery. *Color should return within 3 to 5 seconds in both the ulnar and the radial arteries.*	■ The normal ulnar artery may or may not have a palpable pulse. ■ Persistent pallor with the Allen test suggests ulnar artery occlusion.
Inspect and palpate each leg, noting size, shape, and symmetry; arterial pattern; skin color, temperature, and texture; hair pattern; pigmentation; rashes; ulcers, sensation; and capillary refill. *Legs should be symmetric in size and shape, arterial pattern, appropriate color, warm, without lesions. Capillary refill on toenails should be immediate.*	■ Chronic arterial insufficiency may be due to arteriosclerosis or autonomic dysfunction, or to acute occlusion resulting from thrombosis, embolus, or aneurysm. ■ Signs of arterial disruption include pallor, dependent rubor (dusky redness); cool to cold temperature; and atrophic changes, such as hair loss with shiny and smooth texture, thickened nails, sensory loss, slow capillary refill, and muscle atrophy. ■ Ulcers with symmetric margins, a deep base, black or necrotic tissue, and absence of bleeding may occur at pressure points on or between the toes, on the heel, on the lateral malleolar or tibial area, over the metatarsal heads, or along the side or sole of the foot. ■ Gangrene due to complete arterial occlusion presents as black, dry, hard skin; pregangrenous color changes include deep cyanosis and purple-black discoloration.

Lower Extremity Assessment

With the client supine, assess the venous pattern of the legs. Repeat with the client standing. *Venous pattern on both legs should be symmetric, and there should be no edema, cyanosis, or lesions.*	■ Signs of venous insufficiency include swelling, thickened skin, cyanosis, stasis dermatitis (brown pigmentation, erythema, and scaling), and superficial ankle ulcers located predominantly at the medial malleolus with uneven margins, ruddy granulation tissue, and bleeding. ■ Varicose veins appear as dilated, tortuous, and thickened veins, which are more prominent in a dependent position.

Technique/Normal Findings	Abnormal Findings
Palpate the femoral, popliteal, posterior tibial, and dorsalis pedis pulses for volume, amplitude, and symmetry (see Figure 33–12). *All lower extremity pulses should be strong and equal in amplitude.*	■ Diminished or absent leg pulses suggest partial or complete arterial occlusion of the proximal vessel and are often due to arteriosclerosis obliterans. ■ Increased and widened femoral and popliteal pulsations suggest aneurysm. ■ Absence of a posterior tibial pulse with signs and symptoms of arterial insufficiency is usually due to acute occlusion by thrombosis or embolus. ■ Diminished or absent pedal pulses are often due to popliteal occlusion associated with diabetes mellitus.
If pulses are diminished, observe for postural color changes. Elevate both legs 60 degrees, and observe the color of the soles of the feet. Have the client sit and dangle the legs; note the return of color to the feet.	■ Extensive pallor on elevation is suggestive of arterial insufficiency. ■ Rubor (dusky redness) of the toes and feet along with delayed venous return (over 45 seconds) suggests arterial insufficiency.
If arterial insufficiency is suspected, auscultate the femoral arteries. *No bruits should be heard.*	■ Femoral bruits suggest arterial narrowing due to arteriosclerosis.
Inspect and gently palpate the calves. *There should be no redness or swelling, heat, or pain in the calves of the legs.*	■ Redness, warmth, swelling, tenderness, and cords along a superficial vein suggest thrombophlebitis or deep venous thrombosis.
Inspect and palpate for edema. Use your thumb to compress the dorsum of the client's foot, around the ankles, and along the tibia (Figure 33–13A ■). A depression in the skin that does not immediately refill is called pitting edema. *Normally, there is no edema.*	Edema can be graded on a scale from 1+ to 4+ (Figure 33–13B): 1+ (–2 mm depression) No visible change in the leg; slight pitting 2+ (–4 mm depression) No marked change in the shape of the leg; pitting slightly deeper 3+ (–6 mm depression) Leg visibly swollen; pitting deep 4+ (–8 mm depression) Leg very swollen; pitting very deep ■ Edema may be caused by disease of the cardiovascular system such as CHF; by renal, hepatic, or lymphatic problems; or by infection. ■ Venous distention suggests venous insufficiency or incompetence.

Figure 33–13 ■ Evaluation of edema. *A*, Palpating for edema over the tibia. *B*, Four-point scale for grading edema.

Technique/Normal Findings	Abnormal Findings

Abdominal Assessment

Inspect and palpate the abdominal aorta. Note size, width, and any visible pulsations or bulging. *Abdominal aorta should be of appropriate size without visible pulsations or bulging.*

- A pulsating mass in the upper abdomen suggests an aortic aneurysm, particularly in the older adult.
- An aorta greater than 2.5 to 3 cm in width reflects pathologic dilation, most likely due to arteriosclerosis.

Auscultate the epigastrium and each abdominal quadrant, using the bell of the stethoscope (Figure 33–14 ■). *No bruits should be heard over the abdominal aorta.*

- Abdominal bruits reflect turbulent blood flow associated with partial arterial occlusion.
- A bruit heard over the aorta suggests an aneurysm.
- A bruit heard over the epigastrium and radiating laterally, especially with HTN, suggests renal artery stenosis.
- Bruits heard in the lower abdominal quadrants suggest partial occlusion of the iliac arteries.

Aorta
Renal artery
Iliac artery
Femoral artery

Figure 33–14 ■ Auscultation sites of the abdominal aorta and its branches.

Lymph Node Assessment

Palpate the regional lymph nodes of the head and neck, axillae, arms, and groin. Use firm, circular movements of the finger pads and note size, shape, symmetry, consistency, delineation, mobility, tenderness, sensation, and condition of overlying skin. *Nodes should not be enlarged or painful.*

- **Lymphadenopathy** refers to the enlargement of lymph nodes (over 1 cm) with or without tenderness. It may be caused by inflammation, infection, or malignancy of the nodes or the regions drained by the nodes.
- Lymph node enlargement with tenderness suggests inflammation (*lymphadenitis*). With bacterial infection, the nodes may be warm and matted with localized swelling.
- Malignant or metastatic nodes may be hard, indicating lymphoma; rubbery, indicating Hodgkin's disease; or fixed to adjacent structures. Usually they are not tender.
- Ear infections and scalp and facial lesions, such as acne, may cause enlargement of the preauricular and cervical nodes.
- Anterior cervical nodes are enlarged and infected with streptococcal pharyngitis and mononucleosis.
- Lymphadenitis of the cervical and submandibular nodes occurs with herpes simplex lesions.
- Enlargement of supraclavicular nodes, especially the left, is highly suggestive of metastatic disease from abdominal and thoracic cancer.
- Axillary lymphadenopathy is associated with breast cancer.
- Lesions of the genitals may produce enlargement of the inguinal nodes.
- Persistent generalized lymphadenopathy is associated with acquired immune deficiency syndrome (AIDS) and AIDS-related complex.

Technique/Normal Findings	Abnormal Findings

Spleen Assessment

Palpate for the spleen, in the upper left quadrant of the abdomen. *The spleen is normally not palpable.*

- A palpable spleen in the left upper abdominal quadrant of an adult may indicate abnormal enlargement (splenomegaly) and may be associated with cancer, blood dyscrasias, and viral infection, such as mononucleosis.

Percuss for splenic dullness in the lowest left intercostal space (ICS) at the anterior axillary line or in the ninth to tenth ICS at the midaxillary line (Figure 33–15 ■). *Normally, tympany is heard.*

- A dull percussion note in the lowest left ICS at the anterior axillary line or below the tenth rib at the midaxillary line suggests splenic enlargement.

Figure 33–15 ■ Percussing the spleen.

EXPLORE MediaLink

Prentice Hall Nursing MediaLink DVD-ROM
Audio Glossary
NCLEX-RN® Review

Animation
Oxygen Transport

COMPANION WEBSITE www.prenhall.com/lemone
Audio Glossary
NCLEX-RN® Review
Care Plan Activity: Peripheral Vascular System
Case Study: Arterial Blood Pressure
MediaLink Application: Blood Pressure
Links to Resources

TEST YOURSELF NCLEX-RN® REVIEW

1 What part of the peripheral vascular system has the major control of blood pressure?
1. veins
2. capillaries
3. arteries
4. arterioles

2 Your client has a very low RBC count. What subjective manifestation would you expect to find during a health history?
1. sore throat
2. chest pain
3. fatigue
4. nausea

3 A client has a low platelet count. What would you likely find on physical assessment?
1. enlarged lymph nodes
2. excessive bruising
3. varicose veins
4. changes in pulse pressure

4 What physiologic difference from the veins accounts for the ability of the arteries to dilate and constrict?
1. veins have smooth muscle
2. veins are larger in diameter
3. arteries are more distensible
4. arteries have smooth muscle

5 An older client is severely dehydrated and, as a result, has increased blood viscosity. How will this affect the peripheral vascular resistance (PVR)?
   1. increased PVR
   2. decreased PVR
   3. no change
   4. depends on gender

6 What is the source of lymph?
   1. the respiratory system
   2. the cardiovascular system
   3. the central nervous system
   4. the integumentary system

7 What method would be most appropriate to assess the carotid arteries?
   1. Inspect for absence of movement.
   2. Auscultate with the bell of the stethoscope.
   3. Palpate with firm pressure.
   4. Percuss lightly over each artery.

8 When auscultating the abdominal aorta, you hear a murmuring or blowing sound. You would document this sound as a:

   1. hypokinetic pulse.
   2. bigeminal pulse.
   3. bruit.
   4. dysrhythmia.

9 Swelling of a body part as a result of lymphatic obstruction is labeled:
   1. lymphedema.
   2. lymphadenopathy.
   3. atrophic change.
   4. central cyanosis.

10 You are assessing a man who has severe leg pain. The leg is cool and cyanotic. You are unable to palpate a femoral pulse. What would be your priority intervention based on these assessments?
   1. Document your findings.
   2. Ask the family about this problem.
   3. Teach the man relaxation techniques.
   4. Notify the physician immediately.

See Test Yourself answers in Appendix C.

BIBLIOGRAPHY

Amella, E. (2004). Presentation of illness in older adults: If you think you know what you're looking for, think again. *American Journal of Nursing, 104*(10), 40–52.

Benbow, M. (2004). Doppler readings and leg ulceration. *Practice Nurse, 28*(4), 16, 18, 21.

Bench, S. (2004). Clinical skills: Assessing and treating shock. A nursing perspective. *British Journal of Nursing, 13*(12), 715–721.

Bickley, L., & Szilagyi, P. (2007). *Bates' guide to physical examination and history taking* (9th ed.). Philadelphia: Lippincott.

Board, J., & Harlow, W. (2002). Lymphoedema 1: Components and function of the lymphatic system. *British Journal of Nursing, 11*(5), 304–309.

Day, M. (2004). Action stat. Hypertensive emergency. *Nursing, 34*(7), 88.

Eliopoulos, E. (2005). *Gerontological nursing* (6th ed.). Philadelphia: Lippincott Williams & Wilkins.

Jarvis, C. (2004). *Physical examination & health assessment.* St. Louis, MO: Mosby.

Kee, J. (2005). *Prentice Hall handbook of laboratory & diagnostic tests with nursing implications.* Upper Saddle River, NJ: Prentice Hall.

Millard, F. (2004). The lymphatic system: Applied anatomy. *AAO Journal, 14*(1), 9–15.

Murray, J. (2004). Leg ulceration part 2: Patient assessment. *Nursing Standard, 19*(2), 45–54.

National Institutes of Health. (2003). *Genes and disease. Blood and lymph diseases.* Retrieved from http://www.ncbi.nlm.nih.gov/books/bv.fcgi?rid=gnd.section98

Porth, C., (2005). *Pathophysiology: Concepts of altered health states* (7th ed.). Philadelphia: Lippincott.

Reilly, P. (2004). How to check perfusion lickety-split. *Nursing, 34*(4), 64.

Rice, K. (2005). How to measure ankle/brachial index. *Nursing, 35*(1), 56–57.

Rushing J. (2004). Taking blood pressure accurately. *Nursing, 43*(11), 26.

_____. (2005). Assessing for orthostatic hypotension. *Nursing, 35*(1), 30.

Tanabe, P., Steinmann, R., Kippenhan, M., Stehman, C., & Beach, C. (2004). Undiagnosed hypertension in the ED setting—an unrecognized opportunity by emergency nurses. *Journal of Emergency Nursing, 30*(3), 225–229, 292–297.

Weber, J., & Kelley, J. (2006). *Health assessment in nursing* (3rd ed.). Philadelphia: Lippincott.

Willis, K. (2001). Gaining perspective on peripheral vascular disease. *Nursing, 31*(2), Hospital Nursing, 32hn1–4.

Woodrow, P. (2003). Assessing pulse in older people. *Nursing Older People, 15*(6), 38–40.

Young, T. (2001). Leg ulcer assessment. *Practice Nurse, 21*(7), 50, 52.

CHAPTER 34
Nursing Care of Clients with Hematologic Disorders

LEARNING OUTCOMES

- Relate the physiology and assessment of the hematologic system and related systems to commonly occurring hematologic disorders.

- Describe the pathophysiology of common hematologic disorders.

- Explain nursing implications for medications and other treatments prescribed for clients with hematologic disorders.

- Discuss indications for and complications of bone marrow or stem cell transplantation, as well as related nursing care.

- Compare and contrast the pathophysiology, manifestations, and management of bleeding disorders.

- Describe the major types of leukemia and the most common treatment modalities and nursing interventions.

- Differentiate Hodgkin's disease from non-Hodgkin's lymphomas.

CLINICAL COMPETENCIES

- Assess effects of hematologic disorders and prescribed treatments on clients' functional health status.

- Monitor and document continuing assessment data, including laboratory test results, subjective and objective information, reporting data outside the normal or expected range.

- Based on knowledge of pathophysiology, prescribed treatment, and assessed data, identify and prioritize nursing diagnoses for clients with hematologic disorders.

- Use nursing research and evidence-based practice to identify and implement individualized nursing interventions for the client with a hematologic disorder.

- Safely and knowledgeably administer prescribed medications and treatments for clients with hematologic disorders.

- Collaborate with the interdisciplinary care team to plan and provide coordinated, effective care for clients with hematologic disorders.

- Provide appropriate teaching for clients with hematologic disorders, evaluating learning and the need for continued reinforcement of information.

- Use continuing assessment data to revise the plan of care as needed to restore, maintain, or promote functional health in the client with a hematologic disorder.

MEDIALINK

Resources for this chapter can be found on the Prentice Hall Nursing MediaLink DVD-ROM accompanying this textbook, and on the Companion Website at http://www.prenhall.com/lemone

Disorders affecting the blood and blood-forming organs have effects that range from minor disruptions in daily activities to major life-threatening crises. Clients with hematologic disorders need holistic nursing care, including emotional support and care for problems involving major body systems.

This chapter focuses on health changes resulting from changes in red cells, white cells, platelets, and clotting factors. Before proceeding with this chapter, read Chapter 33 ∞, which provides a review of the physiology of blood and its formation, as well as important information about assessing clients with hematologic disorders.

RED BLOOD CELL DISORDERS

Red blood cells (RBCs) transport oxygen to body tissues and help return carbon dioxide to the lungs for excretion. Alterations in the number, size, shape, or composition of RBCs affect their ability to effectively carry out these functions. Anemia, the most common RBC disorder, is an abnormally low RBC count or reduced hemoglobin content. Polycythemia is an abnormally high RBC count.

THE CLIENT WITH ANEMIA

Anemia is an abnormally low number of circulating RBCs, low hemoglobin concentration, or both. Decreased numbers of circulating RBCs is the usual cause of anemia. This may result from blood loss, inadequate RBC production, or increased RBC destruction. Insufficient or defective hemoglobin within RBCs contributes to anemia. Depending on its severity, anemia may affect all major organ systems.

FAST FACTS
- Iron deficiency anemia, a nutritional anemia, is the most common type of anemia.
- Blood loss anemia may be either acute, resulting from hemorrhage, or chronic, resulting from chronic blood loss (e.g., menstrual flow, slow GI bleeding).

Physiology Review

As blood flows through the pulmonary vascular system, oxygen diffuses from alveoli into capillary blood. The majority of the oxygen binds reversibly with the hemoglobin in red blood cells; only about 3% of the oxygen remains in solution in the blood. When the blood reaches the capillaries serving body tissues, oxygen is released from the hemoglobin molecule, and diffuses out of the capillary to reach the cells. The amount of oxygen that reaches the tissues depends on a number of factors, including:
- Available oxygen in the alveoli
- The diffusing surface and capacity of the lungs

- The number of red blood cells and the amount and type of hemoglobin they contain
- The ability of the cardiovascular system to transport blood and oxygen to the tissues.

For more information about red blood cells, hemoglobin, and their production and function, see Chapter 33 ∞.

Physiology and Manifestations

A number of different pathologic mechanisms can lead to anemia (Box 34–1). Regardless of the cause, every type of anemia reduces the oxygen-carrying capacity of the blood due to a deficiency of RBCs or hemoglobin, leading to tissue hypoxia. The resulting manifestations depend on the severity of the anemia, how quickly it develops, and other factors such as age and health status.

When anemia develops gradually and the RBC reduction is moderate, successful compensatory mechanisms may result in few symptoms except when the oxygen needs of the body increase due to exercise or infection. Symptoms develop as RBCs and hemoglobin levels are further reduced. Pallor of the skin, mucous membranes, conjunctiva, and nail beds develops as a result of blood redistribution to vital organs and lack of hemoglobin (Figure 34–1 ■). As tissue oxygenation decreases, the heart and respiratory rates rise in an attempt to increase cardiac output and tissue perfusion. Tissue hypoxia may cause angina, fatigue, dyspnea on exertion, and night cramps. It also stimulates erythropoietin release; increased erythropoietin activity stimulates RBC production in the bone marrow, and may lead to bone pain. Cerebral hypoxia can lead to headache, dizziness, and dim vision. Heart failure may develop in severe anemia.

With rapid blood loss, blood volume is decreased as well as the oxygen-carrying capacity of the blood. Initial manifestations include tachycardia and tachypnea; the skin may be pale, cool, and clammy as peripheral vessels constrict to maintain blood flow to the heart and brain. With significant blood loss, signs of circulatory shock may occur, including hypotension,

BOX 34–1 Pathophysiologic Mechanisms of Anemia

Decreased RBC Production
- Altered hemoglobin synthesis
  - Iron deficiency
  - Thalassemias
  - Chronic inflammation
- Altered DNA synthesis
  - Vitamin B_{12} or folic acid malabsorption or deficiency
- Bone marrow failure
  - Aplastic anemia (stem cell dysfunction)
  - Red cell aplasia
  - Myeloproliferative leukemias
  - Cancer metastasis, lymphoma
  - Chronic infection or inflammation, physical and emotional fatigue

Increased RBC Loss or Destruction
- Acute or chronic blood loss
  - Hemorrhage or trauma
  - Chronic gastrointestinal bleeding, menorrhagia
- Increased hemolysis
  - Hereditary cell membrane disorders
  - Defective hemoglobin—sickle cell anemia or trait
  - Pyruvate kinase (PK) or G6PD deficiency affecting glycolysis or cell oxidation
  - Immune mechanisms and disorders (e.g., blood reaction, hypersensitivity responses, autoimmune disorders)
  - Splenomegaly and hypersplenism
  - Infection
  - Erythrocyte trauma (e.g., due to cardiopulmonary bypass, hemolytic uremic syndrome)

tachycardia, decreased level of consciousness, and oliguria. With chronic bleeding, fluid shifts from the interstitial spaces into the vessels, maintaining blood volume. Blood viscosity is reduced, which may result in a systolic heart murmur. See page 1104 for *Multisystem Effects of Anemia.*

Anemia is categorized by cause: blood loss, nutritional, hemolytic, and bone marrow suppression. The pathophysiology and specific manifestations of these types of anemias follow.

Blood Loss Anemia

When anemia results from acute or chronic bleeding, RBCs and other blood components (such as iron) are lost from the body. With acute blood loss, circulating volume decreases. As a result, the cardiac output falls. Compensatory mechanisms are activated to maintain the cardiac output: the heart rate increases, and peripheral blood vessels constrict. Vessels in the liver, a blood storage organ, also constrict, increasing circulating volume. Fluid shifts from the interstitial spaces into the vascular compartment to maintain blood volume, diluting the cellular components of the blood and reducing its viscosity. If

Figure 34–1 ■ The skin of the client with anemia appears pale beside that of a person with a normal hemoglobin and hematocrit.
Source: Westminster Hospital, Photo Researchers, Inc.

hemorrhage continues, compensatory mechanisms become less effective, increasing the risk for shock and circulatory failure (see Chapter 11 ∞).

In acute blood loss, circulating RBCs are of normal size and shape (*normocytic*). Early in the hemorrhage, the RBC count, hemoglobin, and hematocrit may be normal; as fluid shifts from the interstitial space into the vascular space to maintain circulating volume, the RBC count, hemoglobin, and hematocrit fall. If sufficient iron is available, the number of circulating RBCs and hemoglobin levels return to normal within 3 to 4 weeks after the bleeding episode. Chronic blood loss, on the other hand, depletes iron stores as RBC production attempts to maintain the RBC supply. The resulting RBCs are *microcytic* (small) and *hypochromic* (pale).

Nutritional Anemias

A number of different nutrients are required for normal red blood cell development (erythropoiesis). Iron is a key nutrient necessary for hemoglobin synthesis. In addition, adequate supplies of protein (and its building blocks, amino acids), vitamins, and other minerals are required. The B vitamins, particularly B_{12} (cobalamin) and folate, play a key role in RBC development. Vitamins C and E also are necessary. Nutritional anemias result from nutrient deficits that affect RBC formation or hemoglobin synthesis. The nutrient deficit may be caused by inadequate diet, malabsorption of the nutrient, or an increased need for the nutrient. The most common types of nutritional anemias are iron deficiency anemia, vitamin B_{12} anemia, and folic acid deficiency anemia. Vitamin B_{12} and folic acid anemias are sometimes called *megaloblastic* anemias, because enlarged nucleated RBCs called megaloblasts are seen in these anemias.

IRON DEFICIENCY ANEMIA **Iron deficiency anemia** is the most common type of anemia. It develops when the supply of iron is inadequate for optimal RBC formation. The body cannot synthesize hemoglobin without iron. Normally, the body efficiently recycles and stores iron, reusing much of the iron contained in RBCs that are removed from circulation due to age or damage. However, small amounts of iron continually are lost

MULTISYSTEM EFFECTS **of Anemia**

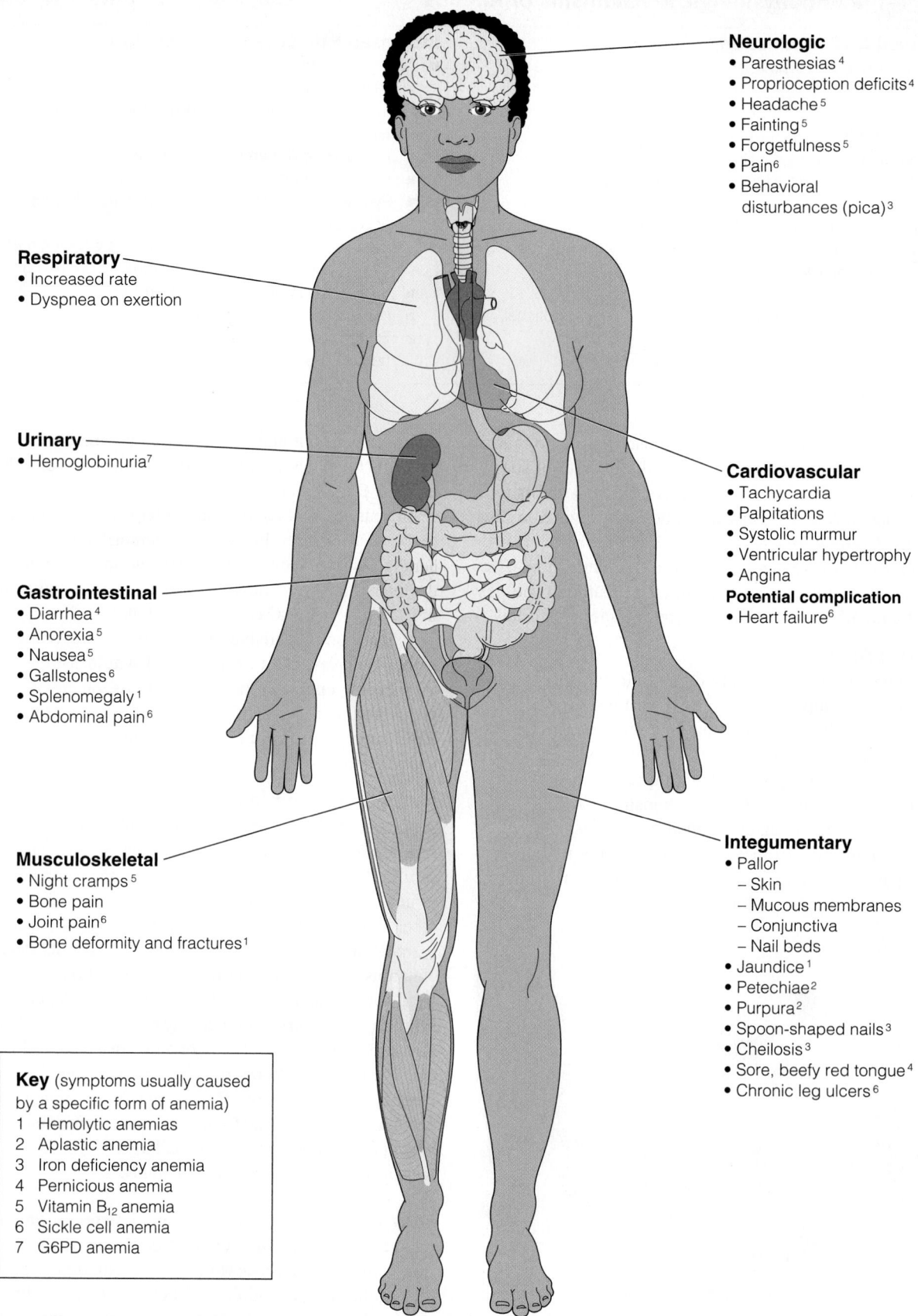

Neurologic
- Paresthesias [4]
- Proprioception deficits [4]
- Headache [5]
- Fainting [5]
- Forgetfulness [5]
- Pain [6]
- Behavioral disturbances (pica) [3]

Respiratory
- Increased rate
- Dyspnea on exertion

Urinary
- Hemoglobinuria [7]

Cardiovascular
- Tachycardia
- Palpitations
- Systolic murmur
- Ventricular hypertrophy
- Angina

Potential complication
- Heart failure [6]

Gastrointestinal
- Diarrhea [4]
- Anorexia [5]
- Nausea [5]
- Gallstones [6]
- Splenomegaly [1]
- Abdominal pain [6]

Musculoskeletal
- Night cramps [5]
- Bone pain
- Joint pain [6]
- Bone deformity and fractures [1]

Integumentary
- Pallor
  - Skin
  - Mucous membranes
  - Conjunctiva
  - Nail beds
- Jaundice [1]
- Petechiae [2]
- Purpura [2]
- Spoon-shaped nails [3]
- Cheilosis [3]
- Sore, beefy red tongue [4]
- Chronic leg ulcers [6]

Key (symptoms usually caused by a specific form of anemia)
1. Hemolytic anemias
2. Aplastic anemia
3. Iron deficiency anemia
4. Pernicious anemia
5. Vitamin B_{12} anemia
6. Sickle cell anemia
7. G6PD anemia

in the feces; therefore, adequate iron intake is necessary for normal hemoglobin synthesis and RBC production. Iron deficiency anemia results in fewer numbers of RBCs, microcytic and hypochromic RBCs, as well as malformed RBCs (*poikilocytosis*) (Figure 34–2 ■).

Excessive iron loss due to chronic bleeding is the usual cause of iron deficiency anemia in adults. Menstrual blood loss is the most common cause in adult females. Iron deficiency anemia also may result from inadequate dietary iron intake (less than 1 mg/day), malabsorption syndromes, or the increased iron requirements associated with pregnancy and lactation. Box 34–2 summarizes common causes of iron deficiency anemia.

Iron deficiency anemia is particularly common in older adults. Chronic, occult (hidden) blood loss may occur from slowly bleeding peptic ulcers, gastrointestinal inflammation, hemorrhoids, and cancer. Inadequate dietary iron intake also contributes to anemia in the older adult. Access to transportation may limit fresh food consumption, a factor contributing to poor iron intake among all adults, especially people with limited or fixed incomes.

Manifestations In addition to the general manifestations of anemia described earlier, chronic iron deficiency may lead to brittle, spoon-shaped nails; cheilosis (cracks at the corners of the mouth); a smooth, sore tongue; and *pica* (a craving for unusual substances, such as clay or starch).

VITAMIN B₁₂ DEFICIENCY ANEMIA Vitamin B₁₂ is necessary for DNA synthesis and is almost exclusively found in foods derived from animals. Vitamin B₁₂ deficiency occurs when inadequate vitamin B₁₂ is consumed or, more commonly, when it is poorly absorbed from the gastrointestinal tract. Deficiency of this vitamin impairs cell division and maturation of the cell nucleus, especially in rapidly proliferating red blood cells. As a result, macrocytic (large), misshapen (oval rather than concave) RBCs with thin membranes are produced. Great numbers of these large, immature RBCs enter the circulation. These

Figure 34–2 ■ A blood smear showing RBCs characteristically seen in iron deficiency anemia. Note the pale color of the RBCs (hypochromic). Many of the cells also are smaller than normal (microcytic) and misshapen, reducing their oxygen-carrying capacity.
Source: Dr. E. Walker, Photo Researchers, Inc.

BOX 34–2 Causes of Iron Deficiency Anemia

- Dietary deficiencies
  - Vegetarian diet
  - Inadequate protein intake
- Decreased absorption
  - Partial or total gastrectomy
  - Chronic diarrhea
  - Malabsorption syndromes
- Increased metabolic requirements
  - Pregnancy
  - Lactation
- Blood loss
  - Gastrointestinal bleeding (especially due to ulcers or chronic aspirin use)
  - Menstrual losses
- Chronic hemoglobinuria

---

cells are fragile, incapable of carrying adequate amounts of oxygen, and have a shortened life span.

Failure to absorb dietary vitamin B₁₂ is called **pernicious anemia**. It develops due to lack of *intrinsic factor*, a substance secreted by the gastric mucosa. Intrinsic factor binds with vitamin B₁₂ and travels with it to the ileum, where the vitamin is absorbed. In the absence of intrinsic factor, vitamin B₁₂ cannot be absorbed into the body.

Vitamin B₁₂ deficiency may also result from other malabsorption disorders and dietary factors. Resection of the stomach or ileum, loss of pancreatic secretions, and chronic gastritis can affect vitamin B₁₂ absorption. Dietary deficiencies of vitamin B₁₂ are rare, usually occurring only among strict vegetarians.

Manifestations Manifestations of vitamin B₁₂ deficiency anemia develop gradually as bodily stores of the vitamin are depleted. Pallor or slight jaundice and weakness develop. In pernicious anemia, a smooth, sore, beefy red tongue and diarrhea may occur. Because vitamin B₁₂ is important for neurologic function, *paresthesias* (altered sensations, such as numbness or tingling) in the extremities and problems with *proprioception* (the sense of one's position in space) develop. These manifestations may progress to difficulty maintaining balance due to spinal cord damage. Central nervous system (CNS) manifestations of relatively short duration (6 months or less) are reversible with treatment, but may be permanent if treatment is delayed (Tierney et al., 2005).

FOLIC ACID DEFICIENCY ANEMIA Like vitamin B₁₂, folic acid is required for DNA synthesis and normal maturation of red blood cells. Folic acid deficiency anemia is characterized by fragile, megaloblastic (large and immature) cells. Folic acid is found in green leafy vegetables, fruits, cereals, and meats, and is absorbed from the intestines.

Folic acid deficiency anemia due to inadequate intake is more common among people who are chronically undernourished. This includes older adults, alcoholics, and the drug addicted. Alcoholics are especially at risk because alcohol suppresses folate metabolism, which forms folic acid. Increased folic acid requirements also may lead to anemia. Pregnant women are at the greatest risk. Infants and teenagers can develop temporary folic acid deficiencies during periods of rapid growth. Impaired folic acid absorption and metabolism can cause folic acid deficiency anemia. Malabsorption disorders such as celiac sprue (a hereditary gastrointestinal disorder characterized by inability to metabolize amino acids found in gluten), and certain medications, such as methotrexate and some chemotherapeutic agents, may be implicated. Causes of folic acid deficiency anemia are summarized in Box 34–3.

Manifestations The manifestations develop gradually as folic acid stores are depleted. Signs and symptoms may include pallor, progressive weakness and fatigue, shortness of breath, and heart palpitations. Manifestations similar to those associated with vitamin B_{12} anemia, such as glossitis, cheilosis, and diarrhea, are common. No neurologic symptoms occur with folic acid deficiency anemia, helping differentiate it from vitamin B_{12} deficiency anemia. These two nutritional anemias do, however, sometimes coexist.

Maternal folic acid deficiency is strongly associated with neural tube defects such as meningomyelocele. The neural tube develops early in the process of fetal development, often before pregnancy is recognized.

Hemolytic Anemias

Hemolytic anemias are characterized by premature destruction (*lysis*) of RBCs. When RBCs break down, iron and other by-products of their destruction remain in the plasma. RBC lysis (hemolysis) may occur within the circulatory system or due to phagocytosis by WBCs such as circulating monocytes and macrophages in the spleen. In response to hemolysis, the hematopoietic activity of bone marrow increases, leading to increased reticulocytes (immature RBCs) in circulating blood. Most types of hemolytic anemia are characterized by normocytic and normochromic RBCs.

There are many different causes of hemolytic anemias (Box 34–4). The cause may be *intrinsic,* arising from disorders within the RBC itself, or *extrinsic,* originating outside the RBC.

BOX 34–4 Causes of Hemolytic Anemia

Intrinsic
- RBC cell-membrane defects
- Hemoglobin structure defects (e.g., sickle cell anemia, thalassemia)
- Inherited enzyme defects (e.g., G6PD deficiency)

Extrinsic
- Drugs, chemicals
- Toxins and venoms
- Bacterial and other infections
- Trauma, burns
- Mechanical damage (prosthetic heart valves)

Intrinsic disorders include cell membrane defects, defects in hemoglobin structure and function, and inherited enzyme deficiencies. See the accompanying Focus on Cultural Diversity box for more information about inherited intrinsic RBC disorders associated with hemolytic anemia. Extrinsic causes of hemolytic anemia include drugs, bacterial and other toxins, and trauma. This section discusses sickle cell anemia, thalassemia, acquired hemolytic anemia, and glucose-6-phosphate dehydrogenase anemia.

SICKLE CELL ANEMIA **Sickle cell anemia** is a hereditary, chronic hemolytic anemia. It is characterized by episodes of *sickling,* during which RBCs become abnormally crescent shaped. The disorder is transmitted as an autosomal recessive genetic defect (Figure 34–3 ■). This defect causes synthesis of an abnormal form of hemoglobin (HbS) within red blood cells. Sickle cell anemia can significantly shorten life span, with most deaths occurring due to infection (McCance & Huether, 2006).

The disease is most common among people of African descent (see Focus on Cultural Diversity box below). In the

---

BOX 34–3 Causes of Folic Acid Deficiency Anemia

- Inadequate dietary intake
  At risk:
  a. Older adults
  b. Alcoholics
  c. Clients receiving total parenteral nutrition
- Increased metabolic requirements
  At risk:
  a. Pregnant women
  b. Infants and teenagers
  c. Clients undergoing hemodialysis
  d. Clients with forms of hemolytic anemia
- Folic acid malabsorption and impaired metabolism
  a. Celiac sprue
  b. Chemotherapeutic agents, folate antagonists (methotrexate, pentamidine), or anticonvulsants
  c. Alcoholism

FOCUS ON CULTURAL DIVERSITY
Inherited Hemolytic Anemias

- Sickle cell anemia affects about 72,000 people in the United States
  - In African Americans, sickle cell anemia occurs in 1 out of every 600 births.
  - People from Central and South America, Cuba, Saudi Arabia, India, and Mediterranean countries such as Turkey, Greece, and Italy also may be at risk; sickle cell anemia occurs in 1 of every 1000 to 1400 Hispanic American births.
- Thalassemia is less common than sickle cell anemia.
  - Alpha-thalassemia primarily affects people of Southeast Asian, Indian, Chinese, or Filipino ancestry.
  - Beta-thalassemia is seen primarily in people of Mediterranean, Asian, and African origin.
- G6PD anemia primarily affects people of African or Mediterranean descent.
  - This hereditary defect is carried on the X chromosome and affects more men than women.

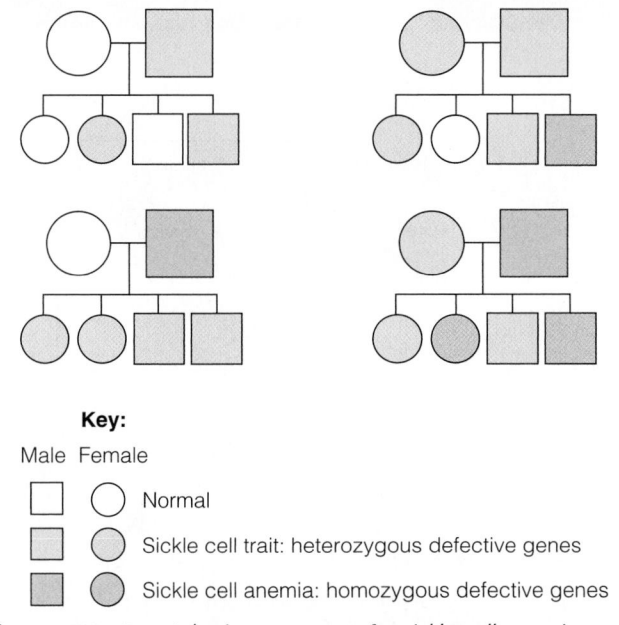

Key:

Male Female

□ ○ Normal

▨ ◍ Sickle cell trait: heterozygous defective genes

▩ ◓ Sickle cell anemia: homozygous defective genes

Figure 34–3 ■ Inheritance pattern for sickle cell anemia.

FOCUS ON CULTURAL DIVERSITY
Sickle Cell Anemia

Sickle cell anemia tends to affect people whose origins are in equatorial countries, particularly those in central Africa, the Near East, the Mediterranean region, and parts of India. Hispanics from the Caribbean and Central and South America also may have the HbS gene. This gene may protect against lethal forms of malaria, an endemic disease in many equatorial regions.

The gene for HbS is transmitted in an autosomal recessive pattern from parent to offspring. A parent with one HbS gene (heterozygous) has a 50% risk of transmitting the gene to each child (see Figure 34–3). If both parents carry the gene, each child has a 25% risk of inheriting the gene from both parents. A person who carries both HbS genes (homozygous) is likely to develop sickle cell disease.

Sickle cell anemia is a serious chronic and recurrent disease. The stress of the disease is compounded by the risk for its transmission to offspring. Recommend that all clients with sickle cell trait or disease obtain genetic counseling as part of their family planning process.

United States, 7% to 13% of blacks carry the defective gene, having inherited it from one parent (McCance & Huether, 2006). These people have *sickle cell trait.* About 40% of their hemoglobin is HbS (Porth, 2005). They are likely to remain asymptomatic unless stressed by severe hypoxia. Less than 1% of African Americans are homozygous for the disorder; that is, they have inherited a defective gene from both parents. These people have *sickle cell disease;* nearly all their hemoglobin is HbS (Porth, 2005). They are at risk for **sickle cell crisis**, severe episodes of fever and intense pain that are the hallmark of this disorder.

The HbS gene changes the structure of the beta chain of the hemoglobin molecule. When hypoxemia develops and HbS is deoxygenated, it crystallizes into rodlike structures. Clusters of these rods form long chains that deform the erythrocyte into a crescent or sickle shape (Figure 34–4 ■). The sickled cells tend to clump together and obstruct capillary blood flow, causing ischemia and possible infarction of surrounding tissue. See *Pathophysiology Illustrated: Sickle Cell Anemia* on page 1108.

When normal oxygen tension is restored, the sickled RBCs resume their normal shape; that is, they "unsickle." Repeated episodes of sickling and unsickling weaken RBC cell membranes. The weakened RBCs are hemolyzed and removed. Consequently, the normal life span of RBCs is greatly reduced in sickle cell anemia, increasing the demand for RBC production. Conditions likely to trigger sickling include hypoxia, low environmental or body temperature, excessive exercise, anesthesia, dehydration, infections, or acidosis.

Manifestations and Complications The acute and chronic manifestations of sickle cell anemia arise from episodes of RBC sickling. Sickling causes general manifestations of hemolytic anemia, including pallor, fatigue, jaundice, and irritability. Extensive sickling can precipitate a crisis due to occluded circulation, impaired erythropoiesis, or sequestration of large amounts of blood in the liver or spleen.

A vasoocclusive or thrombotic crisis occurs when sickling develops in the microcirculation. Obstruction of blood flow triggers vasospasm that halts all blood flow in the vessel. Lack of blood flow leads to tissue ischemia and infarction. Vasoocclusive crises are painful and last an average of 4 to 6 days. Infarction of small vessels in the extremities causes painful swelling of the hands and feet; large joints also may be affected. Priapism (persistent, painful erection of the penis) may develop. Abdominal pain may signal infarction of abdominal organs and structures. Infarction may affect bone marrow or lead to aseptic necrosis of affected bones. Stroke may result from cerebral vessel occlusion (McCance & Huether, 2006). Skin ulcers may develop as the result of

Figure 34–4 ■ Blood smear containing normal red blood cells and sickle cells.

Source: Oliver Meckes and Nicole Ottawa, Photo Researchers, Inc.

MEDIALINK Sickle Cell Anemia Animation

Sickle Cell Anemia

Hemoglobin S and Red Blood Cell Sickling

Sickle cell anemia is caused by an inherited autosomal recessive defect in Hb synthesis. Sickle cell hemoglobin (HbS) differs from normal hemoglobin only in the substitution of the amino acid valine for glutamine in both beta chains of the hemoglobin molecule.

When HbS is oxygenated, it has the same globular shape as normal hemoglobin. However, when HbS off-loads oxygen, it becomes insoluble in intracellular fluid and crystallizes into rodlike structures. Clusters of rods form polymers (long chains) that bend the erythrocyte into the characteristic crescent shape of the sickle cell.

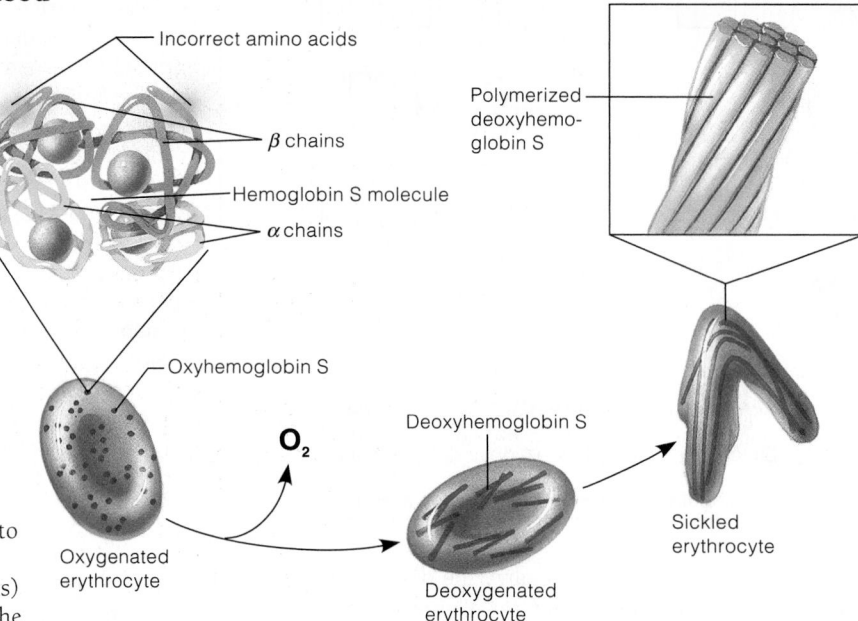

The Sickle Cell Disease Process

Sickle cell disease is characterized by episodes of acute painful crises. Sickling crises are triggered by conditions causing high tissue oxygen demands or that affect cellular pH. As the crisis begins, sickled erythrocytes adhere to capillary walls and to each other, obstructing blood flow and causing cellular hypoxia. The crisis accelerates as tissue hypoxia and acidic metabolic waste products cause further sickling and cell damage.

Sickle cell crises cause microinfarcts in joints and organs, and repeated crises slowly destroy organs and tissues. The spleen and kidneys are especially prone to sickling damage.

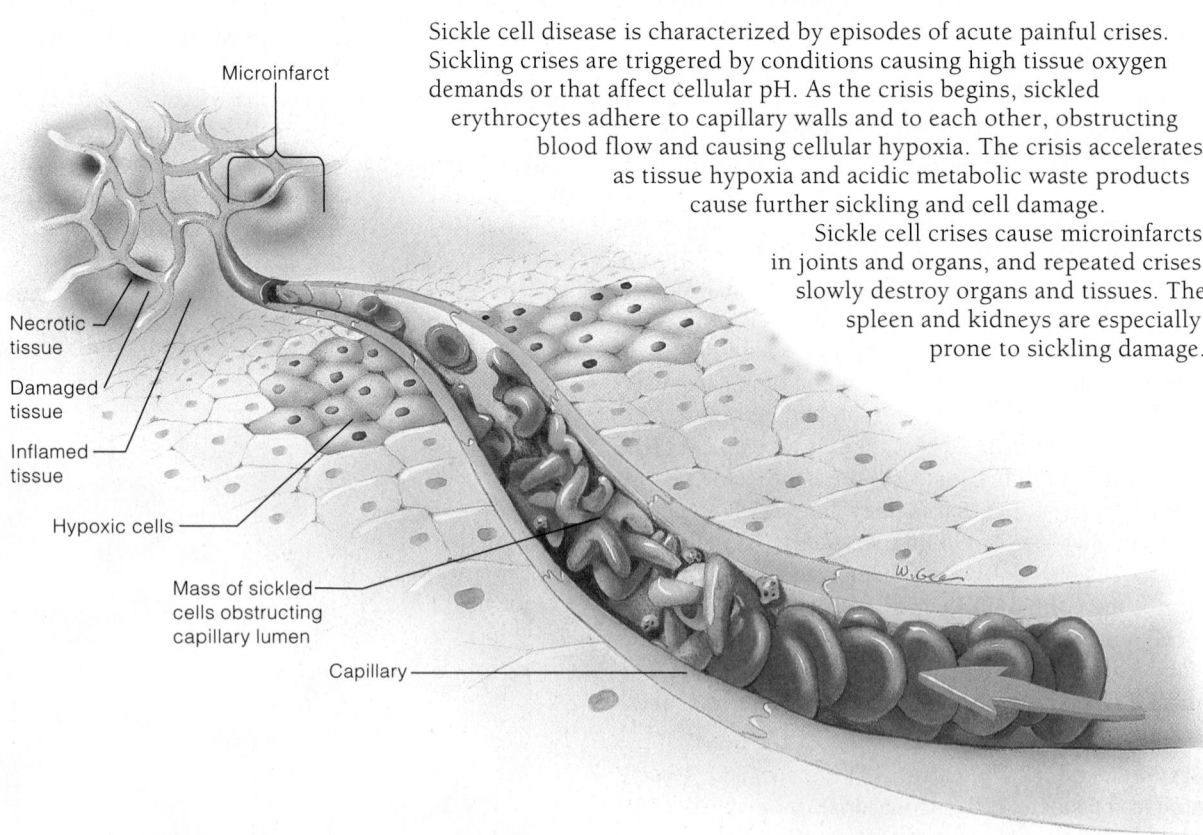

occluded vessels supplying the dermis. Repeated infarcts associated with sickling can affect the structure and function of nearly every organ system. People with sickle cell disease may develop an enlarged spleen and liver, renal insufficiency, gallstones, and other manifestations of organ dysfunction. *Acute chest syndrome*, a symptom complex that includes fever, chest pain, an increasing WBC count, and pulmonary infiltrates, may develop, as well as other pulmonary complications such as pneumonia, pulmonary infarction, and pulmonary embolism (Porth, 2005).

The shortened RBC life span and compromised erythropoiesis can lead to profound *aplastic anemia* in sickle cell disease. *Sequestration crises* are marked by pooling of large amounts of blood in the liver and spleen. This sickle cell crisis only occurs in children, but is thought to be the cause of sickle cell disease-related deaths in early childhood (Porth, 2005).

THALASSEMIA The **thalassemias** are inherited disorders of hemoglobin synthesis in which either the alpha or beta chains of the hemoglobin molecule are missing or defective. This leads to deficient hemoglobin production and fragile hypochromic, microcytic RBCs called *target cells* because of their distinctive bull's-eye appearance.

Thalassemia usually affects certain populations. People of Mediterranean descent (southern Italy and Greece) are more likely to have beta-defect thalassemias (often called *Cooley's anemia* or *Mediterranean anemia*). People of Asian ancestry, especially from Thailand, the Philippines, and China, more often have alpha-defect thalassemia. Africans and African Americans may have both alpha- and beta-defect thalassemia. As with sickle cell anemia, only one defective beta chain-forming gene may be present (*beta-thalassemia minor*), causing mild symptoms, or both may be defective (*beta-thalassemia major*), leading to more severe symptoms. Children with thalassemia major rarely reach adulthood, although repeated blood transfusions may extend their life span (McCance & Huether, 2006). Four genes are responsible for alpha chain formation; one, two, three, or all four may be defective. In the latter case (*alpha-thalassemia major*), death is inevitable and usually occurs *in utero*. Genetic studies and counseling are recommended for people at risk for this illness.

Manifestations and Complications People with thalassemia minor often are asymptomatic. When manifestations do occur, they include mild to moderate anemia, mild splenomegaly, bronze skin coloring, and bone marrow hyperplasia. The major form of the disease causes severe anemia, heart failure, and liver and spleen enlargement from increased red cell destruction. Fractures of the long bones, ribs, and vertebrae may result from bone marrow expansion and thinning due to increased hematopoiesis. Jaundice may develop due to hemolysis, as well as hepatomegaly and splenomegaly. Accumulation of iron in the heart, liver, and pancreas following repeated transfusions for treatment may eventually cause failure of these organs.

ACQUIRED HEMOLYTIC ANEMIA Acquired hemolytic anemia results from hemolysis due to factors outside of the RBC. Causes of acquired hemolytic anemias include:

- Mechanical trauma to RBCs produced by prosthetic heart valves, severe burns, hemodialysis, or radiation
- Autoimmune disorders

- Bacterial or protozoal infection
- Immune-system-mediated responses, such as transfusion reactions
- Drugs, toxins, chemical agents, or venoms.

The manifestations of acquired hemolytic anemia depend on the extent of hemolysis and the body's ability to replace destroyed RBCs. The anemia itself often is mild to moderate as erythropoiesis increases to replace the destroyed RBCs. The spleen enlarges as it removes damaged or destroyed RBCs. If the breakdown of heme units exceeds the liver's ability to conjugate and excrete bilirubin, jaundice develops. When the condition is severe, bone marrow expands, and bones may be deformed or may develop pathologic fractures. The severity of generalized manifestations of anemia (tachycardia, pallor, etc.) depends on the degree of anemia and deficiency of tissue oxygenation.

GLUCOSE-6-PHOSPHATE DEHYDROGENASE (G6PD) ANEMIA *Glucose-6-phosphate dehydrogenase (G6PD) anemia* is caused by a hereditary defect in RBC metabolism. It is relatively common in people of African and Mediterranean descent. The defective gene is located on the X chromosome and therefore affects more males than females. There are many variations of this genetic defect.

G6PD is an enzyme that catalyzes glycolysis, the process in which an RBC derives cellular energy. A defect in G6PD action causes direct oxidation of hemoglobin, damaging the RBC. Hemolysis usually occurs only when the affected person is exposed to stressors (e.g., drugs such as aspirin, sulfonamides, or vitamin K derivatives) that increase the metabolic demands on RBCs. The G6PD deficiency impairs the necessary compensatory increase in glucose metabolism and causes cellular damage. Damaged RBCs are destroyed over a period of 7 to 12 days.

When exposed to a stressor triggering G6PD anemia, symptoms develop within several days. These may include pallor, jaundice, hemoglobinuria (hemoglobin in the urine), and an elevated reticulocyte count. As new RBCs develop, counts return to normal.

Aplastic Anemia

In **aplastic anemia**, the bone marrow fails to produce all three types of blood cells, leading to *pancytopenia*. Normal bone marrow is replaced by fat. Fortunately, aplastic anemia is rare. *Fanconi anemia* is a rare aplastic anemia caused by defects of DNA repair. The underlying cause of about 50% of acquired aplastic anemia is unknown (*idiopathic aplastic anemia*). Other cases follow stem cell damage caused by exposure to radiation or certain chemical substances such as benzene, arsenic, nitrogen mustard, certain antibiotics (especially chloramphenicol), and chemotherapeutic drugs (McCance & Huether, 2006). Aplastic anemia also may occur with viral infections such as mononucleosis, hepatitis C, and HIV disease (Porth, 2005).

In aplastic anemia, the number of stem cells in the bone marrow is significantly reduced. The stem cell pool may be less than 1% of normal when the disease is recognized. Anemia develops as the bone marrow fails to replace RBCs that have reached the end of their life span. Remaining RBCs may be normochromic and normocytic or may be large with increased mean corpuscular volume.

Manifestations Manifestations of aplastic anemia vary with the severity of the pancytopenia. Its onset usually is insidious, but may be sudden. Manifestations include fatigue, pallor, progressive weakness, exertional dyspnea, headache, and ultimately tachycardia and heart failure. Platelet deficiency leads to bleeding problems; bleeding gums, excessive bruising, and nosebleeds may be the initial symptoms. A deficiency of white blood cells increases the risk of infection, causing manifestations such as sore throat and fever.

INTERDISCIPLINARY CARE

Ensuring adequate tissue oxygenation is the priority of care in treating anemia. Specific therapy is determined by the underlying cause of the disorder. Usual treatments include medications, dietary modifications, blood replacement, or supportive interventions. Table 34–1 outlines interdisciplinary care measures for selected types of anemia.

Diagnosis

When anemia is suspected, the following laboratory and diagnostic tests may be ordered:

- *Complete blood count (CBC)* is done to determine blood cell counts, hemoglobin, hematocrit, and red blood cell indices. The severity of the anemia, shape, volume, and iron content of the RBCs can help determine the cause of anemia.
- *Iron levels* and *total iron-binding capacity* are performed to detect iron deficiency anemia. A low serum iron concentration and elevated total iron-binding capacity are indicative of iron deficiency anemia.
- *Serum ferritin* is low due to depletion of the total iron reserves available for hemoglobin synthesis. Ferritin is an iron-storage protein produced by the liver, spleen, and bone marrow. Ferritin mobilizes stored iron when metabolic needs are higher than dietary intake.
- *Sickle cell test* is a screening test to evaluate hemolytic anemia and detect HbS.
- *Hemoglobin electrophoresis* separates normal hemoglobin from abnormal forms. It is used to evaluate hemolytic ane-

TABLE 34–1 Interdisciplinary Care Focus for Major Anemias

TYPE OF ANEMIA	INTERDISCIPLINARY CARE
Iron deficiency anemia	■ Increased dietary intake of iron-rich foods ■ Oral or parenteral iron supplements
Vitamin B_{12} deficiency	■ Increased dietary intake of foods containing vitamin B_{12} (e.g., meats, eggs, and dairy products) ■ Oral or parenteral vitamin B_{12} supplements ■ Parenteral vitamin B_{12} for deficiency due to malabsorption or lack of intrinsic factor
Folic acid deficiency	■ Increased dietary intake of foods rich in folic acid (folate) ■ Oral folic acid supplements ■ Folic acid supplements recommended for women who are pregnant or may become pregnant to prevent neural tube defects

Sickle cell anemia	■ Treatment is primarily supportive
	■ Hydroxyurea 10–30 mg/kg per day
	■ Sickle cell crisis:
	  ■ Rest
	  ■ Oxygen therapy to maintain SaO_2
	  ■ Narcotic analgesia
	  ■ Vigorous hydration
	  ■ Treatment of precipitating factors
	■ Acute chest syndrome:
	  ■ Careful hydration; hemodynamic monitoring
	  ■ Oxygen therapy
	  ■ Transfusion
	■ Folic acid supplements
	■ Blood transfusions during surgery or pregnancy as necessary
	■ Genetic counseling recommended

Thalassemia	■ Regular blood transfusions ■ Folic acid supplements ■ Possible splenectomy ■ Genetic counseling
Aplastic anemia	■ Withdrawal of the causative agent, if known ■ Blood transfusions ■ Bone marrow transplant as indicated

mia, diagnose thalassemia, and differentiate sickle cell trait from sickle cell disease.

- *Schilling test* measures vitamin B_{12} absorption before and after intrinsic factor administration to differentiate between pernicious anemia and intestinal malabsorption of the vitamin. A 24-hour urine sample is collected following administration of radioactive vitamin B_{12}. Lower than normal levels of the tagged B_{12} when intrinsic factor is given concurrently indicate malabsorption rather than pernicious anemia.
- *Bone marrow examination* is done to diagnose aplastic anemia. In aplastic anemia, normal marrow elements are significantly decreased as they are replaced by fat cells. Nursing implications for bone marrow collection are described in the Diagnostic Tests box in Chapter 33 ∞.
- *Quantitative assay of G6PD* may be performed to confirm a diagnosis of glucose-6-phosphate dehydrogenase deficiency.

Medications

Medications used to treat anemia depend on its cause. Iron replacement therapy is ordered for iron deficiency anemia. Supplemental iron may be given by mouth or parenterally. Intravenous administration of iron is becoming more common, particularly in clients with an acute deficiency and in anemia associated with chronic GI blood loss, chronic renal failure, and other chronic conditions that increase the need for blood cell production (e.g., cancers). The risk of anaphylaxis is a major concern when iron dextran is given intravenously. Other parenteral iron solutions, including intravenous sodium ferric gluconate (Ferrlecit) and iron sucrose (Venofer), carry a much lower risk of adverse and allergic reactions (Kasper et al., 2005).

Parenteral vitamin B_{12} is given when malabsorption or lack of intrinsic factor leads to vitamin B_{12} deficiency anemia. Folic acid is ordered for women of childbearing age, pregnant women, and clients with folic acid deficiency or sickle cell anemia to meet the increased demands of the bone marrow. Hydroxyurea, a drug that promotes fetal hemoglobin production, may be prescribed for clients with sickle cell disease, particularly those with frequent crises or severe disease. Resulting increased levels of fetal hemoglobin interfere with the sickling process and reduce the incidence of painful crises (Kasper et al., 2005). Nursing implications for clients receiving iron, vitamin B_{12}, and folic acid are found in the Medication Administration box on page 1112.

Erythropoietin may be ordered for clients with low erythropoietin levels (e.g., clients with chronic renal failure) and people with anemia associated with other chronic diseases. Erythropoietin is given subcutaneously, and may be given as often as three times a week in chronic renal failure. Because erythropoietin stimulates RBC production, adequate iron must be present. Clients receiving erythropoietin may require regular intravenous iron therapy as well (Kasper et al., 2005).

Immunosuppressive therapy with antithymocyte globulin (ATG), corticosteroids, and cyclosporine may be used to treat aplastic anemia. Androgens may stimulate blood cell production in some clients with aplastic anemia. See Chapter 13 ∞ for more information about immunosuppression.

Nutrition

Dietary modifications are recommended for nutritional deficiency anemias, such as iron deficiency anemia, vitamin B_{12} deficiency anemia, or folic acid deficiency anemia. Box 34–5 identifies good sources of dietary iron, vitamin B_{12}, and folic acid.

Blood Transfusion

Blood transfusions may be indicated to treat anemias resulting from major blood loss, such as from trauma or major surgery, and severe anemia regardless of cause. In acute hemorrhage, whole blood may be given to replace both blood cells and volume. A unit of packed red blood cells may be given when anemia is severe and the client demonstrates cardiovascular instability or compromise. Blood transfusions are fully discussed in Chapter 11 ∞.

Complementary Therapies

Complementary healthcare practitioners may recommend specific plant enzymes to treat nutritional anemias. Plant enzymes are believed to aid digestion of proteins, fats, and carbohydrates, facilitating absorption of their nutrients. Therapy is determined by the specific type of anemia. Plant enzymes should

---

BOX 34–5 **Dietary Sources of Iron, Folic Acid, and Vitamin B_{12}**

Iron

Iron in the diet comes from two sources. *Heme iron* makes up about one-half of the iron from animal sources. *Nonheme iron* includes the remaining iron from animal sources and all the iron from plants, legumes, and nuts. Heme iron promotes absorption of nonheme iron from other foods when both forms are consumed at the same time. Absorption of nonheme iron is also enhanced by vitamin C and inhibited by tea and coffee.

Sources of Heme Iron

- Beef
- Chicken
- Egg yolk
- Clams, oysters
- Pork loin
- Turkey
- Veal

Sources of Nonheme Iron

- Bran flakes
- Brown rice
- Whole-grain breads
- Dried beans
- Dried fruits
- Greens
- Oatmeal

Sources of Folic Acid

- Green leafy vegetables
- Broccoli
- Organ meats
- Eggs
- Wheat germ
- Asparagus
- Liver
- Milk
- Yeast
- Kidney beans

Sources of Vitamin B_{12}

- Liver
- Fresh shrimp and oysters
- Eggs
- Milk
- Kidney
- Meats (muscle)
- Cheese

MEDICATION ADMINISTRATION Drugs to Treat Anemia

IRON SOURCES
Ferrous sulfate (Feosol, Fer-in-sol)
Ferrous gluconate (Fergon, Ferralet, Fertinic)
Iron dextran injection (Imferon)
Iron polysaccharide
Iron sucrose (Venofer)
Sodium ferric gluconate (Ferrlecit)

Iron preparations are normally taken by mouth and are absorbed from the gastrointestinal tract. They are given to treat anemias resulting from iron deficiency or blood loss. When absorbed, iron combines with transferrin. This complex then is transported to the bone marrow and incorporated into hemoglobin.

Nursing Responsibilities
- Prior to giving the drug, assess for use of drugs that might interact with iron (e.g., antacids, allopurinol, chloramphenicol, tetracyclines, vitamin E), gastrointestinal bleeding, and manifestations of anemia.
- Administer iron preparations with orange juice to enhance absorption.
- If using an elixir, give it through a straw to prevent staining the teeth.
- Monitor for manifestations of iron toxicity: nausea, diarrhea, or constipation; symptoms of anaphylactic shock (extreme cases).
- Monitor hemoglobin and reticulocyte counts.
- If the client is also taking tetracyclines, schedule the dose of iron 2 hours before tetracycline (iron reduces the absorption of tetracycline).
- When administering IM or IV, monitor closely for anaphylaxis.

Health Education for the Client and Family
- Gastrointestinal side effects may be reduced by taking iron with food (but not milk, which decreases absorption).
- Stools may be dark green or black; this is harmless.
- Increase fluids and fiber in diet to decrease constipation.

VITAMIN B$_{12}$ SOURCES
Cyanocobalamin (Kaybovite [oral], Anacobin [parenteral], Bedoz)

Cyanocobalamin is used to treat vitamin B$_{12}$ deficiencies or malabsorption and pernicious anemia. It is rapidly absorbed when administered orally or by injection, and it is stored in the liver. Intrinsic factor is necessary for absorption from the gastrointestinal tract.

Nursing Responsibilities
- Do not expose crystalline injection to light.
- Assess for other drugs that might interfere with the therapeutic response: chloramphenicol, cimetidine, colchicine, and timed-release potassium decrease its effectiveness.
- Do not mix cyanocobalamin in a syringe with other medications.
- Administer parenteral doses intramuscularly or deep subcutaneously to decrease local irritation.
- Monitor hemoglobin, RBC counts, reticulocyte counts, and potassium levels.

Health Education for the Client and Family
- A burning sensation with injection is temporary.
- Avoid alcohol, which interferes with absorption.
- If used to treat pernicious anemia, the medication must be taken for life.

FOLIC ACID SOURCES
Folic acid (Folvite)
Synthetic folic acid is used to treat folic acid deficiency and megaloblastic or macrocytic anemia. It is absorbed from the gastrointestinal tract and stored in the liver.

Nursing Responsibilities
- Prior to giving the medication, assess for use of drugs that alter its effect: corticosteroids, methotrexate, oral contraceptives, phenytoin, sulfonamides.
- Do not mix folic acid with other medications in the same syringe.
- Monitor for possible hypersensitivity response of skin rash.

Health Education for the Client and Family
- Large doses of folic acid may cause the urine to become darker yellow.
- Excess alcohol intake increases folic acid requirements.

---

not be used alone to treat anemia, and it is important to check for possible interactions with prescribed medications before starting therapy.

NURSING CARE

For nursing care specific to the client with a nutritional anemia see the accompanying Nursing Care Plan.

Health Promotion

Nursing measures to prevent anemia focus on teaching good dietary habits to all clients, regardless of age. Stress the importance of consuming adequate amounts of iron, folate, and the B vitamins. Provide a list of dietary sources of these nutrients. Discuss alternate iron sources with vegetarian clients, and teach them that foods high in vitamin C enhance the absorption of iron from grains, legumes, and other sources. Emphasize the importance of adequate iron intake in women of childbearing age and older adults. Stress the increased need for these nutrients during pregnancy, and discuss strategies to ensure an adequate intake.

Assessment

Assessment data to collect for clients with suspected anemia includes:
- *Health history:* Complaints of shortness of breath with activity, fatigue, weakness, dizziness or fainting, palpitations; history of previous anemia, bleeding episodes; menstrual history (if appropriate); medications; chronic diseases; usual diet and patterns of alcohol intake or cigarette smoking.
- *Physical Examination:* General appearance, skin color; vital signs including temperature; heart and lung sounds; peripheral pulses, capillary refill; abdominal tenderness; obvious bleeding or bruising.

NURSING CARE PLAN   A Client with Folic Acid Deficiency Anemia

Sheri Matthews is a 76-year-old widow who lives alone. She tells Lisa Apana, RN, the nurse in her care provider's office, that she liked to cook when her husband was alive, but preparing an entire meal just for herself seems senseless. She relates that her typical day's menu includes coffee for breakfast, a bologna sandwich and coffee for lunch, and a hot dog or two, a few cookies, and a glass of milk for dinner.

ASSESSMENT

Mrs. Matthews's nursing history includes a 20-lb (9-kg) weight loss since her husband died 8 months ago. She states that she sometimes has heart palpitations and always feels weak. Physical assessment shows: T 98.8°F (37.1°C), P 110, R 22, BP 90/52. Skin warm, pale, and dry. Diagnostic tests indicate folic acid deficiency anemia, and Mrs. Matthews is started on an oral folic acid supplement and instructed about foods containing folic acid.

DIAGNOSES

- *Activity Intolerance* related to weakness secondary to decreased tissue oxygenation
- *Imbalanced Nutrition: Less than Body Requirements* related to lack of motivation to cook and understanding of nutritional needs, as manifested by weight loss of 20 lb and folic acid deficiency
- *Deficient Knowledge* related to lack of information about a well-balanced diet and foods containing folic acid

EXPECTED OUTCOMES

- Verbalize the importance of taking folic acid supplements and eating a balanced diet.
- Gain at least 1 lb (0.45 kg) per week.
- Return to previous level of physical energy.
- Consume a balanced diet, including foods containing folic acid.

PLANNING AND IMPLEMENTATION

- Discuss foods required for a well-balanced diet, as well as dietary sources of folic acid.
- Develop a dietary plan with Mrs. Matthews that includes food preferences and foods that are easy and quick to prepare.
- Discuss the importance of taking the folic acid supplement. Advise to continue taking it even after she begins to feel better.
- Help Mrs. Matthews develop a schedule of activities that provides adequate rest and energy for cooking.

EVALUATION

Mrs. Matthews gained 1 lb (0.45 kg) during the first week of treatment. She has met with a nutritionist and has a better understanding of nutritional needs. She states that she can prepare hot meals when she schedules a rest period before and after lunch. Ms. Apana has provided written and verbal information about the folic acid supplement and diet. Mrs. Matthews verbalizes understanding, stating, "I will continue to take the folic acid until the doctor tells me to stop. I'm beginning to enjoy cooking again, now that I have a reason to cook!" Ms. Apana contacts the local senior services representative to determine if Mrs. Matthews is able to participate in the local Meals-on-Wheels program.

CRITICAL THINKING IN THE NURSING PROCESS

1. What is the pathophysiologic basis for Mrs. Matthews's abnormal vital signs during her initial assessment?
2. Design a week's menu that includes foods high in folic acid.
3. Why was Mrs. Matthews placed on a folic acid supplement in addition to dietary modifications?
4. Why is the older adult at increased risk for developing folic acid deficiency anemia? Consider physiologic, economic, and social factors.

See Evaluating Your Response in Appendix C.

- *Diagnostic tests:* CBC, hemoglobin, and hematocrit; bone marrow studies; specialized tests (e.g., hemoglobin electrophoresis, Schilling test).

Nursing Diagnoses and Interventions

Anemia affects circulating oxygen levels and tissue oxygenation. Priority nursing diagnoses include activity intolerance, altered oral mucous membranes, and self-care deficits. With acute blood-loss anemia, risk for insufficient cardiac output also is a priority. Clients with sickle cell disease have specific needs related to the effects of the disease on tissue perfusion; see the section on disseminated intravascular coagulation later in this chapter for nursing interventions appropriate to ineffective tissue perfusion, associated pain, and maintaining oxygenation.

Activity Intolerance

Anemia causes weakness and shortness of breath on exertion. These symptoms are due to decreased circulating oxygen levels secondary to low hemoglobin levels. Weakness, fatigue, and/or vertigo may occur even during activities of daily living, including those associated with self-care, home life, job performance, and social roles.

- Help identify ways to conserve energy when performing necessary or desired activities. *Modifying the approach to a particular activity may reduce cardiorespiratory symptoms and activity-related fatigue. Alternative ways of performing tasks (e.g., sitting when performing hygiene care and kitchen tasks) may reduce oxygen demands. In some cases, assistance from others is necessary to conserve energy and reduce symptoms.*
- Help the client and family establish priorities for tasks and activities. *Because family members may need to assume responsibility for additional tasks, the plan's success depends on mutually established goals.*
- Assist to develop a schedule of alternating activity and rest periods throughout the day. *Rest periods decrease oxygen needs, reducing strain on the heart and lungs, and allowing restoration of homeostasis before further activities.*
- Encourage 8 to 10 hours of sleep at night. *Rest decreases oxygen demands and increases available energy for morning activities.*
- Monitor vital signs before and after activity. *Vital signs provide a measure of activity tolerance. Increased heart and respiratory rates or a change in blood pressure may indicate intolerance of the activity.*

- Discontinue activity if any of the following occurs:
  a. Complaints of chest pain, breathlessness, or vertigo
  b. Palpitations or tachycardia that does not return to normal within 4 minutes of resting
  c. Bradycardia
  d. Tachypnea or dyspnea
  e. Decreased systolic blood pressure.

  These changes may signify cardiac decompensation due to insufficient oxygenation. The intensity, duration, or frequency of the activity needs to be reduced.

- Instruct the client not to smoke. *Smoking causes vasoconstriction and increases carbon monoxide levels in the blood, interfering with tissue oxygenation.*

Impaired Oral Mucous Membrane

Glossitis and cheilosis may occur with nutritional deficiencies of iron, folate, and vitamin B_{12}. The tongue and lips become very red, and fissures or cracks may form at the corners of the mouth.

- Monitor condition of lips and tongue daily. *Glossitis and cheilosis increase the risk for bleeding and infection and may require medical treatment. Pain and discomfort may interfere with oral intake, further worsening the nutritional deficiency.*

- Use a mouthwash of saline, saltwater, or half-strength peroxide and water to rinse the mouth every 2 to 4 hours. Avoid alcohol-based mouthwashes. *This cleanses and soothes oral mucous membranes. Alcohol-based mouthwashes further irritate and dry oral tissues.*

- Provide frequent oral hygiene (after each meal and at bedtime) with a soft bristle toothbrush or sponge. *Removing food debris from painful fissures promotes comfort. A soft toothbrush reduces irritation or bleeding of oral mucosa. Keeping the oral cavity clean also reduces the risk of infection.*

- Apply a petroleum-based lubricating jelly or ointment to the lips after oral care. *Lubricating ointment helps to retain moisture, facilitate healing, and protect the lips from other drying agents.*

- Instruct to avoid hot, spicy, or acidic foods. *Such foods may further irritate and dry mucous membranes.*

- Encourage soft, cool, bland foods. *Foods that are soothing to the mucous membranes promote comfort and help maintain adequate food and fluid intake. Minimizing oral pain may also promote compliance with oral care routines.*

- Encourage eating four to six small meals daily with high protein and vitamin content. *Small, frequent meals may be better tolerated, increasing intake. Nutrient-rich meals promote healing of the mucous membranes.*

Risk for Decreased Cardiac Output

Cardiac output may be affected by acute bleeding and volume loss or by heart failure resulting from severe anemia. In addition, impaired tissue oxygenation leads to an increased respiratory rate and dyspnea.

- Monitor vital signs, breath sounds, and apical pulse. *Increased cardiac workload can affect the blood pressure, heart, and respiratory rates. Increased blood flow can lead to heart murmur or abnormal heart sounds such as S_3 or S_4. Tachypnea and dyspnea may affect the depth of respirations, alveolar ventilation, and blood and tissue oxygenation.*

- Assess for pallor, cyanosis, and dependent edema. *Blood is shunted to the vital organs, causing vasoconstriction of skin vessels. This, in addition to lower levels of hemoglobin, causes pallor. Cyanosis, especially of the lips and nail beds, indicates inadequate oxygenation of blood. Dependent edema occurs in response to right ventricular failure.*

> **PRACTICE ALERT**
> Report signs of decreased cardiac output to the physician. Severe anemia can lead to heart failure, necessitating additional treatment.

- Closely monitor for manifestations of anaphylaxis (urticaria, erythema or flushing, edema, wheezing, dyspnea, nausea and vomiting, anxiety) when administering parenteral iron preparations, particularly iron dextran. Immediately notify the physician, and prepare to administer prescribed drugs such as diphenhydramine (Benadryl) or epinephrine as ordered. Institute cardiopulmonary resuscitation measures as necessary. *Anaphylaxis, a systemic type I hypersensitivity (allergic) reaction, is a risk when administering parenteral iron preparations, iron dextran in particular. Anaphylaxis can lead to severe cardiopulmonary compromise, necessitating emergency measures to preserve life.*

Self-Care Deficit

Energy expenditures for activities of daily living (ADLs) may cause oxygen demands to exceed supply in the client with severe anemia.

- Assist with ADLs, such as bathing, grooming, and eating, as needed. *Assistance decreases energy expenditures and tissue requirements for oxygen, reducing cardiac workload.*

- Discuss the importance of rest periods prior to such activities as dressing. *Rest reduces oxygen demand and cardiac workload. The person who is able to perform self-care in activities of daily living maintains independence, self-esteem, and morale.*

NANDA, NIC, and NOC Linkages

See Chart 34–1 for linkages between NANDA nursing diagnoses, nursing interventions, and nursing outcomes for the client with anemia.

Community-Based Care

With the exception of anemia resulting from acute hemorrhage, most clients with anemia are treated in the home and community setting. Include the following topics when preparing the client and family for home care:

- Nutritional strategies to address deficiencies
- Prescribed medications, vitamins, or mineral supplements and their appropriate use, intended effect, possible adverse effects, and interactions with food or other medications
- Energy conservation strategies
- Other recommended treatment measures and follow-up
- If the anemia is genetically transmitted, such as sickle cell anemia, include inheritance patterns of the disorder, symptoms of crisis, and manifestations to report to the physician.

Provide referrals for counseling to facilitate decisions about pregnancy as indicated. Also refer for nutritional assistance and

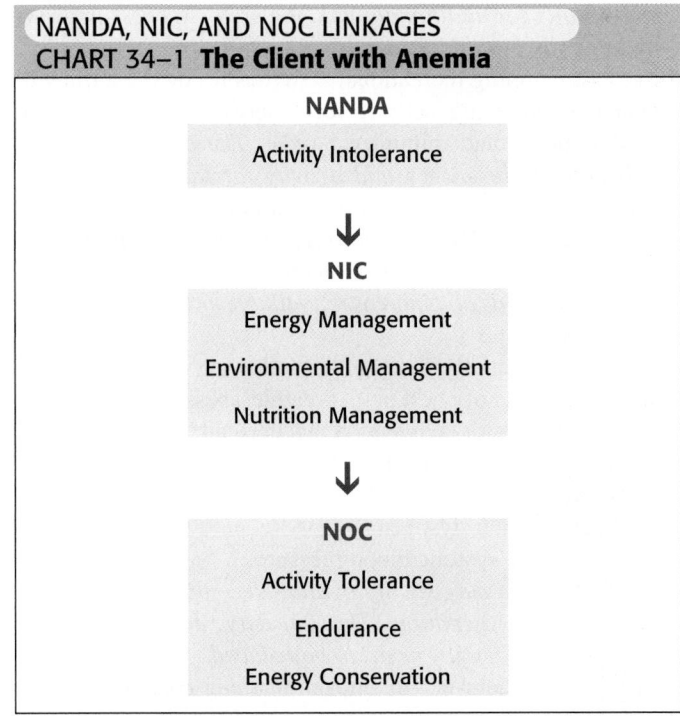

NANDA, NIC, AND NOC LINKAGES
CHART 34–1 **The Client with Anemia**

NANDA

Activity Intolerance

↓

NIC

Energy Management

Environmental Management

Nutrition Management

↓

NOC

Activity Tolerance

Endurance

Energy Conservation

Data from *NANDA's Nursing Diagnoses: Definitions & Classification 2005–2006* by NANDA International (2005), Philadelphia; *Nursing Interventions Classification (NIC)* (4th ed.) by J. M. Dochterman & G. M. Bulechek (2004), St. Louis, MO: Mosby; and *Nursing Outcomes Classification (NOC)* (3rd ed.) by S. Moorhead, M. Johnson, and M. Mass (2004), St. Louis, MO: Mosby.

teaching, home health care, or assistance with self-care and home maintenance activities as indicated. Older adults with nutritional anemias may benefit from community services such as senior meals or Meals-on-Wheels.

THE CLIENT WITH MYELODYSPLASTIC SYNDROME

Myelodysplastic syndrome (MDS) is a group of blood disorders characterized by abnormal-appearing bone marrow and cytopenia (low numbers of circulating blood cells). MDS is not a single disease; at least five variations of the disorder have been identified. Anemia that does not respond to treatment (*refractory anemia*) is a characteristic of most forms of myelodysplasia.

Idiopathic MDS primarily affects older adults; men have a slightly higher incidence of the disorder than women. Risk factors for secondary MDS include exposure to environmental toxins such as cigarette smoke, benzene, radiation, radiation therapy or chemotherapy for cancer treatment, and other anemias such as aplastic anemia or Fanconi's anemia (Demakos & Linebaugh, 2005; Kasper et al., 2005).

FAST FACTS

- Idiopathic or primary MDS accounts for 70% to 80% of all identified cases.
- Twenty percent to 30% of MDS cases occur as a secondary condition, related to factors such as smoking or exposure to environmental toxins, radiation, chemotherapy, or other risk factors (Demakos & Linebaugh, 2005).

Pathophysiology

MDS is a stem cell disorder in which stem cells fail to reproduce and differentiate into the various types of blood cells. The genetic components of stem cells (nuclear DNA and/or mitochondrial DNA) are altered. The bone marrow loses its ability to produce normal blood cells, instead producing abnormal (*dysplastic*) cells. With significant alterations, leukemia (proliferation of abnormal white blood cells) may develop in people with MDS.

Manifestations

Anemia is the predominant early manifestation of MDS. The client may develop symptoms of the anemia with increasing fatigue, weakness, dyspnea and pallor. In many cases, the disorder is asymptomatic, identified when a routine blood count shows anemia. Splenomegaly may develop, leading to discomfort and a feeling of fullness in the left upper quadrant of the abdomen. Hepatomegaly also may develop, leading to right upper quadrant discomfort. Thrombocytopenia can lead to abnormal bleeding tendencies, and neutropenia increases the risk for infection (Demakos & Linebaugh, 2005).

INTERDISCIPLINARY CARE

Clients with MDS require long-term supportive care and therapy to maintain their quality of life. Stem cell transplant offers the only real hope for cure in MDS. See the Interdisciplinary Care section of the client with leukemia later in this chapter for more information about stem cell transplant and associated nursing care.

Diagnosis

- The *CBC* reveals anemia. Although anemia may be the only abnormality of the blood count, the white blood cell (WBC) count also may be low, as may be the platelet count. Abnormalities of size and shape may be noted in all blood cells.
- The *bone marrow* often appears normal, although precursor cells may have an abnormal appearance. Increased numbers of myeloblasts (granulocyte precursor cells) may be present in the bone marrow.
- *Serum erythropoietin, vitamin B$_{12}$, serum iron, total iron-binding capacity, ferritin levels,* and *RBC folate levels* are drawn to help guide supportive therapy.

Treatment

Management of MDS is based on the severity of the disease. Several classification systems are available, including the French-American-British (FAB) classification system, the International Prognostic Scoring System (IPSS), and the World Health Organization (WHO) classification system (National Comprehensive Cancer Network [NCCN], 2006). These systems are used to guide therapy for the client with MDS.

All clients with MDS require monitoring, with regular physician visits and laboratory evaluations. Psychosocial support is provided to assist the client and family dealing with a chronic, progressive, and ultimately fatal disease.

Clients with MDS may require frequent red blood cell transfusions to treat the predominant anemia. Each unit of packed

RBCs contains 250 to 300 mg of iron. The body is unable to excrete this excess iron, so it accumulates, leading to problems such as endocrine dysfunction, cirrhosis, pericarditis, and heart failure. *Iron chelation therapy* is used to remove excess iron from the body. Desferrioxamine (Desferal) is administered by slow intravenous infusion or continuous subcutaneous infusion using an infusion pump to maintain a normal or negative iron balance. This drug is relatively safe, although local skin reactions such as rash and urticaria may develop. An oral form of the drug, deferasirox, is available, but not widely used.

Blood cell growth factors may be administered to stimulate stem cell development in MDS, although the response rate is low. Platelet transfusions are given when bleeding occurs due to low platelet levels. Antibiotic therapy is initiated for bacterial infections (NCCS, 2006). Chemotherapy regimens similar to those employed to treat leukemia may be used, but rarely are effective in treating MDS. Azacitidine (Vidaza), an antileukemic agent that acts on abnormal blood-forming cells in the bone marrow, may be more effective in treating MDS than standard chemotherapy regimens (Demakos & Linebaugh, 2005). As previously noted, stem cell transplant offers the only hope for cure. This high-risk therapy, however, is reserved for higher risk clients. Factors such as age, functional ability, and other existing disease conditions help guide the decision to undergo stem cell transplant (NCCN, 2006).

NURSING CARE

Nursing Diagnoses and Interventions

Activity intolerance and the need for education about this disorder are the priorities of nursing care for the client with MDS being managed in a community-based setting. Although neutropenia and thrombocytopenia may accompany the anemia of MDS, these problems are less common. See the section of this chapter on leukemia for additional potential nursing diagnoses and interventions for the client with MDS.

Activity Intolerance

The client with MDS experiences fatigue, weakness, and shortness of breath on exertion related to the lack of RBCs and ineffective oxygen transport. These symptoms may affect the client's ability to maintain self-care, home life, job performance, and social roles.

■ Monitor vital signs, breath sounds, and apical pulse. *Increased cardiac workload due to anemia and impaired oxygen transport can affect the blood pressure, heart, and respiratory rates. Increased blood flow can lead to heart murmur or abnormal heart sounds such as S_3 or S_4. Accumulated iron can lead to pericarditis and a pericardial friction rub.*

■ Help identify energy-conserving ways of performing necessary or desired activities. *Alternative ways of performing tasks (e.g., sitting while performing hygiene measures) may reduce oxygen demands and fatigue.*

■ Help the client and family establish priorities for tasks and activities. *Because family members may need to assume responsibility for additional tasks, the plan's success depends on mutually established goals.*

■ Suggest planning recreational activities following a transfusion and adjusting activity level between transfusions to match energy and minimize fatigue. *The client with MDS will have more energy and activity tolerance following a transfusion when RBC counts, hemoglobin, and hematocrit approach normal levels and oxygen transport is optimal.*

■ Encourage 8 to 10 hours of sleep at night. *Rest decreases oxygen demands and increases available energy for morning activities.*

■ Discontinue activity if any of the following occurs:
  a. Complaints of chest pain, breathlessness, or vertigo
  b. Palpitations or tachycardia that does not return to normal within 4 minutes of resting
  c. Bradycardia
  d. Tachypnea or dyspnea
  e. Decreased systolic blood pressure.
  These changes may signify cardiac decompensation due to insufficient oxygenation. The intensity, duration, or frequency of the activity needs to be reduced.

■ Instruct the client not to smoke. *Smoking causes vasoconstriction and increases carbon monoxide levels in the blood, interfering with tissue oxygenation.*

Risk for Ineffective Health Maintenance

MDS is a chronic, usually progressive disorder, requiring active management to maintain functional status and quality of life. Regular visits to the physician or clinic may be necessary. In addition, the client or family members may need to learn to administer iron chelation therapy or chemotherapy drugs and measures to prevent complications. The chronic nature of the disorder and the often advanced age of the client and family caregivers may interfere with effective management of the disorder.

■ Assess knowledge of the disorder and the related treatments. *Assessment allows identification of knowledge gaps and provides a basis on which to provide additional information. Impaired disease management may be due to lack of knowledge or an inability to learn and perform psychomotor skills (e.g., administration of parenteral drug therapy).*

■ Provide information about the disorder, its effects, and prescribed medications and treatments. *Individualized instruction is more effective than general, possibly irrelevant information. The client and caregivers need to be able to identify and manage possible adverse effects of drug therapy, as well as recognize potential complications to be reported to the physician.*

■ Provide emotional support, expressing confidence in the client's and caregivers' abilities to manage care. *Emotional support helps the client and family caregivers incorporate the care regimen into their lifestyle.*

■ Provide supervised learning and practice opportunities for administering parenteral medications if ordered. *Successful practice sessions instill confidence in the ability to manage care and provide an opportunity for questions and exploring alternatives.*

Community-Based Care

The client with myelodysplastic syndrome needs information about this chronic and ultimately fatal disease. Provide information about treatment options, including management of the infusion pump if ordered. Discuss the timing of and options for stem cell transplant, and assist the client to evaluate the potential benefits and risks of this treatment option.

THE CLIENT WITH POLYCYTHEMIA

Polycythemia, or *erythrocytosis*, is an excess of red blood cells characterized by a hematocrit higher than 55%. The two major types of polycythemia are primary and secondary. A third type of polycythemia, relative polycythemia, results from a fluid volume deficit, not excess RBCs.

FAST FACTS

- *Primary polycythemia (polycythemia vera)* is uncommon.
  - In primary polycythemia, RBC production is increased.
  - Primary polycythemia more commonly affects men of European Jewish ancestry between age 40 and 70.
- *Secondary polycythemia (erythrocytosis)* is the most common form of polycythemia.
  - Secondary polycythemia occurs when erythropoietin levels are elevated.
  - It may affect clients of any age or origin.
  - It usually develops in response to hypoxia (living at a high altitude, smoking, or chronic lung disease).
- *Relative polycythemia* occurs due to fluid deficit, not excess RBCs.
  - In relative polycythemia the total RBC count is normal.
  - The hematocrit is elevated because of increased cell concentration.
  - It is corrected by rehydration.

Pathophysiology

Primary Polycythemia

Primary polycythemia, or polycythemia vera (PV), is a neoplastic stem cell disorder characterized by overproduction of RBCs and, to a lesser extent, white blood cells and platelets. It is classified as a myeloproliferative disorder. Its cause is unknown. In PV, colonies of endogenous erythroid stem cells develop. These colonies produce RBCs in the absence of erythropoietin, leading to excess RBC production.

MANIFESTATIONS Initially, PV is asymptomatic, and the diagnosis may be made during routine blood tests. Its manifestations are caused by increased blood volume and viscosity. Hypertension is common, and may lead to complaints of headaches, dizziness, and vision and hearing disruptions. Venous stasis causes *plethora*, a ruddy, red color of the face, hands, feet, and mucous membranes. This often is accompanied by severe, painful itching of the fingers and toes. Retinal and cerebral vessels may be engorged. Hypermetabolism develops, causing weight loss and night sweats. Mental status may be altered, leading to drowsiness or delirium.

Thrombosis and hemorrhage are potential complications of PV. Thrombosis may cause transient ischemic attacks, angina,

or manifestations of peripheral vascular disease. Gastrointestinal bleeding may occur, and portal hypertension may develop.

Secondary Polycythemia

Secondary polycythemia, or erythrocytosis, is increased numbers of RBCs in response to excess erythropoietin secretion or prolonged hypoxia. Secondary polycythemia is the most common form of polycythemia.

Abnormally high erythropoietin levels can result from kidney disease or erythropoietin-secreting tumors (e.g., renal cell carcinoma). Chronic hypoxia that stimulates erythropoietin release is a more common cause of secondary polycythemia. People living at high altitudes where the atmospheric oxygen pressure is lower develop a degree of polycythemia, as do people with chronic heart or lung disease and smokers. Abnormal hemoglobin that forms tighter bonds with oxygen also may lead to secondary polycythemia.

MANIFESTATIONS The manifestations of secondary polycythemia are similar to those of primary polycythemia. Splenomegaly, however, does not develop. Early symptoms often are overshadowed by the manifestations of the underlying disorder. For the manifestations of polycythemia see the box below.

INTERDISCIPLINARY CARE

Diagnosis

In PV, serum erythropoietin levels are low. Bone marrow studies show hyperplasia of all hematopoietic elements. With secondary polycythemia, serum erythropoietin levels usually are high, and bone marrow studies show only red stem cell hyperplasia.

Treatments

For secondary polycythemia, treatment focuses on the underlying cause of the disorder. It is a physiologic response in people living at high altitudes, and unless the hematocrit is too high or oxygen saturation levels are low, no treatment is usually necessary. Smokers are urged to quit. Measures to raise oxygen saturation levels and reduce tissue hypoxia often will relieve the polycythemia. Clients with both primary and secondary polycythemia benefit from periodic phlebotomy, removing 300 to 500 mL of blood, to keep blood volume and viscosity within normal levels. For PV, chemotherapeutic agents such as hydroxyurea may be used to suppress marrow function but may

---

MANIFESTATIONS of Polycythemia

- Hypertension
- Headache, tinnitus, blurred vision
- Plethora: dark redness of the lips, feet, ears, fingernails, and mucous membranes
- Splenomegaly (polycythemia vera)
- Severe pruritus, extremity pain
- Weight loss, night sweats
- Gastrointestinal bleeding
- Intermittent claudication
- Symptoms from thrombosis within various organs

increase the risk of developing leukemia (discussed later in this chapter). Pruritus may be relieved by antihistamines, or may require more aggressive treatment with interferon alpha or other treatments. One 325-mg aspirin tablet daily may be ordered to control thrombosis without increasing the risk of bleeding.

NURSING CARE

Preventing polycythemia begins with educating children and adults about the dangers of smoking. Measures to reduce risk factors for cardiovascular disease also may be beneficial.

This chronic condition is managed in community-based settings unless a complication develops. Teach the client and family the importance of maintaining adequate hydration, and increasing fluid intake during hot weather and when exercising. Discuss measures to prevent blood stasis: elevating legs and feet when sitting, using support stockings, and continuing treatment measures. Instruct to report manifestations of thrombosis (leg or calf pain, chest pain, neurologic symptoms) or bleeding (black, tarry stools, vomiting of blood or coffee-grounds emesis) immediately. Monitor the hematocrit and cell counts throughout treatment.

Examples of nursing diagnoses appropriate for the client with polycythemia follow:
- *Decisional Conflict Regarding Smoking Cessation* related to addictive effects
- *Pain* related to effects of altered blood flow in distal extremities
- *Risk for Ineffective Tissue Perfusion* related to sluggish blood flow and increased risk for thrombosis.

WHITE BLOOD CELL AND LYMPHOID TISSUE DISORDERS

Disorders of the white blood cells and lymphoid tissue include infectious mononucleosis, the leukemias, multiple myeloma, and malignant lymphomas (Hodgkin's disease and non-Hodgkin's lymphoma). Review the physiology of WBCs and lymphoid tissues and assessment of their function in Chapter 33 ∞ before proceeding with this section.

THE CLIENT WITH LEUKEMIA

Leukemia (literally, "white blood") is a group of chronic malignant disorders of white blood cells and white blood cell precursors. In leukemia, the usual ratio of red to white blood cells is reversed. Leukemias are characterized by replacement of bone marrow by malignant immature white blood cells, abnormal immature circulating WBCs, and infiltration of these cells into the liver, spleen, and lymph nodes throughout the body.

Incidence and Risk Factors

Although leukemia is often thought of as a childhood disease, it is diagnosed 10 times more often in adults than in children. An estimated 34,810 new cases of leukemia occur annually; slightly more than half are acute leukemia and less than half are chronic leukemia. In 2005, the ACS (2005) estimated that approximately 22,570 people died of leukemia. The highest incidence of leukemia is found in the United States, Canada, Sweden, and New Zealand (McCance & Huether, 2006).

Although the cause of most leukemias is unknown, certain risk factors have been identified. Men are affected more frequently than are women. People with certain genetic disorders such as Down syndrome have a higher incidence of leukemia. Environmental risk factors play a role as well. Risk factors for myeloid leukemia include cigarette smoking and chemicals such as benzene (present in cigarette smoke and gasoline). Exposure to ionizing radiation increases the risk for several types of leukemia. Clients who have undergone treatment for cancer have an increased risk. The human T-cell leukemia/lymphoma virus-1, a retrovirus, is known to cause certain leukemias and lymphomas (ACS, 2005).

Physiology Review

White blood cells are the most diverse of the cellular components of the blood. White blood cells arise from three different precursor cells: myeloblasts, which further differentiate into the granular leukocytes (granulocytes), neutrophils, eosinophils, and basophils; monoblasts, which mature into circulating monocytes, and ultimately into macrophages; and lymphoblasts, which become lymphocytes and mature in lymphoid tissue to B cells and T cells.

As a whole, the primary function of WBCs is to help maintain the body's immune defenses. Neutrophils, the most numerous WBC in circulation, are active phagocytes, the first cells to arrive to injured tissue. Monocytes and macrophages also are phagocytic cells that dispose of foreign and waste material from tissues. Eosinophils and basophils are more specialized. Eosinophils are primarily involved in allergic responses and parasitic infections. Basophils are actively involved in the inflammatory response, releasing substances such as histamine and heparin into inflamed tissues. Lymphocytes, the smallest of the WBCs, are an integral part of the immune system. B cells are part of the humoral immune response, producing antibodies to specific antigens. T cells are part of the cell-mediated immune response. For more information about the inflammatory and immune responses, see Chapter 12 ∞. The normal WBC count and differential are presented in Table 34–2.

TABLE 34–2 Normal White Blood Cell Count and Differential

LABORATORY TEST	VALUE
WBC count	5000–10,000/mm³
Differential WBC count	
Neutrophils	60–70% or 3000–7000/mm³
Eosinophils	1–3% or 50–400/mm³
Basophils	0.3–0.5% or 25–200/mm³
Lymphocytes	20–30% or 1000–4000/mm³
Monocytes	3–8% or 100–600/mm³

Pathophysiology

Leukemia begins with malignant transformation of a single stem cell. Leukemic cells proliferate slowly, but do not differentiate normally. They have a prolonged life span and accumulate in the bone marrow. As they accumulate, they compete with the proliferation of normal cells. Leukemic cells do not function as mature WBCs, and are ineffective in the inflammatory and immune processes. Leukemic cells replace normal hematopoietic elements in the marrow. Because erythrocyte- and platelet-producing cells are crowded out, severe anemia, splenomegaly, and bleeding difficulties result.

Leukemic cells leave the bone marrow and travel through the circulatory system, infiltrating other body tissues such as the CNS, testes, skin, gastrointestinal tract, and the lymph nodes, liver, and spleen. Death usually is due to internal hemorrhage and infections.

Manifestations

The general manifestations of leukemia (regardless of type) result from anemia, infection, and bleeding. These include pallor, fatigue, tachycardia, malaise, lethargy, and dyspnea on exertion. Infection may cause fever, night sweats, oral ulcerations, and frequent or recurrent respiratory, urinary, integumentary, or other infections. Increased bleeding due to thrombocytopenia leads to bruising, petechiae, bleeding gums, and bleeding within specific organs and tissues. *Multisystem Effects of Leukemia* can be seen on page 1120.

Other manifestations result from leukemic cell infiltration, increased metabolism, and increased leukocyte destruction. Infiltration of the liver, spleen, lymph nodes, and bone marrow causes pain and tissue swelling in the involved areas. Meningeal infiltration may cause manifestations of increased intracranial pressure, such as headache, altered level of consciousness, cranial nerve impairment, nausea, and vomiting. Infiltration of the kidneys may affect renal function, with decreased urine output and increased blood urea nitrogen and creatinine. Increased metabolism causes heat intolerance, weight loss, dyspnea on exertion, and tachycardia. Destruction of large numbers of WBCs releases substantial amounts of uric acid into the circulation; uric acid crystals may obstruct renal tubules, causing renal insufficiency.

Without treatment, leukemia is invariably fatal, usually due to complications of leukemic cell infiltration of bone marrow or vital organs. With treatment, prognosis varies. The overall 5-year survival rate is 46%. Survival rates differ by type of leukemia: People with acute myeloid leukemia have a 20% 5-year survival rate, whereas the rate is 73% for people with chronic lymphocytic leukemia (American Cancer Society, [ACS], 2005). The types, pathology, manifestations, and treatment for the major leukemias are outlined in Table 34–3.

Classifications

Leukemias are classified by their acuity and by the predominant cell type involved. The *acute* leukemias are characterized by an acute onset, rapid disease progression, and immature or undifferentiated blast cells. *Chronic* leukemias, on the other hand, have a gradual onset, prolonged course, and abnormal mature-appearing cells. *Lymphocytic* (or *lymphoblastic*) leukemias involve immature lymphocytes and their precursor cells in the bone marrow. Lymphocytic leukemias infiltrate the spleen, lymph nodes, CNS, and other tissues. *Myeloid* (also called *myelogenous, myelocytic,* or *myeloblastic*) leukemias involve myeloid stem cells in the bone marrow, interfering with the maturation of all types of blood cells, including granulocytes, RBCs, and thrombocytes (Porth, 2005). Acute lymphoblastic leukemia is the most common type of leukemia in children. In adults, acute myeloid leukemia and chronic lymphocytic leukemia are the most common types (McCance &

TABLE 34–3 Major Types of Leukemia

CLASSIFICATION	CHARACTERISTICS	MANIFESTATIONS	TREATMENT
Acute lymphoblastic leukemia (ALL)	Primarily affects children and young adults; leukemic cells may infiltrate CNS	Recurrent infections; bleeding; pallor, bone pain, weight loss, sore throat, fatigue, night sweats, weakness	Chemotherapy; bone marrow transplant (BMT), or stem cell transplant (SCT)
Chronic lymphocytic leukemia (CLL)	Primarily affects older adults; insidious onset and slow, chronic course	Fatigue; exercise intolerance; lymphadenopathy and splenomegaly; recurrent infections, pallor, edema, thrombophlebitis	Often requires no treatment; chemotherapy; BMT
Acute myeloid leukemia (AML)	Common in older adults, may affect children and young adults. Strongly associated with toxins, genetic disorders, and treatment of other cancers	Fatigue, weakness, fever; anemia; headache; bone and joint pain; abnormal bleeding and bruising; recurrent infection; lymphadenopathy, splenomegaly, and hepatomegaly	Chemotherapy; SCT
Chronic myeloid leukemia (CML)	Primarily affects adults; early course slow and stable, progressing to aggressive phase in 3–4 years	*Early:* weakness, fatigue, dyspnea on exertion; possible splenomegaly *Later:* fever, weight loss, night sweats	Interferon alpha; chemotherapy with imatinib mesylate (Gleevec), SCT

MULTISYSTEM EFFECTS of Leukemia

Neurologic
- Headache
- Altered LOC
- Cranial nerve impairment

Potential complications
- Subarachnoid hemorrhage
- Retinal hemorrhage
- Seizures, coma

Respiratory
- Dyspnea on exertion
- Pharyngitis, sore throat
- Frequent respiratory infections

Potential complication
- Pulmonary bleeding

Gastrointestinal
- Anorexia, nausea
- Oral ulcerations, infection
- Bleeding gums
- Gingival hyperplasia
  (gum overgrowth)
- Abdominal pain
- Hepatomegaly
- Occult GI bleeding

Urinary
- Urinary tract infection
- Hematuria

Potential complication
- Renal insufficiency or failure

Musculoskeletal
- Weakness
- Bone tenderness, pain
- Joint pain

Metabolic Processes
- Malaise, lethargy
- Heat intolerance
- Diaphoresis
- Chills, fever
- Night sweats
- Weight loss

Cardiovascular
- Tachycardia, palpitations
- Orthostatic hypotension
- Heart murmurs
- Hematomas
- Edema

Potential complications
- Hemorrhage
- Thrombophlebitis

Hematologic
- Anemia
- Thrombocytopenia
- Leukopenia
- Bleeding (epistaxis)
- Splenomegaly

Potential complication
- DIC

Immunologic
- Frequent or recurrent infections
- Lymphadenopathy

Potential complications
- Abscesses
- Septicemia

Integumentary
- Skin and mucous membrane pallor
- Petechiae
- Bruising, purpura
- Ulcerations
- *Chloromas* (skin infiltrations near
  bony prominences)

Huether, 2006). In summary, the general types of leukemia are as follows:

- Acute lymphocytic (lymphoblastic) leukemia (ALL)
- Chronic lymphocytic leukemia (CLL)
- Acute myeloid (myeloblastic) leukemia (AML)
- Chronic myeloid (myelogenous) leukemia (CML).

This general system of classifying leukemias does not differentiate subtypes of acute leukemias. The FAB system for classifying acute leukemias further differentiates acute leukemias by the predominant cell involved and the degree of cell differentiation (Table 34–4).

Acute Myeloid Leukemia

Acute myeloid leukemia is characterized by uncontrolled proliferation of myeloblasts (the precursors of granulocytes) and hyperplasia of the bone marrow and spleen (Figure 34–5 ■). AML accounts for 80% of acute leukemia cases in adults (Copstead & Banasik, 2005). Treatment induces complete remission in 66% of clients, although only about 30% to 40% achieve cure or long-term remission (Porth, 2005).

The manifestations of AML result from neutropenia and thrombocytopenia. Decreased neutrophils lead to recurrent severe infections, such as pneumonia, septicemia, abscesses, and mucous membrane ulceration. The manifestations of thrombocytopenia include petechiae, purpura, ecchymoses (bruising), epistaxis (nosebleeds), hematomas, hematuria, and gastrointestinal bleeding. Bone infarctions or subperiosteal infiltrates of leukemic cells may cause bone pain. Anemia is a late manifestation, causing fatigue, headaches, pallor, and dyspnea on exertion. Death usually results from infection or hemorrhage.

Bone marrow aspiration shows a proliferation of immature WBCs. The CBC shows thrombocytopenia and normocytic, normochromic anemia.

Chronic Myeloid Leukemia

Chronic myeloid leukemia is characterized by abnormal proliferation of all bone marrow elements. This type of leukemia constitutes approximately 15% of adult leukemias. It affects men more frequently than women. The onset of CML typically is between ages 30 or 40 and 50, although it is seen in children and adolescents as well (Copstead & Banasik, 2005; Porth 2005).

Figure 34–5 ■ A blood smear from the bone marrow of a client with acute myeloid leukemia. Note the abnormally large number of myelocyte WBCs (stained purple) among the small RBCs.

Source: Dr. Gopal Murti, Photo Researchers, Inc.

CML is usually associated with a chromosome abnormality called the Philadelphia chromosome, a balanced translocation of chromosome 22 to chromosome 9 (Figure 34–6 ■). The fusion gene produced by this translocation, known as *bcr/abl,* is an *oncogene* capable of initiating a malignancy. Very large doses of ionizing radiation also may induce CML in some clients (Kasper et al., 2005).

People with CML are often asymptomatic in the early stages and, in fact, are often diagnosed when a routine blood test reveals abnormal cell counts. Anemia causes weakness, fatigue, and dyspnea on exertion. The spleen often is enlarged, causing abdominal discomfort. Within 3 to 4 years, disease progresses to a more aggressive phase. Rapid cell proliferation and hypermetabolism cause fatigue, weight loss, sweating, and heat intolerance. The spleen enlarges, leading to a sensation of abdominal fullness and discomfort. Platelet function is affected in this stage, leading to bleeding and increased bruising. Finally, the disease evolves to acute leukemia, with blast cell proliferation. This stage, known as the *terminal blast crisis phase,* is characterized by significant constitutional manifestations, splenomegaly, and infiltration of leukemic cells into the skin, lymph nodes, bones, and CNS

TABLE 34–4 FAB Classification of Acute Leukemia

TYPE	CLASS	PREDOMINANT CELLS	PROGNOSIS
Acute lymphocytic leukemia	L_1	Immature lymphoblasts	>90% remission rate in children
	L_2	Mature lymphoblasts	Relapse common after 2 or more years of remission
Acute myeloid leukemia	M_0	Undifferentiated cells	Poor
	M_1	Immature myeloblasts	Good; complete response in 65% or more
	M_2	Mature myeloblasts	Good for 2 or more years of remission
	M_3	Promyelocytes	Good in adults
	M_4	Myelocytes and monocytes	Poorest in adults
	M_5	Poorly or well-differentiated monocytes	Poor
	M_6	Predominant erythroblasts	Variable
	M_7	Megakaryocytes	

Figure 34–6 ■ The Philadelphia chromosome. Note the chromosomes of pairs 9 and 22. In each instance, the left-hand chromosome of the pair is normal, whereas an exchange of material between chromosomes has made the right-hand chromosome 9 larger and the right-hand chromosome 22 smaller. In stem cells within the bone marrow, the chromosome 22 defect leads to chronic myeloid leukemia.

Source: Addenbrookes Hospital, Photo Researchers, Inc.

Figure 34–7 ■ A blood smear from the bone marrow of a client with acute lymphocytic leukemia. Note the abnormally large number of lymphocytes (stained purple) crowding the bone marrow. As a result, normal production of RBCs, functional WBCs, and platelets is suppressed.

Source: Dr. Gopal Murti, Photo Researchers, Inc.

(Porth, 2005). Survival following the onset of this final stage averages only 2 to 4 months.

Acute Lymphocytic Leukemia

Acute lymphocytic leukemia is the most common type of leukemia in children and young adults. In adults, ALL is rarely seen until late middle age, and then its incidence increases with aging. Genetic factors may play a role in its development, particularly the *bcr/abl* translocation also implicated in CML (Copstead & Banasik, 2005).

Most (80%) cases of ALL result from malignant transformation of B cells, with the remaining 20% arising from T cells. The malignant cells resemble immature lymphocytes (*lymphoblasts*); however, they do not mature or function effectively to maintain immunity. These lymphoblasts accumulate in the bone marrow, lymph nodes, and spleen, as well as in circulating blood. Some types of lymphoma (discussed later in this chapter) are thought to represent a later stage of the same disease.

The onset of ALL is usually rapid. Lymphoblasts proliferating in bone marrow and peripheral tissues crowd the growth of normal cells (Figure 34–7 ■). Normal hematopoiesis is suppressed, leading to thrombocytopenia, leukopenia, and anemia. Manifestations of infections, bleeding, and anemia develop. Bone pain resulting from rapid generation of marrow elements, lymphadenopathy, and liver enlargement are also common. Infiltration of the CNS causes headaches, visual disturbances, vomiting, and seizures.

The CBC shows an elevated WBC count with increased lymphocytes on the differential. RBC and platelet counts are decreased. Bone marrow studies reveal a hypercellular marrow with growth of lymphoblasts. Combination chemotherapy produces complete remission in 80% to 90% of adults with ALL.

Chronic Lymphocytic Leukemia

Chronic lymphocytic leukemia is characterized by proliferation and accumulation of small, abnormal, mature lymphocytes in the bone marrow, peripheral blood, and body tissues. The abnormal cells are usually B lymphocytes that are unable to produce adequate antibodies to maintain normal immune function. Only about 5% of CLL involves T cells (Copstead & Banasik, 2005). CLL occurs more commonly in adults, especially in older adults (median age 65). CLL is the least common type of the major leukemias.

CLL has a slow onset and is often diagnosed during a routine physical examination. If symptoms are present, they usually include vague complaints of weakness or malaise. Possible clinical findings include anemia, infection, and enlarged lymph nodes, spleen, and liver. As in other leukemias, bone marrow hyperplasia is present. Erythrocyte and platelet counts are reduced. Leukocyte counts may either be elevated or reduced, but abnormal cells are always present. In CLL, years may elapse before treatment is required. Survival of this disease averages approximately 7 years.

INTERDISCIPLINARY CARE

Treatment for leukemia focuses on achieving remission or cure and relieving symptoms. The methods of treatment may include chemotherapy, radiation therapy, and bone marrow or stem cell transplantation. Cure is more often achieved in children with acute leukemia than in adults, although long-term remissions (disease-free periods with no signs or symptoms) often can be achieved.

Diagnosis

The following diagnostic tests are ordered when leukemia is suspected:

- *CBC* with differential is done to evaluate cell counts, hemoglobin and hematocrit levels, and the number, distribution, and morphology (size and shape) of WBCs.

TABLE 34–5 Diagnostic Findings by Type of Leukemia

TEST	AML	CML	ALL	CLL
RBC count	Low	Low	Low	Low
Hemoglobin	Low	Low	Low	Low
Hematocrit	Low	Low	Low	Low
Platelet count	Very low	High early, low late	Low	Low
WBC count	Varies	Increased	Varies	Increased
Myeloblasts	Present			
Neutrophils	Decreased	Increased	Decreased	Normal
Lymphocytes		Normal		Increased
Monocytes		Normal/low		
Blasts	Present	Present (crisis)	Present	
Bone Marrow	Hypercellular		Hypercellular	
Myeloblasts	Present			
Lymphoblasts			Present	
Lymphocytes				Present

- *Platelets* are measured to identify possible thrombocytopenia secondary to the leukemia and the risk of bleeding.
- *Bone marrow examination* provides information about cells within the marrow, the type of erythropoiesis, and the maturity of erythropoietic and leukopoietic cells.

Table 34–5 outlines usual diagnostic test results in the various forms of leukemia.

Chemotherapy

Single agent or combination chemotherapy is the treatment of choice for most types of leukemia, with the goal of eradicating leukemic cells and producing remission. Table 34–6 outlines typical chemotherapy regimens for different types of leukemia. Combination chemotherapy reduces drug resistance and toxicity, and interrupts cell growth at various stages of the cell cycle, producing a complementary effect of the drugs used. Cancer treatment with chemotherapy is discussed in detail in Chapter 14 ∞ .

Chemotherapy for leukemia generally is divided into the induction phase and postremission therapy. During *induction*, drug doses are high to eradicate leukemic cells from the bone marrow. These high doses often also damage stem cells and interfere with production of normal blood cells. Circulating mature blood cells are not affected because they are no longer dividing. The degree of bone marrow suppression is influenced by a number of factors, including age, nutritional status, concurrent chronic diseases such as impaired liver or renal function, the drug and drug dose, and prior treatment.

Colony-stimulating factors (CSFs), also called hematopoietic growth factors, often are administered to "rescue" the bone marrow following induction chemotherapy. CSFs are cytokines that regulate the growth and differentiation of blood cells. Factors that support neutrophil maturation, *granulocyte-macrophage CSF (GM-CSF)* and *granulocyte CSF (G-CSF)*, are commonly used. Bone pain is a common side effect of therapy with these agents. Clients also may experience fevers, chills, anorexia, muscle aches, and lethargy (Kasper et al., 2005).

Once remission has been achieved, postremission chemotherapy is continued to eradicate any additional leukemic cells, prevent relapse, and prolong survival. A single chemotherapeutic agent, combination therapy, or bone marrow transplant may be used for postremission treatment.

Radiation Therapy

Radiation therapy damages cellular DNA. While the cell continues to function, it cannot divide and multiply. Cells that divide rapidly, such as bone marrow and cancer cells (radiosensitive cells), respond quickly to radiation therapy.

TABLE 34–6 Chemotherapeutic Regimens Used to Treat Leukemia

Acute myeloid leukemia	■ Cytarabine (Cytoxan, an alkylating agent), *with* daunorubicin (Cerubidine, an antitumor antibiotic) *or* idarubicin (Idamycin, an antitumor antibiotic)
	■ All-*trans* retinoic acid (ATRA) added for clients with promyelocytic leukemia
Chronic myeloid leukemia	■ Imatinib mesylate (Gleevec), a *bcr/abl* tyrosine kinase (enzyme) inhibitor
	■ Hydroxyurea (a DNA inhibitor) *or* homoharringtonine (HHT, a plant alkaloid) if imatinib not tolerated
Acute lymphocytic leukemia	■ Daunorubicin (Cerubidine, an antitumor antibiotic) *with* vincristine (Oncovin, a plant alkaloid) *with* prednisone *with* asparaginase (Elspar)
Chronic lymphocytic leukemia	■ Fludarabine (Fludara, an antimetabolite) *or* chlorambucil (Chloromycetin, an antitumor antibiotic)
	■ Cyclophosphamide (Cytoxan, an alkylating agent), vincristine, and prednisone
	■ Cyclophosphamide, doxorubicin (Adriamycin, an antitumor antibiotic), vincristine, and prednisone

Although normal cells are affected, they are better able to recover from the damage caused by the radiation than are cancer cells. The types of delivery, effects, and toxicities of radiation are discussed in greater detail in Chapter 14 ∞.

Bone Marrow Transplant

Bone marrow transplant (BMT) is the treatment of choice for some types of leukemia (see Table 34–3). BMT often is used in conjunction with or following chemotherapy or radiation. There are two major categories of BMT: In allogeneic BMT, the bone marrow of a healthy donor is infused into the client with the illness; in autologous BMT, the client is infused with his or her own bone marrow.

ALLOGENEIC BMT *Allogeneic BMT* uses bone marrow cells from a donor (often from a sibling with closely matched tissue antigens; closely matched unrelated donors also may be used). Prior to allogeneic BMT, high doses of chemotherapy and/or total body irradiation are used to destroy leukemic cells in the bone marrow. The donor's bone marrow is aspirated (Figure 34–8 ■) and infused through a central venous line into the recipient. Prior to BMT and reestablishment of bone marrow function, the client is critically ill and at significant risk for infection and bleeding due to depletion of WBCs and platelets.

AUTOLOGOUS BMT *Autologous BMT* uses the client's own bone marrow to restore bone marrow function after chemotherapy or radiation. This procedure is often called *bone marrow rescue.* In autologous BMT, about 1 L of bone marrow is aspirated (usually from the iliac crests) during a period of disease remission. The bone marrow is then frozen and stored for use after treatment. If relapse occurs, lethal doses of chemotherapy or radiation are given to destroy the immune system and malignant cells, and to prepare space in the bone marrow for new cells. The filtered bone marrow is then thawed and infused intravenously through a central line. The infused marrow cells slowly become a part of the client's bone marrow, the neutrophil count increases, and normal hematopoiesis takes place.

As in allogeneic BMT, the client is critically ill during the period of bone marrow destruction and immunosuppression. The client is hospitalized in a private room for 6 to 8 weeks or more. Potential complications include malnutrition, infection, and bleeding.

Stem Cell Transplant

Allogeneic **stem cell transplant (SCT)** is an alternative to bone marrow transplant. SCT results in complete and sustained replacement of the recipient's blood cell lines (WBCs, RBCs, and platelets) with cells derived from the donor stem cells.

Donors must have tissue that is closely matched with that of the recipient. Prior to harvesting, hematopoietic growth factors, including G-CSF and GM-CSF, are administered to the donor for 4 to 5 days. This increases the concentration of stem cells in peripheral blood, allowing it to be used for the transplant instead of bone marrow. Peripheral blood is removed and white cells are separated from the plasma, then administered via a large central venous catheter. Large concentrations of stem cells also are present in umbilical cord blood. This may be stored and used in some cases (Kasper et al., 2005).

The recipient undergoes similar treatment prior to SCT as for BMT. The risks for infection and other complications, as well as graft-versus-host disease, are similar.

Graft-Versus-Host Disease

Allogeneic BMT or SCT may precipitate *graft-versus-host disease (GVHD),* which develops in up to 60% of all clients receiving an allogeneic BMT or SCT (Kasper et al., 2005). In GVHD, immune cells of the donated bone marrow identify the recipient's body tissue as foreign. Consequently, T lymphocytes in the donated marrow attack the liver, skin, and GI tract, causing skin rashes progressing to desquamation (loss of skin), diarrhea, GI bleeding, and liver damage. *Acute GVHD* develops within days or weeks of the transplant and is usually marked by a pruritic, maculopapular rash that begins on the palms and soles of the feet, and may extend over the entire body. Vaso-occlusive disease of the liver affects up to 25% of allogeneic bone marrow transplant recipients, with jaundice and elevated liver function tests (Porth, 2005). *Chronic GVHD* develops later, 100 or more days after the transplant, affecting 20% to 50% of clients who survive 6 months or more following allogeneic BMT or SCT (Kasper et al., 2005). It may follow acute GVHD or develop in clients with no prior symptoms. GVHD is treated with antibiotics and steroids; immunosuppressant drugs such as thalidomide and immunotoxin (XomaZyme) may be used if necessary.

Biologic Therapy

Cytokines such as interferons and interleukins are biologic agents that may be used to treat some leukemias. These agents modify the body's response to cancer cells; in some cases they are cytotoxic as well. Interferons are a complex group of messenger pro-

Figure 34–8 ■ Allogeneic bone marrow transplant. Bone marrow from the donor is aspirated, then filtered and infused into the recipient.

Source: Simon Fraser, Photo Researchers, Inc.

teins normally produced in response to antigens such as viruses (see Chapter 12 ∞). They have multiple effects, including moderating immune function and inhibiting abnormal cell proliferation and growth. Interferon alpha may be used to treat some leukemias, particularly CML. Side effects commonly associated with interferon therapy include flulike symptoms, persistent fatigue and lethargy, weight loss, and muscle and joint pain.

Complementary Therapies

Although many complementary and alternative medicine therapies have been purported to treat cancer in general, at this time none have been shown to have sustained benefit in treating leukemia. Clinical trials have demonstrated the efficacy of both

coping skills training (relaxation and imagery) and hypnosis to significantly reduce oral discomfort associated with leukemia and its treatment (Spencer & Jacobs, 2003).

NURSING CARE

For nursing care specific to the client undergoing diagnostic testing for leukemia, see the accompanying Nursing Care Plan.

Health Promotion

Health promotion activities related to leukemia include teaching about leukemia risk factors, particularly those that can be controlled. Discuss the potential dangers of exposure to ionizing

---

NURSING CARE PLAN A Client with Acute Myelocytic Leukemia

Catherine Cole is a 37-year-old secretary who lives with her husband, Ray, and teenage daughter, Amy, in an apartment in a large metropolitan area. About 2 months ago, Mrs. Cole began to tire easily and experience night sweats several times a week. She also noted that she was pale, bruised easily, and was having heavier menstrual periods. Blood tests ordered by her primary care provider are abnormal. She is admitted for a bone marrow biopsy.

ASSESSMENT

Mary Losapio, RN, obtains a nursing history and physical assessment for Mrs. Cole. Mrs. Cole tells her, "I'm so tired, and I have these bruises all over me. I'm so afraid of the results of the bone marrow examination. I don't know what we will do if I have cancer." Mrs. Cole clutches her husband's hand and then begins to cry. Physical assessment data include height, 64 inches (156 cm); weight, 106 lb (48.1 kg); vital signs: T 100°F, P 102, R 22, BP 130/82. Numerous petechiae scattered over trunk and arms; ecchymoses noted on lower right arm and right calf. Oral mucosa is red, with several small ulcerations in buccal areas.

Blood count shows reduced RBCs, hemoglobin, and hematocrit levels. The WBC is high, with myeloblasts seen on differential. The platelet count is very low. A tentative diagnosis of acute myelogenous leukemia is made.

DIAGNOSES

- *Risk for Infection* related to altered WBC production and immune function
- *Ineffective Protection* related to reduced platelet count and risk for bleeding
- *Impaired Oral Mucous Membrane* secondary to anemia and reduced platelets
- *Fatigue* related to anemia
- *Anxiety* related to fear of leukemia diagnosis

EXPECTED OUTCOMES

- Remain free of infection.
- Experience no significant bleeding.
- Have intact oral mucous membranes.
- Manage self-care activities despite fatigue.
- Verbalize decreased anxiety.

PLANNING AND IMPLEMENTATION

- Place in a private room.
- Limit visitors to immediate family for the present.

- Instruct all staff, the family, and client to carefully wash hands. Post a sign over the washbasin in the room as a reminder.
- Record vital signs every 4 hours.
- Avoid invasive procedures unless absolutely necessary.
- Monitor for bleeding every 4 hours, including skin, oral mucosa, abdominal assessment, body fluids, and menstrual pad count.
- Instruct to perform oral hygiene every 2 to 4 hours, using a soft-bristle toothbrush.
- Ask the dietitian to work with Mrs. Cole to identify preferred foods. Instruct to avoid foods that may damage oral mucosa, such as very hot, very cold, or highly acidic or spicy foods.
- Provide for periods of rest alternating with activity.
- Teach about the bone marrow biopsy. Allow time for questions and to verbalize fears.
- Refer to the oncology nurse specialist for further teaching and support.

EVALUATION

The bone marrow biopsy confirms the diagnosis of acute myelogenous leukemia. Mrs. Cole is very upset, but calms as the physician and the oncology nurse discuss treatment plans and the possibility of remission. She decides to have outpatient chemotherapy. During her hospital stay, Mrs. Cole remained free of infection or further bleeding. She tells Ms. Losapio that her mouth feels better, although it is still painful. During routine assessment, Mrs. Cole remarks, "You know, I was so scared when I came here, but I think I am a little less so now. Sometimes not knowing what is wrong is worse than knowing."

CRITICAL THINKING IN THE NURSING PROCESS

1. Describe how alterations in WBCs can increase a person's susceptibility to infection.
2. List sources of potential infection for the hospitalized client.
3. What is the rationale for having the client do her own oral and physical hygiene?
4. Outline a teaching plan for this client and her family for home care to prevent infection.
5. Develop a care plan for Mrs. Cole for the nursing diagnosis *Activity Intolerance*.

See Evaluating Your Response in Appendix C.

radiation and certain chemicals such as benzene. Encourage all clients to avoid smoking cigarettes. Discuss genetic counseling with clients at high risk for having a child with Down syndrome (over age 35).

Assessment

Focused assessment data related to leukemia include:

- *Health history:* Complaints of fatigue, weakness, dyspnea on exertion, frequent infections, sore throat, night sweats, bleeding gums, or nose bleeds; recent weight loss; exposure to ionizing radiation (multiple x-rays, residence near a site of radiation or atomic testing) or chemicals (occupational); prior treatment for cancer; history of an immune disorder.
- *Physical examination:* Skin and mucous membranes for bruising, purpura, petechiae, ulcers or lesions; pallor; vital signs including orthostatic vitals; heart and lung sounds; abdominal examination; stool for occult blood.
- *Diagnostic tests:* Blood count with differential; bone marrow studies.

Nursing Diagnoses and Interventions

When caring for the client with leukemia, the nurse considers the chronic and life-threatening nature of the disease as well as the effects of treatment. See the Nursing Research box below. Priority nursing problems may include *Risk for Infection, Imbalanced Nutrition: Less than Body Requirements, Impaired Oral Mucous Membranes, Ineffective Protection (Bleeding),* and *Anticipatory Grieving.*

Risk for Infection

Changes in white blood cell function impair the immune and inflammatory responses in leukemia, increasing the risk for infection. WBCs may be immature and ineffective or, in some cases, deficient. Chemotherapy or radiation therapy further depresses bone marrow function and increases the risk for infection.

- Promptly report manifestations of infection: fever, chills, throat pain, cough, chest pain, burning on urination, purulent drainage, and itching and burning in vaginal or rectal areas. *Prompt reporting allows timely intervention to prevent overwhelming infection and sepsis.*
- Institute infection protection measures:
  a. Maintain protective isolation as indicated.
  b. Ensure meticulous hand washing among all people in contact with the client.
  c. Assist as needed with appropriate hygiene measures.
  d. Restrict visitors with colds, flu, or infections.
  e. Provide oral hygiene after every meal.
  f. Avoid invasive procedures when possible, including injections, intravenous catheters, catheterizations, and rectal and vaginal procedures. When necessary, use strict aseptic technique for all invasive procedures and monitor carefully for infection.

These precautions minimize exposure to bacterial, viral, and fungal pathogens. Infection is the major cause of death in clients with leukemia. Mucous membranes are especially susceptible to breakdown and infection as a result of tissue damage from chemotherapy or radiation.

NURSING RESEARCH Evidence-Based Practice for Clients with Acute Leukemia and Lymphoma

Clients with acute leukemia and malignant lymphoma experience a number of distressing manifestations of their disease, including malaise and fatigue, fever, night sweats, infections, and possible hemorrhage. Treatments such as radiation therapy and chemotherapy often have numerous adverse effects as well, including anorexia and nausea, stomatitis, lethargy, malaise, and fatigue. In these studies, clients in remission from acute leukemia or malignant lymphoma were surveyed regarding physical problems, their view of help they received and who was of most help during treatment, and the impact of the disease and treatment on their current life (Persson, Hallberg, & Ohlsson, 1997; Persson & Hallberg, 2004).

Clients identified energy loss and nutritional problems as being most troublesome during disease treatment. In general, clients with more physical problems were less satisfied with the nursing care they received, suggesting that nurses were less effective in meeting the needs of the sickest clients. Clients continued to experience reduced psychologic and sexual energy and a significant need for intimate help and counseling during remission. While family relationships improved, work and finances were negatively impacted by their disease.

IMPLICATIONS FOR NURSING

This study points out the need for nurses to actively focus their care on the physical problems experienced during treatment, es-

pecially energy loss and nutritional problems. Overwhelming fatigue interferes with the client's ability to provide self-care, but its effects may not be readily apparent to nurses. The long-term effects of reduced psychologic and sexual energy, as well as continued susceptibility to infections, indicate a need for continued follow-up care, teaching, and possibly referral to counseling services.

CRITICAL THINKING IN CLIENT CARE

1. Explain the physiologic responses to malignancies and cancer treatments that cause fatigue, malaise, and nutritional problems.
2. Clients undergoing treatment for leukemia, malignant lymphoma, and other cancers may have few outward manifestations of their disease or responses to treatment. Discuss how this apparent well-being may affect the nurses' perception of care needs.
3. How may continued problems of fatigue and lack of psychologic and sexual energy affect family relations?
4. Develop a nursing care plan for a client with acute leukemia to address the nursing diagnosis *Ineffective Sexuality Patterns* related to fatigue and lack of energy.

- Monitor vital signs including temperature and oxygen saturation every 4 hours. Report temperature spikes with chilling, tachypnea, tachycardia, restlessness, change in PaO_2, and hypotension. *The inflammatory response may be impaired in leukemia, masking signs of infection until sepsis develops, indicated by manifestations such as those above.*
- Monitor neutrophil levels (measured in cubic millimeters) for relative risk for infection:
  2000 to 2500: no risk
  1000 to 2000: minimal risk
  500 to 1000: moderate risk
  Below 500: severe risk.
  Neutrophils are the first line of defense against infection. As levels decrease, the risk for infection increases.
- Explain infection precautions and restrictions and their rationale; explain that these measures are usually temporary. *Client and family understanding increases compliance and lowers the risk of infection.*

Imbalanced Nutrition: Less than Body Requirements

The client with leukemia may have difficulty meeting nutritional needs due to increased metabolism, fatigue, loss of appetite from radiation, nausea and vomiting from chemotherapy, or painful oral mucous membranes that make chewing and swallowing difficult and/or painful.

- Weigh regularly and evaluate weight loss over time to determine degree of malnutrition. A weight loss of 10% to 20% may indicate malnutrition. *A minimum intake of nutrients is necessary for health and tissue repair; cancer increases metabolic needs over this basal requirement. Weight loss occurs when metabolic requirements are not met. Both the disease process and its treatment can interfere with nutrient intake.*
- Address causative or contributing factors to inadequate food and fluid intake.
  a. Provide mouth care before and after meals; use a soft toothbrush or sponges as necessary.
  b. Provide liquids with different textures and tastes.
  c. Increase liquid intake with meals.
  d. Reduce intake of milk and milk products, which makes mucus more tenacious.
  e. Assist to a sitting position for eating.
  f. Ensure that the environment is clean and odor free.
  g. Provide medications for pain or nausea 30 minutes before meals, if prescribed.
  h. Provide rest periods before meals.
  i. Offer small, frequent meals including low-fat, high-kilocalorie foods throughout the day.
  j. Provide commercial supplements, such as Ensure.
  k. Avoid painful or unpleasant procedures immediately before or after meals.
  l. Suggest measures to improve food tolerance, such as eating dry foods when arising, consuming salty foods if allowed, and avoiding very sweet, rich, or greasy foods.

Anorexia, nausea and vomiting, diarrhea, stomatitis, taste changes, and dysphagia often make eating difficult during cancer treatment when good nutrition is most important.

Maintaining nutritional status decreases morbidity and mortality by preventing weight loss, improving the response to treatment, minimizing adverse effects, and improving quality of life. Small, frequent meals are often better tolerated, especially high-protein, high-kilocalarie foods.

Impaired Oral Mucous Membrane

Stomatitis, inflammation and ulceration of the oral mucous membrane, is common in leukemia. Chemotherapy can further impair the integrity of constantly dividing oral tissues.

- Inspect the buccal region, gums, sublingual area, and the throat daily for swelling or lesions. Ask about oral pain or burning. *Breakdown of the oral mucous membrane increases the risk of infection and bleeding, causes pain and discomfort with eating and swallowing, and may cause swelling that interferes with the airway.*
- Culture any oral lesions. *Herpes simplex virus and* Candida *(yeast) are more common in clients with neutropenia. Herpes lesions are usually red, raised, fluid-filled blisters;* Candida *causes a white coating and patches of white plaque.*
- Assist with mouth care and oral rinses with saline or a solution of hydrogen peroxide and water (1:1 or 1:3 hydrogen peroxide and water) every 2 to 4 hours. Apply petroleum jelly to the lips to prevent dryness and cracking. *These measures help prevent infection and increase comfort.*
- Encourage use of soft-bristle toothbrush or sponge to clean teeth and gums. *Toothbrushes with hard bristles may abrade inflamed mucosa, causing bleeding and increasing the risk of infection.*
- Administer medications as ordered to treat infection or relieve pain. *Topical antifungal agents such as nystatin may be prescribed to treat* Candida *infections. Topical anesthetics such as lidocaine may be prescribed to relieve comfort and facilitate good oral care.*
- Instruct to avoid alcohol-based mouthwashes, citrus fruit juices, spicy foods, very hot or very cold foods, alcohol, and crusty foods. Suggest bland, cool foods and cool liquids at least every 2 hours. *Avoiding mucosa-traumatizing foods and liquids increases comfort; bland, cool foods and liquids cause the least pain. Intake of adequate fluids is necessary to prevent dehydration.*

Ineffective Protection

Bleeding is the second most common cause of leukemia deaths. As platelet counts decrease, the risk of bleeding increases (see the section later in this chapter on thrombocytopenia). Tumor lysis syndrome also is a risk in clients with leukemia who are undergoing their initial treatment with chemotherapy. Tumor lysis syndrome develops when a large number of malignant cells are destroyed by treatment with chemotherapy or radiation. The resultant by-products of cell lysis can overwhelm the body's ability to effectively eliminate them, leading to hyperkalemia, hyperphosphatemia with secondary hypocalcemia, and hyperuricemia (Cantril & Haylock, 2004).

- Assess vital signs every 4 hours and body systems every shift for bleeding:
  a. Skin and mucous membranes for petechiae, ecchymoses, and purpura

b. Gums, nasal membranes, and conjunctiva for bleeding
c. Vomitus, stool, and urine for visible or occult blood
d. Vaginal bleeding
e. Prolonged bleeding from puncture sites
f. Neurologic changes such as headache, visual changes, altered mentation, decreased level of consciousness, seizures
g. Abdomen for complaints of epigastric pain, diminished bowel sounds, increasing abdominal girth, rigidity or guarding.

Early identification of bleeding helps prevent significant blood loss and potential shock. Internal hemorrhage may lead to tachycardia, hypotension, pallor, and diaphoresis. Bleeding into the lungs may cause dyspnea; bleeding into the abdomen causes increased girth, pain, and guarding. Intracranial bleeding affects mental status and level of consciousness.

- Avoid invasive procedures such as rectal temperatures and suppositories, vaginal douches, suppositories, tampons, urinary catheterization, and parenteral injections if possible. Diagnostic procedures such as biopsy or lumbar puncture should not be done if the platelet count is less than 50,000. *Invasive procedures can cause tissue trauma and bleeding. Procedures that use large-bore needles should be delayed until the platelet count is increased.*
- Apply pressure to injection sites for 3 to 5 minutes, and to arterial punctures for 15 to 20 minutes. *Pressure prevents prolonged bleeding by prompting hemostasis and clot formation.*
- Instruct to avoid forcefully blowing or picking the nose, forceful coughing or sneezing, and straining to have a bowel movement. *These activities can damage mucous membranes, increasing the risk for bleeding.*
- Monitor and promptly report abnormal blood levels of electrolytes, uric acid, urea nitrogen, and creatinine, or manifestations of tumor lysis syndrome. *Significant alterations in electrolyte levels can lead to complications such as cardiac dysrhythmias, muscle weakness or tetany, paresthesias, and mental status changes. Excess uric acid can compromise renal function, and lead to metabolic acidosis and gout.*
- Maintain adequate hydration and administer prescribed medications such as allopurinol and diuretics as ordered. *Hydration is vital to maintain renal function and promote elimination of tumor lysis by-products. Allopurinol reduces the risk of uric acid crystallization in the kidneys and other tissues* (Cantril & Haylock, 2004).

Anticipatory Grieving

The diagnosis of cancer and a potentially life-threatening illness causes actual or perceived losses, such as loss of function, independence, normal appearance, friends, self-esteem, and self. Grieving is the emotional response to those losses. The adaptive process of mourning a loss and resolving grief is called grief work; grief work cannot begin until a loss is acknowledged. See Chapter 5 ∞ for a detailed discussion of grief and loss.

- Discuss roles of the client and family and ways in which they managed stressful situations in the past. Assess coping strategies and their effectiveness. Help identify sources of strength and support. Discuss changing roles resulting from leukemia diagnosis, and its effect on spiritual, social, and

economic status and usual lifestyle. Evaluate cultural or ethnic factors that affect grief reactions. *Grieving is a normal response to a real or potential loss that begins at the time of diagnosis. The timing, duration, and intensity of grief and responses to grief may differ among family members. Share information on diagnosis, role change, and physical loss among all family members to build the foundation for mutual understanding and trust.*

- Use therapeutic communication skills to facilitate open discussion of losses and provide permission to grieve. *Encouraging discussion of the meaning of the loss helps decrease some of the anxiety associated with loss. This in turn allows the client and family to examine the current situation and compare it with past situations that they have coped with successfully.*
- Provide information about agencies that may help in resolving grief, and make referrals as indicated. Consider self-help groups, cancer support groups, and bereavement groups. *Participating in support groups with others who are anticipating or experiencing a similar loss can decrease feelings of isolation.*

Linking NANDA, NIC, and NOC

Chart 34–2 shows links between NANDA nursing diagnoses, NIC, and NOC for the client with leukemia.

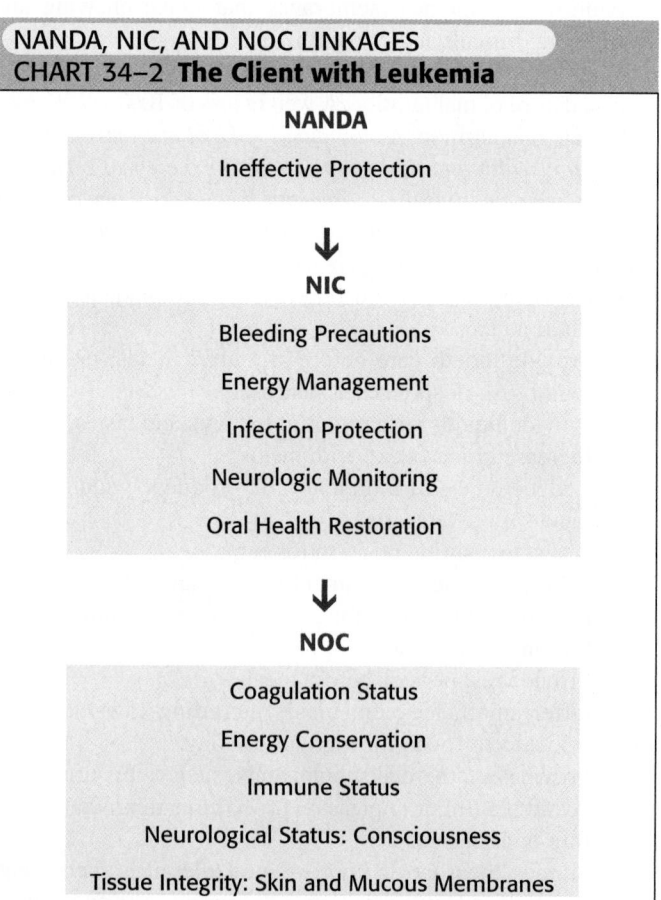

NANDA, NIC, AND NOC LINKAGES
CHART 34–2 The Client with Leukemia

NANDA

Ineffective Protection

↓

NIC

Bleeding Precautions

Energy Management

Infection Protection

Neurologic Monitoring

Oral Health Restoration

↓

NOC

Coagulation Status

Energy Conservation

Immune Status

Neurological Status: Consciousness

Tissue Integrity: Skin and Mucous Membranes

Data from *NANDA's Nursing Diagnoses: Definitions & Classification 2005–2006* by NANDA International (2005), Philadelphia; *Nursing Interventions Classification (NIC)* (4th ed.) by J. M. Dochterman & G. M. Bulechek (2004), St. Louis, MO: Mosby; and *Nursing Outcomes Classification (NOC)* (3rd ed.) by S. Moorhead, M. Johnson, and M. Mass (2004), St. Louis, MO: Mosby.

Community-Based Care

Client and family teaching for home care after treatment for leukemia focuses on encouraging self-care, providing information about the disease and the treatment, preventing infection and injury, and promoting nutrition. Teaching topics for each of these areas are as follows.

Encouraging Self-Care

- Hygiene measures and energy conservation during self-care activities
- Oral hygiene including using a soft-bristle toothbrush several times daily; avoiding flossing
- Reporting lesions, bleeding, or signs of infection promptly
- Maintaining a balance of rest and activity.

Information about Leukemia and Treatment

- Bone marrow function, the pathophysiology of leukemia, and potential complications of leukemia
- Prognosis for the specific type of leukemia
- Treatment measures such as chemotherapy, radiation, bone marrow or stem cell transplant, their purpose and effects, where treatment is available, and potential adverse effects or risks
- Community, regional, and national resources for people with leukemia.

Preventing Infection and Injury

- Hand washing and other measures to reduce exposure to pathogens such as avoiding people who are ill and avoiding crowds
- Avoiding foodborne illnesses by washing fruits and vegetables, proper food storage
- Dental hygiene measures
- Avoiding immunizations
- Manifestations to report: fever, chills, burning on urination, foul-smelling urine, vaginal or rectal discharge, skin lesions
- Avoiding contact sports or strenuous exercise if platelet count is low
- Using an electric razor for shaving, avoiding rectal or vaginal suppositories, vaginal tampons, or enemas
- Increasing dietary fiber and using a bulk-forming laxative as needed to prevent straining
- Avoiding over-the-counter or prescription drugs that interfere with platelet function (see Box 34–6 on page 1140)
- The importance of reporting any bleeding (nosebleeds, rectal bleeding, vomiting blood, excessive menstrual periods, blood in the urine, bleeding gums, bruises, or collections of blood under the skin) or changes in behavior to the healthcare provider.

Promoting Nutrition

- Eating several small, low-fat, high-calorie meals and drinking five to eight glasses of water daily
- Reporting continued weight loss, loss of appetite, or inability to eat for 24 hours
- Discussing dietary needs with the dietitian.

Assistance with physical care, finances, and transportation may be required following discharge. Refer the client and family to social services, support groups, home care services as needed, and other agencies that can provide needed services (such as local chapters of the American Cancer Society, which can provide hospital beds and transportation for outpatient cancer treatment).

THE CLIENT WITH MALIGNANT LYMPHOMA

Lymphomas are malignancies of lymphoid tissue. They are characterized by the proliferation of lymphocytes, histiocytes (resident monocytes or macrophages), and their precursors or derivatives. Lymphomas are closely related to lymphocytic leukemias. Some experts consider them to be different forms or stages of the same disease processes.

Although there are many types of malignant lymphoid cells, at this time lymphomas commonly are identified as Hodgkin's disease or non-Hodgkin's lymphoma.

Incidence and Risk Factors

Malignant lymphomas are the seventh leading cause of cancer deaths in the United States. Approximately 63,740 new cases of lymphoma were diagnosed in 2005, and 20,600 deaths were attributed to the disease. The incidence of non-Hodgkin's lymphoma has nearly doubled since 1970, but currently has stabilized, primarily due to a fall in its incidence related to HIV infection and AIDS. The incidence of Hodgkin's disease has significantly declined since 1990 (ACS, 2005).

While the cause of lymphoma is unknown, some risk factors have been identified. See the accompanying Genetics Considerations box for information about identified genetic links for lymphoma development. Immunosuppression due to drug therapy following organ transplant or to HIV disease increases the risk for non-Hodgkin's lymphoma. Infectious agents such as HTLV-1 and EBV also have been identified as risk factors. Others may include occupational herbicide or chemical exposure (ACS, 2005).

Pathophysiology

Hodgkin's Disease

Hodgkin's disease is a lymphatic cancer, occurring most often in people between the ages of 15 and 35 or over age 50. It is somewhat more common in men than women. Approximately

---

GENETIC CONSIDERATIONS
Focus on Lymphoma

Although specific genetic alterations have not been identified for all types of lymphoma, recurring genetic abnormalities associated with lymphomas point to a genetic link in disease development. Three distinct genetic abnormalities have been identified in non-Hodgkin's lymphomas: gross chromosomal changes such as translocations, rearrangements of specific genes, and altered expression of specific oncogenes (overexpression, underexpression, or mutation). Consistent genetic changes are associated with some lymphomas; in other cases, several genetic abnormalities may be seen. Hodgkin's disease is unique from other lymphomas in that no specific genetic abnormalities have been identified (Kasper et al., 2005). For more information about genetics and disease, see Chapter 8 ∞ .

7350 new cases of Hodgkin's disease were diagnosed in 2005 (ACS, 2005). The exact cause of Hodgkin's disease is unknown, but both Epstein-Barr virus (EBV) infection and genetic factors appear to play a role in its development. Hodgkin's disease is one of the most curable cancers. As many as 60% to 90% of people with localized disease achieve cure with a normal life span (Porth, 2005).

Hodgkin's disease develops in a single lymph node or chain of nodes, spreading to adjoining nodes. Involved lymph nodes contain *Reed-Sternberg cells* (malignant cells) surrounded by host inflammatory cells. These malignant cells secrete inflammatory mediator substances, attracting inflammatory cells to the tumor site. They may invade almost any tissue in the body. The spleen often is involved; as the disease progresses, the liver, lungs, digestive tract, and CNS may be affected (Porth, 2005). Rapid proliferation of abnormal lymphocytes impairs the immune response, especially cell-mediated immune responses. Infections are common.

Hodgkin's disease is classified as classic Hodgkin's disease or as nodular lymphocyte-predominant Hodgkin's disease. The classic form of the disease accounts for 95% of all cases; nodular lymphocyte-predominant Hodgkin's is rare. Classic Hodgkin's can be further divided into four subtypes by cells identified within the tumor, but the subtype does not affect the prognosis (Copstead & Banasik, 2005; Kasper et al., 2005).

MANIFESTATIONS The most common symptom of Hodgkin's disease is one or more painlessly enlarged lymph nodes, usually in the cervical or subclavicular region. Systemic manifestations such as persistent fever, night sweats, fatigue, and weight loss are associated with a poorer prognosis for the disease. Late symptoms such as malaise, pruritus, and anemia indicate spread of the disease (Porth, 2005). The spleen may be enlarged, and other organ systems such as the lungs and gastrointestinal tract are occasionally involved.

Non-Hodgkin's Lymphoma

Non-Hodgkin's lymphoma is a diverse group of lymphoid tissue malignancies that do not contain Reed-Sternberg cells. Non-Hodgkin's lymphomas tend to arise in peripheral lymph nodes and spread early to tissues throughout the body. Non-Hodgkin's lymphoma is more common than Hodgkin's disease, affecting an estimated 56,390 people annually and causing about 19,200 deaths in 2005 (ACS, 2005). Older adults are more often affected, and it occurs more frequently in men than in women. Like Hodgkin's disease, its cause is unknown, although both genetic and environmental factors (e.g., viral infections such as EBV, human T-cell leukemia/lymphoma virus-1 [HTLV-1] and HTLV-2, and HIV) are thought to play a role.

As in most malignancies, non-Hodgkin's lymphoma begins as a single transformed cell; it may arise from T cells, B cells, or tissue macrophages (histocytes). The primary types of non-Hodgkin's lymphoma are identified in Table 34-7. Although non-Hodgkin's lymphoma usually arises in a lymph node, it can originate in any lymphoid tissue. It tends to spread early and unpredictably to other lymphoid tissues and organs. Extra-

TABLE 34-7 Subtypes of Non-Hodgkin's Lymphoma

SUBTYPE	INCIDENCE	COURSE AND PROGNOSIS
B-Cell Lymphomas		
Diffuse large B-cell lymphomas	Most common adult type (40%–50% of adult lymphomas) More common in males Incidence increases with aging	Aggressive tumor 45%–50% cure rate
Follicular lymphoma	Accounts for 40% of adult lymphomas, rare in children Incidence increases with aging	Bone marrow frequently involved Course slow, indolent; 72% 5-year survival
Extranodal marginal zone lymphoma (MALT lymphoma)	Accounts for about 5% of adult lymphomas, rare in children Incidence increases with aging More common in Italy	Presents with tumors outside lymphatic system: GI tract, lung, thyroid, urinary tract, skin, CNS Slow, indolent course; 74% 5-year survival
Mantle cell lymphoma	Accounts for 3% to 4% of adult lymphomas, rare in children Predominantly affects older men (74%)	Aggressive, difficult to cure 27% 5-year survival
Burkitt lymphoma	Rare in adults (<1% of lymphomas), more common in children (~30% NHL)	Rapidly progressive but responds well to therapy 45% 5-year survival
T-Cell Lymphomas		
Precursor T-cell lymphoblastic leukemia/lymphoma	More common in children and young adults More common in males than females	Can present either as ALL or lymphoma Aggressive disease; 26% 5-year survival
Peripheral T-cell lymphoma	Most common T-cell lymphoma in adults	Often presents as disseminated disease 25% 5-year survival
Mycosis fungoides/cutaneous T-cell lymphoma	Onset typically during mid-50s; more common in African Americans	Cutaneous lymphoma Slow course, progressing from patchy skin lesions to plaque to cutaneous tumors

nodal spread may involve the nasopharynx, gastrointestinal tract, bone, CNS, thyroid, testes, and soft tissue.

The prognosis for non-Hodgkin's lymphoma ranges from excellent to poor, depending on the identified cell type and grade of differentiation. Low-grade tumors (better differentiated) tend to be less aggressive and more curable. Higher grade tumors often are disseminated at the time of diagnoses, and have a poorer prognosis (Copstead & Banasik, 2005).

MANIFESTATIONS The early manifestations of non-Hodgkin's lymphoma are similar to those for Hodgkin's disease. Painless lymphadenopathy may be localized or widespread (Figure 34–9). Systemic manifestations such as fever, night sweats, fatigue, and weight loss may be present, but are less common in non-Hodgkin's lymphoma. Organ system involvement may cause symptoms such as abdominal pain, nausea, and vomiting. Headaches, peripheral or cranial nerve symptoms, altered mental status, or seizures may signal CNS involvement.

The manifestations and clinical features of Hodgkin's disease and non-Hodgkin's lymphoma are compared in Table 34–8.

Course

In both Hodgkin's disease and non-Hodgkin's lymphoma, the stage of the disease, the presence of systemic manifestations, and factors such as age help determine the prognosis. The prognosis is good when the disease is localized to one or two node regions. Factors such as anemia, thrombocytopenia, and older age reduce the likelihood of disease cure.

INTERDISCIPLINARY CARE

Chemotherapy and radiation therapy, either alone or in combination, are the primary treatments for Hodgkin's and non-Hodgkin's lymphomas. Use of monoclonal antibodies to target lymphoma cells, and bone marrow and peripheral stem cell transplants are under investigation for treating lymphomas as well. See the previous section on treatment of leukemia for more information about these transplants.

Diagnosis

The following diagnostic tests may be ordered for lymphomas:
- *CBC* often shows a mild normochromic, normocytic anemia in Hodgkin's disease; other findings in Hodgkin's disease

Figure 34–9 ■ Cervical lymphadenopathy in a client with lymphoma of the neck.
Source: Centers for Disease Control and Prevention (CDC)

may include leukocytosis with high neutrophil and eosinophil counts, and an elevated erythrocyte sedimentation rate (ESR). In non-Hodgkin's lymphoma, the CBC typically remains normal until late in the disease, when pancytopenia may develop.
- An ESR is done to identify possible inflammatory causes of lymph node enlargement.
- *Chemistry studies* of major organ function (including liver function tests and renal function studies) are performed to identify possible organ involvement. *Serum LDH levels* and *protein electrophoresis* also may be done when Hodgkin's disease is suspected.
- *Chest x-ray* is done to identify possible enlarged mediastinal lymph nodes and pulmonary involvement.
- *CT scans* of the chest, abdomen, and pelvis are performed to identify abnormal or enlarged nodes.
- *Positron emission tomography (PET or gallium scans)* may be performed in diagnosing the disease, as well as to evaluate the effectiveness of treatment.
- *Biopsy* of the largest, most central enlarged lymph node and of the bone marrow is done to establish the diagnosis for both

---

TABLE 34–8 Features and Manifestations of Hodgkin's Disease and Non-Hodgkin's Lymphoma

FEATURE OR MANIFESTATION	HODGKIN'S DISEASE	NON-HODGKIN'S LYMPHOMA
Lymphadenopathy	Localized to a single node or chain, often cervical, subclavicular, or mediastinal	Multiple peripheral nodes, nodes of the mesentery often involved
Spread	Orderly and continuous	Diffuse and unpredictable
Extranodal involvement	Rare	Early and common
Bone marrow involvement	Uncommon	Common
Fever, night sweats, weight loss	Common	Uncommon until disease is extensive
Other manifestations	Fatigue, pruritus, splenomegaly; anemia, neutrophilia	Abdominal pain, nausea, vomiting; dyspnea, cough; CNS symptoms; lymphocytopenia

Hodgkin's disease and non-Hodgkin's lymphoma. The presence of Reed-Sternberg cells confirms the diagnosis of Hodgkin's disease.

Staging

Staging is used to determine the extent of the disease and appropriate treatment. The Ann Arbor Staging System is used to assess the extent and severity of lymphomas. The stages are:

Stage I: involvement of a single lymph node region or lymphoid structure (e.g., spleen, thymus, lymphoid tonsillar tissue)

Stage II: involvement of two or more lymph node regions on the same side of the diaphragm

Stage III: involvement of lymph node regions or structures on both sides of the diaphragm

■ III₁: limited to upper abdomen (spleen, splenic, celiac, or portal nodes)

■ III₂: involvement of lower abdominal nodes (para-aortic, iliac, or mesenteric)

Stage IV: involvement of an extranodal site (not proximal or contiguous with an involved node) such as the liver, lung or pleura, bone or bone marrow, or skin.

The presence or absence of systemic symptoms is indicated by either an A (no systemic symptoms) or B (systemic symptoms of fever, night sweats, weight loss).

Chemotherapy

Combination chemotherapy is used to treat both Hodgkin's disease and non-Hodgkin's lymphoma. In both cases, chemotherapy often is followed by radiation therapy to involved lymph node regions. The choice of drug combination depends on the stage of the disease as well as the client's age and general condition. Combination regimens used in the United States include CHOP (cyclophosphamide, doxorubicin, vincristine, and prednisone); ABVD (doxorubicin, bleomycin, vinblastine, and dacarbazine); MOPP (nitrogen mustard, vincristine, procarbazine, and prednisone); and ChlVPP (chlorambucil, vinblastine, procarbazine, and prednisone). These regimens also may be combined in alternating months to reduce the adverse effects and improve tumor cell kill. More than 75% of clients with Hodgkin's disease who do not have systemic symptoms achieve complete remission with treatment. The prognosis for clients with non-Hodgkin's lymphoma varies by the type and stage of the disease. For more information about nursing care of the client receiving combination chemotherapy, see Chapter 14 ∞.

Radiation Therapy

Radiation therapy may be the primary treatment for early-stage Hodgkin's disease, although early chemotherapy is becoming more common. In later stages and in non-Hodgkin's lymphoma it usually is combined with chemotherapy. Many lymphomas are highly responsive to radiation. The involved lymph node region is treated, with careful shielding to protect unaffected areas and minimize the extent of radiation burn and normal cell destruction (Figure 34–10 ■). If the disease is advanced, total nodal irradiation may be done. See Chapter 14 ∞ for nursing care of the client receiving radiation therapy.

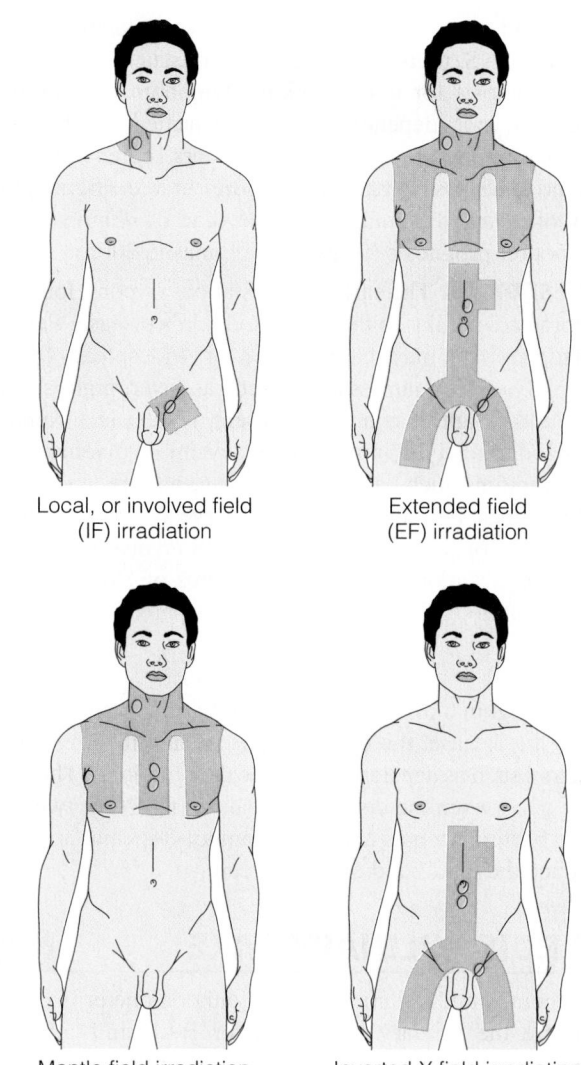

Local, or involved field (IF) irradiation

Extended field (EF) irradiation

Mantle field irradiation

Inverted-Y field irradiation

Figure 34–10 ■ Patterns of radiation therapy used to treat lymphoma based on the location and extent of the disease.

Stem Cell Transplant

Autologous peripheral blood stem cell transplant (PBSCT) is a treatment option for clients who experience remission of malignant lymphoma. Autologous PBSCT uses the client's own stem cells to restore bone marrow function after chemotherapy or radiation. In autologous PBSCT, stem cells are obtained from peripheral blood following chemotherapy and treatment with colony-stimulating factors to promote development of normal blood cells. The blood containing these normal stem cells is then frozen and stored for use after treatment. If relapse occurs, lethal doses of chemotherapy or radiation are given to destroy the immune system and malignant cells. The blood is then thawed and infused intravenously through a peripheral line. The infused stem cells become a part of the client's bone marrow and normal hematopoiesis takes place.

The client is critically ill during the period of bone marrow destruction and immunosuppression. The client is hospitalized in a private room for 6 to 8 weeks or more. See the accompanying nursing research box for discussion of fatigue related to autologous PBSCT.

NURSING RESEARCH   Evidence-Based Practice: Client Undergoing Stem Cell Transplant

Fatigue and depression are common adverse effects of chemotherapy and radiation therapy in clients undergoing cancer treatment. Fatigue is prevalent, affecting 80% to 100% of people undergoing standard chemotherapy and often leading to lost work time and difficulty maintaining functional roles within the family and society. A study by El-Banna and colleagues (2004) sought to describe patterns of fatigue and depression and their relationship to one another among clients undergoing autologous PBSCT. Three time periods during therapy were selected for evaluation: prior to the initiation of chemotherapy, during chemotherapy just prior to transplant, and following the transplant. The setting for this study allowed transplant clients to reside in a hotel-like suite with a designated caregiver (family member or friend).

This study revealed that, among study participants, total fatigue and all its identified dimensions (behavioral, cognitive/mood, sensory, and affective) increased sharply at the time of the transplant, peaking at 7 days post-transplant. Depression followed the same pattern as fatigue, peaking at post-transplant day 7. Peak depression scores were indicative of major depression using the tool employed in this study.

IMPLICATIONS FOR NURSING

This study suggests that nurses should assess for fatigue and depression in clients following stem cell transplant. Nursing measures to help conserve the client's energy are appropriate to manage fatigue. Early detection and intervention for fatigue may actually reduce the intensity of fatigue at its peak. Nurses can use this information to prepare clients for common symptom patterns following SCT, thus reducing anxiety and concern that their condition may be declining rather than improving after SCT. Additionally, assessment tools to measure fatigue and depression among clients undergoing SCT should be incorporated into nursing care.

CRITICAL THINKING IN CLIENT CARE

1. The average age of participants ($N=27$) in this study was 49 years (range: 19 to 71 years); 56% were male, 44% female. Does this sample reflect the demographic of clients with malignant lymphoma and those undergoing autologous PBSCT? How can information about the sample be used to guide application of study findings to the general population of clients undergoing this treatment? To older adults? To adolescents and young adults?
2. In this study, participants resided in a hotel-like setting with a family member or friend who participated in care. How might you expect the results to differ had the clients been unable to closely interact with a caregiver of their own choosing?
3. Can the results of this study be applied when caring for clients undergoing allogeneic BMT or SCT? Why or why not?

Complications of Treatment

Both chemotherapy and radiation therapy may have long-term effects. Permanent sterility is common, especially in older adults. Bone marrow depression can lead to immunosuppression, anemia, and bleeding. Secondary cancers and cardiac injury are the most serious late adverse effects of treatment. Chemotherapy regimens using the MOPP or a related protocol carry a risk of acute leukemia. Cancers such as breast or lung cancer may develop 10 or more years after thoracic radiation. Thoracic radiation also increases the risk for coronary heart disease and hypothyroidism (Kasper et al., 2005).

NURSING CARE

Assessment and priority nursing care for the client with lymphoma follows. See also the Nursing Care Plan at the end of this section for application of nursing care strategies for a specific client with Hodgkin's disease.

Assessment

Focused assessment of the client with Hodgkin's disease or non-Hodgkin's lymphoma includes:

- *Health history:* Complaints of enlarged lymph node(s), fever, night sweats, weight loss, fatigue or general malaise, abdominal pain, respiratory symptoms, numbness or tingling of extremities, visual changes, or changes in mentation; history of infectious mononucleosis, HIV disease, or other immunosuppressive disorders.
- *Physical examination:* Mental status exam; inspect and palpate lymph nodes (cervical, subclavicular, axillary, and inguinal) for enlargement, tenderness; heart and lung sounds; abdominal examination for tenderness, masses, liver or spleen enlargement.
- *Diagnostic tests:* CBC, hemoglobin and hematocrit, ESR; serum chemistry results; x-ray, scan, and biopsy results.

Nursing Diagnoses and Interventions

Nursing care of the client with malignant lymphoma involves both physical and emotional support during diagnosis and treatment. Common nursing care problems include impaired protection due to bone marrow suppression, fatigue, nausea, and altered body image. See the nursing care section for leukemia for specific nursing interventions for *Ineffective Protection*.

Fatigue

General malaise and fatigue may accompany malignant lymphoma and are side effects of chemotherapy. In addition, the physical and psychologic stress of dealing with a chronic, debilitating disease and its treatment may cause fatigue.

- Inquire about feelings of malaise (a vague feeling of body weakness or discomfort) and fatigue (a pervasive, drained feeling that cannot be eliminated). *Both malaise and fatigue are subjective experiences with physiologic, situational, and psychologic components.*
- Encourage verbalization of feelings about the impact of the disease and fatigue on lifestyle. *Discussion of feelings helps the client clarify values and may assist in identifying priorities.*
- Encourage enjoyable but quiet activities, such as reading, listening to music, or hobbies. *Enjoyable activities help decrease feelings of fatigue. Quiet activities conserve energy while yielding a sense of accomplishment.*

NURSING CARE PLAN   A Client with Hodgkin's Disease

Albin Quito, age 28, is the nurse manager of a thoracic intensive care unit in a large teaching hospital. Lately he has been more tired than usual, often wakes up at night covered with sweat, and just does not feel well. He had thought that his symptoms were due to a viral illness and his busy work schedule. However, yesterday morning Albin noticed a large swollen area on the right side of his neck. He made an appointment with his primary health provider who found a large cervical lymph node. A biopsy of the node and a CT scan of the chest were scheduled.

ASSESSMENT

David Herzog, the nurse in charge of the outpatient clinic, obtains a nursing history and assessment on Mr. Quito. His physical examination is essentially normal, with the exception of the enlarged node, which is not tender to palpation. When Mr. Quito is weighed, he tells Mr. Herzog that he has lost 7 lb (3.2 kg) in the past 2 months. In reviewing the results of the blood studies, Mr. Herzog notes mild anemia and an increased neutrophil count. The lymph node biopsy shows Reed-Sternberg cells. The clinic physician and Mr. Herzog tell Mr. Quito that the findings indicate stage 1-B Hodgkin's disease but that the prognosis is very good. The physician recommends a short course of combination chemotherapy followed by radiation therapy to involved sites.

DIAGNOSES

- *Anxiety* related to the diagnosis of Hodgkin's disease and effects of treatment on job performance
- *Risk for Infection* related to potential bone marrow depression due to chemotherapy
- *Fatigue* related to effects of cancer, chemotherapy, and radiation therapy

EXPECTED OUTCOMES

- Verbalize reduced anxiety.
- Remain free of infection.
- Identify and use methods to preserve energy.

PLANNING AND IMPLEMENTATION

- Encourage to consider a leave of absence from work during course of treatment.
- Discuss joining a support group for people with cancer.
- Provide information about the illness, combination chemotherapy, and radiation therapy.
- Reinforce knowledge of actions to decrease the risk of infection.
- Discuss ways to decrease fatigue and maintain energy:
  - Take a 1- to 2-hour nap once or twice a day.
  - Avoid overexertion during weekends and time off.
  - Maintain a well-balanced diet.

EVALUATION

When Mr. Quito returns the following week to begin chemotherapy, he brings his friend Nancy to meet Mr. Herzog and asks him to discuss his treatment with her. Mr. Quito says, "I am still really scared, but being able to talk about this with Nancy will help a lot." Mr. Quito has made arrangements to take a 4-month leave from work, with the understanding that his job will be held for him. He states that he will have some problems with money but is working them out. He also says he feels that taking a nap is silly but that he will rest to maintain his energy level. Mr. Quito and Nancy express confidence that he will be cured and say they plan to be active members of the cancer support group—even after recovery.

CRITICAL THINKING IN THE NURSING PROCESS

1. Discuss the rationale for treating Hodgkin's disease with chemotherapy and radiation.
2. Design a teaching plan to help Mr. Quito prevent infection while he is at home.
3. What effect does the diagnosis of cancer have on the developmental tasks of a young adult?
4. Develop a care plan for Mr. Quito for the nursing diagnosis *Ineffective Role Performance*.

See Evaluating Your Response in Appendix C.

- Encourage to establish priorities and include rest periods or naps when scheduling daily activities. *This provides a sense of control over activities and helps maintain self-esteem. Scheduled rest periods help restore energy and decrease fatigue.*
- Encourage delegation of some responsibilities to family members. *Delegation helps maintain the client's involvement and role in family decisions and responsibilities, while conserving energy for those activities identified as high priority by the client.*
- Identify and encourage the client to use energy-saving equipment. *Performing tasks with less exertion and in less time helps conserve energy.*
- Encourage a diet high in carbohydrates and fluids. *A high-carbohydrate diet helps maintain muscle glycogen stores. A liberal fluid intake promotes excretion of metabolic by-products that may contribute to malaise and fatigue.*

Nausea

The effects of malignant lymphoma and its treatment with chemotherapy and/or radiation therapy can contribute to nausea and interfere with nutritional status. Nausea, a sensation of abdominal fullness, and fear of vomiting often limit food intake. See also the nursing diagnosis *Imbalanced Nutrition* in the section on leukemia for additional interventions.

- Assess precipitating factors for nausea and/or vomiting, the frequency of vomiting, and relief measures used by the client. *Careful assessment allows development of interventions tailored to the client's situation and needs.*

PRACTICE ALERT

Provide ordered antiemetics before chemotherapy is started. Administering prescribed antiemetics before chemotherapy helps prevent nausea and the psychologic association of nausea with chemotherapy.

- Teach measures to prevent or relieve nausea and vomiting.
  a. Eat soda crackers and suck on hard candy.
  b. Eat soft, bland foods that are cold or at room temperature.
  c. Avoid unpleasant odors, and get fresh air.
  d. Eat prior to but not immediately before chemotherapy.

e. Use distraction or progressive muscle relaxation when nauseated.

f. If vomiting occurs, gradually resume oral intake with frequent sips of clear liquids or ice, progressing to bland foods.

Crackers and hard candy often relieve queasiness, whereas hot, spicy, sweet, or strong smelling foods may increase nausea. Alternative nausea relief measures may be effective.

■ Provide small feedings of high-kilocalorie, high-protein foods and fluids. *This increases nutritional intake.*

■ Assist with oral care, general hygiene, and environmental control of temperature, appearance, and odors. *These measures enhance appetite.*

■ Identify and provide preferred foods. *This promotes nutritional intake.*

■ Assist to a sitting position during and immediately after meals. *The sitting position helps decrease early feelings of fullness.*

Disturbed Body Image

The diagnosis of cancer is often devastating to the sense of trust in and the perception of one's body. Radiation and chemotherapy lead to changes in appearance and body function (e.g., hair loss, reduced libido, and infertility), further altering body image. Reactions to this diagnosis vary and may include refusal to look in a mirror or discuss the effects of the disease or treatment, unwillingness to participate in rehabilitation, inappropriate treatment decisions, increasing dependence on others or refusal to provide self-care, hostility, withdrawal, and signs of grieving.

■ Assess perception of body image through subjective information such as:

a. What the client likes most and least about his or her body

b. Preillness perception of people who are sick or have a disability

c. Current understanding of health and limitations imposed by illness or treatment

d. Feelings about the illness and its effect on perception of self and others.

Body image is one's mental idea or picture of the body. It is based on past and present experiences and includes components of one's actual body and emotional responses to that body. Body image changes constantly. There is often a time lag between an actual body change and the changed body image; during this time, the diagnosis, teaching, and treatment may be rejected.

■ Discuss the risk for and measures to cope with alopecia. Suggest wearing wigs, scarves, hats, or caps. Teach proper scalp care using baby shampoo or mild soap, a soft brush, sunscreen, and mineral oil to reduce itching. If eyelashes and eyebrows are lost, teach eye protection, such as wearing eyeglasses and caps with wide brims. *Chemotherapeutic agents attack rapidly dividing cells such as those responsible for hair growth. Hair loss usually begins 1 to 2 weeks after initiation of chemotherapy, with maximum loss 1 to 2 months later. Alopecia may range from thinning to total hair loss. Regrowth depends on the treatment schedule and doses; however, it usually begins 2 to 3 months after treatment ends. New hair may be softer, more curly, and slightly different in color. Teaching and emotional support help the client antic-*

ipate hair loss, discuss its potential effect on body image, and learn self-care techniques.

■ Discuss available resources for financial assistance with purchase of wigs, including local American Cancer Society chapters and insurance plans. *A well-matched wig (or one the color the client has always wished for!) can help maintain a positive body image.*

Sexual Dysfunction

Sexual dysfunction may result from the malignancy and the effects of radiation and chemotherapy. Reproductive tissues are made of rapidly dividing cells, and cancer treatment may cause temporary or permanent sterility, changes in menstruation, and changes in libido.

■ Encourage discussion of actual or potential sexual dysfunction or sterility with the client and significant other. *Clients may be reluctant to discuss this unintended effect of treatment unless encouraged.*

■ Assess knowledge, provide information, and clarify misconceptions. Discuss realistic measures for coping (e.g., sperm banking prior to chemotherapy or radiation therapy). *Clients and their partners may be unclear about expected effects on sexuality, reproduction, and the permanency of these effects.*

■ Refer for counseling as indicated. *Sexual counseling can help the client and partner develop alternative strategies for expressing their sexuality.*

Risk for Impaired Skin Integrity

Malignant lymphomas may cause significant pruritus and drenching night sweats. As a result, skin integrity may be impaired. In addition, radiation therapy can cause superficial burns, which also may affect skin integrity.

■ Frequently assess skin, especially in areas undergoing radiation. *Early identification of lesions allows timely treatment and can prevent further disruption of this important line of defense against infection.*

■ Provide and teach measures to promote comfort and relieve itching: Use cool water and a mild soap to bathe; blot (rather than rub) dry skin; apply plain cornstarch or nonperfumed lotion or powder to the skin unless contraindicated; use lightweight blankets and clothing; maintain adequate humidity and a cool room temperature; wash bedding and clothes in mild detergent, and put them through second rinse cycle. *Pruritus is aggravated by excessive warmth, excessive dryness, rough fabrics, fatigue, and stress. Lotions and some powders may be contraindicated during radiation therapy.*

Linking NANDA, NIC, and NOC

Chart 34–3 shows linkages between nursing diagnoses, nursing interventions, and nursing outcomes for the client with malignant lymphoma.

Community-Based Care

When teaching the client and family for home care, include the following topics in addition to those previously identified for specific nursing diagnoses:

■ Information about the illness, planned treatment, and anticipated side effects of treatment

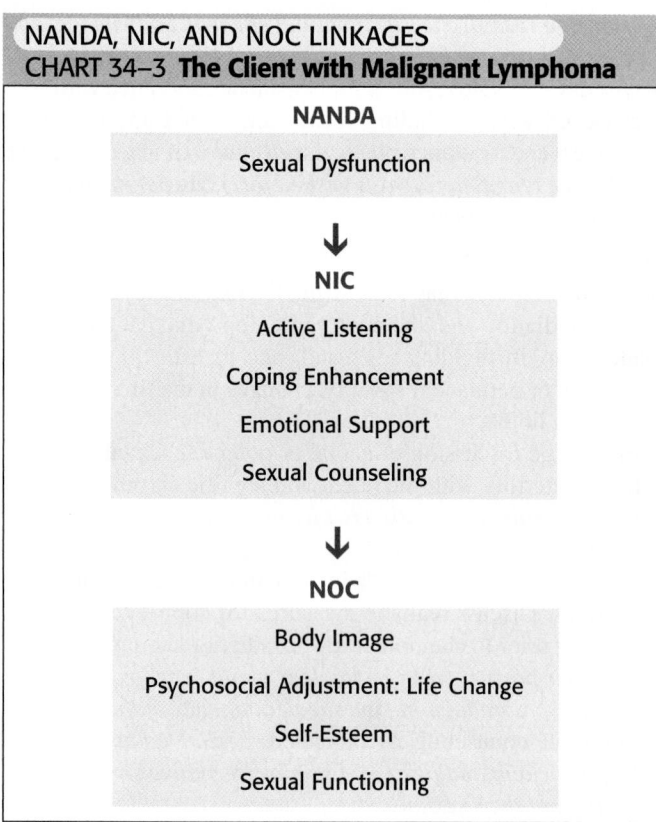

NANDA, NIC, AND NOC LINKAGES
CHART 34-3 The Client with Malignant Lymphoma

NANDA

Sexual Dysfunction

↓

NIC

Active Listening

Coping Enhancement

Emotional Support

Sexual Counseling

↓

NOC

Body Image

Psychosocial Adjustment: Life Change

Self-Esteem

Sexual Functioning

Data from *NANDA's Nursing Diagnoses: Definitions & Classification 2005–2006* by NANDA International (2005), Philadelphia; *Nursing Interventions Classification (NIC)* (4th ed.) by J. M. Dochterman & G. M. Bulechek (2004), St. Louis, MO: Mosby; and *Nursing Outcomes Classification (NOC)* (3rd ed.) by S. Moorhead, M. Johnson, and M. Mass (2004), St. Louis, MO: Mosby.

- Skin care and measures to relieve itching and protect areas of radiation
- Symptoms to report to the physician, including those of vertebral compression (decreased sensation or strength in lower extremities)
- Use of analgesics and alternative relief strategies for abdominal pain and peripheral neuropathies
- Respiratory care if mediastinal nodes are enlarged or lungs or pleurae are involved
- Planning activities of daily living to ensure adequate rest and exercise
- Measures to relieve nausea and maintain adequate nutrition.

Refer clients and family members to the local chapter of the American Cancer Society for information, assistance, and counseling. A list of state and local agencies that offer information about malignant lymphoma and financial assistance can be obtained from the Leukemia Society of America.

THE CLIENT WITH MULTIPLE MYELOMA

Multiple myeloma is a malignancy in which plasma cells multiply uncontrollably and infiltrate the bone marrow, lymph nodes, spleen, and other tissues. *Plasma cells* are B-cell lymphocytes that develop to produce antibodies (immunoglobins).

Incidence and Risk Factors

The incidence of multiple myeloma is increasing slightly, with an estimated 15,980 cases diagnosed and 11,300 deaths due to the disease in 2005 (ACS, 2005). It affects blacks nearly twice as often as whites, and men slightly more frequently than women. The incidence of multiple myeloma increases with age, rarely occurring before age 40 (Kasper et al., 2005). Its cause is unknown. Possible contributing factors include genetic alterations, radiation exposure, oncogenic virus, inflammatory stimuli, and chronic antigenic stimulation. The risk for developing multiple myeloma is higher in people of lower socioeconomic status. This increased risk may relate to environmental factors such as poor housing, occupational hazards, poor nutritional status, and other physical and psychosocial stressors such as exposure to infectious agents (Mangan, 2005).

Pathophysiology

Malignant plasma cells arise from one clone (*monoclonal*) of B cells that produce abnormally large amounts of a particular immunoglobin called the *M protein*. This abnormal protein interferes with normal antibody production and impairs the humoral immune response. It also increases blood viscosity and may damage kidney tubules. As myeloma cells proliferate, they replace the bone marrow and infiltrate the bone itself. Cortical bone is progressively destroyed by tumor growth and enzymes produced by myeloma cells. These enzymes facilitate bone destruction, its infiltration by tumor cells, development of new blood vessels to sustain the tumor, and growth of myeloma cells (McCance & Huether, 2006). Affected bones (primarily the vertebrae, ribs, skull, pelvis, femur, clavicle, and scapula) are weakened and may break without trauma (*pathologic fracture*). With disease progression, malignant cells spread via the bloodstream to invade other organs (Figure 34–11 ■).

Manifestations

The disease develops slowly, with up to 30% of clients diagnosed during evaluation for unrelated problems (Mangan, 2005). Manifestations of multiple myeloma are due to its effects on the bone and the impaired immune response due to M-protein production. Bone pain is the most common presenting symptom. With progression of the disease, the pain may increase in severity and become more localized. Rapid bone destruction releases calcium from the bone, leading to hypercalcemia and manifestations of neurologic dysfunction, such as lethargy, confusion, and weakness.

As functional antibody formation decreases and the humoral immune response is suppressed, recurrent infections develop. Cell-mediated immunity remains intact. *Bence Jones proteins* are found in the urine in multiple myeloma. These proteins are toxic to the renal tubules, and may lead to renal failure with azotemia and uremia. (See Chapter 29 ∞ for more information about renal failure.)

About 15% of clients with multiple myeloma die within 3 months of the diagnosis. More frequently, the disease course is chronic, progressing more rapidly with each relapse after remission. The acute terminal stage of the disease is marked by pancytopenia and widespread organ infiltration by myeloma cells (Kasper et al., 2005).

Figure 34–11 ■ An illustration of the progress of multiple myeloma in an African American male. Abnormal plasma cells proliferate uncontrollably, gradually replacing bone marrow and infiltrating bone itself. As the disease progresses, these cells spread to other organs via the bloodstream.

Source: Kevin A. Somerville, Phototake NYC

INTERDISCIPLINARY CARE

Diagnosis and Staging

Diagnostic tests for multiple myeloma include the following:

- *X-rays* and other radiologic studies of the bone may reveal multiple punched-out lesions.
- *Bone marrow examination* shows an abnormal number of immature plasma cells.
- *CBC* shows moderate to severe anemia, and the *ESR* usually is elevated.
- *Protein electrophoresis* shows a spike of one type of antibody, usually IgG.
- *Serum calcium, creatinine, uric acid,* and *BUN* levels often are elevated.
- *Urinalysis* shows Bence Jones protein in the urine.
- *Biopsy* of myeloma lesions confirms the diagnosis of multiple myeloma.

Staging of multiple myeloma is based on the hemoglobin and serum calcium levels, the amount of abnormal protein present, and the degree of bone involvement.

Treatment

There is no cure for multiple myeloma. In some clients, active observation is indicated, as the disease may continue with a slow, *indolent* (sluggish, not developing or progressing) course for many years (Mangan, 2005). When indicated by disease stage or progression, standard treatment includes induction chemotherapy followed by stem cell transplant and maintenance chemotherapy to control progression of the disease. Supportive care is provided to reduce complications of the disease and their effects.

Combination chemotherapy with an alkylating agent (melphalan [Alkeran], cyclophosphamide [Cytoxan], or chlorambucil [Chloromycetin]) and prednisone administered for 4 to 7 days every 4 to 6 weeks is commonly used. Chemotherapy typically reduces bone pain, hypercalcemia, anemia, and the number of infections (Kasper et al., 2005). Localized radiation therapy may be used to treat painful bone lesions. High-dose chemotherapy followed by peripheral allogeneic stem cell transplant may be more effective in achieving a cure, but is associated with a high mortality rate. When autologous SCT is used, granulocyte colony-stimulating factor is administered prior to harvesting and preserving peripheral stem cells for transplant.

Supportive care may include treatment of hypercalcemia with hydration, possible bisphosphonate therapy to reduce bone loss (see Chapter 42), and calcium, vitamin D, and fluoride supplements to support bone structure. Plasma exchange therapy (plasmapheresis) to remove circulating M proteins is used as needed to treat acute renal failure. Infections are treated promptly when they develop.

NURSING CARE

Assessment

Focused assessment data for the client with multiple myeloma include the following:

- *Health history:* Complaints of back or bone pain, onset, duration, and intensity; complaints of weakness, fatigue, anorexia; history of frequent or recurrent infections; neurologic symptoms such as numbness and tingling or clumsiness.
- *Physical examination:* Level of consciousness and mental status; mobility, gait; localized tenderness or pain, bony crepitus with movement or palpation; movement and sensation in extremities.

Nursing Diagnoses and Interventions

Nursing care of the client with multiple myeloma focuses on problems of chronic pain, impaired mobility, and the risk for injury. Risk for infection is a major nursing care focus; see the previous section on leukemia for specific interventions to reduce this risk. Other nursing care needs are similar to those of clients with other cancers and chronic pain. See Chapters 9 and 14 for additional specific nursing interventions for these problems.

Chronic Pain

Clients with multiple myeloma typically experience chronic back pain and deep bone pain as myeloma cells saturate the bone marrow and invade the bone structure. Pathologic fractures are a common and reoccurring problem.

- Assess pain, including intensity (use a standard pain scale), onset, duration, precipitating factors, and effective relief measures. *Identifying the intensity, causes, and precipitating factors of pain helps determine and evaluate effective pain relief measures.*

- Determine position of greatest comfort, and assist as needed into this position. *The client is best able to identify positions that minimize pain, but may need assistance with repositioning.*
- Support position with pillows. *Bony prominences may be painful due to infiltrates. Pillows can help relieve pressure on these prominences, thus reducing pain.*
- Provide uninterrupted rest periods. *Adequate rest facilitates pain relief and improves pain tolerance.*
- Teach adjunctive pain relief strategies such as relaxation or guided imagery. *A combination of pharmacologic and non-pharmacologic methods provides better management of chronic pain, especially bone pain.*
- Teach effective analgesic use, including the family in instruction. *Analgesics are most effective when taken before pain becomes severe. Clients and their families may be reluctant to use prescription analgesics on a regular basis.*
- Report unrelieved pain to the physician. *A different analgesic or addition of an adjunctive medication such as a nonsteroidal anti-inflammatory drug (NSAID) may be needed to effectively control pain.*

Impaired Physical Mobility

Painful bony infiltrates and pathologic fractures may limit mobility. A brace or splint may be used to protect extremities or support the back. In addition, persistent weakness associated with the cancer and anemia may limit the client's ability to participate in usual activities.

- Assist to change position at least every 2 hours. *Assistance with repositioning is necessary due to weakness. Frequent repositioning improves comfort and reduces the risk for impaired skin and tissue integrity.*

PRACTICE ALERT
Gently support extremities during repositioning. Weakened extremities due to infiltration of bone by myeloma cells and muscle atrophy from lack of use increase the risk for pathologic fractures.

- Provide a trapeze to assist in repositioning. *A trapeze provides better leverage, allowing the client to assist with repositioning and providing a degree of independence. The ability to participate in self-care improves self-esteem.*

Risk for Injury

The bone involvement of multiple myeloma places the client at high risk for pathologic and traumatic fractures. Pathologic fractures can occur with simple activities such as turning or reaching for an item. The spine usually is affected; the ribs and bones of the extremities also may be at risk for fracture.

- Place needed items close at hand. *Straining to reach objects increases the risk of falling or sustaining other injury.*
- Provide safety measures to prevent falls from bed: Place the bed in a low position, use side rails as indicated, and place the call bell within reach. *Safety measures help prevent acci-*

dental injury. *A secure environment minimizes risk and helps prevent falls.*

- Provide shoes with nonskid soles, a clear pathway, adequate lighting, and a level surface free of scatter rugs or other hazards when ambulating. Provide a walker as needed for support and security. *Weight-bearing exercise promotes bone repair. Safety measures, such as an unobstructed pathway and a firm walking surface, help prevent falls.*

Community-Based Care

When teaching clients and their families for home care, include the following topics:

- Strategies for home maintenance management
- Signs and symptoms of complications to be reported to the physician (e.g., symptoms of vertebral and extremity fractures)
- Manifestations of infection to report: fever and chills; increased malaise, fatigue, or weakness; cough with or without sputum; sore throat; dysuria, nocturia, frequency, urgency, or malodorous urine.

Provide referrals for home health and home maintenance services, physical or occupational therapy, social services, and hospice care as appropriate.

THE CLIENT WITH NEUTROPENIA

Leukopenia is a decrease in the total circulating white blood cell count. Although any type of WBC may be affected, neutrophils, which make up the majority of WBCs, are affected most often. *Neutropenia* is a decrease in circulating neutrophils, usually less than 1500 cells/mm³. Neutropenia may be either congenital or acquired, developing secondarily to prolonged infection, hematologic disorders, starvation, or autoimmune disorders (such as rheumatoid arthritis). Chemotherapy and other drugs can suppress the bone marrow. Neutropenia develops in approximately half of clients undergoing chemotherapy to treat cancer (Eggenberger et al., 2004). *Agranulocytosis* is severe neutropenia, with less than 200 cells/µm. Numbers of other granulocytes also are reduced. It is usually due to impaired leukocyte formation in the bone marrow or increased cell destruction in circulating blood. Agranulocytosis significantly increases the risk for infection. *Aplastic anemia* affects production of all blood cells, resulting in anemia, thrombocytopenia, and agranulocytosis.

Pathophysiology and Manifestations

Neutrophils are an integral component of the immune response. They are phagocytes, drawn to and activated by infection and inflammation to engulf and degrade invading microorganisms. Their life span in peripheral blood is short, less than 1 day. When *granulopoiesis* (the development and maturation of granulocytes) in the bone marrow is suppressed, the number of circulating neutrophils falls rapidly. As a result, the body's ability to defend itself against infection is significantly reduced.

The manifestations of neutropenia reflect the resulting impaired immunity and inflammatory response. Opportunistic bacterial, fungal, and protozoal infections develop, commonly affecting the respiratory tract and mucosa of the mouth, GI tract, and vagina. Malaise, chills, and fever with extreme weakness and fatigue are common manifestations.

INTERDISCIPLINARY CARE

The diagnosis of neutropenia is made based on the client's manifestations, risk factors, and the CBC. The total white blood count is low, often less than 1000/mm³.

Hematopoietic growth factors such as GM-CSF are administered to stimulate granulocyte maturation and differentiation. Infections are treated with antibiotic therapy. Protective isolation procedures may be initiated to prevent exposure to pathogens. When neutropenia is related to chemotherapy, cancer treatment often must be halted, at least temporarily, to allow the bone marrow to recover.

NURSING CARE

The primary nursing care focus is early identification of neutropenia and protecting the client from infection. The WBC count is monitored on a regular basis, and any decline reported to the physician. Protective isolation may be indicated, including restricting the number of visitors and people with apparent illness. See *Risk for Infection* in the earlier section on leukemia for specific nursing interventions for the client with neutropenia.

THE CLIENT WITH INFECTIOUS MONONUCLEOSIS

Infectious mononucleosis is characterized by invasion of B cells in the oropharyngeal lymphoid tissues by the Epstein-Barr virus. This disease is usually benign and self-limiting. It often affects young adults between the ages of 15 and 30. Although many children are infected with EBV, symptomatic infectious mononucleosis is uncommon in early childhood. The virus is present in saliva, which appears to be the primary mode of transmission. As a result, infectious mononucleosis is often called the "kissing disease."

EBV also is associated with some cancers, including Burkitt's lymphoma and Hodgkin's disease, B-cell lymphoma, and nasopharyngeal carcinoma (Kasper et al., 2005).

Pathophysiology and Manifestations

When the virus enters the body, unaffected B cells produce antibodies against the virus, and T cells directly attack the virus. Infected B cells are destroyed as the virus replicates. The proliferation of B and T cells, as well as the removal of dead and damaged leukocytes, is responsible for the swelling of lymphoid tissues.

The incubation period for infectious mononucleosis is 4 to 8 weeks. Its onset is insidious, with headache, malaise, and fatigue. Fever, sore throat, and cervical lymphadenopathy (lymph node enlargement and pain) lasting 1 to 3 weeks is common. Symptom severity varies from person to person. Lymph node involvement may be generalized; about 50% of people with infectious mononucleosis develop an enlarged spleen (splenomegaly).

INTERDISCIPLINARY CARE

Laboratory findings include increased lymphocytes and monocytes, with about 20% of the cells atypical in form. Early in the infection, the WBC count usually is normal or low, but by the second week it increases and remains elevated for 4 to 8 weeks. Platelet counts are often low during the illness.

Recovery occurs in 2 to 3 weeks; however, debility and lethargy may last for up to 3 months. The treatment includes bed rest and analgesic agents to alleviate the symptoms. Nursing care is primarily educational to prevent further spread of the disease.

PLATELET AND COAGULATION DISORDERS

Platelet and coagulation disorders affect **hemostasis**, control of bleeding. Hemostasis maintains a relatively steady state of blood volume, blood pressure, and blood flow through injured vessels. Bleeding disorders result from deficient platelets, disruption of the clotting cascade, or a combination of factors

THE CLIENT WITH THROMBOCYTOPENIA

Thrombocytopenia is a platelet count of less than 100,000 per milliliter of blood. It can lead to abnormal bleeding. A continuing decline in circulating platelets to less than 20,000/mL can lead to spontaneous bleeding and hemorrhage from minor trauma (Figure 34–12 ■). Bleeding due to platelet deficiency usually occurs in small vessels, causing manifestations such as *petechiae* and *purpura*. The mucous membranes of the nose, mouth, GI

Figure 34–12 ■ Significant ecchymosis of the eyelid associated with minor trauma in a client with thrombocytopenia.

Source: Scott Camazine, Photo Researchers, Inc.

tract, and vagina often bleed. Serious and potentially fatal bleeding occurs when the platelet count is less than 10,000/mL.

Thrombocytopenia results from one of three mechanisms: decreased production, increased sequestration in the spleen, or accelerated destruction. Primary thrombocytopenia that leads to increased platelet destruction is discussed below. Secondary thrombocytopenia may be caused by aplastic anemia, bone marrow malignancy, infection, radiation therapy, or drug therapy (Box 34–6). Heparin therapy is the most common drug-induced thrombocytopenia; it is included in the discussion that follows. Platelet sequestration usually is due to an enlarged spleen. Up to 80% of platelets may be removed from circulation with significant splenomegaly (Porth, 2005). Finally, thrombocytopenia may result from premature platelet destruction associated with disseminated intravascular coagulation (DIC).

Physiology Review

Effective control of bleeding requires a series of complex interactions between the damaged tissue and blood vessel, platelets, clotting factors, and processes to dissolve clots once bleeding has been controlled (see Figures 33–5, 33–6, and 33–7 ∞). Platelets are formed in the bone marrow under control of thrombopoietin, a protein produced by the liver, kidney, smooth muscle, and bone marrow. Platelets are attracted to the damaged vessel wall, where they aggregate and release mediators that activate the clotting process. See Chapter 33 ∞ for a more complete discussion about platelets, clotting, and hemostasis.

Pathophysiology

The two types of primary thrombocytopenia are immune thrombocytopenic purpura and thrombotic thrombocytopenic purpura.

Immune Thrombocytopenic Purpura

Immune thrombocytopenic purpura (ITP), also known as *idiopathic thrombocytopenic purpura,* is an autoimmune disorder in which platelet destruction is accelerated. In ITP, proteins on the platelet cell membrane stimulate autoantibody production, usually IgG antibodies. These autoantibodies adhere to the platelet membrane. Although the platelets function normally, the spleen reacts to them as being foreign and destroys the altered platelets after only 1 to 3 days of circulation.

MANIFESTATIONS The manifestations of ITP are due to bleeding from small vessels and mucous membranes. Petechiae and purpura develop, often on the anterior chest, arms, neck, and oral mucous membranes. Bruising also may be apparent. As bleeding progresses, epistaxis (nosebleed), hematuria, excess menstrual bleeding, and bleeding gums occur. Spontaneous intracranial bleeding is rare but does occur. Associated symptoms include weight loss, fever, and headache.

INCIDENCE AND COURSE Acute ITP affects people of any age following a viral illness (Copstead & Banasik, 2005). Acute ITP typically lasts only 1 to 2 months, resolving without long-term consequences. In its chronic form, ITP typically affects adults between ages 20 and 50; women are affected more often than men. Its onset is insidious. Chronic (or adult) ITP often occurs in people with other immune-associated disorders such as systemic lupus erythematosus or HIV disease (Copstead & Banasik, 2005).

Thrombotic Thrombocytopenic Purpura

Thrombotic thrombocytopenic purpura (TTP) is a rare disorder in which thrombi occlude arterioles and capillaries of the microcirculation. Many organs are affected, including the heart, kidneys, and brain. The incidence of TTP is increasing (McCance & Huether, 2006). Its cause is unknown. Platelet aggregation is a key feature of the disorder. As RBCs circulate through partially occluded vessels, they fragment, leading to hemolytic anemia (Porth, 2005).

MANIFESTATIONS TTP may be acute, the more common and severe form, or chronic. Acute idiopathic TTP may be fatal within months if untreated. The manifestations of TTP include purpura and petechiae, and neurologic symptoms such as headache, seizures, and altered consciousness.

Heparin-Induced Thrombocytopenia

Heparin-induced thrombocytopenia (HIT) develops as a result of an abnormal response to heparin therapy. Unfractionated heparin carries a greater potential to precipitate HIT; it can, however, develop in clients receiving low-molecular-weight heparin who have previously been treated with unfractionated heparin. See Chapter 35 ∞ for further discussion of heparin therapy and the forms of heparin.

Heparin is a protein that occurs naturally in human tissues and inflammatory cells. It can react directly with platelets, causing them to agglutinate (clump) and be removed from circulation by phagocytosis. This form of HIT, called type I HIT, typically causes mild thrombocytopenia. The more severe form, type II HIT, results from an immune reaction to heparin. In type II HIT, heparin forms an immune complex with a platelet protein known as platelet factor 4 (PF4). This complex acts as a foreign antigen in some clients, stimulating antibody production. The antibody binds with the heparin-PF4 complex, and these antibody-heparin-PF4 complexes subsequently bind with circulating

---

BOX 34–6 Selected Causes of Secondary Thrombocytopenia

Diseases
- Vitamin B$_{12}$ anemia
- Folic acid anemia
- Aplastic anemia
- Leukemia
- Alcoholism
- DIC
- Infectious mononucleosis
- Viral infections
- HIV disease

Drugs
- Thiazide diuretics
- Aspirin
- Ibuprofen
- Indomethacin
- Naproxen
- Sulfonamides
- Phenytoin
- Cimetidine
- Digoxin
- Furosemide
- Heparin
- Morphine

Treatments
- Radiation therapy
- Chemotherapy
- Massive transfusion of stored blood

platelets, causing them to aggregate. As affected platelets aggregate, they are removed from circulation, leading to thrombocytopenia. In addition, small pieces of platelets can break loose, stimulating the clotting cascade and the development of thrombosis (clotting) (Francis & Drexler, 2005). The thrombocytopenia and the thrombosis can be reversed by prompt withdrawal of heparin therapy (Kasper et al., 2005).

MANIFESTATIONS Despite thrombocytopenia, bleeding is usually a manifestation of HIT, probably because of the increased tendency to form clots that deplete clotting factors. The client may develop manifestations of an arterial thrombosis (severe pain, paresthesias, pallor and cool skin temperature, and pulselessness distal to the arterial occlusion) or of venous thrombosis (edema, redness, and warmth of the affected area). On rare occasion, an intravenous bolus of unfractionated heparin can precipitate an acute inflammatory response with manifestations that may mimic an acute pulmonary embolism: fever, chills, hypertension, tachycardia, dyspnea, chest pain, and cardiopulmonary arrest (Francis & Drexler, 2005).

INTERDISCIPLINARY CARE

The diagnosis of thrombocytopenia is based on history, manifestations, and diagnostic test results. Management focuses on treating or removing any causative factors and treating the platelet deficiency.

Diagnosis

The following diagnostic tests are used to identify thrombocytopenia:

- *CBC with platelet count* is done to evaluate blood cell counts, hemoglobin, and hematocrit.
- *Antinuclear antibodies (ANA)* are measured to assess for autoantibodies and identify possible contributing disorders such as systemic lupus erythematosus.
- *Serologic studies* for hepatitis viruses, cytomegalovirus (CMV), EBV, toxoplasma, and HIV may be done. Serologic testing also may be performed when HIT is suspected.
- *Bone marrow examination* evaluates for aplastic anemia and megakaryocyte production.

Medications

Oral glucocorticoids, such as prednisone, are prescribed to suppress the autoimmune response. Many clients who respond to glucocorticoid treatment relapse when the drug is withdrawn, however. Immunosuppressive drugs such as azathioprine, cyclophosphamide, and cyclosporine may be used.

Prompt withdrawal of heparin therapy is vital when HIT is the cause of thrombocytopenia. All sources of heparin are removed, including heparin used to flush intravenous or other catheters and heparin-coated catheters (Francis & Drexler, 2005). A non-heparin anticoagulant such as lepirudin (Refludan) or argatroban may be substituted. Lepirudin is a thrombin inhibitor. It is a recombinant form of hirudin, originally isolated from the salivary glands of leeches. Its primary adverse effect is bleeding; as a protein, it also can stimulate antibody development, resulting in rare instances of anaphylaxis. Argatroban is a synthetic direct thrombin inhibitor with a short half-life. It clears quickly when the in-

fusion is discontinued, an advantage if excessive bleeding develops or invasive procedures must be performed (Rice et al., 2002).

Treatments

Platelet transfusions may be required to treat acute bleeding due to thrombocytopenia. Platelets are prepared from fresh whole blood; one unit contains 30 to 60 mL of platelet concentrate. The expected increase in platelets after one unit is infused is 10,000/mL. *Plasmapheresis,* or *plasma exchange therapy,* is the primary treatment for acute thrombotic thrombocytopenic purpura. The client's plasma is removed and replaced with fresh frozen plasma to remove autoantibodies, immune complexes, and toxins.

Surgery

A *splenectomy* (surgical removal of the spleen) is the treatment of choice if the client with ITP relapses when glucocorticoids are discontinued. The spleen is the site of platelet destruction and antibody production. This surgery often cures the disorder, although relapse may occur years after splenectomy.

 # NURSING CARE

Assessment

- *Health history:* Complaints of bruising with minor or no trauma, bleeding gums, nosebleed, heavy or prolonged menstrual periods, black, tarry, or bloody stools, hematemesis, headache, fever, or neurologic symptoms; recent weight loss; recent viral or other illness; current and recent medications; exposure to toxins; previous exposure to heparin.
- *Physical examination:* Skin and mucous membranes for color, temperature, petechiae, purpura, or bruises; vital signs; weight; mental status and level of consciousness; heart and breath sounds; abdominal exam; body fluids for occult blood.
- *Diagnostic tests:* CBC, hemoglobin and hematocrit, platelet count; serologic and ANA test results; bone marrow examination results.

Nursing Diagnoses and Interventions

Inadequate platelets impair hemostasis, placing the client at risk for bleeding. Bleeding gums, an early sign of the disorder, affects oral mucous membrane integrity as well.

Ineffective Protection

Bleeding is a serious complication associated with thrombocytopenia. As platelet counts (measured in cubic millimeters) decrease, the risk of bleeding increases. The risk is minimal with counts greater than 50,000 mm³; moderate when the count is between 20,000 and 50,000 mm³; and significant when the count falls below 20,000 mm³.

- Monitor vital signs, heart and breath sounds every 4 hours. Frequently assess for other manifestations of bleeding:
  a. Skin and mucous membranes for petechiae, ecchymoses, and hematoma formation
  b. Gums, nasal membranes, and conjunctiva for bleeding
  c. Overt or occult blood in emesis, urine, or stool

d. Vaginal bleeding
e. Prolonged bleeding from puncture sites
f. Neurologic changes: headache, visual changes, altered mental status, decreasing level of consciousness, seizures
g. Abdominal: epigastric pain, absence of bowel sounds, increasing abdominal girth, abdominal guarding or rigidity.

Early identification of bleeding is important to prevent serious blood loss and shock.

> ### PRACTICE ALERT
> Avoid invasive procedures such as rectal temperatures, urinary catheterization, and parenteral injections to the extent possible. Diagnostic procedures such as biopsy or lumbar puncture should be avoided if the platelet count is less than 50,000 mm^3. Invasive procedures can cause tissue trauma and bleeding. Procedures that use large-bore needles should be delayed until the platelet count is increased.

- Apply pressure to puncture sites for 3 to 5 minutes; apply pressure to arterial puncture sites for 15 to 20 minutes. *Pressure promotes hemostasis and clot formation.*
- Instruct to avoid forcefully blowing the nose or picking crusts from the nose, straining to have a bowel movement, and forceful coughing or sneezing. *These activities increase the risk of external and internal bleeding.*

Impaired Oral Mucous Membranes

Thrombocytopenia frequently leads to bleeding of the gums and oral mucosa. As a result, risk for infection and impaired nutrition increases.

- Frequently assess the mouth for bleeding. Inquire about oral pain or tenderness. *Breakdown of oral mucous membranes increases the risk of infection and bleeding, and causes discomfort with eating.*
- Encourage use of a soft-bristle toothbrush or sponge to clean teeth and gums. *Hard bristles may abrade oral mucosa, causing bleeding and increasing the risk of infection.*
- Instruct to rinse the mouth with saline every 2 to 4 hours. Apply petroleum jelly to lips as needed to prevent dryness and cracking. *Saline mouth rinses and petroleum jelly help maintain oral tissue integrity and promote cleansing and healing.*
- Instruct to avoid alcohol-based mouthwashes, very hot foods, alcohol, and crusty foods. Teach to drink cool liquids at least every 2 hours. *Avoiding foods and liquids that traumatize oral mucosa increases comfort; fluid intake prevents dehydration and helps maintain mucous membrane integrity.*

Community-Based Care

In the adult, ITP often is a chronic disorder that the client and family must learn to manage. Secondary thrombocytopenia may be either acute or chronic. Discuss the following topics when preparing the client and family for home care:

- Nature of the disorder, its usual course, and the treatment plan
- Use of and desired and potential adverse effects of prescribed medications
- Risks and benefits of surgery or treatments such as plasma replacement therapy

- The importance of follow-up tests and visits for care
- Measures to reduce the risk of bleeding: safety measures such as a soft-bristle toothbrush, electric razor, avoidance of contact sports and hazardous activities, and avoiding medications that further interfere with platelet function (Box 34–7)

Refer for home health or other community services (e.g., housekeeping, shopping) as indicated.

THE CLIENT WITH HEMOPHILIA

Hemophilia is a group of hereditary clotting factor disorders that lead to persistent and sometimes severe bleeding (see the accompanying Genetic Considerations box). Although often considered a disease of children, hemophilia may be diagnosed in adults. Deficiencies of three clotting factors, VIII, IX, and XI, account for 90% to 95% of the bleeding disorders collectively called hemophilia (McCance & Huether, 2006).

Physiology Review

When tissue injury occurs, platelets collect at the site, adhering to the damaged vessel wall (the platelet plug). Activation of the clotting cascade, a sequential process of interactive reactions of clotting factors, is vital to form a stable clot. Clotting factors are plasma proteins primarily produced by the liver. A number of these factors require the presence of vitamin K for synthesis and activation. Once the clot has been formed and stabilized, it begins to retract, pulling together the edges of the damaged blood vessel to initiate the healing process.

Pathophysiology

Hemophilia A (or *classic hemophilia*) is the most common type of hemophilia, caused by deficiency or dysfunction of clotting factor VIII. It is transmitted as an X-linked recessive disorder from mothers to sons (Figure 34–13 ■). The genetic defect of hemophilia A on the X chromosome may cause deficient factor VIII production or a defective form of the pro-

---

BOX 34–7 Medications That May Interfere with Platelet Function

Over-the-Counter Medications
- Aspirin and salicylates, including:
  - Alka-Seltzer
  - Bufferin
  - Doan's pills
  - Ecotrin
  - Excedrin
  - Midol
  - Pepto-Bismol
  - Vanquish
- NSAIDs such as
  - Advil
  - Aleve
  - Nuprin
  - Pamprin IB

Prescription Medications
- Aspirin-containing analgesics
- Chemotherapy drugs
- Antibiotics such as penicillin
- Carbamazepine (Tegretol)
- Colchicine
- Dipyridamole (Persantine)
- Gold salts
- Heparin
- Quinine derivatives
- Sulfonamides
- Thiazide diuretics

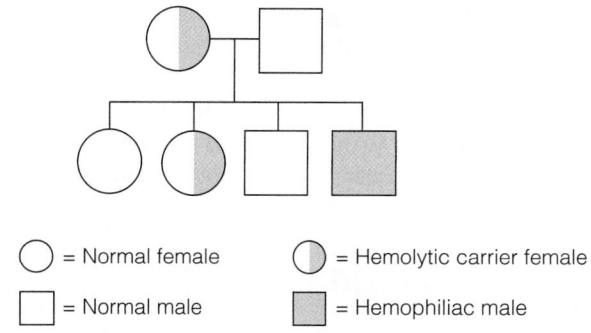

GENETIC CONSIDERATIONS
Focus on Hemophilia

The incidence and pattern of inheritance for the forms of hemophilia differ.

- Hemophilia A occurs in about 1 in 10,000 male births, transmitted on the X chromosome: Each male offspring has a 50% risk of inheriting the defective gene; each female offspring has a 50% risk of becoming a carrier.
- Hemophilia B occurs in about 1 in 100,000 male births, transmitted on the X chromosome.
- Von Willebrand's disease affects about 1 in 100 to 500 people, usually inherited as an autosomal dominant trait: Offspring of an affected person have a 50% risk of inheriting the trait and the disorder.
- Factor XI deficiency inherited as an autosomal recessive trait: Each offspring of a carrier and an unaffected individual has as 50% risk of inheriting the trait; each offspring of two carriers has a 50% risk of being a carrier and a 25% risk of having the disorder. This deficiency is common in Ashkenazi Jews.

○ = Normal female   ◐ = Hemolytic carrier female
□ = Normal male   ▨ = Hemophiliac male

Figure 34–13 ■ The inheritance pattern of hemophilia A and B. Both are transmitted as X-linked recessive disorders. Females may be carriers, but males develop these disorders.

tein. When the concentration of the clotting factor is 5% to 35% of normal, the disease is *mild*. Bleeding is infrequent, and usually associated with trauma. Concentrations of 1% to 5% of normal result in *moderate* disease. Again, bleeding usually occurs secondarily to trauma. *Severe* hemophilia occurs when concentrations are less than 1% of normal. Bleeding is frequent, often occurring without trauma (Kasper et al., 2005; McCance & Huether, 2006).

Hemophilia B (also called *Christmas disease*) accounts for about 15% of cases, and is caused by a deficiency in Factor IX. Despite the difference in clotting factor deficits, hemophilia A and B are clinically identical.

Von Willebrand's disease, often considered a type of hemophilia, is the most common hereditary bleeding disorder (Porth, 2005). It is caused by a deficit of or defective von Willebrand (vW) factor, a protein that mediates platelet adhesion (Tierney et al., 2005). Reduced levels of Factor VIII often also are present, because vW factor carries Factor VIII. This clotting disorder affects men and women equally. Bleeding associ-

ated with von Willebrand's disease rarely is severe. It often is diagnosed when prolonged bleeding follows surgery or a dental extraction.

Factor XI deficiency (or *hemophilia C*) is usually a mild disorder, identified when postoperative bleeding is prolonged. A comparison of the types of hemophilia is found in Table 34–9.

People with hemophilia form a platelet plug at the site of bleeding, but the clotting factor deficit impairs formation of a stable fibrin clot. The effect of vW factor deficiency is somewhat different, in that platelet aggregation at the site of injury is impaired. In either case, prolonged or extensive bleeding may result. Often bleeding occurs in response to injury or as a result of surgery. However, a severe clotting factor deficit can lead to spontaneous bleeding into the joints (*hemarthrosis*), deep tissues, and CNS. Hemarthrosis often causes joint deformity and disability, usually of the elbows, hips, knees, and ankles.

Manifestations

The following are manifestations of hemophilia:
- Hemarthrosis
- Easy bruising and cutaneous hematoma formation with minor trauma (e.g., an injection)
- Bleeding from the gums and prolonged bleeding following minor injuries or cuts

TABLE 34–9 Types of Hemophilia

TYPE/NAME	DEFICIENCY	CHARACTERISTICS	TREATMENT
Hemophilia A (classic hemophilia)	Factor VIII	Transmitted by females; occurs primarily in males; bleeding time normal; coagulation time prolonged	Factor VIII concentrate or cryoprecipitate
Hemophilia B	Factor IX	Transmitted by females; occurs primarily in males; bleeding time normal; coagulation time prolonged	Factor IX (Christmas disease concentrate)
Von Willebrand's disease	vW factor Factor VIII	Occurs in both females and males; bleeding time and coagulation time are both prolonged	Cryoprecipitate and DDAVP
Factor XI deficiency	Factor XI	Occurs in both males and females; the activated partial thromboplastin time is prolonged	Fresh frozen plasma

- Gastrointestinal bleeding, with hematemesis (vomiting blood), occult blood in the stools, gastric pain, or abdominal pain
- Spontaneous hematuria or epistaxis (nosebleed)
- Pain or paralysis due to the pressure of hematomas on nerves
- Intracranial hemorrhage is a potentially life-threatening manifestation of hemophilia.

INTERDISCIPLINARY CARE

Treatment of hemophilia focuses on preventing and/or treating bleeding, primarily by replacing deficient clotting factors. Specific treatment depends on the severity of the disorder and the specific factor deficiency. Care may be complicated by hepatitis or HIV disease in people with hemophilia treated with clotting factor concentrates prepared from multiple units of donated blood. Today, routine testing of all blood, improved blood donor screening, and current methods of treating hemophilia have significantly reduced the risk for these bloodborne diseases.

Diagnosis

The following laboratory tests may be ordered:

- *Serum platelet levels* are measured and are usually normal.
- *Coagulation studies* such as APTT, bleeding time, and prothrombin time are used to screen for hemophilia when abnormal bleeding occurs. APTT is increased in all types of hemophilia. Prothrombin time is unaffected in these disorders but may be measured to rule out other disorders. Bleeding time is prolonged in von Willebrand's disease but normal in hemophilia A and B.
- *Factor assays* are performed; Factor VIII is decreased in hemophilia A and often in von Willebrand's disease, Factor IX is decreased in hemophilia B, and Factor XI in hemophilia C.
- *Amniocentesis* or *chorionic villus sampling* is used to identify the genetic defect of hemophilia when there is a known family history of the disease.

Medications

Deficient clotting factors are replaced regularly, as a prophylactic measure before surgery and dental procedures, and to control bleeding. Clotting factors may be given as fresh-frozen plasma, cryoprecipitates, or concentrates. Factor levels are measured on a regular basis to determine whether the treatment is adequate. Clotting factors are often self-administered and may be taken either on a regular or intermittent schedule.

Fresh-frozen plasma replaces all clotting factors (including both Factor VIII and Factor IX) except platelets. When the cause of bleeding is not yet determined, fresh-frozen plasma may be administered intravenously until a definitive diagnosis is made.

Hemophilia A is usually treated with either heat-treated Factor VIII concentrate (heat treating reduces the risk of transmitting disease) or recombinant Factor VIII. Although recombinant Factor VIII, produced using recombinant DNA technology, eliminates the risk of viral disease transmission, its use is limited by cost. The dose of Factor VIII is determined by the severity of the deficit and the presence or prospect of active bleeding (e.g., planned surgery).

Desmopressin acetate (DDAVP, Stimate) may be given to people with mild hemophilia A or von Willebrand's disease prior to minor surgeries. This drug causes release of Factor VIII and will raise blood levels by two- or threefold for several hours, reducing the risk of bleeding and the need for clotting factor concentrate (Tierney et al., 2005).

Factor IX concentrate (administered intravenously) is used to treat hemophilia B. Because Factor IX concentrates also contain a number of other proteins, there is risk of thrombosis with recurrent use. They are used judiciously, only when needed. Products produced by recombinant technology or that are monoclonally purified carry a lower risk of stimulating thrombus formation (Kasper et al., 2005). Fresh-frozen plasma replaces Factor XI and is used when necessary. It may be given daily until the risk for bleeding decreases.

Factor VIII concentrates contain functional vW factor, and may be used to treat von Willebrand's disease. Aspirin is avoided in all types of hemophilia.

NURSING CARE

Although primary responsibility for care falls to the client and family, nursing care presents challenges. For additional assessment and nursing care strategies, see the accompanying Nursing Care Plan.

Health Promotion

Encourage clients with a family history of hemophilia or bleeding disorders to seek genetic counseling during their family planning process. Although tests are available for the hemophilia gene, the technology to correct the disorder *in utero* does not yet exist. See Chapter 8 ∞.

Assessment

While severe hemophilia usually is diagnosed in childhood, milder cases may not be identified until surgery, invasive dental work, or a traumatic injury causes extensive or prolonged bleeding. Focused assessment related to hemophilia includes the following:

- *Health history:* Previous bleeding episodes with or without trauma; history of easy bruising, hematomas, epistaxis, bleeding gums, hematuria, vomiting blood, or joint pain; aspirin use; family history of hemophilia or bleeding disorders.
- *Physical examination:* Vital signs; bruising or bleeding of skin or mucous membranes; mental status; abdominal assessment; presence of joint deformity, decreased range of motion.
- *Diagnostic tests:* CBC including hemoglobin, hematocrit, and platelet count; clotting factor assays; tests for occult blood (urine, stool, emesis); x-ray and scan results for evidence of bleeding.

Nursing Diagnoses and Interventions

Impaired blood clotting, the need for continuing care and disease management, and the risk for genetic transmission of hemophilia are priority problems for the client with hemophilia.

NURSING CARE PLAN A Client with Hemophilia

Jermiel Cruise is a 20-year-old student at the community college. He is admitted to the emergency department with a nosebleed that began when he fell during a touch football game. It has continued to bleed for over an hour.

ASSESSMENT

Mr. Cruise states that he has hemophilia and realizes that playing contact sports "is probably a dumb thing to do." He adds that he has not had any recent bleeding episodes. An icebag and manual pressure are applied in the emergency department. The physician orders Factor VIII concentrate to be administered. Physical assessment findings are T 97.2°F (36.2°C), BP 118/64, R 18. Skin pale but warm. Laboratory tests reveal a prolonged APTT and a normal bleeding time and PT. Following treatment, Mr. Cruise's bleeding subsides.

DIAGNOSES

- *Risk for Aspiration* related to uncontrolled nosebleed
- *Noncompliance* with activity recommendations
- *Ineffective Protection* related to lack of clotting factor VIII

EXPECTED OUTCOMES

- Exhibit no further signs of bleeding.
- Maintain vital signs within his usual range.
- Maintain an open airway.
- Identify sports and recreation activities in which he can safely participate.
- Verbalize self-care measures to control bleeding.

PLANNING AND IMPLEMENTATION

- Monitor vital signs and for further signs of bleeding.
- Assess airway and auscultate breath sounds.

- Review emergency measures to help stop bleeding.
- Reiterate the importance of seeking prompt medical attention if bleeding should occur.
- Advise regarding the importance of wearing a Medic-Alert bracelet identifying him as a hemophiliac.
- Discuss alternative noncontact sports and recreational activities.

EVALUATION

On discharge, Mr. Cruise has no further signs of bleeding, shock, or aspiration. He is able to verbalize methods to help stop local bleeding and the importance of seeking medical attention promptly when bleeding continues. Mr. Cruise agrees to stop at a local drug store on the way home to order a Medic-Alert bracelet. In addition, Mr. Cruise verbalizes an understanding of the importance of avoiding contact sports and has identified swimming and golf as alternative leisure activities that he might enjoy.

CRITICAL THINKING IN THE NURSING PROCESS

1. What is the pathophysiologic basis for the bleeding that occurs in hemophilia A and B?
2. What was Mr. Cruise's priority nursing diagnosis? Why?
3. Why is family planning a special consideration with a client who has hemophilia?
4. Outline a plan to teach the family of a client diagnosed with hemophilia how to administer an intravenous infusion.
5. Develop a care plan for Mr. Cruise for the nursing diagnosis *Impaired Social Interaction*. Consider Mr. Cruise's age and developmental level in creating the plan.
   See Evaluating Your Response in Appendix C.

Ineffective Protection

The inability to form stable clots and stem bleeding from injured blood vessels creates a significant risk for the client with hemophilia. Nursing care measures focus on preventing injury and protecting the skin from damage.

- Monitor for signs of bleeding, including hematomas, ecchymoses, and purpura, as well as surface oozing or bleeding. Check emesis and stool for occult blood. *Bleeding may occur in cutaneous tissues as well as internal organs. Bleeding in the upper gastrointestinal tract may not be readily apparent in the stool.*
- Notify the physician of any apparent bleeding. *Prompt intervention with administration of clotting factor concentrate decreases the risk of hemorrhage and subsequent hypovolemia.*
- Avoid intramuscular injections, rectal temperatures, and enemas. *These can pose a risk of tissue and vascular trauma, which can precipitate bleeding.*
- Use safety measures in personal care. For example, use an electric razor rather than a razor blade to shave. *Use of an electric razor minimizes the opportunity to develop superficial cuts that may result in bleeding.*
- If bleeding occurs, control blood loss using gentle pressure, ice, or a topical hemostatic agent, such as an absorbable gelatin sponge, microfibrillar collagen hemostat, or topical thrombin. *Direct pressure occludes bleeding vessels. Ice, a*

vasoconstrictor, may facilitate bleeding control, as do topical hemostatic agents.
- Instruct to avoid activities that increase the risk of trauma, including contact sports, physical exertion associated with job performance, and to eliminate safety hazards in the home. *Depending on the severity of the clotting factor deficit, even minor trauma can lead to serious bleeding episodes. Safer activities such as noncontact sports (e.g., swimming, golf) and occupations that do not require physical labor may be substituted.*

Risk for Ineffective Health Maintenance

Hemophilia is a chronic disorder, requiring active management to prevent and control bleeding and complications. Frequent visits to the physician or clinic may be necessary. In addition, the client may need to learn to self-administer clotting factors and measures to prevent complications. The lifelong nature of the disorder may interfere with compliance, especially during early adulthood.

- Assess knowledge of disorder and the related treatments. *Assessment allows identification of knowledge gaps and provides a basis on which to provide additional information. Impaired disease management may be due to lack of knowledge or a conscious decision not to follow the recommendations of the healthcare provider.*

- Provide information about the bleeding disorder and pre-scribed medications and treatments. *Individualized instruction is more effective than general, possibly irrelevant information.*
- Provide emotional support, expressing confidence in the client's self-care abilities. *Emotional support helps the client incorporate the care regimen into his or her lifestyle.*
- Provide supervised learning and practice opportunities for administering clotting factors and topical hemostatic agents. *Successful practice sessions instill confidence in the ability to manage care and provide an opportunity for questions and exploring alternatives.*

Linking NANDA, NIC, and NOC

Linkages between NANDA nursing diagnoses, nursing interventions, and nursing outcomes for the client with hemophilia are illustrated in Chart 34–4.

Community-Based Care

Discuss the following topics when preparing the client with a bleeding disorder and the family for home care:

- Recognizing the manifestations of internal bleeding: pallor, weakness, restlessness, headache, disorientation, pain, swelling. These manifestations require emergency medical care and should be reported immediately.
- Applying cold packs and immobilizing the joint for 24 to 48 hours if hemarthrosis occurs.
- Using analgesics for pain; avoiding prescription and over-the-counter drugs containing aspirin.

NANDA, NIC, AND NOC LINKAGES
CHART 34–4 The Client with Hemophilia

NANDA

Ineffective Health Maintenance

↓

NIC

Health Education

Self-Responsibility Facilitation

Teaching: Procedure/Treatment

↓

NOC

Health-Seeking Behavior

Knowledge: Health Behaviors

Knowledge: Treatment Regimen

Data from *NANDA's Nursing Diagnoses: Definitions & Classification 2005–2006* by NANDA International (2005), Philadelphia; *Nursing Interventions Classification (NIC)* (4th ed.) by J. M. Dochterman & G. M. Bulechek (2004), St. Louis, MO: Mosby; and *Nursing Outcomes Classification (NOC)* (3rd ed.) by S. Moorhead, M. Johnson, and M. Mass (2004), St. Louis, MO: Mosby.

- Ensuring a safe home environment (e.g., padding sharp edges of furniture, using transition lighting or a night light; avoiding scatter rugs, and wearing protective gloves when working in the house or yard).
- Using safe grooming practices such as electric razors.
- Wearing a Medic-Alert bracelet in case of accident.
- Practicing good dental hygiene to decrease potential tooth decay and extractions. If dental procedures are necessary, discuss the need for prophylactic factor administration with the dentist and physician.
- Following safer sex practices.
- Preparing and administering intravenous medications.

Refer the client and family to a local hemophilia or bleeding disorders support group. Provide contact information for national organizations and information clearinghouses, such as the National Hemophilia Foundation.

THE CLIENT WITH DISSEMINATED INTRAVASCULAR COAGULATION

Disseminated intravascular coagulation (DIC) is a disruption of hemostasis characterized by widespread intravascular clotting and bleeding. It may be acute and life threatening or relatively mild. DIC is a clinical syndrome that develops as a complication of a wide variety of other disorders (Box 34–8). Sepsis is the most common cause of DIC. Gram-negative and gram-positive bacteria as well as viruses, fungi, and protozoal infections may lead to DIC (McCance & Huether, 2006).

Pathophysiology

DIC is triggered by endothelial damage, release of tissue factors into the circulation, or inappropriate activation of the clotting cascade by an endotoxin. Both the intrinsic and the extrinsic clotting cascade may be activated, although the extrinsic cascade usually is the one activated. Extensive thrombin

---

BOX 34–8 Conditions That May Precipitate Disseminated Intravascular Coagulation

Tissue Damage
- Trauma: burns, gunshot wounds, frostbite, head injury
- Obstetric complications: septic abortion, abruptio placentae, amniotic fluid embolus, retained dead fetus
- Neoplasms: acute leukemia, adenocarcinomas
- Hemolysis
- Fat embolism

Vessel Damage
- Aortic aneurysm
- Acute glomerulonephritis
- Hemolytic uremic syndrome

Infections
- Bacterial infection or sepsis
- Viral or mycotic infections
- Parasitic or rickettsial infection

entering the systemic circulation overwhelms natural anticoagulants, leading to unrestricted clot formation (McCance & Huether, 2006). Clotting may be localized to an individual organ, or widespread with deposition of small thrombi and emboli throughout the microvasculature (Kasper et al., 2005). The widespread clotting consumes clotting factors (prothrombin, platelets, factor V, and factor VIII in particular) and activates fibrinolytic processes with anticoagulant production. As a result, hemorrhage occurs (Figure 34–14 ■).

The sequence of DIC follows:

1. Endothelial damage, tissue factors, or toxins stimulate the clotting cascade.
2. Excess thrombin within the circulation overwhelms naturally occurring anticoagulants.
3. Widespread clotting occurs within the microvasculature.
4. Thrombi and emboli impair tissue perfusion, leading to ischemia, infarction, and necrosis.
5. Clotting factors and platelets are consumed faster than they can be replaced.
6. Clotting activates fibrinolytic processes, which begin to break down clots.
7. Fibrin degradation products (FDPs, potent anticoagulants) are released, contributing to bleeding.
8. Clotting factors are depleted, the ability to form clots is lost, and hemorrhage occurs.

Manifestations

The manifestations of DIC result from both clotting and bleeding, although bleeding is more obvious, especially in acute DIC. Bleeding ranges from oozing blood following an injection to frank hemorrhage from every body orifice (see box below). Chronic DIC may be asymptomatic, or may present with peripheral cyanosis, thrombosis, and pregangrenous changes in the fingers and toes, nose, and genitalia (Kasper et al., 2005).

MANIFESTATIONS of DIC

- Frank hemorrhage from incisions
- Oozing of blood from punctures, intravenous catheter sites
- Purpura, petechiae, bruising
- Cyanosis of extremities
- Gastrointestinal bleeding or hemorrhage
- Dyspnea, tachypnea, bloody sputum
- Tachycardia, hypotension
- Hematuria, oliguria, acute renal failure
- Manifestations of increased intracranial pressure: decreased level of consciousness, papillary, motor, and sensory changes
- Mental status changes

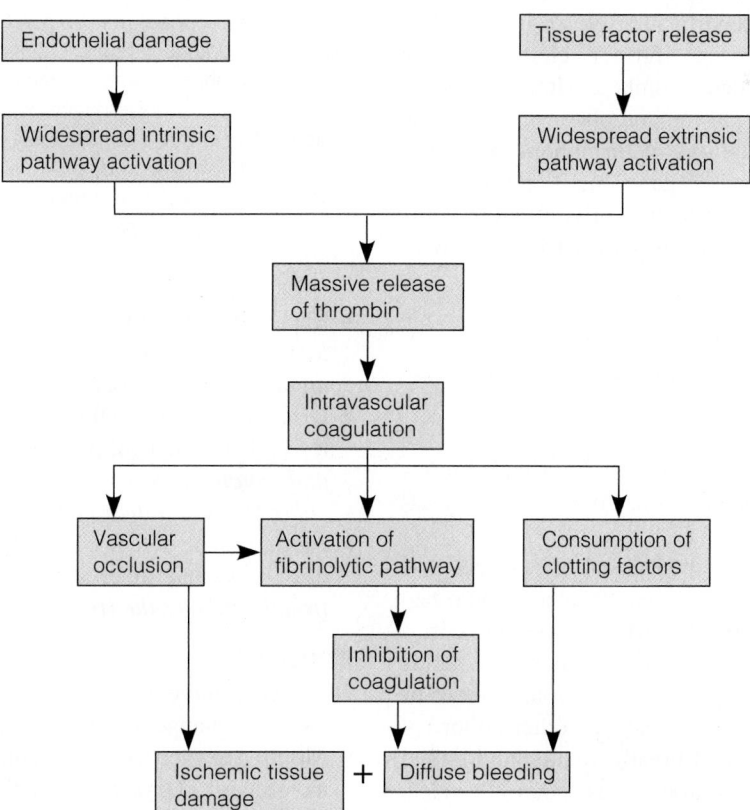

Figure 34–14 ■ Disseminated intravascular coagulation (DIC). Endothelial cell injury or release of tissue factors activate the intrinsic or extrinsic clotting pathway (or both). As a result, numerous microthrombi form throughout the vasculature, causing ischemic tissue damage. Simultaneously, rapid consumption of clotting factors and activation of fibrinolytic mechanisms trigger widespread bleeding.

INTERDISCIPLINARY CARE

Treatment of DIC is directed toward treating the underlying disorder and preventing further bleeding or massive thrombosis. Treatment stabilizes the client, reduces complications, and allows recovery to occur; it does not cure DIC (Kasper et al., 2005).

Diagnosis

Diagnostic tests are used to confirm the diagnosis of DIC and evaluate the risk for hemorrhage.

- *CBC* and *platelet count* are used to evaluate the hemoglobin, hematocrit, and number of circulating platelets. *Schistocytes,* fragmented RBCs, may be noted due to cell trapping and damage within fibrin thrombi. The platelet count is decreased.
- *Coagulation studies* show prolonged *prothrombin time (PT), partial thromboplastin time (PTT),* and *thrombin time,* and a low *fibrinogen level* due to depletion of clotting factors. The fibrinogen level helps predict bleeding in DIC: As it falls, the risk of bleeding increases (Kasper et al., 2005).
- *Fibrin degradation products (FDPs)* or *fibrin split products (FSPs)* are increased due to the fibrinolysis that occurs with DIC.

Treatments

When bleeding is the major manifestation of DIC, fresh frozen plasma and platelet concentrates are given to restore clotting factors and platelets. Heparin, although controversial, may be administered. Heparin interferes with the clotting cascade and may prevent further clotting factor consumption due to uncontrolled thrombosis. It is used when bleeding is not controlled by plasma and platelets, as well as when the client has manifestations of thrombotic problems such as acrocyanosis and possible gangrene. Long-term heparin therapy (administered by injection or continuous infusion using a portable pump) may be necessary for clients with chronic DIC.

NURSING CARE

Assessment

Nurses can be instrumental in identifying early manifestations of DIC, facilitating timely intervention. Focused nursing assessment for DIC includes:

- *Health history:* Recent abortion (spontaneous or therapeutic) or current pregnancy; presence of a known malignant tumor; history of abnormal bleeding episodes or a hematologic disorder.
- *Physical examination:* Bleeding from puncture wounds (e.g., injections), IV sites, incisions; hematuria, obvious or occult blood in emesis or stool, epistaxis, other abnormal bleeding; vital signs; heart and breath sounds; abdominal assessment including girth, contour, bowel sounds, tenderness or guarding to palpation; color, temperature, skin condition of hands, feet, and digits; petechiae or purpura of skin, mucous membranes.

- *Diagnostic tests:* CBC with hemoglobin, hematocrit; platelet count; coagulation studies; evaluations of organ system function (e.g., liver and renal function tests); CT scans of the head and abdomen.

Nursing Diagnoses and Interventions

Clients with acute DIC often are critically ill, with multiple nursing care needs. Priority nursing diagnoses discussed in this section focus on impaired tissue perfusion and gas exchange, pain, and fear. Septic shock may precipitate DIC; hemorrhagic shock may occur as a complication of DIC. See Chapter 11 ∞ for nursing diagnoses and interventions related to these problems.

Ineffective Tissue Perfusion

Thrombi and emboli forming throughout the microcirculation affect the perfusion of multiple organs and tissues. Additionally, bleeding due to clotting factor consumption affects cardiac output and blood flow to these tissues.

- Assess extremity pulses, warmth, and capillary refill. Monitor level of consciousness (LOC) and mental status. *Monitoring central and peripheral tissue perfusion facilitates early treatment of impaired perfusion.*

> **PRACTICE ALERT**
> Promptly report complaints of chest pain, changes in mental status, LOC, tissue perfusion, respirations, gastrointestinal function, and urinary output. Chest pain or respiratory changes (tachypnea, dyspnea, orthopnea) may be due to angina, pulmonary embolism, or bleeding into lung tissue. Changes in mentation or LOC can indicate cerebral ischemia. A painful, pale, and cold extremity with no or diminished pulses indicates arterial occlusion. Prompt intervention is critical to save the extremity. Acute abdominal pain, decreased bowel sounds, and GI bleeding may indicate mesenteric occlusion, a surgical emergency. Decreased urine output may signify renal artery thrombosis; renal failure may develop.

- Carefully reposition at least every 2 hours. *Position changes facilitate circulation and tissue perfusion and also provide an opportunity to assess for purpura, pallor, and bleeding.*
- Discourage crossing the legs, and do not elevate the knees on the bed or with a pillow. *These positions may impair arterial and venous flow to the lower legs and feet, increasing vascular stasis and the risk for thrombosis.*
- Minimize use of tape on the skin, using binders, nonadhesive dressings, and other devices as needed. *Preventing skin trauma reduces the risk for bleeding and potential infection.*

Impaired Gas Exchange

Microclots in the pulmonary vasculature are likely to interfere with gas exchange in the client with DIC.

- Monitor oxygen saturation continuously. Administer oxygen as ordered. *Oxygen saturation levels are a noninvasive means of assessing gas exchange. Supplemental oxygen promotes gas exchange and reduces cardiac work, relieving dyspnea.*

Monitor arterial blood gas results; report abnormal results to the physician. Low Pao₂ and rising Paco₂ levels indicate impaired gas exchange and may signify the need for additional treatment.

- Place in Fowler's or high-Fowler's position as tolerated. *Elevating the head of the bed improves diaphragmatic excursion and alveolar ventilation.*
- Maintain bed rest. *Bed rest reduces oxygen demands and cardiac work.*
- Encourage deep breathing and effective coughing. *Increased respiratory depth and clearance of secretions from airways improves alveolar ventilation and oxygenation.*
- Cautious nasotracheal suctioning may be instituted if cough is ineffective or an endotracheal tube is in place. *Removal of secretions facilitates ventilation and oxygenation. However, care must be used to minimize suction-induced hypoxia and airway trauma.*
- Administer analgesics and antianxiety drugs as needed to control pain and anxiety. Provide reassurance and comfort measures. *Pain and anxiety increase the respiratory rate and decrease the depth of respirations, reducing effective ventilation and gas exchange.*

Pain

Both the underlying cause of DIC and tissue ischemia from microvascular clots can cause pain. Identifying the etiology of pain is important to identify potential complications or harmful effects of DIC and to institute effective treatment.

- Use a standard pain scale to evaluate and monitor pain and analgesic effectiveness. *Monitoring pain and response to medication facilitates development of an appropriate and effective treatment plan.*

Notify the physician promptly of new or a sudden increase in pain, especially when accompanied by changes in assessment findings. New or increased complaints of pain may signify increased circulatory impairment and ischemic changes in tissues such as the heart, bowel, or extremities. Circulation to a painful, pale or cyanotic, or cold extremity may be occluded by an arterial clot. Prompt intervention is necessary to save the extremity. Acute abdominal pain may signify mesenteric occlusion, a surgical emergency. Anginal pain may indicate occlusion of coronary arteries.

- Handle extremities gently. *Gentle handling reduces the risk of further injury to and pain in ischemic tissues.*
- Apply cool compresses to painful joints. *Application of cold decreases pain through the gate-control mechanism, inhibiting the dorsal horn of the spinal cord and reducing the sensation of pain.*

Continuously monitor effects of analgesics, mental and respiratory status. Analgesics may mask manifestations of neurologic impairment due to thromboembolism, and may depress the respiratory center, further impairing gas exchange. Judicious analgesic administration with careful monitoring is vital to safely provide effective pain relief.

Fear

The underlying serious illness and a complication such as DIC result in an uncertain prognosis, often accompanied by fear.

- Encourage the client and family to verbalize concerns. *This helps the client and family identify their concerns and frame questions.*
- Answer questions truthfully. *Providing honest answers is vital to developing a therapeutic nurse–client relationship. Accurate responses allow the client and family to set priorities as they plan for an uncertain future.*
- Help the client and family identify coping strategies to manage this significant situational stressor. *Implementing past effective coping methods may provide the skills to manage the current crisis.*
- Provide emotional support. *The presence of a caring nurse helps reduce the fear and anxiety associated with a crisis.*
- Maintain a calm environment. *A calm environment provides reassurance that the situation is in control, reduces anxiety, and promotes rest.*
- Respond promptly when the client calls for help. *Prompt response to expressed needs helps develop a trusting relationship and a sense of security that assistance is readily available.*
- Teach relaxation techniques. *Relaxation techniques can reduce muscle tension and other signs of anxiety. Gaining control over physical responses can help the client gain a sense of control over the situation.*

Community-Based Care

Although the immediate crisis of acute DIC is resolved prior to discharge, the client may have some continuing effects of the disorder, such as impaired tissue integrity of distal extremities. Teach the client and family about specific care needs, such as foot care (see Box 35–4 ∞) or dressing changes. Provide instruction about any continuing medications and follow-up care.

Clients with chronic DIC may require continuing heparin therapy, using either intermittent subcutaneous injections or a portable infusion pump. Teach the client and family members how to administer the injection or manage the infusion pump. Provide a referral to home health care or a home intravenous management service for assistance. Discuss the manifestations of excessive bleeding or recurrent clotting that need to be reported to the physician.

EXPLORE MEDIALINK

Prentice Hall Nursing MediaLink DVD-ROM
Audio Glossary
NCLEX-RN® Review

Animation/Video
Sickle Cell Anemia

COMPANION WEBSITE www.prenhall.com/lemone
Audio Glossary
NCLEX-RN® Review
Care Plan Activity: Acute Myelocytic Leukemia
Case Studies
Disseminated Intravascular Coagulation
Immune Thrombocytopenic Purpura
MediaLink Applications
Blood Alternatives
Sickle Cell Anemia
Stem Cell Transplant
Synthetic Blood Products
Links to Resources

CHAPTER HIGHLIGHTS

- Anemia is the most common disorder of the red blood cells; nutritional deficiencies are the most common causes of anemia. Its manifestations relate to the function of RBCs and hemoglobin, transporting oxygen to the cells: fatigue, increased respiratory and heart rates, shortness of breath with activity, and pallor.

- Genetically transmitted disorders such as sickle cell disease and thalassemia can cause significant anemia and associated problems in affected populations. These clients require teaching and episodic acute care for crises such as vaso-occlusive crisis in sickle cell disease.

- Nursing care related to anemia is primarily educational to prepare the client for effective self-care, including diet, prescribed medications, and measures to prevent sickling episodes (for clients with sickle cell disease).

- Leukemia and lymphomas are the primary disorders of white blood cells and lymphoid tissues.

- Manifestations of the leukemias reflect the altered ability of abnormal WBCs to perform effective immune surveillance and crowding of the bone marrow and other organs by rapidly proliferating cells. Frequent sore throats, increased risk for infection, and manifestations of anemia and thrombocytopenia are seen, as well as an enlarged spleen and abdominal pain.

- Four major subgroups of leukemia are identified, acute and chronic myeloid leukemias, and acute and chronic lymphocytic (or lymphoblastic) leukemias. The primary population affected differs for each of these leukemias, as does their course.

- Genetic alterations and certain viruses are linked to the development of leukemia, as are exposure to chemotherapy drugs, environmental toxins, and ionizing radiation.

- Lymphocytic leukemias and lymphomas are closely related disorders.

- Nursing care for clients with leukemia and lymphoma focuses on reducing the risk for infection and bleeding, managing the effects of chemotherapy and radiation therapy, and, in some cases, caring for clients before and after bone marrow or stem cell transplant.

- The major risks associated with bone marrow and stem cell transplant are infection prior to and immediately following the transplant and graft-versus-host disease, a potentially fatal condition. A pruritic rash and desquamation of the palms and soles; abdominal pain, nausea, and diarrhea; and jaundice and elevated liver enzymes are common early manifestations of GVHD.

- The treatment of and nursing care for clients with lymphomas (including Hodgkin's lymphoma and non-Hodgkin's lymphomas) is similar to that provided for clients with leukemia.

- Multiple myeloma is a malignancy of plasma cells, B lymphocytes that produce antibodies. Circulating M proteins and Bence Jones proteins in the urine are seen in multiple myeloma. The usual presenting manifestation is bone pain. Pathologic fractures and hypercalcemia are common complications of multiple myeloma as bone is destroyed.

- Bleeding and clotting disorders can result from either inadequate platelets (thrombocytopenia) or disruption of the clotting mechanisms (hemophilia, DIC). Petechiae and purpura are common manifestations of bleeding/clotting disorders.

- Hemophilias are genetically transmitted disorders. Hemophilia A and B are transmitted on the X chromosome (sex-linked) from mother to son. Von Willebrand's disease, the most common bleeding disorder, is transmitted as an autosomal dominant disorder and affects men and women equally.

- Hemophilias are treated by replacement of the missing clotting factor and measures to prevent injury and bleeding.

- Disseminated intravascular coagulation is a disorder of widespread microvascular clotting. It commonly is precipitated by sepsis, but also may occur with conditions such as major trauma, malignancy, or as an obstetric emergency.

- In DIC, platelets and clotting factors are consumed by the abnormal clotting processes, leading the manifestations of bleeding, including frank hemorrhage, hematuria, oozing blood from parenteral and intravenous injection sites, and GI bleeding. Blood flow to organs and tissues is compromised by clot formation, leading to manifestations such as cyanosis of extremities, abdominal pain, renal failure, and changes in mental status and level of consciousness. Nursing care is supportive, focusing on administering prescribed treatments and monitoring and supporting cardiovascular, respiratory, and renal function.

TEST YOURSELF NCLEX-RN® REVIEW

1. In assessing a female client with moderate anemia, the nurse would expect to find which of the following?
   1. hematocrit 45%
   2. pulse rate 140
   3. complaints of shortness of breath with exercise
   4. WBC 14,000/μL

2. The nurse following a client after gastric resection observes carefully for evidence of nutritional deficiency anemia related to malabsorption, including:
   1. numbness and tingling of extremities.
   2. steatorrhea.
   3. dark yellow or bronze skin color.
   4. bone pain.

3. Which of the following nursing diagnoses would be of highest priority for the client hospitalized for a bone marrow transplant to treat relapse of acute myelocytic leukemia?
   1. *Disturbed Body Image*
   2. *Ineffective Protection*
   3. *Anxiety*
   4. *Imbalanced Nutrition: Less than Body Requirements*

4. The nurse caring for a client with acute myeloid leukemia plans which of the following nursing interventions during hospitalization? (Select all that apply.)
   1. Place in a private room.
   2. Implement airborne infection control precautions.
   3. Assist with oral hygiene after meals.
   4. Monitor rectal temperature q4h.
   5. Request soft, bland diet.

5. A client with non-Hodgkin's lymphoma tells the nurse, "I might as well give up on dating. No woman will want me now." What is the most appropriate response?
   1. "It sounds like you are concerned about the effects of this disease and the proposed treatment plan."
   2. "Don't worry. Malignant lymphomas are very treatable when caught in an early stage of the disease."
   3. "Well, you may never be able to have children all right, but there are other ways to have a satisfying relationship with a woman."
   4. "Lots of women find bald men attractive; besides, your hair may grow back soft and curly."

6. The nurse caring for a client with lymphoma who is being started on the CHOP chemotherapy regimen understands that chemotherapy drugs are used in combination to:
   1. target malignant cells in different organs.
   2. prevent the development of adverse effects.
   3. target different phases of the cell cycle.
   4. support growth and development of normal cells.

7. A client with multiple myeloma calls the home health nurse complaining of severe back pain of new onset. The appropriate response by the nurse is to:
   1. reassure the client that bone pain is expected with this disease.
   2. inquire about the client's use of NSAIDs and analgesics to manage pain.
   3. suggest use of a back brace to reduce pain.
   4. notify the physician of the onset of new pain.

8. The nurse observes reddish-purple spots and areas of purple bruising on a newly admitted client. Which laboratory results support this assessment finding?
   1. hematocrit 28%
   2. platelets 6000/mm^3
   3. INR 4.0
   4. WBC 4500/mm^3

9. A client whose husband has hemophilia asks if her newborn baby girl could have the disease. The nurse's response is based on the knowledge that:
   1. the most common forms of hemophilia are transmitted as sex-linked recessive disorders; her daughter is at risk for carrying the defective gene.
   2. because hemophilia is a sex-linked recessive disorder carried on the Y chromosome, her daughter has no risk of having or carrying the disease.
   3. hemophilia is an autosomal dominant disorder; therefore, her daughter has a 50% chance of having the disorder.
   4. although hemophilia is genetically transmitted, its pattern of inheritance is unknown, and her daughter will need to be tested for the defective gene.

10. The nurse administering platelets to a client with disseminated intravascular coagulation (DIC) understands that the intended effect of this treatment is to:
    1. replace specific clotting factors.
    2. promote intravascular clotting.
    3. restore tissue oxygenation.
    4. replace depleted platelets.

See Test Yourself answers in Appendix C.

BIBLIOGRAPHY

American Cancer Society. (2002). *Gleevec's new successes show growing promise of targeted therapies.* Retrieved from http://www.cancer.org/eprise/main/docroot/NWS/content/NWS_1_1x_Gleevec
_____. (2005). *Cancer facts and figures 2005.* Atlanta: Author.
Barcelona, R. (2001). Type II heparin-induced thrombocytopenia: New treatment options. Retrieved from http://www.cleavelandclinicmeded.com/medical_info/pharmacy/septoct2001

Bennett, L. (2005). Understanding sickle cell disorders. *Nursing Standard, 19*(32), 52–63.
Beser, N. G., & Öz, F. (2005). Quality of life in lymphoma patients. *Clinical Excellence for Nurse Practitioners, 9*(3), 153–161.
Blackhouse, R. (2004). Understanding disseminated intravascular coagulation. *Nursing Times, 100*(36), 38–42.
Breed, C. D. (2003). Diagnosis, treatment, and nursing care of patients with chronic leukemia. *Seminars in Oncology Nursing, 19*(2), 109–117.

Brewster, B. (2003). Achieving optimal patient outcomes with intravenous iron. *Nursing Times, 99*(29), 30–32.
Burruss, N., & Holz, S. (2005). Managing the risks of thrombocytopenia. *Nursing, 35*(6), 32hn1–32hn2, 32hn4–32hn5.
Cantril, C. A., & Haylock, P. J. (2004). Tumor lysis syndrome. *American Journal of Nursing, 104*(4), 49–52.
Cashion, A. (2002) Genetics in transplantation. *Medsurg Nursing, 11*(2), 91–94.
Coleman, E. A., Coon, S., Hall-Barrow, J., Richards, K., Gaylor, D., & Stewart, B. (2004). Feasibility of exercise during

treatment for multiple myeloma. *Cancer Nursing, 26*(5), 410–419.

Coleman, E. A., Hutchins, L., & Goodwin, J. (2004). An overview of cancer in the older adult. *Medsurg Nursing, 13*(2), 75–80, 109.

Colfer, M. (2003). Achieving optimal patient outcomes with intravenous iron. *Nephrology Nursing, 30*(4), 449–453.

Coon, S. K., & Coleman, E. A. (2004). Exercise decisions within the context of multiple myeloma, transplant, and fatigue. *Cancer Nursing, 27*(2), 108–118.

Cope, D. (2004). Tumor lysis syndrome. *Clinical Journal of Oncology Nursing, 8*(4), 415–416.

Copstead, L. C., & Banasik, J. L. (2005). *Pathophysiology* (3rd ed.). St. Louis, MO: Elsevier/Saunders.

_____. (2004a). Chronic myelogenous leukemia. *Clinical Journal of Oncology Nursing, 9*(5), 535–538, 561–563.

D'Antonio, J. (2004b). You can lessen leukemia's toll. *Nursing, 34*(7), 32hn1–32hn2, 32hn4.

Demakos, E. P., & Linebaugh, J. A. (2005). Advances in myelodysplastic syndrome: Nursing implications of azacitidine. *Clinical Journal of Oncology Nursing, 9*(4), 417–423.

Devenney, B., & Erickson, C. (2004). Multiple myeloma: An overview. *Clinical Journal of Oncology Nursing, 8*(4), 401–405.

Devine, H., & DeMeyer, E. (2003) Hematopoietic cell transplantation in the treatment of leukemia. *Seminars in Oncology Nursing, 19*(2), 118–132.

Dochterman, J., & Bulechek, G. (2004). *Nursing interventions classification (NIC)* (4th ed.). St. Louis, MO: Mosby.

Dolan, S., Crombez, P., & Murnoz, M. (2005). Neutropenia management with granulocyte colony-stimulating factors: From guidelines to nursing practice protocols. *European Journal of Oncology Nursing, 9*(Suppl 1), S14–S23.

Dowsett, C. (2005). Managing leg ulceration in patients with sickle cell disorder. *Nursing Times, 101*(16), 48–49.

Dressler, D. K. (2004). DIC: Coping with a coagulation crisis. *Nursing, 34*(5), 58–62.

Druker, B. J., Sawyers, C. L., Capdeville, R., Ford, J. M., Baccarani, M., & Goldman, J. M. (2001). Chronic myelogenous leukemia. *Hematology (American Society of Hematology Education Program)*, pp. 87–113. Abstract from National Cancer Institute. Retrieved from http://www.nci.nih.gov/cancerinformation/doc_cit.aspx?args= 22; 11722980

Dyson, S. (2005). Sickle cell and thalassaemia screening. *Practice Nurse, 29*(10), 17–18, 20.

Eggenberger, S. K., Krumwiede, N., Meiers, S. J., Bliesmer, M., & Earle, P. (2004). Family caring strategies in neutropenia. *Clinical Journal of Oncology Nursing, 8*(6), 617–621, 638–640.

El-Banna, M. M., Berger, A. M., Farr, L., Foxall, M. J., Friesth, B., & Schreiner, E. (2004). Fatigue and depression in patients with lymphoma undergoing autologous peripheral blood stem cell transplantation. *Oncology Nursing Forum, 31*(5), 937–944.

Fischbach, F. (2002). *Nurses' quick reference to common laboratory and diagnostic tests* (3rd ed.). Philadelphia: Lippincott.

Fontaine, K. L. (2005). *Healing practices: Alternative therapies for nursing* (2nd ed.). Upper Saddle River, NJ: Prentice Hall Health.

Francis, J. L., & Drexler, A. J. (2005). Striking back at heparin-induced thrombocytopenia. *Nursing, 35*(9), 48–51.

Gever, M. P. (2005). Lepirudin: Test your drug IQ. *Nursing, 35*(11), 32cc4.

Holcomb, S. S. (2005). Anemia. *Nursing, 35*(3), 53.

Iovino, C. S., & Camacho, L. H. (2003). Acute myeloid leukemia: A classification and treatment update. *Clinical Journal of Oncology Nursing, 7*(5), 535–540.

Kasper, D. L., Braunwald, E., Fauci, A. S., Hauser, S. L., Longo, D. L., & Jameson, J. L. (Eds.). (2005). *Harrison's principles of internal medicine* (16th ed.). New York: McGraw-Hill.

Krimmel, T. (2003). Disseminated intravascular coagulation. *Clinical Journal of Oncology Nursing, 7*(4), 479–481.

Lea, D. H., & Williams, J. K. (2002). Genetic testing and screening. *American Journal of Nursing, 102*(7), 36–43.

Mangan, P. (2005). Recognizing multiple myeloma. *Nurse Practitioner, 30*(3), 14–18, 23–24, 26–29.

Maningo, J. (2002). Peripheral blood stem cell transplant: Easier than getting blood from a bone. *Nursing, 32*(12), 52–55,

McCance, K. L., & Huether, S. E. (2006). *Pathophysiology: The biologic basis for disease in adults & children* (4th ed.). St. Louis, MO: Mosby.

McCloskey, J. C., & Bulechek, G. M. (Eds.). (2000). *Nursing interventions classification (NIC)* (3rd ed.). St. Louis, MO: Mosby.

McGrath, P. (2004). Positive outcomes for survivors of haematological malignancies from a spiritual perspective. *International Journal of Nursing Practice, 10*(6), 280–291.

Medoff, E. (2000). Oncology today: Leukemia. *RN, 63*(9), 42–49.

Moorhead, S., Johnson, M., & Maas, M. (2004). *Nursing Outcomes Classification (NOC)* (3rd ed.). St. Louis, MO: Mosby.

NANDA International. (2005). *Nursing Diagnoses: Definitions and Classification 2005–2006.* Philadelphia: Author.

National Comprehensive Cancer Network. (2006). *Clinical practice guidelines in oncology. Myelodysplastic syndromes* (Version 3). Retrieved from http://www.nccn.org/professionals/physician_gls/PDF/mds.pdf

National Heart, Lung, and Blood Institute, National Institutes of Health. (2002). *Morbidity & mortality: 2002 chart book of cardiovascular, lung, and blood diseases.* Bethesda, MD: Author.

Navuluri, R. (2001). Understanding hemostasis. *American Journal of Nursing, 101*(9), Hospital extra: 24B, 24C.

Persson, L., & Hallberg, I. R. (2004). Lived experience of survivors of leukemia or malignant lymphoma. *Cancer Nursing, 27*(4), 303–313.

_____ , Hallberg, I. R., & Ohlsson, O. (1997). Survivors of acute leukemia and highly malignant lymphoma—retrospective views of daily life problems during treatment and when in remission. *Journal of Advanced Nursing, 25*(1), 68–78.

Porth, C. M. (2005). *Pathophysiology: Concepts of altered health states* (7th ed.). Philadelphia: Lippincott.

Redaelli, A., Laskin, B. L., Stephens, J. M., Botteman, M. F., & Pashos, C. L. (2004). The clinical and epidemiological burden of chronic lymphocytic leukemia. *European Journal of Cancer Care, 13*(3), 279–289.

_____, (2005). A systematic literature review of the clinical and epidemiological burden of acute lymphoblastic leukaemia (ALL). *European Journal of Cancer Care, 14*(1), 53–62.

Rempher, K. J., & Little, J. (2004). Assessment of red blood cell and coagulation laboratory data. *AACN Clinical Issues, 15*(4), 622–637.

Rice, L., Nguyen, P. H., & Vann, A. R. (2002). Preventing complications in heparin-induced thrombocytopenia. *Postgraduate Medicine online.* Retrieved from http://www.postgradmed.com/issues/2002/09_02/rice.htm

Rogers, B. (2005). Looking at lymphoma & leukemia. *Nursing, 35*(7), 56–64.

Sadler, G. R., Wasserman, L., Fullerton, J. T., & Romero, M. (2004). Supporting patients through genetic screening for cancer risk. *Medsurg Nursing, 13*(4), 233–246.

Shelton, B. K. (2003). Evidence-based care for the neutropenic patient with leukemia. *Seminars in Oncology Nursing, 19*(2), 133–141.

Simmons, P. (2003). A primer for nurses who administer blood products. *Medsurg Nursing, 12*(3), 184–190.

Spahis, J. (2002). Human genetics: Constructing a family pedigree. *American Journal of Nursing, 102*(7), 44–49.

Spencer, J. W., & Jacobs, J. J. (2003). *Complementary and alternative medicine: An evidence-based approach* (2nd ed.). St. Louis, MO: Mosby.

Tariman, J. D., & Estrella, S. M. (2005). The changing treatment paradigm in patients with newly diagnosed multiple myeloma: Implications for nursing. *Oncology Nursing Forum, 32*(6), Online Exclusive: E127–38.

Tierney, L. M., Jr., McPhee, S. J., & Papadakis, M. A. (Eds.). (2005). *Current medical diagnosis & treatment* (44th ed.). New York: McGraw-Hill.

Treating the older patient with leukemia, lymphoma, and myeloma. (2004). *ONS News, 19*(9 Suppl), 77–78.

U.S. Food and Drug Administration, Center for Drug Evaluation and Research. (2001). *Drug information. Gleevec (imatinib mesylate) questions and answers.* Retrieved from http://www.fda.gov/cder/drug/infopage/gleevec/qa.htm

Viele, C. S. (2003). Diagnosis, treatment and nursing care of acute leukemia. *Seminars in Oncology Nursing, 19*(2), 109–117.

Waldman, A. R. (2003). Understanding non-Hodgkin's lymphomas. *Clinical Journal of Oncology Nursing, 7*(1), 93–96.

Wilkinson, J. M. (2005). *Nursing diagnosis handbook* (8th ed.). Upper Saddle River, NJ: Prentice Hall.

Wilson, C., & Sylvanus, T. (2005). Graft failure following allogeneic blood and marrow transplant: Evidence based nursing care study review. *Clinical Journal of Oncology Nursing, 9*(2), 151–159.

Wuicik, D. (2003). Molecular biology of leukemia. *Seminars in Oncology Nursing, 19*(2), 83–89.

CHAPTER 35 Nursing Care of Clients with Peripheral Vascular Disorders

LEARNING OUTCOMES

- Describe the etiology, pathophysiology, and manifestations of common peripheral vascular and lymphatic disorders.

- Compare and contrast the manifestations and effects of disorders affecting large and small vessels, arteries and veins.

- Explain risk factors for and measures to prevent peripheral vascular disorders and their complications.

- Explain the nursing implications for medications and other interdisciplinary treatments used for clients with peripheral vascular disorders.

- Describe preoperative and postoperative nursing care of clients having vascular surgery.

CLINICAL COMPETENCIES

- Assess clients with peripheral vascular disorders, using data to select and prioritize appropriate nursing diagnoses and identify desired outcomes of care.

- Identify the effects of peripheral vascular disorders on the functional health status of assigned clients.

- Use research and an evidence-based plan to provide individualized care for clients with peripheral vascular disorders.

- Collaborate with the interdisciplinary care team in planning and providing care for clients with peripheral vascular disorders.

- Safely and knowledgeably administer medications and prescribed treatments for clients with peripheral vascular disorders.

- Provide client and family teaching to promote, maintain, and restore health in clients with common peripheral vascular disorders.

MEDIALINK

Resources for this chapter can be found on the Prentice Hall Nursing MediaLink DVD-ROM accompanying this textbook, and on the Companion Website at http://www.prenhall.com/lemone

KEY TERMS

aneurysm, *1170*
atherosclerosis, *1176*
blood pressure, *1154*
chronic venous insufficiency, *1194*
deep venous thrombosis (DVT), *1186*
diastolic blood pressure, *1154*
dissection, *1172*
embolism, *1184*
hypertension, *1154*
intermittent claudication, *1172*

lymphedema, *1199*
mean arterial pressure (MAP), *1154*
peripheral vascular disease (PVD), *1176*
primary hypertension, *1155*
pulse pressure, *1154*
Raynaud's disease/phenomenon, *1182*
secondary hypertension, *1167*
systolic blood pressure, *1154*

thromboangiitis obliterans, *1180*
thromboembolus, *1184*
thrombus, *1184*
varicose veins, *1195*
vasoconstriction, *1176*
vasodilation, *1176*
venous thrombosis, *1186*

The major processes that interfere with peripheral blood flow and that of lymphatic fluid include constriction, obstruction, inflammation, and vasospasm. These conditions lead to disorders of blood pressure regulation, peripheral artery function, aortic structure, venous circulation, and lymphatic circulation.

A holistic approach is important when caring for clients with disorders of the peripheral vascular and lymphatic systems. The focus of care is on teaching long-term care measures, pain relief, improving peripheral blood and lymphatic circulation, preventing tissue damage, and promoting healing. The prescribed treatment may have emotional, social, and economic effects on the client and family.

DISORDERS OF BLOOD PRESSURE REGULATION

Blood flows through the circulatory system from areas of higher pressure to areas of lower pressure. The amount of pressure in any portion of the vascular system is affected by a number of factors, including blood volume, vascular resistance, and cardiac output. The **blood pressure** is the tension or pressure exerted by blood against arterial walls. A certain amount of pressure within the system is necessary to maintain open vessels, capillary perfusion, and oxygenation of all body tissues. Excess pressure, however, has harmful effects, increasing the workload of the heart, altering the structure of the vessels, and affecting sensitive body tissues such as the kidneys, eyes, and central nervous system (CNS).

This section focuses on **hypertension**, or excess pressure in the arterial portion of systemic circulation. Excessively low blood pressure, *hypotension,* is discussed in the shock section of Chapter 11 ∞. Altered pulmonary vascular pressures are discussed in Chapter 39 ∞.

Physiology Review

Blood flow through the circulatory system requires *sufficient blood volume* to fill the blood vessels and *pressure differences* within the system that allow blood to move forward. The arterial, or supply, side of the circulation has relatively high pressures created by the thick elastic walls of the arteries and arterioles. The venous, or return, side of the system, on the other hand, is a low-pressure system of thin-walled, distensible veins. Blood flows through the capillaries linking these two systems from the higher pressure arterial side to the lower pressure venous side.

The arterial blood pressure is created by the ejection of blood from the heart during systole (*cardiac output* or *CO*) and the tension, or resistance to blood flow, created by the elastic arterial walls (*systemic vascular resistance* or *SVR*). The blood pressure rises as the heart contracts during systole, ejecting its blood. This pressure wave, or the **systolic blood pressure**, is felt as the peripheral pulse and heard as the Korotkoff's sounds during blood pressure measurement. In healthy adults the average systolic pressure is less than 120 mmHg. During diastole, or cardiac relaxation and filling, elastic arterial walls maintain a minimum pressure, the **diastolic blood pressure**, to maintain blood flow through the capillary beds. The average diastolic pressure in a healthy adult is less than 80 mmHg. The difference between the systolic and diastolic pressure, normally about 40 mmHg, is known as the **pulse pressure**. The **mean arterial pressure (MAP)** is the average pressure in the arterial circulation throughout the cardiac cycle. It can be calculated using the formula [systolic BP + 2 (diastolic BP)] / 3.

PRACTICE ALERT
- Cardiac output and systemic (or peripheral) vascular resistance are the primary factors that determine blood pressure.
- A decrease in cardiac output (e.g., due to hemorrhage) or decreased peripheral vascular resistance (e.g., systemic vasodilation) cause the blood pressure to fall.
- Increased cardiac output (e.g., during exercise) or increased peripheral vascular resistance (e.g., vasoconstriction due to drug administration) cause the blood pressure to rise.

Cardiac output is determined by the blood volume and the ability of the ventricles to fill and effectively pump that blood. A number of factors contribute to systemic vascular resistance, including vessel length, blood viscosity, and vessel diameter and distensibility (compliance). While vessel length and blood viscosity remain relatively constant, vessel diameter and compliance are subject to normal regulatory activities and disease.

The arterioles normally determine the SVR as their diameter changes in response to a variety of stimuli:

- *Sympathetic nervous system (SNS)* stimulation. Baroreceptors in the aortic arch and carotid sinus signal the SNS via the cardiovascular control center in the medulla when the MAP changes. A drop in MAP stimulates the SNS, increasing the heart rate and cardiac output, and constricting arterioles (except in skeletal muscle). As a result, BP rises. A rise in MAP has the opposite effect, decreasing the heart rate and cardiac output, and causing arteriolar vasodilation.
- *Circulating epinephrine and norepinephrine* from the adrenal cortex (e.g., the fight-or-flight response) have the same effect as SNS stimulation.
- *Renin–angiotensin–aldosterone system* responds to renal perfusion. A drop in renal perfusion stimulates renin release. Renin converts angiotensinogen to angiotensin I, which is subsequently converted to angiotensin II in the lungs by angiotensin-converting enzyme (ACE). Angiotensin II is a potent vasoconstrictor. It also promotes sodium and water retention both directly and by stimulating the adrenal medulla to release aldosterone. Both SVR and CO increase, raising BP.
- *Atrial natriuretic peptide (ANP)* and *brain natriuretic peptide (BNP)* are released from atrial cells in response to stretching by excess blood volume. These hormones promote vasodilation and sodium and water excretion, lowering BP.
- *Adrenomedullin* is a peptide synthesized and released by endothelial and smooth muscle cells in blood vessels. It is a potent vasodilator.

- *Vasopressin* or *antidiuretic hormone* (from the posterior pituitary gland) promotes water retention and vasoconstriction, raising BP.
- *Local factors* such as inflammatory mediators and various metabolites can promote vasodilation, affecting BP.

In addition to the preceding, the primary factor affecting vessel compliance is the extent of arteriosclerosis (hardening of the arteries) and atherosclerosis (plaque accumulation). Figure 35–1 ■ summarizes the interrelationships of major factors regulating blood pressure.

FAST FACTS

- Sympathetic nervous system stimulation, epinephrine and norepinephrine, and the hormones angiotensin II and vasopressin (antidiuretic hormone or ADH) are *vasoconstrictors,* increasing the blood pressure.
- Parasympathetic nervous system stimulation and the hormones ANP, BNP, and adrenomedullin are *vasodilators,* decreasing the blood pressure.
- The hormones aldosterone and ADH promote sodium and water retention, increasing the blood pressure.

THE CLIENT WITH PRIMARY HYPERTENSION

Primary hypertension, also known as *essential hypertension,* is a persistently elevated systemic blood pressure. About 50 to 65 million people in the United States have hypertension (American Heart Association [AHA], 2005; National Heart, Lung, and Blood Institute [NHLBI], 2004b). More than 90% of these have primary hypertension, which has no identified cause.

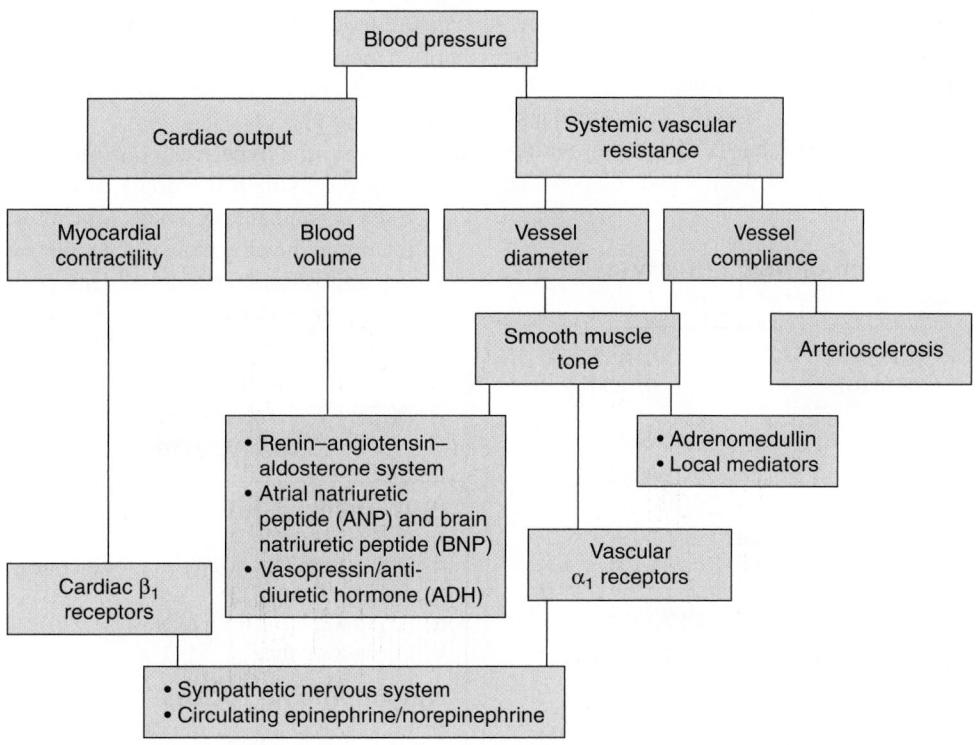

Figure 35–1 ■ Factors affecting blood pressure.

Hypertension is defined as systolic blood pressure of 140 mmHg or higher, or diastolic pressure of 90 mmHg or higher, based on the average of three or more readings taken on separate occasions (NHLBI, 2004b). Exceptions include clients being treated for hypertension and an initial reading of a systolic pressure of 210 mmHg or higher and/or a diastolic blood pressure of 120 mmHg or higher. Table 35–1 identifies classifications of blood pressure for adults age 18 and older as defined by the Joint National Committee.

Hypertension is an important public health issue: While it rarely causes symptoms or noticeably limits the client's functional health, hypertension is a major risk factor for coronary heart disease, heart failure, stroke, and renal failure. Hypertension and its consequences are not unique to the United States. The World Health Organization identifies blood pressure above optimal levels (a systolic BP > 115 mmHg) as responsible for 62% of cerebrovascular disease and 49% of ischemic heart disease worldwide (NHLBI, 2004b).

While the identification and treatment of hypertension in the United States has improved significantly in the past 25 years, approximately 30% of hypertensive adults remain unaware of their condition. Although 59% of hypertensive adults are being treated for the disorder, effective blood pressure control is achieved in only about 34% (NHLBI, 2004b).

Incidence and Risk Factors

Hypertension primarily affects middle-aged and older adults: More than 50% of people ages 60 to 69 and about 75% of those age 70 and older are hypertensive (NHLBI, 2004b). An age-related increase in the systolic blood pressure is the primary factor leading to the high incidence of hypertension in older adults. Unlike the diastolic blood pressure, which tends to rise until approximately age 50, then level off, the systolic blood pressure continues to rise with aging (NHLBI, 2004b).

The prevalence of hypertension is significantly higher in blacks than in whites and Hispanics. Nearly 40% of black adults are hypertensive, whereas less than 30% of adult white and Hispanic people are affected. In whites and Hispanics, more males than females are hypertensive; in blacks, more women than men are affected (NHLBI, 2004a). Essential hypertension affects people of all income groups, having great financial effects because of its effects on other body systems.

FAST FACTS

- Almost one-third of the adult population in the United States has hypertension.
- The prevalence of hypertension is highest in African American females and lowest in people of Asian ancestry.
- The prevalence of hypertension is higher among people who live in the southeastern United States.
- Up until age 55, more men than women are affected by hypertension; after that it affects more women than men.
- Hypertension increases the risk of stroke to about four times that of people with normal blood pressure, and the risk for heart failure by two to three times that of people with normal blood pressure (AHA, 2005).

A number of risk factors have been identified for primary hypertension (Box 35–1). Genetics plays a role, as do environmental factors.

- *Family history.* Studies show a genetic link in about 30% of people with primary hypertension (Kasper et al., 2005). Genes involved in the renin–angiotensin–aldosterone system and others that affect vascular tone, salt and water transportation in the kidney, obesity, and insulin resistance are likely involved in the development of hypertension, although no consistent genetic linkages have been found.
- *Age.* The incidence of hypertension rises with increasing age. Aging affects baroreceptors involved in blood pressure regulation as well as arterial compliance. As the arteries become less compliant, pressure within the vessels increases. This is often most apparent as a gradual increase in the systolic pressure with aging. See the Nursing Care of the Older Adult box on page 1157.
- *Race.* Essential hypertension is more common and more severe in blacks than in people of other ethnic backgrounds (see the accompanying Focus on Cultural Diversity box). It also tends to develop at an earlier age, and is associated with more cardiovascular and renal damage. More African Americans with hypertension have low renin levels and altered re-

TABLE 35–1 Classification of Blood Pressure for Adults[a]

CATEGORY	SYSTOLIC (mmHG)		DIASTOLIC (mmHG)
Normal	<120	and	<80
Prehypertension	120–139	or	80–89
Hypertension[b]			
Stage 1	140–159	or	90–99
Stage 2	≥160	or	≥100

[a]When systolic and diastolic blood pressures fall into different categories, the higher category is used to classify blood pressure status.
[b]Based on the average of two or more readings taken at each of two or more visits after an initial screening.
Source: Adapted from *The Seventh Report of the Joint National Committee on Prevention, Detection, Education, and Treatment of High Blood Pressure,* NIH Publication No. 04-5250 by NHLBI, 2004b, Bethesda, MD: National Institutes of Health. Retrieved from http://www.nhlbi.nih.gov/guidelines/hypertension.

BOX 35–1 Factors Contributing to Hypertension

Modifiable Factors
- High sodium intake
- Low potassium, calcium, and magnesium intake
- Obesity
- Excess alcohol consumption
- Insulin resistance

Nonmodifiable Factors
- Genetic factors
- Family history
- Age
- Race

NURSING CARE OF THE OLDER ADULT Hypertension

Controlling high blood pressure is as important in the older adult as in younger adults. In the United States, the lifetime risk of hypertension is about 90% in men and women who live to age 80 to 85 (NHLBI, 2004b). Systolic hypertension is common, as is an elevated pulse pressure (systolic BP minus diastolic BP), indicating decreased compliance of large arteries. Despite this fact, less than two-thirds of people over age 80 who have high blood pressure are being treated and only 38% of men and 23% of women undergoing treatment had blood pressures that met established targets (NHLBI, 2005).

The Framingham Heart Study shows that cardiovascular deaths are two to five times more common in older adults with isolated systolic hypertension than in people with normal blood pressures. Stroke also is more common in older adults with sys-

tolic hypertension. These findings appear to relate to changes in blood vessels associated with aging: decreased compliance and decreased baroreceptor sensitivity. Decreased compliance impairs the ability of the vessels to expand and contract with varying amounts of blood, increasing peripheral vascular resistance and decreasing renal blood flow.

To obtain accurate blood pressure readings for older clients, slightly different procedures may be required. Palpation of the artery during cuff inflation is recommended to prevent inaccurate systolic readings due to an auscultatory gap, present in many older adults. The reflexes that maintain blood pressure during position changes diminish with aging. Allow the older client to sit upright or stand for 2 to 5 minutes before evaluating the blood pressure for true orthostatic readings.

---

nal excretion of sodium at normal blood pressure levels. This genetic tendency to conserve salt may have developed as an adaptation to working in a warm environment, when salt and water conservation are beneficial (Porth, 2005).

- *Mineral intake.* High sodium intake often is associated with fluid retention. Hypertension related to sodium intake involves a number of different physiologic mechanisms, including the renin–angiotensin–aldosterone system, nitric oxide, catecholamines, endothelin, and ANP (Copstead & Banasik, 2005). Low potassium, calcium, and magnesium intakes also contribute to hypertension by unknown mechanisms. The ratio of sodium to potassium intake appears to play a role, possibly through the effects of increased potassium intake on sodium excretion. Potassium also promotes vasodilation by reducing responses to catecholamines and angiotensin II. Calcium also has a vasodilator effect. While magnesium has been shown to reduce the blood pressure, the mechanism of action is unclear.

- *Obesity.* Central obesity (fat cell deposits in the abdomen), determined by an increased waist-to-hip ratio, has a stronger correlation with hypertension than body mass index or skinfold thickness. Although a clear correlation exists between obesity and hypertension, the relationship may be one of com-

mon cause: Genetic factors appear to play a role in the common triad of obesity, hypertension, and insulin resistance.

- *Insulin resistance.* Insulin resistance with resulting hyperinsulinemia is linked with hypertension by its effects of excess circulating insulin on the sympathetic nervous system, vascular smooth muscle, renal regulation of sodium and water, and ion transport across cell membranes. Insulin resistance may be a genetic or an acquired trait. Although it is more commonly seen in obese individuals, insulin resistance also has been found in people of normal weight.

- *Excess alcohol consumption.* Regular consumption of three or more drinks a day increases the risk of hypertension. Decreasing or discontinuing alcohol consumption reduces the blood pressure, particularly systolic readings. Lifestyle factors associated with excessive alcohol intake (obesity and lack of exercise) may contribute to hypertension as well.

- *Stress.* Physical and emotional stress cause transient elevations of blood pressure, but the role of stress in primary hypertension is less clear. Blood pressure normally fluctuates throughout the day, increasing with activity, discomfort, or emotional responses such as anger. Frequent or continued stress may cause vascular smooth muscle hypertrophy or affect central integrative pathways of the brain (Porth, 2005).

Pathophysiology

Primary hypertension is thought to develop from complex interactions among factors that regulate cardiac output and systemic vascular resistance. These interactions may include:

- Excess sympathetic nervous system with overstimulation of α- and β-adrenergic receptors, resulting in vasoconstriction and increased cardiac output.

- Altered function of the renin–angiotensin–aldosterone system and its responsiveness to factors such as sodium intake and overall fluid volume. The renin–angiotensin–aldosterone system affects vasomotor tone and salt and water excretion. Chronically high levels of angiotensin II lead to arteriolar remodeling, which permanently increases SVR. In approximately 20% of people with primary hypertension, renin levels are lower

FOCUS ON CULTURAL DIVERSITY
Hypertension in African Americans

- The prevalence of hypertension among African Americans living in the United States is among the highest in the world: in African American adults, 41.8% of males and 45.4% of females are hypertensive.
  - African Americans with the highest risk for hypertension tend to be:
    - Middle aged or older
    - Less educated
    - Overweight or obese
    - Physically inactive
    - Affected by diabetes (AHA, 2005).

than normal. Increased sodium intake increases the blood pressure in these clients. Low plasma renin levels are more commonly seen in African Americans than in whites. Another 15% of clients with hypertension have higher than normal plasma renin levels. For these clients, salt intake has less of an effect on blood pressure (Kasper et al., 2005). Most people with hypertension have normal levels of renin activity.

- Other chemical mediators of vasomotor tone and blood volume such as atrial natriuretic peptide also play a role by affecting vasomotor tone and sodium and water excretion. Vascular endothelium itself produces hormones (*endothelins*) that also affect vasomotor tone. Endothelin-1 is a potent vasoconstrictor (Copstead & Banasik, 2005).
- The interaction between insulin resistance, hyperinsulinemia, and endothelial function may be a primary cause of hypertension. Excess insulin has several effects that potentially contribute to hypertension: (1) sodium retention by the kidneys, (2) increased SNS activity, (3) hypertrophy of vascular smooth muscle, and (4) changes in ion transport across cell membranes (Kasper et al., 2005).

The result is sustained increases in blood volume and peripheral resistance. The cardiovascular system adapts to increased blood volume by increasing cardiac output. Autoregulatory mechanisms in the systemic arteries react to the increased volume, causing vasoconstriction. The increased systemic vascular resistance causes hypertension.

It appears unlikely that one single cause and pathologic process will be found to account for essential hypertension. Increasingly, evidence points to hypertension as a diverse group of pathophysiologic mechanisms resulting in the common manifestation of elevated blood pressure.

Manifestations

The early stages of primary hypertension typically are asymptomatic, marked only by elevated blood pressure. Blood pressure elevations are initially transient but eventually become permanent. When symptoms do appear, they are usually vague. Headache, usually in the back of the head and neck, may be present on awakening, subsiding during the day. Other symptoms result from target organ damage, and may include nocturia, confusion, nausea and vomiting, and visual disturbances. Examination of the retina of the eye may reveal narrowed arterioles, hemorrhages, exudates, and *papilledema* (swelling of the optic nerve).

Complications

Sustained hypertension affects the cardiovascular, neurologic, and renal systems. The rate of atherosclerosis accelerates, increasing the risk for coronary heart disease and stroke. The workload of the left ventricle increases, leading to ventricular hypertrophy, which then increases the risk for coronary heart disease, dysrhythmias, and heart failure. The diastolic blood pressure is a significant cardiovascular risk factor until age 50; the systolic pressure then becomes the more important factor contributing to cardiovascular risk (NHLBI, 2004b). Most deaths due to hypertension result from coronary heart

disease and acute myocardial infarction or heart failure (Kasper et al., 2005).

Accelerated atherosclerosis associated with hypertension increases the risk for cerebral infarction (stroke). Increased pressure in the cerebral vessels can lead to development of microaneurysms and an increased risk for cerebral hemorrhage. *Hypertensive encephalopathy,* a syndrome characterized by extremely high blood pressure, altered level of consciousness, increased intracranial pressure, papilledema, and seizures, may develop. Its etiology is unclear.

Hypertension also can lead to nephrosclerosis and renal insufficiency. Proteinuria and microscopic hematuria develop, as well as signs of chronic renal failure. Blacks experience hypertensive kidney disease more frequently than whites. Renal failure causes about 10% of deaths attributed to hypertension (Kasper et al., 2005).

INTERDISCIPLINARY CARE

Hypertension management focuses on reducing the blood pressure to less than 140 mmHg systolic and 90 mmHg diastolic. The ultimate goal of hypertension management is to reduce cardiovascular and renal morbidity and mortality. The risk of cardiovascular complications (coronary heart disease, heart failure, stroke) decreases when the average blood pressure is less than 140/90; when the client also has diabetes or renal disease, the treatment goal is a blood pressure of less than 130/80. It now is recognized that most people with hypertension will require a combination of two or more drugs along with lifestyle changes to achieve recommended blood pressure levels (NHLBI, 2004b). Although there is no cure for hypertension, it can be controlled. Figure 35–2 ■ shows the recommended algorithm for hypertension management.

Diagnosis

The client with hypertension is evaluated for the presence of identifiable causes of hypertension, cardiovascular risk factors, and the presence or absence of target organ damage (heart, brain, kidneys, peripheral vascular systems, and retina of the eye). Before treatment is started, the following diagnostic tests are performed:

- Electrocardiogram (ECG)
- Urinalysis
- Blood glucose
- Hematocrit
- Serum potassium, creatinine, and calcium
- Cholesterol and lipoprotein profile, including HDL, LDL, and triglycerides.

Additional tests that may be done include urinary albumin excretion, evaluation of the glomerular filtration rate (such as the creatinine clearance), and tests for emerging cardiovascular risk factors such as C-reactive protein and homocystine levels.

Lifestyle Modifications

Lifestyle modifications are recommended for all clients whose blood pressure falls within the prehypertension range (120–139/80–89) and everyone with intermittent or sustained

Figure 35–2 ■ Algorithm for treating hypertension.

Source: Adapted from *The Seventh Report of the Joint National Committee on Prevention, Detection, Evaluation, and Treatment of High Blood Pressure* (2004b). National Heart, Lung, and Blood Institute, Bethesda, MD: National Institutes of Health.

hypertension. These modifications include weight loss, dietary changes, restricted alcohol use and cigarette smoking, increased physical activity, and stress reduction (Box 35–2).

BOX 35–2 Lifestyle Modifications for Hypertension

- Maintain normal body weight; lose weight if overweight.
- Dietary modifications:
  - Eat a diet rich in fruits, vegetables, and low-fat dairy products.
  - Reduce sodium intake.
  - Reduce intake of cholesterol, total and saturated fat.
- Limit alcohol intake to no more than 1 oz of ethanol (1/2 oz for women and lighter weight people) per day.
- Engage in aerobic exercise for 30 minutes most days of the week (5 to 6).
- Stop smoking.
- Use stress management techniques such as relaxation therapy.

DIET Dietary approaches to managing hypertension focus on reducing sodium intake, maintaining adequate potassium and calcium intakes, and reducing total and saturated fat intake. A mild to moderate sodium restriction (no added salt) lowers blood pressure and potentiates the effect of antihypertensive drugs for most hypertensive clients. The DASH (Dietary Approaches to Stop Hypertension) diet has proven beneficial effects in lowering blood pressure. This diet (Box 35–3) focuses on whole foods rather than individual nutrients. It is rich in fruits and vegetables (up to 10 servings per day), and low in total and saturated fats.

Weight loss is recommended for clients who are obese. Loss of as little as 10 pounds (4.5 kg) reduces blood pressure in many people (NHLBI, 2004b). A balanced diet such as the DASH diet is recommended for weight loss.

PHYSICAL ACTIVITY Regular exercise (such as walking, cycling, jogging, or swimming) reduces blood pressure and contributes to weight loss, stress reduction, and feelings of overall

BOX 35-3 DASH Diet Recommendations

- Grains—7 to 8 servings per day
- Vegetables—4 to 5 servings per day
- Fruits—4 to 5 servings per day
- Nonfat/low-fat dairy products—2 to 3 servings per day
- Meats, poultry, and fish—2 or less 3-oz servings per day
- Nuts, seeds, and dry beans—4 to 5 servings per week
- Fats and oils—2 to 3 servings per day
- Sweets—5 servings per week (should be low in fat)

well-being. Previously sedentary clients are encouraged to engage in aerobic exercise for 30 to 45 minutes per day most days of the week (5 to 6 days). Isometric exercise (such as weight training) may not be appropriate, because it can raise the systolic blood pressure.

ALCOHOL AND TOBACCO USE The recommended alcohol intake for clients with hypertension is no more than 1 oz of ethanol or two drinks per day. A drink is 12 oz of beer, 5 oz of wine, or 1.5 oz of 80-proof whiskey. Women and lighter weight people should reduce this limit by half. Although alcohol withdrawal may increase blood pressure, this is usually temporary and diminishes as abstinence or restricted intake continues.

Although nicotine is a vasoconstrictor, substantial data linking smoking to hypertension are lacking. A definitive link exists between smoking and heart disease, however. Clients who smoke are strongly urged to quit. Smoking also reduces the effect of some antihypertensive medications such as propranolol (Inderal). Smoking cessation aids such as nicotine patches and gum contain lower amounts of nicotine and usually do not raise blood pressure.

STRESS REDUCTION Stress stimulates the sympathetic nervous system, increasing vasoconstriction, systemic vascular resistance, cardiac output, and the blood pressure. Regular, moderate exercise is the treatment of choice for reducing stress in hypertensive clients. Relaxation techniques such as biofeedback, therapeutic touch, yoga, and meditation to relax both mind and body may also lower blood pressure, although their effect has not been proven in hypertension management.

Medications

Current pharmacologic treatment of hypertension involves using one or more of the following drug classes: diuretics, beta-adrenergic blockers, centrally acting sympatholytics, vasodilators, ACE inhibitors, angiotensin II receptor blockers (ARBs), and calcium channel blockers. For most clients, two or more antihypertensive drugs selected from different drug classes are necessary to achieve effective control. These drug classes have different sites of action (Figure 35–3 ■). Nursing implications for administration of antihypertensive drugs (other than diuretics) are outlined on pages 1161–1162.

DRUG CLASSES Diuretics are the preferred treatment for systolic hypertension in older adults. Diuretics are relatively safe and well-tolerated drugs; in addition, most are relatively inexpensive. Thiazide diuretics, such as hydrochlorothiazide (HydroDIURIL),

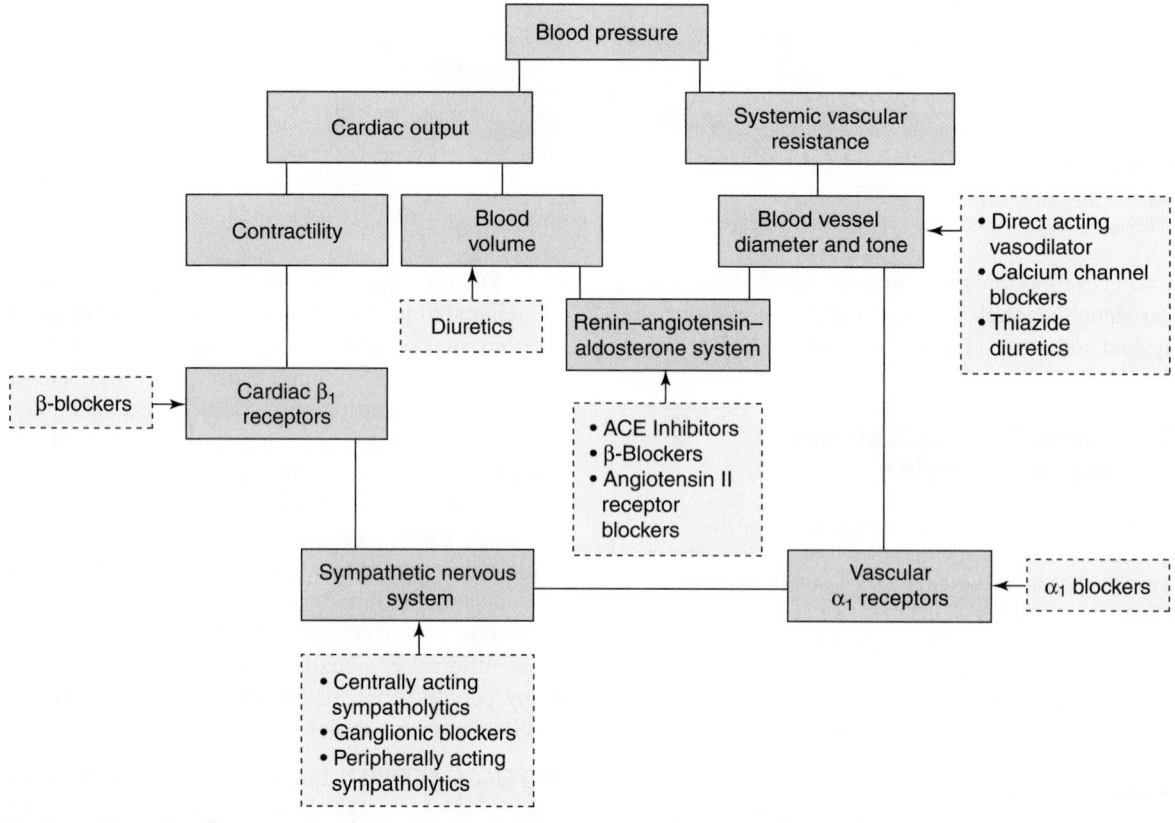

Figure 35–3 ■ Sites of antihypertensive drug action.

MEDICATION ADMINISTRATION Antihypertensive Drugs

ALPHA-ADRENERGIC BLOCKERS
Doxazosin (Cardura)
Prazosin (Minipress)
Terazosin (Hytrin)
Alpha-adrenergic blocking agents block alpha-receptors in vascular smooth muscle, decreasing vasomotor tone and vasoconstriction. They also reduce serum levels of low-density lipoproteins (LDL) and very low-density lipoproteins (VLDL). However, vasodilation may cause orthostatic hypotension and reflex stimulation of the heart, resulting in tachycardia and palpitations. A beta-blocker may be ordered to minimize this effect.

Nursing Responsibilities
- Give the first dose at bedtime to minimize risk of fainting (called "first-dose syncope"). If the first dose is given in the daytime (or if the dose is increased), instruct to remain in bed for 3 to 4 hours.
- Assess blood pressure and apical pulse before each dose and as indicated thereafter.

Health Education for the Client and Family
- There is a risk of fainting after taking the first dose of this drug. Take the drug at bedtime to reduce this risk, and do not drive or engage in other hazardous activities for 12 to 24 hours after the first dose.
- This drug may cause dizziness or light-headedness. Change positions slowly, and sit down if you become dizzy or light-headed.
- Notify your primary care provider if you develop nasal congestion or impotence while taking this drug.
- Notify your primary care provider before discontinuing this medication.

ANGIOTENSIN-CONVERTING ENZYME (ACE) INHIBITORS
Benazepril (Lotensin)	**Moexipril (Univasc)**
Captopril (Capoten)	**Perindopril (Aceon)**
Enalapril (Vasotec)	**Quinapril (Accupril)**
Fosinopril (Monopril)	**Ramipril (Altace)**
Lisinopril (Prinivil, Zestril)	**Trandolapril (Mavik)**

ANGIOTENSIN II RECEPTOR BLOCKERS (ARBS)
Candesartan (Atacand)	**Olmesartan (Benicar)**
Eprosartan (Teveten)	**Telmisartan (Micardis)**
Irbesartan (Avapro)	**Valsartan (Diovan)**
Losartan (Cozaar)	

The ACE inhibitors lower blood pressure by preventing conversion of angiotensin I to angiotensin II. This in turn prevents vasoconstriction and sodium and water retention. ARBs have the same effect, but they act by blocking the effect of angiotensin II on receptors. Both ACE inhibitors and ARBs are less effective in black clients and are contraindicated in pregnancy (Lehne, 2004). Their primary adverse effects are persistent cough, first-dose hypotension, and hyperkalemia.

Nursing Responsibilities
- Assess blood pressure and WBC before giving the first dose. Monitor blood pressure for 2 hours after the first dose and regularly thereafter.
- Administer PO 1 hour before meals; tablets may be crushed.
- Report changes in WBC or differential, hyperkalemia, or changes in BUN or serum creatinine to the primary care provider.

- Do not administer to clients with renal artery stenosis or who are pregnant.
- Immediately report and treat manifestations of angioedema (giant wheals and edema of the tongue, glottis, and pharynx). Initiate resuscitation measures as needed. Discontinue drug immediately and do not use in the future.

Health Education for the Client and Family
- Report peripheral edema, signs of infection, or difficulty breathing to your primary care provider.
- Change position (lying to sitting and sitting to standing) slowly to prevent dizziness; sit down if dizziness or light-headedness develops.
- Do not take a potassium supplement or use a potassium-based salt substitute while taking this drug unless prescribed by your physician.
- Notify your physician if you become pregnant while taking this drug. Although it is safe early in pregnancy, taking the drug during the second and third trimesters may harm the fetus.

BETA-ADRENERGIC BLOCKING AGENTS
Acebutolol (Sectral)	**Nadolol (Corgard)**
Atenolol (Tenormin)	**Penbutolol (Levatol)**
Betaxolol (Kerlone)	**Pindolol (Visken)**
Bisoprolol (Zebeta)	**Propranolol (Inderal)**
Metoprolol tartrate (Lopressor)	**Timolol (Blocadren)**

Combined with an alpha-blocker:
Carvedilol (Coreg)	**Labetalol (Normodyne)**

Beta-adrenergic blockers are commonly used to control hypertension. Beta-blockers reduce blood pressure by preventing beta-receptor stimulation in the heart, thereby decreasing heart rate and cardiac output. Beta-blockers also interfere with renin release by the kidneys, decreasing the effects of angiotensin and aldosterone. Potential adverse effects of beta-blockers include bronchospasm, fatigue, sleep disturbances, nightmares, bradycardia, heart block, worsening of heart failure, gastrointestinal disturbances, impotence, and increased triglyceride levels.

Nursing Responsibilities
- Before giving initial dose, assess for contraindications to beta-blockers such as asthma, chronic lung disease, bradycardia, or heart block.
- Assess blood pressure and apical pulse before giving; notify primary care provider if vital signs are outside established parameters.
- Report adverse effects such as bradycardia, decreased cardiac output (fatigue, dyspnea with exertion, hypotension, decreased level of consciousness), heart failure, heart block, bronchoconstriction (wheezing, dyspnea), or altered blood glucose levels (in diabetic clients).
- Carefully monitor responses of the older client.

Health Education for the Client and Family
- Monitor blood pressure and pulse daily as instructed.
- Change position (lying to sitting and sitting to standing) slowly to prevent dizziness and possible falls.
- Report effects such as fatigue, lethargy, and impotence to your primary care provider.
- Notify your physician if you become short of breath or develop a cough or swelling of your extremities.

(continued)

MEDICATION ADMINISTRATION   Antihypertensive Drugs (continued)

- If you have diabetes, check blood glucose levels more frequently because hypoglycemia may develop with few symptoms.
- Talk to your primary care provider before taking any over-the-counter medications.
- Carry an adequate supply of the drug when traveling. Do not stop taking this drug without notifying your primary care provider.

CALCIUM CHANNEL BLOCKERS

Amlodipine (Norvasc)	Nicardipine (Cardene)
Diltiazem (Cardizem)	Nifedipine (Procardia)
Felodipine (Plendil)	Nisoldipine (Sular)
Isradipine (DynaCirc)	Verapamil (Isoptin)

Calcium channel blockers inhibit the flow of calcium ions across the cell membrane of vascular tissue and cardiac cells. In doing so, they relax arterial smooth muscle, lowering peripheral resistance through vasodilation. Calcium channel blockers can cause reflex tachycardia, and some (e.g., verapamil and diltiazem) may impair cardiac function, worsening heart failure.

Nursing Responsibilities

- Assess blood pressure, apical pulse, and liver and renal function tests prior to giving these drugs.
- Calcium channel blockers may be given orally or intravenously.
- Do not administer verapamil or diltiazem to clients with severe hypotension, sinus, or atrioventricular blocks. Administer with caution to clients also taking digoxin or a beta-blocker.
- Periodically monitor blood pressure and apical pulse during therapy. Promptly report signs of bradycardia, AV block, or heart failure to the physician.

Health Education for the Client and Family

- Take blood pressure and pulse daily as taught. Notify your physician if your pulse is less than 60 bpm or your blood pressure is not within the specified range.
- This drug may cause constipation. Drink six to eight glasses of water each day, and increase fiber in diet.
- Report shortness of breath, weight gain, or swelling in feet or ankles to your primary care provider.

CENTRALLY ACTING SYMPATHOLYTICS

Clonidine (Catapres)	Methyldopa (Aldomet)
Guanfacine (Tenex)	Reserpine (generic)

The centrally acting sympatholytics stimulate the α_2-receptors in the CNS to suppress sympathetic outflow to the heart and blood vessels. A fall in cardiac output and vasodilation result, reducing blood pressure. Dry mouth and sedation are common adverse effects. Severe reflex hypertension may occur if abruptly discontinued. Clonidine is contraindicated during pregnancy; methyldopa is contraindicated for clients with active liver disease.

Nursing Responsibilities

- Assess for contraindications to therapy. Obtain baseline blood pressure, CBC, Coombs' test, and liver function studies.
- Administer oral doses at bedtime to minimize effects of sedation.
- Methyldopa may be given intravenously for hypertensive emergencies.

- Apply transdermal clonidine patch to dry, hairless area of intact skin on the chest or upper arm. Assess for rash, which indicates allergy, at area of application.
- Promptly report changes in laboratory values to the physician. Discontinue methyldopa if manifestations of liver dysfunction develop.

Health Education for the Client and Family

- Relieve dry mouth by sipping water or chewing sugarless gum.
- Take with meals if gastric upset or nausea develop.
- Change position (lying to sitting and sitting to standing) slowly to prevent dizziness and possible falls.
- Do not suddenly discontinue medication or skip doses; this could cause serious hypertension.
- Report mental depression or decreased mental acuity to your healthcare provider.
- Side effects (such as dry mouth, nausea, and dizziness) tend to diminish over time.
- Do not drive a car if the medications cause drowsiness.

VASODILATORS

Hydralazine (Apresoline)	Minoxidil (Loniten)

Vasodilators reduce blood pressure by relaxing vascular smooth muscle (especially in the arterioles), and decreasing peripheral vascular resistance. These drugs are often prescribed in combination with a diuretic or beta-blocker, because they can cause reflex tachycardia and fluid retention. Because these drugs can have significant toxic effects, they are not routinely used to manage chronic hypertension.

Nursing Responsibilities

- Hydralazine may be given orally or intravenously; minoxidil is given orally.
- Assess blood pressure and pulse before giving the drug and monitor during therapy as indicated. Report tachycardia or hypotension to the physician.
- Report peripheral edema and manifestations of volume overload and heart failure.
- Immediately report muffled heart sounds or paradoxical pulse because pericardial effusion and possible cardiac tamponade may develop during minoxidil therapy.
- Discontinue hydralazine and report manifestations of a systemic lupus erythematosus (SLE) like syndrome: muscle or joint pain, fever, or symptoms of nephritis or pericarditis.

Health Education for the Client and Family

- Change position (lying to sitting and sitting to standing) slowly to prevent dizziness and possible falls.
- Report muscle, joint aches, and fever to your healthcare provider.
- Headache, palpitations, and rapid pulse may develop but should abate in about 10 days.
- Do not discontinue the medication without talking to your healthcare provider.
- Minoxidil may cause excessive hair growth. Contact your physician if this becomes troublesome.

are widely used. In major clinical studies, treatment with a single diuretic controlled blood pressure in about 50% of the clients and reduced hypertension-linked morbidity and mortality related to coronary heart disease. Diuretics control hypertension primarily by preventing tubular reabsorption of sodium, thus promoting sodium and water excretion and reducing blood volume. Thiazide diuretics also reduce systemic vascular resistance through an unknown mechanism. Diuretics are particularly effective in blacks and in clients who are obese, older, or who have increased plasma volume or low renin activity. The adverse effects of diuretics generally are dose related. In addition to hypokalemia, diuretics may affect serum levels of glucose, triglycerides, uric acid, LDLs, and insulin. More information about diuretics can be found in Chapters 10 and 29 ∞.

Clients with heart failure, coronary heart disease (CHD), or diabetes may initially be treated with a beta-blocker. These drugs lower blood pressure, apparently by reducing peripheral vascular resistance. They may also reduce the amount of renin released by the kidneys by blocking $beta_1$-receptors in the kidney. Beta-blockers reduce the risk of complications such as heart failure and stroke. They are, however, relatively contraindicated for clients with asthma or chronic obstructive pulmonary disease, because they promote bronchial constriction.

ACE inhibitors and ARBs also are commonly used in initial treatment of hypertension, particularly for clients who are diabetic or who have heart failure, a history of myocardial infarction (MI), or chronic kidney disease. ACE inhibitors block formation of angiotensin II by inhibiting the action of angiotensin-converting enzyme. Angiotensin II is a potent vasoconstrictor that also stimulates aldosterone release from the adrenal gland; blocking its action prevents vasoconstriction and sodium and water retention resulting from aldosterone release. ARBs have a very similar effect, although their action is to block angiotensin II receptors, thus preventing its vasoconstrictive and volume expansion effects.

Several drug classes work through their ability to promote vasodilation and reduce peripheral vascular resistance. Alpha-blockers such as prazosin and terazosin block stimulation of $alpha_1$-receptors on arterioles and veins, preventing vasoconstriction. Because of their ability to dilate both arterioles and veins, alpha-blockers can cause significant orthostatic hypotension, particularly following the initial dose. Calcium channel blockers promote dilation of arterioles, the primary regulators of peripheral vascular resistance. These drugs can cause reflex tachycardia. Some calcium channel blockers, verapamil and diltiazem in particular, also suppress heart function, reducing stroke volume and cardiac output. Reflex tachycardia is minimal with these calcium channel blockers. Direct-acting vasodilators such as hydralazine and minoxidil also directly affect the arterioles, reducing peripheral vascular resistance. These drugs have little effect on veins, so the risk of orthostatic hypotension is minimal. They are, however, associated with reflex tachycardia and fluid retention, so rarely are administered as in single-drug treatment regimens.

Other factors considered in selecting drugs for treating hypertension include demographic characteristics of the client, concurrent conditions, quality of life, cost, and possible interactions among prescribed drugs. In general, diuretics and calcium channel blockers are more effective for treating hypertension in blacks than beta-blockers or ACE inhibitors. Beta-blockers are preferred to treat hypertension with concurrent coronary heart disease and angina, but are contraindicated for clients who have asthma or depression. Beta-blockers also reduce exercise tolerance and may adversely affect lifestyle for some clients.

DRUG REGIMENS Treatment usually is initiated using a single antihypertensive drug at a low dose. Unless otherwise indicated, a diuretic is recommended as the initial drug of choice. The dose is slowly increased until optimal blood pressure control is achieved. If the drug does not effectively lower the blood pressure or has troubling side effects, a different drug from another class of antihypertensive medications is substituted. If, on the other hand, the drug is tolerated well but has not lowered blood pressure to the desired level, a second drug from another class may be added to the treatment regimen.

Treatment of clients with stage 2 hypertension generally is more aggressive to minimize the risk of MI, heart failure, or stroke. When the average blood pressure is greater than 200/120, immediate therapy, and possible hospitalization, is vital.

After a year of effective hypertension control, an effort may be made to reduce the dosage and number of drugs. This is known as step-down therapy. It is more successful in clients who have made lifestyle modifications. Careful blood pressure monitoring is necessary during and after step-down therapy, because the blood pressure often rises again to hypertensive levels.

Complementary Therapies

Behavioral and mind–body therapies may be helpful for some clients in lowering blood pressure (see the Nursing Research box on page 1164). The blood pressure increases in response to physiologic and psychologic stress and anxiety. Mind–body therapies such as yoga and t'ai chi, meditation, and guided imagery are designed to modify both physiologic and cognitive aspects of the stress response. In a study of older African American men and women with moderate hypertension, transcendental mediation was shown to reduce the blood pressure. Eastern exercises such as yoga and t'ai chi, which often combine imagery, meditation, and physical exercise, have been shown to reduce sympathetic nervous system activity, blood pressure, and heart and respiratory rates (Spencer & Jacobs, 2003). A nursing research study of hypertensive clients in Thailand demonstrated the effectiveness of yoga to reduce blood pressure, heart rate, and body mass index (McCaffrey et al., 2005).

 NURSING CARE

Health Promotion

Health promotion teaching and activities focus on the modifiable risk factors for hypertension. Advise all clients (as well as children and adolescents) to stop or never start smoking. Discuss the risks of obesity, excess alcohol intake, and a sedentary lifestyle with clients. Encourage all clients to eat a diet rich in fruits and vegetables and low in total and saturated fat. Discuss the potential benefits of following the DASH diet or a similar

NURSING RESEARCH Evidence-Based Practice: The Client with Primary Hypertension

Standard therapies for hypertension include lifestyle changes and medications. Clients often are advised to reduce stress levels in their lives, but rarely are provided with the tools to do so. A study by Yucha and colleagues (2005) sought to identify those clients who were most likely to benefit (reduced blood pressure in both clinic and ambulatory settings) from biofeedback-assisted relaxation training. Participants, all of whom had stage 1 or 2 hypertension, received 8 weeks of relaxation training with biofeedback provided by measurements of finger temperature, muscle tension, and respiratory sinus arrhythmia. The most benefit (greatest reduction in BP) occurred in participants who were not taking antihypertensive medication, had lower starting finger temperatures, had less daytime blood pressure variation, and who had a more external health locus of control.

IMPLICATIONS FOR NURSING

Predicting which clients would benefit from biofeedback-assisted relaxation training to lower blood pressure could potentially reduce the risk that these clients will go on to develop stage 1 or 2 hypertension. While biofeedback-assisted relaxation training is expensive and may not be covered by insurance, its benefits in reducing the overall costs of treating hypertension and its potential consequences are significant.

Nurses are in a position to identify clients with prehypertension through blood pressure screening. It is very appropriate to suggest mind–body therapies such as relaxation training with biofeedback to these clients, most of whom do not require medication.

CRITICAL THINKING IN CLIENT CARE

1. This study found that clients who were not taking antihypertensive medications were more likely to benefit from training in biofeedback-assisted relaxation. Think about the different ways in which antihypertensive medications work. Why do you think more benefit was seen in those clients who were not taking drugs?
2. Another finding of the study showed more benefit in clients with a more external health locus of control. Compare characteristics of clients with an internal health locus of control and those with an external health locus. What differences in these clients might account for this finding?
3. While you are discussing lifestyle modifications and the use of mind–body therapies with a client with prehypertension, he tells you that he thinks all this is nonsense. How would you respond?

eating plan. Advise all clients to remain active and engage in aerobic exercise 5 or more days a week. Discuss the stress-reducing benefits of exercise.

Offer blood pressure screening, and refer clients for follow-up as indicated (Table 35–2).

Assessment

Focused assessment of the client with hypertension includes:

- *Health history:* Complaints of morning headache, cervical pain; cardiovascular or central nervous system manifestations; history of hypertension, renal disease, diabetes; family history of high blood pressure, heart failure, or kidney disease; current medications.
- *Physical examination:* Vital signs including blood pressure in both arms, apical and peripheral pulses; ophthalmologic exam of retinal fundus as appropriate.
- *Diagnostic tests:* Serum electrolytes, glucose, and creatinine; cholesterol and lipoprotein profile; urinalysis.

Nursing Diagnoses and Interventions

All clients with primary hypertension and their families need significant teaching to manage this chronic condition. Health maintenance is a high-priority problem. Depending on the stage of hypertension and concurrent illnesses, other appropriate nursing diagnoses may include *Imbalanced Nutrition, Fluid Volume Excess,* and *Risk for Noncompliance.*

Ineffective Health Maintenance

Unhealthy lifestyle and behaviors can contribute to health problems such as hypertension. When hypertension has been identified, knowledge of the disease and its management is vital for the client. Willingness to take responsibility for hypertension management is central to effective blood pressure control. Adopting healthy lifestyle changes enhances drug therapy; in some cases, the need for medications may be eliminated or reduced. Because hypertension is often an asymptomatic disease and many antihypertensive drugs have unpleasant side effects, it

TABLE 35–2 Recommended Blood Pressure Follow-Up

CATEGORY	BLOOD PRESSURE (mmHG)	RECOMMENDED FOLLOW-UP
Normal	<120/80	Recheck in 2 years.
Prehypertension	120–139/80–89	Recheck in 1 year.
Stage 1 hypertension	140–159/90–99	Confirm within 2 months.
Stage 2 hypertension	≥160/≥100	Evaluate or refer to care provider within 1 month; for higher pressures (e.g., ≥180/≥110), evaluate or refer to care provider immediately or within 1 week as indicated.

Source: Adapted from *The Seventh Report of the Joint National Committee on Prevention, Detection, Education, and Treatment of High Blood Pressure,* NIH Publication No. 04-5250, by NHLBI, 2004b, Bethesda, MD: National Institutes of Health. Retrieved from http://www.nhlbi.nih.gov/guidelines/hypertension.

is vital that the client understand the chronic progressive nature of the disease and its long-term consequences.

- Assist with identifying current behaviors that contribute to hypertension. *The client must first identify contributory behaviors before he or she can change them. Using knowledge of hypertension risk factors, the nurse can help identify behaviors and factors contributing to hypertension that can be changed. Including the family in this process is important to reduce potential sabotage of the client's efforts to adopt healthier behaviors.*
- Assist in developing a realistic health maintenance plan. *Preparing a health maintenance plan for the client does little to encourage personal responsibility for health. However, nurses can guide clients in developing realistic goals and expectations for the treatment plan and modifying risk factors such as smoking, exercise, diet, and stress.*
- Help the client and family identify strengths and weaknesses in maintaining health. *Discussing areas of the health maintenance plan that are working well and those that present difficulties can help to identify necessary changes in the plan and additional strategies for implementing it.*

Risk for Noncompliance

Noncompliance, or failure to follow the identified treatment plan, is a continuing risk for any client with a chronic disease. Recommended lifestyle changes such as diet, exercise, restricted alcohol intake, stress reduction, and smoking cessation often are difficult to maintain on a continuing basis. In addition, prescribed medications may have undesirable effects whereas hypertension itself often has no symptoms or noticeable effects.

- Inquire about reasons for noncompliance with recommended treatment plan. Listen openly and without judging. *Nonthreatening discussion of factors contributing to noncompliance validates the client's self-esteem and partnership in the treatment plan.*

PRACTICE ALERT
Assess factors contributing to noncompliance, such as adverse drug effects. Suggest measures to manage adverse effects or, if indicated, contact the primary care provider about possible alternative drugs. Some adverse effects of antihypertensive drugs, such as gastric upset, light-headedness, or nocturia, may be easily managed by changing the timing of the drug dose. Others, such as fatigue, decreased exercise tolerance, or impotence may interfere with lifestyle and life roles to the extent that the client finds them intolerable.

- Evaluate knowledge of hypertension, its long-term effects, and treatment. Provide additional information and reinforce teaching as needed. *Knowledge increases the sense of control, which also increases the likelihood of compliance with treatment.*
- Assist to develop realistic short-term goals for lifestyle changes. *Attempting to lose weight, exercise daily, stop smoking, and dramatically change the diet all at the same time may be overwhelming, leading to a sense of failure. Smaller, gradual changes are more easily incorporated into lifestyle and daily activities, improving compliance.*

PRACTICE ALERT
Work with the client to develop mutual outcomes for the treatment plan. Discuss measures to improve compliance. The client has absolute control over compliance with the treatment plan. Demonstrating respect and involving the client in decision making and planning can improve compliance.

- Help the client identify cues and develop reminders (e.g., written notes, a medication box filled weekly) to assist with maintaining a schedule for exercise and medications. *Cues and other devices provide helpful reminders of activities and schedules until they are incorporated into habits.*
- Reassure the client that relapse into old habits and behaviors is common. Encourage avoiding feelings of guilt associated with relapse, and use the circumstance to renew efforts to comply with treatment. *Guilt and feelings of failure can lead to further noncompliance unless the event is used to identify reasons for noncompliance and ways to prevent it from recurring in the future.*

Imbalanced Nutrition: More than Body Requirements

The relationship between obesity, excess alcohol intake, and hypertension is well documented. Hypertension is particularly associated with central obesity, identified by waist circumference greater than hip circumference. Although weight loss is difficult and takes commitment to changing eating and exercise habits, it is possible for most clients to achieve.

- Assess usual daily food intake, and discuss possible contributing factors to excess weight, such as sedentary lifestyle, or using food as a reward or stress reliever. Inquire about diversional activities, exercise patterns, and previous weight reduction efforts (e.g., participation in weight reduction programs or using fad or crash diets). *Assessment data provide clues about contributing factors to obesity, the client's knowledge base about the relationship between eating and exercise habits and weight, and safe weight loss strategies. This provides direction for further teaching and for developing a realistic weight reduction plan.*
- Mutually determine with the client a realistic target weight (e.g., loss of 10% of current body weight over a 6-month period). Regularly monitor weight. Encourage a system of nonfood rewards for achieving small, incremental goals. *Setting weight loss goals helps formalize the process and provides motivation for continued progress. Developing realistic goals may be difficult; unrealistic goals, however, set the client up for failure. Continuous incremental weight loss provides reassurance that it can be achieved and promotes permanent weight reduction.*
- Refer to a dietitian for information about low-fat, low-calorie foods and eating plans. Focus on changing eating habits as opposed to "following a diet." *Focusing on changing eating habits promotes the sense that low-fat, low-calorie eating patterns should become a part of lifestyle rather than a short-term measure to be endured until the weight loss goal is achieved.*

- Recommend participating in an approved weight loss program such as Weight Watchers, Overeaters Anonymous, or Take off Pounds Sensibly (TOPS). *Organized weight loss programs provide structure for a balanced weight reduction program, as well as mutual support from others trying to lose weight.*

Excess Fluid Volume

Excess fluid volume often contributes to hypertension by increasing the cardiac output. A number of factors associated with hypertension can cause excess fluid volume, including sodium retention and disruption of the renin–angiotensin–aldosterone system. In addition, some antihypertensive drugs, such as calcium channel blockers and vasodilators, can contribute to excess fluid in the interstitial spaces and peripheral edema.

> **PRACTICE ALERT**
> Monitor blood pressure and other vital signs as indicated: every 1 to 2 hours or more frequently during acute hypertensive states; once a week or more frequently during initial treatment in the community. Vital signs are an indicator of fluid balance and the effectiveness of treatment. An elevated blood pressure, pulse, and respiratory rate may indicate fluid retention, whereas orthostatic hypotension and tachycardia may indicate fluid volume deficit.

- Monitor intake and output, and weigh daily (if in an acute or long-term care facility) or weekly (in the community). *Rapid weight changes (over days) more accurately reflect fluid balance than intake and output records. One liter of fluid weighs 1 kg (2.2 lb). Weight changes and intake and output records help monitor the effects of therapy.*
- Monitor for peripheral edema (sacral edema in the bedridden client). *Drugs such as vasodilators can cause fluid accumulation in interstitial tissues, leading to peripheral or dependent edema. Adding a diuretic to the treatment plan may be necessary.*
- Refer to a dietitian for teaching about a restricted sodium diet. Discuss the relationship between sodium intake and fluid retention. Provide opportunities to choose low-sodium foods from simulated menus. Support efforts, and reassure that lifestyle changes such as consuming less sodium take time. *Knowledge provides the power to take control of sodium intake. Patience and perseverance are needed to succeed; positive reinforcement of efforts to change long-standing dietary patterns is important.*

> **PRACTICE ALERT**
> Monitor laboratory values, such as blood urea nitrogen (BUN), urine specific gravity, creatinine, electrolytes, and hematocrit and hemoglobin. Hypertension can alter renal perfusion and function, leading to fluid retention and altered laboratory values. Changes in BUN and creatinine indicate impaired renal function, whereas changes in hematocrit and hemoglobin often reflect changes in fluid volume.

- Discuss the importance of adhering to treatment plans such as dietary restrictions and medication schedules. *Understanding the rationale for treatment measures promotes the client's sense of control and encourages compliance with the treatment regimen.*

Using NANDA, NIC, and NOC

See Chart 35–1 for linkages between NANDA nursing diagnoses, nursing interventions, and nursing outcomes for the client with hypertension.

Community-Based Care

Effective control of hypertension requires the client to not only participate in the plan of care, but also to take an active role in managing the disease. Treatment is managed in community settings, with regular visits to a clinic or office to monitor blood pressure and effects of treatment measures. Include the following topics when teaching the client and family about hypertension:

- Specific lifestyle changes recommended for the client and suggestions for implementing them. For example:
  - Increase activity gradually. Develop a realistic exercise program that is enjoyable and fits into lifestyle. Identify an exercise buddy for additional motivation. Activity and exercise, through a gradual conditioning of muscles and blood vessels, lower blood pressure by reducing peripheral vascular resistance. As the heart becomes conditioned and pumps more efficiently, kidney perfusion improves and intravascular volume falls, further reducing blood pressure. Exercise also reduces stress and contributes to weight loss and maintenance. Aerobic exercise, such as walking, jogging, swimming, and cycling, are appropriate; isometric activities (such as weight lifting) should be avoided without physician approval.

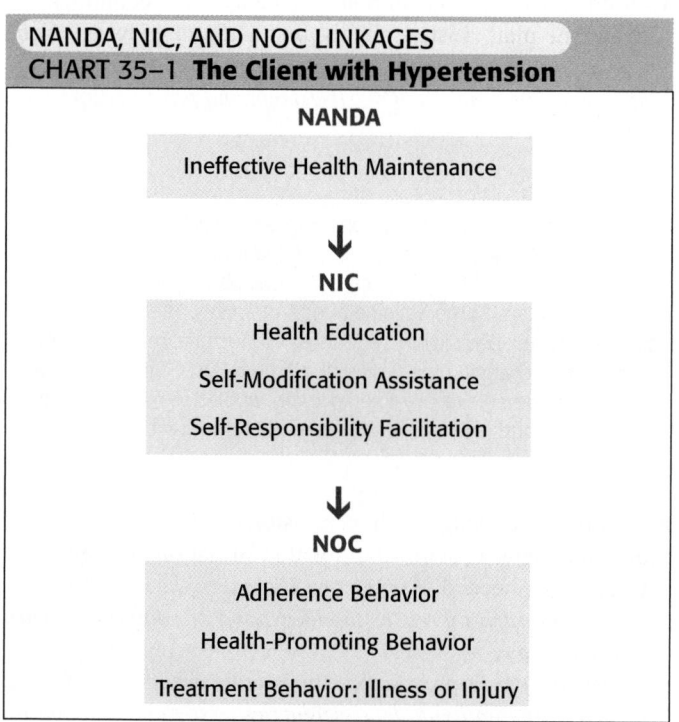

NANDA, NIC, AND NOC LINKAGES
CHART 35–1 The Client with Hypertension

NANDA

Ineffective Health Maintenance

↓

NIC

Health Education

Self-Modification Assistance

Self-Responsibility Facilitation

↓

NOC

Adherence Behavior

Health-Promoting Behavior

Treatment Behavior: Illness or Injury

Data from *NANDA's Nursing Diagnoses: Definitions & Classification 2005–2006* by NANDA International (2005), Philadelphia; *Nursing Interventions Classification (NIC)* (4th ed.) by J. M. Dochterman & G. M. Bulechek (2004), St. Louis, MO: Mosby; and *Nursing Outcomes Classification (NOC)* (3rd ed.) by S. Moorhead, M. Johnson, and M. Maas (2004), St. Louis, MO: Mosby.

- Adopt healthy eating patterns, following a low-fat, low-cholesterol, moderate sodium diet that also is rich in fruits and vegetables and includes at least two servings of low-fat milk or milk products daily. Do not give up if you slip into old eating habits on occasion; use such occasions to identify ways to avoid future lapses.
- Stop smoking. Participating in organized smoking cessation programs or using aids such as nicotine patches can help.
- Use alcohol in moderation if at all, consuming no more than 1.5 oz of hard liquor, 5 to 10 oz of wine, or 12 to 20 oz of beer per day.
- Use stress-reducing techniques such as meditation, relaxation, deep breathing, and exercise to manage stress. Anger and hostility intensify vasoconstriction; channeling these emotions into more positive responses such as using a change process to modify factors that provoke these emotions can reduce their harmful effects on blood pressure.
- Prescribed medications, their intended effect, dose and timing, interactions, and possible adverse effects. Discuss effects that should be reported to the physician, and those that can be managed by the client or that will diminish over time.
- The importance of monitoring blood pressure and regular visits to the primary care provider or hypertension clinic to monitor treatment. During follow-up visits, assess the blood pressure and specific laboratory work (such as serum creatinine, BUN, and/or serum electrolytes) to evaluate the disease and the effects of antihypertensive medications.

Refer the client to community blood pressure clinics, and to home health services as needed for regular follow-up and reinforcement of teaching. Refer to a dietitian or to an organized weight loss program as indicated for further teaching and weight loss support. The Nursing Care Plan on page 1168 provides additional information about community-based care for the client with high blood pressure.

THE CLIENT WITH SECONDARY HYPERTENSION

Secondary hypertension is elevated blood pressure resulting from an identifiable underlying process. It accounts for only 5% to 10% of identified cases of hypertension. Kidney disease is the most common identifiable cause of high blood pressure in both adults and children (Copstead & Banasik, 2005). Other common identifiable causes of hypertension in adults include renovascular disease (reduced blood flow to the kidneys), disorders of the adrenal cortex, pheochromocytoma, coarctation of the aorta, and sleep apnea. The pathophysiology of selected causes of high blood pressure are summarized here:

- *Kidney disease.* Any disease that affects renal blood flow (e.g., renal artery stenosis) or renal function (e.g., glomerulonephritis, renal failure) can lead to hypertension. Disruption of the blood supply stimulates the renin–angiotensin–aldosterone system, with resulting vasoconstriction and sodium and water retention. Altered kidney function affects the elimination of water and electrolytes, leading to hypertension.
- *Coarctation of the aorta.* Coarctation of the aorta is narrowing of the aorta, usually just distal to the subclavian arteries.

Reduced renal and peripheral blood flow stimulates the renin–angiotensin–aldosterone system and local vasoconstrictive responses, raising the blood pressure. A marked difference between pressures in the upper and lower extremities is common, with weak pulses and poor capillary refill in the lower extremities.

- *Endocrine disorders.* Adrenal gland disorders such as Cushing's syndrome and primary aldosteronism can cause hypertension. A rare tumor of the adrenal medulla, *pheochromocytoma,* causes persistent or intermittent hypertension. Other endocrine disorders such as hyperthyroidism and pituitary disorders also can lead to hypertension.
- *Neurologic disorders.* Increased intracranial pressure causes an elevated blood pressure as the body attempts to maintain cerebral blood flow. Disorders that interfere with autonomic nervous system regulation (such as high spinal cord injury) may allow the sympathetic nervous system to predominate, increasing systemic vascular resistance and blood pressure.
- *Drug use.* Estrogen and oral contraceptive use may lead to hypertension, possibly by prompting sodium and water retention and affecting the renin–angiotensin–aldosterone system. Stimulant drugs, such as cocaine and methamphetamines, increase systemic vascular resistance and cardiac output, resulting in hypertension.
- *Pregnancy.* About 10% of all pregnant women are hypertensive. Hypertension may predate pregnancy or occur as a direct response to the pregnancy. The mechanism of pregnancy-induced hypertension (PIH) is unclear. It is a significant cause of maternal and fetal morbidity and mortality and requires careful perinatal management.

The pattern of secondary hypertension varies, depending on its cause. Pheochromocytoma may cause attacks of hypertension that last for minutes to hours, accompanied by anxiety, palpitations, diaphoresis, pallor, and nausea and vomiting. Primary aldosteronism may cause hypertension, weakness, paresthesias, polyuria, and nocturia (see Chapter 18 ∞). Symptoms of kidney disease accompany hypertension when a renal disorder is the cause.

The following diagnostic tests may be ordered to differentiate primary from secondary hypertension:

- *Renal function studies* and *urinalysis* to identify renal causes of hypertension. Elevated serum creatinine and BUN, reduced creatinine clearance, and hematuria, proteinuria, and casts often indicate kidney disease.
- *Serum potassium* is decreased in hyperaldosteronism.
- *Blood chemistries,* including serum electrolytes, glucose, and lipid studies, are done to detect abnormalities indicative of endocrine or cardiovascular disease.
- *Intravenous pyelography (IVP), renal ultrasonography, renal arteriography,* and *CT or MRI* may be done when secondary hypertension is suspected.

Interdisciplinary and nursing care for the client with secondary hypertension is the same as that for primary hypertension, discussed in the previous section. In addition, the underlying process is treated. See chapters covering specific disorders for more information about treatment measures.

NURSING CARE PLAN   A Client with Hypertension

Margaret Spezia is a married, 49-year-old Italian American with eight children whose ages range from 3 to 18 years. For the past 2 months, Mrs. Spezia has had frequent morning headaches, and occasional dizziness and blurred vision. At her annual physical examination 1 month ago, her blood pressure was 168/104 and 156/94. She was instructed to reduce her fat and cholesterol intake, to avoid using salt at the table, and to start walking for 30 to 45 minutes daily. Mrs. Spezia returns to the clinic for follow-up.

ASSESSMENT

While escorting Mrs. Spezia to the exam room and obtaining her weight, blood pressure, and history, Lisa Christos, RN, notices that Mrs. Spezia seems restless and upset. Ms. Christos says, "You look upset about something. Is everything OK?" Mrs. Spezia responds, "Well, my head is throbbing, and I'm sort of dizzy. I think I'm just overdoing it and not getting enough rest. You know, raising eight children is a lot of work and expense. I just started working part time so we wouldn't get behind in our bills. I thought the extra money might relieve some of my stress, but I'm not so sure that's really happening. I'm not getting any better and I'm worried that I'll lose my job or become disabled and that my husband won't be able to manage the children by himself. I really need to go home, but first, I want to get rid of this awful headache. Would you please get me a couple of aspirin or something?"

Mrs. Spezia's history shows a steady weight gain during the past 18 years. She has no known family history of hypertension. Physical findings include height 63 inches (160 cm), weight 225 lb (102 kg), T 99°F (37.2°C), P 100 regular, R 16, BP 180/115 (lying), 170/110 (sitting), 165/105 (standing), average 10-point difference in readings between right and left arm (lower on left). Skin cool and dry, capillary refill 4 seconds right hand, 3 seconds left hand. Mrs. Spezia's total serum cholesterol is 245 mg/dL (normal <200 mg/dL). All other blood and urine studies are within normal limits. Based on analysis of the data, Mrs. Spezia is started on enalapril 5 mg and hydrochlorothiazide 12.5 mg in a combination drug (Vaseretic), and placed on a low-fat, low-cholesterol, no-added-salt diet.

DIAGNOSES

- *Fatigue* related to effects of hypertension and stresses of daily life
- *Imbalanced Nutrition: More than Body Requirements* related to excessive food intake
- *Ineffective Health Maintenance* related to inability to modify lifestyle
- *Deficient Knowledge* related to effects of prescribed treatment

EXPECTED OUTCOMES

- Reduce blood pressure readings to less than 150 systolic and 90 diastolic by return visit next week.
- Incorporate low-sodium and low-fat foods from a list provided into her diet.

- Develop a plan for regular exercise.
- Verbalize understanding of the effects of prescribed drug, dietary restrictions, exercise, and follow-up visits to help control hypertension.

PLANNING AND IMPLEMENTATION

- Teach to take own blood pressure daily and record it, bringing the record to scheduled clinic visits.
- Teach name, dose, action, and side effects of her antihypertensive medication.
- Instruct to walk for 15 minutes each day this week, and to investigate swimming classes at the local pool.
- Discuss strategies for achieving a realistic weight loss goal.
- Refer for a dietary consultation for further teaching about fat and sodium restrictions.
- Discuss stress-reducing techniques, helping identify possible choices.

EVALUATION

Mrs. Spezia returns to the clinic 1 week later. Her average blood pressure is now 148/88 mmHg. She has lost 1.5 lb, and states that her oldest daughter has suggested that they join a weight reduction program together. Mrs. Spezia is walking for an average of 20 minutes at a local mall each day. She verbalizes an understanding of her medication, and is taking it in the morning and before dinner each day. She met with the dietitian and discussed ways to reduce the sodium and fat in her diet. The dietitian provided a list of low-fat, low-sodium foods and recommended cookbooks to help Mrs. Spezia modify her cooking. Mrs. Spezia tells Ms. Christos, "I just can't believe how much better I feel already. My headaches are gone, and I've actually lost some weight—and I feel motivated to keep going. If I had only known how much better I could feel! I don't expect I'll ever go back to my old habits again; it's just not worth it!"

CRITICAL THINKING IN THE NURSING PROCESS

1. Identify the factors that contributed to Mrs. Spezia's hypertension. Which were modifiable and which were not?
2. What is the rationale for reducing sodium and fat in Mrs. Spezia's diet?
3. Suppose your hypertensive client is homeless and has no source of income. How could you help ensure your client would follow the treatment plan? What would you do if the client did not follow it?
4. Discuss the role of stress in hypertension. What factors in Mrs. Spezia's life contribute to her stress level?
5. Develop a plan of care for the nursing diagnosis *Low Self-Esteem* related to obesity.
   See Evaluating Your Response in Appendix C.

THE CLIENT WITH HYPERTENSIVE CRISIS

Some clients with hypertension may, for reasons not clearly understood, develop rapid, significant elevations in systolic and/or diastolic pressures. In a *hypertensive emergency* (or *malignant hypertension*), the systolic pressure is greater than 180 mmHg

and the diastolic pressure higher than 120 mmHg. Immediate treatment (within 1 hour) is vital to prevent cardiac, renal, and vascular damage, and reduce morbidity and mortality. Intense cerebral artery spasms help protect the brain from excess pressure; however, cerebral edema often develops. Prolonged severe hypertension damages walls of the arterioles and renal blood vessels, and may lead to intravascular coagulation and acute renal failure.

Clients presenting with a hypertensive emergency may have manifestations such as headache, confusion, swelling of the optic nerve (papilledema), blurred vision, restlessness, and motor and sensory deficits. Manifestations of hypertensive emergencies are listed in the accompanying box.

Most hypertensive emergencies occur when clients suddenly stop taking their medications or their hypertension is poorly controlled. Younger clients (30 to 50 years old), African American men, pregnant women with preeclampsia, and people with collagen and/or renal disease also are at higher risk for a hypertensive emergency (Porth, 2005).

The goal of care in hypertensive emergencies is to reduce the blood pressure by no more than 25% within minutes to 1 hour, then toward 160/100 within 2 to 6 hours. It is important to avoid rapid or excessive blood pressure decreases that may lead to renal, cerebral, or cardiac ischemia (NHLBI, 2004b). Blood pressure is monitored frequently (every 5 to 30 minutes)

MANIFESTATIONS of Hypertensive Emergencies

- Rapid onset
- Blurred vision, papilledema
- Systolic pressure > 180 mmHg
- Diastolic pressure > 120 mmHg
- Headache
- Confusion
- Motor and sensory deficits

during a hypertensive emergency. The BUN, serum creatinine, calcium, and total protein levels are carefully monitored to help determine the prognosis for recovery. Drug treatment for malignant hypertension includes parenteral administration of a rapidly acting antihypertensive, such as the potent vasodilator sodium nitroprusside (Nipride). Other medications that may be used are outlined in Table 35–3. Management also focuses on

TABLE 35–3 Intravenous Drugs Used to Treat Hypertensive Emergencies

CLASS/DRUG	ONSET	DURATION	NURSING IMPLICATIONS
Vasodilator			
Sodium nitroprusside (Nipride)	seconds	1 to 2 min	■ Effective, easy to titrate ■ May cause nausea, vomiting, muscle twitching, sweating ■ Use with caution in increased intracranial pressure
Nitroglycerin	2 to 5 min	5 to 10 min	■ Used when coronary ischemia accompanies hypertension ■ May cause headache, vomiting ■ Tolerance may develop with prolonged use
Diazoxide (Hyperstat)	1 to 2 min	4 to 24 h	■ Avoided in clients with coronary artery disease ■ Used with beta-blockers and diuretics ■ Painful if it enters tissues
Fenoldopam (Corlopam)	<5 min	30 min	■ Use with caution in clients with glaucoma ■ May cause tachycardia, headache, nausea, flushing ■ Do not use concurrently with beta-blockers ■ Monitor for heart failure, ischemic heart disease
Hydralazine (Apresoline)	10 to 30 min	2 to 6 h	■ May be used for hypertension associated with eclampsia ■ Avoided in clients with CHD ■ May cause tachycardia, flushing, headache, vomiting, angina
Calcium Channel Blocker			
Nicardipine (Cardene)	5 to 10 min	15 to 30 min; up to 4 h	■ Use with caution in CHD ■ Avoid in clients with heart failure ■ May cause tachycardia, headache, flushing, local phlebitis
ACE Inhibitor			
Enalaprilat (Vasotec)	15 to 30 min	6 to 12 h	■ Monitor for hypotension ■ Used in acute left heart failure ■ Avoid in acute myocardial infarction
Adrenergic Blockers			
Labetalol (Trandate)	5 to 10 min	3 to 6 h	■ Avoid in clients with acute heart failure and asthma ■ May cause nausea, vomiting, dizziness ■ Monitor for dyspnea, wheezing, heart block, orthostatic hypotension
Esmolol (Brevibloc)	1 to 2 min	10 to 30 min	■ Avoided in clients with heart failure and asthma ■ May cause nausea ■ Monitor for hypotension, dyspnea, wheezing, heart failure, first-degree heart block
Phentolamine (Regitine)	1 to 2 min	10 to 30 min	■ May cause tachycardia, flushing, headache

treating any underlying or coexisting heart, kidney, and CNS disorders.

Nursing care for the client with a hypertensive emergency focuses on continuous monitoring of the blood pressure and titrating drugs (administered by intravenous bolus or infusion) as ordered to achieve desired blood pressure. Avoiding excessive or very rapid blood pressure reductions is as important as achieving the desired blood pressure readings. Reassure the client and family of the rapid effect of prescribed drugs. Provide psychologic and emotional support as needed. Maintain an attitude of confidence that the treatment will achieve the desired effect. Following resolution of the hypertensive crisis, review causes of the crisis. Teach the client and family measures to effectively manage hypertension and prevent future hypertensive emergencies.

DISORDERS OF THE AORTA AND ITS BRANCHES

The aorta and its branches may be affected by occlusions, aneurysms, and inflammations. These disorders may be chronic or acute and life threatening (e.g., a thoracic dissection). This section focuses on aneurysms of the aorta and its branches.

THE CLIENT WITH AN ANEURYSM

An **aneurysm** is an abnormal dilation of a blood vessel, commonly at a site of a weakness or tear in the vessel wall. Aneurysms commonly affect the aorta and peripheral arteries, because of the high pressure in these vessels. An aneurysm also may develop in the ventricular wall, usually affecting the left ventricle. Most arterial aneurysms are caused by arteriosclerosis or atherosclerosis; trauma also may lead to aneurysm formation.

Arterial aneurysms are most common in men over age 50, most of whom are asymptomatic at the time of diagnosis. Hypertension is a major contributing factor in the development of some types of aortic aneurysms.

FAST FACTS
- The incidence of aortic aneurysm is an estimated 5.9 per 100,000 persons per year.
- Aortic dissection affects an estimated 5 to 30 per 1 million people per year.
- Although aortic aneurysm and aortic dissection can occur concurrently, this is rare (Wung & Aouizerat, 2004).

Pathophysiology and Manifestations

Aneurysms form due to weakness of the arterial wall. The major structural proteins of the aorta are collagen and elastin. Collagen provides tensile strength of the vessel, preventing excessive dilation. Elastin allows vessel recoil, during which the vessel returns to its original size following systole. This recoil provides continued propulsion of the bolus of blood expelled from the ventricle. Elastin is a primary component of internal elastic lamina, which separates the intimal and medial layers of the aorta, and of the media, the smooth muscle layer of the aorta. Destruction of elastin can lead to abnormal dilation of the vessel; collagen destruction can allow the vessel to rupture (Wung & Aouizerat, 2004).

True aneurysms are caused by slow weakening of the arterial wall due to the long-term, eroding effects of atherosclerosis and hypertension. True aneurysms affect all three layers of the vessel wall, and most are fusiform and circumferential. *Fusiform aneurysms* are spindle shaped and taper at both ends. *Circumferential aneurysms* involve the entire diameter

Figure 35–4 ■ A magnetic resonance angiogram (MRA) showing a circumferential aneurysm of the lower abdominal aorta.
Source: Zephyr, Photo Researchers, Inc.

of the vessel (Figure 35–4 ■). They generally grow slowly but progressively. Their length and diameter vary considerably among clients. A large fusiform aneurysm may affect most of the ascending aorta as well as a large portion of the abdominal aorta.

False aneurysms, also known as traumatic aneurysms, are caused by a traumatic break in the vessel wall rather than weakening of the vessel. They often are *saccular,* shaped like small outpouchings (sacs) on a portion of the vessel wall (Figure 35–5 ■). A *berry aneurysm* is a type of saccular aneurysm. They are often small (less than 2 cm in diameter), caused by congenital weakness in the tunica media of the artery. Berry aneurysms are commonly found in the circle of Willis in the brain.

Dissecting aneurysms are unique, developing when a break or tear in the tunica intima and media allows blood to invade or *dissect* the layers of the vessel wall. The blood usually is contained by the adventitia, forming a saccular or longitudinal aneurysm).

Aneurysms affect different segments of the aorta and its branches. Their manifestations generally are due to pressure of the aneurysm on adjacent structures. Table 35–4 summarizes the manifestations and complications of various types of aortic aneurysms.

Figure 35–5 ■ An angiogram showing a saccular (berry) aneurysm in the carotid artery of a 50-year-old man.

Source: Simon Fraser/RNC, Newcastle, Photo Researchers, Inc.

Thoracic Aortic Aneurysms

Thoracic aortic aneurysms account for about 10% of aortic aneurysms, with an annual incidence of about 6 per 100,000 people (Klein, 2005). See Figure 35–6 ■. They usually result from weakening of the aortic wall by arteriosclerosis and hypertension (Tierney et al., 2005). Other causes include trauma, coarctation of the aorta, tertiary syphilis, fungal infections, and Marfan syndrome. The syphilis spirochete can invade and weaken aortic smooth muscle, causing an aneurysm to develop as long as 20 years after the primary infection. Marfan syndrome fragments elastic fibers of the aortic media, weakening the vessel wall. The box on page 1172 discusses genetic links associated with thoracic aortic aneurysms.

Thoracic aneurysms frequently are asymptomatic. When present, manifestations are caused by the effects of the aneurysm on blood flow (e.g., to the coronary arteries and

Figure 35–6 ■ An angiogram showing a large aneurysm of the ascending aorta and aortic arch.

great vessels of the head and upper body) and pressure placed by distended aorta on surrounding structures. Consequently, manifestations vary by the location, size, and growth rate of the aneurysm. Substernal, neck, or back pain may occur. Pressure on the trachea, esophagus, laryngeal nerve, or superior vena cava may cause dyspnea, stridor, cough, difficult or painful swallowing, hoarseness, edema of the face and neck, and distended neck veins.

Aneurysms of the ascending aorta typically cause angina due to disruption of blood flow into the coronary arteries. Heart failure may develop as a result of disruption of the aortic valve and

TABLE 35–4 Manifestations and Complications of Aortic Aneurysms

TYPE OR LOCATION	MANIFESTATIONS	COMPLICATIONS
Thoracic	■ May be asymptomatic ■ Back, neck, or substernal pain ■ Dyspnea, stridor, or brassy cough if pressing on trachea ■ Hoarseness and dysphagia if pressing on esophagus or laryngeal nerve ■ Edema of the face and neck ■ Distended neck veins	■ Rupture and hemorrhage
Abdominal	■ Pulsating abdominal mass ■ Aortic calcification noted on x-ray ■ Mild to severe midabdominal or lumbar back pain ■ Cool, cyanotic extremities if iliac arteries are involved ■ Claudication (ischemic pain with exercise, relieved by rest)	■ Peripheral emboli to lower extremities ■ Rupture and hemorrhage
Aortic dissection	■ Abrupt, severe, ripping or tearing pain in area of aneurysm ■ Mild or marked hypertension early ■ Weak or absent pulses and blood pressure in upper extremities ■ Syncope	■ Hemorrhage ■ Renal failure ■ MI, heart failure, cardiac tamponade ■ Sepsis ■ Weakness or paralysis of lower extremities

GENETIC CONSIDERATIONS
Thoracic Aortic Aneurysms

About 20% of clients with aortic aneurysms have a family history of the disorder.

A condition known as *cystic medial necrosis* is prevalent in clients with Marfan syndrome and Ehlers-Danlos syndrome, inherited disorders involving connective tissues. In cystic medial necrosis, collagen and elastic fibers of the tunica media of the aorta degenerate. This loss of collagen and elastic tissues weakens the wall of the proximal aorta, leading to circumferential dilation of the ascending aorta and development of a fusiform aneurysm. In many other clients with thoracic aortic aneurysm (up to 20%), genetic syndromes affecting collagen and elastin are not recognized, but a strong family history of the disorder is present (Wung & Aouizerat, 2004).

regurgitation of blood back into the left ventricle. Aneurysms of the aortic arch often cause dysphagia, dyspnea, hoarseness, confusion, and dizziness (due to disrupted cerebral blood flow). Thrombi that form within a thoracic aneurysm can embolize, causing a stroke, renal or mesenteric ischemia, or ischemia of the lower extremities (Klein, 2005). Aneurysms of the thoracic aorta tend to enlarge progressively and may rupture, causing death.

Abdominal Aortic Aneurysms

Abdominal aortic aneurysms are associated with arteriosclerosis and hypertension. Increasing age and smoking are believed to contribute as well. Most abdominal aortic aneurysms are found in adults over age 70. The vast majority (over 90%) develop below the renal arteries, usually where the abdominal aorta branches to form the iliac arteries (see Figure 35–4).

Most abdominal aneurysms are asymptomatic, but a pulsating mass in the mid and upper abdomen and a bruit over the mass are found on exam. When pain is present, it may be constant or intermittent, usually felt in the midabdominal region or lower back. Its intensity may range from mild discomfort to severe pain. Pain intensity often correlates with the size and severity of the aneurysm. Severe pain may indicate impending rupture.

Sluggish blood flow within the aneurysm may cause thrombi (blood clots) to form. These can become emboli (circulating clots), traveling to the lower extremities and occluding peripheral arteries. The aneurysm may also rupture, with hemorrhage and hypovolemic shock. The risk of rupture increases as the size of the aneurysm increases; 20% to 40% of aneurysms more than 5 cm in diameter rupture. After acute rupture, the mortality rate is greater than 50%, even when emergency surgery is performed (Kasper et al., 2005).

Popliteal and Femoral Aneurysms

Most popliteal and femoral aneurysms are due to arteriosclerosis. They are often bilateral and usually affect men.

Popliteal aneurysms may be asymptomatic (Figure 35–7 ■). Manifestations, if any, are due to decreased blood flow to the lower extremity and include **intermittent claudication** (cramping or pain in the leg muscles brought on by exercise and relieved by rest), rest pain, and numbness. A pulsating mass may be palpable in the popliteal fossa (behind the knee). Thrombo-

Figure 35–7 ■ An angiogram showing several popliteal aneurysms.
Source: Zephyr, Photo Researchers, Inc.

sis and embolism are complications; gangrene may result, often necessitating amputation.

A *femoral aneurysm* usually is detected as a pulsating mass in the femoral area. The manifestations are similar to those of popliteal aneurysms, resulting from impaired blood flow. Femoral aneurysms may rupture.

Aortic Dissections

Dissection is a life-threatening emergency caused by a tear in the intima of the aorta with hemorrhage into the media. The hemorrhage dissects or splits the vessel wall, forming a blood-filled channel between its layers. Dissection can occur anywhere along the aorta. *Type A dissection* (also called *proximal dissection*) affects the ascending aorta; *type B dissection* (*distal dissection*) is limited to the descending aorta.

Hypertension is a major predisposing factor for aortic dissection, accounting for 70% of aortic dissections. Cystic medial necrosis (see the Genetic Considerations box above) also is a major risk factor. Other risk factors include male gender, advancing age, pregnancy, congenital defects of the aortic valve, coarctation of the aorta, and inflammatory aortitis (Kasper et al., 2005).

Dissection of the thoracic aortic walls progresses along the length of the vessel, moving both proximally and distally. As the aneurysm expands, pressure may prevent the aortic valve from closing or may occlude the branches of the aorta. Descending aortic dissection may extend into the renal, iliac, or femoral arteries.

The primary symptom of an aortic dissection is sudden, excruciating pain. The pain, often described as a ripping or tearing sensation, is usually over the area of dissection. Thoracic dissections cause chest or back pain. Other symptoms may include syncope, dyspnea, and weakness. The blood pressure may initially be increased, but rapidly falls and is often inaudible as the dissection occludes blood flow. Peripheral pulses are absent for the same reason.

Complications develop if major arteries are affected. Obstruction of the carotid artery causes neurologic symptoms such as weakness or paralysis. The myocardium, kidneys, or bowel may become ischemic or infarct if blood flow to the coronary arteries, renal arteries, or mesenteric artery is affected. Acute aortic regurgitation may develop with dissection of the ascending aorta. With treatment, the long-term prognosis is generally good, although the in-hospital mortality rate following surgery is 15% to 20% (Kasper et al., 2005).

INTERDISCIPLINARY CARE

Most aneurysms are asymptomatic, detected through a routine physical examination. Treatment depends on the size of the aneurysm. Small, asymptomatic aneurysms may not be treated or are medically managed; large aneurysms (>5 cm) at risk for rupture require surgery.

Diagnosis

Diagnostic studies done to establish the diagnosis and determine the size and location of the aneurysm may include:

- *Chest x-ray* to visualize thoracic aortic aneurysms.
- *Abdominal ultrasonography* to diagnose abdominal aortic aneurysms.
- *Transesophageal echocardiography* to identify the specific location and extent of a thoracic aneurysm and to visualize a dissecting aneurysm.
- *Contrast-enhanced CT* or *MRI* allows precise measurements of aneurysm size.
- *Angiography* uses contrast solution injected into the aorta or involved vessel to visualize the precise size and location of the aneurysm.

Medications

Thoracic aortic aneurysms may be treated with long-term beta-blocker therapy and additional antihypertensive drugs as needed to control heart rate and blood pressure.

Clients with aortic dissection are initially treated with intravenous beta-blockers such as propranolol (Inderal), metoprolol (Lopressor), or esmolol (Brevibloc) to reduce the heart rate to about 60 bpm. Sodium nitroprusside (Nipride) infusion is started concurrently to reduce the systolic pressure to 120 mmHg or less. Calcium channel blockers (verapamil and diltiazem) also may be used. Direct vasodilators such as diazoxide (Hyperstat) and hydralazine (Apresoline) are avoided because they may actually worsen the dissection (Kasper et al., 2005). Constant monitoring of vital signs, hemodynamic pressures (via Swan-Ganz catheter; see Chapter 32 ∞ for more information about hemodynamic pressure monitoring), and urine output are vital to ensure adequate perfusion of vital organs.

Following surgical correction of an aneurysm, anticoagulant therapy may be initiated. Heparin therapy is used initially, with conversion to oral anticoagulation prior to discharge. Many clients are maintained indefinitely on anticoagulant therapy; others may use lifelong, low-dose aspirin therapy to reduce the risk of clot formation.

Surgery

Operative repair of aortic aneurysms is indicated when the aneurysm is symptomatic or expanding rapidly. Thoracic aneurysms more than 6 cm in diameter are surgically repaired; asymptomatic abdominal aneurysms greater than 5 cm in diameter may be repaired, depending on the client's operative risk factors. Type A dissections are repaired as soon as feasible; type B dissections may be surgically repaired, depending on the extent of involvement and risk for rupture (Kasper et al., 2005).

Endovascular stent grafts (EVSGs) are increasingly being used to treat abdominal and thoracic aortic aneurysms. The use of EVSG to treat aortic dissections is in investigational stages. The stent, which consists of a metal sheath covered with polyester fabric or a woven polyester tube, usually is placed percutaneously via the femoral artery. Fluoroscopy is used to guide its placement. Both straight and bifurcated grafts are available. Endovascular stent placement results in a shorter hospital stay and lower treatment cost. EVSG is associated with fewer pulmonary, renal, and cardiovascular complications than open surgical aneurysm repair (Jones, 2005). This option generally is preferred for clients who have a high surgical risk. The most common complication of endovascular aneurysm repair is persistent perfusion of the aneurysm (*endoleak*) caused by an ineffective seal at the proximal or distal end of the graft (Way & Doherty, 2003). Regular follow-up with abdominal CT scans is necessary to detect this complication, which can develop at any time postoperatively. Because stent grafts are handcrafted to fit the individual, repeated CT scans with contrast media are required preoperatively, increasing the risk for kidney damage and renal failure. On rare occasions, the graft may be malpositioned or may migrate from the desired location (Jones, 2005).

An open surgical procedure in which the aneurysm is excised and replaced with a synthetic fabric graft is the standard treatment for expanding abdominal aortic aneurysms (Figure 35–8 ■). Although the aneurysm walls may be excised, they usually are left intact and used to cover the graft. Surgical repair of thoracic aneurysms is similar but more complex due to major vessels exiting at the aortic arch. Cardiopulmonary bypass is required if the ascending aorta is involved. The aortic valve also may be replaced during surgery. See the box on page 1174 for nursing care of the client having surgery of the aorta.

NURSING CARE

Assessment

Focused assessment for the client with a suspected aortic aneurysm includes:

- *Health history:* Complaints of chest, back, or abdominal pain; extremity weakness; shortness of breath, cough, difficult or painful swallowing, hoarseness; history of hypertension, coronary heart disease, heart failure, or peripheral vascular disease.
- *Physical examination:* Vital signs including blood pressure in upper and lower extremities; peripheral pulses; skin color

Figure 35–8 ■ Repair of an abdominal aortic aneurysm. The aorta is exposed and clamped between the renal and iliac arteries. Atherosclerotic plaque and thrombotic material are removed. A synthetic graft is used to replace the aneurysm. The aneurysm walls are then sutured around the graft.

Source: Stevie Grand, Photo Researchers, Inc.

and temperature; neck veins; abdominal exam including gentle palpation for masses and auscultation for bruits; neurologic exam including level of consciousness (LOC), sensation, and movement of extremities.

Nursing Diagnoses and Interventions

Nursing care for clients with an aneurysm of the aorta or its branches focuses on monitoring and maintaining tissue perfusion, relieving pain, and reducing anxiety. Nursing care usually is acute, precipitated by a complication or surgical repair of the aneurysm.

Risk for Ineffective Tissue Perfusion

Clients with aortic aneurysms are at risk for impaired tissue perfusion due to aneurysm rupture with resulting hemorrhage and lack of blood flow to tissues distal to the rupture. In addition, thrombi often form within the aneurysm and may become emboli, obstructing distal arterial blood flow.

NURSING CARE OF THE CLIENT HAVING Surgery of the Aorta

PREOPERATIVE CARE

■ As time permits, provide routine preoperative care and teaching as outlined in Chapter 4 ∞. *Clients having vascular surgery have similar preoperative nursing care needs to other clients having major abdominal or thoracic surgery. If emergent surgery is required, time for preoperative care and teaching may be limited.*

■ Implement measures to reduce fear and anxiety:
   a. Orient to the intensive care unit, if appropriate.
   b. Describe and explain the reason for all equipment and tubes, such as cardiac monitors, ventilators, nasogastric tubes, urinary catheters, intravenous lines and fluids, and intra-arterial lines.
   c. Explain what to expect following surgery (sights, sounds, frequency of taking vital signs, dressings, pain relief measures, communication strategies).
   d. Allow time for questions and expression of fears and concerns.
   These explanations provide a sense of control for the client and family.

■ Monitor for and implement care to reduce the risk of aneurysm rupture (see the following section). *Clients with a rapidly expanding or symptomatic aneurysm are at risk for rupture prior to surgical repair.*

POSTOPERATIVE CARE

■ Provide routine postoperative care and specific measures as ordered by the physician. *Clients undergoing aneurysm repair require nursing care similar to that provided to all clients with major thoracic or abdominal surgery, in addition to specific measures related to vascular surgery.*

■ Maintain fluid replacement and blood or volume expanders as ordered. Promptly report changes in vital signs, level of consciousness, and urine output. *Hypovolemic shock may develop due to blood loss during surgery, third spacing, inadequate fluid replacement, and/or hemorrhage if graft separation or leakage occurs.*

PRACTICE ALERT

Monitor for and report manifestations of graft leakage:

   a. Ecchymoses of the scrotum, perineum, or penis; a new or expanding hematoma
   b. Increased abdominal girth
   c. Weak or absent peripheral pulses; tachycardia; hypotension
   d. Decreased motor function or sensation in the extremities
   e. Fall in hemoglobin and hematocrit
   f. Increasing abdominal, pelvic, back, or groin pain
   g. Decreasing urinary output (less than 30 mL/h)
   h. Decreasing CVP, pulmonary artery pressure, or pulmonary artery wedge pressure.

These manifestations may signal graft leakage and possible hemorrhage. Pain may be due to pressure from an expanding hematoma or bowel ischemia. Decreased renal perfusion causes the glomerular filtration rate and urine output to fall.

■ Report manifestations of lower extremity embolism: pain and numbness in lower extremities, decreasing pulses, and pale, cool, or cyanotic skin. *Pulses may be absent for 4 to 12 hours postoperatively due to vasospasm; however, absent pulses with pain, changes in sensation, and a pale, cool extremity are indicative of arterial occlusion.*

■ Report manifestations of bowel ischemia or gangrene: abdominal pain and distention, occult or fresh blood in stools, and diarrhea. *Bowel ischemia may result from an embolism or occur as a complication of surgery.*

■ Report manifestations of impaired renal function: urine output less than 30 mL/h, fixed specific gravity, increasing BUN and serum creatinine levels. *Hypovolemia or clamping of the aorta during surgery may impair renal perfusion, leading to acute renal failure.*

■ Report manifestations of spinal cord ischemia: lower extremity weakness or paraplegia. *Impaired spinal cord perfusion may lead to ischemia and impaired function.*

PRACTICE ALERT
Immediately report manifestations of impending rupture, expansion, or dissection of the aneurysm: increased pain; discrepancy between upper and lower extremity blood pressures and peripheral pulses; increased mass size; change in LOC or motor or sensory function; laboratory results. Rapid expansion may indicate increased risk for rupture, with resulting hemorrhage, shock, and possible death. Elective or planned surgery may rapidly become emergency surgery to prevent complications.

■ Implement interventions to reduce the risk of aneurysm rupture:
  a. Maintain bed rest with legs flat.
  b. Maintain a calm environment, implementing measures to reduce psychologic stress.
  c. Prevent straining during defecation and instruct to avoid holding the breath while moving.
  d. Administer beta-blockers and antihypertensives as prescribed.
  Activity, stress, and the Valsalva maneuver increase blood pressure, increasing the risk of rupture. Elevating or crossing the legs restricts peripheral blood flow and increases pressure in the aorta or iliac arteries. Beta-blockers and antihypertensives often are ordered to reduce pressure in the dilated vessel.

PRACTICE ALERT
Report manifestations of arterial thrombosis or embolism: absent peripheral pulses; a pale or cyanotic, cool extremity; severe, diffuse abdominal pain with guarding; or increased groin, lumbar, or lower extremity pain. Sluggish blood flow within the aneurysm often causes thrombi to form. These thrombi can break loose, becoming emboli that can occlude peripheral arteries or arteries to the kidneys or mesentery. Arterial occlusion may necessitate emergency surgery to restore blood flow and prevent tissue infarct or gangrene.

■ Continuously monitor cardiac rhythm. Report complaints of chest pain or changes in ECG tracing. Administer oxygen as indicated. *Aortic dissection and repair place the client at significant risk for MI, a major cause of postoperative mortality and morbidity (Kasper et al., 2005). Rapid identification and treatment of this complication can reduce the risk of death or long-term adverse effects of MI.*

PRACTICE ALERT
Immediately report changes in mental status or symptoms of peripheral neurologic impairment (weakness, paresthesias, paralysis). The expanding aneurysm or dissection can affect carotid and cerebral blood flow or spinal cord perfusion, leading to neurologic symptoms. Immediate restoration of blood flow is vital to prevent permanent neurologic deficits.

Risk for Injury
Potent antihypertensive drugs often are given intravenously to reduce the pressure on an expanding or dissecting aneurysm. Continuous monitoring of infusions and hemodynamic parameters such as arterial pressure, pulmonary pressures, and cardiac output is vital to ensure that adequate tissue perfusion is maintained during infusions of these potent drugs.

PRACTICE ALERT
Use an infusion control device for all drug infusions. These devices prevent accidental or inadvertent changes in the rate of the infusion and dose of the drug.

■ Continuously monitor arterial pressure and hemodynamic parameters as indicated. Promptly report results outside the specified parameters to the physician. *Many of the drugs used are effective within minutes. Responses vary among individuals, particularly in the older adult, necessitating continuous monitoring.*
■ Monitor urine output hourly. Report output less than 30 mL/h. *The kidneys are very sensitive to reduced perfusion pressure; inadequate renal blood flow can lead to acute renal failure.*

Anxiety
Clients with aortic aneurysms often are highly anxious because of the urgent nature of the disorder. The nurse must manage the anxiety levels of both the client and family members to effectively address physiologic care needs. Stress reduction also is necessary to help maintain the blood pressure within desired limits.

■ Explain all procedures and treatments, using simple and understandable terms. *Simplified explanations are necessary when anxiety levels interfere with learning and understanding.*
■ Respond to all questions honestly, using a calm, empathetic, but matter-of-fact manner. *Honesty with the client and family promotes trust and provides reassurance that the true nature of the situation is not being "hidden" from them.*
■ Provide care in a calm, efficient manner. *Using a calm manner even during preparations for emergency surgery reassures the client and family that although the situation is critical, the staff is prepared to handle things effectively.*
■ Spend as much time as possible with the client. Allow supportive family members to remain with the client when possible. *The presence of a health professional and supportive family member reassures the client that he or she is not alone in facing this crisis.*

Community-Based Care
Topics to discuss when preparing clients and their families for home care or care in a community-based setting depend on the treatment plan. Discuss the following topics when surgical repair is not immediately planned and the aneurysm will be monitored:
■ Measures to control hypertension, including lifestyle and prescribed drugs
■ The benefits of smoking cessation
■ Manifestations of increasing aneurysm size or complications to report to the physician.
  Following surgery, discuss the following topics in preparing the client and family for home care:
■ Wound care and preventing infection; manifestations of impaired healing or infection to be reported
■ Prescribed antihypertensive and anticoagulant medications and their expected and unintended effects

- The importance of adequate rest and nutrition for healing
- Measures to prevent constipation and straining at stool (such as increasing fluid and fiber in the diet)
- The importance of avoiding prolonged sitting, lifting heavy objects, engaging in strenuous exercise, and having sexual intercourse until approved by the physician (usually 6 to 12 weeks)

- Signs and symptoms of complications to report to the physician.

Provide referrals to a home health agency or community health service as necessary. Referrals are especially important for older adults and their caregivers, who may require additional assistance with the complex care needs.

DISORDERS OF THE PERIPHERAL ARTERIES

Disorders that impair peripheral arterial blood flow may be *acute* (e.g., arterial thrombosis) or *chronic* (e.g., peripheral arteriosclerosis). Chronic occlusive disorders may be due to structural defects of the arterial walls or spasm of affected arteries. Impaired peripheral arterial circulation limits the availability of oxygen and nutrients to the tissues, and can have significant adverse effects. This section focuses on acute and chronic disorders affecting peripheral arteries. The nurse's role in caring for clients with peripheral arterial disorders focuses on maintaining tissue perfusion and educating the client and family about the disorder and its management.

Physiology Review

Peripheral arteries are the part of the systemic circulation that delivers oxygen and nutrients to the skin and the extremities. Arterial walls have three layers: the intima, which includes the endothelium and a layer of connective tissue and the basement membrane; the media, composed of smooth muscle and elastic fibers; and the adventitia, a thin layer of connective tissue that contains collagen and elastic fibers. The smooth muscle of peripheral arteries controls blood flow as it contracts and relaxes. Contraction narrows the vessel lumen (**vasoconstriction**), whereas smooth muscle relaxation expands the vessel (**vasodilation**). Peripheral arteries become progressively smaller; arterioles are less than 0.5 mm in diameter and are composed primarily of smooth muscle. The arterioles control blood flow through the capillary beds where gas, nutrient, and waste product exchange occurs. Capillary walls are very thin, consisting of a single layer of endothelial cells surrounded by a thin basement membrane.

Blood flows from an area of higher pressure to an area of lower pressure. *Resistance* opposes blood flow. Resistance is created by friction of the blood itself, although the primary determinants of vascular resistance are the diameter and length of the blood vessel. See the physiology review section earlier in this chapter under "Disorders of Blood Pressure Regulation" for more information about factors that determine vessel resistance.

THE CLIENT WITH PERIPHERAL VASCULAR DISEASE

Arteriosclerosis is the most common chronic arterial disorder, characterized by thickening, loss of elasticity, and calcification of arterial walls. **Atherosclerosis** is a form of arteriosclerosis in which deposits of fat and fibrin obstruct and harden the arteries. In the peripheral circulation, these pathologic changes impair the blood supply to peripheral tissues, particularly the lower extremities. This is known as **peripheral vascular disease (PVD)** or peripheral artery disease (PAD).

Incidence and Risk Factors

PVD usually affects people in their 60s and 70s; men are more often affected than women. Deaths attributed to peripheral arterial disease are about the same for black and white males, but are higher among black women than white women (NHLBI, 2004a).

Risk factors for PVD are similar to those for atherosclerosis and CHD (see Chapter 30 ∞). Diabetes mellitus, hypercholesterolemia, hypertension, cigarette smoking, and high homocystine levels are risk factors for PVD (Kasper et al., 2005).

> **FAST FACTS**
> - PVD is a common manifestation of atherosclerosis, particularly in older men.
> - PVD interferes with arterial blood flow to the lower extremities, increasing the risk for neuropathy and paresthesias, ulcers that do not heal, necrosis, gangrene, and amputation.
> - Regular daily exercise is a primary intervention for all types of peripheral arterial disease to promote development of collateral circulation and maintain tissue perfusion.

Pathophysiology

The pathophysiology of atherosclerosis is detailed in Chapter 31 ∞. Atherosclerotic lesions involve both the intima and the media of the involved arteries. Lesions typically develop in large and midsize arteries, particularly the abdominal aorta and iliac arteries (30% of symptomatic clients), the femoral and popliteal arteries (80% to 90% of clients), and more distal arteries (40% to 50% of clients) (Kasper et al., 2005). Arteriosclerosis in the abdominal aorta leads to the development of aneurysms as plaque erodes the vessel wall.

Plaque tends to form at arterial bifurcations. The vessel lumen is progressively obstructed, decreasing blood flow to the lower extremities. Tissue hypoxia or anoxia results. With gradual obstruction of the vessel, collateral circulation often develops. However, it is usually not adequate to supply tissue needs, especially when metabolic demand increases (e.g., during exercise). Manifestations typically develop only when the vessel is occluded by 60% or more.

Manifestations and Complications

Pain is the primary symptom of peripheral atherosclerosis. **Intermittent claudication,** a cramping or aching pain in the calves of the legs, the thighs, and the buttocks that occurs with a predictable level of activity, is characteristic of PVD. The pain is often accompanied by weakness and is relieved by rest.

Rest pain, in contrast, occurs during periods of inactivity. It is often described as a burning sensation in the lower legs. Rest pain increases when the legs are elevated and decreases when the legs are dependent (e.g., hanging over the side of the bed). The legs also may feel cold or numb along with the pain. Sensation is diminished and the muscles may atrophy.

Peripheral pulses may be decreased or absent. A bruit may be heard over large affected arteries, such as the femoral artery and the abdominal aorta. The legs are pale when elevated, but often are dark red (*dependent rubor*) when dependent. The skin often is thin, shiny, and hairless, with discolored areas. Toenails may be thickened. Areas of skin breakdown and ulceration may be evident. Edema may develop with severe PVD. See the box below for manifestations of peripheral atherosclerosis.

Complications of peripheral atherosclerosis include gangrene and extremity amputation, rupture of abdominal aortic aneurysms, and possible infection and sepsis.

INTERDISCIPLINARY CARE

Management of peripheral vascular disease focuses on slowing the atherosclerotic process and maintaining tissue perfusion.

Diagnosis

Although PVD often can be diagnosed by the history and physical examination, diagnostic tests may be ordered to evaluate its extent. Noninvasive studies often are sufficient.

- *Segmental pressure measurements* use sphygmomanometer cuffs and a Doppler device to compare blood pressures between the upper and lower extremities (normally similar) and within different segments of the affected extremity. In PVD, the BP may be lower in the legs than in the arms.
- *Stress testing* using a treadmill provides functional assessment of limitations. In PVD, pressure at the ankle may decline even further with exercise, confirming the diagnosis. Evaluation for coronary heart disease may be done simultaneously during exercise testing (Kasper et al., 2005).
- *Doppler ultrasound* uses sound waves reflected off moving red blood cells within a vessel to evaluate blood flow. The impulses may be translated into an audible signal or a graphic waveform. With significant PVD, the waveform becomes progressively flatter as the transducer is moved distally along the affected vessel. Segmental pressures may be used to locate the site of obstruction.

- *Duplex Doppler ultrasound* combines the audible or graphic Doppler ultrasound with ultrasound imaging to identify arterial or venous abnormalities. Ultrasonic imaging provides views of the affected vessel while Doppler ultrasound evaluates blood flow. *Color-flow Doppler ultrasound (CDU)* provides color images of the vessel and blood flow.
- *Transcutaneous oximetry* evaluates oxygenation of tissues.
- *Angiography* or *magnetic resonance angiography* is done before revascularization procedures to locate and evaluate the extent of arterial obstruction. For angiography, a contrast medium is injected and vessels are visualized using fluoroscopy and x-rays. MRA does not require injection of a contrast medium and may replace angiography.

See Chapter 33 for more information on diagnostic testing for PVD.

Medications

Drug treatment of peripheral atherosclerosis is less effective than with coronary heart disease. Medications to inhibit platelet aggregation, such as aspirin or clopidogrel (Plavix), are ordered to reduce the risk of arterial thrombosis. Cilostazol (Pletal), a platelet inhibitor with vasodilator properties, improves claudication. Pentoxifylline (Trental) decreases blood viscosity and increases red blood cell flexibility, increasing blood flow to the microcirculation and tissues of the extremities. Parenteral vasodilator prostaglandins may be given on a long-term basis to decrease pain and facilitate healing in clients with severe limb ischemia (Kasper et al., 2005).

Treatments

Smoking cessation is vital. Nicotine not only promotes atherosclerosis, but also causes vasospasm, further reducing blood flow to the extremities.

Meticulous foot care is vital to prevent ulceration and infection (Box 35–4). Elastic support hose, which reduce circulation to the skin, are avoided. Elevating the head of the bed on blocks may help relieve rest pain. Regular, progressively strenuous exercise, such as 30 to 45 minutes of walking daily, is important. The client is taught to rest at the onset of claudication, resuming activity when the pain resolves.

Other measures to slow the process of atherosclerosis, such as controlling diabetes and hypertension, lowering cholesterol levels, and weight loss, also are recommended (see Chapter 30). See the box on page 1178 for care of the older adult.

Revascularization

Revascularization may be performed if symptoms are progressive, severe, or disabling. Other indications for surgery include symptoms that significantly interfere with activities of daily living (ADLs), rest pain, and pregangrenous or gangrenous lesions. Either nonsurgical revascularization procedures or surgery may be performed.

Nonsurgical procedures include percutaneous transluminal angioplasty (PTA), stent placement, or atherectomy. Techniques may include balloon angioplasty to dilate the narrowed lumen, mechanical atherectomy to remove plaque, or laser or thermal angioplasty to vaporize the occluding material. In either case, a stent typically is placed at the time of PTA to maintain vessel

---

MANIFESTATIONS of Peripheral Atherosclerosis

- Intermittent claudication
- Rest pain
- Paresthesias (numbness, decreased sensation)
- Diminished or absent peripheral pulses
- Pallor with extremity elevation, dependent rubor when dependent
- Thin, shiny, hairless skin; thickened toenails
- Areas of discoloration or skin breakdown

BOX 35–4 Foot Care for the Client with Peripheral Atherosclerosis

1. Keep legs and feet clean, dry, and comfortable.
   - Wash legs and feet daily in warm water, using mild soap.
   - Pat dry using a soft towel; be sure to dry between the toes.
   - Apply moisturizing cream to prevent drying.
   - Use powder on the feet and between the toes.
   - Buy shoes in the afternoon (when feet are largest); never buy shoes that are uncomfortable. Be sure toes have adequate room.
   - Wear a clean pair of cotton socks each day.
2. Prevent accidents and injuries to the feet.
   - Always wear shoes or slippers when getting out of bed.
   - Walk on level ground and avoid crowds, if possible.
   - Do not go barefoot.

- Inspect legs and feet daily; use a mirror to examine backs of legs and bottoms of feet.
- Have a professional foot care provider trim toenails and care for corns, calluses, ingrown toenails, or athlete's foot.
- Always check the temperature of the water before stepping into the tub.
- Do not get the legs or tops of the feet sunburned.
- Report leg or foot problems (increased pain, cuts, bruises, blistering, redness, or open areas) to your healthcare provider.

3. Improve blood supply to the legs and feet.
   - Do not cross legs.
   - Do not wear garters or knee stockings.
   - Do not swim or wade in cold water.

---

patency. Iliac and femoral-popliteal PTA initially reestablish good blood flow and relieve symptoms in more than 80% of clients. While the 3-year success rate is lower, stent placement improves the duration of symptom relief (Kasper et al., 2005). See Chapter 31 ∞ for more information about revascularization procedures.

Surgical options include endarterectomy to remove occlusive plaque from the artery and bypass grafts. Knitted Dacron bypass grafts are commonly used. Both immediate and long-term graft patency is better with bypass grafting than with nonsurgical revascularization procedures, but the risk for operative complications such as myocardial infarction, stroke, infection, and peripheral embolization is higher (Kasper et al., 2005). Nursing care for the client having revascularization surgery is similar to that provided for clients having an aortic aneurysm repair (see the box on page 1174).

Complementary Therapies

Complementary therapies for peripheral vascular disease include interventions to improve circulation and to reduce stress. A number of complementary therapies may improve peripheral circulation, including aromatherapy with rosemary or vetiver; biofeedback; healing or therapeutic touch and massage; herbals such as ginkgo, garlic, cayenne, hawthorn, and bilberry; and exercise including yoga. Aromatherapy and yoga also may reduce stress, as can breathing exercises, meditation, and counseling. In addition, complementary therapies to reduce atherosclerosis and lower cholesterol levels may slow the progress of PVD. Measures such as a very low-fat or vegetarian diet, including antioxidant nutrients or using vitamin C, vitamin E, or garlic supplements, and traditional Chinese medicine may be useful.

NURSING CARE

Health Promotion

Discuss healthy lifestyle habits with community and religious groups, schoolchildren (grades K through 12), and through the print media to reduce the incidence and slow the progression of atherosclerosis.

Strongly encourage all clients to avoid smoking in the first place, and to stop all forms of tobacco use. Discuss the adverse effects of smoking and the benefits of quitting. Provide information about dietary recommendations to maintain a healthy weight and optimal cholesterol levels. Discuss the benefits and importance of regular exercise. Finally, encourage clients with cardiovascular risk factors to undergo regular screening for hypertension, diabetes, and hyperlipidemia.

Assessment

Focused assessment related to peripheral atherosclerosis includes the following:
- *Health history:* Complaints of pain, its relationship to exercise or rest, timing, associated symptoms, and relief measures; history of coronary heart disease, peripheral vascular disease, hyperlipidemia, hypertension, or diabetes; current medications; smoking history; usual diet and activity patterns.
- *Physical examination:* Vital signs; strength and equality of peripheral pulses of all extremities; capillary refill; skin color, temperature, hair distribution, presence of any discolorations or lesions; movement and sensation of lower extremities.

NURSING CARE OF THE OLDER ADULT
Peripheral Vascular Disease

With aging, blood vessels thicken and become less compliant. These changes reduce oxygen delivery to the tissues and impair carbon dioxide and waste product removal from the tissues. When normal effects of aging combine with an increased risk of atherosclerosis, the risk of peripheral vascular disease is high.

The older adult with peripheral vascular disease requires the same care and teaching as other clients. However, visual deficits and osteoarthritis may make foot care more difficult. Long-standing smoking habits are difficult to break. Mobility may be impaired by arthritis or the effects of neurologic disorders. The client who lives alone may resist walking. Periodic visits by a community or home health nurse may be helpful, as may be encouraging the client to join a support group for stopping smoking, changing eating habits, and taking part in regular activity.

Nursing Diagnoses and Interventions

Impaired tissue perfusion is an obvious problem in peripheral atherosclerosis. Acute and chronic pain may interfere with ADLs, and ambulation may be limited. The possibility of losing a lower extremity is frightening.

Ineffective Tissue Perfusion: Peripheral

Impaired blood flow to the lower extremities affects gas, nutrient, and waste product exchange between the capillaries and cells. Oxygen and nutrient deprivation impairs cell function and tissue integrity, causing pain and impaired healing. Pain develops with exercise and when extremities are elevated.

- Assess peripheral pulses, pain, color, temperature, and capillary refill every 4 hours and as needed. Use a Doppler device if pulses are not palpable. Mark pulse locations with an indelible marker. *Assessment data provide a baseline for evaluating the effectiveness of interventions and identifies changes in arterial blood flow.*
- Position with extremities dependent. *Gravity promotes arterial flow to the dependent extremity, increasing tissue perfusion and relieving pain.*

> **PRACTICE ALERT**
> Instruct to avoid smoking. If necessary, obtain an order for a nicotine patch or gum from the physician. Nicotine is a potent vasoconstrictor that further impairs arterial blood flow. Smoking cessation is a vital component of care. Nicotine patches and gum contain less nicotine than cigarettes, and can help reduce the stress of smoking cessation.

- Discuss the benefits of regular exercise. *Exercise promotes development of collateral circulation to ischemic tissues and slows the process of atherosclerosis.*
- Use a foot cradle and lightweight blankets, socks, and slippers to keep extremities warm. Avoid electric heating pads or hot water bottles. *Keeping extremities warm conserves heat, prevents vasospasm, and promotes arterial flow. External heating devices are avoided to reduce the risk of burns in the client with impaired sensation. The foot cradle protects tissues from compression by linens.*
- Encourage frequent position changes. Instruct to avoid crossing legs or using a pillow under the knees. *Position changes promote blood flow and reduce damage caused by pressure. Leg crossing and excessive flexion of the hip or knee joints can compress partially obstructed arteries and impair blood flow to distal tissues.*

Pain

Impaired blood flow results in tissue ischemia. Metabolism shifts from an efficient aerobic process to an anaerobic process. Lactic acid and metabolic waste products accumulate in tissues, causing pain. Severe and cramping pain generally occurs with exercise early in the disease. Rest initially produces relief, similar to the process of angina (see Chapter 31 ∞). As the disease progresses, pain develops with less exercise and often occurs even at rest. Rest pain disrupts sleep, the sense of well-being, and has significant disruptive effects on life roles.

- Assess pain at least every 4 hours, using a standard pain scale. *Pain is a subjective experience. Using a standard pain scale allows evaluation of treatment mea-sures in relieving pain and restoring blood flow.*
- Keep extremities warm. *Cooling leads to vasoconstriction, increasing pain. Warming the extremities promotes vasodilation and improves arterial flow, reducing pain.*
- Teach pain relief and stress reduction techniques such as relaxation, meditation, and guided imagery. *Pain increases stress. The stress response leads to vasoconstriction, increasing pain. Stress reduction techniques, when combined with other measures to promote blood flow, can help reduce pain.*

Impaired Skin Integrity

Clients with PVD are at risk for impaired skin integrity as a result of oxygen and nutrient deprivation. Chronic tissue ischemia leads to dry, scaly, and atrophied skin. Pruritus can lead to scratching; minor injuries may go unnoticed due to impaired sensation. Impaired tissue healing can lead to ulceration, infection, and potential gangrene.

> **PRACTICE ALERT**
> Assess and document skin condition at least every 8 hours or with each home visit; more frequently as indicated. Tissue ischemia increases the risk for damage, even with minor trauma such as pressure from poorly fitting shoes or bed linens. Frequent inspection and documentation of skin condition is vital to identify early indicators of impaired skin integrity and reduce the risk of complications such as infection.

- Provide meticulous daily skin care, keeping the skin clean and dry. Apply a moisturizing cream to dry or scaly areas. *Intact skin is the body's first defense against bacterial invasion. Ischemic tissues of the injured extremity provide an excellent medium for microorganism growth. Clean, dry, supple skin decreases the risk of breakdown.*
- Apply a bed cradle. *The bed cradle suspends bed linens over the legs, preventing them from placing pressure on extremities and injured tissues. Minimizing pressure on the tissues promotes capillary blood flow.*
- Provide an egg-crate mattress, flotation pad, sheepskin, or heel protectors. *Ischemic tissues may be damaged by minor trauma such as that created by the shearing forces of skin against bed linens.*

Activity Intolerance

Pain and impaired perfusion of peripheral tissues may limit the client's ability to engage in desired activities, even impairing self-care.

- Assist with care activities as needed. *Severe claudication or rest pain may limit activities. Muscle atrophy of affected extremities is common, leading to fatigue and weakness.*
- Unless contraindicated, encourage gradual increases in duration and intensity of exercise. Teach to rest with extremities dependent when claudication develops, resuming activity after pain has abated. *Gradual increases in the duration and intensity of exercise promote development of collateral circulation,*

improve exercise tolerance, provide a sense of well-being, and support self-esteem.

■ Provide diversional activities during periods of prescribed bed rest. Encourage relaxation techniques to reduce muscle tension. *Diversional activities help prevent boredom and stress associated with enforced rest. Relaxation techniques reduce vasoconstriction induced by stress, improving peripheral circulation.*

■ Encourage frequent position changes and active range-of-motion exercises. Encourage self-care to the extent possible. *Position changes relieve pressure on tissues, improving capillary circulation and reducing tissue ischemia. Range-of-motion exercises help prevent muscle atrophy and joint contractures. Self-care supports self-esteem.*

Using NANDA, NIC, and NOC

Chart 35–2 shows links between NANDA nursing diagnoses, NIC, and NOC for the client with peripheral vascular disease.

Community-Based Care

Discuss the following topics when preparing the client and family for home and community-based care. See the accompanying Nursing Care Plan for additional community-based nursing interventions.

■ Smoking cessation strategies and ways to avoid second-hand smoke

---

NANDA, NIC, AND NOC LINKAGES
CHART 35–2 The Client with Peripheral Vascular Disease

NANDA

Ineffective Tissue Perfusion: Peripheral

↓

NIC

Circulatory Care: Arterial Insufficiency

Exercise Promotion

Positioning

Skin Surveillance

↓

NOC

Tissue Integrity: Skin and Mucous Membranes

Activity Tolerance

Tissue Perfusion: Peripheral

Data from *NANDA's Nursing Diagnoses: Definitions & Classification 2005–2006* by NANDA International (2005), Philadelphia; *Nursing Interventions Classification (NIC)* (4th ed.) by J. M. Dochterman & G. M. Bulechek (2004), St. Louis, MO: Mosby; and *Nursing Outcomes Classification (NOC)* (3rd ed.) by S. Moorhead, M. Johnson, and M. Maas (2004), St. Louis, MO: Mosby.

■ Prescribed medications and anticoagulants, their purpose, doses, desired and adverse effects
■ Signs of excess bleeding to report to the physician
■ Skin surveillance and foot care (see Box 35–4)
■ Recommended diet and exercise
■ Weight loss strategies if appropriate.

If revascularization or surgery has been performed, include the following topics as appropriate:

■ Incision care
■ Manifestations of complications (e.g., infection, graft leakage, or thrombosis) to be reported to the physician
■ Activity limitations.

Provide referrals to home health services, physical or occupational therapy, and home maintenance assistance services as indicated. Consider resources such as Meals-on-Wheels for clients who are severely limited by their disease.

THE CLIENT WITH THROMBOANGIITIS OBLITERANS

Thromboangiitis obliterans (also called *Buerger's disease*) is an occlusive vascular disease in which small and midsize peripheral arteries become inflamed and spastic, causing clots to form. This disease may affect either the upper or lower extremities; it often affects a leg or foot. Its exact etiology is unknown.

Incidence and Risk Factors

Thromboangiitis obliterans primarily affects men under age 40 who smoke. Cigarette smoking is the single most significant cause of the disease. The disease is more prevalent in Asians and people of Eastern European descent. The incidence of HLA-B5 and 2A9 antigens is higher in people with thromboangiitis obliterans, suggesting a genetic link.

Pathophysiology and Course

Inflammatory cells infiltrate the wall of small and midsize arteries in the feet and possibly the hands. This inflammatory process is accompanied by thrombus formation and vasospasms of arterial segments that impair blood flow. Adjacent veins and nerves also may be affected. As the disease progresses, affected vessels become scarred and fibrotic.

The course of the disease is intermittent with dramatic exacerbations and marked remissions. The disease may remain dormant for periods of weeks, months, or years. As the disease progresses, collateral vessels are more extensively involved. Consequently, subsequent episodes are more intense and prolonged. Prolonged periods of tissue hypoxia increase the risk for tissue ulceration and gangrene.

Manifestations and Complications

Pain in the affected extremities is the primary manifestation of thromboangiitis obliterans. Both claudication, cramping pain in calves and feet or the forearms and hands, and rest pain in

NURSING CARE PLAN   **A Client with Peripheral Vascular Disease**

William Duffy, age 69, is retired. His wife convinces him to see his primary care provider for increasing leg pain with walking and other exercise.

ASSESSMENT

Katie Kotson, RN, obtains Mr. Duffy's history before he sees his physician. He states that he can only walk about a block before the pain in his calves gets so bad that he has to stop and rest. As a result, he has been less and less active, spending most of his time the past few months watching sports on television. He denies rest pain. He was diagnosed with type 2 diabetes about 15 years ago, which he manages with daily glyburide (DiaBeta), an oral hypoglycemic. He also has stable angina, for which he takes atenolol (Tenormin) and an occasional nitroglycerin tablet. His alcohol intake is moderate, averaging one to two beers per day, and he smokes about a pack of cigarettes per day. He states he tried to quit smoking after developing angina, but "after nearly 50 years of smoking, I think that's impossible!"

Physical exam findings include height 68 inches (173 cm), weight 235 lb (107 kg), BP 168/78, P 66, R 16, T 97.6°F (36.5°C); upper extremities warm and pink, normal hair distribution, pulses strong and equal; lower extremities below knees cool and ruddy when dependent, pale to pink when elevated, skin shiny, scant hair; posterior tibial pulses weak bilaterally; weak pedal pulse on R, unable to palpate on L; 1+ to 2+ edema both feet and ankles.

The physician finds that Mr. Duffy's systolic blood pressure in his legs is an average of 28 mmHg lower than in his arms. He makes the diagnosis of peripheral atherosclerosis, and schedules Mr. Duffy for an exercise stress test with ankle pressure measurements before and after exercise and a color-flow Doppler ultrasound. Mr. Duffy is to return in 3 weeks after these studies have been completed.

DIAGNOSES

- *Activity Intolerance* related to poor blood flow to lower extremities
- *Ineffective Health Maintenance* related to smoking and lack of information about disease management
- *Risk for Impaired Skin Integrity* related to ischemic tissues of legs and feet
- *Risk for Peripheral Neurovascular Dysfunction* related to impaired peripheral blood flow to lower extremities

EXPECTED OUTCOMES

- Walk for at least 15 minutes three to four times per day, gradually increasing his pace and duration of exercise.
- Relate the benefits of smoking cessation.
- Identify strategies to improve chances for success in stopping smoking.
- Meet with dietitian before next visit to discuss dietary measures to promote weight loss and slow atherosclerosis.

- Verbalize an understanding of appropriate foot care measures.
- Identify measures to prevent inadvertent injury of feet and legs.

PLANNING AND IMPLEMENTATION

- Teach about peripheral atherosclerosis and its relationship to Mr. Duffy's symptoms.
- With Mr. and Mrs. Duffy, plan strategies to start and maintain a program of regular exercise.
- Instruct to warm up slowly, and to stop exercise and rest for 3 minutes (or until pain is relieved) when claudication develops, then resume exercising.
- Discuss the effects of smoking on blood vessels.
- Help Mr. Duffy identify smoking cessation strategies such as support groups, clinics, and nicotine patches.
- Schedule an appointment with the dietitian to develop a low-calorie, low-fat, and low-cholesterol ADA diet that includes preferred foods and considers usual eating patterns.
- Reinforce and supplement previous foot care teaching.
- Discuss effects of impaired circulation on sensation in feet and legs and measures to prevent injury.

EVALUATION

When Mr. Duffy returns to the office 3 weeks later, his diagnosis has been confirmed by the diagnostic studies. The physician decides to continue conservative therapy, now prescribing atorvastatin (Lipitor) to lower Mr. Duffy's serum cholesterol level, and cilostazol (Pletal) to reduce the risk of thrombosis and improve symptoms of claudication. Mr. Duffy also asks his physician for a prescription for nicotine patches, saying he is ready to quit smoking, but thinks he needs help to be successful. Mr. and Mrs. Duffy tell Miss Kotson that they are walking before every meal and really enjoying being outside more. They plan to walk in the local shopping mall when the weather gets worse. Mrs. Duffy has bought an American Heart Association cookbook, and is carefully planning their meals. Both Mr. and Mrs. Duffy have lost 5 lb since the previous visit. Mr. Duffy's skin on his legs and feet remains intact, and he identifies the measures he is using to protect his lower extremities from injury.

CRITICAL THINKING IN THE NURSING PROCESS

1. What additional lifestyle changes related to peripheral atherosclerosis might be appropriate to suggest to Mr. Duffy at this time? Why?
2. Explain the relationship between physical exercise and pain in the client with peripheral atherosclerosis. Compare this relationship to that between exercise and angina.
3. Mr. Duffy uses a beta-blocker, atenolol, to prevent angina. Why is this drug not effective in preventing claudication?
4. Develop a nursing care plan for the nursing diagnosis *Imbalanced Nutrition: More than Body Requirements*.
See Evaluating Your Response in Appendix C.

---

the fingers and toes may occur. Sensation is diminished. Eventually, the skin becomes thin and shiny and the nails are thickened and malformed. On examination, the involved digits and/or extremities are pale, cyanotic, or ruddy, and cool or cold to touch. Distal pulses (e.g., the dorsalis pedis, posterior tibial,

ulnar, or radial) are either difficult to locate or absent, even with a Doppler device.

Painful ulcers and gangrene may develop in the fingers and toes as a result of severely impaired blood flow. Amputation may be necessary to remove necrotic tissue.

INTERDISCIPLINARY CARE

Thromboangiitis obliterans usually is diagnosed by the history and physical examination. Doppler studies may be used to locate and determine the extent of the disease. Angiography and magnetic resonance imaging may also be used to evaluate the extent of the disease, but usually are unnecessary.

The one most important component in managing this disease is smoking cessation. While stopping smoking does not cure the disease, it may slow its extension to other vessels. With continued smoking, attacks become increasingly intense and last much longer, significantly increasing the risk for ulcerations and gangrene.

Additional conservative measures are used to prevent vasoconstriction, improve peripheral blood flow, and prevent complications of chronic ischemia. These measures include keeping extremities warm, managing stress, keeping affected extremities in a dependent position, preventing injury to affected tissues, and regular exercise. Walking for 20 or more minutes several times a day is recommended.

There are no specific drugs for thromboangiitis obliterans. A calcium channel blocker such as diltiazem (Cardizem) or verapamil (Isoptin), or pentoxifylline (Trental), which decreases blood viscosity and increases red blood cell flexibility to improve peripheral blood flow, may provide some symptom relief.

Surgical approaches for thromboangiitis obliterans include sympathectomy or arterial bypass graft. Sympathectomy interrupts sympathetic nervous system input to affected vessels, reducing vasoconstriction and spasm. Arterial bypass grafts may be useful when larger vessels are affected by the disease. Amputation of an affected digit or extremity may be necessary if gangrene develops (see Chapter 41 ∞ for more information about amputation). Only portions of digits or of limbs (e.g., below the knee) are usually amputated, to preserve as much healthy tissue as possible.

The prognosis for thromboangiitis obliterans depends significantly on the client's ability and willingness to stop smoking. With smoking cessation and good foot care, the prognosis for saving the extremities is good, even though no cure is available.

NURSING CARE

Health promotion activities to prevent thromboangiitis obliterans focus on preventing smoking, especially in high-risk populations. Nursing assessment and care for clients with this disease are similar to those provided for clients with other arterial occlusive diseases. Nursing care focuses on promoting arterial circulation and preventing prolonged tissue hypoxia. Because inflammatory, spastic episodes may be unpredictable, care focuses on smoking cessation and relieving acute manifestations. In addition, postsurgical care is necessary if surgery has been performed. See the nursing care section for peripheral atherosclerosis as well as nursing care of the postsurgical client (Chapter 4 ∞) and following amputation (Chapter 41 ∞).

Community-Based Care

Discuss the following topics when preparing clients with thromboangiitis obliterans and their families for home or community-based care:

- Absolute necessity of smoking cessation
- Foot care
- Protecting affected extremities from injury
- Purpose, dose, desired and adverse effects, interactions, and any precautions associated with prescribed medications
- Signs and symptoms to report to the physician.

THE CLIENT WITH RAYNAUD'S DISEASE

Raynaud's disease and **phenomenon** are characterized by episodes of intense vasospasm in the small arteries and arterioles of the fingers and sometimes the toes (Porth, 2005). Raynaud's disease and phenomenon differ only in terms of cause. Raynaud's disease has no identifiable cause; Raynaud's phenomenon occurs secondarily to another disease (such as collagen vascular diseases such as scleroderma and rheumatoid arthritis), other known causes of vasospasm, or long-term exposure to cold or machinery (McCance & Huether, 2006; Porth, 2005).

Raynaud's disease primarily affects young women between the ages of 20 and 40. Genetic predisposition may play a role in its development, although the actual cause is unknown. Table 35–5 compares thromboangiitis obliterans and Raynaud's disease.

Pathophysiology and Manifestations

Raynaud's disease and phenomenon are characterized by spasms of the small arteries in the digits. The arterial spasms limit arterial blood flow to the fingers and possibly the toes. Initial attacks may involve only the tips of one or two fingers; with disease progression, the entire finger and all fingers may be affected.

The manifestations of Raynaud's occur intermittently when spasms develop. Raynaud's disease has been called the "blue-white-red disease," because affected digits initially turn blue as blood flow is reduced due to vasospasm, then white as circulation is more severely limited, and finally very red as the fingers are warmed and the spasm resolves (Figure 35–9 ■). Sensory changes may occur during attacks, including numbness, stiffness, decreased sensation, and aching pain.

The attacks tend to become more frequent and prolonged over time. With repeated attacks (and resultant decrease in oxygenation), the fingertips thicken and the nails become brittle. Ulceration and gangrene are serious complications that rarely occur.

INTERDISCIPLINARY CARE

Raynaud's disease and phenomenon are primarily diagnosed by the history and physical examination. There are no specific diagnostic tests for these disorders.

Vasodilators may be prescribed to provide symptomatic relief. Low doses of a sustained release calcium channel blocker

TABLE 35–5 Comparison of Raynaud's Disease and Thromboangiitis Obliterans

TOPIC	RAYNAUD'S DISEASE	THROMBOANGIITIS OBLITERANS
Etiology	■ Unknown ■ Possible genetic predisposition	■ Cigarette smoking most probable single cause ■ Possible autoimmune response
Incidence/course of the disease	■ Onset commonly between 15 and 45 years of age ■ Usually affects young women ■ Becomes progressively worse over time	■ Occurs predominantly in men under age 40 ■ More common in Asians and people of European heritage ■ Intermittent course with exacerbations and remissions ■ Increased severity and duration of attacks over time
Triggering stimuli	■ Emotional stress ■ Exposure to cold	■ Cigarette smoking
Assessment findings	■ Usually affects hands, sometimes toes ■ Pain becomes more severe and prolonged as disease progresses ■ "Blue-white-red" changes in color of hands with accompanying changes in skin temperature	■ Claudication and pain ■ Numbness or diminished sensation ■ Cool, pale, or cyanotic skin ■ Shiny, thin skin and white, malformed nails in affected extremities ■ Distal pulses difficult to find or absent ■ Trophic changes to nail beds ■ Ulceration and gangrene in later stages ■ Small, red, tender vascular cords in affected extremities
Management	■ Avoid unnecessary cold exposure ■ Emphasize smoking cessation ■ Medications such as calcium channel or alpha-adrenergic blockers as indicated ■ Teach stress management	■ Stop smoking (crucial) ■ Regular exercise ■ Protect extremities from cold injury ■ Teach stress management

such as nifedipine (Procardia) or diltiazem (Cardizem) may be prescribed. The alpha-adrenergic blocker prazosin (Minipress) also may reduce the frequency and severity of attacks. Transdermal nitroglycerin (or longer acting oral nitrates) helps some clients by decreasing the amount of time necessary for the hands to return to normal following an attack (Tierney et al., 2005).

Conservative measures are a mainstay of treatment. Clients are instructed to keep their hands warm, wearing gloves when outside in cold weather and kitchen gloves when handling cold items (for instance, when preparing and serving cold foods and cleaning the refrigerator). Measures to avoid injury to the hands

are taught. Sometimes attacks can be stopped by swinging the arms back and forth, increasing perfusion pressure in the small arteries by centrifugal force.

Smoking cessation is important. Stress reduction measures such as exercise, relaxation techniques, massage therapy, hobbies, aroma therapy, and counseling are taught or suggested. Additional lifestyle habits that contribute to vascular health are encouraged, such as reducing dietary fat, increasing activity level, and maintaining normal body weight.

NURSING CARE

Nursing care for the client with Raynaud's disease or phenomenon is primarily educative and supportive. Protecting the hands and feet from exposure to cold and trauma is the major teaching topic. Nursing diagnoses and interventions previously outlined for peripheral atherosclerosis also are appropriate for clients with Raynaud's.

Community-Based Care

Reassure clients with Raynaud's phenomenon that most people with the disorder experience only mild, infrequent episodes. Discuss the following topics in preparing the client for managing the disorder:

■ Dress warmly, keeping the trunk and hands warm.
■ Avoid unnecessary exposure to cold.
■ Stop smoking or do not start.
■ The use, purpose, desired and potential adverse effects of prescribed medications, if any.

Figure 35–9 ■ Hands of a client with Raynaud's phenomenon. Note cyanosis of fingers on the right hand and the left thumb and the extreme pallor of the other digits of the left hand.

Source: Bart's Medical Library, Phototake NYC.

THE CLIENT WITH ACUTE ARTERIAL OCCLUSION

A peripheral artery may be acutely occluded by development of a thrombus (blood clot) or by an embolism. Blood flow to tissues supplied by the artery is impaired, resulting in acute tissue ischemia and a risk for necrosis and gangrene.

Pathophysiology

Arterial Thrombosis

A **thrombus** is a blood clot that adheres to the vessel wall. Thrombi tend to develop in areas where intravascular factors stimulate coagulation (e.g., where a vessel lumen is partially obstructed and its wall is damaged and roughened by atherosclerosis). Other disorders, such as infection or inflammation of the vessel wall or pooling of blood (e.g., in an aneurysm) also can prompt coagulation and thrombus formation (McCance & Huether, 2006). A developing thrombus can occlude arterial blood flow through the vessel, leading to ischemia of tissues supplied by that artery. The extent of ischemia depends on the size of the affected artery and the degree of collateral circulation. In gradual processes of arterial occlusion such as atherosclerosis, collateral vessels often develop to compensate for impaired arterial flow. The extent of collateral circulation affects the degree of tissue ischemia distal to the thrombus.

Arterial Embolism

An **embolism** is sudden obstruction of a blood vessel by debris. A thrombus can break loose from the arterial wall to become a **thromboembolus**. Other substances also can become emboli: atherosclerotic plaque, masses of bacteria, cancer cells, amniotic fluid, bone marrow fat, and foreign objects such as air bubbles or broken intravenous catheters. Regardless of cause, an embolus eventually lodges in a vessel that is too small to allow it to pass.

Arterial emboli often originate in the left side of the heart. They are associated with myocardial infarction, valvular heart disease, left-sided heart failure, atrial fibrillation, or infectious heart diseases. Emboli from the left heart often enter the carotid arteries and become trapped in the cerebral circulation, causing neurologic deficits (see Chapter 43 ∞). Thromboemboli that develop in the aorta or peripheral arterial circulation tend to lodge in areas where the arterial lumen is narrowed by atherosclerotic plaque and at arterial bifurcations.

Manifestations

The manifestations of arterial thrombosis and embolism are those of tissue ischemia. Ischemic tissues are painful, pale, and cool or cold. Distal pulses are absent. Paresthesias (numbness and tingling) develop in the extremity. Cyanosis and mottling are common. Paralysis and muscle spasms may develop in the affected extremity. A line of demarcation between normal and ischemic tissue may be seen, particularly with embolism. Tissue below the line is cool or cold, and pale, cyanotic, or mottled. See the Manifestations box that follows.

Arterial occlusion can result in permanent vessel and limb damage. Complete arterial occlusion leads to tissue necrosis and gangrene unless blood flow is promptly restored.

MANIFESTATIONS **of Acute Arterial Occlusion**

- Pain
- Pallor or mottling
- Paresthesias (numbness and tingling)
- Cool or cold skin
- Pulselessness distal to the blockage
- Possible paralysis, weakness, or muscle spasms
- Possible line of demarcation; with pallor, cyanosis, and cooler skin distal to the blockage (especially with arterial embolism)

INTERDISCIPLINARY CARE

Acute arterial occlusions may require emergency treatment to preserve the limb if the obstructed vessel is large or collateral circulation is minimal. If the limb is not in jeopardy, more conservative management may be initiated.

Diagnosis

The diagnosis of acute arterial occlusion often is apparent by the signs and symptoms. *Arteriography* is used to confirm the diagnosis, locate the occlusion, and determine its extent.

Medications

Anticoagulation with intravenous heparin is initiated to prevent further clot propagation and recurrent embolism. Anticoagulation is continued with oral anticoagulants after discharge. See the section on venous thrombosis later in this chapter for more information about anticoagulant therapy.

Arterial thrombosis may be treated with intra-arterial fibrinolytic therapy using streptokinase, urokinase, or tissue plasminogen activator (t-PA) (see Chapter 31 ∞). Lysis of the thrombus or embolus is achieved in 50% to 80% of the cases (Tierney et al., 2005). Local intra-arterial injection of the fibrinolytic drug allows use of lower doses and reduces the bleeding risk associated with fibrinolytic drugs.

Surgery

Immediate *embolectomy* (within 4 to 6 hours) is the treatment of choice for acute arterial occlusion by an embolus to prevent tissue necrosis and gangrene. When the involved vessel is in an extremity, local anesthesia and a special balloon-tipped catheter known as a Fogarty catheter may be used for high surgical risk clients (Tierney et al., 2005). An embolus in the mesenteric circulation necessitates emergency laparotomy. The risk of complications and limb loss increases significantly if surgery is delayed by 12 or more hours. Potential major complications include compartment syndrome (see Chapter 41 ∞), acute respiratory distress syndrome (Chapter 39 ∞), or acute renal failure (Chapter 28 ∞).

Arterial thrombosis also may be treated surgically, although the required surgery may be more extensive due to the length of the vessel involved. *Thromboendarterectomy* is done to remove the thrombus and plaque in the artery. An arterial graft may be required. Nursing care for clients who have undergone embolectomy or thrombus removal is discussed in the nursing care section that follows.

NURSING CARE

Assessment

Nursing assessment for the client with an acute arterial occlusion is highly focused due to the emergency nature of the problem.

- *Health history:* Complaints of pain, numbness, tingling, or weakness in the involved extremity; history of atherosclerotic vessel disease, heart disease, or recent invasive procedure (e.g., angiography, percutaneous revascularization procedure).
- *Physical examination:* Vital signs; peripheral pulses in both extremities; color, temperature, sensation, and movement of involved extremity; skin condition; presence of a line of demarcation.

Nursing Diagnoses and Interventions

Nursing care related to acute arterial occlusion focuses on protecting the affected extremity, managing anxiety, and reducing the risk of complications related to anticoagulant therapy.

Ineffective Tissue Perfusion: Peripheral

Protecting ischemic tissue from injury prior to surgery or medical thrombolysis is vital. Following surgery, there is a risk for thrombosis at the graft site or impaired perfusion due to edema of the surgical site.

> **PRACTICE ALERT**
> Monitor extremity perfusion, comparing affected and unaffected extremities. Assess peripheral pulses (using the Doppler stethoscope as needed), skin temperature and color, capillary refill, movement, and sensation every 1 to 4 hours. Promptly report changes or complaints of increased or unrelieved pain. Propagation of a thrombus can further obstruct arterial flow, increasing tissue ischemia. Following surgery, arterial spasms may cause a cyanotic, pulseless extremity; normal color and pulses should return within 12 hours. A thrombus may form at the surgical site or within a graft, causing tissue ischemia with pain and other manifestations of arterial occlusion. Further measures to restore circulation may be necessary.

- Maintain intravenous fluids as ordered. *Adequate circulating blood volume is necessary to maintain cardiac output and tissue perfusion.*
- Protect the extremity, keeping it horizontal or lower than the heart. Use a cradle to keep bedclothes off the extremity and sheepskin or foam pad to protect it from hard or abrasive surfaces. Do not apply heat or cold. *Keeping the extremity lower than the heart promotes collateral blood flow. Ischemic tissue is easily damaged by minimal trauma such as shearing by bed linens, or heat or cold application.*
- Following surgery, avoid raising the knee gatch, placing pillows under the knees, or sitting with 90-degree hip flexion. *These activities may impair blood flow through the affected vessel.*

Anxiety

Clients with an acute arterial occlusion often are very anxious. The rapid and intense nature of preoperative activities can be overwhelming, increasing anxiety about the disorder and its out-come. Manifestations of anxiety may include trembling, palpitations, restlessness, dry mouth, helplessness, inability to relax, irritability, forgetfulness, and lack of awareness of surroundings. Nursing measures focus on establishing trust and minimizing the effects of anxiety to decrease surgical risk and improve recovery.

- Spend as much time as possible with the client. Provide opportunities to verbalize anxiety; offer reassurance and support. Support adaptive coping mechanisms. *The presence of a caring nurse provides a safe environment for expressing fears and anxieties. Coping mechanisms reduce the immediate perceived threat and increase the ability to deal with the situational crisis.*
- Perform required measures in an expedient but calm manner. *Calm, confident performance of treatment measures reassures the client and family that appropriate care is being given to treat the problem at hand.*
- Assess anxiety level at least every 8 hours; more often as needed. Intervene as indicated to reduce anxiety. *Assessment helps determine the intensity of anxiety, the client's ability to control it, and directs interventions to reduce it.*
- Decrease sensory stimuli as much as possible. *Reducing environmental stimuli provides the client a degree of control over anxiety.*
- Speak slowly and clearly and avoid unnecessary interruptions when listening. Give concise directions, focusing on the present. Involve the client in simple tasks and decisions to the extent possible. *High levels of anxiety interfere with learning. Keeping interactions focused on the present situation directs the client's focus and provides reassurance that it is the most important focus of the nurse as well. Providing opportunities for self-care and decision making reinforces the client's importance and power to control the situation.*

Altered Protection

Fibrinolytic and/or anticoagulant therapy used to dissolve existing clots and prevent further clot formation increase the risk for bleeding. Close monitoring of physical status and laboratory data is vital, as are measures to reduce the risk for injury and bleeding.

> **PRACTICE ALERT**
> Assess for and report manifestations of impaired clotting, including excessive incisional bleeding; prolonged oozing from injection sites; bleeding gums, nosebleed, or hematuria; petechiae, bruising, or purpura. Anticoagulants and fibrinolytics interfere with the clotting cascade and may cause abnormal bleeding.

- Monitor activated partial thromboplastin time (aPTT) during heparin therapy and prothrombin time (PT) or International Normalized Ratio (INR) during oral anticoagulant therapy. Report values outside desired range. *The APTT, PT, and INR are prolonged by anticoagulant therapy. Values higher than the desired range may indicate an increased risk for bleeding; values below the target may indicate inadequate anticoagulation.*
- Protect from injury: Use side rails or other measures as needed to prevent falls; avoid parenteral injections and other invasive procedures as much as possible; hold firm pressure over injection and intravenous sites for 5 minutes and over

arterial punctures for 20 minutes; use a soft toothbrush or sponge for oral care; use an electric razor for shaving. *Minor trauma can lead to extensive bleeding, particularly in the client who has received a fibrinolytic drug.*

Community-Based Care

When preparing the client and family for home or community-based care related to an acute arterial occlusion, discuss the following topics as indicated:

- Care of the incision
- Manifestations of complications to be reported, including symptoms of infection or occlusion of the graft or artery

- Long-term anticoagulant therapy, including the reason, prescribed dose, follow-up laboratory testing and appointments, interactions with other drugs, and manifestations of excessive bleeding
- Any activity restrictions or dietary modifications
- Lifestyle modifications to slow atherosclerosis and control hypertension
- Measures to promote peripheral circulation and maintain tissue integrity (see the discussion of peripheral atherosclerosis earlier in the chapter).

Refer for home care services (nursing care, physical therapy, housekeeping services) as indicated.

DISORDERS OF VENOUS CIRCULATION

The two primary categories of venous system disorders are occlusive disorders and those related to ineffective venous blood flow. Impaired venous blood flow can lead to stasis and clotting, as well as tissue changes associated with venous congestion.

Physiology Review

The venous system is a low-pressure system in comparison with the arterial circulation. Veins and venules are thin-walled, distensible vessels. While they contain smooth muscle that allows them to contract or expand, the media (muscle layer) of veins is significantly thinner than that of arteries. The low pressures in the venous system allow it to serve as a reservoir for blood. Stimulation by the sympathetic nervous system causes veins to contract, helping maintain vascular volume. The low-pressure venous system relies on skeletal muscle contractions and pressure changes in the abdomen and thorax to facilitate blood return to the heart. Unlike arteries, veins of the extremities contain valves to prevent retrograde blood flow.

THE CLIENT WITH VENOUS THROMBOSIS

Venous thrombosis (also known as *thrombophlebitis*) is a condition in which a blood clot (thrombus) forms on the wall of a vein, accompanied by inflammation of the vein wall and some degree of obstructed venous blood flow.

Venous thrombi are more common than arterial thrombi because of lower pressures and flow within the venous system (McCance & Huether, 2006). Thrombi can form in either superficial or deep veins. **Deep venous thrombosis (DVT)** is a common complication of hospitalization, surgery, and immobilization. Obstetric and orthopedic procedures carry a higher risk for venous thrombosis; it may develop in more than 50% of clients having orthopedic surgery, particularly surgeries involving the hip or knee (Kasper et al., 2005). Other significant risk factors for venous thrombosis include abdominal or thoracic surgery, certain cancers, trauma, pregnancy, and use of oral contraceptives or hormone replacement therapy. See Box 35–5.

BOX 35–5 Factors Associated with Venous Thrombosis

- Immobilization: myocardial infarction, heart failure, stroke, postoperative
- Surgery: orthopedic, thoracic, abdominal, genitourinary
- Cancer: pancreatic, lung, ovary, testes, urinary tract, breast, stomach
- Trauma: fractures of the spine, pelvis, femur, tibia; spinal cord injury
- Pregnancy and delivery
- Hormone therapy: oral contraceptives, hormone replacement therapy
- Coagulation disorders

FAST FACTS

- DVT is a common complication of surgery and immobility. It usually develops in the deep veins of the calf (80%).
- Venous stasis (sluggish blood flow), altered blood coagulation, and damage (e.g., inflammation) to blood vessels are precipitating factors for DVT.
- A thrombus or a portion of a thrombus may break loose, traveling through the venous system to the right side of the heart and into the pulmonary circulation, where it ultimately becomes lodged (pulmonary embolus).

Pathophysiology

Three pathologic factors, called *Virchow's triad,* are associated with thrombophlebitis: stasis of blood, vessel damage, and increased blood coagulability. Vessel trauma stimulates the clotting cascade. Platelets aggregate at the site, particularly when venous stasis is present. Platelets and fibrin form the initial clot. Red blood cells are trapped in the fibrin meshwork, and the thrombus propagates (grows) in the direction of blood flow. The inflammatory response is triggered, causing tenderness, swelling, and erythema in the area of the thrombus. Initially the thrombus floats within the vein. Pieces of the thrombus may break loose and travel through the circulation as emboli. Fibroblasts eventually invade the thrombus, scarring the vein wall and destroying venous valves. Although patency of the vein may be restored, valve damage is permanent, affecting directional flow (Tierney et al., 2005).

Deep Venous Thrombosis

The deep veins of the legs, primarily in the calf, and the pelvis provide the most hospitable environment for venous thrombosis. Approximately 80% of deep vein thromboses begin in the deep veins of the calf, often propagating into the popliteal and femoral veins (Figure 35–10 ■) (Tierney et al., 2005). DVT usually is asymptomatic; in some clients, a pulmonary embolism may be the first indication.

MANIFESTATIONS When present, the manifestations of DVT are primarily due to the inflammatory process accompanying the thrombus. Calf pain, which may be described as tightness or a dull, aching pain in the affected extremity, particularly upon walking, is the most common symptom. Tenderness, swelling, warmth, and erythema may be noted along the course of involved veins. The affected extremity may be cyanotic and often is edematous. Rarely, a cord may be palpated over the affected vein. A positive Homan's sign (pain in the calf when the foot is dorsiflexed) is an unreliable indicator of DVT. See the Manifestations box for a summary of the manifestations of deep and superficial venous thrombosis.

COMPLICATIONS The major complications of DVT are chronic venous insufficiency (see the next section of this

---

MANIFESTATIONS of Venous Thrombosis

Deep Venous Thrombosis
- Usually asymptomatic
- Dull, aching pain in affected extremity, especially when walking
- Possible tenderness, warmth, erythema along affected vein
- Cyanosis of affected extremity
- Edema of affected extremity

Superficial Venous Thrombosis
- Localized pain and tenderness over the affected vein
- Redness and warmth along the course of the vein
- Palpable cordlike structure along the affected vein
- Swelling and redness of surrounding tissue

---

chapter) and pulmonary embolism. Pulmonary embolism occurs when the clot fragments or breaks loose from the vein wall. As the clot travels, it moves through progressively larger veins and into the right side of the heart. From there it enters the pulmonary circulation, where it eventually occludes arterial flow to a portion of the lungs. The result is a mismatch between ventilation (air flow) and perfusion (blood flow) in a portion of the lungs. The effect on gas exchange depends on the size of the embolism and the vessel it

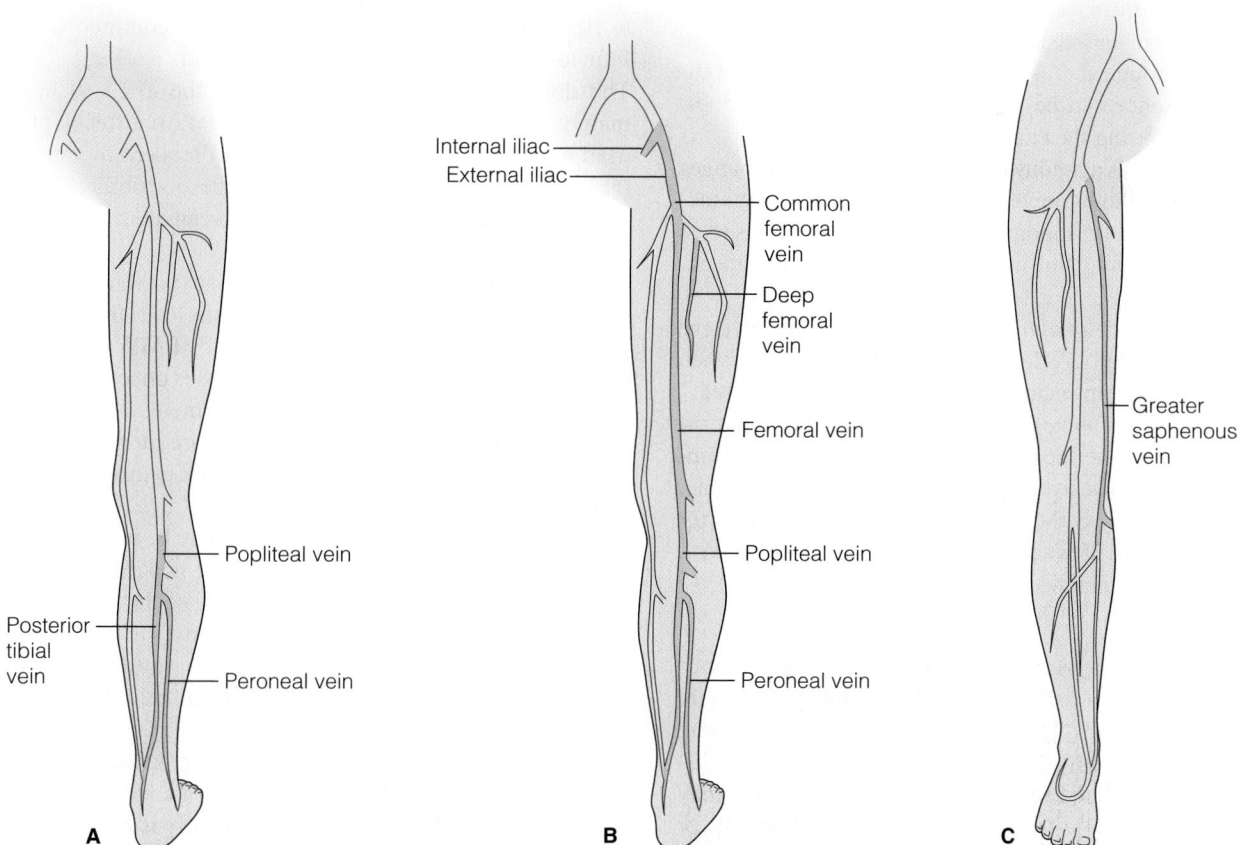

Figure 35–10 ■ Common locations of venous thrombosis. *A,* The most common sites of DVT. *B,* DVT extending from the calf to the iliac veins. *C,* Superficial venous thrombosis.

occludes. See Chapter 39 ∞ for more information about pulmonary emboli.

Superficial Venous Thrombosis

Venous catheters and infusions are the primary risk factors for superficial venous thrombosis. Superficial venous thrombosis also may develop in conjunction with thromboangiitis obliterans, varicose veins, or DVT. It may develop spontaneously in pregnant women or following delivery. In some cases, superficial venous thrombosis of the long saphenous vein is the earliest sign of an abdominal cancer such as pancreatic cancer (Tierney et al., 2005).

Superficial venous thrombosis is marked by pain and tenderness at the site of the thrombus. A reddened, warm, tender cord extending along the affected vein can be palpated. The area surrounding the vein may be swollen and red (see the Manifestations box).

INTERDISCIPLINARY CARE

It is important to differentiate venous thrombosis from other causes of extremity pain, such as cellulitis, muscle strain, contusion, and lymphedema. The history, physical examination, and diagnostic tests are used to establish the diagnosis. Treatment focuses on preventing further clotting or extension of the clot and addressing underlying causes.

Diagnosis

- *Duplex venous ultrasonography* is a noninvasive test used to visualize the vein and measure the velocity of blood flow in the veins. Although the clot often cannot be visualized directly, its presence can be inferred by an inability to compress the vein during the examination.
- *Plethysmography* is a noninvasive test that measures changes in blood flow through the veins. It is often used in conjunction with Doppler ultrasonography. Plethysmography is most valuable in diagnosing thromboses of larger or more superficial veins.
- *Magnetic resonance imaging (MRI)* is another noninvasive means of detecting DVT. It is particularly useful when thrombosis of the venae cavae or pelvic veins is suspected.
- *Ascending contrast venography* uses an injected contrast medium to assess the location and extent of venous thrombosis. Although invasive, expensive, and uncomfortable, contrast venography is the most accurate diagnostic tool for venous thrombosis. It is used when the results of less invasive tests leave the diagnosis unclear (Tierney et al., 2005).

Prophylaxis

Medications and other measures are used to prevent venous thrombosis when the risk is high. Low-molecular-weight (LMW) heparins prevent DVT in clients who are undergoing general or orthopedic surgery, experiencing acute medical illness, or on prolonged bed rest. Oral anticoagulation also may be used as a prophylactic measure in clients with fractures or who are undergoing orthopedic surgery.

Elevating the foot of the bed with the knees slightly flexed promotes venous return. Early mobilization and leg exercises

such as ankle flexion and extension assist venous flow by muscle compression. Intermittent pneumatic compression devices applied to the legs are effective to prevent DVT. They also are used when anticoagulation is contraindicated due to the increased risk for bleeding (Kasper et al., 2005). Elastic stockings are also used to prevent venous thrombosis in clients at risk.

Medications

Anticoagulants to prevent clot propagation and enable the body's own lytic system to dissolve the clot are the mainstay of treatment for venous thrombosis. Fibrinolytic drugs such as streptokinase or t-PA may accelerate the process of clot lysis and prevent damage to venous valves. There is, however, no evidence that fibrinolytic therapy is more effective in preventing pulmonary embolism in clients with existing DVT than anticoagulants (Kasper et al., 2005). It also significantly increases the risk for bleeding and hemorrhage.

Nonsteroidal anti-inflammatory agents (NSAIDs) such as indomethacin (Indocin) or naproxen (Naprosyn) may be ordered to reduce inflammation in the veins and provide symptomatic relief, particularly for clients with superficial venous thrombosis.

ANTICOAGULANTS Anticoagulants are given to prevent clot extension and reduce the risk of subsequent pulmonary embolism. See the Medication Administration box on pages 1189–1190 for the nursing implications for anticoagulant therapy.

Anticoagulation is initiated with unfractionated heparin or LMW heparin. Following an initial intravenous bolus of 7500 to 10,000 units of unfractionated heparin, a continuous heparin infusion of 1000 to 1500 international units per hour is started. The dosage is calculated to maintain the aPTT at approximately twice the control or normal value. An infusion pump is used to deliver the prescribed dosage. Frequent monitoring of the infusion is an important nursing responsibility. Subcutaneous heparin injections may be used as an alternative to intravenous infusion in some instances.

LMW heparins are increasingly used to prevent and treat venous thrombosis. They do not require the close laboratory monitoring of unfractionated heparins. LMW heparin is administered subcutaneously in fixed doses once or twice daily, allowing the option of outpatient treatment. LMW heparins have additional advantages, in that they are more effective and carry lower risks for bleeding and thrombocytopenia than conventional, unfractionated heparins.

Oral anticoagulation with warfarin may be initiated concurrently with heparin therapy. Overlapping heparin and warfarin therapy for 4 to 5 days is important because the full anticoagulant effect of warfarin is delayed, and it may actually promote clotting during the first few days of therapy (Tierney et al., 2005). Warfarin doses are adjusted to maintain the INR at 2.0 to 3.0 (Kasper et al., 2005).

Once this level is achieved, the heparin is discontinued and a maintenance dose of warfarin is prescribed to prevent recurrent thrombosis. Anticoagulation generally is continued for at least 3 months. When DVT is recurrent or risk factors such as altered coagulability or cancer are present, anticoagulant therapy may be prolonged. Regular follow-up is necessary to

MEDICATION ADMINISTRATION   Anticoagulant Therapy

HEPARIN

Heparin interferes with the clotting cascade by inhibiting the effects of thrombin and preventing the conversion of fibrinogen to fibrin. This prevents the formation of a stable fibrin clot. At therapeutic levels, heparin prolongs the thrombin time, clotting time, and activated partial thromboplastin time. When given intravenously, its effect is immediate. Given subcutaneously, its onset of action is within 1 hour. When heparin is discontinued, clotting times return to normal within 2 to 6 hours (Spratto & Woods, 2003). *Heparin-induced thrombocytopenia (HIT)* is a potential complication of therapy with unfractionated heparin. See Chapter 34 ∞ for more information about HIT and nursing responsibilities in monitoring for this dangerous potential complication.

Nursing Responsibilities

■ Assess for history of unexplained or active bleeding. Assess laboratory results for abnormal clotting profile or evidence of active bleeding.
■ Give a test dose as indicated to clients with a history of multiple allergies or a history of asthma.
■ Administer by deep subcutaneous injection; abdominal sites are preferred. Avoid injecting within 2 inches of the umbilicus. Rotate sites. Do not aspirate prior to injecting or massage after the injection.
■ Intravenous solutions may be diluted with dextrose, normal saline, or Ringer's solution. Use an infusion pump.
■ Keep protamine sulfate, a heparin antagonist, available to treat excessive bleeding.
■ Monitor and report abnormal laboratory results and aPTT values outside the desired range.
■ Promptly report evidence of bleeding such as hematemesis, hematuria, bleeding gums, or unexplained abdominal or back pain.

Health Education for the Client and Family

■ Report unusual bleeding or excessive menstrual flow.
■ Use an electric razor and a soft-bristle toothbrush; prevent injury by clearing pathways, using a night light, and other measures. Do not consume alcohol.
■ Avoid contact sports while on anticoagulant therapy.
■ Do not consume large amounts of food rich in vitamin K (yellow and dark green vegetables).
■ Do not use aspirin or NSAIDs while on heparin therapy unless advised to do so by your physician.
■ Wear a Medic-Alert tag and advise all healthcare providers (including dentists and podiatrists) of therapy.

LOW-MOLECULAR-WEIGHT HEPARINS

Ardeparin (Normiflo)
Dalteparin (Fragmin)
Enoxaparin (Lovenox)
Tinzaparin (Innohep)

LMW heparins are the most bioavailable fraction of heparin. They provide a more precise and predictable anticoagulant effect than unfractionated heparins. Like unfractionated heparin, LMW heparin prevents conversion of prothrombin to thrombin, liberation of thromboplastin from platelets, and formation of a stable clot. LMW heparins cannot be used interchangeably with each other or with unfractionated heparin. Although the risk of heparin-induced thrombocytopenia is significantly lower with LMW heparin, clients who were previously treated with unfractionated heparin may develop HIT when treated with LMW heparin.

Nursing Responsibilities

■ Assess for evidence of active bleeding, a history of bleeding disorders or thrombocytopenia, or sensitivity to heparin, sulfites, or pork products.
■ Monitor for unusual or masked bleeding. PT and aPTT levels may be within normal levels even in the presence of hemorrhage.
■ Administer by deep subcutaneous injection into abdominal wall, thigh, or buttocks. Rotate sites. Do not aspirate or massage.

Health Education for the Client and Family

■ Subcutaneous self-administration technique, timing of doses, and site rotation. Do not rub site after administering to minimize bruising.
■ Do not take aspirin, NSAIDs, or other over-the-counter drugs unless recommended by your physician.
■ Promptly report excessive bruising or bleeding, chest pain, difficulty breathing, itching, rash, or swelling to your healthcare provider.
■ Keep follow-up appointments as scheduled.

ORAL ANTICOAGULANT
Warfarin (Coumadin)

Warfarin interferes with synthesis of vitamin K–dependent clotting factors by the liver, leading to depletion of these factors. It has no effect on already circulating clotting factors or on existing clots. Warfarin inhibits extension of existing thrombi and the formation of new clots. Its action is cumulative and more prolonged than that of heparin.

Nursing Responsibilities

■ Assess laboratory results and history for evidence of abnormal bleeding.
■ Multiple drugs affect the metabolism and protein binding of warfarin; note all medications and assess for interactions with warfarin.
■ Do not give during pregnancy because warfarin may cause congenital malformations.
■ Oral tablets may be crushed and given without regard to meals.
■ Dilute intravenous warfarin with supplied diluent; administer within 4 hours by direct intravenous injection at a rate of 25 mg/min.
■ Keep vitamin K available to reverse effects of warfarin in the event of excessive bleeding or hemorrhage.
■ Monitor PT or INR; report values outside the desired range.

Health Education for the Client and Family

■ If bleeding occurs (hematemesis, bright red or black tarry feces, hematuria, bleeding gums, excessive bruising, etc.), do not take your prescribed dose and notify your physician immediately. Report rash or manifestations of hepatitis (dark urine, malaise, yellow skin or sclera).
■ Take your warfarin at the same time every day; do not change brands because their effects may differ.

(continued)

be sure prothrombin times (INR) remain within the desirable range for anticoagulation.

Treatments

Treatment of venous thrombosis also includes measures to relieve symptoms and reduce inflammation. With superficial venous thrombosis, applying warm, moist compresses over the affected vein, extremity rest, and anti-inflammatory agents usually provide relief of symptoms.

Bed rest may be ordered for deep venous thrombosis. The duration of bed rest typically is determined by the extent of leg edema. The legs are elevated 15 to 20 degrees, with the knees slightly flexed, above the level of the heart to promote venous return and discourage venous pooling. Elastic antiembolism stockings (TEDS) or pneumatic compression devices are also frequently ordered to stimulate the muscle-pumping mechanism that promotes the return of blood to the heart. When permitted, walking is encouraged while avoiding prolonged standing or sitting. Crossing the legs also is avoided, as are tight-fitting garments or stockings that bind.

Surgery

Venous thrombosis usually is effectively treated with conservative measures and anticoagulation. In some cases, however, surgery is required to remove the thrombus, prevent its extension into deep veins, or prevent the effects of embolization.

Venous thrombectomy is done when thrombi lodge in the femoral vein and their removal is necessary to prevent pulmonary embolism or gangrene. Successful thrombus removal rapidly improves venous circulation. The duration of this effect varies.

When venous thrombosis is recurrent and anticoagulant therapy is contraindicated, a filter may be inserted into the vena cava to capture emboli from the pelvis and lower extremities, preventing pulmonary embolism. Several different filters are available (Figure 35–11 ■). The Greenfield filter is widely used for its ability to trap emboli within its apex while maintaining patency of the vena cava. The filter can be inserted under fluoroscopy with local anesthesia. Mortality and morbidity associated with the filter are very low.

Extensive thrombosis of the saphenous vein may necessitate ligation and division of the saphenous vein where it joins the femoral vein to prevent clot extension into the deep venous system. A vein affected by septic venous thrombosis

Figure 35–11 ■ Venal caval filters. *A,* Greenfield filter. *B,* Nitinol filter.

is excised to control the infection. Antibiotic therapy also is initiated.

 NURSING CARE

Health Promotion

Prevention of venous thrombosis is an important component of nursing care for all at-risk clients. Position clients to promote venous blood flow from the lower extremities, with the feet elevated and the knees slightly bent. Avoid placing pillows under the knees and positions in which the hips and knees are sharply flexed. Use a recliner chair or footstool when sitting. Ambulate clients as soon as possible, and maintain a regular schedule of ambulation throughout the day. Teach ankle flexion and extension exercises, and frequently remind clients to perform them. Apply elastic hose and pneumatic compression devices when appropriate. Instruct clients to avoid crossing legs when in bed or sitting. Inquire about possible prophylactic heparin or warfarin therapy for clients undergoing orthopedic surgery or other high-risk procedures. Frequently assess intravenous sites. Change the site and catheter as dictated by agency protocol and if evidence of local inflammation is noted.

Assessment

Assess clients at risk for venous thrombosis for manifestations and risk factors.

- *Health history:* Complaints of leg or calf pain, its duration and characteristics, and the effect of walking on the pain; history of venous thrombosis or other clotting disorders; current medications.
- *Physical examination:* Inspect affected extremity for redness, edema; palpate for tenderness, warmth, cordlike structures; body temperature.
- *Diagnostic tests:* Clotting studies (aPTT, protime, INR).

See the accompanying Nursing Care Plan for an example of an assessment of a client with deep venous thrombosis.

Nursing Diagnoses and Interventions

In addition to the preventive measures identified earlier, priority nursing diagnoses for the client with venous thrombosis relate to pain, maintenance of tissue perfusion and integrity, and the potential adverse effects of prescribed treatments.

Pain

The pain associated with venous thrombosis results from inflammation of the involved vein. It may be aggravated by use

---

NURSING CARE PLAN   A Client with Deep Venous Thrombosis

Mrs. Opal Hipps, age 75, lives alone with her dog, Chester, in her family home in the suburbs. She retired from her job as a postal clerk 10 years ago and now spends a lot of time reading and watching television. Over the past week she has developed a vague aching pain in her right leg. She ignored the pain until last night when it developed into a much more severe pain in her right calf. She noticed that her right lower leg seemed larger than the left, and it was very tender to the touch. After seeing her physician and undergoing Doppler ultrasound studies, Mrs. Hipps is admitted to the hospital with the diagnosis of deep venous thrombosis in the right leg. She is placed on bed rest, and intravenous heparin. Michael Cookson, RN, is assigned to admit and care for Mrs. Hipps.

ASSESSMENT

Mr. Cookson notices that Mrs. Hipps was admitted 14 months ago for repair of a fractured femur. Mrs. Hipps says, "This business about a blood clot really has me worried." She also tells Mr. Cookson that she is worried about who will care for her dog while she is in the hospital. Physical findings include height 62 inches (157 cm), weight 149 lb (68 kg), T 99.2°F (37.3°C); vital signs within normal limits otherwise. Her left leg is warm and pink, with strong peripheral pulses and good capillary refill. Her right calf is dark red, very warm, and dry to touch. It is tender to palpation. The right femoral and popliteal pulses are strong, but the pedal and posterior tibial pulses are difficult to locate. The right calf diameter is 0.5 inch (1.27 cm) larger than the left.

DIAGNOSES

- *Pain* related to inflammatory response in affected vein
- *Anxiety* related to unexpected hospitalization and uncertainty about the seriousness of her illness
- *Ineffective Tissue Perfusion: Peripheral* related to decreased venous circulation in the right leg
- *Risk for Impaired Skin Integrity* related to pooling of venous blood in the right leg

EXPECTED OUTCOMES

- Verbalize relief of right leg pain by day of discharge.
- Verbalize reduced anxiety by the second day of her hospitalization.
- Demonstrate reduced right leg diameter by 0.25 inch (0.64 cm) by the fifth day of hospitalization.
- Maintain intact skin in the right foot throughout the hospital stay.

PLANNING AND IMPLEMENTATION

- Elevate legs, maintaining slight knee flexion, while in bed.
- Apply warm, moist compresses to right leg using a 2-hour-on, 2-hour-off schedule around the clock.
- Administer prescribed analgesics and evaluate effectiveness.
- Spend time with Mrs. Hipps to explain venous thrombosis and its treatment.
- Arrange for a friend or neighbor to care for Mrs. Hipps's dog.
- Apply antiembolism stockings as ordered; remove for 30 minutes every 8 hours.
- Monitor laboratory values to assess effect of anticoagulant therapy; report values outside desired range.
- Assist with progressive ambulation when allowed.
- Inspect legs and feet and record findings every 8 hours.

EVALUATION

Seven days after admission, the pain in Mrs. Hipps's right leg has subsided and the diameter of her right calf is equal to that of her left calf. Mrs. Hipps admits to Mr. Cookson that her fears really relate to a cousin who was hospitalized for a similar problem and had his leg amputated. After talking about her condition and the steps she can take to prevent its recurrence, she is much less anxious. Before discharge, Mr. Cookson reviews instructions for antiembolism stockings, daily walking, warfarin schedule, and scheduled follow-up appointment. Her neighbor, Kate, came to pick her up. As Mr. Cookson was helping Mrs. Hipps into the car, Kate handed her a small brown dog and said, "I took good care of Chester for you, but he's missed you." Mrs. Hipps smiled, and assured Mr. Cookson that she would call the number he provided if she had any questions.

CRITICAL THINKING IN THE NURSING PROCESS

1. Describe the pathophysiologic reasons for the pain in Mrs. Hipps's right leg.
2. How would you respond if Mrs. Hipps tells you she does not have the money to buy the prescribed anticoagulant when she goes home?
3. How would you change your teaching and discharge planning if Mrs. Hipps had difficulty caring for herself?
4. Design a plan of care for Mrs. Hipps for the nursing diagnosis *Activity Intolerance.*

See Evaluating Your Response in Appendix C.

of the involved extremity. Associated edema and swelling may contribute to discomfort. Measures to reduce the inflammation often help relieve the pain.

- Regularly assess pain location, characteristics, and level using a standardized pain scale. Report increasing pain or changes in its location or characteristics. *Tissue substances released during the inflammatory process can stimulate pain receptors. In addition, localized swelling presses on pain-sensitive structures in the area of the inflammation, contributing to discomfort. As inflammation and swelling are reduced, pain should abate. Continued or increasing pain may indicate extension of the thrombosis. Sudden chest pain may indicate a pulmonary embolism, necessitating immediate intervention.*
- Measure calf and thigh diameter of the affected extremity on admission and daily thereafter. Report increases promptly. *The inflammatory process causes vasodilation and increases vessel permeability, causing edema of the affected extremity. Baseline and subsequent measurements provide a measure of treatment effectiveness.*
- Apply warm, moist heat to affected extremity at least four times daily, using warm, moist compresses or an aqua-K pad. *Moist heat penetrates tissues to a greater depth. Warmth promotes vasodilation, allowing reabsorption of excess fluid into the circulation. Vasodilation also reduces resistance within the affected vessel, reducing pain. As edema subsides, pressure on surrounding tissues is relieved, thereby reducing pain.*
- Maintain bed rest as ordered. *Using leg muscles during walking exacerbates the inflammatory process and increases edema. This, in turn, increases venous compression and pain.*

Ineffective Tissue Perfusion: Peripheral

As thrombi develop, they occlude the lumen of the vein and obstruct blood flow. In addition, the accompanying inflammatory response may precipitate vessel spasms, further impairing arterial and venous blood flow and tissue perfusion. Impaired tissue perfusion, in turn, deprives tissues of nutrients and oxygen. As a result, distal tissues of the affected extremity are at risk for ulceration and infection.

PRACTICE ALERT

Assess peripheral pulses, skin integrity, capillary refill times, and color of extremities at least every 8 hours. Report changes promptly. Assessment of both extremities allows comparison of the affected and unaffected limbs. Weak or absent pulses, impaired capillary refill, or significant color changes in the affected extremity may indicate extension of the thrombus or a possible complication.

- Assess skin of the affected lower leg and foot at least every 8 hours; more often as indicated. *Frequent assessment is important to rapidly detect early signs of tissue breakdown and implementation of measures to protect vulnerable tissues. Early intervention allows healing and restoration of tissue integrity; allowed to continue, the process can lead to necrosis and potential gangrene.*

- Elevate extremities at all times, keeping knees slightly flexed and legs above the level of the heart. *Elevation of the extremities promotes venous return and reduces peripheral edema. Knee flexion promotes muscle relaxation.*

PRACTICE ALERT

Remove antiembolic stockings or pneumatic compression device for 30 to 60 minutes during daily hygiene. Antiembolic stockings (e.g., TED hose) and pneumatic compression devices exert pressure on the extremity and promote venous return. They can, however, impair perfusion of the dermis. Removing them periodically allows assessment of the underlying tissue and restores perfusion of the dermis, reducing the risk for skin breakdown. Their use may be continued following discharge to reduce the risk of recurrent venous thrombosis.

- Use mild soaps, solutions, and lotions to clean the affected leg and foot daily. Pat dry after washing, and apply a non-alcohol-based lotion or moisturizing cream. *Daily hygiene with nondrying soaps and solutions removes potential pathogens from the skin surface, and maintains skin integrity and the first line of defense against infection. Caustic or harsh soaps or solutions can dry and crack the skin. Dry, cracked skin permits bacteria and other microorganisms to enter and infect the tissue, potentially leading to ulceration and venous gangrene.*
- Use egg-crate mattress or sheepskin on the bed as needed. *Egg-crate mattresses and sheepskins distribute weight more evenly, preventing excess pressure on affected tissues.*
- Encourage frequent position changes, at least every 2 hours while awake. *Frequent position changes reduce pressure on bony prominences and edematous tissue, reducing the risk of tissue breakdown.*

Ineffective Protection

Anticoagulant therapy interferes with the body's normal clotting mechanisms, increasing the risk for bleeding and hemorrhage.

PRACTICE ALERT

Assess for and promptly report evidence of bleeding, such as petechiae, bruising, bleeding gums, obvious or occult blood in vomitus, stool, or urine, unexplained back or abdominal pain. Anticoagulants interfere with the ability to form a stable clot and prevent excessive bleeding. Even minor trauma such as toothbrushing or bumping into furniture can result in bleeding.

- Monitor laboratory results, including the INR (prothrombin time), aPTT, hemoglobin, and hematocrit as indicated. Report values outside the normal or desired range. *Coagulation studies are used to monitor the effect of anticoagulant medications. Values within the desired range prevent further clot development while carrying a low risk for bleeding and hemorrhage. A fall in the hemoglobin and hematocrit may indicate undetected bleeding.*

Impaired Physical Mobility

Although prolonged bed rest rarely is required, it is associated with many problems, including constipation, joint contractures, muscle atrophy, and boredom. Nursing care goals include maintaining joint range of motion, minimizing muscle atrophy, and reducing boredom.

■ Encourage active range-of-motion (ROM) exercises at least every 8 hours. Provide passive range of motion as needed. *ROM exercises maintain joint mobility and prevent contractures. Active range of motion (performed by the client) also helps prevent muscle atrophy and preserve function. While passive ROM exercises do not prevent muscle atrophy, they do maintain joint mobility.*

■ Encourage frequent position changes, deep breathing, and coughing. *Prolonged immobility can lead to impaired airway clearance and respiratory complications, such as atelectasis or pneumonia. Turning, coughing, and deep breathing facilitate expulsion of secretions from the respiratory tract, airway clearance, and alveolar ventilation.*

■ Encourage increased fluid and dietary fiber intake. *Constipation is a frequent complication of immobility due to decreased gastrointestinal motility and loss of abdominal muscle strength. Increasing fluid and fiber intake helps maintain soft, easily expelled stools.*

■ Assist with and encourage ambulation as allowed. *Ambulation promotes venous blood flow, helps maintain muscle tone and joint mobility, and increases the sense of well-being.*

■ Encourage diversional activities such as reading, handiwork or other hobbies, television or video games, and socializing. *Boredom may lead to dozing and inertia, with little physical movement or mental stimulation, increasing the risk for complications of immobility.*

Risk for Ineffective Tissue Perfusion: Cardiopulmonary

A thrombus that forms in the deep veins of the legs or pelvis may break loose or fragment, becoming an embolism. Emboli that originate in the venous system usually become trapped in the pulmonary circulation (pulmonary embolism). Gas exchange in the affected area is impaired as blood flow ceases or is reduced to an area of the lungs that is well ventilated (see Chapter 38 ∞).

■ Frequently assess respiratory status, including rate, depth, ease, and oxygen saturation levels. *A mismatch of ventilation and perfusion can significantly affect gas exchange, leading to rapid, shallow respirations, dyspnea and air hunger, and a fall in oxygen saturation levels.*

PRACTICE ALERT
Immediately report complaints of chest pain and shortness of breath, anxiety, or a sense of impending doom. The manifestations of pulmonary embolism are similar to those of myocardial infarction. Prompt intervention to restore pulmonary blood flow can reduce the risk of significant adverse effects.

■ Initiate oxygen therapy, elevate the head of the bed, and reassure the client who is experiencing manifestations of pulmonary embolism. *Oxygen therapy and elevating the head of*

the bed promote ventilation and gas exchange in those alveoli that are well perfused, helping maintain tissue oxygenation. Reassurance helps reduce anxiety and slow the respiratory rate, promoting greater respiratory depth and alveolar ventilation.*

Using NANDA, NIC, and NOC

Chart 35–3 illustrates linkages between nursing diagnoses, nursing interventions, and nursing outcomes for the client with deep venous thrombosis.

Community-Based Care

Treatment measures for venous thrombosis may be initiated and carried out on an outpatient basis or continued for an extended period of time following hospital discharge. Include the following topics when teaching for home care:

■ Explanation of the disease process
■ Treatment measures, including laboratory tests and their purposes, medications and adverse effects that should be reported
■ Appropriate methods of heat application
■ Prescribed activity restrictions
■ Measures to prevent future episodes of venous thrombosis
■ The importance of follow-up visits and laboratory tests as scheduled.

Refer clients for community nursing services for continued assessment and reinforcement of teaching. Provide referrals for assistance with ADLs and home maintenance services as indicated. Consider referral for physical therapy if needed.

NANDA, NIC, and NOC Linkages
CHART 35–3 The Client with DVT

NANDA

Ineffective Tissue Perfusion: Peripheral

↓

NIC

Circulatory Care: Venous Insufficiency

Positioning

Teaching: Prescribed Activity/Exercise

↓

NOC

Knowledge: Health Behaviors

Tissue Integrity: Skin and Mucous Membranes

Tissue Perfusion: Peripheral

Data from *NANDA's Nursing Diagnoses: Definitions & Classification 2005–2006* by NANDA International (2005), Philadelphia; *Nursing Interventions Classification (NIC)* (4th ed.) by J. M. Dochterman & G. M. Bulechek (2004), St. Louis, MO: Mosby; and *Nursing Outcomes Classification (NOC)* (3rd ed.) by S. Moorhead, M. Johnson, and M. Maas (2004), St. Louis, MO: Mosby.

THE CLIENT WITH CHRONIC VENOUS INSUFFICIENCY

Chronic venous insufficiency is a disorder of inadequate venous return over a prolonged period. Deep venous thrombosis is the most frequent cause of chronic venous insufficiency. Other conditions, such as varicose veins or leg trauma, may contribute; in some instances, it develops without an identified precipitating cause (Kasper et al., 2005; Tierney et al., 2005).

Pathophysiology

Following DVT, large veins may remain occluded, increasing the pressure in other veins of the extremity. This increased pressure distends the veins, separating valve leaflets and impairing their ability to close. DVT also damages valve leaflets, causing them to thicken and contract. The result is impaired unidirectional blood flow and deep vein emptying (Porth, 2005).

When venous valves are incompetent, the muscle-pumping action produced during activity cannot propel blood back to the heart. Venous blood collects and stagnates in the lower leg (*venous stasis*). Venous pressures in the calf and lower leg increase, particularly during ambulation. This increased pressure impairs arterial circulation to the lower extremities as well. The body's ability to provide sufficient oxygen and nutrients to the cells and remove metabolic waste products diminishes. Eventually, there is so little oxygen and nutrients that cells begin to die. The skin atrophies, and subcutaneous fat deposits necrose. Breakdown of red blood cells in the congested tissues causes brown skin pigmentation (Porth, 2005). Venous stasis ulcers develop. Congested tissues impair the body's ability to increase the supply of oxygen, nutrients, and metabolic energy to heal the ulcer. As a result, the condition worsens and, over time, the ulcers enlarge. The congested venous circulation also prevents the blood from mounting effective inflammatory and immune responses, significantly increasing the risk for infection in the ulcerated tissue (McCance & Huether, 2006).

Manifestations

Manifestations of chronic venous insufficiency include lower leg edema, itching, and discomfort of the affected extremity that increase with prolonged standing. The extremity is cyanotic. Recurrent stasis ulcers develop (Figure 35–12 ■), usually forming just above the ankle, on the medial or anterior aspect of the leg. They heal poorly, forming scar tissue that breaks down easily. Tissue surrounding the ulcer is shiny, atrophic, and cyanotic, and there is a brownish pigmentation to the skin. Other skin changes may develop as well, such as eczema or stasis dermatitis. Necrosis and fibrosis of subcutaneous tissue causes the affected area of the leg to feel hard and somewhat leathery to the touch, but even the slightest trauma to the area can produce serious tissue breakdown. See the box on this page for the manifestations of chronic venous insufficiency. Table 35–6 compares venous and arterial ulcers.

INTERDISCIPLINARY CARE

Collaborative care for the client with venous insufficiency focuses on relieving symptoms, promoting adequate circulation, and healing and preventing tissue damage.

Figure 35–12 ■ Chronic venous insufficiency. Note the discoloration of the ankle and the stasis ulcer.
Source: Dr. P. Marazzi, Photo Researchers, Inc.

The history and physical examination often establish the diagnosis of chronic venous insufficiency. Because a history of DVT is a major risk factor, careful evaluation of the past medical history and questioning of the client is important. There are no specific diagnostic tests to confirm the diagnosis of chronic venous insufficiency.

Conservative management of venous insufficiency focuses on reducing edema and treating ulcerations. Prolonged standing or sitting is discouraged. Graduated compression hosiery is ordered for daytime use, and frequent elevation of the legs and feet during the day is recommended. At night, the legs and feet should be elevated above the level of the heart by raising the foot of the mattress.

Treatment of associated stasis dermatitis varies, based on the duration of the condition. Wet compresses of boric acid, buffered aluminum acetate (Burow's solution), or isotonic saline solution are applied to acute weeping dermatitis four times a day for 1-hour periods. Following the compress, a topical corticosteroid (such as 0.5% hydrocortisone cream) is applied. Bed rest is prescribed during the acute period. Stasis dermatitis that is subsiding or chronic may be treated with a topical corticosteroid, zinc oxide ointment, or a topical broad-spectrum antifungal cream such as clotrimazole (Lotrimin) cream or miconazole (Monistat) cream (Tierney et al., 2005).

Isotonic saline compresses or wet-to-dry dressings are applied to stasis ulcers to promote healing. A dilute topical an-

---

MANIFESTATIONS **of Chronic Venous Insufficiency**

- Lower extremity edema that worsens with standing
- Itching, dull leg discomfort or pain that increases with standing
- Thin, shiny, atrophic skin
- Cyanosis and brown skin pigmentation of lower leg and foot
- Possible weeping dermatitis
- Thick, fibrous (hard) subcutaneous tissue
- Recurrent ulcerations of medial or anterior ankle

TABLE 35–6 Comparison of Arterial and Venous Leg Ulcers

FACTOR	ARTERIAL ULCERS	VENOUS ULCERS
Location	Toes, feet, shin	Over medial or anterior ankle
Ulcer appearance	Deep, pale	Superficial, pink
Skin appearance	Normal to atrophic	Brown discoloration
	Pallor on elevation	Stasis dermatitis
	Rubor on dependency	Cyanosis on dependency
Skin temperature	Cool	Normal
Edema	Absent or mild	May be significant
Pain	Usually severe	Usually mild
	Intermittent claudication	Aching pain
	Rest pain	
Gangrene	May occur	Does not occur
Pulses	Decreased or absent	Normal

tibiotic solution also may be used (Kasper et al., 2005). The ulcer may be treated by using a semirigid boot applied to the foot and lower leg. This device may be made of Unna's paste or Gauzetex bandage. Bony prominences must be well padded. The boot must be changed every 1 to 2 weeks, depending on the amount of drainage from the ulcer. This device often allows ambulatory treatment.

A very large, chronic ulcer may require surgery. In this case, the incompetent veins are ligated, the ulcer is excised, and the area is covered with a skin graft (see Chapter 17 ∞).

NURSING CARE

Nursing care for the client with chronic venous insufficiency is primarily educative and supportive. Client teaching includes the following recommendations:

- Elevate the legs while resting and during sleep. See the box on page 1196 for a nursing research study that suggests the supine position for resting.
- Walk as much as possible, but avoid sitting or standing for long periods of time.
- When sitting, do not cross your legs or allow pressure on the back of the knees (such as sitting on the side of the bed).
- Do not wear anything that pinches your legs (such as knee-high hose, garters, or girdles).
- Wear elastic hose as prescribed. The elastic hose should be tighter over the feet than at the top of the leg. Be sure the tops of the elastic hose do not cut into your legs. Put on the hose after you have had your legs elevated.
- Keep the skin on your feet and legs clean, soft, and dry.
- Follow guidelines in Box 35–4 for care of the legs and feet.

The following nursing diagnoses may apply to the client with chronic venous insufficiency.

- *Disturbed Body Image* related to edema and stasis ulcers on lower leg
- *Ineffective Health Maintenance* related to lack of knowledge about disorder and prescribed treatments
- *Risk for Infection* related to ulcerations

- *Impaired Physical Mobility* related to pain and edema in lower legs
- *Impaired Skin Integrity* related to presence of stasis ulcers
- *Ineffective Tissue Perfusion: Peripheral* related to incompetent venous valves.

See other sections of this chapter for specific nursing interventions related to many of these diagnoses. See the box on page 1196 for nursing care for the older adult with chronic venous stasis.

THE CLIENT WITH VARICOSE VEINS

Varicose veins are irregular, tortuous veins with incompetent valves. Varicosities may develop in any vein, and may be called by other names, such as hemorrhoids in the rectum and varices in the esophagus. Varicosities usually affect the veins of the lower extremities; the long saphenous vein is often affected, and they also may develop in the short saphenous vein.

Incidence and Risk Factors

Varicose veins affect about 2% of people in industrialized nations. They are more common in women over age 35. Studies also suggest that the increased risk for varicose veins in women may relate to venous stasis during pregnancy. Aging is a risk factor, possibly related to decreased exercise and other factors that contribute to venous stasis. People in occupations that involve prolonged standing (such as beauticians, salespeople, and nurses) also have an increased incidence of varicose veins. Race is a risk factor: Whites are more frequently affected than blacks. The majority of people with primary varicose veins (those affecting superficial veins) have a family history of the disorder, suggesting a genetic link (Porth, 2005).

Most varicosities occur in the deep veins of the legs. Contributing causes include obesity, venous thrombosis, congenital arteriovenous malformations, or sustained pressure on abdominal veins (as in pregnancy and/or the presence of abdominal tumors). The effects of gravity, produced by long periods of standing, are a major causative factor.

NURSING RESEARCH   Evidence-Based Practice for the Client with Venous Leg Ulcers

Chronic leg ulcers due to venous insufficiency are a challenge to treat and heal. Oxygen is necessary for tissue repair and to prevent infection; however, peripheral perfusion to deliver oxygen to the tissues is impaired in clients with chronic venous insufficiency. Using measurements of transcutaneous tissue oxygen (TcPo$_2$), a group of nurse researchers evaluated the effects of four different positions and supplemental oxygen on a small group of subjects with venous ulcers (Wipke-Tevis et al., 2001). Not surprisingly, these researchers found lower extremity resting TcPo$_2$ levels in clients with venous ulcers than in healthy adults. Changes in position resulted in minimal TcPo$_2$ changes in tissue surrounding the ulcer. When supplemental oxygen was given, TcPo$_2$ levels were higher in the supine position than with the legs elevated, sitting, or standing. These results suggest that control of peripheral circulation and tissue oxygenation may be impaired in clients with venous ulcers.

IMPLICATIONS FOR NURSING
The results of this study support advising clients with chronic venous ulcers to stay off their feet and rest in bed as much as possible to promote healing of venous ulcers. Remove compression stockings and devices while the client is in bed to promote perfusion of subcutaneous tissues and of the region surrounding the ulcer itself. Discuss the effects of position on peripheral tissue perfusion with clients, and encourage frequent rest periods during the day. Consider discussing the option of supplemental oxygen therapy for a client with delayed ulcer healing with the primary care provider.

CRITICAL THINKING IN CLIENT CARE
1. What is the usual response of blood vessels to changing positions from supine or sitting to standing? How does this compare with the results found here?
2. What is required for tissue healing? What measures can the nurse take to promote tissue healing in a client with impaired peripheral tissue perfusion?
3. How do the measures used to treat arterial and venous ulcers compare? Explain the rationale for differing treatment measures.

Pathophysiology

Varicose veins are classified as primary (with no involvement of deep veins) or secondary (caused by the obstruction of deep veins). In both cases, long-standing increased venous pressure stretches the vessel wall. This sustained stretching impairs the ability of the venous valves to close, causing them to become incompetent.

The erect position produces a twofold negative effect on the veins. When standing, the leg veins resemble vertical columns and must withstand the full force of venous blood pressure. Prolonged standing, the force of gravity, lack of leg exercise, and incompetent venous valves all weaken the muscle-pumping mechanism, reducing venous blood return to the heart. As standing continues, the amount of blood pooled in the veins increases, further stretching the vessel wall. The venous valves become increasingly incompetent.

Manifestations
Although varicose veins may be asymptomatic, most cause manifestations such as severe aching leg pain, leg fatigue, leg heaviness, itching, or feelings of heat in the legs. The degree of valvular incompetence does not seem to correlate well with the extent of symptoms. The menstrual cycle tends to worsen symptoms, suggesting a possible correlation with hormonal factors in women. Assessment reveals obvious dilated, tortuous veins beneath the skin of the upper and lower leg. If varicose veins are long standing, the skin above the ankles may be thin and discolored, with a brown pigmentation. See the Manifestations box below.

Complications
Complications of varicose veins include venous insufficiency and stasis ulcers. Chronic stasis dermatitis may also develop. Superficial venous thrombosis may develop in varicose veins, especially during and after pregnancy, following surgery, and in clients on estrogen therapy (oral contraceptives or hormone replacement therapy).

NURSING CARE OF THE OLDER ADULT
Chronic Venous Stasis

Disorders of venous stasis are common after the fifth decade of life. Aging affects vessels and tissues, increasing the risk for venous insufficiency and varicose veins. In addition, mobility frequently declines with aging, reducing the effect of the muscle pump in promoting venous return.

Regular exercise, walking in particular, is an important part of the treatment plan. Safety when walking is an important issue for older clients. Assess the client's mobility and stability during ambulation. If appropriate, suggest using a walker and quadcane as needed. Assist older clients holding jobs that require prolonged standing to identify strategies to minimize standing and incorporate periods of activity into their work.

Following surgery or during treatment for stasis ulcers, older clients may need additional assistance with home care and maintenance. Initiate referral to social services as needed to arrange for home nursing care, meals, assistance with ADLs, and home maintenance services as indicated. In some instances, temporary placement in an extended care facility is necessary until the client and family can assume care.

MANIFESTATIONS   of Varicose Veins

- Severe, aching pain in the leg
- Leg fatigue, heaviness
- Itching of the affected leg (stasis dermatitis)
- Feelings of warmth in the leg
- Visibly dilated veins
- Thin, discolored skin above the ankles
- Stasis ulcers

INTERDISCIPLINARY CARE

Varicose veins usually can be managed using conservative measures, although surgery may be required if symptoms are severe, when complications develop, or for cosmetic reasons.

Diagnosis

While varicose veins often are diagnosed by the history and physical examination, diagnostic tests may be ordered.

- *Doppler ultrasonography* or *duplex Doppler ultrasound* may be performed to identify specific locations of incompetent valves. This test is particularly useful before surgery to identify valves that allow reflux of blood from the femoral, popliteal, or peripheral deep veins into the superficial veins (Tierney et al., 2005).
- *Trendelenburg test* may be performed to determine the underlying cause of superficial venous insufficiency. The leg is elevated, then an elastic tourniquet is placed around the distal thigh. The varicosities then are observed as the client stands. When valves of the deep veins are incompetent, the veins remain flat on standing; they rapidly distend when the superficial venous valves are the underlying cause.

Treatments

Although there is no real cure, conservative measures are the core of treatment for most clients with uncomplicated varicose veins. These measures often relieve symptoms and prevent complications by improving venous circulation and relieving pressure on venous tissues. Properly fitted graduated compression stockings are commonly prescribed. They compress the veins, propelling blood back to the heart. Compression stockings augment the muscle pumping action of the legs. When worn during times of prolonged standing and in combination with frequent leg elevation, compression stockings often prevent progression of the condition and development of complications.

Regular, daily walking also is important. Prolonged sitting and standing are discouraged, although elevating the legs for specified periods during the day is beneficial. Leg elevation promotes venous return, prevents venous stasis, and decreases leg heaviness and fatigue.

Compression Sclerotherapy

In compression sclerotherapy, a sclerosing solution is injected into the varicose vein and a compression bandage is applied for a period of time. This obliterates the vein. Venous blood is rerouted through healthy vessels whose valves are not compromised. Compression sclerotherapy may be used to treat small, symptomatic varicosities. It may be the primary treatment, or it may be used in conjunction with varicose vein surgery. While compression sclerotherapy may be done for cosmetic reasons, complications such as phlebitis, tissue necrosis, or infection may occur and need to be considered prior to the procedures.

Surgery

Surgical treatment of varicose veins generally is reserved for clients who are very symptomatic, experience recurrent superficial venous thrombosis, and/or develop stasis ulcers. The objective of surgery is to remove the diseased veins. It may be considered for cosmetic reasons.

Surgery usually involves extensive ligation and stripping of the greater and lesser saphenous veins (Kasper et al., 2005). The evening before surgery, the surgeon marks all incompetent superficial and perforating varicose veins with a permanent ink marker. Under either regional or general anesthesia, the greater saphenous vein is removed and the connected smaller tributaries that have not naturally clotted off are tied off. Multiple small incisions may be made over the varicosities, allowing removal of the affected segments of the vein. Incompetent tributaries that communicate with larger vessels also are ligated. For clients with less extensive disease or clients seeking cosmetic improvement, surgery may involve only the removal of the lesser saphenous vein through an incision in the popliteal fossa.

Postoperative care includes applying pressure bandages for a minimum of 6 weeks, elevating the extremities to minimize postoperative edema, and gradually increasing amounts of ambulation. Sitting and standing are prohibited during the initial recovery period, and are gradually reintroduced as deemed appropriate by the surgeon.

NURSING CARE

Health Promotion

Health promotion activities to reduce the incidence of varicose veins include teaching all clients, particularly young women, the benefits of regular exercise continued over the lifetime. Discuss the effect of prolonged sitting or standing on the legs, and encourage the client whose occupation involves these activities to periodically get up and move or to sit with the legs elevated. Encourage all clients to maintain normal weight for their height.

Assessment

Focused assessment of the client with varicose veins includes the following:

- *Health history:* Complaints of leg pain, aching, heaviness, or fatigue; ankle swelling; history of venous thrombosis.
- *Physical examination:* Visible, dilated, tortuous superficial veins in lower extremities.

Nursing Diagnoses and Interventions

In planning and providing nursing care for clients with varicose veins, emphasis is placed on the importance of health teaching to manage the symptoms of varicose veins, particularly because there is no cure for the disease. Nursing care for clients who have undergone surgical treatment for varicose veins focuses on assessing and promoting wound healing and preventing infection. Nursing diagnoses may include those related to pain, impaired tissue perfusion and skin integrity, and a risk for impaired neurovascular function.

Chronic Pain

Varicose veins can lead to pooling of venous blood in the lower extremities. Venous congestion can cause a dull ache or feeling of pressure in the legs, particularly after prolonged standing. As venous pressure rises, arterial circulation and delivery of oxygen and nutrients to tissues is impaired. Tissue ischemia contributes to the pain. The pain associated with varicose veins tends to be chronic, developing and progressing gradually over a long period of time.

- Assess pain, including its intensity, duration, and aggravating and relieving factors. *Pain assessment allows collaborative planning with the client to identify appropriate interventions.*
- Inquire about current measures being used by the client to manage pain and its effects. Ask about the effectiveness of current management strategies and the desire to change. *Chronic pain management ultimately falls to the client. Strategies to address the pain must meet the client's needs.*

> **PRACTICE ALERT**
> Suggest keeping a diary of pain intensity, timing, precipitating events, and effectiveness of relief measures. Systematic tracking of pain is an important measure in improving its management.

- Teach and reinforce nonpharmacologic pain management strategies such as progressive relaxation, imagery, deep breathing, distraction, and meditation. *The effectiveness of such strategies is well documented. Nonpharmacologic measures provide a variety of options for controlling pain while maintaining independence. These measures also can reduce reliance on analgesics.*
- Collaborate with the client to establish a pain control plan. *Collaborative planning for pain management increases the client's sense of control and reduces powerlessness. This, in turn, enhances the ability to cope with pain and its effects.*
- Regularly evaluate the effectiveness of planned interventions and pain management strategies. *Regular evaluation allows modification of the care plan as needed, as well as providing a measure of disease progression. Increasing or poorly controlled pain may necessitate additional collaborative interventions to manage the disorder.*

Ineffective Tissue Perfusion: Peripheral

Varicose veins and venous stasis impair delivery of nutrients and oxygen to peripheral tissues as elevated venous pressures interfere with blood flow through the capillary beds. Improving venous blood flow reduces venous pressures and promotes arterial flow to peripheral tissues.

- Assess peripheral pulses, capillary refill, skin color and temperature, and extent of edema. *Assessment of arterial flow and tissue perfusion provides baseline and continuing data for evaluating the effectiveness of interventions.*
- Teach application and use of properly fitted elastic graduated compression stockings. *Elastic compression stockings compress the veins, promoting venous return from the lower extremities. During ambulation, the stockings enhance the blood-pumping action of the muscles. Because elastic stockings inhibit blood flow through small superficial ves-*

sels, they should be removed at least once each day for at least 30 minutes.

> **PRACTICE ALERT**
> Instruct to maintain a program of regular exercise, such as walking for 20 to 30 minutes several times a day. Exercise stimulates circulation and promotes blood flow through the vascular system. When ambulation is restricted, active ROM exercises help maintain muscle tone, joint mobility, and venous return.

- Advise to elevate the legs for 15 to 20 minutes several times a day and to sleep with the legs elevated above the level of the heart. *Elevating the legs promotes venous return, reducing tissue congestion and improving arterial circulation. Improved venous return also increases the cardiac output and renal perfusion, promoting elimination of excess fluid and decreasing peripheral edema.*

Risk for Impaired Skin Integrity

Ineffective venous valve function impairs venous return and increases venous pressures. These increased pressures oppose arterial blood flow and the delivery of oxygen and nutrients to the cells. As a result, tissues are vulnerable to any additional insult, and may break down.

- Assess lower extremity color, temperature, moisture, and for evidence of pressure or breakdown on admission and at each visit. *Initial and continuing assessment allows timely detection of early signs of skin and tissue breakdown. This, in turn, allows early institution of measures to prevent further tissue damage and promote healing.*
- Teach foot and skin care measures such as daily cleansing with nondrying soap, gentle drying, and lotions to prevent skin dryness and cracking. *Cleansing removes potentially harmful microorganisms and stimulates circulation. Care is taken to keep the skin moist and supple, promoting its function as the first line of defense against infection.*
- Discuss the importance of adequate nutrition and fluid intake. *Adequate nutrients are necessary to maintain tissue integrity and promote healing. A diet high in protein, carbohydrates, and vitamins and minerals promotes growth and maintenance of skin cells, provides energy, and helps prevent skin breakdown. Adequate hydration helps maintain the moisture and turgor of skin, reducing the risk of drying and breakdown.*

Risk for Peripheral Neurovascular Dysfunction

Severe varicose veins can lead to chronic venous insufficiency, impaired arterial circulation, and ultimately, disrupted sensation in the affected extremity. Impaired neurologic function increases the client's risk for injury and infection of the extremity, because minor trauma may go unnoticed.

- Assess circulation, sensation, and movement of the lower extremities. *Disrupted circulation and venous congestion may interfere with sensory and motor function of the affected extremity. The potential for nerve and muscle involvement is especially high in clients with venous stasis ulcers.*

PRACTICE ALERT

Instruct to report signs of neurovascular dysfunction, such as numbness, coldness, pain, or tingling of an extremity. Early recognition of neurovascular dysfunction facilitates institution of interventions to prevent complications. Because the postoperative hospital stay following varicose vein surgery or venous stasis ulcer repair is brief, manifestations of neurovascular dysfunction may initially be detected by the client. Careful assessment and prompt reporting help prevent potential complications such as skin breakdown, infection, and nerve damage.

■ Teach measures to protect the extremities from injury, such as always wearing shoes or firm slippers, cotton socks to absorb moisture, and testing the temperature of bath water with a thermometer or the upper extremities before stepping in. *Sensation in the lower extremities may be affected by poor circulation, necessitating additional measures to protect the legs and feet from injury.*

Community-Based Care

Most clients with varicose veins provide self-care at home. Include the following topics when preparing the client and family for home care:

■ Leg elevation and exercise program
■ Application and use of graduated elastic compression stockings
■ Foot and leg care (see Box 35–4)
■ Measures to avoid injury and skin breakdown
■ Symptoms or potential complications to report to the physician.

Provide information about suppliers for elastic stockings and any other required supplies. If venous stasis ulcers have developed, consider referral to home health services for regular assessment of healing and additional teaching.

DISORDERS OF THE LYMPHATIC SYSTEM

The lymphatic system, which includes the lymphatic vessels and the lymph nodes, is a unique part of the circulatory system. The lymphatic system returns plasma and plasma proteins filtered out of the capillaries from interstitial tissues to the bloodstream. This fluid is called *lymph*. The lymphatic system consists of closed capillaries leading to larger lymphatic venules and lymphatic veins. These vessels contain smooth muscle and one-way valves that help move fluid toward the heart. Lymphatic vessels share the same sheath as arteries and veins; arterial pulsations and skeletal muscle contractions compress the lymphatic vessels to assist in maintaining lymph flow. As lymph moves through the lymphatic system, it is filtered through thousands of bean-shaped lymph nodes clustered along the vessels. Within these nodes, phagocytes remove foreign material from the lymph, preventing it from entering the bloodstream.

THE CLIENT WITH LYMPHADENOPATHY

Lymphadenopathy, enlarged lymph nodes, may be localized or generalized. Localized lymphadenopathy usually results from an inflammatory process (e.g., streptococcal pharyngitis or an infected wound). The node enlarges as lymphocytes and monocytes proliferate within the node to destroy infectious material. Palpable lymph nodes often develop in response to minor trauma or a localized infection. Generalized lymphadenopathy usually is associated with malignancy or disease. Malignant cells or other abnormal cells invade the node, causing it to enlarge.

Lymphangitis, inflammation of the lymph vessels draining an infected area of the body, is characterized by a red streak along the inflamed vessels, pain, heat, and swelling. Fever and chills also may be present. Local lymph nodes are swollen and tender.

Treatment for lymphadenopathy and lymphangitis focuses on identifying and treating the underlying condition. Elevating the body part and applying heat to inflamed lymphatic vessels help reduce swelling and promote blood flow to the affected area.

THE CLIENT WITH LYMPHEDEMA

Lymphedema may be a primary or a secondary disorder, resulting from inflammation, obstruction, or removal of lymphatic vessels. It is characterized by extremity edema due to accumulation of lymph. *Primary lymphedema* is uncommon, affecting about 1 in 10,000 people. It affects females more frequently than males, and may be associated with a genetic disorder such as Turner syndrome or Klinefelter syndrome. See the accompanying Genetic Considerations box.

Secondary lymphedema is an acquired condition, resulting from damage, obstruction, or removal of lymphatic vessels. The most common worldwide cause of secondary lymphedema is *filariasis*, infestation of the lymphatic vessels by filaria, a nematode worm. Other important causes of secondary lymphedema include recurrent episodes of bacterial lymphangitis, obstruction of lymph vessels by tumors, and surgical or radiation treatment for breast cancer (Kasper et al., 2005).

GENETIC CONSIDERATIONS
Primary Lymphedema

■ Primary lymphedema develops as a result of agenesis, hypoplasia, or obstruction of lymphatic vessels.
■ *Congenital lymphedema* appears shortly after birth; two other forms of lymphedema develop later, one at the time of puberty (*lymphedema praecox*), the other usually after age 35 (*lymphedema tarda*).
■ Congenital lymphedema and lymphedema praecox may be inherited as an autosomal dominant trait with variable penetrance.
■ Lymphedema also may be inherited (although less commonly) as an autosomal or sex-linked recessive disorder (Kasper et al., 2005).

Pathophysiology and Manifestations

Obstruction of lymph drainage prevents fluid and protein molecules from interstitial tissues from returning to the circulation. The protein molecules increase the osmotic pressure in interstitial tissues, drawing in additional fluid that causes edema in the soft tissues. One or both extremities may be affected.

The edema begins distally, progressing up the limb to involve the entire extremity. Initial edema is soft and pitting; with chronic congestion, subcutaneous tissues become fibrotic, causing thick, rough skin and a woody texture of the limb (*brawny edema*). In contrast, the edema associated with venous disorders is softer, and the skin often is hyperpigmented with evidence of stasis dermatitis. Lymphedema generally is painless, although the limb may feel heavy.

INTERDISCIPLINARY CARE

Interdisciplinary care for the client with lymphedema focuses on relieving edema and preventing or treating infection. The disorder may be difficult to treat effectively, and can lead to progressive disability due to the weight and awkwardness of the affected extremity.

Diagnosis

Abdominal or pelvic ultrasound and CT scans are used to detect obstructing lesions. MRI can show edema and identify lymph nodes and enlarged lymphatic vessels. More invasive procedures such as lymphangiography and radioactive isotope studies may occasionally be necessary to identify the lymphatic defect causing lymphedema.

- *Lymphangiography* uses injected contrast media to illustrate lymphatic vessels on x-rays. Organic dyes are used to identify a distal lymphatic vessel, and then a contrast medium is injected into the vessel for visualization of the lymphatic system of the limb. In primary lymphedema, lymph vessels are absent or hypoplastic (underdeveloped). In secondary lymphedema, lymph channels often are dilated; it may be possible to determine the level of obstruction (Kasper et al., 2005).
- *Lymphoscintigraphy* involves injecting a radioactively tagged substance into distal subcutaneous tissues of the extremity, then mapping its flow through the lymphatic system. The pattern of lymph fluid distribution and transport is abnormal in clients with lymphedema.

Treatments

Meticulous skin and foot care is vital to prevent infection in the affected extremity. Shoes should always be worn to reduce the risk of injury. Careful cleansing and use of emollient lotions are recommended to prevent drying of the skin. Exercise is encouraged, as are frequent periods of leg elevation. The foot of the bed is raised by 15 to 20 degrees at night to promote lymph flow. Elastic graduated compression stockings may be ordered for use during the day. In some cases, an intermittent pneumatic compression device to reduce edema may be prescribed for home use.

Antibiotics are given to prevent and treat infection, which can be recurrent and difficult to eradicate. Diuretic therapy may be used intermittently, particularly when primary lymphedema is exacerbated by the menstrual cycle or seasonal variability (Tierney et al., 2005).

Clients who do not respond to conservative treatment measures or who experience recurrent episodes of cellulitis and lymphangitis may require surgical treatment. Microvascular techniques may be used to create anastomoses between obstructed lymphatic vessels and adjacent veins, providing channels to redirect lymph into the venous system. Successful surgery may improve both extremity function and its cosmetic appearance (Tierney et al., 2005).

NURSING CARE

Nursing care for clients with lymphatic disorders focuses on reducing edema, preventing tissue damage related to the edema, and promoting effective coping with the effect of the disorder on body image and function.

Nursing Diagnoses and Interventions

Nursing diagnoses for the client with lymphedema may include *Impaired Tissue Integrity, Excess Fluid Volume,* and *Disturbed Body Image.*

Impaired Tissue Integrity

Obstructed lymphatic flow leads to fluid congestion of the interstitial spaces of subcutaneous tissue. The resulting edema compresses and damages tissues of the affected extremity. Subcutaneous tissues become fibrotic, reducing their protective functions of shock absorption and insulation. In addition, obstructed lymphatic flow reduces the effectiveness of lymph nodes in filtering and removing foreign material and pathogens from the body. This increases the risk for local tissue infection such as *cellulitis,* a diffuse bacterial infection of the skin. Cellulitis increases the risk for skin and tissue breakdown and, if not effectively treated, can lead to sepsis.

> **PRACTICE ALERT**
> Frequently inspect the skin of the affected extremity, documenting condition with each assessment. Promptly report areas of pallor, redness, or apparent inflammation. Breaks in the skin surface allow microbial invasion, and increase the risk for infection. Prompt identification and treatment of any lesions is vital to prevent further tissue breakdown and infection.

- Apply well-fitting elastic graduated compression stockings or intermittent pneumatic pressure devices as ordered. *Elastic stockings and/or pneumatic pressure devices oppose the movement of fluid out of capillaries and improve its reabsorption into vascular spaces for transportation back to the heart.*

> **PRACTICE ALERT**
> Remove elastic stockings and intermittent pressure devices every 8 hours or at each home visit to inspect the underlying skin for evidence of redness, irritation, dryness, or breakdown. Elastic graduated compression stockings, antiembolic stockings, and pneumatic compression devices compress small vessels nourishing the skin and subcutaneous tissue. Periodic removal not only allows inspection of the underlying skin, but also allows restoration of blood flow to these small vessels and the tissues.

- Instruct to elevate the extremities while seated and during sleep. *Elevation of the extremities diminishes venous congestion, promotes venous return, facilitates arterial circulation and tissue perfusion, and helps reduce the accumulation of excess fluids in interstitial spaces of the affected extremity.*

PRACTICE ALERT
Use preventive skin care devices as indicated. Collected fluid in the affected extremity increases its weight and interferes with regular movement. The increased weight places greater pressure on surfaces of the limb that come in contact with furniture. Protective devices such as egg-crate foam, sheepskin, pillows, or padding help prevent tissue compression, promoting circulation and reducing the risk of skin and tissue breakdown.

- Keep skin clean and dry, especially in interdigital spaces. Teach skin and foot care to the client and family. *Clean, dry skin provides the first line of defense against infection. Significant limb edema can interfere with reaching the distal extremity and cleaning interdigital spaces. The dark, moist spaces between the toes are an excellent environment for bacterial growth. Teaching fosters self-care and independence, as well as preparing the client and family to manage this often chronic condition.*
- Discuss the importance of adhering to the therapeutic regimen. *Lymphedema generally is a chronic condition; effective management requires active client participation in planning and implementing care to reduce edema and maintain tissue integrity.*

Excess Fluid Volume
In lymphedema, obstruction, destruction, or congenital malformation of lymphatic vessels interferes with the normal circulation of lymphatic fluid. As a result, lymph collects in the subcutaneous tissues of the affected extremity, causing excess fluid volume of that extremity. Some clients may benefit from intermittent diuretic therapy and dietary sodium restriction.

PRACTICE ALERT
Monitor intake and output and/or weight (daily or weekly). Use consistent scales, timing, and clothing for accurate weight measurements. Intake and output records and short-term changes in weight reflect fluid balance. Measures of fluid balance permit evaluation of the effectiveness of interventions such as restricted sodium intake and diuretic therapy.

- Discuss the rationale for restricted sodium intake if ordered. Teach ways to maintain the recommended sodium restriction, and assist to choose foods that are low in sodium. *Sodium causes retention of extracellular water; restricting dietary sodium may help prevent additional fluid accumulation in interstitial spaces.*
- During acute periods, assess the affected extremity daily for increased edema; measure girth of the extremity using consistent technique. *The size of the affected extremity provides a measure of the effectiveness of ordered interventions and progression of the disorder.*

Disturbed Body Image
The disproportionate size of an extremity or extremities due to lymphedema can profoundly affect body image. During early stages of the disease, conservative measures may effectively reduce the edema and size of the affected limb. However, as the disease progresses, conservative measures may become less effective, leading to more permanent disfigurement. Mobility may be impaired, and the client may develop an increasingly negative self-perception.

- Encourage discussions about usual coping patterns and perception of self. *Knowledge of existing coping patterns and behaviors helps the nurse assess the client's ability to cope with the current situation. This knowledge is then used to reinforce effective coping mechanisms and help develop more effective coping strategies. This exchange also allows the client to voice feelings related to actual or perceived changes in body image.*
- Accept the client's perception of self and of the impact of the changes in appearance. *Nonjudgmental acceptance of the client's view of self and of the effects of changes in appearance builds trust and promotes rapport. A trusting relationship promotes the client's ability to take an active role in managing the disorder, participate in healthcare decisions, and adhere to the plan of care. Nonjudgmental listening also promotes mutual respect and demonstrates caring and compassion.*
- Encourage active participation in self-care. Assist with identifying alternative self-care strategies when the extent of edema interferes with performing some aspects of self-care such as trimming toenails or washing feet. *The client initially may have difficulty viewing or touching the affected body part. Gentle encouragement and support from the nurse helps the client assume self-care and accept the affected body part. Brainstorming to identify alternative care strategies promotes the client's independence even when total self-care is not feasible.*

Community-Based Care
When preparing the client with chronic lymphedema and family to manage the disorder, include the following teaching topics:
- Recommended program of exercise and elevation of the extremity
- Foot and skin care
- Use of elastic graduated compression stockings and/or intermittent pressure devices
- Importance of wearing elastic stockings during the majority of waking hours, removing them once during the daytime and while sleeping
- Measures to prevent infection in the affected extremity, such as wearing gloves while gardening
- Signs and symptoms to report to the healthcare provider (e.g., manifestations of tissue breakdown or infection, increasing edema, or evidence of compromised circulation)
- Use and precautions associated with any prescribed medications
- Sodium-restricted diet if ordered.

Provide information about contacts for questions, and make referrals as needed. Evaluate the need for home health, home maintenance assistance, and other services such as physical or occupational therapy.

EXPLORE MEDIALINK

Prentice Hall Nursing MediaLink DVD-ROM
Audio Glossary
NCLEX-RN® Review

COMPANION WEBSITE www.prenhall.com/lemone
Audio Glossary
NCLEX-RN® Review
Care Plan Activity: Lymphedema
Case Study: Abdominal Aortic Aneurysm
MediaLink Application
 Calcium Channel Overdose
 Peripheral Vascular Disease
Links to Resources

CHAPTER HIGHLIGHTS

- Essential hypertension, blood pressure of 140/90 or higher with no clearly identified cause, rarely causes symptoms but is a major risk factor for coronary heart disease, heart failure, stroke, and renal insufficiency.

- Prehypertension, a newly identified category, is an average blood pressure of 120–139/80–89. Clients with prehypertension are advised to make lifestyle changes indicated for hypertension (weight loss, exercise, dietary changes, limited alcohol intake, and stress reduction), but generally are not treated with medications unless other risk factors such as diabetes or kidney disease are present.

- Systolic hypertension, an elevated systolic blood pressure without elevation of the diastolic pressure, is common in older adults and contributes to complications such as coronary heart disease and stroke.

- Medications to treat hypertension include diuretics, alpha- and beta-adrenergic blockers, ACE inhibitors and angiotensin II blockers, calcium channel blockers, and vasodilators. A combination of two or more drugs often is required for effective blood pressure control.

- Aneurysms, abnormal dilation of a blood vessel, commonly affect the aorta and the iliac arteries, particularly in older men. A slowly expanding abdominal aortic aneurysm that does not produce symptoms or impair flow through the renal arteries may not be repaired, particularly in an older client. Percutaneously inserted endovascular splints provide an alternative to surgery for abdominal aortic aneurysms.

- Peripheral vascular disease, obstruction or occlusion of peripheral arteries by atherosclerotic plaque, is common and a leading cause of disability and amputation.

- Smoking cessation and regular daily exercise are key components of treatment for peripheral vascular disorders such as atherosclerosis, thromboangiitis obliterans, and Raynaud's disease.

- Venous thrombosis, particularly of the deep veins of the legs and pelvis, develops as a result of venous stasis, blood vessel damage, and increased coagulability of the blood. The developing clot may fragment or break loose, becoming an embolus that typically lodges in the pulmonary circulation (pulmonary embolus). Chronic venous insufficiency and venous stasis may develop as a result of deep venous thrombosis.

- Prophylactic anticoagulation and mobilization of the client are the primary preventive measures for venous thrombosis. Monitoring coagulation studies and assessing for evidence of bleeding (overt or covert) are important nursing measures for the client on anticoagulant therapy.

- Lymphadenopathy (enlarged lymph nodes), lymphangitis (inflammation of the lymph vessels), and lymphedema are the most common disorders affecting the lymph system.

TEST YOURSELF NCLEX-RN® REVIEW

1 A potential blood donor whose blood pressure is found to average 180/106 on two different readings tells the nurse, "I don't understand how it could be so high—I feel just fine." The appropriate response by the nurse is:
1. "This is probably just a false reading due to 'white coat syndrome.' Don't worry about it."
2. "It is unusual that you are not having some symptoms such as severe headaches and nosebleeds."
3. "High blood pressure often has few or no symptoms; that's why it is called the 'silent killer.'"
4. "You probably should have your blood pressure rechecked in 3 months or so and then follow up with your primary care provider if it is still high."

2 The nurse teaching a client about the DASH diet determines that additional teaching is necessary when the client states:
1. "I'm glad I can still eat as much pasta as usual; I was afraid I would have to give up my weekly lasagna."
2. "It will be a challenge to incorporate all those servings of fruits and vegetables into my diet."
3. "Having a handful of nuts when the pre-dinner 'munchies' hit is a good idea."
4. "I will enjoy having frozen yogurt as my bedtime snack on occasion."

3 The nurse teaching a client about his new prescription for Diovan HCT, a combination angiotensin II receptor blocker and thiazide diuretic, includes which of the following in his instructions? (Select all that apply.)
1. Use a potassium-based salt substitute to prevent hypokalemia while taking this drug.
2. Use caution when rising from bed or a chair to prevent dizziness.
3. Take the drug at bedtime to reduce the risk of falling due to light-headedness.
4. Report a persistent disruptive cough to your physician.
5. You may stop taking this drug once your blood pressure is within the normal range for 2 months.

4 A client is complaining of new-onset calf and foot pain. The nurse notes that the leg below the knee is cool and pale, and that dorsalis pedis and posterior tibial pulses are absent. The priority nursing intervention is to:
1. notify the physician.
2. place a cradle over the leg to prevent pressure from bedding.
3. position the leg flat, supported in anatomic position.
4. prepare to initiate heparin therapy.

5 An 86-year-old client with a newly diagnosed abdominal aortic aneurysm wonders if he will need surgery to repair the aneurysm, even though he feels fine. The nurse's response is based on the knowledge that:
1. the risk of surgical repair is lower than the risk that the aneurysm will rupture.
2. opening the abdomen for the surgical procedure greatly increases the risk of rupture.
3. surgery is indicated for type A aneurysms.
4. a percutaneously inserted endovascular stent may be considered because of his age.

6 An expected assessment finding in a client with peripheral atherosclerosis would be:
1. pallor of the legs and feet when dependent.
2. increased hair growth on the affected extremity.
3. higher blood pressure readings in the affected extremity.
4. impaired sensation in the affected extremity.

7 All of the following are appropriate home care measures for the client with peripheral vascular disease. Place them in order of priority.
1. foot and leg care
2. smoking cessation
3. daily inspection of feet and legs
4. regular daily exercise
5. weight loss strategies

8 The nurse evaluates her teaching of a client admitted with deep venous thrombosis as effective when the client states:
1. "I'll use a hard-backed, upright chair when sitting instead of my recliner."
2. "I'll get my blood drawn as scheduled and notify the doctor if I have any unusual bleeding or bruising."
3. "I understand why I am not allowed to exercise for the next 6 weeks and will take it easy."
4. "I'll have my wife buy a low-cholesterol cookbook and we'll make an appointment with the dietician to learn about a low-fat, low-cholesterol diet."

9 A client with visible varicose veins tells the nurse that she wants to have surgery to remove them, because "my legs ache every evening and they are really ugly!" The most appropriate response would be:
1. "Often measures such as elevating your legs and elastic stockings can relieve the discomfort associated with varicose veins."
2. "Surgery will have a good cosmetic effect, but will not relieve the discomfort associated with varicose veins."
3. "All varicose veins should be surgically removed to restore adequate blood flow to your legs and prevent gangrene."
4. "Surgery is never indicated unless the varicose veins are interfering with circulation. Have you tried cosmetic measures to cover them up?"

10 Which of the following nursing interventions is of highest priority for the client with lymphedema?
1. Elevate affected extremities at night.
2. Assist to don elastic compression stockings during the day.
3. Carefully dry and apply emollient lotion to affected extremities after bathing.
4. Reinforce the importance of taking prescribed diuretics.

See Test Yourself answers in Appendix C.

BIBLIOGRAPHY

American Heart Association. (2005). *Heart disease and stroke statistics–2005 update.* Dallas, TX: Author.

Aortic aneurysms: Synthetic graft prevents ruptures. (2005). *Nursing, 35*(6), 34.

Applying antiembolism stockings isn't just pulling on socks. (2004). *Nursing, 34*(8), 48–49.

Bartley, M. K. (2006). Preventing venous thromboembolism. *Nursing, 36*(1), Critical Care 64cc1, 64cc3–64cc4.

Beese-Bjurstrom, S. (2004). Hidden danger: Aortic aneurysms & dissections. *Nursing, 34*(2), 36–42.

Bonner, L. (2004). Clinical. The preventions and treatment of deep vein thrombosis. *Nursing Times, 100*(29), 38–42.

Canadian Hypertension Society. (2005). Management of hypertension. *Canadian Nurse, 101*(5), 25.

Chant, T. (2004). Clinical update: Peripheral vascular disease. *Primary Health Care, 14*(8), 29–34.

Copstead, L. C., & Banasik, J. L. (2005). *Pathophysiology* (3rd ed.). St. Louis, MO: Elsevier/Saunders.

Crowther, M., & McCourt, K. (2004). Get the edge on deep vein thrombosis: Head off progression of this deadly condition by knowing when to assess and what to look for during patient screening. *Nursing Management, 35*(1), 21–30.

_____. (2005). Venous thromboembolism: A guide to prevention and treatment. *Nurse Practitioner, 30*(8), 26–29, 32–34, 39–45.

Dee, R. (2003). Issues in geriatrics. Getting a leg up on varicose veins. *Clinical Advisor, 6*(1), 65–67.

Deglin, J. H., & Vallerand, A. H. (2003). *Davis's drug guide for nurses* (8th ed.). Philadelphia: F. A. Davis.

Dochterman, J., & Bulechek, G. (2004). *Nursing interventions classification (NIC)* (4th ed.). St. Louis, MO: Mosby.

Dunn, D. (2005). Preventing perioperative complications in special populations. *Nursing, 35*(11), 36–45.

Elton, G. (2004). Review: Elastic compression stockings prevent post-thrombotic syndrome in patients with deep venous thrombosis. *Evidence-Based Nursing, 7*(3), 86.

Fontaine, K. L. (2005). *Healing practices: Alternative therapies for nursing* (2nd ed.). Upper Saddle River, NJ: Prentice Hall Health.

Foxton, J. (2004). Actions to identify and reduce the risk of atherothrombosis in susceptible patients. *Professional Nurse, 19*(11), 30–33.

Gendreau-Webb, R. (2005). Is it a kidney stone . . . or abdominal aortic aneurysm? *Nursing Made Incredibly Easy, 3*(1), 44–47, 49.

Glover, A. J. (2005). How to detect and defend against DVT. *Nursing, 35*(10), Hospital Nursing 32hn1–32hn2, 32hn4.

Goldhaber, S. Z., McRae, S. J., & Wang, J. (2005, April 1). How to use low-molecular-weight heparin to prevent DVT. *Patient Care for the Nurse Practitioner.*

Gould, S. D., & Spandorfer, J. M. (2005, May 1). Unilateral leg swelling: Clues to cause and ways to treat. *Patient Care for the Nurse Practitioner.*

Graham, J. (2005). Heel pressure ulcers and ankle brachial pressure index. *Nursing Times, 101*(4), 47–48.

Jones, L. E. B. (2005). Endovascular stent grafting of thoracic aortic aneurysms: Technological advancements provide an alternative to traditional surgical repair. *Journal of Cardiovascular Nursing, 20*(6), 376–384.

Kasper, D. L., Braunwald, E., Fauci, A. S., Hauser, S. L., Longo, D. L., & Jameson, J. L. (Eds.). (2005). *Harrison's principles of internal medicine* (16th ed.). New York: McGraw-Hill.

King, M. J., & DiFalco, E. G. (2004). Addressing the pain. Lymphedema: Skin and wound care in an aging population. *Ostomy/Wound Management, 50*(5), 10–12.

Klein, D. G. (2005). Thoracic aortic aneurysms. *Journal of Cardiovascular Nursing, 20*(4), 245–250.

Lehne, R. A. (2004). *Pharmacology for nursing care* (5th ed). St. Louis: Saunders.

McCaffrey, R., Ruknui, P., Hatthakit, U., & Kasetsomboon, P. (2005). The effects of yoga on hypertensive persons in Thailand. *Holistic Nursing Practice, 19*(4), 173–180.

McCance, K. L., & Huether, S. E. (2006). *Pathophysiology: The biologic basis for disease in adults and children* (5th ed.). St. Louis, MO: Mosby.

Miller, E. R., III, & Jehn, M. L. (2004). New high blood pressure guidelines create new at-risk classification: Changes in blood pressure classification by JNC 7. *Journal of Cardiovascular Nursing, 19*(6), 367–373.

Moll, S., & Severson, M. A. (2004). Deep vein thrombosis: The hidden threat. *Care Management* (Suppl), 5–47.

Moore, J. (2005). Hypertension: Catching the silent killer. *Nurse Practitioner, 30*(10), 16–18, 23–24, 26–27+.

Moorhead, S., Johnson, M., & Maas, M. (2004). *Nursing outcomes classification (NOC)* (3rd ed.). St. Louis, MO: Mosby

Morris, C. M. (2005). Comorbidities increase hypertension dangers. *Clinical Advisor for Nurse Practitioners, 8*(3), 46–48.

Nadeau, C., & Varrone, J. (2003). Treat DVT with low molecular weight heparin. *Nurse Practitioner: American Journal of Primary Health Care, 28*(10), 22–23, 26, 29–31.

NANDA International. (2005). *NANDA nursing diagnoses: Definitions & classification 2005–2006.* Philadelphia: Author.

National Heart, Lung, and Blood Institute. (2003). *Facts about the DASH eating plan* (NIH Publication No. 03-4082). Retrieved from http://nhlbi.hih.gov

_____. (2004a). *Morbidity & mortality: 2004 chart book of cardiovascular, lung, and blood diseases.* Bethesda, MD: National Institutes of Health.

_____. (2004b). *The seventh report of the Joint National Committee on prevention, detection, evaluation, and treatment of high blood pressure.* Bethesda, MD: National High Blood Pressure Education Program, National Institutes of Health.

_____. (2005). NHLBI study: High blood pressure not well controlled among older men and women. *NIH News.* Retrieved from http://www.nhlbi.nih.gov/new/press/05-07-26.htm

Porth, C. M. (2005). *Pathophysiology: Concepts of altered health states* (7th ed.). Philadelphia: Lippincott.

Rice, K. L. (2005). How to measure ankle/brachial index. *Nursing, 35*(1), 56–57.

Rothrock, J. C. (2003). *Alexander's care of the patient in surgery* (12th ed.). St. Louis, MO: Mosby.

Ruff, D. (2005). Conservative management of varicose veins. *Nursing Times, 101*(4), 51–52, 54.

Skulski, C. (2004). Endovascular stent insertion for abdominal aortic aneurysm: A nursing perspective. *Canadian Operating Room Nursing Journal, 22*(3), 6, 9–10, 12.

Spencer, J. W., & Jacobs, J. J. (2003). *Complementary and alternative medicine: An evidence-based approach* (2nd ed.). St. Louis, MO: Mosby.

Spratto, G. R., & Woods, A. L. (2003). *2003 edition PDR® nurse's drug handbook™.* Clifton Park, NY: Delmar Learning.

Then, K. L., & Ranking, J. A. (2004). Hypertension: A review for clinicians. *Nursing Clinics of North America, 39*(4), 793–814.

Tierney, L. M., McPhee, S. J., & Papadakis, M. A. (2005). *Current medical diagnosis & treatment* (44th ed.). New York: McGraw-Hill.

Townsend, E., Griffiths, G., Rocker, M., Winter, R., & Lewis, M. (2005). Clinical. Setting up a screening service for abdominal aortic aneurysm. *Nursing Times, 101*(5), 36–38.

U.S. Preventive Services Task Force. (2004). Screening for high blood pressure: Recommendations and rationale. *American Journal of Nursing, 104*(11), 82–85, 87.

_____. (2005). Screening for abdominal aortic aneurysm: Recommendation statement. *The American Journal for Nurse Practitioners, 9*(5), 55–60.

Van Blerk, D. (2004). Evaluating an intermittent compression system for thromboembolism prophylaxis. *Professional Nurse, 20*(4), 48–49.

Way, L. W., & Doherty, G. M. (2003). *Current surgical diagnosis & treatment* (11th ed.). New York: McGraw-Hill

Widmar, B. (2005). When cure is care: Diagnosis and management of pulmonary arterial hypertension. *Journal of the American Academy of Nurse Practitioners, 17*(3), 104–112.

Wilkinson, J. M. (2005). *Nursing diagnosis handbook* (8th ed.). Upper Saddle River, NJ: Prentice Hall.

Wipke-Tevis, D. D., Stotts, N. A., Williams, D. A., Froelicher, E. S., & Hunt, T. K. (2001). Tissue oxygenation, perfusion, and position in patients with venous leg ulcers. *Nursing Research, 50*(1), 24–32.

Wong, J., & Wong, S. (2005). Evidence-based care for the elderly with isolated systolic hypertension. *Nursing & Health Sciences, 7*(1), 67–75.

Woods, A. (2004). Loosening the grip of hypertension. *Nursing, 34*(12), 36–45.

Woods, S. L., Froelicher, E. S., Motzer, S. A., & Bridges, E. (2004). *Cardiac nursing* (5th ed.). Philadelphia: Lippincott.

Wung, S., & Aouizerat, B. E. (2004). Newly mapped gene for thoracic aortic aneurysm and dissection. *Journal of Cardiovascular Nursing, 19*(6), 409–416.

Yang, J. C. (2005). Prevention and treatment of deep vein thrombosis and pulmonary embolism in critically ill patients. *Critical Care Nursing Quarterly, 28*(1), 72–79.

Yucha, C. B., Tsai, P. S., Calderon, K. S., & Tian, L. (2005). Biofeedback-assisted relaxation training for essential hypertension: Who is most likely to benefit? *Journal of Cardiovascular Nursing, 20*(3), 198–205.

Responses to Altered Peripheral Tissue Perfusion

FUNCTIONAL HEALTH PATTERN: Activity-Exercise

■ Think about clients with altered activity-exercise patterns and hematologic or peripheral vascular disorders for whom you have cared during your clinical experiences, and how the disease/disorder affected their activities.

■ What were the clients' major medical diagnoses (e.g., hypertension, anemia, leukemia, aneurysm, peripheral vascular disease, chronic venous insufficiency)?

■ What kinds of manifestations did each of these clients have? How were these manifestations similar or different among clients with different health conditions?

■ How did the clients' patterns of activity and exercise contribute to their health problems? Conversely, how did the clients' health status interfere with their daily activities and ability to exercise? Did the clients exercise regularly? Were the clients' symptoms affected by exercise, temperature changes, or changes in position? Did you observe changes in skin color, condition or temperature, hair distribution, or sensation? What other chronic medical conditions were present? What was your clients' history of alcohol or tobacco use?

■ The Activity-Exercise Pattern describes patterns of activity, exercise, leisure, and recreation. Disorders that affect the blood or vascular system can lead to insufficient physiologic energy for activities, disrupting the activity-exercise pattern.

Blood transports oxygen, nutrients, hormones, and metabolic wastes; is vital to immune function; maintains hemostasis and contributes to homeostasis. Changes in the amount or composition of blood affect its function and ability to meet cellular metabolic demands, leading to manifestations such as:

■ Fatigue (low RBC or hgb levels ▶ reduced oxygen-carrying capacity ▶ tissue hypoxia ▶ decreased cellular energy production ▶ weakness, fatigue, shortness of breath with activity)

■ Frequent infections (impaired WBC production or increased WBC destruction ▶ impaired immune surveillance ▶ increased incidence of infections)

■ Bruising, petechiae, bleeding tendency (impaired bone marrow function ▶ decreased platelet production ▶ impaired ability to form stable clots ▶ bleeding into tissues and external)

■ With each heartbeat, blood moves through a system of vessels that transport oxygenated blood to organs and tissues and return deoxygenated blood to the heart and lungs. The lymphatic system filters and returns excess tissue fluid (lymph) to the bloodstream.

Disorders of peripheral blood and lymphatic flow include constriction, obstruction, inflammation, and spasm. Arterial obstruction leads to tissue ischemia and insufficient oxygen to meet metabolic needs. Obstruction of a vein or lymph vessel increases pressure behind the obstruction, pushing fluid into interstitial spaces (edema), and interfering with oxygen delivery to the tissues. Manifestations often associated with peripheral vascular disorders include:

■ Intermittent claudication and impaired sensation (arterial occlusion ▶ decreased blood flow ▶ tissue ischemia ▶ pain, neuron damage ▶ paresthesias, impaired sensation)

■ Edema (venous or lymphatic vessel obstruction ▶ increased fluid pressure in capillary beds ▶ imbalance between capillary fluid loss and resorption ▶ increased interstitial fluid)

■ Priority nursing diagnoses within the Activity-Exercise Pattern that may be appropriate for clients with hematologic or peripheral vascular disorders include:

■ *Ineffective Peripheral Tissue Perfusion* as evidenced by changes in skin color and temperature, lack of hair growth, skin irritations or ulcers

■ *Activity Intolerance* as evidenced by weakness, fatigue, vital sign changes with activity

■ *Fatigue* as evidenced by difficulty completing usual daily activities, frequent desire to rest

■ *Impaired Home Maintenance* as evidenced by inability to maintain family roles

■ *Risk for Peripheral Neurovascular Dysfunction* as evidenced by changes in color, temperature, sensation of extremities.

■ Two nursing diagnoses from other functional health patterns often are of high priority for the client with altered hemotologic or peripheral tissue perfusion:

■ *Impaired Tissue Integrity* (Nutritional-Metabolic)

■ *Effective Therapeutic Regimen Management* (Health Perception-Health Management)

CLINICAL SCENARIO

You have been assigned to work with the following four clients for the 0700 shift on a cardiac medical-surgical unit. Significant data obtained during report are as follows:

- Theresa Cartwright is a 34-year-old female admitted for anticoagulant therapy after developing a deep venous thrombosis after a fall down the steps and hitting her calf. She was started on heparin yesterday and needs blood drawn for an activated partial thromboplastin time (aPTT) to determine her morning dose of heparin.
- Bessie Gregg is a 56-year-old with a 10-year history of alcoholism. She was admitted 2 days ago with pallor, shortness of breath, heart palpitations, weakness, and fatigue. She is agitated and requesting to be discharged.

- Scott Jacoby is a 25-year-old with Down syndrome. He was admitted yesterday with an upper respiratory infection. On assessment he was pale, T 101°F, P 100, R 30 with dyspnea on exertion, BP of 118/86, and multiple bruises and petechiae on his arms and legs. He is scheduled for a bone marrow examination this morning.
- Robert Tucker is a 65-year-old admitted 3 hours ago with moderate pain in the midabdominal region. On admission, a pulsating mass was felt in the midabdomen and a bruit was found over the same area. He is now complaining of severe pain in the midabdominal area.

Questions

In what order would you visit these clients after report?

1. _____
2. _____
3. _____
4. _____

2. What top two priority nursing diagnoses would you choose for each of the clients presented above? Can you explain, if asked, the rationale for your choices?

	Priority Nursing Diagnosis #1	Priority Nursing Diagnosis #2
Theresa Cartwright		
Bessie Gregg		
Scott Jacoby		
Robert Tucker		

3. Mrs. Cartwright needs further teaching regarding anticoagulant therapy when she makes which statement?
   1. "The heparin will be continued for four to five days for the Coumadin to reach a good effect."
   2. "I need to continue to have blood drawn to watch my drug levels as long as I am taking these drugs."
   3. "I cannot continue to take birth control pills while I am taking these drugs."
   4. "I need to take the medication at the same time every day for the drug to be effective."

4. The nurse explains to Mrs. Gregg that she needs a diet high in folic acid to treat her manifestations. Mrs. Gregg understands this diet when she picks which meal plan?
   1. chili with kidney beans, roll, and milk
   2. pork roast with baked potato and lemonade
   3. spaghetti with meat sauce and iced tea
   4. chicken and dumplings with coffee

5. Which is the most important for the client with leukemia to report?
   1. constipation and straining with bowel movements
   2. fever and burning on urination
   3. weight loss and decreased appetite
   4. dyspnea and shortness of breath with exercising

6. Which nursing interventions should reduce the risk of rupture of an aneurysm?
   1. Administer anticoagulant therapy medications.
   2. Instruct patient to hold the breath while moving.
   3. Maintain the patient on bed rest with the legs flat.
   4. Place the patient in a room near the nurse's station.

7. Which discharge instructions does the nurse teach the hypertensive client? (Select all that apply.)
   1. Maintain normal body weight.
   2. Eat a diet rich in fruits and vegetables.
   3. Reduce potassium intake.
   4. Limit alcohol to no more than 20 oz. of beer or 6 oz. of wine per day.
   5. Engage in aerobic exercise for 1 hour three times a week.
   6. Stop smoking.

8. Which nursing diagnosis has the highest priority for the client with varicose veins?
   1. *Body Image Disturbance*
   2. *Impaired Tissue Perfusion*
   3. *Activity Intolerance*
   4. *Risk for Infection*

9. With a history of Raynaud's disease, which is a priority teaching instruction for the client?
   1. Enter a smoking cessation program.
   2. Reduce dietary fats and carbohydrates.
   3. Wear gloves and socks in cold weather.
   4. Begin an exercise program.

10. A prescription for the calcium channel blocker diltiazem (Cardizem) is ordered for the client with hypertension. What will the nurse instruct the client regarding administration of the medication?
    1. Limit fluids to decrease the development of peripheral edema.
    2. Notify the physician for a pulse of less than 60 beats per minute.
    3. Increase fiber in the diet because diarrhea may be a side effect.
    4. Report tachycardia and an increase in blood pressure.

11. When the client is placed on warfarin (Coumadin) therapy, which laboratory studies would you expect to draw? (Select all that apply.)
    1. activated partial thromboplastin time (aPTT)
    2. international normalized ratio (INR)
    3. partial thromboplastin time (PTT)
    4. complete blood cell count (CBC)
    5. white blood cell count (WBC)
    6. prothrombin time (PT)

12. A client with history of hemophilia fell and cut his leg while hiking in the woods. Which intervention should the client do until help arrives?
    1. Apply a tourniquet above the cut.
    2. Splint the leg to prevent movement.
    3. Apply pressure to the femoral artery.
    4. Apply gentle pressure over the cut.

CASE STUDY

Grace Schmidt is a 49-year-old female who works as a teaching assistant at an elementary school. She comes to the medical clinic complaining of a throbbing headache and dizziness. Her height and weight are 5'6" and 245 pounds. Upon assessment her vital signs are P 100, R 16, BP lying is 180/115, sitting is 170/110, and standing is 165/105. Her skin is cool and dry. Her capillary refill is 4 seconds. She denies smoking, drinks an occasional glass of wine, and does not participate in a regular exercise program. She states that her job can be stressful at times. Nutrition assessment indicates a diet high in fats and sodium. She denies any family history of hypertension or heart disease. She is married and has a daughter and son who live in the same town. A medical diagnosis of hypertension is determined.

Based on Mrs. Schmidt's assessment, blood pressure readings, and weight, the priority nursing diagnosis of *Ineffective Health Maintenance* is identified for planning nursing care.

UNIT 11

Responses to Altered Respiratory Function

CHAPTER 36 Assessing Clients with Respiratory Disorders

LEARNING OUTCOMES

- Describe the anatomy, physiology, and functions of the respiratory system.
- Explain the mechanics of ventilation.
- Compare and contrast factors affecting respiration.

- Identify specific topics for consideration during a health history interview of the client with health problems involving the respiratory system.
- Describe normal variations in assessment findings for the older adult.
- Identify manifestations of impairment of the respiratory system.

CLINICAL COMPETENCIES

- Conduct and document a health history for clients having or at risk for alterations in the respiratory system.
- Conduct and document a physical assessment of respiratory structures and functions.

- Monitor the results of diagnostic tests and report abnormal findings.

EQUIPMENT NEEDED

- Tongue blade
- Penlight
- Nasal speculum

- Metric ruler
- Marking pen
- Stethoscope with diaphragm

The respiratory system provides the cells of the body with oxygen and eliminates carbon dioxide, formed as a waste product of cellular metabolism. The events in this process, called respiration, are:

- *Pulmonary ventilation:* Air is moved into and out of the lungs.

- *External respiration:* Exchange of oxygen and carbon dioxide occurs between the alveoli and the blood.
- *Gas transport:* Oxygen and carbon dioxide are transported to and from the lungs and the cells of the body via the blood.
- *Internal respiration:* Exchange of oxygen and carbon dioxide is made between the blood and the cells.

ANATOMY, PHYSIOLOGY, AND FUNCTIONS OF THE RESPIRATORY SYSTEM

The respiratory system functions as a whole, but is divided into the upper respiratory system and the lower respiratory system for discussion of respiratory disorders in the following chapters.

The Upper Respiratory System

The upper respiratory system serves as a passageway for air moving into the lungs and carbon dioxide moving out to the external environment (Figure 36–1 ■). As air moves through these structures, it is cleaned, humidified, and warmed.

The Nose

The nose is the external opening of the respiratory system. The external nose is given structure by the nasal, frontal, and maxillary bones as well as plates of hyaline cartilage. The nostrils (also called the external nares) are two cavities within the nose,

separated by the nasal septum. These cavities open into the nasal portion of the pharynx through the internal nares. The nasal cavities just behind the nasal openings are lined with skin that contains hair follicles, sweat glands, and sebaceous glands. The nasal hairs filter the air as it enters the nares. The rest of the cavity is lined with mucous membranes that contain olfactory neurons and goblet cells that secrete thick mucus. The mucus not only traps dust and bacteria but also contains lysozyme, an enzyme that destroys bacteria as they enter the nose. As mucus and debris accumulate, mucosal ciliated cells move it toward the pharynx, where it is swallowed. The mucosa is highly vascular, warming air that moves across its surface.

Three structures project outward from the lateral wall of each nasal cavity: the superior, middle, and inferior turbinates. The turbinates cause air entering the nose to become turbulent

Figure 36–1 ■ The upper respiratory system.

and also increase the surface area of mucosa exposed to the air. As air moves through this area, heavier particles of debris drop out and are trapped in the mucosa of the turbinates.

The Sinuses

The nasal cavity is surrounded by paranasal sinuses (Figure 36–2 ■), located in the frontal, sphenoid, ethmoid, and maxillary bones. Sinuses lighten the skull, assist in speech, and produce mucus that drains into the nasal cavities to help trap debris.

The Pharynx

The pharynx, a funnel-shaped passageway about 5 inches (13 cm) long, extends from the base of the skull to the level of the C6 vertebra. The pharynx serves as a passageway for both air and food. It is divided into three regions: the nasopharynx, the oropharynx, and the laryngopharynx.

The nasopharynx serves only as a passageway for air. Located beneath the sphenoid bone and above the level of the soft palate, the nasopharynx is continuous with the nasal cavities. This segment is lined with ciliated epithelium, which continues to move debris from the nasal cavities to the pharynx. Masses of lymphoid tissue (the tonsils and adenoids) are located in the mucosa high in the posterior wall; these tissues trap and destroy infectious agents entering with the air. The auditory (eustachian) tubes also open into the nasopharynx, connecting it with the middle ear.

The oropharynx lies behind the oral cavity and extends from the soft palate to the level of the hyoid bone. It serves as a passageway for both air and food. An upward rise of the soft palate prevents food from entering the nasopharynx during swallowing. The oropharynx is lined with stratified squamous epithelium that protects it from the friction of food and damage from the chemicals found in food and fluids.

The laryngopharynx extends from the hyoid bone to the larynx. It is also lined with stratified squamous epithelium, and serves as a passageway for both food and air. Air does not move into the lungs while food is being swallowed and moved into the esophagus.

The Larynx

The larynx is about 2 inches (5 cm) long. It opens superiorly at the laryngopharynx and is continuous inferiorly with the trachea. The larynx provides an airway and routes air and food into the proper passageway. As long as air is moving through the larynx, its inlet is open; however, the inlet closes during swallowing. The larynx also contains the vocal cords, necessary for voice production.

The larynx is framed by cartilages, connected by ligaments and membranes. The thyroid cartilage is formed by the fusion of two cartilages; the fusion point is visible as the Adam's apple. The cricoid cartilage lies below the thyroid cartilage; other pairs of cartilages form the walls of the larynx. The epiglottis, also a cartilage, normally projects upward to the base of the tongue; however, during swallowing, the larynx moves upward and the epiglottis tips to cover the opening to the larynx. If anything other than air enters the larynx, a cough reflex expels the foreign substance before it can enter the lungs. This protective reflex does not work if the person is unconscious.

The Trachea

The trachea begins at the inferior larynx and descends anteriorly to the esophagus to enter the mediastinum, where it divides to become the right and left primary bronchi of the lungs. The trachea is about 4 to 5 inches (12 to 15 cm) long and 1 inch (2.5 cm) in diameter. It contains 16 to 20 C-shaped rings of cartilage joined by connective tissue. The mucosa lining the trachea consists of pseudostratified ciliated columnar epithelium containing seromucous glands that produce thick mucus. Dust and debris in the inspired air are trapped in this mucus, moved toward the throat by the cilia, and then either swallowed or coughed out through the mouth.

The Lower Respiratory System

The lower respiratory system includes the lungs and the bronchi (Figure 36–3 ■ and Figure 36–4 ■).

The Lungs

The center of the thoracic cavity is filled by the mediastinum, which contains the heart, great blood vessels, bronchi, trachea, and esophagus. The mediastinum is flanked on either side by the lungs (see Figure 36–3). Each lung is suspended in its own pleural cavity, with the anterior, lateral, and posterior lung surfaces lying close to the ribs. The hilus, on the mediastinal surface of each lung, is

Frontal view

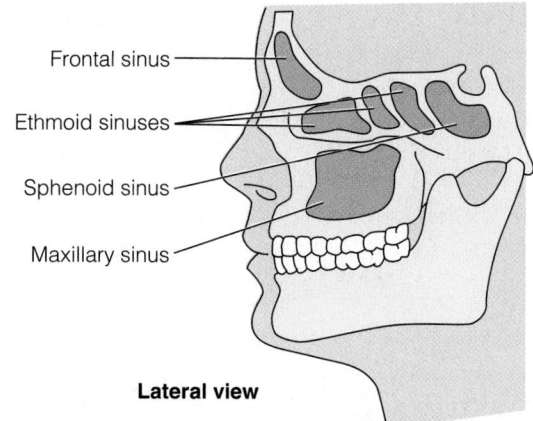

Lateral view

Figure 36–2 ■ Sinuses, frontal and lateral views.

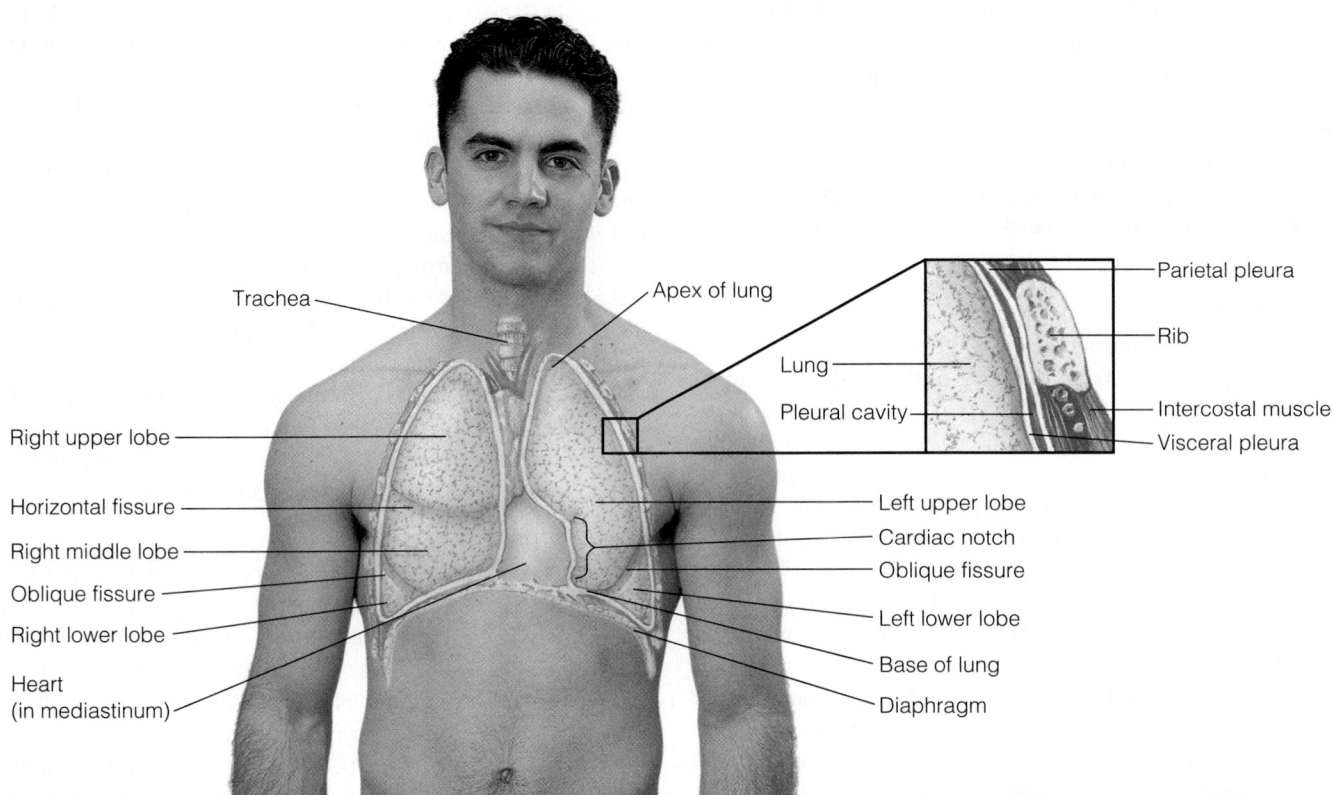

Figure 36–3 ■ The lower respiratory system, showing the location of the lungs, the mediastinum, and layers of visceral and parietal pleura.

where blood vessels of the pulmonary and circulatory systems enter and exit the lungs. The primary bronchus also enters in this area. The apex of each lung lies just below the clavicle, whereas the base of each lung rests on the diaphragm. The lungs are elastic connective tissue, called stroma, and are soft and spongy.

The two lungs differ in size and shape. The left lung is smaller and has two lobes, whereas the right lung has three lobes. Each of the lung lobes contains a different number of bronchopulmonary segments, separated by connective tissue.

There are 8 segments in the two lobes of the left lung and 10 segments in the three lobes of the right lung.

The vascular system of the lungs consists of the pulmonary arteries, which deliver blood to the lungs for oxygenation, and the pulmonary veins, which deliver oxygenated blood to the heart. Within the lungs, the pulmonary arteries branch into a pulmonary capillary network that surrounds the alveoli. Lung tissue receives its blood supply from the bronchial arteries and drains by the bronchial and pulmonary veins.

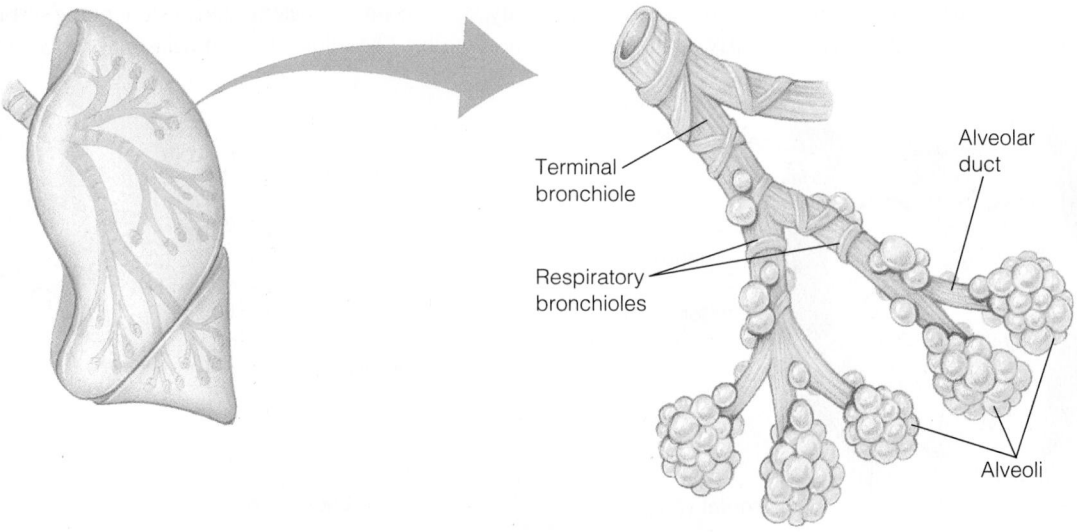

Figure 36–4 ■ Respiratory bronchi, bronchioles, alveolar ducts, and alveoli.

The Pleura

The pleura is a double-layered membrane that covers the lungs and the inside of the thoracic cavities (see Figure 36–3). The parietal pleura lines the thoracic wall and mediastinum. It is continuous with the visceral pleura, which covers the external lung surfaces. The pleura produces pleural fluid, a lubricating, serous fluid that allows the lungs to move easily over the thoracic wall during breathing. The pleura's two layers also cling tightly together and hold the lungs to the thoracic wall. The structure of the pleura creates a slightly negative pressure in the pleural space (which is actually a potential rather than an actual space), necessary for lung function.

The Bronchi and Alveoli

The trachea divides into right and left primary bronchi; in comparison to the left primary bronchus, the right primary bronchus is shorter, wider, and situated more vertically (making aspiration of foreign bodies into the right primary bronchus more likely). The point where the trachea divides is innervated with sensory neurons; activities such as tracheal suctioning may induce coughing and bronchospasm from stimulation of these neurons. These main bronchi subdivide into the secondary (lobar) bronchi, with the right middle lobe bronchus being smaller in diameter and length, and sometimes it bends sharply near its bifurcation. The secondary bronchi then branch into the tertiary (segmental) bronchi, and then into smaller and smaller bronchioles, ending in the terminal bronchioles, which are extremely small (see Figure 36–4). These branching passageways collectively are called the bronchial or respiratory tree. From the terminal bronchioles, air moves into air sacs (called respiratory bronchioles), which further branch into alveolar ducts that lead to alveolar sacs and then to the tiny alveoli. During inspiration, air enters the lungs through the primary bronchus and then moves through the increasingly smaller passageways of the lungs to the alveoli, where oxygen and carbon dioxide exchange occurs in the process of external respiration. During expiration, the carbon dioxide is expelled.

Alveoli cluster around the alveolar sacs, which open into a common chamber called the atrium. The adult lung has approximately 300 million alveoli, providing an enormous surface for gas exchange (Porth, 2005). Alveoli have extremely thin walls of a single layer of squamous epithelial cells over a very thin basement membrane. The external surface of the alveoli are covered with pulmonary capillaries. The alveolar and capillary walls form the respiratory membrane. Gas exchange across the respiratory membrane occurs by simple diffusion. The alveolar walls also contain cells that secrete a surfactant-containing fluid, necessary for maintaining a moist surface and reducing the surface tension of the alveolar fluid to help prevent collapse of the lungs.

The Rib Cage and Intercostal Muscles

The lungs are protected by the bones of the rib cage and the intercostal muscles. There are 12 pairs of ribs, which all articulate with the thoracic vertebrae (Figure 36–5 ■). Anteriorly, the first 7 ribs articulate with the body of the sternum. The 8th, 9th, and 10th ribs articulate with the cartilage immediately above the ribs. The 11th and 12th ribs are called floating ribs, because they are unattached.

The sternum has three parts: the manubrium, the body, and the xiphoid process. The junction between the manubrium and the body of the sternum is called the manubriosternal junction or the angle of Louis. The depression above the manubrium is called the suprasternal notch.

The spaces between the ribs are called the intercostal spaces. Each intercostal space is named for the rib immediately above it (e.g., the space between the third and fourth ribs is designated as the third intercostal space). The intercostal muscles between the ribs, along with the diaphragm, are called the inspiratory muscles.

FACTORS AFFECTING VENTILATION AND RESPIRATION

Many factors affect ventilation and respiration. Those discussed here include changes in volume and capacity; air pressures; oxygen, carbon dioxide, and hydrogen ion concentrations in the blood; airway resistance, lung compliance, and elasticity; and alveolar surface tension.

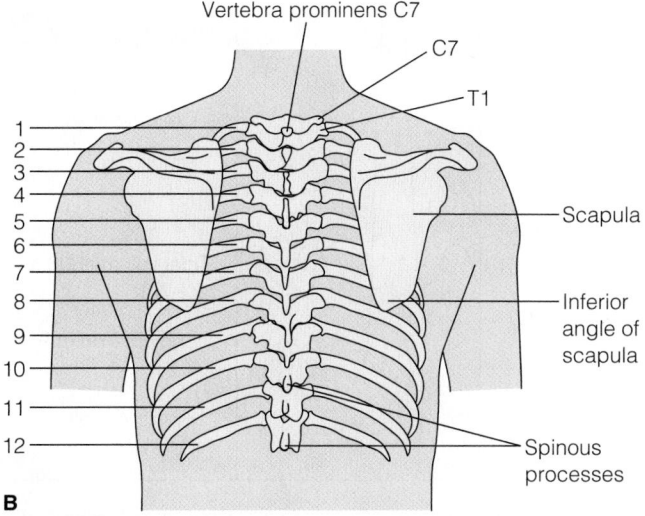

Figure 36–5 ■ *A*, Anterior rib cage, showing intercostal spaces. *B*, Posterior rib cage.

Respiratory Volume and Capacity

Respiratory volume and capacity are affected by gender, age, weight, and health status.

- **Tidal volume (TV)** is the amount of air (approximately 500 mL) moved in and out of the lungs with each normal, quiet breath.
- *Inspiratory reserve volume (IRV)* is the amount of air (approximately 2100 to 3100 mL) that can be inhaled forcibly over the tidal volume.
- *Expiratory reserve volume (ERV)* is the approximately 1000 mL of air that can be forced out over the tidal volume.
- The *residual volume* is the volume of air (approximately 1100 mL) that remains in the lungs after a forced expiration.

- **Vital capacity (VC)** refers to the sum of TV + IRV + ERV and is approximately 4500 mL in the healthy client.
- About 150 mL of air never reaches the alveoli (the amount remaining in the passageways) and is called anatomic dead space volume.

Pulmonary function tests measure these and other respiratory volumes and capacities, and are described and illustrated in Box 36–1.

Air Pressures

Pulmonary ventilation depends on volume changes within the thoracic cavity. A change in the volume of air in the thoracic

---

BOX 36–1 Pulmonary Function Tests

Pulmonary function tests (PFTs) are performed in a pulmonary function laboratory. After preparing the client, a nose clip is applied and the unsedated client breathes into a spirometer or body plethysmograph, a device for measuring and recording lung volume in liters versus time in seconds. The client is instructed how to breathe for specific tests: for example, to inhale as deeply as possible and then exhale to the maximal extent possible. Using measured lung volumes, respiratory capacities are calculated to assess pulmonary status. The specific values determined by PFT and illustrated in the figure include the following.

- *Total lung capacity (TLC)* is the total volume of the lungs at their maximum inflation. Four values are used to calculate TLC.
  - a. *Total volume (TV)*, the volume inhaled and exhaled with normal quiet breathing (also called tidal volume)
  - b. *Inspiratory reserve volume (IRV)*, the maximum amount that can be inhaled over and above a normal inspiration
  - c. *Expiratory reserve volume (ERV)*, the maximum amount that can be exhaled following a normal exhalation.
  - d. *Residual volume (RV)*, the amount of air remaining in the lungs after maximal exhalation.
- *Vital capacity (VC)* is the total amount of air that can be exhaled after a maximal inspiration. It is calculated by adding together the IRV, TV, and the ERV.

- *Inspiratory capacity* is the total amount of air that can be inhaled following a normal quiet exhalation. It is calculated by adding the TV and IRV.
- *Functional residual capacity (FRC)* is the volume of air left in the lungs after a normal exhalation. The ERV and RV are added to determine the FRC.
- *Forced expiratory volume (FEV_1)* is the amount of air that can be exhaled in 1 second.
- *Forced vital capacity (FVC)* is the amount of air that can be exhaled forcefully and rapidly after maximum air intake.
- *Minute volume (MV)* is the total amount or volume of air breathed in 1 minute.

In older clients, residual capacity is increased, and vital capacity is decreased. These age-related changes result from the following:

- Calcification of the costal cartilage and weakening of the intercostal muscles, which reduce movement of the chest wall
- Vertebral osteoporosis, which decreases spinal flexibility and increases the degree of kyphosis, further increasing the anterior-posterior diameter of the chest
- Diaphragmatic flattening and loss of elasticity.

The relationship of lung volumes and capacities. Volumes (mL) shown are for an average adult male.

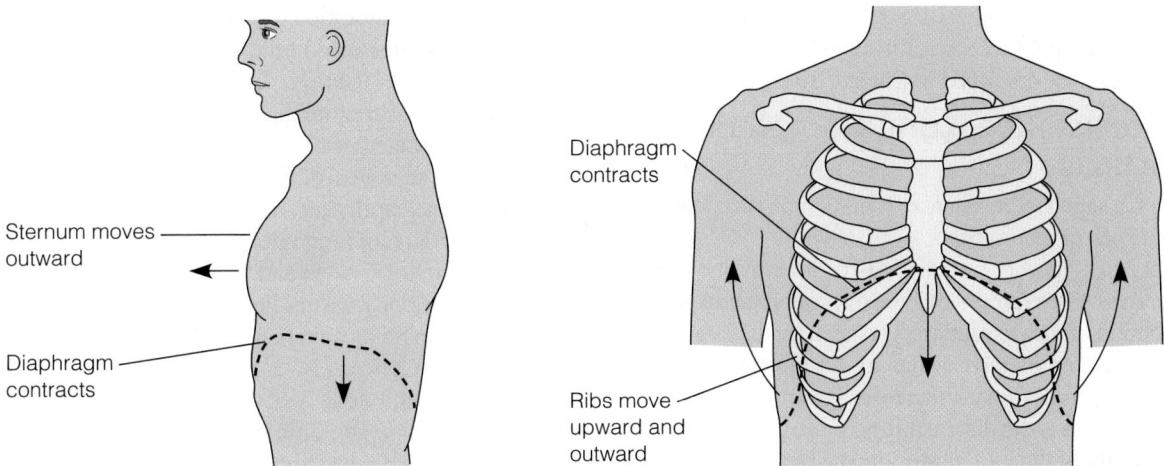

Figure 36–6 ■ Respiratory inspiration: lateral and anterior views. Note the volume expansion of the thorax as the diaphragm flattens.

cavity leads to a change in the air pressure within the cavity. Because gases always flow along their pressure gradients, a change in pressure results in gases flowing into or out of the lungs to equalize the pressure.

The pressures normally present in the thoracic cavity are the intrapulmonary pressure and the intrapleural pressure. The intrapulmonary pressure, within the alveoli of the lungs, rises and falls constantly as a result of the acts of ventilation (inhalation and exhalation). The intrapleural pressure, within the pleural space, also rises and falls with the acts of ventilation, but it is always less than (or negative to) the intrapulmonary pressure. Intrapulmonary and intrapleural pressures are necessary not only to expand and contract the lungs, but also to prevent their collapse.

Pulmonary ventilation has two phases: inspiration, during which air flows into the lungs; and expiration, during which gases flow out of the lungs. The two phases make up a single breath, and normally occur from 12 to 20 times each minute. A single inspiration lasts for about 1 to 1.5 seconds, whereas an expiration lasts for about 2 to 3 seconds.

During inspiration, the diaphragm contracts and flattens out to increase the vertical diameter of the thoracic cavity (Figure 36–6 ■). The external intercostal muscles contract, elevating the rib cage and moving the sternum forward to expand the lateral and anteroposterior diameter of the thoracic cavity, decreasing intrapleural pressure. The lungs stretch and the intrapulmonary volume increases, decreasing intrapulmonary pressure slightly below atmospheric pressure. Air rushes into the lungs as a result of this pressure gradient until the intrapulmonary and atmospheric pressures equalize.

Expiration is primarily a passive process that occurs as a result of the elasticity of the lungs (Figure 36–7 ■). The inspiratory muscles relax, the diaphragm rises, the ribs descend, and the lungs recoil. Both the thoracic and intrapulmonary pressures increase, compressing the alveoli. The intrapulmonary pressure rises to a level greater than atmospheric pressure, and gases flow out of the lungs.

Oxygen, Carbon Dioxide, and Hydrogen Ion Concentrations

The rate and depth of respirations are controlled by respiratory centers in the medulla oblongata and pons of the brain and by chemoreceptors located in the medulla and in the carotid and aortic bodies. The centers and chemoreceptors respond to changes in the concentration of oxygen, carbon dioxide, and hydrogen ions

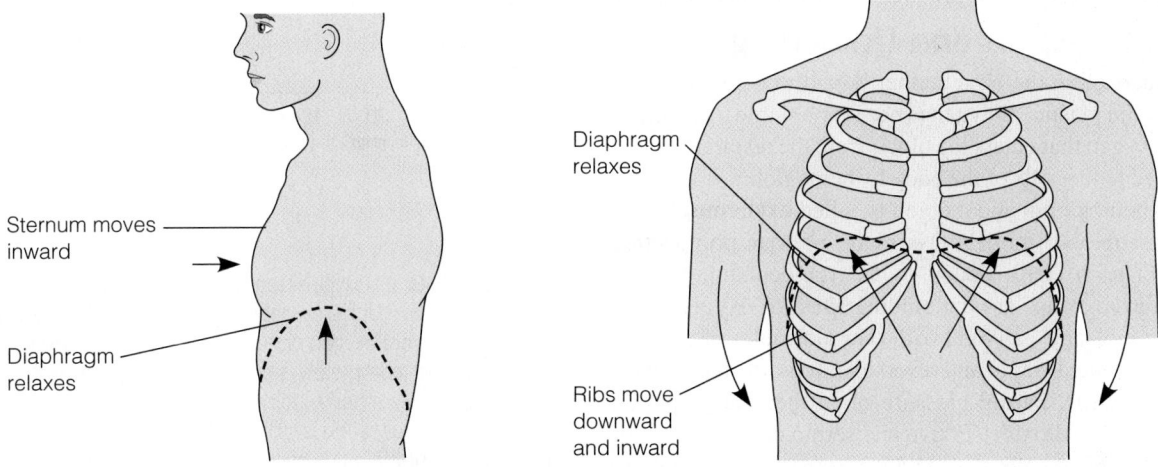

Figure 36–7 ■ Respiratory expiration: lateral and anterior views.

in arterial blood. For example, when carbon dioxide concentration increases or the pH decreases, the respiratory rate increases. This process is further described in Chapter 10 ∞.

Airway Resistance, Lung Compliance, and Elasticity

Respiratory passageway resistance, lung compliance, and lung elasticity also affect respiration.

- Respiratory passageway resistance is created by the friction encountered as gases move along the respiratory passageways, by constriction of the passageways (especially the larger bronchioles), by accumulations of mucus or infectious material, and by tumors. As resistance increases, gas flow decreases.
- **Lung compliance** is the distensibility of the lungs. It depends on the elasticity of the lung tissue and the flexibility of the rib cage. Compliance is decreased by factors that decrease the elasticity of the lungs, block the respiratory passageways, or interfere with movement of the rib cage.
- Lung elasticity is essential for lung distention during inspiration and lung recoil during expiration. Decreased elasticity from disease such as emphysema impairs respiration.

Alveolar Surface Tension

A liquid film of mostly water covers the alveolar walls. At any gas–liquid boundary, the molecules of liquid are more strongly attracted to each other than to gas molecules. This produces a state of tension, called surface tension, that draws the liquid molecules even more closely together. The water content of the alveolar film compacts the alveoli and aids in the lungs' recoil during expiration. In fact, if the alveolar film were pure water, the alveoli would collapse between breaths.

Surfactant, a lipoprotein produced by the alveolar cells, interferes with this adhesiveness of the water molecules, reducing surface tension, and helping expand the lungs. With insufficient surfactant, the surface tension forces can become great enough to collapse the alveoli between breaths, requiring tremendous energy to reinflate the lungs for inspiration.

BLOOD GASES

Gases are transported by the blood to provide cells with oxygen and to remove carbon dioxide produced during cellular activities.

Oxygen Transport and Unloading

Oxygen is carried in the blood either bound to hemoglobin or dissolved in the plasma. Oxygen is not very soluble in water, so almost all oxygen that enters the blood from the respiratory system is carried to the cells of the body by hemoglobin. This combination of hemoglobin and oxygen is called **oxyhemoglobin**.

Each hemoglobin molecule is made of four polypeptide chains, with each chain bound to an iron-containing heme group. The iron groups are the binding sites for oxygen; each hemoglobin molecule can bind with four molecules of oxygen.

Oxygen binding is rapid and reversible. It is affected by temperature, blood pH, partial pressure of oxygen (PO₂), partial pressure of carbon dioxide (PCO₂), and serum concentration of an organic chemical called 2,3-DPG. These factors interact to ensure adequate delivery of oxygen to the cells.

The relative saturation of hemoglobin depends on the P_{O_2} of the blood, as illustrated in the oxygen-hemoglobin dissociation curve (Figure 36–8 ■).

- Under normal conditions, the hemoglobin in arterial blood is 97.4% saturated with oxygen. Hemoglobin is almost fully saturated at a P_{O_2} of 70 mmHg. As arterial blood flows through the capillaries, oxygen is unloaded, so that the oxygen saturation of hemoglobin in venous blood is 75%.
- The affinity of oxygen and hemoglobin decreases as the temperature of body tissues increases above normal. As a result, less oxygen binds with hemoglobin, and oxygen unloading is enhanced. Conversely, as the body is chilled, oxygen unloading is inhibited.
- The oxygen-hemoglobin bond is weakened by increased hydrogen ion concentrations. As blood becomes more acidotic, oxygen unloading to the tissues is enhanced. The same process occurs when the partial pressure of carbon dioxide increases because this decreases the pH.
- The organic chemical 2,3-DPG is formed in red blood cells and enhances the release of oxygen from hemoglobin by binding to it during times of increased metabolism (as when body temperature increases). This binding alters the structure of hemoglobin to facilitate oxygen unloading.

Carbon Dioxide Transport

Active cells produce about 200 mL of carbon dioxide each minute; this amount is exactly the same as that excreted by the lungs each minute. Excretion of carbon dioxide from the body requires transport by the blood from the cells to the lungs. Carbon dioxide is transported in three forms: dissolved in plasma, bound to hemoglobin, and as bicarbonate ions in the plasma (the largest amount is in this form).

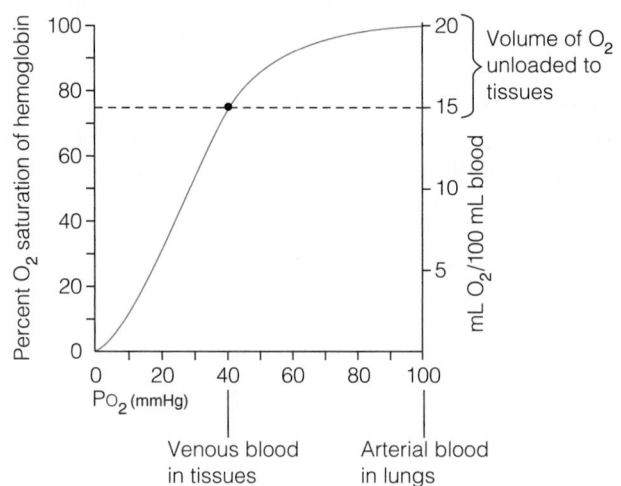

Figure 36–8 ■ Oxygen-hemoglobin dissociation curve. The percent O₂ saturation of hemoglobin and total blood oxygen volume are shown for different oxygen partial pressures (Po₂). Arterial blood in the lungs is almost completely saturated. During one pass through the body, about 25% of hemoglobin-bound oxygen is unloaded to the tissues. Thus, venous blood is still about 75% saturated with oxygen. The steep portion of the curve shows that hemoglobin readily off-loads or on-loads oxygen at Po₂ levels below about 50 mmHg.

The amount of carbon dioxide transported in the blood is strongly influenced by the oxygenation of the blood. When the P_{O_2} decreases, with a corresponding decrease in oxygen saturation, increased amounts of carbon dioxide can be carried in the blood. Carbon dioxide entering the systemic circulation from the cells causes more oxygen to dissociate from hemoglobin, in turn allowing more carbon dioxide to combine with hemoglobin and more bicarbonate ions to be generated. This situation is reversed in the pulmonary circulation, where the uptake of oxygen facilitates the release of carbon dioxide.

ASSESSING RESPIRATORY FUNCTION

Function of the respiratory system is assessed by findings from diagnostic tests, a health assessment interview to collect subjective data, and a physical assessment to collect objective data. Sample documentation of an assessment of the respiratory system is included in the box on this page.

Diagnostic Tests

The results of diagnostic tests of respiratory function are used to support the diagnosis of a specific disease, to provide information to identify or modify the appropriate medications or therapy used to treat the disease, and to help nurses monitor the

SAMPLE DOCUMENTATION
Assessment of the Lungs

57-year-old male, history of smoking 2 packs cigarettes/day for 37 years; continues to smoke despite previous discussions. Works as a dry-wall installer. No family history of cancer or TB. States he has trouble breathing, especially at night. Often sleeps on a recliner "to breathe better." Complains of a cough, but denies sputum production. Diagnosed 3 years ago with emphysema. Color of face is dusky red. Fingernails pink. Respirations 30, unlabored, regular (R varies from 26 to 32 on visits to the clinic). Thoracic assessment = intercostal bulging, barrel chest, diminished lung sounds bilaterally in lower lobes. Crackles present in upper lobes, not cleared by coughing. Discussed possible use of low-flow nasal oxygen at night to help with breathing; will check with primary provider.

client's responses to treatment and nursing care interventions. Diagnostic tests to assess the structures and functions of the respiratory system are described in the Diagnostic Tests table below and summarized in the bulleted list that follows. More information is included in the discussion of specific disorders in Chapters 37, 38, and 39 ∞ .

DIAGNOSTIC TESTS of the Respiratory System

NAME OF TEST Sputum Studies

- Culture and sensitivity
- Acid-fast smear and culture
- Cytology

PURPOSE AND DESCRIPTION Culture and sensitivity of a single sputum specimen is done to diagnose bacterial infections, identify the most effective antibiotic, and evaluate treatment.

Sputum is examined for presence of acid-fast bacillus, specifically tuberculosis. A series of three early morning sputum specimens is used.

Sputum is examined for presence of abnormal (malignant) cells. A single sputum specimen is collected in a special container of fixative solution.

RELATED NURSING CARE See Procedure 36–1 on page 1220 for obtaining a sputum specimen. Sputum specimens may also be obtained during bronchoscopy (described later) if the client is unable to provide a specimen.

NAME OF TEST Arterial blood gases (ABGs)

PURPOSE AND DESCRIPTION This test of arterial blood is done to assess alterations in acid–base balance caused by a respiratory disorder, a metabolic disorder, or both. A pH of less than 7.35 indicates acidosis and a pH of more than 7.45 indicates alkalosis (see Chapter 10 ∞). To determine a respiratory cause, assess the Pa_{CO_2}: If pH is decreased and Pa_{CO_2} is increased, respiratory acidosis is indicated.

Normal values:
pH: 7.35–7.45
Pa_{CO_2}: 35–45 mmHg

Pa_{O_2}: 75–100 mmHg
HCO_3: 24–28 mEq/L
BE: ± 2 mEq/L

RELATED NURSING CARE Arterial blood is collected in a heparinized needle and syringe. Sample is placed on an icebag and taken immediately to the lab. If client is receiving oxygen, indicate on lab slip. Apply pressure to puncture site for 2–5 minutes, or longer if needed. Do not collect blood from the same arm used for an IV infusion.

NAME OF TEST Pulse oximetry

PURPOSE AND DESCRIPTION This noninvasive test is used to evaluate or monitor oxygen saturation of the blood. A device that uses infrared light is attached to an extremity (most commonly the finger, but can also be used on the toe, earlobe, or nose) and light is passed through the tissues or reflected off bony structures.

Normal value: 90%–100%

RELATED NURSING CARE Assess for factors that may alter findings, including faulty placement, movement, dark skin color, and acrylic nails.

(continued)

DIAGNOSTIC TESTS of the Respiratory System (continued)

NAME OF TEST Chest x-ray

PURPOSE AND DESCRIPTION Chest x-rays are used to identify abnormalities in chest structure and lung tissue, for diagnosis of diseases and injuries of the lungs, and to monitor treatment.

RELATED NURSING CARE No special preparation is needed.

NAME OF TEST Computed tomography (CT)

PURPOSE AND DESCRIPTION CT of the thorax may be performed when x-rays do not show some areas well, such as the pleura and mediastinum. It is also done to differentiate pathologic conditions (such as tumors, abscesses, and aortic aneurysms), to identify pleural effusion and enlarged lymph nodes, and to monitor treatment. Images are shown in cross section.

RELATED NURSING CARE No special preparation is needed.

NAME OF TEST Magnetic resonance imaging (MRI)

PURPOSE AND DESCRIPTION An MRI of the thorax is used to diagnose alterations in lung tissue more difficult to visualize by CT scan and to identify abnormal masses and fluid accumulation.

RELATED NURSING CARE Assess for any metallic implants (such as pacemaker, pacemaker wires, or implant). Test will not be performed if present.

NAME OF TEST Positron emission tomography (PET)

PURPOSE AND DESCRIPTION This relatively noninvasive test, when used to examine the lungs, is performed to identify lung nodules (cancers). The client is given a radioactive substance and cross-sectional images are displayed on a computer. Radiation from PET is only 25% of that from a CT scan.

RELATED NURSING CARE No alcohol, coffee, or tobacco is allowed for 24 hours prior to the test. Encourage increased fluid intake post-test to help eliminate the radioactive material.

NAME OF TEST Pulmonary angiography

PURPOSE AND DESCRIPTION This test is done to identify pulmonary emboli, tumors, aneurysms, vascular changes associated with emphysema, and pulmonary circulation. A catheter is inserted into the brachial or femoral artery, threaded into the pulmonary artery, and dye is injected. ECG leads are applied to the chest for cardiac monitoring. Images of the lungs are taken.

RELATED NURSING CARE Monitor injection site and pulses distal to the site after the test.

NAME OF TEST Pulmonary ventilation/perfusion scan (V/Q scan)

PURPOSE AND DESCRIPTION This test is performed with two nuclear scans to measure breathing (ventilation) and circulation (perfusion) in all parts of the lungs. A perfusion scan is performed by injecting radioactive albumin into a vein and scanning the lungs. A ventilation scan is performed by scanning the lungs as the client inhales radioactive gas. A decreased uptake of radioisotope during the perfusion scan indicates a blood flow problem, such as from a pulmonary embolus or pneumonitis. A decreased uptake of gas during the ventilation scan may indicate airway obstruction, pneumonia, or chronic pulmonary obstructive disease (COPD).

RELATED NURSING CARE No special preparation is needed.

NAME OF TEST Bronchoscopy

PURPOSE AND DESCRIPTION A bronchoscopy is the direct visualization of the larynx, trachea, and bronchi through a bronchoscope to identify lesions, remove foreign bodies and secretions, obtain tissue for biopsy, and improve tracheobronchial drainage (Figure 36–9 ■). During the test, a catheter brush or biopsy forceps can be passed to obtain secretions or tissue for examination for cancer.

RELATED NURSING CARE

- Provide routine preoperative care as ordered. *Bronchoscopy is an invasive procedure requiring conscious sedation or anesthesia. Care provided prior to the procedure is similar to that provided before many minor surgical procedures.*
- Provide mouth care just prior to bronchoscopy. *Mouth care reduces oral microorganisms and the risk of introducing them into the lungs.*
- Bring resuscitation and suction equipment to the bedside. *Laryngospasm and respiratory distress may occur following the procedure. The anesthetic suppresses the cough and gag reflexes, and secretions may be difficult to expectorate.*

Figure 36–9 ■ Fiberoptic bronchoscopy.

DIAGNOSTIC TESTS of the Respiratory System (continued)

- Following the procedure, closely monitor vital signs and respiratory status. *Possible complications of bronchoscopy include laryngospasm, bronchospasm, bronchial perforation with possible pneumothorax or subcutaneous emphysema, hemorrhage, hypoxia, pneumonia or bacteremia, and cardiac stress.*
- Instruct to avoid eating or drinking for approximately 2 hours or until fully awake with intact cough and gag reflexes. *Suppression of the cough and gag reflexes by systemic and local anesthesia used during the procedure increase the risk for aspiration.*
- Provide an emesis basin and tissues for expectorating sputum and saliva. *Until reflexes have returned, the client may be unable to swallow sputum and saliva safely.*
- Monitor color and character of respiratory secretions. Secretions normally are blood tinged for several hours following bronchoscopy, especially if biopsy has been obtained. Notify the physician if sputum is grossly bloody. *Grossly bloody sputum may indicate a complication such as perforation.*

- Collect postbronchoscopy sputum specimens for cytologic examination as ordered. *Cells in the sputum may be examined if a tumor is suspected.*

Health Education for the Client and Family

- Fiber-optic bronchoscopy requires 30 to 45 minutes to complete. It may be done at the bedside, in a special procedure room, or in the surgical suite.
- The procedure usually causes little pain or discomfort, because an anesthetic is given. You will be able to breathe during the bronchoscopy.
- Some voice hoarseness and a sore throat are common following the procedure. Throat lozenges or warm saline gargles may help relieve discomfort.
- You may develop a mild fever within the first 24 hours following the procedure. This is a normal response.
- Persistent cough, bloody or purulent sputum, wheezing, shortness of breath, difficulty breathing, or chest pain may indicate a complication. Notify your physician if they develop.

NAME OF TEST Lung biopsy

PURPOSE AND DESCRIPTION Done to obtain tissue to differentiate benign from malignant tumors of the lungs. May be done during a bronchoscopy, or by surgical procedure.

RELATED NURSING CARE Same as bronchoscopy or the same as a thoracotomy (incision through the chest wall) if a surgical biopsy is performed.

NAME OF TEST Thoracentesis

PURPOSE AND DESCRIPTION Done to obtain a specimen of pleural fluid for diagnosis (and used as a procedure to remove pleural fluid or instill medication). A large-bore needle is inserted

through the chest wall and into the pleural space. Following the procedure, a chest x-ray is taken to check for a pneumothorax.

RELATED NURSING CARE Nursing care of the client having a thoracentesis is provided in Chapter 38 ∞.

- Sputum tests include a culture and sensitivity to identify organisms causing infections as well as the most effective antibiotic to treat the infection, an acid-fast smear and culture to identify the tuberculosis bacillus, and cytology to identify malignancies. See Procedure 36–1.
- Arterial blood gases are conducted to evaluate alterations in acid–base balances.
- Pulse oximetry is used to evaluate or monitor the oxygen saturation of the blood.
- Many different radiologic examinations are used to diagnose respiratory disorders, including a chest x-ray to evaluate structures and tissues, a CT scan to differentiate pathologic conditions, an MRI to more accurately identify abnormal masses and fluid accumulation, a PET to identify lung cancers, and a pulmonary angiogram to identify various disorders including pulmonary emboli and emphysema.
- A bronchoscopy is a direct visualization of the larynx, trachea, and bronchi. During the test, lesions can be identified, foreign bodies or mucous plugs removed, and tissue taken for biopsy. In addition, a biopsy of lung tissue may be done through an incision through the chest wall.

- A thoracentesis, when done for diagnostic purposes, is conducted to obtain a specimen of pleural fluid.

Regardless of the type of diagnostic test, the nurse is responsible for explaining the procedure and any special preparation needed, for assessing for medication use that may affect the outcome of the tests, for supporting the client during the examination as necessary, for documenting the procedures as appropriate, and for monitoring the results of the tests.

Genetic Considerations

When conducting a health assessment interview and a physical assessment, it is important for the nurse to consider genetic influences on health of the adult. During the health assessment interview, ask about family members with health problems affecting respiratory function. In addition, ask about a family history of emphysema, asthma, cystic fibrosis, or lung cancer. During the physical assessment, assess for any manifestations that might indicate a genetic disorder (see the Genetic Considerations box on page 1220). If data are found to indicate genetic risk factors or alterations, ask about genetic testing and refer for appropriate genetic counseling and evaluation. Chapter 8 ∞ provides further information about genetics in medical-surgical nursing.

PROCEDURE 36–1 OBTAINING A SPUTUM SPECIMEN

GATHER SUPPLIES

- Sterile sputum container, specimen cup, or mucous trap
- Mouth care supplies
- Sterile suction kit, if necessary
- Gloves

BEFORE THE PROCEDURE

If the sputum specimen is to establish the initial diagnosis, obtain the specimen before starting oxygen and/or antibiotic therapy. Antibiotics reduce the bacterial count, making it difficult to identify the infecting organism. Oxygen therapy dries mucous membranes, making it more difficult to obtain a specimen. Unless otherwise instructed, obtain the specimen early in the morning, just after awakening. Respiratory secretions tend to pool during sleep; it is easier to obtain a specimen before normal coughing and daily activity has cleared them.

Provide for privacy, and explain the procedure. Emphasize the importance of coughing deeply to obtain sputum from the lower respiratory tract, avoiding expectoration of saliva. Increasing fluid intake prior to obtaining the specimen can help liquefy secretions, making them easier to expectorate.

DURING THE PROCEDURE

1. Use standard precautions.
2. Provide for mouth care prior to obtaining the specimen to reduce contamination by oral flora.
3. Instruct to cough deeply several times, expectorating mucus into the container.
4. Close the container securely.
5. Label the container with name and other identifying data, time and date, and any special conditions, such as antibiotic or oxygen therapy. Enclose specimen container in a clean plastic bag, and take to the laboratory or refrigerate as ordered to preserve the specimen.
6. To obtain a specimen by suctioning:
   - Provide mouth care.
   - Obtain a sterile mucous trap. Using aseptic technique, attach the trap to the suction apparatus between the suction catheter and tubing.
   - Preoxygenate for suctioning as needed.
   - Perform tracheal suctioning using aseptic technique via either the nasotracheal route, endotracheal tube, or tracheostomy. Lubricate the catheter with sterile normal saline. Apply no suction as the catheter is being inserted into the trachea; apply suction for no longer than 10 seconds while withdrawing the catheter.
   - Detach the mucous trap; close and label. Clear the suction catheter and tubing with normal saline after removing the mucus trap. Dispose of equipment appropriately.
7. A sputum specimen also may be obtained during bronchoscopy procedure.

AFTER THE PROCEDURE

Provide mouth care as needed. Teach the importance of completing all ordered antibiotic prescriptions to ensure complete eradication of microorganisms. Document the time and date that the specimen was obtained; and note color, consistency, and odor of sputum.

GENETIC CONSIDERATIONS
Respiratory Disorders

- Deficiency of alpha$_1$-antitrypsin (a protein that protects the body from damage by its immune cells) is caused by a mutation of a gene located on chromosome 14. Deficiency of this protein leaves the lung susceptible to emphysema.
- Asthma, a disease that affects more than 5% of the population, is an inheritable disease with a number of responsible genes. (There are also other causes of asthma.)
- Cystic fibrosis is the most common fatal genetic disease in the United States today. All gene defects result in defective transport of chloride and sodium by epithelial cells. As a result, the amount of sodium chloride is increased in body secretions. Thick mucus is produced that clogs the lungs, leads to infection, and blocks pancreatic enzymes from reaching the intestines to digest food.
- A familial history of lung cancer increases the risk of developing lung cancer, and small-cell lung cancer has a definite genetic component. In addition, researchers have found that lung cancer patients who never smoked are more likely than smokers to have one of two genetic mutations linked to the disease.

Health Assessment Interview

A health assessment interview to determine problems with respiratory structure and function may be conducted during a health screening, may focus on a chief complaint (such as shortness of breath), or may be part of a total health assessment. If the client has a problem with respiratory function, analyze its onset, characteristics, course, severity, precipitating and relieving factors, and any associated symptoms, noting the timing and circumstances. For example, ask the client:

- Describe the problems you are having with your breathing. Is your breathing more difficult if you lie flat? Is it painful to breathe in or out?
- When did you first notice that your cough was becoming a problem? Do you cough up mucus? What color is the mucus?
- Have you had nosebleeds in the past?

During the interview, carefully observe the client for difficulty in breathing, pausing to breathe in the middle of a sentence, hoarseness, changes in voice quality, and cough. Ask about present health status, medical history, family health history, and risk factors for illness, These areas of the client's health status include information about the nose, throat, and lungs.

To determine present health status, ask about pain in the nose, throat, or chest. Information about cough includes what type of cough, when it occurs, and how it is relieved. The client should describe any sputum associated with the cough. Is the client experiencing any dyspnea (difficult or labored breathing)? How is the dyspnea associated with activity levels and time of day? Is the client having chest pain? How is this related to activity and time of day? Note the severity, type, and location of the pain. Explore problems with swallowing, smelling, or taste. Also ask about nosebleeds and nasal or sinus stuffiness or pain, and about current medication use, aerosols or inhalants, and oxygen use.

Document past medical history by asking questions about a history of allergies, asthma, bronchitis, emphysema, pneumonia, tuberculosis, or congestive heart failure. Other questions include a history of surgery or trauma to the respiratory structures and a history of other chronic illnesses such as cancer, kidney disease, and heart disease. If the client has a health problem involving the respiratory system, ask about medications used to relieve nasal congestion, cough, dyspnea, or chest pain. Document a family history of allergies, tuberculosis, emphysema, and cancer.

The client's personal lifestyle, environment, and occupation may provide clues to risk factors for actual or potential health problems. Question the client about a history of smoking and/or exposure to environmental chemicals (including smog), dust, vapors, animals, coal dust, asbestos, fumes, or pollens. Other risk factors include a sedentary lifestyle and obesity. Also ask the client about use of alcohol and substances that are injected (such as heroin) or inhaled (such as cocaine or marijuana).

Interview questions categorized by functional health patterns follow.

FUNCTIONAL HEALTH PATTERN INTERVIEW: Respiratory System

Functional Health Pattern	Interview Questions and Leading Statements
Health Perception–Health Management	■ Describe any respiratory problems (such as allergies, asthma, bronchitis, frequent cold, pneumonia, tuberculosis, emphysema), injuries or surgery of the nose, throat, or lungs you have had. ■ If you had such problems, how were they treated (for example, medications, surgery, breathing treatments, oxygen, environmental control of allergens, other)? ■ Do you use oxygen for your respiratory problem? If so, how and when do you use it and at what flow rate? ■ Do you now or have you ever smoked tobacco? If so, what type, how long, and how much? If you no longer smoke, when did you quit? ■ Do you notice more respiratory problems at certain seasons of the year? Explain. ■ Do you do anything to decrease environmental irritants in your home or at work? Describe if so. ■ When was your last chest x-ray and TB skin test? What were the results of those tests? ■ Do you have annual flu shots? Have you had a pneumonia shot (if over age 65)? ■ Do certain foods, pollens, dust, or animals seem to increase your difficulty breathing? Explain. ■ Do you work or do hobbies in an area where you are exposed to paints, glues, dust, pollen, fumes, or chemicals that might irritate your respiratory system? If so, describe.
Nutritional–Metabolic	■ Describe your usual 24-hour intake of food and fluids. ■ Has your appetite been affected by your respiratory problem? Is it difficult for you to eat because of your breathing problems? Explain. ■ Has there been a recent change in your weight? Explain.
Elimination	■ Has having this health problem made it more difficult for you to have a bowel movement? ■ *For women:* Have you had difficulty controlling your urine when you cough?
Activity–Exercise	■ Describe your usual activities in a 24-hour period. ■ What type of exercise do you usually do? Has this changed, and if so, how? ■ Has your ability to care for yourself changed with this respiratory problem? Explain. ■ Has your energy level decreased since you have had this problem with breathing? If so, how has it affected your daily life? ■ How many flights of stairs can you climb before you become short of breath? ■ Do certain activities make you very tired? Explain. ■ Are your activities interrupted by frequent coughing? Explain. ■ Do you cough up phlegm or sputum? If so, describe its amount, color, odor, and the presence of blood.
Sleep–Rest	■ Does having this problem interfere with your ability to rest and sleep? Explain. ■ How many pillows do you use at night to breathe more easily? Has this changed? ■ Do you ever wake up coughing?

(continued)

FUNCTIONAL HEALTH PATTERN INTERVIEW: Respiratory System (continued)

Cognitive–Perceptual	■ Do you have any pain in your sinuses, nose, chest, with breathing? If so, using a scale from 0 to 10, with 10 being the most severe pain, how would your rate that pain? Describe where and when you have the pain, how often you have it, what makes it worse, and what you do to relieve it. ■ Are there times when you feel anxious, restless, apprehensive, confused, or faint? Describe what you do if you have these feelings. ■ Do you know how to use the medications, inhalers, or oxygen prescribed for your respiratory problem?
Self-Perception–Self-Concept	■ How does having this condition make you feel about yourself?
Role–Relationships	■ How has having this condition affected your relationships with others? ■ Has having this condition interfered with your ability to work? Explain. ■ Is there a history of lung disease in your family? Explain.
Sexuality–Reproductive	■ Has this condition interfered with your usual sexual activity?
Coping–Stress-Tolerance	■ Has having this condition created stress for you? If so, does your breathing seem to be more difficult when you are stressed? ■ Have you experienced any kind of stress that makes the condition worse? Explain. ■ Describe what you do when you feel stressed.
Value–Belief	■ Describe how specific relationships or activities help you cope with this problem. ■ Describe specific cultural beliefs or practices that affect how you care for and feel about this problem. ■ Are there any specific treatments (such as being on a machine that breathes for you) that you would not use to treat this problem?

Physical Assessment

Physical assessment of the respiratory system may be performed either as part of a total assessment, or alone for a client with known or suspected problems. The techniques used to assess the respiratory system are inspection, palpation, percussion, and auscultation. In addition, note the client's level of consciousness, restlessness, and anxiety level, and assess the color of the lips and nail beds. Normal age-related findings for the older adult are summarized in Table 36–1.

The room should be warm and well lighted. Ask the client to remove all clothing above the waist; give women a gown to wear during the examination. Conduct the examination with the client in the sitting position. Prior to the examination, collect all necessary equipment and explain the techniques to the client to decrease anxiety.

TABLE 36–1 Age-Related Changes in the Respiratory System

AGE-RELATED CHANGE	SIGNIFICANCE
■ ↓ elastic recoil of lungs during expiration because of less elastic collagen and elastin. ■ Loss of skeletal muscle strength in the thorax and diaphragm. ■ Alveoli are less elastic, more fibrotic, and have fewer functional capillaries. ■ Cough is less effective. ■ Po_2 reduces as much as 15% by age 80.	The older adult often has an increased anterior-posterior chest diameter, with kyphosis and barrel chest. There is a reduction in vital capacity and an increase in residual volume, with decreased effectiveness in coughing up phlegm or sputum. All of these changes greatly increase the risk of respiratory infections (such as pneumonia), especially if the person becomes immobile. They also mean that respiratory infections are more difficult to treat.

RESPIRATORY ASSESSMENTS

Technique/Normal/Findings	Abnormal Findings

Nasal Assessment

Inspect the nose for changes in size, shape, or color. *The nose should be midline in the face, of the same color as the face, and the nares should be symmetric.*	■ The nose may be asymmetrical as a result of previous surgery or trauma. ■ The skin around the nostrils may be red and swollen in allergies or upper respiratory infections.

Technique/Normal/Findings	Abnormal Findings
Inspect the nasal cavity. Use an otoscope with a broad, short speculum. Gently insert the speculum into each of the nares and assess the condition of the mucous membranes and the turbinates. *The septum should be midline with pink mucosa and without drainage.*	■ The septum may be deviated. ■ Perforation of the septum may occur with chronic cocaine abuse. ■ Red mucosa indicates infection. ■ Purulent drainage indicates nasal or sinus infection. ■ Allergies may be indicated by watery nasal drainage, pale turbinates, and polyps on the turbinates.
Assess ability to smell (cranial nerve I, olfactory). Ask the client to breathe through one nostril while pressing the other one closed. Ask the client to close his or her eyes. Place a substance with an aromatic odor under the client's nose (use ground coffee or alcohol) and ask the client to identify the odor. Test each nostril separately. *This test is usually done only if the client has problems with the sense of smell, but the client should be able to distinguish different odors.*	■ Changes in the ability to smell may be the result of damage to the olfactory nerve or to chronic inflammation of the nose. ■ Zinc deficiency may cause a loss of the sense of smell.

Sinus Assessment

Palpate the frontal and maxillary sinuses. *The sinuses should not be tender to palpation.*	■ Frontal and maxillary sinuses are tender to palpation with allergies or sinus infections.

Thoracic Assessment

Assess respiratory rate. *The normal respiratory rate is 12 to 20 breaths per minute.*	■ **Tachypnea** (rapid respiratory rate) is seen in **atelectasis** (collapse of lung tissue following obstruction of the bronchus or bronchioles), pneumonia, asthma, pleural effusion, pneumothorax, congestive heart failure, anxiety, and in response to pain. ■ Damage to the brainstem from a stroke or head injury may result in either tachypnea or **bradypnea** (low respiratory rate). ■ Bradypnea is seen with some circulatory disorders, lung disorders, and as a side effect of some medications. ■ **Apnea**, cessation of breathing lasting from a few seconds to a few minutes, may occur following a stroke or head trauma, as a side effect of some medications, or following airway obstruction.
Inspect the anteroposterior diameter of the chest. The anteroposterior diameter of the chest should be less than the transverse diameter. *Normal ratio is 1:2.*	■ The anteroposterior diameter is equal to the transverse diameter in barrel chest, which typically occurs with emphysema.
Inspect for intercostal retraction or bulging. *There should be no retraction or bulging.*	■ Retraction of intercostal spaces may be seen in asthma. ■ Bulging of intercostal spaces may be seen in pneumothorax.

Technique/Normal/Findings	Abnormal Findings

Inspect and palpate for chest expansion. Place your hands with the fingers spread apart palm down on the client's posterolateral chest. Gently press the skin between your thumbs (Figure 36–10 ■). Ask the client to breathe deeply. As the client inhales, watch your hands for symmetry of movement. *Chest expansion should be bilaterally symmetric, with the examiner's hands moving 5 to 10 cm apart.*

- Thoracic expansion is decreased on the affected side in atelectasis, pneumonia, pneumothorax, and pleural effusion.
- Bilateral chest expansion is decreased in emphysema.

Figure 36–10 ■ Palpating for chest expansion.

Gently palpate the location and position of the trachea. *The trachea should be midline.*

- The trachea shifts to the unaffected side in pleural effusion and pneumothorax and shifts to the affected side in atelectasis.

Palpate for tactile fremitus. Ask the client to say "ninety-nine" as you palpate at three different levels for a vibratory sensation called tactile fremitus, which occurs as sound waves from the larynx travel through patent bronchi and lungs to the chest wall. *Fremitus is symmetric and easily palpated in the upper regions of the lungs.*

- Tactile fremitus is decreased in atelectasis, emphysema, asthma, pleural effusion, and pneumothorax. It is increased in pneumonia if the bronchus is patent.

Percuss the lungs for dullness over shoulder apices and over anterior, posterior, and lateral intercostal spaces (Figure 36–11 ■). *The normal percussion tone over normal lung tissue is resonance.*

- Dullness is heard in clients with atelectasis, lobar pneumonia, and pleural effusion.
- Hyperresonance is heard in those with chronic asthma, emphysema, and pneumothorax.

Figure 36–11 ■ Sequence for lung percussion.

Technique/Normal/Findings	Abnormal Findings

Percuss the posterior chest for diaphragmatic excursion. Systematic percussion of the posterior chest from a level of lung resonance to the level of diaphragmatic dullness reveals *diaphragmatic excursion,* a measurement of the level of the diaphragm. First percuss downward over the posterior thorax while the client exhales fully and holds the breath. Mark the spot at which the sound changes from resonant to dull. Then ask the client to inhale and hold the breath while you percuss downward again to note the descent of the diaphragm. Again mark the spot where the sound changes. *Measure the difference in diaphragmatic excursion which normally varies from about 3 to 5 cm (Figure 36–12 ■).*

- Diaphragmatic excursion is decreased in emphysema, ascites, on the affected side in pleural effusion, and in pneumothorax.
- A high level of dullness or a lack of excursion may indicate atelectasis or pleural effusion.

Figure 36–12 ■ Measuring diaphragmatic excursion.

Breath Sound Assessment

Auscultate the lungs for breath sounds with the diaphragm of the stethoscope by having the client take slow deep breaths through the mouth. Listen over anterior, posterior, and lateral intercostal spaces (Figure 36–13 ■). *The three different types of normal breath sounds are vesicular, bronchovesicular, and bronchial (Table 36–2).*

- Bronchial breath sounds (expiration > inspiration) and bronchovesicular breath sounds (inspiration = expiration) are heard over lungs filled with fluid or solid tissue.
- Breath sounds are decreased or diminished over atelectasis, emphysema, asthma, pleural effusion, and pneumothorax.
- Breath sounds are increased over lobar pneumonia.
- Breath sounds are absent over collapsed lung, surgical removal of lung, pleural effusion, and primary bronchus obstruction.

Figure 36–13 ■ Sequence for lung auscultation.

TABLE 36–2 Normal Breath Sounds

TYPE OF BREATH SOUND	CHARACTERISTICS
Vesicular	■ Soft, low-pitched, gentle sounds ■ Heard over all areas of the lungs except the major bronchi ■ Have a 3:1 ratio for inspiration and expiration, with inspiration lasting longer than expiration
Bronchovesicular	■ Medium pitch and intensity of sounds ■ Have a 1:1 ratio, with inspiration and expiration being equal in duration ■ Heard anteriorly over the primary bronchus on each side of the sternum, and posteriorly between the scapulae
Bronchial	■ Loud, high-pitched sounds ■ Gap between inspiration and expiration ■ Have a 2:3 ratio for inspiration and expiration, with expiration longer than inspiration ■ Heard over the manubrium

Technique/Normal/Findings	Abnormal Findings
Auscultate for crackles, wheezes, and friction rubs. If crackles or wheezes are heard, ask the client to cough and note if adventitious sound is cleared. *Normally, there are no crackles, wheezes, or friction rubs.*	■ **Crackles** (short, discrete, crackling or bubbling sounds) may be noted in pneumonia, bronchitis, and congestive heart failure. ■ **Wheezes** (continuous, musical sounds) may be heard in clients with bronchitis, emphysema, and asthma. ■ A **friction rub** is a loud, dry, creaking sound that indicates pleural inflammation.
Auscultate voice sounds where any abnormal breath sound is noted by having client say "ninety-nine" (bronchophony); whisper "one, two, three" (whispered pectoriloquy); and say "ee" (egophony). *Normally, these sounds are heard by the examiner, but are muffled.*	■ Voice sounds are decreased or absent over areas of atelectasis, asthma, pleural effusion, and pneumothorax. ■ Voice sounds are increased and clearer over lobar pneumonia. ■ When testing egophony, the sound becomes louder and changes to "a" over areas of consolidation or compression.

EXPLORE MEDIALINK

Prentice Hall Nursing MediaLink DVD-ROM
Audio Glossary
NCLEX-RN® Review

Animation/Video
Carbon Dioxide Transport
Oxygen Transport

COMPANION WEBSITE www.prenhall.com/lemone
Audio Glossary
NCLEX-RN® Review
Case Study: Respiratory Assessment
MediaLink Applications
Pulmonary Function Testing
Wheezes and Crackles
Links to Resources

TEST YOURSELF NCLEX-RN® REVIEW

1 Where is the apex of each lung located?
1. in the mediastinum
2. resting on the diaphragm
3. within the parietal pleura
4. just below the clavicle

2 What physiologic process is involved in gas exchange at the respiratory membrane?
1. facilitated transport
2. active transport
3. simple diffusion
4. hydrostatic pressure

3 What structures cover the external surface of the alveoli?
1. terminal bronchioles
2. pulmonary arteries
3. pulmonary veins
4. pulmonary capillaries

4 What process is initiated between oxygen and hemoglobin as the temperature of body tissues increases?
1. Oxygen unloading is enhanced.
2. Oxygen unloading is inhibited.
3. Respiratory rate decreases.
4. Lung compliance increases.

5 You are teaching a client about a thoracentesis. How would you best describe this procedure?
1. "You will be asleep when they make the incision."
2. "Fluid will be drawn off the area around your lung."
3. "It involves lying very still in a large, noisy machine."
4. "The doctor will be able to see inside your lung."

6 Which of the following questions should be included when conducting a health history to identify a genetic risk of respiratory disease?
1. "Tell me how many colds you have each year."
2. "Has anyone in your family had a stroke or heart attack?"
3. "Has lung cancer ever been diagnosed in your family?"
4. "Do your children have trouble breathing at night?"

7 While auscultating your client's breath sounds, you note continuous musical sounds. You document these sounds as:
1. murmurs.
2. wheezes.
3. crackles.
4. rales.

8 Your client has had a lung removed. What type of breath sound would you expect to assess over the affected side?
1. resonance
2. crackles
3. bronchovesicular
4. absent

9 What would you ask the client to do as you auscultate the lungs?
1. "Hold your breath."
2. "Repeat the number 99 several times."
3. "Take slow deep breaths through your mouth."
4. "Breathe in and out through your nose."

10 While assessing your client with a left pneumothorax you note decreased diaphragmatic excursion on the left. What would you do next?
1. Notify the physician immediately.
2. Document the assessment.
3. Repeat the assessment several times.
4. Tell the client to hold his or her breath.

See Test Yourself answers in Appendix C.

BIBLIOGRAPHY

Amella, E. (2004). Presentation of illness in older adults: If you think you know what you're looking for, think again. *American Journal of Nursing, 104*(10), 40–52.

Benham, L., Benbow, H., & Hansen, C. (2003). Respiratory care. The development of a respiratory assessment tool. *Nursing Times, 99*(23), 52–53, 55.

Bickley, L., & Szilagyi, P. (2007). *Bates' guide to physical examination and history taking.* (9th ed.). Philadelphia: Lippincott.

Bokhari, F., Brakenridge, S., Nagy, K., Roberts, R., Smith, R., Joseph, K., et al. (2002). Prospective evaluation of the sensitivity of physical examination in chest trauma. *Journal of Trauma: Injury, Infection, and Critical Care, 53*(60), 1135–1138.

Connolly, M. (2001). Chest x-rays: Completing the picture. *RN, 64*(6), 56–62, 64.

Eliopoulos, E. (2005). *Gerontological nursing* (6th ed.). Philadelphia: Lippincott Williams & Wilkins.

Finsilver, C. (2003). Pulmonary assessment: What you need to know. *Progress in Cardiovascular Nursing, 18*(2), 83–92.

Jarvis, C. (2004). *Physical examination & health assessment.* St. Louis, MO: Mosby.

Kee, J. (2005). *Prentice Hall handbook of laboratory & diagnostic tests with nursing implications.* Upper Saddle River, NJ: Prentice Hall.

Kleinpell, R., & Elpern, E. (2004). Community-acquired pneumonia: Updates on assessment and management. *Critical Care Nursing Quarterly, 27*(3), 231–240.

Mehta, M. (2003). Assessing respiratory status: Learn how to evaluate your patient's lungs through sight, sound and touch. *Nursing, 33*(2), 54–56.

Meng, A., & McConnell, S. (2003). Symptom perception and respiratory sensation: Clinical applications. *Nursing Clinics of North America, 38*(4), 737–748.

National Institutes of Health. (2003). *Genes and disease. Respiratory diseases.* Retrieved from http://www.ncbi.nlm.nih.gov/books/bv.fcgi?rid=gnd.section98.243

Porth, C. (2005). *Pathophysiology: Concepts of altered health states* (7th ed.) Philadelphia: Lippincott.

Simpson, H. (2004). Interpretation of arterial blood gases: A clinical guide for nurses. *British Journal of Nursing, 13*(9), 522–528.

United Press International. (2005). *Lung cancer linked to mutations.* Retrieved from http://www.nlm.nih.gov/medlineplus/news/fullstory_23290.html (not available after April 1, 2005).

Weber, J., & Kelley, J. (2006). *Health assessment in nursing* (3rd ed.). Philadelphia: Lippincott.

CHAPTER 37 Nursing Care of Clients with Upper Respiratory Disorders

LEARNING OUTCOMES

- Relate anatomy and physiology of the upper respiratory tract to commonly occurring disorders and risk factors for these disorders.

- Describe the pathophysiology of common upper respiratory tract disorders, relating their manifestations to the pathophysiologic process.

- Discuss nursing implications for medications and other interdisciplinary care measures to treat upper respiratory disorders.

- Describe surgical procedures used to treat upper respiratory disorders and their implications for client care and recovery.

- Identify health promotion activities related to reducing the incidence of upper respiratory disorders, describing the appropriate population and setting for implementing identified measures.

- Discuss treatment options for oral and laryngeal cancers with their implications for the client's body image and functional health.

CLINICAL COMPETENCIES

- Assess functional health status of clients with upper respiratory disorders, using data to identify and prioritize holistic nursing care needs.

- Use nursing research and evidence-based practice to plan and implement nursing care for clients with upper respiratory disorders.

- Provide safe and effective nursing care for clients having surgery involving the upper respiratory system and/or with a tracheostomy.

- Safely and knowledgeably administer medications and prescribed treatments for clients with disorders of the upper respiratory tract.

- Provide appropriate teaching for the client and family affected by upper respiratory tract disorders.

- Evaluate the effectiveness of care, reassessing and modifying the plan of care as needed to achieve desired client outcomes.

MEDIALINK

Resources for this chapter can be found on
the Prentice Hall Nursing MediaLink DVD-ROM
accompanying this textbook, and
on the Companion Website at
http://www.prenhall.com/lemone

Upper respiratory disorders may affect the nose, paranasal sinuses, tonsils, adenoids, larynx, and pharynx. Upper respiratory disorders may be minor, such as the common cold. However, a patent upper airway is necessary for effective breathing. Acute and even life-threatening problems develop when upper airway patency is affected (e.g., by laryngeal edema). Upper respiratory disorders can affect breathing, communication, and body image. When breathing is compromised because of swelling, bleeding, or accumulation of secretions, fear and anxiety develop.

Nursing care focuses on maintaining the airway, managing pain and symptoms, promoting effective communication, and providing psychologic support for the client and family. Prior to proceeding with this chapter, review the anatomy and physiology, diagnostic tests, and assessment of the upper respiratory system in Chapter 36 ∞ as needed.

INFECTIOUS OR INFLAMMATORY DISORDERS

Constant exposure of the upper respiratory tract to the environment makes it vulnerable to a variety of infectious and inflammatory conditions. Although most upper respiratory infections and inflammations are minor, complications may result. In the frail older adult, the risk of serious problems following an upper respiratory infection can be significant.

Rhinitis, inflammation of the nasal cavities, is the most common upper respiratory disorder. Rhinitis may be either acute or chronic. *Acute viral rhinitis,* or the common cold, is discussed below. Chronic rhinitis includes allergic, vasomotor, and atrophic rhinitis. *Allergic rhinitis,* or hay fever, results from a sensitivity reaction to allergens such as plant pollens. It tends to occur seasonally. The etiology of *vasomotor rhinitis* is unknown. Although its manifestations are similar to those of allergic rhinitis, it is not linked to allergens. *Atrophic rhinitis* is characterized by changes in the mucous membrane of the nasal cavities.

THE CLIENT WITH VIRAL UPPER RESPIRATORY INFECTION

Viral upper respiratory infections (URIs or the common cold) are the most common respiratory tract infections and are among the most common human diseases. URIs are highly contagious and are prevalent in schools and work environments. The incidence of acute URI peaks during September and late January, coinciding with the opening of schools, as well as toward the end of April. Most adults experience two to four colds each year (Porth, 2005).

FAST FACTS
- Rhinoviruses are the most common cause of viral URIs.
- Colds due to rhinovirus are more common in early fall and late spring.
- More than 100 different serotypes of rhinovirus have been identified.
- Parainfluenza viruses, respiratory syncytial viruses (RSV), coronaviruses, and adenoviruses also can cause URIs.
- Colds due to RSV, coronavirus, and adenovirus peak in winter and spring (Porth, 2005).

Pathophysiology

More than 200 strains of virus cause URI, including rhinoviruses, adenoviruses, parainfluenza viruses, coronaviruses, and respiratory syncytial virus (see the section that follows for more information about RSV). Occasionally, more than one virus may be present. Viruses causing acute URIs spread by aerosolized droplet nuclei during sneezing or coughing or by direct contact. The virus usually spreads when the hands and fingers pick it up from contaminated surfaces and carry it to the eyes and mucous membranes of the susceptible host. Infected clients are highly contagious, shedding virus for a few days prior to and after the appearance of symptoms. Although immunity is produced to the individual virus strain, the number of viruses causing URI ensures that most people continue to experience colds throughout their lifetimes.

Viscous mucous secretions in the upper respiratory tract trap invading organisms, preventing contamination of more vulnerable areas. Cells of the upper respiratory tract are infected when the virus attaches to receptors on the cell. Local immunologic defenses, such as secretory IgA antibodies in respiratory secretions, then attempt to inactivate the antigen, producing a local inflammatory response. The mucous membranes of the nasal passages swell and become hyperemic and engorged. Mucus-secreting glands become hyperactive. These responses to the virus produce the typical manifestations of viral URI.

Manifestations and Complications

Acute viral upper respiratory infection often presents as the common cold. Nasal mucous membranes appear red (*erythematous*) and *boggy* (swollen). Swollen mucous membranes, local vasodilation, and secretions cause nasal congestion. Clear, watery secretions lead to **coryza,** profuse nasal discharge. Sneezing and coughing are common. Sore throat is common, and may be the initial symptom. Systemic manifestations of acute viral URI may include low-grade fever, headache, malaise, and muscle aches. Symptoms generally last for a few days up to 2 weeks. Although acute viral URI is typically mild and self-limited, its effects on the immune defenses of the upper respiratory tract can increase the risk for more serious bacterial infections, such as sinusitis or otitis media.

INTERDISCIPLINARY CARE

Because most acute viral upper respiratory infections are self-limiting, self-care is appropriate and encouraged. Medical treatment is usually required only when complications such as sinusitis or otitis media develop.

Diagnosis of acute viral URI is usually based on the history and physical examination. Diagnostic testing may be indicated if a complication such as bacterial infection is suspected. A white blood count (WBC) may be ordered to assess for leukocytosis (an elevated WBC). Cultures of purulent discharge may also be obtained.

Treatment is symptomatic. Adequate rest, maintaining fluid intake, and avoiding chilling help relieve systemic symptoms such as fever, malaise, and muscle ache. Instruct clients to cover the mouth and nose with tissue when coughing or sneezing, and to dispose of soiled tissues properly. Additionally, avoiding crowds helps prevent spread of the infection to others.

Medications

Medications may be recommended to shorten the duration of the illness and relieve symptoms. Mild decongestants or over-the-counter (OTC) antihistamines may help relieve coryza and nasal congestion. Nasal sprays such as phenylephrine (Neo-Synephrine) rapidly relieve nasal congestion, but may lead to dependence and rebound congestion if used for more than a few days at a time. Warm saltwater gargles, throat lozenges, or mild analgesics may be used for sore throat. Although no specific antiviral therapy has been shown to be effective in shortening the duration of a URI, experimental vaccines to prevent acute viral URI are in developmental stages. For the nursing implications of decongestants and common antihistamines see the box below.

MEDICATION ADMINISTRATION **Decongestants and Antihistamines**

DECONGESTANTS
Phenylephrine (Neo-Synephrine, others)
Phenylpropanolamine (Comtrex, Ornade, Triaminic, others)
Pseudoephedrine (Sudafed, Actifed, others)

Decongestants promote vasoconstriction, reducing the inflammation and edema of nasal mucosa and relieving nasal congestion. They are very effective when applied topically (by nasal spray) because of their rapid onset of action. However, the duration of effect is short, followed by vasodilation and rebound congestion. Because of their rapid effect and short duration, these preparations are habit forming. Chronic use may lead to *rhinitis medicamentosa*, a rebound phenomenon of drug-induced nasal irritation and inflammation.

Nursing Responsibilities
- Assess for contraindications, such as hypertension or chronic heart disease. These drugs stimulate the sympathetic nervous system, increasing peripheral vascular resistance, blood pressure, and heart rate.
- Evaluate medication regimen for potential interactions such as antihypertensive medications and monoamine oxidase (MAO) inhibitors.

Health Education for the Client and Family
- Do not use more than the recommended dose.
- Check with the physician before taking decongestants if you are taking any prescription medications or are being treated for high blood pressure or heart disease.
- Use nasal sprays for no more than 3 to 5 days.
- Increase fluid intake to relieve mouth dryness.
- These drugs may cause nervousness, shakiness, or difficulty sleeping. Stop the drug if these effects occur.
- In some states, drugs containing pseudoephedrine may require a prescription or be kept behind the counter to reduce its use in preparing methamphetamine.

ANTIHISTAMINES
Brompheniramine (Dimetane, others)
Chlorpheniramine (Chlor-Trimeton, others)
Clemastine (Tavist)
Dexchlorpheniramine (Dexchlor, others)
Diphenhydramine (Benadryl, others)
Triprolidine (Actidil, Myidil)
Nonsedating
Cetirizine (Zyrtec)
Fexofenadine (Allegra)
Loratadine (Claritin)

Antihistamines are widely available with and without a prescription. They are frequently combined with decongestants in over-the-counter cold and allergy preparations. Antihistamines relieve the systemic effects of histamine and dry respiratory secretions through an anticholinergic effect. Most antihistamines cause drowsiness; nonsedating forms are less likely to interfere with alertness. Diphenhydramine is used in numerous over-the-counter sleep aids as well as in cold and allergy preparations.

Nursing Responsibilities
- Before administering or recommending these drugs, assess for possible contraindications, including the following:
  - Acute asthma or lower respiratory disease that may be aggravated by drying of secretions
  - Hypersensitivity to antihistamines
  - Glaucoma (increased intraocular pressure)
  - Impaired gastrointestinal motility or obstruction
  - Prostatic hypertrophy or other urinary tract obstruction
  - Heart disease.
- For clients who must remain alert while on antihistamine therapy, recommend nonsedating forms.

Health Education for the Client and Family
- Do not drive or operate machinery while taking over-the-counter or prescription forms of antihistamines known to be sedating.
- Stop the drug and notify your doctor immediately if you develop confusion, excessive sedation, chest tightness, wheezing, bleeding, or easy bruising while taking antihistamines.
- Do not use alcohol or other CNS depressants while taking antihistamines.
- Hard candy, gum, ice chips, and liquids help relieve mouth dryness caused by antihistamines.

Complementary Therapies

Complementary therapies are appropriate for treating most acute viral URI. Herbal remedies such as echinacea and garlic may have antiviral and antibiotic effects (Fontaine, 2005). Echinacea also is thought to stimulate the immune system, improving the body's response to infection. Taken at the first sign of infection, echinacea may reduce the duration and symptoms, although clinical trials have shown no consistent benefit (National Center for Complementary and Alternative Medicine, 2005). The recommended dose of echinacea varies, depending on the part of the plant used in the preparation. It should not be used for longer than 2 weeks. It is contraindicated for use during pregnancy and lactation, and in people who have an autoimmune disease such as rheumatoid arthritis.

Dietary supplements such as vitamin C and zinc also are promoted as measures to reduce the severity and duration of URI. Again, however, no consistent benefit is demonstrated in clinical trials. Although selected studies have shown a beneficial effect of zinc gluconate lozenges to reduce the duration of an induced URI, no such benefit was found when zinc was compared with placebo to treat naturally occurring URI (National Institutes of Health, 2002).

Aromatherapy with essential oils such as basil, cedarwood, eucalyptus, frankincense, lavender, marjoram, peppermint, or rosemary can reduce congestion and promote comfort and recovery. Teach clients that these essential oils are to be used only for inhalation, not for internal consumption.

Acupuncture and acupressure have been shown to be effective in treating URI in adults, particularly when combined with use of Chinese herbs (Spencer & Jacobs, 2003). Their beneficial effect is most likely related to stimulation of the immune response by acupuncture and acupressure.

 ## NURSING CARE

Health Promotion

Clients can limit their incidence of acute viral URI by frequent hand washing and avoiding exposure to crowds. Maintaining good general health and stress-reducing activities support the immune system and help prevent acute viral URI. Teach the client that becoming chilled or going out in the rain do not cause colds, and that URI are more likely to occur during periods of physical or psychologic stress.

Community-Based Care

The primary nursing role in caring for clients with acute viral URI is educational. Self-care is appropriate for most clients unless the problem is recurrent or a complication occurs. Acute viral URI may interfere with work and recreational activities. Unless limited by symptoms, normal daily activities and roles usually can be maintained. Additional rest during the acute phase of illness is recommended. Additional fluid intake and a well-balanced diet help support the immune response, hastening recovery.

Include the following topics in teaching for home care:
- Using disposable tissues to cover the mouth and nose while coughing or sneezing to reduce airborne spread of the virus

- Blowing the nose with both nostrils open to prevent infected matter from being forced into the eustachian tubes
- Washing hands frequently, especially after coughing or sneezing, to limit viral transmission
- Using OTC preparations for symptomatic relief; precautions related to the sedating effects of antihistamines
- Limiting use of nasal decongestants to every 4 hours for only a few days at a time to prevent rebound effect.

THE CLIENT WITH RESPIRATORY SYNCYTIAL VIRUS

Respiratory syncytial virus (RSV) is a common virus that is the primary cause of respiratory illnesses in young children and the majority of lower respiratory disease in infants. Older children and adults also are commonly and repetitively infected by RSV, but the disease is milder, usually presenting as a common cold. However, the elderly and people who are immunocompromised may develop severe pneumonitis when exposed to RSV (Kasper et al., 2005). The disease may be fatal among people who have undergone or are preparing to undergo bone marrow transplant (Tierney et al., 2005).

RSV is transmitted in much the same way as other URI: via contaminated hands or objects and by coarse droplets spread by coughing and sneezing. The incubation period is 4 to 6 days.

In adults, the manifestations of RSV are those of other common URI, including rhinorrhea, sore throat, and cough. Headache, malaise, and low-grade fever may occur. In older adults, RSV may present as lower respiratory infection with fever or pneumonia (Kasper et al., 2005). While the illness also presents as URI in infants, it is more likely to progress to pneumonia, bronchiolitis, and tracheobronchiolitis in this population.

Treatment for adults with upper respiratory RSV is symptomatic (see the preceding section on URI). When the lower respiratory tract is involved, hydration and other measures to mobilize respiratory secretions are important. Intubation and mechanical ventilation may be necessary if hypoxia develops. Aerosolized ribavirin (Virazole, an antiviral drug) may be prescribed for older adults and immunocompromised clients with RSV pneumonia.

Nursing care is supportive. The focus of nursing care for the adult with URI manifestations of RSV is on teaching for self-care, identification of complications, and prevention of viral spread. When lower respiratory symptoms are present, nursing care is similar to that provided for clients with pneumonia (see Chapter 38 ∞).

THE CLIENT WITH INFLUENZA

Influenza, or *flu,* is a highly contagious viral respiratory disease characterized by coryza, fever, cough, and systemic symptoms such as headache and malaise. Influenza usually occurs in epidemics or pandemics, although sporadic cases do occur. Localized outbreaks of influenza usually occur about every 1 to 3 years. Global epidemics (pandemics) are less frequent, developing every 10 to 15 years until the past two decades. A recently identified strain of avian (bird) influenza has raised concerns about a potential future pandemic. This strain of influenza virus has not yet demonstrated the ability to spread between humans; however, concerns are that it will mutate to allow person-to-person spread. This viral strain has a mortality rate of greater than 50% in people who have been infected due to close association with infected birds. See Box 37–1 for more information about avian influenza.

Although influenza tends to be mild and self-limited in healthy adults, older adults and people with chronic heart or pulmonary disease have a high incidence of complications (such as pneumonia) and a higher risk for mortality related to the disease and its complications (Kasper et al., 2005).

Pathophysiology

Influenza virus is transmitted by airborne droplet and direct contact. Three major strains of the virus have been identified as influenza A virus, influenza B virus, and influenza C virus. Influenza A is responsible for most infections and the most severe outbreaks of influenza. This is primarily due to its ability to alter its surface antigens, bypassing previously developed immune defenses to the virus. New strains of influenza virus are named according to the strain, geographic origin, and year the strain was identified (e.g., A/Taiwan/89). Surface antigens of the specific virus may be used to further differentiate influenza A viruses. Outbreaks of influenza B virus are generally less extensive and less severe than those caused by

influenza A virus. Illness associated with influenza C virus is mild and often goes unrecognized.

The incubation period for influenza is short, only 18 to 72 hours. The virus infects the respiratory epithelium. It rapidly replicates in infected cells and is released to infect neighboring cells. Inflammation leads to necrosis and shedding of serous and ciliated cells of the respiratory tract. This allows extracellular fluid to escape, producing rhinorrhea. With recovery, serous cells are replaced more rapidly than ciliated cells, leading to continued cough and coryza. Systemic manifestations of influenza likely are caused by release of inflammatory mediators such as tumor necrosis factor alpha, interleukin alpha, and interleukin 6 (Kasper et al., 2005). The humoral and cell-mediated immune responses

BOX 37–1 Focus on Avian Influenza

Influenza viruses are common in nature, found in wild birds such as ducks and shore birds. Although these birds carry the virus, they usually are not harmed by it. Movement of the virus into domesticated flocks of ducks and chickens can not only devastate populations of these birds, but can also spread the virus to other domestic animals such as pigs.

Avian influenza is caused by a type A influenza virus identified as H5N1. Type A influenza viruses are subclassified by two proteins found on the surface of the virus, hemagglutinin (HA) and neuraminidase (NA). HA allows the virus to attach to a cell and initiate an infection, whereas NA allows the virus to exit the host cell after replicating. Currently, there are only three known subtypes of influenza A circulating among humans (H1N1, H1N2, and H3N2). The H5N1 virus, which is particularly virulent and spread by migratory birds, raises fears of a potential human pandemic should it evolve to become transmissible from human to human. Influenza viruses are very changeable, undergoing small, continuous changes as well as occasional large and abrupt changes. *Antigenic drift* is the term for small changes that occur continuously as a virus makes copies of itself. These changes help the virus elude the immune system, and necessitate the production of new vaccines every year. Sudden, dramatic changes occur when two different strains of influenza virus (for example, avian influenza and human influenza) infect the same cell and exchange genetic material. These changes, called *antigenic shift*, create a new subtype of the virus to which people have little or no immunity.

As of March 2006, the World Health Organization (WHO) reported a cumulative total of 186 confirmed human cases of avian

influenza A, with the majority of these cases occurring in Viet Nam. Among these confirmed cases, more than half of the people infected died (105 deaths) (WHO, 2006). It is important to note that the cases being reported probably represent the most seriously ill people and milder infections may not be reflected in reported numbers. Most reported cases of avian influenza A have occurred in previously healthy children and young adults.

Symptoms of avian influenza include typical flulike manifestations such as fever, cough, sore throat, and myalgias. In addition, affected people may develop eye infections, pneumonia, and respiratory distress, including acute respiratory distress syndrome (ARDS; see Chapter 39 ∞ for more information about ARDS and its manifestations).

No vaccine to protect against H5N1 virus has yet been developed for commercial use. Measures are being taken, however, to develop pre-pandemic vaccines based on current strains of H5N1 influenza virus, to increase the capacity for vaccine production in the United States, and to research new types of vaccines. Some currently available antiviral medications may effectively treat avian influenza; however, the virus implicated in deaths in southeast Asia was found to be resistant to amantadine and rimantadine, two commonly used drugs to treat influenza (General information, 2006).

A severe pandemic of avian influenza could disrupt all aspects of life, not only causing severe illness and death, but also overwhelming the healthcare system, impacting social services, and causing significant economic loss. Advance preparations such as those currently being undertaken by the WHO and the United States and other countries can reduce the impact of a pandemic.

are activated by influenza infection, and are supplemented by other local and systemic responses (such as interferons).

Manifestations

Infection with influenza virus produces one of three syndromes: uncomplicated nasopharyngeal inflammation, viral upper respiratory infection followed by bacterial infection, or viral pneumonia. The onset is rapid; profound malaise may develop in a matter of minutes.

Manifestations of influenza include abrupt onset of chills and fever, malaise, muscle aches, and headache. Respiratory manifestations include dry, nonproductive cough, sore throat, substernal burning, and coryza (see the box below). Acute symptoms subside within 2 to 3 days, although fever may last as long as a week. The cough may be severe and productive. Along with fatigue and weakness, the cough can persist for days or several weeks.

Complications

The respiratory epithelial necrosis caused by influenza increases the risk for secondary bacterial infections. Sinusitis and otitis media are frequent complications of influenza. Tracheobronchitis, inflammation of the trachea and bronchi, may develop. Although tracheobronchitis is not a serious health risk, its manifestations may persist for up to 3 weeks.

Influenza is clearly linked to an increased risk for pneumonia, particularly in older adults. Changes in respiratory function associated with aging, including decreased effectiveness of cough and increased residual lung volume, pose little risk in the healthy older adult but greatly increase the risk for pneumonia associated with influenza. Primary influenza viral pneumonia, while uncommon, is a serious complication that may be fatal. It typically develops within 48 hours of the onset of influenza, often in clients with preexisting heart valve or pulmonary disease. Influenza pneumonia progresses rapidly and can cause hypoxemia and death within a few days. Bacterial pneumonia is more likely to occur in older at-risk adults but also may affect otherwise healthy adults. It usually presents as a relapse of influenza, with a productive cough and evidence of pneumonia on the chest x-ray. See Chapter 38 ∞ for more information about pneumonia.

Other respiratory complications of influenza include exacerbation of chronic obstructive pulmonary disease (COPD),

chronic bronchitis, or asthma. Sinusitis (discussed later in this chapter) also may develop.

Reye's syndrome is a rare but potentially fatal complication of influenza. Although it is more likely to affect children, it also has been identified in older adults. It is most often associated with influenza B virus. Reye's syndrome develops within 2 to 3 weeks after the onset of influenza. It has a 30% mortality rate. Hepatic failure and encephalopathy develop rapidly in clients with Reye's syndrome.

While uncommon, other potential complications of influenza include myositis (inflammation of skeletal muscles), myocarditis (inflammation of the heart muscle), and central nervous system (CNS) disorders such as encephalitis and Guillain-Barré syndrome.

INTERDISCIPLINARY CARE

Preventing community outbreaks and protecting vulnerable populations (e.g., older adults and people with chronic diseases) are the primary focus for interdisciplinary care related to influenza. Medical treatment of influenza focuses on establishing the diagnosis, providing symptomatic relief, and preventing complications.

Prevention

Preventing influenza by immunizing at-risk populations is an important aspect of care. Immunization with polyvalent (containing antigens of several viral strains) influenza virus vaccine is about 85% effective in preventing influenza infection for several months to a year (Tierney et al., 2005). Annual immunization is recommended for at-risk clients, including people over the age of 65, residents of nursing homes, adults and children with chronic cardiopulmonary disorders (e.g., asthma) or chronic metabolic diseases such as diabetes, and healthcare workers who have frequent contact with high-risk clients. Additionally, family members of at-risk clients should be vaccinated to reduce the client's risk of exposure. The vaccine is given in the fall, prior to the annual winter outbreak. Live attenuated vaccine, administered by intranasal spray, is available for healthy people under age 50.

Diagnosis

The diagnosis of influenza is based on history, clinical findings, and knowledge of an influenza outbreak in the community. A chest x-ray and WBC count may be done to rule out complications such as pneumonia. The WBC count is commonly decreased in influenza; bacterial infections usually cause increased WBCs.

Medications

Yearly immunization with influenza vaccine is the single most important measure to prevent or minimize symptoms of influenza. Although the vaccine is readily available and inexpensive, only about 30% of at-risk clients are vaccinated each year. Many may fear a reaction from the vaccine, although the vaccines are highly purified and reactions are rare. About 5% of people experience mild symptoms of low-grade fever, malaise, or myalgia for up to 24 hours after vaccination. Because the vaccine is produced in eggs, it should not be given to people who are allergic to

---

MANIFESTATIONS of Influenza

RESPIRATORY MANIFESTATIONS
- Coryza
- Cough, initially dry becoming productive
- Substernal burning
- Sore throat

SYSTEMIC MANIFESTATIONS
- Fever and chills
- Malaise
- Muscle aches
- Fatigue

egg protein. Serious adverse reactions to influenza vaccine are rare. Guillain-Barré syndrome, an acute neurologic disorder characterized by muscle weakness and distal sensory loss, has been associated with certain batches of vaccine.

Amantadine (Symmetrel) or rimantadine (Flumadine) may be used for prophylaxis in unvaccinated people who are exposed to the virus. If the drug is given before or within 48 hours of exposure, it inhibits viral shedding and prevents or decreases the symptoms of influenza. If possible, unvaccinated people should receive the vaccine along with the antiviral drug. The drug is continued for several weeks or for the duration of the influenza outbreak. Some strains of type A influenza virus have been found to be resistant to amantadine and rimantadine, potentially limiting their effectiveness in preventing or treating an influenza outbreak.

Amantadine, rimantadine, and the antiviral drugs zanamivir (Relenza), oseltamivir (Tamiflu), and ribavirin (Virazole) also may be used to reduce the duration and severity of flu symptoms. Both zanamivir and ribavirin are administered by inhalation; the other drugs are given orally. Zanamivir can precipitate bronchospasm in clients with a history of asthma or COPD, so it is not recommended for use in these clients (Food and Drug Administration, 2000). See Chapter 12 ∞ for nursing implications for antiviral drugs.

Over-the-counter analgesics such as aspirin, acetaminophen, or nonsteroidal anti-inflammatory drugs (NSAIDs) provide symptomatic relief of fever and muscle ache. Antitussives may decrease cough, promoting rest. Antibiotics are not indicated unless secondary bacterial infection occurs.

 NURSING CARE

Health Promotion

Stress the importance of yearly influenza vaccination for clients in high-risk groups and their families. Teach about spread of the disease, including measures to reduce the risk of contracting influenza, such as avoiding crowds and people who are ill.

Assessment

Unless there is a known outbreak of influenza in the community, it can be difficult to differentiate the manifestations of influenza from those of other URI.

- *Health History:* Known exposure to virus; current symptoms, their onset and duration; presence of dyspnea, chest pain, productive cough, facial pain or pressure in sinus areas; current medications, history of influenza vaccine; chronic diseases such as heart disease, COPD, or diabetes; known medication allergies.
- *Physical Examination:* General appearance; vital signs including temperature; skin color; lung sounds; abdominal exam.
- *Diagnostic Tests:* WBC, throat and sputum cultures, and chest x-ray for evidence of bacterial infection or pneumonia.

Nursing Diagnoses and Interventions

Although the symptoms of influenza are distressing, most people with the illness provide self-care and do not contact a

healthcare provider. Recommendations to rest in bed during the acute phase of the illness and limit activities until recovery are appropriate for influenza.

Severe disease or complications of influenza may necessitate hospitalization for respiratory support and management. For these clients, nursing care focuses on maintaining airway clearance, breathing patterns, and adequate rest.

Ineffective Breathing Pattern

Muscle aches, malaise, and elevated temperature may increase the respiratory rate and alter the depth of respirations, decreasing effective alveolar ventilation. Shallow respirations also increase the risk of *atelectasis* (lack of ventilation in an area of lung).

> **PRACTICE ALERT**
> Monitor respiratory rate and pattern. Tachypnea and/or rapid, shallow respirations may impair effective alveolar ventilation and gas exchange.

- Pace activities to provide for periods of rest. *Tachypnea increases the work of breathing, causing fatigue; fatigue, in turn, can further impair ventilation and reduce the effectiveness of coughing.*
- Elevate the head of the bed. *The upright position improves lung excursion and reduces the work of breathing by lowering the diaphragm, moving abdominal contents downward, creating less resistance to diaphragmatic excursion, and slightly decreasing venous return.*

Ineffective Airway Clearance

Swelling and congestion of mucous membranes, extracellular fluid exudate, and impaired ciliary action due to cell damage increase the risk of impaired airway clearance in influenza. The older adult is at particular risk because of normally reduced ciliary activity and increased lung compliance.

> **PRACTICE ALERT**
> Monitor the effectiveness of cough and ability to remove airway secretions. Fatigue and general malaise may impair the ability to cough effectively and mobilize secretions.

- Maintain adequate hydration. Assess mucous membranes and skin turgor for evidence of dehydration. *Fever and decreased oral fluid intake may lead to dehydration and increased viscosity of secretions. Thick, viscous secretions are more difficult to expectorate.*
- Increase the humidity of inspired air with a bedside humidifier. *Increasing the water content of inhaled air helps loosen thick secretions and soothe mucous membranes.*
- Teach effective cough techniques. Administer analgesics as ordered. *The huff cough is effective to maintain open airways and it spares energy. (See Box 39–5 for client teaching of this technique.) Relieving muscle ache increases the ability to cough effectively.*

Disturbed Sleep Pattern

Airway congestion, malaise, muscle aches, and persistent cough may interfere with the ability to rest, increasing fatigue and prolonging recovery.

- Assess sleep patterns using subjective and objective information. *The client may appear to be sleeping but not achieving normal sleep patterns because of influenza symptoms. Both subjective and objective data are important to accurately assess sleep.*
- Provide antipyretic and analgesic medications at or shortly before bedtime. *These drugs promote comfort by reducing fever and relieving muscle aches.*

> **PRACTICE ALERT**
> If necessary, request a cough suppressant for nighttime use. Cough suppressants are not recommended during the day because coughing promotes airway clearance. They may, however, be necessary at night to allow rest.

Risk for Infection

Infection control measures are recommended to prevent person-to-person transmission of influenza and control influenza outbreaks in healthcare facilities.

- Use standard precautions and encourage all staff and visitors to frequently wash hands. *Hand washing is a primary infection control measure for infections transmitted via respiratory secretions.*
- Instruct clients and visitors to control respiratory secretions by using tissues, and to maintain a distance of at least 3 feet from others when coughing or sneezing. Provide masks for clients and visitors who are unable to control secretions. *Limiting the spread of aerosolized secretions by covering the nose and mouth and maintaining distance from other people can reduce the spread of the disease to vulnerable populations.*
- Use droplet precautions for clients with suspected or confirmed influenza: private room, masks for caregivers and visitors, and a mask for the client when transporting within the facility. *These measures limit the spread of respiratory secretions.*

Using NANDA, NIC, and NOC

Chart 37–1 illustrates linkages between NANDA nursing diagnoses, nursing interventions, and nursing outcomes for the client with influenza.

Community-Based Care

Encourage appropriate self-care for clients with influenza. Discuss the following topics related to home care:

- Increase rest during the acute, febrile phase of the illness.
- Maintain a liberal fluid intake even if anorexic.
- Appropriately use OTC medications for symptom relief.
- Employ hygiene measures such as using disposable tissues and frequent hand washing to reduce spread of the disease.
- Know manifestations of potential complications of influenza to report to the primary care provider.

THE CLIENT WITH SINUSITIS

Sinusitis is inflammation of the mucous membranes of one or more of the sinuses (see Figure 36–2). Sinusitis is a common condition that usually follows an upper respiratory infection

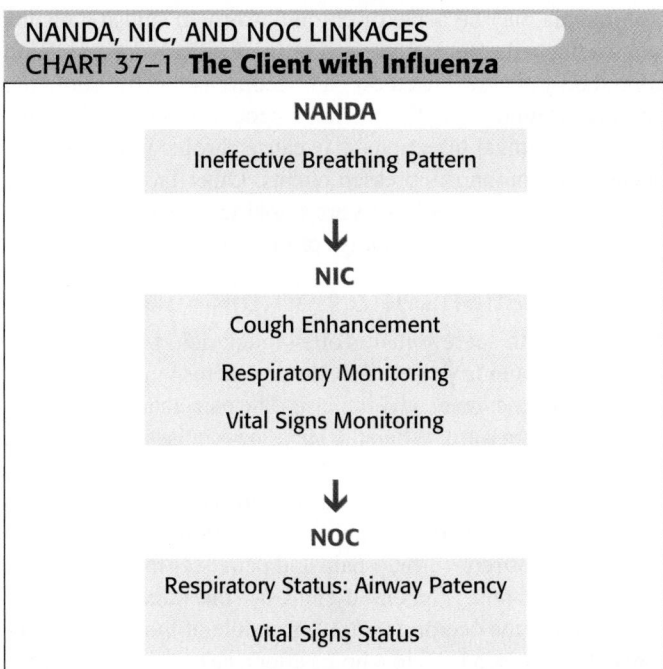

NANDA, NIC, AND NOC LINKAGES
CHART 37–1 The Client with Influenza

NANDA

Ineffective Breathing Pattern

↓

NIC

Cough Enhancement

Respiratory Monitoring

Vital Signs Monitoring

↓

NOC

Respiratory Status: Airway Patency

Vital Signs Status

Data from *NANDA's Nursing Diagnoses: Definitions & Classification 2005–2006* by NANDA International (2005), Philadelphia; *Nursing Interventions Classification (NIC)* (4th ed.) by J. M. Dochterman & G. M. Bulechek (2004), St. Louis, MO: Mosby; and *Nursing Outcomes Classification (NOC)* (3rd ed.) by S. Moorhead, M. Johnson, and M. Maas (2004), St. Louis, MO: Mosby.

such as acute viral upper respiratory infection or influenza. Common causative organisms include streptococci, *S. pneumoniae, Haemophilus influenzae,* and staphylococci. The risk of sinusitis is higher when the immune system is suppressed by immunosuppressive drugs or HIV infection. Sinusitis is common and difficult to treat in people who have AIDS.

Physiology Review

The sinuses (or *paranasal sinuses*) are air-filled cavities in the facial bones that open into the turbinates of the nasal cavity. They are lined with ciliated mucous membranes that help move fluid and microorganisms out of the sinuses into the nasal cavity. The sinuses normally are sterile. Air within the sinuses has a lower oxygen content than inspired air.

Pathophysiology

Sinusitis develops when nasal mucous membranes swell or other disorders obstruct sinus openings, impairing drainage. Mucous secretions collect in the sinus cavity, serving as a medium for bacterial growth. The nasal and sinus mucous membranes are continuous; therefore, bacteria generally spread to the sinuses via the opening into the nasal turbinates. The inflammatory response provoked by bacterial invasion draws serum and leukocytes to the area to combat the infection, increasing swelling and pressure.

Any process that impairs drainage from the sinuses may precipitate sinusitis. These include nasal polyps, deviated septum, rhinitis, tooth abscess, or swimming or diving trauma. In hospitalized clients, sinusitis may develop following prolonged nasotracheal intubation. Usually more than one sinus is infected. The frontal and maxillary sinuses are usually involved in adults.

Sinusitis may be acute or chronic. Chronic sinusitis results when acute sinusitis is untreated or inadequately treated. With continued infection, bacteria can become isolated, producing chronic inflammation. Over time, mucous membranes become thickened. Fungal infections may cause chronic infections, especially in immunosuppressed clients. Other factors that may contribute to chronic sinusitis are smoking, a history of allergy, and habitual use of nasal sprays or inhalants.

Manifestations and Complications

The client with acute sinusitis often looks sick. Manifestations of sinusitis include pain and tenderness across the infected sinuses, headache, fever, and malaise. The pain usually increases with leaning forward. When the maxillary sinuses are involved, pain and pressure are felt over the cheek. The pain may be referred to the upper teeth. Frontal sinusitis causes pain and tenderness across the lower forehead. Infection of the ethmoid sinus produces retro-orbital pain and pain over the high lateral aspect of the nose. Sphenoid sinusitis, the rarest form, may cause pain in the occiput, vertex, or middle of the head. Symptoms often worsen for 3 to 4 hours after awakening and then become less severe in the afternoon and evening as secretions drain. The intensity and location of headache pain may change as sinuses drain. In acute sinusitis, the pain is usually constant and severe. In chronic sinusitis, the pain is described as dull and may be constant or intermittent.

Other symptoms include nasal congestion, purulent nasal discharge, and bad breath. The nasal mucous membrane is red and swollen. Purulent drainage may be noted at the opening to the middle turbinate. This may be the only sign of chronic sinusitis. Swallowed secretions irritate and inflame the throat, and may cause nausea or vomiting.

Complications develop when the infection spreads to surrounding structures (Box 37–2). These include periorbital abscess or cellulitis, cavernous sinus thrombosis, meningitis, brain abscess, or sepsis. Eustachian tube edema may lead to hearing loss.

INTERDISCIPLINARY CARE

Treatment of sinusitis focuses on restoring drainage of obstructed sinuses, controlling infection, relieving pain, and preventing complications.

BOX 37–2 Potential Complications of Sinusitis

Local Complications
- Orbital cellulitis
- Subperiosteal abscess
- Orbital abscess
- Cavernous sinus thrombosis
- Mucocele
- Osteomyelitis

Intracranial Complications
- Meningitis
- Epidural abscess
- Subdural abscess
- Brain abscess
- Venous sinus thrombosis

Diagnosis

The diagnosis of acute sinusitis usually can be made using the history and physical exam. Diagnostic studies such as CT scan or sinus x-rays generally are done only when sinusitis is persistent, chronic, or recurrent. See Chapter 36 for more information about diagnostic studies and their nursing implications.

- *Sinus x-rays* are evaluated. Sinuses are normally translucent because they are filled with air; affected sinuses appear cloudy or opaque. A visible air-fluid level or thickening of the sinus mucosa may be seen in infected sinuses.
- *CT scan* is a more sensitive indicator of acute and chronic sinusitis and often is performed without preceding x-rays.
- *Magnetic resonance imaging (MRI)* may be ordered if malignancy of the sinus is suspected.

Medications

Antibiotic therapy directed at the usual organisms causing sinusitis typically is prescribed. Amoxicillin (possibly combined with clavulanate [Augmentin]), trimethoprim-sulfamethoxazole (Bactrim, Septra), cefuroxime (Ceftin), cefaclor (Ceclor), ciprofloxacin (Cipro), or clarithromycin (Biaxin) are commonly used antibiotics for sinusitis. Antibiotic therapy is continued for 10 to 14 days; occasionally a longer course is prescribed to prevent relapse. If the sinusitis does not respond to treatment with oral antibiotics, hospitalization and intravenous antibiotic therapy may be required. See Chapter 12 for nursing care related to antibiotic therapy.

Oral or topical (in the form of nasal sprays) decongestants such as pseudoephedrine or phenylephrine are also prescribed to reduce mucosal edema and promote sinus drainage. Antihistamines may decrease nasal congestion and facilitate sinus drainage, but they also tend to increase the viscosity of secretions and hinder drainage. For this reason, they may not be as effective as decongestants. Saline nose drops or sprays promote sinus drainage, as does inhalation of warm steam.

PRACTICE ALERT
To administer topical drugs, the client's head is tilted backward and to the side on which the drops are to be instilled. The client may need to remain in position for 5 minutes to allow the drops to reach the posterior nares.

Systemic mucolytic agents such as guaifenesin may be useful to liquefy secretions, promoting sinus drainage. Aerobic exercise also promotes mucous flow and may be recommended.

Surgery

Clients who do not respond to pharmacologic measures and who experience persistent facial pain, headache, or nasal congestion may require *endoscopic sinus surgery*. Detailed evaluation of the sinuses by CT scan is done prior to surgery. Under local or general anesthesia, a fiberoptic nasal endoscope is inserted to visualize the sinus opening. If obstruction is present, it can be removed, restoring patency and drainage. This surgery is most effective for local disease, recurrent acute sinusitis, and for removing anatomic obstructions (Way & Doherty,

2003). Clients who have endoscopic sinus surgery usually do not require nasal packing postoperatively. Instead, frequent nasal cleaning and irrigation with normal saline are performed. The client is instructed to sneeze with the mouth open and avoid blowing the nose, lifting, or straining for a week following surgery.

Antral irrigation can be done in the physician's office under local anesthesia. A 16-gauge needle is inserted under the inferior turbinate of the nose into the maxillary sinus on the affected side. Saline solution is instilled to irrigate the area and wash out the sinus of purulent exudate. The client is seated with the head forward and mouth open to allow drainage of the solution through the nose and mouth. A culture of the exudate may be obtained to determine appropriate antibiotic therapy.

The *Caldwell-Luc procedure* may be necessary if endoscopic sinus surgery is unsuccessful. It is performed under local or general anesthesia. An incision is made under the upper lip into the maxillary sinus, and diseased mucous membrane and periosteum are removed. An opening between the maxillary sinus and lateral nasal wall, a "nasal antral window," is created to increase aeration of the sinus and promote drainage into the nasal cavity. The area is packed with gauze for 24 to 48 hours postoperatively. The gauze packing obstructs nasal breathing while it is in place. As the maxillary sinus heals, exposed bone is covered by mucosa. The upper lip and teeth may be numb for several months after the procedure because of nerve trauma. Chewing may be impaired on the affected side. Only liquids are given for the first 24 hours, followed by a soft diet. The client is instructed to avoid wearing dentures and the Valsalva maneuver (no blowing the nose, coughing, or straining at stool) for about 2 weeks after the packing has been removed to prevent bleeding.

In *external sphenoethmoidectomy,* an incision along the side of the nose from the middle of the eyebrow is used to open and remove diseased tissue from the sphenoid or ethmoid sinuses (Figure 37–1 ■). Nasal polyps may also be removed using this approach. Nasal packing is inserted, and an eye pressure patch is applied to decrease periorbital edema. Care is similar to that following the Caldwell-Luc procedure.

Complementary Therapies
Complementary therapies may help relieve symptoms of sinusitis and promote comfort. Aromatherapy using herbs such as

Figure 37–1 ■ Incision to access ethmoid and frontal sinuses. Resulting scar is nearly invisible in folds of the eye.

basil, marjoram, or eucalyptus in a vaporizer or on a handkerchief, herbal teas made from goldenseal, yarrow, or coltsfoot, hot or cold compresses or steam inhalation, and acupressure may be employed (Fontaine, 2005).

 ## NURSING CARE

Health Promotion
Measures to prevent sinusitis are those that promote nasal drainage: encouraging liberal fluid intake, judicious use of nasal decongestants as needed, and treating any obstructive process. Encourage clients with URI to blow their nose with both nares open. Advise clients that use of saline nasal sprays can help maintain patency of the opening to the sinuses, promoting drainage and reducing the risk of obstruction and infection.

Assessment
Focused assessment of the client with suspected sinusitis includes the following:
- *Health History:* Complaints of frontal or periorbital headache, cheek, teeth, or ear pain; timing of pain and changes in intensity over course of the day; nasal discharge or postnasal drip; other symptoms; previous sinus problems; current medications, known medication allergies.
- *Physical Examination:* General appearance; vital signs including temperature; inspect nasal and pharyngeal mucous membranes; percuss sinuses for tenderness.
- *Diagnostic Tests:* WBC and differential, cultures of sinus drainage, sinus x-rays or other imaging studies.

Nursing Diagnoses and Interventions
The client with sinusitis is often acutely uncomfortable. Obstructed and congested sinuses cause pain and pressure that increase with position changes and leaning forward. Treatment usually is community based, making education the key nursing role. When the client is hospitalized for intravenous antibiotic therapy or sinus surgery, *Pain* and *Imbalanced Nutrition* are priority nursing diagnoses.

Pain
Although sinus surgery is relatively minor, both the incision and postoperative swelling can cause discomfort. Nasal packing, if used, contributes to the discomfort.
- Assess pain using a standardized pain scale. Administer analgesics as ordered. *Relief of pain promotes a feeling of well-being and enhances recovery.*
- Apply ice packs to the nose. *Cold compresses reduce swelling, control bleeding, and provide local analgesia.*
- Elevate the head of the bed to Fowler's or high-Fowler's position for 24 to 48 hours after surgery. *Elevating the operative site minimizes tissue swelling and promotes comfort.*

Imbalanced Nutrition: Less than Body Requirements
Postoperatively, the sense of smell, an appetite stimulus, is diminished by nasal packing. Mouth discomfort from the

incision and numbness of the upper teeth also may impact appetite and eating.

- Provide clear liquid diet progressing to soft foods as tolerated. High-calorie dietary supplements may be used. *A progressive diet is used to assess the ability to swallow without choking and allay fears. Foods high in calories and nutritional value provide for metabolic and healing requirements.*
- Monitor intake, output, and weight. *This information allows assessment of overall fluid balance and the adequacy of dietary intake.*
- Elevate the head of the bed during meals. *The upright position facilitates swallowing and minimizes risk of aspiration.*

Community-Based Care

Teaching for clients with sinusitis and their families focuses on following through with appropriate treatment and promoting comfort. Discuss the following topics when preparing for home care:

- The importance of completing the entire course of prescribed antibiotics to achieve cure and prevent the development of antibiotic-resistant bacteria. Assist in developing a schedule that helps ensure all doses are taken.
- Measures to prevent superinfections (such as vaginitis or oral thrush) during the prolonged course of treatment (e.g., consume 8 oz of yogurt containing live bacterial cultures daily while on antibiotics).
- Use of systemic or topical decongestants to promote sinus drainage.
- Maintaining a liberal fluid intake to reduce the viscosity of mucous drainage.
- Use of a humidifier or steam inhalation to promote sinus drainage.
- Sleeping with the head of the bed elevated to a 45-degree angle and on the unaffected side to promote drainage of affected sinuses.
- Application of a warm, moist pack to the area of pain and tenderness to promote comfort.
- Notify the physician if symptoms do not improve with treatment or if signs of a complication develop, such as increased pain, and redness and swelling on the side of the nose or around the eyes.
- Postoperative instructions to prevent bleeding, such as avoiding blowing the nose for 7 to 10 days and avoiding strenuous activity such as heavy lifting for about 2 weeks.
- Use of saline nasal sprays postoperatively to keep the nasal mucosa moist.

THE CLIENT WITH PHARYNGITIS OR TONSILLITIS

Pharyngitis, acute inflammation of the pharynx, is one of the most commonly identified clinical problems. Although it is usually viral in origin, pharyngitis may also be caused by bacterial infection. *Group A beta-hemolytic streptococcus* (strep throat) is the most common cause of bacterial pharyngitis. Other bacteria that may cause pharyngitis include *Neisseria gonorrhoeae,* a gram-negative diplococcus that is sexually transmitted, *Mycoplasma,* and *Chlamydia trachomatis.*

Tonsillitis is acute inflammation of the palatine tonsils. Although it is sometimes viral in origin, tonsillitis is usually due to streptococcal infection. The incidence of streptococcal infections is greatest between late fall and spring, especially in cold climates. Viral tonsillitis may occur in epidemics in people living in crowded conditions, such as military recruits.

Pathophysiology and Manifestations

Pharyngitis and tonsillitis are contagious and spread by droplet nuclei. Incubation varies from a few hours to several days, depending on the organism. Viral infections are communicable for 2 to 3 days. Symptoms usually resolve within 3 to 10 days after onset.

Viral pharyngitis may be attributed to the same viruses causing the common cold: rhinovirus, coronavirus, or parainfluenza virus. Pharyngitis caused by adenovirus, influenza virus, or Epstein-Barr virus (associated with infectious mononucleosis) may be particularly severe.

Acute pharyngitis causes pain and fever. The pain may vary from a scratchy sore throat to one so painful that swallowing is difficult. Streptococcal pharyngitis is usually marked by an abrupt onset, with fever of 101°F (38.3°C) or higher, severe sore throat with dysphagia, malaise, and often arthralgias and myalgias. Anterior lymph nodes are often enlarged and tender. Exudate (pus) may be seen on the pharynx and tonsils (Figure 37–2 ■). In contrast, the onset of viral pharyngitis is often gradual, with manifestations of low-grade fever, sore throat, mild hoarseness, headache, and rhinorrhea. The pharyngeal membranes appear mildly red with vascular congestion. Infectious mononucleosis, caused by the Epstein-Barr virus, often presents as acute pharyngitis, with visible patches of exudate on the pharynx or tonsils (Kasper et al., 2005). The cervical lymph nodes are enlarged and tender as well. See the accompanying box for the manifestations of pharyngitis and tonsillitis.

In tonsillitis, the tonsils appear bright red and edematous. White exudate is present on the tonsils; pressing on a tonsil may produce purulent drainage. The uvula may also be reddened and swollen. Cervical lymph nodes are usually tender and enlarged.

Figure 37–2 ■ The appearance of the oral pharynx and tonsils in acute pharyngitis and tonsillitis.

MANIFESTATIONS of Pharyngitis and Tonsillitis

LOCAL
- Sore throat
- Possible dysphagia and otalgia
- Tender, swollen anterior cervical lymph nodes
- Hoarse voice
- Red, swollen pharyngeal mucous membranes and/or tonsils
- Possible visible exudate on pharyngeal membranes and/or tonsils

GENERAL
- Fever
- General malaise
- Arthralgia, myalgia

The client with tonsillitis complains of a sore throat, difficulty swallowing, general malaise, fever, and otalgia (pain referred to the ear). Manifestations are often more severe in adolescents and adults than in children. Infection may extend via the eustachian tubes to cause acute otitis media. This may lead to further damage such as spontaneous rupture of the eardrums and mastoiditis. See Chapter 48 ∞ for more information about otitis media.

Complications

Although bacterial pharyngitis may be mild and indistinguishable from viral pharyngitis by its signs and symptoms, it can lead to significant complications such as abscess, scarlet fever, toxic shock syndrome, rheumatic fever, or acute poststreptococcal glomerulonephritis.

Peritonsillar abscess, or *quinsy,* is a potential complication of tonsillitis. It usually results from group A beta-hemolytic streptococcus infection extending from the tonsils to the surrounding tissue. The abscess causes pus formation behind the tonsil with marked swelling and asymmetric deviation of the uvula. The degree of swelling may make it difficult to swallow anything other than liquids. The client may exhibit thickening of the voice, drooling, and a tonic contraction of the muscles of mastication, called trismus.

Rare (1% to 3%) but serious complications of streptococcal pharyngitis and tonsillitis include acute glomerulonephritis and rheumatic fever, abnormal immune responses to the infection. Acute glomerulonephritis generally presents with sudden onset of hematuria, proteinuria, and less commonly, hypertension and edema within 7 to 10 days after the acute infection. Rheumatic fever typically presents 3 to 5 weeks after acute infection with fever, painful or swollen joints, rash, and heart murmur. Other complications of bacterial infection include sinusitis, otitis media, mastoiditis, and cervical adenitis.

INTERDISCIPLINARY CARE

Both viral and bacterial pharyngitis are usually self-limited diseases. However, because of the risk for serious complications associated with streptococcal sore throat, an effort is usu-

ally made to establish an accurate diagnosis and treat bacterial pharyngitis.

- *Throat swab* is obtained and examined for streptococcus antigen using the latex agglutination (LA) antigen test or enzyme immunoassay (ELISA) testing. These tests allow rapid identification of the antigen (in as little as 10 minutes for the LA test) but are not highly sensitive. When the test is positive, treatment for strep throat is initiated. If the test is negative, the swab is cultured to ensure that streptococcus organisms are not present. Even throat cultures are not always accurate, with approximately 10% false negative and 20% false positive results. See Chapter 36 ∞ for nursing care related to obtaining a throat swab.
- *Complete blood count (CBC)* may be done on severely ill clients or to rule out other causes of pharyngitis. The WBC count is usually normal or low in viral infections and elevated in bacterial infections.

Antipyretics and mild analgesics such as aspirin or acetaminophen provide symptomatic relief for throat pain and associated myalgias. Penicillin is the drug of choice for group A streptococci. Erythromycin, amoxicillin, or cefuroxime (Ceftin, Kefurox) may be used if the client is allergic to penicillin. Antibiotic therapy is continued for at least 10 days. The client is no longer contagious after 24 hours of antibiotic therapy.

A peritonsillar abscess is drained by needle aspiration or by incision and drainage. The area is first sprayed with a topical anesthetic such as Cetacaine and then injected with a local anesthetic. The sitting position is preferred for the procedure, because it enables expectoration of blood and pus. (See the accompanying Nursing Care Plan for nursing care of the client with a peritonsillar abscess.) Tonsillectomy is done either immediately or 6 weeks after incision and drainage of peritonsillar abscess.

Tonsillectomy (surgical removal of the tonsils) is indicated for recurrent or chronic infections that have not responded to antibiotic therapy, hypertrophy of the tonsils with risk of airway obstruction, peritonsillar abscess, repeated attacks of purulent otitis media, and tonsil malignancy. Adenoid tissue usually is removed at the same time. Bleeding is the most significant postoperative complication of tonsillectomy, and may develop up to 2 weeks following the surgery.

NURSING CARE

Because of the risk of significant complications associated with streptococcal pharyngitis, encourage all clients with symptoms that persist for several days or that include fever, lymphadenopathy, and myalgias to seek evaluation and treatment.

Home care is appropriate for acute uncomplicated pharyngitis. Treatment focuses on adequate rest and relief of symptoms. A liquid or soft diet is useful when swallowing is difficult. Increased fluid intake is encouraged, especially when febrile. Warm saline gargles, moist inhalations, and application of an ice collar are soothing to the sore throat.

Following tonsillectomy, ensure a patent airway by placing the client in semi-Fowler's position with the head turned to the side to allow secretions to drain from the mouth and pharynx.

NURSING CARE PLAN A Client with Peritonsillar Abscess

Monica Wunderman, age 27, was recently treated for tonsillitis caused by infection by group A streptococcus. She presents to the emergency department 10 days later appearing acutely ill. She states that her throat is so sore that she has difficulty swallowing even liquids. Barbara Ironhorse, the ED nurse, completes an assessment of Ms. Wunderman.

ASSESSMENT

Findings include T 102°F (38.8°C). An acutely swollen and reddened area of the soft palate is noted in her mouth, half occluding the orifice from the mouth into the pharynx. Yellow exudate is present. CBC reveals an elevated WBC of 16,000/mm^3. A diagnosis of peritonsillar abscess is made. Needle aspiration of the abscess is performed.

DIAGNOSES

- *Acute Pain* related to swelling
- *Risk for Ineffective Airway Clearance* related to pain and swelling
- *Deficient Fluid Volume* related to fever and difficulty in swallowing fluids

EXPECTED OUTCOMES

- Have minimal or no pain.
- Maintain a patent airway as demonstrated by normal respiratory rate and rhythm.
- Maintain optimal fluid intake as evidenced by consumption of fluids and semiliquid foods, moist mucous membranes, normal skin turgor, and normal temperature.

PLANNING AND IMPLEMENTATION

- Teach that ice-cold fluids may be easier to swallow than hot or room temperature beverages and may provide a local analgesic effect.
- Advise to avoid citrus juices, hot or spicy foods, and rough-textured foods for 1 week.
- Teach pain management strategies such as applying an ice collar as desired and gargling with warm saline or mouthwash solution every 1 to 2 hours for the first 24 to 48 hours after aspiration of the abscess.
- Instruct to take medications as prescribed.

EVALUATION

When Ms. Ironhorse contacts Ms. Wunderman by telephone 2 days after her visit to the emergency department, she reports complete relief of symptoms. She is afebrile, taking fluids without difficulty, and has had no difficulty breathing. She has not experienced any pain.

CRITICAL THINKING IN THE NURSING PROCESS

1. Describe common symptoms of infectious or inflammatory diseases of the upper airway and discuss methods of symptom relief.
2. Describe common pharmacologic interventions for these disorders.
3. What themes of nursing diagnoses emerge for clients with these types of disorders?
See Evaluating Your Response in Appendix C.

Keep the airway in place until the gag and swallowing reflexes have returned. Apply an ice collar to reduce swelling and pain. Notify the surgeon immediately if excessive bleeding or hemorrhage occurs. If there is no bleeding, allow water and cracked ice as desired. Warm saline mouthwashes are helpful in managing thick oral secretions following tonsillectomy. A liquid or semiliquid diet is recommended for several days.

Community-Based Care

Discuss the following topics when preparing the client for home care:

- The importance of completing the full 10 days of antibiotic therapy if prescribed
- Using warm saline gargles or throat lozenges for symptomatic relief
- Signs and symptoms of possible complications of streptococcal infection such as glomerulonephritis or rheumatic fever
- Monitoring temperature in the morning and evening until well to ensure that the infection has not spread to deeper tissues
- Proper use and disposal of tissues and frequent hand washing to prevent spreading the infection to others.

For the client who has had a peritonsillar abscess drainage or tonsillectomy, provide the following instructions:

- Postoperative mouth and throat care
- Avoiding use of aspirin for 2 weeks to reduce the risk of postoperative bleeding

- Manifestations of bleeding to report to the physician (delayed hemorrhage may occur for up to 1 week postsurgery).

THE CLIENT WITH A LARYNGEAL INFECTION

The larynx, located between the upper airways and the lungs, protects the lower respiratory tract from inhaled substances other than air, and allows speech. The larynx includes the epiglottis, which covers the larynx during swallowing, and the glottis, or vocal cords. Either portion of the larynx may become inflamed.

Epiglottitis

Epiglottitis, inflammation of the epiglottis, is an uncommon disorder that presents as a medical emergency. *H. influenzae* infection is the most common cause of epiglottitis. Epiglottitis is a rapidly progressive cellulitis that begins between the base of the tongue and the epiglottis. The epiglottis itself becomes swollen and inflamed; swelling of adjacent tissues pushes the epiglottis posteriorly. This swelling and edema threaten the airway. Adults usually present with a 1- to 2-day history of sore throat, *odynophagia* (painful swallowing), dyspnea, and possibly drooling and stridor.

Using a tongue blade to view the oropharynx is avoided; this may precipitate laryngospasm and airway obstruction. The epiglottis is visualized using a flexible fiberoptic laryngoscope to establish the diagnosis. The epiglottis appears red, swollen, and edematous. Nasotracheal intubation may be required to ensure airway patency. The client is admitted to a critical care unit and intravenous antibiotic therapy is initiated. Ceftriaxone (Rocephin), cefuroxime (Ceftin), or ampicillin/sulbactam (Unasyn) may be prescribed. If allergic to penicillin, a combination of clindamycin (Cleocin) and either trimethoprim-sulfamethoxazole (TMP-SMZ) or ciprofloxacin (Cipro) may be used. Dexamethasone, a systemic corticosteroid, is also given to suppress the inflammatory response and rapidly reduce swelling of the epiglottis.

Nursing care for the client with acute epiglottitis focuses on monitoring and maintaining airway patency. Monitor oxygen saturation continuously. Observe closely for signs of airway obstruction, including nasal flaring, restlessness, stridor, use of accessory muscles, and decreased oxygen saturation measurements. If the client is not intubated, supplies for emergency intubation should be kept in the unit. Epiglottitis is frightening for both the client and the nurse. Maintaining a calm, reassuring manner is an essential nursing role.

Laryngitis

Laryngitis, inflammation of the larynx, is a common disorder that may occur alone or in conjunction with other upper respiratory infections. It is commonly associated with a viral URI such as influenza. It may also occur with bronchitis, pneumonia, or other respiratory infections. Excessive use of the voice, sudden changes in temperature or exposure to dust, irritating fumes, smoke, or other pollutants can also cause acute or chronic laryngitis. It is more common in the winter and in colder climates.

In laryngitis, the mucous membrane lining the larynx becomes inflamed; the vocal cords also may become edematous. The primary symptom of laryngitis is a change in the voice. Hoarseness or *aphonia,* complete loss of the voice, may occur. The throat is often sore and scratchy, and a dry, harsh cough may be present.

There is no specific treatment for viral laryngitis. Any identified precipitating factors such as overuse of the voice and exposure to irritants should be eliminated. Voice rest is advised, as is abstinence from tobacco and alcohol, which are chemical irritants. Treatment may also include inhaling steam or spraying the throat with antiseptic solutions. Identifying and eliminating irritants are helpful to prevent future attacks.

Impaired verbal communication is the priority nursing problem for clients with laryngitis. The meaning of messages is conveyed not only by the words used, but also by the tone and loudness of voice. Instruct to rest the voice as much as possible. Encourage speaking in short sentences or using alternate methods of communication, such as writing. Resting the voice hastens recovery and decreases throat discomfort. Advise to use soothing throat lozenges, sprays, or other comfort measures such as gargling with a warm antiseptic solution. Help identify potential irritants, such as fumes, chemicals, or cold temperature, to prevent future bouts of laryngitis.

THE CLIENT WITH DIPHTHERIA

Diphtheria is an acute, contagious disease caused by *Corynebacterium diphtheriae,* a small aerobic pathogen. This disease, which primarily affects adults, is uncommon in the United States. Waning immunity due to lack of periodic booster immunizations is the primary risk factor for diphtheria in the United States.

The disease is spread through droplet nuclei and by contamination of articles such as eating utensils. Asymptomatic carriers can be a factor in spreading this infection. People who have recovered from diphtheria can harbor bacteria in their throats for up to 4 weeks. Diphtheria is easily spread in areas where sanitation is poor, living conditions are crowded, and access to health care is limited. Immunization is readily available, and infants and children are usually immunized against diphtheria, pertussis, and tetanus concurrently.

Pathophysiology and Manifestations

C. diphtheriae infects the mucous membranes of the respiratory tract and can invade skin lesions. The tonsils and pharynx are common sites of infection. Toxins released by the organism inflame mucosal surfaces of the pharynx. Exudate from inflamed tissues forms a thick, grayish, rubbery pseudomembrane over the posterior pharynx and sometimes into the trachea. This pseudomembrane adheres to inflamed, eroded surfaces and interferes with eating, drinking, and breathing. The airway may be obstructed, necessitating tracheostomy to maintain respirations. The toxins damage the heart and CNS and may cause myocarditis and paralysis of cranial or peripheral nerves.

Clients with diphtheria develop fever, malaise, sore throat, and malodorous breath. In severe cases, the neck may be warm and swollen because of lymphadenopathy. Isolated patches of gray or white exudate grow and extend to form a gray membrane that becomes progressively thicker. Dislodging the membrane often causes bleeding. Symptoms of airway obstruction, such as stridor and cyanosis, can develop quickly.

INTERDISCIPLINARY CARE

Collaborative care goals for diphtheria are to prevent its transmission, treat the infection, neutralize toxins, and provide respiratory support. The diagnosis is confirmed by a throat culture. Gram-stain or immunofluorescent antibody stains may also be used.

Strict isolation procedures are instituted, and all contacts are screened and immunized. Booster shots are given to people who were immunized 5 or more years previously. Unimmunized contacts are treated with immunization and antibiotics.

Diphtheria antitoxin is given to neutralize free toxin and prevent further toxin production. Diphtheria antitoxin is produced in horses; a skin test for sensitivity to horse serum should precede immunization. Anaphylaxis is a risk during antitoxin therapy; epinephrine must be readily available. Antibiotics such as penicillin or erythromycin are administered to eliminate the organism.

NURSING CARE

Clients with diphtheria require intensive nursing care. The client is placed on bed rest and monitored closely for airway obstruction, cardiac manifestations, and CNS complications. Nutrition and fluid balance may be affected by difficulty swallowing. Upright positioning can promote fluid intake during the acute phase of the disease. Equipment for suction, emergency intubation, and tracheostomy are kept at the bedside.

> **PRACTICE ALERT**
> Diphtheria is a reportable disease. Immediately contact the local health department and the Centers for Disease Control and Prevention (CDC) concerning all suspected and confirmed cases.

Preventing further cases of diphtheria is a nursing responsibility. Symptomatic clients are isolated and treated until two negative throat cultures are obtained. Nasopharyngeal and throat cultures are also obtained from all close contacts. Asymptomatic disease carriers are confined to home until at least 3 days of antibiotic therapy have been completed. All contacts, including hospital personnel, receive tetanus and diphtheria toxoids (Td).

THE CLIENT WITH PERTUSSIS

Pertussis, or *whooping cough,* is a highly contagious acute upper respiratory infection caused by the bacterium *Bordetella pertussis.* Although it is thought to be a childhood disease that has been virtually eliminated by aggressive immunization of infants, pertussis still occurs in North America. Up to 45% of people affected by pertussis are adolescents and adults. Adults are thought to be an important reservoir for this disease (Kasper et al., 2005).

Pathophysiology

B. pertussis is a gram-negative rod that is spread by respiratory droplets. The bacteria attach to ciliated epithelial cells of the nasopharynx, multiplying and invading respiratory tissues. The damage and effects of pertussis are not due to the infection itself, but to toxins produced by the bacteria. These toxins damage the mucosa and paralyze the cilia. As a result, clearance of respiratory secretions is impaired, increasing the risk for pneumonia. The toxins also prompt an inflammatory response and inhibit immune defenses.

Although immunization does not appear to confer lifetime immunity, the disease tends to be milder in adolescents, adults, and people who have been immunized. These infected individuals can, however, transmit the disease to other susceptible people, including unimmunized or underimmunized infants (Atkinson et al., 2000).

Young infants have the highest risk for complications of the disease, such as pneumonia and neurologic complications. Neurologic complications are thought to result from hypoxia due to prolonged paroxysms of coughing. Complications in adolescents and adults may occur as a result of increased intrathoracic pressure during prolonged coughing spells. These may include pneumothorax, weight loss, inguinal hernia, rib fracture, and *cough syncope* (fainting due to hypoxia) (Kasper et al., 2005).

Manifestations

Classic pertussis follows a predictable pattern, with typical URI symptoms (coryza, sneezing, low-grade fever, and mild cough) beginning 7 to 10 days after exposure. After 1 to 2 weeks, the cough becomes more frequent, occurring in paroxysms or bursts of rapid coughs, often ending with an audible whoop caused by rapid inspiration. This whoop is less common in adolescents and adults, often delaying diagnosis. Vomiting commonly follows an episode of coughing. Coughing paroxysms vary in frequency from several per hour to 5 to 10 per day, interfering with eating and sleep. This stage of the disease, called the *paroxysmal stage,* usually lasts no more than 6 weeks, after which coughing becomes less severe and gradually resolves over a period of up to 3 months.

In adolescents and adults, pertussis is suspected when an upper respiratory infection produces a cough that persists longer than 7 days, is accompanied by vomiting, and is worse at night. See the Manifestations box below.

INTERDISCIPLINARY CARE

Active immunization with pertussis vaccine is the primary preventive strategy for pertussis. Acellular pertussis vaccines that are effective but produce fewer adverse reactions than traditional whole-cell vaccines are available and preferred for immunization.

The diagnosis of pertussis is established by culture of nasopharyngeal secretions. However, nasopharyngeal secretions may remain positive for the organism for only about 3 weeks after the onset of symptoms, so blood tests for antibodies to the organism may be necessary to confirm the diagnosis. Lymphocytosis (elevated lymphocyte count) may be present.

Erythromycin is the antibiotic of choice to eradicate *B. pertussis* infection. TMP-SMZ may be used as an alternate to erythromycin. Hospitalization rarely is required for adults, although children and infants with severe disease often are hospitalized to prevent complications such as neurologic effects of hypoxia and malnutrition. Respiratory isolation is instituted for 5 days after antibiotic therapy is started. Prophylactic erythromycin or TMP-SMZ is prescribed for all household and close contacts of the infected client.

> **MANIFESTATIONS** **of Pertussis**
>
> **CLASSIC**
> - *Catarrhal phase:* coryza, malaise, low-grade fever, sneezing, cough
> - *Paroxysmal phase:* frequent spasms of sometimes violent coughing, worse at night; characteristic whoop on inspiration following cough paroxysm; vomiting, fatigue, weight loss resulting from severe cough
> - *Convalescent phase:* gradually decreasing frequency and severity of coughing episodes
>
> **ATYPICAL (OFTEN SEEN IN ADOLESCENTS AND ADULTS)**
> - Severe, prolonged cough that may not be paroxysmal; whoop uncommon
> - Vomiting with cough
> - Cough at night

NURSING CARE

Nurses are instrumental in promoting effective immunization of all infants and young children against pertussis. Education is a key nursing role related to immunization, as significant controversy currently exists about potential long-term adverse consequences of the vaccine. Recommend that all parents request acellular vaccine due to its lower risk of adverse effects.

Recommend nasopharyngeal culture for clients complaining of persistent cough, especially when the cough is accompanied by vomiting or significantly worse at night, or if other members of the household or close contacts have a similar illness.

PRACTICE ALERT
Pertussis is a reportable communicable disease. Report all probable and confirmed cases to the local health department and the CDC.

Education is a primary nursing role related to pertussis. Adult clients usually remain in the community for treatment.

Teach respiratory isolation measures to be used until the disease is no longer communicable. Discuss ways to control respiratory secretions, and the importance of disposing of tissues and secretions personally to prevent exposure of others. Stress the importance of prophylactic treatment for all household and close contacts. Discuss measures to maintain fluid and nutrient intake, and use of a cough suppressant at night to promote rest. Encourage increased fluid intake to promote expectoration of respiratory secretions. Teach about the prescribed antibiotic, including its potential adverse effects and measures to reduce them, such as taking erythromycin with meals to prevent gastric upset. Contact the local county health department for follow-up of contacts and compliance with prescribed treatment.

PRACTICE ALERT
Adults should receive a diphtheria vaccine booster immunization every 10 years (usually given in combination with tetanus vaccine). A newly available diphtheria-tetanus-acellular pertussis vaccine is available for adults (CDC, 2005b).

UPPER RESPIRATORY TRAUMA OR OBSTRUCTION

Obstruction of the upper airway due to trauma (fracture of the nasal septum or the larynx), bleeding (e.g., epistaxis), or a tumor is not only frightening for the client, it also may interfere with the ability to breathe.

THE CLIENT WITH EPISTAXIS

The nose has a rich blood supply, receiving major arterial vessels from both the internal and external carotid artery systems. **Epistaxis**, or nosebleed, may be precipitated by a number of factors. Trauma (picking the nose or blunt trauma) can cause epistaxis, as can drying of nasal mucous membranes, infection, substance abuse (e.g., cocaine), arteriosclerosis, or hypertension. Epistaxis may also indicate a bleeding disorder related to acute leukemia, thrombocytopenia, aplastic anemia, or severe liver disease. Additionally, treatment with an anticoagulant or antiplatelet drug may cause nosebleed. In adults, men more frequently have nosebleeds than women.

Pathophysiology and Manifestations

Ninety percent of all nosebleeds arise in the anterior nasal septum from Kiesselbach's area, a rich vascular plexus. Because of their location, these vessels are susceptible to trauma from nose picking, drying, and infection. Posterior epistaxis more often develops secondarily to systemic disorders such as blood dyscrasias, hypertension, or diabetes. In posterior epistaxis, bleeding is from the terminal branches of the sphenopalatine and internal maxillary arteries. Posterior epistaxis tends to be more severe and occurs more frequently in the older adult.

Anterior nosebleeds usually produce obvious bleeding from the nares, as well as bleeding into the posterior nasal and oral pharynx. The bleeding from a posterior nosebleed may be less apparent, with most of the blood draining into the posterior nasopharynx and swallowed by the client. Nausea and vomiting may occur due to swallowed blood.

INTERDISCIPLINARY CARE

The goal of treatment for epistaxis is to identify and control the source of bleeding.

Anterior bleeding can usually be managed by simple first-aid measures, such as applying pressure (pinching the nose toward the septum) for 5 to 10 minutes and applying ice packs to the nose and forehead to cause vasoconstriction. The client is placed in a sitting position to decrease blood flow to the head and reduce venous pressure. Leaning forward reduces drainage of blood backward into the nasopharynx and decreases swallowing of blood. The client is instructed to spit out the blood to help estimate the amount of bleeding and to prevent nausea and vomiting as a result of swallowed blood.

If applying pressure does not control the bleeding, medications, nasal packing, or surgery may be necessary.

Medications

Topical vasoconstrictors such as cocaine (0.5%), phenylephrine (Neo-Synephrine) (1:1000), or adrenaline (1:1000) may be used to control anterior bleeding. These medications may be applied by nasal spray or on a cotton swab held against the bleeding site. Chemical cauterization of the bleeding vessel may be done using agents such as silver nitrate or Gelfoam. A topical anesthetic such as tetracaine, lidocaine, or cocaine may be used prior to nasal packing. If posterior nasal packing is required, prophylactic antibiotic therapy is initiated to prevent sinusitis or possible toxic shock syndrome.

Nasal Packing

If bleeding cannot be controlled with pressure and local medications, a nasal tampon (a soft balloon filled with air) may be used to apply direct pressure to the bleeding vessel, or the nasal cavity may be packed with 0.25-inch petroleum gauze. For an anterior pack, several feet of packing are placed carefully and systematically along the floor of the nasal cavity and then into the vault of the nose. Anterior nasal packs are usually left in place for 24 to 72 hours. If epistaxis is caused by a bleeding disorder, the packing may be left in place for 4 to 5 days while the disorder is treated.

Posterior nosebleeds are more difficult to control, requiring both anterior and posterior packing (Figure 37–3 ■). Posterior packs are usually left in place for 2 to 5 days. A loose anterior nasal pack may also be inserted. Posterior nasal packing is very uncomfortable, and can cause respiratory and cardiovascular complications. Hypoxemia is common; supplementary oxygen is administered. Endotracheal intubation may be necessary to maintain adequate ventilation and gas exchange. Narcotic analgesics are prescribed to manage the discomfort. Hypertension, dysrhythmias, and even acute myocardial infarction may occur in clients with severe cardiovascular disease. Toxic shock syndrome is another potential complication of posterior nasal packing. The pack may occlude the eustachian tube and sinus openings, resulting in ear discomfort, possible otitis media, or sinusitis. Oral and nasal dryness can be minimized by use of a high-humidity face tent. Nursing care of the client with nasal packing is outlined in the box on the next page.

A Foley catheter or inflatable nasal balloon may be used as an alternative to posterior nasal packing for effective tamponade. The catheter or nasal balloon is inserted through the nose into the nasopharynx, inflated, and left in place for 2 to 3 days.

Surgery

Chemical or surgical cautery procedures may be used to sclerose involved vessels in the anterior aspect of the nose. The resulting scab must be left undisturbed until the mucosa has healed, or further bleeding may occur.

Surgical procedures to control bleeding are often preferred to posterior nasal packing for posterior bleeding. The bleeding vessel may be cauterized using an endoscopic approach. In some cases, surgery is required to occlude the internal maxillary artery by ligation (tying off) or embolization. These procedures may be done under either conscious sedation and local anesthesia or general anesthesia. Facial paralysis, paresthesias, facial pain, and dental injury are potential complications (Way & Doherty, 2003).

NURSING CARE

Assessment

Nursing assessment of the client with a nosebleed focuses on the immediate problem and possible underlying conditions.

- *Health history:* Duration of current bleed; any identified precipitating factors such as trauma; history of prior nosebleeds; current medications; chronic conditions such as hypertension, bleeding disorders, and so on.
- *Physical examination:* Estimated amount of bleeding; presence of blood in oropharynx; vital signs; evidence of facial or nasal trauma.
- *Diagnostic tests:* Hemoglobin, hematocrit, and CBC as indicated; oxygen saturation; tests of organ function such as liver function tests (bilirubin, AST, ALT, LDH) or kidney function tests (serum creatinine, BUN).

Nursing Diagnoses and Interventions

Nosebleeds can be frightening, particularly when they occur without preceding trauma. Nurses provide care for clients with

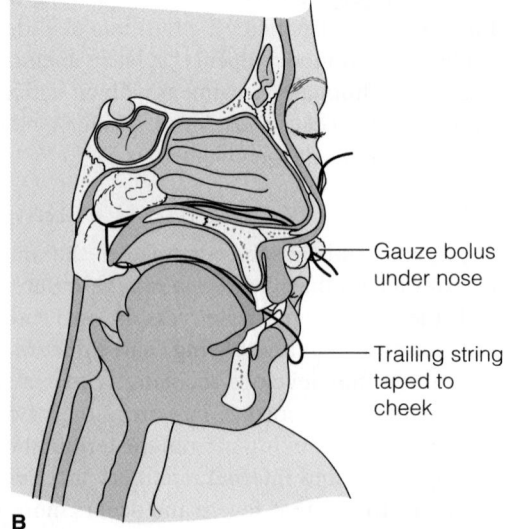

Gauze bolus under nose

Trailing string taped to cheek

Figure 37–3 ■ Posterior nasal packing. *A,* A rubber catheter is inserted through the nose and out the mouth and attached to the packing. *B,* The catheter is withdrawn through the nose to position the packing in the posterior nasopharynx. Ties exiting through the nose and mouth are used to stabilize the packing in position and remove it when it is no longer needed.

NURSING CARE OF THE CLIENT WITH   Nasal Packing

- Continuously monitor oxygen saturation. Administer supplementary oxygen as ordered. *Posterior nasal packing causes hypoxemia. Supplemental oxygen is given to maintain tissue oxygenation.*
- Frequently monitor vital signs and respiratory rate or pattern. *Posterior nasal packing increases the risk for respiratory and cardiovascular complications. Tachycardia and tachypnea may be early signs of cardiac or respiratory compromise.*
- Inspect the mouth and oropharynx. Notify the physician if the packing is seen in the oropharynx. *Misplacement of nasal packing can obstruct the upper airway.*
- Elevate the head of the bed. *Elevating the head of the bed facilitates ventilation.*
- Encourage deep, slow breathing through the mouth. Provide psychologic support, reassurance, and teaching. *Inability to breathe through the nose causes anxiety and fear.*

- Check for blood at the back of the throat and frequent swallowing. *Visible blood or frequent swallowing could indicate posterior bleeding.*
- Report hematemesis. *Bleeding from the posterior portion of the nose often drains down the nasopharynx and is swallowed. Hematemesis may indicate continued bleeding.*
- Apply cold compresses to nose. *An ice or cold compress decreases pain and promotes vasoconstriction, decreasing bleeding and swelling.*
- Provide for rest. *Rest reduces the metabolic demands and oxygen consumption.*
- Ensure adequate oral fluid intake. *Fluid intake helps maintain fluid balance and decreases dryness of oral mucous membranes because of mouth breathing.*
- Provide frequent oral hygiene. Use a bedside humidifier. *These measures reduce drying of oral mucous membranes and promote comfort.*

epistaxis in outpatient and emergency settings, and may care for hospitalized clients with nasal packing. Support, reassurance, and education are important nursing roles related to epistaxis. Priority nursing diagnoses include *Anxiety* and *Risk for Aspiration*.

Anxiety

The amount of blood lost in a nosebleed can be frightening. The sensation of blood draining down the throat and inability to breathe through the nose contribute to anxiety. Spontaneous epistaxis may lead to fear of a major health problem such as high blood pressure.

PRACTICE ALERT
Maintain an attitude of calm reassurance. By remaining calm and confident, the nurse reassures the client that the nosebleed is not a life-threatening event.

- Instruct the client to pinch the nares together at the bridge of the nose. *Most nosebleeds are anterior in origin; direct pressure usually stops the bleeding. Having the client place pressure on the nose provides a focus and helps restore a sense of control, reducing anxiety.*
- Encourage slow, deep breathing through the mouth. *Controlled mouth breathing maintains lung ventilation and reduces anxiety.*
- Provide a basin and tissues; encourage the client to expectorate blood, not swallow it. *These measures give the client greater control and reduce the fear of choking on blood.*

PRACTICE ALERT
Assess the client with nasal packing frequently for adequate oxygenation. Maintain supplemental oxygen as ordered. Cerebral hypoxia produces a sense of apprehension and fear.

Risk for Aspiration

Anxiety and blood draining into the nasopharynx increase the risk for aspiration of blood into the trachea. When nasal packing is in place, the client is unable to breathe through the nose, increasing the risk of aspiration when food or fluids are consumed.

PRACTICE ALERT
Position upright with the head forward. Provide a basin for expectorating blood. These measures minimize the amount of blood draining down the nasopharynx and swallowed, reducing the risk of aspiration and minimizing nausea from swallowed blood. Vomiting of swallowed blood increases the risk of aspiration.

- Apply ice or a cold compress to the nose. *Cold causes vasoconstriction, reducing bleeding.*

PRACTICE ALERT
Position the client with nasal packing with the head elevated and on the side when asleep. This position reduces the risk of aspiration of oral secretions.

Community-Based Care

Following an episode of epistaxis, teaching for home care focuses on measures to prevent further bleeding. Include the following teaching topics:

- Avoid strenuous exercise for several days or weeks, depending on the severity of the nosebleed and its treatment.
- Do not blow the nose or engage in activities such as heavy lifting or bending that could increase pressure and dislodge the crust; sneeze with the mouth open to avoid increasing pressure in nasal vessels.
- For an anterior nosebleed, use petroleum jelly, a water-soluble lubricant, or bacitracin ointment to lubricate nasal mucosa and reduce the risk of spontaneous bleeding.
- Use a humidifier or vaporizer to minimize dryness of the mucous membranes.
- Do not forcefully blow the nose or pick the nose.

- For spontaneous nosebleed, seek medical evaluation for any possible underlying problem, such as hypertension or a bleeding disorder.

THE CLIENT WITH NASAL TRAUMA OR SURGERY

The nose is the most commonly broken bone of the face. A nasal fracture (broken nose) usually is caused by a sports injury or trauma related to violence or motor vehicle crashes. The nasal septum normally divides the nose into two equal parts. Deviation of the septum can result from nasal trauma. Soft-tissue trauma commonly accompanies nasal fracture.

Pathophysiology and Manifestations

One or both sides of the nose may be broken. A *unilateral fracture* involves only one side of the nose. It causes little displacement or cosmetic deformity. It is usually not serious, but septal deviation and swelling can obstruct the airway. *Bilateral fractures* are more common, with depression or displacement of both nasal bones to one side. The nose appears flattened or deviated with an S or C configuration. *Complex fractures* may also involve the septum, ascending processes of the maxilla, and frontal bones of the face.

Soft-tissue trauma commonly accompanies nasal fracture. Mucous membrane tears cause epistaxis. Soft-tissue hematomas (black eye) are also frequent. Swelling develops rapidly following the injury and may obscure the fracture. Boney crepitus may be felt on gentle palpation. Septal hematoma may develop, increasing the risk for infection. The manifestations of nasal fracture are listed in the box below.

Complications

Potential complications of nasal fracture include septal hematoma and abscess formation, septal perforation or deviation, and cerebrospinal fluid (CSF) leakage. Septal hematoma can lead to complete and bilateral nasal obstruction. If undrained, hematoma increases the risk of staphylococcal abscess, which can lead to necrosis of septal cartilage and *saddle nose deformity.*

Septal deviation causes varying degrees of nasal obstruction. The septal cartilage bulges or deviates to one side, partially or totally obstructing the nares. Mild deviation is generally asymptomatic. Partial obstruction of air flow through one side may cause noisy breathing while awake and snoring during sleep. Major deviations can cause pain because of sinus

MANIFESTATIONS of Nasal Fracture

- Epistaxis
- Deformity or displacement to one side
- Crepitus
- Periorbital edema and ecchymosis
- Nasal bridge instability

obstruction or infection. They may also cause nosebleeds due to dryness of the nasal mucosa. Occasionally, the defect is severe enough to cause cosmetic deformity. Perforations are usually not serious and do not usually require repair unless obstruction or external deformity occur.

Fractures of other facial bones may accompany a broken nose, particularly when facial trauma is severe. Fractures in the nasoethmoidal or frontal region can disrupt the dura, causing CSF leakage or rhinorrhea. CSF rhinorrhea is suspected if watery nasal drainage tests positive for glucose.

INTERDISCIPLINARY CARE

The major treatment goals for nasal fractures are to maintain a patent airway and prevent deformity. Respirations are closely monitored.

Diagnosis

Head and facial x-rays are done to identify the fracture and assess for other facial fractures. The intranasal cavity is examined using a nasal speculum to rule out septal hematoma. If a CSF leak is suspected, a CT scan is done. A radiopaque substance or fluorescein dye may be instilled into the intrathecal or lumbar subarachnoid space to identify the site of leakage.

Treatments

Ideally, the fracture is reduced early, before significant edema develops. Nasal fractures heal rapidly. Simple reduction may be done in the emergency department with local anesthesia. An external splint may be applied for 7 to 10 days to maintain proper alignment until healing occurs. The splint is padded to prevent skin breakdown. Ice may be gently applied to the face and nose to control edema and bleeding. Nasal packing may be used to control epistaxis.

Surgery

Complex nasal fractures, nasal septal deviation, or persistent CSF leakage may require surgical repair or realignment of nasal bones. Rhinoplasty with concurrent septoplasty is the most common procedure used to repair nasal fracture or a deviated nasal septum.

Rhinoplasty is surgical reconstruction of the nose. It is done to relieve airway obstruction and repair visible deformity of the nose following fracture. If edema is excessive after nasal fracture, surgery is delayed for 7 to 10 days to allow swelling to subside. Using an intranasal incision, the nasal skin is lifted and the framework of the nose reshaped by removing, rearranging, or augmenting bone or cartilage. The skin is then repositioned over the reconstructed frame. Prosthetic implants may help reshape the nose. Either local or general anesthesia may be used; hospitalization is often unnecessary. Following surgery, nasal packing is left in place for up to 72 hours to minimize bleeding and provide tissue support. A temporary plastic splint molded to the shape of the nose is removed in 3 to 5 days. The splint protects the reshaped nose and helps to control swelling. Most swelling and bruising subside within 10 to 14 days; normal sensation returns within several months following surgery. Rhinoplasty generally has few complications.

Either a septoplasty or a submucous resection may be done under local anesthesia to correct a deviated septum. *Septoplasty* involves incising one side of the septum, elevating the mucous membrane, and removing or straightening the deviated portion of septal cartilage. In a *submucous resection,* bone and cartilage are removed. In both procedures, packing is applied to both sides of the nose to prevent bleeding and to keep the septal mucosa in the midline position.

Small defects in the cribriform plate, fovea ethmoidalis, or sphenoid sinus associated with persistent CSF leakage may require endoscopic repair. Either a tissue graft or fibrin glue may be used to repair the defect. The graft or glue is held in place with absorbable packing. Large defects may require craniotomy for repair (Way & Doherty, 2003).

 ## NURSING CARE

Health Promotion

Teach all people, children and adolescents in particular, about the importance of wearing helmets and facial protectors when participating in high-risk sports such as football, hockey, and baseball catching. Promote the use of seat belts with shoulder harness and air bags in vehicles to reduce the risk of facial injury in motor vehicle crashes.

Assessment

Focused nursing assessment for the client with a suspected nasal fracture includes:

- *Health History:* Nature and circumstances of the injury; pain; ability to breathe through the nose.
- *Physical Examination:* Evident trauma, swelling, ecchymosis, or deformity of the nose; vital signs, respiratory rate and ease; gently palpate nose and facial bones for crepitus; inspect oropharynx for drainage; test nasal discharge for glucose.

Nursing Diagnoses and Interventions

Nursing care for clients with nasal fracture focuses on controlling pain, bleeding, and swelling. Airway management is a priority. Most nasal fractures are managed on an outpatient basis, and education is a vital nursing function. See the accompanying Nursing Care Plan for additional nursing diagnoses and interventions for the client with nasal trauma.

Ineffective Airway Clearance

Immediately following nasal trauma and fracture, the airway is at risk for obstruction by bleeding and edema. Deformity resulting from inappropriate fracture position during healing also can impair nasal airway clearance. This is a consideration when inserting nasogastric tubes or suctioning clients with septal deviation.

NURSING CARE PLAN | A Client with Nasal Trauma

Clifton Kavanaugh is a 36-year-old mailman who broke his nose when he was hit in the face by a baseball. He is admitted to the emergency department accompanied by a friend.

ASSESSMENT

Mr. Kavanaugh presents with obvious deformity of the nose. It is swollen, bloody, and deviated to one side. The nose is bleeding slightly. Mr. Kavanaugh rates the pain as a 6 on a scale of 1 to 10. Vital signs are BP 132/70, P 120 and regular, R 22, T 98.6°F (37°C) axillary.

Mr. Kavanaugh is breathing through his mouth and holding an ice compress to his nose. Bony crepitus and edema are felt on palpation. There is no evidence of CSF leak from either nose or ears. X-ray confirms a nasal fracture.

DIAGNOSES

- *Acute Pain* related to nasal fracture
- *Ineffective Breathing Pattern* related to nasal swelling and bleeding
- *Anxiety* related to pain and need for emergency care
- *Disturbed Body Image* related to nasal deformity

EXPECTED OUTCOMES

- Verbalize relief of pain.
- Maintain a patent airway and normalize the breathing pattern.
- Demonstrate reduced anxiety.
- Express concerns about potential body image change.

PLANNING AND IMPLEMENTATION

- Administer analgesics as ordered.
- Apply ice compress to nose.
- Inspect oropharynx for evidence of bleeding.
- Encourage deep, slow breathing through the mouth.
- Provide oral hygiene.
- Discuss concerns regarding injury.
- Assist with nasal splint application.

EVALUATION

Following treatment, Mr. Kavanaugh reports his pain has decreased to a level of 2 on a scale of 1 to 10. He appears more relaxed, no longer grimacing and with a relaxed posture. His respirations are easy at 18. The nasal splint is intact. Mr. Kavanaugh is able to look in a mirror and state with a laugh, "I look like a raccoon." He is admitted to the hospital for rhinoplasty.

CRITICAL THINKING IN THE NURSING PROCESS

1. A client in the emergency department with nasal trauma becomes extremely panicky because of blood draining down his throat. How would you intervene to reduce this client's anxiety without using nasal suction? Why is it important to avoid suctioning the nasopharynx in the client with nasal trauma?
2. Develop a plan of care for the client with a leak of CSF from a nasal fracture.
3. Compare immediate versus delayed rhinoplasty for the client with nasal fracture.

See Evaluating Your Response in Appendix C.

PRACTICE ALERT

Monitor airway patency. Edema and bleeding may obstruct the airway, causing signs of respiratory distress such as tachypnea, dyspnea, shortness of breath, tachycardia, and use of accessory muscles.

■ Monitor cough effectiveness and ability to clear airway secretions. *Pain, edema, and nasal bleeding may impair the ability to cough effectively.*

PRACTICE ALERT

Have suction equipment available. Airway patency is a priority; oropharyngeal suctioning may be necessary to remove secretions and maintain a clear airway. Suctioning of the nasopharynx is avoided to prevent additional tissue trauma.

■ Maintain adequate hydration. Assess mucous membranes and skin turgor for evidence of dehydration. *Decreased oral fluid intake may lead to dehydration and thick, viscous secretions that are more difficult to expectorate.*

■ Assess patency of both nares before inserting a nasogastric tube or feeding tube. If airflow is obstructed through one side, insert the tube through the unobstructed nare. Carefully monitor respiratory status following tube insertion. *The nasogastric tube is inserted through the unobstructed nare to avoid mucosal trauma; however, a large gastric tube may interfere with nasal breathing, necessitating close monitoring.*

Risk for Infection

The client with a nasal fracture is at increased risk for infection. The nasal mucosa is a natural barrier to infection, and trauma increases the risk for invasion by pathogens. Septal hematoma can lead to abscess formation and staphylococcal infection. A CSF leak indicates disruption of the dura, increasing the risk of ascending infection and meningitis.

PRACTICE ALERT

Test watery, clear fluid dripping from the ear or nose for glucose. CSF will test positive for glucose on a glucose test strip.

■ Avoid suctioning if possible. *Suctioning catheters could introduce microorganisms and cause additional trauma to tissues.*

■ Monitor vital signs every 4 hours. *A rise in temperature may indicate infection.*

■ Administer antibiotics as ordered. *Antibiotics may be prescribed to prevent abscess formation, and, if CSF leakage is present, to prevent meningitis.*

Using NANDA, NIC, and NOC

Linkages between NANDA nursing diagnoses, nursing interventions, and nursing outcomes for the client with nasal trauma are demonstrated in Chart 37–2.

Community-Based Care

Provide the following teaching when preparing the client with a nasal fracture for home care:

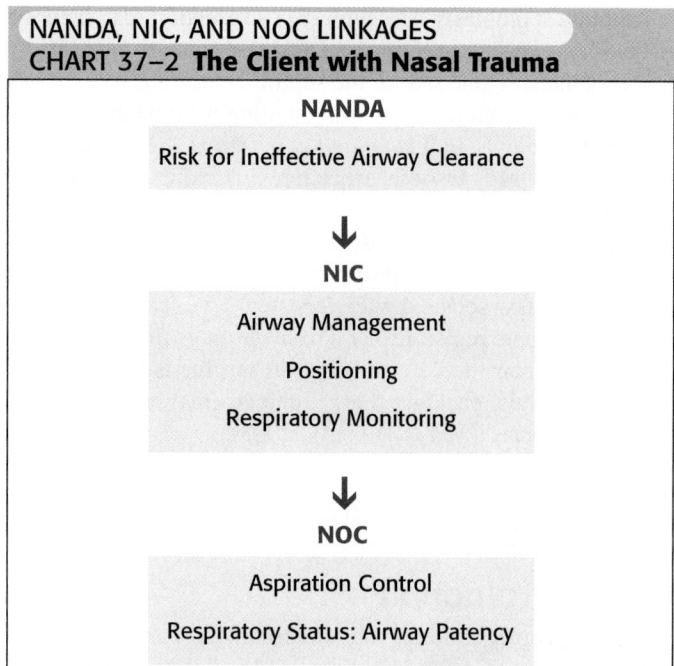

NANDA, NIC, AND NOC LINKAGES
CHART 37–2 The Client with Nasal Trauma

NANDA

Risk for Ineffective Airway Clearance

↓

NIC

Airway Management

Positioning

Respiratory Monitoring

↓

NOC

Aspiration Control

Respiratory Status: Airway Patency

Data from *NANDA's Nursing Diagnoses: Definitions & Classification 2005–2006* by NANDA International (2005), Philadelphia; *Nursing Intervention Classification (NIC)* (4th ed.) by J. M. Dochterman & G. M. Bulechek (2004), St. Louis, MO: Mosby; and *Nursing Outcomes Classification (NOC)* (3rd ed.) by S. Moorhead, M. Johnson, and M. Maas (2004), St. Louis, MO: Mosby.

■ Elevate the head of the bed with blocks and apply ice or cold packs to the nose for 20 minutes four times a day to reduce swelling.

■ Swelling usually subsides in several days; bruising may persist for several weeks.

■ It is difficult to determine the final cosmetic outcome until swelling has subsided.

■ If indicated by delayed fracture reduction or malformation, discuss rhinoplasty and its potential benefits.

If CSF leakage is present, also include the following instructions:

■ Rest in bed with the head of the bed elevated to 30 to 45 degrees.

■ Restrict fluid intake as ordered and take the prescribed diuretic to reduce intracranial pressure and CSF leakage.

■ Distribute allowed fluids throughout the day.

■ List name, purpose, effects, and precautions for any prescribed medication.

■ Avoid straining, blowing the nose, sneezing, or vigorous coughing until allowed by the physician.

■ Immediately report manifestations of infection, including stiff neck, headache, and fever, to the physician.

Following rhinoplasty or septoplasty, provide the following instructions:

■ Apply ice packs to the nose to relieve discomfort and reduce swelling.

■ Elevate the head of the bed on blocks to decrease local edema.

■ Do not blow the nose for 48 hours after the packing is removed to prevent bleeding.

■ Vigorous coughing or straining at stool may cause bleeding and should be avoided.

- Clean teeth and mouth frequently and increase fluid intake to decrease oral dryness due to mouth breathing.
- Bruising around the eyes and nose will last for several days.

THE CLIENT WITH LARYNGEAL OBSTRUCTION OR TRAUMA

The larynx is the narrowest portion of the upper airway. As such, it is at risk for obstruction. Laryngeal obstruction is a life-threatening emergency. Blows to the neck or other traumatic injuries may damage the larynx, interfering with its patency and function.

Pathophysiology and Manifestations
Laryngeal Obstruction

The larynx may be partially or fully obstructed by aspirated food or foreign objects, or by laryngospasm or edema due to inflammation, injury, or anaphylaxis. Anything that occludes the larynx can obstruct the airway. The most common cause of obstruction in adults is ingested meat that lodges in the airway (the so-called *café coronary*). Risk factors for food aspiration include ingesting large boluses of food and chewing them insufficiently, consuming excess alcohol, and wearing dentures. A foreign body in the larynx causes pain, laryngospasm, dyspnea, and inspiratory stridor. Aspirated foreign bodies may pass through the larynx into the trachea and lungs, causing pneumonitis.

Laryngospasm occurs due to repeated or traumatic intubation attempts, chemical irritation, or hypocalcemia. An acute type I hypersensitivity response may cause anaphylaxis with release of inflammatory mediators, leading to angioedema of upper airways and severe laryngeal edema.

The most common manifestations of laryngeal obstruction are coughing, choking, gagging, obvious difficulty breathing with use of accessory muscles, and inspiratory stridor. As the airway is obstructed, signs of asphyxia become apparent. Respirations are labored and noisy with wheezing and stridor. Cyanosis may develop. Respiratory arrest and death may result without prompt treatment.

Laryngeal Trauma

Trauma to the larynx can occur in motor vehicle crashes or assaults (e.g., blows to the neck or attempted strangulation). The larynx also may be traumatized during endotracheal intubation or tracheotomy. Trauma may fracture thyroid and/or cricoid cartilage, resulting in loss of airway patency. Soft-tissue injuries can cause swelling that further impairs the airway. Manifestations of laryngeal trauma may include subcutaneous emphysema or crepitus, voice change, dysphagia and pain with swallowing, inspiratory stridor, hemoptysis, and cough.

INTERDISCIPLINARY CARE

The treatment goal is to maintain an open airway. If airway obstruction is partial and the client is able to cough and move air in and out of the lungs, radiologic and laryngoscopic examination may be done to locate the foreign body. An endotracheal tube may be inserted to maintain airflow through the larynx in spasm or an edematous larynx. For anaphylaxis, epinephrine may be administered to reduce laryngeal edema and relieve obstruction.

When airway obstruction due to a foreign body is complete, the Heimlich maneuver is performed immediately to clear the obstruction. For the conscious person, the rescuer wraps his or her arms around the victim from behind, places one fist between the umbilicus and xiphoid process, covers the fist with the other hand, and forcefully thrusts the hands upward (Figure 37–4A ■). For the unconscious victim, the rescuer straddles the victim's thighs and delivers thrusts upward and inward on the upper abdomen (Figure 37–4B). These moves are continued until the

A

B

Figure 37–4 ■ Administering abdominal thrusts (the Heimlich maneuver) to *A,* a conscious victim, and *B,* an unconscious victim.

obstruction is relieved or more definitive care can be given. Endotracheal intubation may be attempted. If intubation is unsuccessful, an immediate cricothyrotomy or tracheotomy must be performed to open the airway.

CT scan is used to identify laryngeal fractures; however, emergency treatment may be required prior to diagnosis to ensure airway patency and preserve life. Soft-tissue injuries may be managed conservatively with bedside humidifier, intravenous fluids, antibiotics, and corticosteroids to reduce edema. More severe injuries require endotracheal intubation or immediate tracheostomy. Nursing care related to caring for the client with a tracheostomy is presented later in this chapter. See Chapter 39 ∞ for more information about endotracheal intubation and nursing care for the intubated client.

 ## NURSING CARE

PRACTICE ALERT
The priority of nursing care in laryngeal obstruction or trauma is restoring a patent airway to prevent cerebral anoxia and death. Laryngeal obstruction and trauma are medical emergencies requiring immediate intervention.

Closely monitor clients at risk for laryngeal obstruction (e.g., following neck trauma, newly extubated clients, and people receiving medications with a high risk of anaphylaxis, such as intravenous antibiotics or radiologic dyes) for manifestations of obstruction, including dyspnea, nasal flaring, tachypnea, anxiety, wheezing, and stridor. Suction the airway as needed; small aspirated foreign bodies might possibly be removed by suctioning. If obstruction is complete, initiate a cardiopulmonary arrest procedure and perform the Heimlich maneuver until the obstruction is relieved or the emergency response team arrives. Prepare to assist with emergency intubation or tracheotomy as needed. Provide emotional support, reassurance, and teaching for the client and family to reduce anxiety.

Community-Based Care
Health promotion and teaching for home care focus on preventing laryngeal obstruction and early intervention techniques. Everyone should be aware of the risk factors for adult aspiration. Caution clients who wear dentures to take small bites, chewing each bite carefully before swallowing. Discuss the relationship between excess alcohol intake and food aspiration. Participate in promoting training of the general public in CPR and the Heimlich maneuver. The more people who are adequately trained in emergency procedures, the more likely it is that emergency procedures will be initiated in a timely manner. Clients with a known risk for anaphylaxis, such as people with a previous anaphylactic response and those allergic to bee venom, should wear a Medic-Alert tag and carry a bee-sting kit to allow early intervention to prevent severe laryngeal edema and spasm.

THE CLIENT WITH OBSTRUCTIVE SLEEP APNEA

Sleep apnea, intermittent absence of airflow through the mouth and nose during sleep, is a serious and potentially life-threatening disorder. It affects at least 2% of middle-aged women and 4% of middle-aged men. Sleep apnea is a leading cause of excessive daytime sleepiness, and may contribute to other problems such as poor work performance and motor vehicle crashes (Kasper et al., 2005; McCance & Huether, 2006). Recent studies have linked sleep apnea with an increased risk for hypertension, ischemic heart disease, and exacerbation of heart failure.

Types of sleep apnea include obstructive and central. In *obstructive sleep apnea*, the more common type, the respiratory drive remains intact, but airflow ceases due to occlusion of the oropharyngeal airway. *Central sleep apnea* is a rare neurologic disorder that involves transient impairment of the neurologic drive to respiratory muscles.

Risk Factors
In addition to male gender, risk factors for obstructive sleep apnea include increasing age and obesity. Large neck circumference (>17 inches in men and >16 inches in women) also is a known risk factor for obstructive sleep apnea (Porth, 2005). Use of alcohol and other CNS depressants may contribute to sleep apnea.

Pathophysiology
During sleep, skeletal muscle tone decreases (except the diaphragm). The most significant decrease occurs during rapid eye movement (REM) sleep (Porth, 2005). Loss of normal pharyngeal muscle tone permits the pharynx to collapse during inspiration as pressure within the airways becomes negative in relation to atmospheric pressure. The tongue is also pulled against the posterior pharyngeal wall by gravity during sleep, causing further obstruction. Obesity or skeletal or soft-tissue changes that decrease inspiratory tone, such as a relatively large tongue in a relatively small oropharynx, contribute to the problem. Airflow obstruction causes the oxygen saturation, P_{O_2}, and pH to fall, and the P_{CO_2} to rise. This progressive asphyxia causes brief arousal from sleep, which restores airway patency and airflow. Sleep can be severely fragmented because these episodes may occur hundreds of times each night.

Manifestations
Narrowed upper airways produce loud snoring during sleep, often years before obstructive sleep apnea occurs. Excessive daytime sleepiness, headache, irritability, and restless sleep also are common manifestations. See the box on the next page.

Complications
Recurrent episodes of apnea and arousal during sleep have secondary physiologic effects. Sleep fragmentation and loss of slow-wave sleep are thought to contribute to neurologic and behavior problems such as excessive daytime sleepiness, impaired intellect, memory loss, and personality changes. Recurrent nocturnal asphyxia and negative intrathoracic pressure due to airway

Chapter 36 ∞. See Chapter 43 ∞ for more information about electroencephalography.

> ### MANIFESTATIONS of Obstructive Sleep Apnea
>
> - Loud, cyclic snoring
> - Periods of apnea lasting 15 to 120 seconds during sleep
> - Gasping or choking during sleep
> - Restlessness, thrashing during sleep
> - Daytime fatigue and sleepiness
> - Morning headache
> - Personality changes, depression
> - Intellectual impairment
> - Impotence
> - Hypertension

obstruction increase the workload of the heart. People with coronary heart disease may develop myocardial ischemia and angina. Dysrhythmias such as significant bradycardia and dangerous tachydysrhythmias may develop. Left ventricular function may be impaired and heart failure may occur. Systemic blood pressure remains high during sleep and may contribute to systemic hypertension that affects more than 50% of people with obstructive sleep apnea (Kasper et al., 2005). Pulmonary hypertension also may develop. Sudden cardiac death is believed to be a potential fatal complication of obstructive sleep apnea.

Obstructive sleep apnea is a common condition in people who are morbidly obese. When these clients undergo gastric bypass surgery to treat their obesity, sleep apnea places them at significant risk for postoperative respiratory complications. Not only does the obesity interfere with chest movement and ventilation, it increases metabolic demands and carbon monoxide production. Anesthetic and analgesics used during surgery and in the postoperative period can lead to hypoxemia due to muscle relaxation and depression of the respiratory drive (Deutzer, 2005).

INTERDISCIPLINARY CARE

The goal of care for obstructive sleep apnea is to restore airflow and prevent the adverse effects of the disorder. Sustained weight loss may cure obstructive sleep apnea.

Diagnosis

The diagnosis of obstructive sleep apnea is based on *polysomnography,* an overnight sleep study. Several variables are recorded during the study, including:

- Electroencephalogram and measurements of ocular activity and muscle tone
- Recordings of ventilatory activity and airflow
- Continuous arterial oxygen saturation readings
- Heart rate.

Transcutaneous arterial P_{CO_2} readings also may be monitored during the study. Because sleep studies are time consuming and expensive, overnight monitoring of oxygen saturation by pulse oximetry may be used to confirm the diagnosis of sleep apnea when symptoms indicate a high probability of the disorder (Kasper et al., 2005). Nursing implications for pulmonary function studies and pulse oximetry are presented in

Treatments

Mild to moderate obstructive sleep apnea may be treated by weight reduction, alcohol abstinence, improving nasal patency, and avoiding the supine position for sleep. Although weight reduction often cures the disorder, maintaining optimal weight is difficult. Oral appliances designed to keep the mandible and tongue forward also may be prescribed.

Nasal continuous positive airway pressure (CPAP) is the treatment of choice for obstructive sleep apnea. Positive pressure generated by an air compressor and administered through a tight-fitting nasal mask (Figure 37–5 ■) splints the pharyngeal airway, preventing collapse and obstruction. With proper training, this device is well tolerated by the client. Nasal airways can become dry and irritated with CPAP, so an in-line humidifier or a room humidifier is recommended. A newer device, the BiPAP ventilator, delivers higher pressures during inhalation and lower pressures during expiration, providing less resistance to exhaling.

Surgery

Tonsillectomy and adenoidectomy may relieve upper airway obstruction in some clients. Excision of obstructive tissue from the soft palate, uvula, and posterior lateral pharyngeal wall may be accomplished by *uvulopalatopharyngoplasty (UPPP).* Although only about 50% of these surgeries are successful in treating sleep apnea, UPPP is useful in selected cases. In severe cases, tracheostomy may also be performed to bypass the area of obstruction.

NURSING CARE

Obstructive sleep apnea usually is treated in the home. Nursing care focuses on teaching the client and family about equipment use and strategies to decrease contributing factors such as obesity and alcohol intake. The following nursing diagnoses are appropriate for clients with sleep apnea:

- *Disturbed Sleep Pattern* related to repeated apneic episodes
- *Fatigue* related to interrupted sleep patterns

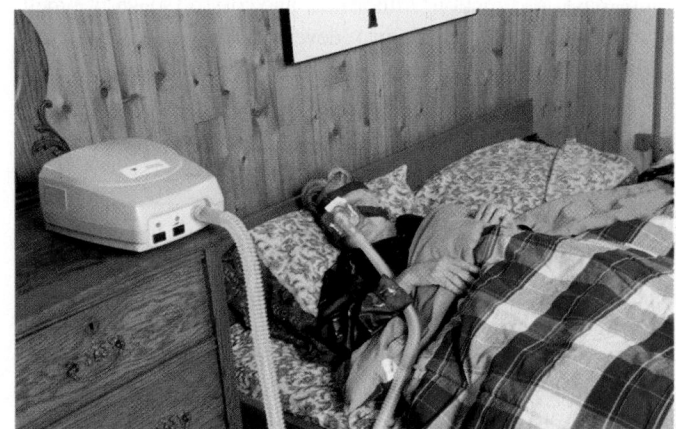

Figure 37–5 ■ A client using a nasal mask and CPAP to treat sleep apnea.

Source: Custom Medical Stock Photo, Inc.

- *Ineffective Breathing Pattern* related to obstruction of upper airway during sleep
- *Impaired Gas Exchange* related to altered lung ventilation during obstructive episodes
- *Risk for Injury* related to daytime somnolence and altered judgment
- *Risk for Sexual Dysfunction* related to impotence resulting from sleep apnea.

Community-Based Care

Effective sleep apnea management depends on the client's willingness to participate in care. Provide teaching about the following topics:

- Relationship between obesity and sleep apnea
- Plans, resources, and referrals as needed for weight loss (e.g., programs such as Weight Watchers to provide additional support)
- Relationship of alcohol and sedatives to sleep apnea; referral to an alcohol treatment program or Alcoholics Anonymous as indicated
- How to use CPAP if ordered
- The importance of using CPAP continuously at night
- Measures to reduce airway dryness, including supplemental humidity and an adequate fluid intake to maintain moist mucous membranes.

If a support group for people with sleep apnea syndrome is available in the local area, refer the client and family to the group.

UPPER RESPIRATORY TUMORS

Although tumors of the upper respiratory tract are relatively uncommon, they have the potential to impair the upper airways and interfere with breathing and ventilation of the lungs. Of the upper respiratory tract structures, the larynx is affected by abnormal growths most often.

THE CLIENT WITH NASAL POLYPS

Nasal polyps are benign grapelike growths of the mucous membrane lining the nose. These benign tumors can interfere with air movement through nasal passages or obstruct sinus openings, leading to sinusitis. They usually affect people who have chronic allergic rhinitis or asthma.

Pathophysiology and Manifestations

Chronic irritation and swelling of the mucous membranes from allergic rhinitis may cause slow polyp formation. Polyps form in areas of dependent mucous membrane, presenting as pale, edematous masses covered with mucous membrane. They are usually bilateral and have a stemlike base, making them fairly movable. Polyps can continue to enlarge, eventually becoming larger than a grape. Polyps may be asymptomatic, although large polyps may cause nasal obstruction, rhinorrhea, and loss of sense of smell. Manifestations of sinusitis may develop. The voice may have a nasal tone. Asthmatics who have nasal polyps may have an associated aspirin allergy of which they are not aware.

INTERDISCIPLINARY CARE

When polyps occur in conjunction with an acute upper respiratory infection, they may regress spontaneously with resolution of the infection. When symptomatic, polyps may be managed with topical corticosteroid nasal sprays or low-dose oral corticosteroids to shrink the edematous polyps and manage allergic symptoms. However, polyps continue to enlarge when corticosteroid therapy is discontinued.

Surgery may be required to restore normal breathing. Surgical removal of polyps (*polypectomy*) often is done in the physician's office under local anesthesia. A wire snare is used to clip the polyps from their stemlike base. Nasal packing is inserted to control bleeding after removal. Alternatively, laser surgery may be used to remove polyps. Healing is more rapid following laser intervention, and the risk of bleeding is reduced. Because polyps tend to recur, repeated surgeries may be necessary.

NURSING CARE

Teaching about home care following polypectomy is the primary nursing responsibility for the client with nasal polyps. Provide postoperative care instructions, and discuss measures to reduce the risk of bleeding.

- Apply ice or cold compresses to the nose to decrease swelling, promote comfort, and prevent bleeding.
- Avoid blowing the nose for 24 to 48 hours after nasal packing is removed.
- Avoid straining at stool, vigorous coughing, and strenuous exercise.

Discuss manifestations of possible bleeding, such as frequent swallowing or visible blood at the back of the throat. Swallowed blood may cause nausea and vomiting. Encourage the client to rest for 2 to 3 days after surgery to reduce the risk of bleeding. Instruct to increase fluid intake and clean mouth frequently to reduce oral dryness associated with mouth breathing while nasal packing is in place.

THE CLIENT WITH A LARYNGEAL TUMOR

Laryngeal tumors may be either benign or malignant. Benign tumors of the larynx include papillomas, nodules, and polyps. People who chronically shout, project, or vocalize in an abnormally high or low tone, abusing the voice, are at risk for developing benign laryngeal tumors. In adults, vocal cord nodules are often referred to as "singer's nodules"; cheerleaders and public speakers may also develop them. Voice abuse also contributes to the development of vocal cord polyps, as does cigarette smoking and chronic irritation from industrial pollutants. Malignant tumors of the larynx, although uncommon, can have devastating effects if diagnosis and treatment is delayed.

FAST FACTS

- Malignancy, or cancer, of the larynx is uncommon and is often curable if detected early.
- An estimated 3770 people died from laryngeal cancer in 2005; and 9880 new cases were diagnosed (ACS, 2005a).

Risk Factors

Men are affected by laryngeal cancer more than four times as often as women. Cancer of the larynx usually develops between ages 50 and 70. Tobacco use is the major risk factor for laryngeal cancer: The risk of developing laryngeal cancer is significantly greater in smokers (cigarette, pipe, or cigar) than in nonsmokers. Alcohol consumption is a significant cofactor in increasing the risk. When combined with smoking, the risk increases significantly, perhaps as much as 100 times (ACS, 2005b). Other risk factors include poor nutrition, human papillomavirus infection, exposure to asbestos and other occupational pollutants, and race (laryngeal cancer is more common in African Americans than among whites).

Pathophysiology and Manifestations

Benign Tumors

Papillomas are small, wartlike growths believed to be viral in origin. Polyps and nodules may develop on the vocal cords of the larynx as a result of voice abuse (Figure 37–6 ■). Nodules occur as paired lesions on the free edges of the vocal cords. Hoarseness and a breathy voice quality are manifestations of benign vocal cord tumors.

Laryngeal Cancer

Squamous cell carcinoma is the most common malignancy of the larynx. Changes in the laryngeal mucosa occur over time as it is subjected to noxious irritants such as cigarette smoke. White, patchy, precancerous lesions known as *leukoplakia* appear. Red, velvety patches, called *erythroplakia,* are thought to represent a later stage of carcinoma development. The initial cancerous lesion, carcinoma *in situ* (CIS), is superficial. Malignant cells replace the lining layer, but do not invade into deeper tissues. Untreated, most CIS lesions develop into squamous cell cancer (ACS, 2005b). Laryngeal cancer spreads by both direct invasion of surrounding tissues and by metastasis.

Figure 37–6 ■ Laryngoscopy showing a polyp on the left vocal cord.

Figure 37–7 ■ Cancer of the larynx and epiglottis.

It may metastasize to the lungs; however, metastases of other cancers to the larynx are rare.

Laryngeal cancer may develop in any of the three areas of the larynx: the glottis, the supraglottis, and the subglottis. Manifestations vary according to site of the lesion.

Lesions of the true vocal cords or glottis account for nearly 60% of all laryngeal cancers. Fortunately, these cancers tend to be well differentiated and slow growing. Metastasis occurs late in the course of the disease because of a limited lymphatic supply. The usual symptom of glottic cancer is hoarseness, or a change in the voice because the tumor prevents complete closure of the vocal cords during speech.

Approximately 35% of laryngeal cancers develop in the supraglottic area, which includes the epiglottis, aryepiglottic folds, arytenoid muscles and cartilage, and false vocal cords (Figure 37–7 ■). Lymphatic supply to this region of the larynx is rich; tumors often invade locally and metastasize early. Symptoms often do not develop until the tumor is relatively large, delaying diagnosis. Manifestations of supraglottic cancer include painful swallowing, sore throat, or a feeling of a lump in the throat. Later manifestations include dyspnea, foul breath, and pain that radiates to the ear.

Subglottic tumors (below the vocal cords) are the least common, accounting for the remaining 5% of laryngeal tumors. They often are asymptomatic until the enlarging tumor obstructs the airway. Common manifestations of laryngeal cancer are listed below.

MANIFESTATIONS of Laryngeal Cancer

- Hoarseness
- Change in the voice
- Painful swallowing
- Dyspnea
- Foul breath
- Palpable lump in neck
- Earache

INTERDISCIPLINARY CARE

Benign laryngeal tumors may resolve with correction of the underlying problem, such as voice training with a speech therapist or smoking cessation. Treatment of laryngeal malignancy varies with the extent of the cancer. Early diagnosis and treatment are important: 80% to 95% of early stage tumors can be cured, whereas 50% to 80% of people with advanced laryngeal cancer die of the disease.

Diagnosis

- *Direct* or *indirect laryngoscopy* is used for initial evaluation when laryngeal cancer is suspected. A fiberoptic laryngoscope is used for direct laryngoscopy; mirrors are used to visualize the larynx in indirect laryngoscopy.
- *Biopsy* is obtained from suspicious lesions to examine the cells. Biopsy is usually obtained under general anesthesia or conscious sedation. Tissue may be obtained via endoscopy or by fine-needle aspiration of the mass.
- *Imaging studies* such as CT scan, MRI, and chest x-ray are obtained to evaluate the size of the mass, possible extension into deeper tissues, involvement of lymph nodes, and possible metastasis to the lungs. A barium swallow may be done to evaluate the effects of the tumor on swallowing. A PET scan also may be done (possibly in conjunction with CT scan) to detect tumor metastasis.

Treatments

An inhaled steroid spray may be used for vocal cord polyps. In some cases, surgical excision of benign nodules or polyps is required. This usually is performed via laryngoscopy, using microforceps or a laser. A biopsy of the tumor is done to rule out malignancy.

Laryngeal cancer treatment is determined by *staging* the cancer. Information such as tumor size and location (T), number of involved lymph nodes (N), and presence or absence of metastases (M) is combined to assign a stage, designated by Roman numerals I to IV. Table 37–1 outlines laryngeal cancer stages.

RADIATION THERAPY Radiation therapy is often the treatment of choice for early laryngeal cancer. Radiation disrupts the DNA of the cell, causing it to die. External radiation commonly is used; brachytherapy, implants of iridium seeds placed into hollow plastic needles that are inserted directly into or near the tumor site during surgery to deliver radiation, is less frequently used for laryngeal or hypopharyngeal cancer. Radiation therapy is extremely effective for treating glottic cancer, with cure rates equal to those achieved by surgery. Radiation therapy preserves the voice, although the tone or timber of the voice may be affected.

Radiation therapy may be used in combination with chemotherapy (*chemoradiotherapy*) to treat more advanced laryngeal cancers. Nearly two-thirds of clients with locally invasive cancers can avoid total laryngectomy when treated with combination radiation and chemotherapy. Survival rates are equal to those achieved with total laryngectomy (Way & Doherty, 2003).

Radiation therapy also may be used in conjunction with surgery to destroy any remaining cancerous cells, or as a palliative treatment for advanced tumors. See Chapter 14 ∞ for more information about radiation therapy and its nursing implications.

CHEMOTHERAPY Chemotherapy is used in combination with radiation therapy as the primary treatment for some laryngeal cancers. It also is used to treat distant metastasis and for palliation when the tumor is unresectable. The most commonly used chemotherapy drugs to treat laryngeal cancer are cisplatin (Platinol) and 5-fluorouracil (5-FU). Other drugs that may be used include methotrexate (Mexate), bleomycin sulfate (Blenoxane), and carboplatin (Paraplatin). A multiple-drug treatment regimen may be employed to maximize therapeutic effects. See Chapter 14 ∞ for the nursing implications for chemotherapy.

Surgery

The type of surgery used to treat laryngeal cancer is based on site, size, and invasiveness of the tumor into the larynx and surrounding tissues. The goals of surgery are to remove the malignancy, maintain airway patency, and achieve optimal cosmetic appearance.

Carcinoma *in situ,* vocal cord polyps, and early vocal cord cancers may be removed by laser during a laryngoscopy procedure. The cure rate for early tumors using this method is excellent. This surgery may be performed on an outpatient basis. The degree of trauma to the vocal cords varies, depending on the size of the lesion. The voice is preserved, but total voice rest with whispering only may be ordered for a week or more following surgery. In some cases, a temporary tracheostomy may

---

TABLE 37–1 Staging of Laryngeal Tumors

Stage 0	■ Carcinoma *in situ* ■ No lymph node involvement or metastasis
Stage I	■ Tumor confined to site of origin with normal vocal cord mobility ■ No lymph node involvement or metastasis
Stage II	■ Tumor involves adjacent tissues ■ No lymph node involvement or metastasis
Stage III	■ Tumor confined to larynx with fixation of vocal cords; immediately surrounding supraglottic tissues may be involved ■ No lymph node involvement or a single positive node on the side of the tumor ■ No metastasis
Stage IV	■ Massive tumor that extends beyond boundaries of larynx to involve surrounding tissues ■ Single or multiple lymph nodes may be involved ■ Distant metastasis may be present

be done at the time of surgery to ensure that swelling does not interfere with airway patency. Once the tracheostomy tube is removed and the opening is closed, the client can eat, speak, and breathe normally.

Laryngectomy, removal of the larynx, may be necessary. A *partial laryngectomy* (hemilaryngectomy, vertical partial laryngectomy) may be used for tumors localized to a portion of the larynx with limited extension beyond the larynx. In a partial laryngectomy, 50% or more of the larynx is removed. The voice generally is well preserved, although it may be changed by the surgery. A tracheostomy tube may be inserted for early postoperative airway management. It is usually removed in 5 to 7 days as postoperative swelling subsides, and the stoma is allowed to close. Normal speaking, breathing, and swallowing are restored. If the epiglottis has been removed, careful monitoring for aspiration is necessary. Enteral tube feedings or parenteral nutrition may be required for several weeks after surgery. Swallowing techniques to prevent aspiration are taught.

A *total laryngectomy* is required for cancers that extend beyond the vocal cords. The entire larynx is removed, along with the epiglottis, thyroid cartilage, several tracheal rings, and the hyoid bone. Because the trachea and the esophagus are permanently separated by this surgery (Figure 37–8 ■), there is no risk of aspiration during swallowing. Normal speech is lost, and a permanent tracheostomy is created. The tracheostomy tube inserted during surgery may be left in place for several weeks and then removed, leaving a natural stoma, or it may be left in place permanently. See page 1256 for nursing care of the client undergoing a total laryngectomy. Procedure 37–1 on page 1257 outlines tracheostomy care.

If cervical lymph nodes are involved but there is no evidence of distal metastasis, *radical* or *modified neck dissection* may be performed along with total laryngectomy. In a radical neck dissection, all soft tissue from the lower edge of the mandible down to the clavicle is removed, including cervical lymph nodes, the sternocleidomastoid muscle, internal jugular vein, cranial nerve XI (spinal accessory), and submaxillary salivary gland. Extensive tissue dissection can result in significant deformity. Skin grafts or flaps may be used to close the wound. Hemovac drains are placed in the wound to prevent hematoma and extensive edema formation. After surgery, the client may have difficulty lifting and turning the head because of muscle loss. Resection of the spinal accessory nerve causes shoulder drop on the affected side. In a modified neck dissection, neck contents are removed, with the exception of the sternocleidomastoid muscle, internal jugular vein, and spinal accessory nerve.

A gastrostomy also may be performed to maintain nutrition in the client with laryngeal or hypopharyngeal cancer. See Chapter 23 ∞ for more information about caring for the client with a gastrostomy tube.

Speech Rehabilitation

Various techniques may be used to restore speech after total laryngectomy. *Tracheoesophageal puncture (TEP)* is the usual method used to restore speech. A small fistula is created between the posterior tracheal wall and the anterior esophagus. A small, one-way shunt valve is fitted into the fistula (Figure 37–9 ■). Occluding the tracheostomy stoma with a

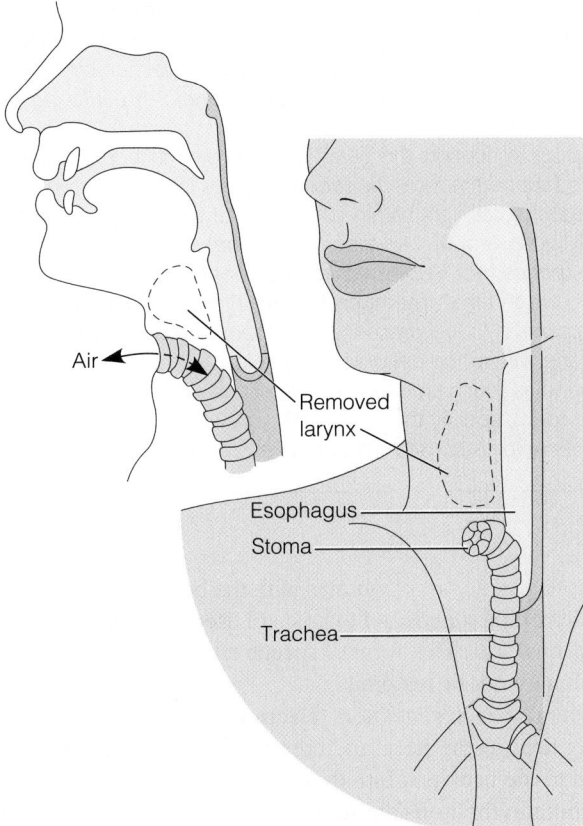

Figure 37–8 ■ Following a total laryngectomy, the client has a permanent tracheostomy. No connection between the trachea and esophagus remains.

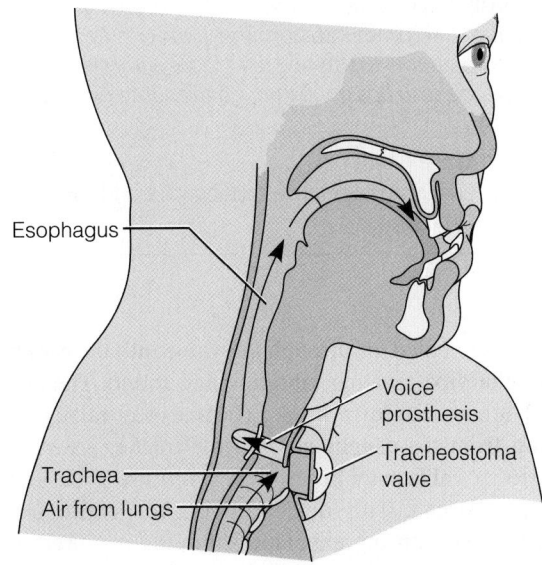

Figure 37–9 ■ The tracheoesophageal prosthesis allows diversion of air from the trachea through a one-way valve into the esophagus and oropharynx, producing speech when the tracheostomy stoma is occluded. The one-way valve prevents food from entering the trachea.

NURSING CARE OF THE CLIENT HAVING A Total Laryngectomy

PREOPERATIVE CARE

- Provide routine preoperative care and teaching as explained in Chapter 4 ∞.
- Assess knowledge and understanding of the diagnosis and proposed surgery. Clarify information and reinforce previous teaching as needed. *A clear understanding by the client and family of the purpose, anticipated benefits, and consequences of total laryngectomy prior to surgery is vital to promote postoperative recovery.*
- Assess anxiety levels of the client and family related to the diagnosis and proposed surgery. *High levels of anxiety interfere with learning and the ability to cooperate in care. Interventions to reduce anxiety may be required prior to teaching and providing preoperative instructions.*
- Without increasing fear, emphasize that total laryngectomy results in a loss of speech and that the client will breathe through a permanent stoma in the neck. *Although clients and family members may verbalize an understanding of the loss of speech following surgery, they may believe that verbal communication will still be possible through the stoma.*
- Establish a means of communicating postoperatively, using a magic slate, alphabet board, eye or hand signals, or other strategies. *Learning techniques for communicating preoperatively decreases the client's and family's postoperative anxiety. Long-term speech rehabilitation measures, such as the tracheoesophageal puncture, are not appropriate for use in the immediate postoperative period.*
- Point out that surgery will affect the senses of taste and smell and hence eating in the initial postoperative period. Reassure that nutritional and fluid needs will be met with intravenous or enteral feedings until eating can be resumed. *The client may not be prepared for the effect of surgery on taste and smell and, therefore, the enjoyment of food.*
- If possible and desired by the client and family, arrange a visit by a postlaryngectomy client who effectively uses an alternate form of verbal communication. *The client and family may feel more comfortable expressing their fears and asking questions of someone who has gone through the same experience they are facing.*

POSTOPERATIVE CARE

- Provide routine postoperative nursing care and monitoring as explained in Chapter 4 ∞.

- Frequently monitor airway patency and respiratory status, including respiratory rate and pattern; lung sounds; oxygen saturation. *Excessive or retained respiratory secretions can impair gas exchange, increase the work of breathing, and lead to complications such as pneumonia.*
- Encourage deep breathing and coughing. *Deep breathing helps ensure adequate ventilation of lower airways; coughing helps to move secretions out of airways.*
- Elevate the head of the bed. *The upright position promotes effective ventilation of the lungs, and reduces edema and swelling of the neck.*
- Maintain humidification of inspired gases. *With a tracheostomy, humidification of inspired air in the upper airways is lost. Humidified air helps maintain moist mucous membranes and secretions, promoting secretion removal by coughing or suctioning.*
- Maintain an adequate fluid intake (intravenously, enterally, and orally when allowed). *Adequate hydration keeps secretions liquid and mucous membranes moist.*
- Suction via tracheostomy using sterile technique as needed. *Surgery, impaired nutrition, and the effects of radiation therapy may cause fatigue and a weak cough effort. Suctioning may be necessary to clear secretions and maintain airway patency.*
- Provide tracheostomy care as needed. See Procedure 37–1. *Periodic cleaning of the tracheostomy tube is necessary to remove accumulated secretions and maintain airway patency.*
- Teach to protect the stoma from particulate matter in the air with a gauze square or other stoma protector. *Permanent tracheostomy results in loss of the protective mechanisms of the upper airway that prevent foreign material from entering the lungs.*
- Instruct to support the head when moving in bed. *Additional head support reduces the strain on tissues in the operative area.*
- Place the call light within easy reach at all times; answer the call light promptly. *The client who is unable to speak needs reassurance that help is within reach at all times.*
- Encourage family members to remain present when possible. *Supportive family presence helps reassure the client that he or she will not be left alone or helpless.*
- Spend as much time as possible with the client. When leaving the room, specify the time when you will return. *These measures help establish trust and relieve anxiety.*

---

finger forces exhaled air through the valve into the esophagus and hypopharynx, creating vibration and sound. The muscles of speech are used to form words. The one-way valve prevents aspiration from the esophagus into the trachea. An external tracheostoma valve may be used to avoid using the hand to occlude the stoma. This device covers the entire tracheal stoma and closes during exhalation, forcing air directly into the voice prosthesis. Not all postlaryngectomy clients are candidates for this device, because its use requires motivation and manual dexterity.

Esophageal speech uses swallowed air to create sound and form words as it is expelled in a controlled belch. The pharyn-

goesophageal segment vibrates with the belch, creating sound. Muscles of the mouth and tongue are used to control the sound and form words. This form of speech takes practice, and fluent speech may not be restored.

Several speech generators (electrolarynx) are available. One type is held to the neck and creates vibrations that are transmitted to the neck and into the mouth (Figure 37–10A ■). The transmitted vibrations are formed into words using the normal muscles of speech. Another device delivers a tone into the mouth via a plastic tube inserted into the corner of the mouth (Figure 37–10B ■). The lips, tongue, and mouth muscles are used to form the sound into words.

PROCEDURE 37-1 PROVIDING TRACHEOSTOMY CARE

GATHER SUPPLIES

- Tracheostomy cleaning kit
- Sterile suction catheter and glove kit
- Sterile disposable replacement inner cannula, if appropriate
- Cleaning solutions (e.g., hydrogen peroxide and sterile normal saline)

- Sterile 4 × 4 gauze dressings (not cotton-filled) or precut dressing
- Sterile cotton-tipped applicators
- Single-use tracheostomy tube holder or cotton twill ties
- Scissors
- Clean exam gloves

BEFORE THE PROCEDURE

Provide for privacy. Explain the procedure. Provide for a means of communication (e.g., eye blinking or raising a finger to indicate distress). If the client's condition permits, provide a pencil and paper or magic slate for questions. Place in semi-Fowler's or Fowler's position to facilitate lung ventilation. Assess lung sounds; suction the tracheostomy using sterile technique as needed.

DURING THE PROCEDURE

- Use standard precautions.
- Wearing a clean disposable glove, remove the tracheostomy dressing. Dispose of the glove and dressing.
- Open sterile supplies, pouring hydrogen peroxide and normal saline into separate containers. Don sterile gloves.
- Using sterile applicators or gauze dressings moistened with normal saline, clean around the incision, using each applicator or gauze dressing only once. Hydrogen peroxide may be used to remove crusted secretions; thoroughly rinse the area with gauze moistened with normal saline afterward to prevent skin irritation from hydrogen peroxide.
- If the tracheostomy tube has an inner cannula that can be removed for disposal or cleaning, remove the tube and set it aside for disposal or place it in the hydrogen peroxide. Cleanse the flange of the outer cannula in the same manner as the incision.
- Clean reusable inner cannulas using a small brush, pipe cleaners (provided in the tracheostomy care kit), or cotton-tipped applicators.
- Rinse the inner cannula thoroughly in normal saline. Tap it gently against the inner aspect of the sterile bowl to remove excess liquid.
- Suction the outer cannula using sterile technique.
- Replace the inner cannula (using a new disposable cannula or the cleaned cannula) into the tracheostomy tube.
- Replace the dressing, using either a commercially prepared tracheostomy dressing or an opened gauze 4 × 4 refolded into a V shape (see the accompanying figure). Do not cut the dressing or use a cotton-filled dressing to prevent aspiration of foreign material into the respiratory tract.
- Apply a clean tracheostomy holder or clean ties using either the one- or two-strip method.
  One-Strip Method
  a. Cut a length of twill tape 2.5 times the length needed to go around the client's neck from one tube flange to the other.
  b. Thread one end of the tape through one flange of the tracheostomy tube. Bring the other end around the back of the client's neck, then thread it through the other flange and back around the back of the neck to meet the first end. Tie the loose ends securely using a square knot and allowing one or two fingers' breadth of slack between the tie and the client's neck.

Two-Strip Method
  a. Cut a length of twill tape about 1.5 times the distance from flange to flange under the client's neck. Divide this into two unequal pieces (approximately one-third and two-thirds).
  b. Make a small slit approximately 2 to 3 cm from one end of each piece. Thread the end of the tape with the slit through the flange, then thread the other end of the tape through the slit to secure it. Repeat with the other portion of tape.
  c. Position the longer tape behind the client's neck and tie the free ends of tape securely, using a square knot and allowing a small amount of slack as before.
- Once the clean ties are secured, remove the old ties.
- Pad the knot to reduce skin irritation.

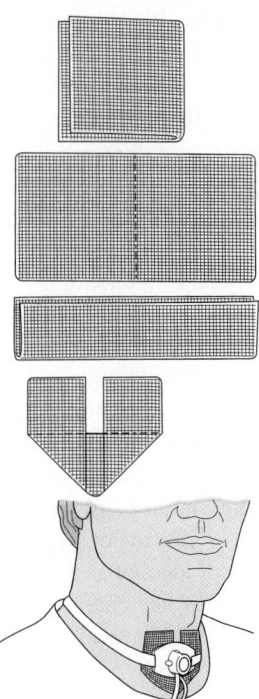

Steps for folding a gauze 4 × 4 into a tracheostomy dressing.

AFTER THE PROCEDURE

Assess breathing and tolerance of the procedure. Dispose of supplies and used solutions. Wash hands. Chart the procedure and any observations made during the procedure such as amount, color, and consistency of sputum and appearance of the incision.

A

Speech generator

Control button

B

Figure 37–10 ■ Speech generators. *A*, The client holds the vibrating tip of the speech generator against the throat, using the mouth to form words. *B*, A plastic handpiece of the generator is held in the corner of the mouth. The audible tone produced by the generator is formed into words.

NURSING CARE

Nurses can be instrumental in early identification and treatment of laryngeal disorders by emphasizing the need for clients with new chronic hoarseness to seek treatment.

Health Promotion

Health promotion activities to prevent laryngeal cancer focus on preventing smoking among children, adolescents, and young adults, and promoting smoking cessation in people who do smoke. Activities to promote abstinence or moderate alcohol use also are beneficial in reducing a significant risk factor for laryngeal cancer.

Assessment

Nurses can be instrumental in identifying early signs of laryngeal cancer, facilitating early diagnosis and treatment.
- *Health history:* Current symptoms, including voice change, difficulty swallowing, throat pain; risk factors such as voice abuse, family history of cancer, occupational exposures; smoking history, use of alcohol and amount.
- *Physical examination:* Voice character; general appearance and apparent state of health; swallowing ability; visible or palpable mass in neck.

Nursing Diagnoses and Interventions

Nursing care for the client with a benign tumor of the larynx focuses on maintaining a patent airway and teaching about the disorder and strategies to prevent its recurrence. The client with laryngeal cancer has multiple nursing care needs. The risk for impaired verbal communication is significant. Dysphagia may interfere with swallowing and nutrition. Nutrition also may be impaired by radiation, chemotherapy, and surgery. The diagnosis of cancer is frightening for most clients, no matter what the potential for cure is with treatment. See the Nursing Care Plan that follows for additional nursing diagnoses and interventions.

Risk for Impaired Airway Clearance

Following resection of a benign or malignant vocal cord nodule, local tissue edema may interfere with airway patency.

PRACTICE ALERT
During the immediate postoperative period, closely monitor for signs of airway obstruction, such as labored breathing or inspiratory stridor. The larynx is the narrowest portion of the upper airways. Tissue edema following surgery can further restrict the airway, interfering with lung ventilation and gas exchange.

- Apply cold packs to the neck as ordered or indicated. *Cold application constricts local blood vessels and reduces edema development.*
- Withhold food and fluids until the cough and gag reflexes have returned. *Local anesthesia used during removal of benign tumors and nodules impairs the cough and gag reflexes, increasing the risk for aspiration.*

Impaired Verbal Communication

Treatment of laryngeal cancer often alters the quality of the voice, results in short-term restriction of speaking, or, in the case of total laryngectomy, causes loss of the voice. The client ultimately determines treatment choices for laryngeal cancer; some choose to forgo laryngectomy to avoid voice loss when the chance for long-term success and cancer cure is minimal.

NURSING CARE PLAN   A Client with Total Laryngectomy

David Tom is a 61-year-old accountant who is divorced and has two adult children. He has smoked two packs of cigarettes daily since high school, and usually has three or four cocktails each evening. After several months of persistent sore throat and hoarseness, Mr. Tom was diagnosed with cancer of the larynx. He has been admitted to the surgical care unit from the ICU 2 days post total laryngectomy.

ASSESSMENT

Mr. Tom's vital signs are stable: BP 146/84, P 92 and regular, R 18, T 98°F (36.7°C) axillary. A tracheostomy tube is sutured in place, and he is receiving humidified oxygen at 28% per tracheostomy collar. Pulse oximetry is 94%. He is receiving continuous tube feeding per nasogastric feeding tube. Two Hemovac wound drains are present in the right neck area. A moderate amount of edema is noted in the right facial and submandibular area. Mr. Tom is ambulatory within the room.

DIAGNOSES

- *Risk for Ineffective Airway Clearance* related to postoperative edema
- *Risk for Ineffective Breathing Pattern* related to pain and anxiety
- *Disturbed Body Image* related to total laryngectomy and presence of tracheostomy stoma
- *Impaired Verbal Communication* related to total laryngectomy
- *Pain* related to surgical procedure
- *Risk for Imbalanced Nutrition: Less than Body Requirements* related to difficulty eating after surgery

EXPECTED OUTCOMES

- Maintain clear airways and lung sounds.
- Maintain oxygen saturation level greater than 92%.
- Demonstrate interest in providing incision and stoma care.
- Accept information about potential communication strategies.

- Communicate effective pain management.
- Maintain appropriate body weight, intake, and output.

PLANNING AND IMPLEMENTATION

- Assess respiratory status including rate, pattern, lung sounds, and cough effectiveness at least every 4 hours.
- Monitor quantity, color, and odor of secretions.
- Assess vital signs and pain at least every 4 hours. Administer analgesics as ordered.
- Schedule time to sit with Mr. Tom and discuss his concerns and feelings at least three times per day.
- Provide written information as requested.
- Monitor intake, output, and daily weight.
- Arrange dietary consultation to determine caloric requirements.

EVALUATION

Mr. Tom reports in writing that his pain is adequately controlled. His respiratory status is stable with clear breath sounds throughout and an oxygen saturation of 94%. He is afebrile. Mr. Tom is tolerating tube feedings well and expresses a desire to begin eating. The dietitian has visited and assisted in planning to begin oral feedings. Intake and output are stable, as is his weight. Mr. Tom has been receptive to receiving information about follow-up care and exploration of various modalities of speech.

CRITICAL THINKING IN THE NURSING PROCESS

1. Compare and contrast advantages and disadvantages of various methods to allow speech following total laryngectomy.
2. Develop a plan of care for Mr. Tom for the nursing diagnosis *Disturbed Body Image.*
3. Discuss nursing interventions to provide wound care for the client with laryngectomy and radical neck dissection.
4. List strategies to optimize ventilation.
   See Evaluating Your Response in Appendix C.

- Prior to surgery, assess for additional obstacles to communication. *Communication may be impaired by hearing loss, illiteracy, or weakness associated with the disease process, altering the ability to use alternative communication strategies.*
- Assess the importance of verbal communication to self-concept, occupation, and lifestyle. *Many factors influence adaptation to the loss of normal verbal communication. If the ability to speak is central to an occupation (e.g., elementary school teacher, singer) or self-concept (e.g., a politician or attorney), adapting to a total laryngectomy may be difficult. For these clients, laryngectomy may mean a loss of employment or career.*

PRACTICE ALERT

Prior to surgery, introduce nonverbal communication strategies such as pencil and paper, magic slate, or an alphabet board. Encourage the client to practice using each method and to choose the most acceptable one. Having the client determine a means of communication prior to surgery helps to alleviate anxiety and increases the sense of control.

- Arrange consultation with a speech therapist about alternate forms of oral communication prior to surgery if possible. *Determining a means of communicating on a continuing basis prior to surgery helps to relieve fear of inability to communicate and may guide the choice of a surgical procedure.*

PRACTICE ALERT

After surgery, assess frequently. Place the call bell at hand. The presence of a caring nurse helps to decrease anxiety and promotes communication. Knowing that help is readily available enhances feelings of security and decreases anxiety.

- Reinforce teaching about alternative communication strategies. *Anxiety or information overload may impair the ability to retain information; reinforcement facilitates learning.*
- Maintain a positive attitude about postoperative communication, but do not promote unrealistic expectations. *Not all clients are able to use all alternative methods of verbal communication after the laryngectomy. Some clients remain nonverbal.*

- If desired, arrange a visit by a rehabilitated laryngectomy client who has mastered an alternative form of verbal communication and has a positive attitude about rehabilitation. *Many clients and their families find that they are better able to communicate their fears with someone who has gone through the same experience they are facing.*

See the accompanying nursing research box for more information about assistive devices for use in the early postoperative period.

Impaired Swallowing

Disruption of laryngeal structures by the tumor itself or due to radiation or surgery can impair the swallowing mechanism. Additionally, even when a total laryngectomy has been performed and a connection between the oropharynx and trachea no longer exists, swallowing may cause fear of choking.

- Maintain intravenous fluids and enteral feedings or parenteral nutrition until adequate food and fluids can be ingested orally. *It is important to maintain nutritional and fluid balance until normal eating can be resumed.*
- Postoperatively, initiate oral intake with soft foods, not liquids. *Soft foods are easier to handle and swallow initially. As recovery progresses, thickened liquids can be swallowed and, eventually, a normal diet can be resumed.*
- Following total laryngectomy, reassure that choking is not possible, because there is no connection between the esophagus and trachea. *Clients often fear that swallowing will result in choking and they will be unable to cough effectively.*
- Instruct to initiate a swallow by placing a small amount of food on the back of the tongue, flex the head forward, and then think "swallow." *Swallowing is no longer an automatic function and needs to be relearned.*

PRACTICE ALERT

Provide for privacy during initial attempts at eating. Eating in the presence of others may cause embarrassment until confidence in eating is regained. Privacy also reduces distractions, allowing concentration on swallowing.

Imbalanced Nutrition: Less than Body Requirements

Large laryngeal tumors often place pressure on the esophagus and may cause dysphagia (difficulty swallowing) or odynophagia (painful swallowing). In either case, difficulty eating may ultimately impair nutrition. Additionally, cancer often produces a hypermetabolic state, increasing calorie requirements. If surgery is performed, difficulty swallowing and a fear of aspiration in the early postoperative period also interfere with eating. Enteral or parenteral feedings are usually needed initially to meet nutritional status. After a total laryngectomy, the senses of taste and smell are disrupted. Although the sense of taste may be partially recovered, clients may complain that eating no longer is pleasurable.

- Assess nutritional status using height and weight charts, reported weight loss, and anthropometric measurements such as skin folds. *Thorough assessment of nutritional status is important in planning to meet current and anticipated calorie needs.*

PRACTICE ALERT

Monitor food and fluid intake and urinary output. Pain or fatigue, rather than a sensation of fullness, may prompt the decision to stop eating, resulting in inadequate intake.

- Evaluate current and preferred eating habits and foods, as well as understanding of nutrition. *This evaluation provides additional information about nutrition as well as a basis for future planning.*

NURSING RESEARCH   Evidence-Based Practice: The Client Undergoing Laryngectomy

Communication methods and content among clients who had undergone surgery for head or neck cancer were evaluated in this pilot study of the use of electronic speech-generating devices (SGDs) (Happ et al., 2005). The researchers also looked at the quality (ease and client satisfaction) of communications among study participants, as well as barriers to SGD use and the effect of client factors such as age and illness severity on communications. All study participants were alert and able to write legibly; the majority had at least some experience using a computer.

Although 60% of study participants were found to be able to use SGDs with minimal assistance and instruction, the devices were used in only 17% of observed communications; writing and nonverbal communications were used the majority of the time. Barriers to use of the devices included placement of the device out of the client's reach, mechanical malfunctions, and impatience of caregivers with the time required for typed communications. Clients expressed frustration with the lack of a standard keyboard and with the impersonality of the computerized voice. Overall, the devices were found to be useful as one of several methods of communication used by the client.

IMPLICATIONS FOR NURSING

Speech-generating devices can facilitate communication for selected clients, particularly when the content of the message is complex. Training of clients, caregivers, and family members is necessary for effective use of these devices, however. Preoperatively, clients scheduled for laryngectomy should be instructed in communication methods to use after surgery, including use of gestures, written messages (including predeveloped messages, such as "I am in pain"), and use of any assistive communication devices.

CRITICAL THINKING IN CLIENT CARE

1. In this study, SGDs often were found out of the client's reach. What planning should the nurse do to help ensure that assistive communication devices are accessible to the client?
2. Clients in this study were literate and many had at least some experience using computers. Do you think results of the study would differ if the study population had less education, was illiterate, or had minimal English language proficiency? Why or why not?
3. Develop a teaching plan for a preoperative laryngectomy client using the nursing diagnosis *Deficient Knowledge: Postoperative Communication Strategies.*

- Refer to a dietitian for further evaluation, planning, and education. *A professional can identify nutritional needs and help plan a diet that will meet them.*
- Encourage experimentation with foods of different textures and temperatures. *Very cold foods or foods of a soft texture may be easier to swallow.*
- Encourage frequent, small meals rather than three large meals per day. *Frequent, small quantities of food improve overall intake when dysphagia, odynophagia, or fatigue interfere with nutrition.*
- Recommend liquid supplements such as Ensure when calorie needs are not being met. Provide information about where to obtain nutritional supplements. *Liquid dietary supplements provide balanced nutrition as well as additional calories and are an effective way of increasing intake. They are available without prescription in major supermarkets.*
- Provide mouth care before meals and supplemental feedings. Provide a topical anesthetic such as viscous lidocaine before eating for stomatitis or esophagitis related to radiation or chemotherapy. *The tumor or its treatment may cause bad breath or a foul taste in the mouth, which suppresses appetite. Inflamed mucosa may make eating uncomfortable. A topical anesthetic may relieve this discomfort and thus promote food intake.*
- Provide an antiemetic 30 minutes before eating as needed to relieve nausea. *Nausea interferes with food intake. An antiemetic can relieve nausea and make eating possible.*
- Suggest enteral (tube) feedings via nasogastric or gastrostomy tube if the client is unable to consume enough food to maintain weight and nutritional status. *Both cancer and surgery increase calorie needs. Supplemental enteral feedings may be necessary to prevent catabolism and to promote healing and recovery.*

- Instruct to perform mouth rinses before initiating feeding postoperatively. *Rinsing helps clean the mouth and also provides practice in using tongue and cheek muscles to control fluid in the mouth.*
- Refer to a physical or speech therapist for swallowing rehabilitation following laryngectomy. *Because surgery changes the relationship of the trachea, esophagus, and oropharynx, swallowing needs to be relearned before eating.*
- Reinforce swallowing instructions. *Reinforcement promotes learning.*

Anticipatory Grieving

The client with laryngeal cancer faces not only the diagnosis of cancer, which is often perceived as a death sentence, but also the prospect of mutilating surgery. If laryngectomy is necessary, the client grieves the loss of both a body part and an important function, speech, a vital aspect of social interaction and often necessary for one's career. It also enables people to express their needs when they cannot meet them alone. The loss of speech, therefore, is a major loss. In addition, the tracheal stoma changes the manner in which the client breathes. If radical neck dissection is required, loss of neck musculature and function also alters body image and self-concept.

- Provide opportunities for expressing feelings of grief, anger, or fear about the diagnosis of cancer, the impending surgery, and the anticipated loss of speech. *The client with laryngeal cancer needs the opportunity (and may need permission) to grieve anticipated losses. A cancer diagnosis may precipitate grieving for unfulfilled plans and expectations, even though a cure may be anticipated. Laryngectomy causes a major change in body image, with loss of a vital body part and creation of a stoma. The client also grieves the loss of speech. This loss can have a significant impact on occupation and social interaction.*

- Help the client and family discuss the potential impact of the loss on family structure and function. *Discussion helps family members understand each other's feelings and support one another.*
- Refer for psychologic or spiritual counseling as appropriate. *Counseling and spiritual guidance can help the client and family deal with the diagnosis and proposed treatment, and help prevent a sense of defeat and hopelessness.*
- Help identify additional resources, such as coping strategies that have been successfully used in the past to deal with crises. *This exercise helps the client and family identify strengths they can use to deal with the present situation.*

Using NANDA, NIC, and NOC

Chart 37–3 shows links between NANDA nursing diagnoses, NIC, and NOC for the client with laryngeal cancer.

Community-Based Care

Teaching for the client with a benign laryngeal tumor emphasizes management of contributing factors. Stress the importance of not yelling or screaming. Refer clients, particularly singers, to a speech therapist for voice training. Emphasize the need to keep the voice within its normal range to reduce vocal cord stress. Encourage smoking cessation, particularly if the client is also a singer. Discuss the relationship of industrial pollutants to laryngeal tumors and help explore ways of reducing pollutant exposure.

Teaching the client and family about laryngeal cancer, treatment options, and home care related to those treatments is an important nursing responsibility. Include the following topics when teaching:

- Clarification of treatment options, including risks and benefits.
- Importance of early intervention to reduce the risk of local spread and metastasis.

NANDA, NIC, AND NOC LINKAGES
CHART 37–3 The Client with Laryngeal Cancer

NANDA

Impaired Verbal Communication

↓

NIC

Communication Enhancement: Speech Deficit

Anxiety Reduction

Aspiration Precautions

Support System Enhancement

↓

NOC

Communication Ability

Communication: Expressive Ability

Coping

Aspiration Control

Data from *NANDA's Nursing Diagnoses: Definitions & Classification 2005–2006* by NANDA International (2005), Philadelphia; *Nursing Interventions Classification (NIC)* (4th ed.) by J. M. Dochterman & G. M. Bulechek (2004), St. Louis, MO: Mosby; and *Nursing Outcomes Classification (NOC)* (3rd ed.) by S. Moorhead, M. Johnson, and M. Maas (2004), St. Louis, MO: Mosby.

- If a total laryngectomy is proposed, options for communication after surgery, including the pros and cons of each:
  a. The tracheoesophageal puncture device requires some manual dexterity to manipulate.
  b. Only about 30% of clients are able to master esophageal speech.

  c. A trial of the speech generator prior to surgery may reduce frustration in learning to use it postoperatively.
- Care related to radiation therapy, including skin and mouth care, management of secretions (see Chapter 14 for more information about radiation therapy and its effects).
- Strategies and resources for smoking cessation and alcohol abstinence.
- Ways to achieve and maintain optimal nutrition.
- Tracheostomy stoma care and preventing respiratory infection. Provide opportunities to practice and redemonstrate techniques. Clean technique (rather than sterile) is used; the tracheostomy tube may not be needed once the stoma is fully healed. Discuss these additional measures:
  a. Using a humidifier or vaporizer to add humidity to inspired air.
  b. Increasing fluid intake to maintain mucosal moisture and loosen secretions.
  c. Shielding the stoma with a stoma guard, such as a gauze square on a tie around the neck, to prevent particulate matter from entering the lower respiratory tract.
  d. Promptly removing secretions from skin surrounding the stoma to prevent irritation and skin breakdown.
  e. Water sports are contraindicated with a permanent tracheostomy; there is no restriction on other activities although lifting may be more difficult because of inability to hold the breath (the Valsalva maneuver).
  f. Showering and bathing (without submerging the neck or head) are allowed; protect the stoma with a cupped hand or washcloth.
- Manifestations of potential complications of laryngectomy to be reported to the physician, including loss of hearing or facial expression due to auditory or facial nerve injury, or shoulder drop due to damage to the spinal accessory nerve.

The client and family need emotional and motivational support through this trying time. Refer to local support groups such as a laryngectomy club or lost cord club. If the client and family are having difficulty adjusting to the diagnosis of cancer and the effects of treatment, provide referral to counseling.

EXPLORE MediaLink

Prentice Hall Nursing MediaLink DVD-ROM

   Audio Glossary
   NCLEX-RN® Review

COMPANION WEBSITE www.prenhall.com/lemone

   Audio Glossary
   NCLEX-RN® Review
   Care Plan Activity: Epistaxis
   Case Study: Sleep Apnea
   MediaLink Applications
     Laryngectomy
     Pulse Oximetry
   Links to Resources

CHAPTER HIGHLIGHTS

- Upper respiratory infections (the common cold) are caused by a multitude of different viruses. Most are mild, self-limiting infections, appropriate for self-care; some viruses, however, such as RSV can cause serious lower respiratory illness in the very young or very old.

- Three different strains of influenza virus are identified; type A causes most outbreaks of influenza. Because this disease increases the risk of pneumonia in older adults, people with chronic diseases, and people who are immunocompromised, annual immunization is important for these populations and their caregivers.

- Influenza is differentiated from URI primarily by the presence of systemic manifestations, the duration and degree of fever, and the presence of persistent cough.

- Pharyngitis (sore throat) may be either viral or bacterial in origin; manifestations are similar. Clients with persistent or severe symptoms that include fever, enlarged lymph nodes, and myalgias should be evaluated to rule out streptococcal pharyngitis, which can have significant complications such as rheumatic fever or post-streptococcal glomerulonephritis.

- The incidence of pertussis, a highly contagious reportable disease, is increasing due to waning immunity and improved identification of the infection among adults. In adults, it is often recognized by prolonged and persistent coughing spells. Pertussis is treated in community settings with antibiotic therapy (usually erythromycin or TMP-SMZ).

- Epistaxis (nosebleed) and nasal fracture are relatively common, and pose a risk only when airway clearance is impaired. Emergency care for epistaxis includes pinching the nares or bridge of the nose, sitting upright and leaning forward, and applying ice to the nose. When nasal packing is required to control bleeding, close monitoring of respiratory status (respiratory rate and effort, oxygen saturation) is critical.

- Persistent voice hoarseness is the primary manifestation of laryngeal cancer. When identified and treated early, the rate of cure for laryngeal cancer is high. Some laryngeal tumors, however, have few manifestations until advanced. They may be treated by radiation therapy, chemotherapy, or surgery (laryngectomy and neck dissection).

- Following total laryngectomy, a permanent tracheostomy is created and the upper trachea and esophagus are separated, preventing aspiration when feedings are resumed. A tracheoesophageal puncture may be created to allow verbal communication following total laryngectomy.

TEST YOURSELF NCLEX-RN® REVIEW

1 A client with hypertension asks the nurse what he can do to relieve the symptoms of an acute URI. The nurse recommends that he
  1. ask his physician for an antibiotic prescription.
  2. use an over-the-counter decongestant such as pseudoephedrine to relieve symptoms.
  3. take 1000 mg of vitamin C and use zinc lozenges on a regular basis.
  4. use an over-the-counter nasal spray for no more than 3 days to relieve congestion.

2 Which of the following health promotion activities planned by a nurse working with a group of community-dwelling senior citizens would be most likely to prevent influenza and pneumonia?
  1. indoor exercise programs during winter months
  2. influenza vaccine clinics at the senior center
  3. teaching effective hand washing
  4. advising seniors to avoid crowds

3 In teaching a client with bacterial sinusitis about home care, the nurse stresses the importance of
  1. completing the antibiotic prescription as ordered.
  2. sleeping with the head of the bed elevated to 45 degrees.
  3. using a humidifier to promote sinus drainage.
  4. maintaining a liberal fluid intake to help liquefy secretions.

4 Which of the following nursing interventions for the client with posterior nasal packing is of highest priority?
  1. Elevate the head of the bed.
  2. Apply cold compresses to the nose.
  3. Maintain oxygen therapy.
  4. Provide frequent oral hygiene.

5 A client in the emergency department following facial trauma complains that his nose "just keeps dripping." The drainage appears like watery blood. The most appropriate nursing action would be to:
  1. provide a box of tissues.
  2. reassure the client that this is expected with a nasal fracture.
  3. suction the nasopharynx.
  4. obtain a specimen for glucose testing.

6 Expected findings in a client with obstructive sleep apnea would include: (Select all that apply.)
  1. confusion and signs of dementia.
  2. enlarged tongue.
  3. complaints of daytime sleepiness.
  4. decreased oxygen saturation levels while awake.
  5. elevated blood pressure.
  6. complaints of morning headache.

7 The nurse in a physician's office notes that a regular client's voice is hoarse, a change from previous visits. The most appropriate question to ask the client would be:
  1. "How long has your voice been hoarse?"
  2. "Do you smoke?"
  3. "Do you have a sore throat?"
  4. "Would you like a prescription for throat lozenges?"

8 The nurse evaluates his teaching as effective when a client with stage I laryngeal cancer states:
  1. "I'm glad I don't have to worry about treating this cancer now because it is so early."
  2. "I hate to think about eventually losing the ability to speak, but I'd rather treat it aggressively than lose my life to cancer."
  3. "I'm glad this was diagnosed early, when it can be treated with radiation so I won't lose my voice."
  4. "Thank goodness this type of cancer usually doesn't spread anywhere else."

9 Place the following nursing interventions for the client who has undergone total laryngectomy and radical neck dissection in order of priority. 4 5 2 1 3
1. Arrange consultation with speech therapist.
2. Provide small, frequent meals.
3. Encourage to express feelings regarding loss of voice.
4. Suction via tracheostomy as needed.
5. Instruct to support head when moving.

10 When providing tracheostomy care, the nurse
1. cuts the dressing using sterile scissors.
2. secures clean ties before removing soiled ones.
3. uses clean technique to cleanse the outer cannula.
4. cleanses the incision with an iodine-based antiseptic.

See Test Yourself answers in Appendix C.

BIBLIOGRAPHY

Alper, B. S. (2005a). Evidence-based medicine. Antiviral resistance in influenza may be increasing. *Clinical Advisor for Nurse Practitioners, 8*(12), 125.

_____. (2005b). Evidence-based medicine. Ginseng may reduce incidence of upper respiratory infection in adults. *Clinical Advisor for Nurse Practitioners, 8*(12), 126, 128.

American Cancer Society. (2005a). *Cancer facts and figures 2005*. Atlanta: Author.

_____. (2005b). *Laryngeal and hypopharyngeal cancer*. Retrieved from http://www.cancer.org

Atkinson, W., Wolfe, C., Humiston, S., & Nelson, R. (Eds.). (2000). *Epidemiology and prevention of vaccine-preventable diseases* (6th ed.) Atlanta: Centers for Disease Control and Prevention.

Centers for Disease Control and Prevention. (2005a). *CDC guidelines and recommendations. Updated infection control measures for the prevention and control of influenza in health-care facilities.* Atlanta: Author.

_____. (2005b). *Recommended adult immunization schedule, by vaccine and age group. United States, October 2005–September 2006.* Atlanta: Author.

Chasens, E. R., Pack, A. I., Maislin, G., Dinges, D. F., & Weaver, T. E. (2005). Claustrophobia and adherence to CPAP treatment. *Western Journal of Nursing Research, 27*(3), 307–321.

Conn, V. (1991). Self-care actions taken by older adults for influenza and colds. *Nursing Research, 40*(3), 176–181.

Copstead, L. C., & Banasik, J. L. (2005). *Pathophysiology* (3rd ed.). St. Louis, MO: Elsevier/Saunders.

Dash, G. P., & 2004 APIC Immunization Practices Working Group Association for Professionals in Infection Control and Epidemiology. (2004). APIC position paper: Improving health care worker influenza immunization rates. *American Journal of Infection Control, 32*(3), 123–125.

Davey, M. J. (2003). Understanding obstructive sleep apnoea. *Nursing Times, 99*(22), 26–27.

deCastro, A. B. (2005). Health and safety. Preventing exposure to influenza: Steps health care workers can take. *American Journal of Nursing, 105*(1), 112.

Desbiens, N. A. (2005). A 5-year experience with influenza prevention and containment in a program of all-inclusive care for elderly adults. *American Journal of Infection Control, 33*(4), 238–242.

Deutzer, J. (2005). Potential complications of obstructive sleep apnea in patients undergoing gastric bypass surgery. *Critical Care Nursing Quarterly, 28*(3), 293–299.

Dochterman, J., & Bulechek, G. (2004). *Nursing interventions classification (NIC)* (4th ed.). St. Louis, MO: Mosby.

Dworkin, M. S. (2005, October 1). Pertussis and its comeback—in persons of all ages. *Patient Care for the Nurse Practitioner.*

Ecklund, M. M. (2005). Caring for the bariatric patient with obstructive sleep apnea. *Critical Care Nursing Clinics of North America, 16*(3), 311–317.

Edgtton-Winn, M., & Wright, K. (2005). Clinical update. Tracheostomy: A guide to nursing care. *Australian Nursing Journal, 13*(5), 17–20.

Fischbach, F. (2002). *Nurses' quick reference to common laboratory and diagnostic tests* (3rd ed.). Philadelphia: Lippincott.

Fontaine, K. L. (2005). *Healing practices: Alternative therapies for nursing* (2nd ed.). Upper Saddle River, NJ: Prentice Hall Health.

Food and Drug Administration. (2000). *Relenza consumer information.* Retrieved from http://www.fda.gov/cder/consumerinfo/druginfo/relenza.HTM

General information. (2006). Retrieved from http://www.pandemicflu.gov/general

Goldrick, B. A. (2004). Emerging infections. Influenza 2004–2005: What's new with the flu. *American Journal of Nursing, 104*(10), 34–36.

_____. (2005). Emerging infections. Pertussis on the rise: Clinicians should be aware of its signs and symptoms until vaccination recommendations are changed. *American Journal of Nursing, 105*(1), 69–71.

Gupta, N. E. (2005). How worried should you be about avian flu? *Clinical Advisor for Nurse Practitioners, 8*(12), 31–32, 34–35.

Happ, M. B., Roesch, T. K., & Kagan, S. H. (2005). Patient communication following head and neck cancer surgery: A pilot study using electronic speech-generative devices. *Oncology Nursing Forum, 32*(6), 1179–1187.

Holman, M. L. (2005). Obstructive sleep apnea syndrome: implications for primary care. *Nurse Practitioner, 30*(9), 38–45.

Jull, A. (2003). Review: Specific signs and symptoms can help practitioners to diagnose acute purulent sinusitis in general practice. *Evidence-Based Nursing, 6*(1), 24.

Kasper, D. L., Braunwald, E., Fauci, A. S., Hauser, S. L., Longo, D. L., & Jameson, J. L. (Eds.). (2005). *Harrison's principles of internal medicine* (16th ed.). New York: McGraw-Hill.

Larsson, M., Hedelin, B., Johansson, I., & Athlin, E. (2005). Eating problems and weight loss for patients with head and neck cancer: A chart review from diagnosis until one year after treatment. *Cancer Nursing, 28*(6), 425–435.

Lewis, T., & Oliver, G. (2005). Improving tracheostomy care for ward patients. *Nursing Standard, 19*(19), 33–37.

Malcolm, A. (2005). The nurse role in managing and treating sleep disorders. *Nursing Times, 101*(23), 34–37.

McCance, K. L., & Huether, S. E. (2006). *Pathophysiology: The biologic basis for disease in adults and children* (5th ed.). St. Louis, MO: Mosby.

McErlane, K., & Pence, C. (2004). Action stat. Epistaxis. *Nursing, 34*(8), 88.

Merritt, S. L., & Johnson, J. (2004). Beats & breath. Obstructive sleep apnea-hypopnea syndrome: Nurses may detect a problem often overlooked by other providers. *American Journal of Nursing, 104*(7), 49–52.

Moorhead, S., Johnson, M., & Maas, M. (2004). *Nursing outcomes classification (NOC)* (3rd ed.). St. Louis, MO: Mosby.

NANDA International. (2005). *Nursing diagnoses: Definitions and classification 2005–2006.* Philadelphia: Author.

National Center for Complementary and Alternative Medicine, National Institutes of Health. (2005). *Herbs at a glance. Echinacea.* Retrieved from http://nccam.nih.gov/health/echinacea/

National Institute of Allergy and Infectious Diseases, National Institutes of Health. (2006). Focus on the flu. Retrieved from http://www3.niaid.nih.gov/news/focuson/flu/research/primer/default.htm

National Institutes of Health (NIH). (2002). *Facts about dietary supplements. Zinc.* Clinical Nutrition Service, Warren Grant Magnuson Clinical Center, Office of Dietary Supplements.

Retrieved from http://ods.od.nih.gov/factsheets/cc/zinc.html

Nosing into flu season: Learn how to administer influenza vaccine intranasally in a few steps. (2004). *Nursing, 34*(9), 49.

Oliver, L. T. (2005). Improving tracheostomy care for ward patients. *Nursing Standard, 19*(19), 33–37.

Pierrynowski-Gallant, D. M. (2004). Influenza vaccination choices. *Canadian Nurse, 100*(2), 16–21.

Porth, C. M. (2005). *Pathophysiology: Concepts of altered health states* (7th ed.). Philadelphia: Lippincott.

Roman, M. (2005). Clinical "how to". Tracheostomy tubes. *MEDSURG Nursing, 14*(2), 143–145.

Rothrock, J. C. (2003). *Alexander's care of the patient in surgery* (12th ed.). St. Louis, MO: Mosby.

Rutledge, B. J. (2005). Avian flu: What to look for, who's at risk. *Healthcare Traveler, 13*(1), 24–31

Schweon, S., & Mangan, D. (2003). Don't underestimate group A strep. *RN, 66*(8), 28–33.

Sheff, B. (2006). Avian influenza: Poised to launch a pandemic? *Nursing, 36*(1), 51–53.

Spencer, J. W., & Jacobs, J. J. (2003). *Complementary and alternative medicine: An evidence-based approach* (2nd ed.). St. Louis, MO: Mosby.

St. John, R. E. (2004). Contemporary issues in adult tracheostomy management. *Critical Care Nursing Clinics of North America, 16*(3), 413–430.

Stafanski, A. M. (2005). Obstructive sleep apnea: A primary care approach. *American Journal for Nurse Practitioners, 9*(10), 21–24, 27–28.

Tierney, L. M., McPhee, S. J., & Papadakis, M. A. (2005). *Current medical diagnosis & treatment* (44th ed.). New York: Lange Medical Books/McGraw-Hill.

Trupp, R. J. (2004) The heart of sleep: Sleep-disordered breathing and heart failure. *Journal of Cardiovascular Nursing, 19*(6S), S67–S74.

Urden, L. D., Stacy, K. M., & Lough, M. E. (2002). *Thelan's critical care nursing: Diagnosis and management* (4th ed.). St. Louis, MO: Mosby.

The Voice Center. (2002). *Speech after a total laryngectomy.* Retrieved from http://www.voice-center.com/alaryngeal_speech.htm

Way, L. W., & Doherty, G. M. (2003). *Current surgical diagnosis and treatment* (11th ed.). New York: McGraw-Hill.

Wilkinson, J. M. (2005). *Nursing diagnosis handbook with NIC interventions and NOC outcomes* (8th ed.). Upper Saddle River, NJ: Prentice Hall Health.

Willard, R. M., & Dreher, H. M. (2005). Wake-up call for sleep. *Nursing, 35*(3), 46–49.

Wilson, T., & Olson-Burgess, C. (2004). Are you up to date on immunizations? *The Nurse Practitioner, 29*(9), 33–34, 36, 38–38, 43.

World Health Organization. (2006). Cumulative number of confirmed human cases of avian influenza A/(H5N1) reported to WHO. Retrieved from http://www.who.int/csr/disease/avian_influenza/country/cases_table_2006_03_24

Yantis, M. A. (2002). Pain control. Obstructive sleep apnea syndrome. *American Journal of Nursing, 102*(6), 83, 85.

CHAPTER 38 Nursing Care of Clients with Ventilation Disorders

LEARNING OUTCOMES

- Relate the pathophysiology and manifestations of lower respiratory infections and inflammation, lung cancer, chest wall disorders, and trauma to the ability to maintain effective ventilation and respiration (gas exchange).

- Compare and contrast the etiology, risk factors, and vulnerable populations for lower respiratory infections, lung cancer, chest wall disorders, and trauma.

- Describe interdisciplinary care and the nursing role in health promotion and caring for clients with lower respiratory infections, lung cancer, chest wall disorders, and trauma.

- Discuss surgery and other invasive procedures used to treat lung cancer, chest wall disorders, and trauma, and nursing responsibilities in caring for clients undergoing these procedures.

- Describe the nursing implications for oxygen therapy and medications used to treat respiratory disorders.

CLINICAL COMPETENCIES

- Assess functional health status and the effects of lower respiratory and chest wall disorders on ventilation and gas exchange.

- Use assessed data and knowledge of the effects of the disorder and prescribed treatment to identify priority nursing diagnoses and plan care for clients with lower respiratory disorders.

- Use the nursing process and evidence-based nursing research to plan and implement individualized nursing care, including measures to promote ventilation and gas exchange, for clients with lower respiratory disorders.

- Plan and provide appropriate teaching for health promotion among vulnerable populations and to prepare clients and families for community-based care.

- Evaluate the effectiveness of nursing interventions and teaching, revising strategies and teaching plans as needed.

- Safely and knowledgeably coordinate interdisciplinary care and administer prescribed medications and treatments for clients with lower respiratory disorders.

MEDIALINK

Resources for this chapter can be found on the Prentice Hall Nursing MediaLink DVD-ROM accompanying this textbook, and on the Companion Website at http://www.prenhall.com/lemone

Disorders affecting the lower respiratory system (below the larynx), pleural cavity, and chest wall can affect the ability to effectively move air into and out of the lungs (ventilation) and the exchange of oxygen and carbon dioxide across the alveolar-capillary membrane (respiration). The disorders discussed in this chapter—respiratory infections and inflammation, trauma and disorders of the chest wall or pleural cavity, and neoplasms of the lung—all affect the ability to maintain clear and patent airways and ventilate the lungs. While these disorders can also affect gas exchange, nursing care for clients with these disorders generally focuses on maintaining airway patency and an effective breathing pattern. Disorders that primarily affect gas exchange are discussed in Chapter 39 ∞.

The lower respiratory and chest wall disorders discussed in this chapter and Chapter 39 have both local and systemic effects. Local effects include cough, excess mucous production, shortness of breath or **dyspnea** (difficult or labored breathing), **hemoptysis** (bloody sputum), and chest pain. Systemic effects may include fever, anorexia and malaise, **cyanosis** (gray to blue or purple skin color caused by deoxygenated hemoglobin), and other manifestations of impaired gas exchange. Before continuing, review the anatomy, physiology, and assessment of the lower respiratory system in Chapter 36 ∞.

INFECTIONS AND INFLAMMATORY DISORDERS

Infections and inflammation of the lower respiratory system are common. The respiratory tree is constantly exposed to the environment as air moves into and out of the lower respiratory tract. In addition, the oropharynx is colonized by huge numbers of microorganisms that may be aspirated into the bronchial tree. Both anatomic and physiologic defenses help maintain the sterility of the lower respiratory tract. When these defenses are impaired, the risk for infection increases. For example, drugs, alcohol, or neuromuscular disease may suppress the cough reflex, and the influenza virus can leave the respiratory epithelium vulnerable to bacterial infection. Even in healthy people, microorganisms and other foreign material occasionally enter the bronchial tree and lung parenchyma.

THE CLIENT WITH ACUTE BRONCHITIS

Bronchitis, inflammation of the bronchi, may be either an acute or a chronic condition. Acute bronchitis is relatively common in adults. Impaired immune defenses and cigarette smoking increase the risk for acute bronchitis. In otherwise healthy adults, it typically follows a viral upper respiratory infection (URI). Chronic bronchitis is a component of chronic obstructive pulmonary disease (COPD) and is discussed in Chapter 39 ∞.

Pathophysiology and Manifestations

Infectious bronchitis can be caused by either viruses or bacteria that damage the respiratory mucosa. In healthy adults, bacterial bronchitis generally only occurs as a complication of viral infection. Inhalation of toxic gases or chemicals can lead to inflammatory bronchitis.

The inflammatory response to infection or tissue damage from inhaled substances causes capillary dilation and edema of the mucosal lining of the bronchi. Inflammatory cells infiltrate the affected mucosa, leading to exudate formation and increased mucous production. Ciliated epithelium is damaged by the inflammatory response and ciliary function is impaired. The immune response of lymphocytes and tissue macrophages is inhibited by some viruses and mycobacteria, increasing the risk for bacterial infection. Mucosal irritation and increased mucous production initiate the cough reflex. The respiratory tract may become hyperirritable for an extended period of time, leading to paroxysms of coughing and bronchospasm (Copstead & Banasik, 2005).

Acute bronchitis is typically heralded by a nonproductive cough that later becomes productive. The cough often occurs in paroxysms, and may be aggravated by cold, dry, or dusty air. Chest pain, often substernal, is common. Other manifestations include moderate fever and general malaise.

INTERDISCIPLINARY CARE

The diagnosis of acute bronchitis typically is based on the history and clinical presentation. A chest x-ray may be ordered to rule out pneumonia, because the presenting manifestations can be similar. Other diagnostic testing is rarely indicated. Treatment is symptomatic and includes rest, increased fluid intake, and the use of aspirin or acetaminophen to relieve fever and malaise. Many physicians prescribe a broad-spectrum antibiotic such as erythromycin or penicillin, because approximately 50% of acute bronchitis is bacterial in origin. An expectorant cough medication is recommended for use during the day and a cough suppressant at night to facilitate rest.

NURSING CARE

Nursing interventions for clients with acute bronchitis are primarily educational. Include the following teaching topics:

- Increase fluid intake to keep mucus thin and meet increased needs related to fever.
- Use over-the-counter (OTC) analgesics and cough preparations containing dextromethorphan for symptom relief.
- Describe use and effects of any prescribed medications.
- Stress the importance of smoking cessation (as appropriate).

THE CLIENT WITH PNEUMONIA

Inflammation of the lung parenchyma (the respiratory bronchioles and alveoli) is known as **pneumonia**. Despite significant advances in antibiotic therapy, pneumonia remains the seventh leading cause of death in the United States, and the leading cause of death from infectious disease (Porth, 2005). In 2003, more than 65,000 deaths in the United States were attributed to pneumonia and influenza (Hoyert et al., 2006). Its incidence and mortality are highest in older adults and people with debilitating diseases. Pneumonia currently accounts for about 10% of adult hospital admissions in the United States.

FAST FACTS
- The age-adjusted death rate for influenza and pneumonia per 100,000 population declined from 53.7 in 1960 to 22.4 in 2003.
- Overall, men have a higher death rate (27.0 per 100,000) attributed to influenza and pneumonia than women (19.9 per 100,000).
- The differences in death rates attributed to influenza and pneumonia among different races and ethnicity are relatively small; Asian/Pacific Islanders have the lowest rate at 17.5 per 100,000, and African Americans have the highest rate at 24 per 100,000 (National Center for Health Statistics, 2005).

Pneumonia may be either infectious or noninfectious. Bacteria, viruses, fungi, protozoa, and other microbes can lead to infectious pneumonia. Noninfectious causes include aspiration of gastric contents and inhalation of toxic or irritating gases. Pneumonias often are classified as community acquired, nosocomial (hospital acquired), or opportunistic. Different organisms are implicated in each of these classifications (Table 38–1). The most common causative organism for community-acquired pneumonia is *Streptococcus pneumoniae* (also called pneumococcus), a gram-positive bacterium. This organism causes about 50% of cases of community-acquired pneumonia leading to hospital admission. *Mycoplasma pneumoniae, Chlamydia pneumoniae, Haemophilus influenzae*, and the influenza virus are also leading causes of community-acquired pneumonia (Kasper et al., 2005). *Staphylococcus aureus* and gram-negative bacteria such as *Klebsiella pneumoniae, Pseudomonas aeruginosa*, and enteric bacilli, including *Escherichia coli*, are often implicated as nosocomial causes of pneumonia. Organisms such as *Pneumocystis* generally cause infections only in immunocompromised people (opportunistic infections).

Physiology Review

The lower respiratory tract normally is sterile. A number of defense mechanisms help maintain this sterile environment. Infectious particles trapped by the mucous membranes of the nose are removed by sneezing, while those deposited in the nasopharynx usually are swallowed or expectorated. Reflex closure of the epiglottis and the branching bronchial tree present anatomic barriers to entry of microorganisms and other possible contaminants. The cilia and mucus that line the respiratory tract and the cough reflex serve to trap and eliminate foreign matter that enters the lower respiratory tract. Organisms that make it past these barriers usually are rapidly phagocytized in the alveolus by resident macrophages, then attacked by the inflammatory and immune defenses of the body. Aging impairs these immune responses, increasing the risk for pneumonia (see the box on page 1268).

Pathophysiology

The most common means of entry of pathogens into the lung is aspiration of oropharyngeal secretions containing microbes. Microorganisms also may be inhaled after having been released when an infected person coughs, sneezes, or talks. Contaminated aerosolized water also may be inhaled, an important means of spread for viral and some other types of pneumonia. Finally, bacteria may spread to the lungs through the bloodstream from infection elsewhere in the body. Host defenses must be overwhelmed either by the number of organisms or their *virulence* (disease-causing ability) in order for an infection to develop.

TABLE 38–1 Common Organisms Causing Pneumonia in Adults

COMMUNITY ACQUIRED	HOSPITAL ACQUIRED	OPPORTUNISTIC
Streptococcus pneumoniae	*Staphylococcus aureus*	*Pneumocystis carinii*
Mycoplasma pneumoniae	*Pseudomonas aeruginosa*	*Mycobacterium tuberculosis*
Haemophilus influenzae	*Klebsiella pneumoniae*	Cytomegalovirus (CMV)
Influenza virus	*Escherichia coli*	Atypical mycobacteria
Chlamydia pneumoniae		Fungi
Legionella pneumophila		

NURSING CARE OF THE OLDER ADULT
Pneumonia

Several changes associated with aging and disease affect respiratory function and airway clearance. The number of cilia decreases, and the cough weakens. Gag and cough reflexes diminish. The older adult is at greater risk for dehydration, leading to thick, viscous mucus that is difficult to expectorate. Immune function declines with aging. These factors increase the risk of pulmonary infection and reduce the older adult's ability to respond effectively to infectious processes.

Other factors also may increase the risk for and severity of lower respiratory infections in the older adult: immobility, smoking history, surgical procedures, use of multiple medications, malnutrition, and such diseases as COPD and heart disease.

Figure 38–1 ■ In pneumonia, the inflammatory response causes fluid to accumulate in the alveoli and edema to form as alveolar capillaries dilate and allow fluid to leak into interstitial tissues.
Source: Kevin A. Somerville, Phototake NYC.

When the invading microorganisms colonize the alveoli, an inflammatory and immune response is initiated. The antigen–antibody response and endotoxins released by some organisms damage bronchial and alveolar mucous membranes, causing inflammation with vascular congestion and edema. Infectious debris and exudate can fill alveoli, interfering with ventilation and gas exchange (Figure 38–1 ■). Pneumonia may develop in four distinct patterns: lobar pneumonia, bronchopneumonia, interstitial pneumonia, and miliary pneumonia (Table 38–2).

The pathologic process, anatomic location, and manifestations of pneumonias vary according to the infective organism.

Acute Bacterial Pneumonia

Of the bacterial pneumonias, the pathogenesis of pneumococcal (*Streptococcus pneumoniae*) pneumonia is best understood (Figure 38–2 ■). These bacteria reside in the upper respiratory tract of up to 70% of adults. They may be spread by direct person-to-person contact via droplets. In many cases, infection results from aspiration of resident bacteria. In the lower respiratory tract, the inflammatory response initiated by these organisms causes alveolar edema and the formation of exudate. As alveoli and respiratory bronchioles fill with serous exudate, blood cells, fibrin, and bacteria, *consolidation* (solidification) of lung tissue occurs. The lower lobes of the lungs are usually affected because of gravity. Consolidation of a large portion of an entire lung lobe is known as *lobar pneumonia*. This is the typical pattern for pneumococcal pneumonia. *Bronchopneumonia* is patchy consolidation involving several lobules. Other bacterial pneumonias often present with the patchy involvement of bronchopneumonia; pneumococcal pneumonia may also follow this pattern. The process resolves when macrophages predominate, digesting and removing inflammatory exudate from the infected lung.

TABLE 38–2 Patterns of Lung Involvement in Pneumonia

PATTERN OF INVOLVEMENT	DESCRIPTION
Lobar pneumonia	Typically involves an entire lobe of a lung. Early in the process, when the immune response is minimal, bacteria spread throughout the affected lobe by rapid accumulation of fluid exudate. As the immune and inflammatory responses develop, RBCs and neutrophils, damaged epithelial cells, and fibrin accumulate in the alveoli. Purulent exudate containing neutrophils and macrophages forms. As alveoli and respiratory bronchioles fill with exudate, blood cells, fibrin, and bacteria, *consolidation* (solidification) of lung tissue occurs. Finally, the process resolves as enzymes destroy the exudate and residual debris is reabsorbed, phagocytized, or coughed out.
Bronchopneumonia	Usually involves dependent portions of lung tissue, characterized by patchy consolidation. Exudate tends to remain primarily in the bronchi and bronchioles, with less edema and congestion of the alveoli than in lobar pneumonia.
Interstitial pneumonia	The inflammatory process primarily involves the interstitium: the alveolar walls and connective tissue supporting the bronchial tree. Involvement may be patchy or diffuse as lymphocytes, macrophages, and plasma cells infiltrate the alveolar septa. While alveoli typically do not contain significant exudates, protein-rich hyaline membranes may line the alveoli, interfering with gas exchange.
Miliary pneumonia	In miliary pneumonia, numerous discrete inflammatory lesions develop as a result of spread of the pathogen to the lungs via the bloodstream. Miliary pneumonia is primarily seen in people who are severely immunocompromised. As a result, the immune response is poor and damage to pleural tissue may be significant.

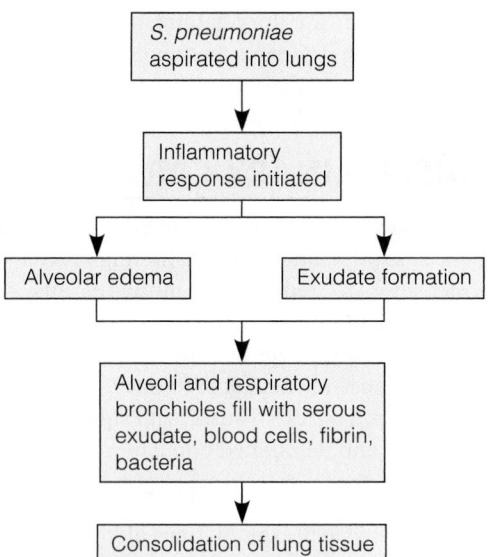

Figure 38–2 ■ The pathogenesis of pneumococcal pneumonia.

MANIFESTATIONS The presentation of bacterial pneumonia is usually acute, with rapid onset of shaking chills, fever, and cough productive of rust-colored or purulent sputum. Chest aching or *pleuritic pain* (sharp localized chest pain that increases with breathing and coughing) is common. Limited breath sounds and fine crackles or rales are heard over the affected area of lung. A pleural friction rub may be audible. If the involved area is large and gas exchange is impaired, dyspnea and cyanosis may be noted.

A more insidious onset with low-grade fever, cough, and scattered crackles is more typical of bronchopneumonia. Dyspnea is less commonly seen. The older adult or debilitated client may have atypical manifestations of pneumonia, with little cough, scant sputum, and minimal evidence of respiratory distress. Fever, tachypnea, and altered mentation or agitation may be the primary presenting symptoms. Confusion 1st

COMPLICATIONS Pneumococcal pneumonia typically resolves uneventfully; normal lung structure is restored on completion of the process. Local extension of the infection to involve the pleura (*pleuritis*) is the most common complication. Pneumonias caused by *Staphylococcus aureus* and gram-negative bacteria often cause extensive parenchymal damage with necrosis, lung abscess, and empyema or pleural effusion. Progressive destruction of lung tissue and functional impairment is a possible consequence of *Klebsiella* pneumonia.

A *lung abscess* is a local area of necrosis and pus formation within the lung itself. They are relatively uncommon. The manifestations of lung abscess develop slowly, and include weight loss, malaise, night sweats, fever, and a productive cough. Sputum is foul smelling and tasting. Rupture of the abscess into a larger airway is heralded by production of copious amounts of purulent sputum.

Empyema is accumulation of purulent exudate in the pleural cavity. It is identified by chest x-ray or CT scan. Thoracentesis may be done or a chest tube inserted to remove purulent exudates. (Nursing care of the client undergoing thoracentesis or with a chest tube is discussed later in this chapter.)

Bacteremia can spread the infection to other tissues, leading to meningitis, endocarditis, or peritonitis, and increasing the risk of mortality.

Legionnaires' Disease

Legionnaires' disease is a form of bronchopneumonia caused by *Legionella pneumophila*, a gram-negative bacterium widely found in water, particularly warm, standing water. Legionnaires' disease occurs sporadically and in outbreaks, such as that which occurred at an American Legion convention in 1976, when the disease was first recognized. Contaminated water-cooled air conditioning systems and other water sources have been implicated in its spread.

Smokers, older adults, and people with chronic diseases or impaired immune defenses are most susceptible to Legionnaires' disease. Symptoms develop gradually, beginning 2 to 10 days after exposure. Dry cough, dyspnea, general malaise, chills and fever, headache, confusion, anorexia and diarrhea, myalgias, and arthralgias are common manifestations. Consolidation of lung tissue is patchy or lobar. The mortality rate in Legionnaires' disease is up to 31% without treatment in otherwise healthy people and up to 80% in people who are immunocompromised (Kasper et al., 2005).

Primary Atypical Pneumonia

Pneumonia caused by *Mycoplasma pneumoniae* is generally classified as *primary atypical pneumonia*, because its presentation and course significantly differ from other bacterial pneumonias. Mycoplasma infection often causes pharyngitis or bronchitis. When pneumonia develops, patchy inflammatory changes in the alveolar septum and interstitial tissue of the lung occur. Alveolar exudate and consolidation of lung tissue are not features of atypical pneumonia.

Young adults—college students and military recruits in particular—are the primary affected population. Primary atypical pneumonia is highly contagious. Its manifestations resemble those of viral pneumonia; systemic manifestations of fever, headache, myalgias, and arthralgias often predominate. The cough associated with atypical pneumonia is dry, hacking, and nonproductive. Because of the typically mild nature and predominant systemic manifestations, mycoplasmal and viral pneumonia are often referred to as "walking pneumonias."

Viral Pneumonia

Approximately 10% of pneumonias in adults are viral. Influenza and adenovirus are the most common organisms; however, the incidence of cytomegalovirus (CMV) pneumonia is increasing in immunocompromised people. Other viruses such as herpesviruses and measles virus also may cause viral pneumonia. As in primary atypical pneumonia, lung involvement in viral pneumonia is limited to the alveolar septum and interstitial spaces.

Viral pneumonia is typically a mild disease that often affects older adults and people with chronic conditions. It usually occurs in community epidemics. Flulike symptoms of headache, fever, fatigue, malaise, and muscle aching are common, along with a dry cough.

Pneumocystis Pneumonia

People with acquired immune deficiency syndrome (AIDS) and others with significant immunocompromise are at risk for developing an opportunistic pneumonia caused by *Pneumocystis*, a common parasite found worldwide. Immunity to *Pneumocystis* is nearly universal, except in immunocompromised people. Opportunistic infection may develop in people treated with immunosuppressive or cytotoxic drugs for cancer or organ transplant and in people with genetic or acquired immunodeficiency. People with AIDS account for most cases (60%) of *Pneumocystis* pneumonia (PCP) (Copstead & Banasik, 2005).

Infection with *Pneumocystis* produces patchy involvement throughout the lungs, causing affected alveoli to thicken, become edematous, and fill with foamy, protein-rich fluid. Gas exchange is severely impaired as the disease progresses.

PCP has an abrupt onset with fever, tachypnea and shortness of breath, and a dry, nonproductive cough. Respiratory distress can be significant, with intercostal retractions and cyanosis.

Table 38–3 compares the manifestations of infectious pneumonias.

Aspiration Pneumonia

Aspiration of gastric contents into the lungs results in a chemical and bacterial pneumonia known as *aspiration pneumonia*. Major risk factors for aspiration pneumonia include emergency surgery or obstetric procedures, depressed cough and gag reflexes, and impaired swallowing. Older surgical clients are at significant risk. Enteral nutrition by either nasogastric or gastric tube also increases the risk for aspiration pneumonia. Vomiting is not always apparent; silent regurgitation of gastric contents may occur when the level of consciousness is decreased. Measures to reduce the risk for aspiration pneumonia include minimizing the use of preoperative medications, promoting anesthetic elimination from the body, and preventing nausea and gastric distention.

The low pH of gastric contents causes a severe inflammatory response when aspirated into the respiratory tract. Pulmonary edema and respiratory failure may result. Common complications of aspiration pneumonia include abscesses, bronchiectasis (chronic dilation of the bronchi and bronchioles), and gangrene of pulmonary tissue.

INTERDISCIPLINARY CARE

Prevention is a key component in managing pneumonia. Identifying vulnerable populations and instituting preventive strategies are measures to reduce the mortality and morbidity associated with pneumonia. With early identification of the infecting organism, appropriate treatment, and support of respiratory function, most clients recover uneventfully. However, pneumonia remains a serious disease with significant mortality, especially in aged and debilitated populations.

Diagnosis

The history and physical examination, along with diagnostic testing, are used to establish the diagnosis, determine the extent of lung involvement, and identify the causative organism. See Chapter 36 ∞ for more information about the following tests and their nursing implications:

- *Chest x-ray* is obtained to determine the extent and pattern of lung involvement. Fluid, infiltrates, consolidated lung tissue, and atelectasis (areas of alveolar collapse) appear as densities on the film. The *CT scan* provides a more detailed image of pulmonary tissue and may be used when the chest x-ray is not diagnostic.
- *Sputum Gram stain* rapidly identifies the infecting organisms as gram-positive or gram-negative bacteria. Antibiotic therapy can then be directed at the predominant type of organism until culture and sensitivity results are obtained.
- *Sputum culture and sensitivity* is ordered to identify the infecting organism and determine the most effective antibiotic therapy. When obtaining sputum for culture, it is important to obtain secretions from the lower respiratory tract, not the mouth and nasal passages. See Procedure 36–1 on page 1220.

TABLE 38–3 Manifestations of Infectious Pneumonias

TYPE	ONSET	RESPIRATORY MANIFESTATIONS	SYSTEMIC MANIFESTATIONS
Pneumococcal or lobar pneumonia	Abrupt	Cough productive of purulent or rust-colored sputum; pleuritic or aching chest pain; decreased breath sounds and crackles over affected area; possible dyspnea and cyanosis	Chills and fever
Bronchopneumonia	Gradual	Cough, scattered crackles; minimal dyspnea and respiratory distress	Low-grade fever
Legionnaires' disease	Gradual	Dry cough; dyspnea	Chills and fever; general malaise; headache; confusion; anorexia and diarrhea; myalgias and arthralgias
Primary atypical pneumonia	Gradual	Dry, hacking, nonproductive cough	Fever, headache, myalgias, and arthralgias predominate
Viral pneumonia	Sudden or gradual	Dry cough	Flulike symptoms
Pneumocystis pneumonia	Abrupt	Dry cough; tachypnea and shortness of breath; significant respiratory distress	Fever

- *Complete blood count (CBC) with white blood cell (WBC) differential* shows an elevated WBC (11,000/mm³ or higher) with increased circulating immature leukocytes (a left shift) in response to the infectious process. White blood cell changes are minimal in viral and other pneumonias.
- *Serology testing*, blood tests to detect antibodies to respiratory pathogens, may be used to identify the infecting organism when blood and sputum cultures are negative.
- *Pulse oximetry*, a noninvasive method of measuring arterial oxygen saturation, is ordered to continuously monitor gas exchange. The SaO_2 normally is 95% or higher. An SaO_2 of less than 95% may indicate impaired alveolar gas exchange.
- *Arterial blood gases (ABGs)* may be ordered to evaluate gas exchange. Respiratory secretions or pleuritic pain can interfere with alveolar ventilation. Alveolar inflammation can interfere with gas exchange across the alveolar-capillary membrane, especially if exudate or consolidation is present. An arterial oxygen tension (PaO_2) of less than 75 to 80 mmHg indicates impaired gas exchange or alveolar ventilation. See Chapters 10 and 36 ∞ for more information about gas transport, ABGs, and normal or expected values.
- *Fiberoptic bronchoscopy* may be done to obtain a sputum specimen or remove secretions from the bronchial tree (Figure 36–9). Nursing responsibilities related to bronchoscopy are summarized in the Diagnostic Tests box in Chapter 36 ∞.

Immunization

Vaccines offer some degree of protection against the most common bacterial and viral pneumonias.

Pneumococcal vaccine, made of antigens from 23 types of pneumococcus, usually imparts lifetime immunity with a single dose. The vaccine is recommended for people who have a high risk of adverse outcome from bacterial pneumonias: people over age 65; those with chronic cardiac or respiratory conditions, diabetes mellitus, alcoholism, or other chronic diseases; and immunocompromised people. A one-time revaccination is recommended for selected populations, including people over age 65 who were immunized more than 5 years previously and before age 65, people with chronic renal failure or immunosuppressive conditions (e.g., malignancy), and people receiving chemotherapy with selected agents (CDC, 2005).

Influenza vaccine is also recommended for high-risk populations. The predominant strain of influenza virus varies from year to year. A new vaccine formulation is prepared yearly, incorporating antigens of the influenza strains predicted to be the most prevalent for the upcoming flu season (typically the winter months). Vulnerable populations for whom yearly vaccine is recommended include those listed above as well as healthcare workers and residents of long-term care facilities. The vaccine contains egg protein, and is not recommended for people who have a severe allergy to eggs or who have previously experienced a severe hypersensitivity response to the vaccine.

Medications

Medications used to treat pneumonia may include antibiotics to eradicate the infection and bronchodilators to reduce bronchospasm and improve ventilation.

Initial antibiotic therapy is based on the results of sputum Gram stain and the pattern of lung involvement shown on a chest x-ray. Considerations such as the presence of cardiovascular disease or residence in a long-term care facility also are considered in the initial antibiotic choice. Typically, a broad-spectrum antibiotic such as a macrolide (e.g., clarithromycin, azithromycin, or erythromycin), a penicillin or a second- or third-generation cephalosporin, or a fluoroquinolone (e.g,. ciprofloxacin) is ordered until the results of sputum culture and sensitivity tests are available. Table 38–4 lists commonly prescribed antibiotics for selected pneumonias; nursing implications for selected antibiotics are summarized in Chapter 12 ∞.

When an inflammatory response to the infection causes bronchospasm and constriction, bronchodilators may be ordered to improve ventilation and reduce hypoxia. Bronchodilators generally belong to one of two major groups: the

TABLE 38–4 Antibiotic Therapy for Selected Pneumonias

CAUSATIVE ORGANISM	ANTIBIOTIC OF CHOICE	ALTERNATIVE ANTIBIOTICS
Streptococcus pneumoniae	Penicillin G; amoxicillin	Erythromycin, cephalosporins, doxycycline, fluoroquinolone, clindamycin, vancomycin, trimethoprim-sulfamethoxazole (TMP-SMZ), linezolid
Haemophilus influenzae	Second- or third-generation cephalosporins, doxycycline, azithromycin, TMP-SMZ	Fluoroquinolones, clarithromycin
Staphylococcus aureus	Penicillinase-resistant penicillin (e.g., nafcillin); vancomycin for methicillin-resistant organisms	Cephalosporins, vancomycin, clindamycin; ciprofloxacin, fluoroquinolones, TMP-SMZ
Mycoplasma pneumoniae	Erythromycin, doxycycline	Clarithromycin, azithromycin, fluoroquinolone
Klebsiella pneumoniae	Third-generation cephalosporin (with aminoglycoside if severe); metronidazole	Aztreonam, imipenem-cilastatin, fluoroquinolone
Legionella pneumophila	Macrolide + rifampin; fluoroquinolone	TMP-SMZ, doxycycline + rifampin
Pneumocystis	TMP-SMZ, pentamidine + prednisone	Dapsone + trimethoprim, clindamycin + primaquine, trimetrexate + folinic acid
Chlamydia pneumoniae	Doxycycline	Macrolide, fluoroquinolone

sympathomimetic drugs, such as albuterol sulfate (Proventil) and metaproterenol (Alupent); or the methylxanthines, such as theophylline and aminophylline. Use of these drugs and related nursing implications are discussed in detail in the section on asthma in Chapter 39 ∞.

An agent to "break up" mucus or reduce its viscosity may be prescribed. Acetylcysteine (Mucomyst), potassium iodide, and guaifenesin (a common ingredient in expectorant cough syrups) help to liquefy mucus, making it easier to expectorate. For many clients, however, increasing fluid intake is an effective means of liquefying mucus.

Treatments

When mucous secretions are thick and viscous, increasing fluid intake to 2500 to 3000 mL per day helps liquefy secretions, making them easier to cough up and expectorate. If the client is unable to maintain an adequate oral intake, intravenous fluids and nutrition may be required.

Incentive spirometry may be used to promote deep breathing, coughing, and clearance of respiratory secretions. Endotracheal suctioning may be required if the cough is ineffective. This invasive technique is discussed in Chapter 39 ∞ in the section describing nursing care for the client with acute respiratory failure. On occasion, bronchoscopy is used to perform pulmonary toilet and remove secretions.

OXYGEN THERAPY Oxygen therapy may be indicated for the client who is tachypneic or hypoxemic.

Inflammation of the alveolar-capillary membrane interferes with diffusion of gases across the membrane. Diffusion is affected by several other factors, including the partial pressure of gases on each side of the membrane. Increasing the percentage of inspired oxygen above that of room air (21%) increases the partial pressure of oxygen in the alveoli and enhances its diffusion into the capillaries. Supplemental oxygen therefore improves oxygenation of the blood and tissues in clients with pneumonia.

Depending on the degree of hypoxia, oxygen may be administered by either a low-flow or high-flow system. Low-flow systems include the nasal cannula, simple face mask, partial rebreathing mask, and nonrebreathing mask (Figure 38–3 ■). A nasal cannula can deliver 24% to 45% oxygen concentrations with flow rates of 2 to 6 L/min. The nasal cannula is comfortable and does not interfere with eating or talking. A simple face mask delivers 40% to 60% oxygen concentrations with flow rates of 5 to 8 L/min. Up to 100% oxygen can be delivered by the nonrebreather mask, the highest concentration possible without mechanical ventilation. When the amount of oxygen delivered must be precisely regulated, a high-flow system such as a Venturi mask is used (Figure 38–4 ■). The Venturi mask regulates the ratio of oxygen to room air, allowing precise regulation of the oxygen percentage delivered, from 24% to 50%. Severe hypoxia may necessitate intubation and mechanical ventilation. Endotracheal intubation and methods of mechanical ventilation are discussed in Chapter 39 ∞.

CHEST PHYSIOTHERAPY Chest physiotherapy, including percussion, vibration, and postural drainage, may be prescribed to reduce lung consolidation and prevent atelectasis.

Figure 38–3 ■ Low-flow oxygen delivery devices: *A,* nasal cannula; *B,* simple face mask; *C,* nonrebreather mask.

Source: A, C, Michal Heron, Pearson Education/PH College; *B,* Tony McConnell, Photo Researchers, Inc.

Percussion is performed by rhythmically striking or clapping the chest wall with cupped hands (Figure 38–5A ■), using rapid wrist flexion and extension. Cupping traps air between the palm and the client's skin, setting up vibrations through the chest wall that loosen respiratory secretions. The trapped air also provides a cushion, preventing injury. When per-

Figure 38–4 ■ Venturi mask, a high-flow oxygen delivery system.
Source: Michal Heron, Pearson Education/PH College

formed correctly, percussion produces a hollow, popping sound. Percussion may also be done using a mechanical percussion cup. The breasts, sternum, spinal column, and kidney regions are avoided during percussion.

Vibration facilitates secretion movement into larger airways. It usually is combined with percussion, although it may be used when percussion is contraindicated or poorly tolerated. Vibration is performed by repeatedly tensing the arm and hand muscles while maintaining firm but gentle pressure over the affected area with the flat of the hand (Figure 38–5B).

Percussion and vibration are done in conjunction with *postural drainage*, which uses gravity to facilitate removal of secretions from a particular lung segment. The client is positioned with the segment to be drained superior to or above the trachea or mainstem bronchus. Drainage of all lung segments requires a variety of positions (Figure 38–6 ■); rarely do all segments require drainage. Bronchodilators or nebulizer treatments are administered as ordered prior to postural drainage. It is best to perform postural drainage before meals to avoid nausea and vomiting.

Complementary Therapies

Although complementary therapies do not replace conventional treatment for pneumonia, they often promote comfort and speed recovery. The herb echinacea is widely used to stimulate immune function and treat URIs. Because viral URIs often precede pneumonia, echinacea may be helpful in preventing pneumonia. Recent research, however, shows mixed results for the effectiveness of echinacea in reducing the duration and severity of URI (National Center for Complementary and Alternative Medicine [NCCAM], 2005). Goldenseal, which often is sold in combination with echinacea, is used to treat bacterial, fungal, and protozoal infections of the mucous membranes of the respiratory tract.

A

B

Figure 38–5 ■ *A,* Percussing (clapping) the upper posterior chest. Notice the cupped position of the nurse's hands. *B,* Vibrating the upper posterior chest.

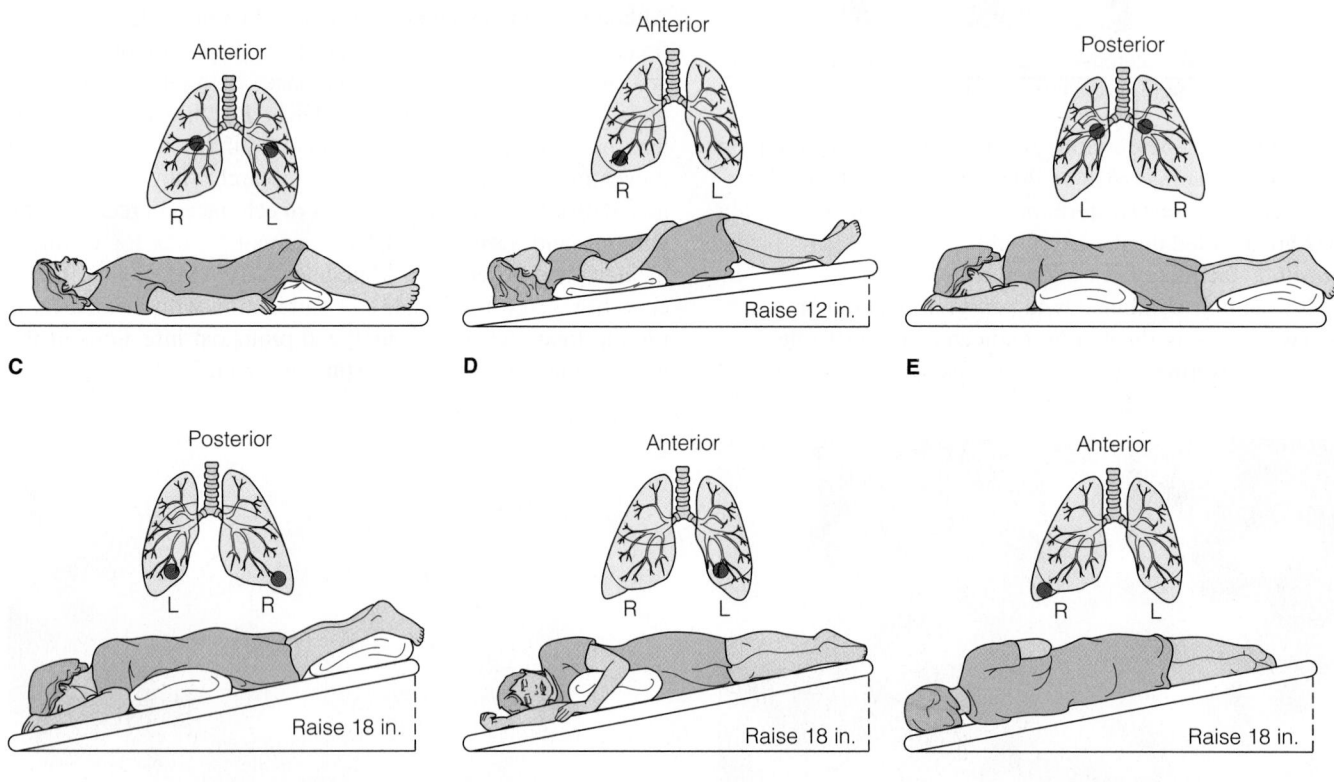

Figure 38–6 ■ Positions for postural drainage. *A,* Left and right anterior apical. *B,* Left and right posterior apical. *C,* Left and right anterior upper. *D,* Right middle lobe. *E,* Superior lower lobes. *F,* Left and right lower posterior. *G,* Left lower lateral. *H,* Right lower lateral.

Ma huang contains the active ingredient ephedra, which has been used to relieve bronchospasm and ease breathing. The primary active ingredient in ephedra is epinephrine, a cardiac and CNS stimulant. Because of the dangers associated with its use, sale of herbal products containing ephedra has been banned (NCCAM, 2004). Advise clients inquiring about the use of Chinese herbal remedies to reduce pneumonia symptoms to inquire if any recommended product contains ma huang or ephedra, and to avoid such products.

 NURSING CARE

Health Promotion

Health promotion activities focus on pneumonia prevention. Make clients in high-risk groups aware of the benefits of immunizations against influenza and pneumococcal pneumonia. A single dose of pneumococcus vaccine usually produces immunity to most strains of pneumococcal pneumonia, although repeat doses may be needed for older adults and people who are immunosuppressed. (Pneumococcus vaccine is contraindicated for people receiving immunosuppressive therapy.) Annual influenza vaccine helps prevent pneumonia, because pneumonia often occurs as a sequela to influenza.

PRACTICE ALERT
Inquire about allergic responses to eggs or previous influenza vaccinations prior to administering influenza vaccine. A significant hypersensitivity response may occur in clients who are allergic to egg protein.

Additional measures to screen for and detect pneumonia in older adults are appropriate. Frequent pulmonary assessment and aggressive interventions help prevent problems. Restoring and maintaining mobility improves ventilation and helps mobilize secretions. Promoting adequate fluid intake is necessary because fluid helps liquefy secretions, making them easier to expectorate.

Assessment

Focused assessment of the client with pneumonia includes the following:

- *Health History:* Current symptoms and their duration; presence of shortness of breath or difficulty breathing, chest pain and its relationship to breathing; cough, productive or nonproductive, color, consistency of sputum; other symptoms; recent upper respiratory or other acute illness; chronic diseases such as diabetes, chronic lung disease, or heart disease; current medications; medication allergies.
- *Physical Examination:* Presentation, apparent distress; level of consciousness; vital signs including temperature; skin color, temperature; respiratory excursion, use of accessory muscles of respiration; lung sounds.
- *Diagnostic Tests:* WBC with differential, sputum Gram stain, culture and sensitivity, chest x-ray or CT scan.

Nursing Diagnoses and Interventions

Clients with lower respiratory disorders such as pneumonia may have multiple nursing care needs, depending on the severity of the illness. Alveolar ventilation and the process of alveolar respiration can be affected by inflammation and secretions. **Hypoxemia**, low levels of oxygen in the blood, and tissue hypoxia may result. Nursing care focuses on supporting optimal respiratory function and promoting rest to reduce metabolic and oxygen needs. Priority nursing diagnoses include *Ineffective Airway Clearance, Ineffective Breathing Pattern*, and *Activity Intolerance*.

Ineffective Airway Clearance

The inflammatory response to infection causes tissue edema and exudate formation. In the lungs, the inflammatory response can narrow and potentially obstruct bronchial passages and alveoli. Assessment findings supporting this nursing diagnosis include adventitious breath sounds such as crackles (rales), rhonchi, and wheezes; dyspnea and tachypnea; coughing; and indicators of hypoxia such as cyanosis, reduced SaO_2 levels, anxiety, and apprehension.

- Assess respiratory status, including vital signs, breath sounds, SaO_2, and skin color at least every 4 hours. *Early identification of respiratory compromise allows intervention before tissue hypoxia is significant.*
- Assess cough and sputum (amount, color, consistency, and possible odor). *Assessment of the cough and nature of sputum produced allows evaluation of the effectiveness of respiratory clearance and the response to therapy.*
- Monitor ABG results; report increasing hypoxemia and other abnormal results to the physician. *Blood gas changes may be an early indicator of impaired gas exchange due to airway narrowing or obstruction.*
- Place in Fowler's or high-Fowler's position. Encourage frequent position changes and ambulation as allowed. *The upright position promotes lung expansion; position changes and ambulation facilitate the movement of secretions.*

- Assist to cough, deep breathe, and use assistive devices. Provide endotracheal suctioning using aseptic technique as ordered. *Coughing, deep breathing, and suctioning help clear airways.*
- Provide a fluid intake of at least 2500 to 3000 mL per day. *A liberal fluid intake helps liquefy secretions, facilitating their clearance.*
- Work with the physician and respiratory therapist to provide pulmonary hygiene measures, such as postural drainage, percussion, and vibration. *These techniques help mobilize and clear secretions.*
- Administer prescribed medications as ordered, and monitor their effects. *If the infecting organism is resistant to the prescribed antibiotic, little improvement may be seen with treatment. Bronchodilators help maintain open airways but may have adverse effects such as anxiety and restlessness.*

Ineffective Breathing Pattern

Pleural inflammation often accompanies pneumonia, causing sharp localized pain that increases with deep breathing, coughing, and movement, which can lead to rapid and shallow breathing. Distal airways and alveoli may not expand optimally with each breath, increasing the risk for atelectasis and decreasing gas exchange. Fatigue from the increased work of breathing is an additional problem in pneumonia. This, too, can lead to decreased lung inflation and an ineffective breathing pattern.

> **PRACTICE ALERT**
> Assess respiratory rate, depth, and lung sounds at least every 4 hours. Tachypnea and diminished or adventitious breath sounds may be early indicators of respiratory compromise.

- Provide for rest periods. *Rest reduces metabolic demands, fatigue, and the work of breathing, promoting a more effective breathing pattern.*
- Assess for pleuritic discomfort. Provide analgesics as ordered. *Adequate pain relief minimizes splinting and promotes adequate ventilation.*
- Provide reassurance during periods of respiratory distress. *Hypoxia and respiratory distress produce high levels of anxiety, which tends to further increase tachypnea and fatigue and decrease ventilation.*
- Administer oxygen as ordered. *Oxygen therapy increases the alveolar oxygen concentration and facilitates its diffusion across the alveolar-capillary membrane, reducing hypoxia and anxiety.*
- Teach slow abdominal breathing. *This breathing pattern promotes lung expansion.*
- Teach use of relaxation techniques, such as visualization and meditation. *These techniques help reduce anxiety and slow the breathing pattern.*

Activity Intolerance

Impaired airway clearance and gas exchange interfere with oxygen delivery to body cells and tissues. At the same time, the infectious process and the body's response to it increase metabolic demands on the cells. The net result of this imbalance between oxygen delivery and oxygen demand is a lack of physiologic energy to maintain normal daily activities.

■ Assess activity tolerance, noting any increase in pulse, respirations, dyspnea, diaphoresis, or cyanosis. *These assessment findings may indicate limited or impaired activity tolerance.*

PRACTICE ALERT
Activity intolerance may be an early sign of cardiorespiratory compromise, particularly in the older adult or client with preexisting heart disease. New or worsening manifestations of activity intolerance should be reported to the physician.

■ Assist with self-care activities, such as bathing. *Assistance with ADLs reduces energy demands.*
■ Schedule activities, planning for rest periods. *Rest periods minimize fatigue and improve activity tolerance.*
■ Provide assistive devices, such as an overhead trapeze. *These assistive devices facilitate movement and reduce energy demands.*
■ Enlist the family's help to minimize stress and anxiety levels. *Stress and anxiety increase metabolic demands and can decrease activity tolerance.*
■ Perform active or passive range-of-motion (ROM) exercises. *Exercises help maintain muscle tone and joint mobility, and prevent contractures if bed rest is prolonged.*
■ Provide emotional support and reassurance that strength and energy will return to normal when the infectious process has resolved and the balance of oxygen supply and demand is restored. *The client may be concerned that activity intolerance will continue to be a problem after the acute infection is resolved.*

Using NANDA, NIC, and NOC
Links between NANDA nursing diagnoses, NIC, and NOC for the client with pneumonia are outlined in Chart 38–1.

Community-Based Care
Clients with pneumonia usually are treated in the community, unless their respiratory status is significantly compromised (e.g., altered mental status, tachypnea, tachycardia, hypotension, hypo- or hyperthermia, and altered blood gases) or if risk factors such as advanced age and/or coexisting heart, kidney, or liver disease are present.

Discuss the following topics when preparing the client and family for home care:
■ The importance of completing the prescribed medication regimen as ordered; potential drug side effects and their management, including manifestations that necessitate stopping the drug and notifying the physician
■ Recommendations for limiting activities and increasing rest
■ Maintaining adequate fluid intake to keep mucus thin for easier expectoration
■ Ways to maintain adequate nutritional intake, such as small, frequent, well-balanced meals
■ The importance of avoiding smoking or exposure to secondhand smoke to prevent further irritation of the lungs

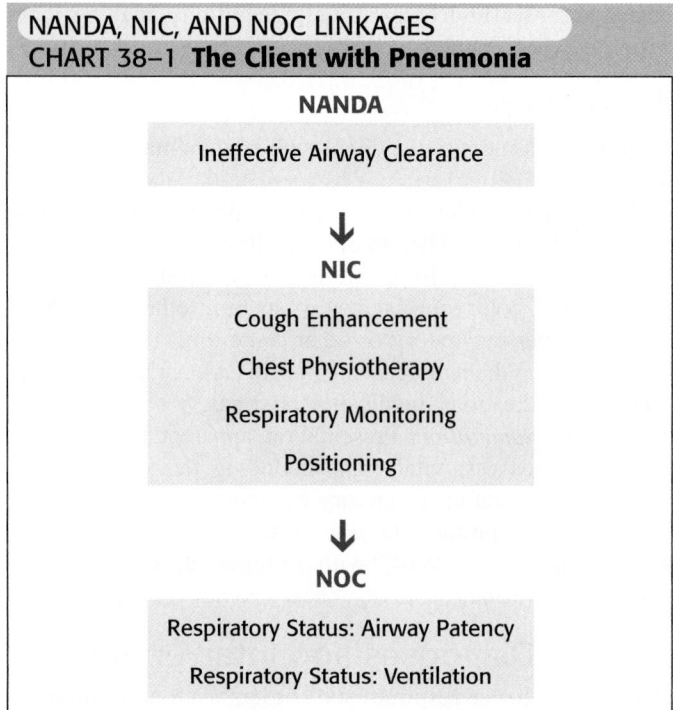

NANDA, NIC, AND NOC LINKAGES
CHART 38–1 **The Client with Pneumonia**

NANDA

Ineffective Airway Clearance

↓

NIC

Cough Enhancement

Chest Physiotherapy

Respiratory Monitoring

Positioning

↓

NOC

Respiratory Status: Airway Patency

Respiratory Status: Ventilation

Data from *NANDA's Nursing Diagnoses: Definitions & Classification 2005–2006* by NANDA Interational (2005), Philadelphia; *Nursing Interventions Classification (NIC)* (4th ed.) by J. M. Dochterman & G. M. Bulechek (2004), St. Louis, MO: Mosby; and *Nursing Outcomes Classification (NOC)* (3rd ed.) by S. Moorhead, M. Johnson, and M. Maas (2004), St. Louis, MO: Mosby.

■ Manifestations to report to the physician, such as increasing shortness of breath, difficulty breathing, increased fever, fatigue, headache, sleepiness, or confusion
■ The importance of keeping all follow-up appointments to ensure disease cure.

The accompanying Nursing Care Plan provides further nursing interventions for clients treated in the community.

Clients with respiratory compromise or who are elderly or debilitated may require home care assistance to remain at home. Provide referrals to home intravenous services, home health nursing services, and home maintenance services as indicated. Community services such as Meals-on-Wheels can provide support to reduce the energy demands of meal preparation.

THE CLIENT WITH SEVERE ACUTE RESPIRATORY SYNDROME

Severe acute respiratory syndrome (SARS) is a lower respiratory illness of unknown etiology first described in people in Asia in the fall of 2002. Since then, this emerging disease has been identified in clients in North America, Australia, and Europe, although the majority of identified cases are in China (including Hong Kong and Singapore) (World Health Organization, 2003). The primary population affected by SARS is previously healthy adults ages 25 to 70 years.

Pathophysiology
The infective agent responsible for SARS is a coronavirus not previously identified in humans. This virus appears to spread

NURSING CARE PLAN   A Client with Pneumonia

Mary O'Neal is a 35-year-old executive assistant and a part-time college student. On returning home from class one evening, she begins to chill. She alternates between chills and sweats all night. Staying home from work, she remains in bed most of the next day. Her fever continues, and she develops a cough and dull aching chest pain. When the cough becomes productive of rust-colored sputum the following day, she seeks medical treatment from her family doctor.

ASSESSMENT

Debby Kowalski, RN, the family practice clinic nurse, admits Mrs. O'Neal to the clinic and obtains the nursing assessment. Mrs. O'Neal denies any previous history of respiratory diseases "other than the usual colds, flu, and such." She also denies any history of smoking or medication allergies. She says her symptoms began abruptly with the onset of the chills. She describes her chest pain as a dull ache that was initially substernal but now is localized in her lower lateral right chest. The pain increases with deep breathing, coughing, and moving. Her cough is increasing in frequency and severity, and her sputum appears rusty brown. Her vital signs are BP 116/74, P 104 and regular, R 26, T 101.8°F (38.7°C). Skin warm and flushed, with no evidence of cyanosis. Respirations shallow, unlabored; respiratory excursion equal. Diminished breath sounds in bases bilaterally, crackles noted in right posterior and lateral base. Faint pleural rub heard at right midaxillary line.

A STAT CBC shows a WBC of 18,900/mm³; differential shows increased numbers of neutrophils and immature WBCs (bands). Ms. Kowalski has Mrs. O'Neal rinse with an antiseptic mouthwash and then collects a sputum specimen for culture and Gram stain prior to seeing the physician.

The physician orders a chest x-ray after examining Mrs. O'Neal. Based on her history, examination, and the chest x-ray, he makes the diagnosis of acute bacterial pneumonia, probably pneumococcal. He prescribes oral penicillin V, 500 mg every 6 hours for 10 days. He asks Mrs. O'Neal to return for a follow-up appointment in 10 days and refers her back to Ms. Kowalski for appropriate teaching.

DIAGNOSES

- *Ineffective Breathing Pattern* related to pleuritic chest pain
- *Hyperthermia* related to inflammatory process
- *Deficient Knowledge* about pneumonia and its treatment

EXPECTED OUTCOMES

- Maintain normal pulmonary function.
- Describe measures to minimize elevations in body temperature.
- Identify a schedule for taking her medication that will facilitate compliance with the regimen.

- Describe manifestations that should be reported to the physician.

PLANNING AND IMPLEMENTATION

- Assess knowledge and understanding of pneumonia and its effects.
- Assist to develop a medication schedule that coordinates with normal daily routine.
- Teach about the following:
  a. Importance of avoiding use of a cough suppressant except at night to facilitate rest
  b. Ways to increase fluid intake to reduce fever and maintain thin mucus for easy expectoration
  c. Beneficial effects of rest, especially during the acute phase of her illness
  d. Safe use of aspirin and acetaminophen to reduce fever
  e. Importance of taking all prescribed medication doses as scheduled
  f. Common side effects of penicillin V and their management
  g. Early manifestations of penicillin allergy that necessitate stopping the medication and notifying the physician
  h. Signs of complications of pneumonia or worsening pneumonia to report.

EVALUATION

The sputum culture confirms *S. pneumoniae* as the cause of Mrs. O'Neal's pneumonia. When she returns for her follow-up appointment, she reports that she began to feel better after 2 days on the penicillin and returned to work the following Monday. Her examination reveals good breath sounds throughout with no adventitious sounds. The follow-up sputum culture is free of pathogens.

CRITICAL THINKING IN THE NURSING PROCESS

1. Do any of the factors identified in the case study increase Mrs. O'Neal's risk for acute bacterial pneumonia?
2. Mrs. O'Neal's WBC differential showed increased neutrophil and band counts. Describe the reason for and effect of this change.
3. Even though Mrs. O'Neal has no history of medication allergies, anaphylactic shock remains a potential risk. Describe the sequence of events leading to anaphylactic shock, its initial symptoms, and immediate nursing interventions.
4. Had Mrs. O'Neal required hospitalization to treat her acute pneumonia, interruption of her usual activities and responsibilities could lead to anxiety. Develop a care plan for this situation, using the nursing diagnosis *Ineffective Role Performance* related to hospitalization.

See Evaluating Your Response in Appendix C.

---

primarily by contact with respiratory secretions. Other potential sources of the infection are through direct contact with an infected person or contaminated object, and exposure of the eyes or mucous membranes to respiratory secretions (CDC, 2004). Contact with contaminated water or sewage may transmit the disease, suggesting fecal–oral transmission as well (Kasper et al., 2005).

The virus infects cells of the respiratory tract, leading to surface necrosis and sloughing of pneumocytes in the alveolar spaces and formation of hyaline membranes (a fibrin and protein "film" that interferes with gas exchange within the alveoli). The alveolar damage is accompanied by inflammation of interstitial pulmonary tissues with infiltration by lymphocytes and monocytes. The virus also is found in the blood, urine, and feces.

Manifestations and Complications

The incubation period for SARS is generally 2 to 7 days, although it may be as long as 10 days in some people. Fever higher than 100.4°F (38°C) is typically the initial manifestation of the disease. The high fever may be accompanied by chills, headache, malaise, and muscle aches. After 1 to 2 days, respiratory manifestations of SARS develop, including nonproductive cough, shortness of breath, dyspnea, and possible hypoxemia. Respiratory symptoms may worsen, progressing to respiratory distress, during the second week of the illness.

Although the majority of people with SARS recover, up to 20% of affected clients require intubation and mechanical ventilation (see Chapter 39 ∞). Acute respiratory distress syndrome (ARDS) or multiorgan dysfunction (see Chapter 11 ∞) may develop. The overall mortality rate for SARS is about 11%. The disease is less severe in children than in adults (Kasper et al., 2005).

INTERDISCIPLINARY CARE

Prompt identification of SARS, infection control measures, and reporting of the disease are vital to control this potentially fatal disease. Healthcare providers and public health personnel should report cases of SARS to state and local health departments.

Diagnosis

Diagnostic testing for SARS may include the following:

- *Serology tests* (including enzyme-linked immunosorbent assay [ELISA] or immunofluorescence tests) for antibodies to the coronavirus may performed, but often are undetectable during the acute stage of the illness.
- *Reverse-transcriptase polymerase chain reaction (RT-PCR)* testing of respiratory and blood samples provides a rapid mechanism for identifying the virus, but only about 33% of early samples are positive.
- *Chest x-ray* may be normal or show interstitial infiltrates in a focal or generalized patchy pattern. In late stages of SARS, consolidation may be evident.
- *Pulse oximetry (oxygen saturation)* often shows hypoxemia in the respiratory phase of the illness.
- *CBC* often demonstrates a low lymphocyte count early in the disease. Leukopenia and thrombocytopenia may develop at the peak of the respiratory illness.
- *Creatinine phosphokinase (CPK or CK), ALT,* and *AST* levels may be markedly increased in SARS.
- *Sputum specimen* is obtained. Gram stain and culture are performed on the specimen to rule out other causes of pneumonia.
- *Blood culture* may be done to identify possible bacteremia.

Medications

At this time, no medications have been shown to be consistently effective in treating SARS. Antibiotic and/or antiviral therapy targeted at community-acquired forms of pneumonia may be administered if the diagnosis is unclear.

Infection Control

Because healthcare workers are at risk for developing SARS after caring for infected clients, infection control precautions should be immediately instituted when SARS is suspected. Standard precautions (see Appendix A ∞) are implemented along with contact and airborne precautions. The CDC (2005) recommends hand hygiene, gown, gloves, eye protection, and an N95 respirator to prevent transmission of SARS in healthcare settings.

When clients with SARS are managed in the community, they are advised to remain home for 10 days after the fever has resolved and until respiratory symptoms are absent or minimal. Members of the household are advised to wash hands frequently or use alcohol-based hand rubs. The client is advised to cover the mouth and nose with tissue when coughing or sneezing and to wear a surgical mask during close contact with uninfected people. Sharing of utensils, towels, and bedding should be avoided. Routine cleaning (e.g., washing with soap and hot water) is adequate to disinfect objects and no special precautions are necessary for disposing of waste.

Treatments

Care of the client with SARS is supportive. Oxygen may be administered to treat hypoxemia. Intubation and mechanical ventilation may be required if respiratory failure or ARDS develops.

NURSING CARE

Nursing care of the client with SARS focuses on preventing spread of the disease to others and providing respiratory support.

Health Promotion

Use respiratory and contact infection control precautions in addition to standard precautions when caring for all clients with suspected SARS to prevent spread of the disease to healthcare workers or other clients.

Assessment

Focused assessment data for the client with suspected SARS include the following. For more complete respiratory assessment, see Chapter 36 ∞.

- *Health History:* Current symptoms, including fever, malaise, shortness of breath, and cough; onset of symptoms; recent international travel or exposure to a person known to have SARS.
- *Physical Assessment:* Vital signs including temperature; respiratory status, including respiratory rate, depth, and effort; presence of cough; adventitious lung sounds.

Nursing Diagnoses and Interventions

The client with SARS poses a risk for spread of the infection to healthcare workers and others. In addition, while many people with this disease experience only mild symptoms and recover fully and uneventfully, others develop severe respiratory distress and may require significant respiratory support. Gas exchange may be impaired, leading to significant hypoxemia. In addition to the nursing diagnoses discussed in the previous section on pneumonia, *Impaired Gas Exchange* and *Risk for Infection* are priority nursing diagnoses.

Impaired Gas Exchange

SARS causes hypoxemia of varying degrees in affected clients. Significant hypoxemia may necessitate intubation and mechanical ventilation to support cellular function until recovery occurs.

- Monitor vital signs, color, oxygen saturation, and ABGs. Assess for manifestations such as anxiety or apprehension, restlessness, confusion, lethargy, or complaints of headache. *These assessment data alert the nurse and care providers to potential hypoxemia or hypercapnia due to impaired gas exchange.*

PRACTICE ALERT
Promptly report signs of respiratory distress, including tachypnea, tachycardia, nasal flaring, use of accessory muscles, intercostal retractions, cyanosis, increasing restlessness, anxiety, or decreased level of consciousness (LOC). These may be early manifestations of respiratory failure and inability to maintain ventilatory effort.

- Promptly report worsening ABGs and oxygen saturation levels. *Close assessment of these values allows timely intervention as needed.*
- Maintain oxygen therapy and mechanical ventilation as ordered. Hyperoxygenate prior to suctioning. *Oxygen and mechanical ventilation support alveolar gas exchange. Hyperoxygenation prior to suctioning reduces the degree of hypoxemia that occurs during suctioning.*
- Place in Fowler's or high Fowler's position. *Sitting positions decrease pressure on the diaphragm and chest, improving lung ventilation and decreasing the work of breathing.*
- Minimize activities and energy expenditures by assisting with activities of daily living (ADLs), spacing procedures and activities, and allowing uninterrupted rest periods. *Rest is vital to reduce oxygen and energy demands.*

PRACTICE ALERT
Avoid sedatives and respiratory depressant drugs unless mechanically ventilated. These medications can further depress the respiratory drive, worsening respiratory failure.

- If intubation and mechanical ventilation are necessary, explain the procedure and its purpose to the client and family, providing reassurance that this *temporary* measure improves oxygenation and reduces the work of breathing. Alert that talking is not possible while the endotracheal tube is in place, and establish a means of communication. *Thorough explanation is important to relieve anxiety.*

See the section in Chapter 39 ∞ on respiratory failure for more information about caring for a client who is intubated and mechanically ventilated.

Risk for Infection

The spread of SARS is a risk both in the healthcare facility and the community in which the client resides. Respiratory and contract precautions are recommended to prevent the spread of SARS via respiratory secretions or contact with the virus.

- Place the client in a private room with airflow control that prevents air within the room from circulating into the hall-

way or other rooms. A negative flow room in which air is diluted by at least six fresh-air exchanges per hour is recommended. *A negative flow room and multiple fresh-air exchanges dilute the concentration of virus within the room and prevent its spread to adjacent areas.*

- Use standard precautions and respiratory and contact isolation techniques as recommended by the CDC, including wearing respirators, gowns, and eye protection when caring for clients with SARS. *These measures are important to prevent the spread of SARS to others.*
- Discuss the reasons for and importance of respiratory and contact isolation procedures during treatment. *Maintenance of infection control precautions during and immediately following the febrile and respiratory phases of SARS is vital to prevent its spread to healthcare workers and the community.*
- Place a mask on the client when transporting to other parts of the facility for diagnostic or treatment procedures. *Covering the client's nose and mouth during transport minimizes air contamination and the risk to visitors and personnel.*
- Inform all personnel having contact with the client of the diagnosis. *This allows personnel to take appropriate precautions.*
- Assist visitors to mask prior to entering the room. *Providing visitors with appropriate masks or respirators reduces their risk of infection.*
- Teach the client how to limit transmitting the disease to others:
  a. Always cough and expectorate into tissues.
  b. Dispose of tissues properly, placing them in a closed bag.
  c. Wear a mask if sneezing or unable to control respiratory secretions.
  d. Do not share eating utensils, towels, bedding, or other objects with others, because this disease may also be spread by contact with contaminated objects.

Teaching appropriate precautions helps prevent the spread of SARS to others while allowing as much freedom from restraints as possible.

Community-Based Care

Many clients with SARS experience only mild symptoms and are appropriately cared for in the community. Teaching about home care and infection control precautions is vital to prevent spread of this disease to the community. Include the following topics when teaching for home care:

- The disease, its origin, and how it is spread
- Manifestations of impaired respiratory status to report to the physician
- Preventing spread of the disease to others:
  - Cover the mouth and nose with tissues when coughing or sneezing. Personally dispose of tissues in a paper bag or the garbage. Wear a surgical mask during close contact with other members of the household.
  - Limit interactions outside the home; do not go to work, school, or other public areas until you have been free of fever for 10 days and your respiratory symptoms are resolving.
  - Remind all members of the household to wash hands (or use an alcohol-based hand sanitizer) frequently, particularly after direct contact with body fluids.

- Do not share eating utensils, towels, or bedding with others. These items can be cleaned with soap and hot water between uses. Clean contaminated surfaces with a household disinfectant.
- Monitoring uninfected members of the household for signs of the illness (Instruct to report fever or respiratory symptoms to the physician.)

THE CLIENT WITH LUNG ABSCESS

A **lung abscess** is a localized area of lung destruction or necrosis and pus formation. The most common cause of lung abscess is aspiration and resulting pneumonia. Risk factors, therefore, are those for aspiration: decreased LOC due to anesthesia, injury or disease of the central nervous system (CNS), seizure, excessive sedation, or alcohol abuse; swallowing disorders; dental caries; and debilitation secondary to cancer or chronic disease. Lung abscess also may occur as a complication of some types of pneumonia, including those due to *S. aureus, Klebsiella,* and *Legionella.*

Pathophysiology and Manifestations

A lung abscess forms after lung tissue becomes consolidated (i.e., after alveoli become filled with fluid, pus, and microorganisms). Consolidated tissue becomes necrotic. This necrotic process can spread to involve the entire bronchopulmonary segment and progress proximally until it ruptures into a bronchus. With rupture, the contents of the abscess empty into the bronchus, leaving a cavity filled with air and fluid, a process known as *cavitation.* If purulent material from the abscess is not expectorated, the infection may spread, leading to diffuse pneumonia or a syndrome similar to acute respiratory distress syndrome (discussed in Chapter 39 ∞).

Manifestations of lung abscess typically develop about 2 weeks after the precipitating event (aspiration, pneumonia, and so on). Their onset may be either acute or insidious. Early symptoms are those of pneumonia: productive cough, chills and fever, pleuritic chest pain, malaise, and anorexia. The temperature may be significantly elevated, 103°F (39.4°C) or higher. When the abscess ruptures, the client may expectorate large amounts of foul-smelling, purulent, and possibly blood-streaked sputum. Breath sounds are diminished, and crackles may be noted in the region of the abscess. A dull percussion tone is also present.

INTERDISCIPLINARY CARE

The diagnosis of lung abscess usually is based on the history and presentation. The CBC may indicate leukocytosis. Sputum culture may not show the organism involved unless rupture occurs. Chest x-ray shows a thick-walled, solitary cavity with surrounding consolidation, although differentiating lung abscess from consolidation can be difficult until cavitation occurs.

Lung abscess is treated with antibiotic therapy, usually intravenous clindamycin (Cleocin), amoxicillin-clavulanate (Augmentin), or penicillin (Tierney et al., 2005). Postural drainage may be ordered to relieve obstruction and promote drainage. In some cases, bronchoscopy is used to drain the ab-

scess. If the pleural space becomes involved, a chest tube (*tube thoracostomy*) may be used to drain the abscess. See the section on pneumothorax later in this chapter for further discussion of chest tubes.

NURSING CARE

Although most clients with lung abscess recover fully with appropriate antibiotic treatment, rupture and drainage of the abscess into a bronchus is a frightening experience. Nursing care needs of the client relate primarily to maintaining a patent airway and adequate gas exchange. The following nursing diagnoses may be appropriate for the client with lung abscess:

- *Risk for Ineffective Airway Clearance* related to large amounts of purulent drainage in bronchi
- *Impaired Gas Exchange* related to necrotic and consolidated lung tissue
- *Hyperthermia* related to infectious process
- *Anxiety* related to copious amounts of purulent sputum.

Health education for the client and family focuses on the importance of completing the prescribed antibiotic therapy. Most lung abscesses are successfully treated with antibiotics; however, treatment may last up to 1 month or more. Emphasize the importance of completing the entire course of therapy to eliminate the infecting organisms. Teach about the medication, including its name, dose, and desired and adverse effects. Stress the need to contact the physician if symptoms do not improve or if they become worse. Infection from lung abscess can spread not only to lung and pleural tissue but systemically, causing sepsis. If postural drainage is ordered, teach the client and family how to perform this procedure. When procedures such as bronchoscopy or thoracostomy are performed to drain the abscess, provide preoperative teaching and instruction on postoperative care.

THE CLIENT WITH TUBERCULOSIS

Tuberculosis (TB) is a chronic, recurrent infectious disease that usually affects the lungs, although any organ can be affected. This disease, caused by *Mycobacterium tuberculosis,* is uncommon in the United States, especially among young adults of European descent.

M. tuberculosis is a relatively slow-growing, slender, rod-shaped, acid-fast organism with a waxy outer capsule, which increases its resistance to destruction. Although the lungs are usually infected, tuberculosis can involve other organs as well. It is transmitted by *droplet nuclei,* airborne droplets produced when an infected person coughs, sneezes, speaks, or sings. The tiny droplets can remain suspended in air for several hours. Infection may develop when a susceptible host breathes in air containing droplet nuclei and the contaminated particle eludes the normal defenses of the upper respiratory tract to reach the alveoli.

Incidence and Prevalence

The incidence of tuberculosis fell steadily until the mid-1980s, thanks to improved sanitation, surveillance, and treatment of people with active disease. The late 1980s and early 1990s saw a resurgence of the disease, attributed primarily to the HIV/AIDS epidemic, the emergence of multiple-drug-resistant (MDR) strains of TB, and social factors such as immigration, poverty, homelessness, and drug abuse. Today, the number of people affected by TB in the United States continues to decline, with a total of 14,093 cases reported in 2005, the lowest number recorded since national reporting began in 1953 (CDC, 2006b). This decline can be attributed to TB-control programs that emphasize promptly identifying new cases and initiating and completing appropriate therapy.

Worldwide, TB continues to be a significant health problem, with an estimated 2 billion people (one-third of the world's population) infected by *M. tuberculosis*. An estimated 9 million cases of TB develop annually, with the vast majority (95%) occurring in developing countries of Asia, Africa, the Middle East, and Latin America. TB accounts for an estimated 2 million deaths each year (CDC, 2006c).

Today, TB in the United States is a disease primarily affecting immigrants, those infected with HIV, and disadvantaged populations. See the Focus on Cultural Diversity box on the primary populations affected by TB. Poor urban areas are hit the hardest—areas that are also affected by the epidemics of injection drug use, homelessness, malnutrition, and poor living conditions. Overcrowded institutions also contribute to the spread of TB; transmission in hospitals, homeless shelters, drug treatment centers, prisons, and residential facilities has been documented. People with altered immune function, including older adults (see the box on page 1282) and people with AIDS are at particular risk for tuberculosis. Some strains of *M. tuberculosis* have become resistant to the primary drugs used to treat the disease (isoniazid and rifampin), with the number of MDR cases of TB increased by 13.3% between 2004 and 2005 (CDC, 2006a).

> ### FOCUS ON CULTURAL DIVERSITY
> **Tuberculosis**
>
> - The TB case rate for foreign-born U.S. residents is 8.7 times higher than that for people born in the United States (CDC, 2006b).
> - Asians and Pacific Islanders living in the United States have the highest case rates, nearly 20 times higher than that for whites.
> - Case rates for blacks and Hispanics in the United States are 7 to 8 times that for whites.

FAST FACTS
- Worldwide, approximately 39% of identified *M. tuberculosis* strains are MDR, demonstrating resistance to at least isoniazid and rifampin.
- Of MDR tuberculosis strains identified worldwide, 7% are extensively drug resistant (XDR). XDR tuberculosis is resistant to isoniazid and rifampin, as well as at least three of the six main classes of second-line tuberculosis drugs (CDC, 2006a).
- The prevalence of MDR and XDR tuberculosis in the United States is lower, with 1.6% of cases reported from 1993 through 2004 identified as MDR. Of these, 4.1% were resistant to three or more classes of antituberculosis drugs, qualifying as XDR tuberculosis (CDC, 2006a).

Risk Factors

The risk for infection by *M. tuberculosis* is affected by characteristics of the infectious person, the extent of air contamination, duration of exposure, and susceptibility of the host. The number of microbes in the sputum, frequency and force of coughing, and behaviors such as covering the mouth when coughing affect the production of droplet nuclei. In a small, closed, or poorly ventilated space, droplet nuclei become more concentrated, increasing the risk of exposure. Prolonged contact, such as living in the same household, increases the risk. Less-than-optimal immune function, a problem for people in lower socioeconomic groups, injection drug users, the homeless, alcoholics, and people with HIV infection, increases the susceptibility of the host.

Pathophysiology
Pulmonary Tuberculosis
Minute droplet nuclei containing one to three bacilli that elude upper airway defense systems to enter the lungs implant in an alveolus or respiratory bronchiole, usually in an upper lobe. As the bacteria multiply, they cause a local inflammatory response. The inflammatory response brings neutrophils and macrophages to the site. These phagocytic cells surround and engulf the bacilli, isolating them and preventing their spread. *M. tuberculosis* continues to slowly multiply; some enter the lymphatic system to stimulate a cellular-mediated immune response. (See Chapter 12 ∞ for a review of immune responses.) Neutrophils and macrophages isolate the bacteria but cannot destroy them. A granulomatous lesion called a *tubercle*, a sealed-off colony of bacilli, is formed. Within the tubercle, infected tissue dies, forming a cheeselike center, a process called *caseation necrosis*.

If the immune response is adequate, scar tissue develops around the tubercle, and the bacilli remain encapsulated. These lesions eventually calcify and are visible on x-ray. The client, while infected by *M. tuberculosis*, does not develop tuberculosis disease. If the immune response is inadequate to contain the bacilli, the disease of tuberculosis can develop. Occasionally, the infection can progress, leading to extensive destruction of lung tissue. In *primary tuberculosis*, granulomatous tissue may erode into a bronchus or into a blood vessel, allowing the disease to spread throughout the lung or other organs. This severe form of tuberculosis is uncommon in adults (Kasper et al., 2005).

A previously healed tuberculosis lesion may be reactivated. *Reactivation tuberculosis* occurs when the immune system is suppressed due to age, disease, or use of immunosuppressive drugs. The extent of lung disease can vary from small lesions to extensive cavitation of lung tissue. Tubercles rupture, spreading bacilli into the airways to form satellite lesions and produce tuberculosis pneumonia. Without treatment, massive lung involvement can lead to death, or a more chronic process of tubercle formation and cavitation may

NURSING CARE OF THE OLDER ADULT　Tuberculosis

The prevalence of active tuberculosis is significantly higher among older Caucasian adults in the United States than it is in young adults (Kasper et al., 2005). Of cases among older adults, approximately 90% occur due to reactivation of a dormant bacterium. Older adults are at increased risk for reactivation tuberculosis due to age-related decreases in cell-mediated immunity. Chronic illnesses, poor nutrition, gastrectomy, alcoholism, or the long-term use of steroids and immunosuppressive agents may also reactivate dormant TB lesions.

Presenting symptoms of tuberculosis in the older adult are often vague, including coughing, weight loss, anorexia, or periodic fevers. These signs and symptoms should not be dismissed as a normal part of aging.

Residents of nursing homes are at increased risk for acquiring tuberculosis because of group living. Yearly tuberculin skin testing with purified protein derivative (PPD) is often required by state health departments. If the initial test is negative, a repeat PPD in 1 to 2 weeks is recommended. This improves sensitivity to the test so that silent cases of tuberculosis are not missed. A chest x-ray and sputum culture for acid-fast bacilli are obtained if the PPD is positive.

Successful treatment for tuberculosis includes taking at least two drugs for at least 6 to 9 months to totally eradicate the organism. Older adults usually do not develop drug-resistant forms of tuberculosis, because they acquired the disease prior to emergence of drug-resistant strains.

Assessing for Home Care

Community-dwelling older adults are susceptible to tuberculosis as well as those in care facilities. The older adult with respiratory symptoms often is treated presumptively for pneumonia, without a sputum smear and Gram stain. Older adults living in the community may not have had a tuberculin test or chest x-ray for many years.

Assess risk factors for tuberculosis:
- General health and nutritional status, including intake of specific nutrients such as vitamin D (lack of vitamin D is associated with a higher risk of developing active tuberculosis)
- Presence of a chronic disease such as silicosis, diabetes, alcoholism, or HIV infection; past history of a gastrectomy
- Past history of a positive tuberculin test that now has converted to negative
- Medications such as corticosteroids or other immunosuppressive drugs.

Assess living and social situation:
- Natural light and ventilation in the home
- Access to clean water, cooking facilities, grocery stores, and other services
- Possible exposure to infected people, for example, sharing a household with someone with active TB, crowded living facilities, homelessness, frequent participation in senior activities,

volunteer work in residential care facilities or other institutional settings
- Access to health care

Tuberculosis is typically treated in the community; hospitalization or institutionalization rarely is necessary or desirable. For the older adult being treated for active TB in the community, assess:
- Knowledge and understanding of the disease and the prescribed treatment regimen
- Mental status and ability to follow prescribed regimen and precautions to avoid exposing others to the disease
- Transportation and ability to access healthcare services on a regular basis
- Financial resources to complete treatment and follow-up care
- Need for home health or social services to ensure adequate treatment.

Health Education for the Client and Family

Teaching focuses on improving the older adult's ability to self-manage the disease and treatment. Teach about tuberculosis and how it is spread. Emphasize the importance of taking all medications as prescribed and complying with follow-up appointments and testing. Discuss the importance of:
- Using disposable tissues to contain respiratory secretions, especially during the first 2 weeks of treatment when the disease may be transmitted to others
- Avoiding exposure to crowds or people with infectious diseases
- Eating a well-balanced diet with adequate nutrients
- Getting adequate rest, sleep, and exercise to maintain good general health
- Ensuring that housemates or others having frequent contact with the client are tested and receive prophylactic treatment if indicated.

Teach about possible side effects of the prescribed medications and the importance of reporting these to healthcare providers:
- Peripheral neuropathy (numbness, tingling, or a burning sensation of the extremities) may occur with isoniazid (INH). Pyridoxine (vitamin B$_6$) often is prescribed to prevent this adverse effect.
- Both INH and rifampin may cause hepatitis. Avoid alcohol while taking these drugs, and report any manifestations such as nausea and anorexia, jaundice, a change in urine or stool color, or pain in the upper right quadrant.
- Rifampin may cause an orange-red coloration of saliva and urine.
- Streptomycin can affect hearing and balance; promptly report any changes, because they may be irreversible.
- Ethambutol may affect red-green color discrimination and visual acuity. Use caution when driving or walking in unfamiliar areas and promptly report any vision changes.

result. People with chronic disease continue to spread *M. tuberculosis* into the environment, potentially infecting others. *Pathophysiology Illustrated: Tuberculosis* on pages 1284–1285 illustrates the pathogenesis of tuberculosis.

Clients with HIV disease are at high risk for developing active tuberculosis, due to primary infection or reactivation. HIV infection suppresses cellular immunity, which is vital to limiting the replication and spread of *M. tuberculosis*.

FAST FACTS

- The organism causing tuberculosis, *Mycobacterium tuberculosis*, is spread through droplet nuclei that remain suspended in air for several hours.
- A tubercle is a sealed-off colony of bacilli; if it ruptures, organisms spread, leading to tuberculosis pneumonia.
- Primary or secondary tuberculosis lesions may affect other body systems such as the kidneys, genitalia, bone, and brain.

MANIFESTATIONS AND COMPLICATIONS The initial infection causes few symptoms and typically goes unnoticed until the tuberculin test becomes positive or calcified lesions are seen on chest x-ray. Manifestations of primary progressive or reactivation tuberculosis often develop insidiously and are initially nonspecific (see the box below). Fatigue, weight loss, anorexia, low-grade afternoon fever, and night sweats are common. A dry cough develops, which later becomes productive of purulent and/or blood-tinged sputum. It is often at this stage that the client seeks medical attention.

Tuberculosis empyema and bronchopleural fistula are the most serious complications of pulmonary tuberculosis. When a tuberculosis lesion ruptures, bacilli may contaminate the pleural space. Rupture also may allow air to enter the pleural space from the lung, causing pneumothorax.

Extrapulmonary Tuberculosis

When primary disease or reactivation allows live bacilli to enter the bronchi, the disease may spread through the blood and lymph system to other organs. These distant disease metastases may produce an active lesion, or they may become dormant and reactivate at a later time. Extrapulmonary tuberculosis is especially prevalent in people with HIV disease.

MILIARY TUBERCULOSIS *Miliary tuberculosis* results from hematogenous spread (through the blood) of the bacilli throughout the body. Miliary tuberculosis causes chills and fever, weakness, malaise, and progressive dyspnea. Multiple lesions evenly distributed throughout the lungs are noted on x-ray. The sputum rarely contains organisms. The bone marrow is usually involved, causing anemia, thrombocytopenia, and leukocytosis. Without appropriate treatment, the prognosis is poor.

GENITOURINARY TUBERCULOSIS The kidney and genitourinary tract are common extrapulmonary sites for tuberculosis. The organism spreads to the kidney through the blood, initiating an inflammatory process similar to that which occurs in the lungs. Reactivation can occur years after the original infection.

MANIFESTATIONS of Pulmonary Tuberculosis

- Fatigue
- Weight loss
- Anorexia
- Low-grade afternoon fever and night sweats
- Cough: initially dry, later productive of purulent and/or blood-tinged sputum

As the lesion then enlarges and caseates, a large portion of the renal parenchyma is destroyed. The infection then can spread to the rest of the urinary tract, including the ureters and bladder. Scarring and strictures commonly result. In men, the prostate, seminal vesicles, and epididymis may be involved. In women, tuberculosis may affect the fallopian tubes and ovaries.

Manifestations of genitourinary tuberculosis develop insidiously. Symptoms of a urinary tract infection, including malaise, dysuria, hematuria, and pyuria, develop. Flank pain may be present. Men may develop manifestations of epididymitis or prostatitis: perineal, sacral, or scrotal pain and tenderness; difficulty voiding; and fever. Women may have manifestations of pelvic inflammatory disease, impaired fertility, or ectopic pregnancy.

TUBERCULOSIS MENINGITIS Tuberculosis meningitis results when tuberculosis spreads to the subarachnoid space. In the United States, this complication most often affects older adults, usually from reactivation of latent disease. Manifestations develop gradually, with listlessness, irritability, anorexia, and fever. Headache and behavior changes are common early symptoms in the older adult. As the disease progresses, the headache increases in intensity, vomiting develops, and the level of consciousness decreases. Convulsions and coma may follow. Without appropriate treatment, neurologic effects may become permanent.

SKELETAL TUBERCULOSIS Tuberculosis of the bones and joints is most likely to occur during childhood, when bone epiphyses are open and their blood supply is rich. The organisms spread via the blood to vertebrae, the ends of long bones, and joints. Immune and inflammatory processes isolate the bacilli, and the disease often becomes evident years or decades later.

Tuberculous spondylitis usually involves the thoracic vertebrae, eroding vertebral bodies and causing them to collapse. Significant kyphosis develops, and the spinal cord may be compressed. The large, weight-bearing joints (hips and knees) are most often affected by tuberculous arthritis, although other joints may be affected, particularly if they have been previously damaged. The involved joint is painful, warm, and tender.

INTERDISCIPLINARY CARE

Tuberculosis was a major public health concern earlier in this century, before the development of effective sanitation measures and drug treatment. Developing drug-resistant strains, susceptibility of people with HIV disease, and inadequate access to health care for high-risk populations contribute to the continuing significance of tuberculosis as a significant public health threat. Interdisciplinary care, therefore, focuses on the following:

- Early detection
- Accurate diagnosis
- Effective disease treatment
- Preventing tuberculosis spread to others.

Hospitalization is rarely required to treat tuberculosis. With appropriate treatment, clients become noninfective to others fairly rapidly. However, a client with active tuberculosis may be admitted for a concurrent problem or a complication of the disease. Nurses and other healthcare workers are at risk for exposure if the disease has not yet been diagnosed. When a client

Pulmonary arteriole

Terminal bronchiole

Pulmonary venule

Alveolus

Alveolar duct

Alveolar macrophages

Tubercle bacillus

Infiltrating macrophage (not activated)

Pulmonary capillary

Infiltrating neutrophils

M. tuberculosis, a rod-shaped aerobic bacterium, is spread via droplet nuclei from an infected person to a susceptible host. Droplet nuclei are tiny droplets of respiratory secretions spread via coughing, sneezing, or speaking. When dried, they can remain suspended in air for several hours. Most inhaled bacilli are trapped in the upper airways; those reaching distal airways implant in the respiratory bronchioles and alveoli. Rarely, these tubercle bacilli multiply unchecked to cause primary tuberculosis. In most cases, activated alveolar macrophages ingest the bacilli. The bacilli may be destroyed; however, unique characteristics of the tuberculosis bacillus resist its destruction by the macrophage. The bacilli multiply within the macrophage, eventually killing the macrophage.

Bronchiole

Ingested tubercle bacillus

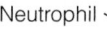

Early tubercle

Neutrophil

The dead macrophages lyse, releasing various chemotaxic factors into the bloodstream. Neutrophils and non-activated macrophages are attracted to the site. These phagocytic cells ingest the tubercule bacilli released from the lysed macrophages.

Caseous center

Tubercle bacilli

Activated
macrophages

Lymphocyte

After several weeks, a delayed hypersensitivity response to bacterial antigens destroys many of the macrophages. Concurrently, a cell-mediated immune response activates additional macrophages, which ingest and destroy the bacilli. The lysed macrophages and bacilli are surrounded by a mass of live, activated macrophages and lymphocytes. Scar (granulomatous) tissue forms, encapsulating the primary lesion. Most lesions calcify and are visible on x-ray. These lesions may remain dormant for a year or more (in some cases, many years) before being reactivated to produce secondary or reactivation tuberculosis.

When the immune and macrophage-activating responses are weakened by age or disease (e.g., HIV disease), the tuberculosis bacilli continue to multiply within the lesion. The caseous material at the center of the lesion liquefies, and the lesion grows.

Outer scar tissue
layer of mature
tubercle

Tubercle bacilli

Tuberculous cavity

Rupture of
bronchiole wall

Rupture of
capillary wall

The enlarging lesion damages surrounding bronchial walls and blood vessels. Granulomatous tissue surrounding the lesion can erode into a bronchus, forming an air-filling cavity. Within this cavity, the bacilli multiply, spreading into the airways and the environment via infected sputum. Bacilli multiply, spreading into the airways and the environment via infected sputum. Bacilli also spread via the blood and within macrophages to regional lymph nodes, and from there to many organs and tissues. Resulting extrapulmonary lesions evolve in the same sequence as pulmonary lesions.

with tuberculosis is institutionalized, maintain respiratory isolation to minimize the risk of infection to other clients and to the healthcare workers.

Noncompliance with prescribed treatment is a major problem in treating active tuberculosis: The client can continue transmitting the disease to others, and drug-resistant strains of bacteria can develop when treatment is incomplete. Tuberculosis must be reported to local and state public health departments; contacts are identified and examined. People who share living or work environments with the client are tested and receive prophylactic treatment. Continuing contact with clients who have active TB is vital to ensure effective cure.

Screening

The tuberculin test is used to screen for tuberculosis infection. A cellular, or delayed hypersensitivity, response to *M. tuberculosis* develops within 3 to 10 weeks after the infection. Injecting a small amount of *purified protein derivative (PPD)* of tuberculin any time thereafter activates this response, attracting macrophages to the area and causing a pronounced local inflammatory response. The amount of induration surrounding the injection site is used to determine infection (see Table 38–5 and Figure 38–7 ■). It is important to remember that a positive response indicates that infection and a cellular (T-cell) response have developed; however, it does not mean that active disease is present or that the client is infectious to others.

Several methods are currently available for tuberculin testing:

- *Intradermal PPD (Mantoux) test:* 0.1 mL of PPD (5 tuberculin units, or TU) is injected intradermally into the dorsal aspect of the forearm. This test is read within 48 to 72 hours (the peak reaction period) and recorded as the diameter of induration (raised area, not erythema) in millimeters.
- *Multiple-puncture (tine) test:* A multiple-puncture device is used to introduce tuberculin into the skin. This test is less accurate than other testing methods. A vesicular reaction is considered positive; any other reaction must be confirmed using a Mantoux test.

Figure 38–7 ■ *A,* Intradermal injection for tuberculin testing. *B,* The injection causes a local inflammatory response (wheal). *C,* Measurement of induration following tuberculin testing.

Although it is impractical and unnecessary to screen the entire population, the CDC recommend screening people in the following risk groups:

- People with or at high risk for HIV infection
- Close contacts of people who have or are suspected of having infectious TB

TABLE 38–5 Interpreting Tuberculin Test Results

AREA OF INDURATION	SIGNIFICANCE
Less than 5 mm	Negative response; does not rule out infection.
5 to 9 mm	Positive for people who: ■ Are in close contact with a client with infective TB. ■ Have an abnormal chest x-ray. ■ Have HIV infection or are immunocompromised. ■ Have an organ transplant. Negative for all others.
10 to 15 mm	Positive for people who have other risk factors: ■ Birth in a high-incidence country. ■ African American, Hispanic, Asian American in poverty areas. ■ Injection drug use. ■ Residence in a long-term care facility, correctional institution, residential care setting, homeless shelter. ■ Medical risk factors (e.g., malnutrition, diabetes, others).
Greater than 15 mm	Positive for all people.

- People with medical risk factors, such as silicosis, chronic malabsorption, end-stage renal failure, diabetes mellitus, immunosuppression, and hematologic and other malignancies
- People born in countries with a high prevalence of TB
- Medically underserved low-income populations, including racial and ethnic minorities
- Alcoholics and injection drug users
- Residents and staff of long-term residential facilities, such as long-term care facilities, correctional institutions, and mental health facilities.

False-negative responses are common in people who are immunosuppressed. A two-step procedure may be necessary to elicit a positive response. If the first test elicits a negative response, a second PPD test is given 1 week later. If the second test also is negative, the client either is free of infection or is *anergic* (unable to react to common antigens). This two-step procedure is recommended for long-term care residents and workers.

Diagnosis

A positive tuberculin test alone does not indicate active disease. Sputum tests for the bacillus and chest x-rays are routinely used to diagnose and evaluate active disease. A series of three consecutive early morning sputum specimens is typically examined for bacilli (see Procedure 36–1). Use special procedures or personal protective devices when obtaining sputum specimens. If possible, collect specimens in a room equipped with airflow control devices, ultraviolet light, or both. Alternatively, have the client step outside to collect the specimen. Wear a mask capable of filtering droplet nuclei when collecting sputum specimens. Aerosol therapy, percussion, and postural drainage may help the client produce sputum. Occasionally, endotracheal suctioning, bronchoscopy, or gastric lavage may be necessary to obtain a specimen. See the Diagnostic Tests box in Chapter 36 ∞ for nursing care related to bronchoscopy.

- *Sputum smear* is microscopically examined for *acid-fast bacilli. M. tuberculosis* resists decolorizing chemicals after staining. This property is called *acid fast*. The acid-fast smear provides a rapid indicator of the tubercle bacillus.
- *Sputum culture* positive for *M. tuberculosis* provides the definitive diagnosis. However, *M. tuberculosis* is slow growing, requiring 4 to 8 weeks before it can be detected using traditional culture techniques. Automated radiometric culture systems (such as Bactec) allow detection of *M. tuberculosis* in several days.
- Once the organism is detected, *sensitivity testing* is performed to identify appropriate drug therapy.
- *Polymerase chain reaction (PCR)* permits rapid detection of DNA from *M. tuberculosis.*
- *Chest x-ray* is ordered to diagnose and evaluate TB. Typical findings in pulmonary TB include dense lesions in the apical and posterior segments of the upper lobe and possible cavity formation.

Prior to initiating antituberculosis drug therapy, several additional diagnostic tests may be done to establish baseline data for monitoring potential adverse effects of the drugs.

- *Liver function tests* are obtained prior to treatment with isoniazid (INH) because this drug is hepatotoxic.

- A thorough *vision examination* is done prior to treatment with ethambutol, a commonly used antituberculosis medication. Optic neuritis is a potential adverse effect of this drug. Periodic eye examinations are scheduled during the course of therapy.
- *Audiometric testing* is performed before streptomycin therapy is initiated. Ototoxicity is a significant adverse effect of streptomycin and other aminoglycoside antibiotics. Hearing also is evaluated periodically during the course of therapy to detect any hearing loss.

Medications

Chemotherapeutic medications are used both to prevent and treat tuberculosis infection. Goals of the pharmacologic treatment of TB are to:

- Make the disease noncommunicable to others.
- Reduce symptoms of the disease.
- Effect a cure in the shortest possible time.

Prophylactic treatment is used to prevent active tuberculosis. Clients with a recent skin test conversion from negative to positive are often started on prophylactic therapy, especially when other risk factors are present. Prophylactic therapy also is used for people in close household contact with a person whose sputum is positive for bacilli. Single-drug therapy is effective for prophylactic treatment, whereas treatment of active disease always involves two or more chemotherapeutic medications. For adults, INH, 300 mg per day for a period of 6 to 12 months, is commonly used to prevent active TB.

When INH prophylaxis is contraindicated, bacilli Calmette-Guérin (BCG) vaccine may be prescribed. This vaccine is widely used in developing countries. BCG is made from an attenuated strain of *M. bovis,* a closely related bacillus that causes tuberculosis in cattle. In the United States, BCG vaccine is recommended only for infants, children, and healthcare workers with a negative tuberculin test who are repeatedly exposed to untreated or ineffectively treated people with active disease. After vaccination with BCG, a positive reaction to tuberculin testing is common. Periodic chest x-rays may be required for screening purposes.

The tuberculosis bacillus mutates readily to drug-resistant forms when only one anti-infective agent is used. Active disease is always treated with concurrent use of at least two antibacterial medications to which the organism is sensitive. The primary antituberculosis drugs can prevent development of resistance because all act by different mechanisms. However, the organism is protected within the tubercle, and 6 or more months of treatment is necessary to eradicate it.

Newly diagnosed tuberculosis is typically treated with an initial regimen of four oral antitubercular drugs, isoniazid, rifampin, and pyrazinamide, and ethambutol daily (or several times per week on a decreasing schedule of frequency) for the first 2 months of treatment. This initial regimen is followed by at least 4 additional months of therapy with isoniazid and rifampin, given daily, twice per week, or weekly. In the presence of HIV infection, treatment is continued for at least 9 months. The most common antituberculosis drugs are outlined in Table 38–6; their nursing implications are outlined in the Medication Administration box on pages 1288–1289.

TABLE 38–6 Antituberculosis Medications

DRUG AND DOSAGE	ADVERSE EFFECTS	NURSING IMPLICATIONS
Isoniazid (INH), oral: 300 mg daily or 900 mg one, two, or three times weekly	Peripheral neuropathy Hepatitis	Administer pyridoxine (vitamin B$_6$) concurrently. Monitor liver function studies (AST and ALT); avoid other hepatotoxins.
Rifampin (RMP), oral: 600 mg daily or two or three times weekly	Hepatitis Flulike syndrome; fever	As for INH. Do not miss or skip doses; flulike syndrome and fever occur when drug is resumed.
	Colors body fluids—including sweat, urine, saliva, tears, and cerebrospinal fluid (CSF)—orange-red	Contact lenses may become discolored and should not be worn.
Pyrazinamide (PZA), oral: 1 to 2 g daily; or 2 to 4 g twice weekly	Hyperuricemia Hepatotoxicity	Monitor uric acid levels. Monitor AST and ALT; avoid other hepatotoxins.
Ethambutol (EMB), oral: 800 mg to 1600 mg daily; or 2 to 4 g twice weekly	Optic neuritis	Monitor red-green color discrimination and visual acuity.
Streptomycin (SM), intramuscular: 15 mg/kg, up to 1 g daily; or 25 to 30 mg/kg twice weekly	Ototoxicity, vertigo Nephrotoxicity	Have periodic audiometric examinations conducted. Monitor renal function studies, including BUN and serum creatinine.

If a drug-resistant strain is suspected, therapy is tailored to the resistance. In some cases, four or more anti-infective drugs may be used.

Antitubercular medications have many adverse and toxic effects. Close monitoring during therapy is necessary. Most have some degree of, or risk for, hepatotoxicity. For this reason, clients should avoid using alcohol and other drugs (such as acetaminophen) or chemicals that can damage the liver. Baseline liver and renal function studies are done prior to initiating therapy. Audiometric testing also may be done before treatment is started, because several commonly used medications can affect hearing. Regular visits to a healthcare provider are necessary to evaluate regularly for adverse effects. Although none of these drugs have been proved to be teratogenic, potential adverse effects on the fetus are weighed against the benefit to the mother before they are prescribed during pregnancy.

Compliance with the prescribed regimen also is evaluated during follow-up visits. The urine can be examined for color changes characteristic of rifampin and tested for metabolites of INH. When compliance is a problem, medications are administered under direct supervision. Twice-weekly therapy is more cost effective in this instance, with a public health nurse watching the client take and swallow the prescribed medication.

MEDICATION ADMINISTRATION **Antituberculosis Drugs**

ISONIAZID (INH, LANIAZID, NYDRAZID)

Isoniazid is the drug of choice for tuberculosis prophylaxis and a first-line drug for treating active disease. It is effective against both intracellular and extracellular organisms. Isoniazid is used alone as a prophylactic medication and in combination with rifampin, ethambutol, or both. A fixed-dose combination form with 150 mg of INH and 300 mg of rifampin (Rifamate) is available as well.

Nursing Responsibilities

- Administer on an empty stomach 1 hour before or 2 hours after meals for maximal effect if tolerated; may be given with meals to reduce gastrointestinal effects.
- Monitor for adverse effects:
  - a. Numbness and tingling of the extremities (most likely to occur in malnourished, alcoholic, or diabetic clients)
  - b. Hepatotoxicity, as evidenced by abnormal liver function studies and scleral jaundice
  - c. Hypersensitivity reactions, such as rash, drug fever, or evidence of anemia, bruising, bleeding, or infection related to agranulocytosis.
- Isoniazid interferes with the metabolism of diazepam (Valium), phenytoin (Dilantin), and carbamazepine. Doses of these drugs may need to be reduced to prevent toxicity.

Health Education for the Client and Family

- Take the medication as prescribed for the entire treatment period to prevent incomplete eradication of the bacteria and development of resistant strains.
- Take the medication on an empty stomach. If nausea and vomiting occur, take with meals.
- If anorexia, nausea, vomiting, and jaundice (yellowing of the skin and the whites of the eyes) develop, notify your doctor immediately.
- Take pyridoxine as prescribed to prevent peripheral neuropathy.
- Avoid alcohol and other agents that may be harmful to the liver.
- Notify your doctor if you develop signs of an allergic reaction, such as rash, fever, easy bruising, bleeding gums, or fatigue.

MEDICATION ADMINISTRATION Antituberculosis Drugs (continued)

■ Use measures to prevent pregnancy while taking INH; this drug may be harmful to the developing fetus.

RIFAMPIN (RIFADIN, RIMACTANE)

Rifampin is commonly used in combination with INH and other antitubercular drugs. It is relatively low in toxicity, although it can cause hepatitis, a flulike immune response, and, rarely, renal failure. Rifampin stimulates the microsomal enzymes of the liver, increasing the rate of metabolism of many drugs and decreasing their effectiveness.

Nursing Responsibilities

■ Administer on an empty stomach.
■ Monitor CBC, liver function studies, and renal function studies for evidence of toxicity.
■ Rifampin reduces the effect of oral contraceptives, quinidine, corticosteroids, warfarin, methadone, digoxin, and hypoglycemics. Monitor for the effectiveness of these drugs.

Health Education for the Client and Family

■ Rifampin causes body fluids, including sweat, urine, saliva, and tears, to turn red-orange. This is not harmful. Avoid wearing soft contact lenses because they may be permanently stained.
■ Aspirin may interfere with rifampin absorption and should not be taken concurrently.
■ Fever, flulike symptoms, excessive fatigue, sore throat, or unusual bleeding may indicate an adverse reaction to the drug and should be reported to your doctor.

PYRAZINAMIDE (TEBRAZID)

Pyrazinamide typically is given with INH and rifampin for the first 2 months of tuberculosis treatment. Concurrent use of pyrazinamide allows a shorter course of therapy. As with many of the antitubercular agents, pyrazinamide is toxic to the liver. Its other principal adverse effect is hyperuricemia. Gout, however, rarely develops.

Nursing Responsibilities

■ Administer with meals to reduce gastrointestinal side effects.
■ Monitor liver function studies and serum uric acid levels. Notify the physician if changes are noted.

Health Education for the Client and Family

■ Notify your doctor if you develop loss of appetite, nausea, vomiting, jaundice, or symptoms of gout (a painful, red, hot, swollen joint, often the great toe or elbow).
■ While taking this drug, avoid using alcohol or other substances that may be harmful to the liver.

ETHAMBUTOL (MYAMBUTOL)

Ethambutol is added to the initial treatment regimen or substituted for INH when an INH-resistant strain of TB is suspected. Ethambutol is a bacteriostatic drug that reduces the development of resistance to the bactericidal first-line agents. Its principal toxic effect is optic neuritis; fortunately, this is reversible. Early signs of optic neuritis include decreased visual acuity and loss of red-green discrimination. This drug may be safe for use in pregnancy.

Nursing Responsibilities

■ Record a baseline visual examination prior to therapy. Schedule periodic eye exams during the course of treatment.
■ Administer with meals to reduce gastrointestinal side effects.
■ Monitor liver and renal function studies and neurologic status while taking this drug. Notify the physician of abnormal findings or significant changes.

Health Education for the Client and Family

■ Monitor vision daily by reading newspapers and looking at the same blue object (using usual corrective lenses, if appropriate). Notify your doctor if changes in vision or color perception occur.

STREPTOMYCIN

An aminoglycoside antibiotic, streptomycin is highly effective in treating most mycobacterial infection. Resistance may develop if it is used alone. There are two primary drawbacks to streptomycin: (1) It must be administered parenterally because it is not absorbed in the gastrointestinal tract, and (2) it has toxic effects on the kidneys and ears.

Nursing Responsibilities

■ Administer by deep intramuscular injection into a large muscle mass, rotating sites to minimize tissue trauma.
■ Monitor urine output, weight, and renal function studies (including BUN and serum creatinine) to detect early signs of nephrotoxicity. Report significant changes to the physician.
■ Maintain fluid intake at 2000 to 3000 mL per day to minimize the concentration of drug in the kidney tubules.
■ Assess hearing and balance frequently. Have audiometric testing performed as indicated.

Health Education for the Client and Family

■ Maintain a daily fluid intake of at least 2.5 to 3 quarts.
■ Weigh yourself on the same scale at least twice a week; report any significant weight gain to your doctor.
■ Notify your doctor if hearing acuity decreases, ringing or buzzing sensations in the ear develop, or dizziness occurs.

Repeat sputum specimens and chest x-rays are used to evaluate the effectiveness of therapy. In most cases, sputum cultures for *M. tuberculosis* are negative within 2 months of therapy; virtually all clients have negative sputum cultures within 3 months. If cultures remain positive at 3 months and beyond, treatment failure and drug resistance are suspected. In this case, cultures of the organism are tested for susceptibility to antitubercular agents, and two or three previously unused drugs are added to the treatment regimen (Kasper et al., 2005).

With adherence to prescribed treatment, virtually all clients should have negative sputum cultures for *M. tuberculosis*

within 3 months. The relapse rate for current treatment regimens is less than 5%. The principal cause of treatment failure is noncompliance (Tierney et al., 2005).

NURSING CARE

Health Promotion

Tuberculosis today presents a greater threat to public health than it does to individuals. Nurses play a key role in maintaining public health. Education and tuberculosis screening are major nursing strategies to prevent TB. See the accompanying Nursing Research box regarding tuberculosis screening for a homeless population.

Public health teaching includes increasing awareness of tuberculosis as a reemerging threat. Teach clients in all settings how to reduce the spread of TB by covering their mouths when coughing or sneezing and disposing of sputum appropriately. The benefit of screening programs to identify infected (though not necessarily infective) people also needs to be included in public health education.

The best tuberculosis prevention is early diagnosis of infections and appropriate treatment to achieve cure. BCG vaccine is recommended for infants born in countries where tuberculosis is prevalent, but is not widely used in the United States. It may be administered to healthcare workers in settings where the risk of infection with MDR strains of *M. tuberculosis* is high despite rigorous infection control measures (Kasper et al., 2005).

The primary preventive strategy used in the United States is treating people with latent tuberculosis infection demonstrated by a positive tuberculin test. A 9- to 10-month course of treatment with isoniazid reduces the risk of active TB by 90% or more (Kasper et al., 2005). Isoniazid also is prescribed prophylactically for people with HIV infection who have been exposed to TB.

ASSESSMENT

Focused assessment for the client with suspected TB includes the following:

- *Health history:* Complaints of fatigue, weight loss, night sweats, difficulty breathing, cough (productive or nonproductive), bloody sputum, or chest pain; known exposure to TB; most recent tuberculin test and results; living circumstances; alcohol and other recreational drug use.
- *Physical examination:* Vital signs including temperature; general appearance; respiratory rate and lung sounds.
- *Diagnostic tests:* Tuberculin test results, presence of acid-fast bacilli in sputum, chest x-ray.

Nursing Diagnoses and Interventions

Nursing care related to tuberculosis focuses primarily on infection control and compliance with prescribed treatment. See the accompanying Nursing Care Plan on the next page.

Deficient Knowledge

Adequate knowledge and information are necessary to manage the disease and prevent its transmission to others. The client needs to understand reasons for prolonged drug therapy and the importance of complying with treatment and follow-up. Antituberculosis drugs are relatively toxic. The client needs to know how to minimize toxicity.

- Assess knowledge about the disease process; identify misperceptions and emotional reactions. *Teaching based on previous learning enhances understanding and retention of information.*
- Assess ability and interest in learning, developmental level, and obstacles to learning. *Assessment allows presentation of information in a manner tailored to the learning needs and style of the client, promoting learning.*

NURSING RESEARCH   Evidence-Based Practice: Clients with Risk for Tuberculosis

Homeless people and those living in homeless shelters have several identified risk factors for TB: high incidence of drug and alcohol abuse, lowered immune status, and crowded living conditions. Access to and participation in TB screening, however, often is problematic. Swigart and Kolb (2004) identified factors contributing to homeless persons' decisions to participate in free TB screening. Contrary to the beliefs of many healthcare providers, many homeless people chose to participate in the screening out of a desire to maintain good health and a recognition that homelessness and shelter life increased their risk of developing TB. The desire to maintain good health was particularly noted as a reason among those participants in early recovery from drug or alcohol addiction. Other major factors cited for participating included a history of lung problems, a desire to identify possible problems related to smoking, and encouragement by shelter personnel. Fear of the results and a desire "not to be bothered" had negative effects on participation. Women with children were least likely to participate in screening in this study, citing fear of being identified as ill that could result in loss of child custody.

IMPLICATIONS FOR NURSING

Outreach to homeless populations for health services, while difficult, has personal and public health benefits. The homeless often lack access to preventive and health promotion services, instead interacting with healthcare providers only intermittently when urgent care is needed. This study suggests, however, that a portion of this population desires to maintain good health and is receptive when screening and health promotion services are accessible. Shelter personnel were instrumental in getting many of the study participants to the screening. Recruiting the support of these workers can improve resident participation. Regularly scheduling a nurse in a shelter can allow trust to develop and can also improve participation in health promotion activities. This may be a particularly important strategy in shelters for women with children—bringing services to the residents to reduce the fear of being perceived as unable to care for dependent children.

CRITICAL THINKING IN CLIENT CARE

1. What factors contribute to the perception of many healthcare providers that homeless people and shelter residents do not care about maintaining good health?
2. The participants in this study were screened for their ability to understand English and to read or hear and comprehend the interview and process. How might the healthcare team need to alter its approach to reach homeless people who have mental illnesses that affect thinking and cognition?
3. Design a TB screening program using a multidisciplinary team to reach a specific population. Identify members of the team and discuss your rationale for their inclusion on the team.

NURSING CARE PLAN   A Client with Tuberculosis

Harry Facée, age 53, arrives at a metropolitan public health clinic complaining of aching chest pain that has lasted for the past few days. He says that his sputum also is bloody. He is afraid he might have lung cancer, so he came in to see a doctor.

ASSESSMENT

Raj Kamil, RN, the public health nurse at the clinic, obtains an admission history and physical examination of Mr. Facée. Mr. Kamil notes that Mr. Facée is a homeless person who has lived on the streets and in various shelters for the past "10 years or so." He usually prefers to sleep outdoors, taking refuge in shelters only during very cold or very wet weather. He has a small disability income, but usually scrounges for food or eats with other homeless people at soup kitchens. Mr. Facée states that he has had a cough for a long time, which has become worse recently. It is now productive, especially in the mornings. He also admits that he has recently been waking up drenched with sweat in the middle of the night and is more tired than usual.

Although Mr. Facée's clothes are tattered, he is fairly clean. He answers questions appropriately and intelligently. Mr. Kamil does not detect any odor of alcohol on his breath. He is very thin, almost emaciated. Mr. Facée's vital signs are BP 152/86, P 92, R 20, and T 100.2°F (37.8°C).

Suspecting tuberculosis, Mr. Kamil obtains a sputum specimen for Gram stain and culture, administers a tuberculin test, and sends Mr. Facée for a chest x-ray before he sees the clinic physician. Although the chest x-ray is inconclusive, the Gram stain is positive for acid-fast bacilli. The diagnosis of probable active pulmonary tuberculosis is made. The physician prescribes isoniazid, 300 mg orally; rifampin, 600 mg orally; and pyrazinamide, 1500 mg orally daily for 2 months, to be followed by twice weekly isoniazid 900 mg orally and rifampin 600 mg orally. The physician also orders weekly sputum cultures for the first month.

DIAGNOSES

- *Ineffective Health Maintenance* related to homelessness
- *Risk for Noncompliance with Prescribed Treatment* related to lack of understanding and resources
- *Imbalanced Nutrition: Less than Body Requirements* related to increased metabolic needs associated with infection
- *Risk for Disturbed Sensory Perception: Kinesthetic* related to effects of isoniazid therapy

EXPECTED OUTCOMES

- Keep all follow-up appointments as scheduled.
- Verbalize an understanding of his disease and its treatment.

- Follow the prescribed plan of care.
- Demonstrate measures to prevent spread of the organism to others.
- Gain 1 to 2 lb of weight per week.
- Promptly report symptoms of peripheral neuropathy, including numbness, tingling, or burning sensations.

PLANNING AND IMPLEMENTATION

- Teach about tuberculosis, and provide a client education pamphlet about the disease.
- Instruct about the prescribed medications, potential adverse effects, and the importance of completing the entire prescribed regimen.
- Emphasize the importance of continued follow-up.
- Teach and demonstrate sputum and droplet control measures.
- Escort to the local incentive shelter program for directly observed medical therapy and meals.
- Identify verbally and in writing manifestations to report to the physician.

EVALUATION

Mr. Kamil successfully enrolls Mr. Facée in the local incentive shelter program. In this program, a healthcare worker administers Mr. Facée's medications daily, watching him swallow them. He is assigned a small individual room and can eat three daily meals at the shelter. He still prefers to sleep outside when the weather permits, but he complies with the requirement for supervised medication administration because he "likes the food there." Always a clean person, Mr. Facée is able to demonstrate appropriate sputum control measures and practices them faithfully. The sputum culture done after 2 months of treatment is negative for tubercle bacilli, and his chest x-ray indicates no disease progression.

CRITICAL THINKING IN THE NURSING PROCESS

1. Many homeless people have schizophrenia or other mental diseases. How would you adapt the care plan for a homeless schizophrenic client with active tuberculosis?
2. Mr. Kamil was fortunate in having access to an incentive shelter with healthcare workers to supervise medication compliance. Identify available resources in your area for homeless clients infected with tuberculosis.
3. Develop a care plan for the nursing diagnosis *Ineffective Airway Clearance* related to mucopurulent sputum and weak cough.

See Evaluating Your Response in Appendix C.

- Identify support systems, and include significant others in teaching. *A knowledgeable significant other provides reinforcement of learning, confirmation of understanding, and encouragement for the client. Including significant others also reduces the risk of inadvertent sabotage of the treatment plan.*
- Establish a relationship of mutual trust with the client and significant others. *An atmosphere of trust increases receptiveness to teaching and learning.*
- Develop mutually acceptable learning goals with the client and significant other. *Working together to identify learning*

needs and establish goals increases the client's "ownership" and interest in the process.

- Select appropriate teaching strategies, using learning aids such as literature and visual materials that are appropriate for age, level of education, and intellect. *Teaching tailored to the client is more effective and results in better learning.*
- Teach about tuberculosis and the prescribed treatment, including:
  a. Nature of the disease and its spread
  b. Purpose of treatment and follow-up procedures

c. Measures to prevent spreading the disease to others

d. Importance of maintaining good general health by eating a well-balanced, high-protein, high-carbohydrate diet; balancing exercise with rest; and avoiding crowds and people with upper respiratory infections

e. Names, doses, purposes, and adverse effects of prescribed medications

f. Importance of avoiding alcohol and other substances that may damage the liver while taking chemotherapeutic drugs

g. Fluid intake needs of 2.5 to 3.0 quarts of fluid per day

h. Manifestations to report to the physician: chest pain, hemoptysis, difficulty breathing; anorexia, nausea, or vomiting; yellow tint to skin or sclera; sudden weight gain, swollen feet, ankles, legs, or hands; hearing loss, tinnitus, or vertigo; change in vision or difficulty discriminating colors.

Tuberculosis is a chronic disease requiring lengthy treatment with antitubercular medications. A good understanding of the disease, its treatment, and potential adverse effects of therapy prepares the client to manage care.

■ Document teaching and level of understanding. Reinforce teaching and learning as needed. *Teaching is not complete until the client can demonstrate learning of the information.*

Ineffective Therapeutic Regimen Management

The populations at highest risk for developing active tuberculosis—the homeless and members of lower socioeconomic groups—are also at high risk for being unable to manage its complex treatment regimen. Three or more costly medications that may have unpleasant or even dangerous side effects are prescribed. Frequent medical follow-up is required. Infectious diseases such as TB carry a stigma that may lead to denial of the disease or its seriousness. Alcoholics and IV drug users need to withdraw from their addiction to be successful in treating the disease. The client with HIV infection faces a potentially fatal disease and costly treatment that may well override concerns about tuberculosis management.

■ Assess self-care abilities and support systems. *Assessment is used to help determine the client's ability to follow the prescribed regimen.*

■ Assess knowledge and understanding of the disease, its complications, treatment, and risks to others. Provide additional teaching and reinforcement as indicated. *Lack of understanding is a barrier to compliance with and management of the treatment regimen.*

■ Work collaboratively to identify barriers or obstacles to managing the prescribed treatment. *Working collaboratively with the client and other members of the healthcare team provides insight for overcoming identified barriers to effective treatment.*

■ Assist the client, significant others (if available), and healthcare team members to develop a plan for managing the prescribed regimen. *Including the client in developing a plan to manage care increases the sense of control and ownership and helps ensure that personal, cultural, and lifestyle factors are considered. This increases the likelihood of compliance.*

■ Provide verbal and written instructions that are clear and appropriate for level of literacy, knowledge, and understanding. *Clearly written directions provide support and reinforcement for the client.*

■ Provide active intervention for homeless people, including shelter placement or other housing and ongoing follow-up by easily accessed healthcare providers (clinics and public health workers in the neighborhood that do not present transportation or access problems, either real or perceived). *Simple referral will not ensure compliance, especially among disenfranchised populations. Active intervention is needed to help ensure treatment compliance.*

■ Refer clients who are unlikely to comply with the treatment regimen to the public health department for management and follow-up. *Because tuberculosis presents a significant public health risk, public health follow-up is essential. In some cases, it is necessary for nurses to administer medications, observing the client swallow all pills.*

Risk for Infection

The spread of tuberculosis is a risk in any facility housing many people. It is especially high in residential care facilities for older clients and for people with AIDS. The increasing incidence of TB among homeless people and members of lower socioeconomic groups increases the risk in hospitals, emergency departments, and public and urgent care clinics. Respiratory precautions are necessary to prevent the spread of TB via microscopic airborne droplets to other clients and to healthcare workers.

■ Place the client in a private room with airflow control that prevents air within the room from circulating into the hallway or other rooms. A negative flow room in which air is diluted by at least six fresh-air exchanges per hour is recommended. *A negative flow room and multiple fresh-air exchanges dilute the concentration of droplet nuclei within the room and prevent their spread to adjacent areas.*

■ Use standard precautions and tuberculosis isolation techniques as recommended by the CDC, including wearing masks and gowns when caring for clients who do not reliably cover the mouth when coughing. *These measures are important to prevent the spread of tuberculosis to others.*

> ### PRACTICE ALERT
> Use personal protective devices to reduce the risk of transmission during client care. The Occupational Safety and Health Administration (OSHA) requires use of a HEPA-filtered respirator for protection against occupational exposure to tuberculosis. Surgical masks are ineffective to filter droplet nuclei, necessitating the use of protective devices capable of filtering bacteria and particles smaller than 1 micron.

■ Discuss the reasons for and importance of respiratory isolation procedures during initial hospitalization. When treatment is provided as an outpatient, instruct to avoid crowds and close physical contact and maintain ventilation in living facilities, particularly during the first 3 weeks of treatment. *These measures help protect others during initial treatment, when sputum is still likely to contain significant numbers of bacilli.*

- Place a mask on the client when transporting to other parts of the facility for diagnostic or treatment procedures. *Covering the client's nose and mouth during transport minimizes air contamination and the risk to visitors and personnel.*
- Inform all personnel having contact with the client of the diagnosis. *This allows personnel to take appropriate precautions.*
- Assist visitors to mask prior to entering the room. *Providing visitors with appropriate masks or respirators reduces their risk of infection.*
- Teach the client how to limit transmitting the disease to others:
  a. Always cough and expectorate into tissues.
  b. Dispose of tissues properly, placing them in a closed bag.
  c. Wear a mask if you are sneezing or unable to control respiratory secretions.
  d. The disease is not spread by touching inanimate objects, so no special precautions are required for eating utensils, clothing, books, or other objects used.

  Teaching appropriate precautions helps prevent the spread of tuberculosis to others while allowing as much freedom from restraints as possible.
- Teach how to collect sputum specimens. If necessary, have the client step outside to collect a sputum specimen. *This minimizes the risk of exposure to healthcare personnel and provides for rapid dilution of any droplet nuclei produced and their exposure to ultraviolet light (which kills the bacteria).*
- Teach the importance of complying with the prescribed treatment for the entire course of therapy. *Completion of the entire treatment regimen is important to reduce the risk of relapse and creation of drug-resistant organisms.*

Using NANDA, NIC, and NOC

Linkages between NANDA nursing diagnoses, nursing interventions, and nursing outcomes for the client with tuberculosis are illustrated in Chart 38–2.

Community-Based Care

Most clients with TB are managed in community settings; few require institutionalization. In addition to the teaching topics and strategies identified above, discuss the following topics when preparing the client and significant others for home care:

- Importance of screening close contacts for infection and possibly prophylactic treatment
- Effect, dose, and timing for all medications, and potential side effects and their management
- Importance of long-term therapy in eradicating the disease
- Principles of good nutrition, dietary guidelines for a client with TB, and other measures to help maintain good health, such as balancing rest with exercise
- Signs and symptoms of complications to report to the physician or healthcare provider.

Provide referrals as appropriate:
- Smoking cessation clinics or support groups
- Alcohol treatment facilities, Alcoholics Anonymous, other treatment programs or support groups

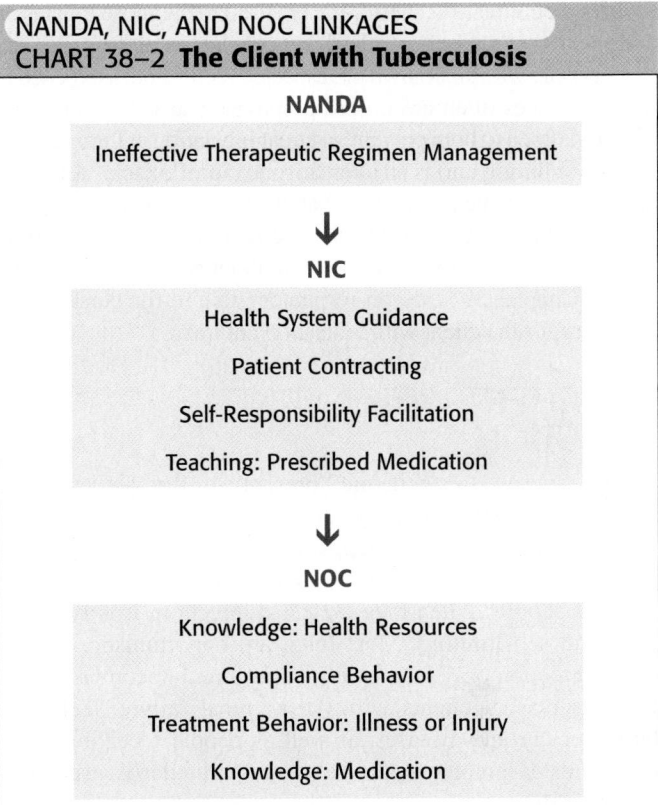

NANDA, NIC, AND NOC LINKAGES
CHART 38–2 The Client with Tuberculosis

NANDA

Ineffective Therapeutic Regimen Management

↓

NIC

Health System Guidance

Patient Contracting

Self-Responsibility Facilitation

Teaching: Prescribed Medication

↓

NOC

Knowledge: Health Resources

Compliance Behavior

Treatment Behavior: Illness or Injury

Knowledge: Medication

Data from *NANDA's Nursing Diagnoses: Definitions & Classification 2005–2006* by NANDA International (2005), Philadelphia; *Nursing Interventions Classification (NIC)* (4th ed.) by J. M. Dochterman & G. M. Bulechek (2004), St. Louis, MO: Mosby; and *Nursing Outcomes Classification (NOC) (3rd ed.)* by S. Moorhead, M. Johnson, and M. Maas (2004), St. Louis, MO: Mosby.

- Drug treatment facilities, Narcotics Anonymous, other outpatient or inpatient treatment programs or support groups
- Low-cost community clinics and incentive programs for people with TB
- Counseling, support groups, and other community resources that provide additional assistance and support.

THE CLIENT WITH INHALATION ANTHRAX

Inhalation anthrax is a relatively new potential threat in the United States. This disease rarely affects humans in nature, even though both wild and domestic animals can be infected. However, *Bacillus anthracis*, the spore-forming rod responsible for causing anthrax, has been identified as an agent likely to be used as a biologic weapon. Anthrax spores can be aerosolized so they remain suspended in the air, allowing them to be inhaled into the lungs. Person-to-person transmission does not occur.

Inhalation anthrax causes initial flulike symptoms, including malaise, dry cough, and fever. This is followed by an abrupt onset of severe dyspnea, stridor, and cyanosis. Lymph nodes in the mediastinum and thorax become inflamed and enlarged. Septic shock and/or meningitis may develop. Untreated, death results from hemorrhagic thoracic lymphadenitis and hemorrhagic mediastinitis with resultant hypotension and hypoxemia (Kasper et al., 2005).

Blood cultures and chest x-ray are used to diagnose inhalation anthrax. However, because death can quickly result from the disease, people who are known or suspected to have been exposed to anthrax spores often are treated prophylactically. Ciprofloxacin (Cipro) is used to both prevent and treat inhalation anthrax. Doxycycline (Vibramycin) is an alternative to ciprofloxacin. Although an anthrax vaccine exists, its use at this time is considered experimental (Persell et al., 2002). See the section on bioterrorism in Chapter 7 ∞ for more information about anthrax and the section in Chapter 39 ∞ on respiratory failure for nursing care measures for the client with inhalation anthrax.

THE CLIENT WITH A FUNGAL INFECTION

Fungal spores are endemic, present in the air everyone breathes. Normal respiratory defense mechanisms allow few of these spores to reach the lungs. If they reach the lungs, pulmonary macrophages and neutrophils efficiently remove them in most people. When they do cause infection, it is typically mild and self-limiting. Most fungi are opportunistic, able to cause infection only in people who are immunocompromised. For this reason, clients with AIDS, renal failure, leukemia, burns, or chronic diseases, as well as people receiving corticosteroids or immunosuppressants, are particularly susceptible to fungal diseases.

Many fungal lung diseases have a geographic distribution pattern. Histoplasmosis and blastomycosis are more common in the southeastern, mid-Atlantic, and central states. California, Arizona, and western Texas are the primary sites for coccidioidomycosis, also known as San Joaquin valley fever (Kasper et al., 2005).

The course and manifestations of fungal lung diseases resemble those of tuberculosis. Lung lesions are slow to develop, and symptoms are mild. The fungus can disseminate from the lung to other organs.

Pathophysiology

Histoplasmosis

Histoplasmosis, an infectious disease caused by *Histoplasma capsulatum*, is the most common fungal lung infection in the United States. The organism is found in the soil and is linked to exposure to bird droppings and bats. Infection occurs when the spores are inhaled and reach the alveoli. Most infections develop into *latent asymptomatic disease*, much like tuberculosis, or *primary acute histoplasmosis*, a mild, self-limiting influenza-like illness. Initial chest x-rays are nonspecific; later ones show areas of calcification. *Chronic progressive disease*, usually seen in older adults, typically is limited to the lung but may involve any organ. Progressive lung changes and cavitation occur, with increasing dyspnea and eventual disabling pulmonary disease.

Regional lymph vessels spread the organism from the lungs to other parts of the body, much like the process that occurs in tuberculosis. In the healthy host, normal immune responses inactivate and remove the organism. In the immunocompromised host, however, macrophages remove the fungi but are unable to destroy them, resulting in *disseminated histoplasmosis*. This type of histoplasmosis is often fatal. Manifestations of fever, dyspnea, cough, weight loss, and muscle wasting are usual. Ulcerations of the mouth and oropharynx may be present, and the liver and spleen are enlarged.

Coccidioidomycosis

Coccidioidomycosis is an infectious disease caused by the fungus *Coccidioides immitis*. This mold grows in the soil of the arid Southwest, Mexico, and Central and South America. When inhaled, the fungus typically causes an acute, self-limiting pulmonary infection that often is asymptomatic and goes unrecognized. If manifestations do occur, they resemble those of influenza, with malaise, fever, body aches, and cough. Pleuritic pain, skin rash, and arthritis of the knees and ankles also may develop. Disseminated disease, which may affect the lymph nodes, meninges, spleen, liver, kidney, skin, and adrenal glands, is rare in immunocompetent people. When it does occur, the mortality rate is high. Meningitis is the usual cause of death.

Blastomycosis

The fungus *Blastomyces dermatitidis* causes the infectious disease blastomycosis. It occurs primarily in the south central and midwestern regions of the United States and in Canada. Men are affected more frequently than women. The lungs are the primary site for the disease, although it may spread to involve the skin, bones, genitourinary system, and, rarely, the CNS. Pulmonary symptoms include fever, dyspnea, pleuritic chest pain, and cough, which may become productive of bloody or purulent sputum. If untreated, the disseminated disease is slowly progressive and ultimately fatal.

Aspergillosis

Aspergillus spores are common in the environment, but rarely cause disease except in the immunocompromised. When they do cause infection, *Aspergillus* species invade blood vessels and produce hyphae that branch at acute angles, frequently causing venous or arterial thrombosis. In the lungs, aspergillosis can cause an acute, diffuse, self-limited pneumonitis. The manifestations of pulmonary aspergillosis include dyspnea, nonproductive cough, pleuritic chest pain, chills, and fever. If the organism invades a pulmonary blood vessel, hemoptysis or massive pulmonary hemorrhage can occur. In clients with underlying lung disease, balls of *Aspergillus* hyphae may form within cysts or cavities, usually in the upper lobes of the lung. When this occurs, symptoms often are milder and more insidious in onset, with fever, weight loss, night sweats, and cough (Kasper et al., 2005).

INTERDISCIPLINARY CARE

Most fungal lung infections can be diagnosed by microscopic examination of a sputum specimen for the fungus. (See Chapter 36 ∞ for nursing responsibilities related to collecting a sputum specimen.) Blood cultures also may be done, as well as cultures of cerebrospinal fluid if indicated. Chest x-ray may show typical changes in lung tissue or widening of the mediastinum, depending on the infecting organism.

Acute pulmonary histoplasmosis and acute pulmonary coccidioidomycosis usually resolve without treatment, although antifungal drugs may be given to shorten the disease course.

Oral itraconazole (Sporanox), a broad-spectrum antifungal agent, is commonly prescribed to treat histoplasmosis. Other fungal lung diseases and clients who are immunocompromised are often treated with intravenous amphotericin B. Surgery (lobectomy) may be indicated for clients with severe hemoptysis associated with aspergillosis.

NURSING CARE

Clients with fungal lung infections have different nursing care needs, depending on the disease and their immune status. For most clients, nursing care focuses on education. People living in high-prevalence areas or who have specific risk factors such as exposure to bird droppings (for example, by cleaning chicken coops, pigeon lofts, or barns where birds roost), decomposed vegetation, rotting wood, or stored grain need to be aware

of the risk, common symptoms, and measures to reduce the risk. Clients with latent histoplasmosis may need education to maintain good general health to prevent reactivation. Teach clients receiving antifungal drugs about the specific drug, its intended and adverse effects, the duration of therapy, and symptoms to report to the physician. Include teaching about any specific precautions such as drug or food interactions. Itraconazole interacts with many medications; verify the safety of concurrent usage with all other prescribed drugs. Its use is contraindicated during pregnancy and lactation; emphasize the importance of effective birth control and of notifying the physician immediately if pregnancy occurs. Amphotericin B is a toxic drug. Administer the initial intravenous dose slowly after premedicating with an antihistamine and antiemetic as ordered to manage its adverse effects. Monitor carefully during infusion and therapy for changes in vital signs, hydration, nutrition, weight, or urine output.

DISORDERS OF THE PLEURA

The *pleura* is a thin membrane with two layers: the visceral pleura, which overlies the lung surface, and the parietal pleura, which lines the inner chest wall. Between the layers of pleura is a potential space, the *pleural cavity*, which contains a thin layer of serous fluid. As the thoracic cavity expands during inspiration, the pressure in this space becomes negative in relation to atmospheric and alveolar pressure. The expansible lung is drawn out, and air rushes into the alveoli. When the pleura is inflamed or affected by disease or injury, air or fluid can collect in the pleural cavity, restricting lung expansion, air movement, and ventilation.

THE CLIENT WITH PLEURITIS

Pleuritis (*pleurisy*), inflammation of the pleura, irritates sensory fibers of the parietal pleura, causing characteristic pain. Pleural inflammation usually occurs secondarily to another process, such as a viral respiratory illness, pneumonia, or rib injury.

The onset of pleuritis is typically abrupt. The pain is unilateral and well localized; it is usually sharp or stabbing in nature. Pain may be referred to the neck or the shoulder. Deep breathing, coughing, and movement aggravate the pain. Respirations are rapid and shallow, and chest wall movement is limited on the affected side. Breath sounds are diminished, and a pleural friction rub may be heard over the site.

The diagnosis of pleuritis is based on its manifestations. Chest x-ray and ECG may be ordered to rule out other causes of chest pain. Treatment for pleuritis is symptomatic. Analgesics and nonsteroidal anti-inflammatory drugs (NSAIDs), indomethacin (Indocin) in particular, help relieve the pain. Codeine may be ordered, both to relieve pain and to suppress the cough.

Nursing care for the client with pleuritis is directed toward promoting comfort, including administration of NSAIDs and analgesics. Positioning and splinting the chest while coughing also are helpful. Although wrapping the chest with 6-inch-wide elastic bandages may help relieve pain, this may excessively restrict chest motion, increasing the risk of impaired airway clearance.

Teach the client and family that pleuritis is generally self-limited and of short duration. Discuss symptoms to report to

the physician: increased fever, productive cough, difficulty breathing, or shortness of breath. Provide information about prescription and nonprescription NSAIDs and analgesics, including the drug ordered, how to use it, and its desired and possible adverse effects.

THE CLIENT WITH A PLEURAL EFFUSION

The pleural space normally contains only about 10 to 20 mL of serous fluid. **Pleural effusion** is collection of excess fluid in the pleural space. Pleural effusions result from either systemic or local disease. Systemic disorders that may lead to pleural effusion include heart failure, liver or renal disease, and connective tissue disorders, such as rheumatoid arthritis and systemic lupus erythematosus (SLE). Pneumonia, atelectasis, tuberculosis, lung cancer, and trauma are local conditions that may cause pleural effusion.

Pathophysiology and Manifestations

Excess pleural fluid may be either *transudate*, formed when capillary pressure is high or plasma proteins are low, or *exudate*, the result of increased capillary permeability. Heart failure is the most common precipitating factor in transudate formation; it also may accompany renal failure, nephrosis, liver failure, and malignancy. Exudate, a protein-rich fluid, is seen with inflammatory processes such as infections, systemic inflammation (e.g. rheumatoid arthritis or SLE), pulmonary infarction (leading to tissue necrosis and an inflammatory response), and malignancy (Porth, 2005). Other pleural fluid collections include *empyema*, pus in the pleural cavity; *hemothorax*, the presence of blood in the cavity; *hemorrhagic pleural effusion*, a mixture of blood and pleural fluid; and *chylothorax*, a collection of lymph in the pleural space. In adults, chylothorax may result from thoracic surgery or placement of a central catheter in one of the great veins (Porth, 2005).

A large pleural effusion compresses adjacent lung tissue. This causes the characteristic manifestation of dyspnea. Pain may develop, although with inflammatory processes pleuritic pain often is relieved by formation of an effusion, as the fluid reduces friction between inflamed visceral and parietal pleura. Breath sounds are diminished or absent, and a dull percussion tone is heard over the affected area. Chest wall movement may be limited.

INTERDISCIPLINARY CARE

Chest x-ray often provides the first evidence of a pleural effusion. Because fluid typically collects in dependent regions, it is seen at the base of the affected lung on an upright chest x-ray, and along the lateral wall when the client is positioned on the affected side. CT scans and ultrasonography also are used to localize and differentiate pleural effusions.

Thoracentesis

If the cause of pleural effusion is not apparent, a thoracentesis is done. **Thoracentesis** is an invasive procedure in which fluid (or occasionally air) is removed from the pleural space with a needle. Aspirated fluid is analyzed for appearance, cell counts, protein and glucose content, the presence of enzymes such as LDH and amylase, abnormal cells, and culture.

When pleural effusion is significant and interferes with respirations, thoracentesis is the treatment of choice to remove the fluid (Figure 38–8 ■). Thoracentesis may be performed at the bedside, in a procedure room, or in an outpatient setting. Local anesthesia is used, and the procedure requires less than 30 minutes to complete. Percussion, auscultation, radiography, or ultrasonography are used to locate the effusion and needle insertion site. The amount of fluid removed is limited to 1200 to 1500 mL at one time to reduce the risk of cardiovascular collapse from rapid removal of too much fluid. Pneumothorax is a possible complication of thoracentesis if the visceral pleura is punctured or a closed drainage system is not maintained during the proce-

dure. Nursing care for the client undergoing a thoracentesis is outlined in the box on the next page.

Treatments

Because pleural effusion usually occurs secondarily to another disease or disorder, medical management also focuses on treating the underlying condition to prevent further fluid accumulation. An empyema may require repeated drainage, as well as high doses of parenteral antibiotics. Occasionally, thoracotomy and surgical excision may be necessary. See the box on page 1313 for nursing care of the client undergoing thoracic surgery. Recurrent pleural effusions, often due to cancer, may be prevented by instilling an irritant, such as doxycycline bleomycin, or talc, into the pleural space to cause adhesion of the parietal and visceral pleura (*pleurodesis*). Water-seal chest tube drainage is often employed for hemothorax.

NURSING CARE

Nursing care for the client with a pleural effusion is directed toward supporting respiratory function and assisting with procedures to evacuate collected fluid. With a large pleural effusion and partial lung collapse, impaired gas exchange and activity intolerance are high-priority nursing problems. Risk for impaired gas exchange is also a priority problem during the initial period following thoracentesis.

Teaching for home care focuses on symptoms of recurrent effusion or complications following a thoracentesis to report to the physician: increasing dyspnea or shortness of breath, cough, and hemoptysis. Pleuritic pain may be an early sign of effusion and also should be reported. Further teaching about an underlying condition also may be necessary; for example, the client with heart failure may need teaching about a salt-restricted diet.

Figure 38–8 ■ Thoracentesis. With the client seated, a needle is inserted between the ribs into the pleural space to withdraw accumulated fluid.

NURSING CARE OF THE CLIENT HAVING A **Thoracentesis**

BEFORE THE PROCEDURE

- Verify a signed informed consent for the procedure. *This invasive procedure requires informed consent.*
- Assess knowledge and understanding of the procedure and its purpose; provide additional information as needed. *An informed client will be less apprehensive and more able to cooperate during the thoracentesis.*
- Preprocedure fasting or sedation is not required. *Only local anesthesia is used in this procedure, and the gag and cough reflexes remain intact.*
- Administer a cough suppressant if indicated. *Movement and coughing during the procedure may cause inadvertent damage to the lung or pleura.*
- Obtain a thoracentesis tray, sterile gloves, injectable lidocaine, povidone-iodine, dressing supplies, and an extra overbed table or Mayo stand. *These supplies are used by the physician performing the procedure.*
- Position the client upright, leaning forward with arms and head supported on an anchored overbed table. *This position spreads the ribs, enlarging the intercostal space for needle insertion.*
- Inform the client that although local anesthesia prevents pain as the needle is inserted, a sensation of pressure may be felt. *A pressure sensation occurs as the needle punctures the parietal pleura to enter the pleural space.*

AFTER THE PROCEDURE

- Monitor pulse, color, oxygen saturation, and other signs during thoracentesis. *These are indicators of physiologic tolerance of the procedure.*
- Apply a dressing over the puncture site, and position on the unaffected side for 1 hour. *This allows the pleural puncture to heal.*
- Label obtained specimen with name, date, source, and diagnosis; send specimen to the laboratory for analysis. *Fluid obtained during thoracentesis may be examined for abnormal cells, bacteria, and other substances to determine the cause of the pleural effusion.*
- During the first several hours after thoracentesis, frequently assess and document vital signs; oxygen saturation; respiratory status, including respiratory excursion, lung sounds, cough, or hemoptysis; and puncture site for bleeding or crepitus. *Frequent assessment is important to detect possible complications of thoracentesis, such as pneumothorax.*
- Obtain a chest x-ray. *Chest x-ray is ordered to detect possible pneumothorax.*
- Normal activities generally can be resumed after 1 hour if no evidence of pneumothorax or other complication is present. *The puncture wound of thoracentesis heals rapidly.*

THE CLIENT WITH PNEUMOTHORAX

Accumulation of air in the pleural space is called **pneumothorax**. Pneumothorax can occur spontaneously, without apparent cause, as a complication of preexisting lung disease, as a result of blunt or penetrating trauma to the chest, or from an iatrogenic cause (e.g., following thoracentesis).

Pathophysiology

Pressure in the pleural space is normally negative in relation to atmospheric pressure. This negative pressure is vital to the process of breathing. Contraction of the diaphragm and the intercostal muscles enlarges the thoracic space. Negative intrapleural pressure draws the lung outward, increasing its volume so air rushes in to fill the expanded lung space.

When either the visceral or parietal pleura is breached, air enters the pleural space, equalizing this pressure. Lung expansion is impaired, and the natural recoil tendency of the lung causes it to collapse to a greater or lesser extent, depending on the size and rapidity of air accumulation. Table 38–7 illustrates the classifications of pneumothorax.

Spontaneous Pneumothorax

Spontaneous pneumothorax develops when an air-filled bleb, or blister, on the lung surface ruptures. Rupture allows air from the airways to enter the pleural space. Air accumulates until pressures are equalized or until collapse of the involved lung section seals the leak. Spontaneous pneumothorax may be either *primary* (*simple*) or *secondary* (*complicated*).

Primary pneumothorax affects previously healthy people, usually tall, slender men between ages 16 and 24 (Way & Doherty, 2003). The cause of primary pneumothorax is unknown. Risk factors include smoking and familial factors. Air-filled blebs tend to form in the apices of the lungs. This is considered to be a benign condition, although recurrences are common. Certain activities also increase the risk of spontaneous pneumothorax, such as high-altitude flying and rapid decompression during scuba diving.

Secondary pneumothorax, generally caused by overdistention and rupture of an alveolus, is more serious and potentially life threatening. It develops in clients with underlying lung disease, usually COPD. Middle-age and older adults are primarily affected. Secondary pneumothorax also may be associated with asthma, cystic fibrosis, pulmonary fibrosis, tuberculosis, acute respiratory distress syndrome (ARDS), and other lung diseases. Rarely, a form of secondary pneumothorax called *catamenial pneumothorax* can develop in affected women within 24 to 48 hours of the onset of menstrual flow.

MANIFESTATIONS The manifestations of spontaneous pneumothorax depend on the size of pneumothorax, extent of lung collapse, and any underlying lung disease. Typically, pleuritic chest pain and shortness of breath begin abruptly, often while at rest. The respiratory and heart rates increase as gas exchange is affected. Chest wall movement may be asymmetrical, with less movement on the affected side than the unaffected side. The affected side is hyperresonant to percussion, and breath sounds may be diminished or absent. Hypoxemia may develop, although normal mechanisms that shunt

TABLE 38–7 **Types of Pneumothorax**

TYPE	PATHOPHYSIOLOGY	MANIFESTATIONS
A. Spontaneous 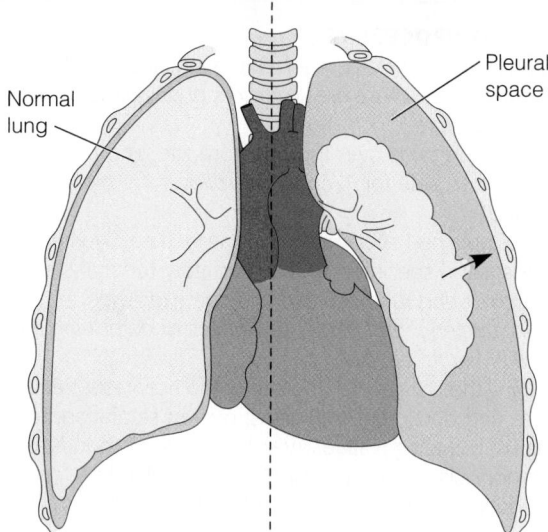	Rupture of a bleb on the lung surface allows air to enter pleural space from airways. ■ *Primary pneumothorax* affects previously healthy people. ■ *Secondary pneumothorax* affects people with preexisting lung disease (e.g., COPD).	■ Abrupt onset ■ Pleuritic chest pain ■ Dyspnea, shortness of breath ■ Tachypnea, tachycardia ■ Unequal lung excursion ■ Decreased breath sounds and hyperresonant percussion tone on affected side
B. Traumatic 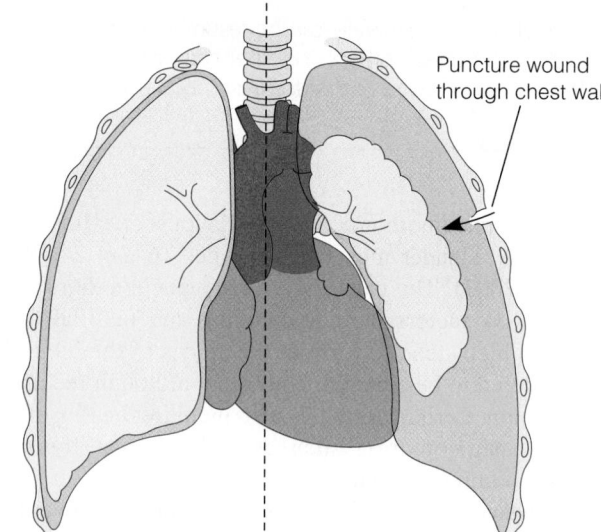	Trauma to the chest wall or pleura disrupts the pleural membrane. ■ *Open* occurs with penetrating chest trauma that allows air from the environment to enter the pleural space. ■ *Closed* occurs with blunt trauma that allows air from the lung to enter the pleural space. ■ *Iatrogenic* involves laceration of visceral pleura during a procedure such as thoracentesis or central-line insertion.	■ Pain ■ Dyspnea ■ Tachypnea, tachycardia ■ Decreased respiratory excursion ■ Absent breath sounds in affected area ■ Air movement through an open wound
C. Tension 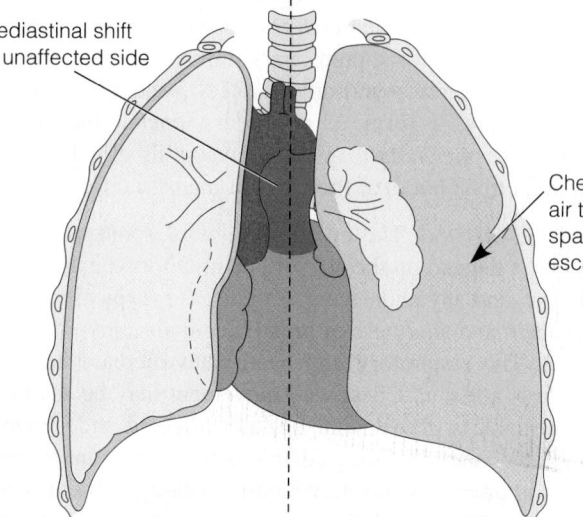	Air enters pleural space through chest wall or from airways but is unable to escape, resulting in rapid accumulation. Lung on affected side collapses. As intrapleural pressure increases, heart, great vessels, trachea, and esophagus shift toward the unaffected side.	■ Hypotension, shock ■ Distended neck veins ■ Severe dyspnea ■ Tachypnea, tachycardia ■ Decreased respiratory excursion ■ Absent breath sounds on affected side ■ Tracheal deviation toward unaffected side

Figure labels:
- A. Spontaneous: Normal lung; Pleural space
- B. Traumatic: Puncture wound through chest wall
- C. Tension: Mediastinal shift to unaffected side; Chest wound allows air to enter pleural space but prevents escape.

blood flow to the unaffected lung often maintain normal oxygen saturation levels. Hypoxemia is more pronounced in secondary pneumothorax.

Traumatic Pneumothorax

Blunt or penetrating trauma of the chest wall and pleura can cause pneumothorax. Blunt trauma, for example, due to a motor vehicle crash, fall, or during cardiopulmonary resuscitation (CPR), can lead to a *closed pneumothorax*. Fractured ribs penetrating the pleura are the leading cause of pneumothorax due to blunt trauma (Yamamoto et al., 2005). Fracture of the trachea and a ruptured bronchus or esophagus also may result from blunt trauma, leading to closed pneumothorax.

Open pneumothorax (*sucking chest wound*) results from penetrating chest trauma such as a stab wound, gunshot wound, or impalement injury. With open pneumothorax, air moves freely between the pleural space and the atmosphere through the wound. Pressure on the affected side equalizes with the atmosphere, and the lung collapses rapidly. The result is significant hypoventilation.

Iatrogenic pneumothorax may result from puncture or laceration of the visceral pleura during central-line placement, thoracentesis, or lung biopsy. During bronchoscopy, bronchi or lung tissue can be disrupted. Alveoli can become overdistended and rupture during anesthesia, resuscitation procedures, or mechanical ventilation.

MANIFESTATIONS With traumatic pneumothorax, manifestations of pain and dyspnea may be masked or missed due to other injuries. Tachypnea and tachycardia may be attributed to the primary injury. Focused assessment for evidence of pneumothorax is vital. Chest wall movement on the affected side is diminished, and breath sounds are absent. If a penetrating wound is present, air may be heard and felt moving through it with respiratory efforts. Hemothorax frequently accompanies traumatic pneumothorax. The manifestations of iatrogenic pneumothorax are similar to those of spontaneous pneumothorax.

Tension Pneumothorax

Tension pneumothorax develops when injury to the chest wall or lungs allows air to enter the pleural space but prevents it from escaping. Pressure within the pleural space becomes positive in relation to atmospheric pressure as air rapidly accumulates with each breath. The lung on the affected side collapses, and pressure on the mediastinum shifts thoracic organs to the unaffected side of the chest, placing pressure on the opposite lung as well. Ventilation is severely compromised, and venous return to the heart is impaired. Tension pneumothorax is a medical emergency requiring immediate intervention to preserve respiration and cardiac output.

MANIFESTATIONS In addition to manifestations of pneumothorax, hypotension and distended neck veins are evident as venous return and cardiac output are affected. The trachea is displaced toward the unaffected side as a result of the mediastinal shift. Signs of shock may be present. See Chapter 11 ∞ for the manifestations and treatment of shock.

INTERDISCIPLINARY CARE

Treatment for pneumothorax depends on the severity of the problem. A small simple pneumothorax may require no treatment other than monitoring with serial x-rays. Air is absorbed from the pleural space, allowing most small pneumothoraces to resolve spontaneously. A large pneumothorax with significant symptoms usually requires treatment with *thoracostomy*, or the placement of chest tubes. Surgical intervention may be necessary to prevent recurrent spontaneous pneumothorax.

Diagnosis

Oxygen saturation measurements are obtained to evaluate the effect of pneumothorax on gas exchange. ABGs may be obtained to further assess gas exchange.

The chest x-ray is an effective diagnostic tool for pneumothorax. In tension pneumothorax, air is evident on the affected side, and mediastinal structures are shifted toward the opposite or unaffected side.

Treatments

CHEST TUBES The treatment of choice for significant pneumothorax is placement of a closed-chest catheter to allow the lung to reexpand. When a tube is placed in the pleural cavity to remove air or fluid, it must be sealed to prevent air from also entering the tube and, in essence, creating an open pneumothorax. Chest tubes are sealed with a Heimlich (one-way) valve (Figure 38–9 ■) or connected to a closed drainage system with a "water seal." The valve or water seal prevents air from entering the chest cavity during inspiration and allows air to escape during expiration. Applying a low level of suction to the system helps to reestablish negative pressure in the pleural space, allowing the lung to reexpand.

A number of closed-drainage chest tube systems are available. Most are self-contained disposable systems (Figure 38–10 ■). Drainage from the chest tube is collected in the first collection chamber. This sealed chamber is connected to a water seal chamber, which is in turn connected to the suction control chamber. Nursing care of the client with chest tubes is discussed in the box on page 1300.

A large-bore needle or plastic intravenous catheter may be inserted through the chest wall as emergency treatment of a tension pneumothorax. This allows air to escape from the affected side, relieving pressure on mediastinal structures and the opposite lung.

PLEURODESIS Although controversial, *pleurodesis*, or creation of adhesions between the parietal and visceral pleura, may be used to prevent recurrent pneumothorax. This procedure involves instilling a chemical agent such as doxycycline into the

Figure 38–9 ■ The Heimlich one-way valve allows air to escape from the pleural space, helping to reestablish negative pressure and allowing the lung to reexpand.

Connect to external
suction source

Connect to
chest tube

Atmosphere vent

Suction
control
chamber

Collection
chamber

Water seal
chamber

Figure 38–10 ■ A closed-chest drainage system.

pleural space. The subsequent inflammatory response creates scar tissue and adhesions between the pleural layers. This procedure reduces the recurrence rate to as low as 2% but can make subsequent surgery more difficult (Way & Doherty, 2003).

Surgery

The risk for recurrence of spontaneous pneumothorax increases with each attack. Clients at high risk for recurrent pneumothorax may have surgery to reduce the risk of future ruptures. A thoracotomy is done to excise or oversew blebs (usually at the apices of the lungs). The overlying pleura is then roughened or irritated to induce scarring and adhesion to the surface of the lung. In some cases, the parietal pleura may be partially excised. These procedures can be done using video-assisted thoracoscopic surgery (VATS), a minimally invasive surgical technique (Way & Doherty, 2003).

NURSING CARE

Health Promotion

Health promotion activities to prevent spontaneous and traumatic pneumothorax primarily involve health teaching. Initiate

---

NURSING CARE OF THE CLIENT WITH Chest Tubes

BEFORE THE PROCEDURE

■ Ensure a signed informed consent for chest tube insertion. *This invasive procedure requires informed consent.*

■ Provide additional information as indicated. Explain that local anesthesia will be used but that pressure may be felt as the trocar is inserted. Reassure that breathing will be easier once the chest tube is in place and the lung reexpands. *The client may be extremely dyspneic and anxious and may need reassurance that this invasive procedure will provide relief.*

■ Gather all needed supplies, including thoracostomy tray, injectable lidocaine, sterile gloves, chest tube drainage system, sterile water, and a large sterile catheter-tipped syringe to use as a funnel for filling water seal and suction chambers. *These supplies are used during the insertion procedure to establish a water seal drainage system.*

■ Position as indicated for the procedure. *Either an upright position (as for thoracentesis) or side-lying position may be used, depending on the site of the pneumothorax.*

■ Assist with chest tube insertion as needed. The procedure may be performed in a procedure room, in the surgical suite, or at the bedside. *Although chest tube insertion is a relatively simple procedure, nursing assistance is necessary to support the client and rapidly establish a closed drainage system.*

AFTER THE PROCEDURE

■ Assess respiratory status at least every 4 hours. *Frequent assessment is necessary to monitor respiratory status and the effect of the chest tube.*

■ Maintain a closed system. Tape all connections, and secure the chest tube to the chest wall. *These measures are important*

to prevent inadvertent tube removal or disruption of system integrity.

■ Keep the collection apparatus below the level of the chest. *Pleural fluid drains into the collection apparatus by gravity flow.*

■ Check tubes frequently for kinks or loops. *These could interfere with drainage.*

■ Check the water seal frequently. The water level should fluctuate with respiratory effort. If it does not, the system may not be patent or intact. Periodic air bubbles in the water seal chamber are normal and indicate that trapped air is being removed from the chest. *Frequent assessment of the system is important to ensure appropriate functioning.*

■ Measure drainage every 8 hours, marking the level on the drainage chamber. Report drainage that is cloudy, in excess of 70 mL per hour, or red, warm, and free flowing. *Red, free-flowing drainage indicates hemorrhage; cloudiness may indicate an infection. Emptying the drainage would disrupt integrity of the closed system.*

■ Periodically assess water level in the suction control chamber, adding water as necessary. *Adequate water in the suction control chamber prevents excess suction from being placed on delicate pleural tissue.*

■ Assist with frequent position changes and sitting and ambulation as allowed. *Chest tubes should not prevent performance of allowed activities. Care is needed to prevent inadvertent disconnection or removal of the tubes.*

■ When the chest tube is removed, immediately apply a sterile occlusive petroleum jelly dressing. *An occlusive dressing prevents air from reentering the pleural space through the chest wound.*

and participate in programs to prevent smoking among children and teenagers. Teach safe behaviors such as always wearing a seat beat in an automobile, driving safely, and using precautions to prevent falls when working or recreating in high places.

Assessment

The client with pneumothorax may be in acute respiratory distress, necessitating rapid and focused assessment.

- *Health History:* Current symptoms and their duration; precipitating factors or activities if known; previous episodes of pneumothorax; smoking history; chronic pulmonary diseases such as COPD.
- *Physical Assessment:* General appearance and degree of apparent respiratory distress; evidence of chest trauma; vital signs, oxygen saturation, skin color, LOC; respiratory excursion, percussion tone, and breath sounds anterior and posterior chest; neck vein inspection, position of trachea; peripheral pulses.
- *Diagnostic Tests:* Chest x-ray, ABGs.

Nursing Diagnoses and Interventions

Maintaining or restoring adequate alveolar ventilation and gas exchange is of highest priority for the client with a pneumothorax. Chest tubes may interfere with physical mobility, contributing to a high risk for injury.

Impaired Gas Exchange

Loss of negative pressure in the pleural cavity and the resulting collapse of lung tissue can cause poor chest expansion and loss of alveolar ventilation. As the pneumothorax is removed or reabsorbed, ventilation and gas exchange improve.

- Assess and document vital signs and respiratory status, including rate, depth, lung sounds, and oxygen saturation at least every 4 hours. *Frequent assessment is important to monitor the adequacy of respirations and lung expansion.*

PRACTICE ALERT
Evaluate chest wall movement, position of the trachea, and neck veins frequently. Early identification of tension pneumothorax and appropriate interventions are vital to preserve cardiorespiratory function.

- Place in Fowler's or high-Fowler's position. *This position facilitates lung expansion.*
- Administer oxygen as ordered. *Supplemental oxygen is given to improve oxygenation of the blood and tissues.*

PRACTICE ALERT
Provide emotional support, particularly in early stages and during chest tube insertion. Dyspnea and hypoxemia can cause extreme anxiety and apprehension, impairing the ability to cooperate with procedures.

- Assess chest tube, system function, and drainage at least every 2 hours. *The system must remain patent and intact to function effectively.*
- Provide for rest. *Adequate rest is important to conserve energy and reduce oxygen demand.*

Risk for Injury

Pain and the presence of chest tubes can reduce the perceived ability to ambulate and provide self-care. Moderate activity is encouraged unless respiratory function is significantly impaired. Caution is taken to maintain integrity of the chest tube system. If the tube is inadvertently pulled out or system integrity is disrupted, the pneumothorax may increase or infection may develop.

PRACTICE ALERT
Avoid placing tension on chest tubes during positioning, ambulation, and care activities. The chest tubes are minimally secured to the chest wall and can be dislodged if tension is placed on them.

- Secure a loop of drainage tubing to the sheet or gown. *Looping the drainage tubing prevents direct pressure on the chest tube itself.*
- When turning to the affected side, ensure that neither the chest tube nor drainage tubing is kinked or occluded under the client. *This maintains patency of the system.*
- Teach the client how to ambulate with the drainage system, keeping the system lower than the chest. In most cases, suction can be discontinued during ambulation. *Ambulation facilitates lung ventilation and expansion. Drainage systems are portable to allow ambulation while chest tubes are in place. Keeping the drainage system lower than the chest promotes drainage and prevents reflux.*
- Observe insertion site for redness, swelling, pain, or drainage. Report any signs of infection, including fever, to the physician. *Interruption of skin integrity by chest tube insertion increases the risk for infection.*
- If a connection comes loose, reconnect it as soon as possible. *A closed, sealed system is vital to prevent air from entering the pleural space and an open pneumothorax.*

PRACTICE ALERT
Seal the wound of an open pneumothorax or a wound from inadvertent tube removal as soon as possible with a sterile occlusive dressing, such as gauze impregnated with petroleum jelly. If a sterile dressing is not available, other occlusive material such as foil or plastic wrap can be used. Tape the dressing on three sides only. An occlusive dressing taped on three sides prevents the development of a tension pneumothorax by inhibiting air from entering the wound during inhalation but allowing it to escape during exhalation.

Community-Based Care

Clients who have experienced spontaneous pneumothorax need education about their future risk. After a single episode of spontaneous pneumothorax, the risk of recurrence is 40% to 50%. This risk increases with subsequent episodes (Way & Doherty, 2003). Stress the importance of quitting smoking to reduce the risk. Other activities that can precipitate recurrent episodes include mountain climbing or those involving exposure to high altitudes, flying in unpressurized aircraft, and scuba diving (Tierney et al., 2005). The client may be advised to avoid contact sports.

Following a pneumothorax, instruct the client to gradually increase exercise and activity to previous levels. Stress the importance of follow-up care and monitoring. Discuss manifestations to report to the physician: upper respiratory infections; fever, cough, or difficulty breathing; sudden, sharp chest pain; or redness, pain, swelling, tenderness, or drainage from the chest tube puncture wound.

THE CLIENT WITH HEMOTHORAX

Hemothorax, or blood in the pleural space, usually occurs as a result of chest trauma, surgery, or diagnostic procedures. Hemothorax develops in about 25% of clients with chest trauma, usually due to laceration of the lung, an intercostal vessel, or the internal mammary artery. If a major thoracic vessel is disrupted, hemorrhage can be massive (Yamamoto et al., 2005). Tumors, pulmonary infarction, and infections such as tuberculosis also can cause hemothorax. When blood collects in the pleural space, pressure on the affected lung impairs ventilation and gas exchange. With significant hemorrhage, a risk of shock exists.

Hemothorax causes symptoms similar to those of pneumothorax or pleural effusion. Lung sounds are diminished, and a dull percussion tone is noted over the collected blood, typically at the base of the lung. Chest x-ray is used to confirm the diagnosis of hemothorax.

Thoracentesis or thoracostomy with chest tube drainage is used to remove blood from the pleural space. With significant hemorrhage (e.g., due to trauma or surgery), the blood may be collected for subsequent autotransfusion. Blood for autotransfusion should be collected and reinfused within 4 hours. Strict aseptic technique is used in collecting the blood. It is collected through a gross particulate filter into a container primed with anticoagulant and reinfused when the container is full or when transfusion is necessary. Air is removed from the blood container prior to reinfusion and a filter used to eliminate debris, such as degenerating blood cells, fat particles, and fibrin.

Priority nursing care for the client with hemothorax focuses on assessing and maintaining adequate respiratory function and cardiac output. The priority of care depends on the rate and extent of hemothorax. In a large, slow-developing hemothorax, ventilatory status may be affected significantly. In this instance, *Impaired Gas Exchange* and *Ineffective Breathing Pattern* are priority nursing diagnoses. When hemothorax develops rapidly and hemorrhage is significant, additional priority nursing diagnoses include *Decreased Cardiac Output* and *Risk for Deficient Fluid Volume*.

When preparing the client for home care following a hemothorax, discuss the importance of avoiding smoking and preventing respiratory infection. Include symptoms to report to the physician. If trauma or infection caused the hemothorax, discuss measures to prevent future trauma and continuing treatment for the infection as indicated.

TRAUMA OF THE CHEST OR LUNG

Chest injury is a leading cause of death from trauma. It is commonly associated with motor vehicle crashes, violent crime, and falls. Chest injuries can range from mild, such as a simple rib fracture, to severe and fatal. Traumatic injury to the chest may involve both the chest wall and underlying thoracic structures, including the lungs, heart, great vessels, and esophagus. Chest and lung injury can result from several different mechanisms: penetrating trauma, such as a stab or gunshot wound; blunt trauma, such as a fall, motor vehicle crash (MVC), vehicle–pedestrian impact, or crush injury; or inhalation injury, such as smoke inhalation or near drowning.

Rapid and continuing assessment of the airway, breathing, and circulation (ABCs) is vital in chest or lung injuries. Chest trauma can disrupt any or all of these functions. Chest injuries that may be life threatening include airway obstruction, tension pneumothorax, open pneumothorax, massive hemothorax, and flail chest with pulmonary contusion.

THE CLIENT WITH A THORACIC INJURY

Thoracic injuries may be minor and have little effect on respiratory status, for example, simple rib fracture in a previously healthy client. When pain or chest wall instability impair breathing or the underlying lung tissue is damaged, the risk is more significant. Thoracic trauma usually is caused by motor vehicle crashes or falls.

Pathophysiology and Manifestations

Acceleration–deceleration injury and direct mechanisms of injury (e.g., crush injuries) are the most common mechanisms of thoracic injuries. Acceleration–deceleration injuries are caused by a rapid change in velocity such as occurs in a MVC or fall. The body stops suddenly, but the tissues and organs within the chest cavity continue to move forward until they impact with the chest wall. Injuries sustained can be significant, depending on the velocity (speed) of the vehicle or body at the point of impact, the surface with which the body impacts, and individual characteristics (e.g., size and bone structure).

Rib Fracture

Simple rib fracture, usually involving a single rib, is the most common chest wall injury. Rib fracture generally is tolerated well and heals rapidly in a young, previously healthy person. In an older adult or person with preexisting lung disease, however, a fractured rib may lead to significant complications, such as pneumonia, atelectasis, and, potentially, respiratory failure. Displaced fractured ribs can penetrate the pleura, leading to pneumothorax and possible hemothorax. Fractures of certain ribs are more frequently associated with underlying tissue damage. Intrathoracic vessels may be damaged or torn with fractures of the first and second ribs. Fractures of the seventh through tenth ribs may cause liver or spleen injuries.

Rib fracture causes pain on inspiration and coughing. This leads to voluntary splinting, with rapid, shallow respirations and inhibited cough. Bruising may be seen over the fracture, and crepitus may be palpated with respiratory movement. Breath sounds are diminished, especially in the bases, due to splinting. If pneumothorax develops, chest wall movement on the affected side may be reduced, and breath sounds absent or significantly diminished. A hyperresonant percussion tone usually is noted. Hemothorax also causes diminished or absent breath sounds on the affected side, with a dull percussion note.

Flail Chest

Multiple rib fractures may impair chest wall stability and normal chest wall function. When two or more consecutive ribs are fractured in multiple places, a free-floating segment of the chest wall, or **flail chest**, results. Physiologic function of the chest wall is impaired as the flail segment is sucked inward during inhalation and moves outward with exhalation. This is known as *paradoxic movement* (Figure 38–11 ■).

Flail chest can significantly affect ventilation and, consequently, gas exchange. Lung expansion is impaired and the work of breathing increases. Flail chest is frequently associated with underlying pulmonary contusion, which may lead to respiratory failure.

Flail chest causes dyspnea and pain, especially on inspiration. Paradoxic chest movement is evident with inspection. Chest expansion is unequal, and palpable crepitus is present. Breath sounds are diminished, and crackles may be heard on auscultation.

Pulmonary Contusion

Pulmonary contusion, or lung tissue injury, is frequently associated with flail chest and other blunt chest trauma. It may occur unilaterally or bilaterally. Pulmonary contusion often results from abrupt chest compression followed by sudden decompression, as can occur with MVC, significant fall, or crush injury. Alveoli and pulmonary arterioles rupture, causing intraalveolar hemorrhage and interstitial and bronchial edema. The resulting inflammatory response increases capillary permeabil-ity, leading to edema, which may be localized to the damaged lung tissue or more generalized. Inflammation and edema impair the production of surfactant within the alveoli, decreasing compliance. Pulmonary vascular resistance increases and blood flow decreases. Airway obstruction, atelectasis, and impaired gas diffusion result. Associated chest wall injury impairs the ability to clear secretions effectively, and the work of breathing is significantly increased.

Manifestations of pulmonary contusion may not be apparent until 12 to 24 hours after the injury. Increasing shortness of breath, restlessness, apprehension, and chest pain are early signs. Copious sputum, which may be blood tinged, is present. Later manifestations include tachycardia, tachypnea, dyspnea, and cyanosis. Even with appropriate treatment, pulmonary contusion can lead to acute respiratory distress and potential death.

INTERDISCIPLINARY CARE

Chest x-ray is used to identify most chest wall injuries. Rib fractures are evident on x-ray. Pulmonary contusion may show as initial patchy opacifications progressing to diffuse opacification, or "white-out." Changes in oxygen saturation and ABGs depend on the degree to which ventilation and gas exchange are affected by the injury.

Simple rib fractures typically heal uneventfully. Providing adequate analgesia to promote breathing, coughing, and movement is the primary intervention. With multiple rib fractures, an intercostal nerve block may be used to ensure adequate ventilation. Rib belts, binders, and taping to stabilize the rib cage are not recommended, because they may interfere with ventilation and lead to atelectasis. Even with simple rib fracture, older clients and clients with preexisting lung disease require close monitoring to prevent and detect atelectasis, pneumonia, and other complications.

Intercostal nerve blocks or continuous epidural analgesia may be employed to manage the pain associated with flail chest. For a small flail chest, analgesia combined with supplemental

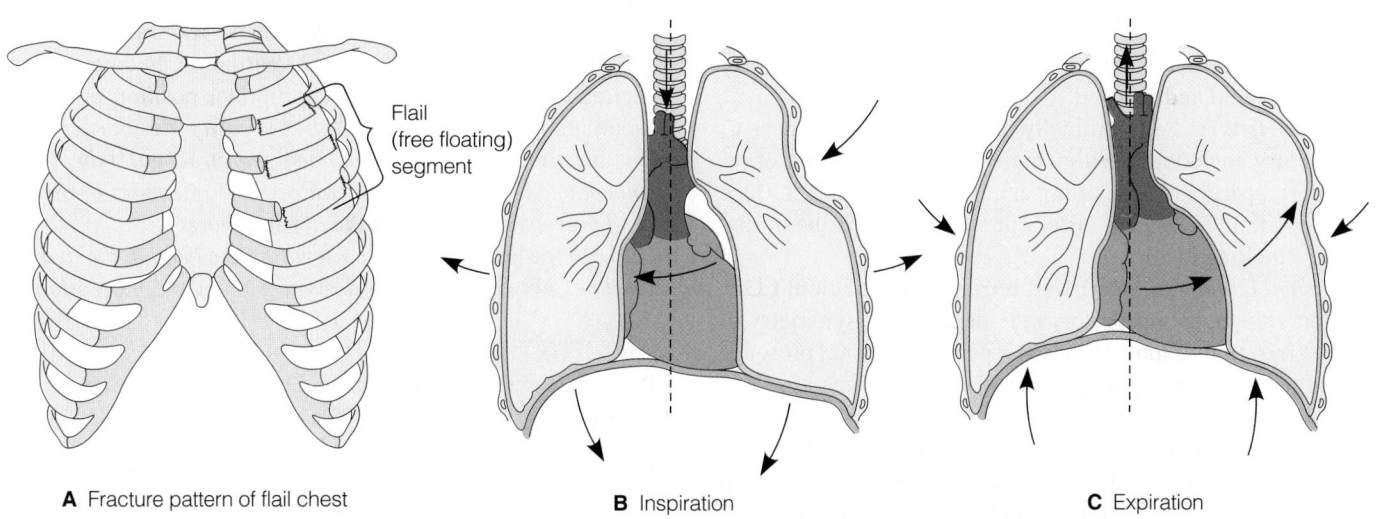

A Fracture pattern of flail chest   **B** Inspiration   **C** Expiration

Figure 38–11 ■ Flail chest with paradoxic movement.

oxygen therapy may be adequate. In some cases, internal or external fixation of the flail segment may be done.

The preferred treatment for flail chest is intubation and mechanical ventilation. Positive-pressure ventilation provides support and stabilization of the flail segment and improves ventilation and gas exchange. The work of breathing is decreased and healing improved.

Clients with pulmonary contusion often are critically ill, requiring intensive care management. Treatment is supportive, directed at maintaining adequate ventilation and alveolar gas exchange. Endotracheal intubation and mechanical ventilation are necessary in most cases. Repeated bronchoscopy may be done to remove secretions and cellular debris, preventing atelectasis. Although adequate hydration is necessary to prevent shock, overhydration can increase pulmonary edema. Pulmonary arterial pressure monitoring with a Swan-Ganz catheter and frequent ABG measurement is required for optimal fluid replacement and management of ventilatory support. See Chapter 32 ∞ for more information about pulmonary artery pressure monitoring, and Chapter 39 ∞ for nursing care of the client who is intubated and ventilated.

Unilateral pulmonary contusion may present a unique management problem. Mechanical ventilation with positive end-expiratory pressure (PEEP) to maintain open alveoli and adequate gas exchange can damage the unaffected lung. Intubation with a double-lumen endotracheal tube that permits independent ventilation of each lung may be used.

 ## NURSING CARE

Health Promotion

Encourage the use of seat belts, shoulder harnesses, and supplemental restraint systems such as air bags to significantly reduce the incidence of thoracic injury associated with motor vehicle crashes. Discuss the importance of appropriate protective equipment and gear for people engaging in potentially hazardous activities such as contact sports, mountain climbing, and occupations such as roofing or house painting.

Assessment

The nursing assessment of the client with a thoracic injury may need to be rapid and focused.
- *Health History:* Pain, difficulty breathing; circumstances of the injury, including position in the motor vehicle, use of restraints, speed and type of impact; distance of a fall, surface and position on impact; history of chronic lung or heart disease; smoking history.
- *Physical Examination:* Airway, breathing, circulation; LOC; color, vital signs; respiratory rate, depth, ease; symmetry of chest movement; lung sounds and percussion tone; presence of bruising, crepitus, or paradoxical chest movement.

Nursing Diagnoses and Interventions

Chest wall trauma can interfere with adequate chest expansion and alveolar ventilation. When a pulmonary contusion is also present, gas exchange is affected as well. Priorities for nursing management include controlling pain, ensuring adequate ventilation, and promoting gas exchange.

Acute Pain

With many thoracic injuries, pain interferes with lung expansion and coughing, leading to such complications as pneumonia and atelectasis. Adequate pain management is a key component of medical and nursing management for these clients.
- Frequently assess pain, using a standard pain scale and objective data. *Increased respiratory rate, shallow respirations, diminished breath sounds, and reluctance to move and cough may indicate inadequate pain control in a thoracic injury.*
- Administer analgesics by patient-controlled analgesia or on a schedule to maintain pain control. *Analgesics are more effective when pain is not allowed to become intense.*

> **PRACTICE ALERT**
> Assess for possible respiratory depression due to narcotic analgesia. Respiratory depression can further compromise ventilation in the client with thoracic injury.

- Notify the physician if pain relief is inadequate or excess sedation and respiratory depression occur. *An intercostal nerve block may be done to reduce the need for narcotic analgesia. Assess for bleeding and adequate ventilation following a nerve block.*

Ineffective Airway Clearance

Aggressive respiratory hygiene may be necessary to maintain open airways and adequate ventilation.
- Assess lung sounds and respiratory rate, depth, and effort frequently. Encourage to cough, deep breathe, and change position every 1 to 2 hours, and use the incentive spirometer. *Frequent assessment and measures to maintain airway patency are vital to prevent complications in the client with thoracic injury.*
- Teach how to splint the affected area with a blanket or pillow when coughing. *Splinting reduces movement and discomfort of the affected area.*
- Suction airway as indicated. Work with respiratory therapy to maintain optimal mechanical ventilation. Secure the endotracheal tube to maintain appropriate position and lung ventilation. *Endotracheal tube security is particularly important when a double-lumen endotracheal tube is in place, because malposition can occlude one main bronchus and prevent ventilation of the affected lung.*
- Elevate the head of the bed. *Elevating the head of the bed facilitates lung expansion and reduces the work of breathing.*

> **PRACTICE ALERT**
> Promptly report to the physician signs of complications, such as diminished breath sounds, increasing crackles (rales) or rhonchi, dull or hyperresonant percussion tones, unequal chest movement, hemoptysis, chills or fever, or changes in vital signs. Prompt intervention for complications is vital to promote healing and recovery.

Impaired Gas Exchange

Impaired gas exchange is of particular concern in pulmonary contusion. Alveolar damage and pulmonary edema can significantly impair oxygenation of the blood and removal of carbon dioxide.

- Monitor vital signs, color, oxygen saturation, and ABGs. Assess for manifestations such as anxiety or apprehension, restlessness, confusion, lethargy, or complaints of headache. *These assessment data alert the nurse and care providers to potential hypoxemia or hypercapnia due to impaired gas exchange.*
- Maintain oxygen therapy and mechanical ventilation as ordered. Hyperoxygenate prior to suctioning. *Oxygen and mechanical ventilation support alveolar gas exchange. Hyperoxygenation prior to suctioning reduces the degree of hypoxemia that occurs during suctioning.*
- Monitor intake and output, weigh daily, and monitor central venous pressure and pulmonary artery pressure as ordered. Maintain any ordered fluid restriction. *Fluid volume status is monitored to reduce the effects of pulmonary edema on lung tissues.*
- Maintain bed rest or activity restriction as ordered. Space activities to allow periods of uninterrupted rest. *Rest reduces the metabolic rate and oxygen consumption.*

Community-Based Care

Simple rib fracture and minor chest wall injuries often are managed on an outpatient basis. Include the following topics when teaching for home care:

- Pain management and its importance in preventing respiratory complications
- Importance of coughing and deep breathing; how to splint the rib cage during coughing
- Reasons for not taping or wrapping the chest continuously
- Symptoms to report to the physician: chills and fever, productive cough, purulent or bloody sputum, shortness of breath or difficulty breathing, and increasing chest pain
- Importance of avoiding respiratory irritants, such as cigarette smoke and occupational or environmental pollutants.

Significant pulmonary contusion can result in long-term respiratory insufficiency. Discuss activity modifications and occupational changes with the client and family as indicated. Refer to home care services such as respiratory therapy and home health if needed.

THE CLIENT WITH INHALATION INJURY

The internal environment of the lungs normally is protected from noxious substances by respiratory defense mechanisms. If these defenses are breached, inhaled agents, such as gases, fumes, toxins, and water, can cause internal trauma to the lungs.

Pathophysiology and Manifestations

Smoke Inhalation

Pulmonary injury due to inhalation of hot air, toxic gases, or particulate matter is the leading cause of death in burn injury (Kasper et al., 2005). Smoke inhalation affects up to one-third of clients admitted to burn units. Smoke inhalation can significantly affect normal respiratory function through three different mechanisms:

- Thermal damage to the airways, leading to impaired ventilation
- Carbon monoxide or cyanide poisoning, resulting in tissue hypoxia
- Chemical damage to the lung from noxious gases, which can impair gas exchange.

Smoke inhalation is suspected whenever a burn occurs in a closed space; if there are burns to the face or upper torso or singed nasal hairs; if sputum contains ashlike material; and when manifestations such as dyspnea, wheezing, rales, or rhonchi develop.

The lower airways of the lungs typically are protected from thermal damage by cooling of the inhaled gases in the upper airway and laryngeal spasm. Upper airway obstruction due to tissue edema and laryngeal spasm can occur quickly, however, resulting in **asphyxiation**, or oxygen deprivation, without lung damage. Steam inhalation can cause thermal damage to tissues of the lower respiratory tract.

Inhalation of carbon monoxide or cyanide gas poses an immediate threat to life. Carbon monoxide is a colorless, odorless gas produced in a fire. It binds readily with hemoglobin. The affinity of carbon monoxide for hemoglobin is 200 to 250 times stronger than that of oxygen. Hemoglobin bound to carbon monoxide reduces the oxygen-carrying capacity of blood and oxygen delivery to cells of the body. Carbon monoxide poisoning is suspected if the burn occurred in a closed space, if there is evidence of inhalation injury, or if dyspnea develops.

The manifestations of carbon monoxide poisoning depend on the level of carboxyhemoglobin saturation. When hemoglobin is 10% to 20% saturated with carbon monoxide, symptoms include headache, dizziness, dyspnea, and nausea. A characteristic "cherry-red" color of the skin and mucous membranes may be seen. With increasing levels, confusion, visual disturbances, irritability, hallucinations, hypotension, seizures, and coma develop. Permanent neurologic deficit can occur in survivors of severe, acute carbon monoxide poisoning.

Many other toxic chemicals may be present in smoke, especially in a house fire or industrial plant fire. Hydrogen cyanide can be lethal when inhaled. Inhalation of toxic chemicals causes bronchospasm and edema of the airways and alveoli. Acute respiratory distress syndrome may develop within 1 to 2 days. Sloughing of damaged mucosa leads to airway obstruction and atelectasis. Pneumonia is common following smoke inhalation.

Near-Drowning

Drowning is a leading preventable cause of accidental death in the United States. Approximately 5500 people die of drowning every year in the United States. Alcohol ingestion is a factor in about 25% of adult drowning deaths. Other circumstances that may contribute to drowning and near-drowning include excessive fatigue, a sudden acute condition such as seizure or myocardial infarction, and head or spinal cord injury associated with diving (Tierney et al., 2005).

Asphyxiation and aspiration are the primary problems associated with drowning and near-drowning. About 10% of victims do not aspirate water; instead, laryngeal spasm causes asphyxia. This is known as "dry drowning." In most cases, however, asphyxia and hypoxemia are the result of fluid aspiration. The effects of hypoxemia occur rapidly; loss of consciousness can occur within 3 to 5 minutes after total immersion. Circulatory impairment, brain injury, and brain death can occur within 5 to 10 minutes. Immersion in very cold water and the *dive reflex,* a protective mechanism that slows the heartbeat, constricts peripheral vessels, and shunts blood to the brain and heart, may prolong survival.

Water aspiration can cause delayed death from near-drowning. Respiratory and systemic effects differ, depending on whether freshwater or saltwater has been aspirated. Freshwater is hypotonic; when aspirated, it is rapidly absorbed from the alveoli, leading to hypervolemia and hemodilution. Hemolysis occurs as blood cells are subjected to a hypotonic environment, and serum electrolytes are diluted. Electrolyte imbalances can cause cardiac dysrhythmias and death. Hemolysis can lead to acute tubular necrosis and acute renal failure. Aspiration of freshwater impairs pulmonary surfactant and damages the alveolar-capillary membrane. Respiratory failure can result.

Nearly the opposite effects occur with saltwater aspiration. As a hypertonic fluid, saltwater draws fluid into the alveoli, resulting in hypovolemia and hemoconcentration. Hemolysis is insignificant, and small elevations in serum sodium and chloride levels rarely cause life-threatening effects. With either type of near-drowning episode, inhaled microorganisms and debris can lead to pneumonia. The pathophysiologic changes associated with freshwater and saltwater near-drowning are illustrated in Figure 38–12 ■.

Manifestations of near-drowning may include altered LOC, restlessness, and apprehension. The client may complain of headache or chest pain. Other signs include vomiting, possible cyanosis, apnea, tachypnea, and wheezing. If pulmonary edema is present, pink froth may be visible in the mouth and nose. Other manifestations include tachycardia, dysrhythmias, hypotension, shock, and cardiac arrest. Hypothermia may be present.

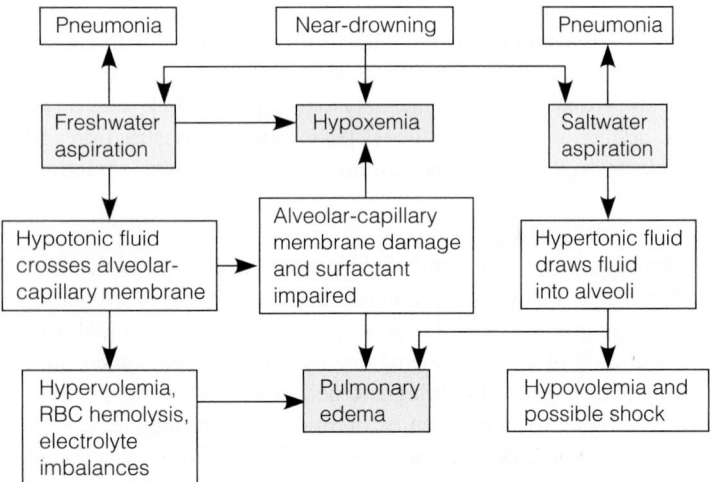

Figure 38–12 ■ The pathogenesis of near-drowning, freshwater and saltwater.

The near-drowning victim who never loses consciousness or is conscious on admission to the emergency department has a good prognosis for recovery. The prognosis is less optimistic when neurologic damage has occurred.

INTERDISCIPLINARY CARE

With inhalation injuries, the most effective treatment is prevention. A working smoke detector (with functioning batteries) could prevent the majority of deaths from smoke inhalation occurring in the home. The statement "A smoke detector was found, but the batteries had been removed" is all too familiar in news reports of fire-related deaths.

To prevent drowning, life preservers and flotation vests or jackets should be worn on the body, not stored in the hold of the boat. These devices are designed to keep the head above water. Even accomplished swimmers should never enter the water alone in unguarded areas. Just as alcohol and driving do not mix, neither do alcohol and boating or other water sports.

The second most important line of defense against death or permanent injury from inhalation injuries is removing the victim from the area of the fire or water and administering effective CPR. In many cases, immediate restoration of effective breathing and circulation is key to preserving life. Hypoxemia progresses rapidly until breathing is restored; reversal of tissue hypoxia depends on adequate circulation. In both smoke inhalation and near drowning, intubation may be necessary to establish an airway. Oxygen is administered as soon as possible. Attempts to drain water from the lungs of the near-drowning victim waste time and are generally ineffective in restoring alveolar ventilation. External cardiac defibrillation may be necessary to reestablish an effective cardiac rhythm and circulation. When the victim is hypothermic, resuscitation measures are continued until the core body temperature reaches approximately 90°F (32°C). The basic rule in hypothermia is that the client is not declared dead until the body has been rewarmed and life signs remain absent.

Diagnosis

When inhalation injury is known or suspected, the following diagnostic tests may be done:
- *ABGs* are drawn to evaluate gas exchange and the degree of hypoxemia. Combined respiratory and metabolic acidosis may be apparent. With effective ventilation and supplemental oxygen, acidosis may reverse quickly. With carbon monoxide poisoning, arterial Po_2 may be normal, but oxyhemoglobin saturation is less than normal.
- *Carboxyhemoglobin levels* are drawn in suspected carbon monoxide poisoning. Normal levels are less than 5% in nonsmokers and less than 10% in smokers. Higher levels indicate carbon monoxide poisoning. Levels less than 20% are considered mild poisoning; between 20% and 40% is moderate poisoning; and 40% to 60% is severe poisoning. Levels higher than 60% are generally fatal.
- *Serum electrolytes* and *osmolality levels* vary in near-drowning, depending on the type of water aspirated. In freshwater drowning, serum electrolyte levels and osmolal-

ity may be significantly reduced. With saltwater drowning, serum sodium and chloride may be somewhat high, and osmolality is increased because of hypovolemia.

- *Chest x-ray* is done, but may not show changes until 12 or more hours after the insult. Evidence of ARDS may be seen 24 to 48 hours after inhalation injury.
- *Bronchoscopy* may be ordered to inspect damaged lung tissue, particularly with smoke inhalation and possible thermal injury.

Treatments

Treatment of inhalation injury is generally supportive. Endotracheal intubation and mechanical ventilation often are required to maintain the airway and provide adequate alveolar ventilation and oxygenation. All clients with inhalation injury require supplemental oxygen, even when intubation and ventilation are not required. *Hyperbaric oxygen therapy,* the delivery of 100% oxygen at increased atmospheric pressure, may be used to treat carbon monoxide poisoning. This treatment carries some risks, such as oxygen toxicity and potential trauma to lung tissues, sinuses, and ears due to the increased pressures.

Other treatment measures may include bronchodilator therapy to manage bronchospasm. Bronchodilators can be administered by aerosol inhalation or intravenous infusion. Coughing and suctioning are important to remove secretions and debris. Chest physiotherapy with percussion and postural drainage may be performed.

Intravenous fluids may be ordered; if significant hemolysis has occurred, packed red blood cells may be given to improve the oxygen-carrying capacity of the blood. Fluid therapy is monitored carefully, using pulmonary artery or central venous pressures to reduce the risk of pulmonary edema.

With near-drowning victims, measures such as inducing hypothermia or barbiturate-induced coma and administering corticosteroids and osmotic diuretics may be employed to help prevent neurologic damage.

Careful monitoring for complications such as pneumonia and ARDS is vital throughout the course of treatment. Respiratory status, vital signs, and other data are frequently assessed to identify complications and allow early intervention.

 NURSING CARE

Health Promotion

Prevention of inhalation injuries is an important nursing responsibility. Teach everyone the value of a working smoke detector, especially in the sleeping areas of the house. Encourage families to develop an escape plan in case of fire and to use fire drills to rehearse getting out of the house. Smoldering cigarettes are a leading cause of house fires; help clients develop a plan to stop smoking. Teach people to drop and roll should clothing catch fire. (Flames rise, increasing the risk of respiratory injury when upright.)

Learning to swim safely is important to prevent drowning. Teach clients never to swim alone, when fatigued, or immediately following a meal. Remind clients that knowing how to swim will not prevent drowning in very cold water or in large bodies of water, such as lakes, rivers, or the ocean. Instruct to always wear flotation devices while boating, water-skiing, surfing, or wind-surfing. Wet suits help prevent hypothermia during activities in very cold water. Advise covering or fencing swimming pools, hot tubs, and ponds to prevent inadvertent entry and drowning.

A population well trained in effective, safe CPR provides the best second line of defense against inhalation injury. Rapid restoration of breathing is essential to prevent hypoxia and brain damage. Encourage all people to be trained and regularly update CPR skills. Work with communities to increase the number of trained people. Refer clients to local chapters of the American Red Cross or American Heart Association for classes.

Assessment

Inhalation injuries may be a medical emergency, necessitating focused and timely nursing assessment.

- *Health History:* Circumstances of the injury, including duration of exposure to smoke or time under water, explosion or fire in a closed area, type and temperature of water immersed in; resuscitation measures used; allergies, and current medical problems.
- *Physical Examination:* Airway, breathing, circulation; LOC; color, oxygen saturation level; vital signs; heart and lung sounds; urine output; evidence of burns or soot around nares or mouth.
- *Diagnostic Tests:* Carboxyhemoglobin levels, serum electrolytes and osmolality; ABGs; chest x-ray.

Nursing Diagnoses and Interventions

Nursing care priorities for the client with an inhalation injury are determined by the type of injury or tissue damage. Airway clearance is a major concern in all inhalation injuries, as is impaired gas exchange. Tissue hypoxia also can be a significant problem.

Ineffective Airway Clearance

Nursing measures to maintain an adequate airway begin with careful and frequent assessment of respiratory status, including rate, depth, and effort as well as breath sounds. Note amount, color, and consistency of sputum. Assist to cough frequently; suction the intubated client as needed to remove secretions. Elevate the head of the bed to facilitate alveolar ventilation unless otherwise ordered. Stabilize the endotracheal tube to prevent displacement into a mainstem bronchus, which could lead to ventilation of only one lung. Report changes in the character of secretions that may indicate complications: pink, frothy sputum suggesting pulmonary edema, or purulent sputum suggestive of pneumonia. Administer bronchodilators as ordered. Perform percussion and postural drainage as ordered.

Impaired Gas Exchange

Support gas exchange by administering supplemental oxygen, with or without mechanical ventilation. Frequently assess oxygen saturation, skin color, and mental status. Decreasing level of consciousness may be an early sign of hypoxemia. Monitor exhaled carbon dioxide, ABGs, and pulmonary artery pressures as ordered and indicated. Report changes to the physician. Maintain oxygen flow rates as ordered. Provide frequent mouth care to reduce the discomfort of dry mucous membranes and prevent tissue breakdown. Work with respiratory therapy to maintain effective oxygen delivery with mechanical ventilation. Administer sedation as required. Maintain fluid restriction if ordered.

Ineffective Tissue Perfusion: Cerebral

Impaired cerebral tissue perfusion is a priority problem, especially with near-drowning. Hypoxia and possible hypervolemia can lead to cerebral edema and increased intracranial pressure (IICP), further impairing blood flow. Monitor vital signs and neurologic status frequently. A change in level of consciousness or behavior is typically the earliest sign of IICP. Changes noted on an intracranial pressure monitor also provide early evidence of IICP. Increasing systolic blood pressure and pulse pressure and slowed heart rate are late signs. Other manifestations may include pupillary changes and decreasing muscle strength. Report changes promptly to the physician. Elevate the head of the bed and keep the head in neutral position to promote drainage

from the cranial vault. Maintain effective ventilation and oxygenation; hypercapnia and hypoxemia increase cerebral edema. Administer sedation, osmotic diuretics, or corticosteroids as ordered to reduce cerebral edema. Maintain fluid restriction. Space activities and promote rest to reduce metabolic demands.

Community-Based Care

Teach clients who do not require hospitalization for inhalation injury about symptoms that may indicate a complication and should be reported to the physician: increasing dyspnea, cough productive of purulent or pink frothy mucus, confusion, or other changes. Manifestations of respiratory damage may not be apparent for 24 to 48 hours following the injury.

Significant hypoxia due to near-drowning or carbon monoxide poisoning may cause permanent neurologic effects. Work with the family to develop communication techniques and identify remaining strengths. Help the family identify future care needs and means for meeting them, such as home health, personal care aides, or long-term care facilities. Provide social services and support group referrals.

LUNG CANCER

THE CLIENT WITH LUNG CANCER

Lung cancer is the leading cause of cancer deaths among all racial groups in the United States, accounting for 31% of all cancer deaths in men and 27% of all cancer deaths in women. In 2005, more than 168,000 people died from lung cancer in the United States; an estimated 184,800 new cases were diagnosed in that same year (American Cancer Society [ACS], 2005). It is a major health problem with a grim prognosis: Most people with lung cancer die within 1 year of the initial diagnosis.

Incidence and Risk Factors

The incidence of lung cancer varies from state to state and among nations. It increases with age, occurring most commonly in clients over age 50. Family clusters of lung cancer suggest a genetic predisposition; however, exposure to tobacco smoke may be necessary for expression of the trait. Cigarette smoke, which contains 43 known chemical carcinogens and cancer promoters, is clearly the most significant cause of lung cancer (ACS, 2005). More than 80% of lung cancer cases are related to smoking, and the disease is 10 times more common in smokers than nonsmokers. There is a dose–response relationship between smoking and lung cancer; the more the person smokes and the longer the person smokes, the greater the risk. Even former smokers who have abstained for a number of years have a higher risk of developing lung cancer than nonsmokers. Exposure to ionizing radiation and inhaled irritants, asbestos in particular, is also recognized as a risk factor for lung cancer (Porth, 2005). Exposure to radon, a radioactive gas, also is identified as a lung cancer risk factor (ACS, 2005). Radon forms as radium, an element present in the earth's crust, disintegrates. Radon tends to accumulate in closed spaces where air circulation is poor, such as caves, mines, and energy-efficient houses.

FAST FACTS

- In the United States, the incidence of lung cancer is second to prostate cancer in men and breast cancer in women.
- Lung cancer is, however, the leading cause of cancer deaths in the United States, responsible for 31% of cancer deaths in men and 27% of cancer deaths in women.
- Tobacco use and exposure to cigarette smoke are the leading risk factors for lung cancer.

Pathophysiology

Lung cancer develops as damaged bronchial epithelial cells mutate over time to become neoplastic. The genetic abnormality commonly seen is on chromosome 3, with loss of genetic material. Alterations of tumor suppressor genes also are seen in some types of lung cancer.

The vast majority of primary lung lesions are *bronchogenic carcinoma*, tumors of the airway epithelium. These tumors are further differentiated by cell type: small-cell carcinoma, adenocarcinoma, squamous cell carcinoma, and large-cell carcinoma. For clinical purposes, the latter three cell types frequently are classified together as non–small-cell carcinomas. *Small-cell carcinomas*, which account for approximately 25% of lung cancers, grow rapidly and spread early. These tumors have paraneoplastic properties; that is, they produce manifestations at sites that are not directly affected by the tumor. Small-cell lung carcinomas can synthesize bioactive products and hormones such as adrenocorticotropic hormones (ACTH), antidiuretic hormone (ADH), a parathormone-like hormone, and gastrin-releasing peptide. *Non–small-cell carcinoma* accounts for about 75% of lung cancers. Each cell type differs in its incidence, presentation, and manner of spread. Table 38–8 outlines the incidence and unique characteristics of each cell type.

TABLE 38–8 Comparison of Lung Cancer Cell Types

	CELL TYPE AND PREVALENCE	PRESENTATION AND ASSOCIATED MANIFESTATIONS	SPREAD
	Small-cell (oat cell) carcinoma: 20% to 25% of all lung cancers	Central lesion with hilar mass common, early mediastinal involvement, no cavitation; SIADH, Cushing's syndrome, thrombophlebitis	Aggressive tumor; more than 40% of clients have distant metastasis at time of presentation
	Adenocarcinoma: 20% to 40% of all lung cancers	Peripheral mass involving bronchi; few local symptoms; hypertrophic pulmonary osteoarthropathy	Early metastasis to CNS, skeleton, and adrenal glands
	Squamous cell carcinoma: 30% to 32% of all lung cancers	Central lesion located in large bronchi; client presents with cough, dyspnea, atelectasis, and wheezing; hypercalcemia common	Spreads by local invasion
	Large-cell carcinoma: 10% to 15% of all lung cancers	Usually, peripheral lesion that is larger than that associated with adenocarcinoma and tends to cavitate; gynecomastia, thrombophlebitis	Early metastasis

Bronchogenic cancer, regardless of cell type, tends to be aggressive, locally invasive, and have widespread metastatic lesions. Tumors begin as mucosal lesions that grow to form masses that obstruct the bronchi or invade adjacent lung tissue. All types frequently spread via the lymph system to nodes and other organs such as the brain, bones, and liver.

Manifestations

The manifestations of lung cancer are related to the location and spread of the tumor. Clients may present with symptoms related to the primary tumor, manifestations of metastatic disease, or with systemic symptoms. Initial symptoms often are attributed to smoking or chronic bronchitis. Chronic cough is common, as is hemoptysis. Wheezing and shortness of breath occur as a result of airway obstruction. Dull, aching chest pain occurs as the tumor spreads to the mediastinum; pleuritic pain occurs when the pleura is invaded. Hoarseness and/or dysphagia indicates pressure of the tumor on the trachea or esophagus.

Systemic and paraneoplastic manifestations of lung cancer include weight loss, anorexia, fatigue, and weakness; bone pain, tenderness, and swelling; clubbing of the fingers and toes; and various endocrine, neuromuscular, cardiovascular, and hematologic symptoms. The *Multisystem Effects of Lung Cancer* are illustrated on the next page.

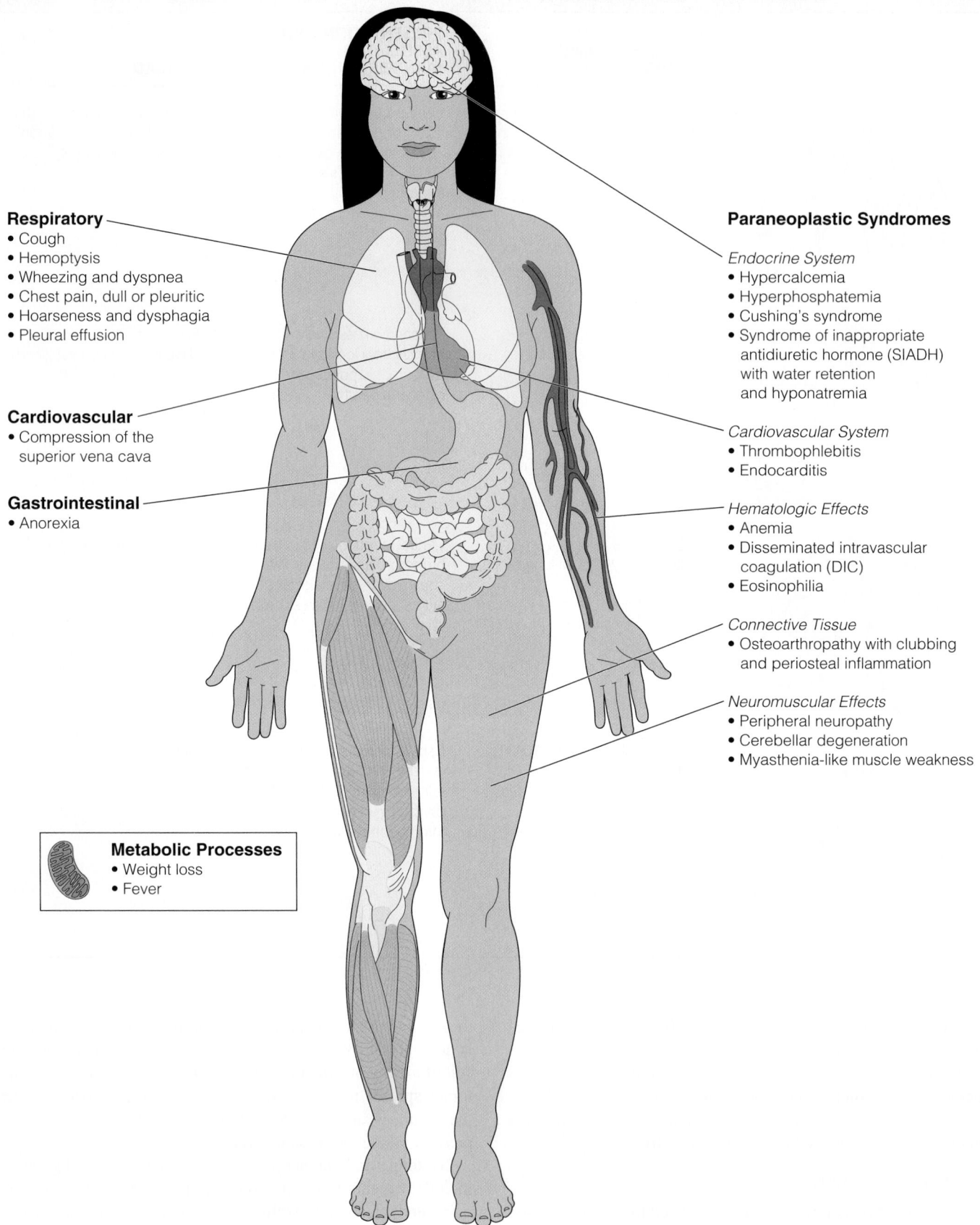

Respiratory
- Cough
- Hemoptysis
- Wheezing and dyspnea
- Chest pain, dull or pleuritic
- Hoarseness and dysphagia
- Pleural effusion

Cardiovascular
- Compression of the superior vena cava

Gastrointestinal
- Anorexia

Metabolic Processes
- Weight loss
- Fever

Paraneoplastic Syndromes

Endocrine System
- Hypercalcemia
- Hyperphosphatemia
- Cushing's syndrome
- Syndrome of inappropriate antidiuretic hormone (SIADH) with water retention and hyponatremia

Cardiovascular System
- Thrombophlebitis
- Endocarditis

Hematologic Effects
- Anemia
- Disseminated intravascular coagulation (DIC)
- Eosinophilia

Connective Tissue
- Osteoarthropathy with clubbing and periosteal inflammation

Neuromuscular Effects
- Peripheral neuropathy
- Cerebellar degeneration
- Myasthenia-like muscle weakness

Confusion, impaired gait and balance, headache, and personality changes may indicate brain metastasis. Bone metastases cause bone pain, pathologic fractures, and possible spinal cord compression, as well as thrombocytopenia and anemia if bone marrow is invaded. When the liver is affected, symptoms of liver dysfunction and biliary obstruction—including jaundice, anorexia, and upper right quadrant pain—are evident.

Complications and Course

Superior vena cava syndrome, partial or complete obstruction of the superior vena cava, is a potential complication of lung cancer, particularly when the tumor involves the superior mediastinum or the mediastinal lymph nodes. Obstructed venous flow from the head and neck produces the symptoms of superior vena cava syndrome (edema of the neck and face, headache, dizziness, vision disturbances, and syncope) and may develop acutely or more gradually. Veins of the upper chest and neck are dilated; flushing occurs, followed by cyanosis. Cerebral edema may affect the level of consciousness; laryngeal edema may impair respirations.

Paraneoplastic syndromes commonly associated with lung cancer include syndrome of inappropriate ADH secretion (SIADH) with fluid retention, hyponatremia, and edema, Cushing's syndrome (see Chapter 19 ∞) related to abnormal ACTH production, and hypercalcemia. Lung tumors also may produce procoagulation factors, increasing the risk for venous thrombosis, pulmonary embolism, and thrombotic endocarditis. In lung cancer, neuromuscular symptoms such as muscle weakness and wasting of the limbs may be the first indication of the disease (Porth, 2005).

At the time of diagnosis, cancer of the lung typically is well advanced, with distant metastasis present in 55% of clients and regional lymph node involvement in another 25%. The prognosis is generally poor: The overall 5-year survival rate is only 15% (ACS, 2005).

INTERDISCIPLINARY CARE

Because lung cancer typically is advanced when diagnosed and the prognosis generally is poor, prevention of the disease must be a primary goal for all healthcare providers. With 80% of lung cancer related to cigarette smoking, reducing tobacco use can have a significant impact on the death rate from lung cancer—a far greater impact than advances in treatment.

Establishing an accurate diagnosis is the first step in treating lung cancer. Treatment decisions are based on the tumor location, type of cancer cell, staging of the tumor, and the client's ability to tolerate treatment. Lung cancer is staged by the tumor size, location, degree of invasion of the primary tumor, and the presence of metastatic disease. Lung cancer staging is summarized in Table 38–9. Surgery is the treatment of choice for most forms of lung cancer.

Diagnosis

- *Chest x-ray* usually provides the first evidence of lung cancer. It is particularly reliable as a diagnostic tool when compared with previous chest x-ray. In high-risk populations, the chest x-ray may be used as a screening tool for lung cancer.
- *Sputum specimen* is sent for *cytologic examination* to establish the diagnosis of lung cancer. The sputum sample is collected on arising in the morning. If malignant cells are found in the sputum, more expensive and invasive examinations may be unnecessary. However, a sputum sample negative for malignant cells does not rule out lung cancer; it may simply indicate that the tumor is not shedding cells into mucous secretions.

TABLE 38–9 Lung Cancer Staging

	PRIMARY TUMOR (T STAGE)	REGIONAL LYMPH NODES (N)	DISTANT METASTASIS (M)
Stage 0	T_0—No evidence of primary tumor T_X—Malignant cells in bronchopulmonary secretions, but no tumor visualized		M_X—Presence of distant metastasis cannot be assessed
Stage I	T_1S—Carcinoma *in situ*	N_0—No regional lymph node metastasis	M_0—No distant metastasis
	T_1—Tumor that is 3 cm in diameter or less, with no evidence of invasion		
Stage II	T_2—Tumor that is greater than 3 cm in diameter, or invades visceral pleura, or has associated atelectasis or pneumonitis	N_1—Metastasis or direct extension to peribronchial or ipsilateral hilar nodes	
Stage III	T_3—Tumor with direct extension into an adjacent structure, or any tumor with associated pleural effusion or atelectasis or pneumonitis of entire lung	N_2—Metastasis to ipsilateral mediastinal or subcarinal nodes	
Stage IV	T_4—Tumor that invades mediastinum or involves the heart, great vessels, trachea, esophagus, vertebral body, or carina; presence of malignant pleural effusion	N_3—Metastasis to contralateral mediastinal, scalene, or supraclavicular nodes	M_1—Distant metastasis present

- *Bronchoscopy* is frequently done to visualize and obtain tissue for biopsy from the tumor. When a tumor mass or suspicious tissue is identified visually, a cable-activated instrument is used to obtain a biopsy specimen. If the tumor cannot be seen, the airways may be flushed with a saline solution (bronchial washing) to obtain cells for cytologic examination. Nursing care of the client undergoing a bronchoscopy is included in the Diagnostic Tests box in Chapter 36 ∞.
- *CT scan* is used to evaluate and localize tumors, particularly tumors in the lung parenchyma and pleura. It also is done prior to needle biopsy to localize the tumor. CT scanning can also detect distant tumor metastasis and evaluate tumor response to treatment.
- Cells or tissue for *cytologic examination and biopsy* may be obtained by aspirating fluid from a pleural effusion, percutaneous needle biopsy, and lymph node biopsy. These procedures may be done in an outpatient or a surgical setting.
- *CBC, liver function studies,* and *serum electrolytes* including calcium are obtained to evaluate for evidence of metastatic disease or paraneoplastic syndromes.
- *Tuberculin test (PPD)* is performed to rule out tuberculosis as the cause of symptoms and abnormalities seen on chest x-ray.
- *Pulmonary function tests (PFTs)* and *ABGs* may be performed prior to the initiation of treatment if the client has manifestations of respiratory insufficiency (e.g., dyspnea, activity intolerance, low oxygen saturation levels).

See Chapter 36 ∞ for nursing care related to commonly used diagnostic tests for lung cancer.

Medications

Combination chemotherapy (often combined with radiation therapy and/or surgery) is the treatment of choice for small-cell lung cancer because of its rapid growth, dissemination, and sensitivity to cytotoxic drugs. Used in combination, chemotherapeutic drugs allow tumor cells to be attacked at different parts of the cell cycle and in different ways, increasing the effectiveness of therapy. Fifty percent of clients with tumors at early stages achieve complete tumor remission with combination chemotherapy. When a complete tumor response is achieved in the first few cycles of chemotherapy, the chances for long-term survival are much greater.

Combination chemotherapy is used also as an adjunct to surgery or radiation therapy for other types of lung cancer. It may be used to reduce the size of advanced local tumors prior to surgery, and to lengthen survival when distant metastases are present. See Chapter 14 ∞ for further discussion of chemotherapy.

Bronchodilators may be prescribed to reduce airway obstruction. Analgesics and pain management strategies are vital when the cancer is advanced. See Chapter 9 ∞ for more information about postoperative and cancer pain management.

Surgery

Surgery offers the only real chance for a cure in non–small-cell lung cancer. Unfortunately, most tumors are inoperable or only partially resectable at the time of diagnosis. The 5-year survival rate following curative surgery in clients with resectable tumors is about 30%, with most clients succumbing to metastatic disease within 5 years (Kasper et al., 2005). The type of surgery performed depends on the location and size of the tumor, as well as the client's pulmonary and general health. The goal of surgery is to remove all involved tissue while preserving as much functional lung as possible. Table 38–10 outlines various surgical procedures used to treat lung cancer. Nursing care for the client having lung surgery is outlined in the box on page 1313.

Radiation Therapy

Radiation therapy is used alone or in combination with surgery or chemotherapy for lung cancer. The treatment goal may be either cure or symptom relief (palliative). Prior to surgery, radiation therapy is used to "debulk" tumors. When cancer has spread by direct extension to other thoracic structures and surgery is not feasible, radiation therapy may be the treatment of choice. It also may be used to relieve manifestations such as cough, hemoptysis, pain due to bone metastasis, and dyspnea from bronchial obstruction. Complications of lung cancer, such as superior vena cava syndrome, may be treated with radiation.

TABLE 38–10 Types of Surgery for Lung Cancer

PROCEDURE	DESCRIPTION	USED FOR
Laser bronchoscopy	Bronchoscopy-guided laser used to resect tumor	Tumors localized in a main bronchus
Mediastinoscopy	Visualization of the mediastinum using an endoscope passed through a suprasternal incision	Evaluation and biopsy of a mediastinal tumor and lymph nodes
Thoracotomy	Incision into the chest wall	Access the lung and thoracic cavity for surgery
Wedge resection	Removal of a small section (wedge) of peripheral lung tissue	Small, peripheral lung tumors
Segmental resection	Removal of an individual bronchovascular segment of a lobe	Peripheral lung tumor with no evidence of extension to the chest wall or metastasis
Sleeve resection (bronchoplastic reconstruction)	Resection of a section of a major bronchus with reconstruction of remaining normal bronchus	Small lesion of a major bronchus
Lobectomy	Removal of a single lung lobe	Tumors confined to a single lobe
Pneumonectomy	Removal of an entire lung	Tumor widespread throughout the lung, involving the main bronchus, or fixed to the hilum

NURSING CARE OF THE CLIENT HAVING Lung Surgery

PREOPERATIVE CARE

- Provide routine preoperative nursing care as outlined in Chapter 4 ∞.
- Note any history of smoking, respiratory and cardiac diseases, and other chronic conditions in the nursing history. *These factors may affect the response to surgery and the risk for postoperative complications.*
- Provide emotional and psychologic support for the client and family. *In addition to facing surgery, the client may be adjusting to a new diagnosis of cancer and the possibility that surgical intervention will be only partially successful.*
- Instruct about postoperative procedures, including respiratory therapy, breathing exercises, and coughing techniques. Allow practice time. *Learning will be easier in the preoperative period, when pain and analgesia are not affecting mental function.*
- If the client will return from surgery with an endotracheal tube and mechanical ventilation, establish a means of communication using hand or eye signals or a magic slate. *Establishing a means of communication prior to surgery reduces postoperative anxiety at being unable to speak.*
- If the client will return to the ICU, introduce the client and family to the unit and any machines, such as ventilators and monitors, that will be used. *The knowledge that this is an expected part of surgical recovery reduces the client's and family's postoperative anxiety.*

POSTOPERATIVE CARE

- Assess and provide routine postoperative care as outlined in Chapter 4 ∞.
- Assess for adequate pain control, and provide analgesics as needed. *Incisional pain commonly causes altered breathing patterns in the client who has undergone lung surgery.*
- Frequently assess respiratory status, including color, oxygen saturation, respiratory rate and depth, chest expansion, lung sounds, percussion tone, and ABGs. *Maintaining adequate ventilation and gas exchange postoperatively is vital to reduce mortality and morbidity. Gas exchange may be impaired*

by complications of lung surgery, including pneumothorax, atelectasis, bronchospasm, pulmonary embolus, bronchopleural fistula, and ARDS.

- Assist with effective coughing techniques, postural drainage, and incentive spirometry. Perform endotracheal suctioning as needed while intubated. *Surgical manipulation and anesthesia can increase the mucous production, leading to airway obstruction. Aggressive pulmonary hygiene is important to prevent this complication.*
- Monitor and maintain effective mechanical ventilation. *This is vital to ensure adequate ventilation and gas exchange in the early postoperative period.*
- Maintain patent chest tubes and a closed drainage system. Monitor chest tube output every hour initially, then every 2 to 4 or 8 hours as indicated. Notify the physician if chest tube output exceeds 70 mL per hour and/or is bright red, warm, and free flowing. *Maintaining a patent, intact chest drainage system is vital to reestablish negative pressure within the chest cavity and reexpansion of the lungs. Increased amounts of warm, free-flowing blood indicate intrathoracic hemorrhage that may necessitate surgical intervention.*
- Assess for signs of infection involving the incision or chest tube site(s). Use strict aseptic technique in caring for incisions and invasive monitoring devices. *The postoperative client is at risk for incisional infections, empyema in the chest cavity, and pneumonia.*
- Assist with turning and to ambulate as soon as possible. *Early mobility is important to prevent possible complications, such as pneumonia or pulmonary embolus.*
- Assess and maintain nutritional status. Initiate enteral or parenteral nutrition early if intubation and mechanical ventilation will be required for an extended period. Provide frequent small feedings once extubated. *Maintaining nutritional status promotes wound healing and prevents negative nitrogen balance. Giving frequent small feedings reduces the fatigue associated with eating.*

Radiation therapy may be delivered by external beam to the primary tumor site or by intraluminal radiation, or brachytherapy. Radiation therapy and related nursing care are discussed further in Chapter 14 ∞. Specific nursing measures for the client undergoing radiation therapy for lung cancer are outlined in the Nursing Care box on page 1314.

Complementary Therapies

Research indicates that a significant number of clients diagnosed with lung cancer use complementary and alternative medicine (CAM). In one study of clients with lung cancer in eight European nations, 23.6% used CAM therapies (Molassiotis et al., 2006). The CAM remedies used included herbal medicines, medicinal teas, homeopathy, animal extracts, and spiritual therapies. While these therapies may be safe when used alone, the potential for interactions with conventional medical treatment must be considered. Inquire of clients about their use of complementary and alternative therapies, and inform members of the healthcare team when present.

NURSING CARE

Health Promotion

The incidence of lung cancer is decreasing as the use of tobacco products declines. Teach people of all ages, particularly children and teenagers, about the link between cigarette smoking and lung cancer. Not smoking and avoiding exposure to secondhand smoke is the primary preventive measure for lung cancer. In addition, explain the risk of lung cancer to clients with occupational risk factors, exposure to asbestos products in particular.

Assessment

Nursing assessment related to lung cancer focuses on identifying risk factors for the disease, early manifestations of lung cancer, and respiratory function in the client undergoing treatment.

- *Health History:* Current symptoms, including chronic cough, shortness of breath, blood-tinged sputum; systemic

NURSING CARE OF THE CLIENT RECEIVING Radiation Therapy

Although radiation therapy is well controlled and specifically directed toward the tumor cells, some normal cells are also damaged in the process of treatment. Nursing care and client teaching help the client cope with uncomfortable side effects associated with radiation therapy.

Nursing Responsibilities

- Monitor for potential complications:
  a. Radiation pneumonitis—dyspnea on exertion, dry cough, fever
  b. Pericarditis—chest pain, pericardial friction rub; muffled heart sounds, paradoxical pulse, ECG abnormalities (Notify the physician if symptoms develop.)
  c. Esophagitis—pain, sore throat, difficulty swallowing.
- Encourage adequate fluid intake to liquefy respiratory secretions.
- Provide local analgesics and local anesthetics such as viscous lidocaine as ordered to relieve dysphagia and sore throat.
- Offer small frequent meals of soft, cool foods and liquids to maintain nutritional status.

Health Education for the Client and Family

- If dyspnea or pneumonitis develop, teach positioning, pursed-lip techniques, and relaxation exercises to facilitate breathing.
- Reassure that pneumonitis is generally a self-limiting process and should resolve when the course of radiotherapy is completed.
- Teach the manifestations of pericarditis, which may develop during treatment or up to 1 year after its completion. Chest pain or pressure, rapid heartbeat, and fever may signal pericarditis; increasing fatigue, dyspnea, and light-headedness can indicate a chronic process with pericardial effusion and possible cardiac tamponade.
- Instruct to eliminate hot, spicy, or acidic foods from the diet if esophagitis is a problem. Alcohol and tobacco should also be avoided.
- Adequate rest and nutrition are important to alleviate the symptoms of radiation fatigue, which is common in clients receiving radiation therapy for lung cancer. The fatigue is generally temporary.

---

manifestations such as recent weight loss, fatigue, anorexia, bone pain; smoking history; occupational exposure to carcinogens; chronic diseases such as COPD.

- *Physical Examination:* General appearance; skin color, evidence of clubbing; weight and height; vital signs; respiratory rate, depth, excursion; lung sounds to percussion and auscultation.
- *Diagnostic Tests:* CBC and coagulation studies, serum electrolytes and osmolality, liver and renal function studies; chest x-ray and CT scan results; ABGs and oxygen saturation levels.

Nursing Diagnoses and Interventions

The client with lung cancer is facing invasive treatments with undesirable side effects, possibly surgery, and typically a poor prognosis for long-term survival. Nursing care needs are diverse, related to respiratory status, the cancer itself and possible metastases, and the treatment plan. Priority nursing diagnoses related to respiratory function include *Ineffective Breathing Pattern* and *Activity Intolerance. Pain* and *Anticipatory Grieving* also are likely to be high-priority problems. See the accompanying Nursing Care Plan on page 1315.

Ineffective Breathing Pattern

Breathing pattern and ventilation may be affected by the tumor itself or by treatment of the tumor. Thoracic surgery increases the risk due to the incision and disruption of the muscles of respiration. Maintaining effective lung ventilation is particularly important postoperatively to reexpand remaining lung tissue and prevent surgical complications.

- Assess and document respiratory rate, depth, and lung sounds at least every 4 hours; evaluate more frequently in the immediate postoperative period or as indicated by condition. *Early detection of signs of respiratory compromise or adventitious lung sounds is vital for effective intervention.*

PRACTICE ALERT
Monitor oxygen saturation, exhaled carbon dioxide, and/or blood gas results, reporting changes from normal. Changes in levels of blood oxygen or exhaled CO_2 may be early indications of respiratory compromise.

- Frequently assess and document pain level (using a standard pain scale); provide analgesics as needed. *Pain and attempting to avoid chest movement to prevent additional pain can lead to rapid, shallow respirations and ineffective ventilation.*
- Elevate the head of the bed to 60 degrees. *Elevating the head of the bed reduces pressure on the diaphragm and permits optimal lung expansion.*
- Assist to turn, cough, and deep breathe and use incentive spirometry. Help splint the chest with a pillow or blanket when coughing. *These measures promote airway clearance.*
- Suction airway as needed. *Suctioning may be required to remove secretions that the client is unable to cough up and expectorate.*

PRACTICE ALERT
Maintain chest tube integrity and patency by ensuring uninterrupted gravity flow. Chest tubes help reestablish negative pressure in the thoracic cavity, allowing the lung to fully reexpand.

- Provide chest physiotherapy with percussion and postural drainage as needed or ordered. *Percussion and postural drainage help maintain airway patency and effective respirations.*
- If mechanical ventilation is instituted, work with respiratory therapy and use analgesia or sedation as needed to synchronize respirations with the ventilator. *Coordination of the*

NURSING CARE PLAN A Client with Lung Cancer

After coughing up bloody sputum one morning, James Mueller, a 68-year-old retired mill worker, sees his physician. A chest x-ray shows a suspicious density in the central portion of his right lung. Mr. Mueller is admitted to the hospital the following Monday for diagnostic tests.

ASSESSMENT

Anita Sarros, RN, admits Mr. Mueller to the oncology unit and obtains a nursing history. Mr. Mueller is married and has three grown children. He worked in a local paper mill for 35 years before retiring at age 62. He describes himself as "pretty healthy," except for a chronic smoker's cough. He started smoking as a young man in the army. He has a 50 pack-year smoking history, having smoked a pack a day for 50 years, since age 18. Mr. Mueller says he briefly quit smoking following a small heart attack 3 years ago, but started again after 4 months. On further questioning, Mr. Mueller says his cough has been productive for the past few months, especially in the morning, and that he is shorter of breath than usual with activity.

Mr. Mueller's examination data include BP 162/86, P 78 and regular, R 20, and T 98.4°F (36.9°C). Color good, skin warm and dry. Inspiratory and expiratory wheezes noted in right chest but good breath sounds throughout. No other abnormal findings are noted on examination. The physician orders early morning sputum specimens times 3 days for cytologic examination and schedules a CT scan of the chest the morning after admission.

Mr. Mueller's CBC shows mild anemia, but remaining routine laboratory tests are essentially normal. Sputum cytology is positive for small-cell bronchogenic cancer. The CT scan shows a central mass approximately 4 cm in diameter with involved mediastinal and subclavicular lymph nodes. A small mass is also noted on the lumbar spine. After conferring with his physician and an oncologist, Mr. Mueller decides to undergo a trial course of chemotherapy.

DIAGNOSES

- *Ineffective Airway Clearance* related to tumor mass
- *Risk for Imbalanced Nutrition: Less than Body Requirements* related to effects of chemotherapy
- *Risk for Compromised Family Coping* related to new diagnosis of lung cancer
- *Deficient Knowledge* about lung cancer and aids to smoking cessation

EXPECTED OUTCOMES

- Maintain a patent airway.
- Maintain current weight.
- Express feelings and concerns about the effect of cancer on the family unit.
- Participate in care.
- Contact appropriate support groups.
- Verbalize an understanding of the disease, its treatment, and prognosis.

- Develop a plan to stop smoking.

PLANNING AND IMPLEMENTATION

- Teach coughing, deep breathing, and hydration measures to facilitate airway clearance.
- Discuss symptoms to report to the physician: increased dyspnea or hemoptysis, severe stridor or wheezing, chest pain.
- Discuss measures to relieve nausea associated with chemotherapy, including premedication with a prescribed antiemetic.
- Have dietitian consult with Mr. and Mrs. Mueller to develop a diet plan for maintaining ideal weight.
- Discuss possible effects of lung cancer with Mr. and Mrs. Mueller.
- Encourage Mr. and Mrs. Mueller to call a family conference to discuss the disease with their children and grandchildren.
- Evaluate family members' knowledge and understanding of lung cancer, correcting misinformation and teaching as needed.
- Have an American Cancer Society volunteer contact the family.
- Refer to local cancer support group.
- Refer to home health department for follow-up and further teaching.
- Work with Mr. Mueller to develop a plan to stop smoking.
- Ask the physician for a prescription for nicotine patches or gum for Mr. Mueller.

EVALUATION

Mr. Mueller had his first chemotherapy treatment in the hospital and was discharged 4 days after admission. After 3 months of chemotherapy, his tumor shows little regression, and a liver scan reveals further metastasis. He and his wife decide to stop chemotherapy, a decision with which the children reluctantly agree. Mr. and Mrs. Mueller are referred to hospice services. With the help of hospice nurses and volunteers, Mr. Mueller is able to remain at home. His pain is managed initially with oral MS Contin, a sustained-release form of morphine sulfate, and later with an intravenous morphine infusion. Mr. Mueller dies at home with his family at his side 9 months after his diagnosis of lung cancer.

CRITICAL THINKING IN THE NURSING PROCESS

1. The oncologist prescribed a chemotherapy regimen of cyclophosphamide, doxorubicin, and vincristine. Describe how each of these drugs works against cancer cells, and discuss the rationale for using this combination.
2. Develop a care plan to deal with the specific side effects for the above treatment regimen.
3. Mr. Mueller had small-cell (oat cell) cancer. How would his presentation and treatment differ if the diagnosis had been non–small-cell adenocarcinoma, stage $T_2N_2M_0$?

See Evaluating Your Response in Appendix C.

---

client's respiratory effort with ventilator-delivered breaths is important for fully effective mechanical ventilation.

- Provide reassurance and emotional support. *These measures help relieve anxiety and promote an effective breathing pattern.*

Activity Intolerance

Both resectional lung surgery and inoperable lung cancer reduce the amount of functional lung tissue and surface area for gas diffusion. This can lead to activity intolerance if the oxygen supply is insufficient to meet the body's oxygen demand.

> **PRACTICE ALERT**
> Assess and document physiologic responses to activity, including pulse, respiratory rate, dyspnea, and fatigue. These assessments are good indicators of activity tolerance.

- Plan rest periods between activities and procedures. *Rest periods reduce oxygen demands and fatigue.*
- Assist the postoperative client to increase activities gradually. *Increasing activity levels gradually improves exercise tolerance.*
- Teach measures to conserve energy while performing ADLs, such as sitting while showering and dressing and wearing slip-on shoes. *These energy-conserving measures reduce oxygen demand and allow the client to remain independent as long as possible.*
- Keep frequently used objects within easy reach. *This helps conserve energy.*
- Administer oxygen as prescribed. Teach the client and family about home oxygen use if appropriate. *Supplemental oxygen can help improve activity and exercise tolerance.*
- Encourage maintenance of physical activity to tolerance. *Maintaining activity levels to the degree possible improves physical and emotional well-being.*
- Allow family members to provide assistance as needed. *This helps the client conserve energy and allows the family to retain a sense of usefulness.*

Pain

Pain is a priority problem in both the postoperative period as well as in the terminal stages of cancer. Poorly managed pain prolongs recovery from surgery. In the terminal cancer client, chronic and acute pain must be managed effectively to allow a peaceful death.

- Assess and document pain using a standardized pain scale and objective data. *Pain is a subjective experience, best evaluated by the client. Changes in vital signs, guarded movement, or unwillingness to move may indicate unreported pain.*
- Provide analgesics as needed to maintain comfort. *Postoperative recovery and restoration of function is facilitated by adequate pain management.*
- For cancer pain, maintain an around-the-clock medication schedule using narcotic, nonsteroidal anti-inflammatory drugs, and other medications as ordered. *Addiction is not a concern in terminal cancer; providing adequate pain relief that does not allow "breakthrough" pain is important.*
- Provide or assist with comfort measures, such as massage, positioning, distraction, and relaxation techniques. *These techniques promote relaxation and enhance pain relief.*
- Assist the client and family to plan and engage in activities that distract from pain such as reading, watching television, and engaging in social interactions. *Distraction helps the client focus away from the pain.*
- Spend as much time with the client as possible; allow family members to remain with the client. *Physical presence of the nurse and family provides emotional support for the client.*

Anticipatory Grieving

Because lung cancer often is advanced when diagnosed, the client faces the very real prospect of dying from the disease. Grieving for the anticipated loss of life is a normal response as the client and family begin to adapt to the diagnosis. Nursing care goals are to promote expression of feelings and thoughts about the loss, and to help the client and family initiate grief work, make decisions, and use appropriate resources and coping mechanisms to deal with the loss.

- Spend time with the client and family. *Time is necessary to develop a trusting, therapeutic relationship.*
- Answer questions honestly; do not deny the probable outcome of the disease. *Honesty reinforces reality and provides a sense of control over decisions to be made.*
- Encourage the client and family to express their feelings, fears, and concerns. *Open expression of feelings helps to promote understanding and acceptance.*
- Assist with understanding the grieving process and acceptance of feelings as normal. *Feelings of guilt, anger, or depression may cause the client to withdraw from others. Explanation of the grieving process enhances understanding and ability to cope.*
- Help identify strengths and coping measures that have been used effectively in the past. Provide positive reinforcement for effective coping behavior. *Past effective coping measures can help the client and family deal with the present situation and regain a sense of control.*
- Help the client and family make decisions regarding treatment and care. *This also is important to give them a sense of control.*
- Encourage use of other support systems, such as spiritual and social groups. Refer the client and family to support groups, social support services, and hospice care as indicated. Provide American Cancer Society literature and information as appropriate. *These support systems provide emotional support and help the client and family cope with the diagnosis.*
- Discuss advance directives (the Living Will) and power of attorney for health care with the client and family. *These documents give the client and family a sense of control over medical care provided if the client is no longer able to express his or her own wishes.*

Using NANDA, NIC, and NOC

Linkages between NANDA nursing diagnoses, nursing interventions, and nursing outcomes for the client with lung cancer are illustrated in Chart 38–3.

Community-Based Care

A primary teaching need to prepare the client and family affected by lung cancer for home care is information about the disease itself, expected prognosis, and planned treatment strategies. Provide honest information; do not promote false hope. Include the following additional topics in teaching for home care:

- Importance of quitting smoking, especially if surgery has been performed. (The client with lung cancer may have dif-

NANDA, NIC, AND NOC LINKAGES
CHART 38–3 The Client with Lung Cancer

NANDA

Ineffective Coping

↓

NIC

Coping Enhancement

Decision-Making Support

Support System Enhancement

NOC

Coping

Decision Making

Social Support

Data from *NANDA's Nursing Diagnoses: Definitions & Classification 2005–2006* by NANDA Interational (2005), Philadelphia; *Nursing Interventions Classification (NIC)* (4th ed.) by J. M. Dochterman & G. M. Bulechek (2004), St. Louis, MO: Mosby; and *Nursing Outcomes Classification (NOC)* (3rd ed.) by S. Moorhead, M. Johnson, and M. Maas (2004), St. Louis, MO: Mosby.

ficulty recognizing the need to stop smoking. Include information about the effects of nicotine and the tars in cigarette smoke on healing and already compromised lung tissue.)

- Planned treatments such as chemotherapy or radiation therapy, including expected effects and usual side effects of each
- Strategies to cope with noxious effects of radiation or chemotherapy
- Activities and exercises to improve strength and regain function for the postoperative client
- The need to continue coughing and deep-breathing exercises at home
- Symptoms to report to the physician: fever, increasing or continued shortness of breath, cough, increased or purulent sputum, redness, pain, swelling, or incisional drainage
- Use of prescribed medications, including desired and potential side effects and interactions with other drugs or foods
- Use of analgesics and other pain relief measures for postoperative or cancer pain
- Information about hospice services, home health, local cancer support groups for clients and caregivers, and American Cancer Society services.

Refer the client and family for home health services including nursing care, assistance with ADLs, respiratory care, and respite care as needed.

EXPLORE MEDIALINK

Prentice Hall Nursing MediaLink DVD-ROM
   Audio Glossary
   NCLEX-RN® Review

Animation
   Tuberculosis

COMPANION WEBSITE www.prenhall.com/lemone
   Audio Glossary
   NCLEX-RN® Review
   Care Plan Activity: Pneumonia
   Case Study: TB Medication and Compliance
   MediaLink Applications
      Health Promotion Among Vulnerable Populations
      SARS
   Links to Resources

CHAPTER HIGHLIGHTS

- Pneumonia, inflammation of the respiratory bronchioles and alveoli, usually is bacterial in origin. Different organisms are usually found in hospital-acquired pneumonia than in community-acquired pneumonia. Nursing care focuses on promoting airway clearance, supporting effective gas exchange, and promoting rest.
- Infection control measures, including standard, airborne, and contact precautions, are vital to prevent the spread of viral severe acute respiratory syndrome.

- Tuberculosis affects many people worldwide; in the United States, the primary affected populations are immigrants, people with compromised immunity, and people living in crowded or unsanitary conditions.
- The tuberculin test (PPD) detects a cellular immune response to *M. tuberculosis*, indicating infection, but not necessarily active disease.
- Effective tuberculosis treatment is a public health concern, requiring therapy and compliance monitoring, contact follow-up, and assessment for adverse treatment effects.

■ Fungal lung infections tend to have a geographic pattern of distribution. People with compromised immune status are more likely to be affected. Their manifestations resemble those of pneumonia or tuberculosis.

■ Disorders of the pleura, such as pleural effusion and pneumothorax, can affect lung expansion, ventilation, and gas exchange when significant.

■ Tension pneumothorax develops when air enters the pleural space but is unable to escape, collapsing the lung on the affected side and placing pressure on the unaffected lung and mediastinum. Ventilation, gas exchange, venous return, and cardiac output can be significantly affected.

■ Trauma may affect the chest wall (rib fracture, flail chest), the surface of the lungs (pulmonary contusion), or the airways and alveoli (smoke inhalation and near-drowning). Flail chest and pulmonary contusion often occur concurrently; hemothorax also frequently develops with chest trauma. Chest trauma (chest wall or airways) can endanger effective ventilation and gas exchange.

■ Lung cancer, the leading cause of cancer deaths, typically is advanced when diagnosed. Surgery, radiation therapy, and chemotherapy are used to treat lung cancer, often in combination.

■ Superior vena cava syndrome (impaired venous drainage from the head and neck) and paraneoplastic syndromes (abnormal hormone production, fluid and electrolyte imbalance, and altered clotting with possible venous thrombosis and pulmonary emboli) may complicate lung cancer.

TEST YOURSELF NCLEX-RN® REVIEW

1 Admitting orders for a client with acute bacterial pneumonia include an intravenous antibiotic every 8 hours, oxygen per nasal cannula at 5 L/min, continuous pulse oximetry monitoring, bed rest with bathroom privileges and chair at bedside as desired, diet as tolerated, sputum specimen for C&S, CBC, urinalysis, and chemistry panel. Which order should the nurse carry out first?
1. Start the oxygen per nasal cannula.
2. Insert an intravenous catheter and start the prescribed antibiotic.
3. Provide a dinner tray to the client.
4. Obtain the sputum specimen.

2 When assessing a client with bacterial pneumonia, the nurse notes that the client's overall skin tone is somewhat gray and there is a bluish tinge around the client's lips. The nurse should: (Place the following in the correct order of priority.)
1. start oxygen.
2. assess breath sounds.
3. notify the physician.
4. raise the head of the bed.
5. obtain oxygen saturation level.

3 The nurse evaluating a tuberculin test result 72 hours after it was administered notes an area of induration 9 mm in diameter. What additional information would indicate to the nurse that this is a positive result? The client
1. resides in a long-term care facility.
2. was born in Southeast Asia.
3. has HIV disease.
4. is an injection drug user.

4 The nurse teaching a client taking prophylactic daily isoniazid (INH) following tuberculin test conversion includes which of the following in the instructions?
1. This drug turns your urine red-orange. This is harmless.
2. Report numbness and tingling of your extremities to your doctor.
3. You will need to have periodic eye examinations during treatment.
4. Do not use aspirin while taking this drug because abnormal bleeding may occur.

5 Which of the following statements made by a client with a new diagnosis of lung cancer would indicate that the nurse's teaching has been effective?
1. "Well, since I'm going to die anyway, I may as well go home, put my affairs in order, and spend the rest of my time in the easy chair."

2. "I understand that because the cancer has already spread, I will be undergoing aggressive cancer treatment for the next several years to beat this thing."
3. "Even though I can't undo the damage caused by cigarette smoking, I will try to quit to prevent further damage to my lungs."
4. "Having the 'big C' is very scary; I'm just glad it is one of the more curable forms of cancer."

6 The nurse caring for a client following a lobectomy notes 100 mL of red drainage in the chest drainage container since checking it 30 minutes previously. The nurse should: (Select all that apply.)
1. empty the chest-tube drainage system.
2. note the finding and reevaluate drainage in 30 minutes.
3. notify the surgeon.
4. assess vital signs and level of consciousness.
5. apply pressure to the chest tube insertion site.

7 The nurse caring for a client having a thoracentesis appropriately assists the client to:
1. sit upright leaning forward during the procedure.
2. breathe deeply as the needle is inserted.
3. remain on quiet bed rest for 4 hours following the procedure.
4. cough as the fluid is withdrawn.

8 The nurse teaches a client being discharged from the emergency department with a diagnosis of fractured rib to:
1. avoid using pain medications to prevent respiratory depression.
2. use elastic roller bandages (ACE wraps) to stabilize the chest wall and promote comfort.
3. remain on bed rest for a week to allow the fracture to stabilize.
4. use a small pillow to splint the area when coughing.

9 Which of the following assessment findings of a client with smoke inhalation does the nurse find of greatest concern?
1. ash-like material in the sputum
2. respiratory rate of 36
3. skin and mucous membranes pink
4. fine crackles in bilateral bases

10 Which of the following nursing diagnoses does the nurse identify as of highest priority for a client with tension pneumothorax?
1. *Decreased Cardiac Output*
2. *Ineffective Breathing Pattern*
3. *Acute Pain*
4. *Risk for Aspiration*

See Test Yourself answers in Appendix C.

BIBLIOGRAPHY

Ahrens, T., Kollef, M., Stewart, J., & Shannon, W. (2004). Effect of kinetic therapy on pulmonary complications. *American Journal of Critical Care, 13*(5), 376–383.

Ailinger, R. L., Armstrong, R., Nguyen, N., & Lasus, H. (2004). Latino immigrants' knowledge of tuberculosis. *Public Health Nursing, 21*(6), 519–523.

American Cancer Society. (2005). *Cancer facts and figures 2005.* Atlanta: Author.

American Thoracic Society, CDC, & Infectious Diseases Society of America. (2003). Treatment of tuberculosis. *MMWR Recommendations and Reports, 55*(RR11), 1–77. Retrieved from: http://cdc.gov/mmwr/preview/mmwrhtml/rr5211al.htm

Banning, M. (2005). Community acquired pneumonia: Common causes, treatment and resistance. *Nurse Prescribing, 3*(5), 195–200.

Barry, M. (2004). Penetrating chest wounds. *RN, 67*(5), 36, 42.

Carlisle, D. (2005). Targeted TB prevention. *Community Practitioner, 78*(11), 385–386.

Cava, M. A., Fay, K. E., Beanlands, H. J., McCay, E. A., & Wignall, R. (2005). Risk perception and compliance with quarantine during the SARS outbreak. *Journal of Nursing Scholarship, 37*(4), 343–347.

Centers for Disease Control and Prevention (CDC). (2004). Fact sheet. Basic information about SARS. Retrieved from www.cdc.gov/ncidod/sars/pdf/factsheet.pdf.

_____. (2005). Public health guidance for community-level preparedness and responses to severe acute respiratory syndrome (SARS) Version 2/3. Retrieved from www.cdc.gov/ncidod/sars/guidance/index.htm

_____. (2006a). Emergence of *Mycobacterium tuberculosis* with extensive resistance to second-line drugs—worldwide, 2000–2004. *MMWR, 55*(11), 301–305.

_____. (2006b). Trends in tuberculosis—United States, 2005. *MMWR, 55*(11), 305–308.

_____. (2006c). World TB day—March 24, 2006. *MMWR, 55*(11), 301.

Chatterjee, M. (2005). Vulnerable TB patents slipping through the net. *Nursing Times, 101*(6), 7.

Chernecky, C., Sarna, L., Waller, J. L., & Bracht, M. L. (2004). Assessing coughing and wheezing in lung cancer: A pilot study. *Oncology Nursing Forum, 31*(6), 1095–1101.

Clinical rounds: Bioterrorism. How to identify inhalation anthrax. (2004). *Nursing, 34*(10), 34–35.

Coleman, P. R. (2004). Pneumonia in the long-term care setting: Etiology, management and prevention. *Journal of Gerontological Nursing, 30*(4), 14–23, 54–55.

Copstead, L. C., & Banasik, J. L. (2005). *Pathophysiology* (3rd ed.). St. Louis, MO: Elsevier/Saunders.

Darlison, L. (2005). Respiratory care. Lung cancer: An update on current diagnostic techniques and treatment. *Nursing Times, 101*(14), 42–44, 46.

DeBoer, S., & O'Connor, A. (2004). Prehospital and emergency department burn care. *Critical Care Nursing Clinics of North America, 16*(1), 61–73.

Dent, M. (2004). Hospital-acquired pneumonia: The "gift" that keeps on taking. *Nursing, 34*(2), 48–51.

Dick, J., Lewin, S., Rose, E., Zwarenstein, M., & van der Walt, H. (2004). Changing professional practice in tuberculosis care: An educational intervention. *Journal of Advanced Nursing, 48*(5), 434–442.

Dochterman, J., & Bulechek, G. (2004). *Nursing interventions classification (NIC)* (4th ed.). St. Louis, MO: Mosby.

Dreher, H. M., Dean, J. L., Moriarty, D. M., Kaiser, R., Willard, R., O'Donnell, S., et al. (2004). What you need to know about SARS now. *Nursing, 34*(1), 58–63.

Dunn, L. (2005). Pneumonia: Classification, diagnosis and nursing management. *Nursing Standard, 19*(42), 50–54.

Fontaine, K. L. (2005). *Healing practices: Alternative therapies for nursing* (2nd ed.). Upper Saddle River, NJ: Prentice Hall Health.

Gift, A. G., Jablonski, A., Stommel, M., & Given, C. W. (2004). Symptom clusters in elderly patients with lung cancer. *Oncology Nursing Forum, 31*(2), 203–210.

Grap, M. J., Munro, C. L., Hummel, R. S. III, Elswick, R. K., McKinney, J. L., & Sessler, C. N. (2005). Effect of backrest elevation on the development of ventilator-associated pneumonia. *American Journal of Critical Care, 14*(4), 325–333.

Hilton, P. (2004). Clinical. Evaluating the treatment options for spontaneous pneumothorax. *Nursing Times, 100*(28), 32–33.

Hoyert, D. L., Heron, M., Murphy, S. L., & Kung, H. C. (2006). Deaths: Final data for 2003. Health & Stats. Retrieved from www.cdc.gov/nchs/products/pubs/pubd/hestats/finaldeaths03

Jantarakupt, P., & Porock, D. (2005). Dyspnea management in lung cancer: Applying the evidence from chronic obstructive pulmonary disease. *Oncology Nursing Forum, 32*(4), 785–797.

Joseph, H. A., Shrestha-Kuwahara, R., Lowry, D., Lambert, L. A., Panlilio, A. L., Raucher, B. G., et al. (2004). Factors influencing health care workers' adherence to work site tuberculosis screening and treatment policies. *American Journal of Infection Control, 32*(8), 456–461.

Kasper, D. L., Braunwald, E., Fauci, A. S., Hauser, S. L., Longo, D. L., & Jameson, J. L. (Eds.). (2005). *Harrison's principles of internal medicine* (16th ed.). New York: McGraw-Hill.

Kim, S., & Crittenden, K. S. (2005). Risk factors for tuberculosis among inmates: A retrospective analysis. *Public Health Nursing, 22*(2), 108–118.

Kleinpell, R. M., & Elpern, E. H. (2004). Community-acquired pneumonia: Updates in assessment and management. *Critical Care Nursing Quarterly, 27*(3), 231–240.

Ladd, E. (2005). The use of antibiotics for viral upper respiratory tract infections: An analysis of nurse practitioner and physician prescribing practices in ambulatory care, 1997–2001. *Journal of the American Academy of Nurse Practitioners, 17*(10), 416–424.

Lakasing, E., & Tester, M. (2006). How to manage lung cancer in primary care. *Practice Nursing, 17*(1), 35–39.

Lehne, R. A. (2004). *Pharmacology for nursing care* (5th ed.). St. Louis, MO: Saunders.

Leonard, M. K., Osterhlot, D., Kourbatova, E. V., Del Rio, C., Wand, W., & Blumberg, H. M. (2005). How many sputum specimens are necessary to diagnose pulmonary tuberculosis? *American Journal of Infection Control, 33*(1), 58–61.

McCance, K. L., & Huether, S. E. (2006). *Pathophysiology: The biologic basis for disease in adults & children* (5th ed.). St. Louis, MO: Mosby.

McInnes, K., & Safian, L. (2005). Keeping SARS out: An education program for SARS screeners in one Ontario hospital. *Journal for Nurses in Staff Development, 21*(2), 73–78.

Merrel, P., & Mayo, D. (2004). Inhalation injury in the burn patient. *Critical Care Nursing Clinics of North America, 16*(1), 27–38.

Molassiotis, A., Panteli, V., Patiraki, E., Ozden, G., Platin, N., Madsen, E., et al. (2006). Complementary and alternative medicine use in lung cancer patients in eight European countries. *Complementary Therapies in Clinical Practice, 12*(1), 34–39.

Montgomery, S. S., Burke, E. M., Wissman, S. A., Feldman, D. S., & Leier, C. V. (2005). Natural course of large spontaneous pneumothorax. *Heart & Lung, 34*(5), 332–334.

Moorhead, S., Johnson, M., & Maas, M. (2004). *Nursing outcomes classification (NOC)* (3rd ed.). St. Louis, MO: Mosby.

Myrianthefs, P. M., Kalafati, M., Samara, I., & Baltopoulos, G. J. (2004). Nosocomial pneumonia. *Critical Care Nursing Quarterly, 27*(3), 241–257.

NANDA International. (2005). *Nursing diagnoses: Definitions and classification 2005–2006.* Philadelphia: Author.

National Center for Complementary and Alternative Medicine. (2004). Consumer advisory. Ephedra. Retrieved from http://www.nccam.nih.gov/health/alerts/ephedra/consumeradvisory

_____. (2005). Herbs at a glance. Echinacea. Retrieved from http://www.nccam.nih.gov/health/echinacea/

National Center for Health Statistics. (2005). *Health, United States, 2005 with Chartbook on trends in the health of Americans.* Hyattsville, MD: U.S. Government Printing Office.

Neafsey, P. J. (2005). Medication news. Ketolides: New antimicrobials for community-acquired pneumonia. *Home Healthcare Nurse, 23*(3), 141–143.

Nyamathi, A., Berg, J., Jones, T., & Leake, B. (2005). Predictors of perceived health status of tuberculosis-infected homeless. *Western Journal of Nursing Research, 27*(7), 896–914.

Porth, C. M. (2005). *Pathophysiology: Concepts of altered health states* (7th ed.). Philadelphia: Lippincott.

Pruitt, B., & Jacobs, M. (2006). Best-practice interventions: How can you prevent ventilator-associated pneumonia? *Nursing, 36*(2), 36–42.

Ross, J. L. (2005). Near drowning. *RN, 68*(7), 36, 42.

Rothrock, J. C. (2003). *Alexander's care of the patient in surgery* (12th ed.). St. Louis, MO: Mosby.

Ryan, B. (2005). Pneumothorax: Assessment and diagnostic testing. *Journal of Cardiovascular Nursing, 20*(4), 251–253.

Sarna, L., Brown, J. K., Cooley, M. E., Williams, R. D., Chernecky, C., Padilla, G., et al. (2005). Quality of life and meaning of illness in women with lung cancer. *Oncology Nursing Forum, 32*(1), E9–E19.

Schleder, B. J. (2004). Taking charge of hospital-acquired pneumonia. *The Nurse Practitioner, 29*(3), 50–53.

Spencer, J. W., & Jacobs, J. J. (2003). *Complementary and alternative medicine: An evidence-based approach* (2nd ed.). St. Louis, MO: Mosby.

Swigart, V., & Kolb, R. (2004). Homeless persons' decisions to accept or reject public health disease-detection services. *Public Health Nursing, 21*(2), 162–170.

Tierney, L. M. Jr., McPhee, S. J., & Papadakis, M. A. (Eds.). (2005). *Current medical diagnosis & treatment* (44th ed.). New York: McGraw-Hill.

Todd, B. (2005). Emerging infections. Legionella pneumonia: Many cases of Legionnaire disease go unreported or unrecognized. *American Journal of Nursing, 105*(11), 35–36, 38.

Tolomiczenko, G. S., Kahan, M., Ricci, M., Strathern, L., Jeney, C., Patterson, K., et al. (2005). SARS: Coping with the impact at a community hospital. *Journal of Advanced Nursing, 50*(1), 101–110.

Toth, A., Fackelmann, J., Pigott, W., & Tolomeo, O. (2004). Tuberculosis prevention and treatment: Occupational health, infection control, public health, general duty staff, visiting, parish nursing or working in a physician's office—all nursing roles are key in improving tuberculosis control. *Canadian Nurse, 100*(9), 27–30.

Tseng, H., Chen, T., & Chou, S. (2005). SARS: Key factors in crisis management. *Journal of Nursing Research, 13*(1), 58–64.

Understanding pleural effusion. (2004). *Nursing, 34*(8). 64.

Vecchiarino, P., Bohannon, R. W., Ferullo, J., & Malijanian, R. (2004). Short-term outcomes and their predictors for patients hospitalized with community-acquired pneumonia. *Heart & Lung, 33*(5), 301–307.

Way, L. W., & Doherty, G. M. (2003). *Current surgical diagnosis & treatment* (11th ed.). New York: McGraw-Hill.

Wilkinson, J. M. (2005). *Nursing diagnosis handbook* (8th ed.). Upper Saddle River, NJ: Prentice Hall.

Williams, V. G. (2006). Tuberculosis: Clinical features, diagnosis and management. *Nursing Standard, 20*(22), 49–53.

Willis, D., VanSickle, D., Van Riper, S., & Valerio, C. (2005). Pneumonia: Bringing JCAHO and CMS to the bedside. *American Journal of Nursing, 105*(3), 72A, 72C–72D.

Wing, S. (2004). Pleural effusion: Nursing care challenge in the elderly. *Geriatric Nursing, 25*(6), 348–354.

Withy, K., & Alper, B. S. (2005). Stat consult. Acute bronchitis. *Clinical Advisor for Nurse Practitioners, 8*(1), 73–74, 77.

Woods, A., & Hathaway, L. (2004). Treating community-acquired pneumonia. *Nurse Practitioner, 29*(6), 11.

World Health Organization. (2003). Cumulative number of reported probable cases of severe acute respiratory syndrome (SARS). *Communicable Disease Surveillance & Response (CSR).* Author.

Yamamoto, L., Schroeder, C., Morley, D., & Beliveau, C. (2005). Thoracic trauma: The deadly dozen. *Critical Care Nursing Quarterly, 28*(1), 22–40.

CHAPTER 39
Nursing Care of Clients with Gas Exchange Disorders

LEARNING OUTCOMES

- Relate the pathophysiology and manifestations of obstructive, pulmonary vascular, and critical respiratory disorders to their effects on ventilation and respiration (gas exchange).

- Compare and contrast the etiology, risk factors, and vulnerable populations for disorders affecting ventilation and gas exchange within the lungs.

- Describe interdisciplinary care and the nursing role in health promotion and caring for clients with disorders that affect the ability to ventilate the lungs and exchange gases with the environment.

- Discuss interdisciplinary interventions to provide airway and ventilatory support for the client with respiratory failure, and nursing responsibilities in caring for clients requiring airway and ventilatory support.

- Describe the nursing implications for medications used to promote ventilation and gas exchange.

CLINICAL COMPETENCIES

- Assess functional health status of clients with disorders affecting ventilation and gas exchange.

- Use assessed data and knowledge of the effects of the disorder and prescribed treatment to identify priority nursing diagnoses and plan care for clients with disorders affecting ventilation and gas exchange.

- Use the nursing process and evidence-based nursing research to plan and implement individualized nursing care for clients, including measures to promote ventilation and gas exchange.

- Plan and provide appropriate teaching for health promotion among vulnerable populations and to prepare clients and families for community-based care.

- Evaluate the effectiveness of nursing interventions and teaching, revising strategies and teaching plans as needed.

- Safely and knowledgeably coordinate interdisciplinary care and administer prescribed medications and treatments for clients with disorders affecting ventilation and gas exchange.

MEDIALINK

Resources for this chapter can be found on the Prentice Hall Nursing MediaLink DVD-ROM accompanying this textbook, and on the Companion Website at http://www.prenhall.com/lemone

acute respiratory distress syndrome (ARDS), *1365*
asthma, *1321*
atelectasis, *1343*
bronchiectasis, *1344*
chronic bronchitis, *1331*

chronic obstructive pulmonary disease (COPD), *1330*
cor pulmonale, *1352*
cystic fibrosis (CF), *1340*
emphysema, *1332*
pulmonary embolism, *1347*

pulmonary hypertension, *1352*
respiratory failure, *1353*
sarcoidosis, *1346*
status asthmaticus, *1323*
weaning, *1360*

Normal function of the lower respiratory system depends on several organ systems: the central nervous system, which stimulates and controls breathing; chemoreceptors in the brain, aortic arch, and carotid bodies, which monitor the pH and oxygen content of blood; the heart and circulatory system, which provide for blood supply and gas exchange; the musculoskeletal system, which provides an intact thoracic cavity capable of expanding and contracting; and the lungs and bronchial tree, which allow air movement and gas exchange. Impaired function of any of these systems affects ventilation and respiration. As a result, tissues may become *hypoxic,* with inadequate oxygen to support metabolic activity.

Although some of the disorders discussed in this chapter can affect ventilation (air movement into and out of the airways and alveoli), all can have significant effects on gas exchange. The mechanisms by which they affect gas exchange differ:

- In reactive airway disease (asthma) and obstructive disorders, air trapping reduces the amount of oxygen available to drive gas exchange.
- Interstitial lung disorders affect the ability of the lungs to expand and the work of breathing, again, reducing alveolar oxygenation and gas exchange.
- Pulmonary vascular disorders affect blood flow to the lungs or a portion of the lungs, reducing gas exchange through their effects on perfusion of the lungs.
- Respiratory failure is the ultimate consequence of impaired gas exchange; the lungs cannot adequately oxygenate the blood or eliminate carbon dioxide.

With a few exceptions, the disorders discussed in this chapter are relatively common, chronic lung diseases.

FAST FACTS

- Chronic lower respiratory diseases are the fourth leading cause of death in the United States.
- The death rate for chronic lower respiratory diseases is higher for men than women.
- Whites have a higher death rate due to chronic lower respiratory diseases than blacks, Native Americans, or Hispanics; people of Asian heritage have the lowest death rate due to chronic lower respiratory diseases.
- Adults age 45 and older have the greatest risk: Chronic lower respiratory diseases are not among the leading causes of death for adults ages 25 to 44; in the 45- to 64-year-old age grouping, however, they are the sixth leading cause of death, jumping to the fourth leading cause of death for people 65 years old and older.

Source: National Center for Health Statistics, 2005.

Disorders of other body systems, such as neurologic disorders (e.g., head injury, spinal cord trauma or disorders, amyotrophic lateral sclerosis, myasthenia gravis) also can affect gas exchange through their effects on the central or peripheral nervous systems. These disorders and their effects on the respiratory system are discussed in subsequent chapters of this text.

Aging affects pulmonary ventilation and gas exchange as well. The number of alveoli decrease, and emphysematous changes (senile emphysema) reduce the surface area for gas exchange. Alveoli become less elastic, causing increased air trapping and dead space. For most older adults who remain active, these changes have minimal effect on exercise tolerance and activities of daily living (ADLs). When combined with lung disease, however, age-related pulmonary changes increase the client's risk for developing respiratory failure.

REACTIVE AIRWAY DISORDERS

In reactive airway disorders, the airways narrow in response to a stimulus. Airway narrowing limits airflow both into and out of the alveoli. Limited airflow increases the work of breathing and the residual volume of the lungs as air is trapped behind narrowed airways. Inspired air mixes with an abnormally large volume of residual air, effectively reducing the amount of oxygen available in the alveoli. Decreased alveolar ventilation further reduces oxygen available for exchange.

THE CLIENT WITH ASTHMA

Asthma is a chronic inflammatory disorder of the airways characterized by recurrent episodes of wheezing, breathlessness, chest tightness, and coughing. Inflammation causes increased responsiveness of the airways to multiple stimuli. The widespread airflow obstruction that occurs during acute episodes usually reverses either spontaneously or with treatment. While most episodes or asthma "attacks" are relatively brief, some clients with asthma may experience longer episodes with some degree of airway impairment daily. In rare cases, an acute episode of asthma is so severe that respiratory failure and death result.

Incidence and Risk Factors

In the United States, approximately 11 million people experienced at least one asthma attack in the year 2003. After several

MEDIALINK

Asthma Animation

years of increase, the prevalence of asthma currently is relatively stable. Hospitalizations and deaths due to asthma have decreased in recent years, likely as a result of better disease management. Asthma is a serious disease, causing more than 4000 deaths in the United States in 2002 (American Lung Association [ALA], 2005a).

FAST FACTS

- Although asthma is more common in children than adults, 5.5% to 10% of adults are affected (National Heart, Lung, and Blood Institute [NHLBI], 2004).
- Across races, the mortality rate associated with asthma is higher in women than in men.
- The asthma mortality rate of blacks is nearly three times that of whites and is higher than that of Hispanics and other ethnic groups.
- Deaths due to asthma are rare in children and increase with age, particularly in middle and late adulthood and old age (ALA, 2005a).

A number of risk factors can be identified for asthma, although many clients develop the disease in the absence of known risk factors. Allergies play a strong role in childhood asthma, a lesser role in adults. There is a strong genetic component to the disease, although a specific pattern of inheritance has not been identified. Multiple regions on several chromosomes appear to contribute to asthma-related factors such as airway hyperreactivity and high IgE levels (Kasper et al., 2005). Environmental factors, including air pollution and occupational exposure to industrial compounds, may contribute. Respiratory viruses such as rhinovirus and influenza can precipitate asthma attacks. Other contributory factors include exercise (particularly in cold air) and emotional stress.

Physiology Review

Airways within the lungs contain crisscrossing strips of smooth muscle that control their diameter. This muscle is innervated by the autonomic nervous system. Parasympathetic (cholinergic) stimulation leads to bronchoconstriction, or narrowing of the airways. Sympathetic stimulation through β_2-adrenergic receptors causes bronchodilation, or expansion of the airways. Slight bronchoconstriction normally predominates. However, when increased airflow is necessary (e.g., during exercise), the parasympathetic system is inhibited, and stimulation of the sympathetic system causes bronchodilation. Inflammatory mediators (such as histamine) released during an antigen–antibody response act directly on bronchial smooth muscle to produce bronchoconstriction.

Pathophysiology

In asthma, the airways are in a persistent state of inflammation. During symptom-free periods, airway inflammation in asthma is subacute or quiet. Even during these periods, however, inflammatory cells such as eosinophils, neutrophils, and lymphocytes may be found in airway tissues and edema may be present. An acute inflammatory response, during which resident inflammatory cells interact with inflammatory mediators, cytokines, and additional infiltrating inflammatory cells, may be triggered by a variety of factors. Common triggers for an acute asthma attack include exposure to allergens, respiratory tract infection, exercise, inhaled irritants, and emotional upsets.

Attack Triggers

Childhood asthma (which may continue into adulthood) is most often linked to inhalation of allergens such as pollen, animal dander, or household dust. Clients with allergic asthma often have a history of other allergies. Environmental pollutants, such as tobacco smoke and irritant gases (e.g., sulfur dioxide, nitrogen dioxide, and ozone), can provoke asthma. Exposure to secondhand smoke as a child is associated with a higher risk for and increased severity of asthma. Agents found in the workplace, such as noxious fumes and gases, chemicals, and dusts, may cause occupational asthma.

Respiratory infections, viral in particular, are a common internal stimulus for an asthmatic attack. Exercise-induced asthma attacks also are common, affecting 40% to 90% of people with bronchial asthma (Porth, 2005). Loss of heat or water from the bronchial surface may contribute to exercise-induced asthma. Exercising in cold, dry air increases the risk of an asthma attack in susceptible people.

Emotional stress is a significant etiologic factor for attacks in as many as half of clients with asthma. Common pharmacologic triggers include aspirin and other nonsteroidal anti-inflammatory drugs, sulfites (which are used as preservatives in wine, beer, fresh fruits, and salad), and beta-blockers.

Responses

When a trigger such as inhalation of an allergen or irritant occurs, an *acute* or *early response* develops in the hyperreactive airways predisposed to bronchospasm. Sensitized mast cells in the bronchial mucosa release inflammatory mediators such as histamine, prostaglandins, and leukotrienes. Resident and infiltrating inflammatory cells also produce inflammatory mediators such as cytokines, bradykinin, and growth factors. These mediators stimulate parasympathetic receptors and bronchial smooth muscle to produce bronchoconstriction. They also increase capillary permeability, which allows plasma to escape and leads to mucosal edema. Mucous production is stimulated; excess mucus collects in the narrowed airways.

The attack is prolonged by the *late phase response*, which develops 4 to 12 hours after exposure to the trigger. Inflammatory cells such as basophils and eosinophils are activated, and they damage airway epithelium, produce mucosal edema, impair mucociliary clearance, and produce or prolong bronchoconstriction. The degree of hyperreactivity depends on the extent of inflammation. Together, bronchoconstriction, edema and inflammation, and mucous secretion narrow the airway. Airway resistance increases, limiting airflow and increasing the work of breathing (Figure 39–1 ■).

Limited expiratory airflow traps air distal to the spastic, narrowed airways. Trapped air mixes with inspired air in the alveoli, reducing its oxygen tension and gas exchange across the alveolar-capillary membrane. Distended alveoli compress alveolar capillaries, reducing blood flow and further affecting

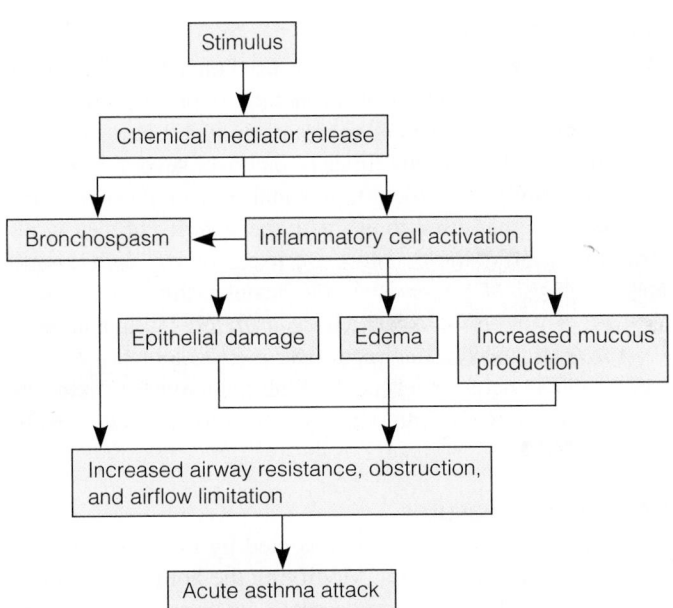

Figure 39–1 ■ The pathogenesis of an acute episode of asthma.

MANIFESTATIONS **of Acute Asthma**

- Chest tightness
- Cough
- Dyspnea
- Wheezing
- Tachypnea and tachycardia
- Anxiety and apprehension

gas exchange. As a result, hypoxemia develops. Hypoxemia and increased lung volume due to trapping stimulate the respiratory rate. Hyperventilation causes the $PaCO_2$ to fall, leading to respiratory alkalosis. (See Chapter 10 ∞ for more information about acid–base imbalances.)

To summarize, in an acute asthma attack, inflammatory mediators are released from sensitized airways followed by activation of inflammatory cells. These events lead to bronchoconstriction, airway edema, and impaired mucociliary clearance. Airway narrowing limits airflow and increases the work of breathing; trapped air mixes with inhaled air, impairing gas exchange.

Manifestations and Complications

An asthma attack is characterized by a subjective sensation of chest tightness, cough, dyspnea, and wheezing (see the Manifestations box above). The onset of symptoms may be either abrupt or insidious, and an attack may subside rapidly or persist for hours or days. A sense of chest constriction and nonproductive cough are common early manifestations of an attack. During an attack, tachycardia, tachypnea, and prolonged expiration are common. Diffuse wheezing is heard on auscultation. With more severe attacks, use of the accessory muscles of respiration, intercostal retractions, loud wheezing, and distant breath sounds may be noted. Fatigue, anxiety, apprehension, and severe dyspnea that allows speaking only one or two words between breaths may occur with persistent severe episodes. The onset of respiratory failure is marked by inaudible breath sounds with reduced wheezing and an ineffective cough. Without careful assessment, this apparent relief of symptoms can be misinterpreted as an improvement.

The frequency of attacks and severity of symptoms vary greatly from person to person. Although some people have infrequent, mild episodes, others have nearly continuous manifestations of cough, dyspnea on exertion, and wheezing with periodic severe exacerbations (Table 39–1).

Status asthmaticus is severe, prolonged asthma that does not respond to routine treatment. Without aggressive therapy, status asthmaticus can lead to respiratory failure with hypoxemia, hypercapnia, and acidosis. Endotracheal intubation, mechanical ventilation, and aggressive drug treatment may be necessary to sustain life.

TABLE 39–1 Classification of Asthma Severity

CLASSIFICATION	SYMPTOM FREQUENCY	NIGHTTIME SYMPTOMS
Mild intermittent	■ No more than twice a week ■ Brief attacks (hours to days) of varied intensity ■ Asymptomatic and normal peak expiratory flow rate between attacks	No more than twice a month
Mild persistent	■ More than twice a week but less than once a day ■ Exacerbations may affect activity	More than twice a month
Moderate persistent	■ Daily symptoms ■ Daily short-acting bronchodilator use ■ Exacerbations affect activity ■ Exacerbations more than twice a week; may last for days	More than once a week
Severe persistent	■ Continual symptoms ■ Limited physical activity ■ Frequent exacerbations	Frequent

Source: Adapted from *Expert Panel Report 2: Guidelines for the Diagnosis and Management of Asthma,* Publication No. 97-4051 by National Education and Prevention Program, 1997, Bethesda, MD: National Institutes of Health.

In addition to acute respiratory failure, other complications associated with acute asthma include dehydration, respiratory infection, atelectasis, pneumothorax, and cor pulmonale.

Cough-Variant Asthma

Asthma is one of the three most common causes of chronic cough (the other two being postnasal drip and gastroesophageal reflux disease [GERD]) (Kasper et al., 2005; Martin, 2003). Cough can be initiated by either upper airway irritants (e.g., postnasal drip or GERD) or by inflammation or constriction of the lower airways. Most commonly, cough associated with asthma is accompanied by classic asthma symptoms such as chest constriction, dyspnea, and wheezing. Clients with *cough-variant asthma*, however, have persistent cough without wheezing or dyspnea, often delaying diagnosis. These clients do have significant airway inflammation and demonstrate the pathophysiologic features of asthma.

INTERDISCIPLINARY CARE

The diagnosis of asthma is based primarily on the history and manifestations. Treatment goals are twofold. Daily management focuses on controlling symptoms and preventing acute attacks. During an acute attack, therapy is directed toward restoring airway patency and alveolar ventilation.

Diagnosis

Diagnostic tests are used to determine the degree of airway involvement during and between acute episodes and identify causative factors such as allergens. See Chapter 36 ∞ for more information about and the nursing care related to these diagnostic tests.

- *Pulmonary function tests (PFTs)* are used to evaluate the degree of airway obstruction. Pulmonary function testing done before and after use of an aerosolized bronchodilator helps determine the reversibility of airway obstruction. The residual volume of the lungs may be increased and vital capacity decreased or normal even during periods of remission. The forced expiratory volume and peak expiratory flow rate are the most valuable pulmonary function studies to evaluate the severity of an asthma attack and the effectiveness of treatment measures. See Box 36–1.
- *Challenge* or *bronchial provocation testing* uses an inhaled substance such as methacholine or histamine with PFTs to confirm the diagnosis of asthma by detecting airway hyperresponsiveness.
- *Arterial blood gases (ABGs)* are drawn during an acute attack to evaluate oxygenation, carbon dioxide elimination, and acid–base status. ABGs initially show hypoxemia with a low Pao_2, and mild respiratory alkalosis with an elevated pH and low $Paco_2$ due to tachypnea. Severe airflow obstruction causes significant hypoxemia and respiratory acidosis (pH less than 7.35 and $Paco_2$ greater than 42 mmHg), indicative of respiratory failure and the need for mechanical ventilation. See Chapter 10 ∞ for more information about arterial blood gases and their interpretation.
- *Skin testing* may be done to identify specific allergens if an allergic trigger is suspected for asthma attacks.

Disease Monitoring

Peak expiratory flow rate (PEFR) is used on a day-to-day basis to evaluate the severity of bronchial hyperresponsiveness. Small, inexpensive meters to measure PEFR are available. Readings taken at varying times of day over several weeks are used to establish the client's personal best or normal PEFR. This value is then used to evaluate the severity of airway obstruction. Traffic signal colors are used for simplicity: *green* (80% to 100% of personal best) indicates asthma that is under control; *yellow* (50% to 80%) is caution, indicating a need for further medication or treatment; and *red* (50% or less) signals an immediate need for a bronchodilator and medical treatment if the level does not immediately return to the yellow range (Porth, 2005).

Preventive Measures

Asthma attacks often can be prevented by avoiding allergens and environmental triggers. Modifying the home environment by controlling dust, removing carpets, covering mattresses and pillows to reduce dust mite populations, and installing air filtering systems may be useful. Pets may need to be removed from the household. Eliminating all tobacco smoke in the home is vital. Wearing a mask that retains humidity and warm air while exercising in cold weather may help prevent attacks of exercise-induced asthma. Early treatment of respiratory infections is vital to prevent asthma exacerbations.

Medications

Medications are used to prevent and control asthma symptoms, reduce the frequency and severity of exacerbations, and reverse airway obstruction. Drugs used for long-term control of asthma are taken daily to maintain control of the disease. The primary drugs in this group are anti-inflammatory agents, long-acting bronchodilators, and leukotriene modifiers. Quick-relief medications provide prompt relief of bronchoconstriction and airflow obstruction with associated wheezing, cough, and chest tightness. Short-acting adrenergic stimulants (rapid-acting bronchodilators), anticholinergic drugs, and methylxanthines fall into this category.

A stepwise approach for managing asthma is recommended. This approach is based on the severity of disease (see Tables 39–1 and 39–2). For all clients, a short-acting inhaled β_2-agonist is recommended for quick relief of acute symptoms. Up to three treatments at 20-minute intervals or a single nebulizer treatment may be used as needed. Strategies for long-term control may need to be modified if a short-acting bronchodilator is needed more than twice a week (NHLBI, 2003).

Many of the drugs used for continued asthma management and relief of an acute attack can be administered by a metered-dose inhaler (MDI), dry powder inhaler (DPI), or nebulizer. The advantages of administering medications locally by inhalation include rapid onset and reduced systemic effects of the drugs. In an MDI, a chemical propellant is used to deliver the medication when the canister is depressed. DPI, in contrast, contain no propellant. Instead, the medication is released by inhaling rapidly through the mouthpiece. Box 39–1 outlines client teaching for use of an MDI or DPI.

TABLE 39–2 Stepwise Approach to Asthma Management for Adults

STEP/DISEASE SEVERITY	PREFERRED TREATMENT	ALTERNATE OR AS NEEDED TREATMENT
Step 1: mild intermittent	No daily medication needed	Systemic corticosteroids for severe exacerbations
Step 2: mild persistent	Low-dose inhaled corticosteroids	Cromolyn, leukotriene modifier, nedocromil, or sustained-release theophylline
Step 3: moderate persistent	Low-to-moderate dose inhaled corticosteroids *and* long-acting inhaled β₂-agonist	Increase inhaled corticosteroid dose *or* combine inhaled corticosteroid with leukotriene modifier or theophylline
Step 4: severe persistent	High-dose inhaled corticosteroid *and* long-acting inhaled β₂-agonist	Add systemic corticosteroid

Source: Adapted from *Expert Panel Report 2: Guidelines for the Diagnosis and Management of Asthma, Update on Selected Topics 2002,* Publication No. 02-5074 by National Education and Prevention Program, 2003, Bethesda, MD: National Institutes of Health.

BRONCHODILATORS Most asthmatics need bronchodilator therapy to control their symptoms. Inhalation of nebulized medication is the preferred means of administration. The primary bronchodilators used include adrenergic stimulants, methylxanthines, and anticholinergic agents. These drugs often are administered in combination with an anti-inflammatory agent.

Adrenergic stimulants (β₂-agonists) affect receptors on smooth muscle cells of the respiratory tract, causing smooth muscle relaxation and bronchodilation. Long-acting adrenergic stimulants such as inhaled salmeterol and oral sustained-release albuterol are used in conjunction with anti-inflammatory drugs to control symptoms, but are not appropriate to treat an acute episode of asthma. Inhaled short-acting beta-adrenergic agonists such as albuterol, bitolterol, pirbuterol, and terbutaline, administered by MDI or DPI, are the treatment of choice for quick relief. They act within minutes, but their duration generally is short, lasting only 4 to 6 hours. Tachycardia and muscle tremors, common side effects of adrenergic agonists, are minimal with inhalation therapy.

BOX 39–1 Client Teaching: Using a Metered-Dose Inhaler or Dry Powder Inhaler

Metered-Dose Inhaler

- Firmly insert a charged metered-dose inhaler canister into the mouthpiece unit or spacer (if used).
- Remove mouthpiece cap. Shake canister vigorously for 3 to 5 seconds.
- Exhale slowly and completely.
- Holding the canister upside down, place the mouthpiece in the mouth, closing lips around it if a spacer is being used. When no spacer is used, hold the mouthpiece directly in front of the mouth.
- Press and hold the canister down while inhaling deeply and slowly for 3 to 5 seconds (see figure).

Source: Michal Heron, Pearson Education/PH College

- Hold breath for 10 seconds, release pressure on the container, remove from mouth, and exhale. Wait 20 to 30 seconds before repeating the procedure for a second puff.

- Rinse the mouth after using the inhaler to minimize systemic absorption and drying of the mucous membranes.
- Rinse the inhaler mouthpiece and spacer after use; store in a clean location.

Dry Powder Inhaler

- Keep the inhaler and medication in a clean, dry location. Do not refrigerate or store in a humid place (for example, the bathroom).
- Remove the cap and hold the inhaler upright. Inspect to be sure that the mechanism is clean and the mouthpiece is clear.
- If necessary, load the dose into the inhaler, following manufacturer's directions.
- Hold the inhaler level with the mouthpiece end facing down.
- Breathe slowly and completely. Tilt your head back slightly.
- Place the mouthpiece in your mouth with your teeth over the mouthpiece. Seal your lips around the mouthpiece. Do not block the inhaler with your tongue.
- Breathe in rapidly and deeply through your mouth over 2 to 3 seconds to activate the flow of medication.
- Remove the inhaler from your mouth and hold your breath for 10 seconds.
- Exhale slowly through pursed lips to allow the medication to enter distal airways. Never exhale into the inhaler mouthpiece to prevent clogging.
- Rinse your mouth or brush your teeth after using the inhaler to avoid a bad taste from the medication and to prevent a yeast infection (if a corticosteroid medication is being used).
- Store the inhaler in a clean, sealed plastic bag; do not wash the inhaler unless so directed by the manufacturer. The mouthpiece should be cleaned weekly using a dry cloth.

Anticholinergic medications prevent bronchoconstriction by blocking parasympathetic input to bronchial smooth muscle. Ipratropium bromide, an anticholinergic drug administered by MDI, is useful when asthma symptoms are poorly controlled by adrenergic stimulants alone. Anticholinergic drugs act more slowly than adrenergic stimulants, requiring up to 60 to 90 minutes to achieve maximal effect.

Theophylline is a methylxanthine used as adjunctive treatment for asthma. It relaxes bronchial smooth muscle and may also inhibit the release of chemical mediators of the inflammatory response. Monitoring of serum theophylline levels is necessary because of wide individual variations in metabolism and elimination of the drug and its toxic effects. Serum levels of 10 to 20 mcg/mL or lower are recommended. Theophylline may be used as a long-term bronchodilator, given once or twice daily. A related drug, aminophylline, may be administered intravenously to treat an acute, severe exacerbation of the disease.

ANTI-INFLAMMATORY AGENTS Corticosteroids and two nonsteroidal anti-inflammatory agents, cromolyn sodium and nedocromil, are used to suppress airway inflammation and reduce asthma symptoms.

Corticosteroids block the late response to inhaled allergens and reduce bronchial hyperresponsiveness. The preferred route of administration is by MDI or DPI to minimize systemic absorption and reduce the adverse effects of prolonged steroid use (cushingoid effects). For a severe acute attack, corticosteroids may be given systemically to alleviate symptoms and induce remission.

Cromolyn sodium and nedocromil are used to prevent acute episodes of asthma. They reduce airway hyperreactivity and inhibit the release of mediator substances. These drugs are used for long-term control of asthma, not quick relief. They have a wide margin of safety and few side effects.

LEUKOTRIENE MODIFIERS Leukotriene modifiers, montelukast (Singulair), zafirlukast (Accolate), and zileuton (Zyflo Filmtab), are oral medications that reduce the inflammatory response in asthma. They appear to improve lung function, diminish symptoms, and reduce the need for short-acting bronchodilators. These drugs affect the metabolism and excretion of other medications such as warfarin and theophylline and may cause liver toxicity.

Nursing implications for medications used to treat asthma are outlined in the Medication Administration box on pages 1327–1328.

Complementary Therapies

A number of herbal preparations and other complementary therapies have been shown to be helpful in treating asthma. Dietary therapies, environmental medicine, and nutritional supplements are the complementary therapies most widely recommended by healthcare professionals for asthma (Spencer & Jacobs, 2003). Nutritional and dietary therapies may include elimination of certain foods or food additives (e.g., sulfite) from the diet, often in the absence of a documented food allergy or relationship between consumption and the onset of asthma symptoms. Although the evidence is inconsistent, some studies suggest that increasing intake of ascorbic acid, an antioxidant,

zinc, and magnesium may help alleviate manifestations of asthma. People with mild asthma may benefit from addition of omega-3 polyunsaturated fatty acids to the diet, experiencing less severe and fewer acute attacks (Spencer & Jacobs, 2003).

Herbal preparations may include atropa belladonna (the natural form of atropine) or ephedra (also called ma huang), an herb that contains ephedrine. These herbals have effects similar to those of drugs used to treat asthma, and should not be used in combination with sympathetic stimulants or anticholinergic preparations. Because of the dangers associated with its use, sale of herbal products containing ephedra has been banned (National Center for Complementary and Alternative Medicine, 2004). Advise clients asking about the use of Chinese herbal remedies to treat asthma to inquire if any recommended product contains ma huang or ephedra, and to avoid such products. Capsaicin also may relieve acute asthma symptoms. Other herbal preparations include quercetin and grape seed extract. Refer clients interested in using natural preparations to a qualified herbalist, and emphasize the importance of talking to the physician before using these preparations along with conventional treatment.

In addition to herbals, other complementary therapies such as biofeedback, yoga, breathing techniques, acupuncture, homeopathy, and massage have been found to alleviate or help control asthma symptoms.

NURSING CARE

Nurses encounter clients with asthma both in the acute care setting during an acute exacerbation and as outpatients or in homes. The priority nursing care needs differ with each setting.

Health Promotion

Although specific measures to prevent asthma have not yet been identified, the link between parental smoking and childhood asthma is strong. Discuss this link with young people and families with children. Encourage all clients to not start smoking, and if they do smoke, to quit. Provide referrals to smoking cessation clinics, help groups, or a care provider for nicotine patches as needed to facilitate quitting. Additional evidence suggests that early exposure to certain infectious diseases and to other children and limited use of antibiotics reduces the risk for developing asthma (NHLBI, 2003).

Assessment

Assessment of the client experiencing an acute asthma attack must be very focused and timely.

- *Health History:* Current symptoms, including chest tightness, shortness of breath, dyspnea; duration of current attack; measures used to relieve symptoms and their effect; identified precipitating factors for the attack; frequency of attacks; current medications; known allergies.
- *Physical Examination:* Apparent level of distress; color; vital signs; respiratory rate and excursion, breath sounds throughout lung fields; apical pulse.
- *Diagnostic Tests:* Forced expiratory volume, peak expiratory flow rate; arterial blood gases.

MEDICATION ADMINISTRATION Asthma

ADRENERGIC STIMULANTS
Epinephrine
Isoproterenol (Isuprel)
Metaproterenol (Alupent, Metaprel)
Terbutaline (Brethaire, Brethine)
Isoetharine (Bronkosol, Bronkometer)
Albuterol (Proventil, Ventolin)
Bitolterol (Tornalate)
Pirbuterol (Maxair)
Salmeterol (Serevent)
Formoterol (Foradil)
***Combination products:* albuterol/ipratropium**
(Combivent); salmeterol/fluticasone (Advair)
Adrenergic stimulants affect sympathetic receptors in the respiratory tract. Administered by metered-dose inhalers or dry powder inhalers, these drugs are the treatment of choice for acute bronchial asthma. Nearly all of the drugs in this class (epinephrine and isoproterenol being the exceptions) selectively activate β_2-receptors at the doses typically used to treat asthma. β_2-receptor activation results in smooth muscle relaxation and bronchodilation. Formoterol and salmeterol are highly selective to β_2-receptors, resulting in fewer adverse effects. Formoterol and salmeterol have been shown to increase the risk of serious asthma exacerbations and death, however. The U.S. Food and Drug Administration (FDA, 2005b) recommends using these drugs only when the disease cannot be adequately controlled with other medications.

Oral forms of adrenergic agonists may be used for prophylaxis but are not effective in treating an acute attack because of their slow onset. When administered orally or parenterally, their effect on sympathetic nervous system receptors can produce undesirable side effects such as nervousness, irritability, tachycardia, and cardiac dysrhythmias.

Nursing Responsibilities
- Use with caution in clients with hypertension, cardiovascular disease or dysrhythmias, hyperthyroidism, or diabetes.
- When given to a client who is hypoxemic and acidotic, these drugs may cause potentially dangerous cardiac stimulation.
- When given by MDI, wait 1 to 2 minutes between puffs to allow airways to dilate, permitting the second dose to reach distal airways.
- Observe for desired effect of reduced dyspnea and wheezing. Central nervous system stimulation (anxiety, irritability, and insomnia) and tremor are common side effects.

Health Education for the Client and Family
- Use the prescribed inhaler or nebulizer as directed.
- If you are taking a bronchodilator along with another medication by inhalation, use the bronchodilator first to open airways and enhance the effectiveness of the second medication.
- Rinse the mouth after using inhalers to reduce systemic absorption of the medication.
- Keep a log to track your bronchodilator use. If the drug becomes less effective, or if you need a higher dosage or more frequent doses than prescribed, contact your physician.
- Report palpitations, irregular pulse, and other side effects to the physician.

METHYLXANTHINES
Theophylline (Bronkotabs, Quibron, Slo-Phyllin Theolair, Theo-Dur, others)
Aminophylline (Somophyllin)
The methylxanthines are central nervous system (CNS) stimulants chemically related to caffeine. These drugs produce bronchodilation through relaxation of bronchial smooth muscle. As CNS stimulants, they produce adverse effects such as nervousness, insomnia, and tremors. When administered in large doses, convulsions may result.

Once the drugs of choice for preventing and treating asthma attacks, they are now used primarily to prevent nocturnal asthma in affected adult clients. Theophylline has a narrow margin of safety and high potential for toxicity. Because the metabolism and excretion of theophylline vary significantly from person to person—affected by such factors as age, smoking, genetic factors, alcoholism, and other chronic diseases—monitoring of serum levels is vital.

Nursing Responsibilities
- The therapeutic blood level for theophylline is 10 to 20 mcg/mL.
- Monitor for manifestations of toxicity. Anorexia, nausea, vomiting, restlessness, insomnia, cardiac dysrhythmias, and seizures are early manifestations. Other manifestations include epigastric pain, hematemesis, diarrhea, headache, irritability, muscle twitching, palpitations, tachycardia, flushing, and circulatory failure.
- Administer with meals or a full glass of water or milk to minimize gastric irritation.
- Monitor effect closely when administering concurrently with other medications such as barbiturates, anticonvulsants, thyroid hormone, beta blockers, bronchodilators, and others.
- Aminophylline is incompatible with many other intravenous drugs. Use a separate line or flush the line with normal saline before and after administering any other preparation.

Health Education for the Client and Family
- Oral methylxanthines are ineffective to treat an acute asthma attack; do not delay other treatment by using these drugs.
- Check with the physician before taking any over-the-counter medications or other prescription drugs while on theophylline.
- Do not smoke while using this drug.
- Report adverse effects to the physician.

ANTICHOLINERGICS
Atropine
Ipratropium bromide (Atrovent)
Tiotropium bromide (Spiriva)
Combination products: albuterol/ipratropium
(Combivent)
Anticholinergics are potent bronchodilators, blocking muscarinic receptors of the parasympathetic nervous system. Activation of muscarinic receptors produces smooth muscle contraction and bronchoconstriction; blockade of these receptors facilitates smooth muscle relaxation and bronchodilation. Atropine is used infrequently because of its tendency to dry secretions of the mucous membranes and other side effects. Ipratropium and tiotropium bromide are available as inhalers and have fewer side effects than atropine.

(continued)

Nursing Responsibilities

- Assess for possible contraindications to the drug, including hypersensitivity, glaucoma, prostatic hypertrophy, or bladder-neck obstruction.
- Assess for desired and/or adverse effects: improving or worsening symptoms; nausea, vomiting, abdominal cramping, anxiety, dizziness; headache.
- Provide ice chips, fluids, or hard candy to relieve dry mouth.

Health Education for the Client and Family

- To prevent overdose, take no more than the prescribed number of doses per day.
- If the drug becomes less effective over time, notify the physician; an adjustment in dosage may be needed.

CORTICOSTEROIDS

Beclomethasone dipropionate (Vanceril, Beclovent)
Triamcinolone acetonide (Azmacort)
Flunisolide (AeroBid)
Fluticasone propionate (Flovent)
Dexamethasone sodium phosphate (Decadron Phosphate Respihaler)
***Combination products:* salmeterol/fluticasone (Advair)**

The anti-inflammatory effect of corticosteroids helps both prevent and treat acute episodes. Corticosteroids are used to reduce the frequency and severity of asthma attacks and allow reduced dosages of other drugs. The beneficial effects of corticosteroids for asthma result from their ability to decrease the synthesis and release of inflammatory mediators (such as histamine and leukotrienes), reduce inflammatory cell activation and infiltration, and decrease airway edema. Corticosteroids also decrease mucous production in the airways and increase the number and receptivity of β_2-receptors (Lehne, 2004). The cushingoid side effects of corticosteroids, always a major concern with their use, are minimized when they are inhaled. Note that the combination product salmeterol/fluticasone is associated with an increased risk of serious asthma exacerbations and death. It is a second-line drug, recommended for use only when asthma is inadequately controlled using other preparations (FDA, 2005a).

Nursing Responsibilities

- Administer inhaler doses after bronchodilators to facilitate transit of the medication to distal airways.
- Assess for common side effects: sore throat; hoarseness; and oropharyngeal or laryngeal *Candida albicans* infection.
- Administer antifungal medications or gargles as ordered.

Health Education for the Client and Family

- Rinse the mouth after using the inhaler and maintain good oral hygiene to reduce the risk of fungal infections.
- These medications should not be used to alleviate the symptoms of an acute attack.
- Several weeks of continued therapy may be required before a beneficial effect is noticed.
- Notify the physician if you develop weight gain, fluid retention, muscle weakness, redistribution of fat, or mood changes.

MAST CELL STABILIZERS

Cromolyn sodium (Intal, NasalCrom)
Nedocromil (Tilade)

Cromolyn sodium and nedocromil inhibit inflammatory cells in the airway, blocking early and late responses to inhaled antigens. Both drugs also prevent bronchoconstriction in response to inhaling cold air. These drugs act primarily by stabilizing the cytoplasmic membrane of mast cells, preventing the cells from releasing inflammatory mediators such as histamine (Lehne, 2004). These drugs are used only for preventing asthma attacks, not to treat an acute attack. They are administered by metered-dose inhaler, and have a wide margin of safety. Clients using nedocromil may complain of an unpleasant taste.

Nursing Responsibilities

- Evaluate for potential adverse effects of wheezing and bronchoconstriction.

Health Education for the Client and Family

- Gargling or sipping water can decrease the throat irritation associated with nebulizer treatment.
- Use appropriate technique. Inhale deeply with head tipped back to open airways, hold breath, and then exhale. Repeat until all of the drug has been inhaled.
- These drugs are used only to prevent asthma attacks; they are not effective in treating an acute attack.
- Several weeks may be required before a beneficial effect is noted.

LEUKOTRIENE MODIFIERS

Montelukast (Singulair)
Zafirlukast (Accolate)
Zileuton (Zyflo)

Leukotriene modifiers interfere with the inflammatory process in the airways by suppressing the effects of leukotrienes, a group of inflammatory mediators. Leukotrienes are powerful bronchoconstrictors and vasodilators; blocking their synthesis or their receptors improves airflow, decreases symptoms, and reduces the need for short-acting bronchodilators. They are used for maintenance therapy in adults and children over the age of 12 as an alternative to inhaled corticosteroid therapy. They are not used to treat an acute attack.

Nursing Responsibilities

- Administer at least 1 hour before or 2 hours after meals.
- These drugs inhibit some liver enzymes, affecting the metabolism of warfarin and possibly terfenadine and theophylline. Monitor prothrombin times and theophylline blood levels.
- Monitor liver enzymes, because these drugs may be toxic to the liver.

Health Education for the Client and Family

- Take the drugs as prescribed on an empty stomach.
- Notify the physician if a change in color of stools or urine is noted or if jaundice develops.

Nursing Diagnoses and Interventions

An acute asthma attack causes fear as breathing becomes increasingly difficult and hypoxemia develops. Anxiety in turn tends to increase the severity and manifestations of the attack. Priority nursing care needs during an acute attack focus on improving airway clearance and reducing fear and anxiety. Teaching about prevention of future attacks and home management must be postponed until adequate ventilation is restored.

Ineffective Airway Clearance

Bronchospasm and bronchoconstriction, increased mucous secretion, and airway edema narrow the airways and impair airflow during an acute attack of asthma. Both inspiratory and expiratory volume are affected, decreasing the oxygen available at the alveolus for the process of respiration. Narrowed air passages increase the work of breathing, increasing the metabolic rate and tissue demand for oxygen.

PRACTICE ALERT

Frequently assess respiratory status (at least every 1 to 2 hours): respiratory rate and depth, chest movement or excursion, breath sounds, and peak expiratory flow rate. Respiratory status can change rapidly during an acute asthma attack and its treatment. Decreasing PEFRs indicate worsening airflow restriction. Slowed, shallow respirations with significantly diminished breath sounds and decreased wheezing may indicate exhaustion and impending respiratory failure. Immediate intervention is necessary.

- Monitor skin color and temperature and level of consciousness (LOC). *Cyanosis, cool clammy skin, and changes in LOC (agitation, lethargy, or confusion) indicate worsening hypoxia.*
- Assess ABG results and pulse oximetry readings; notify the physician of abnormal values or changes in status. *These values provide information about gas exchange and the adequacy of alveolar ventilation. A fall in oxygen saturation levels is an early indicator of impaired gas exchange.*

PRACTICE ALERT

Assess cough effort and sputum for color, consistency, and amount. Ineffective cough may also signal impending respiratory failure.

- Place in Fowler's, high-Fowler's, or orthopneic (with head and arms supported on the overbed table) position to facilitate breathing and lung expansion. *These positions reduce the work of breathing and increase lung expansion, especially of basilar areas.*
- Administer oxygen as ordered. If a mask is used, monitor closely for feelings of claustrophobia or suffocation. *Supplemental oxygen reduces hypoxemia. Although the mask is a very effective oxygen delivery system, it may increase anxiety.*
- Administer nebulizer treatments and provide humidification as ordered. *Nebulizer treatments are used to administer bronchodilators and other medications; humidity helps loosen secretions.*
- Initiate or assist with chest physiotherapy, including percussion and postural drainage. *Percussion and postural drainage facilitate the movement of secretions and airway clearance.*

- Increase fluid intake. *Increasing fluids helps keep secretions thin.*
- Provide endotracheal suctioning as needed. *Endotracheal suctioning may be necessary to remove secretions and improve ventilation if the client is unable to clear secretions by coughing.*

Ineffective Breathing Pattern

The physiologic changes in lung ventilation that occur during an acute asthma attack impair both lung expansion and emptying. Anxiety caused by hypoxia and dyspnea compounds the problem by increasing the respiratory rate. Collaborative and nursing interventions can help restore a more normal breathing pattern and adequate lung ventilation.

PRACTICE ALERT

Frequently assess respiratory rate, pattern, and breath sounds. Note manifestations of ineffective breathing, including rapid rate, shallow respirations, nasal flaring, use of accessory muscles, intercostal retractions, and diminished or absent breath sounds. Early identification of ineffective respirations allows timely initiation of interventions.

- Monitor vital signs and laboratory results. *Tachypnea, tachycardia, an elevated blood pressure, and increasing hypoxemia and hypercapnia are signs of compromised respiratory status.*
- Assist with ADLs as needed. *This conserves energy and reduces fatigue.*
- Provide rest periods between scheduled activities and treatments. *Scheduled rest is important to prevent fatigue and reduce oxygen demands.*
- Teach and assist to use techniques to control breathing pattern:
   a. Pursed-lip breathing
   b. Abdominal breathing
   c. Relaxation techniques including visualization and meditation.
   Pursed-lip breathing helps keep airways open by maintaining positive pressure, and abdominal breathing improves lung expansion. Relaxation techniques reduce anxiety and its effect on the respiratory rate.
- Administer medications, including bronchodilators and anti-inflammatory drugs, as ordered. Monitor for desired and possible adverse effects. *Medications are used to improve airway status and facilitate breathing.*

Anxiety

Acute exacerbations of asthma can produce significant anxiety. Fear of being unable to breathe and feelings of suffocation associated with acute asthma are significant. Financial or other concerns may cause the client to want to avoid hospitalization. Increasingly frequent and severe episodes may cause fear for the future. Hypoxia contributes to anxiety as well, stimulating the sympathetic nervous system and the fight-or-flight response.

- Assess level of anxiety. *Interventions for severe anxiety or panic differ from those for mild or moderate anxiety.*
- Assist to identify coping skills that have been successful in the past. *Successful coping helps the client regain control of the situation, reducing anxiety.*

PRACTICE ALERT

Provide physical and emotional support. Remain with the client during episodes of severe anxiety; schedule time every 1 to 2 hours to be with the mildly or moderately anxious client. Answer call lights promptly. The severely anxious client may fear being alone or believe that he or she will die if someone is not on hand. Knowing that the nurse is readily available and will return regardless if help is needed reduces anxiety.

■ Listen actively to concerns; do not deny or negate the fear of dying or of being unable to breathe. *Active listening promotes trust and helps the client express concerns.*

PRACTICE ALERT

Provide clear, concise directions and explanations about procedures. Avoid presenting more information than the client is able to assimilate. Anxiety interferes with the ability to learn. Explanations may need to be repeated frequently.

■ Include the client in care planning and decisions as appropriate, without making excessive demands. *Participating in decision making increases the client's sense of control. Because high levels of anxiety interfere with the ability to make decisions, it is important to avoid placing demands on the client that may further increase the level of anxiety.*
■ Reduce excessive environmental stimuli, and maintain a calm demeanor. *This promotes rest.*
■ Allow supportive family members to remain with the client. *Significant others provide additional support and can help reduce anxiety.*
■ Assist to use relaxation techniques, such as guided imagery, muscle relaxation, and meditation. *These techniques help restore psychologic balance and reduce sympathetic stimulation and responses.*

Ineffective Therapeutic Regimen Management

Once acute asthma is under control and effective respirations have been reestablished, it is important to help the client identify contributing factors to the attack. This helps the client prevent future episodes.

■ Assess level of understanding about asthma and the prescribed treatment regimen. Provide additional information and teaching as indicated. *Assessment helps to identify and clarify misperceptions and difficulties with disease management.*
■ Discuss the client's perception of the illness and its effect on his or her lifestyle. *Open discussion can help identify conflicts between lifestyle and the treatment regimen.*

PRACTICE ALERT

Assist to identify factors that contributed to the acute episode. Identifying contributing factors increases the client's awareness of the disease and strategies to prevent future exacerbations.

■ Assist the client and significant others to identify problems or difficulties integrating the treatment regimen into their lifestyle. *Asthma and its management may necessitate lifestyle modifications to prevent acute exacerbations. This can significantly impact family members, for example, elim-*inating cigarette smoking or pets from the household, removing carpets, or daily damp-dusting to remove dust mites.
■ Assess knowledge and understanding of prescribed medications and use of over-the-counter (OTC) preparations. *This is important to determine misperceptions or possible misuse of medications.*
■ Provide verbal and written instructions. *Written instructions reinforce teaching and allow future reference.*
■ Refer to counseling, support groups, or self-help organizations. *Counseling, support groups, and self-help organizations can help the client and family adapt to living with asthma and the treatment regimen.*

Community-Based Care

Asthma is a chronic disease that is best managed by the client with assistance from medical personnel. Teaching for home care focuses on promoting the highest level of wellness and preventing and managing acute episodes and exacerbations of the disease. Topics to include in teaching are as follows:

■ Suggestions for lifestyle changes to avoid specific triggers for asthma attacks, for example:
  ■ Warm up slowly before exercising in cold weather; wear a special mask or scarf to retain air warmth and humidity while exercising.
  ■ Substitute indoor exercises during cold, dry weather.
  ■ Reduce the risk for respiratory infections (e.g., adequate rest, good nutrition, and stress management to maintain immune function, yearly influenza vaccines and immunization against pneumococcal pneumonia).
  ■ Use techniques to reduce or manage physical and psychologic stress.
■ Using PEFR meter to monitor airway status; how to manage the disease based on results
■ Using prescribed medications, including:
  ■ Name, frequency, dose, and desired effect
  ■ Potential adverse effects and their management, including effects to report to the physician
  ■ Potential interactions with other drugs (including OTC herbal preparations) or foods
  ■ If tolerance is a potential risk, how to identify it and steps to take.

Provide referrals to local or regional resources for further teaching and support as needed. Consider the need for home health services, home respiratory care services, and others as needed.

THE CLIENT WITH CHRONIC OBSTRUCTIVE PULMONARY DISEASE

Clients with chronic airflow obstruction due to chronic bronchitis and/or emphysema are said to have **chronic obstructive pulmonary disease (COPD)**.

Incidence and Risk Factors

In 2003, approximately 10.7 million Americans were affected by COPD (ALA, 2006). It is more common among whites than blacks and affects men more frequently than women. It is the fourth leading cause of death in the United States. The death rate from COPD continues to rise among black and American Indian males and among females of all ethnic groups; the death rate is stable in whites, Hispanics, and Asians. In 2002, COPD and other chronic obstructive lung diseases accounted for more than 125,500 deaths (NHLBI, 2004). In addition, COPD morbidity is significant. In people under age 65, COPD is second only to heart disease as a cause of disability, resulting in an estimated 250 million lost work-hours yearly.

> **FAST FACTS**
> - Since 2000, the number of deaths due to COPD in women has exceeded the number of men who have died due to COPD.
> - Chronic bronchitis affected an estimated 8.6 million Americans in 2003.
> - Women are now more than twice as likely to be diagnosed with chronic bronchitis as men.
> - Approximately 3.1 million Americans have emphysema.
> - While more men than women have emphysema, its prevalence is increasing in women and decreasing in men.
>
> *Source: Lung Disease Data: 2006 by the American Lung Association, 2006; retrieved from at http://www.lungusa.org.*

Obstructive lung disease typically affects middle-aged and older adults. Cigarette smoking is clearly implicated as the primary cause of COPD. Even though COPD develops in a minority of smokers, smokers are 12 to 13 times more likely to die from COPD than nonsmokers (ALA, 2006). Cigarette smoke and the irritants it contains impair ciliary movement, inhibit the function of alveolar macrophages, and cause mucus-secreting glands to hypertrophy. It also produces emphysema or airway destruction and constricts smooth muscle, increasing airway resistance. Other contributing factors include air pollution, occupational exposure to noxious dusts and gases, airway infection, and familial and genetic factors (see the accompanying Genetic Considerations box).

Pathophysiology

COPD is characterized by slowly progressive obstruction of the airways. The disease is one of periodic exacerbations, often re-

> ### GENETIC CONSIDERATIONS
> ### Chronic Obstructive Pulmonary Disease
>
> Severe α_1-antitrypsin (α_1AT or ATT) deficiency, present in about 1% to 2% of clients with COPD, is a proven risk factor for COPD. Normal α_1AT levels are associated with the common M allele. Two other alleles, the S allele and the Z allele, lead to reduced α_1AT levels. An estimated 25 million Americans carry a single gene associated with α_1AT deficiency and can pass that gene on to their offspring (ALA, 2006). People who inherit two Z alleles or one Z allele and one null allele have severe α_1AT deficiency. Approximately 1 in 3000 people in the United States inherit severe α_1AT deficiency (Kasper et al., 2005). An estimated 100,000 people in the United States have emphysema related to α_1AT deficiency (ALA, 2006). Although studies suggest additional genetic factors in the development of COPD, at this time none have been proven (Kasper et al., 2005).

lated to respiratory infection, with increased symptoms of dyspnea and sputum production. Unlike acute processes in which lung tissues recover, airways and lung parenchyma do not return to normal following an exacerbation; instead, they demonstrate progressive destructive changes.

Although one or the other may predominate, COPD typically includes components of both chronic bronchitis and emphysema, two distinctly different processes. Small airways disease, narrowing of small bronchioles, is also part of the COPD complex. Through different mechanisms, these processes cause airways to narrow, resistance to airflow to increase, and expiration to become slow or difficult (Figure 39–2 ■). The result is a mismatch between alveolar ventilation and blood flow or perfusion, leading to impaired gas exchange.

Chronic Bronchitis

Chronic bronchitis is a disorder of excessive bronchial mucous secretion. It is characterized by a productive cough lasting 3 or more months in 2 consecutive years (Porth, 2005). Cigarette smoke is the major factor implicated in the development of chronic bronchitis.

Inhaled irritants lead to a chronic inflammatory process with vasodilation, congestion, and edema of the bronchial mucosa. Goblet cells increase in size and number, and mucous glands enlarge. Thick, tenacious mucus is produced in increased amounts. Changes in bronchial squamous cells impair the ability to clear mucus (Kasper et al., 2005). Narrowed airways and excess secretions obstruct airflow; expiration is affected first, then inspiration. Because ciliary function is impaired, normal defense mechanisms are unable to clear the mucus and any inhaled pathogens. Recurrent infection is common in chronic bronchitis.

Figure 39–2 ■ The pathogenesis of chronic obstructive pulmonary disease.

An imbalance between ventilation and perfusion leads to hypoxemia, hypercapnia, and pulmonary hypertension. Pulmonary hypertension often leads to right-sided heart failure.

Emphysema

Emphysema is characterized by destruction of the walls of the alveoli, with resulting enlargement of abnormal air spaces. As in chronic bronchitis, cigarette smoking is strongly implicated as a causative factor in most cases of emphysema. Deficiency of α_1-antitrypsin, an enzyme that normally inhibits the activity of proteolytic enzymes and tissue destruction in the lungs, contributes to the development of emphysema, especially when combined with exposure to cigarette smoke.

Inflammatory cells that collect in distal airway tissues appear to lead to destruction of elastic fibers in the respiratory bronchioles and alveolar ducts. Alveolar wall destruction causes alveoli and air spaces to enlarge with loss of corresponding portions of the pulmonary capillary bed. As a result, the surface area for alveolar-capillary diffusion is reduced, affecting gas exchange. Elastic recoil is lost, reducing the volume of air that is passively expired. The loss of support tissue also affects airways, increasing the risk of expiratory collapse and further air trapping. Anatomically, either respiratory bronchioles or alveoli may be the primary tissue involved.

To summarize, COPD is a progressive, nonreversible process of airway narrowing and loss of supporting tissue. Three separate processes typically are involved:

- Chronic bronchitis with persistent airway edema, excessive mucous production, and impaired airway clearance
- Emphysema with loss of interstitial membranes and airway support tissue, resulting in airway collapse and loss of alveolar surface area for gas exchange
- Small airways disease with bronchoconstriction.

The result of these processes and their combined effects is increased work of breathing, impaired expiration with air trapping, and impaired gas exchange.

Manifestations

The clinical presentation of COPD varies from simple chronic bronchitis without disability to chronic respiratory failure and

---

BOX 39–2 Classification of COPD by Severity

Stage 0— At risk. Lung function normal, but chronic cough and sputum production are present

Stage 1—Mild COPD. Mild airflow limitation, usually with chronic cough and sputum production

Stage 2—Moderate COPD. Worsening airflow limitation, usually with progressing manifestations including dyspnea on exertion

Stage 3—Severe COPD. Further worsening of airflow limitation, increased shortness of breath, and repeated exacerbations impacting quality of life

Stage 4—Very severe COPD. Severe airflow limitation with significantly impaired quality of life and potentially life-threatening exacerbations

Source: Adapted from *Global Initiative for Chronic Obstructive Lung Disease. Pocket Guide to COPD Diagnosis, Management, and Prevention: A Guide for Health Care Professionals*, 2005, by the National Heart, Lung, and Blood Institute and the World Health Organization.

---

severe disability. Box 39–2 outlines the classifications of COPD severity. Manifestations are typically absent or minor early in the disease. When the client finally seeks care, productive cough, dyspnea, and exercise intolerance often have been present for as long as 10 years. The cough typically occurs in the mornings and often is attributed to "smoker's cough." Initially, dyspnea occurs only on extreme exertion; as the disease progresses, dyspnea becomes more severe and accompanies mild activity. Manifestations characteristic of chronic bronchitis and emphysema develop. The clinical features and manifestations of COPD are summarized in Table 39–3.

Manifestations of chronic bronchitis are a cough productive of copious amounts of thick, tenacious sputum, cyanosis, and evidence of right-sided heart failure, including distended neck veins, edema, liver engorgement, and an enlarged heart. Adventitious lung sounds, including loud rhonchi and possible wheezes, are prominent on auscultation.

Emphysema is insidious in onset. Dyspnea is the initial symptom. Initially occurring only with exertion, dyspnea may progress to become severe even at rest. Cough is minimal or absent. Air trapping and hyperinflation increase the anterior-posterior chest

---

TABLE 39–3 Clinical Features and Manifestations of COPD

	FEATURE	CHRONIC BRONCHITIS	EMPHYSEMA
History	Onset	After age 35; recurrent respiratory infections	After age 50; insidious progressive dyspnea
	Smoking	Usual	Usual
	Cough	Persistent, productive of copious mucopurulent sputum	Absent or mild with scant clear sputum, if any
Physical Examination	Appearance	Often obese; edematous and cyanotic; distended neck veins and other symptoms of right-sided heart failure	Usually thin and cachectic; barrel chest; prominent accessory muscles of respiration
	Chest	Adventitious sounds with wheezing and rhonchi; normal percussion note	Distant or diminished breath sounds; hyperresonant percussion note
Other Features	Blood gases	Hypercapnia and hypoxemia; respiratory acidosis	Normal or mild hypoxemia; normal pH
	Pulmonary function studies	Normal or decreased total lung capacity; moderately increased residual volume	Increased total lung capacity; markedly increased residual volume
	Pulmonary hypertension	May be severe	Only when advanced

diameter, causing *barrel chest*. The client often is thin, tachypneic, uses accessory muscles of respiration, and often assumes a position of sitting and leaning forward (Figure 39–3 ■). The expiratory phase of the respiratory cycle is prolonged. On auscultation, breath sounds are diminished, and the percussion tone is hyperresonant.

INTERDISCIPLINARY CARE

Although COPD can be prevented in most people, it cannot be cured. Smoking abstinence is the only certain way to prevent COPD and to slow its progression. To a certain extent, airway obstruction can be reversed and disability minimized early in the disease. Treatment generally focuses on relieving symptoms, minimizing obstruction, and slowing disability.

Diagnosis

Diagnostic tests are used to help establish the diagnosis of chronic obstructive pulmonary disease and identify the predominant component, emphysema or chronic bronchitis. These procedures also are used to assess respiratory status and monitor treatment effectiveness. See Chapter 36 ∞ for more information about these diagnostic procedures and related nursing care.

■ *Pulmonary function testing* is performed to establish the diagnosis and evaluate the extent and progress of COPD (see Box 36–1). Results are based on calculated norms for each person by age, height, sex, and weight; note these as well as all current medications on the requisition. In COPD, the total lung capacity and residual volume typically are increased. The forced expiratory volume (FEV_1) and forced vital capacity (FVC) are decreased due to narrowed airways and resistance to airflow.

Figure 39–3 ■ Typical appearance of a client with emphysema. Note the client's anxious expression and assumption of the tripod position, leaning forward with the hands on the knees.
Courtesy of Michal Heron/Pearson Education/PH College

■ *Ventilation-perfusion scanning* may be performed to determine the extent of ventilation-perfusion mismatch—that is, the extent to which lung tissue is ventilated but not perfused (dead space), or perfused but inadequately ventilated (physiologic shunting) (Figure 39–4 ■). A radioisotope is injected or inhaled to illustrate areas of shunting and absent capillaries.

■ *Serum α_1-antitrypsin (α_1AT) levels* may be drawn to screen for deficiency, particularly in clients with a family history of obstructive airway disease, those with an early onset,

Figure 39–4 ■ Ventilation-perfusion relationships. *A*, Normal alveolar-capillary unit with an ideal match of ventilation and blood flow. Maximum gas exchange occurs between alveolus and blood. *B*, Physiologic shunting: A unit with adequate perfusion but inadequate ventilation. *C*, Dead space: A unit with adequate ventilation but inadequate perfusion. In the latter two cases, gas exchange is impaired.

women, and nonsmokers. Normal adult serum α_1AT levels range from 80 to 260 mg/dL. Fasting is not required prior to this test.

- *ABGs* are drawn to evaluate gas exchange, particularly during acute exacerbations of COPD. Clients with predominant emphysema often have mild hypoxemia and normal or low carbon dioxide tension. Respiratory alkalosis may be present due to an increased respiratory rate. Predominant chronic bronchitis and airway obstruction may cause marked hypoxemia and hypercapnia with respiratory acidosis. Oxygen saturation levels are low due to marked hypoxemia. See page 240 for steps to interpret ABGs.

PRACTICE ALERT

Hypercapnia (elevated $Paco_2$ levels) often is chronic in clients with COPD (CO_2 retainers). In these clients, administering oxygen can actually increase the $Paco_2$, leading to somnolence and acute respiratory failure. While oxygen is the drug of choice for treating clients with COPD, close monitoring is necessary during oxygen therapy.

- *Pulse oximetry* is used to monitor oxygen saturation of the blood. Marked airway obstruction and hypoxemia often cause oxygen saturation levels of less than 95%. Pulse oximetry may be continuously monitored to assess the need for supplemental oxygen.
- *Exhaled carbon dioxide (capnogram or ETco$_2$)* may be measured to evaluate alveolar ventilation. The normal $ETco_2$ reading is 35 to 45 mmHg; it is elevated when ventilation is inadequate, and decreased when pulmonary perfusion is impaired. $ETco_2$ monitoring can reduce the frequency of ABG determinations.
- *Complete blood count (CBC) with white blood cell (WBC) differential* often shows increased red blood cells (RBCs) and hematocrit (erythrocytosis) as chronic hypoxia stimulates increased erythropoiesis to improve the oxygen-carrying capacity of the blood. *Polycythemia,* increased numbers of all blood cells, may be evident. Increased WBC count and a higher percentage of immature WBCs (bands) are often indicative of bacterial infection.
- *Chest x-ray* may show flattening of the diaphragm due to hyperinflation and evidence of pulmonary infection if present.

Smoking Cessation

Smoking cessation can not only prevent COPD from developing, but also can improve lung function once the disease has been diagnosed. FEV$_1$ improves, and survival is prolonged, largely due to lower rates of lung cancer and heart disease. Sustained quitting is difficult; only 6% of smokers succeed in long-term abstinence from smoking (Kasper et al., 2005). Use of nicotine patches or gum and an antidepressant such as bupropion (Wellbutrin, Zyban) improve the chances of success.

Medications

Immunization against pneumococcal pneumonia and yearly influenza vaccine are recommended to reduce the risk of respiratory infections. A broad-spectrum antibiotic is prescribed if infection is suspected. Recent studies indicate that clients with

purulent sputum and increased dyspnea will likely benefit from antibiotic therapy, even if no other signs of infection are present. Prophylactic antibiotics may be ordered for clients who experience four or more disease exacerbations per year (Kasper et al., 2005).

Bronchodilators improve airflow and reduce air trapping in COPD, resulting in improved dyspnea and exercise tolerance. Bronchodilators may be given by MDI, DPI, by nebulizer, or orally. Oral administration may promote adherence, but is associated with much higher rates of adverse effects. A spacer or holding chamber may facilitate effective use of an MDI. Ipratropium bromide, an anticholinergic agent administered by MDI, is frequently prescribed. It has a longer duration of action than the short-acting β_2-adrenergic stimulant bronchodilators and few side effects. Salmeterol, a longer acting β_2-agonist, may be used in combination therapy. Oral theophylline, a methylxanthine, is a weak bronchodilator and has a narrow therapeutic range, but often is prescribed for its other effects. Theophylline stimulates the respiratory drive, strengthens diaphragmatic contractions, and improves cardiac output. As a result, dyspnea, exercise tolerance, and quality of life improve for the client with COPD. Bronchodilators are discussed in further detail in the section on asthma, and their nursing implications are outlined in the Medication Administration box on pages 1327–1328.

Corticosteroid therapy may be used when asthma is a major component of COPD. It also improves symptoms and exercise tolerance, and may reduce the severity of exacerbations and the need for hospitalization. Oral corticosteroids, such as prednisone, are used initially. If a beneficial response occurs, the amount is reduced to the lowest effective dose. Every-other-day dosing or administration by inhaler is preferred to minimize steroid side effects, such as cushingoid effects and an increased risk for osteoporosis and vertebral fractures.

α_1AT replacement therapy is available for clients with emphysema due to a genetic deficiency of the enzyme. Although expensive and inconvenient (α_1AT is administered weekly by intravenous infusion), it has been shown to reduce the rate of airflow decline and mortality.

Treatments

In addition to refraining from smoking, exposure to other airway irritants and allergens should be avoided. The client should remain indoors during periods of significant air pollution to prevent exacerbations of the disease. Air filtering systems or air conditioning may be useful.

Pulmonary hygiene measures, including hydration, effective coughing, percussion, and postural drainage, are used to improve clearance of airway secretions. Maintaining adequate systemic hydration is essential to keep secretions thin. Forceful coughing is often less effective than leaning forward and repeatedly "huffing," with relaxed breathing between huffs. Percussion and postural drainage may be necessary if the client is unable to clear secretions by usual means. Cough suppressants and sedatives generally are avoided because they may cause retention of secretions.

Unless disabling cardiac disease is present, a regular exercise program is beneficial for:

- Improving exercise tolerance.
- Enhancing ability to perform ADLs.
- Preventing deterioration of physical condition.

A program of regular aerobic exercise (e.g., walking for 20 minutes at least three times weekly) designed to gradually increase exercise tolerance is recommended. Activities that strengthen the muscles used for breathing and ADLs, such as swimming and golf, also are beneficial. See the Nursing Research box below.

Breathing exercises are used to slow the respiratory rate and relieve accessory muscle fatigue. Pursed-lip breathing slows the respiratory rate and helps maintain open airways during exhalation by keeping positive pressure in the airways. Abdominal breathing relieves the work of accessory muscles of respiration.

Oxygen

Long-term oxygen therapy is used for severe and progressive hypoxemia. Oxygen therapy improves exercise tolerance, mental functioning, and quality of life in advanced COPD. It also reduces the rate of hospitalization and increases length of survival. Oxygen may be used intermittently, at night, or continuously. For severely hypoxemic clients, the greatest benefit is seen with continuous oxygen. Home oxygen may be supplied as liquid oxygen, compressed gas cylinders, or oxygen concentrators.

An acute exacerbation of COPD may necessitate oxygenation and inspiratory positive-pressure assistance with a face mask or intubation and mechanical ventilation. Oxygen administered without intubation and mechanical ventilation requires caution: Administering oxygen to clients with chronic elevated carbon dioxide levels in the blood can actually increase the $PaCO_2$, leading to increased somnolence and even respiratory failure. Close monitoring of LOC and ABGs during oxygen therapy is vital (Simmons & Simmons, 2004).

Surgery

When medical therapy is no longer effective, lung transplantation may be an option. Both single and bilateral transplants have been performed successfully, with a 2-year survival rate of 75%. Lung reduction surgery is an experimental surgical intervention for advanced diffuse emphysema and lung hyperinflation. The procedure reduces the overall volume of the lung, reshapes it, and improves elastic recoil. As a result, pulmonary function and exercise tolerance improve and dyspnea is reduced. See the box on page 1313 for nursing care of the client undergoing lung surgery. Special nursing care considerations related to lung or heart-lung transplant are summarized in Box 39–3.

Complementary Therapies

Complementary therapies may be useful to help manage symptoms of COPD. Dietary measures such as minimizing intake of dairy products and salt may help reduce mucous production and keep mucus more liquefied. Be sure to recommend measures to replace the protein and calcium in dairy products to help maintain nutritional balance.

Herbal teas made with peppermint and yarrow, coltsfoot, or comfrey may act as expectorants to help relieve chest congestion. Licorice root, which may be taken in several forms, also has expectorant and anti-inflammatory effects that may be beneficial. Licorice root can, however, cause toxicity when used for extended periods of time (Spencer & Jacobs, 2003). Refer clients to a qualified herbalist for treatment.

Acupuncture may help the client with smoking cessation, and also has been used to treat asthma and other respiratory

---

NURSING RESEARCH   Evidence-Based Practice: Client with COPD

The correlation between physical activity and performance of essential ADLs, quality of life, and higher level functioning is well established. This is particularly true for the elderly and people with disease-related impairment in physical abilities. Physical inactivity is both a cause and an effect of declining physical function in the elderly as well as in clients with chronic obstructive pulmonary disease.

A study by Yang and Chen (2005) looked at change processes involved in moving from inactivity to activity in clients with COPD. This study found that those who adopted more behavioral change processes (counter-conditioning, helping relationships, reinforcement management, and self-liberation) were more likely to engage in and maintain regular exercise (defined as at least 20 minutes of exercise of any intensity performed more than three times a week), usually walking. Most of these clients were aware of exercise benefits and the link between exercise and illness. Even so, 15% of study participants who achieved exercise maintenance returned to a more sedentary, inactive lifestyle.

IMPLICATIONS FOR NURSING
This study and others support a program of regular physical activity to maintain functional status and reduce symptom progression. Additionally, this study suggests the importance of providing support and tools to help the client incorporate exercise into daily routines, rather than simply recommending an exercise program and discussing the benefits of exercise. Strategies such as regular telephone follow-ups and creation of support groups help promote self-care responsibility. Encourage COPD clients to enroll in a pulmonary rehabilitation program if one is available. If there is no organized program in the area, work with the client, family, and social support network to develop an exercise routine that can and will be maintained.

CRITICAL THINKING IN CLIENT CARE
1. Consider other populations for whom regular exercise is recommended (e.g., clients who are overweight, clients with heart failure). What strategies have been shown to improve compliance with recommendations for regular exercise in these groups? How could these strategies be adapted for clients with COPD?
2. Use the physiologic and psychologic effects of regular exercise to explain its correlation with improved symptoms in the client with COPD.
3. Consider the age of most clients with COPD. What other physical or psychosocial factors commonly limit physical activity in this population? How can you use this information in designing an appropriate exercise program?

BOX 39–3 Nursing Considerations Related to Lung Transplant

While immediate postoperative care for clients undergoing lung or heart-lung transplant is provided by specially trained interdisciplinary teams in transplant centers, increased survival following transplant means that these clients increasingly are seen in community-based settings, non-transplant hospitals, and on general nursing care units. An understanding of common post-transplant complications and care needs of the post-transplant client facilitates appropriate nursing care.

Common Post-Transplant Complications

In the early post-transplant period, the most common complications relate to the surgical procedure itself or to rejection of the transplanted organ(s).

- *Rejection.* Acute organ rejection can occur at any time following the transplant. An acute change in FEV_1 and FVC on home spirometry often is the first indication of acute rejection. Other manifestations of rejection include fever, shortness of breath, and an elevated WBC count. Because these manifestations are similar to those of infection, the client is instructed to return to the transplant clinic or center for a transbronchial biopsy (Petty, 2003). Acute rejection is treated with increased corticosteroids and adjustment of the immunosuppressive regimen (see Chapter 13 ∞). Chronic rejection is less amenable to therapy, ultimately necessitating retransplant.
- *Infection.* Prevention of infection is vital in lung transplant clients. Clients are encouraged to reduce their risk of infection by avoiding contact with people who have an infectious disease (e.g., URI, shingles, diseases of childhood). Prophylactic trimethoprim-sulfamethoxazole (TMP-SMZ) is administered weekly to prevent *Pneumocystis* pneumonia (see Chapter

38 ∞). Bacterial endocarditis prophylaxis also is provided as needed (see Chapter 32 ∞). The post-transplant client may not have typical manifestations of infection due to immunosuppression. Any vague symptoms with or without fever or leukocytosis are investigated. Recurrent viral infections such as CMV have been associated with chronic rejection; hence, they are aggressively treated with antiviral therapy. Treatment of other infections is targeted to the infectious organism.

Nursing Considerations for the Post-Transplant Client

Reverse isolation procedures are not necessary unless the neutrophil count is very low ($<500/mm^3$). Use good hand washing and standard precautions at all times, and aseptic technique for dressing changes, IV starts and site care, and other invasive procedures (such as urinary catheterization). Do not allow caregivers or visitors with URI to have contact with the client; a mask may be provided for short visits if contact is unavoidable. Skin surveillance and care is vital following transplant. Intact skin reduces the risk of infection; however, corticosteroid therapy increases the risk for skin tears and breakdown.

The effect of all medications on immunosuppressive therapy and the transplanted organ(s) should be carefully investigated prior to administration. Some antibiotics and other drugs can affect blood levels of immunosuppressants (Petty, 2003).

Particular attention must be paid to pulmonary hygiene. Denervation of the transplanted lung eliminates the usual cough stimuli. Regularly scheduled coughing and deep breathing, and the use of vibration, percussion, and postural drainage, are important to prevent accumulation of secretions (Petty, 2003).

---

conditions. Hypnotherapy and guided imagery are used to assist with smoking cessation. These techniques also can help the client control anxiety and breathing patterns. Refer clients to a trained professional. Nurses, physicians, psychologists, counselors, social workers and others can take professional training in hypnotherapy and guided imagery (Fontaine, 2005).

 ## NURSING CARE

Health Promotion

Not smoking—never starting, or quitting—is the best preventive measure for chronic obstructive pulmonary disease. Even in clients with COPD, smoking cessation improves lung function and increases survival. Educate all clients, including preschool and school-age children, about the risks of smoking. See Box 39–4.

Assessment

Focused assessment for the client with chronic obstructive pulmonary disease includes:

- *Health History:* Current symptoms, including cough, sputum production, shortness of breath or dyspnea, activity tolerance; frequency of respiratory infections and most recent episode; previous diagnosis of emphysema, chronic bronchitis, or asthma; current medications; smoking history (in pack-years—

packs per day times number of years smoked), history of exposure to secondhand smoke, occupational or other pollutants.
- *Physical Examination:* General appearance, weight for height, mental status; vital signs including temperature; skin color and temperature; anterior-posterior:lateral chest diameter, use of accessory muscles, nasal flaring or pursed-lip breathing; respiratory excursion and diaphragmatic excursion; percussion tone; breath sounds throughout; neck veins, apical pulse and heart sounds, peripheral pulses, edema.
- *Diagnostic Tests:* FVC and FEV_1, ABGs, hematocrit.

Nursing Diagnoses and Interventions

Clients with chronic obstructive pulmonary disease, whether hospitalized or in the community, have multiple nursing care needs. Because of the obstructive nature of the disease, airway clearance is a high priority. Nutritional deficit is common, particularly when emphysema is predominant. Because this chronic disease affects all functional health patterns, psychosocial issues are also of concern in planning nursing care. In addition to the nursing diagnoses presented here, see the Nursing Care Plan that follows.

Ineffective Airway Clearance

Both chronic bronchitis and emphysema affect the ability to maintain open airways. In chronic bronchitis, copious

BOX 39–4 Cigarette Smoking and Tobacco Use

The use of tobacco reaches back to early civilizations, when it was used in religious ceremonies and as an offering of friendship. At one time, tobacco was thought to have medicinal qualities effective against all common diseases. Widespread use of tobacco among the male population of the industrialized world began during World War I.

Tobacco is now recognized as the leading cause of preventable illness in the world. Diseases directly related to tobacco use are responsible for the deaths of more than 438,000 Americans every year. Smoking will lead to the deaths of about half of all regular cigarette smokers (ALA, 2006). In spite of this knowledge, aggressive marketing of the product continues, and its worldwide use is increasing, especially in underdeveloped countries.

The link between tobacco use and lung cancer was reported as early as 1912. In 1987, lung cancer became the leading cause of cancer-related death in the United States among both men and women.

Cigarette smoke contains over 4800 chemicals (69 of which are known to cause cancer), including nicotine (ALA, 2006). Nicotine is a highly addictive psychoactive substance that is relatively cheap and readily available. It produces euphoria, which acts as a positive reinforcer for continued use. In North American society, tobacco is more acceptable than many other dependency-producing drugs.

Tar is the particulate matter in cigarette smoke that is responsible for most of its carcinogenic and pathologic effects on the lungs. Smoke also paralyzes the cilia, reducing their ability to remove tars from contact with the respiratory epithelium. The risk for cancer and other lung diseases is dose related, affected by the age at which smoking began, the number of cigarettes smoked per day, and the number of years smoked. Smoking cessation reduces the risks associated with tobacco use. For some, such as those at risk for coro-

nary heart disease, quitting smoking yields rapid benefits. For others, the degree of risk reduction is less immediate, but still significant.

Nurses need to do more than simply advise clients to quit smoking and talk about the risks of smoking. Nurses can take an active role in smoking cessation. Identify smoking habits, smoking-related illnesses, and previous efforts to quit. Work with the client to identify barriers and obstacles to quitting. Educate about the addictive nature of nicotine, and explain the manifestations of nicotine withdrawal (anxiety, irritability, headache, and disturbed sleep). Develop a plan with the client that specifies a target date to quit and includes ways to deal with obstacles to quitting, withdrawal symptoms, and the temptation to resume smoking. Offer self-help material at an appropriate reading level. Refer to a counselor, physician, self-help group, or smoking cessation clinic. If a relapse occurs, accept it as a normal part of rehabilitation from any addictive substance. Continue to provide support and encouragement, helping the client avoid further relapses.

Nurses can be especially effective in primary prevention of cigarette smoking and the diseases associated with it. Just as tobacco companies direct advertising at women and teens, nurses can target these populations and younger children for programs to prevent smoking. In addition, nurses need to become active in reducing minors' access to tobacco products, especially cigarettes and chewing tobacco (often the first product used by teens).

Nursing diagnoses that may be appropriate related to smoking include the following:

- *Ineffective Health Maintenance* related to tobacco use
- *Decisional Conflict* related to tobacco use
- *Ineffective Denial* related to acknowledgment of substance abuse and dependence.

---

amounts of thick, tenacious mucus are produced. Ciliary action is impaired, making it difficult to clear mucus from the airways. The loss of supporting tissue caused by emphysema increases the risk for airway collapse. In both cases, air is trapped distally, and less oxygen is available to the alveoli for diffusion. Normal respiratory defense mechanisms are impaired, and mucous-plugged airways provide an ideal environment for bacterial growth. Respiratory infection further impairs airway clearance and is often the cause of an acute exacerbation.

- Assess respiratory status every 1 to 2 hours or as indicated. Assess rate and pattern; cough and secretions (color, amount, consistency, and odor); and breath sounds, both normal and adventitious. *Frequent assessment is vital to monitor current status and response to treatment. Adventitious sounds should decrease with effective intervention. Diminished or absent breath sounds may indicate increasing airway obstruction and possible atelectasis.*

PRACTICE ALERT

Promptly report changes in oxygen saturation, skin color, or mental status. A drop in oxygen saturation levels, increasing cyanosis, or altered LOC indicate hypoxemia, possibly related to airway obstruction.

- Monitor ABG results. *Increasing hypoxemia, hypercapnia, and respiratory acidosis may indicate increasing airway obstruction.*
- Weigh daily, monitor intake and output, and assess mucous membranes and skin turgor. *Dehydration causes respiratory secretions to become thicker, more tenacious, and difficult to expectorate; fluid overload can further compromise respiratory status.*
- Encourage a fluid intake of at least 2000 to 2500 mL per day unless contraindicated. *Adequate fluid intake helps keep mucous secretions thin.*
- Place in Fowler's, high-Fowler's, or orthopneic position; encourage movement and activity to tolerance. *Upright positions improve ventilation and reduce the work of breathing. Activity helps mobilize secretions and prevent them from pooling.*
- Assist with coughing and deep breathing at least every 2 hours while awake. Position seated upright, leaning forward during coughing. *The upright position promotes chest expansion, increasing the effectiveness of coughing and reducing the work involved.*
- Provide tissues and a paper bag to dispose of expectorated sputum. *This important infection control measure reduces the spread of respiratory organisms to other people.*
- Refer to a respiratory therapist, and assist with or perform percussion and postural drainage as needed. *Percussion helps*

NURSING CARE PLAN   A Client with COPD

Anna Mercurio, known as "Happy" to all her friends, is an 83-year-old widow who lives with her two adult sons. During the past 15 years, Mrs. Mercurio has become increasingly short of breath while gardening and walking, two favorite activities. She also has developed a chronic cough that is particularly bad in the mornings. Ten years ago, her family physician told her that she had emphysema. She is admitted to the hospital with possible pneumonia and acute exacerbation of COPD.

ASSESSMENT

Jeff Harris, RN, admits Mrs. Mercurio to the medical unit. In the nursing history, Mr. Harris notes that she denies ever smoking, but says that her husband and two sons have been smokers "for practically their whole lives." She says she lived an active life before developing lung disease, but now her breathing and cough have progressed so that she now must rest after just a few minutes of housework or other activity. Her cough is productive of moderate to large amounts of sputum, particularly in the mornings. She developed increasing shortness of breath and sputum 2 days ago; this morning, she could not complete her morning activities without resting, so she contacted her doctor.

On physical examination, Mr. Harris notes the following: skin very warm and dry, color dusky. Pauses frequently while speaking to breathe. Respiratory rate 36, fairly shallow; coughs frequently, producing large amounts of thick, tenacious green sputum. Other vital signs: P 115 and irregular, BP 186/60, T 102.4°F (39°C). Appears very thin; weight 96 lb (43.6 kg), height 63 inches (160 cm). Anteroposterior:lateral chest diameter approximately 1:1; moderate kyphosis noted. Chest hyperresonant to percussion. Auscultation reveals distant breath sounds with scattered wheezes and rhonchi throughout lung fields. Chest x-ray shows flattening of diaphragm, slight cardiac enlargement, prominent vascular and bronchial markings, and patchy infiltrates. Initial laboratory work reveals moderate erythrocytosis, leukocytosis, and low serum albumin. Arterial blood gas results: pH 7.19; PaO_2 54 mmHg; $PaCO_2$ 59 mmHg; HCO_3^- 30 mg/dL, and O_2 saturation 88%. Admitting orders include sputum specimen for culture; intravenous penicillin G, 2 million units every 4 hours; albuterol/ipratropium (Combivent) inhaler, two puffs every 6 hours; salmeterol/fluticasone (Advair) dry powder inhaler, twice a day; bed rest with bathroom privileges; oxygen per nasal cannula at 2 L continuously; and regular diet.

DIAGNOSES

- *Ineffective Airway Clearance* related to pneumonia and COPD
- *Impaired Gas Exchange* related to acute and chronic lung disease
- *Risk for Impaired Spontaneous Ventilation* related to loss of hypoxemic respiratory drive and respiratory muscle fatigue
- *Impaired Home Maintenance* related to activity intolerance

EXPECTED OUTCOMES

- Expectorate secretions effectively.
- Return to level of pulmonary function prior to acute exacerbation.
- Demonstrate improved ABG and oxygen saturation values.
- Maintain spontaneous respirations without excess fatigue.
- Verbalize willingness to allow sons or a housekeeper to assist with daily household tasks.

PLANNING AND IMPLEMENTATION

- Assess respiratory status and LOC every 1 to 2 hours until stable, then at least every 4 hours.
- Closely monitor response to oxygen therapy, including skin color, oxygen saturation, sputum consistency, and respiratory drive.
- Increase fluid intake to at least 2500 mL per day and provide bedside humidifier.
- Elevate head of bed to at least 30 degrees at all times.
- Teach "huff" coughing technique.
- Administer medications as ordered, providing ipratropium inhaler before beclomethasone inhaler. Provide mouth care after inhalers.
- Contact respiratory therapy for percussion and postural drainage following inhaler treatments.
- Provide for uninterrupted rest periods following treatments and procedures.
- Meet with Mrs. Mercurio and her sons to develop a postdischarge care plan.
- Refer to home health department for nursing follow-up.
- Refer to social services for possible assistance with home maintenance.

EVALUATION

After the first day in the hospital, Mrs. Mercurio's condition begins to improve slowly. On discharge 6 days later, she is able to provide self-care with less fatigue and dyspnea. She is using oxygen at night only, admitting that it is just for security. Although a few scattered wheezes and rhonchi are still present in her lungs, Mrs. Mercurio's sputum is thinner, white, and easily expectorated. She will continue taking oral penicillin V for an additional 10 days at home. She will also continue using the Advair and Combivent inhalers as prescribed at home. Although Mrs. Mercurio's sons admit they will probably never be able to quit smoking, they have agreed to smoke only in the garage or outside. A home health nurse will initially evaluate Mrs. Mercurio's progress three times weekly. Arrangements have been made for a housekeeper to come twice a week for cleaning and laundry. Mrs. Mercurio is glad to be returning home and grateful for the arrangements that have been made.

CRITICAL THINKING IN THE NURSING PROCESS

1. Mrs. Mercurio has never been a smoker but had long-term exposure to secondhand smoke. How does secondhand smoke contribute to lung diseases in adults and children?
2. Mr. Harris's nursing care plan included the nursing diagnosis *Risk for Impaired Spontaneous Ventilation* related to loss of hypoxemic respiratory drive and respiratory muscle fatigue. Identify the normal physiologic events that stimulate breathing, and describe how these differ for the client with chronic hypoxemia and hypercapnia.
3. The client with an acute exacerbation of COPD is at risk for respiratory failure. What changes in Mrs. Mercurio's assessment findings could indicate this complication?
4. Develop a nursing care plan for Mrs. Mercurio for the nursing diagnosis *Deficient Diversional Activities* related to inability to continue preferred activities.

See Evaluating Your Response in Appendix C.

loosen secretions in airways; postural drainage facilitates movement of these secretions out of the respiratory tract.

> **PRACTICE ALERT**
> Provide endotracheal, oral, or nasopharyngeal suctioning as necessary. Suctioning may be necessary to stimulate cough and help clear secretions.

- Provide rest periods between treatments and procedures. *The client with COPD fatigues easily; adequate rest is important to conserve energy and reduce fatigue.*
- Administer expectorant and bronchodilator medications as ordered. Correlate timing with respiratory treatments. *Using expectorants and bronchodilators prior to coughing, percussion, and postural drainage increases their effectiveness in clearing airways.*
- Provide supplemental oxygen as ordered. *Supplemental oxygen helps maintain adequate blood and tissue oxygenation.*

> **PRACTICE ALERT**
> Prepare for intubation and mechanical ventilation if respiratory status deteriorates (increasing hypoxemia and hypercapnia, decreased LOC, cyanosis, or worsening airway obstruction). Respiratory failure is a possible complication of an acute exacerbation of COPD and requires immediate intervention to preserve life.

Imbalanced Nutrition: Less than Body Requirements

With advanced COPD, minimal activity, including eating, can cause fatigue and dyspnea. The client may be unable to consume a full meal without resting. At the same time, the increased work of breathing increases metabolic demands, and more calories are required. The client may appear cachectic (thin and wasted). Poor nutritional status further impairs immune function and increases the risk of a complicating infection.

- Assess nutritional status, including diet history, weight for height (use reference tables of desired weights), and anthropometric (skinfold) measurements. *It is important to differentiate nutritional status from body type rather than assume a nutritional impairment.*
- Observe and document food intake, including types, amounts, and caloric intake. *This information can provide direction for supplementation, if needed.*
- Monitor laboratory values, including serum albumin and electrolyte levels. *These values provide information about the adequacy of nutritional intake, including protein.*
- Consult with a dietitian to plan meals and nutritional supplements that meet caloric needs. *More concentrated sources of high-energy foods may be required to maintain caloric intake without excess fatigue. A diet high in proteins and fats without excess carbohydrates is recommended to minimize carbon dioxide production during metabolism (carbohydrates are metabolized to form CO_2 and water).*
- Provide frequent, small feedings with between-meal supplements. *Frequent, small meals help maintain intake and reduce fatigue associated with eating.*

- Place seated or in high-Fowler's position for meals. *An upright position promotes lung expansion and reduces dyspnea.*
- Assist to choose preferred foods from the menu; encourage family members to bring food from home if allowed. *Providing preferred foods encourages eating.*
- Keep snacks at the bedside. *Snacks provide additional caloric intake.*
- Provide mouth care prior to meals. *This helps enhance the appetite.*
- If unable to maintain oral intake, consult with the physician about enteral or parenteral feedings. *Maintenance of caloric and nutrient intake is vital to prevent catabolism.*

Compromised Family Coping

Chronic illness affects the entire family structure. Roles and relationships change; additional demands are placed on the family. Family members may blame the client for causing the illness or have distorted perceptions about it, even denying its existence. They may refuse to assist or participate in care. The client may develop an attitude of helplessness or dependence or may demonstrate anger, hostility, or aggression.

- Assess interactions between client and family. *Assessment helps identify desired and potential destructive behaviors.*
- Assess the effect of the illness on the family. *Assessment of family interactions, roles, and relationships assists in planning appropriate interventions.*
- Help the client and family identify strengths for coping with the situation. *Identifying personal and family strengths helps the family regain a sense of control.*
- Provide information and teaching about COPD. *Education helps the family gain an understanding of the client's condition and needs.*
- Encourage expression of feelings. Avoid judging feelings expressed or family members as "good" or "bad," "right" or "wrong." *It is important that the nurse remain objective to maintain the therapeutic relationship.*
- Help family members recognize behaviors and attitudes that may hinder effective treatment, such as continuing to smoke in the house. *Family members may be unaware of the effect of their behavior on the client's ability to change habits and cope with a disabling disease.*
- Encourage family members to participate in care. *This helps develop skills for use at home.*
- Initiate a care conference involving the client, family, and healthcare team members from a variety of disciplines. *A wide range of perspectives and areas of expertise aids in problem solving and facilitates communication.*
- If dysfunctional family relationships interfere with measures to enhance coping, advocate for the client, reaffirming his or her right to make decisions. *Dysfunctional family relationships are not likely to change simply because of illness. The nurse can better meet the client's needs by accepting his or her limitations in dealing with family members.*
- Refer the client and family to support groups and pulmonary rehabilitation programs, as available. *Support groups and structured rehabilitation programs enhance coping abilities.*

- Arrange a social services consultation. *This can help the client and family identify care and support service needs.*
- Refer community agencies or services such as home health, homemaker services, or Meals-on-Wheels as appropriate. *Agencies or community services can provide additional support beyond the family's means or capability.*

Decisional Conflict: Smoking

Smoking is more than a habit; it is an addiction. The client who must quit is facing a significant loss, not only of nicotine but also of a lifestyle. Although the client may fully comprehend the consequences of continuing to smoke, the decision to give up a part of his or her life is not easy. This fear may be expressed in such concerns as "I'll gain weight" or "What will I do with my hands?" In addition to providing practical information, a plan, and assistance with nicotine withdrawal, the nurse must support the client's decision-making process to comply with an order to stop smoking.

- Assess knowledge and understanding of the choices involved and possible consequences of each. *The decision to quit smoking ultimately belongs to the client. He or she needs a full understanding of the consequences of quitting or continuing to smoke.*
- Acknowledge concerns, values, and beliefs; listen nonjudgmentally. *The nurse needs to avoid imposing his or her values and beliefs about smoking on the client.*
- Spend time with the client, encouraging expression of feelings. *This demonstrates acceptance of the client and his or her right to make the decision.*
- Help plan a course of action for quitting smoking and adapt it as necessary. *When the client develops the plan, he or she has more ownership in it and interest in making it work.*
- Demonstrate respect for decisions and the right to choose. *Respect supports self-esteem and the ability to cope.*
- Provide referral to a counselor or other professional as needed. *Counselors or other people trained to assist with smoking cessation can help with decision making.*

Using NANDA, NIC, and NOC

Chart 39–1 shows links between NANDA nursing diagnoses, NIC, and NOC for the client with COPD.

Community-Based Care

As with any chronic disease, the client and family will have primary responsibility for disease management. Teaching is vital to promote optimal health and slow disease progression. Teaching for home care focuses on effective coughing and breathing techniques (Box 39–5), preventing exacerbations, and managing prescribed therapies.

THE CLIENT WITH CYSTIC FIBROSIS

Cystic fibrosis (CF) is an autosomal recessive disorder that affects epithelial cells of the respiratory, gastrointestinal, and reproductive tracts and leads to abnormal exocrine gland secretions (see the accompanying box). Although it can affect many organ systems, CF is particularly damaging to the lungs, leading to COPD

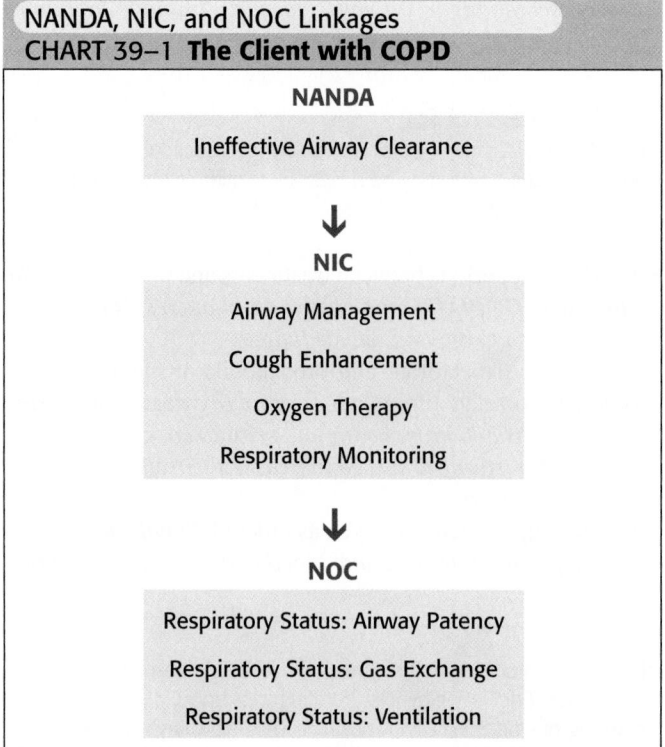

NANDA, NIC, and NOC Linkages
CHART 39–1 The Client with COPD

NANDA

Ineffective Airway Clearance

↓

NIC

Airway Management

Cough Enhancement

Oxygen Therapy

Respiratory Monitoring

↓

NOC

Respiratory Status: Airway Patency

Respiratory Status: Gas Exchange

Respiratory Status: Ventilation

Data from *NANDA's Nursing Diagnoses: Definitions & Classification 2005–2006* by NANDA International (2005), Philadelphia; *Nursing Interventions Classification (NIC)* (4th ed.) by J. M. Dochterman & G. M. Bulechek (2004), St. Louis, MO: Mosby; and *Nursing Outcomes Classification (NOC)* (3rd ed.) by S. Moorhead, M. Johnson, and M. Maas (2004), St. Louis, MO: Mosby.

in childhood and early adulthood. Respiratory manifestations of CF are the usual cause of morbidity and death from this disease. The gastrointestinal tract also is affected significantly; exocrine pancreatic insufficiency is characteristic of CF. Abnormally high sweat electrolytes also occur in CF.

Incidence and Prevalence

CF is the most common lethal genetic disease in Caucasian Americans, affecting about 1 in 2500 live births. It is less common in African Americans and rare in Asians. About 5% of

GENETIC CONSIDERATIONS
Cystic Fibrosis

The gene responsible for cystic fibrosis is at a single locus on the long arm of chromosome 7. This gene codes for a protein known as the *cystic fibrosis transmembrane conductance regulator* (CFTR). More than 1000 mutations of this gene have been identified. The most common mutation, identified as △F508, accounts for about 66% of cystic fibrosis (Aronson & Marquis, 2004). Cystic fibrosis is an autosomal recessive disorder: It is not transmitted as a sex-linked trait, and the normal gene is dominant. People with one abnormal gene do not have the disorder but can transmit this abnormal gene to their offspring. When a child inherits an abnormal gene from both parents, the disorder is seen. Genetic screening of family members of a CF client can detect 70% to 75% of carriers of the CF gene. Screening for the CF gene is not recommended for the general population.

BOX 39-5 Client Teaching: Effective Coughing and Breathing Techniques

Pursed-lip and diaphragmatic breathing techniques help minimize air trapping and fatigue. Pursed-lip breathing helps maintain open airways by maintaining positive pressures longer during exhalation. Teach the client to:

1. Inhale through the nose with the mouth closed.
2. Exhale slowly through pursed lips, as though whistling or blowing out a candle, making exhalation twice as long as inhalation.

Diaphragmatic or abdominal breathing helps conserve energy by using the larger and more efficient muscles of respiration. Teach the client to:

1. Place one hand on the abdomen, the other on the chest.
2. Inhale, concentrating on pushing the abdominal hand outward while the chest hand remains still.
3. Exhale slowly, while the abdominal hand moves inward and the chest hand remains still.

Repeat these exercises as often as necessary until the techniques become incorporated into normal breathing.

Several different coughing techniques may be useful. For controlled cough technique, teach the client to:

1. Following prescribed bronchodilator treatment, inhale deeply, and hold breath briefly.
2. Cough twice, the first time to loosen mucus, the second to expel secretions.
3. Inhale by sniffing to prevent mucus from moving back into deep airways.
4. Rest. Avoid prolonged coughing to prevent fatigue and hypoxemia.

For huff coughing, teach the client to:

1. Inhale deeply while leaning forward.
2. Exhale sharply with a "huff" sound, to help keep airways open while mobilizing secretions.

In addition, include the following topics when teaching for home care:

- Maintaining adequate fluid intake, at least 2.0 to 2.5 quarts of fluid daily
- Avoiding respiratory irritants, including cigarette smoke, both primary and secondary, other smoke sources, dust, aerosol sprays, air pollution, and very cold dry air
- Preventing exposure to infection, especially upper respiratory infections
- Importance of pneumococcal vaccine and annual influenza immunization
- Prescribed exercise program, maintaining ADLs, and balancing rest and exercise
- Maintaining nutrient intake (e.g., eating small frequent meals and using nutritional supplements to provide adequate calories)
- Ways of reducing sodium intake if prescribed
- Identifying early signs of an infection or exacerbation and the importance of seeking medical attention for the following: fever, increased sputum production, purulent (green or yellow) sputum, upper respiratory infection, increased shortness of breath or difficulty breathing, decreased activity tolerance or appetite, increased need for oxygen
- Prescribed medications, including purpose, proper use, and expected effects
- Avoiding use of OTC medications unless approved by the physician
- Other prescribed therapies, such as use of home oxygen, percussion, postural drainage, and nebulizer treatments
- Use, cleaning, and maintenance of any required special equipment
- Importance of wearing an identification band and carrying a list of medications at all times in case of an emergency.

Provide referrals to home care services such as home health, assistance with ADLs as needed, home maintenance services, respiratory therapy and home oxygen services, and other agencies such as Meals-on-Wheels and senior services as indicated.

Caucasians in the United States carry the CF trait. Although the manifestations of CF usually develop in childhood, about 7% of clients with CF are diagnosed as adults. Adults now make up just over one-third of the CF population in the United States, with about 13% surviving into their 30s (Kasper et al., 2005).

Pathophysiology

The CFTR protein is involved in membrane transport of chloride and sodium in cells lining the ducts of exocrine glands (sweat glands, pancreas, liver, and reproductive systems). The genetic abnormality of CF leads to a lack or abnormality of this protein, with resulting abnormal electrolyte transport across epithelial cell membranes. Defective chloride transport causes more water and sodium reabsorption than normal. Secretions in affected organs become thick and viscous, obstructing glands and ducts. This obstruction causes dilation of secretory glands and damage to exocrine tissue. The hallmark pathophysiologic effects of CF include:

- Excess mucous production in the respiratory tract with impaired ability to clear secretions and progressive COPD
- Pancreatic enzyme deficiency and impaired digestion

- Abnormal elevation of sodium and chloride concentrations in sweat.

In the lungs, viscous mucus plugs small airways and impairs mucociliary clearance, leading to atelectasis, infection, bronchiectasis, and dilation of distal airways. Lower respiratory infections with *Staphylococcus aureus* and *Pseudomonas* are common (Porth, 2005). Acute and chronic damage to lung parenchyma causes tissue loss and extensive scarring and fibrosis. The upper lobes are involved to a greater extent than the lower lobes. Severe airway obstruction and chronic hypoxemia lead to pulmonary hypertension, right ventricular hypertrophy, and eventual cor pulmonale. Death usually results from a combination of cardiovascular changes and respiratory failure.

Pancreatic insufficiency is a frequent component of CF. It can range from slight pancreatic dysfunction to complete absence of function due to obstruction of pancreatic ducts with thick mucus and degenerative and fibrotic changes. Pancreatic insufficiency and impaired enzyme secretion lead to impaired digestion and absorption of proteins, carbohydrates, and fats.

About 8% of clients with CF develop diabetes mellitus (Porth, 2005). Liver failure is another potential complication of the disease (McCance & Huether, 2006). Because the genetic defect also affects cells of the reproductive tract, males with CF usually are sterile. Although females may have difficulty conceiving, pregnancies usually are carried to term (Kasper et al., 2005).

Manifestations

Manifestations of CF in a young adult include a history of chronic lung disease. Recurrent pneumonia, exercise intolerance, and chronic cough are typical. Other pulmonary manifestations include *clubbing* of the fingers and toes (Figure 39–5), increased anteroposterior chest diameter (barrel chest), hyperresonant percussion tone, and basilar crackles on auscultation. Distended neck veins, ascites, and peripheral edema accompany right-sided heart failure. Abdominal pain and *steatorrhea* (excess fat in the stools, causing frequent, bulky, foul-smelling stool) commonly result from associated pancreatic insufficiency. Growth and development are often retarded, resulting in small stature.

INTERDISCIPLINARY CARE

The treatment plan for cystic fibrosis is multidisciplinary, with the goals of preventing or treating respiratory complications and maintaining adequate nutrition. Psychosocial care is vital, as is genetic and occupational counseling.

Diagnosis

Although evidence of lung disease and pancreatic insufficiency suggests CF, analysis of Cl^- concentration in sweat is used to confirm the diagnosis. In CF, the Cl^- concentration is >70 mEq/L. Pilocarpine (a parasympathomimetic agent) and a small electric current are used to increase sweat production on the forearm. Absorbent paper or gauze is used to collect the sweat for analysis.

ABGs and oxygen saturation levels show hypoxemia. Pulmonary function studies reveal reduced airflow, reduced forced vital capacity (see Box 36–1 on page 1214), and reduced total lung capacity. Alveolar-capillary diffusion also is typically reduced.

Figure 39–5 ■ Clubbing of fingers caused by chronic hypoxemia.
Source: John Radcliffe Hospital/Science Photo Library/Photo Researchers, Inc.

Medications

Immunization against respiratory infections is vital to promote optimal health. Yearly influenza vaccine is recommended, along with measles and pertussis boosters as needed.

Bronchodilator inhalers may be used to control airway constriction. Acute pulmonary infections are treated with appropriate antibiotic therapy as determined by sputum culture and sensitivity tests. A prolonged treatment course or multiple antibiotics may be required to eradicate pulmonary infections. Antibiotics may be administered by several routes, including inhalation, to achieve the desired concentration in large airways (Aronson & Marquis, 2004). Dornase alfa, recombinant human DNase, breaks down the excess DNA in the sputum of clients with CF, decreasing its viscosity and making it easier to clear. Dornase alfa, administered by aerosol, reduces the frequency of hospitalizations and the need for antibiotics for some clients.

Treatments

Chest physiotherapy with percussion and postural drainage is used to promote airway clearance. Newer airway clearance techniques include the use of the "huff" cough technique with specified breathing cycles or patterns. In one technique, a valved mask or mouthpiece is used to maintain positive expiratory pressure (PEP) for approximately 20 breaths, followed by three to five "huff" coughs. This cycle is repeated for a total of 20 minutes. The autogenic drainage technique, a form of biofeedback, involves controlled breathing at specific lung volumes and patterns to facilitate the movement of mucus into larger airways, where it can be cleared with the "huff" cough. A flutter valve device, which looks like a fat pipe, contains a steel ball within an inner cone. The weight of the ball provides intermittent PEP, which vibrates airway walls to loosen secretions.

Oxygen therapy may be required for hypoxemia. A liberal fluid intake helps reduce the viscosity of mucous secretions. A diet high in protein, fat, and calories may be necessary to maintain weight. Vitamins and minerals are supplemented to counteract excess losses in the sweat and stools. Enteral or parenteral nutrition may be required during acute exacerbations of the disease.

Surgery

Lung transplantation currently offers the only definitive treatment for CF. Lung transplantation lengthens life span and improves quality of life. Single-lung, double-lung, and heart-lung transplants have been successfully completed. Because the donor lungs do not have the CF gene, they do not develop the pathophysiologic changes of CF. Although the other defects characteristic of CF remain, these can be managed with pharmacologic therapy.

NURSING CARE

Nursing care for the client with cystic fibrosis is much the same as that for any chronic obstructive lung disease. Promoting airway clearance is the priority of nursing care. The genetic component of the disease and the client's age are important considerations. Adults with CF are just entering their productive years and face a life span that is likely to be shortened significantly. Females who do conceive face the prospect of transmitting the defective gene to their offspring.

Nursing Diagnoses and Interventions

Ineffective Airway Clearance

Bronchial hygiene measures, including vibration, percussion, and postural drainage, are the mainstay of treatment for clients with CF.

- Assess respiratory status, including vital signs, breath sounds, SaO₂, and skin color, at least every 4 hours. *Early identification of respiratory compromise allows intervention before tissue hypoxia is significant.*
- Assess cough and sputum (amount, color, consistency, and possible odor). *Assessment of the cough and nature of sputum produced allows evaluation of the effectiveness of respiratory clearance and the response to therapy.*
- Monitor ABG results; report increasing hypoxemia and other abnormal results to the physician. *Blood gas changes may be an early indicator of impaired gas exchange due to airway obstruction.*
- Place in Fowler's or high-Fowler's position. Encourage frequent position changes and ambulation as allowed. *The upright position promotes lung expansion; position changes and ambulation facilitate the movement of secretions.*
- Assist to cough, deep breathe, and use assistive devices. Provide endotracheal suctioning using aseptic technique as ordered. *Coughing, deep breathing, and suctioning help clear airways.*
- Provide a fluid intake of at least 2500 to 3000 mL per day. *A liberal fluid intake helps liquefy secretions, facilitating their clearance.*
- Work with the physician and respiratory therapist to provide pulmonary hygiene measures, such as postural drainage, percussion, and vibration. *These techniques help mobilize and clear secretions.*
- Administer prescribed medications as ordered, and monitor their effects. *If the infecting organism is resistant to the prescribed antibiotic, little improvement may be seen with treatment. Bronchodilators help maintain open airways but may have adverse effects such as anxiety and restlessness.*

Anticipatory Grieving

The client with CF and family members face the knowledge that life span is likely to be short: The median survival for males is over 32 years; for females it is 29 years (Kasper et al., 2005).

- Spend time with the client and family. *Time is necessary to develop a trusting, therapeutic relationship.*
- Answer questions honestly; do not deny the probable outcome of the disease. *Honesty reinforces reality and provides a sense of control over decisions to be made.*
- Encourage the client and family to express their feelings, fears, and concerns. *Open expression of feelings helps to promote understanding and acceptance.*
- Assist with understanding the grieving process and acceptance of feelings as normal. *Feelings of guilt, anger, or depression may cause the client to withdraw from others.*

Explanation of the grieving process enhances understanding and ability to cope.

- Help the client and family make decisions regarding treatment and care. *This also is important to give them a sense of control.*
- Encourage use of other support systems, such as spiritual and social groups. Refer the client and family to support groups, social support services, and hospice care as indicated. *These support systems provide emotional support and help the client and family cope with the diagnosis.*
- Discuss advance directives (the living will) and power of attorney for health care with the client and family. *These documents give the client and family a sense of control over medical care provided if the client is no longer able to express his or her own wishes.*

Community-Based Care

Education of the client and family affected by cystic fibrosis is essential to maintaining optimal health. The adult whose disease was diagnosed in infancy or childhood has grown up with the disease and often has a much greater knowledge level than many caregivers. However, when the initial diagnosis is made as an adolescent or young adult, teaching needs are significant. Include the following topics when teaching for home care:

- Respiratory care techniques, including percussion, postural drainage, and controlled cough techniques
- Specific breathing and coughing exercises and procedures
- The importance of avoiding respiratory irritants, such as cigarette smoke, air pollution, and occupational dusts and gases
- Measures to prevent respiratory infection, such as maintaining immunizations and optimal general health, and avoiding exposure to large crowds and infected people.

Refer to a dietitian for planning and teaching to maintain adequate nutrition and minimize gastrointestinal symptoms. Referral to community agencies and support groups is also helpful.

Discuss the genetic transmission of cystic fibrosis and refer for counseling and possible genetic testing. Help the client and family sort through the impact of the disease on future pregnancies and generations. Remember that the possibility of CF may present an ethical dilemma regarding future pregnancies. Provide support as needed.

THE CLIENT WITH ATELECTASIS

Atelectasis is not a disease but a condition associated with many respiratory disorders. It is a state of partial or total lung collapse and airlessness. It may be acute or chronic. The most common cause of atelectasis is obstruction of the bronchus ventilating a segment of lung tissue. The affected segment may be small or an entire lobe. Other causes include compression of the lung by pneumothorax, pleural effusion, or tumor; or loss of pulmonary surfactant and inability to maintain open alveoli.

The manifestations of atelectasis depend on its size. Diminished breath sounds over the affected area may be the only sign of a small atelectasis. If a large lung segment is affected, manifestations may include tachycardia, tachypnea, dyspnea, cyanosis, and other signs of hypoxemia. Chest expansion may be reduced and breath sounds absent on the affected side. Fever and other manifestations of infection may be present.

Chest x-ray shows an area of airless lung. CT scan may help determine the cause of atelectasis.

The primary therapy for atelectasis is prevention. High-risk clients, such as those with COPD, smokers undergoing surgery, and people on prolonged bed rest or mechanical ventilation, should have vigorous chest physiotherapy to maintain open airways. Frequently assess respiratory status, including rate, breath sounds, and spirometry readings for early detection and treatment.

When atelectasis develops, treatment focuses on the underlying cause. Vigorous coughing and chest therapy may relieve obstruction by a mucous plug. Bronchoscopy may be necessary to remove the obstruction. Antibiotic therapy is ordered to treat infectious causes.

Nursing care to prevent and treat atelectasis is directed toward airway clearance. Position the client with atelectasis on the unaffected side to promote gravity drainage of the affected segment. Encourage frequent position changes, ambulation, coughing, and deep breathing. Unless contraindicated, encourage fluids to help liquefy secretions. Teach the client at high risk for developing atelectasis about pulmonary care measures, fluid intake, and preventing pulmonary infections.

THE CLIENT WITH BRONCHIECTASIS

Bronchiectasis is characterized by permanent abnormal dilation of one or more large bronchi and destruction of bronchial walls. Infection often is present. The destructive process of bronchiectasis is initiated by inflammation, usually due to recurrent airway infections. About half of all cases of bronchiectasis are related to cystic fibrosis. Other causes include infections, such as severe pneumonia, tuberculosis, or fungal infections; lung abscess; exposure to toxic gases; abnormal lung or immunologic defenses; and localized airway obstruction due to a foreign body or tumor. Inflammation and airway obstruction are common to all of these processes. Bronchial walls become weakened and dilated as a result, leading to pooling of secretions and further infection and inflammation.

A chronic cough productive of large amounts of mucopurulent sputum is characteristic. Other manifestations of bronchiectasis include hemoptysis, recurrent pneumonia, wheezing and shortness of breath, malnutrition, right-sided heart failure, and cor pulmonale.

Collaborative care for bronchiectasis focuses on maintaining optimal pulmonary function and preventing progression of the disorder. The diagnosis is typically based on the history and physical examination. Chest x-ray and CT scan may be ordered to help confirm the diagnosis and determine the extent of lung damage.

Antibiotics are prescribed at the first indication of infection and may also be used prophylactically. Inhaled bronchodilators may be ordered. Chest physiotherapy is a vital component of continuing care for bronchiectasis. Percussion and postural drainage help mobilize secretions. Oxygen may be prescribed. Bronchoscopy may be used to clear retained secretions or obstruction or to evaluate hemoptysis. If lung destruction is localized and unresponsive to conservative management, surgical lung resection may be necessary.

Nursing care of the client with bronchiectasis is similar to that for clients with other obstructive lung diseases. Airway clearance is a primary problem, as is ineffective breathing pattern. Other applicable nursing diagnoses may include *Impaired Gas Exchange, Imbalanced Nutrition: Less than Body Requirements,* and *Self-Care Deficit.*

INTERSTITIAL PULMONARY DISORDERS

Many lung diseases damage the interstitial or connective tissue of the lung. Occupational lung diseases and sarcoidosis are interstitial lung diseases. Toxic drugs and radiation also cause interstitial damage. Table 39–4 identifies common causes of interstitial lung disorders. These disorders may be acute or insidious. Their rate of progression varies from person to person, as does the degree of disability they produce.

The Client with an Occupational Lung Disease

Occupational lung diseases are a diverse group of disorders directly related to inhalation of noxious substances in the work environment. There are two major classifications of occupational lung diseases:

- *Pneumoconioses:* chronic fibrotic lung diseases caused by inhalation of inorganic dusts and particulate matter
- *Hypersensitivity pneumonitis:* allergic pulmonary diseases caused by exposure to inhaled organic dusts.

FAST FACTS
- In the United States, occupational illnesses and injuries account for more than $170 billion per year in direct and indirect costs.
- The U.S. Department of Energy estimates that $30 billion to $150 billion annual savings could result from improvement of buildings and indoor environments.
- Of this amount, an estimated $6 billion to $19 billion annual savings in healthcare costs and increased productivity could be attributed to reduced lung disease (ALA, 2006).

Physiology Review

Lung tissue contains elastin and collagen fibers. Elastin fibers are easily stretched, facilitating lung expansion. Collagen fibers, in contrast, resist stretching. This increases the work of breathing. Both elastin and collagen affect lung compliance, or the ease with which the lungs are inflated. Other factors affecting compliance include the water content of lung tissue and surface tension (Porth, 2005).

TABLE 39-4 Selected Causes of Interstitial Lung Disorders

CAUSE	EXAMPLES
Inorganic dusts	Silica (silicosis), asbestos (asbestosis), coal (coal worker's pneumoconiosis), talc (talcosis)
Organic dusts	Cotton (byssinosis), sugar cane (bagassosis), moldy hay (farmer's lung)
Drugs	Antineoplastic agents, antibiotics, gold salts, phenytoin
Radiation	External radiation or inhaled radioactive materials
Infections	Widespread TB or fungal infections, viral or *Pneumocystis carinii* pneumonia
Poisons and noxious gases	Paraquat, nitrogen dioxide, chlorine, ammonia, sulfur dioxide
Systemic diseases	Uremia, pulmonary edema
Unknown causes	Sarcoidosis, idiopathic pulmonary fibrosis, connective tissue disorders

Pathophysiology and Manifestations

When a noxious substance is inhaled, the response to that substance depends on:

- The size of particulates
- Its nature (organic or inorganic)
- Where it deposits in the respiratory tract
- The susceptibility of the individual.

Relatively large particles, larger than 6 microns, are too big to reach lower airways and often are deposited in the nose. Smaller particles can be carried with inspired air into the alveoli. Normal lung defenses, including alveolar macrophages, lymph channels, and the mucociliary escalator, attempt to remove particulate matter from the alveoli. Cigarette smoking, alcohol ingestion, or hypersensitivity reactions can impair these defenses.

The inhaled substance damages alveolar epithelium, leading to an inflammatory process of the alveoli and interstitial tissue of the lung. The inflammatory response produces further damage, and abnormal fibrotic (scar) tissue replaces the elastin fibers of normal lung tissue. As a result, the lungs become stiff and noncompliant. Lung volumes decrease, the work of breathing increases, and alveolar-capillary diffusion is impaired, leading to hypoxemia.

Asbestosis

Inhalation of asbestos fibers is a common cause of occupational lung disease. *Asbestosis* is a diffuse interstitial fibrotic disease involving the terminal airways, alveoli, and pleurae. Exposure to asbestos fibers occurs during mining, milling, manufacturing, and application of asbestos products. Although symptoms may not become apparent until 20 years after exposure, they tend to progress, even when further exposure has been halted. Asbestosis is also associated with an increased risk of bronchogenic carcinoma, especially in cigarette smokers. Mesothelioma, a rare cancer of the pleural membrane, is also associated with asbestos exposure. The period between asbestos exposure and tumor development in mesothelioma is long, ranging from 20 to 30 years (ALA, 2006). People exposed to asbestos prior to imposition of strict environmental controls may only now be developing manifestations of this disease.

The manifestations of asbestosis include exertional dyspnea, exercise intolerance, and inspiratory crackles. Diffuse, small, irregular or linear opacities appear on chest x-ray, primarily in the lower lobes. As the disease progresses, respiratory failure and marked hypoxemia may develop.

Silicosis

Inhalation of silica dust by hard-rock miners, foundry workers, sandblasters, pottery makers, and granite cutters can lead to *silicosis*, a nodular pulmonary fibrosis. Silicosis affects 1.2 to 3 million workers in the United States. Although generally associated with long-term exposure to silica, it can develop in as little as 10 months of intense exposure (Kasper et al., 2005). In silicosis, macrophages are destroyed as they engulf silica particles, releasing substances that damage lung tissue and lead to fibrosis and scarring.

Simple silicosis is asymptomatic with no demonstrable respiratory impairment. Complicated silicosis, in contrast, is characterized by large conglomerate densities in the upper lungs. These clients may be severely dyspneic and have a productive cough. Pulmonary function testing shows both restrictive and obstructive changes. Increasing size of conglomerate masses can lead to severe disability, cor pulmonale, and death.

Coal Worker's Pneumoconiosis

Ingestion of coal dust by alveolar macrophages causes "coal macules" to form, leading to *coal worker's pneumoconiosis*, or *black lung disease*. This occupational lung disease affects 12% of all miners, with a higher incidence in the eastern United States than in the West (Kasper et al., 2005). Coal macules appear on chest x-ray as diffuse, small opacities primarily affecting the upper lungs.

Simple coal worker's pneumoconiosis (CWP) generally is asymptomatic. A small percentage of clients (1% to 2%) develop progressive massive fibrosis, which destroys the pulmonary vascular bed and airways of the upper lungs. This progressive form of the disease causes symptoms similar to those of complicated silicosis.

Hypersensitivity Pneumonitis

Workers exposed to organic dusts and gases may develop *hypersensitivity pneumonitis*, an allergic pulmonary disease affecting the airways and alveoli. Byssinosis, resulting from cotton dust exposure; bagassosis, due to exposure to moldy sugar cane fiber; farmer's lung, and bird-fancier's lung are examples of hypersensitivity pneumonitis.

Either acute or subacute illness can occur. Acute illness occurs 4 to 8 hours after exposure and is heralded by sudden onset of malaise, chills and fever, dyspnea, cough, and nausea. The subacute syndrome is characterized by an insidious onset of chronic cough, progressive dyspnea, anorexia, and weight loss. Diffuse fibrosis occurs after repeated exposure to the organic material, leading to respiratory insufficiency.

INTERDISCIPLINARY CARE

Prevention is a key strategy for all occupational lung diseases. Containing dust and wearing personal protective devices that limit the amount of inhaled particles are essential for people who work in industries with known risks.

Chest x-ray, pulmonary function studies, bronchoscopy, and possibly lung biopsy are used to establish the diagnosis of pneumoconioses. Characteristic patterns are seen for each disorder on x-ray. Pulmonary function testing shows restrictive impairment of lung ventilation, with reduced vital capacity and reduced total lung capacity. The diffusing capacity of the lungs is also decreased. Blood gas analysis reveals hypoxemia, especially with exercise. Bronchoscopy may be performed to obtain tissue for biopsy. Specialized lung scans may be used to determine the extent of fibrosis.

Eliminating further exposure to the offending agent is an important part of disease management. There is no specific therapy. Anti-inflammatory drugs, such as corticosteroids, may reduce the inflammatory response and slow the progression of the disease. Preventing exposure to other damaging substances such as cigarette smoke and pollution is vital. Pneumococcal vaccine and annual influenza immunizations are recommended to reduce the risk of lower respiratory infections. Other care is supportive, similar to that for COPD.

NURSING CARE

Health Promotion

Teaching about the dangers of occupational lung diseases and ways to reduce their risk needs to begin early, before the disease develops. Nurses in industrial and public health settings can begin by recognizing potential dangers and teaching workers about measures to reduce dust in their work area and the use of personal protective devices such as masks. Nurses working with affected families have an excellent opportunity to begin educating children about the risks associated with the occupation.

Nursing Diagnoses and Interventions

Nursing care for clients with occupational lung diseases is similar to that for clients with COPD. Activity intolerance is a high-priority problem for many clients. Severe dyspnea can significantly interfere with ADLs. Nursing measures to reduce energy expenditures and provide for rest are essential. Caregiver role strain, either actual or potential, must be considered when the client with severe disability is being cared for at home.

Both client and family coping may be compromised. Many of these diseases develop after 20 to 30 years of exposure to the hazardous material. Clients who entered the industry following high school may develop evidence of disease in their 40s and face the possibility of changing their occupation or developing significant disability. The resulting role strain affects all members of the family.

Other nursing diagnoses to consider for the client with an occupational lung disease follow:
- *Ineffective Breathing Pattern* related to restrictive lung disease
- *Anticipatory Grieving* related to potential loss of employment and income
- *Low Self-Esteem: Situational* related to change of occupation.

Community-Based Care

The affected client and family need teaching in preparation for home care, including:
- Prevention of further lung damage, for example, avoiding cigarette smoke and heavy air pollution
- Recommendations for pneumococcal and annual influenza immunizations; yearly tuberculin testing for clients with silicosis
- Pulmonary hygiene measures, such as liberal fluid intake, coughing, and deep-breathing exercises
- Use and care of oxygen therapy equipment if required
- Use and effects of any prescribed or recommended OTC medications.

THE CLIENT WITH SARCOIDOSIS

Sarcoidosis is a chronic, multisystem disease characterized by an exaggerated cellular immune response in involved tissues. This abnormal immune response leads to granuloma formation in the lungs, lymph nodes, liver, eyes, skin, and other organs. Its cause is unknown. Sarcoidosis primarily affects young adults between the ages of 20 and 40. In the United States, the incidence is highest in African Americans. Women are affected at a slightly higher rate than men (Kasper et al., 2005).

In sarcoidosis, multiple granulomas form; these lesions may resolve spontaneously or proceed to fibrosis. The lungs are affected in about 90% of clients with sarcoidosis. Sarcoidosis has a low mortality rate—less than 3%—but a relatively high rate (approximately 10%) of serious disability from ocular, respiratory, or other organ damage. Pulmonary hemorrhage and cardiac and respiratory failure from pulmonary fibrosis are the leading causes of death from sarcoidosis.

The manifestations of sarcoidosis vary, depending on the organ system affected. It may be asymptomatic, diagnosed by characteristic findings on routine chest x-ray. Symptoms may be insidious, with anorexia, fatigue, weight loss, fever, dyspnea, arthralgias, and myalgias. Skin lesions, uveitis, lymphadenopathy, hepatomegaly, or other manifestations may also develop.

Leukopenia, eosinophilia, and an elevated erythrocyte sedimentation rate (ESR) typically are noted in sarcoidosis. The chest x-ray helps to determine the extent of pulmonary involvement. Biopsy of a granulomatous lesion may be required to confirm the diagnosis. Pulmonary function tests reveal decreased compliance and impaired diffusing capacity.

Sarcoidosis often resolves spontaneously; therefore, treatment is indicated only when symptoms are severe or disabling.

Corticosteroid therapy is prescribed to suppress the inflammatory process when indicated. Relapse frequently occurs when corticosteroids are discontinued. Other anti-inflammatory or immune-modifier medications may also be used, including chloroquine, indomethacin, azathioprine, and methotrexate.

Nursing care for clients with sarcoidosis is directed by involved organ systems and related manifestations. Respiratory care is supportive and includes avoiding respiratory irritants and maintaining adequate ventilation. Refer for smoking cessation assistance as needed.

Teach clients with limited symptoms about the disease and symptoms to report to a healthcare provider, including shortness of breath, tearing and eye inflammation, chest pain or irregular pulse, skin lesions, and swollen and painful joints. If corticosteroid therapy is prescribed, teach the importance of taking the drug as prescribed and not stopping it abruptly. Include information about managing the side effects of corticosteroids by limiting sodium and increasing potassium in the diet, taking the medication with food or milk to minimize gastric irritation, and identifying early signs of infection.

PULMONARY VASCULAR DISORDERS

The cardiovascular and respiratory systems are closely interrelated. As blood flows through the capillary network of the pulmonary vascular system, oxygen diffuses into it, and carbon dioxide diffuses out. An effective match of alveolar ventilation and capillary perfusion is essential to maintain this process and, ultimately, tissue oxygenation and function of all organ systems. Both vascular and alveolar changes can alter gas exchange. Arteriosclerotic changes in pulmonary vasculature reduce blood flow to the alveolus. Nearly all lower respiratory system disorders potentially can affect ventilation. Many also have a secondary effect on lung perfusion, because breakdown or fibrosis of alveolar walls destroys the capillary network as well. This section focuses on primary disorders of the pulmonary vascular system.

THE CLIENT WITH PULMONARY EMBOLISM

A **pulmonary embolism** (or *thromboembolism*) is obstruction of blood flow in part of the pulmonary vascular system by an embolus. Thromboemboli, or blood clots, that develop in the venous system (deep venous thrombosis or DVT) or right side of the heart are the most frequent cause of pulmonary embolism. Other sources of emboli include tumors that have invaded venous circulation, fat or bone marrow entering the circulation due to fracture or other trauma, amniotic fluid released into the circulation during childbirth, and intravenous injection of air or other foreign substances.

Pulmonary embolism is a medical emergency. Fifty percent of deaths from pulmonary embolism occur within the first 2 hours following embolization. In many cases, DVT has not been recognized or treated; often embolization also goes undetected. Prevention is the most effective treatment strategy for pulmonary embolism.

Incidence and Risk Factors

Pulmonary embolism causes an estimated 200,000 deaths annually, making it the third leading cause of death in hospitalized clients (Tierney et al., 2005). Although many substances can become emboli, thrombus arising from the deep veins of the legs is the leading cause of pulmonary embolism. *Deep venous thrombosis* develops in approximately 5 million people per year in the United States. The risk factors for pulmonary embolus are those for DVT: stasis of venous blood flow, vessel wall damage, and altered blood coagulation.

Prolonged immobility; trauma, including hip and femur fractures; surgery (orthopedic, pelvic, and gynecologic surgery in particular); myocardial infarction and heart failure; obesity; and advanced age are risk factors for DVT. Women who use oral contraceptives or estrogen therapy are at risk, as are women during pregnancy and childbirth. See Chapter 35 ∞ for more information about DVT.

Physiology Review

The right heart receives deoxygenated blood from the systemic venous circulation. The entire output of the right ventricle enters the pulmonary circulation via the pulmonary artery. This artery branches into successively smaller arteries, arterioles, and capillaries of the pulmonary vascular system. Each alveolus of the lungs is surrounded by a meshwork of capillaries. Oxygen and carbon dioxide readily diffuse across the alveolar-capillary membrane, driven by a concentration gradient. The partial pressure of oxygen in the alveolus is greater than in the capillary; therefore, it diffuses into the blood. Carbon dioxide diffuses from the capillaries into the alveoli, driven by the higher pressure of dissolved carbon dioxide in venous blood.

A match between blood flow through the pulmonary vascular system (perfusion) and lung ventilation is necessary for effective *respiration* (gas exchange) (see Figure 39–4). Local factors regulate ventilation and perfusion to maintain this match. A low alveolar P_{O_2} constricts alveolar capillaries, directing blood flow to better ventilated areas of the lung. High alveolar P_{CO_2} levels cause local bronchodilation, increasing airflow and eliminating excess carbon dioxide.

Pathophysiology

Thrombi affecting only the deep veins of the calf rarely embolize to the pulmonary circulation. However, thrombi often propagate proximally to the popliteal and ileofemoral veins. From there, they may break loose to become an embolus. As vessels of the venous system become progressively larger, the embolus moves freely until it enters the pulmonary arterial system with its progressively smaller vessels leading to the pulmonary capillary beds (Figure 39–6 ■).

The impact of a pulmonary embolus depends on the extent to which pulmonary blood flow is obstructed, the size of the embolus, its nature, and secondary effects of the obstruction. The effects can range widely:

Figure 39–6 ■ A thromboembolism lodged in a pulmonary vessel.

Source: Steve Oh, M. S., Phototake NYC

- Occlusion of a large pulmonary artery with sudden death. Gas exchange is significantly reduced or prevented, and cardiac output falls dramatically as blood fails to move through the pulmonary vascular system and return to the left heart.
- Lung tissue infarction due to occlusion of a significant portion of pulmonary blood flow. Fewer than 10% of pulmonary emboli result in pulmonary infarction.
- Obstruction of a small segment of the pulmonary circulation with no permanent lung injury.
- Chronic or recurrent, possibly multiple, small emboli with recurring symptoms.

Obstruction of pulmonary blood flow by an embolus affects both perfusion and ventilation. Neurohumoral reflexes triggered by obstruction cause vasoconstriction, increasing pulmonary vascular resistance. In severe cases, this can lead to pulmonary hypertension and right ventricular heart failure. Systemically, hypotension and a drop in cardiac output may develop. Bronchoconstriction occurs in the affected area of lung. Dead space (areas of the lung that are ventilated but not perfused) increases. Alveolar surfactant decreases, increasing the risk for atelectasis.

If infarction does not occur, the fibrinolytic system (see Chapter 33 ∞) ultimately dissolves the clot, and pulmonary function returns to normal. Infarcted tissue becomes scarred and fibrotic.

Fat emboli are the most common nonthrombotic pulmonary emboli. A fat embolism usually occurs after fracture of long bone (typically the femur) releases bone marrow fat into the circulation. Adipose tissue or liver trauma may also lead to fat emboli.

Manifestations

The manifestations of pulmonary embolism depend on its size and location. Small emboli may be asymptomatic. Manifestations usually develop abruptly, over a period of minutes. The most common symptoms are dyspnea and pleuritic chest pain. Anxiety, a sense of impending doom, and cough are also common. See the box below. Diaphoresis and hemoptysis may develop. Massive pulmonary embolus can cause syncope and cyanosis. On examination, tachycardia and tachypnea are noted. Crackles may be heard on auscultation of the chest, and a cardiac gallop (S_3 and possibly S_4) may be noted. A low-grade fever may develop. It is difficult to differentiate pulmonary embolism from myocardial infarction or pneumonia by manifestations.

Characteristic manifestations of fat emboli include sudden onset of cardiopulmonary and neurologic symptoms: dyspnea, tachypnea, tachycardia, confusion, delirium, and decreased LOC. Petechiae often develop on the chest and arms.

INTERDISCIPLINARY CARE

Because deep venous thrombosis may not be identified until pulmonary embolism occurs, prevention is the primary goal in treating pulmonary embolism.

Early ambulation of medical and surgical clients is an effective means of preventing venous stasis and reducing the incidence of pulmonary embolism. External pneumatic compression of the legs is also effective for clients undergoing neurosurgery, urologic surgery, or major surgery of the hip or knee, or when anticoagulant therapy is contraindicated. Other preventive measures include elevating the legs and active and passive leg exercises.

When pulmonary embolism occurs, treatment is supportive. Oxygen therapy is initiated, and analgesics may be ordered to relieve severe pleuritic pain and anxiety. Pulmonary artery and wedge pressures are monitored with a balloon (Swan-Ganz) catheter. Cardiac outputs also may be assessed. Cardiac rhythm is monitored to detect dysrhythmias.

MANIFESTATIONS **of Pulmonary Embolism**

Common
- Dyspnea and shortness of breath
- Chest pain
- Anxiety and apprehension
- Cough
- Tachycardia and tachypnea
- Crackles (rales)
- Low-grade fever

Less Common
- Diaphoresis
- Hemoptysis
- Syncope
- Cyanosis
- S_3 and/or S_4 gallop

Diagnosis

The studies performed to identify DVT differ from those used to diagnose a pulmonary embolism. See Chapter 35 ∞ for diagnostic studies for venous thrombosis.

- *Plasma D-dimer levels* are highly specific to the presence of a thrombus. D-Dimer is a fragment of fibrin formed during lysis of a blood clot; elevated blood levels indicate thrombus formation and lysis (e.g., DVT and pulmonary embolism).
- *Chest CT with contrast* is the principal test used to diagnose pulmonary embolism. Chest CT effectively shows large, central PE; newer generation scanners also can detect peripheral emboli.
- *Lung scans,* including perfusion and ventilation scans, may be used. In a perfusion lung scan, radiotagged albumin is injected intravenously and distributed in the lungs by the pulmonary blood flow. The lungs are then scanned for distribution of the isotope. An area of lung in which the isotope is undetectable is suggestive of occluded blood flow and pulmonary embolism. For a ventilation scan, a radiotagged gas is inhaled and the lungs are scanned for gas distribution. Combined perfusion and ventilation scans allow identification of areas of the lungs that are ventilated but not perfused, a characteristic of pulmonary embolism.
- *Pulmonary angiography* is the definitive test for pulmonary embolism when other, less invasive tests are inconclusive. It is possible to detect very small emboli with angiography. A contrast medium injected into the pulmonary arteries illustrates the pulmonary vascular system on x-ray.
- *Chest x-ray* often shows pulmonary infiltration and occasionally pleural effusion.
- *Electrocardiogram (ECG)* is ordered to rule out acute myocardial infarction as the cause of symptoms. ECG findings commonly associated with pulmonary embolism include tachycardia and nonspecific T-wave changes.
- *ABGs* usually show hypoxemia (PaO_2 less than 80 mmHg) and often respiratory alkalosis (pH > 7.45, $PaCO_2 < 38$ mmHg) due to tachypnea and hyperventilation.
- *$ETCO_2$* may be measured to evaluate alveolar perfusion. The normal $ETCO_2$ reading is 35 to 45 mmHg; it is decreased when pulmonary perfusion is impaired.
- *Coagulation studies* are ordered to monitor the response to therapy. The *activated partial thromboplastin time (aPTT or PTT)* is used to assess the intrinsic clotting pathway and the response to heparin therapy. Desired levels with anticoagulant therapy are 1.5 to 2 times the control value. The risk of recurrent thromboembolism is high at lower levels; the risk of bleeding increases at higher levels. The *International Normalized Ratio (INR)* is used to assess the extrinsic clotting system and oral anticoagulation with warfarin (Coumadin). The goal of anticoagulant therapy is to achieve a therapeutic range of 2.0 to 3.0.

Medications

Anticoagulant therapy is the standard treatment to prevent pulmonary emboli. It is often instituted in high-risk clients who have no evidence of pulmonary embolism, to prevent possible devastating effects. In the client with DVT or a pulmonary embolus, anticoagulants are administered to prevent further clotting and embolization. See Chapter 35 ∞ for more information about anticoagulant therapy to prevent and treat DVT. See the Medication Administration box on pages 1189–1190 for the nursing implications for anticoagulant therapy.

For pulmonary embolus, heparin therapy is initiated with an intravenous bolus of 5000 to 10,000 units of heparin, followed by continuous infusion at the rate of 1000 to 1500 units per hour. The aPTT or PTT is monitored frequently until stabilized. Heparin therapy is typically continued for about 5 days or until oral anticoagulant therapy has become fully effective.

Oral anticoagulant therapy with warfarin sodium (Coumadin) is initiated at the same time as heparin. Warfarin alters the synthesis of vitamin K–dependent clotting factors and requires 5 to 7 days to be fully effective. Anticoagulant therapy is continued for 2 to 3 months when few risk factors for thromboemboli exist; long-term therapy is used when chronic disorders that increase the risk of thromboemboli are present.

Bleeding is a risk associated with anticoagulant therapy. Although major hemorrhage is uncommon, it occurs in approximately 5% of clients receiving intravenous heparin. Cardiac, hepatic, and renal disease increase the risk of significant bleeding, as does age over 60 years. Protamine, a protein that combines with heparin to inactivate it, is used to stop its anticoagulant effect if major bleeding occurs. Vitamin K is given to treat bleeding associated with Coumadin therapy.

Fibrinolytic therapy may be used to treat massive pulmonary embolus and hypotension. Streptokinase, urokinase, or tissue plasminogen activator (tPA) are used to *lyse* (disintegrate) the embolus, restore pulmonary blood flow, and reduce pulmonary artery and right heart pressures. Although fibrinolytic therapy may not reduce mortality associated with pulmonary embolus, it may reduce the incidence of pulmonary hypertension, which develops 3 to 5 years after an embolism. Fibrinolysis significantly increases the risk of bleeding, particularly cerebral bleeding. Contraindications to fibrinolysis include intracranial disease, recent stroke, active bleeding or a bleeding disorder, pregnancy, severe hypertension, and recent surgery or trauma. Because of the increased risk of hemorrhage, invasive procedures are avoided after fibrinolysis. See Chapter 31 ∞ for further discussion of fibrinolytic therapy and its nursing implications.

Surgery

When anticoagulant therapy fails to prevent recurrent emboli or is contraindicated, an umbrella-like filter may be inserted into the inferior vena cava to trap large emboli while allowing continued blood flow (see Figure 35–11). The filter usually is inserted percutaneously, via either the femoral or jugular vein.

 NURSING CARE

Health Promotion

Nurses are key in preventing pulmonary embolism. Encouraging clients to ambulate after surgery or illness, applying compression stockings or pneumatic compression devices, teaching and encouraging leg exercises, discouraging the use of pillows under the knees—all of these measures help prevent DVT and subsequent pulmonary emboli.

Teach clients to reduce the risks associated with long periods of immobility, stopping every 1 to 2 hours during long automobile trips for a brief stretch and walk, getting up every hour or so and doing leg exercises while seated during long flights, and avoiding crossing the legs to prevent venous stasis and pooling. Regular exercise such as walking also reduces the risk of DVT. Instruct clients who stand for long periods to use well-fitted elastic stockings, being careful to avoid hose that bind around the knee or thigh.

Assessment

Because pulmonary embolus can be a medical emergency, assessment may be very focused. In other instances, when emboli are small and not life threatening, a more extensive nursing assessment may be done.

- *Health History:* Chest pain, shortness of breath, other symptoms, including onset, severity, precipitating factors; history of recent surgery, venous thrombosis, or other risk factor such as childbirth or malignancy; current medications.
- *Physical Examination:* Level of consciousness, presence of respirations and pulse; color, skin temperature and moisture; vital signs including apical pulse and temperature; breath sounds and heart sounds; oxygen saturation level; neck vein distention, peripheral edema.
- *Diagnostic Tests:* Plasma D-dimer levels, coagulation studies; chest x-ray and other imaging studies; oxygen saturation and ABGs; ECG.

Nursing Diagnoses and Interventions

A large pulmonary embolus can cause a significant mismatch between pulmonary ventilation and circulation. Impaired gas exchange is a priority problem and focus for interventions. Cardiac output may be significantly affected by obstructed pulmonary blood flow. Fibrinolytic and anticoagulant therapy affect the clotting process, increasing the risk for bleeding. Anxiety accompanies pulmonary embolism almost universally.

Impaired Gas Exchange

Pulmonary embolism results in areas of the lung that are ventilated but not perfused; they receive no capillary blood flow. If the embolus is large and a major segment of the lung is unperfused, gas exchange is significantly affected. Nursing interventions are directed toward compensating for impaired gas exchange.

- Frequently assess respiratory status, including rate, depth, effort, lung sounds, and oxygen saturation. *Impaired ventilation will further compromise gas exchange and worsen hypoxemia. Oxygen saturation can be monitored continuously and noninvasively to evaluate gas exchange.*

PRACTICE ALERT
Monitor and record LOC, mental status, and skin color. Hypoxemia often causes confusion and agitation; hypercapnia may reduce LOC. Cyanosis indicates significant hypoxemia.

- Place in Fowler's or high-Fowler's position, with the lower extremities dependent. *This position facilitates maximal lung expansion and reduces venous return to the right side of the heart, lowering pressures in the pulmonary vascular system.*

PRACTICE ALERT
Start oxygen per nasal cannula or mask. Obtain a physician's order if one has not been written. Supplemental oxygen increases alveolar and arterial oxygenation. Oxygen is a drug and must be prescribed by the physician. It may, however, be initiated by the nurse in an emergency to prevent tissue hypoxia.

- Monitor ABG results, reporting abnormal findings as indicated. *ABGs are used to assess gas exchange and tissue oxygenation. An arterial line may be inserted for monitoring arterial pressure and arterial blood sampling.*
- Maintain bed rest. *Bed rest reduces metabolic demands and tissue needs for oxygen.*

Decreased Cardiac Output

The impact of a large pulmonary embolus on hemodynamic status can be significant. Pressures in the pulmonary vascular system and right heart increase; blood return to the left heart and cardiac output may significantly decrease. Nursing interventions focus on preserving an adequate blood pressure and organ function until cardiopulmonary status stabilizes. A central line for hemodynamic monitoring may be instituted. (See Chapter 32 ∞ for nursing care related to hemodynamic monitoring.)

PRACTICE ALERT
Assess and record vital signs and cardiopulmonary status every 15 to 30 minutes initially, then every 2 to 4 hours as condition stabilizes. Frequent assessment facilitates timely interventions to maintain cardiovascular status and preserve organ function.

- Auscultate heart sounds every 2 to 4 hours, reporting any abnormalities. *Sounds such as an S_3 or S_4 gallop may indicate cardiac compromise.*

PRACTICE ALERT
Record intake and output hourly. Decreased urinary output often is an early indicator of decreased cardiac output. Maintaining renal perfusion is vital to preserve renal function and prevent acute renal failure.

- Assess skin color and temperature. *These assessments monitor tissue perfusion.*
- Monitor cardiac rhythm. *A drop in cardiac output and other hemodynamic alterations resulting from pulmonary embolism can precipitate dysrhythmias. Dysrhythmias, in turn, can further impair cardiac output.*
- Administer vasopressors and other medications as ordered. Carefully monitor the response to prescribed medications. *Drugs may be prescribed to maintain adequate arterial pressure and tissue perfusion. Potent drugs such as vasopressors require careful monitoring for desired and adverse effects.*

- Monitor pulmonary artery pressures, neck vein distention, and peripheral edema. Report findings as indicated. *Right-sided heart failure is a potential complication of pulmonary embolism because of increased pulmonary artery pressures.*
- Maintain intravenous and arterial access sites as well as central lines. *The client may be in unstable and critical condition, potentially needing immediate interventions to maintain life.*

PRACTICE ALERT
Provide frequent skin care. Impaired tissue perfusion and oxygenation increase the risk of skin and tissue breakdown.

- Instruct to report chest pain or other symptoms. *Decreased cardiac output and an increased workload due to pulmonary hypertension may cause anginal pain.*

Ineffective Protection

Fibrinolytics and anticoagulant therapy impair normal clotting mechanisms, increasing the risk for bleeding and hemorrhage. This risk is particularly acute during the first 24 to 48 hours following fibrinolytic drug administration.

- Assess frequently for overt and covert signs of bleeding: bleeding gums; hematuria; obvious or occult blood in stool or vomitus; incisional bleeding, bleeding or bruising of injection sites or with minor trauma; joint pain or immobility; abdominal or flank pain. *Careful monitoring is necessary to identify early signs of abnormal bleeding and prevent potential hemorrhage.*

PRACTICE ALERT
Promptly report changes in neurologic status. Although cerebral bleeding is not evident externally, changes in LOC and other neurologic signs suggest it and should be reported immediately.

- Report coagulation study results outside the desired range for anticoagulant therapy. *Levels less than the target range may indicate an increased risk for further clot development and pulmonary emboli; levels above the target range indicate an increased risk for bleeding.*
- Keep protamine sulfate available for heparin therapy and vitamin K available for warfarin (Coumadin) therapy. *Bleeding or hemorrhage due to excess anticoagulant may require antidote administration to rapidly reverse anticoagulant effects.*
- Assess medication regimen for possible drug interactions that could potentiate or inhibit anticoagulant effects. *Drug interactions can increase the risk for hemorrhage or further embolus formation.*
- Avoid invasive procedures, injections, and venous punctures when possible, particularly during and following fibrinolytic therapy. *Invasive procedures increase the risk of tissue trauma and bleeding.*
- Maintain firm pressure on injection and venipuncture sites. Maintain pressure for 30 minutes following arterial puncture. *Firm pressure reduces the risk for bleeding into the tissues.*

PRACTICE ALERT
Use an infusion device to administer heparin infusion. Using an infusion pump or device helps prevent administration of excess medication.

- Maintain adequate fluid intake. Administer stool softeners as ordered. *These measures help prevent constipation and straining, which may precipitate bleeding of hemorrhoids.*

Anxiety

Pulmonary embolism is a physiologic and psychologic threat to safety and integrity. It is a major physiologic stressor, eliciting a strong neuroendocrine stress response. The feeling of suffocation and inability to catch one's breath that accompanies a pulmonary embolus is also a strong psychologic stressor. Fear, anxiety, and apprehension are common responses.

- Assess anxiety level. *Appropriate interventions are determined by the level of anxiety.*

PRACTICE ALERT
Provide reassurance and emotional support, listening to fears. Do not negate the fear of dying, but reassure that treatment usually restores effective respiratory function. The fear of death is very real and must not be discounted; however, it is important to provide reassurance to alleviate excess anxiety.

- Remain with the client as much as possible. *The presence of a caring nurse helps reduce fear.*
- Explain procedures and treatments, using short, simple sentences. *Providing clearly understood, simple instructions reduces fear of the unknown.*
- Reduce environmental stimuli, and use a calm, reassuring manner. *These measures help reduce anxiety (for both the nurse and the client).*
- Allow supportive family members to remain with the client as much as possible. *Calm, supportive family members provide further reassurance.*
- Administer morphine sulfate as ordered. *Morphine is given to reduce pain and anxiety.*

Using NANDA, NIC, and NOC

Linkages between NANDA nursing diagnoses, nursing interventions, and nursing outcomes for the client experiencing a pulmonary embolism are illustrated in Chart 39–2.

Community-Based Care

Discuss the following topics when preparing the client with pulmonary embolism and family members for home care:

- Use of prescribed anticoagulant, including drug interactions, scheduled laboratory testing, and manifestations of bleeding to report to the primary care provider
- Using a soft toothbrush and electric razor to reduce the risk of bleeding
- Avoiding aspirin (unless prescribed) and other OTC medications unless approved by the physician
- Importance of wearing a Medic-Alert tag for anticoagulant use

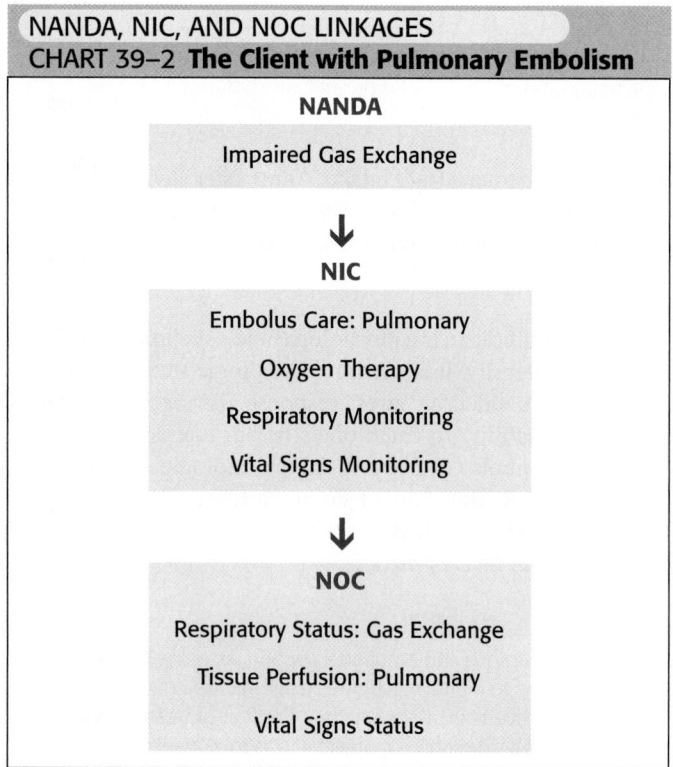

NANDA, NIC, AND NOC LINKAGES
CHART 39-2 The Client with Pulmonary Embolism

NANDA

Impaired Gas Exchange

↓

NIC

Embolus Care: Pulmonary

Oxygen Therapy

Respiratory Monitoring

Vital Signs Monitoring

↓

NOC

Respiratory Status: Gas Exchange

Tissue Perfusion: Pulmonary

Vital Signs Status

Data from *NANDA's Nursing Diagnoses: Definitions & Classification 2005–2006* by NANDA International (2005), Philadelphia; *Nursing Interventions Classification (NIC)* (4th ed.) by J. Dochterman & G. M. Bulechek (2004), St. Louis, MO: Mosby; and *Nursing Outcomes Classification (NOC)* (3rd ed.) by S. Moorhead, M. Johnson, and M. Maas (2004), St. Louis, MO: Mosby.

■ Health promotion measures to reduce the risk of recurrent pulmonary embolism
■ Symptoms of recurrent pulmonary embolism, such as sudden chest pain, shortness of breath, and possibly bloody sputum.

THE CLIENT WITH PULMONARY HYPERTENSION

The pulmonary vascular system is normally a high-flow, low-pressure, low-resistance system that can accommodate large increases in blood flow when necessary (e.g., during exercise). The normal mean arterial pressure in the pulmonary system is 12 to 15 mmHg (25 to 28 systolic/8 diastolic). **Pulmonary hypertension** is abnormal elevation of the pulmonary arterial pressure.

Pathophysiology

Pulmonary hypertension can develop as a primary disorder, but usually occurs secondarily to another condition. In both instances, changes in the pulmonary artery lead to abnormal growth and remodeling of pulmonary vessels. Smooth muscle cells and fibroblasts proliferate, leading to abnormal vasoconstriction and fibrosis of pulmonary vessels. Once initiated, pulmonary vascular changes are progressive and nonreversible. Vasoconstrictive substances such as endothelin 1 and thromboxane A_2 are produced in excess, while the production of va-

sodilating substances such as nitric oxide is reduced. This further contributes to vasoconstriction and increased pulmonary artery pressures. Thromboxane A_2 also stimulates platelet aggregation, promoting clot formation in pulmonary vessels. Inflammation may contribute to progression of the disease. Vasoconstriction and increased pressures in the pulmonary system increase the workload of the right ventricle, ultimately leading to right ventricular failure (Sims, 2003; Steinbis, 2004).

Primary Pulmonary Hypertension

Primary pulmonary hypertension is an uncommon disorder without identified cause. It occurs in both familial and sporadic patterns. In the familial form, a gene transmitted in an autosomal dominant pattern affects a protein receptor in the walls of pulmonary arteries, leading to abnormal vessel growth and remodeling (Sims, 2003; Steinbis, 2004). Primary pulmonary hypertension affects primarily women in their 30s or 40s.

FAST FACTS
■ An estimated 300 new cases of primary pulmonary hypertension are diagnosed annually.
■ Median survival after being diagnosed with primary pulmonary hypertension is 3 years (ALA, 2006).

Secondary Pulmonary Hypertension

Secondary pulmonary hypertension is more common than primary. HIV infection and collagen diseases such as scleroderma and lupus may lead to secondary pulmonary hypertension. However, its usual cause is reduced size of the pulmonary vascular bed, which may be due to vasoconstriction or widespread vessel destruction or obstruction. Hypoxemia is a potent pulmonary vasoconstrictor and a common initiating factor in pulmonary hypertension. Chronic lung diseases, sleep apnea, and hypoventilation due to obesity or neuromuscular disease can lead to hypoxemia. Alveolar wall destruction associated with emphysema leads to loss of pulmonary capillaries. Large or multiple pulmonary emboli may cause significant vessel obstruction. Other factors such as left ventricular failure or mitral stenosis also can lead to elevated pulmonary pressures. Once initiated, pulmonary hypertension becomes self-sustaining, as pulmonary vessels undergo changes that further narrow the pulmonary bed.

Manifestations

The manifestations of pulmonary hypertension are progressive dyspnea, fatigue, angina, and syncope with exertion. In secondary pulmonary hypertension, the signs and symptoms often are masked by those of the underlying disease. Dull, retrosternal chest pain may occur in addition to the manifestations of the primary disease. Primary pulmonary hypertension is a progressive disorder that generally causes a steady decline to death within 3 to 4 years.

Complications

Cor pulmonale is a condition of right ventricular hypertrophy and failure resulting from long-standing pulmonary hypertension. Chronic obstructive pulmonary disease is the most common cause of cor pulmonale.

The manifestations of cor pulmonale are those of the underlying pulmonary disorder and right-sided heart failure. Chronic productive cough, progressive dyspnea, and wheezing are common. With right-sided heart failure, peripheral edema and distended neck veins are seen. Skin is warm, moist, and both ruddy and cyanotic because of increased numbers of RBCs and hypoxemia.

INTERDISCIPLINARY CARE

The CBC commonly shows *polycythemia,* increased numbers of red blood cells. ABGs and oxygen saturation measurements reveal hypoxemia. The chest x-ray shows right heart enlargement and dilation of central pulmonary arteries. Typical ECG changes are those of right ventricular hypertrophy. An echocardiogram may be done to identify cardiac changes occurring either as a cause or result of pulmonary hypertension. Doppler ultrasonography is a noninvasive means of estimating pulmonary artery pressure, but cardiac catheterization may be required for definitive diagnosis. See Chapter 30 ∞ for nursing care of the client undergoing cardiac catheterization.

Treatment for pulmonary hypertension focuses on slowing the course of the disease, preventing thrombus formation, and reducing pulmonary vasoconstriction. Oxygen is administered to reduce hypoxemia and improve activity tolerance. If polycythemia is present, phlebotomy is performed to reduce the viscosity of the blood.

The calcium channel blockers nifedipine (Procardia) or diltiazem (Cardizem) may be given to reduce pulmonary vascular resistance and improve cardiac output. Short-acting direct vasodilators such as intravenous epoprostenol (Flolan) or treprostinol (Remodulin) or oral bosentan (Tracleer) may be used for clients who do not respond to calcium channel blockers. An oral anticoagulant (Coumadin) is given to prevent clotting (Steinbis, 2004).

Bilateral lung or heart-lung transplant is the most effective long-term treatment for primary pulmonary hypertension.

When cor pulmonale is present, salt and water restrictions as well as diuretic therapy are added to the above regimen to manage the right-sided heart failure.

NURSING CARE

Nursing care for the client with pulmonary hypertension or cor pulmonale is largely supportive. The focus is toward the underlying lung disease. Impaired gas exchange due to contraction of the pulmonary vascular system is a significant problem that causes many secondary problems, such as activity intolerance, anxiety, fatigue, and others. Nursing interventions for impaired gas exchange are directed toward maintaining adequate alveolar ventilation, oxygenation, and perfusion. The following measures may be included:

- Monitoring breath sounds, respiratory rate, skin color, and use of accessory muscles
- Positioning for optimal lung expansion
- Coughing, deep breathing, and chest physiotherapy
- Administering prescribed vasodilators.

It is important to assess fatigue and dyspnea with activities and to plan frequent rest periods. Assist with self-care as needed to conserve energy.

With primary pulmonary hypertension, *Anticipatory Grieving* and *Hopelessness* are additional potential nursing diagnoses. When cor pulmonale is present, *Decreased Cardiac Output, Excess Fluid Volume,* and *Ineffective Individual Coping* must be considered.

Community-Based Care

Most care for these chronic conditions is provided in the home and community settings. Teaching is directed both at the underlying lung disease, if present, and the resulting hypertensive process. Refer to the section on COPD for teaching related to this disease, the most frequent underlying cause of cor pulmonale. In addition, provide teaching about the following topics for the client and family:

- Disease process, its management, and the prognosis
- Manifestations or changes in condition to report to the physician, such as a change in activity tolerance, increased edema, and signs of respiratory infection or exacerbation
- Importance of planned rest periods between activities and measures to conserve energy, such as using a shower chair
- Importance of not smoking due to its irritant and vasoconstrictive effects
- Prescribed medications, including their use and effects.

RESPIRATORY FAILURE

Many of the conditions discussed in this chapter and in Chapter 38, from pneumonia to acute respiratory distress syndrome, can lead to respiratory failure. In **respiratory failure**, the lungs are unable to oxygenate the blood and remove carbon dioxide adequately to meet the body's needs, even at rest.

THE CLIENT WITH ACUTE RESPIRATORY FAILURE

Respiratory failure is not a disease but a consequence of severe respiratory dysfunction. It is often defined by ABG values. An arterial oxygen level (PaO_2) of less than 50 to 60 mmHg and an arterial carbon dioxide level ($PaCO_2$) of greater than 50 mmHg are generally accepted as indicators of respiratory failure. However, clients with advanced COPD may be alert and functional with blood gas values that would indicate respiratory failure in someone whose respiratory function was previously normal. In clients with COPD, respiratory failure is indicated by an acute drop in blood oxygen levels along with increased carbon dioxide levels.

Respiratory failure can result from inadequate alveolar ventilation (hypoventilation), impaired gas exchange, or a

TABLE 39–5 Selected Causes of Respiratory Failure

TYPE OF DYSFUNCTION	EXAMPLES
Impaired Ventilation	
■ Airway obstruction	Laryngospasm, foreign body aspiration, airway edema
■ Respiratory disease	Asthma, COPD
■ Neurologic causes	Spinal cord injury, poliomyelitis, Guillain-Barré syndrome, drug overdose, stroke
■ Chest wall injury	Flail chest, pneumothorax
Impaired Diffusion	
■ Alveolar disorders	Pneumonia, pneumonitis, COPD
■ Pulmonary edema	Heart failure, ARDS, near-drowning
Ventilation-perfusion mismatch	Pulmonary embolism

significant ventilation-perfusion mismatch. COPD is the most common cause of respiratory failure. Other lung diseases, chest injury, inhalation trauma, neuromuscular disorders, and cardiac conditions can also lead to respiratory failure. Selected causes of acute respiratory failure are identified in Table 39–5.

Pathophysiology

Respiratory failure may be characterized by primary hypoxemia or a combination of hypoxemia and hypercapnia (Figure 39–7 ■). In hypoxemic respiratory failure, PaO_2 is significantly reduced, whereas $PaCO_2$ remains normal or is low due to stimulation of the respiratory center and tachypnea. Impaired diffusion across the alveolar-capillary membrane, and a ventilation-perfusion mismatch can cause a drop in arterial oxygen levels that is more rapid than the rise in carbon dioxide. Metabolic acidosis results from tissue hypoxia. The increased work of breathing can eventually lead to respiratory muscle fatigue and hypoventilation.

Hypoventilation, or reduced movement of air into and out of the lung, causes carbon dioxide retention. With significant hypoventilation, the carbon dioxide level in the blood rises rapidly, leading to respiratory acidosis. Hypoxemia develops more slowly, and responds readily to administration of oxygen unless gas exchange also is impaired.

In summary, hypoxemia without a corresponding rise in carbon dioxide levels indicates a failure of oxygenation; hypoxemia with hypercapnia is the result of lung hypoventilation.

Manifestations and Course

The manifestations of respiratory failure are caused by hypoxemia and hypercapnia, as well as the underlying disease process. Hypoxemia causes dyspnea and neurologic symptoms such as restlessness, apprehension, impaired judgment, and motor impairment. Tachycardia and hypertension develop as the cardiac output increases in an effort to bring more oxygen to the tissues. Cyanosis is present. As hypoxemia progresses, dysrhythmias, hypotension, and decreased cardiac output may develop.

Increased carbon dioxide levels depress CNS function and cause vasodilation. Dyspnea and headache are early signs. Other manifestations include peripheral and conjunctival va-

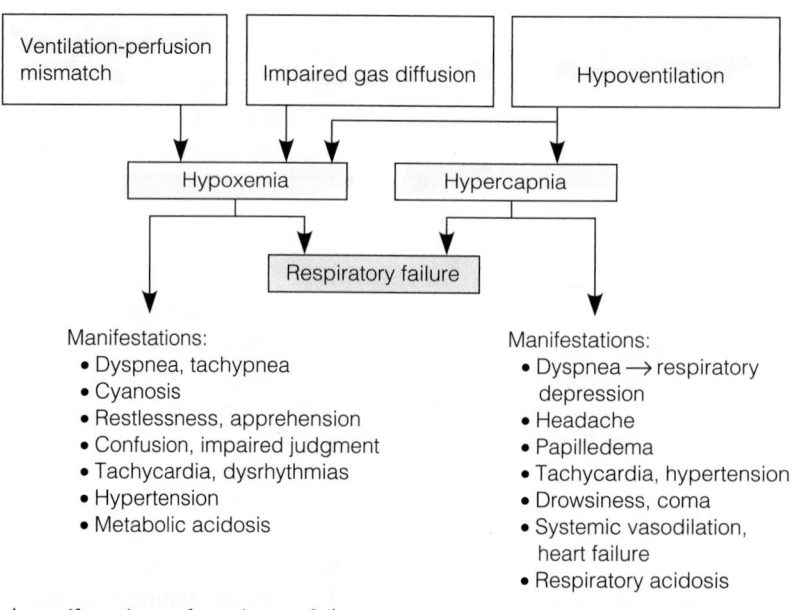

Figure 39–7 ■ Causes and manifestations of respiratory failure.

sodilation, papilledema, neuromuscular irritability, and decreased LOC. As hypercapnia worsens, the respiratory center may be depressed, reducing dyspnea and slowing respirations. Increased carbon dioxide and hydrogen ion concentrations no longer stimulate the respiratory center; hypoxemia provides the primary active breathing stimulus. Administering oxygen without ventilatory support may further reduce the drive to breathe, leading to respiratory arrest.

The prognosis for acute respiratory failure varies, depending on the underlying disease process. Respiratory failure resulting from uncomplicated drug overdose generally resolves quickly without long-term effects. When respiratory failure results from underlying lung disease, the course may be prolonged and the outcome less favorable.

FAST FACTS

Among adults requiring mechanical ventilation for acute respiratory failure:

- An estimated 62% survive to be weaned from the ventilator
- Only 43% survive to be discharged from the hospital
- About 30% remain alive at 1 year after discharge (Tierney et al., 2005).

INTERDISCIPLINARY CARE

Treatment of respiratory failure focuses on correcting the underlying cause or disease, supporting ventilation, and correcting hypoxemia and hypercapnia. Care related to disorders that can precipitate respiratory failure is discussed in the sections specific to each disorder.

Diagnosis

Exhaled carbon dioxide and ABGs are used to diagnose and monitor treatment of respiratory failure.

- *ETCO_2* is used to evaluate alveolar ventilation. The normal ETCO_2 is 35 to 45 mmHg; it is elevated when ventilation is inadequate, and decreased when pulmonary perfusion is impaired.
- *ABGs* also are used to evaluate alveolar ventilation and gas exchange. With hypoxemic respiratory failure, the PaCO_2 may be normal, 38 to 42 mmHg, or even low due to tachypnea. A pH of less than 7.35 and low bicarbonate levels indicate metabolic acidosis, typical of hypoxemic respiratory failure.

In respiratory failure due to hypoventilation, the PaCO_2 is elevated, usually greater than 50 mmHg. The pH is low due to respiratory acidosis. Acidosis develops rapidly in hypoxemia and hypercapnia because of increased acid production (metabolic) and decreased acid elimination (respiratory).

Medications

Drugs used in treating respiratory failure depend on the underlying cause of the failure and the need for intubation and mechanical ventilation.

Beta-adrenergic (sympathomimetic) or anticholinergic medications may be administered by inhalation to promote bronchodilation. If mechanical ventilation is required, the drugs may be given by nebulizer attached to the ventilator. Methylxanthine

bronchodilators (theophylline derivatives) may be given intravenously. See the box on pages 1327–1328 and the asthma section of this chapter for more information about bronchodilators and their nursing implications. Corticosteroids, administered by inhalation or intravenously, may be ordered to reduce airway edema. Antibiotics are given to treat any underlying infection.

Sedation and analgesia often are required during mechanical ventilation to decrease pain and anxiety. Benzodiazepines such as diazepam (Valium), lorazepam (Ativan), or midazolam (Versed) may be used for sedation and to inhibit the respiratory drive. Intravenous morphine or fentanyl provides analgesia and also inhibits the respiratory drive, allowing more effective mechanical ventilation. Occasionally, the client's respiratory drive competes with the ventilator despite sedation, decreasing its effectiveness and increasing the work of breathing. A neuromuscular blocking agent may be necessary to induce paralysis and suppress the ability to breathe. Nursing implications of neuromuscular blockers are described in the Medication Administration box on page 1356.

Oxygen Therapy

Oxygen is administered to reverse hypoxemia in acute respiratory failure. In general, the goal is to achieve an oxygen saturation of 90% or greater without oxygen toxicity. A PaO_2 of about 60 mmHg usually is adequate to meet the oxygen needs of body tissues. Higher levels do not significantly increase oxygen saturation and may lead to hypoventilation in clients with chronic hypercapnia. As little as 1 to 3 L of oxygen per nasal cannula or 28% oxygen per Venturi mask may correct hypoxemia in advanced COPD. Oxygen concentrations of 40% to 60% may be required when diffusion is impaired (e.g., in pneumonia or ARDS). High concentrations are used only for short periods to avoid oxygen toxicity. Both the oxygen concentration and duration of therapy contribute to oxygen toxicity. Continued high oxygen concentrations impair the synthesis of surfactant, reducing lung compliance (ease of inflation). ARDS or absorption atelectasis may develop.

When respiratory failure is caused by hypoventilation or usual oxygen delivery systems do not correct hypoxemia, a tight-fitting mask to maintain *continuous positive airway pressure* (CPAP) may be used. CPAP increases lung volume, opening previously closed alveoli, improving ventilation of underventilated alveoli, and improving ventilation-perfusion relationships.

Airway Management

If the upper airway is obstructed or positive-pressure mechanical ventilation is necessary to correct hypoxemia and hypercapnia, an endotracheal tube that extends from the mouth or nose into the trachea is inserted (Figure 39–8 ■). To maintain positive-pressure ventilation, the tube is cuffed with an air-filled or foam sac just above the end of the tube. When the cuff is inflated, it obstructs the upper airway, preventing air from escaping back into the nose or mouth. Excess pressure of the cuff can cause tissue ischemia and necrosis of the trachea. To minimize this risk, high-volume, low-pressure ("floppy") cuffs are used. Tubes with low-pressure cuffs may be left in place for 3 to 4 weeks.

MEDICATION ADMINISTRATION   Neuromuscular Blockers

NONDEPOLARIZING NEUROMUSCULAR BLOCKERS
Rocuronium (Zemuron)
Pancuronium bromide (Pavulon)
Atracurium besylate (Tracrium)
Cisatracurium (Nimbex)

Nondepolarizing neuromuscular blockers competitively block the action of acetylcholine (ACh) at skeletal muscle receptors, preventing muscle depolarization and contraction. Complete muscle paralysis is achieved within minutes. Facial muscles are affected first, followed by muscles of the limbs, neck, and trunk. The muscles of respiration (the diaphragm and intercostal muscles) are least sensitive to the effects of neuromuscular blockers and are paralyzed last. When the drug is discontinued or an antagonist is given, muscles recover in reverse order; respiratory function is recovered first.

Nursing Responsibilities
- Prior to administering, assess endotracheal tube placement and ensure effective mechanical ventilator function. The risk of hypoxemia and organ damage is significant if respiratory muscles are paralyzed without adequate ventilatory support in place.
- Administer the drug by slow intravenous injection and/or intravenous infusion as prescribed.

- Keep an acetylcholinesterase (AChE) inhibitor such as neostigmine (Prostigmin) available at the bedside to rapidly reverse neuromuscular effects if needed.
- Administer morphine sulfate, diazepam (Valium), or other antianxiety agent or sedative as ordered. Neuromuscular blockers provide no sedation or pain relief; muscle paralysis produces extreme anxiety.
- Instill artificial tears every 2 to 4 hours.
- Suction oral cavity as needed to remove saliva.
- *Never* turn off ventilator alarms when administering neuromuscular blockers. Should the tubing become disconnected or plugged, the client is unable to breathe independently or call for help.
- Treat the client as though awake and alert. Although unable to respond, mental function is unaffected.

Health Education for the Client and Family
- Reassure that the ability to move and communicate will return when the drug is discontinued.
- Teach the family about the effects of the drug and the reason for its use. Explain that the client can hear and understand what is going on.

A tracheostomy may be performed if long-term ventilatory support is required. Although a tracheostomy is more comfortable and easier to secure in place, complications such as cuff necrosis and increased risk of infection are associated with tracheostomy as well as endotracheal intubation. Table 39–6 compares the advantages, disadvantages, and possible complications of endotracheal tubes and tracheostomy.

When the client is able to maintain effective respirations and ventilatory support is no longer required, the endotracheal tube is removed (*extubation*). Gag, cough, and swallow reflexes must be intact to prevent aspiration. After oxygenation and suctioning, the cuff is deflated and the tube removed. Humidified oxygen is provided immediately following removal. Close observation for respiratory distress is vital following extubation. Inspiratory stridor within the first 24 hours indicates laryngeal edema, which may necessitate reintubation. Sore throat and a hoarse voice are common after extubation. Oral intake is reinitiated slowly, with careful assessment of swallowing.

Mechanical Ventilation
Mechanical ventilation is indicated when alveolar ventilation is inadequate to maintain blood oxygen and carbon dioxide levels. Specific indications for mechanical ventilation include:
- Apnea or acute ventilatory failure
- Hypoxemia unresponsive to oxygen therapy alone
- Increased work of breathing with progressive client fatigue.

The most common indicator for ventilation support is respiratory muscle fatigue or its potential (Fenstermacher & Hong, 2004). Drug overdose, neural disorders, chest wall injury, and airway problems such as severe asthma or COPD can lead to acute ventilatory failure. Disorders that affect alveolar-capillary diffusion, such as pulmonary contusion, pneumonia, and ARDS, may necessitate mechanical ventilation to attain adequate oxygenation. Positive-pressure ventilation increases lung volume, helps redistribute fluid from the alveolar to the interstitial space, and helps reduce the oxygen demand caused by increased work of breathing.

TYPES OF VENTILATORS   Two broad general classifications of mechanical ventilators are available. Negative-pressure ventilators create negative (subatmospheric) pressure externally to draw the chest outward and air into the lungs, mimicking spontaneous breathing. The iron lung, cuirass ventilator, and PulmoWrap are examples of negative-pressure ventilators. Negative-pressure ventilators primarily are used by clients with neuromuscular disorders (e.g., post-polio syndrome, amyotrophic lateral sclerosis) that interfere with the ability to maintain adequate ventilation. They also may be used by clients who primarily require ventilator support during sleep.

Figure 39–8 ■ Nasal endotracheal (nasotracheal) intubation.

TABLE 39–6 A Comparison of Endotracheal Tubes and Tracheostomy

	ADVANTAGES	DISADVANTAGES	POTENTIAL COMPLICATIONS
Oral endotracheal tube	■ More easily inserted ■ Larger tube can be used, facilitating work of breathing, suctioning	■ More difficult to secure ■ Can be obstructed by biting ■ Communication and mouth care more difficult ■ Increased risk of lower respiratory infection	■ Obstruction or displacement ■ Pressure necrosis of lip ■ Tracheoesophageal fistula
Nasal endotracheal tube	■ More easily secured and stabilized ■ Well tolerated by client ■ Facilitate communication and oral hygiene	■ Necessitates smaller tube, which may impede removal of secretions ■ Increased risk of lower respiratory infection	■ Obstruction or displacement ■ Pressure necrosis of nares ■ Obstruction of sinus drainage, possible sinusitis ■ Tracheoesophageal fistula
Tracheostomy	■ Easily secured and stabilized ■ Enable swallowing, speech, and oral hygiene ■ Avoid upper airway complications	■ Require surgical incision ■ Increased risk of lower respiratory infection	■ Hemorrhage due to incision or vessel erosion by tube ■ Wound infection ■ Subcutaneous emphysema ■ Tracheoesophageal fistula ■ Tracheal infarction and stenosis

Positive-pressure ventilators are used more often than negative-pressure ones, especially in treating acute respiratory failure (Figure 39–9 ■). These ventilators push air into the lungs, rather than drawing it in like negative-pressure ventilators. Either invasive ventilation using an endotracheal tube or tracheostomy or noninvasive positive-pressure ventilation may be used. Increasingly, noninvasive techniques, which use a nasal or face mask, nasal plugs, or an oral mouthpiece, are being used (Fenstermacher & Hong, 2004).

Noninvasive ventilation (NIV) provides ventilator support using a tight-fitting face mask, thus avoiding intubation. Its primary use is to support clients with obstructive sleep apnea, neu-

Figure 39–9 ■ *A,* Positive-pressure ventilator and *B,* the control panel used to set the mode, rate, limits, and percentage of oxygen delivered.

romuscular disease, or impending respiratory failure (e.g., advanced COPD). NIV also may be used for clients in respiratory failure who refuse intubation. The degree of success varies, primarily limited by client intolerance due to the physical and psychologic discomfort of wearing a mask when dyspneic (Kasper et al., 2005). NIV tends to be more successful in clients without significant underlying lung disease (e.g., respiratory failure related to neuromuscular disease).

Several variables are used to trigger, cycle, and limit airflow with positive-pressure ventilators. The *trigger* prompts the ventilator to deliver a breath. The client's inspiratory effort triggers *ventilator-assisted breaths*. *Ventilator-controlled breaths* usually are triggered by a preset time interval (e.g., a breath is delivered every 5 seconds for a rate of 12 breaths per minute). The ventilator *cycle*, or duration of inspiration, can be limited by volume, pressure, flow, or time. *Volume-cycled ventilators* deliver air until a preset volume is delivered. *Pressure-cycled ventilators* cycle off when a preset pressure is achieved within the airways. *Flow-cycled ventilators* are cycled by a preset inspiratory flow rate, and *time-cycled ventilators* deliver air for a set time interval. Airflow delivered by the ventilator also can be limited by factors such as airway pressure (e.g., a volume-cycled ventilator can be set to immediately stop inspiratory flow if airway pressure exceeds a preset value).

MODES OF VENTILATION A number of different *modes* or patterns of ventilation may be used with positive-pressure ventilators. The mode determines whether a breath is initiated by the client or the ventilator and the pattern of airway support provided by the ventilator. CPAP, bilevel airway pressure support, assist-control mode ventilation, synchronized intermittent mandatory ventilation, positive end-expiratory pressure, pressure support ventilation, and pressure-control ventilation are common modes of ventilation in use today (Table 39–7).

Continuous positive airway pressure applies positive pressure to the airways of a spontaneously breathing client. CPAP may be used with either endotracheal intubation or a tight-fitting face mask. All breathing is spontaneous (client triggered) and pressure controlled. CPAP is used to help maintain open airways and alveoli, decreasing the work of breathing. *Bilevel ventilators* (BiPAP) provide inspiratory positive airway pressure as well as airway support during expiration. Bilevel ventilation is primarily used at night with a tight-fitting mask (nasal, facial, or oral). Three modes of ventilation can be used with BiPAP: spontaneous breathing (S); timed mode (T), in which pressure-supported breaths are delivered at a predetermined rate; and spontaneous/timed (S/T), in which the ventilator switches to timed mode if spontaneous breathing falls below a preset rate (International Ventilator Users Network, 2006).

Assist-control mode ventilation (ACMV or AC) is frequently used to initiate mechanical ventilation and when the client is at risk for respiratory arrest (e.g., overdose or head injury). Assisted breaths are triggered by inspiratory effort; however, if the respiratory rate falls below a preset number (e.g., 14 per minute), ventilator-controlled breaths are delivered. All

breaths, assisted and controlled, are delivered at a specific tidal volume or pressure and inspiratory flow rate.

Synchronized intermittent mandatory ventilation (SIMV) allows the client to breathe spontaneously, without ventilator assistance, between delivered ventilator breaths. Mandatory or ventilator-controlled breaths are delivered at a preset rate, volume, and/or pressure, coordinated with the client's inspiratory efforts. This mode of ventilation is used to support ventilation, to exercise respiratory muscles between ventilator-assisted breaths, and during the weaning process (Kasper et al., 2005).

Positive end-expiratory pressure (PEEP) requires intubation and can be applied to any of the previously described ventilator modes. With PEEP, a positive pressure is maintained in the airways during exhalation and between breaths. Keeping alveoli open between breaths improves ventilation-perfusion relationships and diffusion across the alveolar-capillary membrane. This reduces hypoxemia and allows use of lower percentages of inspired oxygen. PEEP is particularly useful for treating ARDS.

In *pressure support ventilation* (PSV), ventilator-assisted breaths are delivered when the client initiates an inspiratory effort. The cycle is flow limited; inspiration is terminated when inspiratory airflow falls below a preset rate. This mode decreases the work of breathing. It can be used in combination with SIMV when the respiratory drive is depressed. Ventilator support can be gradually withdrawn during weaning.

Pressure-control ventilation (PCV), in contrast, controls pressure within the airways to reduce the risk of airway trauma (e.g., following thoracic surgery). Ventilation is time triggered and time cycled, but pressure is limited. The ventilator maintains a preset airway pressure throughout inspiration. Because all breaths are controlled by the ventilator, heavy sedation may be required to prevent competition between inspiratory effort and ventilator control.

VENTILATOR SETTINGS In addition to choosing the mode of ventilation, other parameters are set to meet individual client needs when positive-pressure ventilation is used (Table 39–8).

For most adult clients, the rate is initially set between 12 and 15 breaths per minute. With ACMV or SIMV, the client's respiratory rate often is higher than the ventilator setting due to spontaneous breathing. Exhaled carbon dioxide ($ETco_2$) or the $Paco_2$ may be used to determine the rate. A $Paco_2$ of less than 38 mmHg indicates hyperventilation and respiratory alkalosis; the set rate is reduced. A $Paco_2$ above 42 mmHg or an $ETco_2$ greater than 45 mmHg indicates hypoventilation and a need to increase the rate.

The tidal volume setting controls the amount of gas delivered with each ventilator breath. The normal adult tidal volume at rest is about 7 mL/kg of body weight, or 400 to 550 mL. The tidal volume delivered by mechanical ventilation is slightly higher (500 to 750 mL) to compensate for tubing dead space. Higher tidal volumes can cause lung tissue trauma.

The percentage of oxygen delivered with ventilator breaths is adjusted to maintain the oxygen saturation and Pao_2 within acceptable ranges. Because prolonged delivery of high oxygen concentrations increases the risk of oxygen toxicity and

TABLE 39–7 Modes of Positive-Pressure Ventilator Operation

MODE	DESCRIPTION	PATTERN
Spontaneous breathing	Client has full control of rate, tidal volume, pressures.	
Assist-control mode ventilation (ACMV)	Client can trigger ventilator to deliver breaths at preset volume or pressure and inspiratory flow rate; breaths will be delivered at preset rate if client does not initiate.	
Synchronized intermittent mandatory ventilation (SIMV)	Mandatory breaths delivered by ventilator are synchronized with client's inspiratory effort.	
Continuous positive airway pressure (CPAP)	Positive pressure is maintained in airways; all breaths are spontaneous.	
Positive end-expiratory pressure (PEEP)	Used in conjunction with other ventilator modes; positive airway pressure is maintained throughout respiratory cycle.	
Pressure support ventilation (PSV)	Pressurized inspiratory flow supports the client's inspiratory effort, decreasing the work of breathing.	

TABLE 39–8 Ventilator Settings

PARAMETER	DESCRIPTION
Rate (f)	Number of ventilator-delivered breaths per minute: usually 12 to 15 in adults using ACMV; may be lower in SIMV
Tidal volume (V_t)	Amount of gas delivered with each ventilator breath: usually 8 to 10 mL/kg of body weight
Oxygen concentration (FIo_2)	Percentage of oxygen delivered with ventilator breaths; can be set between 21% (room air) and 100%
I:E ratio	Duration of inspiration to expiration: usually 1:2 to 1:1.5
Flow rate	Speed at which air is delivered
Sensitivity	Effort required by client to initiate a ventilator-assisted breath
Pressure limit	Maximal pressure within airways that will terminate a ventilator breath

pulmonary fibrosis, the FIo_2 is set at the lowest possible level for adequate tissue oxygenation. For most clients, the goal is to maintain an oxygen saturation level of greater than 90%. Lower oxygen saturation levels may be appropriate for clients with long-standing COPD.

COMPLICATIONS Although endotracheal intubation and mechanical ventilation can be lifesaving in respiratory failure, they are not without risk. Improper endotracheal tube placement or advancement of the tube into a mainstem bronchus can result in ventilation of one lung only. The inflated lung becomes overdistended and traumatized, and the uninflated lung develops atelectasis. In noninvasive ventilation, associated complications include gastric dilation, aspiration, facial skin necrosis, drying of the eyes and mucous membranes, stress, and claustrophobia (Fenstermacher & Hong, 2004).

Nosocomial Pneumonia Infection is a significant risk associated with intubation and mechanical ventilation. Normal upper respiratory tract defense mechanisms are bypassed, with loss of air humidification and trapping of pathogens. Oral secretions and gastric contents can enter the respiratory tree through the open epiglottis. Frequent, meticulous oral hygiene is vital in preventing ventilator-associated pneumonia. Often the cough reflex is inhibited or impaired by the underlying disease process and the continued presence of the endotracheal tube. Even when strict asepsis is used for suctioning and other respiratory procedures, the lower airways are contaminated within 24 hours of intubation (Urden et al., 2006). Secretions often become thick and tenacious, increasing the risk of atelectasis.

Barotrauma *Barotrauma* (also called *volutrauma*) is lung injury due to alveolar overdistention. Both the volume of delivered gas and the pressures under which it is delivered can contribute to barotraumas. As a result, overdistended alveoli rupture, allowing air to escape into the pulmonary interstitial spaces and the mediastinum, pleural space, and other tissues. Subcutaneous emphysema, pneumothorax, and pneumomediastinum are possible results of barotrauma. *Subcutaneous emphysema,* or air in the subcutaneous tissue, causes tissue swelling of the chest, neck, and face. A "crackling" or air-bubble-popping sensation is felt on palpation of subcutaneous emphysema. Swelling may be massive. Once the cause is corrected, the air is gradually reabsorbed.

Pneumothorax is identified by signs of unequal chest expansion, a sudden loss or significant decrease in breath sounds on the affected side, and a hyperresonant percussion tone. Rapid chest tube insertion is necessary to prevent tension pneumothorax and cardiovascular compromise. *Pneumomediastinum* is the presence of air in the mediastinum, the space between the lungs that contains the heart, great vessels, trachea, and esophagus. Air in the mediastinal space can interfere with the function of all of these organs and lead to such complications as pneumopericardium (air in the pericardial sac). Pneumomediastinum may have few manifestations, but the chest x-ray shows widening of the mediastinal space.

Cardiovascular Effects Positive-pressure ventilation increases intrathoracic pressure, which can interfere with venous return to the heart and ventricular filling. As a result, cardiac output falls. Use of PEEP increases the effects of mechanical ventilation on cardiac output. The decreased cardiac output can affect liver and kidney function secondarily.

Gastrointestinal Effects Gastrointestinal complications are commonly associated with prolonged mechanical ventilation. Stress ulcers (erosive gastritis) may develop, leading to painless gastrointestinal hemorrhage. Histamine H_2-receptor blockers or sucralfate are often used to prevent stress ulcers. Air leaks around the endotracheal tube can cause gastric distention; a nasogastric tube often is inserted to prevent vomiting. Sedation and other medications used during mechanical ventilation can slow intestinal motility, leading to constipation.

WEANING The process of removing ventilator support and reestablishing spontaneous, independent respirations is called **weaning**. Weaning begins only after the underlying process causing respiratory failure has been corrected or stabilized. The process and time required for weaning depend on factors such as preexisting lung condition, duration of mechanical ventilation, and the client's general condition, both physical and psychologic. In all cases, the vital signs, respiratory rate, extent of dyspnea, blood gases, and clinical status are used to evaluate weaning and its progress.

Following a brief period of mechanical ventilation, T-piece or CPAP may be used for weaning. In T-piece weaning, the ventilator is removed for brief periods during which oxygen is delivered using a T-piece (Figure 39–10 ■). The duration of periods off the ventilator is gradually increased until the client can

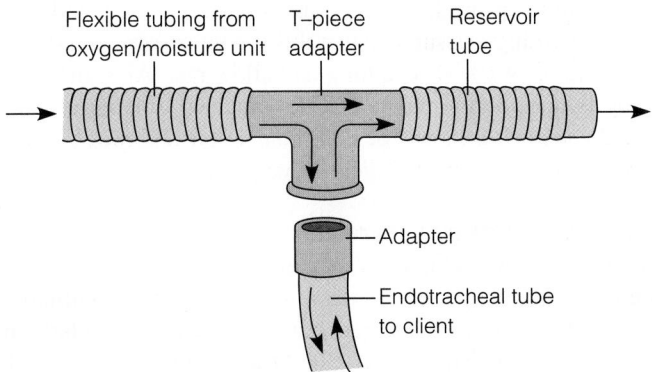

Figure 39–10 ■ A T-piece, or "blow-by" unit, for weaning from mechanical ventilation.

maintain adequate independent respirations for several hours. Vital signs, oxygen saturation, $ETCO_2$, and PaO_2 are carefully monitored during the process. The client is placed back on the ventilator at previous settings if signs of respiratory distress develop. When mechanical ventilation is no longer needed, the endotracheal tube is removed. CPAP weaning follows a similar process, with trials of spontaneous breathing supported by the ventilator in CPAP mode.

SIMV and PSV are used for weaning when the duration of mechanical ventilation has been longer and reconditioning of respiratory muscles is needed. When SIMV is used, the number of mandatory ventilator-assisted breaths is gradually decreased as ABGs, $ETCO_2$, and the respiratory rate are monitored. When the client is able to tolerate SIMV at 4 breaths per minute without rest periods of greater ventilatory support, CPAP or T-piece weaning is attempted prior to extubation (Kasper et al., 2005).

Weaning is the primary use for pressure-support ventilation. Initially, PSV is set slightly below peak inspiratory pressures required during volume-cycled ventilation. Pressure support levels are gradually decreased, often in a cyclic pattern of periods of minimal support alternating with higher support to recondition respiratory muscles. When the PSV level is just enough to overcome endotracheal tube resistance, support is discontinued and the client is extubated (Kasper et al., 2005).

Terminal Weaning When an illness is terminal or irreversible with a poor prognosis, terminal weaning may be requested by the client or family. *Terminal weaning* is the gradual withdrawal of mechanical ventilation when survival without assisted ventilation is not expected. Unlike weaning when recovery is expected, which usually occurs in an intensive care unit, the client is moved to a quiet medical-surgical or hospice room or even home prior to initiating terminal weaning. Family members are encouraged to remain with the client throughout the process. If possible, decisions about sedation and analgesia prior to and during weaning are made with the client, as are decisions about hydration and nutritional support following weaning. Ventilator support is gradually withdrawn using the same modes described earlier (SIMV, PSV). Analgesia and sedation are given to promote comfort during weaning.

Nutrition and Fluids

Attention also must be paid to fluid and electrolyte status and adequate nutrition. Mechanical ventilation promotes sodium and water retention due to its effects on cardiac output. Renal perfusion is decreased, stimulating the renin–angiotensin–aldosterone system to retain sodium and water. A Swan-Ganz catheter is often inserted to monitor pulmonary artery pressures and cardiac output. An arterial line allows repeated blood gas analysis and continuous arterial pressure monitoring. Serum electrolytes are drawn frequently, and intake, output, and daily weight are carefully monitored.

Enteral or parenteral nutrition are provided during mechanical ventilation, because the endotracheal tube prohibits eating. A nasogastric, gastrostomy, or jejunostomy feeding tube is placed for enteral nutrition. A jejunostomy tube may be used to reduce the risk of regurgitation and aspiration.

NURSING CARE

Health Promotion

Education is a primary strategy to prevent respiratory failure. Teach all clients and the public about the risks of smoking, water safety, the value of a working smoke detector, and measures to prevent smoke inhalation in a fire. Discuss the importance of pneumococcal vaccine and annual influenza immunizations for people who are at high risk, including those over age 65 and people with chronic diseases. Teach clients with spinal cord injury or neuromuscular disease to use effective breathing and coughing techniques to maintain airway patency. Work with clients addicted to narcotic drugs to attain and maintain drug-free status. Teach clients with COPD about measures to reduce their risk of respiratory infection and symptoms to report to the physician.

Assessment

Focused assessment data related to respiratory failure include the following:
- *Health History:* Current manifestations, their duration, and identified precipitating factors (may need to be obtained from family members if mental status is affected); history of previous episodes; chronic diseases such as COPD, occupational lung disease; current medications.
- *Physical Examination:* LOC, mental status; vital signs; color and oxygen saturation; respiratory assessment including rate and depth, use of accessory muscles, respiratory excursion, auscultation; cardiovascular assessment including heart rate and sounds, neck vein distention, peripheral pulses, evidence of clubbing.
- *Diagnostic Tests:* ABGs, chest x-ray, pulmonary artery pressure and wedge pressure readings, cardiac output.

Nursing Diagnoses and Interventions

Clients in respiratory failure are often unstable and critically ill. They require both intensive medical care and intensive nursing care. Priority nursing needs relate to maintaining ventilation and a patent airway. Perhaps less obvious, but no less critical, nursing care needs relate to preventing injury and managing anxiety.

Impaired Spontaneous Ventilation

In acute respiratory failure, fatigue from the work of breathing may impair the ability to maintain adequate ventilation. This is a concern both prior to initiation of mechanical ventilation and during the weaning process.

- Assess and document respiratory rate, vital signs, and oxygen saturation every 15 to 30 minutes. *Close monitoring is vital to detect early signs of increasing respiratory distress and inability to sustain adequate breathing.*

PRACTICE ALERT
Promptly report signs of respiratory distress, including tachypnea, tachycardia, nasal flaring, use of accessory muscles, intercostal retractions, cyanosis, increasing restlessness, anxiety, or decreased LOC. These may be early manifestations of respiratory failure and inability to maintain ventilatory effort.

- Promptly report worsening ABGs and oxygen saturation levels. *Close assessment of these values allows timely intervention as needed.*
- Administer oxygen as ordered, monitoring response. Observe closely for respiratory depression, especially in the client with COPD. *Oxygen administration reduces the hypoxemic respiratory drive. Chronically high $PaCO_2$ levels depress the respiratory center; hypoxemia may provide the only respiratory drive.*
- Place in Fowler's or high-Fowler's position. *Sitting positions decrease pressure on the diaphragm and chest, improving lung ventilation and decreasing the work of breathing.*
- Minimize activities and energy expenditures by assisting with ADLs, spacing procedures and activities, and by allowing uninterrupted rest periods. *Rest is vital to reduce oxygen and energy demands.*

PRACTICE ALERT
Avoid sedatives and respiratory depressant drugs unless mechanically ventilated. These medications can further depress the respiratory drive, worsening respiratory failure.

- Prepare for endotracheal intubation and mechanical ventilation:
  a. Obtain an intubation tray with a selection of sterile endotracheal tubes and laryngoscope with a variety of adult blades.
  b. Check laryngoscope lamp; replace battery pack or bulb as needed.
  c. Set up for endotracheal suction, bringing continuous suction head, container, tubing, sterile catheter and glove kits, and sterile normal saline to the bedside.
  d. Notify respiratory therapy to set up the ventilator.
  e. Notify radiology that a portable chest x-ray will be needed on completion of intubation to verify correct placement of the endotracheal tube.

Intubation and mechanical ventilation may be required to maintain ventilation and gas exchange.

- Explain the procedure and its purpose to the client and family, providing reassurance that this is a temporary measure to reduce the work of breathing and allow rest. Alert that talking is not possible while the endotracheal tube is in place, and establish a means of communication. *Thorough explanation is important to relieve anxiety.*

Ineffective Airway Clearance

Ineffective airway clearance may either cause respiratory failure or occur as a result of interventions. Impaired ventilation frequently leads to acute respiratory failure, particularly in clients with COPD or asthma. Chest trauma also can impair airway patency as a result of pulmonary contusion and ineffective cough. Although intubation and mechanical ventilation can be lifesaving measures, they also increase the risk of respiratory infection and ineffective secretion management.

PRACTICE ALERT
Frequently assess respiratory rate, chest movement, lung sounds, oxygen saturation, $ETCO_2$, and ABGs. Intubation and mechanical ventilation do not ensure adequate oxygenation and ventilation. Displacement of the endotracheal tube or obstruction by respiratory secretions impairs ventilation.

- Suction as needed to maintain a patent airway. Indicators for suctioning include crackles and rhonchi on auscultation, frequent coughing or setting off of the high-pressure alarm, and increasing restlessness or anxiety. Procedure 39–1 outlines endotracheal suctioning. *Although clients with a tracheostomy can usually cough up secretions, the length and diameter of endotracheal tubes makes this extremely difficult. Even with humidification, secretions often become thick and tenacious, further inhibiting their removal.*
- Obtain sputum for culture if it appears purulent or is odorous. *Culture is necessary to identify pathogens and guide antibiotic therapy.*
- Perform percussion, vibration, and postural drainage as ordered. *These techniques help loosen secretions and move them into larger airways for removal by coughing or suctioning.*

PRACTICE ALERT
Evaluate endotracheal tube cuff pressure by measurement (should have no more than 20 to 25 mmHg of pressure) or by auscultating the suprasternal notch for a hissing sound at the end of inspiration. The minimum effective cuff pressure to maintain alveolar ventilation is used to reduce the risk of tracheal ischemia and necrosis.

- Firmly secure endotracheal or tracheostomy tube. Provide adequate slack on ventilator tubing to prevent tension on the tube when turning, positioning, or transferring to chair or stretcher. If necessary, loosely restrain hands. *These measures are important to ensure proper airway placement and prevent its inadvertent removal.*
- Assess fluid balance and maintain adequate hydration. *Adequate hydration helps liquefy secretions.*

PROCEDURE 39–1   ENDOTRACHEAL SUCTIONING

GATHER SUPPLIES

- Suction unit with connecting tubing and connector at the bedside
- If an in-line suction catheter is not present
  a. Sterile suction catheter (size 12 to 16 Fr) and glove-kit or suction catheter and sleeve
  b. Sterile normal saline
- Personal protective devices as indicated: goggles, mask, gown

BEFORE THE PROCEDURE

Explain the procedure and why it is being done. Tell the client that although suctioning is not painful, it is uncomfortable. While suction is being applied, breathing is difficult but these periods last only 10 seconds. Stress that suctioning allows removal of secretions and stimulates coughing, which helps clear secretions from smaller airways. Establish a means of communicating; for example, tell the client to raise a finger or rapidly blink if unable to tolerate suctioning.

DURING THE PROCEDURE

1. Use standard precautions.
2. Prepare the suction unit by turning it on and regulating it to no more than −80 to −120 mmHg.
3. Open sterile saline bottle, leaving the cap loosely in place.

With an In-Line Catheter

- Wearing exam gloves, attach the catheter to suction tubing.
- Adjust the oxygen (FIo$_2$) to 100%; allow three breaths.
- Manipulating the catheter through the plastic shield (to maintain its sterility), insert the catheter without applying suction until resistance is met; apply suction while slowly withdrawing the catheter with a twirling motion (see figure).
- Suction for no longer than 10 seconds (count the seconds or watch the clock—the time passes more quickly than you think), then allow to rest for three to five breaths. Repeat the procedure as needed for a total of no more than three times.
- Remove suction tubing from the catheter, clear the tubing, turn off suction, and remove and discard gloves.

With a Separate Catheter-and-Glove Kit

- Open suction catheter/glove kit. Remove saline cup, and fill with sterile normal saline.
- Put on sterile gloves, and attach catheter to suction tubing, keeping dominant hand sterile; lubricate catheter tip with sterile saline.
- Use the nondominant hand to adjust oxygen (FIo$_2$) to 100%; allow three breaths.
- Using the nondominant hand, disconnect ventilator tubing from the endotracheal tube. Manipulating the suction catheter with the dominant (sterile) hand and the suction control valve with the nondominant (nonsterile) hand, insert the catheter, without applying suction until resistance is met. Then, apply suction while slowly withdrawing the catheter, using a twirling motion.

- Suction for no longer than 10 seconds. Reconnect the ventilator, and allow to rest for three to five breaths; clear suction tubing with sterile saline.
- Repeat the preceding two steps as needed for a total of three times.
- Reconnect ventilator tubing to the endotracheal tube.
- Clear suction tubing, turn off suction, and remove the catheter, discarding it with the gloves.
4. Provide three additional breaths at 100% oxygen, then readjust to the previous ordered level.
5. Note color, quantity, consistency, and odor of sputum.
6. Assess lung sounds and tolerance of the procedure.
7. Wash hands.

AFTER THE PROCEDURE

Document assessment before and after suctioning, along with the character of the sputum and the client's tolerance of the procedure.

Report changes in sputum character, such as purulence or an odor that may indicate infection.

Risk for Injury

Many factors increase the risk for injury in acute respiratory failure. Hypoxemia and hypercapnia affect the level of consciousness and may impair mental status. Endotracheal intubation and mechanical ventilation carry risks of tracheal damage and trauma to the lungs. Neuromuscular blockade, if used, presents a significant risk for injury as the client is unable to breathe spontaneously, communicate, and move.

- Assess frequently, noting the following:
  a. LOC, orientation, and awareness
  b. Condition of mucosa of mouth and nose

c. Respiratory: lung sounds, chest excursion, and ventilator pressures
d. Cardiovascular: vital signs, skin color, capillary refill, and peripheral pulses
e. Gastrointestinal: bowel sounds; test gastric secretions and feces for occult blood
f. Genitourinary: urine output, daily weight
g. Skin and extremities

Complications associated with respiratory failure and mechanical ventilation can affect many body systems. Frequent assessment allows early detection and intervention.

PRACTICE ALERT
Do not bypass or turn off any ventilator alarms. The intubated client is unable to communicate verbally and cannot call for help. If neuromuscular blockers are used, the client is also unable to breathe without ventilator support.

- Report condition changes such as increasing air leak around the cuff and decreased breath sounds or chest movement. *These may be manifestations of a complication of intubation and ventilation, such as tracheal necrosis, displacement of the endotracheal tube into the right mainstem bronchus, pneumothorax, or atelectasis.*
- Turn and reposition frequently, taking care to stabilize endotracheal tube during movement. *Repositioning helps maintain tissue perfusion and prevent skin and tissue breakdown.*
- Keep skin and linens clean, dry, and wrinkle-free. Protect pressure areas with padding, egg-crate, or heel and elbow protectors. *The client may not be able to perceive and report pain, and move voluntarily to reduce pressure, necessitating excellent skin care.*
- Perform passive range-of-motion exercises every 4 to 8 hours. *These exercises maintain joint flexibility and help prevent contractures associated with long-term immobility.*

- Keep side rails up and use soft restraints as needed. *These safety measures are important to prevent falls, inadvertent disconnection of the ventilator, or dislodging of the endotracheal tube.*
- Administer histamine H_2-blockers and sucralfate as ordered. *Stress gastritis and possible gastrointestinal hemorrhage are common, preventable complications of mechanical ventilation.*

Anxiety

Critical illness creates anxiety for any client. In acute respiratory failure, this anxiety is compounded by the presence of an endotracheal tube or tracheostomy, mechanical ventilator, numerous monitors and equipment, and, potentially, neuromuscular blockade and paralysis of voluntary muscles. Fear of continued dependence on the mechanical ventilator and inability to return to a normal life may compound this anxiety.

PRACTICE ALERT
Frequently monitor anxiety level. High levels of anxiety increase oxygen use and often interfere with the ability to work with the respirator. This can increase hypoxemia and further increase anxiety; intervention is necessary to break this cycle.

See the accompanying Nursing Research box for information about assessing and managing pain in clients who are intubated.

- Remain with the client as much as possible. *The frequent and continuing presence of a caregiver provides reassurance that help is readily available.*
- Explain all monitors, procedures, unusual sounds, and machinery. *Understanding of the environment and various sounds and alarms reduces anxiety.*
- Provide a simple means of communication, such as a slate, picture board, or alphabet board. If neuromuscular blockade is used, use methods such as looking to the right for "yes" and left for "no." Reassure that endotracheal tube removal re-

---

NURSING RESEARCH   Evidence-Based Practice for the Client Who Is Intubated

Clients who are intubated cannot communicate verbally. Subjective experiences, then, such as pain may not be recognized and effectively treated in these clients. This retrospective study by Gélinas and colleagues (2004) used a standardized instrument to look at the assessment and management of pain as documented in the records of 52 clients undergoing mechanical ventilation. A total of 183 pain episodes were analyzed. In the majority of episodes, observable indicators of pain (such as restlessness, changes in vital signs, muscle tension) were recorded. Subjective reports were recorded only 29% of the time. Following intervention, pain was reassessed only about 60% of the time, usually using objective data and rarely (8%) using subjective information. The study concluded that documentation of pain and its management was incomplete or inadequate for intubated clients.

IMPLICATIONS FOR NURSING
Pain is now considered as the fifth vital sign, necessitating frequent assessment and monitoring. Unrelieved pain is known to reduce healing and prolong recovery. Observable indicators of

pain are not always present; some clients deal with pain by attempting to relax muscles and doze. When neuromuscular blockers or other anesthetic agents are administered to clients who are intubated and mechanically ventilated, objective pain indicators are lost in addition to the ability to subjectively report pain. However, it is important to remember that nursing practice standards dictate that pain level be assessed regularly and both before and following interventions to reduce or relieve pain.

CRITICAL THINKING IN CLIENT CARE
1. What tools are available to assist the nurse in evaluating the client's subjective perception of pain?
2. How can the nurse adapt these tools to use for a client under neuromuscular blockade (consciousness intact but unable to move voluntary muscles)?
3. What factors might contribute to pain in the client who is intubated and mechanically ventilated?
4. Identify five nonpharmacologic measures the nurse could implement to reduce or relieve pain in intubated and ventilated clients.

stores the ability to speak. *The inability to speak and call out for help is frightening for the client. Providing an alternate means of communication helps reduce anxiety.*

- Encourage frequent family visits, especially if the time of visitations is being limited. Encourage family participation in care. *Family visits help reduce anxiety and feelings of abandonment. Allowing family members to participate in care helps reduce their anxiety as well.*
- Explain to the family that the client can hear and understand. Emphasize the importance of talking to the client, not over or about the client. *The family may not understand that the client may be mentally alert although unable to respond. Talking to the client about everyday things reduces the client's sense of isolation and fear.*
- Provide distraction with radio or television if allowed. *Distraction helps reduce the focus on machines and unusual sounds of monitors and alarms.*
- Attend to physical needs promptly and completely. *This provides reassurance that needs will be met even though the client is unable to ask for assistance.*
- Reassure that intubation and mechanical ventilation is a temporary measure to allow the lungs to rest and heal. Reinforce that the client will be able to breathe independently again. *The client may fear continued dependence on mechanical ventilation.*

> **PRACTICE ALERT**
> Provide sedation and antianxiety medications as needed, especially when neuromuscular blockade is used. Although neuromuscular blockade paralyzes voluntary muscles, the level of consciousness is unimpaired.

Using NANDA, NIC, and NOC

Linkages between NANDA nursing diagnoses, nursing interventions, and nursing outcomes for the client with respiratory failure are illustrated in Chart 39–3.

Community-Based Care

Prior to hospital discharge, teach the client and family about the following topics:

- Factors that precipitated respiratory failure and measures to prevent it in the future (e.g., the impact of respiratory irritants on compromised lungs)
- Measures to prevent future episodes such as remaining indoors with an air filter or air conditioning when pollution levels are high, obtaining influenza and pneumonia immunizations, and avoiding exposure to cigarette smoke
- Effective coughing and pulmonary hygiene measures such as percussion, vibration, and postural drainage.

Acute respiratory failure resulting from an acute insult such as pneumonia or near-drowning often resolves with few long-term sequelae. When respiratory failure results from an underlying disease such as COPD, the prognosis is less optimistic. Clients with end-stage COPD may have repeated episodes of respiratory failure, with a gradual loss of respiratory function and reserve. These clients may choose terminal weaning rather

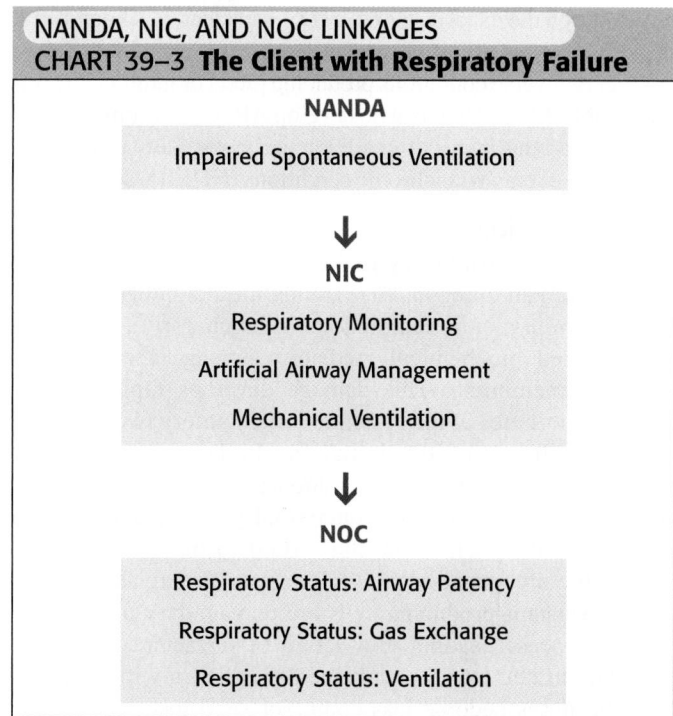

NANDA, NIC, AND NOC LINKAGES
CHART 39–3 The Client with Respiratory Failure

NANDA

Impaired Spontaneous Ventilation

↓

NIC

Respiratory Monitoring

Artificial Airway Management

Mechanical Ventilation

↓

NOC

Respiratory Status: Airway Patency

Respiratory Status: Gas Exchange

Respiratory Status: Ventilation

Data from *NANDA's Nursing Diagnoses: Definitions & Classification 2005–2006* by NANDA International (2005), Philadelphia; *Nursing Interventions Classification (NIC)* (4th ed.) by J. M. Dochterman & G. M. Bulechek (2004), St. Louis, MO: Mosby; and *Nursing Outcomes Classification (NOC)* (3rd ed.) by S. Moorhead, M. Johnson, and M. Maas (2004), St. Louis, MO: Mosby.

than a future of increasing disability. Discuss what to expect during the terminal weaning process with the client and family. Discuss use of sedation prior to and during the weaning process. Explain that medications are used to reduce respiratory distress and dyspnea during weaning. Assure the client and family that nursing support is continuously available during the weaning process and that family and other supporters such as clergy are allowed to remain with the client.

THE CLIENT WITH ACUTE RESPIRATORY DISTRESS SYNDROME

Acute respiratory distress syndrome (ARDS) is characterized by noncardiac pulmonary edema and progressive refractory hypoxemia. First identified in 1967, ARDS has been known by various names, such as shock lung and adult hyaline membrane disease. It is widely recognized as a severe form of acute respiratory failure. The mortality rate associated with acute respiratory distress syndrome, while declining, remains around 30% to 40% (ALA, 2006).

> **FAST FACTS**
> - Approximately 150,000 Americans are affected by ARDS annually (NHLBI, 2006).
> - Most clients recover near-normal lung function within 6 months of developing ARDS.
> - Mortality associated with ARDS often is due to multiple-organ system dysfunction related to ineffective tissue oxygenation (ALA, 2006).

Although the exact cause of ARDS is unclear, it is known that ARDS does not occur as a primary process but may follow a number of diverse conditions producing direct or indirect lung injury (Table 39–9). Clients who develop ARDS as a complication of an acute lung injury or condition are more likely to fully recover than clients with chronic conditions (NHLBI, 2006).

Pathophysiology

The underlying pathology in ARDS is acute lung injury resulting from an unregulated systemic inflammatory response to acute injury or inflammation. Inflammatory cellular responses and biochemical mediators damage the alveolar-capillary membrane. This damage develops rapidly, often within 90 minutes of the systemic inflammatory response and within 24 hours of the initial insult. Damaged capillary membranes allow plasma and blood cells to escape into the interstitial space. Increased interstitial pressure and damage to the alveolar membrane allow fluid to enter the alveoli. Within the alveolus, the fluid dilutes and inactivates surfactant. Surfactant-producing cells are damaged by the inflammatory process, leading to a deficit of surfactant, increased alveolar surface tension, and alveolar collapse with atelectasis. The lungs become less compliant, and gas exchange is impaired. As the syndrome progresses, hyaline membranes form, further reducing gas exchange and compliance. Finally, fibrotic changes occur in the lungs. Intra-alveolar septa thicken, and alveolar surface area for gas exchange is reduced. Hypoxemia becomes refractory or resistant to improvement with supplemental oxygen, and the $Paco_2$ rises as diffusion is further impaired. Figure 39–11 and the *Pathophysiology Illustrated* figure on pages 1368–1369 illustrate the pathophysiology of ARDS.

As ARDS progresses, tissue hypoxia becomes significant, and metabolic acidosis develops. Carbon dioxide exchange is impaired as well as oxygen exchange, leading to combined respiratory and metabolic acidosis. Sepsis and multiple organ system dysfunction of the kidneys, liver, gastrointestinal tract, CNS, and cardiovascular system are the leading causes of death in ARDS. If the process is halted before this occurs, the long-term prognosis for recovery is good.

Manifestations

Initial manifestations of ARDS typically develop 24 to 48 hours after the initial insult. Dyspnea, tachypnea, and anxiety

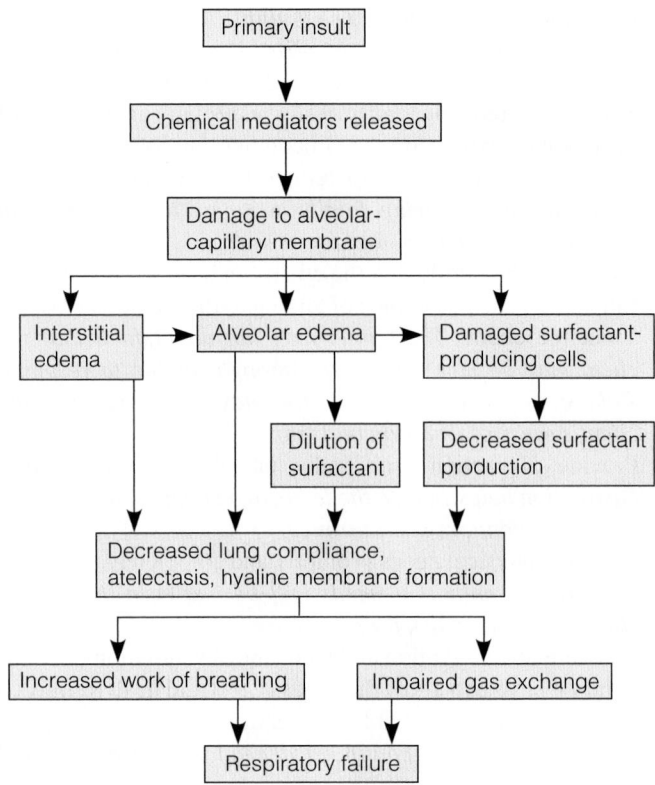

Figure 39–11 ■ The pathogenesis of ARDS.

are early manifestations. Progressive respiratory distress develops, with increasing respiratory rate, intercostal retractions, and use of accessory muscles of respiration. Cyanosis develops that may not improve with oxygen administration. Breath sounds are initially clear, but crackles (rales) and rhonchi develop later. As respiratory failure progresses, mental status changes such as agitation, confusion, and lethargy occur.

INTERDISCIPLINARY CARE

ARDS management is directed toward identifying and treating its underlying cause and providing aggressive respiratory support.

Diagnosis

Refractory hypoxemia (hypoxemia that does not improve with oxygen administration) is the hallmark of ARDS.

TABLE 39–9 Conditions Associated with the Development of ARDS

CONDITIONS	EXAMPLES
Shock	Hemorrhagic shock, septic shock
Inhalation injuries	Aspiration of gastric contents, smoke and toxic gases, near-drowning, oxygen toxicity
Infections	Gram-negative sepsis, viral pneumonias, *Pneumocystis carinii* pneumonia, miliary tuberculosis
Drug overdose	Heroin, methadone, propoxyphene, aspirin
Trauma	Burns, head injury, lung contusion, fat emboli
Other	Disseminated intravascular coagulation, pancreatitis, uremia, amniotic fluid and air emboli, multiple transfusions, open heart surgery with cardiopulmonary bypass

- *ABGs* initially show hypoxemia with a PaO_2 of less than 60 mmHg and respiratory alkalosis due to tachypnea.
- *Chest x-ray* changes may not be evident for as long as 24 hours after the onset of ARDS. Diffuse infiltrates are seen initially, progressing to a "white out" pattern. Chest *CT scan* provides a better illustration of the pattern of alveolar consolidation and atelectasis in ARDS (Kane & Galanes, 2004).
- *Pulmonary function testing* shows decreased lung compliance with reduced vital capacity, minute volume, and functional vital capacity (see Box 36–1).
- *Pulmonary artery pressure monitoring* shows normal pressures in ARDS, helping distinguish ARDS from cardiogenic pulmonary edema.

Medications

Although there is no definitive drug therapy for ARDS, a number of medications may be used. Inhaled nitric oxide reduces intrapulmonary shunting and improves oxygenation by dilating blood vessels in better ventilated areas of the lungs. Surfactant therapy may be prescribed. Surfactant is a complex mixture of phospholipids, neutral lipids, and proteins that forms a thin layer atop a thin layer of water on the inner surface of the alveolus, reducing the surface tension within the alveoli. Surface tension tends to pull the walls of the alveoli together, increasing the likelihood of collapse during exhalation. Surfactant, by reducing surface tension, helps maintain open alveoli, decreasing the work of breathing, improving compliance and gas exchange, and preventing atelectasis.

Interventions to block the inflammatory response are under investigation, such as using nonsteroidal anti-inflammatory agents and corticosteroids. Corticosteroids may be used late in the course of ARDS to improve oxygenation and lung mechanics when fibrotic changes occur.

Mechanical Ventilation

The mainstay of ARDS management is endotracheal intubation and mechanical ventilation. With ARDS, it is rarely possible to maintain adequate tissue oxygenation with oxygen therapy alone.

With mechanical ventilation, the FIO_2 is set at the lowest possible level to maintain a PaO_2 higher than 60 mmHg and oxygen saturation of approximately 90%. When the PaO_2 cannot be maintained with less than 50% inspired oxygen, there is a risk that oxygen toxicity will accentuate ARDS. Often it is necessary to add CPAP, BiPAP, or PEEP to mechanical ventilation settings to maintain blood and tissue oxygenation. Maintaining open airways and alveoli enhances gas diffusion and reduces ventilation-perfusion mismatch. PEEP decreases cardiac output and increases the risk of barotrauma, necessitating close monitoring. Either assist-control or SIMV may be used along with PEEP or CPAP in treating ARDS.

It is important to remember that mechanical ventilation does not cure ARDS; it simply supports respiratory function while the underlying problem is being identified and treated.

Treatments

Atelectasis frequently occurs in dependent lung regions in ARDS. Prone positioning in conjunction with mechanical ventilation reduces the pressure of surrounding tissue on dependent regions and improves oxygenation.

Other management strategies include careful fluid replacement, attention to nutrition, treatment of any infection, and correction of the underlying condition. A Swan-Ganz line is placed to monitor pulmonary artery pressures and cardiac output. Fluid replacement is carefully tailored to these measurements to avoid fluid imbalances, which may worsen hypoxia and ARDS. Enteral or parenteral feeding is necessary to maintain nutritional status and prevent tissue catabolism. Infections are treated with intravenous antibiotic therapy tailored to the causative organism. Low-molecular-weight heparin may be ordered to prevent thrombophlebitis and possible pulmonary embolus or disseminated intravascular coagulation, a possible complication of ARDS.

NURSING CARE

The nursing care needs of the client with ARDS are very similar to those of any client with acute respiratory failure. Maintaining adequate ventilation and respirations are of highest priority, along with preventing injury and managing anxiety. See the section on acute respiratory failure for nursing care related to these diagnoses. Additional high-priority nursing care concerns for the client with ARDS are related to the effects of PEEP on cardiac output and potential problems of weaning ventilatory support. See the Nursing Care Plan that follows for additional nursing interventions for the client with ARDS.

Nursing Diagnoses and Intervention

Decreased Cardiac Output

With positive pressure ventilation, increased intrathoracic pressure decreases cardiac output. When PEEP is applied, intrathoracic pressure increases further; this can significantly decrease venous return, ventricular filling, stroke volume, and cardiac output. Manifestations of decreased cardiac output include hypotension and compensatory tachycardia as the heart attempts to maintain cardiac output despite decreased stroke volume. In the client who is already hypoxic because of ARDS, this drop in cardiac output can increase tissue damage. Urine output falls, and dysrhythmias may develop.

- Monitor and record vital signs, including apical pulse, at least every 2 hours; more frequently immediately following initiation of mechanical ventilation or addition of PEEP. *Frequent assessment is vital to detect early signs of decreased cardiac output.*

> **PRACTICE ALERT**
> Record urine output hourly. Because a significant portion of the cardiac output goes directly to the kidneys, a fall in urine output to less than 30 mL per hour is often the first sign of decreased cardiac output.

- Assess level of consciousness at least every 4 hours. *Altered LOC, confusion, and restlessness are early signs of cerebral hypoxia due to decreased cardiac output.*
- Monitor pulmonary artery pressures, central venous pressure, and cardiac output readings every 1 to 4 hours. *Changes in these measurements may indicate worsening cardiac status.*

Acute Respiratory Distress Syndrome

Acute respiratory distress syndrome (ARDS) is a severe form of acute respiratory failure that occurs in response to pulmonary or systemic insults. ARDS is characterized by noncardiogenic pulmonary edema caused by inflammator damage to alveolar and capillary walls. Many disorders ma precipitate ARDS, although sepsis is the most common.

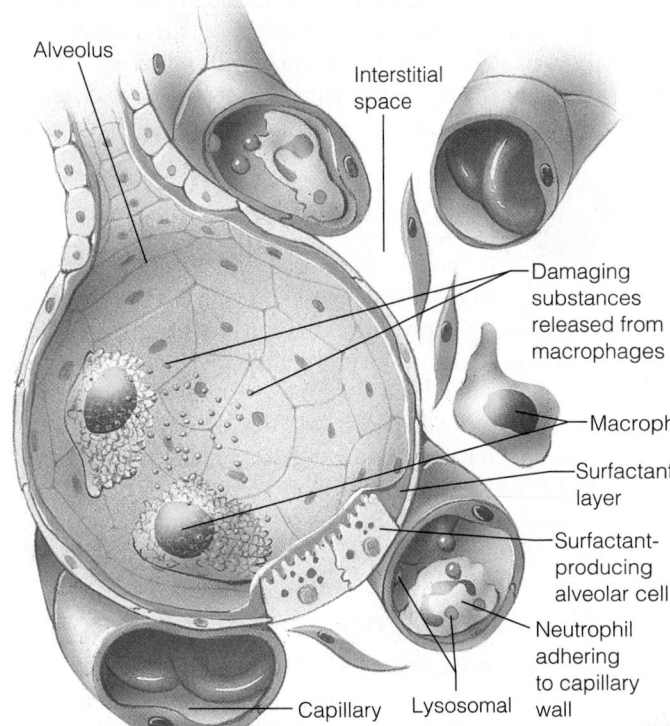

1. Initiation of ARDS

In sepsis-induced ARDS, bacterial toxins cause macrophages and neutrophils to adhere to endothelial surfaces of the alveoli and capillaries. The macrophages release oxidants, inflammatory mediators, enzymes, and peptides that damage the capillary and alveolar walls. In response, neutrophils release lysosomal enzymes causing further damage.

2. Onset of Pulmonary Edema

The damaged capillary and alveolar walls become more permeable, allowing plasma, proteins, and erythrocytes to enter the interstitial space. As interstitial edema increases, pressure in the interstitial space rises and fluid leaks into alveoli. Plasma proteins accumulating in the interstitial space lower the osmotic gradient between the capillary and interstitial compartment. As a result, the balance is disrupted between the osmotic force that pulls fluid from the interstitial space into the capillaries and the normal hydrostatic pressure that pushes fluid out of the capillaries. This imbalance causes even more fluid to enter alveoli.

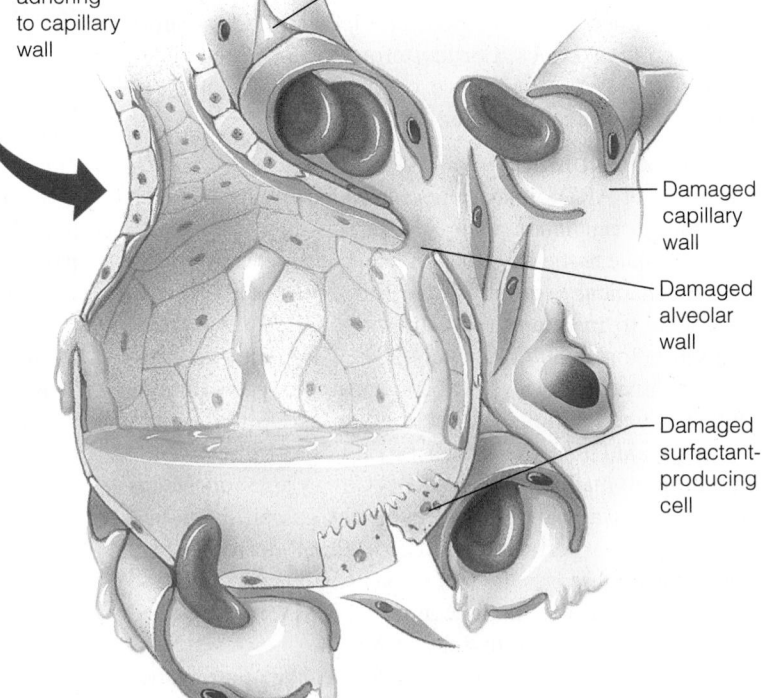

4. End-Stage ARDS

Fibrin and cell debris from necrotic cells combine to form hyaline membranes, which line the interior of the alveoli and further reduce alveolar compliance and gas exchange. Because CO_2 cannot diffuse across hyaline membranes, $PaCO_2$ levels now begin to rise while PaO_2 levels continue to fall. Rising $PaCO_2$ levels can lead to respiratory acidosis. Without respiratory support, respiratory failure will develop.
Even with aggressive treatment, almost 50% of clients with ARDS die.

O_2

Hyaline membrane

CO_2

O_2

CO_2

3. Alveolar Collapse

Protein-rich fluid accumulates in the alveoli, inactivating surfactant and damaging type II alveolar cells that produce surfactant. (Surfactant is important in maintaining alveolar compliance—the ability of tissue to stretch or distend.) As active surfactant is lost, the alveoli stiffen and collapse, leading to atelectasis, which increases breathing effort.

Decreased alveolar compliance, atelectasis, and fluid-filled alveoli interfere with gas exchange across the alveolar-capillary membrane. Blood oxygen (PaO_2) levels fall. Because carbon dioxide diffuses more readily than oxygen, however, blood carbon dioxide ($PaCO_2$) levels also fall initially as tachypnea causes more CO_2 to be expired.

NURSING CARE PLAN A Client with ARDS

Peggy Adamson is a 36-year-old single woman admitted to the hospital following a near-drowning in a local lake. On admission to the emergency department, Ms. Adamson is alert and oriented, having been rescued and resuscitated within 2 minutes of the accident. Rescuers report that she seemed to have aspirated "a lot" of water as she was water-skiing when the accident occurred. She is admitted to the intensive care unit for observation. Oxygen is started per nasal cannula at 6 L/min, intravenous fluids are administered to correct electrolyte imbalances, and 40 mg of furosemide (Lasix) is given intravenously for hypervolemia.

ASSESSMENT

Nadia Mucha cares for Ms. Adamson the evening of the day after her admission. Throughout her stay, Ms. Adamson has remained alert and oriented with stable vital signs. Her respiratory rate has been 20 to 24 per minute, with scattered crackles, oxygen saturations of around 94%, and a PaO_2 of 75 to 80 mmHg on 6 L/min of oxygen. Her pulse has been 96 to 100 and regular. On her initial assessment, Ms. Mucha notes that Ms. Adamson seems apprehensive and anxious. Although her blood pressure is 116/74, unchanged from previous levels, her heart rate is up to 106 and respiratory rate is 28 per minute. Her lungs have scattered crackles but good breath sounds throughout, unchanged from previous assessments. Ms. Adamson's oxygen saturation has dropped to 84%, so Ms. Mucha orders ABGs and increases the oxygen to 8 L/min. ABG results show PaO_2, 65 mmHg; respiratory alkalosis, pH, 7.48; and $PaCO_2$, 32 mmHg.

Ms. Mucha orders a portable chest x-ray and notifies the physician of the ABG results and the change in Ms. Adamson's status. The physician orders a nonrebreather mask at 8 L/min and repeat ABGs in 1 hour. The chest x-ray reveals scattered infiltrates and a normal heart size.

Ms. Adamson's oxygen saturation continues to fall, and subsequent blood gases show a PaO_2 of 55 mmHg. The attending physician diagnoses probable ARDS and orders nasotracheal intubation and mechanical ventilation.

DIAGNOSES

- *Ineffective Breathing Pattern* related to anxiety
- *Impaired Gas Exchange* related to effects of near-drowning
- *Anxiety* related to hypoxemia
- *Risk for Decreased Cardiac Output* related to mechanical ventilation
- *Risk for Injury* related to endotracheal intubation

EXPECTED OUTCOMES

- Breathe effectively with the mechanical ventilator.
- Demonstrate improved oxygen saturation, $ETCO_2$, and ABG values.
- Express fears related to intubation and mechanical ventilation.
- Demonstrate reduced anxiety levels (relaxed facial expression, ability to rest).
- Maintain adequate cardiac output and tissue perfusion.
- Tolerate endotracheal intubation and mechanical ventilation without evidence of infection or barotrauma.

PLANNING AND IMPLEMENTATION

- Obtain all necessary supplies and notify respiratory therapy and radiology in preparation for intubation and mechanical ventilation.
- Explain the purpose and procedure of intubation.
- Provide an opportunity to express fears related to intubation and mechanical ventilation; answer questions and provide reassurance.
- Discuss communication strategies while intubated; obtain a magic slate.
- Administer analgesics and/or sedatives as ordered.
- Monitor oxygen saturation and $ETCO_2$ levels every 30 to 60 minutes initially after instituting mechanical ventilation; report changes to the physician.
- Obtain ABGs as ordered or indicated; monitor and report results.
- Suction via endotracheal tube as needed to maintain clear airways.
- Allow periods of uninterrupted rest.
- Monitor vital signs every 1 to 2 hours.
- Assess skin color, capillary refill, and the presence of edema every 4 hours.
- Monitor urine output hourly; report output of less than 30 mL per hour.
- Assess lung sounds and chest excursion every 1 to 2 hours.

EVALUATION

Ms. Adamson is intubated and placed on a volume-cycled ventilator at 50% FIO_2 and a tidal volume of 700 mL in the assist-control mode at 16 breaths per minute. She has difficulty working with the ventilator initially, so a fentanyl drip is ordered to reduce her anxiety. Ms. Adamson's oxygen saturation, $ETCO_2$, and ABG results do not begin to improve until 5 mmHg of PEEP is added to ventilator settings. After 3 days of mechanical ventilation with PEEP and aggressive fluid and diuretic therapy, Ms. Adamson begins to improve. She is placed on SIMV, and over the course of another 3 days she is gradually weaned off the ventilator to a face mask with CPAP. She eventually recovers fully, with minimal apparent long-term effects.

CRITICAL THINKING IN THE NURSING PROCESS

1. Endotracheal intubation and mechanical ventilation were effective in supporting Ms. Adamson's respiratory status as she recovered from ARDS. Discuss a possible sequence of events had it not been possible to wean her from the ventilator.
2. How might the presentation and management of an acute episode of respiratory failure due to ARDS differ from respiratory failure related to COPD?
3. What measures can nurses take to prevent the development of ARDS?
4. Develop a nursing care plan for Ms. Adamson for the nursing diagnosis *Powerlessness* related to endotracheal intubation and mechanical ventilation.

See Evaluating Your Response in Appendix C.

- Assess heart and lung sounds frequently. *Increasing crackles or abnormal heart sounds may indicate heart failure.*
- Weigh daily at the same time. *Accurate daily weights are the best indicator of fluid volume status.*

- Frequently provide good skin care, keeping skin clean and dry and protecting pressure points. *Tissue hypoxia increases the risk of skin breakdown, which in turn increases the risk of infection and sepsis.*

- Maintain intravenous fluids as ordered. *Intravenous fluids are given to maintain vascular volume and prevent dehydration.*
- Administer analgesics, sedatives, and neuromuscular blockers as needed. *These medications may be prescribed to decrease cardiac workload.*

Dysfunctional Ventilatory Weaning Response

The client with dysfunctional ventilatory weaning response has difficulty adjusting to reduced mechanical ventilator support, prolonging the weaning process. Airway congestion, inadequate rest or nutrition, pain, anxiety, and a nonsupportive environment are factors that can contribute to difficulty weaning. With ARDS, the pathologic processes of the disease and its effects on gas exchange may be responsible for a prolonged or ineffective weaning process.

Assessment findings indicative of dysfunctional weaning include:

- Dyspnea, apprehension, or agitation
- Decreasing oxygen saturation level
- Cyanosis or pallor, diaphoresis
- Increased blood pressure, pulse, and respiratory rate
- Diminished or adventitious breath sounds, use of accessory muscles
- Decreased LOC
- Deteriorating ABG values
- Shallow, gasping breaths or paradoxic abdominal breathing.

Nursing interventions for dysfunctional weaning include the following:

- Assess vital signs every 15 to 30 minutes following changes in ventilator settings and during T-piece trials. *Vital signs, heart and respiratory rates in particular, can provide early signs of hypoxemia and poor tolerance of the weaning process.*

PRACTICE ALERT
Frequently monitor oxygen saturation, ETco₂, and ABGs following changes in ventilator settings. These values are used to assess the adequacy of ventilation and gas exchange during the weaning process.

- Place in Fowler's or high-Fowler's position. *Fowler's position facilitates lung expansion and reduces the work of breathing.*
- Fully explain all weaning procedures, along with expected changes in breathing. *Adequate explanations help reduce anxiety and improve the ability to cooperate.*
- Remain with the client during initial periods following changes of ventilator settings or T-piece trials. *This provides reassurance and allows close monitoring of the response.*
- Limit procedures and activities during weaning periods. *Reducing energy expenditures and cardiac work facilitates the weaning process.*
- Provide diversion, such as television or radio. *Diversion helps distract the focus from breathing.*
- Begin weaning procedures in the morning, when the client is well rested and alert; weaning may be discontinued overnight to provide rest. *The work of breathing increases during the weaning process; adequate rest is important.*
- When SIMV is used for weaning, decrease the SIMV rate by increments of two breaths per minute. *Slow reduction of ven-*

tilator support allows respiratory muscle reconditioning and gradual resumption of the work of breathing.

- Avoid administering drugs that may depress respirations during the weaning process (except as ordered at night to facilitate rest when ventilator support is provided). *Sedatives or analgesics that depress respirations can impair the weaning process.*

PRACTICE ALERT
Frequently assess respiratory status following weaning and extubation. Keep an intubation kit readily available following extubation; be prepared for emergency reintubation. Laryngeal spasm or laryngeal edema may develop following extubation, necessitating reintubation to maintain respirations.

- Keep oxygen at the bedside following weaning and extubation. *Supplemental oxygen may be necessary to maintain adequate blood and tissue oxygenation.*
- Provide pulmonary hygiene with percussion and postural drainage. *Maintaining patent airways and adequate alveolar ventilation is vital during the weaning process.*

Using NANDA, NIC, and NOC

Linkages between NANDA nursing diagnoses, nursing interventions, and nursing outcomes for the client with ARDS are illustrated in Chart 39–4.

NANDA, NIC, AND NOC LINKAGES
CHART 39–4 The Client with ARDS

NANDA

| Dysfunctional Ventilatory Weaning Response |

NIC

Anxiety Reduction

Energy Management

Mechanical Ventilatory Weaning

Respiratory Monitoring

NOC

Anxiety Control

Respiratory Status: Gas Exchange

Respiratory Status: Ventilation

Energy Conservation

Data from *NANDA's Nursing Diagnoses: Definitions & Classification 2005–2006* by NANDA International (2005), Philadelphia; *Nursing Interventions Classification (NIC)* (4th ed.) by J. M. Dochterman & G. M. Bulechek (2004), St. Louis, MO: Mosby; and *Nursing Outcomes Classification (NOC)* (3rd ed.) by S. Moorhead, M. Johnson, and M. Maas (2004), St. Louis, MO: Mosby.

Community-Based Care

When preparing the client who has recovered from ARDS and the family for home care, discuss the following topics:

- ARDS did not result from something they did or did not do, but developed as a consequence of serious illness. Provide factual information about ARDS.
- Maximal respiratory function following ARDS is usually achieved within 6 months; respiratory function may remain significantly impaired. This may necessitate changes in occupation, lifestyle, and family roles.

- Avoiding smoking and exposure to secondhand smoke and environmental pollutants is vital to prevent further lung damage.
- Obtain immunization for pneumococcal pneumonia and annual influenza immunizations to prevent further episodes of serious respiratory disease.

Provide referrals to home health and respiratory care services as indicated, as well as for occupational therapy and counseling as needed.

EXPLORE MEDIALINK

Prentice Hall Nursing MediaLink DVD-ROM
Audio Glossary
NCLEX-RN® Review

Animation/Video
ARDS
Asthma
Metered-Dose Inhalers
Using a Nebulizer

COMPANION WEBSITE www.prenhall.com/lemone
Audio Glossary
NCLEX-RN® Review
Care Plan Activity: Acute Asthma Attack
Case Study: Acute Asthma Attack
Exercise: Compare and Contrast
MediaLink Application: Respiratory Disorders
Links to Resources

CHAPTER HIGHLIGHTS

- Obstructive disorders of the lower respiratory system, including asthma, COPD, and cystic fibrosis, impair airflow into and out of the lungs, often affecting the outflow of air to a greater extent than inflow. As a result, air trapped in the alveoli increases the residual volume of the lungs and reduces functional residual capacity. Alveolar ventilation is reduced as well. The net result is less available oxygen in the alveoli and impaired gas exchange.
- In many instances, acute episodes of asthma can be avoided through the use of inhaled steroids to reduce airway inflammation, inhaled long-acting bronchodilators, and frequent self-monitoring of expiratory flow rate. Nursing care focuses on teaching for self-management, and providing care during acute episodes of airway constriction.
- Chronic obstructive pulmonary disease (COPD) is a long-term process of progressive lung dysfunction. COPD involves two different disease processes: chronic bronchitis, characterized by airway edema and excessive mucous production, and emphysema, characterized by destruction of supporting tissue with enlargement of respiratory bronchioles and alveolar spaces and loss of surface area for gas exchange.
- Smoking and exposure to tobacco smoke is the single greatest risk factor for COPD. A small percentage of cases result from an inherited deficiency of α_1-antitripsin, an enzyme that inhibits lung

tissue destruction. Although smoking cessation does not reverse COPD, it does slow the progress of the disease.
- Cystic fibrosis, inherited as an autosomal recessive disorder, causes thick, viscous secretions in affected organs, primarily the lungs, pancreas, sweat glands, and reproductive tract. In the lungs, small airway clearance is impaired, leading to atelectasis, bronchiectasis, infection, and dilation of distal airways with air trapping and impaired gas exchange. Chest physiotherapy and early treatment of respiratory infections are key components of disease management. Ultimately, lung or heart-lung transplant may be required.
- Occupational lung diseases, pneumoconiosis and hypersensitivity pneumonitis, damage interstitial tissues of the lungs, leading to fibrosis and scarring that causes the lungs to become stiff and noncompliant. Lung volumes decrease, the work of breathing increases, and gas diffusion is impaired. Most occupational lung diseases are progressive and nonreversible. Interdisciplinary care is similar to that provided for clients with COPD.
- Pulmonary vascular disorders affect blood flow through the pulmonary vascular system and gas exchange. Pulmonary embolism, obstruction of pulmonary blood flow, is a potentially critical condition usually resulting from deep venous thrombosis. Sudden onset of chest pain and dyspnea with changes in

hemodynamic status are possible manifestations of pulmonary embolism. Prevention through early ambulation, lower extremity exercises, and sequential compression devices is the most effective treatment for pulmonary embolism.

- In primary and secondary forms of pulmonary hypertension, constriction of pulmonary vessels and remodeling of the pulmonary vascular bed increase pressure in the pulmonary system and right heart, ultimately leading to right-sided heart failure (cor pulmonale). Treatment focuses on slowing disease progression through oxygen therapy, administration of vasodilators and anticoagulants, and supporting client function.

- Hypoventilation, impaired gas exchange, and significant ventilation-perfusion mismatch (e.g., pulmonary embolism) can lead to respiratory failure. Hypoventilation leads to hypoxemia and hypercapnia, whereas in impaired gas exchange or ventilation-perfusion mismatch, hypoxemia predominates.

- The manifestations of respiratory failure relate directly to the effects of hypoxemia (dyspnea, restlessness, apprehension, impaired judgment, motor impairment, tachycardia, hyper- or hypotension, and cyanosis) and hypercapnia (dyspnea, headache, peripheral and conjunctival vasodilation, papilledema, neuromuscular irritability, and decreased LOC).

- Respiratory support often is required, using positive-pressure ventilators. Variables of mechanical ventilation include the mode or cycle of ventilation, the flow rate and amount, pressures delivered, and the oxygen concentration. Either invasive or noninvasive techniques may be used.

- Complications of mechanical ventilation include lung and mucous membrane trauma and infection, reduced cardiac output, gastric dilation, impaired communication, and stress.

- ARDS is noncardiac pulmonary edema caused by a diffuse inflammatory response with increased pulmonary capillary permeability leading to interstitial and alveolar edema and impaired gas exchange. As the process continues, lung compliance decreases, increasing the work of breathing, and atelectasis and consolidation of lung tissue develop. Respiratory failure with refractory hypoxemia result.

- Mechanical ventilation and measures to support physiologic function are the primary treatments for ARDS. The mortality rate, however, remains high at about 50%.

TEST YOURSELF NCLEX-RN® REVIEW

1 All of the following nursing diagnoses are appropriate for a client with an acute asthma attack. Which is of highest priority?
1. *Anxiety* related to difficulty breathing
2. *Ineffective Airway Clearance* related to bronchoconstriction and increased mucous production
3. *Ineffective Breathing Pattern* related to anxiety
4. *Ineffective Health Maintenance* related of lack of knowledge about attack triggers and appropriate use of medications

2 The nurse caring for a client with asthma notices that the client's respirations have slowed and he is no longer coughing. Breath sounds are diminished throughout his lung fields and absent in the bases. The nurse should:
1. notify the physician.
2. allow the client to rest undisturbed.
3. obtain a chest x-ray.
4. ask family members to leave.

3 When teaching use of a metered-dose inhaler (MDI), the nurse instructs her client to:
1. take quick shallow breaths in rapid succession while holding the canister down.
2. use the inhaler containing the anti-inflammatory drug first, then the bronchodilator.
3. use the anti-inflammatory drug as needed to treat acute episodes of wheezing.
4. rinse the mouth after using the inhaler to reduce systemic absorption of the drug.

4 Which of the following would be an expected assessment finding in a client admitted with chronic obstructive airway disease?
1. AP chest diameter equal to or greater than lateral chest diameter
2. mental confusion and lethargy
3. 3+ pitting edema of ankles and lower legs
4. oxygen saturation readings of 85% or less

5 An appropriate goal for a client admitted with an acute exacerbation of COPD would be:
1. will verbalize self-care measures to regain lost lung function.
2. arterial blood gases will be within normal limits by discharge.
3. will maintain SaO_2 of 90% or higher.
4. will identify strategies to help reduce number of cigarettes smoked per day.

6 Which of the following statements best represents a nurse's understanding of use of supplemental oxygen in clients with COPD?
1. Because oxygen is flammable, the client should not smoke.
2. Oxygen is used only at night for clients with COPD.
3. Oxygen is never used for clients with COPD because they may become dependent on it.
4. The client needs to be closely monitored for signs of respiratory depression.

7 The home care nurse working with a client who has cystic fibrosis specifically directs the home care aide to report which of the following? (Select all that apply.)
1. thick, tenacious milky white sputum
2. fever
3. bulky, fatty stools
4. difficulty clearing mucous secretions
5. increasing shortness of breath and fatigue

8 A client in skeletal traction suddenly develops right-sided chest pain and shortness of breath. The nurse should:
1. check for Homans' sign.
2. start oxygen per nasal cannula.
3. administer the prescribed analgesic.
4. elevate the head of the bed to 45 degrees.

9 The nurse caring for a client with COPD recognizes which of the following as an early sign of possible respiratory failure?
1. restlessness and tachypnea
2. deep coma
3. hypotension and tachycardia
4. decreased urine output

10 The nurse caring for a client undergoing mechanical ventilation for acute respiratory failure plans and implements which of the following measures to help maintain effective alveolar ventilation?

1. Keeps the client in supine position.
2. Increases the tidal volume on the ventilator.
3. Maintains ordered oxygen concentration.
4. Performs endotracheal suctioning as indicated.

See Test Yourself answers in Appendix C.

BIBLIOGRAPHY

American Lung Association (ALA). (2005a). *Asthma in adults fact sheet.* Retrieved from http://www.lungusa.org
_____. (2005b). *Chronic obstructive pulmonary disease (COPD) fact sheet.* Retrieved from http://www.lungusa.org
_____. (2005c). Trends in asthma morbidity and mortality. American Lung Association Epidemiology & Statistic Unit, Research and Program Services. Retrieved from http://www.lungusa.org
_____. (2006). *Lung disease data: 2006.* Retrieved from http://www.lungusa.org
Aronson, B. S., & Marquis, M. (2004). Care of the adult patient with cystic fibrosis. *Medsurg Nursing, 13*(3), 143–154.
Barnett, M. (2006). COPD: The role of the nurse. *Journal of Community Nursing, 20*(2), 18–20, 22.
Belza, B., Steele, B. G., Hunziker, J., Lakshminaryan, S., Holt, L., & Buchner, D. M. (2001). Correlates of physical activity in chronic obstructive pulmonary disease. *Nursing Research, 50*(4), 195–202.
Berkowitz, D. S., & Coyne, N. G. (2003). Understanding primary pulmonary hypertension. *Critical Care Nursing Quarterly, 26*(1), 28–34.
Bialous, S. A., & Sarna, L. (2004). Sparing a few minutes for tobacco cessation. *American Journal of Nursing, 104*(12), 54–62.
Boyle, A. H., & Locke, D. L. (2004). Update on chronic obstructive pulmonary disease. *Medsurg Nursing, 13*(1), 42–48.
Burns, S. M. (2004). The science of weaning: When and how? *Critical Care Nursing Clinics of North America, 16*(3), 379–386.
_____. (2005). Mechanical ventilation of patients with acute respiratory distress syndrome and patients requiring weaning: The evidence guiding practice. *Critical Care Nurse, 25*(4), 14–16, 18, 20–24.
Capriotti, T. (2005). Changes in inhaler devices for asthma and COPD. *Medsurg Nursing, 14*(3), 185–194.
Cardin, T., & Marinelli, A. (2004). Pulmonary embolism. *Critical Care Nursing Quarterly, 27*(4), 310–324.
Carlson, B. W., & Mascarella, J. J. (2003). Living with illness. Changes in sleep patterns in COPD. *American Journal of Nursing, 104*(12), 71–72, 74.
Caroci, A. D. S., & Lareau, S. C. (2005). Descriptors of dyspnea by patients with chronic obstructive pulmonary disease versus congestive heart failure. *Heart & Lung, 33*(2), 102–110.
Charlebois, D. (2005). Early recognition of pulmonary embolism: The key to lowering mortality. *Journal of Cardiovascular Nursing, 20*(4), 254–259.
Cheever, K. H. (2005). An overview of pulmonary arterial hypertension: Risks, pathogenesis, clinical manifestations, and management. *Journal of Cardiovascular Nursing, 20*(2), 108–118.
Copstead, L. C., & Banasik, J. L. (2005). *Pathophysiology* (3rd ed.). St. Louis, MO: Elsevier/Saunders.
Covey, M. K., & Larson, J. L. (2004). Beats & breaths. Exercise and COPD. *American Journal of Nursing, 104*(5), 40–43.
DeJong, S. R., & Veltman, R. H. (2004). The effectiveness of a CNS-led community-based COPD screening and intervention program. *Clinical Nurse Specialist, 18*(2), 72–79.
Dochterman, J., & Bulechek, G. (2004). *Nursing interventions classification (NIC)* (4th ed.). St. Louis, MO: Mosby.
Esmond, G., Butler, M., & McCormack, A. M. (2006). Comparison of hospital and home intravenous antibiotic therapy in adults with cystic fibrosis. *Journal of Clinical Nursing, 15*(1), 52–60.
Farquhar, S. L., & Fantasia, L. (2005). Pulmonary anatomy and hysiology and the effects of COPD. *Home Healthcare Nurse, 23*(3), 167–176.
Fenstermacher, D., & Hong, D. (2004). Mechanical ventilation: What have we learned? *Critical Care Nursing Quarterly, 27*(3), 256–294.
Fontaine, K. L. (2005). *Healing practices: Alternative therapies for nursing* (2nd ed.). Upper Saddle River, NJ: Prentice Hall Health.

Frazier, S. C. (2005). Implications of the GOLD report for chronic obstructive lung disease for the home care clinician. *Home Healthcare Nurse, 23*(3), 109–116.
Gélinas, C., Fortier, M., Viens, C., Fillion, L., & Puntillo, K. (2004). Pain assessment and management in critically ill intubated patients: A retrospective study. *American Journal of Critical Care, 13*(2), 126–135.
Gronkiewicz, C., & Borkgren-Okonek, M. (2004). Acute exacerbation of COPD: Nursing application of evidence-based guidelines. *Critical Care Nursing Quarterly, 27*(4), 336–352.
Grossman, S., & Grossman, L. C. (2005). Pulmonary care. Pathophysiology of cystic fibrosis: Implications for critical care nurses. *Critical Care Nurse, 25*(4), 46–51.
Higgins, P. A. (1998). Patient perception of fatigue while undergoing long-term mechanical ventilation: Incidence and associated factors. *Heart & Lung, 27*(3), 177–183.
Hoyert, D. L., Heron, M., Murphy, S. L., & Kung, H. C. (2006). Deaths: Final data for 2003. Health E-Stats. Retrieved from http://www.cdc.gov/nchs/products/pubs/pubd/hestats/finaldeaths03/finaldeaths03.htm
International Ventilator Users Network (IVUN). (2006). *Home ventilator guide.* Post-Polio Health International (PHI). Retrieved from http://www.post-polio.org/IVUN/HomeVentGuide05S.pdf
Jacobs, M. (2005). Ease the stress of managing ARDS. *Nursing Made Incredibly Easy! 3*(1), 6–15, 17–18.
Kane, C., & Galanes, S. (2004). Adult respiratory distress syndrome. *Critical Care Nursing Quarterly, 27*(4), 325–335.
Kapella, M. C., Larson, J. L., Patel, M. K., Covey, M. K., & Berry, J. K. (2006). Subjective fatigue, influencing variables, and consequences in chronic obstructive pulmonary disease. *Nursing Research, 55*(1) 10–17.
Kasper, D. L., Braunwald, E., Fauci, A. S., Hauser, S. L., Longo, D. L., & Jameson, J. L. (Eds.). (2005). *Harrison's principles of internal medicine* (16th ed.). New York: McGraw-Hill.
Khan, N. U. A., & Novahed, A. (2005). Pulmonary embolism and cardiac enzymes. *Heart & Lung, 34*(2), 142–146.
Koschel, M. J. (2004). Emergency. Pulmonary embolism. *American Journal of Nursing, 104*(6), 46–50.
Lehne, R. A. (2004). *Pharmacology for nursing care* (5th ed.). Philadelphia: Saunders.
Lenaghan, N. A. (2000). The nurse's role in smoking cessation. *Medsurg Nursing, 9*(6), 298–302.
Lindgren, V. A., & Ames, N. J. (2005). Caring for patients on mechanical ventilation: What research indicates is best practice. *American Journal of Nursing, 105*(5), 50–61.
Markou, N. K., Myrianthefs, P. M., & Baltopoulos, G. J. (2004). Respiratory failure: An overview. *Critical Care Nursing Quarterly, 27*(4), 353–379.
Martin, R. J. (2003). Cough-variant asthma. Retrieved from http://www.medscape.com/viewarticle/465233.
McCance, K. L., & Huether, S. E. (2006). *Pathophysiology: The biologic basis for disease in adults and children* (5th ed.). St. Louis, MO: Mosby.
Meek, P. M. (2005). Patients with acute exacerbations of COPD saw anxiety as a sign, rather than cause, of breathlessness. *Evidence-Based Nursing, 8*(2), 61.
Moorhead, S., Johnson, M., & Maas, M. (2004). *Nursing outcomes classification (NOC)* (3rd ed.). St. Louis, MO: Mosby.
Mukherjee, R., & Burge, P. S. (2006). Occupational asthma. *Practice Nursing, 17*(2), 77–80.
National Center for Complementary and Alternative Medicine. (2004). Consumer advisory. Ephedra. Retrieved from http://www.nccam.nih.gov/health/alerts/ephedra/consumeradvisory.
National Center for Health Statistics. (2005). *Health, United States, 2005 with Chartbook on trends in the health of Americans.* Hyattsville, MD: U.S. Government Printing Office.
National Heart, Lung, and Blood Institute. (2006). ARDS. Retrieved from: www.nhlbi.nih.gov/health/dci/Diseases/Ards.

_____. (2003). *Expert panel report: Guidelines for the diagnosis and management of asthma. Update on selected topics 2002.* (NIH Publication No. 02-5074). Bethesda, MD: Author.
_____. (2004). *Morbidity & mortality: 2004 chart book of cardiovascular, lung, and blood diseases.* Bethesda, MD: Author.
_____. (2005). *Global initiative for chronic obstructive lung disease. Pocket guide to COPD diagnoses, management, and prevention.* Bethesda, MD: Author.
NANDA International. (2005). *Nursing diagnoses: Definitions and classification 2005–2006.* Philadelphia: Author.
O'Leary-Kelley, C. M., Puntillo, K. A., Barr, J., Stotts, N., & Douglas, M. K. (2005). Nutritional adequacy in patients receiving mechanical ventilation who are fed enterally. *American Journal of Critical Care, 14*(3), 222–231.
O'Neill, P. (2004). Hospital nursing. Nutrition series: Nutrition for a patient with COPD can be complicated. *Nursing, 34*(12), 32hn6, 32hn8.
Petty, M. (2003). Lung and heart-lung transplantation: Implications for nursing care when hospitalized outside the transplant center. *Medsurg Nursing, 12*(4), 250–259.
Porth, C. M. (2005). *Pathophysiology: Concepts of altered health states* (7th ed.). Philadelphia: Lippincott.
Roman, M. (2005). Clinical "how to." Tracheostomy tubes. *Medsurg Nursing, 14*(2), 143–144.
Simmons, P., & Simmons, M. (2004). Informed nursing practice: The administration of oxygen to patients with COPD. *Medsurg Nursing, 13*(2), 82–85.
Sims, J. M. (2003). What's new in pulmonary artery hypertension. *Dimensions of Critical Care Nursing, 22*(4), 167–170.
Smyth, M. (2005a). Acute respiratory failure, part 1. Failure in oxygenation. *American Journal of Nursing, 105*(5), Critical Care Extra, 72GG–72JJ, 72MM, 7200.
_____. (2005b). Acute respiratory failure, part 2. Failure of ventilation: Exploring the other cause of acute respiratory failure. *American Journal of Nursing, 105*(6), Critical Care Extra 72AA–72DD.
Spencer, J. W., & Jacobs, J. J. (2003). *Complementary and alternative medicine: An evidence-based approach* (2nd ed.). St. Louis, MO: Mosby.
Steinbis, S. (2004). What you should know about pulmonary hypertension. *The Nurse Practitioner, 29*(4), 8–10, 13–15, 19.
Theander, K., & Unosson, M. (2004). Fatigue in patients with chronic obstructive pulmonary disease. *Journal of Advanced Nursing, 45*(2), 172–177.
Tierney, L. M., McPhee, S. J., & Papadakis, M. A. (2005). *Current medical diagnosis & treatment* (44th ed.). New York: Lange Medical Books/McGraw-Hill.
Urden, L. D., Stacy, K. M., & Sough, M. E. (2006). *Thelan's critical care nursing* (5th ed.). St. Louis: Mosby.
U.S. Food and Drug Administration (FDA). (2005a). *Alert for healthcare professionals. Fluticasone propionate; salmeterol xinafoate (marketed as Advair Diskus).* Retrieved from http://www.fda.gov/cder/drug/InfoSheets/HCP/fluticasonelHCP.htm.
U.S. Food and Drug Administration. (2005b). *Alert for healthcare professionals. Formoterol fumarate (marketed as Foradil).* Retrieved from: http://www.fda.gov/cder/drug/InfoSheets/HCP/formoterolHCP.htm.
Wilkinson, J. M. (2005). *Nursing diagnosis handbook with NIC interventions and NOC outcomes* (8th ed.). Upper Saddle River, NJ: Prentice Hall Health.
Winters, A. C. (2004). Management of acute severe asthma. *Critical Care Nursing Clinics of North America, 16*(3), 285–291.
Yang, J. C. (2005). Prevention and treatment of deep vein thrombosis and pulmonary embolism in critically ill patients. *Critical Care Nursing Quarterly, 28*(1), 72–79.
Yang, P. S., & Chen, C. H. (2005). Exercise stage and processes of change in patients with chronic obstructive pulmonary disease. *Journal of Nursing Research, 13*(2), 97–104.

UNIT 11 BUILDING CLINICAL COMPETENCE
Responses to Altered Respiratory Function

FUNCTIONAL HEALTH PATTERN: Activity-Exercise

■ Think about clients with respiratory disorders and altered patterns of activity and exercise for whom you have cared in your clinical experiences.

- ■ What were the clients' major medical diagnoses affecting the respiratory system (e.g., upper respiratory infection, laryngeal cancer, pneumonia, tuberculosis, asthma, pleural effusion, pneumothorax, chronic obstructive pulmonary disease, respiratory failure)?
- ■ What manifestations did each of these clients have? Were these manifestations similar or different?
- ■ How did the clients' health status interfere with their activity and exercise? Was their breathing difficult or painful? Did the clients experience shortness of breath with activity or at rest? How many pillows did they use to sleep? Did your clients have a dry or productive cough? What color, odor, and consistency was the sputum? Did they smoke? Had they been exposed to environmental smoke or pollution? Did your clients have a history of respiratory disorders? Were they taking any medications or using oxygen? Had they had a chest x-ray and a tuberculosis skin test?

■ The Activity-Exercise Pattern describes the client's usual patterns of exercise and activity. Disorders that affect physiologic energy production affect the Activity-Exercise Health Pattern. The respiratory system provides oxygen to support cellular metabolism and eliminates carbon dioxide (a metabolic waste product) with each breath. This occurs through ventilation, the movement of air into and out of the lungs, and respiration, the exchange of oxygen and carbon dioxide between air and blood that occurs in the alveoli, respiratory bronchioles, and tissues.

The upper respiratory system cleans, humidifies, and warms air entering the lungs. Upper respiratory disorders affect breathing, communication, and body image.

Lower respiratory system disorders affect air movement (ventilation) and gas exchange across the alveolar-capillary membrane (respiration).

- ■ Rhinorrhea (antigen [a viral pathogen or allergen] ► inflammation and release of chemical mediators ► mucosal vasodilation and release of WBCs and fluid from capillaries ► mucosal edema and watery discharge from the nose)
- ■ Cough (irritants or excess secretions in respiratory tract ► stimulation of cough receptors in tracheobronchial wall ► impulses transmitted to medullary center ► rapid inhalation of large volume of air ► closure of glottis and rapid contraction of abdominal and expiratory muscles ► increased intrathoracic pressure ► sudden opening of glottis and explosive air expulsion)
- ■ Dyspnea (discrepancy between respiratory muscle strength, stretch; bronchial smooth muscle contraction; decreased lung compliance or inspiratory capacity ► stimulation of receptors in lungs, thorax, or cerebral cortex ► dyspnea, a subjective perception of difficulty breathing)
- ■ Cyanosis (decreased oxygen tension in alveoli ► decreased diffusion of oxygen into capillaries ► decreased blood oxygen tension ► increased amount of deoxygenated hemoglobin ► gray to blue or purple color of skin and mucous membranes)
- ■ Wheezing (bronchoconstriction, airway inflammation or obstruction ► turbulent airflow through narrowed airway ► high- or low-pitched musical breath sounds).

■ Priority nursing diagnoses within the Activity-Exercise Pattern that may be appropriate for clients with respiratory disorders include:

- ■ *Ineffective Breathing Pattern* as evidenced by shortness of breath, dyspnea, orthopnea, retractions, nasal flaring, altered chest excursion
- ■ *Ineffective Airway Clearance* as evidenced by ineffective cough, diminished or abnormal breath sounds, cyanosis, restlessness
- ■ *Impaired Gas Exchange* as evidenced by cyanosis, abnormal respiratory rate and rhythm, nasal flaring, tachycardia, diaphoresis, confusion
- ■ *Impaired Spontaneous Ventilation* as evidenced by dyspnea, use of accessory muscles, tachycardia, apprehension.

■ Two nursing diagnoses from other functional health patterns often are of high priority for the client with altered respiratory function:

- ■ *Disturbed Sleep Pattern* (Sleep-Rest)
- ■ *Anxiety* (Self-Perception-Self-Concept)

Directions: Read the clinical scenarios below and answer the questions that follow. To complete this exercise successfully, you will use not only knowledge of the content in this unit, but also principles related to setting priorities and maintaining client safety.

CLINICAL SCENARIO

You have been assigned to work with the following clients on a respiratory unit. Significant data obtained during report are as follows:

■ Jack Holt, a 65-year-old male, has bacterial pneumonia. Vital signs are T 101°F, P 94, R 30, BP 146/88. He is complaining of chest pain with breathing and has a productive cough of rusty-colored sputum. His SaO2 is 90% in room air.

■ Maggie Sawyer, an 82-year-old female, is being discharged today following treatment for a deep venous thrombosis. She has congestive obstructive pulmonary disease. Suddenly she complains of difficulty breathing, chest pain, coughing, restlessness, and a feeling that she is going to die.

■ James Mohr, a 25-year-old male, sustained head, neck, and chest injuries and has a tracheostomy from a motor vehicle crash. His vital signs were stable at the last assessment. He begins coughing and puts on his call light.

■ Amy Campbell, a 30-year-old female, is being treated after having a severe asthma attack. Her current vital signs are T 99°F, P 64, R 26, BP 124/84. She has inspiratory and expiratory wheezing. Her O2 sat reading is 94% on 4 L O2 via nasal cannula.

Questions

1 In what order would you visit these clients after report?
1. _____
2. _____
3. _____
4. _____

2 What top two priority nursing diagnoses would you choose for each of the clients presented above? Can you explain, if asked, the rationale for your choices?

	Priority Nursing Diagnosis #1	Priority Nursing Diagnosis #2
Jack Holt		
Maggie Sawyer		
James Mohr		
Amy Campbell		

3 The older adult is prone to respiratory problems due to which age-related changes in the respiratory system? (Select all that apply.)
1. loss of skeletal muscle strength in the thorax
2. increased elastic recoil of lungs during expiration
3. alveoli that are less elastic and more fibrotic
4. decreased residual volume of lung
5. decreased effectiveness of coughing

4 Bacterial pneumonia is spread by droplets. When using standard precautions, which equipment is necessary to prevent its spread?
1. Wear a gown when bathing the client.
2. Wear a gown and gloves when touching the client.
3. Wear a mask and gloves when suctioning the client.
4. Wear a cap to keep hair from touching the client.

5 For the client receiving percussion and vibration with postural drainage for left lower lobe pneumonia, which position most facilitates removal of secretions?
1. semi-Fowler's position with arms elevated
2. right Sims' position with head in Trendelenberg
3. high-Fowler's position leaning on a bedside tray
4. left Sims' position with head flat

6 On discharge, the nurse teaches Mrs. Sawyer ways to prevent pulmonary embolism. Which instruction is appropriate?
1. Use pillows under the knees when in bed.
2. Apply knee-high elastic stockings when ambulating.
3. Exercise the legs vigorously to encourage blood flow.
4. Stop every 1 to 2 hours to stretch legs when traveling.

7 Mr. Mohr will be discharged with a tracheostomy. What should the nurse teach the client about tracheostomies?
1. The tracheostomy will not interfere with lifting when returning to work.

2. Water skiing is allowed, but swimming in a pool or lake is not allowed.
3. Showering is allowed as long as the tracheostomy is covered with a washcloth.
4. A small amount of alcohol is allowed but smoking is not allowed.

8 Amy Campbell is instructed to take her asthma medications in which order?
1. atrovent, cromolyn, and albuterol
2. albuterol, atrovent, and cromolyn
3. cromolyn, atrovent, and albuterol
4. albuterol, cromolyn, and atrovent

9 When admitted to the emergency department, which laboratory studies would you expect to obtain on a client with an inhalation injury?
1. arterial blood gases, carboxyhemoglobin levels, electrolytes
2. sputum cultures and sensitivity, serology testing, sputum Gram stain
3. methemoglobin levels, venous blood gases, white blood cell count
4. complete blood cell count, oxygen saturation, sputum specimen

10 Arterial blood gases results are ordered on a client with acute respiratory distress. The results are: pH, 7.22; PaO_2, 50 mmHg; $PaCO_2$, 58 mmHg; HCO_3^-, 29 mEq/L. How would a nurse interpret these results?
1. respiratory acidosis
2. respiratory alkalosis
3. metabolic acidosis
4. metabolic alkalosis

11 Corticosteroids are ordered to decrease the inflammatory process of asthma. Which comment indicates the client understands how to take corticosteroids?
1. "Corticosteroids have very few side effects to worry about."
2. "I understand that I cannot stop taking the medication abruptly."
3. "I can stop taking the corticosteroids as soon as I feel better."
4. "I can take an over-the-counter medication if I develop a cold."

12 Which are early manifestations of pulmonary tuberculosis?
1. tachypnea, tachycardia, activity intolerance
2. bradypnea, foul-smelling sputum, weight gain
3. blood-tinged sputum, high-grade fever, fatigue
4. low-grade fever, night sweats, dry cough

CASE STUDY

Gladys Hamer is an 83-year-old female who is seen in the emergency department with complaints of shortness of breath and fever. Her vital signs are T 102.4°F, P 115 and irregular, R 35 and shallow, BP 168/66. Her height is 63″ and weight is 96 pounds. On assessment, her skin is very dry and warm. Her color is dusky. Scattered wheezes and rhonchi are heard throughout all lung fields. Her chest is hyperresonant to percussion. A pulse oximeter is applied and the O_2 sat reading is 88%. Mrs. Hamer has a past medical history of emphysema for 10 years, complaints of shortness of breath on exertion, and has a chronic cough productive of thick, grayish sputum. Her spouse passed away 5 years ago and she has lived with her two adult sons since then.

Blood is drawn for arterial blood gases and results are pH, 7.19; Pao_2, 54 mmHg, $Paco_2$, 55 mmHg; HCO_3^-, 30 mEq/L. These results indicate respiratory acidosis. Based on her current assessment, arterial blood gas results, and past medical history, a medical diagnosis of chronic obstructive pulmonary disease (COPD) is determined.

When planning nursing care for Mrs. Hamer, the nursing diagnosis of *Impaired Gas Exchange* related to acute and chronic lung disease is appropriate for implementing nursing interventions.

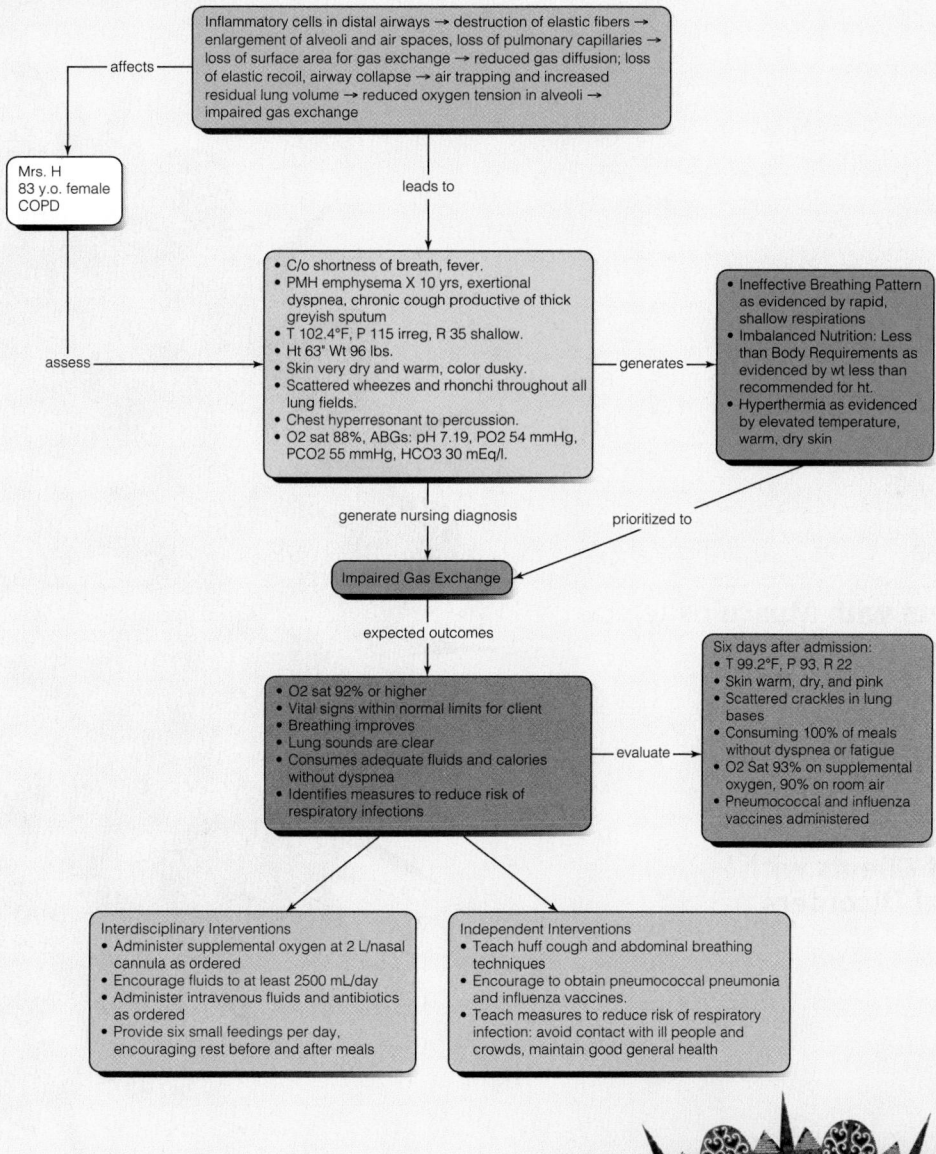

UNIT 12

Responses to Altered Musculoskeletal Function

CHAPTER 40 Assessing Clients with Musculoskeletal Disorders

LEARNING OUTCOMES

- Describe the anatomy, physiology, and functions of the musculoskeletal system.
- Explain the normal movements allowed by synovial joints.
- Identify specific topics for consideration during a health history interview of the client with health problems involving the musculoskeletal system.
- Describe normal variations in assessment findings for the older adult.
- Identify manifestations of impairment of the musculoskeletal system.

CLINICAL COMPETENCIES

- Conduct and document a health history for clients having or at risk for alterations in the musculoskeletal system.
- Conduct and document a physical assessment of musculoskeletal structures and functions.
- Monitor the results of diagnostic tests and report abnormal findings.

EQUIPMENT NEEDED

- Tape measure
- Goniometer

MEDIALINK

Resources for this chapter can be found on the Prentice Hall Nursing MediaLink DVD-ROM accompanying this textbook, and on the Companion Website at http://www.prenhall.com/lemone

The tissues and structures of the musculoskeletal system perform many functions, including support, protection, and movement. The musculoskeletal system has two subsystems: the bones and joints of the skeleton, and the skeletal muscles.

These subsystems work together to allow the body to perform both gross, simple movements such as closing a door, and fine, complex movements such as repairing a watch.

ANATOMY, PHYSIOLOGY, AND FUNCTIONS OF THE MUSCULOSKELETAL SYSTEM

The musculoskletal system is composed of bones of the skeletal system; ligaments, tendons, and muscles of the muscular system; and joints. The bones serve as the framework for the body and for the attachment of muscles, tendons, and ligaments. Innervated by the nervous system, contraction and relaxation of muscles permit movement at joints.

The Skeleton

Bones form the body's structure and provide support for soft tissues. They also protect vital organs from injury and serve to move body parts by providing points of attachment for muscles. Bones also store minerals and serve as a site for **hematopoiesis** (blood cell formation).

The human skeleton is made up of 206 bones (Figure 40–1 ■). Bones of the skeletal system are divided into the axial skeleton and the appendicular skeleton. The axial skeleton includes the bones of the skull, the ribs and sternum, and the vertebral column. The appendicular skeleton consists of all the bones of the limbs, the shoulder girdles, and the pelvic girdle.

Bone Structure

Bone cells include osteoblasts (cells that form bone), osteocytes (cells that maintain bone matrix), and osteoclasts (cells that resorb bone). Bone matrix is the extracellular element of bone tissue; it consists of collagen fibers, minerals (primarily calcium and phosphate), proteins, carbohydrates, and ground substance. Ground substance is a gelatinous material that facilitates diffusion of nutrients, wastes, and gases between the blood vessels and bone tissue. Bones are covered with periosteum, a double-layered connective tissue. The outer layer of the periosteum contains blood vessels and nerves; the inner layer is anchored to the bone.

Bones consist of a rigid connective tissue called osseous tissue, of which there are two types: Compact bone is smooth and dense; spongy bone contains spaces between meshworks of bone. Both types contain the same elements and are found in almost all bones of the body.

The basic structural unit of compact bone is the Haversian system (also called an osteon). The Haversian system consists of a central canal, called the Haversian canal; concentric layers of bone matrix, called lamellae; spaces between the lamellae, called lacunae; osteocytes within the lacunae; and small channels, called canaliculi (Figure 40–2 ■).

Spongy bone has no Haversian systems. Instead, the lamellae are arranged in concentric layers called trabeculae that branch and join to form meshworks. The spongy sections of long bones and flat bones contain tissue for hematopoiesis. In the adult, these sections, called red marrow cavities, are present in the spongy center of flat bones (especially the sternum) and in only two long bones: the humerus and the head of the femur. This red marrow is active in hematopoiesis in adults.

Bone Shapes

Bones are classified by shape (Figure 40–3 ■):

- *Long bones* are longer than they are wide. They have a midportion, or shaft, called a diaphysis and two broad ends, called epiphyses (Figure 40–4 ■). The diaphysis is compact bone and contains the marrow cavity, which is lined with endosteum. Each epiphysis is spongy bone covered by a thin layer of compact bone. Long bones include the bones of the arms, legs, fingers, and toes.
- *Short bones,* also called cuboid bones, are spongy bone covered by compact bone. They include the bones of the wrist and ankle.
- *Flat bones* are thin and flat, and most are curved. Their disklike structure consists of a layer of spongy bone between two thin layers of compact bone. Flat bones include most bones of the skull, the sternum, and the ribs.
- *Irregular bones* are of various shapes and sizes and, like flat bones, are plates of compact bone with spongy bone between. Irregular bones include the vertebrae, the scapulae, and the bones of the pelvic girdle.

Bone Remodeling in Adults

Although the bones of adults do not normally increase in length and size, constant remodeling of bones, as well as repair of damaged bone tissue, occurs throughout life. In the bone remodeling process, bone resorption and bone deposit occur at all periosteal and endosteal surfaces. Hormones and forces that

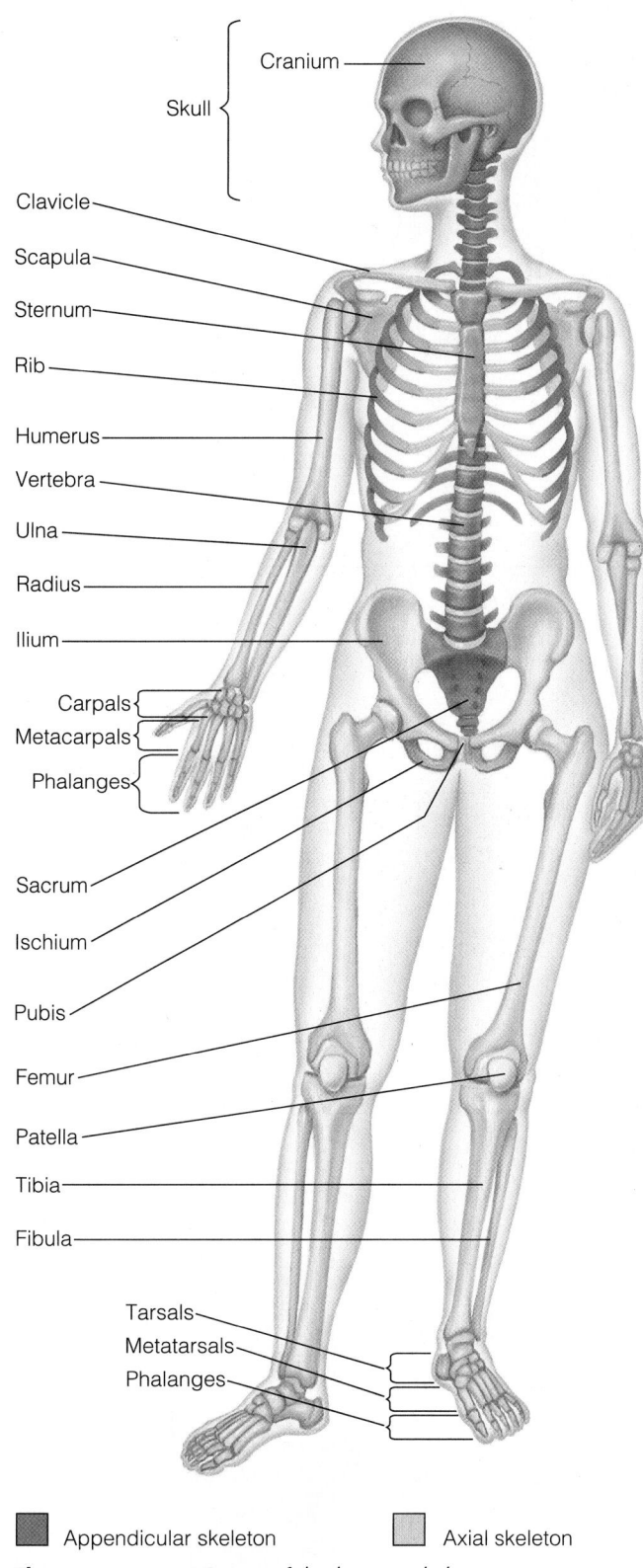

Cranium

Skull

Clavicle

Scapula

Sternum

Rib

Humerus

Vertebra

Ulna

Radius

Ilium

Carpals

Metacarpals

Phalanges

Sacrum

Ischium

Pubis

Femur

Patella

Tibia

Fibula

Tarsals

Metatarsals

Phalanges

▨ Appendicular skeleton   ▨ Axial skeleton

Figure 40–1 ■ Bones of the human skeleton.

put stress on the bones regulate this process, which involves a combined action of the osteocytes, osteoclasts, and osteoblasts. Bones that are in use, and are therefore subjected to stress, increase their osteoblastic activity to increase **ossification** (the development of bone). Bones that are inactive undergo increased osteoclast activity and bone resorption.

The hormonal stimulus for bone remodeling is controlled by a negative feedback mechanism that regulates blood calcium levels. This stimulus involves the interaction of parathyroid hormone (PTH) from the parathyroid glands and calcitonin from the thyroid gland. When blood levels of calcium decrease, PTH is released; PTH then stimulates osteoclast activity and bone resorption so that calcium is released from the bone matrix. As a result, blood levels of calcium rise, and the stimulus for PTH release ends. Rising blood calcium levels stimulate the secretion of calcitonin, inhibit bone resorption, and cause the deposit of calcium salts in the bone matrix. Thus, bones are necessary to regulate blood calcium levels. Calcium ions are necessary for the transmission of nerve impulses, the release of neurotransmitters, muscle contraction, blood clotting, glandular secretion, and cell division. Of the body's 1200 to 1400 g of calcium, over 99% is present as bone minerals.

Bone remodeling is also regulated by the response of bones to gravitational pull and to mechanical stress from the pull of muscles. Although the exact mechanism is not fully understood, it is known that bones that undergo increased stress are heavier and larger. This finding supports Wolff's law, which states that bone develops and remodels itself to resist the stresses placed on it.

The process of bone repair following a fracture is discussed in Chapter 41.

Muscles

The three types of muscle tissue in the body are skeletal muscle, smooth muscle, and cardiac muscle (Table 40–1). This discussion focuses on skeletal muscle, the only muscle that allows musculoskeletal function. Skeletal muscles attach to and cover the bones of the skeleton. Skeletal muscles promote body movement, help maintain posture, and produce body heat. They may be moved by conscious, voluntary control or by reflex activity. The body has approximately 600 skeletal muscles (Figure 40–5 ■).

Skeletal muscles are thick bundles of parallel multinucleated contractile cells called fibers. Each single muscle fiber is itself a bundle of smaller structures called myofibrils. The myofibrils have alternating light and dark bands that give skeletal muscle its striated (striped) appearance under an electron microscope. Myofibrils are strands of smaller repeating units called sarcomeres, which consist of thick filaments of myosin and thin filaments of actin, proteins that contribute to muscle contraction.

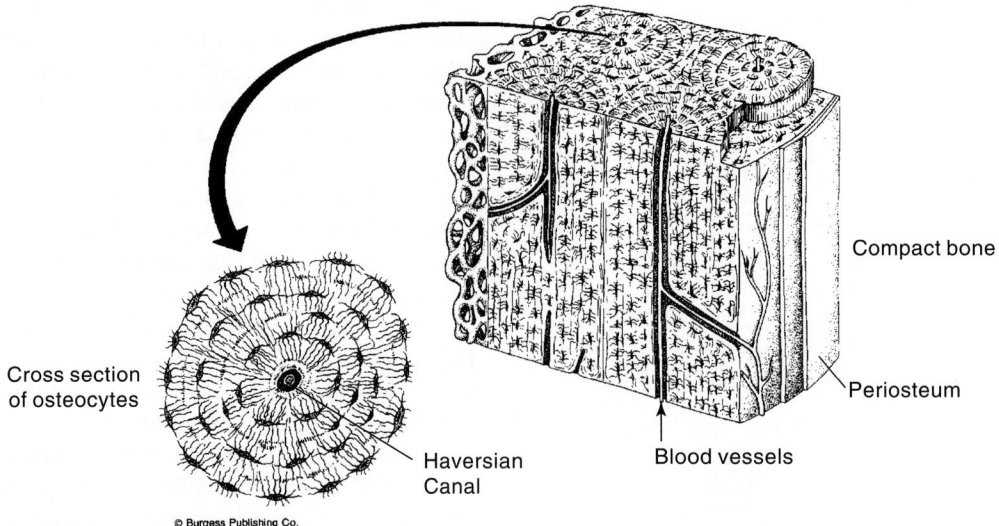

Cross section
of osteocytes

Haversian
Canal

Compact bone

Periosteum

Blood vessels

© Burgess Publishing Co.

Figure 40–2 ■ The microscopic structure (Haversian system) of compact bone.

Epiphysis

Diaphysis

Long bones
(e.g., humerus)

Short bones
(e.g., carpals)

Flat bones
(e.g., parietal bone)

Irregular bones
(e.g., vertebra)

Figure 40–3 ■ Classification of bones according to shape.

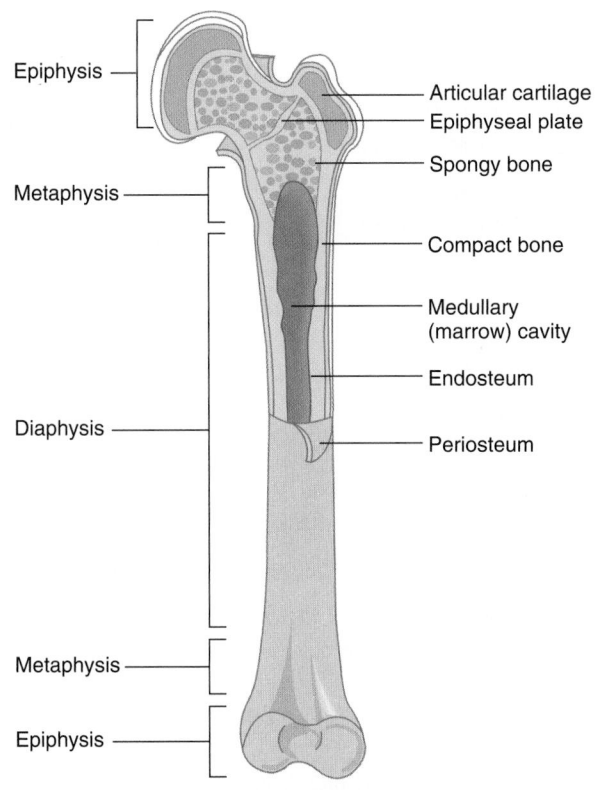

Epiphysis

Articular cartilage
Epiphyseal plate
Spongy bone

Metaphysis

Compact bone

Medullary
(marrow) cavity

Endosteum

Diaphysis

Periosteum

Metaphysis

Epiphysis

Figure 40–4 ■ Parts of a long bone.

Skeletal muscle cells have typical functional properties:

- *Excitability:* the ability to receive and respond to a stimulus. The stimulus is usually a neurotransmitter released by a neuron, and the response is the generation and transmission of an action potential along the plasma membrane of the muscle cell. (Chapter 41 ∞ discusses action potentials.)
- *Contractibility:* the ability to respond to a stimulus by forcibly shortening.
- *Extensibility:* the ability to respond to a stimulus by extending and relaxing; muscle fibers shorten when they contract and extend when they relax.
- *Elasticity:* the ability to resume its resting length after it has shortened or lengthened.

Skeletal muscle movement is triggered when motor neurons release acetylcholine, a neurotransmitter that crosses the neu-

romuscular junction and alters the permeability of the muscle fiber. Sodium ions enter the fiber, producing an action potential that causes muscle contraction. The more fibers that contract, the stronger the contraction of the entire muscle.

Prolonged strenuous activity causes continuous nerve impulses and eventually results in a buildup of lactic acid and reduced energy in the muscle, or muscle fatigue. However, continuous nerve impulses are also responsible for maintaining muscle tone. Lack of use results in muscle atrophy, whereas regular exercise increases the size and strength of muscles.

Joints, Ligaments, and Tendons

Joints, or articulations, are regions where two or more bones meet. Joints hold the bones of the skeleton together while allowing the body to move. Joints may be classified by function as synarthroses, amphiarthroses, or diarthroses. Table 40–2 describes each of these types. Joints are also classified by structure as fibrous, cartilaginous, or synovial.

Fibrous Joints

Fibrous joints permit little or no movement, because the articulating bones are joined either by short connective tissue fibers that bind the bones together, as with the sutures of the skull, or by short cords of fibrous tissue called ligaments, which permit slight give but no true movement.

Cartilaginous Joints

Some cartilaginous joints, such as the sternocostal joints of the rib cage, are composed of hyaline cartilage growths that fuse together the articulating bone ends. These joints are immobile. In other cartilaginous joints, such as the intervertebral disks, the hyaline cartilage fuses to an intervening plate of flexible fibrocartilage. This structural feature accounts for the flexibility of the vertebral column.

Synovial Joints

Bones in synovial joints are enclosed by a cavity that is filled with synovial fluid, a filtrate of blood plasma (Figure 40–6 ■). Synovial joints are freely movable, allowing many kinds of movements, as listed and described in Table 40–3. Synovial

TABLE 40–1 **Types of Body Muscle**

TYPE	DESCRIPTION	EXAMPLES
Skeletal	Striated, voluntary muscle (can consciously move)	Biceps, triceps, deltoid, gluteus maximus
Smooth	Nonstriated, involuntary muscle (cannot consciously move)	Muscles in the walls of the bladder, stomach, and bronchi
Cardiac	Striated, involuntary muscle	Heart muscle

TABLE 40–2 **Functional Classification of Joints**

TYPE	DESCRIPTION	EXAMPLES
Synarthrosis	Immovable joint	Skull sutures Epiphyseal plates Joint between first rib and manubrium of sternum
Amphiarthrosis	Slightly movable joint	Vertebral joints Joint of the public symphysis
Diarthrosis	Freely movable joint	Joints of the limbs Shoulder joints Hip joints

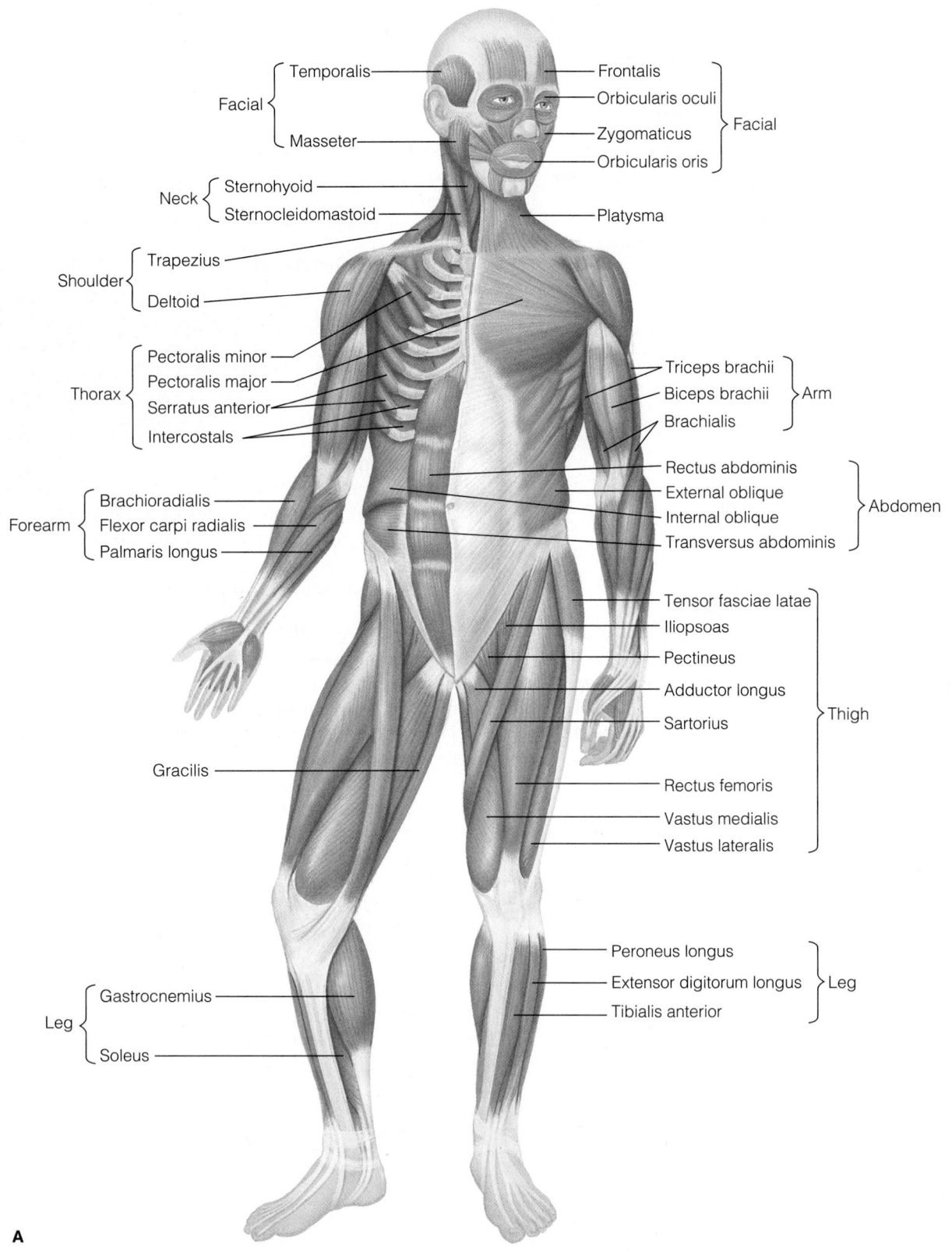

A

Figure 40–5 ■ *A,* Muscles of the anterior body. *B,* Muscles of the posterior body.

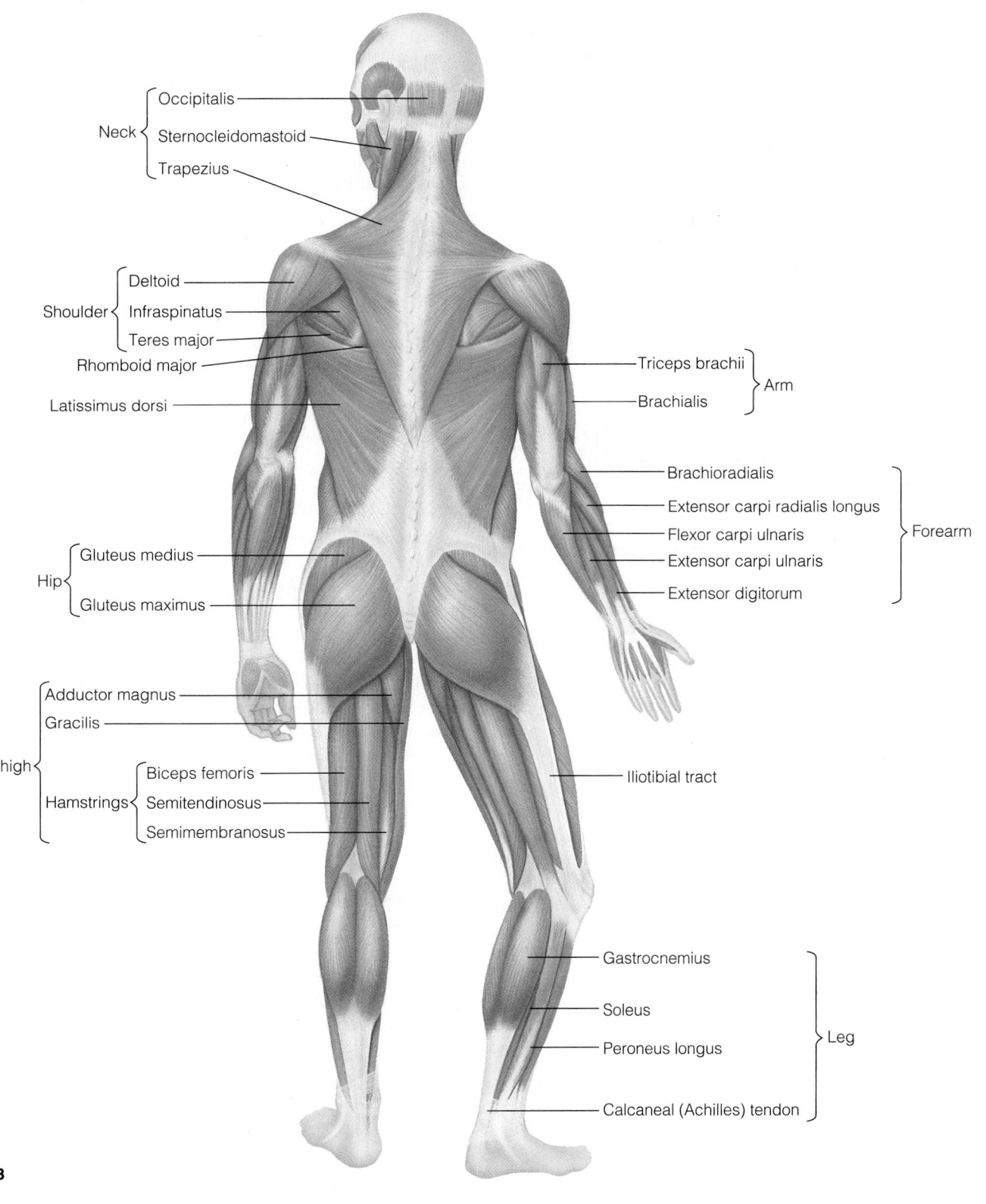

B

Figure 40–5 ■ Continued

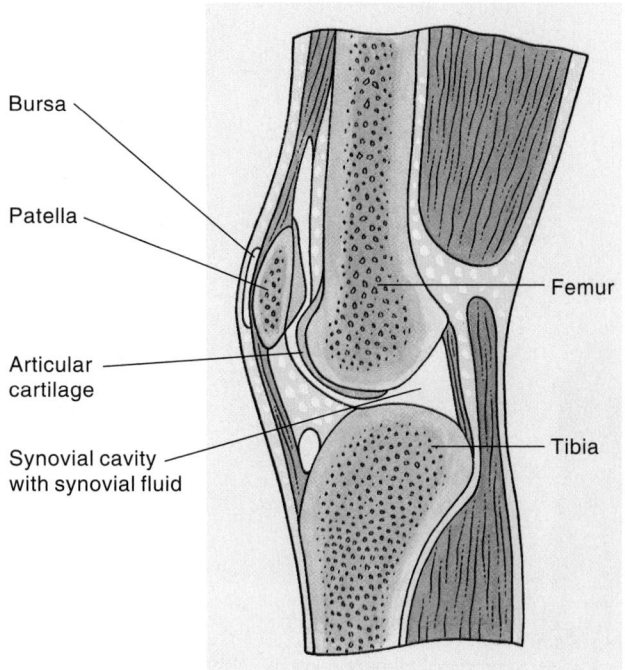

Figure 40–6 ■ Structure of a synovial joint (knee).

Labels: Bursa, Patella, Articular cartilage, Synovial cavity with synovial fluid, Femur, Tibia

joints are found at all articulations of the limbs. They have several characteristics:

- The articular surfaces are covered with articular cartilage.
- The joint cavity is enclosed by a tough, fibrous, double-layered articular capsule; internally, the cavity is lined with a synovial membrane that covers all surfaces not covered by the articular cartilage.
- Synovial fluid fills the free spaces of the joint capsule, enhancing the smooth movement of the articulating bones.

Bursae are small sacs of synovial fluid that cushion and protect bony areas that are at high risk for friction, such as the knee

TABLE 40–3 Movements Allowed by Synovial Joints

MOVEMENT	DESCRIPTION
Abduction	Move limb away from body midline
Adduction	Move limb toward body midline
Extension	Straighten limbs at joint
Flexion	Bend limbs at joint
Dorsiflexion	Bend ankle to bring top of foot toward shin
Plantar flexion	Straighten ankle to point toes down
Pronation	Turn forearm to place palm down
Supination	Turn forearm to place palm up
Eversion	Turn out
Inversion	Turn in
Circumduction	Move in circle
Internal rotation	Move inward on a central axis
External rotation	Move outward on a central axis
Protraction	Move forward and parallel to ground
Retraction	Move backward and parallel to ground

and the shoulder. Tendon sheaths are a form of bursae, but they are wrapped around tendons in high-friction areas.

The fibrous capsules that surround synovial joints are supported by ligaments, dense bands of connective tissue that connect bones to bones. Ligaments limit or enhance movement, provide joint stability, and enhance joint strength. Tendons are fibrous connective tissue bands that connect muscles to the periosteum of bones and enable the bones to move when skeletal muscles contract. When muscles contract, increased pressure causes the tendon to pull, push, or rotate the bone to which it is connected.

ASSESSING MUSCULOSKELETAL FUNCTION

Structures and functions of the musculoskeletal system are assessed by findings from diagnostic tests, a health assessment interview to collect subjective data, and a physical assessment to collect objective data. Sample documentation of an assessment of the musculoskeletal system is given in the accompanying box.

Diagnostic Tests

The results of diagnostic tests of musculoskeletal structure and function are used to support the diagnosis of a specific injury or disease, to provide information to identify or modify the appropriate medications or therapy used to treat the disease, and to help nurses monitor the client's responses to treatment and nursing care interventions. Diagnostic tests to assess the structures and functions of the musculoskeletal system are described in the table on the next page and summarized in the bulleted list that follows. More information is included in the discussion of specific injuries or diseases in Chapter 41 and 42 ∞.

- Blood tests are used to monitor levels of alkaline phosphatase, calcium, uric acid, and creatine kinase, commonly increased in bone and joint diseases and muscle trauma (Table 40–4).
- Radiologic examinations, including x-rays, CT scans, MRIs, and bone scans, are done to identify and evaluate bone density and structure in conditions such as arthritis, interverte-

---

SAMPLE DOCUMENTATION
Assessment of the Musculoskeletal System

58-year-old Hispanic male, employed as a roofer, comes to the orthopedic clinic for evaluation of chronic knee pain. Client states "The pain in my knees is worse when I get up in the morning and when I carry something heavy at work." Posture erect, gait even without obvious limp. Bones of lower extremities appear equal in size and shape bilaterally. No swelling noted, bulge test negative for fluid around knee. Crepitus heard in both knees during flexion and extension. ROM in both knees slightly decreased. No obvious decrease in muscle mass. Client states knee pain during ROM is a 3 on a 1 to 10 scale. Referred to clinic physician for further evaluation, including x-rays of both knees.

DIAGNOSTIC TESTS of the Musculoskeletal System

NAME OF TEST Blood chemistry

PURPOSE AND DESCRIPTION See Table 40–4

RELATED NURSING CARE No special preparation is needed.

NAME OF TEST X-ray

PURPOSE AND DESCRIPTION X-rays are done to identify and evaluate bone density and structure. Injection of contrast medium with an accompanying x-ray may be done to visualize joint structures, intervertebral disks, and wounds deep in muscle.

RELATED NURSING CARE No special preparation needed for standard x-rays. If contrast medium is used, assess for allergy to shellfish, iodine, or contrast medium used in previous tests. If allergy is present, test will not be performed.

NAME OF TEST Computed tomography (CT) scan

PURPOSE AND DESCRIPTION Provides a three-dimensional picture used to evaluate musculoskeletal trauma and bony abnormalities.

RELATED NURSING CARE No special preparation is needed.

NAME OF TEST Magnetic resonance imaging (MRI)

PURPOSE AND DESCRIPTION Used in diagnosis and evaluation of avascular necrosis, osteomyelitis, tumors, disk abnormalities, and tears in ligament or cartilage. Uses radio waves and magnetic fields; gadolinium may be injected to increase visualization of bony or muscular structures.

RELATED NURSING CARE Assess for metallic implants or metal on clothing (metallic implants, such as clips on aneurysms, pacemakers, or shrapnel, will prohibit having an MRI).

NAME OF TEST Bone scan

PURPOSE AND DESCRIPTION Degree of uptake of a radioisotope (based on blood supply to bone) is measured with a Geiger counter and recorded on paper. Uptake is increased in osteomyelitis, osteoporosis, cancers of the bone, and in some fractures. Uptake is decreased in avascular necrosis.

RELATED NURSING CARE No special preparation is needed; tell client to increase oral fluids after the test to aid in excretion of the radioisotope.

NAME OF TEST Bone density (BD)
- Dual energy x-ray absorptiometry (DEXA)
- Quantitative ultrasound (QUS)
- Bone mineral density (BMD)
- Bone absorptiometry

PURPOSE AND DESCRIPTION Bone density examinations are done to evaluate bone mineral density and to evaluate degree of osteoporosis. DEXA can calculate the size and thickness of bone. Osteoporosis is diagnosed if the peak bone mass level is below >2.5 standard deviations.

Normal Value: 1 standard deviation below peak bone mass.

RELATED NURSING CARE No special preparation is needed. Assess for previous fractures, which may increase bone density.

NAME OF TEST Arthroscopy

PURPOSE AND DESCRIPTION An endoscopic examination of the interior surfaces of a joint, used to perform surgery and diagnose diseases of the patella, meniscus, and synovial and extrasynovial membranes. In addition, fluid may be drained from the joint and tissue removed for biopsy. A fiber-optic endoscope is inserted into the joint, either with local anesthesia or general anesthesia.

RELATED NURSING CARE If general anesthesia is used, client is NPO after midnight. Following the procedure, assess for bleeding and swelling, apply ice to the area if prescribed, and teach client to avoid excessive use of the joint for 2 to 3 days.

NAME OF TEST Arthrocentesis

PURPOSE AND DESCRIPTION Done to obtain synovial fluid from a joint for diagnosis (such as infections) or to remove excess fluid. A needle is inserted through the joint capsule and fluid is aspirated.

RELATED NURSING CARE
No special preparation is needed. Apply compression dressing and assess for bleeding and leakage of fluid following the procedure.

(continued)

DIAGNOSTIC TESTS **of the Musculoskeletal System (continued)**

NAME OF TEST Electromyogram (EMG)

PURPOSE AND DESCRIPTION Measures the electrical activity of skeletal muscles at rest and during contraction; useful in diagnosing neuromuscular diseases. Needle electrodes are inserted into skeletal muscle (as on the legs) and electrical

activity can be heard, viewed on an oscilloscope, and recorded on graph paper. Normally, there is no electrical activity at rest.

RELATED NURSING CARE Tell client not to drink fluids containing caffeine or to smoke for 3 hours before the test, and not to take medications such as muscle relaxants, anticholinergics, or cholinergics.

NAME OF TEST Somatosensory evoked potential (SSEP)

PURPOSE AND DESCRIPTION Measures nerve conduction along pathways to evaluate evoked potential of muscle contractions. Used to identify dysfunction of lower motor

neurons as well as muscle disease. Transcutaneous or percutaneous electrodes are applied to the skin and provide recordings.

RELATED NURSING CARE No special preparation is needed.

---

bral disk disease, musculoskeletal trauma, muscle tears, osteomyelitis, and bone tumors.

- Bone density examinations (dual energy x-ray absorptiometry [DEXA], quantitative ultrasound [QUS], and bone mineral density [BMD]) are done to evaluate bone mineral density and evaluate the degree of osteoporosis.
- An arthroscopy uses a fiber-optic endoscope to examine the joint interior, to diagnose diseases, and to perform surgery. An arthrocentesis is done to withdraw fluid from a joint by needle aspiration.
- Both electromyogram (EMG) and somatosensory evoked potential (SSEP) are tests of the electrical activity of skeletal muscle.

Regardless of the type of diagnostic test, the nurse is responsible for explaining the procedure and any special preparation needed, for assessing for medication use that may affect the outcome of the tests, for supporting the client during the examination as necessary, for documenting the procedures as appropriate, and for monitoring the results of the tests.

Genetic Considerations

When conducting a health assessment interview and a physical assessment, it is important for the nurse to consider genetic influences on health of the adult. During the health assessment interview, ask about family members with health problems affecting musculoskeletal structure or function. In addition, ask about a family history of arthritis, abnormally long bones, children with muscular dystrophy, and amyotrophic lateral sclerosis (ALS). During the physical assessment, assess for any manifestations that might indicate a genetic disorder (see the box on the next page). If data are found to indicate genetic risk factors or alterations, ask about genetic testing and refer for appropriate genetic counseling and evaluation. Chapter 8 ∞ provides further information about genetics in medical-surgical nursing.

Health Assessment Interview

A health assessment interview to determine problems with musculoskeletal structure and/or function may be conducted

---

TABLE 40–4 Blood Tests with Purposes Specific to the Musculoskeletal System

NAME OF TEST	PURPOSE	NORMAL VALUE
Alkaline phosphatase (ALP)	To identify bone diseases. Increased in bone cancer, Paget's disease, healing fractures, rheumatoid arthritis, osteoporosis.	42–136 unit/L ALP[1] 20–130 unit/L ALP[2] (increases slightly with aging)
Calcium (Ca)	To monitor calcium levels and detect calcium imbalances. Decreased with lack of calcium and vitamin D intake, and malabsorption from the gastrointestinal tract. Increased in bone cancer and multiple fractures.	4.5–5.5 mEq/L or 9–11 mg/dL (serum)
Phosphorus (P), phosphate (PO_4)	To assess phosphorus levels. Increased with bone tumors and healing fractures.	1.7–2.6 mEq/L or 2.5–4.5 mg/dL
Rheumatoid factor (RF)	To diagnose rheumatoid arthritis (RA) (positive for RA at >1:80) Also increased in lupus erythematosus and scleroderma.	<1:20 titer
Uric acid	To diagnose and monitor the treatment of gout. Panic level considered >12 mg/dL.	Male: 3.5–8.0 mg/dL Female: 2.8–6.8 mg/dL
Human leukocyte antigen (HLA)	To diagnose diseases such as juvenile RA or ankylosing spondylitis.	Match or no match; no normal values
Creatine kinase (CK)	To diagnose muscle trauma or disease. Increased in muscular dystrophy and traumatic injuries (specifically, CPK-MM isoenzyme).	94%–100%

- Myotonic dystrophy is an inherited disorder in which the muscles become weak, have a decreased ability to relax, and eventually waste away. Other parts of the body affected are mental deficiency, hair loss, and cataracts. Although rare, the disease does increase in severity with each successive generation.
- Marfan's syndrome, an autosomal dominant disorder of connective tissue, affects the bones, lungs, eyes, heart, and blood vessels. It is characterized by abnormally long extremities, and is believed to have affected Abraham Lincoln. The aspect of the disease that is most life threatening is the effect on the cardiovascular system. The average life span of a person with Marfan's syndrome is 30 to 40 years (Porth, 2005).
- Ellis-van Creveld syndrome is a rare genetic disorder characterized by a variety of physical alterations, including short-limb dwarfism, additional fingers or toes, malformed wrists, cardiac abnormalities, and partial tooth eruption.
- Duchenne muscular dystrophy, an X-linked disorder, affects primarily males. It is one of the most common muscular dystrophies, and is characterized by rapid muscle degeneration early in life.
- Amyotropic lateral sclerosis (ALS) is a neurologic disease that affects the motor neurons in the spinal cord and brain, eventually resulting in paralysis and death.
- Other musculoskeletal diseases believed to have a genetic component include rheumatoid arthritis, osteoarthritis, gout, muscular dystrophy, ankylosing spondylitis, lupus erythematosus, and scleroderma.

during a health screening, may focus on a chief complaint (such as joint pain), or may be part of a total health assessment. Health problems affecting the neurologic system may manifest as problems with musculoskeletal function and an assessment of both systems may be necessary. (See Chapter 43 ∞ for assessment of the neurologic system.) If the client has problems with musculoskeletal structure or function, analyze its onset, characteristics, course, severity, precipitating and relieving factors, and any associated symptoms, noting the timing and circumstances. For example, ask the client:

- Describe the pain you have had in your elbow. Does the pain increase with movement? Have you noticed any redness or swelling?
- Did you injure your ankle before you began to experience difficulty walking?
- Is your pain worse in the morning, or does it get worse throughout the day?

The primary manifestations of altered function of the musculoskeletal system are pain and limited mobility. Specific descriptors of the pain, its location, and its nature are important. Other significant information includes associated manifestations, such as fever, fatigue, changes in weight, rash, and/or swelling. Also collect information about the client's lifestyle: type of employment, ability to carry out activities of daily living (ADLs) and provide self-care, exercise or participation in sports, use of alcohol or drugs, and nutrition. Explore past injuries and measures to self-treat pain (such as over-the-counter [OTC] medications, prescribed medications, application of heat or cold, splinting, wrapping, or rest).

Interview questions categorized by functional health patterns are listed in the Functional Health Pattern Interview table on page 1390.

Physical Assessment

Physical assessment of the musculoskeletal system may be performed either as part of a total assessment, or alone for a client with known or suspected problems. The techniques used to assess the musculoskeletal system are inspection, palpation, and measurement of muscle mass and range of motion (ROM). The client should be comfortably dressed in clothing that lets you see the movement of all joints clearly. The client may be standing, sitting, or lying down; the sequence of the examination should be such that the client does not have frequent position changes. An assessment of the older adult, the client in pain, or the client who is weak may take extra time. Normal age-related findings for the older adult are summarized in Table 40–5.

TABLE 40–5 Age-Related Changes in the Musculoskeletal System

AGE-RELATED CHANGE	SIGNIFICANCE
Bones and Joints: ■ ↓ bone mass and minerals. ■ ↓ calcium reabsorption, a slow resorption of the interior of long bones, and slower production of new bone on the outside surface of bones. ■ Vertebrae shorten and intervertebral disks thin, and kyphosis often occurs. ■ Cartilage on bone surfaces in joints deteriorates and bone spurs may occur.	Decreased bone mass as well as decreased calcium absorption contributes to bones that are often thinner and weaker, with an increased risk of fractures with trauma. As the spinal column shortens, height decreases. Loss of joint cartilage and formation of bone spurs makes movement more painful and may even limit mobility.
Muscles ■ Muscle fibers atrophy and fibrous tissue slowly replaces muscle tissue. ■ ↓ muscle mass and strength. ■ ↓ muscle movements, especially in the arms and legs. ■ Range of motion decreases. ■ Tendons shrink and harden. ■ Muscle cramping is common.	Regular exercise is very important in decreasing the loss associated with aging in terms of maintaining muscle mass, strength, and agility.

FUNCTIONAL HEALTH PATTERN INTERVIEW   Musculoskeletal System

Functional Health Pattern	Interview Questions and Leading Statements
Health Perception-Health Management	■ Have you ever had any muscle or bone diseases or injuries? If so, describe them. ■ Describe any surgery, physical therapy, heat, or other treatments you have received for problems with your muscles or bones. ■ List any medications, such as muscle relaxants or prescribed or over-the-counter (OTC) medications and ointments you use for musculoskeletal problems. ■ Do you take any herbal or nutritional supplements for musculoskeletal problems? If so, what and how often?
Nutritional-Metabolic	■ Describe your dietary intake in a typical 24-hour period. Does your diet include milk, cheese, cottage cheese, and vegetables? If so, how often? ■ Do you take vitamins and/or additional calcium supplements? If so, what type and how often? ■ Have you had a recent weight gain or loss? What do you see as your ideal weight? ■ Have you had any redness or swelling in your joints?
Elimination	■ Does your musculoskeletal problem make it difficult for you to get to the bathroom?
Activity-Exercise	■ Describe your usual activities for a 24-hour period. ■ Describe any musculoskeletal problems (such as weakness, stiffness, pain) that limit your activities of daily living (ADLs), such as driving, gardening, dressing, bathing, walking, climbing stairs, cooking, or cleaning. ■ Has there been a change in your usual ability to move around? Describe. ■ Do you regularly exercise, or take part in strenuous activities such as heavy lifting? Describe. If you have to lift heavy objects at work, do you use any type of special equipment? Describe. ■ Do you use any assistive devices (such as a cane or walker) to help move around?
Sleep-Rest	■ Does having this problem with your musculoskeletal system interfere with your ability to rest and sleep? If so, how and what do you do?
Cognitive-Perceptual	■ Describe any muscle, bone, or joint pain that you have. What relieves it or makes it worse? ■ Describe any changes in the color, temperature, or sensations in your extremities. ■ Describe any muscle weakness you are experiencing. ■ Do you have stiffness in your joints when you wake up? Does it get better with movement? ■ Do you ever have muscle cramps?
Self-Perception-Self-Concept	■ How does having this condition make you feel about yourself?
Role-Relationships	■ How has having this condition affected your relationships with others? ■ Has having this condition interfered with your ability to work? Explain. ■ Has anyone in your family had problems with bone, joint, or muscle disease? Explain.
Sexuality-Reproductive	■ Has this condition interfered with your usual sexual activity?
Coping-Stress-	■ Has having this condition created stress for you? ■ Have you experienced any kind of stress that makes the condition worse? Explain. ■ Describe what you do when you feel stressed.
Value-Belief	■ Describe how specific relationships or activities help you cope with this problem. ■ Describe specific cultural beliefs or practices that affect how you care for and feel about this problem. ■ Are there any specific treatments that you would not use to treat this problem?

Prior to the examination, collect all equipment and explain the techniques to decrease the client's anxiety. The sequence for a musculoskeletal examination follows:

1. Begin the examination with an assessment of gait and posture. Observe how the client walks, sits, and/or moves about in bed.
2. Inspect and palpate the bones for any obvious deformity or changes in size or shape. Palpation also will elicit tenderness or pain.
3. Measure the extremities for length and circumference. Before taking measurements, make sure the client is lying in a comfortable position. Remember to compare limbs bilaterally.
4. Assess muscle mass by first inspecting for obvious increase or decrease in size. Assess and document muscle strength on a scale of 0 to 5 (Table 40–6). Box 40–1 provides instructions for testing the strength of various muscles.

BOX 40–1 Guidelines for Assessing Muscle Strength

In adults, muscles are usually strong and equally strong bilaterally. However, neuromuscular diseases, disuse, metabolic disorders, or infections can cause muscle weakness. Muscle strength is expected to be greater in the dominant arm and leg. In most instances (and especially when moving digits and extremities), the nurse provides resistance by pushing in the opposite direction.

The muscles listed below are routinely tested. Instructions for clients are also provided.

MUSCLE	CLIENT INSTRUCTIONS
Ocular muscles and lids	Close eyes tightly.
Finger muscles	Shake hands.
	Make a fist.
	Spread fingers.
Facial muscles	Blow out cheeks.
	Stick out tongue.
Hip muscles	Raise straight leg while supine.
Neck muscles	Bend head forward and backward.
Gluteal and leg muscles	Alternately cross legs while sitting.
Deltoid muscles	Hold arms up.
Biceps muscle	Bend the arm.
Quadriceps muscle	Straighten leg.
Triceps muscle	Straighten the arm.
Wrist muscles	Bend hand forward and backward.
Ankle and foot muscles	Bend foot up and down.

TABLE 40–6 Muscle Grading Scale

GRADING SCALE	ASSESSMENT DESCRIPTION
0	(No visible) contraction; paralysis
1	Can feel contraction of muscle but there is no movement of limb
2	Passive ROM
3	Full ROM against gravity
4	Full ROM against some resistance
5	Full ROM against full resistance

Figure 40–7 ■ Using a goniometer to measure joint ROM.

5. Assess joints for swelling, pain, redness, warmth, crepitus, and ROM. Only assess the ROM of every joint if the client has a specific musculoskeletal problem; however, assessing one or more joints is a common part of nursing care. Use a goniometer for precise measurements of joint ROM (Figure 40–7 ■).

This device has a pointer joined to a protractor at 0 degrees. These two arms are placed along articulating bones, and the angle of joint movement is recorded in degrees.

MUSCULOSKELETAL ASSESSMENTS

Technique/Normal Findings	Abnormal Findings

Gait and Body Posture Assessment

Inspect body posture and gait. *Body posture should be upright, gait should be smooth and steady.*

- Joint stiffness, pain, deformities, and muscle weakness can cause changes in gait and posture.

Inspect the spine for curvature. Ask the client to stand and bend back slowly as far as possible, bend slowly to the right and then to the left as far as possible, turn slowly to the right and left in a circular motion, and bend forward slowly and try to touch fingers to toes. *When viewed from the back, the cervical and lumbar spine are concave, the thoracic spine is convex, and the spine is straight.*

- With herniated lumbar disks, the lumbar curve flattens and spinal mobility is decreased.
- An increased lumbar curve, called **lordosis**, may be seen in obesity or pregnancy.
- A lateral, S-shaped curvature of the spine is called **scoliosis**. Functional scoliosis usually is a compensatory response to painful paravertebral muscles, herniated disks, or discrepancy in leg length. It disappears with forward flexion. Structural scoliosis is often congenital and tends to appear during adolescence. It is accentuated with forward bending. These disorders are discussed and illustrated in Chapter 42.
- **Kyphosis** is an exaggerated thoracic curvature of the spine common in older adults.

Technique/Normal Findings	Abnormal Findings

Joint Assessment

Inspect the joints for deformity, swelling, and redness. *There should be no visible deformity, swelling, or redness of joints.*

- Diseases of the joints may be manifested by such deformities as tissue loss, tissue overgrowth, contractures, or irreversible shortenings of muscles and tendons.
- Edema in a joint may cause obvious bulging.
- Redness, swelling, and pain are evidence of an inflammation or infection in the joint.

Palpate the joints for tenderness, warmth, crepitation, consistency, and muscle mass. *Joints should be nontender and consistent bilaterally, and without visible or palpable excess warmth, crepitation, or masses.*

- Inflammation and injury cause joint pain.
- Arthritis, bursitis, tendonitis, and osteomyelitis (infection of a bone) result in painful, hot joints.
- **Crepitation** (a grating sound) is present in a joint when the articulating surfaces have lost their cartilage, such as in arthritis.

Range-of-Motion Assessment

Assess joint ROM by asking the client to perform activities specific to each joint, as follows: *All bilateral joints should move through full range of motion.* *Temporomandibular joint:* **"Open your mouth wide, and then close your mouth." (As the client opens and closes the mouth, palpate the temporomandibular joints with your index and middle fingers, as shown in Figure 40–8 ■.)**

- Clicking or popping noises, decreased ROM, pain, and swelling may indicate temporomandibular joint syndrome or, in rare cases, osteoarthritis.

Figure 40–8 ■ Palpating the temporomandibular joints.

Cervical spine:
45-degree flexion: "Touch your chin to your chest."
55-degree extension: "Look at the ceiling."
40-degree lateral bending: "Try to touch your right ear to your right shoulder." Repeat with the left side.
70-degree rotation: "Try to touch your chin to each shoulder."

- Neck pain and limited extension with lateral bending are seen with herniated cervical disks and in cervical spondylosis.
- An immobile neck with head and neck thrust forward is seen with ankylosing spondylitis.

Lumbar spine:
75- to 90-degree flexion: "Touch your toes with your fingers" (Figure 40–9A ■).
30-degree extension: "Bend backward slowly."
35-degree lateral bending: "Bend right and left" (Figure 40–9B).
30-degree rotation: "Twist your shoulders right and left" (Figure 40–9C).

- Decreased movement or pain with movement may indicate an abnormal spinal curvature, arthritis, herniated disk, or spasm of paravertebral muscles.

Figure 40–9 ■ *A,* Forward flexion of spine. *B,* Lateral flexion of spine. *C,* Rotation of spine.

Technique/Normal Findings	Abnormal Findings
Fingers: Flexion: "Make a fist." Extension: "Open your hand." Abduction: "Spread your fingers." Adduction: "Close your fingers."	■ Flexion and extension of fingers are decreased in arthritis. ■ Heberden's nodes and Bouchard's nodes are hard, nontender nodules on the dorsolateral parts of the distal and proximal interphalangeal joints, respectively. They are common in osteoarthritis. ■ Stiff, painful, swollen finger joints are seen in acute rheumatoid arthritis. ■ Boutonnière and swan-neck deformities are seen in chronic rheumatoid arthritis. ■ Swollen finger joints with a white chalky discharge may be seen in chronic gout.
Wrists: 90-degree flexion: "Bend wrist down." 70-degree extension: "Bend wrist up." 55-degree ulnar deviation: "Bend wrist toward little finger." 20-degree radial deviation: "Bend wrist toward thumb."	■ Bilateral chronic swelling in the wrist is seen in arthritis.
Elbows 160-degree flexion: "Touch your hands to your shoulders." 180-degree extension: "Straighten your elbows." 90-degree supination: "Bend your elbows 90 degrees, and turn hands palm up." 90-degree pronation: "Bend your elbows 90 degrees, and turn fists down."	■ Swollen, tender, inflamed elbows are apparent in gouty arthritis and rheumatoid arthritis. ■ Pain and tenderness at the lateral epicondyle occur in tennis elbow.

Technique/Normal Findings	Abnormal Findings
Shoulders: 180-degree flexion: "Hold your arms straight up and out." 50-degree hyperextension: "Put your straight arm behind your back." 90-degree internal rotation: "Put your forearm behind your lower back." 180-degree abduction: "Raise your straight arm up and out to your side." 50-degree adduction: "Put your straight arm across your chest."	▪ Pain and tenderness over the biceps tendon occurs with **tendonitis** (inflammation of a tendon). ▪ The arm cannot be abducted fully when the supraspinatus tendon of the shoulder is ruptured. ▪ Pain and limited abduction is also seen with **bursitis** (inflammation of a bursa) and calcium deposits in this area.
Toes: 90-degree flexion: "Walk on your toes."	▪ The great toe is excessively abducted in hallux valgus. ▪ The joint above the great toe is swollen, inflamed, and painful in gouty arthritis. ▪ There is hyperextension of the metatarsophalangeal joint and flexion of the proximal interphalangeal joint with hammer toes.
Ankles: 20-degree dorsiflexion: "Point your foot to the ceiling." 45-degree plantar flexion: "Point your foot to the floor." 30-degree inversion: "Walk on the outside of your feet." 20-degree eversion: "Walk on the inside of your feet."	▪ Contractures of the Achilles tendon may occur in clients with rheumatoid arthritis or following prolonged bed rest.
Knees: 130-degree flexion: "Do a deep knee bend." 180-degree extension: "Sit down and hold your legs straight out in front of you."	▪ Swelling over the suprapatellar pouch is seen with inflammation and fluid in the articular capsule of the knee. **Synovitis** is inflammation of the synovial membrane lining the articular capsule of a joint. It is common with knee trauma. ▪ Swelling over the patella is seen in bursitis.
Hips: (The client is lying down.) 120-degree flexion: "Bring bent knee up to your chest." 30-degree hyperextension: "Lie on the abdomen, and lift up one leg at a time." 45-degree abduction: "Hold your leg straight, and move it out to the side." 40-degree internal rotation: "Bend your knee, and swing it toward your other leg." 45-degree external rotation: "Bend your knee, and swing it out to the side."	▪ Movement of the hip is limited and/or painful in arthritis.

Technique/Normal Findings	Abnormal Findings

Special Assessments

Perform Phalen's test. Ask the client to hold the wrist in acute flexion for 60 seconds (Figure 40–10 ■). *There should be no tingling, numbness, or pain.*

- Numbness and burning in the fingers during Phalen's test may indicate carpal tunnel syndrome.

Figure 40–10 ■ Phalen's test.

Check for small amounts of fluid on the knee by conducting the bulge test. Milk upward on the medial side of the knee, and then tap the lateral side of the patella (Figure 40–11 ■). *No bulge of fluid should appear on the medial side of the knee.*

- A fluid bulge indicates increased fluid in the knee joint rather than soft tissue swelling.

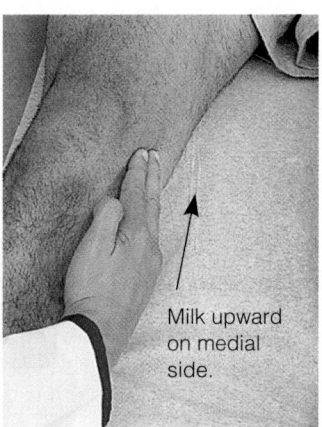

Milk upward on medial side.

Press lateral side.

Look here for swelling.

Figure 40–11 ■ Checking for the bulge sign.

Check for larger amounts of fluid by conducting the ballottement test, to detect large amounts of fluid in the knee. Apply downward pressure on the knee with one hand while pushing the patella backward against the femur with the other hand (Figure 40–12 ■). *There should be no movement of the patella. The patella should rest firmly over the femur.*

- Increased fluid will cause a tapping sound as the patella displaces the fluid and hits the femur.

Tap the patella; if it rebounds against your fingers, fluid is present.

Press here to milk fluid behind patella.

Figure 40–12 ■ Checking for ballottement.

Technique/Normal Findings	Abnormal Findings

Perform McMurray's test. While reclining, ask the client to turn the flexed knee toward the center of the body. Stabilize the knee with one hand, and apply pressure on the lower leg with the other hand (Figure 40–13 ■). *There should be no pain or clicking.*

- Pain, locking (inability to fully extend the knee), or a popping sound may indicate an injury to a meniscus, a disk of cartilaginous tissue in the knee.

Figure 40–13 ■ McMurray's test.

Perform the Thomas test. Ask the client to lie down and extend one leg while bringing the knee of the opposite leg to the chest (Figure 40–14 ■). *The extended leg should not rise off the table.*

- A hip flexion contracture will cause the extended leg to rise off the table.

Figure 40–14 ■ Thomas test for hip contracture.

EXPLORE MEDIALINK

Prentice Hall Nursing MediaLink DVD-ROM
Audio Glossary
NCLEX–RN® Review

Animation
Joint Movement

COMPANION WEBSITE www.prenhall.com/lemone
Audio Glossary
NCLEX-RN® Review
Care Plan Activity: Musculoskeletal Disorders
Case Study: Knee Pain
MediaLink Application: Musculoskeletal Injuries of
  Health Care Providers
Links to Resources

TEST YOURSELF NCLEX-RN® REVIEW

1 Your client has an epiphyseal fracture. Based on this information, what classification of bone is involved?
   1. irregular
   2. flat
   3. long
   4. short

2 When asking a client to move an extremity away from the body midline, you are assessing:
   1. abduction.
   2. adduction.
   3. extension.
   4. flexion.

3 Your client asks you, "Why is blood being examined for uric acid?" What would be your most accurate response?
   1. "A uric acid test is done to see if your gout medication is effective."
   2. "A uric acid test is done to diagnose rheumatoid arthritis."
   3. "Do you have a family history of muscle or bone disease?"
   4. "Tell me how you got that big bruise on your hip."

4 What age woman would be most likely to have a bone density examination?
   1. teenager
   2. a woman in her 20s
   3. a woman in her 40s
   4. a woman in her 60s

5 With aging, bone mass and calcium absorption decrease. What risk is increased as a result?
   1. obesity
   2. weakness
   3. fractures
   4. deformity

6 What would you ask the client to do in order to assess facial muscle strength?
   1. "Close your eyes tightly."
   2. "Stick out your tongue."
   3. "Bend your head forward."
   4. "Open your eyes widely."

7 What term is used to document a grating sound when a joint is moved?
   1. crackles
   2. arthritis
   3. synovitis
   4. crepitation

8 While conducting the ballottement test, you note the patella rebounds against your fingers. What does this finding indicate?
   1. deformity of the elbow
   2. infection of the metatarsals
   3. fluid in the knee joint
   4. crepitus in the hip joint

9 During the physical assessment of a young adult, you note a lateral, S-shaped curve of the spine. What is the name of this condition?
   1. lordosis
   2. scoliosis
   3. kyphosis
   4. musclosis

10 What are the most common manifestations of musculoskeletal disorders?
   1. pain and limited mobility
   2. swelling and exaggerated reflexes
   3. cyanosis and decreased pulses
   4. pallor and decreased ROM

See Test Yourself answers in Appendix C.

BIBLIOGRAPHY

Abdelhafiz, A., Lowles, R., Alam, N., Adebajo, A., & Philp, I. (2003). Clinical assessment of symptomatic osteoarthritis in older people. *Age and Aging, 32*(3), 359–360.

Amella, E. (2004). Presentation of illness in older adults: If you think you know what you're looking for, think again. *American Journal of Nursing, 104*(10), 40–52.

Asrani, C. (2003). Assessment of a patient with joint pain. *National Journal of Homeopathy, 5*(4), 245–246.

Assessment of a limb in a cast. (2003). *Nursing Times, 99*(31), 27.

Bickley, L., & Szilagyi, P. (2005). *Bates' guide to physical examination and history taking* (9th ed.). Philadelphia: Lippincott.

Burrow, J., & McLarnon, N. (2004). Foot assessment: Recognizing potential problems. *Nursing & Residential Care, 6*(2), 68–71.

Cole, E. (2004). Assessment and management of the trauma patient. *Nursing Standard, 18*(41), 45–52, 54.

Della-Giustina, D., & Nolan, R. (2004). Evaluation and management of low back pain. *Emergency Medicine, 36*(7), 20–26, 27–28.

Eliopoulos, E. (2005). *Gerontological nursing* (6th ed.). Philadelphia: Lippincott Williams & Wilkins.

Fredericson, M., & Wun, C. (2003). Differential diagnosis of leg pain in the athlete. *Journal of the American Podiatric Medical Association, 93*(4), 321–324.

Jarvis, C. (2004). *Physical examination & health assessment.* St. Louis, MO: Mosby.

Kasper, C., Talbot, L., & Gaines, J. (2002). Skeletal muscle damage and recovery. *AACN Clinical Issues: Advanced Practice in Acute and Critical Care, 13*(2), 237–247.

Kee, J. (2005). *Prentice Hall handbook of laboratory & diagnostic tests with nursing implications.* Upper Saddle River, NJ: Prentice Hall.

Leclercq, C. (2003). General assessment of the upper limb. *Hand Clinics, 19*(4), 557–564.

McConnell, E. (2002). Clinical do's & don'ts. Assessing neurovascular status in a casted limb. *Nursing, 32*(9), 20.

National Institutes of Health. (2003). *Genes and disease. Muscle and bone diseases.* Retrieved from http://www.ncbi.nlm.nih.gov/books/bv.fcgi?rid=gnd.section.59

Porth, C. (2005). *Pathophysiology: Concepts of altered health states* (7th ed.). Philadelphia: Lippincott.

Schultz, J. (2004). Clinical evaluation of the shoulder. *Physical Medicine and Rehabilitation Clinics of North America, 15*(2), 351–371.

Watson, R. (2001). Assessing the musculoskeletal system in older people. *Nursing Older People, 13*(5), 29–30.

Weber, J., & Kelley, J. (2006). *Health assessment in nursing* (3rd ed.). Philadelphia: Lippincott.

CHAPTER 41 Nursing Care of Clients with Musculoskeletal Trauma

LEARNING OUTCOMES

- Compare and contrast the causes, risk factors, pathophysiology, manifestations, interdisciplinary care, and nursing care of contusions, strains, sprains, joint dislocations, and fractures.

- Describe the stages of bone healing.

- Explain the pathophysiology, manifestations, and related treatment for complications of bone fractures: compartment syndrome, fat embolism syndrome, deep venous thrombosis, infection, delayed union and nonunion, and reflex sympathetic dystrophy.

- Discuss the purposes and related nursing interventions for casts, traction, and stump care.

- Explain the causes, levels, types, and potential complications (infection, delayed healing, chronic stump pain, phantom pain, and contractures) of an amputation.

- Describe the pathophysiology, interdisciplinary care, and nursing care for repetitive use injuries: carpal tunnel syndrome, bursitis, and epicondylitis.

CLINICAL COMPETENCIES

- Assess functional health status of clients with musculoskeletal injuries, and monitor, document, and report abnormal manifestations.

- Use evidence-based research to plan and implement nursing care for clients with skeletal pin sites.

- Determine priority nursing diagnoses, based on assessed data, to select and implement individualized nursing interventions for clients with musculoskeletal injuries.

- Provide skilled cast care, traction care, and stump care.

- Integrate interdisciplinary care into care of clients with musculoskeletal trauma.

- Provide teaching appropriate for prevention and self-care of traumatic injuries of the musculoskeletal system.

- Revise plan of care as needed to provide effective interventions to promote, maintain, or restore functional health status to clients with traumatic injuries of the musculoskeletal system.

MEDIALINK

Resources for this chapter can be found on the Prentice Hall Nursing MediaLink DVD-ROM accompanying this textbook, and on the Companion Website at http://www.prenhall.com/lemone

Musculoskeletal trauma is an injury to muscle, bone, or soft tissue that results from excessive external force. The external force transmits more kinetic energy than the tissue can absorb, and injury results. The severity of the trauma depends not only on the amount of force but also on the location of the impact, because different parts of the body can withstand different amounts of force. A wide variety of external forces can cause trauma, and the force involved can vary in severity (e.g., a step off the curb, a fall, being tackled in a football game, and a motor vehicle crash). See Chapter 11 ∞ for a detailed discussion of the results of different forces and types of injury from trauma.

Traumatic musculoskeletal injuries include blunt tissue trauma, alterations in tendons and ligaments, and fractures of bones. Various forces that cause musculoskeletal trauma are typical for a specific environment, activity, or age group. For example, motorcycle crashes resulting in fractures of the distal tibia, midshaft femur, and radius are common in young men.

Sports injuries, resulting from either overuse or acute trauma, are seen more often in adolescents and young adults. Falls are the most common cause of injury in people age 65 or older, with fractures of the vertebrae, proximal humerus, and hip seen most often (Porth, 2005). Regardless of the cause, the injury may require rehabilitation and temporary or permanent changes in lifestyle.

Musculoskeletal trauma can result in mild or severe injuries. A client may experience a soft tissue injury, a fracture, and/or a complete amputation. In addition, trauma to one part of the musculoskeletal system often produces dysfunction in adjacent structures. For example, a fracture of the femur prevents the adjacent muscles from abducting and adducting. Nursing care helps minimize the effects of trauma, prevents complications, and hastens restoration of function. This chapter discusses fractures, amputations, soft tissue injuries, dislocations, and repetitive use injuries.

TRAUMATIC INJURIES OF THE MUSCLES, LIGAMENTS, AND JOINTS

THE CLIENT WITH A CONTUSION, STRAIN, OR SPRAIN

Contusions, strains, and sprains are among the most commonly reported injuries. They account for about 50% of work-related injuries, with lower back injuries being the most commonly reported occupational injury. However, many sprains and strains are not work related and often are not reported. The lower back and cervical region of the spine are the most common sites for muscle strains; the ankle is the most commonly sprained joint, usually caused by forced inversion of the foot.

Pathophysiology and Manifestations

A **contusion,** the least serious form of musculoskeletal injury, is bleeding into soft tissue that results from a blunt force, such as a kick or striking a body part against a hard object. The skin remains intact, but small blood vessels rupture and bleed into soft tissues. A contusion with a large amount of bleeding is referred to as a hematoma. The manifestations of a contusion include swelling and discoloration of the skin. The blood in the soft tissue initially results in a purple and blue color commonly referred to as a *bruise*. As the blood begins to reabsorb, the area involved becomes brown and then yellow until it disappears.

A **strain** is a stretching injury to a muscle or a muscle-tendon unit caused by mechanical overloading. A muscle that is forced to extend past its elasticity will become strained. Lifting heavy objects without bending the knees, or

a sudden acceleration-deceleration, as in a motor vehicle crash, can cause strains. The most common sites for a muscle strain are the lower back and cervical regions of the spine. The manifestations of a strain include pain, limited motion, muscle spasms, swelling, and possible muscle weakness. Severe strains that partially or completely tear the muscle or tendon are painful and disabling.

A **sprain** is a stretch and/or tear of one or more ligaments surrounding a joint. Forces going in opposite directions cause the ligament to overstretch and/or tear. The ligaments may be partially or completely torn. Although any joint may be involved, sprains of the ankle and knee are most common, with more than 25,000 people spraining an ankle each day in the United States (National Institute of Arthritis and Musculoskeletal and Skin Diseases [NIAMS], 2004). Manifestations include loss of the ability to move or use the joint, a feeling of a "pop" or tear, discoloration, pain, and rapid swelling. Motion increases the joint pain. The intensity of the manifestations depends on the severity of the sprain. A comparison of sprains and strains is presented in Box 41–1.

INTERDISCIPLINARY CARE

The goal of the initial stage of treating soft tissue trauma is to reduce swelling and pain. Clients should follow a regimen of rest, ice, compression, and elevation (RICE) for the first 24 to 48 hours (see Table 41–1 for RICE therapy). Severe sprains may require

---

BOX 41–1 Comparison of Sprains and Strains

Sprain
- Defined as an injury to a ligament that results from a twisting motion.
- Can cause joint instability.
- Pain, edema, and swelling are present.
- Motion increases the joint pain.

Strain
- Defined as a microscopic tear in the muscle.
- Sharp or dull pain is present.
- Pain increases with isometric contraction of the muscle.
- Swelling and local tenderness are present.

---

surgical repair. Ankle sprains may be immobilized with an air cast, with no limitations on weight bearing. A knee injury often requires a knee immobilizer. If an upper extremity is injured, a sling is provided. Physical therapy may be recommended for rehabilitation. Time required for healing depends on the severity of the injury; for example, a mild ankle sprain may require up to 3 to 6 weeks of rehabilitation, whereas a severe sprain may require up to 8 to 12 months to return to full activities (NIAMS, 2004).

When soft tissue trauma is suspected, x-rays are taken to rule out soft tissue injury, and magnetic resonance imaging (MRI) may be done if further assessment is necessary. Medications used to treat soft tissue trauma include nonsteroidal anti-inflammatory drugs (NSAIDs) and analgesics.

NURSING CARE

The nursing care of each client is individualized. A strain or sprain may not be as devastating to an attorney as it is to a professional athlete; therefore, the nurse should determine what the injury means to the particular client.

Nursing Diagnoses and Interventions

Nursing diagnoses focus on providing information about self-care to decrease pain and return physical mobility to preinjury levels.

Acute Pain

The pain that results from soft tissue trauma is due primarily to the injury to the muscle or ligament and secondarily to bleeding and edema at the injury site.

- Teach the client to use RICE (rest, ice, compression, elevation) therapy to care for the injury. *The interventions included in RICE therapy allow the injured muscle, ligament or tendon to heal (rest), cause vasoconstriction and reduce pain (ice), decrease edema formation and pain (compression), and promote venous return to decrease edema and pain (elevation).*

Impaired Physical Mobility

Pain causes the client to avoid using or bearing weight with the injured extremity. Always observe the client's use of assistive devices; if the device is inappropriate, the client can face a greater risk of falling. Also consider that the device may be appropriate, but the client may not be using it correctly or safely. As a person ages, muscle mass in the upper extremities declines. As a result, the older client with a sprained ankle may not be able to use crutches, because crutches require that the person distribute body weight along the upper extremities. Older clients may therefore find a walker more useful.

- Teach the correct use of crutches, walkers, canes, or slings if prescribed. *Use of the correct technique increases safety and encourages use of these devices.*
- Encourage follow-up care. *Severe sprains may require further evaluation to determine if surgical intervention is indicated.*

THE CLIENT WITH A JOINT DISLOCATION

A **dislocation** is an injury of a joint in which the ends of bones are forced from their normal position. Dislocations usually follow trauma such as a fall or blow, with the bone ends displaced or separated from their normal position in the joint capsule. They commonly are seen in people who take part in contact sports such as football or from falls during activities such as skiing. Although dislocations may occur in any joint, they occur most frequently in the shoulder and acromioclavicular joints. Dislocations may

---

TABLE 41–1 RICE Therapy for Musculoskeletal Injuries

ACTION	CLIENT AND FAMILY EDUCATION
Rest	■ Decrease regular activities of daily living and exercise as needed. ■ If advised by your healthcare provider, do not put weight on the injured area for 48 hours. ■ Crutches may help if you can't put weight on an ankle or knee. ■ If you use a cane or crutch for an ankle injury, use it on the uninjured side so you can lean away from and relieve weight on the injured ankle.
Ice	■ Apply an ice pack to the injured area for 20 minutes at a time, four to eight times a day. ■ An ice bag, cold pack, plastic bag filled with ice, or a bag of frozen peas may be used. ■ Do not apply the ice pack for longer than 20 minutes to avoid cold injury and frostbite.
Compression	■ Compression often helps reduce swelling. The kind you use will depend on the recommendation of your healthcare provider. ■ Examples of compression bandages include Ace wraps, special boots, air casts, and splints.
Elevation	■ Keep the injured extremity elevated on a pillow above heart level, to help reduce swelling and pain.

also result from a disease such as rheumatoid arthritis. A **subluxation** is a partial dislocation in which the bone ends are still partially in contact with each other.

Pathophysiology

Dislocations may be congenital, traumatic, or pathologic. Congenital dislocations are present at birth and are seen in the hip and knee. Traumatic dislocations result from falls, blows, or rotational injuries. Pathologic dislocations result from disease of the joint, including infection, rheumatoid arthritis, paralysis, and neuromuscular diseases.

Manifestations

The manifestations of a dislocation include pain, deformity, and limited motion.

INTERDISCIPLINARY CARE

Care of the client with a dislocation focuses on relieving pain, correcting the dislocation, and preventing complications. The dislocation is diagnosed by physical examination and x-rays. The joint is most often reduced (bone ends realigned) by means of manual traction.

Treatment of a shoulder joint dislocation depends on the severity of the dislocation. Immobilization is no longer recommended, and only the most severe dislocations are surgically reduced. A dislocated hip requires immediate reduction in the emergency room to prevent necrosis of the femoral head and injury to the sciatic and femoral nerves. After reduction, the client is placed on bed rest. In some cases, traction is needed for several weeks. If a hip dislocation is accompanied by a fracture, the client will undergo surgery to increase mobility, decrease complications, and rapidly stabilize the joint.

NURSING CARE

Nursing care of the client with a dislocation or subluxation is individualized to the cause of injury, the type of dislocation, and the age of the client. It is important to teach clients to seek im-

mediate medical attention, to splint the joint to prevent further damage, and to put ice on the injured joint (Mayo Clinic, 2006).

Nursing Diagnoses and Interventions

Nursing diagnoses focus on relieving pain and preventing complications.

Risk for Injury

The client with a dislocation requires frequent assessments to ensure that neurovascular compromise does not develop.

- Monitor neurovascular status by assessing the 5 "P's": pain, pulses, pallor, paralysis, and paresthesia. *Neurovascular compromise is indicated by increased pain, decreased or absent pulses, pale skin, inability to move a body part or extremity, and changes in sensation (such as "pins and needles" sensations, or loss of sense of sharp/dull touch).*
- Maintain immobilization after reduction. *Immobilization prevents the joint from dislocating again.*

Community-Based Care

Joint dislocations often tend to be recurring injuries for clients actively participating in contact sports and other vigorous physical activities. Prolonged immobilization (for several weeks after the injury) and aggressive rehabilitation following the initial dislocation can reduce the risk of recurrent dislocation. The following topics should be addressed in preparing the client for community-based care:

- Importance of complying with the prescribed length of immobilization
- Skin care and ways to prevent skin-to-skin contact, particularly in the axillary area
- Prescribed rehabilitation exercises that will strengthen muscles and other supportive structures in the shoulder, decreasing the risk of future dislocations
- Alternatives to activities that precipitate recurrent dislocations
- Instructions or referrals to physical therapy if needed for further teaching about using assistive devices
- Referrals to physical and occupational therapy and home health services as needed.

TRAUMATIC INJURIES OF BONES

THE CLIENT WITH A FRACTURE

A **fracture** is any break in the continuity of a bone. Fractures vary in severity according to the location and the type of fracture. Although fractures occur in all age groups, they are more common in people who have sustained trauma and in older clients.

Pathophysiology

Any of the 206 bones in the body can be fractured. A fracture occurs when the bone is subjected to more kinetic energy than it can absorb. Fractures may result from a direct blow, a crushing force (compression), a sudden twisting motion (torsion), a severe muscle contraction, or disease that has weakened the bone (called a *stress* or *pathologic fracture*). Two basic mechanisms produce

fractures: direct force and indirect force. With direct force, the kinetic energy is applied at or near the site of the fracture. The bone cannot withstand the force. With indirect force, the kinetic energy is transmitted from the point of impact to a site where the bone is weaker. The fracture occurs at the weaker point.

Fractures in adults are classified in the following ways:

- If the skin is intact, the fracture is considered a *closed (simple) fracture.* If the skin integrity is interrupted, the fracture is considered an *open (compound) fracture* (Figure 41–1 ■). An open fracture allows bacteria to enter the injured area and increases the risk of complications.
- The fracture line may be *oblique* (at an angle to the bone) or *spiral* (curves around the bone). An *avulsed* fracture occurs when the fracture pulls bone and other tissues away from the point of

Figure 41–1 ■ *A,* An open fracture. *B,* A closed fracture.

attachment. It may also be described as *comminuted* (the bone breaks in many pieces), *compressed* (the bone is crushed), *impacted* (the broken bone ends are forced into each other), or *depressed* (the broken bone is forced inward) (Figure 41–2 ■).

■ *Complete* fractures involve the entire width of the bone, whereas *incomplete* fractures involve only a part of the width of the bone.

■ A *stable* (nondisplaced) fracture is one in which the bones maintain their anatomic alignment. An *unstable* (displaced) fracture occurs when the bones move out of correct anatomic alignment. If a fracture is displaced, immediate interventions are required to prevent further damage to soft tissue, muscle, and bone.

Fractures may also be classified by point of reference on the bone, such as midshaft, middle third, and distal third. The point of reference may also be specific, such as intra-articular or diaphyseal.

Fracture Healing

Regardless of classification or type, fracture healing progresses over three phases: the inflammatory phase, the reparative phase,

and the remodeling phase. (See *Pathophysiology Illustrated* on pages 1404–1405). The bleeding and inflammation that develop at the site of the fracture initiate the inflammatory phase. A hematoma forms between the fractured bone ends and around the bone surfaces. The osteocytes at the bone ends die as the hematoma clots, obstructing blood flow and depriving them of oxygen and nutrients. Necrosis of the cells heightens the inflammatory response, which in turn leads to vasodilation and edema. In addition, fibroblasts, lymphocytes, macrophages, and even osteoblasts from the bone migrate to the fracture site. Fibro-blasts form a fibrin meshwork and promote the growth of granulation tissue and capillary buds. The lymphocytes and macrophages wall off the area, localizing and containing the inflammation. The capillary buds invade the fracture site and supply a source of nutrients to promote the formation of collagen. The collagen allows calcium to be deposited.

Once calcium is deposited, a callus begins to form. In this reparative phase, osteoblasts promote the formation of new bone, and osteoclasts destroy dead bone and assist in the synthesis of new bone. Collagen formation and calcium deposition continue. During the remodeling phase, excess callus is removed and new bone is laid down along the fracture line. Eventually, the fracture site is calcified, and the bone is reunited.

The age, physical condition of the client, and the type of fracture sustained influence the healing of fractures. Other factors influence bone healing either positively or negatively and may be grouped according to their local or systemic influence (Box 41–2). Healing time varies with the individual. An uncomplicated fracture of the arm or foot can heal in 6 to 8 weeks. A fractured vertebra will take at least 12 weeks to heal. Healing of a fractured hip may take from 12 to 16 weeks.

Manifestations

Fractures are often accompanied by soft tissue injuries that involve muscles, arteries, veins, nerves, or skin. The degree of soft tissue involvement depends on the amount of energy or

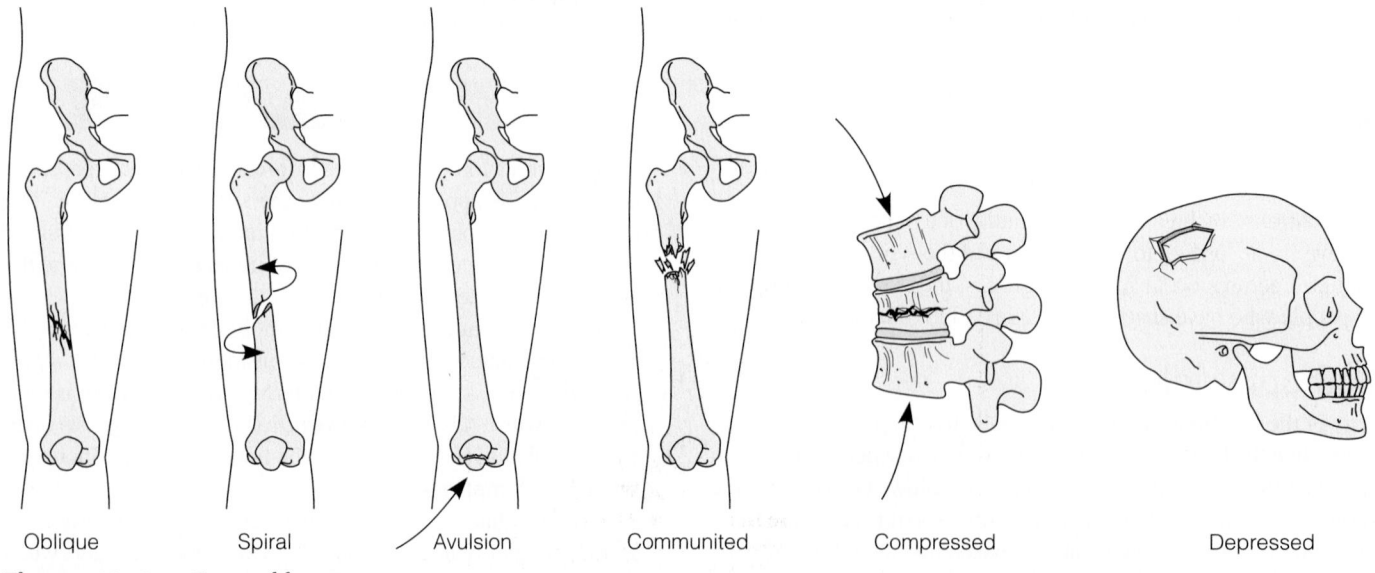

| Oblique | Spiral | Avulsion | Communited | Compressed | Depressed |

Figure 41–2 ■ Types of fractures.

BOX 41–2 Factors Influencing Bone Healing

Positive Factors

Local
- Immobilization
- Timely correction of displacement
- Application of ice
- Electrical stimulation

Systemic
- Adequate amounts of growth hormone, vitamin D, and calcium
- Adequate blood supply
- Absence of infection or diseases
- Younger age
- Moderate activity level prior to injury

Negative Factors

Local
- Delay in correction of displacement
- Open fracture (increases risk of infection)
- Presence of foreign body at fracture site

Systemic
- Immunocompromised status
- Decreased circulation (as in diabetes or peripheral vascular disease)
- Malnutrition
- Osteoporosis
- Advanced age

MANIFESTATIONS of Fracture

MANIFESTATION	CAUSE
Deformity	Abnormal position of bones secondary to fracture and muscles pulling on fractured bone
Swelling	Edema from localization of serous fluid and bleeding
Pain/tenderness	Muscle spasm, direct tissue trauma, nerve pressure, movement of fractured bone
Numbness	Nerve damage or nerve entrapment
Guarding	Pain
Crepitus	Grating of bones or entrance of air in an open fracture. *Note:* Do not manipulate the extremity to elicit crepitus; doing so may cause additional damage.
Hypovolemic shock	Blood loss or associated injuries
Muscle spasms	Muscle contraction near the fracture
Ecchymosis	Extravasation of blood into the subcutaneous tissue

force transmitted to the area. Fracture manifestations and their causes are outlined in the Manifestations box on this page.

Complications

Complications of musculoskeletal trauma are associated with pressure from edema and hemorrhage, development of fat emboli, deep venous thrombosis, infection, loss of skeletal integrity, or involvement of nerve fibers. Bone fragments may also result in further injury or complications.

Compartment Syndrome

A compartment is a space enclosed by a fibrous membrane or fascia. The fascia lines the compartment within the limbs and is nonexpandable. Compartments within the limbs may enclose and support bones, nerves, and blood vessels. **Compartment syndrome** occurs when excess pressure in a limited space constricts the structures within a compartment, reducing circulation to muscles and nerves. Acute compartment syndrome may result from hemorrhage and edema within the compartment following a fracture or from a crush injury, or from external compression of the limb by a cast that is too tight. Increased pressure within the confined space of the compartment results in entrapment of nerves, blood vessels, and muscles.

Entrapment of the blood vessels limits tissue perfusion, beginning a cycle of events that may result in the loss of the limb. Inadequate oxygen supply causes cellular acidosis, which intensifies as cellular energy requirements are met

through anaerobic metabolism. The capillaries inside the compartment dilate in an attempt to increase the supply of blood and oxygen. Additional blood and oxygen are not available, and plasma proteins leak out into the interstitial tissues. The interstitial tissue then pulls fluid in to balance the protein load. As a result, edema within the compartment increases. The edema causes further compression of the vascular network, and the cycle continues. Uninterrupted, this cycle threatens the client's limb and increases the risk of sepsis. Compartment syndrome usually develops within the first 48 hours of injury, when edema is at its peak. Manifestations of compartment syndrome are listed in the box below. It is important to note that arterial pulses may remain normal, even when pressure within the compartment is high enough to significantly impair tissue perfusion.

MANIFESTATIONS of Compartment Syndrome

EARLY MANIFESTATIONS
- Pain
- Normal or decreased peripheral pulse

LATER MANIFESTATIONS
- Cyanosis
- Tingling, loss of sensation (paresthesias)
- Weakness (paresis)
- Severe pain, especially when the extremity is passively flexed
- Eventual renal failure (due to release of myoglobin into the bloodstream; myoglobin molecule is too large for effective filtration and excretion by kidney, and renal failure results)

Bone Healing

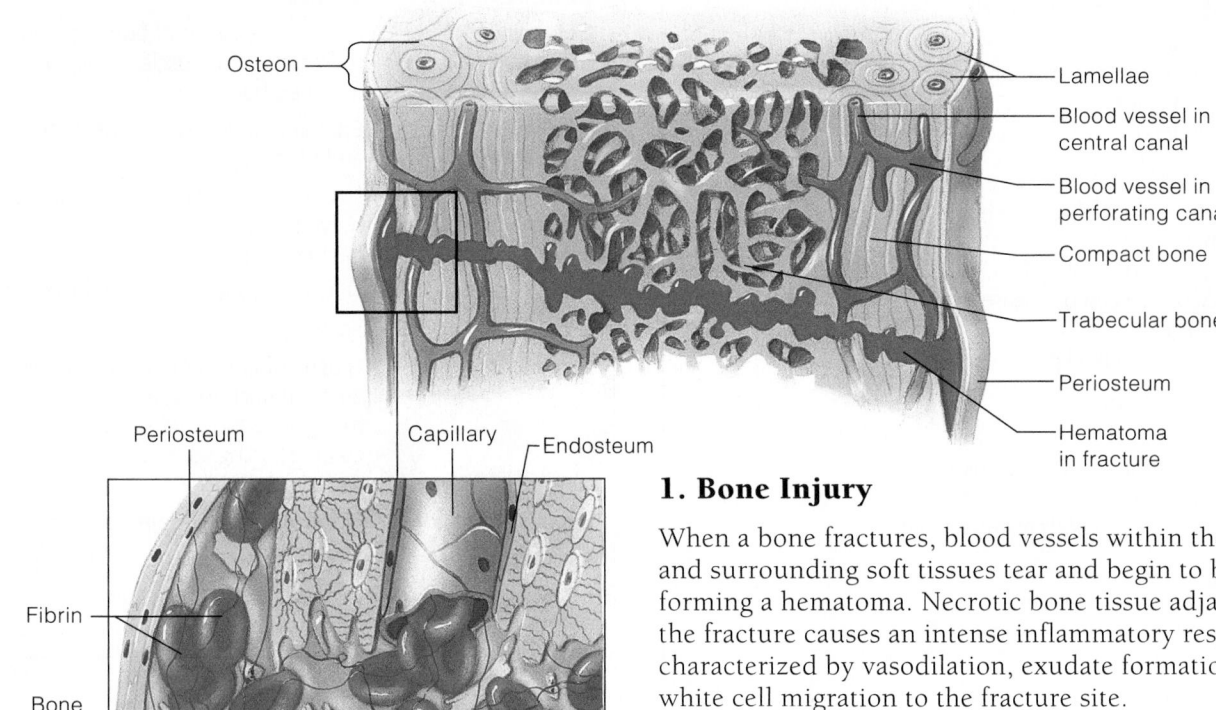

Osteon — Lamellae
Blood vessel in central canal
Blood vessel in perforating canal
Compact bone
Trabecular bone
Periosteum
Hematoma in fracture

Periosteum — Capillary — Endosteum
Fibrin
Bone fragment
Osteocyte

1. Bone Injury

When a bone fractures, blood vessels within the bone and surrounding soft tissues tear and begin to bleed, forming a hematoma. Necrotic bone tissue adjacent to the fracture causes an intense inflammatory response characterized by vasodilation, exudate formation, and white cell migration to the fracture site.

2. Fibrocartilaginous Callus Formation

Clotting factors within the hematoma form a fibrin meshwork. Within 48 hours, fibroblasts and new capillaries growing into the fracture form granulation tissue that gradually replaces the hematoma. Phagocytes begin to remove cell debris.

Osteoblasts, bone-forming cells, proliferate and migrate into the fracture site, forming a fibrocartilaginous callus. The osteoblasts build a web of collagen fibers from both sides of the fracture site that eventually unites to connect bone fragments, thus splinting the bone. Chondroblasts lay down patches of cartilage that provide a base for bone growth.

Phagocyte
Osteoblast
Fibroblast
Collagen
Chondroblast
Cartilage

4. Bone Remodeling

Osteoblasts continue to form new woven bone, which is in turn organized into the lamellar structures of compact bone. Osteoclasts resorb excess callus as it is replaced by mature bone.

As the bone heals and is subjected to the mechanical stress of everyday use, osteoblasts and osteoclasts respond by remodeling the repair site along the lines of force. This ensures that the repaired section of bone eventually resembles the structure of the uninjured part.

Osteoclast   New compact bone

3. Bony Callus Formation

Osteoblasts continue to proliferate and synthesize collagen fibers and bone matrix, which are gradually mineralized with calcium and mineral salts to form a spongy mass of woven bone. The trabeculae of woven bone bridge the fracture. Osteoclasts migrate to the repair site and begin removing excess bone in the callus. Bony callus formation usually continues for 2 to 3 months.

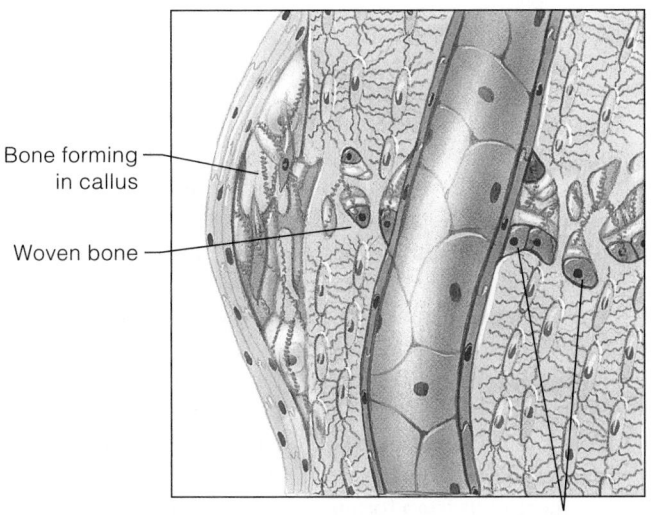

Bone forming in callus

Woven bone

Osteoblasts

MediaLink · Bone Healing Animation

If compartment syndrome develops, interventions to alleviate pressure will be implemented; these may include removal of a tightly fitting cast. If the pressure is internal, a *fasciotomy,* a surgical intervention in which muscle fascia is cut to relieve pressure within the compartment, may be necessary. After a fasciotomy, the incision is left open, and passive ROM exercises are performed on the extremity.

Volkmann's contracture, a common complication of elbow fractures, can result from unresolved compartment syndrome. Arterial blood flow decreases, leading to ischemia, degeneration, and contracture of the muscle. Arm mobility is impaired, and the client is unable to completely extend the arm.

Fat Embolism Syndrome

Fat emboli occur when fat globules lodge in the pulmonary vascular bed or peripheral circulation. **Fat embolism syndrome (FES)** is characterized by neurologic dysfunction, pulmonary insufficiency, and a petechial rash on the chest, axilla, and upper arms. Long bone fractures and other major trauma are the principal risk factors for fat emboli; hip replacement surgery also poses a risk for FES.

When a bone is fractured, pressure within the bone marrow rises and exceeds capillary pressure; as a result, fat globules leave the bone marrow and enter the bloodstream. Another contributing factor may be the stress-induced release of catecholamine, which causes the rapid mobilization of fatty acids. Once the fat globules are released, they combine with platelets and travel to the brain, lungs, kidneys, and other organs, occluding small blood vessels and causing tissue ischemia.

Manifestations usually develop within a few hours to a week after injury. The manifestations result from the occlusion of the blood supply and the presence of fatty acids. Altered cerebral blood flow causes confusion and changes in level of consciousness. Pulmonary circulation may be disrupted, and free fatty acids damage the alveolar-capillary membrane. Pulmonary edema, impaired surfactant production, and atelectasis can result in significant respiratory insufficiency and manifestations of acute respiratory distress syndrome (see Chapter 39 ∞). Fat droplets activate the clotting cascade, causing thrombocytopenia. Petechiae (pin-sized purplish areas from bleeding under the skin) appearing on the skin, buccal membranes, and conjunctival sacs are thought to result from either microvascular clotting or the accompanying thrombocytopenia.

Early stabilization of long bone fractures is preventive for FES. Prompt identification and treatment of the syndrome are necessary to maintain adequate pulmonary function. In severe cases, the client may require intubation and mechanical ventilation to prevent hypoxemia. Fluid balance is closely monitored. Corticosteroids may be administered to decrease the inflammatory response of lung tissues, stabilize lipid membranes, and reduce bronchospasm (Porth, 2005).

Deep Venous Thrombosis

A *deep venous thrombosis (DVT)* is a blood clot that forms along the intimal lining of a large vein. Three precursors linked to DVT formation are (1) venous stasis, or decreased blood flow; (2) injury to blood vessel walls; and (3) altered blood coagulation (Table 41–2). Any or all of these precursors can cause a DVT to

TABLE 41–2 Precursors of Deep Venous Thrombosis

PRECURSOR	IMPLICATIONS FOR FRACTURES
Decreased blood flow	Common in fracture clients, who are immobilized and less active. Bed rest alone can decrease venous flow by 50%.
Injury to blood vessel wall	May occur as a direct result of the force that caused the fracture or from surgical manipulation.
Altered blood coagulation	May result from active blood loss. The body's attempt to maintain homeostasis leads to increased production of platelets and clotting factor.

form. Damage to the lining of the vein causes the platelets to aggregate or clump together, forming the thrombus. Fibrin, white blood cells (WBCs), and red blood cells (RBCs) begin to cling to the thrombus, and a tail forms. This tail or the entire thrombus may dislodge and move to the brain, lungs, or heart. Five percent of DVTs dislodge and enter the pulmonary circulation to form a pulmonary embolus. If the thrombus remains in the vein, venous insufficiency may result from scarring and valve damage.

If a DVT is present, there may be swelling, leg pain, tenderness, or cramping. Not all clients experience manifestations, however. For this reason, diagnostic tests, such as a venogram or Doppler ultrasound of lower extremities, may be required. A venogram requires intravenous administration of dye in the radiology department, whereas a Doppler ultrasound study is noninvasive and can be performed at the client's bedside. Doppler ultrasonography uses sound waves to form an image on a computer screen.

The best treatment for DVT is prevention. Early immobilization of the fracture and early ambulation of the client are imperative. The extremity should be elevated above the level of the heart. Frequent assessments of the injured extremity may lead to early recognition of DVT and prevent the formation of pulmonary embolus. Prophylactic anticoagulant administration is beneficial. Antiembolism stockings and compression boots increase venous return and prevent stasis of blood. Constrictive clothing should be avoided.

The diagnosis of DVT requires rapid intervention. The client is placed on bed rest for 5 to 7 days to prevent dislodgment of the clot. Fibrinolytic agents, which dissolve the clot, may be administered. Heparin may be administered intravenously to prevent more clots from forming. A vena cava filter may be placed to prevent the existing clot from entering the pulmonary circulation and forming a pulmonary embolus. In extreme cases in which anticoagulation therapy is contraindicated, a thrombectomy (surgical removal of the clot) may be necessary. See Chapter 35 ∞ for further discussion of DVT.

Infection

Infection is more likely to occur in an open fracture than a closed fracture, but any complication that decreases blood supply increases the risk of infection. Infection may result from contamination at the time of injury or during surgery.

Pseudomonas, Staphylococcus, or *Clostridium* organisms may invade the wound or bone. *Clostridium* infection is particularly serious because it may lead to severe gas gangrene and cellulitis, but any infection may delay healing and result in osteomyelitis, infection within the bone that can lead to tissue death and necrosis. (See Chapter 42 ∞ for a discussion of osteomyelitis.)

Delayed Union and Nonunion

Delayed union is the prolonged healing of bones beyond the usual time period. Many factors may inhibit bone healing, including poor nutrition, inadequate immobilization, prolonged reduction time, infection, necrosis, age, immunosuppression, and severe bone trauma resulting in multiple fragments. Delayed union is diagnosed by means of serial x-ray studies. It is important to note that x-ray findings may lag 1 to 2 weeks behind the healing process; for example, a client may be completely healed by week 13, but this fact may not be apparent on the x-ray until week 14.

Delayed union may lead to **nonunion**, which can cause persistent pain and movement at the fracture site. Nonunion may require surgical interventions, such as internal fixation and bone grafting. If infection is present, the bones are surgically debrided. Electrical stimulation of the fracture site may be as effective as bone grafting.

Reflex Sympathetic Dystrophy

Reflex sympathetic dystrophy may occur after musculoskeletal or nerve trauma. This term refers to a group of poorly understood post-traumatic conditions involving persistent pain, hyperesthesias, swelling, changes in skin color and texture, changes in temperature, and decreased motion. Diagnosis is made by the client's history and physical examination. X-rays may demonstrate spotty osteoporosis, and bone scans may reveal increased uptake of radionuclide. Treatment with a sympathetic nervous system blocking agent often alleviates the manifestations.

INTERDISCIPLINARY CARE

A fracture requires treatment to stabilize the fractured bone(s), maintain bone immobilization, prevent complications, and restore function. The diagnosis of a fracture is primarily based on physical assessments and x-rays.

Emergency Care

Emergency care of the client with a fracture includes immobilizing the fracture, maintaining tissue perfusion, and preventing infection. In the case of serious trauma, normal body alignment must be maintained and may involve cervical immobilization. Once the client is in a secure location, he or she is assessed for instability or deformity of the bone. If any deformity or instability is detected, the extremity is rapidly immobilized. Open wounds are covered with sterile dressings, and bleeding may be controlled with a pressure dressing. The extremities are assessed for the presence of pulses, movement, and sensation. The joint above and below the deformity is immobilized. Pulses, movement, and sensation are reevaluated after splinting.

The fracture is splinted to maintain normal anatomic alignment and prevent the fracture from dislocating. Splinting relieves pain and prevents further damage to the arteries, nerves, and bones. Splinting can be accomplished with air splints. If equipment is not available, the limb may be secured to the body. For example, an arm may be secured to the torso with a sling, or one leg may be strapped to the other leg.

Diagnosis

Diagnosis of a fracture begins with the history and initial assessment and usually is confirmed by radiographic tests. X-rays and bone scans are used to identify fractures (Figure 41–3 ■). Blood chemistry studies, complete blood count (CBC), and coagulation studies may be used to assess blood loss, renal function, muscle breakdown, and the risk of excessive bleeding or clotting. Diagnostic tests are described in Chapter 40 ∞.

Figure 41–3 ■ X-ray of an oblique fracture of the femur.

Source: Charles Stewart and Associates.

Medications

Most clients with a fracture require pharmacologic interventions. The priority intervention focuses on relieving pain. In the case of multiple fractures or fractures of large bones, narcotics are administered initially. As healing progresses, the client begins to take oral medication for pain. Pain management for the client with a fracture is described in Box 41–3.

Stool softeners may be administered to decrease the risk of constipation secondary to narcotics and immobility. Clients who have sustained trauma are often placed on antiulcer medications or antacids. NSAIDs may be prescribed to decrease inflammation. Antibiotics may be administered prophylactically, particularly to clients with open or complex fractures. Anticoagulants may be prescribed to prevent DVT.

Treatments

Fracture treatment may involve a closed reduction and the application of a cast, or may include one or more of the following: traction, casts, surgery, and electrical bone stimulation.

TRACTION Muscle spasms usually accompany fractures and may pull bones out of alignment. Traction is the application of a straightening or pulling force to return or maintain the fractured bones in normal anatomic position. Weights are applied to maintain the necessary force (Figure 41–4 ■). Types of traction are as follows:

- In *manual traction,* the hand directly applies the pulling force.
- *Skin traction* (also called straight traction) is used to control muscle spasms and to immobilize a part of the body before surgery, with traction exerting its grabbing and pulling force through the client's skin. The most common type of skin traction is Buck's traction, in which traction tape or a foam boot is applied to the lower portion of a client's leg and a free-hanging weight is attached to the taped or booted area (Figure 41–4A). Buck's traction is used to immobilize the leg before surgery to repair a fracture of the proximal femur. The advantage of skin traction is the relative ease of use and ability to maintain comfort. The disadvantage is that the weight required to maintain normal body alignment or fracture alignment cannot exceed the tolerance of the skin, about 6 lb per extremity. It is important to ensure that the weights remain hanging freely; they should never rest on the bed or the floor. The nurse may have to reposition the client or the weights if this occurs.

- *Balanced suspension traction* involves more than one force of pull. Several forces work in unison to raise and support the client's injured extremity off the bed and pull it in a straight line away from the body (Figure 41–4B). The advantage of this type of traction is that it increases mobility without threatening joint continuity. The disadvantage is that the increased use of multiple weights makes the client more likely to slide down in the bed.

- *Skeletal traction* is the application of a pulling force through placement of pins into the bone (Figure 41–4C). The client may receive a local, spinal, or general anesthetic, and the pins are inserted into the bone. This type of traction must be applied under sterile conditions because of the increased risk of infection. One or more pulling forces may be applied with skeletal traction. The advantage of this type of traction is that more weight can be used to maintain the proper anatomic alignment if necessary. The disadvantages include increased anxiety, increased risk of infection, and increased discomfort. The weights used for skeletal traction are not removed by the nurse. Nursing interventions for clients receiving traction are described in Box 41–4.

BOX 41–3 Pain Management in the Client with a Fracture

The client who has had musculoskeletal trauma experiences pain from many different causes:

- The interruption in the continuity of the bone itself
- Damage to ligaments and tendons
- Swelling of tissues around the trauma site
- Muscle spasms
- Tissue anoxia from swelling inside a cast, splint, or the muscle fascia sheath
- Hematoma formation
- Pressure over bony prominences from casts or splints.

The pain is often severe and may be described as sharp, aching, or burning. Carefully assess any complaint of pain; pain may be an indication of a serious complication, such as compartment syndrome, decreased tissue perfusion and neurovascular impairment, or pressure ulcers. Do not administer analgesics until the location, character, and duration of pain have been carefully assessed. After the cause of the pain has been identified, the following nursing interventions may be implemented:

1. Administer prescribed analgesics, which may include NSAIDs and narcotic analgesics. For serious fractures or following orthopedic surgery, patient-controlled analgesia (PCA) or epidural methods of providing pain relief may be used. If medications are used on an as-needed basis, tell the client to request the medication before the pain is severe; alternatively, offer the medications at regular intervals for the first 24 to 48 hours. Reassure the client that addiction does not result from taking medications to relieve fracture or surgical pain. Most clients require only oral analgesics by the third or fourth day after orthopedic surgery.

2. Elevate the involved extremity, and apply cold (if prescribed) to help decrease swelling.

3. Monitor and drain the accumulated fluids in any drainage devices to ensure patency and to decrease the possibility of hematoma formation.

4. Encourage the client to wiggle fingers or toes on an extremity in a cast or traction to improve venous return and decrease edema.

5. Assist the client to change positions to relieve pressure and use pillows to provide support.

6. Teach the client alternative methods of pain management, such as relaxation and guided imagery.

7. Notify the physician of unrelieved pain, which may indicate a serious complication such as compartment syndrome or neurovascular impairment.

Figure 41–4 ■ Traction is the application of a pulling force to maintain bone alignment during fracture healing. Different fractures require different types of traction. *A*, Skin traction (also called straight traction) such as Buck's traction shown here, is often used for hip fractures. *B*, Balanced suspension traction is commonly used for fractures of the femur. *C*, Skeletal traction, in which the pulling force is applied directly to the bone, may be used to treat fractures of the humerus.

BOX 41–4 Nursing Interventions for Clients in Traction

- In skeletal traction, never remove the weights.
- In skin traction, remove weights only when intermittent skin traction has been ordered to alleviate muscle spasm.
- For traction to be successful, a countertraction is necessary. In most instances, the countertraction is the client's weight. Therefore, do not wedge the client's foot or place it flush with the footboard of the bed.
- Maintain the line of pull:
  a. Center the client on the bed.
  b. Ensure that weights hang freely and do not touch the floor.
- Ensure that nothing is lying on or obstructing the ropes. Do not allow the knots at the end of the rope to come into contact with the pulley.
- If a problem is detected, assist in repositioning. The area of the fracture must be stabilized when the client is repositioned.
- In skin traction:

  a. Frequently assess skin for evidence of pressure, shearing, or pending breakdown.
  b. Protect pressure sites with padding and protective dressings as indicated.
- In skeletal traction:
  a. Frequent skin assessments should include pin care per policy.
  b. Report signs of infection at the pin sites, such as redness, drainage, and increased tenderness.
  c. The client may require more frequent analgesic administration.
- Perform neurovascular assessments frequently.
- Assess for common complications of immobility, including formation of pressure ulcers, formation of renal calculi, deep venous thrombosis, pneumonia, paralytic ileus, and loss of appetite.
- Teach the client and family about the type and purpose of the traction.

CASTS A cast is a rigid device applied to immobilize the injured bones and promote healing. The cast immobilizes the joint above and the joint below the fractured bone so that the bone will not move during healing. A fracture is first reduced manually (by hand) and a cast is then applied. Casts are applied on clients who have relatively stable fractures

The cast, which may be composed of plaster or fiberglass, is applied over a thin cushion of padding and molded to the normal contour of the body. The cast must be allowed to dry before any pressure is applied to it; simply palpating a wet cast with the fingertips will leave dents that may cause pressure ulcers. A plaster cast may require up to 48 hours to dry, whereas a fiberglass

A Short arm cast

B Shoulder spica cast

C Long leg cast

D One-and-one half hip spica cast

Figure 41–5 ■ Examples of types of casts used to immobilize fractures

cast dries in less than 1 hour. The type of cast applied is determined by the location of the fracture (Figure 41–5 ■). Nursing care of the client with a cast is discussed in the box below. During follow-up appointments, the physician may x-ray the bone to assess alignment and healing, and possibly remove the cast for skin assessment.

SURGERY Surgery is indicated for a fracture that requires direct visualization and repair, a fracture with common long-term complications, or a fracture that is severely comminuted and threatens vascular supply.

The simplest form of surgery is done by external fixation with an external fixator device. An external fixator consists of a frame connected to pins that are inserted perpendicular to the long axis of the bone (Figure 41–6 ■). The number of pins inserted varies with the type and site of the fracture, but in all cases the same number of pins is inserted above and below the

---

NURSING CARE OF THE CLIENT WITH A   Cast

NURSING INTERVENTIONS
- Perform frequent neurovascular assessments.
- Palpate the cast for "hot spots" that may indicate the presence of underlying infection.
- Report any drainage promptly.

HEALTH EDUCATION FOR THE CLIENT AND FAMILY
- Do not place any objects in the cast.
- If the cast is made of plaster, keep it dry.
- If the cast is made of fiberglass, dry it with a blow dryer on the cool setting if it becomes wet.
- Assess the injured extremity for coolness, changes in color, increased pain, increased swelling, and/or loss of sensation.

- Use a blow dryer on the cool setting to relieve itching by blowing cool air into the cast.
- If a sling is used, it should distribute the weight of the cast evenly around the neck. Do not roll the sling; this can impair circulation to the neck.
- If crutches are used, arrange for physical therapist to teach correct crutch walking.
- When the cast is removed, an oscillating cast remover will be used. A guard prevents the cast remover from penetrating past the depth of the cast, so it will not cut the client. It is noisy, and the client will feel vibration.

Figure 41–6 ■ In external fixation, pins are placed through the bone above and below the fracture site to immobilize the bone. External fixation rods hold the pins in place.

fracture line. The pins require care similar to that of skeletal traction pins. The client is monitored for infection, and frequent neurovascular assessment is performed. The fixator increases independence while maintaining immobilization.

Internal fixation can be accomplished through a surgical procedure called an *open reduction and internal fixation (ORIF)*. In this procedure, the fracture is reduced (placed in correct anatomic alignment) and nails, screws, plates, or pins are inserted to hold the bones in place (Figure 41–7 ■). Open fractures of the arms and legs are most commonly repaired in this way. Hip fractures in older clients are almost always repaired with ORIF to prevent

complications and to allow early rehabilitation. Interventions for postoperative nursing care are presented in Box 41–5.

ELECTRICAL BONE STIMULATION Electrical bone stimulation is the application of an electrical current at the fracture site. It is a painless method of treating fractures that are not healing appropriately. The electrical stress increases the migration of osteoblasts and osteoclasts to the fracture site. Mineral deposition increases, promoting bone healing. Electrical bone stimulation can be accomplished invasively or noninvasively (Figure 41–8 ■). In invasive stimulation, the surgeon inserts a cathode and a lead

Figure 41–7 ■ Internal fixation hardware is entirely within the body. *A,* Fixation of a short oblique fracture using a plate and screws above and below the fracture. *B,* Fixation of a long oblique fracture using screws through the fracture site. *C,* Fixation of a segmental fracture using a medullary nail.

BOX 41–5 Nursing Interventions for Clients with Internal Fixation

- Expect the client to have sutures and at least one Hemovac drain.
- Perform neurovascular assessments frequently.
- Assess the following:
  a. Wounds for drainage
  b. Hemovac for drainage of serosanguineous fluid
  c. Bowel sounds
  d. Lung sounds.

- Administer medications, such as analgesics and antibiotics, per physician's orders.
- In hip fractures, place an abductor pillow between client's legs to prevent dislocation of the hip joint.
- Arrange for physical and occupational therapy, as ordered.
- Assist with weight-bearing program, if ordered.
- Encourage early mobilization, coughing, and deep breathing, as appropriate to help prevent complications.

---

wire at the fracture site. The lead wire is attached to an internal or external generator, which delivers electricity through the lead wire to the cathode 24 hours a day. In noninvasive inductive stimulation, a treatment coil encircles the cast or skin directly over the fracture site. The coil is attached to an external generator that runs on batteries. The electricity goes through the skin to the fracture site. The time period for external stimulation can vary from 3 to 10 hours per day. The client may be taught to self-administer the noninvasive electrical stimulation. Electrical bone stimulation is contraindicated in the presence of infection and for upper extremities if the client has a pacemaker.

Fractures of Specific Bones or Bony Areas

Causes, manifestations, complications, treatment and selected nursing interventions are described for the following fractures: skull, face, spine, clavicle, humerus, elbow, radius/ulna, wrist/hand, ribs, pelvis, femur, hip, tibia/fibula, and ankle/foot.

Fracture of the Skull

The skull may be fractured as a result of either a fall or a direct blow. The client must be assessed for neurologic damage and any loss of consciousness (LOC) must be documented. A complete neurologic assessment is conducted: Pupillary reaction to light, movement and strength of all extremities, complaints of nausea and vomiting, LOC, and orientation to person, place, and time are noted. A displaced skull fracture, which is referred to as depressed, may press on the brain and cause neurologic damage. Brain injuries related to skull fractures are discussed in Chapter 44 ∞.

Fracture of the Face

Fracture of the facial bones may result from a direct blow. The client presents with hematomas, pain, edema, and bony deformity. Nondisplaced fractures are monitored to ensure the airway is not compromised. The client is observed for any neurologic deficits. Severely displaced or multiple facial fractures are treated with ORIF with wires or plates.

Nursing care focuses on maintaining the airway by helping the client clear secretions from the oropharynx. The nurse monitors the client's breathing for increased effort or tachypnea and notifies the physician immediately if these findings are noted. Pain is treated with analgesics, and body image disturbances are addressed. If the client asks to see his or her face, the nurse should plan to stay with the client and answer questions while the client looks in a mirror.

Fracture of the Spine

The spine can be injured in many ways, including sports injuries, falls, and motor vehicle crashes. The spine can be fractured in the cervical, thoracic, lumbar, or sacral area. The most severe complication of spine fracture is injury to the spinal cord (discussed in Chapter 45 ∞). A fracture to the vertebrae may cause the bones to become displaced and apply pressure on the spinal cord. This pressure on the spinal cord may result in permanent paralysis.

A nondisplaced cervical spinal fracture may be treated with a cervical collar or a halo immobilizing brace. The displaced cervical fracture is reduced by manual or skeletal traction and, eventually, application of a brace and/or surgical stabilization of the bones with plates and screws. Immobilization after a spinal fracture may last as long as 6 months.

Fracture of the Clavicle

A fracture of the clavicle commonly results from a direct blow or a fall. The most common location is midclavicular. A person with a midclavicular fracture typically assumes a protective slumping position to immobilize the arm and prevent shoulder movement. A less common fracture occurs along the distal third of the clavicle. This type of fracture may be associated with ligament damage. Injuries to the clavicle may be associated with skull or cervical fractures. The fractured bone, if displaced, may lacerate

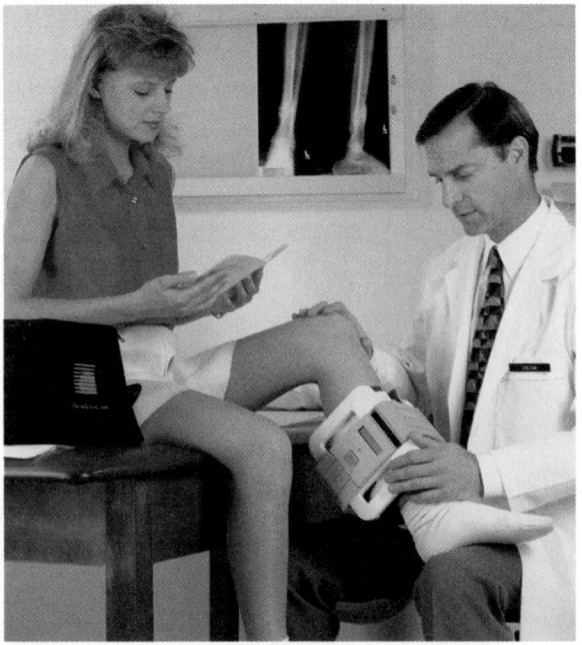

Figure 41–8 ■ External electrical bone growth stimulator.

the subclavian vessels and result in hemorrhage. The fractured bone may also puncture the lung, resulting in a pneumothorax. Malunion may occur at the fracture site and result in asymmetry of the clavicles. Injury to the brachial plexus may result in numbness and decreased movement of the arm on the affected side.

A deformity may be observed or palpated along the clavicle. Treatment focuses on immobilizing the fractured bone in normal anatomic position by applying a clavicular strap, or a surgical repair may be necessary.

Fracture of the Humerus

The exact location of the fracture, the presence of displacement, and the results of the neurovascular examination determine the severity of a fracture of the humerus and the appropriate interventions. Treatment focuses on immobilizing the fractured bone in normal anatomic position. Common complications of humeral fracture include nerve and ligament damage, frozen or stiff joints, and malunion. Early interventions may prevent permanent damage.

Fractures of the proximal humerus are common in older adults. A simple nondisplaced fracture of the proximal humerus (near the humeral head) with a normal neurovascular assessment can be safely treated with immobilization. A more complicated displaced fracture of the proximal humerus with bone fragmentation requires surgical intervention. The more severe the fracture and damage to soft tissue, the more likely it is that the range of motion (ROM) of the shoulder will be impaired. Rehabilitative measures focus on increasing ROM.

The humerus may also fracture along the shaft, usually as a direct result of trauma. If the humeral shaft fracture is simple and nondisplaced, a hanging arm cast is applied. This cast maintains alignment of the fracture by using the pulling force of gravity; therefore, the client must be instructed not to rest the cast on anything to alleviate the weight. If the client is on bed rest, a hanging arm cast is not applied, because the arm would not be able to hang freely. Instead, the fracture is immobilized with external skeletal traction. This traction places the injured arm in an upright position over the face, and weights are hung off the distal portion of the humerus (see Figure 41–4C). Nursing interventions for clients with fractures of the humerus are presented in Box 41–6.

Fracture of the Elbow

The most common location of an elbow fracture is the distal humerus. Elbow fractures usually result from a fall or direct blow to the elbow. The client guards the injured extremity, holding the arm rigidly in a flexed position or an extended position. Because the radius, ulna, or humerus may be involved in the elbow fracture, all three bones must be visualized by x-ray.

Complications of an elbow fracture include nerve or artery damage and hemarthrosis, a collection of blood in the elbow joint. The most serious complication of an elbow fracture is Volkmann's contracture, which results from arterial occlusion and muscle ischemia. The client complains of forearm pain, impaired sensation, and loss of motor function. Rapid interventions are aimed at relieving pressure on the brachial artery and nerve and preventing muscle atrophy.

Nondisplaced elbow fractures are treated by immobilizing the fracture with a posterior splint or cast. The displaced frac-

---

> ### BOX 41–6 Nursing Interventions for Clients with Fractures of the Humerus
>
> - Perform neurovascular assessments frequently.
> - Administer prescribed medications to alleviate pain.
> - Encourage exercises for clients with a hanging cast:
>   a. Finger exercises: Move each finger of the affected arm through complete range of motion.
>   b. Pendulum shoulder exercises: Dangle the affected arm at the side, and move it forward and backward about 30 degrees in each direction.
> - If client is discharged, instruct the client and family in cast care and sling application, neurovascular assessments, exercises, prescribed pain medications, and manifestations of complications.
> - If client is admitted to the hospital, provide preoperative teaching.

ture is first reduced and then immobilized. Nursing interventions focus on alleviating pain, maintaining immobilization, and educating clients in neurovascular assessments.

Fracture of the Radius and/or Ulna

Fractures of the radius and ulna may occur as a result of either indirect injury, such as twisting or pulling on the arm, or direct injury, such as that resulting from a fall. The usual treatment of radius fractures depends on the location. The proximal radial head may be fractured from a fall on an outstretched hand. Blood commonly collects in the elbow joint and must be aspirated. If the fracture is nondisplaced, a sling is applied. If the fracture is displaced, surgical intervention is required. After surgical repair of a displaced fracture, the arm is splinted with a posterior plaster splint. The client avoids movement for the first week and then initiates movement gradually.

When both bones are broken, the fracture is usually displaced. The client complains of pain and inability to turn the palm of the hand up. A nondisplaced fracture is casted for about 6 weeks, and either a shorter cast or a brace is then applied for 6 more weeks. If the fracture is displaced, surgical intervention is performed. The physician reduces the fracture and may insert pins or screws to keep the bones in alignment. After the surgery, a cast is applied, and the client is encouraged to exercise the fingers.

Complications after a radius and/or ulnar fracture include compartment syndrome, delayed healing, and decreased wrist and finger movement. After surgery, the client also has an increased risk of infection. Nursing interventions focus on alleviating pain, maintaining immobilization, and educating clients in neurovascular assessments, the importance of elevation, and the need to inform the physician of changes in sensation or an increase in pain.

Fractures in the Wrist and Hand

Wrist fractures often result from a fall onto an outstretched hand or onto the back of the hand. A common type of wrist fracture is *Colles's fracture,* in which the distal radius fractures after a fall onto an outstretched hand. The client with a wrist fracture presents with a bony deformity, pain, numbness, weakness, and decreased ROM of the fingers. The capillary refill and sensation of the hand must be assessed.

The hand is composed of many bones. Most commonly, the metacarpals and phalanges are involved in a hand fracture. The injuring mechanism in a hand fracture varies from striking an object with a closed fist to closing a hand in a door. The client presents with complaints of pain, edema, and decreased ROM.

Comparative x-rays may be obtained to compare left and right wrists and hands. Complications of wrist and hand fractures are compartment syndrome, nerve damage, ligament damage, and delayed union. A wrist fracture is commonly treated with closed reduction, cast application, and elevation of the injured extremity. A hand fracture is splinted and elevated.

Nursing interventions focus on alleviating pain and educating the client in neurovascular assessments, the importance of elevation, and how to exercise the fingers to prevent stiffness. If the dominant hand is injured, the client will require assistance in performing activities of daily living (ADLs).

Fracture of the Ribs

Rib fractures commonly result from blunt chest trauma. The location of the fracture and involvement of underlying organs determine the severity of the injury. Fractures of the first through third ribs may result in injury to the subclavian artery or vein. Fractures of the lower ribs may result in spleen and liver injuries.

The client presents with a history of recent chest trauma. Typically, the client complains of pain along the lateral portion of the rib. Palpation of the rib reveals a bony deformity and increases pain. Deep inspiration also increases pain. The skin over the fracture site may be ecchymotic (bruised).

A complication of rib fractures is a **flail chest**, which results from the fracture of two or more adjacent ribs in two or more places and the formation of a free-floating segment that moves in the opposite direction of the rib cage. The bony instability impairs respirations. Treatment is aimed at stabilizing the flail segment and supporting respirations. Other complications of rib fractures include pneumothorax and/or hemothorax. The fractured rib may pierce the lung and injure it. The lower ribs may pierce the liver or spleen, resulting in intra-abdominal bleeding. Pneumonia may also develop from ineffective clearing of respiratory secretions.

A simple rib fracture is treated with pain medication and instructions for coughing, deep breathing, and splinting. The client is also instructed to return to the emergency room if shortness of breath develops. Nursing interventions focus on alleviating pain and teaching the client about splinting. Because deep inspiration increases pain, clients frequently avoid it. The client may be instructed to splint the injured rib with the hand or a pillow and take deep breaths and cough to decrease the chance of developing pneumonia and/or atelectasis. Incentive spirometry is encouraged.

Fracture of the Pelvis

Pelvic fractures are often caused by trauma, such as a fall or an automobile crash. The client with a pelvic fracture presents with pain in the back or hip area. A single fracture in the pelvis is treated conservatively with bed rest on a firm mattress. Log rolling increases client comfort. A pelvic fracture with two fracture sites is considered unstable and treated with surgery. An external fixator may be applied to stabilize the pelvis. In the client who is not stable for surgery, a pelvic sling may be used. The pelvic sling stabilizes the pelvis and allows the client to move in bed with less pain. Common complications include hypovolemia, spinal injury, bladder injury, urethral injury, kidney damage, and gastrointestinal trauma.

Nursing care focuses on alleviating discomfort, maintaining immobilization, and preparing the client for surgery if necessary. The nurse monitors the client for increased heart rate, decreased blood pressure, and decreasing hemoglobin levels. These findings may indicate impending hypovolemia due to bleeding into the pelvis. Any blood in the urine should be reported to the physician; this may indicate kidney, bladder, or urethral damage.

Fracture of the Shaft of the Femur

A large amount of force, such as from motor vehicle crashes, falls, or acts of violence, is required to fracture the shaft of the femur. Clients with femoral shaft fractures often have associated multiple traumas. A fracture of the femoral shaft is manifested by an edematous, deformed, painful thigh. The client is unable to move the hip or knee. Initial assessment focuses on the circulation and sensation present in the affected extremity. Pedal pulses and capillary refill in the affected extremity are compared to the unaffected extremity. Complications of a femoral shaft fracture include hypovolemia due to blood loss (which may be as great as 1.0 to 1.5 L), fat embolism, dislocation of the hip or knee, muscle atrophy, and ligament damage.

Treatment of fractures of the shaft of the femur initially includes skeletal traction to separate the bony fragments and reduce and immobilize the fracture. Depending on the location and severity of the fracture, traction may be followed by either external or internal fixation. Strength in the affected extremity is maintained through gluteal and quadricep exercises. ROM exercises for unaffected extremities are critical in preparation for ambulation. Although full weight bearing is usually restricted until x-rays demonstrate bone union, the client may be allowed to carry out non-weight-bearing activities with an assistive device.

The nurse assesses pulses in the extremity and compares them bilaterally. Sensation is evaluated by asking whether the client can feel touch and discriminate sharp from dull objects. Nursing interventions include providing pain medication, providing reassurance and decreasing anxiety, and assisting with exercises of the lower legs, feet, and toes.

Fracture of the Hip

A hip fracture refers to a fracture of the femur at the head, neck, or trochanteric regions (Figure 41–9 ■). Hip fractures are classified as intracapsular or extracapsular. *Intracapsular fractures* involve the head or neck of the femur; *extracapsular fractures* involve the trochanteric region. The majority of hip fractures involve the neck or trochanteric regions. The femoral head and neck lie within the joint capsule and are not covered in periosteum; thus, they do not have a large blood supply. Fractures at this location usually fragment, further decreasing blood supply and increasing the risk of nonunion and avascular necrosis. The trochanteric region is covered in periosteum and therefore has more blood supply than the head or neck.

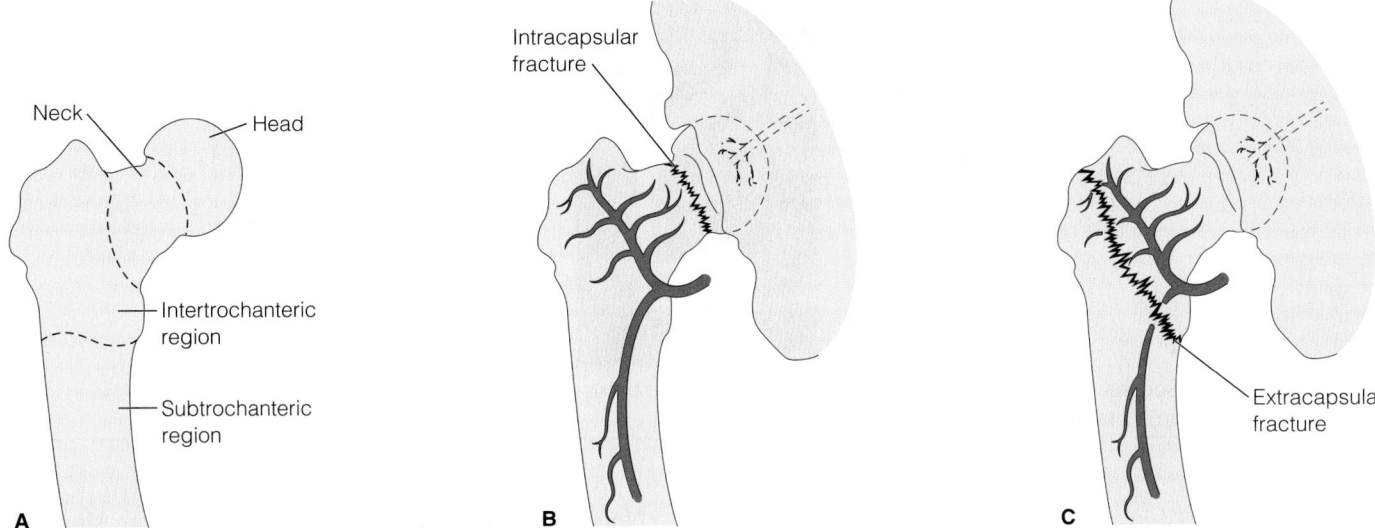

Figure 41–9 ■ Regions where hip fractures may occur: *A*, the head of the femur, the neck of the femur, and the trochanteric regions of the femur. *B*, Intracapsular fractures occur across the head or neck of the femur. *C*, Extracapsular fractures occur across the trochanteric regions. Note how both intracapsular and extracapsular fractures disrupt the blood supply to the bone.

Hip fractures result from falls and are the most common injury in the older population, requiring hospitalization of more than 300,000 older adults each year in the United States. They result in the greatest number of deaths and most serious health problems of all fractures for people 65 years or older (Centers for Disease Control and Prevention, [CDC], 2006). By the year 2040, the number of hip fractures is expected to exceed 500,000, which reflects society's increasing older population. Factors contributing to falls include problems with gait and balance, neurologic and musculoskeletal impairments, dementia, psychoactive medications, and visual impairments. Modifiable risk factors, identified through research, include lower body weakness, problems with walking and balance, and taking four or more medications or any psychoactive medications.

Hip fractures are common in older adults as a result of decreases in bone mass and the increased tendency to fall. Whether the femur breaks spontaneously and causes the fall or whether the fall causes the fracture is not always clear; regardless of the cause of the fracture, rapid interventions are required to prevent bone necrosis. Assessment findings commonly associated with a hip fracture are pain, inability to walk, and shortening and external rotation of the affected lower extremity. Rarely, the fracture dislocates posteriorly; if that occurs, the extremity may internally rotate. However, some patients with a hip fracture have only vague pain in the buttocks, knees, thighs, groin, or back and their ability to walk is unaffected. If the fracture is not visible on x-ray, a bone scan or MRI may be done to confirm the presence of the fracture.

A hip fracture may be treated with traction to decrease muscle spasms, followed by surgery; or surgery may be performed immediately or within the first 24 hours. The goal of surgery is to reduce and stabilize the fracture, thereby increasing mobility, decreasing pain, and preventing complications. Surgery usually consists of ORIF of the fracture. Fixation is accomplished by securing the femur in place with pins, screws, nails, or plates (Figure 41–10A ■). An ORIF works well for fractures in the trochanteric area. Fractures of the femoral neck frequently disrupt blood supply to the femoral head. If blood supply is disrupted, the surgeon will replace the femoral head with a prosthesis (Figure 41–10B). If the acetabulum has been damaged, the surgeon may insert a metal cup. Replacement of either the femoral head or the acetabulum with a prosthesis is called a *hemiarthroplasty*. Replacement of both the femoral head and the acetabulum is a *total hip arthroplasty (THA)*, discussed in Chapter 42 ∞.

Nursing care for a client with a hip fracture focuses on maintaining skin integrity, preventing infection, alleviating pain, maintaining circulation to the injured extremity, and increasing mobility, and is discussed in more detail in the following nursing care section.

FAST FACTS

Hip Fracture in Older Adults

- More than one-third of all adults over the age of 65 fall each year. Of those, white men have the highest fall-related death rates, followed by white women, black men, and black women.
- Older adults most often fracture the hip from falls; in contrast, motor vehicle crashes are the most common cause in young and middle adults.
- The risk for a fractured hip increases with each decade of life, especially in white postmenopausal women, who have the highest incidence of osteoporosis. Women have about 80% of all hip fractures. Women who smoke are at greater risk, because smoking reduces bone density among menopausal women.
- Complications are related both to the fracture and to the resulting treatment. Only a small number of clients retain their previous mobility, while about 20% require nursing home care.
- Half of all older adults hospitalized for a hip fracture cannot return home or live independently after the fracture.

Data from CDC (2006).

Figure 41–10 ■ Surgical fixation of hip fractures. *A,* A surgical nail or screw used to stabilize an intertrochanteric fracture. *B,* Use of a hip prosthesis (artificial hip) to replace a damaged femoral head.

Fracture of the Tibia and/or Fibula

Fractures of the lower extremities often result from a fall on a flexed foot, a direct blow, or a twisting motion. The client presents with edema, pain, bony deformity, and a hematoma at the level of injury.

Circulation and sensation are assessed to rule out common complications of the fracture, including damage to the peroneal nerve or tibial artery, compartment syndrome, hemarthroses, and ligament damage. Peroneal nerve damage may be indicated by the client's inability to point the toe on the affected side upward. Tibial artery damage may be the cause of an absent dorsalis pedis pulse on the affected side. Compartment syndrome may be present if the client develops pain on passive movement and paresthesias. An edematous knee may indicate a collection of blood in the knee joint. Ligament damage may be present if the client cannot move the knee and/or ankle.

If the fracture is closed, a closed reduction and casting are frequently performed. A long leg cast that allows for partial weight bearing is used. Partial weight bearing usually is prescribed by the physician within 10 days of the fracture. A short leg cast will be applied in 3 to 4 weeks. If the fracture is open, either external fixation or ORIF will be performed. After surgery, a cast may be applied, and weight bearing begins according to the physician's orders, usually in about 6 weeks.

Nursing care is designed to increase comfort, monitor neurovascular status, and prevent complications. The nurse instructs the client in cast care, on the use of assistive devices, how to perform neurovascular assessment, and when to follow up with the physician.

Fracture in the Ankle and Foot

The client with an ankle fracture presents with pain, limited ROM, hematoma, edema, and difficulty ambulating. Most ankle fractures are treated by closed reduction and casting. Open fractures are treated by surgical intervention and splinting.

The client with a foot fracture presents with similar symptoms; however, ROM of the ankle is not usually affected. Most foot fractures are nondisplaced and treated with closed reduction and casting. More severe displaced foot fractures may require surgery and the placement of wires to maintain reduction of the fracture.

Nursing care focuses on increasing comfort, increasing mobility, and educating the client. Analgesia is given for pain. The extremity should be elevated, and ice can be applied. The client is taught cast care, neurovascular assessment, and crutch walking.

NURSING CARE

In planning and implementing nursing care for the client with fractures, the nurse should consider the client's response to the traumatic experience. Although each client has individual needs, nursing care commonly focuses on client problems with pain, impaired physical mobility, impaired tissue perfusion, and neurovascular compromise.

Health Promotion

Trauma prevention can save lives. Many communities are educating people of all ages, from grade-schoolers to older adults, in trauma prevention. Young adults face a high risk of sustaining trauma. They need to be taught the importance of safety equipment—such as automobile seat belts, bicycle and motorized vehicle helmets, football pads, proper footwear, protective eyewear, and hard hats—in preventing or decreasing the severity of injury from trauma. Older adults should have regular screenings for osteoporosis (with a bone density test), activity levels, cognitive and affective disorders, vision impairments, and risk for falls. Older adults can reduce their risk of falling by increasing lower body strength and balance through regular physical activity, and by asking their healthcare provider or pharmacist to review their medications. Educational programs about workplace and farm safety, including information about ergonomic principles, can also help prevent musculoskeletal injuries.

Having a regular exercise program and avoiding obesity are important factors in maintaining good bone health in all adults. An adequate intake of calcium is essential to ensure proper growth, development, and maintenance of strong bones throughout life. It is important that women ensure good bone health prior to menopause, because the loss of estrogen during and after menopause decreases calcium use and increases the risk of osteoporosis. Strong bones are formed by calcium intake and weight-bearing exercise, both of which are equally important in the postmenopausal woman.

Older clients are at higher risk for musculoskeletal trauma due to falls. For these clients, home assessments must be performed and potential hazards removed. Specific teaching topics for preventing falls in older adults are outlined in the Meeting Individualized Needs box below.

Assessment

Collect the following data through the health history and physical examination (see Chapter 40 ∞).

- *Health History:* Age, history of traumatic event, history of chronic illnesses, history of prior musculoskeletal injuries, medications (ask the older adult specifically about anticoagulants and calcium supplements).
- *Physical Assessment:* Pain with movement, pulses, edema, skin color and temperature, deformity, range of motion, touch. These assessments include the 5 P's of neurovascular assessment, as follows, included in both the initial assessment and ongoing focused assessments:
- *Pain.* Assess pain in the injured extremity by asking the client to grade it on a scale of 0 to 10, with 10 as the most severe pain.
- *Pulses.* Assess distal pulses beginning with the unaffected extremity. Compare the quality of pulses in the affected extremity to those of the unaffected extremity.
- *Pallor.* Observe for pallor and skin color in the injured extremity. Paleness and coolness may indicate arterial compromise, whereas warmth and a bluish tinge may indicate venous blood pooling.
- *Paralysis/Paresis.* Assess ability to move body parts distal to the fracture site. Inability to move indicates paralysis. Loss of muscle strength (weakness) when moving is paresis. A finding of limited range of motion may lead to early recognition of problems such as nerve damage and paralysis.
- *Paresthesia.* Ask the client if any change in sensation such as burning, numbness, prickly feeling, or stinging (all these are paresthesias) has occurred.

Nursing Diagnoses and Interventions

Nursing care for clients with fractures ranges from teaching for home care treatments provided in the emergency or urgent care department (such as manual reduction and cast application) to providing interventions to maintain health and decrease the risk of complications in clients with complex or multiple fractures. Teaching is also necessary for caregivers of the older adult who is discharged home or to a long-term care or rehabilitation facility following a fractured hip. A Nursing Care Plan is included on page 1418.

Acute Pain

Pain is caused by soft tissue damage and is compounded by muscle spasms and swelling.

- Monitor vital signs. *Some analgesics decrease respiratory effort and blood pressure.*
- Ask the client to rate the pain on a scale of 0 to 10 (with 10 as the most severe pain) before and after any intervention. *This facilitates objective assessment of the effectiveness of the chosen pain relief strategy. Pain that increases in intensity or remains unrelieved with analgesics can indicate compartment syndrome.*
- For the client with a hip fracture, apply Buck's traction per physician's orders. Keep the traction weights hanging freely. *Buck's traction immobilizes the fracture and decreases pain and additional trauma.*

> **PRACTICE ALERT**
> Do not let weights lie on the bed or the floor. The weights can be removed long enough to move the client up or down in bed to ensure freely hanging weights.

- Move the client gently and slowly. *Gentle moving helps prevent the development of severe muscle spasms.*
- Elevate the injured extremity above the level of the heart. *Elevating the extremity promotes venous return and decreases edema, which decreases pain.*
- Encourage distraction or other noninvasive methods of pain relief, such as deep breathing and relaxation. *Distraction, deep breathing, and relaxation help decrease the focus on the pain and may lessen the intensity of pain.*

MEETING INDIVIDUALIZED NEEDS Teaching Older Adults to Prevent Falls

- Begin a regular exercise program; lack of exercise leads to weakness and an increased chance of falling. Exercises that improve balance and coordination (such as t'ai chi) are the most helpful.
- Make your home safer:
  - Remove any items in your pathway, including from stairs, to avoid tripping.
  - Remove small throw rugs or use double-sided tape to keep rugs from slipping.
  - Place frequently used items within easy reach to avoid use of a step stool.
  - Install grab bars next to your toilet and in the tub or shower.
  - Use nonslip mats in the bathtub and on shower floors.

- Improve lighting, using lamp shades or frosted bulbs to reduce glare.
- Install handrails and lights in all staircases.
- Wear shoes that give good support and have thin, nonslip soles. Avoid wearing slippers and athletic shoes with deep treads.
- Ask your healthcare provider to review your medications, including prescriptions and over-the-counter medications. Some medications or a combination of medications may cause dizziness or drowsiness, leading to falls.
- Have your vision checked by an eye doctor. Your glasses may no longer have the correct prescription, or you may have developed an eye condition such as cataracts or glaucoma that limits your vision.

NURSING CARE PLAN   A Client with a Hip Fracture

Stella Carbolito is a 74-year-old Italian American with a history of osteoporosis. She is a widow and lives alone in a two-story row home. Mrs. Carbolito is retired and depends on a pension check and social security for her income. She takes pride in making all her own food from scratch.

While walking to the market one day, Mrs. Carbolito falls and fractures her left hip. She is transported by ambulance to the nearest hospital emergency department.

ASSESSMENT

During the initial assessment at the ED, abnormal findings are that Mrs. Carbolito's left leg is shorter than her right leg and is externally rotated. Distal pulses are present and bilaterally strong; both legs are warm. Mrs. Carbolito complains of severe pain but states that no numbness or burning is present. She is able to wiggle the toes on her left leg and has full movement of her right leg. Initial vital signs are as follows: T 98.0°F (36.6°C), P 100, R 18, BP 120/58. Diagnostic tests include CBC, blood chemistry, and x-ray studies of the left hip and pelvis. The CBC reveals a hemoglobin of 11.0 g/dL and a normal WBC count. Blood chemistry findings are within normal limits. The x-ray reveals a fracture of the left femoral neck. Mrs. Carbolito is admitted to the hospital with an order for 10 lb of straight leg traction. An open reduction and internal fixation (ORIF) is planned for the following day.

DIAGNOSES

- *Acute Pain* related to fractured left femoral neck and muscle spasms
- *Impaired Physical Mobility* related to bed rest and fractured left femoral neck
- *Risk for Ineffective Tissue Perfusion* related to unstable bones and swelling
- *Risk for Disturbed Sensory Perception: Tactile* related to the risk of nerve impairment

EXPECTED OUTCOMES

- Verbalize a decrease in pain.
- Verbalize the purpose of traction and surgery.

- Maintain normal neurovascular status.
- Demonstrate postoperative exercises.

PLANNING AND IMPLEMENTATION

- Assess pain on a scale of 0 to 10 before and after implementing measures to reduce pain.
- Administer narcotics per the physician's order.
- Perform neurovascular assessment every 2 to 4 hours, and document findings.
- Apply straight leg traction per physician's order.
- Encourage deep breathing and relaxation techniques.
- Teach the purpose of traction and surgery.
- Teach the purpose of and the procedure for performing isometric and flexion/extension exercises.

EVALUATION

Three days after surgery, Mrs. Carbolito is out of bed and in a chair. She verbalizes a decrease in pain. There have been no abnormal neurovascular assessments. She is able to independently perform isometric and flexion/extension exercises in both lower extremities. Discharge planning includes referrals for home care. A home health nurse will visit, and the social worker at the hospital has ordered a trapeze for her bed, an elevated toilet seat, an elevated cushion for her chair, and a walker.

CRITICAL THINKING IN THE NURSING PROCESS

1. What factors placed Mrs. Carbolito at risk for a hip fracture?
2. Mrs. Carbolito says, "I don't understand why they had to put that heavy thing on my leg before I went to surgery to get my hip fixed." What would you tell her? What preoperative factors might have decreased teaching effectiveness?
3. Describe how each of the following, if manifested by Mrs. Carbolito, would increase her risk for postoperative complications: urinary incontinence, weight more than 20% under normal for her height, chronic constipation. What nursing diagnoses and interventions would you include in her plan of care to decrease the risk?

See Evaluating Your Response in Appendix C.

- Administer pain medications as prescribed. For home care, explain the importance of taking pain medications before the pain is severe. *Analgesics alleviate pain by stimulating opiate receptor sites.*

PRACTICE ALERT
In the case of fracture in an extremity, supporting the extremity above and below the fracture can also decrease pain and muscle spasms.

Risk for Peripheral Neurovascular Dysfunction

In the client with a fracture, compartment syndrome or deep venous thrombosis can impair circulation and, in turn, tissue perfusion.

- Assess the 5 P's every 1 to 2 hours. Report abnormal findings immediately. *Unrelenting pain, pallor, diminished distal pulses, paresthesias, and paresis are strong indicators of compartment syndrome.*

PRACTICE ALERT
Pulses may remain strong, even in the presence of compartment syndrome.

- Assess nail beds for capillary refill. If nails are too thick or discolored, assess the skin around the nail. *Delayed capillary refill may indicate decreased tissue perfusion.*

PRACTICE ALERT
It may not be possible to accurately assess capillary refill in older adults who often have thickened, discolored nails. If so, test nearby skin.

- Monitor the extremity for edema and swelling. *Excessive swelling and hematoma formation can compromise circulation.*
- Assess for deep, throbbing, unrelenting pain. *Pain that is not relieved by analgesics may indicate neurovascular compromise.*

- Encourage independence in ADLs:
  - Explain that the client should sit only on high chairs to prevent excess flexion of the hip; a high toilet seat can be added to a regular toilet seat.
  - Encourage the client and family to equip the shower with a rail to aid stability and prevent falls.
  - If a walker is needed, teach the client its proper use: Do not carry the walker, but lift it, advance it, and then take two steps, or use a rolling walker.
  - If a cane is needed, instruct the client to use it on the affected side.
- Stress the importance of well-balanced meals, and explain all prescribed medications.

Clients who have experienced a fracture or who have had orthopedic surgery often have a cast and require an extended period of immobilization or limited activities. Address the following topics for home care:

- Do not try to scratch under a cast with a sharp object.
- Do not get a plaster cast wet.
- Follow the physician's order for weight bearing.
- Physical therapy departments or offices often can evaluate the home environment for safety and suggest modifications as needed. Physical therapists also teach crutch walking, limited weight bearing, transferring, and other activities.
- Home care agencies can teach wound care and provide ongoing monitoring of wound healing.
- Local medical equipment and supply sources rent or sell durable equipment such as crutches, walkers, wheelchairs, overhead trapeze units, shower chairs, elevated toilet seats, grab bars, and bedside commodes. Slings or braces may be purchased through medical equipment dealers.
- Local pharmacies are good resources for dressing supplies such as antiseptic solutions or ointments, dressings, and tape.
- Fitness equipment suppliers may be able to provide rehabilitation equipment such as hand or ankle weights for strengthening exercises.

THE CLIENT WITH AN AMPUTATION

An **amputation** is the partial or total removal of an extremity. Amputation may be the result of an acute process, such as a traumatic event, or a chronic condition, such as peripheral vascular disease or diabetes mellitus. Regardless of the cause, an amputation is devastating to the client.

FAST FACTS
Amputation
- It is estimated that 350,000 people with amputations live in the United States, and that 135,000 new amputations occur each year.
- In the United States, the most common causes of lower extremity amputations are disease (70%), trauma (22%), congenital or birth defects (4%), and tumors (4%).
- Upper extremity amputation is usually due to trauma or birth defect.

Data from Moss Rehab Resource Net (2005).

The loss of all or part of an extremity has a significant physical and psychosocial effect on the client and family. Adaptation may take a long time and require much effort. Interdisciplinary health care is always important, but is especially necessary to meet the client's physical, spiritual, cultural, and emotional needs after an unexpected or planned amputation.

Causes of Amputation

Peripheral vascular disease (PVD) is the major cause of amputation of the lower extremities (see Chapter 35 ∞). Common risk factors for the development of PVD include hypertension, diabetes, smoking, and hyperlipidemia. Peripheral neuropathy also places the person with diabetes at risk for amputation. In peripheral neuropathy, loss of sensation frequently leads to unrecognized injury and infection. Untreated infection may lead to gangrene and the need for amputation. These risks are discussed in Chapter 20 ∞.

The incidence of traumatic amputations is highest among young men. Most amputations in this group result from motor vehicle crashes or accidents involving machinery at work. The client presents to the trauma center with an injury that may be life threatening; significant loss of blood and tissue may have already occurred, and shock may develop. (See Chapter 11 ∞ for a discussion of shock and trauma.) Other traumatic events that may necessitate an amputation are frostbite, burns, or electrocution.

Amputations result from or are necessitated by interruption in blood flow, either acute or chronic. In acute trauma situations, the limb is partially or completely severed, and tissue death ensues. However, replantation of fingers, small body parts, and entire limbs has been successful. In chronic disease processes, circulation is impaired, venous pooling begins, proteins leak into the interstitium, and edema develops. Edema increases the risk of injury and further decreases circulation. Stasis ulcers develop and readily become infected because impaired healing and altered immune processes allow bacteria to proliferate. The presence of progressive infection further compromises circulation and ultimately leads to gangrene (tissue death), which requires amputation.

Levels of Amputation

The level of amputation is determined by local and systemic factors. Local factors include ischemia and gangrene; system factors include cardiovascular status, renal function, and severity of diabetes mellitus. The goals are to alleviate symptoms, to maintain healthy tissue, and to increase functional outcome. When possible, the joints are preserved because they allow greater function of the extremity. Figure 41–12 ■ illustrates common sites of amputation.

Types of Amputation

Amputations may be open (*guillotine*) or closed (*flap*). Open amputations are performed when infection is present. The wound is not closed but remains open to drain. When infection is no longer present, surgery is performed to close the wound.

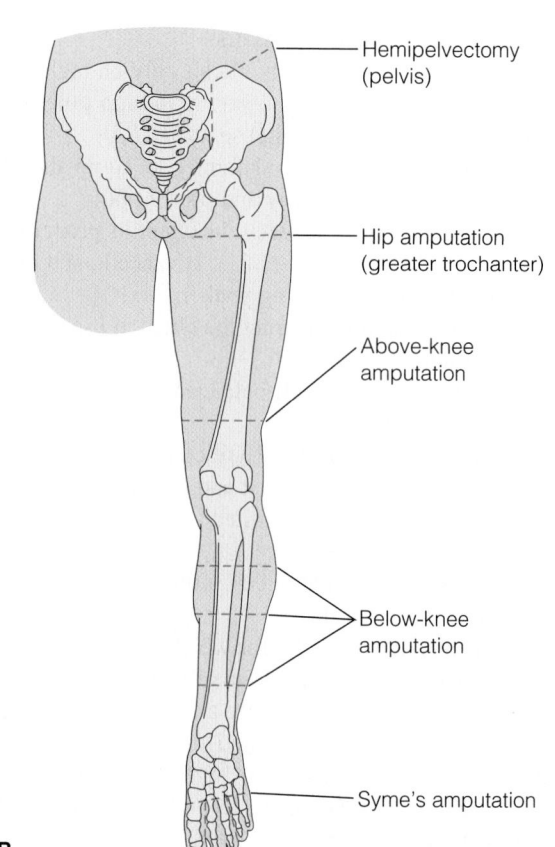

Figure 41–12 ■ Common sites of amputation. *A,* The upper extremities. *B,* The lower extremities. The surgeon determines the level of amputation based on blood supply and tissue condition.

In closed amputations, the wound is closed with a flap of skin that is sutured in place over the stump. Terms used to refer to amputations are defined in Table 41–3.

TABLE 41–3 **Amputation Terms**

TERM	MEANING
Arm	Amputation of a portion of the arm, either above or below the elbow
Disarticulation	Amputation through a joint
Forequarter	Removal of the entire arm and disarticulation of the shoulder
Closed (flap)	Amputation in which a flap of skin is formed to cover the end of the wound
Open (guillotine)	Perpendicular cutting of the extremity in which the wound is left open; used when infection is present
Leg	Amputation below the knee (BK)
Thigh	Amputation above the knee (AK)
Finger or toe	Amputation of one or all of the fingers or toes
Syme	Modified disarticulation of the ankle
Foot	Amputation of part of the foot and toes

Amputation Site Healing

For the prosthesis to fit well, the amputation site must heal properly. To promote healing, a rigid or compression dressing is applied to prevent infection and minimize edema. A rigid dressing is made by placing a cast on the stump and molding the stump to fit a prosthesis. A soft compression dressing is applied when frequent wound checks are necessary. When this type of dressing is used, a splint is sometimes applied to help mold the extremity to fit the prosthesis. After the wound is dressed, the client is encouraged to toughen the stump skin by pushing it into first soft and then harder surfaces. The stump is wrapped in an Ace bandage to allow a conical shape to form and to prevent edema. The bandage is applied from the distal to the proximal extremity (Figure 41–13 ■).

Complications

Complications that may occur after an amputation include infection, delayed healing, chronic stump pain and phantom pain, and contractures.

Infection

Generally, the client who suffers a traumatic amputation has a greater risk of infection than the person who has a planned amputation. However, even planned amputations carry a risk of infection. The client who is older, has diabetes mellitus, or suffers peripheral neurovascular compromise is at a particularly high

Figure 41–13 ■ Stump dressings increase venous return, decrease edema, and help shape the stump for a prosthesis. With an above-knee amputation, a figure-eight bandage is started by bringing the bandage down over the stump and back up around the hips.

risk for infection. Infection may present itself locally or systemically. Local manifestations of infection include drainage, odor, redness and increased discomfort at the suture line. Systemic manifestations include fever, an increased heart rate, a decrease in blood pressure, chills, and positive wound or blood cultures.

Delayed Healing

If infection is present or if the circulation remains compromised, delayed healing (occuring at a slower rate than expected) will result. In older clients, other preexisting conditions can increase the risk of delayed healing. In clients of any age, electrolyte imbalances can contribute to delayed healing processes, as can a diet that lacks the proper nutrients to meet the body's increased metabolic demands during healing. Smoking compromises healing by causing vasoconstriction and decreasing blood flow to the stump. Deep venous thrombosis and compromised venous return, which may result from prolonged immobilization, are other potential factors. Decreased cardiac output decreases blood flow and thus also delays healing.

Chronic Stump Pain and Phantom Pain

Chronic stump pain is the result of neuroma formation, causing severe burning pain. Interventions to relieve this pain include medications, nerve blocks, transcutaneous electrical nerve stimulation (TENS), and surgical stump reconstruction. **Phantom limb pain** is not the same as phantom limb sensation. A majority of amputees experience phantom limb sensation (sensations such as tingling, numbness, cramping, or itching in the phantom foot or hand) early in the postoperative period. It is often self-limited, but may last for decades in some clients. When phantom limb sensation is painful, it is referred to as phantom limb pain. Although various theories have been proposed, the exact cause of this experience is unknown. Treatments include pain management, TENS, and a variety of surgical procedures. The management of phantom limb pain is difficult for both clients and

healthcare professionals. Clients with phantom limb pain often benefit from referral to a pain clinic for a comprehensive pain management program.

Contractures

A **contracture** is an abnormal flexion and fixation of a joint caused by muscle atrophy and shortening. Contracture of the joint above the amputation is a common complication. The client needs to be taught to extend the joint. The client with an above-the-knee amputation should lie prone for periods throughout the day. The client with a below-the-knee amputation should elevate the stump, keeping the knee extended. The same principles apply to the upper extremities. All joints should receive either active or passive ROM exercises every 2 to 4 hours. A trapeze frame should be added to the bed to encourage the client to change position every 2 hours. The client who has an upper extremity amputation should exercise both shoulders. Postural exercises can help prevent the client from hunching over secondary to the loss of weight on the affected side. The client with an above-the-knee amputation should not sit for prolonged periods of time; prolonged sitting can lead to hip contracture.

INTERDISCIPLINARY CARE

Interdisciplinary care is essential for the client who has sustained an amputation. Physical therapy and occupational retraining are necessary, and the client may also benefit from the presence of clergy. The entire healthcare team must view both the positive and the negative effects of amputation; that is, they must see amputation as a means to increase the client's independence and to relieve symptoms. The client should be able to become familiar with the members of the healthcare team and their roles; this allows the client greater control over his or her care and rehabilitation and promotes independence.

Diagnosis

Preoperatively, the client has routine laboratory and diagnostic tests (see Chapter 4 ∞ for care of the client having surgery). Preoperative tests, including Doppler flowmetry, segmental blood pressure determination, transcutaneous partial pressure oxygen readings, and angiography, are performed to assess the circulation present in the limb at different levels and to determine the level of viable tissue. Postoperative tests include CBC to monitor for hemorrhage, WBC count to monitor for infection, blood chemistries to evaluate electrolytes and fluid balance, and a vascular Doppler ultrasonography if a DVT is suspected.

Medications

The client receives medications preoperatively, intraoperatively, and postoperatively. Preoperatively, the physician may prescribe intravenous antibiotics. Intraoperatively, anesthetic agents are administered. It also may be necessary to administer agents to control blood pressure during the surgery. Postoperatively, the client resumes any routinely prescribed medications and in addition may receive antibiotics and analgesics. Steroids may be administered to decrease swelling. A histamine H_2 antagonist may also be ordered to decrease the risk of peptic ulcer formation. Stool softeners may be administered to prevent constipation.

Prosthesis

The type of prosthesis selected for the client with an amputation depends on the level of the amputation as well as the client's occupation and lifestyle. Each prosthesis is based on a detailed prosthetic prescription and is custom made for the client based on the specific characteristics of the stump. Most are made of plastic and foam materials. Many factors influence the client's use of the prosthesis, including the status of the remaining limb, cognitive status, cardiovascular status, preoperative activity level, and motivation to use the prosthesis.

Clients with a lower extremity amputation are often fitted with early walking aids. Pneumatic devices that fit over the stump are used in the immediate postoperative period to allow early ambulation, decreased postoperative swelling, and improved morale. Clients may begin weight bearing as soon as 2 weeks after surgery. Clients with upper extremity amputations may be fitted for a prosthesis immediately after surgery. Rehabilitation of the client with an amputation is a team effort, involving the client, nurse, physician, physical therapist, occupational therapist, social worker, prosthetist, and vocational counselor.

 ## NURSING CARE

Health Promotion

The goals of health promotion activities focus on preventing the progression of chronic diseases such as PVD and diabetes mellitus, and on safety. Clients with PVD from any cause need education about foot care and early recognition of decreased circulation. Education within both urban and rural populations should provide knowledge about working safely with lawn care equipment as well as farm and occupational machinery.

In addition, it is important that the public know what to do if a traumatic amputation occurs in the home, community, or workplace. The following guidelines may help preserve the amputated part until it can be surgically reattached:

- Keep the person in a prone position with the legs elevated.
- Apply firm pressure to the bleeding area, using a towel or article of clothing.
- Wrap the amputated part in a clean cloth. If possible, soak the cloth in saline (such as contact lens solution).
- Put the amputated part in a plastic bag and put the bag on ice. Do not let the amputated part come into direct contact with the ice or water.
- Send the amputated part to the emergency department with the injured person, and be sure the emergency personnel know what it is.

Assessment

Collect the following data through the health history and physical examination. Further focused assessments are described in the following nursing interventions sections.

- *Health History:* Mechanism of injury, current and past health problems, pain, occupation, ADLs, changes in sensation in the feet, cultural and/or religious guidelines for handling the amputated part.
- *Physical Examination:* Bilateral neurovascular status of the extremities, bilateral capillary refill time, skin over the lower extremities (discoloration, edema, ulcerations, hair, gangrene).

Nursing Diagnoses and Interventions

The goals of nursing care for a person with an amputation are to relieve pain, promote healing, prevent complications, support the client and family during the process of grieving and adaptation to alterations in body image, and restore mobility. Care is individualized, and the circumstances that led to the amputation (e.g., traumatic injury or disease) also must be addressed. (See the accompanying Nursing Care Plan on page 1425.) Applying rehabilitation principles to nursing care is also important.

Acute Pain

Pain from the surgical procedure can be compounded by muscle spasms, swelling, and phantom limb pain.

- Ask the client to rate the pain on a scale of 0 to 10 (with 10 as the most severe pain) before and after any intervention. *This facilitates objective assessment of the effectiveness of the chosen pain relief strategy. Pain that increases in intensity or remains unrelieved with analgesics can indicate compartment syndrome.*
- Splint and support the injured area. *Splinting prevents additional injury by immobilizing the stump and decreasing edema while molding the stump for a good prosthetic fit.*
- Unless contraindicated, elevate the stump on a pillow for the first 24 hours after surgery. *Elevating the stump promotes venous return and decreases edema, which will decrease pain.*

> **PRACTICE ALERT**
> Elevating the stump for long periods after the immediate postoperative period increases the risk for hip contractures.

- Move and turn the client gently and slowly. *Gentle moving and turning prevents the development of severe muscle spasms.*
- Administer pain medications as prescribed. A PCA pump may be ordered by the physician. *Analgesics alleviate pain by stimulating opiate receptor sites. PCA pumps increase client control over and allow early relief of pain before it intensifies.*
- Encourage deep breathing and relaxation exercises. *These techniques increase the effectiveness of analgesics and modify the pain experience.*
- Reposition client every 2 hours; turn from side to side and onto abdomen. *Repositioning alleviates pressure from one area and distributes it throughout the body and helps prevent cramping of muscles.*

> **PRACTICE ALERT**
> Lying prone prevents hip contracture.

Risk for Infection

The client who has an amputation is at risk for wound infection. Early recognition of infection can lead to early treatment and prevent wound dehiscence.

NURSING CARE PLAN A Client with a Below-the-Knee Amputation

John Rocke is a 45-year-old divorcee with no children. He has a history of type 1 diabetes mellitus and poor control of blood glucose levels. Mr. Rocke is unemployed and currently receives unemployment compensation. He lives alone in a second-floor apartment. Mr. Rocke had developed gangrene in the foot and failed to seek prompt medical attention; as a result, a left below-the-knee amputation was necessary.

Mr. Rocke is in his second postoperative day and his vital signs are stable. The stump is splinted and has a soft dressing. The wound is approximating well without signs of infection. He has not performed ROM exercises or turning since his surgery, complaining of severe pain. When the nurse goes into the room, he yells, "Get out! I don't want anyone to see me like this." No one has visited him since his hospitalization. He is tolerating an 1800-kcal diabetic diet and is using a urinal independently. He has an order for meperidine (Demerol), 100 mg IM every 4 hours prn for pain, and cefazolin (Ancef), 1 g IV every 8 hours. He is on blood glucose coverage with regular insulin subcutaneously.

ASSESSMENT

Jane Simmons, RN, has just come on duty. She notes that the client is upset and angry. Mr. Rocke will not let anyone enter the room to give him medication or assess his vital signs.

DIAGNOSES

- *Disturbed Body Image* related to amputation of left lower leg
- *Dysfunctional Grieving* related to anger and loss of left lower leg
- *Situational Low Self-Esteem* related to appearance
- *Risk for Injury from Infection and Contractures* related to refusal of care
- *Acute Pain* related to surgery

EXPECTED OUTCOMES

- Verbalize his feelings about the amputation.
- Allow the staff to monitor his vital signs and administer medications.
- Be allowed to control his pain with a PCA pump.
- Verbalize a decrease in pain.
- Verbalize the importance of turning.
- Turn every 2 hours.

PLANNING AND IMPLEMENTATION

- Encourage verbalization of feelings.
- Actively listen to the client.
- Offer to arrange a visit with a fellow amputee.
- Ask the physician if the client can be placed on a PCA pump.
- Teach the client the importance of turning every 2 hours to prevent contractures.
- Encourage turning and lying prone.
- Teach the importance of antibiotics in preventing and treating infection.

EVALUATION

One week after his surgery, Mr. Rocke is actively participating in his care. He has apologized for his behavior and has explained to Ms. Simmons that he was angry about the loss of his leg. He states, "I thought I knew what to expect but I didn't."

CRITICAL THINKING IN THE NURSING PROCESS

1. Once Mr. Rocke is ready to assist with his stump care, how would you proceed? Would you give him full responsibility for care and dressings, or would you gradually increase his participation? Why?
2. What factors in Mr. Rocke's home environment and medical history may make self-care more difficult? Do you expect Mr. Rocke to follow up on care after his discharge? Why or why not?
3. Mr. Rocke states, "Why should I exercise this leg—it was already cut off!" How would you respond? What is the purpose of exercising the stump?

See Evaluating Your Response in Appendix C.

- Assess the wound for redness, drainage, temperature, edema, and suture line approximation. *Redness is normal in the immediate postoperative period; if it persists, however, it can indicate infection. A hot area that is palpated over the incision or increased drainage may also indicate infection.*
- Take the client's temperature every 4 hours. *Increased body temperature may indicate infection.*
- Monitor WBC count. *The WBC count rises in the presence of infection.*
- Use aseptic technique to change the wound dressing. *Aseptic technique prevents the contamination of the wound with bacteria.*
- Administer antibiotics as ordered. *Antibiotics inhibit bacterial cell replication and help prevent or eradicate infection.*
- Teach the client stump-wrapping techniques. *Correctly wrapping the stump from the distal to proximal extremity increases venous return and prevents pooling of fluid, thereby reducing the chance of infection.*

Risk for Impaired Skin Integrity

Stump care is essential, not only in the postoperative healing period, but also throughout life with a prosthesis. A variety of skin problems may be caused by a prosthesis, including epidermoid cysts, abrasions, blisters, and hair follicle infections. The client must be taught stump care prior to discharge.

- Each day, preferably at night, wash the stump with soap and warm water and dry thoroughly. Inspect the stump for redness, irritation, or abrasions. *It is essential to maintain intact skin to ensure successful use of the prosthesis.*
- Massage the end of the stump, beginning 3 weeks after surgery. *Massage helps desensitize the remaining part of the limb and prevents scar tissue formation. If the skin adheres to the underlying tissue, it will tear when stressed by wearing a prosthesis.*
- Expose any open areas of skin on the remaining part of the limb for 1 hour four times a day. *Air exposure promotes healing.*

■ Change stump socks and elastic wraps each day. Wash these in mild soap and water, and allow to completely dry before using again. *Stump socks and elastic wraps must be kept clean and dry to prevent skin breakdown.*

Risk for Dysfunctional Grieving

The client who has lost an extremity is at risk for dysfunctional grieving. Denial of the need for surgery and the inability to discuss feelings compound this risk.

■ Encourage verbalization of feelings, using open-ended questions. *Asking open-ended questions allows the client to discuss feelings and communicates the listener's willingness to listen.*

■ Actively listen and maintain eye contact. *Active listening and eye contact communicate respect for what the client is expressing.*

■ Reflect on the client's feelings. *Reflection statements such as "You seem angry" allow the client to recognize feelings and perhaps develop a plan for resolution.*

■ Allow the client to have unlimited visiting hours, if possible. *Unlimited visiting hours allow increased social support.*

■ If desired by the client, provide spiritual support by encouraging activities such as visits from a spiritual leader, prayer, and meditation. *These activities often provide support during the grieving process.*

Disturbed Body Image

Although amputation is a reconstructive surgery, the client's body image will be disturbed. Risk for body image disturbance is higher in young trauma clients, in whom body image is a particularly important component of self-image.

■ Encourage verbalization of feelings. *This allows the client to communicate concerns and fears and lets the client know the nurse is willing to listen.*

■ Allow the client to wear clothing from home. *Familiar clothing provides emotional comfort and helps the client retain a sense of his or her own identity.*

■ Encourage the client to look at the stump. *Looking at and touching the stump helps the client face his or her fear of the unknown and move from denial to acceptance.*

■ Encourage the client to care for the stump. *Active participation in care increases self-esteem and independence.*

■ Offer to have a fellow amputee visit the client. *A support person who has experienced the same change gives the client the hope that he or she can regain independence.*

■ Encourage active participation in rehabilitation. *Active participation in rehabilitation increases independence and mobility.*

Impaired Physical Mobility

If time allows, the client should begin strengthening muscles preoperatively. If the amputation is the result of an emergency, exercises begin within 24 to 48 hours of surgery. The return of independent mobility boosts self-esteem and promotes adaptation to amputation.

■ Perform ROM exercises on all joints. *ROM exercises help prevent the development of joint contractures that limit mobility.*

■ Maintain postoperative stump shrinkage devices. These may be elastic bandages, shrinker socks, an elastic stockinette, or

a rigid plaster cast. *Postoperative dressings decrease edema and shape the stump for prosthetic wear.*

■ Turn and reposition the client every 2 hours. *The client with a lower extremity amputation should lie prone every 4 hours. Repositioning increases blood flow to muscles, forces synovial fluid into joints, and helps prevent contractures.*

■ Reinforce teaching by the physical therapist in crutch walking or the use of assistive devices. *These devices increase mobility by balancing the client and facilitating ambulation.*

■ Encourage active participation in physical therapy. *Physical therapy will fatigue the client in the early stage of healing. Encouragement may increase the client's participation in the physical therapy regimen and thereby increase activity tolerance.*

Using NANDA, NIC, and NOC

Chart 41–2 shows links between NANDA nursing diagnoses, NIC, and NOC when caring for the client with an amputation.

Community-Based Care

Client and family teaching includes stump care, prosthesis fitting and care, medications, assistive devices, exercises, rehabilitation, counseling, support services, and follow-up appointments. The depth of teaching depends on the cause and site of the amputation and the needs of the client. See the Meeting Individualized Needs box on the next page.

Holistic nursing care is especially important for the older client with an amputation. The normal aging process decreases

NANDA, NIC, and NOC LINKAGES
CHART 41–2 The Client with an Amputation

NANDA

Disturbed Body Image

↓

NIC

Amputation Care

Wound Care

Grief Work Facilitation

Coping Enhancement

Body Image Enhancement

↓

NOC

Grief Resolution

Body Image

Data from *NANDA's Nursing Diagnoses: Definitions & Classification 2005–2006* by NANDA International (2005), Philadelphia; *Nursing Interventions Classification (NIC)* (4th ed.) by J. M. Dochterman & G. M. Bulechek (2004), St. Louis, MO: Mosby; and *Nursing Outcomes Classification (NOC)* (3rd ed.) by S. Moorhead, M. Johnson, and M. Maas (2004), St. Louis, MO: Mosby.

MEETING INDIVIDUALIZED NEEDS The Client with an Amputation

Amputation of a limb has significant long-term consequences for the client. The client will grieve the loss of a body part and must adjust to a new self-image. The client's ability to perform normal ADLs and to maintain his or her usual family and social roles may be significantly affected, at least initially. Depending on the client's occupation, job performance may be affected, necessitating a change of career.

The nurse may be responsible for involving multiple members of the healthcare team in the client's care and rehabilitation and coordinating their activities. Following an amputation, the client may need the services of any or all of the following:

- Social services to help with rehabilitative and financial arrangements
- Physical therapists to teach ambulation techniques, and to provide deep heat or massage
- Occupational therapists to assist the client in developing adaptive techniques to deal with the loss of a limb
- Prosthetists to develop a prosthesis for the missing limb that will meet the client's needs for ADLs and other activities
- Home health services for nursing care such as assessments and wound care
- Support group services to assist in adapting to the body image change and effects of amputation on ADLs.

ASSESSING FOR HOME CARE
Preparing the amputee for home care includes a careful assessment of the client family and support services, and the home for possible barriers to the client's safety and independence.

Assess the client's acceptance of the amputation and knowledge base about care needs, any activity restrictions or special needs, and resources for home care. Discuss home management—who is responsible for household activities such as cleaning and cooking. Inquire about arrangements that have been made for home care activities and ADLs. Evaluate the client's use of prescription and nonprescription medications, paying particular attention to possible in-

teractions and drugs that may affect the client's balance, mental alertness, or appetite. Ask about social habits, such as cigarette smoking, alcohol use, or other drug use, that may affect healing or the client's ability to provide self-care.

Assess the client's home environment for possible safety hazards or barriers to ambulation, such as:

- Scatter rugs
- Stairs between living areas of the house
- Presence of grab bars to facilitate toileting and bathing
- Access to clean water and other needs for wound care.

TEACHING FOR HOME CARE
The new amputee needs a great deal of teaching to learn to adapt to loss of a limb, whether it is an upper or lower extremity that has been lost. Because the client must be ready to learn before teaching can be effective, use therapeutic communication techniques to encourage the client to verbalize feelings about the amputation and its effects. Use active listening and teach the client ways to reduce anxiety and deal with feelings of helplessness and loss. Encourage the client to participate in care of the stump to build self-esteem and reinforce teaching. Include the following in teaching for home care:

- Teach the client to wrap the stump appropriately in preparation for fitting the prosthesis.
- Discuss positioning of the stump. Contractures are a particular problem for clients with an above-knee amputation, and can interfere with ability to effectively use a prosthesis.
- Teach the client how to perform stump exercises to maintain joint mobility and muscle tone of the affected limb.
- Encourage the client to resume physical activities as soon as possible. This improves the client's health and well-being, as well as the client's self-esteem.
- Discuss household modifications to promote independence, such as grab bars in the bathroom, faucets with single-handle controls for water flow and temperature, and handheld shower heads and shower chairs for bathing.

---

renal and liver function; hence, medications have longer half-lives. Altered circulation prolongs wound healing, and slowing of reflexes and alterations in gait may disrupt balance. A walker may be more appropriate than crutches, because older clients have less strength in the upper extremities. Safety issues, such as decreasing the risk for recurrent falls, must be addressed. The nurse should also assess the client's need for in-home assistance and make appropriate referrals to visiting nurses and home health aides.

In addition, suggest the following resources:
- The Amputee Coalition of America
- Amputee Resource Foundation of America.

THE CLIENT WITH A REPETITIVE USE INJURY

Repeatedly twisting and turning the wrist, pronating and supinating the forearm, kneeling, or raising arms over the head can result in repetitive use injuries. Clients with repetitive use injuries

pose a challenge to the healthcare team. Often these clients appear puzzled as they relate a history of manifestations that have worsened over time. They deny abrupt trauma and often worry about the ability to return to work. Repetitive use injuries are common. The number of worker's compensation claims for repetitive use injuries is steadily growing. The increase is believed to be a result of technology advances in the workplace.

Pathophysiology

Common repetitive use injuries include carpal tunnel syndrome, bursitis, and epicondylitis.

Carpal Tunnel Syndrome
The carpal tunnel is a canal through which flexor tendons and the median nerve pass from the wrist to the hand. The syndrome develops from narrowing of the tunnel and irritation of the median nerve. Carpal tunnel syndrome involves compression of the median nerve as a result of inflammation and swelling of the synovial lining of the tendon sheaths. The client complains of numbness and tingling of the thumb, index finger,

and lateral ventral surface of the middle finger. The client may also complain of pain in this area that interferes with sleep and is alleviated by shaking or massaging the hand and fingers. The affected hand may become weak and the client may be unable to hold utensils or perform activities that require precision.

Carpal tunnel syndrome is one of the three most common work-related injuries. The incidence is believed to be related directly to the number of people using computers. The incidence of carpal tunnel syndrome is higher in women, especially postmenopausal women.

Bursitis

Bursitis is an inflammation of a bursa. A bursa is an enclosed sac found between muscles, tendons, and bony prominences. The bursae that commonly become inflamed are in the shoulder, hip, knee, and elbow. Constant friction between the bursa and the musculoskeletal tissue around it causes irritation, edema, and inflammation. Manifestations develop as the sac becomes engorged. The area around the sac is tender, and extension and flexion of the joint near the bursa produce pain. The inflamed bursa is hot, red, and edematous. The client guards the joint to decrease pain and may point to the area of the bursa when identifying joint tenderness.

Epicondylitis

Epicondylitis is the inflammation of the tendon at its point of origin into the bone. Epicondylitis is also referred to as *tennis elbow* or *golfer's elbow*. The exact pathophysiology of epicondylitis is unknown. Current theories attribute inflammation of the tendon to microvascular trauma. Tears, bleeding, and edema are thought to cause avascularization and calcification of the tendon. Manifestations of epicondylitis include point tenderness, pain radiating down the dorsal surface of the forearm, and a history of repetitive use.

INTERDISCIPLINARY CARE

Medical management of repetitive use disorders focuses on relieving pain and increasing mobility. Once the diagnosis is made, treatment can range from conservative measures, such as rest and pharmacologic agents, to aggressive measures such as surgery.

Diagnosis

Carpal tunnel syndrome is diagnosed by the client's history and physical examination. The history may reveal an occupation that involves areas such as computer work, jackhammer operation, mechanical work, or gymnastics. History of a radial bone fracture or rheumatoid arthritis also increases the risk of carpal tunnel syndrome. Tests specific for carpal tunnel include the Phalen test (see Chapter 40). Bursitis and epicondylitis are diagnosed by history and physical examination.

Medications

The client with a repetitive use injury usually receives NSAIDs. Narcotics also may be administered for acute flare-ups and severe pain. For the client who has epicondylitis or carpal tunnel syndrome, corticosteroids may be injected into the joint.

Treatments

Treatment of repetitive use injuries is performed first by conservative management, followed, if necessary, by surgery.

CONSERVATIVE MANAGEMENT The first steps in the care of all repetitive use injuries are to immobilize and rest the involved joint. The joint may be splinted, and ice may be applied (as described in Table 41–1) in the first 24 to 48 hours to decrease pain and inflammation. Ice application may be followed by heat application every 4 hours.

SURGERY Surgery is usually reserved for the client who does not obtain relief with conservative treatment. Surgery for carpal tunnel syndrome includes resection of the carpal ligament to enlarge the tunnel. In epicondylitis and bursitis, calcified deposits may be removed from the area surrounding the tendon or bursa.

NURSING CARE

The nursing care of a client with a repetitive use injury focuses on relieving pain, teaching about the disease process and treatment, and improving physical mobility.

Nursing Diagnoses and Interventions

Acute Pain

Swelling and nerve inflammation cause pain in the client with a repetitive use injury.

- Ask the client to rate the pain on a scale of 0 to 10 (with 10 being the most severe pain) before and after any intervention. *This facilitates objective assessment of the effectiveness of the chosen pain relief strategy.*
- Encourage the use of immobilizers. *Splinting maintains joint alignment and prevents pain due to movement of inflamed tissues.*
- Teach the client to apply ice and/or heat as prescribed. *Ice causes vasoconstriction and decreases the pooling of blood in the inflamed area. Ice may also numb the tender area. Heat decreases swelling by increasing venous return.*
- Encourage use of NSAIDs as prescribed. *NSAIDs decrease swelling by inhibiting prostaglandins.*
- Explain why treatment should not be abruptly discontinued. *Abrupt discontinuation of treatment may cause reinflammation of the injured area.*

Impaired Physical Mobility

Joint pain and swelling can impair mobility.

- Suggest interventions to alleviate pain (such as using an immobilizer and taking pain medications). *If the joint is pain free, the client will be more likely to take an active role in therapy.*
- Refer to a physical therapist for exercises. *The physical therapist can assist the client with exercise to prevent joint stiffness.*
- Suggest consultation with an occupational therapist. *Occupational therapy can help the client learn new ways to perform tasks to prevent recurring symptoms.*

Community-Based Care

Address the following topics for home care:

- Causes of and treatments for repetitive use injury.
- Rehabilitation to allow the client to return to a state of independence.
- Ways to avoid unnecessary exposure to the activities that increase risk of redeveloping the injury. Suggest evaluation of

the client's work environment by an environmental risk manager who can prescribe measures to reduce the risk of repetitive use injuries. Wrist supports or an ergonomic keyboard may be useful for the client who uses a computer extensively. Appropriate desk and chair height also are important in maintaining the correct anatomic position while working.

- Information about sources for braces or other assistive devices.

EXPLORE MediaLink

Prentice Hall Nursing MediaLink DVD-ROM
Audio Glossary
NCLEX-RN® Review

Animation/Video
Bone Healing
Crutch Instruction

COMPANION WEBSITE www.prenhall.com/lemone
Audio Glossary
NCLEX-RN® Review
Care Plan Activity: Below-the-Knee Amputation
Case Study: A Client with Fractures
MediaLink Applications
  Compartment Syndrome
  Preventing Musculoskeletal Injuries
Links to Resources

CHAPTER HIGHLIGHTS

- The most commonly reported musculoskeletal injuries are contusions, strains, and sprains. Immediate treatment includes RICE (rest, ice, compression, elevation) therapy.
- Dislocations may be congenital, traumatic, or pathologic. Nursing assessments include monitoring neurovascular status by assessing for increased pain, decreased or absent pulses, pale skin, inability to move a body part or extremity, and changes in sensation.
- Any of the 206 bones of the body may sustain a fracture. Fractures are closed or simple (skin is intact) or open or compound (skin integrity is interrupted); open fractures are at risk for infection. Other fracture descriptors include oblique or spiral, avulsed, comminuted, compressed, impacted, or depressed.
- Fractures heal through three phases: inflammatory, reparative, and remodeling. Healing is influenced by the age and physical condition of the client and by the type of fracture.
- Fracture complications include compartment syndrome, fat embolism syndrome, deep venous thrombosis, infection, delayed union and nonunion, and reflex sympathetic dystrophy.

- Fractures are treated with surgery, traction, and/or casts to stabilize the fractured bone, maintain bone immobilization, prevent complications, and restore function.
- Fractures of the hip are most often sustained by older adult women, and are usually the result of a fall. They are the most common injury in the older population, resulting in the greatest number of deaths and most serious health problems of all fractures for people age 65 years and older.
- Nursing care for the client with a fracture focuses on interventions for acute pain, risk for peripheral vascular dysfunction, risk for infection, impaired physical mobility, and risk for disturbed tactile sensory perception.
- An amputation is the partial or total removal of an extremity. This loss has a significant physical and psychosocial effect on the client and on the family. The most common cause for amputation of a lower extremity is peripheral vascular disease. Trauma is the most common cause for upper extremity amputation.
- Complications that may follow an amputation include infection, delayed healing, chronic stump pain, phantom pain, and

contractures. Stump care is necessary to prevent complications and to prepare the stump for a prosthesis.

■ Nursing care for the client with an amputation is provided as part of the interdisciplinary team, and is focused on a return to functional health, with interventions to meet needs for acute pain,

impaired skin integrity, grieving, disturbed body image, and impaired physical mobility.

■ Repetitive use injuries, especially common in the workplace, include carpal tunnel syndrome, bursitis, and epicondylitis.

TEST YOURSELF NCLEX-RN® REVIEW

1 You are teaching a young adult how to provide self-care for a sprained ankle. You explain that the reason for applying ice immediately after the injury is based on the principle that ice:
1. increases the diameter of blood vessels.
2. decreases the diameter of blood vessels.
3. is helpful in increasing white blood cells.
4. lowers the blood pressure and pulse.

2 A client with a compound, open fracture has been admitted to the emergency department and is scheduled for immediate surgery. Which of the following nursing diagnoses would be most appropriate in the immediate postoperative period?
1. *Risk for Post-Trauma Syndrome*
2. *Impaired Transfer Ability*
3. *Risk for Infection*
4. *Risk for Falls*

3 While providing care to an older woman with a cast on her left lower arm (from below the elbow to above the fingers), you perform a neurovascular assessment. Which of the following assessments indicates a possible complication?
1. slightly edematous fingers
2. warm, pink skin above the cast
3. pale, cold fingers
4. pain rating of 2 on a 1 to 10 scale

4 Which of the following minerals is essential to bone healing?
1. potassium
2. magnesium
3. sodium
4. calcium

5 You are assessing a young man with a newly applied long-leg cast. He complains of extreme pain in his leg, and his toes are cyanotic and lack sensation. What is your priority intervention?
1. Document the assessments carefully and accurately.
2. Notify the healthcare provider who applied the cast.
3. Elevate the leg on at least three pillows.
4. Apply an ice bag over the painful area.

6 Your assigned client has been diagnosed with DVT of the left lower extremity. What body system would require very careful monitoring?
1. hematologic
2. respiratory
3. digestive
4. renal

7 Although nursing diagnoses are always individualized, what is one nursing diagnosis common to all musculoskeletal injuries?
1. *Disturbed Body Image*
2. *Acute Pain*
3. *Chronic Pain*
4. *Risk for Infection*

8 At what position would you place the remaining extremity following a below-the-knee amputation during the first 24 hours after surgery?
1. elevated above the level of the heart
2. lower than the rest of the body
3. crossed over the intact extremity
4. level with the rest of the body

9 The day following a below-the-knee amputation, your client tells you that he feels as though his toes are cramping in the amputated foot. What is this experience called?
1. chronic stump pain
2. contractures
3. attention-seeking
4. phantom limb pain

10 Your husband is cutting wood with a circular saw. He suddenly screams that he has cut off his finger. What would you do with the amputated finger?
1. Don't worry about it; the important thing is to get him to the hospital.
2. Put it in a storage bag filled with warm water.
3. Tape it to his hand so the emergency personnel will know where it is.
4. Wrap it in a towel, put it in a plastic bag, and lay it on ice.

See Test Yourself answers in Appendix C.

BIBLIOGRAPHY

Altizer, L. (2003a). Forearm and humeral fractures. *Orthopaedic Nursing, 22*(4), 266–273.

_____. (2003b). Hand and wrist fractures. *Orthopaedic Nursing, 22*(3), 232–239.

_____. (2004a). Casting for immobilization. *Orthopaedic Nursing, 23*(2), 1135–1141.

_____. (2004b). Compartment syndrome. *Orthopaedic Nursing, 23*(6), 391–396.

Assessment of a limb in a cast. (2003). *Nursing Times, 99*(31), 27.

Bergland, A., & Wyller, T. (2004). Risk factors for serious fall related injury in elderly women living at home. *Injury Prevention, 10*(5), 308–313.

Bongiovanni, M., Bradley, S., & Kelley, D. (2005). Orthopedic trauma: Critical care nursing issues. *Critical Care Nursing Quarterly, 28*(1), 60–71.

Brunner, L., Eshilian-Oates, L., & Kuo, T. (2003). Hip fractures in adults. *American Family Physician, 67*(3). Retrieved from http://www.aafp.org/afp/wooeoeow/53l7.html

Burgess, B., & Sennett, B. (2003). Traumatic shoulder instability: Nonsurgical management versus surgical intervention. *Orthopaedic Nursing, 22*(5), 345–352.

Centers for Disease Control and Prevention. (2005). Bone health. Retrieved from http://www.cdc.gov/nccdphp/dnpa/bonehealth/

Childs, S. (2003). Stimulators of bone healing: Biologic and biomechanical. *Orthopaedic Nursing, 22*(6), 421–428.

Cole, E. (2004). Assessment and management of the trauma patient. *Nursing Standard, 18*(41), 45–52, 54.

Clontz, A., Annonio, D., & Walker, L. (2004). Trauma nursing: Amputation. *RN, 67*(7), 38–44.

Davis, P. (2004). Venous thromboembolism prevention—an update. *Journal of Orthopaedic Nursing, 8*(1), 50–56.

Dochterman, J., & Bulechek, G. (2004). *Nursing interventions classification (NIC)* (4th ed.). St. Louis, MO: Mosby.

Feury, K. (2003). Injury prevention: Where are the resources? *Orthopaedic Nursing, 22*(2), 124–130.

Harris, H. (2004). Action stat. Fat embolism. *Nursing, 34*(6), 96.

Harvey, C. (2005). Wound healing. *Orthopaedic Nursing, 24*(2), 143–160.

Hip fracture. Information about a broken hip. (2004). Retrieved from http://orthopedics.about.com/cs/hipsurgery/a/brokenhip.htm

Holmes, S., & Brown, S. (2005). Skeletal pin site care. National Association of Orthopaedic Nurses guidelines for orthopaedic nursing. *Orthopaedic Nursing, 24*(2), 99–108.

Houghton, K., Peregrina, M., Gillies, D., & Herden, J. (2003). A small trial of the nursing care of patients immobilized with a Thomas splint. *Journal of Orthopaedic Nursing, 7*(4), 201–204.

Kasper, C., Talbot, L., & Gaines, J. (2002). Skeletal muscle damage and recovery. *AACN Clinical Issues: Advanced Practice in Acute and Critical Care, 13*(2), 237–241.

Kass-Wolff, J. (2004). Calcium in women: Healthy bones and much more. *Journal of Obstetrics, Gynecologic, and Neonatal Nursing, 33*(1), 21–33.

Little, D., & Alper, B. (2004). Ankle sprain. *Clinical Advisor, 7*(11), 56, 61–62.

Love, C. (2003). Carpal tunnel syndrome. *Journal of Orthopaedic Nursing, 7*(1), 33–42.

Mayo Clinic. (2006). *Dislocation; first aid.* Retrieved from http://health/first-aid-dislocation/FA0009www.mayoclinic.com

McConnel, E. (2002). Assessing neurovascular status in a casted limb. *Nursing, 32*(9), 20.

Miller, R. L. S. (2003). Reflex sympathetic dystrophy. *Orthopaedic Nursing, 22*(2), 91–101.

Moorhead, S., Johnson, M., & Maas, M. (2003). *Nursing outcomes classification (NOC)* (3rd ed.). St. Louis, Mo: Mosby.

Moss Rehab Resource Net. (2005). *Amputation fact sheet.* Retrieved from http://www.mossresourcenet.org/amputa.htm

_____. (2004). *Falls and hip fractures among older adults.* Retrieved from http://www.cdc.gov/ncipc/factsheets/falls.htm

National Center for Injury Prevention and Control. (2006). *Falls and hip fractures among older adults.* Retrieved from http://www.cdc.gov/ncipc/factsheets/falls.htm

National Institute of Arthritis and Musculoskeletal and Skin Diseases. (2004). *Questions and answers about sprains and strains.* Retrieved from http://www.niams.nih.gov/hi/topics/strain_sprain/strain_sprain.htm

NANDA International. (2005). *Nursing diagnoses: Definitions & classification 2005–2006.* Philadelphia: Author.

Porth, C. M. (2005). *Pathophysiology: Concepts of altered health states* (7th ed.). Philadelphia: Lippincott.

Proehl, J. (2004). Emergency. Accidental amputation: A frightening injury requiring quick action. *American Journal of Nursing, 104*(2), 50–53.

Reed, D. (2004). Understanding and meeting the needs of farmers with amputations. *Orthopaedic Nursing, 23*(6), 397–405.

Ruddick, S., & Scollen, C. (2003). Fracture prevention in the frail elderly. *Practice Nurse, 14*(8), 361–366.

Shannon, M., Wilson, B., & Stang, C. (2005). *Nurse's drug guide 2005.* Upper Saddle River, NJ: Prentice Hall.

Siddle, L. (2004). The challenge and management of phantom limb pain after amputation. *British Journal of Nursing, 13*(11), 664–667.

Taggart, H., Mincer, A., & Thompson, A. (2004). Caring for the orthopaedic patient who is obese. *Orthopaedic Nursing, 23*(3), 204–210.

Tierney, L., McPhee, S., & Papadakis, M. (Eds.). (2004). *Current medical diagnosis & treatment* (43rd ed.). Stamford, CT: Appleton & Lange.

Vestergaard, P., Emborg, C., Stoving, R., Hagen, C., Mosekilde, L., & Briken, K. (2003). Patients with eating disorders: A high-risk group for fractures. *Orthopaedic Nursing, 22*(5), 325–331.

Walls, M. (2002). Orthopedic trauma. *RN, 65*(7), 53–56.

Wilkinson, J. (2005). *Prentice Hall nursing diagnosis handbook with NIC interventions and NOC outcomes* (8th ed.). Upper Saddle River, NJ: Prentice Hall.

Wilson, B., Shannon, M., & Stang, C. (2005). *Prentice Hall nurse's drug guide 2005.* Upper Saddle River, NJ: Prentice Hall.

Young, T. (2004). The healing of amputation wounds. *Nursing Standard, 18*(45), 74, 76, 78.

CHAPTER 42 Nursing Care of Clients with Musculoskeletal Disorders

LEARNING OUTCOMES

- Explain the pathophysiology, manifestations, complications, inter-disciplinary care, and nursing care of metabolic, degenerative, autoimmune, inflammatory, infectious, neoplastic, connective tissue, and structural musculoskeletal disorders.

- Compare and contrast the pathophysiology, manifestations, diagnosis, and treatments for osteoporosis, osteoarthritis, Paget's disease, and rheumatoid arthritis.

- Discuss the purposes, nursing implications, and health education for the client and family for medications used to treat osteoporosis, Paget's disease, gout, osteomalacia, osteoarthritis, rheumatoid arthritis, systemic lupus erythematosus, osteomyelitis, bone tumors, scleroderma, and low back pain.

- Describe the surgical procedures used to treat clients with arthritis.

CLINICAL COMPETENCIES

- Assess functional status of clients with musculoskeletal disorders, and monitor, document, and report abnormal manifestations.

- Use evidence-based research to assess clients at risk for osteoporosis and to evaluate the effectiveness of Internet use to teach older adults with rheumatoid arthritis.

- Determine priority nursing diagnoses, based on assessed data, to select and implement individualized nursing interventions for clients with musculoskeletal disorders.

- Administer topical, oral, and injectable medications used to treat musculoskeletal disorders knowledgeably and safely.

- Provide skilled care of clients having a surgical debridement for osteomyelitis and a total joint replacement.

- Integrate interdisciplinary care into care of clients with musculoskeletal disorders.

- Provide teaching appropriate for community-based self-care of musculoskeletal disorders.

- Revise plan of care as needed to provide effective interventions to promote, maintain, or restore functional health status to clients with musculoskeletal disorders.

MEDIALINK

Resources for this chapter can be found on the Prentice Hall Nursing MediaLink DVD-ROM accompanying this textbook, and on the Companion Website at http://www.prenhall.com/lemone

Various metabolic, degenerative, autoimmune, inflammatory, infectious, neoplastic, connective tissue, and structural disorders may affect the musculoskeletal system. Many of these diseases have significant physical, psychosocial, and financial consequences. When these problems occur, clients experience a variety of individualized responses to their altered health status. Nursing care is directed toward meeting physiologic needs, providing education, and ensuring psychologic support for the client and family.

Arthritis refers to inflammation of the joints, while **rheumatic disorders** refer to diseases of the muscles and bones as well as the joints. These diseases affect not only the joints but also the connective tissues of the body. The various types of arthritis are discussed in this chapter in different sections, depending on the primary etiology of the disorder. Arthritis and other rheumatic disorders are widespread, affecting about 70

million people in the United States (Flynn & Johnson, 2005). Arthritic disorders are a leading cause of disability; however, their very prevalence may lead the public and healthcare professionals to treat them as normal aging processes or discount the validity of the pain and disability experienced by the person with arthritis.

There are more than 100 different types of arthritis, but the most common are osteoarthritis, rheumatoid arthritis, systemic lupus erythematosus, and gout (Moss Rehab Resource Net, 2005). The etiology of most rheumatic disorders is not clear; in many cases, the pathophysiologic processes involved are often complex and poorly understood. Many are primary disorders; others occur as secondary processes associated with another disease. The wear and tear of aging, autoimmune processes, metabolic disorders, genetic factors, and infection are also implicated as causative factors in some forms of rheumatic disease.

METABOLIC BONE DISORDERS

Metabolic bone disorders originate in the bone remodeling process, which normally involves a sequence of events of bone reabsorption and formation. In the adult, this process is primarily internal remodeling through replacement of trabecular bone. Adults replace about 25% of trabecular bone every 4 months through reabsorption of old bone by osteoclasts and formation of new bone by osteoblasts (Porth, 2005). Metabolic bone disorders may result from a variety of factors, including aging, calcium and phosphate imbalances, genetics, and changes in levels of hormones.

THE CLIENT WITH OSTEOPOROSIS

Osteoporosis, literally defined as "porous bones," is a metabolic bone disorder characterized by loss of bone mass, increased bone fragility, and an increased risk of fractures. The reduced bone mass is caused by an imbalance of the processes that influence bone growth and maintenance. Although osteoporosis may result from an endocrine disorder or malignancy, it is most often associated with aging.

The National Osteoporosis Foundation (2006) has found that osteoporosis is a health threat for an estimated 44 million Americans; 10 million people have osteoporosis and 34 million have low bone mass, increasing their risk for the disease. Although osteoporosis can occur at any age and in both men and women, 80% of those with osteoporosis are women. One in two women

and one in four men over age 50 will have an osteoporosis-related fracture in his or her remaining lifetime.

Risk Factors

The risk of developing osteoporosis depends on how much bone mass is achieved between ages 25 and 35, and how much is lost later. Certain diseases, lifestyle habits, and ethnic backgrounds increase the risk of developing osteoporosis (see Focus on Cultural Diversity on page 1434). Different variables affect one's risk of osteoporosis—some can be modified and others cannot. The risk factors are summarized in Box 42–1.

BOX 42–1 Risk Factors for Osteoporosis

- A family history of osteoporosis
- Personal history of fracture after age 50
- Current low bone mass
- History of fracture in a first-degree relative
- Being female, especially Caucasian or Asian
- Being thin and/or having a small frame
- Menopause-associated low estrogen levels
- Low testosterone levels in men
- Dietary: low lifetime calcium intake, vitamin D deficiency
- Medication use: anticonvulsants, corticosteroids
- Lifestyle: inactivity, cigarette smoking, excess alcohol
- Presence of certain chronic diseases

Unmodifiable Risk Factors

Both men and women are susceptible to osteoporosis as they age, because the osteoblasts and osteoclasts undergo alterations that diminish their activity. Women have a significantly higher risk for manifestations and complications of osteoporosis because their peak bone mass is 10% to 15% less than that of men. In addition, age-related bone loss begins earlier and proceeds more rapidly in women, beginning in their 30s and accelerating before menopause. Estrogen in women and testosterone in men appear to help prevent bone loss; decreasing levels of these hormones associated with aging contribute to bone loss. Age-related bone loss in men occurs 15 to 20 years later than in women and at a slower rate.

European Americans and Asians are at a higher risk for osteoporosis than African Americans, who have greater bone density (bone mass positively correlates with the amount of skin pigmentation). Premature osteoporosis is increasing in female athletes, who have a greater incidence of eating disorders and amenorrhea. Poor nutrition and intense physical training can result in a deficient production of estrogen. Decreased estrogen, combined with a lack of calcium and vitamin D, results in a loss of bone density (Porth, 2005).

Clients who have an endocrine disorder such as hyperthyroidism, hyperparathyroidism, Cushing's syndrome, or diabetes mellitus are at high risk for osteoporosis. These disorders affect the metabolism, in turn affecting nutritional status and bone mineralization.

Modifiable Risk Factors

Modifiable risk factors include behaviors that place a person at risk for developing osteoporosis, as well as physical changes such as menopause whose contribution to osteoporosis can be modified by preventive strategies. Calcium deficiency is an important modifiable risk factor contributing to osteoporosis. Calcium is an essential mineral in the process of bone formation and other significant body functions. When there is an insufficient intake of calcium in the diet, the body compensates by removing calcium from the skeleton, weakening bone tissue. Acidosis, which may result from a high-protein diet, contributes to osteoporosis in two ways. Calcium is withdrawn from the bone as the kidneys attempt to buffer the excess acid. Acidosis also may directly stimulate osteoclast function. A high intake of diet soda with a high phosphate content also can deplete calcium stores.

With menopause and decreasing estrogen levels, bone loss accelerates in women. Estrogen promotes the activity of osteoblasts, increasing new bone formation. In addition, estrogen enhances calcium absorption and stimulates the thyroid gland to secrete calcitonin, a hormone that suppresses osteoclast activity and increases osteoblast activity.

Both cigarette smoking and excess alcohol intake are risk factors for osteoporosis. Smoking decreases the blood supply to bones. Nicotine slows the production of osteoblasts and impairs the absorption of calcium, contributing to decreased bone density. Alcohol has a direct toxic effect on osteoblast activity, suppressing bone formation during periods of alcohol intoxication. In addition, heavy alcohol use may be associated with nutritional deficiencies that contribute to osteoporosis. Interestingly, moderate alcohol consumption in postmenopausal women actually may increase bone mineral content, possibly by increasing levels of estrogen and calcitonin.

Sedentary lifestyle is another modifiable risk factor that can cause osteoporosis. Weight-bearing exercise, such as walking, influences bone metabolism in several ways. The stress of this type of exercise causes an increase in blood flow to bones, which brings growth-producing nutrients to the cells. Walking causes an increase in osteoblast growth and activity.

Prolonged use of medications that increase calcium excretion, such as aluminum-containing antacids and anticonvulsants, increase the risk of developing osteoporosis. Heparin therapy increases bone resorption, and its prolonged use is associated with osteoporosis. Antiretroviral therapy for people with AIDS or HIV infection may cause decreased bone density and osteoporosis (Porth, 2005).

Anyone who takes a glucocorticoid medication for more than 3 months is at risk for glucocorticoid-induced osteoporosis. These medications, often prescribed to control many rheumatic diseases, include prednisone (Deltasone, Orasone), prednisolone (Prelone), dexamethasone (Decadron, Hexadrol), and cortisone (Cortisone Acetate). These medications can directly affect bone cells, slowing the rate of bone formation. They also interfere with how the body uses calcium and affect levels of sex hormones, leading to bone loss. Problems that result, such as an increased possibility of fractures, can be prevented by taking a daily regimen of calcium supplements with added vitamin D and one multivitamin (American College of Rheumatology [ACR], 2004a).

Pathophysiology

Although the exact pathophysiology of osteoporosis is unclear, it is known to involve an imbalance of the activity of osteoblasts that form new bone and osteoclasts that resorb bone. Until age 35, when peak bone mass occurs, formation occurs more rapidly than does reabsorption. After peak bone mass is achieved, slightly more is lost than is gained (about 0.3% to 0.5% per year); this loss is accelerated if the diet is deficient in vitamin D and calcium. In women, bone loss increases after menopause (with loss of estrogen), then slows but does not stop at about age 60. Older women may have lost between 35% and 50% of their bone mass, older men may have lost between 20% and 35% (Mayo Clinic, 2002).

Osteoporosis affects the diaphysis (shaft of the bone) and the metaphysis (portion of the bone between the diaphysis and the epiphysis). The diameter of the bone increases, thinning the outer supporting cortex. As osteoporosis progresses, trabeculae are lost from cancellous bone (the spongy tissue of bone), and the outer cortex thins to the point that even minimal stress will fracture the bone (Porth, 2005).

Manifestations

The most common manifestations of osteoporosis are loss of height, progressive curvature of the spine, low back pain, and fractures of the forearm, spine, or hip. Osteoporosis is often called the "silent disease," because bone loss occurs without symptoms.

The loss of height occurs as vertebral bodies collapse. Acute episodes generally are painful, with radiation of the pain around the flank into the abdomen. Vertebral collapse can occur with little or no stress; minimal movements such as bending, lifting, or jumping may precipitate the pain. In some clients, vertebral collapse may occur slowly, accompanied by little discomfort. Along with loss of height, characteristic dorsal kyphosis and cervical lordosis develop, accounting for the "dowager's hump" often associated with aging. The abdomen tends to protrude and knees and hips flex as the body attempts to maintain its center of gravity (Figure 42–1 ■).

Complications

Fractures are the most common complication of osteoporosis, with the disease being responsible for more than 1.5 million fractures each year. These include 700,000 vertebral compression fractures, 300,000 hip fractures, 250,000 wrist fractures, and 300,000 fractures at other sites (National Osteoporosis Foundation, 2006). There may be no obvious manifestations of osteoporosis until fractures occur. Some fractures are spontaneous; others may result from everyday activities. While wrist and vertebral fractures have not been shown to increase disability or mortality, persistent pain and associated posture changes may restrict the client's activities or interfere with activities of daily living (ADLs).

INTERDISCIPLINARY CARE

Care of the client with osteoporosis focuses on stopping or slowing the process, alleviating the symptoms, and preventing complications. Proper nutrition and exercise are important components of the treatment program.

Figure 42–1 ■ Spinal changes caused by osteoporosis. As the condition progresses, height can be reduced by as much as 7 inches.

Diagnosis

The manifestations of osteoporosis can mimic those of other bone disorders, so diagnostic tests are needed to differentiate osteoporosis from other problems.

Dual-energy x-ray absorptiometry (DEXA) measures bone density in the lumbar spine or hip and is considered to be highly accurate. Ultrasound transmits painless sound waves through the heel of the foot to measure bone density. This 1-minute test is not as sensitive as DEXA, but is accurate enough for screening purposes. These tests are described in Chapter 40 ∞.

Laboratory tests include alkaline phosphatase (AST), which may be elevated following a fracture, and serum bone Glaprotein (osteocalcin), which can be used as a marker of osteoclastic activity and therefore is an indicator of the rate of bone turnover. This test is most useful to evaluate the effects of treatment, rather than as an indicator of the severity of the disease. A comparison of laboratory tests for metabolic bone diseases is outlined in Table 42–1.

Medications

Estrogen replacement therapy reduces bone loss, increases bone density in the spine and hip, and reduces the risk of fractures in postmenopausal women. It is particularly recommended for women who have undergone surgical menopause before age 50, and often is prescribed for women with other osteoporosis risk factors. Estrogen therapy alone is associated with an increased risk of endometrial cancer, so it usually is prescribed in combination with progestin (hormone replacement therapy or HRT). The choice of using HRT to prevent osteoporosis is one that must be made between the woman and her healthcare provider.

Raloxifene (Evista) is a selective estrogen receptor modulator (SERM) that appears to prevent bone loss by mimicking estrogen's beneficial effects on bone density in postmenopausal women. It does not have the risks of estrogen. Hot flashes are a common side effect, and this drug should not be taken by a woman with a history of blood clots.

Alendronate (Fosamax) and risedronate (Actonel) are from the class of drugs known as bisphosphonates. Bisphosphonates are potent inhibitors of bone resorption that may be used to prevent and treat osteoporosis. They inhibit bone breakdown, preserve bone mass, and increase bone density in the hip and vertebrae. Alendronate is especially useful for men and young adults and to prevent or treat glucocorticoid-induced osteoporosis. The nursing implications of bisphosphonates are found in the Medication Administration box on page 1437. Teriparatide (Forteo) is a synthetic parathyroid hormone, administered subcutaneously to stimulate new bone formation and mass. It is used to decrease the risk of bone fracture from osteoporosis in postmenopausal women and in men with primary or secondary hypogonadism.

Ibandronate sodium (Boniva) is the first monthly osteoporosis medication to be approved by the U.S. Food and Drug Administration (FDA). It is used for both treatment and prevention of postmenopausal osteoporosis, and reduces the number of vertebral fractures in women with osteoporosis as well as increases bone density in women who do not have the disease.

Calcitonin (Miacalcin) is a hormone that increases bone formation and decreases bone resorption. Calcitonin increases spinal bone density and reduces the risk of compression fractures; it may reduce the risk of hip fracture as well. Calcitonin usually is prescribed as a nasal spray, although it also is available in parenteral form. Because calcitonin is a protein, it can precipitate anaphylactic-type allergic responses.

Sodium fluoride stimulates osteoblast activity, increasing bone formation. When used to treat osteoporosis, bone mass of the spine increases and the risk of spinal fractures may be reduced. Fluoride therapy may, however, be associated with an increased risk of hip and other nonvertebral fractures.

Medications being investigated include vitamin D metabolites and other bisphosphonates and SERMS. See the Medication Administration Box on page 1437 for information about calcium, calcitonin, and fluoride.

TABLE 42–1 Differential Features of Osteoporosis, Osteomalacia, and Paget's Disease

DIFFERENTIATING FEATURES	OSTEOPOROSIS	OSTEOMALACIA	PAGET'S DISEASE
Pathophysiology	Resorption greater than bone formation	Inadequate mineralization of bone matrix	Excessive osteoclastic activity and formation of poor-quality bone
Calcium level (serum)	Normal	Low or normal	Normal or elevated (especially in immobilized clients)
Phosphate level (serum)	Normal	Low or normal	Normal
Parathyroid hormone level (serum)	Normal	High or normal	Normal
Alkaline phosphatase level (serum)	Normal	Elevated	Increased; not a reliable test for clients who have liver disease or are pregnant
Hydroxyproline (urine)	Not applicable	Not applicable	Increased
Radiographic findings	Osteopenia, fractures	Decreased bone density, radiolucent bands known as Looser's zones, or pseudofractures	"Punched-out" appearance of bone, increase in bone thickness, linear fractures, mosaic pattern of bone matrix

MEDICATION ADMINISTRATION The Client with Osteoporosis

CALCIUM

Postmenopausal women, regardless of whether they take replacement estrogens, are encouraged to take calcium to prevent osteoporosis.

Nursing Responsibilities

- Help clients maintain an adequate dietary intake of calcium. The best dietary source is milk and other dairy products, including yogurt.
- Postmenopausal women who take estrogens need 1000 mg of calcium daily. Those who do not take estrogens need about 1500 mg daily to minimize osteoporosis.
- Identify alternate sources, such as skim milk and low-fat yogurt, oysters, canned sardines or salmon, beans, cauliflower, and dark-green leafy vegetables.

Health Education for the Client and Family

- Take calcium carbonate in divided doses 30 to 60 minutes before meals to allow for absorption.
- Take calcium citrate with meals to minimize gastrointestinal distress.

CALCITONIN

Calcitonin-salmon injection, synthetic
Calcimar
Miacalin (injection or nasal spray)

In postmenopausal osteoporosis, calcitonin prevents further bone loss and increases bone mass if the client consumes adequate amounts of calcium and vitamin D. Calcitonin may be used in postmenopausal women who cannot or will not take estrogen.

Nursing Responsibilities

- Calcitonin is protein in nature; both the parenteral and nasal spray forms may cause an anaphylactic-type allergic response. Observe the client for 20 minutes after administration; have appropriate emergency equipment and drugs available to treat anaphylaxis.
- Alternate nostrils daily when administering calcitonin nasal spray.
- Review medical history for conditions that contraindicate use of calcitonin products: hypersensitivity to salmon calcitonin

and lactation (calcitonin is secreted in breast milk and may inhibit lactation).

- Observe for side effects: nausea and vomiting, anorexia, mild transient flushing of the palms of the hands and the soles of the feet, and urinary frequency.
- Teach the client the proper technique for handling and injecting the drug at home.

Health Education for the Client and Family

- Take the medication in the evening to minimize side effects.
- Warm nasal spray to room temperature before using.
- Rhinitis (runny nose) is the most common side effect with calcitonin nasal spray. Other possible side effects include sores, itching, or other nasal symptoms. Report nosebleeds to your primary care provider.
- Nausea and vomiting may occur during initial stages of therapy; they disappear as treatment continues.
- While taking the medication, be sure to consume adequate amounts of calcium and vitamin D.

FLUORIDE

Fluoride is a mineral long recognized as essential for the normal formation of dentin and tooth enamel. Fluoride appears to decrease the solubility of bone mineral and therefore the rate of bone reabsorption. Its use in preventing and treating osteoporosis is relatively new but promising.

Nursing Responsibilities

- Monitor serum fluoride levels every 3 months.
- Have bone mineral density studies conducted at 6-month intervals to document progress of bone growth.

Health Education for the Client and Family

- Take sodium fluoride tablets after meals, and avoid milk or dairy products; these reduce gastrointestinal absorption of the medication.
- While taking fluoride, be sure to maintain an adequate calcium intake.
- Use fluoride mouth rinse immediately after brushing teeth and just before retiring at night. Do not swallow the rinse, and avoid eating or drinking for at least 30 minutes after use.
- Notify the physician if teeth become stained or mottled after repeated use of fluoride mouth rinse.

NURSING CARE

Osteoporosis is both preventable and treatable; therefore, nursing care focuses primarily on planning and implementing interventions to prevent the disease, its manifestations, and the resulting injuries. An important aspect of preventing osteoporosis is educating clients under age 35. A Nursing Care Plan for a client with osteoporosis is found on page 1438.

Health Promotion

Health promotion activities to prevent or slow osteoporosis focus on calcium intake, exercise, and health-related behaviors.

Nutrition

For clients of all ages, stress the importance of maintaining a daily calcium intake that meets National Institutes of Health

(NIH) recommendations (see Chapter 10 ∞). This is particularly important for adolescent girls and young adult women who may avoid eating many high-calcium foods such as dairy products because of concerns about weight. Optimal calcium intake before ages 30 to 35 probably increases peak bone mass. Emphasize that low-fat (or nonfat) dairy products also contain calcium, although some fat in the product may enhance calcium absorption.

Milk and milk products are the best sources of calcium. The lactose in milk facilitates calcium absorption as well. Other food sources of calcium include sardines, clams, oysters, and salmon, as well as dark green, leafy vegetables such as broccoli, collard greens, bok choy, and spinach. For clients who avoid dairy products because of lactose intolerance or a vegetarian diet, suggest alternate sources.

NURSING CARE PLAN A Client with Osteoporosis

Nancy Bauer is a 53-year-old schoolteacher. She has been married for 36 years and has two children. Mrs. Bauer is 65 inches tall. She has smoked one pack of cigarettes a day for 30 years and drinks one to two glasses of wine with dinner each evening. She does not routinely exercise. Mrs. Bauer has had symptoms of menopause for 8 years, including hot flashes in the early years and mood swings of late. She has never been on hormone replacement therapy.

Mrs. Bauer is currently seeking medical advice for continuous low back pain. The pain is not relieved with an over-the-counter analgesic, and she frequently wakes up during the night because of the pain. She is diagnosed with osteoporosis.

ASSESSMENT

The nurse practitioner notes that Mrs. Bauer's vital signs are within normal limits. She has full range of motion of all extremities and is able to stand and bend over, but she reports discomfort when returning to the upright position. Mrs. Bauer has a slightly pronounced "hump" on her upper back and is 1 inch shorter than her stated height on admission. Her muscle strength is symmetric and strong.

DIAGNOSIS

- *Acute Pain* of the lower spine related to vertebral compression
- *Deficient Knowledge* related to osteoporosis and treatment to prevent further damage
- *Imbalanced Nutrition: Less than Body Requirements* related to inadequate intake of calcium
- *Risk for Injury* related to effects of change in bone structure secondary to osteoporosis

EXPECTED OUTCOMES

- Verbalize a decrease in back pain.
- Be able to describe ways to treat her osteoporosis and prevent further complications.
- Verbalize an understanding of the current research and treatment regarding osteoporosis.
- Verbalize how stopping smoking can help prevent further progression of osteoporosis.
- Seek consultation for supplements and medications to prevent further bone loss.
- Design a program of physical activity to prevent complications of osteoporosis.
- Verbalize safety precautions to prevent fractures due to falls.

PLANNING AND IMPLEMENTATION

- Teach back strengthening exercises.
- Refer to an osteoporosis support group, if available.
- Provide realistic, yet optimistic, feedback about loss of height and bone integrity and the potential outcomes of treatment.
- Assess current knowledge base, and correct misconceptions regarding treatment of osteoporosis.
- Provide current educational literature regarding treatment of osteoporosis.
- Instruct in dietary and calcium supplements that help prevent effects of osteoporosis.
- Discuss physical exercises that help prevent complications due to osteoporosis.
- Review safety and fall precautions, and provide literature regarding how to create a safe home environment.

EVALUATION

On her return visit 6 months later, Mrs. Bauer reports that she feels much better. She is no longer irritable and does not experience mood swings, because she has been taking her prescribed hormone replacements for 6 months: She is eating products rich in calcium and taking a daily supplement of calcium with vitamin D. Mrs. Bauer has reduced her wine intake to one glass in the evening and now drinks decaffeinated coffee and tea. She also states that since she stopped smoking, she has been walking 30 to 45 minutes every day.

CRITICAL THINKING IN THE NURSING PROCESS

1. What is the rationale for stopping smoking and limiting caffeine and alcohol intake in the treatment of osteoporosis?
2. What foods would you encourage for clients at high risk for osteoporosis whose serum cholesterol and LDL/HDL ratios indicate a high risk for cardiovascular disease?
3. What physical activities would you consider beneficial in helping to prevent the effects of osteoporosis in the female client who is wheelchair bound or has limited mobility?
4. Develop a care plan for Mrs. Bauer for the nursing diagnosis *Risk for Trauma*

See Evaluating Your Response in Appendix C.

Calcium supplements are available in many forms. Most supplements (including Tums) provide calcium carbonate in the range of 200 to 600 mg per tablet. Other forms of calcium, including citrate, gluconate, and lactate, generally provide a lower amount of elemental calcium per tablet. A combination of calcium with vitamin D is recommended, particularly for older adults who may have a vitamin D deficiency that impairs their ability to absorb and use calcium.

Exercise

Teach clients the importance of physical activity and weight-bearing exercises in preventing and slowing bone loss. Suggest that clients participate in regular exercise such as walking for at least 20 minutes four or more times a week. Inform clients that swimming and pool aerobic exercises are not as beneficial for maintaining bone density because of the lack of weight-bearing activity.

Healthy Behaviors

Behaviors that help prevent osteoporosis include not smoking, avoiding excessive alcohol intake, and limiting caffeine intake to two or three cups of coffee each day.

Assessment

Collect the following data through the health history and physical examination (see Chapter 40 ∞):

- *Health History:* Age, risk factors, history of fractures, smoking history, alcohol intake, medications, usual diet, menstrual history including menopause, usual exercise/activity level (see the Nursing Research box below), low back pain.

■ *Physical Examination:* Height, spinal curves.

Nursing Diagnoses and Interventions

Nursing care of clients who have osteoporosis focuses on teaching about the disease process, helping maintain physical mobility and nutrition, and solving problems associated with pain and injury.

Health-Seeking Behaviors

At multiple points in the client's lifetime, nurses can provide vital information that will help clients use self-care strategies to reduce their risk of developing osteoporosis:

■ Assess the client's health habits, including diet, exercise, smoking, and alcohol use. *The risk of developing osteoporosis in later life is affected by such things as diet, regular participation in weight-bearing exercise, and personal habits such as smoking and alcohol consumption.*

■ Teach women and men of all ages the importance of maintaining an adequate calcium intake. Provide a list of calcium-rich foods, and discuss the use of calcium supplements with clients who do not consume adequate dietary calcium. *Calcium needs vary during the course of a lifetime; however, many clients never consume adequate amounts of calcium. This affects their peak bone mass and the rate of bone loss with aging. Calcium in foods is more completely absorbed than that supplied by calcium supplements.*

■ Discuss the importance of maintaining a regular schedule of weight-bearing exercise, either through an exercise program or regular physical activity. *Weight-bearing exercise promotes osteoblast activity, helping maintain bone strength and integrity.*

■ Refer clients to smoking-cessation programs and alcohol treatment programs as appropriate. *Smoking interferes with*

estrogen's protective effects on bones, promoting bone loss. Excess alcohol intake affects the nutritional status of the client, increasing the risk of calcium and vitamin D deficiency.

■ Refer clients with significant risk factors for osteoporosis to primary care providers or clinics for bone-density evaluation. *Early identification and treatment of osteoporotic changes in bones can reduce the risk and possible long-term consequences of falls and fractures.*

Risk for Injury

Falls that would result in little or no injury in the healthy adult may cause fractures in the client with osteoporosis. Even normal movements such as twisting, bending, lifting, or rising from bed can precipitate a vertebral fracture.

■ Implement safety precautions as necessary for the client who is hospitalized or in a long-term care facility. Maintain the bed in low position; use side rails if indicated to prevent the client from getting up alone; provide nighttime lighting to toilet facilities. *Most falls are preventable, particularly in hospitals and long-term care facilities.*

■ Avoid using restraints (if hospitalized or a resident in a long-term care facility) if at all possible. *Restraints may actually increase the client's risk of falling and increase the risk of injury associated with a fall.*

> **PRACTICE ALERT**
> Clients may fracture osteoporotic bones when pulling against restraints.

■ Teach clients who are able to participate in weight-bearing exercises to perform exercises at least three times a week for a sustained period of 30 to 40 minutes. The mechanical force of weight-bearing exercises promotes bone growth. *Bones weaken and demineralize without exercise. Walking is an*

NURSING RESEARCH **Evidence-Based Practice for the Client with Osteoporosis**

Osteoporosis is a major health problem in the United States. Risk factors for osteoporosis include being white, having a small body frame, not doing weight-bearing exercises, and having a family history of osteoporosis. Nursing can do much to prevent the development of osteoporosis by assessing risk factors and teaching about diet, exercise, and lifestyle. A study by Schoen (2004) was conducted to determine the validity of items on a risk assessment screening questionnaire called the Osteoporosis Risk Assessment Tool (ORAT).

IMPLICATIONS FOR NURSING

Assessment is a critical component of the nursing process, enabling nurses to identify clients at risk for diseases, to monitor ongoing interventions, and to design teaching specific to client needs. Based on review of items contained in the ORAT, the following were retained: age, gender, body mass index, previous fractures, diagnosis of thyroid disease, use of thyroid replacement medication, estrogen replacement therapy, weight-bearing exer-

cise, family history of fractures, age at onset of menopause, use of calcium supplements, diet of calcium-rich foods, and alcohol and tobacco use. This tool is a useful means of quickly assessing clients for osteoporosis risk factors and for identifying and teaching about the prevention, diagnosis, treatment, and complications of osteoporosis.

CRITICAL THINKING IN CLIENT CARE

1. At what age do women develop maximum bone mass? (Review information in a text or on the Internet.) Based on this information, what type of teaching would be most effective?

2. Compare and contrast your teaching for a 24-year-old black woman who has a calcium-poor diet but is a nonsmoker and a thin, white 64-year-old woman who is postmenopausal and smokes.

3. While screening clients in a clinic for health risks, including osteoporosis, a man in his 70s says "Oh, I can't have bad bones . . . I'm a man!" How would you respond?

Data from Schoen, D. C. (2004). Osteoporosis. *Orthopaedic Nursing, 23*(4), 261–267.

easy, low-impact form of exercise. Swimming (including walking on the bottom of the pool) does not provide the needed weight-bearing activity.

- Encourage older adults to use assistive devices to maintain independence in ADLs. *Walking sticks, canes, and other assistive devices encourage client independence and support activities that promote bone growth.*
- Teach older clients about safety and fall precautions. *An assessment of the client's home for safety and fall risks may reduce the risk of fractures and, in turn, the cost of hospitalization and potential disability and/or death.*

Imbalanced Nutrition: Less than Body Requirements

Most Americans do not maintain their recommended daily intake of calcium. Clients must therefore be made aware of the relationship between an adequate calcium intake and maintaining strong bones.

- Teach adolescents, pregnant or lactating women, and adults through age 35 to eat foods high in calcium and to maintain a daily calcium intake of 1200 to 1500 mg. *The NIH recommends a daily calcium intake of 1200 to 1500 mg per day for adolescents and young adults, as well as for pregnant and lactating women.*
- Encourage postmenopausal women to maintain a calcium intake of 1000 to 1500 mg daily, either through diet or a calcium supplement. *Calcium needs for postmenopausal women vary, depending on age.*
- Teach clients taking calcium supplements the importance of taking the medication at the proper time and the side effects that may occur. *Free hydrochloric acid is needed for calcium absorption. Calcium carbonate supplement (e.g., Tums) should be taken 30 to 60 minutes before meals to allow adequate absorption. Calcium citrate supplements should be taken with meals to prevent gastrointestinal distress.*

> **PRACTICE ALERT**
> Calcium supplements should be taken in divided doses (two to three times daily) for improved distribution.

Acute Pain

Advanced stages of osteoporosis can result in pain and immobilization. Acute pain usually results from a complicating fracture, especially a compression fracture of the vertebrae.

- Suggest anti-inflammatory pain medications for treatment of both acute and chronic phases of pain. Clients should be instructed in the amount and frequency as noted on the manufacturer's labels. *Continuous administration of ibuprofen or other nonsteroidal anti-inflammatory, drugs (NSAIDs) can be useful to provide relief from pain, but clients must be cautioned not to exceed dosage recommendations.*

> **PRACTICE ALERT**
> Teach clients on long-term anti-inflammatory medications to watch for bright red bleeding from the stomach (in vomitus) or dark black bowel movements.

- Suggest the application of heat to relieve pain. *A heating pad may offer temporary pain relief. To avoid the "rebound effect," the heat should be removed every 20 to 30 minutes.*

Using NANDA, NIC, and NOC

Chart 42–1 shows links between NANDA nursing diagnoses, NIC, and NOC when caring for the client with osteoporosis.

Community-Based Care

The client who has osteoporosis needs education on safety and preventing falls. In addition to home safety, outdoor safety is important, too. Clients should be taught to use assistive devices for added stability, to wear rubber-soled shoes for traction, to walk on the grass when sidewalks are slippery, and to sprinkle salt or kitty litter on icy sidewalks in the winter.

Address the following topics when discussing home care:

- Resources for medical supplies and assistive devices
- Diet, exercise, and medications
- Pain management
- Maintaining good posture to help prevent stress on the spine
- Helpful resources:
  - National Osteoporosis Foundation
  - Osteoporosis and Related Bone Diseases National Resource Center (NIH)
  - National Women's Health Resource Center
  - Older Women's League
  - American College of Rheumatology

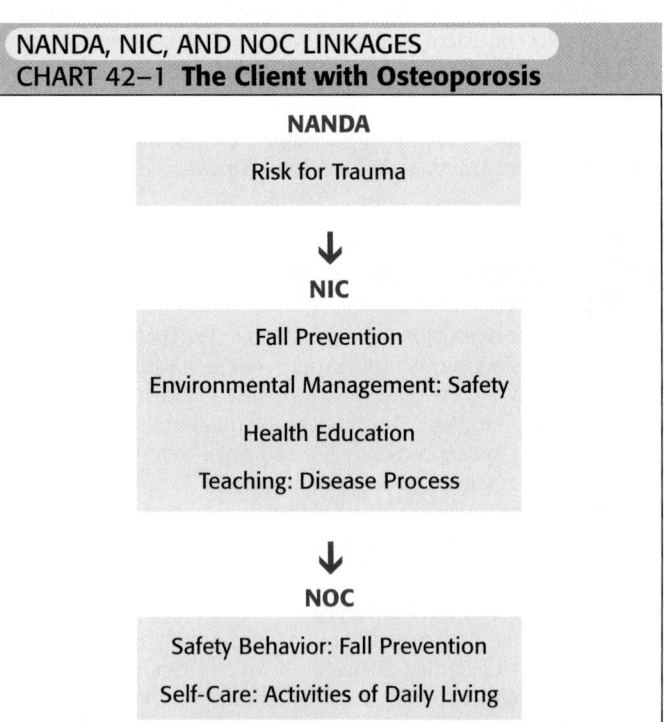

NANDA, NIC, AND NOC LINKAGES
CHART 42–1 The Client with Osteoporosis

NANDA

Risk for Trauma

↓

NIC

Fall Prevention

Environmental Management: Safety

Health Education

Teaching: Disease Process

↓

NOC

Safety Behavior: Fall Prevention

Self-Care: Activities of Daily Living

Data from *NANDA's Nursing Diagnoses: Definitions & Classification 2005–2006* by NANDA International (2005), Philadelphia; *Nursing Interventions Classification (NIC)* (4th ed.) by J. M. Dochterman & G. M. Bulechek (2004), St. Louis, MO: Mosby; and *Nursing Outcomes Classification (NOC)* (3rd ed.) by S. Moorhead, M. Johnson, and M. Maas (2004), St. Louis, MO: Mosby.

THE CLIENT WITH PAGET'S DISEASE

Paget's disease, also called *osteitis deformans*, is a progressive metabolic skeletal disorder that results from excessive metabolic activity in bone, with excessive bone resorption followed by excessive bone formation. This chronic remodeling results in the affected bones being larger and softer, with manifestations of bone pain, arthritis, obvious skeletal deformities, and fractures. The disorder affects bones of the axial skeleton, especially the femur, pelvis, vertebrae, and skull. The disease may affect one bone or multiple bones. The cause is unknown; however, several theories have been proposed, including hormonal imbalance, vascular disorder, neoplasm, autoimmune disorder, and inborn error of connective tissue. It is the second most common bone disease in the United States.

Paget's disease occurs in both men and women, affecting 1.5% to 8% of the population over the age of 50 in many countries. It is less common in people of Asian, Indian, and Scandinavian descent. It has a familial tendency as a result of mutations in several genes. The measles virus has been found in bone lesions, and the relevance of that finding is under investigation (Paget Foundation, 2004a).

Pathophysiology

Paget's disease progresses slowly. It usually follows a two-stage process: an excessive amount of osteoclastic bone resorption, followed by excessive osteoblastic bone formation. The initial phase presents with an abnormal increase in osteoclasts. The bones increase in size and thickness because of the acceleration in bone resorption and regeneration, resulting in a thick layer of coarse bone with a rough and pitted outer surface (Porth, 2005). Resorption of cancellous bone occurs rapidly. As new bone tissue tries to replace the loss, fibrous tissue forms in the bone marrow. The bone is at first hyperemic and soft, and bowing occurs. When this excessive bone cell activity decreases, the result is a gain in bone mass, but the newly formed bone becomes hard and brittle. This brittleness may lead to fractures.

Manifestations

Most clients with Paget's disease are asymptomatic for years, and the disease often is discovered when typical changes are seen on an incidental x-ray. Manifestations are often vague and depend on the specific area involved (see the box on this page). The most common manifestation is localized pain of the long bones, spine, pelvis, and cranium. The pain is described as a mild to moderate deep ache that is aggravated by pressure and weight bearing. It is more noticeable at night or when the client is resting. The pain usually is due to metabolic bone activity, secondary degenerative osteoarthritis, fractures, or nerve impingement. Because of the increase in blood flow to pagetic bone, flushing and warmth of the overlying skin may be apparent.

Complications

Complications of Paget's disease are as follows:
- Nerve palsy syndromes from involvement of the upper extremities

---

MANIFESTATIONS of Paget's Disease

MUSCULOSKELETAL EFFECTS
- Pain (in the long bones of lower extremities or joints)
- Deformity (enlargement of skull, bowing of lower extremities, and deformity of elbows and knees)
- Fractures of lower extremities
- Pathologic fractures (especially of the tibia)
- Compression fractures
- Collapse of the vertebrae, resulting in kyphosis and loss of height
- Muscle weakness

NEUROLOGIC EFFECTS
- Hearing loss
- Spinal cord injuries
- Dementia
- Pain from spinal stenosis
- Bladder and/or bowel dysfunction

CARDIOVASCULAR EFFECTS
- Congestive heart failure

METABOLIC EFFECTS
- Symptoms of hypercalcemia in immobilized clients
- Hypercalciuria and renal calculi
- Increased skin temperature over affected extremities

- Pathologic fractures from loss of bone structure
- Mental deterioration from compression of the brain when the skull is involved
- Compression of the spinal cord from affected cervical vertebrae causing quadraplegia
- Cardiovascular disease, resulting from vasodilation of the vessels in the skin and subcutaneous tissues overlying the affected bones
- Osteogenic sarcoma, seen in 5% to 10% of people with severe disease (Porth, 2005).

INTERDISCIPLINARY CARE

Care of the client with Paget's disease focuses on relieving pain, suppressing bone cell activity if necessary, and preventing or minimizing the effects of complications. Many clients with Paget's disease are asymptomatic and do not require treatment. For more severely affected clients, pharmacologic agents are usually effective. Occasionally, surgery may be required.

Diagnosis

Many of the diagnostic tests that are useful for the diagnosis of osteoporosis are equally useful for clients with Paget's disease (see Table 42–1). These include x-rays and bone scans to illustrate localized areas of demineralization in the early stages, seen as "punched-out" areas that lend a coarse, irregular appearance to the bone. In the later phase, x-rays show enlargement of the bones, tiny cracks in the long bones, and/or bowing of the weight-bearing bones. Computed tomography (CT) scans and magnetic resonance imaging (MRI) help identify possible causes of pain, including degenerative problems, spinal stenosis, or nerve root impingement. Diagnostic tests are described in Chapter 40 .

Laboratory tests used in diagnosis include a serum alkaline phosphatase, which will show a steady rise as the disease progresses; the normal level (30 to 115 international units/L) may be elevated from high normal to over 3000 international units/L. A urinary collagen pyridinoline test is a sensitive indicator of the rate of bone resorption.

Medications

Clients who have mild symptoms often find relief using aspirin or NSAIDs, such as ibuprofen (Motrin) and indomethacin (Indocin). Clients who are experiencing manifestations and whose diagnostic test results are elevated are usually treated with an agent that retards bone resorption, such as calcitonin or a bisphosphonate.

Bisphosphonates such as alendronate (Fosamax), pamidronate (Aredia), and tiludronate (Skelid) are the primary treatments used for severe Paget's disease. These drugs inhibit bone resorption, possibly by attaching to the surface of the calcium/phosphate phase of bone and inhibiting osteoclast activity. They are safe and usually are well tolerated by the client. Alendronate is available as an oral preparation, and pamidronate is available for intravenous administration. Oral preparations are poorly absorbed from the GI tract, and may cause gastric or esophageal irritation. Alendronate should be given with a full glass of water on an empty stomach, at least 30 minutes before other medications or food. Pamidronate is given

as an intravenous infusion in D_5W or normal saline. It is given for 3 successive days, generally promoting a rapid response with reduced urinary excretion of hydroxyproline and pyridinium and a fall in alkaline phosphatase. Intravenous pamidronate may cause flulike symptoms, but these generally are brief. Calcium supplements also are prescribed for clients receiving bisphosphonates. After bisphosphonate treatment, clients often experience remission of symptoms for a year or more. See the Medication Administration box below for nursing implications.

Calcitonin inhibits osteoclastic resorption of bone. It also works as an analgesic for bone pain. The two derivatives of this medication are salmon (fish) and human. Salmon calcitonin (Calcimar) is generally preferred because it is inexpensive and widely available. Human calcitonin (Cibacalcin) is derived from human thyroid glands, which makes it more expensive and difficult to obtain. The parenteral form of calcitonin is used in treating Paget's disease. (Refer to the Medication Administration Box on page 1437 for nursing implications.)

Surgery

Different surgical interventions may be used to treat clients with Paget's disease, such as repairing a complete fracture through pagetic bone, realigning a knee through tibial osteotomy to decrease pain, or replacing a hip and/or knee for osteoarthritis. Because increased bleeding is a manifestation of Paget's disease, it is important to administer a potent bisphosphonate prior to surgery to decrease hypervascularity and reduce the risk of increased operative blood loss (Paget Foundation, 2004a).

MEDICATION ADMINISTRATION | **The Client with Paget's Disease**

BISPHOSPHONATES
Alendronate (Fosamax) **Etidronate (Didronel)**
Pamidronate (Aredia) **Risedronate (Actonel)**
Tiludronate (Skelid)

The bisphosphonates inhibit bone resorption, increasing the mineral density of bones and reducing the incidence of fractures. They are also used both in the prevention and treatment of osteoporosis: When used for Paget's disease, bisphosphonates slow the accelerated bone turnover associated with this disease. Bone pain is relieved, and the incidence of pathologic fractures is reduced. Cardiac and vascular manifestations of the disease also improve.

Nursing Responsibilities
- Administer alendronate with water 30 minutes before food or other medications.
- Do not give foods high in calcium, vitamins with mineral supplements, or antacids within 2 hours of administering alendronate.
- Instruct the client to avoid lying down for 30 minutes after taking the drug.
- Assess renal function studies before initiating therapy; alendronate is not recommended for use in clients with renal insufficiency.
- Dilute the prescribed dose of pamidronate in 1000 mL of D_5W or normal saline; infuse over at least 4 hours. Do not

add to calcium-containing solutions such as Ringer's or lactated Ringer's solutions.
- Monitor the IV site for signs of thrombophlebitis.
- Assess the client for signs of electrolyte imbalance or other adverse responses such as a drug fever.

Health Education for the Client and Family
- Take the medication as directed with clear water only. Consuming other beverages or food within 30 minutes of taking alendronate may interfere with its absorption and effectiveness.
- Do not lie down until after you have eaten. Alendronate can irritate the esophagus.
- Report symptoms such as new or worsening heartburn, difficulty swallowing, or painful swallowing.
- Fever with or without chills may occur while receiving intravenous pamidronate; this will subside without treatment. Flulike symptoms also may occur; these will subside within a week or so.
- Report any abnormal symptoms such as tingling around the mouth or numbness and tingling of the fingers or toes, which may indicate an imbalance of electrolytes in the blood.
- Take calcium and vitamin D supplements as instructed by your primary care provider.
- Response to these medications is gradual, and continues for months after the drug is stopped.

NURSING CARE

Nursing Diagnoses and Interventions

The nursing interventions for the client with symptomatic Paget's disease focus on pain control, prevention of injury or fractures, and education regarding the disease process and prescribed therapies.

Chronic Pain

The most common manifestation of Paget's disease is bone pain. This usually is the manifestation that prompts the client to seek health care.

- Assess the location and extent of the pain to determine the bone areas involved. *Bone pain in Paget's disease is poorly localized and is frequently described as "aching and deep."*
- Teach the client to take NSAIDs or aspirin on a regular basis as prescribed. *Pain is most noticeable at night or when the client is resting. The pain can become evident when it is aggravated by pressure and weight bearing.*
- Ensure correct placement of prescribed brace or corset. The client may be required to wear a light brace or corset to relieve back pain and provide support when assuming an upright position. *The client may need instruction in the correct application of the device and in the evaluation of pressure areas that may result from wearing the device.*
- Suggest referral for heat therapy and massage. *Heat therapy and massage can alleviate mild discomfort. Care should be taken when applying massage over areas prone to pathologic fractures.*

Impaired Physical Mobility

Clients with Paget's disease need to maintain or improve mobility so that they can perform necessary self-care activities and prevent complications of immobility.

- Provide an assistive device for use when ambulating. *During the active phase of Paget's disease, the client is prone to fractures. Bone deformities, activity intolerance, fear of falling, and pain are all factors that may make the client more prone to falls. An assistive device can provide both physical and psychologic support during ambulation, permit the client to ambulate further, and provide a device for resting during ambulation.*
- Teach good body mechanics. *The client with bone deformities should avoid activities that require lifting and twisting.*

> **PRACTICE ALERT**
> Activities as seemingly simple as lifting a heavy box may result in a fracture in the client with Paget's disease.

- Reinforce information about exercise protocols and activity regimens. *Exercise and activity protocols should be planned carefully to prevent injury and to minimize fatigue.*

Community-Based Care

A diagnosis of Paget's disease can be frightening for the client and family. It is important that they understand that this is a treatable disease, and that many manifestations of the disease will be relieved with treatment. Inform the client that remissions of the disease often last for a year or more after effective treatment. The Paget Foundation should be suggested as a resource. Discuss the following topics:

- The importance of following the prescribed treatment regimen and keeping scheduled follow-up appointments
- Because it may take several weeks to notice a response to treatment, the importance of continuing therapy during this time and after a response is obtained
- If bisphosphonates such as alendronate or pamidronate are ordered, the importance of taking supplemental calcium to prevent low blood calcium levels
- The importance of remaining active
- Safety in the home and outdoor environment to prevent falls
- The need to report to the primary care provider any sudden pain or disability, even if no trauma has occurred, because pathologic fractures are possible.

THE CLIENT WITH GOUT

Gout is a metabolic disease that occurs from an inflammatory response to the production or excretion of uric acid resulting in high levels of uric acid in the blood (hyperuricemia) and in other body fluids, including synovial fluid. The disorder is characterized by deposits of urates (insoluble precipitates) in the connective tissues of the body. Gout has an acute onset, usually at night, and often involves the first metatarsophalangeal joint (great toe). The initial acute attack is usually followed by a period of months or years without manifestations. As the disease progresses, urates are deposited in various other connective tissues. Deposits in the synovial fluids cause acute inflammation of the joint (*gouty arthritis*). Over time, urate deposits in subcutaneous tissues cause the formation of small white nodules (called **tophi**). Deposits of crystals in the kidneys can form urate kidney stones and result in kidney failure.

Gout may occur as either a primary or secondary disorder. Primary (inherited) gout is characterized by elevated serum uric acid levels resulting from either an inborn error of purine metabolism or a decrease in renal uric acid excretion due to an unknown cause. Purines are part of the structure of the nuclear compounds DNA and RNA; they also may be synthesized by the body. Impaired uric acid excretion leads to hyperuricemia in the majority of people with primary gout. In secondary gout, hyperuricemia occurs as a result of another disorder or treatment with certain medications. Disorders associated with rapid cell turnover, such as some malignancies (leukemia in particular), hemolytic anemia, and polycythemia, can increase purine metabolism. Chronic renal disease, hypertension, starvation, and diabetic ketoacidosis can interfere with uric acid excretion, as can certain drugs, including some diuretics (such as furosemide, ethacrynic acid, and chlorothiazide), pyrazinamide, cyclosporin, ethambutol, and low-dose salicylates. Alcohol ingestion appears to interfere with uric acid excretion and to accelerate its synthesis. In addition, hospitalized clients with gout are at risk for an acute attack from changes in their diet, abdominal surgery, or medications (Tierney et al., 2004).

Gout affects more than 84% of all Americans (ACR, 2005). Gout occurs more often in men, usually after age 30 years. In women, attacks of gout are rarely seen until after menopause. Obesity increases the risk of gout; about half of those with the disorder are 15% or more above their ideal weight (Flynn & Johnson, 2005).

Pathophysiology

Uric acid is the breakdown product of purine metabolism. Normally, a balance exists between its production and excretion, with approximately two-thirds of the amount produced each day excreted by the kidneys and the rest in the feces. The serum uric acid level is normally maintained between 3.4 and 7.0 mg/dL in men and 2.4 and 6.0 mg/dL in women. At levels greater than 7.0 mg/dL, the serum is saturated, and monosodium urate crystals may form. It is not known exactly how crystals of monosodium urate crystals are deposited in joints. Several mechanisms may be involved:

- Crystals tend to form in peripheral tissues of the body, where lower temperatures reduce the solubility of the uric acid.
- A decrease in extracellular fluid pH and reduced plasma protein binding of urate crystals are evident.
- Tissue trauma and a rapid change in uric acid levels may also lead to crystal deposition. A rapid increase in uric acid may occur with tissue trauma and release of cellular components.

The monosodium urate crystals may form in the synovial fluid or in the synovial membrane, cartilage, or other joint connective tissues. They may also form in the heart, earlobes, and kidneys. These crystals stimulate and continue the inflammatory process, during which neutrophils respond by ingesting the crystals. The neutrophils release their phagolysosomes, causing tissue damage, which perpetuates the inflammation.

Manifestations

The manifestations of gout are hyperuricemia, recurrent attacks of inflammation of a single joint, tophi, renal disease, and renal stones. Unless treated, the manifestations of gout appear in three stages: asymptomatic hyperuricemia, acute gouty arthritis, and tophaceous gout. See the Manifestations box on this page.

Asymptomatic Hyperuricemia

The first stage is asymptomatic hyperuricemia, with serum levels averaging 9 to 10 mg/dL. Most people with hyperuricemia do not progress to further stages of the disease.

Acute Gouty Arthritis

The second state is acute gouty arthritis. The acute attack (called a "flare"), usually affecting a single joint, occurs unexpectedly, often beginning at night. It may be triggered by trauma, alcohol ingestion, dietary excess, or a stressor such as surgery. It is often precipitated by an abrupt or sustained increase in uric acid levels. The affected joint becomes red, hot, swollen, and exquisitely painful and tender.

Approximately 50% of initial attacks of acute gouty arthritis occur in the metatarsophalangeal joint of the great toe. Other sites for acute attacks include the instep of the foot, ankles, heels, knees, wrists, fingers, and elbows. The pain, often intense, peaks within several hours and may be accompanied by fever and an elevated white blood cell (WBC) count and sedimentation rate. The affected joints are swollen, and the skin over the joint is warm and dusky red.

Acute attacks of gouty arthritis last from several hours up to several weeks and typically subside spontaneously. There are no long-lasting sequelae, and the client enters an asymptomatic period called the intercritical period. The intercritical period may last up to 10 years; however, approximately 60% of people experience a recurrent attack within 1 year. Successive attacks tend to last longer, occur with increasing frequency, and resolve less completely than the initial attack.

Tophaceous (Chronic) Gout

Tophaceous or chronic gout occurs when hyperuricemia is not treated. The urate pool expands, and monosodium urate crystal deposits (tophi) develop in cartilage, synovial membranes, tendons, and soft tissues. They are seen most often in the helix of the ear; in tissues surrounding joints and bursae (especially around the elbows and knees); along tendons of the finger, toes, ankles, and wrists; on ulnar surfaces of the forearms; along the shins of the legs; and on other pressure points. The skin over tophi may ulcerate, exuding chalky material containing inflammatory cells and urate crystals. Tophi can also develop in the tissues of the heart and spinal epidura. Although tophi themselves are not painful, they may restrict joint movement and cause pain and deformities of the affected joints. Tophi may also compress nerves and erode and drain through the skin.

Complications

Kidney disease may occur in clients with untreated gout, particularly when hypertension is also present. Urate crystals are deposited in renal interstitial tissue. Uric acid crystals also form in the collecting tubules, renal pelvis, and ureter, forming stones. The stones can range in size from a grain of sand to a massive structure filling the spaces of the kidney. Uric acid stones can potentially obstruct urine flow and lead to acute renal failure.

> ### MANIFESTATIONS of Gout
>
> **ACUTE GOUTY ARTHRITIS**
> - Usually monoarticular, affecting metatarsophalangeal joint of great toe, instep, ankle, knee, wrist, or elbow
> - Acute pain
> - Red, hot, swollen, and tender joint
> - Fever, chills, malaise
> - Elevated WBC and sedimentation rate
>
> **TOPHACEOUS (CHRONIC) GOUT**
> - Tophi evident on joints, bursae, tendon sheaths, pressure points, helix of ear
> - Joint stiffness, limited ROM, and deformity
> - Ulceration of tophi with chalky discharge

INTERDISCIPLINARY CARE

The classic presentation of acute gouty arthritis is so distinctive that the diagnosis can often be based on the client's history and physical examination. Treatment is directed toward terminating an acute attack, preventing recurrent attacks, and reversing or preventing complications resulting from crystal deposition in tissues and formation of uric acid kidney stones.

Diagnosis

Diagnostic testing is performed to establish an accurate diagnosis and direct long-term therapy. Diagnostic tests are described in Chapter 40 ∞.

Serum uric acid is nearly always elevated (usually above 7.5 mg/dL). The WBC count shows significant elevation, reaching levels as high as 20,000/mm^3 during an acute attack. Eosinophil sedimentation rate (ESR or sed rate) is elevated during an acute attack from the acute inflammatory process that accompanies deposits of urate crystals in a joint. In addition, a 24-hour urine specimen is analyzed to determine uric acid production and excretion, and analysis of fluid aspirated from the acutely inflamed joint or material aspirated from a tophus shows typical needle-shaped urate crystals, providing the definitive diagnosis of gout.

Medications

Medications are used to terminate an acute attack, prevent further attacks, and reduce serum uric acid levels to prevent long-term sequelae of the disease. It is important to treat the acute attack of gouty arthritis before initiating treatment to reduce serum uric acid levels, because an abrupt decrease in serum uric acid may lead to further acute manifestations. Pharmacologic therapy is a mainstay of treatment in achieving these goals.

ACUTE ATTACK NSAIDs are the treatment of choice for an acute attack of gout. Indomethacin (Indocin) is the most frequently used NSAID for gout, although others are equally effective. Other NSAIDs that may be prescribed include ibuprofen (Motrin), naproxen (Naprosyn, Anaprox), tolmetin sodium (Tolectin), piroxicam (Feldene), and sulindac (Clinoril). Although extremely effective, NSAIDs are contraindicated for clients with active peptic ulcer disease, impaired renal function, or a history of hypersensitivity reactions to the drugs. As with other anti-inflammatory drugs, clients should be aware of possible risks and follow recommended doses carefully.

Colchicine can dramatically affect the course of an acute attack. Joint pain begins to diminish within 12 hours of the initiation of treatment and disappears within 2 days. Colchicine apparently acts by interrupting the cycle of urate crystal deposition and inflammation in an acute attack of gout. It has no anti-inflammatory effect in other forms of arthritis, and its use is limited to gout. The use of colchicine is limited by significant side effects. When administered orally, many clients develop abdominal cramping, diarrhea, nausea, or vomiting. Intravenous administration is limited by potential toxic effects including local pain, tissue damage if extravasation occurs during injection, bone marrow suppression, and disseminated intravascular coagulation (DIC). It is contraindicated for clients who have significant gastrointestinal, renal, hepatic, or cardiac disease.

Corticosteroids may also be prescribed for the client with acute gouty arthritis. If possible, the intra-articular route is preferred for monoarticular arthritis to avoid the multiple systemic effects of steroid therapy. When gout is polyarticular, corticosteroids may be administered either orally or intravenously.

Analgesics may also be prescribed during an acute episode of gouty arthritis. Either codeine or meperidine (Demerol) may be administered orally to manage the client's pain. Aspirin is avoided because it may interfere with uric acid excretion.

PROPHYLACTIC THERAPY In clients at high risk for future attacks of acute gout, prophylactic therapy with daily colchicine may be initiated. Prophylaxis is particularly useful during the first 1 to 2 years of treatment with antihyperuricemic agents. Although colchicine does not affect the serum uric acid directly, it reduces the frequency of attacks by preventing crystal deposition within the joint. The doses required to achieve this effect are small, and few side effects are associated with therapy.

Treatment to reduce serum uric acid levels is typically initiated for clients with recurring gout, tophi, or renal damage. Asymptomatic hyperuricemic clients require no treatment. Uricosuric agents are used for clients who do not eliminate uric acid adequately; allopurinol is prescribed for clients who produce excessive amounts of uric acid. Uricosuric drugs block the tubular reabsorption of uric acid, promoting its excretion and reducing serum levels. These drugs reduce the frequency of acute attacks, particularly when administered with colchicine. Probenecid (Benemid) and sulfinpyrazone (Aprazone, Anturane, Zynol) are the primary uricosuric drugs employed.

Allopurinol (Zyloprim) is a xanthine oxidase inhibitor that lowers plasma uric acid levels and facilitates the mobilization of tophi. Because of its effectiveness in lowering serum uric acid levels, it may trigger an attack of acute gout. The nursing implications for medications used to treat gout are included in the Medication Administration box on page 1446.

Complementary and Alternative Therapy

A variety of nutritional and herbal supplements may be used to help prevent gout or decrease the onset of manifestations. These include:
- Vitamin E and selenium may decrease tissue inflammation.
- Amino acids (alanine, aspartic acid, glutamic acid, and glycine) increase the ability of the kidneys to excrete uric acid.
- Dark reddish-blue berries (such as cherries and blackberries) are good sources of flavonoids, which help lower uric acid levels, decrease inflammation, and prevent or repair joint tissue damage.
- Acupuncture can provide pain relief.

Treatments

Treatments for gout, in addition to medications, include dietary management and rest.

NUTRITION Dietary purines contribute only slightly to uric acid levels in the body, and no specific diet may be recommended. If a low-purine diet is recommended, the client should be taught that

MEDICATION ADMINISTRATION   The Client with Gout

COLCHICINE

Colchicine is used to terminate an acute attack of gouty arthritis and to prevent recurrent episodes of the disease. Colchicine does not alter serum uric acid levels, but appears to interrupt the cycle of urate crystal deposition and inflammatory response. It may be administered either by mouth or intravenously. Colchicine is also available as a fixed-dose combination with a uricosuric agent, probenecid (Benemid). Only plain colchicine is used to treat an acute attack of gout; combination therapy is employed to prevent further attacks.

Nursing Responsibilities

- Assess for possible contraindications to colchicines therapy, including serious gastrointestinal, renal, hepatic, or cardiac disease.
- Administer the following as ordered:
  - *Intravenous doses*: Give undiluted or diluted in up to 20 mL sterile normal saline for injection. Administer over a period of 2 to 5 minutes.
  - *Oral doses:* Give on an empty stomach to facilitate absorption.
  - Evaluate for adverse effects, including abdominal cramping, nausea, vomiting, and diarrhea, and report promptly, because these side effects may necessitate discontinuation of the drug.

Health Education for the Client and Family

- Drink 3 to 4 quarts of liquid per day.
- Report adverse responses, including gastrointestinal problems, fatigue, bleeding, easy bruising, or recurrent infections, to the physician.
- Do not drink alcohol.

URICOSURIC DRUGS
Probenecid (Benemid)
Sulfinpyrazone (Anturane)

Probenecid is a uricosuric drug that inhibits the tubular reabsorption of urate, promoting the excretion of uric acid and decreasing serum uric acid levels. Sulfinpyrazone is a uricosuric drug that potentiates the renal excretion of uric acid, reducing serum uric acid levels. It is used to prevent recurrent attacks of acute gouty arthritis and treat chronic gout.

Nursing Responsibilities

- Assess for prior hypersensitivity responses to this drug.
- Administer after meals or with milk to minimize gastric distress.
- Increase fluid intake to at least 3 L/day to prevent the formation of uric acid kidney calculi.
- Administer sodium bicarbonate or potassium citrate as ordered to maintain an alkaline urine.
- Do not administer aspirin to clients receiving probenecid because salicylates interfere with the action of the drug.
- Monitor clients receiving the following drugs concurrently with probenecid for increased or toxic effects: penicillin and related antibiotics, indomethacin, acetaminophen, naproxen, ketoprofen, meclofenamate, lorazepam, and rifampin.
- Monitor for possible adverse effects of probenecid, including headache, dizziness, hepatic necrosis, nausea and vomiting, renal colic, bone marrow depression, anaphylaxis, fever, hives, and pruritus.
- Administer sulfinpyrazone with meals or antacid to minimize gastric distress.

- Monitor clients taking sulfinpyrazone with other sulfa drugs for increased or toxic effects; monitor for hypoglycemia in clients receiving insulin or oral hypoglycemics concurrently, and monitor for bleeding or increased anticoagulant effect in clients receiving warfarin concurrently.
- Assess for contraindications to therapy with sulfinpyrazone, including active peptic ulcer disease, a history of hypersensitivity to phenylbutazone or other pyrazoles, or blood dyscrasias.

Health Education for the Client and Family

- Do not take aspirin or products containing aspirin while taking probenecid. Use acetaminophen for relief of mild pain.
- Drink at least 3 quarts of fluids per day to minimize the risk of kidney stone formation.
- Take sulfinpyrazone with meals to minimize gastric distress, and report epigastric pain, nausea, or black stools to the physician promptly

ALLOPURINOL (ZYLOPRIM)

Allopurinol acts on purine metabolism, reducing the production of uric acid and decreasing serum and urinary concentrations of uric acid. It is used for clients with manifestations of primary or secondary gout, including acute attacks, tophi, joint destruction, urinary stones, and nephropathy. It is not indicated for use in the treatment of asymptomatic hyperuricemia.

Nursing Responsibilities

- Monitor intake and output and increase fluid intake to approximately 3 L/day.
- Monitor for desired effect of decreased serum uric acid levels, and for adverse effects such as nausea, diarrhea, and rash.
- Assess BUN and creatinine levels prior to the initiation of and during treatment with allopurinol. Report signs of impaired renal function such as an elevated BUN and creatinine, decreased urine output, and dilute or frothy urine to the physician.
- Administer with meals to minimize gastric distress.
- Monitor CBC periodically because allopurinol therapy may cause bone marrow depression.
- In clients receiving warfarin concurrently, monitor prothrombin times and be alert to evidence of bleeding, because allopurinol prolongs the half-life of warfarin.
- Monitor clients receiving chlorpropamide, cyclophosphamide, hydantoin, theophylline, vidarabine, or ACE inhibitors concurrently for increased drug effects.
- Discontinue the drug and notify the physician immediately if the client develops a rash. Rash and hypersensitivity responses occur more frequently in clients receiving ampicillin, amoxicillin, or thiazide diuretics.

Health Education for the Client and Family

- Stop taking the drug and report any skin rash, painful urination, blood in the urine, eye irritation, or swelling of the lips or mouth to the physician immediately.
- Take the medication after meals to minimize gastric distress.
- Drink 3 to 4 quarts of fluid daily to maintain a urinary output greater than 2 L/day.
- Acute gouty attacks may occur during the initial stages of allopurinol therapy; continue therapy prescribed for attacks (such as colchicine) to minimize acute episodes.
- Do not take a double dose of medication if you miss a dose.

high purine foods include all meats and seafood, yeast, beans, peas, lentils, oatmeal, spinach, asparagus, cauliflower, and mushrooms. The obese client is advised to lose weight, but fasting is contraindicated for clients with gout. Alcohol intake and specific foods that tend to precipitate attacks are avoided.

A liberal fluid intake to maintain a daily urinary output of 2000 mL or more is recommended to increase urate excretion and reduce the risk of urinary stone formation. Urinary alkalinizing agents, such as sodium bicarbonate or potassium citrate, may be prescribed as well to minimize the risk of uric acid stones. It is important to monitor clients receiving these preparations carefully for signs of fluid and electrolyte or acid–base imbalances.

REST During an acute attack of gouty arthritis, bed rest is prescribed. It is continued for approximately 24 hours after the attack has subsided, because early ambulation may bring about recurrence of acute manifestations (Tierney et al., 2004). The affected joint may be elevated and hot or cold compresses may be applied for comfort.

NURSING CARE

Clients with gout provide self-care at home. Teaching focuses on self-management of pain and altered mobility.

Nursing Diagnoses and Interventions

Pain is a primary focus for nursing interventions in the client experiencing an acute attack of gout. The client's mobility is also impaired during an acute attack, both because of pain and prescribed activity limitations.

Acute Pain

The pain associated with an attack of acute gouty arthritis is intense and accompanied by exquisite tenderness of the affected joint. Measures to alleviate the pain are vital in the initial period until anti-inflammatory medications become effective and the acute inflammatory response is relieved. The following are important in teaching about pain relief:

- Position the affected joint for comfort. Elevate the joint or extremity (usually the foot) on a pillow, maintaining alignment. *Elevation and normal body alignment facilitate blood return from the affected joint, alleviating some of the edema.*
- Protect the affected joint from pressure, placing a foot cradle on the bed to keep bed covers off the foot. *A foot cradle keeps bed linens from applying pressure on the affected joint.*
- Take anti-inflammatory and antigout medications as prescribed. In the initial period, colchicine may be given hourly. *These medications reduce the acute inflammatory response, gradually relieving discomfort.*

PRACTICE ALERT
The affected joints are so painful that even the weight of a sheet can be unbearable.

- Take analgesics as prescribed. *Supplemental analgesia may be necessary in the acute period until the inflammatory response is mediated.*

- Maintain bed rest. *It is important to immobilize the affected joint and promote rest to prevent exacerbation of joint inflammation.*

Community-Based Care

Discuss the following topics with the client:
- *The disease and its manifestations.* Tell the client that initial attacks cause no permanent damage but that recurrent attacks can lead to permanent damage and joint destruction. Discuss other potential effects of continued hyperuricemia, including tophaceous deposits in subcutaneous and other connective tissues. Discuss the potential for kidney damage and kidney stones.
- *The rationale for and use of prescribed medication.* Stress the need to continue the medication until the physician discontinues it, even though the client is free of manifestations of gout. Tell the client to avoid drugs that increase uric acid blood levels: hydrochlorothiazide (HydroDIURIL), cyclosporine (Neoral, Sandimmune), furosemide (Lasix), and high dose of aspirin. Clients who need to reduce their risk of heart attacks may safely take one baby aspirin each day (Flynn & Johnson, 2005).
- The importance of a high intake of fluids each day and avoiding the use of alcohol.

THE CLIENT WITH OSTEOMALACIA

Osteomalacia, often referred to as *adult rickets,* is a metabolic bone disorder characterized by inadequate or delayed mineralization of bone matrix in mature compact and spongy bone, resulting in softening of bones. Bone mineralization requires adequate calcium and phosphate ions in extracellular fluid. When either of these ions is insufficient due to (1) inadequate calcium intake or decreased calcium absorption from the intestines because of insufficient vitamin D, or (2) increased renal losses or decreased intestinal absorption of phosphate, the bone matrix is not mineralized and cannot sustain weight bearing. Marked deformities of weight-bearing bone and pathologic fractures occur. The primary causes of osteomalacia are vitamin D deficiency and hypophosphatemia. Osteomalacia can be corrected with treatment.

Osteomalacia has been almost nonexistent in the United States because many foods are fortified with vitamin D, but its incidence is increasing among older adults, and people who adhere to strict vegetarian diets. It is a significant health problem in cultures whose diets tend to be deficient in calcium and vitamin D. Women in northern China, Japan, and northern India have a higher incidence of the disorder (Porth, 2005).

The major risk factors for vitamin D deficiency are a diet low in vitamin D, decreased endogenous production of vitamin D because of inadequate sun exposure, impaired intestinal absorption of fats (vitamin D is a fat-soluble vitamin), and disorders that interfere with the metabolism of vitamin D to its active forms. Gastrectomy and small-bowel disorders may reduce the absorptive surface of the bowel to the extent that nutrients are not completely or adequately absorbed.

Both vitamin D and calcium absorption may be affected. Hepatobiliary disorders that interfere with bile production and release, and chronic pancreatic insufficiency with inadequate pancreatic enzyme production can affect the absorption of fats and vitamin D from the bowel. Once absorbed, vitamin D is metabolized in the liver and the kidney to its active form; therefore, liver disorders such as cirrhosis and renal disorders can affect this activation. Certain drugs, such as isoniazid, rifampin, and anticonvulsants, accelerate vitamin D metabolism, resulting in less availability to the tissues. Renal excretion of vitamin D is increased in some kidney disorders such as nephrotic syndrome (Box 42–2).

Hypophosphatemia can be the result of insufficient dietary intake, excessive losses through the urine or stool, or a shift into the cells. Alcohol abuse is the most common cause of hypophosphatemia, because of related dietary deficiencies, vomiting, antacid use, and increased renal excretion of phosphate. Ingesting large amounts of nonabsorbable antacids causes increased phosphate losses in the stool. Several acquired and genetic disorders cause increased losses of phosphate in the urine.

Pathophysiology

The two main causes of osteomalacia are insufficient calcium absorption in the intestine due to a lack of calcium or resistance to the action of vitamin D and increased losses of phosphorus through the urine (Porth, 2005). In its natural form, vitamin D is obtained from certain foods and ultraviolet radiation of the sun. Vitamin D maintains adequate serum levels of calcium and phosphate for normal mineralization of the bone. Vitamin D deficiency or resistance to its action disrupts the normal mineralization of the bone, causing softening of the bone.

Vitamin D is inactive when it is absorbed from the intestine or synthesized from exposure to ultraviolet light. For vitamin D to become active, a two-step process must occur. Vitamin D (and its metabolites) is transported in the blood to the liver, where it is converted to calcidiol. Calcidiol is then transported to the kidney and transformed to an active form, calcitriol.

The active form of vitamin D is needed for optimal absorption of calcium and phosphorus from the intestine. Calcium and phosphorus are transported in the blood to the bones for normal mineralization. If there is a lack of vitamin D, calcium and phosphorus are not absorbed from the intestine, and serum calcium and phosphorus levels therefore fall. A deficiency in these minerals in turn activates the parathyroid glands, with loss of calcium and phosphorus from bone. The continued loss of calcium and phosphate in the bone disrupts bone mineralization.

Impaired bone mineralization causes abnormalities in both spongy and compact bone. The osteoid (the soft, noncalcified part of the matrix) continues to be produced but is not mineralized. This abnormal buildup of demineralized bone leads to gross deformities of the long bones, spine, pelvis, and skull, because the bone is soft and unable to bear the weight and stress of body movement.

Manifestations

The manifestations of osteomalacia include bone pain and tenderness (see the box below). As the disease progresses, fractures occur. In contrast to osteoporosis, osteomalacia is not associated with a significant occurrence of hip fractures. Instead, pathologic fractures occur in the commonly weakened areas (e.g., distal radius and proximal femur).

INTERDISCIPLINARY CARE

Osteomalacia may be difficult to differentiate from osteoporosis because the manifestations are very similar; however, once the specific cause is determined, appropriate therapy will correct the disorder.

Diagnosis

A history of inadequate dietary intake, renal failure, or some malabsorption states may suggest osteomalacia. Diagnostic

---

BOX 42–2 Causes of Osteomalacia

Vitamin D Deficiency
- Inadequate dietary intake
- Lack of sun exposure
- Malabsorption from intestines: gastrectomy, small-bowel disorders, gallbladder disease, chronic pancreatic insufficiency
- Renal or liver disorders
- Drug effects: isoniazid, rifampin, anticonvulsants

Phosphate Depletion
- Inadequate intake
- Impaired absorption due to chronic antacid use
- Impaired renal tubular reabsorption due to either acquired or genetic disorders

Systemic Acidosis
- Renal tubular acidosis
- Ureterosigmoidostomy
- Fanconi's syndrome

Bone Mineralization Inhibitors
- Hypophosphatasia
- Sodium fluoride or disodium etidronate (Didronel)
- Aluminum intoxication

Chronic Renal Failure

Calcium Malabsorption

MANIFESTATIONS of Osteomalacia

- Bone pain: May be vague and generalized at first, becoming more intense with activity as the disease progresses; occurs most frequently in the pelvis; long bones of the extremities, spine, and ribs.
- Difficulty changing from lying to sitting position and sitting to standing position.
- Muscle weakness: Frequently an early sign in severe cases.
- Waddling gait: May be due to pain and muscle weakness.
- Dorsal kyphosis: May occur in severe cases.
- Pathologic fractures.

tests are described in Chapter 40 ∞. Table 42–1 compares the diagnostic findings of osteomalacia with those of osteoporosis and Paget's disease. X-rays demonstrate the effects of generalized bone demineralization: trabecular bone loss, cyst formation, compression fractures, bowing and bending deformities of the long bones, and osteoid deposits, particularly in the vertebral bodies and pelvis.

Laboratory tests include serum calcium, parathyroid hormone, and alkaline phosphatase levels. Calcium may be normal or low, depending on the cause of the disease. Calcium levels may be reduced when calcium absorption is impaired or in severe vitamin D deficiency. Secondary hypoparathyroidism may shift calcium from the bone into extracellular fluid, maintaining a normal serum calcium level. Parathyroid hormone is frequently elevated as a compensatory response to hypocalcemia in renal failure or vitamin D deficiency. Alkaline phosphatase usually is elevated.

Medications

Therapeutic management of osteomalacia depends on the cause of the disease. Because the causes are so diverse, it is difficult to generalize treatment. Most clients are placed on vitamin D therapy. Calcium and phosphate supplements may be indicated. Radiologic evidence of healing often is apparent within weeks of initiating therapy.

NURSING CARE

Managing the client with osteomalacia includes assessing the client's current dietary intake of vitamin D, calcium, and phosphorus and exposure to ultraviolet light. It also includes managing client responses to bone pain and tenderness, fractures, and muscle weakness.

Teaching is important not only for the client with osteomalacia, but also for people at risk for developing the disease.

When milk and other dairy products began to be fortified with vitamin D, the incidence of childhood rickets decreased dramatically. Now many clients are unaware of the importance of vitamin D, calcium, and phosphorus to bone health.

Older adults as a group are at high risk for osteomalacia because of dietary deficiencies, age-related intestinal malabsorption, and possible physical mobility limitations that restrict their exposure to sunlight. Teach older adults about the importance of maintaining an adequate intake of milk and other dairy products that are not only rich in calcium and phosphorus, but also are fortified with vitamin D. Few other food sources provide enough vitamin D to meet recommended levels. Cod liver oil may be used as a supplement, because it contains significant amounts of vitamin D. Supplements are not recommended, however, for clients who get adequate vitamin D through dietary sources and sun exposure, because this fat-soluble vitamin may become toxic at high levels. Instruct clients who are taking supplements to report to their primary care provider symptoms such as anorexia, nausea and vomiting, frequent urination, muscle weakness, and constipation that may be indicative of hypervitaminosis D.

Teach the client with osteomalacia about safety measures to prevent falls. Discuss the importance of eliminating scatter rugs and clutter from living areas to prevent tripping. Teach the client to place a night-light in hallways and the bathroom to prevent falls associated with nighttime toileting. Suggest installing grab bars in the shower and tub and next to the toilet for safety.

Teach clients with bone pain and muscle weakness to use assistive devices such as walkers, canes, or crutches when ambulating. Provide referrals to physical therapy for teaching clients how to safely use these devices. Encourage clients to participate in a supervised exercise program such as water aerobics or t'ai chi to improve muscle strength and balance.

DEGENERATIVE DISORDERS

Degenerative disorders, especially degenerative joint disease, are the most common form of arthritis in the older adult. Both primary and secondary forms are seen in adults of all ages. Primary or idiopathic osteoarthritis, the most common type, occurs without a clear precipitating factor. Secondary osteoarthritis is associated with an identifiable cause. For instance, it may be related to trauma to a joint, inflammation, skeletal disorders such as congenital hip dysplasia, or metabolic disorders. Regardless of cause, degenerative disorders of the joints and muscles can lead to impaired mobility and chronic pain. These problems may in turn cause disability, especially in the performance of ADLs by older adults.

THE CLIENT WITH OSTEOARTHRITIS

Osteoarthritis (OA) (also labeled *degenerative joint disease*) is the most commonly occurring of all forms of arthritis, and a leading cause of pain and disability in older adults (Porth, 2005). This disease is characterized by loss of articular cartilage in articulating joints and hypertrophy of the bones at the articular margins. OA may be idiopathic (without known

cause) or secondary (associated with known risk factors). OA affects more than 12% of Americans between the ages of 25 and 74 years, with about 90% of people having x-ray evidence of OA in the weight-bearing joints by age 40 (ACR, 2005; Flynn & Johnson, 2005). Men are affected more than women at an earlier age, but the rate of OA in women exceeds men by the middle adult years. The joints most affected are in the hand, wrist, neck, lower back, hip, knee, ankle, and feet. Men are more likely than women to have hip OA, whereas postmenopausal women more often have hand OA. Racial and ethnic effects on the development of OA are outlined in the box below.

FOCUS ON DIVERSITY
The Client with Osteoarthritis

- White women are more likely to have hand OA.
- Black women are more likely to have knee OA.
- Hip OA incidence is less in Chinese people.

Localized OA affects only one or two joints. Generalized OA affects three or more joints. Generalized OA may also be classified as nodal (involving the hand) or nonnodal (no hand involvement). Nodal OA may also affect the knees, hips, cervical spine, and lumbar spine. Idiopathic OA most commonly affects the terminal interphalangeal joints (*Heberden's nodes*), and less often the proximal interphalangeal joints (*Bouchard's nodes*) (Figure 42–2 ■), the joints of the thumb, the hip, the knee, the metatarsophalangeal joint of the big toe, and the cervical and lumbar spine. Secondary OA may occur in any joint from an articular injury.

Risk Factors

Idiopathic OA is associated with increasing age. It has been suggested that OA may be inherited as an autosomal recessive trait, with genetic defects causing premature destruction of the joint cartilage. The causes of secondary OA include trauma, mechanical stress, and inflammation of joint structures, joint instability, neurologic disorders, endocrine disorders, and selected medications.

Excessive weight contributes to the development of OA, especially in the hip and knee. Excess fat may have a direct metabolic effect in the development of the disease. Primary OA of the knee is almost four times more common in obese women and five times more common in obese men (Flynn & Johnson, 2005). Inactivity is another risk factor. Moderate recreational exercise has been shown to both decrease the chance of developing OA and the progression of manifestations when OA is present. People involved in strenuous, repetitive exercise (such as participating in sports) have an increased risk of developing secondary OA.

Other risk factors that are linked to OA are hormonal factors such as decreased estrogen in menopausal women, excessive growth hormone, and increased parathyroid hormone.

Pathophysiology

The cartilage that lines joints provides a smooth surface, so that the bones of the joint glide over one another without friction, and it distributes the load from one bone to the next, dissipat-ing the mechanical stress that occurs with joint loading. This cartilage normally contains more than 70% water. More than 90% of its dry weight is collagen, which provides strength, and proteoglycans, which provide elasticity and stiffness to compression. Cartilage cells, the chondrocytes, nest in this meshwork of collagen and proteoglycans. Normal articular cartilage exudes some of its water with compression, providing lubrication for joint surfaces. This water is reabsorbed during relaxation of the joint.

In OA, proteoglycans and collagen are lost from the cartilage as a result of enzymatic degradation. The water content of the cartilage increases as the collagen matrix is destroyed. With the loss of proteoglycans and collagen fibers, the cartilage becomes yellow or brownish gray and loses its tensile strength. Surface ulcerations occur, and fissures develop in deeper layers of the cartilage. Eventually, large areas of articular cartilage are lost, and underlying bone is exposed. The bone thickens in exposed areas, reducing its ability to absorb energy in joint loading. Cysts can also develop in the bone. Cartilage-coated *osteophytes* (bony outgrowths often called "joint mice") change the anatomy of the joint. As these spurs or projections enlarge, small pieces may break off, leading to mild synovitis (inflammation of the synovial membrane).

Manifestations

The onset of OA is usually gradual and insidious, and the course slowly progressive. Pain and stiffness in one or more joints (usually weight bearing) are the first manifestations of OA. The pain is localized to the affected joints and may be described as a deep ache. It typically is aggravated by use or motion of the joint and relieved by rest, although it may become persistent as the disease progresses. Pain at night may be accompanied by paresthesias (numbness, tingling). Pain may also be referred to other parts of the body; for example, OA of the lumbosacral spine may cause severe pain along the path of the sciatic nerve. Following periods of immobility, such as sleeping all night or after a long automobile ride, involved joints may stiffen. Usually only a few minutes of activity are necessary to relieve the stiffness. Range of motion (ROM) of the joint decreases as the disease progresses, and grating or crepitus may be noted during movement. Bony overgrowth may cause joint enlargement, and flexion contractures may occur because of joint instability. In OA, enlarged joints are characteristically bony-hard and cool on palpation. Manifestations specific to affected joints are outlined in the box on the next page.

Complications

OA of the spine may involve the vertebral bodies and intervertebral disks, the diarthrodial joints, or both. *Spondylosis* is degenerative disk disease. As the intervertebral disks degenerate, disk space between the vertebrae is lost. Degenerative disk disease may be complicated by herniated disk, the protrusion of the nucleus pulposus of the disk. Herniation usually occurs in a lateral direction, potentially compressing nerve roots and causing radicular (distributed along the nerve) pain and muscle weakness. See Chapter 45 ∞ for further discussion of disk disorders.

Figure 42–2 ■ Typical interphalangeal joint changes associated with osteoarthritis.

Source: L. Samsuri/Custom Medical Stock Photo.

MANIFESTATIONS of Osteoarthritis

Affected Site	Manifestations
Interphalangeal joints	■ *Heberden's nodes*—bony enlargements of distal joints; may cause pain, redness, swelling ■ *Bouchard's nodes*—bony enlargement of proximal joints
First carpometacarpal	■ Swelling, tenderness at base of thumb ■ Crepitus with movement ■ "Squared" appearance of joint
Spine	■ Localized pain and stiffness ■ Muscle spasm ■ Limited range of motion ■ Nerve root compression with radicular pain and motor weakness
Hips	■ Pain referred to inguinal area, buttock, thigh, or knee ■ Loss of internal rotation ■ Limited extension, adduction, and flexion
Knees	■ Pain and bony enlargement ■ Effusions ■ Crepitus ■ Instability and deformity with advanced disease

Disk degeneration and joint space narrowing alter the mechanics of the spinal column, promoting osteoarthritic changes in the articular processes (the facet joints) of the vertebrae. The cartilage covering the inferior and superior articular processes degenerates, causing localized pain, stiffness, muscle spasm, and limited range of motion. Osteophytes may form on articular processes, further contributing to pain and muscle spasm.

The presentation of OA in older clients is similar to that in younger adults. However, in this population, the risk of debilitation because of OA is greater, and the disease may progress faster. In addition, pain, stiffness, and limited ROM increase the risk of falls and fractures in the older adult.

INTERDISCIPLINARY CARE

At this time, no treatment is available to arrest the process of joint degeneration. Appropriate management, however, is important to relieve pain and maintain the client's function and mobility. Research is also ongoing on a new class of medications called disease-modifying osteoarthritis drugs (DMOADs) and gene therapy.

Diagnosis

The diagnosis of OA is generally based on the client's history, physical examination, and x-rays of affected joints. Diagnostic tests are described in Chapter 40 ∞.

Characteristic changes of OA are visible in x-ray studies of affected joints. Initially, irregular joint space narrowing is seen. Progressive changes include increased density of subchondral

(under cartilage) bone, osteophyte formation at the joint periphery, and the formation of cysts in the bone. Examination of synovial fluid from involved joints can identify the type of arthritis. In addition, research of the blood level of hyaluronic acid (HA) (a lubricating substance in cartilage and joint synovial fluid) suggests that HA may be a useful biochemical marker indicating the presence and severity of OA (National Institute of Arthritis Musculoskeletal and Skin Diseases, 2005c).

Medications

The pain of OA often can be managed through the use of analgesics such as aspirin or acetaminophen. Acetaminophen (Tylenol) is generally preferred for use in older clients because it has fewer toxic side effects. NSAIDs such as ibuprofen (Motrin), naproxen (Aleve), or ketoprofen (Orudis KT) may also be prescribed. See information with medications for rheumatoid arthritis for FDA actions concerning these drugs. These medications are discussed in more detail in Chapter 9 .

Topical medications include counterirritants, salicylates, and capsaicin, sold without prescription as creams, gels, sprays, patches, or ointments to relieve pain. Counterirritants include Flexall 454 Maximum Strength Gel, ArthriCare, Bengay, and Icy Hot; salicylates include Aspercreme and Sportscreme, and capsaicin is included in Capzasin and Zostrix. The client should be taught to keep the medications away from their eyes, nose, mouth, or any open skin, and not to bandage or apply heat to the treated area. The products should be used no more than three or four times a day and discontinued immediately if severe irritation occurs.

Medications that are effective in decreasing the pain and stiffness of OA are the NSAID COX-2 inhibitors. However, because of the increased risk of adverse cardiovascular (heart attack and strokes) and gastrointestinal (bleeding) effects of most drugs in this category, several have been recalled by the FDA and the only COX-2 inhibitor being prescribed as of 2006 was celecoxib (Celebrex).

Potent anti-inflammatory medications, such as systemic corticosteroids, are seldom prescribed for clients with OA, although intra-articular corticosteroid injections may be used. With intra-articular injections, a long-acting corticosteroid medication, often mixed with a local anesthetic such as lidocaine, is injected directly into the joint space of the affected joints. Although this procedure may provide marked pain relief, it can hasten the rate of cartilage breakdown if performed more frequently than every 4 to 6 months.

Treatments

OA is initially treated conservatively, but as pain increases and joint function decreases, surgery often becomes necessary.

CONSERVATIVE TREATMENT The goals of OA treatment are to relieve pain and maintain as much normal joint function as possible. Conservative treatment may include any or all of the following:

■ ROM exercises, muscle strengthening exercises, aerobic exercises
■ Heat and ice
■ A balance between exercise and rest

- Use of a cane, crutches, or a walker
- Weight loss, if indicated
- Analgesic and anti-inflammatory medications.

VISCOSUPPLEMENTATION Viscosupplementation is a new treatment for OA of the knee. Hyaluronan, a natural component of synovial fluid, is injected directly into the knee joint. Four hyaluronan derivatives have been approved for use: Hyalgan, Supartz, Orthovisc, and Synvisc. The injection may provide pain relief and improvement in knee function for up to 1 year, but its long-term effects are unknown (Flynn & Johnson, 2005).

SURGERY Surgical procedures can provide dramatic results for clients with significant chronic pain and loss of joint function. Although elective surgical procedures are frequently avoided in the older adult, even older clients can benefit significantly if they do not have a chronic medical condition that contraindicates surgery.

Arthroscopy An *arthroscopy* is a surgical procedure in which an arthroscope (a thin tube that is lighted and has a camera in one end) is inserted into a joint. It may be done to diagnose the type of arthritis or to perform debridement by smoothing rough cartilage and flushing out the joint to remove debris. Although arthroscopic debridement and lavage of involved joints have been used, arthroscopy has not proven effective in the treatment of knee OA. It may be useful to remove large pieces of debris or repair a torn cartilage (Flynn & Johnson, 2005).

Osteotomy An *osteotomy*, an incision into or transection of the bone, may be performed to realign an affected joint, particularly when significant bony overgrowth or osteophyte formation has occurred. This procedure may also be used to shift the joint load toward areas of less severely damaged cartilage. Although osteotomy does not halt the process of OA, it may have a beneficial effect on joint function and pain, delaying the need for a joint replacement by several years.

Joint Arthroplasty A *joint arthroplasty* is the reconstruction or replacement of a joint. Arthroplasty is usually indicated when the client has severely restricted joint mobility and pain at rest. Pain is virtually eliminated, and the function of the joint is generally improved. Arthroplasty may involve partial joint replacement or reshaping of the bones of a joint. For most clients with OA, both surfaces of the affected joint are replaced with prosthetic parts in a procedure known as a *total joint replacement*. Joints that may be replaced include the hip, knee, shoulder, elbow, ankle, wrist, and joints of the fingers and toes.

In a total joint replacement, some or all of the synovium, cartilage, and bone on both sides of the joint are removed. A metallic prosthesis is inserted to replace one joint surface (generally the load-end or distal portion of a weight-bearing joint). The other joint surface is replaced by a silicone-lined ceramic or plastic prosthesis.

Most prosthetic joints are uncemented, that is, made of porous ceramic and metal components inserted so that they fit tightly into existing bone. The implant is secured by new bone growth into the prosthesis, a process that requires approximately 6 weeks. Although a longer non-weight-bearing period is necessary initially until the prosthesis is fixed in place by the bony growth, the implant appears to have a longer useful life span than cemented prostheses. In a cemented joint replacement, methyl methacrylate (a pliable polymer that hardens to hold the prosthesis in place) is used to secure the prosthesis to existing bone. Although the client is able to resume normal activities more rapidly following a cemented joint replacement, methyl methacrylate initiates an inflammatory response, and the joint eventually loosens.

- In a *total hip replacement,* the articular surfaces of the acetabulum and femoral head are replaced. The entire head of the femur and part of the femoral neck are removed and replaced with a prosthesis (Figure 42–3 ■). The acetabulum is remodeled, and a prosthesis of high-molecular-weight polyethylene is inserted. The success rate for total hip replacement is reported to be greater than 90%. Approximately 150,000 total hip replacements are done each year in the United States; most are for treatment of OA (Boston Total Joint Association, 2004). Most hip replacements last 10 to 15 years, after which a second joint replacement, called a revision, can be performed. Potential problems associated with a total hip replacement include blood clots in leg veins, dislocation within the prosthesis, loosening of joint components from surrounding bone, and infection. If recurrent or ineffectively treated, these complications may necessitate removal of the prosthesis, resulting in severe shortening of the extremity and an unstable hip joint.

- *Total knee replacement* is performed if the client has intractable pain and x-ray films show evidence of arthritis of the knee. More than 350,000 knee replacements are performed in the United States each year (Flynn & Johnson, 2005). Several prosthetic devices involving removal of varying amounts of bone are available for knee joint replacement (Figure 42–4 ■). The femoral side of the joint is replaced with a metallic surface, and the tibial side with polyethylene. More than 80% of clients obtain significant or total relief of pain with a total knee replacement. They must, however, engage in a vigorous program of rehabili-

Porous socket mounted in acetabulum

Shaft mounted into femur

Figure 42–3 ■ Total hip prosthesis.

Femoral component

Tibial component

Figure 42–4 ■ Total knee replacement.

tation to achieve the best results. Joint failure is more common with knee replacement than with a total hip replacement. Loosened joint components, often on the tibial side, are the most common cause of failure. The possible complications following a total knee replacement are the same as for a total hip replacement.

■ *Total shoulder replacement* is indicated for unremitting pain and marked limitation of range of motion because of arthritic involvement of both the humeral and glenoid joint surfaces of the shoulder. The joint is immobilized in a sling or abduction splint for 2 to 3 weeks following arthroplasty. Dislocation, loosening of the prosthesis, and infection are potential problems associated with total shoulder replacement.

■ *Total elbow replacement* involves replacement of the humeral and ulnar surfaces of the elbow joint with a metal and poly-ethylene prosthesis. Pain and disabling stiffness of the joint are indications for an elbow arthroplasty. Complications, including dislocation, fracture, tricep weakness, loosening, and infection, occur frequently.

Infection is the major complication associated with total joint replacement. Not only does infection interfere with healing and prolong recovery, but it may also necessitate removal of the prosthesis and may lead to loss of joint function. Other potential complications include circulatory impairment to the affected limb, thromboembolism, nerve damage, and dislocation of the joint.

Nursing care for the client undergoing total joint replacement is outlined in the box below. Refer to Chapter 4 ∞ for further discussion of care for the client undergoing surgery.

NURSING CARE OF THE CLIENT HAVING Total Joint Replacement

PREOPERATIVE CARE

■ Assess the client knowledge and understanding of the planned operative procedure. Provide further explanations and clarification as needed. *It is important that the client have a clear and realistic understanding of the surgical procedure and expected results. Knowledge decreases anxiety and increases the client's ability to assist with postoperative care procedures.*

■ Obtain a health history and physical assessment, including range of motion of the affected joints. *This information not only allows nurses to tailor care to the needs of the individual but also serves as a baseline for comparison of postoperative assessment data.*

■ Explain necessary postoperative activity restrictions. Teach how to use the overhead trapeze for changing positions. *The client who learns and practices moving techniques before surgery can use them more effectively in the postoperative period.*

■ Provide or reinforce teaching of postoperative exercises specific to the joint on which surgery is to be performed. *Exercises are prescribed postoperatively to (a) strengthen muscles providing joint stability and support, (b) prevent muscle atrophy and joint contractures; and (c) prevent venous stasis and possible thromboembolism.*

■ Teach respiratory hygiene procedures such as the use of incentive spirometry, coughing, and deep breathing. *Adequate respiratory hygiene is imperative for all clients undergoing joint replacement to prevent respiratory complications associated with immobility and the effects of anesthesia. In addition, many clients undergoing total joint replacement are elderly and may have reduced mucociliary clearance.*

(continued)

NURSING CARE OF THE CLIENT HAVING Total Joint Replacement (continued)

- Discuss postoperative pain control measures, including use of patient-controlled analgesia (PCA) or epidural infusion as appropriate. *It is important for the client to understand the purpose and use of postoperative pain control measures to allow early mobility and reduce complications associated with immobility.*
- Teach or provide prescribed preoperative skin preparation such as shower, shampoo, and skin scrub with antibacterial solution. *These measures help reduce transient bacteria that may be introduced into the surgical site.*
- Administer intravenous antibiotic as ordered. *Antibiotic therapy is initiated before or during surgery and continued postoperatively to further reduce the risk of infection.*

POSTOPERATIVE CARE

- Monitor vital signs, including temperature and level of consciousness, every 4 hours or more frequently as indicated. Report significant changes to the physician. *These routine assessments provide information about the client's cardiovascular status and can give early indications of complications such as excessive bleeding, fluid volume deficit, and infection.*
- Perform neurovascular checks (color, temperature, pulses and capillary refill, movement, and sensation) on the affected limb hourly for the first 12 to 24 hours, then every 2 to 4 hours. Report abnormal findings to the physician immediately. *Surgery can disrupt the blood supply to or innervation of the affected extremity. If so, rapid intervention is important to preserve the function of the extremity.*
- Monitor incisional bleeding by emptying and recording suction drainage every 4 hours and assessing the dressing frequently. *Significant blood loss can occur with a total joint replacement, particularly a total hip replacement.*
- Reinforce the dressing as needed. *The dressing is usually changed 24 to 48 hours after surgery but may need reinforcement if excess bleeding occurs.*
- Maintain intravenous infusion and accurate intake and output records during the initial postoperative period. *The client is at risk for fluid volume deficit in the initial postoperative period because of blood and fluid loss during surgery, as well as the effects of the anesthetic.*
- Maintain bed rest and prescribed position of the affected extremity using a sling, abduction splint, brace, immobilizer, or other prescribed device. *Proper positioning of the affected extremity is vital in the initial postoperative period so that the joint prosthesis does not become dislocated or displaced.*
- Help the client shift position at least every 2 hours while on bed rest. *Shifting of position helps prevent pressure ulcers and other complications of immobility.*
- Remind the client to use the incentive spirometer, to cough, and to breathe deeply at least every 2 hours. *These measures are important to prevent respiratory complications such as pneumonia.*

- Assess the client's level of comfort frequently. Maintain PCA, epidural infusion, or other prescribed analgesia to promote comfort. *Adequate pain management promotes healing and mobility.*
- Help the client get out of bed as soon as allowed. Teach and reinforce the use of techniques to prevent weight bearing on the affected extremity, such as the overhead trapeze, pivot turning, and toe touch. *Early mobility prevents complications such as pneumonia and thromboembolism, but appropriate techniques must be used to prevent injury to the operative site.*
- Initiate physical therapy and exercises as prescribed for the specific joint replaced, such as quadriceps setting, leg raising, and passive and active ROM exercises. *These exercises help prevent muscle atrophy and thromboembolism and strengthen the muscles of the affected extremity so that it can support the prosthetic joint.*
- Use sequential compression devices, or antiembolism stockings, as prescribed. *These help prevent thromboembolism and pulmonary embolus for the client who must remain immobile following surgery.*
- For the client with a total hip replacement, prevent hip flexion of greater than 90 degrees or adduction of the affected leg. Provide a seat riser for the toilet or commode. *These measures prevent dislocation of the joint.*
- Assess the client with a total hip replacement for signs of prosthesis dislocation, including pain in the affected hip or shortening and internal rotation of the affected leg.
- For the client with a total knee replacement, use a continuous passive range-of-motion (CPM) device or ROM exercises as prescribed. *Dislocation is not a problem with a knee replacement, and more emphasis is placed on range-of-motion exercises in the early postoperative period.*
- Maintain fluid intake and encourage a high-fiber diet. Administer stool softeners or rectal suppositories as needed. *Immobility contributes to the potential problem of constipation; these measures help maintain regular fecal elimination.*
- Encourage consumption of a well-balanced diet with adequate protein. *Adequate nutrition promotes tissue healing.*
- Teach or reinforce postdischarge exercises and activity restrictions. Emphasize the importance of scheduled follow-up physician visits. *Clients are discharged from the acute care facility before healing is complete. Exercises are prescribed and activities are resumed gradually to protect the integrity of the joint replacement and prevent contractures.*
- For those clients needing additional direct care after discharge, arrange placement in a long-term care or rehabilitation facility. *Activity restrictions may preclude discharge to home for some clients.*
- Make referrals as needed to home health agencies and physical therapy. *Clients often require home health care for both nursing care needs and continued physical therapy following discharge from acute or long-term care.*

PHYSICAL THERAPY AND REHABILITATION Recovery from all types of joint replacement requires postoperative physical therapy, focusing on building strength and regaining joint flexibility. Rehabilitation begins in the hospital, most often the day following surgery, and may be continued during home care. Recovery from a hip replacement is 80% complete in 4 weeks and 100% complete in 6 months. Recovery from a knee replacement is 80% complete in 4 weeks and 100% complete after 1 year. During rehabilitation, the client must follow a regimen of exercise, rest, and medication (Flynn & Johnson, 2005).

COMPLEMENTARY AND ALTERNATIVE THERAPIES The following complementary therapies are examples of those that may be used by people with OA to relieve pain and stiffness. These same therapies are also used by people with rheumatoid arthritis.

- Biomagnetic therapy
- Acupuncture
- Eliminating nightshade foods such as potatoes, tomatoes, peppers, eggplant, tobacco
- Taking nutritional supplements, such as glucosamine, chondroitin, boron, zinc, copper, selenium, manganese, flavonoids, and/or SAM-e
- Herbal therapy
- Massage therapy
- Osteopathic manipulation
- Vitamin therapy
- Yoga.

NURSING CARE

OA is a chronic process for which there is no cure. The focus of nursing care for the client with OA is providing comfort, helping maintain mobility and ADLs, and assisting with adaptations to maintain life roles. A Nursing Care Plan for a client with OA is found on the next page.

Health Promotion

Although OA cannot be prevented, maintaining a normal weight and having a program of regular, moderate exercise will reduce risk factors. Glucosamine and chondroitin are nutritional supplements for OA that are increasingly popular and have been found to be of benefit in reducing manifestations. Clients should discuss these supplements with their healthcare provider before using them.

Assessment

Collect the following data through the health history and physical examination (see Chapter 40 ∞):

- *Health History:* Family history of OA, occupation, recreational activities, joint pain and stiffness, ability to carry out ADLs and self-care activities.
- *Physical Assessment:* Height/weight; gait; joints: symmetry, size, shape, color, appearance, temperature, pain, crepitus, range of motion, Heberden's nodes, Bouchard's nodes.

Nursing Diagnoses and Interventions

The priority nursing interventions for clients with OA are directed toward managing chronic pain, facilitating physical mobility, and improving ability to provide self-care.

Chronic Pain

Pain is a primary manifestation of OA. As joint tissues degenerate and changes in joint structure occur, the amount of discomfort generally increases. The pain associated with OA increases with activity and tends to be relieved with rest. Nonpharmacologic comfort measures are appropriate, with mild analgesics used to supplement these as needed.

- Monitor the level of pain, including intensity, location, quality, and aggravating and relieving factors. *Accurate assessment of pain provides a basis for evaluation of the effect of interventions.*
- Teach clients to take prescribed analgesic or anti-inflammatory medication as needed. *Analgesics reduce the perception of pain and may decrease muscle spasm as well. Anti-inflammatory medication may be ordered to decrease local inflammatory response in affected joints.*
- Encourage rest of painful joints. *The pain of OA is often relieved by joint rest.*
- Suggest applying heat to painful joints using the shower, a tub or sitz bath, warm packs, hot wax baths, heated gloves, or diathermy, which uses high-frequency electrical currents to generate heat. *Heat application reduces accompanying muscle spasm, relieving pain. Moist heat penetrates deeper than dry heat; diathermy delivers heat directly to lesions in deeper body tissues.*
- Emphasize the importance of proper posture and good body mechanics for walking, sitting, lifting, and moving. *Good body mechanics and posture reduce stress on affected joints.*
- Encourage the overweight client to reduce weight. *Excess weight places abnormal stress on joints, particularly the knees.*
- Encourage the use of nonpharmacologic pain relief measures such as progressive relaxation, meditation, visualization, and distraction. *These adjunctive pain relief measures can reduce the client's reliance on analgesics and increase comfort.*

Impaired Physical Mobility

As intra-articular cartilage degenerates and joint structures are altered, the client with OA experiences pain, stiffness, and decreased range of motion in affected joints. When the spine, large weight-bearing joints of the hips and knees, or the ankles and feet are affected, physical mobility can be significantly reduced.

- Assess the range of motion of affected joints. *Assessing joint mobility is important as a basis for planning appropriate interventions.*
- Perform a functional mobility assessment, evaluating gait, ability to sit and rise from sitting position, ability to step into and out of the tub or shower, and negotiation of stairs. *The functional assessment provides vital data about the client's ability to maintain ADLs.*

NURSING CARE PLAN A Client with Osteoarthritis

Robert Cerulli is a 72-year-old retired commercial fisherman who has experienced arthritic pain in his hips for the past 10 to 15 years. During the past year, the pain in his right hip has become severe, prompting him to seek medical attention. Significant degenerative changes in both hip joints are noted on x-ray films. The physician recommends a total replacement of the right hip, and total replacement of the left hip to follow in 6 to 12 months. Mr. Cerulli has preoperative teaching and tests the afternoon prior to his surgery, scheduled for 0800 the following morning.

ASSESSMENT

Christie Phlaugh, RN, completes a health history and examination of Mr. Cerulli on admission. Reviewing his medical record, she notes that Mr. Cerulli has mild Parkinson's disease and is taking carbidopa/levodopa (Sinemet 25-100) four times a day to control his symptoms. No other chronic medical conditions have been reported. Mr. Cerulli says he has been essentially healthy his entire life. He has no known allergies to medications, has never smoked, and consumes only small amounts of alcohol.

On examination of Mr. Cerulli, Ms. Phlaugh notes that he is alert and oriented. His vital signs are BP 116/64, P 68 regular, R 18, T 97.4°F (36.3°C) PO. Peripheral pulses are strong and equal in the upper extremities, and slightly weaker but equal in the lower extremities. His feet are cool to touch but have immediate capillary refill. He has full ROM of his shoulders, elbows, and wrists. The ROM of both hips is significantly restricted. Hip flexion beyond 90 degrees prompts pain on both sides. Both flexion and extension of the knees are limited slightly. Mr. Cerulli walks with a limp, favoring his right hip, and has a shuffling gait.

Preoperative laboratory studies including CBC, coagulation studies, chemistry panel, and urinalysis show a serum creatinine of 1.7 mg/dL and BUN of 30 mg/dL, with no other abnormal values noted. His ECG and chest x-ray show no apparent pathologies. Cefazolin (Ancef) 500 mg is to be administered intravenously at 0600 prior to surgery, and Mr. Cerulli is to shower and shampoo with antibacterial soap at bedtime. The physical therapist meets with Mr. Cerulli to evaluate his mobility and begin teaching him about postoperative weight-bearing restrictions.

DIAGNOSES (POSTOPERATIVE)

- *Acute Pain* related to surgical incision
- *Impaired Physical Mobility* related to activity and weight-bearing restrictions
- *Risk for Infection* related to disruption in skin integrity
- *Risk for Ineffective Tissue Perfusion, Right Leg* related to vascular disruption and edema

EXPECTED OUTCOMES

- Maintain an adequate level of comfort postoperatively as demonstrated by:
  - The ability to move easily within restrictions
  - Compliance with instructions to cough and breathe deeply
  - Verbal expressions of comfort.
- Remain free of adverse consequences of immobility such as pneumonia, pressure areas, thromboembolism, or contracture.
- Remain free of infection.

- Maintain adequate perfusion of affected leg.
- Remain free of injury postoperatively.

PLANNING AND IMPLEMENTATION

- Assess pain at least hourly during first 24 to 48 hours postoperatively, and as needed thereafter.
- Instruct in the use of PCA and monitor its effectiveness.
- Help change position at least every 2 hours; encourage the use of the overhead trapeze to shift positions frequently.
- Maintain sequential compression device and antiembolic stocking as ordered; remove for 1 hour daily.
- Encourage the use of the incentive spirometer hourly for first 24 hours, then at least every 2 hours while awake.
- Assist out of bed three times a day after the first 24 hours.
- Maintain abduction of the right hip with pillows.
- Perform passive ROM exercises of unaffected extremities every shift.
- Encourage frequent quadriceps-setting exercises and plantar and dorsiflexion of feet.
- Assess the surgical site frequently; report signs of excess bleeding or inflammation.
- Monitor temperature every 4 hours.
- Assess pulses, color, movement, and sensation of right foot hourly for the first 24 hours, then every 2 hours for 24 hours, then every 4 hours.

EVALUATION

Mr. Cerulli returns to the orthopedic unit from the postanesthesia care unit. He becomes confused and disoriented during the first 36 hours after surgery, but his orientation and thought processes gradually clear. His family has stayed with him, and he has not experienced injury or other adverse consequences from his confusion. Otherwise, Mr. Cerulli has had an uneventful postoperative recovery. Six days after surgery, he is transferred to an extended care rehabilitation facility for further therapy until he is able to ambulate with partial weight bearing on his affected leg. He returns home 5 weeks after surgery, able to use a walker for ambulation. Arrangements are made for an overbed trapeze, elevated toilet seat, and shower chair in his home. A home health nurse and physical therapist visit Mr. and Mrs. Cerulli weekly for a month following his discharge. During this time he gradually resumes full weight bearing. Mr. Cerulli expresses pleasure with the relief of his hip pain and says he has no fear of having his left hip replaced in the future.

CRITICAL THINKING IN THE NURSING PROCESS

1. Mr. Cerulli's preoperative laboratory work showed a modest elevation in his serum creatinine and BUN. What do these studies indicate? How might these changes affect nursing responsibilities related to medication administration for Mr. Cerulli?

2. Mr. Cerulli became confused postoperatively. What factors in his history might have alerted the nurses to this possibility? How might anesthesia and postoperative analgesics have contributed to his confusion?

3. Develop a care plan for Mr. Cerulli using the nursing diagnosis *Acute Confusion*.

See Evaluating Your Response in Appendix C.

Nursing Diagnoses and Interventions

Self-Care Deficit

The progressive muscle weakness that is associated with MD impairs the client's ability to perform self-care.

- Provide clients and family with supportive care during the progress of the disease. *The goal of treatment is to prolong each functional stage and delay or prevent deformity. When transition from ambulation to a wheelchair occurs, depression and grief may occur.*
- Promote independence. Encourage tasks that can be accomplished rather than letting the client struggle with tasks that may prove frustrating. *All forms of MD result in progressive muscle weakness. Management of the disease is directed toward keeping the client as functional as possible while preventing any deformities.*

Community-Based Care

Teaching the client with MD focuses on maintaining function and independence and preventing deformities. Teach prescribed exercises such as stretching and counterposturing exercises. For the client with braces, discuss skin care and ways to prevent irritation under the brace. Because the client may have weakness involving muscles of respiration, teach the client how to prevent respiratory infections, such as avoiding crowds during flu season and being immunized against pneumococcal pneumonia and influenza. Provide information about support services and organizations such as the Muscular Dystrophy Association.

AUTOIMMUNE AND INFLAMMATORY DISORDERS

Autoimmune and inflammatory disorders of the musculoskeletal system are chronic systemic rheumatic disorders, characterized by diffuse inflammatory lesions and degenerative changes in connective tissues. The disorders have similar clinical features and may affect many of the same structures and organs.

THE CLIENT WITH RHEUMATOID ARTHRITIS

Rheumatoid arthritis (RA) is a chronic systemic autoimmune disease that causes inflammation of connective tissue, primarily in the joints. Its course and severity are variable, and the range of manifestations is broad. Manifestations of RA may be minimal, with mild inflammation of only a few joints and little structural damage, or relentlessly progressive, with multiple inflamed joints and marked deformity. Most clients exhibit a pattern of symmetric involvement of multiple peripheral joints and periods of remission and exacerbation.

FAST FACTS
RA
- RA is found worldwide, affecting 1% to 2% of the total population and all races.
- RA affects 3 times as many women as men.
- The onset of RA occurs most frequently between the ages of 20 and 40 years.

The cause of RA is unknown. A combination of genetic, environmental, hormonal, and reproductive factors is thought to play a role in its development. It is speculated that infectious agents, such as bacteria, mycoplasmas, and viruses (especially Epstein-Barr virus), may play a role in initiating the autoimmune processes present in RA. Several studies have found that heavy smokers are at increased risk for developing RA. It is known that the incidence of RA has decreased during the past 40 years, supporting the theory that environmental factors may change and either promote or protect against RA (Flynn & Johnson, 2005).

The course of RA is variable and fluctuating. Remissions are most likely to occur in the first year of the disease. The rate at which joint deformities develop is not constant. Disease progression is fastest during the first 6 years, slowing thereafter. RA contributes to disability and a tendency to shorten life expectancy. About 10% of people with RA go into long-term remission within 1 year; and another 50% to 60% go into remission within 2 years (Flynn & Johnson, 2005).

RA is less common than OA, with RA affecting 1% to 2% of the population (about 2.1 million people) (Flynn & Johnson, 2005). The incidence of RA increases with age up to about 70 years. Although the onset and manifestations of RA are much the same in older and younger clients, differentiating between RA and OA in the older adult may be difficult at times. It is important to establish an accurate diagnosis, however, because the management of these disorders differs significantly. Clinical features distinguishing RA from OA are listed in Table 42–3.

For older clients, RA is managed much as it is for younger people. However, prolonged bed rest or inactivity is not prescribed for acute episodes, because it may result in irreversible immobility in the older adult. Also, medications are used with greater caution because of the increased risk of toxicity. In many cases, less emphasis is placed on preventing joint deformity and more emphasis on maintaining functional status for the older client with RA.

Pathophysiology

It is believed that long-term exposure to an unidentified antigen causes an aberrant immune response in a genetically susceptible host. As a result, normal antibodies (immunoglobulins) become autoantibodies and attack host tissues. These transformed antibodies, usually present in people with RA, are called *rheumatoid factors (RFs).* The self-produced antibodies bind with their target antigens in blood and synovial membranes, forming immune complexes (see Chapter 13 ∞ for further information about autoimmune processes).

The damage to cartilage that occurs in RA is the result of at least three processes:

- Neutrophils, T cells, and other synovial fluid cells are activated and degrade the surface layer of the articular cartilage.
- Cytokines, especially interleukin-1 (IL-1) and tumor necrosis factor alpha (TNF-α), cause the chondrocytes to attack the cartilage.

MEDIALINK ... Case Study: Rheumatoid Arthritis

TABLE 42–3 Comparison of the Manifestations of Rheumatoid Arthritis and Osteoarthritis

FEATURE	RHEUMATOID ARTHRITIS	OSTEOARTHRITIS
Onset	Usually insidious, may be abrupt	Insidious
Course	Generally progressive, characterized by remissions and exacerbations	Slowly progressive
Pain and stiffness	Predominant on arising, lasting >1 hour; also occurs after prolonged inactivity	Pain with activity; stiffness following periods of immobility generally relieved within minutes
Affected joints	■ Appear red, hot, swollen; "boggy" and tender to palpation; decreased ROM, weakness ■ Multiple joints affected in symmetric pattern; PIP, MCP, wrists, knees, ankles, and toes often involved	■ Affected joints may appear swollen; cool and bony hard on palpation; decreased ROM ■ One or several joints affected including hips, knees, lumbar and cervical spine, PIP and DIP, wrist, and 1st MTP joint
Systemic manifestations	Fatigue, weakness, anorexia, weight loss, fever; rheumatoid nodules; anemia	Fatigue

■ The synovium digests nearby cartilage, releasing inflammatory molecules containing IL-1 and TNF-α.

Leukocytes are attracted to the synovial membrane from the circulation, where neutrophils and macrophages ingest the immune complexes and release enzymes that degrade synovial tissue and articular cartilage. Activation of B and T lymphocytes results in increased production of rheumatoid factors and enzymes that increase and continue the inflammatory process.

The synovial membrane is damaged by the inflammatory and immune processes. It swells from infiltration of the leukocytes and thickens as cells proliferate and abnormally enlarge. The inflammation spreads and involves synovial blood vessels. Small venules are occluded, and vascular flow to the synovial tissue decreases. As blood flow decreases and metabolic needs increase (from the increased number and size of cells), hypoxia and metabolic acidosis occur. Acidosis stimulates synovial cells to release hydrolytic enzymes into surrounding tissues, starting erosion of the articular cartilage and inflammation of the supporting ligaments and tendons.

The inflammation also causes hemorrhage, coagulation, and deposits of fibrin on the synovial membrane, in the intracellular matrix, and in the synovial fluid. Fibrin develops into granulation tissue (*pannus*) over denuded areas of the synovial membrane. The formation of pannus leads to scar tissue formation that immobilizes the joint (Figure 42–5 ■).

Joint Manifestations

The onset of RA is typically insidious, although it may be acute (precipitated by a stressor such as infection, surgery, or trauma). Joint manifestations are often preceded by systemic manifestations of inflammation, including fatigue, anorexia, weight loss, and nonspecific aching and stiffness. Clients report joint swelling with associated stiffness, warmth, tenderness, and pain. The pattern of joint involvement is typically polyarticular (involving multiple joints) and symmetric. The proximal interphalangeal (PIP) and metacarpophalangeal (MCP) joints of the fingers, the wrists, the knees, the ankles, and the toes are most frequently involved, although RA can af-fect any joint. Stiffness is most pronounced in the morning, lasting more than 1 hour. It may also occur with prolonged rest during the day and may be more severe following strenuous activity. Swollen, inflamed joints feel "boggy" or spongelike on palpation because of synovial edema. Range of motion is limited in affected joints, and weakness may be evident.

The persistent inflammation of RA causes deformities of the joint itself and supporting structures such as ligaments, tendons, and muscles. As the joint is destroyed, ligaments, tendons, and the joint capsule are weakened or destroyed. Joint cartilage and bone are also destroyed. Weakening or destruction of these supporting structures results in lack of opposition to muscle pull, causing deformity.

Characteristic changes in the hands and fingers include ulnar deviation of the fingers and subluxation at the MCP joints. Swan-neck deformity is characterized by hyperextension of the PIP joint with compensatory flexion of the distal interpha-

Pannus with areas of eroded cartilage and bone

Increased joint fluid

Inflamed synovium

Figure 42–5 ■ Joint inflammation and destruction in rheumatoid arthritis. Note synovial inflammation with pannus formation and the erosion of cartilage and underlying bone.

langeal (DIP) joints. A flexion deformity of the PIP joints with extension of the DIP joint is called a boutonniére deformity (Figure 42–6 ■). The ability to effect a pinch is limited by hyperextension of the interphalangeal joint and flexion of the MCP joint of the thumb.

Wrist involvement is nearly universal, leading to limited movement, deformity, and carpal tunnel syndrome. Inflammation of the elbows often causes flexion contracture.

The knees are frequently affected in RA, with visible swelling often obliterating normal contours. Instability of the knee joint along with quadriceps atrophy, contractures, and valgus (knock-knee) deformities can lead to significant disability. Ambulation may be limited by pain and deformities when the ankles and feet are involved. Typical deformities of the feet and toes include subluxation, hallux valgus (deviation of the great toe toward the other digits of the foot), lateral deviation of the toes, and cock-up toes (turned-up toes).

Spinal involvement is usually limited to the cervical vertebrae. Neck pain is common, and neurologic complications can occur.

Extra-Articular Manifestations

RA is a systemic disease with a variety of extra-articular manifestations. These are seen particularly in clients with high levels of circulating rheumatoid factor. Fatigue, weakness, anorexia, weight loss, and low-grade fever are common when the disease is active. Anemia resistant to iron therapy frequently affects clients with RA. Skeletal muscle atrophy is common, usually most apparent in the musculature around affected joints.

Rheumatoid nodules may develop, usually in subcutaneous tissue in areas subject to pressure: on the forearm, olecranon bursa, over the MCP joints, and on the toes. Rheumatoid nodules are granulomatous lesions that are firm and either movable or fixed. They may also be found in viscera, including the heart, lungs, intestinal tract, and dura.

Other possible extra-articular manifestations of RA include subcutaneous nodules, pleural effusion, vasculitis, pericarditis, and splenomegly (enlargement of the spleen). The *Multisystem Effects of RA* are illustrated on page 1462.

Increased Risk of Coronary Heart Disease

People with rheumatoid arthritis have an increased risk of developing coronary heart disease (CHD). In turn, CHD increases the risk of myocardial infarction and death; in fact, RA is associated with a shortened life expectancy (Flynn & Johnson, 2005). RA affects the heart by:

■ Direct effects on the blood vessels, with measures of C-reactive proteins (inflammatory markers) being more predictive of future cardiovascular disease than are low-density lipoprotein (LDL) levels.
■ Increased risk of having low high-density lipoprotein, high cholesterol and triglyceride levels, high blood pressure, and high levels of homocysteine—all of which increase the risk for CHD.
■ The damaging side effects that many medications, such as methotrexate and steroids, often have on coronary vessels.

INTERDISCIPLINARY CARE

The diagnosis of RA is based on the client's history, physical assessment, and diagnostic tests. Diagnostic criteria developed by the American Rheumatism Association are used as well (Box 42–3). At least four of seven criteria must be present to establish the diagnosis.

Once the diagnosis of RA has been established, the goals of therapy are to relieve pain, reduce inflammation, slow or stop joint damage, and improve well-being and ability to function. No cure currently exists for RA; the goal of treatment is to relieve its manifestations. An interdisciplinary approach is used, with a balance of rest, exercise, physical therapy, and suppression of the inflammatory processes.

Because a cure is not available and traditional therapies are not always fully effective, the client with RA is vulnerable to quackery. Many nontraditional treatments, including diets, topical preparations, vaccines, hormones, plant extracts, and copper bracelets, have been put forth. These treatments are often costly, and none has been shown to be effective.

Figure 42–6 ■ Typical hand deformities associated with rheumatoid arthritis.

— Ulnar deviation

— Swan neck deformity

— Boutonnière deformities

Source: Biophoto Associates/Photo Researchers, Inc.

BOX 42–3 Diagnostic Criteria for Rheumatoid Arthritis

■ Morning stiffness lasting for at least 1 hour and persisting for at least 6 weeks
■ Arthritis with swelling or effusion of three or more joints persisting for at least 6 weeks
■ Arthritis of wrist, MCP, or PIP joints persisting for at least 6 weeks
■ Symmetric arthritis with simultaneous involvement of corresponding joints on both sides of the body
■ Rheumatoid nodules
■ Positive serum rheumatoid factor
■ Characteristic radiologic changes of rheumatoid arthritis noted in hands and wrists

MULTISYSTEM EFFECTS OF **Rheumatoid Arthritis**

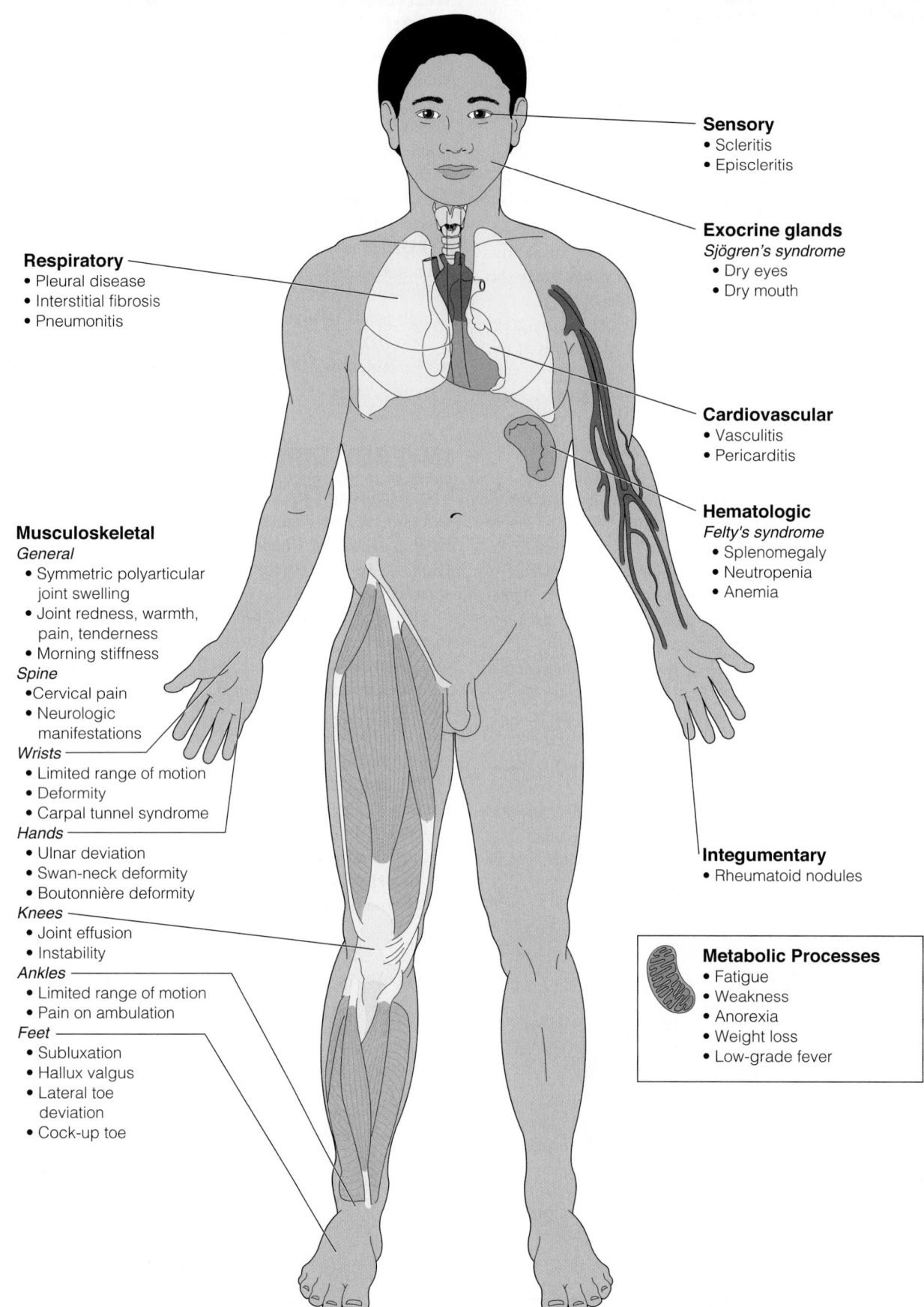

Sensory
- Scleritis
- Episcleritis

Exocrine glands
Sjögren's syndrome
- Dry eyes
- Dry mouth

Respiratory
- Pleural disease
- Interstitial fibrosis
- Pneumonitis

Cardiovascular
- Vasculitis
- Pericarditis

Hematologic
Felty's syndrome
- Splenomegaly
- Neutropenia
- Anemia

Musculoskeletal
General
- Symmetric polyarticular
  joint swelling
- Joint redness, warmth,
  pain, tenderness
- Morning stiffness
Spine
- Cervical pain
- Neurologic
  manifestations
Wrists
- Limited range of motion
- Deformity
- Carpal tunnel syndrome
Hands
- Ulnar deviation
- Swan-neck deformity
- Boutonnière deformity
Knees
- Joint effusion
- Instability
Ankles
- Limited range of motion
- Pain on ambulation
Feet
- Subluxation
- Hallux valgus
- Lateral toe
  deviation
- Cock-up toe

Integumentary
- Rheumatoid nodules

Metabolic Processes
- Fatigue
- Weakness
- Anorexia
- Weight loss
- Low-grade fever

Diagnosis

Diagnostic tests are used to help establish the diagnosis of RA. Testing is also used to rule out other forms of arthritis and connective tissue disorders. Diagnostic tests are described in Chapter 40.

Laboratory tests are used to measure rheumatoid factors and the ESR, which is typically elevated. A complete blood count (CBC) is done to identify anemia. Diagnosing RA in the early stages is often difficult, but a new test is highly effective. In this blood test, clients are tested for antibodies to cyclic citrullinated peptide (CCP) with accurate detection of early RA.

Synovial fluid examination will demonstrate changes associated with inflammation, including increased turbidity (cloudiness), decreased viscosity, and increased protein and WBC levels. X-rays of affected joints are the most specific test for diagnosis of RA. Early in the disease, few changes may be evident other than soft tissue swelling and joint effusions. As the disease progresses, joint space narrowing and erosions are seen.

Medications

Four general approaches are used in the pharmacologic management of clients with RA:

- Aspirin and other NSAIDs and mild analgesics are used to reduce the inflammatory process and manage the manifestation of the disease. Although these drugs may relieve manifestations of RA, they appear to have little effect on disease progression.
- The second approach uses low-dose oral corticosteroids to reduce pain and inflammation. Recent studies suggest that low-dose oral corticosteroids also may slow the development and progression of bone erosions associated with RA.
- A diverse group of drugs classified as disease-modifying or slow-acting antirheumatic drugs are employed in the third approach to treating RA. These drugs, which include gold compounds, D-penicillamine, antimalarial agents, infliximab (Remicade), and sulfasalazine, appear to alter the course of the disease, reducing its destruction of joints. Immunosuppressive and cytotoxic drugs are included in this category as well.
- Intra-articular corticosteroids may be used to provide temporary relief in clients for whom other therapies have failed to control inflammation.

ASPIRIN Aspirin is often the first drug prescribed in the treatment of RA unless its use is contraindicated for the client. Aspirin is an inexpensive and effective anti-inflammatory and analgesic agent. The dose of aspirin required to achieve a therapeutic blood level of 15 to 30 mg/dL and its full anti-inflammatory effect is approximately 4 g per day in divided doses (three or four 5-g [325-mg] tablets qid). This effective dose is just under the toxic dose, which produces tinnitus and hearing loss. The client may be instructed to increase the dose of aspirin gradually until either maximal improvement or toxicity occurs. If tinnitus develops, the client reduces the dose by two to three tablets per day until the tinnitus stops.

Gastrointestinal side effects and interference with platelet function are the greatest hazards of aspirin therapy. Clients are instructed to take aspirin with meals, milk, or antacids to minimize gastrointestinal distress and reduce the risk of GI bleeding.

Enteric-coated forms of aspirin and nonacetylated salicylate compounds produce less gastric distress than plain or buffered aspirin and reduce the risk of gastric ulceration, but they are more expensive. Salsalate (Disalcid, Mono-Gesic, Salflex) and choline magnesium trisalicylate (Trilisate, Tricosal) are examples of nonacetylated salicylate products. All salicylate products are contraindicated for clients with a history of aspirin allergy.

OTHER NONSTEROIDAL ANTI-INFLAMMATORY DRUGS A number of other NSAIDs are available for use in the management of RA if aspirin is not tolerated or effective. All NSAIDs act by inhibiting prostaglandin synthesis. Although the efficacy of all NSAIDs, including aspirin, is equivalent, client responses are individual. Several trials of different NSAIDs may be necessary to find the most effective drug.

Some NSAIDs are considerably more expensive than aspirin but may cause less gastrointestinal distress and require fewer doses per day. Gastric irritation, ulceration, and bleeding remain the most common toxic effects of NSAIDs. They can also affect the lower intestinal tract, leading to perforation or aggravation of inflammatory bowel disorders. All NSAIDs can also be toxic to the kidneys.

NSAIDs commonly prescribed for clients with RA are listed in Table 42–4. The FDA (2005) has issued planned regulatory actions for both prescription and over-the-counter (OTC) nonselective NSAIDs. These actions include increased label warnings about the potential serious adverse cardiovascular and gastrointestinal effects of these drugs; the nonprescription drugs include those containing ibuprofen, naproxen, and ketoprofen. Nursing implications for the administration of NSAIDs are described in Chapter 12 ∞.

CORTICOSTEROIDS Systemic corticosteroids can dramatically relieve the symptoms of RA and appear to slow the progression of joint destruction. The long-term use of corticosteroids is associated with multiple side effects, such as poor wound healing, increased risk of infection, osteoporosis, and gastrointestinal bleeding. Severe rebound manifestations can occur when these medications are discontinued. For these reasons, the use of systemic corticosteroids is limited to low dosages daily. The nursing implications for corticosteroid therapy are discussed in Chapter 13 ∞.

DISEASE-MODIFYING DRUGS Disease-modifying drugs are a diverse group of medications including drugs that modify immune and inflammatory responses, gold salts, antimalarial agents, sulfasalazine, and D-penicillamine (Table 42–5). They share characteristics that make them useful in the treatment of RA. Although beneficial effects are not apparent for several weeks or months following the initiation of therapy, they can produce not only clinical improvement but also evidence of decreased disease activity. Because their anti-inflammatory effect is minimal, NSAIDs are continued during therapy. As many as two-thirds of clients taking disease-modifying drugs show improvement, although these drugs have not been shown to slow bone erosion or facilitate healing. All of these drugs are fairly toxic, and close monitoring is necessary during the course of therapy.

Drugs that modify the autoimmune and inflammatory responses in clients with RA include leflunomide (Arava) and

TABLE 42–4 Examples of Nonsteroidal Anti-Inflammatory Drugs Used to Treat Rheumatoid Arthritis

DRUG	AVERAGE DOSE	COMMENTS AND PRECAUTIONS
Aspirin	600–900 mg 4 to 6 times daily	Least expensive NSAID; associated with risk of GI ulceration, bleeding, and possible hemorrhage; may cause hepatotoxicity
Diclofenac (Voltaren)	50 mg tid or qid; or 75 mg bid	Expensive; risk of hepatotoxicity
Etodolac (Lodine)	200-400 mg q6h	Expensive; may have less gastrointestinal toxicity
Fenoprofen (Nalfon)	300-600 mg tid or qid	Should not be administered to clients with impaired renal function; risk of GU effects such as dysuria, cystitis, hematuria, acute interstitial nephritis, and nephrotic syndrome
Flurbiprofen (Ansaid)	50-100 mg tid or qid, not to exceed 300 mg/day	Expensive
Ibuprofen (Motrin, Advil, others)	300 mg qid; 400-800 mg tid or qid	Available in prescription and OTC forms; less gastric distress reported than with aspirin or indomethacin; discontinue if visual disturbances develop
Indomethacin (Indocin)	25-50 mg bid or tid	A potent NSAID used for moderate to severe RA and acute episodes of chronic disease; higher incidence of adverse GI effects and CNS effects such as headache, dizziness, and depression
Ketoprofen (Orudis)	50-75 mg tid or qid	Expensive; older adults and clients with renal insufficiency require lower doses
Meclofenamate sodium (Meclomen)	100 mg bid to qid	Increased risk of adverse effects in older adults; GI effects include diarrhea and abdominal pain; anemia may develop during therapy
Nabumetone (Relafen)	1000-2000 mg per day	Most common adverse effects include diarrhea, dyspepsia, and abdominal pain
Naproxen (Aleve, Anaprox, Naprosyn)	250-500 mg bid	Available in prescription and OTC preparations
Oxaprozin (Daypro)	1200 mg daily	Expensive; risk of severe hepatotoxicity; rash may occur
Piroxicam (Feldene)	20 mg daily in a single or divided dose	Expensive; GI side effects including stomatitis, anorexia, and gastric distress may occur more frequently than with other NSAIDs
Sulindac (Clinoril)	150-200 mg bid	May be safer for use than other NSAIDs in clients with chronic renal disease; rare fatal hypersensitivity reaction with fever, liver function abnormalities, and severe skin reaction
Tolmetin (Tolectin)	200-600 mg tid	Expensive; may have higher rate of side effects including GI distress, headache, dizziness, elevated blood pressure, edema, and weight gain

etanercept (Enbrel). Leflunomide reversibly inhibits an enzyme involved in the autoimmune process, and etanercept inhibits the binding of tumor necrosis factor to receptor sites. Infliximab (Remicade) is a biologic response modifier and TNF-α receptor antagonist. Given by intravenous infusion, the drug is administered to reduce infiltration of inflammatory cells and TNF-α production. Adalimumab (Humira) is a biologic response modifier that is given to people with RA to reduce the inflammatory events of polyarthritis and slow the progression of joint damage. Given by subcutaneous injection, the drug cannot be administered if the person has an acute or chronic infection in any part of the body. Prior to initiating the drug, the person should be tested for tuberculosis.

Gold salts may be administered by mouth, but the intramuscular route is preferred because it is more effective. The mode of action of gold is unknown, but it may produce clinical remission in some clients and decrease new bony erosions. Weekly therapy is continued until significant improvement is noted unless toxic reactions occur. Clients experiencing benefit from gold therapy may be continued on monthly injections for several years. About one-third of clients on gold therapy ex-

perience toxic reactions, including dermatitis, stomatitis, bone marrow depression, and proteinuria. Mild skin reactions do not always necessitate discontinuation of therapy. CBC and urinalysis are monitored throughout treatment with gold to assess for more severe toxic responses.

Hydroxychloroquine (Plaquenil) is an antimalarial agent sometimes employed in the treatment of RA. Three to 6 months of therapy is required to achieve the desired response, and many clients do not experience significant benefit. Although hydroxychloroquine has a relatively low toxicity, it can cause pigmentary retinitis and vision loss. Clients receiving this drug require a thorough vision examination every 6 months.

Sulfasalazine, a drug regularly prescribed for chronic inflammatory bowel disease, may also be prescribed for RA. See Chapter 26 ∞ for further discussion of this drug and its nursing implications. For clients not responding to the above preparations, penicillamine may be prescribed. Although this agent may be effective in the management of RA, toxic reactions are common and can be severe, including bone marrow suppression, proteinuria, and nephrosis.

TABLE 42–5 Disease-Modifying Drugs Used to Treat Rheumatoid Arthritis

CLASS/MEDICATIONS	USUAL DOSE	ADVERSE EFFECTS	COMMENTS/NURSING RESPONSIBILITIES
Gold salts: Gold sodium thiomalate (Myochrysine) Aurothioglucose (Solganal) Auranofin (Ridaura Capsules)	Parenteral: 1st dose 10 mg; 2nd dose 25 mg, then 50 mg weekly IM Oral: 6 mg daily	■ Pruritus, dermatitis ■ Stomatitis, metallic taste ■ Renal toxicity ■ Blood dyscrasias ■ Gastrointestinal distress	■ Frequent UA and CBC ■ Monitor client after injection for flushing, fainting, dizziness, sweating, possible anaphylactic reaction
Antimalarial: Hydroxychloroquine (Plaquenil)	200-600 mg daily with meals	■ CNS reactions including irritability, nightmares, psychoses ■ Retinopathy ■ Alopecia, pruritus ■ Blood dyscrasias ■ GI disturbances	■ Should not be used during pregnancy ■ Regular ophthalmologic examination required
Sulfasalazine (Azulfidine)	2 g/day in divided doses with meals	■ Anorexia, nausea, vomiting, gastric distress ■ Decreased sperm count ■ Headache ■ Rash ■ Blood dyscrasias ■ Hypersensitivity responses including Stevens-Johnson syndrome ■ CNS, liver, and renal toxicity	■ Administer in evenly divided doses ■ Maintain high fluid intake ■ May cause yellow-orange skin or urine discoloration ■ Regular CBCs necessary
Penicillamine (Cuprimine, Depen Titratable)	125-250 mg/day initially, slowly increased to a total of 1000-1500 mg/day	■ Skin rashes ■ Fever ■ Gastrointestinal distress ■ Oral ulcers, loss of taste ■ Fever ■ Bone marrow depression with thrombocytopenia, leukopenia, anemia ■ Renal toxicity ■ May induce immune complex disorders such as Goodpasture's syndrome and myasthenia gravis	■ Regular CBC and UA necessary ■ Administer on an empty stomach ■ Discontinue during pregnancy ■ May require 2 to 3 months of therapy before benefit is seen

IMMUNOSUPPRESSIVE THERAPY Immunosuppressive or cytotoxic drugs are increasingly employed in the management of RA. Indeed, many now consider methotrexate the treatment of choice for clients with aggressive RA. Methotrexate may be used along with NSAIDs in the initial treatment plan. A weekly dose can produce a beneficial effect in as few as 2 to 4 weeks. Gastric irritation and stomatitis are the most frequent side effects associated with methotrexate, but side effects may be better controlled if folic acid is taken at the same time. Alcoholism, diabetes, obesity, advanced age, and renal disease increase the risk of toxic effects (hepatotoxicity, bone marrow suppression, interstitial pneumonitis).

Other immunosuppressive agents such as cyclosporine, azathioprine, and monoclonal antibodies have also been employed in the treatment of clients with severe, progressive, crippling disease who have failed to respond to other measures.

Treatments

The primary objectives in treating RA are to reduce pain and inflammation, preserve function, and prevent deformity.

REST AND EXERCISE A balanced program of rest and exercise is an important component in the management of clients with RA. During an acute exacerbation of the disease, the client may be hospitalized, or a short period of complete bed rest may be prescribed. For most clients, regular rest periods during the day are beneficial to reduce manifestations of the disease. Additionally, splinting of inflamed joints reduces unwanted motion and provides local joint rest. A variety of orthotic devices are available to reduce joint strain and help maintain function.

Rest must be balanced with a program of physical therapy and exercise to maintain muscle strength and joint mobility. ROM exercises are prescribed to maintain joint function and prevent contractures. Isometric exercises are used to improve muscle strength without increasing joint stress. Isotonic exercises also help improve muscle strength and preserve function. Low-impact aerobic exercises, such as swimming and walking, have been shown to benefit clients with RA without adversely affecting joint inflammation or prompting acute episodes.

PHYSICAL AND OCCUPATIONAL THERAPY Physical and occupational therapists can design and monitor individualized activity and rest programs.

HEAT AND COLD Heat and cold are used for their analgesic and muscle-relaxing effects. Moist heat is generally the most effective, and can be provided by a tub bath. Joint pain is relieved in some clients through the application of cold.

ASSISTIVE DEVICES AND SPLINTS Assistive devices, such as a cane, walker, or raised toilet seat, are most useful for clients with significant hip or knee arthritis. Splints provide joint rest and prevent contractures. Night splints for the hands and/or wrists should maintain the extremity in a position of maximum function. The best "splint" for the hip is lying prone for several hours a day on a firm bed. In general, splints should be applied for the shortest period needed, should be made of lightweight materials, and should be easily removed to perform ROM exercises once or twice a day.

NUTRITION For most clients with RA, an ordinary, well-balanced diet is recommended. Some clients may benefit from substitution of usual dietary fat with omega-3 fatty acids found in certain fish oils.

SURGERY Surgical intervention may be employed for the client with RA at a variety of disease stages. Early in the course of the disease, synovectomy (excision of synovial membrane) can provide temporary relief of inflammation, relieve pain, and slow the destructive process, helping to preserve joint function. Arthrodesis (joint fusion), may be used to stabilize joints such as cervical vertebrae, wrists, and ankles. Arthroplasty, or total joint replacement, may be necessary in cases of gross deformity and joint destruction. Total joint replacement and nursing care of clients undergoing this surgery are discussed in the preceding section on OA.

OTHER THERAPIES Several newer treatments that are not yet in widespread use may be employed in clients with progressive RA. Plasmapheresis has been used to remove circulating antibodies, moderating the autoimmune response. Total lymphoid irradiation decreases total lymphocyte levels, although serious adverse effects are associated with this treatment, and its continued efficacy has not been established.

NURSING CARE

Clients with chronic, progressive, systemic disorders such as RA have multiple nursing care needs involving many functional health patterns. Physical manifestations of the disease often result in acute and chronic pain, fatigue, impaired mobility, and difficulty performing routine tasks. The disease also has many psychosocial effects. The client has an incurable chronic disease that may lead to severe crippling. Pain and fatigue can interfere with the client's ability to perform expected roles, such as home maintenance or job responsibilities. Even though the client's hands may appear swollen or deformed, other people may not understand the systemic nature of the disease or realize the difference between RA and OA. A Nursing Care Plan for a client with RA is found on the next page.

Health Promotion

People with RA have control of their lives by becoming arthritis self-managers. They can help prevent deformities and the effects of arthritis by following prescriptions for exercise, rest, weight management, posture, and positioning. The following suggestions are outlined by the Moss Rehab Resource Net (2005):

- Never attempt an activity that cannot be stopped immediately if it proves to be beyond your power to complete it.
- Respect pain as a warning signal. When you experience pain, change your method of doing things, use equipment or tools if necessary, and take intermittent rest periods.
- Use the strongest joints available for an activity. For example, use the palm of your hand or the crook of your elbow instead of fingers for grasping while carrying.
- Avoid stress toward a position of deformity, such as when the fingers drift toward the little finger. For example, open a jar with your right hand and close a jar with your left hand.
- Avoid activities that need a tight grip, such as writing, wringing, and unscrewing.

Assessment

Collect the following data through the health history and physical examination (see Chapter 40 ∞):

- *Health History:* Pain, stiffness, fatigue, joint problems: location, duration, onset, effect on function, fever, sleep patterns, past illnesses or surgery, ability to carry out ADLs and self-care activities.
- *Physical Assessment:* Height/weight; gait; joints: symmetry, size, shape, color, appearance, temperature, range of motion, pain; skin: nodules, purpura; respiratory: cough, crackles; cardiovascular: pericardial friction rub, apical bradycardia, S_3.

Nursing Diagnoses and Interventions

Many nursing diagnoses may be appropriate for the client with RA. This section focuses on those related to its predominant manifestations and their effect on the client's life.

Chronic Pain

Pain is a constant feature of RA when the disease is active. Pain accompanies both acute inflammation and lower levels of chronic inflammation. Some clients say the pain in joints and surrounding tissue is like a deep, constant toothache. Pain can significantly affect the client's ability to provide self-care and maintain daily activities. It also contributes to the client's fatigue.

- Monitor the level of pain and duration of morning stiffness. *Pain and morning stiffness are indicators of disease activity. Increased pain may necessitate changes in the therapeutic treatment plan.*
- Encourage the client to relate pain to activity level and adjust activities accordingly. Teach the importance of joint and whole-body rest in relieving pain. *Pain is an indicator of excess stress on inflamed joints. Increasing pain indicates a need to decrease activity levels.*
- Teach the use of heat and cold applications to provide pain relief. The client may apply heat by showering or taking tub

NURSING CARE PLAN A Client with Rheumatoid Arthritis

Janice James is a 42-year-old high school science teacher who began noticing vague joint pain, fatigue, poor appetite, and general malaise, which she initially attributed to a case of the flu. However, her symptoms continued, and she reports feeling very stiff in the mornings, often taking until 10:00 or 11:00 A.M. to begin to feel "normal." She then began to notice aching in her hands and wrists, which she attributed to the quilting she loves to do in the evenings. She made an appointment with her family physician when she noticed that her knuckles and finger joints are not just achy but also swollen and hot. Noting that Mrs. James has lost 10 lb since her last visit and has mild anemia and a significantly elevated ESR, the physician refers her to the rheumatology clinic for further evaluation. Following examination, laboratory, and radiologic testing, the rheumatologist establishes a diagnosis of rheumatoid arthritis and initiates a multidisciplinary team conference to plan the management of Mrs. James's rheumatoid arthritis.

ASSESSMENT

Cathy Greenstein, RN, completes an assessment of Mrs. James. She notes that Mrs. James is well groomed and answers questions readily but appears fatigued and ill. Mrs. James relates that her job has been extremely stressful because teacher layoffs have resulted in larger class sizes and fewer teaching assistants. Despite symptoms, she continues to teach full time, but says she feels unable to keep up with all her responsibilities due to her fatigue.

Mrs. James states that she is allergic to penicillin. Her past medical history reveals only the usual childhood diseases and three uncomplicated pregnancies, resulting in the births of her children, ages 14, 11, and 9. Physical assessment findings include BP 124/78, P 82 regular, R 18, T 100.2°F (37.8°C) PO. Hands: swelling of the proximal interphalangeal (PIP) and metacarpophalangeal (MCP) joints of both hands; second and third PIP and second MCP joints on right hand are red, shiny, hot, spongy, and tender to palpation; able to extend fingers to 180 degrees but cannot make a complete fist with either hand, with flexion limited to less than 90 degrees; grip strength is weak bilaterally; wrist ROM is limited in all directions. Knees are swollen, and flexion is slightly limited; positive bulge sign in the right knee. Diagnostic findings are an ESR of 52 mm/h, a hematocrit of 30% and positive for rheumatoid factor. Few changes other than soft tissue swelling are evident on hand and wrist x-rays.

DIAGNOSES

- *Chronic Pain* related to joint inflammation
- *Impaired Home Maintenance* related to fatigue
- *Activity Intolerance* related to the effects of inflammation
- *Deficient Knowledge: Therapeutic Regimen*

EXPECTED OUTCOMES

- Verbalize effective pain management strategies:
  - Use assistive devices to minimize joint stress with ADLs:

- Verbalize a plan to reduce responsibilities for home maintenance.
- Express a willingness to plan rest breaks during the day.
- Demonstrate understanding of the prescribed therapeutic regimen and its importance for both short- and long-term benefit.

PLANNING AND IMPLEMENTATION

- Teach techniques for relieving pain and morning stiffness, including:
  - Schedule NSAIDs at equal intervals throughout the day
  - Take morning NSAID dose with milk and crackers approximately 30 minutes before rising
  - Perform ROM exercises in shower or bathtub
  - Apply local heat with paraffin dip or compress, use cold packs as needed.
  - Teach techniques to minimize joint stress while performing ADLs.
- Provide Arthritis Foundation literature and information.
- Discuss ways to delegate household tasks to other family members.
- Explore ways to incorporate 30-minute rest breaks into work schedule.
- Provide information about the disease process and its manifestations, prescribed medications with desired and adverse effects, and the importance of balancing rest and activity.

EVALUATION

The initial treatment regimen of aspirin, rest, exercise, and physical therapy succeeded in partially relieving the acute manifestations of rheumatoid arthritis in Mrs. James. However, complete remission has not been achieved. She has had difficulty scheduling rest periods at work and has had to struggle to delegate household tasks. "I don't look sick to the kids, and they seem to think housecleaning is a terrible imposition on their time. It's often easier to just do it myself than to fight about it. Besides, that way it gets done right." Mrs. James has faithfully followed the prescribed medication regimen and exercise routines, and she has kept her scheduled appointments and maintained contact with the treatment team.

CRITICAL THINKING IN THE NURSING PROCESS

1. Mrs. James is 42 years old. Would your nursing interventions differ if she were 72 years old? If so, how.
2. Rheumatoid arthritis is a chronic illness. What are the physical, emotional, and economic implications of a chronic illness that results in chronic pain and deformity?
3. Develop a nursing care plan for Mrs. James using the nursing diagnosis *Ineffective Role Performance*.
   See Evaluating Your Response in Appendix C.

---

baths, or using warm compresses or other local applications such as paraffin dips. For clients who find that heat increases pain and swelling during periods of acute inflammation, cold packs may be more effective. *Both heat and cold have analgesic effects and can help relieve associated muscle spasms.*

- Teach about the use of prescribed anti-inflammatory medications and the relationship of pain and inflammation. *Anti-inflammatory agents reduce chemical mediators of inflammation and swelling, relieving pain.*
- Encourage using other nonpharmacologic pain relief measures such as visualization, distraction, meditation, and progressive

relaxation techniques. *These techniques can reduce muscle tension and help the client focus away from the pain, decreasing the intensity of the pain experience.*

Fatigue

The pain and chronic inflammatory processes associated with RA lead to fatigue. Other factors contribute as well. Discomfort often disrupts the client's sleep patterns. Anemia, muscle atrophy, and poor nutrition also play a role in the development of fatigue. The client with RA may experience depression or hopelessness, with associated manifestations of fatigue.

- Encourage a balance of periods of activity with periods of rest. *Both joint and whole-body rest are important to reduce the inflammatory response.*
- Stress the importance of planned rest periods during the day. *Rest is vital during acute exacerbations of the disease but also important to maintain the client in remission.*
- Help in prioritizing activities, performing the most important ones early in the day. *Assigning priorities helps the client avoid performing relatively unimportant activities at the expense of more meaningful and important ones.*
- Encourage regular physical activity in addition to prescribed ROM exercises. *Aerobic exercise promotes a sense of well-being and restful sleep patterns.*
- Refer to counseling or support groups. *Counseling and support groups can help the client develop effective coping strategies and deal with depression and hopelessness.*

Ineffective Role Performance

Fatigue, pain, and the crippling effects of RA can interfere with the client's ability to pursue a career and fill other life roles, such as parent, spouse, or homemaker. As the client's role changes, so must the roles of other family members. This can contribute to changes in family processes, increased stress in the family, and further difficulty coping with the effects of the disease.

- Discuss the effects of the disease on the client's career and other life roles. Encourage the client to identify changes brought on by the disease. *Discussion helps the client to accept the changes and begin to identify strategies for coping with them.*
- Encourage the client and family to discuss their feelings about role changes and grieve lost roles or abilities. *Verbalization allows family members to validate and accept feelings about losses and changes, thus helping them to move into new roles.*
- Listen actively to concerns expressed by the client and family members; acknowledge the validity of concerns about the disease, prescribed treatment, and the prognosis. *Demonstrating acceptance of these feelings and concerns promotes trust and validates their reality.*

> **PRACTICE ALERT**
> Remember that grief resolution takes time and that clients may respond to loss with anger.

- Help the client and family identify strengths they can use to cope with role changes. *Identifying strengths helps the client and family to consider role changes that maintain self-esteem and dignity.*

- Encourage the client to make decisions and assume personal responsibility for disease management. *Clients who assume a personal and active role in managing their disease maintain a greater sense of self-control and self-esteem.*

Disturbed Body Image

The acute and long-term effects of RA can affect the client's body image, leading to feelings of hopelessness and powerlessness, social withdrawal, and difficulty adapting to changes. When inflammation and joint deformity occur despite compliance, the client may have difficulty accepting the need to continue therapeutic measures, particularly those that have side effects or are costly or time consuming. In addition, unproven alternative treatment strategies and quackery may become increasingly attractive to the client.

- Demonstrate a caring, accepting attitude toward the client. *This attitude helps the client accept the physical changes brought on by the disease.*
- Encourage the client to talk about the effects of the disease, both physical effects and effects on life roles. *Verbalization helps the client identify feelings and gives the nurse opportunity to validate these feelings.*
- Encourage the client to maintain self-care and usual roles to the extent possible. Discuss the use of clothing and adaptive devices that promote independence. *Independence enhances the client's self-esteem.*
- Provide positive feedback for self-care activities and adaptive strategies. *Positive reinforcement encourages the client to continue adaptive measures and maintain independence.*
- Refer to self-help groups, support groups, and other agencies that provide assistive devices and literature. *These groups and agencies can help the client develop adaptive strategies to cope with the effects of RA, enhancing the client's self-concept, body image, and independence.*

Using NANDA, NIC, and NOC

Chart 42–3 shows links between NANDA nursing diagnoses, NIC, and NOC when caring for the client with RA.

Community-Based Care

RA is typically a chronic, progressive disease. As with most diseases of this nature, involvement of the client and family in its management is vital. Education is an important nursing role in caring for clients with RA and their families. (See the Nursing Research box on page 1469). Address the following topics for home care of the client and for family members:

- Disease process and treatments, including rest and exercise
- Medications
- Management of stiffness and pain
- Energy conservation
- Use of assistive devices to maintain independence, including self-care aids such as handheld showers, long-handled brushes and shoehorns, and eating utensils with oversized or special handles
- Clothing options such as elastic waist pants without zippers, Velcro closures, zippers with large pull-tabs, and slip-on shoes
- How to apply splints and take care of skin

NANDA, NIC, AND NOC LINKAGES
CHART 42-3 The Client with Rheumatoid Arthritis

NANDA

Powerlessness

↓

NIC

Self-Esteem Enhancement

Support Group

Emotional Support

Environmental Management

Self-Care Assistance

↓

NOC

Health Beliefs: Perceived Control

Health Beliefs: Perceived Resources

Social Support

Data from *NANDA's Nursing Diagnoses: Definitions & Classification 2005–2006* by NANDA International (2005), Philadelphia; *Nursing Interventions Classification (NIC)* (4th ed.) by J. M. Dochterman & G. M. Bulechek (2004), St. Louis, MO: Mosby; and *Nursing Outcomes Classification (NOC)* (3rd ed.) by S. Moorhead, M. Johnson, and M. Maas (2004), St. Louis, MO: Mosby.

- Home and equipment modifications, such as a raised toilet seat, grab bars in the bathroom, a bath chair, or adapted counter heights for clients in a wheelchair
- Physical therapy, occupational therapy, home health and homemaker services
- Helpful resources:
  - National Institute of Arthritis and Musculoskeletal and Skin Diseases
  - American College of Rheumatology
  - Arthritis Foundation.
  - The Arthritis Society
  - American Physical Therapy Foundation
  - American Chronic Pain Association.

THE CLIENT WITH ANKYLOSING SPONDYLITIS

Ankylosing spondylitis (AS) is a chronic inflammatory arthritis that primarily affects the axial skeleton, leading to pain and progressive stiffening and fusion of the spine. The typical age of onset is between 17 and 35, with at least half a million people with AS in the United States (Spondylitis Association of America, 2006). The incidence is greater in men than women and men have more severe disease. AS is difficult to diagnose in the early stages, but may be a major cause of persistent back pain in young adults.

The cause of ankylosing spondylitis is unknown. As with the other spondyloarthropathies, there is a strong genetic component. Approximately 90% of people with ankylosing spondylitis have the HLA-B27 antigen; about 8% of the general population has this antigen (Porth, 2005).

 NURSING RESEARCH | **Evidence-Based Practice: Teaching the Client with Rheumatoid Arthritis**

Rheumatoid arthritis (RA) is a disease that can occur at any age, but is seen most often in older adults. RA causes physical, emotional, and economic difficulties, but appropriate management can do much to reduce pain and disability, improve a sense of control, and improve quality of life. With recent advances in computer technology, the Internet has become a convenient means of providing information to people with RA. However, little is known about how many older adults use the computer to gain access to information. This study was conducted to examine the use of computers and the Internet by older adults with arthritis and to describe the characteristics of those who did use the Internet to find health information. Although one of every four older adults who participated in the study owned a computer, only slightly more than half actually used the Internet. Lack of knowledge about using the computer or about accessing the Internet were given as possible reasons.

IMPLICATIONS FOR NURSING

The Internet is a powerful method for providing health information to older adults. Although health history questions rarely contain questions about availability and use of the computer and the Internet, it may be equally as important as asking about other components of one's dwelling. If older adults have but do not use a computer, referral to community resources that provide computer learning classes can facilitate their success in using the computer and doing online searches of the Internet for health information. In addition, prior to recommending an Internet-based health resource, nurses should review the site for content, readability, navigation features, credibility, organization, and graphic appearance.

CRITICAL THINKING IN CLIENT CARE

1. You are designing an Internet site to teach older adults about RA. What topics would you include? How would your presentation be most effective for this age group?
2. You are conducting a computer-literacy course for older adults with RA at a local library. All of them have computers, but none of them have used the Internet to find out about the disease. What sites would you recommend, and why?
3. Develop a plan to include assessment about computers on an agency's health history. What would you include to convince the agency personnel that this is important?

Data from Tak, S. H., & Hong, S. H. (2005). Use of the Internet for health information by older adults with arthritis. *Orthopaedic Nursing, 24*(2), 134-139.

Pathophysiology

Early inflammatory changes often are first noted in the sacroiliac joints. As the cartilage erodes, joint margins ossify and are replaced by scar tissue. The joints of the spine are also affected, with inflammation of the cartilaginous joints, and gradual calcification and ossification that leads to ankylosis, or joint consolidation and immobility. Other organ systems may be affected as well, including the eyes, lungs, heart, and kidneys.

Manifestations

The onset of ankylosing spondylitis is usually gradual and insidious. Clients may have persistent or intermittent bouts of low back pain. The pain is worse at night, followed by morning stiffness that is relieved by activity. Pain may radiate to the buttocks, hips, or down the legs. As the disease progresses, back motion becomes limited, the lumbar curve is lost, and the thoracic curvature is accentuated. In severe cases, the entire spine becomes fused, preventing any motion. Clients with ankylosing spondylitis may also experience peripheral arthritis, primarily affecting the hip, shoulders, and knee joints. Systemic manifestations include anorexia, weight loss, fever, and fatigue. Many clients develop uveitis (inflammation of the iris and the middle, vascular layer of the eye).

For most clients with ankylosing spondylitis, the disease is intermittent with mild to moderate acute episodes. These clients have a good prognosis with little risk of severe disability.

INTERDISCIPLINARY CARE

Diagnostic testing shows an elevated ESR during periods of active disease and typically a positive HLA-B27 antigen. The diagnosis of ankylosing spondylitis is usually confirmed with x-ray examination of the sacroiliac joints and spine. The sacroiliac joint becomes blurred and gradually obliterated. As the disease progresses, vertebrae become squared, and disk spaces narrow.

As with other forms of arthritis, the management of ankylosing spondylitis is multidimensional. Physical therapy and daily exercises are important to maintain posture and joint ROM. NSAIDs relieve pain and stiffness and allow the client to perform necessary exercises. Indomethacin (Indocin) is the NSAID most commonly used to treat ankylosing spondylitis. It may, however, have many adverse effects, including headache, nausea and vomiting, depression, and psychosis. Other drugs that may be prescribed include sulfasalazine (Azulfidine) and topical or intra-articular corticosteroids. Severe hip joint arthritis may necessitate total hip arthroplasty.

NURSING CARE

The primary nursing role in ankylosing spondylitis is to provide supportive care and education. To promote mobility, teach the client to take NSAIDs at regular intervals throughout the day with food, milk, or antacid. Encourage the client to maintain a fluid intake of 2500 mL or more per day. Suggest that the client perform exercises in the shower because warm, moist heat prompts mobility. Stress the importance of following the prescribed physical therapy and exercise program to maintain mobility.

Teach the client that proper positioning and posture are important. When sleeping, a bed board may be used to provide firmness, and the person should sleep in the supine position using either no pillow or only one small pillow. Other important self-care activities include losing weight if applicable, avoiding smoking, and using muscle-strengthening exercises. Suggest occupational counseling if pain and deformity are severe enough to cause work-related problems.

THE CLIENT WITH REACTIVE ARTHRITIS

Reactive arthritis (ReA) (*Reiter's syndrome*) is an acute, nonpurulent inflammatory arthritis that is believed to be a response to an exposure or infection with certain types of bacteria, including *Chlamydia* (a bacterium contracted during sexual activity) or *Salmonella, Shigella, Yersinia, or Campylobacter* (which cause dysentery from contaminated or spoiled food). This type of arthritis most often affects young men who have an inherited HLA-B27 antigen. Reactive arthritis is often found in clients with HIV infection, although the reason for the association is not clear. Reactive arthritis is typically self-limited, although it can be recurrent or progressive. About 15% to 20% of people with ReA develop a chronic arthritis or spondylitis (Spondylitis Association of America, 2006).

Manifestations

Nonbacterial urethritis is often the initial manifestation of Reiter's syndrome. In women, urethritis and cervicitis may be asymptomatic. Conjunctivitis and inflammatory arthritis follow. The arthritis is usually asymmetric, affecting large weight-bearing joints such as the knees and ankles, the sacroiliac joints, or the spine. Mouth ulcers, inflammation of the glans penis, and skin lesions may occur. The heart and aorta may also be affected.

INTERDISCIPLINARY CARE

The diagnosis of reactive arthritis is based on the client's history and presenting symptoms. Manifestations of ReA typically occur 2 to 4 weeks after the infection, and subside in 3 to 12 months. The condition has a tendency to recur. No test is specific for the disorder. Urethral or cervical cultures are obtained to rule out gonococcal infection. When *Chlamydia* is suspected, the client and sexual partner are treated with tetracycline or erythromycin. Reactive arthritis is treated symptomatically, usually with NSAIDs.

NURSING CARE

Clients with reactive arthritis usually are seen in primary care settings such as a clinic or physician's office, making the nursing role primarily one of education. Teach the client about the association of the arthritis with the precipitating infection (if identified). Stress the importance of treating the infection effectively if it is still present. Use this opportunity to provide information about sexually transmitted infections and protective measures to prevent their transmission (see Chapter 52 ∞). Discuss the usual self-limited nature of reactive arthritis, the appropriate use of prescribed NSAID preparations, and symptomatic relief measures such as application of heat and rest.

THE CLIENT WITH SYSTEMIC LUPUS ERYTHEMATOSUS

Systemic lupus erythematosus (SLE) is a chronic inflammatory connective tissue disease. It affects almost all body systems, including the musculoskeletal system. The manifestations of SLE are widely variable and are thought to result from cell and tissue damage caused by deposition of antigen–antibody complexes in connective tissues. SLE affects multiple body systems, and it can range from a mild, episodic disorder to a rapidly fatal disease process.

FAST FACTS
SLE

- Approximately 1 person in 2000 is affected by SLE (about 500,000 in the United States), with women predominating by a ratio of 9:1 over men.
- SLE usually affects women of childbearing age (when the incidence is 30 times greater than in men) but it can occur at any age.
- SLE is more common in African Americans, Hispanics, and Asians than it is in Caucasians (Porth, 2005).
- The incidence of SLE is higher in some families.

Although the exact etiology of SLE is unknown, genetic, environmental, and hormonal factors play a role in its development. Twin studies and a familial pattern of the disease point to a genetic component, as does an increased incidence of other connective tissue diseases in relatives of people with SLE. Certain human leukocyte antigen (HLA) genes are seen more frequently in people with SLE. Environmental factors such as viruses, bacterial antigens, chemicals, drugs, or ultraviolet light may play a role in activation of the pathologic mechanisms of the disease. In addition, it is felt that sex hormones may influence the development of SLE. Women with SLE have reduced levels of several active androgens that are known to inhibit antibody responses. Estrogens have been shown to enhance antibody responses and have an adverse effect in clients with SLE.

The course of SLE is mild in most clients, with periods of remission and exacerbation. The number and severity of exacerbations tend to decrease with time. In some clients, however, SLE is a virulent disease with significant organ system involvement.

Clients with active disease have an increased risk for infections, which are often opportunistic and severe. Infections such as pneumonia and septicemia are the leading cause of death in clients with SLE, followed by the effects of renal or central nervous system (CNS) involvement. See the Multisystem Effects of SLE on the next page.

Pathophysiology

The pathophysiology of SLE involves the production of a large variety of autoantibodies against normal body components such as nucleic acids, erythrocytes, coagulation proteins, lymphocytes, and platelets. Autoantibody production results from hyperreactivity of B cells (humoral response) because of disordered T-cell function (cellular immune response). The most characteristic autoantibodies in SLE are produced in response to nucleic acids, including DNA, histones, ribonucleoproteins, and other components of the cell nucleus.

SLE autoantibodies react with their corresponding antigen to form immune complexes, which are then deposited in the connective tissue of blood vessels, lymphatic vessels, and other tissues. The deposits trigger an inflammatory response leading to local tissue damage. The kidneys are a frequent site of complex deposition and damage; other tissues affected include the musculoskeletal system, brain, heart, spleen, lung, GI tract, skin, and peritoneum. The autoantibodies produced and their target tissue determine the manifestations of SLE.

A number of drugs can cause a syndrome that mimics lupus in clients with no other risk factors for the disease. Procainamide (e.g., Procan-SR, Pronestyl) and hydralazine (Apresoline, Hydralyn) are the most common drugs implicated, along with isoniazid (INH).

Renal and CNS manifestations of SLE rarely occur with drug-induced lupus, but arthritic and other systemic symptoms are common. Manifestations of drug-induced lupus usually resolve when the medication is discontinued.

Manifestations

Typical early manifestations of SLE mimic those of rheumatoid arthritis, including systemic manifestations of fever, anorexia, malaise, and weight loss, and musculoskeletal manifestations of multiple arthralgias and symmetric polyarthritis. Joint symptoms affect more than 90% of clients with SLE. Although synovitis may be present, the arthritis associated with SLE is rarely deforming.

Most people affected by SLE have skin manifestations at some point during their disease. In fact, SLE was originally described as a skin disorder and named for the characteristic red butterfly rash across the cheeks and bridge of the nose (Figure 42–7 ■).

Figure 42–7 ■ The butterfly rash of systemic lupus erythematosus.

MULTISYSTEM EFFECTS of Systemic Lupus Erythematosus

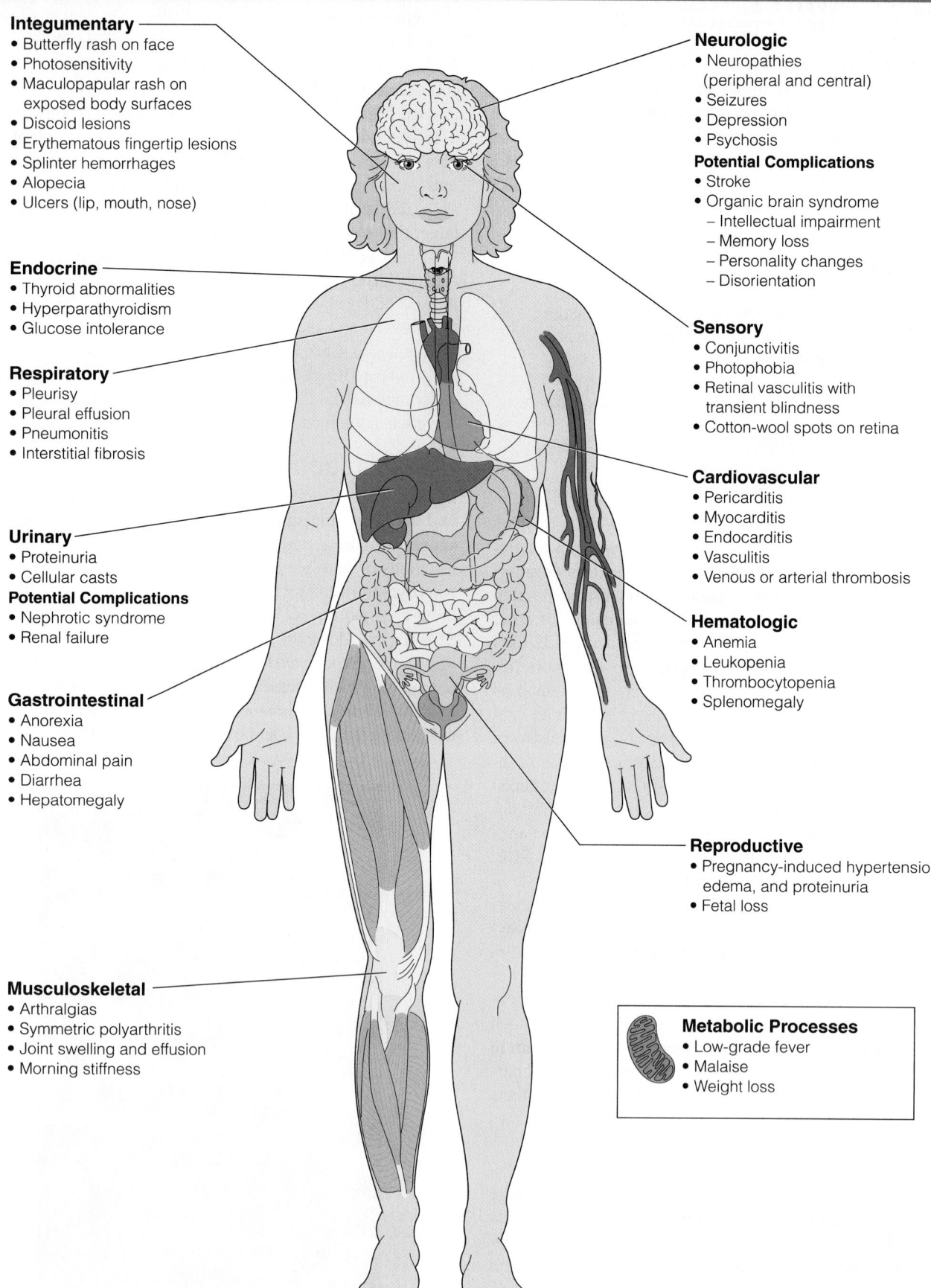

Integumentary
- Butterfly rash on face
- Photosensitivity
- Maculopapular rash on exposed body surfaces
- Discoid lesions
- Erythematous fingertip lesions
- Splinter hemorrhages
- Alopecia
- Ulcers (lip, mouth, nose)

Endocrine
- Thyroid abnormalities
- Hyperparathyroidism
- Glucose intolerance

Respiratory
- Pleurisy
- Pleural effusion
- Pneumonitis
- Interstitial fibrosis

Urinary
- Proteinuria
- Cellular casts

Potential Complications
- Nephrotic syndrome
- Renal failure

Gastrointestinal
- Anorexia
- Nausea
- Abdominal pain
- Diarrhea
- Hepatomegaly

Musculoskeletal
- Arthralgias
- Symmetric polyarthritis
- Joint swelling and effusion
- Morning stiffness

Neurologic
- Neuropathies (peripheral and central)
- Seizures
- Depression
- Psychosis

Potential Complications
- Stroke
- Organic brain syndrome
  - Intellectual impairment
  - Memory loss
  - Personality changes
  - Disorientation

Sensory
- Conjunctivitis
- Photophobia
- Retinal vasculitis with transient blindness
- Cotton-wool spots on retina

Cardiovascular
- Pericarditis
- Myocarditis
- Endocarditis
- Vasculitis
- Venous or arterial thrombosis

Hematologic
- Anemia
- Leukopenia
- Thrombocytopenia
- Splenomegaly

Reproductive
- Pregnancy-induced hypertension, edema, and proteinuria
- Fetal loss

Metabolic Processes
- Low-grade fever
- Malaise
- Weight loss

Many clients with SLE are photosensitive; a diffuse maculopapular rash on skin exposed to the sun is common. Other cutaneous manifestations include discoid lesions (raised, scaly, circular lesions with an erythematous rim), hives, erythematous fingertip lesions, and splinter hemorrhages. Alopecia is common in clients with SLE, although the hair usually grows back. Painless mucous membrane ulcerations may occur on the lips or in the mouth or nose. Common manifestations of SLE are listed in the box below.

Approximately 50% of people with SLE experience renal manifestations of the disease, including proteinuria, cellular casts, and nephrotic syndrome. Up to 10% develop renal failure as a result of the disease.

Hematologic abnormalities such as anemia, leukopenia, and thrombocytopenia are common with SLE. Cardiovascular disorders such as pericarditis, vasculitis, and Raynaud's phenomenon often occur. Less frequently, myocarditis, endocarditis, and venous or arterial thrombosis may develop. Pleurisy, pleural effusions, and lupus pneumonitis are common pulmonary manifestations of SLE.

Many clients with SLE develop transient nervous system involvement, often within the first year of the disease. Organic brain syndrome manifestations include decline in intellect, memory loss, and disorientation. Other possible neurologic manifestations include psychosis, seizures, depression, and stroke. Ocular manifestations of SLE include conjunctivitis, photophobia, and transient blindness due to retinal vasculitis.

Gastrointestinal manifestations of SLE, such as anorexia, nausea, abdominal pain, and diarrhea, may affect up to 45% of clients with the disease. The liver may be enlarged, and liver function tests may yield abnormal results.

INTERDISCIPLINARY CARE

Because of the diversity of organ system involvement and manifestations of SLE, diagnosis can be difficult. No one specific test is available to confirm the presence of this disease in all people suspected of having it. Instead, the diagnosis is based on the client's history and physical assessment, as well as laboratory studies.

As with rheumatoid arthritis, effective management of SLE requires teamwork, with active participation by both the client and members of the healthcare team. Although there is no cure for

---

MANIFESTATIONS of SLE

- Painful or swollen joints and muscle pain
- Unexplained fever
- Red rash, especially on the face
- Unusual loss of hair
- Pale, cyanotic fingers or toes
- Sensitivity to the sun
- Edema in legs and around eyes
- Ulcers in the mouth
- Enlarged glands
- Extreme fatigue

SLE, the 10-year survival rate is greater than 70% among clients with this disease, which was once considered fatal in most cases.

Diagnosis

The multiple autoantibodies produced in SLE cause a number of abnormalities in laboratory tests. Diagnostic tests for the musculoskeletal system are described in Chapter 40 .

- *Anti-DNA antibody testing* is a more specific indicator of SLE, because these antibodies are rarely found in any other disorder.
- *ESR* is typically elevated, occasionally to >100 mm/h.
- *Serum complement levels* are usually decreased as complement is consumed or "used up" by the development of antigen-antibody complexes.
- *CBC* abnormalities include moderate to severe anemia, leukopenia and lymphocytopenia, and possible thrombocytopenia.
- *Urinalysis* shows mild proteinuria, hematuria, and blood cell casts during exacerbations of the disease when the kidneys are involved. Renal function tests including *serum creatinine* and *blood urea nitrogen (BUN)* may also be ordered to evaluate the extent of renal disease.
- *Kidney biopsy* may be performed to assess the severity of renal lesions and guide therapy (see Chapter 27).

Medications

The client with mild or remittent SLE may need little or no therapy other than supportive care. Arthralgias, arthritis, fever, and fatigue can often be managed with aspirin or other NSAIDs. Aspirin is particularly beneficial for clients with SLE because its antiplatelet effects help prevent thrombosis. It may, however, cause liver toxicity and hepatitis.

Skin and arthritic manifestations of SLE may be treated with antimalarial drugs such as hydroxychloroquine (Plaquenil). Hydroxychloroquine has also been shown to be effective in reducing the frequency of acute episodes of SLE in people with mild or inactive disease. Retinal toxicity and possibly irreversible blindness are the primary concerns with this drug. For this reason, the client taking hydroxychloroquine undergoes ophthalmologic exam every 6 months.

Clients with severe and life-threatening manifestations of SLE (such as nephritis, hemolytic anemia, myocarditis, pericarditis, or CNS lupus) require corticosteroid therapy in high doses. Such clients may require 40 to 60 mg of prednisone per day initially. The dosage is tapered as rapidly as the client's disease allows, although lowering the dosage may precipitate an acute episode. Some clients with SLE require long-term corticosteroid therapy to manage symptoms and prevent major organ damage. These clients are at increased risk for corticosteroid side effects, such as cushingoid effects, weight gain, hypertension, infection, accelerated osteoporosis, and hypokalemia.

Immunosuppressive agents such as cyclophosphamide or azathioprine may be used, alone or in combination with corticosteroids, to treat clients with active SLE or lupus nephritis (see the Medication Administration box on the next page). When these agents are used in combination, lower, less toxic doses of each drug can be used. The client receiving immunosuppressive agents is at increased risk for infection, malignancy, bone marrow depression, and toxic effects specific to the drug prescribed.

MEDICATION ADMINISTRATION **Immunosuppressive Agents for SLE**

CYTOTOXIC AGENTS
Azathioprine (Imuran)
Cyclophosphamide (Cytoxan)
Cyclosporine (Sandimmune)
Certain cytotoxic or antineoplastic drugs are effective as immunosuppressive agents. They act by decreasing the proliferation of cells within the immune system and are widely used to prevent rejection following a tissue or organ transplant. They are usually administered concurrently with corticosteroid therapy, allowing lower doses of both preparations, and resulting in fewer side effects.

Nursing Responsibilities
- Monitor blood count, with particular attention to the WBC and platelet counts. Notify the physician if WBCs fall below 4000 or platelets below 75,000.
- Monitor renal and liver function studies including creatinine, BUN, creatinine clearance, and liver enzyme levels. Report any abnormal levels to the physician.
- Oral preparations should be administered with food to minimize gastrointestinal effects. Antacids may be ordered.
- Increase fluids to maintain good hydration and urinary output.
- Monitor intake and output.

- Monitor for signs of abnormal bleeding: bleeding gums, bruising, petechiae, joint pain, hematuria, and black or tarry stools.
- Use meticulous hand washing and other appropriate measures to protect the client from infection. Assess for signs of infection.
- Pulmonary fibrosis is a potential adverse effect of cyclophosphamide. Therefore, monitor the results of pulmonary function studies and be alert to clinical signs of dyspnea or cough.

Health Education for the Client and Family
- Avoid large crowds and situations where you might be exposed to infections.
- Report signs of infection such as chills, fever, sore throat, fatigue, or malaise to the physician.
- Use contraceptive measures to prevent pregnancy while you are taking these drugs because they cause birth defects.
- Avoid the use of aspirin or ibuprofen while taking these drugs. Report any signs of bleeding to the physician.
- You may stop menstruating while you are taking cyclophosphamide. The menses will resume after the drug is discontinued.
- If you are taking cyclophosphamide, be sure to report difficulty breathing or cough to the physician.

Treatments

Because of the photosensitivity associated with SLE, the client should be cautioned to avoid sun exposure. Clients should use sunscreens with a sun protection factor (SPF) rating of 15 or higher when out of doors. Topical corticosteroids may be used to treat skin lesions. Some physicians recommend avoiding the use of oral contraceptives, because estrogen can trigger an acute episode.

Clients with lupus nephritis who progress to develop end-stage renal disease are treated with dialysis (hemodialysis or peritoneal dialysis) and kidney transplantation, discussed in Chapter 29 ∞.

NURSING CARE

Nursing care for the client with mild SLE may be limited to teaching. The client with severe disease, however, has many diverse nursing needs, which vary according to the organ systems involved. Because of the close link between rheumatoid arthritis and SLE, many of the nursing diagnoses and interventions identified for the client with arthritis may be appropriate for the client with lupus. The client with lupus nephritis or end-stage renal disease has the nursing care needs outlined in the sections of Chapter 29 ∞ related to glomerulonephritis and chronic renal failure. This section focuses on the needs of the client related to the dermatologic manifestations of lupus, an increased risk for infection, and health maintenance.

Nursing Diagnoses and Interventions

The priority nursing interventions for the client with SLE are focused on problems with impaired skin integrity, ineffective protection, and impaired health maintenance.

Impaired Skin Integrity

Skin lesions are a common manifestation of SLE. A rash or discoid lesion interrupts the integrity of the skin and the first line of protection against infection, increasing the client's already high risk of infection. These lesions, which usually appear on exposed parts of the skin, can also be disfiguring and cause the client emotional distress.

- Assess knowledge of SLE and its possible effects on the skin. *Assessment allows the nurse to base teaching and information on the client's existing knowledge, improving learning and retention.*
- Discuss the relationship between sun exposure and disease activity, both dermatologic and systemic. *It is important for the client to understand that sun exposure may not only cause dermatologic manifestations but also trigger an acute episode.*
- Suggest the following strategies to limit sun exposure:
  - Avoid being out of doors during hours of greatest sun intensity (10:00 A.M. to 3:00 P.M.).
  - Use sunscreen with an SPF of 15 or higher when sun exposure cannot be avoided. Apply it 30 minutes before going out into the sun.
  - Reapply sunscreen after swimming, exercising, or bathing.
  - Wear loose clothing with long sleeves and wide-brimmed hats when out of doors.
  These strategies can help the client maintain a normal lifestyle while helping to prevent acute episodes.
- Keep skin clean and dry; apply therapeutic creams or ointments to lesions as prescribed. *These measures promote healing and reduce the risk of infection.*

Ineffective Protection

Ineffective protection can be a problem for the client with SLE, who is at increased risk for infection and multiple organ system problems because of the disease. In addition, treatment with corticosteroids or immunosuppressive agents further impairs immune responses and the ability to fight infection. The following interventions are for the client who is hospitalized.

- Wash hands before and after providing direct care. *Hand washing removes transient organisms from the skin, reducing the risk of transmission to the client.*

> **PRACTICE ALERT**
> Hands must be washed before and after providing direct care, even if gloves are worn. A decrease in this type of medical asepsis is contributing to the increasing number of hospital-acquired infections that are resistant to antibiotics.

- Use strict aseptic technique in caring for intravenous lines and indwelling urinary catheters or performing any wound care. *Aseptic technique offers protection against external and resident host microorganisms.*
- Assess frequently for infection. Monitor temperature and vital signs every 4 hours. Assess for signs of cellulitis, including tenderness, redness, swelling, and warmth. Report signs of infection to the physician promptly. *Therapy can suppress usual responses, such as elevated temperature and inflammation. The fever of infection may be mistaken for the fever commonly associated with lupus. The client receiving immunosuppressive therapy for the disease has an even higher risk for infection.*
- Monitor laboratory values, including CBC and tests of organ function; report changes to the physician. *An elevation in the WBC count with a shift to the left (increased numbers of immature leukocytes in the blood) may be an early indication of infection. Changes in liver function studies, renal function studies, myocardial enzymes, or other laboratory values may indicate organ system involvement.*
- Initiate reverse or protective isolation procedures as indicated by the client's immune status. *These procedures provide further protection from infection for the severely immunocompromised client.*
- Ensure an adequate nutrient intake, offering supplementary feedings as indicated or maintaining parenteral nutrition if necessary. *Adequate nutrition is important for healing and immune system function.*
- Teach the client the importance of good handwashing after using the bathroom and before eating. *Hand washing reduces the risk of infection with endogenous organisms.*
- Monitor for potential adverse effects of medications including thrombocytopenia and possible bleeding, fluid retention with edema and possible hypertension, loss of bone density, osteoporosis, and possible pathologic fractures, renal or hepatic toxicity, and cardiac effects, particularly in the client with fluid retention and hypervolemia. *Medications used to treat SLE have many potential adverse effects that can impair normal protective and homeostatic mechanisms.*

Impaired Health Maintenance

As with other chronic diseases, much of the responsibility for maintaining optimal health rests with the client. Disease manifestations such as fatigue, arthralgias, arthritis, and increased risk for infection can interfere with the client's ability to maintain health. Psychosocial issues can also be a significant factor in health maintenance for the client with lupus. These issues may include denial of the significance of the disease, poor coping, lack of financial and other resources, and an inadequate support system.

- Assess the ability to maintain optimal health, identifying physical and psychosocial factors that may affect health maintenance. *Before intervening to improve the client's health maintenance, the nurse must identify and understand factors affecting it.*
- Provide care and teaching in a nonjudgmental manner. *To intervene effectively, the nurse must accept the client and family as they are.*
- Encourage the client and family members to discuss the effect of the disease on their lives. *Open discussion helps the client and the nurse identify barriers to health maintenance and begin exploring alternative strategies.*
- Initiate an interdisciplinary care conference with the client and family. *In this care conference, a number of perspectives can be expressed, improving the planning of strategies for health maintenance activities.*
- Refer the client and family to counseling as needed. *Counseling may help the client and family develop the necessary coping skills to accept and deal with the disease.*
- Refer the client and family to community and social service agencies, and local support groups. *These groups and agencies are valuable resources for the client and family.*

Community-Based Care

Teaching is a critical factor in preparing clients with SLE for self-care at home. Address the following topics:

- The disease and its potential effects. Promote an optimistic outlook, stressing that the majority of clients do not require long-term corticosteroid therapy and that the disease may improve over time.
- The importance of skin care.
- The importance of avoiding exposure to infection.
- The need to follow the prescribed treatment plan, including rest and exercise, medications, and follow-up appointments. Discuss manifestations of an acute episode (often called a *flare*) and stress the importance of contacting the physician promptly if any of these manifestations occur.

> **PRACTICE ALERT**
> **Warning Signs of a Flare**
> - Increased fatigue
> - Pain, abdominal discomfort
> - Rash
> - Headache
> - Fever
> - Dizziness

- The significance of wearing a Medic-Alert tag identifying their condition and therapy such as corticosteroids or immunosuppressives.
- Family planning with the client and spouse. The use of oral contraceptives may be contraindicated for the client; if appropriate,

provide information about alternative means of birth control. Pregnancy is not contraindicated for most women with lupus. However, the pregnant client requires close monitoring because acute episodes sometimes accompany pregnancy.

- The need for preventive health care for both men and women with SLE. Women should have gynecologic and breast examinations and men should have prostate examinations each year. Both men and women should have regular screenings for cholesterol and blood pressure. Annual influenza vaccinations are important, as is pneumococcal vaccinations for older clients. If clients are taking corticosteroids or antimalarial medications, annual eye examinations should be conducted to screen for and treat any eye problems.
- Helpful resources:
  - National Institute of Arthritis and Musculoskeletal and Skin Diseases
  - Lupus Foundation of America.

THE CLIENT WITH POLYMYOSITIS

Polymyositis is a systemic connective tissue disorder characterized by inflammation of connective tissue and muscle fibers leading to muscle weakness and atrophy. When muscle fiber inflammation is accompanied by skin lesions, the disease is known as dermatomyositis. Polymyositis is an autoimmune disorder of unknown cause that affects more women than men. The onset of the disease typically occurs between the ages of 40 and 60 years, although a childhood-onset form is also seen.

The immune mechanism causing the inflammatory response in polymyositis is not clear, but autoantibodies can be identified in the majority of people with the disease. The activation of complement is thought to contribute to the inflammatory process. Inflammation leads to muscle fiber necrosis and degeneration.

Manifestations

Initial manifestations of polymyositis include muscle pain, tenderness, and weakness; rash; arthralgias; fatigue; fever; and weight loss. Skeletal muscle weakness is the predominant manifestation. Its onset may be either insidious or abrupt. Muscle weakness tends to progress over weeks to months. Muscles of the shoulder and pelvic girdles are particularly affected, making it difficult for the client to get out of chairs, climb stairs, and reach overhead. Weakness of neck flexor muscles may make it difficult to raise the head from a pillow. Affected muscles may also be tender and painful. A characteristic dusky red rash may be present on the face and upper trunk. Other manifestations include Raynaud's phenomenon, dysphagia, dyspnea, and cough (due to interstitial pneumonitis). The risk of malignancy is increased, particularly in clients with dermatomyositis.

INTERDISCIPLINARY CARE

There is no specific test to diagnose polymyositis. Autoantibodies may be identified in blood serum. Serum levels of muscle enzymes are elevated, particularly creatine kinase (CK) and aldolase levels. Biopsy of involved muscle shows patchy muscle fiber necrosis and the presence of inflammatory cells.

A combination of rest and corticosteroid therapy is prescribed for the client with polymyositis. Long-term corticosteroid therapy may be necessary to manage the disease. Immunosuppressive agents such as methotrexate, cyclophosphamide, and azathioprine may be used for clients who do not respond well to treatment with corticosteroids.

NURSING CARE

The nursing role in caring for the client with polymyositis is supportive. Measures to promote comfort are important. Muscle weakness may interfere with the client's ability to provide self-care and manage health and home. The client may have difficulty with speech because of pharyngeal muscle weakness. Provide alternate means of communication as needed, and use patience in listening. Observe closely while the client eats, because aspiration is a potential problem. Modify the client's diet as needed to maintain nutrition and safety.

Education of the client and family is an important component of care. Emphasize the need to balance periods of rest and activity. Discuss skin care to prevent dryness and infection. Teach the client about prescribed medications and their short- and long-term side effects. Provide information about safety measures while eating. Encourage family members to become trained in performance of the Heimlich maneuver and CPR. Discuss signs of respiratory infection and other possible complications of polymyositis, including renal failure and malignancy.

THE CLIENT WITH LYME DISEASE

Lyme disease is an inflammatory disorder caused by the spirochete *Borrelia burgdorferi,* which is transmitted primarily by ticks. It is the most commonly reported tick-borne illness in the United States. Geographically, Lyme disease is more prevalent in the areas where the ticks are found: in the coastal Northeast, the upper Midwest, and coastal California regions of the United States (ACR, 2004b). It has also been reported throughout Europe, Asia, and Australia. Ticks that act as vectors for Lyme disease, primarily *Ixodes dammini, I, pacificus,* and *I. scapularis* in the United States, are usually carried by mice or deer, although other animals may be infected. The most frequent time of onset is the summer months.

> **FAST FACTS**
> **Lyme Disease**
> - Lyme disease is the most common tick-transmitted disease in the United States.
> - Lyme disease occurs most often in children and young adults living in rural areas.
> - All stages of Lyme disease can be cured by antibiotics, but some people with late neurologic or arthritic involvement may not improve.

Pathophysiology

Borrelia burgdorferi enters the skin at the site of the tick bite. After an incubation period of up to 30 days, it migrates outward in the skin, forming a characteristic lesion called erythema migrans. It may also spread via lymph or blood to other skin sites, nodes, or organs. The inflammatory joint changes associated with Lyme disease closely resemble those of rheumatoid arthritis (vascular congestion, tissue infiltration by inflammatory cells, possible pannus formation, and erosion of cartilage and bone).

Manifestations

Manifestations often are seen in the skin, musculoskeletal system, and CNS. Lyme disease begins with flulike manifestations and a skin rash, followed weeks or months later by Bell's palsy or meningitis, and months to years later, by arthritis. This progression is highly individualized.

Erythema migrans is the initial manifestation of Lyme disease. This flat or slightly raised red lesion at the site of the tick bite expands over several days (up to a diameter of 50 cm), with the central area clearing as it expands. Systemic symptoms such as fatigue, malaise, fever, chills, and myalgias often accompany the initial lesion. As the disease spreads, secondary skin lesions develop, as do migratory musculoskeletal symptoms, including arthralgias, myalgias, and tendinitis. Persistent fatigue is common during this stage of the disease. Headache and stiff neck are characteristic neurologic manifestations.

Complications

With untreated infection, complications can develop months to years after the initial infection. Chronic recurrent arthritis, primarily affecting large joints (especially the knee), is common. Permanent disability may result. Other effects that may be seen weeks to months after the initial infection include meningitis, encephalitis, and neuropathies, as well as cardiac complications including myocarditis and heart block.

INTERDISCIPLINARY CARE

Both manifestations and laboratory studies are used to establish the diagnosis of Lyme disease. Culture of the organism from tissues and body fluids is difficult and slow. Antibodies to *B. burgdorferi* can be detected by either enzyme-linked immunosorbent assay (ELISA) or Western blot methods within 2 to 4 weeks of the initial skin lesion.

The early diagnosis and proper antibiotic treatment of Lyme disease are important to preventing the complications of infection. A number of antibiotics may be used to treat Lyme disease, including doxycycline (Doxy-Caps, Vibramycin), tetracycline, amoxicillin (Amoxil), cefuroxime axetil (Ceftin), or erythromycin. Therapy may be continued for up to 1 month to ensure eradication of the organism from affected tissues. The nursing implications for various classes of antibiotics are summarized in Chapter 12 ∞ .

In addition to antibiotic treatment, aspirin or another NSAID may be prescribed for relief of arthritic symptoms. The affected joint may be splinted to rest the joint. When the knee is involved, weight bearing may be restricted and the use of crutches indicated.

NURSING CARE

Nursing care focuses on prevention of the disease. Many people do not protect themselves from tick bites. This protection is becoming increasingly important with a higher incidence of Lyme disease, due in part to an overpopulation of deer and the encroachment of the suburbs on once rural areas. Simple measures that can help prevent tick bites are as follows:

- Avoid tick-infested areas, especially in spring and summer, such as woods and rural areas with brush and tall weeds.
- Cover exposed skin with long-sleeved shirts and tuck pants into socks. Wearing high rubber boots may provide additional protection.
- Use insect repellents that contain DEET on clothing and exposed skin and apply permethrin to clothing prior to exposure.
- Inspect skin, especially in areas of tight-fitting clothing, after exposure.
- Remove attached ticks with fine-tipped tweezers. Grasp the tick firmly as close to the skin as possible and pull the tick's body away from the skin. If the tick's head remains in the skin, it will not cause Lyme disease (the bacteria are in the tick's midgut). Most cases occur when the tick has been feeding for at least 24 hours (Tierney et al., 2004). Clean the area with an antiseptic.

INFECTIOUS DISORDERS

Infectious disorders of bone and joints are caused by a pathogen, and are often difficult to treat. Chronic infections may result in pain, deformity, and disability.

THE CLIENT WITH OSTEOMYELITIS

Osteomyelitis is an infection of the bone. Osteomyelitis may occur as an acute, subacute, or chronic process. It occurs as a consequence of bacteremia (hematogenous osteomyelitis), invasion from a contiguous focus of infection, or skin breakdown in the presence of vascular insufficiency (Tierney et al., 2004).

Osteomyelitis can occur at any age, but adults over age 50 are more commonly affected. The older adult is at risk for osteomyelitis for several reasons. Immune function tends to decline with aging; the older adult also is more likely to have a chronic disease process that affects immune function. Circulatory status in

older adults often is compromised by atherosclerotic processes, impairing blood flow to the bone. Older adults have a higher risk of pressure ulcers because of circulatory, skin, sensation, and mobility changes associated with aging. Pressure ulcers that cannot be staged and treated because of eschar formation pose a particular risk. In addition, the older adult may not demonstrate the typical signs of infection and inflammation, which allows an infectious process to become well established before it is detected.

Pathophysiology

The cause of osteomyelitis is usually bacterial; however, fungi, parasites, and viruses can also cause bone infection. *Staphylococcus aureus* is the most common infecting organism. Other organisms include *Escherichia coli, Pseudomonas, Klebsiella, Salmonella,* and *Proteus.*

Direct contamination of bone from an open wound, such as an open fracture or a gunshot or puncture wound, is the most common cause of osteomyelitis; osteomyelitis also may occur as a complication of surgery. The third mode of entry for microorganisms that invade bone tissue is the extension from adjacent soft tissue infection. Clients with venous stasis or arterial ulcers of the lower extremities or long-term complications of diabetes mellitus are at risk for this type of bacterial invasion.

After entry, bacteria lodge and multiply in the bone, resulting in the inflammatory and immune system response. Phagocytes attempt to contain the infection, releasing enzymes in the process that destroy bone tissue. Pus forms, followed by edema and vascular congestion. The Haversian canals in the medullary (marrow) cavity of the bone allow the infection to travel to other segments of the bone. If the infection reaches the outer margin of the bone (Figure 42–8 ■), it raises the periosteum of the bone, spreading along the surface. Lifting of the periosteum from the cortex disrupts the blood vessels that enter the bone. Pressure increases, further compromising the vascular supply and leading to ischemia and eventual necrosis of the bone. Blood and antibiotics cannot reach the bone tissue once the pressure compromises the vascular and arteriolar systems. In addition, bacteria adhere to damaged bone, coating the underlying bone with a protective film that further impedes host defenses.

Hematogenous Osteomyelitis

Hematogenous infections are caused by pathogens that are carried in the blood from sites of infection elsewhere in the body. Hematogenous osteomyelitis primarily affects older adults, people with sickle cell anemia, and intravenous drug users. The spine is the usual site of infection in adults. Pathogens enter the well-perfused vertebral bodies of adults via the spinal arteries. From there, the infection spreads into the disk space. The lumbar spine is involved more frequently than the thoracic or cervical spine. Urinary tract infections, soft tissue infection, endocarditis, and infected intravenous sites are sources of pathogens.

Clients with acute hematogenous osteomyelitis experience an acute onset of pain, tenderness, and fever. Soft tissue swelling over the affected bone may be noted. The course of vertebral osteomyelitis in intravenous drug users often is subacute, with vague, dull pain in the affected region and a normal or low-grade fever. The pain intensifies over 2 to 3 months, and is accompanied by tenderness, muscle spasm, and limited range of motion.

Osteomyelitis from a Contiguous Infection

Infections caused by an extension of infection from adjacent soft tissues fall into this category of osteomyelitis. The infection is a result of or complication of direct penetrating wounds, joint replacements, decubitus ulcers, and neurosurgery. This is the most common cause of osteomyelitis in adults.

The diagnosis of osteomyelitis often is not made until the infection has become chronic because the signs of acute infection may be masked by local tissue inflammation. Failure to heal a surgical wound or fracture or a developing sinus tract may be initial indicators of a bone infection.

Osteomyelitis Associated with Vascular Insufficiency

People with diabetes and peripheral vascular disease are at risk for developing osteomyelitis involving the feet. Diabetic neuropathy exposes the foot to trauma and pressure ulcers. The client may be unaware of the infection as it spreads into the bone. When tissue perfusion is poor, normal inflammatory responses and wound healing are impaired. The infection often is diagnosed when the client seeks treatment for a nonhealing sore, swollen toe, or acute cellulitis.

Manifestations

Manifestations of osteomyelitis vary according to the age of the client, the cause and site of involvement, and whether the infection is acute, subacute, or chronic (see the box on page 1479).

INTERDISCIPLINARY CARE

The care of the client with osteomyelitis focuses on relieving pain, eliminating the infection, and preventing or minimizing complications. Early diagnosis is important to prevent bone necrosis by early administration of the appropriate antibiotic.

A Initial infection

B Acute phase

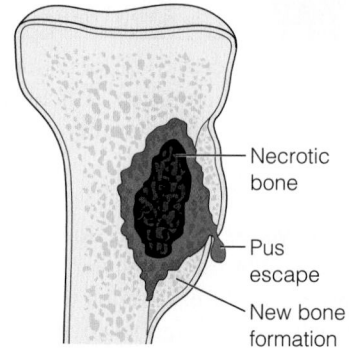

C Chronic phase

Figure 42–8 ■ Osteomyelitis. *A,* Site of initial infection. Bacteria enter and multiply in the bone, and the inflammatory response is initiated. *B,* Acute phase, in which infection spreads to other parts of the bone. Pus forms, edema occurs, and the vascular supply is compromised. If the infection reaches the outer margin of the bone, the periosteum is lifted, and ischemia and necrosis eventually occur. *C,* Chronic phase. Necrotic bone separates, a new layer of bone forms around the necrotic bone, and a sinus develops to allow the wound to drain.

MANIFESTATIONS of Osteomyelitis

CARDIOVASCULAR EFFECTS
- Tachycardia

GASTROINTESTINAL EFFECTS
- Nausea and vomiting
- Anorexia

MUSCULOSKELETAL EFFECTS
- Limp in involved extremity
- Localized tenderness, especially in epiphyseal area

INTEGUMENTARY EFFECTS
- Drainage and ulceration at involved site
- Swelling, erythema, and warmth at involved site
- Lymph node involvement, especially in the involved extremity

OTHER EFFECTS
- High temperature with chills
- Abrupt onset of pain
- Malaise

Most clients require both debridement of bone and a long period of antibiotic administration.

Diagnosis

The diagnosis of osteomyelitis is based on bone scans, MRI, blood tests, and biopsy. As described in Chapter 40 ∞, an MRI, CT scan, and bone scan may be conducted to identify abscesses, sinus tracts, and bone changes. An ultrasound can detect subperiosteal fluid collections, abscesses, and periosteal thickening and elevation associated with osteomyelitis. During an acute infection, ESR and WBC are elevated. Blood and tissue cultures (from affected bone or soft tissue) are obtained to identify the infecting organism and direct antibiotic therapy.

Medications

Antibiotic therapy is mandatory to prevent acute osteomyelitis from progressing to the chronic phase. Parenteral antibiotic therapy begins as soon as cultures (blood and/or wound) are obtained. A penicillinase-resistant semisynthetic penicillin (e.g., methicillin, oxacillin) may be given until the culture and sensitivity results are known. These antibiotics are used initially because many cases of osteomyelitis are caused by *Staphylococcus aureus*. When the detailed sensitivity report is obtained from the cultures, more definitive antibiotics are prescribed.

For the client with acute or chronic osteomyelitis, antibiotics are continued for 4 to 6 weeks. Intravenous antibiotic administration or oral therapy is common. Oral therapy with twice-daily ciprofloxacin has been shown to be as effective as parenteral therapy for treating adult clients with chronic osteomyelitis caused by susceptible organisms (Tierney et al., 2004).

Surgery

Surgical debridement is the primary treatment for the client with chronic osteomyelitis. The periosteum is excised and the cortex is drilled to release the pressure from accumulated pus. During this procedure, cultures may be obtained and sent to the laboratory for analysis. The wound holes are irrigated, and the wound is then closed. The cavity may be kept clean by inserting drainage tubes that are connected to an irrigation and suction system. Postoperatively, the nurse is responsible for instilling and removing dilute antibiotic solutions through the drainage tubes. See the box below for related nursing care.

A musculocutaneous (myocutaneous) flap is another approach used for the treatment of the dead space caused by extensive debridement of the infected site. The procedure involves moving or rotating a muscle and the section of skin fed by the arteries from that muscle into the cavity created by the surgery. A skin graft is performed later.

NURSING CARE OF THE CLIENT UNDERGOING Surgical Debridement for Osteomyelitis

PREOPERATIVE CARE
- Discuss the impending surgery, the client's concerns regarding surgery and its risks, and what steps will be taken if surgery is ineffective. *Open discussion and active listening are important means of gaining the client's trust and encouraging the client to express concerns about the outcome of the surgery. Surgery is frequently performed when 36 to 48 hours of antimicrobial therapy yields no improvement and when prolonged bacteremia and evidence of an abscess formation are present. The periosteum is excised, allowing access to the purulent material in the infected area. If pus is not apparent, several holes may be drilled into the bone. In some cases, irrigation tubes are inserted and connected to an elaborate system for postoperative antimicrobial therapy.*
- Clients may need extensive antimicrobial treatment postoperatively if an irrigation system is surgically implanted. Before the procedure, explain to the client that bed rest and an extended period of treatment in the hospital are imperative. *Clients who understand the events that may occur postoperatively may be more accepting of the required restrictions.*

POSTOPERATIVE CARE
- Provide meticulous care of the dressing and/or irrigation setup. *Frequently, the irrigation tubes are connected to a three-way stopcock, which allows irrigation and drainage of the debrided area without separating the tube from the collection device. Nurses need to be extremely coutious and adhere to strict sterile technique.*
- Assess the client for manifestations of further infection. *Although the client will receive antimicrobial agents, it is important to monitor the client continually for sudden spikes in temperature, pain at the involved site, and other indications of superinfection.*

HEALTH EDUCATION FOR THE CLIENT AND FAMILY
- While receiving antimicrobial agents, be sure to drink adequate amounts of fluid and eat a high-calorie diet to minimize the risks for damage to the kidneys, yeast infection, and adverse gastrointestinal effects.

NURSING CARE

The client with chronic osteomyelitis faces frequent and lengthy hospitalizations and/or treatment modalities. The prognosis is uncertain, and functional deficits and amputation are a constant concern. The ongoing expenses, loss of financial support, and role changes within the family are also client concerns.

Nursing Diagnoses and Interventions

Nursing diagnoses associated with acute osteomyelitis focus on preventing the transmission of infection and problems due to immobility. Providing comfort and client teaching are also very important.

Risk for Infection

Compromised immune status places the client with osteomyelitis at risk for superinfection. An inadequate kilocalorie intake is an additional factor that contributes to the risk.

- Maintain strict hand washing practices. *Meticulous hand washing helps prevent the spread of infection by minimizing the entry of organisms into susceptible clients.*

> **PRACTICE ALERT**
> Careful hand washing before and after direct care is essential even if gloves are worn.

- Administer antimicrobial therapy at specified time intervals. *Optimal blood levels of antibiotic therapy are mandatory in clients with infectious processes.*
- Maintain the client's optimal dietary kilocalorie and protein intake. *High kilocalorie and protein intake provide the client with sufficient nutritional support for the body's needs during the stressful event of the inflammatory process.*

Hyperthermia

The infection and associated inflammatory process can cause fever in the client with osteomyelitis.

- Monitor temperature every 4 hours and when client reports chills and/or fever. Blood cultures are frequently ordered when an acute elevation of temperature occurs. *A sudden rise in temperature in clients with either acute or chronic osteomyelitis may indicate inadequate antimicrobial management.*
- Maintain a cool environment and provide light clothing and bedding during temperature elevation. *Proper environmental conditions and clothing enhance the evaporative process during acute temperature elevation and promote comfort.*
- Ensure a daily fluid intake of 2000 to 3000 mL. Dehydration may result from evaporative fluid losses during acute temperature elevations. Furthermore, clients taking large doses of antibiotic therapy may experience fluid loss through excessive diarrhea as a side effect of the therapy. *Fluid replacement is necessary during this time to prevent further dehydration.*

Impaired Physical Mobility

Pain, infection, inflammation, and the use of immobilizers can all impair the mobility of the client with osteomyelitis.

- Maintain the affected limb in functional position when immobilized. *The client may hesitate to move the involved extremity*

because of continuous pain; therefore, the extremity must be maintained in functional position to avoid flexion contracture.

- Maintain rest, and avoid subjecting the affected extremity to weight-bearing activities. *The involved extremity must be immobilized to avoid pathologic fractures caused by stress on the weakened bone.*
- Ensure active or passive ROM exercises every 4 hours. *Flexion contracture occurs when the client remains immobile or when there is only minimal joint movement. Consult a physical therapist for plan of exercises to avoid contracture.*

Acute Pain

The client with osteomyelitis experiences pain due to swelling.

- Use a splint or immobilizer when the client experiences acute pain from swelling. *Splinting or immobilizing the involved extremity provides support and reduces pain caused by movement.*
- Ask the physician to order scheduled administration of narcotic and nonnarcotic analgesics on a 24-hour basis rather than as needed. *The use of 24-hour administration allows blood levels of pain-relieving medications to remain constant.*

> **PRACTICE ALERT**
> Clients are often reluctant to ask for a prn pain medication, allowing the pain to reach a level that is difficult to manage.

- Use nonpharmacologic strategies (e.g., heat distraction, relaxation techniques) for pain management. *Pain of the muscles and joints may be controlled through nonpharmacologic interventions. Warm moist packs, warm baths, or heating pads to the involved extremity provide comfort due to vasodilation.*
- Avoid excessive manipulation of the involved area; handle the area gently. Carefully assess the client for guarding, limping, or unwillingness to move the affected part. Communicate to other healthcare professionals the client's preferences for assistive devices and means of manipulating the involved area. *Gentle handling and minimal manipulation help reduce pain.*

Community-Based Care

Although clients may be hospitalized for acute treatment and surgery, most care is provided at home. Home health services can provide intravenous medications, if prescribed. Discuss the following topics for home care:

- The importance of careful hand washing, especially after toileting and dressing changes.
- The importance of taking all antibiotics as prescribed. Include information about helping prevent the yeast infections (of the mouth or vagina) often associated with prolonged antibiotic therapy by eating 8 oz of live-culture yogurt each day.
- The need to take pain medications on a regular basis to prevent pain from becoming severe. Provide information about how to deal with side effects, such as constipation, by increasing fluid and fiber intake.
- How to perform wound care and sources for needed equipment and supplies.
- Rest or limited weight bearing for the affected extremity or body part. Teach how to avoid complications associated with

prolonged immobilization, such as frequently shifting position, keeping skin and linens clean and dry, and doing active ROM exercises for unaffected joints.

- The importance of maintaining good nutrition. An adequate supply of kilocalories, protein, and other nutrients is necessary for immune function and healing. Suggest frequent small meals and using nutritional supplements such as Ensure to help maintain nutritional intake.

THE CLIENT WITH SEPTIC ARTHRITIS

Septic arthritis can develop if a joint space is invaded by a pathogen. The primary risk factors for septic arthritis are persistent bacteremia (bacteria in the blood) (e.g., due to use of injectable drugs, endocarditis) and previous joint damage (e.g., due to trauma or rheumatoid arthritis). Arthroscopic surgery and total joint replacements that allow potential direct contamination of the joint are additional risk factors (Tierney et al., 2004).

Pathophysiology

The most common bacteria implicated in septic arthritis include *gonococci, S. aureus,* and streptococci. Infections by gram-negative bacteria such as *E. coli* and *Pseudomonas* are seen with increasing frequency, particularly in people who inject recreational drugs or are immunocompromised (Tierney et al., 2004).

Infection of the joint leads to inflammation with resulting synovitis and joint effusion. Abscesses may form in synovial tissues or bone underlying joint cartilage. If not treated promptly and effectively, septic arthritis can lead to destruction of the affected joint. A single joint, often the knee, is usually affected. Septic arthritis may also affect other joints such as the shoulder, wrist, hip, fingers, or elbow.

Manifestations

The onset of septic arthritis is typically abrupt, marked by pain and stiffness of the infected joint. The joint appears red and swollen, and is hot and tender to the touch. Effusion (increased fluid within the joint space) is usually present. Systemic manifestations of infection, such as chills and fever, often accompany local manifestations, although these may be muted if the client is taking anti-inflammatory medications.

INTERDISCIPLINARY CARE

Septic arthritis is a medical emergency requiring prompt treatment to preserve joint function. When it is suspected, fluid from the affected joint is aspirated and sent for Gram stain and culture. Cultures also are obtained from all likely sources of the infection, including blood, sputum, or wounds. The synovial fluid culture is always positive in nongonococcal septic arthritis but often is negative for bacteria in early gonococcal arthritis. Infected synovial fluid usually is cloudy, with a high WBC count and a low glucose level. Joint x-ray films are often normal in the initial stages, but soon show demineralization, bony erosions, and joint space narrowing.

The infected joint is treated with rest, immobilization, elevation, and systemic antibiotics. Treatment with a broad-spectrum parenteral antibiotic is initiated before the results of culture are obtained. The medication may be changed or adjusted once the organism has been identified. Antibiotic therapy is continued for at least 2 weeks after inflammatory manifestations have abated. Frequent joint aspirations may be performed to remove excess fluid and pus, and to evaluate for the continued presence of bacteria. Surgical drainage may be performed if the hip joint is involved (because of the difficulty of aspirating this joint) or when medical therapy does not rapidly eliminate bacteria from the synovial fluid. Physical therapy is implemented during the recovery period to ensure maintenance of optimal joint function.

 NURSING CARE

Septic arthritis can be frightening to the client who experiences a sudden onset of joint pain and swelling and is faced with the possibility of rapid functional loss of movement. Nursing care is both supportive and educative. Clients may be hospitalized for initial treatment with intravenous antibiotics. It is important to monitor the client's response to therapy, including systemic manifestations such as fever. Position the affected joint appropriately, using pillows to elevate it as needed. Splints or traction may be used to immobilize the joint. Warm compresses may be ordered for comfort. Active ROM exercises preserve joint mobility and should be initiated as soon as the physician allows.

The client with septic arthritis needs information about the disorder, its etiology, and its treatment. Teach the client how organisms may gain entry into the joint space. Discuss the role that the use of injected drugs and sexually transmitted infections play in septic arthritis, and means to prevent infection as appropriate (e.g., using clean "works," practicing safer sex). Refer the client to a drug treatment program if necessary. Emphasize the importance of complying with all aspects of the treatment plan to prevent joint destruction and disability.

NEOPLASTIC DISORDERS

Bone tumors may be either primary (arising in the bone itself) or metastatic (seeded from a tumor elsewhere in the body). Like other tumors, bone tumors can be either benign or malignant.

THE CLIENT WITH BONE TUMORS

Benign bone tumors tend to grow slowly and do not often destroy surrounding tissues. Primary malignant tumors of the bone are rare, accounting for only about 1% of all adult cancers (Porth, 2005). Malignant tumors grow rapidly and metastasize. Virtually every malignant tumor can metastasize to bone. However, the most common metastatic bone tumors originate from primary tumors of the prostate, breast, kidney, thyroid, and lung.

Primary bone tumors arise from bone tissue itself, that is, cartilage (chondrogenic), bone (osteogenic), collagen (collagenic), and bone marrow cells (myelogenic). The tissue type, neoplasm classification, sites, and incidence of the most common primary bone tumors are summarized in Table 42–6. The focus for discussion in this section is care of the client with a primary bone tumor.

Pathophysiology

The etiology of bone tumors is unknown, but there is a connection between increased bone activity and the development of primary bone tumors. Bone tumors frequently occur when primary bone growth is at its peak in adolescence or is over-stimulated during disease, such as Paget's disease.

Primary tumors cause bone breakdown, called *osteolysis*, which weakens the bone, resulting in bone fractures. Normal bone adjacent to the tumor responds to tumor pressure by altering its normal pattern of remodeling. The bone's surface becomes altered, and the contours enlarge in the area of the tumor growth.

Malignant bone tumors invade and destroy adjacent bone tissue by producing substances that promote bone resorption or by interfering with a bone's blood supply. Benign bone tumors, unlike malignant ones, have a symmetric, controlled growth pattern. As they grow, they push against neighboring bone tissue. This weakens the bone's structure until it becomes unable to withstand the stress of ordinary use and frequently causes pathologic fracture.

Manifestations

The three main manifestations of bone tumors are pain, a mass, and impaired function. Bone pain usually comes on slowly and lasts for as long as a week, is constant or intermittent, and may be worse at night. The mass is described as a swelling or lump on the bones that is firm, slightly tender, and may be felt through the skin. The mass may interfere with normal movement and/or cause the bone to break. The manifestations of bone tumors are usually associated with a history of a fall or blow to the extremity that brings the mass to the client's attention. The injury, rather than the growth itself, usually causes the client to seek medical attention. Manifestations of bone tumors are listed in the box on the next page.

INTERDISCIPLINARY CARE

Treatment and care of the client with bone tumors focuses on prompt diagnosis, removal of the tumor, prevention of complications, and client education.

Diagnosis

The diagnosis of bone tumors is critical to the survival of the client and possible preservation of the affected limb. Diagnostic tests are described in Chapter 40 ∞.

Radiologic studies include x-rays, CT scans, and MRI. X-rays show the location of the tumors and the extent of bone involvement. Benign tumors are characterized by sharp margins that are clearly separate from the surrounding normal bone. Metastatic bone destruction has a characteristic "moth-eaten" pattern in which the growth has a less-defined margin that cannot be separated from the normal bone. CT scan and MRI are useful in evaluating the extent of tumor invasion into bone, soft tissues, and neurovascular structures. Percutaneous needle biopsy or needle biopsy at the time of surgery is used to determine the exact type of bone tumor.

TABLE 42–6 Description of Common Primary Bone Tumors

TISSUE TYPE	BENIGN	MALIGNANT	SITE	INCIDENCE
Chondrogenic (cartilage-forming tumors)	Osteochondroma— most common benign tumor		Pelvis, scapula, ribs	Higher in males
	Chondroma		Hands, feet, ribs, spine, sternum, or long bones	Ages 30 to 50 Higher in males
		Chondrosarcoma	Femur, pelvis, ribs, head (epiphysis) of long bones	13% of malignant bone tumors Middle age and older Higher in males
Osteogenic (bone-forming tumors)	Osteoid Osteoma		Shaft (diaphysis) of long bones (i.e., femur, tibia)	Ages 20 to 30 Higher in males
		Osteosarcoma— most common malignant tumor	Long bones, knee	38% of malignant bone tumors Predominant in adolescents and people ages 50 to 60
Collagenic (collagen-forming tumors)		Fibrosarcoma	Femur, tibia	4% of malignant bone tumors Wide age distribution, but usually occurs in people ages 40 to 50 Higher in females
Myelogenic (tumors of bone marrow cells)	Giant cell tumor		Shaft (diaphysis) of long bones (i.e., femur, tibia, radius, humerus)	4% to 5% of bone tumors Wide age distribution Higher in females

MANIFESTATIONS of Neoplasms of the Musculoskeletal System

BONY SARCOMAS

Site
Upper or lower extremity or pelvis

Metaphysis of distal femur, proximal tibia, proximal humerus, and pelvis

Manifestations
- Worsening deep bony pain
- Pain at night or during rest that may radiate and become severe
- Muscular weakness or atrophy
- Soft tissue mass extending from bone with erythematous or warm skin over tissue mass
- Change in ability to perform ADLs
- Fever

SOFT TISSUE SARCOMAS

Site
Upper or lower extremity and pelvis

Thigh; shoulder, and pelvis

Pelvis

Manifestations
- Enlarging firm mass with irregular borders, which causes pain in surrounding soft tissue structures
- Erythema or warmth and venous dilation over skin
- Muscular weakness and atrophy with limited range of motion change in ability to perform ADLs and change in gait
- Paresthesia with neurologic involvement and distal swelling
- Palpable local lymph nodes
- Altered bowel and bladder habits or pain with intercourse

Laboratory tests include an alkaline phosphatase (elevated with malignant bone tumor) and a calcium level (increased with massive bone destruction).

Treatments

As with other malignant tumors, bone tumors are treated with chemotherapy, radiation therapy, and surgery.

CHEMOTHERAPY Chemotherapeutic agents are administered to shrink the malignant tumor before surgery, to control recurrence of tumor growth after surgery, or to treat metastasis of the tumor. Chemotherapeutic agents used to treat bone tumors are listed in Box 42-4. See Chapter 14 ∞ for further discussion of chemotherapy and its nursing implications.

RADIATION THERAPY Radiation therapy may be used in combination with chemotherapy. Radiation therapy is frequently applied to metastatic bone carcinomas as a method of pain control. It is also used to eliminate bony tumors or to eliminate any remaining tumor after a surgical procedure. Radiation therapy is discussed in Chapter 14 ∞.

SURGERY The goal of surgery for the treatment of primary bone tumors is to eliminate the tumor completely. Tumors are removed either by excising the tumor itself or by amputating the affected limb. The type of procedure varies from removing the tumor only, to removing the tumor along with a small margin of normal tissue surrounding the tumor, to removing the tumor and a wide zone of normal tissue, to removing the tumor and part or all of the bone in which it lies. Cadaver allografts or metal prostheses often are used to replace missing bone, avoiding amputation. Care of the client undergoing amputation is discussed in Chapter 41 ∞.

NURSING CARE

Nursing care for the client with bone tumors requires innovative interventions from the time of diagnosis through the rehabilitation phase. In the acute phase, problems associated with pain, lack of knowledge, immobility, coping, and anxiety are foremost. If the client develops complications from treatment or if a malignancy metastasizes, problems related to home health maintenance management, self-concept, and prevention of further complications take priority.

Nursing Diagnoses and Interventions

The client with a bone tumor requires nursing care to meet many health problems, including prevention of injury, relief of pain, assistance with mobility, and teaching about the disease process and treatment.

Risk for Injury

In the client with a bone tumor, changes in bone tissue can cause pathologic fractures.
- Teach how to avoid falls or injury to the tumor site, such as by using assistive devices when walking and ensuring the home environment is not conducive to falling (for example, remove throw rugs and use night-lights). *Pathologic fractures may occur at the tumor site because bone destruction can weaken the area.*

BOX 42–4 Chemotherapeutic Agents Used for Musculoskeletal Neoplasms

Alkylating Agents
Ifosfamide
Cyclophosphamide

Antibiotics
Doxorubicin
Bleomycin

Antimetabolites
Methotrexate

Plant Alkaloids
Vincristine

Synthetic Agents
Cisplatin

- Provide referral to physical or occupational therapy for fitting of and teaching about assistive devices for ambulating, such as a cane, crutches, or a walker. *Assistive devices can reduce the risk of falling when the client has significant weakness of an extremity or when balance has been affected by treatment of the disease.*

Acute Pain, Chronic Pain

In the client with a bone tumor, pain may be related to direct invasion of the tumor or to pathologic fractures. Clients may experience both acute and chronic pain.

- Develop strategies for controlling both acute pain (from surgery, fracture, or inflammation) and chronic pain (from progression of the disease). *Analgesics combined with nonpharmacologic methods of pain control provide optimum relief of pain. Chronic pain, when mild in nature, is best managed with NSAIDs or aspirin. Moderate pain is best managed with a combination of codeine and NSAIDs. Severe pain is best relieved with long-acting or sustained-relief narcotic analgesics.*
- Provide assistive devices (e.g., canes, walkers, crutches) when the client ambulates. *Assistive devices lessen the pain by supporting weight bearing during ambulation.*

Impaired Physical Mobility

Pain, muscle wasting, or surgical procedures can impair the physical mobility of the client with a bone tumor.

- Begin muscle strengthening and active and passive ROM exercises immediately after surgery. A continuous passive motion (CPM) machine may be used after surgical procedures to either upper or lower extremities. *Muscle strengthening exercises must be encouraged as soon as possible to prevent muscle wasting and shorten the rehabilitation period.*
- Encourage exercises that help strengthen the triceps muscles. *The triceps are the major muscles in the arms and must be strengthened to assist in use of crutches or other assistive devices.*

- For the client who has undergone an amputation of a lower extremity, encourage quadriceps and gluteal setting exercises and leg raises. *These exercises will benefit the client when the rehabilitation period begins.*

Decisional Conflict

A lack of knowledge about the diagnosis and treatment regimen can impair the client's ability to make informed decisions about the treatment plan.

- Discuss issues related to diagnosis, radiologic evaluation, biopsy, surgery, chemotherapy, radiation therapy, potential complications, alternative therapies, risks, benefits, nursing management, discharge plans, home care, and long-term treatment and follow-up. *The client requires this information in order to make informed decisions about treatment.*

Community-Based Care

The client with a primary bone tumor needs information about the disease, its potential consequences, and treatment options. Present information in a matter-of-fact manner, taking time to listen to and address the client's and family's concerns. Discuss expected effects and potential side effects of surgery, chemotherapy, and radiation therapy. Provide information about how to minimize side effects. Teach the postsurgical client about wound care, demonstrating dressing changes and stump care (if amputation has occurred). Provide the client with a list of local resources for obtaining supplies. Discuss activity and weight-bearing restrictions. Refer the client to physical therapy for teaching about ambulation and appropriate muscle-group strengthening exercises. Ensure that the client who has experienced an amputation is working with or has a referral to a prosthetic specialist. For the client with metastatic disease, discuss hospice services and support groups for clients with cancer.

CONNECTIVE TISSUE DISORDERS

Connective tissue is the most abundant and widely distributed body tissue. It not only connects body parts but also provides support; forms bones, cartilage, and the walls of blood vessels; and attaches muscles to bones. Connective tissue consists of three elements: (1) long fibers embedded in a (2) noncellular ground substance, and (3) cells specific to the class of connective tissue. Fibers made up primarily of collagen, a protein, are the most abundant in connective tissue.

Connective tissue disorders, also known as collagen diseases, are a group of immune-mediated disorders. Although they appear to have a genetic component, their cause is unknown. Because connective tissue and collagen are widely distributed in many varied tissues, these are systemic diseases with diverse manifestations.

THE CLIENT WITH SYSTEMIC SCLEROSIS (SCLERODERMA)

Systemic sclerosis, also known as **scleroderma** ("hardening of the skin"), is a chronic disease characterized by the formation of excess fibrous connective tissue and diffuse fibrosis of the skin and internal organs. The cause of scleroderma is unknown, but genetic, immune, and environmental factors are thought to play a role. Although this uncommon disease is distributed worldwide, a higher incidence is noted in coal and gold miners and in people exposed to certain chemicals such as polyvinyl chloride, epoxy resins, and aromatic hydrocarbons.

FAST FACTS
Scleroderma

- Scleroderma affects approximately 300,000 people in the United States, with about one-third having the systemic form and the rest the localized form.
- Scleroderma affects women more often than men by a ratio of approximately 3:1.
- Although it can occur at any age from infants to older adults, the onset of scleroderma typically occurs between the ages of 25 and 55 years (Scleroderma Foundation, 2006).

Pathophysiology

Abnormalities in cellular immune function are believed to contribute to the development of scleroderma. Abnormal proliferation of fibrous connective tissue occurs in affected tissues, including the skin, blood vessels, lungs, kidneys, and other organs.

Scleroderma may be either localized, affecting the skin only, or generalized (systemic sclerosis), with both skin and visceral organ involvement. Localized involvement may occur as irregularly shaped patches of skin (morphea) or a line of disease on the arm, leg, or side of the face (linear scleroderma) (International Scleroderma Network, 2004). Eighty percent of people with generalized disease have limited involvement, frequently manifested by CREST syndrome, a combination of calcinosis (abnormal calcium salt deposition in the tissues), Raynaud's phenomenon, esophageal dysfunction, sclerodactyly (localized scleroderma of the fingers), and telangiectasia (dilated, superficial blood vessels). The remainder of clients with generalized systemic sclerosis have a diffuse form of the disease and a higher risk of visceral organ involvement. Infections and diseases of the cardiovascular, renal, pulmonary, and CNS are the most common causes of death in people with systemic sclerosis.

Manifestations

The initial manifestations of systemic sclerosis are usually noted in the skin, which thickens markedly. Diffuse, nonpitting swelling also is noted. As the disease progresses, the skin begins to atrophy, becoming taut, shiny, and hyperpigmented (Figure 42–9 ■). Facial skin tightening leads to loss of skin lines and a pursed-lip appearance. Skin tightness may limit mobility, particularly of the face and hands. Other skin manifestations include telangiectasias (flat, red areas caused by dilation of small blood vessels, usually noted on the face, hands, and in the mouth) and calcium deposits, usually noted around joints.

Arthralgias and Raynaud's phenomenon are common early manifestations of systemic sclerosis. Raynaud's phenomenon (intermittent attacks of small artery vasospasm) is characterized by pallor of the fingers followed by cyanosis, and then reactive hyperemia with redness. Attacks are usually triggered by cold temperatures.

Figure 42–9 ■ Characteristic skin changes of scleroderma.
Source: Logical Images/Custom Medical Stock Photo.

The client with visceral organ involvement may have varied symptoms. Dysphagia is common, because the motility of the esophagus is affected. Pulmonary involvement can lead to exertional dyspnea due to impaired gas exchange and right-sided heart failure due to pulmonary hypertension. Involvement of the heart may cause manifestations of pericarditis and dysrhythmias. Diarrhea or constipation, abdominal cramping, and malabsorption can occur when the GI tract is affected. Renal effects can lead to proteinuria, hematuria, hypertension, and renal failure.

The prognosis for localized and limited scleroderma is good; many clients have a normal life span. The course of diffuse systemic sclerosis is highly variable. This disease is usually progressive; complete remission is rare.

INTERDISCIPLINARY CARE

The manifestations of systemic sclerosis often allow diagnosis with little or no testing. No cure is currently available; treatment is symptomatic and supportive.

Diagnosis

No single diagnostic test is specific for systemic sclerosis, although a titer of 1:40 or higher for antinuclear antibody (ANA) is the most sensitive for diagnosis. Other laboratory studies that are done include an ESR, which is typically elevated from the chronic inflammatory process and a CBC, which will demonstrate anemia. A skin biopsy may be done to confirm the diagnosis.

Medications

Medications to treat systemic sclerosis are chosen based on the client's symptoms. Immunosuppressive agents and corticosteroids are of limited benefit, but may be used to slow or prevent pulmonary fibrosis and in life-threatening disease. Penicillamine may be used to treat scleroderma and pulmonary fibrosis. Calcium channel blockers such as nifedipine (Procardia) or alpha-adrenergic blockers such as prazosin (Minipress) may be prescribed for clients with Raynaud's phenomenon. When manifestations of esophagitis accompany systemic sclerosis, H_2-receptor blockers such as cimetidine (Tagamet) or ranitidine (Zantac), antacids, or omeprazole (Prilosec), which blocks all gastric secretion, may be ordered. Tetracycline or another broad-spectrum antibiotic may be prescribed to suppress intestinal flora and relieve symptoms of malabsorption. Clients with kidney disease are usually treated with angiotensin-converting enzyme (ACE) inhibitors such as captopril (Capoten) to control hypertension and preserve renal function. End-stage kidney disease is managed with dialysis and transplantation.

Physical Therapy

Physical therapy is an important part of the management of systemic sclerosis to maintain mobility of affected tissues, the hands and face in particular. Because the mouth opening, if involved, becomes increasingly smaller as the disease progresses, stretching and strengthening of facial muscles can be vital to maintaining oral food intake.

NURSING CARE

Nursing care needs of clients with systemic sclerosis are individualized to the effects and manifestations of the disease, with interventions summarized in the following discussion.

Nursing Interventions

Skin manifestations are present to some degree in nearly all clients with scleroderma. Nursing care related to the skin focuses on maintaining skin integrity and flexibility. Measures to maintain supple skin are important, because elasticity cannot be regained once it is lost. Apply moisturizers to prevent dryness and cracking. Protect the skin where it is stretched taut over joints or bony prominences. Perform ROM exercises to help prevent joint contractures due to increasingly tight skin.

Difficulty swallowing and recurrent esophagitis may interfere with the client's nutritional status. Provide small, frequent meals. Consult with the dietitian and the client to determine which foods are easy to swallow. Keep the client in a sitting or Fowler's position after meals and elevate the head of the bed at night to minimize esophageal reflux.

The dermatologic and systemic effects of the disease may have significant psychologic effects on the client, leading to feelings of helplessness and hopelessness, and self-esteem disturbance. Establish an atmosphere of trust with the client. Listen actively and acknowledge concerns about the disease and its effects on the client's life and appearance. Encourage the client to share these concerns with family members and significant others. Provide referral to social services or counseling as appropriate.

The client with predominant pulmonary disease has nursing care needs similar to those of other clients with restrictive respiratory disorders . If the client with systemic sclerosis has impaired renal function, nursing care is similar to that for clients with chronic renal failure (see Chapter 29 ∞).

Community-Based Care

Teach the client with systemic sclerosis about the disease and introduce measures to help manage its effects. Stress the importance of good skin care and physical therapy exercises to maintain mobility, particularly of the hands and face. Discuss the need to avoid chilling (local and whole body) to prevent episodes of Raynaud's phenomenon. Teach the role of proper dress in the winter: loose, warm clothing, gloves, and warm stockings. If needed, stress the need to stop smoking because of the vasoconstrictive effect of nicotine and the respiratory effects of the disease. Provide the client with information about manifestations of disease progression and organ involvement. Teach the client to report new or worsening symptoms to the physician. In addition, suggest the following resources:

- National Institute of Arthritis and Musculoskeletal and Skin Diseases
- Scleroderma Foundation
- Scleroderma Research Foundation
- International Scleroderma Network.

THE CLIENT WITH SJÖGREN'S SYNDROME

Sjögren's syndrome is an autoimmune disorder that causes inflammation and dysfunction of exocrine glands throughout the body. Sjögren's syndrome primarily affects women, with a ratio of women to men at 9:1 The highest incidence is between the ages of 40 and 60 years. Although it can occur as a primary disorder, Sjogren's syndrome is often associated with other rheumatic disease, including rheumatoid arthritis, SLE, primary biliary cirrhosis, scleroderma, Hashimoto's thyroiditis, and interstitial pulmonary fibrosis (Tierney et al., 2004).

Pathophysiology

In this disease, exocrine glands in many areas of the body are destroyed by infiltration of lymphocytes and deposits of immune complexes. The salivary and lacrimal glands are particularly affected, leading to the characteristic manifestations of *xerophthalmia* (dry eyes) and *xerostomia* (dry mouth). Clients often experience dry, gritty-feeling eyes and may develop corneal ulcerations. Mucosal dryness affects taste, smell, chewing, and swallowing and leads to increased dental caries. Parotid gland enlargement is common. Excess dryness can also affect the nose, throat, larynx, bronchi, vagina, and skin. Systemic effects of Sjögren's syndrome include arthritis, dysphagia, pancreatitis, pleuritis, neurologic manifestations including migraine, and vasculitis. Nephritis may occur, but renal failure rarely results. Clients with Sjögren's syndrome have a greatly increased risk of developing malignant lymphoma.

INTERDISCIPLINARY CARE

The diagnosis of Sjögren's syndrome is often based on the client's history and clinical presentation. Schirmer's test, which measures the quantity of tears secreted in a 5-minute period in response to irritation, ocular staining, and slit-lamp examination of the eye, may be performed. A definitive diagnosis can be made by biopsy of either the lacrimal or salivary gland.

Treatment is supportive. Artificial tears are used to decrease eye irritation and dryness. The client can keep the mouth moist by drinking fluids, using a saliva substitute, and chewing sugarless gum. Medications that increase mouth dryness, such as atropine and decongestants, should be avoided.

NURSING CARE

Nurses caring for clients with Sjögren's syndrome need to teach measures to protect the client's eyes and oral mucosa. Instill artificial tears as needed. Encourage the client to sip fluids throughout the day. Provide frequent oral hygiene, particularly before and after meals. Ensure that the client has sufficient fluids to drink during meals, because fluids help with chewing and swallowing.

THE CLIENT WITH FIBROMYALGIA

Fibromyalgia is a common rheumatic syndrome characterized by musculoskeletal pain, stiffness, and tenderness. Fibromyalgia affects more than 6 million Americans, 90% of them women between 20 and 50 years of age (National Fibromyalgia Research Association, 2004). The cause is unknown, but possible etiologies include sleep disorders, depression, infections, and an altered perception of normal stimuli. Fibromyalgia can be a complication of hypothyroidism, rheumatoid arthritis, or (in men) sleep apnea. It closely resembles chronic fatigue syndrome, except that musculoskeletal pain is predominant in fibromyalgia, whereas fatigue is a more significant feature of chronic fatigue syndrome.

Pathophysiology

No inflammatory, structural, or physiologic muscle changes have been demonstrated in fibromyalgia. A connection between fibromyalgia and the central nervous system is being studied.

Manifestations

A gradual onset of chronic, achy muscle pain is typical, although the onset may be sudden, occasionally following a viral illness. The pain may be localized or involve the entire body. The neck, spine, shoulders, and hips are often affected. Pain is produced by palpating localized "tender points" (Figure 42–10 ■). Local tightness or muscle spasm may also occur. Systemic manifestations of fibromyalgia include fatigue, sleep disruptions, headaches, morning stiffness, painful menstrual periods, and problems with thinking and memory (called the "fibro fog"). Pain and fatigue are aggravated by exertion.

INTERDISCIPLINARY CARE

The diagnosis of fibromyalgia is based on the history and physical assessment. The criteria developed by the American College of Rheumatology that are used for diagnosis are a history of widespread pain that has been present for at least 3 months and pain at 11 of the 18 tender points on palpation. There are no laboratory or diagnostic tests for the disorder, although tests may be performed to rule out other rheumatic disorders, such as rheumatoid arthritis or SLE. Fibromyalgia also may occur as a complication of hypothyroidism, so thyroid function studies are performed.

This disorder may resolve spontaneously or become chronic and recurrent. The client with fibromyalgia needs reassurance of the benign nature of the disorder along with validation of its reality. Therapeutic measures include local heat applications, massage, stretching exercises, and sleep improvement. Amitriptyline, a tricyclic antidepressant, has been shown to promote better sleep and relieve manifestations of fibromyalgia. NSAIDs have not been effective in its treatment.

The National Institute of Arthritis and Musculoskeletal and Skin Diseases (2005a) is conducting research to better understand

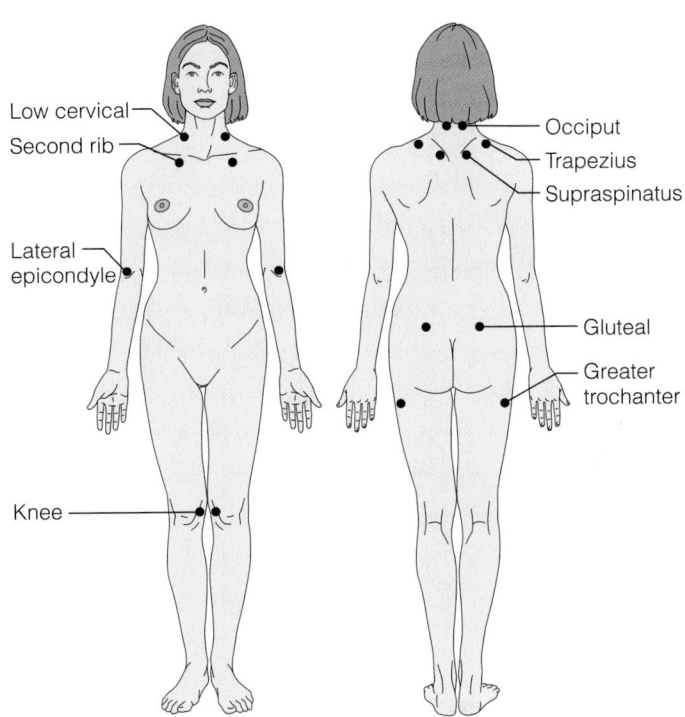

Figure 42–10 ■ Location of "tender points" in fibromyalgia.

why people with fibromyalgia have increased sensitivity to pain, the role of stress hormones in the body, the effect of genetics, and what medications or behavioral treatments are most effective.

NURSING CARE

Nursing care for clients with fibromyalgia is supportive and educational, provided in community settings such as clinics and other primary care settings. It is important to validate clients' concerns and reassure them that their symptoms are not "all in the head." This syndrome is recognizable and manageable; its course is not progressive. Teach clients about the disorder, and reassure them that it resolves uneventfully in most instances. Provide verbal and written instructions about the use of heat, exercise, stress-reduction techniques, and prescribed medications to relieve manifestations. In addition, suggest the following resources:

- Fibromyalgia Network
- National Fibromyalgia Research Association
- American College of Rheumatology
- National Institute of Arthritis and Musculoskeletal and Skin Diseases.

STRUCTURAL DISORDERS

Structural disorders of the musculoskeletal system most commonly affect the spine. The disorders discussed in this section are spinal deformities and low back pain.

THE CLIENT WITH SPINAL DEFORMITIES

Scoliosis and kyphosis are the two most common deformities of the spinal column. *Scoliosis* is a lateral curvature of the spine. *Kyphosis* is excessive angulation of the normal posterior curve of the thoracic spine (Figure 42–11 ■).

An estimated 500,000 adults in the United States are affected by scoliosis. It usually is diagnosed in adolescence, with girls affected more than boys by an 8:1 margin. Idiopathic scoliosis is the most common form of the disorder, accounting for approximately 75% of cases. Congenital and neuromuscular

Figure 42–11 ■ Common deformities of the spinal column: *A,* Scoliosis is a lateral curvature of the spine. *B,* Kyphosis is an exaggerated posterior curvature of the thoracic spine.

disorders such as cerebral palsy, poliomyelitis, and MD account for the rest (Porth, 2005).

Pathophysiology

Detailed discussions of the causes and treatment of scoliosis and kyphosis in younger clients can be found in pediatric nursing textbooks. This discussion focuses on the nursing care of adults with these disorders. The manifestations of scoliosis and kyphosis are listed in the box on below.

Scoliosis

Scoliosis is classified as *postural* when the small curve corrects with bending, and *structural* when the curve does not

---

MANIFESTATIONS of Scoliosis and Kyphosis

SCOLIOSIS
- Asymmetry of shoulders, scapulae, waist creases
- Prominence of the thoracic ribs or paravertebral muscles on forward bend
- Lateral curvature and vertebral rotation on posteroanterior x-ray film

SEVERE SCOLIOSIS
- Back pain
- Shortness of breath
- Anorexia, nausea

KYPHOSIS
- Posterior rounding at the thoracic level
- Kyphotic curve of over 45 degrees on x-ray film

---

correct with bending (Porth, 2005). Most clients requiring treatment have structural scoliosis, a curve caused by a fixed deformity.

The lateral curve that occurs in scoliosis is usually evident in the thoracic, lumbar, or thoracolumbar regions of the spine. The vertebral bodies in these spinal regions can be rotated as well as curved to one side or the other.

As scoliosis emerges, the soft tissues (muscles and ligaments) shorten on the concave side of the curvature. Over time, progressive deformities of the vertebral column and ribs develop, causing one-sided compression of the vertebral bodies. The degree of compression and twisting varies according to the location of each vertebra within the curved portion of the spine.

If the lateral curvature is less than 40 degrees when the client's spine reaches maturity, the risk of further progression during adult life is small. However, the spine becomes unstable if the lateral curvature is greater than 50 degrees, and curvature likely will worsen throughout the client's lifetime.

Scoliosis is usually first noted by the deformity it causes, such as one shoulder that is higher than the other, a prominent hip, or a projecting scapula. Pain is present in severe cases, usually in the lumbar region. Pain also may be caused by pressure on the ribs or the crest of the ilium. Shortness of breath may result from diminished chest expansion, and gastrointestinal disturbances may occur because of crowding of the abdominal organs.

Kyphosis

Like scoliosis, kyphosis is classified as postural or structural. Postural kyphosis is caused by a slumping posture. Structural kyphosis may result from congenital malformations or pediatric disorders such as rickets or poliomyelitis. However, kyphosis also may occur during adulthood from vertebral tuberculosis and Paget's disease or from metabolic disorders such as osteoporosis and osteomalacia. The condition can also result from the surgical removal or radiation of intervertebral disks for the treatment of spinal cord tumors or cysts.

The manifestations of kyphosis include moderate back pain and increased curvature of the thoracic spine as viewed from the side ("hunchback"). Impaired mobility and respiratory problems may occur in cases of severe curvature.

INTERDISCIPLINARY CARE

Diagnosis of scoliosis and kyphosis is important to prevent severe spinal deformity in the adult. The client stands with the arms relaxed and hanging freely at the sides while the examiner evaluates the client from both the back and the front for symmetry of the shoulders, scapulae, waist creases, and the length of the arms. The client then bends forward, and the examiner observes for prominence of the thoracic ribs or vertebral muscles. The client is then viewed from the side while the screener looks for increased thoracic rounding or lumbar swayback.

A scoliometer is used to quantify the prominence of any curvatures noted during the examination. The scoliometer is placed at the apex of the curvature. A reading of greater than 10 degrees requires referral to a physician (Porth, 2005).

Diagnosis

Upright posteroanterior and lateral x-rays are used to confirm the diagnosis of curvature of the spine. For the client with scoliosis, the degree of curvature is measured by determining the amount of lateral deviation to the left or right. For the client with kyphosis, anteroposterior and lateral views typically reveal wedging of the vertebrae.

Treatments

Scoliosis and kyphosis may be treated conservatively or with surgery.

CONSERVATIVE TREATMENT Braces, electrical stimulation, and traction may be used to prevent progression of scoliosis and kyphosis in younger clients whose skeletons have not yet matured. Unfortunately, these approaches are ineffective in the adult client. Conservative treatment for adults with scoliosis and kyphosis may include weight reduction, active and passive exercises, and the use of braces for support.

SURGERY The use of surgery to correct spinal deformities depends on factors such as the degree of curvature and the client's overall physical, emotional, and neurologic status. Even with surgery, it is not possible to correct the abnormal curvature completely. The surgical procedure involves attaching metal reinforcing rods to the vertebrae, and is usually performed using an anterior approach, although more severe curvature may require both an anterior and a posterior approach. The types of straightening devices used most frequently use bilateral rods with wire hooks or screws that stabilize the spine and correct the deformity.

NURSING CARE

Nursing Diagnoses and Interventions

Nursing interventions focus on minimizing the risk for injury and neurologic impairment.

Risk for Injury

Clients with spinal deformities are at risk for injury from several sources, including structural aspects of bracing both before and after surgical intervention, dislocation of hooks and rods resulting from improper alignment or movement of the back, and changes in body position after prolonged immobilization.

- Assess the environment for safety hazards. *The client needs to learn to use handrails on stairways and take precautions when walking on slippery surfaces or areas with throw rugs.*

> **PRACTICE ALERT**
> Some braces do not allow the client to flex or hyperextend the spinal column.

- Teach the client ways to reduce irritation of skin surfaces beneath the brace: wearing a smooth cotton t-shirt or cotton tube under the brace at all times, changing undergarments at least once daily, and washing them with a mild soap. Undergarments should be changed more frequently in warmer weather. *The client wearing a brace is especially prone to skin breakdown and must take precautions to prevent it.*

> **PRACTICE ALERT**
> Teach the client to avoid lotion and body powders; they may irritate the skin.

- Teach the client to loosen the brace during meals and for the first 30 minutes after each meal. *Clients have difficulty eating if the brace is tight. Loosening the brace during and after each meal will allow adequate nutritional intake and promote comfort.*
- Teach clients how to apply the brace, and explain ambulatory restrictions. *Clients requiring a brace need to learn how to apply the brace prior to ambulating. Ambulation is frequently restricted to walking rather than sitting for long periods.*
- Turn clients who have undergone spinal surgery by using the log-rolling technique. Clients require a position change at least every 2 hours. *The use of a turn sheet and sufficient assistance allow the nurse to maintain the client's proper body alignment during the turning procedure.*
- Use a fracture bedpan following surgery. *The fracture bedpan provides minimal misalignment of spine and is more comfortable.*

Risk for Peripheral Neurovascular Dysfunction

Surgical procedures can lead to neurologic impairment in the client with a spinal deformity.

- Monitor the movement and sensation of lower extremities every 2 hours for the first 8 hours then every shift and as needed. *Neurologic assessment related to sensation and movement of the lower extremities is necessary because the surgical procedure is in close proximity to spinal nerves. Swelling of the surgical site can impinge on the spinal nerves and cause a loss of sensation and movement.*

Community-Based Care

Clients with structural scoliosis or kyphosis need reassurance that the condition was not caused by poor posture. If a brace is prescribed to relieve pain and other symptoms associated with the disorder, provide verbal and written instructions for wearing the brace, such as the number of hours per day it is to be worn and activity restrictions to follow when wearing or not wearing the brace. Teach the client how to protect and care for skin under the brace.

Surgical clients need postoperative teaching regarding site care and activities. Clients who have spinal surgery often are allowed to ambulate fairly soon after surgery, but sitting may be restricted because of the stresses it places on the spine. Instruct the client to notify the physician if numbness, tingling, pain, or weakness of an extremity develops after surgery.

Discuss the importance of not smoking and of avoiding respiratory infections for clients with scoliosis or kyphosis that restricts respiratory excursion. Encourage these clients to obtain pneumococcal pneumonia and influenza immunizations.

THE CLIENT WITH LOW BACK PAIN

Acute or chronic low back pain involves the lumbar, lumbosacral, or sacroiliac areas of the back. In most cases, low back pain is due to strains in the muscles and tendons of the back caused by abnormal stress or overuse. Low back pain caused by degenerative disk disease and herniated vertebral disks is covered in Chapter 45 ∞.

Pathophysiology

The pathophysiology of back pain varies with its many causes (Box 42–5). In general, the five causes and types of back pain are as follows:

- Local pain is caused by compression or irritation of sensory nerves. Fractures, strains, and sprains are common causes of local pain; tumors also may press on pain-sensitive structures.
- Referred pain may originate from abdominal or pelvic viscera.
- Pain of spinal origin, that is, pain associated with pathology of the spine such as disk disease or arthritis, may be referred to other structures such as the buttocks, groin, or legs.
- Radicular back pain is sharp, radiating from the back to the leg along a nerve root. This pain may be aggravated by movements such as coughing, sneezing, or sitting.
- Muscle spasm pain is associated with many spine disorders, although its origin may be unclear. This type of back pain is dull and may be accompanied by abnormal posture and taut spinal muscles.

Manifestations

Clients with low back pain report pain ranging from mild discomfort lasting a few hours to chronic debilitating pain. Acute

---

BOX 42–5 Factors Associated with Back Pain

Mechanical Injury or Trauma
- Muscle strain or spasm
- Compression fracture
- Lumbar disk disease

Degenerative Disorders
- Spondylosls
- Spinal stenosis
- Osteoarthritis

Systemic Disorders
- Osteomyelitis
- Osteoporosis or osteomalacia
- Neoplasms, primary or metastatic

Referred Pain
- Gastrointestinal disorders
- Genitourinary disorders
- Gynecologic disorders
- Abdominal aortic aneurysm
- Hip pathology

Other
- Fibromyalgia
- Psychiatric syndromes
- Chronic anxiety
- Depression

---

pain is usually caused when the client participates in an activity that is not usually pursued, such as unusual lifting or bending, playing an active sport, or shoveling snow. Manifestations are presented in the box below.

MANIFESTATIONS of Low Back Pain

ALTERATIONS IN GAIT AND FLEXION
- Walking in a stiff, flexed state
- Inability to bend at waist
- Limp, which may indicate impairment of the sciatic nerve

NEUROLOGIC INVOLVEMENT
- When tested for light and deep touch with a pin and cotton ball, may feel sensations in both limbs but experience a stronger sensation in the unaffected side
- Loss of both bowel and bladder control due to involvement of the sacral nerve

PAIN
- Pain in the affected leg when walking on heel or toes
- Continuous, knifelike localized pain in muscles close to the affected disk
- Pain that radiates down posterior of leg
- Sharp, burning pain in the posterior thigh or calf
- Pain in middle of buttock
- Tenderness when muscle close to the affected disk is palpated
- Severe pain with straight leg-raising maneuver

INTERDISCIPLINARY CARE

Care of the client with low back pain focuses on relieving pain, correcting the condition if possible, preventing complications, and educating the client.

Diagnosis

The choice of diagnostic tests for the client with low back pain depends on the suspected diagnoses, clinical findings, and history. Current guidelines for care recommend that radiography, CT scans, and MRI be used only with clinical signs of a potentially serious underlying condition. Diagnostic testing may be considered if pain and other manifestations continue to limit the client after 4 weeks of conservative treatment. Diagnostic tests are described in Chapter 40 ∞.

Medications

The medications of choice for low back pain include NSAIDs and analgesics. NSAIDs block prostaglandin production and reduce inflammation, thus relieving the pain. Muscle relaxants, such as cyclobenzaprine (Flexeril), methocarbamol (Robaxin), or carisoprodol (Soma), may be used, but little evidence supports their efficacy.

Epidural steroid injections may be used to help reduce intense, intractable pain. A steroid solution is injected into the epidural space, which helps decrease the swelling and inflammation of the spinal nerves.

Conservative Treatment

The majority of clients with acute low back pain need only a short-term treatment regimen. Limited rest, combined with appropriate exercise and education, is often the primary method of treatment. There is no evidence that activity is harmful or aggravating to the source of pain. In fact, activity promotes bone and muscle strength and may increase endorphin levels. Therefore, active rehabilitation helps to restore function and reduce pain.

Pain may be relieved by an ice bag or hot water bottle (or heating pad) applied to the back. Exercise programs are helpful provided that the client begins gradually and increases activity gradually as the recovery process continues. Physical therapy procedures include diathermy (deep heat therapy), ultrasonography, hydrotherapy, and transcutaneous electrical nerve stimulation (TENS) units. These therapies reduce the muscle spasms and pain temporarily. They are frequently used in combination with exercise to provide early mobilization for the client.

NURSING CARE

Nursing care of the client with low back pain focuses on relieving the pain. In addition, most clients have very little understanding of the anatomy of the spine, the reasons for the pain, the choices for treatment, and the importance of self-management. Therefore, education is another essential aspect of treating low back pain.

Health Promotion

Recommendations for preventing back pain from the National Institute of Neurological Disorders and Stroke include the following:

- Have a regular exercise program.
- Stretch before working in the yard, jogging, and playing sports.
- Quit smoking.
- Lose weight, if needed.
- Maintain a correct posture.
- Use supportive seats when driving.
- Lift by bending at the knees rather than at the waist.
- Reduce emotional stress that causes muscle tension.

In industrial and work settings, nurses should be alert for situations that increase the risk of back pain and injury. Office workers should have chairs with appropriate seat height and length and back support. Modifications of work space or machinery may be necessary for industrial workers to avoid excess stresses on back muscles. Finally, it is important to remember that back pain is a leading cause of lost work time for nurses themselves. Remind coworkers to use good body mechanics and to seek help when lifting or moving clients.

Nursing Diagnoses and Interventions

Nursing interventions for the client with low back pain are based on problems with acute pain, deficient knowledge, and risk for impaired adjustment.

Acute Pain

Muscle spasms and inflammation are among the contributing factors of low back pain.

- Teach the client appropriate comfort measures. *Clients with low back pain have discomfort due to muscle spasms and/or inflammation due to nerve compression, surgery, or irritation from a brace.*
- Instruct the client to take NSAIDs or analgesics on a routine schedule rather than as needed. *Maintaining a constant blood level of the NSAIDs or analgesics reduces inflammation and provides continuous pain relief.*

Deficient Knowledge

The client with low back pain requires information regarding treatment modalities.

- Encourage clients to stay active. *There is little scientific evidence to show that bed rest is beneficial, but there is ample evidence about the adverse effects of bed rest. Staying in bed for more than one to two days can actually increase pain, and cause joint stiffness and muscle weakness.*
- Teach the client about the "rebound phenomenon" of prolonged heat or ice therapy. *Ice remaining on the skin longer than 15 minutes or heat longer than 30 minutes causes a reverse effect known as the rebound phenomenon. For example, heat produces maximum vasodilation in 20 to 30 minutes. Continuation of the application beyond 30 to 45 minutes causes tissue congestion, and the blood vessels constrict. Likewise, with cold application, maximum vasoconstriction occurs when the skin reaches a temperature of 60°F (15°C). Prolonged cold can create a drop in temperature, at which time vasodilation occurs.*
- Provide instructions about appropriate back exercises such as partial sit-ups with the knees bent and knee-chest exercises to stretch hamstrings and spinal muscles. Each exercise

should be done 5 times and gradually increased to 10 times. Advise the client to discontinue any exercise that is painful and to seek professional advice before continuing the exercise. *Repetition of prescribed back exercises, such as the pelvic tilt, partial sit-ups, and back rolls, will strengthen the muscles that protect the spine and thus prevent back strain.*

Risk for Impaired Adjustment
The need for lifestyle changes may lead to impaired adjustment in people with back pain.

- Teach the use of appropriate body mechanics in lifting and reaching. The client should be instructed to plan the lift, keep the object being lifted close to the body, and avoid twisting when lifting. Encourage the client to obtain help when lifting. *An item is considered excessively heavy if it equals 35% of the lifter's body weight.*
- Instruct the client to modify the workplace or environment to minimize stress to the lower back. *Lumbar supports in chairs, adjustment of chair or table height, and rubber floor mats help prevent back strain or injury.*
- Encourage obese clients to lose weight. *The trunk of the body must carry excess weight when the client is obese. Obese people are farther away from the objects they lift because of their greater abdominal girth. They may also have more difficulty squatting to lift. The greater the distance between an object and the client's center of gravity, the higher the risk for straining the lower back.*

Community-Based Care
Back pain is a common problem in the United States and other industrialized countries. Nurses can have an effect on this significant problem by teaching health practices to prevent back injury to clients of all ages. Teach clients how to safely lift, bend, and turn when engaging in physical activity. Stress the importance of using large muscle groups of the legs to lift rather than bending and lifting with the smaller muscles of the back. Teach other aspects of good body mechanics, including posture, sleeping on a firm mattress, and sitting in chairs that provide good support. Discuss the positive effect of maintaining optimal body weight and good physical fitness.

THE CLIENT WITH COMMON FOOT DISORDERS

Hallux valgus, hammertoe, and Morton's neuroma are common foot disorders that cause pain or difficulty in walking. All three disorders may be caused by wearing poorly fitting or confining shoes. These disorders are more prevalent among women.

Pathophysiology

Hallux Valgus
Hallux valgus, commonly called a *bunion*, is the enlargement and lateral displacement of the first metatarsal (the great toe) (Figure 42–12 ■). Hallux valgus develops when chronic pres-

Figure 42–12 ■ Hallux valgus (bunion).

sure against the great toe causes the connective tissue in the sole of the foot to lengthen so that the stabilizing action of the great toe is gradually lost. The toe bends laterally away from the midline of the body, and the metatarsophalangeal joint (MTP) is exposed to friction during walking and becomes enlarged. As the deformity progresses, calluses form over the metatarsal head, and bursitis develops in the MTP. In severe cases, the lateral displacement of the great toe may approach 70 to 90 degrees, and the second toe may be forced upward, causing hammertoe. Although bunions may be a congenital disorder, most are caused by wearing pointed, narrow-toed shoes or high heels.

Hallux valgus is obvious on physical examination of the foot. The client may report an inability to fit into shoes. Often, the client may report joint pain or pain around calluses. In advanced or severe cases, the first metatarsal joint may have limited range of motion, particularly in dorsiflexion, and crepitus (crackling or popping) may occur during joint movement.

Hammertoe
Hammertoe (claw toe) is the dorsiflexion of the first phalanx with accompanying plantar flexion of the second and third phalanges. The condition may affect any toe, but the second toe is most commonly affected. Clients initially experience mild inflammation of the synovial membranes of the involved joints. As the deformity progresses, the dorsiflexed joint rubs against the overlying shoe, causing painful corns to develop.

Morton's Neuroma
Morton's neuroma is a tumorlike mass formed within the neurovascular bundle of the intermetatarsal spaces (Figure 42–13 ■). The neuromas usually occur in only one foot, most frequently in the third web space. Like other common foot disorders, Morton's neuroma usually is caused by wearing tight, confining shoes. The condition develops when repeated compression of the toes causes irritation and scarring of tissues surrounding the plantar digital nerve. The affected nerve becomes inflamed and swells. After repeated episodes of inflammation, the nerve fibers become fibrotic, and a neuroma forms.

Manifestations include a burning pain at the web space of the affected foot that radiates into the tips of the involved toes.

Figure 42–13 ■ Morton's neuroma.

Weight bearing usually worsens any symptoms; removing the shoe and massaging the foot often relieves the pain. The neuroma may present as a palpable mass between the affected toes. The area over the neuroma usually is tender.

INTERDISCIPLINARY CARE

Care of the client with common foot disorders such as hallux valgus, hammertoe, and Morton's neuroma focuses on relieving pain, correcting the structural deformity, and preventing reoccurrence. In most cases, all three conditions are diagnosed by inspection. X-ray films of the affected foot are taken if the need for surgery arises.

Conservative treatment for common foot disorders usually involves the use of corrective shoes. Orthotic devices that cushion and stretch the affected joints may be placed within shoes or between the client's toes. For Morton's neuroma, metatarsal pads are used to spread the client's toes and decompress the affected nerve. Analgesics may be prescribed to relieve pain and inflammation. In severe cases, corticosteroid drugs may be injected into the affected joints or surrounding tissue to relieve acute inflammation.

Surgery is reserved for clients with intractable toe deformities or pain. Hallux valgus is treated with bunionectomy; ligaments are lengthened or shortened as needed, and pins are drilled into place so the toe remains in position. Similarly, the correction of hammertoe also involves straightening the affected toe and inserting pins to retain the correction. A cast may be applied over the foot following surgery to correct toe deformities. Surgery for Morton's neuroma causes loss of sensation to a portion of the foot because removing the neuroma involves cutting out a portion of the plantar nerve.

NURSING CARE

Nursing care for clients with these foot deformities focuses on the same areas because the conservative treatment and preoperative and postoperative interventions are similar.

Nursing Diagnoses and Interventions

Pain relief, prevention of infection, and client education are important components of the nursing care of clients with foot disorders.

Chronic Pain

In the client with a foot deformity, constant pressure of footwear over the involved joint can cause pain.

■ Instruct clients to wear corrective footwear to assist in the conservative treatment of foot problems. *Pain related to foot problems can result from improper footwear that does not provide proper toe room; in addition, heels higher than 1 inch can cause constant flexion and hyperextension problems. In some instances, the client must purchase special shoes or orthotics to ensure correct fit and relief of symptoms.*

■ Suggest purchasing appropriate pads to wear over painful bunions, calluses/corns, and the ball of the foot. *Protective pads are manufactured for specific foot problems; these include bunion pads, corn pads, and metatarsal pads.*

■ Instruct clients to remove pads and inspect the skin every other day. Clients who have difficulty reaching or observing the involved foot should ask another person to do the inspection for them. *It is especially important to emphasize the need for inspection to clients who have experienced loss of sensation of the feet due to such disorders as diabetes and chronic peripheral vascular disease.*

Risk for Infection

Like all surgeries, foot surgery carries a risk of infection. This risk may be increased because of impaired peripheral circulation and exposure of the feet to the environment.

■ Teach clients proper care and cleaning of exposed pins implanted during the surgical procedure. *Pins inserted into soft tissue of the toes and bones are prone to becoming infected and can potentially result in osteomyelitis.*

■ Teach clients how to keep pins and casts dry while bathing or ambulating in inclement weather. Clients must wear a plastic bag over the cast or pins when bathing or walking in rain or snow. *When casts or pins are exposed in water, infection may result.*

Community-Based Care

For clients in all age groups, teach the importance of well-fitting footwear. Discuss the long-term effects of wearing high-heeled shoes with constricting toes with women in particular. Suggest alternatives for stylish footwear, and encourage clients to wear supportive and nonrestrictive footwear at all times. Discuss the possible effects of bunions on balance, and talk about safety measures to prevent falls and injury. Teach clients techniques to relieve pressure on affected joints.

EXPLORE MediaLink

Prentice Hall Nursing MediaLink DVD-ROM
Audio Glossary
NCLEX-RN® Review

Animations
Arthritis
Carpal Tunnel
Muscular Dystrophy
Osteoporosis

COMPANION WEBSITE www.prenhall.com/lemone
Audio Glossary
NCLEX-RN® Review
Care Plan Activity: Lower Back Pain
Case Studies:
Diet and Gout
Hip Replacement
Rheumatoid Arthritis
MediaLink Applications
Compartment Syndrome
Osteoporosis Prevention
Links to Resources

CHAPTER HIGHLIGHTS

- Metabolic bone disorders begin in the bone remodeling process, and may result from aging, calcium and phosphate imbalances, genetics, and changes in hormone levels. The disorders include osteoporosis, Paget's disease, gout, and osteomalacia.

- Osteoporosis is a major health problem in the United States, with fractures being the most common complication. Health promotion activities to prevent development of the disease include a calcium-rich diet, weight-bearing exercise, and a healthy lifestyle.

- Gout is characterized by hyperuricemia and the deposit of tophi in the subcutaneous tissues. Attacks of the disease typically begin with an acutely painful inflammation of the first joint of the great toe.

- Degenerative musculoskeletal disorders include osteoarthritis (OA) and muscular dystrophy (MD). OA is the most commonly occurring of all forms of arthritis, and a leading cause of pain and disability in older adults. The disease is characterized by loss of cartilage in articulating joints and hypertrophy of bone at the articular margins. Pain and inflammation are most often conservatively managed with NSAIDs.

- If pain and disability are not controlled in clients with arthritis, total joint replacements may be performed.

- Autoimmune and inflammatory disorders of the musculoskeletal system include rheumatoid arthritis (RA), ankylosing spondylitis (AS), reactive arthritis (ReA), systemic lupus erythematosus (SLE), polymyositis, and Lyme disease.

- Although the cause of RA is unknown, it is believed to be a combination of genetic, environmental, hormonal, and reproductive factors. RA is a systemic disease, affecting one or many joints with the risk for severe contractures and deformity, and also causing fatigue, weakness, anorexia, weight loss, and

fever. The primary objectives of treatment and care are to reduce pain and inflammation, preserve function, and prevent deformity.

- SLE is a chronic inflammatory connective tissue disease, affecting almost all body systems, including the musculoskeletal system. Skin lesions are a common manifestation, exhibited by a characteristic rash on the face. The client with SLE is at increased risk for infection.

- Lyme disease is caused by the spirochete *Borrelia burgdorferi*, carried and transmitted primarily by ticks. The disease can be treated effectively with antibiotics.

- Osteomyelitis and septic arthritis are infectious musculoskeletal disorders. Osteomyelitis may be the result of a bloodborne pathogen, a contiguous infection, or a complication of vascular insufficiency. Septic arthritis is a medical emergency, requiring immediate treatment to preserve joint function.

- Bone tumors may be benign or malignant, primary or metastatic. The primary manifestations of a bone tumor are pain, a mass, and impaired function. Nursing care is directed toward teaching to prevent injury and interventions to relieve pain.

- Scleroderma is a chronic disease characterized by the formation of excess connective tissue and diffuse fibrosis of the skin and internal organs. It may be either localized or generalized. Other connective musculoskeletal disorders are Sjögren's syndrome and fibromyalgia.

- Structural musculoskeletal disorders affecting the spine are manifested by scoliosis, kyphosis, and low back pain. Those commonly affecting the feet are hallux valgus, hammertoe, and Morton's neuroma.

TEST YOURSELF NCLEX-RN® REVIEW

1 Although all of the following nursing diagnoses are important when planning care for the client with osteoporosis, which is most significant in terms of long-term disability?
1. *Chronic Pain*
2. *Risk for Falls*
3. *Activity Intolerance*
4. *Acute Pain*

2 You are preparing a teaching plan for a woman with osteoarthritis. Which group of medications should you prepare to discuss?
1. opioids
2. antibiotics
3. hormones
4. NSAIDs

3 You are monitoring the laboratory reports for a client with an acute attack of gout. Which of the following measurements would you expect to be increased?
1. hematocrit
2. uric acid
3. alkaline phosphatase
4. creatinine

4 What is a potential complication of both osteoporosis and osteomalacia?
1. infection
2. blood clots
3. fractures
4. contractures

5 You are assessing a woman who has come to an orthopedic clinic complaining of knee pain. Which of the following assessments you made would indicate an increased risk for osteoarthritis?
1. being overweight by 30 pounds
2. having a history of falls
3. eating a diet high in calcium
4. walking 30 minutes each day

6 A postoperative nursing care plan for a client who has had a total knee replacement includes monitoring vital signs and laboratory results. The rationale for these interventions is to:

1. teach the client the importance of these assessments.
2. promote rapport between the client and the healthcare providers.
3. ensure adequate circulation to the involved extremity.
4. prevent the progression of infection.

7 When comparing osteoarthritis and rheumatoid arthritis, what assessment finding would be different in the client with rheumatoid arthritis?
1. Health history includes weight loss and fever.
2. Abnormal joint findings are limited to the hands.
3. Stiffness is relieved by activity.
4. Heberden's nodes are located on the finger joints

8 *Ineffective Protection* is an appropriate nursing diagnosis for the client with SLE. What would be your most important intervention for the hospitalized client?
1. Monitor laboratory findings.
2. Provide appropriate skin care.
3. Practice careful hand washing.
4. Administer prescribed medications.

9 How is the causative organism for Lyme disease spread?
1. through the bite of an infected mosquito
2. by brief contact with an infected tick
3. primarily by droplets from infected people
4. by an infected tick embedded for >24 hours

10 Of the different types of arthritis, which one is considered a medical emergency, requiring immediate diagnosis and treatment?
1. osteoarthritis
2. septic arthritis
3. reactive arthritis
4. gouty arthritis

See Test Yourself answers in Appendix C.

BIBLIOGRAPHY

Abdelhafiz, A., Lowles, R., Alam, N., Abebajo, A., & Philp, I. (2003). Clinical assessment of symptomatic osteoarthritis in older people. *Age and Aging, 32*(3), 359–360.
_____. (2005a). *FDA actions on COX-2 inhibitors & NSAIDs (Non-steroidal anti-inflammatory drugs)*. Retrieved from http://arthritis.about.com/od/arthritismedications/a/qufdaactions_p.htm
About Arthritis. (2005b). *FDA announces changes for all NSAIDSs; Bextra withdrawn from market*. Retrieved from http://arthritis.about.com/od/nsaids/fadaaction.htm
Altizer, L. (2004). Patient education for total hip or knee replacement. *Orthopedic Nursing, 23*(4), 383–388.
American College of Rheumatology. (2004a). *Glucocorticoid-induced osteoporosis*. Retrieved from http://www.rheumatology.org/public/factsheets/gi_osteopor_new.asp?aud=mem
_____. (2004b). *Lyme disease*. Retrieved from http://www.rheumatology.org/public/factsheets/lyme.asp?aud=mem
_____. (2005). *Background information on arthritis and rheumatology: Prevalence statistics*. Retrieved from http://www.rheumatology.org/press/index.asp?uad=mem
Arthritis Foundation. (2004). *Disease center: Osteoarthritis treatment*. Retrieved from http://www.arthritis.org/conditions/DiseaseCenter/OA/oa_treatment1.asp

Berarducci, A. (2004). Osteoporosis education: A health-promotion mandate for nurses. *Orthopaedic Nursing, 23*(2), 118–120.
Boston Total Joint Association. (2004). *Total hip replacement surgery*. Retrieved from http://www.bostontotaljoint.com/thr.html
Brown, S. (2005). Managing systemic lupus erythematosus. *Nurse 2 Nurse, 4*(11), 28–30.
Capriotti, T. (2004). The 'alphabet' of rheumatoid arthritis treatment. *Medsurg Nursing, 13*(6), 420–428.
Centers for Disease Control and Prevention. (2005). *Bone health*. Retrieved from www.cdc.gov/nccdphp/dnpa/bonehealth/
Cornell, T. (2004). Factfile. Ankylosing spondylitis: An overview. *Professional Nurse, 19*(8), 431–432.
Dochterman, J., & Bulechek, G. (2004). *Nursing interventions classification (NIC)* (4th ed.). St. Louis, MO: Mosby.
Easterbrook, L. (2003). Explaining about ... arthritis. *Working with older people, 7*(3), 7–9.
Flynn, J., & Johnson, T. (2005). *The Johns Hopkins white papers: Arthritis*. Baltimore, MD: Johns Hopkins Medicine.
Gill, J., Quisel, A., Rocca, P., & Walters, D. (2003). Diagnosis of systemic lupus erythematosus. *American Family Physician, 68*(11). Retrieved from http://www.aafp.org/afp/20031201/2179.html

Harvey, C. (2005). Wound healing. *Orthopaedic Nursing, 24*(2), 143–160.
International Scleroderma Network. (2004). *What in the world is scleroderma?* Retrieved from http://www.sclero.org
Kass-Wolff, J. (2004). Calcium in women: Healthy bones and much more. *Journal of Obstetrics, Gynecologic, and Neonatal Nursing, 33*(1), 21–33.
Kee, J. (2004). *Handbook of laboratory and diagnostic tests with nursing implications* (5th ed.). Upper Saddle River, NJ: Prentice Hall.
Lange, R., & Nies, M. (2004). Benefits of walking for obese women in the prevention of bone and joint disorders. *Orthopedic Nursing, 23*(3), 211–215.
Lucas, B. (2004). Does a pre-operative exercise programme improve mobility and function post-total knee replacement: A mini-review. *Journal of Orthopaedic Nursing, 8*(1), 25–33.
Mayo Clinic. (2002). *Osteoporosis*. Retrieved from www.mayocli8nic.com/invoke.cfm?id=DS00128
Moorhead, S., Johnson, M., & Maas, M. (2003). *Nursing outcomes classification (NOC)*. (3rd ed.). St. Louis, MO: Mosby.
Morrow, M. (2004). Duchenne muscular dystrophy—A biopsychosocial approach. *Physiotherapy, 90*, 145–150.
Moss Rehab Resource Net. (2005). *Arthritis fact sheet*. Retrieved from http://www.mossresourcenet.org/arthritis/htm

NANDA International. (2005). *Nursing diagnoses: Definitions & classification 2005–2006*. Philadelphia: Author.

National Fibromyalgia Research Association. (2004). *Fibromyalgia syndrome*. Retrieved from http://www.nfra.net/

National Institute of Arthritis and Musculoskeletal and Skin Diseases. (2003). *Systemic lupus erythematosus; lupus and quality of life*. Retrieved from http://www.niams.nih.gov/hi/topics/lupus/slehandout/

_____. (2004a). *Questions and answers about arthritis and rheumatic diseases*. Retrieved from http://www.niams.nih.gov/hi/topics/arthritis/arthrheu.htm

_____. (2004b). *Questions and answers about knee problems*. Retrieved from http://www.niams.nih.gov/hi/topics/kneeprobs/kneeqa.htm

_____. (2005a). *Fibromyalgia*. Retrieved from http://www.niams.nih.gov/hi/topics/fibromyalgia/ffibro.htm

_____. (2005b). *Hyaluronic acid shows potential as biomarker for osteoarthritis*. Retrieved from http://www.niams.nih.gov/ne/highlights/spotlight/2005/hyaluronic_acid.htm

_____. (2005c). *What is gout?* Retrieved from http://www.niams.nih.gov/hi/topics/gout/ffgout.htm

National Osteoporosis Foundation. (2006). *Fast facts*. Retrieved from http://www.nof.org/osteoporosis/diseasefacts.htm

Nivens, A. (2004). Paget's disease: A case in point. *Orthopedic Nursing, 23*(6), 355–363.

Overstreet, M. (2005). Lyme disease: The dangerous hitchhiker. *Nursing Made Incredibly Easy, 3*(3), 38–44.

Paget Foundation. (2004a). *A health professional's guide to the management of Paget's disease of the bone*. Retrieved from http://www.Paget's.org/Information/FactSheet/mgmt_of_pdisbone.html

_____. (2004b). *A nurse's guide for assessment and management of patients diagnosed with Paget's disease of bone*. New York: The Paget Foundation.

Porth, C. M. (2005). *Pathophysiology: Concepts of altered health states* (7th ed.). Philadelphia: Lippincott.

Pullen, R., Jr. (2004). Caring for a patient on Plaquenil therapy. *Nursing, 34*(6), 32hn4, 32hn16.

_____, Cannon, J., & Rushing, J. (2003). Managing organ-threatening systemic lupus erythematosus. *Medsurg Nursing, 12*(6), 368–379.

Roberts, D. (2003). Alternative therapies for arthritis treatment: Part 1. *Orthopedic Nursing, 22*(5), 335–344.

Risley, S., Thomas, M., & Bray, V. (2004). Rheumatoid arthritis, new standards of care: Nursing implications of infliximab. *Journal of Orthopaedic Nursing, 8*(1), 41–49.

Schoen, D. C. (2004). Osteoporosis. *Orthopaedic Nursing, 23*(4), 261–267.

Scleroderma Foundation. (2006). *What is scleroderma?* Retrieved from http://scleroderma.org/medical/overview.shtm

Spondylitis Association of America. (2006). *Reactive arthritis/Reiter's syndrome, (ReA), Fast facts about ankylosing spondylitis (AS)*. Retrieved from http://www.spondylitis.org/about/reative.aspx

Taggart, H., Mincer, A., & Thompson, A. (2004). Caring for the orthopaedic patient who is obese. *Orthopaedic Nursing, 23*(3), 204–210.

Tak, S. H., & Hong, S. H. (2005). Use of the Internet for health information by older adults with arthritis. *Orthopaedic Nursing, 24*(2), 134–139.

Temple, J. (2004). Total hip replacement. *Nursing Standard, 19*(3), 44–51, 53.

Tierney, L., McPhee, S., & Papadakis, M. (Eds.). (2004). *Current medical diagnosis & treatment* (43rd ed.). Stamford, CT: Appleton & Lange.

Tretheway, P. (2004). Systemic lupus erythematosus. *DCCN: Dimensions of Critical Care Nursing, 23*(3), 111–115.

U. S. Food and Drug Administration (FDA). (2005). *COX-2 selective (includes Bextra, Celebrex, and Vioxx) and non-selective non-steroidal anti-inflammatory drugs (NSAIDs)*. Retrieved from http://www.fda.gov/cder/drug/infopage/COX2/

Vestergaard. P., Emborg, C., Stoving, R., Hagen, C., Mosekilde, L., & Briken, K. (2003). Patients with eating disorders: A high-risk group for fractures. *Orthopaedic Nursing, 22*(5), 325–331.

Wilkens, R. (2004). Making the most of antirheumatic drugs in older patients. *Journal of Musculoskeletal Medicine, 21*(6), 317–322.

Wilkinson, J. (2005). *Prentice Hall nursing diagnosis handbook with NIC interventions and NOC outcomes* (8th ed.). Upper Saddle River, NJ: Prentice Hall.

Wilson, B., Shannon, M., & Stang, C. (2005). *Prentice Hall nurse's drug guide 2005*. Upper Saddle River, NJ: Prentice Hall.

Responses to Altered Musculoskeletal Function

FUNCTIONAL HEALTH PATTERN: Activity-Exercise

■ Think about clients with altered activity-exercise patterns for whom you have cared in your clinical experiences.

- What were the clients' major medical diagnoses (e.g., sprain, joint dislocation, fracture, amputation, carpal tunnel syndrome, osteoporosis, Paget's disease, gout, osteomalacia, osteoarthritis, muscular dystrophy, rheumatoid arthritis, ankylosing spondylitis, systemic lupus erythematosus, polymyositis, Lyme disease, osteomyelitis, bone tumors, systemic sclerosis, scoliosis, low back pain, hammertoe)?
- What manifestations did each of these clients have? Were these manifestations similar or different?
- How did the clients' altered activity-exercise patterns interfere with their health status? Did pain increase with movement? Was the pain worse in the morning or did the pain increase throughout the day? Did they complain of muscle weakness or muscle cramps? Did they notice any redness or swelling of the joints? Had they ever had any muscle or bone diseases or injuries? Did they have any surgery or physical therapies for muscle or bone problems? Did they take any medications or herbal supplements for musculoskeletal disorders? Did they include foods with calcium in the diet? Did they have any family history of bone, joint, or muscle problems? Did they exercise regularly? Did they take part in strenuous activity or heavy lifting? Did they use assistive devices to move around?

■ The Activity-Exercise Pattern includes disorders that result in insufficient physiologic movement to carry out activities of daily living. Activity and exercise are affected by the ability of the musculoskeletal system to allow movement of the body and by perceived health status in two primary ways:

- Factors that result from trauma or surgery to tissues (e.g., contusion), tendons (e.g., strain, epicondylitis), ligaments (e.g., sprain), or bones (e.g., dislocation, fracture, amputation).
- Factors that result from medical disorders or deformities of joints (e.g., arthritis, gout, hammertoe), bones (e.g., osteoporosis, Paget's disease, osteomalacia, osteomyelitis, tumors, scoliosis), or muscles (e.g., muscular dystrophy, polymyositis).

■ The tissues and structures of the musculoskeletal system perform many functions, including support, protection, and movement. The bones form the body's structure and provide support for soft tissues. The bones protect vital internal organs from injury. The bones also store minerals and serve as a site for hematopoiesis (blood cell formation). The bones and joints of the skeleton and the skeletal muscles work together to allow the body to perform both gross, simple movements and fine, complex movements. Musculoskeletal disorders affect a client's perceived activity-exercise patterns, leading to manifestations such as:

- Pain (tissue damage ▶ stimulates sensory nerve endings ▶which release chemical mediators such as bradykinin and histamine ▶resulting in transmission of pain sensation to brain and nerve fibers)
- Limited mobility (disease or injury ▶causes excessive loss of movement to muscles and joints ▶resulting in reduction or restriction of range of motion to a body part)
- Edema (inflammation or infection ▶causes impaired circulation, venous pooling, and proteins leaking into the interstitium ▶resulting in edema).

■ Priority nursing diagnoses within the activity-exercise pattern that may be appropriate for clients include:

- *Risk for Disuse Syndrome* related to decreased range of motion, pain with movement, use of functional positioning splints
- *Risk for Falls* related to impaired balance, difficulty with gait, numbness of feet, decreased lower extremity strength
- *Impaired Physical Mobility* as evidenced by limited ability to perform gross/fine motor skills, uncoordinated or jerky movements, postural instability
- *Risk for Peripheral Neurovascular Dysfunction* related to musculoskeletal pain, pallor, diminished pulses, paralysis, and paresthesia.

■ Two nursing diagnoses from other functional health patterns often are of high priority for the client with altered activity-exercise patterns:

- *Impaired Skin Integrity* (Nutritional-Metabolic)
- *Risk for Disturbed Sensory Perception: Tactile (Cognitive-Perceptual)*

CLINICAL SCENARIO

You have been assigned to work with the following four clients for the 0700 shift on an orthopedic unit. Significant data obtained during report are as follows:

- Jesse Drummond is a 70-year-old African American man with type 2 diabetes mellitus who is 3 days postoperative with bilateral below-the-knee amputations. Vital signs are T 99°F, P 88, R 24, BP 150/92. He is complaining of feeling pain in his feet.
- Joyce Stevens is an 84-year-old who is 2 days postoperative for hip replacement surgery. Her vital signs are T 99.6°F, P 100, R 30 and shallow, BP 110/86. She is confused when spoken to. Petechiae have been noted on her arms and legs. She is complaining of difficulty breathing.

- José Rivera, a 21-year-old, was admitted with osteomyelitis of the upper right leg. He has a history of a gunshot wound to the leg. Vital signs are T 102.6°F, P 98, R 22, BP 138/80. He is scheduled for surgical debridement of the wound this morning. He is complaining of pain and requesting pain medication.
- Kim Wong is a 30-year-old who was admitted with manifestations of painful and swollen joints, muscle pain, pale and cyanotic fingers and toes, and edema of the legs and periorbital areas. Her vital signs are T 100.6°F, P 78, R 16, BP 108/72. She is complaining of extreme fatigue. She is to have blood drawn for complete blood count (CBC), anti-DNA antibody testing, and serum complement levels.

Questions

1 In what order would you visit these clients after report?
1. _____
2. _____
3. _____
4. _____

2 What top two priority nursing diagnoses would you choose for each of the clients presented above? Can you explain, if asked, the rationale for your choices?

	Priority Nursing Diagnosis #1	Priority Nursing Diagnosis #2
Jesse Drummond		
Joyce Stevens		
José Rivera		
Kim Wong		

3 After the amputation wound is dressed, what is the client taught to do to toughen the stump?
1. Dangle the stump for 20 minutes every hour while awake.
2. Push the stump into soft and then harder surfaces.
3. Elevate the stump on two pillows, keeping the knee straight.
4. Apply prosthesis over the compression dressing.

4 To prevent hip contractures in the client with an above-the-knee amputation, what does the nurse instruct the client to do?
1. Lie supine for short periods throughout the day.
2. Elevate the stump above the level of the heart.
3. Perform active range-of-motion exercises every 8 hours.
4. Avoid sitting in a chair for prolonged periods of time.

5 The nurse explains to the client with gout that a low-purine diet is recommended. The client understands a low-purine diet when which meal is ordered?
1. ham and asparagus casserole
2. chicken and dumplings
3. chili and spinach salad
4. shrimp and scallop pasta

6 The client's laboratory results are hematocrit of 28%, hemoglobin of 8 g/dL, WBC count of 4000/mm³, platelet count of 98,000/mL, eosinophil sedimentation rate of 100 mm/h, positive anti-DNA antibodies. What medical diagnosis is supported by these lab values?
1. systemic lupus erythmatosus
2. rheumatoid arthritis
3. ankylosing spondylitis
4. polymyositis

7 Clients who have autoimmune diseases such as systemic lupus erythematosus are at increased risk for developing what disease?
1. chronic renal failure
2. hypertension
3. liver insufficiency
4. coronary heart disease

8 A prescription for ibuprofen (Advil) is given on discharge to the client with rheumatoid arthritis. Which toxic effects of the medication does the nurse instruct the client about?
1. diarrhea, nausea, and vomiting
2. blurred vision, tinnitus, and headache
3. gastric irritation, ulceration, and bleeding
4. dizziness, dry mouth, and abdominal cramps

9 When performing a neurovascular assessment, which are included in the initial and focused assessments? (Select all that apply.)
1. pain
2. paroxysm
3. pallor
4. pulses
5. paresis
6. pallesthesia
7. paresthesia

10 Which client is at greatest risk for developing osteoporosis?
1. menopausal, Caucasian woman who smokes one pack of cigarettes a day
2. menopausal, African American woman who has diabetes and hypertension
3. premenopausal, underweight Asian woman who is allergic to dairy products
4. premenopausal, obese African American woman who has a sedentary lifestyle

11 An older adult sprained an ankle after tripping on an uneven sidewalk. Which is the MOST important intervention?
1. Use a walker when ambulating.
2. Take anti-inflammatory and pain medications to reduce ankle pain.
3. Follow a regimen of rest, ice, compression, and elevation.
4. Immobilize the ankle with an air splint.

12 Which actions by the nurse need to be followed when caring for the client with osteomyelitis?
1. Place the client in a private room and use gloves and gown with wound care and good hand washing.
2. Place the client in a semiprivate room with another infected client and use isolation precautions for both clients.
3. Place the client near the nurse's station and use standard precautions when caring for the client.
4. Place the client at the end of the hall away from other clients to prevent spread of infection and teach the client to use good hand washing.

CASE STUDY

William Comfort is a 24-year-old Caucasian male admitted with a compound fracture of the left femur. He states he was riding a four-wheeler on a hill-side path and was thrown from the vehicle. He slid approximately 50 feet down the hill on his left side. His fall was stopped when his foot became tangled in some brush. On admission, his vital signs were T 99.8°F, P 100 and thready, R 24, BP 116/70. His height is 74" and weight is 198 pounds. Assessment revealed an open fracture of the left leg with bleeding and edema around the open site and severe pain on movement of the leg. Popliteal and pedal pulses are difficult to palpate. His left leg is pale and cool to touch with a capillary refill of 4 seconds. He states his leg feels numb. Multiple lacerations and abrasions are noted on his left trunk and arm. He states he does not have any medical problems and has not seen a doctor in the past 5 years. He is employed as a computer repairman. He lives in an apartment with two friends.

Blood is drawn for a baseline compete blood count (CBC) and urine is obtained for a urinalysis. An intravenous line is started in the right arm with lactated Ringer's infusing at 150 mL/h. He is given a tetanus toxoid immunization and is medicated with morphine sulfate for pain. X-rays are taken of the left leg, left arm, and abdomen. The wounds are cleansed with an antibacterial solution and antibiotic ointment is applied. He went to surgery for an open reduction of the left leg fracture and has been placed in skeletal traction to separate the bony fragments and reduce and immobilize the left leg fracture.

The pathophysiology of a femur fracture is a large amount of force applied to the shaft of the femur, resulting in breaking of the bone. An open fracture is diagnosed when the bone is broken with bone fragments protruding through the skin. Manifestations of a femur fracture are edema, and a deformed and painful thigh. The client is unable to move the hip or knee. Popliteal and pedal pulses are difficult to palpate. Capillary refill time is increased. Pallor and coolness indicate arterial compromise. Sensations to the leg may be burning, numbness, prickly feeling, or stinging. Complications of a femur fracture include hypovolemia, fat embolism, dislocation of the hip or knee, muscle atrophy, and ligament damage.

Skeletal traction is the application of a pulling force through placement of pins into the bone. Pins are inserted under sterile conditions into the bone. One or more pulling forces may be applied to maintain alignment of the femur fracture. The disadvantages of skeletal traction are increased anxiety, increased risk of infection, and increased discomfort.

When planning nursing care for Mr. Comfort, the nursing diagnosis of *Impaired Physical Mobility* related to fracture of the left femur with skeletal traction is appropriate for implementing nursing interventions.

affects ——

- Trauma resulted in application of direct force, fracturing the bone
- Compound (open) fracture is diagnosed when the skin integrity is interrupted by parts of the fractured bone

Mr. W.C.
24 y.o. male
Trauma/fracture

leads to

assess ——

- Compound fracture left femur
- Open reduction of fracture in surgery
- Left leg immobilized in skeletal traction

— generates —

- Acute Pain related to fractured femur
- Risk for Infection related to open fracture sustained in dirty area
- Risk for Peripheral Neurovascular Dysfunction related to fracture and traction
- Risk for Constipation related to immobility

generate nursing diagnosis

Impaired Physical Mobility

— prioritized to —

expected outcomes

- Actively participates in physical therapy and in-room exercises to maintain muscle strength
- Normal neurovascular status, left leg
- Able to transfer and ambulate after fracture is healed

— evaluate —

- Physical therapy at bedside twice a day; client is active participant
- Neurovascular status normal
- On discharge, could transfer to chair and walk with non-weight-bearing assistive devices

Interdisciplinary Interventions
- Request physical therapy consult to establish goals for transfer and ambulation after fracture healing
- Ask physical therapy to provide information to client and staff for in-bed exercises to strengthen gluteals, quadriceps, triceps, and biceps

Independent Interventions
- Monitor neurovascular status of left foot and leg q 4 to 8 hours (use 5Ps)
- Provide ROM exercises to unaffected extremities twice a day

PART
V

Cognitive and Perceptual Patterns

Functional Health Patterns with Related Nursing Diagnoses

HEALTH PERCEPTION-HEALTH MANAGEMENT

- Perceived health status
- Perceived health management
- Healthcare behaviors: health promotion and illness prevention activities, medical treatments, follow-up care

VALUE-BELIEF

- Values, goals, or beliefs (including spirituality) that guide choices or decisions
- Perceived conflicts in values, beliefs, or expectations that are health related

COPING-STRESS-TOLERANCE

- Capacity to resist challenges to self-integrity
- Methods of handling stress
- Support systems
- Perceived ability to control and manage situations

NUTRITIONAL-METABOLIC

- Daily consumption of food and fluids
- Favorite foods
- Use of dietary supplements
- Skin lesions and ability to heal
- Condition of the integument
- Weight, height, temperature

PART V
COGNITIVE-PERCEPTUAL PATTERNS
NANDA NURSING DIAGNOSES

- Acute Confusion
- Decreased Intracranial Adaptive Capacity
- Autonomic Dysreflexia
- Risk for Autonomic Dysreflexia
- Chronic Confusion
- Impaired Verbal Communication
- Acute Pain
- Chronic Pain
- Impaired Memory
- Unilateral Neglect
- Risk for Peripheral Neurovascular Dysfunction
- Risk for Post-Trauma Syndrome
- Ineffective Protection
- Disturbed Sensory Perception
- Disturbed Thought Processes
- Decisional Conflict
- Risk for Trauma
- Wandering
- Impaired Environmental Interpretation Syndrome

SEXUALITY-REPRODUCTIVE

- Satisfaction with sexuality or sexual relationships
- Reproductive pattern
- Female menstrual and perimenopausal history

ELIMINATION

- Patterns of bowel and urinary excretion
- Perceived regularity or irregularity of elimination
- Use of laxatives or routines
- Changes in time, modes, quality or quantity of excretions
- Use of devices for control

ROLE-RELATIONSHIPS

- Perception of major roles, relationships, and responsibilities in current life situation
- Satisfaction with or disturbances in roles and relationships

ACTIVITY-EXERCISE

- Patterns of personally relevant exercise, activity, leisure, and recreation
- ADLs that require energy expenditure
- Factors that interfere with the desired pattern (e.g., illness or injury)

SELF-PERCEPTION–SELF-CONCEPT

- Attitudes about self
- Perceived abilities, worth, self-image, emotions
- Body posture and movement, eye contact, voice and speech patterns

SLEEP-REST

- Patterns of sleep and rest-/relaxation in a 24-h period
- Perceptions of quality and quantity of sleep and rest
- Use of sleep aids and routines

COGNITIVE-PERCEPTUAL

- Adequacy of vision, hearing, taste, touch, smell
- Pain perception and management
- Language, judgment, memory, decisions

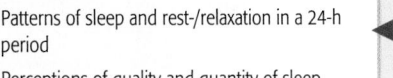

UNIT 13

Responses to Altered Neurologic Function

CHAPTER 43 Assessing Clients with Neurologic Disorders

LEARNING OUTCOMES

- Describe the anatomy, physiology, and functions of the nervous system.
- Identify specific topics for consideration during a health history assessment interview of the client with neurologic disorders.
- Explain techniques for assessment of neurologic function, including examinations of mental status, cranial nerves, sensory nerves, motor nerves, cerebellar function, and reflexes.
- Identify manifestations of impairment of neurologic function.
- Describe normal variations in assessment findings for the older adult.

CLINICAL COMPETENCIES

- Conduct and document a health history for clients having or at risk for alterations in the neurologic system.
- Conduct and document a physical assessment of neurologic structures and functions.
- Perform specific neurologic assessments for clients with suspected meningeal irritation and for disoriented or comatose clients.
- Monitor the results of diagnostic tests and report abnormal findings.

EQUIPMENT NEEDED

- Cotton balls
- Safety pin
- Tongue depressor
- Tuning fork
- Reflex hammer
- Pencil and paper
- Penlight
- Printed materials
- Substances to test the senses of smell and taste

MEDIALINK

Resources for this chapter can be found on the Prentice Hall Nursing MediaLink DVD-ROM accompanying this textbook, and on the Companion Website at
http://www.prenhall.com/lemone

The nervous system regulates and integrates all body functions, muscle movements, senses, mental abilities, and emotions. It collects information from the internal and external environ-ments as sensory input, processes and interprets the input, and causes responses that are manifested as motor or sensory output.

ANATOMY, PHYSIOLOGY, AND FUNCTIONS OF THE NERVOUS SYSTEM

The nervous system is divided into two regions: the central nervous system (CNS), which consists of the brain and spinal cord, and the peripheral nervous system (PNS), which consists of the cranial nerves, the spinal nerves, and the autonomic nervous system.

Nerve Cells, Action Potentials, and Neurotransmitters

The highly integrated CNS and PNS consist of just two types of cells: neurons, which receive impulses and send them on to other cells, and neuroglia, which protect and nourish the neurons.

Neurons

Each neuron consists of a dendrite, a cell body, and an axon (Figure 43–1 ■). The dendrite is a short process (projection) from the cell body that conducts impulses toward (afferent) the cell body. Cell bodies, most of which are located within the CNS, are clustered in ganglia or nuclei. The cell bodies and dendrites comprise what is often called the gray matter of the CNS. The axon, a long process, conducts impulses away (efferent) from the cell body. Many axons are covered with a myelin sheath, a white lipid substance. It is interrupted at intervals in unmyelinated areas called nodes of Ranvier, which allow movement of ions between the axon and the extracellular fluid. The myelin sheath serves to increase the speed of nerve impulse conduction in axons and is essential for the survival of larger nerve processes. Myelinated nerve fibers comprise the white matter of the brain and spinal cord.

Action Potentials

Action potentials are impulses (movements of electrical charge along an axon membrane) that allow neurons to communicate with other neurons and body cells. They are initiated by stimuli and propagated by the rapid movement of charged ions through the cell membrane. When a neuron reaches a certain level of stimulation, an electrical impulse is generated and conducted along the length of its axon. The movement of impulses to and from the CNS is made possible by afferent and efferent neurons. Afferent, or sensory, neurons have receptors in skin, muscles, and other organs and relay impulses to the CNS. Ef-ferent, or motor, neurons transmit impulses from the CNS to cause some type of action.

Nerve impulses occur when a stimulus reaches a point great enough to generate a change in electrical charge across the cell membrane of a neuron. A neuron that is not involved in impulse conduction is in a resting, or polarized, state, in which the number of positive ions in the fluid outside of the cell membrane is greater than in the fluid within the cell. The chief regulators of membrane potential are sodium and potassium: Sodium is the major positive ion in the extracellular fluid, and potassium is the major positive ion in the intracellular fluid. In response to an electrical stimulus, the cell membrane becomes permeable to sodium, which moves into

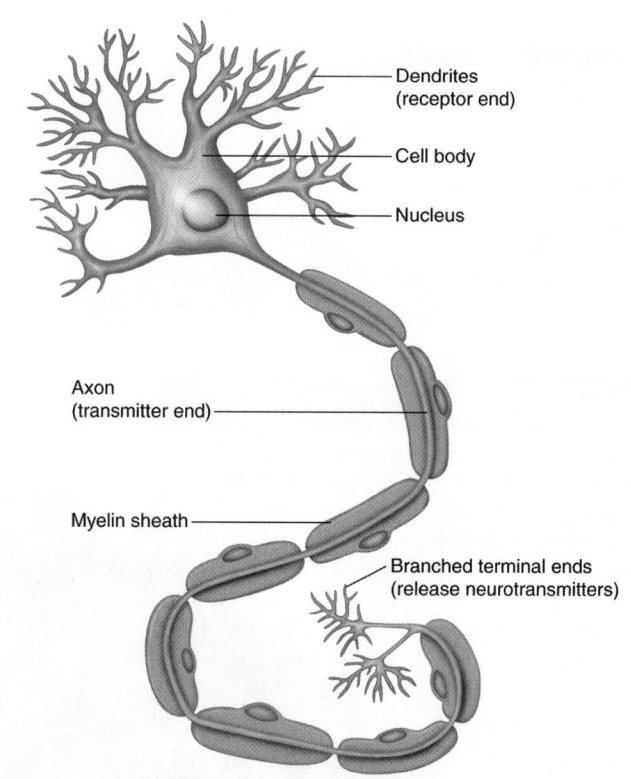

Figure 43–1 ■ A typical neuron.

the cell. This changes the polarity of the cell membrane, and the neuron is said to depolarize. This event stimulates an action potential, or a nerve impulse, to travel down the axon. When the charges and ions return to their original resting state, the neuron is repolarized. The events in an action potential are as follows:

1. Initially, sodium permeability increases. As the membrane is depolarized, sodium channels open and sodium rushes into the cell to a point of depolarization (the inside of the cell becomes less negative in comparison to the outside of the cell).
2. This is followed by a decrease in sodium permeability, lasting only about 1 millisecond. The sodium gates close and the sodium influx stops.
3. The final event is an increase in potassium permeability. The potassium gates open, potassium rushes out of the cell, and the cell interior becomes progressively less positive. The membrane potential moves back to its resting state and is repolarized.

The action potential is generated only at the point of the stimulus; but once generated, it is propagated along the entire length of the axon regardless of whether the stimulus continues. Conduction of the impulse is rapid in myelinated fibers, with the action potential "jumping" from one node of Ranvier to the next. The conduction of the impulse is slower in unmyelinated fibers.

Neurotransmitters

Neurotransmitters are the chemical messengers of the nervous system. When the action potential reaches the end of the axon at the presynaptic terminal, a neurotransmitter is released and travels across the synaptic cleft to bind with receptors in the postsynaptic neuron dendrite or cell body. The neurotransmitter may either be inhibitory or excitatory. The excitatory neurotransmitter is almost always acetylcholine (ACh), which is rapidly degraded by the enzyme acetylcholinesterase. Norepinephrine (NE), which may be either excitatory or inhibitory, is another major neurotransmitter.

Nerves that transmit impulses through the release of ACh are called *cholinergic*. Receptors that bind ACh are found in the viscera, skeletal muscle cells, and the adrenal medulla (where they stimulate the release of epinephrine). The effect of ACh binding may be either to stimulate or to inhibit a response.

Nerves that transmit impulses through the release of NE are called *adrenergic*. Receptors that bind NE are found in the heart, lungs, kidneys, blood vessels, and all target organs stimulated by the sympathetic division except the heart. Adrenergic receptors are further divided into alpha and beta types. Alpha-adrenergic receptors help control such varied functions as arterial vasoconstriction and pupil dilation. Beta-adrenergic fibers may be either beta₁- or beta₂-receptors. Beta₁-receptors are found in the heart, where they regulate the rate and force of contraction. Beta₂-receptors are found in receptor cells of the lungs, arteries, liver, and uterus; they help regulate bronchial diameter, arterial diameter, and glycogenesis. Generally, binding of NE to alpha-receptors stimulates a response, whereas binding to beta-receptors inhibits a response.

Other neurotransmitters include gamma aminobutyric acid (GABA), which inhibits CNS function; dopamine, which may be inhibitory or excitatory and helps control fine movement and emotions; and serotonin, which is usually inhibitory and controls sleep, hunger, and behavior and also affects consciousness.

The Central Nervous System

The central nervous system (CNS) consists of the brain and spinal cord, highly evolved clusters of neurons that act to accept, interconnect, interpret, and generate a response to nerve impulses originating throughout the body.

The Brain

The brain is the control center of the nervous system and also generates thoughts, emotions, and speech. Averaging 3 to 4 lb in weight, the brain is surrounded by the skull, a bony structure that provides support and protection. The brain has four major regions: the cerebrum, the diencephalon, the brainstem, and the cerebellum (Figure 43–2 ■). The general functions of these regions are summarized in Table 43–1.

The two hemispheres of the cerebrum account for almost 60% of brain weight. The surface of the cerebrum is folded into elevated ridges of tissue called gyri, which are separated by shallow grooves called sulci. Deep grooves called fissures further divide the surface of the cerebrum. The longitudinal fissure separates the hemispheres, and the transverse fissure separates the cerebrum from the cerebellum. In addition, each cerebral hemisphere is divided into frontal, parietal, temporal, and occipital lobes (Figure 43–3 ■).

The cerebral hemispheres are connected by a thick band of nerve fibers called the corpus callosum, which allows communication between the two hemispheres. Each hemisphere receives sensory and motor impulses from the opposite side of the body. One of the cerebral hemispheres tends to develop more than the other. Most people have a more highly developed left hemisphere, which is responsible for the control of language. The right hemisphere has greater control over nonverbal perceptual functions.

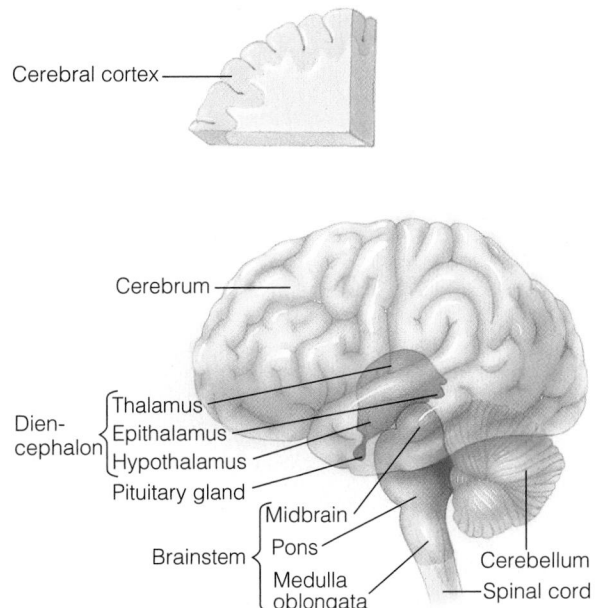

Figure 43–2 ■ The four major regions of the brain.

TABLE 43–1	General Functions of the Four Regions of the Brain
REGION	**FUNCTIONS**
Cerebrum	Interprets sensory input. Controls skeletal muscle activity. Processes intellect and emotions. Contains skills memory.
Diencephalon	Conducts sensory and motor impulses. Regulates autonomic nervous system. Regulates and produces hormones. Mediates emotional responses.
Brainstem	Serves as conduction pathway. Serves as site of decussation of tracts. Contains respiratory nuclei. Helps regulate skeletal muscles.
Cerebellum	Processes information. Provides information necessary for balance, posture, and coordinated muscle movement.

TABLE 43–2	Functions of Lobes of the Cerebrum and Areas of the Cerebral Cortex
AREA	**FUNCTIONS**
Parietal lobe (somatic sensory area of cerebral cortex)	Promotes recognition of pain, coldness, and light touch. The left side receives input from the right side of the body, and vice versa.
Occipital lobe	Receives and interprets visual stimuli.
Temporal lobe	Receives and interprets olfactory and auditory stimuli.
Frontal lobe	Controls movements of voluntary muscles.
Primary motor area	Facilitates voluntary movement of skeletal muscles.
Speech area	Promotes understanding of spoken and written words.
Motor speech area (Broca's area)	Promotes vocalization of words.

The cerebral cortex is the outer surface of the cerebrum. It consists of neuron cell bodies, unmyelinated fibers, neuroglia, and blood vessels. The functions of the different lobes of the cerebrum and the specific areas of the cerebral cortex are shown in Figure 43–3 and listed in Table 43–2.

The diencephalon is embedded in the cerebrum superior to the brainstem. It consists of the thalamus, hypothalamus, and epithalamus (see Figure 43–2). The thalamus begins to process sensory impulses before they ascend to the cerebral cortex. It serves as a sorting, processing, and relay station for input into the cortical region. The hypothalamus, located inferior to the thalamus, regulates temperature, water metabolism, appetite, emotional expressions, part of the sleep–wake cycle, and thirst. The epithalamus forms the dorsal part of the diencephalon and includes the pineal body, which is part of the endocrine system that affects growth and development.

BRAINSTEM The brainstem consists of the midbrain, pons, and medulla oblongata (see Figure 43–2). The midbrain is a center for auditory and visual reflexes. In addition, it functions as a nerve pathway between the cerebral hemispheres and lower brain. The pons is located just below the midbrain. It consists mostly of fiber tracts, but it also contains nuclei that control respiration. The medulla oblongata, located at the base of the brainstem, is continuous with the superior portion of the spinal cord. Nuclei of the medulla oblongata play an important role in controlling cardiac rate, blood pressure, respiration, and swallowing.

The cerebellum is connected to the midbrain, pons, and medulla. Its functions include coordinating skeletal muscle activity, maintaining balance, and controlling fine movements.

VENTRICLES The brain contains four ventricles, which are chambers filled with cerebrospinal fluid (CSF). They are linked by ducts that allow the CSF to circulate. One lateral ventricle is located within each hemisphere. These communicate with the third ventricle through the foramen of Monro. The third ventricle communicates with the fourth ventricle through the cerebral aqueduct that runs through the midbrain. The cerebral aqueduct is continuous with the central canal of the spinal cord.

CEREBROSPINAL FLUID Cerebrospinal fluid, a clear and colorless liquid, is formed by the choroid plexus, which are groups of specialized capillaries located in the brain ventricles. Derived from blood plasma, CSF consists of 99% water and contains protein, sodium, chloride, potassium, bicarbonate, and glucose (see Table 43–3 for normal laboratory values for CSF). The usual amount of CSF ranges from 80 to 200 mL, averaging about 150 mL, and is replaced several times each day. It is absorbed by arachnoid villi. CSF is normally produced and absorbed in equal amounts. CSF circulates from the lateral ventricles of the cerebral hemispheres into the third ventricle, through the midbrain, and into the fourth ventricle. Some CSF flows down the center of the spinal cord as the rest of it circulates into the subarachnoid space and returns to the

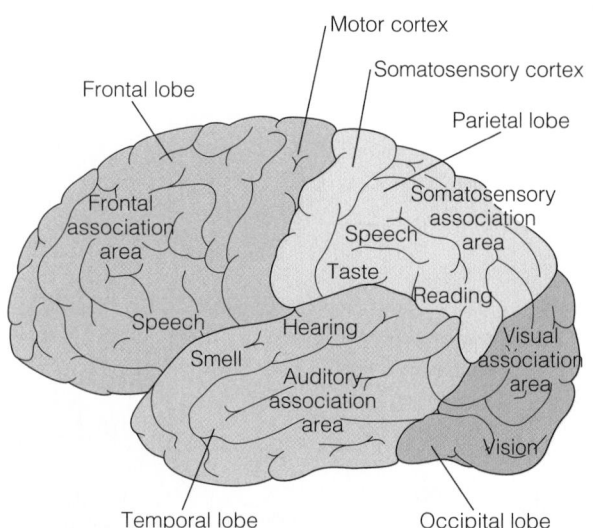

Figure 43–3 ■ Lobes of the cerebrum and functional areas of the cerebral cortex.

TABLE 43–3 Normal Laboratory Values for Cerebrospinal Fluid

COMPONENT	NORMAL VALUE
Appearance	Clear and colorless
pH	7.35
Specific gravity	1.007
WBCs	0–8 mm³
Protein	15–45 mg/dL
Glucose	40–80 mg/dL
Chloride	118–132 mEq/L
Pressure	<200 mmH₂O

blood through the arachnoid villi. CSF forms a cushion for the brain tissue, protects the brain and spinal cord from trauma, helps provide nourishment for the brain, and removes waste products of cerebrospinal cellular metabolism.

Meninges The brain and spinal cord are covered and protected by three connective tissue membranes called meninges. The meninges form divisions within the skull, enclose venous sinuses, and contain CSF. The meninges have three layers (Figure 43–4 ■). The outermost double layer, the dura mater, is attached to the inner surface of the skull. The middle layer is the arachnoid mater, which encloses the entire CNS. It forms the subarachnoid space that contains CSF. The innermost layer, the pia mater, clings to the brain, spinal cord, and segmental nerves and is filled with small blood vessels.

CEREBRAL CIRCULATION AND THE BLOOD–BRAIN BARRIER
The brain receives about 750 mL of blood each minute and uses 20% of the body's total oxygen uptake. The large amount of oxygen is necessary for metabolism of glucose, which is the brain's sole source of energy. Blood flow to the brain is mostly controlled by autoregulatory or local mechanisms that respond

to the brain's metabolic needs. Autoregulation is defined as the ability of the brain to maintain constant cerebral blood flow despite changes in systemic blood pressure. At least three metabolic factors affect cerebral blood flow: carbon dioxide, hydrogen ion, and oxygen concentrations. Of these, increased carbon dioxide is the major stimulus for vasodilatation with resultant increased cerebral blood flow.

The anterior part of the brain is supplied with blood by the two internal carotid arteries, and the posterior part of the brain is supplied with blood by the vertebral arteries. The internal carotid artery branches into further arteries: the ophthalmic, posterior communicating, anterior choroidal, anterior cerebral, and middle cerebral. The brainstem and cerebellum receive their blood supply from the basilar artery. These major arteries are connected by small anterior and posterior communicating arteries, which form a circle of connected blood vessels called the circle of Willis (Figure 43–5 ■). This circle serves as a protective device, providing alternative routes for brain tissues to receive their blood supply.

The capillaries in the brain have low permeability because the cells that compose their walls join at very tight junctions and are surrounded by a basement membrane and by the processes of supporting cells in the brain (called astrocytes). As a result, the brain is protected from many harmful substances in the blood. This blood–brain barrier allows lipids, glucose, some amino acids, water, carbon dioxide, and oxygen to pass through it, thus maintaining a controlled environment. Substances such as urea, creatinine, proteins, some toxins, and most antibiotics cannot pass this barrier and enter brain tissue. However, injury to or infection of the brain may cause increased permeability of the blood–brain barrier, altering concentrations of proteins, water, and electrolytes.

THE LIMBIC SYSTEM AND THE RETICULAR FORMATION The
limbic system and the reticular formation are functional brain systems. These systems, made of networks of neurons, communicate across areas of the brain.

The limbic system consists of structures that form a ring of tissue in the medial side of each hemisphere, surrounding the upper portion of the brainstem and corpus callosum. The limbic system integrates and modulates input to make up the affective part of the brain, providing emotional and behavioral responses to environmental stimuli.

The reticular formation is located through the central core of the medulla oblongata, pons, and midbrain. This system has widespread connections throughout the brain and relays sensory input from all body systems to all levels of the brain. The reticular formation includes the reticular activating system (RAS). The RAS is a stimulating system for the cerebral cortex, keeping it alert and responsive to incoming sensory stimuli while filtering out repetitive or unwanted stimuli. The sleep center inhibits activity of the RAS, and drugs and alcohol may depress it. Other parts of the reticular formation include motor nuclei that help maintain muscle tone and coordinated movements through interconnections with spinal nerves, and the vasomotor and cardiovascular regulatory centers, which are part of autonomic regulation of the cardiovascular system.

Scalp
Periosteum
Skull
Dura mater
Arachnoid mater ⟩ Meninges
Pia mater
Subdural space
Subarachnoid space
Brain

Figure 43–4 ■ Anatomy of the meninges.

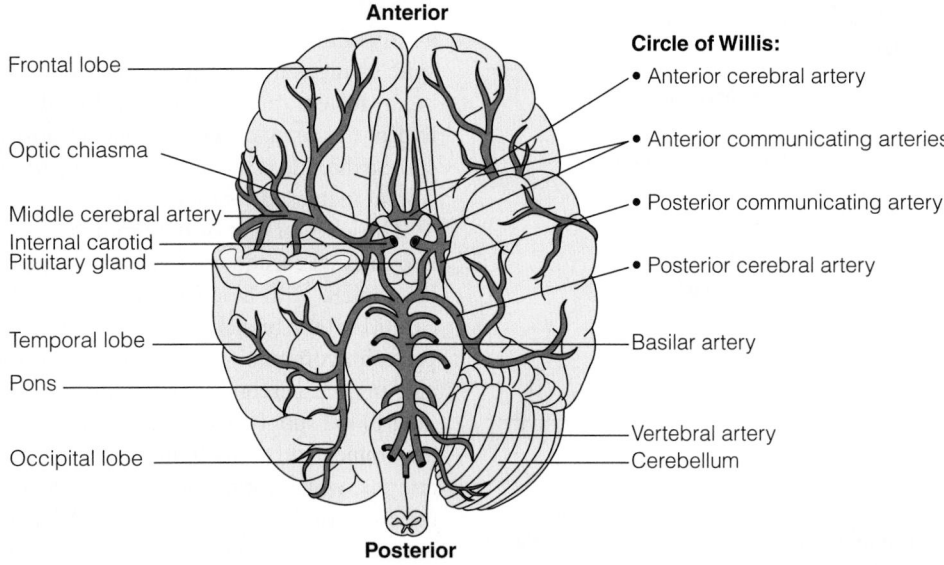

Figure 43–5 ■ Major arteries serving the brain and the circle of Willis.

The Spinal Cord

The spinal cord extends from the medulla to the level of the first lumbar vertebra (Figure 43–6 ■). It serves as a center for conducting messages to and from the brain and as a reflex center. The spinal cord is about 17 inches (42 cm) long and 0.75 inch (1.8 cm) thick. The cord is protected by the vertebrae, the meninges, and CSF. The gray matter of the cord is on the inside, and the white matter is on the outside (the reverse of the arrangement in the brain).

The spinal cord is surrounded and protected by 33 vertebrae: 7 cervical, 12 thoracic, 5 lumbar, 5 sacral, and 4 fused vertebrae, which form the coccyx. Each vertebra consists of a body and a vertebral arch formed by projections from the body. This arch encloses a space called the vertebral foramen. The vertebral foramina of all the vertebrae form the vertebral canal through which the spinal cord passes. Intervertebral foramina are spaces between the vertebrae through which spinal nerve roots pass as they exit the vertebral column.

Intervertebral disks are located between each of the movable vertebrae. Each disk is made of a thick capsule surrounding a gelatinous core called the nucleus pulposus. Ligaments that provide mobility and protection surround the vertebral column, discussed in greater detail in Chapter 45 ∞.

The roots of 31 pairs of spinal nerves, divided into the cervical, thoracic, lumbar, sacral, and coccygeal nerves, arise from the cord (see Figure 43–6). Each separates into posterior (sensory) and anterior (motor) roots. Damage to the posterior roots results in loss of sensation, whereas damage to the anterior root results in flaccid paralysis.

FUNCTIONS OF THE SPINAL CORD AND SPINAL ROOTS

Messages to and from the brain are conducted via ascending (sensory) pathways and descending (motor) pathways (Figure 43–7 ■). The major ascending tracts are the lateral and anterior spinothalamic tracts, which carry sensations for pain, temperature, and crude touch; and the posterior tracts, which carry sensations for fine touch, position, and vibra-

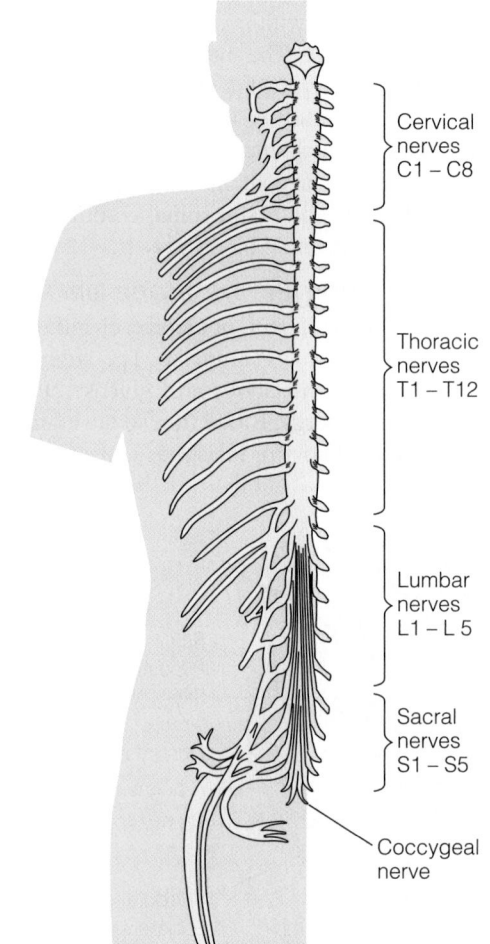

Figure 43–6 ■ Distribution of spinal nerves.

tion. The lateral and anterior corticospinal (pyramidal) tracts are descending tracts consisting of fibers that originate in the motor cortex of the brain and travel to the brainstem and then down the spinal cord. They mediate voluntary purposeful

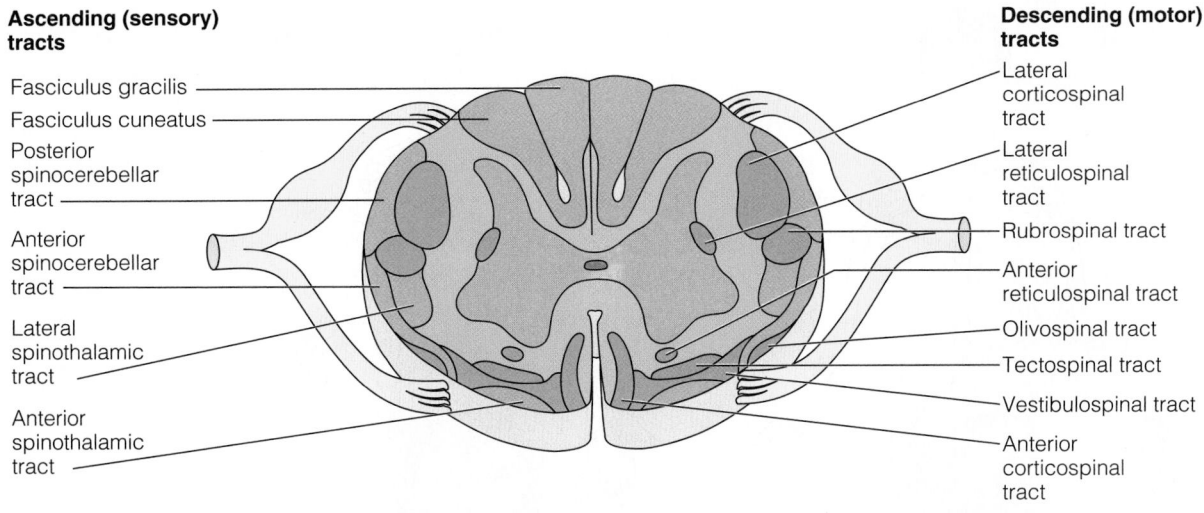

Figure 43–7 ■ Ascending and descending tracts of the spinal cord.

movements and stimulate certain muscular actions while inhibiting others. They also carry fibers that inhibit muscle tone. The rubrospinal, anterior and lateral reticulospinal, and tectospinal (extrapyramidal) tracts include the pathways between the cerebral cortex, basal ganglia, brainstem, and spinal cord outside the pyramidal tract. They maintain muscle tone and gross body movements.

UPPER AND LOWER MOTOR NEURONS Upper motor neurons, such as those of the corticospinal and extrapyramidal tract, carry impulses from the cerebral cortex to the anterior gray column of the spinal cord. Damage to upper motor neurons results in increased muscle tone, decreased muscle strength, decreased coordination, and hyperactive reflexes. Lower motor neurons begin in the anterior gray column of the spinal cord and end in the muscle. Damage to lower motor neurons results in decreased muscle tone, muscle atrophy, fasciculations, and loss of reflexes.

The Peripheral Nervous System

The peripheral nervous system links the CNS with the rest of the body. It is responsible for receiving and transmitting information from and about the external environment. The PNS consists of nerves, ganglia (groups of nerve cells), and sensory receptors located outside—or peripheral to—the brain and spinal cord. The PNS is divided into a sensory (afferent) division and a motor (efferent) division. Most nerves of the PNS contain fibers for both divisions and all are classified regionally as either spinal nerves or cranial nerves.

Spinal Nerves

The 31 pairs of spinal nerves (see Figure 43–6) are named by their location:

- Cervical nerves: 8 pairs
- Thoracic nerves: 12 pairs
- Lumbar nerves: 5 pairs
- Sacral nerves: 5 pairs
- Coccygeal nerves: 1 pair

Spinal nerves exit the vertebral column through intervertebral foramina to travel to the body regions they serve. The spinal cord does not reach the end of the vertebral column; as a result, the lumbar and sacral nerve roots travel inferiorly through the vertebral canal for some distance before exiting the vertebral column through their associated intervertebral foramina. This collection of descending nerve roots is called the cauda equina.

Each spinal nerve contains both sensory and motor fibers. The sensory fibers are located in the dorsal root, and their cell bodies are located within the dorsal root ganglion. The motor fibers are located in the ventral root, and their cell bodies are located within the spinal cord. The dorsal and ventral roots merge outside the vertebral canal just past the dorsal root ganglion, forming a spinal nerve. Each spinal nerve further divides into branches called rami.

The ventral rami of the cervical, brachial, lumbar, and sacral regions form complex clusters of nerves called plexuses. The main spinal nerve plexuses innervate the skin and the underlying muscles of the arms and legs. For example, the cervical plexus innervates the diaphragm through the phrenic nerve; the brachial plexus innervates the upper extremities through the median, ulnar, and radial nerves; and the lumbar plexus innervates the anterior thigh through the femoral nerve.

An area of skin innervated by cutaneous branches of a single spinal nerve is called a dermatome. The dorsal roots of the spinal nerves carry sensations from these specific dermatomes. Dermatomes provide anatomic landmarks that are useful for locating neurologic lesions (Figure 43–8 ■).

Cranial Nerves

Twelve pairs of cranial nerves originate in the forebrain and brainstem (Figure 43–9 ■). The vagus nerve extends into the ventral body cavity, but the 11 other pairs innervate only head and neck regions. Although most are mixed nerves, three pairs (olfactory, optic, and acoustic) are solely sensory. The cranial nerves and their related functions are listed in Table 43–4.

Reflexes

A reflex is a rapid, involuntary, predictable motor response to a stimulus. Reflexes are categorized as either somatic or autonomic.

Figure 43–8 ■ A, Anterior, and B, posterior dermatomes of the body.

Key

☐ Cervical spinal nerves

☐ Thoracic spinal nerves

☐ Lumbar spinal nerves

☐ Sacral spinal nerves

Figure 43–9 ■ Cranial nerves.

TABLE 43–4 **Cranial Nerves**

NAME	FUNCTION
I Olfactory	Sense of smell
II Optic	Vision
III Oculomotor	Eyeball movement Raising of upper eyelid Constriction of pupil Proprioception
IV Trochlear	Eyeball movement
V Trigeminal	Sensation of the upper scalp, upper eyelid, nose, nasal cavity, cornea, and lacrimal gland Sensation of the palate, upper teeth, cheek, top lip, lower eyelid, and scalp Sensation of the tongue, lower teeth, chin, and temporal scalp Chewing
VI Abducens	Lateral movement of the eyeball
VII Facial	Movement of facial muscles Secretions of lacrimal, nasal, submandibular, and sublingual glands Sensation of taste
VIII Acoustic	Sense of equilibrium Sense of hearing
IX Glossopharyngeal	Swallowing Gag reflex Secretions of parotid salivary gland Sense of taste Touch, pressure, and pain from pharynx and posterior tongue Pressure from carotid arteries Receptors to regulate blood pressure
X Vagus	Swallowing Regulation of cardiac rate Regulation of respirations Digestion Sensation from thoracic and abdominal organs Proprioception Sense of taste
XI Accessory	Movement of head and neck Proprioception
XII Hypoglossal	Movement of tongue for speech and swallowing

Figure 43–10 ■ A typical reflex arc of a spinal nerve. In the two-neuron reflex arc, the stimulus is transferred from the sensory neuron directly to the motor neuron at the point of synapse in the spinal cord.

Deep tendon reflexes (DTRs) occur in response to muscle contraction and cause muscle relaxation and lengthening. DTRs depend on intact sensory and motor nerve roots, functional synapses in the spinal cord, a functional neuromuscular junction, and a competent muscle. Thus, an abnormal DTR could indicate a variety of health problems, including a lesion of a spinal nerve. Flexor, or withdrawal, reflexes are caused by actual or perceived painful stimuli and result in withdrawal of the part of the body that is threatened. Superficial responses result from gentle cutaneous stimulation. These responses depend on functional upper motor pathways and on an intact reflex arc.

The Autonomic Nervous System

The autonomic nervous system (ANS) is a division of the PNS that regulates the internal environment of the body. It is also called the general visceral motor system, because it consists of motor neurons that innervate the body's viscera. Whereas skeletal muscle activity and reflexes are regulated by a division of the PNS called the somatic nervous system, the ANS regulates the activity of cardiac muscle, smooth muscle, and glands.

The ANS is primarily controlled by the reticular formation in the brainstem. Stimulation of centers in the medulla initiates reflexes that regulate cardiac rate, blood vessel diameter, and gastrointestinal function.

The ANS has sympathetic and parasympathetic divisions. Although fibers from both divisions affect the same structures, the actions of the two divisions are opposite in effect, and they serve to counterbalance each other. The major neurotransmitters for impulse transmission in the ANS are acetylcholine and norepinephrine. Acetylcholine is the primary neurotransmitter of the parasympathetic division. Norepinephrine is the primary neurotransmitter of the sympathetic division.

Sympathetic Division

The sympathetic division of the ANS prepares the body to handle situations that are perceived as harmful or stressful and to participate in strenuous activity. Cell bodies for this division arise in the lateral horns of the spinal cord in the area from

Somatic reflexes result in skeletal muscle contraction. Autonomic reflexes activate cardiac muscle, smooth muscle, and glands. A reflex occurs over a pathway called a reflex arc.

The essential components of a reflex arc are a receptor, a sensory neuron to carry afferent impulses to the CNS, an integration center in the spinal cord or brain, a motor neuron to carry efferent impulses, and an effector (the tissue that responds by contracting or secreting) (Figure 43–10 ■).

Somatic reflexes mediated by the spinal cord are called *spinal reflexes.* Many spinal reflexes occur without impulses traveling to and from the brain, with the cord serving as the integration center, whereas others require brain activity and modulation.

T1 through L2. The fibers separate after leaving the cord and form a chain of ganglia that extends from the neck to the pelvis. Long fibers then extend to the organs that are supplied by the sympathetic division. Stimulation of the sympathetic division can exert the following effects on target organs or tissues:

- Dilated pupils
- Inhibited secretions
- Copious production of sweat (**diaphoresis**)
- Increased rate and force of heartbeat
- Vasodilation of the coronary arteries
- Dilation of the bronchioles
- Decreased digestion
- Increased release of glucose by the liver
- Decreased urine output
- Vasoconstriction of arteries
- Vasoconstriction of abdominal and skin blood vessels
- Increased blood clotting
- Increased metabolic rate
- Increased mental alertness.

Parasympathetic Division

The parasympathetic division of the ANS operates during non-stressful situations. Cell bodies for this division are located in the brainstem (for the cranial nerves) and in the lateral gray matter of S2 through S4. Other than the fibers supplying the cranial nerves III, VII, IX, and X, the fibers are carried by the vagus nerve to body tissues, thoracic organs, and visceral organs. Stimulation of the parasympathetic division of the ANS produces the following effects:

- Constriction of pupils
- Stimulation of glandular secretions
- Decreased heart rate
- Vasoconstriction of coronary arteries
- Constriction of the bronchioles
- Increased peristalsis and secretion of gastrointestinal fluid.

ASSESSING NEUROLOGIC FUNCTION

Structures and functions of the neurologic system are assessed by findings from diagnostic tests, a health assessment interview to collect subjective data, and a physical assessment to collect objective data. Sample documentation of an assessment of the neurologic system is included in the box on this page.

Diagnostic Tests

The results of diagnostic tests of neurologic structure and function are used to support the diagnosis of a specific injury or disease, to provide information to identify or modify the appropriate medications or therapy used to treat the disease, and to help nurses monitor the client's responses to treatment and nursing care interventions. Diagnostic tests to assess the structures and functions of the neurologic system are described in table beginning on page 1514 and summarized in the following bulleted list. More information is included in the discussion of specific injuries or diseases in Chapters 44, 45, and 46 ∞ .

- Radiologic examinations of the skull and spine include standard x-rays, computed tomography (CT) scans, magnetic resonance imaging (MRI), magnetic resonance angiography (MRA), and

---

SAMPLE DOCUMENTATION
Assessment of the Neurologic System

45-year-old male having annual physical examination. No history of injury or infection involving the head or spine. No history of seizures, dizziness, headaches, memory loss, or problems with speaking, or swallowing. Alert, oriented to person, place, and time. Able to follow directions, explain simple proverbs, and compare unlike objects. Cranial nerve testing results:

I = Identifies scents correctly.

II = Vision 40/20 in both eyes. Has full visual fields bilaterally.

III, IV, VI = Bilateral full extraocular movements, pupils are equally round, react to light and accommodation. No ptosis present in either eye.

V = Able to identify sharp, dull, and light touch to forehead, cheek, and chin. Corneal reflex present bilaterally, but decreased (wears contact lenses).

VII = Able to smile, frown, wrinkle forehead, show teeth, puff out cheek, purse lips, raise eyebrows, and close eyes against resistance.

VIII = Heard whispered words with both ears.

IX, X = Gag reflex present. Swallows without difficulty.

XI = Equal strength when shrugging both shoulders.

XII = Able to protrude tongue midline without tremors.

All extremities have full range of motion without tremors, tics, or weakness. No atrophy of muscles noted. Can perform repetitive alternating movements without difficulty. Gait is steady. Negative Romberg test. All reflexes are 2+ bilaterally. Abdominal reflex present. No Babinski's present.

---

magnetic resonance spectroscopy (MRS). Findings from these examinations are used to diagnose and evaluate fractures, vertebral displacements, tumors, hemorrhage, aneurysms, cysts, edema, ischemia, atrophy, necrosis, seizures, multiple sclerosis, Alzheimer's disease, coma, and vascular lesions.

- Both positron emission tomography (PET) and single-photon emission computed tomography (SPECT) are used to assess brain function and blood flow, to differentiate types of dementia, to evaluate the stage of a brain tumor, and to identify brain tumors, strokes, and seizure disorders.
- Occlusion of the carotid arteries is evaluated by measuring velocity of blood flow with a carotid duplex study; and extracranial blood vessels are evaluated with a transcranial Doppler study.
- Electrical activity of the brain is measured with an electroencephalogram (EEG) to diagnose brain disease and brain death. A magnetoencephalogram (MEG) measures electrical activity of neurons to pinpoint the area of the brain affected by a stroke, brain trauma, brain disorders, or seizures.
- Cerebrospinal fluid, removed through a lumbar puncture (LP), is examined in the laboratory to diagnose a variety of brain diseases and infections.
- A myelogram is used to identify lesions of the spinal cord, such as tumors or herniated intervertebral disks.

Regardless of the type of diagnostic test, the nurse is responsible for explaining the procedure and any special preparation needed, assessing for medication use that may affect the outcome of the tests, supporting the client during the examination as necessary, documenting the procedures as appropriate, and monitoring the results of the tests.

Genetic Considerations

When conducting a health assessment interview and a physical assessment, it is important for the nurse to consider genetic influences on the health of the adult. Several neurologic diseases that directly affect the nervous system have a genetic component; some are due to mutation of a single gene while others have a more complex method of inheritance (National Institutes of Health, 2003). During the health assessment interview,

GENETIC CONSIDERATIONS
Neurologic Disorders

- In all types of spinocerebellar ataxia, there is degeneration of the spinal cord and cerebellum, resulting in loss of muscular coordination and spasticity.
- One recently confirmed risk factor for Parkinson's disease is a positive family history of the disease. This neurodegenerative disease affects more than half a million people, manifested by tremor, muscular stiffness, and difficulty with balance and walking.
- Although multiple sclerosis (MS) is not directly inherited, genetic factors may influence a predisposition to MS within families as well as the severity and course of the disease.
- Narcolepsy, a sleep disorder, does have a familial connection.
- Huntington's disease is an inherited degenerative disorder that leads to dementia. It currently affects approximately 30,000 Americans, with an additional 150,000 at risk for inheriting the disease from their parents.
- Friedreich's ataxia is a rare inherited disease that causes a progressive loss of voluntary muscle coordination and enlargement of the heart.
- Essential tremor, as a primary disorder, affects as many as 3 to 4 million people. In more than half of cases, essential tremor is inherited as an autosomal dominant trait, meaning that children of an individual with the disease have a 50% chance of also developing the disorder.
- Epilepsy is one of the most common neurologic diseases, characterized by abnormal cell firing in the brain that causes recurring seizures. Recent evidence suggests that there may be a genetic predisposition in up to 70% of cases.
- Charcot-Marie-Tooth syndrome is the most common inherited peripheral neuropathy in the world, characterized by a slowly progressive degeneration of the muscles of the foot, lower leg, hand, and forearm.
- Alzheimer's disease (AD) is a leading cause of death in adults, increasing in incidence with age and more common in women. AD tends to run in families, with mutations in 4 genes believed to be responsible for the disease.
- Amyotrophic lateral sclerosis (ALS) is a neurologic disease that causes progressive degeneration of motor neurons in the brain and spinal cord, resulting in paralysis and death. Chromosome abnormalities have been linked to familial ALS.
- Although Tay-Sachs disease is most often considered a disease of children, there is a chronic adult form that causes neuron dysfunction and psychosis.

ask about family members with health problems affecting neurologic structure or function. In addition, ask about a family history of problems with muscular coordination, Parkinson's disease, narcolepsy, tremor, seizures, Alzheimer's disease, or amyotrophic lateral sclerosis (ALS). During the physical assessment, assess for any manifestations that might indicate a genetic disorder (see the box on this page). If data is found to indicate genetic risk factors or alterations, ask about genetic testing and refer for appropriate genetic counseling and evaluation. Chapter 8 ∞ provides further information about genetics in medical-surgical nursing.

Health Assessment Interview

A health assessment to determine problems with neurologic structure and/or function may be conducted during a health screening, may focus on a chief complaint (such as headaches), or may be part of a total health assessment. Health problems affecting the neurologic system may manifest as problems with musculoskeletal function and an assessment of both systems may be necessary. If the client's level of consciousness is altered, the nurse may need to rely on family members for information. The client's level of consciousness may be assessed by using the Glasgow Coma Scale (Table 43–5).

If the client has problems with neurologic structure or function, analyze its onset, characteristics, course, severity, precipitating and relieving factors, and any associated symptoms, noting the time and circumstances. For example, ask the client the following:

- Describe the location and intensity of the pain you have experienced in your left leg. Is it made worse by coughing, sneezing, or walking?
- When did you first notice that you were having numbness in your fingers?
- Describe the difficulty you have when you try to walk.

Questions about present health status include information about numbness, tingling sensations, tremors, problems with

TABLE 43–5 Glasgow Coma Scale

ASSESSMENT	RESPONSE	SCORE*
Eyes open (Record C if eyes are closed by swelling.)	Spontaneously	4
	To speech	3
	To pain	2
	No response	1
Best motor response (Record best upper arm response.)	Obeys commands	6
	Localizes pain	5
	Flexion-withdrawal	4
	Abnormal flexion	3
	Abnormal extension	2
	No response	1
Best verbal response (Record T if an endotracheal or tracheostomy tube is in place.)	Oriented	5
	Confused	4
	Inappropriate words	3
	Incomprehensible sounds	2
	No response	1
Total Score:		___

*A higher score indicates a higher level of functioning.

DIAGNOSTIC TESTS of the Neurologic System

NAME OF TEST X-rays of skull and spine

PURPOSE AND DESCRIPTION Standard x-rays of the skull and spine are done to identify fractures, displacement of vertebrae, spinal curves, and tissue displacement (as by tumors).

RELATED NURSING CARE No special preparation is needed.

NAME OF TEST Computed tomography (CT) scan

PURPOSE AND DESCRIPTION Used to identify intracerebral hemorrhage, tumors, cysts, aneurysms, edema, ischemia, atrophy, and tissue necrosis. May also be used to evaluate a shift in intracranial contents and differentiate type of stroke. Involves computer assisted x-rays of several levels of cross sections of the body part being examined; may be done with or without contrast.

CLIENT PREPARATION

- Ensure a signed consent form.
- Check hospital policy on withholding food and fluids. Clients are usually on NPO status (except for the medications ordered as part of the test) for 8 hours before the test if it is done in the morning. If the test is done in the afternoon, the client may have a liquid breakfast.
- Give medications up to 2 hours before test.
- Assess for possible reaction to iodine dye (by asking about allergy to seafood). Document any allergy and inform the physician and radiology department.
- Remove metal hairpins, clips, and earrings.

HEALTH EDUCATION FOR THE CLIENT AND FAMILY

- (*If applicable*) Do not drink or eat anything before the test except for the ordered medications.
- You may be given an intravenous infusion. When the contrast dye is injected, you may feel warm and have a metallic taste in the mouth.
- The exam lasts from 30 to 90 minutes.
- Your head will be positioned in a cradle, and a wide rubber strap will be applied snugly across the forehead during the test (to keep your head immobilized).
- The CT scanner is circular with a round opening. You are strapped to a special table, and the scanner revolves around the body part to be examined. The scanner makes a clicking noise.
- The test is painless.
- Someone is always immediately available during the test.

NAME OF TEST Magnetic Resonance Imaging (MRI) Functional MRI

PURPOSE AND DESCRIPTION An *MRI* is done to identify and monitor conditions of the brain and spinal cord, including stroke, tumors, trauma, seizures, and multiple sclerosis. Uses magnetic energy to provide images. Gadolinium contrast media may be used to enhance visualization. A *functional MRI* is done to evaluate metabolic or blood flow responses of the brain to specific tasks, such as activity and rest.

RELATED NURSING CARE Assess for metal implants (such as a pacemaker or defibrillator), body piercings, and shrapnel, which would contraindicate tests.

NAME OF TEST Magnetic Resonance Angiography (MRA)

PURPOSE AND DESCRIPTION Can provide information about the blood vessels of the brain and identify vascular lesions. Uses the signals from blood vessels to reconstruct only those vessels with blood flow. Can also be done using contrast media.

RELATED NURSING CARE Assess for metal implants (such as a pacemaker) and shrapnel, which would contraindicate tests.

NAME OF TEST Magnetic Resonance Spectroscopy (MRS)

PURPOSE AND DESCRIPTION Uses a scanner to confirm the presence of Alzheimer's disease, determine the extent of head injury from trauma or stroke, and identify the causes of coma.

RELATED NURSING CARE Assess for metal implants, as for an MRI, which would contraindicate tests.

NAME OF TEST Positron Emission Tomography (PET) Single-Photon Emission Computed Tomography (SPECT)

PURPOSE AND DESCRIPTION When used to study the brain, a *PET* can assess normal brain function and cerebral blood flow and volume; can differentiate different types of dementia; and can identify stages of brain tumors. A substance containing a radionuclide is given by gas or by injection and cross sections of tissue are detected and displayed by computer. A *SPECT* is similar to a PET, but uses different substances. It can be used to diagnose strokes, brain tumors, and seizure disorders.

RELATED NURSING CARE Tell the client not to drink coffee or alcohol or to smoke for 24 hours before the test. Assess glucose levels pretest. Post-test, encourage oral fluids to facilitate excretion of the radioactive substance.

NAME OF TEST Cerebral Angiogram

PURPOSE AND DESCRIPTION The definitive diagnostic procedure for aneurysms, arteriovenous malformations, blood vessel patency and stenosis, thrombosis, vasospasm, aneurysm, and space-occupying lesions (such as tumors or hematomas). May be performed either as part of a surgical procedure or with local anesthesia. In radiology, a contrast medium is injected and films are taken at various time intervals.

RELATED NURSING CARE Obtain informed consent, inform about need to remain NPO for 8 hours prior to the procedure, explain that a burning sensation may be felt for a few (4 to 6) seconds behind the eyes or in the jaw, teeth, tongue, or lips. Bed rest is maintained for 8 hours after the procedure, vital signs are monitored, and fluids are forced to clear the contrast medium.

DIAGNOSTIC TESTS of the Neurologic System (continued)

NAME OF TEST Carotid Duplex Study
Transcranial Doppler Study

PURPOSE AND DESCRIPTION A *carotid duplex study* evaluates the velocity of blood flow through the carotid arteries and identifies occlusive disease. Uses sound waves produced by the blood flow to produce an image. A *transcranial Doppler study* follows the same procedure, but is used to evaluate intracranial blood vessels.

RELATED NURSING CARE No special preparation is needed.

NAME OF TEST Electroencephalogram (EEG)
Magnetoencephalogram (MEG)

PURPOSE AND DESCRIPTION An *EEG* is used to measure the electrical activity of the brain to diagnose brain disease and brain death. Electrodes are applied to the scalp with skin clips and a graphic picture is obtained (similar to an ECG of the heart). A *MEG* can identify the area of the brain affected by a stroke, brain disorders or trauma, or seizures. MEG detects magnetic fields generated by activity of neurons.

CLIENT PREPARATION

- Explain the procedure, emphasizing the importance of cooperation.
- Withhold fluids, foods, and medications (as prescribed) that may stimulate or depress brain waves. These include anticon-vulsants, tranquilizers, depressants, and caffeine-containing foods (e.g., coffee, tea, colas, and chocolate). Medications are usually withheld for 24 to 48 hours before the test.
- Help the client wash the hair before the test.

HEALTH EDUCATION FOR THE CLIENT AND FAMILY

- The test takes about 1 hour.
- The test is painless and will be performed while sitting in a comfortable chair or lying on a stretcher.
- The electrodes are applied to the scalp with a thick paste.
- During the test, you will first be asked to breathe in and out deeply for a few minutes. Then, you will close your eyes while a light is flashed on them and, finally, you will lie quietly with your eyes closed.
- After the test, the nurse will help you wash the paste out of your hair.

NAME OF TEST Evoked Potentials

PURPOSE AND DESCRIPTION Measures nerve conduction along pathways to evaluate evoked potential of muscle contractions. Used to diagnose and evaluate neuromuscular diseases and identify nerve damage. Transcutaneous or percutaneous electrodes are applied to the skin and provide recordings.

RELATED NURSING CARE No special preparation is needed.

NAME OF TEST Electromyogram (EMG)

PURPOSE AND DESCRIPTION Measures the electrical activity of skeletal muscles at rest and during contraction; useful in diagnosing neuromuscular diseases. Needle electrodes are inserted into skeletal muscle (as on the legs) and electrical activity can be heard, viewed on an oscilloscope, and recorded on graph paper. Normally, there is no electrical activity at rest.

RELATED NURSING CARE Tell client not to drink fluids containing caffeine or to smoke for 3 hours before the test, and not to take medications such as muscle relaxants, anticholinergics, and cholinergics.

NAME OF TEST Lumbar Puncture (LP)

PURPOSE AND DESCRIPTION Used to measure CSF pressure and to obtain a sample of CSF to use in diagnosis of multiple sclerosis, or increased intracranial pressure from meningitis, subarachnoid hemorrhage, brain tumor, brain abscess, encephalitis and viral infections. A needle is inserted in L3–L4 or L4–L5 and fluid is aspirated.

RELATED NURSING CARE Related nursing care for the client having a lumbar puncture is described below.

CLIENT PREPARATION

- Ensure a signed consent form (this consent may be obtained as part of the general consent given on admission to the hospital or agency).
- Ask the client to empty the bladder before the procedure begins.
- Help the client to assume a lateral recumbent position near the side of the bed. The client should assume the fetal position (knees flexed toward the head, head bent toward the chest), with the hands clasped around the knees.

CLIENT AND FAMILY TEACHING

- A local anesthetic is injected into the skin over the area of the needle insertion. This medication may cause a burning sensation.
- A long, thin needle is inserted into the lower back below the level of the spinal cord. Cerebrospinal fluid is withdrawn.
- The cerebrospinal fluid pressure is measured with a calibrated tube called a manometer.
- There may be slight pain down one leg during the procedure.
- It is important to remain still during the procedure.
- A small dressing is used to cover the place where the needle was inserted.
- After the procedure, remain flat in bed for the number of hours prescribed by the physician (this ranges from 4 to 24 hours). The nurses will take your vital signs and look under the small dressing at regular intervals.
- Drink fluids so that your body can replace the fluid that was withdrawn.
- If you have a headache or backache, take medications for pain.
- Notify your healthcare provider if you notice increased pain or drainage from the area where the procedure was done.

(continued)

DIAGNOSTIC TESTS of the Neurologic System (continued)

POSTPROCEDURE NURSING CARE (LP)

- Take and record vital signs as indicated by agency standards.
- Monitor neurologic status at least every 4 hours for 24 hours.
- Monitor the puncture site for leakage of cerebrospinal fluid or hematoma formation.

NAME OF TEST Myelogram

PURPOSE AND DESCRIPTION Used to identify lesions of the spinal cord, such as tumors or herniated intervertebral disk. A lumbar puncture is done, a contrast medium is injected into the subarachnoid space, and x-rays are taken.

CLIENT PREPARATION

- Ensure a signed informed consent.
- The meal prior to the procedure is usually omitted.
- The client should be well hydrated.
- Administer enemas or laxatives as ordered to ensure visualization of lumbar spine.
- Administer prescribed pretest medications, such as a sedative or diazepam (Valium).

HEALTH EDUCATION FOR THE CLIENT AND FAMILY

- Remain NPO several hours before the test.
- The examination lasts about 1 hour.
- The position used to perform the examination will depend on the physician. You may have to lie on your stomach, sit and lean forward, or sit with the knees to the chest.
- A strap may be used to prevent falls, and the table will be tilted during the examination.
- A lumbar puncture ("spinal tap") is performed to inject the dye. A local anesthetic is used where the needle will be inserted. There may be a feeling of pressure during needle insertion. The needle is inserted below the level of the spinal cord.
- Tell the physician if you experience pain.
- Stay in bed with the head of the bed elevated for at least 6 to 12 hours (the length of time will depend on physician preference and hospital policy).

- Ensure that the client voids within 8 hours of the procedure.
- Encourage increased intake of fluids (up to 3000 mL in 24 hours).
- Administer analgesics as prescribed for pain.

- The nurse will check your blood pressure, pulse, and respirations. The nurse will also check your ability to feel and move at least every 4 hours (or more often) after the examination.

POSTPROCEDURE NURSING CARE

- Take and record vital signs and assess neurologic status as prescribed (and at least every 4 hours) for 24 hours postexamination. Record and report any changes.
- Assess the site of the lumbar puncture for leakage of cerebrospinal fluid or bleeding every 4 hours. Notify the physician of leakage or bleeding.
- Encourage increased intake of oral fluids to replace that withdrawn during the examination. (This may also help decrease a postmyelogram headache.)
- Make sure that the client voids within 8 hours after the examination. If policy permits, allow male clients to stand at the beside, or clients of either gender to use the bathroom. Notify the physician if the client has not voided within 8 hours.
- Administer analgesics as prescribed for postexamination pain, headache, or muscle spasms.
- Keep the client's head elevated at least 30 degrees (in bed or in a chair) for 12 hours, or as ordered.
- Resume diet if there is no nausea or vomiting.
- Force oral fluids to 2400 to 3000 mL in 24 hours, beginning immediately after the procedure.
- Administer prescribed medications for nausea.
- Do not give any phenothiazine derivatives for 48 hours (to reduce the possibility of seizures).

---

coordination or balance, or loss of movement in any part of the body. Ask the client about difficulty with speaking, seeing, hearing, tasting, or detecting odors. In addition, elicit information about memory, feeling state (such as anxiety or depression), recent changes in sleep patterns, ability to perform self-care and activities of daily living, sexual activity, and weight. If the client is taking prescribed medications, over-the-counter medications, or herbal supplements, ask about the type and purpose, as well as the frequency and duration of use.

Ask about any past history of seizures, fainting, dizziness, headaches, and any trauma, tumors, or surgery of the brain, spinal cord, or nerves. Discuss illnesses that may cause neurologic manifestations, including cardiac disease, strokes, pernicious anemia, sinus infections, liver disease, and/or renal failure. Also ask the client about family history of neurologic health problems, diabetes mellitus, hypertension, seizures, or mental health problems.

Question the client about occupational hazards, such as exposure to toxic chemicals or materials, use of protective head-

gear, and the amount of time spent performing repetitive motions (e.g., data entry and assembly). Ask questions about self-care to assess the client's diet and use of tobacco, drugs, or alcohol, and ask whether the client wears a helmet when riding a bike or motorcycle or participating in contact sports or uses seat belts when driving a vehicle.

Interview questions categorized by functional health patterns are listed in the Functional Health Pattern Interview table on the following page.

Physical Assessment

Physical assessment of the client begins when the nurse first meets the client and makes an overall evaluation of the client's mental and physical status. The mental status examination is conducted with both the nurse and the client seated. The rest of the neurologic examination may be performed with the client either sitting or standing. A thorough neurologic examination is discussed here, but in most instances,

FUNCTIONAL HEALTH PATTERN INTERVIEW Neurologic System

Functional Health Pattern	Interview Questions and Leading Statements
Health Perception-Health Management	■ Have you ever had a surgery, injury, or illness of the neurologic system, such as seizures, stroke, tumor, meningitis? If so, describe the problem and how it was treated. ■ Do you have high blood pressure? If so, how is it treated? ■ Have you ever had problems with the ability to move body parts? Describe. ■ Would you say you think clearly? If not, how and when did the change occur? ■ Are you having any problems with the ability to see, hear, taste, or smell? Explain. ■ Have you ever had any diagnostic tests for a neurologic problem, such as an MRI or spinal tap? If so, what were the results? ■ Do you take medications for seizures, headaches, or other neurologic problems? If so, what are they and how often do you take them? ■ Do you now or have you ever smoked, used street drugs, or drank alcohol? If so, what type, how much, and for how long? ■ Where were you born and raised as a child?
Nutritional-Metabolic	■ Describe your usual food and fluid intake for a 24-hour period. ■ Have you noticed any problems with chewing or swallowing your food? ■ Do you have trouble with coughing when you eat or drink?
Elimination	■ Has there been any change in your urinary or bowel elimination? If so, describe the change. ■ Do you use laxatives, suppositories, or enemas to assist with bowel elimination? If so, what type and how often? ■ Are you able to go to the bathroom without assistance? If not, describe your usual routine.
Activity-Exercise	■ Describe your usual activities in a 24-hour period. ■ Do you have any problems with balance, coordination, or walking? Do you use any assistive device when you walk, such as a cane or walker? ■ Have you noticed any weakness in your arms or legs? If so, describe. ■ Are you able to move all of your body parts? If not, explain. ■ Do you trip or fall easily? ■ Have you experienced any shakiness or tremors? Where? ■ If you have seizures, what type do you have? Can you tell when they are going to happen? Does anything specific make you have a seizure? How do you feel after the seizure is over?
Sleep-Rest	■ Does this health problem interfere with your ability to sleep and rest? If so, how? ■ Do you take any medication to help you sleep? If so, what? ■ Describe your energy level. Do rest and sleep restore your energy?
Cognitive-Perceptual	■ Describe any headaches you experience, including frequency, type, location, and precipitating/relieving factors. ■ Do you ever feel dizzy or have you fainted? Do you ever feel the room is spinning? Explain. ■ Do you ever experience any numbness, burning, or tingling sensations? If so, where and when? ■ Do you have any visual problems, such as double vision, blurring, or blind spots? ■ Do you have any problems with hearing? Explain. ■ Has there been any change in your ability to taste or smell? If so, explain. ■ Do you have any difficulty remembering things? If so, describe what you do.
Self-Perception-Self-Concept	■ How does having this condition make you feel about yourself?
Role-Relationships	■ How has having this condition affected your relationships with others? ■ Has having this condition interfered with your ability to work? Explain. ■ Has anyone in your family had problems with neurologic disease? Explain.
Sexuality-Reproductive	■ Has this condition interfered with your usual sexual activity?
Coping-Stress-Tolerance	■ Has having this condition created stress for you? If so, does your health problem seem to be more difficult when you are stressed? ■ Have you experienced any kind of stress that makes the condition worse? Explain. ■ Describe what you do when you feel stressed.
Value-Belief	■ Describe how specific relationships or activities help you cope with this problem. ■ Describe specific cultural beliefs or practices that affect how you care for and feel about this problem. ■ Are there any specific treatments that you would not use to treat this problem?

the nurse will conduct a focused assessment specific to the client's health status.

The neurologic system is assessed through inspection, palpation, and percussion (with a reflex hammer). When conducting the mental status and cognitive portions of the examination, be aware that fatigue or illness may alter findings. Provide rest periods for the client as needed. When interpreting findings, consider the client's age, educational background, and cultural orientation. Normal age-related findings for the older adult are summarized in Table 43–6.

The assessment should take place in a private, comfortable setting. Ask the client to remove outer clothing, shoes, and stockings. Provide a gown for the client to wear. It is important to explain that the neurologic examination is lengthy and may consist of questions and requests that seem strange to the client. Explain the rationale for each part of the examination.

A brief version of this physical assessment, often referred to as a *neuro check,* may be performed in a shorter time period when a client requires frequent ongoing assessments of neurologic status (Box 43–1).

BOX 43–1 Abbreviated Neurologic Assessment (Neuro Check)

1. Assess level of consciousness (response to auditory and/or tactile stimulus).
2. Obtain vital signs (BP, P, R).
3. Check pupillary response to light.
4. Assess strength of hand grip and movement of extremities bilaterally.
5. Determine ability to sense touch/pain in extremities.

TABLE 43–6 Age-Related Changes in the Neurologic System

AGE-RELATED CHANGE	SIGNIFICANCE
■ ↓ number of brain cells, cerebral blood flow, and metabolism. ■ Slower nerve conduction velocity. ■ Slower retrieval of information from long-term memory.	Delayed response to multiple stimuli and slower reflexes; may need additional time to process and respond to verbal stimuli. There is some age-related forgetfulness, which can be improved by using memory aids such as making lists.
■ Slower response to changes in balance. ■ May exhibit less readiness to learn and depend on prior experiences to solve problems. ■ Is more easily distracted and has a decrease in the ability to maintain attention.	May contribute to increased risk for falls. Learning new skills or knowledge is improved when they are related to previously learned information and when limits are set on times for learning (for example, no more than 30 minutes at one time).

NEUROLOGIC ASSESSMENTS

Technique/Normal Findings	**Abnormal Findings**

Mental Status Assessment

Assess appearance, including dress, hygiene, grooming, gait, and posture. *The client should be appropriately dressed and clean, with normal gait and posture.*

- Unilateral neglect (inattention to one side of body) may occur with some strokes. Poor hygiene and grooming may be seen in clients with dementing disorders.
- Abnormal gait and posture may be seen in transient ischemic attacks (TIAs), strokes, and Parkinson's disease.

Assess behavior, including actions and affect, content and quality of speech, and level of consciousness (LOC). Use the Glasgow Coma Scale (see Table 43–5) to document findings. *A score of 15 on the Glasgow Coma Scale indicates the client is alert and oriented.*

- Emotional swings or changes in personality may be observed in clients who have had a stroke.
- The face appears masklike (very little expressive movement of facial muscles) in clients with Parkinson's disease.
- Apathy is seen in dementing disorders.
- **Aphasia** (defective or absent language function) may occur in TIAs and strokes. Aphasias are seen with damage to the left cerebral cortex. Aphasias are more often seen with strokes of the left hemisphere than the right hemisphere.
- **Dysphonia** (change in the tone of the voice) is common in strokes. Dysphonia is seen with paralysis of the vocal cords (cranial nerve X).
- **Dysarthria** (difficulty speaking) is seen with lesions of upper and lower motor neurons, the cerebellum, and the extrapyramidal tract.
- Damage to the brainstem and/or cerebral cortex may alter LOC.
- Drowsiness and decreased LOC may be associated with brain trauma, infections, TIAs, stroke, and brain tumors.
- Level of consciousness, ranging from confusion to coma, is usually altered with a stroke.

Technique/Normal Findings	Abnormal Findings
Assess cognitive function. Note orientation to time, place, and person. Note attention span and recent and remote memory. Ask the client to: 1. Repeat five to seven numbers. 2. Recall three items after 5 minutes. 3. Recall his or her address, breakfast, or birthday. Assess thought processes (both content and perceptions) by noting responses to questions. Note ability to understand what is said and to express thoughts. Note ability to make logical and safe judgments. *The client should be oriented to time, place, and person; demonstrate attention and ability to remember recent and past events; respond appropriately to questions; and be able to make judgments.*	■ Disorientation to time and place may occur in clients with stroke of the right cerebral hemisphere. ■ Memory deficits are often seen in clients with a stroke. ■ Perceptual deficits may be seen in strokes. These same deficits may occur following brain trauma and in dementing disorders. ■ Impaired cognition is often noted with strokes, cerebral trauma, and brain tumors.

Cranial Nerve Assessments

Test CN I (olfactory). Note client's ability to smell scents (e.g., soap, coffee) with each nostril. This test is usually done only if a problem with the ability to smell is reported. *Sense of smell should be equal in both nostrils.*	■ **Anosmia** (an inability to smell) may be seen with lesions of the frontal lobe and may also occur with impaired blood flow to the middle cerebral artery.
Test CN II (optic). Assess vision in each eye with Snellen chart (see Chapter 47 ∞ for guidelines). *Based on previous ability to see and use of visual aids, client should be able to see with both eyes.*	■ Blindness in one eye may be seen with strokes or with TIAs. Impaired vision or blindness in one side of both eyes (homonymous hemianopia) is associated with stroke. ■ Impaired vision may be seen with strokes and brain tumors. ■ Blindness or double vision may be noted with stroke and TIAs.
Test CN III, IV, and VI (oculomotor, trochlear, and abducens). Assess extraocular movements by asking the client to follow your finger as you write an *H* in the air (see Chapter 47 ∞). Assess PERRL ("pupils equally round and reactive to light") by covering one eye at a time and shining a bright light directly into the uncovered eye (use a penlight or the ophthalmoscope). See Chapter 47 ∞ for more detailed assessment guidelines. *Extraocular movements should be present bilaterally, and pupils should be equally round and reactive to light.*	■ **Nystagmus** (involuntary eye movement) may be seen with strokes. ■ Constricted pupils are associated with impaired blood flow from a stroke.

Technique/Normal Findings	Abnormal Findings
Assess for **ptosis** (drooping eyelids). *Eyelids should not droop.*	▪ Ptosis (also called Horner syndrome) occurs with strokes, myasthenia gravis, and palsy of CN III.
Test CN V (trigeminal). Assess ability to feel light, dull, and sharp sensations on the face. With the client's eyes closed, check whether sensation is the same on both sides of the face. Stroke the cheek with a wisp of cotton for light touch, with a closed safety pin for dull touch, and with a tongue depressor for sharp touch. If the sharp point of a safety pin is used to assess sharp touch, be sure to avoid scratching the surface of the skin, and discard the pin after it is used. Assess the corneal reflex by touching the corneal surface with a wisp of cotton. The reflex may be absent or decreased in clients who wear contact lenses. *Ability to feel light, dull, and sharp sensations should be intact. Normally the client blinks.*	▪ Changes in facial sensations are noted with impaired blood flow to the carotid artery. ▪ Decreased sensations to the face and cornea on the same side of the body, as well as numbness of the lip and mouth, occur with strokes. ▪ Loss of facial sensation or contraction of the masseter and temporal muscles is seen with lesions of CN V. ▪ Severe facial pain is seen with trigeminal neuralgia (tic douloureux). ▪ The corneal reflex may be impaired with lesions of CN V or VII.
Test CN VII (facial). Assess ability to taste sweet, sour, and salt on the anterior two-thirds of the tongue by asking the client to stick out the tongue and applying a salty, sweet, or sour substance. Assess ability to frown, show teeth, blow out cheeks, raise eyebrows, smile, and close eyes tightly. *Ability to taste sweet, sour, and salt is intact. Should be able to frown, show teeth, blow out cheeks, raise eyebrows, smile, and close eyes tightly. Muscle movement should be equal bilaterally.*	▪ Loss of ability to taste may occur with brain tumors or with nerve impairment. ▪ Asymmetry or decreased movement of facial muscles is noted with lesions of the upper and lower motor neurons. ▪ Paralysis of the lower motor neurons from injury to CN VII results in the inability to close eyes, a flat nasolabial fold, paralysis of lower face, and inability to wrinkle forehead. ▪ Paralysis of the upper motor neurons from a stroke results in weakness of eyelids and paralysis of lower face. ▪ Pain, paralysis, and sagging of facial muscles is seen on the affected side in Bell's palsy.
Test CN VIII (acoustic). Assess ability to hear the ticking of a watch and whispered and spoken words (see Chapter 47 ∞). *Client should be able to hear with both ears.*	▪ Decreased hearing or deafness may occur with strokes and/or tumors of CN VIII.
Test CN IX and X (glossopharyngeal and vagus). If gag reflex is intact, observe client swallowing a small drink of water. Observe for a symmetrical rise of the soft palate and uvula as the client says "ah."	▪ **Dysphagia** (difficulty swallowing) is common with impaired blood flow to the brain. ▪ Unilateral loss of the gag reflex occurs with lesions of CN IX and X.

Technique/Normal Findings	Abnormal Findings
Assess gag reflex by touching back of client's throat with tongue depressor. Assess ability to taste salty, sweet, and sour substances on the posterior third of the tongue (see previous description). *Client should be able to swallow without difficulty, have symmetrical rise of the soft palate, have intact gag reflex, and taste appropriately.*	
Test CN XI (spinal accessory). Assess the client's ability to shrug the shoulders and turn head against resistance: Ask the client to turn the head to one side against the resistance of your hand; ask the client to shrug the shoulders while you exert downward pressure. Observe symmetry, strength, and size of muscles. *Client should be able to shrug shoulders and turn head against resistance.*	■ Muscle weakness is noted with lower motor neuron disease. Contralateral hemiparesis is seen with strokes.
Test CN XII (hypoglossal). Assess the client's ability to stick out the tongue and move the tongue from side to side against resistance of a tongue depressor. *Client should be able to stick out tongue, and move it from side to side against resistance.*	■ Atrophy and **fasciculations** (twitches) of the tongue are seen in lower motor neuron disease. The tongue may deviate toward involved side of the body.

Sensory Function Assessments Findings

Assess ability to perceive various sensations. Touch both sides of various parts of the body (the chest, abdomen, arms, and legs) with one or more of the following: ■ Cotton wisp ■ Sharp object ■ Dull object ■ Vibrating tuning fork placed on bony prominences. *Client can differentiate between soft and sharp, and can feel vibrations appropriately.*	■ Decreased sensation of pain occurs with injury to the spinothalamic tract. ■ Decreased vibratory sensations are seen with injuries to the posterior column tract. ■ Transient numbness of face, arm, or hand is seen with TIAs. ■ Sensory loss on one side of the body is seen with lesions of higher pathways to the spinal cord. ■ Bilateral sensory loss is seen in polyneuropathy (a disease in which multiple peripheral nerves are affected, such as Guillain-Barré syndrome or diabetes mellitus). Sensations are impaired with strokes, brain tumors, and spinal cord trauma or compression.
Assess sense of position (**kinesthesia**). Move the client's finger or big toe up or down. Ask the client to describe the movement. *Client can accurately describe position of finger or toe when moved up or down.*	■ Lesions of the posterior column of the spinal cord may affect sense of position.

Technique/Normal Findings	**Abnormal Findings**

Assess ability to discriminate fine touch.
Ask the client to identify:
1. Object in hand, such as a coin or key (tests stereognosis).
2. Number written on hand (tests graphesthesia) (Figure 43–11 ■).
3. Two points of simultaneous pinpricks on the hand (tests two-point discrimination) (Figure 43–12 ■).
4. Where he or she is being touched (tests localization).
5. How many sensations are felt when touched simultaneously on both sides of the body (tests extinction). *Client can identify and discriminate fine touch.*

- Inability to discriminate fine touch (stereognosis, graphesthesia, two points, point localization, and extinction) may occur with injury to the posterior columns or sensory cortex.

Figure 43–11 ■ Testing graphesthesia.

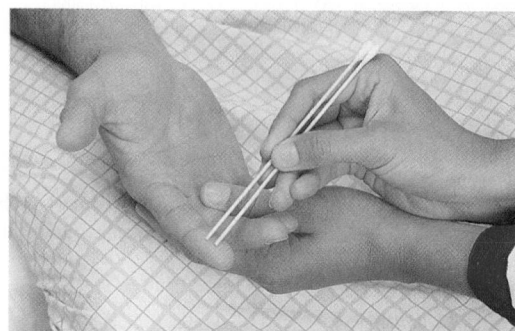

Figure 43–12 ■ Testing two-point discrimination.

Motor Function Assessments

Assess bilateral symmetry and size of muscles.
Assess for **tremors** (rhythmic movements) and fasciculations (irregular movements). Observe movements as client is at rest (not making a purposeful movement) and with activity (making a purposeful movement, such as reaching for a glass of water). *Muscles are bilaterally symmetrical and of equal size. Tremors or fasciculations are not present.*

- Atrophy of muscles is seen with disease of the lower motor neurons.
- Tremors that occur with activity are seen in multiple sclerosis and diseases of the cerebellar system.
- Tremors that occur at rest and disappear with movement are common in Parkinson's disease.
- Fasciculations occur in disease or trauma to the lower motor neurons, as a side effect of medications, in fever, in sodium deficiency, and in uremia.

Assess muscle tone. *Muscle tone is appropriate.*

- Muscle tone is decreased (**flaccidity**) in disease or trauma of the lower motor neurons and early stroke.
- Muscle tone is increased (**spasticity**) in disease of the corticospinal motor tract.
- Muscles are rigid in disease of the extrapyramidal motor tract.
- Muscles move in small, regular jerky movements (cogwheel rigidity) in Parkinson's disease.

Assess bilateral muscle strength and movement.
Ask the client to:
1. Squeeze your hands.
2. Push feet against the resistance of your hands.
3. Raise both legs off the bed.
See Chapter 40 ∞ for a scale to grade muscle strength. Muscle strength and movement are bilaterally equal and strong.

- Weakness of the arms, legs, or hands is often seen with TIAs.
- Hemiplegia (paralysis of one-half of the body vertically) is noted with strokes.
- Flaccid paralysis is noted with strokes.
- Paralysis or decreased movement is seen in multiple sclerosis and myasthenia gravis.
- There is total loss of motor function below the level of injury in complete spinal cord transection and in injuries to the anterior portion of the spinal cord.
- Spasticity of muscles may occur as a result of incomplete spinal cord injuries.

Cerebellar Function Assessments

Assess the gait. Ask the client to walk normally, then in a heel-to-toe fashion, then on toes, and finally on heels.

- **Ataxia** is a lack of coordination and a clumsiness of movements, with staggering, wide-based, and unbalanced gait. Ataxia is often seen with strokes and cerebellar tumors. Swaying and falling are seen in cerebellar ataxia. Inability to walk on toes, then heels, may indicate disease of the upper motor neurons.

Technique/Normal Findings	Abnormal Findings

Client has appropriate gait, and can walk heel-to-toe, on toes, and on heels.

Perform Romberg's test: Ask the client to stand with the feet together and eyes closed. (Stand close to client to prevent falling). *There should be minimal swaying for up to 20 seconds.*

- Spastic hemiparesis is often associated with strokes or upper motor neuron disease. The client walks with one leg stiffly dragging while the other leg circles out and forward. One arm is held flexed and close to the side.
- Steppage gait is noted with disease of the lower motor neurons. The client drags or lifts the foot high, then slaps the foot onto the floor. The client cannot walk on the heels.
- Sensory ataxia may be associated with polyneuropathy or damage to the posterior columns. The client walks on the heels before bringing down the toes and the feet are held wide apart. Gait worsens with the eyes closed.
- Parkinsonian gait is often seen in Parkinson's disease. The client stoops over while walking and shuffles the feet. The arms are held close to the side.
- A positive Romberg's test may be seen in cerebellar ataxia.

Assess coordination.
Observe ability to pat knees, alternating front and back of hands and increasing speed. Observe ability to touch each finger of one hand to the thumb. Observe ability to touch the nose, then one of your fingers, then the nose again. Observe ability to run each heel down each shin, while in a supine position (Figure 43–13 ■). *Client demonstrates coordinated movements.*

- Ataxic movements are apparent in cerebellar disease.

Figure 43–13 ■ Heel-to-shin test.

REFLEX ASSESSMENTS

A reflex hammer is used to strike the tendon of various reflex sites. To test deep tendon reflexes, ask the client to lock the fingers of both hands together and then pull; this encourages relaxation and promotes reflexes of lower extremities. Superficial reflexes are assessed by lightly stroking the area with the end of a tongue depressor. The following criteria for recording reflexes are often used:

0 = absent or no response
1 = hypoactive; weaker than normal (+)
2 = normal (++)
3 = stronger than normal (+++)
4 = hyperactive, sustained clonus (++++)
A score of 2 is considered normal.

Technique/Normal Findings	Abnormal Findings

Assess the patellar, biceps, brachioradialis, triceps, and Achilles deep tendon reflexes (Figure 43–14 ■).

- Hyperactive reflexes are present with lesions of upper motor neurons.
- Decreased reflexes are present with lower motor neuron involvement.

Assess for clonus by dorsiflexing the client's foot.

- Clonus, a hyperactive, rhythmic dorsiflexion and plantar flexion, is noted with upper motor neuron disease.

A   **B**   **C**   **D**   **E**

Figure 43–14 ■ Deep tendon reflexes. *A,* Using reinforcement technique to test the patellar reflex. *B,* Biceps reflex. *C,* Brachioradialis reflex. *D,* Triceps reflex. *E,* Achilles reflex.

MediaLink

Testing Reflexes Video

Technique/Normal Findings	Abnormal Findings

Assess the superficial abdominal and cremasteric reflexes.
Abdominal reflex: Lightly stroke the abdomen with a tongue depressor from the side to the midline. Normally the side of the abdomen being stroked will contract toward the umbilicus (Figure 43–15 ■).
Cremasteric reflex: Lightly stroke the inner thigh of the male client with a tongue depressor. Normally, the testicle on the side being stroked will rise.

- Superficial reflexes may be absent with disease of the lower and upper motor neurons.

Figure 43–15 ■ Location of superficial abdominal reflexes.

Assess the Babinski reflex (Figure 43–16 ■).

- Dorsiflexion of the big toe and fanning of the other toes is seen with upper motor neuron disease of the pyramidal tract.

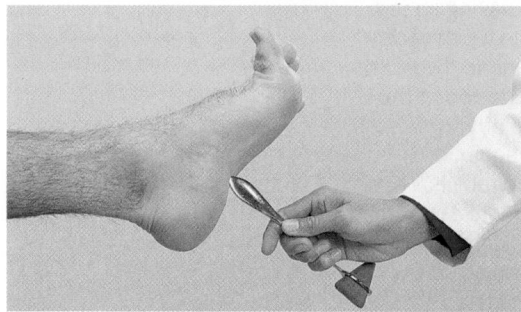

Figure 43–16 ■ Assessing the Babinski reflex.

Special Neurologic Assessments

Assess for Brudzinski's sign. With the client supine, flex the head to the chest (Figure 43–17 ■). *There should be no pain, resistance, or flexion of the hips or knees.*
Assess for Kernig's sign. With the client supine, flex the knees and hips, then straighten the knee (Figure 43–18 ■). *There should be no pain or resistance.*

- Pain, resistance, and flexion of hips and knees occur with meningeal irritation.
- Excessive pain and/or resistance occurs with meningeal irritation.

Figure 43–17 ■ Assessing Brudzinski's sign.

Figure 43–18 ■ Assessing Kernig's sign.

Technique/Normal Findings	Abnormal Findings
Assess for abnormal postures in clients who are unconscious. *There should be no abnormal posturing.*	Observe for **decorticate posturing**, in which the upper arms are close to the sides; the elbows, wrists, and fingers are flexed; the legs are extended with internal rotation; and the feet are plantar flexed (Figure 43–19 ■). Observe for **decerebrate posturing**, in which the neck is extended, with the jaw clenched; the arms are pronated, extended, and close to the sides; the legs are extended straight out; and the feet are plantar flexed (Figure 43–20 ■). ■ Decorticate posturing occurs with lesions of the corticospinal tracts. ■ Decerebrate posturing occurs with lesions of the midbrain, pons, or diencephalon.

Figure 43–19 ■ Decorticate posturing.

Figure 43–20 ■ Decerebrate posturing.

EXPLORE MEDIALINK

Prentice Hall Nursing MediaLink DVD-ROM
Audio Glossary
NCLEX-RN® Review

Animation/Video
Testing Reflexes

COMPANION WEBSITE www.prenhall.com/lemone
Audio Glossary
NCLEX-RN® Review
Care Plan Activity: Neurologic Disorders
Case Study: Assessing an Unconscious Client
MediaLink Application: NIH Stroke Scale
Links to Resources

TEST YOURSELF NCLEX-RN® REVIEW

1 What component of the brain protects it from harmful substances?
1. the circulation of cerebrospinal fluid
2. the large oxygen demand
3. the structure of neurons
4. the blood-brain barrier

2 What pathophysiology results from damage to the lower motor neurons?
1. loss of cognitive ability
2. inability to communicate verbally
3. loss of reflexes
4. decreasing levels of consciousness

3 Which of the following statements about cerebrospinal fluid (CSF) is true?
1. If CSF contains glucose, the person has a metabolic disorder.
2. CSF circulates through the brain via the meninges.
3. CSF protects the brain and spinal cord from trauma.
4. A lumbar puncture is done to withdraw CSF from the brain.

4 Following a motorcycle crash, a client has damage to the posterior spinal roots. What assessment would you expect to find?
1. loss of sensation to dull and sharp
2. flaccid paralysis of the legs
3. changes in peripheral vision in both eyes
4. decreased sense of smell and taste

5 You narrowly miss having an automobile crash while merging onto the freeway. Your body responses to this stress are caused by which division of the autonomic nervous system?
1. sympathetic
2. parasympathetic
3. cholinergic
4. adrenergic

6 Which of the physical assessment techniques is **not** used in the neurologic examination?
1. inspection
2. auscultation
3. percussion
4. palpation

7 What would you need to assess function of cranial nerve V (trigeminal)?
1. cotton ball and safety pin
2. stethoscope with bell and diaphragm
3. measuring tape and pencil
4. various scents, such as coffee and vanilla

8 In which of the following clients would assessing the corneal reflex be appropriate?
1. anyone over the age of 50
2. people who wear contact lenses
3. a client with spinal cord trauma
4. an unconscious client

9 You have been asked to assess a client's gag reflex. What equipment would you need to do this?
1. safety pin
2. cotton ball
3. tongue depressor
4. stethoscope

10 Which position best describes decorticate posturing?
1. neck extended, arms extended and pronated, feet plantar flexed
2. arms close to sides, elbows and wrists flexed, legs extended
3. in prone position with arms and knees sharply flexed
4. in supine position, spine extended, legs extended

See Test Yourself answers in Appendix C.

BIBLIOGRAPHY

Aird, T., & McIntosh, M. (2004). Nursing assessment. Nursing tools and strategies to assess cognition and confusion. *British Journal of Nursing, 13*(10), 621–625.

Amella, E. (2004). Presentation of illness in older adults: If you think you know what you're looking for, think again. *American Journal of Nursing, 104*(10), 40–52.

Arbour, R. (2004). Intracranial hypertension: Monitoring and nursing assessment. *Critical Care Nurse, 24*(5), 19–20, 22–26, 28–34.

Arnold, E. (2004). Sorting out the 3 D's: Delirium, dementia, depression. *Nursing, 34*(6), 36–43.

Bickley, L., & Szilagyi, P. (2005). *Bates' guide to physical examination and history taking* (9th ed.). Philadelphia: Lippincott.

Buck, A. (2004). Assessment and management of dementia. *Practice Nurse, 28*(3), 39–43.

Chaudhuri, A., & Behan, P. (2004). Fatigue in neurological disorders. *Lancet, 363*(9413), 978–988.

Cole, E. (2004). Assessment and management of the trauma patient. *Nursing Standard, 18*(41), 45–52, 54.

Cox, C., Boswell, G., McGrath, A., Reynolds, T., & Cole, E. (2004). Cranial nerve damage. *Emergency Nurse, 12*(2), 14–21.

Crimlisk, J., & Grande, M. (2004). Neurologic assessment skills for the acute medical surgical nurse. *Orthopaedic Nursing, 23*(1), 3–11.

Don't overlook mental status changes in elderly. (2003). *ED Nursing, 6*(10), 117–118.

Eliopoulos, E. (2005). *Gerontological nursing* (6th ed.). Philadelphia: Lippincott Williams & Wilkins.

Jarvis, C. (2004). *Physical examination & health assessment.* St. Louis, MO: Mosby.

Kee, J. (2005). *Prentice Hall handbook of laboratory & diagnostic tests with nursing implications.* Upper Saddle River, NJ: Prentice Hall.

Maher, L. (2000). A quick neurologic examination. *Patient Care, 34*(3), 161–162, 165–168, 171–172.

Mooney, G., & Comerford, D. (2003). Neurological observations. *Nursing Times, 99*(17), 24–25.

National Institutes of Health. (2003). *Genes and disease. The nervous system.* Retrieved from http://www.ncbi.nlm.nih.gov/books/bv.fcgi?rid=gnd.section.75

Nick, J. (2003). Deep tendon reflexes: The what, why, where, and how of tapping. *Journal of Obstetric, Gynecologic, and Neonatal Nursing, 32*(3), 297–306.

Porth, C. (2005). *Pathophysiology: Concepts of altered health states* (7th ed.). Philadelphia: Lippincott.

Pullen, R. (2004a). Assessing for signs of meningitis. *Nursing, 34*(5), 18.

Pullen, R. (2004b). Neurologic assessment for pronator drift. *Nursing, 34*(3), 22.

Weber, J., & Kelley, J. (2006). *Health assessment in nursing* (3rd ed.). Philadelphia: Lippincott.

CHAPTER 44 Nursing Care of Clients with Intracranial Disorders

LEARNING OUTCOMES

- Compare and contrast the pathophysiology, manifestations, interdisciplinary care, and nursing care of clients with alterations in level of consciousness and increased intracranial pressure.

- Explain the pathophysiology, manifestations, complications, interdisciplinary care, and nursing care of intracranial disorders, including headaches, epilepsy, traumatic brain injury, central nervous system infections, and brain tumors.

- Describe criteria for diagnosing persistent vegetative state and brain death.

- Discuss the purposes, nursing implications, and health education for the client and family for medications used to treat altered cerebral function, headaches, epilepsy, traumatic brain injury, central nervous system infections, and brain tumors.

- Discuss surgical options for the treatment of increased intracranial pressure, epilepsy, traumatic brain injury, and brain tumors.

CLINICAL COMPETENCIES

- Assess functional status of clients with intracranial disorders and monitor, document, and report abnormal manifestations.

- Determine priority nursing diagnoses, based on assessed data, to select and implement individualized nursing interventions for clients with intracranial disorders.

- Administer oral and injectable medications used to treat intracranial disorders knowledgeably and safely.

- Provide skilled care to clients having intracranial pressure monitoring, tonic-clonic seizures, and intracranial surgery.

- Integrate intradisciplinary care into care of clients with intracranial disorders.

- Provide appropriate teaching and evidence-based practice to facilitate community-based care to promote safety and prevent injury, and to provide information and support necessary for long-term care of clients with intracranial disorders.

- Revise plan of care as needed to provide effective interventions to promote, maintain, or restore functional health status to clients with intracranial disorders.

The client with an intracranial disorder presents a unique nursing challenge. Problems the client experiences in the acute stage of the disorder are often a prelude to long-term problems requiring ongoing management. These long-term problems range from alterations in the body's basic functioning to dysfunctions in the complex processes of the human mind. Systemic problems may accompany or develop sec-ondary to an intracranial disorder. Intracranial disorders may affect both the client's quality of life and that of the client's family. This chapter first discusses altered level of consciousness and increased intracranial pressure, followed by intracranial disorders that may manifest these and other health problems. Information specific to the client with a stroke is provided in Chapter 45 ∞.

ALTERED CEREBRAL FUNCTION

The manifestations of altered cerebral function occur as a result of illness or injury. Assessment of the patterns of those manifestations helps determine the extent of the cerebral dysfunction and improvement or deterioration of cerebral function. Except in the case of direct damage to the brainstem and reticular activating system (RAS), brain function deterioration usually follows a predictable progression, that is, a pattern in which higher levels of function are impaired initially, pro-gressing to impairment of more primitive functions. Altered level of consciousness (LOC) and behavior changes are early manifestations of the deterioration of the function of the cerebral hemispheres. Structures in the midbrain and brainstem are affected sequentially, with characteristic changes in LOC; patterns of respiration, pupillary, and oculomotor responses; and motor function. Manifestations of progressive deterioration of cerebral function are outlined in Table 44–1.

TABLE 44–1 Progression of Deteriorating Brain Function

LEVEL OF CONSCIOUSNESS	PUPILLARY RESPONSE	OCULOMOTOR RESPONSES	MOTOR RESPONSES	BREATHING
Alert; oriented to time, place, and person	Brisk and equal; pupils regular	Eyes move as head turns Caloric testing (ear irrigation) produces nystagmus	Purposeful movement; responds to commands	Regular pattern with normal rate and depth
Responds to verbal stimuli; decreased concentration; agitation, confusion, lethargy; disoriented	Small and reactive	Roving eye movements; doll's eyes positive, with gaze fixed straight ahead; eye deviation away from cold caloric stimulus and toward warm stimulus	Purposeful movement in response to pain stimulus	Yawning, sighing respirations
Requires continuous stimulation to rouse			Decorticate posturing with upper extremity flexion	Cheyne-Stokes respirations with crescendo–decrescendo pattern in rate and depth followed by period of apnea
Reflexive positioning to pain stimulus	Pupils fixed (nonreactive) in midposition	Caloric testing produces nystagmus	Decerebrate posturing with adduction and rigid extension of upper and lower extremities	Central neurogenic hyperventilation with rapid, regular, and deep respirations; apneustic breathing with prolonged inspiration and pauses at full inspiration and following expiration
No response to stimuli	Pupils fixed in midposition	No spontaneous eye movement or nystagmus	Extension of upper extremities with flexion of lower extremities; flaccidity	Cluster or ataxic breathing with irregular pattern and depth of respirations; gasping respirations or apnea

THE CLIENT WITH ALTERED LEVEL OF CONSCIOUSNESS

Consciousness is a condition in which the person is aware of self and environment and is able to respond appropriately to stimuli. Full consciousness requires both normal arousal and full cognition.

- *Arousal*, or alertness, depends on the RAS, a diffuse system of neurons in the thalamus and upper brainstem.
- *Cognition* is a complex process involving all mental activities controlled by the cerebral hemispheres, including thought processes, memory, perception, problem solving, and emotion.

These two components of consciousness depend on the normal physiologic functions of and connections between the arousal mechanisms of the reticular formation and the cognitive functions of the cerebral hemispheres. Because arousal and cognition are independent components of consciousness, each can act separately on stimuli. For example, the RAS reacts to the discomfort caused by a full bladder by waking the person in the middle of the night. Once awake, however, the frontal cortex alerts the person that the bladder is full and prompts the person to go to the bathroom and empty it.

Conditions that affect either the RAS or the function of the cerebral hemispheres can interfere with the normal level of consciousness. Terms describing altered LOC are listed and defined in Table 44–2. Nurses should remember that consciousness is a dynamic state: A client may pass from full consciousness to coma within hours or experience a slow diminishment of consciousness that does not become evident for weeks or months. The nurse can help provide effective care for a client with an altered LOC by looking beyond the diagnostic labels of consciousness and accurately assessing the client's behavior and response to stimuli.

Pathophysiology

Level of consciousness may be altered by processes that affect the arousal functions of the brainstem, the cognitive functions of the cerebral hemispheres, or both. The major causes are (1) lesions or injuries that affect the cerebral hemispheres directly and widely or that compress or destroy the neurons of the RAS and (2) metabolic disorders.

Arousal and Cognition

The physiologic seat of consciousness, the reticular formation, is a mass of nerve cells and fibers that make up the core of the brainstem, extending from the medulla to the midbrain. The axons of reticular neurons are exceptionally long and branch outward to cells in the hypothalamus, thalamus, cerebellum, and spinal cord. A system of reticular neurons within the RAS passes steady streams of impulses through thalamic relays in order to stimulate the cerebral cortex into wakefulness. The body's sensory tracts interact with RAS neurons; this interrelationship helps control the strength of the RAS's rousing effect on the cerebrum.

Damage to the RAS impairs the person's ability to maintain wakefulness and arousal. Stroke is the most common cause of RAS destruction. Other causes include demyelinating diseases

TABLE 44–2	**Terms Used to Describe Level of Consciousness**
TERM	**CHARACTERISTICS OF CLIENT**
Full consciousness	Alert; oriented to time, place, and person; comprehends spoken and written words
Confusion	Unable to think rapidly and clearly; easily bewildered, with poor memory and short attention span; misinterprets stimuli; judgment is impaired
Disorientation	Not aware of or not oriented to time, place, or person
Obtundation	Lethargic, somnolent; responsive to verbal or tactile stimuli but quickly drifts back to sleep
Stupor	Generally unresponsive; may be briefly aroused by vigorous, repeated, or painful stimuli; may shrink away from or grab at the source of stimuli
Semicomatose	Does not move spontaneously; unresponsive to stimuli, although vigorous or painful stimuli may result in stirring, moaning, or withdrawal from the stimuli, without actual arousal
Coma	Unarousable; will not stir or moan in response to any stimulus; may exhibit nonpurposeful response (slight movement) of area stimulated but makes no attempt to withdraw
Deep coma	Completely unarousable and unresponsive to any kind of stimulus, including pain; absence of brainstem reflexes, corneal, papillary, and pharyngeal reflexes and tendon and plantar reflexes

such as multiple sclerosis, tumors, abscesses, and head injury. Function of the RAS may be suppressed by compression of the brainstem, which produces edema and ischemia. Pressure and compression of the brainstem may be due to tumors, increased intracranial pressure, hematomas or hemorrhage, or aneurysm. Although it is possible to assess LOC or arousal in the client with RAS damage, the impairment in arousal may make it impossible to assess cognitive function.

The function of the brain, especially the cerebral hemispheres, depends on continuous blood flow with unimpeded supplies of oxygen and glucose. Processes that disrupt this flow of blood and nutrients may cause widespread damage to the cerebral hemispheres, impairing arousal and cognition. Bilateral hemispheric lesions (such as global ischemia), or metabolic disorders (such as hypoglycemia), are the most common causes of altered LOC related to cerebral dysfunction of the hemispheres. Localized masses, such as a hematoma or cerebral edema, that displace normal structures and cause direct or indirect pressure on the opposite hemisphere or brainstem can also affect LOC. The client who has widespread damage to the cerebral hemispheres but an intact RAS has sleep–wake cycles and may rouse in response to stimuli; the client cannot be said to be alert, however, because cognition is impaired.

Both localized neurologic processes and systemic disorders can alter LOC. Processes occurring within the brain, which may directly destroy or compress neurologic structures, include the following:

- Increased intracranial pressure
- Stroke
- Hematoma
- Intracranial hemorrhage
- Tumors
- Infections
- Injury from excitatory amino acids
- Demyelinating disorders.

Any systemic condition that affects the delivery of blood, oxygen, and glucose to the brain or alters cell membranes may also alter LOC. If cerebral blood flow is impaired or the client becomes hypoxic or hypoglycemic, cerebral metabolism is impaired and level of consciousness declines rapidly. Severe hypoxia quickly leads to ischemia. Ischemia may be focal (for example, following a stroke) or global (as from cardiac arrest or hypovolemic shock). Widespread global ischemia causes almost immediate unconsciousness (Porth, 2005). Clients at particular risk include those with poorly controlled diabetes and those with cardiac or respiratory failure.

Other metabolic alterations that can affect LOC include fluid and electrolyte imbalances, such as hyponatremia or hyperosmolality, and acid–base alterations, such as hypercapnia (an elevated arterial carbon dioxide level). Accumulated waste products and toxins from liver or renal failure can affect neuronal and neurotransmitter function, altering LOC. Drugs that depress the central nervous system (e.g., alcohol, analgesics, anesthetics) suppress metabolic and membrane activities in the RAS and cerebral hemispheres, thereby affecting LOC. Glutamate, the main excitatory neurotransmitter in the brain, may accumulate during prolonged ischemia, resulting in acute glutamate toxicity and cell death.

Seizure activity, with abnormal electrical discharges from a local area of the brain or from the entire brain, commonly affects LOC. It appears that the spontaneous, disordered discharge of activity that occurs during a seizure exhausts energy metabolites or produces locally toxic molecules, altering LOC for a time after the seizure. Consciousness returns when the metabolic balance of the neurons is restored.

As the impairment of brain function progresses, more stimuli are required to elicit a response from the client. Initially, the client may rouse to verbal stimuli and respond appropriately to questions, remaining oriented to time, place, and person. With deterioration of neurologic function, the client becomes more difficult to rouse and may become agitated and confused when awakened. Orientation to time is lost initially, followed by orientation to place and then to person. Continuous stimulation or vigorous shaking is required to maintain wakefulness as LOC decreases. Eventually, the client does not respond, even with deep painful stimuli.

Patterns of Respirations

Progressive impairment of neural function also causes predictable changes in respiratory patterns as respiratory centers are affected. In normal respirations, a rhythmic pattern is maintained by neural centers in the pons and medulla that respond to changes in arterial levels of oxygen (Pao_2) and carbon dioxide ($Paco_2$). When there is damage to the RAS or cerebral hemispheres, neural control of these centers is lost, and lower brainstem centers regulate breathing patterns by responding only to changes in $Paco_2$, resulting in irregular respiratory patterns. The initial manifestations of deteriorating brain function are yawning and sighing. As outlined in Table 44–1 and illustrated in Table 44–3, progressive deterioration in brain function is accompanied by decreasing LOC and changes in breathing patterns. The type of respirations, by area of cerebral damage, are as follows:

- Diencephalon: *Cheyne-Stokes respirations* (alternating regular periods of deep, rapid breathing followed by periods of apnea)
- Midbrain: *neurogenic hyperventilation* (may exceed 40 per minute), the result of uninhibited stimulation of the respiratory centers
- Pons: *apneustic respirations*, characterized by sighing on midinspiration or prolonged inhalation and exhalation; results from excessive stimulation of the respiratory centers
- Medulla: *ataxic/apneic respirations* (totally uncoordinated and irregular), probably as a result of the loss of responsiveness to CO_2.

TABLE 44–3 Breathing Patterns Characteristic of Altered Level of Consciousness

PATTERN		DESCRIPTION
Cheyne-Stokes respirations		A regular crescendo–decrescendo pattern with increasing then decreasing rate and depth of respirations followed by a period of apnea
Central neurogenic hyperventilation		A sustained pattern of rapid, regular, deep respirations (hyperapnea)
Apneustic breathing		Prolonged inspiration with a pause at full inspiration followed by expiration and a possible pause following expiration
Cluster breathing		Clusters of several breaths with irregular periods of apnea between clusters
Ataxic respirations		Respirations that are completely irregular in pattern and depth with irregular periods of apnea

Head in neutral position

Eyes midline

Head rotated to client's left

Doll's eyes present:
Eyes move right in
relation to head.

Doll's eyes absent:
Eyes do not move
in relation to head.
Direction of vision follows
head to left.

Figure 44–1 ■ Doll's eye movements characteristic of altered LOC.

Pupillary and Oculomotor Responses

The brainstem areas that control arousal are adjacent to areas that control the pupils. A predictable progression of pupillary and oculomotor responses occurs as level of consciousness deteriorates toward coma (see Table 44–1). If the lesion or process affecting neurologic function is localized, effects may initially be seen in the ipsilateral pupil (the pupil on the same side as the lesion). With generalized or systemic processes, pupils are affected equally. If the pupils are small and equally reactive, metabolic processes affecting LOC may be present. With compression of cranial nerve III at the midbrain, the pupils may become oval or eccentric (off center). As the level of functional impairment progresses, the pupils become fixed (unresponsive to light) and, eventually, dilated.

In deteriorating LOC and coma, spontaneous eye movement is lost and reflexive ocular movements are altered. Normally, both eyes move simultaneously in the same direction; injury to the cranial nerve nuclei in the midbrain and pons can impair normal movement. *Doll's eye movements* are reflexive movements of the eyes in the opposite direction of head rotation; they are an indicator of brainstem function (Figure 44–1 ■). As a result of the oculocephalic reflex, the eyes move upward with passive flexion of the neck and downward with passive neck extension. As brainstem function deteriorates, this reflex is lost. The eyes fail to turn together and, eventually, remain fixed in the midposition as the head is turned.

Motor Responses

The level of brain dysfunction and the side of the brain affected may be assessed by motor responses. These responses are the most accurate identifier of changes in mental status. In altered LOC, motor responses to stimuli range from an appropriate response to a command (e.g., "squeeze my hand" or "push my hands away with your feet") to flaccidity (see Table 44–1). Initially, the client may be able to move purposefully away from a noxious stimulus, for example, to brush the examiner's hand away from the face. As function declines, movements become more generalized (withdrawal, grimacing) and less purposeful.

Reflexive motor responses may occur, including decorticate posturing with flexion of the upper extremities accompanied by extension of the lower extremities. With further decline, decerebrate posturing is seen, with adduction and rigid extension of the upper and lower extremities. Without intervention, the client eventually becomes flaccid, with little or no motor response to stimuli.

Coma States and Brain Death

Possible outcomes of altered LOC and coma include full recovery with no long-term residual effects, recovery with residual damage (such as learning deficits, emotional difficulties, or impaired judgment), or more severe consequences such as persistent vegetative state (cerebral death) or brain death. Resources for families are listed in Box 44–1.

BOX 44–1 Organizations Providing Information for Families of Clients in a Coma

Coma Recovery Association
807 Carman Avenue
Westbury, NY 11590
Tel: 516-997-1826

Brain Injury Association of America, Inc.
8201 Greensboro Drive, Suite 611
McLean, VA 22102
FamilyHelpline@blausa.org
Tel: 800-444-6443

Brain Trauma Foundation
523 East 72nd Street, 8th Floor
New York, NY 10021
www.braintrauma.org
Tel: 212-772-0608

Family Caregiver Alliance/National Center on Caregiving
180 Montgomery Street, Suite 1100
San Francisco, CA 94104
Tel: 800-445-8106

PERSISTENT VEGETATIVE STATE **Persistent vegetative state** (also called irreversible coma) is a permanent condition of complete unawareness of self and the environment and loss of all cognitive functions. Usually the result of severe brain trauma or global ischemia, this condition results from death of the cerebral hemispheres with continued function of the brainstem and cerebellum. While the homeostatic regulatory functions of the brain continue, the ability to respond meaningfully to the environment is lost. The diagnosis of persistent vegetative state requires that the condition has continued for at least 1 month (Porth, 2005).

The client has sleep–wake cycles and retains the ability to chew, swallow, and cough but cannot interact with the environment. When awake, the eyes may wander back and forth across the room, but they cannot track an object or person. In a minimally conscious state, the client is aware of the environment and can follow simple commands, manipulate objects, gesture or verbalize to indicate "yes/no" responses, and make meaningful movements (such as blinking or smiling) in response to a stimulus. With appropriate supportive care, the client may remain in this state for years.

LOCKED-IN SYNDROME **Locked-in syndrome** is distinctly different from persistent vegetative state in that the client is alert and fully aware of the environment and has intact cognitive abilities, but is unable to communicate through speech or movement because of blocked efferent pathways from the brain. Motor paralysis affects all voluntary muscles, although the upper cranial nerves (I through IV) may remain intact, allowing the client to communicate through eye movements and blinking. In essence, the client is "locked" inside a paralyzed body while remaining fully conscious of self and environment. Infarction or hemorrhage of the pons that disrupts outgoing nerve tracts but spares the RAS is the usual cause of locked-in syndrome. This condition may also result when the corticospinal tracts between the midbrain and pons are interrupted. Disorders of the lower motor neurons or muscles, such as acute polyneuritis, myasthenia gravis, or amyotrophic lateral sclerosis (ALS), may also paralyze motor responses, leading to locked-in syndrome.

BRAIN DEATH **Brain death** is the cessation and irreversibility of all brain functions, including the brainstem. Although the exact criteria for establishing brain death may vary somewhat from state to state, it is generally agreed that brain death has occurred when there is no evidence of cerebral or brainstem function for an extended period (usually 6 to 24 hours) in a client who has a normal body temperature and is not affected by a depressant drug or alcohol poisoning. Generally recognized criteria are:

- Unresponsive coma with absent motor and reflex movements
- No spontaneous respiration (apnea)
- Pupils fixed (unresponsive to light) and dilated
- Absent ocular responses to head turning and caloric stimulation (Caloric stimulation is performed by irrigating the ear with ice-cold water to test the oculovestibular reflex, a reflex controlled by the brainstem. Normally, the cold causes the eyes to first move toward the irrigated side, followed by a return to midline.)

- Flat electroencephalogram (EEG) and no cerebral blood circulation present on angiography (if performed)
- Persistence of these manifestations for 30 minutes to 1 hour and for 6 hours after onset of coma and apnea.

Apnea in the comatose client is determined by the apnea test. The ventilator is removed while maintaining oxygenation by tracheal cannula and allowing the P_{CO_2} to increase to 60 mmHg or higher. This level of carbon dioxide is high enough to stimulate respiration if the brainstem is functional. The EEG may be used to establish the absence of brain activity when brain death is suspected. A flat (isoelectric) EEG over a period of 6 to 12 hours in a client who is not hypothermic or under the influence of drugs that depress the central nervous system (CNS) is generally accepted as an indicator of brain death.

Prognosis

The prognosis for clients with altered levels of consciousness and coma varies according to the underlying cause and pathologic process. Age and general medical condition also play a role in determining outcome. Young adults may fully recover following deep coma from head injury, drug overdose, or other cause. Recovery of consciousness within 2 weeks is associated with a favorable outcome. In general, the prognosis is poor for clients who lack pupillary reaction or reflex eye movements 6 hours after the onset of coma.

INTERDISCIPLINARY CARE

Management of the client with an altered LOC or coma must begin immediately. The focus of management is to identify the underlying cause, preserve function, and prevent deterioration if possible. Airway and breathing must be maintained during the initial acute stage until the diagnosis and prognosis can be established. Intravenous fluids are used to support circulation and to correct fluid, electrolyte, and acid–base imbalances. Treatment protocols to reduce increased intracranial pressure or control seizure activity (discussed later in this chapter) may be initiated. Changes in LOC associated with craniocerebral trauma, such as hematomas, often require immediate surgical intervention.

Diagnosis

Although the client's history and physical examination findings often indicate the cause of alterations in LOC, several diagnostic tests may be useful in establishing the diagnosis. The tests used to evaluate for possible metabolic, toxic, or drug-induced disorders include both radiologic and laboratory tests.

CT and MRI scanning are done to detect neurologic damage due to hemorrhage, tumor, cyst, edema, myocardial infarction, or brain atrophy. These tests may also identify displacement of brain structures by large or expanding lesions. Radioisotope brain scan is performed to identify abnormal lesions in the brain and evaluate cerebral blood flow. Cerebral angiography allows radiographic visualization of the cerebral vascular system. This exam can identify lesions such as aneurysms, occluded vessels, or tumors, and may also be used to determine cessation of cerebral blood flow and brain death. Transcranial Doppler studies use an ultrasound velocity detector that records sound waves reflected from RBCs in blood vessels to assess cerebral blood flow. Lumbar puncture with cerebrospinal fluid (CSF) analysis is performed when infection and possible meningitis are suspected as a cause of altered LOC. EEG is used to evaluate the electrical activity of the brain. (See Chapter 43 ∞ for further information and nursing implications of neurologic tests.)

Laboratory tests are used to identify and monitor altered LOC. These may include any or all of the following:

- *Blood glucose* is measured immediately when coma is of unknown origin and hypoglycemia is suspected or possible. When the blood glucose falls to less than 40 to 50 mg/dL, cerebral function declines rapidly. The client with type 1 diabetes is at particular risk for hypoglycemia-induced coma.
- *Serum electrolytes*—sodium, potassium, bicarbonate, chloride, and calcium in particular—are measured to assess for metabolic disturbances and guide intravenous therapy. Hyponatremia, in which serum sodium levels are below 115 mEq/L (normal level: 135 to 145 mEq/L), is associated with coma and convulsions, especially if it develops rapidly.
- *Serum osmolality* is evaluated. Both hyperosmolar and hypo-osmolar states may be associated with coma. Hyperosmolality (above 320 mOsm/kg H_2O) causes cellular dehydration of brain tissue as fluid is drawn into the vascular system by osmosis. Hypo-osmolality (less than 250 mOsm/kg H_2O), by contrast, leads to cerebral edema and swelling, impairing consciousness.
- *Arterial blood gases* (ABGs) are drawn to evaluate arterial oxygen and carbon dioxide levels as well as acid–base balance. Hypoxemia is a frequent cause of altered LOC; increased levels of carbon dioxide are also toxic to the brain and can induce coma, particularly when the onset of hypercapnia is acute.
- *Liver function tests*, including bilirubin, AST, ALT, LDH, serum albumin, and serum ammonia levels, are determined to evaluate hepatic function. High ammonia levels seen in hepatic failure interfere with cerebral metabolism and neurotransmitters, affecting LOC.
- *Toxicology screening* of blood and urine is done to determine if altered LOC is the result of acute drug or alcohol toxicity. Serum alcohol levels are measured and the blood is assessed for the presence of substances such as barbiturates, carbon monoxide, or lead.

Medications

Medications are used to support homeostasis and normal function for the client with altered LOC, as well as to treat specific underlying disorders. An intravenous catheter is inserted, and fluid balance is maintained using isotonic or slightly hypertonic solutions, such as normal saline or lactated Ringer's solution. The client's response to fluid administration is monitored carefully for evidence of increased cerebral edema.

If hypoglycemia is present, 50% glucose is administered intravenously to restore cerebral metabolism rapidly. Conversely, insulin is administered to the client with hyperglycemia to reduce the blood glucose level and thus the serum osmolality. With narcotic overdose, naloxone is administered. Naloxone is a narcotic antagonist that competes for narcotic receptor sites, effectively blocking the depressant effect of the narcotic. Thiamine may be administered with glucose, particularly if the client is malnourished or known to abuse alcohol, to prevent exacerbation of Wernicke's encephalopathy, a hemorrhagic encephalopathy due to thiamine deficiency that is associated with chronic alcoholism (Tierney et al., 2005).

Any underlying fluid and electrolyte imbalance is corrected by administering medications or appropriate electrolytes. For the client who is hyponatremic and has a low serum osmolality, furosemide (Lasix) or an osmotic diuretic such as mannitol may be administered to promote water excretion. Appropriate antibiotics are administered intravenously to the client with suspected or confirmed meningitis.

Surgery

Although surgery is not indicated for most clients with altered LOC, it may be necessary if the cause of coma is an intracerebral tumor, hemorrhage, or hematoma. Surgical intervention is discussed later in this chapter, in the section on brain tumors. When there is a risk of increased intracranial pressure, the client is monitored continuously. These measures are discussed in the section on increased intracranial pressure that follows.

Other Treatments

Support of the airway and respirations is vital in the client with an altered LOC. The client who is drowsy but rousable may need little more than an oral pharyngeal airway. With more severe alterations in consciousness, the client may need endotracheal intubation to maintain airway patency, particularly if the cough and gag reflexes are absent. Mechanical ventilation is indicated when hypoventilation or apnea is present. Unless a do-not-resuscitate (DNR) order is in effect, mechanical ventilation should be initiated even if it has not been established that the disorder is reversible; without ventilatory support, cerebral anoxia develops rapidly, and brain death may ensue. ABGs are monitored frequently to determine the adequacy of ventilation. Cautious hyperventilation may be used to reduce $PaCO_2$ and promote cerebral vasoconstriction to reduce cerebral edema.

Nutrition

In clients with long-term alterations in consciousness, such as vegetative state or locked-in syndrome, measures to maintain nutritional status are initiated. Enteral feedings with a gastrostomy tube are preferred if the client is unable to take enough food by mouth without aspirating. In some cases, total parenteral nutrition may be used.

NURSING CARE

Nursing care of the client with an altered LOC is planned and implemented for a variety of responses of both the client and the family of the client.

Support of the Family

Family members of a client with an altered level of consciousness are often very anxious. It is difficult for the family to deal with the client's uncertain prognosis. They may experience various conflicting emotions, such as guilt and anger. Reinforce information provided by the physician, and encourage the family to talk to the client as though he or she were able to understand. Explain that this communication may initially seem awkward, but in time it will feel appropriate. Evaluate the family's readiness to receive explanations regarding the client's treatment and care. The presence of many tubes (e.g., intravenous line, catheter, ventilator) may be overwhelming to the family. They may not perceive the seriousness of the situation if a thorough explanation is not given. Include family members in the client's care as much as they wish to be involved.

Allow significant others to stay with the client when possible. Reinforce the need for family members to care for themselves by encouraging adequate meals and rest. Offer to contact support services such as friends, neighbors, and social services that the hospital may provide. Ask family members to leave a telephone number where they can be reached, and assure them that they will be called if any significant changes occur. Encourage family members to call if they have questions or concerns.

Nursing Diagnoses and Interventions

Nursing diagnoses and interventions discussed in this section are directed toward the unconscious client and focus on problems with airway maintenance, skin integrity, contractures, and nutrition.

Ineffective Airway Clearance

Ineffective airway clearance related to loss of the cough reflex and the inability to expectorate is a major problem for the unconscious client. The cough reflex may be absent or impaired when conditions that produce coma depress the function of the medullary centers.

- Assess ability to clear secretions. Monitor breath sounds, rate and depth of respirations, dyspnea, pulse oximeter, and the presence of cyanosis. *The client's ability to clear secretions serves as the initial assessment base for developing further interventions.*
- In unconscious clients or those without an intact cough reflex, maintain an open airway by periodic suctioning, limiting the time of suctioning to 10 to 15 seconds or less. Periodic suctioning may be necessary to clear the airway of mucus, blood, or other drainage. *Suctioning for more than 15 seconds in the client with increased intracranial pressure may cause hypercapnia, which in turn vasodilates cerebral vessels, increases cerebral blood volume, and increases intracranial pressure.*

PRACTICE ALERT
If the client has a basilar skull fracture or CSF draining from the ears or nose, never suction nasally.

- Turn from side to side every 2 hours, and maintain a side-lying position with the head of the bed elevated approximately 30 degrees. Do not position the unconscious client on the back. *Turning the client from side to side facilitates respirations, prevents the tongue from obstructing the airway, and helps prevent pooling of secretions in one area of the lungs (thus decreasing the risk of pneumonia).*

- If the client has a tracheostomy, provide tracheostomy care every 4 hours and suction when secretions are present (see Chapter 37 ∞) *to maintain an open airway.*
- Monitor the results of arterial blood gas analysis and pulse oximetry. Maintain records of trends. *ABGs and pulse oximetry directly measure the oxygen content of blood and are good indicators of the lungs' ability to oxygenate the blood.*

Risk for Aspiration

The unconscious client with a depressed or absent gag and swallowing reflex is at high risk for aspiration. Drainage, mucus, or blood may obstruct the airway and interfere with oxygenation. Pooling of aspiration secretions in the lungs also increases the risk of pneumonia.

- Assess swallowing and gag reflexes every shift as appropriate to the client's level of consciousness. *Deepening levels of unconsciousness may cause a loss in swallow and gag reflexes.*
- Monitor for and report manifestations of aspiration: crackles and wheezes, dullness to percussion over an area of the lungs, dyspnea, tachypnea, and cyanosis. *Early recognition facilitates prompt intervention.*
- Provide interventions to prevent aspiration:
  - Maintain NPO status.
  - Place in the side-lying position.
  - Provide oral hygiene and suctioning as needed.
  The side-lying position allows secretions to drain from the mouth rather than into the pharynx. Oral hygiene and suctioning remove secretions that might otherwise be aspirated.

PRACTICE ALERT
Never give unconscious clients oral food and fluids because of the risk of aspiration.

Risk for Impaired Skin Integrity

The unconscious client is at risk for impaired skin integrity as a result of immobility and the inability to provide self-care. On average, healthy people change positions during sleep every 11 minutes; the unconscious client often cannot maintain the movement needed to prevent pressure on the skin, especially over bony prominences. As a result, the skin and subcutaneous tissues may become ischemic and prone to develop pressure ulcers. Perspiration and incontinence of urine and stool may exacerbate the problem. Nursing interventions are directed to maintaining the integrity not only of the skin, but also of the lips and mucous membranes.

- Assess skin every shift, especially over bony prominences, the back of the scalp, and around genitals and buttocks. *The large surface area of the skin bears weight and is in constant contact with the surface of the bed. The skin, subcutaneous tissue, and muscles, especially those tissues over bony prominences, undergo constant pressure. This impairs normal capillary blood flow, which interferes with the exchange of nutrients and waste products. Tissue ischemia and necrosis may result and lead to the development of pressure ulcers.*
- Provide proper positioning. Reposition bed-ridden clients at least every 2 hours if this is consistent with the overall treatment goals. Keep the head of the bed elevated no higher than

30 degrees unless prescribed differently. Provide special pads and mattresses that distribute weight more evenly (e.g., silicone-filled pads, egg-crate cushions, turning frames, flotation pads). Consider requesting/using a special thera-peutic bed that automatically turns the client at regular inter-vals. Lift the client instead of dragging the client across the sheet. *When the head of the bed is elevated above 30 degrees, the client's torso tends to slide down toward the foot of the bed. Friction and perspiration cause the skin and superficial fascia to remain fixed against the bed linens while the deep fascia and skeleton slide downward. When a person is pulled rather than lifted, the skin remains fixed to the sheet while the fascia and muscles are pulled upward. These shearing forces promote tissue breakdown.*

- Provide interventions to prevent breakdown of the skin and mucous membranes:
  - Keep bed linens clean, dry, and wrinkle free.
  - Provide daily bath with mild soap.
  - Cleanse the skin after urine and fecal soiling with a mild cleansing agent.
  - Provide oral care and lubricate the lips every 2 to 4 hours.
  - Maintain accurate intake and output records.
  - Keep the cornea moist by instilling methyl cellulose solution (0.5% to 1%) and apply protective eye shields or close the eyelids with adhesive strips if the corneal reflex is absent.

  Keeping linens clean, dry, and wrinkle free decreases the risk of injury from the shearing force of bed rest and protects against environmental factors that cause drying. Adequate hy-dration of the stratum corneum appears to protect the skin against mechanical insult. Preventing dehydration maintains circulation and decreases the concentration of urine, thereby minimizing skin irritation in people who are incontinent. Proper eye care prevents corneal abrasion and irritation.

Impaired Physical Mobility

Clients who are unconscious are unable to maintain normal musculoskeletal movement and are at high risk for contrac-tures related to decreased movement. Because the flexor and adductor muscles are stronger than the extensors and abduc-tors, flexor and adductor contractures develop quickly with-out preventive measures. Passive ROM exercises must be performed routinely to maintain muscle tone and function, to prevent additional disability, and to help restore impaired mo-tor function.

- Maintain extremities in functional positions by providing proper support devices. Remove support devices every 4 hours for skin care and passive ROM exercises. Provide pil-lows for the axillary region; rolled washcloths may be placed in elevated hands; use splints to prevent plantar flexion (foot drop). *Pillows in the axillary region help prevent adduction of the shoulder. Rolled washcloths help decrease edema and flexion contracture of the fingers. Splints are useful in pre-venting plantar flexion.*
- Collaborate with a physical therapist to develop and implement passive range-of-motion (ROM) exercises (unless contraindi-cated, as for the client with increased intracranial pressure) at least four times a day, keeping the following principles in mind:

  - Place one hand above the joint being exercised. The other hand gently moves the joint through its normal range of motion.
  - Move the body part to the point of resistance, and stop.

  Placing one hand above the joint provides support against gravity and prevents unwanted movement. ROM exercises help prevent contractures by stretching muscles and tendons and maintaining joint mobility.

Risk for Imbalanced Nutrition: Less than Body Requirements

The unconscious client is at risk for an alteration in nutrition re-lated to a reduced or complete inability to eat. This is especially true for the client who is unconscious as the result of an infec-tion or trauma, both of which increase metabolic requirements.

- Monitor nutritional status through daily weights (on bed scales) and laboratory data. For accuracy, weigh the client at the same time each day, using the same scales. Ensure that the client wears the same clothing. *Changes in laboratory data with decreased nutrition include a decrease in the lev-els of serum prealbumin and serum transferrin.*
- Assess the need for alternative methods of nutritional support (tube feeding or total parenteral nutrition) through collabora-tion with dietitian. *Clients unable to take oral food require parenteral nutrition or liquid feedings through a nasogastric, gastrostomy, or jejunostomy tube. Needs for protein, calories, zinc, and vitamin C increase during wound healing.*

THE CLIENT WITH INCREASED INTRACRANIAL PRESSURE

Increased intracranial pressure (IICP) (also labeled *intracranial hypertension*) is sustained elevated pressure (10 mmHg or higher) within the cranial cavity (Wilensky & Bloom, 2005). Transient in-creases in ICP occur with normal activities such as coughing, sneezing, straining, or bending forward. These transient increases are not harmful; however, sustained IICP can result in significant tissue ischemia and damage to delicate neural tissue. Cerebral edema is the most frequent cause of sustained increases in ICP. Other causes include head trauma, tumors, abscesses, stroke, in-flammation, and hemorrhage.

Pathophysiology

In the adult, the rigid cranial cavity created by the skull is normally filled to capacity with three essentially noncompressible elements: the brain (80%), cerebrospinal fluid (8%), and blood (12%). A state of dynamic equilibrium exists; if the volume of any of the three components increases, the volume of the others must de-crease to maintain normal pressures within the cranial cavity. This is known as the *Monro-Kellie hypothesis.* The normal intracranial pressure is 5 to 10 mmHg (measured intracranially with a pressure transducer while the client is lying with the head elevated 30 de-grees) or 60 to 180 cm H_2O (measured with a water manometer while the client is lying in a lateral recumbent position).

Cerebral blood flow and perfusion are important concepts for understanding the development and effects of increased intracranial pressure. Whereas blood and CSF contribute an equal percentage to normal intracranial volume, vascular factors account for twice the amount of increase in ICP that CSF does. The brain requires a constant supply of oxygen and glucose to meet its metabolic demands; 15% to 20% of the resting cardiac output goes to the brain to meet its metabolic needs. Interruption of the cerebral blood flow leads to ischemia and disruption of the cerebral metabolism.

Pressure and chemical autoregulation are compensatory mechanisms in which cerebral arterioles change diameter to maintain cerebral blood flow when ICP increases. In pressure autoregulation, stretch receptors within small blood vessels of the brain cause smooth muscle of the arterioles to contract. Increased arterial pressure stimulates these receptors, leading to vasoconstriction; when arterial pressure is low, stimulation of these receptors decreases, causing relaxation and vasodilation. Chemical, or metabolic, autoregulation works in much the same way as pressure autoregulation. In this case, the stimulus is a buildup of metabolic by-products of cell metabolism, including lactic acid, pyruvic acid, carbonic acid, and carbon dioxide. Carbon dioxide and increased hydrogen ion concentration are potent cerebral vasodilators that may act locally or systemically to increase cerebral blood flow. Conversely, a fall in $PaCO_2$ causes cerebral vasoconstriction. Arterial oxygen tension (PaO_2) also affects cerebral blood flow, although it is a less powerful mechanism than that exerted by carbon dioxide and hydrogen ions.

IICP may result from an increase in intracranial contents from a space-occupying lesion, hydrocephalus, cerebral edema (swelling), excess cerebrospinal fluid, or intracranial hemorrhage. Displacement of some CSF to the spinal subarachnoid space and increased CSF absorption are early compensatory mechanisms. The low-pressure venous system is also compressed, and cerebral arteries constrict to reduce blood flow. Brain tissue's ability to accommodate change is relatively restricted. The relationship between the volume of the intracranial components and intracranial pressure is known as *compliance*. When the capacity to compensate for increased intracranial pressure is exceeded, increased intracranial pressure (hypertension) develops. Intracranial hypertension is a sustained state of IICP and is potentially life threatening.

Autoregulatory mechanisms have a limited ability to maintain cerebral blood flow. When autoregulation fails, cerebrovascular tone is reduced and cerebral blood flow becomes dependent on changes in blood pressure. Autoregulation may be lost either locally or globally because of several factors, including increasing intracranial pressure, local or diffuse cerebral tissue ischemia or inflammation, prolonged hypotension, and hypercapnia or hypoxia.

Manifestations

With loss of autoregulation, intracranial pressure continues to rise and cerebral perfusion falls. Cerebral tissue becomes ischemic, and manifestations of cellular hypoxia appear. The manifestations of IICP are listed in the box on this page.

Level of Consciousness

Because the neurons of the cerebral cortex are most sensitive to oxygen deficit, changes in cortical function are the earliest man-

---

MANIFESTATIONS of Increased Intracranial Pressure

- Decreased level of consciousness. *Early*: Confusion; restlessness, lethargy; disorientation, first to time, then to place and person. *Late:* Comatose with no response to painful stimuli.
- Pupillary dysfunction. Sluggish response to light progressing to fixed pupils; with a localized process, pupillary dysfunction is first noted on the ipsilateral side.
- Oculomotor dysfunction. Inability to move eye(s) upward; ptosis (drooping) of the eyelid.
- Visual abnormalities. Decreased visual acuity, blurred vision, diplopia.
- Papilledema. May be late sign.
- Motor impairment. *Early*: Hemiparesis or hemiplegia of the contralateral side. *Late*: Abnormal responses such as decorticate or decerebrate positioning; flaccidity.
- Headache. Uncommon but may occur with processes that slowly increase ICP; worse on rising in the morning and with position changes.
- Projectile vomiting without nausea.
- Cushing's response. Increased systolic blood pressure, widening pulse pressure, bradycardia.
- Respirations. Altered respiratory pattern related to level of brain dysfunction.
- Temperature. May be significantly elevated as compensatory mechanisms fail.

---

ifestations of increasing ICP (Porth, 2005). Behavior and personality changes occur; the client may become irritable and agitated. Memory and judgment are impaired, and speech pattern changes may be noted. The client's LOC decreases. As cerebral hypertension and hypoxia progress, the LOC continues to decrease in a predictable pattern to coma and unresponsiveness.

Motor Responses

Pressure on the pyramidal tract often causes weakness (hemiparesis) on the contralateral side early in IICP. As ICP continues to increase, hemiplegia and abnormal motor responses, such as decorticate or decerebrate posturing, develop (see Chapter 43 ∞ for an illustration of these postures).

Vision and Pupils

Altered vision is an early manifestation of IICP; it is caused by pressure on the visual pathways and cranial nerves. Blurred vision, decreased visual acuity, and diplopia are common. Pupillary and oculomotor responses are affected as well. Because the cause of IICP is often localized at first, pupillary changes, including gradual dilation and sluggish response to light, may initially be limited to the ipsilateral side.

Vital Signs

Ischemia of the vasomotor center in the brainstem triggers the CNS ischemic response, a late sign of IICP. Neuronal ischemia in the vasomotor center causes a marked increase in the mean arterial pressure (MAP), with a significant increase in systolic blood pressure and increased pulse pressure. The increased

MAP causes reflexive slowing of the cardiac rate. This trio of manifestations (increased MAP, increased pulse pressure, and bradycardia) is known as *Cushing's response* (or triad), and represents the brainstem's final effort to maintain cerebral perfusion (Porth, 2005). The respiratory pattern also changes, often in the predictable progression outlined earlier in Table 44–1. Although the temperature is usually normal in early stages, as ICP continues to increase, hypothalamic function is impaired and the temperature may rise dramatically.

Other Manifestations

Additional manifestations of IICP include headache, particularly on rising, that worsens with position changes. Headache is more common with slowly developing IICP and occurs because of pressure on pain-sensitive structures, such as the middle meningeal arteries, the venous sinuses, and the dura at the base of the skull. Papilledema (edema and swelling of the optic disk) may be noted on funduscopic examination. Vomiting, often projectile and occurring without warning, may develop.

Cerebral Edema

Cerebral edema is an increase in the volume of brain tissue due to abnormal accumulation of fluid. Cerebral edema is often associated with increased intracranial pressure; it may occur as a local process in the area of a tumor or injury, or it may affect the entire brain. Two types of cerebral edema have been identified and are described as follows (Porth, 2005):

- *Vasogenic edema*, an increase in the capillary permeability of cerebral vessels, occurs with impairment of the blood–brain barrier, allowing diffusion of water and protein into the interstitial spaces of the brain. A variety of pathologies, such as ischemia, hemorrhage, brain tumors and injuries, and infections (such as meningitis), may cause the increase in capillary permeability. The site of the brain injury, the level of increase in capillary permeability, and the client's systemic blood pressure influence the rate and extent of the edema's spread. Vasogenic edema is manifested by focal (localized) neurologic deficits, altered levels of consciousness, and severe intracranial hypertension.
- *Cytotoxic edema*, actual swelling of the brain cells from an increase in intracellular fluid, involves changes in the functional or structural integrity of cell membranes due to pathologies such as water intoxication (such as from the syndrome of inappropriate secretion of antidiuretic hormone [SIADH]) or severe ischemia, intracranial hypoxia, acidosis, and brain trauma. With abnormally low cerebral perfusion, oxygen and nutrients are depleted, intracranial cells switch to anaerobic metabolism, and the sodium-potassium pump in the cell walls is impaired. Sodium diffuses into the cells, pulling fluid with it. The cells swell, and intracranial pressure rises. Accumulated metabolic waste products, such as lactic acid, contribute to a rapid deterioration of cell function. Cytotoxic edema is a slowly progressive process that results in altered consciousness. The edema may be so severe that it causes cerebral infarction with brain tissue necrosis.

Cerebral edema tends to be proportional to the extent of the pathology precipitating it. Brain function is not disrupted by cerebral edema unless the edema causes an increase in ICP. When it does, a vicious cycle can ensue: Cerebral edema increases ICP, which in turn decreases cerebral blood flow. Brain tissue becomes hypoxic and ischemic, increasing toxic metabolic by-products, hydrogen ion concentration, and carbon dioxide levels in the tissue. Autoregulatory mechanisms cause vasodilation and increase cerebral blood flow, further increasing cerebral edema and intracranial pressure. Without effective intervention, the client's condition can deteriorate rapidly; intracranial pressure increases to the point where brain structures herniate.

Hydrocephalus

Hydrocephalus refers to a progressive dilatation of the ventricular system, which becomes dilated as the production of CSF exceeds its absorption (Hickey, 2003). Hydrocephalus may increase ICP when it develops acutely. It is generally classified as either noncommunicating or communicating hydrocephalus. Noncommunicating hydrocephalus occurs when CSF drainage from the ventricular system is obstructed. It may develop when a mass or tumor, inflammation or hemorrhage, or congenital malformation obstructs the ventricular system. Communicating hydrocephalus is a condition in which CSF is not effectively reabsorbed through the arachnoid villi. It may occur secondarily to subarachnoid hemorrhage or scarring from infection. In *normal pressure hydrocephalus*, seen most often in adults age 60 or older, ventricular enlargement causes cerebral tissue compression but the CSF pressure on lumbar puncture is normal. This condition may follow cerebral trauma or surgery, or the cause may not be known.

Manifestations of hydrocephalus depend on the rate of its development. They may be mild and insidious in onset, presenting as progressive cognitive dysfunctions, gait disruptions, and urinary incontinence. If the process causing hydrocephalus is an acute one, the manifestations are those of IICP.

Brain Herniation

If IICP is not treated, cerebral tissue is displaced toward a more compliant area. This can result in brain herniation, the displacement of brain tissue from its normal compartment under dural folds of the falx cerebri or through the tentorial notch or incisura of the tentorium cerebelli (Porth, 2005). Herniation of the cerebellum through the tentorium exerts pressure on the brainstem, with subsequent herniation through the foramen magnum. This is a lethal complication of IICP because it puts pressure on the vital centers of the medulla.

Brain herniation syndromes are generally categorized as supratentorial or infratentorial, depending on their location above or below the tentorium cerebelli (Figure 44–2 ■). Supratentorial herniation syndromes include cingulate herniation, central or transtentorial herniation, uncal or lateral transtentorial herniation, and infratentorial.

- *Cingulate herniation* (Figure 44–2A) occurs when the cingulate gyrus is displaced under the falx cerebri. Local blood supply and cerebral tissue are compressed, resulting in ischemia and further increases in intracranial pressure.

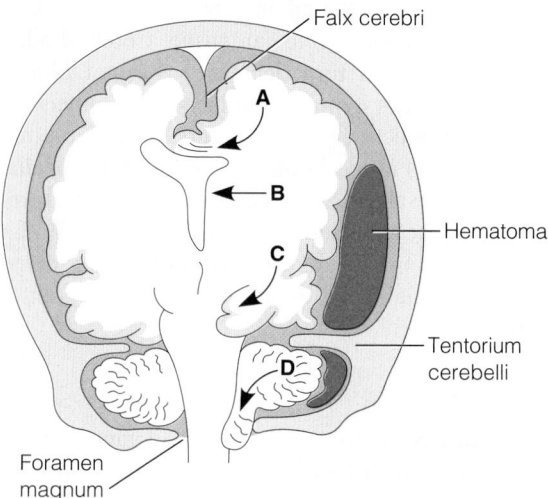

Figure 44–2 ■ Forms of brain herniation due to intracranial hypertension. *A,* Cingulate herniation occurs when the cingulate gyrus is compressed under the falx cerebri. *B,* Central herniation occurs when a centrally located lesion compresses central and midbrain structures. *C,* Lateral herniation occurs when a lesion at the side of the brain compresses the uncus or hippocampal gyrus. *D,* Infratentorial herniation occurs when the cerebellar tonsils are forced downward, compressing the medulla and top of the spinal cord.

- *Central or transtentorial herniation* is the downward displacement of brain structures, including the cerebral hemispheres, basal ganglia, diencephalon, and midbrain through the tentorial incisura (Figure 44–2B). The client's neurologic signs may deteriorate rapidly, with decreased LOC progressing to coma, Cheyne-Stokes respirations progressing to central neurogenic hyperventilation, and pupils progressing from small and reactive to midsize and fixed. The client may demonstrate abnormal motor responses with unilateral decorticate posturing.
- *Uncal or lateral transtentorial herniation* occurs when a lateral mass displaces cerebral tissue centrally, forcing the medial aspect of the temporal lobe under the edge of the tentorial incisura (Figure 44–2C). The oculomotor nerve (cranial nerve III) often becomes trapped between the uncus and the tentorium, causing ipsilateral pupillary dilation. Other manifestations include alterations in LOC, motor deficits (which may occur on the same side as the herniation because of compression of the cerebral peduncle on the opposite side), decreased sensation, respiratory changes, abnormal positioning, and eventual respiratory arrest.
- *Infratentorial herniation* results from increased pressure within the infratentorial compartment. Herniation may occur either upward, with structures displaced through the tentorial incisura, or downward, with displacement through the foramen magnum (Figure 44–2D). Downward displacement compresses the medulla, including its centers for controlling vital functions. Manifestations associated with medullary compression include coma, altered respiratory patterns, fixed pupils, and decorticate or decerebrate posturing. Respiratory or cardiac arrest may occur.

INTERDISCIPLINARY CARE

Management of the client with IICP is directed toward identifying and treating the underlying cause of the disorder, and controlling ICP to prevent herniation syndrome. IICP is a medical emergency, and there is little time to complete lengthy diagnostic tests. The diagnosis must be made on the basis of observation and neurologic assessment; even subtle changes may be clinically significant.

Diagnosis

Diagnostic tests focus on identifying the presence of IICP and its underlying cause. A CT scan or MRI is generally the initial test used to identify the possible causes of IICP (such as space-occupying lesions or hydrocephalus) and to evaluate therapeutic options. In general, a lumbar puncture is not performed when IICP is suspected because the sudden release of the pressure in the skull may cause cerebral herniation.

In addition to the diagnostic tests listed in the previous section for altered LOC, the following specific tests are usually ordered and their results closely monitored:

- Serum osmolality is an indicator of hydration status in the client with IICP. The test measures the number of dissolved particles (electrolytes, urea, glucose) in the serum. The normal range for the adult is 280 to 300 mOsm/kg H_2O. In addition to the restriction of fluids in the client with IICP, serum osmolality is maintained at a slightly elevated level (325 mOsm/kg H_2O) to draw excess intracellular fluid into the vascular system.
- ABGs are monitored frequently to assess pH and levels of oxygen and carbon dioxide. Hydrogen ions and carbon dioxide are both potent vasodilators; hypoxemia also causes vasodilation, although to a lesser degree.

Medications

Medications play an important role in the management of IICP. Diuretics, particularly osmotic diuretics, are commonly used to reduce ICP and are the mainstays of pharmacologic treatment. Nursing implications for these medications are described in the Medication Administration box on the next page.

Osmotic diuretics work by increasing the osmolarity of the blood, thereby drawing water out of edematous brain tissue and into the vascular system for elimination via the kidneys. The effects of these drugs vary with the type of injury. Regardless of the agent used, the optimal dose is the lowest that reduces ICP. Mannitol is the most commonly employed osmotic diuretic. Glucose, urea, and glycerol are other osmotic diuretics that may be used. Urine output by Foley catheter is monitored. Electrolyte levels are carefully assessed and potassium is replaced as indicated.

Loop diuretics, such as furosemide (Lasix) (the drug of choice) and ethacrynic acid (Edecrin), may be prescribed for some clients with IICP. These diuretics act on the renal tubule and are extremely effective in promoting diuresis. Additionally, loop diuretics may be used to manage the rebound effect that may occur with mannitol administration.

Sedation and paralysis are used as chemical restraints to control restlessness and agitation, because these movements increase blood pressure, ICP, and cerebral metabolism. Paralysis

MEDICATION ADMINISTRATION   Increased Intracranial Pressure

OSMOTIC DIURETICS
Mannitol (Osmitrol)
Urea
Glucose

Osmotic diuretics (hyperosmotic agents) draw fluid out of brain cells by increasing the osmolality of the blood. The effects of these drugs vary with the type of injury. Mannitol therapy is often initiated if the client's ICP has exceeded 15 to 20 mmHg for at least 10 minutes. Both intravenous bolus and continuous infusion techniques are used. Repeated use of mannitol can lead to continual elevations in serum osmolality, with attendant risk of seizures and serious fluid and electrolyte imbalance. Urea is seldom administered intravenously because a severe local reaction may result if leakage occurs at the injection site. Mannitol and urea are used cautiously if renal disease is present.

Note: Because the client with increased intracranial pressure often has an altered level of consciousness, client and family teaching are not discussed in this box.

Nursing Responsibilities
- Monitor vital signs, urinary output, central venous pressure (CVP), and pulmonary artery pressures (PAP) before and every hour throughout administration.
- Assess client for manifestations of dehydration.
- Assess client for muscle weakness, numbness, tingling, paresthesia, confusion, and excessive thirst.
- Assess client for pulmonary edema while administering the medication.
- Monitor neurologic status and intracranial pressure readings.
- Monitor renal function and serum electrolytes throughout therapy.
- Do not administer the medication if crystals are present in solution. Administer with an in-line filter. Observe infusion site frequently for infiltration.
- Do not administer mannitol solution with blood.
- Do not discontinue medication abruptly. Rebound migraine headaches may occur.

LOOP DIURETICS
Furosemide (Lasix)
Ethacrynic acid (Edecrin)

Loop diuretics such as furosemide and ethacrynic acid inhibit sodium and chloride reabsorption at the ascending loop of Henle. They cause a reduction in the rate of CSF production, thus reducing the ICP.

Nursing Responsibilities
- Monitor vital signs and electrolyte values closely.
- Assess fluid status throughout therapy.
- Monitor blood pressure and pulse before and during administration.
- Monitor renal laboratory studies closely.
- Use infusion pump to ensure accurate dosage.

INTRAVENOUS FLUIDS
Keeping the client moderately dehydrated to maintain serum osmolality can be effective in reducing cerebral edema. When giving intravenous fluids, closely monitor the osmolality of the solutions; if clients with increased ICP are given hypo-osmolar solutions, increased cerebral edema can occur. Preferred solutions include 0.45% to 0.9% sodium chloride solutions.

Nursing Responsibilities
- Monitor fluid status closely.
- Monitor neurologic status closely.
- Avoid administering hypo-osmolar solutions, such as 5% dextrose in water.
- Half-strength normal saline (0.45% sodium chloride) is considered a suitable fluid for a client who has increased intracranial pressure.
- Take care not to restrict fluids excessively in clients receiving dehydrating agents (such as osmotic or loop diuretics).

OTHER PHARMACOLOGIC INTERVENTIONS FOR ICP
- Antipyretics, such as acetaminophen, are used to reduce hyperthermia, thereby decreasing the high cerebral metabolism that contributes to ICP.
- Antiulcer drugs, such as histamine H_2 antagonists (for example, ranitidine [Zantac]) or sucralfate (Carafate), are used in clients with ICP to decrease the development of stress ulcers.
- Antihypertensive agents, such as beta-adrenergic blocking agents, may be used if the mean arterial pressure is high.
- Vasopressors may be used if the mean arterial pressure is low.
- Anticonvulsants may be given to prevent or treat seizures.

---

with neuromuscular blockage is most often accomplished with pancuronium. Clients must be closely monitored during treatment for residual muscle weakness and signs of respiratory distress. A peripheral nerve stimulator may be used for this purpose.

Antipyretics, such as acetaminophen, are used alone or in combination with a hypothermia blanket to treat hyperthermia. Hyperthermia increases the cerebral metabolic rate and exacerbates an existing increase in ICP. Anticonvulsants are often required to manage seizure activity associated with brain injury and IICP. Gastrointestinal prophylaxis with intravenous histamine H_2 antagonists or proton pump inhibitors are often used, because clients with IICP are at increased risk for the development of stress gastritis and ulcers (Tierney et al., 2005).

Intravenous fluids are usually necessary to maintain the client's fluid and electrolyte balance as well as vascular volume. If the client's blood pressure is unstable, vasoactive medications may be administered to maintain the MAP in a range that supports cerebral perfusion while minimizing increases in ICP. When enteral feeding is not possible, total parenteral nutrition may be administered.

Surgery

Clients with IICP may undergo various intracranial surgical techniques to treat the underlying cause (see the discussion in the later section on brain tumors). In addition, infarcted or necrotic tissue may be resected to reduce brain mass. A drainage catheter or shunt may be inserted laterally via a burr hole into a ventricle to drain excess cerebrospinal fluid and reduce hydrocephalus. The removal of even a small amount of CSF may dramatically reduce IICP and restore cerebral perfusion pressure.

ICP Monitoring

Critical to preserving brain function and preventing secondary brain damage from IICP are careful assessments and monitoring with ICP monitors, measuring cerebral blood flow and cerebral perfusion pressure, and measuring oxygen levels of brain tissue. Intracranial pressure monitors facilitate continual assessment of ICP and the effects of medical therapy and nursing interventions on ICP. In addition, cerebral perfusion pressure (the difference between MAP and ICP) can be readily calculated, allowing more precise manipulation of therapeutic measures to maintain cerebral perfusion and thereby prevent ischemia. The criteria for ICP monitoring depends on the client, but in general, clients who are comatose and have a Glasgow Coma Score (described in Chapter 43 ∞) of 8 or less should be monitored.

Basic monitoring systems include an intraventricular catheter, subarachnoid bolt or screw, and epidural probe (Figure 44–3 ■). Intraventricular fluid-filled catheters are placed in the anterior horn of the lateral ventricle (most often in the right side). Ventricular catheters can both drain CSF and measure ICP. The ICP value is measured deep in the brain and is considered the most reflective of the whole brain pressure. Subarachnoid devices are placed in the subarachnoid space. A fiber-optic transducer-tipped catheter can be placed in the epidural, subdural, or parenchymal space, with ICP values considered very accurate. Once the intracranial sensor is implanted, it is connected to a transducer that converts the impulses to a signal that the recording device can translate into an oscilloscope tracing, digital value, or graphic recording. Factors that increase the risk for infection during ICP monitoring are listed in Table 44–4.

Transcranial blood flow is monitored with transcranial Doppler studies (TCD) to measure the velocity of blood flow in the cerebral vessels. Cerebral perfusion pressure (CPP) is the pressure it takes for the heart to provide the brain with blood, calculated by subtracting the ICP from mean arterial pressure (normal CPP is 70 to 95 mmHg). Brain oxygenation monitoring may be conducted by using a jugular bulb oxygen saturation (SjO_2) monitor connected to a small fiber-optic catheter inserted into the jugular vein. (Normal SjO_2 is 50% to 75%.) Another device used to monitor brain tissue oxygenation is the LICOX system, which includes information about oxygen status and temperature status within the brain tissue itself (Brettler, 2004). In addition, cerebral microdialysis catheters can provide information about the nature of the cerebral interstitial fluid.

Figure 44–3 ■ Types of intracranial pressure monitoring. *A*, Epidural probe. *B*, Subarachnoid screw. *C*, Intraventricular catheter.

Mechanical Ventilation

Clients with ICP often require intubation and are placed on a ventilator for respiratory management. Mechanical ventilation may be used to maintain partial pressure of oxygen and carbon dioxide, thus preventing hypoxemia and hypercapnia, both of which can increase intracranial pressure. It is important to maintain adequate oxygenation with a partial pressure of arterial oxygen at about 100 mmHg and a partial pressure of arterial carbon dioxide of about 35 mmHg. The client with IICP and signs of impending herniation may be judiciously hyperventilated to cause cerebral vasoconstriction; however, this also increases cerebral ischemia.

TABLE 44–4 **Risk Factors for Infection with Intracranial Pressure Monitoring**

FACTOR	RATIONALE
Intraventricular catheter	Is more invasive than other monitoring devices
Open head trauma or neurosurgery	Disrupts protective skin and skeletal barriers
Intracranial hemorrhage	Necessitates frequent flushing of catheter to maintain patency
Older adult	Tends to have impaired immune defenses
Monitoring for more than 3 to 5 days; or open system or frequent irrigation	Offers increased opportunity for pathogens to enter and grow

NURSING CARE

The nursing care of clients with IICP involves identifying those at risk and managing factors known to increase intracranial pressure. A major focus is protecting the client from sudden increases in ICP or a decrease in cerebral blood flow.

Nursing Diagnoses and Interventions

Nursing interventions include performing neurologic assessments, maintaining the patency of the airway, ensuring adequate ventilation, positioning and moving, instituting seizure precautions, and monitoring fluids and electrolytes. Additionally, both client and family need emotional support during this period. The client with IICP has varied responses to actual or potential changes in physiologic processes.

Ineffective Tissue Perfusion: Cerebral

A number of disorders may lead to IICP, including cerebral edema, hydrocephalus, space-occupying lesions and hemorrhage, herniation syndromes, and changes in carbon dioxide concentrations. Increasing intracranial pressure alters cerebral perfusion and oxygenation of brain cells. The client with IICP requires intensive care, and often needs ventilator assistance.

- Assess for and report manifestations of IICP every 15 minutes to 1 hour and as necessary. Assessment areas include LOC, behavior, motor/sensory functions, pupillary size and reaction to light, and vital signs, including temperature. Look for trends, because vital signs alone do not correlate well with early deterioration. *Assessment of neurologic status establishes the client's clinical condition and provides a baseline to measure changes. Sudden changes in neurologic signs often indicate deterioration. An elevated temperature with increased oxygen consumption further increases intracranial pressure. Pupillary responses mirror the status of the midbrain and pons. Pressure on the brainstem may compromise the function of cranial nerves IX and X and protective mechanisms, such as the gag and cough reflexes.*

> **PRACTICE ALERT**
> Often, the earliest manifestations of a change in intracranial pressure are alterations in the level of consciousness and respirations.

- For the client on a ventilator: Maintain patency of the airway; preoxygenate with 100% oxygen before suctioning; limit suctioning to 10 seconds; suction gently. *Preoxygenation helps maintain oxygen levels during suctioning. Suctioning stimulates the cough reflex and Valsalva maneuver. Correct suctioning minimizes the risk of hypoxemia.*
- Monitor ABGs. *ABGs provide a reliable indicator of oxygen and carbon dioxide levels. If oxygen concentration is low, oxygen may be given or increased.*
- Elevate head of the bed to 30 degrees or keep flat, as prescribed; maintain the alignment of the head and neck to avoid hyperextension or exaggerated neck flexion; avoid prone position. *Keeping the head of the bed elevated facilitates venous drainage from the cerebrum. Obstruction of jugular veins can impede venous drainage from the brain.*

- Monitor bladder distention and bowel constipation. Administer stool softeners and use the Credé technique (applying pressure to the suprapubic region with the fingers of one or both hands) to empty the bladder. If the Credé technique is not effective, evaluate the pros and cons of urinary catheterization if the bladder remains distended. *Constipation and bladder distention increase intrathoracic or intra-abdominal pressure and place the client at risk for impaired venous drainage from the brain.*
- If alert, assist in moving up in bed. Do not ask to push with heels or arms or push against a footboard. Avoid a footboard and restraints. *Moving up in bed requires pushing. Helping the client move prevents initiation of the Valsalva maneuver, which increases intracranial pressure.*
- Plan nursing care so that activities are not clustered together; avoid turning the client, getting the client on the bedpan, or suctioning within the same time period. Schedule nursing care to provide rest periods between procedures. *Multiple procedures, including certain nursing care activities, can increase ICP. Constant stimulation tends to increase ICP. Individualized nursing care ensures optimal spacing of activities and rest.*
- Provide a quiet environment, limiting noxious stimuli. Avoid jarring the bed. Try to limit situations that cause emotional upset; maintain a calm, reassuring manner; caution family members to refrain from unpleasant conversations or conversations that may be emotionally stimulating to the client. *Noxious stimuli and emotional upsets cause an elevation in ICP.*
- Maintain fluid limitations, if prescribed. *Restricting fluids helps decrease cerebral edema by reducing total body water.*

Risk for Infection

Although any client with an open head wound is at risk for infection, the interventions discussed here are for the client with an intracranial monitoring device. Most clinical units have written protocols for managing these systems. The following nursing actions serve only as a general guide.

- Keep dressings over the catheter dry, and change dressings on a prescribed basis (usually every 24 to 48 hours). *Wet dressings are conducive to bacterial growth.*
- Monitor the insertion site for leaking CSF, drainage, or infection. Monitor for manifestations of infection, including changes in vital signs, chills, increased WBC counts, and positive cultures of drainage. *Close monitoring helps detect the earliest signs of infection and helps prevent major complications. Fever is usually considered the key assessment. However, fever in a client with a neurologic disorder may be due to damage to the hypothalamus. Headache, generalized muscle aches, shivering, and chills may also be seen in the client with infection.*
- Use strict aseptic technique when in contact with the device. Check drainage system for loose connections. *The use of aseptic technique and monitoring drainage systems for loose connections help prevent nosocomial infections. Most nosocomial infections are transmitted by healthcare workers who fail to wash their hands properly, to change gloves between clients, or to follow aseptic technique protocols. Invasive procedures provide an excellent opportunity for microbes to enter the body.*

Client and Family Education

Teach the client at risk for or having IICP (and able to follow instructions) to avoid coughing, blowing the nose, straining to have a bowel movement, pushing against the bed rails, or performing isometric (muscle contracting) exercises. Advise the client to maintain head and neck alignment when turning in bed and to take rest periods.

Encourage the family to talk to the client, but maintain a quiet environment with a minimum of stimuli. Inform family members that upsetting the client may increase intracranial pressure and that they should avoid discussions that may distress the client. For clients unable to make decisions about treatment and to sign informed consent, the family must carry out these functions.

THE CLIENT WITH A HEADACHE

Headache, one of the most frequent manifestations of a health problem people experience, is pain within the cranial vault. Headaches may occur as a result of benign or pathologic conditions, intracranial or extracranial conditions, diseases of other body systems, stress, musculoskeletal tension, or a combination of these factors.

Most headaches are mild, transient, and relieved by a mild analgesic. However, some headaches are chronic, intense, and recurrent. Manifestations of headache vary according to the cause, type, and precipitating symptoms.

Pathophysiology

The bones and brain tissue itself lack pain-sensitive nerve fibers, but selected structures within the cranial vault are sensitive to pain. Headache is experienced when there is traction, pressure, displacement, inflammation, or dilation of nociceptors (nerve endings that are receptors of noxious stimuli) in areas sensitive to pain (Hickey, 2003). Pain-sensitive structures include supporting structures, such as the skin, muscles, and periosteum; the nasal cavities and sinuses; portions of the meninges, cranial nerves II, III, IV, V, VI, IX, and X; and cerebral vessels, including extracranial arteries and the venous sinuses. Most facial and scalp structures are sensitive to pain. The most common types of headaches are migraine, cluster, and tension headaches (Table 44–5).

Migraine Headache

Migraine headache is a recurring vascular headache lasting from 4 to 72 hours, often initiated by a triggering event and usually accompanied by a neurologic dysfunction. It affects about 15% of the population, with three times as many women as men having migraines (eMedicine Health, 2006). It is more common between the ages of 25 and 55 years. More than 80% of people with migraines (called *migraineurs*) have family members with them too. Migraine headaches may occur daily or as infrequently as once a year.

> **FAST FACTS**
> **Migraine Headache**
> - Eight out of 10 migraineurs have severe or extremely severe attacks.
> - One out of 4 migraineurs seek emergency room treatment.
> - Fifty-one percent of migraineurs say that the headache reduces their work and/or school productivity by at least 50%.
> - The direct and indirect annual costs of migraines is approximately $13 billion (National Headache Foundation, 2005).

There are two types of migraine headaches: common migraine (without an aura) and classic migraine (with an aura; most often experienced as a visual disturbance prior to the

TABLE 44–5 Comparison of Migraine, Cluster, and Tension Headaches

TYPE	RISK FACTORS	FREQUENCY AND DURATION	DESCRIPTION	PRODROMAL AND ASSOCIATED MANIFESTATIONS
Migraine	Female Family history of migraine headache.	Episodic: - Tends to occur with stress and crisis. - Often correlates with menstrual cycle. - Can last hours to days.	Slow onset; pain becomes more severe, involving one side of head more than other.	Prodromal manifestations: visual defects, confusion, paresthesias. Associated manifestations: nausea, vomiting, chills, fatigue, irritability, sweating.
Cluster	Male Use of alcohol or nitrates. May begin in early childhood.	Episodes are clustered together in rapid succession for a few days or weeks with remissions that last for months. Can last a few minutes to a few hours.	May begin in infraorbital region and spread to head and neck; throbbing, deep pain, often unilateral.	Prodromal manifestations: uncommon. Associated manifestations: flushing, tearing of eyes, nasal congestion, sweating and swelling of temporal vessels.
Tension	Related to tension and anxiety. No family history. Often begins in adolescence.	Episodic: - Varies with amount of stress. - Duration also varies; can be constant.	Tight, pressing, viselike; may involve neck and shoulders.	Prodromal manifestations: uncommon. Associated manifestations: sustained contraction of neck muscles.

pain). Common migraines occur in 80% of the people who are affected by this disorder. Headaches classified as migraines may differ in intensity, duration, and frequency. The exact causes of migraine are not fully understood, but they are believed to be the result of abnormalities in cerebrovascular blood flow, a reduction in brain and electrical activity, or increased release of sensory substances such as serotonin, norepinephrine, substance P, nitric oxide, or glutamate.

A variety of factors are believed to trigger the onset of a migraine headache. Rapid changes in blood glucose levels, stress, emotional excitement, fatigue, hormonal changes due to menstruation, stimuli such as bright lights, and food high in tyramine or other vasoactive substances (e.g., aged cheese, nuts, chocolate, and alcoholic beverages) have been associated with migraine attacks. Hypertension and fever may make the disorder worse.

COMMON MIGRAINE This type is the most common and is associated with hereditary factors. The aura stage is absent; clients are aware only that a headache is eminent. The headache develops gradually, lasting hours to days, and may occur in women during periods of premenstrual tension and fluid retention. Chills, nausea and vomiting, fatigue, and nasal congestion are often present.

CLASSIC MIGRAINE The classic migraine headache has several stages, as follows:

- The aura stage is characterized by sensory manifestations, usually visual disturbances such as bright spots or flashing lights zigzagging across the visual fields. This stage lasts from 5 to 60 minutes. Less common sensory symptoms include numbness or tingling of the face or hand, weakness of an arm or leg, mild aphasia, confusion, drowsiness, and lack of coordination. Additionally, some clients experience a premonition the day prior to an attack. They may feel nervous or have other mood changes. The aura period corresponds with the initial physiologic change of vasoconstriction.
- The headache stage is characterized by vasodilation, a decline in serotonin levels, and the onset of throbbing headache. It appears that the pain is related to increased vessel permeability and polypeptide exudation by perivascular nerve endings rather than the vasodilation itself. Cerebral arteries are dilated and distended, with walls that are edematous and rigid. Beginning unilaterally, the headache eventually may involve both sides as it increases in intensity during the next several hours. Nausea and vomiting often occur. The client may be acutely ill and is often extremely irritable. The sensory organs often become hypersensitive, and the client withdraws from sound and light. The scalp is tender. The headache may last from several hours to a day or two.
- During the post-headache phase, the headache area is sensitive to touch, and a deep aching is present. The client is exhausted. Vessel size and serotonin levels return to normal.

Cluster Headache

A *cluster headache* is an extremely severe, unilateral, burning pain located behind or around the eyes. The cluster headache is predominantly experienced by men between the ages of 20 and 40 years. The headaches occur in groups or "clusters" of one to eight each day for several weeks or months, followed by remission lasting months to years (Hickey, 2003). The physiologic mechanism underlying cluster headaches is not well understood, but involves a vascular disorder, a disturbance of serotonergic mechanisms, a sympathetic defect, or dysregulation of the hypothalamus.

Although the headache may occur at any time, it typically begins 2 to 3 hours after falling asleep, awakens the person, and then lasts from 15 to 180 minutes. Prodromal signs are absent. Intense unilateral pain around or behind one eye is accompanied by rhinorrhea, lacrimation, flushing, sweating, facial edema, and possible miosis or ptosis on the affected side. The same side of the head is involved in each cluster of attacks.

The headaches often occur in the spring and fall and then disappear for an extended period. Attacks may be triggered by drinking alcohol, eating specific foods, medications such as nitroglycerin, or there may be no known precipitating event.

Tension Headache

Tension headache is characterized by bilateral pain, with a sensation of a band of tightness or pressure around the head. Sharply localized painful spots (trigger points) may be present. The onset is gradual, and the intensity, frequency, and duration of the attack vary greatly. This type of headache is caused by sustained contraction of the muscles of the head and neck. It is often precipitated by stressful situations and anxiety. Secondary causes include prolonged computer use and disorders of the eyes, ears, sinuses, or cervical vertebrae. Abnormal posture associated with occupations that require bending over a desk (e.g., office workers, students) often precipitates tension-type headache. Additionally, slouching while reading or watching television can lead to muscle contraction. Most headaches are tension-type headaches.

INTERDISCIPLINARY CARE

Identifying the underlying cause(s) of the headache is the initial focus of interdisciplinary care. If the underlying cause is treatable, the headache will often decrease or disappear. An accurate diagnosis of the type of headache is key to the treatment.

Therapeutic management for migraine headache includes a combination of client teaching, medications, and measures to control contributing factors. Dietary changes such as eliminating caffeine, cured meats, monosodium glutamate (MSG), and foods containing tyramine (red wine, aged cheese, and others) may be necessary. Stress management or biofeedback is also part of the overall strategy. Treatment protocols for cluster headache include eliminating aggravating factors (e.g., consumption of alcohol) and using medications and oxygen inhalation. The management of tension headaches is directed toward reducing the client's level of stress and relieving pain with ice and aspirin or nonsteroidal anti-inflammatory drugs (NSAIDs).

Diagnosis

Diagnosis and treatment are based on history, identifying triggering or precipitating events, and the type of headache. A thorough history and physical examination are integral parts of the assessment. Neurodiagnostic testing may be done to rule out a structural disease process. Testing may include a brain scan,

MRI, x-ray studies of the skull and cervical spine, EEG, or lumbar puncture for CSF if inflammation is suspected. Serum metabolic screens and hypersensitivity testing also may be performed if systemic problems are suspected.

Medications

Pharmacologic management depends on the type of headache. The goals of treatment are to reduce the frequency and severity of headaches and to limit or relieve a headache that is beginning or in progress.

The management of migraine headache includes administering medications to prevent pain (prophylactic therapy) as well as drugs to stop (or abort) a headache in progress. The client with frequent migraine headaches is a candidate for prophylactic therapy. Drugs used to reduce the frequency and severity of migraine follow:

- Methysergide maleate (Sansert) is a serotonin antagonist that competitively blocks serotonin receptors in the CNS and is also a potent vasoconstrictor.
- Propranolol hydrochloride (Inderal) is a beta-blocker that prevents dilation of vessels in the pia mater and inhibits serotonin uptake.
- Topiramate (Topamax) and valproic acid (Depakote) are CNS agents and anticonvulsants. They have been approved by the FDA for use to prevent migraines (National Headache Foundation, 2005).

When the manifestations of migraine are recognized early, several medications may be used to abort or limit the severity and duration of the headache. Ergotamine tartrate (Cafergot) is a complex drug that reduces extracranial blood flow, decreases the amplitude of cranial artery pulsation, and decreases basal artery hyperperfusion. Administered at the onset of an attack, ergotamine controls up to 70% of acute attacks. Sumatriptan (Imitrex) is available in oral, nasal spray, or subcutaneous injection forms. It binds with serotonin$_1$ receptors and is rapidly effective. Zolmitriptan (Zomig), a selective serotonin$_1$ receptor agonist, is administered orally and is effective in the treatment of acute headache. Once a migraine is in progress, a narcotic analgesic such as codeine or meperidine (Demerol) may be required. Antiemetics may be prescribed to control nausea and vomiting.

Many of the same medications used for migraine also prevent or treat cluster headache. Because the onset of cluster headaches is abrupt, abortive therapy is not possible. Medications such as ergotamine tartrate may be given in suppository form at bedtime to prevent headache during the episodic attacks. Clients may find that inhaling 100% oxygen at 7 L/min for 15 minutes at the onset of an attack relieves their headache (Tierney et al., 2005).

Nonnarcotic analgesics such as aspirin or acetaminophen may relieve tension headaches. Additionally, tranquilizers such as diazepam may reduce muscle tension.

Nursing implications for drugs commonly prescribed for headaches are described in the Medication Administration on the next page.

Alternative and Complementary Therapies

The following alternative and complementary therapies are used to relieve the pain of headaches.

- Vitamin D, elemental calcium, riboflavin (vitamin B), and magnesium
- Acupuncture
- Relaxation, guided imagery, massage
- Melatonin, 5-HTP, CoQ10
- Magnetic field therapy
- Herbal therapy
- Osteopathic manipulation

NURSING CARE

In addition to the nursing care discussed in this section, a Nursing Care Plan for a client with migraine headaches is found on page 1547.

Health Promotion

Teach clients with tension headaches relaxation techniques, such as massage and biofeedback. Counseling for chronic anxiety may also be helpful. Triggers for migraine or cluster headache should be identified and, if possible, eliminated. For example, avoiding physical and emotional stress, having regular and consistent sleep patterns, eating meals regularly, and avoiding specific foods or alcohol can be incorporated into daily life and are helpful. Specific suggestions are outlined in Box 44–2.

Assessment

Collect the following data through the health history and physical examination.

- *Health history:* History of intracerebral trauma, tumor, or infection; detailed history and description of headache characteristics; family history; triggering factors; usual diet; effects of recurring headaches on lifestyle, activities of daily living (ADLs), and role performance.
- *Physical assessment:* Skin (diaphoresis, pallor, flushing), eyes (sensitivity to light, tearing), muscle strength and movement.

Nursing Diagnoses and Interventions

The primary response of the client requiring nursing interventions is acute pain. Develop nursing interventions to help the client identify strategies for controlling the pain and discomfort of the headache.

BOX 44–2 Suggestions to Decrease Incidence of Migraine Headaches

- Wake up at the same time each morning.
- Exercise at least three times a week.
- No smoking or caffeine after 3 P.M.
- No artificial sweeteners.
- No MSG.
- Reduce or eliminate red wine, cheese, alcohol, chocolate, and caffeine.
- Try a gluten-free diet.

MEDICATION ADMINISTRATION Headaches

BETA-BLOCKERS
Propanolol hydrochloride (Inderal)
Nadolol (Corgard)
Atenolol (Tenormin)
Timolol maleate (Blocadren)
Beta-blockers are effective in the prophylactic treatment of headache. They act by combining with beta-adrenergic receptors to block the response to sympathetic nerve impulses, circulating catecholamines, or adrenergic drugs.

Nursing Responsibilities
- Before beginning therapy, determine pulse and blood pressure in both arms with client lying, sitting, and standing.
- Assess baseline and monitor serum glucose level, CBC, electrolytes, and liver and renal function studies.
- Note any history of diabetes or impaired renal function.
- Note the rate and quality of respirations; drugs in this category may cause dyspnea and bronchospasm.
- Administer the drug with meals to prevent gastrointestinal disturbances.
- Be alert that beta-blockers cause bradycardia and the heart rate may not rise in response to stress, such as exercise or fever. Notify the primary healthcare provider if pulse falls below 50 or if blood pressure changes significantly.
- Teach the client or family member how to take a pulse and blood pressure reading.

Health Education for the Client and Family
- Take the medication with meals to provide a coating for the gastrointestinal tract and prevent gastrointestinal disturbances.
- Return for blood work as prescribed.
- Take the last dose of the day at bedtime.
- Rise from a sitting or lying position to a standing position slowly to avoid dizziness and falls.
- Take pulse and blood pressure each day and maintain a record of readings.
- Avoid excessive intake of alcohol, coffee, tea, or cola. Consult with the healthcare provider before taking any over-the-counter medications.
- Report any cough, nasal stuffiness, or feelings of depression to the healthcare provider.

TRICYCLIC ANTIDEPRESSANTS
Imipramine hydrochloride (Tofranil)
Amitriptyline hydrochloride (Elavil)
The tricyclic antidepressants have been successful in the prophylaxis of cluster and migraine headaches. Although the exact mechanism is not known, they do prevent the reuptake of norepinephrine or serotonin, or both. They are chemically related to the phenothiazines, and as such they exhibit many of the same pharmacologic effects (e.g., anticholinergic, antiserotonin, sedative, antihistaminic, and hypotensive effects).

NURSING RESPONSIBILITIES
- Assess baseline CBC and liver function studies, heart sounds, and neurologic status before initiating prescribed therapy.

Health Education for the Client and Family
- Make position changes slowly.
- Chew sugarless gum to relieve dry mouth.
- Do not abruptly quit taking the medication.

ERGOT ALKALOID DERIVATIVES
Methysergide maleate (Sansert)
Methysergide is an ergot alkaloid derivative structurally related to LSD. It acts by stimulating smooth muscle, leading to vasoconstriction. It is thought that methysergide prevents headaches by blocking the effects of serotonin, a powerful vasodilator believed to play a role in vascular headaches. It also inhibits the release of histamine from mast cells and prevents the release of serotonin from platelets.

Nursing Responsibilities
- Note any history of renal or hepatic disease.
- Assess baseline eosinophil and neutrophil counts before beginning therapy.
- Administer the drug with meals or milk to minimize gastrointestinal irritation due to increased hydrochloric acid production.
- Assess for renal, CNS, and cardiovascular complications.
- Drug dosage should be gradually reduced over 2 to 3 weeks to prevent rebound headaches. A drug-free interval of 3 to 4 weeks is required with each 6-month course of therapy to prevent complications.
- Monitor for signs of ergotism, such as coldness or numbness of the fingers and toes, nausea, vomiting, headache, muscle pain, and weakness. Vasoconstriction may further impair peripheral circulation and increase blood pressure.

Health Education for the Client and Family
- Take the medication with meals or milk to minimize gastrointestinal upset.
- Report to the primary care provider nervousness, weakness, rashes, hair loss, or swelling of the extremities.
- Weigh daily and report any unusual weight gain to the primary care provider.
- Return to the primary care provider for a checkup at least every 6 months or as instructed. Do not take the drug on a regular basis for longer than 6 months, but do not abruptly stop taking it.
- Return for follow-up blood work as ordered.

SEROTONIN SELECTIVE AGONIST
Sumatriptan succinate (Imitrex)
Zolmitriptan (Zomig)
Rizatriptan Benzoate (Maxalt)
Binds to vascular receptors to vasoconstrict cranial blood vessels and relieve migraine headache.

Nursing Responsibilities
- Assess for history of peripheral vascular disease, renal or hepatic problems, and pregnancy.
- Evaluate relief of migraine headache, and assess for side effects of photophobia, sound sensitivity, and nausea and vomiting.

Health Education for the Client and Family
- Do not use more than two injections in a 24-hour period, and allow at least 1 hour between injections.
- Use the autoinjector to administer the medication, and follow instructions for proper method of giving the injection and disposing of the syringe.
- Report wheezing, heart palpitations, skin rash, swelling of the eyelids or face, or chest pain to the healthcare provider immediately.

CALCIUM CHANNEL BLOCKERS
Verapamil (Isoptin)
Nifedipine (Procardia)

(continued)

MEDICATION ADMINISTRATION Headaches (continued)

The calcium channel blockers may have value in controlling cerebral vasospasms by two mechanisms: inhibiting the influx of calcium into the cerebral artery and interfering with the destruction of erythrocytes and aggregation of platelets.

Nursing Responsibilities
- These drugs cause peripheral vasodilation. Therefore, monitor blood pressure and pulse during the initial administration of the drug. Any excessive hypotensive response and tachycardia may precipitate angina. Request written parameters for safe drug administration.
- Monitor intake and output and daily weights. Assess for manifestations of congestive heart failure: weight gain, peripheral edema, dyspnea, rales, and jugular vein distention.
- Teach client and family members how to take pulse and blood pressure readings.

Health Education for the Client and Family
- Take the medication with meals to reduce gastrointestinal irritation.
- Take pulse and blood pressure before taking medications each day at the same time, and follow instructions regarding when to withhold medication and when to contact the provider. Keep a record of pulse and blood pressure readings.
- Report any side effects, such as dizziness, vertigo, unusual flushing, facial, warmth, or headaches, to the primary care provider.
- Report immediately any swelling of the hands or feet, pronounced dizziness, or chest pain accompanied by sweating, shortness of breath, or severe headaches.

NONSTEROIDAL ANTI-INFLAMMATORY DRUG (NSAID): SALICYLATE

Acetylsalicylic acid (Ecotrin, Bufferin)
Acetylsalicylic acid, or aspirin, is a nonnarcotic analgesic, antipyretic, anti-inflammatory agent used to relieve headache pain.

Nursing Responsibilities
- Determine the type and pattern of pain. If aspirin was used in the past for pain control, note its effectiveness.

- Note any history of peptic ulcers or other conditions that may suggest potential problems with the use of salicylates.
- Assess clients receiving anticoagulant therapy for bruises, bleeding of the mucous membranes, or blood in the urine or stool.

Health Education for the Client and Family
- Take aspirin after meals or before meals with an antacid and a full glass of water to minimize gastric irritation.
- Report ringing in the ears, unusual bleeding of gums, bruising, or black tarry stools to the primary healthcare provider.
- Monitor blood glucose levels carefully (if you have diabetes), and report hypoglycemia if it occurs.

ERGOTAMINE

Caffeine-ergotamine tartrate combination (Cafergot)
Ergotamine tartrate (Gynergen)
Ergot alkaloids vasoconstrict the cerebral blood vessels, decreasing the amplitude of the pulsations of the cranial arteries. The major use of ergot alkaloids is the treatment of migraine headaches. Cafergot has the same actions as Gynergen, in addition, the caffeine it contains provides a vasoconstrictive action, enhancing the effects of ergotamine.

Nursing Responsibilities
- Because the drug accumulates in the body and is eliminated slowly, ergotamine poisoning may occur. Sepsis, renal and vascular disease, heavy smoking, malnutrition, pregnancy, contraceptive hormones, and fever can increase the risk of ergotamine poisoning.
- These drugs are contraindicated in clients with diabetes mellitus, sepsis, hepatic or renal disease, peripheral and coronary artery disease, hypertension, and pregnancy.

Health Education for the Client and Family
- Take the drug immediately at onset of headache.
- Report the following to your healthcare provider: pain in the leg muscles, weakness, and coldness or numbness of fingers or toes.
- A dose of Cafergot taken late in the day may prevent sleep because of the effects of caffeine.

Acute Pain

Headaches originate from both intracranial and extracranial sources and range in severity from benign, transient discomfort to severe, incapacitating pain. Interventions focus on teaching the client self-care measures to control or relieve the pain, and reducing any associated problems, such as nausea and vomiting or anxiety.

- Teach to maintain a diary of headaches, including duration, onset, location, relation to menstruation or food intake, and related manifestations such as factors that relieve or intensify the pain. *A thorough assessment of the headache is essential for both the client and the healthcare provider to identify the circumstances and patterns of headache occurrence.*
- Ask the client to rate the pain or discomfort on a scale of 0 to 10 (with 10 being the worst pain). *Using a scale to rate the pain provides an objective measure of the client's subjective experience of the pain or discomfort. The scale can also be used to evaluate the effectiveness of pain relief measures.*

- Teach to minimize light, noise, and activity and rest in a quiet, nonstimulating environment when experiencing a headache. *Manipulating the environment helps reduce noxious stimuli that may increase pain.*
- Teach to use noninvasive and nonpharmacologic pain relief measures such as deep breathing or relaxation to facilitate self-management of pain (see Chapter 9 ∞). *Alternative strategies to control pain can help reduce tension and may help to increase the client's sense of control over the pain.*
- Suggest application of cold compresses or dry heat to the head and neck. *The application of cold causes vasoconstriction, which helps reduce pain in vascular headaches. Application of heat can reduce muscle tension and improve circulation.*
- Teach to follow good nutrition guidelines, get regular exercise and sleep, and minimize stress. *Headaches are more likely to occur when ill, tired, or under stress.*

NURSING CARE PLAN   A Client with a Migraine Headache

Betty Friedman is a 25-year-old grade-school teacher. Her friends and the other teachers regard Ms. Friedman as an enthusiastic person who sets high standards for herself and strives for perfection. During the spring semester, Ms. Friedman begins to miss work and sometimes appears very nervous. One day, another teacher notices Ms. Friedman running down the hall and into the restroom; the teacher finds Ms. Friedman vomiting. As she washes up, Ms. Friedman tells the other teacher that she has been having headaches since she began menstruating, but that they have never been as intense and frequent as during this past year. Ms. Friedman agrees to see the nurse practitioner, Jane Schickadanz, at the school clinic for evaluation.

ASSESSMENT

During her health history, Ms. Friedman relates that each month before her menstrual cycle she becomes nervous and sees flashing lights. She also has difficulty expressing herself and thinking clearly. The next day she develops a "sick headache." She states that the headache can last 1 to 2 days and that afterwards she cannot brush her hair because her scalp hurts. Ms. Friedman attributes these symptoms to PMS and adds that she thinks she is allergic to cheese and nuts because she gets sick after eating them. After assessment, and in consultation with the physician, Ms. Schickadanz diagnoses Ms. Friedman's problem as a migraine with aura headache. Sumatriptan succinate (Imitrex) is prescribed.

DIAGNOSES

- *Acute Pain* related to vasodilation of cerebral vessels and a decreased serotonin level
- *Deficient Knowledge* of pain management
- *Altered Role Performance* related to pain

EXPECTED OUTCOMES

- Experience reduced frequency and duration of pain.

- Identify available resources for helping with self-management of pain.

PLANNING AND IMPLEMENTATION

- Ask to keep a diary of her headaches for the next month, noting times of their occurrence, location and duration of pain, and factors that trigger the onset, such as her menstrual period or certain foods.
- Teach to take medication at the first awareness of an impending attack.
- Suggest an appointment with a counselor to learn methods of relaxation and stress relief.
- Request dietary referral for elimination of foods that might precipitate headaches.

EVALUATION

Four weeks after beginning medication therapy with Imitrex and relaxation techniques, Ms. Friedman has noted a decrease in the intensity of the headaches. She reports that the medication has stopped the headaches, which, she has noted, tend to occur more frequently immediately before her menstrual period. She is walking for 30 minutes each day and has made changes in her usual diet. Ms. Friedman states, "I feel good about going to work with my kids at school and knowing I can control my pain."

CRITICAL THINKING IN THE NURSING PROCESS

1. List the questions you would include in a health history that would identify stressors consistent with migraine headaches.
2. Develop a teaching plan for Ms. Friedman that includes methods of reducing fluid retention before her menstrual period, as well as a suggested diet based on the food guide pyramid.
3. Design a plan of care for Ms. Friedman for the nursing diagnosis *Disturbed Sleep Pattern.*
See Evaluating Your Response in Appendix C.

Community-Based Care

In addition to implementing comfort measures, client education has a high priority. Develop a teaching plan to help the client learn how to limit attacks (e.g., by avoiding precipitating factors) and reduce the effects of the headache. Provide specific information about prescribed medications. Referrals for methods of stress reduction may be necessary for clients with long-term or migraine headaches.

THE CLIENT WITH EPILEPSY

Epilepsy (also called *seizure disorder*) is a chronic disorder of abnormal recurring, excessive, and self-terminating electrical discharge from neurons. Epilepsy is characterized by recurring seizures accompanied by some type of change in behavior. A **seizure** (sometimes called a convulsion) is a single event of abnormal electrical discharge in the brain resulting in an abrupt and temporary altered state of cerebral function (Hickey, 2003). This abnormal neuronal activity, which may involve all or part of the brain, disturbs skeletal motor function, sensation,

autonomic function of the viscera, behavior, and/or consciousness. Epilepsy is categorized as a paroxysmal disorder because its manifestations are discontinuous; that is, minutes, days, weeks, or even years may elapse between seizures.

Incidence and Prevalence

Epilepsy is one of the most common neurologic conditions, affecting up to 2.5 million people in the United States. There is a strong genetic component. Although people of any age may be affected, the prevalence and incidence of epilepsy increases dramatically in older adults (see the Meeting Individualized Needs box on page 1548).

FAST FACTS
Epilepsy
- Epilepsy affects people of all ages, races, and ethnic backgrounds.
- Every year, more than 181,000 people develop epilepsy for the first time (Epilepsy Foundation, 2005a).
- Epilepsy is not a mental disorder.

For years, epilepsy was believed to be a disease that only affected children. Research has now found that the incidence of epilepsy in adults age 75 and over is higher than in the first 10 years of life, with 7% of all older adults having epilepsy (Spitz, 2005). These data have important implications for nursing assessments and care.

- The most common cause of epilepsy in older adults is arteriosclerosis of the cerebrovascular system (with up to 80% of the older population having arteriosclerosis).
- The manifestations of epilepsy in older adults are different than in younger adults and children. Although 60% of younger people have generalized tonic-clonic seizures, only 30% of older adults have generalized tonic-clonic seizures. The most common type of seizure in older adults is a complex partial seizure.
- Older adults tend to have longer postseizure manifestations than do younger adults.
- Epilepsy that begins in older adults is often easier to control with antiepileptic drugs (AEDs) than that in younger people. However, some AEDs decrease the effect of statins used to treat arteriosclerosis (the most common cause of epilepsy in the elderly).

The incidence of epilepsy is increasing. Researchers have suggested that the increase may be due to technologic advances in obstetric and pediatric care that allow extremely high-risk neonates to survive and to other technologic advances that have improved survival rates after craniocerebral trauma.

Isolated seizure episodes may occur in otherwise healthy people for a variety of reasons, including an acute febrile state, infection, metabolic or endocrine disorder (such as hypoglycemia), or exposure to toxins. Epilepsy may be idiopathic (that is, it may have no identifiable cause), or it may be secondary to birth injury, infection, vascular abnormalities, trauma, or tumors.

Pathophysiology

Normally, when the mind is actively working, electrical activity in the brain is unsynchronized; when the mind is at rest, electrical activity is mildly synchronized. It is believed that most seizures arise from a few unstable, hypersensitive, and hyperreactive neurons in the brain. During a seizure, these neurons produce a rhythmic and repetitive hypersynchronous discharge. Although the exact initiating factor for seizure activity has not been identified, several theories have been proposed (Porth, 2005):

- Alterations in the permeability of, or ion distribution across, cell membranes
- Alterations in the excitability of neurons resulting from neuroglia (neuroglia are CNS connective or supporting cells; they include astrocytes, oligodendroglia, and microglia)
- Scarring or decreased inhibition of activity in the cerebral cortex or thalamic region
- Imbalances of excitatory and inhibitory neurotransmitters such as acetylcholine (ACh) or gamma aminobutyric acid (GABA).

All people have a seizure threshold; when this threshold is exceeded, a seizure may result. In some people, the seizure threshold may be abnormally low, increasing their risk for seizure activity; in other people pathologic processes may alter the seizure threshold (Porth, 2005). The neurons that initiate seizure activity are called the *epileptogenic focus*. Abnormal neuronal activity may remain localized, causing a partial or focal seizure, or it may spread to involve the entire brain, causing generalized seizure activity.

Seizures may also be provoked or unprovoked. Unprovoked (primary or idiopathic) seizures have no identifiable cause, with multiple episodes diagnosed as a seizure disorder. Provoked (secondary) seizure etiologies include febrile seizures in children, toxemia of pregnancy, rapid withdrawal from alcohol or barbiturates, systemic metabolic conditions (such as hypoglycemia, hypoxia, uremia, and electrolyte imbalances), and pathologies of the brain (such as meningitis, cerebral bleeding, or cerebral edema).

Metabolic needs of the brain increase dramatically during seizure activity. The demand for adenosine triphosphate (ATP), the energy source of the brain, increases by approximately 250%. Consequently, the demand for glucose and oxygen (which are needed to produce ATP) increases, and oxygen consumption increases by about 60%. To supply this increased oxygen need and remove carbon dioxide and other metabolic by-products, cerebral blood flow increases to about 2.5 times that of the normal rate. As long as oxygenation, blood glucose levels, and cardiac function remain normal, cerebral blood flow can respond to this increased metabolic demand of the brain. If cerebral blood flow cannot meet these needs, however, cellular exhaustion and cellular destruction may result.

Manifestations

Although seizures may be categorized in several different ways, the classification developed by the International League Against Epilepsy is the most useful clinically (Tierney et al., 2005). In this classification, seizures are divided into those that affect only part of the brain (partial seizures) and those that are generalized (affect all of the brain). An individual may have more than one type, in what are called mixed seizures.

Partial Seizures

Partial seizures involve the activation of only a restricted part of one cerebral hemisphere. A partial seizure accompanied by no alteration in consciousness is called a *simple partial seizure*; one in which consciousness is impaired is called a *complex partial seizure*.

SIMPLE PARTIAL SEIZURES The manifestations of simple partial seizures depend on the involved area of the brain. Manifestations may include alterations in motor function, sensory signs, or autonomic or psychic symptoms. Typically, the motor portion of the cortex is affected, causing recurrent muscle contractions of the face or a contralateral part of the body, such as a finger or hand. This motor activity may stay confined to one area or spread sequentially to adjacent parts, a phenomenon known as a *Jacksonian march* or *Jacksonian seizure*. Manifestations of a simple partial seizure involving the sensory portion of the brain may include abnormal sensations or hallucinations. Disruptions in the function of the autonomic nervous system, with resulting tachycardia, flushing, hypotension, and hypertension, or psychic manifestations, such as a sense of déjà vu (a feeling that "this has happened before") or inappropriate fear or anger, may also be experienced during a simple partial seizure.

COMPLEX PARTIAL SEIZURES During a complex partial seizure, consciousness is impaired and the client may engage in repetitive, nonpurposeful activity, such as lip smacking, aimless walking, or picking at clothing. These behaviors are known as *automatisms*. During the seizure, the client loses conscious contact with the environment; amnesia is common after the seizure, and several hours may elapse before the client regains full consciousness. Complex partial seizures usually originate in the temporal lobe and may be preceded by an aura, such as an unusual smell, a sense of déjà vu, or a sudden intense emotion.

Generalized Seizures

Generalized seizures involve both hemispheres of the brain as well as deeper brain structures, such as the thalamus, basal ganglia, and upper brainstem. Consciousness is always impaired with generalized seizures. Absence and tonic-clonic seizures are the common forms of generalized seizure activity; they occur more frequently (especially in children) than partial seizures.

ABSENCE SEIZURES Absence *(petit mal) seizures* are characterized by a sudden brief cessation of all motor activity accompanied by a blank stare and unresponsiveness. Absence seizures are more common in children than in adults. The seizure typically lasts only 5 to 10 seconds, although some may last for 30 seconds or more. Movements such as eyelid fluttering or automatisms such as lip smacking may occur during an absence seizure. Seizure activity may vary from occasional episodes to several hundred per day.

TONIC-CLONIC SEIZURES *Tonic-clonic seizures* (grand mal) are the most common type of seizure activity in adults. This type of seizure activity follows a typical pattern. A warning *aura* may precede generalized seizure activity. The aura may be a vague sense of uneasiness or an abnormal gustatory, visual, auditory, or visceral sensation (such as a metallic taste in the mouth, a smell of burning rubber, or seeing a bright light). Often, however, the seizure occurs without warning.

The seizure begins with a sudden loss of consciousness and sharp tonic muscle contractions (the tonic phase of the seizure). With the muscle contraction, air is forced out of the lungs, and the client may cry out. Postural control is lost, and the client falls to the floor in the opisthotonic posture (Figure 44–4A ■). Muscles are rigid, with the arms and legs extended and the jaw clenched. Urinary incontinence is common; bowel incontinence may also occur. Breathing ceases and cyanosis develops during the tonic phase of a seizure. The pupils are fixed and di-

Figure 44–4 ■ Tonic-clonic seizures in grand mal seizures. *A,* Tonic phase. *B,* Clonic phase.

lated. The tonic phase lasts an average of 15 seconds, although it may persist for up to a minute.

The clonic phase, which follows the tonic phase, is characterized by alternating contraction and relaxation of the muscles in all the extremities along with hyperventilation (Figure 44–4B). The eyes roll back, and the client froths at the mouth. The clonic phase varies in duration and subsides gradually. The entire tonic-clonic portion of the seizure generally lasts no more than 60 to 90 seconds.

Following the clonic phase of seizure activity, the client remains unconscious and unresponsive to stimuli. This period is known as the postictal period or phase. The client is relaxed and breathes quietly. The client regains consciousness gradually and may be confused and disoriented on waking. Headache, muscle aches, and fatigue often follow the seizure, and the client may sleep for several hours. Amnesia of the seizure is usual; the client also may not recall events just prior to the seizure activity.

Because of the lack of warning with tonic-clonic seizures, the client may experience injury. Head injury, fractures, burns, or motor vehicle crashes may occur secondarily to seizure activity.

Status Epilepticus

Status epilepticus can develop during seizure activity. In this case, the seizure activity becomes continuous, with only very short periods of calm between intense and persistent seizures. The repetitive seizures may be of any type, although they are usually generalized tonic-clonic (Porth, 2005). Repeated seizures have a cumulative effect, producing muscular contractions that can interfere with respirations. The client is in great danger of developing hypoxia, acidosis, hypoglycemia, hyperthermia, and exhaustion if the convulsive activity is not halted. Status epilepticus is considered a life-threatening medical emergency that requires immediate treatment.

INTERDISCIPLINARY CARE

Initial treatment focuses on controlling the seizure; the long-term goal is to determine the cause and prevent future seizures.

Interdisciplinary care includes diagnostic testing, medications, and, in some cases, surgery.

Diagnosis

Diagnostic testing is performed to confirm the seizure diagnosis and to determine any treatable causes and precipitating factors. (See Chapter 43 ∞ for a description of neurologic tests and related nursing care.) Radiologic examinations include an MRI or CT scan to determine abnormalities in the brain and a skull x-ray to identify any bony abnormalities. An electroencephalogram (EEG) helps localize any brain lesions and confirm the diagnosis. A lumbar puncture may be performed to assess spinal fluid for CNS infections (increased WBCs) or tumors (increased protein levels). Blood studies are used to assess blood count, electrolytes, blood urea, and blood glucose.

Medications

Antiepileptic drugs (AEDs) (also called anticonvulsant drugs) can reduce or control most seizure activity. More than 20 drugs are used in the treatment of epilepsy. These medications do not cure the disorder; they only manage its manifestations. AEDs generally act in one of two ways: by raising the seizure threshold or by limiting the spread of abnormal activity within the brain.

The goals of medications for epilepsy are to protect the client from harm and to reduce or prevent seizure activity without impairing cognitive function or producing undesirable side effects. Ideally, the lowest possible dose of a single medication that will control the client's seizures is prescribed; often, however, several medications must be tried before the most effective is identified, and a combination of drugs may be needed to manage the client's seizures. Therapy is individualized, based on the type of seizure activity and the client's response to the medication. Four drugs are recommended by the American Academy of Neurology as monotherapy (taking one drug at a time) for newly diagnosed adults with either partial or mixed seizures. These are gabapentin (Neurontin), lamotrigine (Lamictal), oxcarbazepine (Trileptal), and topiramate (Topamax). Examples of, and nursing implications for AEDs are described in the Medication Administration below; drug interactions are listed in Box 44–3.

If the client has been seizure free for at least 3 years, withdrawal of medications may be considered, with the dose of one drug at a time reduced over weeks or months. There is no way to predict which clients can remain seizure free without medication, but if seizures reoccur, the same medications usually provide good control.

Status epilepticus requires immediate intervention to preserve life. Establishing and maintaining the airway is a priority. A solution of 50% dextrose is administered intravenously to prevent hypoglycemia. Diazepam (Valium) or lorazepam (Ativan) is given intravenously, and the dose repeated in 10 minutes

---

MEDICATION ADMINISTRATION **Seizures**

ANTIEPILEPTIC DRUGS (AEDS)
Examples of AEDs are:

Phenytoin (Dilantin)
Phenobarbital
Primidone (Mysoline)
Carbamazepine (Tegretol)
Valproic acid (Depakene)
Ethosuximide (Zarontin)
Clonazepam (Klonopin)
Gabapentin (Neurontin)
Lamotrigine (Lamictal)
Tiagabine HCL (Gabitril)

AEDs are used to control chronic seizures and involuntary muscle spasms or movements characteristic of certain neurologic diseases. These drugs act in the motor cortex of the brain to reduce the spread of electrical discharges from the rapidly firing epileptic foci in this area. These agents control seizures without impairing the normal functions of the CNS. Drugs effective against one type of seizure may not be effective against another; anticonvulsant therapy must be individualized.

Nursing Responsibilities
- Monitor blood pressure, pulse, and respirations.
- Note evidence of CNS side effects, such as blurred vision, dimmed vision, slurred speech, nystagmus, or confusion. Gingival hyperplasia may be noted in clients taking phenytoin.
- Recognize that if clients are to be on prolonged therapy, they may need a diet rich in vitamin D.
- Monitor the serum calcium level as ordered; phenytoin can contribute to demineralization of bone.

- When administering anticonvulsants intravenously, monitor closely for respiratory depression and cardiovascular collapse.
- Administer gabapentin 2 hours after antacids.
- Administer tiagabine HCL with food.

Health Education for the Client and Family
- Take the exact dosage prescribed. Do not increase, decrease, or discontinue the dosage without obtaining the primary care provider's approval; doing so may lead to convulsions.
- Avoid hazardous tasks until the drug has been regulated. AEDs may at first decrease mental alertness and cause drowsiness, headache, dizziness, and incoordination of muscles. These effects are usually dose related and may disappear with a change of dosage or continued therapy.
- If you are taking phenytoin (Dilantin), maintain good oral hygiene: Use a soft toothbrush, massage the gums, and floss daily.
- It is very important to obtain liver function studies regularly as ordered by the primary care provider. This will help detect early signs of hepatitis and other liver problems. Report for all scheduled laboratory studies, including complete blood count, kidney and liver function studies, and drug levels.
- Carry identification indicating the type of seizures for which you are being treated.
- Do not take gabapentin 1 hour before or less than 2 hours after an antacid.
- If you are taking lamotrigine and develop a rash, tell your healthcare provider.
- Take tiagabine HCL (Gabitril) with food.

BOX 44–3 Drug Interactions with AEDs

- *Valproic acid (Depakene) and phenobarbital.* Blood levels of phenobarbital may rise significantly when valproic acid is added to the client's medication regimen.
- *Phenobarbital and digoxin.* This combination may increase the metabolism of digoxin, resulting in decreased digoxin levels.
- *Phenobarbital and sodium warfarin (Coumadin).* Phenobarbital may decrease the absorption of sodium warfarin from the gastrointestinal tract and decrease the drug's anticoagulant response.
- *Disulfiram (Antabuse) and phenobarbital.* This combination may inhibit the metabolism of the anticonvulsant drug and increase the incidence of side effects associated with the anticonvulsant drug.
- *Carbamazepine and oral contraceptives.* Carbamazepine decreases the effectiveness of oral contraceptives.
- *Other drugs.* Other drugs reported to interact with anticonvulsant drugs include aspirin, certain antibiotics, isoniazid, acetazolamide (Diamox), antacids, folic acid, and narcotics.

if necessary to stop seizure activity. Phenytoin (Dilantin) is administered intravenously for longer term control of seizures. Phenobarbital may also be administered to clients in status epilepticus.

Surgery

Resective surgery, with removal of the epileptogenic focus, is an option that is still in its early stages. Candidates for this type of surgery include those who are unresponsive to medical management, who have a unilateral focus, and who have impaired quality of life from seizures. Resections of the temporal lobe are most commonly performed and are most effective for partial complex seizures. An estimated 5% of clients with epilepsy may be candidates for surgery. The goal of surgery is to reduce the client's uncontrollable seizures.

To be selected as a candidate for surgery, the client must be highly motivated and psychologically prepared. A psychologic screening is required because the preoperative preparation is extensive and time consuming and because the surgery is long and requires that the client remain awake during surgery so that he or she can cooperate and respond to commands. The EEG is monitored during surgery to identify the epileptogenic focus and evaluate the effect of surgical intervention.

General postoperative care for the client with intracranial surgery follows the nursing management guidelines outlined later in the chapter. Specific preoperative and postoperative care for a client with a seizure disorder is described in the box below.

Vagal Nerve Stimulation Therapy

Vagal nerve stimulation (VNS) therapy is approved as a treatment for clients with partial-onset seizures who do not respond to AEDs. The therapy does not stop the seizures, but rather reduces the number and improves the client's quality of life. It is almost always necessary to continue taking AEDs. The therapy is designed to prevent seizures by sending regular small pulses of electrical energy to the brain via the vagus nerve. A flat, round battery (about the size of a silver dollar) is implanted in the chest wall, and electrodes are threaded under the skin and wound around the vagus nerve in the neck. The battery is programmed to deliver a few seconds of electrical energy every few seconds. If the person feels that a seizure is about to happen, a discharge can be activated by passing a small magnet over the battery. In some people this stops the seizures. Side effects are hoarseness and throat discomfort.

 NURSING CARE

See the next page for a Nursing Care Plan for a client with seizures.

Health Promotion

Health promotion activities for the client with seizures focus on teaching to reduce the incidence of seizure activity and to promote safety. Stress the following:

- Know the importance of follow-up care, of keeping medical appointments, and of continuing to take AEDs as prescribed even when no seizures are experienced.
- Review any state and local laws that apply to people with seizure disorders. Driving a motor vehicle is usually prohibited for 6 months to 2 years after a seizure episode. Usually, a driver's license can be reinstated or obtained after a seizure-free period and a letter from the nurse practitioner or physician.

NURSING CARE OF THE CLIENT WITH Seizures Who Is Having Surgery

PREOPERATIVE CARE

- For most clients, AEDs are withheld the morning or evening of the day before surgery. *AEDs may interfere with intraoperative EEG monitoring.*
- For clients with frequent and/or severe seizures, however, a partial dose of medication may be administered. *This prevents seizures or status epilepticus during surgery.*
- A low dose of analgesics is administered before surgery. *The client must remain awake throughout the lengthy procedure to respond to commands during EEG recording.*

POSTOPERATIVE CARE

- AEDs are administered parenterally until the client can tolerate oral fluids; medications are then continued orally. *It is common for the client to have seizures in the early postoperative period.*
- Steroids are administered for the first 3 days after surgery and are tapered and then discontinued during the following week. *Steroids are given to decrease cerebral edema.*

NURSING CARE PLAN A Client with a Seizure Disorder

Janet Carlson is a 19-year-old college student who lives with her parents and one younger sister. Although Janet had seizures while she was in grade school, they have been controlled with medication. However, she had a tonic-clonic seizure yesterday and immediately made an appointment with her family physician. She is currently taking phenytoin (Dilantin) 300 mg/day as a maintenance medication to prevent seizures.

ASSESSMENT

Evita Farias, RN, completes a health history for Ms. Carlson. During the history, she tells Ms. Farias that she has been under stress because of difficulties in completing her course requirements this semester. She has not been sleeping as many hours per night, and sometimes she forgets to take her medication. Janet's serum phenytoin level is 8 mg/mL. Therapeutic level is 10 to 20 mg/mL.

DIAGNOSES

- *Risk for Injury* related to recurrence of generalized tonic-clonic seizure activity and low serum phenytoin levels
- *Deficient Knowledge* of activities that may trigger seizure occurrence, the effect of stress on seizures, and medication information

EXPECTED OUTCOMES

- Verbalize precipitating and triggering factors related to the onset of seizures.
- Verbalize the relationship between emotional and physical stress and seizures.
- Verbalize the importance of taking AEDs.

PLANNING AND IMPLEMENTATION

- Teach client and her family the following:
  - Current information about seizures

  - Care during and after a seizure
  - Medication protocols
  - Factors and activities that can trigger seizures
  - The importance of follow-up care.
- Refer client and her family to a local epilepsy support group.
- Recommend that she purchase and wear a Medic-Alert bracelet.

EVALUATION

Ms. Carlson is instructed to continue taking Dilantin 300 mg/day. She states the importance of nutrition, rest, and measures to reduce stress. She also discusses the importance of maintaining the proper blood levels of her medication, stating that too little or too much of the medication could cause problems. Ms. Carlson recognizes that the seizures had recurred during a busy time in school during which she had forgotten to take her medication. She is now wearing a Medic-Alert bracelet. Ms. Farias provides the Carlsons with the telephone number of the Epilepsy Foundation of America.

CRITICAL THINKING IN THE NURSING PROCESS

1. If you were Ms. Carlson's nurse, would your teaching differ if she were living alone? If so, how?
2. Ms. Carlson tells you that although she knows she should not drive a car, she often drives her friend to work. How would you approach this problem?
3. Ms. Carlson states that "it's embarrassing to wear a Medic-Alert bracelet." How would you respond, and what recommendation(s) would you make?

See Evaluating Your Response in Appendix C.

- Know drug interactions with other prescribed drugs, over-the-counter (OTC) drugs, street drugs, and alcohol.
- Teach family members first aid for a seizure:
  - Cushion the head.
  - Loosen anything tight around the neck.
  - Turn on the side.
  - Nothing in the mouth.
  - Don't hold down.
- Teach family members when to call for medical assistance:
  - If the seizure lasts for more than 5 minutes
  - If there is slow recovery, a second seizure, or difficulty breathing after the seizure
  - If there are signs of injury (such as bleeding from the mouth).

Assessment

Collect the following data through the health history and physical examination:

- *Health history:* Past seizures; age when the first seizure occurred, most recent seizure, factors precipitating a seizure, any warning signs (aura), prophylactic anticonvulsant therapy, and specific concerns the client may have about the seizures.
- *Physical assessment:* Important data used in determining an accurate diagnosis describes manifestations obtained from

nursing assessments before, during, and after a seizure. (Table 44–6 lists nursing assessments with rationale.)

Nursing Diagnoses and Interventions

Nursing care of clients with a seizure disorder focuses on providing care during and immediately after the seizure and on client/family teaching. The client with seizures has a wide variety of responses to actual or potential changes in health status; interventions discussed in this section focus on facilitating physical and psychologic comfort and safety.

Risk for Ineffective Airway Clearance

During a seizure, the tongue may fall back and obstruct the airway, the gag reflex may be depressed, and secretions may pool at the back of the throat. These may put the client at risk for an obstructed airway. Most seizures occur in the home or community; therefore, teach these interventions to the client's family:

- Provide interventions to maintain a patent airway:
  - Loosen clothing around the neck.
  - Turn on the side.
  - Do not force anything into the mouth.
  - If prescribed and available, administer oxygen by mask.

TABLE 44–6 Nursing Assessments Before, During, and After a Seizure

ASSESSMENT	RATIONALE
What was the client's level of consciousness? If consciousness was lost, at what point?	Indicates area of brain involved and type of seizure.
What was the client doing just before the attack?	May suggest precipitating factors.
In what part of the body did the seizure start?	May indicate the site of seizure activity in the brain tissue; for example, if jerking movements were first observed in right hand, the seizure focus may be in left motor cortex.
Was there an epileptic cry?	Usually indicates the tonic stage of a generalized tonic-clonic seizure.
Were any automatisms such as eyelid fluttering, chewing, lip smacking, or swallowing observed?	Often seen in complex, partial, and absence seizures.
How long did movements last? Did the location or character change (tonic to clonic)? Did movements involve both sides of the body or just one?	Indicates areas in which focal activity originated.
Did the head and/or eyes turn to one side and, if so, which side?	Helps localize the focus of the seizure. During the seizure, the head and eyes typically will turn away from the side of the epileptogenic focus.
Were there changes in pupillary reactions?	Indicates involvement of the autonomic nervous system.
If the client fell, was the head hit?	Skull x-ray studies may be needed to rule out subdural hematoma or fracture.
Was there foaming or frothing from the mouth?	Usually indicates a tonic-clonic seizure.

Although it was at one time believed that it was necessary to place a padded tongue blade in the client's mouth during a seizure, this is no longer recommended; an improperly placed tongue blade can obstruct the airway. Turning the client on the side allows secretions to drain from the mouth.

■ Teach family members or significant others how to care for the client during a seizure to prevent airway obstruction. *Family members are often the only people present to provide this emergency intervention.*

Anxiety

The client with a seizure disorder is understandably anxious about the future, with questions about ability to go to school, work, have a family, and drive a car. Feelings of embarrassment about having a seizure in public and rejection by others are common and also increase the client's anxiety.

■ Provide support by explaining that concerns are normal. *It is important to be sensitive to the effect of seizures on the*

client's self-concept and body image; alterations in these areas not only increase anxiety but also cause withdrawal from socialization with others. Demonstrating acceptance of the client's concerns allows further discussion.

■ Help identify safe leisure activities. *Worrying about being hurt if a seizure occurs may cause withdrawal from social activities that are pleasurable.*

■ Provide information about sources and support groups. *Sharing information with other people with similar health problems allows for a more realistic viewpoint; accurate information can clear up misconceptions that cause anxiety.*

■ Provide accurate information about hiring practices and legal limitations on driving or operating heavy or dangerous machinery. *Accurate information decreases anxiety about the unknown. The Americans with Disabilities Act prohibits discrimination; however, there are legal limitations on driving until the person is proved free of seizures.*

Using NANDA, NIC, and NOC

Chart 44–1 shows links between NANDA nursing diagnoses, NIC, and NOC when caring for the client with a seizure disorder.

Community-Based Care

Teaching follows a systematic assessment of the needs of both the client and family. Include family members so that they can learn seizure management, including the care and observations necessary before and during a seizure. Stress the importance of safety and keeping the airway patent.

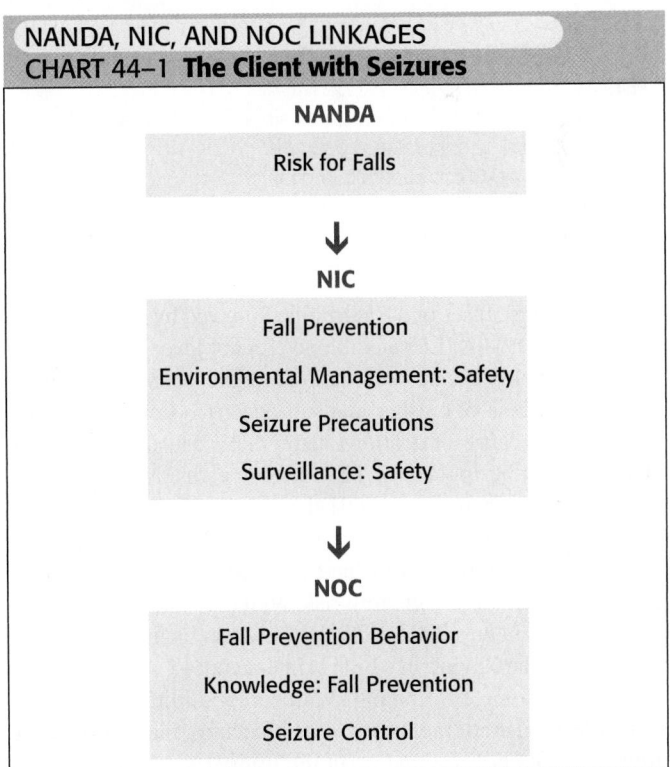

NANDA, NIC, AND NOC LINKAGES
CHART 44–1 The Client with Seizures

NANDA

Risk for Falls

↓

NIC

Fall Prevention

Environmental Management: Safety

Seizure Precautions

Surveillance: Safety

↓

NOC

Fall Prevention Behavior

Knowledge: Fall Prevention

Seizure Control

Data from *NANDA's Nursing Diagnoses: Definitions & Classification 2005–2006* by NANDA International (2005), Philadelphia; *Nursing Interventions Classification (NIC)* (4th ed.) by J. M. Dochterman & G. M. Bulechek (2004), St. Louis, MO: Mosby; and *Nursing Outcomes Classification (NOC)* (3rd ed.) by S. Moorhead, M. Johnson, and M. Maas (2004), St. Louis, MO: Mosby.

Help both the client and family adjust to a diagnosis of epilepsy. Address the following topics:

- The importance of wearing a Medic-Alert band or carrying a medical alert card at all times
- Avoiding alcoholic beverages and limiting coffee intake
- Taking showers versus tub baths, because of safety issues during a generalized seizure

- Factors that may trigger a seizure, such as abrupt withdrawal from medication, constipation, fatigue, excessive stress, fever, menstruation, sights and sounds such as television, flashing video, and computer screens
- Helpful resources include:
  - American Epilepsy Society
  - Epilepsy Foundation.

TRAUMATIC BRAIN INJURY

Traumatic brain injury (TBI) (also called *craniocerebral trauma*) refers to any injury of the scalp, skull (cranium or facial bones), or brain. TBI is a leading cause of death and disability in the United States. The National Head Injury Foundation defines TBI as a traumatic insult to the brain capable of causing physical, intellectual, emotional, social, and vocational changes. A TBI may be classified as a penetrating (open) head injury (e.g., resulting from a knife, bullet, or baseball bat) or a closed head injury (a blunt injury to the brain that does not result in an open skull fracture). TBI may cause problems with cognition, movement, sensation, and emotions. Even mild brain injuries, if repeated over an extended period of time, can result in cumulative neurologic and cognitive deficits.

Each year, 1.5 million Americans sustain a TBI. Of those who survive, one of every six people is unable to return to school or work when discharged from the hospital (Centers for Disease Control and Prevention [CDC], 2004b).

The leading causes of TBI are falls, followed by motor vehicle crashes and assaults. Elevated blood alcohol levels, not wearing motorcycle helmets, and not wearing seat belts contribute significantly to the risk of crashes and subsequent injury. Firearm use is the leading cause of death related to TBI, causing 10% of all TBI but resulting in 44% of TBI-related deaths. Nine out of 10 people with firearm-related TBI die; of those, nearly 66% are classified as suicidal in intent (CDC, 2004). Other causes of head injury include sports injuries and occupational injuries. Adults ages 15 to 44 are at the greatest risk, with the male-to-female ratio of 3-to-1 (Hickey, 2003). Other risk factors include being over the age of 75 and living in a high-crime area.

Specific damage following craniocerebral injuries is related to the mechanism of the injury (how it occurs), the nature of the injury (type), and the location of the injury (where it occurs).

Head injuries may be classified as blunt or penetrating, and can occur through several mechanisms:

- Acceleration injury is sustained when the head is struck by a moving object, such as a swinging bat.

- Deceleration injury occurs when the head hits a stationary object, such as a concrete wall.
- Acceleration-deceleration injury (also called a *coup-contrecoup* phenomenon) occurs when the head hits an object and the brain "rebounds" within the skull (Figure 44–5 ■). The brain is injured at the point of impact (the coup) and on the opposite side of the impact (the contrecoup). Two or more areas of the brain can be injured as a result of this phenomenon.
- Deformation injuries are those in which the force deforms and disrupts the integrity of the impacted body part (e.g., skull fracture).

Types of craniocerebral trauma include injuries to the skull (including fractures), injuries to the brain (including concussion and contusion), and intracranial hemorrhage (including hematomas). Brain injury can result either from the direct effects of the trauma on brain tissue or from secondary responses to trauma, such as cerebral edema, hematoma (blood clot), swelling, or increased intracranial pressure.

THE CLIENT WITH A SKULL FRACTURE

A *skull fracture* is a break in the continuity of the skull. It may occur with or without damage to the brain; however, intracranial trauma often results from skull fractures. The considerable force of impact significantly increases the risk of underlying hematoma formation. Disruption of the skull can also cause cranial nerve injury, allow bacteria to enter the cranial vault, and/or allow CSF to leak out.

Figure 44–5 ■ Coup-contrecoup head injury. Following the initial injury (coup), the brain rebounds within the skull and sustains additional injury (contrecoup) in the opposite part of the brain.

Pathophysiology

Skull fractures are classified as open or closed. In an open fracture, the dura is torn, and in a closed fracture, the dura is not torn. Skull fractures are further classified into one of four categories: linear, comminuted, depressed, or basilar (Table 44–7).

Linear Fractures

Linear fractures are the most common, accounting for 80% of all skull fractures. They typically extend from the point of impact toward the base of the skull. Although the risk of infection or CSF leakage is minimal with this type of fracture because the dura usually remains intact, subdural or epidural hematomas (a collection of blood) frequently underlie the fracture. A hematoma (discussed later in this chapter) places pressure on underlying brain tissue, increasing both intracranial pressure and the risk of brain damage.

Comminuted and Depressed Fractures

Comminuted and depressed skull fractures increase the risk of direct damage to brain tissue from bruising (contusion) and bone fragments. However, the risk of secondary brain injury may be reduced in these fractures, because in breaking the bone, the traumatic impact energy is distributed and dissipated. If the skin overlying the fracture is lacerated or the dura is torn, the risk of infection is increased.

Basilar Fractures

Basilar skull fractures involve the base of the skull and usually are extensions of adjacent fractures, although they may occur independently. Although most basilar skull fractures are uncomplicated, they may involve the sinuses of the frontal bone or the petrous portion of the temporal bone (middle ear). If the dura is disrupted, CSF may leak through the tear. CSF leakage may include *rhinorrhea* (CSF leakage through the nose) or *otorrhea* (CSF leakage from the ear). Blood may be visible behind the tympanic membrane (hemotympanum), or ecchymosis may be noted over the mastoid process (Battle's sign). Bilateral periorbital ecchymosis ("raccoon eyes") is another possible manifestation. If CSF leakage is present, the risk of infection is high. Other complications of basilar skull fractures include injury to the internal carotid artery and compression of cranial nerve I, II, III, IV, V, VII, or VIII.

INTERDISCIPLINARY CARE

Treatment of a client with a skull fracture depends on the type and location of the fracture. Skull fracture may be only one of several head injuries.

A simple linear fracture generally requires bed rest and observation for underlying injury to brain tissue or hematoma formation. No specific treatment is required. Depressed skull fractures require surgical intervention, usually within 24 hours of the injury, to debride the wound completely and remove bone fragments, which may become embedded in brain tissue or cerebral blood vessels. If depressed deeply, the bone may be elevated. If cerebral edema is not present, a cranioplasty with insertion of acrylic bone may be performed. Basal skull fractures do not require surgery unless CSF leakage persists. Regular neurologic assessments and observation for manifestations of meningitis are required for the hospitalized client. Antibiotics may be administered prophylactically.

NURSING CARE

The client with a craniocerebral trauma may have a variety of responses and healthcare needs, depending on the location and extent of the trauma. Many of those problems with related nursing interventions are discussed in other sections of this chapter, including seizures, increased intracranial pressure, and bleeding within the brain.

Risk for Infection

The client with a skull fracture is at increased risk for infection related to access to the cranial contents through a tear in the dura. In an open, depressed fracture, the wound may be contaminated by dirt, hair, or other debris.

- Monitor for otorrhea or rhinorrhea. *Open fractures of the skull increase the possibility of leakage of CSF from the ears or nose.*
- Test drainage of clear fluid from ear and nose for glucose by using a glucose reagent strip, such as Dextrostix. *Clear drainage that tests positive for glucose indicates leakage of CSF; however, be aware that false positives may occur.*
- Observe blood-tinged fluid for "halo" sign. *CSF dries in concentric rings on gauze or tissues This sign is suggestive of CSF leakage.*
- Keep the nasopharynx and the external ear clean. Place a piece of sterile cotton in the ear, or tape a sterile cotton pad loosely under the nose; change dressings when they become wet. *Wet dressings facilitate movement of organisms.*
- Instruct client not to blow nose, cough, or inhibit sneeze; sneeze through open mouth. *Blowing the nose and coughing increase ICP. Withholding a sneeze forces bacteria backward.*
- Use aseptic technique at all times when changing head dressings or ICP monitor dressings and insertion sites. *Using aseptic technique reduces the possibility of introducing infection.*

TABLE 44–7 Types of Skull Fractures

TYPE	DESCRIPTION
Linear (simple)	Simple, clean break in skull. Occurs with low-velocity injuries.
Comminuted	Bone is crushed into small, fragmented pieces. Usually seen with high-impact injuries.
Depressed	Inward depression of bone fragments. Usually due to a powerful blow to the skull. The dura may or may not be intact. Bone fragments may penetrate into the brain tissue.
Basilar	Occurs at the base of the skull. May be linear, comminuted, or depressed.

Knowledge Deficit: Skull Fracture

The client and family need to be informed about the degree of injury that has occurred with the skull fracture. The client with a linear fracture, who may not be hospitalized, will need teaching that focuses on the need to monitor progress closely. To prevent complications, advise the client and family to go to the emergency room if the client experiences any of the following:

- Growing drowsiness or confusion
- Difficulty waking (instruct a family member to wake the client every 2 hours during the first night home)
- Vomiting (especially if projectile)
- Blurred vision
- Slurred speech
- Prolonged headache
- Blood or clear fluid leaking from the ears or nose
- Weakness in an arm or leg
- Stiff neck
- Seizure.

THE CLIENT WITH A FOCAL OR DIFFUSE TRAUMATIC BRAIN INJURY

Even when the skull and other structures overlying the brain remain intact, a blow to the head can cause significant brain injury. Closed head injuries may result in either focal or diffuse damage to the brain. They range in severity from mild to severe.

Pathophysiology

Brain injury results from both primary and secondary mechanisms. Primary injury results from the impact. A blow to the head, even with no break in the skull, can cause serious and diffuse brain injury. Injury to axons disrupts oligodendroglia, and direct mechanical disruption is caused by debris and leakage.

The immediate vascular response to the injury results in increased capillary permeability to solutes.

Secondary injury is the progression of the initial injury resulting from events that affect perfusion and oxygenation of brain cells. These events include intracranial edema, hematoma, infection, hypoxia, or ischemia. Cerebral ischemia is the most common cause of secondary brain injury (Porth, 2005). Ischemia leads to cerebral hypoxia, with consequences of increased glial permeability to sodium (cytotoxic edema), an influx of calcium with changes in electrophysiology, and release of free fatty acids and lactic acidosis.

Acute brain injury affects all body systems as well as the central nervous system. Systemic effects of acute brain injury are listed in Table 44–8.

Focal Brain Injuries

Focal brain injuries are specific, grossly observable brain lesions confined to one area of the brain. They include contusions, lacerations, and intracranial hemorrhage. The force of an impact produces contusions from direct contact with the inside of the skull that in turn may cause epidural hemorrhage and subdural and intracerebral hematomas. The mechanisms of injury are coup and/or contrecoup damage to the brain at the point of the impact and the rebound effect. The damaged brain area is surrounded by edema, contributing to IICP. Infarction and necrosis, multiple hemorrhages, and edema are found within the contused areas. The maximum effects of the injury peak in 18 to 36 hours.

Intracranial hemorrhage can result directly from the trauma (e.g., beneath a fracture) or from shearing forces on cerebral arteries and veins that occur with acceleration–deceleration. Depending on the site and rate of bleeding, manifestations may appear immediately or may not become evident for hours or even weeks. Intracranial hemorrhages and the hematomas they cause place pressure on surrounding structures, causing manifestations of an expanding focal lesion. They also cause IICP, leading to altered

TABLE 44–8 Systemic Effects of Acute Brain Injury

CAUSE	EFFECT
■ Stimulation of the sympathetic nervous system, which stimulates the adrenal cortex and medulla to increase glucocorticoid and mineralocorticoid levels	■ Increased metabolism of carbohydrates, fats, and proteins ■ Retention of sodium and water
■ Stimulation of the sympathetic nervous system, increasing the serum catecholamine levels	■ Hypertension ■ EEG changes ■ Dysrhymias (bradycardia, sinus tachycardia)
■ Altered release of ADH from the posterior pituitary ■ Neurogenic pulmonary dysfunction	■ Retention of water or diuresis and diabetes insipidus ■ Abnormal respiratory patterns ■ Reduced residual capacity with retention of CO_2, vasodilation, and increased ICP ■ Pulmonary edema
■ Stress response to trauma ■ Increased platelet, plasma fibrinogen, and thromboplastin levels	■ Hyperglycemia ■ Decreased clotting and prothrombin times ■ Vascular occlusion ■ Disseminated intravascular coagulation ■ Anemia
■ Immunosuppression ■ Decreased gastric motility and increased gastric acidity	■ Infection ■ Gastritis ■ Gastric ulcers

TABLE 44–9 Comparison of Intracranial Hematomas

TYPE/FREQUENCY	LOCATION/COMMON SITE	PRECIPITATING FACTORS	MANIFESTATIONS
Epidural Hematoma 2% to 6% of all types of head injuries	Located in the space between the skull and the dura mater Common site: the temporal bone (over the middle meningeal artery)	Skull fractures Contusion	Momentary loss of consciousness followed by a lucid period lasting from a few hours to 1 to 2 days Rapid deterioration in level of consciousness (drowsiness to confusion to coma) Seizures Headache Hemiparesis (may be ipsilateral or contralateral) Fixed dilated ipsilateral pupil Rise in blood pressure with decreases in pulse and respirations indicates a rapidly increasing hematoma
Subdural Hematoma Approximately 29% of all types of head injuries	Located in the space below the dural surface (between the dura and arachnoid and pia mater layers of meninges) Common site: may occur any place in cranium	Closed head injury Acceleration–deceleration injury Cerebral atrophy (seen in older adults) Chronic alcoholism Use of anticoagulants Contusion	Acute: ■ Headache ■ Drowsiness ■ Agitation ■ Slowed thinking ■ Confusion Subacute: ■ Same as those of acute subdural hematoma but develop more slowly Chronic: ■ Manifestations may not appear until weeks to months after injury ■ Confusion, slowed thinking, drowsiness
Intracerebral Hematoma 14% to 15% of all types of head injuries	Located directly in the brain tissue Common sites: frontal or temporal region	Gunshot wounds Depressed bone fractures Stab injury Long history of systemic hypertension Contusions	Headache Deteriorating consciousness to deep coma Hemiplegia on contralateral side Dilated pupil on the side of the clot

levels of consciousness and potential herniation syndromes. Intracranial hematomas are classified by their location as epidural, subdural, or intracerebral. Table 44–9 compares the frequency, locations, common sites, precipitating factors, and manifestations of intracranial hematomas; Figure 44–6 ■ illustrates their locations.

Figure 44–6 ■ Three types of hematomas: epidural hematoma, subdural hematoma, and intracerebral hematoma.

CONTUSION A *contusion* is a bruise of the surface of the brain, typically accompanied by small, diffuse venous hemorrhages. Both white and gray matter may have a bruised, discolored appearance. A decrease in pH, with accumulation of lactic acid and decreased oxygen consumption, may hinder cell function. Contusions (and other focal brain injuries) occur when the brain strikes the inner skull, often with a coup (point of impact) lesion and a contrecoup lesion on the opposite side of the brain. Contusions occur most frequently near bony prominences of the skull. Cerebral edema can follow contusion, resulting in IICP. Contusions; small, diffuse venous hemorrhages; and brain swelling are at their peak 12 to 24 hours after injury.

Manifestations of the contusion depend on the size and location of the brain injury. An initial loss of consciousness occurs; LOC may remain altered, and behavior changes such as combativeness may persist for an extended period. Full consciousness may be regained extremely slowly, and residual deficits may persist; in some clients, full LOC never really returns. Focal effects of the contusion may cause loss of reflexes, hemiparesis (muscular weakness of one-half of the body), or abnormal posturing. Manifestations of IICP may occur if cerebral edema develops. Regaining full LOC may take an extended period of time and residual deficits may persist.

EPIDURAL HEMATOMA An **epidural hematoma** (also called an *extradural hematoma*) develops in the potential space between the dura and the skull, which normally adhere to one another. As the blood collects, the expanding hematoma strips the dura away from the skull. Epidural hematomas affect young to middle-aged adults more frequently than older adults, because the dura becomes more tightly attached to the skull with aging.

Epidural hematomas usually result from a skull fracture that tears an artery, often the middle meningeal artery. Because epidural hematomas are arterial in origin, they tend to develop rapidly. The client may lose consciousness with the initial injury, and then have a brief lucid period before the LOC rapidly declines from drowsiness to coma as the hematoma expands, stripping the dura away from the skull and placing pressure on brain tissue. Other manifestations include headache; vomiting; a fixed, dilated pupil on the same side (ipsilateral) as the hematoma; contralateral (opposite side) hemiparesis or hemiplegia; and possible seizures. Because epidural hematomas usually develop rapidly, timely intervention is vital to prevent significant increases in ICP and herniation.

SUBDURAL HEMATOMA **Subdural hematomas**, in which a localized mass of blood collects between the dura mater and the arachnoid mater, are more common than epidural hematomas. Acute subdural hematomas are usually located at the top of the head, and develop within 48 hours of the initial head injury. Chronic subdural hematomas develop over weeks or months. The chronic type is seen most often in the older adult and people who have some brain atrophy with subsequent enlarged epidural space. These hematomas are often venous in origin, although they may involve bleeding from small arteries as well. Subdural hematomas may form without direct trauma or contusion; acceleration–deceleration forces may tear the bridging veins that connect veins on the surface of the cerebral cortex to the dural sinuses. As blood collects, it places direct pressure on underlying brain tissue.

Acute subdural hematomas develop rapidly following head injury. Although a lucid period may occur, the client commonly develops drowsiness, confusion, and enlargement of the ipsilateral pupil within minutes or hours of the injury. If responsive, the client may complain of a unilateral headache. Hemiparesis and respiratory pattern changes may occur.

Chronic subdural hematomas are often associated with relatively minor trauma such as a fall. Weeks to months may elapse before manifestations of the hematoma occur; the initial trauma may have been forgotten. Chronic subdural hematomas may also occur spontaneously in the older adult or in clients with bleeding disorders. Manifestations of the hematoma develop slowly and may be mistaken for the onset of dementia in the older adult. Slowed thinking, confusion, drowsiness, or lethargy are common early manifestations. Other manifestations include headache, dilation and sluggishness of the ipsilateral pupil, and possible seizures.

INTRACEREBRAL HEMATOMA Intracerebral hematomas may be single or multiple, and are associated with contusions. They may occur in any location but usually are found in the frontal or temporal lobes. They may result from closed head trauma, particularly contusion or shearing of small blood vessels deep within the hemispheres. Intracerebral hematomas can also accompany other types of head trauma such as lacerations. Older adults are particularly vulnerable to intracerebral hemorrhage because cerebral blood vessels are more fragile and easily torn.

The manifestations of intracerebral hematoma vary according to the location of the hematoma. Headache may develop, along with decreasing LOC, hemiplegia, and dilation of the ipsilateral pupil. The expanding clot increases intracranial pressure, and herniation may occur.

Diffuse Brain Injury

A diffuse brain injury (DBI) affects the entire brain and is caused by a shaking motion, with twisting movement (rotational acceleration) as the primary mechanism of injury. DBIs include concussions and diffuse axonal injuries. Shearing stresses on brain tissue cause axonal damage from shearing, tearing, or stretching of nerve fibers. The most serious axonal injuries are located farthest from the brainstem, with the frontal and temporal axonal tracts being most vulnerable to injury. Physical deficits resulting from DBIs include spastic paralysis, peripheral nerve injury, swallowing disorders, visual and hearing impairments, and taste and smell disorders. Damage decreases the speed of information processing and responding and disrupts attention, resulting in serious cognitive and affective impairments. Cognitive deficits that may result include disorientation and confusion, short attention span, problems with memory and learning, perceptual problems, and poor judgment. Possible behavioral deficits include agitation, impulsivity, depression, and social withdrawal.

Initially, the damage involves tearing of axons, blood vessels, and brain tissue (visible only by electron microscope). The number of damaged axons progressively increases, with pathology involving the nuclei and axons. The damaged axons, which resemble sausage links, regress into round balls called retraction balls (visible with light microscopy). After several weeks, the retraction balls are replaced by clusters of microglia. In the final phase, astrocytosis (equivalent to scarring) occurs at the site of axonal damage, accompanied by demyelination of long axon tracts.

The categories of DBI include mild concussion, classic cerebral concussion, and diffuse axonal injury. Manifestations of a concussion are listed in the box below.

MANIFESTATIONS of Concussion

- Immediate loss of consciousness (lasting usually no longer than 5 minutes)
- Amnesia for events surrounding injury
- Headache
- Drowsiness, confusion, dizziness
- Visual disturbances
- Possible brief seizure activity with transient apnea, bradycardia, pallor, and hypotension

Postconcussion Syndrome
- Persistent headache
- Dizziness
- Irritability and insomnia
- Impaired memory and concentration, learning problems

MILD CONCUSSION The word **concussion** means violent shaking. A concussion involves temporary axonal disturbances. It is defined as a momentary interruption of brain function. A concussion is associated with an immediate, brief loss of consciousness on impact. Altered consciousness may last only seconds or persist for several hours. Amnesia for events immediately preceding (antegrade amnesia) and following (retrograde amnesia) the injury is common. Other manifestations of concussion include headache, drowsiness, confusion, dizziness, and visual disturbances such as diplopia or blurred vision.

CLASSIC CEREBRAL CONCUSSION A classic cerebral concussion involves diffuse cerebral disconnection from the brainstem RAS. An immediate loss of consciousness occurs, lasting less than 6 hours. Both retrograde and anterograde amnesia occur. Cerebral contusions may be present. In a severe concussion, a brief seizure and respiratory arrest may occur; transient pallor, bradycardia, and hypotension may accompany loss of consciousness.

Following concussion, clients may develop postconcussion syndrome with persistent headache, dizziness, irritability, insomnia, impaired memory and concentration, and learning problems. Postconcussion syndrome may last for several weeks or, rarely, up to a year.

DIFFUSE AXONAL INJURY Diffuse axonal injury (DAI) is a brain injury in which a high-speed acceleration–deceleration injury, typically associated with motor vehicle crashes, causes widespread disruption of axons in the white matter. Focal lesions may be found in the corpus callosum, midbrain, and brainstem. An immediate loss of consciousness occurs. The prognosis is poor; most clients with severe DAI either die or remain in a persistent vegetative state.

DAIs may range from mild to severe. In mild DAI, coma lasts 6 to 24 hours, and cognitive, psychologic, and sensorimotor deficits may persist. In moderate DAI, injury and impairment is spread throughout the cerebral cortex and diencephalon. There is axonal tearing, coma lasting more than 24 hours, and often incomplete recovery. In severe DAI, axonal injury occurs in both cerebral hemispheres, the diencephalon, and the brainstem. Immediate autonomic dysfunction occurs, and IICP is manifested. Profound cognitive and sensorimotor deficits occur, involving movement, verbal and written communication, ability to learn and reason, and ability to modulate behavior.

INTERDISCIPLINARY CARE

The client with a brain injury may receive medical and/or surgical treatment. Specific guidelines for the medical management of head injury have been developed by the Brain Trauma Foundation (2003) for concussion and acute TBI:

- *Concussion* Following a concussion, the client may be observed for 1 to 2 hours in the emergency department (ED), and then discharged home with instructions for further observation to detect manifestations of secondary injury. If the

loss of consciousness extended more than 2 minutes, the client may be admitted to the hospital for observation.
- *Acute TBI* Recognition and management of acute TBI with transport to an ED is essential to client outcomes. Morbidity and mortality increase with hypotension (systolic pressure less than 90 mmHg) and hypoxia (PaO_2 less than 60 mmHg), so fluids are given to support a mean systolic arterial blood pressure at more than 90 mmHg (Hickey, 2003). Assessment of the client's airway, breathing, and circulation (ABCs), with management of dysfunction, is necessary to decrease the secondary effects of the brain injury. The fluid of choice for intravenous fluids is hypertonic saline, because it reduces intracranial hypertension. An intracranial pressure monitor probe may be inserted to assess ICP and monitor therapy to reduce cerebral edema and maintain cerebral perfusion. Osmotic diuretics such as mannitol also may be administered to reduce cerebral edema. Adequate oxygenation is vital to maintain cerebral metabolism; carbon dioxide is a potent vasodilator, and increased levels may contribute to cerebral edema and IICP.

On admission to the ICU from the ED, the client may be placed on a special bed and connected to various monitoring devices. Invasive lines are inserted, including a central venous pressure (CVP) catheter, arterial line, pulmonary catheter, ventriculostomy, ICP monitor, and perhaps a retrograde jugular catheter. In most instances, an endotracheal tube is inserted and connected to a mechanical ventilator, cardiac monitoring is initiated, bilateral sequential pressure boots are applied, pulse oximetry is started, and a rectal temperature probe is inserted. All values are monitored for changes to ensure early detection of cerebral hypoxia and impending ischemia to prevent secondary brain injury. The values that are monitored are outlined in Table 44–10.

Diagnosis

Diagnostic testing may be done to monitor hemodynamic status and detect conditions that may contribute to cerebral edema. Radiologic examinations include skull x-rays (to identify skull fractures and assess penetrating objects) and CT scan or MRI to detect contusions and lacerations associated with diffuse axonal injury. ABGs are analyzed, with particular attention to oxygen and carbon dioxide levels.

Managing IICP

IICP is managed (as described in a previous section) to reestablish equilibrium of the intracranial contents and prevent secondary brain damage. Treatments include airway management, hyperventilation (used if signs of herniation appear), fluid resuscitation, positioning, temperature regulation, and medications. Medications other than those previously discussed include a category of drugs called neuroprotectants. These drugs are used to treat or alter some of the pathologic pathways that occur in ischemia, and must be administered within a short time of the injury to be effective. Classifications of the drugs include lipid peroxidase inhibitors, free radical scavengers, receptor antagonists, calcium channel blockers, and gangliosides.

TABLE 44–10 Monitoring Cerebral Oxygenation with Laboratory Values

ASSESSMENT	NORMAL RANGE OR VALUE	ABNORMAL FINDINGS
Partial pressure of oxygen in brain tissue (PbtO$_2$)	25–50 mmHg	<15 mmHg = ischemia
Intracranial pressure (ICP)	<10 mmHg	10–20 mmHg = mild to moderate increase in IICP >20 mmHg = severe increase in IICP
Mean arterial pressure (MAP)	70–110 mmHg	<60 mmHg = decreased cerebral perfusion pressure
Cerebral perfusion pressure (CPP)	70–100 mmHg	<50 mmHg = compromised cerebral blood flow
PaCO$_2$	35–45 mmHg	<35 mmHg may result in cerebral vasoconstriction, further decreasing oxygenation of brain tissue
PaO$_2$	80–100 mmHg	If decreased, can cause tissue hypoxia and decrease oxygenation of brain tissue

Source: Data from Wilensky, E., & Bloom, S. (2005). Monitoring brain tissue oxygenation after severe brain injury. *Nursing, 35*(2), 32cc1–32cc4.

Surgery

Small subdural hematomas can frequently be reabsorbed and may be treated conservatively, with close observation and supportive care. However, the treatment of choice for epidural hematomas and large acute subdural hematomas is surgical evacuation of the clot. This can often be performed through burr holes made into the skull (Figure 44–7 ■). In an epidural hematoma, the bleeding vessel can also be ligated during this procedure, preventing further bleeding. Rebleeding may occur following evacuation of an acute subdural hematoma in older adults and clients with chronic alcoholism. A craniotomy is necessary to evacuate chronic subdural hematomas because the hematoma tends to solidify, making it difficult or impossible to remove through burr holes. Surgery is less successful in treating intracerebral hematomas because of widespread tissue damage. Supportive care to manage intracranial pressure and prevent complications is provided.

NURSING CARE

In addition to the nursing care discussed in this section, a Nursing Care Plan for a client with a subdural hematoma is found on the next page.

Health Promotion

The best way to treat any injury is to prevent it from happening. Public education must continue to stress the importance of safe driving, the dangers of driving under the influence of alcohol or drugs, and the necessity of wearing seat belts and cycle helmets. Legislation has mandated such motor vehicle changes as seat belts, child safety seats, and air bags. Other behaviors that can reduce the morbidity and mortality associated with TBI are following gun safety rules, promoting farm safety, and teaching older adults about safety (such as preventing falls) in the home.

Assessment

Collect the following data through the health history and physical examination (see Chapter 43 ∞):
- *Health history:* A history of the injury is helpful in understanding the nature of the craniocerebral trauma; knowledge about loss of consciousness assists the nurse in planning care.
- *Physical examination:* Neurologic assessment, including pupils, LOC, Glasgow Coma Scale, brainstem reflexes (cornea, cough, gag, extraocular movements), vital signs; skull and face (deformity, lacerations, bruising, bleeding); movement of extremities.

Nursing Diagnoses and Interventions

Nursing care of the client in the acute care phase initially focuses on maintaining an effective airway and breathing pattern. Nursing care is also directed toward continuous assessment and monitoring of neurologic function as well as other body systems.

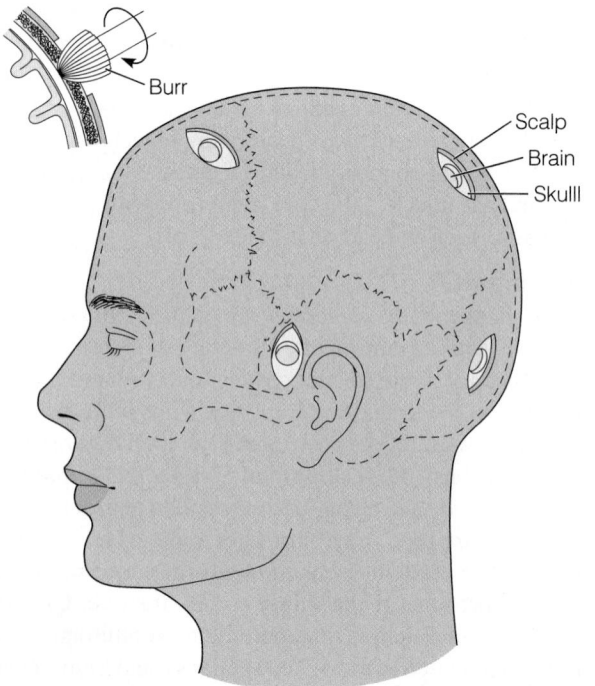

Figure 44–7 ■ Possible locations of burr holes.

NURSING CARE PLAN A Client with a Subdural Hematoma

Wong Lee is a 50-year-old tug boat mechanic who is married and has three sons. Although Mr. Lee has been through rehabilitation twice for alcoholism, he has not been able to quit drinking. His physician has explained the physical consequences and the possible interaction between alcohol and the anticoagulant Mr. Lee is taking for chronic atrial fibrillation. While attending a family reunion, during which he eats a large meal and drinks several beers, Mr. Lee joins a game of softball. Mrs. Lee is concerned that Mr. Lee has consumed too much alcohol to play ball in the heat, but Mr. Lee is adamant and states that he wants to pitch. During the end of the second inning, the batter hits a ball that strikes Mr. Lee in the head. Mr. Lee stumbles and drops to the ground, holding his head. He does not lose consciousness and gets up on his own. His sons and wife try to persuade him to go to the hospital, but Mr. Lee insists he feels fine.

Two weeks later, after an evening of consuming several mixed drinks, Mr. Lee develops a headache. He attributes the headache to a hangover, but instead of improving the next day, the headache becomes steadily worse. He becomes confused and disoriented. His wife, concerned that his drinking is increasing again, calls the physician, who admits Mr. Lee to the detoxification center at the local hospital. A CT scan is performed. The diagnosis of a subdural hematoma is made, and Mr. Lee is transferred to the neurosurgical unit.

ASSESSMENT

When Saundra Knight, the nurse on the neurosurgical unit, enters the room, she notices that Mr. Lee is sitting in bed, laughing and giddy. As she begins to talk to Mr. Lee, he states, "Don't ask me anything—I can't think. My headache is getting worse." Over the next few hours, the giddiness subsides, and Mr. Lee becomes drowsy. Ms. Knight reports a Glasgow Coma Scale score of 11. An ICP monitor is inserted and reveals increased intracranial pressure. Mr. Lee is scheduled to have burr holes and hematoma evacuation that afternoon.

DIAGNOSES

- *Risk for Ineffective Breathing Pattern* related to pressure on respiratory center by intracranial hematoma
- *Ineffective Cerebral Tissue Perfusion* related to increased intracranial pressure secondary to cerebral edema

EXPECTED OUTCOMES

- Maintain a respiratory rate and rhythm within normal limits.
- Maintain adequate cerebral perfusion, as evidenced by stable vital signs, stable neurologic status, and no decrease in level of consciousness.

PLANNING AND IMPLEMENTATION

- Perform neurologic assessment every 2 hours or as needed.
- Monitor vital signs every 2 hours or as needed.
- Explain to the family the procedure for intracranial surgery.

EVALUATION

The first day postoperatively, Mr. Lee begins breathing on his own without ventilatory support. His respiratory rate and rhythm are within normal limits, with no signs of abnormal breath sounds. The ICP monitor readings are appropriate, and Mr. Lee shows significant improvement in level of consciousness, with a Glasgow Coma Scale score of 15. Mr. Lee continues to improve and is discharged to home 5 days after surgery.

CRITICAL THINKING IN THE NURSING PROCESS

1. Describe the similarities and differences between Mr. Lee's disorder and the manifestations of other types of intracranial hematomas.
2. Mr. Lee kept trying to pull out his ICP line. You know he should not be restrained, because pulling against restraints increases restlessness and increases intracranial pressure. What would you do?
3. Write a care plan for Mr. Lee for the nursing diagnosis *Acute Confusion.*

See Evaluating Your Response in Appendix C.

This close monitoring provides early recognition and treatment of problems and complications, and initiation of aggressive forms of therapy that may be needed.

Many nursing diagnoses associated with traumatic brain injury correspond with those outlined previously in the sections on the client with altered LOC and IICP. Specific nursing diagnoses discussed in this section focus on problems with intracranial adaptive capacity, airway clearance, and breathing patterns.

Decreased Intracranial Adaptive Capacity

The client with a traumatic brain injury has or is at high risk for IICP. As the mechanisms that normally compensate for changes in intracranial pressure are compromised, intracranial pressure increases in disproportional response to a variety of stimuli. (See the discussion earlier in the chapter for other nursing diagnoses and interventions for the client with IICP.)

- Monitor for manifestations of IICP, including eye opening response, motor response, and verbal response. *These responses evaluate the ability to integrate commands with conscious and involuntary movement.*
- Monitor for changes in vital signs: bradycardia or tachycardia, varying breathing patterns, hypertension, and/or widening pulse pressure. Vital signs vary depending on the site of impairment. *Cushing's triad (bradycardia, increased systolic blood pressure, and increased pulse pressure) indicates brainstem ischemia leading to cerebral herniation.*
- Monitor for vomiting, headache, lethargy, restlessness, purposeless movements, and changes in mentation. *These manifestations may be early indicators of intracranial pressure changes.*
- Monitor temperature and initiate hypothermia treatment as prescribed. *Impaired hypothalamic function can interfere with temperature regulation. Hyperthermia may increase ICP.*
- Monitor fluid status: Regularly compare intake and output, review serum osmolality, and use infusion pump to administer IV fluids (if prescribed). *Osmotic diuretics, if used to treat cerebral edema, may cause hypotension and decreased cardiac output.*

PRACTICE ALERT
Overhydration from rapid infusion of IV fluids may cause or further increase IICP.

Ineffective Airway Clearance

The primary objective in the care of any trauma client is maintaining a patent airway to prevent hypoxia. However, in the initial acute care phase, the risk of cervical vertebral fractures and spinal cord injury may complicate the process of establishing a patent airway. In addition, other multisystem injuries may complicate the interpretation of vital signs. In general, all unconscious people with a head injury should be intubated with an endotracheal tube to prevent aspiration. Clients with head trauma may also require a tracheostomy to provide an airway and be placed on a ventilator.

- Monitor neurologic manifestations on a regular schedule. *Changes in neurologic manifestations may indicate IICP, with the risk of further depression of the respiratory system and respiratory arrest.*
- Maintain head and neck in neutral alignment, immobilized until injury is determined. *Head rotation and neck flexion are associated with IICP, decreased jugular venous outflow, and localized changes in cerebral blood flow. Immobilization prevents spinal cord injury in suspected or actual fractures of the cervical spine; spinal cord injury at this level would further impair respiratory function.*
- Clear the nose and mouth of mucus and blood. *This helps maintain patency of the upper airway.*
- Suction the airway as needed, limiting suctioning time to no more than 10 seconds at one time. Do not suction the nasal passages until a dural tear has been ruled out. *Suctioning is usually necessary to maintain a patent airway.*

Ineffective Breathing Pattern

The client with a traumatic brain injury and hematoma is at high risk for ineffective breathing pattern related to IICP. If ICP increases dramatically, tentorial herniation may occur, leading to sudden respiratory arrest.

- Monitor the respiratory pattern for rate, depth, and rhythm every 2 hours or as needed if the client is not on a ventilator. Assess breath sounds, presence of cyanosis, restlessness, and use of accessory respiratory muscles. Monitor pulse oximetry and blood gas levels. *Head injuries may cause alterations in respirations. An increased respiratory rate may indicate hypoxia. A decrease in respiratory rate may be the result of depression of the medullary respiratory center.*

PRACTICE ALERT
In general, an initial increase in intracranial pressure causes respirations to slow; as the pressure continues to increase, respirations become rapid.

- Monitor ICP readings. Continuous measurement of ICP is used to diagnose and monitor increased intracranial pressure. *As ICP increases, herniation may occur, leading to respiratory arrest and death.*

- If the client is not intubated, prepare for oxygen administration and/or tracheal intubation if respiratory distress occurs. *Supplying oxygen prevents hypoxia until a hematoma can be evacuated, relieving pressure on the respiratory center.*
- Prepare for cranial surgery if deteriorating respiratory pattern and neurologic changes are noted. *Surgical intervention usually consists of placing several burr holes in the skull or performing a craniotomy to remove the hematoma. (Intracranial surgery is discussed later in the chapter.) However, the cerebral edema and increased intracranial pressure may cause death even if surgery is performed.*

Using NANDA, NIC, and NOC

Chart 44–2 shows links between NANDA nursing diagnoses, NIC, and NOC when caring for the client with an acute brain injury.

Community-Based Care
Concussion

Inform the client and family that a postconcussion syndrome sometimes occurs. If the client experiences persistent headaches and dizziness, is uncharacteristically emotional, seems overly tired, or has difficulty paying attention or remembering, the healthcare provider should be notified. Explain that these manifestations may persist for some time. Rehabilitation may help the client compensate for memory impairment and attention deficits.

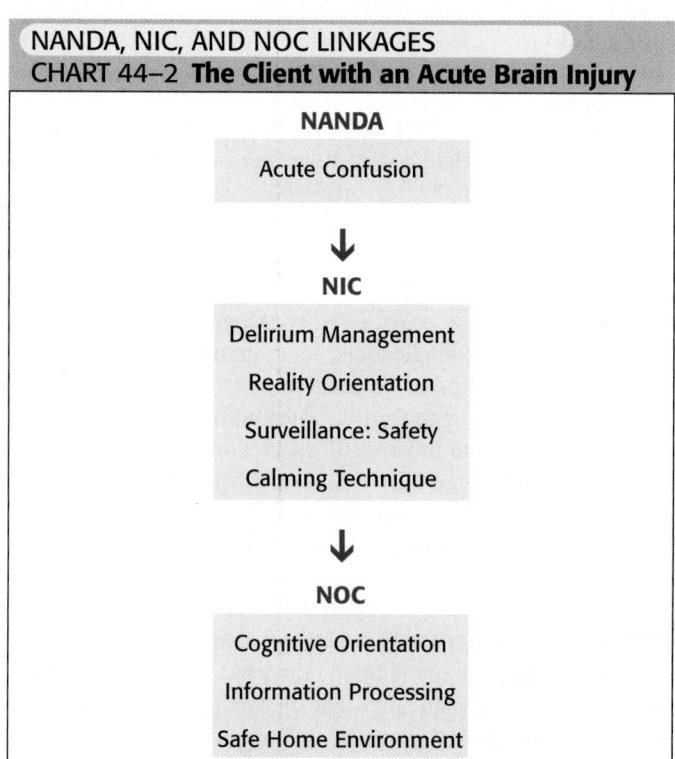

NANDA, NIC, AND NOC LINKAGES
CHART 44–2 The Client with an Acute Brain Injury

NANDA

Acute Confusion

↓

NIC

Delirium Management
Reality Orientation
Surveillance: Safety
Calming Technique

↓

NOC

Cognitive Orientation
Information Processing
Safe Home Environment

Data from *NANDA's Nursing Diagnoses: Definitions & Classification 2005–2006* by NANDA International (2005), Philadelphia; *Nursing Interventions Classification (NIC)* (4th ed.) by J. M. Dochterman & G. M. Bulechek (2004), St. Louis, MO: Mosby; and *Nursing Outcomes Classification (NOC)* (3rd ed.) by S. Moorhead, M. Johnson, and M. Maas (2004), St. Louis, MO: Mosby.

Acute Brain Injury

Clients who survive an acute brain injury will require long-term physical care and rehabilitation. Although recovery is highly individualized, many clients who regain consciousness require lifelong care; others remain in a coma or vegetative state. The family often expects the client to recover fully after the coma subsides, and they need information about the real possibility of residual deficits in self-care, emotional responses, cognition, communication, and movement (see the Nursing Research box below). Topics that should be addressed for home care include:

- The need to encourage self-care and independence as much as possible
- Information to enhance recovery (CDC, 2006):
  - Get lots of rest. Don't rush back to work or school.
  - Avoid anything that could cause another blow or jolt to the head.

- Consult with physician about when it will be safe to drive a car, ride a bike, or use heavy equipment (reaction time is often slower after a TBI).
- Take only prescribed drugs and don't drink alcohol.
- Write things down if you are having problems remembering.
- If the injury was severe, therapy may be needed to learn lost skills, such as speaking, walking or reading.
- Safety issues
- Equipment needs, such as a wheelchair and hospital bed
- Vocational counseling and services
- Referral to community resources and support groups
- Helpful resources:
  - National Head Injury Foundation
  - Brain Injury Association of America
  - Brain Trauma Foundation
  - International Center for Individuals with Disabilities.

NURSING RESEARCH   Evidence-Based Practice: Caregivers of Young Adults with TBI

TBI is a leading cause of death and disability across all age groups, but the age group most affected is young adults, and especially young men. This is the result of increased risk-taking behavior in the age group, including drinking alcohol and using drugs while operating a motor vehicle. This population of TBI survivors is large and caring for them is expensive. Most research of TBI survivors has focused on problems of the survivor, but few have examined the burden placed on the family. This is especially true for the experience of the survivors' mothers, who are in almost all cases the primary caregiver. A study was conducted by Kao and Stuifben (2004) to describe the meaning of the experience of the relationship between young adult TBI survivors and their mothers. Both the survivors and the mothers were interviewed and the data were analyzed to describe the experience. The survivors described having a sense of being abnormal; the mothers struggled with a balance of protecting their children and letting them become independent. The mothers also struggled to maintain relationships inside and outside of the family. All of these experiences resulted in ongoing stress for the mothers.

IMPLICATIONS FOR NURSING

The findings of this study have implications for community-based teaching and interventions for TBI survivors and their caregivers. Each year a significant number of TBI survivors leave the acute care setting and return to their homes, where caregivers are often

unprepared for the lifelong multiple disabilities and problems they will face.

Developing an appropriate tool to measure family caregiver burden for those with disabilities from TBI is recommended, so as to be able to design and implement individualized interventions and teaching. The teaching and interventions should be developed as part of a systematic and integrated discharge plan, a community-based program, and a follow-up approach to assist TBI survivors and their families to effectively decrease the stressors that are a part of caregiver load.

CRITICAL THINKING IN CLIENT CARE

1. You are making a home visit to a 22-year-old woman who has recently been discharged from acute care following a serious automobile crash resulting in mild diffuse axonal injury. She says to you "I had my accident on the way home from spring break. This is my third year in nursing school. Will I be able to be a nurse?" How would you respond?
2. On discharge from the hospital, a nursing diagnosis for a young adult TBI survivor who would be cared for at home by his single mother was *Risk for Parental Role Conflict*. Do you think this is an appropriate diagnosis? Why or why not?
3. If you were to outline topics for a program to reduce the incidence of TBI in a rural community, how would it differ from one for residents of a large urban city?

Source: Data from Kao, H., & Stuifbergen, A. (2004). Love and load: The lived experience of the mother–child relationship among young adult traumatic brain-injured survivors. *Journal of Neuroscience Nursing, 36*(2), 73–81.

CENTRAL NERVOUS SYSTEM INFECTIONS

THE CLIENT WITH A CENTRAL NERVOUS SYSTEM INFECTION

The central nervous system, including the meninges, neural tissues, and blood vessels, may be directly affected by bacteria, viruses, fungi, protozoans, and rickettsiae. The CNS may also be affected by toxins from bacterial infections. In general, or-

ganisms enter the brain in two ways: through the bloodstream by crossing the blood–brain barrier or by direct invasion through a skull fracture or bullet hole. Very rarely, a CNS infection occurs as a result of contamination of a surgical field or lumbar puncture. The major CNS infections include meningitis, encephalitis, and brain abscesses.

The incidence of pathogenic infections of the CNS increases with the onset of AIDS. Clients who are HIV positive may have CNS infections caused by toxoplasmosis, cryptococcus, tuberculosis, herpes simplex, cytomegalovirus (CMV), or a polyoma virus (resulting in progressive multifocal leukoencephalopathy).

Pathophysiology

When pathogens enter the CNS and the meninges, an inflammatory process results. The pathology of CNS infections includes the invading pathogens, the subsequent inflammation, and the increase in intracranial pressure that may result from the inflammatory processes. Both the pathogenic damage and the IICP may result in brain damage and life-threatening complications.

Meningitis

Meningitis is an inflammation of the pia mater, the arachnoid, and the subarachnoid space. Inflammation spreads rapidly throughout the CNS because of the circulation of CSF around the brain and spinal cord. Meningitis may be acute or chronic, and it may be bacterial, viral, fungal, or parasitic in origin. Meningococcal meningitis may occur in epidemics among people who are in close contact with one another, such as military recruits and students living in dormitories. Pneumococcal meningitis, in contrast, primarily affects the very young and very old.

The organism responsible for meningitis must overcome nonspecific and specific host defense mechanisms to invade and replicate in the CSF. These defenses include the skin barrier, the blood–brain barrier, the nonspecific inflammatory response, and the immune response. Host response to the particular pathogen is responsible for the manifestations of clinical meningitis. The organisms that initiate the host response in meningitis demonstrate an affinity for the nervous system. They colonize and invade the nasopharyngeal mucosa, survive intravascularly, and penetrate the CNS if the blood–brain barrier is damaged, as can happen during surgery, the inflammatory response, or cerebral edema.

Infection of the CSF and meninges causes an inflammatory response in the pia, arachnoid, and CSF. Because the meninges and subarachnoid space are continuous around the brain, spinal cord, and optic nerves, the infection and inflammatory response are always cerebrospinal, involving both the brain and the spinal cord. Inflamed blood vessels in the area leak fluids as cell permeability increases. Purulent exudate infiltrates cranial nerve sheaths and blocks the choroid plexus and subarachnoid villi. IICP occurs as brain tissue responds to the pathogen. With an increase in ICP, cerebral perfusion decreases and cerebral autoregulation is lost.

BACTERIAL MENINGITIS The causative organisms of bacterial meningitis include *Neisseria meningitis*, meningococcus, *Streptococcus pneumoniae*, *Haemophilus influenzae*, and *Escherichia coli*. Risk factors include head trauma with a basal skull fracture, otitis media, mastoiditis, sinusitis, neurosurgery, systemic sepsis, or immunocompromise (Porth, 2005). Even when appropriate antibiotics are used, the mortality rate for adults remains at approximately 25%.

Once the pathogen enters the central nervous system, it or its toxic products (free radicals) initiate an inflammatory response in the meninges, CSF, and ventricles. Meningeal vessels become engorged, and their permeability increases. Phagocytic white blood cells migrate into the subarachnoid space, forming a purulent exudate that thickens and clouds the CSF and interferes with its flow. Rapid exudate formation causes further inflammation and edema of meningeal cells. Blood vessel engorgement, exudate formation, impaired CSF flow, and cellular edema cause the intracranial pressure to increase.

Manifestations The client with bacterial meningitis typically presents with fever and chills, headache, back and abdominal pain, and nausea and vomiting. (The older adult may not have a high fever, but may instead exhibit confusion.) Meningeal irritation causes nuchal rigidity (stiff neck) and positive Brudzinski's sign (flexion of the neck that causes the hip and knee to flex) and positive Kernig's sign (inability to extend the knee while the hip is flexed at a 90-degree angle). Photophobia is present; the client may also experience diplopia. With meningococcal meningitis, a rapidly spreading petechial rash involving the skin and mucous membranes may be noted. The client may also have IICP, manifested by decreased LOC, seizures, changes in vital signs and respiratory pattern, and papilledema. The manifestations of bacterial meningitis are listed in the box below.

Complications Complications of bacterial meningitis include arthritis, cranial nerve damage, and hydrocephalus. Cranial nerve VIII, the auditory nerve, is frequently affected, with resulting nerve deafness. Thrombophlebitis may develop in cerebral vessels, with infarction of surrounding tissues (Porth, 2005).

VIRAL MENINGITIS Acute viral meningitis, also called *aseptic meningitis*, is a less severe disease than bacterial meningitis. It can be caused by numerous viruses, such as herpes simplex, herpes zoster, Epstein-Barr virus, or cytomegalovirus (CMV). Viral meningitis most often appears after a case of mumps. Although viral infection also triggers the inflammatory response, the course of the disease is benign and of short duration. Recovery is uneventful.

Manifestations The manifestations of viral meningitis are similar to those of bacterial meningitis, although usually milder. The client may have a mild flulike illness prior to the onset of meningitis. Headache is intense and is accompanied by malaise, nausea, vomiting, and lethargy. Photophobia may be present. The

---

MANIFESTATIONS of Bacterial Meningitis

- Restlessness, agitation, and irritability
- Severe headache
- Signs of meningeal irritation:
  a. Nuchal rigidity
  b. Positive Brudzinski's sign
  c. Positive Kernig's sign
- Chills and high fever
- Confusion, altered LOC
- Photophobia (aversion to light), diplopia
- Seizures
- Signs of increased ICP (widened pulse pressure and bradycardia, respiratory irregularity, decreased LOC, headache, and vomiting)
- Petechial rash (in meningococcal meningitis)

client generally remains oriented, although possibly drowsy. Temperature is mildly elevated. Neck stiffness, positive Brudzinski's sign, and positive Kernig's sign are usually present.

Encephalitis

Encephalitis is an acute inflammation of the parenchyma of the brain or spinal cord. It is almost always caused by a virus, but it may also be caused by bacteria, fungi, and other organisms. Other less common causes include ingested lead; postvaccination encephalitis (from vaccines for measles, mumps, and rabies), and HIV (Porth, 2005). See Table 44–11 for a list of the most common causes of encephalitis.

VIRAL ENCEPHALITIS Viruses depend on living tissue for reproduction and become highly destructive when they invade brain tissue. The inflammatory response extends over the cerebral cortex, the white matter, and the meninges, with degeneration of the neurons. The pathology of encephalitis includes local necrotizing hemorrhage, which ultimately becomes generalized, with prominent edema. There is progressive degeneration of nerve cell bodies. The inflammatory response in encephalitis does not cause exudate formation as it does in meningitis. Certain viruses show a propensity for specific areas of the brain (e.g., herpes simplex virus involves frontal and temporal lobes). The virus gains access to the CNS via the bloodstream or along peripheral or cranial nerves, or it may already be present in the meninges in the client with meningitis.

The manifestations of viral encephalitis vary, depending on the organism and area of the brain affected. Usual manifestations are similar to those of meningitis, including fever,

headache, seizures, stiff neck, and altered LOC. The client may be disoriented, agitated and restless, or lethargic and drowsy. As the disease progresses, the LOC deteriorates, and the client may become comatose.

ARBOVIRUS ENCEPHALITIS The arboviruses are arthropod (mosquito or tick)-borne agents that infect humans. They include many different types, including Western equine encephalitis, St. Louis encephalitis, and Rift Valley fever. Adults are most often infected with St. Louis encephalitis, with older adults affected more often. The arthropods may live in small mammals and birds, or may be carried by horses and deer. The newest arboviral encephalitis in the United States is West Nile encephalitis.

The arthropod-borne agents cause widespread degeneration of nerve cells, and edema and necrosis with or without hemorrhage occur. IICP may develop. Manifestations include fever, malaise, sore throat, nausea and vomiting, stiff neck, tremors, paralysis of extremities, exaggerated deep tendon reflexes, seizures, and altered LOC.

Brain Abscess

A brain abscess is an infection with a collection of purulent material within the brain tissue. Approximately 80% are found in the cerebrum and 20% are cerebellar.

The causes of a brain abscess include open trauma and neurosurgery; infections of the mastoid, middle ear, nasal cavity, or nasal sinuses; metastatic spread from distant foci (such as heart, lungs, skin, abscessed teeth, and dirty needles); and arising from other associated areas of infection. The immunocompromised are at increased risk for abscesses. The most common

TABLE 44–11 Causes of Encephalitis

CAUSE	COMMENTS
Arboviruses	Transmitted by bites from ticks and mosquitoes. Bites from ticks occur more frequently in spring. Bites from mosquitoes occur in middle to late summer. Most common types are St. Louis and Eastern and Western equine encephalitis. May destroy major parts of the lobe or hemisphere. Two-thirds of clients who develop Eastern equine encephalitis either die or develop severe residual disabilities (e.g., seizures, blindness, deafness, speech disorders, or mental retardation). The incubation is 5 to 15 days. Mortality rates associated with arboviruses are higher than those associated with enteroviruses.
Enteroviruses, such as echovirus, coxsackievirus, poliovirus, paramyxovirus (the virus that causes mumps), and varicella-zoster (the virus that causes chickenpox)	Infection occurs more frequently in summer (except infection by the mumps virus, which occurs more frequently in early winter). Some degree of protection can be afforded by immunization against measles, mumps, and poliomyelitis. Mortality rates are lower than those associated with herpes simplex type 1 virus.
Herpes simplex type 1 virus	Most common nonepidemic encephalitis in North America. Can occur any time of year and throughout the world. Has an affinity for the frontal and temporal lobes. Prognosis is grave but not hopeless: Mortality rate can be as high as 40%, and client may die within 2 weeks.
Amebic meningoencephalitis due to infection by *Naegleria* and *Acanthamoeba* protozoa	Both protozoa are found in warm freshwater. Enter the nasal mucosa of people swimming in ponds or lakes. May also be found in soil and decaying vegetation. Incidence of infection is increasing in North America.
Exogenous poisoning	May occur after ingestion of lead or arsenic or inhalation of carbon monoxide.

pathogens causing the abscess are streptococci, staphylococci, and bacteroids. Yeast and fungi may also cause brain abscess.

A brain abscess results from the presence of microorganisms in the brain tissue. If the abscess is encapsulated, it has the ability to enlarge and, therefore, behave as a space-occupying lesion within the cranium. This predisposes the client not only to the systemic effects of the inflammatory process but also to the serious consequences of increased intracranial pressure. Occasionally, the abscess does not become encapsulated; instead, it spreads through the brain tissue to the subarachnoid space and ventricular system.

Initially, the client exhibits the general symptoms associated with an acute infectious process, such as chills, fever, malaise, and anorexia. Because brain abscess generally forms after infection, the client may consider these signs to be an exacerbation of that illness. The client may experience seizures, altered LOC, and manifestations of IICP. As the abscess enlarges, specific symptoms are related to location; for example, the client with a frontal lobe abscess may have contralateral hemiparesis, expressive aphasia, focal seizures, and frontal headache.

INTERDISCIPLINARY CARE

Bacterial meningitis is a medical emergency that, if not treated immediately, can be fatal within days. Successful management depends on rapid diagnosis and aggressive treatment with antibiotics and corticosteroids to eradicate the infecting organism and support vital functions. The client may be placed in strict or respiratory isolation until the organism has been identified, depending on hospital policy. Universal precautions apply to CSF as well as blood.

Treatment for viral meningitis focuses on managing client symptoms and is supportive. Antipyretics and analgesics may provide relief. Antibiotic therapy is not indicated, and isolation precautions are not required.

Treatment of the client with a brain abscess focuses on prompt initiation of antibiotic therapy. Other manifestations are treated symptomatically, as with the client diagnosed with meningitis or encephalitis. If pharmacologic management is not effective, the abscess may be drained or, if it is encapsulated, removed.

Diagnosis

The diagnosis of meningitis is based on manifestations and diagnostic tests results. Gram stain and culture of the CSF are used to determine if a bacterial infection is present and to determine the specific infectious agent. Counterimmunoelectrophoresis (CIE) is a laboratory test that may be ordered to determine the presence of viruses or protozoa. Polymerase chain reaction techniques may be used to detect viral DNA or RNA in spinal fluid. CT scan will show an area of increased contrast surrounding a low-density core with brain abscess.

Lumbar puncture with examination of the CSF is the definitive diagnostic measure for bacterial meningitis. Data that indicate bacterial meningitis include turbid, cloudy fluid; a markedly increased white blood cell (WBC) count and protein content; and a decreased glucose content. The opening pressure on the lumbar puncture is elevated. In contrast, the client with encephalitis may have a normal CSF analysis and pressure or

may have some lymphocytes. The client with a brain abscess will have a markedly elevated pressure with elevated protein content and elevated WBC count. Glucose content is normal. (Because a lumbar puncture in the presence of a space-occupying lesion can result in brain herniation and death, a CT scan is performed first if neurologic findings support such a lesion.)

Medications

Immediate intravenous administration of a broad-spectrum antibiotic that crosses the blood–brain barrier into the subarachnoid space is instituted in cases of bacterial meningitis. Once culture reports identify the causative organism, drug therapy is continued from 7 to 21 days, using the most effective drug or drugs specific to that bacterium. The cephalosporin antibiotics are preferred. A major concern in the treatment of CNS infections is penicillin-resistant streptococci. Recommendations for treatment are for a broad-spectrum cephalosporin, such as rifampin (Rifadin), cefotaxime (Claforan), or vancomycin (Vancocin). However, as the bacteria are killed, the toxins they release increase production of inflammatory cytokines, which are potentially lethal. Steroids such as dexamethasone (Decadron) are often given with the antibiotics to suppress inflammation. The CDC recommends that the client remain on isolation for 24 hours after the start of antibiotic therapy.

Treatment for encephalitis consists of administering specific medications and preventing complications. Fungal meningitis is treated with antifungal agents, such as amphotericin-B (Amphotec), flucytosine (Ancobon), and fluconazole (Diflucan). Viral encephalitis is treated with intravenous acyclovir (Zovirax) or vidarabine (Vira-A).

Antibiotic therapy is the primary treatment for brain abscess. A combination of broad-spectrum antibiotics is used if the infecting organism is unknown.

Anticonvulsant medications such as phenytoin (Dilantin) are often prescribed to prevent or control seizure activity. Antipyretic and analgesic medications may provide symptomatic relief; however, analgesics that have a depressant effect on the CNS (such as opiates) are avoided to prevent masking of early manifestations of deteriorating LOC. The client initially may require antiemetics to control nausea and vomiting. Fluid and electrolyte status is maintained through intravenous fluid replacement until the client is able to resume oral intake.

Surgery

Surgical drainage of an encapsulated abscess may be necessary. The decision to perform surgery is based on the client's general condition, the stage of abscess development, and the site of the abscess.

NURSING CARE

Central nervous system infections are serious illnesses, with potentially life-threatening effects and complications. Nursing assessments and interventions are critical in identifying changes in the client's neurologic status and preventing complications from IICP. In addition to the nursing care described in this section, a Nursing Care Plan for a client with bacterial meningitis is found on the next page.

NURSING CARE PLAN   A Client with Bacterial Meningitis

Monty Cook is a 22-year-old musician who plays in a local rock band. He is unmarried and lives with his parents. He is known by everyone in the community as a quiet, low-key, easygoing person and an excellent guitar player. During a performance 2 days ago, he had difficulty playing his guitar, complaining of bright stage lights blazing in his eyes. When he tried to keep his head down to prevent the lights from hurting his eyes, he noticed his neck was very stiff. After the performance, one of the newest members of the band remarked that it certainly was not their best performance. Monty responded angrily that maybe the new members of the group needed more practice. Then he stomped out and went home to bed.

He wakes at 4:00 A.M. with a severe headache, sweating, and chills; his temperature is 102°F, and he cannot bend his neck without severe pain. His mother recognizes that he is agitated and irritable, which is uncharacteristic. Frightened, she rushes him to the hospital emergency room. A lumbar puncture performed in the emergency room reveals turbid, cloudly fluid; a markedly increased WBC count; and protein with a decreased glucose content. Bacterial meningitis is the medical diagnosis. Mr. Cook is admitted to the hospital for treatment and care.

ASSESSMENT

When the nurse, Aisha Aldi, enters Mr. Cook's isolation room, she sees him thrashing about in the bed, talking incoherently, and becoming more agitated. On assessment, Ms. Aldi notes dry mucous membranes, cracked lips, and small petechiae over the upper torso and abdomen. Mr. Cook's temperature is 104°F. Kernig's sign is positive. Intravenous broad-spectrum antibiotics are prescribed and initiated. After the first 2 hours of care, Ms. Aldi notes a decrease in Mr. Cook's level of consciousness.

DIAGNOSES

- *Hyperthermia* related to infection and abnormal temperature regulation by hypothalamus
- *Disturbed Thought Processes* related to intracranial infection
- *Ineffective Protection* related to progression of illness

EXPECTED OUTCOMES

- Have a decrease in body temperature.

- Become less restless and agitated.
- Remain free of injury.

PLANNING AND IMPLEMENTATION

- Monitor vital signs every 2 hours.
- Provide sponge baths if temperature continues to rise.
- Provide a quiet, nonstimulating environment with the shades drawn.
- Provide oral care every 4 hours.
- Measure and compare intake and output every 2 hours.
- Perform neurologic assessments every 2 to 4 hours.
- Monitor for and report seizure activity and decreasing level of consciousness.
- Keep bed in low position with side rails elevated.
- Administer prescribed intravenous antibiotics.

EVALUATION

After 4 days of antibiotic therapy, Mr. Cook's temperature has returned to near normal. Ms. Aldi notes that he has begun opening his eyes and visually tracking her as she moves about the room. Mr. Cook responds to a request to squeeze Ms. Aldi's fingers and after several hours asks her what had happened. On day 5, Mr. Cook states that he feels better and his headache is gone. He ask for sips of juice and begins urinating regularly. Seven days after admission, Mr. Cook is discharged and is able to go home with his mother. He has some weakness in his legs, but otherwise has no evidence of neurologic deficits.

CRITICAL THINKING IN THE NURSING PROCESS

1. What strategies should the nurse use to decrease the environmental stimuli for Mr. Cook, and what is the rationale for doing these?
2. If you were caring for Mr. Cook in the initial phase of the illness and he became combative, what would you do?
3. Develop a plan of care for Mr. Cook for the nursing diagnosis *Acute Pain*. Consider the effect of narcotics on respiratory function in designing the plan.

See Evaluating Your Response in Appendix C.

Health Promotion

As with many other intracranial injuries and disorders, educational activities to promote health by preventing CNS infections are important nursing interventions. The following information should be provided:.

- Vaccinations for meningococcal meningitis are recommended or required for military recruits and college students (groups at increased risk for invasive meningococcal meningitis).
- Administration of prophylactic rifampin (Rifadin) is recommended for people exposed to meningococcal meningitis.
- Mosquito control with repellants, insecticides, and protective clothing.
- Destruction of the insect larvae and elimination of breeding places, such as pools of stagnant water.
- Vaccination against Japanese B encephalitis (recommended for summer travelers to rural East Asia).
- Prompt diagnosis and treatment of infections of the head, neck, and respiratory system.

Assessment

Collect the following data through the health history and physical examination (see Chapter 43 ∞). Further focused assessments are described with nursing interventions below.

- *Health history:* Risk factors (concurrent infections, other illnesses, travel), when manifestations began, severity of manifestations, current nausea and headache, seizures.
- *Physical examination:* Glasgow Coma Scale, level of consciousness, vital signs, motor function, pupillary check, cranial nerves, neck ROM, Brudzinski's sign, Kernig's sign, skin (rash, petechiae, purpura), muscle movement and strength, speech.

Nursing Diagnoses and Interventions

In planning and implementing nursing care for the client with a CNS infection, the prognosis may depend on the supportive care given. The client is often very ill, and the combination of fever, dehydration, and cerebral edema may predispose the client to seizures. Airway obstruction, respiratory arrest, or cardiac dysrhythmias may occur. Nursing diagnoses and interventions previously discussed for the client with an altered LOC, IICP, and seizures are also appropriate for the client with a CNS infection. Nursing interventions in this section focus on ineffective protection and risk for fluid volume deficit.

Ineffective Protection

Clients with CNS infections are less able to protect themselves against insults from both internal and external sources. The effects of the inflammation and resulting pathophysiologic processes may include pain, fever, altered LOC, seizures, IICP, and cranial nerve dysfunction. In addition, pathophysiologic effects on the brain from toxins or thrombosis of a cerebral vessel may lead to permanent neurologic deficits, such as loss of motor function or dementia.

- Monitor neurologic status on a regular basis. *Many complications are evidenced by changes in neurologic manifestations.*
- Monitor vital signs, including temperature, on a regular basis. *The client often has a high temperature throughout the illness, ranging from 101°F (38°C) to 105°F (40.5°C).*

PRACTICE ALERT
Hyperthermia may result from increased intracranial pressure, while an increased temperature can also increase ICP.

- Monitor levels of consciousness. Assess levels of orientation, memory, attention span, and response to stimuli. *Early in the infection, the client often has problems with memory and orientation. There may be problems with following commands, restlessness, irritability, and combativeness. As the illness progresses, the LOC decreases to lethargy and finally into deep coma.*
- Monitor for manifestations of seizure activity, and institute seizure precautions:
  - Monitor twitching of hands or face and tonic-clonic movements.
  - Have an oral airway and suction equipment readily available.
  - Pad side rails, maintain bed in low position, and keep side rails up.
  Irritation of the cerebral cortex secondary to meningeal inflammation may cause seizures. Careful monitoring and seizure precautions are necessary to prevent injury.
- Monitor for manifestations of cranial nerve damage; monitor extraocular movements, facial movement, dizziness, ability to hear, double vision, drooping upper eyelids (ptosis), and pupillary changes. *Cranial nerve dysfunction may result from inflammation or vascular changes in the brain.*
- Monitor for manifestations of increased intracranial pressure: decreased pulse, increased blood pressure, widening pulse pressure, respiratory changes, and vomiting. *Increased intracranial pressure results from infectious or inflammatory exudate, cerebral edema, and hydrocephalus.*
- Administer prescribed medications and maintain prescribed fluid restrictions. *Diuretics are often prescribed to prevent increases in ICP, anticonvulsants are prescribed to prevent or control seizures, and antibiotics are prescribed to eradicate the bacteria. Fluids may be restricted to help prevent IICP.*

Risk for Deficient Fluid Volume

The client is at risk for fluid volume deficit related to increased metabolic rate, diaphoresis, and fluid restrictions.
- Monitor for presence, or worsening, of fluid volume deficit.
  - Measure and compare intake and output every 2 to 4 hours.
  - Monitor daily body weights.
  - Monitor skin turgor.
  - Monitor condition of mucous membranes.
  - Monitor urine amount, color, and odor.
  - Monitor BUN:creatinine ratio.
  The elastic property of the skin depends partially on interstitial fluid volume. If there is a fluid volume deficit, skin flattens more slowly after a pinch is released. Mucous membranes are dry. In fluid volume deficit, urine output is decreased, urine is dark in color and concentrated with a strong odor, and urine specific gravity is greater than 1.020, and BUN will rise out of proportion to serum creatinine.

PRACTICE ALERT
A weight loss of 1 lb represents a fluid loss of approximately 500 mL.

- When administering fluids, either orally or parenterally, consider concurrent illnesses. *Clients with increased intracranial pressure or renal failure require complex management. See Chapter 10 ∞ for a further discussion of fluid volume deficit.*

Using NANDA, NIC, and NOC

Chart 44–3 shows links between NANDA nursing diagnoses, NIC, and NOC when caring for the client with a CNS infection.

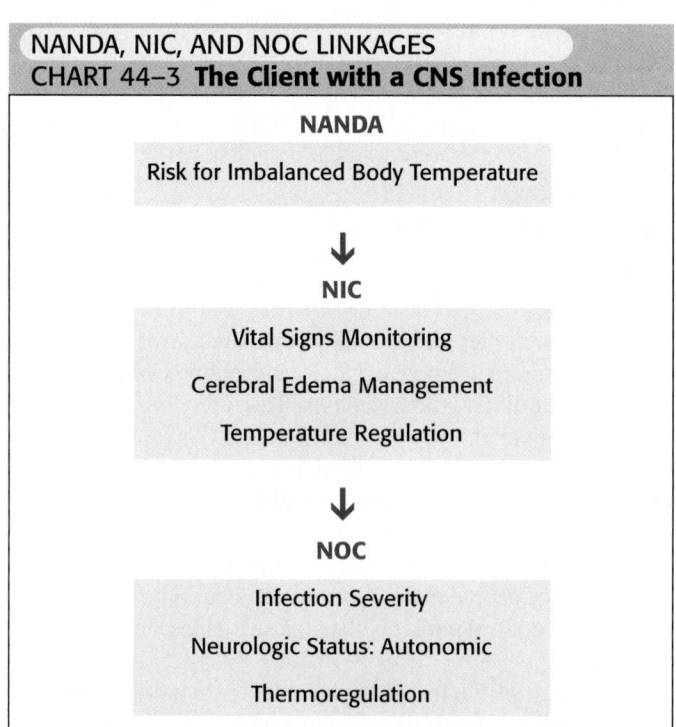

NANDA, NIC, AND NOC LINKAGES
CHART 44–3 The Client with a CNS Infection

NANDA

Risk for Imbalanced Body Temperature

↓

NIC

Vital Signs Monitoring

Cerebral Edema Management

Temperature Regulation

↓

NOC

Infection Severity

Neurologic Status: Autonomic

Thermoregulation

Data from *NANDA's Nursing Diagnoses: Definitions & Classification 2005–2006* by NANDA International (2005), Philadelphia; *Nursing Interventions Classification (NIC)* (4th ed.) by J. M. Dochterman & G. M. Bulechek (2004), St. Louis, MO: Mosby; and *Nursing Outcomes Classification (NOC)* (3rd ed.) by S. Moorhead, M. Johnson, and M. Maas (2004), St. Louis, MO: Mosby.

Community-Based Care

The importance of preventive measures, such as recognizing predisposing conditions, is a major focus for client education. People who have had close contact with the client with meningitis should be monitored for fever, headache, or neck stiffness. Some physicians believe that those closest to the client are candidates for antimicrobial prophylaxis. Also address the following topics:

- The need to report any manifestations of ear infection, sore throat, or upper respiratory infection
- The names and purposes of all medications that may be prescribed
- The importance of taking all medication until completely gone, because some clients may think it is acceptable to stop the medication as soon as they feel better.

TUMORS OF THE BRAIN

THE CLIENT WITH A BRAIN TUMOR

Brain tumors are growths within the cranium, including tumors in brain tissue, meninges, the pituitary gland, or blood vessels. Brain tumors may be benign or malignant, primary or metastatic, and intracerebral or extracerebral. Regardless of type or location, brain tumors are potentially lethal as they grow within a closed cranial vault and displace or impinge on CNS structures.

Incidence and Prevalence

An estimated 19,000 new cases of malignant brain tumors are diagnosed annually in the United States, and approximately 13,000 people die each year (American Cancer Society, 2006). Although brain tumors can occur in any age group, the highest incidence in adults is in those ages 50 to 70. In the adult population, the most common tumor is glioblastoma multiforme, followed by meningioma and cytoma. Glioblastomas represent more than 50% of all primary intracranial lesions.

The cause of many brain tumors is unknown. Although a number of chemical and viral agents can cause brain tumors in laboratory animals, there is no evidence that these agents cause tumors in humans. Other factors associated with brain tumors include heredity, cranial irradiation, and exposure to some chemicals (Porth, 2005).

Pathophysiology

Brain tumors may be classified as benign or malignant, based on the tissue type and characteristics of the cells. The use of the term *benign* may be misleading. A tumor that is benign by histologic examination but is surgically inaccessible may continue to grow and expand, increasing intracranial pressure and causing neurologic deficits, herniation, and finally death. In discussions of brain tumors, the term *malignant* is used to describe the lack of cell differentiation, the invasive nature of the tumor, and its ability to metastasize.

Brain tumors also may be classified as primary or metastatic, depending on their origin (Table 44–12). Primary tumors of CNS tissue arise from the cells and structures that are found within the brain, for example, neurons and neuroglia. The primary intracranial tumors that originate in the skull cavity but not from brain tissue itself arise from the supporting structures, including the meninges, pituitary gland, and pineal gland. Primary brain tumors rarely metastasize outside the CNS. Metastatic brain tumors originate from structures outside the brain, such as the breasts, lungs, and prostate gland.

Focal disturbances take place when there is compression of brain tissue and infiltration or direct invasion of brain parenchyma with destruction of neural tissue. As the tumor grows, edema develops in adjacent tissues. The mechanism is not completely understood, but it is thought that an osmotic gradient causes the tumor to absorb fluid. Some tumors may cause hemorrhage. Venous obstruction and edema due to breakdown of the blood–brain barrier increase intracranial volume and intracranial pressure. Obstruction of the circulation of CSF from the lateral ventricles to the subarachnoid space causes hydrocephalus.

An estimated 25% of people with cancer develop brain metastasis. Metastatic brain tumors present in the same way as primary brain tumors, with IICP, and focal and/or diffuse cerebral dysfunction. The most common source of intracranial metastasis is cancer of the lung. Other common primary sites are the breast, kidney, and gastrointestinal tract. The metastasis reaches the brain through the circulation. In most cases, the tumors are multiple and are scattered through the cerebellum and cerebrum.

Manifestations

Multiple manifestations can develop as a result of the growth of the tumor, while others are related to the location of the lesion (see the box below). Some of the more common mani-

MANIFESTATIONS of Brain Tumors

Frontal Lobe Tumors
- Inappropriate behavior
- Personality changes
- Inability to concentrate
- Impaired judgment
- Recent memory loss
- Headache
- Expressive aphasia
- Motor dysfunctions

Parietal Lobe Tumors
- Sensory deficits: paresthesia, loss of two-point discrimination, visual field deficits

Temporal Lobe Tumors
- Psychomotor seizures

Occipital Lobe Tumors
- Visual disturbances

Cerebellum Tumors
- Disturbances in coordination and equilibrium

Pituitary Tumors
- Endocrine dysfunction
- Visual deficits
- Headache

TABLE 44–12 Classification on Brain Tumors

TUMOR TYPE	TUMOR NAME	CHARACTERISTICS
Primary Tumors Intracerebral tumors Account for 40%–50% of all brain tumors Originate from neuroglia and invade brain tissue Most common type of brain tumor	*Glioma* ■ Astrocytoma ■ Glioblastoma multiforme ■ Ependymoma ■ Oligodendroglioma ■ Astroblastoma	Most common glioma Graded I to IV according to degree of cell differentiation Most malignant form Fast growing Tumor that develops from lining of ventricles Graded I to IV according to degree of cell differentiation Slow growing Rare, slow growing May be encapsulated Benign
Extracerebral tumors Tumors arising from the supporting structures of the nervous system Account for 10% to 15% of all brain tumors	Medulloblastoma Meningioma Acoustic neuroma	Fast growing and malignant Occurs primarily in children; can occur in adults Found in cerebellum Slow growing Develops in meninges (especially dura) Firm and encapsulated Slow growing Benign Originates from Schwann cells of the cranial nerve XIII May also affect cranial nerves V, VII, IX, and X Also called neurofibromatosis Genetic origin due to autosomal dominant mendelian trait Firm, encapsulated lesions attached to nerve
Congenital (developmental) tumors Account for 4% to 8% of all brain tumors	Hemangioblastoma Craniopharyngioma	Vascular tumor Slow growing Originates from Rathke's pouch Solid or cystic tumor Compresses pituitary gland Presses on the third ventricle and may cause blockage of cerebrospinal fluid (CSF)
Pituitary adenomas Account for 8% to 12% of all brain tumors	Chromophobic Eosinophilic Basophilic	Account for 90% pituitary tumors Nonsecreting tumor Slow growing Secreting tumors that produce growth hormone Secreting tumors that produce adrenocorticotropic hormone Fast growing
Secondary Tumors Metastastic brain tumors Account for 10% of all brain tumors		Slow-growing tumors that arise from other parts of the body Usually well differentiated from the brain Spread from tumors of the lung, breast, lower gastrointestinal tract, pancreas, kidney, skin

festations include changes in cognition or consciousness, a headache that is usually worse in the morning, seizures, and vomiting. Compression of brain tissue and the invasion of the brain tumor into the cerebral tissue may lead to changes typically seen with cerebral edema and IICP. Cerebral blood supply may diminish as the tumor compresses blood vessels. Shifts in brain tissue can occur, leading to brain herniation syndromes and, if untreated, death.

INTERDISCIPLINARY CARE

Treatment for a brain tumor may involve chemotherapy, radiation therapy, surgery, or any combination of these. Several variables are considered when selecting the appropriate treatment modality: the size and location of the tumor, the type of tumor, related symptoms (such as neurologic deficits), and the client's overall condition.

Diagnosis

The following diagnostic tests may be ordered.

- A CT scan or an MRI with gadolinium enhancement can locate the tumor and define its size, shape, extent to which normal anatomy is distorted, and the degree of any associated cerebral edema.
- Arteriography may show stretching or displacement of cerebral vessels by the tumor, as well as the presence of tumor vascularity.
- EEG provides information about cerebral function, may demonstrate focal or diffuse changes, and is useful if seizures are present.
- Endocrine studies are conducted if a pituitary tumor is suspected.

Medications

The choice of drug for treatment is based on the type of tumor, its location, and the client's response to therapy. The use of chemotherapy to treat brain tumors is still emerging. An intraventricular method of medication administration uses an Ommaya reservoir that has been surgically implanted into a lateral ventricle of the brain (Figure 44–8 ■). Other medications that may be prescribed include corticosteroids and anticonvulsants.

Surgery

Surgery is used to remove tumors, to reduce the size of the tumor, or for symptom relief (palliation). The type of procedure, the surgical approach, and the timing of surgery (emergency versus planned procedure) influence the overall nursing management of the client having intracranial surgery.

Some of the more common intracranial neurosurgical procedures follow:

- *Burr hole.* A hole made in the skull with a special drill. The hole may facilitate the evacuation of an extracerebral clot, or a series of holes may be made in preparation for craniotomy (see Figure 44–7).
- *Craniotomy.* A surgical opening into the cranial cavity (Figure 44–9 ■). For a craniotomy, a series of burr holes are made. The bone between the holes is then cut with a special saw called a craniotome. The tumor is excised, and the bone flap is returned to the opening. A craniotomy may also be performed to repair defects associated with traumatic head injuries or to repair a cerebral aneurysm.

  A supratentorial craniotomy refers to surgery above the tentorium. It provides access to the frontal, temporal, parietal, and occipital lobes. The incision for this procedure is usually within the hairline over the area involved.

  An infratentorial craniotomy refers to surgery below the tentorium. Access is provided to lesions in the cerebellum and the brainstem. The incision is made at the nape of the neck, around the occipital lobe.
- *Craniectomy.* An excision of a portion of the skull and complete removal of the bone flap. This procedure may be done to provide decompression after cerebral edema. Pressure on the brain structures is lessened by providing space for expansion.
- *Cranioplasty.* Plastic repair to the skull in which synthetic material is inserted to replace the cranial bone that was removed. This procedure may be performed after a large craniectomy. The plastic repair restores the contour and integrity of the cranium.

Figure 44–8 ■ Ommaya reservoir for medication administration.

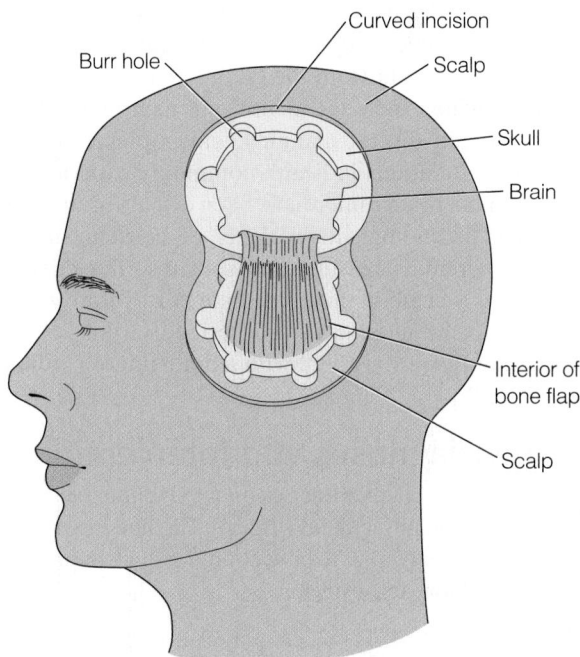

Figure 44–9 ■ In a craniotomy, a portion of the skull and overlying scalp is removed to allow access to the brain.

Radiation Therapy

Radiation therapy may be administered alone or as adjunctive therapy with surgery. Radiation is often the treatment of choice for surgically inaccessible tumors; it may also be used to decrease the size of a tumor prior to surgery. Tumors that were not completely excised by surgery may also be treated with radiation.

Specialty Procedures

Technologic advances—including the development of special instruments, the use of stereotaxic techniques for localizing a specific target, and the use of the laser beam—have greatly advanced neurosurgical practice. Microsurgery involves an operating microscope with microinstruments and supportive illumination equipment. Using stereotaxic techniques to precisely locate a specific target point allows for location of discrete areas of the brain that control specific functions and exact locations of deep brain lesions. The use of a laser beam for excision of a tumor results in less damage to surrounding tissue and less postoperative swelling. The gamma knife, which is not actually a knife but a gamma unit, consists of a heavily shielded helmet containing 201 sources of cobalt-60, which is capable of destroying deep and otherwise inaccessible lesions in a single treatment session. A new area of chemotherapy is that of biodegradable anhydrous wafers, which are impregnated with the chemotherapy drug and implanted into the tumor at the time of surgery. The wafers are made so they slowly release the drug over a period of many months (Porth, 2005).

NURSING CARE

The nursing care of the client with a brain tumor includes support during the diagnostic period and specific management as directed by the selected treatment. The foundation for care is data from the health history and physical assessment, which includes identifying neurologic deficits. This information directs planning and implementing care. Many of the alterations in health commonly experienced by the client with a brain tumor have been discussed throughout this chapter, including altered level of consciousness, increased intracranial pressure, and seizures. The client will require intensive care in the immediate postoperative period. In addition to the nursing care described in this section, a Nursing Care Plan for a client with a brain tumor is found on page 1573.

Nursing Diagnoses and Interventions

This section of the chapter focuses on nursing interventions for the client who has intracranial surgery. The nursing diagnoses discussed are anxiety, risk for infection, ineffective protection, acute pain, and low self-esteem.

Anxiety

The diagnosis of a brain tumor brings anxiety and feelings of uncertainty about the future. Both the client and family members are likely to be apprehensive and require education and emotional support.

- Explain routine medical procedures, including blood work and radiologic studies. *Baseline laboratory and radiologic studies are needed to ensure that the client has no other preexisting medical condition. Explaining the procedures and assisting the client through this process help decrease anxiety.*
- Reinforce, clarify, and repeat information. *Both client and family may have limited understanding of the scheduled diagnostic tests, procedures, and treatment modalities. The client may be confused or have altered thought processes as a result of the tumor. Information may need to be repeated or reexplained.*
- Encourage client and family to verbalize feelings, questions, and fears; provide realistic information appropriate to their level of understanding. *Verbalization helps reduce anxiety and fear.*
- Review client and family strengths and effective coping skills. *Personal strengths, support systems, and coping skills can aid in the development of appropriate strategies to reduce anxiety.*
- Arrange for a member of the clergy to visit if desired. *Faith in a higher being is often a strong source of strength and support.*
- Provide preoperative teaching, including the following information.
  - Type of anesthesia and surgery
  - Time surgery will begin and expected length of procedure and recovery room stay
  - Where the client will be taken after surgery (CCU, ICU) (If possible, show the client and family the CCU or ICU and introduce them to the nurse who will be in charge of care after the surgery.)
  - Where family can wait during and following surgery
  - Appearance of the client after surgery, which may include swollen, bruised eyelids and other facial features; a large dressing covering the head; a partially or fully shaved head; and a tracheostomy or endotracheal tube
  - Behavior of the client after surgery, which will differ depending on the site of surgery, although cognitive and behavioral changes are common.
  Information about what to expect reduces anxiety.
- Allow time for client and family to be together. *Clients and families need quiet time together to support each other and prepare emotionally for surgery.*

Risk for Infection

The client who has had intracranial surgery is at risk for infection from multiple invasive lines, the scalp wound, and the risk of introduction of bacteria into the operative area. The nurse provides interventions to monitor for and prevent infection.

- Monitor for leakage of CSF:
  - Presence of glucose in clear drainage from ears, nose, or wound
  - Complaints of "something dripping down the back of the throat"
  - Constant swallowing.
  These manifestations indicate an opening in the dura, which provides an avenue for an ascending infection.
- Provide interventions to prevent contamination of area leaking CSF:

NURSING CARE PLAN   A Client with a Brain Tumor

Claire Lange is a 44-year-old television announcer. During one night's broadcast, she confuses several major news items so badly that her co-anchor tries to correct her. Ms. Lange responds angrily that she does not need any help and then rises and storms off the set. As she leaves the camera area, she limps noticeably and appears to drag her left leg. The show's producer asks her what is wrong; she screams that nothing is wrong—she simply has another headache. He follows her to her dressing room and inquires about her headaches. She tells him that they come and go but have been getting worse lately. He then asks her if she has injured her left leg; she responds that the leg was weak because she was tired. As the producer leaves the dressing room, Ms. Lange begins to shake and collapses on the floor. The producer recognizes that she is having a seizure and calls for an ambulance.

Ms. Lange is admitted to the neurology floor of the local hospital for evaluation. A CT scan, MRI, and EEG are completed and identify an intracranial mass. A biopsy of the mass is positive for malignant cells. A glioma in the frontal lobe is identified, and surgery is scheduled for that week.

ASSESSMENT

When Clara Rosetti, RN, enters Ms. Lange's room, she sees Ms. Lange looking at her shoulder-length hair in the mirror. Ms. Lange tells Ms. Rosetti that she has never in her life worn her hair any shorter, and "Now you're going to cut it all off!" She paces the room and makes the statement, "I guess the hair isn't really important if I survive this situation." She also says that she has a headache.

DIAGNOSES

- *Acute Pain* (headache) related to tumor and increase in intracranial pressure
- *Disturbed Body Image* related to upcoming hair loss and cranial incision
- *Anxiety* related to unknown future following surgery

EXPECTED OUTCOMES

- Verbalize the causes of pain.
- Verbalize an understanding of the changes in body appearance that are associated with the scheduled intracranial surgery (e.g., shaving of the head prior to surgery, cranial incision, facial swelling postoperatively).
- Identify measures that will help minimize the effect of the hair loss.
- Verbalize a reduction in anxiety.

PLANNING AND IMPLEMENTATION

- Assess level of discomfort using a rating scale of 0 to 10.
- Provide a quiet, nonstimulating environment.
- Position the client for comfort, keeping the head of the bed elevated to promote venous drainage.
- Assess level of consciousness for potential increases in ICP.
- Encourage to verbalize feelings about the surgery.
- Suggest measures that may help minimize the hair loss, such as the use of turbans, scarves, hats, and wigs.
- Suggest relaxation techniques to decrease anxiety.

EVALUATION

By the time of surgery, Ms. Lange has recognized the relationship between the brain tumor and the headache. She states that lying in a flat position and coughing increase the headache. The head of the bed is kept at a 30- to 45-degree angle. Daily activities are spaced to provide periods of rest. Ms. Lange demonstrates no significant changes in level of consciousness. She has talked about the effect of the hair loss and her television responsibilities. Ms. Lange has learned that the hair preparation would be done in surgery and that the hair would be saved for her. She states she has already consulted her hair stylist and that "scarves and turbans are on the way."

CRITICAL THINKING IN THE NURSING PROCESS

1. Outline interventions to decrease intracranial pressure both before and after surgery.
2. When making your initial assessments on the morning of surgery, you find that Ms. Lange has a decreased pulse and increased blood pressure. She tells you her headache is worse and suddenly vomits. What do you do now?
3. Ms. Lange asks you to be sure that she has absolutely no visitors after surgery, because she knows how ugly she will look. How would you respond?
4. Design a plan of care for Ms. Lange for the nursing diagnosis of *Powerlessness*.
See Evaluating Your Response in Appendix C.

- If leaking from the nose: Keep head of bed elevated 20 degrees unless contraindicated; do not suction nasally; do not clean nose; tell client not to put finger in nose; do not insert packing.
- If leaking from the ear: Position client on side of leakage unless contraindicated; do not clean ear; tell client not to put finger in ear; do not insert packing.
- Place a sterile dressing over the area of drainage and change as soon as it becomes damp.
Leakage of CSF indicates a break in the dura and increases the risk of an ascending infection. Surgery may be necessary to repair the break; however, the leak usually heals spontaneously in about 1 week.
- Monitor for and report manifestations of infection:
  - Take and record temperature on a regular basis.

- Assess IV insertion sites for redness, swelling, drainage, and pain.
- Assess scalp wound for redness, swelling, bulging, drainage, and pain.
- Assess for manifestations of meningitis: fever and chills, increasing headache, neck stiffness, positive Kernig's or Brudzinski's sign, photophobia.
- Monitor laboratory reports for increased WBC count.
Intact skin is the first line of defense against infection. Any break in the skin increases the risk of infection. Intracranial surgery increases the risk of meningitis, with infectious agents ascending into the brain.
- Implement interventions to prevent infection:
  - Use strict aseptic technique when changing dressings and when caring for wound drains and ICP monitor lines.

- Keep the client's hands away from drains and dressings; use mitten restraints if necessary.
- Administer prescribed antibiotics.

Sterile technique decreases the risk of introducing infection into a wound. Antibiotics are usually prescribed prophylactically to prevent infection.

Ineffective Protection

The client who has intracranial surgery does not have normal human defenses against changes in intracranial pressure and is also at risk from cerebral edema and a shift of intracerebral contents. In addition, the surgery may cause cerebral bleeding or hematoma formation.

- Monitor for manifestations of increased intracranial pressure:
  - Restlessness, agitation, and decreasing level of consciousness
  - Headache
  - Vomiting
  - Seizures
  - Decreasing sensory and motor function
  - Changes in pupil size and reaction
  - Changes in vital signs: altered respiratory rate or depth, increasing pulse pressure, decreasing pulse rate, increasing blood pressure
  - Abnormal posturing

Increasing intracranial pressure is manifested by alterations in the functions and centers controlled by the brain.

- Implement interventions to decrease the risk of increased intracranial pressure:
  - Elevate the head of the bed 15 to 30 degrees as prescribed (unless contraindicated).
  - Avoid neck flexion or rotation; keep head in midline position unless a large bone flap or mass was removed; then position the client on unoperated side to decrease venous congestion in the operative area.
  - Do not take rectal temperatures.
  - Avoid clustering activities that increase intracranial pressure: suctioning, turning, bathing.
  - Administer medications to prevent vomiting.
  - Do not suction for more than 10 seconds at one time.
  - Teach the client (if possible) to avoid coughing, sneezing, and straining to have a bowel movement.
  - Maintain fluid restrictions as prescribed.
  - For internal shunts: Avoid pressure on the shunt, reservoir, or tubing. Pump the shunt only if prescribed.
  - For external shunts: Avoid kinks in tubing, and maintain the drainage collecting device and client's head at the prescribed levels.

Keeping the head of the bed slightly elevated facilitates venous drainage from the brain. Neck flexion or rotation disrupts circulation to and from the brain. Rectal stimulation, suctioning, turning, bathing, coughing, sneezing, and straining to have a bowel movement all initiate Valsalva's maneuver, which constricts the jugular veins and impairs venous return from the brain. Fluid restriction may be prescribed to dehydrate the client slightly and lessen ICP.

- Maintain (as much as possible) a quiet, calm, softly lighted environment. Avoid excessive sensory stimulation. *These interventions promote rest and decrease stimulation, thereby reducing ICP.*
- Implement interventions to prevent seizures or, if they occur, to prevent injury to the client:
  - Pad side rails of the bed.
  - Place bed in lowest position, and keep side rails up.
  - Carry out interventions to prevent and treat increased intracranial pressure.
  - Have an oral airway and suction equipment immediately available.
  - Administer prescribed anticonvulsants.
  - If a seizure occurs: Maintain a patent airway; do not restrain client; do not force anything into the client's mouth; provide physical and emotional support.

These interventions promote safety and help prevent injury. Anticonvulsants are often prescribed prophylactically to prevent seizures after intracranial surgery.

- Carefully monitor hydration status. Compare trends in intake and output, laboratory results of serum osmolality, and urine specific gravity and osmolality. *Changes in fluid balance and osmolality may result from excess intravenous fluids, osmotic diuretics, surgically induced diabetes insipidus or syndrome of inappropriate antidiuretic hormone secretion, fever, diarrhea, tube feedings, or hyperglycemia.*

Acute Pain

The client who has intracranial surgery has pain, manifested as a headache, as a result of either compression or displacement of brain tissue or from increased intracranial pressure. A headache may also be a manifestation of meningitis.

- Assess the location, duration, and intensity of the pain, using a scale from 0 (no pain) to 10 (worst pain) in the client who can verbally communicate. *The client is the best source of information about pain.*
- Implement interventions to reduce the pain:
  - Raise the head of the bed slightly.
  - Reduce noise and bright lights in the room.
  - If allowed, loosen head dressing.
  - Administer narcotic analgesics with caution.

Nonpharmacologic measures may be used to reduce increased intracranial pressure and headache.

> ### PRACTICE ALERT
> Narcotic analgesics mask changes in eye signs and depress respirations.

Situational Low Self-Esteem

The client who has intracranial surgery has many alterations that affect self-esteem and body image. Physical changes include a loss of hair on the scalp, swelling and bruising in the eyelids and face, and perhaps an indentation in the skull. The client is no longer independent in self-care, but must depend on others to meet basic needs. There are often long-term neurologic deficits, affecting areas such as speech, vision, and motor abilities, which require changes in roles and relationships.

■ Assess for verbal and nonverbal manifestations of negative self-esteem:

- ■ Denial of changes
- ■ Preoccupation with changes
- ■ Refusal to look in the mirror
- ■ Withdrawal from family and friends
- ■ Expressions of grief and loss (see Chapter 5 ∞).

Low self-esteem can be initiated by stressful situations and changes in body image.

■ Provide interventions to improve self-concept:

- ■ Limit negative self-assessment.
- ■ Help focus on positive areas of life.
- ■ Help identify sources of support and strength.
- ■ Help identify and use helpful coping methods.
- ■ Encourage significant others to visit.
- ■ Encourage independence in self-care.

Self-esteem is derived from one's own perceptions of competence and from the responses of others. When one's self-concept and self-ideal are congruent, self-esteem is enhanced.

Using NANDA, NIC, and NOC

Chart 44–4 shows links between NANDA nursing diagnoses, NIC, and NOC when caring for the client with a brain tumor.

Community-Based Care

The effect of the possible outcomes following the surgery produces fear in both client and family, interfering with their ability to retain information. The client may have cognitive or neurologic deficits that interfere with learning. Family members also must be assessed for their ability to cope with the stress of the surgery. Information may have to be repeated several times.

Clients and their families who have experienced intracranial surgery require emotional support. The process of recovery is often extended and may involve adaptation to changes in body image and management of any motor or sensory deficits. The family should be involved in the care of the client. If family members are willing, they may begin to assist with ADLs while the client is in the hospital, such as assisting with personal hygiene and meals. Clients should also be encouraged to take an active role in their own care. Discharge planning includes a discussion of the following topics: medication information; wound care; the use of wigs, turbans, hats, or colorful scarves; and the importance of follow-up visits. In addition, emphasize the importance of reporting manifestations such as stiff neck, increasing headache, elevated temperature, new motor or sensory deficits, vision changes, or seizures.

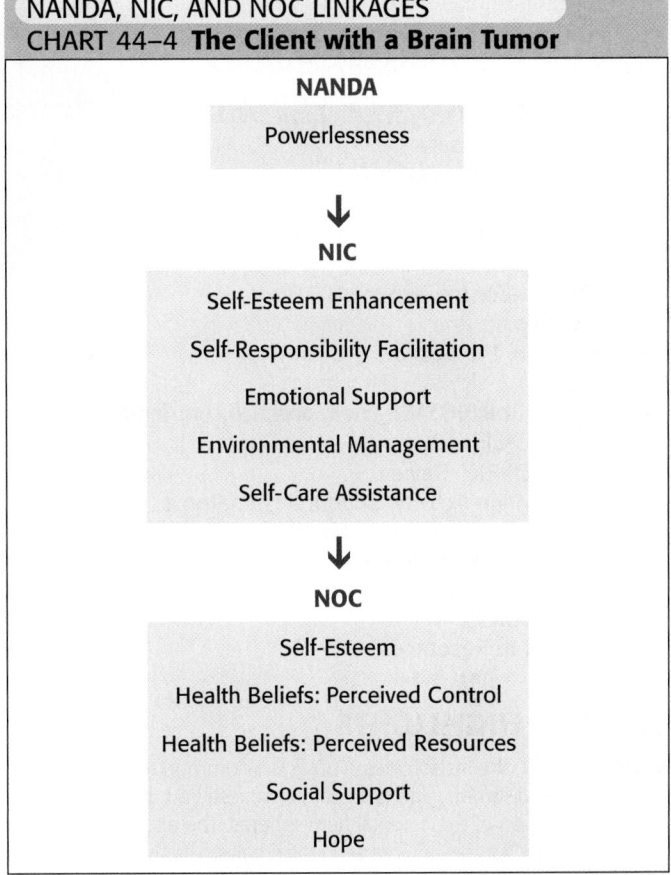

NANDA, NIC, AND NOC LINKAGES
CHART 44–4 The Client with a Brain Tumor

NANDA

Powerlessness

↓

NIC

Self-Esteem Enhancement

Self-Responsibility Facilitation

Emotional Support

Environmental Management

Self-Care Assistance

↓

NOC

Self-Esteem

Health Beliefs: Perceived Control

Health Beliefs: Perceived Resources

Social Support

Hope

Data from *NANDA's Nursing Diagnoses: Definitions & Classification 2005–2006* by NANDA International (2005), Philadelphia; *Nursing Interventions Classification (NIC)* (4th ed.) by J. M. Dochterman & G. M. Bulechek (2004), St. Louis, MO: Mosby; and *Nursing Outcomes Classification (NOC)* (3rd ed.) by S. Moorhead, M. Johnson, and M. Maas (2004), St. Louis, MO: Mosby.

Provide information about the overall treatment plan, management of deficits and/or disabilities, and future needs. Specific teaching topics are as follows:

■ Safety measures for motor deficits, sensory deficits, lack of coordination, seizures, and cognitive deficits
■ Comfort measures for nausea, vomiting, and pain
■ Measures for communication if aphasia is present
■ Measures to improve vision if visual deficits are present
■ How to buy wigs and hairpieces
■ Referrals to support groups and community resources
■ Helpful resources:

- ■ American Cancer Society
- ■ American Brain Tumor Association
- ■ National Brain Tumor Foundation
- ■ Brain Tumor Society.

EXPLORE MediaLink

Prentice Hall Nursing MediaLink DVD-ROM
Audio Glossary
NCLEX-RN® Review

Animations
Complex Seizure
Coup-Contrecoup Injury
Epilepsy
Grand Mal Seizure

COMPANION WEBSITE www. prenhall.com/lemone
Audio Glossary
NCLEX-RN® Review
Care Plan Activity: Subdural Hematoma
Case Study: Bacterial Meningitis
MediaLink Applications
   Meningitis Prevention
   Paralysis
Links to Resources

CHAPTER HIGHLIGHTS

- Altered level of consciousness (LOC) is a common response to intracranial disorders, and is an early manifestation of deterioration of the function of the cerebral hemispheres. The alteration in cerebral function occurs in a sequential pattern, with characteristic changes in LOC, respiratory patterns, pupillary and oculomotor responses, and motor function. Coma states include persistent vegetative state and locked-in syndrome.

- Increased intracranial pressure (IICP) is a sustained elevated pressure (≥10 mmHg) within the cranial cavity. IICP may result from cerebral edema, hydrocephalus, head trauma, tumors, abscesses, inflammation, hemorrhage, or stroke.

- The manifestations of IICP include a decreasing LOC, abnormal motor weakness and responses, altered vision, altered vital signs, headache, papilledema, and projectile vomiting. If untreated, IICP causes a displacement (herniation) of cerebral tissue, herniation of the cerebellum through the tentorium, followed by herniation of the brainstem through the foramen magnum. This is a lethal complication of IICP because it puts pressure on the vital centers in the medulla. IICP is primarily managed with osmotic diuretics and monitored with continuous intracranial pressure monitors.

- Headaches, a common type of intracranial pain, are categorized as tension, migraine, and cluster. A classic migraine is characterized by an aura; a common migraine does not have an aura.

- Epilepsy is a chronic disorder of abnormal, recurring, excessive, and self-terminating electrical discharges from neurons. A seizure is a single event of abnormal electrical discharge. Seizures are categorized into those that affect only a part of the brain (partial seizures) and those that affect all of the brain (generalized). The

most common type of seizure in adults is a tonic-clonic generalized seizure. Seizures are treated medically with antiepileptic drugs (AEDs), surgery, and/or vagal nerve stimulation therapy.

- Traumatic brain injury (TBI) refers to any injury of the scalp, skull, or brain, and is a leading cause of death and disability. TBIs include skull fractures and focal or diffuse brain injury. An acute brain injury affects all body systems, and carries the risk of secondary injury to the brain from hypoxia and ischemia.

- An epidural hematoma develops in the potential space between the dura and the skull. A subdural hematoma collects between the dura mater and the arachnoid mater. Diffuse brain injuries include contusions, concussions, and diffuse axonal injury. Clients with an acute TBI must have immediate transport and treatment in an ED, followed by care in an ICU. They will require long-term physical care and rehabilitation.

- Central nervous system infections may be caused by bacteria, bacterial toxins, viruses, fungi, protozoans, and rickettsiae. Organisms may enter the brain through the bloodstream or by direct invasion. The major CNS infections are meningitis, encephalitis, and brain abscess. CNS infections are treated with broad-spectrum antibiotics and antifungal agents.

- Brain tumors are growths within the cranium, including on or in brain tissue, the meninges, the pituitary gland, or blood vessels. Brain tumors may be benign or malignant, primary or metastatic, and intracerebral or extracerebral. Regardless of the type or location, brain tumors are potentially lethal because they displace or impinge on CNS structures within a closed bony system.

TEST YOURSELF NCLEX-RN® REVIEW

1 Which of the following pathophysiologic events results in irregular respiratory patterns as LOC decreases?
1. pressure on the meninges
2. reflexive motor responses
3. loss of the oculocephalic reflex
4. brainstem responses to changes in $Paco_2$

2 The unconscious client has depressed or absent gag and swallowing reflexes. Which nursing diagnosis would be appropriate?
1. *Decreased Intracranial Adaptive Capacity*
2. *Risk for Aspiration*
3. *Imbalanced Nutrition: Less than Body Requirements*
4. *Ineffective Breathing Pattern*

3 What is the rationale for the use of osmotic diuretics to treat IICP?
1. Hyperthermia increases the cerebral metabolic rate and exacerbates IICP.
2. Increased blood osmolality draws edematous fluid into the vascular system.
3. Clients with ICP are at increased risk for gastrointestinal hemorrhage.
4. Brain injury and IICP often cause seizures.

4 You are monitoring the neurologic status of a client in a coma. Which of the following commands would be most accurate in identifying changes in mental status?
1. "Tell me your name."
2. "Look at this light when I shine it in your eyes."
3. "Squeeze my hand."
4. "Are you having trouble breathing?"

5 On admission to the ED, a client who has altered LOC has a variety of laboratory tests to facilitate the diagnosis of the etiology of the condition. Which tests would likely be performed? (Select all that apply.)
1. blood glucose
2. serum electrolytes
3. blood and urine toxicology
4. urine for WBCs
5. spinal fluid osmolarity

6 Of the following diagnostic tests, which one is the most accurate indicator of hydration status in the client with altered LOC?
1. CBC
2. urinalysis
3. serum osmolality
4. blood culture

7 What manifestation is consistently assessed in clients with generalized seizures?
1. loss of consciousness
2. repetitive nonpurposeful activity
3. tonic movements
4. clonic movements

8 When assessing a client with a head injury, you test fluid dripping from one ear for glucose. What are you assessing for?
1. infection
2. blood
3. CSF
4. serum

9 You are administering an antiepileptic drug to a newly diagnosed seizure client. The client says, "Will this cure my convulsions?" What would you say?
1. "No, but it will relieve your headache."
2. "No, but it will help decrease the aura you experience."
3. "No, not for the first year."
4. "No, but it may reduce or control them."

10 Which of the following statements is true of brain tumors?
1. All brain tumors are potentially lethal.
2. Only malignant tumors are lethal.
3. Metastatic brain tumors are benign tumors.
4. Benign brain tumors rarely require treatment.

See Test Yourself answers in Appendix C.

BIBLIOGRAPHY

American Academy of Neurology. (2004). *Efficacy and tolerability of the new antiepileptic drugs for treatment of new onset epilepsy.* Retrieved from http://www.neurology.org/cgi/reprint/62/8/1252.pdf

American Cancer Society. (2006). *Brain/CNS tumors in adults.* Retrieved from http://www.cancer.org

Brain Trauma Foundation, Inc., American Association of Neurological Surgeons, Congress of Neurological Surgeons, & Joint Section of Neurotrauma and Critical Care. (2003). *Guidelines for the management of severe traumatic head injury.* New York: The Brain Trauma Foundation.

Brettler, S. (2004). *Trauma nursing:* Traumatic head injury. *RN, 67*(4), 32–38.

Celik, S., Aksoy, G., & Akyolcu, N. (2004). Nursing role in preventing secondary brain injury. *Accident and Emergency Nursing, 12*(2), 94–98.

Centers for Disease Control and Prevention. (2003). *CDC answers your questions about St. Louis encephalitis.* Retrieved from http://www.cdc.gov/ncidod/dvbid/arbor/sle_qa.htm

_____. (2004). *Meningococcal disease.* Retrieved from http://www.cdc.gov/ncidod/dbmd/diseaseinfo/meningococcal_t.htm

_____. (2006). *Traumatic brain injury (TBI); incidence & distribution; risks & groups at risk; causes & characteristics; prevention, control & elimination; outcomes & consequences.* Retrieved from http://cdc.gov/node/doid/0900f3ec8000dbdc/aspectId

Cook, N. (2003). Respiratory care in spinal cord injury with associated traumatic brain injury: Bridging the gap in critical care nursing interventions. *Intensive & Critical Care Nursing, 19*(3), 143–153.

Cree, C. (2003). Acquired brain injury: Acute management. *Nursing Standard, 18*(11), 45–56.

Dandan, I. (2004). Altered consciousness. *Topics in Emergency Medicine, 26*(3), 242–245.

Dochterman, J., & Bulechek, G. (2004). *Nursing interventions classification (NIC)* (4th ed.). St. Louis, MO: Mosby.

EMedicineHealth. (2006). *Migraine headache FAQs.* Retrieved from http://www.emedicinehealth.com/migraine_headache_faqs/article_em.htm

Epilepsy Foundation. (2005a). *Epilepsy: An introduction.* Retrieved from http://www.epilepsyfoundation.org/answerplace/About-Epilepsy.cfm

_____. (2005b). *Overview: Vagus nerve stimulation therapy.* Retrieved from http://epilepsyfoundation.org/answerplace/Medical/treatment/vns/treatvns.cfm

Fan, J. (2004). Effect of backrest position on intracranial pressure and cerebral perfusion pressure in individuals with brain injury: A systematic review. *Journal of Neuroscience Nursing, 36I*(5), 278–288.

Freeborn, K. (2004). Neurotrauma—The role of the nurse practitioner in traumatic brain injury. *Topics in Emergency Medicine, 26*(3), 225–230.

Giacino, J., & Whyte, J. (2005). The vegetative and minimally conscious states: Current knowledge and remaining questions. *Journal of Head Trauma Rehabilitation, 20*(1), 30–50.

Hickey, J. (2003). *The clinical practice of neurological and neurosurgical nursing* (4th ed.). Philadelphia: Lippincott.

Kao, H., & Stuifbergen, A. (2004). Love and load: The lived experience of the mother–child relationship among young adult traumatic brain-injured survivors. *Journal of Neuroscience Nursing, 36*(2), 73–81.

Kee, J. (2006). *Handbook of laboratory and diagnostic tests with nursing implications* (6th ed.). Upper Saddle River, NJ: Prentice Hall.

Lam, P., & Beaulieu, M. (2004). Experience of families in the neurological ICU: A "bedside phenomenon." *Journal of Neuroscience Nursing, 36*(3), 142–146, 151–155.

Lammi, M., Smith, V., Tate, R., & Taylor, C. (2005). The minimally conscious state and recovery potential: A follow-up study 2 to 5 years after traumatic brain injury. *Archives of Physical Medicine and Rehabilitation, 86*(4), 746–754.

Martin, D., & Smith, M. (2004). Medical management of severe traumatic brain injury. *Hospital Medicine, 65*(11), 674–680.

Mateo, M., & Glod, C. (2003). Mild traumatic brain injury and psychiatric disorders. *Journal of the American Psychiatric Nurses Association, 9*(4), 129–135.

McCleod, A. (2004). Traumatic injuries to the head and spine 2; Nursing considerations. *British Journal of Nursing, 13*(17), 1041–1049.

Moorhead, S., Johnson, M., & Maas, M. (2003). *Nursing outcomes classification (NOC)* (3rd ed.). St. Louis, MO: Mosby.

Mukherjee, D., Reis, J., & Heller, W. (2003). Women living with traumatic brain injury: Social isolation, emotional functioning and implications for psychotherapy. *Women & Therapy, 26*(1/2), 3–26.

NANDA International. (2005). *Nursing diagnoses: Definitions & classification 2005–2006.* Philadelphia: Author.

National Headache Foundation. (2005). *Migraine prevention: A guide to the latest methods and treatments.* Retrieved from http://www.headaches.org/consumer/educationalmodules/migrain_module/page_home.htm

National Institute of Neurological Disorders and Stroke. (2005a). *NINDS brain and spinal tumors information page.* Retrieved from http://www.ninds.nih.gov/disorders/brainandspinaltumors/brainandspinaltumors.htm

_____. (2005b). *NINDS coma and persistent vegetative state information page.* Retrieved from http://www.ninds.nih.gov/disorders/coma/coma_pr.htm

_____. (2005c). *Headache: Hope through research.* Retrieved from http://www.ninds.nih.gov/disorders/headache/detail_headache_pr.htm

Porth, C. M. (2005). *Pathophysiology: Concepts of altered health states* (7th ed.). Philadelphia: Lippincott.

Roberts, I., Schierhout, G., & Wakai, A. (2005). Mannitol for acute traumatic injury. *The Cochrane Library (Oxford)* (2) (ID#CD001049).

Spitz. M. (2005). *Review and commentary on epilepsy and the elderly.* Retrieved from http://professionals.epilepsy.com/page/ar_1110476473.html

Tierney, L., McPhee, S., & Papadakis, M. (Eds.). (2005). *Current medical diagnosis & treatment* (44th ed.). New York: McGraw-Hill.

Wagner, K., Johnson, K., & Kidd, P. (2006). *High acuity nursing* (4th ed.). Upper Saddle River, NJ: Prentice Hall.

Wilensky, E., & Bloom, S. (2005). Monitoring brain tissue oxygenation after severe brain injury. *Nursing, 35*(2), 32cc1–32cc4.

Wilkinson, J. (2005). *Prentice Hall nursing diagnosis handbook with NIC interventions and NOC outcomes* (8th ed.). Upper Saddle River, NJ: Prentice Hall.

Wilson, B., Shannon, M., & Stang, C. (2006). *Prentice Hall nurse's drug guide 2006.* Upper Saddle River, NJ: Prentice Hall.

Yarbo, C., Frogge, M., & Goodman, M. (2005). *Cancer nursing: Principles and practice* (6th ed.). Sudbury, MA: Jones & Bartlett.

CHAPTER 45
Nursing Care of Clients with Cerebrovascular and Spinal Cord Disorders

LEARNING OUTCOMES

- Identify prevalence, incidence, and risk factors responsible for disorders of cerebral blood flow and spinal cord structure and function.

- Explain the pathophysiology, manifestations, complications, interdisciplinary care, and nursing care of clients with stroke, ruptured intracranial aneurysm, arteriovenous malformation, spinal cord injury, herniated intervertebral disk, and spinal cord tumor.

- Compare and contrast the acute treatment and care of the client with a stroke or ruptured intracranial aneurysm and a spinal cord injury.

- Discuss the pathophysiologic effects of injuries and tumors of the spinal cord by level of injury.

- Discuss the purposes, nursing implications, and health education of the client and family for medications used to treat stroke, ruptured intracranial aneurysm, and spinal cord injury.

- Describe the methods used to stabilize and immobilize spinal cord injuries.

- Describe the surgical procedures used to treat cerebrovascular and spinal cord disorders.

CLINICAL COMPETENCIES

- Assess functional status of clients with cerebrovascular and spinal cord disorders, and monitor, document, and report abnormal manifestations.

- Use evidence-based research to promote early recognition and treatment of the warning signs of a stroke.

- Determine priority nursing diagnoses, based on assessed data, to select and implement individualized nursing interventions for clients with cerebrovascular and spinal cord disorders.

- Administer oral and injectable medications used to treat cerebrovascular and spinal cord disorders knowledgeably and safely.

- Provide skilled care to clients having a carotid endarterectomy, halo fixation, and a posterior laminectomy.

- Integrate interdisciplinary care into care of clients with cerebrovascular and spinal cord disorders.

- Provide appropriate teaching to facilitate self-catheterization, self-care of a ruptured intervertebral disk, and community-based self-care of disabilities resulting from cerebrovascular and spinal cord disorders.

- Revise plan of care as needed to provide effective interventions to promote, maintain, or restore functional health status to clients with cerebrovascular and spinal cord disorders.

MEDIALINK

Resources for this chapter can be found on the Prentice Hall Nursing MediaLink DVD-ROM accompanying this textbook, and on the Companion Website at http://www.prenhall.com/lemone

The health problems discussed in this chapter result from alterations in cerebral blood flow and disorders of the spinal cord. Clients with disorders of cerebral blood flow and the spinal cord experience a wide variety of neurologic deficits that affect cognitive and perceptual functional health patterns. They also require treatment and care for both acute and long-term health problems.

Nursing care for clients with these disorders is tailored to meet the needs of the client and is individualized according to the client's responses to alterations in intracranial and spinal cord structure and function. This chapter's discussion of nursing care includes consideration of both acute and long-term healthcare needs. The disabilities and long-term effects resulting from cerebrovascular disorders and spinal cord injuries almost always cause loss and grief, not only in the client but also in the family of the client. Chapter 5 ∞ provides information about client responses to loss and nursing interventions to help reduce grieving.

CEREBROVASCULAR DISORDERS

THE CLIENT WITH A STROKE

A **stroke** (*cerebral vascular accident [CVA]*, or *brain attack*), is a condition in which neurologic deficits result from a sudden decrease in blood flow to a localized area of the brain. Strokes may be *ischemic* (when blood supply to a part of the brain is suddenly interrupted by a thrombus [blood clot], embolus [foreign matter traveling through the circulation], or stenosis [narrowing]), or *hemorrhagic* (when a blood vessel breaks open, spilling blood into spaces surrounding neurons). The neurologic deficits caused by ischemia and the resultant necrosis of cells in the brain vary according to the area of the brain involved, the size of the affected area, and the length of time blood flow is decreased or stopped. A major loss of blood supply to the brain can cause severe disability or death. When the duration of decreased blood flow is short and the anatomic area involved is small, the person may not be aware that damage has been done.

Incidence and Prevalence

On average, someone in the United States has a stroke every 45 seconds and dies of a stroke every 3 minutes. Stroke is the third leading cause of death and disability in North America, where approximately 700,000 people suffer a stroke each year. Of those, 160,000 die, and many clients who survive are left with some type of functional impairment. Although strokes occur in every age group, the highest incidence occurs in people over 65 years of age; 28% of strokes occur in people under the age of 65. Strokes occur more frequently in men than women, although the risk of stroke may be greater in women during pregnancy and for the 6 weeks following birth (American Heart Association [AHA], 2005a).

FAST FACTS
Estimated Cost of Stroke in the United States
- Total costs: about $57 billion/year.
- Direct costs for medical care and therapy: $28 billion/year.
- Indirect costs from lost productivity and other factors: $15 million/year.
- Costs within 30 days: depending on type, ranges from $13,000 to $20,000.

Source: AHA, 2005a.

Risk Factors

Certain diseases, lifestyle habits, and ethnic backgrounds increase the risk of a stroke (see the box on the next page), including the following (National Institute of Neurological Disorders and Stroke [NINDS], 2005d):

- *Hypertension.* Hypertension is the greatest risk factor for a stroke. Increased systolic and diastolic blood pressure is associated with damage to all blood vessels, including the cerebral vessels. People with hypertension have a four to six times greater risk for stroke than do those without hypertension. One-third of the adult American population has hypertension.

- *Heart disease.* Atrial fibrillation is the second greatest risk factor for stroke. Affecting as many as 2.2 million people, fibrillation increases the risk for stroke by 4% to 6% (AHA, 2005a). Other cardiovascular problems that increase the risk for a stroke are mitral valve stenosis, patent foramen ovale, and cardiac surgery.

- *Diabetes mellitus.* Diabetes leads to vascular changes in both the systemic and cerebral circulation and increases the risk of hypertension (the prevalence of hypertension is 40% higher in people with diabetes). People with diabetes are three times more likely to have a stroke compared to those without diabetes.

- *Sleep apnea.* Considered a major risk for stroke, sleep apnea increases blood pressure and causes decreased oxygen and increased carbon dioxide in the blood.
- *Blood cholesterol levels.* Increased blood cholesterol levels contribute to the risk of atherosclerosis, including arteries in the cerebral circulation.
- *Smoking.* Cigarette smoking doubles a person's risk for ischemic stroke and increases the risk for cerebral hemorrhage by up to 3.5%. Smoking is directly responsible for more strokes in young adults.
- *Sickle cell disease.* Changes in the shape of the red blood cells (RBCs) increase blood viscosity and produce erythrocyte clumps that may occlude small cerebral vessels.
- *Substance abuse.* The injection of unpurified substances increases the risk for a stroke, and abuse of certain drugs can decrease cerebral blood flow and increase the risk for intracranial hemorrhage. Substances associated with strokes include marijuana, anabolic steroids, heroin, amphetamines, and cocaine.
- *Living in the stroke belt.* People living in the southeastern United States have the highest stroke mortality rate in the country. The cause has not been identified.

Other risk factors include a family history of stroke, obesity, a sedentary lifestyle, recent viral and bacterial infections, and previous transient ischemic attacks (TIAs). Risk factors specific to women are oral contraceptive use, pregnancy, childbirth, menopause, migraine headaches with aura, autoimmune disorders (such as diabetes and lupus), and clotting disorders.

FOCUS ON DIVERSITY
Risk Factors for Stroke

African Americans
- African Americans have almost twice the number of first-ever strokes compared to Caucasians.
- The prevalence of hypertension in African Americans is the highest in the world.
- Among African Americans age 20 and older, 62.9% of men and 77.2% of women are overweight or obese.

Hispanics
- Mexican Americans have an increased incidence of intracerebral hemorrhage, subarachnoid hemorrhage, ischemic stroke, transient ischemic attack and TIA at a younger age when compared to non-Hispanic whites.
- Diabetes is more common among Hispanics than Caucasians, with estimates that 30% or more of Hispanic adults have the disease.
- Hispanics have a greater proportion of hypertension than do Caucasians.
- Obesity is more prevalent among Hispanics than among non-Hispanic whites.
- As a result of language barriers and lack of transportation, Hispanics are more likely to delay or drop out of care.

(American Stroke Association, 2003).

In addition, having a stroke is a major risk factor for having another stroke (called recurrent stroke); about 5% to 14% of people who have a stroke and recover have another stroke within 1 year (AHA, 2005a). The risk is highest immediately after a stroke, then decreases with time. About 3% of clients with a stroke have another stroke within 30 days and one-third of recurrent strokes occur within 2 years of the first stroke (NINDS, 2005a).

Pathophysiology

The brain, which makes up only 2% of total body weight, receives approximately 20% of the cardiac output each minute (about 750 mL) and accounts for 20% of the body's oxygen consumption. Cerebral blood flow, especially in the deep cerebral vessels, is largely self-regulated by the brain to meet metabolic needs. This self-regulation (also called *autoregulation*) allows the brain to maintain a constant blood flow despite changes in systemic blood pressure. However, autoregulation is not effective when systemic blood pressure falls below 50 mmHg or rises above 160 mmHg. In the latter case, the increased systemic pressure (as in hypertension) causes an increase in cerebral blood flow with resultant overdistention of cerebral vessels. Cerebral blood flow also increases in response to increased carbon dioxide concentrations, increased hydrogen ion concentrations, and decreased oxygen concentrations.

When blood flow to and oxygenation of cerebral neurons are decreased or interrupted, pathophysiologic changes at the cellular level take place in 4 to 5 minutes. Cellular metabolism ceases as glucose, glycogen, and adenosine triphosphate (ATP) are depleted and the sodium-potassium pump fails. Cells swell as sodium draws water into the cell. Cerebral blood vessel walls also swell, further decreasing blood flow. Even if circulation is restored, vasospasm and increased blood viscosity can continue to impede blood flow. Severe or prolonged ischemia leads to cellular death. A central core of dead or dying cells is surrounded by a band of minimally perfused cells, called the *penumbra*. Although cells in the penumbra have impaired metabolic activities, their structural integrity is maintained. The survival of these cells depends on a timely return of adequate circulation, the volume of toxic products released by adjacent dying cells, the degree of cerebral edema, and alterations in local blood flow. The potential survival of cells in the penumbra has led to the use of fibrinolytic agents in the early treatment of ischemic stroke (Porth, 2005).

The neurologic deficits that occur as a result of a stroke can often be used to identify its location. Because the motor pathways cross at the junction of the medulla and spinal cord (decussation), strokes lead to loss or impairment of sensorimotor functions on the side of the body opposite the side of the brain that is damaged. This effect, known as a **contralateral deficit**, causes a stroke in the right hemisphere of the brain to be manifested by deficits in the left side of the body (and vice versa).

A stroke is characterized by a gradual or rapid onset of neurologic deficits due to compromised cerebral blood flow.

Strokes may result from a variety of problems, including cerebral thrombosis, cerebral embolism, and cerebral hemorrhage.

Ischemic Stroke

Ischemic strokes result from blockage and/or stenosis of a cerebral artery, decreasing or stopping blood flow and ultimately causing a brain infarction. This type of stroke accounts for about 80% of all strokes (NINDS, 2005a). The blockage may result from a blood clot (either as a thrombus or an emboli), or from stenosis of a vessel resulting from a buildup of plaque. Plaque may cause stenosis in large blood vessels (called large vessel disease) or small blood vessels (called small vessel disease). Large vessel disease usually is the result of thrombi. Small vessel strokes, called lacunar infarcts, are small to very small infarcts in the deep, noncortical areas of the brain or the brainstem. Ischemic strokes are classified as transient, thrombotic, or embolic.

TRANSIENT ISCHEMIC ATTACK   A **transient ischemic attack (TIA)**, sometimes called a mini-stroke, is a brief period of localized cerebral ischemia that causes neurologic deficits lasting for less than 24 hours (usually less than 1 to 2 hours) (Porth, 2005). The deficits may be present for only minutes or may last for hours. TIAs are often warning signals of an ischemic thrombotic stroke. One or many TIAs may precede a stroke, with the time between the TIA and a stroke ranging from hours to months. Of the 50,000 Americans who have a TIA each year, approximately one-third will have an acute stroke some time in the future (NINDS, 2005a). The etiology of TIA includes inflammatory artery disorders, sickle cell anemia, atherosclerotic changes in cerebral blood vessels, thrombosis, and emboli. Neurologic manifestations of a TIA vary according to the location and size of the cerebral vessel involved. Manifestations have a sudden onset and often disappear within minutes or hours. Commonly occurring deficits include contralateral numbness or weakness of the leg, hand, forearm, and corner of the mouth (due to middle cerebral artery involvement); aphasia (due to ischemia of the left hemisphere); and visual disturbances such as blurring (due to involvement of the posterior cerebral artery) (Porth, 2005). The client may also experience a visual disturbance called *amaurosis fugax* (a fleeting blindness of one eye, described as a shade coming down over vision with the affected eye).

THROMBOTIC STROKE   A thrombotic stroke is caused by occlusion of a large cerebral vessel by a thrombus (blood clot). Thrombotic CVAs most often occur in older people who are resting or sleeping. The blood pressure is lower during sleep, so there is less pressure to push the blood through an already narrowed arterial lumen, and ischemia may result.

Thrombi tend to form in large arteries that bifurcate and have narrowed lumens as a result of deposits of atherosclerotic plaque. The plaque involves the intima of the arteries, causing the internal elastic lamina to become thin and frayed with exposure of underlying connective tissue. This structural change causes platelets to adhere to the rough surface and release the enzyme adenosine diphosphate. This enzyme initiates the clotting sequence, and the thrombus forms. A thrombus may remain in place and continue to enlarge, completely occluding

the lumen of the vessel, or a part of it may break off and become an embolus.

The most common locations of thrombi are the internal carotid artery, the vertebral arteries, and the junction of the vertebral and basilar arteries. Thrombotic strokes affecting the smaller cerebral vessels are called lacunar strokes, because the infarcted areas slough off, leaving a small cavity or "lake" in the brain tissue. A thrombotic stroke usually affects only one region of the brain that is supplied by a single cerebral artery.

A thrombotic stroke occurs rapidly but progresses slowly. It often begins with a TIA, and continues to worsen over 1 to 2 days; the condition is called a *stroke-in-evolution*. When maximum neurologic deficit has been reached, usually in 3 days, the condition is called a *completed stroke*. At that time, the damaged area of brain tissue is edematous and necrotic.

EMBOLIC STROKE   An embolic stroke occurs when a blood clot or clump of matter traveling through the cerebral blood vessels becomes lodged in a vessel too narrow to permit further movement. The area of the brain supplied by the blocked vessel becomes ischemic. The most frequent sites of cerebral emboli are at bifurcations of vessels, particularly those of the carotid and middle cerebral arteries. This type of stroke is typically seen in clients who are younger than those experiencing thrombotic strokes and occurs when the client is awake and active.

Many embolic strokes originate from a thrombus in the left chambers of the heart, formed during atrial fibrillation. These are referred to as *cardiogenic embolic strokes*. Emboli result when parts of the thrombus break off and are carried through the arterial system to the brain. Cerebral emboli may also be due to carotid artery atherosclerotic plaque, bacterial endocarditis, recent myocardial infarction, rheumatic heart disease, and ventricular aneurysm.

An embolic stroke has a sudden onset and causes immediate deficits. If the embolus breaks up into smaller fragments and is absorbed by the body, manifestations will disappear in a few hours to a few days. If the embolus is not absorbed, manifestations will persist. Even if the embolus is absorbed, the vessel wall where the embolus lodges may be weakened, increasing the potential for cerebral hemorrhage.

Hemorrhagic Stroke

A hemorrhagic stroke, or intracranial hemorrhage, occurs when a cerebral blood vessel ruptures. It occurs most often in people with sustained increase in systolic-diastolic blood pressure. Intracranial hemorrhage usually occurs suddenly, often when the affected person is engaged in some activity. Although hypertension is the most common cause, a variety of factors may contribute to a hemorrhagic stroke, including rupture of a brittle plaque-encrusted artery wall, ruptured intracranial aneurysms, trauma, erosion of blood vessels by tumors, arteriovenous malformations, anticoagulant therapy, and blood disorders. Of all forms of stroke, this form is most often fatal and occurs in about 20% of all strokes (NINDS, 2005d). There are two types of hemorrhagic strokes: intracerebral hemorrhage and subarachnoid hemorrhage. Hemorrhagic strokes that result from ruptured cerebral aneurysm or an arteriovenous malformation are discussed in the following sections of the chapter.

As a result of the blood vessel rupture, blood enters the brain tissue, the cerebral ventricles, or the subarachnoid space, compressing adjacent tissues and causing blood vessel spasm and cerebral edema. Blood in the ventricles or subarachnoid space irritates the meninges and brain tissue, causing an inflammatory reaction and impairing absorption and circulation of cerebrospinal fluid (CSF).

The onset of manifestations from a hemorrhagic stroke is rapid. Manifestations depend on the location of the hemorrhage, but may include vomiting, headache, seizures, hemiplegia, and loss of consciousness. Pressure on the brain tissue from increased intracranial pressure (discussed in Chapter 44 ∞) may cause coma and death.

Manifestations

Manifestations of a stroke vary according to the cerebral artery involved and the area of the brain affected. Manifestations are always sudden in onset, focal, and usually one sided. The most common manifestation is weakness involving the face and arm, and sometimes the leg. Other common manifestations are numbness on one side, loss of vision, speech difficulties, a sudden severe headache, and difficulties with balance. The various deficits associated with involvement of a specific cerebral artery are collectively referred to as stroke syndromes, although the deficits often overlap, as shown in the box below.

MANIFESTATIONS of a Stroke by Involved Cerebral Vessel

INTERNAL CAROTID ARTERY
- Contralateral paralysis of the arm, leg, and face
- Contralateral sensory deficits of the arm, leg, and face
- If the dominant hemisphere is involved: aphasia
- If the nondominant hemisphere is involved: apraxia, agnosia, unilateral neglect
- Homonymous hemianopia

MIDDLE CEREBRAL ARTERY
- Drowsiness, stupor, coma
- Contralateral hemiplegia of the arm and face
- Contralateral sensory deficits of the arm and face
- Global aphasia (if dominant hemisphere involved)
- Homonymous hemianopia

ANTERIOR CEREBRAL ARTERY
- Contralateral weakness or paralysis of the foot and leg
- Contralateral sensory loss of the toes, foot, and leg
- Loss of ability to make decisions or act voluntarily
- Urinary incontinence

VERTEBRAL ARTERY
- Pain in face, nose, or eye
- Numbness and weakness of the face on involved side
- Problems with gait
- Dysphagia

Complications

Typical complications include sensoriperceptual deficits, cognitive and behavioral changes, communication disorders, motor deficits, and elimination disorders. These may be transient or permanent, depending on the degree of ischemia and necrosis as well as time of treatment. As a result of the neurologic deficits, the client with a stroke has complications that involve many different body systems (see the box on the next page). The disabilities resulting from a stroke often cause serious alterations in functional health status.

Sensoriperceptual Deficits

A stroke may involve pathologic changes in neurologic pathways that alter the ability to integrate, interpret, and attend to sensory data. The client may experience deficits in vision, hearing, equilibrium, taste, and sense of smell. The ability to perceive vibration, pain, warmth, cold, and pressure may be impaired, as may proprioception (the body's sense of its position). The loss of these sensory abilities increases the risk for injury. Deficits may include:

- **Hemianopia**: the loss of half of the visual field of one or both eyes; when the same half is missing in each eye, the condition is called *homonymous hemianopia* (Figure 45–1 ■)
- **Agnosia**: the inability to recognize one or more subjects that were previously familiar; agnosia may be visual, tactile, or auditory
- **Apraxia**: the inability to carry out some motor pattern (e.g., drawing a figure, getting dressed) even when strength and coordination are adequate

Another form of sensory-perceptual deficit is the **neglect syndrome** (or *unilateral neglect*), in which the client has a disorder of attention. In this syndrome, the person cannot integrate and use perceptions from the affected side of the body or from the environment on the affected side, and ignores that part. In severe cases, the client may even deny the paralysis. This deficit is more common following a stroke of the right hemi-

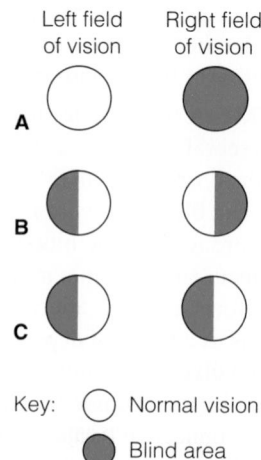

Left field of vision | Right field of vision

A

B

C

Key: ○ Normal vision
● Blind area

Figure 45–1 ■ Abnormal visual fields. *A,* Normal left field of vision with loss of vision in right field. *B,* Loss of vision in temporal half of both fields (bitemporal hemianopia). *C,* Loss of vision in nasal field of right eye and temporal field of left eye (homonymous hemianopia).

MANIFESTATIONS and Complications of Stroke by Body System

INTEGUMENT
- Decubitus (pressure) ulcers

NEUROLOGIC
- Hyperthermia
- Neglect syndrome
- Seizures
- Agnosias
- Communication deficits
  a. Expressive aphasia
  b. Receptive aphasia
  c. Global aphasia
  d. Agraphia
- Visual deficits
  a. Homonymous hemianopia
  b. Diplopia
  c. Decreased acuity
- Cognitive changes
  a. Memory loss
  b. Short attention span
  c. Distractibility
  d. Poor judgment
  e. Poor problem-solving ability
  f. Disorientation
- Behavioral changes
  a. Emotional lability
  b. Loss of social inhibitions
  c. Fear

  d. Hostility
  e. Anger
  f. Depression
- Increased intracranial pressure
- Alterations in consciousness
- Sensory loss (touch, pain, heat, cold, pressure)

RESPIRATORY
- Respiratory center damage
- Airway obstruction
- Decreased ability to cough

GASTROINTESTINAL
- Dysphagia
- Constipation
- Stool impaction

GENITOURINARY
- Incontinence
- Frequency
- Urgency
- Urinary retention
- Renal calculi

MUSCULOSKELETAL
- Hemiplegia
- Contractures
- Bony ankylosis
- Disuse atrophy
- Dysarthria

sphere where damage to the parietal lobe (a center for mediation of directed attention) results in perceptual deficits.

Pain and discomfort may accompany a stroke, with the client experiencing acute pain, numbness, or strange sensations. Although not common, damage to the thalamus may cause *central stroke pain* or *central pain syndrome (CPS)*. The pain in this syndrome includes hot and cold, burning, tingling, and sharp stabbing pain, most often in the extremities. It is worsened by movement and temperature changes. The painful sensations are not relieved by pain medications, nor are there any specific treatments.

Cognitive and Behavioral Changes

A change in consciousness, ranging from mild confusion to coma, is a common manifestation of a stroke. It may result from tissue damage following ischemia or hemorrhage involving either the carotid or vertebral arteries. Altered consciousness may also be the result of cerebral edema or increased intracranial pressure.

Behavioral changes include emotional lability (in which the client may laugh or cry inappropriately), loss of self-control (manifested by behavior such as swearing or refusing to wear clothing), and decreased tolerance for stress (resulting in anger or depression). Intellectual changes may include memory loss, decreased attention span, poor judgment, and an inability to think abstractly.

Communication Disorders

Communication is a complex process, involving motor functions, speech, language, memory, reasoning, and emotions. Communication disorders are usually the result of a stroke affecting the dominant hemisphere. The left hemisphere is dominant in about 95% of right-handed people and 70% of left-handed people (Porth, 2005).

Many different impairments may occur, and most are partial. Disorders of communication affect both speech (the mechanical act of articulating language through the spoken word) and language (the vocal or written formulation of ideas to communicate thoughts and feelings). Language involves oral and written expression and auditory and reading comprehension. Among these disorders are:

- **Aphasia**: the inability to use or understand language; aphasia may be expressive, receptive, or mixed (global).
- *Expressive aphasia:* a motor speech problem in which one can understand what is being said but can respond verbally only in short phrases; also called *Broca's aphasia.*
- *Receptive aphasia:* a sensory speech problem in which one cannot understand the spoken (and often written) word. Speech may be fluent but with inappropriate content; also called *Wernicke's aphasia.*
- *Mixed or global aphasia:* language dysfunction in both understanding and expression.
- *Dysarthria:* any disturbance in muscular control of speech.

Motor Deficits

Body movement results from a complex interaction between the brain, spinal cord, and peripheral nerves. The motor areas of the cerebral cortex, the basal ganglia, and the cerebellum initiate voluntary movement by sending messages to the spinal cord, which then transmits the messages to the peripheral nerves. A stroke may interrupt the central nervous system (CNS) component of this relay system and produce effects in the contralateral side ranging from mild weakness to severe limitation of any kind of movement.

Depending on the area of the brain involved, strokes may cause weakness, paralysis, and/or spasticity. The deficits include:

- **Hemiplegia**: paralysis of the left or right half of the body (Figure 45–2 ■).
- **Hemiparesis**: weakness of the left or right half of the body.
- **Flaccidity:** absence of muscle tone (hypotonia).
- **Spasticity**: increased muscle tone (hypertonia), usually with some degree of weakness. The flexor muscles are usually more strongly affected in the upper extremities, and the extensor muscles are more strongly affected in the lower extremities.

When the corticospinal tract is involved, the affected arm and leg almost always are initially flaccid and then become spastic within 6 to 8 weeks. Spasticity often causes characteristic body positioning: adduction of the shoulder, pronation of the forearm, flexion of the fingers, and extension of the hip and knee. There is often foot drop, outward rotation of the leg, and dependent edema in the involved extremities.

The motor deficits may result in altered mobility, further impairing body function. The complications of immobility involve multiple body systems and include orthostatic hypotension, increased thrombus formation, decreased cardiac output, impaired respiratory function, osteoporosis, formation of renal calculi, contractures, and decubitus ulcer formation.

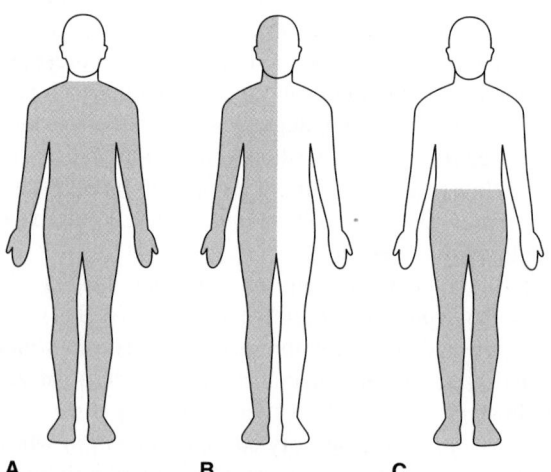

Figure 45–2 ■ Types of paralysis. *A,* Quadriplegia is complete or partial paralysis of the upper extremities and complete paralysis of the lower part of the body. *B,* Hemiplegia is paralysis of one-half of the body when it is divided along the median sagittal plane. *C,* Paraplegia is paralysis of the lower part of the body.

Elimination Disorders

Disorders of bladder and bowel elimination are common. A stroke may cause partial loss of the sensations that trigger bladder elimination, resulting in urinary frequency, urgency, or incontinence. Control of urination may be altered as a result of cognitive deficits. Changes in bowel elimination are common, resulting from changes in level of consciousness (LOC), immobility, and dehydration (Hickey, 2003).

INTERDISCIPLINARY CARE

The type of treatment a client with a stroke receives depends on the stage of the disease. In general there are three treatment stages: stroke prevention, acute care immediately after a stroke, and rehabilitation after a stroke. The client with an acute stroke may receive medical and/or surgical treatment. The focus in the acute care phase is on diagnosing the type and cause of the stroke, supporting cerebral circulation, and controlling or preventing further deficits. The goals of stroke care, defined by the American Heart Association (2005b), are to minimize brain injury and maximize client recovery by:

- Rapid recognition and reaction to stroke warning signs
- Rapid emergency medical services (EMS) dispatch
- Rapid EMS system transport and hospital prenotification
- Rapid diagnosis and treatment in the hospital.

Diagnosis

Diagnosis begins with a complete history and careful physical assessment, including a thorough neurologic examination. The time of the onset of stroke manifestations is a critical part of assessment. The National Institute of Health (NIH) Stroke Scale is a clinical evaluation tool widely used to assess neurologic outcome and degree of recovery. Part of the scale is illustrated in Table 45–1. The tool measures LOC, vision, facial paralysis, motor abilities, ataxia, sensation, language and attention.

Imaging tests are used to identify an increased risk for a stroke or to identify pathophysiologic changes after a stroke has occurred.

Computed tomography (CT) is the first imaging technique used to demonstrate the presence of hemorrhage, tumors, aneurysm, ischemia, edema, and tissue necrosis. A CT scan can also demonstrate a shift in intracranial contents and is useful in distinguishing the type of stroke (e.g., a hemorrhagic stroke results in an increase in density). Cerebral infarctions usually are visible with a CT scan 6 to 8 hours post-stroke; hemorrhage is visible immediately. Other imaging tests that may be used for diagnosis include a cerebral arteriogram, a transcranial ultrasound Doppler, an MRI, an MRA, a PET, and a SPECT (see the Diagnostic Tests box in Chapter 43 ∞).

A lumbar puncture may be performed to obtain CSF for examination if there is no danger of increased intracranial pressure (IICP). (Removal of CSF when intracranial pressure is increased can result in herniation of the brainstem.) A thrombotic stroke may elevate CSF pressure; after a hemorrhagic stroke frank blood may be seen in the CSF.

TABLE 45–1 NIH Stroke Scale: Assessment of Level of Consciousness

INSTRUCTIONS	SCALE DEFINITION	SCORE
1a. **Level of Consciousness:** The investigator must choose a response, even if a full evaluation is prevented by such obstacles as an endotracheal tube, language barrier, orotracheal trauma/bandages. A 3 is scored only if the patient makes no movement (other than reflexive posturing) in response to noxious stimulation.	0 = Alert, keenly responsive. 1 = Not alert, but arousable by minor stimulation to obey, answer, or respond. 2 = Not alert, requires repeated stimulation to attend, or is obtunded and requires strong or painful stimulation to make movements (not stereotyped). 3 = Responds only with reflex motor or autonomic effects or totally unresponsive, flaccid, are flexic.	_____
1b. **LOC Questions:** The patient is asked the month and his/her age. The answer must be correct. There is no partial credit for being close. Aphasic and stuporous patients who do not comprehend the questions will score 2. Patients unable to speak because of endotracheal intubation, orotracheal trauma, severe dysarthria from any cause, language barrier, or any other problem not secondary to aphasia are given a 1. It is important that only the initial answer be graded and that the examiner not "help" the patient with verbal or nonverbal cues.	0 = Answers both questions correctly. 1 = Answers one question correctly. 2 = Answers neither question correctly.	_____
1c. **LOC Commands:** The patient is asked to open and close the eyes and then to grip and release the nonparetic hand. Substitute another one-step command if the hands cannot be used. Credit is given if an unequivocal attempt is made but not completed due to weakness. If the patient does not respond to command the task should be demonstrated to them (pantomime) and score the results (i.e., follows none, one or two commands). Patients with trauma, amputation, or other physical impediments should be given suitable one-step commands. Only the first attempt is scored.	0 = Performs both tasks correctly. 1 = Performs one task correctly. 2 = Performs neither task correctly.	_____

Note: This is a sample of only one part of the NIH Stroke Scale. The entire scale may be viewed as a PDF file at http://www.strokecenter.org/trials/scales/nihss.pdf#search='nih%20STroke%20scale.

In addition to imaging tests, a blood test has recently been approved to screen for recurrent stroke risk. The PLAC test scans the blood for high levels of lipoprotein-associated phospholipase A2 (Lp-Pla2), found to be more common in people who have had strokes.

Medications

Medications are administered to prevent a stroke in clients with TIAs or a previous stroke, and to treat the client during the acute phase of a stroke.

PREVENTION Antiplatelet agents are often used to treat clients with TIAs or who have had a previous stroke. Platelets are concentrated in high blood flow arteries, where they adhere to endothelial tissue damaged by atherosclerosis and occlude the vessel. The drugs used to prevent clot formation and blood vessel occlusion include aspirin, clopidogrel (Plavix), dipyridamole (Persantine), and ticlopidine (Ticlid).

Daily low-dose aspirin reduces TIA occurrence and stroke risk by interfering with platelet aggregation. Ticlopidine (Ticlid) is a platelet-aggregation inhibitor that has shown reduction in thrombotic stroke risk.

ACUTE STROKE Medications are used to treat the client during the acute phase of an ischemic stroke to prevent further thrombosis formation, increase cerebral blood flow, and protect cerebral

neurons. The type of medication used varies according to the type of stroke.

Anticoagulant drug therapy (discussed in Chapter 34 ∞) is often ordered for an ischemic stroke. The most commonly used anticoagulants are warfarin (Coumadin), heparin, and enoxaparin (Lovenox). Anticoagulants are never administered to a client with a hemorrhagic stroke. Anticoagulants do not dissolve an existing clot but prevent further extension of the clot and formation of new clots. Sodium heparin may be given subcutaneously or by continuous IV drip, or warfarin sodium (Coumadin) may be given orally.

Fibrinolytic therapy, using a tissue plasminogen activator such as recombinant tissue plasminogen activator alteplase (rt-PA, tPA), sometimes given concurrently with an anticoagulant, is used to treat thrombotic stroke. The drug converts plasminogen to plasmin, resulting in fibrinolysis of the clot. To be effective, it must be given intravenously within 3 hours of the onset of manifestations, after confirming (with a CT scan) that the client has had an ischemic stroke (Tierney et al., 2005). Antithrombotic drugs, which inhibit the platelet phase of clot formation, have been used as a preventive measure for clients at risk for embolic and thrombotic CVA. Both aspirin and dipyridamole have been used for this purpose. These drugs are sometimes also used in combination with other drugs during acute treatment. Antiplatelet agents are contraindicated in clients with a hemorrhagic stroke.

Management of hypertension is controversial but if the client is eligible for fibrinolytic therapy, blood pressure control is essential to decrease the risk of bleeding. If the blood pressure is sustained at levels >185 mmHg systolic or >110 diastolic, the client cannot be treated with IV tPA (American Heart Association, 2005b).

Corticosteroids, such as prednisone or dexamethasone, have been used to treat cerebral edema, but the results are not always positive. If the client has IICP, hyperosmolar solutions (such as mannitol) or diuretics (such as furosemide) may be administered. Anticonvulsants, such as phenytoin (Dilantin), and barbiturates may be prescribed if IICP causes seizures. Increased intracranial pressure is discussed in Chapter 44 ∞ .

Treatments

The treatments used in the management of a stroke include surgery and rehabilitation.

SURGERY Surgery may be performed to prevent the occurrence of a stroke, to restore blood flow when a stroke has already occurred, or to repair vascular damage or malformations. In people who have had TIAs or are in danger of having another stroke, a carotid endarterectomy at the carotid artery bifurcation may be performed to remove atherosclerotic plaque (Figure 45–3 ■). Nursing care for the client in the initial postoperative period following a carotid endarterectomy is described in the following box.

When an occluded or stenotic vessel is not directly accessible, an extracranial-intracranial bypass may be performed. Bypass of the internal carotid, middle cerebral, or vertebral arteries may be required. The indications for the bypass are manifestations of ischemia caused by TIAs or a mild completed stroke. The procedure reestablishes blood flow to the affected area of the brain.

A carotid angioplasty with stenting is a newer option for treating cerebral stenosis. During the procedure an angioplasty balloon catheter is inserted through an artery in the client's arm or leg. Under fluoroscopy, the catheter is advanced to the area of carotid artery stenosis and a small filter is inserted to catch any clots or pieces of debris that might break loose. The balloon is then inflated to widen the artery, followed by insertion of a permanent stent in the area of the angioplasty (Palmieri, 2006).

REHABILITATION Various types of therapy are necessary for post-stroke rehabilitation. Listed below are the types and goals of therapies used:

- Physical therapy may help prevent contractures and improve muscle strength and coordination. Physical therapists teach exercises to enable the client to relearn how to walk, sit, lie down, and change from one type of movement to another.
- Occupational therapy provides assistive devices and a plan for regaining lost motor skills that greatly improve quality of life after a stroke. These skills include eating, drinking, bathing, cooking, reading, writing, and toileting.
- Speech therapy is provided to help the client relearn language and communication skills, as well as improve swallowing.

NURSING CARE

Even though many people who have a stroke have full recovery, a substantial number are left with disabilities that affect their physical, emotional, interpersonal, and family status.

NURSING CARE OF THE CLIENT HAVING A Carotid Endarterectomy

POSTOPERATIVE CARE

- Position on the unoperated side and either maintain a flat position or elevate the head of the bed 30 degrees as prescribed. Maintain head and neck alignment and avoid rotating, flexing, or hyperextending head. *Pressure on the wound is undesirable. Elevating the head decreases edema in the operative site. Maintaining head and neck alignment prevents additional tension or pressure on the operative side.*
- Support the head when changing position. Teach to support the head with the hands when able to move about. *Supporting the head helps prevent stress on the operative site (which may cause bleeding and hematoma formation); it also helps reduce stress on the suture line.*
- Perform focused assessments to monitor for complications:
  a. *Hemorrhage.* Assess the dressing and the area under the neck and shoulders for drainage. Assess for increased pulse and decreased blood pressure. *The most common cause of respiratory problems is pressure on the trachea from a hematoma formation.*
  b. *Respiratory distress.* Assess respiratory rate, rhythm, depth, and effort. Observe for restlessness. Keep a tracheostomy tray at the bedside. *Respiratory distress, may result from edema and hematoma formation, which may compress the trachea.*
  c. *Cranial nerve impairment.* Observe and record any facial drooping, tongue deviation, hoarseness, dysphagia, or loss of facial sensation. *Cranial nerves may be stretched during surgery, leading to temporary deficits in cranial nerve function.*
  d. *Hypertension or hypotension.* Take and record blood pressure at least hourly. Report any changes immediately and Implement orders for medications to treat hypertension or hypotension. *About one-half of all clients having a carotid endarterectomy develop unstable blood pressure related to surgical denervation of the carotid sinus. Uncontrolled hypertension may precipitate a CVA. The most common problem is hypotension, possibly related to stimulation of the carotid body baroreceptors, which are exposed during surgery. Hypotension may result in myocardial ischemia.*

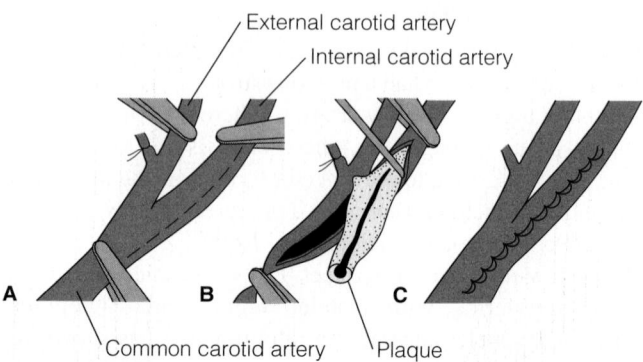

External carotid artery
Internal carotid artery

A   B   C

Common carotid artery   Plaque

Figure 45–3 ■ Carotid endarterectomy. *A,* The occluded area is clamped off and an incision is made in the artery. *B,* Plaque is removed from the inner layer of the artery. *C,* To restore blood flow through the artery, the artery is sutured, or a graft is completed.

The required nursing care is often complex and multidimensional, requiring consideration of continuity of care for clients in acute care settings, long-term care settings, rehabilitation centers, and the home.

Nurses caring for clients who have had a stroke require knowledge and skill to meet client needs during both the acute and the rehabilitative phases of care. The client may have multiple losses: loss of mobility, ability to provide self-care, communications, concept of self, and interpersonal or intimate relationships with others. Holistic, individualized nursing care is essential in all settings and focuses on promoting the achievement of maximum potential and quality of life.

The client's family is often faced with many changes. The young to middle-aged adult with a family member who has had a stroke may be faced with economic difficulties and social isolation. The middle-aged adult family member may become the caretaker for an older parent, in essence switching roles with the parent. An older adult may not be able to care for a spouse and may have to accept nursing home placement. In addition, the older adult who has no family may have to struggle alone to regain the ability to function independently. Although not all of these problems are amenable to nursing solutions, the nurse is most often the healthcare provider who assesses and identifies the needs of each individual and provides information and referrals to clients and families to help meet those needs.

Because a stroke has the potential to cause many different health problems, a wide variety of nursing diagnoses may be appropriate. It is important to remember that each person will be affected differently, depending on the degree of ischemia and the area of the brain involved. Nursing diagnoses discussed in this section focus on problems with cerebral tissue perfusion (specific to nursing care during the acute phase), physical mobility, self-care, communication, sensory-perceptual deficits, bowel and urine elimination, and swallowing (specific to prevention of complications and rehabilitation). A Nursing Care Plan for a client with a stroke is found on the next page.

Health Promotion

Health promotion activities focus on stroke prevention, especially for those people with known risk factors. It is important to discuss, as appropriate, the importance of stopping smoking and drug use with clients of all ages. Maintaining a normal weight through diet and exercise can help reduce obesity, which increases the risk of hypertension and type 2 diabetes mellitus (both in turn increase the risk of a stroke). Cholesterol levels should be screened regularly to monitor for hyperlipidemia. Regular health care to monitor for and treat cardiovascular disorders and to detect and treat infections such as infective endocarditis is important. It is also important to increase public awareness of the signs of a TIA or stroke and of the need to call 911 or to seek care immediately if the following warning signs or symptoms occur:

- Sudden weakness or numbness of the face, arm, or leg, especially on one side of the body
- Sudden confusion, difficulty speaking, or difficulty understanding speech
- Sudden trouble walking, dizziness, loss of coordination

- Sudden difficulty with vision in one or both eyes
- Sudden severe headache without a cause.

Information about public awareness of stroke manifestations and the need for immediate treatment is discussed in the Nursing Research box on page 1589.

Assessment

The following data are collected through the health history and physical examination (see Chapter 43 ∞). Further focused assessments are described with nursing interventions. If the client is a woman, she has risks for stroke different than from a man and should be asked questions specific to her gender (see the box on page 1589).

- *Health history:* Risk factors, previous stroke, drug use (prescribed, over-the-counter, street drugs), smoking history, when manifestations began, severity of manifestations, presence of incontinence, level of consciousness, family support system.
- *Physical assessment:* Level of consciousness, motor strength, coordination, communication, cranial nerves, sensory function.

Nursing Diagnoses and Interventions

The acute phase of a stroke is most often the time from admission to the hospital until the client is stabilized, usually 24 to 72 hours after admission (Hickey, 2003). Depending on the severity of the stroke, the client may be admitted to the intensive care unit. Regardless of the hospital setting, the nurse provides interventions to maintain body functions and prevent complications.

Ineffective Tissue Perfusion: Cerebral

The initial assessment and care of the client admitted for intensive care focuses on identifying changes that may indicate altered cerebral perfusion. The client's airway, breathing, circulation, and neurologic status are monitored and interventions are provided to maintain cerebral perfusion.

- Monitor respiratory status and airway patency. Auscultate pulmonary sounds and monitor respiratory rate and results of studies of arterial blood gases.
- Suction as necessary, using care to suction no longer than 10 seconds at any one time, and using sterile technique.
- Place in a side-lying position.
- Administer oxygen as prescribed.
  The client is often unconscious and breathing may be impaired. Suctioning removes secretions that not only obstruct airflow but also poses the risk for aspiration and pneumonia. Suctioning for longer than 10 seconds at a time may increase intracranial pressure (Hickey, 2003). Respiratory complications develop rapidly, as manifested by crackles and wheezes, rapid respirations, and respiratory acidosis. The administration of oxygen decreases the risk for hypoxia and hypercapnia, which can increase cerebral ischemia and intracranial pressure.

> **PRACTICE ALERT**
> Positioning the client on the side allows secretions to drain out of the mouth, helping to prevent aspiration.

MEDIALINK Care Plan Activity: Hemorrhagic Stroke

NURSING CARE PLAN   A Client with a Stroke

Orville Boren is a 63-year-old African American who had a stroke due to right cerebral thrombosis 1 week ago. He is a history instructor at the local community college. His hobbies are wood carving and gardening. Mr. Boren is also an active member of his church. For the past 2 years, Mr. Boren has been taking medication for hypertension, but his wife Emily reports that he often forgets to take it and that his blood pressure was high at his last physical examination. Mrs. Boren tells the staff that she has never had to worry about her husband's health before and that she wants to learn everything she can to care for him at home. However, she says that her husband was always the one to make the decisions and pay the bills. Mrs. Boren adds that all the children, grandchildren, neighbors, and family pastor want to see Mr. Boren back at home as soon as possible.

ASSESSMENT

Carol Merck, RN, the nurse assigned to Mr. Boren, completes a health history and physical assessment, with Mrs. Boren providing information for the history. Mrs. Boren reports that her husband did have several spells of dizziness and blurred vision the week before his stroke, but they lasted only a few minutes and he believed them to be due to "old age and working out in the sun." On the morning of admission, Mr. Boren woke up and could not move his left arm or leg; he also could not speak sensibly. Mrs. Boren called 911, and an ambulance took her husband to the hospital.

Physical assessment findings include the following: Mr. Boren is drowsy but responds to verbal stimuli. Although he does not respond verbally, he can nod his head to indicate "yes" when asked questions. Flaccid paralysis is present in his left arm and left leg, with no response noted to touch in those extremities (he is left handed). Visual fields are decreased in a pattern consistent with homonymous hemianopia. A CT scan, negative on admission; is repeated on the day after admission and confirms the medical diagnosis of a right-brain stroke due to a thrombus of the middle cerebral artery.

Mr. Boren's medical treatment includes heparin sodium administered by continuous intravenous drip, with clotting studies to be performed every 4 hours and the dose adjusted accordingly.

DIAGNOSES

- *Feeding Self-Care Deficit* related to loss of the ability to use the left hand and arm
- *Impaired Physical Mobility* related to neurologic deficits causing left hemiplegia
- *Risk for Impaired Skin Integrity* related to inability to change position
- *Sensory Perception Disturbed: Visual* related to changes in visual fields
- *Impaired Verbal Communication* related to cerebral injury

EXPECTED OUTCOMES

- Learn to use his right hand to feed himself.
- Participate in exercises necessary to maintain muscle strength and tone.
- Maintain skin integrity.
- Indicate understanding that visual fields may improve in a few weeks.
- Practice and implement speech therapy activities while at the same time using alternative methods of communication.

PLANNING AND IMPLEMENTATION

- Arrange mealtimes so that he is sitting up by the window in a clean and private environment.
- Provide adaptive devices (silverware with thick handles and nonslip plates).
- Encourage Mrs. Boren to visit at mealtimes, to assist with meals, and periodically to bring a favorite food from home.
- Provide passive ROM exercises for his left arm and leg; schedule active ROM exercises for his right extremities as well as quadriceps and gluteal sets every 4 hours during waking hours.
- Keep his skin clean and dry at all times.
- Establish and maintain a regular schedule for turning when he is in bed.
- Place objects (e.g., call bell, tissues) on unaffected side and approach him from that side.
- Support attempts to communicate verbally; when he is not understood, he prefers to use a large marker and tablet.

EVALUATION

Mr. Boren is discharged to his home after being in the hospital for 10 days. During the first 2 months after discharge, Martha Grimes, RN, the home health nurse, visits Mr. and Mrs. Boren at home. At the end of 2 months, Mr. Boren is using his right hand to feed himself. He has regained partial use of his left arm and leg and is using a walker to move around the house and yard; he is even able to work in his flower garden. His skin has remained intact, and his vision is back to normal. He is slowly relearning speech; this has been the most difficult change for him to accept. Once he writes on his tablet, "I think God has forgotten me."

CRITICAL THINKING IN THE NURSING PROCESS

1. Hypertension is sometimes referred to as "the silent killer." Provide justifications for this statement.
2. The functional changes Mr. Boren has experienced may make a return to teaching difficult. What other uses of his knowledge and abilities might you suggest?
3. What would be your reply if, after you had completed passive ROM on Mr. Boren's left arm, he wrote: "I just ignore that part of my body—it doesn't work anyway"?
See Evaluating Your Response in Appendix C.

- Monitor mental status and LOC: restlessness, drowsiness, lethargy, inability to follow commands, unresponsiveness.
- Monitor strength and reflexes, and assess for pain, headache, decreased muscle strength, sluggish pupillary reflexes, absent gag or swallowing reflexes, hemiplegia, Babinski's sign, and decerebrate or decorticate posturing.

Frequent monitoring of neurologic status is necessary to detect changes. Alterations in mental status, LOC, movement, strength, and reflexes indicate increased intracranial pressure, the major cause of death in the acute phase of a stroke.

- Continuously monitor cardiac status, observing for dysrhythmias. *A stroke may cause cardiac dysrhythmias, in-*

NURSING RESEARCH   Evidence-Based Practice: Improve Rapid Treatment of a Stroke

Stroke is the third leading cause of death in the United States and is also a leading cause of severe, long-term disability. The risk of disability and death can be reduced in people who experience a sudden ischemic stroke by the administration of tissue plasminogen activator (tPA). To be effective, tPA must be administered within 3 hours of the warning signs of a stoke, but the public's awareness of stroke manifestations and the need for immediate treatment remain poor. This is especially true for those most at risk: people older than 75 years of age, African Americans, and men. Maze and Bakas (2004) conducted a study to determine (1) the most common manifestations leading to the decision to seek medical care, (2) who makes the decision, (3) the most common mode of transportation, (4) hospital arrival time in relation to onset of warning signs, and (5) factors most associated with hospital arrival time. They found that the most common warning sign leading people to come to the hospital was sudden confusion or trouble speaking or understanding speech, followed by sudden numbness or weakness in one part of the body. In the majority of cases, it was the person having the stroke that decided to come to the hospital, and the most common mode of transportation was by ambulance via the emergency medical system (EMS). The mean arrival time at the hospital after the onset of manifestations was more than 5 hours; only about 29% of those having a stroke arrived within 3 hours. Those that arrived by EMS and reported their incomes as adequate had the shortest arrival times.

IMPLICATIONS FOR NURSING

Nurses provide information to the public in a wide variety of health promotion activities, including stroke awareness and the need for immediate treatment to ensure the best outcomes of care. It is important that the programs be geared toward the specific population most at risk, and targeting people from all socioeconomic and cultural backgrounds. Although not measured in this study, factors that affect behavior, such as perceived risk, benefits and barriers of care, readiness to change, and self-efficacy, are areas that may be effective in designing educational programs to increase stroke awareness.

CRITICAL THINKING IN CLIENT CARE

1. If you were planning a stroke awareness educational program, where would you have it in order to reach the largest number of the population? How would you advertise stroke warning manifestations to reach the most people?
2. How would you change the design of your program for the following groups?
   a. Long-term care or assisted living residents
   b. A men's study group in an African American church
   c. A group of Mexican American women.
3. Think of a slogan for the public that increases awareness of the 3-hour time limit for treatment with tPA.

---

cluding bradycardia, PVCs, tachycardia, and AV block. Characteristic ECG changes include a shortened PR interval, peaked T waves, and a depressed ST segment.
- Monitor body temperature. *Hyperthermia may develop if the hypothalamus is affected.*

MEETING INDIVIDUALIZED NEEDS
Risk Factors for Stroke in Women

Some risk factors for stroke apply only to women, most specifically pregnancy, childbirth, and menopause. These risks are the result of fluctuations in hormones that occur at different stages of life. However, other risks are also more common for women, and information should be collected during a health history. For accurate assessment, ask the following questions, depending on the woman's age:
- How many pregnancies have you had?
- Have you had a miscarriage? If so, how many?
- How many births have you had? When was your last delivery?
- When was your last menstrual cycle?
- Do you take any type of hormone replacement therapy?
- Do you take birth control pills?
- Do you have migraine headaches? If so, do you have an aura?
- Have you ever been diagnosed with diabetes or lupus?
- Have you ever been diagnosed with a clotting disorder? Have you ever had a clot in your leg?

- Maintain accurate intake and output records; measure urinary output via a Foley catheter. *A stroke may damage the pituitary gland, resulting in diabetes insipidus and the possibility of dehydration from greatly increased urinary output.*

PRACTICE ALERT
Diabetes insipidus is indicated by a large output of dilute urine; dehydration is indicated by scanty amounts of dark, concentrated urine.

- Monitor for seizures. Pad the side rails, and administer prescribed anticonvulsants. *Seizures may be the result of cerebral tissue damage or increased intracranial pressure. Padded side rails prevent injury if a seizure occurs. Anticonvulsants prevent or treat seizures.*

Impaired Physical Mobility

The goals of care for clients with impaired mobility are to maintain and improve functional abilities (by maintaining normal function and alignment, preventing edema of extremities, and reducing spasticity) and to prevent complications.
- Encourage active range-of-motion (ROM) exercises for unaffected extremities and perform passive ROM exercises for affected extremities every 4 hours during day and evening shifts and once during the night shift. Support the joint during passive ROM exercises. *Active ROM exercises maintain or improve muscle strength and*

endurance, and help to maintain cardiopulmonary function. Passive ROM exercises do not strengthen muscles but do help maintain joint flexibility.

> ### PRACTICE ALERT
> Both active and passive exercises increase venous return, decreasing the risk of thrombophlebitis.

- Turn every 2 hours around the clock, following a posted schedule for side-to-side and supine-to-prone position changes (verify prone positioning with the physician). Maintain body alignment and support extremities in proper position with pillows. *Turning on a regular basis, accompanied by proper positioning, maintains joint function, alleviates pressure on bony prominences that can lead to skin breakdown, decreases dependent edema in hands and feet, and lessens the risk of complications resulting from immobility* (Figure 45–4 ■).

A

B

C

Figure 45–4 ■ Positioning the client with hemiplegia is important in preventing deformity of the affected extremities. *A,* With the client in a supine position, place a pillow in the axilla (to prevent adduction) and under the hand and arm, with the hand higher than the elbow (to prevent flexion and edema). *B,* When the client is lying supine, use a pillow from the iliac crest to the middle of the thigh to prevent external rotation of the hip. *C,* When the client is in the prone position, place a pillow under the pelvis to promote hip hyperextension.

> ### PRACTICE ALERT
> When lying on the affected side, clients may be restless because they do not have normal sensation and feel as if they may fall.

- Monitor the lower extremities each shift for symptoms of thrombophlebitis. Assess for increased warmth and redness in calves; measure the circumference of the calves and thighs. *Clients on bed rest (especially those with loss of muscle strength and tone) are particularly prone to the development of deep venous thrombosis. Promptly report manifestations of thrombophlebitis.*
- Collaborate with the physical therapist as the client gains mobility, using consistent techniques to move the client from the bed to the wheelchair and to help the client ambulate. *The use of consistent techniques facilitates rehabilitation.*

Self-Care Deficit
The client who has had a stroke may have a self-care deficit as a result of impaired mobility or mental confusion. It is important for clients to perform as much of their own physical care and grooming as possible to promote functional ability, increase independence, decrease feelings of powerlessness, and improve self-esteem.

Before establishing a plan to increase self-care, determine which hand was dominant before the stroke. If the client's dominant side is affected, self-care will be more difficult.

- Encourage use of the unaffected arm to bathe, brush teeth, comb hair, dress, and eat. *Use of the unaffected arm promotes functional ability and independence.*
- Teach the client to put on clothing by first dressing the affected extremities and then dressing the unaffected extremities. *This technique facilitates self-dressing with minimal assistance.*
- Collaborate with the occupational therapist in scheduling times for training for upper extremity functioning necessary for activities of daily living (ADLs). Encourage the use of assistive devices (if required) for eating, physical hygiene, and dressing. *Following a regular schedule in daily routines promotes learning. The use of assistive devices promotes independence and decreases feelings of powerlessness. Optimal grooming facilitates positive self-concept.*

Impaired Verbal Communication
The client who loses communication abilities requires intensive speech therapy and emotional support. It is important to determine the specific nature of the impairment when planning interventions and helping family members understand specific problems. Although the speech therapist is usually most involved with speech rehabilitation, nurses must plan interventions to meet communication needs during all phases of care.

Use the following guidelines:
- Approach and treat the client as an adult.
- Do not assume that the client who does not respond verbally cannot hear. Do not use a raised voice when addressing the client.
- Allow adequate time for the client to respond.
- Face the client and speak slowly.

- When you do not understand the client's speech, be honest and say so.
- Use short, simple statements and questions.
  Accepting the client and providing dignity and respect enhances the nurse–client relationship. Allowing adequate response time and using short verbal statements or questions while facing the client motivates the client to communicate and decreases frustration.
- Accept frustration and anger as a normal reaction to the loss of function. *Anger represents the client's frustration at the inability to control the loss of function.*
- Try alternate methods of communication, including writing tablets, flash cards, and computerized talking boards. *Clients unable to communicate verbally may use other methods effectively.*

Impaired Urinary Elimination and Risk for Constipation

Both urinary and bowel elimination may be altered because of neurologic deficits, impaired mobility, cognitive impairment, communication deficits, or preexisting problems (especially if the client is an older adult). Other causes include changes in food and fluid intake and side effects of medications. Urinary incontinence or retention and constipation and fecal impaction are the usual manifestations.

- Assess for urinary frequency, urgency, incontinence, nocturia, and voiding in small amounts. In addition, assess the client's ability to respond to the need to void, the ability to use the call light, and the ability to use toileting equipment.

> **PRACTICE ALERT**
> Voiding small amounts of urine frequently may be a manifestation of a bladder dysfunction. Assess for a distended bladder.

- Encourage bladder training by having client void on schedule, such as every 2 hours, rather than in response to the urge to void.
- Teach Kegel exercises. To perform Kegel exercises, the client contracts the perineal muscles as though stopping urination, holds the contraction for 5 seconds, and then releases.
- Use positive reinforcement (verbal praise) for successful management of urinary elimination.
  Voiding every 2 hours or on schedule promotes bladder tone and urine storage. Kegel exercises increase pubococcygeal muscle tone and bladder control, decreasing incontinence. Positive reinforcement can be a useful part of the teaching program.
- Discuss prestroke bowel habits, as well as the pattern of bowel elimination since the stroke.
- If the client is able to swallow without difficulty, encourage fluids (up to 2000 mL per day) and a high-fiber diet.
- Increase physical activity as tolerated.
- Assist in using the toilet facilities at the same time each day (based on usual patterns of bowel elimination), ensuring privacy and having client sit in upright position if at all possible.

- Administer prescribed stool softeners if the client is following a bowel elimination routine or is not drinking sufficient fluids.
  Increased fluids, fiber, and activity stimulate intestinal motility. Establishing a regular daily time for bowel movements in the upright position and in privacy promotes normal bowel elimination. Stool softeners help prevent the formation of hard stool that is more difficult to expel.

Impaired Swallowing

A stroke may impair the ability to swallow. Weakness or lack of coordination of the tongue, attention deficits, and deficits involving the swallowing reflex all play a role. Dysphagia (difficulty swallowing) may result in choking, drooling, aspiration, or regurgitation. Nursing care focuses on maintaining safety by preventing aspiration and on ensuring adequate nutrition.

- Monitor results of swallowing studies prior to providing oral food and fluids.
- Ensure safety when eating.
  - Position in upright sitting position with neck slightly flexed.
  - Order puréed or soft food. Liquids should be of the same consistency as honey.
  - Feed or teach client to eat by putting food behind the front teeth on the unaffected side of mouth and tilting the head slightly backward. Teach to swallow one bite at a time.
    - Assess for coughing with eating or drinking. *Coughing may be indicative of dysphagia.*

> **PRACTICE ALERT**
> After eating, check the mouth for "pocketing" of food, especially in the affected cheek.

- Have suction equipment available at the bedside in case of choking or aspiration.
  Sitting upright with the head and neck first slightly flexed and then tilted back helps the client swallow. The client can usually swallow puréed or soft foods more easily than liquid or solid foods. Using the unaffected side of the mouth helps prevent food from collecting in the mouth and makes swallowing safer; in addition, food is less likely to fall out of the mouth.
  - Monitor lung sounds. *Coarse lung sounds heard in the right upper and/or lower lobes may indicate aspiration as the right bronchus is the first division of the bronchi and where the majority of aspirations occur.*
- Minimize distractions and, if necessary, give step-by-step instructions for eating. *Distractions increase the risk of aspiration. Complex activities are easier to perform when broken down into small steps.*

Using NANDA, NIC, AND NOC

Chart 45–1 shows links between NANDA nursing diagnoses, NIC, and NOC when caring for the client with a stroke.

Community-Based Care

Throughout the rehabilitation process, it is important to encourage self-care as much as possible but also to involve family members in the plan of care. Stress that ADLs may take twice as long as they did before the stroke. Emphasize that physical function may continue to improve for up to 3 months,

NANDA, NIC, AND NOC LINKAGES
CHART 45–1 The Client with a Stroke

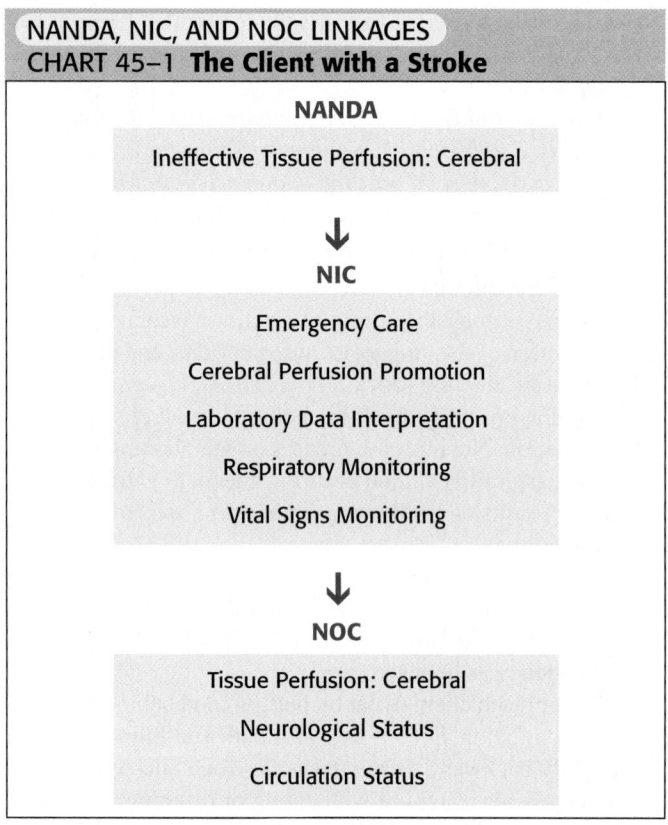

NANDA

Ineffective Tissue Perfusion: Cerebral

↓

NIC

Emergency Care

Cerebral Perfusion Promotion

Laboratory Data Interpretation

Respiratory Monitoring

Vital Signs Monitoring

↓

NOC

Tissue Perfusion: Cerebral

Neurological Status

Circulation Status

Data from *NANDA's Nursing Diagnoses: Definitions & Classification 2005–2006* by NANDA International (2005), Philadelphia; *Nursing Interventions Classification (NIC)* (4th ed.) by J. M. Dochterman & G. M. Bluechek (2004), St. Louis, MO: Mosby; and *Nursing Outcomes Classification (NOC)* (3rd ed.) by S. Moorhead, M. Johnson, and M. Maas (2004), St. Louis, MO: Mosby.

and speech may continue to improve for even longer. Address the following topics in preparing the client and family for community-based care.

- Physical care, medications, physical therapy, occupational therapy, speech therapy
- Realistic expectations
- Time off for the caregiver, respite care services
- Distributors for equipment and supplies
- Home environment conducive to using equipment (e.g., a wheelchair or walker)
- Home and equipment modifications (e.g., a raised toilet seat, grab bars in the bathroom, a bath chair, a vise lid opener, a long-handled shoehorn)
- Home health services
- Community resources, such as Meals-on-Wheels, senior centers, eldercare, large-print telephone dials, stroke clubs, Life-line (emergency alerting systems through a local hospital or agency). Financial assistance may be available within the community for housekeeping and personal care assistance.
- Helpful organizational resources:
  - American Heart Association
  - National Stroke Association
  - Stroke Clubs International
  - The National Institute of Neurological Disorders and Stroke.

THE CLIENT WITH AN INTRACRANIAL ANEURYSM

An *intracranial aneurysm* is a saccular outpouching of a cerebral artery that occurs at the site of a weakness in the vessel wall. The weakness may be the result of atherosclerosis, a congenital defect, trauma to the head, aging, or hypertension. A ruptured cerebral aneurysm is the most common cause of a hemorrhagic stroke.

Incidence and Prevalence

Approximately 5 million North Americans have intracranial aneurysms; most go through life without any manifestations of bleeding. However, it is estimated that 30,000 people will have a rupture of an intracranial aneurysm each year, and two-thirds of the survivors will have serious disabilities. Intracranial aneurysms are most common in adults ages 30 to 60 (Hickey, 2003).

The exact etiology is unknown, but theories of cause include (1) a developmental defect in the vessel wall and (2) degeneration or fragility of the vessel wall due to conditions such as hypertension, atherosclerosis, connective tissue disease, or abnormal blood flow. Hypertension and cigarette smoking may be contributing factors.

Pathophysiology

Intracranial aneurysms tend to occur at the bifurcations and branches of the carotid arteries and the vertebrobasilar arteries at the circle of Willis, with most aneurysms (85%) located anteriorly. They range in size from smaller than 15 mm to larger than 50 mm. Intracranial aneurysms tend to enlarge with time, making the vessel wall thin and increasing the probability of rupture.

There are several different types of intracranial aneurysms: A *berry aneurysm* is probably the result of a congenital abnormality of the tunica media of the artery. The aneurysm usually ruptures without warning. A *saccular aneurysm* is any aneurysm with a saccular outpouching, which distends only a small portion of the vessel wall. This type of aneurysm is often caused by trauma. In a *fusiform aneurysm,* the entire circumference of a blood vessel swells to form an elongated tube. Most aneurysms of this type occur as a result of the changes of arteriosclerosis. Fusiform aneurysms act as space-occupying lesions. In a *dissecting aneurysm,* the tunica intima pulls away from the tunica media of the artery, and blood is forced between the two layers. It may result from atherosclerosis, inflammation, or trauma. *Mycotic aneurysms* are caused by emboli from infections such as bacterial endocarditis.

Intracranial aneurysms typically rupture from the dome rather than the base, forcing blood into the subarachnoid space at the base of the brain. The aneurysm may also rupture and force blood into brain tissue, the ventricles, or the subdural space. This discussion focuses on intracranial hemorrhages due to rupture of a cerebral aneurysm. See Chapter 44 ∞ for further discussion of types of intracranial bleeding and hematomas.

Manifestations

An intracranial aneurysm is usually asymptomatic until it ruptures, although very large aneurysms may cause headache and/or neurologic deficits due to pressure on adjacent intracranial structures. Small leakages of blood may occur periodically, causing headache, nausea, vomiting, and pain in the neck and back. The client may also have prodromal manifestations before the rupture occurs, such as headache, eye pain, visual deficits, and a dilated pupil.

The manifestations of a ruptured intracranial aneurysm (and subsequent subarachnoid hemorrhage) include a sudden, explosive headache; loss of consciousness; nausea and vomiting; a stiff neck and photophobia (due to meningeal irritation); cranial nerve deficits; stroke syndrome manifestations; and pituitary malfunctions (that result primarily from changes in ADH secretion).

The severity of the rupture is often inferred from the manifestations of the subarachnoid hemorrhage. The Hunt-Hess classification of subarachnoid manifestations is frequently used to classify nontraumatic subarachnoid hemorrhages. The grades of severity are:

- Grade 1: Asymptomatic, or minimal headache and slight neck rigidity
- Grade 2: Moderate to severe headache, neck rigidity, cranial nerve deficits
- Grade 3: Drowsy, lethargic, mild neurologic deficits
- Grade 4: Stuporous, moderate to severe hemiparesis, early decerebrate rigidity
- Grade 5: Deep coma, decerebrate rigidity, moribund appearance.

Fibrin and platelets seal off the bleeding point, but the escaped blood forms a clot that irritates the brain tissue. The resulting inflammatory response causes cerebral edema, and both the edema and the hemorrhage increase intracranial pressure (Hickey, 2003). Bleeding into the subarachnoid space causes meningeal irritation. Hypothalamic dysfunction and seizures are also potential complications.

Complications

The major complications of a ruptured intracranial aneurysm are rebleeding, vasospasm, and hydrocephalus.

Rebleeding

The greatest risk for rebleeding is within the first day after the initial rupture, and again in 7 to 10 days (when the initial clot breaks down). Rebleeding is manifested by a sudden severe headache, nausea and vomiting, decreasing levels of consciousness, and new neurologic deficits (Hickey, 2003). The mortality from rebleeding is as high as from the initial rupture.

Vasospasm

Cerebral vasospasm is a common but dangerous complication that occurs between 3 and 10 days after a subarachnoid hemorrhage. It is associated with a large number of deaths and disability. A cerebral vasospasm narrows the lumen of one or more cerebral vessels, causing ischemia and infarction of tissue supplied by the affected vessels. The actual cause is unknown, but it occurs in blood vessels surrounded by thick blood clots, suggesting that some substance in the clot initiates the spasm. The manifestations vary according to the degree of spasm and the area of brain affected. Regional alterations may cause focal

deficits (such as hemiplegia), whereas global alterations cause loss of consciousness.

Hydrocephalus

Hydrocephalus, an abnormal accumulation of CSF within the cranial vault and dilation of the ventricles, is a potential complication of a ruptured intracranial aneurysm. Hydrocephalus is thought to be the result of obstruction of reabsorption of CSF through the arachnoid villi. The obstruction is caused by an increased protein content of the CSF because of lysis of blood in the subarachnoid space (Porth, 2005). The accumulation of cerebrospinal fluid increases intracranial pressure. Initial manifestations of hydrocephalus are typically nonspecific but commonly include decreasing levels of consciousness.

INTERDISCIPLINARY CARE

The care of the client with a ruptured intracranial aneurysm includes determining the location of the aneurysm, treating the manifestations of the hemorrhage, and preventing rebleeding and vasospasm. Interventions using radiology, angiography and a variety of procedures may be used to prevent aneurysm rupture or to stop the bleeding. Surgery is usually the treatment of choice to repair the bleeding artery.

Diagnosis

The diagnostic tests conducted to identify the site and extent of a ruptured intracranial aneurysm, as well as rebleeding, are a CT scan and bilateral carotid and vertebral cerebral angiograms. A cerebral angiogram is the gold standard for evaluating cerebral aneurysm; it can demonstrate the source of the aneurysm in about 80% to 85% of the time (Hickey, 2003). A lumbar puncture will reveal blood-tinged spinal fluid. These tests are described in Chapter 43 ∞.

Medications

Calcium channel blockers, such as nimodipine (Nimotop), are used to improve neurologic deficits due to vasospasm following subarachnoid hemorrhage from ruptured intracranial aneurysms. Administered for 21 consecutive days, it has been found to enhance collateral blood flow and reduce the incidence of ischemic deficits from arterial spasm without side effects (Hickey, 2003; Tierney et al., 2005).

Other medications that may be prescribed include anticonvulsants, such as phenytoin (Dilantin), to prevent seizures if the client has increased intracranial pressure; analgesics for headache; and stool softeners, such as docusate, to prevent constipation and straining with a bowel movement (which increases intracranial pressure and blood pressure and may cause rebleeding).

Procedures Used to Treat Aneurysm

Treatments for an intracranial aneurysm are performed either to prevent rupture or to isolate the vessel to prevent further bleeding. Clients with good neurologic status may have surgery soon after the rupture. In clients with significant neurologic deficits, surgery may be delayed until they are more stable and less at risk for vasospasm; however, the trend is toward surgery as soon as possible.

Several different types of procedures are used to repair a ruptured intracranial aneurysm or to prevent the rupture of an existing large aneurysm. These include:

- The skull is opened (craniotomy), and the aneurysm is located. The neck of the aneurysm may be clipped with a metal clip (preventing the entry of blood into the aneurysm), or the involved artery may be clipped both proximally and distally to the aneurysm to isolate the affected area.
- Endovascular Guglielmi detachable coils (GDCs) are a method used to treat nonruptured aneurysms. One or more small platinum coils are inserted through a microcatheter and threaded through the carotid or femoral artery to the site of the aneurysm, where they are released and fill the body of the aneurysm. The coils initiate the immune response, and the body produces a blood clot inside the aneurysm, strengthening the artery walls and reducing the risk of rupture. After the aneurysm is stabilized, it can be clipped with less risk of hemorrhage and death (NINDS, 2005a). However, endovascular coil procedures are also effective without surgery, especially for smaller aneurysms.
- Stents, which are coil or mesh tubes introduced into the body through a catheter, are used to cover the neck of an aneurysm while coils are deposited within the body of the aneurysm.
- Balloon remodeling is used for large, multiple, or surgically inaccessible aneurysms. A balloon is placed across the neck of the aneurysm and coils are inserted into the body of the aneurysm. The balloon prevents the coils from moving out to the aneurysm.
- Parent vessel occlusion is performed to occlude the parent vessel that supplies blood to the aneurysm. Prior to permanent occlusion, the risk of neurologic impairment is assessed by monitoring motor, sensory, and cognitive functions in an awake client while temporary occlusion is conducted.

NURSING CARE

Nursing care is planned and implemented for the client with a ruptured intracranial aneurysm to prevent rebleeding as well as to meet needs resulting from neurologic deficits.

Nursing Diagnoses and Interventions

Appropriate nursing diagnoses and interventions are described earlier in the chapter in the discussion of nursing care for the client with a stroke. The priority interventions in the acute care stage of a ruptured intracranial aneurysm focus on ineffective cerebral tissue perfusion.

Ineffective Tissue Perfusion: Cerebral

These interventions are for the care of the client immediately after the intracranial aneurysm ruptures. The expected outcome of care is preventing rebleeding and improving cerebral tissue perfusion.

- Institute aneurysm precautions to prevent rebleeding, as follows:
  - Keep the client in a private, quiet, darkened room. Disconnect or remove the telephone. Avoid using bright overhead lights. *A quiet environment helps prevent an increase in blood pressure, which could precipitate rebleeding. The client may experience photophobia (abnormal sensitivity to light) if hemorrhage has damaged the oculomotor nerve.*

- Elevate the head of the bed 30 to 45 degrees; follow prescribed activity orders (usually complete bed rest, but in some cases bathroom privileges may be approved). *Elevating the head of the bed promotes venous return from the brain and thus decreases intracranial pressure. Decreasing activity reduces the likelihood of increases in blood pressure.*
- Limit visitors to two family members at any one time, and limit the duration of visits. Monitor client response to visitors and decrease interactions if the client becomes agitated or upset. *Psychologic stress may increase blood pressure and the risk of rebleeding; however, social isolation may increase anxiety and stress. Each client (and family) must be individually evaluated.*
- Allow reading, watching television, or listening to the radio to promote relaxation. *Although these passive activities were previously contraindicated for the client on aneurysm precautions, current therapy is based on the belief that these activities promote relaxation and help control blood pressure.*
- Prevent constipation and straining to have a bowel movement. Administer stool softeners as prescribed. Collaborate with the client and physician about use of a bedside commode or the bathroom. Do not administer enemas. *The client is at risk for constipation as a result of decreased mobility and the administration of narcotics (such as codeine) for headache. When straining to have a bowel movement, the client uses the Valsalva maneuver, which increases intracranial pressure and may precipitate rebleeding.*

PRACTICE ALERT
Maintaining a daily stool chart is an important assessment in preventing constipation.

- If the client is alert (and depending on physician preferences), allow to feed self and provide own personal care. *In many instances, self-care causes less anxiety and stress than care provided by the nurse. The extent of care provided varies according to client condition and physician preferences.*
- Monitor vital signs and neurologic status as indicated by client condition (frequency of assessments may range from every 15 minutes to every 4 hours). *Vital signs and neurologic assessments provide ongoing data for evaluation of changes indicative of increasing intracranial pressure and decreasing neurologic function. Report any change immediately to the physician.*

PRACTICE ALERT
Restlessness and changes in respirations are often early manifestations of increased intracranial pressure.

- Maintain seizure precautions: Have suction equipment and an oropharyngeal tube at the bedside, maintain the bed in the low position, and keep the side rails padded and raised. *Applying suction and inserting an oropharyngeal airway may be necessary to maintain an open airway in case of seizure. A lowered bed and padded, raised side rails prevent injury if a seizure occurs.*

- Avoid positioning and activities that increase intracranial pressure such as coughing, sneezing, vomiting, sharply flexing the neck, blowing the nose, enemas, or moving self up in bed. *These measures help to prevent increasing intracranial pressure and rebleeding.*

THE CLIENT WITH AN ARTERIOVENOUS MALFORMATION

An arteriovenous (AV) malformation is a congenital intracranial lesion, formed by a tangled collection of dilated arteries and veins that allows blood to flow directly from the arterial into the venous system, bypassing the normal capillary network. Most AV malformations (90%) are located in the cerebral hemispheres; the remainder are found in the cerebellum and brainstem.

Rupture of vessels in the malformations account for 2% of all strokes. Clients with this condition develop manifestations before 40 years of age; it affects men and women equally (Porth, 2005). The manifestations are the result of spontaneous bleeding from the lesion into the subarachnoid space or brain tissue.

Pathophysiology

AV malformations displace rather than encompass normal brain tissue (Hickey, 2003). The pathophysiologic effects of an AV malformation are the result of the shunting of blood from the arterial to the venous system and of altered perfusion of cerebral tissue near the malformation. The shunting of arterial blood directly into the venous system within the malformation transfers the higher arterial pressure directly into the lower pressure venous system. This increased pressure is likely to cause spontaneous bleeding or progressive expansion and rupture of a blood vessel.

Altered cerebral perfusion results when blood flow through a large, high-flow malformation is diverted from the normal cerebral circulation, causing tissue ischemia of the area surrounding the malformation. This is sometimes called a vascular "steal" phenomenon.

AV malformations range in size from very small to very large. Large malformations are usually initially manifested by seizure activity. In contrast, the manifestations of a small malformation are more often due to a hemorrhage that causes neurologic deficits. In both instances, the client may have recurrent headaches that do not respond to treatment.

INTERDISCIPLINARY CARE

AV malformations are diagnosed with the same diagnostic tests used to diagnose an intracranial aneurysm.

If the malformation is accessible, the ideal treatment is excision of the malformation and removal of any hematoma. Large malformations may be treated by embolization. In this procedure, substances such as Gelfoam or metallic pellets are introduced into the involved area of the cerebral circulation, where they form emboli and gradually obstruct blood flow in the malformation. Inaccessible malformations are also treated with radiation therapy or laser therapy, to coagulate blood in the malformation and thicken its vascular elements, eventually obstructing it. When the malformation is excised or obstructed, blood flow is no longer shunted, and cerebral perfusion improves.

NURSING CARE

Nursing care depends on the condition of the malformation. If hemorrhage has not occurred, teach the client to avoid activities that raise blood pressure or could cause injury. The client is usually given medications to control blood pressure and prevent seizures.

If the malformation ruptures and causes an intracranial hemorrhage, nursing care is the same as for any client who has had a hemorrhagic stroke (discussed earlier in this chapter).

SPINAL CORD DISORDERS

THE CLIENT WITH A SPINAL CORD INJURY

Nursing care of clients with a spinal cord injury takes place from the acute management phase through ongoing rehabilitation in a variety of settings. Although priorities of care may change depending on the client and setting, care focuses on maximizing functional health status to preserve quality of life. The nurse provides care and also collaborates with other healthcare professionals in meeting this goal.

Incidence and Prevalence

A **spinal cord injury (SCI)** is usually due to trauma. The major causes of SCI are contusion, laceration, transection, hemorrhage, and damage to blood vessels that supply the spinal cord. If vertebrae are fractured and ligaments are torn, bony fragments can damage the cord and make the spinal column unstable. Injury to blood vessels supplying the cord can cause permanent damage. The injury is identified by vertebral level. For example, a C6 spinal cord injury is at the sixth cervical vertebra.

FAST FACTS
SCI

- Approximately 11,000 people have a SCI each year.
- An estimated 25,000 to 96,000 people are living with SCIs in the United States.
- Although SCIs occur in people of all ages, they are most often seen in young adults ages 16 to 30.
- The majority of the injuries are due to motor vehicle crashes; other causes include acts of violence, falls and sports injuries.

Source: National Spinal Cord Injury Association [NSCIA], 2006.

Risk Factors

The three major risk factors for SCIs are age, gender, and alcohol or drug abuse. Young men are more prone to risk-taking behaviors than are women. Older adults are more likely to have a cord injury from even minor trauma as a result of age-related vertebral degeneration. Motor vehicle crashes while under the influence of alcohol or drugs are a major source of trauma to people of all ages.

MediaLink Case Study: Spinal Cord Injury

Pathophysiology

The spinal cord provides a two-way pathway for the conduction of impulses and information to and from the brain and the body, serves as a major reflex center, and (through its attached spinal nerves) is involved in the sensory and motor innervation of the entire body below the head. It consists of an outer region of white matter and an inner region of gray matter. The gray matter comprises the central canal of the cord, the posterior horns, the anterior horns, and the lateral horns. It is divided into a sensory half (dorsally) and a motor half (ventrally) and innervates somatic and visceral regions of the body. The white matter consists of tracts or pathways that convey information. The ascending (sensory) pathways carry information about proprioception, fine touch, discrimination, pain, temperature, deep pressure, and touch. The descending (motor) pathways carry information about movement. The pyramidal tracts control skilled voluntary movements (such as writing). The extrapyramidal tracts (all tracts other than the pyramidal tracts) bring about all other body movements. See Chapter 43 ∞ for further information.

When the spinal cord is injured, the primary injury causes microscopic hemorrhages in the gray matter of the cord and edema of the white matter of the cord. These initial pathologic changes are followed by the secondary injury, with mechanisms that increase the area of injury. The hemorrhages extend, eventually involving the entire gray matter. Microcirculation to the cord is impaired by edema and hemorrhage. The injured tissue releases norepinephrine, serotonin, dopamine, and histamine; these vasoactive substances cause vasospasm and further decrease microcirculation. As a result, vascular perfusion and oxygen tension of the affected area are decreased, which leads to ischemia.

When ischemia is prolonged, necrosis of both gray and white matter begins within a few hours, and within 24 hours the function of nerves passing through the injured area is lost. Although circulation returns to the white matter of the cord in about 24 hours, decreased circulation in the gray matter continues. Because edema extends the level of injury for two cord segments above and below the affected level, the extent of injury cannot be determined for up to 1 week.

Tissue repair occurs over a period of 3 to 4 weeks. Phagocytes enter the area in 36 to 48 hours after the initial injury. Neurons degenerate and are removed by microphages in the first 10 days after the injury. RBC disintegrate, and the hemorrhages are reabsorbed. Eventually the area of injury is replaced by acellular collagenous tissue, and the meninges thicken.

Forces Resulting in SCI

SCIs are the result of the application of excessive force to the spinal column. The most common cause of abnormal spinal column movements are acceleration and deceleration (forces that are applied to the body, for example, in automobile crashes and falls). *Acceleration* occurs when external force is applied in a rear-end collision; the upper torso and head are forced backward and then forward. *Deceleration* occurs in a head-on collision; the external force is applied from the front. The head and body move forward until they meet a stationary object and then are forced backward. The following forces and movements (Figure 45–5 ■) may cause a variety of spinal cord in-

juries, with the extent of injury depending on the amount and direction of motion, and the rate of application of force:

■ *Hyperflexion,* or forcible forward bending, may compress vertebral bodies and disrupt ligaments and intervertebral disks.

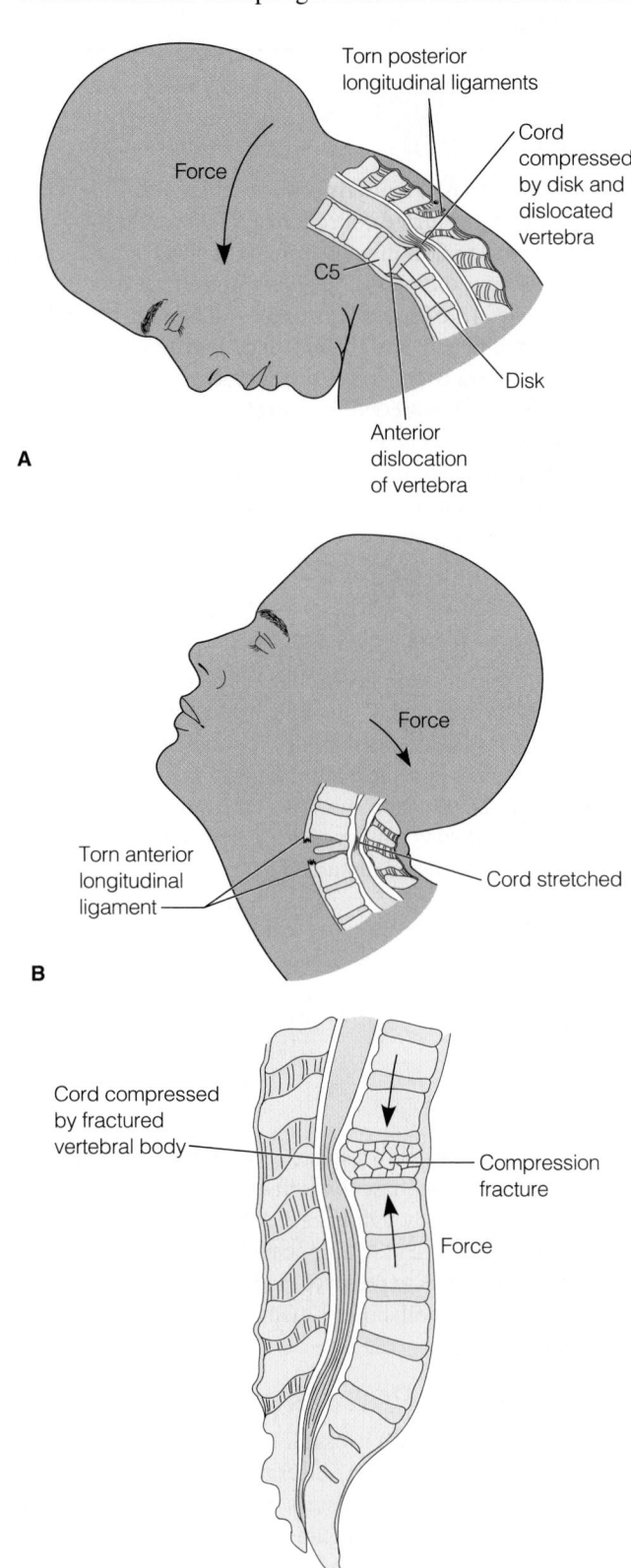

Figure 45–5 ■ Spinal cord injury mechanisms. *A,* Hyperflexion. *B,* Hyperextension. *C,* Axial loading, a form of compression.

- *Hyperextension,* or forcible backward bending, often disrupts ligaments and causes vertebral fractures. A whiplash injury is a less severe form of hyperextension, with injury to soft tissues but no vertebral or spinal cord damage.
- *Axial loading,* a form of compression, is the application of vertical force to the spinal column (for instance, by falling and landing on the feet or buttocks or by diving into shallow water).
- *Excessive rotation,* in which the head is excessively turned, may tear ligaments, fracture articular surfaces, and cause compression fractures.

The alteration of the spinal cord and soft tissues caused by these abnormal movements is called **deformation.** The spinal cord may be penetrated by bullets and other foreign objects (e.g., sharp objects used as weapons, shrapnel from explosions). Penetrating injuries may cause vertebral fractures, tear ligaments and muscles, or cut through a part or all of the spinal cord. Complete severing of the cord is rare.

Sites of Pathology

Injuries occur most often in the lumbar and cervical regions. The most frequent sites of injury of the cord are at the first, second, and fourth to sixth cervical vertebrae (C1, C2, C4 to C6); and the eleventh thoracic to second lumbar vertebrae (T11 to L2). Because the cervical spine has a wider range of movement than the rest of the spine, the cervical portion is more likely to be affected by externally applied forces. In addition, the cord fills most of the vertebral canal in the cervical and lumbar regions and thus is more easily injured. Damage to the vertebrae and ligaments causes the spinal column to become unstable, increasing the possibility of compression or stretching of the spinal cord with any further movement.

Classification of SCI

SCIs are classified according to systems, for instance (1) as complete or incomplete cord injury, (2) by cause of injury, and (3) by level of injury. In clinical practice, these classifications often overlap. In a *complete SCI* (about 45% of all injuries), the motor and sensory neural pathways are completely interrupted (transected), resulting in total loss of motor and sensory function below the level of the injury. However, "complete" does not necessarily mean the spinal cord has been severed. In an *incomplete SCI* (about 55% of all injuries), the motor and sensory pathways are only partially interrupted, with variable loss of function below the level of injury. Incomplete spinal cord injuries are further classified into syndromes as outlined in Table 45–2. Both complete and incomplete injuries can occur in paraplegia and quadriplegia (NSCIA, 2006). The alterations in function that occur as the result of a spinal cord injury vary greatly depending on the amount of tissue damage and the level of injury.

Manifestations

The spinal cord, the vertebrae, the intervertebral disks, the spinal nerves, the ligaments, and the surrounding soft tissue structures are in such close anatomic proximity that any condition or injury affecting one structure may well affect any one or all of the other structures. The conditions with the most critical effects are disorders affecting the spinal cord. Disorders and injuries of the spinal cord have the potential to affect movement, perception, sensation, sexual function, and elimination. Manifestations and complications of SCI by body system are listed in the box on the next page.

TABLE 45–2 Incomplete Spinal Cord Injury Syndromes

TYPE	CAUSE	LOCATION	DEFICITS
Central syndrome	Cord transection Hyperextension	Cervical	Spastic paralysis of the upper extremities Variable paralysis of the lower extremities Variable effects on the bowel, the bladder, and sexual function
Anterior syndrome	Damage to the anterior spinal artery Infarction of the anterior spinal artery Hyperflexion	Anterior two-thirds of the cord	Paralysis below the level of injury Loss of temperature and pain sensation below the level of injury
Posterior syndrome	Vertebral dislocation Herniated disk Compression	Nerve roots	Weakness in isolated muscle groups Tingling, pain Decreased or absent reflexes in the involved area Bowel or bladder dysfunction
Brown-Séquard syndrome	Penetrating trauma	Hemisection of the anterior and posterior cord	Paralysis below the level of injury on the ipsilateral (same) side of the body Contralateral loss of temperature and pain sensation below the level of injury Ipsilateral loss of proprioception below the level of injury
Homer's syndrome	Incomplete cord transection	Cervical sympathetic nerves	Ipsilateral ptosis of the eyelid, constricted pupil, and facial anhidrosis (inability to perspire)

MANIFESTATIONS and Complications of Spinal Cord Injury by Body System

INTEGUMENT
- Decubitus (pressure) ulcers

NEUROLOGIC
- Pain
- Areflexia
- Hypotonia
- Autonomic dysreflexia

CARDIOVASCULAR
- Spinal shock
- Paroxysmal hypertension
- Orthostatic hypotension
- Cardiac dysrhythmias
- Decreased venous return
- Hypercalcemia

RESPIRATORY
- Limited chest expansion
- Decreased cough reflex
- Decreased vital capacity

GASTROINTESTINAL
- Stress ulcers
- Paralytic ileus
- Stool impaction
- Stool incontinence

GENITOURINARY
- Urinary retention
- Urinary incontinence
- Neurogenic bladder
- Impotence
- Testicular atrophy
- Inability to ejaculate
- Decreased vaginal lubrication

MUSCULOSKELETAL
- Joint contractures
- Bone demineralization
- Osteoporosis
- Muscle spasms
- Muscle atrophy
- Pathologic fractures
- Paraplegia
- Quadriplegia

Spinal shock is the temporary loss of reflex function (called *areflexia*) below the level of injury. This response begins immediately after complete transection of the spinal cord, when connections between the brain and the spinal cord are interrupted and the cord does not function at all. The response also occurs (although in varying degrees) after partial transection as well as after spinal cord contusions, compression, and ischemia.

Normal activity of the spinal cord is dependent on constant impulses from the higher centers of the brain. When damage from an injury stops these impulses, spinal shock follows. There is loss of motor function, tendon reflexes, and autonomic function. Spinal shock may begin within 1 hour of the injury. The condition may last from a few minutes to several months (although it usually lasts from 1 to 6 weeks), and then reflex activity returns. Spinal shock ends slowly, with the gradual reappearance of reflexes, hyperreflexia (increased reflex responses), muscle spasticity, and reflex bladder emptying.

The manifestations of acute spinal shock (which vary in degree) include the following:
- Flaccid paralysis of skeletal muscles below the level of injury
- Loss of all spinal reflexes below the level of injury
- Loss of sensations of pain, touch, temperature, and pressure below the level of injury
- Absence of visceral and somatic sensations below the level of injury
- Bowel and bladder dysfunction
- Loss of the ability to perspire below the level of injury.

A person with a cervical or upper thoracic SCI may also have neurogenic shock, resulting in cardiovascular changes. These changes are due to the inability of higher centers in the brainstem to modulate reflexes. As a result, vascular beds below the level of injury dilate, and the cardiac accelerator reflex is suppressed. The client experiences hypotension and bradycardia. Other manifestations may include respiratory insufficiency due to loss of innervation of the diaphragm in C1 to C4 injuries, hypothermia, paralytic ileus, urinary retention, and oliguria.

Both bradycardia and hypotension may persist even after the spinal shock resolves. In addition to losing sympathetic control of the heart rate, the client with a high-level SCI experiences decreased peripheral resistance and loss of muscle activity. These changes result in sluggish blood flow and decreased venous return, increasing the risk for thrombophlebitis.

Complications

The complications of an SCI involve many different body systems and result often in permanent disability and loss of functional health status. The complications include but are not limited to upper and lower motor neuron deficits, paraplegia and quadriplegia, and autonomic dysreflexia. Other complications, depending on the level and severity of the injury, are ineffective respirations; altered skin integrity; increased risk of thrombosis; and alterations in bowel elimination, urinary elimination, and sexual pattern.

Upper and Lower Motor Neuron Deficits

Injuries to the spinal cord are often classified as either *upper motor neuron lesions* or *lower motor neuron lesions*. Motor neurons are functional units that carry motor impulses. The upper motor neurons (located in the cerebral cortex, thalamus, brainstem, and corticospinal and corticobulbar tracts) are responsible for voluntary movement. When these motor pathways are interrupted, the client experiences spastic paralysis and hyperreflexia and may be unable to carry out skilled movement.

Lower motor neurons (located in the anterior horn of the spinal cord, the motor nuclei of the brainstem, and the axons that reach the motor end plate of skeletal muscles) are responsible for innervation and contraction of skeletal muscles. Interruption of lower motor neurons results in muscle flaccidity and extensive muscle atrophy, with loss of both voluntary and involuntary movement. If only some of the motor neurons supplying a muscle are affected, the client experiences partial paralysis (paresis); if all motor neurons to a muscle are affected, the client experiences complete paralysis. Hyporeflexia is also present.

Paraplegia and Quadriplegia

Two common neurologic deficits resulting from an SCI are paraplegia and quadriplegia (see Figure 45–2). **Paraplegia** is paralysis of the lower portion of the body, sometimes involving the lower trunk. Paraplegia occurs when the thoracic, lumbar, and sacral portions of the spinal cord are injured, causing loss or impairment of sensory and/or motor function. **Quadriplegia**, also called *tetraplegia,* occurs when cervical segments of the cord are injured, impairing function of the arms, trunk, legs, and pelvic organs.

Autonomic Dysreflexia

Autonomic dysreflexia (also called *autonomic hyperreflexia*) is an exaggerated sympathetic response that occurs in clients with SCIs at or above the T6 level. This response, which is seen only after recovery from spinal shock, occurs as a result of a lack of control of the autonomic nervous system by higher centers. When stimuli are unable to ascend the cord, mass reflex stimulation of the sympathetic nerves below the level of the injured cord area occurs, triggering massive vasoconstriction. In response, the vagus nerve causes bradycardia and vasodilation above the level of injury. If untreated, autonomic dysreflexia can cause seizures, a stroke, or a myocardial infarction and is potentially fatal (Hickey, 2003).

Autonomic dysreflexia is triggered by stimuli that would normally cause abdominal discomfort (a full bladder is the most common cause), by stimulation of pain receptors, and by visceral contractions (Porth, 2005). Causes include fecal impaction, bladder infections or stones, intrauterine contractions, ejaculation, peritonitis, and stimulation from pressure ulcers or ingrown toenails. The most common precipitating event is a blocked urinary catheter.

The manifestations of this condition include pounding headache; bradycardia; hypertension (with readings as high as 300/160); flushed, warm skin with profuse sweating above the lesion and pale, cold, and dry skin below it; and anxiety (Porth, 2005). Dysreflexia is a neurologic emergency and requires immediate treatment.

INTERDISCIPLINARY CARE

The client with an acute SCI requires emergency assessment and care and medications; sometimes the client also requires immo-

bilization and surgery. The client is first assessed and stabilized at the scene of the accident, initially treated in the emergency room, and then admitted to the hospital intensive care unit.

Emergency Care

The danger of death from SCI is greatest when there is damage to or transection of the upper cervical region. When the injury is at the C1 to C4 level, respiratory paralysis is common, and the client who survives requires ventilator assistance to breathe. Injuries below C4 may increase the risk of respiratory failure if edema ascends the cord. It is of critical importance not to complicate the initial injury by allowing the fractured vertebrae to damage the cord further during transport to the hospital. Although at one time injuries to the high cervical cord were almost always fatal, advances in trauma care have greatly improved the survival rate.

All people who have sustained trauma to the head or spine, or who are unconscious, should be treated as though they have a spinal cord injury. Prehospital management includes rapid assessment of the ABCs (airway, breathing, circulation), immobilizing and stabilizing the head and neck, removing the person from the site of injury, stabilizing other life-threatening injuries, and rapidly transporting the person to the appropriate facility. Guidelines for emergency care are as follows:

- Avoid flexing, extending, or rotating the neck.
- Immobilize the neck, using rolled towels or blankets, or apply a cervical collar before moving the client onto a backboard.
- Secure the head by placing a belt or tape across the forehead and securing it to the stretcher.
- Maintain the client in the supine position.
- Transfer directly from the stretcher with backboard still in place to the type of bed that will be used in the hospital.

Assessment findings at the scene of the accident or in the emergency room vary according to the level of injury. The assessment findings common to the level of injury and spinal shock are outlined in Box 45–1.

The client in the emergency department with a suspected or identified SCI is also treated for respiratory problems, paralytic ileus, atonic bladder, and cardiovascular alterations. Respiratory distress in the client with a cervical-level injury is treated by placing the client on a ventilator. Oxygen is administered to the client with a thoracic-level injury. Paralytic ileus (obstruction of the intestines due to lack of peristalsis) is common in clients with a spinal cord injury and is treated by the insertion of a nasogastric tube with connection to suction. To prevent overdistention of an atonic bladder, an indwelling catheter is inserted and connected to dependent drainage. Cardiovascular status is assessed on a continuous basis by inserting invasive monitoring devices, such as a Swan-Ganz catheter, and attaching the client to a cardiac monitor; or by arterial monitoring to identify hypotension and to draw arterial blood gases (ABGs).

High-dose steroid protocol using methylprednisolone (Medrol) must be implemented within 8 hours of the injury to improve neurologic recovery. Clinical research indicates that the use of this adrenocorticosteroid is effective in preventing secondary spinal cord damage from edema and ischemia. Treatment with G_{MI} ganglioside for 3 to 4 weeks is an experimental approach that has been effective for some clients (Tierney et al., 2005).

BOX 45–1 Assessment Findings in Acute SCI

Cervical Injury

- Paralysis or weakness of extremities
- Respiratory distress manifested by changes in ABG studies, cyanosis, flaring of the nostrils, use of accessory muscles of respiration, and restlessness
- Pulse rate below 60 and systolic BP below 80
- Decreased peristalsis

Thoracic and Lumbar Injury

- Paralysis or weakness of extremities

Spinal Shock

- Loss of skin sensation
- Flaccid paralysis, areflexia
- Absent bowel sounds
- Bladder distention
- Decreasing blood pressure
- Absence of the cremasteric reflex in males (retraction of the left or right testicle in response to stimulation of the skin of, respectively, the inner left or right thigh)

Diagnosis

Diagnostic tests are ordered to identify the level and extent of injury, and to detect any complications. The tests include x-ray of the spine, CT or MRI of the spine, and somatosensory evoked potential studies to locate the level of spinal cord injury by stimulating peripheral nerves and measuring response times. ABG are measured to establish a baseline or to identify problems due to respiratory insufficiency.

Medications

The pharmacologic treatment of the client with SCI is symptomatic. It is directed primarily toward decreasing edema from the injury, treating hypotension and bradycardia, and treating spasticity.

- Corticosteroids, discussed earlier in this section, may be used to decrease or control edema of the cord.

- Vasopressors are used in the immediate acute care phase to treat bradycardia or hypotension due to spinal and neurogenic shock. Examples of drugs are dopamine (Intropin) to treat hypotension in neurogenic shock and dobutamine (Dobutrex) to support cardiac function. Atropine should be available at the bedside to treat bradycardia.
- Antispasmodics are used to treat spasticity in clients with spinal cord injury. Both baclofen (Lioresal) and diazepam (Valium) may be used. A discussion of nursing implications of treatment with antispasmodics is found in the Medication Administration box below.
- Analgesics such as nonsteroidal anti-inflammatory drugs (NSAIDs) and narcotics are administered to reduce pain.
- Proton pump inhibitors, such as omeprazole (Prilosec), rabeprazole (Aciphex), or pantoprazole (Protonix), are often administered to prevent stress-related gastric ulcers, a common complication in SCI.
- Unless contraindicated, anticoagulants (heparin or warfarin) may be given to prevent thrombophlebitis.
- Stool softeners may be administered as part of a bowel training program.

Treatments

The treatments used in the management of an SCI include surgery, stabilization, and immobilization.

SURGERY Early surgical treatment may be necessary if there is evidence of compression of the spinal cord by bone fragments or a hematoma. Surgery may also be done to stabilize and support the spine. However, many clients are treated with stabilization devices and do not require surgery. Surgeries that may be performed include a decompression laminectomy, a spinal fusion, and insertion of metal rods. Surgeries of the spine are discussed later in the chapter.

STABILIZATION AND IMMOBILIZATION As a result of one or more dislocations or fractures of the cervical vertebrae, the client with an SCI may be immobilized in some type of traction or external fixation device to stabilize the vertebral column and

MEDICATION ADMINISTRATION Antispasmodics in Spinal Cord Injury

Baclofen (Lioresal)
Chlorzoxazone (Paraflex)
Cyclobenzaprine hydrochloride (Flexeril)
Diazepam (Valium)
Orphenadrine citrate (Norflex)

These drugs depress the central nervous system and inhibit the transmission of impulses from the spinal cord to skeletal muscle. They are used to control muscle spasm and pain associated with acute or chronic musculoskeletal conditions. They are not always effective in controlling spasticity resulting from cerebral or spinal cord conditions.

NURSING RESPONSIBILITIES

- Assess the client's spasticity and involuntary movements to obtain baseline data for comparison of results of therapy.

- Do not expect therapy to have effects for 1 week.
- Administer oral medications with food to decrease gastrointestinal symptoms.

HEALTH EDUCATION FOR THE CLIENT AND FAMILY

- These drugs may cause drowsiness, diplopia, and impotence.
- Take your medications with meals to decrease gastric irritation.
- Physical improvement may take several weeks.
- Report slurred speech, drooling, or inability to carry out usual functions to the physician.
- Do not stop taking the medication without consulting your healthcare provider.

prevent any further damage (Figure 45–6 ■). Traction may also be used to stabilize the spinal column for clients who are not yet in a condition to have surgery or who have severe bleeding and edema of the injured cord. The physician applies the traction or fixation device; the nurse is responsible for assessments and interventions following the application.

Although used less frequently today, various devices provide cervical traction. For example, Gardner-Wells tongs may be used (Figure 45–7 ■). In this type of traction, the physician applies pins to the skull, approximately 1 cm above each ear, and weights are attached to the device.

The halo external fixation device is often used to provide stabilization if there is no significant involvement of the ligaments (Figure 45–8 ■). It is most often used to provide stability for fractures of the cervical and high thoracic vertebrae without cord damage. This device allows greater mobility, self-care, and participation in rehabilitation programs. The device is

Figure 45–7 ■ Cervical traction may be applied by several methods, including Gardner-Wells tongs.

Figure 45–8 ■ The halo external fixation device.

secured with four pins inserted into the skull, two in the frontal bone and two in the occipital bone. The halo ring is then attached to a rigid plastic vest lined with sheepskin. Nursing interventions for the client using a halo fixation device are described in the box on the next page.

NURSING CARE

Both during the acute phase and the rehabilitative phase, the client with a SCI has complex needs that involve all members of the healthcare team. Because these injuries are more common in younger clients, consideration of lifelong effects on both the client and the family is essential. The nurse coordinates client care and develops and implements a care plan that is individualized to each client and family. The focus of the plan is to prevent the secondary complications of immobility and altered body functions, to promote self-care, and to educate the client and family. A Nursing Care Plan for a client with a SCI is found on page 1603.

Figure 45–6 ■ Examples of traction or external fixation devices.

NURSING CARE OF THE CLIENT IN
Halo Fixation

- Maintain integrity of the halo external fixation device.
  a. Inspect pins and traction bars for tightness; report loosened pins to physician.
  b. Tape the appropriate wrench to the head of the bed for emergency intervention.
  c. Never use the halo ring to lift or reposition the client. *Loosening of the apparatus poses the risk of further damage to the cord. It is the responsibility of the nurse to maintain the integrity of the apparatus and the safety of the client.*
- Assess muscle function and skin sensation every 2 hours in the acute phase and every 4 hours thereafter.
  a. Assess motor function on a scale of 0 to 5, with 0 being no evidence of muscle contraction and 5 being normal muscle strength with full range of motion.
  b. Assess sensation by comparing touch and pain, moving from impaired to normal areas, and testing both the right and left sides of the body.
  Monitoring muscle function and skin sensation allows early identification of potential neurologic deficits.
- Monitor pin sites each shift and follow hospital policy for pin care. Here are some general guidelines.
  a. Assess pin sites for redness, edema, and drainage.
  b. Depending on policy, clean each pin site with a sterile applicator dipped in hydrogen peroxide, apply a topical antibiotic and cover with sterile 2-inch split gauze squares.
  Organisms can enter the body through the pin-insertion site; assessments and care are provided to detect signs of and prevent infection.
- Maintain skin integrity.
  a. Turn the immobile client every 2 hours.
  b. Inspect the skin around edges of the vest every 4 hours.
  c. Change the sheepskin liner when it is soiled and at least once each week.
  These interventions prevent skin injury and irritation.

Health Promotion

Health promotion for SCI primarily involves preventing injuries. Nurses can provide valuable information in the community and in the workplace to prevent SCI. Programs that focus on wearing seat belts and using approved infant seats and child booster chairs in automobiles can do much to help decrease the number of SCIs each year. Educational programs that promote workplace safety and farm safety should include information to prevent falls and how to use heavy equipment safely.

Assessment

The following data are collected through the health history and physical examination (see Chapter 43 ∞). Further focused assessments are described with nursing interventions in the next section.

- *Health history:* Time, location, and type of event-causing injury; location, duration, quality, and intensity of pain; dyspnea; sensation; paresthesia.
- *Physical examination:* Vital signs, motor strength, movement, spinal reflexes, bowel sounds, bladder distention.

Nursing Diagnoses and Interventions

Because an SCI has many possible effects, many nursing diagnoses may be appropriate. Nursing diagnoses discussed in this section focus on problems with physical mobility, respirations, dysreflexia, bowel and bladder elimination, sexual dysfunction, and self-esteem.

Impaired Physical Mobility

After the initial period of spinal shock and areflexia, the client regains spinal reflex activity and muscle tone that is not under the control of higher centers. Clients with injuries above the level of T12 experience involuntary spastic movements of skeletal muscles. These movements reach a peak about 2 years after the injury and then gradually subside (Porth, 2005). Spasms impair the ability to carry out the activities of daily life and work. In addition, the paraplegia or quadriplegia increases the potential for impaired skin integrity, thrombophlebitis, and contractures.

The goals of care for clients with impaired mobility related to a spinal cord injury are to reduce the effects of spasticity and to prevent complications involving the skin, the cardiovascular system, and joint function.

- Perform passive ROM exercises for all extremities at least twice a day. Identify stimuli that cause spastic movements and either avoid the stimuli (such as certain exercises) or teach the client to expect the movements. *ROM exercises help prevent contractures and stretch spastic muscles, promoting rehabilitation.*
- Maintain skin integrity by turning every 2 hours, assessing pressure points at least once each shift, and using a special bed if necessary. The client may be placed on a regular or special bed, such as a kinetic bed. *Immobility compresses soft tissues and promotes the development of decubitus ulcers. The lack of sensory warning mechanisms and of voluntary motor control of skin dermatomes further increases the risk for altered skin integrity. Special beds allow movement or turning while keeping the spinal column in alignment.*
- Assess the lower extremities each shift for manifestations of thrombophlebitis. Observe for redness and for increased heat every shift; measure thigh and calf circumference daily. If antiembolic stockings (TEDs) are ordered, remove for 30 to 60 minutes each shift. Assess for skin impairment and provide skin care while TEDs are removed. *Clients with neurologic deficits are at high risk for deep venous thrombosis as a result of immobility, vasomotor dysfunction, and decreased venous return with venous stasis. Antiembolic stockings help to prevent the pooling of blood in the lower extremities and increase venous return, lessening the risk for venous stasis and thrombus formation.*

NURSING CARE PLAN   A Client with an SCI

Jim Valdez, a 19-year-old college sophomore, is admitted to the hospital by ambulance following an automobile crash. His family (father, mother, and sister) live 100 miles away and cannot visit often, although they are very concerned. On admission to the hospital, a CT scan of the spine shows a fracture and partial laceration of the cord at the C7 level. Mr. Valdez is in halo traction. One night, he tells the nurse, "I wish I had just died when I got hurt. I don't think I can stand to live like this."

ASSESSMENT

When Mr. Valdez is admitted to the intensive care unit, he has flaccid paralysis involving all extremities. He has no sensation below the clavicle or in portions of his arms and legs. His bladder is distended and bowel sounds are absent. Other assessment findings include BP 90/56, P 50, T 97°F (36.1°C), arterial blood gases pH 7.4, PaO_2 96, $PaCO_2$ 37, SaO_2 96%. Oxygen per nasal cannula is given at 2 L/min, and halo traction is applied. A Foley catheter is inserted into his bladder, and a nasogastric tube is inserted and attached to low-pressure continuous suction.

After 7 days, Mr. Valdez is moved from the intensive care unit to the neurosurgical unit for continuing care and planning for transfer to a rehabilitation hospital in his home town. His vital signs have stabilized and are normal for his age; respirations and oxygenation are normal. Other neurologic assessments remain the same.

DIAGNOSES

- *Impaired Physical Mobility* related to paralysis of lower and upper extremities
- *Bowel Incontinence* related to lack of voluntary sphincter control
- *Dysfunctional Grieving* related to denial of loss.

EXPECTED OUTCOMES

- Be actively involved in exercise programs.
- Have a soft, formed stool every second or third day.
- Verbally express his grief to parents and staff.

PLANNING AND IMPLEMENTATION

- Conduct passive exercises on all extremities four times a day.
- Provide progressive mobilization by initially raising the head of the bed 90 degrees (repeat two to three times during the first

day of movement); if blood pressure remains normal, dangle for 5 minutes before transferring him to a chair.
- His usual time for a bowel movement is after breakfast; schedule retraining program for that time.
- Encourage a diet high in fiber and fluids. Likes whole-wheat bread, orange juice, and cola; does not like water.
- Promote grief work by providing time to express feelings. Explain to the family that his denial and anger are part of the grieving process.
- Determine food likes and dislikes and order preferred foods from the menu. Encourage his friends to bring in his favorite foods periodically.
- Take and record weight every third day, using the bed scales.

EVALUATION

By the time Mr. Valdez is transferred to the rehabilitation hospital he is looking forward to learning how to use special equipment and getting his own motorized wheelchair. He is able to sit up in a chair without dizziness or hypotension. The use of ordered stool softeners combined with a high-fiber diet and fluid intake of 2000 to 3000 mL per day has maintained bowel elimination. Mr. Valdez and his parents have spent 3 hours talking about their feelings related to the accident and the future. Although the discussion is emotionally difficult, all three say they now feel much better. Mr. Valdez still has episodes of angry outbursts and tears, but he is more optimistic about what can be done and believes he can finish college. He selects foods from the menu each day and eats most of his meals, but he especially enjoys the times his friends bring in pizza or hamburgers.

CRITICAL THINKING IN THE NURSING PROCESS

1. Considering Mr. Valdez's age and developmental level, do you think his emotional responses to his injury were appropriate?
2. Issues of sexuality are obviously important for the client with a spinal cord injury. How would you approach Mr. Valdez about this topic?
3. What would be your response as a male or female nurse if Mr. Valdez would allow only male nurses to provide care?
4. Outline a teaching program to help Mr. Valdez meet long-term urinary elimination needs.

See Evaluating Your Response in Appendix C.

PRACTICE ALERT
Removing TED stockings each shift not only promotes healthy skin but also lets the nurse assess skin integrity.

Impaired Gas Exchange

Injuries at the level of T1 to T7 leave the phrenic nerve intact, but the innervation of intercostal muscles is affected, compromising respiratory function. In addition, because the abdominal muscles are paralyzed, the client cannot expel secretions by coughing. Clients with cord injuries at C3 or above have paralysis of the respiratory muscles and cannot breathe without a ventilator.

- Monitor vital capacity and respiratory effectiveness, assessing for tachycardia, restlessness, PaO_2 less than 60 mmHg, $PaCO_2$ greater than 50 mmHg, and vital capacity less than 1 L. *Clients with cervical cord injuries frequently require ventilatory support because of reduced vital capacity and inability to expel secretions by coughing.*

PRACTICE ALERT
Changes in ABGs and vital capacity signal respiratory insufficiency.

- Monitor for signs of ascending edema of the spinal cord, including difficulty in swallowing or coughing, respiratory stridor, use of accessory muscles of respiration, bradycardia, and increased motor and sensory loss. *Hemorrhage and edema can further impair respiratory function.*

- Help the client to cough, as follows: Place the hand between the umbilicus and xiphoid process and push in and up as the client exhales and coughs. *The client who is unable to cough effectively and has decreased ventilatory capacity may develop atelectasis, pneumonia, and respiratory failure.*

Ineffective Breathing Patterns

Respiratory function is impaired in the client with SCI in the cervical and thoracic levels if the diaphragm (innervated at C3 to C5), the intercostal muscles (innervated at T1 to T7), and the abdominal muscles are affected. In clients with injury at higher levels, assisted ventilation and a tracheostomy are necessary; when the injury is at lower levels, the client's ability to take a deep breath and cough is diminished. The goal of nursing interventions is to maintain normal respiratory rate (12 to 20 breaths per minute) and to prevent pulmonary complications such as atelectasis and pneumonia.

- Assess respiratory rate, rhythm, and depth every 4 hours (or more frequently if needed). Auscultate breath sounds as a part of respiratory assessment. *Injury to the cord in the cervical or thoracic regions can decrease respiratory function and increase the risk for respiratory problems.*

> **PRACTICE ALERT**
> Auscultate the lungs for crackles and wheezes.

- Monitor results of oxygen saturation with pulse oximetry and ABG studies. *ABG studies provide information about gas exchange; decreasing pH, oxygen, and oxygen saturation levels, and increasing carbon dioxide levels signal respiratory acidosis.*
- Administer supplemental oxygen as prescribed. *Oxygen saturation must be maintained at 100% with supplemental oxygen to prevent hypoxemia and secondary SCI in all acute SCI clients.*
- Help the client turn, cough, and deep breathe at least every 2 hours. Use assisted coughing as necessary. *Paralysis of intercostal or abdominal muscles decreases the ability to expel secretions by coughing; retained secretions increase the risk for pneumonia. The inability to breathe deeply may result in atelectasis.*
- Increase fluids given by mouth to 3000 mL per day (if oral intake is approved), according to client preference for type of liquids and predicated on the client's ability to swallow. *Increased fluid intake thins secretions, which can more easily be expelled and expectorated.*

Dysreflexia

Autonomic dysreflexia is an emergency that requires immediate assessment and intervention to prevent complications of extremely high blood pressure (loss of consciousness, seizure, and even death).

- Elevate the head of the client's bed and remove TEDs or sequential compression boots. *These measures increase pool-*

ing of blood in the lower extremities and decrease venous return, thus decreasing blood pressure.

- Assess blood pressure every 2 to 3 minutes while at the same time assessing for stimuli that initiated the response (such as a full bladder, impacted stool, or skin pressure). *The most serious danger in dysreflexia is elevated blood pressure, which could precipitate a stroke, myocardial infarction, dysrhythmias, or seizures. If the client has a Foley catheter, ensure that there are no kinks in the tubing. If the client does not have a Foley catheter, drain the bladder with a straight catheter. If manifestations persist, assess for a fecal impaction. If an impaction is present, insert Nupercaine cream into the anus, wait 10 minutes, and manually remove the impaction.*

> **PRACTICE ALERT**
> Blood pressure readings may be as high as 300/160.

- If blood pressure remains dangerously elevated, the physician may prescribe intravenous administration of diazoxide (Hyperstat). Other medications that may be used include nifedipine (Procardia) and hydralazine (Apresoline). *Diazoxide is an antihypertensive drug used in emergency situations to lower blood pressure in adults with dangerously high readings. Nifedipine and hydralazine are peripheral vasodilators that are administered to decrease the elevated blood pressure.*

> **PRACTICE ALERT**
> It is important to closely monitor for hypotension following administration of these medications, especially if the stimulus for the dysreflexia has been removed.

Impaired Urinary Elimination and Constipation

Depending on the level of the injury, the client with a SCI may have alterations in bowel and bladder function. Clients with injuries to the cord at or above the S2 to S4 levels will have a neurogenic bladder, with deficits in control of micturition. Voluntary and involuntary bowel control is affected in the client with a lower motor neuron injury. Both bowel and bladder retraining are possible; if not, some form of assisted elimination is necessary. Although an indwelling catheter may be used in the acute phase of care, the goal is to reestablish a catheter-free state.

- Monitor for manifestations of a full bladder. *Overdistention stretches the bladder and can lead to backflow of urine into the ureters and kidney; stasis of urine in an incompletely emptied bladder increases the risk for infection.*

> **PRACTICE ALERT**
> A distended bladder can be palpated over the lower abdomen above the symphysis pubis.

- Teach client to use trigger voiding techniques prior to straight catheterization. These techniques include stroking the inner thigh, pulling the pubic hair, tapping on the abdomen over the bladder, and (in females) pouring warm water over the vulva. *These trigger voiding techniques stimulate parasympathetic nerve fibers to cause reflex activity and may facilitate voiding.*

- Teach self-catheterization to clients who will be able to carry out the procedure alone or with minimal assistance (Procedure 45–1). *Straight catheterization at regular intervals is part of bladder training because periodic distention and relaxation of the muscles of the bladder promote reflex bladder activity. In addition, self-care fosters independence.*

- Monitor residual urine throughout the bladder retraining program. *A residual urine amount of less than 80 mL after a triggered voiding is considered satisfactory.*

- Institute a bowel retraining program as follows:
  - Assess usual patterns of bowel elimination to establish best times for individualized program.
  - Maintain a high-fluid, high-fiber diet.
  - Use stool softeners as prescribed; rectal suppositories and enemas may be used 30 minutes after meals to stimulate stronger peristalsis and facilitate evacuation.
  - Maintain upright position if at all possible and ensure privacy.
  - If client is unable to evacuate, digital stimulation or manual removal on a regular basis may be the most effective long-term management.

  A bowel retraining program to regulate the bowel through reflex activity may be instituted in clients with upper motor neuron injuries. The client with a lower motor neuron injury loses the defecation reflex, and bowel retraining is more difficult (if not impossible).

Sexual Dysfunction

Sexual intercourse is often still possible for the client with an SCI. In men, the general rule is that the higher the level of injury the greater the potential to have reflexogenic erections, although ejaculation or orgasm may not occur, and fertility is usually lower as a result of a lack of temperature control of the testes. However, ejaculation may be stimulated and the sperm used to inseminate the client's partner, so that fatherhood is a possibility. Men who have sacral-level injuries do not have reflexogenic erections but may have psychogenic erections. They are also more likely to remain fertile.

Women with SCI generally do not have sensation during sexual intercourse, but pregnancy is possible. However, pregnant women with an SCI are at increased risk for autonomic dysreflexia during labor and delivery. Birth control options should be discussed prior to discharge from the acute care setting.

A client with an SCI may be deeply concerned about alterations in sexual function. These concerns may lead to lowered self-esteem, altered self-image, or changes in feelings about being an attractive and desirable person. Assess concerns and provide a

---

PROCEDURE 45–1 CLIENT SELF-CATHETERIZATION

Self-catheterization on an intermittent basis (usually a part of self-care at home) is a clean rather than a sterile procedure. The hands should be washed before and after the procedure, and the urinary meatus should be cleaned by washing with soap and water.

FEMALE SELF-CATHETERIZATION

- Attempt to void. If urine is not of sufficient quantity (at least 100 mL) or if you cannot void at all, do self-catheterization. *A large amount of residual urine means that more frequent catheterizations (every 4 to 6 hours) are necessary.*
- While sitting on the wheelchair or the commode, locate the urethra. Visualize the urethra by looking in a mirror, or palpate the urethra with a fingertip. *Visualization or palpation of the meatus is necessary for proper catheter insertion.*
- Lubricate the meatus with a water-soluble lubricant. *Lubrication facilitates the insertion of the catheter and reduces trauma to tissues.*

- Take a deep breath and insert the catheter tip 2 to 3 inches or until urine flows. *The catheter enters the bladder more easily when the sphincter is relaxed. The deep breath relaxes the sphincter. The female urethra is 1½ to 2½ inches long.*
- Hold the catheter securely and allow urine to drain until the flow stops. *Withdrawing and reinserting the catheter increase the risk of infection.*
- Withdraw the catheter and wash it with soap and water. Store the catheter in a clean container. *The catheter can be reused until it is too soft or too hard to be directed into and through the urinary meatus. Clean rather than sterile technique is usually used for self-catheterization at home.*

MALE SELF-CATHETERIZATION

- Attempt to void. If urine is not of sufficient quantity (e.g., less than 100 mL) or if you cannot void at all, do self-catheterization. *A large amount of residual urine means that more frequent catheterizations (every 4 to 6 hours) are necessary.*
- Sit either on the commode or in the wheelchair. Hold the penis with slight upward tension and extend it to its full length. *Extending the penis straightens the urethra.*
- Lubricate the catheter from the tip to about 6 inches downward. *Lubrication is especially important for male catheterization because of the length of the urethra.*
- Take a deep breath and insert the catheter 6 to 7 inches or until urine flows. *The catheter enters the bladder more easily when the*

sphincter is relaxed. The deep breath relaxes the sphincter. The male urethra is about 6 inches long.
- Hold the catheter securely and allow urine to drain until flow has stopped. *Withdrawing and reinserting the catheter increase the risk of infection.*
- Withdraw the catheter and wash it with soap and water. Store the catheter in a clean container. *The catheter can be reused until it is too soft or too hard to be directed into and through the urethra. Clean rather than sterile technique is usually used for self-catheterization at home.*

climate that is receptive to discussion about sexuality. Examples of objectives for sexual counseling for the client with an SCI are that the client will understand how the injury has altered sexual functioning, be aware of alternative ways of achieving sexual pleasure, and have a positive self-concept and body image.

- Include data about sexuality when obtaining the nursing history and database. *Sexuality is a private matter for most people, and the client may not discuss it unless the nurse introduces the topic.*
- Provide accurate information about the effect of the SCI on sexual function. *Accurate information gives the client a realistic picture of how the injury will affect sexuality.*
- Initiate a discussion with the client and partner of alternative means of gaining sexual satisfaction; these include the use of vibrators, and oral–genital and manual stimulation. *Alternatives to intercourse can meet sexual needs and help maintain the relationship with a significant other.*
- Refer for sexual counseling, if appropriate, or to local support groups where questions can be answered by others with similar experiences. *Knowing that others have had similar experiences can decrease social isolation and provide a means of learning alternative methods of sexual functioning.*

Low Self-Esteem

An SCI is often the result of sudden trauma. Within moments, a formerly independent, fully functioning individual is suddenly unable to move and faces enormous adjustments in social, economic, and personal roles and relationships. Body image, self-esteem, and role performance are all affected by the damage. As a result, the client often demonstrates behaviors that may be difficult for the nurse to handle: depression, denial, and anger are seen in the period immediately after the injury. In addition to these responses, the young adult client may act out by making sexually overt statements.

- Encourage talking about all aspects of physical function and care. *Talking provides a safe outlet for fears and frustrations and also increases self-awareness. Acceptance of self facilitates rehabilitation.*
- Encourage self-care and independent decision making. *Participating in self-care can promote positive coping; making decisions decreases feelings of powerlessness.*
- Help identify strategies to increase independence in desired roles; include both short- and long-term goals. Discuss assistive devices (such as hand-operated automobiles). *Identifying strategies to increase independence in the future fosters a positive self-concept and motivates the client to achieve rehabilitation goals.*
- Include family members and important others in discussions. *The realization that others do care and will continue to provide support is important in fostering positive self-regard.*
- Refer the client and family to support groups or for psychologic counseling. *Adjustment to change is more likely when the client and family seek peer and professional assistance.*

Using NANDA, NIC, and NOC

Chart 45–2 shows links between NANDA nursing diagnoses, NIC, and NOC when caring for the client with an SCI.

NANDA, NIC, AND NOC LINKAGES
CHART 45–2 The Client with an SCI

NANDA

Powerlessness

NIC

Self-Esteem Enhancement

Self-Responsibility Facilitation

Support Group

Emotional Support

Environmental Management

Self-Care Assistance

NOC

Self-Esteem

Health Beliefs: Perceived Control

Health Beliefs: Perceived Resources

Social Support

Hope

Data from *NANDA's Nursing Diagnoses: Definitions & Classification 2005–2006* by NANDA International (2005), Philadelphia; *Nursing Interventions Classification (NIC)* (4th ed.) by J. M. Dochterman & G. M. Bluechek (2004), St. Louis, MO: Mosby; and *Nursing Outcomes Classification (NOC)* (3rd ed.) by S. Moorhead, M. Johnson, and M. Maas (2004), St. Louis, MO: Mosby.

Community-Based Care

Rehabilitation of the client with an SCI is an ongoing process that moves from intensive care through intermediate care to rehabilitation and then community-based and home care. Nursing interventions are necessary at all points in the process to prevent the complications of altered physical mobility and body functions, and to teach the client and family measures that promote independence in self-care.

Discharge planning should be addressed even in the initial plan of care while the client is in the critical care setting. Advance planning ensures continuity of care when the client leaves the hospital setting.

The following should be included in teaching the client and family about care at home.

- Self-care activities (ADLs, exercises, bowel and bladder programs, skin care)
- Mobility (use of assistive devices: wheelchair, crutches, special automobiles)
- Preparation of the home environment
    - If the client is in a wheelchair, will steps, stairs, doors, or carpeted floors present physical barriers?

- If a special bed is necessary, have arrangements been made, and is it in the home?
- Psychologic support
- Independent activities
- Community resources, such as Life-line (emergency alerting systems through a local hospital or agency), support groups, career centers for job retraining, counseling
- Coping skills for client and caregiver
- Referral to a home health agency and physical therapist for the client who is returning home
- Helpful resources:
  - The National Spinal Cord Injury Association
  - American Paralysis Association
  - Christopher Reeve Paralysis Foundation
  - Paralyzed Veterans of America
  - Canadian Paraplegic Association
  - Australian Quadriplegic Association.

THE CLIENT WITH A HERNIATED INTERVERTEBRAL DISK

A herniated intervertebral disk, also called a ruptured disk, herniated nucleus pulposus, or a slipped disk, is a rupture of the cartilage surrounding the intervertebral disk with protrusion of the nucleus pulposus (Figure 45–9 ■). Perhaps few neuro-orthopedic disorders are as challenging as those involving the intervertebral disks. Clients with herniation (rupture) of a disk have not only excruciating pain but also limited mobility. These problems may in turn cause alterations in role function, coping, and the ability to perform activities of daily living.

Incidence and Prevalence

A herniated intervertebral disk may occur at any adult age. However, it is more common as people enter middle age and age-related changes occur. The nucleus pulposus loses fluid content, and the disks are less able to absorb shocks. The disks become smaller and slip out of place more easily. Aging causes degeneration in the annulus fibrosus and the posterior longitudinal ligaments, and the vertebrae and disks are less able to respond to movement and are more easily injured.

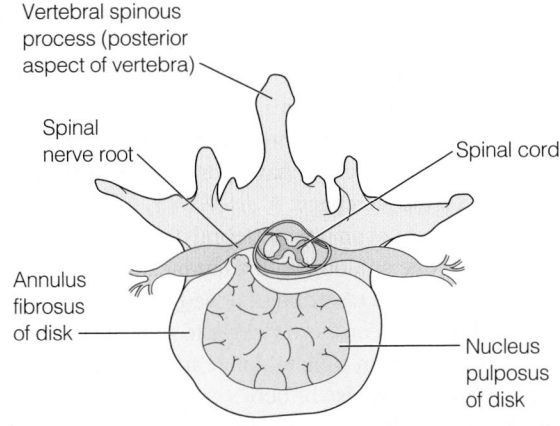

Figure 45–9 ■ A herniated intervertebral disk. The herniated nucleus pulposus is applying pressure against the nerve root.

Labels in figure:
Vertebral spinous process (posterior aspect of vertebra)
Spinal nerve root
Spinal cord
Annulus fibrosus of disk
Nucleus pulposus of disk

Pathophysiology

The intervertebral disks, located between the vertebral bodies, are made of an inner nucleus pulposus and an outer collar (the annulus fibrosus). The disks allow the spine to absorb compression by acting as shock absorbers. A herniated intervertebral disk occurs when the nucleus pulposus protrudes through a weakened or torn annulus fibrosus of an intervertebral disk (see Figure 45-9). This protrusion may occur anywhere along the vertebral column, but herniation of thoracic disks is uncommon. The protrusion may occur spontaneously or as a result of trauma, with trauma (such as lifting heavy objects or falling) causing about half of all cases. Rupture of the disk allows herniation of the nucleus pulposus in a posterolateral direction, with compression of the associated nerve root. The resulting pressure on adjacent spinal nerves causes characteristic manifestations, which vary with the location and the amount of protruding disk material (see the box below). Occasionally the herniation is central rather than posterolateral, with pressure on the spinal cord.

MANIFESTATIONS of a Ruptured Intervertebral Disk

L4 TO L5 LEVEL (AFFECTS FIFTH LUMBAR NERVE ROOT)
- Pain in hip, lower back, posterolateral thigh, anterior leg, dorsal surface of foot, great toe
- Muscle spasms in affected areas
- Paresthesia over lateral leg and web of great toe
- Foot drop (rare)
- Decreased or absent ankle reflex
- Cauda equina syndrome (with complete nerve root compression): bowel and bladder incontinence, paralysis of lower extremities

L5 TO S1 LEVEL (AFFECTS FIRST SACRAL NERVE ROOT)
- Pain in midgluteal region, posterior thigh, calf to heel, plantar surface of the foot to the fourth and fifth toes
- Paresthesias in posterior calf and lateral heel, foot, and toes
- Difficulty walking on toes

C5 TO C6 LEVEL (AFFECTS SIXTH CERVICAL NERVE ROOT)
- Pain in neck, shoulder, anterior upper arm, radial area of forearm, thumb
- Paresthesia of forearm, thumb, forefinger, and lateral arm
- Decreased biceps and supinator reflex
- Triceps reflex normal to hyperactive

The herniation may be abrupt or gradual. Lifting incorrectly or suddenly twisting the spine can cause rupture with immediate intense pain and muscle spasms. Gradual herniation is the result of degenerative changes, osteoarthritis, or ankylosis spondylitis. Clients with a gradual herniation have a slow onset of pain and neurologic deficits.

Lumbar Disk Manifestations

The classic manifestation of a ruptured lumbar disk is recurrent episodes of pain in the lower back. The pain typically radiates across the buttock and down the posterior leg, although it may be experienced only in the leg. **Sciatica** is a term used to describe lumbar back pain that radiates down the posterior leg to the ankle and is increased by sneezing or coughing (the result of pressure on nerve roots L4, L5, S1, S2, or S3, which give rise to the sciatic nerve). Sciatica may be elicited by straight-leg raising: The client feels pain when lifting one leg while dorsiflexing the foot of that leg. Sciatica pain varies in intensity, ranging from mildly uncomfortable to excruciating. It is aggravated by a variety of positions and activities, including sitting, straining, coughing, sneezing, climbing stairs, walking, and riding in a car.

Other manifestations include postural deformity, motor deficits, sensory deficits, and changes in reflexes. In about 60% of clients with ruptured lumbar disks, the normal lumbar lordosis is absent. When standing, the client typically has a slight forward tilt to the trunk, scoliosis of the lumbar spine, slight flexion of the hip and knee on the affected side, and paravertebral muscle spasms (Hickey, 2003). Motor deficits include weakness and in some clients problems with sexual function and urinary elimination. Sensory deficits include paresthesias and numbness. Knee and ankle reflexes are decreased or absent.

Cervical Disk Manifestations

Cervical disks that herniate laterally cause pain in the shoulder, neck, and arm. Other manifestations of lateral cervical herniation include paresthesias, muscle spasms and stiff neck, and decreased or absent arm reflexes. Central cervical herniations result in mild, intermittent pain; however, the client may also experience lower extremity weakness, unsteady gait, muscle spasms, urinary elimination problems, altered sexual function, and hyperactive lower extremity reflexes.

INTERDISCIPLINARY CARE

Considerations for the client with a ruptured intervertebral disk include identifying the location of herniation and determining whether conservative treatment or surgery is indicated. Nursing care is directed toward preparing clients for diagnostic tests and providing teaching and care for the client who has either medical or surgical interventions.

Diagnosis

Diagnostic tests are ordered to differentiate the cause of back pain; for example, back and leg pain is also caused by spinal tumors, degenerative processes, or abdominal diseases. Assessing pain is an important part of diagnosis. The tests include x-rays and CT scans of the lumbosacral or cervical area to identify skeletal deformities and narrowing of the disk spaces (see Chapter 43 ∞). Electromyography (EMG), which measures electrical activity of skeletal muscles at rest and during voluntary contraction, may be conducted to identify specific muscles affected by the pressure of the herniation on the nerve roots.

A myelogram with contrast medium is done to illustrate areas of herniation, although it does not provide the detail found with CT or MRI. However, myelography is diagnostic in 80% to 90% of all cases and is used both to rule out tumors and locate the herniation. Nursing implications for the care of a client having a myelogram are described in Chapter 43 ∞.

Medications

The client with a ruptured intervertebral disk is treated with medications to relieve pain and reduce swelling and muscle spasms. Pain is usually managed with NSAIDs (see Chapter 9 ∞). Muscle spasms are treated with muscle relaxants.

Treatments

A ruptured intervertebral disk may be treated conservatively or with surgery.

CONSERVATIVE TREATMENT A ruptured intervertebral disk is usually managed conservatively unless the client is experiencing severe neurologic deficits. The goals of treatment are pain relief and healing of the involved disk by fibrosis. Conservative treatment is usually prescribed for 2 to 6 weeks. If the client continues to have pain after that time, surgery may be considered. The treatment regimen depends on the severity of the manifestations. Decreasing activity level with bed rest is no longer recommended; and in many cases, the client is advised to continue with normal activities while taking prescribed medications for pain, inflammation, and muscle spasms.

Medications used to treat back pain include nonnarcotic analgesics, anti-inflammatory drugs such as the NSAIDs, muscle relaxants, and sedative-tranquilizers.

SURGERY Surgery is indicated for clients who do not respond to conservative management or have serious neurologic deficits. Several surgical interventions are used to treat a ruptured intervertebral disk. The type of surgery chosen depends on the location of the disk and the stability of the spinal column.

■ A *laminectomy,* the type of surgery most often performed, is the removal of a part of the vertebral lamina. The surgery is done to relieve pressure on the nerves. It is often combined with removal of the protruding nucleus pulposus (*nuclectomy*). Nursing care for the client having a laminectomy is discussed in the box on the next page. A *diskectomy* is the removal of the nucleus pulposus of an intervertebral disk. Diskectomy may be performed alone or along with a laminectomy.

■ Spinal fusion is the insertion of a wedge-shaped piece of bone or bone chips between the vertebrae to stabilize them. The bone is usually taken from a client donor site, such as the iliac crest. A spinal fusion may also be performed through a spinal implant with a device called a BAK (a hollow titanium cylinder with holes), which is packed with grafted bone from a donor site and placed in the space where a disk is removed. Although not

NURSING CARE OF THE CLIENT HAVING A   Posterior Laminectomy

PREOPERATIVE TEACHING

- Demonstrate and ask the client to practice logrolling; explain that it will be done by the nurses for the first day or two, and then the client can do it alone. *To ensure healing, the spinal column must remain in alignment when turning and moving.*
- Explain the importance of taking pain medications regularly and of asking for them before the pain is severe. Include information about the possibility of the pain being much the same after surgery. *Pain is easier to control if medications are taken before the pain is severe. Pain may be the same following surgery for a herniated intervertebral disk because edema due to surgery irritates and compresses the nerve roots.*
- Demonstrate the use of a fracture bedpan and ask the client to practice its use. *The client usually must remain flat in bed for a period of time following surgery. A fracture bedpan is more comfortable for clients who must lie flat.*
- Explain that the client may need to eat while lying flat. *This position prevents flexion of the spine.*
- Demonstrate and ask the client to demonstrate deep breathing, the use of the incentive spirometer, and leg exercises. *These measures prevent respiratory and circulatory complications.*

POSTOPERATIVE CARE

- Maintain the client in a position that minimizes stress on the surgical wound. For clients with cervical laminectomy:
  a. Elevate the head of the bed slightly.
  b. Position a small pillow under the neck.
  c. Maintain the position of the cervical collar.
  For clients with lumbar laminectomy:
  a. Keep the bed flat or elevate the head of the bed slightly.
  b. Place a small pillow under the head.
  c. Place a small pillow under the knees, or use a pillow to support the upper leg when the client lies on one side.
  These positions minimize stress on the surgical wound and suture line. A cervical collar provides stability and prevents flexing or twisting the neck.
- Turn the client every 2 hours, using the logrolling technique. Teach the client **not** to use the side rails to change position. Maintain proper body alignment in all positions. *The client's body is turned as a single unit (usually with a turning sheet) to avoid movement of the operative area. Pulling on the side rails puts stress on the operative area and may also cause misalignment of the vertebral column.*
- Monitor the client for signs of nerve root compression.
  a. Cervical laminectomy: Assess hand grips and arm strength, ability to move the fingers, and ability to detect touch.
  b. Lumbar laminectomy: Assess leg strength, ability to wiggle the toes, and ability to detect touch.
  Compare bilateral findings. Report muscle weakness or sensory impairment to the physician immediately. *Loss of motor and sensory function may indicate nerve root compression.*
- Assess for hematoma formation as manifested by severe incisional pain that is not relieved by analgesics and decreased motor function. Report these findings immediately. *A hematoma may form at the surgical site. If untreated, it may cause irre-*

versible neurologic deficits including paraplegia and bowel/bladder dysfunctions (Hickey, 2003).

- Assess for leakage of cerebrospinal fluid. Assess the dressing for increased moisture. Check the sheets for wetness when the client is lying supine; check for clear liquid running down the back when the client is sitting or standing. Gently palpate the sides of the wound to detect a bulge. Use a Dextrostrix strip to assess any leakage for the presence of glucose, a positive indicator of cerebrospinal fluid. *Although uncommon, leakage of cerebrospinal fluid greatly increases the risk for infection of the wound and of the meninges.*
- Assess for nerve root injury. Assess the client's ability to dorsiflex the foot (lumbar laminectomy) and the client's grip strength (cervical laminectomy). Assess the client who has had a cervical laminectomy for hoarseness. Report hoarseness and further assess the client's ability to swallow. *Nerve root compression may cause permanent damage, resulting in footdrop (in lumbar laminectomy clients) and hand weakness (in cervical laminectomy clients). Damage to the laryngeal nerve may cause permanent hoarseness. Impaired ability to swallow puts the client at risk for aspiration.*
- Assess for urinary retention. The client should void within 8 hours after surgery. If the physician allows, let males stand to void. Compare intake and output for each 8-hour period. *All clients who have received a general anesthetic are at risk for urinary retention. The client who has had a lumbar laminectomy may have even more difficulty voiding as a result of stimulation of sympathetic nerves during surgery.*
- Assess for pain using a scale from 0 (no pain) to 10 (severe pain). Administer prescribed analgesics on a regular basis, or teach the client to use patient-controlled analgesia (PCA), if prescribed. Discuss client concerns about pain that is unrelieved by surgery. *Compression of the nerve root over time results in edema and inflammation. Because of surgery-induced edema, the client is likely to experience either the same pain or perhaps more severe pain in the period immediately after surgery. This pain usually persists for several weeks after surgery. In addition, many clients who have had a lumbar laminectomy have muscle spasms in the lower back, abdomen, and thighs for the first few days after surgery.*
- Assess for infection by taking and recording vital signs at least every 4 hours; report increased body temperature. Assess the wound and dressing for signs of infection: increased redness, drainage, pain, and pus. Use sterile technique to change dressings. *The surgical client is always at risk for infection; the client with a laminectomy is also at risk for arachnoiditis. This inflammation of the arachnoid layer of the spinal meninges results from wound infection or contamination during surgery and may cause the formation of painful adhesions.*
- Encourage deep breathing and the use of the incentive spirometer every 2 hours; coughing may be discouraged. *Anesthesia and immobility depress respiratory function. Coughing may be discouraged because it can disrupt healing tissues, especially in clients having a cervical laminectomy.*
- Increase mobility as prescribed. (The time frame for ambulation is prescribed by the physician; the routine here is

(continued)

NURSING CARE OF THE CLIENT HAVING A Posterior Laminectomy (continued)

representative.) Clients often sit on the side of the bed and dangle their legs the evening after surgery or the first day thereafter. Many clients ambulate the first or second postoperative day. To help the client out of bed, first elevate the head of the bed. Then bring the client's legs over the side of the bed at the same time that the upper body moves into the upright position. Clients should not ambulate without assistance until they are no longer dizzy or weak. *Early ambulation increases respiratory and circulatory function and decreases the risk of thrombophlebitis of the lower extremities. The vertebral column should remain in alignment while the client sits and stands. Safety must be considered throughout care.*

---

appropriate for all clients requiring a spinal fusion, this does facilitate a short hospital stay and convalescence.

- Foraminotomy is an enlargement of the opening between the disk and the facet joint to remove bony overgrowth compressing the nerve. The location and size of the incision vary according to the surgeon's preference and the location and size of the ruptured disk. The posterior approach is taken for lumbar surgery. Either the posterior or the anterior approach may be taken for cervical disks.
- Intradiscal electrothermal therapy (IDET) uses thermal energy to treat pain from a bulging spinal disk. A special needle is inserted into the disk and heated to a high temperature. The heat thickens and seals the disk wall and decreases bulging of the disk.
- A microdiskectomy, in which microsurgical techniques are used, is performed through a very small incision. This type of surgery decreases the possibility of trauma to surrounding structures during surgery and allows early postoperative mobility and a short hospital stay.

NURSING CARE

Nursing care for the client with a ruptured intervertebral disk may be provided through information in community and work settings, during conservative treatment, and during pre- and postoperative treatment. The pain of the ruptured disk is often discouraging and debilitating, and may well affect the client's ability to work.

Health Promotion

Proper body mechanics may help prevent the occurrence of a ruptured intervertebral disk. Teaching the proper method of lifting and moving heavy objects should begin when children enter school. This information should also be given to all workers (including nurses) who have lifting as part of their responsibilities. The guidelines for proper body mechanics are as follows:

- Begin activities by spreading the feet apart to broaden the base of support.
- Use large muscles of the arms to lift and the legs to push when lifting.
- Work as closely as possible to the object that is to be lifted or moved.
- Slide, roll, push, or pull an object rather than lift it.
- When lifting, bend the knees and lift up over your center of gravity.
- When lifting, use a back support belt.

Assessment

The following data are collected through the health history and physical examination (see Chapter 43 ∞).

- *Health history:* Type of employment, risk factors, pain (location, duration, intensity).
- *Physical assessment:* Muscle strength and coordination, sensation, reflexes.

Nursing Diagnosis and Interventions

Nursing care for clients with a herniated intervertebral disk focuses largely on pain management, both during conservative management and after surgery.

Acute Pain

Clients with a ruptured intervertebral disk experience acute back and leg pain. Acute pain may be related to preoperative muscle spasms or nerve root compression. After surgery, the client may have pain at the site of the incision and in the surgical area.

- Assess the degree of pain on a 0 to 10 scale (10 being greatest pain) and identify contributing and relieving factors. *Pain is a subjective experience. The nurse needs to assess it thoroughly before initiating interventions.*
- Use a firm mattress or place a board under the mattress. *A firm bed supports the spinal column and muscles.*
- Teach the client to avoid turning or twisting the spinal column and to assume positions that decrease stress on the vertebral column (e.g., when in the supine position, flex the hips slightly). A small pillow may be placed under the knees (for clients with a herniated lumbar disk) or under the neck (for clients with a herniated cervical disk). *Correct body positions can decrease intradisk pressure.*
- Provide analgesic medications around the clock. *Intense pain can increase muscle spasms; maintaining serum levels of analgesics often prevents severe pain.*

> **PRACTICE ALERT**
> It is important to maintain a constant level of pain relief. Healthcare providers have the responsibility of relieving pain with adequate medications.

Chronic Pain

The client with a ruptured intervertebral disk often has pain for an extended period of time. Despite conservative treatment or previous surgery, pain may be ongoing or intermittent. If previous surgery has not relieved the pain, the client may be depressed or angry. Caring for a client with chronic pain is frustrating, and the client is often regarded as difficult.

- Treat the client's reports of pain with respect. *The client is the person experiencing the pain and is thus the expert about it.*
- Do not refer to the client as being addicted to pain medication. *All types of pain medications may be used legitimately to manage pain.*

PRACTICE ALERT
Although the client may develop tolerance to a narcotic analgesic, tolerance does not imply addiction.

- Monitor the client carefully for any changes in condition. *Significant changes in the client's condition may go unrecognized when pain is present for a prolonged period of time.*
- Maintain written plans of care for pain management that are individualized and ensure continuity of care. *When the client makes several visits (for instance, to an emergency department or a pain clinic), written records help caregivers determine what is effective in managing pain and what is not.*
- Teach the client alternative methods of pain management. *Consider the client's coping style when recommending methods. Clients who have a passive coping style are often better able to manage pain by depending on others, taking medications, and resting. Clients with an active coping style are probably better able to manage pain by learning self-management methods, taking part in activities, and staying busy.*
- Develop effective methods of improving rest and sleep. Problems with rest and sleep make pain management more difficult. *Sleeping poorly at night contributes to decreased motivation, confused thinking, depression, and muscle aches.*
- Refer the client to a physical therapist for an exercise program, if appropriate. *The client needs to know exactly what exercises to do, how many repetitions are recommended, for how long, and how often. The client should not exercise to the point of causing increased pain.*
- Assess the need for referrals (and make them if necessary) for the client who is depressed or anxious. *Anxiety and de-pression often are a part of long-term chronic pain, making pain management more difficult. Suggest that referrals for help with the frustration (rather than "depression") may make a significant difference in the client's ability to manage pain.*

Constipation
The client with a ruptured intervertebral disk often has problems with constipation because of reduced mobility. Nursing interventions to alleviate and prevent constipation are important because straining to have a bowel movement can increase intradisk pressure, thus increasing pain.

- Assess the client's usual bowel routine, including diet, fluid intake, and the use of laxatives or enemas. *Effective interventions are based on individualized needs.*

PRACTICE ALERT
People who use laxatives or enemas for long periods of time may be dependent on those methods of having a bowel movement.

- Encourage a fluid intake of 2500 to 3000 mL per day unless contraindicated by the presence of renal or cardiac disease. *Adequate fluid intake facilitates the passage of feces.*
- Increase fiber and bulk in the diet. If the client is unable to tolerate increased fiber, consult with the physician about the use of stool softeners or bulk-forming agents. *Bulk and fiber promote regularity by retaining water in the large intestine.*

Community-Based Care
It is the nurse's responsibility to teach the client and family about chronic pain control, including specific interventions to alleviate pain. The nurse's role may be that of advocate and creative problem solver (see the Meeting Individualized Needs box below). The following topics should be addressed:

- Often the goal is to control pain so that the client can perform normal ADLs, rather than to reach a pain-free state.

MEETING INDIVIDUALIZED NEEDS   Teaching the Client with a Ruptured Intervertebral Disk

- Sleep on a firm mattress; use a bedboard if necessary.
- When lying in the supine position, flex the knees to approximately a 45-degree angle with a small pillow and use a small pillow under the head.
- Avoid any activities that flex the spine, such as bending or lifting, and do not twist the back.
- Follow your diet to maintain body weight or to lose weight if needed.
- Follow the prescribed exercise program, for example:
  a. Lie flat on your back on the floor. Tighten your abdominal and buttock muscles and tilt your pelvis forward so that your lower back is flat on the floor (this is called a *pelvic tilt*). Hold the position for 3 seconds and repeat for the prescribed number of times.
  b. Lying on the back on a firm surface, press the feet to the floor, tighten the abdominal muscles, and lift the upper

half of the body off the floor. Hold the position for 3 seconds, and repeat as prescribed.
  c. Lying on your back on a firm surface, bring your knees up to the chest. Put your hands around your knees and raise the buttocks off the floor. Repeat as prescribed.
  d. Sit upright on the floor or a firm surface. Keep one leg straight and bend the other knee. Reach for the toes of the straightened leg. Switch legs. Repeat as prescribed.
  e. Stand upright. Squat down, flexing the hips and knees. Straighten your back. Stand upright by straightening the knees. Repeat as prescribed.
- Wear flat-heeled shoes that provide good support.
- Use proper lifting techniques. For instance, squat and use your thigh muscles to lift an object from the floor, and spread your feet to get a wide base of support when you lift while you are standing.

- Nonpharmacologic methods of pain management include relaxation techniques, guided imagery, distraction, hypnosis, and music. Joining a support group may be an effective intervention in coping with and managing pain.
- Clients may be referred to a physical therapist for education about body mechanics and back-strengthening exercises. Nurses should have the client demonstrate the exercises to reinforce teaching.

THE CLIENT WITH A SPINAL CORD TUMOR

Spinal cord tumors may be benign or malignant, primary or metastatic. They may arise at any level of the spinal column. Of all spinal cord tumors, 50% are thoracic, 30% are cervical, and 20% are lumbosacral. They constitute about 0.5% to 1% of all tumors (Hickey, 2003). Tumors of the spinal cord are seen equally in men and in women, and they most often occur between the ages of 20 and 60. They are rarely seen in the older adult.

Classification

Spinal cord tumors are classified by anatomic location as either intramedullary or extramedullary tumors. Intramedullary tumors, which make up about 10% of spinal tumors, arise from within the neural tissues of the spinal cord; those that occur include astrocytomas, ependymomas, glioblastomas, and medulloblastomas (Tierney et al., 2005). Extramedullary tumors arise from tissues outside the spinal cord, with commonly occurring tumors including neurofibromas, meningiomas, sarcomas, chordomas, and vascular tumors.

Extramedullary tumors are further categorized as intradural (arising from the nerve roots or meninges within the subarachnoid space) or extradural (arising from epidural tissue or the vertebrae outside the dura).

Tumors of the spinal cord are also classified as either primary or secondary (metastatic). Primary tumors, arising from the epidural vessels, spinal meninges, or glial cells, have an unknown cause. Secondary tumors are metastatic in origin, most commonly the result of malignancies of the lung, breast, prostate, gastrointestinal tract, or uterus.

Pathophysiology

Depending on their anatomic location, spinal cord tumors result in pathologic changes as a result of compression, invasion, or ischemia secondary to arterial or venous obstruction. Extramedullary tumors (whether benign or malignant) alter normal function through compression of the spinal cord, with destruction of white matter and eventual filling of the space around the spinal cord. Cord compression interferes with normal blood flow and membrane potentials, altering afferent and efferent motor, sensory, and reflex impulses. Compression of the spinal cord also causes edema, which can ascend the cord and cause further neurologic deficits. Intramedullary tumors both compress and invade. As the tumor grows within the cord, the cord also enlarges and distorts the white matter.

Manifestations

The manifestations of a spinal cord tumor depend on the anatomic location, level of occurrence, type of tumor, and spinal nerves involved. General manifestations of a spinal cord tumor include pain, motor and sensory deficits, changes in bowel and/or bladder elimination, and changes in sexual function. Specific manifestations by anatomic level are outlined in the box below.

Pain is often the first manifestation of a spinal cord tumor. It is caused by compression of the spinal cord, tension on the spinal nerves, or tumor attachment to the proximal dura (the covering of the spinal cord). The pain may be either localized or radicular. Localized pain is felt when pressure is applied over the spinous process of the involved area; this type of pain often accompanies metastatic tumors involving the vertebrae. Radicular pain is felt along the course of a nerve as a result of compression, irritation, or tension of a nerve root. The pain is often made worse by any activity that causes intraspinal pressure, such as sneezing or coughing.

Motor manifestations resulting from a spinal cord tumor include paresis and paralysis below the level of the tumor, spasticity, and hyperactive reflexes. The Babinski reflex may be positive. These deficits are the result of involvement of the corticospinal tracts.

Many different sensory manifestations may occur, depending on the location and level of the tumor. Lateral tumor growth and compression affect the lateral spinothalamic tracts, causing pain, numbness, tingling, and coldness. If the tumor involves

---

MANIFESTATIONS **of Spinal Cord Tumors**

CERVICAL CORD TUMORS
- Ipsilateral arm motor involvement, followed by ipsilateral and contralateral leg involvement, followed by contralateral arm involvement
- Paresis of the arms and legs
- Stiffness of the neck
- Paraplegia
- Pain in the shoulders and arms
- Hyperactive reflexes

THORACIC CORD TUMORS
- Paresis and spasticity of one leg, followed by paresis and spasticity of the other leg
- Pain in the back and chest
- Positive Babinski reflex
- Bowel and bladder dysfunction
- Sexual dysfunction

LUMBOSACRAL CORD TUMORS
- Paresis and spasticity of one leg, followed by paresis and spasticity of the other leg
- Pain in the lower back, radiating to the legs and perineal area
- Loss of sensation in the legs
- Bowel and bladder dysfunction
- Sexual dysfunction
- Decreased or absent ankle and knee reflexes

the posterior columns, the senses of vibration and proprioception of body parts are affected.

Bladder and bowel elimination and sexual function are often affected. Bowel elimination deficits include constipation that may progress to paralytic ileus. Initial bladder elimination deficits include frequency, urgency, and difficulty voiding. The deficits may progress to urinary retention and a neurogenic bladder. In addition, the male client may be impotent.

Syringomyelia is a complication of some spinal cord tumors. In this condition, a fluid-filled cystic cavity forms in the central intramedullary gray matter. This syndrome causes pain, motor weakness, and spasticity.

INTERDISCIPLINARY CARE

The medical management of the client with a spinal cord tumor focuses first on diagnosis. Treatment depends on the type of tumor, its location, and the client's condition.

Diagnosis

The client with a spinal cord tumor undergoes many of the same diagnostic tests as does the client with a ruptured intervertebral disk. The tests used to identify the tumor include x-rays, CT scans, MRI, and myelogram (see Chapter 43 ∞). A lumbar puncture of the client with a spinal cord tumor will demonstrate CSF that is commonly xanthochromic (having a yellow color), has increased protein, has few to no cells, and clots immediately (this cluster of findings is called Froin's syndrome).

Medications

The client with a spinal cord tumor is given medications to relieve pain and control edema. If the pain is severe and the result of a metastatic tumor, an epidural catheter may be inserted for narcotic analgesic administration. Pain management for clients with a spinal cord tumor is provided by narcotic analgesics (see Chapter 9 ∞). Steroids, such as dexamethasone (Decadron), are administered to control edema of the cord.

Surgery

Intramedullary and intradural tumors are surgically excised when possible. Advances in microsurgical techniques and laser surgery have increased the possibility of tumor excision. Metastatic tumors may be partially excised to reduce cord compression; rapidly growing metastatic lesions may require surgical decompression to preserve motor, bowel, or bladder function.

The surgical excision is made through a laminectomy. The client with a tumor involving more than two vertebrae often has a spinal fusion and may also have rods inserted to stabilize the spinal column.

Radiation Therapy

Radiation therapy is used to treat metastatic spinal cord tumors for several different reasons. It may be used on an emergency basis to treat the client with rapidly progressing neurologic deficits. It may be used to reduce pain. Radiation may also be used following surgical excision of as much tumor mass as possible.

Radiation of the spinal cord may cause the development of radiation-induced myelopathy. This complication of radiation exposure occurs over time, with manifestations of a *Brown-Séquard syndrome* (weakness or paralysis on one side of the body and loss of sensation on the opposite side) developing 12 to 15 months after therapy. The manifestations may progress to paraplegia, sensory loss, and loss of bowel and bladder control (Hickey, 2003).

NURSING CARE

Nursing care for the client with a spinal cord tumor is individualized in accordance with the type of tumor and the type of treatment. The client with a benign tumor that is removed by surgery has different healthcare needs than the client with a metastatic tumor, even though they may have similar neurologic deficits. The client with a spinal cord tumor (regardless of type) requires nursing care to monitor for neurologic changes, to provide pain management, and to manage motor and sensory deficits in order to preserve quality of life.

The assessments and nursing interventions for the client with a spinal cord tumor are similar to those described for the client with SCI or who is undergoing surgery for a ruptured intervertebral disk. Following surgical treatment, the client may be transferred to a rehabilitation center or may go home for the recovery period. Referrals for home care, occupational therapy, and physical therapy often help the client regain functional abilities. Teach family members how to move the client in the bed and from the bed to a chair. Also teach them how to provide physical care, care for any appliances (such as an indwelling catheter), and prevent or treat constipation.

EXPLORE MediaLink

Prentice Hall Nursing MediaLink DVD-ROM
Audio Glossary
NCLEX-RN® Review

COMPANION WEBSITE www.prenhall.com/lemone
Audio Glossary
NCLEX-RN® Review
Care Plan Activity: Hemorrhagic Stroke
Case Study: Spinal Cord Injury
MediaLink Applications
Intracranial Pressure
Spinal Cord Injury
Stroke
Stroke Lifestyle Changes
Links to Resources

CHAPTER HIGHLIGHTS

- A stroke is a condition in which neurologic deficits result from a sudden decrease in blood flow to a localized area of the brain. Strokes may be ischemic or hemorrhagic. Ischemic strokes result from a blockage of a cerebral artery by formation of a blood clot or by a clot or foreign substance (such as fat or bacteria) lodging in a blood vessel; they include transient ischemic attacks, thrombotic strokes, or embolic strokes. Hemorrhagic strokes occur when a cerebral blood vessel ruptures.

- Depending on the size and location of cerebral tissue damage, strokes may cause cognitive and behavior changes, sensory-perceptual deficits, language disorders, and motor deficits. Treatment of an ischemic stroke with fibrinolytic therapy within 3 hours of the onset of manifestations may reverse damage to cerebral neurons.

- Nursing care is directed toward both prevention of a stroke through community-based educational programs and interventions to promote recovery and decrease complications.

- Intracerebral hemorrhage may follow rupture of an intracranial aneurysm or arteriovenous malformation. Intracranial aneurysms occur at the site of a weakness in a cerebral blood vessel, while AV malformations are a tangled collection of dilated arteries and veins.

- Spinal cord injuries are almost always the result of trauma, with the major risk factors being age (young adults), gender (male), and alcohol or drug abuse. The causes of injury to the spinal cord include contusion, laceration, transection, hemorrhage, and damage to spinal cord blood vessels.

- In a complete SCI, the motor and sensory pathways in the spinal cord are completely interrupted (*transected*), resulting in total loss of motor and sensory function below the level of the injury. In an incomplete SCI, the motor and sensory pathways are only partially interrupted, resulting in variable loss of function below the level of injury. Injuries of the spinal cord have the potential to affect movement, perception, sensation, sexual function, and elimination.

- Spinal shock is the temporary loss of all reflexes (areflexia) below the level of injury. Manifestations of spinal shock include bradycardia, hypotension, and flaccid paralysis.

- Autonomic dysreflexia is an exaggerated sympathetic response in clients with an SCI at or above the T6 level. Triggered by noxious stimuli (such as a blocked urinary catheter or a fecal impaction), this condition results in extreme hypertension and, if untreated, may cause seizures, stroke, or a myocardial infarction.

- Rehabilitation of the client with an SCI is an ongoing process from intensive care to home care. Nursing interventions are necessary in all settings to promote independence in self-care.

- A herniated intervertebral disk is a rupture of the cartilage surrounding the intervertebral disk with protrusion of the nucleus pulposus. The major manifestation of lumbar disks is lower back and sciatic pain on the affected side. Cervical disks cause pain in the shoulder, neck, and arm. A variety of medications, treatments, and surgical procedures are available for the client.

- Spinal cord tumors may be benign or malignant, primary or metastatic. Depending on their size and location, they cause pathologic changes in spinal cord function through compression, invasion, or ischemia.

TEST YOURSELF NCLEX-RN® REVIEW

1 Which of the following manifestations would alert you to the possibility that your client has had a TIA?
1. sudden severe pain over the left eye
2. numbness and tingling in the corner of the mouth
3. complete paralysis of the right arm and leg
4. loss of sensation and reflexes in both legs

2 Although all of the following are risk factors for a stroke, which one is the greatest risk?
1. hypertension
2. heart disease
3. diabetes
4. high cholesterol levels

3 You have been assigned to care for a client who has had an acute ischemic stroke of a left cerebral vessel. You read the chart and realize the client has contralateral deficits. What does this mean?
1. Both sides of the body are involved.
2. The client will have neurologic deficits on the left side of the body.
3. The client will have neurologic deficits on the right side of the body.
4. Deficits will be present below the level of the stroke.

4 What is the rationale for administration of a tissue plasminogen activator within the first 3 hours of a thrombotic stroke?
1. to reduce the risk of vasospasm
2. to decrease the risk of infection
3. to increase platelet aggregation
4. to cause fibrinolysis of the clot

5 Oxygen is often administered to the client who has had a stroke. Preventing hypoxia and hypercapnia through this treatment will lessen the risk of which complication?
1. fluid accumulation in the lungs
2. pulmonary emboli
3. increased intracranial pressure
4. rebleeding

6 What is the primary pathophysiologic process of spinal shock?
1. temporary loss of reflex function below the level of injury
2. loss of control of cardiovascular mechanisms
3. exaggerated sympathetic response
4. damage to the lower motor neurons

7 Your client has manifestations of autonomic dysreflexia. Which of these assessments would indicate a possible cause for this condition?

1. extreme hypertension
2. kinked catheter tubing
3. respiratory wheezes and stridor
4. skin breakdown over the coccyx

8 A client is admitted to the emergency department following an automobile crash. An SCI at the cervical level is identified. What will be done to facilitate respirations?
1. No treatments are necessary.
2. Oxygen per nasal cannula will be administered.
3. The client will be placed on a ventilator.
4. The head of the bed will be elevated.

9 Many different medications may be given to the client with an acute SCI. Which of the following will possibly be administered? (Select all that apply.)
1. corticosteroids
2. vasopressors
3. antibiotics
4. analgesics
5. antihistamines

10 You are conducting a class at a factory to teach methods to prevent a ruptured intervertebral disk. What should be included? (Choose all that apply.)
1. Spread the feet apart to broaden the base of support.
2. Bend from the waist to lift articles from the floor.
3. Use large leg muscles to push when lifting.
4. Always lift articles rather than rolling or pushing them
5. Work as closely as possible to the object to be moved.

See Test Yourself answers in Appendix C.

BIBLIOGRAPHY

American Heart Association. (2005a). *Heart disease and stroke statistics –2005 update.* Dallas: Author.
_____. (2005b). *Part 9: Adult stroke.* Supplement to Circulation. (2005). 112: IV-111-IV-120.
American Stroke Association. (2003). *Stroke among Hispanics.* Retrieved from http://www.strokeassociation.org/presenter.jhtml?identifier=3030389
American Stroke Association. (2005a). *Hidden risk factors for women.* Retrieved from http://www.strokeassociation.org/presenter.jhtml?identifier=3030391
_____. (2005b). *Why me?* Retrieved from http://www.strokeassociation.org/presenter.jhtml?identifier=3030538
Are you putting spinal cord injury patients in danger? (2003). *ED Nursing, 6*(7), 81–83.
Bakas, T., Austin, J., Jessup, S., Williams, L, & Oberst, M. (2004). Time and difficulty of tasks provided by family caregivers of stroke survivors. *Journal of Neuroscience Nursing, 36*(2), 95–106.
Barker, E., & Saulino, M. (2002). First-ever guidelines for spinal cord injuries. *RN, 65*(10), 32–37.
Blissitt, P., Mitchell, P., Newell, D., Woods, S., & Belza, B. (2004). The effect of head of bed elevation on cerebrovascular dynamics in mild or moderate vasospasm following aneurysmal subarachnoid hemorrhage. *Journal of Neuroscience Nursing, 36*(2), 108–109.
Brillhart, B. (2005). A study of spirituality and life satisfaction among persons with spinal cord injury. *Rehabilitation Nursing, 30*(1), 31–34.
Burton, C. (2003). Therapeutic interventions in stroke rehabilitation: A systematic review. *Clinical Effectiveness in Nursing, 7*(3/4), 124–133.
Dochterman, J., & Bulechek, G. (2004). *Nursing interventions classification (NIC)* (4th ed.). St. Louis, MO: Mosby.
Fahey, M. (2002). Spinal shock: A nurse's perspective. *Journal of Orthopaedic Nursing, 6*(1), 18–22.
Finley, J. (2004). Clinical updates. The evolving treatment in acute ischemic stroke. *Journal of Continuing Education in Nursing, 35*(3), 102–103.
Fisher, V. (2004). Manual evacuation can be vital. *Nursing Standard, 18*(34), 30.
Gibson, K. (2003). Caring for a patient who lives with a spinal cord injury. *Nursing, 33*(7), 36–42.

Harvey, J. (2004). Countering "brain attacks." (2004). *Nursing Management, 35*(8), 27–33.
Heath, H. (2004). Stroke: Fact and fiction. *Nursing Older People, 16*(8), 6.
Hickey, J. (2003). *The clinical practice of neurological and neurosurgical nursing* (4th ed.). Philadelphia: Lippincott.
Hughes, R. (2003). The use of NANDA, NIC, and NOC in the identification and measurement of problems, interventions, and outcomes in spinal cord injury. *International Journal of Nursing Terminologies and Classifications, 14*(4), Supplement, 18–19.
Kee, J. (2004). *Handbook of laboratory and diagnostic tests with nursing implications* (5th ed.). Upper Saddle River, NJ: Prentice Hall.
Kelly-Hayes, M. (2004). Stroke outcome measures. *Journal of Cardiovascular Nursing, 19*(5), 301–307.
Mather, D. (2004). A low-tech approach to pain relief. *RN, 67*(3), 41, 43.
Maze, L., & Bakas, T. (2004). Factors associated with hospital arrival time for stroke patients. *Journal of Neuroscience Nursing, 36*(3), 136–141, 155.
Moorhead, S., Johnson, M., & Maas, M. (2003). *Nursing outcomes classification (NOC)* (3rd ed.). St. Louis, MO: Mosby.
The National Spinal Cord Injury Association. [NSCIA]. (2005b). *Autonomic dysreflexia.* Retrieved from http://www.spinalcord.org/html/factsheets/aut_dysreflexia.php
The National Spinal Cord Injury Association. (2006). *More about spinal cord injury.* Retrieved from http://www.spinalcord.org/html/factsheets/spinstat.php
National Institute of Neurological Disorders and Stroke [NINDS]. (2005a). *Low back pain fact sheet.* Available http://www.ninds.nih.gov/disorders/backpain/detail_backpain.htm
National Institute of Neurological Disorders and Stroke [NINDS]. (2005b). *NINDS spinal cord injury information page.* Available http://www.ninds.nih.gov/disorders/sci/sci.htm
National Institute of Neurological Disorders and Stroke [NINDS]. (2005c). *Patent foramen ovale (PFO) and stroke.* Available http://www.stroke.orgt/TemplateSingleHTMLTExtArea.aspx?P=e8af7dba683c4ecbbad686f05ba36fa
National Institute of Neurological Disorders and Stroke [NINDS]. (2005d). *Stroke: Hope through research.* Available

http://www.ninds.nih.gov/disorders/stroke/detail_stroke_pr.htm
NANDA International. (2004). *Nursing diagnoses: Definitions & classification 2003–2004.* Philadelphia: NANDA.
National Stroke Association. (2004a). *All about stroke.* Retrieved from http://www.stroke/org/TemplateSingleHTMLTextArea.aspz?P=270bce9a71e54f6ebf576555f0cc848
National Stroke Association. (2004b). *Controllable stroke risk factors.* Available http://www.stroke.org/HomePage.aspx?P=5885af9240c146e8a4e238f614acac38
Ohshima, H., Murashima, S., & Takahashi, R. (2004). Assessments and nursing care for right brain-damaged stroke patients: Focusing on neglect and related manifestations. *Nursing & Health Sciences, 6*(2), 115–121.
Olinzock, B. (2004). A model for assessing learning readiness for self-direction of care in individuals with spinal cord injuries: A qualitative study. *SCI Nursing, 21*(2), 69–74.
McCleod, A. (2004). Traumatic injuries to the head and spine 2: Nursing considerations. *British Journal of Nursing, 13*(17), 1041–1049.
Palmieri, R. (2006). Cerebral artery stenosis paves the way for a stroke. *Nursing, 36*(6), 36–42.
Phillips, K., Ch'ien, A., Norwood, B., & Smith, C. (2003). Chronic low back pain management in primary care. *Nurses Practitioner: American Journal of Primary Care, 28*(8), 26–28, 31.
Porth, C. M. (2005). *Pathophysiology: Concepts of altered health states* (7th ed.). Philadelphia: Lippincott.
Take these steps if you suspect stroke. (2003). *ED Nursing, 6*(5), 55–57.
Tierney, L., McPhee, S., & Papadakis, M. (Eds.). (2005). *Current medical diagnosis & treatment* (43rd ed.). Stamford, CT: Appleton & Lange.
Virtual Hospital. (2005). *The NIH stroke scale.* Retrieved from http://vh.org/adult/provider/neurology/Stroke/Scaleind.html
Wilkinson, J. (2005). *Prentice Hall nursing diagnosis handbook with NIC interventions and NOC outcomes* (8th ed.). Upper Saddle River, NJ: Prentice Hall.
Williams, J. (2005). Advances on prevention and treatment of stroke and TIA. *Nursing Times, 101*(14), 30–32.
Wilson, B., Shannon, M., & Stang, C. (2005). *Prentice Hall nurse's drug guide 2005.* Upper Saddle River, NJ: Prentice Hall.

CHAPTER 46 Nursing Care of Clients with Neurologic Disorders

LEARNING OUTCOMES

- Identify prevalence, incidence, and risk factors for degenerative neurologic, peripheral nervous system, cranial nerve, and infection- and neurotoxin-caused neurologic disorders.

- Explain the pathophysiology, manifestations, complications, interdisciplinary care, and nursing care of clients with neurologic disorders.

- Compare and contrast the manifestations of the progressive stages of Alzheimer's disease.

- Discuss the purposes, nursing implications, and health education for the client and family for medications used to treat Alzheimer's disease, multiple sclerosis, Parkinson's disease, and myasthenia gravis.

- Describe the procedures (thymectomy, percutaneous rhizotomy, plasmapheresis) used to treat selected neurologic disorders.

CLINICAL COMPETENCIES

- Assess functional status of clients with neurologic disorders, and monitor, document, and report abnormal manifestations.

- Use evidence-based research to design nursing interventions specific to the needs of aging clients with multiple sclerosis.

- Determine priority nursing diagnoses, based on assessed data, to select and implement individualized nursing interventions for clients with neurologic disorders.

- Administer oral and injectable medications used to treat neurologic disorders knowledgeably and safely.

- Provide skilled care to clients having a thymectomy, percutaneous rhizotomy, or plasmapheresis.

- Integrate interdisciplinary care into care of clients with neurologic disorders.

- Provide appropriate teaching to facilitate safety and communication, prevent neurologic infections and toxins (rabies, tetanus, and botulism), and facilitate community-based acute and chronic self-care for healthcare needs resulting from neurologic disorders.

- Revise plan of care as needed to provide effective interventions to promote, maintain, or restore functional health status to clients with neurologic disorders.

This chapter discusses a variety of neurologic disorders. Included are degenerative disorders, peripheral nervous system disorders, cranial nerve disorders, and disorders caused by neurotoxins and viruses. For many of the disorders, nursing care is based on similar nursing diagnoses. To avoid repeating those diagnoses and interventions for each disorder, they have been divided among the nursing care discussions as appropriate.

DEGENERATIVE NEUROLOGIC DISORDERS

Degenerative neurologic disorders affect the central nervous system and the peripheral nerves. By progressively disrupting cognitive processes or motor functions, disorders such as Alzheimer's disease, Parkinson's disease, and multiple sclerosis strike at the core of an individual's sense of personal autonomy and well-being and can be psychologically and emotionally devastating to family members and caregivers.

Ongoing medical research into degenerative neurologic disorders offers an increasing measure of hope to clients and their families. The discovery of genetic or biochemical markers associated with some of these disorders is leading to the development of effective screening and diagnostic methods. In addition, new drugs may make it possible to halt the progression of the disorders in some clients, transforming the disorders into manageable conditions. This chapter begins with a discussion of dementia, which is not a specific disease, but rather a collection of manifestations that are caused by a variety of disorders that affect the brain.

DEMENTIA

Dementia affects multiple cortical functions, calculation, learning capacity, language, and judgment. Impairments of cognitive function are usually accompanied by deterioration in emotional control, social behavior, and motivation. People with dementia lose their ability to solve problems, and may also have personality changes such as agitation and hallucinations. All forms of dementia result from death of neurons and/or the loss of communication among the cells. Although the exact cause is not always known, many forms of dementia are characterized by abnormal structures in the brain called inclusions, and there is clearly a genetic component in the development of some kinds of dementia.

It is estimated that as many as 6.8 million people in the United States have dementia, and at least 1.8 million of those are severely affected. Studies of some communities have found that almost half of all people age 85 and older have some form of dementia. However, despite increased incidence in older people, dementia is not a normal part of aging (National Institute of Neurological Disorders and Stroke [NINDS], 2005i).

Many different diseases and conditions may cause dementia, including Alzheimer's disease, vascular dementia, Huntington's disease, Creutzfeldt-Jakob disease, medications, metabolic disorders, poisoning, and anoxia. Table 46–1 provides an overview of the most common causes of dementia. Doctors do not diagnose dementia unless two or more brain functions (such as memory, language skills, perception, reasoning, or judgment) are significantly impaired without loss of consciousness.

Even though the actual cause of all dementias may not be known, factors that increase the risk of developing one or more kinds of dementia have been identified. These risk factors include advancing age, a family history of a disease that causes dementia, smoking and alcohol use, atherosclerosis, high cholesterol and plasma homocysteine levels, diabetes, mild cognitive impairment, and Down syndrome.

Although sometimes confused with dementia, people often experience other conditions that may mimic dementia. These include the following:

- Age-related cognitive decline, resulting from slower information processing and mild memory impairment. With aging, the brain often decreases in volume and some neurons are lost. These changes are normal and are not considered a part of dementia.
- Mild cognitive impairment, which may progress to dementia, but is not severe enough to be initially diagnosed as such.
- Depression or other emotional problems, causing people to be passive, slow, confused, or forgetful.
- Delirium, characterized by confusion, rapidly altering mental states, disorientation, and possible personality changes. Delirium is usually caused by a treatable physical or mental health illness and, when treated, results in a full recovery.

THE CLIENT WITH ALZHEIMER'S DISEASE

Alzheimer's disease (AD) (also called *dementia of Alzheimer type [DAT]* or *senile disease complex*) is a form of dementia characterized by progressive, irreversible deterioration of general intellectual functioning. Clients with AD live about 8 to 10 years following diagnosis, although some live as long as

TABLE 46–1 Common Causes of Dementia

NAME	CAUSE AND PRIMARY PATHOPHYSIOLOGY
Alzheimer's disease (the most common cause of dementia in people age 65 and older)	Unknown cause; characterized by two abnormalities in the brain: amyloid plaques and neurofibrillary tangles.
Vascular dementia (the second most common cause of dementia)	Caused by brain damage from cerebrovascular and cardiovascular problems (usually strokes). May also be caused by cerebral blood vessel damage from genetic disorders, endocarditis, myeloid angiopathy, vasculitis, and profound hypotension.
Lewy body dementia	Cause usually unknown, although familial cases have been reported. Cells die, and remaining cells in the in substantia nigra contain abnormal structures called Lewy bodies.
Frontotemporal dementia	Nerve cells, especially in the frontal and temporal lobes, degenerate. In many people, abnormal tau protein accumulates in neurofibrillary tangles.

20 years. The cause of death is often aspiration pneumonia because of the loss of the ability to swallow late in the disease (NINDS, 2005i).

Memory loss is usually the first sign of Alzheimer's disease. Memory deficits are initially subtle and family members and friends may not suspect a problem until the disease progresses and manifestations become more noticeable. Family members and clients with AD may also deny the manifestations and hide deficits until the person exhibits unsafe or extremely unusual behavior. Progression of the disease varies, but the course is one of deteriorating cognition and judgment with eventual physical decline and total inability to perform activities of daily living (ADLs). With the loss of the ability to perform even the most basic ADLs, the burden of meeting the client's needs shifts to the caregiver.

Incidence and Prevalence

Alzheimer's disease is the most common degenerative neurologic disorder and the most common cause of cognitive impairment in older adults (Porth, 2005). It accounts for about two-thirds of cases of dementia in America, affecting adults in middle to late life.

Two types of AD exist: *Familial AD* follows an inheritance pattern and *sporadic AD* has no obvious inheritance pattern. AD is further described as early onset (occurring in people younger than 65) and late onset (occurring in people age 65 and older). Early onset AD affects people ages 30 to 60, is relatively rare, and often progresses more rapidly than late-onset AD.

FAST FACTS
Alzheimer's Disease
- Scientists estimate that more than 4.5 million people have AD, usually beginning after age 60, with the risk increasing with age (Alzheimer's Foundation, 2005).
- One in 10 people over the age of 65 and almost one-half of all people over age 85 have AD.
- Each year, at least 360,000 people are diagnosed with AD, and about 50,000 are reported to die from it.
- Early onset forms of AD, which are usually genetic, may appear as early as age 30.

Source: NINDS, 2005i.

Risk Factors and Warning Signs

As one ages, the risk of developing AD increases. With numbers of older people increasing, the incidence of AD is predicted to also increase. The risk factors for AD are older age, family history, and female gender. Warning signs are:
- Memory loss that affects job skills
- Difficulty performing familiar tasks
- Problems with language
- Disorientation to time and place
- Poor or decreased judgment
- Problems with abstract thinking
- Misplacing things
- Changes in mood or behavior
- Changes in personality
- Loss of initiative.

Recognizing early manifestations is important, because the cause of dementia (such as from depression or hypothyroidism) may be reversible. Further information can be obtained from the Alzheimer's Association. Dementia from AD is not reversible. Treatment, however, can maximize quality of life and allow the affected person to plan for the future.

Pathophysiology

Characteristic findings in the brains of AD clients are loss of nerve cells and the presence of *neurofibrillary tangles* and *amyloid plaques* (Figure 46–1 ■). Neurofibrillary tangles result when *tau*, a kind of protein in the neurons, becomes distorted and twisted. Tau normally holds together the microtubules, which guide nutrients and molecules to the end of the axon. In AD, tau changes and twists into pairs of filaments, which then join to form tangles. Because tau no longer maintains the transport system, communication is lost between neurons. Death of neurons may follow, contributing to the development of dementia.

Groups of nerve cells (and especially the terminal axons) degenerate and clump around an amyloid core as plaques, found in the spaces between the neurons of the brain. These plaques, which develop first in areas used for memory and cognition, disrupt transmission of nerve impulses. The plaques consist primarily of insoluble deposits of beta-amyloid, a protein fragment from a larger protein called amyloid precursor protein, mixed with other neurons and nonnerve cells. It is not

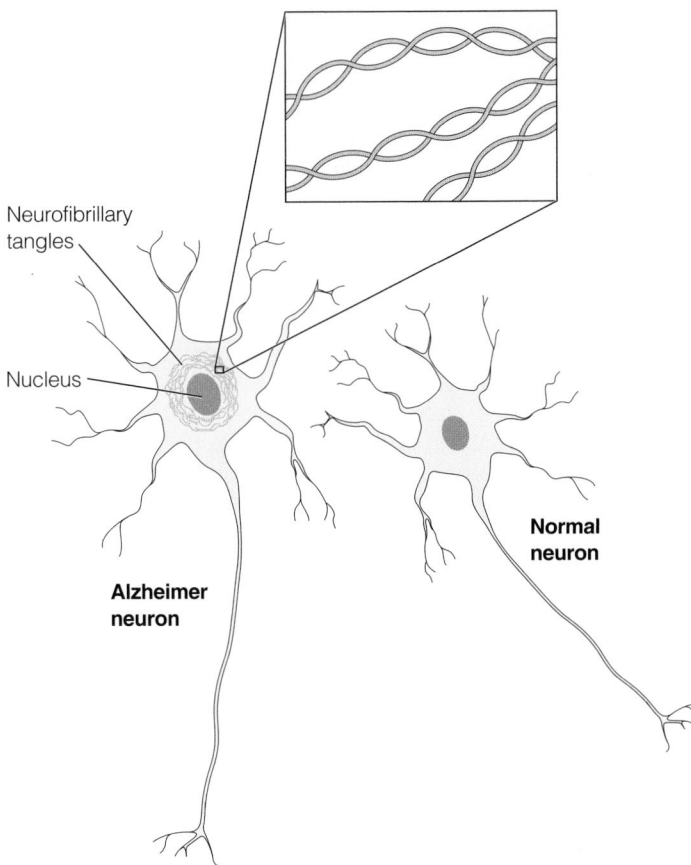

Figure 46–1 ■ Neuron with neurofibrillary tangles seen in Alzheimer's disease.

yet known if plaque formation causes AD or if plaques are a by-product of the AD process.

Blood flow to the affected areas of the brain is decreased. The brain atrophies, and corresponding enlargement of ventricles and sulci is evident (Figure 46–2 ■). As AD progresses, more areas of the brain are affected, with manifestations correlating to those affected areas of the brain. For example, neuronal and neurotransmitter losses in the parietal lobe result in problems with perception and interpretation of environmental stimuli; deficits in the frontal lobe cause changes in personality and emotional lability.

AD is characterized by atrophy of the cortical area of the brain and loss of neurons, especially in the parietal and temporal lobes. With significant atrophy and loss of brain tissue, the ventricles enlarge (a form of hydrocephalus) (Porth, 2005). Several structural and chemical changes in the brain occur with AD, especially in the hippocampus and the frontal and temporal lobes of the cerebral cortex. As AD destroys neurons in the hippocampus and related structures, short-term memory fails and the ability to perform easy and familiar tasks declines. The effect of AD on neurons in the cerebral cortex is loss of language skills and judgment. Emotional outbursts and behavior changes (such as wandering and agitation) begin to occur and become more frequent as the disease progresses. Eventually, other areas of the brain are affected; all affected areas begin to atrophy, and the person becomes totally helpless and unresponsive.

The exact cause of AD is unknown. Theories include a decrease in choline acetyltransferase activity in the cortex and hippocampus. This enzyme is necessary for the synthesis of acetylcholine, a neurotransmitter associated with memory. The decrease in choline acetyltransferase is about equal to the severity of AD. Other theories include a mutation for encoding amyloid precursor protein, and alteration in apolipoprotein E. Other possible causes are gene defects on chromosomes 14, 19, or 21, which may lead to clumping and precipitation of insoluble amyloid as plaques. The role of protein kinase C, the link between AD and aluminum, a viral cause, an autoimmune cause, and mitochondrial defects that alter cell metabolism and protein processing are being studied.

Manifestations

Alzheimer's disease is classified into three stages based on the client's manifestations and abilities, as outlined in the box on page 1620. It is important to note that the progression of AD varies for each individual and may not precisely follow the model.

Stage 1 AD

In stage 1, a client typically appears physically healthy and alert, and cognitive deficits can go undetected unless thorough and periodic evaluations are performed. Clients may seem restless, forgetful, or uncoordinated; they may lack spontaneity, and be disoriented as to time and date. Usually, family members are the first to notice lapses in memory, subtle changes in personality, or problems in doing simple calculations. AD clients and families may consciously or unconsciously compensate for cognitive deficits by adjusting schedules and routines.

Stage 2 AD

In stage 2, memory deficits are more apparent, and the client is less able to behave spontaneously. Clients may wander and get

Figure 46–2 ■ Changes in neuroanatomy associated with Alzheimer's disease. Note areas of cortical atrophy, narrowing of the gyri, enlargement of sulci, and ventricular dilation.

MANIFESTATIONS of Alzheimer's Disease

STAGE 1: APPROXIMATELY 2 TO 4 YEARS

- Short-term memory loss: Forgets location and names of objects and has difficulty learning new information; long-term memory is unaffected.
- Decreased attention span.
- Subtle personality changes: Lacks spontaneity; denial, irritability, and depression are possible.
- Mild cognitive deficits: Attempts to adjust to and cover up memory loss.
- Visuospatial deficits: Some problems with depth perception.

STAGE 2: APPROXIMATELY 2 TO 12 YEARS

- Impaired cognition: Obvious memory deficits and confusion; loss of abstract thinking; astereognosis and agraphia; inability to do math calculations; loss of ability to tell time and time disorientation, manifested as "sundowning"; wandering behavior.

- Personality changes: Becomes easily agitated and irritable; may have delusions or hallucinations.
- Visuospatial deficits: Is unable to dress self; has poor spatial orientation.
- Impaired motor skills: Paces and is restless at times; motor apraxia is evident when using familiar objects.
- Impaired judgment: Diminished social skills; inability to drive a car; inability to make decisions (e.g., choose clothing).

STAGE 3: APPROXIMATELY 2 TO 4 YEARS OR LONGER

- Cognitive abilities grossly decreased or absent: Is usually disoriented to time, place, and person.
- Communication skills usually absent: Is frequently mute.
- Motor skills grossly impaired or absent: Limb rigidity and posture flexion; bowel and bladder incontinence.

---

lost, even in their own homes. Although progression of manifestations continues and orientation to place and time deteriorates, AD clients may still have periods of mental lucidity and engage in time-oriented conversations. Generally, however, clients become more confused and lose their sense of time, leading to changes in sleeping patterns, agitation, and stress. They may demonstrate repetitive behavior and eat ravenously. AD clients are less able to make even simple decisions and to adapt to environmental changes, and are often unable to carry out ADLs. **Sundowning** is another behavioral change, characterized by increased agitation, time disorientation, and wandering behaviors during afternoon and evening hours; it is accelerated on overcast days.

Language deficits are common in stage 2. They include *paraphasia* (using the wrong word), *echolalia* (repetition of words or phrases), and *scanning speech,* in which the client appears to search for words. Eventually, total *aphasia* (absence of speech) may occur. Frustration and depression are common among AD clients as the full extent and implications of the deficits become obvious.

The AD client slowly loses the ability to perform simple tasks required for hygiene or eating because sequencing of tasks is lost. For example, the client may open a can of soup but not remember to pour it into a pan to heat it. Instead, the client might place the can directly on the burner and leave the heat on high even after a smoke alarm sounds. The AD client may falsely interpret the smoke alarm as a telephone ringing, a tornado warning siren, or an ambulance siren. Thus, safety is a high priority for the client in stage 2.

Sensorimotor deficits in stage 2 include *apraxia,* the inability to perform purposeful movements and use objects correctly; *astereognosis,* the inability to identify objects by touch; and *agraphia,* the inability to write properly. Problems related to malnutrition and decreased fluid intake, such as anemia and constipation, may be evident. Sleep pattern disturbances are also common and are related to the loss of time orientation, sundowning phenomenon, and depression.

Stage 3 AD

Stage 3 brings increasing dependence, with inability to communicate, loss of urinary and fecal continence, and progressive loss of cognitive abilities. Common complications include pneumonia, dehydration, malnutrition, falls, depression, delusions, seizures, and paranoid reactions. AD clients are indifferent to food and lose weight. They are unable to recognize family or friends, or even themselves. The average life expectancy is 1 to 2 years from the onset of stage 3, although the individual may live as long as 10 years. Most people with AD are institutionalized during this final stage of the disease. Death frequently occurs from pneumonia secondary to aspiration.

INTERDISCIPLINARY CARE

There is no cure for AD, and the main objective of care is to provide an environment that matches the client's functional abilities. Nurses, physicians, physical therapists, and social workers collaborate with the client's family to provide the least restrictive environment in which the client can safely function.

Diagnosis

Alzheimer's disease is diagnosed by ruling out causes for the client's manifestations. The only definitive method of diagnosis is postmortem examination of brain tissue. An extensive workup is especially important, because the dementia may be due to a reversible or treatable condition. For example, an older client's misuse of medications can lead to overdosing and resulting confusion. Other categories of conditions that may be considered and ruled out include depression, infection, hypothyroidism, dehydration, heart disease, stroke, and chronic obstructive respiratory disease. Mental status is assessed with tests such as the Folstein Mini Mental Status Examination. This examination assesses areas of function such as the client's orientation to time, ability to repeat back a series of words, ability to name objects, and ability to follow written instructions.

MEDICATION ADMINISTRATION The Client with Alzheimer's Disease

CHOLINERGIC (PARASYMPATHOMIMETICS);
CHOLINESTERASE INHIBITORS
Tacrine hydrochloride (Cognex)
Donepezil hydrochloride (Aricept)
Rivastigmine tartrate (Exelon)
In the early stages of AD, the pathologic changes in neurons result in a deficiency of acetylcholine (a key neurotransmitter involved in cognitive functioning). Cholinesterase inhibitors slow the breakdown of acetylcholine release by the remaining intact neurons. In addition, rivastigmine tartrate inhibits the G_1 form of acetylcholinesterase (found in higher levels in the brain of clients with AD), so less acetylcholine is degraded. The drugs are used to improve memory in mild to moderate AD dementia.

Nursing Responsibilities
- Administer tacrine hydrochloride 1 hour before meals, if possible.
- Administer donepezil hydrochloride at bedtime.
- Administer rivastigmine tartrate (both capsules and liquid) with food. Liquid form may be administered undiluted or mixed with water, juice, or soda. Stir to completely dissolve.
- Monitor for jaundice, increased bilirubin levels, and other signs of liver involvement, such as rising serum aminotransferase

(AST, ALT) levels. Therapy is usually decreased when the enzyme level exceeds four times normal limits and discontinued when the level reaches five times normal.
- Observe for gastrointestinal bleeding and gastric ulcer pain.
- Monitor for cholinergic-related problems: bladder outlet obstruction, seizures, and slowed cardiac rate.
- Assist with ambulation because dizziness is a common side effect.
- Monitor glycemic control in clients with diabetes.
- Assess for improvement in AD symptoms, especially in reasoning, memory, and ADLs.

Health Education for the Client and Family
- Notify the physician promptly if jaundice, seizures, slowed heart rate, GI bleeding, or difficulty urinating occurs.
- Follow directions for times and instructions about administration of specific medication.
- Follow your healthcare provider's recommendation for periodic EEG, blood tests, and urine tests.
- These medications do not cure AD, and will at some point become ineffective as the disease progresses.

Guidelines for the early recognition and assessment of AD have been established by the Agency for Healthcare Research and Quality. A diagnosis of Alzheimer's disease requires the documented presence of dementia, onset between age 40 and 90 years (most often after age 65), no loss of consciousness, and absence of systemic or brain disorders that could cause mental changes.

Medications

There is no cure for AD, but some medications are effective in slowing the progression of the disease. Tacrine hydrochloride (Cognex) was the first medication specifically approved for the treatment of AD. Donepezil hydrochloride (Aricept) is used to treat mild to moderate AD dementia with some success. Rivastigmine tartrate (Exelon) is also used to treat mild to moderate AD manifestations. It improves the ability to carry out ADLs, decreases agitation and delusions, and improves cognitive function. Galantamine hydrobromide (Reminyl) is believed to increase the concentration of acetylcholine in the central nervous system (CNS) as treatment of mild to moderate AD. Memantine (Namenda) improves cognitive function in moderate-to-severe AD and mild-to-moderate vascular dementia. Memantine acts by blocking receptors for glutamate, resulting in decreased calcium accumulation into neurons (increased calcium accumulation damages neurons). See the box above for information about selected medications used to treat AD.

Depression often accompanies AD and is treated with the appropriate medication. Antihistamines and tricyclic antidepressants that have high anticholinergic activity are usually avoided because they can increase AD manifestations. Occasionally clients with AD require tranquilizers such as thioridazine (Mellaril) or haloperidol (Haldol) to manage severe agitation. Other

therapies under study to prevent or delay the onset of AD include antioxidants such as vitamin E, anti-inflammatory agents, and antihypertensive drugs to lower hypertension.

Alternative and Complementary Therapy

The following types of alternative and complementary therapies may be used in treating the manifestations of AD.
- Massage, which decreases agitation
- Herbs:
  - Ginkgo biloba and vitamin E, which are thought to improve cognition
  - Huperzine A, a traditional Chinese medicine, which acts as an acetylcholinesterase inhibitor
- Coenzyme Q10, an antioxidant that naturally occurs in the body
- Supplements, such as zinc, selenium, and evening primrose oil
- Therapies involving art, music, sound, and dance.

NURSING CARE

Clients with AD often require intensive, supportive nursing interventions directed at the physical and psychosocial responses to illness. Equally important, the nurse can facilitate the long-term support of these clients by providing teaching and referrals to follow-up care in the community. A Nursing Care Plan for the client with AD is found on the next page.

Health Promotion

Health promotion for the client with AD focuses on maintaining functional abilities and safety. If the client will be cared for at home, address safety considerations (see the box

NURSING CARE PLAN   A Client with AD

Arthur and Ruth Joste, both age 73, have been married for 47 years; he is a retired history teacher, and she has been a home-maker. They have four children; two live in the same town, and two live out of state. Arthur has noticed that he is having problems remembering friends' names and phone numbers; his wife has been asking him if he is driving in the correct direction when they go shopping.

Mrs. Joste has severe osteoarthritis and is unable to lift heavy objects or perform all but light housekeeping tasks. For about 18 months, Mrs. Joste has been aware of her husband's progressive cognitive decline, including forgetting current news from last night's newspaper; miscalculating checkbook balances; neglect-ing his hygiene needs; and confusing their children's and grand-children's names. The Jostes are referred to a neurologist for evaluation.

ASSESSMENT

Martha Spital, RN, assesses Mr. Joste at the neurologist's office. She notes that he is unable to recall his home address without prompting, to name the correct date (although he does know the day of the week), to subtract serial 7s more than twice, and to re-call two of three objects. He is alert to his surroundings. Mrs. Joste states that the problems seem to be getting worse with time and that she has had to "cover up" mistakes for her husband. Mr. Joste seems easily agitated, and his wife reports that his sleep habits are "jumbled"; he has long periods of wakefulness in the night-time hours.

Following a thorough evaluation and diagnostic testing to rule out other possible disorders, the neurologist tells the couple that Mr. Joste has probable dementia of the Alzheimer's type. Both have feared this diagnosis; they want to know how they can be sure that Mr. Joste has this disease and what they can do to pre-vent further decline. Both are obviously much saddened, and they verbalize their feelings of being overwhelmed. The Jostes intend to remain in their home "for as long as we can."

DIAGNOSES

- *Chronic Confusion* related to deterioration of brain function and dementia
- *Self-Care Deficits* related to forgetfulness and declining physi-cal abilities
- *Risk for Injury* related to decreased orientation
- *Disturbed Sleep Pattern* related to time disorientation
- *Caregiver Role Strain* (wife) related to need to care for self and husband

EXPECTED OUTCOMES

- Remain free of injury.
- Navigate home environment with modifications as needed.
- Participate in grooming and hygiene activities with prompting and supervision.
- Obtain a minimum of 7 uninterrupted hours of sleep a night.
- Mrs. Joste will participate in a minimum of two out-of-home activities a week.

PLANNING AND IMPLEMENTATION

The home health nurse, Erick Montane, RN, makes a home visit to evaluate the environment, assess available support, and deter-mine needs. He meets two of the Jostes' children, Dawn and Jay,

who live in the same community and are willing to participate as much as possible in providing care and modifying the home.

Mr. Montane discusses the importance of establishing and maintaining a consistent daily routine. He emphasizes the impor-tance of matching activities to Mr. Joste's mental abilities to avoid frustration and increased agitation. Mr. Montane recommends la-beling drawers with their contents, such as Mr. Joste's sock drawer. Labeling rooms may eventually be necessary.

Because his inability to comprehend and process information distresses and agitates Mr. Joste, Mr. Montane teaches the family to modify their communications to fit Mr. Joste's cognitive ability, such as using simple, direct statements and directions.

Mr. Montane recommends that family members keep back-ground noise to a minimum because this may be a source of confusion.

After assessing the home, Mr. Montane makes the following recommendations about safety:

- Remove throw rugs from hallways, and tack down any re-maining carpets.
- Secure the kitchen, bathroom, and workshop cabinets as well as the controls on the oven and stove.
- Modify the doors so that negotiating locks requires a two-step system of unlocking, such as with a deadbolt and a key.
- Provide extra lighting in dark areas, especially a night-light in the bathroom.

Mr. Montane explains that Mrs. Joste will need assistance with housekeeping as Mr. Joste continues to decline. Mr. Montane pro-vides referrals to community services, including Meals-on-Wheels, which can supply a daily meal. He also suggests that the Jostes obtain the services of a home health aide to provide daily hygiene care. Most of the remaining home maintenance needs can be met with the children's help.

Mr. and Mrs. Joste and the two children attend the weekly lo-cal support group meetings for Alzheimer's disease and related disorders for approximately 3 months; thereafter, Mrs. Joste at-tends with her daughter.

EVALUATION

Six months after the initial home visit and family planning session, Mr. Joste:

- Has not had a fall, burn, or other injury.
- Has periods of confusion when outside his home, but 90% of the time is oriented to place when at home.
- Has attended several support group meetings until 3 months ago. Currently, his wife attends weekly, and a daughter occa-sionally accompanies her. She has continued to participate in their church and maintains contact with a few friends. She is finding it harder to leave her husband unattended for even a few minutes.
- Is able to clean and dress himself with prompting; he is not able to choose his own clothing. If hygiene articles are "set up" (e.g., if the toothpaste is placed on the toothbrush), he re-members to perform the hygiene activity. The children have been replacing buttons and zippers with Velcro closures on his clothing.
- Sleeps an average of 6 hours a night with a 30-minute nap in the afternoon; this pattern is consistent with his previous sleep pattern.

NURSING CARE PLAN   A Client with AD (continued)

- Has seemed to be more easily agitated for the past month. He wanders from room to room, apparently looking for something. These behaviors are worse in the evening and on cloudy days. Mrs. Joste acknowledges her progressive inability to care for her husband.

CRITICAL THINKING IN THE NURSING PROCESS

1. Develop a tool to teach safety needs for the client and family with Alzheimer's disease.

2. List five interventions to decrease agitation in cognitively impaired older adults; give three additional examples of activities suited to an older adult with AD who has osteoarthritis.

3. You are caring for a client in stage 2 Alzheimer's disease. She is 65 inches (165 cm) tall and weighs 132 lb (59.9 kg); she has lost 3 lb within the past month. The client has difficulty focusing on eating and is easily agitated. Describe your plan for ensuring that she has adequate nutrition.
See Evaluating Your Response in Appendix C.

---

below) as well as the caregivers' abilities to meet the client's basic needs, such as maintaining hygiene and other ADLs. Adapt nursing interventions and teaching to the client's stage of Alzheimer's disease. Nurses also promote health in the caregiver; information about caregiver support systems and respite care should be provided.

Assessment

Collect the following data through the health history and physical examination (see Chapter 43 ∞). Further focused assessments are described with nursing interventions below.

- *Health history:* Family member/caregiver support, living arrangements, ability to carry out ADLs, drug use, work history (e.g., exposure to metals), previous history of multiple strokes, brain injury or brain infection, family history of dementia, sleep pattern, changes in cognition and memory, ability to communicate, changes in behavior.
- *Physical assessment:* Height/weight, orientation, abstract reasoning, mental status.

Nursing Diagnoses and Interventions

During the early stage of AD, nursing care focuses on helping the client make minor adaptations to his or her environment. As

the client becomes progressively unable to manage self-care tasks, more adaptations are required. Equally important, the caregiver needs much support—both physical and psychosocial—as the client becomes increasingly dependent.

Impaired Memory

Impaired memory is an appropriate nursing diagnosis in stage 1 AD. At this stage, techniques to help with the memory loss should be included in teaching for both the client and the caregiver.

- Suggest complementary therapies, such as meditation, massage, or exercise. *These activities can help reduce stress; stress can aggravate memory loss.*
- Suggest using a calendar, keeping lists of reminders, or asking someone else to remind of appointments and events. *Written or verbal reminders are helpful if memory is impaired.*
- Recommend using a medication box labeled with days and times. *A medication box is a good way to remember to take medications.*

> **PRACTICE ALERT**
> *It may be necessary to teach the caregiver how to refill the medication box, or to stress the importance of spot-checking if the client fills it.*

MEETING INDIVIDUALIZED NEEDS   Safety Interventions for the Client with AD

DECREASING THE RISK OF FALLS

- Assess usual environment for hazards, such as throw rugs, electrical cords, and slick floors.
- Observe areas of special concern, such as the bathroom, kitchen, and stairs, and modify as needed; for example, provide skidproof surfaces, and mark stairs to show depth.
- Evaluate muscle strength and gait; consult a physical therapist to plan exercises to increase strength and balance.
- Check shoes for fit and support.
- Inquire about alcohol use and medications that affect balance or cause mobility problems; for example, antihypertensive agents can cause dizziness with position changes.
- Use night-lights and increase daytime lighting in dark areas; such as hallways.
- Keep traffic areas free from clutter.

DECREASING THE INJURIES RELATED TO COGNITIVE IMPAIRMENTS

- Secure items that may be mistakenly ingested, such as cleaning preparations and house plants.
- Modify potentially unsafe areas, such as unenclosed porches.
- Provide double lock systems to outside doors and doors to rooms that are off-limits.
- Protect from fire hazards; for example, make matches and cigarettes inaccessible.
- Fence the yard with a locked gate to prevent wandering.
- Modify the controls on the oven and stove.
- Adjust the water heater to a safe temperature.

GENERAL SAFETY CONSIDERATIONS

- Plan a calling system for emergencies; have children call at about the same time every day as a check.
- Ensure that the cognitively impaired family member has no access to objects in the home such as knives and guns.

- If safety is a concern (such as turning on the stove and forgetting it), suggest using alternatives such as a microwave. Program emergency numbers into the telephone. Ask client to consider a Life-Line telephone program. *These measures can increase safety.*
- Suggest using cues, such as an alarm on a watch or a pocket computer, to trigger actions at designated times. *Cues are often helpful when memory loss is a problem.*

Chronic Confusion

Clients with AD often have memory deficits that make functioning in a nonstructured environment difficult. Many of the nursing interventions for this diagnosis need to be modified over time as the client continues to lose cognitive function.

- Label rooms, drawers, and other items as needed. *Visual cues promote the highest possible degree of independence for the client.*
- Remove potential hazards (such as sharp knives or potentially harmful liquids or chemicals) from the environment. *Ensuring safety is a critical factor in providing care.*
- Keep environmental stimuli to a minimum: Decrease noise levels; speak in a calm, low voice; and take an unhurried approach. *Minimizing sensory input and maintaining a calm manner may decrease anxiety.*
- Begin each interaction by identifying self and calling client by name. See Box 46–1 for other communication techniques. *These techniques provide information for the client with memory loss.*
- Limit questions to those that require a simple yes or no response. *Questions need to be appropriate to the client's ability as decision making and verbal skills decline.*
- Orient to the environment, person, and time as able; place large, easy-to-read calendars and clocks in the client's line of vision. Make references to the season or day of the week when conversing with the client. *Orient the client according to his or her level of ability; orienting to precise time may not be possible in the later stages of AD.*
- Provide boundaries by placing red or yellow tape on the floor. *Boundaries help the client stay within safe areas.*

PRACTICE ALERT
Red and yellow are more easily seen by older adults.

- Provide continuity in nursing staff. *This not only promotes consistency of care for the client but also allows the nurse to determine more accurately changes in the client's condition.*
- Repeat explanations simply and as needed to decrease anxiety. *Loss of short-term memory leads to loss of a point of reference; eventually, AD clients think they are experiencing everything for the first time.*

Anxiety

Managing the AD client's behaviors associated with anxiety, restlessness, and confusion is a major challenge confronting nurses and caregivers. Frequently, clients are relatively calm in the morning hours, only to experience increasing periods of agitation in the afternoon and evening hours. The AD client may even waken from the night's sleep with confusion, fearfulness, or panic attacks.

- Monitor for early behaviors of fatigue and agitation. *Early assessment of problems results in prompt intervention to promote rest or to remove the client from the situation causing anxiety.*
- Remove from situations that are causing increased anxiety, such as noisy activities involving large groups. *High-stimulus situations may increase anxious feelings and agitation.*
- Keep daily routine as consistent as possible. *Providing a structured day enhances feelings of familiarity and decreases stress.*
- Schedule rest periods or quiet times throughout the day. *Fatigue contributes to anxiety and lowers the ability to tolerate stress.*
- Provide quiet activities, such as listening to favorite music, in the afternoon or early evening. *Quiet activities may help decrease sundowning.*
- If confusion and agitation persist or escalate, assess for physical causes such as decreased oxygenation, infections, fatigue, constipation, and electrolyte imbalance. *Physical factors can increase agitation in clients with AD.*
- Use therapeutic touch or gentle hand massage. *These activities induce relaxation and have a calming effect.*

Hopelessness

As the client and family recognize the effect of AD on their lives, they may feel a sense of hopelessness. They may not have the coping skills to deal effectively with the diagnosis and anticipated problems. The increasingly degenerative, irreversible nature of the disorder tends to diminish hope; only the ability to adapt to the many problems can restore it.

- Assess the client's and family's response to the diagnosis and understanding of AD; encourage expression of feelings. *Understanding the client/family's perspective enables the nurse to dispel myths about AD.*

BOX 46–1 Communicating with the Client with AD

- Face the client and talk directly to him or her; call the client by name.
- When first approaching the client, identify yourself.
- Use simple sentences and words with few syllables.
- Speak in a calm, low voice.
- Ask one question at a time. Use questions that require only a yes or no response.
- Keep nonverbal communication relaxed and parallel to the verbal communication.
- Avoid giving the impression of being in a hurry; try to have a relaxed approach.
- Observe for anxiety—wringing hands, pacing, darting eye movements—and alter your approach to decrease anxiety.
- Avoid arguing with clients; do not insist on orienting client to reality; the client's point of reference may not be based in reality.
- Give plenty of time for the client with AD to process what you are trying to say; do not expect clients to perform skills beyond their abilities.
- Repeat explanations in simple terms.

- Provide realistic information about the disorder; provide information at the client/family's level of understanding. *Client and family may need to have separate sessions. Factual information provides a foundation for decision making.*
- Avoid criticizing or judging expressed feelings. *An environment accepting of the expression of real feelings promotes both further expression of feelings and willingness to discuss other issues.*
- Support positive family bonds and enhance communication among family members; promote mutual positive regard. *Strong family relationships can provide direction for living and convey a willingness to share the burden.*
- Encourage the client to make as many decisions as possible. *Self-determination enhances a feeling of control over a situation and may give a sense of hope.*
- Encourage the client and family to seek spiritual guidance that previously inspired hope. *The client's church is a legitimate support system. Belief in God can inspire hope beyond present circumstances.*

Caregiver Role Strain

Most caregivers of clients with AD are spouses or other family members. Because AD is a chronic and eventually debilitating disorder, caregivers may feel overwhelmed by their responsibilities. The caregiving spouse faces not only the responsibility for the client's multiple physical demands but also economic and psychosocial stressors. An area that must be discussed is the ability and safety of the client in driving an automobile. Although it may be necessary, the loss of independence represented by the loss of the ability to drive may further trigger anxiety and anger. Fear of the future, loss of income, loss of companionship and a mate—combined with fatigue—make the caregiver vulnerable. Caregivers may become physically and mentally exhausted and socially isolated because of the overwhelming responsibilities of providing total care to the incapacitated family member.

- Teach the caregivers self-care techniques, such as taking rest periods and avoiding fatigue. *Fatigue adds to stress and potentially leads to poor decision making.*
- Have the caregivers list and regularly take part in physical activities they enjoy, such as walking or swimming. *Regular physical exercise decreases stress.*
- Refer the caregivers to local AD support groups. Suggest books pertinent to the subject. *Explicit suggestions in locating support systems and providing specific information promotes coping.*
- Refer the caregivers to Meals-on-Wheels, home health, respite care, and other community services. *Community agencies can relieve some of the daily care burdens, thus providing time for other activities. Programs that support caregivers have been shown to delay nursing home placement.*
- Ensure the family knows that hospice care is available during the end stages of AD. *Hospice services can support the family during this difficult time.*

Using NANDA, NIC, and NOC

Chart 46–1 shows links between NANDA nursing diagnoses, NIC, and NOC when caring for the client with AD.

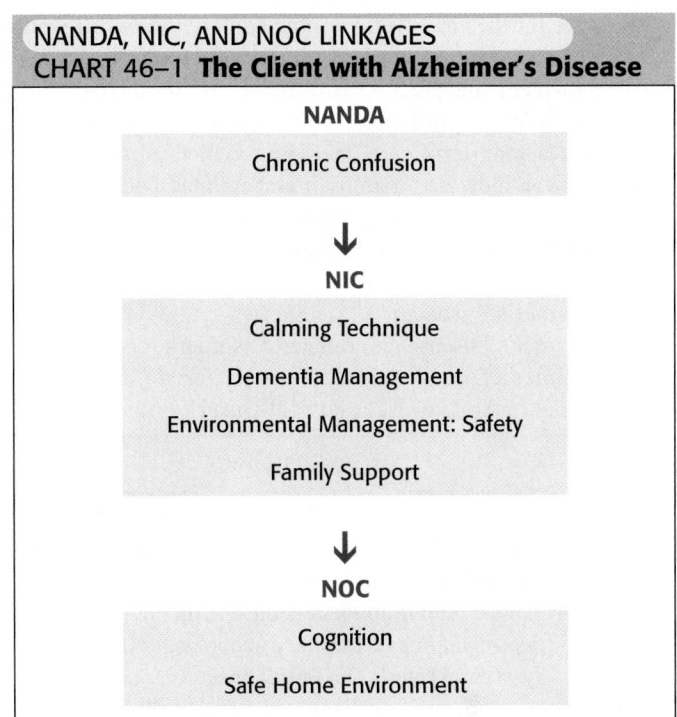

NANDA, NIC, AND NOC LINKAGES
CHART 46–1 The Client with Alzheimer's Disease

NANDA
Chronic Confusion

↓

NIC
Calming Technique
Dementia Management
Environmental Management: Safety
Family Support

↓

NOC
Cognition
Safe Home Environment

Data from *NANDA's Nursing Diagnoses: Definitions & Classification 2005–2006* by NANDA International (2003), Philadelphia; *Nursing Interventions Classification (NIC)* (4th ed.) by J. M. Dochterman & G. M. Bulechek (2004), St. Louis, MO: Mosby; and *Nursing Outcomes Classification (NOC)* (3rd ed.) by S. Moorhead, M. Johnson, and M. Maas (2004), St. Louis, MO: Mosby.

Community-Based Care

Teaching for clients and families centers initially on explaining the disorder and exploring available support systems. Anticipate the need to reexplain the disorder and its consequences, because clients and families may be in shock or denial during the initial period of the disease.

In addition to explaining the anticipated changes with AD, suggest practical solutions to identified problems. It is important to evaluate both the client and caregivers; interventions must be appropriate for the family's situation and resources. Maintaining the least restrictive environment that promotes safety for the client is a major goal of teaching. Using memory cues, such as labeling drawers to indicate the specific types of clothing and labeling rooms, can help orient the client and foster independence. Consistency in the environment and daily routine is an essential part of care. Emphasizing realistic expectations means adjusting care and communication techniques to the client's level of ability.

Address the following topics for home care of the client and for the caregiver:

- Support groups and peer counseling are helpful in handling caregiver stress.
- A person with AD who is confused or agitated is not comfortable and is usually frightened.
- Plan care that matches the person's level of coping, using a consistent routine.
- Provide regular rest periods to decrease the client's stress and fatigue (these do not increase nighttime wandering).

- Plan care for the caregiver. Periodic adult day care or respite care during the initial stages, with plans for increasing assistance to meet the client's daily needs as the disease progresses, may be sufficient. Referrals to the appropriate agency for long-term care, including skilled nursing facilities, may be indicated. Family members may need help adjusting to the idea of extended care but may be relieved to relinquish the physical care needs.
- Suggest the following resources:
  - Alzheimer's Association
  - Alzheimer's Disease and Related Disorders Association
  - Alzheimer's Disease Education and Referral Center
  - National Institute of Neurological Disorders and Stroke.

THE CLIENT WITH MULTIPLE SCLEROSIS

Multiple sclerosis (MS) is a chronic demyelinating neurologic disease of the CNS (brain, optic nerves, and spinal cord), associated with an abnormal immune response to an environmental factor. The manifestations of MS vary according to the area of the nervous system affected. The initial onset may be followed by a total remission, making diagnosis difficult. In about 60% of clients, MS is characterized by periods of exacerbation, when manifestations are highly pronounced, followed by periods of remission, when manifestations are not obvious. The end result, however, is progression of the disease with increasing loss of function.

Incidence and Prevalence

The onset of MS is usually between 20 and 50 years of age, with a peak at age 30. MS is the most prevalent CNS demyelinating disorder, and is a leading cause of neurologic disability in young adults. Although all races are affected, MS is primarily a disease of people of northern European ancestry; however, MS does occur in people of African, Asian, and Hispanic descent. A definite genetic factor has not been established but studies suggest that genetic factors may make some individuals more susceptible than others (National MS Society, 2005).

FAST FACTS
Multiple Sclerosis
- Approximately 400,000 people in the United States have MS; the incidence is 2.5 million worldwide.
- Females are affected two times more often than males, and the incidence is highest in young adults.
- The disease occurs more commonly in temperate climates, including the northern United States. This association is established by approximately age 15, and moving to or from a temperate climate after that age does not change it.

Source: National MS Society, 2005; Porth, 2005.

Pathophysiology

MS is believed to occur as a result of an autoimmune response to a prior viral infection in a genetically susceptible person. The infection, which is thought to occur early in life, activates T cells. T cells usually move in and out of the CNS across the blood–brain barrier, but for an unknown reason, they remain in the CNS in people with MS. The T cells facilitate infiltration by other leukocytes, and an inflammatory process follows. Inflammation destroys myelin and oligodendrocytes (myelin-producing cells), leading to axon dysfunction.

Myelin sheaths are fatty, segmented wrappings that normally protect and insulate nerve fibers and increase the speed of transmission of nerve impulses. In multiple sclerosis, these myelin sheaths of the white matter of the spinal cord, brain, and optic nerve are destroyed in patches, called *plaques,* along the axon (see *Pathophysiology Illustrated* on pages 1628–1629). The demyelination of nerve fibers slows and distorts the conduction of nerve impulses and sometimes results in the total absence of impulse transmission. The neurons usually affected by MS are located in the spinal cord, brainstem, cerebral and cerebellar areas, and the optic nerve.

Both plaques and diffuse lesions form as demyelinating lesions. Plaques typically are scattered through the white matter of the CNS, although they may extend into adjacent gray matter. Early manifestations are the result of inflammatory edema in and around the plaque and partial demyelination. These manifestations typically disappear within weeks after the initial episode. With progression of the disease, the demyelination and plaque formation result in scarring of glia (*gliosis*) and degeneration of axons. Continued loss of function leads to permanent disability, usually over about 20 years.

There are four classifications of MS: relapsing-remitting, primary progressive, secondary progressive, and progressive-relapsing (Box 46–2). Most individuals with MS present with the relapsing-remitting type.

Various stressors have been suggested as triggers for MS. These stressors include febrile states, pregnancy, extreme physical exertion, and fatigue. These precipitating factors can also cause a relapse of the manifestations during the course of the disease.

Manifestations

The manifestations of MS vary according to the areas destroyed by demyelination and the affected body system (see *Multisystems Effects of MS* on page 1630). Fatigue is one of the most disabling manifestations, and affects almost all clients

BOX 46–2 Classifications of Multiple Sclerosis

Relapsing-remitting: The most common clinical course of MS, characterized by exacerbations (acute attacks) with either full recovery or partial recovery with disability.

Primary progressive: Steady worsening of disease from the onset with occasional minor recovery.

Secondary progressive: Begins as with relapsing-remitting, but the disease steadily becomes worse between exacerbations.

Progressive-relapsing: This rare form continues to progress from the onset but also has exacerbations.

with MS. The manifestations, categorized by the established syndromes of MS, are listed in the box below.

Brief attacks of manifestations are described as short lived or paroxysmal. Short-lived attacks of neurologic deficits indicate the appearance or worsening of manifestations. Conditions that cause short-lived attacks include (1) minor increases in body temperature or serum calcium concentrations (both increase the leakage of current through demyelinated neurons) and (2) functional demands that exceed conduction capacity. Paroxysmal attacks are sensory or motor manifestations that occur abruptly and last for only seconds or minutes; the manifestations are paresthesias, dysarthria and ataxia, and tonic head turning. Paroxysmal attacks, which may occur many times a day, result from the direct transmission of nerve impulses between adjacent demyelinated axons.

INTERDISCIPLINARY CARE

Management of the client with MS varies according to the severity of the manifestations. The focus is on retaining the optimal level of functioning possible, given the degree of disability. Rehabilitation—physical, occupational/vocational, and psychosocial—is a cornerstone of an interdisciplinary approach to treatment. During exacerbations, the focus of interventions shifts to controlling manifestations and quickly returning to remission.

Diagnosis

Diagnosis of MS is challenging because the disease does not present uniformly. A diagnosis requires that the client have one of the following: (1) two or more exacerbations separated by 1 month or more and lasting more than 24 hours, followed by recovery; (2) a history of repeated exacerbations and remissions with or without complete recovery, followed by progressively more severe manifestations lasting for 6 months or more; or (3) slowly increasing manifestations for at least 6 months.

Diagnostic tests vary with the presenting complaints. Magnetic resonance imaging (MRI) with findings of lesions is the most definitive test available; however, it is only one of several laboratory and diagnostic tests that may be performed when establishing the diagnosis. Other tests (described in Chapter 43) include:

- Cerebrospinal fluid (CSF) analysis reveals an increased number of T lymphocytes that are reactive with antigens, indicating the presence of an immune response in the client (but is not specific to MS). Of MS patients, 80% have elevated levels of immunoglobulin G (IgG) in the CSF.
- CT scan of the brain shows atrophy and white matter lesions. In about 25% of clients with MS, enlarged ventricles are visible on CT.
- Positron emission tomography (PET) scan measures brain activity. In MS clients, the scan reveals areas with changes in glucose metabolism.
- Evoked response testing of visual, auditory, or somatosensory impulses may show delayed conduction.

Medications

Medications slow the progression of MS and decrease the number of attacks. (See the Medication Administration box on page 1631.) Medications are used for a variety of reasons, including to treat manifestations, to modify the course of the disease, or to interrupt the progression of the disease.

The medications used during an exacerbation are aimed at decreasing inflammation to inhibit manifestations and induce remission. Frequently, a combination of adrenal corticosteroid hormone (ACTH) and glucocorticoids is used to decrease inflammation and suppress the immune system. Immunosuppressive agents, including azathioprine (Imuran) and cyclophosphamide (Cytoxan), are also used. Interferon and glatiramer acetate are used to reduce exacerbations in clients with relapsing-remitting MS. Interferon alpha, beta, and gamma (Roferon-A, Intron A, Wellferon, Infergen, Avonex or Rebif, Betaseron, Actimmune) enhance immune function, while glatiramer acetate (Copaxone) stimulates parts of the myelin basic protein to reduce the relapse rate of MS. Both drugs are given by injection and are usually well tolerated.

Other medications treat the manifestations of MS. Anticholinergics are administered for bladder spasticity; cholinergics

---

MANIFESTATIONS of Multiple Sclerosis

MIXED OR GENERALIZED TYPE (50% OF CASES)
- Visual deficits, with visual blurring, fogginess, or haziness; impaired color perception, decreased central visual acuity, area of diminished vision in the visual fields, acquired color vision deficit (especially to red and green), and an altered pupillary reaction to light.
- Brainstem lesions (cranial nerves III to XII) with nystagmus, dysarthria, deafness, vertigo, vomiting, tinnitus, facial weakness, decreased sensation, diplopia and eye pain; and cognitive dysfunctions involving concentration, short-term memory, word finding, and planning.
- Mood alterations are manifested as depression more often than euphoria.

SPINAL TYPE (25% OF CASES)
- Weakness and/or numbness in one or both extremities (most often the legs).
- Upper motor neuron involvement is manifested by stiffness, slowness, weakness (spastic paresis).
- Bladder dysfunctions include urgency, hesitancy, and incontinence.
- Bowel dysfunction is most often seen as constipation.
- Neurogenic impotence is noted.

CEREBELLAR TYPE (5% OF CASES)
- Manifestations of nystagmus, ataxia, and hyptonia.

AMAUROTIC FORM (5% OF CASES)
- Blindness

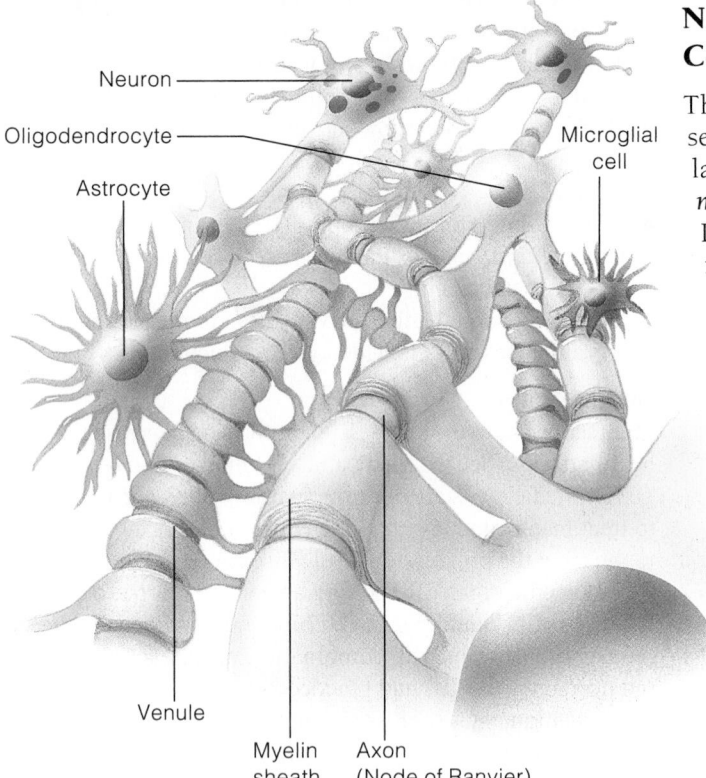

Neuron
Oligodendrocyte
Astrocyte
Microglial cell
Venule
Myelin sheath
Axon (Node of Ranvier)

Normal Anatomy of the Central Nervous System

The central nervous system (CNS) is composed of several cell types arranged in a dense, interconnected lattice. The basic functional cell of the CNS is the *neuron*, which transmits electrochemical impulses. Dendrites, thin projections extending from the neuron body, receive impulses that are passed down the neuronal axon for transmission to other cells. Myelin, a lipid-protein substance, surrounds the axons, insulating them and speeding nerve impulse transmission.

Neurons are surrounded by a network of cells:

- *Astrocytes* support neurons and connnect them to surrounding capillaries and venules.
- *Microglia* are motile phagocytic cells.
- *Oligodendrocytes* wrap concentric layers of myelin around nearby axons.

Acute Attack

Multiple sclerosis (MS) is a demyelinating disease in which axonal myelin in the central nervous system is eroded, destroyed, and replaced by scar tissue.

An autoimmune process apparently triggered by genetic and environmental factors is believed to cause inflammation of venules in the CNS. This disrupts the blood–brain barrier, allowing lymphocytes to enter CNS tissue. These lymphocytes proliferate and produce IgG, an antibody that attacks and damages myelin and causes the release of inflammatory chemicals and edema. As the inflammation subsides, the myelin regenerates and manifestations of the disease subside.

Damaging substances released from macrophages and lymphocytes
Microglial cell ingesting myelin fragment
Macrophage
Lymphocyte
Inflamed myelin sheath

Chronic Lesion

After repeated inflammatory attacks, myelin is irreparably damaged. Segments of axons become totally demyelinated and may degenerate. Astrocytes proliferate in damaged regions of the CNS (a process called *gliosis*), forming plaques. The plaques are scattered throughout the CNS, appearing as gray or pinkish lesions. The relapsing-remitting character of MS and the scattered areas of damage within the CNS account for the variable nature of MS manifestations.

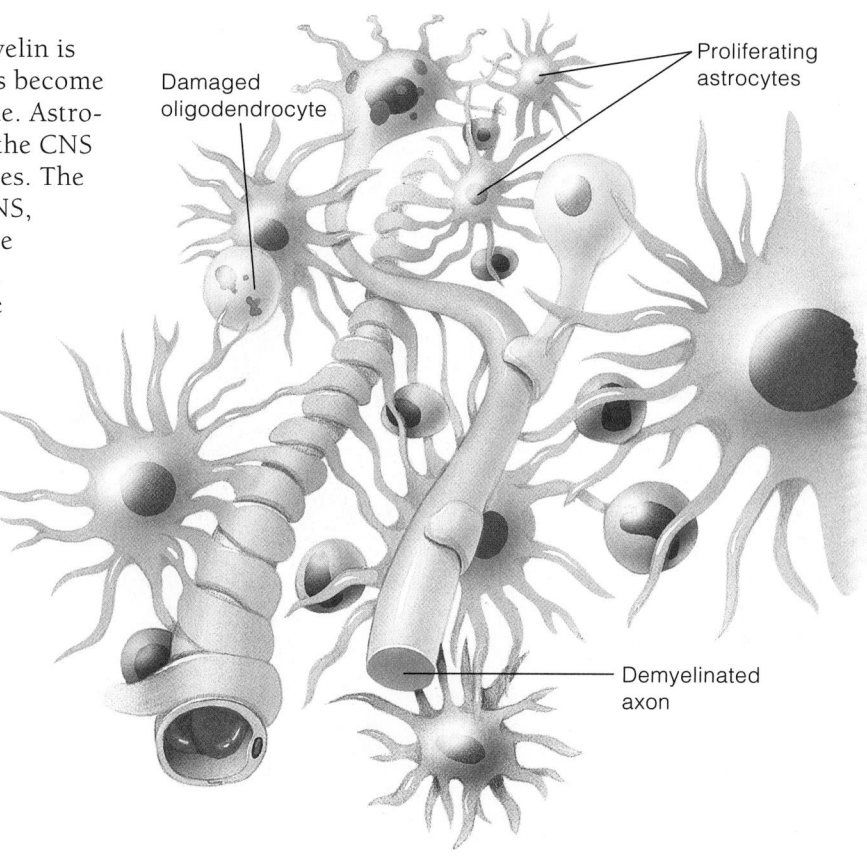

Damaged oligodendrocyte

Proliferating astrocytes

Demyelinated axon

Abnormal Nerve Impulse Transmission

In an undamaged neuron, nerve impulses travel down the axon by "leaping" from one node of Ranvier to the next, thus greatly increasing the speed of impulse transmission. When nerve impulses travel down an axon damaged by MS, they are significantly slowed and weakened as they pass across the surface of demyelin- ated areas. Impulses may be blocked entirely when axons degenerate. The weakening or interruption of the transmission of nerve impulses and plaque formation within the CNS cause the manifestations of MS, including extremity weakness, paresthesias, visual disturbances, bladder dysfunction, and vertigo.

MULTISYSTEM EFFECTS OF **Multiple Sclerosis**

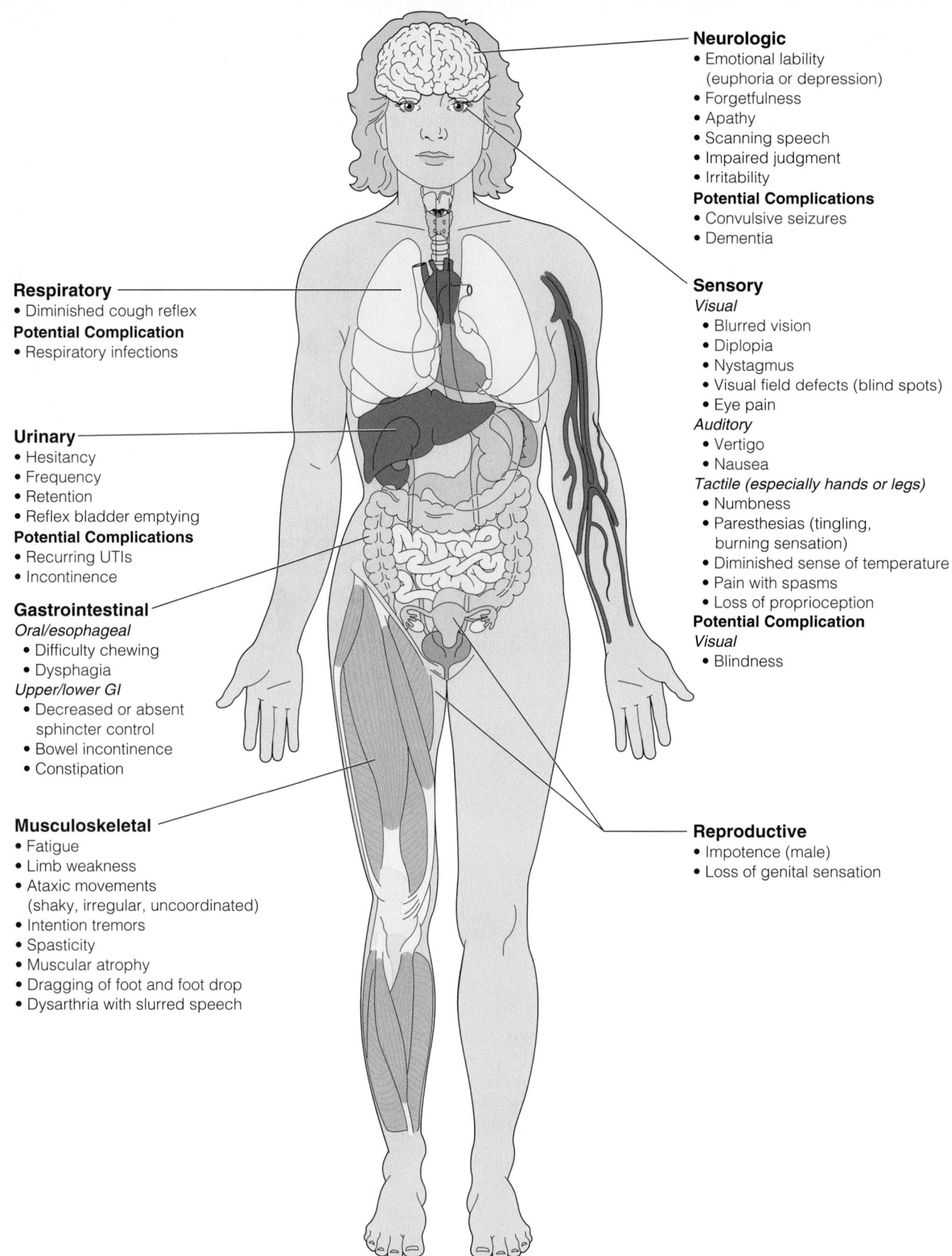

Neurologic
- Emotional lability
  (euphoria or depression)
- Forgetfulness
- Apathy
- Scanning speech
- Impaired judgment
- Irritability

Potential Complications
- Convulsive seizures
- Dementia

Sensory

Visual
- Blurred vision
- Diplopia
- Nystagmus
- Visual field defects (blind spots)
- Eye pain

Auditory
- Vertigo
- Nausea

Tactile (especially hands or legs)
- Numbness
- Paresthesias (tingling,
  burning sensation)
- Diminished sense of temperature
- Pain with spasms
- Loss of proprioception

Potential Complication

Visual
- Blindness

Respiratory
- Diminished cough reflex

Potential Complication
- Respiratory infections

Urinary
- Hesitancy
- Frequency
- Retention
- Reflex bladder emptying

Potential Complications
- Recurring UTIs
- Incontinence

Gastrointestinal

Oral/esophageal
- Difficulty chewing
- Dysphagia

Upper/lower GI
- Decreased or absent
  sphincter control
- Bowel incontinence
- Constipation

Musculoskeletal
- Fatigue
- Limb weakness
- Ataxic movements
  (shaky, irregular, uncoordinated)
- Intention tremors
- Spasticity
- Muscular atrophy
- Dragging of foot and foot drop
- Dysarthria with slurred speech

Reproductive
- Impotence (male)
- Loss of genital sensation

MEDICATION ADMINISTRATION   The Client with Multiple Sclerosis

IMMUNOMODULATORS
Interferon beta-1a (Avonex)
Interferon beta-1b (Betaseron)
Glatiramer acetate (Copaxone, Copolymer-1)

Interferon beta-la, interferon beta-1b, and glatiramer acetate are administered to clients with relapsing-remitting MS to prolong the time of onset to disability. Their use is based on the assumption that MS is an immunologically mediated disease. Interferon beta-1b produces a decrease in the MS lesions in some clients. Some clients, however, develop a decrease in the absolute neutrophil count and increases in the levels of liver enzymes. Anxiety, confusion, and depression with suicidal tendencies also have been reported. Other adverse reactions include pain, inflammation, hypersensitivity at the injection site, and generalized flulike manifestations. Some women experience menstrual disorders. Pregnant women should not take these medications.

Nursing Responsibilities
- Assess baseline parameters to evaluate drug side effects: psychologic profile, liver function tests, and CBC with differential.
- Monitor CBC and liver function tests every 3 months or as prescribed.
- Assess injection site and report ulceration promptly (pain and redness are common reactions).
- Evaluate client's baseline neurologic, sensory, and motor function. Monitor changes in condition and function.
- Report if client is pregnant or breast-feeding.

Health Education for the Client and Family
- These drugs may cause depression and thoughts of suicide; report these feelings immediately to the physician.
- Administer medication within 3 hours of reconstitution. Rotate injection sites, and avoid any areas that are red or show other skin reactions.
- Seek follow-up care to monitor neurologic changes, CBC, and liver function.
- Avoid prolonged exposure to sunlight.

ADRENALCORTICOSTEROID THERAPY
Adrenocorticotropic hormone (ACTH) (Acthar)
Prednisone (Deltasone, Meticorten, Orasone)
Methylprednisolone (Medrol, Solu-Medrol)

Adrenalcorticosteroids are used both to sustain a remission and to treat exacerbations of MS. ACTH is usually given to induce a remission; It is administered intravenously for 1 week and may be followed by oral prednisone therapy. Another protocol involves administering ACTH intravenously for 3 days followed by intramuscular injections every 12 hours for 1 week (Hickey, 2003). The drugs are given to suppress the immune system, implicated in the etiology of MS. If the drug is used long term the usual steroid precautions are indicated, such as monitoring for glucose intolerance, osteoporosis, and cataract formation. The drugs are used with caution in pregnant and lactating women.

MUSCLE RELAXANTS
Baclofen (Lioresal)
Dantrolene (Dantrium)
Diazepam (Valium)

Muscle relaxants are given to clients with MS to relieve muscle spasms. Baclofen and diazepam act by suppressing CNS reflexes that regulate muscle activity; neither drug affects muscle strength. Baclofen therapy should be discontinued over 1 to 2 weeks; sudden withdrawal may cause seizures and paranoid ideation. In contrast to diazepam and baclofen, dantrolene acts directly on skeletal muscles, and it may affect muscle strength. Dantrolene may cause hepatotoxicity and should not be administered when hepatitis or cirrhosis is present.

Nursing Responsibilities
- Evaluate baseline muscle strength and spasticity, ROM, and dexterity.
- Maintain safety or fall precautions; dizziness and drowsiness are common side effects.
- For the client taking dantrolene, monitor liver function tests (enzymes and bilirubin) for signs of hepatotoxicity.

Health Education for the Client and Family
- These drugs may cause sedative effects. Take appropriate safety measures (e.g., avoid driving).
- Avoid CNS depressants (antihistamines, alcohol); they can increase the sedative effects of the medication.
- Continue follow-up care; if you are taking dantrolene, for example, liver function will need to be monitored.
- If you are taking baclofen, do not suddenly stop the medication.
- Increase fiber and fluids in the diet to prevent constipation.
- Change positions slowly to minimize dizziness and other effects of orthostatic hypotension.

IMMUNOSUPPRESSANTS
Azathioprine (Imuran)
Cyclophosphamide (Cytoxan)

Immunosuppressants are given to clients with MS because of the autoimmune component of the disease. Both medications can cause bone marrow suppression and increase the risk of cancer. Azathioprine may produce hepatitis. Toxic effects of cyclophosphamide include hemorrhagic cystitis, sterility, and stomatitis.

Nursing Responsibilities
- Monitor baseline parameters: CBC with platelet count and differential, urinalysis, liver function tests, hepatitis profile.
- Assess for anemia: fatigue, lethargy, pallor.
- Watch for bleeding.
- Protect against and observe for subtle signs of infection.

Health Education for the Client and Family
- Report infection, bleeding, and anemia immediately.
- Drink at least 2 L (2 quarts) of fluid a day, and observe urine for blood.
- Report jaundice immediately.
- Check oral cavity daily for changes or ulcers.
- Avoid becoming pregnant while taking these drugs.
- Obtain follow-up care, including frequent blood tests.

are given if the client has a problem with urinary retention related to flaccid bladder. Depression is treated with antidepressant drugs.

Surgery

Surgery may be indicated for clients who experience severe spasticity and deformity. However, physical therapy can prevent most severe problems. Foot drop from severe plantar flexion can be relieved with an Achilles tenotomy, a surgical procedure in which the Achilles tendon is transected.

Nutrition and Fluids

Several diets involving manipulation of fats are currently under investigation. Clients with MS may be overweight because of their inability to ambulate; depression may contribute to the problem because people who are depressed tend to eat more. Ideally, the client should maintain a weight as close as possible to that recommended for the client's height and body type.

As MS progresses, the client's ability to prepare food and eat is compromised. Changes in muscle tone, tremor, weakness, and ataxia all contribute to nutritional problems. Dysphagia also is a common problem. The diet must be adapted to accommodate changes in the client's ability to chew and swallow.

Rehabilitation

Physical and rehabilitative therapies are tailored to the client's level of functioning. The long-term goal is to enable the client to retain as much independence as possible. One major intervention is to maintain and increase existing muscle strength.

Spasticity is managed with stretching exercises, gait training, and braces, splints, or other assistive devices. To maintain balance, the client is encouraged to widen the base of support by standing with the feet slightly further apart. Walkers and canes may be weighted to provide support and balance for the ataxic client.

An interdisciplinary approach to rehabilitation will provide supportive services: speech therapy for problems with phonation, occupational therapy to maintain strength in the upper extremities and carry out ADLs, and occupational counseling. Referrals to a urologist are indicated for problems with urinary incontinence, urinary tract infections, retention, and impotence. Consultation with a respiratory therapist may be needed if the client develops chronic respiratory infections from inability to cough, move secretions, or breathe deeply, especially with increased debilitation.

✳ NURSING CARE

Because the disease most often affects young adults in the prime of life, the psychosocial and economic effect can be devastating. People with MS have to make adjustments to the body image changes while simultaneously adapting to the altered relationships and decreased earnings usually encountered with the disease. A once-healthy spouse becomes wheelchair bound; a person once independent may eventually become dependent for even the most basic ADLs. The unpredictable course of MS is a challenge for long-term planning. A Nursing Care Plan for the client with MS is given on the next page.

Health Promotion

Following an overview of the disorder, the client needs to understand how to prevent fatigue and exacerbations. Teach the client to avoid stress, extremes of cold and heat, high humidity, physical overexertion, and infections. Because pregnancy can exacerbate manifestations, counseling about this risk is indicated. Also, address preventive measures to avoid risk of respiratory and urinary tract infections.

Assessment

Collect the following data through the health history and physical examination (see Chapter 43 ∞):
- *Health history:* History of childhood viral illnesses, geographical residence when a child, exposure to physical or emotional stressors (pregnancy/delivery, extremes of heat), medications, symptom onset, severity of manifestations.
- *Physical assessment:* Affect, mood, speech, eye movements, gait, tremors, vision and hearing, reflexes, muscle strength and movement, sensation.

Nursing Diagnoses and Interventions

Interventions for the client with MS vary with the acuity of exacerbations and the presenting problems. Many nursing diagnoses relate to the inability to perform ADLs, for example, *Self-Care Deficit* and *Impaired Home Maintenance*. Others reflect problems with musculoskeletal changes or altered nerve conduction, for example, *Impaired Physical Mobility*, *Ineffective Breathing Pattern*, *Constipation*, and *Functional Urinary Incontinence*. The nursing diagnoses discussed in this section are *Fatigue* and *Self-Care Deficit*.

Fatigue

Fatigue is defined by NANDA as an overwhelming sustained sense of exhaustion and decreased capacity for physical and mental work at the usual level. Fatigue affects every aspect of the MS client's life: the ability to remain independent and perform self-care, sexual function, mobility, airway clearance, and ultimately self-concept and coping. A great deal of teaching is needed to help the client and family understand fatigue and how to adapt. Clients and families need assistance managing fatigue in a society in which energy is highly valued.
- Assess degree of fatigue and identify contributing factors. *Fatigue is a subjective experience that needs to be evaluated thoroughly before planning can begin.*
- Arrange daily activities to include rest periods. *Rest is essential to manage feelings of fatigue; periods of relaxation may help replenish energy reserves.*

PRACTICE ALERT
It is important to remember that the fatigue from chronic illnesses such as MS is very different from being "tired," and that rest and sleep may not result in improvement.

- Ask the client to consider which activities are really necessary and to set priorities. *Prioritizing activities promotes independence and self-control.*

NURSING CARE PLAN   A Client with MS

George McMurphy, a 45-year-old from northern Minnesota, was diagnosed with MS approximately 5 years ago. He states that he probably had mild symptoms as long ago as 10 years. He works as a manager for a large grocery store chain near his home. He lives at home with his wife and two children, ages 12 and 15. Recently, Mr. McMurphy has had increasing problems with urinary incontinence, lack of energy, weakness, extreme fatigue, and altered mobility from spasticity in his leg muscles. He also has a fever, chest congestion, and a cough productive of green sputum. He is admitted to the hospital for evaluation and treatment of pneumonia and exacerbation of his MS.

ASSESSMENT

Denise Miller, RN, primary care nurse, is assigned to care for Mr. McMurphy. His major complaint is the inability to "bring up all this sputum; I feel rotten from being so congested. I hate not being able to get to work and for my wife having to tend to my personal needs." Vital signs are as follows: BP 134/84, P 94, R 30, T 102°F (38.8°C). Mr. McMurphy is admitted for an acute exacerbation of the disorder, probably triggered by pneumonia. He will be treated with ACTH and intravenous antibiotics during this admission.

DIAGNOSES

- *Ineffective Airway Clearance* related to lung infection and thick mucus
- *Activity Intolerance* related to fatigue and spasticity
- *Self-Care Deficit: Toileting, Feeding, and Grooming* related to muscle weakness

EXPECTED OUTCOMES

- Be able to clear airway.
- Have breath sounds clear to auscultation and pulse oximetry readings above 95%.
- Be able to ambulate using assistive devices, if needed.
- Perform self-care activities without becoming overly fatigued and tired.
- Verbalize methods to adapt daily routine to his level of tolerance.

PLANNING AND IMPLEMENTATION

- Initiate pulmonary hygiene measures (e.g., incentive spirometry, turning, deep breathing and coughing, breathing exercises, and postural drainage) at least every 2 hours. Assess lung sounds, oxygen saturation, and ability to clear airway.

- Teach the importance of maintaining an oral fluid intake of at least 2000 mL per day to prevent tenacious sputum and urinary tract infections. Teach signs and symptoms of urinary and respiratory infections.
- Encourage participation in decision making about care.
- Assist with ADLs only as needed, based on level of fatigue and muscle weakness.
- Plan self-care activities so that they are performed during periods of peak level of energy; intersperse rest periods throughout the day.
- Refer to an MS support group.
- Refer to physical and occupational therapists for counseling regarding control of spasticity and possible splinting of spastic muscles.
- Consult a urologist for assessment of bladder incontinence; teach intermittent catheterization. Alternatively, the use of an external condom catheter may be indicated.

EVALUATION

Mr. McMurphy is discharged 3 days following admission. He states that he feels stronger; on discharge, he has no problem clearing his airway. Although he continues to pace his activities to avoid fatigue, his muscle strength and "tiredness" have improved. He is able to complete ADLs unassisted.

Pulmonary function has returned to normal prehospitalization levels; ABGs and pulse oximetry are within normal limits. Both Mr. McMurphy and his wife have listed several ways to modify their daily routine to allow more rest and decreased stress. Follow-up visits to his primary care physician have been arranged, and they have been provided with information about the local MS support group.

CRITICAL THINKING IN THE NURSING PROCESS

1. Describe approaches the nurse could take to ensure that Mr. McMurphy does not exceed his activity tolerance.
2. Develop a teaching plan for Mr. McMurphy to help prevent future respiratory infections.
3. Develop a care plan for Mr. McMurphy for the nursing diagnosis *Risk for Injury* related to fatigue, muscle weakness, and spasticity.

See Evaluating Your Response in Appendix C.

- Suggest performing tasks in the morning hours. *Biorhythm studies indicate that people usually have greater energy reserves in the morning hours and diminished reserves in the afternoon.*
- Advise to avoid temperature extremes, such as hot showers or exposure to cold. *Maintaining a relatively constant body temperature may avoid exacerbation of the disorder. Heat can delay impulse transmission across demyelinated nerves, which contributes to fatigue.*
- Refer to the appropriate professionals to manage fatigue: stress management groups, support groups, occupational or physical therapist, as indicated. *Support groups and therapy can facilitate self-management and improve coping.*

Self-Care Deficit

Clients with MS may need assistance with bathing, toileting, dressing, grooming, and feeding. The help needed can range from minimal guidance to total dependence. The client's ability to perform self-care activities is the gauge by which family members and caregivers need to adjust assistance. Self-care encompasses both the decisions about care and the provision of care; most clients are capable of making decisions even after physical limitations prevent physical self-care. The need to maintain self-determination cannot be overemphasized and must be incorporated into each intervention. As the client with MS ages, there may be even more need for teaching to provide self-care, as described in the Nursing Research box on the next page.

NURSING RESEARCH   Evidence-Based Practice for Aging Clients with MS

MS is a chronic debilitating disease, but it does not reduce life expectancy. Most clients are diagnosed with the disease as young to middle adults, and they must learn how to live with the disease for the rest of their lives. However, little research has been published regarding the experiences and health-related concerns of people aging with MS. This study by Finlayson and colleagues (2004) was conducted to initiate dialogue about the role of nurses in addressing those concerns. The study subjects perceived two major differences between their experience of aging with MS and that of people aging without MS: having less freedom (not being able to travel, restriction of social activities, physical accessibility of buildings, and financial limitations) and needing more assistance (with housework, shopping, hygiene, cooking, getting to places).

IMPLICATIONS FOR NURSING
The findings of this study support the need for nurses to include consideration of issues of daily living for clients with chronic disabilities, including MS. Nurses have the knowledge and ability to include information in client teaching that facilitate quality of life, coping with disability, and symptom management. By working closely with members of the interdisciplinary health team, nurses select and implement appropriate interventions to enable clients with MS to age in place, and to continue to be active and involved members of the family and community as they age.

CRITICAL THINKING IN CLIENT CARE
1. How would your teaching differ for the following clients with MS?
   a. A 45-year-old woman, married, with family who lives nearby
   b. A 70-year-old woman, widowed, no family living
   c. A man who has been a farmer all his life and lives in an isolated rural area
   d. A man who has always lived in an urban area with access to public transportation.
2. You are making a home visit to an older woman who has had MS for 30 years. She tells you, "I never leave my condo anymore because I just can't control my urine and I'm so afraid I will have an accident." What can you do to help her resolve this problem?
3. Design a plan of care focused on the nursing diagnosis *Fatigue* for a 73-year-old man who is living independently but says, "Some days I am just too tired to even cook anything to eat."

- Assess the extent of the client's self-care deficit; refer to other health team members for assessment as appropriate. For example, refer to a speech pathologist to assess swallowing and gag reflex, if indicated. *An accurate assessment is crucial to individualizing interventions.*

- Suggest adaptive devices, such as arm or wrist braces, as needed. *Meeting hygiene needs and feeding self are essential for positive self-concept, self-esteem, and socialization.*

- Teach to use assistive devices, such as plate guards; to modify consistency of foods; and to eat when energy level is better. If unable to buy and prepare meals, provide referral to Meals-on-Wheels. *Proper nutrition is basic to health; adapting utensils and foods can facilitate meeting nutritional needs.*

- Teach interventions related to altered bowel and bladder function: fluid intake of at least 2000 mL daily, bowel routine as indicated to prevent constipation, self-catheterization skills as necessary. *Maintaining optimal bowel and bladder function decreases the risk of urinary tract infection and bowel impaction.*

Using NANDA, NIC, and NOC

Chart 46–2 shows links between NANDA nursing diagnoses, NIC, and NOC when caring for the client with MS.

Community-Based Care

The inconsistent and erratic nature of MS can make teaching for self-care difficult. Initial teaching focuses on a realistic explanation of MS. Referral to a support group early in the course of the disease is indicated. Social support can make a positive difference in a client's ability to cope with MS. Address the following topics in preparing the client for home care:

NANDA, NIC, AND NOC LINKAGES
CHART 46–2   The Client with Multiple Sclerosis

NANDA

Disturbed Sensory Perception: Visual

NIC

Communication Enhancement: Visual Deficit

Emotional Support

Environmental Management

NOC

Sensory Function: Vision

Neurological Status: Cranial Sensory/Motor Function

Risk Control: Visual Impairment

Data from *NANDA's Nursing Diagnoses: Definitions & Classification 2005–2006* by NANDA International (2003), Philadelphia; *Nursing Interventions Classification (NIC)* (4th ed.) by J. M. Dochterman & G. M. Bulechek (2004), St. Louis, MO: Mosby; and *Nursing Outcomes Classification (NOC)* (3rd ed.) by S. Moorhead, M. Johnson, and M. Maas (2004), St. Louis, MO: Mosby.

- Various treatment options and their side effects
- Information about medications, particularly steroid use, and about possible interactions with prescription or over-the-counter (OTC) medications

- Ongoing care from nurses, counselors, and physical, occupational, and speech therapists, as well as the physician and community health nurse
- Helpful resources:
  - National MS Society
  - National Institute of Neurological Disorders and Stroke.

THE CLIENT WITH PARKINSON'S DISEASE

Parkinson's disease (PD) is a progressive, degenerative neurologic disease characterized by tremor (shaking), muscle rigidity, and bradykinesia (slowness of movement) (Porth, 2005). People with PD are faced with multiple problems involving independence in ADLs, emotional well-being, financial security, and relationships with caregivers.

Incidence and Prevalence

Parkinson's disease is one of the most common neurologic disorders affecting older adults. The National Parkinson Foundation (2005a) estimates that as many as 60,000 new cases are diagnosed each year, joining the 1.5 million people in the United States who currently have PD. The disorder usually develops after the age of 65 years, but 15% of those diagnosed are under 40 years of age. Men and women are affected equally. Recent discovery of inherited forms of PD suggest a genetic role in the development of this disease.

Parkinson's-like manifestations, called *secondary parkinsonism,* may result from other disorders such as trauma, encephalitis, tumors, toxins, and drugs. Drug-induced parkinsonism, which is usually reversible, may occur in people taking neuroleptics, antiemetics, antihypertensives, and illegal designer drugs containing MPTP, a toxic chemical (Porth, 2005). Carbon monoxide or cyanide poisoning can also cause secondary parkinsonism. This discussion focuses on primary Parkinson's disease, the cause of which is unknown.

Pathophysiology

Coordinated, voluntary body movement is achieved through the actions of neurotransmitters in the basal ganglia of the brain. Some neurotransmitters facilitate the transmission of excitatory nerve impulses, while other neurotransmitters inhibit their transmission. Together, this system allows control of movement. A disturbed balance between excitatory and inhibitory neurotransmitters causes disorders of voluntary motor function, such as PD.

In PD, neurons in the cerebral cortex atrophy and are lost, the dopaminergic nigrostriatal (pigmented) pathway degenerates, and the number of specific dopamine receptors in the basal ganglia decreases. These pathologic processes cause a decrease in the production of dopamine (a neurotransmitter that helps regulate nerve impulses involved in motor function) from the substantia nigra. The usual balance of dopamine (an inhibitory neurotransmitter) and acetylcholine (an excitatory neurotransmitter) in the brain is disrupted, and dopamine no longer inhibits acetylcholine. The failure to inhibit acetylcholine is the underlying basis for the manifestations of the disorder. Parkinson's disease has five stages, outlined in Box 46–3.

BOX 46–3 **Stages of Parkinson's Disease**

  I Unilateral involvement only, usually with minimal or no functional impairment.

 II Bilateral or midline involvement, without impairment of balance.

III First sign of impaired righting reflexes, evidenced as unsteadiness as the client turns or demonstrated when the client is pushed from standing equilibrium with the feet together and eyes closed. Functionally, the client is somewhat restricted in activities but may have some employment potential, depending on the type of employment. Clients are physically capable of leading independent lives, and their disability is mild to moderate.

IV Fully developed, severely disabling disease; the client is still able to walk and stand unassisted but is markedly incapacitated.

 V Client is confined to bed or wheelchair unless aided.

Manifestations

Parkinson's disease begins with subtle manifestations. Clients complain of feeling tired and seem to move more slowly; a slight tremor may accompany the fatigue. Over time, the manifestations progressively increase in severity. The manifestations and complications of PD are presented in the box on the next page.

Tremor

Tremor at rest is usually the first manifestation experienced, with one of the upper extremities more often affected. Resting tremors of the hand show a "pill-rolling" motion of the thumb and fingers. (This name reflects the way in which medicinal pills were formed in the early days of medicine.) The tremor may be controlled with purposeful, voluntary movement, and is worsened by stress and anxiety. Clients have progressive impairment in performing skills that require dexterity and fine muscle control, such as writing and eating.

Rigidity and Bradykinesia

Manifestations related to motor and postural effects include rigidity, bradykinesia, and uncoordinated movements. Rigidity (resulting from involuntary contraction of all skeletal muscles) makes both active and passive movement difficult. It is manifested as increased resistance to passive range of motion (ROM). Although the extremity moves, it does so in a jerky motion, called *cogwheel rigidity.* The first manifestation of rigidity may be muscle cramps in the toes or hands, but most often the client describes stiffness, heaviness, or aching in muscles.

Bradykinesia, experienced as difficulty in starting, continuing, or coordinating movements, is the most common and crippling manifestation. All striated muscles are affected, including those that involve chewing, swallowing, and speaking. Slowed or delayed movements affect the eyes, mouth, and voice, causing a masklike face and softened or muffled voice. Disorders of swallowing result in problems with eating and with drooling. Clients have a staring gaze with minimal

MANIFESTATIONS AND COMPLICATIONS
of Parkinson's Disease

RELATED TO MOTOR DYSFUNCTION
- Nonintention tremor
- Bradykinesia or akinesia
  a. Slowed movements; inability to initiate voluntary movements
  b. Slowed speech, low amplitude
  c. Poor articulation
  d. Decreased eye movements (i.e., blinking)
  e. Masklike, expressionless face
- Rigidity
- Posture and gait disturbances
  a. Trunk tilted forward
  b. Shuffling gait, propulsive at times
  c. Retropulsion
- Complications: falls, fractures, impaired communication, social isolation

RELATED TO AUTONOMIC SYSTEM DYSFUNCTION
- Skin problems
  a. Seborrhea
  b. Excess sweating on face and neck, absence of sweating of trunk and extremities
  c. Mottled skin
- Heat intolerance
- Postural hypotension
- Constipation
- Complications: skin breakdown, dizziness, falls, constipation

RELATED TO COGNITIVE AND PSYCHOLOGIC DYSFUNCTION
- Dementia
  a. Memory loss
  b. Lack of insight and problem-solving ability
  c. Declining intellectual abilities
- Anxiety
- Depression
- Complications: loss of ability to function, social isolation

Figure 46–3 ■ In Parkinson's disease, the client's face lacks expression or animation.
Source: Yoav Levy/Phototake NYC.

change in expression (Figure 46–3 ■). Clients describe being "frozen" in place as voluntary movement is lost, and they sit or lie in one position without movement for long periods of time. Movement is interspersed with freezing, brought about by turning, increasing the effort to move, or making visual or touch contacts.

Abnormal Posture

The loss of normal postural reflexes results in postural abnormalities, including disorders of postural fixation, equilibrium, and righting. Involuntary flexion of the head and shoulders means the person with PD cannot maintain an upright position of the trunk when sitting or standing. This problem of postural fixation results in the characteristic stooped, leaning forward position. Disorders of equilibrium follow loss of postural fixation with an inability to make adjustments when leaning or falling, increasing the risk of injury from falls (the person usually falls backward). The client takes short, accelerated steps to try to maintain an upright position when walking.

Autonomic and Neuroendocrine Effects

Many manifestations result from the loss of functions controlled by the autonomic nervous system. Elimination problems include constipation and urinary hesitation or frequency. Clients may experience problems related to orthostatic hypotension, including dizziness with position change. Eczematous skin changes and seborrhea are related to the increase in sweat gland activity secondary to increased sebotrophic hormone production.

Mood and Cognition

Both depression and dementia are pathologies associated with PD. Depression occurs in half of all clients and a third have dementia. Dementia, resulting from loss of cholinergic cells, loss of neurons, senile plaques, neurofibrillary tangles, and amyloid changes in small blood vessels, occurs in 20% of clients with PD and develops later in the disease (Porth, 2005). The client has manifestations similar to the person with Alzheimer's disease, including confusion, disorientation, memory loss, distractibility, and changes in abstraction and judgment. *Bradyphrenia* may also occur, resulting in slow thinking and a decreased ability to form thoughts, to plan, or to make decisions.

Sleep Disturbances

Clients with PD commonly have sleep disturbances, although they may experience decreased manifestations during sleep in the early stages. The ability to fall and stay asleep is affected by acetylcholine. Muscle rigidity may compromise sleep because of the inability to change position. This lack of muscle movement causes the client to awaken and consciously shift position.

Interrelated Effects

Some of the manifestations that clients with PD experience have multiple contributing factors. For example, constipation is common because of decreased peristalsis. However, decreased peristalsis is not the only cause: immobility, tremors (resulting in being unable to drink from a glass easily), and dietary changes from dysphagia all contribute to the problem of constipation.

Complications

The following complications are associated with Parkinson's disease:

- Oculogyric crisis, in which the eyes become fixed with a lateral and upward gaze
- Paranoia and hallucinations, which may accompany dementia
- Impaired communication due to changes in speech, handwriting, and expressiveness
- Falls from balance, posture, and motor changes
- Infections, such as pneumonia, related to immobility
- Malnutrition related to dysphagia and inability to prepare meals
- Altered sleep patterns due to loss of dopamine, L-dopa side effects (nightmares, dreams), or side effects of anticholinergics (hyperreflexia, muscle twitching), and depression
- Skin breakdown and pressure ulcers associated with urinary incontinence, malnutrition, and sweat reflex changes
- Depression and social isolation.

INTERDISCIPLINARY CARE

Prognosis is poor, owing to the progressive degeneration that ultimately affects multiple physiologic systems and their function. Psychosocial effects are equally devastating, and the fam-ily needs more support as the client's debilitation increases. Total disability is usually seen 10 to 20 years after diagnosis. The leading cause of death is pneumonia.

Diagnosis is based primarily on a thorough history and physical examination, and is made based on having two of the following manifestations: tremor at rest, bradykinesia, rigidity, and postural instability. Interventions vary with the clinical stage of the disorder and include medication, surgery, and rehabilitation to retain the optimal level of functioning possible. An interdisciplinary approach is essential for these clients.

Diagnosis

Diagnostic studies may support a potential diagnosis of Parkinson's disease; no test clearly differentiates Parkinson's disease from other neurologic disorders (Hickey, 2003). However, PET scan will show decreased uptake of 6-[18F]-fluoro-dopa.

Medications

The goal of drug therapy is to control manifestations to the extent possible. Generally, medications vary with the stage of the disease; however, response is individualized and guides the selection of medications. Types of drugs used include monoamine oxidase (MAO) inhibitors, dopaminergics, dopamine agonists, and anticholinergics. Information about these drugs is presented in the Medication Administration box below.

MEDICATION ADMINISTRATION **The Client with Parkinson's Disease**

DOPAMINERGICS
Levodopa (Larodopa, Dopar)
Carbidopa-levodopa (Sinemet)
Amantadine (Symmetrel)

These drugs have their major effect on the akinesia of Parkinson's disease, improving mobility while decreasing muscle rigidity and tremor. Levodopa is a metabolic precursor of dopamine, but unlike dopamine, it can cross the blood–brain barrier. Levodopa is converted to dopamine in the brain by decarboxylase, a catalytic enzyme, and stimulates dopamine receptors to balance the dopamine/acetylcholine concentrations. Carbidopa prevents decarboxylase from converting levodopa to dopamine in the peripheral tissues; therefore, carbidopa is frequently given in combination with levodopa. Amantadine is used to treat dyskinesia and also elevates mood.

Levodopa is avoided in clients with narrow-angle glaucoma, severe angina pectoris, transient ischemic attacks, or melanoma. The "on–off" phenomenon occurs after the client takes levodopa for several years; this phenomenon is characterized by unexpected dyskinesias and lack of symptom control.

Common side effects are nausea and vomiting; darkening of urine and sweat; dyskinesias, especially in the first few months of therapy; dysrhythmias; orthostatic hypotension; and psychologic reactions, such as hallucinations and vivid dreams. Older adults are particularly susceptible to psychologic disturbances.

Nursing Responsibilities

- Establish the client's baseline functional abilities in performing ADLs and administering the medication; assess motor control and coordination.

- To avoid adverse reactions, assess the client's overall health status before initiating therapy.
- Monitor medications known to cause adverse drug interactions: anticholinergics, pyridoxine, and antipsychotic agents alter the effectiveness of levodopa; MAO-B inhibitors can cause severe hypertension because of their vasoconstrictive effects.
- Withhold levodopa for 8 hours prior to administering Sinemet to avoid potentiating the effects of the circulating levodopa.

Health Education for the Client and Family

- Levodopa may not take effect for several weeks to months.
- Do not alter dosages of medications; taking more of a medication may not result in better symptom control and can cause severe side effects.
- Your protein intake should be divided into equal amounts for the day's meals. Avoid foods high in pyridoxine, such as pork, beef, ham, avocado, beans, and oatmeal.
- Levodopa may cause a darker color of urine; this is harmless, however.
- To prevent side effects:
  - Prevent nausea by taking medication with food.
  - Change position slowly to avoid a drop in blood pressure and risk of falling.
  - Prevent constipation by increasing fluid intake and exercising regularly.
- Notify practitioner if you begin to have difficulty making voluntary movements or cardiac or psychologic symptoms develop.

(continued)

MediaLink

Levodopa Animation

MEDICATION ADMINISTRATION The Client with Parkinson's Disease (continued)

■ Watch for the "on–off" phenomenon, in which periods of symptom control alternate with periods when the drug fails to control symptoms.

MONOAMINE OXIDASE INHIBITORS

Selegiline (Eldepryl, Carbex)

Selegiline works by selectively inhibiting the enzyme that inactivates dopamine in the brain. It may be administered alone or as an adjunct therapy with levodopa: Selegiline inhibits the enzyme system that would otherwise break down and destroy dopamine. This synergistic effect lasts approximately 1 to 2 years. The combination of selegiline and levodopa increases the adverse reactions of dopamine; nurses must be alert for orthostatic hypotension, changes in movement, hallucinations, and confusion. These responses can be modified by lowering the dose of levodopa. Because it is highly selective for the MAO-A enzyme, selegiline does not have antidepressant effects like the MAO-B inhibitors. The risk of severe hypertension is low.

Nursing Responsibilities

■ Establish baseline functional abilities: motor control and movements, position changes, mental status.
■ Monitor problems with insomnia.
■ Assess for orthostatic hypotension; look for unsteadiness with position change and complaints of dizziness.
■ Assess for hypertension, which can occur with higher than usual doses.

Health Education for the Client and Family

■ It is very important to take the medication as directed, especially dose and time of administration.
■ Notify the practitioner if insomnia occurs.
■ Report signs of dizziness when changing positions or standing, changes in ability to move, or psychologic changes.
■ Change positions slowly, especially when moving from a sitting to standing position.
■ Keep follow-up appointments for evaluation of the medication's effectiveness.

DOPAMINE AGONISTS

Bromocriptine (Parlodel)
Pergolide (Permax)
Pramipexole (Mirapex)
Ropinirole (Requip)

Dopamine agonists act by directly activating dopamine receptors in the brain. They are frequently used in combination with levodopa therapy: When dopamine agonists are given with levodopa, they increase the therapeutic effects of levodopa and reduce fluctuations in motor symptoms. Adverse reactions are similar to those of levodopa: nausea, orthostatic hypotension, and psychologic disturbances are common. Nursing responsibilities and client and family teaching information are similar to those that apply to the dopaminergics.

COMT INHIBITORS

Tolcapone (Tasmar)
Entacapone (Comtan)

COMT inhibitors inhibit catechol-*O*-methyltransferase (COMT), which is responsible for metabolizing dopamine. The concurrent administration of a COMT inhibitor with levodopa increases the amount of levodopa available to the brain to control Parkinson's disease.

Nursing Responsibilities

■ Monitor liver function test results and manifestations of liver impairment (dark urine, jaundice).
■ Administer with food.
■ If given concurrently with warfarin, monitor PT and INR.

Health Education for the Client and Family

■ Avoid using alcohol and sedatives.
■ Rise slowly from a sitting or lying position to avoid falling.
■ Nausea is common at the beginning of therapy.
■ Do not abruptly stop taking the medication.
■ Report increased loss of muscle control, yellow skin or eyes, dark urine, hallucinations, severe diarrhea.

ANTICHOLINERGICS

Trihexyphenidyl (Artane)
Benztropine (Cogentin)
Biperiden (Akineton)
Cycrimine (Pagitane)
Procyclidine (Kemadrin)
Chlorphenoxamine (Phenoxene)

Anticholinergics are effective in Parkinson's disease because they block the excitatory action of the neurotransmitter acetylcholine. They are frequently used during the early stages of the disease or when the client can no longer take levodopa. They may be given in combination with carbidopa-levodopa therapy. These medications ease drooling, tremors, and rigidity; however, side effects are common and may include blurred vision, dry mouth, constipation, delayed gastric emptying, urinary retention, photophobia, and tachycardia. Older adults are especially susceptible to heat stroke and psychologic side effects, including confusion, depression, delusions, and hallucinations. Anticholinergics should be tapered slowly when discontinued to avoid enhancing parkinsonian symptoms.

Nursing Responsibilities

■ Perform baseline assessment for presence of glaucoma, cardiac dysfunction, and prostatic hypertrophy.
■ Note other medications, including OTC medications that have anticholinergic effects, such as antihistamines and tricyclic antidepressants.
■ Monitor for side effects, especially changes in vision, elimination, gastric emptying, and mentation.

HEALTH EDUCATION FOR THE CLIENT AND FAMILY

■ Inform your practitioner if you begin taking any new medications or notice any new symptoms.
■ Avoid overexposure to heat, and take precautions to avoid heat stroke: Drink fluids, keep cool, and avoid strenuous activity on hot days.
■ Drink adequate amounts of fluid to minimize constipation.
■ Practice home safety to prevent falls associated with blurred vision.
■ Avoid taking OTC antihistamines or sleeping aids; these have anticholinergic activity.
■ Have the eyes examined annually to check for glaucoma; wear dark glasses if photophobia develops.
■ Do not suddenly stop taking anticholinergics.

Initially clients are treated with selegiline (Carbex, Eldepryl), amantadine (Symmetrel), or anticholinergics. As the disease progresses, levodopa (Dopar, Larodopa) in combination with carbidopa (Lodosyn) is used in a medication named carbidopa-levodopa (Sinemet). Because levodopa eventually loses its effectiveness, dopamine agonists are added to increase the effectiveness of levodopa. Eventually, pharmacotherapeutic agents lose their efficacy, and the disease continues to progress despite treatment. Response to the drugs fluctuates; this phenomenon is called the "on–off" response.

Bromocriptine (Parlodel) and pergolide (Permax), agents that inhibit the breakdown of dopamine, are used to delay progression of the disease. Catecholamine-*O*-methyl transferase (COMT) inhibitors (tolcapone [Tasmar] and entacapone [Comtan]) are used in conjunction with carbidopa-levodopa therapy to reduce the metabolism of levodopa, leading to more sustained dopaminergic stimulation of the brain. Selegiline (Deprenyl) increases dopaminergic activity, and is used as an adjunctive therapy for clients who have fluctuations in response, or become unresponsive, to levodopa.

Other medications may be used to treat problems related to Parkinson's disease. Antidepressants may be prescribed. Propranolol (Inderal) may be used to treat tremors; it should be used cautiously when clients have orthostatic hypotension. Botulism toxin injections may be given to treat eyelid spasms and abnormal posturing (dystonia) involving the extremities.

Deep Brain Stimulation

Activa TM tremor control therapy uses an implanted pacemaker-like device to deliver mild electrical stimulation to block the brain impulses that cause tremor, rigidity, stiffness, slowed movement, and problems with walking. In this procedure, an insulated wire is surgically placed in the thalamus and connected to an implanted pulse generator (similar to an advanced cardiac pacemaker) near the clavicle. It is used only for clients who cannot adequately control manifestations with medications (NINDS, 2005c).

Surgery

Pallidotomy is a surgical technique for Parkinson's disease, and its results have been helpful for many clients. In this procedure, the neurosurgeon locates the affected areas of the globus pallidus and destroys the involved tissue. As a result, clients who could not previously ambulate are able to walk, and tremors cease. The long-term effects are still being evaluated.

Stereotaxic thalamotomy (an x-ray is taken during neurosurgery to guide the insertion of a needle into a specific area of the brain) has been used only for clients who do not respond to medications—generally, younger people with extreme unilateral tremor. The surgeon destroys a small amount of tissue by creating a lesion in the ventrolateral nucleus of the thalamus. This surgery decreases tremors and rigidity in the contralateral extremity.

Fetal tissue transplantation is a controversial surgical procedure limited to a few medical centers. In this procedure, brain cells from aborted fetuses are implanted into the brain in the hopes that the new cells will grow and produce enough dopamine to restore some lost mobility.

Rehabilitation

Depending on their individual needs, clients frequently benefit from rehabilitation therapy with a physical therapist, social worker, psychologist, and/or speech therapist.

Physical therapists (PT) can implement an individual exercise program to improve coordination, balance, gait, and transfers. Preventing contractures is an important goal of exercise therapy. It is crucial that family and healthcare personnel permit the client adequate time to perform not only exercise regimens but also ADLs. Activities should not be rushed.

An occupational therapist (OT) helps the client adapt to changing abilities pertinent to work, self-care, and recreational activities. Some rehabilitation centers assign OT personnel the responsibility of addressing the client's upper extremity functions while assigning PT personnel to manage lower extremity problems. For example, skills related to cooking and grooming would be supervised by the OT, whereas mobility and posture skills would be supervised by the PT.

Speech therapists frequently address not only the client's speech but also chewing and swallowing. These therapists evaluate clients and plan treatment regimens. The challenge with clients who have PD is that they not only have vocalization problems, but also dexterity deficits; speech therapists therefore must evaluate the potential benefits of assistive devices, such as a magic slate, voice synthesizer, or computer, for each client.

Nursing Care

The chronic and eventually debilitating nature of PD poses many challenges to clients, families, and healthcare professionals. Dependence due to declining physical and mental abilities is of major concern. In the early stages, most clients are able to remain at home, with the family assisting with or providing many of the client's ADL needs. As the disease progresses and the burden of care increases, the client and family may prefer placement in a long-term care facility. A Nursing Care Plan for the client with PD is given on the next page.

Health Promotion

Teaching preventive measures is extremely important when caring for clients who have Parkinson's disease. Preventing malnutrition, falls and other environmental accidents, constipation, skin breakdown from incontinence or immobility, and joint contracture requires teaching and reinforcement.

In addition to incorporating information about safety needs, teach ways to prevent orthostatic hypotension when the client changes positions; some clients may also benefit from wearing individually fitted compression hose. In addition, address safety considerations about proper administration of medications.

Assessment

Collect the following data through the health history and physical examination (see Chapter 43 ∞). Further focused assessments are described with nursing interventions. When assessing the older client, be aware of normal changes with aging, outlined in Chapter 43 ∞ .

NURSING CARE PLAN   A Client with PD

Walter Avneil, age 78, was diagnosed with PD at age 64. His wife died 5 years ago and he has no other family living. Mr. Avneil worked for more than 40 years as a mechanic in a large factory. He is a resident of a long-term care facility. During his last clinic visit for a review of his medications, the following assessment was made.

ASSESSMENT

White male with history of PD for the past 14 years. Skin oily and damp. Tremors in both hands and the lips. Gait is slow and shuffling, with a forward leaning posture. Speech slow and slurred. Face expressionless. Has lost 10 lb since last visit 3 months ago. Has been on levodopa with carbidopa since diagnosis. States major problems are "eating problems, bowel problems, walking problems."

DIAGNOSIS

- *Constipation* related to lack of exercise, decreased food intake, and effects of medications
- *Impaired Verbal Communication* related to lip tremors, slow/slurred speech, and facial muscle involvement of PD
- *Imbalanced Nutrition: Less than Body Requirements* related to difficulty swallowing and chewing
- *Impaired Physical Mobility* related to rigidity and bradykinesia

EXPECTED OUTCOMES

- Have a soft stool at least every other day.
- Practice exercises provided by speech therapist twice a day.
- Increase number of calories, fluids, and fiber in diet provided at long-term facility.
- Improve joint mobility and ability to ambulate.

PLANNING AND IMPLEMENTATION

- Discuss problems with bowel elimination with staff at long-term facility; suggest increasing fluids to 3000 mL per day and also increasing fiber in the diet with oatmeal for breakfast, and more fruits and vegetables at meals.
- Encourage exercises provided by speech therapist to improve speech and swallowing. If these are not effective, make a referral for another evaluation.
- Discuss diet plan with dietitian at the long-term care facility, including consistency of foods and number of calories. Suggest dietitian be a part of swallowing evaluation by the speech therapist.
- Refer for physical therapy and occupational therapy for a program to improve gait and joint mobility, and to decrease risk of falling.

EVALUATION

In a return visit 3 months later, Mr. Avneil reports that "my bowels are working better." He has gained 7 lb, and the staff report that this is related to multiple factors, including practicing his swallowing exercises, getting more exercise that stimulated his appetite, and changing his diet to six small meals a day of soft or pureed foods. The staff is offering him liquids at meals and snack times, and he usually drinks all they give him. His speech is not much improved. His posture and gait are somewhat better, and he is doing the exercises provided by the physical therapist and occupational therapist. Mr. Avneil's functional abilities have improved so much that the staff is considering training sessions specific to care of residents with PD.

CRITICAL THINKING IN THE NURSING PROCESS

1. Although Mr. Avneil did not mention it, the staff reports that he is frustrated by not being able to dress himself. What suggestions could you make to facilitate his independence?
2. Mr. Avneil spends most of his time alone, although he enjoys the company of the other residents. List assessments and interventions you might provide to increase his diversional activity.
3. The loss of his wife and the debilitating effects of his disease increase Mr. Avneil's risk for the nursing diagnosis of *Chronic Sorrow*. What might you suggest the long-term staff do to reduce this risk?

See Evaluating Your Response in Appendix C.

- *Health history:* Brain trauma, stroke, infection, exposure to heavy metals or carbon monoxide, medication and drug use, incontinence, constipation, weight loss, sweating, sleep problems, muscle pain, mood.
- *Physical assessment:* Affect; appearance; speech, scalp, eyelashes, and skin; drooling; tremor; coordination; posture; gait; muscle rigidity; mental status.

Nursing Diagnoses and Interventions

Clients with PD have complex and, ultimately, multisystem needs. Deficits in mobility and self-care are common. Psychosocial needs may include problems related to *Ineffective Coping, Powerlessness,* and *Disturbed Body Image.* Refer to the nursing care sections throughout this chapter for discussions of fatigue, self-care deficit, ineffective airway clearance, and other pertinent diagnoses. This section focuses on the nursing diagnoses related to impaired physical mobility, impaired verbal communication, imbalanced nutrition, and disturbed sleep pattern.

Impaired Physical Mobility

Clients with PD have impaired mobility for several reasons, including tremors, gait pattern disturbances, and alterations in body positioning, such as forward bending of the trunk. Poor self-esteem may contribute to the client's lack of motivation and willingness to be mobile.

- Suggest referral to a physical therapist to develop an individualized exercise program. *A program specific to the client supplies motivation as well as helping the client maintain muscle tone, flexibility, and mobility.*
- Request the physical therapist teach caregivers how to do ROM exercises at least twice a day, emphasizing the trunk, neck, arms, hips, and legs. *Maintaining joint mobility promotes better function and strength, improving gait pattern. Consistent ROM exercises can prevent contractures.*
- Ask caregivers to ambulate the client at least four times a day if possible. *Exercise fosters independence and self-esteem.*

- Recommend assistive devices, such as lift chairs, canes, splints, or braces, as indicated. *Adaptive equipment improves balance, protects joints, and promotes proper anatomic positioning.*
- To promote mobility and safety:
  - Slightly elevate the back legs of chairs and raise the toilet seat to help rise from a sitting position to a standing position.
  - Wear shoes with Velcro closures.
  - Remove potential hazards, such as unanchored throw rugs.
  - Install handrails and nonskid surfaces in bath tubs and showers.
  - Ensure adequate lighting throughout the home and in outside areas, especially in areas where transfers are common.
  Safety measures prevent potential complications that may result from falls or other accidents and promote self-esteem through self-care.

> ### PRACTICE ALERT
> *Parkinson's disease is a disorder common in older adults, who are at greater risk for falls resulting from orthostatic hypotension, osteoporosis, poor vision, and other problems causing disorientation and confusion, such as Alzheimer's disease.*

Impaired Verbal Communication

Diminished vocal amplitude and loss of muscular control can impair the client's ability to speak. Both caregivers and family members must remember to give clients enough time for self-expression; an unhurried approach is recommended. Seek input from family members when determining alternative methods of communicating with the client.

- Assess current communication abilities in speech, hearing, and writing. *Communication involves both sending and receiving messages.*
- Develop methods of communication appropriate to coordination abilities, such as a magic slate; flash cards with common phrases; pointing to objects. *Individualizing a method of communication decreases anxiety and isolation.*
- Suggest referral to a speech pathologist to develop oral exercises and interventions that will facilitate speaking. *The muscles of speech and swallowing are affected by the Parkinson's disease process.*
- Remind client to speak more loudly, if possible. *A low, monotonous voice is characteristic of the client with Parkinson's disease.*

Imbalanced Nutrition:
Less than Body Requirements

Tremors, altered gait, and impaired chewing and swallowing can cause nutritional problems in the client with PD. As the disorder progresses, interventions for ensuring optimal nutrition need to be adapted to the client's functional abilities. Assess the client's swallow reflex before starting any feeding program. During the initial stages of the disorder, some clients may have the nursing diagnosis *Imbalanced Nutrition: More than Body Requirements* if kilocalorie intake exceeds energy expenditure.

- Assess nutritional status and self-feeding abilities; suggest referral to an occupational or speech therapist, if needed. *An initial assessment of abilities ensures that interventions are personalized to the client's current functional abilities.*
- Teach caregivers how to prepare foods of proper consistency as determined by swallowing function. *The client may aspirate food that is too liquid.*
- Weigh weekly. *Early recognition of weight loss allows for intervention.*
- Teach eating methods to decrease tremors, such as holding a piece of bread in the hand that is not holding an eating utensil. *Nonintention tremor may be reduced through purposeful activity.*
- Encourage diet that is high in bulk and fluids. *Several anti-Parkinson's medications and inactivity can cause constipation.*

Disturbed Sleep Pattern

Rigidity and weakness can cause clients with Parkinson's disease to lose the ability to move and change positions during sleep. The resulting discomfort causes periods of wakefulness. Medications to treat Parkinson's disease contribute to sleep pattern disturbance; for example, levodopa can cause vivid dreams. Nurses can help accurately assess the sleep pattern disturbance and in planning interventions to improve or increase sleep time.

- Assess sleep pattern and existing conditions that may affect sleep, such as depression or pain. *Clients experiencing anxiety, depression, and dementia have a difficult time falling asleep and may wake up more at night.*

> ### PRACTICE ALERT
> Remember to assess pain status; lack of adequate pain control may interfere with sleep.

- Explain the disease process and the effects of decreased dopamine on the sleep–wake cycle. *Depending on the dosage, levodopa causes less REM sleep and deep sleep.*
- Review the client's medication. *Bromocriptine and levodopa, especially if used with an anticholinergic, can cause vivid dreams. Other medications (diuretics, theophylline, hypnotics) also may interfere with sleep.*
- Teach how to modify lifestyle activities that affect sleep:
  - Institute a routine of activities with limited rest periods during the day; avoid napping close to bedtime. Avoid strenuous exercise in the evening. *Daytime sleeping may contribute to decreased nighttime sleeping. Vigorous exercise just before bedtime may act as a stimulant.*
  - Incorporate diet modifications, such as limiting caffeine and alcohol intake. *Caffeine is a stimulant, and alcohol may cause early morning awakenings, increased daytime sleepiness, and nightmares.*
  - Drink a glass of milk before bedtime. *Milk contains L-tryptophan, which produces sedative effects by shortening the time taken to fall asleep (sleep latency).*
  - Adapt the environment to aid in sleep (e.g., darken the room and decrease noises). *Reducing environmental stimuli decreases external sleep disturbances.*

Using NANDA, NIC, and NOC

Chart 46–3 shows links between NANDA nursing diagnoses, NIC, and NOC when caring for the client with PD.

Community-Based Care

It is important for both the client and the family to maintain independence and self-care as long as possible. To maintain function and quality of life, the following topics should be addressed:

- Realistic expectations
- Equipment suppliers
- Home environment conducive to using equipment
- Referrals to speech therapist, occupational therapist, physical therapist, and dietitian
- Gait training and exercises for improving ambulation, speech, swallowing, and self-care
- Increased fluid intake of 3000 mL/day and increased fiber in every meal
- Stool softeners or laxatives as needed for bowel elimination
- Swallowing during eating and taking medications (Have suction equipment available and know the Heimlich maneuver if choking occurs.)
- Foods that can be easily swallowed (such as pureed or soft) and feed six small meals a day if possible

---

NANDA, NIC, AND NOC LINKAGES

CHART 46–3 The Client with Parkinson's Disease

NANDA

Impaired Physical Mobility

↓

NIC

Energy Management

Fall Prevention

Surveillance: Safety

Self-Care Assistance

↓

NOC

Coordinated Movement

Balance

Fall Prevention Behavior

Self-Care: Activities of Daily Living (ADL)

Data from *NANDA's Nursing Diagnoses: Definitions & Classification 2005–2006* by NANDA International (2003), Philadelphia; *Nursing Interventions Classification (NIC)* (4th ed.) by J. M. Dochterman & G. M. Bulechek (2004), St. Louis, MO: Mosby; and *Nursing Outcomes Classification (NOC)* (3rd ed.) by S. Moorhead, M. Johnson, and M. Maas (2004), St. Louis, MO: Mosby.

- Helpful resources:
  - American Parkinson's Disease Association
  - National Parkinson Foundation, Inc.
  - Parkinson's Disease Foundation
  - The National Institute of Neurological Disorders and Stroke.

THE CLIENT WITH HUNTINGTON'S DISEASE

Huntington's disease (HD) is a progressive, degenerative, inherited neurologic disease characterized by increasing dementia and chorea (jerky, rapid, involuntary movements). It is a single-gene autosomal-dominant inherited disease that causes localized death of neurons of the basal ganglia (Porth, 2005). The exact cause is unknown, but postmortem studies have demonstrated a decrease in gamma-aminobutyric acid (GABA), an inhibitory neurotransmitter in the basal ganglia. There is also a decrease in acetylcholine levels, suggesting that the manifestations are the result of an imbalance in dopamine and acetylcholine. HD is a familial disease; each child of an HD parent has a 50% chance of inheriting the HD gene and, if so, will eventually develop the disease (NINDS, 2005f). There is no cure for the disease. Huntington's disease causes progressive chorea, speech problems, and dementia.

Because the client is usually asymptomatic until age 30 to 40, he or she may already have passed the gene to the next generation. The psychologic effect is devastating to clients and their families. The family not only experiences guilt from passing the disease from one generation to the next, but also is faced with the overwhelming long-term care needs of those affected. It is common for several family members to have the disease.

Pathophysiology

Huntington's disease causes destruction of cells in the caudate nucleus and putamen areas of the basal ganglia. Other areas of the brain, such as the frontal lobes, may selectively atrophy. Several neurotransmitters and their receptors are decreased, including GABA and acetylcholine. The neurotransmitter dopamine is not affected in Huntington's disease, but the decrease in acetylcholine results in a relative excess of dopamine in the basal ganglia. Whereas in Parkinson's disease a deficit of dopamine causes slow movement or lack of movement, in Huntington's disease the opposite occurs: There is a relative excess of dopamine, causing excessive, uncontrolled movement.

Manifestations

Manifestations and complications primarily involve abnormal movement and progressive dementia (see the box on the next page). The progression and sequence of manifestations varies somewhat; however, initially the psychologic manifestations are more debilitating than the choreiform (rapid and jerky) movements.

Early signs of personality change include severe depression, memory loss with decreased ability to concentrate, emotional lability, and impulsiveness. The client experiences frequent mood swings ranging from uncontrollable periods of anger to

MANIFESTATIONS AND COMPLICATIONS
of Huntington's Disease

MOTOR EFFECTS

Early
- Restlessness
- "Fidgety" feeling
- Minor gait changes—unsteady on feet
- Posture and positioning disturbances, frequent falls
- Inability to keep the tongue from protruding
- Slurred speech with poor articulation
- Complications: increasing problem with self-care activities, such as bathing, grooming, eating

Late
- Chorea—severely altered gait with irregular, uncontrollable movement; shoulders shrug arrhythmically
- Facial grimacing—raising of eyebrows, uncontrollable protrusion of the tongue
- Dysphagia
- Unintelligible speech
- Impaired diaphragmatic movement
- Complications: immobility, aspiration, choking, and, eventually, total dependence, poor oxygenation, emaciation, and cachexia

PSYCHOSOCIAL EFFECTS

Early
- Irritability
- Outbursts of rage alternating with euphoria
- Depression
- Complication: suicide

Late
- Decreasing memory
- Loss of cognitive skills
- Eventual dementia
- Complication: total dependence

apathy. Eventually, signs of dementia, including disorientation, confusion, and lack of sense of time, become evident and interfere with self-care.

Motor manifestations usually parallel personality and mood changes. The motor manifestations worsen with environmental stimuli and emotional stress but are absent when the client is sleeping. Initially, movement problems are described as "fidgeting" or restlessness, followed by progressive worsening of abnormal movements. The choreiform movements, which begin in the face and arms and then involve the entire body, are manifested by facial grimaces, tongue protrusion, jerky movement of the distal arms or legs, and a rhythmic, lurching gait that almost resembles a dance. (The term *chorea* comes from *choreia*, the Greek word meaning "dance.") Gait changes cause uncoordinated movements and contribute to frequent falls.

The muscles of swallowing, chewing, and speaking are affected, leading to dysphagia and dysarthria and associated problems with communication and nutrition. The client's constant movement and difficulty in swallowing contribute to

weight loss and eventual cachexia. Breathing is impaired because the diaphragm is unable to move effectively.

The manifestations slowly progress over approximately 15 to 20 years after initial manifestations appear. Prognosis is poor, with inevitable debilitation and total dependence. Death usually results from aspiration pneumonia or another infectious process.

INTERDISCIPLINARY CARE

There is no cure for Huntington's disease, and treatment addresses the disease's manifestations. Nurses provide care to clients with Huntington's disease in a variety of community settings. Initially, clients and families can manage care needs at home, but as the disease progresses, the client requires constant supervision, such as that provided in day care facilities. Eventually, skilled long-term care is needed. Clients who develop acute problems may be hospitalized until the crisis is managed. Because of the inevitable total multisystem debilitation of clients with Huntington's disease, nurses and other caregivers face many challenges.

Diagnosis
Genetic testing is the only test available to diagnose clients suspected of having Huntington's disease. Both blood and amniotic fluid may be tested for the presence of a gene mutation on chromosome 4 using DNA analysis. The test can predict with 95% accuracy which offspring have the disease.

Medications
The following medications are given for the manifestations of Huntington's disease:
- Antipsychotics, specifically phenothiazines and butyrophenones, are effective in Huntington's disease because they block dopamine receptors in the brain. The therapeutic goal is to restore the balance among the neurotransmitters.
- Antidepressants are prescribed in the early stage of the disease; however, medications are no substitute for intense follow-up counseling for clients and families.

NURSING CARE

Nurses are faced with a multitude of challenges when caring for families who have Huntington's disease, including physiologic, psychosocial, and ethical problems. Physiologic problems are related to the progressive and eventually debilitating nature of the disease. Psychosocial concerns occur as a result of the client's personality and mental changes, the family's responsibility for providing care, and the guilt implicit in a genetically transmitted disease. Ethical difficulties relate to the genetic nature of the disease: DNA testing for the marker on chromosome 4 can determine whether the person is a carrier of the disease before he or she begins to exhibit manifestations. Children of people with Huntington's disease are thus faced with the choice of finding out whether they will eventually be affected. If they choose not to be tested, they may pass the disease on to yet another generation; and if a fetus is affected, they may face the decision of whether to undergo an abortion.

Nursing Diagnoses and Interventions

Initially, much of the nursing care focuses on teaching about the disease, psychologic support, and genetic counseling. As manifestations become more severe, nursing considerations center on problems related not only to immobility and altered nutrition, but also to the increasing self-care deficits. Families and clients experiencing Huntington's disease face many psychosocial issues. Nurses must be prepared to listen actively as well as to provide comfort and encouragement throughout the lengthy illness. There are many possible nursing diagnoses for the client with Huntington's disease; this section focuses on nursing diagnoses related to aspiration, nutrition, skin integrity, and communication.

Risk for Aspiration

Uncoordinated movements and swallowing and chewing problems put the client at high risk for aspiration.

- Maintain in an upright position while the client eats; support the head. *Proper positioning may prevent aspiration during mealtime.*
- Teach the Heimlich maneuver to caregivers and family members. *Aspiration is a real possibility; caregivers must be prepared to reestablish the client's airway.*
- Provide food that is thick enough to manage, such as thick soups, mashed potatoes, stews, or casseroles. *These foods are more readily tolerated and manipulated by the tongue than liquids.*
- Make sure food is swallowed before giving another spoonful of food. *The automatic phase of swallowing may be disrupted in the client with Huntington's disease; providing adequate time and smaller bites may improve the ability to manipulate foods.*
- Provide a calm, relaxing eating environment. *Stress worsens choreiform movements and inappropriate behaviors.*

Imbalanced Nutrition: Less than Body Requirements

Clients with Huntington's disease have unpredictable choreiform movements of the extremities and decreased ability to control muscles involved with chewing and swallowing. Families and caregivers are challenged to provide sufficient calories to maintain the client in positive nitrogen balance.

- Evaluate current weight and nutritional status, including serum prealbumin and transferrin levels. *Establishing a baseline is crucial for meeting individual caloric, protein, vitamin, and mineral needs.*
- Assess ability to swallow and manipulate eating utensils. *Aspiration is an ever-present danger that must be avoided; utensils may need to be adapted to client's abilities, if client is able to assist at all.*
- Continue feeding even if the client physically turns away from the meal. *Involuntary choreiform movements should not be interpreted as a refusal to eat.*
- Provide high-kilocalorie, nutritious foods and sufficient snacks; request input from a dietitian. *The constant movement of Huntington's disease increases caloric requirements.*

- Avoid milk; provide frequent oral hygiene. *Milk tends to thicken secretions. Decreasing thick secretions may improve ability to swallow and enable the client to ingest more calories.*

Impaired Skin Integrity

Skin integrity is only one component of the client's general need for protection and avoidance of injury. Several factors increase the risk for impaired skin integrity, including poor nutritional status, eventual total immobility, and incontinence.

- Evaluate the skin for actual and potential areas of breakdown. *Establishing a baseline is necessary to modify care and provide prophylactic protection of high-risk pressure areas.*
- Determine nutritional status, especially serum prealbumin level and vitamin, mineral, and kilocalorie intake. *Optimal nutritional status and positive nitrogen balance help prevent skin breakdown and formation of pressure ulcers.*
- Turn and inspect the skin at least every 2 hours, giving special consideration to areas that are most prone to breakdown, such as heels and coccyx. *Pressure points are particularly susceptible to skin breakdown.*
- Provide ROM exercises on a regular schedule in the daytime. *Movement stimulates circulation, which provides oxygenation and allows nutrients to reach muscles and skin.*
- Keep the skin clean and dry; pay particular attention to the perineal area if incontinent. *Skin in close proximity to the perineal area, such as the sacral area, is highly susceptible to breakdown due to exposure to wet, acidic urine and fecal material.*
- Place on an alternating-pressure mattress with foot board. *Decreasing pressure on bony prominences and preventing shearing forces serve to prevent skin breakdown.*
- Pad side rails and headrests of special chairs; have the client wear a football-type helmet. *The client's violent movements can cause trauma to the head and extremities.*

Impaired Verbal Communication

The inability to control muscles related to speech, swallowing, and facial movement contributes to problems of verbal communication. Because Huntington's disease affects fine motor movement, especially the distal portion of the extremities, the hands are not effective in communication. As the disease progresses, mental abilities are also compromised, making both receptive and expressive communication impossible.

- Choose alternative methods of communication while the client is able to participate. *Anticipatory planning may facilitate communication and decrease anxiety.*
- Continue to incorporate therapeutic communication techniques, even though client is not responsive: Maintain eye contact, use touch, and talk directly to the client rather than to others in the room. *These techniques enhance the individual's dignity and worth.*
- Seek input from family about client's usual preferences and how they are communicated; be alert for subtle cues. *Nonverbal communication techniques may be individualized and more readily recognized by the family member or caregiver who usually provides care.*

■ Continue talking to the client, even though there is no apparent response. *Hearing may not be impaired, even though the client cannot speak.*

Community-Based Care

Clients with Huntington's disease and their families may know how devastating the illness is because they may have cared for a parent or other close family member who had the illness. Many families are overwhelmed with just the thought of the physical and psychosocial debilitation that the disease brings. Fear, anxiety, and hopelessness leading to depression are common reactions. Teaching ways to cope effectively with the psychosocial and physical changes is an integral part of the nurse's responsibilities. Referrals to appropriate agencies, such as adult day care centers, the Huntington's Disease Foundation, and local support groups or a psychologist should be part of the nursing plan.

Another aspect of client teaching concerns the genetic transmission of Huntington's disease; refer clients and family members to a geneticist. Nurses are frequently involved with clarifying information, especially concerning the transmission, course of illness, and prognosis. A caring, sensitive approach is crucial. Information about transmission of an autosomal-dominant trait is discussed in Chapter 8 ∞ .

THE CLIENT WITH AMYOTROPHIC LATERAL SCLEROSIS

Amyotrophic lateral sclerosis (ALS), or *Lou Gehrig's disease,* is a rapidly progressive and fatal degenerative neurologic disease characterized by weakness and wasting of muscles under voluntary control, without any accompanying sensory or cognitive changes. The name is derived from the pathophysiologic processes of muscle atrophy (*amyotrophy*) resulting from lower motor neuron involvement and sclerosis of the corticospinal tract in the lateral column of the spinal cord resulting from upper motor neuron involvement. Death results in 2 to 5 years after onset of the manifestations (although some people live 10 years or more), usually due to respiratory failure.

ALS is the most common motor neuron disease in the United States. As many as 20,000 people in the United States have ALS, and approximately 5000 new cases are diagnosed each year. In up to 90% to 95% of cases, the disease occurs at random without clearly associated risk factors. About 5% to 10% of all cases are inherited in what is termed familial ALS (NINDS, 2005a).

Most people are between 40 and 60 years of age at diagnosis; the incidence is higher in men in the earlier ages but becomes equal with women after menopause. Most of the health problems a client with ALS encounters are related to swallowing and managing secretions, communication, and dysfunction of the muscles used in respiration.

Pathophysiology

ALS results from the degeneration and demyelination of both upper and lower motor neurons in the anterior horn of the spinal cord, brainstem, and cerebral cortex. Death of the motor neurons results in axonal degeneration, demyelination, glial proliferation, and scarring along the corticospinal tract. In the early stages of the disease, surviving motor neurons sprout new branches to reinnervate affected muscle fibers, preserving muscle strength. However, when more than half of the lower motor neurons are affected, reinnervation fails and weakness is evidenced.

Although the pathogenesis of ALS is not clear, abnormal glutamate metabolism and hydrogen peroxide production are being studied. Echovirus RNA has also been isolated in spinal cord tissue in some clients with nonfamilial ALS. Environmental factors, excess intracellular calcium, and antibodies to calcium channels are also being researched.

Manifestations

The initial manifestations may relate to dysfunction of upper motor neurons, lower motor neurons, or both. Dysfunction of upper motor neurons results in spastic, weak muscles with increased deep tendon reflexes. Dysfunction of lower motor neurons results in muscle flaccidity, paresis (weakness), paralysis, and atrophy.

Weakness and paresis are common early manifestations. The weakness may initially affect only one muscle group. Manifestations vary according to the particular muscle group involved; *fasciculations* (twitching) of involved muscles are common in the early stage of the disorder. With the loss of muscle innervation, the muscles atrophy, and paralysis results. Muscle mass decreases, and clients complain of progressive fatigue. Typically, the disease first affects the hands, then the shoulders, upper arms, and finally the legs.

Increasing brainstem involvement causes progressive atrophy of the tongue and facial muscles with eventual dysphagia and dysarthria. Emotional lability and loss of control occur, but dementia is not part of the pathologic progression of ALS. Vision, hearing, sensation, and cognitive ability usually remain intact. A summary of manifestations and complications is presented in the box on the next page.

INTERDISCIPLINARY CARE

Because many treatable disorders may cause manifestations similar to those that appear in the initial stage of ALS, a thorough evaluation is required. Once ALS is diagnosed, the primary goal is to support the client and family in meeting physical and psychosocial needs, particularly as the disease progresses.

Medical and nursing care for clients with ALS is primarily supportive. Referral for home health management is indicated. Occupational, physical, speech, and respiratory therapy are major supportive and rehabilitative treatments. As the disorder progresses and swallowing becomes ineffective, a gastrostomy tube may be necessary to provide adequate nutritional intake. Ventilatory assistance should be discussed with clients before the need occurs.

Diagnosis

There is no specific test to diagnose ALS. Rather, diagnosis is made based on manifestations and tests to rule out other diseases. A number of disorders may mimic early ALS, including

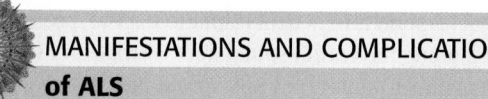

MANIFESTATIONS AND COMPLICATIONS of ALS

MUSCULOSKELETAL SYSTEM
- Weakness and fatigue
- "Heaviness" of legs
- Fasciculations
- Uncoordinated movements, loss of fine motor control in hands
- Spasticity
- Paresis
- Hyperreflexia
- Atrophy
- Problems with articulation
- Complications: paralysis, loss of ability to perform ADLs, total immobility, aspiration, loss of verbal communication

RESPIRATORY SYSTEM
- Dyspnea
- Difficulty clearing airway
- Complications: pneumonia, eventual respiratory failure

NUTRITIONAL EFFECTS
- Difficulty chewing
- Dysphagia
- Complication: malnutrition

EMOTIONAL EFFECTS
- Loss of control, lability
- Complication: depression

hyperthyroidism, hypoglycemia, compression of the spinal cord, toxic agents, infections, and neoplasms.

Medications

Riluzole (Rilutek), an antiglutamate, is the first medication developed to treat ALS. It inhibits the presynaptic release of glutamic acid in the CNS and protects neurons against the excitotoxicity of glutamic acid. This oral medication is administered without food at the same time each day. Clients are regularly monitored for liver function, blood count, blood chemistries, and alkaline phosphatase. They should be warned to report any febrile illness to their healthcare provider and to avoid alcohol.

NURSING CARE

Nursing care focuses on current health problems and on anticipating future difficulties. As with other disorders causing incapacitation and dependence, individualized nursing goals and interventions relate to decreasing complications, especially those associated with loss of muscular function and immobility; promoting independence to the extent possible; initiating referrals, particularly to a support group for both client and family; and providing physical and psychosocial support as indicated.

Of special consideration is planning for the client's eventual inability to communicate. Because the client's eye muscles and movements remain intact, signals can be prearranged before the loss of speech.

Nursing Diagnoses and Interventions

Two nursing diagnoses that frequently apply to clients with ALS are *Risk for Disuse Syndrome* and *Ineffective Breathing Pattern*.

Risk for Disuse Syndrome

Clients with ALS are at risk for developing problems associated with bed rest not only because they cannot move and reposition themselves, but also because they frequently have altered nutritional and hydration status. Nursing interventions focus on preventing skin breakdown and infections, such as urinary tract infections.

- Assess current condition for baseline parameters, particularly skin over bony prominences, lung sounds, and vital signs. *Understanding client's current condition allows accurate future assessment and realistic planning.*
- Assess skin; provide skin care, and obtain an alternating-pressure mattress. *Pressure points are at risk for breakdown; early detection is crucial to instituting appropriate care.*
- Institute active ROM exercises, as the client is able. Perform passive ROM exercises every 2 hours, when the client is turned. *Contractures can develop within a week because extensor muscles are weaker than flexor muscles.*
- Maintain positive nitrogen balance and hydration status: Monitor prealbumin levels, hemoglobin and hematocrit levels, and urine specific gravity. *Adequate protein is required to maintain osmotic pressure and prevent edema; positive nitrogen balance promotes optimal body functioning.*
- Monitor for manifestations of infection; for example, assess urine, especially if a urinary catheter is present. *Urinary catheters place clients at high risk for sepsis; bed rest places the client at greater risk for urinary stasis.*

PRACTICE ALERT
Urinary tract infection is indicated by cloudy, foul-smelling urine, pain on urination, fever, and general malaise.

Ineffective Breathing Pattern

As the muscle weakness of ALS continues, clients become less able to breathe. The respiratory muscles are affected, and clients eventually may require ventilatory assistance. The nurse must initiate measures to support the existing respiratory effort.

- Obtain a baseline assessment of breathing pattern, air movement, and oxygen saturation. *Assessments indicating the client's current condition provide data to plan individualized interventions.*
- Turn at least every 2 hours. *Movement enhances the ability to move pulmonary secretions and prevents stasis.*
- Elevate the head of the bed at least 30 degrees, suction as indicated, and provide oxygen. *This supports ventilation and enhances lung expansion as the client's condition changes.*
- Monitor temperature and lung sounds routinely; obtain sputum culture as indicated. *Early detection of a possible infectious process leads to prompt treatment.*

Community-Based Care

Initial teaching centers on explaining the disease process, expected course, and prognosis. Referral to a social worker to determine home care needs and financial assistance is helpful. Counseling and referrals to a home health agency, dietitian, and physical, speech, and occupational therapists can help the family meet the client's changing needs and abilities. The realistic anticipation of needs cannot be overemphasized.

As the client becomes more debilitated, family members or other care providers focus on preventing complications. For example, family members need to know how to suction the client and perform the Heimlich maneuver to prevent aspiration. Teaching the family how to prevent problems related to immobility is a primary consideration for the nurse.

Another focus of teaching is basic care needs, such as care required to meet elimination needs. Teach families methods to establish a bowel routine, considerations related to a urinary catheter, and the need to promptly report manifestations of an infection.

Throughout the early stage and continued care of the client and family with ALS, much consideration is given to psychosocial concerns. Depression, anger, and denial may be initial reactions; refer the client and family to an ALS support group, social worker, psychologist, or psychiatrist as indicated.

PERIPHERAL NERVOUS SYSTEM DISORDERS

Many etiologic agents are responsible for peripheral nervous system disorders. Autoimmune disorders, viruses, environmental toxins such as heavy metals, and nutritional deficiencies can affect the peripheral nervous system.

THE CLIENT WITH MYASTHENIA GRAVIS

Myasthenia gravis is a chronic autoimmune neuromuscular disorder characterized by fatigue and severe weakness of skeletal muscles. Clients experience periods of remission and exacerbation, and mild forms of the disorder exist. Weakness may remain limited to a few muscle groups, especially the ocular muscles, or may become generalized with all muscles eventually becoming weakened.

Women are affected three times more frequently than men. The age of onset for most clients is between ages 20 and 30 (Porth, 2005). Treatment with anticholinesterase medications has greatly improved the prognosis and symptom management.

Pathophysiology

The axons of motor neurons divide as they enter skeletal muscles, and each axonal ending forms a neuromuscular junction. Although the axonal ending and the muscle fiber are extremely close, they are separated by the synaptic cleft. The transmission of nerve impulses from the nerve to the muscles occurs at the neuromuscular junctions. The neurotransmitter acetylcholine is released from the axonal ending, crosses the synaptic cleft, attaches to acetylcholine receptors on the muscle fiber, and stimulates the muscle.

In myasthenia gravis, antibodies destroy or block neuromuscular junction receptor sites, resulting in a decreased number of acetylcholine receptors. Structural changes also result in diminished acetylcholine uptake. The net result is a decrease in the muscle's ability to contract despite a sufficient amount of acetylcholine. A comparison of a normal neuromuscular junction and one affected by myasthenia gravis is shown in Figure 46–4 ■.

A Normal neuromuscular junction

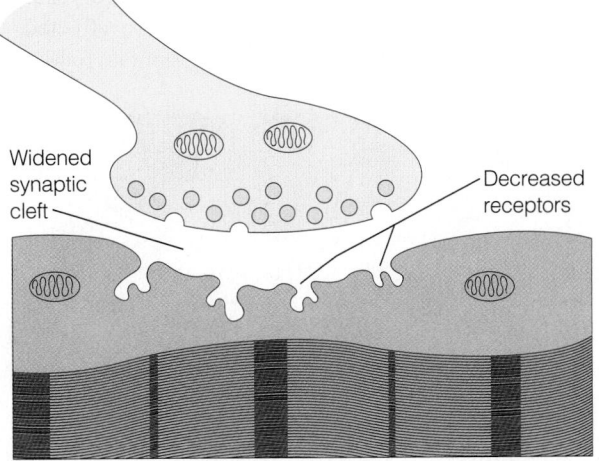

B Myasthenia gravis

Figure 46–4 ■ *A*, A normal neuromuscular junction and *B*, one showing the changes seen in myasthenia gravis. These changes interfere with the transmission of nerve impulses to the muscle.

In about 75% of clients with myasthenia gravis, the thymus gland, which is usually inactive after puberty, continues to produce antibodies because of hyperplasia of the gland or because of tumors. It is believed that the thymus is a source of autoantigen that triggers an autoimmune response in myasthenia gravis. The exact mechanism and reason for the thymus gland's antibody production are unknown.

Myasthenia gravis is sometimes associated with a tumor of the thymus, thyrotoxicosis (hyperthyroidism), rheumatoid arthritis, and lupus erythematosus. The disorder is often diagnosed when a client seeks treatment for a coincidental infection that exacerbates manifestations. Exacerbations may also occur before the menstrual period and during or soon after pregnancy.

Manifestations

The manifestations of myasthenia gravis correspond to the muscles involved. Initially, the eye muscles are affected and the client experiences either diplopia (unilateral or bilateral double vision) or ptosis (drooping of the eyelid) (Figure 46–5 ■). Next, the facial, speech, and mastication muscles become weak, and clients may have periods of dysarthria and dysphagia. Fatigue is evident even when the client tries to eat a meal; the muscles of chewing tire, and the client is forced to stop eating momentarily. A smile becomes a snarl or grimace, and the voice is weak with a muffled nasal quality. Problems performing fine motor movements of the hands, such as writing, appear early in the disease.

As the disease progresses, the muscles of the neck and extremities are affected. When the muscles of the neck become affected, the head juts forward. Deep tendon reflexes are usually normal, however, even in weak muscles. Fatigue and weakness are exacerbated with stress, fever, overexertion, and exposure to heat and are relieved by rest. Manifestations vary on a daily basis. Manifestations and complications of myasthenia gravis are listed in the box on this page.

Complications

Complications are directly related to the degree of muscle weakness and the specific muscles involved. For example, when the pharyngeal and palatal muscles are affected, the client cannot manage swallowing and may aspirate food or flu-

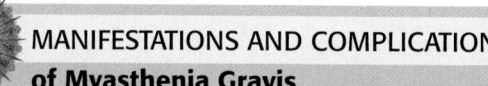

MANIFESTATIONS AND COMPLICATIONS
of Myasthenia Gravis

OCULAR AND FACIAL
- Ptosis
- Diplopia
- Facial weakness
- Dysphagia
- Dysarthria
- Complications: difficulty closing eyes, aspiration, impaired communication and nutrition

MUSCULOSKELETAL
- Weakness and fatigue
- Decreased function of hands, arms, legs, and neck muscles
- Complications: inability to perform ADLs and self-care activities, complications related to immobility, myasthenic and cholinergic crises

RESPIRATORY
- Weakening of intercostal muscles
- Decrease in diaphragm movement
- Breathlessness and dyspnea
- Poor gas exchange
- Complications: decreasing ability to walk, eat, and perform other ADLs, pneumonia

NUTRITIONAL
- Inability to chew and swallow
- Decreasing ability to move tongue
- Impairment of fine motor movements: inability to feed self
- Complications: weight loss, dehydration, malnutrition, aspiration

ids. The client is at increased risk for pneumonia because weakness of the diaphragm and muscles of respiration compromises gas exchange. Clients with myasthenia gravis can develop life-threatening emergencies, including myasthenic crisis and cholinergic crisis.

Myasthenic Crisis
Myasthenic crisis is a sudden exacerbation of motor weakness putting the client at risk of respiratory failure and aspiration. Myasthenic crisis most often is due to undermedication, missed doses of medication, or a developing infection. Manifestations of myasthenic crisis include tachycardia, tachypnea, severe respiratory distress, dysphagia, restlessness, impaired speech, and anxiety.

Cholinergic Crisis
Cholinergic crisis is the result of overdosage with the anticholinesterase (cholinergic) medications used to treat myasthenia gravis. Gastrointestinal manifestations, severe muscle weakness, vertigo, and respiratory distress are signs of cholinergic crisis. Both types of crises are emergency, life-threatening situations; clients frequently require ventilatory assistance. Differentiation is based on the client's response to edrophonium chloride (Tensilon). In myasthenic crisis the test is positive, and in cholinergic crisis the test is negative (see the discussions that follows under Diagnosis).

Figure 46–5 ■ In myasthenia gravis, the client experiences unilateral weakness of the facial muscles. Note the drooping of one eyelid.
Source: Custom Medical Stock Photo, Inc.

INTERDISCIPLINARY CARE

Care of the client with myasthenia gravis focuses on providing appropriate treatment, preventing complications, and supporting the client and family in meeting physical and psychosocial needs, especially as the disease progresses.

Diagnosis

Diagnostic tests are conducted following a thorough history and physical examination, with special attention to the facial, oculomotor, laryngeal, and respiratory muscles. Diagnostic tests include the anticholinesterase (Tensilon) test, nerve stimulation studies, and an analysis of antiacetylcholine receptor antibodies.

In the Tensilon test, the client is injected with edrophonium chloride (Tensilon), a short-acting anticholinesterase. Clients with myasthenia gravis show a significant improvement in muscle strength that lasts approximately 5 minutes. This test is also used to differentiate myasthenic crisis (caused by insufficient medication, so the client shows improvement with the drug) from cholinergic crisis (caused by overmedication, so the client does not show improvement).

Single-fiber electromyography can detect delayed or failed neuromuscular transmission in muscle fibers supplied by a single nerve fiber. Serum assay of circulating acetylcholine receptor antibodies, if increased, is diagnostic of myasthenia gravis with a sensitivity of 80% to 90%.

Medications

The primary group of medications used to treat myasthenia gravis is the anticholinesterases. These drugs act at the neuromuscular junction and allow acetylcholine to concentrate at the receptor sites, thus promoting muscle contraction. Pyridostigmine (Mestinon) is the most commonly used acetylcholinesterase inhibitor for myasthenia gravis. The client's decrease in manifestations guides dosage.

Immunosuppression with glucocorticoids, typically prednisone, is another pharmacologic therapy aimed at improving muscle strength. Clients must be aware of the need to stay on the drug at the prescribed dose to determine the least amount required for efficacy. If clients do not respond to prednisone alone, it may be combined with other immunosuppressive agents, such as cyclosporine or azathioprine (Imuran). Medications used to treat myasthenia gravis are discussed in the Medication Administration box below.

Surgery

Approximately 75% of clients with myasthenia gravis have dysplasia of the thymus gland. Therefore, thymectomy is often

---

MEDICATION ADMINISTRATION   The Client with Myasthenia Gravis

ANTICHOLINESTERASES/CHOLINESTERASE INHIBITORS
Neostigmine (Prostigmin)
Ambenonium (Mytelase Caplets)
Pyridostigmine (Mestinon, Regonol)
For diagnosis: edrophonium chloride (Tensilon)
Cholinesterase inhibitors are used in myasthenia gravis to enhance the effects of acetylcholine at the remaining skeletal muscle receptors. Cholinesterase inhibitors do not cure or change the underlying pathophysiologic processes, but they can provide effective, lifelong improvement of symptoms. Because the cholinesterase inhibitors are nonselective, the neuromuscular, muscarinic, and ganglionic junctions are each affected.

Adjusting the dose to obtain maximum benefit with minimal side effects is a major consideration when administering cholinesterase inhibitors. Initially, small doses are given followed by incremental increases until optimal muscle strength is obtained. The dose may need to be adjusted when activities result in symptoms of undermedication, such as increased ptosis. Severe undermedication results in myasthenic crisis. Although a sustained release form of pyridostigmine is available for bedtime use, it should not be used during the day because of its inconsistent absorption.

Cholinesterase inhibitors should not be administered to clients experiencing obstruction of the intestinal or urinary tract. Caution is advised when administering these drugs to clients with asthma, hyperthyroidism, bradycardia, or peptic ulcer disease. Cholinesterase inhibitors can cross the placenta; reproductive counseling is indicated.

Nursing Responsibilities
- Obtain a baseline assessment of muscle strength and abilities, concentrating on swallowing and ptosis.

- Administer the medication parenterally if the client has dysphagia. Check the dose of the medication carefully when changing from oral to parenteral routes.
- Evaluate the effectiveness of the medication and document the response, for example, time when fatigue occurs in relation to activities.
- Promptly recognize and respond to manifestations of excessive stimulation of muscarinic receptors: excess salivation, urinary urgency, bradycardia, gastrointestinal hypermotility, diaphoresis. Atropine can be administered to combat these manifestations. Respiratory depression and failure can occur and require mechanical ventilation.
- Have a muscarinic antagonist (e.g., physostigmine) readily available to treat poisoning.

Health Education for the Client and Family
- Balancing symptom control with dosage is crucial; record time of dose and response in a journal. Note the time of day when fatigued and any adverse effects, such as excess salivation, sweating, slow heartbeat, and diarrhea.
- Take the medication about 30 minutes prior to meals to enhance swallowing and chewing.
- Report manifestations of myasthenic crisis immediately: severe muscle weakness, fast heartbeat, restlessness, difficulty breathing, increasing difficulty swallowing or speaking.
- Report slow heartbeat, increased salivation or sweating, and/or decreased blood pressure immediately.
- Review possible causes of myasthenic crisis: physical or emotional stress, infection, or reduction in the medication dosage.
- Wear or carry Medic-Alert identification.

NURSING CARE OF THE CLIENT HAVING A   Thymectomy

PREOPERATIVE CARE

- Reinforce the physician's explanation of the procedure, and prepare the client for chest tubes and tracheostomy. *Realistic preparation of what to expect postoperatively encourages compliance and allays anxiety.*
- Anticipate the need for alternative communication. *The client may have a tracheostomy; preoperative planning facilitates communication after surgery.*
- Allow sufficient time for questions. *Thymectomy is a major surgery requiring either a thoracotomy and sternal split or transcervical approach. The client is usually anxious, and adequate time must be allocated to preoperative instruction.*

POSTOPERATIVE CARE

- Provide meticulous pulmonary hygiene: turning, deep breathing, and coughing at least every 2 hours; use an incentive spirometer. *Regardless of surgical approach, measures are aimed at preventing pulmonary complications of atelectasis and pneumonia.*
- Clients with a thoracotomy and sternal split procedure will require care of the anterior chest tube. Observe for complications; such as pneumothorax. *Air may enter the thoracic cavity—be alert for sudden chest pain and dyspnea, decreased breath sounds, and early signs of shock, such as restlessness.*
- Manage pain with scheduled analgesic therapy. *Maintaining a therapeutic blood level of analgesic provides better pain control than waiting until the client requests medication, as on a prn basis.*

recommended for clients younger than 60. The two surgical approaches used are the transcervical approach, which is considered less invasive, and the transsternal approach. The latter approach allows a more extensive removal of the gland; however, it also poses more potential complications because it involves splitting the sternum.

Preoperatively, clients may be tapered from steroid therapy. Usually, pyridostigmine is administered to prevent muscular manifestations during the perioperative period. Postoperative nursing care focuses on preventing complications and controlling pain. Nursing implications for the client undergoing thymectomy are presented in the box on this page. Remission is obtained in about 40% of clients but may take several years to achieve. Refer to Chapter 38 ∞ for care of

the client having a thoracotomy and chest tubes. A tracheostomy may be required when the diaphragm or intercostal muscles are involved.

Plasmapheresis

Plasma exchange in myasthenia gravis may be used in conjunction with other therapies; for example, it may be performed prior to surgical intervention. The goal of therapy is to remove the antiacetylcholine receptor antibodies, thus improving severe muscle weakness, fatigue, and other manifestations. The procedure is frequently performed when respiratory muscle involvement is evident. See Figure 46–6 ■ and the box below for nursing care of the client having a plasmapheresis.

NURSING CARE OF THE CLIENT TREATED WITH   Plasmapheresis

PREPROCEDURE CARE

- Teach about the procedure and what to expect, including what the machine looks like, the need for arterial and venous insertion sites, and the length of time of the procedure (2 to 5 hours). *Giving information, answering questions, and addressing concerns decrease anxiety.*
- Check with physician about holding medications until after the procedure. *Medications may be removed from the body as an incidental part of the plasmapheresis process.*
- Assess vital signs and weight. *Baseline parameters are necessary to evaluate for fluid imbalances and response to therapy.*
- Assess CBC, platelet count, and clotting studies. *Clients undergoing plasmapheresis are at high risk for anemia and coagulation problems secondary to hemolysis of cells.*
- Check blood type and crossmatch for replacement blood products. *Hypersensitivity reactions can occur, and close monitoring is important.*

CARE DURING AND AFTER THE PROCEDURE

- Observe for dizziness or hypotension. *Hypovolemia is a complication of plasma exchange, especially during the proce-*

dure when up to 15% of the client's blood volume is in the cell separator.

- Apply pressure dressing to access site(s). *Direct pressure helps decrease or prevent bleeding.*
- Monitor for infection and bruises at the intravenous port site. *The site of vascular access is at risk for complications and must be routinely and carefully assessed for signs of infection and for bleeding or hematoma formation.*
- Monitor electrolytes and signs of electrolyte loss. Report imbalances, and replace electrolytes as ordered. Observe for circumoral tingling, Chvostek's and Trousseau's signs if calcium levels are low, and cardiac dysrhythmias and leg cramps if potassium levels are low. *Hypocalcemia and hypokalemia may occur. Hypocalcemia occurs because the anticoagulant citrate dextrose binds with calcium.*
- Reevaluate preprocedure laboratory data, especially CBC, platelet count, and clotting times. *The cell-separating process can damage cells; anticoagulation is part of the procedure.*

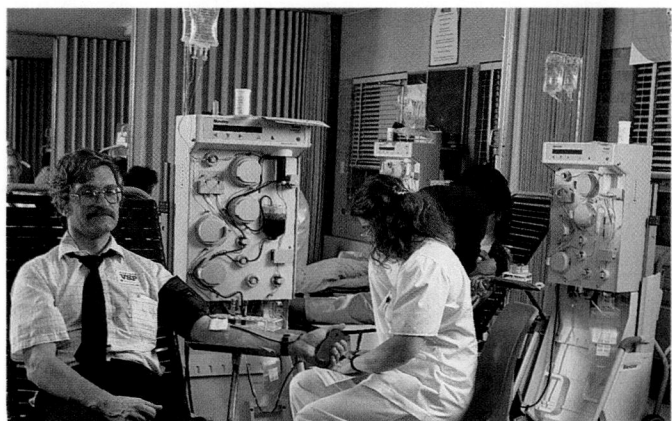

Figure 46–6 ■ Plasmapheresis is a procedure used to separate the blood's cellular components from plasma. About 50 mL per minute is withdrawn to the centrifuge in the plasmapheresis machine. The plasma is replaced with donor plasma or colloids and returned to the client.

Courtesy of Baxter Healthcare Corporation.

NURSING CARE

Because avoiding fatigue is a major part of teaching, it is important to incorporate interventions to enhance rest and conserve energy (Box 46–4). For example, suggest sitting while preparing meals and while performing hygiene and grooming. Anticipating problems, such as impaired communication, and developing alternative solutions can be helpful in promoting independence. A Nursing Care Plan for the client with myasthenia gravis is given on the next page.

Nursing Diagnoses and Interventions

Nursing care of clients with myasthenia gravis focuses not only on present problems but also on anticipated needs. Preventing myasthenic and cholinergic crises and providing psychologic support to clients and families are two important aspects of care. Individualized care depends on the specific therapy instituted. This section discusses the nursing diagnoses related to ineffective airway clearance and impaired swallowing; other nursing diagnoses that commonly

---

BOX 46–4 **Client and Family Teaching: Myasthenia Gravis**

- Schedule periods of rest and avoid stress; conserve energy when possible.
- Avoid cigarette smoke, alcohol, and beverages with quinine (e.g., tonic water).
- Take medications as prescribed. If manifestations change, consult the physician; the dose may need to be adjusted.
- Avoid extremes of temperature; an environment that is too hot or too cold may cause an exacerbation of myasthenia gravis.
- Avoid people with upper respiratory infections; infections can result in an exacerbation and extreme weakness.

---

apply, such as *Fatigue*, are addressed in other sections of this chapter.

Ineffective Airway Clearance

The underlying causes of ineffective airway clearance for the person with myasthenia gravis include poor cough mechanism, decreased rib cage expansion, diminished diaphragm movement, and decreased expiratory effort. The following interventions require particular attention if the client undergoes a thymectomy.

- Assist with turning, deep breathing, and coughing at least every 2 hours. Teach proper coughing techniques; use an incentive spirometer every 2 hours while the client is awake. *Position changes promote lung expansion; coughing helps clear secretions from the tracheobronchial tree.*
- Place in a semi-Fowler's position. *This position expands the lungs and alleviates pressure from the diaphragm, especially important considerations if the client is obese.*
- Maintain hydration status and monitor for dehydration; use a humidifier as needed. If needed, teach family how to perform percussion, postural drainage, and suction. *Interventions to liquefy secretions, such as ensuring a daily fluid intake of up to 2500 mL (perhaps via feeding tube or parenteral route), help the client mobilize and expectorate sputum.*
- Monitor lung sounds, the rate and character of respirations, and pulse oximetry readings at least every 4 hours or as indicated by client's condition. *Frequent assessments are critical to early identification of ineffective respirations and oxygenation of tissues.*

Impaired Swallowing

Clients with myasthenia gravis have weakness of the laryngeal and pharyngeal muscles involved with swallowing. Alterations in swallowing place the client at risk for poor nutrition as well as for possible aspiration. Family members need to be included in teaching, particularly the person who prepares and assists with meals.

- Assess the ability to safely manage various consistencies of foods; consult with a speech therapist for evaluation. *Dysphagic clients are at risk for aspiration; matching food consistency to the client's ability to swallow enhances safety.*
- Plan meals to promote medication effectiveness. *Pyridostigmine should be given 30 minutes before the meal to provide optimal muscle strength for swallowing and chewing.*
- Have the client eat slowly, using small bites of food. Schedule meals during periods when the client is adequately rested; develop a daily schedule incorporating rest periods. *Fatigue may add to dysphagia, putting the client at greater risk for aspiration.*
- If necessary, give cues while eating, such as "Chew your food thoroughly; swallow." *Keeping client focused may enhance swallowing.*
- Teach caregivers the Heimlich maneuver and how to suction. *Knowing specific measures to take in case of aspiration decreases both the client's and family's anxiety and promotes confidence in managing potential problems.*

Community-Based Care

Teaching for the client and family with myasthenia gravis focuses on prevention and recognition of crisis situations,

NURSING CARE PLAN   A Client with Myasthenia Gravis

Kirsten Avis, a 44-year-old homemaker and mother of two teenage sons, was diagnosed with myasthenia gravis 2 years ago. She takes an anticholinesterase medication, pyridostigmine (Mestinon), four times a day. Over the past month she has been experimenting with decreasing the dose of her pyridostigmine because she has "felt so good." She was prescribed 60 mg of pyridostigmine three times a day before meals and one-half of a long-acting 180-mg pyridostigmine tablet at night.

Three days ago, she began having chills and fever and her myasthenic symptoms became markedly worse. Mrs. Avis is easily fatigued and has been experiencing increasing weakness, bilateral ptosis, and mild dysphagia in the late afternoon and evenings. She is admitted to the hospital.

ASSESSMENT

Lela Silva, RN, is caring for Mrs. Avis. Physical examination of Mrs. Avis reveals severe muscle weakness bilaterally in her hands, arms, and thorax. Her voice is nasal, and she speaks slowly; the longer she speaks, the more difficult it becomes to understand her. She is anxious and dyspneic. Her complaints of weakness, dysphagia, dysarthria, problems with mobility, and ptosis are more pronounced later in the day. Vital signs are as follows: BP 138/88, P 88, R 28, T 102.4°F (39°C).

Some improvement in muscle weakness is noted following a restful night's sleep; however, the respiratory distress is more evident, and Mrs. Avis is increasingly restless. She is moved to the intensive care unit for advanced monitoring and possible ventilatory assistance. The medical diagnosis is myasthenic crisis secondary to pulmonary infection.

DIAGNOSES

- *Impaired Gas Exchange* related to ineffective breathing pattern and muscle weakness
- *Risk for Aspiration* related to difficulty swallowing
- *Fatigue* related to increased energy needs from muscular involvement

EXPECTED OUTCOMES

- Pulse oximetry readings will be maintained at 92% or above.
- No aspiration will occur.
- Will verbalize decreasing fatigue when performing ADLs.
- Will state the correct method of medication dosing and demonstrate how she will maintain schedule.

PLANNING AND IMPLEMENTATION

Mrs. Avis's manifestations improve following administration of edrophonium chloride (Tensilon) to verify myasthenic crisis. She is placed on oxygen by mask and suctioned as needed; equipment for possible intubation and ventilation is made readily available. She is placed in a semi-Fowler's position, and vital signs are assessed every 5 minutes during the acute exacerbation. The nurses in the intensive care unit remain in constant attendance throughout the crisis period and provide explanations to Mrs. Avis in an effort to decrease her stress and to avoid further severity of manifestations.

Three days after the crisis period, Mrs. Avis is moved to a progressive nursing care unit. Nurses follow up on teaching her the manifestations of both myasthenic and cholinergic crises. They discuss the need to wear Medic-Alert identification and review medication administration techniques with Mrs. Avis. The nurses emphasize in particular that Mrs. Avis must not split time-released medications.

Within 5 days, Mrs. Avis's condition stabilizes, and her weakness decreases sufficiently to allow discharge home. Although her temperature has returned to normal and her respiratory status has improved, she still has a productive cough. Oral antibiotics are prescribed for 2 weeks, after which she will have a follow-up visit with her primary care provider. She is instructed to seek treatment promptly if respiratory symptoms or temperature indicate recurrence of infection.

EVALUATION

Mrs. Avis is discharged without developing aspiration pneumonia or any symptoms of aspiration. Her airway was maintained throughout the myasthenic crisis, and her pulse oximetry readings remained above 92% once oxygen therapy was initiated. On discharge, pulse oximetry is above 95% without oxygen therapy. Mrs. Avis states that her fatigue and weakness have significantly improved.

Both Mrs. Avis and her husband are able to explain the difference between myasthenic and cholinergic crises and to identify methods to avoid both problems. Mrs. Avis correctly relates her proper medication regimen and makes an appointment for a follow-up visit with her physician.

CRITICAL THINKING IN THE NURSING PROCESS

1. What is the rationale for administering Tensilon to evaluate a myasthenic crisis?
2. Develop a plan to teach Mrs. Avis how to avoid fatigue when preparing and eating meals.
3. Develop a nursing care plan for Mrs. Avis for the nursing diagnosis *Ineffective Role Performance*.

See Evaluating Your Response in Appendix C.

---

understanding the disorder, and methods for coping with both physical and psychosocial problems. Setting realistic goals with the client and family provides opportunities for self-assessment and promotes active participation in rehabilitation.

Address the following topics:

- The importance of maintaining consistency in medication dosage and management
- Realistic expectations

- Methods to avoid fatigue and undue stress; specific measures for avoiding upper respiratory infections and exposure to extreme heat or cold
- Birth control measures or referral for counseling (Pregnancy can exacerbate manifestations; also, medications used to control myasthenia gravis, such as neostigmine bromide [Prostigmin], cross the placenta.)
- Referral to support groups
- Helpful resources such as the Myasthenia Foundation.

THE CLIENT WITH GUILLAIN-BARRÉ SYNDROME

Guillain-Barré syndrome (GBS) is an acute inflammatory demyelinating disorder of the peripheral nervous system characterized by an acute onset of motor paralysis (usually ascending). The classification of Guillain-Barré subtypes includes acute inflammatory demyelinating polyradiculoneuropathy, acute axonal motor neuropathy, and acute motor and sensory axonal neuropathy.

Guillain-Barré syndrome is one of the most common peripheral nervous system disorders, affecting about 3500 people in the United States and Canada each year (Porth, 2005). The cause is unknown, but precipitating events include a respiratory or gastrointestinal viral or bacterial infection 1 to 3 weeks prior to the onset of manifestations, surgery, viral immunizations, and other viral illnesses. In 60% of cases, *Campylobacter jejuni* is identified as the cause of the preceding infection. Approximately 80% to 90% of clients with GBS have a spontaneous recovery with little or no residual disabilities.

The disease is characterized by progressive ascending flaccid paralysis, accompanied by paresthesias and numbness. About 20% of clients have respiratory involvement to the point that ventilatory assistance is required. GBS is often a medical emergency.

Pathophysiology

The primary pathophysiologic process in GBS is the destruction of myelin sheaths covering the axons of peripheral nerves. The demyelination is thought to be the result of both a humoral- and cell-mediated immunologic response. The loss of myelin results in poor conduction of nerve impulses, causing sudden muscle weakness and loss of reflex response. Other manifestations occur when nerve conduction to various muscles is interrupted. The stages of Guillain-Barré syndrome and their usual manifestations are presented in Box 46-5.

Manifestations

Muscles, sensory nerves, and cranial nerves are commonly affected in clients with GBS. Most people experience symmetric muscle weakness, initially in the lower extremities. The weakness and sensory loss then ascends to the upper extremities, torso, and cranial nerves. Sensory involvement includes severe pain, paresthesia, and numbness. Cognition and level of consciousness are not affected. Facial nerve involvement results in the inability to change facial expressions and close the eyes. Muscles involved with chewing, swallowing, and speaking may be affected.

Paralysis of intercostal and diaphragmatic muscles may alter respiratory function. These clients require ventilatory assistance and supportive care. Involvement of the autonomic nervous system is characterized by fluctuating blood pressure, cardiac dysrhythmias and tachycardia, paralytic ileus, syndrome of inappropriate antidiuretic hormone secretion, and urinary retention.

The weakness usually plateaus or improves by the fourth week. Strength then improves slowly over weeks or months. Women who have had Guillain-Barré syndrome are at increased risk for relapse in the first trimester of pregnancy.

BOX 46-5 Stages of Guillain-Barré Syndrome

I. Acute Stage
- Characterized by severe and rapid weakness, especially in the lower extremities; loss of muscle strength progressing to quadriplegia and respiratory failure; decreasing deep tendon reflexes; decreasing vital capacity; paresthesias, numbness; pain, especially nocturnal; facial muscle involvement (inability to wrinkle forehead or change expressions).
- Involvement of the autonomic nervous system manifested by bradycardia, sweating, fluctuating blood pressure (notably hypotension) which may last for 2 weeks.

II. Stabilizing/Plateau Stage
- Occurs 2 to 3 weeks after initial onset.
- Marks the end of changes in condition; characterized by a "leveling off" of symptoms.
- Generally, the labile autonomic functions stabilize.

III. Recovery Stage
- May take from several months to 2 years.
- Marked by improvement in symptoms.
- Generally, muscle strength and function return in descending order.

INTERDISCIPLINARY CARE

Interventions during the acute phase (1 to 3 weeks) focus primarily on ensuring oxygenation via ventilatory assistance and preventing complications from immobility. Rehabilitation time to regain muscle strength and function varies; most people return to full presyndrome muscle function within 6 months to 2 years.

Care of the client with GBS requires a team approach. From the initial acute phase through rehabilitation, many members of the healthcare team are involved. An accurate and rapid diagnosis is needed to ensure prompt supportive treatment, particularly if there is respiratory involvement combined with widespread paralysis.

Diagnosis

Diagnosis of GBS is made after a thorough history and clinical examination. It must be differentiated from several disorders, among them influenza, heavy metal poisoning, Lyme disease, and cranial hemorrhage. Diagnosis is made based on manifestations, history of a recent viral infection, elevated CSF protein levels, and EMG studies reflecting decreased nerve conduction. Although there is no specific test to diagnose this syndrome, several findings support and confirm the diagnosis.

Medications

No medications are available for the specific treatment of Guillain-Barré syndrome. Other medications may be prescribed to provide support or prophylaxis, or to combat concurrent problems; for example, antibiotics may be prescribed for urinary tract or respiratory infections. Morphine is commonly administered to control muscle pain. Anticoagulation therapy is usually instituted to prevent thromboembolic complications, such as deep venous thrombosis and pulmonary embolism, which are associated with prolonged bed rest. If hypotension is a problem, vasopressors are prescribed.

Surgery

Tracheostomy is performed if respiratory failure occurs. Clients who need ventilatory support are usually able to be weaned after 2 to 3 weeks, but the time frame varies greatly. When the client's vital capacity reaches 8 to 10 mL/kg, he or she may be weaned from the ventilator (Hickey, 2003). Insertion of a temporary pacemaker may be indicated for bradycardia.

Plasmapheresis

Plasma exchange has been beneficial, particularly when performed within the first 2 weeks of the syndrome's development. Antibodies are removed, and immunosuppressive agents are administered concurrently. Clients typically have five exchanges during an 8- to 10-day period.

Nutrition and Fluids

Nutritional support for the client who is immobilized for prolonged periods of time is crucial. Maintaining positive nitrogen balance, ensuring sufficient fluid intake and electrolyte balance, and ensuring recommended caloric intake are goals of therapy. When swallowing problems occur, total parenteral nutrition may be indicated if feeding via a nasogastric or gastrostomy tube is ineffective.

Physical and Occupational Therapy

Long-term physical and occupational therapy are crucial to recovery. Clients with Guillain-Barré syndrome usually require prolonged rehabilitation care, which begins during the acute phase and focuses on preventing complications and limiting the effects of immobility. The severe muscle atrophy and loss of muscle tone require that clients relearn many functions and skills, such as walking. Compromise in respiratory function may delay physical rehabilitation; clients need positive reinforcement when they make even small gains in their progress. Continued attention to pain control is essential because paresthesia and pain can interfere with physical therapy.

NURSING CARE

Many of the nursing interventions for clients with this syndrome involve monitoring neurologic function, preventing problems of immobility, ensuring adequate hydration and nutrition, and promoting respiratory function. Anticipating needs of both the client and family is an important aspect of care. For example, developing an alternative method of communication before it is necessary may decrease anxiety. It is important that nursing care focus on preventing complications that may be fatal by following a rigorous predetermined schedule for turning and respiratory care (e.g., coughing, deep breathing, suctioning), using strict aseptic technique, and providing continuous psychosocial support.

Nursing Diagnoses and Interventions

Anxiety and powerlessness are major nursing considerations. The client is almost always admitted to the ICU for care, and is mentally alert but suddenly mute, ventilator dependent, and immobile. Refer to previous nursing care sections in this chapter for interventions related to anxiety, imbalanced nutrition, impaired swallowing, impaired verbal communication, and ineffective airway clearance. This section focuses on the nursing diagnoses related to pain and risk for impaired skin integrity.

Acute Pain

Pain experienced with Guillain-Barré syndrome varies. Frequently, there is a "stocking–glove" pattern, with pain in the hands, feet, and legs. Pain and tenderness in muscles can be severe; interventions must be individualized to client needs. The intense pain combined with altered sensations leads to anxiety; nursing interventions can make a difference in breaking the cycle of increasing pain that leads to increased anxiety and in turn causes more pain.

- Listen to the description of pain; determine presence of triggers or a pattern. *Acknowledging the client's perception of pain is a basis for treatment; listening establishes trust.*
- Use a pain scale for determining extent of pain. *Consistent measurement is essential to evaluate degree of pain and effectiveness of intervention.*
- Use complementary therapies to help manage pain:
  - Application of heat/cold
  - Guided imagery
  - Relaxation techniques
  - Massage.
  Presenting options for managing pain gives the client control over the situation and helps reduce anxiety. Noninvasive interventions may augment the therapeutic benefit of medications.
- Provide analgesics as indicated; administer on a regular schedule rather than waiting until pain becomes severe. *Anticipating and managing pain before it becomes severe decreases anxiety and averts the cycle of increased anxiety leading to increased pain.*
- Monitor for side effects of analgesics, particularly respiratory depression; assess respirations and lung sounds. Perform routine pulmonary care measures and monitor for aspiration. *Clients with Guillain-Barré syndrome have weakened thoracic muscles; frequent respiratory monitoring is indicated.*

Risk for Impaired Skin Integrity

During the acute and plateau stages of Guillain-Barré syndrome, clients are at risk for problems related to immobility and malnutrition. Impaired skin integrity is one such problem. Preventing areas of skin breakdown is important. Prophylactic interventions will help ensure that ingested protein and calories are used to maintain ideal body weight and other body functions rather than to heal an avoidable problem. Implicit in interventions is maintenance of adequate nutrition.

- Inspect bony prominences and provide skin care at least every 2 hours. Reposition the client and clean, dry, and lubricate the skin as needed. *These activities stimulate circulation and ensure even distribution of body weight; baseline observations allow discovery of early signs of altered integrity.*

- Pad bony prominences, such as sacral area, heels, and elbows. *This decreases shearing tears on these pressure points.*
- Use an alternating-pressure mattress or water bed. *Relieving pressure stimulates circulation and promotes oxygenation of tissues.*
- Monitor for incontinence and provide thorough skin care following each episode of incontinence. *Urine is caustic to the skin, and the moisture promotes skin breakdown.*

Community-Based Care

Clients and family members are frequently stunned by the rapid deterioration of function and fear that the paralysis will be permanent. Regularly reinforce teaching because the client's high anxiety level may interfere with listening and understanding. When possible, include the client and family in decision making; for example, seek their input when planning a daily schedule of care that incorporates various therapies.

Teaching the rationales for preventive measures reinforces the client's and family's understanding and may promote compliance during the lengthy rehabilitation. For example, because of autonomic nerve involvement, clients need to be monitored for cardiac dysrhythmias and taught to avoid changing position suddenly to prevent orthostatic hypotension.

Referrals to appropriate therapists are a component of anticipating needs; speech, nutritional, occupational, and physical therapists are an integral part of rehabilitation. Another focus of care is teaching both the client and family; incorporate explanations for interventions aimed at promoting self-care. For further information, refer the client and family to the Guillain-Barré Syndrome Foundation, International.

CRANIAL NERVE DISORDERS

Disorders of the cranial nerves may be caused by intracranial trauma or by pathologic processes. The pairs of cranial nerves, described in Chapter 43 ∞, are numbered in the order in which they arise in the brain and are named according to their anatomic characteristic or primary function. The most common cranial nerve disorders are those affecting the trigeminal (cranial nerve V) and the facial (cranial nerve VII) nerves. These disorders, discussed in the following sections, result primarily in pain or loss of sensory or motor function.

THE CLIENT WITH TRIGEMINAL NEURALGIA

Trigeminal neuralgia, also called *tic douloureux,* is a chronic disease of the trigeminal cranial nerve (V) that causes severe facial pain. The trigeminal nerve has three divisions: the ophthalmic, the maxillary, and mandibular (Figure 46–7 ■). The ophthalmic division supplies the forehead, eyes, nose, temples, meninges, paranasal sinus, and part of the nasal mucosa. The maxillary division supplies the upper jaw, teeth, lip, cheeks, hard palate, maxillary sinus, and part of the nasal mucosa. The mandibular division supplies the lower jaw, teeth, lip, buccal mucosa, tongue, part of the external ear, and the meninges. Sensory fibers of the nerve conduct impulses for touch, pain, and temperature; motor fibers innervate the temporal and masseter muscles used for chewing and lateral movement of the jaw. The maxillary and mandibular divisions are the divisions of the trigeminal nerve affected in almost all cases of this disorder.

Trigeminal neuralgia occurs more commonly in middle-age and older adults and affects women more often than men.

Pathophysiology

The actual cause of trigeminal neuralgia is unknown; however, contributing factors include irritation from flulike illnesses, trauma or infection of the teeth or jaw, and pressure on the nerve by an aneurysm, a tumor, or arteriosclerotic changes of an artery close to the nerve (Hickey, 2003).

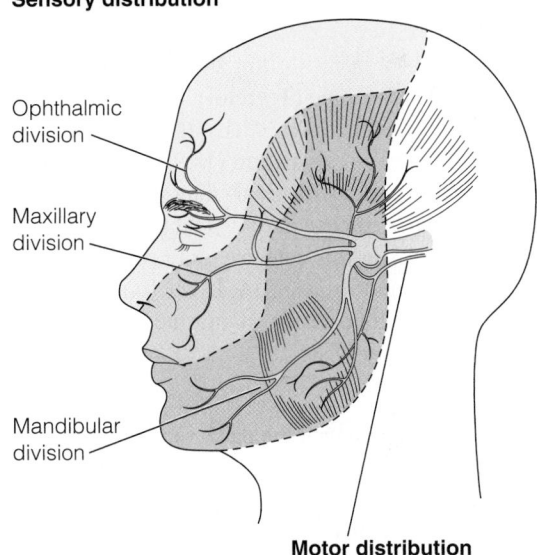

Sensory distribution

Ophthalmic division

Maxillary division

Mandibular division

Motor distribution

Figure 46–7 ■ Sensory and motor distribution of the trigeminal nerve. The three sensory divisions are ophthalmic, maxillary, and mandibular.

Stimulating specific areas of the face, called *trigger zones,* may initiate the onset of pain. These trigger zones usually parallel the distribution of the nerve and typically follow a track leading from just over the eyebrow to the ridge of the cheekbone, along the nasolabial fold, around the corner of the mouth, and down the side of the chin. The episodes of pain are initiated by many factors, including light touch, eating, swallowing, talking, sneezing, shaving, chewing gum, brushing the teeth, or washing the face. Other factors that may trigger a pain episode include changes in temperature and exposure to wind. In an attempt to control the pain, clients may refuse to wash, shave, eat, or talk.

The episodes of pain may recur for several weeks or months. The disease then spontaneously goes into remission, and the client is free of pain for periods lasting from days to years. As the client grows older, the remissions tend to become shorter, and a dull ache may be present between episodes of acute pain.

Manifestations

Trigeminal neuralgia is characterized by brief (lasting a few seconds to a few minutes), repetitive episodes of sudden severe (usually unilateral) facial pain. The pain may occur as often as hundreds of times a day to as infrequently as a few times a year. The pain is experienced over the surface of the skin. It most often begins near one side of the mouth and rises toward the ear, eye, or nostril on the same side of the face. Clients describe the pain as stabbing or lightning-like and often respond to the pain by wincing or grimacing.

INTERDISCIPLINARY CARE

There are no specific diagnostic tests for trigeminal neuralgia. The disorder is diagnosed by the characteristic location and type of pain. The disorder is treated by pharmacologic or surgical interventions.

Medications

The drug most useful in controlling the pain is the tricyclic anticonvulsant carbamazepine (Tegretol). If carbamazepine is ineffective, other medications such as the anticonvulsants phenytoin (Dilantin) or gabapentin (Neurontin) or the skeletal muscle relaxant baclofen (Lioresal) may be used. These drugs are administered to decrease paroxysmal afferent impulses and stop the pain. Drugs in this category may cause side effects of dizziness, nausea, and drowsiness. Liver function, bone marrow function, and blood levels of the medications should be monitored on a regular basis.

Surgery

If medications do not control the pain, surgical procedures may be performed, including various types of *rhizotomy*, the surgical severing of a nerve root. Closed surgical interventions by percutaneous rhizotomy involve inserting a needle through the cheek into the foramen ovale at the base of the brain and partially destroying the trigeminal nerve with glycerol (an alcohol), by radiofrequency-induced heat, or by balloon compression of the trigeminal ganglion. These procedures carry less risk and result in shorter hospital stays than do open procedures, but there is a possibility of recurrence of pain. Following surgery, the client may have some facial numbness, but there usually is no residual paralysis. The involved side of the face is insensitive to pain. The client will have some loss of facial sensation (e.g., to temperature and/or touch) and is at risk for loss of the corneal reflex. Closed procedures provide long-term pain relief and are well tolerated by the older adult. Nursing care of the client undergoing a percutaneous rhizotomy is presented in the box below.

It has been found that some structural abnormalities (such as an artery or vein compressing the nerve) may cause the neuralgia, and if so, decompression and separation of the blood vessel from the nerve root produce lasting relief of the pain (Tierney et al., 2005). The Jannetta procedure involves locating and lifting the involved vessel and placing a small piece of silicone sponge between the vessel and the nerve. Possible complications of the procedure include headache and facial pain.

NURSING CARE

Nursing care for the client with trigeminal neuralgia involves teaching self-management at home after medical or surgical intervention. Primary client concerns are managing pain, maintaining nutrition, and preventing injury.

Nursing Diagnoses and Interventions

Interventions for managing pain and improving nutritional intake are addressed here; teaching to prevent injury following surgery is discussed under client and family teaching.

Acute Pain

The client with trigeminal neuralgia has excruciating pain and often avoids ADLs and socializing with others in an attempt to

---

NURSING CARE OF THE CLIENT HAVING A Percutaneous Rhizotomy

POSTOPERATIVE CARE

- Follow routine postoperative interventions for clients having surgery (see Chapter 4).
- Monitor cranial nerve function every 2 to 4 hours:
  a. Assess the corneal reflex by lightly touching the cornea with a wisp of cotton. If the reflex is intact, the client will blink. *Severing the ophthalmic division of the trigeminal nerve destroys the corneal reflex and leaves the cornea at risk for dryness and injury.*
  b. Assess the facial nerve by asking the client to blow out the cheeks, wrinkle the forehead, frown, wink, and close both eyes tightly. Test taste by placing bitter, salty, and sweet substances on the anterior portion of the tongue. *Facial weakness is evidenced by changes in movement in the involved side of the face. The facial nerve also innervates the anterior two-thirds of the tongue.*
  c. Assess the function of the oculomotor muscles by asking the client to follow your finger through the cardinal positions of vision (see Chapter 47). *The eyes should move together; alterations in movement indicate an abnormal response.*
  d. Assess the motor portion of the trigeminal nerve by asking the client to clench the teeth while you palpate the tightness of the contracted masseter and temporal muscles. *Loss of motor function is indicated by loss of bulk and tightness of these muscles.*
  e. Apply as prescribed; an ice pack to the jaw on the operative site. *Cold decreases bleeding and swelling.*
  f. Teach the client to avoid rubbing the eye on the involved side. *Loss of the corneal reflex removes protection because the client no longer has the sensation of pain in the involved eye. Rubbing the eye could cause corneal abrasions.*

prevent the onset of pain. Pain management is fully discussed in Chapter 9 ∞. Nursing interventions for pain in clients with this disorder focus on strategies for self-management.

- Identify factors that trigger an attack, and discuss strategies to avoid these precipitating factors. *Most clients can clearly identify trigger zones and triggering factors. Identification is the first step in pain control.*
- Determine usual response to pain. *Sensitivity and reaction to pain are influenced by previous experiences with pain and by age, gender, emotional factors, and cultural background.*
- Assess factors that affect the ability to influence pain tolerance, including the knowledge and cause of the pain, the meaning of the pain, the ability to control the pain, cultural background, and support systems. *Pain tolerance, which is the duration and intensity of pain a person is willing to endure, differs greatly among individuals and may also vary within particular clients in different situations.*
- Monitor the effects of the medication prescribed for the neuralgia. *If the prescribed medication does not provide relief, other medications or methods of treatment may be used to control the pain.*

Risk for Altered Nutrition:
Less than Body Requirements

Clients often refuse to eat during periods of pain attacks, fearing that the movements of chewing may precipitate the pain. In addition, the chronic nature of the illness often causes depression, which may depress the appetite.

- Monitor dietary intake and weight at each visit, and ask the client to keep a weekly weight record. *Ongoing assessments are necessary for early detection of nutritional deficiencies.*
- Discuss the temperature and consistency of foods eaten, and suggest referral to a dietitian if necessary. *Hot or cold foods may trigger an attack; soft, warm, or cool foods are less likely to act as triggers.*
- Suggest chewing on the unaffected side of the mouth. *Chewing on the unaffected side is less likely to trigger an attack of pain and so facilitate food intake.*
- If unable to tolerate oral food, tube feedings may be necessary. *Adequate kilocalories and nutrients for metabolic processes are essential.*

Community-Based Care

The client with trigeminal neuralgia who is receiving medical treatment and providing self-care at home requires teaching about the disease process, the medication(s) being taken, and ways to reduce the incidence of attacks or pain. Diet teaching and assistance with self-management of pain are also important. For example, if the home setting is drafty and attacks of pain are triggered by wind blowing across the face, it may be necessary to encourage the client to put weather stripping around windows and doors. To prevent injury to affected areas, the topics in the Meeting Individualized Needs box below should be addressed.

THE CLIENT WITH BELL'S PALSY

Bell's palsy, also called *facial paralysis,* is a disorder of the seventh cranial (facial) nerve, characterized by unilateral paralysis of the facial muscles. The facial nerve is primarily a motor nerve that supplies all the muscles associated with expression on one side of the face. The sensory component innervates the anterior two-thirds of one side of the tongue.

This disorder can occur at any age but is seen most often in adults between 20 and 60. The incidence is equal in men and women. Eighty percent of clients recover completely within a few weeks to a few months (and three-fourths recover without any treatment). Of those remaining, 15% recover some function but have some permanent facial paralysis; these clients are usually older, have diabetes mellitus, or have more severe manifestations, such as vertigo, a sensitivity to noise, and deep head pain.

Pathophysiology

The exact cause of the disorder is unknown, although inflammation of the nerve and a relationship to the herpes simplex virus have been suggested (Tierney et al., 2005).

Manifestations

The onset of Bell's palsy is usually sudden and almost always involves one side of the face. Pain behind the ear or along the jaw may precede the paralysis. The client initially notices

---

MEETING INDIVIDUALIZED NEEDS | **Teaching for Home Care of Trigeminal Neuralgia**

EYE CARE
- Do not rub the eyes; use artificial tears four times a day if the eyes are dry or irritated.
- Wear an eye patch at night.
- Wear protective sunglasses or goggles when outside, when working in dusty areas, when mowing the lawn, and when using any type of spray material (e.g., hair spray, cleaning materials, paint, insecticides).
- Remember to blink frequently.
- Check your eyes for redness or swelling each day.
- Schedule regular eye examinations.

FACE AND MOUTH CARE
- Chew on the unaffected side of the mouth.
- Avoid eating hot foods or drinking hot liquids.
- After every meal, brush your teeth and inspect the inside of your mouth for food that may collect between the gums and cheek.
- Have regular dental examinations; you will not be able to feel pain associated with gum infection or tooth decay.
- Use an electric razor to shave the face.
- Protect your face from very cold or windy conditions.

numbness or stiffness of one side of the face that distorts the appearance. As the disease progresses, the distortion becomes more obvious, and the face appears asymmetric. The facial paralysis causes the entire side of the face to droop, and the client cannot wrinkle the forehead, close the eye, or pucker the lips on the affected side. When the client attempts to smile, the lower facial muscles are pulled to the opposite side of the face. Some clients have only mild manifestations, whereas others have complete facial paralysis (Figure 46–8 ■). Clients often believe they have had a stroke. Manifestations of Bell's palsy are listed in the box on this page.

INTERDISCIPLINARY CARE

There are no definitive laboratory or diagnostic tests for Bell's palsy, nor are there any specific treatments. Treatment includes medications and physical therapy. Recent studies have shown that antiviral drugs such as acyclovir combined with an anti-inflammatory drug such as prednisone may be effective by lim-

Figure 46–8 ■ The client with Bell's palsy shows the typical drooping of one side of the face.
Source: NIH/Phototake NYC.

> **MANIFESTATIONS** **of Bell's Palsy**
>
> - Paralysis of the facial muscles on one side of the face
> - Paralysis of the upper eyelid with loss of the corneal reflex on the affected side
> - Loss or impairment of taste over the anterior portion of the tongue on the affected side
> - Increased tearing from the lacrimal gland on the affected side

iting damage to the nerve. Physical therapy to stimulate the facial nerve and help maintain muscle tone may help prevent permanent contractures before recovery takes place. Moist heat applied to the affected side of the face may decrease pain.

NURSING CARE

Although clients provide self-care at home, the nurse plays a key role in teaching the client and family about the disease and how to prevent injury and maintain nutrition. The client is often anxious about his or her appearance and may require counseling if any deficits in facial expression become permanent. The following topics should be addressed:

- Use artificial tears four times a day to lubricate the eye; wear an eye patch or tape the eye shut at night. Wear sunglasses or goggles when outside, when working in dusty conditions, and when using any type of spray.
- Massage combined with warm, moist heat often is effective in relieving the pain.
- A soft diet that does not require chewing and six small meals a day are helpful. Chew slowly on the unaffected side and avoid hot foods. Clean the mouth and carefully inspect the area between the gums and cheek for food after each meal.
- As function returns, practice wrinkling the forehead, closing the eyes, blowing air out of the puckered mouth, and whistling for 5 minutes three or four times a day.

DISORDERS RESULTING FROM INFECTIONS AND NEUROTOXINS

A variety of disorders of the nervous system may have infectious or toxic causes. Although these disorders are not common, those included here require significant nursing care when they do occur.

THE CLIENT WITH CREUTZFELDT-JAKOB DISEASE

Creutzfeldt-Jakob disease (CJD) (also called *spongiform encephalopathy*) is a rapidly progressive, degenerative, neurologic disease that causes brain degeneration without inflammation. The disease is transmissible and progressively fatal. The causative agent is believed to be an abnormal form of a cellular glycoprotein known as the prion protein. Transmission of the agent is by direct contamination with infected neural tissue, such as during eye and brain surgery. The injection of contaminated human growth hormone from cadaveric pituitaries has also been implicated.

A different form of the disease, called *new variant CJD (vCJD)* is also a rare, degenerative, fatal brain disorder, but is not the same as the classic form of CJD. New variant CJD, referred to as "mad-cow disease," is believed to result from consumption of cattle products contaminated with bovine spongiform encephalopathy (BSE). This form primarily affects young adults. Because the illness is fatal and is associated with infected cattle, severe restrictions have been placed on the importation of cattle, sheep, and goats and on products from these animals from countries in which BSE is known to exist.

The disease occurs worldwide, but clusters occur in several areas, more often in England, Chile, and Italy. The incidence is approximately 1 or 2 cases per 1 million population (Centers for Disease Control and Prevention [CDC], 2005). Classic CJD affects adults over the age of 50; vCJD affects younger adults. The median age of death for people with classic CJD is 68 years. In contrast, the median age of death with vCJD is 28 years.

Pathophysiology

Creutzfeldt-Jakob disease is characterized by degeneration of the gray matter of the brain. The spongiform degeneration (involving the formation of tiny holes and resembling a sponge) produces severe dementia, myoclonus (muscle contractions), and characteristic changes in brain waves. On autopsy or biopsy of brain tissue, the brain shows loss of neurons and a proliferation of astrocytes (indicating destruction of nearby neurons).

Manifestations

The disease has characteristic stages and manifestations. The onset is characterized by memory changes, an exaggerated startle reflex, sleep disturbances, and nervousness. The person then experiences rapid deterioration in motor, sensory, and language function. Tremors, hyperreflexia, rigidity, and a positive Babinski reflex are often present, and confusion progresses to dementia in almost all cases. Clients in the terminal state are comatose and exhibit decorticate and decerebrate posturing. The median duration of illness for CJD is 4 to 5 months; the median duration of illness for vCJD is 13 to 14 months (CDC, 2005).

INTERDISCIPLINARY CARE

No specific treatment is available to stop or slow the progression of CJD. Collaborative interventions focus on the disease's manifestations. The disease is diagnosed by a thorough neurologic examination, specific EEG changes, and a CT scan. However, the final diagnosis of CJD can be made only by postmortem examination. It is often difficult to differentiate this disease from Alzheimer's disease, especially in the early stages.

NURSING CARE

The nurse may identify the manifestations of Creutzfeldt-Jakob disease when conducting a health history and total physical assessment. Include questions about familial history, cultural and geographic risk, and high-risk occupations or procedures in the history. Assessment of mental function, reflexes, and cranial nerve function may provide information to assist in diagnosis.

Nursing care focuses on maximizing comfort, preventing injury, preventing transmission, and providing support. The following guidelines are useful in designing the plan of care:

- Although comfort is difficult to assess in clients with impaired cognitive function, interventions that provide a quiet environment and analgesia are important.
- Communication is essential, even if the client is unable to respond.
- Institute seizure precautions, and pad side rails.
- Provide skin care, changes in position, and pressure-relief mattresses to decrease the risk of pressure ulcers, venous stasis, and pneumonia.
- Use standard precautions for blood and body fluids when providing care. Disinfect surfaces with a solution of 5% bleach. Sterilize contaminated equipment by autoclave, or soak in 5% bleach solution for 1 hour. Label all specimens as biohazardous. Teach staff members and family members

guidelines for care, including careful hand washing. It is not necessary to place the client in isolation, however.
- Provide time for family members to verbalize grief and loss, which may be manifested as anger and frustration with the healthcare system.
- Provide information to family members about all procedures and the plan of care.
- Refer family members to sources of support, such as social services and the appropriate clergy.

THE CLIENT WITH POSTPOLIOMYELITIS SYNDROME

Postpoliomyelitis syndrome is a complication of a previous infection by the poliomyelitis virus. This disease was epidemic in the 1940s and 1950s, but has largely been eradicated through immunization with oral live trivalent virus vaccine. However, it is thought that nearly 50% of the estimated 1.63 million people in the United States who had the disease are reexperiencing manifestations of the acute illness (NINDS, 2005g). These people have struggled for years to rehabilitate themselves and lead productive lives. Now, as they reach retirement age, they are again experiencing manifestations which may be physically and psychologically incapacitating.

The poliomyelitis virus destroys some of the motor cells of the anterior horn cells of the spinal cord, causing neuromuscular effects that range from mild to severe flaccid paralysis and atrophy. The primary cause of death is respiratory arrest (Tierney et al., 2005).

Manifestations of motor neuron degeneration and weakness may emerge 10 to 40 years after the initial infection. Most clients with postpoliomyelitis syndrome initially had a more severe case of polio and required hospitalization, contracted the disease after the age of 10, required ventilator assistance for respiration, and had paralysis in all four extremities. The incidence is slightly higher in women. As the population ages, it is projected that the number of older adults with postpoliomyelitis syndrome will increase.

Pathophysiology

The pathophysiologic process in postpoliomyelitis syndrome is not known.

Manifestations

The manifestations of postpoliomyelitis syndrome include fatigue, muscle and joint weakness, loss of muscle mass, respiratory difficulties, and pain. The manifestations are most often seen in muscles affected by the initial infection, but new muscle groups may also be affected. In addition to neuromuscular manifestations, the client may experience cold intolerance, dizziness, headaches, urinary incontinence, and sleep disorders.

INTERDISCIPLINARY CARE

Postpoliomyelitis syndrome is diagnosed by a previous history of polio and the current manifestations. Diagnostic studies of nerve conduction, muscle strength, and pulmonary function determine current physical status. Treatment addresses the manifestations, and often involves physical therapy and pulmonary rehabilitation programs.

NURSING CARE

The client with postpoliomyelitis syndrome faces the challenge of unexpected physical changes. Clients are often anxious about how others will react or what the future holds. Respiratory dysfunction may result in the need for oxygen. Muscular weakness and decreased pulmonary function may make walking difficult, if not impossible. Activities of daily living, independent self-care, and careers are threatened.

Many clients have not fully recovered psychologically from having polio and may respond to a recurrence of manifestations with denial and disbelief. Older clients may not know they had polio as children. Nurses are responsible for assessing and identifying the manifestations of postpoliomyelitis syndrome. It is essential to question middle to older adults about a past history of polio when conducting the health history and to ask specific questions about manifestations that the client may be experiencing.

The nurse individualizes teaching to meet the physical and psychosocial needs of the client and family. Provide candid explanations, and teach the client how to prevent fatigue, promote optimal respiratory function, meet self-care needs, modify ADLs, and maintain safety. Follow-up care with nurses, physicians, physical therapists, respiratory therapists, and counselors is indicated. Referral to a support group can make a positive difference in the client's and family's ability to cope with the disorder.

THE CLIENT WITH RABIES

Rabies is a rhabdovirus infection of the central nervous system transmitted by infected saliva that enters the human body through a bite or an open wound. If untreated, rabies is a fatal viral encephalitis that causes 30,000 to 70,000 deaths worldwide each year. In the United States, 25,000 to 40,000 people are treated annually for exposure to rabid or potentially rabid animals (Hankins & Rosekrans, 2004). This is a critical illness that almost always causes death if untreated. The rabies virus is carried by both wild and domestic animals, including bats, skunks, foxes, raccoons, cats, and dogs. After an incubation period that may last from 10 days to many years (norm is 3 to 7 weeks), the virus travels to the brain of the infected animal via the nerves. It multiplies and migrates to the salivary glands.

Pathophysiology

The client with rabies usually has a history of an animal bite but may also become infected through an abrasion or open wound that is exposed to the infected saliva. The virus spreads from the wound to local muscle cells and then invades the peripheral nerves. It eventually travels to the central nervous system. The incubation period in humans varies according to the severity and location of the bite. For example, bites on the face may result in manifestations in 10 days to a few weeks, whereas bites on the lower extremities may incubate for as long as 1 year.

Manifestations

The manifestations occur in stages. During the initial, or prodromal, stage, the site of the wound is painful and then exhibits various paresthesias. The infected person is anxious, irritable, and depressed. General manifestations of infection (such as headache, loss of appetite, and sore throat) may appear. The

person may also have increased sensitivity to light and sounds, and the skin is especially sensitive to changes in temperature.

The prodromal stage is followed by an excitement stage. The infected person has periods of excitement that alternate with periods of quiet. Attempts to drink cause such painful laryngospasms that the person refuses to drink (a phenomenon called *hydrophobia*). Large amounts of thick, tenacious mucus are present. The client experiences convulsions, muscle spasms, and periods of apnea. If untreated, death occurs approximately 7 days from the onset of manifestations and is usually due to respiratory failure.

INTERDISCIPLINARY CARE

Animals that bite are kept under observation, if possible, for 7 to 10 days to detect rabies manifestations. Sick animals should be euthanized and their brains examined for presence of the rabies virus, which is detected by fluorescent antibody testing. The blood of an infected person can also be tested with the same diagnostic study to demonstrate the presence of rabies antibodies.

NURSING CARE

Nursing care for clients with rabies is provided in an intensive care unit, with the client in a quiet, darkened room to decrease stimulation as much as possible. The client requires interventions to maintain the airway, maintain oxygenation, and control seizures. Standard precautions are essential, because the rabies virus is present in the saliva of the client. If an open wound of a healthcare provider is contaminated with infected saliva, the provider must receive postexposure immunizations.

Health Promotion

Client and family teaching focuses on the importance of immunizing pets, providing proper care of wounds, seeking immediate medical attention for animal bites, and obtaining treatment after any suspicious bite.

Because the untreated disease is almost always fatal, the best intervention is prevention. Preventive activities follow:

- Immunize household dogs and cats; immunize people who are exposed to animals.
- Local treatment of animal bites and scratches:
  - Carefully and thoroughly clean and flush wounds with soap and water to remove the saliva and dilute the viral exposure.
  - Immediately take the person with the bite for emergency treatment.
- Postexposure care:
  - Rabies immune globulin (RIG) is administered for passive immunization. Up to 50% of the globulin is infiltrated around the wound, and the rest is administered intramuscularly. At the same time, an inactivated human diploid cell vaccine (HDCV) is administered intramuscularly, with 1 mL given on the day of exposure and on days 3, 7, 14, and 28 after exposure (Tierney et al., 2005). RIG and HDCV should never be given in the same syringe or at the same site. Local and mild systemic reactions include itching, tenderness, headaches, muscle aches, and nausea.
  - If RIG is not available, equine rabies antiserum may be administered after testing the client for horse serum sensitivity.

THE CLIENT WITH TETANUS

Tetanus, more commonly called *lockjaw,* is a disorder of the nervous system caused by a neurotoxin elaborated by *Clostridium tetani.* This anaerobic bacillus lives in the soil. Spores of the bacillus enter the body through open wounds contaminated with dirt, street dust, or feces (animal or human). The wounds may result from punctures, scratches or abrasions, bee stings, abortions, surgery, trauma, burns, or intravenous drug use. Incidence is highest among people who have never been immunized, older adults whose immunity has been lost, and women. The majority of cases occur in people over age 50. Tetanus has a high mortality rate, with death occurring in over 40% of all cases. Contaminated lesions of the head and face are more dangerous than those in other parts of the body.

Pathophysiology

When the spores of *C. tetani* enter the open wound, they germinate and produce a toxin called tetanospasmin. The incubation period averages 8 to 12 days but can range from 5 days to 15 weeks (Tierney et al., 2005). The toxins are absorbed by the peripheral nerves and carried to the spinal cord, where they block the action of inhibitory enzymes at spinal synapses and interfere with transmission of neuromuscular impulses. As a result, even minor stimuli cause uncontrolled muscle spasms.

Manifestations

The manifestations begin with pain at the site of the infection. The infected person has stiffness of the jaw and neck and dysphagia. There is often profuse perspiration and drooling from increased salivation. As the infection progresses, the person experiences hyperreflexia, spasms of the jaw muscles (*trismus*) or facial muscles, and rigidity and spasms of the abdominal, neck, and back muscles. Generalized tonic seizures are caused by even minor stimuli, and the person assumes a typical opisthotonic position during the seizures: The head is retracted, the back is arched, and the feet are extended. The muscle spasms are painful. The person may be unable to breathe from spasms of the glottis and respiratory muscles. Despite these physical effects, the client has no change in mental status.

The complications of tetanus include urinary retention and airway obstruction from the spasms. Cardiac and respiratory failure are late, life-threatening complications.

INTERDISCIPLINARY CARE

There are no specific diagnostic tests for tetanus; diagnosis is based on manifestations. Tetanus is completely preventable by active immunization. Immunization for children includes tetanus toxoid, administered as part of the diphtheria-pertussis-tetanus (DPT) immunization series. In adults, immunization is obtained by administering tetanus toxoid as two doses 4 to 6 weeks apart, with a third dose in 6 to 12 months. All individuals should have a booster dose every 10 years throughout life or at the time of a major injury if the last booster dose was given more than 5 years prior to the injury.

If a wound is contaminated or if the person's immunization status is uncertain, passive immunization with tetanus immune globulin is administered. Active immunization with tetanus toxoid is begun at the same time. The wound is carefully and thoroughly debrided and antibiotics administered.

The client with tetanus requires intensive care in an area of minimal stimulation. Penicillin is administered to help destroy the toxin-producing organism. Muscle spasms and seizures are controlled by chlorpromazine (Thorazine) or diazepam (Valium), often combined with a sedative. Anticoagulants may be prescribed to prevent venous thrombosis. In severe cases, seizures and spasms are controlled with paralysis by a curare-like medication, and airway obstruction is managed by mechanical ventilation.

 NURSING CARE

Nursing care for the client with tetanus is intensive and focuses on assessments and interventions to promote safety, prevent injury, maintain nutrition, and maintain pulmonary and cardiovascular function. The client usually requires in-hospital care for 2 to 5 weeks. The nursing care plan commonly includes the following:

- Place in a quiet, darkened room to decrease stimuli that cause muscle spasms and seizures.
- Provide only necessary physical care, and do so during periods of maximal sedation to decrease tactile stimulation that causes muscle spasms.
- Maintain oxygenation through mechanical ventilator and frequent suctioning of secretions.
- Maintain intravenous access for the administration of fluids and medications.
- Administer prescribed antibiotics, anticonvulsants, and sedatives. In the case of cardiovascular complications, administer prescribed beta-adrenergic blocking agents such as propranolol (Inderal).
- Provide adequate nutrition through prescribed nutritional support, such as total parenteral nutrition.
- Monitor respiratory and cardiovascular status and provide immediate interventions for respiratory or cardiovascular failure.
- Monitor fluid and electrolyte status. Ensure adequate fluid intake to maintain hydration and urinary output.
- Monitor urinary output, which should be maintained at 1.5 to 2 L per day.
- Monitor for the hazards of immobility, including constipation, pneumonia, deep venous thrombosis, and pressure ulcers.

Health Promotion

Tetanus is a preventable disorder, and nurses have a major role in promoting immunizations for all children and for educating adults about the need for booster doses. The older population is especially at risk for never having been immunized or for letting immunizations lapse. Information for this age group can be provided through activities such as community health fairs and programs at senior citizen groups.

It is also necessary to teach the proper care of wounds. All wounds, no matter how small, should be thoroughly washed with soap and water. All foreign material should be carefully flushed out or removed from a wound, and medical care should be sought for wounds that are more extensive or contaminated.

THE CLIENT WITH BOTULISM

Botulism is food poisoning caused by ingestion of food contaminated with a toxin produced by the bacillus *Clostridium* *botulinum.* This anaerobic spore-forming bacillus is found in the soil. Most cases of botulism occur from eating improperly canned or cooked foods, especially home-canned vegetables and fruits, smoked meats, and vacuum-packed fish. The mortality rate is high if the disease is untreated.

Pathophysiology

The toxins liberated by *C. botulinum* are absorbed by the gastrointestinal tract and bound to nerve tissues. They block the release of acetylcholine from nerve endings and thus cause respiratory paralysis due to paralysis of skeletal muscles.

Manifestations

Manifestations appear 12 to 36 hours after ingestion of the contaminated food. They usually begin with visual disturbances such as diplopia, loss of accommodation, and fixed, dilated pupils. Ptosis is often present. Gastrointestinal manifestations include nausea and vomiting, diarrhea, dysphagia, and dry mouth. Involvement of the larynx is manifested by dystonia (impaired muscle tone). Paralysis of all muscle groups progresses throughout the body, with respiratory paralysis causing death if the client is not placed on a mechanical ventilator. There is no effect on mental status.

INTERDISCIPLINARY CARE

Infection with the *Clostridium* toxin is verified by laboratory analysis of the serum and stool and of suspected food, if possible. If botulism is suspected, the state health department and the CDC should be notified for assistance with laboratory assays and procuring botulism antitoxin. All people who may have eaten the contaminated food must be located and observed.

Any toxins in the gastrointestinal system are removed by cathartics, enemas, and gastric lavage. The client with respiratory paralysis is placed on a mechanical ventilator and may require a tracheostomy. Botulism antitoxin is administered to eradicate toxins in the circulation. Nutritional support is often provided with total parenteral nutrition. Intravenous fluids are administered to prevent dehydration and renal failure. If ventilation can be maintained, the client often recovers without further neurologic deficits.

NURSING CARE

The client with botulism is hospitalized, and interventions focus on monitoring for respiratory failure and providing ventilatory assistance if necessary. Ongoing assessments are also made for manifestations of paralytic ileus and urinary retention. The client will be NPO until able to swallow and breathe; therefore, hydration and nutritional status are monitored. Teach the client and family that fatigue and weakness may persist for up to a year. During this time, the client may need to modify ADLs and take rest periods throughout the day.

Health Promotion

Education of the public to prevent botulism is important. Address the following topics at health fairs and community programs:

- Home-canned foods must be processed in a pressure cooker rather than in boiling water because the organism is difficult to kill.
- Do not eat home-processed foods that have a change in color, are soft, contain gas bubbles, or have a bad odor.
- Always heat both home-processed and commercial foods at temperatures over 248°F (120°C) or boil for 10 minutes before tasting or eating them.
- Discard home-processed or commercially canned or bottled foods with defective seals.
- Discard commercially prepared canned foods that are damaged or have bulging sides or leaking contents.

EXPLORE MediaLink

Prentice Hall Nursing MediaLink DVD-ROM
Audio Glossary
NCLEX Review

Animations/Videos
Akinesia
Alzheimer's Disease
Bradykinesia
Dopamine
Forward Tremor
Lateral Tremor
Levodopa
Multiple Sclerosis
Parkinson's Disease

COMPANION WEBSITE www.prenhall.com/lemone
Audio Glossary
NCLEX–RN® Review
Care Plan Activity: Guillain-Barré Syndrome
Case Studies
 Huntington's Disease
 Parkinson's Disease
MediaLink Application: Alzheimer's Disease
Links to Resources

CHAPTER HIGHLIGHTS

- Alzheimer's disease (AD) is a form of dementia (a disease of the brain) of older adults with progressive irreversible deterioration of general intellectual functioning. The disease is characterized by atrophy of brain tissue, loss of neurons, neurofibrillary tangles, and amyloid plaques. AD finally leaves the person unable to communicate, maintain continence, and recognize self or others. Caregivers need much teaching and support to not only provide care, but to also avoid caregiver burden.

- Multiple sclerosis (MS) is a chronic demyelinating neurologic disease of the CNS (brain, optic nerves, and spinal cord). Occurring in young to middle-age adults, it is believed to be due to an autoimmune response to a prior viral infection. The loss of myelin leads to axon dysfunction, which slows and distorts nerve impulses. Medications (ACTH, immunosuppressive agents, interferon, and glatiramer acetate) are used to slow the progression of the disease, decrease the number of exacerbations, and treat manifestations.

- Parkinson's disease (PD) is a progressive degenerative neurologic disease characterized by tremor, muscle rigidity, and bradykinesia. The loss of voluntary motor control is the result of pathologic processes resulting in a decrease of dopamine (an inhibitory neurotransmitter) so that it can no longer inhibit acetylcholine (an excitatory neurotransmitter). Medications are used to treat manifestations and include MAO inhibitors, dopaminergics, dopamine agonists, and anticholinergics. Other treatments include deep brain stimulation and surgery.

- Huntington's disease (chorea) is a progressive, degenerative inherited neurologic disease characterized by increasing dementia and chorea. There is an excess of dopamine, causing excessive, uncontrolled movement.

- Amyotrophic lateral sclerosis (ALS) is a rapidly progressive and fatal degenerative motor neuron disease characterized by weakness and wasting of voluntary control muscles, but without sensory or cognitive changes. The client eventually loses the ability to communicate and breathe. Riluzole, antiglutamate medication, is used to treat (but not cure) manifestations.

- Myasthenia gravis (MG) is a chronic autoimmune peripheral nervous system disorder characterized by fatigue and severe skeletal muscle weakness. It results from a decreased number of acetylcholine receptors at the neuromuscular junction, so muscles are unable to contract. Life-threatening emergencies include myasthenic crisis (sudden increase in motor weakness) and cholinergic crisis (from an overdose of the anticholinestease medications used to treat MG).

- Guillain-Barré syndrome (GBS) is an acute inflammatory demyelinating disease of the peripheral nervous system characterized by an acute onset of flaccid motor paralysis that begins in the lower extremities and ascends to involve the upper extremities, torso, and cranial nerves. Paralysis of intercostal and diaphragmatic muscles often necessitates ventilatory assistance. The acute phase lasts from 1 to 3 weeks, followed by recovery, which takes from 6 months to 2 years.

- Cranial nerve disorders include trigeminal neuralgia (tic douloureux) and Bell's palsy. Trigeminal neuralgia is a chronic disorder of cranial nerve V and causes severe facial pain. Bell's palsy is an acute disorder of cranial nerve VII, characterized by unilateral paralysis of the facial muscles. Clients provide self-care at home and require teaching to help prevent complications.

- Neurologic disorders resulting from neurotoxins or viruses include Creutzfeldt-Jakob disease, postpoliomyelitis syndrome, rabies, tetanus, and botulism. Community-based health education can not only provide information but can also prevent illness in the case of rabies, tetanus, and botulism.

TEST YOURSELF NCLEX-RN® REVIEW

1. Which of the following statements is true of dementia? (Choose all that apply.)
   1. Dementia is a general term used to describe manifestations of damage or death of neurons.
   2. Dementia is the term used to describe the cognitive and behavioral manifestations of AD.
   3. Dementia is an acute disorder, resulting from an injury to the brain.
   4. Dementia is the primary manifestation of Guillian-Barré syndrome.

2. What manifestation is usually the first indication of the onset of AD?
   1. inability to perform ADLs
   2. sundowning at night
   3. subtle memory deficits
   4. inability to communicate

3. Which of the following nursing diagnoses is appropriate for clients with MS, regardless of type or severity?
   1. *Fatigue*
   2. *Risk for Aspiration*
   3. *Acute Pain*
   4. *Impaired Gas Exchange*

4. You are preparing information to teach a client about medications for MS. What drugs would you expect to be used?
   1. antibiotics
   2. antihistamines
   3. interferon
   4. levodopa

5. Which of the following topics is important when teaching a young adult with MS?
   1. how to prevent sexually transmitted infections
   2. how pregnancy can improve manifestations
   3. what can be done to cure the disease
   4. why it is important to avoid extremes of heat and cold

6. The manifestations of Parkinson's disease are the result of:
   1. autoimmune responses to a viral infection.
   2. the failure of dopamine to inhibit acetylcholine.
   3. effects of a neurotoxin.
   4. a genetic defect.

7. When teaching care at home for the client with PD, what would be a major area to discuss with caregivers?
   1. preventing an overdose of medications
   2. avoiding daily baths and showers
   3. preventing falling
   4. increasing appetite

8 What drug classification is the medication used to treat ALS?
1. dopamine agonist
2. anticholinergic
3. anti-inflammatory
4. antiglutamate

9 You are preparing a teaching plan for a client with Bell's palsy. What information would you include?
1. "You will experience severe facial pain during attacks."
2. "The disease affects your muscles so you can't walk."
3. "One side of your face will not move normally."
4. "Be sure to boil all home-canned foods before eating them."

10 How can the nurse prevent tetanus?
1. Teach safe food preparation techniques.
2. Promote immunizations for adults and children.
3. Demonstrate proper disposal of soiled dressings.
4. Promote immunization of household pets.

See Test Yourself answers in Appendix C.

BIBLIOGRAPHY

Acello, B. (2003). Handling an unwelcome comeback: Postpolio syndrome. *Nursing, 33*(11), Hospital Nursing: 32hn1–2, 32hn5.

Alzheimer's Disease Education & Referral Center. (2003). *Alzheimer's disease fact sheet.* Retrieved from http://www. alzheimers.org/pubs/adfact.html

Alzheimer's Foundation of America. (2005). *About dementia.* Retrieved from http://alzfdn.org/dementia/index.shtml

American Academy of Neurology. (2005). *Alzheimer's disease guidelines: A summary for patients, family and friends.* Retrieved from http://www.aan.com

Brown, C. (2003). Surgical treatment of trigeminal neuralgia. *AORN Journal, 78*(5), 743–744, 745, 748–750.

Centers for Disease Control and Prevention. (2005). *CJD (Creutzfeldt-Jakob disease, classic; vCJD).* Retrieved from http://cdc.gov/ncidod/dvrd/cjd/index.htm

Cheung, H., & Hocking, P. (2004). The experience of spousal careers of people with multiple sclerosis. *Qualitative Health Research, 14*(2), 153–166.

Dochterman, J., & Bulechek, G. (2004). *Nursing interventions classification (NIC)* (4th ed.). St. Louis, MO: Mosby.

Finlayson, M., Van Denend, T., & Hudson, E. (2004). Aging with multiple sclerosis. *Journal of Neuroscience Nursing, 36*(5), 245–251, 259.

Frock, T., & McCaffrey, R. (2005). Clinical case report. Postauricular pain with Bell's palsy. *Nurse Practitioner: American Journal of Primary Health Care, 30*(4), 58–61.

Gerdner, L., & Hall. G. (2001). Chronic confusion. In M. Maas, K. Buckwalter, M. Hardy, T. Tripp-Reimer, M. Titler, & J. Specht (Eds.), *Nursing care of older adults: Diagnoses, outcomes, & interventions* (pp. 421–441). St. Louis, MO: Mosby.

Hamilton, R., Bowers, B., & Williams, J. (2005). Disclosing genetic test results to family members. *Journal of Nursing Scholarship, 37*(1), 18–24.

Hankins, D., & Rosekrans, J. (2004). Overview, prevention, and treatment of rabies. *Mayo Clinic Proceedings, 79*(5), 671–676.

Hickey, J. (2003). *The clinical practice of neurological and neurosurgical nursing* (4th ed.). Philadelphia: Lippincott.

Holland, J., & Madonna, M. (2005). Nursing grand rounds: Multiple sclerosis. *Journal of Neuroscience Nursing, 37*(1), 15–19.

Huntington's Disease Society of America. (2004). *FAQ's.* Retrieved from http://www.hdsa.org/site/ PageServer?pagename=help_info_ed_faq

Improving the odds for avoiding dementia in advanced age. (2004). *Critical Care Nurse, 24*(5), 8–12.

Kee, J. (2006). *Handbook of laboratory and diagnostic tests with nursing implications* (6th ed.). Upper Saddle River, NJ: Prentice Hall.

Mini-mental state exam. (1975). *Journal of Psychiatric Research, 12,* 189–198.

Moorhead, S., Johnson, M., & Maas, M. (2003). *Nursing outcomes classification (NOC)* (3rd ed.). St. Louis, MO: Mosby.

Moyer, D. (2005). Hallmarks of Alzheimer's advances. *Nursingmatters, 16*(3), 8–9.

NANDA International. (2005). *Nursing diagnoses: Definitions & classification 2005–2006.* Philadelphia: Author.

National Institute of Neurological Disorders and Stroke. (2005a). *Amyotrophic lateral sclerosis fact sheet.* Retrieved from http://www.ninds.nih.gov/disorders/amyotrophiclateral sclerosis/detail_amyotrophiclateralsclerosis_pr.htm

_____. (2005b). *Bell's palsy fact sheet.* Retrieved from http://www.nih.gov/disorders/bells/detail_bells.htm

_____. (2005c). *Deep brain stimulation for Parkinson's disease information page.* Retrieved from http://www. ninds.nih.gov/disorders/deep_brain_stimulation/ deep_brain_stimulation_pr.htm

_____. (2005d). *Multiple sclerosis: Hope through research.* Retrieved from http://www.ninds.nih.gov/ disorders/multiple_sclerosis/detail_multiple_sclerosis.htm

_____. (2005e). *NINDS Guillain-Barré syndrome information page.* Retrieved from http://www.ninds.nih. gov/disorders/gbs?gbs_pr.htm

_____. (2005f). *NINDS Huntington's disease information page.* Retrieved from http://www.ninds/nih. gov/disorders/huntington/huntington.htm

_____. (2005g). *NINDS post-polio syndrome information page.* Retrieved from http://www.ninds. nih.gov/disorders/post_polio/post_polio.htm

_____. (2005h). *Parkinson's disease information page.* Retrieved from http://www.ninds.nikg.gov/disorders/ parkinsons_disease/parkinsons_disease.htm

_____. (2005i). *The dementias: Hope through research.* Retrieved from http://www.ninds.nih.gov/ disorders/alzheimersdisease/detail/alzheimersdisease_ pr.htm

National MS Society. (2005). *Just the facts: 2005–2006.* Retrieved from http://www.nationalmssociety.org/ Brochures-Just%20the.asp

National Parkinson Foundation. (2005a). *About Parkinson disease.* Retrieved from http://www.parkinson.org

_____. (2005b). *Parkinson primer.* Retrieved from http://www.parkinson.org/site/pp.asp?c=9dJFLPwB&b= 71354

O'Maley, K., O'Sullivan, J., Wollin, J., Barras, M., & Brammer, J. (2005). Teaching people with Parkinson's disease about their medication. *Nursing Older People, 17*(1), 14–16, 18, 20.

Parkinson's Disease Foundation, Inc. (2005). *Parkinson's disease: An overview.* Retrieved from http://www.pdf.org/ AboutPD/index.cfm

Porth, C. M. (2005). *Pathophysiology: Concepts of altered health states* (7th ed.). Philadelphia: Lippincott.

Richman, D., & Agius, M. (2003). Treatment of autoimmune myasthenia gravis. *Neurology, 61*(12), 1652–1661.

Rubin, R. (2005). Communication about sexual problems in male patients with multiple sclerosis. *Nursing Standard, 19*(24), 33–37.

Seman, D. (2003). "Listen with the ears of your heart." *Nursing Homes Long Term Care Management, 52*(9), 34, 36–40.

Sheff, B. (2005). Combating infection. Mad cow disease and vCJD: Understanding the risks. *Nursing, 35*(2), 74–75.

Sulton, L. (2001). Caring for the patient with Guillain-Barré syndrome. *Nursing, 31*(10), 32cc1–2, 32cc4, 32cc6.

Tierney, L., McPhee, S., & Papadakis, M. (Eds.). (2005). *Current medical diagnosis & treatment* (45th ed.). New York: McGraw-Hill.

Wilkinson, J. (2005). *Prentice Hall nursing diagnosis handbook with NIC interventions and NOC outcomes* (8th ed.). Upper Saddle River, NJ: Prentice Hall.

Wilson, B., Shannon, M., & Stang, C. (2006). *Prentice Hall nurse's drug guide 2006.* Upper Saddle River, NJ: Prentice Hall.

UNIT 13 BUILDING CLINICAL COMPETENCE
Responses to Altered Neurologic Function

Functional Health Pattern: Cognitive-Perceptual

■ Think about clients with cognitive-perceptual problems for whom you have cared in your clinical experiences.

- ■ What were the clients' major medical diagnoses (e.g., traumatic brain injury, spinal cord injury, stroke, aneurysm)?
- ■ What manifestations did each of these clients have? (Were these manifestations similar or different?
- ■ How did each of these clients respond to interaction with you as you provided care for them? Was it difficult for them to remember the identity of visitors or family members, that they were in a hospital, the correct year? Was their speech affected (aphasia)? Did the family indicate that the client took longer than normal to "find the words" in conversation? Were their words "jumbled" or confused when they spoke?

■ The neurologic system regulates and integrates all body functions, mental abilities, and emotions. It is made up of the central nervous system and peripheral nervous system. These two components are made up of two types of cells: neurons (which receive and transmit information) and neuroglia (which protect and support the neurons). The Cognitive-Perceptual Pattern includes functional abilities such as language, memory, judgment, decision making, and sensation. The pathophysiologic factors affecting cognition and perception are:

- ■ Decreased blood flow to and ischemia of neurons (e.g., stroke, ruptured intracranial aneurysm or arteriovenous malformation, spinal cord injury, increased intracranial pressure, cerebral edema)
- ■ Direct injury to neurologic tissues from trauma or compression (e.g., traumatic brain injury, skull fractures, increased intracranial pressure, spinal cord injury, herniated intervertebral disk, brain tumors, spinal cord tumors)
- ■ Alterations in the electrical activity of cerebral neurons (epilepsy)
- ■ Infections of the neurologic system (e.g., meningitis, encephalitis, rabies, tetanus, botulism)
- ■ Degeneration or alteration of neurons, supporting neurologic structures, or neurotransmitters (e.g., Alzheimer's disease, multiple sclerosis, Parkinson's disease, Huntington's disease, amyotrophic lateral sclerosis, myesthenia gravis, Guillain-Barré syndrome, cranial nerve disorders).

■ One example of the pathophysiologic effects of neurologic disorders, increased intracranial pressure (a response to many disorders of and injuries to the brain) causes cell damage and death and can lead to transient or permanent manifestations such as:

- ■ *Altered level of consciousness* (with decreasing circulation to and oxygenation of neurons → decreased cellular metabolism → Na-K pump failure → edema damage to the RAS)
- ■ *Aphasia or dysphagia* (resulting from changes in the complex neurologic pathways in the speech center through ischemia, decreased oxygen and blood circulation, cell death, and the toxins released by dying cells)
- ■ *Seizures* (seizure threshold is exceeded → abnormal neuronal activity remains localized or spreads to involve the entire brain → causing local or generalized effects).

■ Priority nursing diagnoses within the Cognitive-Perceptual Pattern that may be appropriate for clients with neurologic disease or injury include:

- ■ *Ineffective Tissue Perfusion: Cerebral* as evidenced by level of consciousness changes, cognitive defects, and inaccurate interpretation of stimuli including confusion, comprehension, problem solving, abstraction, and memory deficits
- ■ *Impaired Verbal Communication* as evidenced by inability/difficulty in speaking or understanding spoken or written words
- ■ *Powerlessness* as evidenced by expressions of frustration regarding inability to control their illness, recovery rate, or care
- ■ *Acute Confusion* as evidenced by restlessness, hallucinations, disorientation, anxiety.

■ Two nursing diagnoses from other functional health patterns often are a high priority for the client with neurologic disease or injury:

- ■ *Impaired Swallowing* (Nutritional-Metabolic)
- ■ *Impaired Physical Mobility* (Activity-Exercise)

Directions: Read the clinical scenario below and answer the questions that follow. To complete this exercise successfully, you will use not only knowledge of the content in this unit, but also principles related to setting priorities and maintaining client safety.

CLINICAL SCENARIO

You have been assigned to work with the following clients on a neurologic hospital unit. Significant data obtained during report are as follows:

■ Louie Hernandez is a 74-year-old male who was admitted from the emergency department to the neurologic unit last night. Mr. Hernandez was found by family in his home. He was unable to speak or move the right side of his body and continues to experience paralysis on the right side in both his arm and leg. He is aphasic with facial drooping, but is able to nod his head to communicate. Mr. Hernandez has a known history of hypertension, CHF, and type 2 diabetes controlled by oral hypoglycemic medications. He has smoked a package of cigarettes a day for 40 years. BP is now 140/105, P 98, R 24. Lungs reported to have crackles in the bases. He is receiving 2 liters of oxygen per nasal cannula. A swallowing evaluation has been ordered to be done today.

■ Jane Thomas is a 56-year-old female. She was admitted 4 days ago and underwent a lumbar laminectomy. She was able to ambulate with assistance on day 2 after surgery and now reports no dizziness on ambulation. Her leg strength has progressively increased since surgery. She has equal sensation and is able to wiggle her toes on both feet. Pain is controlled at the client's desired level of 2 to 3 on a scale of 1 to 10 with oral medications.

■ Cesar Phillips is a 39-year-old male, admitted 4 days ago after experiencing paralysis and severe headache at work. He has been diagnosed with stroke following an MRI. He has a history of smoking one package of cigarettes per day and hypertension. His wife reported that he had stopped taking his blood pressure medication due to the side effects of impotence. Mr. Phillips is awake and alert, but has exhibited impulsive behavior and agnosia He also has a difficult time remembering words and neglects the left side of his body in ADLs. BP had been 130/85 at the beginning of last shift but has increased to 170/110. He received an additional prn blood pressure medication 1.5 hours ago.

■ Tonya Walton is a 29-year-old female. She was involved in a car crash 12 hours before her admission 5 days earlier. She developed a headache, drowsiness, confusion, and pupil enlargement several hours after the crash. Following an MRI, Ms. Walton underwent intracranial surgery to evacuate a subdural hematoma. She has been complaining of a headache that has increased in intensity from a 2 to a 6 on a scale of 1 to 10 on the previous shift. She received two Tylenol ES tabs 1 hour ago. BP was 140–150 systolic and 90–100 diastolic for most of the shift. Her BP at the time of the Tylenol administration was 175/115. She has not experienced any changes in her neuro assessment except for the increasing headache and blood pressure elevation.

Questions

1 In what order would you visit these clients after report?
1. _____
2. _____
3. _____
4. _____

2 What two top priority nursing diagnoses would you choose for each of the clients presented above? Can you explain, if asked, the rationale for your choices?

	Priority Nursing Diagnosis #1	Priority Nursing Diagnosis #2
Louis Hernandez		
Jane Thomas		
Cesar Phillips		
Tonya Walton		

3 After completing Mr. Hernandez's beginning-of-shift baseline assessment, what assessment would be your next priority?
1. rhythm strip interpretation
2. intake and output
3. heart sounds
4. level of pain

4 You are completing the beginning-of-shift assessment for Mr. Phillips. What changes would best indicate that the plan initiated by the previous shift was effective?
1. Mr. Phillips no longer has a craving for cigarettes.
2. Mr. Phillips' respiratory rate is 18–20.
3. Mr. Phillips' LOP is now 1–2.
4. Mr. Phillips' blood pressure has decreased to 145/90.

5 What are the top two education priorities for Jane Thomas as you plan for discharge? (Select all that apply.)
1. appropriate exercise
2. pain management
3. weight control
4. incision care
5. importance of rest

6 You review the lab reports for Jane Thomas. You are most interested in the results for which of the following studies? (Select all that apply.)

1. white blood cell count
2. red blood cell indices
3. serum sodium
4. hemoglobin
5. hematocrit
6. osteocalcin
7. prealbumin

7 You are completing the beginning-of-shift assessment for Ms. Walton. What changes would best indicate that the plan initiated by the previous shift was effective?
1. Ms. Walton has no neurologic changes or deterioration.
2. Ms. Walton's BP is 142/94.
3. Ms. Walton's pain level is now 1–2.
4. Ms. Walton's dressing is dry and intact.

8 If you reevaluated Ms. Walton and her headache pain had not decreased, what should be your next priority?
1. Reposition Ms. Walton on her left side with the head of the bed flat.
2. Call the physician about client report of increasing headache.
3. Decrease stimuli in the room by darkening the room and limiting noise.
4. Check the prn orders to evaluate if a stronger pain medication has been ordered.

9 If you were planning an effective team meeting with all disciplines that should be collaborating to provide care and a discharge plan for Mr. Phillips, which six disciplines should be represented and why?
1. _____
2. _____
3. _____
4. _____
5. _____
6. _____

10, 11, 12 Review the five steps of the abbreviated neurologic assessment as outlined in your text. What are three findings you would expect when conducting a neuro check with Mr. Hernandez?
1. _____
2. _____
3. _____

CASE STUDY

Leticia Hays is a 69-year-old African American female. She was admitted 2 days earlier after being diagnosed with a stroke. She lives with her husband of 52 years and her 14-year-old grandson. Her grandson found her lying on the kitchen floor when he got home from school. When he asked her what had happened, she was unable to say words that were clear or understandable. He tried to help her stand up, but was unable to because she was extremely weak in her left side. He called 911 and an ambulance transported her to the emergency department. Her blood pressure when the ambulance arrived was 220/125, P 105, R 24, and she was very anxious and spoke garbled words loudly at the paramedics. She was diagnosed with acute stroke after evaluation at the hospital and was admitted for treatment. Ms. Hays has a history of hypertension and type 2 diabetes. She recently stopped taking her blood pressure medication because it made her feel "tired."

The pathophysiology of a stroke is dependent on location of the causative factor, size of tissue affected, and time of loss of cellular perfusion and oxygenation. Time is critical when it involves compromised perfusion to any organ, and the brain is no exception. Cerebral neuron cellular metabolism is severely affected within 4 to 5 minutes of compromised perfusion. Compromised cellular metabolism leads to glucose, glycogen, and adenosine triphosphate depletion and sodium-potassium pump failure. Wherever sodium goes, water follows. When the sodium-potassium pump fails, the sodium in the cell draws water into the cell, resulting in edema. Additionally, cerebral vessel walls also swell, further compromising blood and oxygen supply. Severe or prolonged ischemia leads to cellular death. The manifestations of a stroke include, but are not limited to, motor deficits, elimination disorders, sensory-perceptual deficits, communication disorders, and behavioral changes. The manifestations are always sudden in onset, focal, and usually unilateral. Typically, a stroke is manifested by weakness of the face, arm, and leg; loss of vision in one eye; speech and swallowing problems; and difficulties with balance. There are many different complications of a stroke, including increased intracranial pressure, coma, death, chronic long-term confusion, and intellectual changes.

The nursing diagnosis of *Ineffective Tissue Perfusion: Cerebral* is appropriate for implementing care for Mrs. Hays.

Ms. H
69 y.o. female
Stroke

— affects →

- Cellular perfusion and oxygenation of area of brain decreased or stopped
- Ischemia of cerebral neurons leads to cellular death

leads to

— assess →

- History of hypertension and type 2 diabetes
- Not taking antihypertensives
- BP 220/125, P 105
- Left side weakness
- Garbled speech
- Confused

— generates →

- Impaired Verbal Communication related to effects of stroke
- Self-Care Deficits related to left-sided weakness and confusion
- Impaired Physical Mobility related to left-sided weakness
- Risk for Impaired Swallowing related to neurologic deficits from stroke

generate nursing diagnosis

prioritized to

Altered Tissue Perfusion: Cerebral

expected outcomes

- Actively participates in rehabilitation, including physical therapy, speech therapy, and occupational therapy
- Demonstrates improved ability to think, speak, carry out self-care, and ambulate
- Verbalizes necessity of taking prescribed medications
- Transfers to rehabilitation facility when health status improves

— evaluate →

- PT, OT and ST initiated twice daily.
- Speech is much improved and understandable
- Alert and oriented to person, place and time
- Able to feed self and walking with the assistance of a walker and another person
- Verbalized need for medications
- Transferred to rehabilitation facility for further care

Interdisciplinary Interventions
- Request referrals to physical therapy, speech therapy, and occupational therapy
- Apply nasal oxygen as prescribed
- Administer prescribed hypoglycemic and antihypertensive medications

Independent Interventions
- Schedule nursing activities for care around rehabilitation times
- Monitor neurologic status, including orientation, LOC, and reflexes
- Monitor pulse oximetry levels
- When appropriate, discuss effects and side effects of medications as well as risks of not taking them
- Discuss future transfer to rehabilitation facility with family members

UNIT 14

Responses to Altered Visual and Auditory Function

CHAPTER 47 Assessing Clients with Eye and Ear Disorders

LEARNING OUTCOMES

- Describe the anatomy, physiology, and functions of the eye and the ear.
- Explain the physiologic processes involved in vision, hearing, and equilibrium.
- Identify specific topics for consideration during a health history interview of the client with health problems of the eye or ear.
- Describe normal variations in assessment findings for the older adult.
- Identify abnormal findings that may indicate impairment in the function of the eye and the ear.

CLINICAL COMPETENCIES

- Conduct and document a health history for clients having or at risk for alterations in the structure or functions of the eye and ear.
- Monitor the results of diagnostic tests and report abnormal findings.
- Conduct and document a physical assessment of the structure or functions of the eye and ear.

EQUIPMENT NEEDED

- Visual acuity charts
- Opaque eye cover
- Pen
- Penlight
- Cotton-tipped applicator
- Ophthalmoscope
- Otoscope
- Tuning fork

MEDIALINK

Resources for this chapter can be found on the Prentice Hall Nursing MediaLink DVD-ROM accompanying this textbook, and on the Companion Website at http://www.prenhall.com/lemone

Vision and hearing allow us to experience the world in which we live. The eyes and ears provide pathways for visual and auditory stimuli to reach the brain. In addition, specialized structures within the ear help maintain position sense and equilibrium. Deficits in vision and hearing may limit self-care, mobility, safety, independence, communication, and relationships with others.

ANATOMY, PHYSIOLOGY, AND FUNCTIONS OF THE EYES

The eyes are complex structures, containing 70% of the sensory receptors of the body. Both extraocular and intraocular structures are considered parts of the eye.

Each eye is a sphere measuring about 1 inch (2.5 cm) in diameter, surrounded and protected by a bony orbit and cushions of fat. The primary functions of the eye are to encode the patterns of light from the environment through photoreceptors and to carry the coded information from the eyes to the brain. The brain gives meaning to the coded information, allowing us to make sense of what we see.

Extraocular Structures

Although the extraocular structures of the eye are outside the eyeball, they are vital to its protection. These structures are the eyebrows, eyelids, eyelashes, conjunctiva, lacrimal apparatus, and extrinsic eye muscles (Figure 47–1 ■).

The eyebrows shade the eyes and keep perspiration away from them. The eyelids are thin, loose folds of skin covering the anterior eye. They protect the eye from foreign bodies, regulate the entry of light into the eye, and distribute tears by blinking. The eyelashes are short hairs that project from the top and bottom borders of the eyelids. An unexpected touch to the eyelashes initiates the blinking reflex to protect the eyes from foreign objects.

The conjunctiva is a thin, transparent membrane that lines the inner surfaces of the eyelids and also folds over the anterior surface of the eyeball. The palpebral conjunctiva lines the upper and lower eyelids, whereas the bulbar conjunctiva loosely covers the anterior sclera (the white part of the eye). The conjunctiva is a mucous membrane that lubricates the eyes. The lacrimal apparatus is composed of the lacrimal gland, the puncta, the lacrimal sac, and the nasolacrimal duct. Together, these structures secrete, distribute, and drain tears to cleanse and moisten the eye's surface.

The six extrinsic eye muscles control movement of the eye, allowing it to follow a moving object and move precisely. The muscles also help maintain the shape of the eyeball. The cranial nerves control the extrinsic muscles (Figure 47–2 ■).

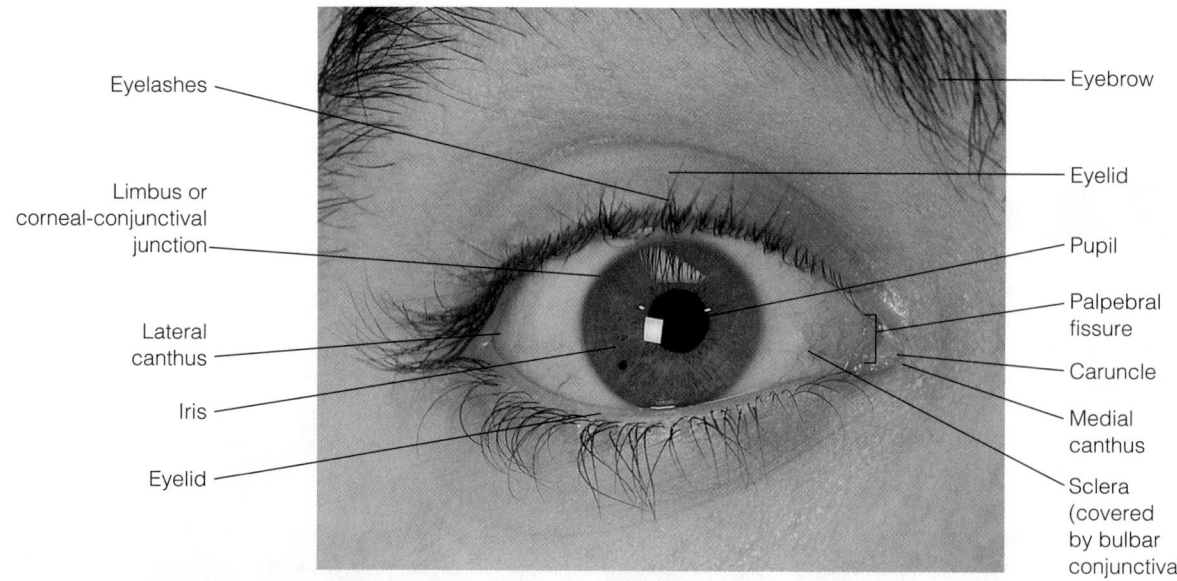

Figure 47–1 ■ Accessory and external structures of the eye.

Source: Todd Buck.

Name	Controlling cranial nerve	Action
Lateral rectus	VI (abducens)	Moves eye laterally
Medial rectus	III (oculomotor)	Moves eye medially
Superior rectus	III (oculomotor)	Elevates eye or rolls it superiorly
Inferior rectus	III (oculomotor)	Depresses eye or rolls it inferiorly
Inferior oblique	III (oculomotor)	Elevates eye and turns it laterally
Superior oblique	IV (trochlear)	Depresses eye and turns it laterally

Figure 47–2 ■ Extraocular muscles. *A,* Lateral view of the right eye. *B,* Superior view of the right eye. *C,* Innervation of the extraocular muscles by the cranial nerves.

Intraocular Structures

The intraocular structures transmit visual images and maintain homeostasis of the inner eye. Those in the anterior portion of each eyeball are the sclera and the cornea (forming the outermost coat of the eye, called the fibrous tunic), the iris, the pupil, and the anterior cavity (Figure 47–3 ■).

Sclera and Cornea

The white sclera lines the outside of the eyeball, and protects and gives shape to the eyeball. The sclera gives way to the cornea over the iris and pupil. The cornea is transparent, avascular, and sensitive to touch. The cornea forms a window that allows light to enter the eye and is a part of its light-bending apparatus. When the cornea is touched, the eyelids blink (**corneal reflex**) and tears are secreted.

Iris

The iris is a disc of muscle surrounding the pupil and lying between the cornea and the lens. The iris gives the eye its color and regulates light entry by controlling the size of the pupil. The pupil is the dark center of the eye through which light enters. The pupil constricts when bright light enters the eye and when it is used for near vision; it dilates when light conditions are dim and when the eye is used for far vision. In response to intense light, the pupil constricts rapidly in the **pupillary light reflex**.

Aqueous Fluid

The anterior cavity is made of the anterior chamber (the space between the cornea and the iris) and the posterior chamber (the space between the iris and the lens). The anterior cavity is filled with aqueous humor. Aqueous humor, a clear fluid, is constantly

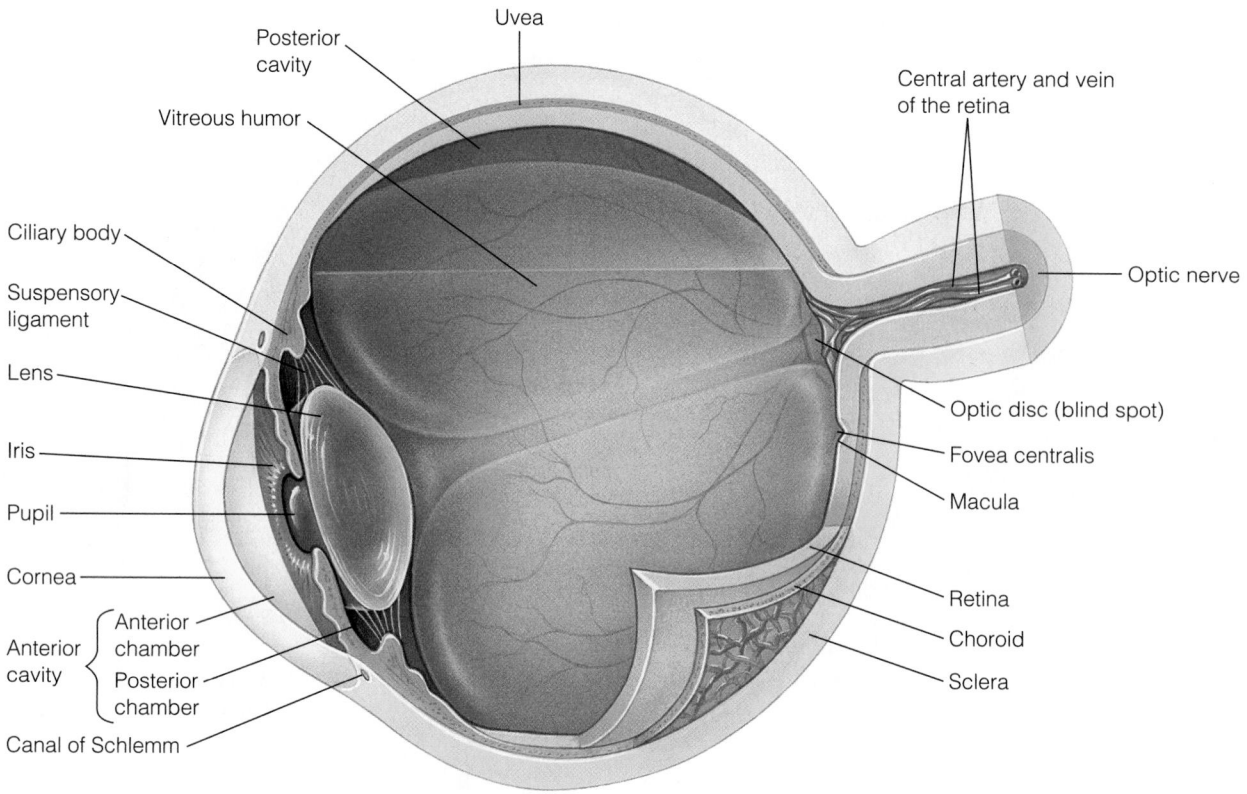

Figure 47–3 ■ Internal structures of the eye.

formed and drained to maintain a relatively constant pressure of from 15 to 20 mmHg in the eye. The canal of Schlemm, a network of channels that circles the eye in the angle at the junction of the sclera and the cornea, is the drainage system for fluid moving between the anterior and posterior chambers. Aqueous humor provides nutrients and oxygen to the cornea and the lens.

Internal Chamber

The intraocular structures that lie in the internal chamber of the eye are the lens, the posterior cavity and vitreous humor, the ciliary body, the uvea, and the retina.

The lens is a biconvex, avascular, transparent structure located directly behind the pupil. It can change shape to focus and refract light onto the retina. The posterior cavity lies behind the lens. It is filled with a clear gelatinous substance, the vitreous humor, which supports the posterior surface of the lens, maintains the position of the retina, and transmits light. The uvea, also called the vascular tunic, is the middle layer of the eyeball. This pigmented layer has three components: the iris, ciliary body, and choroid. The ciliary body encircles the lens, and along with the iris, regulates the amount of light reaching the retina by controlling the shape of the lens. Most of the uvea is made up of the choroid, which is pigmented and vascular. Blood vessels of the choroid nourish the layers of the eyeball. Its pigmented areas absorb light, preventing it from scattering within the eyeball.

The retina is the innermost lining of the eyeball. It has an outer pigmented layer and an inner neural layer. The outer layer, next to the choroid, serves as the link between visual stimuli and the brain. The transparent inner layer is made up of millions of light receptors in structures called rods and cones. Rods enable vision in dim light as well as peripheral vision. Cones enable vision in bright light and the perception of color. The optic disc, a cream-colored round or oval area within the retina, is the point at which the optic nerve enters the eye. The slight depression in the center of the optic disc is called the physiologic cup. Located laterally to the optic disc is the macula, a darker area with no visible blood vessels. The macula contains primarily cones. The fovea centralis is a slight depression in the center of the macula that contains only cones and is a main receptor of detailed color vision.

The Visual Pathway

The optic nerves are cranial nerves formed of the axons of ganglion cells. The two optic nerves meet at the optic chiasma, just anterior to the pituitary gland in the brain. At the optic chiasma, axons from the medial half of each retina cross to the opposite side to form pairs of axons from each eye. These pairs continue as the left and right optic tracts (Figure 47–4 ■). The crossing of the axons results in each optic tract carrying information from both eyes. The left optic tract carries visual information from the lateral half of the retina of the left eye and the medial half of the retina of the right eye, whereas the right optic tract carries visual information from the lateral half of the retina of the right eye and the medial half of the retina of the left eye.

The ganglion cell axons in the optic tracts travel to the thalamus and synapse with neurons, forming pathways called op-

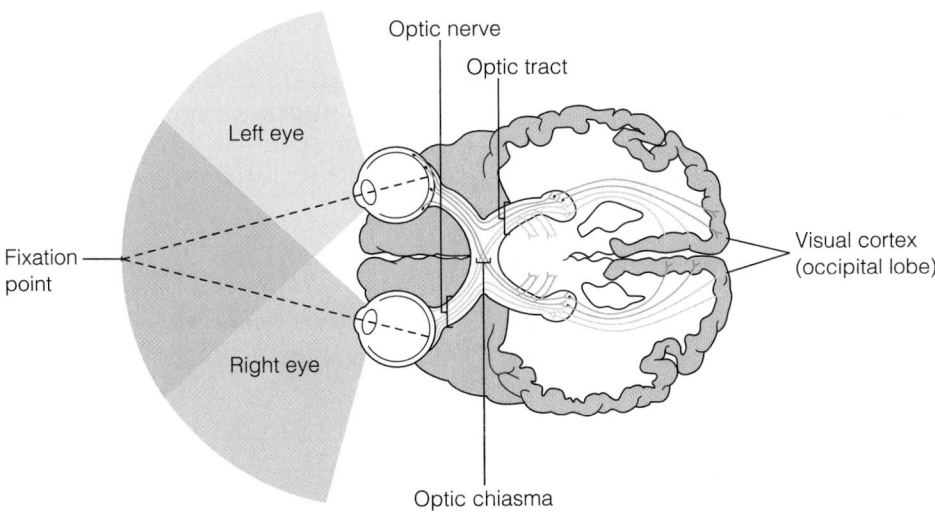

Figure 47–4 ■ The visual fields of the eye and the visual pathways to the brain.

tic radiations. The optic radiations terminate in the visual cortex of the occipital lobe. The nerve impulses that originated in the retina are interpreted here.

The visual fields of each eye overlap considerably, and each eye sees a slightly different view. Because of this overlap and the crossing of the axons, information from both eyes reaches each side of the visual cortex, which then fuses the information into one image. This fusion of images accounts for the ability to perceive depth; however, depth perception depends on visual input from two eyes that both focus well.

Refraction

Refraction is the bending of light rays as they pass from one medium to another medium of different optical density. As light rays pass through the eye, they are refracted at several points: as they enter the cornea, as they leave the cornea and enter the aqueous humor, as they enter the lens, and as they leave the lens and enter the vitreous humor. At the lens, the light is bent so that it converges at a single point on the retina. This focusing of the image is called **accommodation**. Because the lens is convex, the image projected onto the retina (the real image) is upside down and reversed from left to right. This real image is coded as electric signals that are sent to the brain. The brain decodes the image so that the person perceives it as it occurs in space.

The eyes are best adapted to see distant objects. Both eyes fix on the same distant image and do not require any change in accommodation. For people with emmetropic (normal) vision, the distance from the viewed object at which the eyes require no accommodation is 20 ft (6 m). This point is called the far point of vision. To focus for near vision, the eyes must instantly accommodate the lens, constrict the pupils, and converge the eyeballs. Accommodation is accomplished by contraction of the ciliary muscles. This contraction reduces the tension on the lens capsule so that it bulges outward to increase the curvature. This change in shape also achieves a shorter focal length, another requirement for focusing close images on the retina. The closest point on which a person can focus is called the near point of vision; in young adults with normal vision this is usu-

ally 8 to 10 inches (20 to 25 cm). Pupillary constriction helps eliminate most of the divergent light rays and sharpens focus. **Convergence** (the medial rotation of the eyeballs so that each is directed toward the viewed object) allows the focusing of the image on the retinal fovea of each eye.

ASSESSING THE EYES

Structures and functions of the eyes are assessed by findings from diagnostic tests, a health assessment interview to collect subjective data, and a physical assessment to collect objective data.

Diagnostic Tests

The results of diagnostic tests of the structure and functions of the eyes are used to support the diagnosis of a specific injury, disease, or vision problem; to provide information to identify or modify the appropriate medications or assistive devices used to treat the disease or problem; and to help nurses monitor the client's responses to treatment and nursing care interventions. Diagnostic tests of the eye, especially for vision testing, are most often conducted in a healthcare provider's office. Diagnostic tests to assess the structure and functions of the eyes are described in the Diagnostic Tests table on the next page and summarized in the following bulleted list. More information is included in the discussion of specific injuries or diseases in Chapter 48 ∞.

- Refractive errors (with prescription for corrective lenses) are evaluated by retinoscopy and/or refractometry. Pupils must be dilated for accurate diagnosis.
- Tonometry is used to identify and evaluate increased intraocular pressure, characteristic of glaucoma.
- A CT scan may be used to identify foreign objects or tumors of the eye.

Regardless of the type of diagnostic test, the nurse is responsible for explaining the procedure and any special preparation needed, for assessing any medication use that might affect the outcome of the tests, for supporting the client during the examination as necessary, for documenting the procedures as appropriate, and for monitoring the results of the tests.

DIAGNOSTIC TESTS of Eye Disorders

NAME OF TEST Refraction, Retinoscopy, Refractometry

PURPOSE AND DESCRIPTION Used to measure refractive error. Either a handheld retinoscope or an instrument with multiple lenses is used; with latter method, client chooses lenses that provide best vision.

RELATED NURSING CARE No special preparation is needed; tell client that pupils will be dilated with medication and may be enlarged for several hours.

NAME OF TEST Tonometry

PURPOSE AND DESCRIPTION Used to diagnose increased intraocular pressure in glaucoma. A variety of methods are used, ranging from a handheld instrument (tonometer) to a computerized component of the device used to evaluate

refraction. The cornea is anesthetized prior to being touched with the device. **Normal value:** 10–22 mmHg

RELATED NURSING CARE No special preparation is needed.

NAME OF TEST Computed tomography (CT) scan of the eye

PURPOSE AND DESCRIPTION Radiologic examination used to identify foreign objects or tumors within the eyeball or orbit.

RELATED NURSING CARE No special preparation is needed.

Genetic Considerations

When conducting a health assessment interview and a physical assessment, it is important for the nurse to consider genetic influences on health of the adult. Several diseases of the eyes have a genetic component. During the health assessment interview, ask about a family history of glaucoma or blindness.

During the physical assessment, assess for any manifestations that might indicate a genetic disorder (see the Genetic Considerations box below). If data are found to indicate genetic risk factors or alterations, ask about genetic testing and refer for appropriate genetic counseling and evaluation. Chapter 8 ∞ provides further information about genetics in medical-surgical nursing.

Health Assessment Interview

A health assessment interview to determine problems with the eyes and vision may be conducted during a health screening, may focus on a chief complaint (such as blurred vision or an eye infection), or may be part of a total health assessment. If the

GENETIC CONSIDERATIONS
Eye Disorders

- *Glaucoma* is a term used for a group of diseases that damage the optic nerve and cause blindness. About 3 million people have a form of glaucoma, with nearly 100,000 of those in the United States having a form that is a genetic mutation (National Institutes of Health [NIH], 2003a).
- Gyrate atrophy of the choroid and retina is a genetic disorder resulting in a progressive vision loss, with total blindness occurring between ages 40 and 60.
- Best disease is a familial disorder found most often in Caucasians who originated in Europe. The disease causes gradual loss of vision, beginning during the teenage years.

client has a health problem involving one or both eyes, analyze its onset, characteristics and course, severity, precipitating and relieving factors, and any associated symptoms, noting the timing and circumstances. For example, you may ask the client:

- Describe the type of pain you experience in your eyes. When did it begin? How long does it last?
- Have you noticed rings of color around streetlights at night?
- When did you first notice having difficulty reading the paper?

Throughout the interview, be alert to nonverbal behaviors (such as squinting or abnormal eye movements) that suggest problems with eye function. Explore problems such as watery, irritated eyes or changes in vision. Assess the client's use of corrective eyewear and care of eyeglasses or contact lenses. If the client uses eye medications, ask about the type and purpose as well as the frequency and duration of use. When taking the history, find out about eye trauma, surgery, or infections, as well as the date and results of the last eye examination. In addition, ask the client about a medical history of diabetes, hypertension, thyroid disorders, glaucoma, cataracts, and eye infections. Include questions about a family history of nearsightedness or farsightedness, cancer of the retina, color blindness, and any other eye or vision disorders.

Collect information about environmental or work exposure to irritating chemicals, participation in sports or hobbies that pose the risk of eye injury, and the use of protective eyewear during dangerous activities, such as sawing wood or using a grass trimmer.

Interview questions categorized by functional health patterns are listed in the Functional Health Pattern Interview table on the next page.

Physical Assessment of the Eyes and Vision

Physical assessment of the eyes and of visual acuity may be performed as part of a total assessment or separately for clients

FUNCTIONAL HEALTH PATTERN INTERVIEW The Eye

Functional Health Pattern	Interview Questions and Leading Statements
Health Perception-Health Management	■ Describe your vision. Rate it on a scale of 1 to 10, with 10 being excellent vision. Is it the same in both eyes? If not, which eye is better? ■ Describe your current vision problems. How have these been treated? ■ What eye medications do you use? What type and how often? ■ Have you ever had eye surgery? Describe. ■ Describe the type of corrective lens that you use. Are you satisfied with this appliance? How do you care for it? ■ Describe how you care for your eyes each day. ■ Do you wear sunglasses when you are outside? ■ When was your last eye examination? Have you been tested for glaucoma?
Nutritional-Metabolic	■ Do you have any redness, swelling, watering, or dryness of your eyes?
Activity-Exercise	■ Does your vision problem interfere with your usual activities of daily living? Explain. ■ Do you wear protective goggles when you take part in activities that increase the risk of injury to your eyes (such as at work or when operating machinery at home)?
Sleep-Rest	■ Does your eye problem interfere with your ability to rest or sleep (for example, from pain)? If so, what do you do?
Cognitive-Perceptual	■ Do you have any difficulty focusing on objects? If so, do you have more difficulty with near objects or far objects? ■ Is your vision blurry? Do you see halos around lights? Do you see flashes of light or "floaters"? Do you see double? ■ Do you have pain in or around your eyes? If so, describe its location, intensity, what makes it worse, and how long it lasts. How do you treat it?
Self-Perception-Self-Concept	■ Has this problem with your eyes affected how you feel about yourself?
Role-Relationships	■ How has having this condition affected your relationships with others? ■ Has having this condition interfered with your ability to work? Explain. ■ Has anyone in your family had problems with eye disease? Explain.
Sexuality-Reproductive	■ Has this condition interfered with your usual sexual activity?
Coping-Stress-Tolerance	■ Has having this condition created stress for you? If so, does your health problem seem to be more difficult when you are stressed? ■ Have you experienced any kind of stress that makes the condition worse? Explain. ■ Describe what you do when you feel stressed.
Value-Belief	■ Describe how specific relationships or activities help you cope with this problem. ■ Describe specific cultural beliefs or practices that affect how you care for and feel about this problem. ■ Are there any specific treatments that you would not use to treat this problem?

with known or suspected problems of the eyes. The eyes and vision are primarily assessed through inspection of external structures and assessment of visual fields and visual acuity, extraocular muscle function, and internal structures. Palpation (e.g., of a blocked lacrimal duct) may be used if a problem is identified. Prior to the examination, explain the techniques to the client to decrease anxiety. The client may sit or stand during the assessment. Normal age-related findings for the older adult are summarized in Table 47–1.

Assessing Visual Fields

Visual fields are tested to assess the functioning of the macula and peripheral vision. The visual fields of the examiner (which

must be normal to perform this assessment) are used as the standard. To measure visual fields, sit directly opposite the client at a distance of 18 to 24 inches. Ask the client to cover one eye with the opaque cover while you cover your own eye opposite to the client (for example, if the client covers the right eye, you cover your left eye). Ask the client to look directly at you. Move the penlight from the periphery toward the center from right to left, above and below, and from the middle of each of these directions. Both you and the client should see the penlight enter the field of vision at the same time, if the examiner has normal peripheral vision.

The central visual field may be assessed with an Amsler grid (Figure 47–5 ■). The most basic form has black lines on a white

TABLE 47–1 **Age-Related Changes in the Eye**

AGE-RELATED CHANGE	SIGNIFICANCE
The lens: ■ ↓ elasticity, decreasing focus and accommodation for near vision (presbyopia). ■ ↑ density and size, making lens more stiff and opaque. ■ Yellowing of the lens and changes in the retina affect color perception.	Most older adults require corrective lenses to accommodate close and detailed work. Increased opacity leads to the development of cataracts. As cataracts develop, they increase sensitivity to glare and interfere with night vision.
The cornea: ■ Fat may be deposited around the periphery and throughout the cornea. ■ ↓ corneal sensitivity.	A partial or complete white circle may form around the cornea (*arcus senilis*). Lipid deposits in the cornea cause vision to be blurred. Decreased sensitivity increases the risk of injury to the eye.
The pupil: ■ ↓ size and responsiveness to light pupil; sphincter hardens.	Increased light perception threshold and difficulty seeing in dim light or at night means increased light is needed to see adequately.
The retina and visual pathways: ■ Visual fields narrow. ■ Photoreceptor cells are lost. ■ Rods work less effectively. ■ Macular degeneration is a risk. ■ Depth perception is distorted. ■ Adaptation to dark and light takes longer.	Peripheral vision is decreased and central vision may be lost from macular degeneration. Increased risk of falls as a result of changes in depth perception and adaptation to changes in light. Vision progressively declines with age.
The lacrimal apparatus: ■ ↓ reabsorption of intraocular fluid. ■ ↓ production of tears.	Increased risk of developing glaucoma, and eyes feel and look dry.
The posterior cavity: ■ Debris and condensation become visible. ■ Vitreous body may pull away from the retina.	Vision is blurred and distorted, and "floaters" are often seen by the older person.

grid, forming squares (boxes) that measure 5 mm. There is a black dot in the center of the grid. The Amsler grid is useful for identifying early changes in vision from macular degeneration and diabetes mellitus. To use the Amlser grid, ask the client to hold the grid at normal reading distance (about 12 to 14 inches), cover one eye, and stare at the center dot. Ask the client if any of the lines look crooked or bent, if any of the boxes are different in size or shape, and if any of the lines are wavy, missing, blurry, or discolored. Repeat with the other eye. The test should be conducted before the pupils are dilated, and the client should be wearing their best correction.

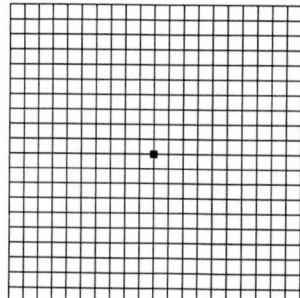

Figure 47–5 ■ The Amsler grid.

EYE AND VISION ASSESSMENTS

Vision Assessment

Visual acuity is assessed with an eye chart such as the Snellen chart or the E chart for testing distance vision and the Rosenbaum chart for testing near vision. The Snellen chart contains rows of letters in various sizes, with standardized numbers at the end of each row. The number at the end of the row indicates the visual acuity of a client who can read the row at a distance of 20 feet. (If the client is unable to read or does not read English, you can use the E chart to test visual acuity.) The top number at the end of the row is always 20, representing the distance between the client and the chart. The bottom number is the distance (in feet) at which a person with normal vision can read the line. A person with normal vision can read the row marked 20/20. To conduct the assessment, ask the person to stand 20 feet from the chart in a well-lit area. Ask the client to cover one eye with an opaque cover (Figure 47–6 ■). Then ask the client to read each row of letters, moving from largest letters to the smallest ones that the client can see. Measure visual acuity in the other eye in the same way, and then assess visual acuity while the client has both eyes uncovered. You may test the client who wears corrective lenses with and without the lenses.

The Rosenbaum chart is held at a distance of from 12 to 14 inches from the eyes, with visual acuity measured in the same manner as with the Snellen chart (Figure 47–7 ■). A gross estimate of near vision may also be assessed by asking the person to read from a magazine or newspaper.

Figure 47–6 ■ Testing distant vision using the Snellen eye chart.

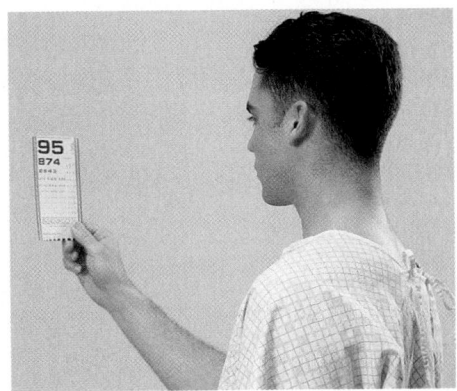

Figure 47–7 ■ Testing near vision using Rosenbaum eye chart.

Technique/Normal Findings	Abnormal Findings
Assess distant vision, using the Snellen or E chart. *When standing 20 feet from the chart, the client can read the smallest line of letters with or without corrective lenses (recorded as 20/20).*	■ Changes in distant vision are most commonly the result of **myopia** (nearsightedness). For example, a reading of 20/100 indicates impaired distance vision. A person has to stand 20 feet from the chart to read a line that a person with normal vision could read 100 feet from the chart.
Assess near vision, using a Rosenbaum chart or a card with newsprint held 12 to 14 inches from the client's eyes. *Normal near visual acuity is 14/14 with or without corrective lenses.*	■ Changes in near vision, especially in clients over age 45, can indicate **presbyopia**, impaired near vision resulting from a loss of elasticity of the lens related to aging. In younger clients, this condition is referred to as **hyperopia** (farsightedness).

Eye Movement Assessment

Assess the cardinal fields of vision to gain information about extraocular eye movements. Ask the client to follow a pen or your finger while keeping the head stationary. Move the pen or your finger through the six fields one at a time, returning to the central starting point before proceeding to the next field (Figure 47–8 ■). *The eyes should move through each field without involuntary movements.*

■ Failure of one or both eyes to follow the object in any given direction may indicate extraocular muscle weakness or cranial nerve dysfunction.
■ An involuntary rhythmic movement of the eyes, **nystagmus**, is associated with neurologic disorders and the use of some medications.

1 Penlight is to nurse's extreme left.

4 Penlight is to nurse's extreme right.

2 Penlight is left and up.

5 Penlight is right and up.

3 Penlight is left and down.

6 Penlight is right and down.

Figure 47–8 ■ The six cardinal fields of vision.

Technique/Normal Findings	Abnormal Findings

The cover–uncover test is a test for strabismus, a weakening of a muscle that causes one eye to deviate from the other when the person is focusing on an object. To conduct the test, hold a pen or your finger about 1 foot from the eyes and ask the person to focus on that object. Cover one of the client's eyes and note any movement in the uncovered eye; as you remove the cover, assess for movement in the eye that was just uncovered. Repeat the procedure with the other eye. *The uncovered eye should remain fixed straight ahead. The covered eye should remain fixed straight ahead after being uncovered.*

Assess convergence. Ask the client to follow an object as you move it toward the client's eyes. *Normally both eyes converge toward the center.*

- Failure of the eyes to converge equally on an approaching object may indicate a neuromuscular disorder or improper eye alignment.

Assess the corneal light reflex. Direct a light source onto the bridge of the nose from 12 to 15 inches. *Observe for equal reflection of the light from each eye.*

- Reflections of the light from different sites on the eyes reveal improper alignment.

Pupillary Assessment

Observe pupil size and equality. *Pupils should be of equal size, 3 to 5 mm.*

- Pupils that are unequal in size may indicate a severe neurologic problem, such as increased intracranial pressure.

Assess direct and consensual pupil response. Ask the client to look straight ahead. Shine a light obliquely into one eye at a time. Observe for constriction of the pupil in the illuminated eye. Test both eyes. To test consensual pupil response, again shine a light obliquely into one eye at a time as the client looks straight ahead. Observe constriction of the pupil in the opposite eye. *The normal direct and consensual pupillary response is constriction.*

- Failure of the pupils to respond to light may indicate degeneration of the retina or destruction of the optic nerve.
- A client who has one dilated and unresponsive pupil may have paralysis of the oculomotor nerve.
- Some eye medications may cause unequal dilation, constriction, or inequality of pupil size. Morphine and narcotic drugs may cause small, unresponsive pupils, and anticholinergic drugs such as atropine may cause dilated, unresponsive pupils.

Technique/Normal Findings	Abnormal Findings

Test for accommodation. Hold an object at a distance of a few feet from the client. The pupils should dilate. Ask the client to follow the object as you bring it to within a few inches of the client's nose. *The pupils should constrict and converge as they change focus to follow the object.*

- Failure of accommodation along with lack of pupil response to light may signal a neurologic problem.
- Lack of response to light with appropriate response to accommodation is often seen in clients with diabetes.

External Eye Assessment

Inspect the eyelids. *Eyelids should be the color of the client's facial skin, without redness, discharge, or drooping. The sclera should not be visible.*

- Unusual redness or discharge may indicate an inflammatory state due to trauma, allergies, or infection.
- Drooping of one eyelid, called **ptosis**, may be the result of a stroke, indicate a neuromuscular disorder, or be congenital (Figure 47–9 ■).
- Unusual widening of the lids may be due to exophthalmos, protrusion of the eyeball. Exophthalmos is often associated with hyperthyroid conditions (see Chapter 19 ∞).
- Yellow plaques noted on or near the lid margins are referred to as xanthelasma and may indicate high lipid levels.
- An acute localized inflammation of a hair follicle is known as a *hordeolum* (sty) and is generally caused by staphylococcal organisms.
- A *chalazion* is an infection or retention cyst of the meibomian glands.

Figure 47–9 ■ Ptosis.
Source: Leonard Lessen/Peter Arnold, Inc.
Source: Custom Medical Stock Photo, Inc.

Inspect the puncta. *The puncta should be free of redness or discharge.*

- Unusual redness or discharge from the puncta may indicate an inflammation due to trauma, infection, or allergies.

Inspect the bulbar and palpebral conjunctiva. *The conjunctiva should be clear, moist, and smooth. The upper and lower palpebral conjunctiva should be clear, without redness or swelling.*

- Increased erythema or the presence of exudate may indicate acute conjunctivitis.
- A cobblestone appearance is often associated with allergies.
- A fold in the conjunctiva, called a *pterygium*, may be seen as a clouded area that extends over the cornea. This is an abnormal growth of the bulbar conjunctiva, usually seen on the nasal side of the cornea. It may interfere with vision if it covers the pupil.

Inspect the sclera. *The sclera is white in Caucasians; people with darker skin normally have yellow sclera.*

- Unusual redness may indicate an inflammatory state as a result of trauma, allergies, or infection.
- Yellow discoloration of the sclera in clients with fair skin may be seen in conditions involving the liver, such as hepatitis.
- Bright red areas in the sclera are often subconjunctival hemorrhages and may indicate trauma or bleeding disorders. They may also occur spontaneously.

Inspect the cornea. *The cornea is normally transparent.*

- Dullness, opacities, or irregularities of the cornea may be abnormal.
- *Corneal arcus* is a thin, grayish white arc seen toward the edge of the cornea. It is normal in older clients.

Assess corneal sensitivity. Lightly touch a wisp of cotton to the client's cornea. *This action should cause a corneal reflex (blinking the eye).*

- Failure of the corneal reflex may indicate a neurologic disorder.

Technique/Normal Findings	Abnormal Findings
Inspect the iris. *The iris is normally round, flat, and evenly colored.*	■ Lack of clarity of the iris may indicate a cloudiness of the cornea. ■ Constriction of the pupil accompanied by pain and circumcorneal redness indicates acute iritis.
Internal Eye Assessment Assess internal structures of the eye by using the ophthalmoscope, an instrument that allows visualization of the lens, the vitreous humor, and the retina. Box 47–1 provides guidelines for using the ophthalmoscope.	
Inspect for the red reflex. *The red reflex should be clearly visible.*	■ Absence of a red reflex often indicates improper position of the ophthalmoscope, but also may indicate total opacity of the pupil by a cataract or a hemorrhage into the vitreous humor.
Inspect the lens and vitreous body. *The lens should be clear.*	■ A cataract is an opacity of the lens, often seen as a dark shadow on ophthalmoscopic examination. It may be due to aging, trauma, diabetes, or a congenital defect.
Inspect the retina. *There should be no visible hemorrhages, exudate, or white patches.*	■ Areas of hemorrhage, exudate, and white patches may be a result of diabetes or long-standing hypertension.
Inspect the optic disc. *The optic disc should be round to oval in shape with clear, well-defined borders.*	■ Loss of definition of the optic disc, as well as an increase in the size of the physiologic cup, is seen in papilledema from increased intracranial pressure.
Inspect the blood vessels of the retina. *The retinal blood vessels should be distinct.*	■ Glaucoma often results in displacement of blood vessels from the center of the optic disc due to increased intraocular pressure. ■ Hypertension may cause a narrowing of the vein where an arteriole crosses over. ■ Engorged veins may occur with diabetes, atherosclerosis, and blood disorders.
Inspect the retinal background. *The retina should be a consistent red-orange color, becoming lighter around the optic disc.*	■ Variations in color or a pale color overall may indicate disease.
Inspect the macula. *The macula should be visible on the temporal side of the optic disc.*	■ Absence of the fovea centralis is common in older clients. It may indicate macular degeneration, a cause of loss of central vision.
Palpate over the lacrimal glands, puncta, and nasolacrimal duct. *There should be no tenderness, drainage, or excessive tearing.*	■ Tenderness over any of these areas or drainage from the puncta may indicate an infectious process. (Wear gloves if you see any drainage.) ■ Excessive tearing may indicate a blockage of the nasolacrimal duct.

ANATOMY, PHYSIOLOGY, AND FUNCTIONS OF THE EARS

As a sensory organ, the ears have two primary functions, hearing and maintaining equilibrium. Anatomically, each ear is divided into three areas: the external ear, the middle ear, and the inner ear (Figure 47–10 ■). Each area has a unique function. All three are involved in hearing, but only the inner ear is involved in equilibrium.

The External Ear

The external ear consists of the auricle (or pinna), the external auditory canal, and the tympanic membrane.

The auricles are elastic cartilage covered with thin skin. They contain sebaceous and sweat glands and sometimes hair. Each auricle has a rim (the helix) and a lobe. The auricle serves to direct sound waves into the ear.

The external auditory canal, which is about 1 inch (2.5 cm) long, extends from the auricle to the tympanic membrane. The canal is lined with skin that contains hair, sebaceous glands, and ceruminous glands. The external auditory canal serves as a resonator for the range of sound waves typical of human speech and increases the pressure that sound waves in this frequency

BOX 47-1 Guidelines for Using the Ophthalmoscope

The ophthalmoscope has a head and a handle. (See the figure below.) The head contains a focus wheel (also called a lens selector dial) located on the side, lenses of varying magnification, and an opening through which the eye structures are visualized. The focus wheel adjusts the lens refraction, which is measured in diopters. The diopter measurements range from 0 to +40 when the lens is rotated clockwise, and from 0 to −25 when the lens is rotated counterclockwise. By moving the focus wheel, the examiner can converge or diverge light rays to visualize the retina.

The handle usually contains batteries that can be recharged.

Before the examination, explain the procedure to the client. Assemble the ophthalmoscope. Wash your hands and wear disposable gloves if the client has any drainage from the eyes. Darken the room (to allow the pupils of the client to dilate), and ask the client to look straight ahead, focusing on a fixed point such as an object on the wall. Hold the ophthalmoscope in one hand, resting the index finger on the focus wheel (see the figure at right).

1. Turn on the ophthalmoscope light, and set focus wheel to 0 diopters. Hold the ophthalmoscope in your right hand with your index finger on the focus wheel. Standing in front of the client, position yourself at a 15-degree angle to the client's line of vision.
2. Hold the opening of the ophthalmoscope up to your right eye and direct the light toward the client's right eye from a distance of about 12 inches.
3. As the beam of light falls on the client's pupil, observe for the red reflex, which appears as a sharply outlined orange glow from within the pupil. This glow is the reflection of the light from the retina.
4. Move closer to the client, turning the focus wheel clockwise toward the positive numbers as needed to maintain clear focus.
5. Examine the lens and the vitreous body, both of which should be clear.
6. Gradually rotate the focus wheel counterclockwise toward the negative numbers as needed, focusing on a structure of the retina (such as the disc or a blood vessel). Turn the focus wheel until the image is clear. Examine the structures of the retina as follows:
   a. The optic disc (see the accompanying figure). Assess for size, shape, color, distinct margins, and the physiologic cup. The disc is round to slightly oval and about 1.5 mm in diameter. It has a yellow to pink color that is lighter than the retina itself. The margins should be sharp and clear. The physiologic cup is a small depression that occupies about one-third of the optic disc, lying temporal to the center of the disc.
   b. The vessels of the retina. Assess for color, arteriolar light reflex, ratio of arterioles to veins, and arteriovenous crossings. The arterioles are red, brighter than the veins,

and about one-fourth smaller. The arterioles normally have a narrow light reflex from the center of each vessel; veins do not have this light reflex. The ratio of arterioles to veins is usually 2:3 or 4:5. The vessels normally cross and become smaller toward the periphery.
   c. The retinal background. Assess color and changes in color. The retina is normally reddish orange and regular in color.
   d. The macula. Assess size and color. To assess the macula, ask the client to look directly into the ophthalmoscope light. The macula is temporal to the optic disc, appears slightly darker than the retina, and has no visible vessels. The fovea centralis may be seen as a bright spot of light. Because looking directly into the light causes some discomfort, conduct this portion of the examination last. The macula is often difficult to visualize.
7. Using the same technique, examine the left eye.

Technique for holding an ophthalmoscope.

An ophthalmoscope.

Blood vessels

Optic disc

Macula

Fovea centralis

The optic disc.

Source: Don Wong/Science Source/Photo Researchers, Inc.

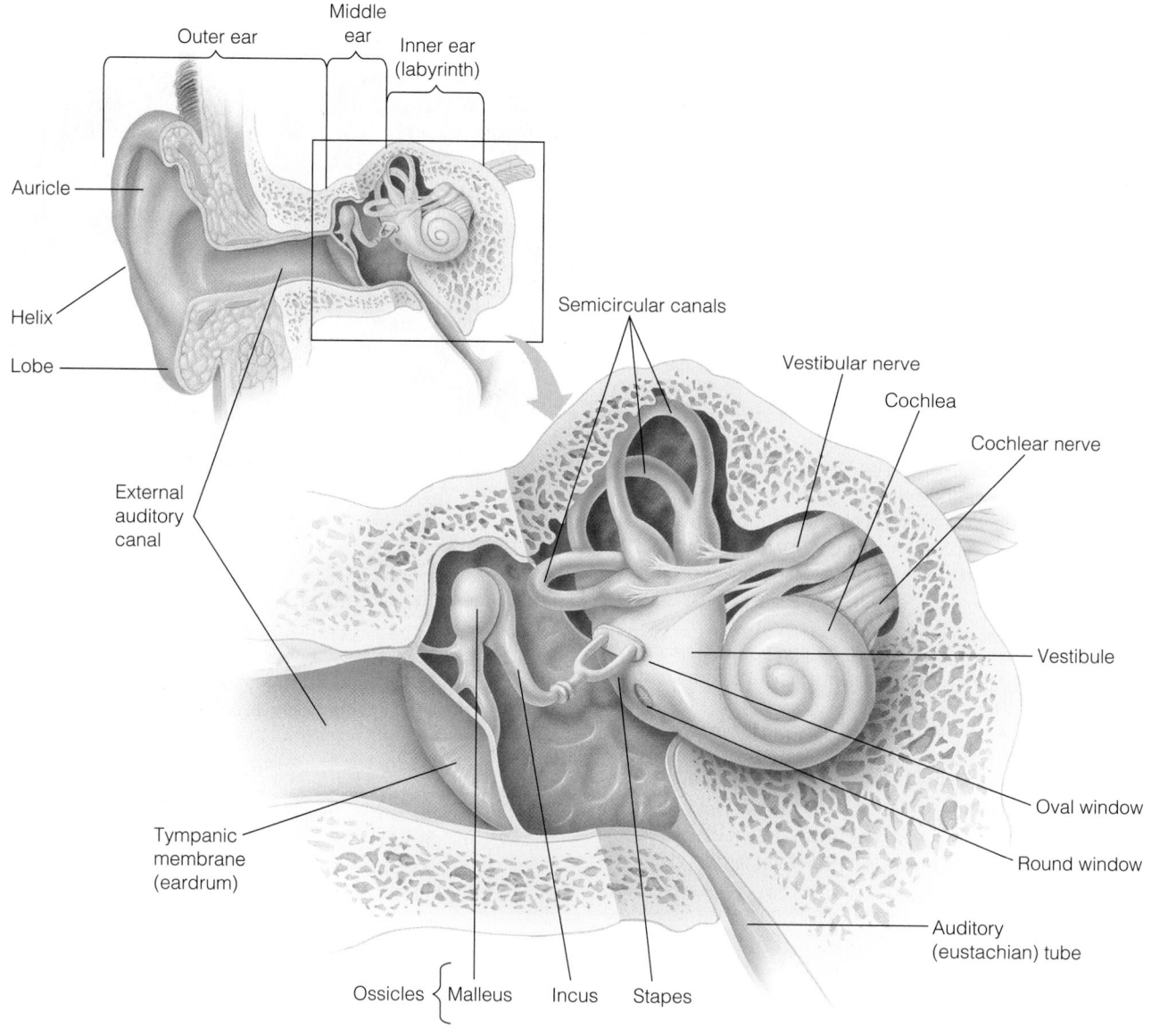

Figure 47–10 ■ Structures of the external ear, middle ear, and inner ear.

Source: Todd Buck.

range place on the tympanic membrane. The canal's ceruminous glands (modified apocrine glands) secrete a yellow to brown waxy substance called **cerumen** (earwax). Cerumen traps foreign bodies; it also has bacteriostatic properties, protecting the tympanic membrane and the middle ear from infections.

The tympanic membrane lies between the external ear and the middle ear. It is a thin, semitransparent, fibrous structure covered with skin on the external side and mucosa on the inner side. The membrane vibrates as sound waves strike it; these vibrations are transferred as sound waves to the middle ear.

The Middle Ear

The middle ear is an air-filled cavity in the temporal bone. The middle ear contains three auditory ossicles: the malleus, the incus, and the stapes. These bones extend across the middle ear. The medial side of the middle ear is a bony wall containing two membrane-covered openings, the oval window and the round

window. The posterior wall of the middle ear contains the mastoid antrum. This cavity communicates with the mastoid sinuses, which help the middle ear adjust to changes in pressure. It also opens into the eustachian tube, which connects with the nasopharynx. The eustachian tube helps to equalize the air pressure in the middle ear by opening briefly in response to differences between middle ear pressure and atmospheric pressure. This action also ensures that vibrations of the tympanic membrane remain adequate. The mucous membrane lining the middle ear is continuous with the mucous membranes lining the throat.

The malleus attaches to the tympanic membrane and articulates with the incus, which in turn articulates with the stapes. The stapes fits into the oval window. When the tympanic membrane vibrates, the vibrations are conducted across the middle ear to the oval window by the ossicles. The vibrations then set in motion the fluids of the inner ear, which in turn stimulate the hearing receptors. Two small muscles attached to the ossicles contract reflexively in response to sudden loud noises, decreasing the vibrations and protecting the inner ear.

The Inner Ear

The inner ear, also called the labyrinth, is a maze of bony chambers located deep within the temporal bone, just behind the eye socket. The labyrinth is further divided into two parts: the bony labyrinth, a system of open channels that houses the second part, the membranous labyrinth. The bony labyrinth is filled with a fluid (similar to cerebrospinal fluid) called perilymph, which bathes the membranous labyrinth. Within the chambers of the membranous labyrinth is a fluid called endolymph.

The bony labyrinth has three regions: the vestibule, the semicircular canals, and the cochlea. The vestibule is the central portion of the inner ear, one side of which is a bony wall containing the oval window. Two sacs within the vestibule (the saccule and the utricle) join the vestibule with the cochlea and the semicircular canals. The saccule and the utricle contain receptors for equilibrium that respond to changes in gravity and changes in position of the head. The three semicircular canals each project into a different plane (anterior, posterior, and lateral). Each canal contains a semicircular duct that communicates with the utricle of the vestibule. Each duct has an enlarged area at one end containing an equilibrium receptor that responds to angular movements of the head.

The cochlea is a tiny bony chamber that houses the organ of Corti, the receptor organ for hearing. The organ of Corti is a series of sensory hair cells, arranged in a single row of inner hair cells and three rows of outer hair cells. The hair cells are innervated by sensory fibers from cranial nerve VIII. The organ of Corti is supported in the cochlea by the flexible basilar membrane, which has fibers of varying lengths that respond to different sound wave frequencies.

Sound Conduction

Hearing is the perception and interpretation of sound. Sound is produced when the molecules of a medium are compressed, resulting in a pressure disturbance evidenced as a sound wave. The intensity or loudness of sound is determined by the amplitude (height) of the sound wave, with greater amplitudes causing louder sounds. The frequency of the sound wave in vibrations per second determines the pitch or tone of the sound, with higher frequencies resulting in higher sounds. The human ear is most sensitive to sound waves with frequencies between 1000 and 4000 cycles per second, but can detect sound waves with frequencies between 20 and 20,000 cycles per second.

Sound waves enter the external auditory canal and cause the tympanic membrane to vibrate at the same frequency. The ossicles not only transmit the motion of the tympanic membrane to the oval window but also amplify the energy of the sound wave. As the stapes moves against the oval window, the perilymph in the vestibule is set in motion. The increased pressure of the perilymph is transmitted to fibers of the basilar membrane and then to the organ of Corti (directly above the basilar

membrane). The up-and-down movements of the fibers of the basilar membrane pull the hair cells in the organ of Corti, which in turn generates action potentials that are transmitted to cranial nerve VIII and then to the brain for interpretation.

Several brainstem auditory nuclei transmit impulses to the cerebral cortex. Fibers from each ear cross, with each auditory cortex receiving impulses from both ears. Auditory processing is so finely tuned that a wide variety of sounds of different pitch and loudness can be heard at any one time. In addition, the source of the sound can be localized.

Equilibrium

The inner ear also provides information about the position of the head. This information is used to coordinate body movements so that equilibrium and balance are maintained. The types of equilibrium are static balance (affected by changes in the position of the head) and dynamic balance (affected by the movement of the head).

Receptors called maculae in the utricle and the saccule of the vestibule detect changes in the position of the head. Maculae are groups of hair cells that have protrusions covered with a gelatinous substance. Embedded in this gelatinous substance are tiny particles of calcium carbonate called otoliths (ear stones), which make the gelatin heavier than the endolymph that fills the membranous labyrinth. As a result, when the head is in the upright position, gravity causes the gelatinous substance to bear down on the hair cells. When the position of the head changes, the force on the hair cells also changes, bending them and altering the pattern of stimulation of the neurons. Thus, a different pattern of nerve impulses is transmitted to the brain, where stimulation of the motor centers initiates actions that coordinate various body movements according to the position of the head.

The receptor for dynamic equilibrium is in the crista, a crest in the membrane lining the ampulla of each semicircular canal. The cristae are stimulated by rotatory head movement (acceleration and deceleration) as a result of changes in the flow of endolymph and of movement of hair cells in the maculae. The direction of endolymph and hair cell movement is always opposite to the motion of the body.

ASSESSING THE EARS

The structure and functions of the ears are assessed by findings from diagnostic tests, a health assessment interview to collect subjective data, and a physical assessment to collect objective data. See the next page for sample documentation of an ear assessment.

Diagnostic Tests

The results of diagnostic tests of the structure and functions of the ears are used to support the diagnosis of a specific injury, disease, or hearing problem; to provide information to identify or modify the appropriate medications or assistive devices used to treat the disease or problem; and to help nurses monitor the client's responses to treatment and nursing care interventions. Diagnostic tests of the ear, especially for hearing, are most often conducted in a healthcare

SAMPLE DOCUMENTATION
Assessment of the Ear

22-year-old male with complaints of "having some problems hearing these days." States he often listens to music in his car "as loud as it will go" and uses ear phones at home so he does not bother other family members. Ears are normally placed bilaterally; skin smooth without lesions. Small amount of dark brown cerumen present in ear canals. Tympanic membranes gray and shiny. No bulging or retraction noted. Whisper test: Unable to repeat back words spoken by examiner. Weber's test: Sound lateralized to left ear. Rinne test: BC ≥ AC. No tenderness noted when mastoids palpated. Referred to ear clinic for further evaluation.

provider's office. Diagnostic tests to assess the structure and functions of the ears are described in the Diagnostic Tests table below and summarized in the following bulleted list. More information is included in the discussion of specific injuries or diseases in Chapter 48 ∞ .

- Audiometry is used to evaluate and diagnose conductive and sensorineural hearing loss.
- Electrical activity of the auditory nerve may be evaluated by using an auditory evoked potential (AEP) or an auditory brainstem response (ABR).
- Vestibular system function is evaluated with a caloric test. If no nystagmus occurs during the test, further testing for brain lesions is conducted.

Regardless of the type of diagnostic test, the nurse is responsible for explaining the procedure and any special preparation needed, for assessing for any medication use that might affect the outcome of the tests, for supporting the client during the examination as necessary, for documenting the procedures as appropriate, and for monitoring the results of the tests.

Genetic Considerations

When conducting a health assessment interview and a physical assessment, it is important for the nurse to consider genetic influences on health of the adult. Several diseases of the ears have a genetic component. During the health assessment interview, ask about a family history of congenital deafness, deafness associated with a thyroid goiter, or tumors of the auditory nerve.

During the physical assessment, assess for any manifestations that might indicate a genetic disorder (see the Genetic Considerations box below). If data are found to indicate genetic risk factors or alterations, ask about genetic testing and refer for appropriate genetic counseling and evaluation. Chapter 8 ∞ provides further information about genetics in medical-surgical nursing.

Health Assessment Interview

The health history assessment to collect subjective data about the ears and hearing may be part of a health screening, may focus on a chief complaint (such as hearing problems or pain in

GENETIC CONSIDERATIONS
Ear Disorders

- Deafness (hearing loss) is a common disorder that is seen from newborns to those of old age. About 1 in 1000 infants have a profound hearing loss, with about half being genetic in origin (NIH, 2003b). Early diagnosis is important to facilitate language and social skill development in adults.
- Penred syndrome is an inherited disorder that accounts for as much as 10% of hereditary deafness. The deafness is usually accompanied by a thyroid goiter.
- Neurofibromatosis, a rare inherited disorder, is characterized by the development of acoustic neuromas (benign tumors of the auditory nerve) and malignant central nervous system tumors.

DIAGNOSTIC TESTS of Ear Disorders

NAME OF TEST Audiometry
PURPOSE AND DESCRIPTION Used to evaluate and diagnose conductive and sensorineural hearing loss. Client sits in soundproof room and responds by raising a hand when sounds are heard.
RELATED NURSING CARE No special preparation is needed.

NAME OF TEST Auditory evoked potential (AEP)
PURPOSE AND DESCRIPTION Used to identify electrical activity of the auditory nerve. Electrodes are placed on various areas of the ear and on the forehead and a graphic recording is made.
RELATED NURSING CARE No special preparation is needed.

NAME OF TEST Auditory brainstem response (ABR)
PURPOSE AND DESCRIPTION Measures electrical activity of the auditory pathway from inner ear to brain to diagnose brainstem pathology, stroke, and acoustic neuroma.
RELATED NURSING CARE No special preparation is needed.

NAME OF TEST Caloric test
PURPOSE AND DESCRIPTION Used to assess vestibular system function. Cold or warm water is used to irrigate the ear canals one at a time and the client is observed for nystagmus (repeated abnormal movements of the eyes). Normally, the nystagmus occurs opposite to the ear being irrigated. If no nystagmus occurs, the client needs further testing for brain lesions.
RELATED NURSING CARE Assess client for use of alcohol, central nervous system depressants, and barbiturates. These chemicals may alter the test results.

the ear), or may be part of a total health assessment. If the client has a problem involving one or both ears, analyze its onset, characteristics and course, severity, precipitating and relieving factors, and any associated symptoms, noting the timing and circumstances. For example, you may ask the following questions:

- Have you noticed any difficulty hearing high-pitched sounds, low-pitched sounds, or both?
- When did you first notice the ringing in your ears?
- Is your workplace very noisy? If so, do you wear protective ear equipment at work?

Throughout the examination, be alert to nonverbal behaviors (such as inappropriate answers or requests to repeat statements) that suggest problems with ear function. Explore changes in hearing, ringing in the ears (*tinnitus*), ear pain, drainage from the ears, or the use of hearing aids. When taking the history, ask about trauma, surgery, or infections of the ear as well as the date of the last ear examination. In addition, ask the client about a medical history of infectious diseases, such as meningitis or mumps, as well as the use of medications that may affect hearing. Because ear problems tend to run in families, ask about a family history of hearing loss, ear problems, or diseases that could result in such problems. If the client has a hearing aid, ascertain the type and assess measures for its care.

Interview questions categorized by functional health patterns are found in the Functional Health Pattern table below.

FUNCTIONAL HEALTH PATTERN INTERVIEW The Ear

Functional Health Pattern	Interview Questions and Leading Statements
Health Perception-Health Management	■ Describe your hearing. Rate it on a scale of 1 to 10, with 10 being excellent hearing. Is it the same in both ears? If not, which ear is better? ■ Describe your current hearing problems. How have these been treated? ■ Do you use ear medications? What type and how often? ■ Have you ever had ear surgery? Describe. ■ Describe the type of hearing aid that you use. Are you satisfied with this appliance? How do you care for it? ■ Describe how you care for your ears each day. ■ When was your last ear examination? Have you ever had your hearing tested? ■ Do you listen to loud music? Do you use ear phones when you listen to loud music?
Nutritional-Metabolic	■ Do you have any swelling or tenderness in the ears or drainage from the ears?
Activity-Exercise	■ Does your hearing problem interfere with your usual activities of daily living? Explain. ■ Do you wear protective earplugs when you take part in activities that increase the risk of injury to your ears (such as at work or when operating machinery at home)?
Sleep-Rest	■ Does your ear problem interfere with your ability to rest or sleep (for example, from pain)? If so, what do you do?
Cognitive-Perceptual	■ Do you have pain in or around your ears? Have you ever had ringing in your ears? If so, describe its location, intensity, what makes it worse, and how long it lasts. How do you treat it? ■ Do you have difficulty hearing conversations, either in person or on the telephone? Do you have trouble hearing the television? Do you have difficulty hearing when you are in crowds or there is background noise? ■ Have you noticed your hearing is different in each ear? ■ Do you have buzzing, ringing, or crackling noises in one or both ears? Explain. ■ Do you ever feel dizzy?
Self-Perception-Self-Concept	■ Has this problem with your ears affected how you feel about yourself?
Role-Relationships	■ How has having this condition affected your relationships with others? ■ Has having this condition interfered with your ability to work? Explain. ■ Has anyone in your family had problems with ear disease? Explain.
Sexuality-Reproductive	■ Has this condition interfered with your usual sexual activity?
Coping-Stress-Tolerance	■ Has having this condition created stress for you? If so, does your health problem seem to be more difficult when you are stressed? ■ Have you experienced any kind of stress that makes the condition worse? Explain. ■ Describe what you do when you feel stressed.
Value-Belief	■ Describe how specific relationships or activities help you cope with this problem. ■ Describe specific cultural beliefs or practices that affect how you care for and feel about this problem. ■ Are there any specific treatments that you would not use to treat this problem?

TABLE 47–2 Age-Related Changes in the Ear

AGE-RELATED CHANGE	SIGNIFICANCE
The inner ear: ■ Loss of hair cells, ↓ blood supply, less flexible basilar membrane, degeneration of spiral ganglion cells, and ↓ production of endolymph result in progressive hearing loss with age (presbycusis). ■ High-frequency sounds are lost; middle and low-frequency sounds may also be lost or decreased. ■ Vestibular structures degenerate, organ of Corti and cochlea atrophy	Older adults may require hearing aids to hear well. With loss of high-frequency sounds, speech may be distorted, contributing to a risk for problems with communication. Degeneration and atrophy of inner ear structures concerned with balance and equilibrium increase the risk for falls.
The middle ear: ■ Muscles and ligaments weaken and stiffen, decreasing the acoustic reflex.	Sounds made from one's own body and speech are louder and may further interfere with hearing, speech, and communications.
The external ear: ■ Cerumen has a higher keratin content, contributing to increased cerumen in the ear canal.	Accumulated cerumen may impair hearing.

Physical Assessment of the Ears and Hearing

Physical assessment of the ears and hearing may be performed as part of a total health assessment or separately for clients with known or suspected problems with the ears. The ears and hearing are assessed primarily through inspection of external structures, the external auditory canal, and the tympanic membrane. Disorders of the middle ear may be identified with tympanom-etry. Hearing acuity is assessed by voice tests and tuning fork tests. The external structures may be palpated. Normal age-related findings for the older adult are summarized in Table 47–2.

The client should be sitting, and the examiner's head should be level with the head of the client. Prior to the assessment, collect all necessary equipment and explain the techniques to the client to decrease anxiety. The auditory canal and tympanic membrane are inspected with the otoscope. Guidelines for use of the otoscope are listed in Box 47–2.

BOX 47–2 Guidelines for Using the Otoscope

The otoscope has a handle that contains batteries for the light and various specula that fit onto the handle. (See the accompanying figure.) This instrument is used to inspect the auditory canal and the tympanic membrane. A pneumatic otoscope is used to determine the mobility of the tympanic membrane. A pneumatic otoscope has an attached rubber bulb that can be squeezed to inject air into the auditory canal, causing a normal tympanic membrane to move in and out.

Before the examination, explain the procedure to the client. Assemble the otoscope, using the largest speculum that will fit into the client's auditory canal without discomfort. Wash your hands; wear disposable gloves if the client has any drainage from the ears. Turn on the otoscope light. Ask the client to tip the head slightly toward the shoulder opposite the ear being examined. When the client is in this position, the auditory canal is aligned with the speculum.

1. Hold the handle of the otoscope in your dominant hand. If the client is restless, hold the otoscope handle upward, resting the hand against the client's head. If the client is cooperative, hold the handle downward.
2. For adult clients, grasp the superior portion of the auricle and pull up, out, and back to straighten the auditory canal. (See the accompanying figure.)
3. Insert the speculum into the ear and advance it gently. Assess the walls of the auditory canal while advancing the speculum, inspecting for color, obstructions, hair growth, and cerumen. Old cerumen is very dark and may obstruct visualization of part or all of the tympanic membrane.

An otoscope.

Technique for using an otoscope.

BOX 47–2 Guidelines for Using the Otoscope (continued)

4. Move the otoscope so that you can see the tympanic membrane. You may need to realign the auditory canal by gently continuing to pull up and back on the auricle. A normal membrane is semitransparent, allowing visualization of a portion of the auditory ossicles. The concave nature of the tympanic membrane and its oblique position in the auditory canal account for the triangular light reflex (cone of light) seen on otoscopic examination.
5. Note the color and surface of the membrane. The normal tympanic membrane is pearly gray, shiny, and semitransparent. The surface should be continuous, intact, and either flat or concave.
6. Identify the landmarks on the tympanic membrane (see the accompanying figure):
   a. The cone of light, located over the anteroinferior quadrant.
   b. The malleus, pars tensa, annulus, pars flaccida, and malleolar folds.
7. Assess movement of the tympanic membrane. If the auditory tube is patent, the membrane moves in and out when air is injected (or when the client performs the Valsalva maneuver).

Structures of the tympanic membrane visible through the otoscope.

8. Gently withdraw the speculum. If the speculum is soiled with drainage or cerumen, use a clean speculum for the other ear.
9. Using the same technique, examine the other ear.

EAR AND HEARING ASSESSMENTS

Hearing Assessment

Tuning forks are used to determine whether a hearing loss is conductive or perceptive (sensorineural). Hold the tuning fork at the base and make it ring softly by stroking the prongs or by lightly tapping them on the heel of the opposite hand. The vibrating tuning fork emits sound waves of a particular frequency, measured in hertz (Hz). Tuning forks with a frequency of 512 to 1024 Hz are preferred for auditory evaluation, because that range corresponds to the range of normal speech.

Technique/Normal Findings	Abnormal Findings	
Perform the Weber test. Place the base of a vibrating tuning fork on the midline vertex of the client's head (Figure 47–11 ■). Ask whether the client hears the sound equally in both ears or better in one than the other. *Sound is normally heard equally in both ears.*	■ Sound heard in, or lateralized to, one ear indicates either a conductive loss in that ear or a sensorineural loss in the other ear. The sound will be louder on the impaired side with a conductive hearing loss. The sound will be softer on the impaired side with a sensorineural hearing loss. Conductive losses may be due to a buildup of cerumen, an infection such as otitis media, or perforation of the eardrum.	**Figure 47–11** ■ Performing the Weber test with a tuning fork.

Technique/Normal Findings	Abnormal Findings

Perform the Rinne test. Place the base of a vibrating tuning fork on the client's mastoid bone. Ask the client to indicate when the sound is no longer heard. When the client does so, quickly reposition the tuning fork in front of the client's ear close to the ear canal. Ask whether the client can hear the sound. If the client says yes, ask the client to indicate when the sound is no longer heard. Repeat over the opposite mastoid bone (Figure 47–12 ■). *The client with no conductive hearing loss will hear the sound twice as long by air conduction as by bone conduction .*

■ Bone conduction is greater than air conduction in the ear with a conductive loss. The normal pattern is AC > BC (air conduction greater than bone conduction).

Figure 47–12 ■ Performing the Rinne test with a tuning fork.

Perform the whisper test. Ask the client to occlude one ear with a finger. Stand 1 to 2 feet away from the client, on the side of the unoccluded ear. Softly whisper numbers and ask the client to repeat them. Repeat the procedure, having the client occlude the other ear. Note whether you need to raise your voice or to stand closer to make the client hear you.

■ This test provides a rough estimate of hearing loss.

Use a tympanogram to measure the pressure of the middle ear and observe the tympanic membrane's response to waves of pressure. Insert the device into the ear canal. Ask the client not to speak, move, swallow, or jump when hearing a sound. Tell the client he or she will hear a loud tone as the measurements are taken. The normal pressure inside the middle ear is a 100 daPa (a very small amount). Repeat for the other ear.

■ Abnormal findings may include fluid in the middle ear, a perforated eardrum, impacted earwax, or a tumor of the middle ear.

External Ear Assessment

Inspect the auricle. *External ears are normally bilaterally equal in size, of equal color with the client's face, without redness or lesions.*

■ Unusual redness or drainage may indicate an inflammatory response to infection or trauma.
■ Scales or skin lesions around the rim of the auricle may indicate skin cancer.
■ Small, raised lesions on the rim of the ear are known as tophi and indicate gout.

Technique/Normal Findings	Abnormal Findings
Inspect the external auditory canal with the otoscope. *Canal walls should be pink and smooth without lesions. Cerumen is normally present in small, odorless amounts.*	■ Unusual redness, lesions, or purulent drainage may indicate an infection. ■ Cerumen varies in color and texture, but hardened, dry, or foul-smelling cerumen may indicate an infection or an impaction of cerumen that requires removal. People with darker skin tend to have darker cerumen.

Inspect the tympanic membrane. *The tympanic membrane should be pearly gray, shiny, and translucent without bulging or retraction.*

- White, opaque areas on the tympanic membrane are often scars from previous perforations (Figure 47–13 ■).
- Inconsistent texture and color may be due to scarring from previous perforations caused by infection, allergies, or trauma.
- Bulging membranes are indicated by a loss of bony landmarks and a distorted light reflex. Such bulges may be the result of otitis media or malfunctioning auditory tubes.
- Retracted tympanic membranes are indicated by accentuated bony landmarks and a distorted light reflex. Such retraction is often due to an obstructed auditory tube.

Figure 47–13 ■ Scarring of the tympanic membrane.

Source: Professor Tony Wright, Institute of Laryngology and Otology/SPL/Photo Researchers, Inc.

Palpate the auricles and over each mastoid process. *There should be no pain or swelling on palpation.*

- Tenderness, swelling, or nodules may indicate inflammation of the external auditory canal or mastoiditis.

EXPLORE MediaLink

Prentice Hall Nursing MediaLink DVD-ROM
  Audio Glossary
  NCLEX-RN® Review

COMPANION WEBSITE www.prenhall.com/lemone
  Audio Glossary
  NCLEX-RN® Review
  Care Plan Activity: Ear Pain
  Case Studies
    Identifying Common Pathologies
    Otitis Media
  MediaLink Applications: Nystagmus
  Links to Resources

TEST YOURSELF NCLEX-RN® REVIEW

1 During an eye assessment, you touch the part of the eye covering the iris and pupil. What normal client response would you expect?
  1. excess tearing
  2. blinking of eyelids
  3. bilateral nystagmus
  4. pupil dilates

2 Which of the following statements would indicate a client has presbyopia? *(near sighted)*
  1. "I just am having so much trouble hearing music."
  2. "I can't seem to remember anything these days."
  3. "I think I have a lot of earwax in my ears."
  4. "My arms just don't seem long enough to read."

3 What equipment would be necessary to test sound conduction during an assessment of the ear?
  1. ophthalmoscope
  2. tuning fork
  3. otoscope
  4. penlight

4 What occurs when light enters the lens of the eye?
  1. accommodation
  2. convergence
  3. pupillary reflex
  4. hyperopia

5 What would you tell a client before a test of refraction is done?
1. "This test is uncomfortable, but it doesn't take long."
2. "You will be blindfolded during the test."
3. "Are you allergic to seafood?"
4. "Your pupils will be dilated for several hours."

6 What function, in addition to hearing, is provided by the inner ear?
1. Coordinates visual pathways.
2. Integrates efferent neuron messages.
3. Provides information about head position.
4. Maintains middle ear structure and function.

7 Why is the Snellen eye chart used during vision assessment?
1. to test distant vision
2. to test near vision
3. to determine visual fields
4. to examine convergence

8 Of the following ear assessments, which one is a rough estimate of the ability to hear?
1. whisper test
2. Rinne test
3. Weber test
4. audiometry

9 What is a high-priority risk for the older adult with age-related changes in the vestibular structures of the ear?
1. infection
2. falls
3. medication errors
4. food intolerance

10 Which criterion is important to accurately assess visual fields?
1. Client must wear corrective lenses.
2. Client must have no less than 20/30 vision.
3. Examiner must not wear glasses.
4. Examiner must have normal visual field.

See Test Yourself answers in Appendix C.

BIBLIOGRAPHY

Bickley, L., & Szilagyi, P. (2007). *Bates' guide to physical examination and history taking* (9th ed.). Philadelphia: Lippincott.

Cox, C., Boswell, G., McGrath, A., Reynolds, T., & Cole, E. (2004). Cranial nerve damage. *Emergency Nurse, 12*(2), 14–21.

Eliopoulos, E. (2005). *Gerontological nursing* (6th ed.). Philadelphia: Lippincott Williams & Wilkins.

Erber, N. (2002). Hearing, vision, communication, and older people. *Seminars in Hearing, 23*(1), 35–42, C1–9.

Ervin, S. (2004). Ménière's disease. Identifying classic symptoms and current treatments. *AAOHN Journal, 52*(4), 156–158.

Hudspeth, A. (2002). How hearing happens. *Hearing Loss, 23*(1), 25–27.

Jarvis, C. (2004). *Physical examination & health assessment.* St. Louis, MO: Mosby.

Kahari, K., Zachau, G., Eklof, M., Sandsjo, L., & Moller, C. (2003). Assessment of hearing and hearing disorders in rock/jazz musicians. *International Journal of Audiology, 42*(5), 179–288.

Kee, J. (2005). *Prentice Hall handbook of laboratory & diagnostic tests with nursing implications.* Upper Saddle River, NJ: Prentice Hall.

Levinson, D. (2003). Many elderly patients with chronic eye disease don't get recommended exams. *Report on Medical Guidelines & Outcomes Research, 14*(20), 1, 5–6.

Mahoney, J. (2000). Hearing loss and assessment: A concern for all. *Nursing Spectrum (Greater Chicago/NE Illinois & NW Indiana Edition), 13*(1), 20–22.

McGrory, A., & Remington, R. (2004). Optimizing the functionality of clients with age-related macular degeneration. *Journal of Rehabilitation Nursing, 29*(3), 90–94.

Meadows, M. (2002). Saving your sight. Early detection is critical. *FDA Consumer, 36*(2), 22–28.

Medline Plus. (2005). *Medical encyclopedia: Tympanometry.* Retrieved from http://www.nlm.nih.gov/medlineplus/print/ency/article/003390.htm

National Institutes of Health. (2003a). *Genes and disease. Diseases of the eye.* Retrieved from http://www.ncbi.nlm.nih.gov/books/bv.fcgi?rid=gnd.section.35

_____. (2003b). *Genes and disease. Ear, nose, and throat.* Retrieved from http://www.ncbi.nlm.nih.gov/books/bv.fcgi?rid=gnd.section.32

Porth, C. (2005). *Pathophysiology: Concepts of altered health states* (7th ed.). Philadelphia: Lippincott.

Smeeth, L., & Iliffe, S. (2005). Community screening for visual impairment in the elderly. *The Cochrane Library (Oxford), 1,* ID#CD001054.

Stuen, C., & Faye, E. (2003). Vision loss: Normal and not normal changes among older adults. *Generations, 27*(1), 8–14.

Wallhagen, M., Pettengill, E., & Whiteside, M. (2006). Sensory impairment in older adults: Part 1: Hearing loss. *American Journal of Nursing, 106*(10), 40–48.

Wandell, B., & Wade, A. (2003). Functional imaging of the visual pathways. *Neurologic Clinics, 21*(2), 417–443.

Weber, J., & Kelley, J. (2006). *Health assessment in nursing* (3rd ed.). Philadelphia: Lippincott.

Whiteside, M., Wallhagen, M., & Pettengill, E. (2006). Sensory impairment in older adults: Part 2: Vision loss. *American Journal of Nursing, 106*(11), 52–61.

CHAPTER 48 Nursing Care of Clients with Eye and Ear Disorders

LEARNING OUTCOMES

- Relate knowledge of normal anatomy, physiology, and sensory functions of the eye and ear to the effects of disorders of these organs on the cognitive/perceptual functional health pattern.

- Describe the pathophysiology of commonly occurring disorders of the eyes and ears, relating their manifestations to the pathophysiologic process.

- Explain the risk factors for selected disorders of the eyes and ears, identifying the nursing implications for these risk factors.

- Identify diagnostic tests used for specific eye and ear disorders.

- Discuss the effects of and nursing implications for medications prescribed to treat eye and ear disorders.

- Describe surgical and other invasive procedures used to treat eye and ear disorders, identifying their implications for nursing care.

- Discuss the nurse's role in caring for clients with impaired vision or hearing loss.

CLINICAL COMPETENCIES

- Assess vision, hearing, and functional health of clients with eye and ear disorders.

- Using assessed data, determine priority nursing diagnoses and interventions for clients with eye and ear disorders.

- Collaborate with other members of the healthcare team to provide effective care for clients with eye and ear disorders.

- Plan and implement appropriate and individualized evidence-based nursing interventions and teaching for the client with an eye or ear disorder.

- Safely and effectively administer eye and ear medications and prescribed treatments.

- Provide appropriate care and teaching for the client having eye or ear surgery.

- Evaluate the effectiveness of nursing care provided for clients with eye and ear disorders, revising plan of care as indicated.

Vision and hearing provide the primary means of input for much of what we know about the world. The ability to receive and organize information orients us to our surroundings. These senses allow us to communicate easily, gain access to information, and derive pleasure from the sights and sounds of the world around us.

This chapter discusses conditions affecting vision and hearing as the result of eye and ear disorders. Nursing care focuses on clients with vision and hearing deficits that can result from the disorders presented.

EYE DISORDERS

Any portion of the eye and its protective structures may be affected by an acute or chronic condition. While many disorders of the eye are minor and have little or no effect on vision, others can and often do result in permanent vision impairment. Disorders and diseases of the outer, visible portion of the eye often cause discomfort and may have cosmetic effects. With appropriate treatment, vision impairment often can be prevented or reversed. Disorders of the cornea present the greatest risk to vision in this group. The client who has had eye surgery or minor trauma may have either temporary or permanent visual impairment. Disorders affecting the internal structures or the function of the eye are more likely to have adverse effects on vision. These disorders are more likely to affect adults over the age of 40, and older adults in particular. More than 3.4 million adults in the United States have some degree of visual impairment (Prevent Blindness America, 2002).

FAST FACTS

Among adults age 40 and older in the United States:

- Nearly 3.3 million or 2.7% of the population are classified as blind or low vision.
- Refractory errors, including myopia (nearsightedness) and hyperopia (farsightedness), are the most common, affecting 25.4% and 9.9% of people age 40 and older.
- Other conditions affecting the vision of middle and older adults, in order of prevalence, are:
  1. Cataracts—17.2%
  2. Macular degeneration—7.6%
  3. Diabetic retinopathy—3.4%
  4. Glaucoma—1.9%.

Source: All data from *Statistics and Data*, National Eye Institute, National Institutes of Health (2004). Retrieved from http://www.nei.nih.gov/eyedata/pbd_tables.asp.

Although disorders that commonly affect vision often cannot be prevented or cured, some can be controlled and vision corrected to normal or near normal. Regardless of the real threat a disorder poses to vision, the client may experience anxiety related to a perceived threat. The box on the next page discusses major causes of significantly impaired vision and nursing care for the client who is blind. These principles of nursing care may apply to clients with many of the disorders discussed in this chapter.

THE CLIENT WITH CONJUNCTIVITIS

The conjunctiva—the thin, transparent membrane that covers the anterior surface of the eye and lines the inner surfaces of the eyelids—is vulnerable to inflammation and infection because of its constant exposure to the environment. **Conjunctivitis**, inflammation of the conjunctiva, is the most common eye disease. Its usual cause is a bacterial or viral infection. These infections can be transmitted to the eye by direct contact (e.g., hands, tissues, towels). Allergens, chemical irritants, and exposure to radiant energy such as ultraviolet light from the sun or tanning devices can also lead to this common condition. Its severity can range from mild irritation with redness and tearing to conjunctival edema, hemorrhage, or a severe necrotizing process with tissue destruction.

Pathophysiology and Manifestations
Acute Conjunctivitis

Infectious conjunctivitis may be bacterial, viral, or fungal in origin. Bacterial conjunctivitis, also known as "pink eye," is highly contagious, and often is caused by *Staphylococcus* and *Haemophilus*. Adenovirus infection is the leading cause of conjunctivitis in adults. Systemic infections that may affect the eyes include herpes simplex and other viral infections. Contact with genital secretions infected with *Gonococcus* can cause gonococcal conjunctivitis, a medical emergency that can lead to corneal perforation.

NURSING CARE OF THE CLIENT WHO IS BLIND

Visual impairment exists on a continuum from blindness to decreased visual acuity that can be corrected with refractive lenses to normal or near normal. *Visual impairment* is defined as 20/40 vision in the better eye, even with corrective lenses. The legal definition of *blindness* is visual acuity no better than 20/200 in the better eye with optimal correction, or a visual field of less than 20 degrees in diameter (compared to the normal of 180 degrees) (Prevent Blindness America, 2002). Total blindness usually indicates that the client has no light perception at all. In practical terms, a person with a visual deficit sufficient to need assistive devices or aid from other people for normal activities of daily living is considered blind.

Ten to 12 million people in the United States have a visual impairment that cannot be corrected. More than 900,000 Americans are legally blind and an additional 2.3 million are visually impaired (National Eye Institute [NEI], 2004). In the United States, blindness affects more blacks than whites and Hispanics, whereas more Hispanics are visually impaired (Prevent Blindness America, 2002). Worldwide, between 40 and 50 million people have visual impairment significant enough to be considered blind.

Although blindness often can be prevented or cured, it remains a significant problem worldwide because of lack of access to care, fear of surgery or treatment, poor sanitation and nutrition, and ignorance of need. In the United States, cataracts, age-related macular degeneration, glaucoma, and diabetic retinopathy remain significant causes of blindness in adults.

Nursing Care

Blind people need to cope not only with the loss of a major sense but often also with societal attitudes that make them feel inferior, helpless, and inadequate. The idea of losing the ability to see is uniformly feared, leaving sighted people often unable to understand the magnitude and impact of the loss in those who have experienced it. Because of this fear and confusion, sighted people are unsure of what the blind expect from them.

The adjustment of the person who is born blind and raised to become an independent member of society differs from that of the person who has been sighted and becomes blind. The person who has been blind from birth has developed numerous adaptive strategies that the newly blind person has yet to learn.

Although adaptation may be easier for the client who experiences a gradual loss of vision than for someone with an abrupt loss, both must grieve the lost sense. The blind client needs to grieve the lost body part as well as the loss of mobility, self-sufficiency, perhaps economic security, and, to a certain extent, contact with reality as it has been perceived. The client's self-concept and self-esteem are threatened. Anger, denial, remorse, and self-pity are not uncommon in the initial period following loss of sight. Interpersonal relationships and roles are affected. Communication patterns change with the loss of the ability to perceive many nonverbal cues. Expressions of sexuality may be impaired.

Acceptance of the change from sighted to blind is characterized by releasing the hope that vision will be regained. Self-esteem increases as the client attempts and masters activities of self-sufficiency such as completing ADLs, cooking, and becoming mobile outside the known home environment.

Health professionals often confuse the role of the blind person with the role of the client, seeing the person as helpless, dependent, and lacking in personal identity and control. Although nurses need to take blindness into account in planning care and maintaining client safety, it is vital to give the blind client the same respect and decision-making power that all clients deserve. Nurses who have dealt with their own emotions and responses to vision loss are better prepared to help the client adapt.

Nurses can foster independence in the hospitalized client with a significant vision deficit by doing the following:

- Orient to the environment verbally and physically. Describe the room using a central point such as the bed. Lead the client around the room, identifying chairs, sink, bathroom, and other landmarks. Be sure that objects such as chairs, personal items, and clothing remain in the same place unless moved by the client. Leave doors either fully open or closed as the client wishes, but, to preserve safety, do not leave doors partially open. Keep the room and hallways free of clutter.
- Use verbal communication freely. Describe activities going on around the client. Introduce yourself as you enter the room and let the client know when you are leaving.
- Provide other sensory stimuli such as radio and television as desired by the client.
- Orient to food trays by using the face of a clock to describe the position of food items on the plate and tray (unless the client has always been blind and cannot visualize a clock face).
- When assisting with ambulation, allow the client to hold your arm as you walk slightly ahead. Do not hold the client's arm. Verbally describe the environment, such as "There will be two steps up five feet ahead."
- Do not hesitate to ask what assistance the client desires.

For the client with a new loss of sight, refer to available services. Counseling can help the client cope with and eventually adapt to the loss of sight. People who are blind can receive mobility training, assistance with relearning self-care activities, education in the use of Braille to communicate, and vocational and other forms of rehabilitation. Local, state, and national agencies such as the American Foundation for the Blind, National Braille Association, and National Federation for the Blind coordinate services for the blind. Many assistive devices are available, including guide or pilot dogs, computer services, talking books and tape players, and low-vision aids.

Redness and itching of the affected eye are common manifestations of acute conjunctivitis (Figure 48–1 ■). The client may also complain of a scratchy, burning, or gritty sensation. Pain is not common; however, photophobia may occur. Tearing and discharge accompany the inflammatory process. The discharge may be watery, purulent, or mucoid, depending on the cause of conjunctivitis. The client may have associated manifestations such as pharyngitis, fever, malaise, and swollen preauricular lymph nodes.

Trachoma

Trachoma, a chronic conjunctivitis caused by *Chlamydia trachomatis*, is a significant preventable cause of blindness worldwide. Trachoma is endemic in sub-Saharan Africa, the Middle

Figure 48–1 ■ The appearance of an eye with conjunctivitis.
Source: Buddy Crofton/Medical Images, Inc.

Figure 48–2 ■ Entropion.
Source: Science Photo Library/Photo Researchers, Inc.

East, and parts of Asia. In the United States, it can be found in Native Americans of the Southwest, but less frequently than in endemic regions. Trachoma is contagious, transmitted primarily by close personal contact (eye-to-eye, hand-to-eye) or by fomites such as towels, handkerchiefs, and flies. Certain forms of trachoma are transmitted during delivery when the newborn is exposed to contaminated genital secretions of the mother (Kasper et al., 2005).

Early manifestations of trachoma include redness, eyelid edema, tearing, and photophobia. Small conjunctival follicles develop on the upper lids. The inflammation also causes superficial corneal vascularization and infiltration with granulation tissue. Scarring of the conjunctival lining of the lid causes entropion (Figure 48–2). The lashes then abrade the cornea, eventually causing ulceration and scarring. The scarred cornea is opaque, resulting in loss of vision.

INTERDISCIPLINARY CARE

Management of the client with conjunctivitis focuses on establishing an accurate diagnosis and prompt treatment.

Diagnosis

Accurate diagnosis of conjunctivitis is especially important, because other potentially vision-threatening conditions, such as acute uveitis or acute angle-closure glaucoma, can also cause a red eye (Table 48–1). Diagnostic procedures may include:

- *Culture and sensitivity* of exudates to determine presence of an infection and identify the infecting organism.
- *Fluorescein stain* with slit-lamp examination to identify possible corneal ulcerations or abrasions, which appear green with staining.
- *Conjunctival scrapings* are examined microscopically or cultured to identify the organisms.

Additional laboratory testing such as blood counts or antibody titers may be used to identify underlying infectious or autoimmune processes.

Medications

Conjunctivitis is treated with antibiotic, antiviral, or anti-inflammatory drugs as appropriate. Topical anti-infectives applied as either eyedrops or ointment may include erythromycin, gentamicin, penicillin, bacitracin, sulfacetamide sodium, amphotericin B, or idoxuridine. For severe infections or cellulitis, anti-infectives may be administered by subconjunctival injection or systemic intravenous infusion. Antihistamines are used to minimize symptoms of conjunctivitis when an allergic response underlies the inflammatory process.

Complementary Therapies

Frequent eye irrigations may be ordered to remove the copious purulent discharge associated with conjunctivitis. Soaking the lids with warm saline compresses prior to cleansing promotes comfort and facilitates the removal of crusts and exudate in conjunctivitis.

TABLE 48–1 Possible Causes of Acute Red Eye

	ACUTE CONJUNCTIVITIS	CORNEAL TRAUMA OR INFECTION	ACUTE UVEITIS	ACUTE ANGLE-CLOSURE GLAUCOMA
Incidence	Very common	Common	Common	Rare
Pain	Mild	Moderate to severe	Moderate	Severe
Vision	Normal	Blurred	Blurred	Markedly blurred
Discharge	May be copious	Watery, may be purulent	None	None
Conjunctival erythema	Diffuse	Primarily around cornea	Primarily around cornea	Primarily around cornea
Cornea	Clear	Depends on cause	Usually clear	Cloudy
Pupils	Normal size, response to light	Normal size, response to light	Small, minimal response to light	Moderately dilated, fixed

NURSING CARE

The nursing role in treating conjunctivitis is primarily one of education to prevent the disorder and to prevent its spread when it does occur.

Health Promotion

Education is a vital strategy for preventing conjunctivitis. Teach all clients about proper eye care, including the importance of not sharing towels, makeup, or contact lenses, and avoiding rubbing or scratching the eyes. Instruct to avoid using old eye makeup, which can cause eye infections. Teach contact lens users appropriate care (Box 48–1). Emphasize the need to follow cleaning instructions precisely to avoid bacterial contamination of lenses. If the eyes become red, irritated, or develop discharge, instruct the client to avoid wearing contact lenses until the inflammatory process has cleared.

Assessment

- *Health history:* Presence of redness, discomfort, tearing, photophobia, and drainage; symptom onset; care measures; use of contact lenses; exposure to "pink eye" or recent travel; allergies; previous history of conjunctivitis; presence of any chronic diseases.
- *Physical assessment:* Visual acuity; inspect eyelids, conjunctiva, sclera, and cornea; vital signs including temperature.

Nursing Diagnoses and Interventions

Nursing care focuses primarily on preventing complications from the disorder. The priority nursing diagnoses include risk for infection and risk of altered vision.

Risk for Infection

Acute conjunctivitis is highly contagious. While most clients experience no more than discomfort from the disease, the infection carries a risk for scarring and damage to the delicate cornea of the eye. Preventing the spread of this infection is a vital nursing role.

- Teach to wash hands thoroughly before instilling eye medications. Instruct to avoid touching or rubbing the eyes. Advise to use a new, clean cotton-tipped swab or cotton ball for cleaning each eye. *Hand washing is the single most important measure to prevent transmission of infection to the eye. Touching or rubbing the eyes increases the risk of infection and corneal trauma. Using a new swab or cotton ball prevents cross-contamination between eyes.*
- Teach to instill prescribed eyedrops as ordered. *Prescribed medications reduce inflammation and eliminate infection.*
- Discuss the importance of avoiding contact lens use until the infectious process has cleared and of completing the prescribed treatment. *Use of contact lenses in the inflamed eyes can lead to further damage and impair healing.*

Risk for Disturbed Sensory Perception: Visual

Conjunctivitis can potentially disrupt the integrity or clarity of the cornea. Because of its vital role in focusing light on the retina, corneal damage can impair visual acuity.

- Assess vision with and without corrective lenses. *Assessment provides a baseline to evaluate possible changes in vision resulting from the infection.*
- Instruct to avoid activities requiring high visual acuity until the infection has cleared. *The inflammatory process, edema of the conjunctiva, and local antibiotic applications can decrease visual acuity and cloud vision.*
- Instruct to use dark sunglasses with appropriate UV protection when out of doors, even on cloudy days. *Photophobia, a common manifestation of conjunctivitis, causes eye pain with increased light intensity.*

Using NANDA, NIC, and NOC

Linkages between nursing diagnoses, nursing interventions, and nursing outcomes for the client with an inflammatory or infectious eye disorder are illustrated in Chart 48–1.

Community-Based Care

Clients with conjunctivitis typically are managed in the community, reinforcing the need for effective teaching for home care. Emphasize to the family ways to prevent transmission of infection. If the client is unable to administer eye medications, involve the family in teaching. Include the following topics:

- Safety and medical asepsis when cleansing the eye
- Instillation of prescribed eyedrops and ointments
- Comfort measures such as reducing lighting intensity and wearing sunglasses
- Avoidance of activities such as excessive reading while eye is inflamed.

THE CLIENT WITH A CORNEAL DISORDER

The clear cornea allows light rays to enter the eye and transmits images onto the retina. It helps to focus light on the retina and protects the internal eye structures. The cornea can be affected by a variety of disorders, including infection and trauma. While the cornea heals quickly after minor injuries or

---

BOX 48–1 Contact Lens Care

- Wash hands thoroughly before handling contact lenses.
- Keep storage case clean.
- Remove lenses before sleep, cleaning and storing as recommended by manufacturer.
- Use cleaning and wetting solutions recommended by eye care professional or lens manufacturer. Do not use water or home-made solutions for wetting or cleaning lenses.
- If eye redness, tearing, vision loss, or pain occurs, remove lenses and contact eye care professional as soon as possible.
- Do not share contact lenses or allow another person to "try on" lenses.

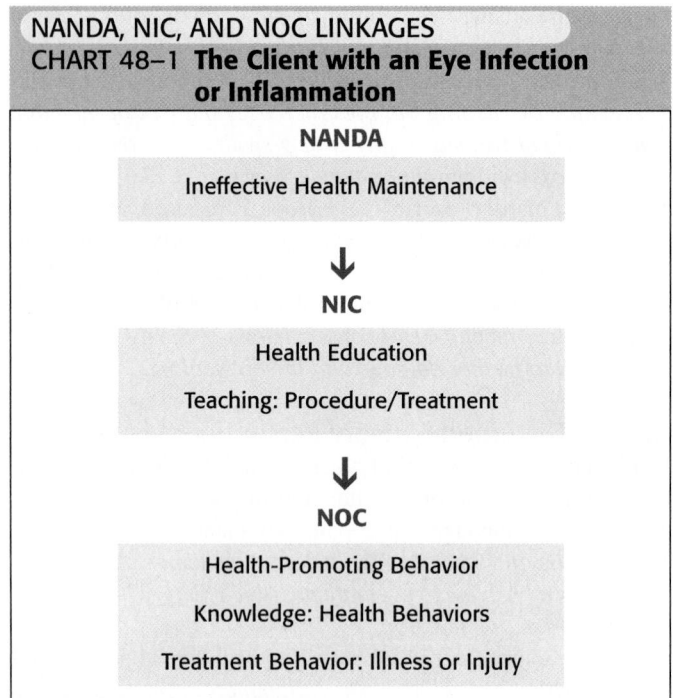

NANDA, NIC, AND NOC LINKAGES

CHART 48-1 **The Client with an Eye Infection or Inflammation**

NANDA

Ineffective Health Maintenance

↓

NIC

Health Education

Teaching: Procedure/Treatment

↓

NOC

Health-Promoting Behavior

Knowledge: Health Behaviors

Treatment Behavior: Illness or Injury

Data from *NANDA's Nursing Diagnoses: Definitions & Classification 2005–2006* by NANDA International (2005), Philadelphia; *Nursing Interventions Classification (NIC)* (4th ed.) by J. M. Dochterman & G. M. Bulechek (2004), St. Louis, MO: Mosby; and *Nursing Outcomes Classification (NOC)* (3rd ed.) by S. Moorhead, M. Johnson, and M. Maas (2004), St. Louis, MO: Mosby.

abrasions, injury to its deeper layers can delay healing or result in scarring.

Physiology Review

The cornea has three major layers: the outermost epithelium, which consists of five or six layers of cells that are constantly being renewed; the stroma, which makes up 90% of corneal tissue; and the single-cell thickness endothelium adjacent to the aqueous humor of the anterior chamber. The cornea is avascular tissue; the central cornea is dependent on atmospheric oxygen to meet its metabolic needs. Because there is no blood supply, immune defenses have difficulty fending off infections of the cornea.

Pathophysiology and Manifestations

Light enters the eye through the normally clear cornea. As light passes through the curved cornea, it is bent or *refracted* onto the lens, which then focuses the light on sensory cells of the retina. A change in the curvature of the cornea or in its clarity affects the ability of the eye to clearly focus; as a result, vision is distorted or blurred. Refractive errors such as nearsightedness, farsightedness, and astigmatism are common. Corneal scarring or ulceration are two major causes of blindness worldwide.

Refractive Errors

Refractive errors are the most common problem affecting visual acuity; they result from an abnormal curvature of the cornea or an altered shape of the eyeball. People with *emmetropia* (normal vision) see near and far objects clearly because light rays focus directly on the retina. In **myopia** (near-

sightedness) the curvature of the cornea is excessive or the eyeball is elongated, causing the image to focus in front of the retina instead of on it. Objects in close range are seen clearly and those at a distance are blurred. The eyeball is too short in **hyperopia** (farsightedness), causing the image to focus behind the retina. People with this condition see objects clearer at a distance than those close to them.

FAST FACTS
- The prevalence of myopia decreases with aging, from an estimated 36.4% of Americans ages 40 to 49 affected (15.5 million) to 17.5% of people ages 80 and older (1.6 million).
- In contrast, the prevalence of hyperopia increases with aging, affecting an estimated 3.1% of Americans ages 40 to 49 (1.5 million) and 23.6% of people ages 80 and older (2.2 million) (NEI, 2004).

Astigmatism develops due to an irregular or abnormal curvature of the cornea. Instead of the round, even curvature of the normal cornea, the cornea curves more in one direction than the other in astigmatism, resembling the back of a spoon. As a result, light rays focus on more than one area of the retina, distorting both near and distance vision.

Keratitis

Keratitis is inflammation of the cornea. When the inflammatory process involves both the conjunctiva and the cornea, the term *keratoconjunctivitis* may be used. Keratitis may be caused by infection, hypersensitivity reactions, ischemia, tearing defects, trauma, and impaired innervation of the cornea. Scarring that occurs as a result of keratitis is a leading cause of blindness worldwide (Porth, 2005).

Keratitis is described as either nonulcerative or ulcerative. In *nonulcerative keratitis,* all layers of corneal epithelium are affected, but remain intact. Viral infections, tuberculosis, and autoimmune disorders such as lupus erythematosus may cause nonulcerative keratitis. *Ulcerative keratitis,* in contrast, affects the epithelium and stroma of the cornea, leading to tissue destruction and ulceration. Bacterial conjunctivitis (e.g., *Staphylococcus, S. pneumoniae, Chlamydia*) may lead to ulcerative keratitis.

Keratitis commonly causes tearing, discomfort ranging from a gritty sensation in the eye to severe pain, decreased visual acuity, and *blepharospasm* (spasm of the eyelid and inability to open the eye). A discharge may be present, especially if the conjunctiva is also inflamed. Corneal ulceration may be visible on direct examination.

Corneal Ulcer

A **corneal ulcer**, local necrosis of the cornea, may be caused by infection, exposure trauma, or the misuse of contact lenses. A frequent cause is bacterial infection following trauma or contact lens overuse. Herpes viruses, including herpes simplex and herpes zoster, are a leading cause of ulcerative corneal disease. Corneal ulcers may also complicate bacterial conjunctivitis, trachoma, gonorrhea, and other acute infections. Clients who are immunosuppressed because of disease or drug therapy are at particular risk for developing corneal ulcers due to infection.

In corneal ulceration, a portion of the epithelium and/or stroma is destroyed. Ulcers may be superficial or deep, penetrating underlying layers and posing a risk of perforation. Fibrous tissue may form during healing, resulting in scarring and opacity of the cornea. Perforation can lead to infection of deeper eye structures or extrusion of eye contents. Partial or total vision loss may result.

Corneal Dystrophies

A corneal dystrophy is accumulation of cloudy material in part or parts of the normally clear cornea, potentially affecting visual acuity. Corneal dystrophies typically are inherited disorders that progress gradually and affect both eyes. *Keratoconus*, progressive thinning of the cornea, is the most common corneal dystrophy. It typically affects teenagers and young adults. In keratoconus, the center of the cornea thins and bulges outward, affecting the shape of the cornea and its ability to focus light on the lens of the eye. In most cases, the thinning stabilizes over time; up to 20% of clients, however, eventually require corneal transplant (NEI, 2005a).

INTERDISCIPLINARY CARE

Management of the client with a disorder of the cornea focuses on establishing an accurate diagnosis and prompt treatment to reduce the risk of permanent vision deficit. The history and physical assessment are key in diagnosing these disorders.

Although many eye disorders can be treated in the community, the client with a severe corneal infection or ulcer may require hospitalization. Corneal ulcers are medical emergencies, requiring prompt referral to an ophthalmologist for treatment. Pressure dressings may be applied to both eyes for comfort and to reduce the risk of perforation and loss of eye contents.

Diagnosis

Visual acuity is tested on all clients presenting with refractory or corneal disorders. See Chapter 47 ∞ for more information about testing visual acuity. The following tests may be ordered to identify the cause and extent of eye infections or inflammations:

- *Fluorescein stain* with slit-lamp examination allows visualization of any corneal ulcerations or abrasions, which appear green with staining.
- *Conjunctival* or *ulcer scrapings* are examined microscopically or cultured to identify the organisms.

Additional laboratory testing such as blood counts or antibody titers may be used to identify any underlying infectious or autoimmune processes.

Medication

Infectious processes are treated with antibiotic or antiviral therapy as appropriate. Topical anti-infectives applied as either eyedrops or ointment may include erythromycin, gentamicin, penicillin, bacitracin, sulfacetamide sodium, amphotericin B, or idoxuridine. For severe infections, central ulcers, or cellulitis, anti-infectives may be administered by subconjunctival injection and/or systemic intravenous infusion. Corticosteroids may be prescribed for keratitis related to systemic inflamma-

tory disorders or trauma; however, it is important to avoid their use with local infections to avoid suppressing the immune and inflammatory responses.

Corrective Lenses

Corrective lenses, either in the form of eyeglasses or contact lenses, generally are prescribed to restore visual acuity for clients with refractive errors such as myopia, hyperopia, and astigmatism. Specially fitted contact lenses to reduce vision distortion are ordered for clients with keratoconus. Because contact lenses are a risk factor for corneal infection and ulcers, teaching appropriate care is vital (see Box 48–1).

Surgery

LASER EYE SURGERY Laser eye surgery is commonly performed to correct refractive errors such as myopia, hyperopia, and astigmatism. In these surgeries, a laser is used to permanently change the shape of the cornea. In most cases, the need to use corrective lenses is reduced or eliminated. Several surgical procedures are available:

- Laser *in situ* keratomileusis (LASIK)
- Photorefractive keratectomy (PRK)
- Laser epithelial keratomileusis (LASEK)
- Laser thermokeratoplasty (LTK).

These procedures reshape the cornea using laser technology to remove a thin layer of epithelial cells or to shrink and reshape the cornea. Candidates for laser vision-correction surgery should be in good health and must have adequate corneal thickness such that perforation is not a risk.

Following surgery, clients may experience a temporary loss of contrast sharpness (images do not appear as crisp as with corrective lenses), over- or undercorrection of visual acuity, dry eyes, or temporarily decreased night vision with halos, glare, and starbursts. Diffuse lamellar keratitis (DLK) is a rare complication of surgery that, while treatable, can lead to vision impairment if not identified and treated early.

Phototherapeutic keratectomy (PTK) provides an alternative to corneal transplant in treating corneal dystrophies, scars, and some infections. In this procedure, diseased corneal tissue is vaporized and surface irregularities corrected with little trauma to surrounding tissue. Healing occurs rapidly.

CORNEAL TRANSPLANT Once the cornea has become scarred and opaque, no treatment can restore its clarity. The first successful corneal transplant (or *keratoplasty*), replacement of diseased cornea by healthy corneal tissue from a donor, was performed in 1906. Current corneal transplant procedures have a success rate of approximately 80% (NEI, 2005a).

Corneas are harvested from the cadavers of uninfected adults who were under the age of 65 and who died as a result of acute trauma or illness. After harvesting, the cornea can be stored in a tissue-culture medium for up to 4 weeks before being used as a graft. Corneal transplantation is usually an elective surgery, although emergency transplantation may be required for perforation of the cornea.

Corneal transplant may be either lamellar or penetrating. In a lamellar keratoplasty, the superficial layer of cornea is removed and replaced with a graft. The anterior chamber remains intact.

In a penetrating keratoplasty, a button or full thickness of cornea is removed and replaced by donor tissue (Figure 48–3 ■). The graft is then sutured in place using suture finer than human hair and a continuous or interrupted stitch. Because the cornea is avascular, these sutures remain in place for up to a year to ensure healing.

Most corneal transplants do not require hospitalization. The eye is patched for 24 hours following surgery. Narcotic analgesia may be required initially, because the cornea is extremely sensitive. Corticosteroid eyedrops are ordered to reduce the inflammatory response and prevent edema of the graft. Antibiotic drops may be prescribed to prevent infection.

The risk of transplant rejection is low. Because the cornea is avascular, there is little exposure of the transplanted corneal tissue to the host's immune defenses (Porth, 2005). Research suggests that matching of blood type (not tissue type, as is required for major organ transplants) between the donor and the transplant recipient may reduce the risk of transplant rejection (NEI, 2005a). When rejection does occur, it occurs within 3 weeks of the transplant, beginning with inflammation at the edge of the grafted tissue and spreading to involve the entire graft.

See the accompanying box for nursing care of the client undergoing eye surgery.

Figure 48–3 ■ Corneal transplant. *A,* The diseased, opaque cornea. *B,* The diseased cornea is removed and a corneal graft is sutured in place using material finer than a human hair.

Source: Custom Medical Stock Photo, Inc.

NURSING CARE

The nursing role in caring for clients with corneal disorders may involve direct care, but more often focuses on prevention and education. Nurses working in clinics and outpatient surgical settings care for clients undergoing corneal transplant and surgeries to correct refractive errors.

Health Promotion

Education is a vital strategy for preventing many corneal disorders. Teach all clients about proper eye care, including the importance of not sharing towels and makeup and avoiding rubbing or scratching the eyes as well as preventing trauma and infection. Teach contact lens users appropriate care and cleaning techniques. Stress the importance of periodic removal of lenses, even extended-wear lenses. In general, lenses should be removed at night, even though manufacturers may claim it is safe to wear them while sleeping. Emphasize the need to follow cleaning instructions precisely to avoid bacterial contamination of lenses and possible corneal infection. If the client experiences a corneal abrasion or keratitis, instruct the client to avoid wearing contact lenses until the cornea has healed completely.

Assessment

Collect the following data through health history and physical examination (see Chapter 47 ∞). Additional focused assessments are described with the interventions below.

- *Health history:* Risk factors; presence of redness, discomfort, tearing, photophobia, edema, and drainage; symptom onset; presence of pain, effect on vision.
- *Physical assessment:* Visual acuity; inspect external eye, including conjunctiva, sclera, and cornea; extraocular movements.

Nursing Diagnoses and Interventions

Nursing care focuses primarily on preventing complications and promoting healing. The priority nursing diagnoses for clients with corneal disorders include risk of altered vision, pain, and risk for injury.

Risk for Disturbed Sensory Perception: Visual

Disorders affecting the cornea may disrupt its integrity or clarity. Because the cornea plays a vital role in focusing light on the retina, corneal damage can affect vision, impairing visual acuity and even causing legal blindness.

- Assess vision with and without corrective lenses. *Assessment provides a baseline to evaluate possible vision changes resulting from the disorder or treatment.*
- Instruct about thorough hand washing before inserting or removing contact lenses or instilling any eye medications. Teach to avoid touching or rubbing the eyes. Instruct to use a new, clean cotton-tipped swab or cotton ball for cleaning each eye. *Hand washing is the single most important measure to prevent transmission of infection to the eye. Touching or rubbing the eyes increases the risk of infection and corneal trauma. Using a new swab or cotton ball prevents cross-contamination between eyes.*
- Emphasize the importance of proper care of contact lenses specific to the type of lens used. *Clients who wear hard con-*

NURSING CARE OF THE CLIENT HAVING Eye Surgery

PREOPERATIVE CARE

- Review Chapter 4 ∞ for routine preoperative care.
- Assess visual acuity of the nonoperative eye prior to surgery. *The client with limited vision in the nonoperative eye may need additional attention and ADL assistance postoperatively to ensure safety.*
- Assess the client's support systems and the possible effect of impaired vision on lifestyle and ability to perform ADLs in the postoperative period. *Safety measures such as installing handrails and removing throw rugs from the home can help promote mobility and safety, especially if the client has limited vision in the unaffected eye.*
- Teach measures to prevent eye injury postoperatively: avoid vomiting, straining at stool, coughing, sneezing, lifting more than 5 lb, and bending over at the waist. *These activities temporarily increase intraocular pressure and may lead to postoperative complications.*
- Remove all eye makeup and contact lenses or glasses prior to surgery. Store corrective lenses in a safe place, and make them readily available to the client on return from surgery. *Maintaining visual acuity in the unaffected eye helps reduce fear and maintain safety.*
- Administer preoperative medications and eyedrops or ointments as prescribed. *Mydriatic (pupil-dilating) or cycloplegic (ciliary-paralytic) drops and drops to lower intraocular pressure may be prescribed preoperatively.*

POSTOPERATIVE CARE

- Review Chapter 4 ∞ for routine postoperative care.
- Assess eye dressing for bleeding or drainage following surgery. *Bleeding or drainage may indicate a surgical complication.*
- Maintain the eye patch or shield in place. *The eye patch or shield helps prevent inadvertent injury to the operative site.*
- Place in semi-Fowler's or Fowler's position on the unaffected side. *Elevating the head of the bed and lying on the unaffected side reduce intraocular pressure in the affected eye.*
- Remind the client to avoid coughing, sneezing, or straining as needed. *These activities increase intraocular pressure.*
- Assess and medicate as necessary for complaints of pain, aching, or a scratchy sensation in affected eye. Immediately report complaints of sudden, sharp eye pain to the physician. *An abrupt increase in or onset of eye pain may indicate hemorrhage or other ocular emergency requiring immediate intervention to preserve sight.*
- Assess for potential complications:
  a. Pain in or drainage from the affected eye

  b. Hemorrhage with blood in the anterior chamber of the eye
  c. Flashes of light, floaters, or the sensation of a curtain being drawn over the eye (indicators of retinal detachment)
  d. Cloudy appearance to the cornea (corneal edema). *Evidence of complications or unusual complaints should be reported to the physician at once. Early intervention is often necessary to preserve sight.*
- Approach the client on the unaffected side. *This approach facilitates eye contact and communication.*
- Place personal articles and the call light within easy reach. *These measures prevent stretching and straining by the client.*
- Administer antibiotic, anti-inflammatory, and other systemic and topical eye medications as prescribed. *Medications are prescribed to prevent infection or inflammation of the operative site, maintain pupil constriction, and control intraocular pressure.*
- Administer antiemetic medication as needed. *It is important to prevent vomiting to maintain normal intraocular pressures.*

Health Education for the Client and Family

- Teach the client and family about home care:
  a. How to instill eyedrops
  b. The name, dosage, schedule, duration, purpose, and side effects of medications
  c. How and when to use the eye patch and eye shield
  d. The importance of avoiding scratching, rubbing, touching, or squeezing the affected eye
  e. Measures to avoid constipation and straining.
  f. Activity limitations, if ordered
  g. Symptoms to report, including eye pain or pressure, redness or cloudiness, drainage, decreased vision, floaters or flashes of light, or halos around bright objects
  h. The need to wear sunglasses with side shields when outdoors to reduce photophobia.
- Remind the client that vision may not stabilize for several weeks following eye surgery. New corrective lenses, if necessary, are not prescribed until vision has stabilized. *Clients may be alarmed that vision seems worse after surgery than before and need reassurance that visual acuity usually improves with time and healing of the affected eye.*
- Emphasize the importance of keeping recommended follow-up appointments. Provide referral to a community home health agency for assistance with home care after discharge as needed.

---

tact lenses must remove them daily, because the central cornea needs exposure to atmospheric oxygen. Although soft and extended-wear lenses allow the cornea to "breathe," improper cleaning carries a major risk for infection.

- Teach the importance of using eye protection when engaging in potentially dangerous activities. *Trauma increases the risk of infection and scarring of the cornea.*
- If corneal perforation is suspected, place in the supine position, close the eye, and cover it with a dry, sterile dressing.

Notify the physician immediately. *Corneal perforation may occur without warning in clients with corneal ulcers. It places the client at risk for loss of eye contents. Emergency measures are taken to reduce intraocular pressure and maintain eye integrity to preserve vision.*

PRACTICE ALERT
Suspect corneal perforation with complaints of sudden, severe eye pain and photophobia.

Acute Pain

The cornea of the eye is extremely sensitive; therefore, corneal disorders frequently cause significant pain. Pain, in turn, increases the stress response and interferes with rest, potentially impairing healing.

- Assess pain, using verbal and nonverbal cues. *Pain is a subjective experience and can be evaluated only by the client's response and in terms of its effect on the client.*
- Administer prescribed analgesia routinely in the first 12 to 24 hours after corneal surgery. *Routine administration of analgesics prevents pain from reaching a level of severity at which it becomes difficult to relieve.*
- Patch both eyes if necessary. *Patching both eyes reduces eye movement and irritation of the affected eye.*
- Teach to apply warm compresses to reduce inflammation and pain. *Warm compresses for 15 minutes, three to four times a day, promote comfort for clients with keratitis or corneal injury.*
- Instruct to use dark sunglasses with appropriate UV protection when out of doors, even on cloudy days. *True photophobia, often associated with corneal disorders, causes eye pain with increased light intensity.*
- Teach to instill prescribed eyedrops as ordered. *Prescribed medications may reduce inflammation and eliminate infection, reducing discomfort.*

Risk for Injury

The client who has undergone corneal transplantation has an increased risk for injury for several reasons. The eye on which surgery was performed is patched for 24 hours after surgery, changing depth perception and increasing the risk for falls. Increased intraocular pressure or trauma to the eye may damage the graft, resulting in graft rejection.

- Instruct to call for help before getting up or ambulating after surgery. Ensure access to the call light. *It may take time for the client to adjust to changes in depth perception caused by the eye patch. Assistance helps prevent falls that may not only injure the client but also traumatize the operative site.*
- Encourage to deep breathe and use the incentive spirometer to promote lung expansion. *These important postoperative measures help prevent pulmonary complications. Coughing is avoided because it increases intraocular pressure.*
- Teach how to apply an eye shield at night after the eye patch is removed. *An eye shield may be recommended at night to prevent inadvertent rubbing or trauma to the eye during sleep.*
- Instruct not to rub or scratch the eye. *Rubbing or scratching may disrupt suture lines or damage the grafted tissue.*
- Reinforce the importance of using eye protection during hazardous activities. *Following a corneal transplant, the client has the same risk of eye injury as other people who perform hazardous activities.*

PRACTICE ALERT

Administer prescribed antiemetics and stool softeners postoperatively to prevent vomiting and straining at stool, activities that increase intraocular pressure, damaging suture lines.

Community-Based Care

Following treatment, teach clients to manage these conditions at home. Emphasize to the family ways to prevent transmission of infection. If the client is unable to administer eye medications or to perform other eye care techniques, involve the family in the teaching session. The following topics should be included:

- Safety and medical asepsis when cleansing the eye
- Instillation of prescribed eyedrops and ointments
- Application of an eye patch and where to obtain supplies
- Avoidance of activities such as excessive reading while eye is inflamed
- Follow-up appointments after corneal transplant surgery
- Signs of graft rejection
- Avoidance of activities that increase intraocular pressure such as straining, coughing, sneezing, bending over, lifting heavy objects
- Helpful resources:
  - National Eye Institute
  - Lighthouse National Center for Vision and Aging

THE CLIENT WITH A DISORDER AFFECTING THE EYELIDS

The eyelids and eyelashes are constantly exposed to the environment as they protect the eye from damage. When these structures are inflamed, deformed, or their function is impaired, it affects both appearance and their protective functions.

Pathophysiology and Manifestations

The most common disorder affecting the eyelids is *marginal blepharitis*, an inflammation of the glands and lash follicles on the margins of the eyelids. This inflammatory disorder can be caused by a staphylococcal infection or it may be seborrheic in origin; commonly, both types are present. Seborrheic blepharitis is usually associated with seborrhea (dandruff) of the scalp or eyebrows. Irritation, burning, and itching of eyelid margins are common manifestations of blepharitis. The eye appears red rimmed with mucous discharge, and there is crusting or scaling of lid margins. Lid margins may ulcerate, resulting in a loss of eyelashes.

Infection of one or more of the sebaceous glands of the eyelid may cause a **hordeolum (sty).** Hordeolum is a staphylococcal abscess that may occur on either the external or internal margin of the lid (Figure 48–4 ■). An external hordeolum is characterized initially by acute pain at the lid margin and redness. A small tender raised area is visible. The client may also experience photophobia, tearing, and the sensation of a foreign body in the affected eye. Internal hordeola are seen on the conjunctival side of the lid and may have more severe manifestations.

Chronic inflammation of a meibomian gland may lead to formation of a **chalazion**, a granulomatous cyst or nodule of the lid (Figure 48–5 ■). It presents as a hard swelling on the lid, and surrounding conjunctival tissue is reddened. Chalazion may also follow a hordeolum that was inadequately treated. Unlike a hordeolum, a chalazion is painless. It may

Figure 48–4 ■ Hordeolum.
Source: Science Photo Library/Photo Researchers, Inc.

Figure 48–6 ■ Ectropion.
Source: Science Photo Library/Photo Researchers, Inc.

slowly increase in size and eventually require removal, but most resolve within several months.

Entropion, inversion of the lid margin (see Figure 48–2), may be associated with the normal aging process (senile entropion) or result from an infectious process such as trachoma. Entropion can lead to corneal irritation and, potentially, scarring as the lashes rub on the conjunctiva and cornea during blinking and sleep. *Ectropion,* or eversion of the lid margin, occurs primarily as an effect of aging (Figure 48–6 ■). Other conditions may also lead to ectropion, including facial nerve paralysis or palsy (Bell's palsy), scarring, or infection. With ectropion, the eye does not close effectively, increasing the risk for drying and damage to conjunctival membrane and the cornea. Both entropion and ectropion have cosmetic effects as well, altering the appearance of the eye and face.

INTERDISCIPLINARY CARE

Disorders affecting the eyelids typically are managed in the community. Diagnosis is typically made through the history and physical examination. Diagnostic tests are rarely required except to identify corneal or conjunctival damage resulting from the condition.

Topical antibiotics (eyedrops or ointments) may be prescribed for the client with hordeolum and to treat infection resulting from irritation of the eye by a deformed lid. Careful cleansing of the lid

margins using a "no-tears" baby shampoo is often recommended for marginal blepharitis. Soaking the lids with warm saline compresses prior to cleansing facilitates the removal of crusts and exudate in blepharitis. Local heat applications may be used to treat hordeolum or chalazion; excision and drainage may be required if this is not effective. In entropion or ectropion, surgery may be performed to correct the defect, reduce the risk of damage to the eye, and improve cosmetic appearance.

NURSING CARE

The nursing role focuses on education and comfort measures. Teach clients about appropriate eye care, including avoiding rubbing or scratching the eyes. Discuss the importance of not using old eye makeup, which can cause lid infections. Instruct to wash hands well before cleansing the eyelids or instilling any eye medications. Instruct to use a new, clean cotton-tipped swab or cotton ball for cleaning each eye. Teach to instill prescribed eyedrops and apply ointments as ordered. If the client is unable to administer eye medications, involve the family in teaching. Teach to apply warm compresses to reduce inflammation and discomfort.

THE CLIENT WITH EYE TRAUMA

More than 2 million eye injuries occur each year. Many eye injuries are minor, but without timely and appropriate intervention, even a minor injury can threaten vision. For this reason, all eye injuries should be considered medical emergencies requiring immediate evaluation and intervention.

Pathophysiology and Manifestations

Any part of the eye, especially the exposed parts, may be affected by trauma. Foreign bodies, abrasions, and lacerations are the most common types of eye injury. Traumatic injury may also be due to a burn, penetrating objects, or blunt force.

Corneal Abrasion

Corneal abrasion is disruption of the superficial epithelium of the cornea. Objects commonly causing corneal abrasion include contact lenses, eyelashes, small foreign bodies such as dust and dirt, and fingernails. Drying of the eye surface and chemical irritants may also result in a corneal abrasion.

Figure 48–5 ■ Chalazion.
Source: Science Photo Library/Photo Researchers, Inc.

Superficial abrasions of the cornea are extremely painful but generally heal rapidly without complication or scarring. Photophobia and tearing are commonly present. When the stroma is damaged by a deep abrasion or laceration, there is an increased risk of infection, slowed healing, and scar formation.

Burns

The outer surface of the eye may be subjected to burns caused by heat, radiation, or explosion, but chemical burns are the most common. Either acid or alkaline substances may burn the eye. Ammonia, products that contain lye (such as oven and drain cleaners), and acids from car batteries or other sources are often implicated in eye injuries. Burns caused by alkaline substances are particularly serious because tiny particles of the chemical may remain in the conjunctival sac, causing progressive damage. Acid causes rapid damage to the eye, but generally causes less serious burns than alkaline substances.

Explosions and flash burn injuries pose the greatest risk for thermal burns of the eye. Ultraviolet rays can also cause corneal damage ranging in severity from mild to extensive. Depending on the source of the ultraviolet light, these burns may be known by various names such as snowblindness, welder's arc burn, or flash burn.

In addition to giving a history of face and eye contact with a caustic substance or other burning agent, the client complains of eye pain and decreased vision. Eyelids are often swollen. Burns may also affect the face or lids. The appearance of the eye may vary, depending on the type of burn. The conjunctiva is reddened and edematous; sloughing may be seen, particularly with chemical burns. The cornea often appears cloudy or hazy, and ulcerations may be evident.

Penetrating Trauma

Perforation of the eye occurs from a variety of causes. Metal flakes or other particles produced by high-speed drilling or grinding, glass shards, or other substances may penetrate the eye. Gunshots (including BBs), arrows, and knives can penetrate the eye. In a penetrating injury, the layers of the eye spontaneously reapproximate after entry of a sharp-pointed object or small missile into the globe. These injuries may not be readily apparent with inspection of the eye. In a perforating injury, the layers of the eye do not spontaneously reapproximate, resulting in rupture of the globe and potential loss of ocular contents (Way & Doherty, 2003).

Penetrating injuries may be hidden because of tissue swelling or missed when the client has other significant injuries that command attention. When the eyelid is lacerated or has a puncture wound, inspection of the underlying eye tissue for possible damage is vital. Eye perforations cause pain, partial or complete loss of vision, and possibly bleeding or extrusion of eye contents.

Blunt Trauma

Sports injuries are a common cause of blunt trauma to the eye: It may be struck with a ball (baseball, tennis, racquetball, and handball are frequently implicated) or injured in contact sports such as basketball, football, boxing, or wrestling. Motor vehicle crashes, falls, and physical assault are examples of other causes of blunt eye trauma.

Blunt trauma may lead to a minor eye injury such as lid ecchymosis (black eye) or subconjunctival hemorrhage, caused by rupture of a blood vessel in the conjunctiva. A well-defined bright area of erythema appears under the conjunctiva. No pain or discomfort is associated with the hemorrhage and no treatment is necessary. The blood typically reabsorbs within 2 to 3 weeks.

Hyphema, bleeding into the anterior chamber of the eye, is a potential result of blunt eye trauma. When the highly vascular uveal tract of the eye is disrupted by blunt force, hemorrhage may result, filling the anterior chamber. The client complains of eye pain, decreased visual acuity, and seeing a reddish tint. Blood is visible in the anterior chamber.

An orbital blowout fracture is another potential result of blunt eye trauma. Although any part of the eye orbit may be fractured, the ethmoid bone on the orbital floor is the most likely site. Orbital contents, including fat, muscles, and the eye itself, may herniate through the fracture into the underlying maxillary sinus. The client complains of diplopia (double vision), pain with upward movement of the affected eye, and decreased sensation on the affected cheek. The eye appears sunken (**enophthalmos**) and has limited movement on examination.

INTERDISCIPLINARY CARE

When trauma to the eye is known or suspected, a thorough examination is conducted to determine the type and extent of the injury. Unless immediate treatment is indicated, as with a chemical burn, vision is evaluated initially. If the client normally wears corrective lenses, vision assessment is performed while glasses are worn. Eye movement is evaluated unless a penetrating object is present, and the lid and eye are inspected for lacerations. Inspection is performed using strong light and magnification with a headband loupe or slit lamp. Topical anesthesia may be used prior to inspection if eye pain and photophobia make eye opening difficult. Fluorescein staining can help identify foreign bodies and abrasions. Any conjunctival or anterior chamber hemorrhage is noted, as is the presence or absence of the red reflex. Ophthalmoscopic examination is used to detect hemorrhage or trauma to the interior chamber.

Facial x-rays and CT scans are used to identify orbital fractures or foreign bodies within the globe. Ultrasonography may be employed to detect a detached retina or vitreous hemorrhage.

Foreign bodies are removed using irrigation, a sterile cotton-tipped applicator, or a sterile needle or other instrument. Antibiotic ointment—erythromycin or sulfacetamide sodium—is applied after their removal. In clients with corneal abrasions and large foreign bodies in the eye, an eye patch is applied firmly after the antibiotic application to keep the eye closed for approximately 24 hours.

The immediate priority of care for clients with chemical burns is flushing the affected eye with copious amounts of fluid. Normal saline is preferred; however, water may be used if saline is not available. A special contact lens irrigating unit (Morgan lens) or a bottle of irrigant with intravenous tubing held to flush all eye surfaces may be useful. The eyelid is everted to identify and remove material from the conjunctival sac. A topical anesthetic, such as tetracaine drops, helps relieve pain, making inspection and irrigation easier. During irrigation, fluid is directed from the inner canthus of the eye to the outer. Tipping the client's head slightly to the affected side prevents contamination of the unaffected eye. Irrigation is continued until the pH of the eye is normal (in the range of 7.2 to 7.4). Following irrigation, a topical antibiotic ointment such as gentamicin ophthalmic is applied.

Penetrating wounds of the eye generally require surgical intervention by an ophthalmic surgeon. Immediate care focuses on relieving pain and protecting the eye from further injury. To prevent loss of intraocular contents, do not place pressure on the eye itself, but gently cover with a sterile gauze or an eye pad. If a foreign body is embedded in or sticking out of the eye, no attempt is made to remove it. The object should be immobilized and the eye protected with a metal eye shield until an ophthalmologist can see the client. A paper cup or other protective device may be used if the object is too large to use an eye shield. Patching the unaffected eye as well decreases ocular movement. Pain is managed using narcotic analgesics such as morphine. The client may also require sedation (e.g., diazepam) and antiemetic medications to prevent vomiting. Antibiotics such as intravenous cefazolin (Ancef) or gentamicin (Garamycin) are prescribed to prevent infection.

Interventions for the client with blunt trauma to the eye include placing the client on bed rest in semi-Fowler's position and protecting the eye from further injury with an eye shield. The unaffected eye is also patched to minimize eye movement. A carbonic anhydrase inhibitor such as acetazolamide (Diamox) or dichlorphenamide (Daranide) may be prescribed to reduce intraocular pressure.

NURSING CARE

The nursing role involves educating people about the prevention of eye injuries and providing direct care to clients with eye injuries.

Health Promotion

Teaching related to eye injuries focuses on prevention and first-aid measures. Teaching individuals and groups how to prevent eye injuries is an important nursing role, especially for people involved in hazardous occupations and activities. Teach employees and participants in high-risk sports or activities how and when to use eye protection devices. Stress the importance of using seat belts and air bags to prevent eye injury in automobile crashes. Instruct clients to immediately flush the eye with copious amounts of water if a chemical splash occurs. Loose, visible foreign bodies can be removed using a clean, moistened cotton-tipped swab. If an abrasion, penetrating, or blunt injury is suspected, the eye should be covered loosely with sterile gauze and medical attention sought immediately. Instruct clients not to remove objects that penetrate the eye.

Nursing Diagnoses and Interventions

Ocular injuries require immediate interventions simultaneously with assessment and accurate history collection. The time, type, and extent of injury and the circumstances under which it occurred are determined. In addition, ask about preexisting visual problems.

Impaired Tissue Integrity: Ocular

All types of eye trauma pose the risk of violating the integrity of the eye, threatening vision. The goals of nursing care, therefore, are preserving vision and the integrity of the eye, and preventing further damage.

- Assess vision in each eye and both eyes, with and without corrective lenses, on entry into the emergency department or primary care setting. *An initial assessment provides valuable information about the effect of the injury on the client's vision and a baseline for future comparisons.*
- Inspect eye(s) carefully for evidence of foreign bodies, burns, penetrating injury, or blunt trauma. Note if lacerations, burns, or other trauma are evident in tissues surrounding the eye. *Eye trauma may be hidden by other injuries and, as a result, remain untreated.*
- If a burn or foreign body is present, anesthetic drops may be instilled and the eye irrigated either before or after the physician evaluates the client. *Blepharism and eye pain may impair assessment of the injured eye. Irrigation to remove the chemical is of higher priority than assessment of the eye.*
- Loose foreign bodies may be removed using a moist, sterile, cotton-tipped applicator. *Prompt removal of foreign bodies may prevent corneal abrasion.*
- For a severe or penetrating injury, promote rest and stabilize the injured eye by applying an eye pad or gauze dressing loosely over both the affected and unaffected eye. Stabilize any penetrating object if possible. *These measures reduce eye movement and can help preserve the client's vision.*
- Following treatment, apply eyedrops or ointment as prescribed and apply an eye pad or shield if ordered. *An eye pad is applied to the affected eye to reduce pain and photophobia and to promote healing.*

Community-Based Care

Following an injury, discuss the following topics with the client and family:

- Prescribed medications and possible adverse effects
- Strategies to prevent further trauma
- Application of the eye pad or shield
- Avoidance of activities that increase intraocular pressure
- Importance of activity restrictions.

THE CLIENT WITH UVEITIS

The middle vascular layer of the eye, including the choroid, the ciliary body, and the iris, is known as the uvea and uveal tract. *Uveitis* is inflammation of all or part of this vascular layer. *Iritis,* inflammation of the iris only, occurs more commonly than uveitis.

Uveitis is usually a disease limited to the eye; it may be idiopathic or caused by an autoimmune process, infection, parasitic disease, or trauma. Many cases can be linked to a systemic disease, often an arthritic or autoimmune disorder such as ankylosing spondylitis, Reiter's syndrome, rheumatoid arthritis, or sarcoidosis (see Chapter 42 ∞). Uveitis has also been linked with tuberculosis and syphilis. Manifestations of uveitis include pupillary constriction and erythema around the limbus. The client may complain of severe eye pain and photophobia, as well as blurred vision.

Immunosuppressive therapy may be used to suppress the inflammatory response in clients with severe uveitis. Atropine may also be prescribed for associated inflammation of the iris. The client may require analgesics such as acetaminophen and/or codeine for pain management. Nursing care is supportive, focusing on promotion of comfort and teaching about the disorder and its management.

THE CLIENT WITH CATARACTS

A **cataract** is an opacification (clouding) of the lens of the eye. This opacification can significantly interfere with light transmission to the retina and the ability to perceive images clearly.

Incidence and Risk Factors

Cataracts are a common and significant cause of visual deficits, affecting nearly 20.5 million people over age 40 in the United States. By age 80, nearly half of the population is affected. In many cases, however, cataract does not significantly impair vision. Cataract affects slightly more women than men, and more whites than people of color. More than a million cataract removal surgeries are performed annually in the United States, costing an estimated 3.4 billion Medicare dollars (Prevent Blindness America, 2002).

FAST FACTS

The prevalence of cataracts in the United States increases rapidly with aging:
- 2.5% (just over 1 million) of adults ages 40 to 49 are affected.
- This increases to more than 2 million (or 6.8%) of those ages 50 to 59, and nearly doubles to over 4 million or 20% of adults ages 60 to 69.
- 68.3% of adults age 80 and older (over 6 million) are affected by cataract (NEI, 2004).

Age is the greatest single risk factor for cataract. Genetics may contribute to the risk, although the link is unclear. Environmental and lifestyle factors play a role: long-term exposure to sunlight (UV-B rays) contributes; cigarette smoking and heavy alcohol consumption are associated with earlier cataract development. Although senile cataracts are by far the most common, cataracts also may be congenital or acquired in origin. Eye trauma, including injury to the lens capsule by a foreign body, blunt trauma, or exposure to heat or radiation, can precipitate cataract formation. Diabetes mellitus is associated with earlier development of cataracts, especially when the blood glucose level is not carefully controlled at or near normal levels. Certain drugs such as systemic or inhaled corticosteroids, chlorpromazine (Thorazine), and busulfan (Myleran) also prompt the formation of cataracts.

Figure 48–7 ■ A scene as viewed by a client with cataracts.
Source: Courtesy of National Eye Institute, National Institutes of Health.

Pathophysiology

The majority of cataracts are senile cataracts, formed as a result of the aging process. As the lens ages, its fibers and proteins change and degenerate. The proteins clump, clouding the lens and reducing light transmission to the retina. This process generally begins at the periphery of the lens, gradually spreading to involve the central portion. As the cataract continues to develop, the entire lens may become opaque. When only a portion of the lens is affected, the cataract is called immature. A mature cataract is opacity of the entire lens. In addition to clouding, the lens may discolor over time, affecting the ability to accurately discriminate colors.

Manifestations

Cataracts tend to occur bilaterally unless related to eye trauma. Fortunately, they tend to develop at different rates, and one cataract generally matures more rapidly than the other. As a cataract interferes with light transmission through the lens, visual acuity decreases, affecting both close and distance vision (Figure 48–7 ■). Light rays are scattered as they pass through the lens, causing complaints of glare. Glare affects the ability to adjust between light and dark environments. Color discrimination is impaired, particularly in the blue to purple range. When the cataract is mature, the pupil may appear cloudy gray or white rather than black.

INTERDISCIPLINARY CARE

The diagnosis of a cataract is made based on the history and eye examination. Ophthalmoscopic examination confirms the diagnosis by identifying the location and extent of a cataract. As the cataract matures, ophthalmoscopy reveals a dark area instead of the red reflex.

Surgery

Surgical removal is the only treatment used at this time for cataracts; no medical treatment is available to prevent or treat them. If the client presents with bilateral cataracts, surgery is only performed on one eye at a time. If an intraocular lens (an artificial lens to replace the diseased lens of the eye) is to be implanted during surgery, the corneal curvature and anteroposterior diameter of the eye are measured prior to surgery to determine the lens power needed for the intraocular lens implant.

Surgical removal of the cataract and lens is indicated when the cataract has developed to the point that vision and activities of daily living are affected. A mature cataract may also be removed when it causes a secondary condition such as glaucoma or uveitis.

Cataract surgery is usually done on an outpatient basis, using local anesthesia. If general anesthesia is required, the client may be hospitalized overnight. The entire lens and its surrounding capsule may be removed in a procedure called intracapsular extraction. Intracapsular extraction is rarely used today (Way & Doherty, 2003). Extracapsular extraction, in which the anterior capsule, nucleus, and cortex of the lens are removed leaving the posterior capsule intact, is the procedure of choice (Figure 48–8 ■). Using an operating microscope, the surgeon makes a small incision at the edge of the cornea and extracts the lens intact or via emulsification and aspiration. In the latter technique, ultrasound vibrations are used to break the lens material into fragments (phacoemulsification), which are then suctioned out of the eye. Phacoemulsification lens removal requires a smaller incision and usually is the procedure of choice (Way & Doherty, 2003). The remaining capsule supports the lens implant and protects the retina.

After removal of the lens, the eye can no longer focus light on the retina, and vision is seriously affected. Usually a poly-methylmethacrylate (PMMA or Plexiglas) intraocular lens is implanted at the time of surgery. This implant rapidly restores binocular vision and depth perception. Following extracapsular lens removal, the intraocular lens is positioned in the posterior capsule behind the iris (see Figure 48–8).

If an intraocular lens cannot be implanted, convex corrective glasses or contact lenses may be used to correct vision after cataract removal. Although contact lenses can provide excellent vision correction following cataract surgery, they may be difficult for some clients to adapt to or manipulate. The client with a preexisting refractive error may continue to require corrective lenses and often needs a prescriptive change after surgery.

Complications of cataract surgery are unusual and occur in less than 1% of the surgeries. Loss of vitreous humor, corneal edema, increased intraocular pressure, hemorrhage, inflammation or infection, retinal detachment, and displacement of the implanted lens are potential complications. Up to 35% of clients who undergo extracapsular extraction may develop opacification of the remaining posterior capsule. Vision can be restored using laser capsulotomy (creating an opening for light to pass through the opacified capsule) or surgical incision into the posterior capsule to allow light to reach the retina (Kasper et al., 2005; Way & Doherty, 2003).

NURSING CARE

Health Promotion

Advise all clients about the importance of protecting the eyes from UVB rays by wearing eye protection during activities such as welding and sunglasses with UVB protection when out of doors. Discuss the link between heavy smoking and cataract development. Provide anti-tobacco use education for young people and resources to stop smoking for people who do smoke.

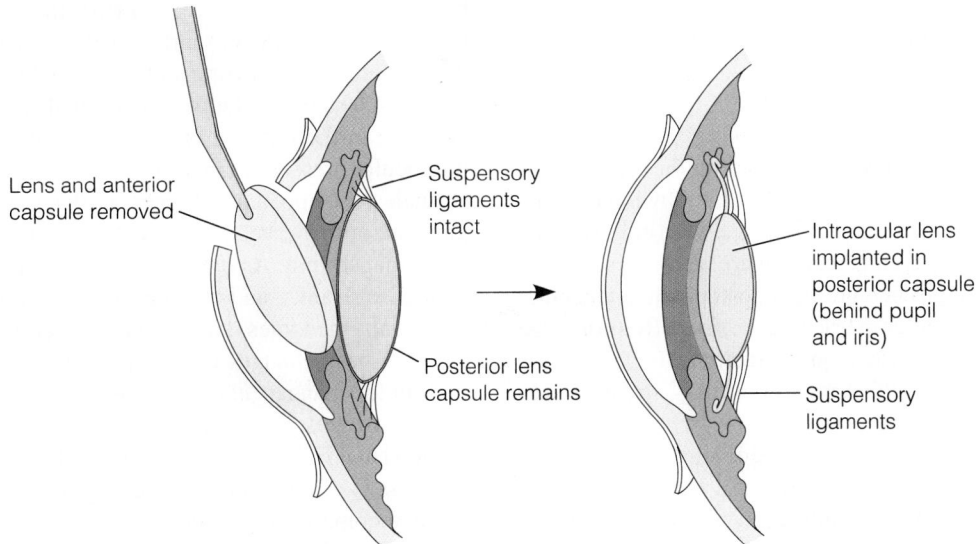

Figure 48–8 ■ Extracapsular cataract extraction with removal of the lens and anterior capsule, leaving the posterior capsule intact. The intraocular lens is implanted within posterior capsule.

Assessment

- *Health history:* Effect of vision changes on lifestyle and activities (e.g., ability to read, watch television, participate in work and recreational activities); history of smoking, diabetes, use of prescription drugs associated with increased risk of cataract.
- *Physical examination:* General health; visual acuity (using corrective lenses and Snellen chart) in each eye; presence of red reflex.

Nursing Diagnoses and Interventions

The client with cataracts has few physical care nursing needs. Patient advocacy, psychologic and emotional support, and teaching/learning needs are typically of higher priority for these clients. Review nursing care of the client having eye surgery as outlined in the box on page 1699.

Decisional Conflict: Cataract Removal

With the initial diagnosis of cataract, the nurse often becomes an important information resource for the client.

- Explain the nonemergent nature of the condition and help the client determine the extent to which the cataract is affecting daily life. *This helps the client decide when to proceed with surgery. Providing information about cataracts and their surgical removal also assists with decision making.*
- Attend to verbalized concerns about surgery and its outcome. Address questions factually and completely. *Fear of blindness is second only to fear of cancer for many clients. Careful listening, teaching, and a caring, understanding attitude can help the client deal with this fear prior to surgery.*

Risk for Ineffective Therapeutic Regimen Management

- Assess for factors that may interfere with the client's ability to provide self-care postoperatively. *A chronic condition such as arthritis that may affect the ability to administer eyedrops may indicate the need to include a family member in teaching.*
- Assess for other care needs that may be impacted by vision changes in the early postoperative period. *Other care needs, such as insulin injections, may suggest the need for home health or nursing care postoperatively.*

Community-Based Care

With the initial diagnosis, teaching focuses on the disorder, indications for surgery, and vision restoration following cataract removal. Teaching adaptive strategies to deal with effects of the cataract on vision and depth perception are also useful. When surgery is scheduled, provide pre- and postoperative teaching, including a significant other in teaching sessions. Reinforce the following information with written instructions:

- Limitations such as avoiding reading, lifting, strenuous activity, and sleeping on operative side
- Importance of not disturbing the eye dressing
- Prescribed medications and side effects
- Importance of follow-up appointments
- Manifestations of postoperative complications such as eye pain, decreased visual acuity or other change in vision, headache, nausea, or itching and redness of the affected eye
- Instillation of eyedrops, and application of eye patch or shield
- Care, insertion, and removal of contact lenses as appropriate
- Visual changes associated with thick-lensed eyeglasses as appropriate.

THE CLIENT WITH GLAUCOMA

Glaucoma is a condition characterized by optic neuropathy with gradual loss of peripheral vision and, usually, increased intraocular pressure of the eye. Glaucoma is a silent thief of vision. The client typically experiences no manifestations other than narrowing of the visual field, which occurs so gradually that it often goes unnoticed until late in the disease process.

Incidence and Risk Factors

Glaucoma affects about 2.2 million people over the age of 40 in the United States; it remains undetected in approximately 25% of these cases. Glaucoma is a leading cause of blindness worldwide and the leading cause of blindness among African Americans. Age and race are the primary identified risk factors; it is more common in blacks and Hispanics than in whites (Prevent Blindness America, 2002).

Glaucoma is usually a primary condition without an identified cause. Primary glaucoma is most common in adults over the age of 60, but may be a congenital condition in infants and children. Secondary glaucoma can develop as a result of infection or inflammation of the eye, cataract, tumor, hemorrhage, or eye trauma.

Pathophysiology

Aqueous humor, a thick fluid, occupies both the anterior and posterior chambers of the eye. The normal intraocular pressure of approximately 12 to 15 mmHg is maintained by a balance between the production of aqueous humor in the ciliary body, its flow through the pupil from the posterior to the anterior chamber of the eye, and its outflow or absorption through the trabecular meshwork and canal of Schlemm (see Figure 47–3). When this balance is disrupted, usually because of a decrease in the outflow or absorption of aqueous humor, the intraocular pressure increases. Although the exact relationship is unclear, it appears that increased intraocular pressure injures the optic nerve. Axons in the periphery of the optic disc are damaged first. As optic fibers are destroyed, the rim of the optic disc shrinks, and the normal depression in its center (the *optic cup*) becomes larger and deeper (called optic "cupping"). These changes to the optic disc are visible before visual field changes can be detected (Porth, 2005). As the disease progresses, there is a painless, progressive narrowing of the visual field (Figure 48–9 ■) and eventual blindness. Vision loss is often significant before the client seeks treatment and glaucoma is diagnosed.

Primary glaucoma in adults has two major forms: open-angle glaucoma and angle-closure glaucoma. Both terms refer to the angle formed at the point where the iris meets the cornea

Figure 48–9 ■ Narrowing of visual fields typical of untreated glaucoma.

Source: Courtesy of National Eye Institute, National Institutes of Health.

A

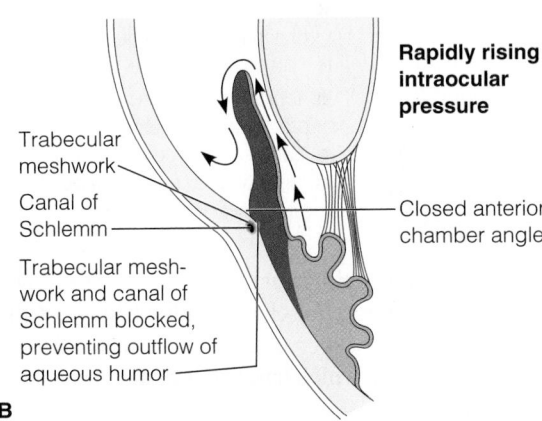

B

Figure 48–10 ■ Forms of primary adult glaucoma. *A,* In chronic open-angle glaucoma, the anterior chamber angle remains open, but drainage of aqueous humor through the canal of Schlemm is impaired. *B,* In acute angle-closure glaucoma, the angle of the iris and anterior chamber narrows, obstructing the outflow of aqueous humor.

in the eye's anterior chamber (Figure 48–10 ■). Forms of primary glaucoma are compared in Table 48–2.

Open-Angle Glaucoma

Open-angle glaucoma, often called chronic simple glaucoma, is the most common form in adults, accounting for approximately 90% of all glaucoma. Its cause is unknown; it is thought to have a hereditary component, but no clear inheritance pattern can be identified. Open-angle glaucoma occurs more frequently and at an earlier age in African Americans than in whites (Tierney et al., 2005).

In open-angle glaucoma, the anterior chamber angle between the iris and cornea is normal (Figure 48–10A), hence the term *open angle.* However, the flow of aqueous humor through the trabecular meshwork and into the canal of Schlemm is relatively obstructed; the cause of this obstruction is unknown. Restricted outflow leads to an increased amount of fluid in the eye and increased intraocular pressure. Open-angle glaucoma tends to be a chronic, gradually progressive disease. The trabecular meshwork increasingly inhibits the outflow of aqueous humor, and the intraocular pressure gradually increases. The result is neuronal ischemia and optic nerve degeneration, leading to gradual loss of vision.

Open-angle glaucoma typically affects both eyes, although the pressures and progression may not be symmetric.

MANIFESTATIONS Open-angle glaucoma is painless, with gradual loss of visual fields. This loss of peripheral vision generally occurs so gradually that the client is often unaware of it and only when it is detected through a comprehensive vision examination is it found. Intraocular pressure usually, but not always, is elevated (Kasper et al., 2005).

Angle-Closure Glaucoma

Acute angle-closure (also called narrow-angle or closed-angle) glaucoma is the other, less common form of primary glaucoma in adults. It accounts for approximately 5% to 10% of all cases of glaucoma (Porth, 2005). Approximately 1% of people over the age of 35 have narrowed anterior chamber angles; the incidence is higher in older adults and in people of Far Eastern, Asian, or Inuit (Alaska native) ancestry (Porth, 2005).

Narrowing of the anterior chamber angle (see Figure 48–10A for an illustration of the normal anterior chamber angle) occurs because of corneal flattening or bulging of the iris into the anterior chamber. When the lens thickens during accommodation or the iris thickens during pupil dilation, this angle can close completely. Closure of the angle blocks the outflow of aqueous humor through the trabecular meshwork and canal of Schlemm, and the intraocular pressure rises abruptly (Figure 48–10B). This abrupt increase in intraocular pressure damages the neurons of the retina and the optic nerve, leading to a rapid and permanent loss of vision if not treated promptly.

Episodes of angle-closure glaucoma are typically unilateral. However, a history of angle-closure glaucoma of one eye increases the risk that it will occur in the other eye.

Because of the effect of pupil dilation on aqueous outflow in angle-closure glaucoma, episodes often occur in association with darkness, emotional upset, or other factors that cause the pupil to dilate. Clients may have intermittent episodes lasting

TABLE 48–2 A Comparison of Open-Angle and Angle-Closure Glaucoma

	OPEN-ANGLE GLAUCOMA	ANGLE-CLOSURE GLAUCOMA
Incidence	■ Common ■ Accounts for 90% of all cases of glaucoma	■ Uncommon
Risk Factors	■ Over age 35 ■ Genetic link ■ African American ancestry	■ Narrow anterior chamber angle ■ Aging ■ Asian ancestry
Pathophysiology	■ Impaired aqueous outflow through the canal of Schlemm ■ Cause unknown ■ Gradual, consistent increase in intraocular pressure ■ Usually bilateral	■ Pupil dilation or lens accommodation causes already narrowed angle to close, blocking aqueous outflow ■ Rapid rise in intraocular pressure ■ Usually unilateral
Manifestations	■ No initial manifestations ■ Frequent lens changes in glasses ■ Impaired dark adaptation ■ Halos around lights ■ Gradual reduction of visual fields with preservation of central vision until late in the disease ■ Mild to severe increased intraocular pressure	■ Abrupt onset of eye pain, headache ■ Decreased visual acuity ■ Nausea and vomiting ■ Reddened conjunctiva ■ Cloudy cornea ■ Fixed pupil ■ Rapid, significant increase in intraocular pressure
Management	■ Topical medications such as miotics, beta-blockers, prostaglandin analogs ■ Carbonic anhydrase inhibitors ■ Laser trabeculoplasty, trabeculectomy	■ Topical miotics or beta-blockers ■ Systemic osmotic agents, carbonic anhydrase inhibitors ■ Laser iridotomy or peripheral iridectomy

several hours before having a more typical prolonged attack of angle-closure glaucoma. For clients with a history of the condition, it is vital to avoid medications such as atropine and other anticholinergics, which have a mydriatic or pupil-dilating effect.

MANIFESTATIONS Symptoms such as severe eye and face pain, general malaise, nausea and vomiting, seeing colored halos around lights, and an abrupt decrease in visual acuity are associated with acute episodes of angle-closure glaucoma. The conjunctiva of the affected eye may be reddened and the cornea clouded with corneal edema. The pupil may be fixed (nonreactive to light) at midpoint.

INTERDISCIPLINARY CARE

Although glaucoma cannot be predicted, prevented, or cured, in most cases it can be controlled and vision preserved if diagnosed early. Because the most prevalent type of glaucoma, open-angle glaucoma, has few symptoms, routine eye examinations are recommended for early detection. Measurement of intraocular pressure, fundoscopy to assess the optic disc, and visual field testing are used for diagnosis and monitoring of treatment effectiveness.

Diagnosis

The following diagnostic studies are used to detect and evaluate for the presence, severity, type, and effects of glaucoma.
■ *Tonometry* indirectly measures intraocular pressure (Figure 48–11 ■). Contact or noncontact tonometry may be used. Routine tonometry screening is recommended for all people over the age of 60. A single elevated pressure reading does not warrant a diagnosis of glaucoma; variations in intraocular pressure

occur throughout the day. See Chapter 47 ∞ for more information about tonometry and related nursing care.
■ *Fundoscopy* (visual inspection of the optic fundus using an ophthalmoscope) identifies pallor and an increase in the size and depth of the optic cup on the optic disc. These changes are significant for diagnosing glaucoma.
■ *Gonioscopy* uses a gonioscope to measure the depth of the anterior chamber. This test differentiates open-angle from angle-closure glaucoma.
■ *Visual field testing* (Figure 48–12 ■) identifies the degree of central visual field narrowing and peripheral vision loss. The client with glaucoma may retain 20/20 central vision even though there is severe peripheral vision loss.

Figure 48–11 ■ An eye professional uses a tonometer to indirectly measure the intraocular pressure of a client's eye.

Source: Courtesy of National Eye Institute, National Institutes of Health.

Figure 48–12 ■ Visual field testing. Peripheral vision or visual fields are assessed by testing the client's ability to detect an object brought into the line of vision from the periphery. The client's peripheral vision is compared to the nurse examiner's. Each eye is tested separately.

Medications

Although medications cannot cure glaucoma, many clients with open-angle glaucoma can control intraocular pressure and preserve vision indefinitely with medications. Medications are used alone or in combination with the timing and dosage individually determined by pressure measurements. The primary pharmacologic agents used to treat glaucoma are topical beta-adrenergic blocking agents, adrenergics (mydriatics), prostaglandin analogs, or carbonic anhydrase inhibitors. An oral carbonic anhydrase inhibitor also may be used.

Topical beta-adrenergic blocking agents decrease the production of aqueous humor in the ciliary body. Beta-adrenergic blockers can be used once or twice a day, depending on the drug and dosage form. When administering beta-blockers or teaching about their use, it is important to remember that ophthalmic preparations can produce systemic effects, including bronchospasm, bradycardia, and heart failure.

Prostaglandin analogs such as latanoprost (Xalatan) are a newer class of ophthalmics prescribed to increase aqueous outflow. They are similar to beta-blockers in their longer duration of action, thus requiring only a daily dose. Although they have fewer systemic effects, these drugs may cause conjunctival hyperemia and permanent changes in the color of the iris and eyebrows.

The adrenergic agonist brimonidine may be prescribed along with a beta-blocker or if beta-blockers are contraindicated (e.g., in a client with heart failure, asthma, or COPD). Another adrenergic agonist, apraclonidine, may be prescribed when other drugs do not sufficiently reduce intraocular pressure, but adverse effects make it inappropriate for long-term use (Tierney et al., 2005).

Dorzolamide (Trusopt), a carbonic anhydrase inhibitor, decreases the production of aqueous humor and reduces intraocular pressure. It is used with other drugs to control pressures and in clients for whom beta-blockers are contraindicated because of heart failure or reactive airway disease. Acetazolamide (Diamox), a systemic carbonic anhydrase inhibitor, also may be used for some clients.

Nursing implications for the medications used to control chronic glaucoma are outlined in the Medication Administration box on the next page.

In acute angle-closure glaucoma, diuretics may be administered intravenously to achieve a rapid decrease in intraocular pressure prior to surgical intervention. Both the carbonic anhydrase inhibitor acetazolamide and osmotic diuretics, such as mannitol, are used. Fast-acting miotic drops, such as acetylcholine, are also administered to constrict the pupil and draw the iris away from the angle and from the canal of Schlemm.

Surgery

Surgical intervention is indicated for clients with acute angle-closure glaucoma and for clients with chronic open-angle glaucoma that is not effectively controlled by medication.

Surgical management of chronic open-angle glaucoma involves improving the drainage of aqueous humor from the anterior chamber of the eye. Trabeculoplasty and trabeculectomy filtration surgery are the most commonly used procedures.

In a *laser trabeculoplasty,* an argon laser is aimed through a gonioscope to create multiple laser burns spaced evenly around the trabecular meshwork. As the burns heal, the scars they create cause tension, stretching and opening the meshwork. This noninvasive technique is the treatment of choice because it requires no incision and can be performed as an outpatient procedure.

Trabeculectomy is a type of filtration surgery in which a permanent fistula is created to drain aqueous humor from the anterior chamber of the eye. A portion of trabecular meshwork is removed, and a flap of sclera is left unsutured to create a channel or fistula between the anterior chamber and the subconjunctival space. Aqueous humor is able to drain into the space under the conjunctiva, where it can be absorbed into the systemic circulation. A trabeculectomy is usually performed under general anesthesia and requires hospitalization.

If these procedures are not fully effective, either photocoagulation using an argon laser (heat) or cyclocryotherapy using a probe to freeze tissue may be employed to destroy portions of the ciliary body. This tissue destruction reduces the production of aqueous humor, subsequently reducing intraocular pressure. Another surgical procedure involves insertion of a glaucoma drainage device that regulates the outflow of aqueous humor.

Surgical procedures used in the treatment of acute angle-closure glaucoma include gonioplasty, laser iridotomy, and peripheral iridectomy. Because of the high risk for a future attack of angle-closure glaucoma in the unaffected eye, these procedures are often performed prophylactically.

In *gonioplasty,* the healing and scarring of microscopic lesions created at the periphery of the iris draw the iris away from the cornea, widening the anterior chamber. This widening of the chamber increases the angle and opens drainage channels for aqueous humor.

Laser iridotomy is a noninvasive procedure using a laser to create multiple small perforations in the iris of the eye. These perforations allow aqueous humor to drain from the posterior chamber to the anterior chamber and out through the trabecular meshwork and the canal of Schlemm. During an *iridectomy,* a small segment of the iris is removed to facilitate the flow of aqueous humor

MEDICATION ADMINISTRATION   The Client with Glaucoma

ADRENERGIC AGONISTS (MYDRIATICS)
Brimonidine (Alphagan)
Apraclonidine
Adrenergic agonists dilate the pupil, reduce the production of aqueous humor, and increase its absorption, effectively reducing intraocular pressure in open-angle glaucoma.

Nursing Responsibilities
- Assess the client for contraindications and adverse reactions to adrenergic agonists, including acute angle-closure glaucoma, hypertension, cardiac dysrhythmias, and coronary heart disease.
- Assess for central nervous system side effects of anxiety, nervousness, and muscle tremors. If these side effects are severe, notify the physician.
- Assess for a hypersensitivity reaction, including itching, lid edema, and discharge from the eyes. Notify the physician if you notice these signs.

Health Education for the Client and Family
- Report any change in visual acuity or eye pain. (Eye pain may indicate an attack of angle-closure glaucoma and must be reported to the physician immediately.)
- Avoid over-the-counter sinus and cold medications containing pseudoephedrine and phenylephrine. They may accentuate the side effects of this drug.

BETA-ADRENERGIC BLOCKERS
Betaxolol (Betoptic)
Carteolol (Cartrol, Ocupress)
Levobunolol (Betagan)
Metipranolol (OptiPranolol)
Timolol (Timoptic)
Selected beta-adrenergic blockers reduce intraocular pressure by decreasing the production of aqueous humor. Because beta-blockers do not affect pupil size and lens accommodation, they do not have the adverse effects on visual acuity that adrenergic agonists do. Their systemic effects, however, may limit their usefulness for certain clients.

Nursing Responsibilities
- Assess the client for allergies or contraindications to beta-blocker therapy, including asthma, chronic obstructive pulmonary disease (COPD), heart block, and heart failure.
- Maintain pressure over the lacrimal sac after administration to prevent systemic absorption.
- Assess for side effects such as bradycardia, hypotension, and depression.
- Teach about the drug, its dose, administration, and desired and side effects.

Health Education for the Client and Family
- Put pressure on the lacrimal sac, at the corner of the eye near the bridge of the nose, to keep the drug from entering your system.
- Your vision may be blurred during the initial period of therapy, but it will improve as you continue to use the drug.
- Report adverse effects, including worsening vision, difficulty breathing, reduced exercise tolerance, and sweating or flushing, to the physician.

CARBONIC ANHYDRASE INHIBITORS
Dorzolamide (Trusopt)
Brinzolamide (Azopt)
Acetazolamide (Diamox)
The carbonic anhydrate inhibitors lower intraocular pressure and are used primarily as adjunctive therapy. Dorzolamide and brinzolamide are administered as eyedrops, whereas acetazolamide may given PO, IM, or IV.

Nursing Responsibilities
- Assess for allergies or other contraindications to the use of carbonic anhydrase inhibitors, including known allergy to sulfa, or severe renal or hepatic disease.
- Monitor for increased drug interactions of amphetamines, procainamide, quinidine, tricyclic antidepressants, and ephedrine and pseudoephedrine.
- Assess daily weight, intake and output, serum electrolytes, and vital signs in clients taking oral or parenteral carbonic anhydrase inhibitors.
- Administer PO in the morning to prevent sleep disruption because of the diuretic effect.
- If used with another topical ophthalmic, administer 10 minutes apart.
- Teach the client about the drug, its dose, administration, and desired and side effects.

Health Education for the Client and Family
- For oral medications, maintain a fluid intake of 2 to 3 L per day and rise slowly from lying or sitting positions because you may feel dizzy when you first stand (orthostatic hypotension).
- For topical medications, notify the physician if you have prolonged eye irritation.

PROSTAGLANDIN ANALOGS
Bimatoprost (Lumigan)
Latanoprost (Xalatan)
Travoprost (Travatan)
The prostaglandin analog drugs relax the ciliary muscle, improving the outflow of aqueous humor and reducing intraocular pressure. These drugs have the advantage of requiring only a single daily dose. They do, however, have some adverse effects such as blurred vision and stinging, and, when used long term, cause permanent darkening of the iris of the eye and eyebrows, increased growth of eyelashes, and conjunctival hyperemia (redness).

Nursing Responsibilities
- Assess and note eye color, presence of inflammation, exudates, or pain.
- Note vital signs and most recent liver function test results because these may be altered by the drug.

Health Education for the Client and Family
- Use once daily at bedtime as directed. This drug may blur vision; use at bedtime minimizes associated safety risks.
- Remove contact lenses before administering this drug.
- Minor eye discomfort, including burning and tearing, may occur with this drug. Notify your doctor if adverse effects are severe or intolerable.
- This drug may cause darkening of your iris, the skin around the eyes, and the eyebrows, as well as increased growth of eyelashes. These color changes are permanent but will not progress if the drug is discontinued by your doctor.

between the posterior and anterior chambers and to open the anterior chamber angle.

NURSING CARE

When planning and providing nursing care for the client with glaucoma, both the specific form of the disease and its actual or potential effects on the client's vision, lifestyle, safety, and psychosocial well-being must be considered. In the hospitalized client, glaucoma is typically a concurrent diagnosis rather than the primary reason for seeking care, unless the diagnosis is acute angle-closure glaucoma. For additional nursing activities for the client with glaucoma, see the accompanying Nursing Care Plan.

NURSING CARE PLAN | A Client with Glaucoma and Cataracts

Lila Rainey is an 80-year-old widow who lives alone in the house she and her late husband built 50 years ago. She has worn glasses for nearsightedness since she was a young girl, and now wears bifocals to correct her near vision as well. She was diagnosed 4 years ago with chronic open-angle glaucoma, for which she takes timolol maleate (Timoptic) 0.5%. Recently she has noticed difficulty reading and watching television despite a new lens prescription. She has stopped driving at night because the glare of oncoming headlights makes it difficult for her to see. Mrs. Rainey's ophthalmologist has told her that she has cataracts but that they do not need to come out until they bother her. Although her glaucoma is still controlled with timolol maleate 0.5%, one drop in each eye twice a day, her intraocular pressure measurements have been gradually increasing. Mrs. Rainey has taken 325 mg of aspirin daily since a transient ischemic attack 8 years ago. She is being admitted to the outpatient surgery unit for a cataract removal and intraocular lens implant in her right eye.

ASSESSMENT

Mrs. Rainey is admitted to the eye surgery unit by Susan Schafer, RN. In her assessment, Ms. Schafer finds Mrs. Rainey to be alert and oriented, though apprehensive about her upcoming surgery. Assessment findings include BP 134/72, P 86, R 18. Mrs. Rainey's neurologic, respiratory, cardiovascular, and abdominal assessments are essentially normal. Her pupils are round and equal, and react briskly to light and accommodation. Her conjunctivae are pink; sclera and corneas, clear. Using the ophthalmoscope, Ms. Schafer notes that the red reflex in Mrs. Rainey's right eye is diminished. Ophthalmic examination shows visual acuity of 20/150 OD (right eye) and 20/50 OS (left eye) with corrective lenses. Her intraocular pressures are 21 mmHg OD and 17 mmHg OS. On fundoscopic exam, no disease of the blood vessels, retina, macula, or disc is found. Ms. Schafer reviews the operative procedure with Mrs. Rainey, answering her questions and telling her what to expect after surgery. Following preoperative protocols, Mrs. Rainey is prepared and transported to surgery.

DIAGNOSES

- *Disturbed Sensory Perception: Visual* related to myopia and lens extraction
- *Anxiety* related to anticipated surgery
- *Deficient Knowledge* related to lack of information regarding postoperative care
- *Impaired Home Maintenance* related to activity restrictions and impaired vision

EXPECTED OUTCOMES

- Regain sufficient visual acuity to maintain ADLs, including reading and watching television for enjoyment.
- Demonstrate a reduced level of anxiety.

- Demonstrate the procedure for instilling eyedrops postoperatively.
- Demonstrate knowledge of the home care she will require after surgery, signs of complications, and actions to take if complications occur.
- Use appropriate resources to assist with home maintenance until vision stabilizes and activity restrictions are lifted.

PLANNING AND IMPLEMENTATION

- Provide a safe environment, placing the call light and personal care items within easy reach.
- Encourage Mrs. Rainey to express her fears about surgery and its potential effect on vision.
- Explain all procedures related to surgery and recovery.
- Instruct her to avoid shutting the eyelids tightly, sneezing, coughing, laughing, bending over, lifting, or straining to have a bowel movement. Teach her to wear glasses during the day and an eye shield at night to prevent injury to the surgical site.
- Explain and demonstrate the procedure for administering eyedrops.
- Provide verbal and written instructions about postoperative care, including a schedule of follow-up examinations, potential complications, and actions to take in response.
- Refer Mrs. Rainey to a discharge planner or social worker to help establish a plan for home maintenance.

EVALUATION

Mrs. Rainey is discharged the morning after her surgery. She is visibly relieved when the eye patch is removed because her vision in the operated eye is better than before surgery, even without her glasses. She is able to relate the recommended activity restrictions. Mrs. Rainey administers her own eyedrops before discharge and relates an understanding of the prescribed postoperative care and safety precautions. Mrs. Rainey's daughter plans to visit her mother two to three times a week to help with laundry and vacuuming until Mrs. Rainey is able to resume all her household activities. Mrs. Rainey says that she won't "be so scared when I need my other eye done." She understands the chronic nature of her glaucoma and says that her vision is too important for her to neglect her timolol drops and routine eye exams.

CRITICAL THINKING IN THE NURSING PROCESS

1. Why did it become more difficult to control Mrs. Rainey's intraocular pressure as her cataract matured?
2. Identify medications that are commonly prescribed following cataract surgery. What are the risks of interactions between these medications and Mrs. Rainey's timolol drops?
3. Develop a care plan for the nursing diagnosis *Self-Care Deficit: Dressing/Grooming,* related to visual impairment and restricted bending.

See Evaluating Your Response in Appendix C.

Health Promotion

Although glaucoma cannot be prevented, its severity and potentially deleterious permanent effects can be limited with early visual screening. The nurse assumes an important role in educating the public about the risk factors for glaucoma such as increased age, and the higher incidence in African Americans and Asians. All people over the age of 40 are encouraged to receive an eye examination every 2 to 4 years, including tonometry screening. Those with a predominant family history should be evaluated more frequently, every 1 to 2 years. After the age of 65, yearly ophthalmologic examinations are recommended.

Assessment

Collect the following data through a health history and physical examination (see Chapter 47 ∞).

- *Health history:* Family history; presence of altered vision, halos, and excessive tearing; sudden, severe eye pain; use of corrective lenses; most recent eye examination.
- *Physical examination:* Distant and near vision, peripheral fields, retina for optic nerve cupping.

Nursing Diagnoses and Interventions

Nursing care planning focuses on problems associated with the temporary or permanent visual impairment, the resultant increased risk for injury, and the psychosocial problems of anxiety and coping.

Disturbed Sensory Perception: Visual

Whether glaucoma and resulting impaired vision is the client's primary problem or a preexisting condition in a client with another disorder, it must be a primary consideration in nursing care planning.

- Address by name and identify yourself with each interaction. Orient to time, place, person, and situation as indicated. State the purpose of your visit. *The client with impaired vision must rely on input from the other senses. A lack of visual cues increases the importance of verbal ones. For example, the client with impaired vision cannot see the nurse checking an intravenous infusion and needs a verbal explanation of who is in the room and why. When the client's normal daily routine is disrupted by illness or hospitalization, additional sensory input such as a radio, television, and explanations of the routine and activities are useful to maintain the client's orientation.*
- Provide any visual aids that are routinely used. Keep them close, making sure that the client knows where they are and can reach them easily. *Easy access encourages the client to use these items and enhances the ability to provide self-care.*
- Orient to the environment. Explain the location of the call bell, personal items, and the furniture in the room. If able, tour client's room, including the bathroom and sink. *Clients with visual impairments are usually very capable of providing self-care in a known environment.*
- Provide other tools or items that can help compensate for diminished vision:
  a. Bright, nonglare lighting
  b. Books, magazines, and instructions in large print
  c. Books on tape
  d. Telephones with oversize pushbuttons
  e. A clock with numbers and hands that can be felt
- Assist with meals by:
  a. Reading menu selections and marking choices.
  b. Describing the position of foods on a meal tray according to the clock system, for example, "On the plate, the peas are at 9 o'clock, the mashed potatoes at 1 o'clock, and the chicken breast at 6 o'clock. The milk glass is at 2 o'clock on the tray above the plate, and coffee is at 11 o'clock."
  c. Placing the utensils in a readily accessible position.
  d. Removing lids from containers, buttering the bread, and cutting meat, as needed.
  e. If the visual impairment is new or temporary, the client may need feeding or continued assistance during the meal.
  Providing assistance during eating is important to maintain the client's nutritional status. The client may be ashamed of needing help or embarrassed to request it and may respond by not eating or by claiming not to be hungry.
- Assist with mobility and ambulation as needed:
  a. Have the client hold your arm or elbow, and walk slightly ahead as a guide. Do not hold the client's arm or elbow.
  b. Describe the surroundings and progress as you proceed. Warn in advance of potential hazards, turns, and steps.
  c. Teach to feel the chair, bed, or commode with the hands and the back of the legs before sitting.
  These measures help ensure the client's safety while providing for mobility and helping prevent complications associated with immobility.
- If the vision loss is unilateral and recent, provide instructions related to unilateral vision loss and change in depth perception:
  a. Caution about the loss of depth perception and teach safety precautions, such as reaching slowly for objects and using visual cues as to distance, especially when driving.
  b. Teach to scan, turning the head fully toward the affected side to identify potential hazards and looking up and down to compensate for the loss of depth perception.
  The client with a unilateral vision loss is often unaware of its effect on peripheral vision and depth perception.

Risk for Injury

Whether the client is experiencing a sudden loss of vision due to acute angle-closure glaucoma or significant visual impairment due to inadequately managed chronic glaucoma, both are at an increased risk for injury. Clients who have had surgical interventions for glaucoma are at even greater risk.

- Assess ability to perform ADLs. *Clients may be reluctant to request assistance, believing that they should be able to perform these familiar tasks. Careful assessment and provision of needed assistance help prevent injury and maintain the client's self-esteem.*
- Notify housekeeping and place a sign on the client's door to alert all personnel not to change the arrangement of the client's room. *The client with impaired vision is at high risk for falling when in an unfamiliar environment. It is important to maintain a safe, familiar room when the client is hospitalized.*

- Raise two or three side rails on the client's bed. *Raised rails remind clients to ask for assistance before ambulating in an unfamiliar environment.*
- Discuss possible adaptations in the home to help the client remain as independent as possible and prevent falls or other injuries. *Often minor changes in the home environment, such as removing scatter rugs and small items of furniture, allow the client to navigate safely in this already familiar environment.*

> **PRACTICE ALERT**
> *Keep traffic area free of clutter to reduce the risk for injury in clients with impaired vision.*

Anxiety

The actual or potential loss of sight threatens the client's self-concept, role functioning, patterns of interaction, and, potentially, environment. The client with impaired vision who functions well in a familiar environment will feel anxious in the unfamiliar setting of a hospital or care facility.

- Assess for verbal and nonverbal indications of level of anxiety and for normal coping mechanisms. Repeated expressions of concern or denial that the vision change will affect the client's life indicate anxiety. Nonverbal indicators include tension, difficulty concentrating or thinking, restlessness, poor eye contact, and changes in vocalization (rapid speech, voice quivering). Physical indicators include tachycardia, dilated pupils, cool and clammy skin, and tremors. *The client may not recognize this feeling as anxiety. Identifying and acknowledging the anxiety state can help the client recognize and deal with it.*
- Encourage to verbalize fears, anger, and feelings of anxiety. *Verbalizing helps externalize the anxiety and allows fears to be addressed.*
- Discuss perception of the eye condition and its effects on lifestyle and roles. *Discussion provides an opportunity to correct misperceptions and introduce alternative activities and assistive devices for clients with visual impairments.*
- Introduce yourself when entering the room, explain all procedures fully before and as they are being performed, and use touch to convey proximity and caring. *The client with impaired vision must rely on the other senses to make up for the loss of sight. Because the client cannot see what you are doing, complete explanations of even simple tasks such as refilling a water glass help to relieve anxiety.*
- Identify coping strategies that have been useful in the past and adapt these strategies to the present situation. *Previously successful coping strategies may be employed to increase the client's sense of control.*

Using NANDA, NIC, and NOC

Chart 48–2 shows links between NANDA nursing diagnoses, NIC, and NOC when caring for the client with glaucoma.

Community-Based Care

Clients with glaucoma require teaching about lifetime strategies for managing the disease at home. They need to under-

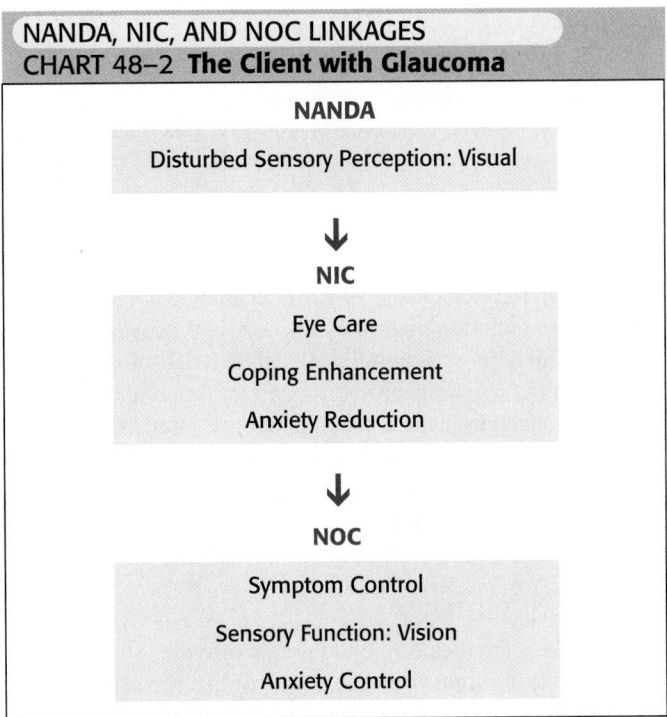

NANDA, NIC, AND NOC LINKAGES
CHART 48–2 The Client with Glaucoma

NANDA

Disturbed Sensory Perception: Visual

↓

NIC

Eye Care

Coping Enhancement

Anxiety Reduction

↓

NOC

Symptom Control

Sensory Function: Vision

Anxiety Control

Data from *NANDA's Nursing Diagnoses: Definitions & Classification 2005–2006* by NANDA International (2005), Philadelphia; *Nursing Interventions Classification (NIC)* (4th ed.) by J. M. Dochterman & G. M. Bulechek (2004), St. Louis, MO: Mosby; and *Nursing Outcomes Classification (NOC)* (3rd ed.) by S. Moorhead, M. Johnson, and M. Maas (2004), St. Louis, MO: Mosby.

stand the importance of lifetime therapy to control the disease and prevent blindness. If a permanent visual impairment has resulted, the client needs information on achieving the maximum possible independence while maintaining safety. The following topics should be discussed with the client and family:

- Prescribed medications including proper way to instill eyedrops
- Importance of not taking certain prescription and over-the-counter medications without consulting a physician
- Periodic eye examinations with intraocular pressure measurement
- Risks, warning signs, and management of acute angle-closure glaucoma
- Possible surgical options
- Community resources, such as Visually Impaired Society, local library, and transportation services
- Helpful resources:
  - National Glaucoma Foundation
  - Young and Under Pressure Glaucoma Foundation
  - Glaucoma Research Foundation
  - Prevention of Blindness Society.

THE CLIENT WITH AGE-RELATED MACULAR DEGENERATION

The leading cause of legal blindness and impaired vision in people over the age of 65 is age-related **macular degeneration** (AMD) (Prevent Blindness America, 2002).

Although the exact cause of AMD is unknown, factors associated with it include aging, smoking, race, and, possibly, genetic factors. Whites have a significantly higher risk of developing AMD than blacks, Hispanics, or people of Asian ancestry. The destructive changes in the macula occur most often as a response to the aging process. It affects males and females equally. Evidence suggests that the risk for developing AMD may be reduced by consumption of certain antioxidant nutrients, including vitamin C, vitamin E, beta-carotene, and zinc (NEI, 2005b).

Pathophysiology

The macula is the area of the retina that provides sharp central vision, receiving light from the center of the visual field. Two forms of age-related macular degeneration are identified, a nonexudative (dry) form and an exudative (wet) form. Although both are progressive disorders, their manifestations and management differ.

Nonexudative, or dry, *macular degeneration* is the more common form of AMD. It is a gradual process that begins with accumulation of deposits called *drusen* beneath the pigment epithelium of the retina. Over time, these deposits enlarge and become more numerous. The pigment epithelium detaches in small areas, and becomes atrophic, interfering with sensory function of the macula. Vision loss typically is not significant, and the disorder progresses slowly. There is, however, a risk that the disorder will progress to an exudative stage of the disease.

Exudative macular degeneration is characterized by the formation of new, weak blood vessels in the potential space between the choroid (vascular layer of the eye) and the retina (neurosensory layer). These new vessels are prone to leak, elevating the retina from the choroid and distorting vision. Although exudative macular degeneration typically is a gradual process, bleeding can lead to acute vision loss in some cases. With significant or repeated bleeding episodes, scar tissue forms, and central vision is permanently lost (Kasper et al., 2005).

Manifestations

When the macula is damaged, central vision becomes blurred and distorted, but peripheral vision remains intact. Distortion of vision in one eye is a common initial manifestation; straight lines appear wavy or distorted. With the loss of central vision, activities that require close central vision, such as reading and sewing, are particularly affected (Figure 48–13 ■).

INTERDISCIPLINARY CARE

AMD is diagnosed through vision and retinal examination. The Amsler grid (see Figure 47–5) may be used to identify distor-

Figure 48–13 ■ Loss of central vision with advanced age-related macular degeneration.
Source: Courtesy of National Eye Institute, National Institutes of Health.

tion of central vision caused by AMD. If treatment for wet AMD is planned, a *fluorescein angiogram* may be done. Pictures are taken as the dye passes through the blood vessels of the retina, allowing detection of leaks.

In its early or intermediate stages, the progress of dry AMD can be slowed through the use of high-dose antioxidants and zinc. Research demonstrated a benefit when vitamin C, vitamin E, beta-carotene (vitamin A), zinc, and copper were administered daily.

Wet AMD is treated with laser surgery or photodynamic therapy. Although these treatments do not cure the disease, they may slow the rate of vision loss. In laser surgery, fragile blood vessels are destroyed, preventing bleeding. There is a risk, however, of damage to surrounding healthy tissue, some vision loss, and continued growth of new vessels. In photodynamic therapy, verteporfin, a drug that tends to adhere to the surface of new blood vessels, is injected systemically. Light is then shined into the affected eye, activating the drug and destroying new blood vessels. This treatment is relatively fast and painless, but does require avoidance of exposure to direct sunlight or bright indoor light for 5 days following treatment (NEI, 2003a).

Large-print books and magazines, the use of a magnifying glass, and high-intensity lighting can help the client to cope with the reduced vision of macular degeneration.

NURSING CARE

Nurses should be alert for clients demonstrating new and rapid onset manifestations of macular degeneration and promptly refer these clients for ophthalmologic evaluation. Early intervention may preserve a greater degree of vision and slow the progress of the disease. For clients with slowly progressive manifestations, the nursing focus is on helping the client and family members adapt to the gradual decline in vision by recommending visual aids and other coping strategies. Client education materials should be in a large-print format. See also the accompanying Nursing Research box.

THE CLIENT WITH DIABETIC RETINOPATHY

Diabetic retinopathy is a vascular disorder affecting the capillaries of the retina. The capillaries become sclerotic and

NURSING RESEARCH **Evidence-Based Practice: The Client with Impaired Vision**

Age-related macular degeneration is the leading cause of significant visual impairment among older adults. However, little research has been done to study the effect of visual impairment on the lives of older adults. Moore and Miller (2003) studied the lived experience of severe visual impairment for a group of older, community-dwelling men with AMD. While the lives of the men in the study tended to be somewhat defined by what they could and could not do, these men tended to express hope and optimism, focusing on remaining abilities and developing strategies to cope with vision loss. However, in contrast to the results of a similar study of older women with AMD, the men in this study expressed skepticism about their disorder and its prognosis, critically questioning treatment and consistency of the care received.

IMPLICATIONS FOR NURSING
Older adults with significant vision deficit continue to cherish their independence and focus on their remaining abilities (as opposed to their disabilities). While it is important to present clear, accurate, and realistic information to clients with irreversible vision impairment, maintenance of hope and optimism also is important to the older adult. Many clients faced with impaired vision make conscious choices to maintain a positive attitude and lifestyle, developing strategies that allow them to continue with activities that are important to them or provide pleasure. The nurse can help support and encourage these choices and selection of positive behaviors to maintain independence and self-worth.

CRITICAL THINKING IN CLIENT CARE
1. The men in this study cherished their freedom and found many ways to maintain it despite impaired vision. Discuss ideas to suggest for a client with impaired vision to continue to engage in activities such as shopping, attending cultural events, and playing golf or participating in other sports.
2. The men participating in this study expressed more skepticism about their diagnosis and prognosis and criticism of their treatment than did older women with AMD who had participated in an earlier study. What factors might account for this difference? What implications could this difference have for nursing assessment and care?
3. Develop a teaching plan for a client with newly diagnosed AMD using the nursing diagnosis *Deficient Diversional Activity* related to recent change in visual acuity.

lose their ability to transport sufficient oxygen and nutrients to the retina.

> **FAST FACTS**
> ■ In the United States, diabetic retinopathy is the leading cause of new blindness in people ages 20 to 74.
> ■ People with diabetes are 25 times more likely to become legally blind than people unaffected by the disease (Kasper et al., 2005).

The risk of developing diabetic retinopathy is related to the duration of the diabetes and the degree of glycemic control. Hypertension also is a risk factor (Kasper et al., 2005). Retinopathy is seen in both type 1 and type 2 diabetes. Nursing care of the client with diabetes is discussed in Chapter 20 ∞.

Pathophysiology and Manifestations

Diabetic retinopathy progresses through four stages: (1) mild *nonproliferative* or background retinopathy, (2) moderate nonproliferative retinopathy, (3) severe nonproliferative retinopathy, and (4) *proliferative* retinopathy (NEI, 2003c). Nonproliferative retinopathy is typically the initial form seen. The venous capillaries of the eye dilate and develop microaneurysms that may then leak, causing retinal edema, or they may rupture, causing small hemorrhages into the retina. On ophthalmoscopic examination, yellow exudates, cotton-wool patches indicative of retinal ischemia, and red-dot hemorrhages are observed (Figure 48–14 ■). When the peripheral retina is involved, the client may experience few symptoms other than light glare. Edema of the macula or a large hemorrhage may cause vision loss.

Diabetic retinopathy may progress to the proliferative form. This disease is marked by large areas of retinal ischemia and the

Figure 48–14 ■ Appearance of the ocular fundus in diabetic retinopathy.
Source: Courtesy of National Eye Institute, National Institutes of Health.

formation of new blood vessels (neovascularization) spreading over the inner surface of the retina and into the vitreous body. These vessels are fine and fragile, making them permeable and easily ruptured. Blood and blood protein leakage contribute to retinal edema, and hemorrhage into the vitreous body may occur. The vessels gradually become fibrous and firmly attached to the vitreous body, increasing the risk of retinal detachment.

INTERDISCIPLINARY CARE

Clients with diabetes should be examined yearly by an ophthalmologist. The development of any new visual manifestations is an additional indication for prompt ophthalmologic examination and possibly retinal angiography.

Laser photocoagulation is used to treat both the nonproliferative and proliferative forms of diabetic retinopathy. Leaking microaneurysms are sealed and proliferating vessels destroyed, reducing the risk of hemorrhage, retinal edema, and retinal detachment. This treatment also slows the progress of aneurysms and new vessel formation; however, it does not cure the disorder. Clients with severe proliferative retinopathy may undergo vitrectomy to remove vitreous hemorrhage or treat associated retinal detachments (Tierney et al., 2005). Although conclusive research is lacking, the diabetic client with retinopathy may be advised to avoid physical activity associated with the Valsalva maneuver (e.g., weight training) (Kasper et al., 2005).

NURSING CARE

As with many other eye disorders, the nursing care focus for diabetic retinopathy is primarily educational. The newly diagnosed diabetic client needs to understand the importance of regular eye examinations beginning approximately 5 years after the onset of type 1 diabetes and at the time of onset of type 2 diabetes. Changes of diabetic retinopathy may already be present when type 2 diabetes is diagnosed.

Teach the client to report promptly any new visual manifestation, including blurred vision; black spots (floaters), cobwebs, or flashing lights in the visual field; or a sudden loss of vision in one or both eyes. Emphasize to the client that careful blood glucose control may help prevent diabetic retinopathy from developing; it may also slow its progress. The client's blood pressure should also be maintained within normal limits to prevent further damage to retinal vessels. Although diabetic retinopathy cannot be halted or cured, its progress can be slowed with aggressive management. Much of the burden for this management falls on the client, increasing the importance of good teaching.

THE CLIENT WITH A RETINAL DETACHMENT

The retina contains the photoreceptors of the eye, which allow the perception of light and initial processing of images and stimuli for transmission to the optic center of the brain. Disruption of this neural layer of the eye by trauma or disease interferes with light perception and image transmission, potentially resulting in blindness.

Both primary eye conditions and systemic diseases can affect the retina and interfere with vision. Retinal tears or detachments can occur either spontaneously or as a result of trauma.

Pathophysiology and Manifestations

Separation of the retina or sensory portion of the eye from the choroid, the pigmented vascular layer, is known as a **retinal detachment.** Although retinal detachment may be precipitated by trauma, it usually occurs spontaneously. The vitreous humor normally adheres to the retina at the optic disc, the macula, and the periphery of the eye. With aging, the vitreous humor shrinks and may pull the retina away from the choroid. Aging therefore is a common risk factor, as are myopia and aphakia, absence of

the lens (e.g., following lens removal for cataracts) (Porth, 2005; Tierney et al., 2005).

The retina may actually tear and fold back on itself, or the retina may remain intact but no longer adhere to the choroid. A break or tear in the retina allows fluid from the vitreous cavity to enter the defect. This, along with fluid that escapes from choroid vessels, the pull of gravity, and traction exerted by the vitreous humor, separates the retina from the choroid. The detached area may rapidly increase in size, increasing loss of vision. Unless contact between the retina and choroid is reestablished, the neurons of the retina become ischemic and die, causing permanent vision loss. For this reason, retinal detachment is a true medical emergency, requiring prompt ophthalmologic referral and treatment.

When the retina detaches, the client experiences floaters, or "spots," and lines or flashes of light in the visual field. Often the client describes the sensation of having a curtain drawn across the vision, much like a curtain being drawn over a window. The area of the visual field affected is directly related to the area of detachment. For example, because light rays cross as they pass through the lens, a retinal tear in the superior portion of the eye results in a deficit in the lower part of the visual field. The client feels no pain, and the eye appears normal to visual inspection. Common manifestations of retinal detachment are listed in the box below.

INTERDISCIPLINARY CARE

Retinal detachment is a medical emergency; prompt treatment is necessary to preserve vision. The manifestations and examination of the ocular fundus by ophthalmoscopy establish the diagnosis of retinal detachment. Early diagnosis and intervention are vital. If the condition is left untreated, the detached portion will become necrotic because of separation from the vascular supply of the choroid. The result is permanent blindness in that portion of the eye. If an ophthalmologist is not readily available, the client's head is positioned so that gravity pulls the detached portion of the retina into closer contact with the choroid.

Interventions are directed toward bringing the retina and choroid back into contact and reestablishing the blood and nutrient supply to the retina. Either cryotherapy, using a supercooled probe, or laser photocoagulation may be used to create an area of inflammation and adhesion to "weld" the layers together.

A surgical procedure called *scleral buckling* also may be used. In this procedure, an indentation or fold is created in the

---

MANIFESTATIONS **of Retinal Detachment**

- Floaters: irregular, dark lines or spots in the field of vision
- Flashes of light
- Blurred vision
- Progressive deterioration of vision
- Sensation of a curtain or veil being drawn across the field of vision
- If the macula is involved, loss of central vision

sclera, bringing the choroid into contact with the retina. Contact is maintained with a local implant on the sclera or an encircling strap or "buckle." Air may also be injected into the vitreous cavity, a procedure called pneumatic retinopexy. The client is positioned so that the air bubble pushes the detached portion of the retina into contact with the choroid.

With a retinal tear, it may be necessary to use surgical instruments to manipulate the detached section of retina into place. Air or a liquid is then injected into the vitreous to maintain retinal contact with the choroid, or laser therapy is used to create a bond.

NURSING CARE

The nursing focus for the client with a detached retina is on early identification and treatment. Because early intervention is vital to preserve the client's sight, nurses must recognize early manifestations of retinal detachment and intervene appropriately to obtain definitive treatment for the client. Retinal detachment can be successfully treated on an outpatient basis, often in an ophthalmologist's office. For these clients, the nursing focus is on education.

Ineffective Tissue Perfusion: Retinal

Restoring contact between the retina and choroid is a priority of nursing and medical care for the client with retinal detachment. Vitreous humor may leak through a retinal tear, and fluid exudate may collect behind the tear, causing further detachment. If the macula is detached, central vision is lost, and the prognosis for full vision restoration is poorer.

> **PRACTICE ALERT**
> Carefully assess anyone who complains of a sudden rapid loss of vision because these are often medical emergencies.

- Assess for other manifestations of eye disease. *Retinal detachment is painless and has no outward manifestations. The client with a red eye or cloudy cornea may be experiencing acute angle-closure glaucoma rather than retinal detachment.*
- Notify physician and the ophthalmologist immediately. *Immediate medical intervention is required in clients with retinal detachment to preserve vision.*
- Position so the area of detachment is inferior. For instance, for a superior temporal retinal detachment of the right eye (with corresponding vision loss in the inferior medial visual field of that eye), place supine with the head turned to the right. *Correct positioning allows the contents of the posterior portion of the eye to place pressure on the detached area, bringing the retina in closer contact with the choroid.*

Anxiety

Retinal detachment causes a rapid decline in vision in the affected eye, often occurring spontaneously and without pain. Unless previous episodes have occurred, the client usually does not know what is causing the problem. Anxiety and fear of complete vision loss are common, expected reactions.

- Maintain a calm, confident attitude while carrying out priority interventions. *Administering care in a calm although urgent manner helps reassure the client that the problem is treatable and that appropriate measures are being taken.*
- Reassure that most retinal detachments are successfully treated, usually on an outpatient basis. *Reassurance can help allay the client's fear of permanent vision loss.*
- For spontaneous detachments, assure the client that he or she did not cause the detachment to occur. *The client may believe that the detachment is related to a specific activity and feel guilty for "causing" this loss of vision.*
- Explain all procedures fully, including the reason for positioning. *Explanations facilitate understanding and help relieve anxiety in unfamiliar settings.*
- Allow supportive family members or friends to remain with the client as much as possible. *Additional support helps lower the client's anxiety level.*

Community-Based Care

Teaching for the client undergoing surgical repair of retinal detachment is similar to that for clients experiencing other types of eye surgery (see page 1699). If the retina remains detached, provide instructions about the change in peripheral vision or other visual fields and changes in depth perception.

Discuss the following topics with the client and family to prepare for home care:
- Limitations on positioning the head before or following repair
- Activity restrictions such as no bending or straining at stool
- Use of eye shield
- Early manifestations and the importance of seeking immediate treatment
- Follow-up treatment with the ophthalmologist.

THE CLIENT WITH RETINITIS PIGMENTOSA

Retinitis pigmentosa is a hereditary degenerative disease characterized by retinal atrophy and loss of retinal function progressing from the periphery to the central region of the retina. It is inherited as an autosomal dominant, autosomal recessive, or X-linked trait and may be associated with other genetic defects (Kasper et al., 2005; Porth, 2005).

In retinitis pigmentosa, the genetic defect appears to cause production of an unstable form of rhodopsin, the receptor protein of rod cells in the retina. Rod cells degenerate, initially at the periphery of the retina. The areas of degeneration and cell death slowly expand, causing vision to narrow. Central vision is finally lost as well.

The initial manifestation of retinitis pigmentosa, difficulty with night vision, is often noted during childhood. As the disease progresses, there is slow loss of visual fields, photophobia, and disrupted color vision. The progression to tunnel vision and blindness is gradual; the client may be totally blind by age 40.

Currently, there is no effective treatment for retinitis pigmentosa. Research into the role that defective rhodopsin plays in the disease holds future promise for the development of therapy that may at least slow its progress.

Clients with retinitis pigmentosa may benefit from low-vision aids, much like those for the client with macular degeneration. Additionally, information about the disease and its progress is vital so the client can plan for the eventual total loss of sight. Clients with retinitis pigmentosa should be referred for genetic counseling prior to starting a family to determine the risk of transmitting the disease to their children.

THE CLIENT WITH HIV INFECTION

More than 50% of people infected with the human immuno-deficiency virus (HIV) develop an infectious or noninfectious ocular condition, generally as a late manifestation of the disease (Kasper et al., 2005).

HIV retinopathy, seen as cotton-wool spots around the optic nerve, is the most common noninfectious ophthalmic lesion in AIDS. Cotton-wool spots indicate areas of retinal ischemia. Microaneurysms and dot-, blot-, or flame-shaped hemorrhages may also be seen in HIV retinopathy.

Neoplasms common in the client with AIDS can also affect the eye. Kaposi's sarcoma may affect the external surface or anterior segment of the eye or the eyelids. Kaposi's lesions vary in color (red, brown, or purple) and in size, shape, and location. Conjunctival lesions resemble a benign subconjunctival hemorrhage. Kaposi's lesions of the lid may cause **ptosis** (drooping of the lid) and abnormal lid function. Vision or eye position and movement may be affected by the tumor or by the effect of increased intracranial pressure on the cranial nerves.

The most serious and frequent opportunistic eye infection associated with HIV infection is cytomegalovirus (CMV) retinitis. CMV retinitis generally develops when CD4 cell counts drop below 50 mL. Initially unilateral, CMV retinitis commonly progresses to become bilateral because of the systemic nature of the infection. CMV invades the retina of the eye directly, producing exudate and cotton-wool spots, hemorrhage, cell death, and necrosis. Visual field deficits develop and can progress to eventual blindness.

Corneal ulcers from opportunistic bacterial, fungal, protozoal, or viral infections are also associated with HIV infection. Toxoplasmic and fungal retinal infections may occur.

The client with an HIV-associated eye disorder may complain of a change in visual acuity, blurring, floaters, or gaps in the field of vision. Extensive retinal damage may cause retinal detachment and symptoms of flashing lights, multiple floaters, and a loss of vision. Because the observed changes in the retina are nonspecific, it is important for the examining physician to know that the client is HIV positive in order to make an accurate diagnosis.

In addition to the general treatment of HIV infection with retroviral medications, specific therapies may be directed toward the ocular manifestations of the disease. CMV retinitis is commonly treated with the antivirals ganciclovir (Cytovene) and foscarnet sodium (Foscavir).

Although treatment of ocular Kaposi's sarcoma is usually not indicated, conjunctival lesions may be excised for comfort or cosmetic reasons. Lid lesions may be treated with radiation or intralesional chemotherapy.

THE CLIENT WITH AN ENUCLEATION

Occasionally surgical removal of an eye is necessary because of trauma, infection, glaucoma, intractable pain, or malignancy. This procedure is known as **enucleation**.

Enucleation is performed under local or general anesthesia. After the globe is removed, the conjunctiva and eye muscles are sutured to a round implant inserted into the orbit to maintain its shape. A pressure dressing is left in place for 24 to 48 hours. The client is permitted out of bed on the day of surgery. Hemorrhage and infection are the most commonly seen complications.

Postoperative nursing care includes teaching, psychologic support, and observation for potential complications. The client may be instructed to apply warm compresses and instill antibiotic ointment or drops postoperatively.

Within 1 week, a temporary prosthesis called a conformer is fitted into the empty socket. The permanent prosthesis is individually designed to closely resemble the client's other eye. The prosthesis can be fitted 1 to 2 months after surgery. Often it is difficult to discern which eye is functional and which is the prosthesis. Procedure 48–1 outlines the proper way to remove and reinsert an eye prosthesis when the client is unable to do so.

EAR DISORDERS

For a person to hear, sound waves must enter the external auditory meatus and travel through the ear canal to vibrate the tympanic membrane and bony structures of the middle ear, which in turn activate the receptors of the cochlea. Trauma or disease involving any portion of this pathway can affect hearing. **Tinnitus**, the perception of sound such as ringing, buzzing, or roaring in the ears, is another potential result of problems affecting the auditory system.

Disorders of the external ear, including the auricle, auditory meatus, and ear canal, can affect the conduction of sound waves and hearing. Obstruction of the external auditory canal or damage to the tympanic membrane, which separates the outer from the middle ear, may lead to conductive hearing loss. Infection or inflammation, trauma, and obstruction of the ear

canal with cerumen (wax) or a foreign body are the most common conditions affecting the external ear.

Disorders of the middle ear may be either acute or chronic. Unless these disorders are treated promptly and effectively, damage and scarring of middle ear structures can result in a permanent conductive hearing loss. Infectious or inflammatory disorders such as otitis media and mastoiditis are the most common conditions affecting the middle ear. Otosclerosis, a genetic condition, may also affect the structures of the middle ear.

THE CLIENT WITH OTITIS EXTERNA

Otitis externa is inflammation of the ear canal. Commonly known as *swimmer's ear,* it is most prevalent in people who

PROCEDURE 48-1 REMOVING AND REINSERTING A PROSTHETIC EYE

GATHER SUPPLIES

- Gloves
- Clean basin or plastic denture cup
- Sterile normal saline or soap and water for cleaning the prosthesis
- Gauze squares or cotton cloth for cleaning the socket
- A bulb syringe for irrigation if necessary

BEFORE THE PROCEDURE

Most clients who have an artificial eye provide self-care and require little assistance. However, it may be necessary for the nurse to remove an eye prosthesis from the unconscious or debilitated client. If the client is conscious, explain the procedure and provide for privacy.

PROCEDURE

- Follow standard precautions.
- Wash the hands and put on clean exam gloves.
- To remove the prosthesis, do one of the following:
  - Pull down the lower lid and gently exert outward and upward pressure on the lower edge of the prosthesis. This pressure usually causes the prosthesis to slip out.
  - Pull down the lower lid and apply a moistened suction cup to the prosthesis by squeezing the device. Twist gently to remove the prosthesis from the socket.
- Wash the prosthesis using mild soap and water or normal saline. Rinse thoroughly. Do not use abrasives or chemicals for cleaning.
- If the prosthesis is not immediately replaced in the eye socket, store it in a clearly labeled plastic container lined with a soft cloth or gauze squares. Avoid scratching or damaging the prosthesis. Store it in a safe place to prevent loss.

- If irrigation of the eye socket is ordered, have the client lean over a sink or basin if possible, or position on the affected side with a clean emesis basin to hold the irrigant as it flows out of the socket. Gently hold the lids open and irrigate the socket using a bulb syringe and clean warm water.
- Reinsert the prosthesis.
  a. Moisten the prosthesis with warm normal saline or water.
  b. Gently hold the lids open. Insert the upper edge of the prosthesis under the upper lid first, then the lower edge under the lower lid using slight pressure.
  c. If a suction device is used, attach it to the cleaned prosthesis over the pupil. Holding the lids open, insert the prosthesis using the above procedure, then remove the suction cup by squeezing it gently and exerting slight pressure on the edge of the cup with the lower lid.

AFTER THE PROCEDURE

Ensure that the client is comfortable. Chart the procedure and any abnormal findings, such as drainage or inflammation.

---

spend significant time in the water. Competitive athletes, including swimmers, divers, and surfers, are particularly prone to otitis externa. Wearing a hearing aid or ear plugs, which hold moisture in the ear canal, is an additional risk factor. Although *Pseudomonas aeruginosa* or other bacterial infection is the most common cause, external otitis may also be due to fungal infection, mechanical trauma (such as cleaning the ear with a toothpick), or a local hypersensitivity reaction.

Pathophysiology and Manifestations

Disruption of the normal environment within the external auditory canal typically precedes the inflammatory process. Retained moisture, cleaning, or drying of the ear canal remove the protective layer of cerumen, an acidic, water-repellent substance with antimicrobial properties. Its removal leaves the skin of the ear canal vulnerable to invasion and infection. For surfers, the presence of *exostoses,* bony growths in the ear canals resulting from prolonged exposure to cold, predisposes to impaction and retained moisture within the canal.

The client with otitis externa often complains of a feeling of fullness in the ear. Ear pain typically is present and may be severe. The pain of otitis externa can be differentiated from that associated with otitis media by manipulation of the auricle. In external otitis, this maneuver increases the pain, whereas the

client with otitis media experiences no change in pain perception. Odorless watery or purulent drainage may be present. The ear canal appears inflamed and edematous on examination.

INTERDISCIPLINARY CARE

Management of the client with an external ear disorder focuses on restoring the normal balance of the external ear and canal and teaching the client how to prevent future problems.

For otitis externa, the following steps are recommended in treatment:

- Thorough cleansing of the ear canal, particularly if drainage or debris is present
- Treatment of the infection with local antibiotics; if cellulitis is present, systemic antibiotics may be necessary
- Medication to relieve the pain and itching
- Teaching on the prevention of future episodes of swimmer's ear.

A topical antibiotic is often prescribed for the treatment of otitis externa. A topical corticosteroid may be ordered in combination with the antibiotic to provide immediate relief of the pain, swelling, and itching. Polymyxin B-neomycin-hydrocortisone (Cortisporin Otic) is a typical combination preparation used to treat external otitis; these antibiotics are effective against

Pseudomonas. It is important to identify known sensitivity to any of the drugs in this preparation prior to initiating therapy. Clients who are sensitive to neomycin may develop dermatitis, in which case the drug must be stopped. Other preparations such as 1% tolnaftate solution (Tinactin) may be prescribed for a fungal infection of the ear canal.

NURSING CARE

External otitis can cause severe pain and discomfort. Although the disorder is rarely serious enough to require hospitalization, the nurse teaches the client about the disorder, comfort measures, and prevention of future episodes.

Nursing Diagnoses and Interventions

Impaired Tissue Integrity

External otitis may result from attempts to clean the ear canal with a toothpick, cotton-tipped applicator, or other implement that damages the skin, allowing an infectious organism to invade the tissue. Even if the canal is not damaged by attempts to clean it, the cleaning process often interrupts normal mechanisms, causing cerumen and debris to collect in the canal. This collected debris, in turn, tends to trap water within the canal, causing maceration of the skin.

- Inform that ear canals rarely need cleansing beyond washing of the external meatus with soap and water. Teach clients of all ages not to clean ear canals with any implement. *"Cleaning" increases the risk of tissue damage and impairs the normal mechanism that clears the canal of accumulated cerumen and debris.*
- Teach client (and, if necessary, a family member) how to instill prescribed eardrops:
  a. Wash the hands.
  b. Warm the medication briefly by holding the container in the hand or placing it in a pocket for approximately 5 minutes before instilling the drops. *Warming the medication promotes comfort.*
  c. Lie on the unaffected side; if sitting, tilt the head toward the unaffected side. *This position allows gravity to assist in moving the medication to the inner portion of the ear canal.*
  d. Partially fill the ear dropper with medication.
  e. Using the nondominant hand, straighten the ear canal by pulling the pinna of the ear up and back. *Straightening helps the medication travel along the length of the canal.*
  f. Administer the prescribed number of drops into the ear canal. *It is important that the full amount of prescribed medication be administered to penetrate the length of the canal and achieve full effectiveness.*
  g. Remain in the side-lying position for approximately 5 minutes after the instillation of drops. *This position allows the medication to penetrate into deeper portions of the canal and prevents it from running out when the head is moved upright.*
  h. Loosely place a small piece of cotton in the auditory meatus for 15 to 20 minutes. *The cotton helps keep the medication in the canal.*
- Teach to avoid getting water in the affected ear until it is fully healed. Cotton balls may be used while showering to prevent water from entering the ear canal. The client should refrain from water sports and activities until approved by the primary care provider. *Retained moisture in the ear canal can further impair skin integrity, increasing inflammation.*

Community-Based Care

The client is ultimately responsible for carrying out the prescribed treatment regimen in external otitis and for implementing measures to prevent future episodes. Teaching is vital. Provide verbal and written instructions on use of the prescribed medications. Teach the client care measures to prevent recurrent episodes especially important in swimmers, divers, and surfers (Box 48–2).

Cellulitis of the surrounding tissue is a possible complication of external otitis. Instruct the client to report to the primary

---

BOX 48–2 **Teaching to Prevent Otitis Externa**

- Stay out of the water until the acute inflammatory process is completely resolved. Ideally, allow 7 to 10 days before resuming water activities.
- Take precautions to keep the ear canal dry while in the water:
  a. Use silicone earplugs, which can keep water out of the ear without reducing hearing significantly.
  b. Wear a tight-fitting swim cap or wet suit hood, especially in cold ocean water. Although these do not prevent water from entering the ear, they protect the ear from the cold and possibly slow the formation of bony growths in the ears. They also protect the ear from sand and other water debris.
- Immediately after swimming, dry the ear canal. Allow water to drain by tilting the head and jumping to shake water out of the ear. Dry the outer ear with a towel, then use a hair dryer on the lowest setting several inches from the ear to dry the canal.
- Do not insert cotton swabs or other objects into the ear canal to dry it. This removes the protective layer of cerumen and may damage the skin of the canal, increasing the risk of bacterial infection. In addition, if debris such as sand is present, the swab may actually push debris further into the canal, forming an impacted mass.
- Use a drying agent in the ear canal after swimming. A 2% acetic acid solution or 2% boric acid in ethyl alcohol is effective in drying the canal and restoring its normal acidic environment.
- If it is necessary to remove impacted debris from the ear canal, irrigate the ear with warm tap water. A bulb syringe available over the counter or a 20-mL syringe attached to a short Teflon intravenous catheter (with the needle removed) is effective. With the head tilted toward the affected side, direct a stream of warm water toward the upper wall of the ear canal, allowing the water to run out into a bowl or sink. Repeated instillations may be necessary to break up and flush out impacted wax and debris.

care provider any increase in pain, swelling, or redness of surrounding tissues; fever; or other manifestations of infection such as malaise or increased fatigue.

THE CLIENT WITH IMPACTED CERUMEN OR A FOREIGN BODY

The external auditory canal can be obstructed by cerumen or foreign bodies. The curved shape and narrow lumen of the canal make it particularly vulnerable to obstruction.

Pathophysiology and Manifestations

As cerumen dries, it moves down and out of the ear canal. In some individuals it tends to accumulate, narrowing the canal. Aging is a risk factor for impaction, because less cerumen is produced and it is harder and drier. The accumulation of cerumen is often aggravated by attempting to remove it using cotton-tipped swabs or hairpins, which pack it more deeply into the ear canal.

A variety of objects become foreign bodies in the ear canal. In adults, implements used to clean the ear canal may break and become lodged. Insects also may enter the ear canal and be unable to exit.

When the ear canal becomes occluded with either cerumen or a foreign body, the client experiences a conductive hearing loss in the affected ear. Manifestations include a sensation of fullness, along with tinnitus and coughing due to stimulation of the vagal nerve. The foreign body or impacted cerumen may be visualized on otoscopy. Impacted cerumen appears as a yellow, brown, or black mass in the canal.

INTERDISCIPLINARY CARE

Treatment focuses on clearing the canal. If there is no evidence of tympanic membrane perforation, irrigation of the canal is often the initial therapy.

Impacted wax, objects, or insects may require physical removal using an ear curet, forceps, or right-angle hook inserted via an otoscope and ear speculum. Mineral oil or topical lidocaine drops are used to immobilize or kill insects prior to their removal from the ear. When an organic foreign body such as a bean or an insect is suspected, water should not be instilled into the ear canal, because it may cause the object to swell, making its removal more difficult. Smooth, round objects present the biggest challenge to remove from the ear canal. Suction applied using a piece of soft intravenous tubing may be effective.

NURSING CARE

Nurses are often involved in identifying and relieving obstructions of the ear canal, especially in outpatient and community settings. Any client with evidence of a new conductive hearing loss or complaints of discomfort and fullness in one ear should be evaluated for possible obstruction. Inability to visualize the tympanic membrane or observation of a dark, shiny mass obstructing the canal may indicate a need for an irrigation or other procedure to clear the canal. It is important to deter-

mine that the tympanic membrane is intact before irrigating; assessment by a physician or advanced practitioner may be necessary if a ruptured membrane is suspected.

Because obstruction of the ear canal with cerumen or a foreign body is generally preventable, teaching is a key component of nursing care. Clients need to know appropriate care measures for the external ear. Although the ear canal rarely needs cleaning, the client prone to cerumen impaction needs teaching about the use of mineral oil or commercial products to soften wax and of irrigation to remove it. All clients should understand the importance of not inserting anything smaller than a finger wrapped with a washcloth into the ear canal to avoid trauma to the canal or eardrum. Stress the risk of impacting cerumen against the tympanic membrane when using cotton-tipped swabs to clean the ear canal. Additionally, the swab may break and lodge in the canal. If eardrops have been prescribed, teach the client and a family member how to instill them.

THE CLIENT WITH OTITIS MEDIA

Otitis media, inflammation or infection of the middle ear, primarily affects infants and young children but may also occur in adults. The tympanic membrane, which separates the middle ear from the external auditory canal, protects the middle ear from the external environment. The eustachian (auditory) tube connects the middle ear with the nasopharynx to help equalize the pressure in the middle ear with the atmospheric pressure. Unfortunately, this connecting tube also provides a route by which infectious organisms enter the middle ear from the nose and throat, causing otitis media, the most common disease of the middle ear.

Pathophysiology

There are two primary forms of otitis media: (1) serous and (2) acute or suppurative. Both forms are associated with upper respiratory infection and eustachian tube dysfunction. The eustachian tube is narrow and flat, normally opening only during yawning and swallowing. Allergies or upper respiratory tract infections can cause edema of the tube lining, impairing its function. Air within the middle ear is trapped and gradually absorbed, creating negative pressure in this space.

Serous Otitis Media

Serous otitis media (also called *otitis media with effusion*) occurs when the eustachian tube is obstructed for a prolonged time, impairing equalization of air pressure in the middle ear. Air within the middle ear space is gradually absorbed; the tube obstruction prevents more air from entering the middle ear. The resulting negative pressure in the middle ear causes sterile serous fluid to move from the capillaries into the space, forming a sterile effusion of the middle ear.

Upper respiratory infection or allergies such as hay fever predispose the client to serous otitis media. In addition, clients with narrowed or edematous eustachian tubes may also be subject to barotrauma or barotitis media. In these clients, the middle ear cannot adapt to rapid changes in barometric pressure such as those that occur during air travel or underwater diving. Barotrauma tends to occur during descent in an airplane, because negative pressure within the middle ear causes the eustachian tube to collapse and lock. However, underwater diving places even greater stress on the eustachian tube and middle ear (Tierney et al., 2005).

MANIFESTATIONS Typical manifestations of serous otitis media include decreased hearing in the affected ear and complaints of "snapping" or "popping" in the ear. On examination, the tympanic membrane demonstrates decreased mobility and may appear retracted or bulging. Fluid or air bubbles are often visible behind the drum. Severe pressure differences such as those occurring with barotrauma may cause acute pain, hemorrhage into the middle ear, rupture of the tympanic membrane, or even rupture of the round window with sensory hearing loss and severe **vertigo** (a sensation of whirling or rotation). *Hemotympanum*, bleeding into or behind the tympanic membrane, may be observed on otoscopic examination.

Acute Otitis Media

The eustachian tube also provides a route for the entry of pathogens into the normally sterile middle ear, resulting in acute or suppurative otitis media. Acute otitis media typically follows an upper respiratory infection. Edema of the eustachian tube impairs drainage of the middle ear, causing mucus and serous fluid to accumulate. This fluid is an excellent environment for the growth of bacteria, which may enter from the oronasopharynx via the eustachian tube. Although a viral upper respiratory infection may predispose the client to a middle ear infection, the bacteria *Streptococcus pneumoniae*, *Haemophilus influenzae*, and *Streptococcus pyogenes* account for most cases of otitis media in adults. Invasion and colonization of the middle ear by bacteria and the resultant migration of white blood cells cause pus formation. Accumulated pus can increase middle ear pressure sufficiently to rupture the tympanic membrane. The bacterial infection may also migrate internally, causing mastoiditis, brain abscess, or bacterial meningitis. A more common complication of otitis media is a persistent conductive hearing loss, which typically resolves when the middle ear effusion clears.

MANIFESTATIONS The client with acute otitis media experiences mild to severe pain in the affected ear. The client's temperature is often elevated. Diminished hearing, dizziness, vertigo, and tinnitus are common associated complaints. Pus within the mastoid air cells often causes mastoid tenderness in acute otitis media. On otoscopic examination, the tympanic membrane appears red and inflamed or dull and bulging (Figure 48–15 ■). Decreased movement of the membrane is demonstrated by tympanometry or air insufflation. Spontaneous rupture of the tympanic membrane releases a purulent discharge. **Myringotomy** (an incision of the tympanic membrane) may be performed to relieve the pressure.

INTERDISCIPLINARY CARE

The diagnosis of otitis media is usually based on the history and the physical examination. The tympanic membrane can be visualized and its mobility evaluated using a pneumatic otoscope that allows a puff of air to be instilled into the ear canal. Generally, the tympanic membrane moves slightly when air is instilled or the client performs the Valsalva maneuver. Less

Figure 48–15 ■ A red, bulging tympanic membrane of otitis media.
Source: Janet Hayes/Medical Images, Inc.

movement is seen in clients with eustachian tube dysfunction and acute otitis media with effusion.

Diagnosis

- *Impedance audiometry,* also known as tympanometry, is an accurate diagnostic test for otitis media with effusion. A continuous tone is delivered to the tympanic membrane by an audiometer with a sealed probe tip. Compliance of the tympanic membrane and middle ear is measured by recording energy reflected from the membrane surface. With middle ear effusion, compliance is reduced.
- A *complete blood count (CBC)* may be done to assess for an elevated WBC count and increased numbers of immature cells indicative of acute bacterial infection.
- If the tympanic membrane has ruptured or a tympanocentesis or myringotomy is performed, drainage is cultured to determine the infecting organism.

Medications

When eustachian tube dysfunction and serous otitis media do not spontaneously resolve or lead to hearing loss, a short course of an anti-inflammatory drug (e.g., oral prednisone for 7 days) is prescribed to reduce mucosal edema of the tube and improve its patency. Although a decongestant or antihistamine may be used, there is little evidence of their effectiveness in treating serous otitis media. See Chapter 13 ∞ for the nursing implications of corticosteroid medications.

The client with eustachian tube dysfunction may be taught to autoinflate the middle ear by performing the Valsalva maneuver or by forcefully exhaling against closed nostrils. Additionally, the client is advised to avoid air travel and underwater diving.

Acute otitis media usually is treated with antibiotic therapy, especially amoxicillin, trimethoprim-sulfamethoxazole, cefaclor, or azithromycin for 5 to 10 days. This course of treatment is long enough to ensure eradication of the infective organism, yet short enough to reduce the incidence of bacterial resistance. (See Chapter 12 ∞ for further discussion of antibiotics.) Symptomatic relief may be provided by analgesics, antipyretics, antihistamines, and local application of heat.

Surgery

A myringotomy or tympanocentesis may be performed to relieve excess pressure in the middle ear and prevent spontaneous rupture of the eardrum. To perform a tympanocentesis, the physician inserts a 20-gauge spinal needle through the inferior portion of the tympanic membrane, allowing aspiration of fluid and pus from the middle ear to relieve pressure and, if necessary, obtain a specimen for culture. Myringotomy may be performed to relieve severe pain or when complications of acute otitis media, such as mastoiditis, are present. As soon as the pressure is released, pain subsides and hearing improves.

Clients who do not respond to antibiotic therapy may require myringotomy with insertion of ventilation (tympanostomy) tubes. Small tubes are inserted into the inferior portion of the tympanic membrane, providing for ventilation and drainage of the middle ear during healing. The tube is eventually extruded from the ear, and the tympanic membrane heals. While the tube is in place, it is important to avoid getting any water in the ear canal because it may then enter the middle ear space.

NURSING CARE

Clients with otitis media are commonly treated in outpatient and community settings. The nursing role is primarily one of support and education.

Health Promotion

Health promotion for otitis media focuses on educating clients about the importance of seeking medical care for prolonged, severe ear pain with or without drainage combined with an upper respiratory tract infection. Untreated or repeated attacks of otitis media can progress to a chronic form of otitis media, acute mastoiditis, or eardrum perforation.

Assessment

Collect assessment data through a health history and physical examination (Chapter 47 ∞).
- *Health history:* Recent upper respiratory infection; presence, intensity, and nature of pain in affected ear; sense of fullness or pressure in the ear; change in hearing; snapping or popping sensation in the affected ear; presence of vertigo.
- *Physical examination:* Temperature; hearing test; inspect tympanic membrane.

Nursing Diagnosis and Interventions

Pain can be a significant problem for clients with otitis media, as can the risk of damage to delicate tissues of the middle ear by the infectious and inflammatory processes.

Pain

Tissue edema, effusion of the middle ear, and the inflammatory response can affect the pain-sensitive tissues of the middle ear in otitis media, causing acute discomfort. This discomfort is increased by pressure changes, such as those that occur during air travel or underwater diving.
- Assess pain for severity, quality, and location. *A thorough assessment is important to determine the source of the pain.*

The pain of otitis media, unlike that of external otitis, is not aggravated by movement of the external ear.
- Encourage the use of mild analgesics such as aspirin or acetaminophen every 4 hours as needed to relieve pain and fever. *These nonprescription medications are effective in reducing the perception of pain. Aspirin also has anti-inflammatory properties that may help relieve the inflammation of the ear.*
- Advise to apply heat to the affected side unless contraindicated. *Heat dilates blood vessels, promoting the reabsorption of fluid and reducing swelling.*
- Instruct to avoid air travel, rapid changes in elevation, or diving. *A rapid change in barometric pressure can increase the client's pain significantly.*
- Instruct to report promptly an abrupt relief of pain to the primary care provider. *Pain that subsides abruptly may indicate spontaneous perforation of the tympanic membrane with relief of pressure within the middle ear.*

Community-Based Care

The client who has otitis media needs teaching about the disorder, its causes and prevention, and any specific treatment recommended or prescribed. Discuss the following topics with the client and family:
- Antibiotic therapy and potential side effects
- Importance of completing all ordered doses
- Follow-up examinations in 2 to 4 weeks
- Avoidance of swimming, diving, or submerging the head while bathing if ventilation tubes are in place.

If surgical intervention is necessary, teach the client and family members about the surgery and postoperative care. Provide instruction about any special postoperative precautions, such as avoiding water in the ear canals or avoiding sudden changes in air pressure.

THE CLIENT WITH ACUTE MASTOIDITIS

The mastoid process is a portion of the temporal bone of the skull lying adjacent to the middle ear. It is full of air cavities called mastoid air cells or mastoid sinuses. The infection of acute otitis media generally extends into the mastoid air cells; effective treatment of acute otitis media eliminates the infection from the mastoid cells as well. When treatment is ineffective, pus remains in the mastoid air cells, and acute **mastoiditis**, bacterial infection of the mastoid process, may develop.

The incidence of acute mastoiditis is low in the United States and in other countries in which the use of antibiotics to treat acute otitis media is similar to that of the United States. Its incidence is higher in countries where antibiotics are less likely to be prescribed for acute otitis media (Kasper et al., 2005).

Pathophysiology and Complications

In acute mastoiditis, the bony septa between mastoid air cells are destroyed and cells coalesce to form large spaces. Portions of the mastoid process are eroded. With chronic infection, an abscess may form, or bony sclerosis of the mastoid may result. Acute mastoiditis increases the risk of meningitis because only a very thin bony plate separates mastoid air cells from the brain. Fortunately, this complication is rare since the advent of effective antibiotic therapy for treating otitis media.

Manifestations

Manifestations of acute mastoiditis usually develop approximately 2 to 3 weeks after an episode of acute otitis media and include recurrent earache and hearing loss on the affected side. The pain is persistent and throbbing; tenderness is present over the mastoid process (behind the ear). It may also be red and inflamed. Swelling of the process can cause the auricle of the ear to protrude more than normal. Fever may be accompanied by tinnitus and headache. Profuse drainage from the affected ear may be noted.

INTERDISCIPLINARY CARE

In addition to the manifestations of acute mastoiditis, loss of septa between mastoid air cells may be noted on radiologic examination. Acute mastoiditis is treated aggressively with antibiotic therapy. Intravenous ticarcillin-clavulanate (Timentin) and gentamicin may be used initially, with therapy tailored to the specific organism once culture results are obtained. Antibiotics are continued for at least 14 days. Infections that do not respond to medical therapy or that pose a high risk of spreading to the brain may necessitate *mastoidectomy*, surgical removal of the infected mastoid air cells, bone, and pus, and inspection of the underlying dura for possible abscess. The extent of tissue destruction determines the extent of surgery required. In a modified mastoidectomy, as much tissue is preserved as possible to avoid disruption of hearing. A radical mastoidectomy involves removal of middle ear structures including the incus and malleus as well as the diseased portions of the mastoid process. Unless reconstruction is performed at the time of surgery, this surgery results in conductive hearing loss. **Tympanoplasty,** surgical reconstruction of the middle ear, can restore or preserve hearing.

NURSING CARE

Prevention is the primary focus of collaborative and nursing care related to mastoiditis. Adequate, effective antibiotic treatment of acute otitis media prevents mastoiditis in nearly all instances.

Following surgical intervention, carefully assess the wound and drainage for evidence of infection or other complications. The client's hearing may be temporarily or permanently affected, depending on the extent of the surgery. If the client has impaired hearing in the unaffected ear as well, develop a means of communication with the client prior to surgery. If the hearing is preserved in the unaffected ear, position the client with that ear toward the door. Speak slowly and clearly; do not shout or speak unusually loudly. Be sure that family and staff know about the client's hearing loss and use appropriate communication techniques. Assist the client with ambulation initially, because dizziness and vertigo are not unusual following surgery.

Nursing care of the client having ear surgery is discussed in the box on the next page.

Community-Based Care

When teaching about acute mastoiditis, stress the importance of complying with the prescribed antibiotic therapy and recommendations for follow-up. Instruct the client and family to report any adverse reactions to the primary care provider so that therapy can be adjusted. Teach the client and family how to change the surgical dressing using aseptic technique. Provide referrals to appropriate community agencies for the client with a new hearing loss resulting from mastoiditis or its treatment.

THE CLIENT WITH CHRONIC OTITIS MEDIA

Chronic otitis media involves permanent perforation of the tympanic membrane, with or without recurrent pus formation. Changes in the mucosa and bony structures (ossicles) of the middle ear often accompany chronic otitis media. It usually is the result of recurrent acute otitis media and eustachian tube dysfunction, but may also result from trauma or other diseases.

Marginal perforations, which usually occur in the posterior-superior portion of the tympanic membrane, are associated with more complications than central perforations. With marginal perforations, squamous epithelium may migrate from the ear canal into the middle ear, where it begins to desquamate and accumulate, forming a *cholesteatoma* (a cyst or mass filled with epithelial cell debris). Its incidence is highest in children and young adults. The desquamating epithelium continues to accumulate and remains infected, producing collagenases (enzymes) that destroy adjacent bone. The inflammatory process impairs the blood supply to the stapes, causing its destruction and conductive hearing loss. Cholesteatomas are benign and slow-growing tumors, which can enlarge to fill the entire middle ear. Untreated, the cholesteatoma can progressively destroy the ossicles and erode into the inner ear, causing profound hearing loss.

Systemic antibiotics are prescribed for exacerbations of purulent otitis media. Tympanic membrane perforation is repaired with a tympanoplasty to restore sound conduction and the integrity of the middle ear. A cholesteatoma may require delicate surgery for its removal. If at all possible, radical mastoidectomy with removal of the tympanic membrane, ossicles, and tumor is avoided.

As with other complications of acute otitis media, a priority of nursing care is prevention of chronic otitis media and cholesteatoma. Clients with chronic otitis media need to understand various treatment options and their risks and benefits, as well as the long-term risk of not treating a perforated tympanic membrane. They are also taught how to instill eardrops, to clean the external auditory meatus, and to not irrigate the ear when the tympanic membrane is perforated or if they think it might be.

If surgical treatment of chronic otitis media will affect the client's hearing, include this information in preoperative teach-

NURSING CARE OF THE CLIENT HAVING Ear Surgery

PREOPERATIVE CARE

- Review Chapter 4 ∞ for routine preoperative care.
- Assess hearing or verify documentation of preoperative hearing assessment. *These data are important in evaluating the results of the surgical procedure.*
- Establish a means of communication to be used after surgery. *Hearing may be impaired after surgery.*
- Explain that blowing of the nose, coughing, and sneezing are restricted postoperatively to prevent pressure changes in the middle ear and potential disruption of the surgical site. Keeping the mouth open during a cough or sneeze minimizes pressure changes in the middle ear. *Providing teaching and the opportunity to practice before surgery promotes cooperation in the postoperative period.*

POSTOPERATIVE CARE

- Review Chapter 4 ∞ for routine postoperative care.
- Assess for bleeding or drainage from the affected ear. *Infection and hemorrhage are possible complications.*
- Administer antiemetics as ordered to prevent vomiting. *Vomiting may increase the pressure in the middle ear, disrupting the surgical site.*
- Elevate the head of bed and position the client on the unaffected side. *This position minimizes the pressure in the middle ear.*
- Assess for vertigo or dizziness, especially with ambulation or movement in bed. Avoid unnecessary movements such as turning. Take measures to ensure safety during ambulation. *Surgery on the ear may disrupt equilibrium, increasing the risk of falling.*

- Assess hearing postoperatively. Stand on the unaffected side to communicate and use other measures such as written messages as needed for effective communication with the client with impaired hearing. Reassure the client that decreased hearing acuity immediately after surgery is expected. *Hearing improvement, if an expected result of the ear surgery, typically does not occur until earplugs are removed and edema and drainage at the operative site have resolved. If no reconstruction of the middle ear is done or the cochlea is involved, permanent hearing loss in the affected ear may be an expected result.*
- Remind to avoid coughing, sneezing, or blowing the nose. *These increase pressure in the middle ear.*

Health Education for the Client and Family

- Provide instructions for home care:
  a. To prevent contamination of the ear canal, avoid showers, shampooing, and immersing the head until the physician says you can do so.
  b. Keep the outer earplug clean and dry, changing it as needed. Do not remove inner ear dressing until instructed to do so by the physician.
  c. Avoid blowing the nose; if you need to cough or sneeze, keep the mouth open.
  d. Do not swim or dive without physician approval. Check with your doctor regarding air travel.
  e. Meclizine hydrochloride (Antivert) or other antiemetic/antihistamine medication may be necessary for up to 1 month following surgery.
  f. Fever, bleeding, increased drainage, increased dizziness, or decreased hearing after discharge may indicate a complication. Notify the physician if any of these occur.

---

ing. Teach the client and family how to use alternative means of communication if this will be necessary postoperatively. When an assistive device is ordered, teach the client and a family member about its use.

THE CLIENT WITH OTOSCLEROSIS

Otosclerosis is a common cause of conductive hearing loss. Abnormal bone formation in the osseous labyrinth of the temporal bone causes the footplate of the stapes to become fixed or immobile in the oval window. The result is a conductive hearing loss.

Otosclerosis is a hereditary disorder with an autosomal dominant pattern of inheritance. It occurs most commonly in Caucasians and in females. The progressive hearing loss typically begins in adolescence or early adulthood and seems to be accelerated by pregnancy. Although both ears are affected, the rate of hearing loss is asymmetric. Because bone conduction of sound is retained, the client may be able to use the telephone but have difficulty conversing in person. Tinnitus may also be associated with otosclerosis.

On examination, a reddish or pinkish-orange tympanic membrane may be noted because of increased vascularity of the middle ear. The Rinne test (Chapter 47 ∞) shows bone

sound conduction to be equal to or greater than air conduction, an abnormal finding.

Clients with otosclerosis may choose conservative treatment, relying on a hearing aid to improve their ability to hear and interact with others. Sodium fluoride may be prescribed to slow bone resorption and overgrowth. Surgical treatment involves a stapedectomy and middle ear reconstruction or a stapedotomy. A *stapedectomy* is a microsurgical technique for removing the diseased stapes. A metallic prosthesis is then inserted, with one end connected to the incus and the other inserted into the oval window. *Stapedotomy* involves creation of a small hole in the footplate of the stapes and insertion of a wire or platinum ribbon prosthesis. An argon, KTP, or CO_2 laser may be used for surgery. Surgery usually restores hearing for the client with otosclerosis.

Education and referral of the client to appropriate community agencies are important nursing care priorities for the client with otosclerosis. For the client who chooses surgical treatment, nursing care is similar to that for other clients undergoing ear surgery. The following nursing diagnoses may be appropriate:

- *Risk for Injury* related to hearing loss or postoperative vertigo
- *Disturbed Sensory Perception: Auditory* related to bony sclerosis of the stapes

- *Impaired Verbal Communication* related to hearing loss
- *Anxiety* related to concern about transmission of a genetic disorder to children.

THE CLIENT WITH AN INNER EAR DISORDER

Disorders affecting the inner ear are much less common than disorders of the outer or middle ear. Inner ear disorders affect equilibrium and may also affect sensorineural hearing, the perception of sound. Labyrinthitis and Ménière's disease are the most common diseases of the inner ear. Vertigo may be a disorder of the inner ear itself or a manifestation of other disorders.

Pathophysiology and Manifestations

The inner ear (also called the labyrinth) contains the cochlea and the semicircular canals. The hair cells and neurons that allow sound perception and transmission to the auditory center of the brain are in the cochlea. The semicircular canals filled with endolymph are the primary organs involved in maintaining equilibrium. Disruption of this portion of the ear by an inflammatory process or excess endolymph not only affects balance but may also result in permanent hearing loss.

Vertigo

Normally, the integration of input from the labyrinths, eyes, muscles, joints, and neural centers maintains balance and posture. This input and integration can be affected by disorders of the labyrinth, vestibular nerve or nuclei, eyes, cerebellum, brainstem, or cerebral cortex, causing vertigo. Vertigo, the sensation of movement when there is none, is a disorder of equilibrium. The sensation of whirling, rotation, or movement is described as either subjective or objective.

Clients with subjective vertigo report the sensation of being in motion in a stable environment. This is not always a sense of spinning; the client may have a sense of tumbling or falling forward or backward. The sensation is reversed in objective vertigo; clients report a sensation of stability in a moving environment. This motion may be perceived as the room spinning around the client or the ground rocking beneath the client's feet. Dizziness, which may be mistaken for vertigo, is a sensation of unsteadiness, lack of balance, light-headedness, or movement within the head. The person who is dizzy does not have the rotational sensation felt with vertigo.

Vertigo may be disabling, resulting in falls, injury, and difficulty walking. Attacks of vertigo are often accompanied by nausea and vomiting, nystagmus, and autonomic symptoms such as pallor, sweating, hypotension, and salivation.

Labyrinthitis

Labyrinthitis, also called otitis interna, is inflammation of the inner ear. It is an uncommon disorder, because the bony protection of the membranous labyrinth makes it difficult for organisms to enter the inner ear. However, bacteria, viruses, and other organisms may enter and infect the inner ear through the oval window during acute otitis media, through the cochlear aqueduct during meningitis, or through the blood. Viral labyrinthitis is suspected when the client has a sudden onset of symptoms after an upper respiratory infection or when there is no evidence of concurrent otitis media. Labyrinthitis also may result from an autoimmune process of unknown etiology.

MANIFESTATIONS Inflammation of the labyrinth typically causes vertigo, sensorineural hearing deficit, and **nystagmus** (rapid involuntary eye movements).

Vertigo is the hallmark manifestation of inner ear disorders. The vertigo of labyrinthitis is severe and often accompanied by nausea and vomiting. Any movement can aggravate the vertigo, and falling is a significant risk if the client attempts to stand. Vertigo lasts days to weeks in labyrinthitis, making client education a vital component of care.

Hearing loss in the ear affected by labyrinthitis may be temporary or permanent. If inflammation destroys tissue of the membranous labyrinth, the hearing loss may be complete and permanent.

The involuntary rhythmic eye movements of nystagmus may not be present in all clients with labyrinthitis. When present, the eye movement is typically horizontal. Applying positive or negative pressure to the tympanic membrane of the affected ear may stimulate nystagmus, as will caloric testing (irrigating the ear canal with warm or cool water). Although nystagmus may also be a symptom of brainstem or cerebellar dysfunction, vertigo and hearing loss are not typically associated with those disorders.

Ménière's Disease

Ménière's disease, also known as endolymphatic hydrops, is a chronic disorder characterized by recurrent attacks of vertigo with tinnitus and a progressive unilateral hearing loss. This disorder affects men and women equally, with adults between the ages of 35 and 60 at highest risk. The cause of Ménière's disease is unclear, although the most common form of the disease is thought to result from viral injury to the fluid transport system of the inner ear. Other factors that may increase the risk for Ménière's disease include trauma, bacterial infections such as syphilis, autoimmune processes, and vascular disorders (Copstead & Banasik, 2005; Porth, 2005). A family history of the disease increases risk, suggesting a possible genetic link in some clients.

Ménière's disease results from an excess of endolymph, the fluid in the membranous labyrinth of the inner ear. Although the precise pathophysiologic mechanism leading to accumulation of endolymph is unclear, it is thought to result from impaired filtration and excretion of the fluid by the endolymphatic sac (Porth, 2005; Tierney et al., 2005). Excessive pressure resulting from the increased fluid volume causes neural organs of the cochlea to degenerate.

COURSE AND MANIFESTATIONS The onset of Ménière's disease may be gradual or sudden. It is characterized by recurrent attacks of vertigo, gradual loss of hearing, and tinnitus. Attacks may be preceded by a feeling of fullness in the ears, and a roaring or ringing sensation. The sensorineural hearing loss and tinnitus are usually unilateral but can become bilateral. Attacks of severe rotary vertigo occur abruptly and often unpredictably, lasting from minutes to hours. An attack may be linked to increased sodium intake, stress, allergies, vasoconstriction, or premenstrual fluid retention. As the disease continues, hearing loss progresses and the vertigo can be severe enough to cause immobility, nausea, and vomiting. Attacks are often accompanied by hypotension, sweating, and nystagmus.

INTERDISCIPLINARY CARE

The manifestations associated with inner ear disorders are similar, making testing necessary to establish a diagnosis. Once the diagnosis is determined, collaborative care is directed toward managing symptoms and preventing permanent hearing loss. Clients with labyrinthitis or an acute attack of Ménière's disease may require hospitalization to manage the vertigo and its effects.

Diagnosis

The following diagnostic studies may be ordered:
- *Caloric testing (electronystagmography)* evaluates the vestibulo-ocular reflex by identifying eye movements (nystagmus) in response to caloric testing. In clients with impaired vestibular function, the normal nystagmus response is blunted or absent. This portion of the test is contraindicated in clients who have a perforated tympanic membrane.
- *Rinne* and *Weber tests* of hearing (Chapter 47 ∞) show decreased air and bone conduction on the affected side if a sensorineural hearing loss is present. In Ménière's disease, audiology shows sensorineural hearing loss involving the low tones.
- *X-rays* and *CT scans* of the petrous bones are used to evaluate the internal auditory canal. In clients with Ménière's disease, the vestibular aqueducts may be shorter and straighter than normal.
- *Glycerol test* is conducted by giving the client oral glycerol to decrease fluid pressure in the inner ear. An acute temporary hearing improvement is considered diagnostic for Ménière's disease.

Medications

A scopolamine patch may be used for clients with recurrent vertigo, although adverse effects such as dry mouth, blurred vision, and urinary retention may limit its use. In Ménière's disease, a diuretic such as hydrochlorothiazide may be prescribed to reduce endolymphatic pressure. A central nervous system depressant such as diazepam (Valium) or lorazepam (Ativan) may halt an attack of vertigo. Parenteral droperidol (Inapsine) provides both a sedative and antiemetic effect, making it a useful drug for acute attacks. Antivertigo/antiemetic medications such as meclizine (Antivert), prochlorperazine (Compazine), or hydroxyzine hydrochloride (Vistaril) are prescribed to reduce the whirling sensation and nausea. If the nausea and vomiting are severe, intravenous fluids may be necessary to maintain fluid and electrolyte balance.

Treatments

Bed rest in a quiet, darkened room with minimal sensory stimuli and minimal movement provides the most comfort for the client experiencing an acute attack of vertigo.

Between acute attacks, management of the client with Ménière's disease is directed at preventing future attacks and pre-

serving hearing. A low-sodium diet helps reduce labyrinthine pressure. The Furstenberg diet, a salt-free neutral ash diet, may be prescribed if moderate sodium restriction is ineffective in controlling attacks. Clients should avoid tobacco, which causes vasoconstriction and can precipitate an attack, along with alcohol and caffeine.

Surgery

When episodes of vertigo are not controlled through medical interventions, surgery may be necessary. Surgical *endolymphatic decompression* relieves the excess pressure in the labyrinth; a shunt is then inserted between the membranous labyrinth and the subarachnoid space to drain excess fluid away from the labyrinths and maintain lower pressure. This procedure preserves hearing for most clients. Vertigo is relieved in approximately 70% of clients, but about half of clients undergoing this procedure continue to experience sensations of fullness and tinnitus.

Destruction of a portion of the acoustic nerve is an alternative to shunting procedures. In a *vestibular neurectomy,* the portion of cranial nerve VIII that controls balance and sensations of vertigo is severed. This procedure relieves vertigo for up to 90% of clients. Although there is a risk of damage to the cochlear portion of the nerve and resultant hearing loss, for most clients hearing loss stabilizes after neurectomy, even improving for some.

The surgery of last resort for Ménière's disease is a *labyrinthectomy.* The labyrinth is completely removed, destroying cochlear function. This procedure is used only when hearing loss is nearly complete and vertigo is persistent. Although labyrinthectomy relieves vertigo in nearly all cases, the client may remain unsteady and have continued problems with balance.

After surgery on the inner ear, the client is positioned to minimize ear pressure and vertigo. Movement is restricted, and assistance is provided when the client gets up. Antiemetics and antivertigo medications are used to manage symptoms resulting from disruption of the inner ear. Complications include infection and leakage of cerebrospinal fluid.

NURSING CARE

The client with an inner ear disorder has multiple nursing care needs related to the manifestations of the disorder.

Health Promotion

Health promotion focuses on identifying clients with potential inner ear disorders. Persistent episodes of dizziness, ringing in the ears, balance problems, or loss of hearing should be reported to a healthcare provider. Clients diagnosed early may have a lower risk for injury and can be taught strategies for maintaining as near normal as possible their work and social life.

Assessment

In addition to the following, assess the older client for other medical causes of imbalance and dizziness, such as neurologic dysfunction, musculoskeletal and cardiovascular disorders, and endocrine problems.

- *Health history:* Medication use; presence of vertigo, tinnitus, nausea and vomiting, and hearing loss; balance problems; frequency and duration of symptoms, precipitating factors for an attack.
- *Physical examination:* Vital signs, general health; hearing, nystagmus, balance.

Nursing Diagnoses and Interventions

The risk for trauma in clients with inner ear disorders is great. Attacks of vertigo may occur without warning and can be so severe that the client is unable to remain upright. If frequent attacks are accompanied by nausea, nutrition may be compromised. Constant or intermittent tinnitus can interfere with sleep and rest. Finally, because nearly all inner ear disorders are associated with some degree of hearing loss, which may be progressive, the client has significant psychosocial needs.

Risk for Trauma

Because of the unpredictable nature of attacks, the client with vertigo due to an inner ear disorder needs to learn strategies for dealing with an acute episode. Because vertigo tends to be chronic except in acute labyrinthitis, the emphasis is on helping the client develop strategies to reduce the frequency of attacks and the risk of injury.

- Monitor for vertigo, nystagmus, nausea, vomiting, and hearing loss. *Monitoring is important to determine the severity of impairment, the duration of attacks, and the client's ability to predict an impending attack.*
- Instruct to not get up without assistance during episodes of vertigo. *During attacks of vertigo, assistance reduces the risk of falling.*

> **PRACTICE ALERT**
> During an acute attack of vertigo, keep on bed rest with the side rails raised and the call light readily accessible.

- Teach to avoid sudden head movements or position changes. *Sudden movement may precipitate an attack of vertigo.*
- Administer prescribed medications as ordered, including antiemetics, diuretics, and sedatives. *These medications may reduce the frequency, severity, and duration of vertigo attacks.*
- Instruct to take the prescribed medication and lie down in a quiet, darkened room when an impending attack is sensed. *These measures help protect the client from injury and may shorten the duration and reduce the severity of the attack.*
- Advise to pull to the side of the road and wait for the symptoms to subside if an attack occurs while driving. *Perception and judgment necessary for safe driving may be impaired during an acute attack; pulling off the road is vital to protect the safety of the client and others.*
- Discuss the effect of unilateral hearing loss on the ability to identify the direction of sounds. To ensure safety, encourage the client to use other senses (e.g., when crossing the street). *Just as depth perception changes when vision is lost in one eye, sound perception and differentiation of direction change when hearing is lost unilaterally.*

Disturbed Sleep Pattern

The tinnitus often associated with inner ear disorders may be loud and continuous, interfering with the client's ability to concentrate, relax, and sleep. It may be perceived as a continuous high-pitched whine, buzzing, ringing, or humming sound. In some clients, it may have a pulsatile quality.

- Refer for a complete hearing and ear examination if one has not been done. *Although most tinnitus is associated with hearing loss, often due to noise exposure, it may also be associated with treatable conditions such as impacted cerumen, hypertension, cerebrovascular disorders, and other conditions.*
- Discuss options for masking tinnitus to promote concentration and sleep:
  a. Ambient noise from a radio or sound system
  b. Masking device or white-noise machine
  c. Hearing aid that produces a tone to mask the tinnitus
  d. Hearing aid that amplifies ambient sound.
  These techniques or devices help mask the subjective perception of tinnitus, allowing the client to focus on something other than the sound.
- Discuss the possible risks and benefits of medications to treat tinnitus. *Many medications have been used to treat tinnitus; oral antidepressants such as nortriptyline (Aventyl, Pamelor) taken at bedtime have been shown to be most effective.*

Using NANDA, NIC, and NOC

Linkages between nursing diagnoses, nursing interventions, and nursing outcomes for the client with an inner ear disorder are illustrated in Chart 48–3.

NANDA, NIC, AND NOC LINKAGES
CHART 48–3 The Client with an Inner Ear Disorder

NANDA

Disturbed Sensory Perception: Auditory

↓

NIC

Communication Enhancement: Hearing Deficit

Environmental Management: Safety

↓

NOC

Hearing Compensation Behavior

Risk Control: Hearing Impairment

Safety Behavior: Fall Prevention

Data from *NANDA's Nursing Diagnoses: Definition & Classification 2005–2006* by NANDA International (2005), Philadelphia; *Nursing Interventions Classification (NIC)* (4th ed.) by J. M. Dochterman & G. M. Bulechek (2004), St. Louis, MO: Mosby; and *Nursing Outcomes Classification (NOC)* (3rd ed.) by S. Moorhead, M. Johnson, and M. Mass (2004), St. Louis, MO: Mosby.

Community-Based Care

Because disorders of the inner ear disrupt balance, safety is a primary focus of teaching. Assist the client to identify possible hazards in the home environment. Discuss the following points during the teaching session:

- Change positions slowly, especially when ambulating.
- Turn the whole body rather than just the head.
- Sit down immediately with the onset of vertigo and lie down if possible.
- Take prescribed antiemetic and antivertigo medications.
- Wear Medic-Alert identification.
- If appropriate, discuss the surgical procedure, the immediate postoperative period, and the long-term effects of the surgery.
- Discuss alternative communication techniques as needed.
- Suggest the following resources:
  - Better Hearing Institute
  - Self-Help for Hard of Hearing People.

THE CLIENT WITH AN ACOUSTIC NEUROMA

An **acoustic neuroma** or schwannoma is a benign tumor of cranial nerve VIII. It typically occurs in adults between the ages of 40 and 50. Acoustic neuromas are common and account for 7% to 8% of intracranial tumors (Way & Doherty, 2003).

These tumors usually occur in the internal auditory meatus, compressing the auditory nerve where it exits the skull to the inner ear. Both the vestibular and cochlear branches are affected; however, the tumor arises from the vestibular division of the auditory nerve twice as often. If allowed to grow, the tumor eventually destroys the labyrinth, including the cochlea and vestibular apparatus. As the tumor expands, it erodes the wall of the internal auditory meatus. The tumor may eventually impinge on the inferior cerebellar artery, which provides blood to the lateral pons and medulla, the brainstem, and the cerebellum. An obstructive hydrocephalus can also occur. Cranial nerves VII (facial) and V (trigeminal) are often affected by the expanding tumor; the tumor frequently wraps around the facial nerve.

Early manifestations of an acoustic neuroma are those associated with disorders of the inner ear: tinnitus, unilateral hearing loss, and nystagmus. Dizziness or vertigo may occur. As the tumor expands and occupies increasing amounts of space in the closed cranium, the client experiences neurologic signs related to the area of the brain affected.

The presence of the tumor can generally be identified on CT or MRI scans. X-ray films of the petrous pyramid of the temporal bone may show erosion caused by the tumor.

The treatment of choice for an acoustic neuroma is surgical excision. In surgery, every effort is made to preserve this nerve and its function as well as other cranial nerves that may be affected. Small tumors of the vestibular division of the acoustic nerve may be excised using microsurgical techniques; hearing can often be preserved. A translabyrinthine approach provides good access to the tumor and allows the facial nerve to be preserved. However, this approach destroys hearing in the affected ear, and it is usually used only when the tumor is large or little

effective hearing remains in the affected ear. Larger tumors require craniotomy for removal; facial nerve paralysis is a common result of surgery.

Postoperative nursing care focuses on preserving cerebral function. Position the client to minimize cerebral edema and monitor frequently for signs of increased intracranial pressure. Because the gag reflex may be affected, assess the client carefully before food and fluids are allowed by mouth. Speech therapy is often prescribed for the client after surgery. Because deficits may not resolve for a long time after surgery, education and support are vital components of nursing care for the client. (See Chapter 44 ∞ for care of the client undergoing craniotomy.)

THE CLIENT WITH HEARING LOSS

Hearing loss is a significant problem, affecting an estimated 10% of adults in the United States (Kasper et al., 2005). The problem of hearing loss is particularly significant in older adults, affecting about 30% to 35% of people between the ages of 65 and 74, and more than 40% of those over age 75 (National Institute on Deafness and Other Communication Disorders, 2005d). As many as 70% of nursing home residents have impaired hearing.

Hearing loss impairs the ability to communicate in a world filled with sound and hearing individuals. A hearing deficit can be partial or total, congenital or acquired. It may affect one or both ears. In some types of hearing loss, the ability to perceive sound at specific frequencies is lost. In others, hearing is diminished across all frequencies.

Clients with a hearing loss often display signs that caregivers can recognize. The voice volume of the client with impaired hearing frequently increases, and the client positions the head with the better ear toward the speaker. The client frequently may ask people to repeat what they have said or respond inappropriately to questions or statements. A question may elicit a blank look if the client has not heard or understood its content.

Pathophysiology and Manifestations

Lesions in the outer ear, middle ear, inner ear, or central auditory pathways can result in hearing loss. The process of aging also can affect the structures of the ear and hearing. Hearing loss is classified as conductive, sensorineural, or mixed, depending on what portion of the auditory system is affected. Profound deafness is often a congenital condition.

Conductive Hearing Loss

Anything that disrupts the transmission of sound from the external auditory meatus to the inner ear results in a conductive hearing loss. The most common cause of conductive hearing loss is obstruction of the external ear canal. Impacted cerumen, edema of the canal lining, stenosis, and neoplasms all may lead to canal obstruction. Other causes of conductive loss include a perforated tympanic membrane, disruption or fixation of the ossicles of the middle ear, fluid, scarring, or tumors of the middle ear.

With conductive hearing loss, there is an equal loss of hearing at all sound frequencies. If the level of sound is greater than the threshold for hearing, speech discrimination is good. Because of this, the client with a conductive hearing loss benefits from amplification by a hearing aid.

Sensorineural Hearing Loss

Disorders that affect the inner ear, the auditory nerve, or the auditory pathways of the brain may lead to a sensorineural hearing loss. In this type of hearing loss, sound waves are effectively transmitted to the inner ear. In the inner ear, however, lost or damaged receptor cells, changes in the cochlear apparatus, or auditory nerve abnormalities decrease or distort the ability to receive and interpret stimuli.

A significant cause of sensorineural hearing deficit is damage to the hair cells of the organ of Corti. In the United States, noise exposure is the major cause. Damage may result from either loud impulse noise (e.g., an explosion) or loud continuous noise (e.g., machinery). Exposure to a high level of noise (e.g., standing close to the stage or speakers at a rock concert) on an intermittent or continuing basis damages the hair and supporting cells of the organ of Corti. Ototoxic drugs also damage the hair cells; when combined with high noise levels, the damage is greater and resultant hearing loss more profound. Ototoxic drugs include aspirin, furosemide (Lasix), aminoglycosides, streptomycin, vancomycin (Vancocin), antimalarial drugs, and chemotherapy such as cisplatin (Platinol). Other potential causes of sensory hearing loss include prenatal exposure to rubella, viral infections, meningitis, trauma, Ménière's disease, and aging.

Tumors such as acoustic neuromas, vascular disorders, demyelinating or degenerative diseases, infections (bacterial meningitis in particular), or trauma may affect the central auditory pathways and produce a neural hearing loss.

Sensorineural hearing losses typically affect the ability to hear high-frequency tones more than low-frequency tones. This loss makes speech discrimination difficult, especially in a noisy environment. Hearing aids are often not useful, because they amplify both speech and background noise. The increased sound intensity may actually cause discomfort for the client.

Presbycusis

With aging, the hair cells of the cochlea degenerate, producing a progressive sensorineural hearing loss. In **presbycusis**, gradual hearing loss associated with aging, hearing acuity begins to decrease in early adulthood and progresses as long as the individual lives. Higher pitched tones and conversational speech are lost initially. Hearing aids and other amplification devices are useful for most clients with presbycusis.

Because the hearing loss of presbycusis is gradual, the client and family may not realize the extent of the deficit. The individual with a hearing impairment may be described as unsociable or paranoid. The family may worry that the person is becoming increasingly forgetful, absentminded, or perhaps "senile." Depression, confusion, inattentiveness, tension, and negativism have been noted in older adults with hearing impairments. Functional problems such as poor general health, reduced mobility, and impaired interpersonal communication are also associated with hearing loss. Caregivers need to be alert for signs of impaired hearing such as cupping an ear, difficulty understanding verbal communication when the person cannot

see the speaker's face, difficulty following conversation in a large group, and withdrawal from social activities.

Tinnitus

Tinnitus is the perception of sound or noise in the ears without stimulus from the environment. The sound may be steady, intermittent, or pulsatile and is often described as a buzzing, roaring, or ringing.

Tinnitus is usually associated with hearing loss (conductive or sensorineural); however, the mechanism producing the sound is poorly understood. It is often an early symptom of noise-induced hearing damage and drug-related ototoxicity. Tinnitus is especially associated with salicylate, quinine, or quinidine toxicity. Other etiologies include obstruction of the auditory meatus, presbycusis, middle or inner ear inflammations and infections, otosclerosis, and Ménière's disease. Most tinnitus, however, is chronic and has no pathologic importance.

Tinnitus that is intermittent or slight enough to be masked by environmental sounds is often well tolerated. When it is loud, continuous, and not responsive to treatment, tinnitus can be a significant stressor. It can interfere with activities of daily living, sleep, and rest.

INTERDISCIPLINARY CARE

The best treatment for hearing loss is prevention. Clients need to know the risk for hearing damage and how to prevent it. Awareness of the effects of noise exposure, especially when combined with the ototoxic effects of aspirin or other drugs, is important to prevent sensorineural hearing loss.

Diagnosis

Hearing evaluation includes gross tests of hearing (such as the whisper test), the Rinne and Weber tests, and audiometry.

- *Rinne* and *Weber tests* compare air and bone sound conduction. When bone conduction of sound is better than air conduction, the hearing deficit is a conductive loss. The Rinne test can identify even mild conductive hearing losses. If both air and bone conduction are impaired, a sensorineural loss is indicated (Chapter 47 ∞).
- *Audiometry* identifies the type and pattern of hearing loss. Specific sound frequencies are presented to each ear by either air or bone conduction.
- *Speech audiometry* identifies the intensity at which speech can be recognized and interpreted. *Speech discrimination* evaluates the ability to discriminate among various speech sounds.
- *Tympanometry* is an indirect measurement of the compliance and impedance of the middle ear to sound transmission. The external auditory meatus is subjected to neutral, positive, and negative air pressure while the resultant sound energy flow is monitored.
- *Acoustic reflex testing* uses a tone presented at various intensities to evaluate movement of the structures of the middle ear.

Amplification

A hearing aid or other amplification device can help many clients with hearing deficits. These assistive devices do nothing to prevent, minimize, or treat the hearing loss itself. They amplify the sound presented to the hearing apparatus of the ear, which may bring the level of sound above the hearing threshold, allowing more accurate perception and interpretation of its meaning. When sound perception is distorted, a hearing aid may be less helpful, because it simply amplifies the distorted sound.

Unfortunately, less than one-fifth of older clients with a hearing deficit have or use a hearing aid. Denial of the deficit, other health problems, poor visual acuity, decreased manual dexterity, and cost all contribute to this low usage. Hearing aids must be individually prescribed by an audiologist. Proper design, proper fit, and regular maintenance are necessary for their effectiveness.

All hearing aids include a microphone, amplifier, speaker, earpiece, and volume control. Many include an option to turn off the microphone when using the telephone, others can be adjusted for the client's pattern of hearing loss. Hearing aids are available in a variety of styles, each with advantages and disadvantages:

- Canal hearing aids (in-the-canal and completely-in-canal) are the least noticeable style, fitting in the ear canal. They are appropriate for mild to moderately severe hearing loss. These small and unobtrusive devices allow use of the telephone and can be worn during exercise. Because of their small size, the client must have good manual dexterity to insert, clean, and change the batteries on canal hearing aids. For this reason, older clients or clients with impaired dexterity may be unable to use them.
- The in-ear style of hearing aid fits into the external ear and is used for mild to severe hearing loss (Figure 48–16 ■). Its larger size makes manipulation somewhat easier, although it still may be difficult for less dexterous individuals. A greater degree of amplification is possible with the in-ear aid. Many have a toggle switch for telephone usage.
- The behind-ear hearing aid allows finer adjustment of the level of amplification and is easier for the client to manipulate (Figure 48–17 ■). They can be used by clients with mild to profound hearing loss. For the client who wears glasses, this style can be modified, with all components fitting into the temple of the eyeglasses.
- Clients with profound hearing loss may require a body hearing aid. The microphone and amplifier of this aid are contained in a pocket-sized case that the client clips on to clothing, slips into a pocket, or carries in a harness. The re-

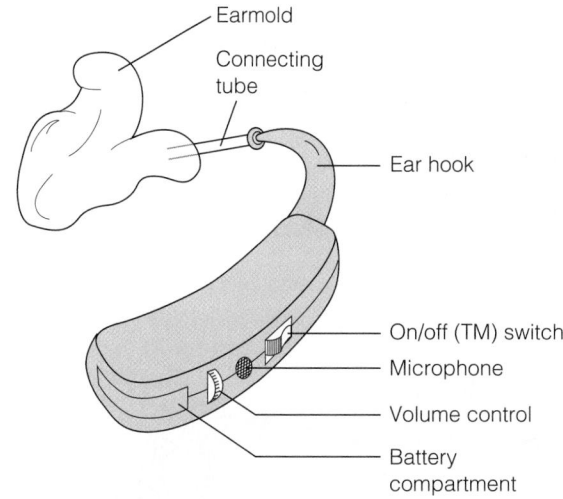

Figure 48–17 ■ A behind-ear hearing aid.

ceiver is attached by a cord to the case and clips onto the ear mold, which delivers the sound to the ear canal.

With both the in-canal and in-ear style, cleaning is important. Small portals may become plugged with cerumen, interfering with sound transmission.

For the client who does not have a hearing aid, an *assistive listening device,* or "pocket talker," with a microphone and "Walkman" type earpieces, is useful. Pocket talkers are available over the counter or through an audiologist and are relatively inexpensive. The earpiece requires no special fitting, and the external microphone allows the client to focus on the desired sound rather than simply amplifying all sounds. Assistive listening devices may also be used in conjunction with a hearing aid.

Clients with tinnitus may find a white-noise masking device helpful to promote concentration and rest. These devices conduct a pleasant sound to the affected ear, allowing the client to block out the abnormal sound.

Surgery

Reconstructive surgeries of the middle ear, such as a stapedectomy or tympanoplasty, may help restore hearing with a conductive hearing loss. Stapedectomy is the removal and replacement of the stapes. This procedure is used to treat hearing loss related to otosclerosis.

In a tympanoplasty, the structures of the middle ear are reconstructed to improve conductive hearing deficits. Chronic otitis media with necrosis and scarring of the middle ear is a common indication for this type of surgery.

For the client with a sensorineural hearing loss, a *cochlear implant* may be the only hope for restoring sound perception. The cochlear implant consists of a microphone, speech processor, transmitter and receiver/stimulator, and electrodes (Figure 48–18 ■). Its function is more similar to the way the ear normally receives and processes sounds than it is to a hearing aid. The microphone picks up sounds, sending them to the speech processor, which selects and processes useful sounds. The transmitter and receiver/stimulator receive signals from the speech processor, convert them to electrical impulses, and

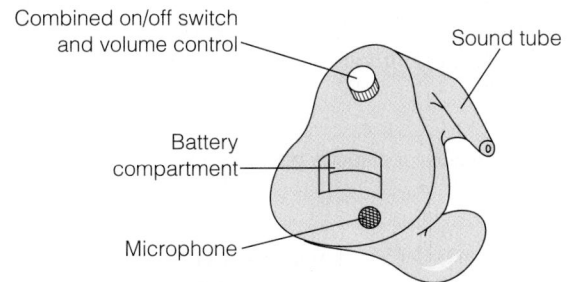

Figure 48–16 ■ An in-ear hearing aid.

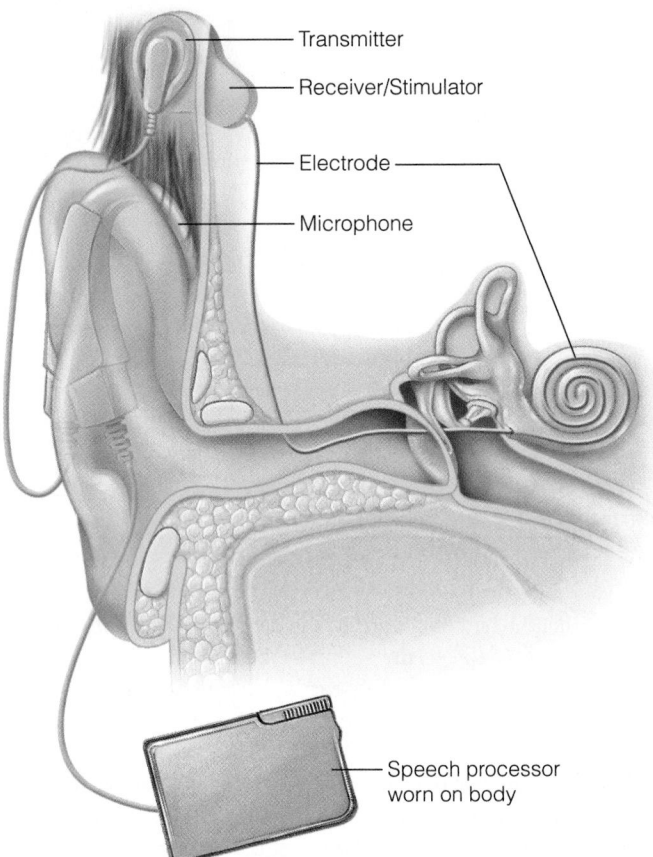

Figure 48-18 ■ A cochlear implant for sensorineural hearing loss.

send these impulses to the electrodes for transmission to the brain.

Cochlear implants provide sound perception but not normal hearing. The client is able to recognize warning sounds such as automobiles, sirens, telephones, and doors opening or closing. They also receive stimuli to alert them to incoming communication so they can focus on the person speaking. Many clients learn to interpret perceived sounds as words, especially when the hearing loss is acquired as an adult.

NURSING CARE

In planning and implementing nursing care for the client with a hearing deficit, the type and extent of hearing loss, the client's adaptation to the loss, and the availability of assistive hearing devices are considered, as well as the client's ability and willingness to use assistive devices.

Health Promotion

Healthcare personnel can be instrumental in preventing hearing loss through education. It is important to promote environmental noise control and the use of ear protection. The Occupational Safety and Health Administration requires ear protection for work environments that consis-

tently exceed 85 decibels. Teaching for primary prevention focuses on the following:
- Care of the ears and ear canals, including cleaning and treatment of infection
- Not placing hard objects into the ear canal
- Use of plugs to protect the ears during swimming or diving
- Avoiding intermittent or frequent exposure to loud noise
- Monitoring for side effects with ototoxic medications
- Hearing evaluation when hearing difficulty is present.

Assessment

- *Health history:* Perceived ability to hear; effect of hearing loss on function and lifestyle; risk factors such as use of ototoxic medications; upper respiratory tract or frequent ear infection; noise exposure; presence of vertigo, tinnitus, unsteadiness, or imbalance.
- *Physical examination:* Apparent perception of normal speech; inspection of external ear, tympanic membrane; whisper, Rinne, and Weber tests; tests of balance and cranial nerve function.

Nursing Diagnoses and Interventions

This section focuses on the problems of having a hearing deficit, impaired communication, and social isolation for the client who is hearing impaired.

Disturbed Sensory Perception: Auditory

Whether the client's hearing deficit is partial or total, impaired sound perception is the primary problem. The client needs to understand what causes the deficit and what to expect for the future. Nursing interventions focus on maximizing available hearing and preventing further deterioration to the extent possible.

- Encourage to talk about the hearing loss and its effect on activities of daily living. *Hearing loss affects each individual in a different way. The client may be denying the extent of the deficit or grieving the loss. Listening and providing support encourage the client to develop coping strategies.*
- Provide information about the type of hearing loss. Refer to an audiologist for evaluation of the hearing loss and possible exploration of amplification devices. *With improved understanding of the deficit, the client can plan ways to compensate.*
- Replace batteries in hearing aids regularly and as needed. *Hearing aid batteries last approximately 1 week. If a battery is old or has been improperly stored, the life may be reduced further.*
- If the hearing aid has a toggle switch for microphone/telephone, be sure it is in the appropriate position. *This ensures proper amplification with the hearing aid.*

> **PRACTICE ALERT**
> Check hearing aids for patency, cleaning out cerumen as necessary.

Impaired Verbal Communication

A hearing deficit impairs the client's ability to receive and interpret verbal communication. A hearing loss affects the client's

Labels in figure: Transmitter; Receiver/Stimulator; Electrode; Microphone; Speech processor worn on body ability to follow conversations, use the telephone, and enjoy television or other forms of entertainment.

- Use the following techniques to improve communication:
  a. Wave the hand or tap the shoulder before beginning to speak.
  b. If the client wears corrective lenses, ensure that they are clean, and encourage the client to wear them.
  c. When speaking, face your client and keep your hands away from your face.
  d. Keep your face in full light.
  e. Reduce the noise in the environment before speaking.
  f. Use a low voice pitch with normal loudness.
  g. Use short sentences and pause at the end of each sentence.
  h. Speak at a normal rate, and do not overarticulate.
  i. Use facial expressions or gestures.
  j. Provide a magic slate for written communication.

Individuals with hearing impairments often lip-read, making good visibility of the speaker's face necessary. Excessive environmental noise interferes with the ability to perceive the message. Higher tones are typically lost with presbycusis and other types of hearing loss. Using short sentences and pausing give the client time to interpret the message. Overarticulating makes it more difficult to follow the flow and to lip-read. Nonverbal cues and written messages enhance the client's understanding.

- Be sure hearing aid is properly placed, is turned on, and has fresh batteries. *The client may not be aware that the hearing aid is not functioning well.*
- Do not place intravenous catheters in the dominant hand. *The client may need to use that hand to write.*
- Rephrase sentences when there is difficulty understanding. *Hearing losses may affect different sound tones, making some words more difficult to comprehend. Using alternative words and phrases may increase the client's ability to perceive the message.*
- Repeat important information. *The nurse makes sure that the client understands the information.*
- Inform other staff about the client's hearing deficit and effective strategies for communication. *Consistent use of effective strategies for communication decreases the client's frustration.*

Social Isolation

The client with impaired hearing often becomes socially isolated. This isolation may be self-imposed because of difficulty communicating, especially in a group. Often, however, the isolation comes about gradually and without intention. The client finds social settings such as family dinners or community gatherings increasingly difficult. Friends and family become frustrated trying to communicate with someone who has a hearing impairment, and invitations to participate in social activities dwindle.

- Identify the extent and cause of the social isolation. Help to differentiate the reality of the isolation and its cause from the client's perception of isolation. *Clients with impaired hearing may be unaware that they are isolated. Identifying factors that contribute to isolation may provide the needed impetus*

to remedy the hearing loss. Clients may also experience paranoid thinking as a result of impaired communication and believe that friends and family have purposely begun to avoid interactions.

- Encourage to interact with friends and family on a one-to-one basis in quiet settings. *Clients with impaired hearing are more successful in understanding conversations that take place in small groups and quiet settings.*
- Treat with dignity and remind friends and family that a hearing deficit does not indicate loss of mental faculties. *Inappropriate responses due to a hearing deficit can cause others to perceive the client as "stupid" or demented.*
- Involve in activities that do not require acute hearing, such as checkers and chess. *The client has an opportunity to interact socially without the stress of straining to hear.*
- Obtain a pocket talker or encourage the client and family to do so.
- Refer the client to an audiologist for evaluation and possible hearing-aid fitting.
- Refer to resources such as support groups and senior citizen centers. *These groups provide new social outlets.*

Using NANDA, NIC, and NOC

Chart 48–4 illustrates linkages between NANDA nursing diagnoses, NIC, and NOC for the client with a hearing deficit.

Community-Based Care

Teaching for home and community-based care for the client with hearing loss focuses on managing the deficit and developing coping strategies. Referral to an audiologist for evaluation of the deficit and the usefulness of a hearing aid may be

NANDA, NIC, AND NOC LINKAGES
CHART 48–4 The Client with a Hearing Deficit

NANDA

Impaired Verbal Communication

↓

NIC

Active Listening

Communication Enhancement, Hearing Deficit

↓

NOC

Communication Ability

Communication: Receptive Ability

Data from *NANDA's Nursing Diagnoses: Definitions & Classification 2005–2006* by NANDA International (2005), Philadelphia; *Nursing Interventions Classification (NIC)* (4th ed.) by J. M. Dochterman & G. M. Bulechek (2004), St. Louis, MO: Mosby; and *Nursing Outcomes Classification (NOC)* (3rd ed.) by S. Moorhead, M. Johnson, and M. Maas (2004), St. Louis, MO: Mosby.

appropriate. In addition, discuss the following topics as appropriate for each client:

- Use, care, and maintenance of a hearing aid
- Strategies for coping with the hearing deficit
- Voicing a preference for individual visits and small group interactions rather than large social functions
- Helpful resources include the following:

- American Academy of Audiology
- American Speech-Language-Hearing Association
- House Ear Institute
- National Institute on Deafness and Other Communication Disorders
- National Deaf Education Center
- Self-Help for Hard of Hearing People.

EXPLORE MEDIALINK

Prentice Hall Nursing MediaLink DVD-ROM

Audio Glossary
NCLEX Review

Animations/Video
Middle Ear Dynamics
Pilocarpine

COMPANION WEBSITE www.prenhall.com/lemone

Audio Glossary
NCLEX-RN® Review
Care Plan Activity: The Client with a Hearing Aid
Case Study: Retinal Detachment
MediaLink Application: Cataracts
Links to Resources

CHAPTER HIGHLIGHTS

- Structures of the external eye are vulnerable to trauma and infection. While usually minor, these problems can cause significant pain, scarring and clouding of the cornea, and loss or impairment of vision.
- Cataracts, glaucoma, age-related macular degeneration, and diabetic retinopathy are leading causes of visual impairment in the United States. While these conditions cannot, in most cases, be prevented, they often can be treated or their progress slowed, preserving vision.
- Age, smoking, diabetes, and long-term use of certain drugs are risk factors for cataract development. Removal of the clouded lens with insertion of an intraocular lens is the treatment of choice for cataracts. Surgery is elective, performed only when the cataract significantly impairs the ability to maintain ADLs and recreational activities.
- Glaucoma is progressive loss of visual fields associated with increased intraocular pressure and impaired aqueous humor drainage. Open-angle glaucoma, the predominant form of the disorder, can be controlled using medications and, as needed, laser surgery to promote aqueous humor drainage.
- Angle-closure glaucoma is a medical emergency requiring immediate treatment to lower intraocular pressure to preserve vision. Angle-closure glaucoma usually affects only one eye; however, the client is at risk for future attacks affecting the other eye.
- Age-related macular degeneration, a leading cause of blindness, cannot be effectively treated, although its progress may be slowed or halted through use of high-dose antioxidant vitamins and zinc if it is identified early. Macular degeneration affects the macula, the area of high-acuity central vision.

- Diabetic retinopathy eventually affects nearly all people with diabetes. It is a disease of the small blood vessels of the retina, leading to formation of aneurysms, retinal ischemia, and growth of fragile new vessels (neovascularization) that easily rupture leading to hemorrhage. It is treated with laser surgery to seal fragile vessels.
- Otitis media is related to eustachian tube dysfunction, with impaired pressure equalization of the middle ear. Otitis media may be either serous (sterile) or infectious (suppurative). Both cause acute discomfort with diminished hearing, snapping, popping, and possible vertigo and systemic symptoms. The risk of complications, including rupture of the tympanic membrane, damage to structures of the middle ear, and spread of infection to surrounding tissues, is greater with acute suppurative otitis media.
- Potential complications of acute otitis media include mastoiditis, chronic otitis media with tympanic membrane perforation, and cholesteatoma formation. Hearing loss in the affected ear is a possibility with these disorders. The primary treatment is prevention through adequate treatment of acute otitis media.
- The primary manifestations of disorders of the inner ear are vertigo and possible hearing loss. Severe vertigo can interfere with safety, nutrition, and the client's ability to maintain ADLs and life roles.
- The two major types of hearing loss are conductive and sensorineural. Presbycusis, hearing loss associated with aging, is a type of sensorineural hearing loss. Hearing loss may be accompanied by tinnitus, the perception of sound without an environmental stimulus. Amplification devices (hearing aids) are the primary treatment for hearing loss.

TEST YOURSELF NCLEX-RN® REVIEW

1 A nurse is working with a group of residents in a long-term care facility. All of the residents have moderate to severe hearing or vision impairment. Which of the following does the nurse identify as the highest priority of care?
1. preventing sensory deprivation
2. encouraging social interaction
3. promoting family relationships
4. maintaining resident safety

2 The nurse teaching a client with newly diagnosed glaucoma emphasizes which of the following instructions?
1. turning the head side to side to compensate for impaired peripheral vision
2. using the prescribed eyedrops as directed on a continuing basis
3. contacting the physician if further decline in vision is noticed
4. avoiding coughing, sneezing, or straining to have a bowel movement

3 A patient with glaucoma has a history of heart failure. Which medication should the nurse discuss with the physician before administering it?
1. brimonidine (Alphagan)
2. dorzolamide (Trusopt)
3. timolol (Timoptic)
4. latanoprost (Xalatan)

4 A client with Ménière's disease experiences frequent attacks of vertigo and tinnitus. Of the following teaching points, which one has the highest priority for this client?
1. Follow a low-sodium diet.
2. Stop smoking.
3. Take prescribed antiemetic medications.
4. Sit down when an attack develops.

5 On a client's return from cataract surgery, the nurse in the ambulatory surgery recovery unit places the client:
1. in semi-Fowler's position.
2. on the affected side.
3. in a private room.
4. in proximity to the nurses' station.

6 A client calls her primary care provider's office with complaints of bright flashing lights to the side of her vision. The appropriate response by the nurse is to:
1. recommend that she lie down until the sensation has passed.
2. advise her to make an appointment to have her blood pressure checked.
3. initiate immediate referral to an ophthalmologist.
4. reassure her that this is not unusual and should resolve without treatment.

7 A client presents at the urgent care clinic with complaints of right ear pain. Which of the following should be included in physical assessment of this client? (Select all that apply.)
1. vital signs with temperature
2. inspection of the oral pharynx
3. manipulation of the ear pinna
4. palpation of cervical lymph nodes
5. inspection of the ear canal and tympanic membrane

8 An elderly resident in an assisted living facility complains to the nurse that his head "feels stuffy" and he has ringing in his ears. The appropriate response by the nurse would be to
1. make an appointment with the resident's primary care physician.
2. refer the client for evaluation by a local audiologist.
3. provide nonprescription eardrops for daily use.
4. inspect the ear canals for patency.

9 The nurse caring for a client with a severe hearing deficit identifies which of the following as an appropriate goal toward improving the client's social interactions?
1. Will plan to have dinner with one or two friends weekly.
2. Will participate in senior center communal lunches at least twice per week.
3. Will engage in activities such as card tournaments and dancing.
4. Will attend religious services of choice.

10 When assessing a client, the nurse notes absence of the red reflex in the client's right eye. On questioning, the client responds "Oh yes, my doctor told me I have cataracts. When do you think I should have them removed?" How should the nurse respond?
1. "It appears that the right eye is due for surgery."
2. "Are you having difficulty reading or doing activities you enjoy?"
3. "Are you starting to experience pain in your right eye or frequent headaches?"
4. "Cataracts can be removed any time that it is convenient for you."

See Test Yourself answers in Appendix C.

BIBLIOGRAPHY

Alper, B. S. (2005a). Evidence-based medicine. Lowering intraocular pressure delays visual-field loss in glaucoma. *Clinical Advisor for Nurse Practitioners, 8*(12), 128.

_____. (2005b). Evidence-based medicine. Lowering intraocular pressure may prevent glaucoma. *Clinical Advisor for Nurse Practitioners, 8*(12), 128.

Bremridge, T. (2005). Caring for those with age-related impaired sight. *Nursing & Residential Care, 7*(11), 507–509.

Browne, M. (2003). The nurse's role in helping patients cope with sight loss. *Nursing Times, 99*(48), 30–31.

Clinical: Glaucoma. (2005). *Nursing Times, 101*(6), 33.

Clinical: What you need to know about infective conjunctivitis. (2004). *Nursing Times, 100*(34), 31.

Cohen, A. S., & Ayello, E. A. (2005). Diabetes has taken a toll on your patient's vision: How can you help? *Nursing, 35*(5), 44–47.

Conley, Y. P., & Gorin, M. B. (2003). The genetics of age-related macular degeneration. *Medsurg Nursing, 12*(4), 238–241, 259.

Copstead, L. E., & Banasik, J. L. (2005). *Pathophysiology* (3rd ed.). Philadelphia: W. B. Saunders.

Davies, S., & de Guzman, A. (2004). Ear drops containing steroids were better than acetic acid for otitis externa. *Evidence-Based Nursing, 7*(2), 43.

Dochterman, J., & Bulechek, G. (2004). *Nursing interventions classification (NIC)* (4th ed.). St. Louis, MO: Mosby.

Ervin, S. E. (2004). Ménière's disease: Identifying classic symptoms and current treatments. *AAOHN Journal, 52*(4), 156–158.

Fontaine, K. L. (2005). *Healing practices: Alternative therapies for nursing* (2nd ed.). Upper Saddle River, NJ: Prentice Hall Health.

Gallacher, R. (2004). Understanding the nursing role in patients who have cataract. *Nursing Times, 100*(21), 31.

Greenlee, E. C. (2005). Laser and surgical treatments for glaucoma: an overview. *Insight: The Journal of the American Society of Ophthalmic Registered Nurses, 30*(4), 32–37.

Halverson, P. (2005). The silent thief. *RN, 68*(3), 41–45, 70–71, 33.

Heimink, A. L., & Sego, S. (2005). Advisor forum. Chronic tinnitus treatment. *Clinical Advisor for Nurse Practitioners, 8*(4), 56.

Holcomb, S. S. (2004). This just in. New guidelines improve treatment of otitis media. *Nurse Practitioner: American Journal of Primary Health Care, 29*(10), 6, 8, 13.

Holman, C., Roberts, S., & Nicol, M. (2005). Promoting good care for people with hearing impairment. *Nursing Older People, 17*(2), 31–32.

Houde, S. C., & Huff, M. A. (2003). Age-related vision loss in older adults: A challenge for gerontological nurses. *Journal of Gerontological Nursing, 29*(4), 25–33, 51–52.

Kasper, D. L., Braunwald, E., Fauci, A. S., Hauser, S. L., Longo, D. L., & Jameson, J. L. (Eds.). (2005). *Harrison's principles of internal medicine* (16th ed.). New York: McGraw-Hill.

Kenny, C. (2003). Taking eye care to the patient. *Nursing Times, 99*(21), 40–41.

Kleinbeck, C., & Williams, A. S. (2004). Disabilities, diabetes, and devices. *Home Healthcare Nurse, 22*(7), 469–475.

Lusk, S. L., Ronis, D. L., Kazanis, A. S., Eakin, B. L., Hong, O., & Raymond, D. M. (2003). Effectiveness of a tailored intervention to increase factory workers' use of hearing protection. *Nursing Research, 52*(5), 289–295.

Malmstrom, J. (2005). National Conference of Gerontological Nurse Practitioners. Gerontologic nurse practitioner care guidelines: assessing and managing hearing deficits in the older adult. *Geriatric Nursing, 26*(1), 57–59.

Marsden, J. (2004a). Clinical. Cataract: The role of nurses in diagnosis, surgery and aftercare. *Nursing Times, 100*(7), 36–40.

_____. (2004b). Clinical. Implications of and treatment options for retinal detachment. *Nursing Times, 100*(37), 44–47.

Moore, L. W., & Miller, M. (2003). Older men's experience of living with severe visual impairment. *Journal of Advanced Nursing, 43*(1), 10–18.

Moore, L. W., & Miller, M. (2005). Driving strategies used by older adults with macular degeneration: Assessing the risks. *Applied Nursing Research, 18*(2), 110–116.

Moorhead, S., Johnson, M., & Maas, M. (2004). *Nursing outcomes classification (NOC)* (3rd ed.). St. Louis, MO: Mosby

National Eye Institutes, National Institutes of Health. (2003a). *Age-related macular degeneration: What you should know* (NIH Publication No. 03-2294). Bethesda, MD: Author.

_____. (2003b). *Cataract: What you should know* (NIH Publication No. 03-201). Bethesda, MD: Author.

_____. (2003c). *Diabetic retinopathy: What you should know* (NIH Publication No. 03-2171). Bethesda, MD: Author.

_____. (2003d). *Glaucoma: What you should know* (NIH Publication No. 03-651). Bethesda, MD: Author.

_____. (2004). *Statistics and data*. Retrieved from http://www.nei.nih.gov/evedata/pbd_tables.asp

_____. (2005a). *Facts about the cornea and corneal disease*. Retrieved from http://www.nei.nih.gov.

_____. (2005c). *Retinal detachment*. Retrieved from http://www.nei.nih.gov

National Guideline Clearinghouse. (2005). *Contact lens care*. Retrieved from http://www.guideline.gov

National Institute on Deafness and Other Communication Disorders, National Institutes of Health. (2005a). *Cochlear implants*. Retrieved February 23, 2005, from http://www.nidcd.nih.gov/health/hearing/coch.asp

_____. (2005b). *Hearing aids*. Retrieved March 1, 2005, from http://www.nidcd.nih.gov/health/hearing/hearingaid.asp

_____. (2005c). *Noise-induced hearing loss*. Retrieved May 4, 2005, from http://www.nidcd.nih.gov/health/hearing/noise.asp

_____. (2005d). *Presbycusis*. Retrieved February 23, 2005, from http://www.nidcd.nih.gov/health/hearing/presbycusis.asp

Neault, G. (2005). Self-care needs of *cataract* patients following ambulatory surgery. *Insight: The Journal of the American Society of Ophthalmic Registered Nurses, 30*(4), 7–11.

Opperwall, B. (2003). Asthma, allergy, and upper airway disease. *Nursing Clinics of North America, 38*(4), 697–711.

Phillips, M. (2003). Genetics of hearing loss. *Medsurg Nursing, 12*(6), 386–390, 411.

Porth, C. M. (2005). *Pathophysiology: Concepts of altered health states* (7th ed.). Philadelphia: Lippincott.

Prevent Blindness America, & National Eye Institute, National Institutes of Health. (2002). *Vision problems in the U.S. Prevalence of adult vision impairment and age-related eye disease in America*. Retrieved from http://www.usvisionproblems.org

Quinlan, K. (2003). The importance of discharge instructions. *Journal of Emergency Nursing, 29*(4), 308.

Rask, E. M. (2004). Recognize cholesteatomas early. *The Nurse Practitioner, 29*(2), 24–27.

Rassin, M., Gorlansky, N., Shahin, E., Hacham, Y., Grant, P., et al. (2005). NT research. Importance of early referral in sudden loss of hearing. *Nursing Times, 101*(49), 34–36.

Rothrock, J. C. (2003). *Alexander's care of the patient in surgery* (12th ed.). St. Louis, MO: Mosby.

Smith, S. C., Lamb, P., & Liu, J. (2005). Age-related macular degeneration: answers to some common questions. *Insight: The Journal of the American Society of Ophthalmic Registered Nurses, 30*(3), 17–23.

Tierney, L. M., McPhee, S. J., & Papadakis, M. A. (Eds.). (2005). *Current medical diagnosis & treatment* (44th ed.). Stamford, CT: Appleton & Lange.

U. S. Preventive Services Task Force. (2005). Screening for glaucoma: Recommendation statement. *American Journal for Nurse Practitioners, 9*(9), 49–50, 52–55.

Watkinson, S. (2005). Visual impairment in older people: The nurse's role. *Nursing Standard, 19*(17), 45–52, 54–55.

Way, L. W., & Doherty, G. M. (2003). *Current surgical diagnosis & treatment* (11th ed.). New York: McGraw-Hill.

Wilkinson, J. M. (2005). *Nursing diagnosis handbook* (8th ed.). Upper Saddle River, NJ: Prentice Hall.

Williams, D. (2005). Does irrigation of the ear to remove impacted wax improve hearing? *British Journal of Community Nursing, 10*(5), 228–232.

Wright, J. (2005). Common ear problems in the primary care setting. *Journal of Community Nursing, 19*(9), 43–44, 46.

UNIT 14 BUILDING CLINICAL COMPETENCE
Responses to Altered Visual and Auditory Function

FUNCTIONAL HEALTH PATTERN: Cognitive-Perceptual

■ Think about clients with impaired vision or hearing for whom you have cared.

- Were their major medical diagnoses related or unrelated to sensory perception?
- How did the clients' sensory disorder interfere with their health status? Did the client have vision changes, eye pain, hearing loss, or vertigo? Did the client wear corrective lenses or use a hearing aid? When was the client's last vision or hearing examination? Did the client use any medications? Did the client have a chronic disease or history of a vision or hearing disorder?

■ The Cognitive-Perceptual Pattern describes the ability to effectively use and interpret input from the five senses: vision, hearing, smell, taste, and touch.

The eyes and ears allow visual and auditory stimuli to reach the brain. The eyes encode patterns of light from the environment through photoreceptors and transmit the information to the brain. The brain gives meaning to the information. Disorders affecting the eyes can lead to manifestations such as:

- Impaired visual acuity (corneal or lens distortion ▶ impaired light ray focus on the retina ▶ distorted or unclear image transmitted to visual centers)
- Vision loss ▶ damage to and loss of retinal sensory receptors ▶ inability to transmit signals from affected retina to visual centers)

■ The primary functions of the ears are hearing and balance. Sound waves vibrate the tympanic membrane, activating structures of the middle and inner ear and generating action potentials. Cranial nerve VIII transmits these signals to the brain for interpretation. The inner ear provides position information used to coordinate body movements, equilibrium, and balance. Ear disorders can lead to manifestations such as:

- Hearing loss (obstruction of or damage to ear structures ▶ impaired sound wave transmission to cochlea ▶ hearing loss cochlear damage impaired transmission of auditory stimuli to auditory centers ▶ hearing loss)
- Vertigo (altered inner ear pressure or circulation ▶ impaired transmission of position sense signals ▶ equilibrium loss and sensations such as whirling or falling)

■ Vision and hearing allow the client to communicate, to gain access to information, and to derive pleasure from sights and sounds in the environment. Priority nursing diagnoses within the cognitive-perceptual health pattern may include:

- *Disturbed Sensory Perception* as evidenced by blurred vision, seeing halos, black spots or floaters, difficulty hearing, altered sense of balance.
- *Impaired Verbal Communication* as evidenced by difficulty comprehending and maintaining communication, inability to articulate speech, absence of eye contact
- *Deficient Knowledge: Vision/Hearing Assistive Devices* as evidenced by expressions of helplessness, lack of health-seeking behaviors
- *Nausea* as evidenced by complaints of queasiness, discomfort associated with movement of the head

■ Two additional nursing diagnoses often are of high priority for the client with altered vision or hearing:

- *Risk for Injury*
- *Ineffective Health Maintenance*

CLINICAL SCENARIO

You have been assigned to work with the following four clients for the 0700 shift on a medical-surgical unit. Significant data obtained during report are as follows:

- Andrew Hardy, a 50-year-old type 1 diabetic with hypertension, is a new admission during the night shift with blood glucose of 600. On assessment, the client reveals that he has been seeing black spot floaters and flashing lights at times. He is now complaining of blurred vision.
- Gladys Harvey is an 84-year-old who had right eye cataract surgery yesterday. Her vital signs have been stable since surgery. She has begun complaining of itching and slight discomfort in the right eye.
- Georgia Stanley is a 45-year-old admitted with complaints of feeling like she is spinning or falling and has ringing and a fullness feeling in her left ear. Her vital signs are T 98.6°F, P 78, R 16, BP 102/68. She is diaphoretic and complains of nausea. She is scheduled for x-rays and a CT scan of her head at 0800.
- Kenneth Koch, a 30-year-old, is a postoperative client who had a right ear tympanoplasty yesterday because of hearing loss due to chronic otitis media. Vital signs are T 99.6°F, P 90, R 20, BP 136/86. The client is requesting medication for ear pain. Pain scale is 9 out of 10 on a scale of 10 being the highest.

Questions

1 In what order would you visit these patients after report?

1. _____
2. _____
3. _____
4. _____

2 What top two priority nursing diagnoses would you choose for each of the clients presented above? Can you explain, if asked, the rationale for your choices?

	Priority Nursing Diagnosis #1	Priority Nursing Diagnosis #2
Andrew Hardy		
Gladys Harvey		
Georgia Stanley		
Kenneth Koch		

3 Which is the correct treatment for a client such as Mr. Hardy who has symptoms of diabetic retinopathy?

1. scleral buckling
2. enucleation
3. photorefractive keratectomy
4. laser photocoagulation

4 After cataract surgery, Ms. Harvey is placed in which position to reduce intraocular pressure?

1. Sims' position on the unaffected side
2. semi-Fowler's position on the unaffected side
3. supine with the head elevated 10 degrees
4. prone position on the affected side

5 A low-sodium diet is ordered for Ms. Stanley, who has Ménière's disease. The client understands this diet when she picks which meal plan?

1. hot dog on a roll with catsup and mustard
2. ham and cheese sandwich with potato salad
3. grilled chicken sandwich with lettuce and tomato
4. hamburger on a roll with potato chips

6 Which assessment data would be most indicative of hyphema, a potential result of blunt eye trauma?

1. eye pain, decreased visual acuity, seeing a reddish tint
2. hypertension, headache, facial pain
3. white eye reflex, pressure and blindness in affected eye
4. double vision, sunken eye, limited eye movement

7 Which techniques may improve communication with the client who has a hearing impairment? (Select all that apply.)

1. Speak loudly to enhance hearing.
2. Speak at a normal rate and avoid overarticulating.
3. Stand in front of a window so client can see the face.
4. Face the client to enhance lip-reading.
5. Turn down the television or radio.
6. Use short sentences and pause frequently.

8 A prescription for gentamicin (Garamycin) is ordered for a client with conjunctivitis. The nurse understands that a serious adverse effect of aminoglycosides is which effect?

1. damage to the eighth cranial nerve resulting in hearing loss
2. vasodilation leading to migraine headaches
3. leg pain caused by thromboembolism
4. stomach irritation leading to gastric ulcers

9 When evaluating for Ménière's disease, which diagnostic studies would you expect to be ordered? (Select all that apply.)

1. caloric testing
2. Rinne and Weber tests
3. troponins
4. complete blood cell count
5. glycerol test
6. blood glucose test

10 After eye surgery, which measures does the nurse instruct the client in?

1. Avoid lifting more than 15 pounds.
2. Avoid coughing or sneezing.
3. Lie on the affected side.
4. Remove the eye patch when sleeping.

11 Which is the correct way to instill eardrops in the adult client with otitis media?

1. Have client hang head over side of bed, pull pinna of the ear straight up, instill eardops and have client turn to instill drops to other ear.
2. Have client tilt head toward unaffected side, pull pinna of the ear down and back, instill eardrops, and have client remain still for 3 minutes.
3. Have client lie on unaffected side, pull the pinna of the ear up and back, instill eardrops, and have client remain still for 5 minutes.
4. Have client lie in Sims' position on unaffected side, pull the pinna of the ear back, instill eardrops, and have the client turn to other side after 1 minute.

12 Which is the appropriate primary prevention to teach Mr. Koch to prevent hearing loss?

1. Cleanse the ear with ear swabs to prevent earwax buildup.
2. Avoid getting water in the ears when showering.
3. Monitor for ringing in the ears when taking acetaminophen.
4. Wear ear protectors when exposed to loud noises.

Case Study

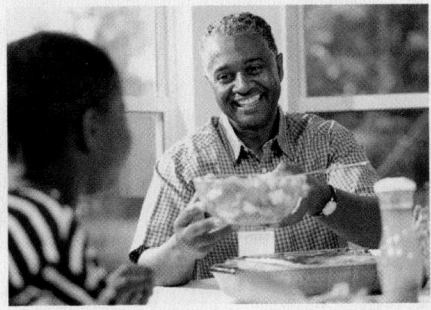

Reggie Madison is a 65-year-old African American male who is seen in the eye clinic for a routine eye examination. He states he has not had any recent eye infections or eye injuries. He denies pain in the eyes. Vital signs are T 98.8°F, P 84, R 16, BP 168/88. His height is 5 '8" and weight is 200 pounds. His medical history indicates that he has hypertension and type 2 diabetes. He is taking hydrochlorothiazide, captopril, and glyburide. He states that he is on a 2000-calorie diabetic diet but he is often noncompliant with the diet. He sees his medical doctor about once a year but has not had an eye exam in about 10 years. He is married with five grown children and six grandchildren. Mr. Madison states he does not know if there is any family history of glaucoma because his father died of a heart attack at age 50 years and his mother died of cancer at 60 years of age.

The ophthalmologist performs a tonometry, which indicates an increase in intraocular pressure. A fundoscopic examination indicates pallor and increase in the size and depth of the optic cup on the optic disc. Visual field testing indicates significant peripheral vision loss. The results of these tests indicate a diagnosis of glaucoma.

Based on the medical diagnosis of open-angle glaucoma and the client's decreased peripheral vision, the nursing diagnosis of *Disturbed Sensory Perception: Visual* is appropriate for planning care for Mr. Madison.

- Obstruction of aqueous humor flow into canal of Schlemm → increased aqueous fluid in eye → increased intraocular pressure
- Increased intraocular pressure → neuronal ischemia → damage to and destruction of optic fibers in the periphery of the optic disc → painless, progressive loss of peripheral vision with narrowing of the visual field and eventual blindness

affects

Mr. R.M.
65 y.o. male
Open-angle glaucoma

leads to

assess →

- 5' 8" tall, 200 lbs.
- T 98.8°F, P 84, R 16
- BP 168/88
- C/o decreased peripheral vision
- History of hypertension, type 2 diabetes
- No known family history of glaucoma
- Current medications: hydrochlorothiazide, captopril, glyburide
- Intraocular pressure 32 mmHg OD, 29 mmHg OS
- Visual field testing reveals significant loss of peripheral vision

generates →

- Risk for Injury r/t loss of vision as evidenced by decreased peripheral visual fields.
- Impaired Home Maintenance r/t impaired vision as evidenced r/t decreased peripheral vision
- Anxiety r/t perceived threat of loss of sight as evidenced by restlessness, poor eye contact, verbalized fears.

generate nursing diagnosis

prioritized to

Disturbed Sensory Perception: Visual

expected outcomes

- Vital signs stable
- Verbalizes understanding of prescribed medications, their administration and side effects
- Able to effectively and appropriately instill eye medications
- Verbalizes understanding of need for continuing follow-up care
- Able to verbalize safety precautions and compensatory measures related to decreased peripheral vision

evaluate →

Follow-up visit 6 weeks later:
- No further loss of peripheral vision, intraocular pressure 15 mm Hg OD and 13 mm Hg OS
- Using eye drops as ordered without adverse effects
- Returns for follow-up examinations as instructed.
- No accidents or injury due to decreased peripheral vision

Interdisciplinary Interventions
- Assess and record vital signs
- Teach how to instill eye medications as prescribed.
- Discuss use and side effects of prescribed medications

Independent Interventions
- Provide psychological support to decrease anxiety
- Teach safety measures and techniques to compensate for loss of peripheral vision
- Discuss possible restrictions such as avoiding sports in which peripheral vision is vital (e.g. contact sports)

PART VI

Sexuality and Reproductive Patterns

UNIT 15
Responses to Altered Reproductive Function

Functional Health Patterns with Related Nursing Diagnoses

HEALTH PERCEPTION-HEALTH MANAGEMENT
- Perceived health status
- Perceived health management
- Healthcare behaviors: health promotion and illness prevention activities, medical treatments, follow-up care

VALUE-BELIEF
- Values, goals, or beliefs (including spirituality) that guide choices or decisions
- Perceived conflicts in values, beliefs, or expectations that are health related

COPING-STRESS-TOLERANCE
- Capacity to resist challenges to self-integrity
- Methods of handling stress
- Support systems
- Perceived ability to control and manage situations

NUTRITIONAL-METABOLIC
- Daily consumption of food and fluids
- Favorite foods
- Use of dietary supplements
- Skin lesions and ability to heal
- Condition of the integument
- Weight, height, temperature

**PART VI
SEXUALITY-REPRODUCTIVE PATTERNS NANDA NURSING DIAGNOSES**
- Rape-Trauma Syndrome
- Sexual Dysfunction
- Ineffective Sexuality Patterns

SEXUALITY-REPRODUCTIVE
- Satisfaction with sexuality or sexual relationships
- Reproductive pattern
- Female menstrual and perimenopausal history

ELIMINATION
- Patterns of bowel and urinary excretion
- Perceived regularity or irregularity of elimination
- Use of laxatives or routines
- Changes in time, modes, quality or quantity of excretions
- Use of devices for control

ROLE-RELATIONSHIPS
- Perception of major roles, relationships, and responsibilities in current life situation
- Satisfaction with or disturbances in roles and relationships

ACTIVITY-EXERCISE
- Patterns of personally relevant exercise, activity, leisure, and recreation
- ADLs that require energy expenditure
- Factors that interfere with the desired pattern (e.g., illness or injury)

SELF-PERCEPTION–SELF-CONCEPT
- Attitudes about self
- Perceived abilities, worth, self-image, emotions
- Body posture and movement, eye contact, voice and speech patterns

SLEEP-REST
- Patterns of sleep and rest/relaxation in a 24-h period
- Perceptions of quality and quantity of sleep and rest
- Use of sleep aids and routines

COGNITIVE-PERCEPTUAL
- Adequacy of vision, hearing, taste, touch, smell
- Pain perception and management
- Language, judgment, memory, decisions

UNIT 15 Responses to Altered Reproductive Function

CHAPTER 49 Assessing Clients with Reproductive System and Breast Disorders

LEARNING OUTCOMES

- Describe the anatomy, physiology, and functions of the male and female reproductive systems, including the breasts.

- Explain the functions of the male and female sex hormones.

- Identify specific topics for consideration during a health history interview of the client with health problems involving the reproductive system and breast structures and/or functions.

- Describe normal variations in assessment findings for the older adult.

- Identify manifestations of impairment in the male and female reproductive system and breast structure or function.

CLINICAL COMPETENCIES

- Conduct and document a health history for men and women having or at risk for alterations of the reproductive system, including the breasts.

- Conduct and document a physical assessment of male and female reproductive system structures and functions, including the breasts.

- Monitor the results of diagnostic tests and report abnormal findings.

EQUIPMENT NEEDED

- Disposable gloves

- Water-soluble lubricant

- A good light source

- Sterile cotton swabs (for culture)

- Culture media (for culture)

- A spatula, cotton swab or endocervical brush, slides, and cytologic fixative (for Pap smear)

- Vaginal speculum of appropriate size

Although the reproductive organs in men and women are very different, they do share common functions: enabling sexual pleasure and reproduction. The reproductive organs, in conjunction with the neuroendocrine system, produce hormones important in biologic development and sexual behavior. Parts of the reproductive organs also enclose and are integral to the function of the urinary system. The assessment of the reproductive and urinary systems is often difficult for both the nurse and the client and requires sensitivity on the part of the nurse when asking questions about topics that the client may be hesitant to talk about. Skill in conducting physical examinations of an area of the body usually considered private is also required.

ANATOMY, PHYSIOLOGY, AND FUNCTIONS OF THE MALE REPRODUCTIVE SYSTEM

The male reproductive system consists of the paired testes, the scrotum, ducts, glands, and penis (Figure 49–1 ■). The breasts are part of the male reproductive system, and are also assessed. The location and functions of the male reproductive organs are summarized in Table 49–1.

The Breasts

The male breast is comprised primarily of an areola (circular pigmented area) and a small nipple. These lie over a thin disk of undeveloped breast tissue that may not be overtly different from surrounding tissue. Approximately one in three men have a firm area of breast tissue 2 cm or larger; the limits of normal size of this area have not been established (Bickley & Szilagyi, 2007).

The Penis

The penis is the genital organ that encloses the urethra (see Figure 49–1). It is homologous to the clitoris of the female. The penis is composed of a shaft and a tip called the glans, which is covered in the uncircumcised man by the foreskin (or prepuce). The shaft contains three columns of erectile tissue: The two lateral columns are called the corpora cavernosa, and the central mass is called the corpus spongiosum.

Erection occurs when the penile masses become filled with blood in response to a reflex that triggers the parasympathetic nervous system to stimulate arteriolar vasodilation. The erection reflex may be initiated by touch, pressure, sights, sounds, smells, or thoughts of a sexual encounter. After ejaculation, the arterioles vasoconstrict, and the penis becomes flaccid.

The Scrotum

The scrotum is a sac or pouch made of two layers. The outer layer is continuous with the skin of the perineum and thighs. The inner layer is made of muscle and fascia. The scrotum hangs at the base of the penis, anterior to the anus, and regulates the temperature of the testes. The optimum temperature for sperm production is about 2 to 3 degrees below body temperature. When the testicular temperature is too low, the scrotum contracts to bring the testes up against the body. When the testicular temperature is too high, the scrotum relaxes to allow the testes to lie further away from the body.

The Testes

The testes develop in the abdominal cavity of the fetus and then descend through the inguinal canal into the scrotum. They are homologous to the female's ovaries. These paired organs are each about 1.5 inches (4 cm) long and 1 inch (2.5 cm) in diameter. They are suspended in the scrotum by the spermatic cord. Each is surrounded by two coverings: an outer tunica vaginalis and an inner tunica albuginea. Each testis is divided into 250 to 300 lobules, with each lobule containing one to four seminiferous tubules. The testes produce sperm and testosterone.

The seminiferous tubules are responsible for sperm production. Leydig's cells (or interstitial cells) lie in the connective tissue surrounding the seminiferous tubules and produce testosterone.

Figure 49–1 ■ The male reproductive system.

TABLE 49–1 Location and Function of the Male Reproductive Organs

MALE REPRODUCTIVE ORGAN	LOCATION	FUNCTION
Penis	Attached to front and sides of the pubic arch. Proximal, ventral surface is directly continuous with the scrotum.	Excretes semen and urine. Deposits sperm in female reproductive tract.
Scrotum	Hangs from body at root of penis.	Contains testes, epididymis, and portions of the vas (ductus) deferens.
Testes	In the scrotal sac.	Produce sperm and testosterone.
Epididymis	Posterolateral to upper aspect of each testis.	Stores sperm. Promotes sperm maturation. Transports sperm to vas deferens.
Vas deferens (ductus deferens)	Between the epididymis and the seminal vesicle forming the ejaculatory duct.	Stores sperm. Transports sperm.
Urethra	Begins at bladder and passes through prostate and penis.	Serves as passageway for urine or semen.
Prostate gland	Encircles the urethra at the neck of the bladder.	Contributes to ejaculatory volume. Enhances sperm motility and fertility.
Seminal vesicles	Lie on posterior bladder wall.	Contribute to ejaculatory volume. Contain nutrients to sustain sperm and prostaglandins to facilitate sperm motility.
Bulbourethral (Cowper's) glands	Inferior to the prostate.	Secrete mucus into urethra. Neutralize traces of acidic urine in the urethra.

The Ducts and Semen

The seminiferous tubules lead into the efferent ducts and become the rete testis. From the rete testis, 10,000 to 20,000 efferent ducts join the epididymis, a long coiled tube that lies over the outer surface of each testis. The epididymis is the final area for the storage and maturation of sperm. When a man is sexually excited, the epididymis contracts to propel the sperm through the vas deferens to the ampulla, where the sperm are stored until ejaculation.

The seminal vesicles at the base of the bladder produce about 60% of the volume of seminal fluid. Seminal fluid is also made of secretions from the accessory sex organs, the epididymis, the prostate gland, and Cowper's glands. Seminal fluid nourishes the sperm, provides bulk, and increases its alkalinity. (An alkaline pH is essential to mobilize the sperm and ensure fertilization of the ova.) Sperm mixed with this fluid is called **semen**. Each seminal vesicle joins its corresponding vas deferens to form an ejaculatory duct, which enters the prostatic urethra. During ejaculation, seminal fluid mixes with sperm at the ejaculatory duct and enters the urethra for expulsion.

The total amount of semen ejaculated is 2 to 4 mL, although the amount varies. The total ejaculate of a healthy male contains from 100 to 400 million sperm.

The Prostate Gland

The prostate gland is about the size of a walnut. It encircles the urethra just below the urinary bladder (see Figure 49–1). It is made of 20 to 30 tubuloalveolar glands surrounded by smooth muscle. Secretions of the prostate gland make up about one-third of the volume of the semen. These secretions enter the urethra through several ducts during ejaculation.

Spermatogenesis

Spermatogenesis is the series of physiologic events that generate sperm in the seminiferous tubules. This process begins with puberty and continues throughout a man's life, with several hundred million sperm produced each day.

The inner layer of the seminiferous tubules consists of sustentacular cells (or Sertoli's cells), which contain the spermatocytes and sperm in different stages of development. Sertoli's cells secrete a nourishing fluid for the developing sperm, as well as enzymes that help convert spermatocytes to sperm. The events in spermatogenesis, which takes 64 to 72 days, are as follows:

1. The spermatogonia (sperm stem cells) undergo rapid mitotic division. As these cells multiply, the more mature spermatogonia divide into two daughter cells. These daughter cells grow and become the primary spermatocytes (and eventually become sperm).
2. Primary spermatocytes divide by meiosis to form two smaller secondary spermatocytes, which in turn divide to form two spermatids. This process occurs over several weeks.
3. The spermatids elongate into a mature sperm cell with a head and a tail. The head contains enzymes essential to the penetration and fertilization of the ova. The flagellar motion of the tail allows the sperm to move. The sperm cells then move to the epididymis to mature further and develop motility.

Male Sex Hormones

The male sex hormones are called **androgens**. Most androgens are produced in the testes, although the adrenal cortex also produces a small amount. **Testosterone**, the primary androgen produced by the testes, is essential for the development and maintenance of sexual organs and secondary sex characteristics, and for spermatogenesis. It also promotes metabolism, growth of muscles and bone, and libido (sexual desire).

ASSESSING THE MALE REPRODUCTIVE SYSTEM

The structures and functions of the male reproductive system are assessed by findings from diagnostic tests, a health assessment interview to collect subjective data, and a physical assessment to collect objective data.

Diagnostic Tests

The results of diagnostic tests of the structures and functions of the male reproductive system are used to support the diagnosis of a specific sexual problem, injury, or disease; to provide information to identify or modify the appropriate medications or treatments used to treat the disease; and to help nurses monitor the man's responses to treatment and nursing care interventions. Diagnostic tests used to assess the male reproductive system are described in the Diagnostic Tests table below and summarized in the bulleted list that follows. More information is included in the discussion of specific health problems or diseases in Chapter 50 ∞.

DIAGNOSTIC TESTS of the Male Reproductive System

NAME OF TEST   Prostate specific antigen (PSA)

PURPOSE AND DESCRIPTION   A blood test used to diagnose prostate cancer and to monitor treatment of prostate cancer.

Normal value:
<4 ng/mL

RELATED NURSING CARE   No special preparation is needed.

NAME OF TEST   Prostate ultrasound

PURPOSE AND DESCRIPTION   Conducted to identify testicular torsion or masses, and to evaluate prostate enlargement. Uses high-frequency sound waves, passed

through tissues of various densities, to produce a visual graphic of tissue being examined.

RELATED NURSING CARE   A full bladder may be required for the study.

NAME OF TEST   Prostate biopsy
- Transrectal biopsy
- Transurethral biopsy

PURPOSE AND DESCRIPTION   Conducted to diagnose prostate cancer. A transrectal ultrasound (TRUS) is often used to guide the placement of the needle during the procedure.
- A transrectal biopsy is performed with a spring-loaded needle, inserted through the rectal wall and into the prostate gland to remove one or more tissue samples.
- A transurethral biopsy is performed by inserting a cystoscope through the urethra and using a cutting loop to remove small samples of prostate tissue.

RELATED NURSING CARE   Advise the man to avoid strenuous activity for 4 hours postprocedure. Explain that there may be some discomfort in the biopsy area for 1 to 2 days, there may be some blood in the urine or from the rectum and semen may appear dark. Following a transurethral biopsy, a urinary catheter may remain in place for a few hours after the procedure and antibiotics will be prescribed. Excess bleeding, pain, or signs of infection should be reported to the physician.

NAME OF TEST   Gonorrhea culture

PURPOSE AND DESCRIPTION   A culture is performed to evaluate for gonorrhea. A swab is used to collect a sample of discharge from the infected area (urethra, penis, anus, or throat), smeared on a slide, and a Gram stain is conducted to

identify the organism (*N. gonorrhoeae*). A urine sample is used in some tests.

RELATED NURSING CARE   No special preparation is needed. If test is positive, request the names of all sexual partners and emphasize need for treatment to eradicate the infection.

NAME OF TEST
- Venereal Disease Research Laboratory (VDRL)
- Rapid plasma reagin (RPR)
- Fluorescent treponemal antibody absorption (FTA-ABS)

PURPOSE AND DESCRIPTION   These blood tests are conducted to screen for syphilis. Positive findings can be made within 1 to 2 weeks after primary lesion appears or 1 to 4

months after the initial infection. The FTA-ABS test is considered the most accurate, and is often used if findings from the VDRL or RPR are questionable.

RELATED NURSING CARE   No special preparation is needed. If test is positive, request the names of all sexual partners and emphasize need for treatment to eradicate the infection.

NAME OF TEST   Semen analysis

PURPOSE AND DESCRIPTION   Done to assess volume, motility and sperm count, and percent of abnormal sperm.

Normal values:
Volume: 2–5 mL

Sperm count: >20 million/mL
Motility: 60% motile
% normal sperm: 60%

RELATED NURSING CARE   Client is asked to bring in a fresh specimen within 2 hours of ejaculation.

- Hormone changes and syphilis are diagnosed with blood tests, discussed in Chapters 50 ∞ and 52 ∞. Gonorrhea, as well as other sexually transmitted infections, is diagnosed by cultures and smears of discharge or mucous membranes.
- Prostate cancer is diagnosed and monitored by measuring prostate specific antigen (PSA).
- The prostate may be examined by ultrasound to identify testicular torsion or masses, and by a prostate biopsy to accurately diagnose cancer.
- Semen analysis is done to evaluate semen volume, sperm count and motility, and percentage of abnormal sperm.

Regardless of the type of diagnostic test, the nurse is responsible for explaining the procedure and any special preparation needed, for assessing for any medication use that might affect the outcome of the tests, for supporting the man during the examination as necessary, for documenting the procedures as appropriate, and for monitoring the results of the tests.

Genetic Considerations

When conducting a health assessment interview and a physical assessment, it is important for the nurse to consider genetic influences on health of the adult. Several diseases of the male reproductive system have a genetic component. During the health assessment interview, it is especially important to ask about a family history of testicular or prostate cancer. During the physical assessment, assess for any manifestations that might indicate a genetic disorder (see the box below). If data are found to indicate genetic risk factors or alterations, ask about genetic testing and refer for appropriate genetic counseling and evaluation. Chapter 8 ∞ provides further information about genetics in medical-surgical nursing.

Health Assessment Interview

A health assessment interview to determine problems with the male reproductive system may be conducted during a health screening, may focus on a chief complaint (such as a discharge from the penis), or may be part of a total health assessment. Men may be embarrassed to discuss health problems or concerns involving their reproductive organs; it is important for the nurse to ask questions in a nonthreatening, matter-of-fact manner. Consider the psychologic, social, and cultural factors that affect sexuality and sexual activity. Use words that the man can

---

GENETIC CONSIDERATIONS
Male Reproductive System Disorders

- Although the exact genetic predisposition for some men to have prostate cancer is unknown, the findings of many studies have identified a family history as a major risk factor.
- A family history of testicular cancer is a risk factor for cancer of the testes.
- Men who have XX chromosomes (instead of XY) often have altered testicular development because they are missing a gene called the sex-determining region Y gene (SRY), which is responsible for the development of secondary sex characteristics in men.

---

understand, and do not be embarrassed or offended by the words he uses. The man may perceive the interview as less threatening if the discussion begins with more general questions and then progresses to specific questions, and if questions are asked in a way that gives him permission to describe behaviors and manifestations. For example, rather than asking a man if he has difficulty achieving or maintaining an erection, ask him to describe any changes he has noticed in his erections.

If the man has a health problem, analyze its onset, characteristics and course, severity, precipitating and relieving factors, and any associated symptoms, noting the timing and circumstances. For example, you may ask the man:

- When did you first notice that you were having difficulty urinating?
- Did you use a different brand of condoms before you noticed the rash on your penis?
- Describe the changes that occurred in your ability to have an erection after you started taking medicine for high blood pressure.

In questioning the man about past medical history, ask about chronic illnesses such as diabetes, chronic renal failure, cardiovascular disease, multiple sclerosis, spinal cord tumors or trauma, or thyroid disease. The effects of these illnesses as well as the treatment of the illnesses may cause **impotence** (inability to achieve or maintain an erection). The following drugs may cause sexual function problems: antihypertensives, antidepressants, antispasmodics, tranquilizers, sedatives, and histamine$_2$-receptor antagonists. Psychosocial stressors also may contribute to impotence.

If the man was born to a woman treated during pregnancy with diethylstilbestrol (DES), a drug used in the 1940s and 1950s to prevent miscarriage, he may have congenital deformities of the urinary tract as well as decreased semen levels. If the man had mumps as a child, sterility is possible. The risk for testicular cancer is greatest in men who have a history of an undescended testicle, an inguinal hernia, testicular swelling with mumps, a history of maternal use of DES or oral contraceptives, and a family history of testicular cancer.

Explore the lifestyle and social history of the man; the use of alcohol, cigarettes, or street drugs may affect sexual function. Frequent sexual intercourse, especially if unprotected, increases the potential for sexually transmitted infections including HIV infection. Ask about sexual preference. Sexual intercourse with same-sex partners further increases the risk for HIV infection. Other questions about sexuality may include number of sexual partners; history of premature ejaculation, impotence, or other sexual problems; any history of sexual trauma; use of condoms or other contraceptives; and current level of sexual satisfaction.

Interview questions categorized by functional health patterns are listed in the Functional Health Pattern Interview table on the next page.

Physical Assessment

Physical assessment of the male reproductive system may be performed as part of a total assessment or separately for men with known or suspected problems. If conducted as part of a total physical assessment, this is usually the final system to be assessed.

FUNCTIONAL HEALTH PATTERN INTERVIEW   The Male Reproductive System

Functional Health Pattern	Interview Questions and Leading Statements
Health Perception-Health Management	■ Have you ever had problems with your reproductive organs (penis, testicles, prostate gland)? Explain. If so, how was the problem treated? ■ Have you ever had surgery on your reproductive organs? If so, what type, when, and what was the outcome? ■ Have you ever noticed any pain or swelling in your breasts? Explain. ■ Do you practice testicular self-examination? How often? ■ Do you smoke? If so, how much and for how long?
Nutritional-Metabolic	■ Describe your usual intake of food and fluids in a 24-hour period.
Elimination	■ Do you now or have you ever had a discharge from your penis? If so, describe the color, odor, consistency, amount, and frequency. ■ Have you ever had any bleeding from your penis? Explain. ■ Have you noticed any change in your urination, such as burning, frequency, urgency, difficulty starting the stream, size of the stream, dribbling, or getting up frequently at night? Explain.
Activity-Exercise	■ Describe your usual activity in a 24-hour period. ■ Do you participate in sports or heavy lifting? If so, do you wear a protective cup or athletic support?
Sleep-Rest	■ Describe the quality of your rest and sleep.
Cognitive-Perceptual	■ Describe any pain you have had in the groin area, testicles, penis, or scrotum. Where is it? Do you experience it in other parts of your body? How long does it last? What makes it worse or relieves it? ■ Has there been a change in the condition or color of the skin on your scrotum or penis? Explain.
Self-Perception-Self-Concept	■ Has this problem affected how you feel about yourself as a man? ■ Do you feel that your needs for intimacy and affection are being met?
Role-Relationships	■ Has having this condition affected your relationships with others? ■ Has having this condition interfered with your ability to work? Explain. ■ Has anyone in your family had problems with prostate cancer? Explain.
Sexuality-Reproductive	■ Are you currently in a sexual relationship? If so, has this condition interfered with your usual sexual activity? How long have you been with your current partner? Have you had any other partners during this time? ■ What is your sexual preference? ■ Has having this problem affected your relationship with your spouse or sexual partner? ■ Are you satisfied with your current level of sexual functioning? ■ Have you ever had any problem with achieving or maintaining an erection or ejaculation? ■ Do you use any medications to facilitate your sexual ability? Describe. ■ Do you use condoms every time you have sexual contact?
Coping-Stress-Tolerance	■ Has having this condition created stress for you? If so, does your health problem seem to be more difficult when you are stressed? ■ Have you experienced any kind of stress that makes the condition worse? Explain. ■ Describe what you do when you feel stressed.
Value-Belief	■ Describe how specific relationships or activities help you cope with this problem. ■ Describe specific cultural beliefs or practices that affect how you care for and feel about this problem. ■ Are there any specific treatments that you would not use to treat this problem?

Problems of the male reproductive system may involve the urinary system, making an assessment of both systems important (see Chapter 27 ∞ for assessment of the urinary system). The nurse must feel comfortable with the examination of clients of the opposite gender; if either the nurse or the client is not comfortable, a nurse of the same gender should be asked to conduct this part of the assessment. Normal age-related findings for the older man are summarized in Table 49–2.

The male reproductive system is assessed by inspection and palpation. Explain the procedures for the examination thoroughly and in a matter-of-fact way to decrease anxiety and embarrassment. If the man is unfamiliar with his internal genitalia, charts may be used to demonstrate the parts that will be examined. Ask the man to empty his bladder (to be more comfortable during the examination), remove his clothing, and put on a gown or drape. The assessment may be done with the man sitting or standing. Expose only those body parts being examined to preserve modesty. Ensure that the examining room is warm and private. Put on gloves before beginning and wear them throughout the examination.

TABLE 49–2 Age-Related Changes in the Male Reproductive System

AGE-RELATED CHANGE	SIGNIFICANCE
Prostate Gland ■ A significant number of older men have some degree of benign prostatic hyperplasia.	Although aging does not cause prostate cancer, its incidence does increase with age.
Penis, Testes, and Scrotum ■ Epithelial tissue and mucosa of seminal vesicles are thinner and have reduced capacity to hold fluid. ■ Sclerosis of penile arteries and veins may occur.	Although men may father children throughout life, the sperm count is reduced in some men. Changes in the vascular system of the penis may mean the aging man takes longer to achieve an erection and ejaculation, or may be impotent.

MALE REPRODUCTIVE SYSTEM ASSESSMENTS

Technique/Normal Findings	Abnormal Findings

Breast and Lymph Node Assessment

Inspect and palpate both breasts, including areola and nipple. *Breast tissue should not be swollen, tender, or enlarged (although soft, fatty, and enlarged breast tissue does occur with obesity in men).*

- A smooth, firm, mobile, tender disk of breast tissue behind the areola indicates **gynecomastia**, abnormal enlargement of the breast(s) in men. Gynecomastia requires additional investigation to determine cause.
- A hard, irregular nodule in the nipple area suggests carcinoma.

Palpate the axillary and supraclavicular lymph nodes. *Lymph nodes should not be palpable.*

- Enlarged axillary nodes are common with infections of the hand or arm but may be caused by cancer.
- Enlarged supraclavicular nodes may indicate metastasis.

External Genitalia Assessment

Inspect and palpate the inguinal and femoral area for bulges. Ask the man to bear down or cough as you palpate (Figure 49–2 ■). *There should be no bulging with coughing or bearing down.*

- A bulge that increases with coughing or straining suggests a hernia.

Figure 49–2 ■ Palpating the male inguinal area for bulges.

Inspect the penis. If the man is uncircumcised, retract the foreskin or ask him to do so. *When nonerect, the penis is normally soft, flaccid, and nontender. The foreskin should be without lesions, of color equal with the penis, and should retract easily. The glans is normally free of lesions.*

- **Phimosis** (tightness of prepuce that prevents retraction of foreskin) may be congenital or due to recurrent balanoposthitis (generalized infection of glans penis and prepuce).
- Narrow or inflamed foreskin can cause paraphimosis, retraction of the foreskin that causes painful swelling of the glans.
- Balanitis (inflammation of the glans) is associated with bacterial or fungal infections.
- Ulcers, vesicles, or warts suggest a sexually transmitted infection.
- Nodules or sores seen in uncircumcised men may be cancer.

Technique/Normal Findings	Abnormal Findings

Inspect the external urinary meatus. Press the glans between the thumb and forefinger (Figure 49–3 ■). Replace the foreskin if appropriate. *The external urinary meatus is normally in the center of the glans, without redness or discharge.*

- Erythema or discharge indicates inflammatory disease. Further assessment is required.

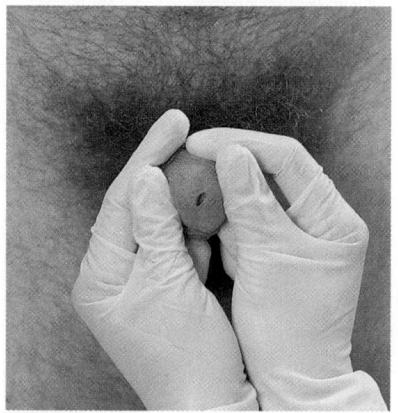

Figure 49–3 ■ Inspecting the external urinary meatus of the male.

Inspect the skin on the shaft of the penis. *The skin on the shaft of the penis should be free of redness or lesions.*

- Excoriation or inflammation suggests lice or scabies.

Palpate the shaft of the penis. *The shaft of the penis should not be tender.*

- Induration with tenderness along the ventral surface suggests urethral stricture with inflammation.

Inspect the scrotum. Further assess any swelling in the scrotum using transillumination: Darken the room and place a lighted flashlight against the skin of the scrotum. *The normal scrotum and epididymis appear as dark masses with regular borders.*

- A unilateral or bilateral poorly developed scrotum suggests cryptorchidism (failure of one or both testes to descend into the scrotum).
- Swelling of the scrotum may indicate indirect inguinal hernia, hydrocele (accumulation of fluid in the scrotum), or scrotal edema. Swellings containing serous fluid will transilluminate. Swellings containing blood or tissue will not transilluminate.

Palpate each testis and epididymis. *The testes should not be tender or swollen.*

- Tender, painful scrotal swelling occurs in acute epididymitis, acute orchitis, torsion of the spermatic cord, and strangulated hernia.
- A painless nodule in the testis is associated with testicular cancer.

Prostate Assessment

The prostate gland is assessed by digital rectal examination (DRE). (See Chapter 25 ∞ for the technique used to palpate the prostrate through the rectal wall.)

With a gloved index finger, palpate the posterior rectal wall for the rounded, two-lobed structure of the posterior prostate. *The prostate is normally nontender, with two lateral lobes that are divided, smooth, and about 2.5 cm long.*

- Enlargement (1-cm protrusion into the rectum) with obliteration of the median sulcus suggests benign prostatic hypertrophy.
- Enlargement with asymmetry and tenderness suggests prostatitis.
- A hard irregular nodule is suspicious of carcinoma.

ANATOMY, PHYSIOLOGY, AND FUNCTIONS OF THE FEMALE REPRODUCTIVE SYSTEM

The female reproductive system consists of the external genitalia (mons pubis, labia, clitoris, vaginal and urethral openings, and glands) and the internal organs (vagina, cervix, uterus, fallopian tubes, and ovaries). The breasts are a part of women's reproductive organs. In women, the urethra and urinary meatus are separated from the reproductive organs; however, they are in so close to each other that a health problem with one often affects the other. The location and function of the female reproductive organs are summarized in Table 49–3.

The Breasts

The breasts (or mammary glands) are located between the third and seventh ribs on the anterior chest wall. They are supported by the pectoral muscles and are richly supplied with nerves, blood, and lymph (Figure 49–4 ■). A pigmented area called the areola is located slightly below the center of each breast and contains sebaceous glands and a nipple. The nipple is usually protrusive and becomes erect in response to cold and stimulation.

The breasts are made of adipose tissue, fibrous connective tissue, and glandular tissue. Cooper's ligaments support the breast and extend from the outer breast tissue to the nipple, dividing the breast into 15 to 25 lobes. Each lobe is made of alveolar glands connected by ducts that open to the nipple.

The External Genitalia

The external genitalia collectively are called the vulva. They include the mons pubis, the labia, the clitoris, the vaginal and urethral openings, and glands (Figure 49–5 ■).

The mons pubis is a pad of adipose (fat) tissue covered with skin. It lies anterior to the symphysis pubis. After puberty, the mons is covered with hair.

The labia are divided into two structures. The labia majora, folds of skin and adipose tissue covered with hair, are outermost; they begin at the base of the mons pubis and end at the

TABLE 49–3 Location and Function of the Female Reproductive Organs

FEMALE REPRODUCTIVE ORGAN	LOCATION	FUNCTION
Mons pubis (mons veneris)	Anterior and superior to the pubis.	Enhances sexual sensations. Protects and cushions pubic symphysis during intercourse.
Labia majora	Extend from mons pubis to perineum.	Protect labia minora, urethral and vaginal openings. Enhance sexual arousal.
Labia minora	Enclosed by the labia majora.	Protect clitoris. Inferiorly, merge to form posterior ring of vaginal introitus (fourchette). Lubricate vulva. Enhance sexual arousal.
Vestibule	Area enclosed by labia minora.	Contains openings for urethra, vagina, Bartholin's glands, and Skene's glands.
Bartholin's (greater vestibular) glands	Posterior on each side of the vaginal orifice. Open onto the sides of the vestibule in the groove between the labia minora and hymen.	Secrete clear, viscid mucus during intercourse.
Skene's (lesser vestibular, paraurethral) glands	Open onto the vestibule on each side of the urethra.	Drain urethral glands. Produce lubricating mucus.
Clitoris	Small bud of erectile tissue just below the superior joining of the labia minora.	Stimulates and elevates levels of sexual arousal.
Perineum	Skin-covered muscular area between vaginal opening and anus.	Provides support for pelvic organs.
Mammary glands	Contained within breasts. Anterior to pectoral muscles of thorax.	Produce human milk. Play a role in sexual arousal.
Ovaries	Lie on each side of the uterus below and behind the uterine tubes.	Produce and secrete ova. Produce the hormones estrogen and progesterone.
Fallopian tubes (uterine tubes, oviducts)	One tube extends medially from the area of each ovary and empties into the upper portion (fundus) of the uterus.	Transport ova.
Uterus (adnexa of the uterus are composed of the uterine tubes and ovaries)	Anterior to the rectum and posterior/superior to the bladder.	Receives, retains, and nourishes the fertilized ovum. Contracts rhythmically to expel infant. Cyclically sheds lining when ovum is not fertilized.
Cervix	Lower portion of uterus extending into the vagina.	Connects uterine cavity with vagina. Opens to allow passage of menstrual flow and infant.
Vagina	Extends from the external orifice in the vestibule to the cervix.	Receives penis and semen during intercourse. Passageway for menstrual flow and expulsion of infant at birth.

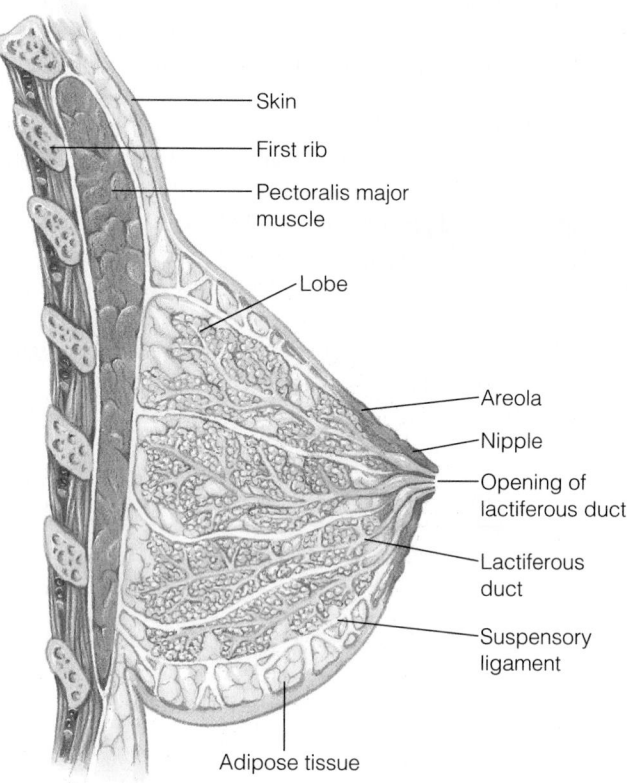

Figure 49–4 ■ Structure of the female breast.

anus. The labia minora, located between the clitoris and the base of the vagina, are enclosed by the labia majora. They are made of skin, adipose tissue, and some erectile tissues. They are usually light pink and hairless.

The area between the labia is called the vestibule, and contains the openings for the vagina and the urethra as well as the

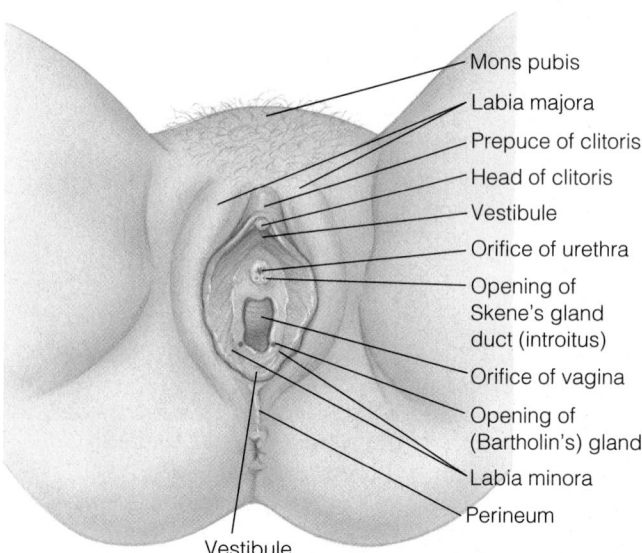

Figure 49–5 ■ The external organs of the female reproductive system.

Bartholin's glands. Skene's glands open onto the vestibule on each side of the urethra. Bartholin's and Skene's glands secrete lubricating fluid during the sexual response cycle prior to menopause.

The clitoris is an erectile organ analogous to the penis in the male. It is formed by the joining of the labia minora. Like the penis, it is highly sensitive and distends during sexual arousal.

The vaginal opening, called the introitus, is the opening between the internal and the external genitals. Prior to intercourse or trauma, the introitus is surrounded by a connective tissue membrane called the hymen.

The Internal Organs

The vagina and cervix, uterus, fallopian tubes, and ovaries are the internal organs of the female reproductive system (Figure 49–6 ■). The ovaries are the primary reproductive organs in women and also produce female sex hormones. The vagina, uterus, and fallopian tubes serve as accessory ducts for the ovaries and a developing fetus.

The Vagina and Cervix

The vagina is a fibromuscular tube about 3 to 4 inches (8 to 10 cm) in length located posterior to the bladder and urethra and anterior to the rectum. The upper end contains the uterine cervix in an area called the fornix. The walls of the vagina are membranes that form folds, called rugae. These membranes are composed of mucous-secreting stratified squamous epithelial cells. The vagina serves as a route for the excretion of secretions, including menstrual fluid, an organ of sexual response, and as a passageway for the birth of an infant.

The walls of the vagina are usually moist and maintain a pH ranging from 3.8 to 4.2. This pH is bacteriostatic and is maintained by the action of estrogen and normal vaginal flora. **Estrogen** stimulates the growth of vaginal mucosal cells so that they thicken and have increased glycogen content. The glycogen is fermented to lactic acid by Döderlein's bacilli (lactobacilli that normally inhabit the vagina), slightly acidifying the vaginal fluid.

The cervix projects into the vagina and forms a pathway between the uterus and the vagina. The uterine opening of the cervix is called the internal os; the vaginal opening is called the external os. The space between these openings, the endocervical canal, serves as a route for the discharge of menstrual fluid, the entrance for sperm, and expulsion of the infant during birth. The cervix is a firm structure, protected by mucus that changes consistency and quantity during the menstrual cycle and during pregnancy.

The Uterus

The uterus is a hollow pear-shaped muscular organ with thick walls located between the bladder and the rectum. It has three parts: the fundus, the body, and the cervix. It is supported in the abdominal cavity by the broad ligaments, the round ligaments, the uterosacral ligaments, and the transverse cervical ligaments. The uterus receives the fertilized ovum and provides a site for growth and development of the fetus.

The uterine wall has three layers. The perimetrium is the outer serous layer that merges with the peritoneum. The my-

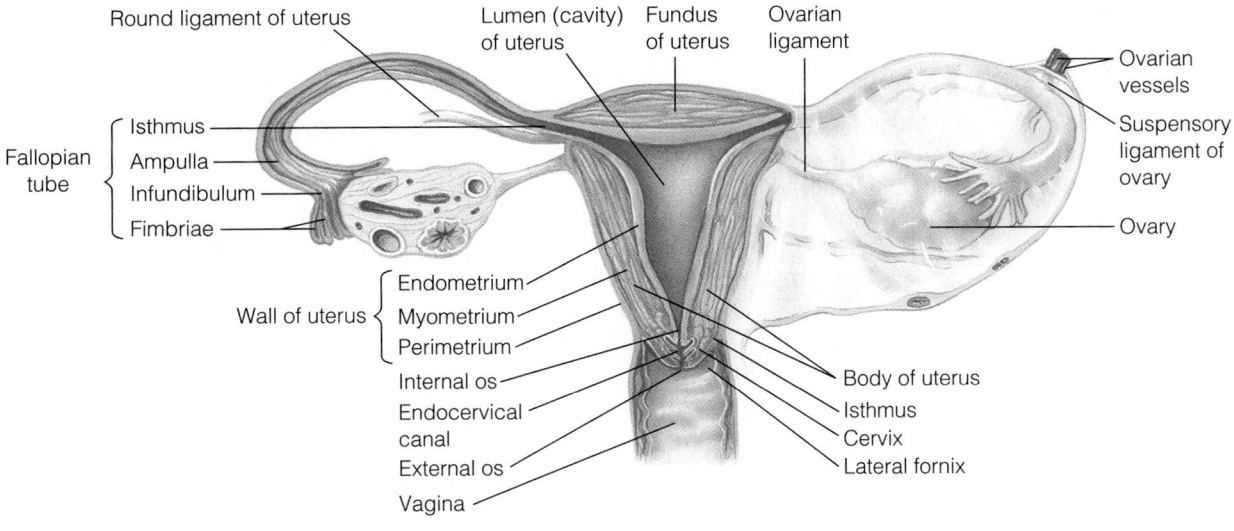

Figure 49–6 ■ The internal organs of the female reproductive system.

ometrium is the middle layer and makes up most of the uterine wall. This layer has muscle fibers that run in various directions, allowing contractions during **menstruation** (the periodic shedding of the uterine lining in a woman of childbearing age who is not pregnant) or childbirth, and expansion as the fetus grows. The endometrium lines the uterus; its outermost layer is shed during menstruation.

The Fallopian Tubes

The fallopian tubes are thin cylindrical structures about 4 inches (10 cm) long and 2.5 inches (1 cm) in diameter. They are attached to the uterus on one end and are supported by the broad ligaments. The lateral ends of the fallopian tubes are open and made of projections called fimbriae that drape over the ovary. The fimbriae pick up the ovum after it is discharged from the ovary.

The fallopian tubes are made of smooth muscle and are lined with ciliated, mucous-producing epithelial cells. The movement of the cilia and contractions of the smooth muscle move the ovum through the tubes toward the uterus. Fertilization of the ovum by the sperm usually occurs in the outer portion of a fallopian tube.

The Ovaries

The ovaries in the adult woman are flat, almond-shaped structures located on either side of the uterus below the ends of the fallopian tubes. They are homologous to the male's testes. They are attached to the uterus by a ligament and are also attached to the broad ligament. The ovaries store the female germ cells and produce the female hormones estrogen and progesterone. A woman's total number of ova is present at her birth.

Each ovary contains many small structures called ovarian follicles. Each follicle contains an immature ovum, called an oocyte. Each month, several follicles are stimulated by follicle-stimulating hormone (FSH) and luteinizing hormone (LH) to mature. The developing follicles are surrounded by layers of follicle cells, with the mature follicles called graafian follicles. The graafian follicles produce estrogen, which stimulates the devel-

opment of endometrium. Each month in the menstruating woman, one or two of the mature follicles eject an oocyte in a process called ovulation. The ruptured follicle then becomes a structure called the corpus luteum. The corpus luteum produces both estrogen and progesterone to support the endometrium until conception occurs or the cycle begins again. The corpus luteum slowly degenerates, leaving a scar on the surface of the ovary.

Female Sex Hormones

The ovaries produce estrogens, progesterone, and androgens in a cyclic pattern. Estrogens are steroid hormones that occur naturally in three forms: estrone (E_1), estradiol (E_2), and estriol (E_3). Estradiol is the most potent and is the form secreted in greatest amount by the ovaries. Although estrogens are secreted throughout the menstrual cycle, they are at a higher level during certain phases of the cycle, as discussed shortly.

Estrogens are essential for the development and maintenance of secondary sex characteristics; and in conjunction with other hormones, they stimulate the female reproductive organs to prepare for growth of a fetus. Estrogens are responsible for the normal structure of skin and blood vessels. They also decrease the rate of bone resorption, promote increased high-density lipoproteins, reduce cholesterol levels, and enhance the clotting of blood. Estrogens also promote the retention of sodium and water.

Menopause, a normal physiologic process, occurs as a result of the gradual decrease and final cessation of estrogen production by the ovaries. Menstruation ceases and the tissues that had been supported by estrogen change. Long-term effects of estrogen deprivation increase the risk of osteoporosis and cardiovascular disease. Menopause is discussed fully in Chapter 51 ∞.

Progesterone primarily affects the development of breast glandular tissue and the endometrium. During pregnancy, progesterone relaxes smooth muscle to decrease uterine contractions. It also increases body temperature. Androgens are responsible for normal hair growth patterns at puberty and may also have metabolic effects.

Oogenesis and the Ovarian Cycle

At her birth, all of a woman's ova are present as primary oocytes in ovarian follicles. Each month from puberty until menopause, the remaining events of oogenesis (the production of ova) occur. Collectively, these events are known as the **ovarian cycle**.

The ovarian cycle has three consecutive phases that occur cyclically each 28 days (although the cycle normally may be longer or shorter), as follows:

- The follicular phase lasts from the 1st to the 10th day of the cycle.
- The ovulatory phase lasts from the 11th to the 14th day of the cycle and ends with ovulation.
- The luteal phase lasts from the 14th to the 28th day.

During the follicular phase, the follicle develops and the oocyte matures. These processes are controlled by the interaction of FSH and LH. On day 1 of the cycle, gonadotropin-releasing hormone (GnRH) from the hypothalamus increases and stimulates increased production of FSH and LH by the anterior pituitary. FSH and LH stimulate follicular growth, and the oocyte increases in size. The structure, now called the primary follicle, becomes a multicellular mass surrounded by a fibrous capsule, the theca folliculi. As the follicle continues to increase in size, estrogen is produced and a fluid-filled space (the antrum) forms within the follicle. The oocyte is enclosed by a membrane, the zona pellucida. By about day 10, the follicle is a mature graafian follicle and bulges out from the surface of the ovary. There are always follicles at different stages of development in each ovary, but usually only one follicle becomes dominant and matures to ovulation, while the others degenerate.

The ovulatory phase begins when estrogen levels reach a level high enough to stimulate the anterior pituitary, and a surge of LH is produced. The LH stimulates meiosis in the developing oocyte, and its first meiotic division occurs. The LH also stimulates enzymes that act on the bulging ovarian wall, causing it to rupture and discharge the antrum fluid and the oocyte. The oocyte is expelled from the mature ovarian follicle in the process called ovulation.

During the luteal phase, the surge in LH also stimulates the ruptured follicle to change into a corpus luteum and then stimulates the corpus luteum to begin immediately producing progesterone and estrogen. The increase of progesterone and estrogen in the blood has a negative feedback effect on the production of LH, inhibiting the further growth and development of other follicles.

If pregnancy does not occur, the corpus luteum begins to degenerate, and its hormone production ceases. The declining production of progesterone and estrogen at the end of the cycle allows the secretion of LH and FSH to increase, and a new cycle begins. The ovarian cycle is compared to the menstrual cycle in Figure 49–7 ■.

The Menstrual Cycle

The endometrium of the uterus responds to changes in estrogen and progesterone during the ovarian cycle to prepare for implantation of the fertilized embryo. The endometrium is recep-

A Fluctuation of gonadotropin levels

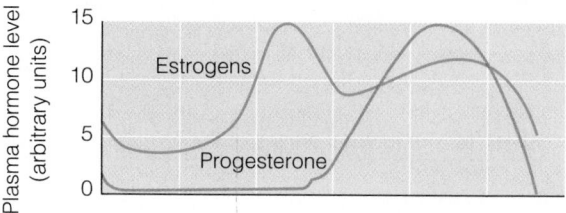

B Fluctuation of ovarian hormone levels

C Ovarian cycle

D Menstrual cycle

Figure 49–7 ■ Comparison of the ovarian and menstrual cycles. *A,* Fluctuating levels of follicle-stimulating hormone (FSH) and luteinizing hormone (LH), the pituitary gonadotropins regulating the ovarian cycle. *B,* Fluctuating levels of ovarian hormones that cause endometrial changes during the menstrual cycle. *C,* Changes in the ovarian follicles during the 28-day menstrual cycle. *D,* Corresponding changes in the endometrium during the menstrual cycle.

tive to implantation of the embryo for only a brief period each month, coinciding with the time when the embryo would normally reach the uterus from the uterine tube (usually 7 days).

The **menstrual cycle** begins with the menstrual phase, lasting from days 1 to 5. The inner endometrial (functionalis) layer detaches and is expelled as menstrual fluid (fluid and blood) for 3 to 5 days. As the maturing follicle begins to produce estrogen (days 6 to 14), the proliferative phase begins. In response, the functionalis layer is repaired and thickens, while spiral arteries increase in number and tubular glands form. Cervical mucus changes to a thin, crystalline substance, forming channels to help the sperm move up into the uterus.

The final phase, lasting from days 14 to 28, is the secretory phase. As the corpus luteum produces progesterone, the rising levels act on the endometrium, causing increased vascularity, changing the inner layer to secretory mucosa, stimulating the secretion of glycogen into the uterine cavity, and causing the cervical mucus again to become thick and block the internal os. If fertilization does not occur, hormone levels fall. Spasm of the spiral arteries causes hypoxia of the endometrial cells, which begin to degenerate and slough off. As with the ovarian cycle, the process begins again with the sloughing of the functionalis layer.

ASSESSING THE FEMALE REPRODUCTIVE SYSTEM

The structures and functions of the female reproductive system are assessed by findings from diagnostic tests, a health assessment interview to collect subjective data, and a physical assessment to collect objective data. Information from the health assessment interview is used to individualize the questions that are asked; for example, the postmenopausal woman would not be asked specific questions about her menstrual cycle, but it would be important to ask about vaginal dryness. Sample documentation of an assessment of the female reproductive system is included in the box below.

Diagnostic Tests

The results of diagnostic tests of the structures and functions of the female reproductive system are used to monitor the health of female reproductive structures; to support the diagnosis of a specific sexual problem, injury, or disease; to provide information to identify or modify the appropriate medications or treatments used to treat the disease; and to help nurses monitor the woman's responses to treatment and nursing care interventions. Diagnostic tests to assess the female reproductive system are described in the Diagnostic Tests table on pages 1756–1758 and summarized in the following bulleted list. More information is included in the discussion of specific health problems or diseases in Chapter 51 ∞.

- Blood tests are used to diagnose a variety of hormone changes and sexually transmitted infections. These tests are discussed in Chapters 51 and 52 ∞.
- Sexually transmitted infections are often diagnosed with cultures and smears of a discharge or mucous membranes.
- A mammogram is used to detect breast tumors, often followed by a breast biopsy for a definitive diagnosis. The type of biopsy conducted depends on many factors, including the size, location, appearance, and characteristics of the breast abnormality.
- The Papanicolaou (Pap) smear and the HPV DNA test are conducted to diagnose premalignant and malignant conditions of the cervix, to monitor positive HPV tests, and may also be used to assess the effects of hormone replacement, identify other infective organisms, and evaluate response to therapy.
- Space-occupying lesions and abnormalities of the vagina, cervix, or uterus may be evaluated with ultrasound, a hysterosalpingogram, a colposcopy, a cervical biopsy, a laparoscopy, and/or an endometrial biopsy.

Regardless of the type of diagnostic test, the nurse is responsible for explaining the procedure and any special preparation needed, for assessing for any medication use that might affect the outcome of the tests, for supporting the woman during the examination as necessary, for documenting the procedures as appropriate, and for monitoring the results of the tests.

Genetic Considerations

When conducting a health assessment interview and a physical assessment, it is important for the nurse to consider genetic influences on health of the adult. Several diseases of the female reproductive system have a genetic component. During the health assessment interview, it is especially important to ask about a family history of ovarian or breast cancer. During the physical assessment, assess for any manifestations that might indicate a genetic disorder (see the box below). If data are found to indicate genetic risk factors or alterations, ask about genetic testing and refer for appropriate genetic counseling and evaluation. Chapter 8 ∞ provides further information about genetics in medical-surgical nursing.

SAMPLE DOCUMENTATION
Assessment of the Female Reproductive System

32-year-old female, first visit to health department for problems with "burning and pain in my crotch area" and "It really hurts to urinate." Also states she had unprotected sex on a date about 2 weeks ago. Oral temperature 101°F. Vaginal examination findings of vesicles and red ulcerations on labia majora and vaginal mucosa. Inguinal lymph nodes enlarged and tender to palpation. Culture of ulcerations taken and specimen sent to the laboratory for analysis.

GENETIC CONSIDERATIONS Female Reproductive System Disorders

- There is a clear genetic link for some of the cases of both breast and ovarian cancer. Two breast cancer susceptibility genes have been identified: BRCA1 and BRCA2. If a woman has either of these genes, she is at increased risk for having breast or ovarian cancer at some point in her life.
- A family history of endometrial, colon, or breast cancer increases a woman's risk for endometrial cancer.
- Turner syndrome is a disorder in a female caused by complete or partial absence of one of the two X chromosomes. The disorder is characterized by short stature and the lack of sexual development at puberty. Other physical effects include a webbed neck, heart defects, and kidney abnormalities.

DIAGNOSTIC TESTS of the Female Reproductive System

SCREENING TESTS, SMEARS, AND CULTURES

NAME OF TEST Papanicolaou smear (Pap test)

PURPOSE AND DESCRIPTION Conducted to diagnose malignant and premalignant lesions of the cervix; assess the effects of hormone replacement; identify viral, bacterial, fungal, and parasitic conditions; and to evaluate response to chemotherapy or radiation therapy to the cervix. Cells are obtained during a pelvic examination, with a wooden spatula, a cotton swab, or an endocervical brush. The sample collected may be smeared on a glass slide or put into a special liquid preservative and then the cells in suspension are processed onto a slide. The cells are then stained and examined.

RELATED NURSING CARE Explain that the test should be done during a time when the woman is not menstruating, and that she should not have intercourse, douche, or use vaginal medications for 36 hours prior to the examination. Ask the woman to void prior to the examination.

NAME OF TEST HPV test
(HPV DNA test, genital human papilloma test)

PURPOSE AND DESCRIPTION Routinely used as a screening tool for human papillomavirus (HPV) in women after the age of 30. Conducted in conjunction with a pelvic examination and Pap smear. A finding of "low-grade changes" on the Pap smear with HPV indicates the likely presence of HPV and the need for further testing. A positive test for HPV indicates the presence of a high risk for cancer type of HPV, but does not specify which type is present.

RELATED NURSING CARE Explain that the test should be done during a time when the woman is not menstruating, and that she should not have intercourse, douche, or use vaginal medications for 36 hours prior to the examination. Ask the woman to void prior to the examination.

NAME OF TEST Chlamydia

PURPOSE AND DESCRIPTION Performed to screen for or diagnose chlamydial infections. A swab of cells from the infected area is taken and either smeared on a slide and analyzed or cultured. Although usually taken from the urethra, vagina, or cervix, cultures may also be taken from the throat and rectum.

RELATED NURSING CARE Assess if the woman is pregnant or has enlargement of inguinal lymph nodes. Withhold antibiotics (if prescribed) until after obtaining the specimen. Instruct not to douche before the examination. If the test is positive, request the names of all sexual partners and emphasize need for treatment to eradicate the infection.

NAME OF TEST Gonorrhea culture

PURPOSE AND DESCRIPTION A culture is performed to evaluate for gonorrhea. A swab is used to collect a sample of discharge from the infected area (cervix, urethra, anus, or throat), smeared on a slide, and a Gram stain is conducted to identify the organism (*N. gonorrhoeae*). A urine sample is used in some tests.

RELATED NURSING CARE No special preparation is needed. Instruct not to douche before the examination. If the test is positive, request the names of all sexual partners and emphasize need for treatment to eradicate the infection.

NAME OF TEST Trichomonas, Bacteria, Candidae (yeast)

PURPOSE AND DESCRIPTION A culture is performed to identify vaginal organisms or blood cells. A specimen of vaginal discharge is obtained with a swab, placed in solution, and examined under the microscope immediately after it is collected (referred to as a wet-mount).

RELATED NURSING CARE Request not to douche before the examination.

NAME OF TEST
■ Venereal Disease Research Laboratory (VDRL)
■ Rapid plasma reagin (RPR)
■ Fluorescent treponemal antibody absorption (FTA-ABS)

PURPOSE AND DESCRIPTION These blood tests are conducted to screen for syphilis. Positive findings can be made within 1 to 2 weeks after primary lesion appears or 1 to 4 months after the initial infection. The FTA-ABS is considered the most accurate, and is often used if findings from the VDRL or RPR are questionable.

RELATED NURSING CARE No special preparation is needed. If test is positive, request the names of all sexual partners and emphasize need for treatment to eradicate the infection.

NAME OF TEST Syphilis (dark-field examination)

PURPOSE AND DESCRIPTION A specimen is obtained from a lesion believed to be caused by syphilis (*Treponema pallidum*) and examined under the microscope.

RELATED NURSING CARE No special preparation is needed. If test is positive, request the names of all sexual partners and emphasize need for treatment to eradicate the infection.

BREAST EXAMINATIONS

NAME OF TEST Mammogram

PURPOSE AND DESCRIPTION Used to detect tumors in the breast. Breasts are flattened in the mammography machine and low-dose x-rays are taken.

RELATED NURSING CARE Ask the woman not to apply body powder or underarm deodorant prior to the test.

DIAGNOSTIC TESTS   of the Female Reproductive System (continued)

NAME OF TEST   Breast ultrasound

PURPOSE AND DESCRIPTION   This examination uses high-frequency sound waves passing through tissues to detect masses in the breast. May be performed if lesions are identified in a mammogram.

RELATED NURSING CARE   No special preparation is needed.

NAME OF TEST   Breast biopsy
- Fine-needle aspiration
- Core needle biopsy
- Vacuum-assisted mammotome
- Large core surgical biopsy
- Open surgical biopsy

PURPOSE AND DESCRIPTION
- A fine-needle aspiration is conducted to withdraw fluid from cysts, and may be used to sample cells from masses in the breast. A 22- to 25-gauge needle is used to collect five to six samples of fluid or cells.
- A core needle biopsy is conducted to obtain a sample of tissue from a solid mass or calcium deposits in the breast. A 10-, 11-, or 12-gauge needle is used to collect five to six tissue samples.
- A vacuum-assisted mammotome is primarily used to evaluate calcifications. An 11- or 14-gauge needle is inserted through a small (1/4-inch) incision and 8 to 10 samples are removed.
- A large core surgical biopsy is performed to evaluate breast masses or calcification identified with a mammogram but nonpalpable. An incision is made and a 5- to 20-mm cylinder of breast tissue (about the size of a wine cork) is removed.
- An open surgical biopsy is performed to evaluate breast masses, hard-to-reach lesions, multiple lesions, and masses with calcifications. A 1.5- to 2-inch incision is made and a golf ball size (or larger) area of tissue is removed.

RELATED NURSING CARE   For all types, wearing a bra, applying ice packs, and mild analgesics decrease discomfort postprocedure.
- Explain that, depending on the physician, some procedures may be performed with or without a local anesthetic.
- Explain that a local anesthetic is used, but no stitches are required for a core needle biopsy or mammatome.
- Explain that a local anesthetic will be administered and stitches will be used to close the incision for a large-core biopsy.
- Explain that a general anesthetic is usually used and that the incision will require stitches and leave a scar for an open surgical biopsy.

TESTS OF THE INTERNAL REPRODUCTIVE SYSTEM

NAME OF TEST   Ultrasound (abdominal, vaginal)

PURPOSE AND DESCRIPTION   Used to detect the presence of space-occupying lesions, such as fibroid tumors, cysts, abscesses, and neoplasms. The abdomen is coated with transducing gel, and a graphic visualization is made. For a vaginal ultrasound, a transducer is covered with a condom or vinyl glove coated with transducer gel and then introduced into the vagina.

RELATED NURSING CARE   Explain need to increase intake of fluids and tell the woman not to void until the test is completed to ensure a full bladder (this lifts the pelvic organs higher in the abdomen and improves visualization).

NAME OF TEST   Hysterosalpingogram

PURPOSE AND DESCRIPTION   Used to diagnose causes of infertility and abnormalities of the uterus or fallopian tubes. A contrast medium is instilled through the cervix, through the uterus, and out the fallopian tubes while x-rays are taken.

RELATED NURSING CARE   Assess for allergy to seafood (iodine) or previous contrast media. Explain that the procedure is briefly painful.

NAME OF TEST   Colposcopy

PURPOSE AND DESCRIPTION   Conducted to further study abnormal Pap tests, and as screening for women exposed to intrauterine DES. A binocular microscope is used to directly visualize the cervix.

RELATED NURSING CARE   No special preparation is needed.

NAME OF TEST   Conization, loop electrosurgical excision of transformation zone (LEETZ), loop electrosurgical excision procedure (LEEP)

PURPOSE AND DESCRIPTION   A conization, LEETZ, or LEEP is performed to remove cervical tissue for evaluation (most often for cervical cancer). A cone-shaped area of tissue surrounding the cervical os is removed.

RELATED NURSING CARE   Explain that the procedure requires general anesthesia. Postoperative self-care includes rest for 2 to 3 days. Explain that minor vaginal bleeding and discharge are expected for several days after the procedures; perineal pads (not tampons) should be used. Sexual intercourse should be avoided until discharge stops. Notify physician of increased bleeding or signs of infection (pain, foul-smelling discharge, fever) occur.

NAME OF TEST   Endometrial biopsy

PURPOSE AND DESCRIPTION   Performed to identify endometrial hyperplasia or endometrial cancer. The cervix is cleaned and tissue is obtained transcervically from the endometrium either by curettage or vacuum aspiration.

RELATED NURSING CARE   Explain that the procedure is briefly painful, and causes vaginal bleeding. Advise to use perineal pads, and avoid tampons and sexual intercourse while bleeding.

(continued)

DIAGNOSTIC TESTS **of the Female Reproductive System (continued)**

NAME OF TEST Cervical biopsy

PURPOSE AND DESCRIPTION Performed for women when Pap test results indicate possible cervical cancer or cervical intraepithelial neoplasia (CIN) and for screening for women at high risk for vaginal and cervical cancers from intrauterine exposure to DES. Cervix is cleaned and a sample of tissue is taken for analysis.

RELATED NURSING CARE Explain that minor vaginal bleeding and discharge are expected for several days after the procedures; perineal pads (not tampons) should be used. Sexual intercourse should be avoided until discharge stops. Notify physician of increased bleeding or signs of infection (pain, foul-smelling discharge, fever) occur.

NAME OF TEST Laparoscopy

PURPOSE AND DESCRIPTION This examination is conducted to visualize the organs in the peritoneal cavity (uterus, fallopian tubes, ovaries); to withdraw fluid for analysis; and to perform a tubal ligation. A fiber-optic scope is inserted through small abdominal incisions and carbon dioxide is inserted into the peritoneal cavity for better visualization.

RELATED NURSING CARE Ask the woman to void prior to the examination and explain that a general anesthetic will be used. Explain that shoulder pain is common after the procedure (referred pain from the retained carbon dioxide gas); that some vaginal bleeding may occur and the woman should use a perineal pad; and to report excess bleeding, pain, or signs of infection to the physician.

Health Assessment Interview

A health assessment interview to determine problems with the female reproductive system may be conducted during a health screening, may focus on a chief complaint (such as severe menstrual cramping), or may be part of a total health assessment. Women may be embarrassed to discuss health problems or concerns involving their reproductive organs; it is important for the nurse to ask questions in a nonthreatening, matter-of-fact manner. Consider the psychologic, social, and cultural factors that affect sexuality and sexual activity. Use words that the woman can understand, and do not be embarrassed or offended by the words she uses. The woman may perceive the interview as less threatening if the discussion begins with more general questions and then progresses to specific questions, and if questions are asked in a way that gives the woman permission to describe behaviors and manifestations. For example, first ask a female client about menstrual and childbirth histories before asking questions about sexually transmitted infections.

The focused interview for the female reproductive system is usually extensive. However, the questions may in many instances be tailored to the specific health problem of the woman. As with the assessment of other body systems, analyze and document the onset of the problem, its duration, frequency, precipitating and relieving factors, any associated symptoms, treatment, self-care, and outcome. For example, ask the woman:

- Have you noticed vaginal bleeding after intercourse?
- Does over-the-counter medication relieve the vaginal itching and discharge?
- Have you had any fever or abdominal pain with this vaginal infection?

Ask about menstrual history, obstetric history, use of contraceptives, sexual history, use of medications, and reproductive system examinations. Also assess the use of condoms during intercourse; unprotected sexual intercourse increases the risk of sexually transmitted infections, including HIV infection. Also ask about smoking; a history of smoking increases the risk of circulatory problems in the woman taking oral contraceptives. Smoking also increases the risk for cancer of the cervix.

Chronic illnesses may affect the function of the female reproductive system. Diabetes mellitus increases the risk of vaginal infections and vaginal dryness, both of which interfere with sexual pleasure. Chronic heavy menstrual flow may result in anemia. Thyroid and adrenal disorders may affect secondary sex characteristics, the menstrual cycle, and the ability to become pregnant.

Obtaining any family history of cancer is important. The risk for endometrial cancer is higher in women with a family history of endometrial, breast, or colon cancer; the risk for ovarian cancer is higher in women with a family history of ovarian or breast cancer; and the risk for breast cancer is higher in women with a family history of breast cancer. Exposure to DES *in utero* increases the risk of cancer of the cervix and vagina. Exposure to asbestos poses a risk of cancer of the ovary. The risk for breast cancer is also greater if the woman has a history of fibrocystic disease.

Carefully explore any history of vaginal bleeding and vaginal discharge. Ask about the onset of vaginal bleeding, any related factors, the color (pink, red, dark red, brown), the character (thin, watery, presence of mucus, size and number of clots), the amount (spotting, how many pads or tampons in a specific amount of time), and relationship to menstrual cycle. Regarding vaginal discharge, ask about the onset, color (white, green, gray), character (thin, thick, curdlike), odor, itching, and rash.

Questions about sexuality may include sexual preference, number of sexual partners; history of **anorgasmia** (absence of orgasm), **dyspareunia** (painful intercourse), or other problems with intercourse; history of sexual trauma; use of condoms or other contraceptives; and current level of sexual satisfaction.

Interview questions categorized by functional health patterns are listed in the Functional Health Pattern Interview table on the next page.

FUNCTIONAL HEALTH PATTERN INTERVIEW The Female Reproductive System

Functional Health Pattern	Interview Questions and Leading Statements
Health Perception-Health Management	■ Have you ever had problems with your reproductive organs (ovaries, tubes, uterus, vagina) or with menstruation or menopause? Explain. If so, how was this problem treated? ■ Do you routinely take any prescribed or herbal medications for symptoms of menopause? If so, what and when do you take it? ■ Did you ever take hormone replacement therapy for menopausal symptoms? ■ Do you practice breast self-examination? When and how often do you do this? ■ Have you noticed any lumps in your breasts or discharge from your nipples? Describe, if so. ■ Have you ever had a breast examination or mammogram? When was your last one? How often do you have these? ■ When was your last gynecologic examination? Pap smear? How often do you have these done? ■ Do you use birth control? If so, what do you use? ■ What do you do to provide self-care if you have mood swings or menstrual cramps? ■ Have you ever had a sexually transmitted infection or an infection of the reproductive organs? What was it? How was it treated? ■ Do you use douches or vaginal sprays? If so, what type and how often? ■ Do you smoke? If so, how much and for how long?
Nutritional-Metabolic	■ Do you notice a change in your appetite right before your menstrual period? ■ Have you gained weight recently? If so, why do think this happened? ■ Describe your usual food intake for a 24-hour period.
Elimination	■ When was your last menstrual period? ■ At what age did you start/end having menstrual periods? ■ Describe the length, amount of flow, and clotting with your menstrual periods. Do you ever have bleeding between your menstrual periods? If so, describe the type and amount. ■ Describe any unusual vaginal discharge you have had (color, consistency, odor, itching, or rash). ■ Have you noticed any changes in urination (frequency, urgency, burning)? ■ Have you noticed changes in bowel elimination during your menstrual periods?
Activity-Exercise	■ Describe your usual activities of daily living. ■ Have you noticed any change in activity or energy during your menstrual period? ■ Have you noticed any change in activity or energy since menopause (if applicable)? If so, how?
Sleep-Rest	■ How long do you sleep at night? ■ Do night sweats wake you? ■ Do menstrual cramps ever wake you at night?
Cognitive-Perceptual	■ Do you have pain or other symptoms (such as headache, mood swings, irritability, bloating, constipation, diarrhea, and/or breast tenderness) before your menstrual period? Describe. What do you do about this? ■ Do you have cramping before or during your menstrual period? Describe the type of cramping, how long it lasts, and what you do to be more comfortable. ■ Do you ever have vaginal itching, pain, burning, or dryness? If so, is it affected by sexual intercourse? Does dryness interfere with intercourse?
Self-Perception-Self-Concept	■ Has this problem affected how you feel about yourself as a woman? ■ Do you believe your needs for intimacy and affection are being met?
Role-Relationships	■ How has having this condition affected your relationships with others? ■ Has having this condition interfered with your ability to work? Explain. ■ Has anyone in your family had problems with breast or ovarian cancer? Explain.
Sexuality-Reproductive	■ Are you currently in a sexual relationship? If so, has this condition interfered with your usual sexual activity? How long have you been with your current partner? Have you had any other partners during this time? ■ What is your sexual preference? ■ Has having this problem affected your relationship with your spouse or sexual partner? ■ Have you ever been pregnant? How many times? Have you ever had a miscarriage? ■ Do you practice birth control? If so, what do you use? ■ Do you ensure that your partner of the opposite gender uses a condom every time you have intercourse? ■ Do you use a vaginal condom?

(continued)

FUNCTIONAL HEALTH PATTERN INTERVIEW The Female Reproductive System (continued)

Functional Health Pattern	Interview Questions and Leading Statements
Coping-Stress-Tolerance	■ Has having this condition created stress for you? If so, does your health problem seem to be more difficult when you are stressed? ■ Have you experienced any kind of stress that makes the condition worse? Explain. ■ Describe what you do when you feel stressed.
Value-Belief	■ Describe how specific relationships or activities help you cope with this problem. ■ Describe specific cultural beliefs or practices that affect how you care for and feel about this problem. ■ Are there any specific treatments that you would not use to treat this problem?

Physical Assessment

Physical assessment of the female reproductive system usually is conducted as part of a scheduled screening (e.g., for an annual Pap smear) or for a specific reproductive health problem. If conducted as part of a total physical assessment, this is usually the final system to be assessed. The nurse must feel comfortable with the examination of clients of the opposite gender; if either the nurse or the client is not comfortable, a nurse of the same gender should be asked to conduct this part of the assessment.

The female reproductive system is assessed by inspection and palpation. Ask the woman to void before having the examination. Prior to the examination, collect all necessary equipment and explain the techniques to the woman to decrease anxiety. Put on disposable gloves before beginning the examination and wear them throughout the examination. Ask the woman to remove her clothing and put on a gown. Ensure that the examining room is private and warm.

The female reproductive system is assessed by inspection and palpation. Explain the procedures for the examination thoroughly and in a matter-of-fact way to decrease anxiety and embarrass-ment. If the woman is unfamiliar with her reproductive organs, charts may be used to demonstrate the parts that will be examined. Carefully explain the procedure for the examination, and show the speculum to the woman. The assessment may be done with the woman in the sitting or supine position to examine the breasts and in the lithotomy position to assess the external genitalia and internal organs. Expose only those body parts being examined to preserve modesty. Normal age-related findings for the older woman are summarized in Table 49–4.

The examination usually begins with examination of the breasts with the woman in the sitting and supine positions. The nurse then helps the woman move to the lithotomy position on the examining table, with the feet in the stirrups and the buttocks even with the foot of the table. Older or frail women may not be able to tolerate this position. In this case, the woman is examined in the supine position. Although the entire examination is described here, the internal examination is conducted only by a nurse with advanced practice in the procedure. However, nurses are often asked to assist with the examination and should be able to explain the examination to a woman.

TABLE 49–4 Age-Related Changes in the Female Reproductive System

AGE-RELATED CHANGE	SIGNIFICANCE
Breasts ■ Atrophy, with sagging of breast tissue ■ Linear strands may appear from shrinkage and fibrotic changes	Although aging does not cause breast cancer, the incidence rises in older women; age-related changes may make finding tumors more difficult.
External Genitalia ■ Labia flatten, and vulvar adipose tissue and hair decrease. ■ ↓ collagen and adipose tissues in the vaginal canal, resulting in loss of rugae, shortening and narrowing of vaginal canal. ■ ↓ vaginal lubrication, epithelium becomes thinner and avascular. ■ More alkaline pH of vagina. ■ Cervix becomes smaller.	Vagina is more easily irritated, increasing the risk of vaginal infections. Lubricants are necessary for comfortable intercourse.
Internal Organs ■ Uterus shrinks. ■ Fallopian tubes shrink and shorten. ■ Ovaries are smaller and thicker. ■ With menopause, hormone production of estrogen decreases. ■ Loss of estrogen may cause pelvic floor muscles to weaken. ■ Loss of estrogen causes changes throughout the body, including loss of skin tone (wrinkling) and growth of facial hair.	With the completion of menopause, the menstrual cycles end and the woman is infertile. Weakening of the pelvic floor muscles may contribute to involuntary incontinence with increased intra-abdominal pressure (as with coughing and sneezing). Skin is dry and thin.

FEMALE REPRODUCTIVE SYSTEM ASSESSMENTS

Technique/Normal Findings	Abnormal Findings

Breast Assessment

Inspect both breasts simultaneously with the woman seated in the following positions: arms at sides, arms overhead, hands pressed on hips, leaning forward. Inspect breast size, symmetry, contour, skin color, texture, venous patterns, and lesions. Lift the breasts, and inspect the lower and lateral aspects. *Breasts normally vary in size and shape, and one breast may normally be larger than the other. Color should be consistent with the skin tone and texture smooth. There should be no redness, swelling, prominent veins, or lesions.*

- Retractions, dimpling, and abnormal contours suggest benign lesions, but may also suggest malignancy.
- Thickened, dimpled skin with enlarged pores (called peau d'orange, orange peel, or pig skin) and unilateral venous patterns are also associated with malignancy.
- Redness may be seen with infection or carcinoma.

Inspect the areolae and nipples. *The color of the areolae should be consistent with the woman's skin color (ranging from dark pink to dark brown), and Montgomery tubercles may be present. The nipples should be equal bilaterally in size, centrally located in each breast, and free of lesions or discharge. Nipples are usually everted, but may normally be inverted or flat.*

- Peau d'orange may be noted first in the areola.
- Recent unilateral inversion of the nipple or asymmetry in the directions in which the nipples point suggests cancer.

Palpate both breasts, axillae, and supraclavicular areas. Figure 49–8 ■ illustrates a possible pattern for breast palpation. Various palpation patterns may be used as long as every part of each breast is palpated, including the axillary tail (also called tail of Spence), which is the breast tissue that extends from the upper outer quadrant toward and into the axillae. Ask the woman to assume a supine position with a small pillow under the shoulder and the arm over the head, and repeat the systematic palpation sequence. Describe identified masses by location, size, shape, consistency, tenderness, mobility, and delineation of borders. *Breasts should feel smooth, firm, and elastic, without palpable masses. Prior to the menstrual cycle, there may be increased nodularity and tenderness.*

- Tenderness may be related to premenstrual fullness, fibrocystic disease, or inflammation. Tenderness may also indicate cancer.
- Nodules in the tail of the breast may be enlarged lymph nodes.
- Hard, irregular, fixed unilateral masses that are poorly delineated suggest carcinoma.
- Bilateral, single or multiple, round, mobile, well-delineated masses are consistent with fibrocystic breast disease or fibroadenoma.
- Swelling, tenderness, erythema, and heat may be seen with mastitis.

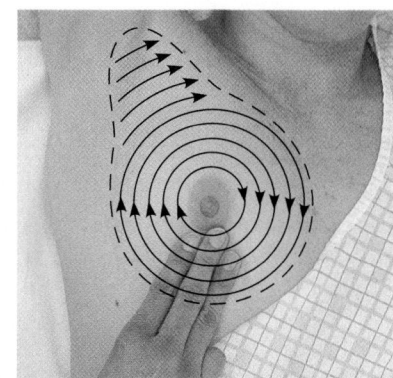

Figure 49–8 ■ Possible pattern for palpation of the breast.

Technique/Normal Findings	Abnormal Findings
Palpate the nipple then compress it between the thumb and index finger. Note the color of any discharge. *Nipples should be firm and elastic, normally without discharge (although some women normally have a clear discharge, and a milky substance may be expressed during pregnancy and lactation).*	■ Loss of nipple elasticity is seen in cancer. ■ Bloody or serous discharge is associated with intraductal papilloma. ■ Milky discharge not due to prior pregnancy and found on both sides suggests galactorrhea (lactation not associated with pregnancy or nursing), which is sometimes associated with a pituitary tumor. ■ Unilateral discharge from one or two ducts can be seen in fibrocystic breast disease, intraductal papilloma, or carcinoma.

Axillary Assessment

Inspect the skin of the axillae. *There should be no redness, irritation, lesions, or enlarged lymph nodes on palpation.*	■ Rash may be due to allergy or other causes. ■ Signs of inflammation and infection may be due to infection of the sweat glands. ■ Palpate all sections of both axillae for palpable nodes (Figure 49–9 ■). ■ Enlarged axillary nodes are most often due to infection of the hand or arm but can be caused by malignancy. ■ Enlarged supraclavicular nodes are associated with lymphatic metastases from abdominal or thoracic carcinoma.

Figure 49–9 ■ Palpating the axillary lymph nodes.

External Genitalia Assessment

Help the woman to the lithotomy position with the knees flexed and separated.

Inspect and palpate the labia majora. *The labia majora should be equal in size and free of lesions or bulging.*	■ Excoriation, rashes, or lesions suggest inflammatory or infective processes. ■ Bulging of the labia that increases with straining suggests a hernia. ■ Varicosities may be present on the labia.
Inspect the labia minora. Separate the labia majora for better visualization. *The labia minora should be symmetrical, dark pink and moist, without redness or lesions.*	■ Inflammation, irritation, excoriation, or caking of discharge in tissue folds suggests vaginal infection or poor hygiene. ■ Ulcers or vesicles may be symptoms of sexually transmitted infection.
Palpate the inside of the labia minora between thumb and forefinger. *There should be no nodules, ulcers, or lesions.*	■ Small, firm, round cystic nodules in labia suggest sebaceous cysts. ■ Wartlike lesions suggest condylomata acuminata (genital warts). ■ Firm, painless ulcers suggest chancre of primary syphilis. ■ Shallow, painful ulcers suggest herpes infection. ■ Ulcerated or red raised lesions in older women suggest vulvar carcinoma.

Technique/Normal Findings	Abnormal Findings
Inspect the clitoris. *The clitoris is normally not enlarged.*	■ Enlargement may be a symptom of a masculinizing condition.
Inspect the vaginal opening. *There should be no swelling, discoloration, lacerations, discharge, or lesions visible in the vaginal opening.*	■ Swelling, discoloration, or lacerations may be caused by trauma. ■ Discharge or lesions may be symptoms of infection. ■ Fissures or fistulas may be related to injury, infection, spreading of a malignancy, or trauma.
Palpate Skene's glands. Using the index finger, "milk" Skene's glands on both sides and over the urethra and inspect for possible discharge (Figure 49–10 ■). *There should be no discharge or tenderness present.*	■ Discharge from Skene's glands and/or tenderness suggests infection.

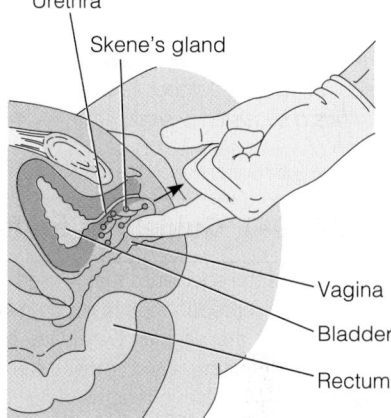

Urethra
Skene's gland
Vagina
Bladder
Rectum

Figure 49–10 ■ Palpating Skene's glands.

Palpate Bartholin's glands at the posterior labia majora (Figure 49–11 ■). *There should be no masses, redness, swelling, or tenderness on palpation.*	■ A nontender mass in the posterolateral portion of the labia majora is indicative of a Bartholin's cyst. ■ Swelling, redness, or tenderness, especially if unilateral, may indicate abscess of Bartholin's glands.

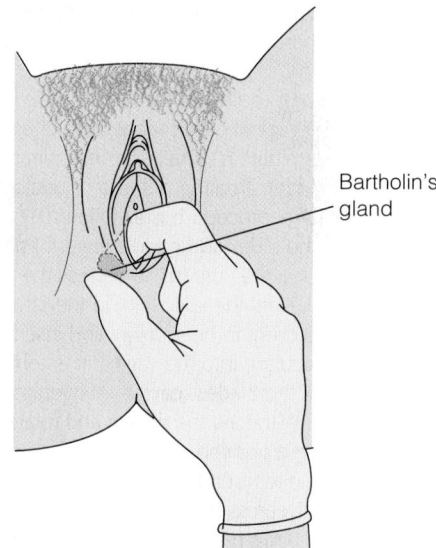

Bartholin's gland

Figure 49–11 ■ Palpating Bartholin's glands.

Inspect the vaginal orifice for bulging and urinary incontinence. Ask the woman to strain or "bear down." *No bulging should be visible with straining.*	■ Bulging of the anterior vaginal wall and urinary incontinence suggest a cystocele. ■ Bulging of the posterior wall suggests a rectocele. ■ Protrusion of the cervix or uterus into the vagina indicates uterine prolapse.
Inspect and palpate the perineum. *The perineum should be free of redness or lesions. Episiotomy scars are a normal finding.*	■ Inflammation, lesions, and growths may be seen in infections or cancer. ■ Fistulas may be the result of injury, trauma, infection, or spreading of a malignancy.

Technique/Normal Findings   **Abnormal Findings**

Vaginal and Cervical Assessment

Use a vaginal speculum to inspect the vaginal walls and cervix. See the guidelines in Box 49–1. *The vaginal opening varies, depending on age, sexual history, and vaginal births. Vaginal mucosa is normally pink and moist, without discharge or odor. There should be no bulging or loss of urine. The cervix is normally smooth and pink, without lesions and has a consistency similar to the tip of the nose.*

- Bluish color of the cervix and vaginal mucosa may be a sign of pregnancy.
- A pale cervix is associated with anemia.
- A cervix to the right or left of the midline may indicate a pelvic mass, uterine adhesions, or pregnancy.
- Projection of the cervix more than 3 cm into the vaginal canal may indicate a pelvic or uterine mass.
- Transverse or star-shaped cervical lacerations reflect trauma causing tearing of the cervix.
- An enlarged cervix is associated with infection.
- Nabothian cysts (small, white, or yellow raised, round areas on the cervix) are considered normal but may become infected.
- Cervical polyps may be cervical or endometrial in origin.

BOX 49–1 Guidelines for Intravaginal Assessment and Use of the Vaginal Speculum

The size of the speculum that is used for an internal examination of the female reproductive system depends on the age of the woman and size of the vagina. Two types of specula are available. The Graves speculum, used most often for examinations of adult women, is available in lengths of 3½ to 5 inches and widths of ¾ to 1½ inches. The Pederson speculum, which is narrower, may be used to examine adolescents or adult woman who are virgins, who have never had a baby, or who are postmenopausal with vaginal atrophy. The speculum should be warm. If cultures or smears are to be obtained, neither water nor gel should be used to warm or to lubricate the speculum.

If cells are to be taken for cytologic studies, the client should not douche, use vaginal medications, or take a tub bath for 24 hours before the examination. Finally, the examination is usually deferred if the client is menstruating or has a vaginal infection.

The general procedure is as follows:

1. Place the index and middle finger of one hand into the vagina, just inside the introitus, and press the fingers toward the rectum. Hold the speculum in the other hand.
2. Ask the client to bear down, and insert the closed blades of the speculum into the vagina at an oblique angle until the ends of the blades reach the fingertips (see the accompanying figure). Withdraw the fingers and rotate the speculum to a transverse position.
3. Continue to insert the speculum until it reaches the end of the vagina. Depress the lever of the speculum to open the blades. If the cervix is not in full view, try closing the blades, withdrawing the speculum about halfway, and inserting it again at a more downward angle. When the cervix is in full view, fix the depressed lever to an open position.
4. Inspect the cervix. The normal cervix is pink and midline. Assess color, position, size, projection into the vagina, surface and shape, and any discharge.

If a Pap smear to collect cervical cells for cytologic studies is done, the following procedure may be used:

1. To collect cells from the vaginal pool, roll a sterile cotton-tipped applicator on the vaginal wall below the cervix. Paint the smear on the slide, and spray the slide with fixative.
2. To collect endocervical cells, place the groove of the spatula snugly against the cervical os, and rotate it 360 degrees. In a single stroke, spread the material from both sides of the spatula on a slide, and immediately spray with fixative.

If cultures are to be done, take a specimen from the vagina and/or cervix with a sterile, cotton-tipped applicator, and then either spread the specimen on a culture plate or place it in a culture container. Follow institutional protocols for preparing specimens for vaginal infections from suspected organisms.

At the end of the examination, loosen the lever control and slowly withdraw the speculum, closing the blades slowly and rotating the speculum while observing all areas of the vaginal wall. Assess the color of the mucosa and the color and appearance of any discharge.

Inserting the vaginal speculum.

Palpate the cervix, uterus, and ovaries. See the guidelines in Box 49–2. *The cervix can be moved slightly without discomfort. The uterus is*

- The uterus may be retroverted (tilted backward) or retroflexed (angled backward).
- Pain on movement of the cervix during manual examination suggests pelvic inflammatory disease (PID).
- Softening of the uterine isthmus (Hegar's sign), softening of the cervix (Goodell's sign), and uterine enlargement may be objective signs of pregnancy.

Technique/Normal Findings	Abnormal Findings

normally at the level of the pubis, moves freely, and is nontender. The ovaries (about the size of a walnut) are firm, smooth, mobile, and slightly tender on palpation. The ovaries are not usually palpable 3 to 5 years after menopause. A small amount of clear drainage is normal.

- Firm, irregular nodules that vary greatly with size and are continuous with the uterine surface are likely to be myomas (fibroids).
- Unilateral or bilateral smooth, compressible adnexal masses are found in ovarian tumors.
- Profuse menstrual bleeding is seen with endometrial polyps, dysfunctional uterine bleeding (DUB), and use of an intrauterine device.
- Irregular bleeding may be associated with endometrial polyps, DUB, uterine or cervical carcinoma, or oral contraceptives.
- Postmenopausal bleeding is seen with endometrial hyperplasia, estrogen therapy, and endometrial cancer.

BOX 49–2 Guidelines for Bimanual Pelvic Examination

The bimanual pelvic examination is done to palpate the cervix, uterus, and ovaries. The examiner's hand that will be used intravaginally is held with the index and middle fingers extended, the thumb abducted, and the fourth and fifth fingers folded on the palm of the hand. The extended fingers are lubricated.

The general procedure is as follows:

1. Spread the labia with the thumb and finger of the opposite hand and insert the lubricated fingers into the vagina with the palm upward.
2. Place the opposite hand on the abdomen; it is used to press on the abdomen and gently move the internal genitals toward the intravaginal fingers (see the accompanying figure).
3. Ask the client to take deep breaths to relax the abdominal wall.
4. Palpate the cervix, assessing size, contour, position, surface, consistency, tenderness, and mobility. The cervix should be freely movable and nontender.
5. Palpate the uterus by pressing downward on the abdomen while placing the intravaginal fingers in the anterior fornix and gently lifting against the abdominal hand. Assess the size, shape, surface, consistency, position, mobility, and tenderness of the uterus. The normal uterus is freely movable and nontender.
6. Palpate the adnexal areas, which surround the uterus and contain the fallopian tubes and ovaries. Because these

Bimanual pelvic examination.

structures are small, palpation may not be possible. If the ovaries are palpable, they should be smooth and firm. The normal ovary is sensitive to touch, firm, and highly movable.

7. Withdraw the fingers. Provide tissues for the client's use in wiping the genital area.

EXPLORE MEDIALINK

Prentice Hall Nursing MediaLink DVD-ROM
Audio Glossary
NCLEX-RN® Review

COMPANION WEBSITE www.prenhall.com/lemone
Audio Glossary
NCLEX-RN® Review
Care Plan Activity: STDs
Case Studies
  Assessing Sexual Function
  Irregular Menstrual Cycle
Exercise: Sexual Function Health History
MediaLink Applications: Breast Cancer Screening
Links to Resources

TEST YOURSELF NCLEX-RN® REVIEW

1 In the male, sperm and testosterone are produced by the:
1. epididymis.
2. seminal vesicles.
3. testes.
4. Cowper's glands.

2 What female structure is analogous to the penis in the male?
1. ovaries
2. labia majora
3. labia minora
4. clitoris

3 You are assessing a 65-year-old man. He says, "I don't understand how having prostate problems can cause me to urinate all the time." What would you say to begin your explanation?
1. "The prostate gland presses on the bladder."
2. "The prostate gland surrounds your urethra."
3. "Your kidneys respond to prostate enlargement."
4. "The prostate glands sit on top of the kidneys."

4 What blood test may be used to diagnose prostate cancer?
1. PSA
2. VDRL
3. CBC
4. WBC

5 Suspected abnormalities of the scrotum may be further assessed through:
1. transillumination.
2. auscultation.
3. palpation.
4. percussion.

6 The loss of estrogen production following menopause may result in elevation of what potentially harmful substance that increases the risk of cardiovascular disease?

1. uric acid
2. glucose
3. cholesterol
4. testosterone

7 Cessation of menstruation in young women is a normal response to what biologic event?
1. implantation of an embryo
2. onset of menopause
3. onset of puberty
4. beginning spermatogenesis

8 Which of the following diagnostic tests may be used to detect cervical cancer?
1. colposcopy
2. mammogram
3. culture
4. Pap smear

9 What assessment technique is **primarily** used to determine abnormalities of the breast?
1. inspection
2. auscultation
3. palpation
4. percussion

10 At what anatomic location would you palpate Bartholin's glands?
1. above the clitoris
2. posterior to the labia majora
3. inferior to the urinary meatus
4. internal vaginal wall

See Test Yourself answers in Appendix C.

BIBLIOGRAPHY

Anderson, M., Klink, K., & Cohrssen, A. (2004). The rational clinical examination. Evaluation of vaginal complaints. *Journal of the American Medical Association, 291*(11), 1368–1379.

Bickley, L., & Szilagyi, P. (2007). *Bates' guide to physical examination and history taking* (9th ed.). Philadelphia: Lippincott.

Buxton-Blake, P. (2003). Recognizing menopausal symptomatology. *Home Health Care Management & Practice, 15*(2), 147–151.

Davis, A., & Calvert, H. (2003). Sexually transmitted diseases in the emergency department. *Topics in Emergency Medicine, 25*(3), 247–255.

Eliopoulos, E. (2005). *Gerontological nursing* (6th ed.). Philadelphia: Lippincott Williams & Wilkins.

Heath, H., & White, I. (2001). Sexuality and older people: An introduction to nursing assessment. *Nursing Older People, 13*(4), 29–31.

Jarvis, C. (2004). *Physical examination & health assessment.* St. Louis, MO: Mosby.

Kee, J. (2005). *Prentice Hall handbook of laboratory & diagnostic tests with nursing implications.* Upper Saddle River, NJ: Prentice Hall.

Kellogg-Spaddt, S., & Albaugh, J. (2003). External genital and dermatologic examination part I: The female patient. *Urologic Nursing, 23*(4), 305–306.

Knight, D. (2004). Health care screening for men who have sex with men. *American Family Physician, 69*(9), 2149–2156.

Mick, J., Hughes, M., & Cohen M. (2004). Using the BETTER model to assess sexuality. *Clinical Journal of Oncology Nursing, 8*(1), 84–86.

National Institutes of Health. (2003a). *Genes and disease. Female-specific diseases.* Retrieved from http://www.ncbi.nlm.nih.gov/books/bv.fcgi?rid=gnd.chapter.39

_____. (2003b). *Genes and disease. Male-specific diseases.* Retrieved from http://www.ncbi.nlm.nih.gov/books/bv.fcgi?rid=gnd.chapter.56

Porth, C. (2005). *Pathophysiology: Concepts of altered health states* (7th ed.). Philadelphia: Lippincott.

Shokar, G., Carlson, C., Davis, B., & Shokar, N. (2003). Testicular cancer screening in a primary care setting. *International Journal of Men's Health, 2*(3), 221–228.

Unber, J. (2004). How to assess and treat erectile dysfunction. *Emergency Medicine, 36*(1), 28–30, 33–37.

Wallace, M. (2003). Try this: Best practices in nursing care to older adults from the Hartford Institute for Geriatric Nursing. Sexuality. *Dermatology Nursing, 15*(6), 570–571.

Weber, J., & Kelley, J. (2006). *Health assessment in nursing* (3rd ed.). Philadelphia: Lippincott.

CHAPTER 50 Nursing Care of Men with Reproductive System and Breast Disorders

LEARNING OUTCOMES

- Explain the pathophysiology, manifestations, complications, interdisciplinary care, and nursing care of disorders of the male reproductive system, including disorders of sexual function, the penis, the testes and scrotum, the prostate gland, and the breast.

- Compare and contrast the risk factors for cancer of the penis, testes, and prostate gland.

- Discuss the purposes, nursing implications, and health education for medications and treatments used to treat disorders of sexual function, the penis, the testes and scrotum, the prostate gland, and the breast.

- Describe the various surgical procedures used to treat disorders of the male reproductive system.

CLINICAL COMPETENCIES

- Assess functional health status of men with reproductive system and breast disorders and monitor, document, and report abnormal manifestations.

- Use evidence-based research to provide appropriate discharge teaching to men having a radical prostatectomy.

- Determine priority nursing diagnoses, based on assessed data, to select and implement individualized nursing interventions for men with disorders of the reproductive system and breast.

- Administer, or teach clients how to administer, topical, oral, and injectable medications used to treat disorders of the male reproductive system knowledgeably and safely.

- Provide skilled care to men having prostate surgery.

- Revise plan of care as needed to provide effective interventions to promote, maintain, or restore functional health status to men with disorders of the reproductive system and breast.

Men are subject to disorders of the penis, scrotum and testes, prostate gland, and breast. These disorders may be inflammatory, structural, benign, or malignant. Young men are at increased risk for testicular cancer. As men age, both benign and malignant conditions of the prostate gland become common. Many of the disorders pose significant risk to the man's fertility and sexual and urinary function, and some are life threatening. This chapter discusses disorders of the male reproductive system, including disorders of sexual expression and the male breast. Because many of the treatments and disorders of the male reproductive system have the potential to affect erection and ejaculation, these problems are discussed first.

DISORDERS OF MALE SEXUAL FUNCTION

THE MAN WITH ERECTILE DYSFUNCTION

Erectile dysfunction (ED) is the inability of the male to attain and maintain an erection sufficient to permit satisfactory sexual intercourse. **Impotence**, a term often used synonymously with erectile dysfunction, may involve a total inability to achieve erection, an inconsistent ability to achieve erection, or the ability to sustain only brief erections. ED has many possible causes (Table 50–1), and may or may not be associated with a loss of **libido** (sexual desire).

The incidence of ED is difficult to estimate because many affected men may not report the disorder. An estimated 15 to 30 million men in the United States have ED, and most are older

TABLE 50–1 Causes of Erectile Dysfunction

MAJOR PATHOLOGIC CAUSES		MAJOR IATROGENIC CAUSES	
		Medications	**Procedures and Infections**
Neurogenic	*Arterial*	*Antihypertensives*	*Surgery*
Spinal cord injury	Atherosclerosis	Hydrochlorothiazide	Coronary artery bypass
Stroke	Hypertension	Spironolactone	Pelvic lymphadenectomy
Parkinson's disease	Aortic aneurysm	Methyldopa	Radical prostatectomy
Multiple sclerosis	Sickle cell anemia	Clonidine	Radical cystectomy
Endocrinologic	*Mechanical*	Prazosin	Abdominal perineal resection
Diabetes mellitus	Decreased penile distensibility	Propranolol	Sympathectomy
Hypogonadism	Congenital disorders	Reserpine	Aortic aneurysm repair
Hypothyroidism	Morbid obesity	*Psychotropic Agents*	Transplant surgeries
Inflammatory	Hydrocele	Phenothiazines	*Other*
Prostatitis	Hip or pelvic fractures	Butyrophenones	Severe nosocomial infection
Cystitis	*Psychogenic*	Tricyclic antidepressants	Radiation therapy to pelvis
Activity Intolerance	Depression	MAO inhibitors	
Pulmonary problems	Stress	Diazepum	
Anemias	Fatigue	Chlorodiazepoxide	
Myocardial infarction	Fear of failure	*Endocrinologic Agents*	
Congestive heart failure	*Compulsive Food Disorders*	LHRH agonists	
Hepatic diseases	Compulsive overeating	Estrogen compounds	
Renal failure	Anorexia nervosa	Progesterone	
Substance Dependency	Bulimia	*Other*	
Alcohol		Antiparkinsonian agents	
Marijuana		Anticholinergic agents	
Narcotics		Immunosuppressive agents	
Sedatives		Antihistamines	
Tobacco			

than age 65 (National Kidney and Urologic Disease Information Clearinghouse [NKUDIC], 2003a). The incidence of the problem increases with age. Most problems with erection are the result of a disease, injury, or chemical substance (such as prescribed medications, alcohol, nicotine, cocaine, or marijuana) that decreases blood flow in the penis (Cleveland Clinic, 2004). Because this is a problem primarily of aging men, the discussion of pathophysiology focuses on this age group.

Pathophysiology

Age-related changes in sexual function involve cellular and tissue changes in the penis, decreased sensory activity, hypogonadism, and the effects of chronic illness. In the penis, a change from elastic collagen to a more rigid collagen results in decreased distensibility (a less rigid erection). This, in turn, interferes with the veno-occlusive mechanism, which prevents blood from "leaking" out of the penis into the general vasculature prematurely. Problems with this mechanism result in incomplete erections. Vibrotactile sensation over the skin of the penis declines with age. This decline may explain why some older men require longer stimulation to achieve an erection. Hypogonadism, common in aging men, results in decreased testosterone levels. There may be a relationship between lower androgen levels and erectile function.

Many illnesses affect erectile function. Damage to arteries, smooth muscles, and fibrous tissues are the most common causes of impotence. Diseases such as diabetes, kidney disease, chronic alcoholism, atherosclerosis, and vascular disease are responsible for organic ED. Innervation and blood flow to the penis may be damaged during surgery, prostate surgery in particular. Given the effects of aging on the vasculature of the penis, the increased incidence of chronic illness, and the multiple medications and treatments required to manage those illnesses, it is not surprising that many older men have problems with ED.

INTERDISCIPLINARY CARE

The management of men with ED is growing in importance and scale, because the population as a whole is aging, so the incidence is increasing proportionately. Another factor is the gradual change in the willingness of men and their partners to discuss sexual concerns. Although sexuality is still a very sensitive and private area for most people, the knowledge that help is available is causing men to seek answers. Many older men are coming to believe that loss of erectile function is not an inevitable part of aging.

Diagnosis

The diagnostic tests that may be ordered include blood studies, penile monitoring, and penile blood flow.

Blood chemistry, testosterone, prolactin, thyroxin, and prostate specific antigen (PSA) levels are measured to identify metabolic and endocrine problems that may be causing the dysfunction. Nocturnal penile tumescence and rigidity (NPTR) monitoring helps differentiate between psychogenic and organic causes. These tests can be performed in a sleep laboratory, although home testing with portable devices is an

alternative. The number and quality of erections occurring during REM sleep can be determined. Cavernosometry and cavernosography of the corpora are used to evaluate arterial inflow and venous outflow of blood in the penis.

Medications

ED can be treated with medications taken orally, injected directly into the penis, or inserted into the urethra at the tip of the penis.

- *Oral medications:* The oral medications used to treat ED include sildenafil citrate (Viagra), vardenafil hydrochloride (Levitra), or tadalafil (Cialis). Viagra and Levitra are taken an hour before sexual activity and enhance the effects of nitrous oxide to facilitate relaxation of the smooth muscle in the penis during sexual stimulation to increase blood flow. Both drugs should be taken no more than once a day, and should not be taken by men who are also taking nitrate-based drugs (for health problems) or alpha-blockers (used to treat hypertension and prostate enlargement). Cialis is a selective phosphodiesterase type 5 inhibitor that allows smooth muscle relaxation to facilitate inflow of blood into the penis. Its action lasts for 36 hours, but an erection only occurs with sexual stimulation. Cialis should not be taken if the man is also taking nitrates, alpha-blockers, erythromycin or rifampicin (antibiotics), ketoconazole or itraconazole (antifungals), or protease inhibitors (for HIV).
- *Injectable medications:* Hormone replacement therapy with testosterone injections (200 mg IM every 3 weeks) or topical patches may be used for men with documented androgen deficiency and who do not have prostate cancer. Injectable medications, including papaverine and prostaglandin E injections, may be used. When injected directly into the penis, papaverine relaxes the arterioles and smooth muscles of the cavernosum, thus inducing tumescence (swelling). An erection usually develops that lasts from 30 minutes to 4 hours. Prostaglandin E functions much as papaverine does, but has fewer side effects. One problem with this treatment is its mode of delivery. There is a high attrition rate, and clients report dissatisfaction with lack of spontaneity, loss of interest in sex, physical limitations, cost, and, occasionally, pain. Alprostadil (Caverject) is another injectable medication that may be used to treat ED. It may be injected into the penis or placed in the urethra as a minisuppository.

Mechanical Devices

A frequently prescribed mechanical device for ED is the vacuum constriction device (VCD). The VCD draws blood into the penis with a vacuum, trapping it there with a constricting band at the base of the penis. After the device is removed for intercourse, a single small band, often called an O-ring, is left at the base of the penis to maintain the erection. If the man can attain an erection but cannot maintain it, then an O-ring alone can be used.

Surgery

Surgical treatment for ED involves either revascularization procedures or implantation of prosthetic devices. Venous or arterial procedures are generally not successful. The result is often temporary, because the underlying cause of the vascular insufficiency is usually not corrected. Implantation of penile prostheses is now common (Figure 50–1 ■). Men are generally satisfied with their prostheses, and they rank the inflatable type highest. Partners are also more likely to report satisfaction with the penile implant, although not to the same degree as clients. Some partners report that the implanted penis is harder than a normal erect penis and therefore causes pain. Also, the man can have intercourse for a prolonged period of time, and some partners do not find prolonged penetration enjoyable. Client and partner teaching is mandatory. Counseling by a sex therapist may be needed to facilitate adaptation to the implant.

NURSING CARE

Nurses in any healthcare setting may encounter men with ED, either through routine examinations or through careful assessment of clients' conditions and treatments that may incidentally cause ED. Nurses employed in clinics, operating rooms, and surgical units with urologic services commonly encounter men being treated for ED. Nurses in a variety of settings, including long-term care, encounter men who have had surgical interventions, such as penile implants.

Nursing Diagnoses and Interventions

Because nurses often complete a client's health history, they are most likely to discover problems of ED (see the Functional Health Pattern Interview guide in Chapter 49 ∞ for appropriate questions to elicit information). Once a problem is known, nurses are involved in giving information, providing emotional support, and referring clients to physicians or counselors. Although there are many possible nursing diagnoses, this section focuses on nursing care related to sexual dysfunction and self-esteem.

Sexual Dysfunction

Many men who lose erectile function are not aware of the cause. Often the man blames the loss on unrelated factors, such as age, a medication for an illness, a dangerous illness, or his sexual partner. Not knowing causes anxiety, which may disrupt the relationship with his partner or lead him to discontinue an important medication.

- Assess for risk factors for ED. Be especially alert to men who have recently begun medications or had recent surgeries that could cause ED. *Awareness of risk factors helps the nurse to prioritize care, although nurses must remember that almost all aging clients have at least one risk factor for ED.*
- Assess for sexual dysfunction. Men have shown increasing willingness to discuss sexual concerns and expect nurses to be aware of the physiologic effects of their disease and side effects of treatment on all aspects of their health. *If a problem exists, information obtained in a sexual assessment guides the nurse in deciding if the next step should be client teaching, referral, or both.*
- Perform a detailed assessment of current sexual practices. *It is essential for healthcare providers to understand the client and partner's sexual pattern in order to provide appropriate, individualized care.*
- Discuss previous methods of coping with ED. *Awareness of coping strategies can provide insight for the nurse and guide teaching.*
- Provide information about treatment options. *The man needs to know the details of the intervention, the chances for success, and the possible complications.*

PRACTICE ALERT
Many men will not volunteer information about sexual function unless asked, but then are open about concerns and appreciate being asked.

A Semirigid

B Self-contained

C Inflatable

Figure 50–1 ■ Types of penile implants. *A,* With semirigid rods implanted in the corpora cavernosa, the penis is always in a state of semi-erection, which may not be acceptable to the man. *B,* With a self-contained penile implant, the penis remains flaccid until the man compresses a pump at the head of the penis, which transfers fluid from a reservoir to a cylinder within the penis to achieve an erection. The man presses a release valve to return the fluid to the reservoir. *C,* With an inflatable penile implant, the penis remains flaccid until the man compresses a pump in the scrotum, which transfers fluid from an abdominal reservoir to cylinders in the corpora cavernosa to achieve an erection. Pressing a release valve returns the fluid to the reservoir.

Situational Low Self-Esteem

The man with ED often believes himself to be "less than a man." In addition, the insertion of a penile implant with a semirigid prosthesis may result in disturbances in body image related to changes in sexual activity as well as the appearance and embarrassment of a permanent semi-erection.

- Collect data during the health history, in a nonjudgmental manner, about physiologic function, other chronic illnesses, and feelings about sexual inadequacy. *This information is necessary to establish the database for individualized interventions.*
- If the man has had a penile implant, teach him and his partner how to use the pump, including how to inflate and deflate the device. Suggest he practice inflation and deflation during the postoperative period. Suggest wearing snug-fitting underwear with the penis placed in an upright position on the abdomen and loose trousers. Provide information about length of healing, and that sexual activity may resume within 6 to 8 weeks following surgery. *Practice using the pump will maintain the pump position and promote tissue growth around the implant. The type of clothing worn can improve the ability to conceal a semirigid prosthesis and decrease embarrassment. Recovery from surgery is necessary before resuming sexual activity.*

Community-Based Care

Many nurses find that men with ED and their partners have lived in isolation with the problem for many years. The partner may even be unaware of the problem. The partner may believe that the man is seeing someone else or that the man has lost his attraction to the partner. The man may have kept his problem a secret because an intense feeling of shame makes him unable to admit that he cannot perform sexually. Many men greet the information about the high incidence of ED with a sense of relief that they are not alone in having this problem. All men and their partners need to be aware of support services available to them. Referral sources include:

- Sexual Function Health Council
- American Urological Association
- American Association of Sex Educators, Counselors, and Therapists.

THE MAN WITH EJACULATORY DYSFUNCTION

There are many types of ejaculatory dysfunction. **Retrograde ejaculation** (seminal fluid discharged into the bladder) may develop in aging men but is usually related to treatment of prostate conditions or testicular cancer. *Premature ejaculation* is usually psychogenic in origin, although diabetes can cause the problem as well. *Delayed ejaculation* can be related to aging changes, such as decreased vibrotactile sensation over the penis or decreased libido secondary to hypogonadism. Delayed ejaculation and inability to ejaculate at all may be caused by certain medications, such as antihypertensives, antidepressants, anxiolytics, and narcotics.

Among these problems, premature ejaculation has proved most responsive to medical management. The man can experiment with ways (such as wearing condoms) to decrease sensitivity. Using relaxation and guided imagery can delay orgasm. Mechanical devices, such as constrictive rings around the base of the penis, can help the man delay ejaculation and sustain an erection.

Nursing care focuses on assessment of the problem and teaching for all types of ejaculatory dysfunction. The man's partner can be taught how to avoid excessive stimulation that would result in premature ejaculation. If the problem persists, the man should be referred to a specialist.

DISORDERS OF THE PENIS

THE MAN WITH PHIMOSIS OR PRIAPISM

Two less common disorders of the penis are phimosis and priapism. Although uncommon, these disorders can cause problems with urination and sexual activity. In some cases, they are considered a medical emergency, because decreased blood flow to the penis may result in tissue ischemia and necrosis.

Pathophysiology

Phimosis is constriction of the foreskin in uncircumcised men so that it cannot be retracted over the glans penis. Phimosis may be congenital, or it may be related to chronic infections under the foreskin, which lead to adhesions. The major problem with this condition is that it prevents adequate hygiene, which may lead to malignant changes of the penis. It also may interfere with urinary elimination and intercourse. In a related disorder, called *paraphimosis,* the foreskin is tight and constricted, and is not able to cover the glans penis. The glans becomes engorged and edematous, and is painful. Paraphimosis may result from long-term retraction of the foreskin, such as occurs in placement of an indwelling catheter in the uncircumcised male (Porth, 2005). The tight foreskin can result in ischemia of the glans.

Priapism is an involuntary, sustained, painful erection that is not associated with sexual arousal. The prolonged erection may result in ischemia and fibrosis of the erectile tissue with high risk of subsequent impotence (Porth, 2005). The disorder, classified as either primary or secondary, is caused by impaired blood flow in the corpora cavernosa. Primary priapism results from conditions such as tumors, infection, or trauma. Secondary priapism is caused by blood disorders (e.g., leukemia, sickle cell anemia, and thrombocytopenia), neurologic disorders (e.g., spinal cord injury or stroke), renal failure, and some medications (Box 50–1). Men who use intracavernous injection therapy or Cialis for ED are at risk for priapism.

INTERDISCIPLINARY CARE

Severe phimosis or paraphimosis may require surgical circumcision. If infection is present, the appropriate antibiotic is administered.

Treatment of priapism includes iced saline enemas, intravenous ketamine (Ketalar) administration to induce anesthesia, and spinal anesthesia. Blood may be aspirated from the corpus through the dorsal glans, followed by catheterization and pressure dressings to maintain decompression. If necessary, more aggressive surgery to create vascular shunts to maintain blood flow is performed. When priapism is prolonged, it increases the risk of subsequent ED.

NURSING CARE

Nursing care for priapism focuses on assessing the penis, monitoring urinary output, and providing pain control. Assessment of the penis includes inspection for degree of erection and changes in color due to ischemia, and palpation of the penis for firmness and degree of rigidity. Monitor urine output, assessing for oliguria or signs of acute urinary retention. Pain is treated with analgesics.

The man usually has moderate to severe anxiety related to pain, the treatment, and the threat to his sexual function. The treatment may sound bizarre and painful, especially since the area is already extremely sensitive. The man may be acutely embarrassed by the erection and needs reassurance that the nurse understands that the erection is not within his control.

THE MAN WITH CANCER OF THE PENIS

Cancer of the penis is a rare cancer in North America, occurring in approximately 1500 men per year (American Cancer Society [ACS], 2005a). It most commonly affects men between the ages of 45 and 60. The cause is unknown. Penile cancer is rare in Jewish and Muslim men, populations in which routine circumcision is practiced, although the correlation between circumcision and this cancer is unclear. Phimosis and poor genital hygiene are risk factors, as are human papillomavirus HPV and HIV infections. Ultraviolet light exposure (such as that used to treat psoriasis) also may play a role (Porth, 2005).

Pathophysiology

Squamous cell carcinoma accounts for 95% of all penile cancers (Porth, 2005). The tumor usually develops as a nodular or wart-like growth or a red velvety lesion on the glans or foreskin. The tumors tend to grow slowly. Penile cancer spreads to the superficial or deep inguinal nodes, and very late in the disease may spread to the bone, liver, or lungs. If the lesion is treated before inguinal node involvement, chances for a cure are good. Most of these lesions are painless but there may be significant ulceration and bleeding. Purulent, foul-smelling discharge may be evident under the foreskin. Occasionally, men with penile cancer may present with enlarged inguinal lymph nodes.

INTERDISCIPLINARY CARE

Cancer of the penis is diagnosed by a biopsy of the lesion, including any suspicious inguinal lymph nodes. The cancer is staged according to the size of the tumor, extent of invasion, status of inguinal lymph nodes, and presence or absence of distant metastasis. Small, localized lesions may be treated with fluorouracil cream, external-beam radiation, laser therapy, or surgical excision. Larger lesions with superficial or deep infiltration of penile structures require partial or total amputation of the penis. Chemotherapy (discussed in Chapter 14 ∞) may be administered to men with distant metastasis.

NURSING CARE

Education can help prevent this disease or provide early detection and cure. Teach men about genital hygiene (including retraction of the foreskin if uncircumcised, and washing the glans penis while bathing or showering) and the risks of unprotected sex, and encourage condom use. Encourage men to shield their genitals when having ultraviolet light therapy or using tanning salons. Discuss the importance of seeking prompt treatment for any lesion or abnormal drainage noted on the penis.

If the man has a penile amputation (*penectomy*), nurses help cope with the problems of a shortened or absent penis, including the potentially devastating effect on body image and self-concept. If a total penectomy is performed, the surgeon creates a perineal urethrostomy, preserving urinary continence. However, the man must void in the sitting position, reinforcing the feeling of loss. Dribbling of urine after voiding may be a problem for a few weeks. The man should be taught to perform careful perineal hygiene following surgery, using mild soap and water. Sitz baths may be helpful to relieve pain and to promote healing. If an inguinal lymph node dissection is performed, the man may experience persistent lymphedema of the lower extremities.

DISORDERS OF THE TESTIS AND SCROTUM

THE MAN WITH A BENIGN SCROTAL MASS

Most scrotal masses are benign and can be managed in a manner that is satisfactory to the client. The most common are hydroceles, spermatoceles, and varicoceles (Figure 50–2 ■).

Pathophysiology

A **hydrocele**, the most common cause of scrotal swelling, is a collection of fluid within the tunica vaginalis. The swelling ranges from slightly larger than the testicle to larger than a grapefruit. The cause of chronic hydrocele in men over the age of 40 years is

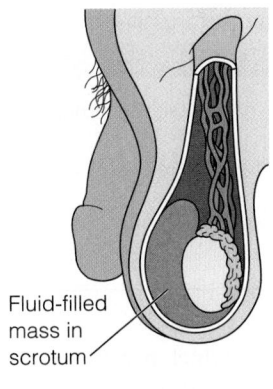

Fluid-filled
mass in
scrotum

Hydrocele

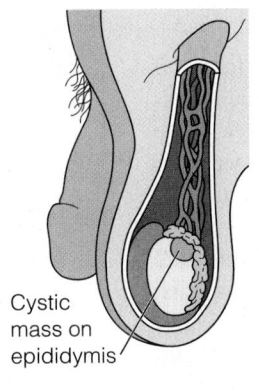

Cystic
mass on
epididymis

Spermatocele

Dilation of
pampiniform
venous
complex

Varicocele

Figure 50–2 ■ Common disorders of the scrotum. Hydroceles and spermatoceles do not usually require treatment unless they become large and cause pain. Varicoceles are usually treated to prevent infertility.

an imbalance between production and reabsorption of fluid within the layers of the scrotum. Hydroceles also may occur secondary to trauma, infection, or a tumor. A hydrocele may be differentiated from a solid mass by transillumination or ultrasound of the scrotum. If the hydrocele becomes large enough to cause embarrassment or significant pain, the fluid is aspirated and an agent is injected into the scrotal sac to sclerose the tunica vaginalis. Hydroceles are not associated with infertility.

A **spermatocele** is a mobile, usually painless mass that forms when efferent ducts in the epididymis dilate and form a cyst. It is thought to result from leakage of sperm due to trauma or infection. Treatment is usually not necessary. Spermatoceles are not associated with infertility.

A **varicocele** is an abnormal dilation of a vein within the spermatic cord. It is caused by incompetent or congenitally missing valves that allow blood to pool in the spermatic cord veins. The dilated vein forms a soft mass that may be painful. Most varicoceles occur after puberty on the left side. A major concern with this condition is that it can decrease blood flow through the testis, interfere with spermatogenesis, and cause infertility. Varicoceles can be felt by scrotal palpation. Sonography is also frequently used for diagnosis. If infertility is a concern, the spermatic vein may be ligated or occluded with a sclerosing agent or balloon catheter. If the varicocele is small and infertility is not a concern, a scrotal support is recommended.

NURSING CARE

Nursing care focuses on reducing anxiety and teaching about comfort measures. Almost all men are aware of the possible pain associated with scrotal manipulation. They need information and reassurance about pain management if surgical treatment is necessary. External bleeding is minimal after surgery; however, some men do develop scrotal hematomas, manifested by scrotal edema and a purple discoloration.

THE MAN WITH EPIDIDYMITIS

Epididymitis is an infection or inflammation of the epididymis, the structure that lies along the posterior border of the testis.

This disorder is more often seen in sexually active men who are less than 35 years of age.

Sexually transmitted urethritis caused by *C. trachomatis* or *N. gonorrhoeae* is the usual precipitating factor for epididymitis in younger men. Men who practice unprotected anal intercourse may acquire sexually transmitted epididymitis from *E. coli, H. influenzae, Cryptococcus,* or tuberculosis. In men older than age 35, epididymitis usually is associated with a urinary tract infection or prostatitis. Chemical epididymitis is associated with an inflammatory response to the reflux of urine into the ejaculatory ducts from urethral strictures, congenital structural anomalies, or increased abdominal pressure from excessive heavy lifting. This type is usually self-limiting and does not require treatment.

Infectious epididymis spreads by ascending the vas deferens from an already infected urethra or bladder. Early manifestations include pain and local edema, which can progress to erythema and edema of the entire scrotum, especially on the side of the involved epididymis. Complications of the disorder include abscess formation, infarction of the testis, and infertility.

INTERDISCIPLINARY CARE

The infection is diagnosed with a specimen culture from a urethral swab or epididymal aspiration. Severe epididymitis may be treated with intravenous antibiotics and hospitalization. Less acute forms of the disease are treated with outpatient antibiotic therapy. The man's sexual partner should be treated with antibiotics if the causative organism is sexually transmitted.

NURSING CARE

Nursing care involves symptomatic relief and teaching. Ice packs and a scrotal support may be applied to the scrotum to relieve pain. Ensure the man knows that complete resolution of the infection may take weeks to months, and that treatment should continue until the infection is gone. Provide information about the possibility of infertility, because the man may wish to seek evaluation for this problem at a later date.

THE MAN WITH ORCHITIS

Orchitis is an acute inflammation or infection of the testes. It most commonly occurs as a complication of a systemic illness or as an extension of epididymitis. Infection may reach the testes through the vas deferens and the lymphatic and vascular channels. Trauma, including vasectomy and other scrotal surgeries, may cause inflammation of the testes.

The most common infectious cause of orchitis in postpubertal men is mumps. Other causes include scarlet fever or pneumonia. The manifestations have a sudden onset, usually within 3 to 4 days after the swelling of the parotid glands. Manifestations include a high fever, increased WBCs, and unilateral or bilateral scrotal redness, swelling, and pain. If both testes are involved, permanent sterility may result, but this is rare (Porth, 2005).

INTERDISCIPLINARY CARE

Treatment is supportive and symptomatic, including antibiotic therapy if urine cultures are positive. Bed rest, scrotal support and elevation, hot or cold compresses, and analgesics for pain are prescribed. If a hydrocele occurs, it is aspirated. Nursing care is similar to that of the client with epididymitis and other scrotal disorders.

THE MAN WITH TESTICULAR TORSION

Testicular torsion, twisting of the spermatic cord with scrotal swelling and pain, is a potential medical emergency. The condition occurs most often between birth and age 20, but can occur at any age. Testicular torsion may occur spontaneously, or it may follow trauma or physical exertion. The torsion of the arteries and veins decreases or stops testicular circulation with resultant vascular engorgement and ischemia.

Testicular torsion is usually diagnosed by history and physical examination. Testicular scanning may be used to determine if blood flow to the testicle is reduced, or a prostate ultrasound may be done to identify masses or torsion. Surgical treatment, which involves detorsion of the testicle and fixation to the scrotum, must begin as quickly as possible. If the testicle is necrotic or has sustained significant damage, an *orchiectomy* (surgical removal of a testes) is performed.

THE MAN WITH TESTICULAR CANCER

Testicular cancer accounts for only 1% of all cancers in men; however, it is the most common cancer in men between the ages of 15 and 40. Annually, an estimated 8000 young men in the United States are diagnosed with this cancer. Although the cause is unknown, white American men are 5 to 10 times more likely to develop testicular cancer than are African American men (ACS, 2005a) (see the Focus on Cultural Diversity box). Survival from testicular cancer has improved dramatically as a result of treatment with effective combination chemotherapy.

The cause of testicular cancer is unknown, but both congenital and acquired factors have been associated with tumor development. About 5% develop in a man with a history of undescended testicle (*cryptorchidism*). Testicular cancer is

---

more common on the right side, which parallels the incidence of cryptorchidism (Tierney et al., 2004).

Risk Factors

Risk factors for testicular cancer are listed below:
- Age
- Cryptorchidism
- Genetic predisposition, especially in identical twins and brothers
- Cancer of the other testicle
- Other risk factors under investigation include occupational risks, presence of multiple atypical nevi, HIV infection, cancer *in situ*, body size, and maternal hormone use (ACS, 2004).

Pathophysiology

Approximately 95% of testicular malignancies are germ cell tumors (Porth, 2005). Germ cell tumors are classified, depending on their origin and ability to differentiate, as seminomas and nonseminomas. Seminomas are the most common type, and are believed to arise from the seminiferous epithelium of the testes. Nonseminomas contain more than one cell type; they include embryonal carcinoma, teratoma, choriocarcinoma, and yolk cell carcinoma. The most common type in men ages 20 to 30 is embryonal carcinomas. Testicular cancer may also arise from specialized cells of the gonadal stroma. These tumors are named for the cells from which they originate: Leydig cell, Sertoli cell, granulosa cell, and theca cell tumors.

Manifestations

The first sign of testicular cancer may be a slight enlargement of one testicle with some discomfort. The man may also have an abdominal ache and a feeling of heaviness in the scrotum. Local spread of the cancer to the epididymis or spermatic cord is inhibited by the outer covering of the testicles, the tunica albuginea. Therefore, spread by lymphatic and vascular channels to other organs often causes distant disease before large masses develop in the scrotum. Lymphatic dissemination usually leads to disease in retroperitoneal lymph nodes, whereas vascular dissemination can lead to metastasis in the lungs, bone, or liver. Bilateral presentation of testicular cancer is unusual. Manifestations of testicular cancer are summarized in the box on the next page. Manifestations of metastasis include lower extremity edema, back pain, cough, hemoptysis, or dizziness. HCG-producing tumors may cause breast enlargement (*gynecomastia*).

MANIFESTATIONS of Testicular Cancer

Common
- Painless swelling on one testicle

Metastatic symptoms
- Neck mass
- Respiratory symptoms
- Gastrointestinal disturbance
- Lumbar back pain

Occasional
- Dull ache in pelvis or scrotum
- Painless nodule on one testicle

Uncommon
- Acute pain in scrotum

Rare
- Infertility
- Gynecomastia

INTERDISCIPLINARY CARE

Care focuses on diagnosis, elimination of the cancer, and prevention or treatment of metastasis. Once testicular cancer is suspected, the man undergoes a number of screening tests to help identify the disease and its stage. If the disease is confined to the testicle, it is classified as stage I. Stage II disease is limited to the testicle and regional lymph nodes. Stage III disease involves metastasis above the diaphragm or extensive visceral involvement. Often, the man does not undergo biopsy before the beginning of treatment, but instead receives a definitive diagnosis after orchiectomy. Most men treated for testicular cancer will live a normal life span.

Diagnosis

Diagnosis may be made by various laboratory tests. Serum studies are done to identify tumor markers. Germ cell tumors produce biochemical markers such as human chorionic gonadotropin (hCG) and alpha-fetoprotein (AFP) that can be measured using radioimmunoassay techniques. Elevated levels provide strong evidence of testicular cancer. These markers are also measured after surgery to help determine the presence of residual disease that remains undetected by other means. Persistent elevation may indicate the need for further therapy. Serum lactic acid dehydrogenase (LDH) levels are elevated in testicular cancer, and may be significantly elevated when metastatic disease is present. The LDH is a less specific indicator of testicular cancer than the hCG and AFP.

Medications

Progress in chemotherapy to treat testicular cancer is one of the chief reasons why most men survive the disease. The client with advanced disease receives platinum-based combination chemotherapy. Two frequently used combinations are (1) cisplatin, bleomycin, and etoposide (BEP), and (2) etoposide plus cisplatin (EP). Toxicity from the BEP regimen can be significant, with nausea, vomiting, hair loss, bone marrow suppression, nephrotoxicity, ototoxicity, and peripheral neuropathy. Decreasing the number of BEP cycles to three (rather than four) or using the EP regimen reduces both the mortality and morbidity associated with chemotherapy. Chemotherapy is discussed in Chapter 14 .

Surgery

Radical orchiectomy is the treatment used in all forms and stages of testicular cancer. A modified retroperitoneal lymph node dissection that preserves the nerves necessary for ejaculation often is performed at the same time.

Radiation Therapy

Radiation therapy is used for stage I seminoma to treat cancer in the retroperitoneal lymph nodes, the most frequent site for distant metastasis. The man may experience temporary diarrhea, nausea, or a decline in bone marrow function, such as thrombocytopenia or leukopenia. These problems are usually mild and respond well to symptomatic treatment or time. Damage to the contralateral testicle is minimized by careful shielding. Pretreatment and posttreatment analysis of sperm number and function is necessary. The most common long-term complication is dyspepsia or ulcer disease. Radiation therapy is discussed in Chapter 14 ∞ .

NURSING CARE

Health Promotion

Unfortunately, most men who develop testicular cancer do not have overt risk factors. Therefore, beginning at the age of 15, all men should perform monthly testicular self-examination, as described in Box 50–2.

Nursing Diagnoses and Interventions

Nursing care of the man with testicular cancer is complex. The nurse must consider the reactions to the diagnosis, the change in body image accompanying treatment, and sexual

BOX 50–2 Testicular Self-Examination

- Examine your testicles when you are taking a warm shower or bath, or just after if you prefer to use a mirror to compare size.
- The scrotum, testicles, and hands should be soapy to allow easy manipulation of the tissue.
- Gently roll each testicle between the thumb and fingers of each hand. If one testicle is substantially larger than the other, or if you feel any hard lumps, consult your physician immediately.
- Normal scrotal contents may be confusing. Just above and behind the testicle is the epididymis. It feels soft and tender overall, although parts of it may be rather firm. This is normal. The spermatic cord, a small, round, movable tube, extends up from the epididymis. It feels firm and smooth. Of greatest concern is any hard lump felt directly on the testicle, even if it is painless.
- Choose a day out of each month on which to examine yourself. Most men choose an easy day to remember, such as the first or last day of the month. Star this day on your calendar to help you remember.

MediaLink

TSE Animation

and reproductive issues. Although chances of a cure are excellent, the long-term effect on quality of life may be extensive, requiring a change in life goals.

Deficient Knowledge

The nurse often initiates and reinforces teaching about what to expect after radical orchiectomy. The man's knowledge about surgery is assessed, and postoperative routines such as early ambulation are explained (see Chapter 4 ∞).

- Explain pain control methods. In addition to the usual analgesics used to control postoperative incisional pain, ice bags may be applied to the scrotum. A scrotal support provides relief, especially when the client ambulates. *Surgery results in incisional pain, and the scrotum is tender and slightly swollen.*
- Teach the manifestations of complications. The incision is closed with Steri-Strips or staples, and, although rare, wound dehiscence is possible. If the incision gapes open, or if there is bleeding beyond slight oozing after 24 hours, the man should call the surgeon. Another rare complication is a hematoma in the scrotum caused by bleeding from the spermatic cord stump. Rapid onset of scrotal edema is a sign of this problem. *Because the man is usually discharged early, complications may not become apparent until he is at home.*

Ineffective Sexuality Patterns

The effect of testicular cancer and its treatment on sexual and reproductive function is varied. If the man has a retroperitoneal lymph node dissection, severing of the sympathetic plexus may result in retrograde ejaculation or failure to ejaculate. Infertility may be caused by ejaculation disorders, surgery, chemotherapy, or radiation therapy.

- Assess the man's prediagnosis sexual function. To assess this area, the nurse must establish an atmosphere of openness and permission to discuss sexual concerns. After the initial shock of the diagnosis, men report intense concern about sexual and reproductive issues, which can be relieved only by information. *Knowledge of the man's usual sexual function can guide teaching.*
- Discuss the possibility of preserving sperm in a bank prior to treatment. *This option may help relieve the man's fears about his ability to father children in the future, but must be completed prior to initiating treatment with surgery, chemotherapy, or radiation therapy.*
- Help coping with feelings about altered sexual function and appearance. Explain that testicular implants can be inserted to preserve appearance. *Many clients, regardless of whether they are in a significant relationship, deeply grieve the loss of the ability to father children. It is important to maintain body image despite disfiguring surgery.*

Community-Based Care

Families need to be included in teaching for a variety of reasons. If the man is of reproductive age, his partner will have significant anxiety and will require information. For the teenager, parents need information about the effect on sexual function and are often very involved in postoperative care. The man needs the support of the people he loves, and knowledgeable loved ones can give effective support.

Provide teaching and reinforcement of the need for follow-up, especially if the retroperitoneal lymph nodes were not surgically explored. For men with a risk for recurrence, surveillance with periodic physical examinations, chest x-ray films, tumor markers, and CT scans of the retroperitoneal nodes could continue for a minimum of 5 years and possibly 10 years after orchiectomy.

DISORDERS OF THE PROSTATE GLAND

THE MAN WITH PROSTATITIS

Prostatitis is a term used to refer to different types of inflammatory disorders of the prostate gland. *Prostatodynia* is a condition in which the client experiences the symptoms of prostatitis but shows no evidence of inflammation or infection. Manifestations of prostatitis and prostatodynia are summarized in the box on the next page.

Pathophysiology and Manifestations

The National Institutes of Health have defined four types of prostatitis: acute bacterial prostatitis, chronic bacterial prostatitis, chronic prostatitis/pelvic pain syndrome, and asymptomatic inflammatory prostatitis. Men with asymptomatic inflammatory prostatitis have no subjective symptoms, but are diagnosed when a biopsy or prostatic fluid examination is conducted.

Acute Bacterial Prostatitis

Acute bacterial prostatitis is most often caused by an ascending infection from the urethra or reflux of infected urine into the ducts of the prostate gland. The organism most often responsible for the infection is *E. coli;* other causative organisms include *Pseudomonas, Klebsiella,* and *Chlamydia.*

Manifestations of acute bacterial prostatitis include increased temperature, malaise, muscle and joint pain, urinary frequency and urgency, dysuria, and urethral discharge. The man often experiences dull, aching pain in the perineum, rectum, or lower back. On rectal examination, the prostate is enlarged and painful.

Chronic Bacterial Prostatitis

Men with chronic bacterial prostatitis often present with a history of recurrent urinary tract infections. The causative organisms are most often *E. coli, Proteus,* or *Klebsiella.* Calculi may form in the prostate and contribute to the chronicity of the problem.

The manifestations of chronic bacterial prostatitis include urinary frequency and urgency, dysuria, low back pain, and perineal discomfort. Epididymitis may be associated with the prostatitis.

Chronic Prostatitis/Chronic Pelvic Pain Syndrome

This type of prostatitis is both the most common and the least understood of the syndromes (NKUDIC, 2003b). The two

MANIFESTATIONS of Prostatitis and Prostatodynia

Acute Bacterial Prostatitis
- Onset (may be abrupt): obstruction, irritation, or pain upon voiding; frequency; and urgency
- Positive cultures of infectious organism
- Nonurinary symptoms: chills, fever, low back and pelvic floor pain

Chronic Bacterial Prostatitis
- Urinary symptoms sometimes similar to those of the acute form, except less sudden, less dramatic, or even absent
- Positive cultures of causative organism not always obtainable

Chronic Prostatitis
- Perineal, suprapubic, low back, or genital pain
- Irritation upon voiding
- Postejaculatory pain
- Negative cultures of organisms

Prostatodynia
- Pelvic, low back, or perineal pain
- Irritation or obstruction upon voiding
- No evidence of inflammation in the prostate
- No urinary tract infection
- Normal prostatic secretions

types (inflammatory and noninflammatory) are based on the presence of white blood cells in the prostatic fluid.

- *Inflammatory prostatitis* is believed to be an autoimmune disorder, but the actual cause is unknown. Men with this type of prostatitis have low back pain; urinary manifestations; pain in the penis, testicles, scrotum, lower back, and rectum; decreased libido; and painful ejaculations. They do not have bacteria in their urine, but do have abnormal inflammatory cells in prostatic secretions.
- *Noninflammatory prostatitis* (prostatodynia) has manifestations similar to those of inflammatory prostatitis, but no evidence of urinary or prostatic infection or inflammation can be found. The cause is not known, but is believed to be the result of a problem outside the prostate gland, such as obstruction of the bladder neck.

INTERDISCIPLINARY CARE

Diagnosis
It is often difficult to diagnose prostatitis. Urine and prostatic secretion examination and cultures are obtained to determine the presence and type of blood cells and bacteria. X-ray studies and ultrasound to visualize pelvic structures also may be useful.

Medications
Bacterial prostatitis is treated with appropriate antibiotics. Men with the chronic form must take antibiotics for a much longer period, often up to 4 months, and may still relapse as soon as the antibiotic is discontinued. Nonbacterial prostatitis does not usually respond satisfactorily to drug therapy, although relief

from symptoms is possible. Nonsteroidal anti-inflammatory drugs are useful for pain, and anticholinergics may reduce voiding symptoms. Prostatodynia is treated symptomatically to relieve muscle tension, usually with alpha-adrenergic blocking agents or muscle relaxants.

NURSING CARE

Teaching for the man with prostatitis focuses on symptom management. Men with acute and chronic bacterial prostatitis should be taught to increase fluid intake to around 3 L daily and to void often. These measures help decrease irritation when voiding. Regular bowel movements help ease the pain associated with defecation. Local heat, such as sitz baths, may be helpful to relieve pain and irritation. It is important to teach the man to finish the course of antibiotic therapy. Men with chronic prostatitis/chronic pelvic pain syndrome need to know that the condition is not contagious and does not cause cancer (Porth, 2005). Referral sources for information include the National Kidney and Urologic Diseases Information Clearinghouse, the American Foundation for Urologic Disease, and the Prostatitis Foundation.

THE MAN WITH BENIGN PROSTATIC HYPERPLASIA

Benign prostatic hyperplasia (BPH), an age-related, nonmalignant enlargement of the prostate gland, is a common disorder of the aging male. The prostate, very small at birth, grows at puberty, and reaches adult size around age 20. Benign hyperplasia (increased number of cells) begins at 40 to 45 years of age, and continues slowly through the rest of life. It is estimated that more than one-half of all men over age 60 have BPH (Porth, 2005). The problem that brings men to a healthcare provider is the associated urinary dysfunction.

Risk Factors
Although the exact cause of BPH is unknown, risk factors include:
- Age
- Family history
- Race (highest in African Americans and lowest in native Japanese)
- Diet high in meat and fats.

Pathophysiology
The two necessary preconditions for BPH are age of 50 or greater and the presence of testes. Men who are castrated before puberty do not develop BPH. The androgen that mediates prostatic growth at all ages is dihydrotestosterone (DHT), which is formed in the prostate from testosterone. Although androgen levels decrease in aging men, the aging prostate appears to become more sensitive to available DHT. Estrogen, produced in small amounts in men, appears to sensitize the prostate gland to the effects of DHT. Increasing estrogen levels associated with aging or a relative increase in estrogen related to testosterone levels may contribute to prostatic hyperplasia.

BPH begins as small nodules in the periurethral glands, which are the inner layers of the prostate. The prostate enlarges through formation and growth of nodules (hyperplasia) and enlargement of glandular cells (hypertrophy). These changes occur over a long period of time. The pathophysiologic effects result from a combination of factors, including urethral resistance to the effects of BPH, intravesical pressure during voiding, detrusor muscle strength, neurologic functioning, and general physical health.

Manifestations

The expanding prostatic tissue compresses the urethra (Figure 50–3 ■) and causes partial or complete obstruction of the outflow of urine from the urinary bladder. The detrusor muscles hypertrophy to compensate for increased resistance to urinary flow; however, eventually decreased bladder compliance and bladder instability result. As a result, the man with BPH has manifestations from obstruction (weak urinary stream, increased time to void, hesitancy, incomplete bladder emptying, and postvoid dribbling) and irritation (frequency, urgency, incontinence, nocturia, dysuria, and bladder pain). Urinary retention may become chronic, resulting in overflow incontinence with any increase in intra-abdominal pressure. There is little correlation between the size of the prostate gland and the urinary manifestations. Manifestations of BPH are summarized in the box on this page.

FAST FACTS
Urinary Problems with BPH
- A hesitant, interrupted weak stream.
- Urgency with leaking or dribbling of urine.
- More frequent urination in small amounts, especially at night (nocturia).

Complications

Unless the enlarging mass is reduced, multiple complications may occur. As urine is retained in the bladder, increasing bladder distention occurs. Diverticula (outpouchings) on the bladder wall result from the distention. The distention may also obstruct the ureters. Infection, more common in retained urine and in diverticula, may ascend from the bladder to the kidneys. Hydroureter, hydronephrosis, and renal insufficiency are possible complications.

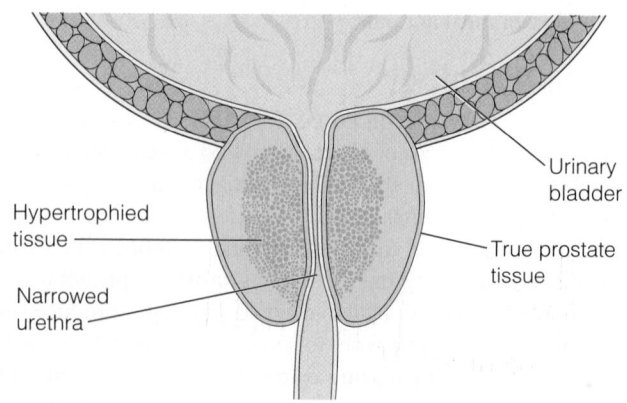

Figure 50–3 ■ Benign prostatic hyperplasia.

Labels: Hypertrophied tissue; Narrowed urethra; Urinary bladder; True prostate tissue

 MANIFESTATIONS **of Benign Prostatic Hyperplasia**

- Diminished force of urinary stream
- Hesitancy in initiating voiding
- Postvoid dribbling
- Sensation of incomplete emptying
- Urinary retention
- Nocturia
- Frequency
- Urgency
- Urge incontinence
- Dysuria

INTERDISCIPLINARY CARE

Care of men with BPH focuses on diagnosing the disorder, correcting or minimizing the urinary obstruction, and preventing or treating complications. There is no way to reverse BPH. Treatment is often determined by the severity of the manifestations and the presence of complications. Mild cases are often monitored over time, and may remain stable or improve.

Diagnosis

A diagnosis of BPH involves both physical examination and laboratory tests to not only diagnose the disease but also to differentiate it from prostate cancer. A digital rectal examination (DRE) is done to examine the external surface of the prostate; in BPH it is asymmetrical and enlarged. Examination of the creatinine levels of the blood is conducted to assess for kidney damage.

The urine is examined for WBCs, RBCs, and bacteria. Urinary function is assessed by measuring residual urine (amount of urine remaining in the bladder after voiding) with ultrasonography or postvoiding catheterization (more than 100 mL is considered high), and through uroflowmetry, which measures urine flow rate; normal is greater than 14 mL/sec. A finding of less than 10 mL/sec indicates obstruction.

Prostate-specific antigen (PSA) levels are obtained to rule out prostate cancer. PSA is a glycoprotein produced only in the cytoplasm of benign and malignant prostate cells; the serum level corresponds with the volume of both benign and malignant prostate tissue. Further information is provided in the next section under diagnosis of prostate cancer.

In addition, the man's own subjective experiences with BPH are included in the diagnosis and treatment. For example, the International Prostate Symptom Score uses a scale of 0 (not at all) to 5 (almost always) to collect data about areas such as feeling as though the bladder did not empty with urinating, need to urinate within 2 hours after urinating, starting and stopping the stream several times while urinating, and straining to urinate. This questionnaire also asks how many times during the night the man gets up to urinate and how the man feels about having the disorder.

Medications

Treatment with medications is based on two considerations: The hyperplastic tissue is androgen dependent, and smooth muscle contraction within the prostate can exacerbate urinary obstruction. The first consideration is usually addressed by treatment for mild prostate enlargement with finasteride (Proscar) or dutasteride (Avodart), antiandrogen agents that inhibit the conversion of testosterone to DHT and cause the enlarged prostate to shrink in size. They may cause impotence, decreased libido, and decreased volume of ejaculate. Client and family education includes the information that crushed tablets should not be handled by pregnant women, because the drug may be absorbed through the skin and be harmful to a male fetus.

Excessive smooth muscle contraction in BPH may be blocked with the alpha-adrenergic antagonists such as terazosin (Hytrin), doxazosin (Cardura), tamsulosin (Flomax), and alfuzosin (Uroxatral). These medications relieve obstruction and increase the flow of urine. They may cause orthostatic hypotension. Client and family teaching includes advice about making position changes slowly to avoid dizziness and accidental falls, how to take and record blood pressure, and to check with the healthcare provider before taking any medication for coughs, colds, or allergies (because these over-the-counter medications may contain an adrenergic agent).

Federal research found that using finasteride and doxazosin together is more effective than using each alone to relieve manifestations and prevent the progression of BPH (NKUDIC, 2004).

Surgery

Men who have urinary retention, recurrent urinary tract infection, hematuria, bladder stones, or renal insufficiency secondary to BPH are candidates for surgical intervention. Surgical treatment may be performed by minimally invasive surgery or through transurethral surgery, open surgery, or by laser surgery.

MINIMALLY INVASIVE SURGERY Because medications are not effective for all men, a number of procedures have been developed to relieve the manifestations of BPH that are less invasive than traditional surgery.

Microwaves are used to heat and destroy excess prostate tissue in a procedure called *transurethral microwave thermotherapy*. During the procedure, a cooling system protects the urinary tract. The procedure takes about an hour and can be performed on an outpatient basis. Although microwave procedures do not cure BPH, they do reduce urinary manifestations. The procedures do not cause impotence or incontinence.

The *transurethral needle ablation (TUNA)* system uses low-level radio frequency through twin needles to burn away a region of the enlarged prostate. Shields protect the urethra. TUNA improves the flow of urine through the urethra. It does not cause impotence or incontinence.

TRANSURETHRAL SURGERY A *transurethral resection of the prostate (TURP)* is the surgical procedure used most often. Obstructing prostate tissue is removed using the wire loop of a resectoscope and electrocautery, inserted through the urethra (Figure 50–4 ■). No external incision is necessary. During the procedure the surgeon uses the resectoscope to remove obstructing tissue one piece at a time. The tissue is flushed into the bladder with fluid and then flushed out at the end of the operation. This surgery has potential risks, however, including postoperative hemorrhage or clot retention, inability to void, and urinary tract infection. Other possible complications are incontinence, impotence, and retrograde ejaculation.

In the *transurethral incision of the prostate (TUIP)* procedure, small incisions are made in the smooth muscle where the prostate is attached to the bladder. The gland is split to reduce pressure on the urethra. No tissue is removed, so this procedure is most appropriate for men with smaller prostate glands. TUIP can be done on an outpatient basis, and has the additional advantage of less risk of postoperative retrograde ejaculation than is associated with TURP or other prostatectomy procedures.

OPEN SURGERY When the prostate gland is very large, an open prostatectomy may be used. These procedures are discussed in the section on prostate cancer that follows. Nursing care for the client having prostate surgery is outlined in the box on the next page.

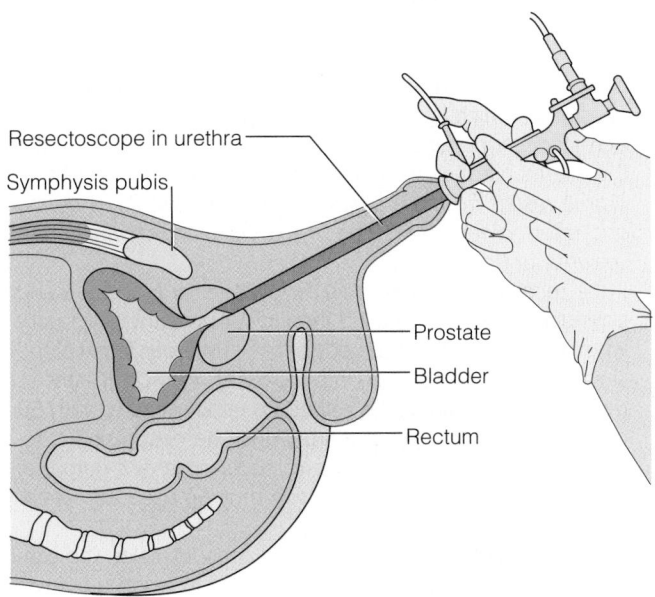

A Transurethral resection of the prostate

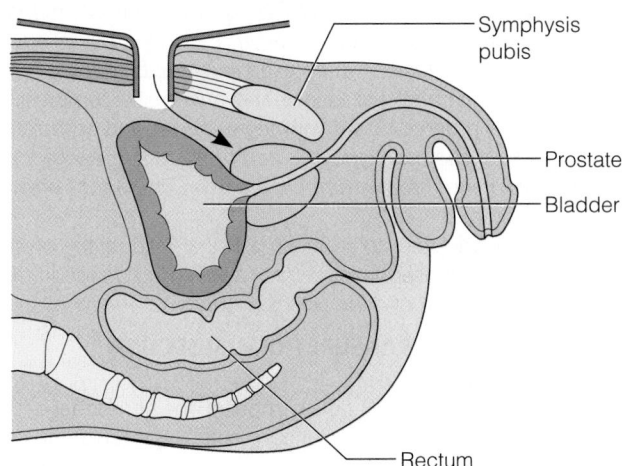

B Retropubic prostatectomy

Figure 50–4 ■ *A,* In a transurethral resection of the prostate, a resectoscope inserted through the urethra is used to remove excess prostate tissue. *B,* In a retropubic prostatectomy, prostate tissue is removed through an abdominal incision.

NURSING CARE OF THE MAN HAVING A Prostatectomy

PREOPERATIVE CARE

- Assess the man's and family's knowledge about the surgery *Some men are confused about the surgical approach because there are several, quite different methods.*
- Inform the man that he will have a urinary catheter when he returns from surgery, and he may have a drain(s) in his incision. He also will be wearing sequential pneumatic compression stockings. *This knowledge can reduce anxiety postoperatively and increase cooperation with postoperative care.*
- Ensure that a signed consent from is in the chart and that all other preoperative tasks outlined in Chapter 4 ∞ are done.
- Bowel preparation with a 2% neomycin enema may be ordered. *This cleanses the bowel if a perineal approach will be used.*
- Communicate willingness to address any concerns of anxiety *Men may be anxious about the outcome of their surgery and potential long-term effects of the surgery of their sexuality. When a prostatectomy is performed for prostate cancer, additional fears include the extent of the cancer and surgery, chances for cure, and possible end-of-life issues.*

POSTOPERATIVE CARE

- Maintain the usual postoperative assessments (see Chapter 4 ∞ and follow aseptic techniques in urinary drainage and irrigation care. Monitor vital signs closely for the first 24 hours and regularly thereafter. *The man who has had prostate surgery is at risk for hemorrhage and infection. Vital sign changes may be early manifestations.*
- Maintain accurate intake and output records, including amounts of irrigating solution used. Frequently assess patency of any catheters and drains. Monitor color and character of urine. *Catheters may become occluded by blood clots or kinks, interfering with urinary drainage and increasing the risk of hemorrhage.*
- Assess and manage the man's pain. *The man may have at least three types of pain: incisional pain, bladder spasms, and abdominal cramps due to intestinal gas. Analgesics and non-steroidal anti-inflammatory drugs (NSAIDs) are administered on a routine and prn basis to control incisional pain. Bladder spasms may be accompanied by strong urges to void and urine leakage around the catheter. Belladonna and opium (B & O) suppositories may be used to relieve bladder spasms.*
- Maintain antiembolic stockings and pneumatic compression devices as ordered. Assist with leg exercises and ambulation as ordered. *The man who has had prostate surgery is at risk for developing thromboemboli; these are important preventive measures.*
- Encourage the man to maintain a liberal fluid intake of 2 to 3 L a day. *Increased fluids reduce burning on urination after catheter removal and the risk of urinary tract infection.*

THE MAN WITH A TRANSURETHRAL RESECTION OF THE PROSTATE (TURP)

- For the first 24 to 48 hours, monitor for hemorrhage, evidenced by frankly bloody urinary output, presence of large blood clots, decreased urinary output, increasing bladder spasms, decreased hemoglobin and hematocrit, tachycardia, and hypotension. Notify the physician if any of these manifes-

tations occur. *Postoperative hemorrhage may be either arterial or venous, and may be precipitated by movement, bladder spasms, or an obstructed urinary drainage system.*

- Instruct the man with a three-way indwelling catheter with traction to keep the leg straight while the traction is applied. *A No. 18- to 22-Fr three-way catheter with a 30- to 45-mL balloon usually is inserted following a TURP. The inflated balloon is pulled down into the prostatic fossa and the catheter tubing is pulled down and taped to the man's leg to apply pressure against the operative site, preventing bleeding.*
- Explain that the presence of a urinary catheter will cause the sensation of needing to void, but it is important not to strain to try to void around the catheter or when having a bowel movement. Explain that bladder spasms; experienced as lower abdominal pressure or pain and a desire to urinate, may occur. Ensure that the man understands that this is an expected sensation, and that medications can help alleviate this discomfort. *Pressure on the urethra by the large catheter and on the internal sphincter by the catheter's balloon stimulate the micturition reflex. Straining to void or to have a bowel movement may stimulate bladder spasms and increase pain; it also may increase the risk for bleeding. Administer pain medications at regular intervals.*
- If the man has a continuous bladder irrigation (CBI), assess the catheter and the drainage tubing at regular intervals. Maintain the rate of flow of irrigating fluid to keep the output light pink or colorless. Assess the urinary output every 1 to 2 hours for color, consistency amount, and presence of blood clots; assess for bladder spasms. *CBI is used to prevent the formation of blood clots which could obstruct urinary output. Bladder distention resulting from output obstruction increases the risk of bleeding. Irrigating fluids are continuously infused and drained at a rate to keep urine light pink or colorless. Urine that is frankly bloody, contains many blood clots, or is decreased in amount, as well as bladder spasms, are indicators of obstruction and bleeding.*
- Assess for fluid volume excess and hyponatremia, called TURP syndrome, which is manifested by hyponatremia, decreased hematocrit, hypertension, bradycardia, nausea, and confusion. If these manifestations occur, notify the physician. *TURP syndrome results from the absorption of irrigating fluids during and after surgery. Untreated, it may result in dysrhythmias, seizures, or both.*
- If the man does not have CBI, follow agency procedure and physician orders for irrigating the indwelling catheter (usually when the urine is frankly bloody or has numerous larger blood clots, or when bladder spasms increase). In most instances, using sterile technique, the catheter is gently irrigated with 50 mL of irrigating solution at a time, until the obstruction is relieved or the urine is clear. Ensure equal input and output of irrigating fluid. *Intermittent irrigation may be used to prevent obstruction of urinary drainage.*
- Following catheter removal, assess the amount, color, and consistency of urine. Explain that the man may experience burning on urination, that dribbling after urination is a common experience, and that the urine may contain small blood clots after catheter removal. *The CBI and catheter usually are removed in*

NURSING CARE OF THE MAN HAVING A   Prostatectomy (continued)

the 24 to 48 hours following surgery. Urinary control may be improved by teaching the man to start and stop the urine stream several times during each voiding and by practicing Kegel exercises. Regaining full control may take up to 1 year.

THE MAN WITH A RETROPUBIC PROSTATECTOMY

- Assess the abdominal incision for the presence of urine. *Because the bladder is not entered during a retropubic prostatectomy, no urine should be found on the dressing.*
- Assess the abdominal incision for increased or purulent drainage, and the man for an increased temperature and pain. *These manifestations indicate the presence of infection.*

THE MAN WITH A SUPRAPUBIC PROSTATECTOMY

- Assess urinary output from both the suprapubic and the urethral catheters. *The man with a suprapubic prostatectomy often has two separate closed drainage systems: one from the suprapubic incision and one from a urethral catheter.*
- Assess the abdominal dressing for urinary drainage, and change saturated dressings frequently. Consult with a skin care specialist if necessary. *Urine is highly irritating to the skin.*
- Following removal of the urethral catheter (usually 2 to 4 days after surgery) and based on physician orders, clamp

the suprapubic catheter and encourage the man to void. Assess residual urine by unclamping the suprapubic catheter and measuring urinary output after voiding. *If residual urine is 75 mL or less with several voidings, the suprapubic catheter is removed.*

THE MAN WITH A PERINEAL PROSTATECTOMY

- Assess perineal incision for drainage and manifestations of infection. *Location of the incision in the perineum increases the risk of infection.*
- Do not take rectal temperatures or administer enemas. *Insertion of a thermometer or enema tubing into the rectum may precipitate bleeding.*
- Use a T-binder or padded scrotal support to hold the dressing in place. Following removal of the dressing and perineal sutures, heat lamps or sitz baths may be used. *The location of the dressing makes application difficult: Heat lamps or sitz baths provide heat and promote healing.*
- Teach the man to perform perineal irrigations with sterile normal saline as ordered and after each bowel movement. *Because of the proximity of the incision to the anus, special wound care is necessary to prevent infection.*

LASER SURGERY In laser surgery, the surgeon uses a cystoscope to pass the YAG laser fiber through the urethra into the prostate and then vaporizes obstructing prostate tissue with several short bursts of energy. An advantage of laser surgery is decreased blood loss and a more rapid recovery time. However, this method may not be as effective for larger prostates.

New Treatments

Newer treatments for BPH include minimally invasive procedures such as balloon urethroplasty and placement of intraurethral stents to maintain patency of the urethra. Balloon urethroplasty is a simple procedure in which a balloon-tipped catheter is inserted into the narrowed portion of the urethra and inflated. Inflation of the balloon widens the urethra, relieving obstruction. These procedures can be done as outpatient surgery.

Alternative and Complementary Therapies

Phytotherapy is the use of plants or plant extracts for medical treatment. Several plant extracts have been used for years in Europe to treat BPH and are being used more often in the United States. The phytotherapy used includes saw palmetto berry, the bark of *Pygeum africanum*, the roots of *Echinacea, purpurea,* and *Hypoxis rooperi,* and the leaves of the trembling poplar. The mechanisms of action of these extracts is unknown, but men report they are effective in relieving manifestations (Tierney et al., 2004).

NURSING CARE

Most men are unsure of the function of the prostate gland and even the prostate's exact location, though its relationship to sexual and urinary function is at least generally known. This lack

of knowledge, coupled with the growing number of treatment options, is confusing to many men. There are many similarities between the nursing care of men with BPH and that of men with prostate cancer (see the section that follows).

Nursing Diagnoses and Interventions

This section provides interventions related to deficient knowledge, urinary retention, risk for infection, and risk for imbalanced fluid volume.

Deficient Knowledge

- Explain the anatomy and physiology of the prostate gland, as well as normal changes that occur with aging. *Men must know about their bodies in order to make accurate decisions about treatment.*
- Discuss treatment options, including information about effects on erectile function, ejaculation, and fertility. Counsel the man to discuss specific concerns with his urologist. *Many different treatment options are available; the choice should be a mutual decision between the man, his partner, and the urologist.*
- Discuss effects of prostate surgery, including urinary retention and urinary incontinence. *These common transient postoperative effects are related to the surgical procedure and the postoperative indwelling catheter.*
- Explain to the man having a TURP that a catheter will be placed into the bladder, with the tubing taped to his inner thigh, and that irrigation fluid will be infusing into and out of the catheter for the first 36 to 72 hours following surgery. *The catheter and irrigation are necessary to remove blood clots from the bladder and allow drainage of urine. Gentle traction is applied to the catheter to apply pressure to the operative site (prostatic fossa) and prevent excessive bleeding.*

- Explain that, following removal of the catheter, he will most likely have urinary frequency and urgency. He may also experience dribbling of urine after voiding. Stress the importance of increasing oral fluid intake and regular Kegel exercises. *Urinary manifestations are related to the surgical procedure and the indwelling catheter. Increased fluid intake helps decrease dysuria. Kegel exercises strengthen periurethral muscles and decrease postvoiding urine leakage.*

Urinary Retention

- Teach the manifestations of acute urinary retention: dysuria, overflow incontinence, bladder pain and distention, no urine output. *Acute urinary retention is a potential complication of BPH, requiring immediate medical attention.*
- Teach that the risk of developing urinary retention increases when the man with BPH takes over-the-counter (OTC) decongestant medications, or prescription medications such as antidepressants, anticholinergics, calcium channel blockers, antipsychotics, and medications to treat Parkinson's disease. *OTC decongestants may contain alpha-adrenergic agonists that increase smooth muscle tone of the prostate, bladder neck, and proximal urethra. The prescribed medications may relax detrusor muscle contractions. Both actions may increase the risk of urinary retention (Gray & Brown, 2002).*
- Suggest avoiding intake of large volumes of liquid at any one time. *A single intake of a large volume of liquid results in rapid bladder filling and increases the risk of urinary retention.*
- Teach how to use the double-voiding technique: Urinate, then sit on the toilet for 3 to 5 minutes, then urinate again. *This technique may relieve mild to moderate urinary retention.*

PRACTICE ALERT
In addition to avoiding a large amount of fluids at one time, it is also important to teach the man to limit liquids that stimulate voiding, such as coffee and alcoholic beverages.

RISK FOR INFECTION

- Monitor WBC and vital signs. *Infection is indicated by an increase in WBCs, body temperature, and pulse rate.*
- Maintain sterile procedures when changing irrigation fluids and emptying Foley catheter draining bag. *Sterile procedures are necessary to prevent infection.*

RISK FOR IMBALANCED FLUID VOLUME
A prostatectomy brings increased risk of imbalanced fluid volume as a result of excessive bleeding from the operative site (prostatic fossa) as well as absorption of irrigating fluid. Report manifestations indicating hypovolemic shock, excess bleeding, and/or TURP syndrome immediately.

- Monitor pulse and blood pressure. *Manifestations of hypovolemic shock include an increasing pulse and a decreasing blood pressure.*
- Monitor color of drainage in urinary drainage bag (Table 50–2). *The appearance of urine and irrigation fluid in the urinary drainage bag is an excellent indicator of bleeding after a prostatectomy.*
- Monitor for manifestations of transurethral resection (TURP) syndrome: nausea and vomiting, confusion, hyper-

TABLE 50–2 Significance of Character of Urine After Prostatectomy and Related Nursing Care

URINE COLOR	NURSING IMPLICATIONS
Light red to red	Normal day of surgery and first postoperative day
Very dark red	May indicate increased venous bleeding or inadequate dilution. Catheter at risk for occlusion. Increase flow rate of irrigant. If urine does not clear, notify physician.
Bright red	May indicate arterial bleeding. Increase flow rate of irrigant, monitor vital signs, and notify physician.
Contains blood clots	Occasional blood clot normal. If clots are frequent, catheter may become obstructed. Increase flow rate of irrigant.
Clear to light pink	Normal throughout hospitalization.

tension, bradycardia, and visual disturbances. *The absorption of isotonic bladder irrigating fluids during and after surgery may cause this hypervolemic, hyponatremic state. Treatment includes diuresis and, in severe cases, hypertonic saline administration (Tierney et al., 2004).*

Community-Based Care

Depending on the man's choice of treatment, the procedure may be performed on an outpatient basis. The man having a TURP, although hospitalized for the surgery, may be discharged within 2 days after surgery if there are no complications. Discharge instructions after prostate surgery are provided in the Meeting Individualized Needs box on the next page. Home care often involves care of an indwelling urinary catheter. Teaching how to care for the catheter and drainage bag includes the following information:

- Change from the daytime leg drainage bag to a larger night drainage bag. A larger bag suspended from the bed frame at night permits gravity drainage of urine and prevents reflux of urine back into the bladder.
- Avoid strapping the leg bag on too tightly, which can decrease venous return and increase risk for thrombophlebitis and embolic complications such as pulmonary emboli.
- Place a soft cloth between the leg bag and thigh to decrease friction and absorb dampness under the bag, reducing the risk of skin irritation.
- Empty the leg bag every 3 to 4 hours during waking hours to prevent overfilling.
- Promptly report any unexpected changes in urine color, consistency, or odor, hematuria, evidence of frank bleeding, or large blood clots, as well as a lack of or significant decrease in urine output to the urologist.

THE MAN WITH PROSTATE CANCER

Cancer of the prostate is the most common type of cancer among men and the second leading cause of death in North America (ACS, 2006). It is primarily a disease of older men, in-

MEETING INDIVIDUALIZED NEEDS Discharge Instructions for Men After Prostate Surgery

ACTIVITY

The healing period lasts from 4 to 8 weeks. Avoid strenuous activity and heavy lifting. Do not drive for 2 weeks, except for short rides. Do take long walks; take stairs slowly and carefully. Continue exercises that you did in the hospital to prevent blood clots in the legs. You can take showers; avoid tub baths while the catheter is in place.

BLEEDING

Bleeding can occur any time after surgery. It is fairly common after a bowel movement, coughing, or increased exercise. If you notice blood in the urine, increase fluids and rest until the urine is clear. If heavy bleeding plugs the channel, call the care provider immediately. Avoid aspirin and NSAIDs for at least 2 weeks.

BOWEL MOVEMENTS

Keep bowel movements regular and soft to avoid pressure on the prostate area. Drink fruit juices and take mild laxatives or stool softeners as ordered.

DIET

Resume your normal diet. Increase fluids to 10 glasses (8 oz) daily. Avoid alcohol unless otherwise advised by your physician.

SEXUAL INTERCOURSE

Do not have sex for 6 weeks after surgery to avoid bleeding. You may still have erections even with the catheter in place. When you resume sex, ejaculate flows back into the bladder, so you will express little or no semen.

URINATION

After your catheter is removed, you may experience some burning, stinging, or leakage for several weeks, and you may pass small blood clots occasionally. These symptoms will disappear as the area heals. It is best to use pads to control leakage.

WORK

If work is not strenuous you may return in 4 weeks; otherwise, wait 6 to 8 weeks.

PLEASE CALL IMMEDIATELY IF:

- You are unable to urinate.
- Bleeding is not controlled by fluids and rest, or is excessive.
- You have chills and fever or severe abdominal pain.
- Your scrotum becomes swollen and tender.
- You have pain in one calf, chest pain, or difficulty breathing.

---

creasing in incidence with age, with the majority of cases diagnosed in men older than 65 years. It is estimated that each year, more than 234,000 men will be diagnosed with prostate cancer, approximately 27,000 will die of it. Prostate cancer is a major health problem for older men, but the death rate is decreasing due to advances in diagnosis and treatment.

When diagnosed early, prostate cancer is curable. When the cancer is confined to the prostate at diagnosis, the 5-year survival rate is 100%. Even when the cancer has spread regionally, approximately 95% of clients are alive after 5 years. More than 75% of prostate cancer diagnoses are made at one of these stages (ACS, 2005b). Many men are found to have prostate cancer on autopsy; usually the cancer has produced no manifestations or complications.

Risk Factors

In addition to age, race is a significant risk factor for prostate cancer (see the Focus on Cultural Diversity box on this page). Other risk factors being investigated are as follows:

- Genetic and hereditary factors, with risk increased in men who have a family history of the disease
- Having a vasectomy, believed to increase the levels of circulating free testosterone
- Dietary factors, including a diet high in animal fat and excessive supplemental vitamin A.

Pathophysiology

The prostate gland consists primarily of glandular epithelial cells. The exact etiology of prostate cancer is unknown, although androgens are believed to have a role in its development. Almost all primary prostate cancers are adenocarcinomas, and they de-

FOCUS ON CULTURAL DIVERSITY
Risk and Incidence of Prostate Cancer

- African Americans have the highest incidence of prostate cancer in the United States and the world, with rates more than twice as high as those of Caucasians.
- African Americans are more likely to be diagnosed later and to die of prostate cancer, with a mortality rate more than double that of other racial and ethnic groups.
- Asians and Native Americans have the lowest incidence of prostate cancer.

velop in the peripheral zones of the prostate gland. This location increases the risk of local spread to the prostatic capsule. Despite its proximity to the rectum, metastasis to the bowel is uncommon because a tough sheet of tissue, Denonvilliers' fascia, acts as an effective physical barrier.

As the tumor enlarges, it may compress the urethra, obstructing urinary flow. The tumor may metastasize and involve the seminal vesicles or bladder by direct extension. Metastasis by lymph and venous channels is common.

Manifestations

Men with early-stage prostate cancer are often asymptomatic. Pain from metastasis to bones is often the initial manifestation noted. Urinary manifestations depend on the size and location of the tumor and the stage of the malignancy. They are often much like manifestations of BPH: urgency, frequency, hesitancy, dysuria, and nocturia. The man may also notice hematuria or blood in the ejaculate (Porth, 2005). Manifestations of prostate cancer are summarized in the box on the next page.

MANIFESTATIONS of Prostate Cancer

Genitourinary
- Dysuria
- Frequency of urination
- Reduction in urinary stream
- Nocturia
- Hematuria
- Abnormal prostate on digital rectal examination

Musculoskeletal
- Bone or joint pain
- Migratory bone pain
- Back pain

Neurologic
- Nerve pain
- Bilateral lower extremity weakness
- Bowel or bladder dysfunction
- Muscle spasms

Systemic
- Weight loss
- Fatigue

Complications

Death usually occurs secondary to debility caused by multiple sites of skeletal metastasis, especially to the vertebrae. Compression fractures of the spine are common, resulting in the possible loss of mobility and bowel and bladder function. Tumors may eventually involve bone marrow, resulting in severe anemias and impaired immune function.

INTERDISCIPLINARY CARE

Care of the man with prostate cancer focuses on diagnosis, elimination or containment of the cancer, and prevention or treatment of complications. There are currently no clinical strategies to prevent the development of prostate cancer. Therefore, early detection remains the major emphasis for control of this disease.

Diagnosis

Although an increasing number of clients are now diagnosed with asymptomatic prostate cancer, many clients with prostate cancer have either locally advanced cancer or distant metastasis at the time of diagnosis. The definitive diagnosis can be made only by biopsy (prostate biopsy is discussed in Chapter 49); however, other tests may suggest the presence of prostate cancer.

A digital rectal examination (DRE) will find the prostate gland nodular and fixed in prostate cancer. Prostate-specific antigen (PSA) levels are used to diagnose and stage prostate cancer, and to monitor response to treatment. Levels depend on age, and there is no specific normal or abnormal level. An increase over time is more significant than one reading. The PSA test is used with a DRE to help detect prostate cancer in men age 50 or older, and is also used to monitor effects of treatment. Many physicians are using the following ranges (National Cancer Institute, 2004):

- 0 to 2.5 ng/mL is low.
- 2.6 to 10 ng/mL is slightly to moderately elevated.
- 10 to 19.9 ng/mL is moderately elevated.
- 20 ng/mL or more is significantly elevated.

Transrectal ultrasonography (TRUS) may be used when the DRE is abnormal or if the PSA is elevated. In this test, a small probe is inserted in the rectum. The probe gives off sound waves that make a picture of the prostate on a video screen. Guided by this picture, the physician inserts a narrow needle through the rectal wall into the prostate gland, and the needle removes a sample of tissue for examination. Other tests that may be ordered include a urinalysis or cystoscopy. Bone scan, MRI, or CT scans may be performed to determine the presence of tumor metastasis.

Grade and stage help to determine prognosis and guide treatment decisions. Grade (cancer cell differentiation) is determined by the pathologist. Prostate cancer is staged with a variety of tests. Table 50–3 outlines treatment options according to the stage of the cancer.

TABLE 50–3 Prostate Cancer Staging and Treatment

STAGE	DESCRIPTION	TREATMENT
I	Confined to prostate, nonpalpable, focal involvement; well differentiated	Observation and follow-up Interstitial or external-beam radiation therapy Prostatectomy
II	Confined to prostate, palpable, involves one or both lobes; poorly differentiated	Careful observation in selected clients Prostatectomy Interstitial or external-beam radiation therapy Ultrasound-guided percutaneous cryosurgery
III	Extension of the tumor outside the prostate capsule, possible seminal vesicle involvement	External-beam radiation therapy Interstitial radiation Radical prostatectomy Adjunctive hormone therapy Palliative surgery (TURP)
IV	Extension of the tumor into surrounding tissues; lymph node involvement or distant metastasis	Hormone therapy External-beam radiation therapy Palliative treatment with radiation therapy and/or TURP Radical prostatectomy with orchiectomy Chemotherapy

Research for Prevention

As reported by the American Society of Clinical Oncology (2005), findings from a study using toremifene (Acapodene) to treat men with abnormal prostate growth might help prevent the growths from becoming malignant. The drug, which blocks some of the effects of estrogen, had previously been used to treat advanced breast cancer in women. Men who have prostate intraepithelial neoplasia (PIN) have about a 30% chance of developing prostate cancer in 1 year and about a 65% chance within 2 years. A larger study is now in progress. In addition, other studies reported that men who took statins (to treat high cholesterol) were less likely to have prostate cancer.

Treatments

The treatment of prostate cancer is complex and depends on the grade and stage of the cancer as well as the age, general health, and preference of the client. In some cases, for example, when the client with a slow-growing tumor is elderly or has a limited life expectancy, watchful waiting is the treatment of choice. Treatments for prostate cancer include surgery, radiation therapy, and hormone manipulation.

SURGERY Surgery for prostate cancer includes several types of prostatectomies. For very early disease in older men, cure may be achieved with a simple prostatectomy (such as TURP), discussed in the section on benign prostate hyperplasia.

- *Radical prostatectomy* involves removal of the prostate, prostate capsule, seminal vesicles, and a portion of the bladder neck. Many clients experience varying degrees of urinary incontinence and ED. Refer to Table 50–4. A fairly new treatment is laparoscopic radical prostatectomy (LRP), in which small incisions are make in the abdomen and a laparoscope is inserted and used to remove the prostate. Some surgeons do

TABLE 50–4 Potential Complications Related to Radical Prostatectomy and Radiation Therapy

RADICAL PROSTATECTOMY	RADIATION THERAPY
Erectile dysfunction	Erectile dysfunction*
Urethral stricture	Urethral stricture
Fistula/rectal injury	Rectal/anal stricture*
Urinary incontinence	Cystitis
Surgical/anesthetic risk	Diarrhea
	Proctitis
	Rectal ulcer
	Bowel obstruction*
	Urinary incontinence

Delayed complications; may appear months or years after completion of therapy.

this from an area other than the operating room by using a robotic interface. Nursing research reporting client satisfaction with a discharge program following a radical prostatectomy is discussed in the evidence-based practice feature on this page.

- *Retropubic prostatectomy* may be performed because it allows adequate control of bleeding, visualization of the prostate bed and bladder neck, and access to pelvic lymph nodes.
- *Perineal prostatectomy* is often preferred for older men or those who are poor surgical risks. This approach requires less time, and involves less bleeding.
- *Suprapubic prostatectomy* is rarely used, usually when problems with the bladder are expected. Control of bleeding is more difficult because the surgical approach is through the bladder.

NURSING RESEARCH   Evidence-Based Practice: Improve Discharge Teaching

The period immediately after hospital discharge for a radical prostatectomy is one that is often a difficult time for men and their families as they cope with the emotional and physical demands of cancer surgery. Deficient knowledge about how long it will take to recover and how to provide care at home can have a major effect on healthy recovery from surgery. Nurses recognize the need to provide discharge teaching prior to hospital discharge, but this need is often not a part of actual practice. A study was conducted by Davison and colleagues (2004) to evaluate a revised program for discharge teaching after a radical prostatectomy for prostate cancer.

IMPLICATIONS FOR NURSING

The discharge teaching program being evaluated was developed based on a review of the literature. It consisted of a printed booklet of information about preoperative and postoperative radical prostate surgery, a patient education checklist, and a discharge bag containing a urinary leg bag, urinary collection bag, wound supplies, incontinence product samples, and a community resources brochure. The patients indicated that they read the entire booklet about surgery and that it helped prepare them for hospital care. Of the patients, almost half indicated catheter care as the most valuable type of information provided, but several of the patients felt even more information would have been useful. This type of information is extremely important as the number of patients having radical prostatectomy increases and hospital stays continue to be shortened. Nurses are now, and will continue to be, challenged to provide the type and amount of information needed for self-care at home.

CRITICAL THINKING IN CLIENT CARE

1. You are caring for a 75-year-old man who has had a radical prostatectomy for prostate cancer. His wife tells you they have always had an active sex life and she hopes this surgery will not change that. What would you say to her?
2. Why would the nursing diagnosis *Risk for Infection* be appropriate for a man providing self-care at home following a radical prostatectomy? What type of interventions would you suggest during discharge teaching to reduce this risk?
3. If you were developing a list of community resources for men following prostate surgery, what would you include? How would your list vary for the following situations?
   - A 64-year-old man with a wife and four married children who all live close
   - A 77-year-old man who lives alone and has no family
   - A 90-year-old man who will go to an assisted living facility after discharge from the hospital.

For clients with stage III, locally advanced (beyond the prostatic capsule) cancer, surgery is controversial because of the likelihood of hidden lymph node metastasis and relapse. TURP is not performed as curative therapy but may be used to relieve urinary obstruction for men with advanced disease (stage III or IV).

Surgical intervention is now available for men with urinary sphincter insufficiency, which is the major cause of incontinence after prostatectomy. An artificial urinary sphincter is surgically implanted (Figure 50–5 ■). To be eligible, the man must

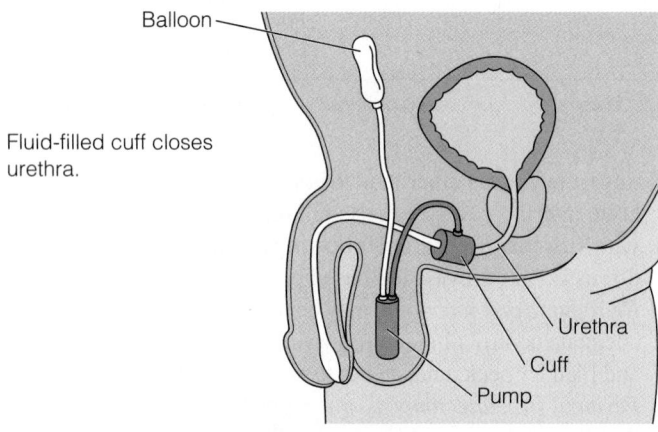

Balloon

Fluid-filled cuff closes urethra.

Urethra

Cuff

Pump

To void, bladder pump is squeezed, drawing fluid from cuff to balloon. Urine drains through open urethra.

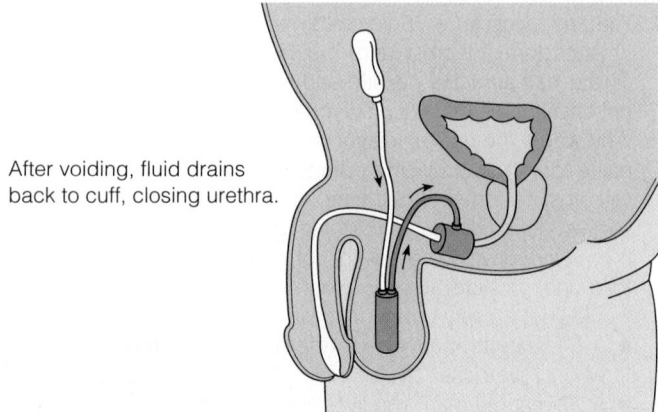

After voiding, fluid drains back to cuff, closing urethra.

Figure 50–5 ■ Method of operation of an artificial urinary sphincter.

be able to manipulate the pump placed in the scrotum and have adequate cognitive function to know when a problem with the appliance occurs.

RADIATION THERAPY Radiation therapy may be used as a primary treatment for prostate cancer. Long-term problems of impotence and urinary incontinence may be avoided, and survival rates often are comparable. Radiation may be delivered either by external beam or interstitial implants of radioactive seeds of iodine, gold, palladium, or iridium (*brachytherapy*). Interstitial radiation has a lower risk of impotence and rectal damage than external-beam radiation. See Chapter 14 ∞ for nursing care of the client receiving radiation therapy.

Radiation therapy has a palliative role for clients with metastatic prostate cancer, reducing the size of bone metastasis, controlling pain, and restoring function, such as continence or the ability to ambulate for clients with spinal cord compression.

HORMONAL MANIPULATION Androgen deprivation therapy is used to treat advanced prostate cancer. Many cells in the growing tumor are androgen dependent and either cease to grow or die if deprived of androgens. Unfortunately, other cancer cells thrive without androgen and are unaffected by therapy to reduce circulating androgens. Therefore, the effects of hormone manipulations vary from complete but temporary regression of the tumor to no response at all. Strategies to induce androgen deprivation vary from orchiectomy to oral administration of hormonal agents. Table 50–5 compares surgical and hormone therapies and the advantages and disadvantages of each. In addition, new drugs are being developed that block the effects of male hormones, and research is being conducted to demonstrate what mix of hormones is best and at what time in the perioperative period they are most effective.

NURSING CARE

Nurses plan and provide interventions to help prevent prostate cancer and to facilitate a return to functional health status. Interventions may range from teaching to using knowledge and skill in physical care following a radical prostatectomy. A Nursing Care Plan for a man having a radical prostatectomy is found on page 1788.

Health Promotion

Nurses are in a unique position to increase public awareness about early detection of prostate cancer. Every encounter with men and their families—in clinics, hospital units, or in the home—is an opportunity to provide information about early detection and identify needs. Several studies have shown a positive correlation between increased awareness of and participation in prostate cancer screening procedures. The American Cancer Society has free pamphlets about early detection of prostate cancer, which are useful in educating the public.

One risk factor that can be easily changed is diet. Men should know that they can lower their risk of prostate cancer by eating less red meat and fat. They should include fruits and vegetables as recommended in the new food pyramid; toma-

TABLE 50–5 Surgical and Hormone* Therapy in the Management of Advanced Prostate Cancer

TREATMENT	ADVANTAGES	DISADVANTAGES
Orchiectomy	Inexpensive Immediate effect; i.e., men report diminished pain from metastasis in the recovery room	Body image problems due to loss of testicles
Estrogen compounds (diethylstilbestrol)	Inexpensive Effects reversible	Increased risk of cardiovascular problems More likely to cause gynecomastia, hypertrophy of breast tissue
Luteinizing hormone-releasing hormone agonist (LHRH) (leuprolide)	Effects reversible No cardiovascular risk Monthly administration	Very expensive Subcutaneous injection route Slow onset: up to 4 weeks
Steroidal antiandrogens (megestrol [Megace])	Effects reversible No cardiovascular risk Inexpensive	May not drop testosterone levels sufficiently Weight gain
Nonsteroidal antiandrogens (flutamide; often used in conjunction with LHRH)	Does not alter circulating androgens Blocks some side effects of LHRH May be effective if other methods fail	Very expensive

*All hormonal manipulations have the potential disadvantage of loss of libido, erectile dysfunction, hot flashes, and gynecomastia.

toes, pink grapefruit, and watermelon are high in lycopenes that help prevent damage to DNA and may help lower prostate cancer risk. Other substances that may help lower the risk are vitamin E and selenium.

All men should be given information about the limitations and benefits of testing for early detection and of treatment so they can make an informed decision. The American Cancer Society (2005a) recommends that the PSA test and DRE should be offered each year, beginning at age 50, to all men with a life expectancy of at least 10 years. Men at high risk (men of African descent and those with a first-degree relative diagnosed at a younger age) should begin testing at age 45.

Assessment

Collect the following data through the health history and physical examination (see Chapter 49 ∞). Note that a digital rectal examination is an advanced nursing assessment.

- *Health history:* Risk factors, urinary elimination patterns and manifestations, hematuria, pain.
- *Physical assessment:* DRE to assess prostate size, symmetry, firmness, and nodules.

Nursing Diagnoses and Interventions

The nursing care of men with prostate cancer must be holistic, sensitive, and individualized. The nursing diagnoses discussed for the man with BPH may also be appropriate. This section focuses on problems with urinary incontinence, sexual function, and pain.

Urinary Incontinence (Reflex, Stress, Total)

Urinary incontinence is a disturbing complication following treatment for prostate cancer. Both radical prostatectomy and external-beam radiation therapy can cause incontinence, ranging from a drop or two when the client lifts a heavy object (*stress incontinence*) to no control at all. Older men may experience *urge incontinence*, the involuntary passage of urine soon after a strong sense of urgency to void. Total and unpredictable loss of urine is classified as total incontinence. The man's reaction to incontinence may be severe even if the incontinence is not great. Many men have significant anxiety at the prospect of an incontinent episode in public, because they feel shame and often guilt about the loss of control.

- Assess the degree of incontinence and its effects on lifestyle. *The nurse needs to determine previous urinary patterns and the type of incontinence currently being experienced to plan appropriate interventions.*
- Teach Kegel exercises to help restore continence. *Pelvic muscle or Kegel exercises can often either eliminate or improve stress incontinence.*
- Teach methods to control dampness and odor from stress incontinence:
  - Do not attempt to prevent accidental voiding by restricting fluids. *Not only will the man continue to have incontinent episodes, but also his urine will become concentrated, exacerbating the problem with odor.*
  - Manage occasional episodes (one to three small-volume accidents per day) with absorbent pads worn inside the underwear and changed as needed. Most pads are made with a polymer gel that controls odor. *Appropriate measures help promote good hygiene, decrease anxiety, and increase comfort.*
- Refer to physical therapy or a continence specialist for additional measures to promote continence. *Special exercises, restricting some types of fluids, and other measures such as bladder training can help the client deal with incontinence.*
- Explore options such as an external collection device (external catheter or Texas catheter) for the man with total incontinence. *This device may improve the man's self-esteem and allow resumption of social activities.*
- Encourage verbalizing feelings about the impact of incontinence on quality of life. *The degree of incontinence does not necessarily correlate with the perceived level of suffering.*

NURSING CARE PLAN   A Man with Prostate Cancer

William Turner, a 71-year-old African American, lives with his wife in a small retirement community in Florida. His wife had a stroke 2 years ago, and Mr. Turner does all the cooking and housework. He has been in good health for most of his life, having only "a small touch" of osteoarthritis in his knees and hands. He has noticed a gradual onset of urinary urgency and frequency over the past 2 years, but has never had incontinence. During a routine checkup, the nurse practitioner at the local health clinic performs a digital rectal examination and palpates a hard nodule on the surface of Mr. Turner's prostate. After his PSA is found to be elevated, he is referred to a urologist, who diagnoses prostate cancer. Mr. Turner chooses to have surgery, and a radical retropubic prostatectomy and lymph node dissection are performed. The lymph nodes are negative for metastasis. Following surgery, his recovery is uncomplicated. However, the nurse caring for Mr. Turner is concerned about his ability to care for his indwelling catheter because of his arthritis and his wife's physical disabilities from the stroke. The nurse makes a referral to a home health agency to ensure Mr. Turner can manage his care at home. An initial home health assessment is scheduled for the day after Mr. Turner is discharged from the hospital.

ASSESSMENT

The home health nurse notes that the house is clean and neat. Mr. Turner is dressed, but still wearing his night urinary drainage bag, even though it is 1300. Mr. Turner tells the nurse that his main problem is going to get groceries, because he is embarrassed to be seen with the drainage bag. He says he has not been able to remove the drainage bag and attach the leg bag because of his arthritis. Physical assessment findings include the pelvic incision to be healing without signs of infection. There is no tenderness in his calves, chest pain, or shortness of breath. The urine is yellow, without odor. Mr. Turner does state that he sees no need for the pelvic exercises since he is no longer in the hospital. He also expresses the belief that he is cured of cancer and questions the need for follow-up care.

DIAGNOSES

- *Risk for stress urinary incontinence* related to surgical procedure
- *Ineffective health maintenance* related to inability to care for the urinary drainage system, not understanding need for postoperative exercises, and questions about follow-up care

EXPECTED OUTCOMES

- Regain urinary continence after catheter removal.
- Change the urinary drainage bag with the appropriate assistance.
- Verbalize the rationale for performing postoperative exercise.
- Verbalize the need for continued follow-up care.

PLANNING AND IMPLEMENTATION

- Discuss the possibility of stress incontinence after the catheter is removed.
- Reinforce the need for Kegel exercises while the catheter is still in place.
- Explore Mr. Turner's support system to identify people who could assist him with catheter care and arrange a teaching session with them.
- Teach Mr. Turner the importance of follow-up care, relating the care to the history of the disease.

EVALUATION

Good friends from Mr. Turner's church have assisted him with care of his drainage bag, and have reminded him to do his Kegel exercises several times a day while the catheter is in place. When the catheter is removed, Mr. Turner has only a small amount of leaking of urine after voiding. He understands that it may take several weeks for this to resolve. Efforts to help him understand the need for continued medical care are less successful. Mr. Turner continues to state that he is cured, his wife needs him, and he sees no need to go back to the doctor.

CRITICAL THINKING IN THE NURSING PROCESS

1. Outline a teaching plan for Mr. Turner for the risk for altered skin integrity related to urinary incontinence.
2. As a result of Mr. Turner's refusal to have ongoing medical-care, he might be labeled as noncompliant. Would you make this nursing diagnosis? Why or why not?
3. If you were the home health nurse making a home visit and found that Mr. Turner had no urinary drainage for 16 hours, what assessments would you make? How would you handle this problem?

See Evaluating Your Response in Appendix C.

Listening to these concerns with sensitivity can help the man work through these feelings and may allow him to move toward a healthy adaptation to his disability.

Sexual Dysfunction

Surgical treatment for prostate cancer may cause ED and changes in ejaculatory function. Hormone therapy for advanced prostate cancer lowers libido and may also cause ED. The diagnosis of cancer and body image changes caused by hormone therapy may lower self-esteem, which in turn can diminish sexual desire and willingness to interact sexually with a partner. Most older men are active sexually and fully capable of sustaining an erection. They are likely to fear the effect of treatment on their sexual health. They may allow this concern to guide their decision about the treatment course, or they may refuse all therapy because of this fear. Reactions vary greatly, and the nurse must maintain a nonjudgmental approach to education and support.

- Assess the man's pretreatment sexual function. *Knowledge of previous sexual function is necessary to plan appropriate interventions.*
- Teach the man about the actual or potential effects of therapy on sexual function. *The incidence of ED varies with different therapies for prostate cancer.*
- Provide an opportunity for the man and his partner to discuss implications of and concerns about the diagnosis and treatment of sexual function. *The treatments for prostate cancer often affect the physiology of erection. The man and his partner need support and counseling during the period of adjustment.*

- Discuss medical and surgical treatments for ED (see first section of this chapter). *Many men are as devastated by the loss of erectile function as they are by the diagnosis of cancer. Information about achieving erection and maintaining sexual intimacy is essential to quality of life.*
- Refer for sexual counseling as appropriate. *The man and his partner may require therapy beyond that provided by nurses.*

> ### PRACTICE ALERT
> A therapeutic approach to assessing how the man feels is to use an opening statement such as "Some men are very concerned about the effects of (type of treatment) on their ability to have an erection. Tell me how you feel about it."

Acute/Chronic Pain

There are many causes of pain in men with advanced prostate cancer. It is not unusual for a client to have three or four distinct pains simultaneously, all from different sources. The most common cause of pain is metastasis to the spinal column, usually the thoracic spine. Other sources of pain include fractures, lymphedema of the lower extremities, and muscle spasms. Because most men with prostate cancer are over the age of 65, many also have pain associated with preexisting conditions, such as osteoarthritis, unrelated to the cancer.

- Assess the intensity, location, and quality of the pain. *A cardinal rule of successful pain management is the importance of reducing or eliminating the cause of pain. Appropriate interventions are based on a careful assessment of the client's pain.*
- Provide optimal pain relief with prescribed analgesics. *It is important that the man and his family understand that pain medications should be used on a regular basis to maintain comfort and should not be delayed until pain is severe.*
- Teach the man and his family noninvasive methods of pain control. *Various modalities can be successful in alleviating pain or reducing its perception, thus enhancing the comfort of the client* (see Chapter 9 ∞).

Using NANDA, NIC, and NOC

Chart 50–1 shows links between NANDA nursing diagnoses, NIC, and NOC when caring for the client with surgical treatment for prostate cancer.

Community-Based Care

Depending on the type of treatment, the following topics should be addressed in preparing the client and his family for home care:
- For the man having a surgical procedure: manifestations of infection and excessive bleeding, catheter care, wound care pain management

> **NANDA, NIC, AND NOC LINKAGES**
> **CHART 50–1 The Client Having Surgery for Prostate Cancer**
>
> **NANDA**
>
> Impaired Urinary Elimination
>
>
>
> **NIC**
>
> Urinary Elimination Management
>
> Bladder Irrigation
>
> Fluid Management
>
> Pain Management
>
> Tube Care: Urinary
>
> Infection Control
>
>
>
> **NOC**
>
> Urinary Elimination
>
> Pain Level
>
> Risk Control

Data from *NANDA's Nursing Diagnoses: Definitions & classification 2005–2006* by NANDA International (2003), Philadelphia; *Nursing Interventions Classification (NIC)* (4th ed.) by J. M. Dochterman & G. M. Bulecheck (2004), St. Louis, MO: Mosby; and *Nursing Outcomes Classification (NOC)* (3rd ed.) by S. Moorhead, M. Johnson, and M. Maas (2004), St. Louis, MO: Mosby.

- For the man receiving radiation therapy:
  - Danger of radiation damage to others (sleep in a room alone for a week, avoid close contact with pregnant women, infants, and children)
  - Condom use during sexual contact (ejaculate may be discolored, distressing sexual partner)
- The importance of keeping appointments with healthcare providers and having yearly PSA and rectal examinations
- If appropriate, community services, such as support groups, home health nurses, and hospice
- Helpful resources:
  - American Cancer Society
  - American Urological Association
  - National Cancer Institute.

MALE BREAST DISORDERS

THE MAN WITH GYNECOMASTIA

Gynecomastia, the abnormal enlargement of the male breast, is thought to result from a high ratio of estradiol to testosterone. It is common during puberty, affecting one breast in as many as 50% of adolescent males, but usually resolves within 1 to 2 years. Any condition that increases estrogen activity or decreases testosterone production can contribute to gynecomastia. Conditions that increase estrogen activity include obesity, testicular tumors, liver disease, and adrenal carcinoma; conditions that decrease testosterone production include chronic illness such as tuberculosis or Hodgkin's disease, injury, and orchitis. Drugs such as digitalis, opiates, and chemotherapeutic agents are also associated with gynecomastia. Gynecomastia after adolescence is usually bilateral. If it is unilateral, biopsy may be necessary to rule out breast cancer.

No treatment is necessary for the transient gynecomastia of puberty. If the condition becomes chronic, however, creating psychologic discomfort, surgery may be necessary to remove the subcutaneous breast tissue. When related to an underlying disorder, treatment of that disorder is required. In severe cases, tamoxifen is given to decrease estrogen activity.

Nursing care for the client with gynecomastia includes education about the cause and treatment of the condition, and emotional support for the psychosocial implications of this feminizing condition.

THE MAN WITH BREAST CANCER

Although male breast cancer is rare, accounting for about 1% of all breast cancer cases, it is as serious to the men who have it as it is to the women. About 1700 men in the United States are estimated to be diagnosed with breast cancer each year, accounting for more than 400 deaths (ACS, 2005a). The etiology of male breast cancer is unclear; hormonal, genetic, and perhaps environmental factors appear to be important.

Male breast cancer is clinically and histologically similar to female breast cancer, although lobular cancer is rare in males. Most tumors are estrogen-receptor positive. Because many men believe that breast cancer is only a woman's disease, they often delay seeking medical attention for symptoms and thus may present with advanced disease.

Treatment of male breast cancer is much like the treatment of female breast cancer, beginning with modified radical mastectomy, node dissection, and staging to determine the therapeutic options. Radiation, chemotherapy, and hormonal therapy (usually tamoxifen) are the conventional adjuncts to surgery. Castration (surgical removal of the testes) is the most successful palliative measure in men with advanced breast cancer, resulting in tumor regression and prolonging life.

Nursing care for the man with breast cancer is essentially the same as for the woman with breast cancer (see Chapter 51 ∞). The nurse has an opportunity to help the man and his family cope with the psychosocial effects of having breast cancer. He may feel embarrassment or shame about his condition as well as fear about the life-threatening nature of the disease. His family may share those feelings. By listening with understanding and empathy, the nurse can help the client and family resolve their feelings and move toward healing.

EXPLORE MEDIALINK

Prentice Hall Nursing MediaLink DVD-ROM
Audio Glossary
NCLEX-RN® Review

Animation/Video
Testicular Self-Examination

COMPANION WEBSITE www.prenhall.com/lemone
Audio Glossary
NCLEX-RN® Review
Care Plan Activity: Radical Prostatectomy
Case Studies
  Benign Prostatic Hyperplasia
  Prostatitis
Teaching Plan: ED Medication and Safety
MediaLink Applications
  Prostate Cancer Prevention
  Sleep Apnea and Erectile Dysfunction
Links to Resources

CHAPTER HIGHLIGHTS

■ Disorders of male sexual function include erectile dysfunction (ED) and ejaculatory dysfunction. Many different illnesses, medications, and surgical procedures may affect male sexual function. Treatments include medications, mechanical devices, and surgical procedures. It is important for nurses to initiate a discussion of sexual concerns during assessments and to recognize that many male reproductive treatments and surgeries may result in sexual dysfunction.

■ Phimosis and priapism are disorders of the penis that can cause problems with urination and sexual activity and may in some cases be considered medical emergencies. The risk of cancer of the penis, although rare, is increased by phimosis, poor genital hygiene, and viral HPV and HIV infections.

- Benign scrotal masses include hydrocele, spermatocele, and varicocele. Epididymitis may be associated with a urinary tract infection, prostatitis, urethral strictures, or a sexually transmitted infection.
- The testes may be infected (orchitis), twisted (testicular torsion), or develop cancer. Testicular cancer is the most common cancer in men between the ages of 15 and 40. Monthly testicular self-examination is critical to early detection and treatment of cancer.
- The prostate gland may be inflamed or infected (prostatitis), enlarged (benign prostatic hyperplasia [BPH]) or develop cancer.

BPH is a common disorder of the aging male that causes problems with urination as the enlarging prostate gland constricts the urethra. Treatments include medications and various types of surgery, depending on the size of the prostate, and the age and health status of the man.

- Cancer of the prostate is the most common type of cancer and the second leading cause of death in American men. When diagnosed early, prostate cancer is curable. Diagnosis is often based on an increasing level of PSA and an abnormal DRE. The cancer is treated with surgery, radiation, or hormonal manipulation.
- The male breast may become enlarged (gynecomastia) or develop cancer.

TEST YOURSELF NCLEX-RN® REVIEW

1 When conducting a health assessment, which of the following statements would most likely elicit information about sexual concerns?
1. "Following your prostate surgery, when did you first notice you had problems with sexual intercourse?"
2. "Why do you think you should be sexually active at your age?"
3. "Do you miss having sex?"
4. "Tell me about your experience with sexual function since you developed prostate enlargement."

2 You are conducting a health teaching session for young men. What topic would be appropriate to reduce the risk of cancer of the penis?
1. wearing a condom during sexual intercourse
2. retracting the foreskin of the penis when showering
3. avoiding tight pants and very hot showers
4. maintaining a regular testicular self-examination schedule

3 What disease of the male reproductive system is a risk if a man also has a sexually transmitted infection (gonorrhea)?
1. epididymitis
2. hydrocele
3. erectile dysfunction
4. gynecomastia

4 Which of the following statements is true of testicular cancer?
1. The incidence increases with age.
2. It occurs most between ages 15 and 40.
3. It rarely occurs in brothers.
4. Severe pain is the initial manifestation.

5 You are teaching a man with chronic prostatitis how to care for himself at home. What simple measures can be used to decrease discomfort?
1. Take cold showers and restrict oral fluids.
2. Wear a scrotal support and take anti-inflammatory drugs.
3. Increase oral fluid intake to 3 L/day and void often.
4. Increase fiber intake and avoid sexual activity.

6 What diagnostic tests are used to differentiate BPH from prostate cancer? (Choose all that apply.)
1. pelvic ultrasound
2. digital rectal examination
3. blood chemistry
4. PSA level
5. sperm count

7 The enlarging prostate in BPH typically is manifested by assessment of problems with:
1. bowel elimination.
2. urinary elimination.
3. peripheral vascular function.
4. skin integrity.

8 You are caring for a man who has returned to the unit from the recovery room following a TURP. His urinary drainage bag is filled with dark red fluid with obvious clots. He is having painful bladder spasms. What would you do first?
1. Assess his intake and output since surgery.
2. Administer pain medication in the form of a B&O suppository.
3. Report your assessments to his urologist.
4. Nothing, because these manifestations are expected following a TURP.

9 What cancer is the most common malignancy in American men?
1. prostate cancer
2. testicular cancer
3. lung cancer
4. colon cancer

10 What nutritional information should be included in a community program to reduce the risk of prostate cancer?
1. Increase fiber intake.
2. Decrease lycopene intake.
3. Avoid foods high in sodium.
4. Decrease red meat and fat intake.

See Test Yourself answers in Appendix C.

BIBLIOGRAPHY

Albaugh, J., & Kellog-Spadt, S. (2003a). Intimacy issues. Man's search for ultimate sex. VIAGRA abuse. *Urologic Nursing, 23*(1), 75–76.

_____. (2003b). Sexuality and sexual health: The nurse's role and initial approach to patients. *Urologic Nursing, 23*(3), 227–228.

American Cancer Society. (2004). *What are the risk factors for testicular cancer?* Retrieved from http://www.cancer.org/docroot/CRI/content/CRI_2_4_2X_What_are_the_risk_factors_for_testicular_can...

American Cancer Society. (2005a). *Cancer facts & figures 2005.* Atlanta: Author.

American Cancer Society (ACS). (2005b). Prostate cancer. Retrieved from http://www.cdc.gov/cancer/prostate/index.htm

American Cancer Society (ACS). (2006). Cancer facts & figures 2006. Atlanta: Author.

American Society of Clinical Oncology. (2005). Breast cancer drug could benefit prostate. Retrieved from http://www.asco.org

Brown, C. (2004). Testicular cancer: An overview. *Urologic Nursing, 24*(2), 83–88, 93–94.

Brown, O. A. (2004). Understanding postoperative hyponatremia. *Urologic Nursing, 24*(3), 197–201.

Calabrese, D. (2004). Prostate cancer in older men. *Urologic Nursing, 24*(4), 258–264, 268–269.

Centers for Disease Control and Prevention. (2004). *Prostate cancer.* Retrieved from http://www.cdc.gov/cancer/prostate/prostate.htm

Cleveland Clinic. (2004). *Erectile dysfunction: Drugs linked to erectile dysfunction*. Retrieved from http://my.webmd.com/content/article/57/66229?printing=true

Davison, B. J., Moore, K., MacMillan, H., Bisaillon, A., & Wiens, K. (2004). Patient evaluation of a discharge program following a radical prostatectomy. *Urology Nursing, 24*(6), 483–489.

Dochterman, J., & Bulechek, G. (2004). *Nursing interventions classification (NIC)* (4th ed.). St. Louis, MO: Mosby.

Dorey, G., Speakman, M., Feneley, R., Swinkels, A., Dunn, C., & Ewings, P. (2004). Pelvic floor exercises for treating post-micturition dribble in men with erectile dysfunction: A randomized trial. *Urologic Nursing, 24*(6), 490–497, 512.

Gray, M., & Brown, K. (2002). Genitourinary system. In J. Thompson, G. McFarland, J. Hirsch, & S. Tucker (Eds), *Mosby's clinical nursing* (5th ed.) (pp. 917–999). St. Louis, MO: Mosby.

Kee, J. (2004). *Handbook of laboratory and diagnostic tests with nursing implications* (5th ed.). Upper Saddle River, NJ: Prentice Hall.

Leonard, B. (2004). Women's conditions occurring in men: Breast cancer, osteoporosis, male menopause, and eating disorders. *Nursing Clinics of North America, 39*(2), 379–393.

Moorhead, S., Johnson, M., & Maas, M. (2003). *Nursing outcomes classification (NOC)* (3rd ed.). St. Louis, MO: Mosby.

Moyad, M. (2003). Complementary and preventive medicine. Lifestyle changes to prevent BPH: Heart healthy = prostate healthy. *Urologic Nursing, 23*(6), 439–441.

Mueller, N., & Mueller, E. (2004). KTP photoselective laser vaporization of the prostate: Indications, procedure, and nursing implications. *Urologic Nursing, 24*(5), 373–379.

NANDA International. (2005). *Nursing diagnoses: Definitions & classification 2005–2006*. Philadelphia: Author.

Nash, M. (2003). Best practice for patient self-cleaning of urinary drainage bags. *Urologic Nursing, 23*(5), 334, 339.

National Cancer Institute. (2004). The prostate-specific antigen (PSA) test: Questions and answers. Retrieved from http://cis.nci.nih.gov/fact/5_29.htm

National Kidney and Urologic Diseases Information Clearinghouse (NKUDIC). (2003a). Erectile dysfunction. Available http://kidney.niddk.nih.gov/kudiseases/pubs/impotence/

_____.(2003b). *Prostatitis: Disorders of the prostate*. Retrieved from http://kidney.niddk.nih.gov/kudiseases/pubs/prostatitis/index.htm

_____.(2004). *Prostate enlargement: Benign prostatic hyperplasia*. Retrieved from http://kidney.niddk.nih.gov/kudiseases/pubs/prostateenlargement/index.htm

Oliffe, J. (2004). Transrectal ultrasound prostate biopsy (TRUS-Bx): Patient perspectives. *Urologic Nursing, 24*(5), 395–400.

Parrott, E. (2003). TUNA of the prostate in an office setting: Nursing implications. *Urologic Nursing, 23*(1), 33–40.

Porth, C. M. (2005). *Pathophysiology: Concepts of altered health states* (7th ed.). Philadelphia: Lippincott.

Scoles, P. (2005). Getting ready for certification. Benign prostatic hyperplasia. *Urologic Nursing, 25*(1), 61.

Tierney, L., McPhee, S., & Papadakis, M. (Eds.). (2004). *Current medical diagnosis & treatment* (43rd ed.). Stamford, CT: Appleton & Lange.

Wilkinson, J. (2005). *Prentice Hall nursing diagnosis handbook with NIC interventions and NOC outcomes* (8th ed.). Upper Saddle River, NJ: Prentice Hall.

Wilson, B., Shannon, M., & Stang, C. (2005). *Prentice Hall nurse's drug guide 2005*. Upper Saddle River, NJ: Prentice Hall.

CHAPTER 51 Nursing Care of Women with Reproductive System and Breast Disorders

LEARNING OUTCOMES

- Explain the pathophysiology, manifestations, complications, interdisciplinary care, and nursing care of disorders of female sexual function, menstrual disorders, structural disorders, reproductive tissue disorders, and breast disorders.

- Describe the physiologic process of menopause.

- Compare and contrast the incidence, risk factors, pathophysiology, manifestations, diagnosis, treatment, and nursing care for cancer of the cervix, endometrium, ovary, vulva, and breast.

- Discuss the purposes, nursing implications, and health education for clients and their families for cancer screening, medications, and treatments for women with disorders of the reproductive system and breast.

- Discuss alternative and complementary therapies used by women to relieve manifestations associated with menopause and menstrual disorders.

- Describe the surgical procedures used to treat female reproductive system and breast disorders.

CLINICAL COMPETENCIES

- Assess functional status of women with reproductive system and breast disorders, and monitor, document, and report abnormal manifestations.

- Use evidence-based research to design interventions to promote early diagnosis and treatment of African American women with breast cancer.

- Determine priority nursing diagnoses, based on assessed data, to select and implement individualized nursing interventions for women with reproductive system and breast disorders.

- Administer medications used to treat female reproductive system and breast disorders knowledgeably and safely.

- Provide skilled care for the woman having a D&C, laparoscopy, hysterectomy, mastectomy, and breast reconstruction.

- Integrate interdisciplinary care into care of women with reproductive system and breast disorders.

- Provide teaching appropriate for community-based self-care of female reproductive and breast disorders.

- Revise plan of care as needed to provide effective interventions to promote, maintain, or restore functional health status to women with reproductive system and breast disorders.

MEDIALINK

Resources for this chapter can be found on the Prentice Hall Nursing MediaLink DVD-ROM accompanying this textbook, and on the Companion Website at http://www.prenhall.com/lemone

KEY TERMS

amenorrhea, *1802*
anorgasmia, *1795*
dysfunctional uterine bleeding
   (DUB), *1802*
dysmenorrhea, *1800*
dyspareunia, *1795*

endometriosis, *1810*
fibrocystic changes (FCC), *1820*
leiomyoma, *1809*
lymphedema, *1825*
menopause, *1795*
menorrhagia, *1802*

metrorrhagia, *1802*
premenstrual syndrome
   (PMS), *1798*

Disorders of the female reproductive system range from a minor discomfort of menstrual cramps to life-threatening diseases such as cancer. Many of these disorders can occur at any point in a woman's adult life. They may affect her ability to bear children, her sexuality, and her sense of well-being as a woman.

Women who experience reproductive system changes and disorders require a holistic approach to meet their physical, emotional, and educational needs. Because the ability to reproduce affects self-esteem, feelings of femininity, and general health, both sensitivity and understanding from caregivers are essential. Providing a medical and family history and undergoing diagnostic tests often require women to disclose personal, intimate information, which they may find embarrassing and uncomfortable. When planning and implementing care, nurses must consider the woman within the context of her culture, socioeconomic and educational level, and lifestyle. It is also important that the nurse not make assumptions or judgments about sexual orientation.

This chapter summarizes disorders of female sexual function and discusses the physiologic process of menopause, menstrual disorders, structural disorders, and disorders of female reproductive tissue, including the breast. Sexually transmitted infections, including vaginal infections and pelvic inflammatory disease, are discussed in Chapter 52 ∞. Many of the disorders result in actual or potential health problems requiring nursing care based on similar nursing diagnoses. To avoid repeating those diagnoses and interventions for each disorder, they have been divided among the nursing care discussions as appropriate. Treatment of cancer with chemotherapy and radiation is discussed in Chapter 14 ∞.

DISORDERS OF FEMALE SEXUAL FUNCTION

The female body maintains the capacity for sexual activity and orgasm long after menopause (see the Meeting Individualized Needs box below). In a typical sexual event, two physiologic sexual responses occur: vasocongestion and myotonia. Sexual stimulation results in vasocongestion of the blood vessels surrounding the vagina, causing engorgement, increased lubrication, and genital swelling and enlargement. Arousal, or myotonia, increases muscular tension, resulting in voluntary and involuntary muscle contraction.

MEETING INDIVIDUALIZED NEEDS   Sexual Function in the Aging Woman

Myths, taboos, and stereotypes held by society may foster the belief that older women are no longer interested in expressing their sexuality. Two commonly held myths are that menopause is the death of a woman's sexuality and that hysterectomy results in the inability to function sexually. Loss of sexual function is not an inevitable result of aging, although physical changes related to aging do affect the female sexual response. These physical changes, along with chronic conditions common in aging women, may alter a woman's sexual function. In addition, some medications used to treat the chronic conditions associated with aging can also alter the sexual response. It is the role of the nurse to educate women about the myths and misinformation about changes in sexual functioning and to provide information about ways to achieve optimal sexual health.

PHYSIOLOGIC CHANGES

Changes in aging women's sexual function begin in the perimenopausal period as estrogen levels decrease. Estrogen-sensitive cells are found throughout the central nervous system and the cardiovascular system. These cells are involved in the female sexual response. With menopause comes a decrease in the levels of estradiol, which affects nerve transmission and the response in the peripheral vascular system. As a result, the timing and degree of vasocongestion during the sexual response are affected.

Specific changes in the female sexual response occur in all phases. During the plateau phase, the capacity for vasocongestion decreases, as does muscle tension. In the orgasmic phase, the contractions are fewer and less intense. During the resolution phase, vasocongestion subsides more quickly.

NURSING CARE

The nurse's role in assisting aging women to reach optimal sexual functioning centers on teaching them about the physiologic and psychologic changes associated with menopause. In addition, the nurse should instruct the woman in how the effects of chronic illness and the medications used to treat these illnesses affect sexual functioning. The woman should be taught the importance of maintaining a healthy lifestyle, which includes a balanced diet, weight-bearing and aerobic exercises, stress management, and routine health examinations.

For problems related to vaginal dryness and dyspareunia, the nurse can recommend water-soluble vaginal lubricants or vaginal gels before intercourse. Intercourse on a regular basis and estrogen replacement therapy can also be recommended for these problems. Women who experience joint pain or other musculoskeletal pain due to conditions such as arthritis can benefit from instruction in how to adapt positions for intercourse.

The sexual response cycle has four phases: excitement, plateau, orgasm, and resolution. These phases always occur in the same sequence; however, the duration of each phase may vary. Sexual arousal typically ends in orgasm (climax), but sometimes fails to do so. A refractory period, or period in which the sexual organs are incapable of responding to stimulus, does not occur in the female. Multiple orgasms are physically possible in all women.

Although nurses may not conduct sexual counseling, they should be able to obtain a sexual history without embarrassment, discuss sexual concerns with women, and make appropriate referrals.

Pathophysiology

Disorders of sexual function include dyspareunia, inhibited sexual desire, and orgasmic dysfunction.

Dyspareunia

The woman with **dyspareunia** (pain during intercourse) may find it difficult to express her feelings to her partner. This condition may manifest itself as decreased desire or inhibited orgasm. The causes of dyspareunia range from organic to psychogenic.

Physical conditions, such as imperforate hymen, vaginal scarring, or vaginismus, may cause dyspareunia. *Vaginismus* is a rare condition in which the vaginal muscles at the introitus contract so tightly that an erect penis cannot be inserted. An early traumatic event, such as sexual abuse, fear of men, or rape, may contribute to this disorder. However, it is estimated that most dyspareunia is psychogenic in origin. The woman develops an anxiety–fear–guilt cycle in which negative thoughts become associated with the act of vaginal penetration, initiating a conditioned involuntary reflex. Other sexual activity may be pleasurable.

Inhibited Sexual Desire

Inhibited sexual desire may be a result of pathophysiologic processes or may be psychogenic in origin. Often, inhibited sexual desire is rooted deeply in childhood teaching or experiences that may be too painful to recall. Cultural and religious values can also affect the processing of sexual stimuli. Fear of pregnancy or sexually transmitted infections (STIs) and depression also contribute to decreased libido.

Orgasmic Dysfunction

Inhibited female orgasm (**anorgasmia**) is the most prevalent sexual problem among women. However, fewer than 20% of cases are physiologic in origin. It is estimated that from 8% to 15% of women have never experienced an orgasm in the waking state. Psychogenically induced anorgasmia may result from unresolved conflicts about sexual activity. Organic causes of anorgasmia include the presence of disease that results in general debilitation or that affects the sexual response cycle, and the use of drugs that depress the central nervous system (CNS).

Primary anorgasmia exists when a woman has never experienced an orgasm during the waking state, either through self-stimulation or intercourse. Secondary anorgasmia exists when a woman who previously experienced orgasms is no longer able to do so.

NURSING CARE

Nursing care focuses on identifying the type of sexual dysfunction with a thorough history, including the onset, duration, frequency, and context or situation in which the problem occurs. The woman's partner should be included in discussions when possible.

Teach the woman and her partner about varied normal sexual responses. The goal is to increase self-awareness and understanding of communication and their relationship to sexual desire. Explain the differences in the behaviors that men and women consider sexually stimulating. Sex therapists may provide training in autostimulation techniques (masturbation) after inhibitions against this practice are discussed. Group therapy may be encouraged to help the woman discuss her problem and to decrease the sense of isolation it gives her.

THE PERIMENOPAUSAL WOMAN

Menopause is the permanent cessation of menses. The *climacteric,* or *perimenopausal,* period denotes the time during which reproductive function gradually ceases. For most women, the perimenopausal period lasts several years. It begins with a decline in the production of the hormone estrogen, includes the permanent cessation of menstruation due to loss of ovarian function, and extends for 1 year after the final menstrual period, at which time a woman is said to be *postmenopausal.* The average woman will live one-third of her life after menopause.

Menopause is neither a disease nor a disorder, but a normal physiologic process. It is included here because it does increase the risk of physical disorders as well as various aspects of women's health. Many women welcome the freedom from monthly menstrual periods and have relatively minor physical effects from the estrogen depletion. However, the hormonal changes that occur can be accompanied by side effects. There is wide variation in how individual women experience these side effects. In the United States, most women stop menstruating between 48 and 55 years of age. Earlier menopause is associated with genetics, smoking, higher altitude, and obesity (Association of Reproductive Health Professionals [ARHP], 2005b). Certain health risks increase after menopause, including heart disease, osteoporosis, macular degeneration, cognitive changes, and breast cancer.

The Physiology of Menopause

The menopausal period marks the natural biologic end of reproductive ability. *Surgical menopause* occurs when the ovaries are removed in premenopausal women, dramatically reducing the production of estrogen and progestins. *Chemical menopause* often occurs during cancer chemotherapy, when cytotoxic drugs arrest ovarian function.

As ovarian function decreases, the production of estradiol (E_2), the most biologically active estrogen, decreases and is ultimately replaced by estrone as the major ovarian estrogen. Estrone is produced in small amounts and has only about one-tenth the biologic activity of estradiol. With decreased ovarian function, the second ovarian hormone, progesterone, which is produced during the luteal phase of the menstrual cycle, also is markedly reduced.

Manifestations

As estrogen decreases, various tissues are affected. The breast tissue, body hair, skin elasticity, and subcutaneous fat decrease. The ovaries and uterus become smaller, and the cervix and vagina also decrease in size and become pale in color. These changes may result in problems with vaginal dryness, dyspareunia, urinary stress incontinence, urinary tract infections (UTIs), and vaginitis. Vasomotor instability often results in hot flashes, palpitations, dizziness, and headaches. Other problems resulting from vasomotor instability include insomnia, frequent awakening, and perspiration (night sweats). The woman may experience irritability, anxiety, and depression as a result of these events.

Long-term estrogen deprivation results in an imbalance in bone remodeling and osteoporosis, leading to fractures and kyphosis. The risk for cardiovascular diseases increases in response to an increase in atherosclerosis (from an increase in the LDL-to-HDL cholesterol ratio). Manifestations of the perimenopausal period are listed in the box below. These manifestations vary widely. Some women experience severe symptoms, others experience moderate symptoms, and some women experience few or no symptoms.

INTERDISCIPLINARY CARE

Care of the woman experiencing menopausal symptoms focuses on relieving symptoms and minimizing postmenopausal health risks.

Diagnosis

As estrogen secretion diminishes, levels of follicle-stimulating hormone (FSH) and luteinizing hormone (LH) rise and remain elevated. A woman who had not menstruated for 1 full year or who has an increased FSH blood level is considered menopausal (Porth, 2005).

MANIFESTATIONS of the Perimenopausal Period

- Menstrual cycles become erratic. Menstrual flow varies widely in amount and duration and eventually ceases.
- Vaginal, vulval, and urethral tissues begin to atrophy.
- Vaginal pH rises, predisposing the woman to bacterial infections.
- Vaginal lubrication decreases, and vaginal rugae decrease in number. This may result in dyspareunia, injury, and fungal infections.
- Vasomotor instability due to a decrease in estrogen may result in hot flashes and night sweats. A hot flash starts in the chest and moves upward toward the face and may last from seconds to several minutes.
- Psychologic symptoms may include moodiness, nervousness, insomnia, headaches, irritability, anxiety, inability to concentrate, and depression.

Medications

Although controversial, hormone replacement therapy (HRT) may be prescribed to alleviate severe manifestations of menopause, but only for a limited amount of time and only after a woman has been provided with known risks. HRT may include estrogen alone for women who have had a hysterectomy, or a combination of estrogen and progestin. The addition of progestin stimulates monthly shedding of the interuterine lining, decreasing the risk of uterine cancer. HRT relieves hot flashes and night sweats and decreases problems of vaginal dryness and urogenital tissue atrophy, which can lead to painful intercourse and urinary incontinence. Long-term HRT may increase the risk for breast cancer, ovarian cancer, stroke, heart attacks, and venous thrombosis (Tierney et al., 2004). However, women who have had a hysterectomy and take estrogen alone do not have an increased risk of breast cancer (Health & Science, 2006).

Selective estrogen receptor modulators (SERMs) such as raloxifene (Evista) and triphenylethylene (Tamoxifen) bind to estrogen receptors and exert site-specific effects in different target tissues. Tamoxifen and toremifene (a derivative of tamoxifen) have a beneficial effect on bone mineral density and serum lipids and decrease the risk of invasive breast cancer in women at high risk. They also provide an alternative to HRT for preventing osteoporosis.

Alternative and Complementary Therapies

As a result of the controversy surrounding the use of HRT, nontraditional or alternative therapies have become more popular. The following complementary therapies are examples of those used by menopausal women to reduce associated discomforts (ARHP, 2005b; Mayo Clinic, 2004):

- Acupuncture
- Biofeedback
- Massage
- Herbs: *Cimcifuga racemosa* (black cohosh), Vitex agnus castii (chaste tree), *Rehmannia*, ginseng, Chinese tonic of He Shou Wu, dong quai, golden seal, flaxseed, and evening primrose
- Supplements: vitamin E, soy protein (soy is high in plant estrogens)
- Meditation and yoga.

NURSING CARE

Nursing care during and after the menopausal period focuses on minimizing the symptoms associated with hormonal changes, reducing the risk of cardiovascular disease, cancer, and osteoporosis, and educating the woman about lifestyle changes important to health and well-being.

Health Promotion

The American Cancer Society recommends a cancer-related checkup every year after the age of 40. This checkup includes examination for cancers of the thyroid, ovaries, lymph nodes, oral cavity, and skin. Other important checkups include screening for cervical, breast, and colorectal cancer. Health counseling should also include information about alcohol and tobacco use, sun exposure, diet and nutrition, exercise, risk factors, sexual practices, and environmental and occupational exposures. It is important to discuss the benefits of rest and exercise, as well as a diet that includes fruits, vegetables, and fiber. In addition, suggest the following resources for further information:

- National Institute on Aging
- Centers for Disease Control and Prevention
- North American Menopause Society
- Association of Reproductive Health Professionals
- Women's Health Initiative
- National Women's Health Information Center.

Assessment

Collect the following data through the health history and physical examination. When assessing the older woman, be aware of normal changes with aging, as outlined in Chapter 49 ∞.

- *Health history:* Problems with urinary frequency, urgency, or incontinence; menstrual history; sexual history; dyspareunia; use of alcohol, nicotine, and drugs; medications, sleep patterns, hot flashes, night sweats, changes in emotional responses.
- *Physical assessment:* Height and weight, posture, vital signs, breast examination, pelvic examination, abdominal assessment.

Nursing Diagnoses and Interventions

Although each nursing care plan must be individualized, interventions often focus on problems with lack of information, sexuality, self-esteem, and a disturbed body image.

Deficient Knowledge

Because menopausal manifestations vary widely, it is difficult to predict their effect on an individual woman. However, the well-informed woman is better prepared to deal with whatever symptoms she experiences.

- Discuss physiologic manifestations, such as hot flashes and night sweats. *The underlying cause of hot flashes is not known (Porth, 2005). Many physiologic effects of menopause are amenable to nonpharmacologic methods of relief, such as lifestyle changes.*

PRACTICE ALERT
When hot flashes occur at night and are accompanied by perspiration, they are called night sweats. Night sweats often interfere with normal sleep patterns, leading to increased fatigue and irritability.

- Provide information about dietary recommendations. The recommended daily intake of calcium for women over 50 is 1200 mg. *Some women need to use calcium supplements or calcium-containing antacid tablets to meet this requirement.*
- Emphasize the importance of weight-bearing exercise. *Weight-bearing exercise reduces the rate of bone loss, helps maintain optimum weight, and reduces cardiovascular risk.*

- Provide information about the benefits and risks of HRT. Not every woman will need or want it. *Every woman needs to understand both the risks and the benefits before deciding whether to use HRT.*
- Encourage the woman to obtain yearly mammograms, clinical breast examinations, and Pap tests, and to perform monthly breast self-examination (BSE) at the same day each month. *The increased risk for cancer of the breast and pelvic reproductive organs makes self-examination and healthcare provider screening during and after menopause even more important.*

Ineffective Sexuality Pattern

Vaginal dryness and atrophy, together with the emotional effect of menopause, can interfere with sexual expression and satisfaction. Suggesting measures to help the woman and her partner cope with these changes can enable them to continue or resume a mutually satisfying sexual relationship.

- Encourage expression of feelings and concerns about how menopause is changing her sex life. *Midlife and older women may not be comfortable in discussing their intimate sexual behavior.*
- Suggest ways to increase vaginal lubrication, such as spending more time in foreplay and/or using water-soluble gels (e.g., Replens) for vaginal lubrication. *A more leisurely approach to sexual activity can be mutually gratifying for both the woman and her partner. Use of water-soluble gels can prevent vaginal pain and irritation and improve the quality of the sexual experience.*

PRACTICE ALERT
Plant estrogens, found in food such as brown rice, corn, green beans, lemon and orange peels, and tofu, are mildly estrogenic and may improve vaginal dryness.

- Explain that as women age, it may take longer for vaginal lubrication and orgasm to occur. *This information is important to prevent the woman from believing something is wrong with her, or her partner believing he or she is no longer interesting or sexually exciting.*

Situational Low Self-Esteem

Each woman responds to the aging process in her own way, and most women have coping skills that adequately equip them to deal with the gradual changes associated with aging. Among the factors that may provoke a self-esteem disturbance are the loss of youth, a sense of emptiness as children leave home, and the need to redefine one's self-concept and roles as parenting becomes less important. Women who place a high value on their physical attractiveness may experience a painful psychologic response to the physical changes of menopause.

- Encourage expression of fears and concerns related to changes in interpersonal and family functions. *Many women associate aging with "uselessness" and unattractiveness.*
- Suggest volunteer activities or employment for the woman who has extra time. *This enables the woman to feel that she is still a contributing member of society. Volunteering for activities involving young people can help reduce anxiety about*

the loss of reproductive ability or any late regrets about not having had children.

■ Discuss the importance of a healthy lifestyle in maintaining physical attractiveness. Identify risk factors and high-risk behaviors. *Lifestyle habits and behaviors affect many body systems and physical appearance. For example, cigarette smoking and overexposure to the sun make the skin age faster, contributing to wrinkles. Active women who exercise and eat a well-balanced diet look and feel better.*

Disturbed Body Image

As women progress through the perimenopausal period, changes in appearance and the loss of childbearing ability may combine to make the woman feel "old, ugly, and useless." Although this is far from the truth, with women living at least one-third of their lives after menopause in productive careers and activities, it nevertheless is the perception of women as well as society. The physical changes the woman often experiences include growth of facial hair, excessive perspiration and flushing of the face, and weight gain.

■ Encourage the woman to describe her perceptions of her own body. *This information is necessary to obtain data to establish an individualized plan of care.*

■ Encourage verbalization of feelings of concern, anger, anxiety, loss, and fear over body changes. *Expressing these emotions can facilitate the grieving process and acceptance of change.*

■ Stress that certain physical characteristics of a person cannot be changed; emphasize the importance of learning to recognize and appreciate one's own special strengths. *These help the woman gain acceptance and a realistic appraisal of self.*

■ Refer, as appropriate, for dietary management, exercise, stress management, and cosmetic assistance (e.g., for aggravating facial hair). *These actions increase wellness and a positive sense of self.*

MENSTRUAL DISORDERS

Monthly menstruation normally involves some minor discomfort, including breast tenderness, a feeling of heaviness and congestion in the pelvic area, uterine cramping, and lower backache. Many women, however, experience more serious effects, both physiologic and psychologic. This section discusses premenstrual syndrome, dysmenorrhea, and abnormal uterine bleeding. (The menstrual cycle is discussed in Chapter 49 .)

THE WOMAN WITH PREMENSTRUAL SYNDROME

Premenstrual syndrome (PMS) is a complex of manifestations (e.g., mood swings, breast tenderness, fatigue, irritability, food cravings, and depression) that are limited to 3 to 14 days before menstruation and relieved by the onset of menses. It is estimated that 25% to 40% of all adult women experience mild to moderate symptoms and 2% to 5% have severe symptoms (Porth, 2005). For a small number of women, PMS is so disabling that it is called by the psychiatric label of *premenstrual dysphoric disorder (PMDD).*

The syndrome is seen less frequently during the teens and 20s, reaching a peak in women in their mid-30s. Major life stressors, age greater than 30, and depression are risk factors associated with PMS. Premenstrual syndrome can be a factor in absenteeism at school or work, decreased productivity, interpersonal relationship difficulties, and lifestyle disruption.

Pathophysiology

Although the pathophysiology of PMS is not clearly understood, it is believed that hormonal changes such as altered estrogen–progesterone ratios, increased prolactin levels, and rising aldosterone levels during the luteal phase of the menstrual cycle contribute to the problem. Increased production of aldosterone results in sodium retention and edema. Decreased levels of monoamine oxidase in the brain are associated with depression, and reduced levels of serotonin can lead to mood swings.

Manifestations

Manifestations of PMS occur during the luteal phase of the menstrual cycle (7 to 10 days prior to the onset of the menstrual flow), abating when the menstrual flow begins. The *Multisystem Effects of PMS* are shown on the next page. Although PMS may produce a variety of physiologic and psychologic manifestations, the exact nature of these manifestations and their intensity are individualized for each woman with this disorder. The manifestations may even differ from month to month in the same woman.

INTERDISCIPLINARY CARE

If no organic cause can be identified, the goals of care are to relieve manifestations and to help develop self-care patterns that will help the woman anticipate and cope more effectively with future episodes of PMS. There are no definitive diagnostic tests for PMS. The regular recurrence of manifestations preceding the onset of menses for at least 3 months leads to a diagnosis of PMS. The treatment of PMS integrates this self-monitored record of manifestations, regular exercise, avoiding caffeine, and a diet low in simple sugars and high in lean proteins (Porth, 2005). Although many different medications, vitamins, and herbal supplements have been used to treat the manifestations of PMS, the most promising appears to be the use of selective serotonin reuptake inhibitors (SSRIs).

Medications

If the manifestations of PMS are severe or incapacitating, ovulation may be suppressed by the use of gonadotropin-releasing hormone (GnRH) agonists, oral contraceptives, or danazol. Progesterone and antiprostaglandin agents such as nonsteroidal anti-inflammatory drugs (NSAIDs) may help relieve cramping. Diuretics may be prescribed to relieve bloating. SSRIs such as fluoxetine (Prozac), sertraline (Zoloft), and paroxetine (Paxil) may be used to manage mood and some physical manifestations of PMS.

MULTISYSTEM EFFECTS OF Premenstrual Syndrome

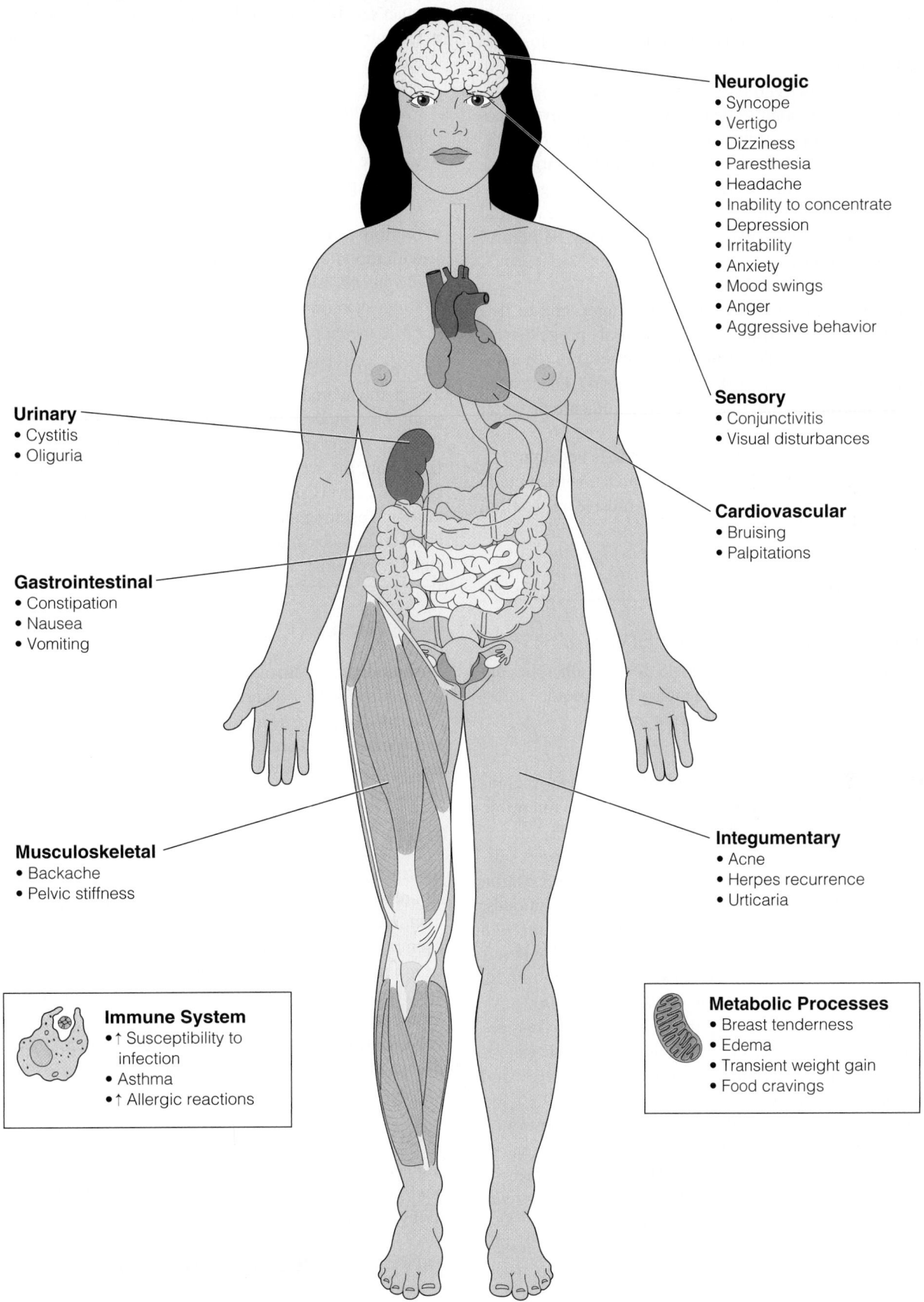

Neurologic
- Syncope
- Vertigo
- Dizziness
- Paresthesia
- Headache
- Inability to concentrate
- Depression
- Irritability
- Anxiety
- Mood swings
- Anger
- Aggressive behavior

Sensory
- Conjunctivitis
- Visual disturbances

Cardiovascular
- Bruising
- Palpitations

Integumentary
- Acne
- Herpes recurrence
- Urticaria

Urinary
- Cystitis
- Oliguria

Gastrointestinal
- Constipation
- Nausea
- Vomiting

Musculoskeletal
- Backache
- Pelvic stiffness

Immune System
- ↑ Susceptibility to infection
- Asthma
- ↑ Allergic reactions

Metabolic Processes
- Breast tenderness
- Edema
- Transient weight gain
- Food cravings

Alternative and Complementary Therapies

Alternative and complementary therapies the woman with PMS may find helpful focus on diet, exercise, relaxation, and stress management:

- A diet high in complex carbohydrates with limited simple sugars and alcohol is recommended to minimize reactive hypoglycemia, which can contribute to the manifestations of PMS.
- Reduced sodium intake helps minimize fluid retention. Increased intake of calcium (1200 mg per day), magnesium (200 mg per day), vitamin B_6 (50 to 100 mg per day), and vitamin E (400 international units per day) may be helpful (Mayo Clinic, 2004).
- Caffeine is restricted to reduce irritability.
- Herbal remedies include black cohosh, ginger, chaste tree berry, and evening primrose oil. Natural progesterone creams, derived from wild yams and soybeans, relieve manifestations in some women (Mayo Clinic, 2004). Discussion about these alternative therapies with the healthcare provider is recommended.
- Exercise is beneficial, but adequate rest also is necessary.
- Techniques for relaxation and stress management include deep abdominal breathing, meditation, muscle relaxation, and guided imagery.

 NURSING CARE

Nursing Diagnoses and Interventions

Nursing care for the woman with PMS focuses on relieving manifestations. Most women experiencing PMS require interventions to manage pain and enhance coping.

Acute Pain

The woman with PMS may have pain from headache (including migraine), menstrual cramps, excessive fluid retention, breast swelling, joint and muscle pain, and backache.

- Teach effective pharmacologic and nonpharmacologic self-care measures to relieve pain: application of heat, relaxation techniques (such as breathing exercises, imagery techniques, or meditation), and exercise. *Heat relieves muscle spasms and dilates blood vessels, increasing blood supply to the pelvis and uterine muscles. Relaxation and exercise aid the release of naturally produced pain relievers called endorphins.*
- Review daily activities and suggest ways to balance rest periods and activity. *During rest periods, energy and oxygen requirements decrease, increasing the amount of energy and oxygen available to muscles.*
- Review manifestations and, if possible, correlate these with dietary patterns and activity levels. Encourage the woman to keep a diary of PMS manifestations. *Maintaining a diary of PMS manifestations, activity, and foods eaten can provide data to identify modifiable causes of discomfort.*
- If appropriate, suggest sexual activity as a way to lessen menstrual cramps. *Orgasm may help relieve dysmenorrhea.*

Ineffective Coping

Many women experience wide mood swings during episodes of PMS, sometimes exhibiting self-destructive or aggressive behaviors toward others. These mood swings can interfere with a woman's ability to manage her responsibilities at home or at work.

- Encourage the woman to keep a journal of her menstrual cycle and to document her mood changes in the 7 to 10 days prior to menstruation. *Recognizing the signs and timing of PMS is the first step in developing methods to cope with the problem.*
- Explore possible ways to rearrange or reschedule activities when experiencing PMS. *Planning ahead enables the woman to assume more control and promotes coping methods.*
- Explore what, if any, self-care measures have helped cope with mood alterations in the past. *Encourage healthful coping mechanisms, such as relaxation techniques and exercise. Some women may rely on alcohol or other drugs during PMS, which only exacerbate the manifestations.*

Community-Based Care

Teach the woman and family that PMS is not caused by a pathologic process but is a physiologic response to hormonal changes of the menstrual cycle. With an understanding of the condition, the woman is better able to manage anxiety and to become actively involved in techniques to reduce the manifestations. Teaching should also include dietary measures, relaxation techniques and exercise, stress reduction techniques, and support systems.

THE WOMAN WITH DYSMENORRHEA

Dysmenorrhea (pain or discomfort associated with menstruation) is experienced by a significant number of menstruating women. *Primary dysmenorrhea* occurs without specific pelvic pathology, and is most often seen in girls who have just begun menstruating, becoming less severe after the mid-20s or giving birth. S*econdary dysmenorrhea* is related to identified pelvic disease.

Pathophysiology

In primary dysmenorrhea, excessive production of prostaglandins stimulates uterine muscle fibers to contract. As the muscles contract, uterine circulation is compromised, resulting in uterine ischemia and pain. These contractions can range from mild cramping to severe muscle spasms. Psychologic factors, such as anxiety and tension, may contribute to dysmenorrhea. Secondary dysmenorrhea is related to underlying organic conditions that involve scarring or injury to the reproductive tract. Endometriosis, fibroid tumors, pelvic inflammatory disease, or ovarian cancer may result in painful menses.

Manifestations

Manifestations of primary dysmenorrhea (see the box on the next page) may be severe enough to disrupt activities of daily living, sexual function, and even fertility.

INTERDISCIPLINARY CARE

Care of the woman with menstrual pain focuses on identifying the underlying cause, reestablishing functional capacity, and managing pain.

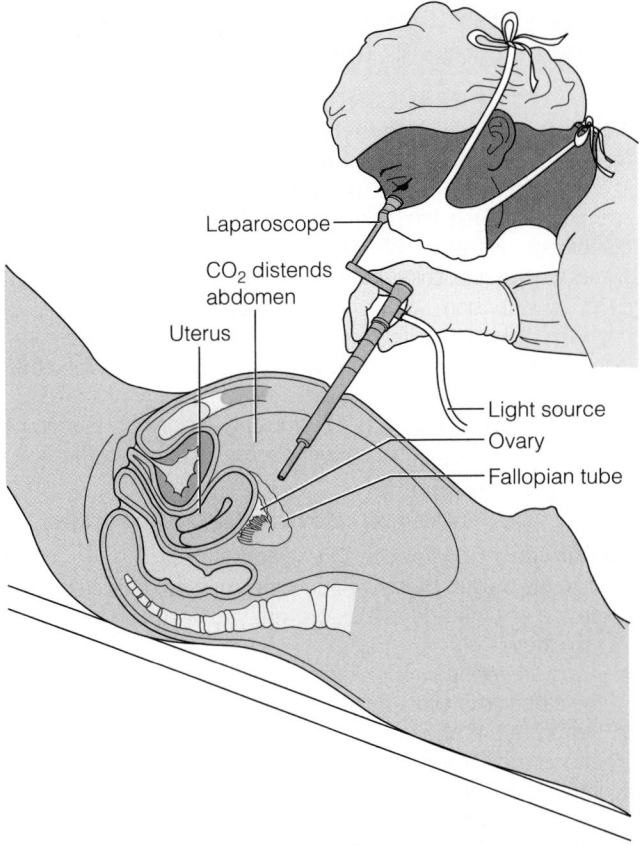

MANIFESTATIONS of Primary Dysmenorrhea

- Abdominal pain beginning with onset of menses and lasting 12 to 48 hours
- Pain radiating to lower back and thighs
- Headache
- Nausea
- Vomiting
- Diarrhea
- Fatigue
- Breast tenderness

A careful history and physical assessment are performed to rule out any underlying organic cause of dysmenorrhea. If no organic cause can be found, the diagnosis is primary dysmenorrhea. In addition, attitudes and expectations about menstruation and lifestyle disruption are identified and explored.

Diagnosis

Various diagnostic tests are performed to identify structural abnormalities, hormonal imbalances, and pathologic conditions that could cause menstrual pain. Diagnostic tests are described in Chapter 49 ∞.

Diagnosis is made based on findings from a pelvic examination and diagnostic procedures, including a Papanicolaou (Pap) smear and cervical and vaginal cultures, ultrasound of the pelvis and vagina, and CT scan or MRI to detect structural abnormalities, malignancy, or infections. Laboratory tests used to assess possible causes of dysmenorrhea are as follows:

- *FSH* and *LH levels* to assess the function of the pituitary gland. The results are correlated with the time of the menstrual cycle.
- Progesterone and estradiol levels to assess ovarian function.
- Thyroid function tests (T_3 and T_4) to assess thyroid function.

Laparoscopy is used to diagnose structural defects and blockages caused by scarring, endometriosis, tumors, and cysts (Figure 51–1 ■). See the box below for nursing care of the woman having a laparoscopy. A dilation and curettage (D&C) of the uterus may be performed to obtain tissue for evaluation

Figure 51–1 ■ Laparoscopy. In this surgical procedure, a flexible, lighted instrument (laparoscope) is inserted through a periumbilical incision. Laparoscopy allows visualization of the pelvic cavity.

or to relieve dysmenorrhea and heavy menstrual bleeding. (This procedure is discussed later in this chapter.)

Medications

Dysmenorrhea may be treated with analgesics, prostaglandin inhibitors such as NSAIDs, or oral contraceptives (see the Medication Administration box on the next page).

Alternative and Complementary Therapies

The complementary therapies listed for the woman with PMS may also be useful for the woman with dysmenorrhea. Other

---

NURSING CARE OF THE WOMAN HAVING A **Laparoscopy**

PREOPERATIVE CARE
- Instruct the woman to empty the bladder prior to the surgical procedure.
- Explain to the woman that referred shoulder pain or expulsion of gas through the vagina may occur postoperatively. *During the procedure, the woman's abdomen is insufflated with carbon dioxide gas to distend the abdomen and facilitate visualization of the pelvic organs. The surgical table is then tilted so that the intestines will fall away from the pelvic organs. Some carbon dioxide gas may remain in the abdomen after the procedure.*

- Explain that pain should be minimal. Instruct the woman to report excessive pain to the nurse or physician at once. *Excessive pain signals infection or other postoperative complication.*

POSTOPERATIVE CARE
- Apply a perineal pad. Teach the woman proper perineal hygiene, emphasizing the need to change pads at least every 4 hours. Keep a pad count. *Proper perineal hygiene reduces the risk of postoperative infection. Pad count is an indication of blood loss.*
- Assess for excessive vaginal bleeding. *Minor bleeding is normal; excessive bleeding may indicate hemorrhage.*

MEDICATION ADMINISTRATION
The Woman with Dysmenorrhea

EXAMPLES OF ORAL CONTRACEPTIVES
Norethindrone and ethinyl estradiol (Brevicon, Norinyl)
Norgestrel and ethinyl estradiol (Ovral)
Oral contraceptives inhibit ovulation and help reduce cramping and bleeding. Side effects of oral contraceptives include breast tenderness, weight gain, nausea, midcycle bleeding, mood swings, depression, chloasma (skin discoloration) on the face and chest, hypertension, vascular complications, vaginal candidiasis, migraines, and glucose intolerance. Oral contraceptives are contraindicated in women with personal or family history of breast cancer in first-degree relatives, hypertension, history of stroke or transient ischemic attack (TIA), smoking, history of estrogen-dependent cancer, pregnancy, liver disease, or thrombophlebitis.

Nursing Responsibilities
- Assess the client for potential contraindications to drug therapy.

Health Education for the Client and Family
- Take the drug as prescribed until the physician indicates otherwise or until side effects prevent you from continuing to take them.
- If you are taking oral contraceptives, be sure to take them at the same time every day.
- Report to the physician suspected pregnancy and any side effects such as nausea, rash, drowsiness, stomach pain, ringing in the ears, tenderness in the calf of the leg, and shortness of breath.
- Do not smoke while taking oral contraceptives.

helpful activities are regular physical exercise, supplementing the diet with zinc and calcium, and using herbal remedies such as *Viburnum prunifolium*, black cohosh, evening primrose oil, and blue cohosh (About Women's Health, 2005). Using a heating pad on the abdomen or taking a warm bath also helps reduce pain.

NURSING CARE

Nursing care for the woman with primary dysmenorrhea focuses on controlling manifestations and providing education about the normal physiology of the menstrual cycle and self-care measures. Care of the woman with secondary dysmenorrhea varies according to the underlying cause and is discussed in this chapter within sections on specific disorders. Nursing interventions previously described for the woman with PMS are also appropriate for the woman with dysmenorrhea.

THE WOMAN WITH DYSFUNCTIONAL UTERINE BLEEDING

Dysfunctional uterine bleeding (DUB) refers to vaginal bleeding that is usually painless but abnormal in amount, duration, or time of occurrence. The types of DUB include primary and secondary amenorrhea, oligomenorrhea, menorrhagia, metrorrhagia, and postmenopausal bleeding.

A number of factors may predispose a woman to DUB. These factors include stress, extreme weight changes, use of oral contraceptive agents or intrauterine devices (IUDs), and

postmenopausal status. Dysfunctional uterine bleeding is usually related to hormonal imbalances or pelvic neoplasms, either benign or malignant.

Pathophysiology

The types of DUB include amenorrhea, oligomenorrhea, menorrhagia, metrorrhagia, and postmenopausal bleeding.

- **Amenorrhea** is the absence of menstruation. Primary amenorrhea, absence of menarche by age 16, or by age 14 if secondary sex characteristics fail to develop, may be caused by structural abnormalities, hormonal imbalances, polycystic ovary disease, or an imperforate hymen. Because a certain percentage of body fat is required for menstruation to occur, anorexia nervosa, bulimia, or excessive athletic training can also cause primary amenorrhea. Secondary amenorrhea, absence of menses for at least 6 months in a previously menstruating female, may also be caused by anorexia nervosa, excessive athletic activity or training, or a large weight loss. Other causes include hormonal imbalances and ovarian tumors. Normal (physiologic) secondary amenorrhea occurs during pregnancy, breast-feeding, and menopause.
- *Oligomenorrhea* (scant menses) usually is related to hormonal imbalances.
- **Menorrhagia** (excessive or prolonged menstruation) may result from thyroid disorders, endometriosis, pelvic inflammatory disease, functional ovarian cysts, or uterine fibroids or polyps. Clotting disorders and anticoagulant medications also can cause menorrhagia. A single heavy or long menses is not in itself a cause for concern; however, repetitive long or heavy menses can lead to hemorrhage, excessive blood loss, fatigue, and anemia.
- **Metrorrhagia** (bleeding between menstrual periods) may be caused by hormonal imbalances, pelvic inflammatory disease, cervical or uterine polyps, uterine fibroids, or cervical or uterine cancer. Because cancer is a possible cause of metrorrhagia, early evaluation and treatment are extremely important. *Mittelschmerz* (midcycle spotting associated with ovulation) occurs in many women and is not considered metrorrhagia.
- *Postmenopausal bleeding* may be caused by endometrial polyps, endometrial hyperplasia, or uterine cancer. The possibility of cancer makes early evaluation and treatment essential.

Hormonal imbalances, especially progesterone deficiency with relative estrogen excess, result in endometrial hyperplasia. Estrogen stimulates endometrial proliferation. However, without the support provided by progesterone, sloughing occurs, resulting in vaginal bleeding that may be irregular, prolonged, or profuse. Defects in the follicular phase shorten the proliferative phase of the menstrual cycle, resulting in spotting and breakthrough bleeding. Defects during the luteal phase result in excessive amount or duration of flow due to persistence of the corpus luteum. This leads to a deficiency of progesterone, resulting in vaginal bleeding. *Anovulation,* absence of ovulation, is associated with both estrogen and progesterone deficiencies. Emotional upsets or stress can cause hormonal imbalances and thus affect menstruation. Pelvic neoplasms, discussed later, also cause abnormal bleeding.

INTERDISCIPLINARY CARE

The care of the woman with DUB focuses on identifying and treating the underlying disease. A careful history and physical examination are performed. Abdominal and pelvic examinations are performed to rule out abdominal masses. The woman may need to keep a menstrual history and basal body temperature chart for several months to determine whether ovulation is occurring.

Diagnosis

A variety of diagnostic tests are used to diagnose the cause of DUB. Diagnostic tests are discussed in Chapter 49 ∞, and include a Pap smear to rule out or identify cervical carcinoma, a pelvic ultrasound to identify luteal cysts, a hysteroscopy to detect abnormalities of the uterine cavity, or an endometrial biopsy to obtain endometrial tissue for histologic examination.

Laboratory studies may include the following:

- A *complete blood count (CBC)* to rule out systemic disease as a contributing factor to DUB and to evaluate its effects.
- *Thyroid function studies,* including measurement of tri-iodothyronine (T_3), thyroxine (T_4), and thyroid-stimulating hormone (TSH) levels, to rule out hyper- or hypothyroidism as a cause of DUB.
- Endocrine studies to evaluate pituitary and adrenal function. Pituitary dysfunction may first be manifested by menstrual irregularities.
- Serum progesterone levels to determine the level of progesterone deficiency.

Medications

For many women, hormonal agents can correct menstrual irregularities. For anovulatory DUB, oral contraceptives may be prescribed for 3 to 6 months. Progesterone or medroxyprogesterone also may be prescribed to regulate uterine bleeding.

Ovulatory DUB may be treated with progestins during the luteal phase. Oral iron supplements may be prescribed to replace iron lost through menstrual bleeding.

Surgery

Surgical intervention emphasizes the least invasive method that proves effective relief, beginning with a therapeutic dilation and curettage (D&C), then endometrial ablation, and, finally, hysterectomy.

THERAPEUTIC D&C In a therapeutic D&C, the cervical canal is dilated and the uterine wall is scraped. D&C, the most frequently performed minor gynecologic surgical procedure, is used to diagnose and treat DUB and other disorders of the female reproductive system. It may be performed to correct excessive or prolonged bleeding. D&C is contraindicated in any woman who has been taking anticoagulant drugs or whose condition precludes the use of regional or general anesthesia. Nursing care of the woman having a D&C is described in the box below.

ENDOMETRIAL ABLATION In an endometrial ablation, the endometrial layer of the uterus is permanently destroyed using laser surgery or electrosurgical resection. It is performed in women who do not respond to pharmacologic management or D&C. The woman needs to understand that this procedure ends menstruation and reproduction.

HYSTERECTOMY Hysterectomy, or removal of the uterus, may be performed when medical management of bleeding disorders is unsuccessful or malignancy is present, particularly if the woman no longer wishes to bear children. In premenopausal women, the ovaries are usually left in place; in postmenopausal women, a total hysterectomy, or panhysterectomy, may be performed; this procedure involves removal of the uterus, fallopian tubes, and ovaries.

FAST FACTS

Hysterectomy

- Approximately 600,000 hysterectomies are performed each year in the United States, and an estimated 20 million women have had a hysterectomy (Centers for Disease Control and Prevention, 2006d).
- This surgery is most often performed in women who are between the ages of 40 and 44.
- The three conditions most associated with hysterectomy are uterine leiomyoma (fibroids), endometriosis, and uterine prolapse.

NURSING CARE OF THE WOMAN HAVING A Dilation and Curettage (D&C)

PREOPERATIVE CARE

- If ordered, ask the woman to come in 24 hours before surgery for insertion of a laminaria tent. *This device absorbs cervical secretions and slowly dilates the cervix.*
- Instruct the woman to remain NPO after midnight on the day of surgery.

POSTOPERATIVE CARE

- Monitor circulation and sensation in the legs, and avoid compression of the popliteal area. *The lithotomy position requires the woman's legs to be elevated in stirrups, which can impair circulation.*

- Instruct the woman to use perineal pads and avoid tampons for 2 weeks. *This reduces the risk of infection and allows tissues to heal.*
- Explain that the onset of the next menstrual period may be delayed.
- Explain that intercourse should be avoided until after the postoperative checkup and after vaginal discharge has ceased. *This precaution reduces the risk of infection.*
- Instruct the woman to rest for several days after surgery, avoid heavy lifting, and report any bleeding that is bright red or exceeds that of a normal menstrual period. *Vigorous activity, lifting, or straining interferes with healing and may cause hemorrhage.*

Hysterectomy may involve either an abdominal or a vaginal approach. The choice depends on the underlying disorder, the need to explore the abdominal cavity, and the preference of the surgeon and woman. Nursing care of the woman undergoing a hysterectomy is described in the box below.

Abdominal hysterectomy is performed when a preexisting abdominal scar is present, when adhesions are thought to be present, or when a large operating field is necessary. For example, the woman with endometriosis is more likely to have an abdominal hysterectomy because endometrial tissue implants that may be present on other abdominal organs need to be removed. The surgical incision may be either longitudinal, made in the midline from umbilicus to pubis, or a *Pfannenstiel incision,* also known as the bikini cut.

Vaginal hysterectomy, removal of the uterus through the vagina, is desirable when the uterus has descended into the vagina or if the urinary bladder or rectum have prolapsed into the vagina. Vaginal hysterectomy leaves no visible abdominal scar. Laparoscopy-assisted vaginal hysterectomy (LAVH) is most often performed.

NURSING CARE

DUB usually causes the woman anxiety. Her self-image, sexuality, or reproductive capacity may be threatened, and she may fear the possibility of cancer. She may be embarrassed to discuss her menstrual history and hygiene practices.

Nursing Diagnoses and Interventions

Interventions for the woman with DUB commonly address problems with anxiety and sexual function.

Anxiety

The anxiety associated with abnormal uterine bleeding can be intense. Until the cause of the bleeding is identified and has been addressed, the woman may fear cancer or other life-threatening conditions.

- Discuss the results of tests and examinations with the woman. *This allows for open exchange of information.*
- Provide information about the causes, treatments, risks, long-term effects of treatments, and prognosis. *This allows the woman to assume responsibility for her own health and become involved in her own treatment plan.*

NURSING CARE OF THE WOMAN HAVING A   Hysterectomy

PREOPERATIVE CARE

- Assess the woman's understanding of the procedure. Provide explanation, clarification, and emotional support as needed. Reassure that the anesthesia will eliminate any pain during surgery and that medication will be administered postoperatively to minimize discomfort. *The woman who understands about the procedure to be performed and what to expect after surgery will be less anxious.*
- Cleanse the abdominal and perineal area, and, if ordered, shave the perineal area.
- If ordered, administer a small cleansing enema and ask the woman to empty her bladder. *This precaution helps prevent contamination from the bowel or bladder during surgery.*
- Administer preoperative medications as ordered.
- Check the chart to ensure that the consent form has been signed.

POSTOPERATIVE CARE

- Assess for signs of hemorrhage. *Hemorrhage is more common after vaginal hysterectomy than after abdominal hysterectomy.*
- Monitor vital signs every 4 hours, auscultate lungs every shift and measure intake and output. *These data are important indicators of hemodynamic status and complications.*
- Once the catheter has been removed, measure the amount of urine voided.
- Assess for complications, including infection, ileus, shock or hemorrhage, thrombophlebitis, and pulmonary embolus.
- Assess vaginal discharge; instruct the woman in perineal care.
- Assess incision and bowel sounds every shift.
- Encourage turning, coughing, deep breathing, and early ambulation.
- Encourage fluid intake.

- Teach to splint the abdomen and cough deeply. Teach the use of the incentive spirometer.
- Instruct to restrict physical activity for 4 to 6 weeks. Heavy lifting, stair climbing, douching, tampons, and sexual intercourse should be avoided. The woman should shower, avoiding tub baths, until bleeding has ceased. *Infection and hemorrhage are the greatest postoperative risks; restricting activities and preventing the introduction of any foreign material into the vagina helps reduce these risks.*
- Explain to the woman that she may feel tired for several days after surgery and needs to rest periodically.
- Explain that appetite may be depressed and bowel elimination may be sluggish. *These are aftereffects of general anesthesia, handling of the bowel during surgery, and loss of muscle tone in the bowel while empty.*
- Teach the woman to recognize signs of complications that should be reported to the physician or nurse:
  a. Temperature greater than 100°F (37.7°C)
  b. Vaginal bleeding that is greater than a typical menstrual period or is bright red
  c. Urinary incontinence, urgency, burning, or frequency
  d. Severe pain.
- Encourage the woman to express feelings that may signal a negative self-concept. Correct any misconceptions. *Some women believe that hysterectomy means weight gain, the end of sexual activity, and the growth of facial hair.*
- Provide information on risks and benefits of hormone replacement therapy, if indicated. *If the ovaries have also been removed, the woman is immediately thrust into menopause and may want or need hormone replacement therapy.*
- Reinforce the need to obtain gynecologic examinations regularly even after hysterectomy.

- Evaluate coping strategies and psychosocial support systems. Teach coping strategies if indicated. *The possibility of surgery or cancer represents a crisis for the woman and her support system. Support groups can provide assistance for the woman through crisis intervention.*

Sexual Dysfunction

The woman with DUB may be unwilling to express herself sexually, particularly if bleeding is frequent or heavy. Additionally, fatigue may prevent her from participating in sexual activity.

- Offer information about engaging in sexual activity during menstruation. Explain that conception is possible during this time and that orgasm may help relieve symptoms. *Some women mistakenly believe that birth control measures are unnecessary during menstruation. Orgasm causes a release of tension and vascular congestion and frequently provides at least temporary relief of symptoms.*
- Provide an opportunity for the expression of concerns related to alterations in lifestyle and sexual functioning. *Some women have had a prolonged period of sexual abstinence related to DUB. Allowing women to verbalize concerns can assist them in working collaboratively with the healthcare provider to minimize the impact of illness and optimize function.*
- Encourage frequent rest periods. *This conserves energy and may allow sexual activities to resume.*

- Provide information about alternative methods of sexual expression. *Methods of sexual expression other than vaginal intercourse may satisfy the needs of both partners.*

> **PRACTICE ALERT**
> If the nurse is not comfortable with frank discussions about sexual activities, referral is indicated.

Community-Based Care

Provide support, appropriate reassurance, and information to help the woman and her family better understand her disorder and the therapeutic interventions indicated. Teaching also includes self-care measures that help minimize the effects of DUB on the daily functioning of the woman. The following topics should be included:

- Administration and side effects of prescribed medications, including iron
- The need to maintain a balanced diet, increasing iron-rich foods such as eggs, beans, liver, beef, and shrimp (Inform the woman that while orange juice may improve the absorption of iron, foods high in calcium and oxalic acid, such as spinach, may reduce its absorption.)
- Importance of maintaining a fluid intake of 2000 to 3000 mL a day
- The need to immediately report recurring episodes of DUB, particularly in postmenopausal women, to the healthcare provider.

STRUCTURAL DISORDERS

Structural disorders of the female reproductive system include displacement disorders and fistulas.

THE WOMAN WITH A UTERINE DISPLACEMENT

The uterus may be displaced within the pelvic cavity or may descend into the vaginal canal. Displacement of the uterus within the pelvic cavity is classified according to the direction of the displacement (Figure 51–2 ■):

- *Retroversion* of the uterus is a backward tilting of the uterus toward the rectum.
- *Retroflexion* involves a flexing or bending of the uterine corpus in a backward manner toward the rectum.
- *Anteversion* is an exaggerated forward tilting of the uterus.
- *Anteflexion* is a flexing or folding of the uterine corpus upon itself.

Prolapse of the uterus into the vaginal canal can vary from mild to complete prolapse outside of the body. First-degree, or mild, prolapse involves a descent of less than half the uterine corpus into the vagina. Second-degree, or marked, prolapse involves the descent of the entire uterus into the vaginal canal, so that the cervix is at the introitus to the vagina. Third-degree prolapse, or *procidentia*, is complete prolapse of the uterus outside the body, with inversion of the vaginal canal (Figure 51–3 ■). Prolapse of the uterus is often accompanied by *cystocele* (herniation of the bladder into the vagina) or *rectocele* (herniation of the rectum into the vagina).

Pathophysiology

Displacement or prolapse of the uterus, bladder, or rectum can be a congenital or an acquired condition. Congenital tilting or flexion of the uterus is rare. More commonly, tilting or flexion disorders in which the uterus remains within the pelvic cavity are related to the scarring and inflammation of pelvic inflammatory disease, endometriosis, pregnancy, and tumors.

Downward displacement of the pelvic organs into the vagina results from weakened pelvic musculature, usually attributable to stretching of the supporting ligaments and muscles during pregnancy and childbirth. Unrepaired lacerations from childbirth, rapid deliveries, multiple pregnancies, congenital weakness, or loss of elasticity and muscle tone with aging may contribute to these disorders.

Manifestations

The manifestations of displacement disorders are listed on page 1807.

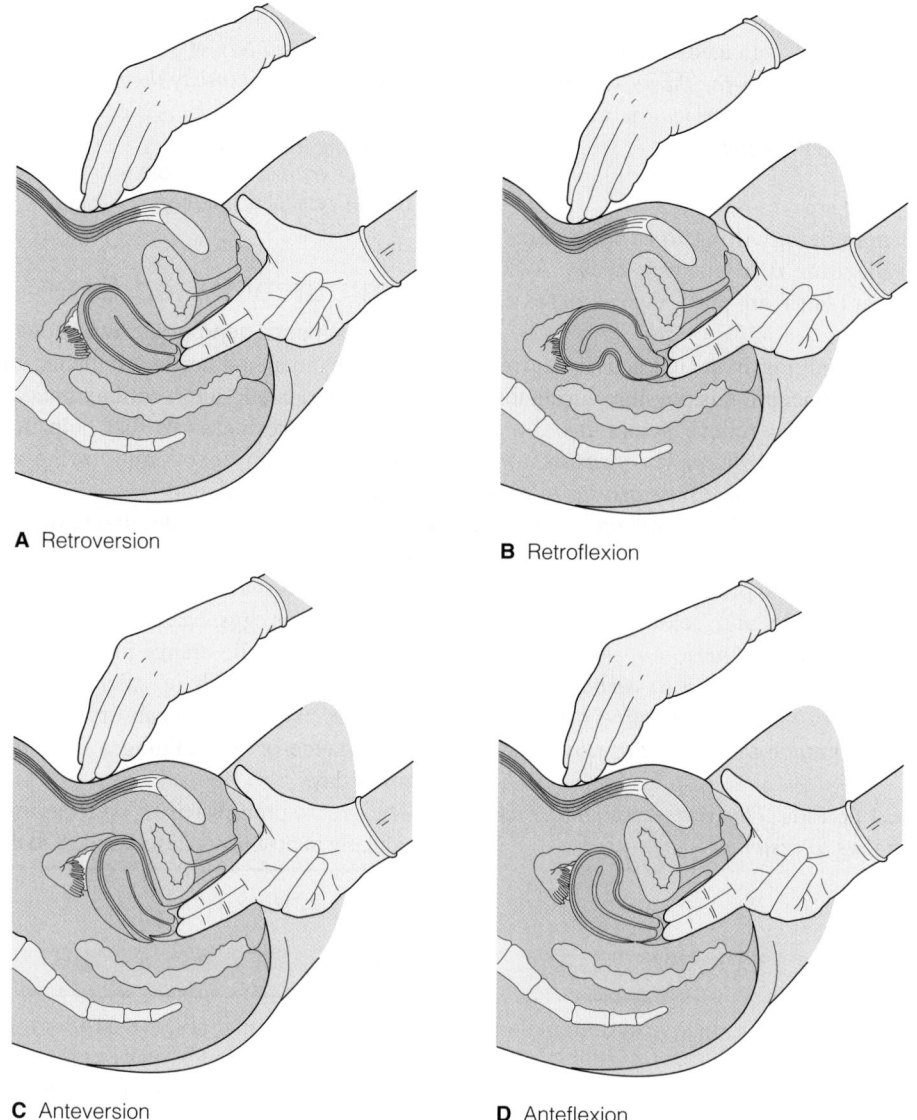

A Retroversion

B Retroflexion

C Anteversion

D Anteflexion

Figure 51–2 ■ Displacements of the uterus within the uterine cavity. *A,* Retroversion is a backward tilting. *B,* Retroflexion is a backward bending. *C,* Anteversion is a forward tilting. *D,* Anteflexion is a forward bending.

INTERDISCIPLINARY CARE

Interdisciplinary care focuses on identifying the cause of the structural disorder, correcting or minimizing the condition, relieving pain, preventing or treating infection, and supporting and educating the woman.

A careful history and physical examination are performed. Diagnosis of uterine displacement is made after physical examination. If herniation of the rectum or bladder is suspected, the woman is asked to bear down or cough during the examination so the prolapse can be palpated and any leakage of urine or feces visualized. A history of infections, multiple pregnancies in rapid succession, and rapid labors support this diagnosis.

Treatment may include Kegel exercises to strengthen weakened pelvic muscles. Kegel exercises can be useful in the early stages of downward displacement. These exercises are discussed in Chapter 28 .

Surgery

Several surgical procedures are used to repair structural disorders. For women presenting with a cystocele, anterior *colporrhaphy* (repair of the cystocele) is the most common procedure. The anterior repair shortens the pelvic muscles, providing tighter support for the bladder. The *Marshall-Marchetti-Krantz procedure* involves resuspension of the urinary bladder in correct anatomic position. A rectocele is repaired with a posterior colporrhaphy, which shortens the pelvic muscles, providing a tighter support for the rectum.

A prolapsed uterus may be surgically repositioned and the supporting muscles shortened to provide greater support. In postmenopausal women or women with procidentia, hysterectomy is the preferred treatment.

Pessary

When surgery is contraindicated, a *pessary* (a removable device) may be inserted into the vagina to provide temporary sup-

Figure 51–3 ■ Prolapse of the uterus can vary from mild to complete. In third-degree uterine prolapse, or procidentia, the uterus prolapses completely outside the body, with inversion of the vagina.

Source: M. English/Custom Medical Stock Photo.

port for the uterus or bladder. At regular intervals, the pessary is removed, cleaned, and reinserted.

NURSING CARE

Nursing care focuses on education about the disorder, proposed treatments, and self-care measures for relief of symptoms.

Nursing Diagnoses and Interventions

Nursing interventions for the woman with a displacement disorder address problems with urinary incontinence and anxiety.

Stress Incontinence

Relaxation of the pelvic floor can lead to stress incontinence. This can prove both troublesome and embarrassing and can increase the incidence of urinary tract infection.

MANIFESTATIONS of Displacement Disorders

Uterine Displacement within the Pelvic Cavity
- Dysmenorrhea
- Dyspareunia
- Backache
- Infertility

Uterine Prolapse
- Backache
- Bearing-down sensation
- Constipation
- Urinary incontinence
- Hemorrhoids
- Dyspareunia

Cytocele/Rectocele
- Bearing-down sensation
- Constipation
- Fecal incontinence
- Hemorrhoids
- Urinary incontinence

- Teach Kegel exercises. *These exercises strengthen perineal muscle tone, minimize urinary leakage, and minimize descent of the bladder and rectum into the vagina. In postmenopausal women, estrogen supplements also can improve muscle tone in the perineal area.*
- Suggest the use of perineal pads (ranging from thin panty liners to full-thickness incontinence pads) or special underwear (such as Depends) to absorb urine leakage. *Using pads or undergarments often allows the woman to once again take part in her usual social activities.*
- Explain perineal care and proper use of perineal pads. *Cleansing the perineum from front to back, and applying and removing perineal pads the same way, minimizes cross infection from the anus to the vaginal and urethral openings. Incontinence pads need to be changed frequently to minimize surface bacterial counts.*
- Suggest reducing or eliminating caffeine intake. *Reducing caffeine intake can reduce urinary frequency and urgency.*
- Stress the importance of cleaning the perineal area. *Urine is very irritating to the skin.*

Anxiety

Anxiety is common among women with a displacement disorder. Many women have only a cursory understanding of their reproductive anatomy. This lack of knowledge often compounds the anxiety. The nurse can use drawings and models to explain structural disorders and treatment options available.

- Encourage questions from the woman and her partner. *This helps assess the level of understanding so that teaching can be more effective.*
- Explain that the relief from discomfort and fatigue may positively influence sexual expression, and reassure the woman that the capacity for orgasm will not be affected. *Many women and their partners have major concerns about the effects of the disorder and its treatment on their sex life and capacity for sexual pleasure.*
- Explore coping mechanisms that have been previously successful. *This can help relieve anxiety and boost self-esteem.*

Community-Based Care

If surgery is the treatment of choice, teaching centers on what to expect in the preoperative and postoperative periods. If medical treatment is used initially, teaching focuses on measures to relieve the manifestations, such as Kegel exercises, use of incontinence pads, or the use, care, and insertion of a pessary.

Because obesity is a risk factor associated with relaxation of the pelvic and abdominal muscles, dietary counseling may be indicated. Preoperatively, a diet high in fiber may alleviate constipation, a particular concern during the postoperative period.

THE WOMAN WITH A VAGINAL FISTULA

A fistula is an abnormal opening or passage between two organs or spaces that are normally separated or an abnormal passage to the outside of the body. Vaginal fistulas may be vesicovaginal or rectovaginal. A *vesicovaginal fistula* is an abnormal opening between the urinary bladder and the vagina, leading to incontinent leakage of urine through the vagina. A *rectovaginal fistula* (less common) is an abnormal opening between the rectum and vagina, causing incontinent leakage of stool or flatus through the vagina.

Fistulas between the bladder and the vagina (vesicovaginal) or between the rectum and the vagina (rectovaginal) may develop as a complication of childbirth, gynecologic or urologic surgery, or radiation therapy for gynecologic cancer. Cancer of the bladder is sometimes involved. The woman with a vaginal fistula often presents with a complaint of involuntary leakage of urine or flatus and symptoms of infection.

Interdisciplinary Care

Fistulas are diagnosed by pelvic examination. Diagnosis of a vesicovaginal fistula can be made by instilling dye into the urinary bladder through a catheter and observing the vagina for leakage. If no leakage is detected, a tampon or vaginal pack is inserted into the vagina, and the woman is asked to ambulate. If an abnormal opening is present, the tampon will absorb the dye. Dye may also be injected intravenously because it is ex-

creted by the kidneys. Urine and vaginal cultures may be performed to rule out infections. Antibiotics are administered if infection is present.

A small vaginal fistula may resolve spontaneously. Otherwise, surgery is performed after inflammation has subsided, often a period of several months. Rarely, in the presence of a large, highly inflamed rectovaginal fistula, a temporary colostomy is performed, allowing inflammation and irritation to subside (see Chapter 26 ∞).

Nursing Care

Nursing care for the woman with repair of a vaginal fistula is similar to that for the woman with a displacement disorder. Teaching is an important component of nursing care. Stress the importance of careful perineal cleansing to reduce irritation and prevent further tissue breakdown. Suggest perineal irrigation or sitz baths for cleansing. Perineal pads or special underwear may be used to absorb urine or fecal drainage. For the woman with a rectovaginal fistula, provide information about avoiding gas-forming foods to minimize embarrassment from odor.

DISORDERS OF FEMALE REPRODUCTIVE TISSUE

Both benign and malignant tissue disorders affect the female reproductive system. Benign tumors and cysts include Bartholin's gland cysts, cervical polyps, endometrial cysts and polyps, ovarian cysts, and uterine leiomyomas (fibroids). Endometriosis is a condition in which endometrial tissue implants outside the uterus in various locations in the pelvic cavity. Malignant tumors of reproductive tissue include cervical cancer, endometrial cancer, ovarian cancer, and vulvar cancer.

THE WOMAN WITH CYSTS OR POLYPS

A *cyst* is a fluid-filled sac. A *polyp* is a highly vascular solid tumor attached by a pedicle or stem. Cysts or polyps of the female reproductive system can occur in the vulva, cervix, endometrium, or ovaries.

Pathophysiology

Following are different types of female reproductive tissue cysts and polyps:
- *Bartholin's gland cysts* are the most common cystic disorder of the vulva. These cysts are caused by the infection or obstruction of Bartholin's gland.
- *Cervical polyps* are the most common benign cervical lesion in women of reproductive age. These polyps tend to occur in women over age 40 who have borne several children and have a history of using oral contraceptives. It is possible that cervical polyps develop from endocervical hyperplasia. The polyp develops at the vaginal end of the cervix, has a stem, and is highly vascular.
- *Endometrial cysts and polyps* are caused by endometrial overgrowth and are often filled with old blood (the dark color leads to the label "chocolate cysts"). Endometrial cysts are the result of endometrial implants on the ovary and are asso-

ciated with endometriosis. Endometrial polyps, in contrast, are intrauterine overgrowths, similar to cervical polyps, and usually have a stalk.
- *Ovarian cysts* are classified as follicular cysts and corpus luteum cysts. Follicular cysts develop as a result of failure of the mature follicle to rupture or failure of an immature follicle to reabsorb fluid after ovulation. Corpus luteum cysts develop as a result of increased hormone secretion by the corpus luteum after ovulation. Most functional cysts regress spontaneously within two or three menstrual cycles.
- *Polycystic ovarian syndrome* (POS, also known as *Stein-Leventhal syndrome*) is an endocrine disorder characterized by an excess of androgens and a long-term lack of ovulation. The exact cause is unknown. As a part of the disease, as many as 8 to 10 cysts form in the ovaries from a failure to release ovum. Manifestations include amenorrhea or irregular menses, hirsutism, obesity, acne, hypertension, sleep apnea, and infertility. Women with POS often have insulin resistance and are at increased risk for early-onset type 2 diabetes, as well as heart disease, breast cancer, and endometrial cancer.

Manifestations and Complications

The causes and manifestations of benign cysts and polyps of the female reproductive system are presented in Table 51–1. Complications associated with these disorders include infection, rupture, infertility, hemorrhage, and recurrence.

INTERDISCIPLINARY CARE

Care focuses on identifying and correcting the disorder and preventing its recurrence. A careful history and physical examination are performed, including inspection and visualization.

TABLE 51–1 Benign Cysts and Polyps of the Female Reproductive System

SITE	TYPE	ETIOLOGIC ORIGIN	MANIFESTATIONS
Ovary	Functional cysts	Ovulation—include follicular cysts and corpus luteum cysts	May resolve spontaneously; can cause pain, menstrual irregularity, or amenorrhea
	Polycystic ovarian syndrome	Unknown; possible hypothalamic-pituitary dysfunction	Hirsutism, obesity; amenorrhea or irregular menses; hyperinsulinemia; infertility
Vulva	Bartholin cysts	Obstruction or infection of Bartholin's gland	Pain, redness, perineal mass, dyspareunia
Endometrium	Chocolate cysts	Endometrial overgrowth; filled with old blood	
	Endometrial polyps	Unknown	Bleeding between periods
Cervix	Cervical polyps	Unknown	Bleeding after intercourse or between periods

Examination of the reproductive tract reveals the presence of most cysts and polyps. The menstrual history may reveal menstrual irregularities.

Diagnosis

Diagnostic tests that may be used to diagnose cysts and polyps of the female reproductive system include a laparoscopy to visualize ovarian cysts, an ultrasound or x-ray to differentiate cysts from solid tumors, and a pregnancy test when luteal cysts are suspected. Laboratory analysis will demonstrate elevated LH and testosterone levels, as well as a reverse in FSH/LH in the woman with polycystic ovary syndrome (POS).

Medications

Antibiotics are used to treat infection or abscess, and oral contraceptives are used to promote regression of functional ovarian cysts. Clomiphene (Clomid, Serophene) may be prescribed to stimulate ovulation in the woman with POS who wishes to become pregnant. Dexamethasone (Decadron) suppresses ACTH and adrenal androgens, and may be added to increase the likelihood of ovulation.

Surgery

Cervical polyps are visible through a vaginal speculum and usually are removed with a clamp, using a twisting motion. To remove endometrial cysts or polyps, a transcervical approach is used. The specimen is sent to the laboratory for evaluation, and chemical or electrical cauterization is applied after cyst removal. For Bartholin's gland cysts and any abscesses, the lesion is incised and drained, and a drainage device is left in place. Follicular cysts may be punctured through laser surgery, or a wedge resection of the ovary may be performed to restore ovulation. Rarely, *oophorectomy* (removal of the ovary) is performed if the cysts are very large.

NURSING CARE

Nursing care focuses on relieving pain and preventing recurrence and complications. Address the following topics for self-care at home:

- The condition, its treatment, and measures to relieve pain
- The importance of keeping follow-up appointments
- Manifestations of infection (for postsurgical care) and the need to notify the physician should they occur

- If cervical polypectomy is performed, advise use of external pads for 1 week. The woman must be able to state the signs of excessive bleeding and recognize that saturating more than one pad in an hour indicates the need for immediate follow-up.
- The importance of long-term follow-up care for the woman with POS.

THE WOMAN WITH LEIOMYOMA

Leiomyomas *(fibroid tumors)* are benign tumors that originate from smooth muscle of the uterus. They are the most common form of pelvic tumor, believed to occur in 1 of every 4 or 5 women older than 35 years of age (Porth, 2005). Fibroids are seen more often and grow more rapidly in African American women.

Pathophysiology

The actual cause of fibroid tumors is not clearly understood, but there is a strong association with estrogen stimulation. Fibroid tumors usually develop in the uterine corpus, and may be intramural, subserous, or submucous (Figure 51–4 ■):

- *Intramural fibroid tumors* (the most common type) are embedded in the myometrium. They usually present as an enlargement of the uterus.
- *Subserous fibroid tumors* lie beneath the serous lining of the uterus and project into the peritoneal cavity. They may become pedunculated (on a stem) and displace or compress other tissues, such as the ureter or bladder.
- *Submucous fibroid tumors* lie beneath the endometrial lining of the uterus. They displace endometrial tissue and are more likely to cause bleeding, infection, and necrosis than the other types.

Manifestations

Small tumors may be asymptomatic. The rate of growth varies, but they may increase in size during pregnancy or with use of oral contraceptives or HRT. Large fibroid tumors can crowd other organs, leading to pelvic pressure, pain, dysmenorrhea, menorrhagia, and fatigue. Depending on the location of the tumor, constipation and urinary urgency and frequency may occur. Most fibroid tumors shrink with menopause.

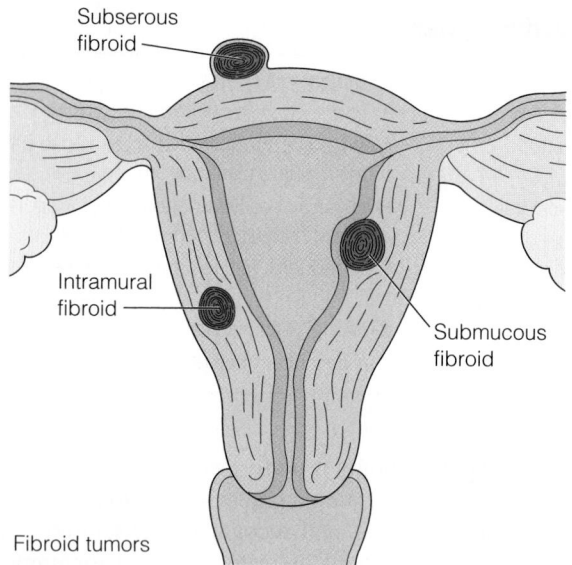

Figure 51–4 ■ Types of uterine fibroid tumors (leiomyomas). Intramural fibroid tumors lie within the uterine wall. Subserous fibroid tumors lie beneath the serous lining of the uterus and project into the peritoneum. Submucous fibroid tumors lie beneath the endometrial lining of the uterus.

INTERDISCIPLINARY CARE

Treatment of the woman with uterine fibroids depends on the size and location of the tumors, the severity of the manifestations, and her age and childbearing status. Tests used to diagnose uterine fibroids may include an ultrasound to differentiate leiomyoma from endometriosis and a laparoscopy to visualize subserosal leiomyomas.

In asymptomatic women who wish to bear children, the fibroid tumors are monitored. Follow-up is recommended two to three times per year to monitor growth.

Medications

Leuprolide acetate (Lupron) is used to decrease the size of the tumor if surgery is contraindicated or not desired. Gonadotropin-releasing hormone (GnRH) agonists are also administered.

Surgery

Myomectomy, removal of the tumor without removing the entire uterus, is the surgical procedure of choice for young women who wish to retain reproductive capability. Laparoscopic laser technique is used for many women. A hysterectomy is performed if tumors are large, and if bleeding or other problems continue in perimenopausal women. A hysterectomy usually requires a hospital stay of 3 to 4 days, and a 6-week recovery time. A nonsurgical method of treatment is a *uterine fibroid embolization.* In this procedure, a catheter is guided through the femoral artery to the uterus, where tiny particles are injected into the artery supplying the fibroid to cut off the fibroid's blood supply. This procedure requires only an overnight hospital stay with a return to normal activities in 1 week.

NURSING CARE

If surgery is deferred, teaching emphasizes the importance of regular follow-up assessments to monitor tumor growth. If a hysterectomy is performed, teaching emphasizes appropriate preoperative and postoperative care. Dietary modifications to increase iron intake, prevent constipation, and promote healing are important.

THE WOMAN WITH ENDOMETRIOSIS

Endometriosis is a condition in which multiple, small, usually benign implantations of endometrial tissue develop most commonly in the pelvic cavity, but may also be found in other areas of the body, such as the lungs. Endometriosis affects from 10% to 15% of women of childbearing age and is more common in women who postpone childbearing. Risk factors for endometriosis include early menarche, regular periods with a cycle of less than 27 days, menses lasting more than 7 days, heavier flow, increased menstrual pain, and a history of the condition in first-degree female relatives (Porth, 2005).

Pathophysiology

The cause of endometriosis is unclear, but several theories have been proposed. The metaplasia theory asserts that endometrial tissue develops from embryonic epithelial cells as a result of hormonal or inflammatory changes. The theory of retrograde menstruation suggests that menstrual tissue backs up through the fallopian tubes during menses, implants on various pelvic structures, and survives. The transplantation theory asserts that endometrial implants spread via lymphatic or vascular routes.

The abnormally located endometrial tissue responds to cyclic ovarian hormone stimulation, and bleeding at the time of menstruation occurs at the sites of implantation. Scarring, inflammation, and adhesions may develop. Endometriosis is a slowly progressive disease, responsive to ovarian hormone stimulation. Thus, the implants regress during pregnancy and atrophy at menopause unless the woman is receiving HRT. Because progressive scarring may interfere with the ability to conceive, women with significant endometriosis are encouraged to have children early if they wish to do so.

Manifestations

Manifestations of endometriosis, which usually occur during the luteal phase of the menstrual cycle, are summarized on the next page.

INTERDISCIPLINARY CARE

Endometriosis may be difficult to diagnose, but a history of dysmenorrhea, dyspareunia, and infertility strongly suggests this diagnosis. Interventions depend on the severity of symptoms, the extent of the disease, and the woman's age and desire for childbearing. Treatment goals focus on pain management and restoring fertility.

Diagnosis

Diagnostic tests are ordered to rule out other medical conditions and identify the endometrial implants. The tests include a pelvic ultrasound and laparoscopy (see Chapter 49) as

MANIFESTATIONS of Endometriosis

- Heavy, throbbing pain of the lower abdomen and pelvis, radiating down the thighs and around the back (The degree of pain, however, is not indicative of the severity of the disease.)
- Feeling of rectal pressure and discomfort when having a bowel movement
- Dyspareunia
- Dysfunctional uterine bleeding
- Infertility

well as a CBC with differential to rule out pelvic abscesses and infectious processes. A low hemoglobin and hematocrit may be noted if menorrhagia accompanies endometriosis or tissue implants bleed significantly during the menses.

Medications

Medications include analgesics to control pain and prostaglandin synthesis inhibitors such as NSAIDs. Hormone therapy may include oral contraceptives or progesterone to induce pseudopregnancy, or danazol (Danocrine) to induce amenorrhea and involution of endometrial tissue. Prolonged use of danazol, however, may result in masculinizing effects. GnRH is used to elevate levels of estrogen and progesterone and minimize bleeding.

Surgery

Surgical interventions include laparoscopy with laser ablation (excision or removal) of endometrial implants. Refractory endometriosis may be treated with total hysterectomy.

NURSING CARE

Nursing care includes providing pain relief, providing education about the condition and the treatment options, and helping the woman cope with treatment outcomes. The severity of the disease and its manifestations are not necessarily related. Advanced disease may exhibit few manifestations, whereas early disease may be quite painful. A Nursing Care Plan for a woman with endometriosis is found below.

NURSING CARE PLAN A Woman with Endometriosis

Angela Hall is a 31-year-old married accountant, who relates a history of severe dysmenorrhea and menorrhagia, a feeling of pelvic heaviness and pain that radiates down her thighs. Because of her discomfort, her husband has complained about the quality of their sex life and has expressed concerns about their plans for having children. Mrs. Hall reports being so tired she doesn't care whether she has sex or not, and, in fact, would really prefer not to: "Sex hurts so much, I just can't stand it." Endometriosis is suspected, and a diagnostic laparoscopy has been scheduled.

ASSESSMENT

Christine Brigham, RN, NP, interviews Mrs. Hall and makes the following assessments: BP 110/70, P 68, R 18, T 98.2°F (36.7°C). Mrs. Hall's weight is 130 lb (59 kg) and within normal limits for her height. Review of laboratory findings indicate a hemoglobin level of 9.8 g/dL (normal range: 12 to 16 g/dL) and a hematocrit of 33.1% (normal range: 35% to 45%). Physical examination reveals pelvic tenderness on manipulation of the cervix, and small masses that are palpable on abdominal/pelvic examination.

DIAGNOSES

- *Chronic Pain* related to endometrial pelvic implants
- *Anxiety* related to effect of endometriosis on fertility
- *Deficient Knowledge* related to diagnosis and treatment options
- *Ineffective Sexuality Pattern* related to the manifestations of endometriosis

EXPECTED OUTCOMES

- Develop effective self-care measures to deal with the pain and discomfort.
- Verbalize decreased anxiety.
- Demonstrate understanding of the disease and treatment options.
- Verbalize an improvement in sexual functioning and a decrease in interpersonal stress between herself and her husband.

PLANNING AND IMPLEMENTATION

- Identify the location, type, duration, and history of the pain.
- Recommend analgesics and heat therapy.
- Provide information on biofeedback, relaxation, and imagery to lessen pain.
- Discuss with Mr. and Mrs. Hall the causes of endometriosis and its manifestations.
- Encourage the Halls to discuss their feelings about the effect of the disease on their sex life, lifestyle, and fertility.
- Refer the couple to the local mental health center if appropriate.

EVALUATION

Two years after the initiation of treatment, Mr. and Mrs. Hall have become parents of a baby girl. Mrs. Hall states that the discomfort and other manifestations of endometriosis have eased. Relaxation and imagery have effectively minimized her pain and brought about improvement in her function as wife, mother, and sexual partner. Counseling has improved the interpersonal and sexual relations between the Halls. Dietary management has improved her anemia, although the menorrhagia persists. The Halls are trying to have a second child, understanding the advantages of rapid succession of pregnancies. They will be followed in the nursing clinic and referred to an infertility clinic if conception does not occur within 1 year.

CRITICAL THINKING IN THE NURSING PROCESS

1. Explain the pathophysiologic basis for Mrs. Hall's anemia.
2. How would you handle the situation if Mr. and Mrs. Hall were extremely uncomfortable and embarrassed about discussing their sexual problems?
3. Develop a plan of care for Mrs. Hall for the nursing diagnosis *Situational Low Self-Esteem* related to the manifestations of endometriosis.

See Evaluating Your Response in Appendix C.

Nursing Diagnoses and Interventions

Interventions for pain, discussed previously, are also appropriate for the woman with endometriosis. A priority diagnosis for the young woman with this disorder is anxiety related to the risk for loss of reproductive function.

Anxiety

Anxiety about the unsure prognosis related to infertility is a particular problem for young women who plan to have a family in the future.

- Encourage expression of fears and anxiety about infertility, and answer questions honestly. *Knowledge helps relieve anxiety and fear.*
- Provide information on fertility awareness methods, including measurement of basal body temperature and other techniques for recognizing ovulation. *Understanding these techniques helps the woman and her partner optimize the conditions for conception.*

Using NANDA, NIC, and NOC

Chart 51–1 shows links between NANDA nursing diagnoses, NIC, and NOC when caring for the client with endometriosis.

Community-Based Care

Explain the cause of the disorder and the various treatment options, including their side effects. Discuss fertility awareness methods and the risks and benefits of long-term use of oral contraceptives. Stress the importance of exercise, smoking cessation, and weight control. If surgical treatment is chosen, provide preoperative and postoperative teaching.

NANDA, NIC, and NOC Linkages
CHART 51–1 The Woman with Endometriosis

NANDA

Deficient Knowledge

↓

NIC

Teaching: Disease Process

Teaching: Sexuality

Preconception Counseling

↓

NOC

Knowledge: Disease Process

Data from *NANDA's Nursing Diagnoses: Definitions & Classification 2005–2006* by NANDA International (2003), Philadelphia; *Nursing Interventions Classification (NIC)* (4th ed.) by J. M. Dochterman & G. M. Bulecheck (2004), St. Louis, MO: Mosby; and *Nursing Outcomes Classification (NOC)* (3rd ed.) by S. Moorhead, M. Johnson, and M. Maas (2004), St. Louis, MO: Mosby.

THE WOMAN WITH CERVICAL CANCER

Cancer of the cervix is the second most common cancer in women worldwide, and the 14th most common in women in the United States (the lower number is primarily the result of screening with Pap tests). The incidence is greater in black women than in white women.

FAST FACTS
Cervical Cancer
- The American Cancer Society (ACS, 2006d) estimates that there will be more than 10,000 new cases of cervical cancer each year, resulting in nearly 4000 deaths annually.
- Nearly 100% of women with cervical cancer have evidence of cervical infection with human papillomavirus (HPV) (see Chapter 52 ∞).
- The FDA recently approved HPV testing as an adjunct to cervical cancer screening.

Effective screening with the Pap smear test and treatment have reduced the death rate by 55% during the last 30 years, although the death rates for blacks continues to be more than two times that of whites (ACS, 2006c). The age of diagnosis is usually between 50 and 55 years; however, cervical cancer begins to appear in women in their 20s.

Risk Factors

Risk factors for cervical cancer include infection of the external genitalia and anus with HPV, first intercourse before 16 years of age, multiple sex partners or male partners with multiple sex partners, a history of sexually transmitted infections, and infection with HIV. The most important risk factor is infection with HPV. Other risk factors include smoking and poor nutritional status, family history of cervical cancer, and exposure to diethylstilbestrol (DES) *in utero*.

Pathophysiology

Most cervical cancers (90%) are squamous cell carcinomas that begin as neoplasia in the cervical epithelium. *Precancerous dysplasia (cervical intraepithelial neoplasia [CIN], cervical carcinoma in situ)* is estimated to occur in one of eight women before the age of 20 and is often associated with HPV infection. Studies have also found a strong association with reproductive infections with *Chlamydia trachomatis*. (These infections are discussed in Chapter 52 ∞ .) The precursor lesions may spontaneously regress (60%), persist (30%), or progress and undergo malignant change (10%). Only about 1% become invasive (Porth, 2005). Systems of grading of dysplastic changes in the cervix use the term *cervical intraepithelial neoplasia (CIN)* or the Bethesda system (Table 51–2). Carcinoma *in situ* is localized; invasive cancer spreads to deeper layers.

Cancer *in situ* most often develops in the transformation zone where the columnar epithelium of the cervical lining meets the squamous epithelium of the outer cervix and vagina. Squamous cell cancers spread by direct invasion of accessory structures, including the vaginal wall, pelvic wall, bladder, and rectum. Although metastasis is most frequently confined to the

TABLE 51–2 Classification Systems for Pap Smears

DYSPLASIA/NEOPLASIA	CIN (CERVICAL INTRAEPITHELIAL NEOPLASIA)	BETHESDA SYSTEM	NUMERICAL
Benign	Benign	■ Normal	1
Benign with inflammation	Benign with inflammation	■ Normal	2
		■ Atypical squamous cells of undetermined significance (ASC-US)	
Moderate dysplasia	CIN I	■ Low-grade squamous intraepithelial lesion (SIL)	3
Severe dysplasia	CIN II	■ High-grade SIL	3
Carcinoma *in situ*	CIN III	■ High-grade SIL	4
Invasive cancer	Invasive cancer	■ Invasive cancer	5

pelvic area, distant metastasis may occur through the lymphatic system.

Manifestations

Preinvasive cancer is limited to the cervix and rarely causes manifestations. Invasive cancer causes vaginal bleeding after intercourse or between menstrual periods, and a vaginal discharge that increases as the cancer progresses. These changes are subtle, and may be more readily noticed by the postmenopausal woman. Manifestations of advanced disease include referred pain in the back or thighs, hematuria, bloody stools, anemia, and weight loss.

INTERDISCIPLINARY CARE

The goals of treatment are to eradicate the cancer and minimize complications and metastasis. The type of treatment depends on the degree of malignant change, the size and location of the lesion, and the extent of metastasis.

Diagnosis

Diagnostic tests used to diagnose cervical cancer include a Pap smear, colposcopy, and cervical biopsy (see Chapter 49 ∞ for further information about these procedures). A loop diathermy technique (loop electrosurgical excision procedure [LEEP]) allows simultaneous diagnosis and treatment of dysplastic lesions found on colposcopy. This procedure is performed in the health provider's office, using a wire for both cutting and coagulation during excision of the dysplastic region of the cervix. An MRI or CT of the pelvis, abdomen, or bones may be performed to evaluate the spread of the tumor.

Medications

Chemotherapy is used for tumors not responsive to other therapy, tumors that cannot be removed, or as adjunct therapy if metastasis has occurred (see Chapter 14 ∞).

Surgery

When combined with colposcopy, laser surgery is a viable treatment method provided that the cancer is limited to the cervical epithelium. Cryosurgery, which involves the use of a probe to freeze tissue, causing necrosis and sloughing, is also used for noninvasive lesions. Conization (Figure 51–5 ■) is performed to treat microinvasive carcinoma when colposcopy cannot define the limits of the invasion. For invasive lesions, hysterectomy or radical hysterectomy (removal of the uterus, fallopian tubes, lymph nodes, and ovaries) is performed.

A *pelvic exenteration*, the removal of all pelvic contents, including the bowel, vagina, and bladder, is performed if the cancer recurs without involvement of the lymphatic system. An anterior exenteration is the removal of the uterus, ovaries, fallopian tubes, vagina, bladder, urethra, and lymphatic vessels and nodes. An ileal conduit is created for excretion of urine (see Chapter 29 ∞). A posterior exenteration is the removal of the uterus, ovaries, fallopian tubes, bowel, and rectum. A colostomy is created for excretion of feces (see Chapter 26 ∞).

Radiation Therapy

Radiation therapy is used to treat invasive cervical cancer. External radiation beam therapy and intracavity cesium irradiation can be used. Radiation is discussed in Chapter 14 ∞ .

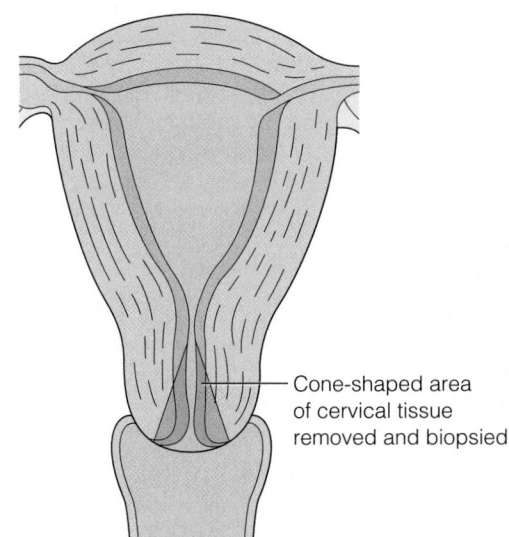

Cone-shaped area of cervical tissue removed and biopsied

Figure 51–5 ■ Conization, the surgical removal of a cone-shaped section of the cervix, is used to treat microinvasive carcinoma of the cervix.

NURSING CARE

Nursing care involves helping the woman deal with the physical and psychologic effects of a potentially life-threatening illness, providing information needed to make informed decisions, and minimizing the adverse effects of therapy. Pain relief measures are important, as is grief work on the part of the woman and family. The woman should be encouraged to perform self-care activities and resume normal everyday activities and sexual functioning to the extent possible. A Nursing Care Plan for a woman with cervical cancer is found below.

Health Promotion

The ACS (2006c) recommends that women should begin annual screening for cervical cancer with the Pap test about 3 years after a woman begins having vaginal intercourse, but no later than 21 years of age. Screening should be done every year with regular Pap tests or every 2 years using liquid-based tests. At or after the age of 30, after three consecutive normal Pap tests, screening can be performed every 2 to 3 years, at the discretion of the healthcare provider. Alternately, cervical cancer screening with HPV DNA tests and Pap tests may be performed every 3 years. Women 70 years of age and older who have had three or more normal Pap smears in the last 10 years may choose to stop cervical cancer screening. Screening for women who have had a total hysterectomy (including the cervix) is not recommended unless the surgery was done as a treatment for cancer. Women who have a hysterectomy without removal of the cervix should continue to follow ACS guidelines (ACS, 2006c).

It is vital that nurses educate women of all ages about controlling risk factors for cervical cancer and about the importance of screening for this cancer throughout the life span. Teach young women about the relationship between early sexual activity, multiple partners, and risk for STIs and cervical cancer. Discuss safer

---

NURSING CARE PLAN A Woman with Cervical Cancer

Anna Eliza Gillam is a 45-year-old divorced mother of four children ranging in age from 16 to 23. She was married at age 18 and had several sexual partners prior to her marriage. She has had three sexual partners since her marriage ended. Last year she was treated with cryosurgery for venereal warts. The Pap smear taken 2 weeks ago showed atypical cells, and she has come in for a repeat test.

ASSESSMENT

Judy Davis, RN, FNP, the admitting nurse, interviews Ms. Gillam and records the following assessment findings: BP 130/80, P 72, R 18, T 99.2°F (37.3°C). Ms. Gillam weighs 142 lb (64.5 kg). Examination of the cervix reveals a large necrotic lesion at the 7 o'clock position. She has reduced her smoking to less than 10 cigarettes per day, and she does not drink alcohol.

Ms. Gillam is extremely fearful and anxious and has told no one about her abnormal Pap smear. She reveals that she has had back pain radiating down her thighs for several months and a foul vaginal discharge that increases after intercourse. Until 2 weeks ago, she had not had a Pap smear for 5 years. Ms. Davis performs the repeat Pap smear, which is positive for squamous cell carcinoma of the cervix. A CT scan and lymphangiography are scheduled. Laparoscopy shows the disease to be widespread in the pelvic cavity.

DIAGNOSES

- *Decisional Conflict* related to treatment options
- *Chronic and Acute Pain* related to metastasis and surgery
- *Risk for Impaired Skin Integrity* related to radiation
- *Fear* related to diagnosis of cervical cancer
- *Anticipatory Grieving* related to potential loss of life

EXPECTED OUTCOMES

- Gain knowledge to make informed decisions about treatment options.
- Develop strategies for pain control.
- Maintain skin and tissue integrity during radiation treatment.
- Express her feelings about the fear of cancer and death.

- Develop effective coping strategies for dealing with life-threatening illness and pain.

PLANNING AND IMPLEMENTATION

- Discuss treatment alternatives, including the prognosis with each option.
- Administer pain medications as prescribed.
- Inspect skin surfaces daily before and after radiation therapy.
- Provide information on biofeedback training and relaxation techniques for control of moderate pain.
- Refer to a local cancer support group so that she can interact with cancer survivors.
- Refer Ms. Gillam to a social worker in preparation for her altered level of functioning.

EVALUATION

Ms. Gillam has begun radiation therapy following pelvic exenteration. She controls her pain with relaxation and imagery techniques, requiring only occasional analgesics. She uses a water-based lotion to soothe the skin surface and is careful not to remove the skin markings. She seems optimistic and has quit smoking. She and her family have continued to attend the cancer support group meetings. Ms. Gillam is planning for the future and has talked with her family about what it means to live with cancer.

CRITICAL THINKING IN THE NURSING PROCESS

1. Compare and contrast your teaching plan for health promotion interventions to decrease the risks of cervical cancer for a young woman of 17 and an older woman of 70. Would they differ and, if so, how?
2. Develop a teaching plan to help Ms. Gillam cope with the effects of radiation.
3. During a home visit, Ms. Gillam tells the nurse that she has been so tired since beginning radiation treatments that all she can do is sit in her chair. Design a plan of care for the nursing diagnosis *Fatigue*.

See Evaluating Your Response in Appendix C.

sex alternatives and using condoms for protection. Emphasize the importance of continued screening exams for the older woman who may not see a gynecologic specialist on a regular basis. Encourage women under the age of 26 to receive Gardasil, the vaccine developed to prevent cervical cancer, precancerous genital lesions, and genital warts due to HPV types 6, 11, 16, and 18. Gardasil is given as three injections over a six-month period and does not protect against HPV in a woman already infected. For this reason, a federal advisory panel is recommending that the vaccine be routinely given to girls ages 11 and 12 (ACS, 2006d).

Assessment

Collect the following data through a health history and physical examination (see Chapter 49 ∞):

- *Health history:* History of STIs, sexual history, partner's sexual history, family history of cervical cancer, vaginal bleeding or discharge, smoking history, maternal treatment with DES.
- *Physical assessment:* Pelvic examination, abdomen, lymph glands.

Nursing Diagnoses and Interventions

This section discusses nursing interventions for the woman who has been diagnosed with cervical cancer and requires surgical and/or radiation treatment. Other nursing diagnoses and interventions that may be appropriate for the woman with cervical cancer are discussed in the sections discussing other female reproductive system cancers.

Fear

Many people believe that cancer equals death; however, this is no longer true in many cases, especially with early diagnosis. For cervical cancer that is diagnosed at an early stage, the 5-year survival rate is 92%. If the disease is *in situ*, the rate is nearly 100% (ACS, 2006a).

- Explain that 71% of all women with cervical cancer survive for 5 years or more and that the earlier the cancer is detected, the better the prognosis. *This gives the woman hope, an essential ingredient in recovery.*
- Allow adequate time for the woman and her partner to express their concerns and to ask questions. *Unexpressed feelings and fears and lack of understanding may cause the woman to view the situation as worse than it is.*
- Refer to cancer counselor or support groups for additional information. *Cancer survivors who visit clients in the hospital provide proof that people can survive the diagnosis and treatment of cancer and lead normal, productive lives.*

Impaired Tissue Integrity

Surgery interrupts the integrity of the skin surface, providing a potential portal of invasion for bacteria. Radiation therapy causes an inflammatory response in the skin and mucous membranes within the field of radiation, creating further risk of tissue reaction and breakdown.

- Teach wound and skin care, particularly if pelvic exenteration is performed. Irrigations with saline or solutions of saline and hydrogen peroxide are performed at intervals, with dry heat applied thereafter to dry the area. *Open and damaged tissue in-*

creases the risk for infection. Meticulous skin and wound care is necessary to prevent infection and further tissue destruction.

- If appropriate, teach stoma care, and care for the skin surrounding the stoma. (These procedures are discussed in Chapters 26 ∞ and 29 ∞.) *Urine and stool are irritating to the skin. Without proper care, the skin surrounding the stoma can become excoriated.*
- Apply non–oil-based lotions to skin surface. This may minimize itching and help maintain integrity. *Oil-based lotions are not recommended for tissue undergoing radiation.*
- Instruct the woman not to remove the markings used to localize the radiation beam to the target area. *Markings are used in future radiation treatments.*
- Monitor for evidence of fistula formation, and teach the woman to do the same. *Fistula formation is a potential complication of radiation to the pelvic or abdominal cavities. Vaginal fistulas may form between the vagina and the bladder or rectum. Fistulas may also develop between the bladder and rectum, resulting in the expulsion of stool in the urine or loss of urine through the anus.*

Using NANDA, NIC, and NOC

Chart 51–2 shows links between NANDA nursing diagnoses, NIC, and NOC when caring for the client with cervical cancer.

Community-Based Care

Teaching varies according to the stage of the cancer and the treatment selected. Provide information concerning radiation,

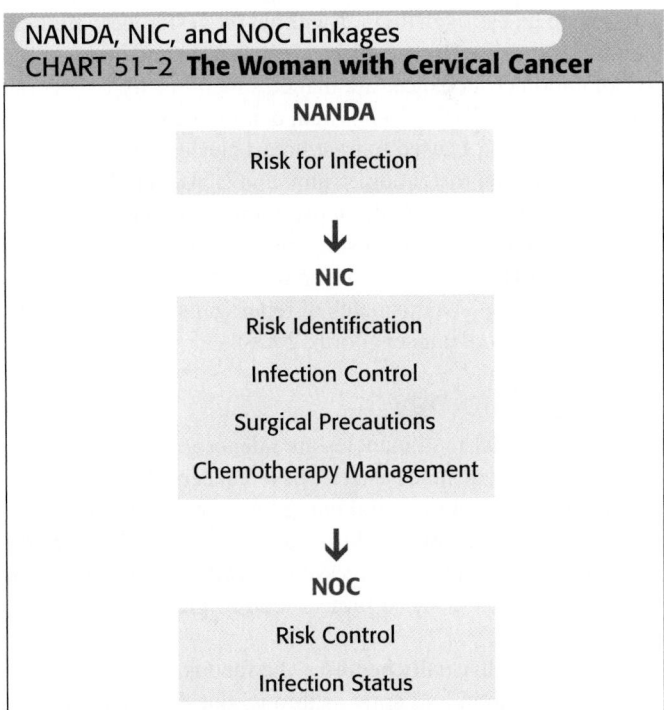

NANDA, NIC, and NOC Linkages
CHART 51–2 The Woman with Cervical Cancer

NANDA

Risk for Infection

↓

NIC

Risk Identification

Infection Control

Surgical Precautions

Chemotherapy Management

↓

NOC

Risk Control

Infection Status

Data from *NANDA's Nursing Diagnoses: Definitions & Classification 2005–2006* by NANDA International (2003), Philadelphia; *Nursing Interventions Classification (NIC)* (4th ed.) by J. M. Dochterman & G. M. Bulecheck (2004), St. Louis, MO: Mosby; and *Nursing Outcomes Classification (NOC)* (3rd ed.) by S. Moorhead, M. Johnson, and M. Maas (2004), St. Louis, MO: Mosby.

chemotherapy, or surgery, as indicated. Preoperative teaching focuses on postoperative expectations, including management of urinary or fecal diversion, if indicated (see Chapter 26 ∞ and 29 ∞). Help the woman and family recognize signs of infection and understand the importance of follow-up care. In addition, suggest the following resources:

- American Cancer Society
- National Cancer Institute
- Women's Cancer Network.

THE WOMAN WITH ENDOMETRIAL CANCER

Endometrial cancer is the most frequently diagnosed pelvic cancer in the United States. The ACS (2006a) estimates that each year approximately 41,000 women are diagnosed with endometrial cancer, and more than 7000 die annually from this disease. The incidence is higher in white women than in black women, but the mortality rate is nearly twice as high in black women. Most endometrial cancer is diagnosed in postmenopausal women, with the peak incidence in the late 50s and early 60s, with only a 2% to 5% incidence in women younger than 40 (Porth, 2005). When diagnosed and treated early in the disease, the 5-year survival rate is about 90%.

Risk Factors

A significant risk factor for endometrial cancer is prolonged estrogen stimulation. Other factors that increase risk are obesity, anovulatory menstrual cycles, decreasing ovarian function (as from menopause), estrogen-secreting tumors, and unopposed estrogen (e.g., estrogen therapy without progesterone). Medical conditions that may alter estrogen metabolism and increase the risk of endometrial cancer are diabetes mellitus, hypertension, and POS (Porth, 2005). Tamoxifen, a drug that blocks estrogen receptor sites and is used to treat breast cancer, has a weak estrogenic effect on the endometrium, and is also a risk factor.

Endometrial cancer is the most commonly inherited gynecologic cancer. A family history of hereditary nonpolyposis colon cancer (HNPCC) may mean that a woman has an inherited mutation that is a mismatch of repair genes, and has a 60% risk of endometrial cancer (Porth, 2005).

Pathophysiology

Most endometrial malignancies are adenocarcinomas that are slow to grow and metastasize. These cancers develop in the glandular cells or endometrial lining of the uterus (the same tissue that is shed each month during a normal menstrual period). Endometrial hyperplasia (excessive growth) is a precursor of endometrial cancer. These tumors tend to grow slowly in the early stages.

Tumor growth usually begins in the fundus, invades the vascular myometrium, and spreads throughout the female reproductive tract. Metastasis occurs by means of the lymphatic system, through the fallopian tubes to the peritoneal cavity, and to the rest of the body via the bloodstream. Target areas for metastasis include the lungs, liver, and bone. The International Federation of Gynecology and Obstetrics (FIGO) classification of endometrial cancer is presented in Table 51–3.

Manifestations

The major manifestation of endometrial hyperplasia or overt endometrial cancer is abnormal, painless vaginal bleeding. In menstruating women, this bleeding is manifested as menorrhagia or metrorrhagia. In postmenopausal women, any bleeding is abnormal. Later manifestations include pelvic cramping, bleeding after intercourse, and lower abdominal pressure. In advanced disease, lymph node enlargement, pleural effusion, abdominal masses, and ascites may be present.

INTERDISCIPLINARY CARE

The goals of care for the woman with endometrial cancer are to eradicate the cancer and minimize complications and metastasis.

Diagnosis

Tests used to diagnose cancer of the endometrium include a vaginal or transvaginal ultrasound, used to determine endometrial thickening, which may indicate hypertrophy or malignant changes, or an endometrial biopsy or a dilation and curettage (D&C) to provide a definitive diagnosis (see Chapter 49 ∞ for further information and nursing care). Other tests to determine the extent of the disease include chest x-ray, intravenous urography, cystoscopy, barium enema, sigmoidoscopy, MRI, and bone scans.

Medications

Although the treatment of choice for primary endometrial carcinoma is surgery, progesterone therapy may be used for recurrent disease. About one-third of women respond favorably, primarily those with well-differentiated tumors. Chemotherapy is less effective than other forms of therapy, although cisplatin or combination chemotherapy may be used for women with disseminated disease.

Surgery

After the diagnosis is confirmed, a total abdominal hysterectomy and bilateral salpingo-oophorectomy is performed for stage I cancer. A radical hysterectomy with node dissection is performed if the disease is stage II or beyond.

TABLE 51–3 FIGO Staging Classification for Endometrial Cancer

STAGE	DESCRIPTION
I	Tumor limited to endometrium or myometrium
II	Endocervical glandular involvement or invasion of cervical stroma
III	Metastasis or invasion of serosa, adnexae, vagina, and pelvic or para-aortic lymph nodes
IV	Tumor invasion of bladder or bowel mucosa; distant metastases

Radiation Therapy

Treatment with external and internal radiation may be performed as a preoperative measure or as adjuvant treatment in advanced cases.

 ## NURSING CARE

Health Promotion

All perimenopausal and postmenopausal women need annual pelvic examinations. The ACS recommends that at the time of menopause all women be informed of the risks and manifestations of endometrial cancer, and strongly encouraged to report any unexpected bleeding or spotting to their healthcare provider. Those in high-risk groups are advised to have endometrial biopsies every 2 years, beginning at age 35. In addition, control of diseases such as diabetes mellitus and hypertension decrease the risk of endometrial hyperplasia.

Assessment

Collect the following data through a health history and physical examination (see Chapter 49 ∞):

- *Health history:* Abnormal vaginal bleeding, menstrual history, use of estrogen (without progesterone) to treat menopausal symptoms, breast cancer treated with tamoxifen, childbearing status, presence of chronic illnesses, family history of hereditary nonpolyposis colon cancer.
- *Physical assessment:* Height and weight, pelvic examination, abdomen, lymph glands.

Nursing Diagnoses and Interventions

Nursing care involves helping the woman deal with the physical and psychologic effects of a potentially life-threatening illness, make informed decisions, and minimize the adverse effects of therapy. Pain relief is a key component of care, as is grief work on the part of the woman and family. Encourage the woman to perform self-care and resume normal activities of daily living.

Acute Pain

Total abdominal hysterectomy can involve severe and prolonged pain, not only from the surgical incision but also from the manipulation of internal organs during surgery. Abdominal viscera are highly vascular and easily bruised by handling.

- Administer analgesics as ordered. *Analgesics provide pain relief and promote early ambulation.*
- Encourage ambulation. *Ambulation facilitates the expulsion of flatus, which can cause distention as well as discomfort.*
- Apply heat to the abdomen, and recommend that the woman use a heating pad at home. *Heat dilates blood vessels, increasing blood supply to the pelvis, decreasing pain.*

Disturbed Body Image

For many women, the side effects of cancer treatment can be almost as difficult and painful as the disease itself. Although side effects of the different therapies vary among individuals, the woman's body image and quality of life are always affected. Such side effects as alopecia (hair loss), nausea, vomiting, fatigue, diarrhea, stomatitis, and surgical scarring disturb body image.

- Review the side effects of the treatment regimen proposed, and assist the woman to develop a plan to deal with these effects. *This promotes a sense of control.*
- Remind the woman and family that side effects are usually manageable and may be temporary. *Over-the-counter agents can be used to alleviate stomatitis. Frequent rest periods can relieve fatigue. Medications can be prescribed for nausea, vomiting, and diarrhea.*

Ineffective Sexuality Pattern

Altered sexuality may result from a feeling of unattractiveness, fatigue, or pain and discomfort. The woman's partner may fear that sexual activity will be harmful.

- Encourage expression of feelings about the effect of cancer on their lives and sexual relationship. *Verbalizing feelings helps relieve stress and maximizes relaxation.*
- Suggest that the couple explore alternative sexual positions and coordinate sexual activity with rest periods and times that are relatively free from pain. *This creates a more favorable environment for satisfying sexual activity.*

Community-Based Care

Provide information about the specific treatment and prognosis for the cancer. Explain the expected side effects of radiation implant therapy (see Chapter 14 ∞). Pain control measures are also an essential part of the teaching plan (see Chapter 9 ∞). The resources listed for the woman with cervical cancer are also appropriate for the woman with endometrial cancer.

THE WOMAN WITH OVARIAN CANCER

Ovarian cancer is the fourth most common gynecologic cancer in women in the United States. Approximately 20,000 women are diagnosed with ovarian cancer and an estimated 15,000 deaths result each year (ACS, 2006a). The incidence increases with age, peaking in women between the ages of 40 and 80 years; half of all cases are in women over 65 years of age (Porth, 2005). Ovarian cancer is more common in white women than in black women, and mortality rate is highest in whites.

Risk Factors

Family history is a significant risk factor, with a 50% risk of developing the disease if two or more first- or second-degree relatives have site-specific ovarian cancer. Other types of inherited risk are breast-ovarian cancer syndrome (first- and second-degree relatives have both breast and ovarian cancer) and family cancer syndrome (Lynch syndrome II), in which male or female relatives have a history of colorectal, endometrial, ovarian, pancreatic, or other types of cancer (Porth, 2005). The breast cancer susceptibility genes *BRAC1* and *BRAC2* are implicated in 5% to 10% of hereditary ovarian cancers.

Risk factors also include having no children or giving birth after age 35, exposure to talc or asbestos, endometriosis, pelvic inflammatory disease, and living in a Western civilized country. Protective factors include long-term contraceptive use, having a child before the age of 25, tubal ligation, breast-feeding, and hysterectomy (Martin, 2005).

Pathophysiology

There are several types of ovarian cancers: epithelial tumors, germ cell tumors, and gonadal stromal tumors. Most ovarian cancers are epithelial tumors, originating from the surface epithelium of the ovary. Ovarian cancer usually spreads by local shedding of cancer cells into the peritoneal cavity and by direct invasion of the bowel and bladder. Cancer cells in peritoneal fluid can implant in the intestines, bladder, and mesentery. Tumor cells also spread through the lymph and blood to such organs as the liver, and across the diaphragm to involve the lungs. Both pelvic and para-aortic lymph nodes may be involved and tumor cells can block lymphatic drainage from the abdomen, resulting in ascites. Staging for ovarian cancer is based on surgical and histologic evaluation (Table 51–4).

Manifestations

In early stages, ovarian cancer generally causes no warning signs or manifestations. When manifestations do develop, they are often vague and mild, such as indigestion, urinary frequency, abdominal bloating, and constipation. Abnormal vaginal bleeding may occur if the endometrium is stimulated by a hormone-secreting tumor or if the tumor erodes the vaginal wall. Pelvic pain sometimes occurs. An enlarged abdomen with ascites signals later stage disease.

Complications

The complications of advanced ovarian cancer, with related nursing assessments and treatment, are outlined in Table 51–5.

INTERDISCIPLINARY CARE

As with other malignancies, care of the woman with ovarian cancer is focused on surgery to determine the stage of the tumor and to remove as much of the tumor as possible. Unfortunately, because there are no early manifestations, the disease is often well advanced prior to diagnosis. In younger women, an ovarian mass may be monitored for several menstrual cycles, but any ovarian mass must immediately be investigated in a postmenopausal woman.

Diagnosis

Tests used in the diagnosis of ovarian cancer may include transvaginal or abdominal ultrasound and a CT scan of the abdomen and pelvis (see Chapter 49 ∞ for further information about diagnostic tests).

The blood test most useful is a CA-125 antigen level. CA-125 is a tumor marker that is highly specific to epithelial ovarian cancer. Transvaginal or transabdominal ultrasonography is used to measure ovarian size and detect small masses. These tests, however, are not appropriate screening measures because they cannot differentiate between cystic or benign ovarian masses and malignancy.

Medications

While surgery is the treatment of choice for ovarian cancer, chemotherapy may be used to achieve remission of the dis-

TABLE 51–4 FIGO Staging Classification for Ovarian Cancer

STAGE	DESCRIPTION
I	Growth limited to the ovaries
II	Growth involving one or both ovaries with pelvic extension
III	Tumor involving one or both ovaries, with peritoneal implants outside the pelvis or positive retroperitoneal or inguinal nodes
IV	Growth involving one or both ovaries with distant metastasis

TABLE 51–5 Complications of Advanced Ovarian Cancer

COMPLICATION	ASSESSMENTS	TREATMENT
Ascites (accumulation of fluid in the abdominal cavity; a form of third spacing)	■ Abdominal distention ■ Everted umbilicus ■ Shiny abdominal skin ■ Dullness on percussion of dependent areas ■ Dyspnea, constipation ■ Abdominal pain	Paracentesis (removing fluid from the abdomen)
Intestinal obstruction	■ Abdominal distention ■ Abdominal pain ■ Projectile vomiting ■ Constipation ■ Hyperactive bowel sounds	Nasogastric tube insertion, NPO
Deep venous thrombosis	■ Leg edema ■ Leg pain ■ Redness, warmth	Anticoagulants
Lymphedema (leg)	■ Edema of leg ■ Decreased range of motion ■ Tight, shiny skin on leg	Skin care, range-of-motion exercises, massage or physical therapy, compression bandaging

ease. Chemotherapy is not curative for ovarian cancer. Combination chemotherapy regimens using cyclophosphamide and cisplatin or other agents may be employed. Combination therapy with a platinum compound (cisplatin or carboplatin) is superior to treatment with a single drug, with paclitaxel/carboplatin the preferred regimen (Martin, 2005). Chemotherapy with paclitaxel (Taxol) may prolong survival. Close monitoring of bone marrow and renal function is vital while the woman is on chemotherapy because these drugs have significant toxic effects.

Surgery

In young women with stage I disease who wish to have children, treatment may be limited to removal of one ovary. Usually, however, total hysterectomy with bilateral salpingo-oophorectomy (removal of the ovaries and fallopian tubes) and removal of the omentum are performed.

Radiation Therapy

Radiation therapy using external-beam or intracavitary implants is performed for palliative purposes only and is directed at shrinking the tumor at selected sites.

NURSING CARE

Nursing care for the woman with ovarian cancer is similar to the nursing care for women with other gynecologic cancers. The side effects of treatment of cancer and generally poor prognosis diminish the woman's quality of life and involve major psychosocial implications (see Chapter 14 ∞).

Community-Based Care

Address the following topics in preparing the woman and her family for self-care:

- If a positive family history of the disease or previous breast cancer exists, stress the importance of obtaining regular pelvic examinations. Inform women in this risk group that annual screening with transvaginal ultrasound and CA-125 measurements may be recommended.
- Long-term use of oral contraceptives may reduce the risk of developing ovarian cancer.
- It is crucial not to ignore manifestations such as indigestion, nausea, or urinary frequency, because these seemingly unrelated manifestations may be early signs of ovarian tumors. Emphasize, however, that ovarian cancer usually is asymptomatic in early stages.
- Discuss treatment options and their side effects and provide information on ways to minimize or manage side effects.
- Refer to hospice services when appropriate. The resources suggested for the woman with cervical cancer are also appropriate for the woman with ovarian cancer.

THE WOMAN WITH CANCER OF THE VULVA

Cancer of the vulva occurs most often in women over 50 years of age. The prognosis of vulvar carcinoma depends on the de-gree of invasion, general health status of the woman, presence of chronic diseases, and ability to withstand treatment.

Pathophysiology

The cause of vulvar cancer is unknown, but there is evidence to associate it with STIs, particularly HPV. Nearly 85% of malignant and premalignant cervical and vulvar lesions have been found to contain HPV DNA, HPV structural antigens, or both. Herpes simplex type 2 (HSV2) infection has also been associated with vulvar cancer. Other risk factors include advanced age, diabetes, and a history of leukoplakia (a precancerous lesion on the vulvar mucous membranes characterized by raised white patches).

Most vulvar cancers are epidermoid or squamous cell carcinomas. The primary site is usually the labia majora, but vulvar cancer is also found on the labia minora, clitoris, vestibule, and occasionally in multiple locations. Metastasis occurs by direct extension into the vagina, perineal skin, anus, and urethra. The cancer also spreads through the lymphatic system via the superficial and deep inguinal and femoral nodes, and to the pelvic lymph nodes.

Manifestations

The woman with vulvar cancer is often asymptomatic, and lesions are discovered on routine examination or self-examination. Discoloration can vary from white macular patches to red painless sores. Lesions may be *exophytic* (proliferating outwardly), *endophytic* (proliferating inwardly), ulcerative, or *verrucous* (resembling a wart).

Pruritus is the most common manifestation, and the woman often has had a history of prolonged vulvar irritation. Perineal pain and bleeding indicate large tumors and advanced disease. In very advanced disease, dysuria related to urethral involvement may be the presenting symptom.

INTERDISCIPLINARY CARE

The report of itching, burning, or a sore on the vulva merits careful investigation and biopsy of any lesions found. Inguinal lymph nodes may be enlarged. The goal of care is to eradicate the lesion and reduce the risk of recurrence. Surgical resection is the preferred treatment. If lymph nodes are involved, radiation therapy is used postoperatively. Chemotherapy is reserved for distant metastases.

Diagnosis is based on the results of an excisional biopsy of the lesion. Metastasis, if suspected, can be evaluated by chest x-ray examination, barium enema, intravenous pyelogram, cystoscopy, CT and MRI scans, and proctoscopy. Lymphangiography can also be used.

Surgery is the most common treatment for vulvar cancer. The specific procedure depends on the stage of the cancer. Early, noninvasive lesions may be treated with laser surgery, cryosurgery, or electrocautery. For more advanced disease, vulvectomy may be performed (Figure 51–6 ■). A simple vulvectomy involves the removal of the vulva, labia majora and minora, clitoris, and prepuce. A radical vulvectomy is

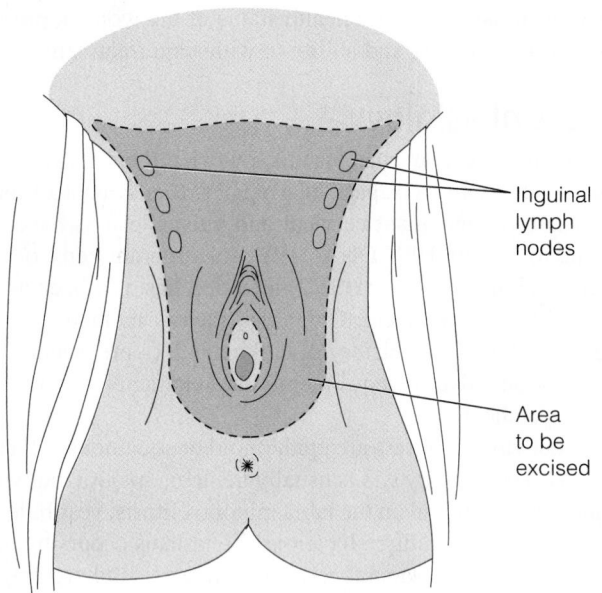

Figure 51–6 ■ Vulvectomy for vulvar carcinoma. A radical vulvectomy involves removal of the vulva, labia majora, labia minora, clitoris, prepuce, subcutaneous tissue, and regional lymph nodes.

performed if invasion is suspected. This procedure involves removal of all the tissue in a simple vulvectomy, as well as the subcutaneous tissue and regional lymph nodes.

NURSING CARE

Nursing care is similar to that for the woman with endometrial cancer. The woman fears death as the ultimate outcome as well as the possible pain and suffering that surgery and other treatments may cause. Radical surgery represents a great loss to women of all ages.

Nursing Diagnoses and Interventions

Disruption of perineal tissues is a priority problem for these women.

Impaired Tissue Integrity

The woman who has undergone a vulvectomy is at high risk for infection and impaired healing because of proximity of the surgical site to urinary and anal orifices. In addition, the women are often older and may have age-related changes in healing and immune function.

■ Teach the woman and/or her partner or other family member the procedure for irrigation of the vulvectomy. If neither is able to perform this procedure, arrange for home health nursing. *Irrigation helps prevent skin breakdown and infection.*

■ After irrigation, apply dry heat using a heat lamp positioned about 18 inches from the area; emphasize safety precautions, including use of a low-wattage bulb (40 to 60 watts). *Dry heat helps promote healing and comfort.*

■ Provide information on maintaining a diet high in protein, iron, and vitamin C. *These nutrients promote collagen formation and wound healing.*

Community-Based Care

Explain the association between STIs such as HPV (genital warts) and cancer of the vulva. Provide information about safer sex practices such as abstinence, limiting the number of sexual partners, and using condoms (male or female). Explain that early diagnosis and treatment of STIs and other irritative conditions of the external genitalia may reduce the risk of developing vulvar cancer. Teaching for the woman undergoing a vulvectomy should emphasize the potential for skin breakdown, particularly with radiation therapy. Explain that removal of lymph nodes leads to lymphedema and that recurrent cellulitis and sexual dysfunction are common complications of vulvar cancer.

DISORDERS OF THE BREAST

Breast disorders are common conditions that primarily affect women (disorders of the male breast are discussed in Chapter 50 ∞). When a woman discovers a breast lump, her first response is often fear: of breast cancer, of losing her breast, and perhaps of losing her life. Because American society views the breast as a significant component of feminine beauty, any problem that threatens the breast often strikes at the core of a woman's self-image.

Nurses play a critical role in the care of women experiencing breast disorders by providing education, support, and advocacy. Part of the nurse's role is educating women about normal breast tissue, common benign breast disorders, available screening techniques and risk factors for breast cancer, and breast self-examination.

THE WOMAN WITH A BENIGN BREAST DISORDER

Benign breast disorders occur frequently in women and may be a source of anxiety. Changes in a woman's breast tissue often correspond to hormonal changes of the menstrual cycle. Most women notice increased tenderness and lumpiness prior to menses. (For this reason, it is best to perform breast self-examination (BSE) 7 to 10 days after the beginning of the menstrual period.) Breast tissue changes in response to hormonal, nutritional, physical, and environmental stimuli. Benign breast disorders include fibrocystic breast changes, fibroadenomas, intraductal papillomas, duct ectasia, fat necrosis, and mastitis (Table 51–6).

Pathophysiology and Manifestations

Fibrocystic Changes

Fibrocystic changes (FCC) (*fibrocystic breast disease*) is the physiologic nodularity and breast tenderness that increases and decreases with the menstrual cycle. An estimated 50% to 80% of all women experience some of these changes, which include fibrosis, epithelial proliferation, and cyst formation. FCC is most common in women 30 to 50 years of age, and is rare in postmenopausal women who are not taking hormone replacement (Porth, 2005).

TABLE 51–6 Summary of Common Breast Disorders

CONDITION	AGE	PAIN	NIPPLE DISCHARGE	LOCATION	CONSISTENCY AND MOBILITY	DIAGNOSIS AND TREATMENT
Duct ectasia	35 to 55 years; median age 40	Burning around nipple	Sticky, multicolored; usually bilateral	No specific location	Retroareolar mass with advanced disease	Open biopsy; local excision of diseased portion of breast
Fibroadenoma	15 to 39 years; median age 20	No	No	No specific location	Mobile, firm, smooth, well-delineated mass	Mammography, surgical or needle biopsy; excision of the tumor
Fibrocystic changes (FCC)	20 to 49 years; median age 30 (may subside with menopause)	Yes	May occur	Upper outer quadrant	Bilateral multiple lumps influenced by the menstrual cycle	Needle aspiration; observation; biopsy if there is an un-resolved mass or mammo-graphic changes
Intraductal papilloma	35 to 55 years; median age 40	Yes	Serous or sanguineous; usually unilateral from one duct	No specific location	Usually soft, poorly delineated mass	Pap smear of nipple discharge; biopsy; wedge resection
Mastitis, acute	Childbearing years	Tenderness, pain	No	No specific location	Generalized redness of overlying skin	Antibiotic therapy; incision and drainage if mastitis progresses to an abscess
Mastitis, chronic	Any age	Tenderness, pain; headache; high fever	No	No specific location	Generalized redness and swelling	Antibiotics, usually penicillin
Fat necrosis	Any age	Tenderness	No	No specific location	Firm, irregular, palpable	Surgical biopsy to rule out cancer

FCC includes many different lesions and breast changes. The more common nonproliferative form does not increase the risk for breast cancer. The proliferative form, accompanied by giant cysts and proliferative epithelial lesions, does increase the risk for breast cancer.

Nonproliferative changes may be cystic or fibrous. Cystic change refers to the dilation of ducts in the subareolar, lobular, or lobe areas. Cysts often go unnoticed unless pain and tenderness is associated with menses. Fibrous changes are infrequent but can occur during the menstrual years. A firm, palpable mass, 2 to 3 cm in size, is typically located in the upper outer breast quadrant following an inflammatory response to ductal irritation.

Women with fibrocystic changes experience bilateral or unilateral pain or tenderness in the upper, outer quadrants of their breasts, and report that their breasts feel particularly thick and lumpy the week prior to menses. Nipple discharge may be present. Pain is due to edema of the connective tissue of the breast, dilation of the ducts, and some inflammatory response; some women report an increase in breast size. Multiple, mobile cysts may form, usually in both breasts (Figure 51–7 ■). Fluid aspirated from these cysts ranges in color from milky white to yellow, brown, or green. If the fluid is tinged with blood, there is reason to suspect malignancy.

Intraductal Disorders

An *intraductal papilloma* is a tiny, wartlike growth on the inside of the peripheral mammary duct that causes discharge from the nipple. The discharge may be clear and sticky or bloody. When more than one of these growths is present, the condition is called *intraductal papillomatosis*. This condition is most common in women in their 30s and 40s. The lesion must be investigated to rule out malignancy.

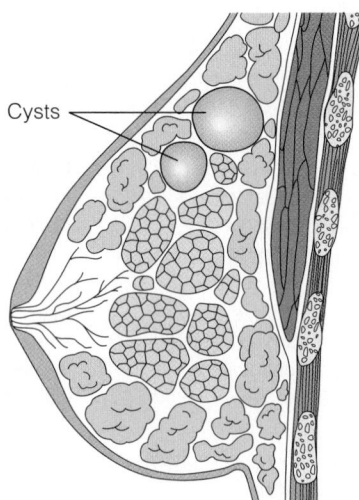

Cysts

Figure 51–7 ■ Fibrocystic breast changes.

Mammary duct ectasia (*plasma cell mastitis*) is a palpable lumpiness found beneath the areola. Duct ectasia involves periductal inflammation, dilation of the ductal system, and accumulation of fluid and dead cells that block the involved ducts. The condition usually occurs in perimenopausal women and is difficult to differentiate from cancer.

Manifestations of mammary duct ectasia include sticky, thick nipple discharge with burning and itching around the nipple, and inflammation. The discharge may be green, greenish brown, or bloody. Nipple retraction often is associated with duct ectasia in postmenopausal women.

INTERDISCIPLINARY CARE

Diagnosis of FCC is based on complete history, physical examination, and imaging studies. A biopsy may be required for diagnosis.

Analysis of nipple discharge, mammography, and possibly ductography may be used to diagnose ductal disorders. The affected duct is excised in an open biopsy procedure. Nursing care for the woman is similar to that for any client with an open biopsy. It also is important to reassure the woman that these disorders are not breast cancer.

The treatment is usually symptomatic. Cyst aspiration may relieve pain, and also allows examination of fluid to confirm the cystic nature of the disease. A well-fitting brassiere ("bra") that provides good support worn day and night helps relieve discomfort. Some women report that eliminating xanthines (found in coffee, tea, cola, and chocolate) from the diet decreases symptoms. Aspirin, mild analgesics, local heat or cold, and vitamin E may help relieve breast pain. Hormone therapy is controversial because of the benign nature of the disease and potential adverse effects of therapy. Danazol, a synthetic androgen, may be prescribed for women with severe pain.

NURSING CARE

When a woman presents with a breast mass, nursing responsibilities include taking a careful history and facilitating

follow-up care. If a palpable mass is present, it is important to ask how long the lesion has been present and whether the woman has noticed any pain associated with the mass, any change in its size, and any changes in association with the menstrual cycle.

In many cases, definitive diagnosis of the breast disorder requires surgical biopsy to rule out cancer. During the diagnostic process, the nurse can provide emotional support and education about diagnostic and therapeutic procedures, self-care and comfort measures, and resources to help the woman cope with the experience.

THE WOMAN WITH BREAST CANCER

Breast cancer is the unregulated growth of abnormal cells in breast tissue. Breast cancer is the most commonly occurring cancer in women and the second leading cause of death in women in the United States. The ACS (2006a) estimates that more than 212,000 women will be diagnosed with breast cancer each year, and approximately 41,000 women will die from it annually. There are racial differences in the incidence and mortality of breast cancer (see the Focus on Cultural Diversity box below).

Risk Factors

Of the various kinds of risk factors for breast cancer, some can be changed and some cannot. Those that cannot be changed are (ACS, 2006e):

■ *Age and gender.* Women are 100 times more likely to have breast cancer than are men, with the risk increasing with age. See the Meeting Individualized Needs on the next page.
■ *Genetic risk factors* (as previously described).
■ *Family history of breast cancer.* Relatives from either the maternal or paternal side of the family. Having a first-degree relative (mother, sister, or daughter) with breast cancer approximately doubles the risk, and having two first-degree relatives increases it fivefold. Having a male family member with breast cancer also poses an increased risk.
■ *Personal history of breast cancer.* A woman with cancer in one breast has a three- to fivefold increase in risk for developing a new cancer in the other breast or in a different part of the same breast.
■ *Previous breast biopsy.* If earlier breast biopsies were diagnosed as proliferative, then breast disease without atypical hyperplasia increases risk by 1.5 to 2 times. A previous biopsy of atypical hyperplasia increases risk by 4 to 5 times.

FOCUS ON CULTURAL DIVERSITY
Incidence and Mortality for Breast Cancer in Women

■ Breast cancer is more prevalent in African American women up to the age of 40 years.
■ Breast cancer is more prevalent in Caucasian women over the age of 40 years.
■ Asian, Hispanic, and American Indian women have a lower risk of developing breast cancer.
■ African American women are more likely to die from the cancer because they are often diagnosed at an advanced stage.

MEETING INDIVIDUALIZED NEEDS Older Women with Breast Cancer

- Although the incidence of breast cancer is increasing among premenopausal women, it is still primarily a disease of older women. However, the needs of older women with breast cancer have been inadequately addressed in the professional literature and in the popular media.
- Women between the ages of 50 and 65 are the group most likely to benefit from annual screening mammography, yet many women in this age group have never had a mammogram. Failure of physicians to refer older women for mammography is the reason most frequently cited for this statistic; nurse practitioners and female physicians are more likely to refer women for mammography. Promotional campaigns for mammography send a confusing message by showing images of women in their 20s and 30s for whom mammography is

largely ineffective, rather than women in older age groups who are more likely to benefit from mammography.
- For too long, mastectomy was perceived as the only treatment option open to most older women with breast cancer, even those with early-stage disease. Slowly that perception is changing as breast-conservation treatment gains greater acceptance. The choice of surgical treatment, particularly for older women, is highly individual. Many older women wish to preserve their breasts.
- Although older women with breast cancer may experience co-existing chronic illnesses and impaired physical function, research suggests that they show lower levels of emotional distress than younger women. Obviously the need for services such as personal care, shopping, housekeeping, and transportation increases as the ages of the woman and the caregiver increase.

- *Previous chest irradiation.* Radiation of the chest as a child or young woman for other cancer (such as Hodgkin's disease) significantly increases the risk.
- *Menstrual history.* Women who begin menstruating before the age of 12 or who have menopause after the age of 50 are at a slightly higher risk.

Lifestyle-related factors and breast cancer risk include using oral contraceptives, not having children or having them after the age of 30, using HRT for more than 5 years, not breast-feeding, drinking alcohol (especially two to five drinks daily), obesity, high-fat diets, physical inactivity, and (possibly) environmental pollution. Lower risk factors for breast cancer include breast-feeding, moderate or vigorous physical activity, and maintaining a healthy body weight.

Pathophysiology

Possible causes of breast cancer include environmental, hormonal, reproductive, and hereditary factors. Two breast cancer susceptibility genes have been identified: *BRCA1* on chromosome 17 and *BRCA2* on chromosome 13. These genes may be responsible for the approximately 10% of women with hereditary breast cancer, with genetic mutations causing up to 80% of breast cancer in women younger than 50 years of age. A woman with identified mutations in *BRCA1* (known to be involved in tumor suppression) has a lifetime risk of 56% to 85% for breast cancer and also has an increased risk for ovarian cancer (Porth, 2005). Mutations of a tumor suppressor gene are also linked to increased risk for breast cancer.

Cancer of the breast begins as a single transformed cell and is hormone dependent. Cancers of the breast are classified as noninvasive (in situ) or invasive, depending on the penetration of the tumor into surrounding tissue. Breast cancer may remain a noninvasive disease, or an invasive disease without metastasis, for long periods of time.

Breast cancer may be categorized as carcinoma of the mammary ducts, carcinoma of mammary lobules, or sarcoma of the breast. Most breast cancers are adenocarcinomas and appear to arise in the terminal section of the breast ductal tissue. There are many histologic types of breast cancer, and only examples are

described here. The most common type is *infiltrating ductal carcinoma*. Two atypical types of breast cancer are inflammatory carcinoma and Paget's disease. Inflammatory carcinoma of the breast, a systemic disease, is the most malignant form of breast cancer. Edema with dimpling of the skin that results in the skin looking like the peel of an orange (*peau d'orange*) is usually present. *Paget's disease* is a rare type of breast cancer involving infiltration of the nipple epithelium.

Breast cancer can metastasize to other sites through the bloodstream or lymphatic system. The common sites of metastasis of breast cancer are bone, brain, lung, liver, skin, and lymph nodes. Staging is a system of classifying cancer according to the size of the tumor, involvement of lymph nodes, and metastasis to distant sites, and the presence/absence of distant metastasis (Table 51–7). The staging of the breast cancer provides important information for making decisions about treatment options and is also used as a basis for prognosis.

Manifestations

The manifestations of breast cancer may include a nontender lump in the breast (most often in the upper outer quadrant, the area with the most glandular tissue), abnormal nipple discharge, a rash around the nipple area, nipple retraction, dimpling of the skin, or a change in the position of the nipple (see the box below). There may also be nipple pain, scaliness, ulceration, skin irritation, or discharge. Breast cancer is usually painless, but

MANIFESTATIONS of Breast Cancer

- Breast mass or thickening
- Unusual lump in the underarm or above the collarbone
- Persistent skin rash near the nipple area
- Flaking or eruption near the nipple
- Dimpling, pulling, or retraction in an area of the breast
- Nipple discharge
- Change in nipple position
- Burning, stinging, or pricking sensation

MEDIALINK Case Study: Breast Cancer

TABLE 51-7 Staging of Breast Cancer

STAGE	TUMOR	NODE	METASTASIS
0	Tis-Carcinoma *in situ* or Paget's disease of the nipple	N0-No regional lymph node metastasis	M0-No evidence of distant metastasis
I	T1-Tumor no larger than 2 cm	N0	M0
IIA	T0-No evidence of primary tumor	N1-Metastasis to movable ipsilateral axillary nodes	M0
	T1		
	T2-Tumor no larger than 5 cm	N0	M0
IIB	T2	N1	M0
	T3-Tumor larger than 5 cm	N0	M0
IIIA	T0	N2-Metastasis to ipsilateral fixed axillary nodes	M0
	T1		
	T2		
	T3	N1	M0
		N2	M0
IIIB	T4-Tumor of any size with direct extension to chest wall or skin	Any N	M0
	Any T	N3-Metastasis to ipsilateral internal mammary lymph nodes	M0
IV	Any T	N0 and N1	M1-Distant metastasis

some women report a burning or stinging sensation. Many women with breast cancer have no manifestations, and their tumors are detected by mammography. However, most breast cancers are found by the women themselves (during BSE or a shower) or by their partners during sexual activity.

INTERDISCIPLINARY CARE

Diagnosis of breast cancer begins with detection, either detection of asymptomatic lesions discovered through screening or symptomatic lesions discovered by the woman. Any palpable mass requires evaluation. Once the diagnosis is made, a number of treatment options are available. The choice of treatment depends on several factors, such as the stage of the cancer, the age of the woman, and the woman's preferences.

Diagnosis

Early detection of breast cancer is possible with clinical breast examination (CBE) and mammogram (see Chapter 49 ∞ for further information). Mammography can detect breast tumors 2 years before they reach palpable size; most of these tumors have been present for 8 to 10 years. Although controversy exists about the ability of screening mammography to improve mortality rates for women under 50, the ACS recommends annual mammograms beginning at age 40 and CBE at least every 3 years for women in their 20s and 30s.

Other diagnostic tests include a percutaneous needle biopsy to define a cystic mass or fibrocystic changes and provide specimens for cytologic examination, and a breast biopsy. In aspiration biopsy or fine-needle aspiration biopsy, a needle is used to remove cells or fluid from the breast lesion (Figures 51-8A and B ■). The types of breast biopsy and related nursing care are described in Chapter 49 ∞. In many

A Aspiration biopsy

B Excisional biopsy

Figure 51-8 ■ Types of breast biopsy. *A,* In an aspiration biopsy, a needle is used to aspirate fluid or tissue from the breast. *B,* In an excisional biopsy, tissue from the breast lesion is removed surgically.

facilities, fine-needle aspiration biopsies are performed using a stereotactic biopsy device; mammography and a computer are used to guide the needle.

Medications

Tamoxifen citrate (Nolvadex) is an oral medication that interferes with estrogen activity. It is used to treat advanced breast cancer, as an adjuvant for early-stage breast cancer, and as a preventive treatment for women at high risk of developing breast cancer. Nursing implications for tamoxifen are presented in the Medication Administration box below.

Immunotherapy, using trastuzumab (Herceptin), is used to stop the growth of breast tumors that express the HER2/neu receptor (which binds an epidermal growth factor that contributes to cancer cell growth) on their cell surface. This drug is a recombinant DNA-derived monoclonal antibody that binds to the receptor, inhibiting tumor cell proliferation.

Chemotherapy has become the standard of care for the majority of breast cancer cases with axillary node involvement. In late metastatic disease, chemotherapy becomes the primary treatment to prolong the woman's life. Chemotherapy is discussed in Chapter 14 ∞. Adjuvant (additional) systemic therapy following primary treatment for early-stage breast cancer refers to the administration of chemotherapy and other pharmacologic agents. This type of therapy has been widely studied; its use reduces the rates of recurrence and death from breast cancer. For example, the drug Avastin, when combined with chemotherapy to treat metastatic breast cancer, has extended cancer-free survival; and Femara (an aromatase inhibitor) has reduced the risk of recurrence after surgery (in some cases more effectively than tamoxifen).

Surgery

Until recently, the treatment of choice for breast cancer was a radical mastectomy. The trend now is toward more conservative surgery combined with chemotherapy, hormone therapy, or radiation, depending on the stage of the tumor and the age of the woman.

MASTECTOMY There are various types of mastectomy for breast cancer. *Radical mastectomy* is the removal of the entire affected breast, the underlying chest muscles, and the lymph nodes under the arms. *Simple mastectomy* is the removal of the complete breast only. *Segmental mastectomy* or *lumpectomy* (Figure 51–9A ■) is the removal of the tumor and the surrounding margin of breast tissues. *Modified radical mastectomy* is the removal of the breast tissue and lymph nodes under the arm (axillary node dissection), leaving the chest wall muscles intact (Figure 51–9B). See the next page for the nursing care of a woman having a mastectomy.

Axillary node dissection is generally performed during surgery for all invasive breast carcinoma to stage the tumor. Because this surgery can cause **lymphedema** (accumulation of fluid in the soft tissues of the arm caused by removal of lymph channels), nerve damage, and adhesions, and because of the role of the lymph nodes in immune system function, nonsurgical methods of detecting lymph node involvement are being used. Sentinel node biopsy prior to a node dissection is conducted by injecting a radioactive substance or dye into the region of the tumor. The dye is carried to the first (sentinel) lymph node to receive lymph from the tumor and would therefore be the node most likely to contain cancer cells if the cancer had metastasized. If the sentinel node is positive, more nodes are removed. If it is negative, further node evaluation is usually not indicated.

LUMPECTOMY Breast conservation surgery (*lumpectomy*) may be defined as excision of the primary tumor and adjacent breast tissue followed by radiation therapy. Many women are candidates for this procedure; however, women who have multicentric breast neoplasms and those who have large tumors in relation to their breast size are examples of unsuitable candidates. Selection of women for this procedure is guided by the need for local control of the lesion, cosmetic results, and personal preference.

BREAST RECONSTRUCTION After a mastectomy, some women may choose to have their breast reconstructed. They report that surgical reconstruction of the breast simplifies their lives and restores a sense of body integrity. Other women choose to use a removable breast prosthesis, and some women are comfortable without reconstruction or a prosthesis.

MEDICATION ADMINISTRATION Tamoxifen

TAMOXIFEN (NOLVADEX)

Tamoxifen is the most widely prescribed breast cancer drug, commonly given to prevent recurrence of estrogen-positive breast cancer in postmenopausal women. It inhibits tumor growth by blocking the estrogen receptor sites of cancer cells. Tamoxifen increases a woman's risk of developing endometrial cancer, deep venous thrombosis (DVT), and pulmonary embolism.

Nursing Responsibilities

■ Assess for potential contraindications to therapy.
■ Assess liver function tests; tamoxifen may interfere with liver function.

Health Education for the Client and Family

■ If in childbearing years, use a nonhormonal, barrier form of contraception; tamoxifen has adverse effects on the developing fetus.
■ Take the drug as prescribed until the physician indicates otherwise.
■ Side effects such as hot flashes, vaginal dryness, irregular periods, and weight gain are commonly experienced by women taking tamoxifen.
■ Do not smoke while taking tamoxifen; smoking further increases the risk of DVT.
■ Promptly report any abnormal vaginal bleeding (nonmenstrual bleeding, bleeding after menopause) to your primary care provider.

A Lumpectomy

B Modified radical mastectomy

Figure 51–9 ■ Types of mastectomy. *A,* In a lumpectomy, only the tumor and a small margin of surrounding tissue are removed. *B,* In a modified radical mastectomy, all breast tissue and the underarm lymph nodes are removed, but the underlying muscles remain.

Breast reconstruction may be performed at the time of the mastectomy or at any time thereafter, depending on the woman's preference. A number of procedures may be used for the breast reconstruction (Figure 51–10 ■). These include placement of a submuscular implant, the use of a tissue expander followed by an implant, the transposition of muscle and blood supply from the abdomen or back, or using (most often) the transverse rectus abdominis myocutaneous (TRAM) free tissue flap. Nursing implications for the care of

women undergoing breast reconstruction surgery are summarized in the box on the next page.

Radiation Therapy

Radiation therapy is typically used following breast cancer surgery to destroy any remaining cancer cells that could cause recurrence or metastasis. If a tumor is unusually large, radiation may be used to shrink the tumor prior to surgery. Radiation therapy is most commonly used in combination with lump-

---

NURSING CARE OF THE WOMAN HAVING A Mastectomy

PREOPERATIVE CARE
- Ensure that the woman or family member signs an informed consent form.
- See Chapter 4 ∞ for preoperative preparation.

POSTOPERATIVE CARE
- Deep-breathing exercises are important because after general anesthesia, it is difficult for air to reach the lungs, particularly with the restrictive surgical dressing that decreases chest expansion.
- A suction apparatus will be placed in the wound to allow drainage of excess body fluids that accumulate when the lymph nodes are removed. This device is usually removed 3 to 5 days after surgery.
- An IV line may be in place for fluid replacement and antibiotics to reduce the risk of postoperative infection.
- Control pain by using the patient-controlled analgesia device or requesting analgesics before pain becomes severe. Take analgesics as needed before performing recommended exercises to facilitate full movement.
- Note any signs of bleeding on the dressing or on the bedding.
- Numbness or feelings of "pins and needles" in the axillary area are common.

- Lying on one's back or on the side not operated on helps fluid drain from the site.
- Moving the arm on the operated side helps regain mobility; specific exercises will be prescribed for increasing mobility after the incisions have healed.
- If fluid builds up after the drains have been removed, it can be aspirated by the surgeon.
- Use caution about lifting heavy objects with the arm on the operated side.
- Be careful about injury and infection on the affected side; wear rubber gloves when washing dishes, garden gloves when working outside. Request that caregivers not perform blood pressures or venipunctures on the operative side to reduce the risk of injury and infection.
- Feelings of anxiety, sadness, and fear of looking at the incision are normal; mastectomy means abrupt change in body image. It is normal to mourn the loss of a breast and to fear the loss of one's life after a cancer diagnosis.
- Sexual intimacy can be affected by mastectomy; it often helps to be able to discuss potential sexual problems with one's partner, with a counselor, or with a breast cancer support group.

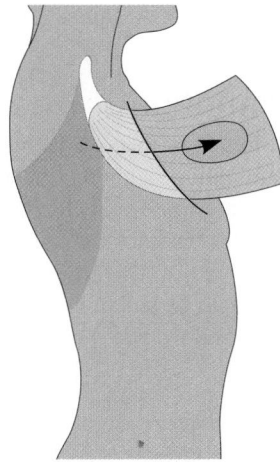

A Implant   **B** Latissimus dorsi musculocutaneous flap

Figure 51–10 ■ Types of breast reconstruction surgeries. *A*, A breast implant is inserted under the pectoris muscle. *B*, Autogenous procedures transfer a flap of skin, muscle, and fat from the donor site on the woman's body to the mastectomy site. The most frequently used donor muscle sites are the latissimus dorsi and the rectus abdominis (the TRAM flap).

ectomy for early stage (I or II) breast cancer. Palliative radiation therapy is also used to treat chest wall recurrences and some bone metastases to help control pain and prevent fractures. Radiation therapy is administered by means of an external-beam or tissue implants (see Chapter 10 ∞).

A new radiation treatment (*intraoperative radiotherapy*) is provided by a single, concentrated dose of radiation. During surgery, a probe is inserted into the cavity created by the lumpectomy and radiation equivalent to 6 weeks of doses is emitted for about 25 minutes. If this proves successful, the treatment could make lumpectomy available to more women and prevent the woman from having 6 weeks of daily radiation treatments following surgery.

NURSING CARE

Breast cancer is not one disease entity, but many, depending on the affected breast tissue, the tissue's estrogen dependency, and the age of the person at onset. The psychosocial impact of breast cancer extends beyond the fear and threat of death. The diagnosis may transform the woman's sense of self and lead to reintegration or negotiation

NURSING CARE OF THE WOMAN HAVING Breast Reconstruction

HEALTH EDUCATION FOR THE CLIENT AND FAMILY

- Controversy exists about the health effects of silicone. While there is no conclusive evidence that silicone implants induce cancer or autoimmune disease, they are associated with hardening and pain due to contracture of the capsule around the implant. The implant may rupture, releasing silicone gel, or infection may occur. Saline-filled breast implants may be an alternative.
- Reconstruction can be done immediately after a mastectomy, or at any time later on. Some surgeons believe that delayed reconstruction offers better cosmetic results.
- Reconstructive surgery can create a natural looking breast that makes clothes fit better. Since it has no nerve endings, however, the reconstructed breast has no feeling or sensations.
- If a simple mastectomy is done, an implant approximately the same size as the other breast is placed under the pectoral muscle on the operative side. This creates a breast mound that closely resembles the natural breast in shape and softness. If the implant is placed over the pectoral muscle, a high degree of firmness may occur.

- With a simple mastectomy or modified radical mastectomy, a tissue expander may be used to replace the breast. The tissue expander is placed under the pectoral muscle and gradually expanded with saline injections every 2 to 3 weeks to stretch the overlying skin and create a pocket. After a period of time, usually 1 to 2 months, the tissue expander is exchanged for a saline implant.
- With more extensive surgery such as radical mastectomy, a flap of skin, fat, or muscle is transferred from a donor site to the operative area. A new nipple may be created by using tissue from the opposite nipple or from the inner thigh.
- Reconstructive surgery may require multiple surgeries, including all the risks associated with anesthesia. As the complexity of the procedures increases, so does the risk of complications such as infection.
- To decrease the risk of a fibrous capsule forming around the implant, it is important to perform breast massage as instructed.

of family relationships. A Nursing Care Plan for a woman with breast cancer is found below.

Health Promotion

The ACS recommends that all women conduct a monthly breast self-examination beginning at age 20, have a clinical breast examination every 3 years from ages 20 to 39 years, and have a clinical breast examination and mammogram each year starting at age 40 years.

All women should be taught to perform BSE monthly (Box 51–1). Premenopausal women should perform BSE 7 to 10 days from the first day of their menstrual period, because hormonal changes increase breast tenderness and lumpiness prior to menses. Postmenopausal women should choose one date of the month (for example, the first day of the month) for BSE.

Educational messages about breast cancer screening need to be culturally sensitive to the intended audience. Media campaigns promoting mammography often show young white women, an approach that has proved ineffective among women of color (see the Nursing Research box on the next page). By working with women of different races and cultures, nurses can help make breast cancer education more meaningful to women in these groups.

NURSING CARE PLAN   A Woman with Breast Cancer

Rachel Clemments is a 42-year-old mother of two, Sarah, age 12, and Jennifer, age 18. Because of a family history of breast cancer, she has been closely monitored (annual mammograms and clinical breast examination, monthly BSE, a needle aspiration biopsy with negative findings) for 4 years prior to her diagnosis. Mrs. Clemments discovers a lump in her left breast during her monthly BSE. An incisional biopsy reveals invasive lobular carcinoma in the left breast. Mrs. Clemments is debating whether to have reconstructive breast surgery. One of her greatest concerns is how her illness will affect her ability to support and care for her daughters. The breast cancer diagnosis seems part of the family legacy. She wonders, "When will it happen to Jennifer? To Sarah?"

ASSESSMENT

During the history, Laura Nelson, RN, the nurse admitting Mrs. Clemments, learns that her mother, two of her aunts, and one sister had been diagnosed with breast cancer. Her mother and one of the aunts died before age 45. Physical assessment findings include T 98.5°F (37.0°C), BP 110/62, P 65, R 14. Her weight is 120 lb (54 kg); she is 66 inches (168 cm) tall. Modified radical mastectomy is performed; histologic examination shows a 3-cm tumor; axillary node dissection shows that 4 of 16 lymph nodes are positive.

DIAGNOSES

- *Risk for Infection* related to surgical incision
- *Acute Pain* related to surgery
- *Disturbed Body Image* related to loss of breast
- *Decisional Conflict* about treatment, related to concerns about risks and benefits
- *Fear* related to disease process/prognosis

EXPECTED OUTCOMES

- Remain free of infection.
- Experience minimal pain or discomfort during her recovery.
- Maintain a positive body image, regardless of her decision about reconstruction.
- Evaluate the treatment options in relation to personal values and decide on a course of action.
- Identify the sources of her fear and demonstrate behaviors that may reduce fears.

PLANNING AND IMPLEMENTATION

- Teach her about hand washing and wound care.
- Assess her pain tolerance and administer analgesics as prescribed.

- Teach her to use caution when moving the arm on the operated side, to avoid lifting heavy objects, and to wear gloves when gardening.
- Encourage her to discuss her thoughts and feelings about her body changes.
- Suggest that she talk with a Reach to Recovery volunteer about her thoughts and feelings.
- Assess her interest in spiritual/religious support and refer if appropriate.
- Discuss the use of a temporary prosthesis and later the fitting of a permanent prosthesis (6 to 8 weeks after surgery), the need to be fitted by an experienced person, and insurance reimbursement for the prosthesis.
- Discuss the possibility of attending a breast cancer support group where she can draw on the experiences of other women who have undergone mastectomy, chemotherapy, or radiation.
- Encourage her to verbalize her fears about her own prognosis and about her daughters' future risk of breast cancer; assess the need/interest for referral to psychologic counseling.

EVALUATION

At discharge, Mrs. Clemments has no signs of physical complications and is looking forward to being at home with her daughters as temporary caregivers. Mrs. Clemments met with a Reach to Recovery volunteer, who brought her a temporary prosthesis and booklets about postmastectomy exercises, chemotherapy, and breast reconstruction. The volunteer also referred her to a local cancer support group. Mrs. Clemments has talked about her concerns related to breast reconstruction. "I want to avoid anything that would increase the risk of complications. The possibility of recurrence and my fear for my daughters' future health are more than enough to worry about."

CRITICAL THINKING IN THE NURSING PROCESS

1. What role could genetic counseling play in helping Mrs. Clemments and her daughters better understand the daughters' risk of breast cancer?
2. Describe the types of mastectomies and their implications for nursing care.
3. What medications might help minimize the side effects of chemotherapy?
4. Develop a plan of care for Mrs. Clemments for the nursing diagnosis *Disturbed Sleep Pattern*.
   See Evaluating Your Response in Appendix C.

BOX 51–1 Breast Self-Examination (BSE)

- Lie down on your back and place your right arm behind your head. (BSE should be done while lying down because this position spreads breast tissue evenly over the chest wall, making it easier to feel all the breast tissue.)
- Use the finger pads of the middle fingers on your left hand to feel for lumps in the right breast. Use overlapping dime-sized circular motions of the finger pads to feel the breast tissue.
- Use three different levels of pressure to feel all the breast tissue. Light pressure is needed to feel the tissue closest to the skin; medium pressure to feel a little deeper; and firm pressure to feel the tissue closest to the chest and ribs. A firm ridge in the lower curve of each breast is normal. Use each pressure level to feel the breast tissue before moving on to the next spot.

- Move around the breast in an up and down pattern starting at an imaginary line drawn straight down your side from the underarm and moving across the breast to the middle of the chest bone (sternum, breastbone). Be sure to check the entire breast area before going down until you feel only ribs and up to the neck or collar bone.
- Repeat the exam on your left breast, using the finger pads of your right hand.
- Stand in front of the mirror with your hands pressing firmly down on your hips. Look at your breasts for any changes in size, shape, contour, or dimpling.
- Examine your underarm while sitting or standing and with your arm only slightly raised.
- If you find any changes, see your healthcare provider as soon as possible.

Assessment

Collect the following data through the health history and physical examination (see Chapter 49 ∞). Further focused assessments are described with nursing interventions.

- *Health history:* Family history of breast cancer, breast changes, nipple discharge, use of HRT, personal history of breast cancer, previous diagnostic tests and treatment for cancer, menstrual history, pregnancies, alcohol intake, physical activity, dietary history.
- *Physical assessment:* Height and weight, breasts, lymph glands.

Nursing Diagnoses and Interventions

Although each woman has individual needs, nursing diagnoses prior to surgery are concerned with anxiety, decisional conflict,

grief, risk for infection, risk for injury, and disturbed body image over the loss of a breast. Because the typical hospital stay is short, usually 2 to 3 days, preoperative teaching is done on an outpatient basis.

Anxiety

The woman with breast cancer is often anxious about the diagnosis, the surgery, the outcome of surgery if nodal involvement is found, and the possible changes in sexual and family relationships. Studies show that young women with breast cancer, a growing population, are particularly vulnerable for anxiety and other psychosocial effects, as are their spouses and their children.

- Provide opportunities to express thoughts and feelings. In this process, the woman can name her fears. *Once the fears*

NURSING RESEARCH Evidence-Based Practice: Improve Diagnosis and Treatment of African American Women with Breast Cancer

Despite efforts to improve both the diagnosis and treatment of women with breast cancer, African American women die more often from breast cancer than other groups of women. It is believed that this statistic is the result of African American women's advanced stage of disease at diagnosis, primarily due to a delay in seeking treatment. Bradley (2005) conducted a study to examine the variables affecting delay in seeking treatment as well as the possible effects of worry about breast cancer manifestations in African American women that might delay seeking treatment. The researcher found that, although delay in some women does exist, one cannot assume that all African American women delay seeking treatment. The researcher recommended that the relationship between worry and delaying treatment for breast cancer in African American women be further studied.

IMPLICATIONS FOR NURSING

Nurses must consider multiple factors when considering what may or may not influence African American women from a delay in seeking diagnosis and treatment for breast cancer, including biologic characteristics and intra- and intercultural differences and similarities, as well as perceptions and health beliefs. It is important that nurses do not assume that a delay in seeking care exists, but rather make assessments and design interventions based on consideration of both individual and group cultural differences.

CRITICAL THINKING IN CLIENT CARE

1. What barriers to breast cancer screening in women of all races can you identify? Do you think these barriers differ based on culture, race, or socioeconomic level? Why or why not?
2. Are there barriers to breast cancer screening that might be unique to African American women? To Hispanic women? To Asian American women?
3. What type of questions would you include in a health assessment to identify women who may be worried about breast cancer, but have not sought diagnosis?

are named, the nurse may simply listen, educate, or dispel fears that stem from lack of understanding.

- Discuss with the woman her knowledge of breast cancer. *Assessing the woman's knowledge of breast cancer helps the nurse plan more effective teaching.*
- Encourage discussion relating to immediate concerns about resuming her life at home and the changes she must make. *Anticipatory guidance can help plan for and cope with changes in her life and relationships.*
- Explain the surgical procedure, including information about preoperative medications, anesthesia, and recovery. *Knowing what to expect helps to decrease anxiety.*
- Explain that it is normal to have decreased sensation in the surgical area. *Severed or damaged nerves reduce sensation.*

Decisional Conflict

The woman with breast cancer must make life-changing decisions about treatment within a relatively brief and highly stressful time. Her age, menopausal status, and stage of cancer are only some of the factors that affect her decisions. Culture, values, lifestyle, socioeconomic status, and self-esteem also are considered.

- Provide an opportunity for the woman to ask questions; answer questions as simply and directly as possible. Make eye contact and pay attention to body language. *During this time, the woman can process information and make informed decisions.*
- Focus on immediate concerns, and provide up-to-date written material for the woman to review. *Written material provides easy reference to information not processed immediately because of anxiety and stress.*
- Listen to the woman in a nonjudgmental manner during her decision-making process. *Nonjudgmental, empathic listening helps the woman process information and make informed decisions. Only she knows the context of her life.*
- If the woman wishes, provide opportunities for her to meet with other women who have had breast cancer surgery. *Not all women are ready to meet others in their situation, but opening the door to this resource is appropriate. The woman may choose to talk with these women after the surgery.*
- Facilitate a team approach with the surgeon, anesthesiologist, oncologist, plastic surgeon, and other health professionals. *Being the woman's advocate during this time of anxiety and decision making reduces the stress of coordinating multiple healthcare provider schedules.*

Anticipatory Grieving

Breast surgery, even lumpectomy, alters the appearance of the breast. This loss is expressed through grief.

- Listen attentively to expressions of grief and watch for nonverbal cues (failure to make eye contact, crying, silence). *Not all women will express grief clearly; sometimes unspoken grief is the most painful. Grief is relieved only when expressed in a nonthreatening environment.*

- Allow time to interact and do not rush interactions. *Taking time to be with the woman communicates caring.*
- Explain that it is normal to have periods of depression, anger, and denial after breast surgery. *All these feelings are appropriate expressions of grief.*
- If the woman wishes to do so, involve the partner in helping the woman cope with her grief. *Remember that the partner may also be grieving. Not all women want to share their grief, and not all partners are interested and supportive.*

Risk for Infection

Like any surgical client, the woman who has breast surgery is at risk for infection. Removal of lymph nodes and the presence of a draining wound increase the risk.

- Assess the surgical dressings for bleeding, drainage, color, and odor every 4 hours for 24 hours and document your findings. Circle any visible bleeding and drainage on the dressing as a baseline for subsequent assessment. *Excessive bleeding or drainage signals postoperative complications that may require emergency attention.*
- Observe the incision and IV sites for pain, redness, swelling, and drainage. Assess the drainage system for patency and adequate suction; note the color and amount of drainage. *Careful observation for any signs of infection is essential because the woman's immune system is compromised. IV catheters should be placed on the uninvolved side only.*
- Change dressings and IV tubing using aseptic technique. *Moist dressings and intravenous tubing provide sites for bacterial growth. Routine dressing and IV tubing changes using aseptic technique reduce the risk for infection.*
- Encourage a protein-rich diet. Discuss the woman's nutritional status with the dietitian and request a consultation for the woman. *Adequate nutrition promotes healing and boosts the immune system.*
- Teach the woman how to care for the drainage system, if present (clean the site, empty the device, and record the amount, color, and type of drainage). *The woman is often discharged prior to removal of the drainage system and dressings and needs teaching to provide self-care.*
- At discharge, teach the woman to watch for and report to her healthcare provider the manifestations of infection: fever, redness or hardness at the surgical site, or purulent drainage. *Any of these manifestations should be reported to the physician/surgeon. Knowing the signs and symptoms of infection prepares the woman to seek prompt treatment if infection occurs.*
- Explain that she may experience scaling, flaking, dryness, itching, rash, or dry desquamation of the skin, particularly after radiation therapy. *Impaired skin integrity increases the risk of infection.*
- Tell the woman to avoid deodorants and talcum powder on the affected side until the incision is completely healed. *These substances may irritate the skin and impede healing.*

Risk for Injury

Removal of the lymph nodes puts the woman at risk for injury and long-term complications such as lymphedema and infection.

- When obtaining blood pressure and starting IVs, use the non-surgical side. *Compression of the arm on the surgical side may cause lymphedema.*
- Elevate the affected arm higher than the shoulder on a pillow, but do not abduct it; the hand should be higher than the elbow. *Elevating the arm permits drainage, prevents swelling, and promotes circulation.*
- Encourage range-of-motion exercises in the affected arm. *Exercise helps develop collateral drainage.*
- Explain that lymphedema massage and an elastic compression bandage may help control the swelling after she has recovered from surgery. *It is important that women know about the resources available after recovery.*

Disturbed Body Image

Breast surgery can change the woman's body image. The surgical changes may be compounded by weight gain and other side effects of chemotherapy or hormone therapy. Self-esteem also affects adjustment to a changed body image.

- Assess how the woman views her body. Discuss with the woman what image of herself she had prior to surgery. *Self-image is related to self-esteem. Discuss whether her self-image has changed.*
- Explain that redness and swelling in the scar will fade with time. *The knowledge that the scar will fade may give the woman a more realistic view of the changes.*

> **PRACTICE ALERT**
> Offer referral to support groups with women experiencing similar problems. Some women may prefer one-on-one counseling.

- Include the partner and family if possible when discussing the plan of care and activities of daily living (ADLs). Request consultation with a psychologist or other professional if the woman is interested. *Discussion with the partner and family can facilitate the woman's emotional healing process.*
- Offer pamphlets and suggest books and videos that might increase knowledge about what lies ahead. *Knowing what to expect can help the woman cope.*
- Encourage the woman to look at her incision when she feels ready; often the reality is not as frightening as the woman had imagined. Explain that it is normal to be afraid to look. *Reassurance that her behavior is normal decreases anxiety.*
- If the woman is interested in breast reconstruction, provide written material and encourage her to talk with a plastic surgeon and with women who have had reconstruction. *It is important for the woman to be fully informed about available options to make an informed decision.*

Using NANDA, NIC, and NOC

Chart 51–3 shows links between NANDA nursing diagnoses, NIC, and NOC when caring for the woman with breast cancer.

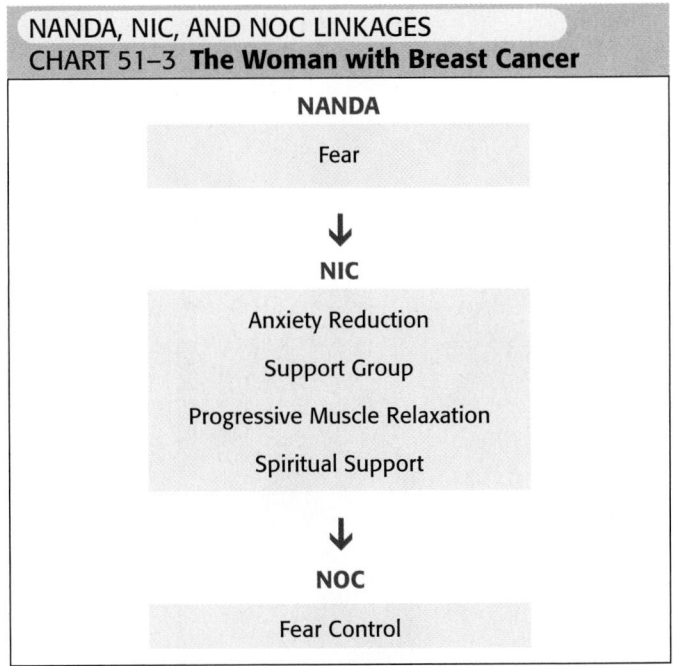

NANDA, NIC, AND NOC LINKAGES
CHART 51–3 The Woman with Breast Cancer

NANDA

Fear

↓

NIC

Anxiety Reduction

Support Group

Progressive Muscle Relaxation

Spiritual Support

↓

NOC

Fear Control

Data from *NANDA's Nursing Diagnoses: Definitions & Classification 2005–2006* by NANDA International (2003), Philadelphia; *Nursing Interventions Classification (NIC)* (4th ed.) by J. M. Dochterman & G. M. Bulecheck (2004), St. Louis, MO: Mosby; and *Nursing Outcomes Classification (NOC)* (3rd ed.) by S. Moorhead, M. Johnson, and M. Maas (2004), St. Louis, MO: Mosby.

Community-Based Care

The woman with breast cancer and her family have much to learn to provide self-care at home. Address the following topics in preparation for home care:

- Manifestations of infection and the need to report any that occur to her healthcare provider
- The importance of ADLs, such as eating, combing her hair, and washing her face
- Postmastectomy exercises and lymphedema care (Figure 51–11 ■) as discussed with physicians and physical therapists
- The need for adequate rest and emotional support
- Participation in a breast cancer support group and online information services and bulletin boards for sources of education and support
- Prosthesis management, if this option is chosen (A temporary lightweight prosthesis may be worn immediately after the drains and sutures have been removed from the surgical site. Because prostheses are expensive, a permanent one should not be purchased until the wound has completely healed. Prostheses are available at medical stores and many larger department stores. Most private and government insurance policies pay for the first prosthesis.)
- Helpful resources:
  - Reach to Recovery
  - American Cancer Society
  - National Breast Cancer Coalition
  - National Lymphedema Network.

Figure 51–11 ■ Postmastectomy exercises. *A*, Wall climbing: Stand facing wall with toes 6 to 12 inches from wall. Bend elbows and place palms against wall at shoulder level. Gradually move both hands up the wall parallel to each other until incisional pulling or pain occurs. (Mark that spot on wall to measure progress.) Work hands down to shoulder level. Move closer to wall as height of reach improves. *B*, Overhead pulley: Using operated arm, toss 6-foot rope over shower curtain rod (or over top of a door that has a nail in the top to hold the rope in place for the exercise). Grasp one end of rope in each hand. Slowly raise operated arm as far as comfortable by pulling down on the rope on opposite side. Keep raised arm close to your head. Reverse to raise unoperated arm by lowering the operated arm. Repeat. *C*, Rope turning: Tie rope to door handle. Hold rope in hand of operated side. Back away from door until arm is extended away from body, parallel to floor. Swing rope in as wide a circle as possible. Increase size of circle as mobility returns. *D*, Arm swings: Stand with feet 8 inches apart. Bend forward from waist, allowing arms to hang toward floor. Swing both arms up to sides to reach shoulder level. Swing back to center, then cross arms at center. Do not bend elbows. If possible, do this and other exercises in front of mirror to ensure even posture and correct motion.

EXPLORE MediaLink

Prentice Hall Nursing MediaLink DVD-ROM
Audio Glossary
NCLEX-RN® Review

Animation
Premenstrual Syndrome

COMPANION WEBSITE www.prenhall.com/lemone
Audio Glossary
NCLEX-RN® Review
Care Plan Activity: Postoperative Hysterectomy Care
Case Studies
   Breast Cancer
   Endometriosis
Teaching Plans
   Breast Cancer
   Mammogram
MediaLink Applications
   Pap Smears
   Post-Menopause Dietary Recommendations
Links to Resources

CHAPTER HIGHLIGHTS

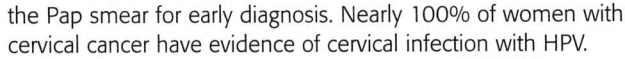

- Disorders of female sexual function include dyspareunia, inhibited sexual desire, and orgasmic dysfunction. Nurses should be able to obtain a sexual history, discuss sexual concerns, and make appropriate referrals without embarrassment.

- Menopause, a normal physiologic event in the life span of a woman, is the permanent cessation of menses. Loss of estrogen results in widespread tissue changes and increases the risk for osteoporosis, fractures, and cardiovascular disease.

- Menstrual disorders encompass PMS, dysmenorrhea, and abnormal uterine bleeding. Nursing interventions are focused on teaching about good health practices and interventions to relieve manifestations. Interdisciplinary care includes a therapeutic D&C and hysterectomy.

- Uterine displacement and vaginal fistulas are structural disorders. Uterine displacements may be treated surgically or with a pessary, and may include teaching Kegel exercises to minimize urinary leakage. Fistulas may spontaneously resolve if small, or may be surgically repaired.

- There are both benign and malignant disorders of female reproductive tissue, including cysts or polyps, leiomyomas, endometriosis, and cancers of the cervix, endometrium, ovaries, and vulva.

- Leiomyomas (fibroid tumors) are benign tumors that originate from smooth muscle of the uterus. Treatment depends on the size and location of the tumors. Both leiomyomas and endometrial implants (benign implants of endometrial tissue in the pelvic cavity) may interfere with the ability to have a child and are reduced in size after menopause.

- Cervical cancer is a common female reproductive system cancer, but the incidence and mortality has been greatly reduced with the Pap smear for early diagnosis. Nearly 100% of women with cervical cancer have evidence of cervical infection with HPV.

- Endometrial cancer is the most frequently diagnosed pelvic cancer in the United States. The major manifestation is abnormal, painless vaginal bleeding (menorrhagia or metrorrhagia in menstruating women). Postmenopausal women should have annual pelvic examinations and report any unexpected vaginal bleeding to their healthcare provider.

- Ovarian cancer increases in incidence with aging; seen most often in women over age 65. In early stages, there are generally no warning signs.

- Benign breast disorders in women include fibrocystic changes and intraductal disorders. Both treatment and nursing care are primarily symptomatic.

- Breast cancer is the most commonly occurring cancer in women and the second leading cause of death in women in the United States. A strong genetic link has been identified, as have a large number of risk factors. Early diagnosis is possible with breast self-examination, clinical breast examination, and mammograms. Treatment includes surgery (one of several types of mastectomy, lumpectomy), radiation therapy, and chemotherapy. Both combination therapies and immunotherapy are proving to be effective in suppressing tumor growth and facilitating longer life. Among other problems, mastectomy and radiation therapy interfere with lymph drainage on the affected side, leading to lymphedema of the arm.

- Appropriate preoperative nursing diagnoses for the woman with breast cancer include anxiety and fear, decisional conflict, and anticipatory grieving. Following surgery, interventions focus on risk for infection, risk for injury, pain, and disturbed body image.

TEST YOURSELF NCLEX-RN® REVIEW

1 During a health assessment at a local clinic, a woman in her 50s tells you that she is having some pain with intercourse. You are uncomfortable discussing this topic with her. What would you say?
1. "I know this can be a problem; please discuss it with your physician."
2. "I don't know anything about that; please ask someone else."
3. "Do you normally enjoy sexual activity?"
4. "What do you think is causing your problem?"

2 Long-term estrogen deprivation results in an increased risk for physical disorders. What are these? (Select all that apply.)
1. colon cancer
2. osteoporosis
3. cardiovascular disease
4. fractures
5. cervical cancer

3 You are conducting an educational seminar for postmenopausal women. When discussing calcium intake, you recommend _____mg per day.

4 An intervention for the woman with a uterine displacement disorder is to teach Kegel exercises. These exercises may help reduce:
1. stress incontinence.
2. menorrhagia.
3. vaginal discharge.
4. retroversion.

5 Which of the following topics would you include in a health-promotion seminar to reduce the risk of cervical cancer?
1. weight loss
2. safer sex methods
3. yearly mammograms
4. a diet high in iron

6 When discussing dietary guidelines with a woman with PMS you recommend she reduce her sodium intake. What is the rationale for this recommendation?

1. Sodium increases reactive hypoglycemia, increasing physical manifestations.
2. Sodium increases thirst, thereby facilitating increased oral fluid intake.
3. In and of itself, sodium is not harmful but it may increase cancer risk.
4. Sodium restriction helps minimize fluid retention.

7 What happens to endometrial implantations after menopause?
1. They tend to become malignant.
2. They tend to atrophy and disappear.
3. The number of implants increases.
4. Each implant enlarges.

8 You are designing a teaching plan for home care for a woman who had an abdominal hysterectomy. What interventions should be included? (Select all that apply.)
1. Restrict heavy lifting for 4 to 6 weeks.
2. Take tub baths until bleeding has stopped.
3. Report an increase in temperature or severe pain.
4. Take regular rest periods.
5. Avoid coughing and deep breathing at home.

9 Of the following women, which one would be most at risk for breast cancer?
1. age 23, two children
2. age 33, never pregnant
3. age 45, very thin
4. age 64, positive family history

10 You are caring for a woman who is scheduled to have a mastectomy for breast cancer. She is crying. What would be an appropriate nursing diagnosis?
1. *Disturbed Body Image*
2. *Fatigue*
3. *Anticipatory Grieving*
4. *Risk for Injury*

See Test Yourself answers in Appendix C.

BIBLIOGRAPHY

Abernathy, K. (2005). Guiding women through menopause—the role of the nurse. *Nurse 2 Nurse, 4*(11), 36–38, 40.

About Women's Health. (2005). *Causes and treatments for menstrual cramps.* Retrieved from http://womenshealth.about.com/cs/crampsmenstrual/a/cramps.htm

Albaugh, J., & Kellog-Spadt, S. (2003). Sexuality and sexual health: The nurse's role and initial approach to patients. *Urologic Nursing, 23*(3), 227–228.

American Cancer Society. (2006a). *Cancer facts & figures 2006.* Atlanta: Author.

_____. (2006b). *HPV vaccine recommended for girls aged 11–12.* Retrieved from http://www.cancer.org

_____. (2006c). *Pap test.* Retrieved from http://www.cancer/org

_____. (2006d). *Role of breast self-examination changes in guidelines.* Retrieved from http://www.cancer.org.docroot/NWS/content/NWS_1_1x_Role_Of_Breast_Self-Examination_Changes_I . . .

_____. (2006e). *What are the risk factors for breast cancer?* Retrieved from http://www.cancer.org/docroot/CRI/content/CRI_what_are_the_risk_factors_for-breast_cancer . . .

Andrist, L., Hoyt, A., Weinstein, D., & McGibbon, C. (2004). The need to bleed: Women's attitudes and beliefs about menstrual suppression. *Journal of the American Academy of Nurse Practitioners, 16*(1), 31–37.

Association of Reproductive Health Professionals. (2005a). *Mature sexuality: Disorders of desire and alternative approaches.* Retrieved from http://www.arhp.org/healthcareproviders/onlinepublications/clinicalproceedings.cfm?ID=178

_____. (2005b). *Physiology of the perimenopause: Treatment options.* Retrieved from http://www.arhp.org/healthcareproviders/onlinepublications/clinicalproceedings.cfm?ID=177

Ausk, K., & Reed, S. (2004). Alternative approaches for treatment of uterine leiomyomas. *Alternative Therapies in Women's Health, 6*(9), 65–70.

Ballantyne, P. (2004). Social context and outcomes for the aging breast cancer patient: Considerations for clinical practitioners. *Journal of Clinical Nursing, 13*(3a); *International Journal of Older People Nursing,* 11–21.

Black Women's Health Imperative. (2005). *Deadlier form of cancer found in black women.* Retrieved from http://www.blackwomenshealth.org/site/News2?page=NewsArticle&id=6644&news_iv_ctrl=1201

Bradley, P. (2005). The delay and worry experience of African American women with breast cancer. *Oncology Nursing Forum, 32*(2), 243–249.

Buxton-Blake, P. (2003). Recognizing menopausal symptomatology. *Home Health Care Management & Practice, 15*(2), 147–151.

Centers for Disease Control and Prevention. (2004). *To be or not to be—on hormone replacement therapy.* Retrieved from http://www.ced.golv/nccdphp/hrt.htm

_____. (2005a). *Breast cancer and mammography information.* Retrieved from http://www.cdc.gov/cancer/nbccedp/info-bc.htm

_____. (2005b). *DES update home.* Retrieved from http://www.cdc.gov/des/

_____. (2005c). *2004/2005 Fact Sheet. Ovarian cancer: Facing the challenge.* Retrieved from http://www.cdc.gov/cancer/ovarian/about2004.htm

_____. (2005d). *Women's reproductive health: Hysterectomy.* Retrieved from http://www.ced.gov/reproductivehealth/WomensRH/Hysterectomy.htm

Coward, D. (2005). Lesson learned in developing a support intervention for African American women with breast cancer. *Oncology Nursing Forum, 32*(2), 261–266.

Dibble, S., Casey, K., Nussey, B., Israel, J., & Luce, J. (2004). Chemotherapy-induced vomiting in women treated for breast cancer. *Oncology Nursing Forum, 31*(1), Online Exclusive: E1–E8.

Dickerson, L., Mazyck, P., & Hunter, M. (2003). Premenstrual syndrome. *American Family Physician, 67*(8), 1743–1752.

Dochterman, J., & Bulechek, G. (2004). *Nursing interventions classification (NIC)* (4th ed.). St. Louis, MO: Mosby.

Donovan, H., & Ward, S. (2005). Representations of fatigue in women receiving chemotherapy for gynecologic cancers. *Oncology Nursing Forum, 32*(1), 113–116.

Endometriosis Association. (2005). *What is endometriosis?* Retrieved from http://www.endometriosisassn.org/endo.html

Endometriosis.org. (2005). *Frequently asked questions about endometriosis.* Retrieved from http://www.endometriosis.org/faq.html

Eversley, R., Estrin, D., Dibble, S., Wardlaw, L., Pedrosa, M., & Favila-Penney, W. (2005). Post-treatment symptoms among ethnic minority breast cancer survivors. *Oncology Nursing Forum, 32*(2), 250–256.

French, L. (2005). Dysmenorrhea. *American Family Physician, 71*(2), 233–235, 285–291.

Greifzu, S. (2004). Breast cancer. *RN, 67*(2), 36–40, 42, 45.

Gynecologic cancer. (2004). *Current Opinions in Oncology, 16*(5), 477–495.

Health & Science. (2006). *Study: Estrogen protects some from breast cancer.* Retrieved from http://cis.nci.nih.gov/fact/5_29.htm

How to treat troublesome fibroids. (2004). *Harvard Women's Health Watch, 12*(4), 4–6.

Institute of Medicine. (2004). *Saving women's lives: Strategies for improving breast cancer detection and diagnosis.* Retrieved from http://www.iom.edu/report/asp?id=20721

Jennings-Sanders, A., & Anderson, E. (2003). Older women with breast cancer: Perceptions of the effectiveness of nurse case managers. *Nursing Outlook, 51*(3), 108–114.

Kee, J. (2004). *Handbook of laboratory and diagnostic tests with nursing implications* (5th ed.). Upper Saddle River, NJ: Prentice Hall.

Keep lymphoedema at arms length. (2003). *Nursing Standard, 17*(49), 9.

Lemaire, G. (2004). More than just menstrual cramps: Symptoms and uncertainty among women with endometriosis. *Journal of Obstetric, Gynecologic and Neonatal Nursing, 33*(1), 71–79.

Lyons, M., & Shelton, M. (2004). Psychosocial impact of cancer in low-income rural/urban women: Phase II. *Online Journal of Rural Nursing and Health Care, 4*(2).

Martin, V. (2005). Straight talk about ovarian cancer. *Nursing, 35*(4), 36–41.

Mayo Clinic. (2004). *Premenstrual syndrome: Complementary and alternative medicines.* Retrieved from http://www.mayoclinic.com/invoke.cfm?objectid=95C74A46-ACOA-405D-AEC831A8CF4&dsect . . .

McCaffrey, R., & Youngkin, E. (2004). Sleep disturbances and remedies for perimenopausal and postmenopausal women. *Clinical Excellence for Nurse Practitioners, 8*(4), 194–202.

McCook, J., Reame, N., & Thatcher, S. (2005). Health-related quality of life issues in women with polycystic ovary syndrome. *Journal of Obstetric, Gynecologic, and Neonatal Nursing, 34*(1), 12–20.

Moorhead, S., Johnson, M., & Maas, M. (2003). *Nursing outcomes classification (NOC)* (3rd ed.). St. Louis, MO: Mosby.

Muscari, E. (2004). Lymphedema: Responding to our patients' needs. *Oncology Nursing Forum, 31*(5), 905–912.

NANDA International. (2005). *Nursing diagnoses: Definitions & classification 2005–2006.* Philadelphia: Author.

National Cancer Institute. (2005a). *Herceptin combined with chemotherapy improves disease-free survival for patients with early-stage breast cancer.* Retrieved from http://www.cancer.gov/newscenter/pressreleases/HerceptinCombination2005=05=28

_____. (2005b). *Study shows link between antibiotic use and increased risk of breast cancer.* Retrieved from http://www.cancer.gov/newcenter/pressreleases/Antibiotics

North American Menopause Society. (2005). *Menopause practice: A clinician's guide.* Retrieved from http://www.menopause.org/edumaterials/cliniciansguide/cliniciansguidetoc.htm

Oakley, E., Buchtel, D., Atanosian, R., & Millar, A. (2004). Relationship of urinary incontinence to hysterectomy and episiotomy. *Journal of the Section on Women's Health, 28*(3), 23–30.

O'Connell, E. (2005). Mood, energy, cognition, and physical complaints: A mind/body approach to symptom management during the climacteric. *Journal of Obstetric, Gynecologic, and Neonatal Nursing, 34*(2), 274–279.

Painful periods should always be investigated. *Nursing Times, 100*(15), 13–19.

Patient notes: Fibrocystic breast disease. (2003). *Postgraduate Medicine, 114*(4), 79–80.

Porth, C. M. (2005). *Pathophysiology: Concepts of altered health states* (7th ed.). Philadelphia: Lippincott.

Stenchever, M. (2003). Diagnosing endometrial pathology in women with postmenopausal bleeding. *ACOG Clinical Review, 8*(2), 10–11.

Tierney, L., McPhee, S., & Papadakis, M. (Eds.). (2004). *Current medical diagnosis & treatment* (43rd ed.). Stamford, CT: Appleton & Lange.

What you need to know about...amenorrhoea. *Nursing Times, 100*(37), 34.

Wilkinson, J. (2005). *Prentice Hall nursing diagnosis handbook with NIC interventions and NOC outcomes* (8th ed.). Upper Saddle River, NJ: Prentice Hall.

Wilson, B., Shannon, M., & Stang, C. (2005). *Prentice Hall nurse's drug guide 2005.* Upper Saddle River, NJ: Prentice Hall.

Yarbo, C., Frogge, M., & Goodman, M. (2005). *Cancer nursing: Principles and practice* (6th ed.). Sudbury, MA: Jones & Bartlett.

CHAPTER 52 Nursing Care of Clients with Sexually Transmitted Infections

LEARNING OUTCOMES

- Explain the incidence, prevalence, characteristics, and prevention/control of sexually transmitted infections (STIs).

- Compare and contrast the pathophysiology, manifestations, interdisciplinary care, and nursing care of genital herpes, genital warts, vaginitis, chlamydia, gonorrhea, syphilis, and pelvic inflammatory disease.

- Explain the risk factors for and complications of STIs.

- Discuss the effects and nursing implications of medications and treatments used to treat STIs.

CLINICAL COMPETENCIES

- Assess functional health status of clients with STIs and monitor, document, and report abnormal manifestations.

- Determine priority nursing diagnoses and select and implement individualized nursing interventions for clients with STIs.

- Administer topical, oral, and injectable medications knowledgeably and safely.

- Integrate interdisciplinary care into care of clients with STIs.

- Provide teaching appropriate for prevention, control, and self-care of STIs.

- Revise plan of care as needed to provide effective interventions to promote, maintain, or restore functional health status to clients with STIs.

bacterial vaginosis, *1842*
candidiasis, *1842*
chancre, *1847*
chlamydia, *1844*
dyspareunia, *1844*

genital herpes, *1838*
genital warts, *1840*
gonorrhea, *1845*
pelvic inflammatory disease (PID), *1850*

sexually transmitted infections (STIs), *1837*
syphilis, *1846*
trichomoniasis, *1843*

Infections transmitted by vaginal, oral, and anal intimate contact and intercourse are referred to as **sexually transmitted infections (STIs)**. Infections transmitted by sexual intercourse are also labeled as *sexually transmitted diseases (STDs)* or *venereal diseases*. STIs also include systemic diseases (such as tuberculosis, hepatitis, and HIV/AIDS) that can be transmitted from an infected person to a partner. This chapter discusses STIs that involve the urogenital system. Vaginal infections are included in this chapter because they are also included in the CDC (2006) treatment guidelines.

OVERVIEW OF SEXUALLY TRANSMITTED INFECTIONS

Sexually transmitted infections include those caused by bacteria, *Chlamydiae*, viruses, fungi, protozoa, and parasites. Portals of entry for these agents of transmission include the mouth, genitalia, urinary meatus, anus, rectum, and skin. STIs have many consequences, and nurses have the responsibility of teaching sexually active clients how to prevent STIs, regardless of their gender, age, or sexual orientation. Nurses have a critical role in the prevention of STIs by teaching clients about these diseases, their prevention, treatment, and potential complications.

Incidence and Prevalence

STIs have reached epidemic proportions in the United States and are on the increase worldwide. They are the most frequent infections encountered by professionals in the field of reproductive health, and occur in more than half of all people at some point in their life (American Social Health Association [ASHA], 2005).

FAST FACTS
STIs
- More than 65 million people in the United States are estimated to have a viral STI; with 15 million new cases occurring each year.
- One in two sexually active persons will contract an STI by age 25.
- More than $8 billion is spent each year to diagnose and treat STIs and their complications. This figure does not include HIV.

Source: American Social Health Association (2005).

Women and infants are disproportionately affected by STIs. Many STIs are more easily transmitted from a man to a woman than from a woman to a man. Women often experience few early manifestations of the infection, delaying diagnosis and treatment. Furthermore, women are at greater risk for complications of STIs such as pelvic inflammatory disease (PID) and genital cancers.

Several factors help explain the escalating incidence of STIs. The so-called sexual revolution of the 1960s and 1970s, fueled by "the pill" and the freedom from unplanned pregnancy, led to a more permissive attitude about sexuality and increases in sexual activity and the number of sexual partners. In addition, since oral contraceptives were introduced to American women in 1961, they have replaced the condom as a birth control method for many couples. However, oral contraceptives do not protect against STIs, a fact of increasing importance.

STIs affect men and women of all ages, backgrounds, and socioeconomic levels. The incidence of STIs is highest in young adults ages 15 to 24 and in minorities. Drug abuse, unprotected sexual activity, and sexual activity with multiple partners also are associated with increased incidence of STIs (Blair, 2004). A further factor in the increasing incidence is that young people are becoming sexually active at an earlier age, marrying later, and divorce is more common. As a result, sexually active people today are more likely to have multiple sex partners in their lifetime and are potentially at risk for STIs (National Institute of Allergy and Infectious Diseases, 2003).

The emergence of HIV/AIDS has created a kind of "epidemiologic synergy" among all STIs. Other STIs, such as syphilis, herpes simplex virus (HSV), and chancroid, facilitate the transmission of HIV/AIDS, and the immune suppression caused by HIV potentiates the infectious process of other STIs. In fact, individuals who are infected with STIs are at greater risk of acquiring HIV if they are exposed to the virus. This is the result of several factors: Genital ulcers create a portal of entry for HIV, nonulcerative STIs increase the concentration of cells in genital secretions that can be targets for HIV, and infection with both an STI and HIV results in an increased likelihood of having HIV in genital secretions and semen.

Characteristics

Although STIs are caused by various organisms, they have several characteristics in common:
- Most can be prevented by the use of latex condoms.
- They can be transmitted during both heterosexual and homosexual activities, including non-penetrating intimate exposure.
- For treatment to be effective, sexual partners of the infected person must also be treated.
- Two or more STIs frequently coexist in the same client.

The complications of STIs in women include PID, ectopic pregnancy, infertility, chronic pelvic pain, neonatal illness and death, and genital cancer. Some bacterial STIs can be cured through appropriate early treatment with antibiotics. Others, such as genital herpes, are chronic conditions that can be managed but not cured because they are caused by viruses. The most serious STI is AIDS, which at this time is incurable. HIV/AIDS is discussed in Chapter 13 ∞. Treatment guidelines for STIs are updated regularly and are available from the Centers for Disease Control and Prevention.

Prevention and Control

The prevention and control of STIs is based on the principles of education, detection, effective diagnosis, and treatment of infected persons; and evaluation, treatment, and counseling of sex partners of people who are infected. The ability of the healthcare provider to obtain an accurate sexual history is essential to prevention and control efforts. One approach to collecting accurate information about key areas of interest has been summarized by the CDC (2006). They include the Five Ps: Partners, Prevention of Pregnancy, Protection from STIs, Practice, and Past History of STIs. Suggested questions to use are found on the CDC website.

The most effective way to prevent sexual transmission of HIV and other STIs is to avoid sexual intercourse with an infected partner. It is recommended that both partners be tested for STIs, including HIV, before beginning to have sexual intercourse. If a person chooses to have intercourse with an infected partner or one whose infection status is unknown, a new condom should be used for each act of intercourse. See Meeting Individualized Needs below for recommended STI barrier guidelines (CDC, 2006).

Prevention teaching for the person who is an injecting-drug user includes:

- Enroll or continue in a drug treatment program.
- Do not use injection equipment that has been used by another person. If equipment is shared, first clean the syringe and needle with bleach and water (to reduce the rate of HIV transmission).
- If needles can legally be obtained in the community, obtain and use clean needles.

Eliminating further transmission and reinfection of STIs is critical to control. For treatable STIs, this means that referral of sex partners for diagnosis, treatment, and counseling is essential. Gonorrhea, syphilis, and AIDS are reportable diseases in every state, and chlamydial infections are reportable in most states. When a healthcare professional refers infected clients to a local or state department of health, every effort is made to identify and contact sex partners. Reports of STI and HIV infections are maintained in strictest confidence, and are protected by law from subpoena. Suggested resources for people with STIs are listed in Box 52–1.

THE CLIENT WITH GENITAL HERPES

Genital herpes are caused by the herpes simplex viruses HSV-1 and HSV-2. Like most STIs, genital herpes are most commonly found in young, sexually active adults and are associated with early onset of sexual activity and multiple sexual partners. Approximately 50 million people ages 12 and older, or 1 out of every 5 teens and adults, have had genital HSV infections (CDC, 2006). There is no cure, and the treatments are primarily symptomatic.

BOX 52–1 Resources for Clients with STIs

- CDC National STD Hotline
- CDC National Prevention Information Network
- National Center for HIV, STD, and TB Prevention
- National HPV and Cervical Cancer Resource Center and Hotline
- National Herpes Hotline
- American Social Health Association

MEETING INDIVIDUALIZED NEEDS   STI Barrier Guidelines

Barrier Protection	Teaching Topics
■ Male condoms	✔ Use a new condom with each act of sexual intercourse.
	✔ Handle carefully to avoid damaging the condom.
	✔ Be sure no air is trapped in the end of the condom.
	✔ Put the condom on when the penis is erect and before genital contact with partner.
	✔ Ensure adequate lubrication exists during intercourse, using only water-based lubricants (e.g., K-y® Jelly, Astroglide®, AquaLube, and glycerine) and latex condoms. Oil-based lubricants, such as petroleum jelly, massage oil, mineral oil, or body lotions can weaken latex.
	✔ Ensure adequate lubrication during vaginal and anal sex.
	✔ Withdraw while the penis is erect and hold the condom firmly against the base of the penis during withdrawal.
■ Female condoms	✔ The female condom (Reality®) is a lubricated polyurethane sheath with a ring on each end that is inserted into the vagina. It is an effective mechanical barrier to viruses.
■ Vaginal spermicides, sponges, diaphragms	✔ Vaginal spermicides used alone without condoms do not reduce the risk for cervical gonorrhea, chlamydia, or HIV infection.
	✔ The diaphragm protects against cervical gonorrhea, chlamydia, and trichomoniasis, but not HIV.

Pathophysiology

One hundred types of HSV viruses have been identified, with more than 30 affecting the urogenital area. HSV-1 is associated with cold sores, but may be transmitted to the genital area by oral intercourse or by self-inoculation through poor hand washing practices. HSV-2 is transmitted by sexual activity or during childbirth from an infected woman, and is the virus that causes genital herpes. HSV infections begin with an exposure to the virus by contact with infectious lesions or secretions. The virus then moves into the stratified squamous epithelium, stimulating the replication of the epithelium and infecting the neurons that innervate the area. HSV viruses are neurotropic viruses, meaning that they grow in neurons and can maintain their disease potential even when there are no manifestations. The virus ascends through the peripheral nerves to the dorsal root ganglia, where it can remain dormant. For unknown reasons, the virus may reactivate and return to the nerve root of the skin, causing lesions. During dormancy, the virus is impervious to treatment. The incubation period ranges from 6 weeks to 8 months (Porth, 2005). Genital HSV-2 infection is more common in women (approximately one in four women) than it is in men (almost one of five) (CDC, 2004).

Manifestations

Within 2 to 10 days after exposure to the herpes virus, painful red papules appear in the genital area. In men, the lesions generally occur on the glans or shaft of the penis. In women, the lesions commonly occur on the labia, vagina, and cervix. Anal intercourse or oral-anal sexual contact may result in lesions in and around the anus.

Soon after the papules appear, they form small painful blisters filled with clear fluid containing virus particles (Figure 52–1 ■). The blisters break, shedding the highly infectious virus and creating patches of painful ulcers that last 6 weeks (or longer if they become infected). Touching these blisters and then rubbing or scratching in another place can spread the infection to other areas of the body (*autoinoculation*).

The first outbreak of herpes lesions is called *first episode infection*, with an average duration of 12 days. Subsequent oc-

currences, usually less severe, are termed *recurrent infections* (average duration of 4 to 5 days). The period between episodes is called *latency,* during which time the person remains infectious even though no symptoms are present. During latency, the virus withdraws into the nerve fibers that lead from the infected site to the lower spine, remaining dormant until recurrence, at which time it retraces its path to the genital area.

The manifestations of genital herpes are presented below. Prodromal symptoms of recurrent outbreaks of genital herpes can include burning, itching, tingling, or throbbing at the sites where lesions commonly appear. These sensations may be accompanied by pain in the legs, groin, or buttocks. Some authorities believe that prodromal symptoms signal increased levels of infectiousness, during which sexual contact should be avoided.

INTERDISCIPLINARY CARE

Presumptive diagnosis of genital herpes is based on history and physical examination of the client, including lesions and patterns of recurrence. Because there is no cure for genital herpes, treatment focuses on relieving symptoms and preventing spread of the infection. Client education is essential to prevent further transmission of the disease and to help clients integrate management of a chronic disease into their lifestyles.

Diagnosis

Definitive diagnosis requires isolation of the virus in tissue culture. Ideally, tissue specimens should be obtained within 48 hours of the appearance of the blisters. Diagnostic tests are described in Chapter 49 ∞.

Medications

Acyclovir (Zovirax) helps reduce the length and severity of the first episode and is the treatment of choice for genital herpes. The oral form is considered most effective for first episode as well as recurrences and is given for 7 to 10 days or until lesions heal. It may also be administered intravenously. Evidence shows that some strains of HSV are becoming resistant to acyclovir, particularly in HIV-positive people. In those cases, foscarnet (Foscavir) is used. Other antivirals used for treatment and prevention are valacyclovir (Valtrex) and famciclovir (Famvir).

Figure 52–1 ■ Genital herpes blisters as they appear on the labia.
Source: Biophoto Associates/Photo Researchers, Inc.

MANIFESTATIONS of Genital Herpes

- Herpetic lesions
- Regional lymphadenopathy
- Headache
- Fever
- General malaise
- Dysuria
- Urinary retention
- Vaginal discharge
- Urethral discharge (men)

NURSING CARE

In planning and implementing nursing care for the client with genital herpes, the nurse needs to consider both short-term and long-term implications. Although the immediate priority is symptom relief and prevention of further transmission, the client needs assistance to deal with the life-changing diagnosis of a chronic disease.

Nursing Diagnoses and Interventions

Nursing diagnoses discussed in this section focus on pain and sexual dysfunction.

Acute Pain

Herpetic lesions are very painful and can become infected. Because the virus resides in the nerve ganglia, pain may also occur in the legs, thighs, groin, or buttocks. Although acyclovir diminishes the pain of herpes and accelerates the healing process, additional measures can relieve the discomfort further.

- Teach how to keep herpes blisters clean and dry. A solution of warm water, soap, and hydrogen peroxide (if lesions are not open) can be used to cleanse the lesions two or three times daily. Burrow's solution (a liquid containing aluminum sulfate, acetic acid, precipitated calcium carbonate, and water) can also be used. Lesions should be dried using a hair dryer turned to a cool setting. It is important to wear loose cotton clothing that will not trap moisture; and to avoid wearing panty hose and tight jeans. *Keeping the lesions clean and dry reduces the possibility of secondary infection and speeds the healing process.*
- For dysuria, suggest pouring water over the genitals while urinating. Drinking additional fluids also helps dilute the acidity of the urine; however, fluids that increase acidity, such as cranberry juice, should be avoided. *These measures dilute the acid content of urine and thereby reduce the burning sensation.*
- Suggest the use of sitz baths (with tepid water) for 15 to 30 minutes several times a day. *The warm water is soothing and decreases pain from ulcers and an irritated urethral meatus. It also facilitates wound healing.*

Sexual Dysfunction

Clients who learn that they are infected with an incurable STI may believe they can no longer have a normal sex life. Fortunately, many people have learned to live with and manage genital herpes without infecting their partners or their children.

- Provide a supportive, nonjudgmental environment for the client to discuss feelings and ask questions about what this diagnosis means to future sexual relationships. *Feelings of guilt, shame, and anger are natural responses to such a diagnosis and can lead to a total avoidance of sexual intimacy.*
- Offer information about support groups and other resources for people with herpes such as the National Herpes Information Hotline. *Information about how others cope with this disease can offset feelings of shame and hopelessness.*

Community-Based Care

Health teaching for clients with genital herpes involves helping them manage this chronic disease with the least possible disruption in lifestyle and relationships. Understanding the disease process and factors that affect it helps the client regain a sense of control and see the potential for future sexual intimacy without transmission of infection. The following topics should be addressed:

- How to recognize prodromal symptoms of recurrence and factors that seem to trigger recurrences (such as emotional stress, acidic food, sun exposure)
- The need for abstinence from sexual contact from the time prodromal symptoms appear until 10 days after all lesions have healed
- If lesions become infected, use of topical acyclovir (Painful lesions can be protected with sterile petroleum jelly or aloe vera gel.)
- Use of latex condoms due to viral shedding at any time and careful hygiene practices (such as not sharing towels or other personal items) even during latency periods.

THE CLIENT WITH GENITAL WARTS

Genital warts (*condylomata acuminata*)**,** caused by the human papillomavirus (HPV) are the most common infectious genital infections in the United States, and are considered epidemic. Genital warts are chronic and, in many people, largely asymptomatic. Currently, they are incurable.

Women are at greater risk for HPV genital infections because they have a larger mucosal surface area exposed in the genital area. Most HPV infections are asymptomatic or unrecognized. An estimated 20 million Americans are infected with the virus, and up to 6.2 million new cases are diagnosed annually (CDC, 2006).

> **FAST FACTS**
> **Genital HPV Infection**
> - At least 50% of sexually active men and women acquire genital HPV infection at some point in their lives.
> - By age 50, at least 80% of women will have acquired genital HPV infection.
> - Most people with a genital HPV infection do not know they are infected; most women are diagnosed by abnormal Pap tests.
>
> *Source:* CDC (2004).

Although the majority of infected people are asymptomatic, others experience frequent recurrences. Other than recurrences, men are not likely to experience serious physical complications of genital warts. Women, however, face concerns about the increased risk of cervical cancer, with HPV DNA having been identified in almost all cervical cancers worldwide and in approximately 50% to 80% of vaginal, vulvar, and anogenital cancers (Porth, 2005).

Pathophysiology

Genital warts are caused by HPV and are transmitted by vaginal, anal, or oral–genital contact. The incubation period is 6 weeks to 8 months (Porth, 2005).

Manifestations

Although some people with HPV may not have manifestations, others exhibit characteristic lesions: single or multiple painless, soft, moist, pink or flesh-colored swellings in the vulvovaginal area, perineum, penis, urethra, anus, groin, or thigh (Figure 52–2). In women, the growths may be in the vagina or on the cervix and be apparent only during a pelvic examination.

The four types of genital warts are as follows:

- *Condyloma acuminata:* cauliflower-shaped lesions that appear on moist skin surfaces such as the vagina or anus
- *Keratotic warts:* thick, hard lesions that develop on keratinized skin such as the labia major, penis, or scrotum
- *Papular warts:* smooth lesions that also develop on keratinized skin
- *Flat warts:* slightly raised lesions, often invisible to the naked eye, that also develop on keratinized skin.

INTERDISCIPLINARY CARE

Treatment is directed at removal of the warts, relief of symptoms, and health teaching to reduce the risk of recurrence and future transmission. Infection with HPV is considered chronic; however, research has shown that for about 90% of women, cervical HPV becomes undetectable within 2 years (CDC, 2004).

Genital and anal warts are diagnosed primarily by clinical appearance. A HPV DNA test is specific for diagnosis in women. There are no HPV tests for men.

Medications

Topical agents used to treat genital warts include podofilox and imiquimod (both can be applied by the client) or podophyllin and trichloroacetic acid (provider-administered treatments). Podophyllin (Condylox, Podofin) is contraindicated during pregnancy and can have side effects in any client, ranging from nausea, diarrhea, and lethargy to paralysis and coma (see the Medication Administration box on the next page). Gardasil is a vaccine developed to prevent genital warts, precancerous genital lesions, and cervical cancer due to HPV. It is administered by 3 intramuscular injections given over a 6-month period. As HPV is so closely associated with cervical cancer, a federal advisory panel has recommended that the vaccine be targeted for females, aged 9 to 26. The vaccine does not protect against an existing HPV infection.

Other Treatments

Genital warts may also be removed by cryotherapy, electrocautery, laser vaporization, or surgical excision. Carbon dioxide laser surgery is becoming increasingly common for removal of extensive warts.

NURSING CARE

Health promotion activities for adults of all ages should include information about the causes, treatments, and prevention of HPV infections.

Nursing Diagnoses and Interventions

Nursing interventions are primarily directed toward problems with deficient knowledge, fear, and anxiety.

Deficient Knowledge

HPV is spread by contact with infectious lesions or secretions, with up to 70% of genital warts spread by people who do not know they have the infection. Although there is no known cure, it is essential to prevent secondary infections.

- Discuss the need for prompt treatment and the necessity for sexual abstinence until lesions have healed, or using a condom while lesions are present. *This reduces the risk of reinfection and further transmission of the disease. Some studies have found that using condoms promotes the regression of HPV lesions in both men and women (ASHA, 2005).*
- Discuss the increased risk of cervical cancer and the importance of an annual Pap smear. *Understanding the risk, the client will be more motivated to seek annual screening.*
- Stress the importance of thorough handwashing. *Handwashing is essential to prevent the spread of HPV.*

Figure 52–2 ■ Genital warts (condyloma acuminatum) on the A, vulva and B, penis.

MEDICATION ADMINISTRATION   The Client with Genital Warts

TOPICAL APPLICATIONS
Podophyllin
Trichloroacetic acid
Although cryotherapy using liquid nitrogen or a cryoprobe is more commonly used to treat genital warts, podophyllum preparations are sometimes used. Podophyllin is applied topically to the warts by the physician once weekly for 3 to 5 weeks.

Podophyllin is contraindicated during pregnancy; the alternative is cryotherapy. Podophyllin is also contraindicated in cervical, urethral, oral, or anorectal warts. It is important to avoid contact of podophyllin resin with the eyes.

Adverse effects of podophyllin include local irritation, severe ulceration of surrounding tissue, nausea, diarrhea, lethargy, paralysis, and coma.

Nursing Responsibilities
- Establish baseline data, including mental status, vital signs, and weight.

- Document and report any existing lesions (genital, anal, or oral).
- Cover the tissue surrounding the warts with petrolatum or a paste of baking soda and water to protect the tissue from the caustic treatment solution.

Health Education for the Client and Family
- Wash off the treated area thoroughly within 1 to 4 hours after the first application; gradually increase this period to 6 to 8 hours after the second and subsequent applications.
- Return for regular treatment until warts are gone.
- Refer partners for examination and any necessary treatment.
- Report any adverse effects (nausea, diarrhea, local irritation, lethargy, numbness)
- Avoid sexual activity until you and your partners have been free of disease for 1 month.
- Use condoms to prevent future infections.
- Return for an annual Pap smear.

Fear

Surgery engenders some degree of fear in most clients: fear of the procedure itself and of pain and possible complications. Surgery or cryotherapy in the genital area involves all of these fears plus fear of possible impaired sexual function.

- Allow the client to express specific fears and feelings about the procedure. Explain the procedure, approximate recovery time, possible complications and ways to avoid them, and ways to cope with complications that do occur. *Knowing what to expect reduces the client's fear and helps the client feel a greater sense of control.*
- Explain that the procedure is performed with a local anesthesia. *Being awake during surgery gives the client a greater sense of participation in the treatment process.*

Anxiety

The woman with an HPV infection faces an increased risk of infection of her neonate during delivery. The neonatal infection can range from asymptomatic to widely disseminated fatal disease. Transmission occurs during passage through the birth canal. The risk is highest during the first episode of infection.

- Discuss with women of childbearing age that cesarean delivery can prevent transmission of infection to the neonate. In women without manifestations of recurrence, vaginal delivery is possible. *Understanding that infection of the neonate can be prevented helps relieve anxiety.*

Community-Based Care

Health teaching emphasizes the need for the client and infected partners to return for regular treatment until lesions have resolved, and to use condoms to prevent reinfection. Because of the increased risk of cervical cancer, annual Pap smears are essential for female clients.

THE CLIENT WITH A VAGINAL INFECTION

The vagina may be infected by yeasts, protozoa, or bacteria. These infections can be sexually transmitted, but the male partner does not usually have manifestations of the infection. Risk factors include the use of hormonal contraceptives or broad-spectrum antibiotics, obesity, diabetes, pregnancy, unprotected sexual activity, and multiple sexual partners. Manifestations of vaginal infections are outlined in Table 52–1.

Preventive measures include educating women about personal hygiene practices and safer sex. Women need to avoid frequent douching and wearing nylon underwear and/or tight pants. Unprotected sexual activity, particularly with multiple partners, increases the risk of vaginal infections.

Pathophysiology and Manifestations

Alterations in pH, changes in the normal flora, and low estrogen levels are conducive to the development of vaginal infections. When conditions are favorable, microorganisms invade the vulva and vagina.

Bacterial Vaginosis

Bacterial vaginosis (nonspecific vaginitis) is the most common cause of vaginal infection in women of reproductive age. *Gardnerella vaginalis* is one of the causative organisms, but others are also implicated. The relationship of sexual activity to this infection is not clear. The primary manifestation is a vaginal discharge that is thin and grayish-white, and has a foul, fishy odor. Complications include PID, preterm labor, premature rupture of the membranes, and postpartum endometritis (Porth, 2005). The infection is treated with oral or intravaginal antibacterial agents.

Candidiasis

Candidiasis (moniliasis or yeast infection) is caused by the organism *Candida albicans*, which has several strains of dif-

TABLE 52–1 Vaginal Infections

INFECTION	TYPE OF DISCHARGE	TYPICAL MANIFESTATIONS	NURSING CARE
Candidiasis (*Monilia,* yeast)	Thick white patches adhering to cervix and vaginal wall, resembling cottage cheese; little odor	Itching of vulva and vaginal area, redness, painful intercourse	Teach perineal hygiene and proper use of vaginal applicators. Instruct the client to complete the entire treatment.
Simple vaginalis (bacterial vaginosis, *Gardnerella* vaginosis)	Thin, white, "milklike," or gray with fishy odor, especially when mixed with potassium hydroxide	None to mild itching or burning in vulvar area; clue cells on microscopic examination	Teach proper perineal hygiene. Instruct client to complete treatment. Teach client relationship of infection to PID.
Trichomoniasis	Frothy, yellow or white, foul odor	Burning and itching of vulva	Teach perineal hygiene.
Atrophic vaginitis (senile vaginitis)	Thin, opaque discharge, occasionally blood tinged, odorless; pale, smooth, thin, dry vaginal walls	Painful intercourse, itching, vaginal dryness	Counsel client on symptoms of menopause and sexual techniques to minimize trauma.

ferent virulence. Candida organisms are part of the normal vaginal environment in up to 50% of women (Porth, 2005), causing problems only when they multiply rapidly. When increased estrogen levels, antibiotics, diabetes mellitus, fecal contamination, or other factors alter the normal vaginal flora, the organism proliferates, resulting in a yeast infection. The manifestations include an odorless, thick, cheesy vaginal discharge. This is often accompanied by itching and irritation of the vulva and vaginadysuria, and dyspareunia (Figure 52–3 ■). Uncircumcised men may develop a yeast infection over the glans penis, manifested by itching and dysuria. The infection is treated with oral or intravaginal antifungal agents.

Figure 52–3 ■ Yeast infection on female genitalia.

Trichomoniasis

Trichomoniasis is caused by *Trichomonas vaginalis,* a protozoan parasite. It is the most common curable STI in young, sexually active women. An estimated 7.4 million new cases occur each year in both men and women (CDC, 2004). Symptoms usually appear in 5 to 28 days of exposure. It most commonly infects the vagina in women and the urethra in men. Most men are asymptomatic, but when symptomatic may complain of dysuria and urethral discomfort. Women have a frothy, green-yellow vaginal discharge with a strong fishy odor, often accompanied by itching and irritation of the genitalia. A woman with HIV who becomes infected has an increased risk of transmitting HIV to her sex partner. Trichomoniasis is treated with a single oral dose of metronidazole or tinidazole.

INTERDISCIPLINARY CARE

Interdisciplinary care focuses on identifying and eliminating the infection and preventing recurrence.

Diagnosis

Diagnostic tests vary with the suspected organism. Cervical cultures are examined to diagnose the causative organism. Trichomonas is identified by microscopically examining a specimen of vaginal discharge in saline. Ten percent potassium hydroxide is used to identify spores and filaments of candida. Diagnostic tests are described in Chapter 49 ∞.

Medications

The pharmacologic treatment varies with the organism as previously described. The sexual partner of a woman with a trichomonas infection must also be treated to prevent reinfection. Some antifungal agents are available without prescription, which can lead to self-medication with the incorrect agent or allow repeated infections to go unreported.

NURSING CARE

Nursing care focuses on teaching the client and, if necessary, her sexual partner to comply with the treatment regimen, use safer sex practices, and prevent future transmission of the infection. Careful history taking may also reveal high-risk sexual practices that require intervention, particularly if the client has had repeated infections. The initial presenting symptom for many HIV-positive women is vaginal candidiasis, which may not respond to over-the-counter treatments. Treatment with some antibiotics destroys normal vaginal flora, resulting in superinfection with yeast.

Nursing Diagnoses and Interventions

Although each nursing care plan must be individualized, nursing diagnoses that often apply to clients with vaginal infections are deficient knowledge and acute pain.

Deficient Knowledge

Many women are unaware of the causes of vaginal infections and the self-care measures to prevent and treat these infections. If possible, both the woman and her sexual partner should be taught the information.

- Explain the transmission of the infection. Many infections are transmitted most easily during menstruation; some can also be transmitted by towels or other inanimate objects, or by certain types of sexual activity. *A frank discussion of disease transmission and prevention with the woman and her partner can reduce the risk of reinfection.*
- The need to complete the course of treatment. *Many infections are asymptomatic in one partner. Incomplete treatment allows for recurrence of the infection and reinfection of the partner.*

Acute Pain

The symptoms of vaginitis can include dysuria, painful excoriation or ulceration of tissue, and painful intercourse (**dyspareunia**). Often these symptoms can be relieved by relatively simple self-care measures. See Box 52–2 for additional comfort measures.

- Suggest the use of cool compresses. *Cool compresses relieve itching.*
- Recommend sitz baths to alleviate discomfort. *Sitz baths cleanse the perineal area and the warmth is soothing to inflamed, irritated skin and membranes.*
- Wear cotton underwear. *Cotton absorbs moisture and allows better air circulation than other types of material.*
- If infected with trichomonas avoid sexual contact until treatment is completed. *Treatment of the infected woman and her partner as well as sexual abstinence are necessary to facilitate healing and to prevent reinfection.*

Community-Based Care

Teaching focuses on eradicating the infection, preventing further disease transmission, and relieving discomfort associated with the condition. Educating the client and her partner(s) about safer sex and improved genital hygiene practices can reduce the incidence of recurrence.

BOX 52–2 Self-Care Comfort Measures

- Do not wear panty hose; wear loose fitting pants or skirts.
- Double-rinse underwear; do not use fabric softener on underwear.
- Do not use bubble bath, perfumed soaps, or feminine hygiene products.
- Use 100% cotton menstrual pads and tampons.
- Use white, unscented toilet paper.
- Use a water-soluble lubricant for intercourse.
- Apply ice or a frozen blue gel pack wrapped in a towel to the vulva after intercourse to relieve burning.
- Rinse vulva with cool water after voiding and intercourse.

THE CLIENT WITH CHLAMYDIA

Chlamydia are a group of STIs, caused by *Chlamydia trachomatis,* a bacterium that behaves like a virus, reproducing only within the host cell. The bacterium is spread by any sexual contact and to the neonate by passage through the birth canal of an infected mother. The infections caused by chlamydia include acute urethral syndrome, nongonococcal urethritis, mucopurulent cervicitis, and PID.

Chlamydia is the most commonly reported bacterial STI in the United States, affecting an estimated 2 to 3 million people each year (CDC, 2004). Of that number, three of every four reported cases occurred in people under age 25. Risk factors for chlamydia are listed in Box 52–3.

Because chlamydia is asymptomatic in most women until the uterus and fallopian tubes have been invaded, treatment may be delayed, resulting in devastating long-term complications. Nearly a third of men with urethral chlamydia are also asymptomatic. Chlamydia is a leading cause of preventable blindness in the newborn.

Pathophysiology

Chlamydia trachomatis is an intracellular bacterial pathogen that resembles both a virus and a bacteria. The organism enters the body as an elementary body, a form in which it is capable of entering uninfected cells. The infection begins when the organism enters a cell and changes into a reticulate body. The reticulate body divides within the cell, bursting the cell and infecting adjoining cells.

Manifestations

The incubation period is from 1 to 3 weeks; however, chlamydia may be present for months or years without producing no-

---

BOX 52–3 Risk Factors for Chlamydial Infection

- Personal or partner history of STI
- Pregnancy
- Adolescent sexual activity
- Oral contraceptive use
- Unprotected sexual activity
- Multiple sexual partners

ticeable symptoms in women. Chlamydia typically invades the same target organs as gonorrhea (cervix and male urethra) and results in similar manifestations (dysuria, urinary frequency, and discharge). Clients may be asymptomatic; however, they are still potentially infectious.

Complications

If a chlamydial infection in women is not treated, it ascends into the upper reproductive tract, causing such complications as PID, which includes endometritis and salpingitis. Chronic pelvic pain may result. These infections are a major cause of infertility and ectopic pregnancy, a potentially life-threatening disorder in women. Complications of chlamydial infections in men include epididymitis, prostatitis, sterility, and Reiter's syndrome. Routine screening for sexually active adolescents and young adults has been suggested by the CDC to minimize these serious complications in asymptomatic people (Porth, 2005).

INTERDISCIPLINARY CARE

C. trachomatis is treated with medications to eradicate the infection. Its prevalence, particularly in younger populations, makes widespread screening necessary if the disease is to be controlled. Because chlamydia is often asymptomatic, treatment is often begun on a presumptive basis.

Diagnosis

The diagnostic tests that may be ordered include Gram stain of discharge from the female endocervix and urethra or from the male urethra to look for poly-morphonuclear leukocytes (considered evidence of infection).

Tests for antibodies to chlamydia such as the direct fluorescent antibody (DFA) test and an enzyme-linked immunosorbent assay (ELISA), as well as polymerase chain reaction (PCR) or ligase chain reaction (LCR) tests, are highly sensitive and specific tests performed on cervical and urethral swab specimens. However, nucleic acid amplification tests (NAATs), also performed on cervical and urethral swab specimens, have become the diagnostic method of choice (Porth, 2005).

Medications

The antibiotic recommended by the CDC for chlamydial infections in men and nonpregnant women is azithromycin (Zithromax), orally in a single dose, or doxycycline (Adoxa, Apo-Doxy), orally for 7 days. Both sexual partners must be treated at the same time or prior to resuming sexual intercourse.

NURSING CARE

Nursing care of the client with chlamydia focuses on eradication of the infection, prevention of future infections, and management of any chronic complications. Nursing diagnoses for the client with chlamydia are the same as for clients with any STI. Interventions are similar to those discussed later in the chapter for gonorrhea and previously for genital herpes.

Community-Based Care

Health teaching for the client with chlamydia centers on the need to comply with the treatment regimen, refer partners for examination and necessary treatment, and the use of condoms to avoid reinfection. If the infection has progressed to PID (discussed later), the client needs additional information on self-care and health promotion. The CDC recommends annual screening for chlamydia for clients who are young, sexually active, and do not use condoms correctly with every act of sexual intercourse.

THE CLIENT WITH GONORRHEA

Gonorrhea, also known as "GC" or "the clap," is caused by *Neisseria gonorrhoeae,* a gram-negative diplococcus. Gonorrhea is the most common *reportable* communicable disease in the United States. The CDC (2004) estimates that approximately 700,000 new cases occur annually, with the rate of reported gonorrhea increasing.

Gonorrhea rates for African Americans are 30% higher than for non-Hispanic whites. Other risk factors include residence in large urban areas, being transients, early onset of sexual activity, multiple serial or consecutive sex partners, drug use, prostitution, and previous gonorrheal or concurrent STI infection.

Pathophysiology

The causative organism of gonorrhea is a pyogenic (pus-forming) bacteria that causes inflammation characterized by purulent exudate. Humans are the only host for the organism. Gonorrhea is transmitted by direct hetero- and homosexual intercourse and during delivery as the neonate passes through the birth canal. The portal of entry can be the genitourinary tract, eyes, oropharynx, anorectum, or skin. The incubation period is 2 to 7 days after exposure. The organism initially targets the female cervix and the male urethra. Without treatment, the disease ultimately disseminates (spreads widely) to other organs. In men, gonorrhea can cause acute, painful inflammation of the prostate, epididymis, and periurethral glands and can lead to sterility. In women, it can cause PID, endometritis, salpingitis, and pelvic peritonitis.

Manifestations

Manifestations of gonorrhea in men include dysuria and serous, milky, or purulent discharge from the penis. Some men also experience regional lymphadenopathy. About 20% of men and 80% of women remain asymptomatic until the disease is advanced. Women with symptoms experience dysuria, urinary frequency, abnormal menses (increased flow or dysmenorrhea), increased vaginal discharge, and dyspareunia.

Anorectal gonorrhea is seen most often in homosexual men. The manifestations include pruritus, mucopurulent rectal discharge, rectal bleeding and pain, and constipation. Gonococcal pharyngitis occurs primarily in homosexual or bisexual men or heterosexual women after oral sexual contact (fellatio) with an infected partner. The manifestations include fever, sore throat, and enlarged lymph glands.

Complications

The complications of untreated gonorrhea in both men and women may be permanent and serious. They include:

- PID in women, leading to internal abscesses, chronic pain, ectopic pregnancy, and infertility
- Blindness, infection of joints, and potentially lethal infections of the blood in the newborn, contracted during delivery
- Epididymitis and prostatitis in men, resulting in infertility and dysuria
- Spread of the infection to the blood and joints
- Increased susceptibility to and transmission of HIV.

INTERDISCIPLINARY CARE

The goals of treatment for the client with gonorrhea include eradication of the organism and any coexisting disease, and prevention of reinfection or transmission. It is important to emphasize the importance of taking all medications as prescribed and abstaining from sexual contact until the infection is cured in both client and partners. Condom use to prevent future infections is essential, particularly for pregnant women whose partners may be infected.

Diagnosis

Diagnosis of gonorrhea is based on cultures from the infected mucous membranes (cervix, urethra, rectum, or throat), examination of urine from an infected person, and a Gram stain to visualize the bacteria under the microscope. Testing for other STIs (especially chlamydia and syphilis) at the same time is recommended. Pregnant women are routinely screened during their first prenatal visit. Diagnostic tests are described in Chapter 49 ∞.

Medications

Because of the many penicillin-resistant strains of *N. gonorrhoeae,* an alternative antibiotic, such as ciprofloxacin (Cipro) or ofloxacin (Floxin), is used to treat gonorrhea. Fluoroquinolone therapy (such as with ciprofloxacin or levofloxacin) is often prescribed because it is inexpensive, oral, and single dose. However, because of increased prevalence of fluoroquinolone-resistant *N. gonorrhoeae* in Asia, the Pacific Islands, and California, this therapy is no longer recommended for use in treating gonorrhea in those areas. A single dose of oral azithromycin (Zithromax) or a 7-day course of oral doxycycline (Vibramycin, Vivox) usually is added to treat any coexisting chlamydial infection. All sexual partners within 60 days before diagnosis of the infection also need to be treated.

NURSING CARE

In planning and implementing care for the client with gonorrhea, the nurse considers the possible coexistence of other STIs such as syphilis and HIV, the impact of the disease and its treatment on the client's lifestyle, and the likelihood of noncompliance. A Nursing Care Plan for the client with gonorrhea is on page 1847.

Nursing Diagnoses and Interventions

Nursing diagnoses discussed in this section focus on noncompliance and impaired social interaction.

Noncompliance

Although one-time treatment with the recommended antibiotic is highly effective in curing gonorrhea, noncompliance with the doxycycline regimen may leave any coexisting chlamydial infection unresolved. Noncompliance with recommendations for abstinence, follow-up, or condom use fosters a high rate of reinfection. Failure to refer partners for examination and treatment also leads to reinfection.

- Reinforce the need to take all medications as directed and keep follow-up appointments to be sure no reinfection has occurred. Discuss the prevalence of gonorrhea and the potential complications if it is not cured. *The client who understands the complications of incomplete or failed treatment is more likely to comply with the medication regimen.*
- Discuss the importance of sexual abstinence until the infection is cured, referral of partners, and condom use to prevent reinfection. *Understanding that cure is possible and reinfection is avoidable helps the client cope with the disease and its treatment and is likely to increase compliance*
- Explain to women that condoms must be used during treatment, even if other methods of birth control are used. *Oral contraceptives increase the alkalinity of the vaginal pH, facilitating the growth of the gonococcal bacteria, and intrauterine devices alter the endometrial barrier, favoring persistent gonococcal infections (Blair, 2004).*

Impaired Social Interaction

Diagnosis of any STI can make clients feel "dirty," ashamed, and guilty about their sexual behaviors, and unworthy to be with others.

- Provide privacy, confidentiality, and a safe, nonjudgmental environment for expression of concerns. Help the client understand that gonorrhea is a consequence of sexual behavior, not a punishment, and that it can be avoided in the future. *Being treated with respect and privacy helps the client realize that the disease does not change an individual's worth as a person. This knowledge enhances the client's ability to relate to others.*

Community-Based Care

Health teaching focuses on helping clients understand the importance of (1) taking any and all prescribed medication, (2) referring sexual partners for evaluation and treatment, (3) abstaining from all sexual contact until the client and partners are cured, and (4) using a condom to avoid transmitting or contracting infections in the future. Clients also need to understand the need for a follow-up visit 4 to 7 days after treatment is completed.

THE CLIENT WITH SYPHILIS

Syphilis is a complex systemic STI caused by the spirochete *Treponema pallidum,* and it can infect almost any body tissue or organ. It is transmitted from open lesions during any sexual

NURSING CARE PLAN **A Client with Gonorrhea**

Janet Cirit, a 33-year-old legal secretary, lives in a suburban Midwestern community. She is unmarried but dating a man named Jim Adkins, who lives in an adjacent suburb. Ms. Cirit visits her gynecologist because her periods have become irregular and she is experiencing pelvic pain and an abnormal amount of vaginal discharge. Recently she has developed a sore throat. The pelvic pain has begun to disrupt her sleeping pattern, and she is concerned that she might have cancer because her mother recently died of ovarian cancer.

ASSESSMENT

When Ms. Cirit arrives for her appointment at the gynecologist's office, Marsha Davidson, the nurse practitioner, interviews her. Ms. Davidson completes a thorough medical and sexual history, including questions about her menstrual periods, pain associated with urination or sexual intercourse, urinary frequency, most recent Pap smear, birth control method, history of STI and drug use, and types of sexual activity. Ms. Cirit reports her symptoms and her concern about ovarian cancer. She also indicates that she is taking oral contraceptives and therefore sees no need for her boyfriend to use a condom because she believes their relationship is monogamous.

Physical examination reveals both pharyngeal and cervical inflammation, and lower abdominal tenderness. Her temperature is 98.5°F (37.0°C). There are no signs or symptoms of pregnancy.

The gynecologist orders a Pap smear and cultures of the cervix, urethra, and pharynx to evaluate for gonorrhea and chlamydial infection. Blood is drawn for WBC. Test results are positive for gonorrhea and negative for chlamydia. The WBC is slightly elevated, indicating possible salpingitis. Because Mr. Adkins has been Ms. Cirit's only sexual partner, it is clear that he is the source of infection and needs to be treated as well.

DIAGNOSES

- *Acute Pain* related to the infectious process
- *Anxiety* related to fear about possible cancer
- *Situational Low Self-Esteem* related to shame and guilt because of having an STI

- *Ineffective Sexuality Patterns* related to the impaired relationship and fear of reinfection

EXPECTED OUTCOMES

- Experience relief of pain, indicating that the infection has been eradicated.
- Verbalize that she has nothing to be ashamed of and that she has been wise to seek treatment as soon as symptoms occurred.
- Verbalize that she will insist her partner use condoms during future sexual activity.

PLANNING AND IMPLEMENTATION

- Administer ceftriaxone IM as ordered.
- Emphasize the need for regular Pap smears and pelvic examinations because of the family history of ovarian cancer.
- Discuss feelings and concerns about the diagnosis of gonorrhea. Stress that such a diagnosis does not reflect on one's self-worth as a person.
- Teach how to talk with a future sexual partner about condom use.

EVALUATION

A week later during her follow-up visit. Ms. Cirit states that she is feeling much better and sleeping well at night since the pain has ended. She has terminated her relationship with Mr. Adkins and is considering joining a health club in the hope of increasing her level of fitness and perhaps meeting someone new.

CRITICAL THINKING IN THE NURSING PROCESS

1. How are Ms. Cirit's manifestations related to the infectious process of gonorrhea?
2. Should the nurse have suggested that Ms. Cirit also be tested for HIV? Why or why not?
3. Develop a care plan for Ms. Cirit for the nursing diagnosis *Impaired Social Interaction*.
   See Evaluating Your Response in Appendix C.

---

contact (genital, oral–genital, or anal–genital). The organism is highly susceptible to heat and drying, but can survive for days in fluids; thus, it may also be transmitted by infected blood or other body fluid such as saliva. The incubation period ranges from 10 to 90 days, averaging 21 days. If not treated appropriately, syphilis can lead to blindness, paralysis, mental illness, cardiovascular damage, and death. Syphilis often occurs with one or more other STIs, such as HIV/AIDS or chlamydial infection.

Although in 1996 the rate of syphilis infection reached its lowest level in many years, it remains a significant problem in certain geographic regions, and among specific populations such as African Americans. Rates also remain high in many urban centers, with higher infection rates found in drug users, transients, and the homeless. The incidence of primary and secondary syphilis is highest in people 20 to 39 years of age, with the incidence in women decreasing. However, the rate of syphilis among men having sex with men (MSM) is increasing (CDC, 2004).

Pathophysiology

Any break in the skin or mucous membrane is vulnerable to invasion by the spirochete. Once it has entered the system, the spirochete is spread through the blood and lymphatic system. Congenital syphilis is transferred to the fetus through the placental circulation.

Manifestations

Syphilis is generally characterized by three clinical stages: primary, secondary, and tertiary. Each stage has characteristic manifestations (see the box on page 1848). The client with syphilis also may experience a latency period when no signs of the disease are evident.

Primary Syphilis

The primary stage of syphilis is characterized by the appearance of a **chancre** (Figure 52–4 ■) and by regional enlargement of lymph nodes; little or no pain accompanies these warning signs. The chancre appears at the site of inoculation (such as the genitals,

MANIFESTATIONS of Syphilis

REPRODUCTIVE

Primary
- Genital chancre (may be internal in female)

Secondary
- Condyloma lata

INTEGUMENTARY SYSTEM

Secondary
- Rash on palms of hands and soles of feet

Tertiary
- Granulomatous lesions involving mucous membranes and skin

GASTROINTESTINAL SYSTEM

Secondary
- Anorexia
- Oral mucous patches

NEUROLOGIC SYSTEM

Secondary
- Asymptomatic
- Headache
- Meningitis
- Cranial neuropathies

Tertiary
- Asymptomatic
- Neurosyphilis
- Personality changes, hyperactive reflexes, Argyll Robertson pupil, decreased memory, slurred speech, optic atrophy
- Tabes dorsalis
- Seizures, hemiparesis, hemiplegia

MUSCULOSKELETAL SYSTEM

Secondary
- Arthralgia
- Bone and joint arthritis
- Myalgia
- Periostitis

Tertiary
- Gummas

CARDIOVASCULAR SYSTEM

Tertiary
- Aortic insufficiency
- Aortic aneurysm
- Stenosis of openings to coronary arteries

RENAL SYSTEM

Secondary
- Glomerulonephritis
- Nephrotic syndrome

OTHER

Primary
- Regional lymphadenopathy

Secondary
- Generalized lymphadenopathy
- Fever
- Malaise
- Hepatitis
- Alopecia

anus, mouth, breast, fingers) 3 to 4 weeks after the infectious contact. In women, a genital chancre may go unnoticed, disappearing within 4 to 6 weeks. In both primary and secondary stages, syphilis remains highly infectious, even if no symptoms are evident.

Secondary Syphilis

Manifestations of secondary syphilis may appear any time from 2 weeks to 6 months after the initial chancre disappears. These symptoms can include a skin rash, especially on the palms of the hands or soles of the feet, mucous patches in the oral cavity; sore throat; generalized lymphadenopathy; condyloma lata (flat, broad-based papules, unlike the pedunculated structure of geni-

tal warts) on the labia, anus or corner of the mouth; flulike symptoms; and alopecia. These manifestations generally disappear within 2 to 6 weeks, and an asymptomatic latency period begins.

Latent and Tertiary Syphilis

The latent stage of syphilis begins 2 or more years after the initial infection and can last up to 50 years. During this stage, no symptoms of syphilis are apparent, and the disease is not transmissible by sexual contact. It can be transmitted by infected blood, however; thus, all prospective blood donors must be screened for syphilis. In two-thirds of all cases, the latent stage persists without further complications. Unless treated, the remaining one-third of infected people progress to late-stage or tertiary syphilis. In the presence of HIV infection, disease progression seems to be more rapid.

Two types of late-stage syphilis occur. Benign late syphilis, of rapid onset, is characterized by localized development of infiltrating tumors (*gummas*) in skin, bones, and liver, generally responding promptly to treatment. Of more insidious onset is a diffuse inflammatory response that involves the central nervous system and the cardiovascular system. Though the disease can still be treated at this stage, much of the cardiovascular and central nervous system damage is irreversible.

INTERDISCIPLINARY CARE

The goals of treatment are to inactivate the spirochete and educate the client about how to prevent reinfection or further transmission. Treatment includes antibiotic therapy and identi-

Figure 52–4 ■ Chancre of primary syphilis on the penis.

fication and referral of partners for testing and treatment if necessary, follow-up testing, and education about condom use to prevent reinfection of self and transmission of disease to partners. In addition, clients should be screened for chlamydial infection and advised to have an HIV test.

Diagnosis

Diagnosis of syphilis is complex because it mimics many other diseases. A careful history and physical examination are obtained, as well as laboratory evaluations of lesions and blood. Diagnostic tests are described in Chapter 49 ∞.

The VDRL (Venereal Disease Research Laboratory) and RPR (rapid plasma reagin) blood tests measure antibody production. People with syphilis become positive about 4 to 6 weeks after infection. However, these tests are not specific for syphilis, and other diseases may also cause positive results. Additional tests are required for definitive diagnosis.

The FTA-ABS (fluorescent treponemal antibody absorption) test is specific for *T. pallidum* and can be used to confirm VDRL and RPR findings. It may be used for clients whose clinical picture indicates syphilis but who have negative VDRL results. In immunofluorescent staining a specimen is obtained from early lesions or aspiration of lymph nodes and is specially treated and examined microscopically for the presence of *T. pallidum*. Darkfield microscopy involves examining a specimen from the chancre for the presence of *T. pallidum* using a darkfield microscope.

Medications

The treatment of choice for all stages of syphilis in adults is penicillin G, given intramuscularly (IM) in a single dose. Clients allergic to penicillin are given oral doxycycline or tetracycline for 28 days.

Treatment of syphilis may result in a severe reaction called the *Jarisch-Herxheimer reaction,* involving fever, musculoskeletal pain, tachycardia, and sometimes hypotension. This is not a reaction to the penicillin itself, but to the sudden and massive destruction of spirochetes by the penicillin and the resulting release of toxins into the bloodstream. The Jarisch-Herxheimer reaction generally begins within 24 hours of treatment and subsides in another 24 hours. Treatment should not be discontinued unless symptoms become life threatening.

NURSING CARE

In planning and implementing nursing care for the client with syphilis, the nurse needs to consider the client's age, lifestyle, access to health care, and educational level. Although each client has individualized needs, nursing diagnoses for the client with syphilis would be the same as for any client with an STI. A Nursing Care Plan for a client with syphilis is on the next page.

Nursing Diagnoses and Interventions

Nursing diagnoses discussed in this section focus on risk for injury, anxiety, and self-esteem.

Risk for Injury

If syphilis is not diagnosed and treated promptly and effectively, it can have devastating effects on all body systems, particularly the neurologic and cardiovascular systems, eventually leading to a painful death.

- Teach the importance of taking any prescribed medication. *Taking the prescribed antibiotic is important to ensure eradication of the infecting organism.*
- Encourage referral of any sexual partners for evaluation and any necessary treatment. *Without treatment of both partners, reinfection can occur or the disease may be transmitted to other people through sexual activity.*
- Teach abstinence from sexual contact until client and partners are cured and to use condoms to prevent future infections. *Abstinence until the organism is eradicated prevents reinfection. Condoms provide barrier protection, reducing the risk of infection during sexual activity.*
- Emphasize the importance of returning for follow-up testing at 3- and 6-month intervals for early syphilis, and 6- and 12-month intervals for late latent syphilis. *Follow-up testing is performed to ensure eradication of the disease.*
- Provide information about manifestations of reinfection. *Successful treatment of the disease does not prevent possible subsequent infections.*

Anxiety

The diagnosis of syphilis understandably causes the client anxiety, not only about personal well-being but about the well-being of partners and, in the expectant woman, her fetus.

- Emphasize that syphilis can be effectively treated, preventing the serious complications of late-stage disease. *This information provides a sense of control and helps decrease anxiety.*
- Teach the pregnant client that taking medications as directed and returning each month for follow-up testing will help ensure the well-being of her baby. *Knowing that treatment can reduce the risk to her baby relieves anxiety and possibly increases compliance.*

Low Self-Esteem

Living with any chronic disease can be damaging to a person's self-esteem. However, the client with syphilis needs additional support to cope with the stigma of this kind of infection. Unfortunately, the populations most affected by STIs often lack family and other social support networks.

- Create an environment where the client feels respected and safe to discuss questions and concerns about the disease and its effect on the client's life. *Being treated with respect helps enhance self-esteem.*
- Provide privacy and confidentiality. *Clients are often embarrassed to discuss the intimate details of their sex lives.*
- Let clients know that the nurse and other healthcare providers care about them and the successful treatment of their disease. *Feeling valued enhances self-esteem.*

Community-Based Care

Education is an essential part of nursing care for the client with any STI, and syphilis is no exception. The nurse emphasizes that

NURSING CARE PLAN **A Client with Syphilis**

Eddie Kratz, age 22, works as bellman at a large hotel. For the past year, he has shared a small apartment with Maria Jones, who is 5 months pregnant with his child. Although he intends to marry Ms. Jones before the baby is born, he has continued a previous relationship with a woman named Justine Simpson. His sexual activities with Ms. Simpson have increased in frequency as Ms. Jones's pregnancy has advanced. Recently Mr. Kratz has noticed a swelling in his groin and a sore on his penis.

ASSESSMENT

When Mr. Kratz comes to the community clinic, he is interviewed by the NP, Sally Morovitz. She takes a thorough medical and sexual history, including questions about drug use, allergies, difficulty with urination, urinary frequency, itching or discharge from the penis, recent sexual activities, precautions taken against infection, history of STIs, and sexual function. She determines that Mr. Kratz has been having unprotected sex with both Ms. Jones and Ms. Simpson. He believes that Ms. Jones is not having sex with anyone except him, but he is not sure.

Physical assessment reveals a classic syphilitic chancre on the shaft of the penis and regional lymphadenopathy. A specimen of exudates from the chancre is sent for darkfield examination. Ms. Morovitz discusses with Mr. Kratz the likelihood that he has syphilis and the need to tell both Ms. Jones and Ms. Simpson so that they can be tested and, if necessary, treated. Ms. Morovitz also suggests that Mr. Kratz be tested for HIV since he has been having unprotected sex with two women, at least one of whom may be sexually active with other partners. He agrees, and blood is drawn for an ELISA test. Darkfield analysis of the chancre exudate confirms the diagnosis of syphilis; the ELISA results are negative for HIV.

DIAGNOSES

- *Risk for Injury* to the client, his partners, and the infant, related to the disease process
- *Ineffective Health Maintenance* related to a lack of knowledge about the disease process, its transmission, and the need for treatment
- *Interrupted Family Processes* related to the effects of the diagnosis of syphilis on the couple's relationship
- *Anxiety* related to the effects of the infection on the unborn child

EXPECTED OUTCOMES

- Prompt treatment will cure the syphilis.

- Verbalize understanding for the need to abstain from sexual contact during treatment, complete all medications, return for follow-up visits, and use condoms to prevent reinfection.
- Verbalize ability to cope with the effect of diagnosis and treatment on the relationship.
- Verbalize decreased anxiety following education and treatment.

PLANNING AND IMPLEMENTATION

- Administer IM injection of penicillin G as ordered.
- Discuss the importance of abstaining from sexual activity until he and his partners are cured, and of using condoms to prevent reinfection.
- Explain the need to return for follow-up testing in 3 months and again at 6 months. Provide a copy of the STI prevention checklist, and document that reminders need to be sent at 3- and 6-month intervals.
- Notify sexual partners that they need to come to the clinic for testing.
- Refer to a social worker for counseling about the effect of the disease on their relationship.
- Teach the couple about the importance of treatment to the health of their infant.

EVALUATION

At the 3-month follow-up visit, the chancre on Mr. Kratz's penis has healed, and he reports that he is using a condom any time he has sex. Ms. Jones has also tested positive for syphilis and negative for HIV, so she, too, is given penicillin G, and verbal and written follow-up instructions, including follow-up until the infant is born. The couple is meeting every other week with the social worker and say that their relationship is improving. Ms. Simpson has received similar test results and is given a prescription for doxycycline because she is allergic to penicillin.

CRITICAL THINKING IN THE NURSING PROCESS

1. What manifestations might a client with early syphilis experience?
2. List some appropriate questions for taking a sexual history when you suspect the presence of one or more STIs.
3. How might you counsel Mr. Kratz to help him break the news of the diagnosis to Ms. Jones?

See Evaluating Your Response in Appendix C.

---

syphilis is a chronic disease that can be spread to others even though no symptoms are evident. Address the following topics:

- Taking all prescribed medication
- Referring sexual partners for evaluation and treatment
- Abstaining from all sexual contact as recommended by CDC guidelines
- Using a condom to avoid transmitting or contracting infections in the future
- The need for follow-up testing (at 3 and 6 months for clients with primary or secondary syphilis, and at 6 and 12 months for those with late-stage disease). If clients are HIV positive,

follow-up visits are recommended 1, 2, 3, 6, 9, and 12 months after treatment.

THE CLIENT WITH PELVIC INFLAMMATORY DISEASE

Pelvic inflammatory disease (PID) is a term used to describe infection of the pelvic organs, including the fallopian tubes (*salpingitis*), ovaries (*oophoritis*), cervix (*cervicitis*), endometrium (*endometritis*), pelvic peritoneum, and the pelvic vascular system. PID can be caused by one or more infectious agents, including *Neisseria gonorrhoeae, Chlamydia trachomatis, Escherichia coli,* and *Mycoplasma hominis. N. gonorrhoeae* and *C. trachomatis* are responsible for as much as 80% of PID; dual infection with both agents is common.

PID is not a reportable disease in the United States; however, it is estimated that about 1 million women experience PID each year. As a result of the infection, more than 100,000 women become infertile and a large proportion of the ectopic pregnancies occurring each year are the result of PID (CDC, 2004). The disease may also cause pelvic abscesses and chronic abdominal pain.

Sexually active women ages 16 to 24 years are most at risk. Risk factors include a history of sexually transmitted infection (especially gonorrhea and chlamydia), bacterial vaginosis, multiple sexual partners, douching, and previous PID. Barrier contraceptive devices such as condoms reduce the risk of PID.

The prognosis depends on the number of episodes, promptness of treatment, and modification of risk-taking behaviors. Prevention includes educating women, especially young women, regarding the causes and transmission of infection and methods of self-protection, such as avoiding unprotected sexual activity.

Pathophysiology

Pelvic inflammatory disease is usually polymicrobial (caused by more than one microbe) in origin, with gonorrhea and chlamydia being common causative organisms. Pathogenic microorganisms enter the vagina and travel to the uterus during intercourse or other sexual activity. They can also gain direct access to the uterus during childbirth, abortion, or surgery of the reproductive tract. The organisms ascend from the endocervical canal to the fallopian tubes and ovaries.

Manifestations

Manifestations of PID include fever, purulent vaginal discharge, severe lower abdominal pain, and painful cervical movement. However, the manifestations may be so mild that the infection is not recognized.

Complications

Complications include pelvic abscess, infertility, ectopic pregnancy, chronic pelvic pain, pelvic adhesions, dyspareunia, and chronic pelvic pain. Abscess formation is common.

INTERDISCIPLINARY CARE

The goals of treatment are to eliminate the infection and prevent complications and recurrence. The physical examination may reveal abdominal, adnexal, and cervical pain.

Diagnosis

Tests used in the diagnosis of PID may include a CBC with differential, which will show a markedly elevated WBC, and an increased sedimentation rate. If a laparoscopy or laparotomy is done, it may reveal inflammation, edema, or hyperemia of the fallopian tubes, or tubal discharge and, possibly, generalized pelvic involvement, abscesses, and scarring.

Medications

Combination antibiotic therapy with at least two broad-spectrum antibiotics administered IV or orally is the typical treatment for PID. If PID is not acute, outpatient antibiotic therapy is prescribed. In acute cases, however, the client may be hospitalized. Analgesics are given, and antibiotics and fluids are administered intravenously. Commonly prescribed antibiotics include parental cefoxitin (Mefoxin), or clindamycin (Cleocin), plus gentamicin (Garamycin) or doxycycline (Vibramcin). Nursing implications for antibiotics are discussed in Chapter 12 ∞.

Surgery

The surgeon may insert a drain into an abscess, if present, and remove any adhesions. If the client does not respond to conservative therapy, surgical removal of the uterus, fallopian tubes, and ovaries may be necessary.

NURSING CARE

The goals of nursing care are to treat the infection and to prevent complications, such as scarring and infertility. The client who is hospitalized maintains bed rest in the semi-Fowler's position to promote drainage and to localize the infectious process in the pelvic cavity.

Nursing Diagnoses and Interventions

Nursing diagnoses that apply to the client with PID include a risk for injury and deficient knowledge.

Risk for Injury

PID can have severe, even life-threatening, complications. Scarring of fallopian tubes can lead to ectopic pregnancy or pelvic abscess. Infertility is a common complication, as are recurrent or chronic PID, chronic abdominal pain, pelvic adhesions, premature hysterectomy, and depression. The woman who has severe infection and manifestations may be hospitalized for treatment.

- Administer antibiotic therapy as ordered, and monitor closely for adverse effects. *Antibiotics used in acute PID are potent agents; some can have serious side effects.*
- Practice thorough hand washing and strict adherence to universal precautions when handling perineal pads and linens. Appropriate disinfection of bedpans, toilet seats, linens, and utensils is also important. *These practices help avoid disseminating the infection to others.*

Deficient Knowledge

PID is most common in young women, who often do not understand their own anatomy and physiology or sexually transmitted infections. Diagnosis and treatment of PID offer an opportunity to increase that understanding, thereby preventing complications and recurrent infection.

- Explain how infection is spread and what measures to take to prevent future infection. *Understanding can improve compliance with treatment regimens and perhaps change high-risk behavior.*

- Explain the need to complete the treatment regimen and the importance of follow-up visits. If the client or partner fails to take all of the medication as prescribed, the infection may not be completely cured. *Noncompliance and recurrence are common, particularly if follow-up appointments are not kept.*
- Teach proper perineal care, especially wiping from front to back. *This reduces transmission of fecal organisms to reproductive tissues and reduces the incidence of urinary tract infections.*
- Caution the client about using tampons. Instruct the client to change tampons or pads at least every 4 hours. *Menstrual flow and other discharges provide a favorable environment for microorganisms to multiply.*
- Provide information about safer sex practices and family planning. Instruct the client to remove diaphragms within 6

hours after use. IUDs are contraindicated. Latex condoms offer the most effective protection against infection. *These measures help prevent recurrence of infection.*
- Teach the client to report any unusual vaginal discharge or odor to the healthcare provider. *Treatment is most effective early in the disease process.*

Community-Based Care

Provide general information related to sexually transmitted infections. Teach measures to eradicate the infection and prevent recurrence, and help the client deal with the physical and psychosocial implications of treatment, including possible infertility. Inform the client that the patency of the fallopian tubes can be evaluated after several menstrual cycles; this delay allows for complete resolution of the inflammatory process.

EXPLORE MediaLink

 Prentice Hall Nursing MediaLink DVD-ROM
    Audio Glossary
    NCLEX-RN® Review

    Animation
       Gonorrhea

 COMPANION WEBSITE www.prenhall.com/lemone
    Audio Glossary
    NCLEX-RN® Review
    Care Plan Activity: Gonorrhea
    Case Studies
       Pelvic Inflammatory Disease
       Syphilis
    Teaching Plans
       Risk of Cancer with HPV
       Singles and Safer Sex
    MediaLink Applications
       HPV
       HPV Prevention
    Links to Resources

CHAPTER HIGHLIGHTS

- Sexually transmitted infections (STIs) are infections transmitted by sexual contact, including vaginal, oral, and anal intercourse. STIs affect women and infants more than men, and are more common in people who have multiple sex partners, abuse drugs, and are of lower socioeconomic status.
- STIs can coexist in the same person and can be transmitted by either heterosexual or homosexual sexual contact. Effective treatment mandates that both sex partners be treated. Most STIs can be prevented by using latex condoms.
- Genital herpes, caused by an infection with an HSV virus, is a commonly occurring STI in teens and young adults. There is no cure and treatment is primarily symptomatic. Nursing care is directed toward relieving the pain of the lesions, mitigating sexual dysfunction, and relieving anxiety.
- Genital warts, caused by the human papilloma virus (HPV), are a chronic, incurable STI. They are manifested by warts of various forms, or may be present without manifestations. Infection with

HPV poses a major risk for cervical cancer. A vaccine against the virus is recommended.
- Urogenital infections include vaginal infections (bacterial vaginosis, candidiasis, and trichomoniasis), chlamydia, gonorrhea, syphilis, and pelvic inflammatory disease (PID).
- Chlamydia, occurring most in young adults under age 25, is a bacterial infection that can spread to the uterus and fallopian tubes in women, causing PID, infertility, and ectopic pregnancy. Untreated chlamydia in men may result in epididymitis, prostatitis, sterility, and Reiter's syndrome.
- Gonorrhea (caused by a bacteria) and syphilis (caused by a spirochete) affect both men and women, and may infect the newborn as it moves through the birth canal in an untreated woman. Syphilis, if untreated, exists in the body in three stages, with the third stage lasting up to 50 years. Both of these STIs are treated with antibiotics. Nursing care focuses on education, preventing injury from complications, relieving anxiety, and supporting self-esteem.

■ PID is an infection of the female pelvic organs, and may be caused by one or more infectious agents. Sexually active young women between the ages of 16 and 24 are most at risk. The prognosis depends on the number of episodes, promptness of treatment, and modification of risk-taking behaviors. The goals of nursing care are to treat the infection and prevent complications.

TEST YOURSELF NCLEX-RN® REVIEW

1 Which population is most often affected by STIs?
  1. men
  2. women and infants
  3. adolescent males
  4. older adults

2 Which of the following statements would indicate a client understands teaching to treat an STI?
  1. "My sex partner and I must both take medications."
  2. "I know I can never have sex again."
  3. "I will douche after every sexual encounter with my partner."
  4. "My sex partner does not have an infection, so won't need medications."

3 You are teaching a male client information about using condoms to prevent STI. What topics would you include? (Select all that apply.)
  1. Use a new condom with each sex act.
  2. Ensure a small amount of air in the tip.
  3. Use oil-based lubricants, such as petroleum jelly.
  4. Handle carefully to ensure no damage.
  5. Withdraw when the penis is erect.

4 You are assessing a young male. He has both blisters and ulcerations on the shaft of his penis. What is his most likely medical diagnosis?
  1. chlamydia
  2. gonorrhea
  3. genital warts
  4. genital herpes

5 Of the following statements about genital warts, which one is **not** true?
  1. The infection is caused by a yeast organism.
  2. The infection can be spread by any type of intercourse.
  3. The infection may be transmitted to the fetus.
  4. The infection cannot be cured.

6 You are counseling a young woman with an HPV genital infection. What screening test would you recommend she have every year?
  1. breast exam and mammogram
  2. stool for occult blood
  3. CBC to detect anemia and infection
  4. pelvic exam and Pap smear

7 Which of the following manifestations would most commonly be elicited during a health history for a woman with a vaginal infection?
  1. pain
  2. itching
  3. nausea
  4. diarrhea

8 You are teaching a woman with an STI who has severe genital discomfort. What is one simple recommendation that may relieve the discomfort?
  1. Wear nylon panty hose.
  2. Cut fingernails short.
  3. Wear cotton underwear.
  4. Have sex more frequently.

9 The infective organism responsible for gonorrhea *initially* targets what body parts?
  1. male urethra and female cervix
  2. female vulva and vagina
  3. male prostate
  4. male and female external genitalia

10 Which of the following would you teach a client about syphilis?
  1. Syphilis is caused by a virus.
  2. Syphilis is a local genital infection.
  3. Syphilis is a systemic infection.
  4. Syphilis has no effect on the developing fetus.

See Test Yourself answers in Appendix C.

BIBLIOGRAPHY

Ali, M., Cleland, J., & Shah, I. (2004). Condom use within marriage. A neglected HIV intervention. *Bulletin of the World Health Organization, 82*(3), 180–186.

American Social Health Association. (2005). *Facts & answers about STDs: Statistics.* Retrieved from http://www.ashastd.org/stdfaqs/statistics.html

Anderson, M., Klink, K., & Cohrssen, A. (2004). The rational clinical examination: Evaluation of vaginal complaints. *Journal of the American Medical Association, 291*(11), 1368–1379.

Ashcroft, T. (2004). Clinical preventative services for men: Information for women's health care providers. *AWHONN LIFELINES, 8*(6), 528–533.

Blair, M. (2004). Sexually transmitted diseases: An update. *Urology Nursing, 24*(6), 467–473.

Centers for Disease Control and Prevention. (2004). *STD general information (PID, syphilis, trichomoniasis, human papillomavirus, genital herpes, HPV, chlamydia).* Retrieved from http://www.cdc.gov/std.htm

_____.(2006). Treatment guidelines for sexually transmitted diseases. Retrieved from http://www.cdc.gov/std/treatment.htm

Drop-in service cuts wait for STI clinic. (2005). *Nursing Times, 101*(10), 9.

Farley, T., Cohen, D., Kahn, R., Lolis, S., Johnson, G., & Martin, D. (2003). The acceptability and behavioral effects of antibiotic prophylaxis for syphilis prevention. *Sexually Transmitted Diseases, 30*(11), 844–849.

Jungmann, E. (2004). Clinical evidence concise. Genital herpes. *American Family Physician, 70*(5), 912–914, 813–815.

Klebanoff, M., Schwebke, J., Zhang, J., Nansel, T., Yu, K., & Andrews, W. (2004). Vulvovaginal symptoms in women with bacterial vaginosis. *Obstetrics and Gynecology, 104*(2), 267–272.

NANDA International. (2005). *Nursing diagnoses: Definitions and classification 2005–2006.* Philadelphia.

National Institute of Allergy and Infectious Diseases, National Institutes of Health. (2003). *An introduction to sexually transmitted infections.* Retrieved from http://niaid.nih.gov/factsheets/stdinfo.htm

Ness, R., Hillier, S., Kip, K., Soper, D., Stamm, C., McGregor, J., et al. (2004). Bacterial vaginosis and risk of pelvic inflammatory disease. *Obstetrics and Gynecology, 104*(4), 761–769.

Phrma. (2005). *New medicines in development.* Retrieved from http://www.phrma.org/newmedicines/

newmedsdb/drugs.cfm?indicationcode=Prevention+of+Human+Pap...

Porth, C. M. (2005). *Pathophysiology: Concepts of altered health states* (7th ed.). Philadelphia: Lippincott.

Snapshot. New trends in STDs in the U.S. (2005). *Contraceptive Technology Update, March.* STD Quarterly, 4.

STD rates soaring: HPA promotes "safe, responsible sex." (2005, January). *RCM Midwives Journal, P.* 2.

Sterk, C., Klein, H., & Elifson, K. (2004). Predictors of condom-related attitudes among at-risk women. *Journal of Women's Health, 13*(6), 676–688.

Tierney, L. M., McPhee, S. J., & Papadakis, M. A. (Eds.). (2004). *Current medical diagnosis & treatment* (43rd ed.). Stamford, CT: Appleton & Lange.

What is the role of herpes virus serology in sexually transmitted disease screening? (2005). *Evidence-Based Practice, 8*(2), 4.

Young men not included in chlamydia testing. (2005). *Practice Nurse, 29*(3), 10l.

Wilson, B., Shannon, M., & Stang, C. (2005). *Nurse's drug guide 2005.* Upper Saddle River, NJ: Prentice Hall.

UNIT 15 BUILDING CLINICAL COMPETENCE
Responses to Altered Reproductive Function

Functional Health Pattern: Sexuality-Reproductive

■ Think about clients with altered sexuality-reproductive patterns for whom you have cared in your clinical experiences.

> ■ What were the clients' major medical diagnoses (e.g., ED, cancer, epididymitis, prostatitis, BPH, PMS, dysmenorrhea, uterine displacement, endometriosis, STI)?
> ■ What manifestations did each of these clients have? Were these manifestations similar or different?
> ■ *For men*: Were there any changes in men in the ability to urinate or achieve or maintain an erection? Did they take any medications to facilitate sexual ability? Did the client have any family history of testicular or prostate cancer? Had they had more than one sexual partner? Had they ever had any sexually transmitted infections? Had the clients ever had surgery on the reproductive organs? Did they perform testicular self-examination?
> ■ *For women*: At what age did they start or end having menstrual periods? Did they complain of menstrual difficulties, vaginal itching, discharge, or bleeding between menstrual periods? Did they take prescribed medication or herbals for menopause? Did they have a family history of endometrial, ovarian, or breast cancer? When were the clients' last mammogram and gynecologic examination? Does the client perform breast self-examination? Had they had more than one sexual partner? Had they ever had any sexually transmitted infections? Had they ever had surgery on the reproductive organs?

■ Male disorders may be inflammatory, structural, benign, or malignant. As men age, benign and malignant conditions of the prostate gland become common. Many of the disorders and treatments pose significant risks to fertility, sexual function, urinary function erection and ejaculation. Disorders of the male reproductive system lead to manifestations such as:

> ■ Phimosis (infection of the glans penis and prepuce ▶ causes tightness of prepuce ▶ resulting in prevention of retraction of foreskin).
> ■ Erectile dysfunction (aging, illness, injury, or medications ▶ cause a decrease in blood flow to the penis ▶ resulting in inability to attain or maintain an erection).

■ Female disorders range from the minor discomfort of menstrual cramps to life-threatening diseases such as cancer. The disorders may affect sexual function and the sense of well-being as a woman. Disorders of the female reproductive system lead to manifestations such as:

> ■ Dysmenorrhea (excessive production of prostaglandins ▶ stimulates uterine muscle fibers to contract ▶ which compromises uterine blood flow ▶ resulting in uterine ischemia and pain)
> ■ PMS (hormonal changes involving estrogen, progesterone, prolactin, and aldosterone along with neurotransmitter changes involving monoamine oxidase and serotonin ▶ cause manifestations prior to the beginning of the menstrual period ▶ resulting in mood swings, breast tenderness, fatigue, irritability, food cravings, and depression).

■ Clients who experience reproductive system changes and disorders require a holistic approach to meet their physical, emotional, and educational needs. Priority nursing diagnoses within the Sexuality-Reproductive Pattern that may be appropriate for clients include:

> ■ *Sexual Dysfunction* as evidenced by loss of sexual function, dyspareunia, vaginismus, inability to achieve or alterations in achieving desired sexual satisfaction
> ■ *Ineffective Sexuality Patterns* evidenced by difficulties or limitations in sexual behaviors, changes in sexual activities, expression of loss

■ Two nursing diagnoses from other functional health patterns often are of high priority for the client with altered reproductive function:

> ■ *Disturbed Body Image* (Self-Perception-Self-Concept)
> ■ *Powerlessness* (Coping-Stress-Tolerance)

CLINICAL SCENARIO

You have been assigned to work with the following four clients for the 0700 shift on a medical-surgical hospital unit. Significant data obtained during report are as follows:

- Daryl Foster, a 22-year-old, is admitted with a diagnosis of sickle cell crisis. Vital signs are T 99.6°F, P 84, R 10 and shallow, BP 140/86. He is complaining of chest pain, back pain, and priapism. He has a PCA with morphine sulfate for pain.
- Barney Green, a 76-year-old, is 3 days postoperative for transurethral resection of the prostate (TURP). Vital signs are T 98.7°F, P 82, R 16, BP 158/82. His urinary catheter was removed at 0600. He is complaining of dribbling of urine after attempting to void.

- Tara Morris is a 21-year-old newly admitted from the ED with complaints of severe lower abdominal pain, purulent vaginal discharge, and cervical pain on pelvic exam. Her vital signs are T 102.6°F, P 88, R 20, BP 110/70. She is to be started on ceftriaxone (Rocephin) and gentamicin (Garamycin) IV as soon as possible.
- Regina Perkins, a 36-year-old, has a history of uterine fibroids. She had a uterine fibroid embolization yesterday. Her vital signs have remained stable throughout the night. Her discharge is written and she is in a hurry to be discharged so her husband can get to work.

Questions

1. In what order would you visit these clients after report?
   1. _____
   2. _____
   3. _____
   4. _____

2. What top two priority nursing diagnoses would you choose for each of the clients presented above? Can you explain, if asked, the rationale for your choices?

	Priority Nursing Diagnosis #1	Priority Nursing Diagnosis #2
Daryl Foster		
Barney Green		
Tara Morris		
Regina Perkins		

3. Mr. Foster asks the nurse about complications due to priapism because he often has this problem with sickle cell crises. Which complication does the nurse discuss with the client?
   1. severe phimosis
   2. erectile dysfunction
   3. penile cancer
   4. urinary retention

4. Mr. Green suddenly develops nausea and vomiting, BP is 170/100, P is 58, and he is confused. What is the probable cause of these manifestations?
   1. allergic reaction to the bladder irrigating fluid solution
   2. anxiety reaction to having prostate surgery
   3. absorption of isotonic bladder irrigating fluids
   4. hypovolemic shock complication of the surgery

5. Which of the following is MOST important to teach Ms. Morris about pelvic inflammatory disease?
   1. Take all medication as prescribed.
   2. Wipe from front to back after urinating.
   3. Use latex condoms when having sex.
   4. Change tampons or pads every 4 hours.

6. Prior to surgery, Ms. Perkins' hematocrit was 34% and hemoglobin was 10 g/dL. She was instructed to increase iron foods in her diet. Which foods are high in iron?
   1. beef, eggs, brown rice
   2. green, leafy vegetables, chicken
   3. fish, broccoli, kidney beans
   4. liver, cheese, asparagus

7. Which is a priority nursing diagnosis for a young female client with endometriosis?
   1. *Acute pain* as manifested by severe abdominal cramping
   2. *Deficient knowledge:* Complications of endometriosis
   3. *Decisional conflict:* Treatment plan options
   4. *Risk for* Anxiety related to loss of reproductive function

8. A prescription for tadalafil (Cialis) is ordered for a man with erectile dysfunction. The client indicates understanding of teaching instructions when he makes which statement?
   1. "I will take Cialis just before intercourse to increase my sex drive."
   2. "I will consult with the doctor before taking other medications."
   3. "I can take a second pill the same day if the first one doesn't work."
   4. "This pill will relieve all of my sex problems."

9. Which laboratory studies would you expect to be conducted to diagnose syphilis? (Select all that apply).
   1. VDRL
   2. Gram stain
   3. RPR
   4. DFA
   5. tissue culture
   6. FTA-ABS

10. Which instructions should be taught to the client who is receiving radiation therapy for prostate cancer?
    1. Eat more red meat to maintain protein for healing.
    2. Avoid close contact with pregnant women, infants, and children.
    3. Avoid sexual contact to prevent stress from dysfunction.
    4. Sleep alone for the first night after radiation therapy.

11. Which symptom would be most significant when assessing a client with possible cervical cancer?
    1. vaginal discharge
    2. weight loss
    3. pain in back and thighs
    4. vaginal bleeding

12. A sexually active woman is being treated for gonorrhea. Which method of birth control does the nurse tell her is safest to use?
    1. oral contraceptives
    2. intrauterine device
    3. condom
    4. estrogen patch

Case Study

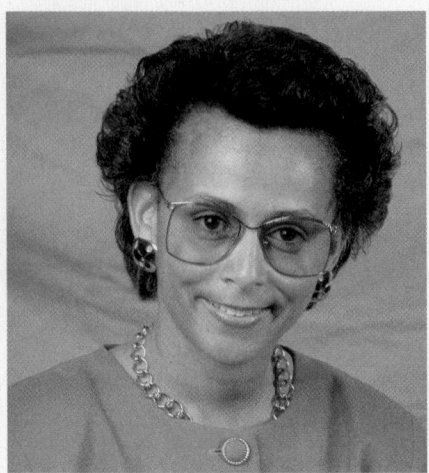

Eva Gibson, a 43-year-old married housewife with two children, had a routine annual mammogram that revealed a mass in the left breast. She has a family history of breast cancer with her mother and a maternal aunt having breast cancer. She was admitted to outpatient surgery for an incisional biopsy, with results of invasive lobular carcinoma. An MRI was performed, which indicated that four axillary glands have been infiltrated with cancer. She was admitted to the hospital and a modified radical mastectomy on the left side is performed. Postoperatively, she is admitted to the chemotherapy unit. Vital signs are T 98.5°F, P 65, R 14, BP 110/68. She has a dressing on the left chest that is dry and intact and the JP drain is intact for suction. Her left arm is elevated on two pillows. The decision has been made to start radiation and chemotherapy treatments as soon as possible.

The pathophysiology of breast cancer is a mutation of breast tissue cells related to hormones and mutations of tumor suppressor genes. Abnormal cell growth occurs. Cancer cells create a factor that stimulates blood vessels to grow into the tumor. Cancer cells invade the blood vessels and travel through the bloodstream or through the lymphatic system to other sites. Manifestations of breast cancer include nontender lump in the breast, abnormal nipple discharge, rash around the nipple area, nipple retraction, edema, dimpling of the skin, or change in position of the nipple. Some women report a burning or stinging sensation in the breast or nipple pain. Complications of breast cancer are metastasis to bone, brain, lung, liver, skin, and lymph nodes, and death.

Based on the client's surgery of modified radical mastectomy and treatment with radiation and chemotherapy, the nursing diagnosis of *Risk for Infection* is appropriate for planning care for Mrs. Gibson.

- Breast tissue cells mutate and grow abnormally
- Cancer cells produce a factor that stimulates growth of blood vessels into tumor
- Cancer cells metastasize

Mrs. E. G.
43 y.o. female
Breast cancer

— affects →

— leads to →

— assess →

- Diagnosis of left breast cancer
- Surgical procedure to remove cancer with thoracic incision and JP drain
- Scheduled to have further treatment with radiation and chemotherapy

— generates →

- Acute Pain related to surgical incision
- Disturbed Body Image related to loss of breast
- Anticipatory Grieving related to diagnosis of cancer
- Anxiety related to concerns about care of children and husband

generate nursing diagnosis

Risk for Infection ← prioritized to

expected outcomes

- Vital signs will remain within normal limits
- WBC findings remain within normal limits
- Incision progressively heals without manifestations of infection
- Consumes increased protein and vitamins

— evaluate →

- Vital signs and WBC remained within normal limits
- Incision healed without evidence of infection
- Verbalized importance of increasing protein in diet

Interdisciplinary Interventions
- Monitor results of lab data and report abnormal findings to surgeon
- Administer prescribed antibiotics

Independent Interventions
- Wash hands before and after each nursing care activity
- Monitor vital signs (especially T) every 4 to 8 hours
- Assess incision each day
- Assess color and amount of drainage on dressing and from JP drain at the end of each shift
- Use sterile procedures to change dressing and empty JP drain
- Discuss importance of diet in wound healing and during treatment for cancer

Standard precautions are designed to reduce the risk of transmission of microorganisms from both recognized and unrecognized sources of infection. They are the primary strategies for preventing nosocomial infections within institutions, and are important to protect healthcare workers as well. Standard precautions apply to (1) blood; (2) all body fluids, secretions, and excretions except sweat, regardless of whether or not they contain visible blood; (3) nonintact skin; and (4) mucous membranes. Standard precautions are applied to all clients receiving care in hospitals, regardless of their diagnosis or presumed infection status. These precautions are specifically designed for hospitals; however, they also may be implemented in extended and long-term care facilities, and to a more limited extent in providing home care or in other community-based care settings.

Hand Washing

- Wash your hands (a) after touching blood, body fluids, secretions, excretions, and contaminated items, whether or not gloves are worn; (b) immediately after removing gloves, even if gloves appear to be intact; (c) between contacts with clients; and (d) when otherwise indicated to prevent transfer of organisms to other clients. You may need to wash your hands between tasks and procedures on the same client to prevent cross-contaminating different body sites.
- Use soap and warm water for hand washing when hands are visibly dirty or contaminated with blood or other body fluids.
- If hands are not visibly soiled, use an alcohol-based hand rub for routinely decontaminating hands in all other situations.

Gloves

- Wear clean, nonsterile gloves when touching blood, body fluids, secretions, excretions, and contaminated items.
- Put on clean gloves just before touching mucous membranes and nonintact skin.
- Change your gloves between tasks and procedures on the same client after contacting material that may contain a high concentration of microorganisms.
- Wear gloves for all invasive procedures such as performing venipuncture or other vascular or surgical procedures.
- Wear gloves if you have cuts, scratches, or other breaks in the skin.
- Remove gloves promptly after use, before touching noncontaminated items and surfaces, and before going to another client; wash hands immediately after removing gloves.

Mask, Eye Protection, Face Shield

Wear a mask and eye protection or a face shield to protect mucous membranes of your eyes, nose, and mouth during procedures and client care activities that are likely to generate splashes or sprays of blood, body fluids, secretions, or excretions.

Gown

Wear a gown (clean, disposable) to protect your skin and prevent soiling of clothing during procedures and client care activities that are likely to generate splashes or sprays of blood, body fluids, secretions, or excretions. Remove soiled gowns promptly, washing your hands immediately after gown removal.

Equipment

Handle used client care equipment that is soiled with blood, body fluids, secretions, and excretions in a way that prevents exposing your skin and mucous membranes, contaminating your clothing, and transferring microorganisms to other clients or environments. Ensure that reusable equipment is cleaned and appropriately reprocessed before using for the care of another client.

Environmental Control

Follow hospital procedures for routine care, cleaning, and disinfecting environmental surfaces, beds, bed rails, bedside equipment, and other frequently touched surfaces.

Linen

Handle and transport linens soiled with blood, body fluids, secretions, and excretions in a manner that prevents exposing your skin and mucous membranes, contaminating your clothing, and transferring microorganisms to other clients and environments. Place soiled linen in leakage-resistant bags at the location where it is used.

Occupational Health and Bloodborne Pathogens

- Take care to prevent injuries when using needles, scalpels, and other sharps; when handling sharp instruments after procedures; when cleaning used instruments; and when disposing of used needles.
- Never recap used needles, manipulate them using both hands, or handle them in a manner that directs the point of a needle toward any part of your body. If it is necessary to protect the needle prior to disposal, use a one-handed "scoop" technique or mechanical device to hold the needle sheath.
- Do not remove used needles from disposable syringes by hand; do not bend, break, or otherwise manipulate used needles by hand.
- Place used disposable syringes and needles, scalpel blades, and other sharp items in appropriate puncture-resistant containers located as close as practical to the area in which the items were used.
- Place reusable syringes and needles in a puncture-resistant container for transport to the reprocessing area.
- Use mouthpieces, resuscitation bags, or other ventilation devices as an alternative to mouth-to-mouth resuscitation methods whenever possible.

Client Placement

Place clients who contaminate the environment or who do not (or are not expected to) assist in maintaining appropriate hygiene or environmental control (e.g., an ambulatory, confused client with fecal incontinence) in a private room.

Sources. *Centers for Disease Control and Prevention. (2002). Guidelines for hand hygiene in health-care settings: Recommendations of the Healthcare Infection Control Practices Advisory Committee and the HICPAC/SHEA/APIC/IDSA Hand Hygiene Taskforce.* MMWR, 51(RR-16), 1–56; *Hospital Infection Control Practices Advisory Committee. (1997). Part II. Recommendations for isolation precautions in hospitals.* Atlanta: Public Health Service, U.S. Department of Health and Human Services, Centers for Disease Control and Prevention.

Activity Intolerance
Activity Intolerance, Risk for
Airway Clearance, Ineffective
Anxiety
Anxiety, Death
Aspiration, Risk for
Attachment, Parent/Infant/Child, Risk for Impaired
Autonomic Dysreflexia
Autonomic Dysreflexia, Risk for
Blood Glucose, Risk for Unstable
Body Image, Disturbed
Body Temperature: Imbalanced, Risk for
Bowel Incontinence
Breastfeeding, Effective
Breastfeeding, Ineffective
Breastfeeding, Interrupted
Breathing Pattern, Ineffective
Cardiac Output, Decreased
Caregiver Role Strain
Caregiver Role Strain, Risk for
Comfort, Readiness for Enhanced
Communication: Impaired, Verbal
Communication, Readiness for Enhanced
Confusion, Acute
Confusion, Acute, Risk for
Confusion, Chronic
Constipation
Constipation, Perceived
Constipation, Risk for
Contamination
Contamination, Risk for
Coping: Community, Ineffective
Coping: Community, Readiness for Enhanced
Coping, Defensive
Coping: Family, Compromised
Coping: Family, Disabled
Coping: Family, Readiness for Enhanced
Coping (Individual), Readiness for Enhanced
Coping, Ineffective
Decisional Conflict
Decision Making, Readiness for Enhanced
Denial, Ineffective
Dentition, Impaired
Development: Delayed, Risk for
Diarrhea
Disuse Syndrome, Risk for
Diversional Activity, Deficient
Energy Field, Disturbed
Environmental Interpretation Syndrome, Impaired
Failure to Thrive, Adult
Falls, Risk for
Family Processes, Dysfunctional: Alcoholism
Family Processes, Interrupted
Family Processes, Readiness for Enhanced
Fatigue
Fear
Fluid Balance, Readiness for Enhanced
Fluid Volume, Deficient
Fluid Volume, Deficient, Risk for
Fluid Volume, Excess
Fluid Volume, Imbalanced, Risk for
Gas Exchange, Impaired
Grieving
Grieving, Complicated
Grieving, Risk for Complicated
Growth, Disproportionate, Risk for
Growth and Development, Delayed
Health Behavior, Risk-Prone

Health Maintenance, Ineffective
Health-Seeking Behaviors (Specify)
Home Maintenance, Impaired
Hope, Readiness for Enhanced
Hopelessness
Human Dignity, Risk for Compromised
Hyperthermia
Hypothermia
Immunization Status, Readiness for Enhanced
Infant Behavior, Disorganized
Infant Behavior: Disorganized, Risk for
Infant Behavior: Organized, Readiness for Enhanced
Infant Feeding Pattern, Ineffective
Infection, Risk for
Injury, Risk for
Insomnia
Intracranial Adaptive Capacity, Decreased
Knowledge, Deficient (Specify)
Knowledge (Specify), Readiness for Enhanced
Latex Allergy Response
Latex Allergy Response, Risk for
Liver Function, Impaired, Risk for
Loneliness, Risk for
Memory, Impaired
Mobility: Bed, Impaired
Mobility: Physical, Impaired
Mobility: Wheelchair, Impaired
Moral Distress
Nausea
Neurovascular Dysfunction: Peripheral, Risk for
Noncompliance (Specify)
Nutrition, Imbalanced: Less than Body Requirements
Nutrition, Imbalanced: More than Body Requirements
Nutrition, Imbalanced: More than Body Requirements, Risk for
Nutrition, Readiness for Enhanced
Oral Mucous Membrane, Impaired
Pain, Acute
Pain, Chronic
Parenting, Impaired
Parenting, Readiness for Enhanced
Parenting, Risk for Impaired
Perioperative Positioning Injury, Risk for
Personal Identity, Disturbed
Poisoning, Risk for
Post-Trauma Syndrome
Post-Trauma Syndrome, Risk for
Power, Readiness for Enhanced
Powerlessness
Powerlessness, Risk for
Protection, Ineffective
Rape-Trauma Syndrome
Rape-Trauma Syndrome: Compound Reaction
Rape-Trauma Syndrome: Silent Reaction
Religiosity, Impaired
Religiosity, Readiness for Enhanced
Religiosity, Risk for Impaired
Relocation Stress Syndrome
Relocation Stress Syndrome, Risk for
Role Conflict, Parental
Role Performance, Ineffective
Sedentary Lifestyle
Self-Care, Readiness for Enhanced
Self-Care Deficit: Bathing/Hygiene
Self-Care Deficit: Dressing/Grooming
Self-Care Deficit: Feeding

Self-Care Deficit: Toileting
Self-Concept, Readiness for Enhanced
Self-Esteem, Chronic Low
Self-Esteem, Situational Low
Self-Esteem, Risk for Situational Low
Self-Mutilation
Self-Mutilation, Risk for
Sensory Perception, Disturbed (Specify: Auditory, Gustatory, Kinesthetic, Olfactory Tactile, Visual)
Sexual Dysfunction
Sexuality Pattern, Ineffective
Skin Integrity, Impaired
Skin Integrity, Risk for Impaired
Sleep Deprivation
Sleep, Readiness for Enhanced
Social Interaction, Impaired
Social Isolation
Sorrow, Chronic
Spiritual Distress
Spiritual Distress, Risk for
Spiritual Well-Being, Readiness for Enhanced
Spontaneous Ventilation, Impaired
Stress, Overload
Sudden Infant Death Syndrome, Risk for
Suffocation, Risk for
Suicide, Risk for
Surgical Recovery, Delayed
Swallowing, Impaired
Therapeutic Regimen Management: Community, Ineffective
Therapeutic Regimen Management, Effective
Therapeutic Regimen Management: Family, Ineffective
Therapeutic Regimen Management, Ineffective
Therapeutic Regimen Management, Readiness for Enhanced
Thermoregulation, Ineffective
Thought Processes, Disturbed
Tissue Integrity, Impaired
Tissue Perfusion, Ineffective (Specify: Cerebral, Cardiopulmonary, Gastrointestinal, Renal)
Tissue Perfusion, Ineffective, Peripheral
Transfer Ability, Impaired
Trauma, Risk for
Unilateral Neglect
Urinary Elimination, Impaired
Urinary Elimination, Readiness for Enhanced
Urinary Incontinence, Functional
Urinary Incontinence, Overflow
Urinary Incontinence, Reflex
Urinary Incontinence, Stress
Urinary Incontinence, Total
Urinary Incontinence, Urge
Urinary Incontinence, Risk for Urge
Urinary Retention
Ventilatory Weaning Response, Dysfunctional
Violence: Other-Directed, Risk for
Violence: Self-Directed, Risk for
Walking, Impaired
Wandering

Source. NANDA Nursing Diagnoses: Definitions and Classification, 2007–2008. Philadelphia: North American Nursing Diagnosis Association. Used with permission.

Test Yourself Answers

Chapter 1: Medical-Surgical Nursing

1. **Answer: 2 Rationale:** This is done in order to standardize the different healthcare professions nationally and develop guidelines of practice.

2. **Answer: 4 Rationale:** Critical thinking is needed in order to perform nursing assessments, prioritize client care, evaluate treatment and education needs, and address any potential safety issues.

3. **Answer: 1 Rationale:** The client is an integral part of developing a care plan. It is very important to include the client in order to establish individualized goals to best meet the needs of the client. Nurses develop a partnership with the client when initiating the plan of care.

4. **Answer: 2, 1, 5, 4, 3 Rationale:** Assessment is the first step to determine the needs of the client. Based on this information, individualized goals and outcomes can be established. Next, the planning stage determines what is necessary to meet the expected outcomes. These expected outcomes should be short-term and realistic, and should be adjusted as necessary. Implementation follows, which is when the plan is put into action. The final step is evaluation. The plan is evaluated to determine the degree of success of the individualized goals and outcomes. The outcomes may be met, partially met, or not met. This is the time when it may be necessary to change the plan and outcomes in order to best meet the client's needs. The client should be involved in each step of the nursing process.

5. **Answer: 3 Rationale:** Although there are many layers of care involved in nursing, the foundation for all aspects of nursing is the knowledge base. Without a strong knowledge base, nurses would not be able to develop clinical competency or practice, or provide holistic care.

6. **Answer: 4 Rationale:** Although nurses function in many capacities that involve health education, including serving as an advocate, caregiver, and researcher, these are not the primary focus. The educator role is the most important function for nurses when developing and providing health information to clients.

7. **Answer: 1 Rationale:** Situations involving a difference of opinion between clients and healthcare providers may arise. The nurse plays an integral part in these situations by assisting and supporting the client's decision making through advocacy.

8. **Answer: 2 Rationale:** When a nurse is responsible for assignments and determining appropriate work activities for other members of the nursing team, this is a leadership or manager role. This role can be formal or informal.

9. **Answer: 2 Rationale:** Critical pathways are developed to address general standards of care and outcomes for a specific client population. This often helps to simplify the nursing process, but the nurse still must individualize the plan for the client.

10. **Answer: 3 Rationale:** The nurse is ultimately responsible for the vital signs performed by unlicensed personnel. If there is any question regarding the readings, it is the nurse's responsibility to evaluate the results, repeat anything in question, and inform the provider as necessary.

Chapter 2: Health and Illness in the Adult Client

1. **Answer: 4 Rationale:** Many clients have underlying disease processes. As a result, daily medications are necessary to assist in maintaining good health. Thus, the definition of wellness is actively practicing healthy behaviors, rather than the absence of disease or illness.

2. **Answer: 1, 2, 4, 5 Rationale:** Height is the only factor listed which does not affect the health of an individual. Genetic makeup can predispose clients for many different chronic illnesses or diseases. Cognitive abilities can affect the understanding, or lack of understanding, a client has regarding how to maintain wellness. Age can affect health as many chronic illnesses become more problematic with age. Age can also affect cognitive abilities and affect other senses necessary to maintain wellness, such as hearing, sight, smell, and taste. Race can also be a factor of health, as many chronic illnesses are more prevalent in particular races and can also be more difficult to manage, such as hypertension in the African-American population.

3. **Answer: 2 Rationale:** Sickle cell disease is an autosomal recessive disease that is primarily found in clients of African-American descent. All other choices are not genetically caused.

4. **Answer: 1 Rationale:** Practicing safer sex is the only choice with a focus on prevention. Any screening tests such as for hypertension or a mammogram are considered secondary prevention, when a client is being screened for a disease process that already may be present in order to recommend treatment. Surgery would serve as tertiary prevention, which is done to minimize, control, or stop progression of symptoms or disease.

5. **Answer: 2 Rationale:** Assuming the sick role is when you take on the responsibility of calling to explain your illness and you do not go to class as a result. Although you may be experiencing symptoms and may seek medical care as a result, these are not part of the action stated above. Finally, you are not assuming a dependent role as you have independently made the decision not to go to class and are not asking for assistance.

6. **Answer: 4 Rationale:** A congenital illness is a disorder that a person is born with, often as a result of a physiological imperfection. Although this may predispose one for an acute illness, this is not how it would be classified. A heart defect is not caused from a malignancy, but from a physical deformity of the heart muscle itself and not from any iatrogenic illness.

7. **Answer: 2 Rationale:** The most important factor when referring to a chronic illness is that it lasts for a lifetime. Although symptoms may wax and wane, and remissions may occur, the underlying disease still exists. Though flares or exacerbations may occur rapidly, be self-limiting, or only last for a short time, the actual disease remains, even if symptoms are not present.

8. **Answer: 1 Rationale:** Although Mr. Jones is at risk for multiple illnesses, the system at greatest risk is the cardiovascular system. He has many risk factors for cardiovascular disease including age, overweight, smoking, and sedentary lifestyle. His renal system is not at great risk. His gastrointestinal system is at mild risk; he should get a colonoscopy for colon cancer screening as he is at increased risk for this due to his age, weight, and smoking history. His nervous system is not at great risk.

9. **Answer: 2 Rationale:** Accident prevention in the home is a very important topic to present to senior citizens. This population is at

greatest risk for falls and injury in the home due to sensory problems including vision loss, unsteady gait, loss of sensation to hot and cold, and loss of sense of smell and taste to identify spoiled food. Substance abuse is more important to address with the young adult and adolescent population, as well as family roles and tasks. Treating acute illness is something all populations may benefit from, but not nearly as vital to seniors as accident prevention in the home.

10. **Answer: 3, 4 Rationale:** Recognizing that dying is a part of living is part of adjusting to aging and recognizing the bodily changes that occur as a result of aging. Coping with loss is part of the grieving process that the widowed spouse must endure as the result of death of a loved one. Although coping with the lack of privacy may occur if they move in with other family members, that is not what is being addressed here. Planning for retirement may be part of what is happening, but is not what is occurring in this setting. Relating to kin may also be occurring, but is not pertinent to this situation.

Chapter 3: Community-Based and Home Care of the Adult Client

1. **Answer: 3 Rationale:** Although all of the choices listed in this question are part of community-based nursing care, the primary focus is individual and family health. Interventions that deal with the function and health of the community are based on individual and family needs.

2. **Answer: 1 Rationale:** Access to healthcare services may be more challenging for rural residents due to transportation issues. Urban residents often have easier access to public transportation to obtain healthcare services. Age and gender of residents, family tasks and values, and ability to follow directions are similar between urban and rural residents.

3. **Answer: 2 Rationale:** Parish nursing is often organized through church services, also known as a faith community. Although some of the services may include respite care, day care, or block nursing, these are not the only services parish nursing may offer clients.

4. **Answer: 4 Rationale:** Respite care provides assistance to full-time caregivers and helps relieve some of the stress associated with this huge responsibility. Although this may be one of the services parishes or block nursing may provide, the official term is respite care. Day care is reserved for children or adults in need of supervision outside of the home, whereas respite care often takes place in the home.

5. **Answer: 1, 3, 4 Rationale:** Mrs. Jones, who cannot live independently at home due to a broken hip, would benefit from home care. A home health aide can assist her with activities of daily living, and a physical therapist may help her with improving her mobility. Miss Ace should not require home care services as her illness is self-limiting and she should be more independent very soon. Mr. Strip would benefit from home care, as he is terminal and wishes to die at home. Hospice care would be an excellent choice. Miss Taylor would benefit from home care as she lives alone and may not be completely independent due to her major abdominal surgery. Mr. Wines is not in need of home care as weakness due to arthritis is not an appropriate reason, further we do not know if he lives alone or not.

6. **Answer: 4 Rationale:** Home care nurses must advocate for their clients by having all necessary paperwork to provide care, which includes advance directives, living wills, and durable power of attorney. Although home care nurses may also func-

tion as providers of direct care, coordinator of services, and educators, these are not part of the role discussed above.

7. **Answer: 4 Rationale:** The registered nurse is the person responsible for care coordination. This is done with the initial visit to assess the individual's need of services and will continue to be evaluated on an ongoing basis. The physician orders services, but leaves the scope of services up to the agency to determine the need. The social worker makes the initial contact with the agency to determine access. The home health aide assists with normal activities.

8. **Answer: 1 Rationale:** Medicare is the largest single reimbursement source for home care. Medicaid, private insurance, and self-pay also provide reimbursement, but not in as great a scope as Medicare.

9. **Answer: 2 Rationale:** Hand washing is the most important factor to help prevent infection in the home. Although it is also important for home care nurses to perform needs assessments regarding fire and smoke detector function, fall prevention, and proper medication administration, the only education factor to prevent the spread of infection is hand washing.

10. **Answer: 4 Rationale:** A treatment form is needed in order to receive reimbursement from insurance. Family member approval is not needed for reimbursement. Completion of agency forms is important for communication between agency personnel, but not for reimbursement. A physician order is needed to start the process of home care, but not for reimbursement of services.

Chapter 4: Nursing Care of Clients Having Surgery

1. **Answer: 2 Rationale:** The nurse's primary responsibility to informed consent is serving as a witness to the client signature on the consent form. It is the physician's responsibility to define the risks and benefits of surgery, as well as explain the right to refuse treatment or withdraw consent, and advise the client and family about what is needed for diagnosis. The nurse may reinforce all of these issues, but they primarily fall under the role of the physician.

2. **Answer: 4 Rationale:** Obtaining a preoperative blood pressure is necessary to provide a baseline for post-operative care. This helps assess for any post-operative blood loss or hemorrhaging. This has no legal requirement issue and is not necessary for induction with anesthesia or preventing atelectasis.

3. **Answer: 3 Rationale:** Nonsteroidal anti-inflammatory drugs potentiate analgesia and reduce inflammation caused from surgery. They do not stimulate appetite, increase amnesia, or improve renal function.

4. **Answer: 2 Rationale:** A high protein diet is important to help with healing post-operatively. Low-fat, high fiber may also be important; however, the most important factor is high protein.

5. **Answer: 4 Rationale:** Neurovascular assessments are important to assess for any complications of surgery such as a blood clot after knee surgery. Urinary pH is not important. Rebound tenderness and Chvostek's sign are not part of post-operative assessments for knee surgery.

6. **Answer: 3 Rationale:** Medications must be reordered post-operatively, as the needs may have changed as a result of surgery. It is not a nursing responsibility to determine if decreasing the dose is needed or to withhold until anesthesia wears off.

7. **Answer: 4 Rationale:** Anesthetic agents cause paralysis and block sympathetic nervous system control. This blocks signs and symptoms of hypoglycemia and could prevent recognition of the condition.

8. **Answer: 3 Rationale:** It is expected that pain is a result of any surgical procedure. Clients may not exhibit signs and symptoms of pain initially due to effects of anesthesia. Medications should be provided regularly to help maintain adequate pain control and help promote rapid recovery.

9. **Answer: 4 Rationale:** The metal OR tables have no cushioning and the OR environment is often kept cooler. The client has to be positioned appropriately for the procedures. This can cause pressure areas to boney prominences. Since the skin of elderly clients is less elastic and more fragile, skin tears may result. The lower temperature in the OR environment can decrease skin circulation. This, compounded with the positioning and the predisposing risks of skin impairment, can cause pressure sores and joint pain.

10. **Answer: 4 Rationale:** Hypothermia can result from the OR environment and prolonged exposure during this period. Anesthesia blocks sympathetic nervous system stimulation, preventing the client from shivering to help increase body temperature. Thus, it is necessary for the nurse to intervene in order to help increase the body temperature.

Chapter 5: Nursing Care of Clients Experiencing Loss, Grief, and Death

1. **Answer: 3 Rationale:** Only the person experiencing loss can evaluate their experiences. This is very individualized and cannot be judged by others. Although cultural values and support of friends and family may impact loss, many other factors affect the ability to cope with loss.

2. **Answer: 4 Rationale:** Denial is often the first stage of grief. Although the different stages of grief do not really go in order, denial is an exception. This is often the first reaction, and the client may go back to denial when going through the grieving process.

3. **Answer: 2 Rationale:** A strong support system of friends and family is extremely important in helping one through the grieving process and to cope with loss. The client does not expect those in their support system to fix their situation but to simply provide moral support and listen for when he/she is ready to talk. Each individual will go through the grieving process in his or her own way and on his or her own time.

4. **Answer: 1 Rationale:** Culture is what dictates the rituals of mourning. This does not replace the grieving process, but is simply part of acceptance in the process. The individual will continue to grieve for the loss in his or her own way. Culture simply provides a pathway to express the loss.

5. **Answer: 2 Rationale:** A living will expresses the exact wishes of a client regarding expectations for medical care. It addresses what the client is willing to or not willing to endure to sustain life. This takes the decision from other family members and provides the client with peace of mind in knowing his/her wishes will be followed.

6. **Answer: 3 Rationale:** Hospice care is for clients suffering from terminal illnesses. Hospice is designed to meet the needs of the client's end-of-life care by providing quality to the time that remains. Although Hospice Homes exist, hospice represents a model of nursing care more than a location.

7. **Answer: 4 Rationale:** We as nurses develop partnerships with our clients regarding their care. End-of-life care is no exception. It is necessary to respect the client's wishes and withhold pain medications. Other methods of pain control can be suggested such as relaxation therapy, therapeutic touch, or positioning for comfort.

8. **Answer: 1 Rationale:** Comatose clients cannot see. As circulation becomes more impaired, sense of touch is diminished. In many near death experiences, clients have recalled hearing the voices of those taking care of them. It is thought that the sense of hearing is the last sense to go before death occurs.

9. **Answer: 3 Rationale:** It is important to continue to manage pain at all times of life, especially in end-of-life care. Terminal illnesses cause great pain and the goal of hospice nursing is to help provide quality to the client's remaining time including helping the client to maintain comfort and be as free of pain as possible.

10. **Answer: 2 Rationale:** The open-ended statement of acknowledging to the woman "This must be a difficult time for you"" is the best choice. This provides the woman to opportunity to express her feelings, recognizing the nurse's willingness to listen.

Chapter 6: Nursing Care of Clients with Problems of Substance Abuse

1. **Answer: 2 Rationale:** The minimum level of alcohol in the blood to consider the individual to be intoxicated is 0.08%. The allowable blood alcohol level for driving in some states is 0.1%, but this has now been lowered to 0.08% in many states.

2. **Answer: 1 Rationale:** Asking a client how many days a week he/she drinks alcoholic beverages is very general. It does not force the client into a defensive "no" answer. It provides an avenue for discussion, which could lead to more specific information.

3. **Answer: 4 Rationale:** Clients suffering from chronic alcoholism have significant malnutrition issues. Thiamine depletion can cause neurological problems and cognitive impairment, known as Wernicke-Korsakoff syndrome. Wernicke's encephalopathy is the acute stage of the disease and Korsakoff's psychosis is the chronic stage of the disease. Thiamine replacement can help prevent this from occurring.

4. **Answer: 3 Rationale:** Alcohol and CNS depressants present the greatest risk during withdrawal due to concerns of seizures and delirium tremens. The brain becomes overly excited since the receptors are no longer being blocked. Delirium tremens from alcohol withdrawal has a mortality rate of 1-5%.

5. **Answer: 2 Rationale:** Clients who suffer from alcoholism feel a sense of enjoyment when they start drinking. Antabuse takes away this pleasant sensation and replaces it, causing physical illness and intense vomiting. Antabuse prevents the breakdown of alcohol if taken while the person is drinking. The goal in taking away the enjoyment of drinking and replacing it with this negative reinforcement is to decrease the desire to drink and help facilitate recovery.

6. **Answer: 3 Rationale:** Clients reporting effective pain control are receiving their needed medications. If clients were consistently reporting poor pain control, this would be more of a cause for concern.

7. **Answer: 2 Rationale:** The smoking rates for women have not steadily declined since the 1950s. In fact, this population has had a rise in the smoking rate.

8. **Answer: 4 Rationale:** It is a good idea for clients to wear a medic alert bracelet while on naltrexone. This medication blocks opiate receptors in the brain that trigger the feelings of pleasure experienced when taking alcohol or narcotics. In case of emergency medical treatment, it is important for caregivers to know the client is taking naltrexone to prevent administration of any narcotics.

9. **Answer: 1 Rationale:** Identifying alternative ways of dealing with stressful situations is key. It is unrealistic to think the craving will

go away. The craving will always be there. It is more important to understand how to cope. Focusing on the past will not help solve the problems of the future, it just causes unnecessary pain and encourages feelings of failure and inadequacy. Avoiding using alcohol or drugs is needed. It is not possible to limit to only one.

10. **Answer: 3 Rationale:** *Ineffective Denial* is the best choice. 1. is not an option since nutrition is often imbalanced due to malnutrition, not excess food intake. 2. is not an option since clients often are not taking vitamins or supplements and even if they do, it would not cause fluid overload. 4. is not an option since there is no infectious process present.

Chapter 7: Nursing Care of Clients Experiencing Disasters

1. **Answer: 3 Rationale:** Emergencies are not controlled. Disasters do not only result from man-made errors, but can be caused by nature. Disasters often involve multiple services and agencies working together.

2. **Answer: 3 Rationale:** Nurses are an integral part in assisting with disasters. However, they do not serve in a leadership role in the command center. Their role is in assisting with triage and in meeting the emergency healthcare needs of those injured or involved in the disaster.

3. **Answer: 4 Rationale:** Reverse triage is necessary when there are limited resources to care for multiple people injured in a disaster. This is so the majority of people can be helped with the resources currently available.

4. **Answer: 3 Rationale:** It is important to recognize that a client whose primary language is not English may not read in his or her primary language. This can create a significant problem when providing health education. It is important to have someone translate all information to the client and have the client explain what has been taught in order to ensure proper understanding of the information.

5. **Answer: 3 Rationale:** PPE should lessen the likelihood of occupational injury and/or illness, but proper precautions also must be taken to ensure safety. This can be as simple as proper hand washing after removing gloves, or following isolation guidelines.

6. **Answer: 2 Rationale:** Decontamination cannot begin in the hot zone as this is the area of greatest contamination. It is important to decontaminate the area outside of the hot zone to prevent its spread.

7. **Answer: 1 Rationale:** A dirty bomb is a bomb that carries a radiological signature and can cause contamination and radiation poisoning.

8. **Answer: 2 Rationale:** Radiation sickness is the direct result of exposure to ionizing radiation, which causes cellular mutation. This condition must be treated rapidly or death may result as the cells continue to mutate and die.

9. **Answer: 3 Rationale:** Older adults have individual needs. Some may be more independent than others regarding the degree of support needed in emergencies, whereas others may require multiple resources and support in an evacuation.

10. **Answer: 4 Rationale:** Nurses often are so involved in caring for others they tend to neglect themselves. In disaster situations, nurses may also suffer from loss while caring for others. As a result the nurse may feel overwhelmed and be as traumatized as those for whom he/she is caring.

Chapter 8: Genetic Implications of Adult Health Nursing

1. **Answer: 2 Rationale:** In an autosomal dominant condition, you only need one of the genotypes to have the condition. An autosomal dominant condition is not a sex-linked disease and is not found on the x or y chromosomes.

2. **Answer: 1, 3 Rationale:** Fabry disease is an x-linked genetic disorder. Since the male provides the y chromosome to a male offspring, the male cannot pass on this disease to male offspring. The female can pass this disorder on. Also, which grandmother (maternal or fraternal) is not stated, and if the grandmother was not affected, she could be a carrier since her brother had the disease.

3. **Answer: 4 Rationale:** It is a nurse's responsibility to explain what is involved in genetic testing. It is not the nurse's responsibility to discuss potential outcomes, as this is the responsibility of the genetic counselor.

4. **Answer: 1, 4 Rationale:** Breast cancer at this early an age is most likely to have a genetic component that makes the client more likely to have this condition. A brother's unexpected infertility can be cause for alarm in many genetic conditions.

5. **Answer: 5 Rationale:** Mitochondrial mutations are only passed from the mother. This is because mitochondria are primarily found in ova and not sperm. This is considered a matrilineal pattern of inheritance. An affected female will pass the condition on to her children; however, an affected male will not.

6. **Answer: 1, 2 Rationale:** Performing a family history assessment helps the nurse know what is important to focus on regarding health promotion and maintenance when planning. This is necessary in order to individualize the treatment plan to best meet the needs of the client and family. This also provides the opportunity to encourage preventative and prophylactic treatments to promote wellness. This is not done to determine specific genotypes, but family and environmental influences on health behavior.

7. **Answer: 3 Rationale:** It is not important to include all details for all those included in the pedigree. It is more important to know cause of death, chronic illness, and age. The paternal side of the family is usually placed on the left and the maternal on the right. A minimum of three generations should be included and labeled appropriately. The proband should be marked with an arrow and a "P" so it is easy to identify.

8. **Answer: 1, 2, 4 Rationale:** Minor physical anomalies are simply visual. However, an ASD is a functional defect, which can impair activity and cause severe complications, as the client gets older.

9. **Answer: 2, 3 Rationale:** Certification status is appropriate as it explains that the results of the testing can be considered reliable. CLIA88 = Clinical Laboratory Improvement Amendment 88 (this is the year the law was amended) is an accreditation for certification, and contains a full list of the certifications for the laboratory. This is done on a yearly basis. It is important to explain that a mutation panel can address the most common gene alterations, but not all.

10. **Answer: 2, 4 Rationale:** Often tests will be ordered at the initial visit to look at chromosome studies. Once the results are received, the client will be informed of the findings. The role of the genetic healthcare provider is to present the client with accurate information to make informed decisions and provide information about the natural history of the condition.

Chapter 9: Nursing Care of Clients Experiencing Pain

1. **Answer: 2 Rationale:** Chronic pain, pain that has been ongoing for more than six months, is the most appropriate answer. Acute pain is sudden in onset and has not been ongoing for

more than six months. Referred pain is pain that originates in another location. Somatic pain is considered to be psychological in origin.

2. **Answer: 1 Rationale:** It is very important to provide medication to prevent pain and to help keep pain from getting worse rather than waiting until it does get bad. Pain causes release of chemical mediators that attach to pain receptors, causing pain to be more intense, difficult to treat, and get in control.

3. **Answer: 2 Rationale:** NSAIDs are known to cause problems with gastric ulcerations. Taking an NSAID for years can cause significant problems with erosion.

4. **Answer: 4 Rationale:** Transdermal pain medications are most effective when placed on the upper torso. This is because the medication is absorbed through the surface of the skin and returned to the heart, where circulation is better than in distal extremities.

5. **Answer: 3 Rationale:** This statement is most appropriate as the nurse is asking for a description of the pain, which addresses the quality.

6. **Answer: 2 Rationale:** An overdose can occur as clients can become over-sedated and develop respiratory depression.

7. **Answer: 2 Rationale:** Constipation, nausea, and sedation are all very common side effects of opioid analgesia. The narcotic slows down peristalsis, causing constipation and nausea. Sedation is caused from the opioids crossing the blood-brain barrier.

8. **Answer: 2 Rationale:** Oral opioid analgesia is the recommended route for chronic pain.

9. **Answer: 4 Rationale:** The equivalent dose of an oral drug compared to the intravenous preparation of the same drug is often significantly less effective. It may take about five times the dose to equal the IV dose.

10. **Answer: 4 Rationale:** Clients treated for chronic pain may need additional pain management strategies to help manage breakthrough pain, acute pain, and end-of-dose pain. In addition to chronic pain, clients often have flares of acute pain. As the pain medication wears off, there may be breakthrough pain or end-of-dose pain.

Chapter 10: Nursing Care of Clients with Altered Fluid, Electrolyte, and Acid-Base Balance

1. **Answer: 1 Rationale:** Ringer's solution is an Isotonic, balanced electrolyte solution that can expand plasma volume and help restore electrolyte balance. Hypertonic solutions such as 10% dextrose and 3% sodium chloride pull interstitial and intracellular fluid into the vascular system, leading to cellular dehydration. A hypotonic solution such as 0.45% sodium chloride may be used to treat cellular dehydration.

2. **Answer: 4 Rationale:** In fluid volume deficit, there is less volume in the vascular system, which decreases venous return and cardiac output, leading to manifestations of dizziness, orthostatic hypotension and flat neck veins. The heart rate increases and the blood pressure falls. Dyspnea and crackles usually are associated with excess fluid volume; headache and muscle cramps are often due to electrolyte imbalance, not fluid loss.

3. **Answer: 1, 3, 4 Rationale:** Frequent neurological checks are necessary as hypernatremia draws water out of brain cells, causing them to shrink. As the brain shrinks, tension is placed on cerebral vessels, which may cause them to tear and bleed. Hypernatremia affects mental status and brain function (including orientation to time, place and person), as can rapid correction of hypernatremia. Fluid replacement is the primary treatment for hypernatremia. Maintaining intravenous access is necessary for administration of fluids and possible emergency medications. There is no reason to limit visit length.

4. **Answer: 2 Rationale:** Hypokalemia affects nerve impulse transmission, including the transmission of cardiac impulses. The client may develop ECG changes and atrial or ventricular dysrhythmias. Although hypokalemia can lead to muscle weakness and activity intolerance, bedrest generally is unnecessary.

5. **Answer: 4 Rationale:** Calcium should be taken with a full glass of water to allow maximum absorption. It is more effectively absorbed when taken on an empty stomach and the prescribed doses spaced throughout the day.

6. **Answer: 1 Rationale:** A positive Chvostek's sign indicates increased neuromuscular excitability, commonly associated with both hypomagnesia and hypocalcemia. Additional manifestations of hypomagnesemia include confusion, hallucinations, and possible psychoses. Administration of magnesium sulfate helps restore magnesium balance and neuromuscular function.

7. **Answer: 1 Rationale:** The pH is indicative of acidosis (less than 7.35), and the bicarbonate level is low (less than 22 mEq/L), indicating bicarbonate deficit as cause of the acidosis. In addition, the $Paco_2$ is low (less than 35 mmHg), indicating respiratory compensation for the excess acid.

8. **Answer: 1, 3, 5 Rationale:** The slow respiratory rate leads to inadequate alveolar ventilation. As a result, carbon dioxide is not effectively eliminated from the blood, causing it to accumulate. This increases carbonic acid levels, leading to respiratory acidosis, as indicated by the low pH and high $Paco_2$. Excess carbon dioxide causes vasodilation, leading to warm, flushed skin, particularly in acute respiratory acidosis.

9. **Answer: 1 Rationale:** Gastric suctioning removes highly acidic gastric secretions, increasing the alkalinity of body fluids. Chloride, the primary anion in extracellular fluid, also is lost through gastric suction, causing the kidneys to retain bicarbonate to restore the balance between positively and negatively charged ions in the body.

10. **Answer: 3 Rationale:** The client is demonstrating classic manifestations of respiratory alkalosis, a potential complication of mechanical ventilation when the rate or volume of ventilations are too high. Arterial blood gases provide the data necessary to confirm and treat this problem.

Chapter 11: Nursing Care of the Client Experiencing Trauma and Shock

1. **Answer: 4 Rationale:** Although all of the choices can be sources of injury or death in adults of all ages, motor vehicle accidents remain the leading cause of injury. As people become more aware of the need for seatbelts and other safety considerations, the fatality rate of motor vehicle accidents decreases.

2. **Answer: 1 Rationale:** Airway obstruction is the first and foremost risk to assess for, as this represents the ABCs of life support. A = airway, B = breathing, C = circulation. Although all of the other choices can also be present, a patent airway must be the number one priority for survival.

3. **Answer: 2 Rationale:** Assessing airway patency is the first step in the ABCs of life support. Although the rest of the choices listed are important to assess also, the first and foremost intervention is the airway patency.

4. **Answer: 3 Rationale:** The most severe reaction is decreasing blood pressure and dyspnea.

5. **Answer: 2 Rationale:** The endotoxins released from bacteria in septic shock stimulate the release of vasoactive proteins causing peripheral vasodilation and decreased peripheral resistance.

6. **Answer: 1 Rationale:** Direct pressure to the wound is the best method to manage uncontrolled bleeding. If 1. is ineffective, then it is necessary to consider the other options. However, in the field, 1. is definitely the first choice.

7. **Answer: 1 Rationale:** Trauma is defined as injury to human tissues from the transfer of energy. It is not specific to intentional or accidental. It simply addresses tissue injury. Knowing the type of energy can help understand the severity of tissue injury.

8. **Answer: 4 Rationale:** Weight gain is not a risk from a blood transfusion.

9. **Answer: 2 Rationale:** Widespread vasodilation can cause distributive shock as the blood pressure drops dangerously due to the very low peripheral vascular resistance. A hypersensitivity reaction will cause anaphylactic shock, not distributive shock.

10. **Answer: 4 Rationale:** Ultimately there is a systemic imbalance between oxygen supply and demand. Sufficient cardiac output is not shock, insufficient cardiac output is. Hemorrhage is a cause of one of the types of shock, but does not define shock. Abnormal blood pressure may be either high or low.

Chapter 12: Nursing Care of Clients with Infections

1. **Answer: 3 Rationale:** Natural passive immunity is the result of a gamma globulin infusion following exposure to hepatitis A. This type of immunity is short-lived and usually lasts only about four weeks. This is considered "borrowed immunity."

2. **Answer: 2 Rationale:** Enlarged lymph nodes are a common physical finding of a systemic infection, as the immune system is actively trying to fight this infection. Lymph node enlargement is stimulated by full activation of the immune system. Pain and erythema can be a symptom of a local infection, but these are not specific to systemic symptoms. A decreased heart rate is a late symptom of shock, not simply a systemic infection.

3. **Answer: 4 Rationale:** Although the exact mechanism of action is unknown, aspirin inhibits prostaglandin synthesis. This can serve many purposes including producing analgesia, anti-inflammatory and anti-pyretic effects, and inhibit platelet aggregation.

4. **Answer: 1 Rationale:** A "left shift" is commonly referred to when there is an increase in band neutrophils. This is to be expected when the body is mounting a response to a bacterial infection. This occurs when the bone marrow is stimulated to rapidly produce more white blood cells. The bone marrow starts churning out increased quantities of immature white blood cells, otherwise known as bands.

5. **Answer: 2 Rationale:** Contact precautions are the form of isolation recommended for an MRSA wound. This requires a gown to be worn for any direct client contact and gloves to be worn upon entering the room. Good hand washing is essential after removing gloves, as the gloves do not ensure cleanliness of the hands.

6. **Answer: 1 Rationale:** The T cells of the immune system adapt to kill intracellular organisms. These can be viral-infected cells, cancer cells, or foreign tissue. This is part of humoral immunity and is a cell-mediated response. All of the other choices are occurring outside of the cells.

7. **Answer: 1 Rationale:** Thrombocytosis is best explained as increased platelets. This causes platelet aggregation and increases clot formation.

8. **Answer: 4 Rationale:** When there is a nursing diagnosis "Risk for Infection," this can pertain to the client, caregivers, or other clients. It addresses the possibility that the client cannot fight infection, the staff is potentially at risk for developing an infection from the infected client, or the other clients are at risk for becoming infected from the infected client.

9. **Answer: 4 Rationale:** When administering antibiotics, the nurse must be aware of potential hypersensitivity reactions. It is important to monitor for any hypersensitivities in addition to providing education about the infection, antibiotic, and any potential side effects of treatment.

10. **Answer: 3 Rationale:** Wearing gloves, gowns, and goggles when coming in contact with contaminated body fluids is considered to be a standard procedure.

Chapter 13: Nursing Care of Clients with Altered Immunity

1. **Answer: 4 Rationale:** Anaphylaxis occurs as the direct result from a Type 1 hypersensitivity reaction. The body has IgE circulating, which is specific to a certain allergen. Allergen re-exposure causes this cascade leading to anaphylaxis.

2. **Answer: 1 Rationale:** An acute tissue rejection episode is the most common and treatable type of rejection. It occurs between four days and three months after the transplant. Symptoms can include fever and tenderness over the liver, and elevated liver enzymes and bilirubin levels.

3. **Answer: 3 Rationale:** These symptoms are indicative of a respiratory infection. Of the choices listed, pneumocystis carinii is the choice that causes the respiratory infection known as PCP.

4. **Answer: 4 Rationale:** When a client tests positive for HIV, this means that antibodies to the AIDS virus are present in the blood. HIV does not equal AIDS. It is important for the nurse to be able to explain the difference between HIV and AIDS to the client. AIDS is diagnosed when the CD4 count drops below 200. The client needs to understand that AIDS could develop in the future, especially without treatment.

5. **Answer: 2 Rationale:** Leukopenia can be an adverse reaction of Retrovir. As Retrovir can cause bone marrow suppression and pancytopenia, CBCs should be done on a routine basis, in addition to other lab work to assess the t-cell levels plus any other warranted lab work.

6. **Answer: 2 Rationale:** Of all of the choices available, the allergen prick testing has the lowest risk of anaphylaxis associated with it. This is because there is the smallest amount of allergen entering the bloodstream. This is also the most accurate way to assess for allergies as the wheal and flare will only occur with the allergens that are positive.

7. **Answer: 2 Rationale:** When hypersensitivity is suspected it is important to avoid any further exposure to the potential cause. The best way to do this is by replacing all tubing and attaching a new line primed with NS.

8. **Answer: 2 Rationale:** Protease inhibitors and nucleoside analogs are associated with serious metabolic problems such as elevated cholesterol and triglycerides, insulin resistance and diabetes mellitus, and changes in body fat composition. These can be very distressing to clients.

9. **Answer: 4 Rationale:** The priority when initiating or changing HIV drug therapy regimens is the client's willingness to adhere

to the drug regimen. This is due to the high resistance to therapy associated when clients choose to discontinue treatment with their anti-viral medications. Since the side effects can be difficult and challenging to overcome, many clients are not willing to continue with their therapy.

10. **Answer: 4 Rationale:** Antithymocyte globulin (ATG) is used to induce immunosuppression immediately following a transplant. Its purpose is to bind with the peripheral lymphocytes and mononuclear cells to remove them from circulation and prevent them from being able to reject the new organ.

Chapter 14: Nursing Care of Clients with Cancer

1. **Answer: 3 Rationale:** Metastasis occurs when cells from a primary tumor site travel through the lymphatic system or bloodstream to find a secondary target.

2. **Answer: 1 Rationale:** One of the many qualities those of us in nursing possess is the ability to listen. Often, when clients are dealing with a difficult diagnosis with a questionable future, this quality helps the client to cope. Encouraging the client to express his feelings about the cancer diagnosis is the most valuable and powerful intervention that could be offered. It is important to document on the chart the client's report of difficulty sleeping and tenseness in order to communicate with other staff, but this is not the primary intervention. It also may be a good idea to obtain an order for medication for sleep from the physician, but again, this is not the best primary intervention. Offering an antianxiety drug may be helpful, but this is not the primary need.

3. **Answer: 3 Rationale:** It is important not to rub or scratch the treated skin areas, as this can cause irritation to the surface of the skin as well as breaks in the skin. Rubbing may also wipe off the ink markings, which are important landmarks to ensure that the radiation treatments are directed to the correct location.

4. **Answer: 2 Rationale:** Providing an antiemetic prior to chemotherapy is an excellent preventative treatment to prevent nausea and vomiting following chemotherapy. This helps to improve the quality of life the client has while in treatment. We know that feeling very ill can increase symptoms of depression; thus, providing the anitemetic prior to the chemotherapy can improve Ms. Smith's general outlook.

5. **Answer: 3 Rationale:** Although all of these choices can be a result of chemotherapy, the one that is directly affected with bone marrow suppression is a low platelet count of 50,000. A fever can also be caused from the degree of neutropenia, as Ms. Smith is not able to fight infection. However, the most correct answer remains c.

6. **Answer: 3 Rationale:** Chemotherapy is not cell type specific. It simply targets cells that are rapidly dividing, which can be both cancer cells and healthy cells. It is important to understand that as normal cells are destroyed, this can cause other symptoms such as mucositis, hair loss, and bone marrow suppression.

7. **Answer: 1 Rationale:** External radiation therapy is when the radiation is initiated outside of the body, directed towards the client, and is set to deliver to a certain depth for a specified period of time. This exposure is meant to destroy the cancer cells the radiation comes into direct contact with.

8. **Answer: 2 Rationale:** Tumor lysis syndrome can cause high levels of uric acid. Clients are often treated with allopurinal to help excrete the uric acid in the urine. Also, electrolyte imbal-

ances may occur and need to be monitored and replaced as needed. Often the client may suffer from low potassium, phosphorus, and calcium levels. This can cause a multitude of problems including severe life-threatening arrhythmias.

9. **Answer: 3 Rationale:** The S phase is when DNA replication occurs. This is when the cell is beginning mitosis and the chromosomes multiply from 23 to 46. They then migrate towards each axis in preparation for division of the cell.

10. **Answer: 1 Rationale:** Oncogenes are genes that stimulate cell growth. These genes require something to activate them in order to cause this reaction to occur.

Chapter 15: Assessing Clients with Integumentary Disorders

1. **Answer: 2 Rationale:** There are many layers to the skin. The layer that has the most glands and hair follicles located in it is the dermis. The epidermis is on top of this layer and the stratum spinosum and stratum basale are beneath the dermis.

2. **Answer: 3 Rationale:** Melanin is the pigment found in skin that protects the skin from the sun. This is the pigment responsible for tanning. It is also the source of malignancy in malignant melanoma.

3. **Answer: 1, 2 Rationale:** Inspection is the first assessment technique to check the skin surface. This is done by simply looking at the skin for any abnormalities or imperfections. The next assessment step is to palpate any areas of the skin that appear abnormal in order to get a better understanding of depth and size of any lesions. This is also a way to assess if the abnormality causes any pain or discomfort.

4. **Answer: 1 Rationale:** Erythema often occurs as a result of increased body temperature. This occurs when the capillaries in the skin dilate to release some of the heat caused from the increased body temperature.

5. **Answer: 3 Rationale:** Often new soap can cause skin irritation and itching. It is important to determine if there is anything that has changed to cause this irritation. This is the easiest variable to assess.

6. **Answer: 1 Rationale:** A decreased skin turgor is a sign of dehydration. This is often referred to as "tenting." By pinching the skin gently, when you release the skin, a small tent remains before flattening out.

7. **Answer: 4 Rationale:** Edema begins in the distal extremities. The best place to assess for this is the ankle area. By pressing the fingertip into the skin and releasing it, you can determine the severity of edema by seeing how deep the pitting goes after removing your fingertips. This is often categorized on a scale of one to four.

8. **Answer: 4 Rationale:** Lichenification is a condition in which the skin cells multiply causing what appears to be thickened and calloused skin. The skin often has a rough and leathery appearance to it. This condition is common in clients suffering from chronic dermatitis.

9. **Answer: 2 Rationale:** Although aging skin is known to bruise easier, a greater concern would be the possibility of elder abuse. It is extremely important for the nurse making the home visit to assess for this in order to provide support and assistance to the older woman and caregiver.

10. **Answer: 3 Rationale:** Head lice cause small white eggs to be found attached to the hair shaft, very close to the scalp. These are called nits and are the eggs of the lice. After using an anti-lice shampoo, it is necessary to carefully comb these out of the hair.

Chapter 16: Nursing Care of Clients with Integumentary Disorders

1. **Answer: 3 Rationale:** Xerosis is a skin condition in which the skin appears very dry and roughened. It is important to help remoisturize the skin. The best way to do this is to apply a moisturizing agent to the skin after bathing. Blotting dry with a towel and then applying a moisturizer will help lock in the moisture from the bath and help nourish the skin.

2. **Answer: 1 Rationale:** Nevi are the skin lesions that need to be monitored for changes. These lesions can become malignant and need to be monitored for any change. The ABCDE of nevi include A-abnormal border, B-black, C-color change, D-diameter, E-elevation.

3. **Answer: 4 Rationale:** Psoriasis causes abnormal growth and division of epidermal cells, causing keratosis. The use of ultraviolet light therapy helps to slow down this cellular division, which decreases the lesions and keratosis associated with psoriasis.

4. **Answer: 2 Rationale:** Pregnancy causes many changes in the body. Included in this is that the vaginal tissue is more prone to yeast infections. During pregnancy there is often an increase in vaginal secretions. Yeast is an opportunistic organism that grows best in warm, dark moist environments such as the vagina.

5. **Answer: 4 Rationale:** This condition is most likely shingles, which is a type of varicella infection. It is important to assess if the client has any degree of natural immunity to varicella. The easiest way to determine this is to know if the client has ever had chickenpox. This can help to determine if the shingles will only be isolated to this dermatome or if the client is at risk for a more severe infection and may need to be started on antiviral therapy.

6. **Answer: 2 Rationale:** It is a myth that only dirty people get lice. Major infestations often occur in areas where many are in close proximity of each other, especially in the public school setting. Lice are a parasite and are found in the hair and scalp of humans.

7. **Answer: 1 Rationale:** People with fair skin, blond hair, and freckles are at increased risk for non-melanoma skin cancers. People meeting this description should have yearly skin checks to assess for any changes in nevi or other lesions.

8. **Answer: 1 Rationale:** A change in the color or size of a nevus is cause for concern when evaluating for the possibility of melanoma. This falls under the ABCDE of skin checks.

9. **Answer: 2 Rationale:** Clients who are bedridden are at increased risk for pressure sores and skin tears. Skin tears may occur as a result of the shearing force of pulling a client up in bed. Skin assessments should be done each shift and appropriate interventions for preventing skin breakdown implemented as needed.

10. **Answer: 3 Rationale:** Dermabrasion is a skin treatment that helps to reduce the appearance of acne scarring and other skin imperfections. Often these treatments are done on a regular basis for clients in a plastic surgery clinic.

Chapter 17: Nursing Care of Clients with Burns

1. **Answer: 3 Rationale:** In the emergent phase of burn management, it is important to monitor electrolyte levels frequently. Initially the client is at risk for fluid and electrolyte imbalances, especially for decreased serum potassium levels. This can cause an increased risk for arrhythmias.

2. **Answer: 4 Rationale:** A full thickness burn is not painful, as the nerves have also been affected from the burn. In this situation, pain is not a good sign. It tells the nurse that the depth of the burn goes beyond the nerves. Superficial, superficial partial thickness, and deep partial thickness burns will still be very painful to the client, as the nerves remain intact or exposed.

3. **Answer: 4 Rationale:** The larger the surface area of the burn and the deeper the burn, the more at risk the client is for burn shock. A high-voltage electrical accident will cause a deeper burn and since this scenario explains that >50% of the body is affected, this places the client at the highest risk.

4. **Answer: 2 Rationale:** Silvadene cream can cause neutropenia. It is important for the nurse to monitor the client's WBC count daily to assess for any changes, which could indicate neutropenia. Although this is the most important intervention, it is also important to keep the client as comfortable as possible. Premedicating is definitely not a bad idea, as burn dressing changes can be very painful and the Silvadene will help debride the burn.

5. **Answer: 2 Rationale:** The Parkland Formula uses lactated Ringer's solution, administered at 4 mL $\times$ kg $\times$ % TBSA burn, with 50% of the total volume infused in the first eight hours, and the remaining 50% over the next 16 hours. This would be $4 \times 70 \times 50\% = 14,000 \times 50\% = 7,000$.

6. **Answer: 1 Rationale:** Urine output is the most sensitive indicator of fluid resuscitation success. A decrease in urine output is seen in dehydration and a recovery from dehydration is seen with an increase in urine output.

7. **Answer: 4 Rationale:** A decreased left radial pulse is cause for alarm in this type and location of burn. This can be the first symptom seen in compartment syndrome and is a surgical emergency.

8. **Answer: 2 Rationale:** The Rule of Nines is a method of quickly estimating the percentage of TBSA affected by a burn injury. It is most useful in emergency situations but is not accurate for estimating TBSA in adults who are short, obese, or very thin. Anterior trunk = 18%, perineum = 1%, left arm = 9%. These are added together to = 28%.

9. **Answer: 1, 3, 5, 6 Rationale:** Teaching injury prevention is a very important job in nursing. Burns are a common injury in the home. It is important to help older adults understand ways to help prevent burns. Wearing close-fitting clothing when cooking can help prevent shirtsleeves or scarves from catching on fire. The water temperature of the water heater should not be set above 120 degrees. This can help prevent burns from water scalding. Installing anti-scald devices can also help prevent water burns. As older adults often have decreased olfactory senses, having a neighbor routinely check for the odor of gas can help prevent fires.

10. **Answer: 3 Rationale:** A 15% carbon monoxide level would cause only mild symptoms of dizziness at this stage. Later stages with higher levels will cause the remaining symptoms of the skin color change, drowsiness, and hypotension.

Chapter 18: Assessing Clients with Endocrine Disorders

1. **Answer: 2 Rationale:** ADH, antidiuretic hormone, helps to concentrate urine, which would decrease the urine output. The ADH causes the distal tubules in the kidney to reabsorb water, which will concentrate the urine.

2. **Answer: 3 Rationale:** Testing for Trousseau's sign is done by inflating a blood pressure cuff above the antecubital area, higher than the systolic blood pressure, for two to five minutes. A positive test causes carpal spasm and the fingers and hand will contract on the arm where the blood pressure cuff is inflated.

3. **Answer: 1 Rationale:** Excessive amounts of glucocorticoids cause symptoms of immunosuppression. The glucocorticoids

are natural steroids, which cause immunosuppression. These are hormones, which affect carbohydrate metabolism. Glucocorticoids include cortisol and cortisone and are released in times of stress. Any significant excess of these can depress the inflammatory response and inhibit the effectiveness of the immune system.

4. **Answer: 3 Rationale:** When assessing the endocrine system, it is important to look for signs and symptoms of diabetes. One of the first symptoms is polydypsia, which is increased thirst. Asking clients if they have noticed any change in their thirst can help to address this symptom.

5. **Answer: 2 Rationale:** Palpating the thyroid gland can assess the size and consistency of the gland. This is important to check when assessing for goiters, enlargement, or nodules.

6. **Answer: 2 Rationale:** Assessment for Chvostek's sign is done by tapping a finger in front of the ear, at the angle of the jaw. A positive sign causes facial grimacing with repeated contractions of the facial muscle. A normal sign shows no grimacing.

7. **Answer: 4 Rationale:** TSH is thyroid-stimulating hormone. This is a hormone, which is supposed to stimulate the thyroid gland to function. When the TSH level is high, the thyroid is not functioning enough, known as hypothyroidism. When the TSH level is very low, this is a condition known as hyperthyroidism.

8. **Answer: 3 Rationale:** The thyroid gland is the only endocrine organ that can be palpated during an exam. It is located behind the thyroid cartilage of the trachea and the edges of the gland can often be palpated on either side of the trachea. The pancreas is found deep in the abdominal cavity. The liver is behind the rib cage, but the edge of the liver can often be palpated at the base of the rib cage. The pituitary gland is located in the brain.

9. **Answer: 2 Rationale:** Rough, dry skin is often found in clients with hypothyroidism. The skin temperature is also often cool.

10. **Answer: 4 Rationale:** Thyroid function can be assessed by testing deep tendon reflexes. Increased deep tendon reflexes are seen in hyperthyroidism. Decreased deep tendon reflexes are seen in hypothyroidism.

Chapter 19: Nursing Care of Clients with Endocrine Disorders

1. **Answer: 1 Rationale:** An antibody attaches to TSH receptors in the thyroid and causes increased production. There is no infectious agent, allergen, or genetic link.

2. **Answer: 3 Rationale:** Oral administration of radioactive iodine concentrates in the thyroid gland and damages or destroys thyroid cells decreasing TH levels. There is no effect on vascularity of the thyroid but hypothyroidism can be created with this therapy.

3. **Answer: 3 Rationale:** The body tries to produce more hormones by simply producing more cells that produce that hormone. TH is not increased, it is decreased. Dietary iodine has no effect on thyroid enlargement.

4. **Answer: 4 Rationale:** Persons who take corticosteroids for treatment of rheumatoid arthritis for long periods are at increased risk for developing Cushing's syndrome since it is the result of increased stimulation of the adrenal cortex.

5. **Answer: 2 Rationale:** A client with the diagnosis of Addison's disease will be stressed by infection and an additional dose of steroids may be needed to prevent crisis. Therefore clients are urged to carry injectable cortisone and a syringe at all times.

6. **Answer: 2 Rationale:** Irritability occurs as the brain and nerve cells become edematous as the blood volume expands.

7. **Answer: 2 Rationale:** Clients with this disorder are at risk for pathological fractures of the bones because of the decreased density of the bone.

8. **Answer: 3 Rationale:** Clients with hypercalcemia will demonstrate decreased bowel sounds related to the decreased neuromuscular excitability with increased calcium. Clients also will have increased urinary output, a negative Chvostek's sign, and decreased deep tendon reflexes.

9. **Answer: 4 Rationale:** In 98% of clients with increased ACTH levels and Addison's disease the exposed and unexposed skin is deeply suntanned or bronzed.

10. **Answer: 1 Rationale:** With a sudden stoppage of steroids, the adrenal cortex cannot recuperate rapidly enough to increase production because it has been suppressed with exogenous steroids. Therefore steroids are gradually decreased and clients weaned to allow endogenous steroid production to resume.

Chapter 20: Nursing Care of Clients with Diabetes Mellitus

1. **Answer: 1 Rationale:** 95% of clients diagnosed with type 1 diabetes mellitus have the genetic markers with DR3 & DR 4 antigens on chromosome 6 of the leukocyte antigen system. This indicates increased susceptibility to develop diabetes type 1. Obesity in adolescence is more indicative of type 2 diabetes. Diabetic women usually produce a baby weighing more than ten pounds, not underweight babies. Elevation of glucagons would occur in hypoglycemia, not hyperglycemia.

2. **Answer: 3 Rationale:** Increased glucagon levels and deficit of insulin increases the liver's production of ketone bodies and increased release of free fatty acids. With this process, bicarbonate production is decreased and it cannot buffer so metabolic acidosis occurs.

3. **Answer: 4 Rationale:** There is an increased risk of developing type 2 diabetes in the older population (over 65) with a decrease in the calorie need and especially with the decrease of exercise.

4. **Answer: 3 Rationale:** With diabetes often the client will state changes in sensation of the feet caused by impaired nerve function. The client may complain of numbness or tingling.

5. **Answer: 3 Rationale:** Checking the feet daily is important. Someone needs to look at all surfaces and between toes for any breaks in skin integrity or changes in cellular makeup. The other three answers are all on the *do not do* list of diabetic foot care.

6. **Answer: 3 Rationale:** Since it is clear, Lantus (glargine) could be confused with regular insulin. Regular insulin is short acting in 4-6 hours and Lantus is long acting in 24-28 hours. Confusing these two insulins could be extremely harmful to client. Lantus should not be mixed with other insulins or given IV.

7. **Answer: 3 Rationale:** Only regular insulin can safely be administered intravenously for diabetic ketoacidosis. Subcutaneous injection is recommended for all other insulins.

8. **Answer: 3 Rationale:** HgbA1C levels 7-9% show that the glucose level has been elevated or erratic over this period of time.

9. **Answer: 3 Rationale:** No intermediate- or long-acting insulin is given the day of surgery since dietary intake post-operatively is uncertain. IV glucose (5%) and regular insulin in equally divided doses will compensate for the increase in serum glucose until the client is eating and drinking normally.

10. **Answer: 4 Rationale:** The abdomen absorbs insulin the fastest. After the abdomen the order is deltoid, thigh, and lastly, hip.

Chapter 21: Assessing Clients with Nutritional and GI Disorders

1. **Answer: 1 Rationale:** Bile is necessary for emulsifying and absorption of fats.

2. **Answer: 3 Rationale:** Catabolism is the breakdown of complex structures into simpler forms. Anabolism is the combining of simple molecules to form complex structures. Metabolism is the biochemical reactions within the cells—anabolism and catabolism.

3. **Answer: 2 Rationale:** Animal products are considered complete proteins in that they meet the body's requirements for tissue building and maintenance. Fruits and vegetables are missing at least one essential amino acid. Butter and oils are sources of fat.

4. **Answer: 2 Rationale:** Vitamin K is an essential element for blood clotting and, without sufficient levels, bleeding can occur. Vitamin K does not affect the other answers.

5. **Answer: 4 Rationale:** A 24-hour dietary intake recall will demonstrate quantities and patterns of food intake that would be important in the nutritional assessment of a client.

6. **Answer: 4 Rationale:** An elevated amylase indicates that the pancreatic enzymes are digesting their own tissues. Cheliosis is the breakdown of tissues of the corner of the mouth due to vitamin B deficiency. Gastric reflux is related to the esophagus and will not produce elevation in enzymes. Gallstones are associated with potential elevation of the bilirubin test.

7. **Answer: 1 Rationale:** The condition of the client's teeth, possible difficulty for her to chew comfortably, and her dry mouth because of decreased production of saliva in the older adult may cause a nutritional deficit because she will tend to eat food that is easier to chew and swallow. She may not eat enough protein.

8. **Answer: 1 Rationale:** The liver is located in the right upper quadrant with the border palpated below the rib cage when the client takes a deep breath.

9. **Answer: 4 Rationale:** In client with ascites of the liver of more than 500 mL, a method of determining fluid presence is palpating dullness in the abdomen in the supine position and then on the right side. The presence of dullness moving in these two positions indicates ascites with shifting dullness pattern.

10. **Answer: 3 Rationale:** Palpation of the abdomen is done last in order to avoid influencing bowel peristalsis or cause pain that could end the exam. The order of assessment is observe, auscultate, percuss, and palpate.

Chapter 22: Nursing Care of Clients with Nutritional Disorders

1. **Answer: 3 Rationale:** The lack of regular exercise in daily life means less expenditure of energy, therefore nutrients are stored as fat. Research has shown that adopted children's weight is related to their biological parents. "Fast foods" are a contributing factor. Allergies are not related to obesity.

2. **Answer: 2 Rationale:** This response informs the client of the calorie-pound relationship and involves the client in the planning strategies to improve and maintain weight loss.

3. **Answer: 1 Rationale:** Recent weight loss is the most prevalent finding in protein-calorie malnutrition. Skinfold thickness is decreased and the client demonstrates lethargy and drowsiness.

4. **Answer: 3 Rationale:** Small-bore feeding tubes displace easily. Accurate placement is evaluated by aspirating contents and checking the pH. In the stomach the pH is <4. None of the other methods are as accurate or supported by research.

5. **Answer: 4 Rationale:** An identified contributing factor to anorexia is family pressure. Family therapy commonly is an important part of the interdisciplinary treatment plan. The caloric intake and weight gain is unrealistic for these clients.

6. **Answer: 2 Rationale:** A BMI greater than 25 and central obesity as indicated by a waist-hip ratio of 1 or greater are associated with a higher risk for hypertension, elevated lipid levels, heart disease and stroke. These conditions have the greatest impact on health over time.

7. **Answer: 4, 5 Rationale:** Because this drug causes dry mouth and potential for constipation, fluids are important to maintain function. The drug is intended to be taken along with a restricted calorie diet for weight loss. The drug is taken only once a day not with each meal, so a skipped meal doesn't matter. There are no guidelines about alcohol consumption in drug reference manuals. Drowsiness is not a problem because this drug will increase stimulation and may in fact interfere with sleep.

8. **Answer: 1, 2, 4, 5 Rationale:** There are many contributing factors that influence nutrition in the home-bound older adult such as inability to shop for nutritional foods, ability to afford and to prepare nutritional food. There are also psychosocial issues of depression and loneliness since eating is a social affair, this could well influence the amount and proportion of caloric intake. Arranging for food to be brought to the client and for the client to be transported to a senior center for a meal may solve the weight loss issue and no further interventions may be necessary.

9. **Answer: 4 Rationale:** Beginning oral intake of nutrients as soon as possible after surgery is the best way to prevent malnutrition. Aggressive pain management may have the opposite effect—it may decrease appetite or sedate the client, interfering with food intake. While IV fluids may be necessary to maintain fluid volume, most do not contain adequate calories to maintain nutritional status. Daily weights often are more reflective of fluid volume status than of nutritional status.

10. **Answer: 1 Rationale:** One of the postoperative complications with gastric bypass surgery is an anastomotic leak causing peritonitis. These symptoms could be related to this condition and the surgeon needs to be notified.

Chapter 23: Nursing Care of Clients Experiencing Upper GI Disorders

1. **Answer: 4 Rationale:** The use of tobacco and drinking alcohol are the two primary risk factors for oral cancers. The others are not risk factors for oral cancer.

2. **Answer: 2, 5 Rationale:** Placing the head of the bed on blocks and avoiding lying down for at least 3 hours after eating will help prevent backflow of gastric content into the esophagus by decreasing the pressure on the lower esophageal sphincter. GERD is a chronic disease that can affect not only lifestyle, but also cause changes in the esophageal mucosa and integrity. Drug therapy may be prolonged. Chocolate and peppermint may aggravate the problem.

3. **Answer: 1 Rationale:** The most common contributing factor to acute stress gastritis is the interruption of the integrity of the gastric lining by gastric irritants such as aspirin and/or NSAIDs. A period of gastric rest, followed by a slow progression to regular dietary intake is advised. There is no indication for bland foods or regular endoscopy. The discussion of consuming fully cooked food is indicated in cases of gastric upset from toxins.

4. **Answer: 4 Rationale:** A peptic ulcer is an interruption of the integrity of the gastric lining; perforation is the most lethal complication of this process. It produces inflammation, infection and possibly shock. While the other nursing diagnoses will be present and need to be addressed at some point, disrup-

tion of the integrity of the gastrointestinal tissue is the highest priority.

5. **Answer: 3 Rationale:** Frequent small meals with solid foods or liquids, not both, are effective in controlling the hyperosmolar problem of dumping syndrome. Proteins and fats slow down the gastric emptying, whereas simple carbohydrates may rapidly enter the duodenum, increasing the risk for dumping syndrome.

6. **Answer: 2 Rationale:** Bright bleeding from the mouth could indicate perforation of the esophageal wall or vessel rupture by invasion of tumor. The other symptoms are manifestations of esophageal cancer but are not an emergency requiring immediate action.

7. **Answer: 1 Rationale:** These symptoms indicate a possible hypersensitivity response to the antibiotics. Anaphylaxis could occur, this is an emergency situation. The other answers are indeed included in the client teaching for taking antibiotics.

8. **Answer: 3 Rationale:** The discomfort of stomatitis is aggravated by eating; viscous lidocaine to reduce mouth pain is important to promote nutrition. Mouthwashes contain alcohol and may produce more pain and damage. Selection of foods that are appealing and smoking cessation are not the priority in this instance.

9. **Answer: 3 Rationale:** Maintaining patency of the nasogastric tube following gastric surgery is vital to prevent pressure gastric distension and pressure on the suture line. Irrigating gently with NS, if ordered, is the appropriate action. If unable to open tube, notify surgeon. Charting the finding without action is harmful to the client. Repositioning nasogastric tubes following gastric surgery is done by the surgeon.

10. **Answer: 3, 4, 5 Rationale:** Severe pain may be a manifestation of perforation of the ulcer. Oral food and fluids are withheld to prevent vomiting and prepare for possible surgery. The client is placed in Fowler's position to localize drainage to the pelvic area, and the physician notified to ensure prompt diagnosis and treatment. Administering additional IV dose of proton pump inhibitor has no benefit. Narcotics may mask the symptoms and should not be administered.

Chapter 24: Nursing Care of the Client Experiencing Gallbladder, Liver, and Pancreatic Disorders

1. **Answer: 1 Rationale:** Right upper quadrant pain following ingestion of a fatty meal is the typical symptom experienced by clients with choleliathiasis. Jaundice and ascites are symptoms of liver failure. Heartburn and acid reflux are symptoms of gastroesophageal reflux disease (GERD).

2. **Answer: 1, 4 Rationale:** Acute cholecystitis usually develops from a stone obstructing the cystic duct preventing release of bile from the gallbladder. High fatty foods like gravies and peanut butter stimulate contraction of the obstructed gallbladder, causing pain. Temperature and severe upper abdominal pain may be symptoms of acute peritonitis resulting from rupture of the necrotic gallbladder.

3. **Answer: 3 Rationale:** Hepatitis A is transmitted by oral-fecal route from an infected person handling food, water, fish or through direct-contact without washing hands before handling food or after using the bathroom. Hepatitis A immunization is not a cost-effective prevention measure. Testing for hepatitis A antigen on employment will not prevent spread of the disease by a newly infected current employee. Hepatitis A rarely is transmitted by blood and body fluids.

4. **Answer: 4 Rationale:** Hepatitis C is transmitted through contact with blood or body fluids. Clients with this disease must understand the importance of refraining from donating blood and using barrier protection (condoms) during sex is important. The client should avoid hepatic toxins such as acetaminophen and alcohol. Biopsies are usually done for cirrhosis. There are antiviral medications used for the treatment of hepatitis but a long life is not guaranteed.

5. **Answer: 2 Rationale:** The hepatitis A virus can be transmitted before manifestations of the disease (including jaundice) develop, therefore it is important to identify people who have had direct contact with the newly diagnosed client. Hepatitis A is not transmitted through sexual contact. Immunization for hepatitis A is only recommended in certain areas, not for the general public.

6. **Answer: 2 Rationale:** Maintaining a patent airway is of highest priority. Placing the client in Fowler's position may prevent aspiration of blood and should be the primary action. The other activities may be needed but are a lesser priority.

7. **Answer: 3 Rationale:** It is important to empty the bladder prior to the paracentesis to make sure the bladder is not punctured during the procedure. It is not necessary for the client to abstain from eating or drinking, rather the client needs to maintain fluid volume prior to the procedure. The physician will do the scrub before inserting the needle. Flatus is not related to paracentesis.

8. **Answer: 1 Rationale:** The nurse should assess bowel sounds and palpate for tenderness since spontaneous bacterial infection can develop with ascites producing fever and worsening encephalopathy. Headache and nuccal rigidity are associated with meningitis. Neck vein distention is associated with right-sided heart failure. Abdominal girth and shifting dullness are important in monitoring progress of ascites, not infection.

9. **Answer: 3 Rationale:** In women, the most common contributing factor to development of acute pancreatitis is a gallstone obstructing the duct, so this is an appropriate response. Pancreatitis usually develops from an immediate toxin or obstruction, not a delayed one. There is no association between pancreatitis and smoking. Clients who use IV drugs are susceptible to hepatitis, not pancreatitis.

10. **Answer: 4 Rationale:** Maintaining a patent nasogastric tube is vital to prevent accumulation of gastric secretions and pressure on the anastomoses created in Whipple's procedure. Smoking cessation is not a priority at this time. Turning and coughing will prevent respiratory complications but this is less important than suture line integrity. Ambulation will prevent thrombosis, but suture line integrity is of utmost importance.

Chapter 25: Assessing Clients with Bowel Elimination Disorders

1. **Answer: 2 Rationale:** The small intestine is where the nutrients and vitamins are absorbed.

2. **Answer: 4 Rationale:** The large intestine's function is to absorb water, salts, and vitamins, and then eliminate undigested substances. Hormones and bile used in digestion come from other parts of the digestive system. Breakdown of lipids, proteins, and carbohydrates occur in the small intestine.

3. **Answer: 1 Rationale:** The appendix is an extension of the surface of the cecum. The others are all parts of the large intestine but not attached to the appendix.

4. **Answer: 3 Rationale:** Internal hemorrhoids occur with impaired venous return during evacuation of stool or increased abdominal pressure in pregnancy causing distension of veins of the anus.

5. **Answer: 4 Rationale:** A client with an ostomy should have questions answered about the consistency of the stool. This

information may indicate location of the opening within the intestinal tract and demonstrate how the bowel is functioning. The other three answers do not give valuable information for a client with an ostomy.

6. **Answer: 4 Rationale:** A stool specimen will supply the opportunity to directly exam the feces and detect presence of intestinal parasites. The other tests are used for other purposes and are invasive and expensive.

7. **Answer: 2 Rationale:** Polyps have been documented as increased risk factors for developing cancer, therefore removal is indicated to prevent neoplastic cell development.

8. **Answer: 4 Rationale:** By listening with a stethoscope, you will hear the soft sounds produced by movement through the intestines every 5-15 seconds. Inspection will identify shapes and contour, palpation will assist with size of masses, and percussion will identify locations of masses.

9. **Answer: 3 Rationale:** Melena is the term used to describe black, tarry stools. Occult blood is the presence of blood in stool that is not obvious. Hematemesis is the vomiting of blood. Steatorrhea is foul smelling, high fat content stool.

10. **Answer: 3 Rationale:** The absence of bowel sounds on the first post operative day after bowel surgery is a normal expectation because the assault during surgery causes peristalsis to stop temporarily. No further action is indicated at this time.

Chapter 26: Nursing Care of Clients with Bowel Disorders

1. **Answer: 2 Rationale:** The nurse must first assess the number, frequency, and water content of stools to confirm the diagnosis of diarrhea, and estimate fluid and electrolyte loss. The client needs to ingest fluids as long as nausea and vomiting are not present, and slowly increase to solid foods. Enterotoxins' possibility should be identified. Anti-diarrhea medications are reserved for use for rectal tissue comfort.

2. **Answer: 3 Rationale:** Once the diagnosis of appendicitis is confirmed, the client should be prepared for surgery quickly before perforation or necrosis develops to decrease chance of complications. The client is kept NPO and no foreign substances are introduced into the intestinal tract. Intravenous fluids will be necessary, since the client is NPO, to maintain vascular volume and electrolyte balance as well as to administer antibiotic solutions.

3. **Answer: 1 Rationale:** Sulfasalazine makes the client susceptible to sunburn so a sunscreen should be used while outside. The drug is best tolerated when taken with meals. Fluid intake is recommended to be around 2000 mL per day. There is no mention of vitamin C supplementation while on this drug.

4. **Answer: 4 Rationale:** The symptoms reported by the client are the definition of steatorrhea. Hematochezia is bright blood in the stool. Frequent, mucus-filled stools are symptomatic of inflammatory bowel disease. These symptoms are not early signs of colorectal cancer; for example, change in bowel habits, narrow stools, diarrhea, or constipation.

5. **Answer: 2 Rationale:** The recommendation for client health with this familial history of cancer is to monitor to identify polyps and tumors early. Research has proven a direct genetic link of polyps and cancer development (20%). CEA is used to monitor treatment and detect reoccurrence and is not a screening tool in early tumor development. Dietary fiber is not the only contributing factor to cancer prevention and should be integrated into the regular diet.

6. **Answer: 4, 5, 7 Rationale:** The documentation and frequent measuring of nasogastric output will help maintain vascular volume with replacement of fluids, and the color will indicate if drainage is normal. Measuring abdominal girth will assist in determining if increased intestinal distension is occurring.

7. **Answer: 4 Rationale:** It is most important to maintain the patency of the nasogastric tube to remove gastric secretions and air that may apply pressure to the anastomosis site and cause failure of the suture line. Keeping the stomach decompressed is important to prevent vomiting that could also cause damage to the anastomosis site.

8. **Answer: 2 Rationale:** Popcorn can cause obstruction to the diverticular opening and set up the environment to initiate diverticulitis. The other foods are recommended for control of stool bulk, decreasing intraluminal pressure, and reduction of spasms associated with diverticular disease.

9. **Answer: 1, 3, 5, 6 Rationale:** Fresh fruits and vegetables, whole wheat bread, and bran cereal supply roughage and fiber in diet that can assist in the evacuation of fecal material and lessen the possibility of developing diverticulum, the incidence of which is high in this age group. Adequate liquid is important to prevent hard, formed stools that are difficult to pass. Taking daily laxatives can decrease the normal bowel reflexes. Colace can be administered safely either in the morning or at nighttime.

10. **Answer: 2 Rationale:** Abdominal adhesions following surgery usually obstruct only one section of the small bowel. The other three do not cause bowel obstruction, they may prevent obstruction.

Chapter 27: Assessing Client with Urinary Disorders

1. **Answer: 4 Rationale:** The nephrons are the working units of the kidney that produce urine. Located within the medulla, the pyramids collect the blood. The ureters transport the urine to the bladder.

2. **Answer: 4 Rationale:** ADH is increased to limit the excretion of water in the urine to maintain fluid balance. The other hormones do not affect fluid balance.

3. **Answer: 3 Rationale:** Creatinine clearance is a test that determines the filtering ability of the glomeruli and the blood circulation to them. Therefore, if the clearance is decreased, the glomeruli are damaged or the circulation is slowed. The other tests do not measure GFR.

4. **Answer: 3 Rationale:** The prostate surrounds the male urethra. The other organs are within the abdominal cavity.

5. **Answer: 2 Rationale:** Nocturia is defined as two or more voidings during the night. Polyuria is excessive urine production. Dysuria is painful urination. Hematuria is blood in the urine.

6. **Answer: 1 Rationale:** The contrast media used in IVPs cause some adverse reactions in clients that are allergic to iodine or products containing iodine. Shellfish contain iodine.

7. **Answer: 3 Rationale:** Collecting a urine specimen allows the examiner to assess the urine for color, odor, and clarity before the exam. By collecting a specimen the client has emptied the bladder. Deep breathing may help the client relax during the exam. The client with a full bladder would possibly make the exam uncomfortable.

8. **Answer: 1 Rationale:** Anesthetic agents used during surgery may cause problems with initiating voiding. Palpation will determine if the bladder is distended. Gastric assessments are not needed here.

9. **Answer: 4 Rationale:** Urinary incontinence is not considered a normal process in aging.

10. **Answer: 2 Rationale:** Skin turgor is the best assessment technique to determine hydration of clients. The other assessment techniques are not measurements of hydration status.

Chapter 28: Nursing Care of Clients with Urinary Disorders

1. **Answer: 2 Rationale:** The form of birth control, especially for those using a diaphragm and spermicidal gel, can alter the vaginal flora and increase the risk of UTIs. The reoccurrence time factor of the UTI is too long to be a failure to complete antibiotic treatment the first time. The other answers are not related to UTIs.

2. **Answer: 1, 3, 4 Rationale:** The nurse needs to inform the client that a urine culture in ten days is done to ensure antibiotic therapy was effective; in a peri-menopausal woman vaginal cream may maintain tissue integrity to prevent bacterial colonization of perineal tissues; instructions on cleansing may prevent further infections. The other two answers are invasive tests and may not be necessary for this client since three UTIs per year in a sexually active woman is considered normal.

3. **Answer: 4 Rationale:** Increasing fluid intake to 3,000 mL per day will produce enough urine to prevent stone-forming salts from concentrating sufficiently to precipitate. Calcium supplement will not prevent stones, it may contribute. Monitoring pH of urine or an indwelling catheter will not prevent stone formation.

4. **Answer: 3 Rationale:** These are manifestations of renal colic and possible ureteral obstruction. Prompt diagnosis and treatment is vital to prevent hydroureter and hydronephrosis should the ureter be completely obstructed. Although pain management and collection of the stone are important, prevention of hydronephrosis is of highest priority. Residual urine is not expected in this scenario.

5. **Answer: 1 Rationale:** Bladder cancer is two times more prevalent in smokers than non-smokers. While occupational exposure to dyes and chemicals are identified as risk factors for bladder cancers, home exposure is not. Caffeine intake and urinary retention are not identified risk factors for bladder cancer.

6. **Answer: 2 Rationale:** Painless hematuria is the usual presenting manifestation of bladder cancers and should be evaluated quickly for best outcome.

7. **Answer: 3 Rationale:** The client with a newly created continent ileal diversion will have to demonstrate self-catheterization since this is the only way to empty the continent ileal diversion. There is no collection device in this surgical procedure. Urine may normally appear cloudy since the ileum continues to produce mucus. Identification of risk factors is not necessary since the bladder has been removed.

8. **Answer: 3 Rationale:** Stress incontinence should not be viewed as a normal result of aging, rather as a treatable problem. Pelvic floor muscle exercises strengthen perineal muscles, increasing urinary sphincter control and will reduce the incidence of incontinence. Artificial sweeteners have been identified as bladder irritants contributing to urge incontinence, but have less impact on stress incontinence.

9. **Answer: 1 Rationale:** Inability to retain urine long enough to reach the toilet following perception of the need to urinate is characteristic of urge incontinence. Caffeine and artificial sweeteners are bladder Irritants, causing instability of the detrusor muscle and aggravating manifestations. Restricting intake of fluids containing these substances in the evening reduces nocturia. While the other measures may be indicated for other types of incontinence, they are of lower priority or not indicated for urge incontinence.

10. **Answer: 4 Rationale:** Catheterizing the client every three to four hours with a straight catheter prevents over distension of the bladder and the increased risk for infection associated with an indwelling catheter. During spinal shock, the bladder does not empty in response to stretch or other reflexes. Measuring residual urine is not indicated at this time.

Chapter 29: Nursing Care of the Client with Kidney Disorders

1. **Answer: 2 Rationale:** The GFR tends to decrease with aging, decreasing drug excretion and increasing the risk for toxicity. Administering smaller doses less frequently reduces the risk, but the client needs continued monitoring for manifestations of digoxin toxicity.

2. **Answer: 3 Rationale:** The adult form of polycystic kidney disease (PKD) is transmitted in an autosomal dominant pattern. Each child has a 50% chance of inheriting the disease. Only 10% of PKD clients are due to new genetic mutation.

3. **Answer: 2 Rationale:** The most common cause of acute glomerulonephritis is an abnormal immune response to beta-hemolytic streptococcus A infection, usually strep throat. Urinary tract infection, contrast media or illicit drug use are not generally implicated in development of glomerulonephritis.

4. **Answer: 1 Rationale:** Soy or animal proteins are complete proteins necessary for growth and tissue maintenance. Complete proteins are preferred when total protein intake is restricted, as in acute glomerulonephritis. Although bed rest may be recommended during the acute phase of the disorder, activities may be resumed during recovery. Dialysis would not be indicated for this client at this time so a device is not needed. Sodium may be restricted if edema is severe or the client is hypertensive, but fluid intake is individually determined, based on fluid volume status.

5. **Answer: 4 Rationale:** Postoperatively, it is important to monitor separately all drainage device volumes to determine function of each catheter or drain, and prevent hydronephrosis. Because of the location of the incision, cough suppression increases the risk of retained respiratory secretions and pneumonia. Catheters may be irrigated only when necessary and by physician's order to reduce the risk of tissue damage and infection.

6. **Answer: 1 Rationale:** Ischemia is the most common cause of acute renal failure (ARF), therefore maintaining fluid volume, cardiac output, and renal output are the highest priority nursing interventions to prevent renal failure.

7. **Answer: 3 Rationale:** Nephrotoxic drugs, including over-the-counter products, can produce further damage to the kidney cells and should be avoided. Depending on urinary output, fluid intake generally is not restricted during the recovery phase of ARF. Vegetable proteins are not complete proteins, therefore are not recommended if protein intake is restricted.

8. **Answer: 1, 3 Rationale:** Weight and orthostatic vital signs are indicators of fluid volume status and electrolyte balance. Laboratory tests are monitored to evaluate the effects of treatment. Restriction of fluid and food during dialysis is not necessary and may contribute to decreased fluid volume.

9. **Answer: 2 Rationale:** The client's ability to state renal replacement therapies indicates understanding of treatment options and the ability to make informed decisions on treatment. Clients may be able to live independently, or with the assistance of a part-time caregiver. Home hemodialysis would require a helper for safety reasons to monitor the client's response. Hospice Care is not necessarily needed for ESRD.

10. **Answer: 4 Rationale:** Cloudy urine could be a symptom of an infection. Prompt treatment is vital to preserve integrity of the transplanted organ in an immunosuppressed client. Recording the finding is insufficient, action must be taken. The nurse does

not increase the intravenous flow rate without a physician's order. Irrigation of the urinary catheter would introduce the possibility of contaminates into an immunosuppressed client.

Chapter 30: Assessing the Client with Heart Disorder

1. **Answer: 3 Rationale:** Coronary circulation supplies the heart with blood. Systemic circulation supplies the body. The pulmonary circulation supplies blood to the lungs and alveoli. The hepatic circulation supplies the liver.
2. **Answer: 4 Rationale:** Definition of cardiac output is the amount of blood pumped by the ventricles in 1 minute. Heart rate is how many times per minute the cardiac cycle occurs. Ventricular contraction is the number of times the ventricles contract. Stroke volume is the measurement of blood volume ejected with each ventricular contraction.
3. **Answer: 2 Rationale:** The coronary arteries are filled during systole when the ventricles contract so it would be prior to ventricular relaxation.
4. **Answer: 3 Rationale:** Hemorrhage would decrease the total volume of blood and venous return, which would decrease stroke volume and likewise cardiac output.
5. **Answer: 1 Rationale:** Action potential is the movement of ions across cell membranes causing electrical impulses that stimulate cardiac muscle contraction.
6. **Answer: 3 Rationale:** Since pain is subjective, a numerical rating scale assesses what the client's perception of pain intensity is. The other answers do not assess intensity.
7. **Answer: 1 Rationale:** This is the only exercise test listed. The others are not conducted during exercise.
8. **Answer: 1 Rationale:** This is the location of the apex of the heart and can be assessed at left midclavicular, 5th intercostals space on most clients.
9. **Answer: 2 Rationale:** Bradycardia is defined as pulse rate < 60 beats per minute. Tachycardia is >100 beats per minute. Hypertension and hypotension relate to blood pressure not pulse rate.
10. **Answer: 2 Rationale:** S1 is the closing of the A-V valves, the mitral, and the tricuspid valves. They are located at the apex of the heart.

Chapter 31: Nursing Care of Clients with Coronary Disorders

1. **Answer: 3 Rationale:** Stopping smoking decreases the risk of coronary heart disease by 50%. The others are contributing factors but the effects are not as significant as smoking cessation.
2. **Answer: 1 Rationale:** These symptoms could indicate myopathy, a serious potential complication of statin drugs that needs to be reported promptly.
3. **Answer: 2 Rationale:** Stable angina is predictable and it is associated with increased activity and relieved by rest and nitrates.
4. **Answer: 4 Rationale:** Re-establishing coronary blood flow and cardiac tissue perfusion within 20–45 minutes is imperative to minimize damage to the myocardium.
5. **Answer: 2 Rationale:** The cardiac catheter used to insert the stent is usually inserted via the femoral artery, a large, high-pressure vessel. The leg is maintained in extension for a prescribed period after the procedure to reduce the risk of bleeding, hematoma formation, or clot formation at the insertion site. No chest tubes are needed as the pleural cavity remains intact. IV lines are maintained for medication administration as indicated. Because the stent re-establishes myocardial blood flow, narcotic analgesics rarely are required.

6. **Answer: 4 Rationale:** Relieving pain in AMI decreases sympathetic nervous system stimulation and cardiac work. Pain relief is of highest priority, although the other goals also are appropriate for the client with AMI.
7. **Answer: 1 Rationale:** Fibrinolytic therapy, administered to restore myocardial perfusion, disrupts the clotting cascade and can lead to potentially serious bleeding. Establishing bleeding precautions is vital to preserve physiologic integrity.
8. **Answer: 3 Rationale:** A CK of 320 U/L, four times the normal level, is indicative of muscle tissue damage; in the client with acute chest pain, it often indicates acute myocardial infarction.
9. **Answer: 2 Rationale:** Mobitz type II AV block often is associated with a large anterior MI and a high mortality rate. Pacemaker therapy may be necessary to maintain effective ventricular contractions and cardiac output.
10. **Answer: 1 Rationale:** Sinus bradycardia may be well tolerated in some clients. Assessment is important before treating. However, if decreased mental status and hypotension is present, intervention is necessary.

Chapter 32: Nursing Care of Clients with Cardiac Disorders

1. **Answer: 1 Rationale:** Normal ejection fraction is 60%; an ejection fraction of 25% indicates severe impairment of ventricular function.
2. **Answer: 3 Rationale:** Interdisciplinary treatment goals for the client with heart failure are to reduce the cardiac workload and improve pump effectiveness. Loss of excess fluid, as indicated by weight loss, reduces cardiac work. The drop in heart rate and reduced pulmonary vascular congestion are indicative of improved cardiac pump.
3. **Answer: 2, 4, 5 Rationale:** In left ventricular failure, the cardiac output falls and pressure in the pulmonary vascular system increases. This leads to fatigue, increasing dyspnea, and crackles in the lung bases. Jugular vein distention is associated with right ventricular heart failure. Chest pain is not a common manifestation of heart failure.
4. **Answer: 4 Rationale:** Calibrating and leveling the system during each shift ensures accuracy and consistency of measurements. The intravenous line should be secured to the client, not the bed linens, to offer movement without tension on the lines. The arterial flush solution will not work with only gravity, it must be under pressure to prevent back-up from high pressure of the artery. Dampening of wave form would be expected during wedge pressure measurements.
5. **Answer: 2 Rationale:** Morphine is given intravenously to relieve anxiety; it also is a venous vasodilator, reducing venous return and cardiac work.
6. **Answer: 1 Rationale:** A pericardial friction rub, a grating sound, is a characteristic sign of pericarditis so it is expected, but should be documented in the client's record. No further action is indicated.
7. **Answer: 4 Rationale:** Effective treatment for acute infective endocarditis requires long-term intravenous antibiotic therapy to eliminate the infecting organisms. One week of treatment is too short for cure, it is a serious condition and potentially life-threatening. Transplantation would not be an option during the infective process since the infection would affect the transplanted organ as well unless eliminated.
8. **Answer: 3 Rationale:** Murmurs are created by turbulant blood flow through valves. The murmur of mitral valve stenosis would be heard during diastole (when blood is flowing through the stenotic valve from the atrium to the ventricle) at the apex of

the heart. Muffled heart sounds are are not characteristic of valvular disorders; S3 and S4 heart sounds are associated with fluid volume overload and heart failure.

9. **Answer: 2 Rationale:** Anticoagulant therapy to prevent clot formation is necessary following insertion of a mechanical valve. Biologic valve replacement does not require anti-rejection medication; these valves, however, are less durable, lasting only 10–15 years. Prosthetic valve endocarditis is a risk following both mechanical and biologic valve replacements.

10. **Answer: 1 Rationale:** In hypertrophic cardiomyopathy, symptoms may not develop until the demand for oxygen increases, such as with athletes during activity, causing sudden death due to a ventricular dysrhythmia. This type of cardiomyopathy is not a filling problem but rather an obstruction to ejection of blood to the body to meet oxygen demand.

Chapter 33: Assessing Clients with Hematologic, Peripheral Vascular, and Lymphatic Disorders

1. **Answer: 4 Rationale:** Arterioles have major control of blood pressure.

2. **Answer: 3 Rationale:** Fatigue would indicate that the body's tissues are not receiving adequate oxygenation. O2 is carried by the hemoglobin molecule on the RBC; if RBC numbers are very low there are insufficient numbers to carry adequate oxygen to meet demands.

3. **Answer: 2 Rationale:** Platelet plug formation is the first step in clotting. If the count is low, fewer platelets are available for clotting, therefore with tissue injury, platelets are not available and bruising occurs.

4. **Answer: 4 Rationale:** The middle layer of the arteries are thicker than in veins, made of smooth muscle that allows the arteries to expand and contract with the heart as it relaxes and contracts with each beat.

5. **Answer: 1 Rationale:** The thickness of the blood will affect the ability of the blood to flow through the vessels thus increasing the peripheral vascular resistance.

6. **Answer: 2 Rationale:** The lymphatic vessels form a network with the cardiovascular system at the capillary beds to collect and drain excess tissue fluid.

7. **Answer: 2 Rationale:** Auscultating with the bell will identify soft sounds such as the carotid arteries and identify any bruits. Inspecting for movement or absence is not precise since carotid movement may not be visible in some clients. Palpation should be done with light pressure so blood flow is not obscured. Percussion of the carotid artery is not recommended.

8. **Answer: 3 Rationale:** A murmuring or blowing sound is the definition of a bruit. The other terms are related to cardiac rhythm assessment.

9. **Answer: 1 Rationale:** The definition of lymphedema is swelling of a body part as the result of obstruction. Lymphadenopathy indicates abnormal enlargement of the lymph nodes, not necessarily a body part. Atrophic change means a change in size. Central cyanosis is oxygen deprivation.

10. **Answer: 4 Rationale:** Notify the physician immediately, these manifestations indicate a severe decrease in perfusion to the leg, and cells are dying from lack of blood flow.

Chapter 34: Nursing Care of Clients with Hematologic Disorders

1. **Answer: 3 Rationale:** Red blood cells and the hemoglobin they contain carry oxygen to the tissues; in anemia, the oxygen-carrying capacity of blood is reduced, leading to exertional dyspnea. Hematocrit of 45% is elevated slightly, not decreased. A pulse rate of 140 would not be expected in moderate anemia. WBC level is unrelated to anemia.

2. **Answer: 1 Rationale:** a. During gastric resection, intrinsic factor production may decrease, leading to vitamin B_{12} deficiency anemia with associated neurologic deficits such as numbness and tingling of extremities. The other answers are not related to nutritional deficiency anemias.

3. **Answer: 2 Rationale:** Prior to bone marrow transplant, chemotherapy or total body irradiation is used to destroy leukemic cells in the bone marrow. Normal blood cells also are destroyed, causing significant risk for infection and bleeding. The other diagnoses, while appropriate, are of lower priority.

4. **Answer: 1, 3, 5 Rationale:** AML causes both neutropenia and thrombocytopenia, with resulting increased risk for infection and bleeding. A private room and oral hygiene help reduce infection risk, and a soft, bland diet reduces trauma to oral mucosal membranes. Leukemia is not communicable; airborne infection control measures are unneccessary. Rectal temperatures are avoided to protect rectal mucosal integrity.

5. **Answer: 1 Rationale:** This question demonstrates a non-verbalized concern. The correct response is open-ended and allows the client to state more specifically what he is concerned about. The other answers assume what the client wishes to discuss.

6. **Answer: 3 Rationale:** Multiple-drug chemotherapy regimes are effective at different phases of the cell cycle, allowing lower doses of individual drugs to decrease adverse effects and more effective tumor destruction. While adverse effects and destruction of normal cells may be reduced, this regime does not eliminate them.

7. **Answer: 4 Rationale:** A new onset of severe pain may signal a pathological fracture and needs to be reported.

8. **Answer: 2 Rationale:** A platelet count of 60,000/mm^3 is significantly low (normal 150,000-450,000/mm^3), increasing the risk of bleeding and bruising with minor trauma.

9. **Answer: 1 Rationale:** The most common form of classic hemophilia is transmitted as an x-linked recessive disorder passed from mother to son, therefore the daughter may be a carrier. The other answers are incorrect.

10. **Answer: 4 Rationale:** A platelet infusion replaces those platelets used in the abnormal clotting process of DIC. Platelets do not replace clotting factors or increase the oxygen-carrying capacity of the blood. Promotion of intravascular clotting is not a desired effect.

Chapter 35: Nursing Care of Clients with Peripheral Vascular Disorders

1. **Answer: 3 Rationale:** Hypertension generally is asymptomatic. Follow-up evaluation and treatment is necessary to reduce long-term effects of the disorder.

2. **Answer: 1 Rationale:** While lasagna made with whole-grain pasta, low-fat cheese, and vegetables or lean meats would be allowed, this answer demonstrates the need for additional teaching.

3. **Answer: 2, 4 Rationale:** First-dose hypotension and orthostatic hypotension are potential adverse effects of this drug, as is persistent cough. The drug should be taken in the morning to reduce potential nocturia. Potassium supplements are not recommended unless prescribed by the physician. Hypertension treatment may be life-long.

4. **Answer: 1 Rationale:** These symptoms indicate a possible arterial occlusion. This is an emergency; immediate intervention is necessary to preserve the extremity.

5. **Answer: 4 Rationale:** Endovascular approach on an 86-year-old client would mean less surgical risk and faster recovery.

6. **Answer: 4 Rationale:** Clients with peripheral atherosclerosis may have paresthesias and decreased hair on the affected extremity. Pallor is associated with elevation of the affected extremity, and the blood pressure may be lower in the affected extremity.

7. **Answer: 2, 3, 1, 4, 5 Rationale:** First, nicotine causes vasoconstriction, further decreasing blood flow; next, daily skin inspections looking for breaks in integrity to prevent infections; then, maintaining feet by regular cleansing, cotton socks, and protecting feet by wearing shoes; fourth, regular daily exercise to develop collateral circulation; and fifth, weight loss if necessary to keep client mobile.

8. **Answer: 2 Rationale:** Anticoagulant therapy will be continued after discharge; understanding the importance of follow-up care and monitoring for adverse effects is vital. Sitting in a straight chair is not recommended as it impairs venous return; progressive exercise is recommended to promote venous return. While a low-fat, low-cholesterol diet is a good idea, it will not prevent future venous thrombosis.

9. **Answer: 1 Rationale:** Elevating the legs and wearing elastic stockings may relieve the discomfort associated wtih varicose veins. Significant symptoms, recurrent superficial venous thrombosis, or stasis ulcers are the primary indications for surgical treatment of varicose veins.

10. **Answer: 3 Rationale:** Careful skin and foot care is a high priority to prevent skin breakdown and potential infection.

Chapter 36: Assessing Clients with Respiratory Disorders

1. **Answer: 4 Rationale:** The apex or top of the lungs is located just below the clavicle.

2. **Answer: 3 Rationale:** Simple diffusion at the respiratory membrane is where gases dissolved in substances move from higher concentration to one of lower concentration.

3. **Answer: 4 Rationale:** Pulmonary capillaries cover the external surface of the alveoli. The other answers are above the alveoli in the lungs.

4. **Answer: 1 Rationale:** As the body temperature rises the bond between oxygen and hemoglobin decreases so less oxygen binds and unloading is enhanced.

5. **Answer: 2 Rationale:** Thoracentesis is the removal of fluid around the lung by placing a needle in the pleural space and extracting the excess fluid.

6. **Answer: 3 Rationale:** To identify a genetic risk of respiratory disease, during an interview the nurse would ask about lung cancer in the family.

7. **Answer: 2 Rationale:** Wheezes are continuous musical sounds heard in the chest. Crackles and rales are discontinuous sounds, and with murmurs, are heard in the cardiac assessment.

8. **Answer: 4 Rationale:** If the client had a lung removed, breath sounds would be absent from that side because without air movement no sound would be generated.

9. **Answer: 3 Rationale:** While auscultating the lungs, the client should take slow deep breaths to allow adequate time for air to go into and out of the lung. Breathing through the mouth amplifies the sound, making it easier to hear.

10. **Answer: 2 Rationale:** Decreased diaphragmatic movement on the left side should be documented; it is an expected outcome with pneumothorax on the left since air movement and diaphragm movement would be decreased.

Chapter 37: Nursing Care of Clients with Upper Respiratory Disorders

1. **Answer: 4 Rationale:** Over-the-counter nasal spray is the best choice to relieve URI symptoms in the client with hypertension, since its effects are local, not systemic. The duration of use is limited to prevent rebound. Many systemic decongestants such as pseudoephedrine elevate the blood pressure. Antibiotics are not effective against viral infections. Vitamin C and zinc lozenges have not been demonstrated to be more effective than placebo in studies.

2. **Answer: 2 Rationale:** Yearly influenza vaccinations are the most effective way of preventing flu and pneumonia in this group. Handwashing will prevent spread to others once the person has developed the flu. The clients should maintain optimum health through exercise all-year-round.

3. **Answer: 1 Rationale:** Completion of the antibiotic medication is the most important in order to cure the bacterial infection and prevent reoccurrence. The other answers will assist but are not the most important.

4. **Answer: 3 Rationale:** Posterior nasal packing obstructs the nares and may compromise oxygenation. While the other interventions are important for comfort, facilitating oxygenation has higher priority.

5. **Answer: 4 Rationale:** Fracture of other facial bones may accompany nasal fracture, damaging the dura and causing spinal fluid leak. A positive glucose indicates the presence of spinal fluid, indicates a need to initiate appropriate treatment to prevent infection. The other responses are inappropriate to preserve physiologic integrity.

6. **Answer: 3, 5, 6 Rationale:** The manifestations of sleep apnea include daytime sleepiness, elevated BP, and complaints of morning headache. Oxygen saturation levels may fall while asleep, not while awake. Confusion, dementia, and an enlarged tongue are not related to obstructive sleep apnea.

7. **Answer: 1 Rationale:** Persistent voice hoarseness may be the first sign of a laryngeal tumor, necessitating follow-up diagnostic testing. While smoking is a risk factor for laryngeal cancer, the question does not help differentiate hoarseness due to an acute infection from laryngeal cancer.

8. **Answer: 3 Rationale:** With stage I laryngeal cancer, radiation can cure the cancer, and preserve the voice. This cancer does metastasize to other areas.

9. **Answer: 4, 5, 2, 1, 3 Rationale:** Maintaining airway patency is of highest priority. The head may need additional support because of the removal of neck muscles. Frequent, small meals help meet metabolic needs; swallowing may be difficult and the effort may produce fatigue. Regaining speech will require practice and assistance from a speech therapist. Loss of the voice will result in grieving; encouraging expression of feelings can facilitate gradual acceptance of the loss.

10. **Answer: 2 Rationale:** When providing tracheostomy care, the nurse secures clean ties before removing soiled ones to prevent accidental dislodgement of the tube. Sterile scissors are not necessary. Sterile technique is used to clean the phlange of the outer cannula; iodine antiseptic interferes with healing, and is avoided.

Chapter 38: Nursing Care of Clients with Ventilation Disorders

1. **Answer: 1 Rationale:** Unless oxygenation is compromised by the inflammatory process, the sputum specimen is obtained first. Oxygen therapy is then initiated, the IV established, and antibiotic therapy started. Providing food is of lower priority.

2. **Answer: 1, 4, 5, 2, 3 Rationale:** Overall gray skin color and bluish tinge to lips indicate hypoxemia; supplemental oxygen is highest priority. Second, raise the head of the bed to promote chest expansion and alveolar ventilation. Assessment of oxygen saturation and breath sounds provide important information to be provided to the physician.

3. **Answer: 3 Rationale:** A 9 mm induration is a positive result in a client with HIV disease. Induration of 10–15 mm would be considered positive in the other instances.

4. **Answer: 2 Rationale:** When teaching a client who is taking INH, the nurse needs to include information on adverse effects such as numbness and tingling of extremities to the doctor. The other answers reflect adverse responses to other drugs used in treatment of TB.

5. **Answer: 3 Rationale:** Smoking cessation is important with the diagnosis of lung cancer to prevent further damage from the chemicals in the cigarettes. The other answers contain statements that either erase all hope or contain unreasonable expectations since lung cancer metastasis early, and survival rates are low at five year interval.

6. **Answer: 3, 4 Rationale:** Chest tube drainage that is red, free-flowing, and exceeds 70mL/hour indicates hemorrhage and must be reported. Vital signs and level of consciousness are measured to evaluate cardiac output and hemodynamic stability. Chest tube drainage devices are never emptied to maintain system integrity; placing pressure on the insertion site will not reduce internal bleeding.

7. **Answer: 1 Rationale:** The client having a thoracentesis needs to sit upright, leaning forward during the procedure to spread the rib cage for easier placement of the needle. The client should hold his breath while needle is inserted to prevent damage to lung tissues. After the procedure, activity may be resumed as tolerated. Coughing during fluid aspiration is not recommended to avoid displacing the needle.

8. **Answer: 4 Rationale:** A client with a fractured rib would be urged to use a small pillow to splint the area when coughing to reduce the movement of rib cage, and pain.

9. **Answer: 2 Rationale:** A respiratory rate of 36 indicates respiratory distress, and is of greatest concern.

10. **Answer: 1 Rationale:** Tension pneumothorax displaces structures in the mediastinum, including the great vessels. Cardiac output may be severely compromised, resulting in inadequate oxygen delivery and nutrients to cells and tissues.

Chapter 39: Nursing Care of Clients with Gas Exchange Disorders

1. **Answer: 2 Rationale:** Ineffective airway clearance is the highest priority because it impairs alveolar ventilation and the exchange of oxygen and carbon dioxide at the capillaries, decreasing the blood and tissue oxygen levels.

2. **Answer: 1 Rationale:** The physician needs to be informed because this indicates increasing fatigue and impending respiratory failure. The other answers do not address the immediate need of the client.

3. **Answer: 3 Rationale:** Rinsing the mouth after using an MDI reduces systemic absorption and adverse effects of the drug. The bronchodilator drug is used before the anti-inflammatory to facilitate its delivery to distal lung tissues.

4. **Answer: 1 Rationale:** Development of a barrel chest due to air trapping is an expected finding in COPD. Confusion, lethargy, and low oxygen saturation levels indicate respiratory failure. Pitting edema may indicate heart failure or an untreated problem.

5. **Answer: 3 Rationale:** During an acute exacerbation of COPD, keeping the SaO_2 above 90% is an appropriate goal. COPD is a progressive disease, lost lung function cannot be regained, nor is it likely ABGs will return to normal values. Smoking cessation, not reduction, is vital.

6. **Answer: 4 Rationale:** In some clients with COPD, decreased arterial oxygen concentrations drive respirations. Administered O_2 may decrease the drive to breathe, however, many clients with COPD require supplemental oxygen.

7. **Answer: 1, 2, 4, 5 Rationale:** Thick, tenacious, milky white sputum and fever indicate possible infection. Difficulty coughing up mucus and increased shortness of breath and fatigue indicate potential early symptoms of respiratory failure. Bulky, fatty stools are an expected finding in clients with cystic fibrosis.

8. **Answer: 2 Rationale:** These symptoms may indicate pulmonary embolism. Oxygen is administered to support gas exchange and tissue oxygenation. While elevating the head of the bed supports ventilation, it may be contraindicated by the type of skeletal traction. Homan's sign may provide information about venous thrombosis, but is not a priority action at this time. The analgesic is of lower priority than oxygen, and may depress the respiratory drive.

9. **Answer: 1 Rationale:** Restlessness and tachypnea are early signs of respiratory failure caused by hypoxemia and stimulation of the respiratory center. The other answers are late symptoms of failure.

10. **Answer: 4 Rationale:** Patent airways are necessary to maintain effective alveolar ventilation and gas exchange. The other options do not promote airway clearance and alveolar ventilation.

Chapter 40: Assessing Clients with Musculoskeletal Disorders

1. **Answer: 3 Rationale:** Long bones have two broad ends that are called epiphyses. The other types of bones do not have the epiphyses.

2. **Answer: 1 Rationale:** Abduction is the term for moving an extremity away from the midline of the body. Adduction is moving the extremity towards the midline of the body. Extension is straightening an extremity. Flexion is bending a joint in an extremity.

3. **Answer: 1 Rationale:** Clients with gout have increased serum uric acid and if medication for treating gout is effective the serum level of uric acid should be decreased. Rheumatoid factor is used to diagnose rheumatoid arthritis. The other answers are not related to gout.

4. **Answer: 4 Rationale:** Women in their 60s are usually postmenopausal, this is when they are at risk for decreased bone density as well as for fractures due to osteoporosis.

5. **Answer: 3 Rationale:** With decreased bone mass and decreased calcium absorption, the bones become brittle and at risk for fractures. The other answers are not related to bone mass or calcium absorption.

6. **Answer: 2 Rationale:** When assessing facial muscle strength the nurse would ask the client to stick out his tongue. This would test cranial nerve IX.

7. **Answer: 4 Rationale:** Crepitation is the grating sound as the joint moves. Arthritis and synovitis are medical conditions. Crackles are lung sounds.

8. **Answer: 3 Rationale:** The ballottement test indicates fluid in the knee joint. The other answers are not in the knee.

9. **Answer: 2 Rationale:** Scoliosis is the term used to describe a lateral curve in the spine. Lordosis is an exaggerated forward curvature of the lumbar spine. Kyphosis is an abnormal protuberance of the thoracic spine.

10. **Answer: 1 Rationale:** Pain and limited mobility are the most common symptoms of musculoskeletal disorders.

Chapter 41: Nursing Care of Clients with Musculoskeletal Trauma

1. **Answer: 2 Rationale:** Ice used on a sprained ankle immediately after injury will cause vasoconstriction of the blood vessels to decrease edema and pain. Ice will not affect WBCs or BP and pulse.
2. **Answer: 3 Rationale:** A client with a compound fracture means bone has broken the skin, which is the first line of defense against bacterial invasion. The client is now at risk for infection either from trauma or during surgery.
3. **Answer: 3 Rationale:** Pale, cold fingers of an older woman with a cast could indicate decreased circulation to the hand. The other answers indicate favorable indications in this situation.
4. **Answer: 4 Rationale:** Calcium deposits in the fracture site allows callus to begin to form and healing occurs.
5. **Answer: 2 Rationale:** The client who is cyanotic and lacks sensation in the toes indicates decreased circulation and pressure on nerve, if not relieved soon permanent damage could occur. While the other answers are usual nursing activities they do not address the emergent need in this situation.
6. **Answer: 2 Rationale:** Clients with deep vein thrombosis of the lower extremity need the respiratory system to be monitored carefully for complications of emboli.
7. **Answer: 2 Rationale:** Clients who have suffered musculoskeletal injuries have soft tissue damage, muscle spasm and swelling causing acute pain. The other nursing diagnoses are not as common.
8. **Answer: 1 Rationale:** During the first 24 hours after amputation the remaining extremity is elevated above the level of the heart to promote venous return and decrease swelling.
9. **Answer: 4 Rationale:** Phantom limb pain is experienced by a majority of amputees especially in the early postoperative period.
10. **Answer: 4 Rationale:** The amputated finger should be wrapped in a clean cloth, put in a plastic bag and place on ice to preserve tissue—not directly on ice, which could cause tissue frostbite. This will preserve the amputated finger so that it can be surgically reattached.

Chapter 42: Nursing Care of Clients with Musculoskeletal Disorders

1. **Answer: 2 Rationale:** Risk for falls is the most significant nursing diagnosis in terms of long-term disability because falls that would result in no injury to the healthy adult may cause fractures in the osteoporotic client.
2. **Answer: 4 Rationale:** Most clients with osteoarthritis use NSAIDs for control of discomfort from disease. The other three categories are not utilized in osteoarthritis.
3. **Answer:2 Rationale:** Clients with gout have increased serum levels of uric acid. The other lab tests are not affected by gout.
4. **Answer: 3 Rationale:** In clients with osteoporosis and osteomalacia, fractures are a potential complication because of lack of calcium intake and vitamin D intake.
5. **Answer: 1 Rationale:** In clients complaining of knee pain, being overweight by thirty pounds is indicative of an increased risk for osteoarthritis. None of the other answers are an increased risk for developing OA.
6. **Answer: 3 Rationale:** By monitoring vital signs, hemoglobin and hematocrit, the nurse can determine early if the fluid volume is deficient, caused by excessive bleeding, or if blood supply to extremity is compromised.

7. **Answer: 1 Rationale:** Fever and weight loss are found in clients with rheumatoid arthritis; not found in osteoarthritis.
8. **Answer: 3 Rationale:** In the nursing diagnosis *ineffective protection*, the most important intervention for the client with SLE would be to practice careful handwashing, since SLE clients are at risk for opportunistic and severe infection.
9. **Answer: 4 Rationale:** Most cases of Lyme disease occur when an infected tick remains embedded for at least 24 hours. Malaria/West Nile Fever are transmitted by mosquitoes. Droplet infection is primarily tuberculosis.
10. **Answer: 2 Rationale:** Septic arthritis is a medical emergency since if not diagnosed quickly and treatment begun, destruction of the affected joint may occur.

Chapter 43: Assessing Clients with Neurologic Disorders

1. **Answer: 4 Rationale:** The blood-brain barrier controls the environment within by allowing oxygen, carbon dioxide, lipids, glucose, and water into the capillaries but preventing urea, creatinine, toxins, proteins, and antibiotic entry.
2. **Answer: 3 Rationale:** The lower motor neurons maintain muscle tone and reflexes, any damage could result in loss of reflexes.
3. **Answer: 3 Rationale:** Cerebrospinal fluid (CSF) cushions the brain tissue and spinal cord, protects them from trauma, provides nourishment to the brain, and removes waste products.
4. **Answer: 1 Rationale:** The posterior spinal roots contain cells that discriminate fine touch sensations such as dull and sharp, therefore damage to these roots would mean the client would be unable to detect dull or sharp sensation.
5. **Answer: 1 Rationale:** The sympathetic division of the ANS has the purpose of preparing the body to handle stressful events, such as a near auto accident, by increasing heart rate, force of contraction, vasodilation of coronary arteries, and increased mental alertness.
6. **Answer: 2 Rationale:** Auscultation is not used in assessing the neurologic examination. Inspection is used to observe physical characteristics and mental condition. Percussion with a hammer checks reflexes. Muscles are palpated.
7. **Answer: 1 Rationale:** A cotton ball and a safety pin would be used to assess sensations of light dull and sharp on the face. The cotton ball would also be used to test corneal reflex.
8. **Answer: 4 Rationale:** In clients that are unconscious the corneal reflex is absent, so when the cornea is touched with a wisp of cotton, the client would not blink the way a conscious client would.
9. **Answer: 3 Rationale:** A tongue depressor is utilized on the posterior section of the tongue to illicit a gag reflex, testing cranial nerve IX.
10. **Answer: 2 Rationale:** In decorticate posturing the upper arms are close to the body, the elbows, wrists, and fingers are flexed, and the legs are extended with internal rotation.

Chapter 44: Nursing Care of Clients with Intracranial Disorders

1. **Answer: 4 Rationale:** Normally the RAS and cerebral hemispheres control respirations with a regular pattern however, when they are damaged, the lower brainstem responds to changes is $PaCO_2$ resulting in irregular respiratory patterns.
2. **Answer: 2 Rationale:** The unconscious client with impaired gag or swallowing reflexes would be at risk for aspiration since saliva and any fluids taken by mouth could not be swallowed normally.
3. **Answer: 2 Rationale:** Osmotic diuretics increase the osmolarity of blood by excreting water and leaving solutes, as a result,

the water in the brain would be drawn into the vascular space. Osmotic diuretics would not be related to other answers.

4. **Answer: 3 Rationale:** Motor responses to a direct stimuli such as "squeeze my hand" are the best way to identify changes in mental status. These other answers would require an alert client, not one in a coma.

5. **Answer: 1, 2, 3 Rationale:** A client with an altered LOC would probably have blood glucose to check for hypoglycemia, electrolytes to check for metabolic disturbances, especially sodium, and toxicology to test for drug or alcohol toxicity. Since testing spinal fluid is invasive, it would not be done unless there were symptoms of meningeal irritation.

6. **Answer: 3 Rationale:** Serum osmolality would assess water and solute balance in the blood indicating the hydration status of the client. The other tests would not tell the hydration status.

7. **Answer: 1 Rationale:** Clients with perceived generalized seizures must have loss of consciousness or they are not considered generalized seizures. Tonic and clonic are movements that may not be present. Repetitive, non-purposeful movements are not associated with seizures.

8. **Answer: 3 Rationale:** In a client with a head injury that has fluid draining from the ear, the nurse must suspect a potential CSF leak and would test the drainage for glucose. That is present in CSF but not fluid from the ear.

9. **Answer: 4 Rationale:** Antiepileptic (AED) drugs are not a cure but rather they provide control of seizures or reduce seizure activity. The other answers are not related to use of AEDs.

10. **Answer: 1 Rationale:** All brain tumors are potentially lethal because they grow within a close, contained space and can produce problems on the CNS.

Chapter 45: Nursing Care of Clients with Cerebrovascular and Spinal Cord Disorders

1. **Answer: 2 Rationale:** Numbness and tingling in the corner of the client's mouth that disappears within minutes or hours is a manifestation of temporary occlusion of the middle cerebral artery. The other manifestations are present with strokes, not TIAs.

2. **Answer: 1 Rationale:** Hypertension is the greatest risk factor for a stroke because it's sustained systolic and diastolic pressure causes damage to cerebral blood vessels with a 4–6X greater risk for stroke than clients without hypertension.

3. **Answer: 3 Rationale:** The motor pathways of the nervous system cross at the medulla and spinal cord meaning damage to the left cerebral vessel will demonstrate neurologic deficits on the right side, an effect called contralateral.

4. **Answer: 4 Rationale:** Tissue plasminogen activator is given within the first 3 hours of the ischemic stroke to cause fibrinolysis of the clot.

5. **Answer: 3 Rationale:** Preventing hypoxia and hypercapnia through administration of oxygen will prevent further ischemia of cerebral tissues and increase of intracranial pressure. The other answers are not related to this question.

6. **Answer: 1 Rationale:** In a client with spinal cord injury no impulses are transmitted between the brain and spinal cord and the cord does not function at all, producing spinal shock that may last from minutes to weeks or months.

7. **Answer: 2 Rationale:** Autonomic dyreflexia can be caused by kinked catheter tubing allowing the bladder to become full, triggering massive vasoconstriction below the injury site, producing the symptoms of this process. The other answers will not cause autonomic dysreflexia.

8. **Answer: 3 Rationale:** SCI at the C1-C4 level produces respiratory paralysis and the client will be unable to breathe on his own, so a ventilator will be necessary to maintain respiratory function.

9. **Answer: 1, 2, 4 Rationale:** Cortiocsteroids will be used to decrease cord edema. Vasopressors will be used to treat bradycardia or hypotension from spinal shock. Analgesics will be used to control pain. There is no reason to use antihistamines or antibiotics.

10. **Answer: 1, 3, 5 Rationale:** In teaching prevention of back injuries the nurse would incorporate principles of proper body mechanics, which are spread feet apart, use large leg muscles, and work as close to the object as possible. Bending from the waist to lift rather than sometimes rolling or pushing, will contribute to back injuries.

Chapter 46: Nursing Care of Clients with Neurologic Disorders

1. **Answer: 1, 2 Rationale:** Dementia is a general term used to describe the outcome of the death of neurons, and the cognitive and behavioral symptoms of AD. The other answers are incorrect.

2. **Answer: 3 Rationale:** Memory deficits are usually the first indication of AD, are subtle and may not be noticed by friends and family until the client exhibits unsafe behaviors. The other answers listed are symptoms in later stages of AD.

3. **Answer: 1 Rationale:** Fatigue affects all clients with MS regardless of type or severity. The other answers are not as pervasive.

4. **Answer: 3 Rationale:** Interferons are used to reduce exacerbations in clients with multiple sclerosis and enhance immune function. The other drugs or category of drugs are not used in treatment of MS.

5. **Answer: 4 Rationale:** When teaching a young adult with MS it is important to stress avoidance of extremes of heat and cold since maintaining a constant body temperature will decrease exacerbations of symptoms, and heat slows down transmission of nerve impulses.

6. **Answer: 2 Rationale:** Parkinson's disease symptoms appear when the brain cells not longer produce enough dopamine to inhibit acetylcholine, this produces uncoordinated motor movement.

7. **Answer: 3 Rationale:** With the gait changes, balance problems and possible orthostatic hypotension, clients with PD are at increased risk for falls. This safety issue needs to be addressed with the caregivers. The other answers are not accurate or not a major concern.

8. **Answer: 4 Rationale:** Antiglutamate is the drug classification used to treat ALS because it prevents the release of glutamic acid and protects against toxicity of neurons. The other drugs are not used to treat ALS.

9. **Answer: 3 Rationale:** When teaching clients about Bell's palsy, the nurse needs to tell the client that one side of the face will not move normally since the affected nerve supplies the muscles that produce expression on one side of the face. Pain in Bell's palsy may be present before the paralysis appears, not during. Bell's palsy affects only the facial area, not walking, and boiling foods is to prevent botulism.

10. **Answer: 2 Rationale:** The nurse can prevent tetanus by promoting tetanus immunization to adults and children, since this is the most effective way to prevent the disease from contaminated wounds. Older adults may not have had the immunization as a child, or may need a booster to keep up immunity. The other answers do not reflect prevention of tetanus.

Chapter 47: Assessing Clients with Eye and Ear Disorders

1. **Answer: 2 Rationale:** When the cornea is touched the client will blink as a mechanism to protect it from foreign objects entering.

2. **Answer: 4 Rationale:** Presbyopia develops in older adults as the lens of the eye looses its ability to adjust, requiring the client to hold papers further away in order to focus and read.

3. **Answer: 2 Rationale:** Tuning forks are used to assess the hearing acuity, if a deficit is present it will tell if the loss is conductive or sensorineural.

4. **Answer: 1 Rationale:** As the light enters the lens, the rays bend and is focused on a single point on the retina; this focusing is called accommodation.

5. **Answer: 4 Rationale:** Clients having a test of refraction will have the pupil dilated for better access to examine the internal structures.

6. **Answer: 3 Rationale:** Receptors within the inner ear maintain equilibrium by responding to changes in head position in order to coordinate body movements and balance.

7. **Answer: 1 Rationale:** The Snellen eye chart measures the client's ability to read letters at a standard distance of twenty feet. The client reads the smallest line, the numbers on the side would indicate visual acuity, e.g., 20/20, 20/30.

8. **Answer: 1 Rationale:** The examiner can whisper a word one or two feet behind the client, asking the client to repeat the word, this may provide a rough estimate of hearing acuity. The other tests are more specific and would be done after the client failed the whisper test.

9. **Answer: 2 Rationale:** The vestibular structures maintain balance. As the person ages this function may decrease and the client may be at risk for loosing balance and falling.

10. **Answer: 4 Rationale:** The examiner must have a normal visual field when assessing the visual field of a client because the examiner's field becomes the standard or norm. If the examiner does not have normal visual field then the results of this part of the exam would be inaccurate.

Chapter 48: Nursing Care of Clients with Eye or Ear Disorders

1. **Answer: 4 Rationale:** The highest priority for residents with moderate to severe hearing or vision impairment is safety.

2. **Answer: 2 Rationale:** In teaching a client with newly diagnosed glaucoma, the nurse emphasizes the importance of taking eye drops as prescribed on a continuing basis to control intraocular pressure and prevent vision loss.

3. **Answer: 3 Rationale:** Timolol is a beta adrenergic blocker that can decrease myocardial contractility and impair cardiac function in the client with heart failure.

4. **Answer: 4 Rationale:** The highest priority for a client with repeated attacks of vertigo and tinnitus is maintenance of safety. Sitting when an attack occurs reduces the risk of injury from falling.

5. **Answer: 1 Rationale:** Following eye surgery, clients are placed in semi-Fowler's or Fowler's position to reduce intraocular pressure and edema.

6. **Answer: 3 Rationale:** Immediate referral to an ophthalmologist is necessary because the symptoms suggest a detached retina. Immediate treatment is necessary to optimize sight restoration. The other answers do not address the seriousness of the situation.

7. **Answer: 1, 2, 3, 4, 5 Rationale:** All the assessments should be included because each provides information about infection and possible location in the ear.

8. **Answer: 4 Rationale:** The client's symptoms could be due to impacted cerumen. The nurse should inspect the ear canal for patency. Aging is a risk factor for cerumen impaction because there is less and it is harder and drier.

9. **Answer: 1 Rationale:** One-on-one social interactions in a quiet environment facilitate effective communication for the client with a severe hearing deficit.

10. **Answer: 2 Rationale:** Cataract removal is elective surgery, generally performed only when visual impairment interferes with activities of daily living.

Chapter 49: Assessing Clients with Reproductive System and Breast Disorders

1. **Answer: 3 Rationale:** In the male the testes produce the sperm and testosterone. The epididymis stores the sperm, the seminal vesicles and Cowper's glands produce the seminal fluid.

2. **Answer: 4 Rationale:** In the female, the clitoris is an erectile organ similar to the penis in the male. The others are not erectile tissue.

3. **Answer: 2 Rationale:** The explanation should begin with the prostate gland surrounding the urethra, as it grows larger it decreases the size of the opening. The client may not empty the bladder and need to urinate more frequently.

4. **Answer: 1 Rationale:** PSA is the diagnostic test used to diagnose and monitor prostate cancer. CBC & WBC monitor blood cells. VDRL is a diagnostic test for sexually transmitted diseases.

5. **Answer: 1 Rationale:** Transillumination is used if any swelling is noted during inspection. None of the other methods will be as helpful in detecting problems in the scrotum.

6. **Answer: 3 Rationale:** Estrogens reduce cholesterol levels but following menopause the estrogen level drops and cholesterol increases, putting the woman at risk for cardiovascular disease.

7. **Answer: 1 Rationale:** When women of reproductive age become pregnant, the embryo implants in the uterus and menstruation stops until after delivery.

8. **Answer: 4 Rationale:** Pap smears are used to detect cervical cancers and precancerous lesions of the cervix. Colposcopy is used after a pap test is abnormal. Mammograms are done to detect breast tumors. Culture is done if an infection is suspected.

9. **Answer: 3 Rationale:** Monthly breast exams done by the client utilize palpation to find any lumps or changes in breast tissues.

10. **Answer: 2 Rationale:** The Bartholin's gland would be palpated at the posterior section of the labia majora.

Chapter 50: Nursing Care of Men with Reproductive System and Breast Disorders

1. **Answer: 4 Rationale:** This is stated in an appropriate way to allow the client to feel free to ask any question about his sexual concerns. The other answers presume problems or contain judgmental attitudes.

2. **Answer: 2 Rationale:** In a health teaching session with young men, the nurse should tell them about retracting the foreskin while showering, and cleaning regularly to decrease the presence of collection of secretions under the foreskin, which has been show to increase the risk of penile cancer.

3. **Answer: 1 Rationale:** Sexually active men who have gonorrhea are especially susceptible to inflammation or infection of the epididymis. A sexually transmitted disease is not associated with the other conditions.

4. **Answer: 2 Rationale:** Testicular cancer commonly occurs between the ages of fifteen and forty. The incidence decreases with age, has a genetic predisposition in brothers and has no associate pain symptoms.

5. **Answer: 3 Rationale:** Men with chronic prostatitis should increase their fluid intake to 3L/day and void often to decrease the irritation when voiding. Cold showers and restricting fluids would be contraindicated, it would not help to relieve symptoms. A scrotal support, increased fiber intake, and avoiding sexual activity would not help discomfort.

6. **Answer: 2, 4 Rationale:** In digital rectal examination for BPH, the prostate is asymmetrical and enlarged while in prostate cancer the exam shows nodules and a fixed position. PSA is specific to the prostate and is released by both benign and malignant cells however, in BPH the amounts of the free form of PSA and complex PSA would be different. The other tests are not helpful in distinguishing cancer from BPH.

7. **Answer: 2 Rationale:** As the prostate enlarges around the urethra it begins to obstruct the outflow of urine from the bladder during urination causing problems with urinary retention, frequency and urgency. The other systems are not affected.

8. **Answer: 3 Rationale:** The nurse needs to notify the surgeon because dark red fluid with obvious clots and painful bladder spasms could indicate that the client may be hemorrhaging postoperatively and the doctor will need to know to direct next actions to keep the client safe. The other answers do not address the need for appropriate action.

9. **Answer: 1 Rationale:** Prostate cancer is the most common type of malignancy in American men and the second leading cause of death in North America.

10. **Answer: 4 Rationale:** Some studies have shown an increase in prostate cancer in societies with diets high in red meats and fats. Informing the community of this relationship could help members change their dietary habits to decrease the risk of prostate cancer.

Chapter 51: Nursing Care of Women with Reproductive System and Breast Disorders

1. **Answer: 1 Rationale:** The nurse acknowledging the problem stated by the client gives credence for the client, but because the nurse is uncomfortable addressing the issue herself, she refers the client to the physician to address her problem. The other answers would not be therapeutic responses.

2. **Answer: 2, 3, 4 Rationale:** Osteoporosis, cardiovascular disease, and fractures are all related to estrogen deprivation. Cervical and colon cancer have not been linked to decreased estrogen levels.

3. **Answer: 1200 Rationale:** This level can be achieved through diet and supplements if necessary.

4. **Answer: 1 Rationale:** Kegel exercises utilized in uterine displacement strengthens perineal muscle tone, minimizes urinary leakage, and the descent of the bladder into the vagina. These exercises do not have an affect on the other conditions.

5. **Answer: 2 Rationale:** A health-promotion seminar for reducing the risk of cervical cancer should contain information about safe sex methods that reduce the incidence of genital infections from HPV, which is the most important risk factor. The other answers are not risk factors of cervical cancer.

6. **Answer: 4 Rationale:** For a woman with PMS, the nurse would recommend a decrease in sodium intake to help minimize the fluid retention due to the increased production of aldosterone, which results in sodium retention and edema.

7. **Answer: 2 Rationale:** Endometrial implantations tend to atrophy and disappear after menopause since ovarian hormones no longer stimulate them.

8. **Answer: 1, 3, 4 Rationale:** A teaching plan for home care of a woman following an abdominal hysterectomy, should include no lifting to decrease chances of hemorrhage, report temperature > 100° F since this may be a sign of infection, and take regular rest periods since she may be tired for several days postoperatively. She should be told to take showers until bleeding stops and should be encouraged to splint abdomen so she may breathe and cough deeply to prevent respiratory complications of atelectasis.

9. **Answer: 4 Rationale:** Risk factors for breast cancer are doubled for the 64-year-old with a positive family history.

10. **Answer: 3 Rationale:** Anticipatory grieving is appropriate ND since she is losing a portion of her body. She is beginning to grieve for that loss by crying.

Chapter 52: Nursing Care of Clients with Sexually Transmitted Infections

1. **Answer: 2 Rationale:** Women and infants are disproportionally affected by STIs because women may not experience symptoms of the disease and pass the infection on to the infant through vaginal birth.

2. **Answer: 1 Rationale:** STIs must be treated by treating both partners to prevent reinfection from one to the other, since symptoms are not always demonstrated when the infection is present.

3. **Answer: 1, 4, 5 Rationale:** Topics of information when teaching a male to prevent an STI should include using a new condom with each sex act, careful handling to prevent damage to condom, and withdrawal from the vagina when the penis is erect, holding the condom against the base of the penis to prevent contamination of the penis. No air should be in the tip and oil-based lubricants should never be used.

4. **Answer: 4 Rationale:** Blisters and ulcers appear on the penis of clients infected with genital herpes. The other STIs do not have these characteristics.

5. **Answer: 1 Rationale:** The statement is untrue about genital warts being caused by a yeast infection, viruses cause them.

6. **Answer: 4 Rationale:** Women with HPV genital infection should be advised to have a pelvic exam and pap smears every year since this infection causes an increased risk in developing cervical cancer, and the annual exams would identify the cancer early.

7. **Answer: 2 Rationale:** Itching is the most common manifestation experienced by a woman with a vaginal infection.

8. **Answer: 3 Rationale:** When teaching a woman with an STI experiencing severe genital discomfort, a simple recommendation is to wear cotton underwear because it absorbs moisture and allows airflow better than other materials. Sex should be avoided until treatment is completed.

9. **Answer: 1 Rationale:** Initially the male urethra and female cervix is affected by the gonorrheal organism.

10. **Answer: 3 Rationale:** Syphilis is a systemic infection that is caused by a spirochete that can affect a developing fetus in multiple places, brain, bone, and eyes.

Evaluate Your Response: Cues for Critical Thinking Questions

Chapter 4: Nursing Care of Clients Having Surgery
A Client Having Surgery

1. Safety concerns include ambulating and not tripping over scatter rugs or clutter. See information in Chapter 3 on safety in the home.

2. Medications used to prevent an occurrence such as infection are called prophylactic medications. Her risks for infection are from the surgical wound and microvascular circulation in bone.

Teach her to take the complete course of antibiotics prescribed and the possible side effects of the antibiotic. Encourage her to notify the physician if side effects or adverse events occur.

3. When blood stops flowing, it clots. Her immobility is a concern and puts her at risk for thrombosis and emboli. She has a risk for bleeding secondary to the anticoagulant and should inform any health care providers such as dentists that she is taking the anticoagulant.

4. Consider the risk for osteoporosis in addition to the degenerative changes Mrs. Overbeck experienced. She will need calcium sources and vitamin D.

Chapter 5: Nursing Care of Clients Experiencing Loss, Grief, and Death
A Client Experiencing Loss and Grief

1. Review the physical manifestations of grief described in the chapter and compare and contrast those with the ones verbalized by Mrs. Rogers.

2. Consider the benefits of including Mrs. Rogers's daughter in a meeting of the staff. What type of questions would be most useful in making the daughter feel a part of the plan of care? Why would a statement such as, "Why don't you do more for your mother," be inappropriate?

3. Consider the losses Mrs. Rogers has experienced. Review the material in the chapter on responses to loss. Think about the reasons you would not say, "Oh, you have a lot to live for." Think of two or three questions or statements that would help you assess the reason why Mrs. Rogers said this to you.

Chapter 6: Nursing Care of Clients with Problems of Substance Abuse

1. Consider the interactions of prescribed or over-the-counter medications with alcohol. What if the client has not taken prescribed medications because of chronic alcoholism?

2. Review the effects of Anatbuse. Make a list of possible interactions and side effects.

3. *Imbalanced nutrition:* Less than body requirements is an appropriate nursing diagnosis when a client does not have sufficient nutritional intake to meet metabolic needs. What in Mr. Russell's history and physical assessment supports this diagnosis? What nutritional information should you provide?

Chapter 7: A Client Experiencing a Disaster

1. What action did Mr. Jones take that probably exacerbated his skin lesions? Review Table 7–1 for injuries related to natural disasters. Consider how Mr. Jones put himself at risk for infection. (See Chapter 12.) How could Mr. Jones have avoided exacerbating his skin lesions?

2. What other testing might you anticipate related to Mr. Jones's delayed healing? Since Mr. Jones has a history of elevated blood pressure that has not been consistently treated or monitored, cardiac status should be evaluated. Which tests are indicated? Also, could his decreased sensation and poor healing be related to cardiac impairment? Mr. Jones also has indentifying data in his history and physical to suggest diabetes. Identify this data, and tests that would be indicated.

3. What were the contributing factors to Mr. Jones's fever? Review risk factors for and causes and manifestations of infection in Chapter 12. Identify the factors that contributed to Mr. Jones's fever.

4. What life situations contributed to Mr. Jones's attitude about life? Consider Mr. Jones's environmental and personal situations. What information do you have about Mr. Jones that indicate a lack of interest in health maintenance? Are there signs of a change in outlook?

Chapter 9: Nursing Care of Clients in Pain
A Client with Chronic Pain

1. Review the factors that affect an individual's response to pain. What have you observed in your own family and friends, as well as clients for whom you have cared?

2. Reflect on the benefits and disadvantages of each alternative. Make your decision based on knowledge about pain and about medications for pain.

3. What factors in Ms. Akers's illness and treatment increase her risk for constipation? What would you include in the plan specific to fluid intake and diet?

Chapter 10: Nursing Care of Clients with Altered Fluid, Electrolyte, or Acid-Base Balance
A Client with Fluid Volume Excess

1. Review the homeostatic mechanisms that control fluid balance and cardiac output. Which mechanisms are employed in this situation?

2. Review the anatomy and physiology of the respiratory system, including cardiopulmonary blood flow. Think about the effects of the upper abdominal organs on respiratory function as well.

3. Use therapeutic communication techniques: What is behind the client's statement? How can you facilitate Mrs. Rainwater's involvement in care decisions?

4. Review the actions and precautions for diuretic therapy. Think about what the client needs to know in terms of timing, possible adverse effects, and other information about diuretic therapy.

A Client with Hypokalemia

1. Review the physiologic effects of potassium, especially its intracellular and neuromuscular effects.

2. Review the potential sites and causes of excess potassium loss.

3. Think about the effects of diuretics on potassium balance and the effects of hypokalemia on digitalis therapy. What is the primary indication for digitalis therapy and how does this contribute to the interaction of these three factors?

4. Review the section in Chapter 26 on constipation and its management.

A Client with Hyperkalemia

1. Review the causes and manifestations of hyperkalemia.

2. What are the potential effects of hyperkalemia on cardiac conduction? At what level of hyperkalemia are these likely to be seen?

3. Review collaborative treatment measures to rapidly reduce potassium levels. Why would these be used with a K1 of 8.5?

4. Think about the effects of anxiety on learning as you develop a plan to provide teaching to avoid future episodes of hyperkalemia. As you develop your plan, remember the potential long-term effects of chronic renal failure.

A Client with Acute Respiratory Acidosis

1. Review normal gas exchange across the alveolar-capillary membrane and the processes that drive this exchange. Then review the role that carbon dioxide plays as a potential acid.

2. Describe the effect of acidosis on mental function.

3. Consider risk factors for choking: alcohol consumption, taking large bites of food, inadequate chewing, and so forth.

Chapter 11: Nursing Care of Clients Experiencing Trauma and Shock
A Client with Multiple Injuries

1. The definition of *Deficient fluid volume* is decreased intravascular, interstitial, and/or intracellular fluid. Which of Mrs. Souza's vital signs would support this definition? What other assessments could you make that would further support this diagnosis?

2. Consider the physiology of cellular metabolism. How long do brain cells live without oxygen? What happens if circulation is improved but the airway is blocked?

3. What can cause restlessness? Consider comfort, elimination, oxygenation, emotional status, and immobility.

4. List the multiple possibilities for entry of pathogens into the human body. Would age and physical condition increase the risk? What about transmission from health care personnel?

A Client with Septic Shock

1. Review the pharmacologic effects of vasopressors. Consider the pathologic basis for septic shock and how these medications may be effective.

2. Review the content on respiratory acidosis in Chapter 10. What do these findings tell you? What is present in Ms. Huang's physical status that would cause these manifestations?

3. Review the content about colloidal intravenous solutions in the chapter. What would you expect them to do when they are administered? How does this correlate to cardiac output? How do you assess increased circulatory volume?

Chapter 12: Nursing Care of Clients with Infection
A Client with Acquired Immunity

1. Review the adult immunizations listed in this chapter. Consider the geographical area in which the client lives. For example, clients living in areas at risk for Lyme disease should check with their physician about the new Lyme disease vaccine.

2. Review the concept of acquired immunity and the discussion of immunization in this chapter. What affect could nonimmunized persons have on their family and community?

3. Identify possible systemic and local reactions associated with immunizations. List manifestations that the client should report to the primary caregiver.

Chapter 13: Nursing Care of Clients with Altered Immunity
A Client with HIV Infection

1. Considering Ms. Lu's age, how effective is her immune system? How could lifestyle factors affect immune status?

2. At this stage of Ms. Lu's diagnosis, would you expect the physician to order a viral load test? Why or why not?

3. You have been asked to discuss AIDS and safe sex practices to a group of high school freshmen. What information would you present to them?

4. What resources could you provide to Ms. Lu and her fiancé regarding their desire to have a child?

Chapter 14: Nursing Care of Clients with Cancer

1. Review content on altered nutrition in Chapter 22 and the content in this chapter on the nursing diagnosis Altered Nutrition: Less than Body Requirements. Make a list of diagnostic tests for malnutrition with normal values.

2. Consider the type of cancers Mr. Casey has been diagnosed as having. Where in the body do these malignancies commonly metastasize? What would cause the pain?

3. Review a pharmacology book for medications that increase appetite and make a list of those appropriate to Mr. Casey.

4. Sepsis is discussed in Chapter 6. Review the content in that chapter on septic shock and outline manifestations. Develop a plan of care for Mr. Casey that is structured by priority of nursing diagnoses.

Chapter 16: Nursing Care of Clients with Integumentary Disorders
A Client with Herpes Zoster

1. Consider environmental, economic, and language barriers. What agencies in your own city or state exist to provide help?

What can you do other than make referrals? If you do make a referral, to whom would it be?

2. Review skin assessment guidelines in Chapter 14. How would you determine that the lesions had not improved? What manifestations would indicate secondary infection of the lesions? What would you do next if the lesions are still very painful and have not improved?

3. *Ineffective role performance* is defined as patterns of behavior and self-expression that do not match the environmental context, norms, and expectations. Related factors include inadequate or inappropriate linkage with the health care system and poverty. Based on this information, what interventions would you use? How would you evaluate the effectiveness of your interventions?

A Client with Malignant Melanoma

1. List reasons why people do not seek health care. Do you believe nurses can effect change? If so, what community activities would be most effective?

2. Consider attitudes toward the possibility of future illnesses. How would this affect your plan? What do you believe would be most effective in teaching this age group?

3. Think about what you know about taking prescribed antibiotics as well as the side effects of antibiotic therapy. What would you suggest that Mr. Sanders do?

4. *Powerlessness* is the perception that one's own actions will not significantly affect an outcome. Is this a common response to the diagnosis of cancer? Consider types of communications and interventions that would allow greater decision making for Mr. Sanders.

Chapter 17: Nursing Care of Clients with Burns
A Client with a Major Burn

1. Review the effects of the major burn wound on the renal and gastrointestinal systems. What assessments would indicate effective fluid resuscitation?

2. What type of burns did Mr. Howard have on his arms? Consider the effect of compression on the peripheral vascular system. What assessments would you make to identify this complication?

3. Consider the type of pain the client has. What do you think might happen if the narcotics were given by other routes, such as oral or intramuscularly?

4. Review the effects of a major burn. Consider the damage to cell wall integrity and capillary beds. What effect does the shift of proteins and sodium have on intravascular volume?

Chapter 19: Nursing Care of Clients with Endocrine Disorders
A Client with Graves' Disease

1. What effect does increased TH have on metabolism and cardiac rate and stroke volume? How does this effect compare to that of sympathetic stimulation?

2. Consider the effect of elevating any body part, such as elevating your leg above heart level for a sprained ankle. How does this affect venous return?

3. You will need to consider Mrs. Manuel from both a medical and a surgical perspective. How would you teach her to care for her incision? With removal of most of the thyroid gland, what symptoms would you be sure she knew about? What should she do if these occur?

A Client with Hypothyroidism

1. Make a list of changes in body systems with aging and with decreased TH levels. How would you determine what assessment findings were abnormal?

2. Consider the effects of the following factors: weakness, fatigue, problems with memory. What would you recommend she do in her home to increase her safety?

3. Prepare a list of manifestations of hyperthyroidism. Be sure they are in terms a client would understand.

A Client with Cushing's Syndrome

1. Review Ms. Domico's lab results and compare them to normal results. What altered the findings in her case?
2. How many ways can you think of to assess fluid balance? Consider weight, I&O, and skin. What other assessments provide information?
3. How does fatigue differ from "just being tired"? Would increasing hours of sleep be an intervention you would include? Why or why not?

A Client with Addison's Disease

1. Review the functions of the hormones of the adrenal cortex in Chapter 18. Consider the effects of stress, and formulate your response with rationale.
2. Review content on fluid imbalance in Chapter 5. Make a list of assessments you might make that would indicate severe dehydration. What is the pathophysiology of fluid loss in the client with Addison's disease?
3. Review content on sodium and potassium in Chapter 5 and make a list of foods you would suggest Mr. Sardoff eat.

Chapter 2: Nursing Care of Clients with Diabetes Mellitus

A Client with Type 1 Diabetes

1. How do the increased urinary output and increased osmolarity of the blood plasma affect the fluid status of the body? What is the response of the body to decreased intravascular volume?
2. Consider the effects of nicotine on blood vessels. How would these effects, when combined with the pathologic effects of long-standing hyperglycemia, affect blood vessel walls?
3. Review the information about chronic illness in Chapter 2. Powerlessness is a perceived lack of control over a situation and/or one's ability to significantly affect an outcome. What types of statements by a client would help you make this nursing diagnosis?
4. Compare and contrast the developmental needs and tasks of the young adult and the older adult (see Chapter 2). Consider the teaching materials that might have to be adapted to physical changes in the older adult.

Chapter 22: Nursing Care of Clients with Nutritional Disorders

A Client with Obesity

1. Review the physiology of cholesterol formation in the body and the factors that affect this process.
2. Consider developmental stages and teaching strategies for adult learners.
3. Think about individual factors, family and support group influences, and cultural factors that may affect recommended weight loss and exercise strategies.

A Client with Malnutrition

1. Review the physiology of albumin and cholesterol formation in the body.
2. Review Mrs. Chow's diet and compare it to the food pyramid or recommendations for food intake to formulate your response.
3. Consider cultural influences and the client's preferred foods as you plan a diet that is high in calories and protein.

Chapter 23: Nursing Care of Clients with Upper Gastrointestinal Disorders

A Client with Oral Cancer

1. Review the major risk factors for oral cancer and identify the populations most likely to have these risk factors.

2. Work with your classmates to plan (and implement) an education program, considering the developmental/teaching needs of this group of young people.
3. Think about the possible causes for Mr. Chavez's refusal to talk (remember that assessment is the first step of the nursing process). How will you identify factors contributing to his behavior?

A Client with Peptic Ulcer Disease

1. Review the physiology of the gastric mucosal barrier and the pathogenesis of peptic ulcer disease, and the effect of *H. pylori* infection on these processes.
2. Review physiologic responses to stress in your physiology or nursing fundamentals text; compare and apply this information with the physiology of the gastric mucosal barrier and the pathophysiology of ulcer development.
3. Consider Mr. O'Donnell's occupation and schedule, as well as the prescribed medications and when each should be taken.
4. Using journal and text resources as well as your classmates, identify as many stress reduction techniques as possible. Then sort your list into those which could be used while working, and identify ways to effectively teach each technique.

A Client with Gastric Cancer

1. Review the healing process and the normal physiology of the stomach as you formulate your answer to this question.
2. Consider the surgery, immediate postoperative care, and what the client and family should expect in developing your teaching plan.
3. Review Chapter 14 and nursing care related to chemotherapy.
4. Again, review Chapter 14 for nursing care measures for clients with cancer; also review Chapter 22 for strategies to prevent and manage malnutrition.

Chapter 24: Nursing Care of Clients with Gallbladder, Liver, and Pancreatic Disorders

A Client with Cholelithiasis

1. Review the composition of gallstones, as well as the physiology of gallbladder function and bile. Research and discuss dietary practices of the Chickasaw tribe (or of Native Americans).
2. Review Chapter 4 for care related to a laparotomy (incision into the abdomen).
3. As you develop your plan, consider Mrs. Red Wing's culture, job, and family obligations.

A Client with Hepatitis A

1. In your plan, consider the transmission and pathophysiology of hepatitis A. Review developmental considerations when teaching clients to adapt your teaching to Mr. Johns's level.
2. Review the hepatitis table in this chapter, as well as the pathophysiology of hepatitis.
3. Review the hepatitis tables as well as standard precautions in Appendix A.
4. In your plan, consider the living situation (group home), the developmental level of the residents, and the resident care managers (largely unskilled). Work with your study or clinical group to develop this plan.

A Client with Alcoholic Cirrhosis

1. Review the anatomy and physiology of the liver and its circulation, as well as the pathophysiology of cirrhosis and its complications.
2. Consult your nutrition textbook as needed for foods that are high in calories but low in protein and sodium. When planning for limited protein intake, be sure to include high-quality proteins and limit intake of lower-quality proteins such as legumes.

3. Review the pathophysiology of hepatic encephalopathy to develop your responses to this question.
4. Review therapeutic communication skills; consult your nursing diagnosis and care planning text book as you develop this care plan.

A Client with Acute Pancreatitis
1. Review Chapter 6 for assessment data indicative of alcohol withdrawal.
2. Review both the pathophysiology of acute pancreatitis and the acute inflammatory process.
3. Consult your nutrition textbook or the American Dietetic Association web site.
4. Consult your nursing care planning textbook to develop this care plan.

Chapter 26: Nursing Care of Clients with Bowel Disorders
A Client with Acute Appendicitis
1. Review the acute inflammatory response to an infectious process and the role WBCs play in the immune response.
2. Review Chapter 4. Consider factors such as incision size, abdominal muscle disruption, and manipulation of the bowel in developing your response.
3. Consider points such as pain management, resumption of activities, incision care, and potential complications in developing your teaching plan. Consider the client's education and developmental stage as well.
4. Review the effects of anxiety on recovery and learning. Identify nursing measures to reduce situational anxiety.

A Client with Ulcerative Colitis
1. Review normal functions of the small and large intestine. Review the usual location of an ileostomy. Review fluid volume deficit in Chapter 10 for manifestations and assessment data.
2. Think about the effect of chronic blood loss and review the effect of malnutrition on the hemoglobin and hematocrit.
3. Review the home care section of inflammatory bowel disease for teaching points to include.
4. Review nursing care for the client with diarrhea, as well as the procedure for ileostomy care.

A Client with Colorectal Cancer
1. Review peripheral innervation and impulse transmission in your anatomy and physiology textbook; think about how nerves in the rectal region are disrupted in an abdominoperineal resection. Also review the phantom pain phenomenon in Chapter 9.
2. Compare elimination through a colostomy with "normal" bowel elimination through the anus. How do they differ in terms of the passage of flatus?
3. Review Procedure 26–1. Also review the procedure for administering an enema in your fundamentals or skills textbook.
4. Review this nursing diagnosis in your nursing diagnosis or nursing care planning handbook; be sure to individualize your plan to Mr. Cunningham's situation and needs.

Chapter 28: Nursing Care of Clients with Urinary Tract Disorders
A Client with Cystitis
1. Consider risk factors for UTI as well as factors affecting Mrs. Waisanen's immune function.
2. Consider the indications for short-course antibiotic therapy and the indications for conventional therapy. Think about factors such as cost, compliance, and the risk for adverse effects, as well as how antibiotics work to eradicate bacteria.
3. Identify why *Ineffective health maintenance* may be an appropriate nursing diagnosis for Mrs. Waisanen and the individual factors contributing to this diagnosis as you plan care.

A Client with Urinary Calculi
1. Review the risk factors for urinary lithiasis.
2/3. Using the medications section of interdisciplinary care for the client with urinary calculi in this chapter and your pharmacology textbook or drug handbook, review analgesia for the client with renal colic and the intended and adverse effects of the drugs given to Mr. Leton.

A Client with a Bladder Tumor
1. Review the physiology of the bladder and the risk factors for urinary tract tumors.
2. Review Mr. Hussain's health history for possible contributing factors.
3. See Chapter 6 for nursing care of clients with problems of substance abuse.
4. Use your nursing care planning and nursing diagnoses textbooks to identify possible outcomes and interventions for Sexual dysfunction.

A Client with Urinary Incontinence
1. Review the desired and adverse effects of the prescribed medications.
2. Review the effects of menopause and estrogen deficiency on perineal tissues.
3. Review Mrs. Giovanni's physical examination findings and risk factors for UTI.
4. Identify factors that may contribute to *Situational low self-esteem* in Mrs. Giovanni and nursing measures to address this diagnosis.

Chapter 29: Nursing Care of Clients with Kidney Disorders
A Client with Acute Glomerulonephritis
1. Review Chapter 12 and the use of antibiotics to treat infection.
2. Review Mr. Chang's history and the risk factors for acute glomerulonephritis.
3. Review the diagnostic tests used to differentiate different forms of glomerulonephritis.

A Client with Acute Renal Failure
1. Review common causes and the pathophysiology of acute renal failure.
2. Review the sections on peptic ulcer disease and stress gastritis in Chapter 23.
3. Consider the position requirements to maintain body and bone alignment in skeletal traction (Chapter 41).

A Client with End-Stage Renal Disease
1. Review the usual onset, pathophysiology, and long-term effects of type 1 and type 2 diabetes (Chapter 20).
2. Consider the effects of urea and ammonia (both neurologic toxins) on brain function.
3. Review the manifestations of uremia.
4. Consider the composition of the dialysate and its possible effect on blood glucose control.

Chapter 31: Nursing Care of Clients with Coronary Heart Disease
A Client with Coronary Artery Bypass Surgery
1. Identify Mr. Clements's modifiable risk factors as you develop your plan. What barriers might need to be overcome to implement strategies to reduce his risk factors?
2. What strategies can you use to overcome denial without creating hostility or impairing the client-nurse relationship?
3. Consider traditional family roles as well as those roles that are unique to these individuals. Identify measures you can use to enlist the spouse's support.

4. Think about therapeutic communications as you formulate your response. Will your age or gender potentially affect your ability to respond effectively to these concerns? Would referral to another health care provider be appropriate?

A Client with Acute Myocardial Infarction

1. Review immediate treatment measures for MI. Are other means available for reestablishing coronary artery perfusion? If you are in a rural area without immediate access to a cardiac catheterization lab, how will this affect your response?
2. Review the section of this chapter on dysrhythmias and their treatment. Research protocols for treating frequent PVCs in the post-MI client at your clinical facility.
3. Review the goals of cardiac rehabilitation and Mrs. Williams's individual risk factors as you develop your teaching plan.
4. Consider the value of using a therapeutic response to Mrs. Williams's statement concerning smoking. Also consider the risks associated with cigarette smoke. How can you respond without supporting Mrs. Williams's desire to smoke and without precipitating anger or resistance? Review Chapter 6.

A Client with Supraventricular Tachycardia

1. Review the effects of sympathetic and parasympathetic nervous system stimulation on cardiac function.
2. Review the section on supraventricular tachycardias, as well as the antidysrhythmic medications for other treatment options.
3. Use your pharmacology textbook as you develop your teaching plan.

Chapter 32: Nursing Care of Clients with Cardiac Disorders
A Client with Heart Failure

1. Review the prescribed medications and their interactions. Do not forget to consider Mr. Jackson's age in assessing his risk for toxicity and interactions.
2. Review therapeutic communications skills and the use of open-ended statements to evaluate the underlying message of Mr. Jackson's statement.
3. Review exercise recommendations for the client with heart failure as well as cardiac rehabilitation principles (Chapter 31).
4. Review the rationale for aspirin therapy in the client with CHD and its effects on platelets and clotting as you formulate your response.
5. Review Chapter 45 for causes of CVA and the section of Chapter 31 on atrial fibrillation.

A Client with Mitral Valve Prolapse

1. Review the pathophysiology and manifestations of MVP, as well as the general treatment measures for valve disorders.
2. Think about the effects of progressive conditioning on cardiac function.
3. Consider the anxiety associated with heart conditions and with a potentially progressive disorder that could affect childbearing and other life activities, as well as ultimately necessitate surgery.
4. Review the manifestations of MVP and of mitral regurgitation.

Chapter 34: Nursing Care of Clients with Hematologic Disorders
A Client with Anemia

1. Consider the effects of Mrs. Matthews's rapid weight loss on fluid balance, as well as the effects of tissue hypoxia on cardiac output.
2. Refer to this chapter and your nutrition text. Be sure to consider Mrs. Matthews's age in designing your menu.
3. Consider factors such as Mrs. Matthews's recent dietary history, the folic acid content of foods, and other pertinent factors in the history and physical assessment

4. In addition to general factors to consider for the older adult (don't forget transportation among other factors), also consider the possible effect of Mrs. Matthews's recent loss and the grieving process.

A Client with Leukemia

1. Review the physiology of white blood cells, and the immune and inflammatory responses.
2. Think about the risks created by hospitalization in terms of exposure to infection and invasive procedures.
3. Think about the effect of inability to perform self care on self-esteem, self-confidence, and perception of power and control.
4. Use information provided in the nursing care and home care sections of this chapter as well as in Chapter 12.
5. Use your nursing care planning and fundamentals texts to develop your care plan.

A Client with Hodgkin's disease

1. Review Chapter 14 and the effects of chemotherapy and radiation on cancerous cells. Think about the advantages of combining these two therapies in terms of short and long-term desired and adverse effects.
2. Consider the primary and potential risks for infection in community settings as you design your teaching plan. What teaching strategies will you use for a young adult with Mr. Quito's education and experience?
3. Review theories of development and the developmental tasks for the young adult.
4. Use your nursing fundamentals and nursing care planning texts for reference in developing your care plan.

A Client with Hemophilia

1. Review the pathophysiology of hemophilia and its effect on the clotting process.
2. Consider both the ABCs and Maslow's hierarchy of needs as you respond to this question.
3. Think about the genetic transmission of hemophilia. How might Mr. Cruise's hemophila affect any children that he has? Grandchildren?
4. Review your nursing fundamentals book, nursing skills book, and intravenous therapy text to develop your teaching plan. Also consider previous learning and developmental levels.
5. Consult your nursing care planning text. Consider why this might be an appropriate nursing diagnosis for Mr. Cruise.

Chapter 35: Nursing Care of Clients with Peripheral Vascular and Lymphatic Disorders
A Client with Hypertension

1. Review Mrs. Spezia's assessment data and the risk factors for primary hypertension.
2. Review the pathophysiology of primary hypertension and of obesity (Chapter 22), as well as the relationship between hypertension and coronary heart disease.
3. Think about resources that are available in your community for homeless people. Talk to community health and social service agencies to identify additional resources.
4. Again, review Mrs. Spezia's assessment data, the pathophysiology of hypertension, and the long-term effects of stress.
5. Use your nursing care planning and nursing diagnosis textbooks to help develop your care plan.

A Client with Peripheral Atherosclerosis

1. Review treatments for peripheral atherosclerosis, as well as lifestyle measures for preventing and treating atherosclerosis and coronary heart disease (Chapter 31).

2. Compare the pathophysiology of peripheral atherosclerosis, intermittent claudication, and coronary heart disease (Chapter 31) to identify similarities and differences.
3. Review the actions of beta blockers and their role in angina prophylaxis.
4. Use your nursing care planning and nutrition textbooks to help develop your care plan.

A Client with Deep Vein Thrombosis
1. Review the pathophysiologic processes of venous thrombosis and inflammation as you develop your answer.
2. Think about questions you could ask for further information as well as potential resources for Mrs. Hipps.
3. Consider assessment data to evaluate Mrs. Hipps's limitations and resources, as well as community resources to help meet her needs.
4. Use your nursing diagnosis and care planning textbooks to develop your plan of care.

Chapter 37: Nursing Care of Clients with Upper Respiratory Disorders
A Client with Peritonsillar Abscess
1/2. Review the manifestations of upper respiratory infections and management of these disorders.
3. Think about the primary uses of the nose, mouth, and pharynx as you consider nursing diagnoses related to upper respiratory disorders.

A Client with Nasal Fracture
1. Consider other measures to restore the client's sense of control over the situation. Consider the potentially traumatic effects of suction on the mucous membranes as well as possible infection control risks.
2. Review the implications and potential dangers of CSF leakage to help you develop your care plan.
3. Think about the benefits and drawbacks of immediate and delayed rhinoplasty.

A Client with Total Laryngectomy
1. Review the options for speech rehabilitation. If available, practice using a speech generator. Practice esophageal speech.
2. Use your nursing care planning and nursing diagnoses handbook to develop your care plan. Consider Mr. Tom's age, occupation, and marital status in your plan of care.
3. Review Chapter 4 for surgical nursing care interventions, as well as your nursing fundamentals textbook for wound care strategies.
4. Consider measures to promote airway clearance and ventilation of all lung fields.

Chapter 38: Nursing Care of Clients with Ventilation Disorders
A Client with Pneumonia
1. Review Mrs. O'Neal's assessment data and compare her history with identified risk factors for pneumonia.
2. Review normal immune and inflammatory responses and the role of white blood cells in these processes.
3. Review Chapter 11 and altered immune responses for the physiology and effects of anaphylactic shock.
4. Use your nursing care planning and nursing diagnosis textbooks to help develop your care plan.

A Client with Tuberculosis
1. Consider available resources for mentally ill clients, as well as community and public health resources. Consider measures to ensure compliance with the prescribed treatment.

2. Contact your local public health department, the discharge planner for your unit, or the social services department in your clinical facility to help identify available resources.
3. Use your nursing fundamentals text, the nursing care section under Pneumonia, and your nursing diagnosis or care planning handbook as you develop your care plan.

A Client with Lung Cancer
1. Review Chapter 14 and use your pharmacology text to research the effects of these drugs and the rationale for combination chemotherapy.
2. Use Chapter 14 and your pharmacology text to identify probable side effects of this treatment regimen. Then use your nursing care planning book to identify appropriate nursing diagnoses and interventions.
3. Review the pathophysiology and collaborative care sections for lung cancer to develop your response to this question.

Chapter 39: Nursing Care of Clients with Gas Exchange Disorders
A Client with COPD
1. Review the processes by which cigarette smoke inflicts damage on lung tissue. Use your pediatric and pathophysiology texts for additional information.
2. Review the physiology of the respiratory drive, as well as the effects of chronic elevated carbon dioxide levels in the blood.
3. Review the manifestations of COPD and its complications as well as the section of this chapter on respiratory failure.
4. Use your nursing diagnosis handbook to help identify appropriate goals and interventions for this nursing diagnosis.

A Client with ARDS
1. As you respond to this question, consider additional treatment measures for ARDS and respiratory failure. Also consider the potential long-term consequences and complications of intubation and mechanical ventilation. Discuss strategies for communicating with Ms. Adamson's family and supporting coping and decision-making by Ms. Adamson and her family in an instance such as this.
2. Think about the precipitating factors for ARDS and the factors that may precipitate respiratory failure in a client with COPD. Consider the probable overall respiratory and general health status of the individual affected by each of these conditions.
3. Review the precipitating factors for ARDS and discuss strategies to prevent them.
4. Use your nursing care planning book to identify appropriate goals and nursing interventions for this nursing diagnosis.

Chapter 41: Nursing Care of Clients with Musculoskeletal Trauma
A Client with a Hip Fracture
1. Consider Mrs. Carbolito's age and the fact that she is postmenopausal. What effect does estrogen have on bone health? What might have increased her risk for falls?
2. Review the principles of traction application. What purpose does it serve prior to surgery? What words could you use that she would understand? Think about the effects of trauma, pain, and suddenly finding oneself in a strange environment on listening and understanding verbal communications.
3. List how each of these manifestations would affect skin integrity, food intake, and bone healing.

A Client with a Below-the-Knee Amputation
1. Design a sequential plan for Mr. Rocke's self-care of the stump. Consider his readiness to learn and the complexity of the care.

Is there a risk in letting him assume total responsibility from the beginning? Why or why not?

2. List the factors used to describe Mr. Rocke. How do these affect his ability or willingness to follow up with medical care? What community agencies are available where you live or go to school that would be good sources of assistance and support for Mr. Rocke?

3. Review the information about exercise. How would Mr. Rocke's choice not to do exercises affect his ability to use a prosthesis to walk?

Chapter 42: Nursing Care of Clients with Musculoskeletal Disorders

A Client with Osteoporosis

1. Review the effects of nicotine and caffeine on blood circulation to bones. What effect does alcohol play in bone loss?

2. Review foods that increase blood cholesterol levels. What is considered a normal cholesterol level? You may need to read content in Chapter 31. Knowing the client needs calcium, what type of dairy products would you recommend?

3. List activities for the client who is not able to be ambulatory. How many of the activities on your list would help prevent osteoporosis?

4. *Risk for trauma* is defined as an increased risk for accidental tissue injury, such as a fracture. What interventions would you teach Mrs. Bauer to reduce this risk?

A Client with Osteoarthritis

1. Review information about serum creatinine and BUN in a laboratory studies textbook or on the web. What medications is Mr. Cerulli taking that may be affecting these findings? Consider what teaching is necessary related to these findings.

2. What assessments are significant for confusion? If necessary, review content related to confusion. Review Mr. Cerulli's history in the case study and determine factors that may have contributed to his risk for confusion before, during, and after surgery.

3. *Acute confusion* is defined as an abrupt onset of a cluster of global, transient changes and disturbances in attention, cognition, psychomotor activity, level of consciousness, and/or sleep/wake cycle. What assessments could you make to support this diagnosis for Mr. Cerulli? What interventions might you design for this diagnosis?

A Client with Rheumatoid Arthritis

1. Think about the role differences in a 42-year-old woman and a 72-year- old woman. On the other hand, consider the effects of a chronic illness that may have been present for 30 years. Would your plan differ? Why or why not?

2. List the possible disabilities that may be caused by rheumatoid arthritis. How do you believe these would affect Mrs. James? What agencies in your community are available for support of people with this type of illness? Where would you go for literature to give Mrs. James?

3. *Ineffective role performance* is defined as behaviors and expressions that do not match norms or expectations. Do you believe this is an appropriate nursing diagnosis for Mrs. James? Why or why not? What interventions could be implemented for this diagnosis?

Chapter 44: Nursing Care of Clients with Intracranial Disorders

A Client with a Migraine Headache

1. Review the content in the chapter on migraine headaches. List questions that you would ask specific to onset, length, manifestations, stages, pain, diet, and factors associated with the headache onset.

2. Consider foods that are high in sodium. What would you suggest if Ms. Friedman eats fast foods at least five times a week? Review the food pyramid in Chapter 2 and outline a weekly meal plan for Ms. Friedman.

3. Discuss with members of your class those factors that interfere with their normal sleep patterns. What suggestions might you give Ms. Friedman to help her improve her sleep? Why is this important?

A Client with a Seizure Disorder

1. List the teaching topics you would include for Ms. Carlson. Consider how her needs (e.g., for safety) would differ if she lived alone.

2. Describe statements you could use to help Ms. Carlson understand not only the dangers but also the legal issues involved. What if Ms. Carlson does not recognize these concerns?

3. What type of questions could you ask Ms. Carlson to determine why she feels this way? Would you personally find it embarrassing? How can you facilitate Ms. Carlson's understanding for this recommendation?

A Client with Subdural Hematoma

1. Review the manifestations of the types of intracranial hematomas. What assessments are specific to a subdural hematoma? Why is it important to know this?

2. What are some other interventions that might be used? How could family help? What if no family members are available?

3. Acute confusion is a sudden onset of changes in attention, cognition, psychomotor activity, level of consciousness, and/or sleep/wake cycle. What would you determine as priority nursing diagnoses and interventions for Mr. Lee?

A Client with Bacterial Meningitis

1. List the environmental stimuli in the hospital setting. How could these be decreased? What effect do these stimuli have on cognition and behavior that is altered by an intracranial infection?

2. Think about how you would feel if Mr. Cook tried to hit you. How would you respond to him? To whom would you report this?

3. Why would Mr. Cook have pain? How would pain be manifested during the initial treatment period for Mr. Cook? Is it important to consider the respiratory effects of narcotics for him? Defend your answer.

A Client with a Brain Tumor

1. Review content in the chapter on increased intracranial pressure and intracranial surgery. List collaborative and nursing interventions to decrease increased intracranial pressure.

2. What do these manifestations indicate? What would be your priority assessment? Who would you notify?

3. Practice the use of therapeutic communications and what response you would make.

4. Consider the reasons Ms. Lange feels powerless. What nursing interventions might decrease this feeling?

Chapter 45: Nursing Care of Clients with Cerebrovascular and Spinal Cord Disorders

A Client with a Stroke

1. What subjective manifestations does the client with hypertension have? (Review content in Chapter 35.)

2. Consider referral to community resources as a volunteer tutor for adult literacy, gardening, and/or woodworking. Tutoring college students is another option.

3. Use statements that will encourage Mr. Boren to talk about his arm and how he feels about being unable to use it.

A Client with a SCI

1. What are the developmental tasks of a 19-year-old? How does the inability to meet these tasks affect emotional responses?
2. Think about questions that explore Mr. Valdez's fears in relation to sexuality. Practice questions and statements with friends until you are not embarrassed to ask them.
3. Consider how your own values and beliefs may differ from those of a client.
4. What baseline assessments and information are necessary before developing a plan for urinary elimination needs? Why would self-catheterization be an option? What are the risks of long-term Foley catheterization?

Chapter 46: Nursing Care of Clients with Neurologic Disorders

A Client with AD

1. Think about what information you would need and how you would collect it. Consider such factors as the age of family members, educational level of family members, and stage of the client's AD. What else would you need to know?
2. Review the suggested activities in this section of the chapter. What others can you think of or have you seen used successfully? Osteoarthritis often results in joint stiffness and pain as well as problems with mobility. Would this affect your interventions? If so, how could they be adapted?
3. Consider the type of foods that might be prepared, the timing of meals, and interventions that might be used to decrease agitation before or during meals.

A Client with MS

1. Outline a typical day's activities for Mr. McMurphy that would provide a balance between activity and rest. What assessments would you make to evaluate the effectiveness of this plan?
2. Consider how respiratory infections are spread. Why is Mr. McMurphy at increased risk?
3. The definition of *Risk for injury* is that one is at risk as a result of environmental conditions interacting with the person's adaptive and defensive resources. What factors in this client's history and physical status would support this diagnosis? What interventions would you include in the care plan and why?

A Client with Parkinson's Disease

1. Consider the adaptations that might be made to clothing and shoes. What adaptive devices might be useful?
2. What information would you need to know before you develop your interventions? Include that from Mr. Avneil and what might be available in the community and the long-term care facility.
3. *Chronic sorrow* is a recurring pattern of sadness in response to continual loss. Consider the type of communications you would need to use with Mr. Avneil to identify his degree of sorrow. What other assessment might provide cues to support this diagnosis (think about eating and sleeping)? How might an activity such as reminiscence help?

A Client with Myasthenia Gravis

1. Review the pathophysiology of myasthenia gravis. What is the action of Tensilon?
2. Consider teaching topics for Mrs. Avis that would assist her in conserving energy while preparing meals. List suggestions to conserve energy while eating.
3. *Ineffective role performance* is the state in which behaviors and self-expression do not match such factors as norms and expectations. What changes occur as a result of this illness? What do you think Mrs. Avis expects of herself? What are some interventions you could implement to facilitate acceptance of the change she is experiencing?

Chapter 48: Nursing Care of Clients with Eye and Ear Disorders

A Client with Glaucoma and Cataracts

1. What is the pathophysiology of glaucoma? How does a cataract affect glaucoma?
2. Consider the effects of corticosteroids on glaucoma. If Mrs. Rainey is to administer several medications at home, identify specific teaching guidelines for her.
3. Consider referral for home health visits. Think about the effect of transferring her for a brief admission to an assisted-living facility.

Chapter 50: Nursing Care of Men with Reproductive System and Breast Disorders

A Man with Prostate Cancer

1. Why would Mr. Turner be at risk for altered skin integrity? Outline the interventions you would include on his teaching plan that would promote skin integrity as he cares for himself at home.
2. Noncompliance is defined as behaviors that do not coincide with the therapeutic plan agreed upon by the person and the health care professional. Do you think Mr. Turner fully understood his treatment and agreed with his follow-up care? What could be done in the preoperative phase of Mr. Turner's care to better ensure his understanding and desire to have continued medical care?
3. What assessments indicate that Mr. Turner does or does not have bladder distention? Would you report this? If so, to whom?

Chapter 51: Nursing Care of Women with Reproductive System and Breast Disorders

A Woman with Endometriosis

1. What is the relationship between Mrs. Hall's manifestations and a decreased RBC count? Review the information in Chapter 34 and list assessments you would make to identify anemia.
2. List nonthreatening questions you would use to begin the discussion. How might it help to ask these questions at the beginning of the interview? Then list questions that you might use to collect data about the couple's sexual history. Would you be embarrassed to ask them? If so, how might this in turn affect their responses?
3. *Situational low self-esteem* is the state in which a person develops a negative perception of self-worth in response to a current situation. What information in Mrs. Hall's history might provide data to support this nursing diagnosis?

A Woman with Cervical Cancer

1. Review the risk factors for cervical cancer. Consider what might differ for a young woman and an older woman.
2. Review the information in Chapter 14 on radiation as a treatment for cancer. What interventions would be appropriate for Ms. Gillam?
3. Based on your review of the information on radiation, explain how radiation might cause fatigue. How does fatigue differ from being tired? What interventions would you include in a plan of care for this nursing diagnosis?

A Woman with Breast Cancer

1. Review the information in the chapter on the genetic factors that pose a risk for developing breast cancer. How could you explain this in terms understandable by Mrs. Clemments and her daughters?
2. List the different types of mastectomies. Consider the implications of the differences, and how this would affect your nursing care.

3. Review the information on chemotherapy in Chapter 14. List the types of chemotherapy and its common side effects. Consider the classifications of medications that are used to treat these side effects.
4. What factors in the treatment of Mrs. Clemments treatment might disrupt the amount and quality of her sleep? What interventions might be used to improve her sleep pattern?

Chapter 52: Nursing Care of Clients with Sexually Transmitted Infections

A Client with Gonorrhea

1. What manifestations does Ms. Cirit have that are typical of the disease? Would you make other assessments? If so, what are they?
2. Review the discussion of HIV in Chapter 13. Do you believe it is true that infection with gonorrhea may increase the risk of HIV? If so, how would you explain this to Ms. Cirit?

3. *Impaired social interaction* is a state of aloneness or rejection experienced by an individual that is perceived as negative. What assessments of Ms. Cirit might support this diagnosis? What interventions and expected outcomes would you develop?

A Client with Syphilis

1. Describe the assessments you would expect to find in a man with early syphilis.
2. Consider topics such as number of sex partners, patterns of sexual activity, and use of safe sex practices. What other topics should be explored? How can you ask these questions without being embarrassed or embarrassing the client?
3. List possible statements you might make. Do you believe this is a nursing responsibility? If you do not feel comfortable with this topic, what could you do?

Abrasion Partial-thickness denudation of an area of integument, generally resulting from falls or scrapes.

Absence seizure (petit mal seizure) A type of generalized seizure characterized by a sudden brief cessation of all motor activity accompanied by a blank stare and unresponsiveness.

Accommodation The ability of the eye to adjust to variations in distance.

Achalasia Absence of peristalsis of the esophagus and high gastroesophageal sphincter pressure resulting in dilation and loss of tone in the esophagus.

Acidosis The condition in which the hydrogen ion concentration increases above normal (reflected in a pH below 7.35).

Acids A substance that releases hydrogen ions in solution.

Acne Disorder of the pilosebaceous (hair and sebaceous gland) structure, resulting in eruption of papules or pustules.

Acoustic neuroma or schwannoma Benign tumor of cranial nerve VIII.

Acquired immune deficiency syndrome (AIDS) A specific group of diseases or conditions that are indicative of severe immunosuppression related to infection with the human immunodeficiency virus.

Acquired immunity Immunity developed after exposure to a pathogen. See *Active immunity.*

Acromegaly Meaning literally "enlarged extremities," this is a condition resulting from excessive growth hormone secretion during adulthood.

Actinic keratosis Also called senile or solar keratosis, this is an epidermal skin lesion directly related to chronic sun exposure and photodamage.

Active immunity Production of antibodies or development of immune lymphocytes against specific antigens.

Active transport Movement of molecules across cell membranes and epithelial membranes against a concentration gradient; requires energy.

Acute coronary syndromes A general term used to describe the effects of coronary heart disease, including angina and myocardial infarction.

Acute gastritis A benign, self-limiting disorder associated with ingestion of gastric irritants such as aspirin, alcohol, caffeine, or foods contaminated with certain bacteria.

Acute illness An illness that occurs rapidly, lasts for a relatively short time, and is self-limiting.

Acute lymphoblastic leukemia (ALL) Abnormal proliferation of lymphoblasts in the bone marrow, lymph nodes, and spleen; the most common type of leukemia in children and young adults.

Acute myeloblastic leukemia (AML) Uncontrolled proliferation of myeloblasts (granulocyte precursors) and hyperplasia of bone marrow and the spleen; the most common acute leukemia in adults.

Acute myocardial infarction (AMI) Necrosis (death) of myocardial cells.

Acute pain Usually temporary, localized, and of sudden onset; it lasts for less than 6 months and has an identifiable cause, such as trauma, surgery, or inflammation.

Acute renal failure Abrupt onset of renal failure, often reversible.

Acute respiratory distress syndrome (ARDS) Noncardiac pulmonary edema and progressive refractory hypoxemia.

Acute tubular necrosis (ATN) A syndrome of abrupt and progressive decline in tubular and glomerular function.

Advance directive Also called a *living will*, this is a document in which a client formally states preferences for health care in the event that he or she later becomes mentally incapacitated and names a person who has durable power of attorney to serve as a substitute decision maker to implement the client's stated preferences.

Aesthetic surgery See *Cosmetic surgery.*

Afterload The force the ventricles must overcome to eject their blood volume; the pressure in the arterial system ahead of the ventricles.

Agnosia The inability to recognize one or more subjects that were previously familiar; agnosia may be visual, tactile, or auditory.

Agranulocytosis Severe neutropenia, with less than 200 cells/µm.

Alcoholic cirrhosis (Laënnec's cirrhosis) The end result of alcoholic liver disease.

Alkalosis The condition where the hydrogen ion concentration decreases below normal (reflected in a pH above 7.45).

Alleles Different forms of a gene or DNA occupying the same place on a pair of chromosomes; an allele for each gene is inherited from each parent.

Allergy A hypersensitivity response to environmental or exogenous antigens.

Allografts Grafts between members of the same species but who have different genotypes and HLA antigens. See also *Homograft.*

Alopecia Loss of hair; baldness.

Alzheimer's disease (AD) A form of dementia characterized by progressive, irreversible deterioration of the general intellectual functioning.

Amenorrhea Absence of menstruation.

Amputation Partial or total removal of a body part.

Amyotrophic lateral sclerosis (ALS) Progressive, degenerative neurologic disease characterized by weakness and wasting of the involved muscles, without any accompanying sensory or cognitive changes; also called *Lou Gehrig's disease.*

Analgesic A medication that reduces or eliminates the perception of pain.

Anaphylactic shock Shock resulting from a widespread hypersensitivity reaction (called *anaphylaxis*). The pathophysiology in this type of shock includes vasodilation, pooling of blood in the periphery, and hypovolemia with altered cellular metabolism.

Anaplasia The regression of a cell to an immature or undifferentiated cell type.

Anasarca Severe, generalized edema.

Androgens Hormones synthesized in the testes, ovaries, and adrenal cortex that promote expression of male sex characteristics.

Anemia An abnormally low number of circulating RBCs, hemoglobin concentration, or both.

Anergy Inability to react to specific antigens.

Anesthesia State produced by medications given intravenously, intraspinally, subcutaneously, or by inhalation to create temporary partial or total loss of sensation and consciousness in a client for invasive procedures such as surgery or painful diagnostic tests.

Aneurysm Abnormal dilation of a blood vessel, commonly at a site of a weakness or tear in the vessel wall.

Angina pectoris (angina) Chest pain resulting from reduced coronary blood flow that causes a temporary imbalance between myocardial blood supply and demand.

Angioma (hemangioma) Benign vascular tumor.

Anion gap The difference between the sum of two measured anions, chloride and bicarbonate, and the principal measured cation, sodium.

Ankylosing spondylitis A chronic inflammatory arthritis that primarily affects the axial skeleton, leading to pain and progressive stiffening and fusion of the spine.

Anorexia Loss of appetite.

Anorexia nervosa An eating disorder characterized by a body weight less than 85% of expected for age and height, and an intense fear of gaining weight.

Anorgasmia Absence of orgasm.

Anosmia Inability to smell.

Anthropometric measurements Measurement of height, weight, triceps skin folds, and midarm circumference.

Antibodies Immunoglobulin molecules that bind with an antigen to inactivate it.

Antibody-mediated (humoral) immune response Activation of B cells to produce antibodies to respond to antigens such as bacteria, bacterial toxins, and free viruses.

Anticipatory grieving A combination of intellectual and emotional responses and behaviors by which people adjust their self-concept in the face of a potential loss.

Antigen A Substance capable of evoking a specific immune response; usually a protein, which the body recognizes as foreign, causing an immune response to be stimulated.

Aortic valve The semilunar valve between the left ventricle of the heart and the aorta in the heart. It prevents blood from flowing backwards into the ventricle.

Aortitis Inflammation of the aorta, usually the aortic arch.

Aphasia Defective or absent language function.

Apical impulse A normal, visible pulsation (thrust) in the area of the midclavicular line in the left fifth intercostal space. It can be seen on inspection in about half of the adult population.

Aplastic anemia A condition manifested by failure of the bone marrow to produce all three types of blood cells.

Apnea Cessation of breathing lasting from a few seconds to a few minutes.

Appendectomy Surgical removal of the appendix.

Appendicitis Inflammation of the vermiform appendix.

Apraxia The inability to carry out a motor pattern (such as drawing a figure) even when strength and coordination are adequate.

Areflexia Lack of normal reflexes.

Arterial blood gas (ABG) A laboratory test used to evaluate acid–base balance and gas exchange.

Arteriovenous (AV) malformation A congenital intracranial lesion, formed by a tangled collection of dilated arteries and veins, that allows blood to flow directly from the arterial into the venous system, bypassing the normal capillary network.

Arthralgia Joint pain.

Arthritis Joint inflammation.

Ascites Excess fluid in the peritoneal cavity.

Asphyxiation Oxygen deprivation.

Asthma Chronic inflammatory disorder of the airways that is characterized by recurrent episodes of wheezing, breathlessness, chest tightness, and coughing.

Astigmatism A condition that develops with abnormal curvature of the cornea or eyeball, causing the image to focus at multiple points on the retina.

Atelectasis Collapse of lung tissue following obstruction of the bronchus or bronchioles.

Atherosclerosis A form of arteriosclerosis in which deposits of fat and fibrin obstruct and harden the arteries.

Atopic dermatitis (eczema) Common inflammatory skin disorder of unknown cause.

Atrial kick Delivery of an additional bolus of blood to the ventricles resulting from atrial systole; occurs just prior to ventricular systole.

Atrial natriuretic factor A hormone released by atrial muscle cells in response to distention from fluid overload.

Ataxia Uncoordinated, irregular gait and muscle movement; weakness.

Aura Sensation preceding generalized seizure activity; may be a vague sense of uneasiness or an abnormal sensation.

Auscultatory gap A temporary disappearance of sound between the systolic and diastolic BP.

Autografting Transplanting of the client's own tissue; the most successful type of tissue transplant.

Autoimmune disorder Failure of immune system to recognize itself, resulting in normal host tissue being targeted by immune defenses.

Autonomic dysreflexia Exaggerated sympathetic response that occurs in clients with spinal cord injuries at or above the T_6 level.

Autosome A single chromosome from any one of the 22 pairs of chromosomes not involved in sex determination (X or Y); humans have 22 pairs of autosomes.

Azotemia Increased blood levels of nitrogenous waste products.

B lymphocytes (B cells) Bursa-equivalent lymphocytes responsible for synthesizing humoral antibody.

Bacterial vaginosis Nonspecific vaginitis.

Bactericidal Capable of killing organisms without immune system intervention.

Bacteriostatic Inhibits growth of microorganisms, leaving the destruction to the host's immune system.

Bacteriuria Bacteria in the urine.

Balanced suspension traction Traction in which several forces of pull work in unison to raise and support the client's injured extremity off the bed and pull it in a straight fashion away from the body.

Balloon tamponade The application of pressure to stop esophageal bleeding using an inflatable balloon.

Basal cell carcinoma Epithelial tumor that is believed to originate either from the basal layer of the epidermis or from cells in the surrounding dermal structures. These tumors are characterized by an impaired ability of the basal cells of the epidermis to mature into keratinocytes, with mitotic division beyond the basal layer.

Basal metabolic rate Test to measure the energy used when the body is at rest; rarely used due to the availability of more accurate thyroid tests.

Base excess A calculated value also known as buffer base capacity. Base excess reflects the degree of acid–base imbalance by indicating the status of the body's total buffering capacity.

Bases (or alkalis) Substances that accept hydrogen ions in solution.

Bell's palsy (facial paralysis) Disorder of the facial nerve (seventh cranial nerve), characterized by unilateral paralysis of the facial muscles.

Benign prostatic hyperplasia (BPH) Enlargement of the prostate gland.

Bereavement The time of mourning experienced after a loss.

Bile A greenish, watery solution containing bile salts, cholesterol, bilirubin, electrolytes, water, and phospholipids.

Biliary colic A severe, steady pain in the epigastric region or upper right quadrant of the abdomen.

Biofeedback An electronic method of measuring autonomic physiologic responses, such as brain waves, muscle contraction, and skin temperature, and then "feeding" this information back to the client.

Bioterrorism Use of an etiologic agent (disease) to cause harm or kill a population, food, and/or livestock.

Biotherapy Treatment that modifies the biologic processes that result in malignant cells, primarily through enhancing the person's own immune responses.

Bivalving Process of splitting a cast down both sides to alleviate pressure on the injured extremity.

Blood clot See *Thrombus.*

Blood flow The volume of blood transported in a vessel, in an organ, or throughout the entire circulation over a given period of time.

Blood pressure The tension or pressure exerted by blood against arterial walls.

Blunt trauma The type of trauma that occurs when there is no communication from the damaged tissues to the outside environment.

Body mass index (BMI) Used to identify excess adipose tissue, BMI is calculated by dividing the weight (in kilograms) by the height (in meters squared, m^2).

Bone marrow transplant (BMT) Infusion of bone marrow cells to restore bone marrow function after chemotherapy or radiation; allogeneic BMT uses donor bone marrow cells from a donor; autologous BMT uses the client's own bone marrow.

Borborygmi Excessive loud and hyperactive bowel sounds.

Botulism A severe, life-threatening form of food poisoning caused by *Clostridium botulinum.*

Brachytherapy A type of radiation therapy in which the source of radiation is placed directly into or adjacent to the tumor, a technique that delivers a high dose to the tumor and a lower dose to normal tissue.

Bradycardia A heart rate of less than 60 beats per minute.

Bradykinesia Slowed movements due to muscle rigidity.

Bradypnea Abnormally low respiratory rate.

Brain abscess Infection with a collection of purulent material within the brain tissue.

Brain death The cessation of cerebral blood flow with global brain infarction and permanent loss of all brain function.

Brain death criteria Clinical signs used to determine whether a comatose client is brain dead.

Breakthrough pain A sudden flare or increase in pain despite comfort with or without baseline analgesia.

Bronchiectasis Permanent abnormal dilation of one or more large bronchi and destruction of bronchial walls, usually accompanied by infection.

Bronchitis Inflammation of the bronchi.

Bruit An adventitious sound heard during auscultation; of venous or arterial origin.

Buffer A substance that prevents major changes in pH by removing or releasing hydrogen ions.

Bulimia nervosa An eating disorder characterized by recurring episodes of binge eating followed by purge behaviors such as self-induced vomiting, use of laxatives or diuretics, fasting, or excessive exercise.

Burn An injury resulting from exposure to heat, chemicals, radiation, or electric current.

Burn shock Hypovolemic shock resulting from the shift of a massive amount of fluid from the intracellular and intravascular compartments into the interstitium following burn injury.

Bursitis Inflammation of the bursa.

Cachexia The wasted physical appearance characteristic of cancer and other chronic illnesses. It is characterized by rapid depletion of the body's protein, particularly in skeletal muscle, with less rapid loss of fat.

Calculi An abnormal concentration in the body, commonly called a stone; occur in the kidneys, ureters, bladder, or urethra.

Cancer A family of complex diseases with manifestations that vary according to body system and type of tumor cells involved; marked by uncontrolled growth and the spread of abnormal cells.

Candidiasis Infection of mucous membranes caused by *Candida albicans*, a yeast-like fungus.

Carbuncle A group of infected hair follicles.

Carcinogen Cancer-causing agent.

Carcinogenesis The production or origin of cancer.

Carcinoma A tumor arising from epithelial tissue.

Cardiac arrest Sudden failure of the heart to pump.

Cardiac cycle The contraction and relaxation of the heart during one heartbeat.

Cardiac index Cardiac output adjusted for body size.

Cardiac output (CO) The amount of blood pumped by the ventricles into the pulmonary and systemic circulations in 1 minute.

Cardiac rehabilitation A long-term program of medical evaluation, exercise, risk factor modification, education, and counseling designed to limit the physical and psychologic effects of cardiac illness and improve the client's quality of life.

Cardiac reserve The ability of the heart to respond to the body's changing need for cardiac output.

Cardiac tamponade Compression of the heart due to pericardial effusion, trauma, cardiac rupture, or hemorrhage.

Cardiogenic shock Shock that occurs when the heart's pumping ability is compromised to the point that it cannot maintain cardiac output and adequate tissue perfusion.

Cardiomegaly Enlargement of the heart.

Cardiomyopathy Primary abnormality of the heart muscle that affects its structural or functional characteristics.

Cardiovascular disease (CVD) Generic term for disorders of the heart and blood vessels.

Carpal tunnel syndrome Compression of the median nerve as a result of inflammation and swelling of the synovial lining of the tendon sheaths.

Carrier Any individual who carries a single copy of an altered gene or mutation for a recessive condition on one chromosome of a chromosome pair and an unaltered form of that gene on the other chromosome; a carrier generally is not affected by the gene alteration; on the average, each person in the general population is a carrier of five or six gene mutations for recessive disorders.

Catabolism Biochemical process involving the breakdown of complex structures into simpler forms.

Cataract Opacification (clouding) of the lens of the eye.

Celiac disease (celiac sprue, nontropical sprue) Chronic hereditary disorder characterized by sensitivity to the gliadin fraction of gluten, a cereal protein.

Cell cycle The four phases that occur during growth and development of a cell.

Cell-mediated (cellular) immune response Direct or indirect inactivation of antigen by lymphocytes.

Cellulitis A localized infection of the dermis and subcutaneous tissue.

Central pain Related to a lesion in the brain that may spontaneously produce high-frequency bursts of impulses that are perceived as pain.

Cerebral concussion Transient, temporary, neurogenic dysfunction caused by mechanical force to the brain.

Cerebral contusion Bruise on the surface of the brain.

Cerebral edema An increase in the volume of brain tissue due to abnormal accumulation of fluid.

Cerumen Earwax.

Chalazion Granulomatous cyst or nodule of the lid.

Chancre Hard, syphilitic primary ulcer.

Cheilosis Chemical peeling; the application of a chemical to produce a controlled and predictable injury that alters the anatomy of the epidermis and superficial dermis.

Chemotherapy Cancer treatment involving the use of cytotoxic medications to decrease tumor size, adjunctive to surgery or radiation therapy; or to prevent or treat suspected metastases.

Chlamydia A group of syndromes caused by *Chlamydia trachomatis,* a bacterium that behaves like a virus spreading within a host cell; spread by sexual contact and to the neonate by passage through the birth canal of an infected mother.

Cholecystectomy Removal of the gallbladder.

Cholecystitis Inflammation of the gallbladder, usually associated with stones in the cystic or common bile duct.

Cholelithiasis Formation of stones (calculi) within the gallbladder or biliary duct system.

Cholera Acute diarrheal illness caused by certain strains of *Vibrio cholerae.*

Chorea Jerky, rapid, involuntary movements.

Chromosome Genetic material carried by each cell; found in the cell nucleus.

Chronic bronchitis Excessive secretion of bronchial mucus characterized by a productive cough lasting 3 or more months in 2 consecutive years.

Chronic gastritis Disorders characterized by progressive and irreversible changes in the gastric mucosa.

Chronic lymphocytic leukemia (CLL) Proliferation and accumulation of small, abnormal, mature lymphocytes in the bone marrow, peripheral blood, and body tissues; least common type of the major leukemias.

Chronic myelogenous leukemia (CML) Abnormal proliferation of all bone marrow elements, usually associated with a chromosome abnormality (the Philadelphia chromosome).

Chronic obstructive pulmonary disease (COPD) Chronic air flow obstruction due to chronic bronchitis and/or emphysema.

Chronic renal failure Progressive renal tissue destruction with loss of entire nephron unit and function; renal mass decreases, and glomerular filtration, tubular secretion, and reabsorption deteriorate.

Chronic otitis media Condition involving permanent perforation of the tympanic membrane, with or without recurrent pus formation and often accompanied by changes in the mucosa and bony structures (ossicles) of the middle ear.

Chronic pain Prolonged pain, usually lasting longer than 6 months. It is not always associated with an identifiable cause and is often unresponsive to conventional medical treatment.

Chronic sorrow A cyclical, recurring, and potentially progressive pattern of pervasive sadness experienced in response to continual loss, throughout the trajectory of an illness or disability.

Chronic stump pain The result of neuroma formation, causing severe burning pain.

Chronic venous insufficiency A chronic disorder of inadequate venous return.

Chvostek's sign Contraction of the lateral facial muscles in response to tapping the face in front of the ear; caused by decreased blood calcium levels.

Chyme Thick, fluid mixture of food and gastric juices formed in the stomach during the digestive process.

Cirrhosis A progressive, irreversible disorder, eventually leading to liver failure; the end stage of chronic liver disease.

Client A term used instead of "patient" that is based on a philosophy that individuals are active participants in health and illness as well as consumers of healthcare services.

Closed fracture (simple fracture) Break in continuity of bone with skin still intact.

Clubbing Enlargement and blunting of the terminal portion of the fingers; associated with chronic hypoxemia.

Cluster headache A form of vascular headache predominantly experienced by men ages 20 to 40. The headache typically begins 2 to 3 hours after the person falls asleep.

Coagulation The process of creating a fibrin meshwork that cements blood components together to form an insoluble clot.

Code of ethics An established and agreed-on group of principles of conduct that provide a professional framework.

Cold sore See *Herpes simplex.*

Cold zone Considered the "safe zone" during a disaster, it is adjacent to the warm zone and is the area where a more in-depth triage of victims would occur; survivors may find shelter in this area, and command and control vehicles would be found here as well as the emergency transport vehicles.

Colectomy Surgical removal of the colon.

Collateral channels Connections between small arteries.

Collateral vessels Accessory pathways connected to the smaller arteries in the coronary system.

Colorectal cancer Malignant tumor arising from the epithelial tissues of the colon or rectum.

Colostomy Ostomy made in the colon.

Comedones Noninflammatory acne lesions.

Community-based care Centers on individual and family healthcare needs. The nurse practicing community-based care provides direct services to individuals to manage acute or chronic health problems and to promote self-care. The care is provided in the local community, is culturally competent, and is family centered.

Compartment A space enclosed by a fibrous membrane or fascia.

Compartment syndrome Condition in which excess pressure constricts the structures within a compartment, and reduces circulation to muscles and nerves.

Concussion Injury resulting from a violent jar, shake, or impact with an object.

Conjunctivitis Inflammation of the conjunctiva.

Consanguinity Related by having a common ancestor; close blood relationship.

Conscious sedation Anesthesia that provides analgesia and amnesia, but in which the client remains conscious. Clients are able to breathe independently and are cardiovascularly stable.

Consciousness A condition in which a person is aware of self and environment and is able to respond appropriately to stimuli; full consciousness requires both normal arousal and full cognition.

Constipation The infrequent (two or fewer bowel movements weekly) or difficult passage of stools.

Contact dermatitis Type of dermatitis caused by a hypersensitivity response or chemical irritation.

Continuous renal replacement therapy (CRRT) A form of hemodialysis in which blood is continuously circulated through a highly porous hemofilter from artery to vein or vein to vein.

Contractility The inherent capability of the cardiac muscle fibers to shorten.

Contracting The negotiation of a cooperative working agreement between the nurse and client that is continuously renegotiated.

Contracture Permanent shortening of connective tissue.

Contralateral deficit Manifestations of a stroke on the side of the body opposite the side of the brain that is damaged.

Contusion Superficial tissue injury resulting from blunt trauma, such as a kick or blow from an object, that causes the breakage of small blood vessels and bleeding into the surrounding tissue.

Conventional weapons Weapons such as bombs and guns that are used more frequently than nonconventional terrorist weapons.

Convergence Moving inward of the eyes to see an object close to the face.

Co-occurring disorders Concurrent diagnosis of a substance use disorder and a psychiatric disorder. One disorder can precede and cause the other, such as the relationship between alcoholism and depression.

Cor pulmonale Condition of right ventricular hypertrophy and failure that results from long-standing pulmonary hypertension.

Core competencies Standards that a profession agrees are essential for a person to be deemed competent in his or her field.

Corneal reflex Closure of eyelids (blinking) due to corneal irritation.

Coronary heart disease (CHD) Heart disease caused by impaired blood flow to the myocardium.

Coryza (rhinorrhea) Profuse nasal discharge.

Cosmetic surgery (aesthetic surgery) One of two fields within plastic surgery. Cosmetic surgery enhances the attractiveness of normal features.

Crackles Discontinuous lung sound heard by auscultation; can be fine or coarse. Produced by air passing over airway secretions or the opening of collapsed airways.

Crepitation A grating sound heard on movement of a joint.

Creutzfeldt-Jakob disease (CJD, spongiform encephalopathy) Rare, progressive neurologic disease that causes brain degeneration without inflammation.

Critical pathway A healthcare plan designed to provide care with a multidisciplinary, managed action focus; developed for specific diagnoses, usually those that are high volume, high risk, and high cost.

Critical thinking Self-directed thinking that is focused on what to believe or do in a specific situation.

CRNA Certified registered nurse anesthetist; a specialty certified nurse in anesthesia administration.

Crohn's disease (regional enteritis) Chronic, relapsing inflammatory disorder affecting the gastrointestinal tract.

Crossing over A process that occurs during meiosis in which homologous maternal and paternal chromosomes break and exchange corresponding sections of DNA and then rejoin; this process can cause an exchange of alleles between chromosomes and provides human diversity.

Cryosurgery The destruction of tissue by cold or freezing with agents such as fluorocarbon sprays, carbon dioxide snow, nitrous oxide, and liquid nitrogen.

Curettage The removal of lesions with a curette, a semisharp cutting instrument.

Curling's ulcers Acute ulcerations of the stomach or duodenum that form following a burn injury.

Cushing's ulcers Stress ulcers occurring as sequelae of head injury or central nervous system surgery.

Cutaneous melanoma See *Malignant melanoma.*

Cyanosis A bluish discoloration of the skin and mucous membranes due to oxygen deficiency.

Cystectomy Complete surgical removal of the urinary bladder and adjacent muscles and tissues.

Cystic fibrosis (CF) Inherited disorder of the exocrine glands that results in the secretion of abnormal amounts of mucus.

Cystitis Inflammation of the urinary bladder.

Cysts of the skin Benign closed sacs in or under the skin surface that are lined with epithelium and contain fluid or a semisolid material. Epidermal inclusion cysts and pilar cysts are the most common types.

Cytokines Hormone-like polypeptides produced primarily by monocytes, macrophages, and T cells. Cytokines act as messengers of the immune system, facilitating communication between the cells to adjust or vary the inflammatory reaction or to initiate immune cell proliferation and differentiation.

Dawn phenomenon A rise in blood glucose between 4 A.M. and 8 A.M. that is not a response to hypoglycemia.

Death Irreversible cessation of circulatory and respiratory functions or irreversible cessation of all functions of the entire brain, including the brainstem.

Death anxiety Worry or fear related to death or dying.

Debridement Process of removing dead tissue from a wound.

Decerebrate posturing Abnormal posture with the neck extended; the jaw clenched; arms pronated, extended, and close to the sides; legs extended and feet plantar flexed. Results from lesions of the midbrain, pons, or diencephalons.

Decorticate posturing Abnormal posture with the upper arms close to the sides; the elbows, wrists, and fingers flexed; the legs extended and internally rotated; and the feet plantar flexed. Results from lesions of the corticospinal tracts.

Deep venous thrombosis (DVT) Blood clot (thrombus) formation and inflammation within a deep vein, usually in the pelvis or lower extremities; a common complication of hospitalization, surgery, and immobilization.

Dehiscence An unintended separation of wound margins due to incomplete healing.

Dehydration Loss of water.

Delayed healing Healing that occurs at a slower rate than expected.

Delegation To effectively assign appropriate work activities to other members of the healthcare team. When the nurse delegates nursing care activities to another person, that person is authorized to act in the place of the nurse, while the nurse retains the accountability for the activities performed.

Delirium tremens (DT) A medical emergency usually occurring 3 to 5 days following alcohol withdrawal and lasting 2 to 3 days; characterized by paranoia, disorientation, delusions, visual hallucinations, elevated vital signs, vomiting, diarrhea, and diaphoresis.

Dementia A global impairment of cognitive function that usually is progressive and may be permanent; interferes with normal social and occupational activities.

Demyelination Destruction or removal of the myelin sheaths of nerves.

Depolarization The rapid inflow of sodium ions, causing an electrical change in which the inside of a cell becomes positive in relation to the outside.

Dermatitis Acute or chronic inflammation of the skin characterized by erythema and pain or pruritus.

Dermatome Area of skin innervated by cutaneous branches of a single spinal nerve.

Dermatophytes Fungi that cause superficial skin infections.

Dermatophytoses Superficial fungal infection of the skin; also called *ringworm.*

Diabetes mellitus (DM) Group of chronic disorders of the endocrine pancreas, all categorized under a broad diagnostic label. The condition is characterized by inappropriate hyperglycemia caused by a relative or absolute deficiency of insulin or by a cellular resistance to the action of insulin.

Diabetic ketoacidosis (DKA) A form of metabolic acidosis induced by stress in a person with type 1 diabetes.

Diabetic nephropathy A disease of the kidneys characterized by the presence of albumin in the urine, hypertension, edema, and progressive renal insufficiency.

Diabetic neuropathies Disorders of the peripheral nerves and the autonomic nervous system manifesting one or more of the following: sensory and motor impairment, muscle weakness and pain, cranial nerve disorders, impaired vasomotor function, impaired gastrointestinal function, and impaired genitourinary function.

Diabetic retinopathy The collective name for the changes in the retina that occur in the person with diabetes. The retinal capillary structure undergoes alterations in blood flow, leading to retinal ischemia and a breakdown in the blood retinal barrier.

Dialysate Dialysis solution.

Dialysis The diffusion of solute molecules across a semipermeable membrane from an area of higher concentration to one of lower concentration.

Diaphoresis Copious production of sweat.

Diarrhea An increase in the frequency, volume, and fluid content of the stool.

Diastolic blood pressure The minimum pressure maintained by elastic arterial walls during diastole (cardiac relaxation) to maintain blood flow through capillary beds; averages 80 mmHg in a healthy adult.

Differentiation A process occurring over many cell cycles that allows cells to specialize in certain tasks.

Diffuse brain injury (DBI) A brain injury from a high-speed acceleration–deceleration accident with widespread disruption of axons in the white matter.

Diffuse esophageal spasm Nonperistaltic contraction of esophageal smooth muscle.

Diffusion The process by which solute molecules move from an area of high solute concentration to an area of low solute concentration to become evenly distributed.

Dilemma A choice between two unpleasant, ethically troubling alternatives.

Diplopia Unilateral or bilateral double vision.

Disability The degree of observable and measurable impairment.

Disaster Event that requires extraordinary efforts beyond those needed to respond to everyday emergencies.

Disease Literally meaning "without ease," this term describes alterations in structure and function of the body or mind. Diseases may have mechanical, biologic, or normative causes.

Dislocation Separation of contact between two bones of a joint.

Dissection (aortic) A life-threatening emergency caused by a tear in the intima of the aorta with hemorrhage into the media.

Disseminated intravascular coagulation (DIC) A disruption of hemostasis characterized by widespread intravascular clotting and bleeding; a syndrome that develops as a complication of many other disorders.

Distributive shock Also called *vasogenic shock,* this includes several types of shock that result from widespread vasodilation and decreased peripheral resistance.

Diverticula Saclike projections of mucosa through the muscular layer of the colon.

Diverticulitis Inflammation in and around the diverticular sac; typically affects only one diverticulum, usually in the sigmoid colon.

Diverticulosis Indicates the presence of diverticula.

Dominant A characteristic or gene that is apparent even when the relevant gene is present in only one copy; a person with a dominant gene usually expresses that gene trait.

Do-not-resuscitate (DNR or "no-code") order Usually written by the physician for the client who has a terminal illness or is near death, this order is usually based on the wishes of the client and family that no cardiopulmonary resuscitation be performed for respiratory or cardiac arrest.

Dual diagnosis The coexistence of substance abuse/dependence and a psychiatric disorder in one individual (used interchangeably with *dual disorder* and *co-occurring disorders*).

Dual disorder See *Dual diagnosis.*

Dumping syndrome Complication of partial gastrectomy characterized by nausea, weakness, sweating, palpitation, syncope, sensation of warmth, and occasionally diarrhea.

Duodenal ulcers Peptic ulcer disease affecting the duodenum.

Durable power of attorney A document that can delegate the authority to make health, financial, and/or legal decisions on a person's behalf. It must be in writing and must state that the designated person is authorized to make healthcare decisions.

Dysarthria Difficulty speaking.

Dysfunctional uterine bleeding (DUB) Vaginal bleeding that is usually painless but abnormal in amount, duration, or time of occurrence.

Dysmenorrhea Pain associated with menstruation.

Dyspareunia Painful intercourse.

Dysphagia Difficulty swallowing.

Dysphonia Change in the tone of voice.

Dysplasia The loss of DNA control over differentiation occurring in response to adverse conditions.

Dyspnea Difficult or labored breathing.

Dysrhythmia Abnormal heart rate or rhythm.

Dysuria Painful urination.

Ecchymosis A flat, irregularly shaped lesion of varying size with no pulsation; cause by blood collecting under skin.

Ectopic beats Impulses originating outside normal conduction pathways of the heart.

Edema Accumulation of fluid in the body's tissues; an excess accumulation of fluid in the interstitial space.

Ejection fraction (EF) The percentage of total blood remaining in the ventricle at the end of diastole (relaxation); normal is 50% to 70%.

Electrical bone stimulation Application of electrical current at the fracture site to treat fractures that are not healing appropriately. The electrical stress increases the migration of osteoblasts and osteoclasts to the fracture site. Mineral deposition increases, promoting bone healing.

Electrocardiography The graphic recording of the heart's electrical activity detected and recorded through electrodes placed on the surface of the body.

Electrolytes Substances that dissociate in solution to form charged particles called ions.

Electrosurgery The destruction or removal of tissue with high-frequency alternating current.

Embolic CVA Cerebrovascular accident occurring when a blood clot or clump of matter traveling through the cerebral blood vessels becomes lodged in a vessel too narrow to permit further movement.

Embolism Sudden obstruction of a blood vessel by debris.

Emergency Encompasses an unforeseen combination of circumstances calling for immediate action for a range of victims from one to many.

Emphysema Destruction of the walls of the alveoli, with resulting enlargement of abnormal air spaces.

Empyema Accumulation of purulent exudate in the pleural cavity.

Encephalitis An acute inflammation of the parenchyma of the brain or spinal cord.

End of life The final days or weeks of life when death is imminent.

Endocarditis Inflammation of the endocardium.

Endometriosis A condition in which multiple, small implants of endometrial tissue develop throughout the pelvic cavity.

Endoscopy Inspection of organs or cavities of the body using an endoscope.

Endotoxins Found in the cell wall of gram-negative bacteria, endotoxins are released only when the cell is disrupted. They act as activators of many human regulatory systems, producing fever, inflammation, and potentially clotting, bleeding, or hypotension when released in large quantities.

End-stage renal disease The final stage of chronic renal failure in which the kidneys are unable to excrete metabolic wastes and regulate fluid and electrolyte balance adequately; characterized by a glomerular filtration rate of less than 5% of normal.

Enophthalmos Sunken appearance of the eyes.

Enteral nutrition Administration of liquid nutritional formulas to meet calorie and protein needs in clients unable to consume adequate food; also called *tube feeding.*

Enucleation Surgical removal of an eye.

Epicondylitis (tennis elbow, golfer's elbow) Inflammation of the tendon at its point of origin into the bone.

Epididymitis Infection or inflammation of the epididymis.

Epidural hematoma (extradural hematoma) A collection of blood between the dura and the skull.

Epilepsy Chronic seizure activity.

Epistaxis Nosebleed.

Erectile dysfunction Inability of the male to attain and maintain an erection sufficient to permit satisfactory sexual intercourse.

Erosive gastritis See *Stress-induced (erosive) gastritis.*

Erysipelas Infection of the skin most often caused by group A streptococci.

Erythema A reddening of the skin.

Erythropoiesis Red blood cell production.

Eschar Hard, leathery crust that covers a burn wound and harbors necrotic tissue.

Escharotomy Surgical removal of eschar from the torso or extremity to prevent circumferential constriction.

Esophageal varices Enlarged, thin-walled veins that form in the submucosa of the esophagus.

Esophagojejunostomy Removal of the entire stomach with anastomosis of the distal esophagus to the jejunum.

Estrogen Hormone produced by the ovary.

Ethics Principles of conduct. Ethical behavior is concerned with moral duty, values, obligations, and the distinction between right and wrong.

Euthanasia From the Greek for painless, easy, gentle, or good death, now commonly used to signify a killing prompted by a humanitarian motive.

Evisceration Protrusion of body contents through a surgical wound.

Exacerbation A period during chronic illness in which symptoms reappear.

Exfoliative dermatitis Inflammatory skin disorder characterized by excessive peeling or shedding of skin.

Exophthalmos Protrusion of the eyeballs.

Exotoxins Soluble proteins secreted into surrounding tissue by the microorganism. Exotoxins are highly poisonous, causing cell death or dysfunction.

External otitis Inflammation of the ear canal.

Extracapsular fractures Fractures of the trochanteric region.

Extracorporeal shock-wave lithotripsy (ESWL, transcutaneous shock-wave lithotripsy) Noninvasive technique for fragmenting kidney stones using shock waves generated outside the body.

Family Two or more persons joined by emotional closeness and shared bonds and who identify themselves as being part of a family.

Fasciculations Involuntary twitching.

Fasciectomy (fascial excision) Process of excising the wound to the level of fascia.

Fat embolism syndrome (FES) Characterized by neurologic dysfunction, pulmonary insufficiency, and a petechial rash on the chest, axilla, and upper arms due to fat globules lodged in the pulmonary vascular bed or peripheral circulation.

Fecal impaction A rock-hard or putty-like mass of feces in the rectum.

Fecal incontinence Loss of voluntary control of defecation.

Fecalith A hard mass of feces.

Fibrocystic changes (FCC) Physiologic nodularity and breast tenderness that increases and decreases with the menstrual cycle.

Fibroid tumors (uterine leiomyomata) Solid, pedunculated benign tumors.

Fibromyalgia (fibrositis) A common rheumatic syndrome characterized by musculoskeletal pain, stiffness, and tenderness.

Filtration The process by which water and dissolved substances (solutes) move from an area of higher hydrostatic pressure to an area of lower hydrostatic pressure.

Fistula Abnormal opening or passage between two organs or spaces that are normally separated or an abnormal passage to the outside of the body.

Flaccidity Decreased muscle tone in disease or trauma of the lower motor neurons.

Flail chest Free-floating segment of the chest wall, resulting from two or more consecutive ribs fractured in multiple places.

Flap A piece of tissue whose free end is moved from a donor site to a recipient site while maintaining a continuous blood supply through its connection at the base or pedicle.

Flatus Gas in the digestive tract.

Fluid resuscitation Replacement of the extensive fluid and electrolyte losses associated with major burn injuries.

Fluid volume deficit (FVD) A decrease in intravascular, interstitial, and/or intracellular fluid in the body.

Fluid volume excess (FVE) Excess extracellular fluid resulting from retention of both water and sodium in the body.

Folic acid deficiency anemia An anemia resulting from folic acid deficiency, a necessary nutrient for DNA synthesis and RBC maturation.

Folliculitis Bacterial infection of the hair follicle, most commonly caused by *Staphylococcus aureus.*

Fracture A break in a bone usually due to trauma.

Freestanding outpatient surgical facilities Surgical units independent of a hospital with or without financial connections to a hospital or healthcare organization.

Friction rub The sound heard when two dry surfaces are rubbed together.

Frostbite An injury of the skin from freezing.

Full-thickness burn A burn that involves all layers of the skin, including the epidermis, dermis, and epidermal appendages.

Fulminant hepatitis Hepatitis with a rapid and severe onset and course.

Furuncle Often called a boil, but also an inflammation of the hair follicle.

Fusiform excision The removal of a full thickness of the epidermis and dermis, usually with a thin layer of subcutaneous tissue.

Galactorrhea Lactation not associated with pregnancy or nursing.

Gastric lavage Irrigation of the stomach with large quantities of normal saline.

Gastric mucosal barrier A protective barrier consisting of lipids, bicarbonate ions, and mucous gel that protects the stomach lining from the damaging effects of gastric juices.

Gastric outlet obstruction Obstruction of the pyloric region of the stomach and duodenum that impairs gastric outflow; a potential complication of peptic ulcer disease.

Gastric ulcers Ulcers of the stomach lining, usually in the lesser curvature and antrum; more common in older adults.

Gastritis Inflammation of the stomach lining.

Gastroduodenostomy (Billroth I) Excision of the pylorus of the stomach with the anastomosis of the upper stomach to the duodenum; commonly used partial gastrectomy procedure.

Gastroenteritis Inflammation of the gastrointestinal tract; not a specific disease, but a group of syndromes or a collection of related manifestations.

Gastroesophageal reflux Backward flow of gastric contents into the esophagus.

Gastrointestinal reflux disease (GERD) The reflux of acidic gastric contents into the lower esophagus.

Gastrojejunostomy (Billroth II) Subtotal excision of the stomach with closure of the duodenum and side-to-side anastomosis of the jejunum to the stomach; commonly used partial gastrectomy procedure.

Gastroparesis Slowed gastrointestinal motility, which causes early satiety.

Gene A sequence of DNA on a chromosome that represents a fundamental unit of heredity; occupies a specific spot on a chromosome (gene locus).

Gene expression When the protein product of a gene is visible (for example, through the presence of a body structure or identifiable through biochemical tests such as insulin or phenylalanine levels).

General anesthesia Deep sedation, which includes analgesia and muscle paralysis. This type of anesthesia requires respiratory maintenance without the aid of the client's respiratory musculature.

Genital herpes (herpes simplex genitalis) An infection of the external genitalia caused by herpes simplex genitalis; transmitted by vaginal, anal, or oral–genital contact.

Genital warts (condyloma acuminatum, venereal warts) A sexually transmitted condition caused by the human papilloma virus.

Genotype The genes and the variations therein that a person inherits from his or her parents.

Germ cells Cells that give rise to a sperm or egg.

Gingivitis Inflamation of the gums, characterized by inflammation, redness, and bleeding.

Gland Tissue that synthesizes hormones.

Glaucoma Condition characterized by increased intraocular pressure of the eye and a gradual loss of vision.

Glomerular filtration rate (GFR) The rate at which plasma is filtered through the glomeruli of the kidney.

Glomerulonephritis Inflammation of the capillary loops of the glomeruli.

Glossitis Inflammation of the tongue.

Glucocorticoid A group of hormones secreted by the adrenal cortex; they regulate carbohydrate levels in the body.

Gluconeogenesis Formation of glucose from fats and proteins.

Glucose-6-phosphate dehydrogenase (G6PD) anemia Anemia due to a hereditary defect in RBC metabolism.

Glucosuria Excessive glucose in urine.

Glycogenolysis Breakdown of liver glycogen to glucose.

Goiter An enlarged thyroid gland. Enlargement results from both inadequate and excessive synthesis of thyroid hormones.

Gonorrhea (GC, clap) An infection caused by *Neisseria gonorrhoeae* that is transmitted by direct sexual contact or by delivery of a neonate by an infected mother.

Gout A syndrome that occurs from an inflammatory response to the production or excretion of uric acid resulting in high levels of uric acid in the blood (hyperuricemia) and in other body fluids, including synovial fluid.

Grief The emotional response to loss and its accompanying changes.

Grieving The internal process the person uses to work through the response to loss.

Guillain-Barré syndrome (GBS) Acute demyelinating disorder of the peripheral nervous system characterized by progressive, usually rapid muscle weakness and paralysis.

Gynecomastia Breast enlargement in men.

Hallucinogens Drugs that produce hallucinations.

Hallux valgus (bunion) The enlargement and lateral displacement of the first metatarsal.

Hammertoe (claw toe) The dorsiflexion of the first phalanx with accompanying plantar flexion of the second and third phalanges.

Handicap The total adjustment to disability that limits functioning at a normal level.

Hazardous materials Substances that pose a potential risk to life, health, or property if they are released because of their chemical, biologic, or physical nature.

Health "A state of complete physical, mental, and social well-being, and not merely the absence of disease or infirmity" (WHO, 1974, p. 1).

Healthcare surrogate An individual selected to make medical decisions when a person is no longer able to make them for his- or herself.

Heart block A block in the normal conduction pathways.

Heart failure Inability of the heart to pump adequate blood to meet the metabolic demands of the body.

Heave An excessive thrust.

Hemangioma See *Angioma*.

Hemarthrosis The collection of blood in the elbow joint.

Hematemesis Blood in the vomit.

Hematochezia Blood in the stool.

Hematoma A contusion with a large amount of bleeding.

Hematopoiesis Blood cell formation.

Hematuria Blood in the urine.

Hemianopia Loss of half of the visual field of one or both eyes.

Hemiparesis Weakness of one side of the body.

Hemiplegia Paralysis in one-half of the body vertically.

Hemodialysis A procedure in which electrolytes, waste products, and excess water are removed from the body by diffusion and ultrafiltration as blood passes by an artificial semipermeable membrane outside the body.

Hemodynamics Study of the forces involved in blood circulation.

Hemoglobin The oxygen-carrying protein within RBCs; composed of the heme molecule and globin, a protein molecule.

Hemolysis The process of RBC destruction.

Hemolytic anemia Premature destruction (lysis) of RBCs.

Hemophilia A group of hereditary clotting factor disorders that lead to persistent and potentially severe bleeding.

Hemophilia A (classic hemophilia) The most common type of hemophilia, caused by clotting factor VIII deficiency.

Hemophilia B (Christmas disease) Hemophilia caused by factor IX deficiency.

Hemoptysis Bloody sputum.

Hemorrhage Rapid or excessive bleeding.

Hemorrhagic CVA (intracranial hemorrhage) Cerebrovascular accident occurring when a cerebral blood vessel ruptures.

Hemorrhoids (piles) Clusters of dilated veins in swollen anal tissue.

Hemostasis Control of bleeding.

Hemothorax Blood in the pleural space.

Hepatic encephalopathy Altered consciousness, mentation, and motor function affecting cirrhotic clients.

Hepatitis Inflammation of the liver, usually caused by a virus; may be acute or chronic.

Hepatorenal syndrome Renal failure accompanied by azotemia, sodium retention, oliguria, and hypotension in clients with cirrhosis and ascites.

Hernia A defect in the abdominal wall that allows abdominal contents to protrude out of the abdominal cavity.

Herniated intervertebral disk Rupture of the cartilage surrounding the intervertebral disk with protrusion of the nucleus pulposus.

Herpes simplex (fever blister, cold sore) Acute viral infections of the skin and mucous membranes caused by two types of herpesvirus: HSV I and HSV II.

Herpes zoster (shingles) Viral infection of a dermatome section of the skin caused by varicella zoster, the same herpesvirus that causes chickenpox.

Heterograft (xenograft) Skin obtained from an animal, usually a pig.

Heterozygous Nonidentical copies of a particular gene (different alleles) on the paired chromosomes.

Hiatal hernia Protrusion of part of the stomach through the esophageal hiatus of the diaphragm into the mediastinal cavity.

Hirsutism Increased growth of coarse hair, usually on the face and trunk.

Histocompatibility The ability of cells and tissues to survive transplantation without immunologic interference by the recipient.

Holistic health care Care in which all aspects of a person (physical, psychosocial, cultural, spiritual, and intellectual) are considered as essential components of individualized care.

Home care Services for clients who are in need of treatment or support to function effectively in the home environment.

Homeostasis The body's tendency to maintain a state of physiologic balance in the presence of constantly changing conditions.

Homograft (allograft) Human skin that has been harvested from cadavers.

Homologous chromosomes Chromosomes that are members of the same pair and normally have the same number and arrangement of genes; usually one copy is from the mother and the other copy is from the father.

Homonymous hemianopia Impaired vision or blindness in one side of both eyes.

Homozygous Identical copies of a particular gene (same alleles) on both paired chromosomes.

Hordeolum (sty) Staphylococcal abscess that may occur on either the external or internal margin of the lid.

Hormone Chemical messengers secreted via body fluids that have specific targets where they increase or inhibit organ functions.

Hospice care A special component of home care, designed to provide medical, nursing, social, psychologic, and spiritual care for terminally ill clients and their families. Hospice care relies on a philosophy of relieving pain and suffering and allowing the client to die with dignity in a comfortable environment.

Hot zone The site of a disaster where a weapon was released or where contamination occurred.

Human genome The total amount of the DNA (genes) in an individual's cells.

Human immunodeficiency virus (HIV) Virus responsible for AIDS.

Huntington's disease Progressive, degenerative, inherited neurologic disease characterized by increasing dementia and chorea; also called *chorea*.

Hydrocele Fluid-filled mass within the scrotum.

Hydrocephalus An abnormal accumulation of cerebrospinal fluid within the cranial vault and dilation of the ventricles.

Hydronephrosis Distention of the urinary tract with urine behind an obstruction.

Hydroureter Distention of the ureter with urine.

Hypercapnia Increased blood levels of carbon dioxide.

Hyperglycemia Elevated blood glucose levels (above 126 mg/dL), which causes osmotic diuresis and, if chronic, damages vessel epithelium and renal glomeruli.

Hyperopia (farsightedness) The condition in which the eyeball is short, causing the image to focus behind the retina.

Hyperosmolar hyperglycemic state (HHS) A condition of very high blood glucose with adequate insulin to prevent ketosis, but which does cause diuresis.

Hyperplasia An increase in the number or density of normal cells.

Hypersensitivity Exaggerated response of the immune system to an antigen.

Hypertension Excess pressure in the arterial portion of systemic circulation.

Hypertrophic scar Overgrowth of dermal tissue that remains within the boundaries of the wound.

Hypervolemia Excess intravascular fluid.

Hyphema Bleeding into the anterior chamber of the eye, possibly as the result of blunt eye trauma.

Hypoglycemia Low blood glucose levels; deficiency of blood sugar.

Hypovolemia Decreased circulating blood volume.

Hypovolemic shock Shock caused by a decrease in intravascular volume of 15% or more. This form of shock is caused by the loss of whole blood, blood plasma, or extracellular fluid.

Hypoxemia Decreased oxygen concentration in the blood, measured by PaO_2.

Hypoxia Insufficient supply of oxygen to the tissues.

Ichthyosis An inherited dermatologic condition in which the skin is dry, fissured, and hyperkeratotic; the surface of the skin has the appearance of fish scales.

Ileostomy An ostomy made in the ileum of the small intestine.

Immunity The protection of the body from disease.

Immunocompetent Possessing an immune system that can identify antigens and effectively destroy or remove them.

Immunocompromised Possessing an immune response that has been weakened by a disease or an immunosuppressive agent.

Immunoglobulin (Ig) A protein that functions as an antibody.

Immunosuppression Inability of the immune system to respond to an antigen. Occurs in response to disease or medications; may be intentional to prevent rejection of transplants or a side effect of some medications.

Impairment A disturbance in structure or function resulting from physiologic or psychologic abnormalities.

Impetigo Infection of the skin caused by either *Staphylococcus aureus* or beta-hemolytic streptococci.

Impotence Inability to achieve or maintain an erection.

Incident pain A type of breakthrough pain that is predictable because it is associated with movement such as turning or coughing.

Increased intracranial pressure (IICP, intracranial hypertension) Sustained elevated pressure (10 mmHg or higher) within the cranial cavity.

Independent nursing care Care provided by nurses within the scope of their practice without the direction or supervision of a physician.

Infection Colonization by and multiplication of an organism within a host. The host can be any organism capable of supporting the nutritional and physical growth requirements of the microorganism, for example, humans.

Inflammation A complex, nonspecific, adaptive response to injury that brings fluid, dissolved substances, and blood cells into the interstitial tissues where the invasion or damage has occurred.

Inflammatory bowel disease (IBD) Chronic inflammation of the bowel common to a group of conditions that includes Crohn's disease and ulcerative colitis.

Influenza Highly contagious viral respiratory disease characterized by coryza, fever, cough, and constitutional manifestations such as headache and malaise.

Informed consent Disclosure of risks associated with the intended procedure or operation to the client. The language of the document varies according to statutory and common law of each state.

Inhalants Inhaled solvents categorized into three types: anesthetics, volatile nitrites, and organic solvents.

Insulin A hormone that facilitates entry of glucose into fat and muscle cells for energy.

Insulin reaction Hypoglycemia in clients with type 1 diabetes mellitus.

Interdisciplinary care Care provided by members of the healthcare team in addition to medical professionals. Usually includes team members who address psychosocial and spiritual issues as well as physical care.

Intermittent claudication Cramping, aching pain in the calves, thighs, and buttocks that occurs with a predictable level of activity and is relieved by rest.

Intracerebral hematomas A collection of blood in the brain tissue, most often located in the frontal or temporal lobes.

Intracranial aneurysm Saccular outpouching of a cerebral artery that occurs at the site of a weakness in the vessel wall.

Intracranial hypertension See *Increased intracranial pressure.*

Intracranial pressure (ICP) The pressure within the cranial cavity, usually measured as the pressure within the lateral ventricles.

Intraductal papilloma A tiny wartlike growth on the inside of the peripheral mammary duct that causes discharge from the nipple.

Intraoperative phase The time during surgery, from beginning to end.

Iron deficiency anemia The most common type of anemia; results from inadequate iron for optimal RBC formation.

Irritable bowel syndrome (IBS) A motility disorder of the gastrointestinal tract characterized by alternating periods of constipation and diarrhea.

Ischemia Deficient blood flow to tissue.

Ischemic Deprived of oxygen.

Islets of Langerhans Hormone-producing cells (alpha cells, beta cells, and delta cells) scattered through the pancreas.

Isograft Tissue transplant where the donor and recipient are identical twins.

Jaundice Yellow-to-orange color visible in the skin and mucous membranes; most often the result of a hepatic disorder.

Joint arthroplasty Reconstruction or replacement of a joint.

Kaposi's sarcoma (KS) A vascular malignancy (a tumor of the endothelial cells lining small blood vessels) that presents as vascular macules, papules, or violet lesions affecting the skin and viscera. It is often the presenting symptom of AIDS.

Keloid Elevated, irregularly shaped, progressively enlarging scar arising from excessive amounts of collagen in the stratum corneum during scar formation in connective tissue repair.

Keratitis Inflammation of the cornea.

Keratosis Any skin condition in which there is a benign overgrowth and thickening of the cornified epithelium.

Ketoacidosis A condition of very high blood glucose and insufficient insulin that results in accumulation of ketones and fatty acids in the blood and urine and diuresis.

Ketonuria The presence of ketones in the urine.

Ketosis An accumulation of ketone bodies produced during the oxidation of fatty acids.

Kindling Long-term changes in brain neurotransmission that occur after repeated detoxifications.

Kinesthesia The ability to perceive movement and sense of position.

Korotkoff's sounds Sounds heard during auscultation of blood pressure.

Korsakoff's psychosis Secondary dementia caused by thiamine (B_1) deficiency that may be associated with chronic alcoholism; characterized by progressive cognitive deterioration, confabulation, peripheral neuropathy, and myopathy.

Kussmaul's respirations Deep, rapid respirations associated with compensatory mechanisms.

Kwashiorkor protein energy undernutrition (protein energy malnutrition, PEM) Chronic protein deficiency with adequate calories to meet body needs.

Kyphosis Exaggerated thoracic curvature of the spine common in older adults.

Labyrinthectomy Surgical removal of the labyrinth.

Labyrinthitis Inflammation of the inner ear.

Laceration Open wound that results from sharp cutting or tearing. Injuries to the integument are at risk for contamination from dirt, debris, or foreign objects.

Lacunar strokes Thrombotic stroke of smaller cerebral blood vessels that causes tissue to slough off, leaving a small cavity in the brain tissue.

Laminectomy Removal of the lamina of the vertebrae.

Laparoscopic cholecystectomy Removal of the gallbladder using an endoscope.

Laryngectomy Removal of the larynx.

Laryngitis Inflammation of the larynx.

Leukemia ("white blood") A group of chronic malignant disorders of white blood cells and WBC precursors; characterized by replacement of bone marrow by malignant immature WBCs, abnormal immature circulating WBCs, and infiltration of malignant cells into other tissues.

Leukocytes Also called white blood cells, these are the primary cells involved in both nonspecific and specific immune system responses. These cells isolate the infecting organism or injury, destroy pathogens, and promote healing.

Leukocytosis An increase in the number of leukocytes in the blood (above 10,000/mm^3), usually caused by infection.

Leukopenia Abnormal decrease of circulating leukocytes, usually below 5000/mm^3; occurs when bone marrow activity is suppressed or when leukocyte destruction increases.

Leukoplakia Formation of white patches or spots on the mucous membranes or tongue; these lesions may become malignant.

Lichen planus Benign inflammatory disorder of the mucous membranes and skin.

Lift A more sustained thrust than normal.

Lipoatrophy Atrophy of subcutaneous tissue.

Liposuction A method of changing the contours of the body by aspirating fat from the subcutaneous layer of tissue.

Lithiasis Stone formation.

Lithotripsy Crushing of renal calculi.

Lobectomy Surgical removal of tumors in a single lobe of lung.

Locked-in syndrome Client is alert and fully aware of the environment, but is unable to communicate through speech or movement as a result of blocked efferent pathways to the brain.

Lordosis Increased lumbar curve.

Lower body obesity (peripheral obesity) A waist-to-hip ratio of less than 0.8.

Lung abscess Localized area of lung destruction or necrosis and pus formation.

Lung compliance Distensibility of the lungs.

Lyme disease An inflammatory disorder caused by a spirochete, *Borrelia burgdorferi,* which is transmitted primarily by ticks.

Lymphadenopathy The enlargement of lymph nodes (over 1 cm) with or without tenderness. It may be caused by inflammation, infection, or malignancy of the nodes or the regions drained by the nodes.

Lymphangitis Inflammation of a lymphatic vessel.

Lymphedema Extremity edema due to accumulated lymph; may be primary or secondary, resulting from inflammation, obstruction, or removal of lymphatic vessels.

Lymphocytes Lymphocytes account for 20% to 40% of circulating leukocytes. Lymphocytes are the principal effector and regulator cells of specific immune responses.

Lymphoid tissues Connective tissues containing lymphocytes; include tissues of the bone marrow, thymus, lymph nodes, and spleen.

Lymphomas Malignancy of lymphoid tissue.

Macrophages Monocytes mature into macrophages after settling into tissue. Macrophages are large phagocytes. They are important in the body's defense against chronic infections.

Macular degeneration Destructive changes in the macula due to injury or gradual failure of the outer pigmented layer of the retina (the retinal layer adjacent to the choroid), which removes cellular waste products and keeps the retina attached to the choroid.

Malabsorption A condition in which nutrients are ineffectively absorbed by the intestinal mucosa, resulting in their excretion in the stool.

Malignant hypertension A hypertensive emergency, marked by a diastolic pressure greater than 120 mmHg.

Malignant melanoma (cutaneous melanoma) Skin cancer that arises from melanocytes.

Malignant pain Pain associated with a life-threatening illness such as cancer but not limited to cancer pain.

Malnutrition Inadequate nutrient intake to meet body needs; may include deficiency of major nutrients (calories, carbohydrates, proteins, and fats) or micronutrients such as vitamins and minerals.

Manifestations Signs and symptoms of a disease or condition caused by alterations in structure or function.

Man-made disasters Either accidental or intentional, they are complex emergencies, technological disasters, material shortages, and other disasters not caused by natural hazards.

Marasmus (protein energy undernutrition) Insufficient protein and calorie intake to meet metabolic needs.

Mass casualty incidents Situations in which 100 or more casualties are involved, significantly overwhelming available emergency medical services, facilities, and resources.

Mastoidectomy Surgical removal of infected mastoid air cells.

Mastoiditis Bacterial infection of the mastoid process.

Maturity-onset diabetes of the young (MODY) Diabetes in young obese adults.

Mean arterial pressure (MAP) The average pressure in the arterial circulation throughout the cardiac cycle; the product of cardiac output and systemic vascular resistance (SVR).

Medical-surgical nursing The health promotion, health care, and illness care of adults, based on knowledge derived from the arts and sciences and shaped by knowledge (the science) of nursing.

Melanin Skin pigment that forms a protective shield to protect keratinocytes and nerve endings in the dermis from the damaging effects of ultraviolet light.

Melena Black, tarry stool that contains blood.

Ménière's disease Chronic disorder of unknown cause characterized by recurrent attacks of vertigo with tinnitus and a progressive unilateral hearing loss.

Meningitis Inflammation of the meninges of the brain and spinal cord.

Menopause Permanent cessation of menses.

Menorrhagia Excessive or prolonged menstruation.

Menstrual cycle Cyclic buildup of the uterine lining, ovulation, and sloughing of the lining occurring approximately every 28 days in nonpregnant females.

Menstruation Periodic shedding of the uterine lining in a woman of childbearing age who is not pregnant.

Metabolism Consisting of the breakdown of complex structures into simpler forms to produce energy (catabolism) and the combination of simpler molecules to produce and maintain more complex structures necessary to living organisms (anabolism).

Metaplasia A change in the normal pattern of differentiation such that dividing cells differentiate into cell types not normally found in that location in the body.

Metastasis Secondary tumor; the process by which spreading of malignant neoplasms occurs; the transfer of disease from one organ or part to another not directly connected with it.

Metrorrhagia Bleeding between menstrual periods; may be caused by hormonal imbalances, pelvic inflammatory disease, cervical or uterine polyps, uterine fibroids, or cervical or uterine cancer.

Microalbuminuria Protein in the urine.

Micturition Releasing urine from the urinary bladder (voiding).

Mild concussion Brain trauma resulting in a brief loss of consciousness that lasts from seconds to hours.

Minor trauma Injury to a single part or system of the body, usually treated in the hospital or emergency department.

Mitigation The action taken to prevent or reduce the harmful effects of a disaster on human health or property, it involves future-oriented activities to prevent subsequent disasters or to minimize their effects.

Mitral valve (bicuspid valve) Valve between the left atrium and ventricle in the heart; prevents blood from flowing backwards into the atrium.

Monosomic (monosomy) When one member of the chromosome pair is missing, for example, Turner syndrome (45, XO).

Morbid obesity Weight greater than 100% over ideal body weight.

Morton's neuroma A tumor-like mass formed within the neurovascular bundle of the intermetatarsal spaces.

Mosaicism A chromosome variation or abnormality that occurs after fertilization during mitosis at an early cell stage so not all cells are affected with the variation; for example, a child who is mosaic for Down syndrome will have some cells with two copies of chromosome 21 and some that have an extra chromosome 21.

Mourning The actions or expressions of the bereaved, including the symbols, clothing, and ceremonies that make up the outward manifestations of grief.

Multifactorial Health conditions determined by multiple factors, including genetic and environmental factors, each having an additive effect.

Multiple casualty incidents Incidents in which more than 2 but fewer than 100 persons are injured.

Multiple myeloma A malignancy in which plasma cells multiply uncontrollably and infiltrate the bone marrow, lymph nodes, spleen, and other tissues.

Multiple sclerosis (MS) A chronic degenerative disease of the central nervous system primarily affecting the white matter.

Multiple trauma Most often the result of a motor vehicle crash, this type of trauma requires immediate intervention specifically focused on ensuring survival.

Murmurs Sounds made by turbulent blood flow through the heart.

Muscular dystrophy (MD) A group of inherited muscle diseases that cause progressive muscle degeneration and wasting.

Myasthenia gravis Chronic, progressive neuromuscular disorder characterized by fatigue and severe weakness of skeletal muscles.

Myocarditis Inflammatory disorder of the heart muscle.

Myopia (nearsightedness) A condition in which the eyeball is elongated, causing the image to focus in front of the retina instead of on it.

Myringotomy Incision of the tympanic membrane.

Myxedema Systemic condition that develops from inadequate levels of thyroid hormone.

Natural disasters Disasters caused by acts of nature or emerging diseases, some are unexpected and some are predictable through advanced meteorological technologies.

Natural killer cells (NK cells, null cells) Large, granular lymphocytes (found in the spleen, lymph nodes, bone marrow, and blood) that provide immune surveillance and resistance to infection, and play an important role in the destruction of early malignant cells.

Nausea An unpleasant sensation usually followed by vomiting.

Necrosis Tissue cell death.

Neglect syndrome (unilateral neglect) A disorder of attention. In this syndrome, the person cannot integrate and use perceptions from the affected side of the body or from the environment on the affected side and, hence, ignores that part.

Neoplasm A mass of new tissue (a collection of cells) that grows independently of its surrounding structures and has no physiologic purpose.

Nephrectomy Removal of the kidney.

Nephrotic syndrome A condition marked by massive proteinuria, hypoalbuminemia, hyperlipidemia, and edema.

Neurogenic bladder Dysfunctional urinary bladder due to lesion of central or peripheral nervous system.

Neurogenic shock Shock resulting from an imbalance between parasympathetic and sympathetic stimulation of vascular smooth muscle. If parasympathetic overstimulation or sympathetic understimulation persists, sustained vasodilation occurs, and blood pools in the venous and capillary beds.

Neuropathy Damage to peripheral nerves causing hyper- or hyposensation and leading to pain and injury.

Neutropenia A decrease in circulating neutrophils.

Nevi (moles) Flat or raised macules or papules with rounded, well-defined borders.

Nociceptors Sensory nerve fibers that conduct pain impulses from the periphery to the central nervous system.

Nocturia Voiding two or more times at night.

Node Elements of the immune system connected by lymphatics; upregulates immune function; does not synthesize hormones.

Nonconventional terrorist weapons Chemical, biological, and nuclear weapons of terrorism; used less frequently than conventional terrorist weapons.

Non-Hodgkin's lymphoma (NHL) Lymphoid tissue malignancies that do not contain Reed–Sternberg cells.

Nonunion A state that exists when the ends of a fracture fail to heal together.

Normal sinus rhythm (NSR) Normal heart rhythm, in which impulses originate in the sinus node and travel through normal conduction pathways without delay.

Nosocomial Pertaining to or occurring in a hospital.

Nosocomial infection Infection contracted during residence in a hospital or extended care facility.

Nuclear terrorism Use of a nuclear device to cause mass murder and devastation.

Nursing process The series of critical thinking activities nurses use as they provide care to clients; this logical approach to care ensures that clients receive comprehensive and effective care.

Nutrients Substances found in food that are used by the body to promote growth, maintenance, and repair.

Nutrition The process by which the body ingests, absorbs, transports, uses, and eliminates food.

Nystagmus Rapid involuntary eye movements.

Obesity An excess of body fat (adipose tissue).

Obstructive shock Shock caused by an obstruction in the heart or great vessels that either impedes venous return or prevents effective cardiac pumping action.

Office-based surgical suites A setting for many elective surgeries, although increasing malpractice insurance premiums have influenced their decline.

Oligomenorrhea Scant menses.

Oliguria Urine output of less than 400 mL in 24 hours.

Oncogene Gene capable of triggering cancerous characteristics.

Oncology The study of cancer.

Onycholysis The separation of the distal nail plate from the nail bed.

Onychomycosis A fungal or dermatophyte infection of the nail plate.

Orchitis Infection or inflammation of the testicle.

Orthopnea Difficulty breathing when supine.

Orthostatic hypotension A decrease in systolic blood pressure of more than 10 to 15 mmHg and a drop in diastolic blood pressure on standing.

Osmosis The process by which water moves across a selectively permeable membrane from an area of lower solute concentration to an area of higher solute concentration.

Ossification The process of bone formation.

Osteitis deformans See *Paget's disease of bone.*

Osteoarthritis (degenerative joint disease) The most commonly occurring of all forms of arthritis. This disease is characterized by loss of articular cartilage in articulating joints and hypertrophy of the bones at the articular margins.

Osteomalacia (adult rickets) Metabolic bone disorder characterized by inadequate mineralization of bone matrix.

Osteomyelitis Infection within the bone that can lead to tissue death and necrosis.

Osteophytes Bony outgrowths often called "joint mice."

Osteoporosis Literally defined as "porous bones," a metabolic bone disorder characterized by loss of bone mass, increased bone fragility, and an increased risk of fractures.

Osteotomy An incision into or transection of the bone.

Ostomy General term for an operation in which an artificial opening is created.

Otitis media Inflammation or infection of the middle ear.

Otorrhea Leakage of cerebrospinal fluid through the ear.

Otosclerosis Abnormal bone formation in the osseous labyrinth of the temporal bone causing the footplate of the stapes to become fixed or immobile in the oval window. The result is a conductive hearing loss.

Ovarian cycle The female cycle that occurs from puberty until menopause in which the production of ova occur.

Oxyhemoglobin The combined form of hemoglobin and oxygen; found in arterial blood, it carries oxygen to body tissues.

Pacemaker A pulse generator used to provide an electrical stimulus to the heart when the heart fails to generate or conduct its own at a rate that maintains the cardiac output.

Paco$_2$ Partial pressure of carbon dioxide in arterial blood.

Paget's disease of bone (osteitis deformans) A skeletal disorder that results from excessive osteoclastic activity. Paget's disease is characterized by bone deformity, especially of the long bones of the lower limbs, the pelvis, the lumbar vertebrae, and the skull.

Pain A subjective response to both physical and psychologic stressors.

Pain tolerance The amount of pain a person can endure before responding to it.

Palliative care An area of care that has evolved out of the hospice experience, but exists outside of hospice programs and is not restricted to the end of life. Palliative care is focused on the relief of physical, mental, and spiritual distress for individuals who have an incurable illness and is used earlier in the disease experience than hospice care. The goal of palliative care is to prevent and relieve suffering by early assessment and treatment of pain and other physical, psychosocial, and spiritual needs to improve the client's quality of life.

Pallor Lack of color; paleness of skin.

Pancreatitis Inflammation of the pancreas.

Pannus Granulation tissue that forms in joints affected by rheumatoid arthritis and leads to the formation of scar tissue that immobilizes the joint.

Pao$_2$ Partial pressure of oxygen in arterial blood.

Papilledema Swelling of the optic nerve.

Paracentesis Aspiration of fluid from the peritoneal cavity.

Paralytic ileus Impaired propulsion or forward movement of bowel contents.

Paraplegia Paralysis of the lower portion of the body, sometimes involving the lower trunk.

Parasites Organisms that live within, on, or at the expense of the client.

Parish nursing A nontraditional, community-based way of providing health promotion and health restoration nursing interventions to a spiritual community.

Parkinson's disease (PD) Progressive, degenerative neurologic disease characterized by nonintention tremor, bradykinesia, and muscle rigidity.

Paronychia An infection of the cuticle of the fingernails or toenails.

Paroxysmal Abrupt onset and termination.

Paroxysmal nocturnal dyspnea Attacks of acute shortness of breath that occur at night, waking up the client.

Partial gastrectomy Removal of a portion of the stomach, usually the distal half to two-thirds.

Partial seizures Seizures that involve a restricted part of one cerebral hemisphere; may be simple partial (without loss of consciousness) or complex partial (with loss of consciousness).

Partial-thickness burn Burn that involves the entire dermis and the papillae of the dermis (superficial partial-thickness burn) or extends into the hair follicles (deep partial-thickness burn).

Passive immunity Temporary protection—provided by antibodies produced by other people or animals—against disease-producing antigens. Protection is gradually lost when these acquired antibodies are used up either by natural degradation or by combining with the antigen.

Pathogens Virulent organisms rarely found in the absence of disease.

Patient-controlled analgesia (PCA) A pump with a control mechanism that allows the client to self-manage pain.

Pediculosis capitis An infestation with head lice.

Pediculosis corporis An infestation with body lice.

Pediculosis pubis An infestation with pubic lice (often called "crabs").

Pelvic inflammatory disease (PID) A term used to describe infection of the pelvic organs.

Pemphigus vulgaris Chronic disorder of the skin and oral mucous membranes characterized by vesicle (blister) formation.

Penetrance The percentage or likelihood that an individual who has inherited a gene mutation will actually express the disease signs and symptoms in his or her lifetime.

Penicillin-resistant Streptococcus pneumoniae (PRSP) Infection transmitted by droplets from the respiratory tract; requires transmission-based droplet precautions.

Peptic ulcer disease (PUD) A break in the mucous lining of the gastrointestinal tract where it comes in contact with gastric juice.

Perforation Penetration of ulcer through mucosal wall.

Pericarditis Inflammation of the pericardium.

Perioperative nursing A specialized area of nursing practice that incorporates the three phases of the surgical experience: preoperative, intraoperative, and postoperative.

Peripheral vascular disease (PVD) Impaired blood supply to peripheral tissues, particularly the lower extremities.

Peripheral vascular resistance (PVR) The opposing forces or impedance to blood flow as the arterial channels become more and more distant from the heart.

Peristalsis Alternating waves of contraction and relaxation of involuntary muscle.

Peritoneal dialysis Procedure in which electrolytes, waste products, and excess water are removed from the body by diffusion using the peritoneum surrounding the abdominal cavity as the dialyzing membrane.

Peritonitis Inflammation of the peritoneum.

Pernicious anemia Anemia resulting from failure to absorb dietary vitamin B_{12} due to lack of intrinsic factor.

Persistent vegetative state (PVS) Condition of complete unawareness of self and the environment.

Personal protective equipment (PPE) Equipment used for the protection of personnel including gloves, masks, goggles, gowns, and biologic disposal bags (red bags); may also include hoods, helmets, head gear, and impermeable suits.

Pertussis (whooping cough) A highly contagious acute upper respiratory infection cause by the bacterium *Bordetella pertussis*.

Phagocytosis A process by which a foreign agent or target cell is engulfed, destroyed, and digested. Neutrophils and macrophages, known as phagocytes, are the primary cells involved in phagocytosis.

Phantom limb syndrome (phantom pain) A confusing pain syndrome that occurs following surgical or traumatic amputation of a limb. The client experiences pain in the missing body part even though there is complete mental awareness that the limb is gone.

Pharyngitis Acute inflammation of the pharynx.

Phenotype The expression of a person's entire physical, biochemical, and physiologic makeup, as determined by the individual's genotype and environmental factors.

Phimosis Constriction of the foreskin so that it cannot be retracted over the glans penis.

Plasmapheresis (plasma exchange) Removal of the plasma component from whole blood.

Plastic surgery The alteration, replacement, or restoration of visible portions of the body, performed to correct a structural or cosmetic defect.

Platelets (thrombocytes) Cell fragments that have no nucleus and cannot replicate.

Pleural effusion Collection of excess fluid in the pleural space.

Pleuritis Inflammation of the pleura.

Pneumonectomy Removal of an entire lung.

Pneumonia Inflammation of the lung parenchyma (the respiratory bronchioles and alveoli).

Pneumothorax Results when air enters the pleural space due to blunt and penetrating injuries to the chest.

Polycystic kidney disease A hereditary disease characterized by cyst formation and massive kidney enlargement.

Polycythemia (erythrocytosis) Excess RBCs characterized by a hematocrit higher than 55%.

Polydipsia Excessive thirst.

Polymyositis A systemic connective-tissue disorder characterized by inflammation of connective tissue and muscle fibers leading to muscle weakness and atrophy.

Polyp Mass of tissue that arises from the bowel wall and protrudes into the lumen.

Polyphagia Excessive eating.

Polysubstance abuse The simultaneous use of many substances.

Polyuria A condition where increased blood volume increases renal blood flow, and the hyperglycemia acts as an osmotic diuretic, thereby increasing urine output.

Portal hypertension Elevated pressure in the portal venous system that causes rerouting of blood to adjoining lower pressure vessels.

Postconcussion syndrome Persistent headache, dizziness, irritability, insomnia, impaired memory and concentration, and learning problems following a concussion; may last for several weeks or up to 1 year.

Postoperative phase Period when a procedure or surgery has been completed and the client is recovering from the stress associated with the surgery.

Postpoliomyelitis syndrome A complication of a previous infection by the poliomyelitis virus.

Preload The amount of cardiac muscle fiber tension or stretch that exists at diastole, just before ventricular contraction.

Premenstrual syndrome (PMS) Complex of symptoms characterized by irritability, depression, edema, and breast tenderness preceding the monthly menses.

Preoperative phase Time when preparation of the client for surgery is conducted and completed.

Presbycusis Age-related loss of the ability to hear high-frequency sounds, may occur because of cochlear hair cell degeneration or loss of auditory neurons in the organ of Corti.

Presbyopia Impaired near vision resulting from a loss of elasticity of the lens related to aging.

Pressure ulcer Ischemic lesion of the skin and underlying tissue caused by external pressure that impairs the flow of blood and lymph.

Priapism Sustained, painful erection that lasts at least 4 hours and is not associated with sexual arousal.

Primary hypertension (idiopathic, essential) A persistently elevated systemic blood pressure.

Primary polycythemia (polycythemia vera) A neoplastic stem cell disorder characterized by overproduction of red blood cells and, to a lesser extent, white blood cells and platelets.

Progesterone Hormone produced by the ovary; works with estrogen to control the menstrual cycle.

Prostatitis Inflammation of the prostate gland.

Protein-calorie malnutrition (PCM) Deficient protein and calories to meet metabolic needs.

Proteinuria Abnormal proteins in the urine.

Pruritus Subjective itching sensation producing an urge to scratch.

Psoriasis Chronic, noninfectious skin disorder that is characterized by raised, reddened, round circumscribed plaques covered by silvery white scales.

Psychogenic pain Pain that is experienced in the absence of any diagnosed physiologic cause or event.

Ptosis Drooping of the eyelid.

Pulmonary edema An abnormal accumulation of fluid in the interstitial tissue and alveoli of the lung.

Pulmonary embolism Sudden occlusion of a pulmonary artery resulting in disruption of blood supply to the lung parenchyma.

Pulmonary hypertension Condition in which the pulmonary arterial pressure is elevated to an abnormal level.

Pulmonic valves One of the semilunar valves, separating the ventricles from the great vessels.

Pulse Rhythmic pressure wave that can be felt over an artery.

Pulse deficit Condition in which the radial pulse is less than the apical pulse, indicating weak, inefficient left ventricular contractions.

Pulse pressure The difference between the systolic and diastolic blood pressure.

Puncture wound Wound that occurs when a sharp or blunt object penetrates the integument.

Pupillary light reflex Reflex in which the pupil contracts in response to a bright light.

Pyelonephritis Upper urinary tract inflammation affecting the kidney and renal pelvis.

Pyoderma Purulent bacterial infection of skin.

Pyuria (bacteriuria) Pus in the urine.

Quadriplegia See *Tetraplegia.*

Quality assurance The process of ensuring quality control activities that evaluate, monitor, or regulate the standard of services provided to the consumer.

Rabies Viral (rhabdovirus) infection of the central nervous system transmitted by infected saliva that enters the human body through a bite or an open wound.

Radiation sickness One of the results of DNA mutation inside cells exposed to ionizing radiation.

Radiation therapy Therapy that uses radiation to kill a tumor, to reduce its size, to decrease pain, or to relieve obstruction.

Radiological dispersion bomb Also called a "dirty bomb," consists of a conventional explosive such as trinitrotoluene (TNT) packed with radioactive waste by-products from nuclear reactors that discharges deadly radioactive particles into the environment.

Raynaud's disease (Raynaud's phenomenon) Disorders characterized by episodes of intense vasospasm in the small arteries and arterioles of the fingers and possibly the toes.

Reactive arthritis (Reiter's syndrome) An acute, nonpurulent inflammatory arthritis that complicates a bacterial infection of the genitourinary or gastrointestinal tracts.

Rebound tenderness Pain that occurs with withdrawal or release of pressure applied during abdominal palpation.

Recessive A characteristic that is apparent only when two copies of the gene encoding it are present, one from the mother and one from the father.

Reconstruction The recovery aspect of disaster response; during this period restoration, reconstitution, and mitigation take place.

Red blood cell (RBCs, erythrocytes) Blood cells shaped like a biconcave disk that contain hemoglobin required for oxygen transport to body tissues; the most common type of blood cell.

Referral source A person recommending home care services and supplying the agency with details about the client's needs. The source may be a physician, nurse, social worker, therapist, or discharge planner.

Referred pain Pain that is perceived in an area distant from the site of the stimuli.

Reflex sympathetic dystrophy A group of poorly understood post-traumatic conditions involving persistent pain, hyperesthesias, swelling, changes in skin color and texture, changes in temperature, and decreased motion.

Reflux, urinary Backflow of urine toward the kidneys.

Refraction The bending of light rays as they pass from one medium to another medium of different optical density.

Refractory period A period in which myocardial cells are resistant to stimulation.

Regional anesthesia Anesthesia that desensitizes the area to be operated but does not involve the full central nervous system or cause sedation.

Regurgitation (valvular) Backflow of blood through an incompletely closed valve into the area it just left.

Rehabilitation The process of learning to live to one's maximum potential with a chronic impairment and its resultant functional disability.

Reiter's syndrome See *Reactive arthritis.*

Remission A period in which symptoms are not experienced even though the disease is still clinically present.

Renal artery stenosis Narrowing of the renal artery.

Renal colic Acute, severe, intermittent pain in the flank and upper outer abdominal quadrant generally associated with acute obstruction of a ureter and resulting ureteral spasm.

Renal failure A condition in which the kidneys are unable to remove accumulated metabolites from the blood, resulting in altered fluid, electrolyte, and acid–base balance.

Renal impairment (decreased renal reserve) A glomerular filtration rate of approximately 50% of normal with normal BUN and serum creatinine levels.

Renal insufficiency A glomerular filtration rate of 20% to 50% of normal with azotemia and some manifestations of renal failure.

Renal transplant The surgical insertion of a functioning kidney.

Renin–angiotensin mechanism Method of controlling the glomerular filtration rate by releasing chemicals that cause intense vasodilation of the afferent arterioles. Conversely, an increase in the flow of filtrate results in the promotion of vasoconstriction, decreasing the glomerular filtration rate.

Repolarization Restoration of the resting cell membrane potential following generation of an action potential.

Respiratory failure Inability of lungs to oxygenate the blood and remove carbon dioxide adequately to meet the body's needs, even at rest.

Respite care Short-term or intermittent home care, often using volunteers. These services exist to give the primary caregiver some relief from the burden of full-time care.

Response Occurs in the emergency stage of disaster response, after the impact of the disaster event has occurred, the community has been rapidly assessed for damage, and the types and extent of injuries suffered as well as the immediate needs of the community have been determined.

Reticular activating system (RAS) A system of reticular neurons within the reticular formation that passes steady streams of impulses through thalamic relays in order to stimulate the cerebral cortex into wakefulness.

Retinal detachment Separation of the retina or sensory portion of the eye from the choroid.

Retinitis pigmentosa Hereditary degenerative disease characterized by retinal atrophy and loss of retinal function progressing from the periphery to the central region of the retina.

Retractions A pulling in of the tissue of the precordium; a slight retraction just medial to the midclavicular line at the area of the apical impulse is normal and is more likely to be visible in thin clients.

Reverse triage Working from the principle of the greatest good for the greatest number, reverse triage is an "upside-down triage" used in mass casualty events in which the victims who are most severely injured, requiring extensive resources with little chance of surviving, are treated last.

Rheumatic fever A systemic inflammatory disease caused by an abnormal immune response to pharyngeal infection by group A beta-hemolytic streptococci.

Rheumatic heart disease (RHD) Slowly progressive valvular deformity following acute or repeated attacks of rheumatic fever; characterized by rigid and deformed valve leaflets; fused valve commissures, and fibrosis of chordae tendineae.

Rheumatoid arthritis A chronic systemic autoimmune disease that causes inflammation of connective tissue, primarily in the joints.

Rhinitis Inflammation of the nasal cavities.

Rhinoplasty Surgical reconstruction of the nose.

Rhinorrhea Leakage of cerebrospinal fluid through the nose.

Ruptured disk See *Herniated intervertebral disk.*

Salmonellosis A form of food poisoning caused by ingestion of foods contaminated with one or more varieties of *Salmonella* bacteria.

Sarcoidosis Systemic disease characterized by granulomas in the lungs, lymph nodes, liver, eyes, skin, and other organs.

Sarcoma A tumor arising from supportive tissues.

Scabies Parasitic infestation caused by the mite *Sarcoptes scabei.*

Sciatica Pain over the sciatic nerve.

Scleroderma Hardening of the skin, a chronic condition characterized by the formation of excess fibrous connective tissue and diffuse fibrosis of the skin and internal organs.

Sclerotherapy The removal of benign skin lesions with a sclerosing agent that causes inflammation with fibrosis of tissue.

Scoliosis A lateral curvature of the spine.

Scrub person Prepares the sterile field, surgical supplies, and equipment for surgical procedures; also assists surgeon and physician assistant by passing instruments, suctioning blood, and maintaining the sterile field.

Seborrheic dermatitis Common and chronic inflammatory disorder of the skin that involves the scalp, eyebrows, eyelids, ear canals, nasolabial folds, axillae, and trunk. The cause is unknown.

Secondary hypertension Elevated blood pressure resulting from an identifiable underlying process.

Seizure An episode of excessive and abnormal discharge of electrical activity within the central nervous system.

Semen Contains sperm and fluids secreted by the male reproductive system glands.

Seminoma A tumor from seminal or germ tissue.

Septic arthritis The type of arthritis that develops when a joint space is invaded by a pathogen.

Septic shock One part of a progressive syndrome called systemic inflammatory response syndrome. Beginning with an infection, septic shock progresses to bacteremia, then sepsis, then septic shock, and finally multiple organ failure syndrome.

Seroconversion Antibody response to a disease or vaccine.

Severe acute respiratory syndrome (SARS) Lower respiratory illness of unknown etiology; spread by close person-to-person contact.

Sexually transmitted infection (STI, sexually transmitted disease, venereal disease) Any infection transmitted by sexual contact, including vaginal, oral, and anal intercourse.

Shigellosis (bacillary dysentery) An acute bowel infection caused by microorganisms of the *Shigella* genus.

Shingles See *Herpes zoster.*

Shock A clinical syndrome characterized by a systemic imbalance between oxygen supply and demand. This imbalance results in a state of inadequate blood flow to the peripheral tissues, causing life-threatening cellular dysfunction, hypotension, and oliguria.

Sickle cell anemia A hereditary, chronic hemolytic anemia characterized by episodes of sickling, during which RBCs become abnormally crescent shaped.

Sickle cell crisis Severe episodes of fever and intense pain that are the hallmark of sickle cell anemia.

Sinusitis Inflammation of the mucous membranes of one or more of the sinuses.

Sjögren's syndrome An autoimmune disorder that causes inflammation and dysfunction of exocrine glands throughout the body.

Skeletal traction Application of a pulling force through placement of pins into the bone.

Skin graft Surgical method of detaching skin from a donor site and placing it in a recipient site, where it develops a new blood supply from the base of the wound.

Skin tags Soft papules on a pedicle.

Skin traction Traction in which the cradle-like sleeve placed around the extremity exerts its pulling force through the client's skin.

Sleep apnea Absence of airflow through the upper airways for 10 or more seconds.

Somatic cell Any cell in the body that is not a sex cell (ova and sperm).

Somatic pain Pain arising from nerve receptors originating in the skin or close to the surface of the body.

Somogyi phenomenon A morning rise in blood glucose to hyperglycemic levels following an episode of nocturnal hypoglycemia and a counterregulatory hormone response.

Spasticity Increased muscle tone in disease of the corticospinal motor tract.

Spermatocele A mobile, usually painless mass containing dead spermatozoa that forms in the epididymis.

Spinal cord injury Injury to spinal cord, usually due to trauma, and classified according to systems.

Spinal cord tumors Benign or malignant, primary or metastatic tumor of the spinal cord.

Spinal shock Temporary loss of reflex function below the level of injury.

Splenomegaly Enlargement of the spleen.

Sprain Tearing or stretching of a ligament that results from a twisting motion.

Sprue A chronic primary disorder of the small intestine in which the absorption of nutrients, particularly fats, is impaired.

Squamous cell carcinoma Malignant tumor of the squamous epithelium of the skin or mucous membranes.

Standard A statement or criterion that can be used by a profession and by the general public to measure quality of practice.

Starvation Inadequate dietary intake; the condition of being without food for long periods of time.

Status asthmaticus Severe, prolonged asthma that does not respond to routine treatment. Without aggressive therapy, status asthmaticus can lead to respiratory failure with hypoxemia, hypercapnia, and acidosis.

Status epilepticus Continuous seizure activity with only very short periods of calm occurring between intense and persistent seizures.

Steatorrhea Greasy, frothy, yellow stools resulting from excess fat in the feces.

Stem cell transplant (SCT) Infusion of donor stem cells to replace the recipient's blood cell lines (WBCs, RBCs, and platelets).

Stem cells (hemocytoblasts) Bone marrow precursor cells for all blood cells.

Stenosis Condition where valve leaflets fuse together and are unable to open or close fully.

Stoma Surface opening.

Stomatitis Inflammation of the oral mucosa.

Straight traction A pulling force applied in a straight line to the injured body part resting on the bed.

Strain Stretching or tearing of muscle fibers that results in bleeding into the tissues.

Stress incontinence Loss of usually less than 50 mL of urine occurring with increased abdominal pressure.

Stress-induced (erosive) gastritis Inflammation and superficial erosions of the gastric mucosa that may occur as a complication of other life-threatening conditions such as shock, severe trauma, major surgery, sepsis, burns, or head injury.

Striae A line above or below tissue that differs in color and texture from surrounding tissue.

Stridor High-pitched, harsh inspiratory sound indicative of upper airway obstruction.

Stroke (brain attack, cerebrovascular accident, CVA) A condition in which neurologic deficits occur as a result of decreased blood flow to a focal (localized) area of brain tissue.

Stroke volume (SV) The amount of blood pumped into the aorta with each contraction of the left ventricle.

Subdural hematoma A localized mass of blood that collects between the dura mater and the arachnoid mater.

Subluxation Partial separation (or dislocation) of the bones of a joint.

Substance abuse The use of any chemical in a fashion inconsistent with medical or culturally defined social norms despite physical, psychologic, or social adverse effects.

Substance dependence A severe condition occurring when the use of a chemical substance is no longer under an individual's control for at least 3 months. Continued use of the substance usually persists despite adverse effects on the person's physical condition, psychologic health, and interpersonal relationships (used interchangeably with addiction).

Sudden cardiac death (SCD) Unexpected death occurring within 1 hour of the onset of cardiovascular symptoms.

Sundowning A behavioral change in Alzheimer's disease characterized by increased agitation, time disorientation, and wandering during afternoon and evening hours.

Superficial burn Burn involving only the epidermal layer of the skin; most often results from damage from sunburn, ultraviolet light, minor flash injury (from a sudden ignition or explosion), or mild radiation burn associated with cancer treatment.

Surfactant A lipoprotein produced by the alveolar cells; interferes with adhesion of water molecules, reducing surface tension and helping to expand lungs.

Surge capacity The healthcare system's ability to rapidly expand beyond normal services to meet the increased demand for qualified personnel, medical care, and public health in the event of a large-scale disaster.

Surgery An invasive medical procedure performed to diagnose or treat illness, injury, or deformity. Although surgery is a medical treatment, the nurse assumes an active role in caring for the client before, during, and after surgery.

Surgical debridement The process of excising a wound to the level of fascia (fascial excision) or sequentially removing thin slices of a burn wound to the level of viable tissue (sequential excision).

Surveillance Collecting and analyzing data to establish a baseline and determine a point at which there is a change or trend in the health of the population.

Synovitis Inflammation of the synovial membrane lining the articular capsule of a joint.

Syphilis A sexually transmitted infection caused by a spirochete that may invade almost any body tissue or organ. It enters the body through a break in the skin or mucous membranes, and can be transferred to the fetus through the placental circulation.

Systemic lupus erythematosus (SLE) A chronic, inflammatory immune complex connective tissue disease.

Systemic sclerosis (scleroderma) Hardening of the skin; a chronic disease characterized by the formation of excess fibrous connective tissue and diffuse fibrosis of the skin and internal organs.

Systole A phase during which the ventricles contract and eject blood into the pulmonary and systemic circuits.

Systolic blood pressure This arterial pressure wave produced by ventricular contraction (systole) averages 120 mmHg in healthy adults.

T lymphocytes (T cells) Type of lymphocyte that matures in the thymus gland.

Tachycardia A heart rate exceeding 100 beats per minute.

Tachypnea Abnormally rapid respiratory rate.

Tendonitis Inflammation of a tendon.

Tension headache Poorly localized headache characterized by ill-defined bilateral head aching, tightness, pressure, or a viselike feeling.

Tension pneumothorax A condition in which an injury to the chest allows air to enter but not escape the pleural cavity.

Testicular torsion Twisting of the testes and spermatic cord.

Testosterone Male hormone produced in the testes.

Tetanus Disorder of the nervous system caused by a neurotoxin elaborated by *Clostridium tetani*.

Tetany Tonic muscular spasms.

Tetraplegia (formerly called quadriplegia) Injury to cervical segments of the cord thus impairing function of the arms, trunk, legs, and pelvic organs.

Thalassemia An inherited disorder of hemoglobin synthesis in which either the alpha or beta chains of the hemoglobin molecule are missing or defective.

Third spacing The accumulation and sequestration of trapped extracellular fluid in an actual or potential body space as a result of disease or injury.

Thoracentesis Invasive procedure in which fluid (or occasionally air) is removed from the pleural space with a needle.

Thoracotomy Incision of the chest wall to gain access to the lung for surgery.

Thrill Palpable vibration over the precordium or an artery.

Thromboangiitis obliterans (Buerger's disease) An occlusive vascular disease involving inflammation, spasm, and clot formation in small- and medium-sized peripheral arteries.

Thrombocytopenia A platelet count of less than 100,000 per milliliter of blood.

Thromboembolus A thrombus that breaks loose from the arterial wall.

Thrombophlebitis See *Venous thrombosis.*

Thrombotic cerebrovascular accident Cerebrovascular accident caused by occlusion of a vessel by a thrombus (a blood clot) on the interior wall of an artery.

Thrombus A blood clot that adheres to a vessel wall.

Tidal volume (TV) The amount of air (approximately 500 mL) moved in and out of the lungs with each normal, quiet breath.

Tinea capitis A fungal infection of the scalp.

Tinea corporis A fungal infection of the body.

Tinea pedis A fungal infection of the toenails and feet.

Tinnitus Perception of sound such as ringing, buzzing, or roaring in the ears.

Titration Administration of analgesics in small increasing or decreasing increments.

Tolerance A cumulative state in which a particular dose of a chemical elicits a smaller response than before. With increased tolerance, the individual needs higher and higher doses to obtain the desired effect.

Tonic-clonic seizures Alternating contraction (tonic phase) and relaxation (clonic phase) of muscles during seizure activity.

Tonsillitis Acute inflammation of the palatine tonsils.

Tophi Small white nodules in subcutaneous tissue composed of urate deposits resulting from gout.

Total colectomy Surgical removal of the entire colon.

Total gastrectomy Removal of the entire stomach.

Total hip arthroplasty (THA) Replacement of both the femoral head and the acetabulum.

Total parenteral nutrition (TPN) Intravenous administration of carbohydrates (high concentrations of dextrose), protein (amino acids), electrolytes, vitamins, minerals, and fat emulsions.

Toxic epidermal necrolysis (TENS) Rare, life-threatening disease in which the epidermis peels off the dermis in sheets, leaving large areas of denuded skin.

Toxic megacolon A condition characterized by acute motor paralysis and dilation of the colon.

Traction The application of a straightening or pulling force to return or maintain the fractured bones in normal anatomic position.

Transcutaneous electrical nerve stimulation (TENS) A unit that consists of a low-voltage transmitter connected by wires to electrodes that are placed by the client as directed by the physical therapist. The client experiences a gentle tapping or vibrating sensation over the electrodes. The client can adjust the voltage to achieve maximum pain relief.

Transdermal Medication absorbed through the skin without injection.

Transfusion An infusion of blood or blood components.

Transient ischemic attack (TIA) Brief period of localized cerebral ischemia that causes neurologic deficits lasting for less than 24 hours.

Transjugular intrahepatic portosystemic shunt (TIPS) Used to relieve portal hypertension and its complications of esophageal varices and ascites. A channel is created through the liver tissue using a needle inserted transcutaneously; an expandable metal stent is inserted into this channel, to allow blood to flow directly from the portal vein into the hepatic vein, bypassing the cirrhotic liver. The shunt relieves pressure in esophageal varices and allows better control of fluid retention with diuretic therapy. Generally is used as a short-term measure until liver transplant is performed.

Translocation The joining of a part of or a whole chromosome to another separate chromosome.

Traumatic brain injury (TBI) A traumatic insult to the brain capable of causing physical, intellectual, emotional, social, and vocational changes.

Tremors Rhythmic movement.

Triage Means "sorting." Triage is a continuous process in which client priorities are reassigned as needed treatments, time, and the condition of the clients change.

Tricuspid valve A valve between the right atrium and ventricle of the heart; prevents blood from flowing backwards into the atrium.

Trigeminal neuralgia (tic douloureux) A chronic disease of the trigeminal cranial nerve (cranial nerve V) that causes severe facial pain.

Triglycerides Molecules of glycerol with fatty acids used to transport and store fats in body tissues.

Trisomy Possessing three chromosomes instead of the usual two as in trisomy 21 or Down syndrome.

Trousseau's sign Contraction of the hand and fingers in response to occlusion of the blood supply by a blood pressure cuff; caused by decreased blood calcium levels.

Tuberculosis (TB) Chronic, recurrent infectious disease caused by *Mycobacterium tuberculosis;* usually affects the lungs, although any organ can be affected.

Tumor marker A protein molecule detectable in serum or other body fluids. This marker is used as a biochemical indicator of the presence of a malignancy.

Tympanoplasty Surgical reconstruction of the middle ear.

Type 1 diabetes One of two types of diabetes characterized by the destruction of beta cells, usually leading to absolute insulin deficiency.

Type 2 diabetes One of two types of diabetes the characteristics of which may range from predominantly insulin resistance with relative insulin deficiency to a predominantly secretory defect with insulin resistance. There is no immune destruction of beta cells.

Ulcer A lesion of the skin or mucous membranes.

Ulcerative colitis Chronic inflammatory bowel disorder of the mucosa and submucosa of the colon and rectum.

Ultrafiltration Removal of excess body water using a hydrostatic pressure gradient.

Uniform Anatomical Gift Act Legislation that requires people to be informed about their options related to organ donation.

Unilateral neglect State in which a client is unaware of and inattentive to one side of body.

Upper body obesity (central obesity) Excess intra-abdominal fat characterized by a waist-to-hip ratio greater than 1 in men and 0.8 in women.

Urea An end product of protein metabolism, and along with water the main constituent of urine.

Uremia Literally "urine in the blood"; the syndrome or group of symptoms associated with end-stage renal failure.

Ureteral stent Thin catheter inserted into the ureter to provide for urine flow and ureteral support.

Ureteroplasty Surgical repair of a ureter.

Urgency A sudden, compelling need to urinate.

Urinary calculi Calculi or "stones" in the urinary tract.

Urinary diversion Procedure to provide for urine collection and drainage following cystectomy. The most common urinary diversion is the ileal conduit.

Urinary drainage system The ureters, urinary bladder, and urethra.

Urinary incontinence Involuntary urination.

Urinary retention Incomplete emptying of the bladder.

Urolithiasis Development of stones within the urinary tract.

Urticaria Hives.

Vaccine Suspensions of whole or fractionated bacteria or viruses that have been treated to make them nonpathogenic.

Valsalva's maneuver Closing the glottis and contracting the diaphragm and abdominal muscles to increase intra-abdominal pressure to facilitate expulsion of feces.

Valvular heart disease Interference of blood flow to, within, and from the heart.

Vancomycin intermediate-resistant *Staphylococcus aureus* (VISA) A form of *S. aureus* with intermediate resistance to vancomycin.

Varicocele Dilation of the pampiniform venous complex of the spermatic cord.

Varicose veins Irregular, tortuous veins with incompetent valves.

Vasectomy Sterilization procedure in which a portion of the spermatic cord is removed.

Vasoconstriction Smooth muscle contraction that narrows the vessel lumen.

Vasodilation Smooth muscle relaxation that expands the vessel lumen.

Vasogenic shock See *Neurogenic shock.*

Venous thrombosis (thrombophlebitis) Blood clot (thrombus) formation on the wall of a vein, accompanied by inflammation of the vein wall and obstructed venous blood flow.

Vertigo Sensation of whirling or rotation.

Very low calorie diet (VLCD) A protein-sparing modified fast (400 to 800 kcal/day or less) under close medical supervision that may be used to treat significant obesity.

Vesicoureteral reflux Condition in which urine moves from the bladder back toward the kidney.

Visceral pain Pain arising from body organs. It is dull and poorly localized because of the low number of nociceptors.

Vital capacity The sum of TV (tidal volume) + IRV (inspiratory reserve volume) + ERV (expiratory reserve volume); approximately 4500 mL in healthy clients.

Vitamin B_{12} deficiency anemia Anemia due to inadequate vitamin B_{12} consumption or impaired absorption.

Vitiligo Abnormal loss of melanin in patches.

Volatile acids Acids eliminated from the body as a gas.

Volkmann's contracture A common complication of elbow fractures, can result from unresolved compartment syndrome. Arterial blood flow decreases, leading to ischemia, degeneration, and contracture of the muscle.

Von Willebrand's disease The most common hereditary bleeding disorder, caused by a deficit of or defective von Willebrand factor.

Warm zone Adjacent to the hot zone of a disaster, the area where decontamination of victims or triage and emergency treatment takes place; also called the control zone.

Warts (verrucae) Lesions of the skin caused by the human papillomavirus.

Weaning Process of removing the client from ventilator support and reestablishing spontaneous, independent respirations.

Weber test A test of hearing; a vibrating tuning fork is placed on the midline of the top of the head and the client is asked to describe where the sound is heard. Normally, sound is heard equally in both ears.

Wernicke's encephalopathy Caused by thiamine (B_1) deficiency and characterized by nystagmus, ptosis, ataxia, confusion, coma, and possible death. Thiamine deficiency is common in chronic alcoholism.

Wheeze Continuous, musical sound caused by narrowing of the lumen in a respiratory passage.

White blood cell (WBCs, leukocytes) The blood cells that contribute to the body's defense against microorganisms.

Wild-type gene The most common type of gene; designated as normal.

Withdrawal Cessation of use of a substance to which an individual has become addicted.

Withdrawal symptoms Constellation of signs and symptoms that occurs in physically dependent individuals when they discontinue drug use.

Xenograft A transplant from an animal species to a human.

Xeroderma A chronic skin condition characterized by dry, rough skin.

Xerosis Dry skin.

X-linked Any gene found on the X chromosome, or traits determined by such genes; also refers to the specific mode of inheritance of such genes; one altered gene on an X chromosome in a male can produce disease, such as hemophilia.

Zollinger–Ellison syndrome Peptic ulcer disease caused by a gastrinoma, or gastrin-secreting tumor of the pancreas, stomach, or intestines.

Page numbers followed by *f* indicate figures and those followed by *t* indicate tables, boxes, or special features. The titles of special features (e.g., Medication Administration; Multisystem Effects; Nursing Care Plan; Nursing Research) are also capitalized.

Excellence in Nursing Skills

Prentice Hall's Real Nursing Skills on CD-ROMs

Prentice Hall Real Nursing Skills series offers you the complete foundation for competency in performing clinical skills. The CD-ROMs provide comprehensive procedures demonstrated in hundreds of videos, animations, illustrations, and photographs. These skills CD-ROMs are designed to help you visualize how to perform each skill and understand the concepts and rationales for each skill.

Basic Nursing Skills:
94 skills on 5 CD-ROMs, 2005, ISBN: 0-13-191526-6

Intermediate & Advanced Nursing Skills:
84 skills on 5 CD-ROMs, 2005, ISBN: 0-13-119344-9

Physical & Health Assessment Nursing Skills:
25 skills on 5 CD-ROMs, 2006, ISBN: 0-13-191525-8

Maternal-Newborn & Women's Health Nursing Skills:
24 skills on 2 CD-ROMs, 2005, ISBN: 0-13-191527-4

Pediatric Nursing Skills:
65 skills on 3 CD-ROMs, 2006, ISBN: 0-13-191524-X

Critical Care Nursing Skills:
35 skills on 2 CD-ROMs, 2005, ISBN: 0-13-119264-7

Excellence in NCLEX-RN® Review

Prentice Hall's Comprehensive NCLEX-RN® Review is designed specifically to help you achieve nursing excellence by simplifying your review and making the most of your valuable study time. This review book is uniquely organized according to the April 2007 NCLEX® Test Plan, providing you with both a comprehensive content review and practice questions in sections covering ✳ Safe, Effective Care Environment ✳ Health Promotion ✳ Physiological Integrity, and ✳ Psychosocial Integrity. Throughout this book, you will find:

- **Memory Aids** that help you remember key concepts.
- **NCLEX® Alerts** that identify critical concepts you are likely to see on the NCLEX-RN®.
- **Check Your NCLEX® IQ** boxes that help you to assess your readiness for the NCLEX-RN® on the topics covered in the chapter.
- **Practice Tests** at the end of the chapter that review the concepts from that chapter and provide comprehensive rationales and test-taking strategies to help you find the right answers.

The **NCLEX-RN® Test Prep CD-ROM** that comes with your book simulates the test-taking environment by allowing you to practice questions on the computer. It contains all the questions in the book PLUS thousands of additional questions. You can choose to practice in Study, Quiz, or Exam modes, and you will receive detailed reports that will help you focus your preparation for NCLEX-RN®.

2008, ISBN 0-13-119599-9

Excellence in Testing

Prentice Hall and the National League for Nursing are pleased to offer you unique practice tests that correlate directly to your Prentice Hall Nursing textbooks. Each test is a comprehensive examination intended for students who have completed their course work and provides feedback regarding comprehension of the course content. The access code gives you access to two unique practice tests—use them to prepare for your course final exams or for NCLEX-RN®. Go to the website below and search for the **National League for Nursing** to find practice tests in any of your core nursing courses or to accompany the **Prentice Hall Reviews & Rationales Series.**

Excellence in Course Review

The **Prentice Hall Nursing Reviews & Rationales Series** will help you achieve nursing excellence by simplifying your review and making the most of your valuable study time for both your nursing courses and for the NCLEX-RN®. Each book in the series provides a comprehensive review of course content across the curriculum, as well as hundreds of practice questions with rationales and test-taking strategies in Pre- and Post-Tests and on the CD-ROM that comes with each book. This is the only review series that offers you a tear-out review card, *Prentice Hall NursingNotes,* and an audio review, *VangoNotes,* for additional purchase to play on your MP3 player.

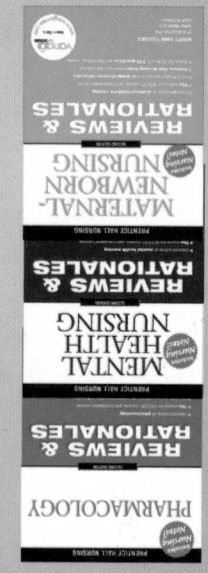

Fundamentals & Nursing Skills, 2nd Ed.	2008	0-13-224078-5
Medical-Surgical Nursing, 2nd Ed.	2008	0-13-178970-8
Nutrition & Diet Therapy, 2nd Ed.	2007	0-13-243712-0
Fluids, Electrolytes, & Acid-Base Balance, 2nd Ed.	2007	0-13-224079-3
Pathophysiology, 2nd Ed.	2008	0-13-178972-4
Pharmacology, 2nd Ed.	2008	0-13-243710-4
Maternal-Newborn Nursing, 2nd Ed.	2007	0-13-178973-2
Child Health Nursing, 2nd Ed.	2007	0-13-243711-2
Mental Health Nursing, 2nd Ed.	2008	0-13-224077-7